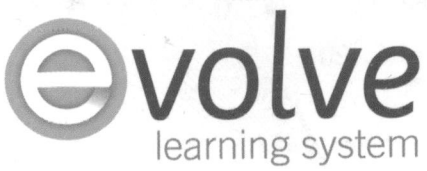
evolve
learning system

To access your Student Resources, visit:

http://evolve.elsevier.com/Wong/ncic/

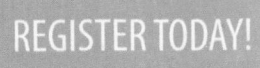

Evolve® Student Resources for Hockenberry & Wilson: Wong's Nursing Care of Infants and Children, *Ninth Edition, include the following:*

- **Prepare for Class, Clinical, or Lab**
  Anatomy Reviews, Animations, Calculators, Care Plan Creator, Case Studies, Critical Thinking Exercises, Evidence-Based Practice Guidelines, Key Points Audio Summaries, Skills Performance Checklists, Videos

- **Prepare for Exams**
  Review Questions for the NCLEX® Examination—More than 400 questions in multiple-choice and alternate-item formats, with rationales for correct and incorrect answers, help you review and apply content and prepare for the NCLEX® Examination!

- **Prepare for Practice**
  Wong on the Web, a unique resource providing access to numerous lectures and studies by Donna Wong that can be used in practice

- **Additional Resources**
  Appendixes, content updates, and WebLinks for further study

ELSEVIER

WONG'S
Nursing Care of Infants and Children

EDITION **9**

WONG'S
Nursing Care of
Infants and Children

EDITION 9

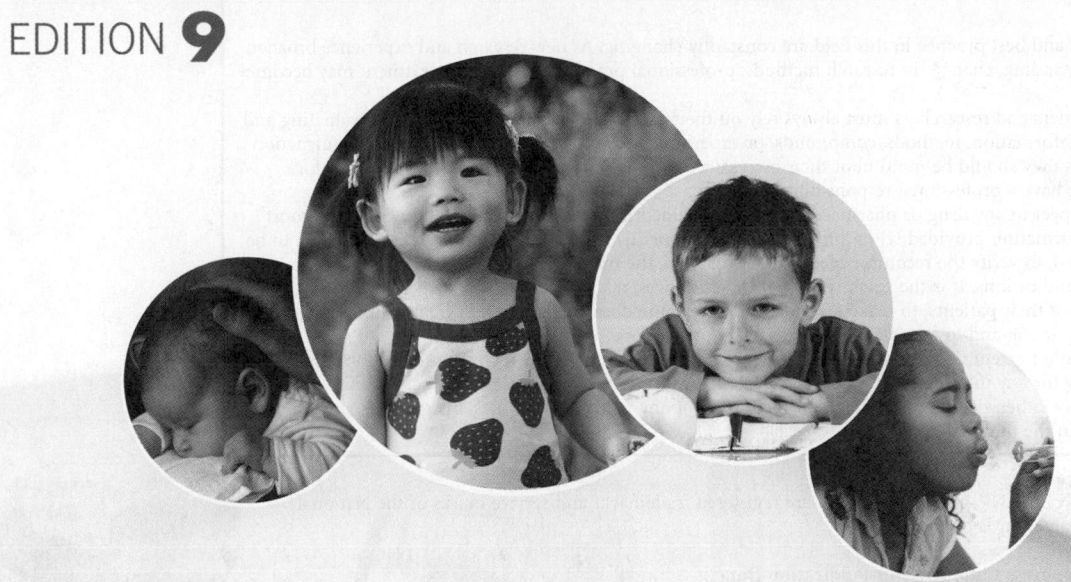

**Marilyn J. Hockenberry,
PhD, RN, PNP-BC, FAAN**
Professor, Department of Pediatrics
Baylor College of Medicine;
Nurse Scientist, Texas Children's Hospital;
Director of Nurse Practitioners
Texas Children's Cancer Center
Houston, Texas

David Wilson, MS, RNC
Faculty
Langston University School of Nursing;
Staff Nurse
Children's Hospital
Saint Francis Hospital
Tulsa, Oklahoma

ELSEVIER
MOSBY

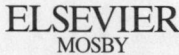

3251 Riverport Lane
St. Louis, Missouri 63043

Library of Congress Cataloging-in-Publication Data
Wong's nursing care of infants and children / [edited by] Marilyn J. Hockenberry, David Wilson.—9th ed.
    p. ; cm.
  Other title: Nursing care of infants and children
  Includes bibliographical references and index.
  ISBN 978-0-323-06912-0 (hardcover : alk. paper) 1. Pediatric nursing. I. Wong, Donna L., 1948-2008. II. Hockenberry, Marilyn J. III. Wilson, David, 1950 Aug. 25- IV. Title: Nursing care of infants and children.
  [DNLM: 1. Pediatric Nursing. 2. Child Care. 3. Infant Care. WY 159]
RJ245.W47 2011
618.92'00231—dc22

2010026203

Managing Editor: Michele D. Hayden
Developmental Editor: Heather Bays
Publishing Services Manager: Deborah L. Vogel
Senior Project Manager: Deon Lee
Design Direction: Kimberly Denando

Printed in the United States of America

Last digit is the print number: 9 8 7 6 5 4 3 2

CONTRIBUTING EDITOR

Patrick Barrera, BS
Assistant Director
Evidence-Based Outcomes Center
Texas Children's Hospital
Houston, Texas

CONTRIBUTORS

Debbie Fraser Askin, MN, RNC-NIC
Associate Professor
Health Studies
Athabasca University
Athabasca, Alberta, Canada
Associate Professor
Centre for Nursing and Health Studies
Athabasa, Alberta, Canada

Annette Baker, MSN, RN, PNP
Nurse Practitioner, Cardiovascular Program
Children's Hospital
Boston, Massachusetts

Rose Ann Urdiales Baker, PhD(c), MSN, RN, PMHCNS-BC
Adjunct Faculty
Kent State University
College of Nursing
Kent, Ohio

Linda Ballard, MSN, RN, CPNP
Pediatric Nurse Practitioner
Aflac Cancer Center and Blood Disorders
    Service
Children's Healthcare of Atlanta
Atlanta, Georgia

Amy Barry, MSN, RN, PNP-BC
Pediatric Nurse Practitioner
Aflac Cancer Center and Blood Disorders
    Service
Children's Healthcare of Atlanta
Atlanta, Georgia

Ashley R. Breland, MSN, RN, CCRN
Research Specialist
Evidence Based Outcomes Center
Texas Children's Hospital
Houston, Texas

Christine A. Brosnan, DrPH, RN
Associate Professor
University of Texas Health Science Center
    at Houston
School of Nursing
Houston, Texas

Terri L. Brown, MSN, RN, CPN
Research Specialist
Texas Children's Hospital
Houston, Texas

Meg Bruening, MPH, RD
University of Minnesota
Minneapolis, Minnesota

Rosalind Bryant, PhD, PNP-BC
Pediatric Nurse Practitioner
Texas Children's Hospital;
Instructor
Baylor College of Medicine
Houston, Texas

Lisa Creamer, BSN, RN
Manager
Child Protection Program
Texas Children's Hospital
Houston, Texas

Martha Curry, MS, RN, CPNP
Pediatric Nurse Practitioner
Rheumatology Service
Texas Children's Hospital;
Instructor
Department of Pediatrics
Baylor College of Medicine
Houston, Texas

Amy Delaney, MSN, RN, CPNP-AC/P
Pediatric Nurse Practitioner
The Cardiovascular Program
The Children's Hospital Boston
Boston, Massachusettes

Angela M. Ethier, PhD, RN, FT
Houston, Texas

Quinn Franklin, MS, CCLS
Research Specialist Texas Children's
    Hospital
Adjunct Faculty University of Alabama
Adjunct Instructor San Jacinto Community
    College
Houston, Texas

Valerie J. Groben, RN, MSN, APRN-BC
Pediatric Nurse Practitioner
St. Jude's Children's Research Hospital
Memphis, Tennessee

Andrea J. Harrison, BSN, RN
Neonatal Intensive Care Unit
Texas Children's Hospital
Houston, Texas

Eufemia Jacob, PhD, RN
Assistant Professor
University of California Los Angeles
Los Angeles, California

Linda M. Kollar, RN, MSN
Clinical Director
Surgical Weight Loss Program for Teens
Cincinnati Children's Hospital Medical
    Center
Cincinnati, Ohio

Caterina Nicole Landry, BSN, RN
Staff Nurse
Progressive Care Unit
Texas Children's Hospital
Houston, Texas

Bonnie L. Magliaro, RN, MS, CNS
Neonatal Clinical Specialist
Newborn Center
Texas Children's Hospital
Houston, Texas

Shannon McCord, MS, RN, CPNP, CNS, WOCN
Director of Patient Care Services
Texas Children's Hospital, West Campus
Houston, Texas

Patricia Barry McElfresh, MN, RN, PNP-BC
Pediatric Nurse Practitioner
Children's Healthcare of Atlanta
Aflac Cancer Center and Blood Disorders
    Service
Neuro Oncology Program
Atlanta, Georgia

Tara Taneski Merck, MS, RN, CPNP
Pediatric Nurse Practitioner
Children's Healthcare of Atlanta
Aflac Cancer Center and Blood Disorders
    Service
Leukemia and Lymphoma Program
Atlanta, Georgia

Mary A. Mondozzi, MSN, PNP-BC
Burn Center Education/Outreach
    Coordinator
Akron Children's Hospital
The Paul and Carol David Foundation Burn
    Institute
The Clifford R. Boeckman, MD Regional
    Burn Center
Akron, Ohio

**Rebecca A. Monroe, MSN, RN, CPNP,
CPON**
Pediatric Nurse Practioner
Pediatrics After Hours
Dallas, Texas

Barbara Montagnino, MS, RN, CNS
Clinical Nurse Specialist
Progressive Care Unit
Texas Children's Hospital
Houston, Texas

**Kim Mooney-Doyle, MSN, CPNP,
CPON**
Lecturer
University of Pennsylvania
School of Nursing
Philadelphia, Pennsylvania

Mary Hershey Pascual, RN, ADN
Registered Nurse
Texas Children's Hospital
Houston, Texas

Cynthia A. Prows, MSN, CNS, FAAN
Clinical Nurse Specialist, Genetics
Children's Hospital Medical Center
Cincinnati, Ohio

Elizabeth Record, DNP, BSN, MSN
Pediatric Nurse Practitioner
Hematology/Oncology Department
Children's Healthcare of Atlanta
Atlanta, Georgia

Patricia A. Ring, MSN, RN, CPNP
Pediatric Nephrology
Children's Hospital of Wisconsin
Milwaukee, Wisconsin

**Cheryl C. Rodgers, PhD, RN, CPNP,
CPON**
Pediatric Nurse Practitioner
Texas Children's Cancer Center
Texas Children's Hospital;
Instructor
Department of Pediatrics
Baylor College of Medicine
Houston, Texas

Elizabeth M. Saewyc, PhD, RN
CIHR/PHAC Chair in Applied Public
    Health
Professor
University of British Columbia
School of Nursing
Vancouver, British Columbia

Jennifer Sanders, MSN, RN
Dayshift Nurse Manager
General Medicine & Transplant Unit
Texas Children's Hospital
Houston, Texas

**Margaret L. Schroeder, MSN, RN,
PNP-BC**
Pediatric Nurse Practitioner
Cardiovascular Surgery
Children's Hospital Boston
Boston, Massachusetts

Rebecca J. Schultz, PhD, RN, CPNP
Pediatric Nurse Practitioner
Comprehensive Epilepsy Program
Texas Children's Hospital;
Instructor
Baylor College of Medicine
Houston, Texas

Jamie Stang, PhD, MPH, RD
Assistant Professor
University of Minnesota School of Public
    Health
Minneapolis, Minnesota

**Annaka G. Thibodeaux, MSN, ARNP,
CPON**
Pediatric Nurse Practitioner
Seattle Children's Hospital
Seattle, Washington

Sandra L. Upchurch, PhD, RN
Associate Professor and Chair
Department of Nursing Systems
School of Nursing
The University of Texas Health Science
    Center at Houston
Houston, Texas

**Barbara J. Wheeler, MN, RN,
IBCLC, RLC**
Neonatal Clinical Nurse Specialist
Lactation Consultant
St. Boniface General Hospital
Winnipeg, Manitoba, Canada

Kristina Wilson, PhD, CCC-SLP
Senior Speech Language Pathologist and
    Clinical Researcher
Texas Children's Hospital;
Adjunct Assistant Professor
Department of Plastic Surgery
Baylor College of Medicine
Houston, Texas

CRITICAL THINKING CASE STUDIES

Terry Delpier, DNP, RN, CPNP
Professor
Department of Nursing
Northern Michigan University
Marquette, Michigan

CURRICULUM GUIDES, INSTRUCTOR'S MANUAL, AND OPEN-BOOK QUIZZES

Jacalyn Peck Dougherty, RN, PhD
Assistant Professor
University of Northern Colorado
Greeley, Colorado

POWERPOINT LECTURE SLIDES WITH AUDIENCE RESPONSE SYSTEM QUESTIONS

Vivian Gamblian, RN, MSN
Professor of Nursing
Collin County Community College
McKinney, Texas

TEST BANK AND NCLEX® REVIEW QUESTIONS

Julie White, RN, MSN
Clinical Instructor, Graduate Entry Program
College of Nursing
University of Illinois at Chicago
Chicago, Illinois

Patricia Ahern, RD, CSP, LD, BS in Nutrition and Dietetics
Senior Pediatric Clinical Dietitian
Texas Children's Hospital
Houston, Texas

Kathleen C. Byington, MSN, RN, FNP, BC
Monroe Carell Jr. Children's Hospital
    at Vanderbilt
Nashville, Tennessee

Patricia Conlon, MS, RN, CNS, CNP
Pediatric Clinical Nurse Specialist
Mayo Eugenio Litta Children's Hospital
Mayo Medical Center
Rochester, Minnesota

Erica Fooshee, MSN, RN, CNE, CPN
Nursing Mentor
Western Governors University
Salt Lake City, Utah

Sarah Gutknecht, DNP, RN, CNP
Pediatric Nurse Practitioner
Pediatric Orthopaedics
Gillette Children's Specialty Healthcare
St. Paul, Minnesota

Suzanne Iniguez, RRT-NPS, AE-C
Respiratory Care Coordinator
Texas Children's Hospital
Houston, Texas

Tricia L. Kinman, BA, MAT
Redability Specialist
St. Louis, Missouri;
Adjunct Instructor
St. Charles Community College
St. Charles, Missouri

Kristie S. Nix, BSN, MS, EdD
Associate Professor
School of Nursing
The University of Tulsa
Tulsa, Oklahoma

Eileen R. O'Shea, DNP, RN-CNS
Assistant Professor
Fairfield University School of Nursing
Fairfield, Connecticut

Ann M. Petersen-Smith, PhD, RN, CPNP-AC
Assistant Professor
PNP Option Coordinator
University of Colorado Denver
College of Nursing
Aurora, Colorado

Tina Reinckens, PhD(c), RN, MA
Assistant Professor
Helene Fuld School of Nursing
Coppin State University
Baltimore, Maryland

Robyn Rice, PhD, RN
Nurse Educator
Lutheran School of Nursing
St. Louis, Missouri;
Home Care Nurse
Gateway Medical Center Home Care
    Department
Granite City, Illinois

Lisa Rinsdale, DNP, RN, CNE, JD
Assistant Professor of Nursing
Florida Southern College
Lakeland, Florida

Sharon Isenhour Sarvey, PhD, RN
Associate Professor
Department of Undergraduate Nursing–
    Junior Division
East Carolina University
Greenville, North Carolina

Cheryl Shell, RN, CNP
Nurse Practitioner
Center for Craniofacial Services
Gillette Children's Specialty Healthcare
St. Paul, Minnesota

Jean C. K. Stansbury, MSN, RN, CNS, CNP
Certified Pediatric Nurse Practitioner
St. Paul, Minnesota

Kerstin West-Wilson, MS, RNC, IBCLC
Assistant Discharge Coordinator in NICU
Certified Lactation Consultant, Newborn
    Nursery
Clinical Nurse III, NICU
Saint Francis Children's Hospital
Tulsa, Oklahoma

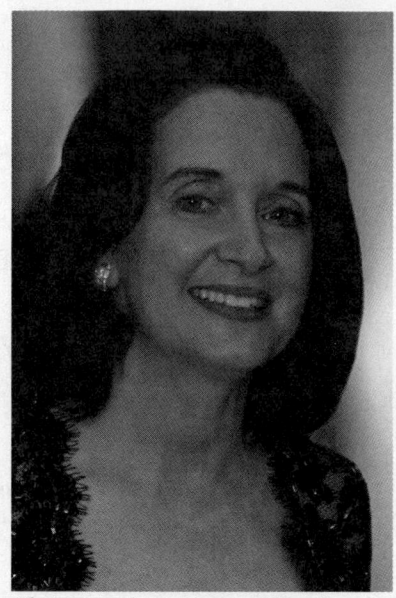

Chris Humphrey, Photographer

We dedicate this edition of *Wong's Nursing Care of Infants and Children* to Donna Lee Wong, PhD, RN, PNP, CPN, FAAN, who passed away on May 4, 2008, following complications of leukemia. Donna was the original coauthor of this book. Among her numerous publications, she is best known as the author of *Wong's Nursing Care of Infants and Children, Wong's Essentials of Pediatric Nursing, Wong's Clinical Manual of Pediatric Nursing,* and the *Pediatric Quick Reference.* She codeveloped the Wong-Baker FACES Pain Rating Scale, a tool used worldwide to assess pain in children and adults and which has been used in extensive research on pain. She was a fellow in the American Academy of Nursing (FAAN) and is listed in *Who's Who in American Nursing* and *The World's Who's Who of Women.* She was awarded many honors and was the first recipient of the Audrey Hepburn/Sigma Theta Tau International (Honorary Nursing Society) Award for Contributions to the Health and Welfare of Children, Rutger's University Outstanding Alumni, and the Society of Pediatric Nursing Barbara Larson Humanitarian Award.

For those of us who had the honor of knowing this remarkable individual, she is most remembered for her outstanding generosity and concern for others. Her commitment to pediatric nursing is reflected in her never-ending pursuit of excellence. Her belief that no child should experience pain when interventions are possible led to the development of the concept of "atraumatic care." Donna taught us that nursing is about providing the best care possible and that our patients will be the better for it. She led by example, always looking for ways to improve care for pediatric patients. Donna Wong was an example for all of us who strive for excellence in our nursing profession. We hold her dear to our hearts and will continue to work to carry on her outstanding legacy. She will never be forgotten.

The ninth edition of *Wong's Nursing Care of Infants and Children* has been revised to keep pace with new innovations in pediatric nursing care. This text has been a landmark in pediatric nursing since it was first published over two decades ago under the leadership of Donna Wong. This kind of recognition places unique accountability and responsibility on us to continue to strive to provide students with the latest information they need to become competent critical thinkers and to attain the sensitivity necessary to become caring pediatric nurses.

Marilyn Hockenberry and David Wilson continue to serve as editors for the Wong textbooks, with Patrick Barrera as a contributing editor. This team has put together an expert panel of more than 60 nurses and multidisciplinary specialists who assisted in reviewing, revising, rewriting, and authoring portions of the text on areas undergoing rapid and complex change, such as immunizations, genetics, home care, high-risk newborn care, adolescent health issues, and numerous diseases. We have carefully preserved aspects of the book that have met with such universal acceptance—its state-of-the-art evidence-based information; its strong, integrated focus on the family and community; its logical and user-friendly organization; and its easy reading style. We have placed additional emphasis on research with concise reviews of important evidence in new Research Focus boxes. This allows students to review new evidence on important topics in a concise way.

New to this edition is the inclusion, throughout the chapters, of quality patient outcomes that focus on serious health problems. Since nurses are the principal caregivers within health care institutions, quality patient outcomes are used as an assessment of the ability to provide excellence in patient care. Pathophysiology review figures have been added throughout the text to provide a concise evaluation of major health care diseases in children. With an understanding of the pathophysiologic process, the nurse is better prepared to develop evidence-based nursing interventions for patient care. In addition, more than 100 new figures have been added, and 30 existing figures have been color enhanced to focus on the importance on visual learning. This update provides the visual learner with a tangible connection to the content of the text for application to clinical practice.

We have tried to meet the increasing demands of faculty and students to teach and to learn in an environment characterized by rapid change, enormous amounts of information, fewer traditional clinical facilities, and less time to teach. To help students quickly locate essential information, most of the features used in the previous edition have been retained. Significant revisions and additions to the Evidence-Based Practice boxes have been made using the PICO approach and GRADE evidence quality assessment criteria. Nursing Care Plans include both NIC and NOC indicators. Most important, this text continues to encourage students to *think critically*.

This book is about families with children, and the philosophy of family-centered care is emphasized. This book has retained the theme which Donna Wong so passionately advocated about providing atraumatic care—care that minimizes the psychologic and physical stress that health promotion and illness can inflict. Features such as Family-Centered Care, Community Focus, and Atraumatic Care boxes bring these philosophies to life throughout the text. Finally, the philosophy of delivering competent pediatric nursing care is addressed. We believe strongly that children and families need consistent caregivers. The establishment of the therapeutic relationship with the child and family is explored as the essential foundation for providing quality nursing care.

This text serves as a reference manual for the practicing nurse. The latest recommendations have been included from authoritative organizations such as the American Academy of Pediatrics, Centers for Disease Control and Prevention, Agency for Healthcare Research and Quality, American Pain Society, American Nurses Association, and National Association of Pediatric Nurse Associates and Practitioners. To expand the universe of available information, websites and e-mail addresses have been included for hundreds of organizations and other educational resources.

ORGANIZATION OF THE BOOK

The same general approach to the presentation of content has been preserved from previous editions, although much content has been added, condensed, and rearranged within this framework to improve flow, minimize duplication, and emphasize health care trends, such as home and community care. This book is divided into two broad parts. The first part of the book, sometimes called the "age and stage" approach, considers infancy, childhood, and adolescence from a developmental context. It emphasizes the importance of the nurse's role in health promotion and maintenance and in considering the family as the focus of care. From a developmental perspective, the care of common health problems is presented, giving readers a sense of what normal problems can be expected in otherwise healthy children and demonstrating when during childhood these problems are most likely to occur. The second part of the book presents the more serious health problems not specific to any particular age group but that frequently require hospitalization or major medical and nursing interventions.

UNIT I (Chapters 1 to 5) provides an overview of the multitude of influences on a child who is developing as a member of a family unit and maturing within a culture, community, and society. Chapter 1 includes a discussion of morbidity and mortality in infancy and childhood and examines child health care from a historical perspective. Because unintentional injury is one of the leading causes of death in children, an overview of this topic is included. The nursing process, with emphasis on nursing diagnosis and outcomes and the importance of developing critical thinking skills, is presented. The critical components of evidence-based practice provide the template for exploring the latest pediatric nursing research or practice guideline throughout the entire book. Discussion of quality patient outcomes and their importance in evaluating the quality of nursing care has been added.

Chapter 2 provides the opportunity to expand the discussion of social, cultural, and religious influences on child development and health promotion, including socioeconomic factors, customs, and health beliefs and practices. The content clearly describes the role of the nurse, with such content as guidelines for culturally sensitive interactions and a table discussing religious beliefs that affect nursing care. Chapter 3, devoted to the family, further emphasizes the importance of this social group to the health and welfare of children. Family strengths and vulnerabilities are addressed, and current findings on adoption, divorce, single parenting, stepfamilies, and dual-earner families have been incorporated. The child in the context of family, culture, and community has been broadened to include discussion in Chapter 4 of the issues involved in community health nursing. This chapter provides important information on community-based nursing care, with emphasis on epidemiology as it applies to the detection and identification of causes of morbidity and mortality in pediatrics. Chapter 5 has been completely revised by a leading genetics nursing expert, who focuses on heredity as it relates to health promotion and the influence of the Human Genome Project on future treatment strategies for inherited diseases.

UNIT II (Chapters 6 and 7) is concerned with the principles of critical nursing assessment by keeping pace with the newest evaluation strategies in nursing. Chapter 6 contains guidelines for communicating with children, adolescents, and their families; telephone triage; and a detailed description of a health assessment, including an extensive discussion of family assessment and nutritional assessment. This chapter provides a comprehensive approach to physical examination and developmental assessment, using the latest literature on temperature measurement and the latest growth charts on how to assess a child's body mass index (BMI).

An important feature in this edition is the chapter devoted to critical assessment and management of pain in children. Although the literature on pain assessment and management in children has grown considerably, this knowledge has not been widely applied in practice. Chapter 7 addresses this concern by presenting detailed pain assessment and management strategies, including discussion of common pain states in children.

UNIT III (Chapters 8 to 11) stresses the importance of the neonatal period, the time of greatest risk to a child's survival, and discusses several health concerns encountered in the vulnerable first month of life. Chapter 8 has been updated and revised to include the latest information on the benefits of breast-feeding, and a new section that discusses the cultural influences on infant feeding is included. Infant formula tables have been revised and simplified, and new additions include the latest vitamin D intake recommendations, as well as the impact of prebiotics and probiotics in infant nutrition. The sections on infant safety, newborn circumcision, and circumcision anal-

gesia have all been revised and updated. Newborn screening guidelines have also been extensively updated. The latest information on preparation for newborn home discharge, newborn skin care and bathing, and umbilical cord care is included. Chapter 9 has been revised and updated in the areas of birth trauma, newborn dermatologic problems, and hyperbilirubinemia, including the latest guidelines for the management of hyperbilirubinemia in late-preterm and term newborns. Guidelines for the management of hyperbilirubinemia in the breastfeeding pair are also included. Updated management protocols and screening guidelines are included for neonatal hypoglycemia and inborn errors of metabolism such as galactosemia and phenylketonuria. Atraumatic care of the newborn remains an important concept in these chapters. Evidence-based practice and critical thinking exercises have been updated as well. Chapter 10 includes an updated section on neurodevelopmental care of the preterm infant, and a new section is devoted to the care of the late-preterm infant. Updated and revised are the sections on care of the preterm infant, including preterm infant nutrition, supplemental oxygen administration, necrotizing enterocolitis, sepsis, discharge planning, retinopathy of prematurity, neonatal skin care guidelines, and bronchopulmonary dysplasia. The most recent information regarding hypoxic ischemic reperfusion injury and therapeutic hypothermia are presented in this chapter. This chapter also contains information regarding maternal conditions that may adversely affect the fetus and newborn, including maternal viruses, fetal alcohol exposure, and neonatal drug exposure. Sections of Chapter 11 have been significantly revised, including the discussion of craniofacial abnormalities including cleft lip, cleft palate, and plagiocephaly. The disorders of sex development (formerly *ambiguous genitalia*) section has been revised according to the latest guidelines and recommendations.

UNITS IV through VII (Chapters 12 to 21) present the major developmental stages in childhood, expanded to provide a broader concept of the stages and the health problems most often associated with each age-group. Special emphasis is placed on the preventive aspects of care. The health promotion chapters follow a standard approach that is used consistently for each age-group.

The chapters on health problems primarily reflect more typical and age-related concerns. The information on many disorders has been revised to reflect recent changes. Examples include the latest information on communicable diseases, childhood immunizations, food allergies, colic, growth failure, child passenger safety, pacifier use, thumb sucking, lead poisoning, wound healing, sexual abuse, Lyme disease, attention deficit hyperactivity disorder, school-related violence, tobacco use, contraception, teenage pregnancy, substance abuse, adolescent suicide, and eating disorders such as obesity. The latest Dietary Reference Intake (DRI) guidelines, American Heart Association dietary guidelines for children, and updated USDA dietary guidelines for children (MyPlate), aimed at decreasing obesity and cardiovascular disease, are presented. The section on sudden infant death syndrome (SIDS) has been extensively updated to include the latest American Academy of Pediatrics considerations for cosleeping and pacifier use.

The chapters on adolescence include the latest information on the management of childhood obesity and other eating disorders, recommendations for preventive health screening in adolescents, rankings of body mass index percentiles, tobacco and substance prevention, as well as current trends in suicide identification and prevention. All psychosocial/physiologic conditions discussed include the latest diagnostic criteria from the *Diagnostic and Statistical Manual of Mental Disorders (DSM-IV-TR)*.

UNIT VIII (Chapters 22 to 25) deals with children who have the same developmental needs as growing children but who, because of congenital or acquired physical, cognitive, or sensory impairment, require alternative interventions to facilitate development. Chapter 22 reflects the latest trends in the care of families and children with chronic illness or disability, such as home care, normalizing children's lives, focusing on developmental needs, enabling and empowering families, and providing early intervention.

Extensive revisions have been made in Chapter 23 to reflect increased awareness of the need for quality nursing care at the end of life. This chapter highlights common fears experienced by the child and family and includes discussion of the nurse's reaction to caring for dying children. The content in Chapter 24 on cognitive, sensory, and communication impairment includes the latest information on mental retardation and learning disorders. Chapter 25 reflects the latest trends in family-centered home care of children with chronic health conditions. This chapter includes guidelines for choosing a pediatric home health care agency, the role of the care coordinator in home care, and parent-professional collaboration in the home.

UNIT IX (Chapters 26 and 27) is concerned with the impact of hospitalization on the child and the family and presents a comprehensive overview of the stressors imposed by hospitalization and nursing interventions available to prevent or eliminate these stressors. Chapter 26 discusses the care of the hospitalized child and family with consideration for increasing care in ambulatory centers. Chapter 27 discusses safe implementation of procedures in children, including emphasis on the use of therapeutic holding. This chapter also includes numerous Evidence-Based Practice boxes designed to provide rationales for the interventions discussed in the chapter. A major focus in this chapter is the evidence related to preparation of the child for procedures commonly performed by nurses. Recommendations for practice are based on the evidence and are concisely presented in Evidence-Based Practice boxes throughout the chapter.

UNITS X through XIV (Chapters 28 to 40) consider serious health problems of infants and children primarily from a biologic system orientation, which has the practical organizational value of permitting health care problems and nursing considerations to relate to specific pathophysiologic disturbances. Important additions and revisions include discussion of hepatitis, all blood disorders, influenza management including H1N1, acute respiratory distress syndrome/acute lung injury (ARDS/ALI), respiratory syncytial virus (RSV), tuberculosis, the latest classification for asthma, effects of tobacco exposure, seizures, chemotherapy, AIDS, diabetes mellitus, and burns. Guidelines for infant and child resuscitation, including automated external defibrillation, have been updated and added. Chapter 39 has sections on considerations for the female athlete as well as childhood injury prevention and management of various sports injuries. Care and management of the child with a fracture has been updated, as have the sections on immobility, mobilization devices, cast care, and orthotics. Conditions such as arthritis and idiopathic scoliosis have been revised and updated. Chapter 40 includes updates on Guillain-Barré syndrome, cerebral palsy, infant botulism, and respiratory management of neuromuscular conditions such as spinal muscular atrophy and muscular dystrophy.

Extensive **Appendixes** are also included and contain information on developmental and sensory assessment; growth measurements, including a complete set of the National Center for Health Statistics growth charts; pediatric laboratory values; and several foreign-language translations of the Wong-Baker FACES Pain Rating Scale. All of the appendixes reflect the most current versions of forms, charts, and measurements.

UNIFYING PRINCIPLES

Several unifying principles have guided the organizational structure of this book since its inception. These principles continue to strengthen the book with each revision to maintain a consistent approach throughout each chapter.

THE FAMILY AS THE UNIT OF CARE

The child is an essential member of the family unit. Nursing care is most effective when it is delivered with the belief that *the family is the patient.* This belief permeates the book. The family is seen as a myriad of structures; each has the potential to provide a caring, supportive environment in which the child can grow, mature, and maximize his or her human potential. In addition to family-centered care being integrated into every chapter, an entire chapter is devoted to understanding the family as the core focus in children's lives. Another chapter discusses the social, cultural, and religious influences on family beliefs. Separate sections in yet another chapter deal in depth with family communication and family assessment. The impact of illness, hospitalization, home care, and the death of a child are covered extensively in three additional chapters. The needs of the family are emphasized throughout the text under Nursing Care Management, with a separate section on family support. Numerous Family-Centered Care boxes are included to assist nurses in understanding and providing helpful information to families.

AN INTEGRATED APPROACH TO DEVELOPMENT

Children are not small adults but are special individuals with unique minds, bodies, and needs. No book on pediatric nursing is complete without extensive coverage of communication, nutrition, play, safety, dental care, sexuality, sleep, self-esteem, and of course, parenting. Nurses promote the healthy expression of development and need to understand how this is observed in children at different ages and stages. Effective parenting depends on the parents' knowledge of development, and it is often the nurse's responsibility to provide parents with a developmental awareness of their children's needs. For these reasons, coverage of the many dimensions of childhood are integrated within each developmental-stage chapter, rather than being presented in a separate chapter. Safety concerns, for instance, are very different for a toddler than for an adolescent. Sleep needs change with age, as do nutritional needs. As a result, the units on each stage of childhood contain complete information on all these subjects as they relate to the specific age. Using the integrated approach, students gain an appreciation for the unique characteristics and needs of children at every age and stage of development.

FOCUS ON WELLNESS AND ILLNESS: CHILD, FAMILY, AND COMMUNITY

In a pediatric nursing text, a focus on illness is expected. Children become ill, and nurses typically are involved in helping children get well. However, it is not sufficient to prepare students to care primarily for sick children. First, health is more than the absence of disease. Being healthy is being whole in mind, body, and spirit. Therefore the majority of the first half of the book is devoted to discussions that promote physical, psychosocial, mental, and spiritual wellness. Much emphasis is placed on anticipatory guidance of parents to prevent injury or illness in the child. Second, more than ever, health care is prevention focused. The objectives set forth in *Healthy People 2020* clearly establish a health care agenda in which solutions to medical/social problems lie in preventive strategies. Competent nursing care flows from this knowledge and is enhanced by an awareness of childhood development, family dynamics, and communication skills.

NURSING CARE

Although this text incorporates information from numerous disciplines (medicine, pathophysiology, pharmacology, nutrition, psychology, sociology), its primary purpose is to provide information on the nursing care of children and families. Discussions of all disorders conclude with a section on Nursing Care Management. Although many aspects of the nursing care of children and families have changed significantly over the last few decades, the focus must continue to be on the quality of care. For the quality of care to be maintained, pediatric nurses must be proactive in staying informed about the strength of evidence that supports specific nursing practices. The Nursing Care Management sections are designed to provide the latest evidence for the implementation of evidence-based nursing practice. In addition, all of the nursing care plans have been updated to current practices. Taken together, they provide coverage of nursing care for numerous diseases, disorders, conditions, and crises of childhood.

The purpose of the care plans, like every other feature of the book, is to teach and convey information. They include all current nursing diagnoses approved by NANDA that have a potential bearing on health problems. The care plans in the text

can be individualized for use with a specific patient in a clinical setting, and as such, individualized nursing interventions should be integrated. For every diagnosis, expected patient outcomes and extensive possible nursing interventions with rationales are included. The care plans include subjective and objective data for the defining characteristics of each nursing diagnosis. NIC and NOC concepts for nursing interventions and expected outcomes are included.

CRITICAL ROLE OF RESEARCH AND EVIDENCE-BASED PRACTICE

This ninth edition is the product of an extensive review of the literature published since the book was last revised. In addition, a new feature, Research Focus boxes, has been added to provide the student with a concise discussion of the latest research on a given topic. So that information is accurate and current, most citations are less than 5 years old, and almost every chapter has entries within 1 year of publication. Examples of current cutting-edge information include recommendations from the American Academy of Pediatrics on immunizations and sleep position. The chapter on pain reflects the latest guidelines from the Agency for Healthcare Research and Quality (AHRQ), formerly known as the Agency for Health Care Policy and Research (AHCPR), and the American Pain Society. The discussions on skin care reflect the AHRQ's guidelines on pressure ulcers. The American Diabetes Association's classification of diabetes mellitus is included, as are the most recent treatment guidelines for asthma.

CANADIAN CONTENT

The ninth edition of this text includes Canadian immunization schedules in Chapter 12. Throughout the text, Canadian resource organizations are also provided. These efforts have been made to make the text as valuable as possible to Canadian readers.

⋯

Just as children and their families bring with them a value system and unique background that affect their role within the health care system, so it is that each nurse brings to each child and family an individual set of characteristics and values that will affect their relationship. Although we have attempted to present a total picture of the child in each age-group, both in wellness and in illness, no one child, family, or nurse will be found in this book. We hope that each page, chapter, and unit builds a foundation on which the nurse can begin to construct an ideal of comprehensive, atraumatic, and individualized nursing care for infants, children, adolescents, and their families.

SPECIAL FEATURES

Much effort has been directed toward making this book easy to teach from and, more important, easy to learn from. In this edition the following features have been included to benefit educators, students, and practitioners.

ATRAUMATIC CARE boxes emphasize the importance of providing competent care without creating undue physical and psychologic distress. Although many of the boxes provide suggestions for managing pain, atraumatic care also considers approaches to promoting self-esteem and preventing embarrassment.

COMMUNITY FOCUS boxes address issues that expand to the community, such as increasing immunization rates, preventing lead poisoning, or decreasing smoking among teens.

COMPLEMENTARY AND ALTERNATIVE THERAPY boxes accentuate different treatment modalities for specific disorders.

CRITICAL THINKING EXERCISES have been revised in this edition to describe brief scenarios of the child-family-nurse interaction that depict real-life clinical situations. From the synthesis of the topical content and a critical analysis of possible options, the reader chooses the best intervention and learns to make clinical judgments. A rationale is offered for the correct answer, and explanations are given for the incorrect options at the end of the chapter.

CULTURAL COMPETENCE boxes integrate concepts of culturally sensitive care throughout the text. Their emphasis is on the clinical application of the information, whether it focuses on toilet training or on male or female circumcision.

DRUG ALERTS highlight critical drug safety concerns for better therapeutic management.

EMERGENCY TREATMENT boxes enable the reader to quickly learn interventions for crisis situations.

EVIDENCE-BASED PRACTICE boxes have been completely revised in this edition to focus the reader's attention on application of both research and critical thought processes to support and guide the outcomes of nursing care and to provide measurable outcomes that nurses can use to validate their unique role in the health care system.

FAMILY-CENTERED CARE boxes present issues of special significance to families who have a child with a particular disorder. This feature is another method of highlighting the needs or concerns of families that should be addressed when family-centered care is provided.

NURSING ALERTS call the reader's attention to considerations that if ignored could lead to a deteriorating or emergency situation. Key assessment data, risk factors, and danger signs are among the kinds of information included.

NURSING CARE GUIDELINES boxes summarize important nursing interventions for a variety of situations and conditions.

NURSING CARE PLANS include nursing diagnoses, defining characteristics of the diagnoses, expected patient outcomes, and rationales for the included nursing interventions that may not be immediately evident to the student. The care plans include NIC and NOC concepts. All care plans include patient and family goals and the most recent NANDA nursing diagnoses.

NURSING TIPS present handy information of a nonemergency nature that makes patients more comfortable and the nurse's job a little easier.

PATHOPHYSIOLOGY REVIEWS have been added to this edition to provide the student with a visual representation of the effects of the disease process on the child. These illustrations provide knowledge required for the nurse to implement appropriate evidence-based nursing interventions and provide independent as well as collaborative care with other health care professionals.

QUALITY PATIENT OUTCOMES are added throughout the text to provide a framework for measuring nursing care performance. Nursing-sensitive outcome measures are integrated into the outcome indicators used throughout the book.

RESEARCH FOCUS boxes review new evidence on important topics in a concise way.

Numerous pedagogic devices that enhance student learning have been retained from previous editions:

- **APPENDIXES** provide additional materials to assist with assessment, including family, developmental, growth, and laboratory evaluation. The translations of the Wong-Baker FACES Pain Rating Scale are found here as well.
- **CHAPTER OUTLINES** with page numbers begin each chapter, which allows readers to quickly locate topics of interest.
- More than 100 **COLOR PHOTOGRAPHS** have been updated or added to this edition to reflect the latest in nursing care. Anatomic drawings are easy to follow, with color appropriately used to illustrate important aspects, such as saturated and desaturated blood. New figures reflecting a **PATHOPHYSIOLOGY REVIEW** of various disorders have

been added throughout the book. As an example, the full-color heart illustrations in Chapter 34 clearly depict congenital cardiac defects and associated hemodynamic changes.

- A functional and attractive **FULL-COLOR DESIGN** visually enhances the organization of each chapter as well as the special features.
- An **INDEX,** detailed and cross-referenced, allows readers to quickly access discussions.
- **KEY POINTS,** located at the end of each chapter, help the reader summarize major points, make connections, and synthesize information.
- **KEY TERMS** are highlighted throughout each chapter to reinforce student learning.
- **MARGINAL NOTES** call readers' attention to the various activities and exercises available on the Evolve website, to aid in their understanding of the material being presented.

- **PRINTED ENDPAPERS** on the inside back cover provide information nurses refer to often, such as vital signs and blood pressure measurements.
- Hundreds of **TABLES** and **BOXES** highlight key concepts and nursing interventions.
- **RELATED TOPICS** and **EVOLVE RESOURCES** at the beginning of each chapter indicate the chapter or chapters where additional discussion of a given topic can be found. On turning to the cross-referenced chapters, readers will find the topic listed in the chapter outline with a page number. Additional exercises and activities included on the Evolve website are listed here to provide further reinforcement to the student.

ACKNOWLEDGMENTS

This ninth edition of *Wong's Nursing Care of Infants and Children* brings with it new contributors to the book. To continue the Wong legacy of excellence in nursing education, we have joined together numerous contributors with diverse expert nursing backgrounds to continue the commitment to providing the latest state-of-the-art information on pediatric nursing practice. We are grateful to the many nursing faculty members, practitioners, and students who have offered their comments, recommendations, and suggestions. We are grateful to the many reviewers who brought constructive criticism, suggestions, and clinical expertise to this edition. We could not have completed the enormous task of updating and adding information without the dedication of these special people.

We are especially thankful to **Patrick Barrera,** Contributing Editor, for his work on the book. His commitment to excellence has provided attention to detail that is essential to maintaining the text's uniqueness and quality. His extensive efforts at searching the literature have provided the book with the most up-to-date information available to pediatric nursing practice. We would like to thank **Scott Murray** in the Health Sciences Library staff at Saint Francis Hospital, Tulsa, for his assistance in obtaining material. No book is ever a reality without the dedication and perseverance of the editorial staff. Although it is impossible to list every individual at Elsevier who has made exceptional efforts to produce this text, we are especially grateful to **Shelly Hayden,** whose commitment to pediatric nursing education over the years is reflective of an outstanding publisher. We appreciate her exceptional leadership skills and devotion to her authors. We also want to acknowledge the exceptional work of **Deon Lee;** her dedication to the Wong textbooks is evident. Special thanks also to **Sally Schrefer, Heather Bays, Meg Brinkley, Deborah Vogel, Kimberly Denando,** and **Susan Copeland** for their support and commitment to excellence.

Marilyn J. Hockenberry
David Wilson

CONTENTS

UNIT IV FAMILY-CENTERED CARE OF THE INFANT, 464

UNIT V FAMILY-CENTERED CARE OF THE YOUNG CHILD, 553

**UNIT XII THE CHILD WITH
PROBLEMS RELATED
TO PRODUCTION AND
CIRCULATION OF
BLOOD, 1340**

UNIT XIII THE CHILD WITH DISTURBANCE OF REGULATORY MECHANISMS, 1461

UNIT XIV THE CHILD WITH A PROBLEM THAT INTERFERES WITH PHYSICAL MOBILITY, 1619

APPENDIXES

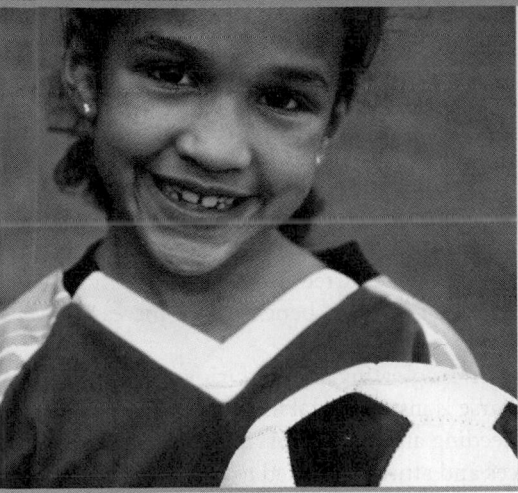

Perspectives of Pediatric Nursing

Marilyn J. Hockenberry and Patrick Barrera

HEALTH CARE FOR CHILDREN

The major goal for pediatric nursing is to improve the quality of health care for children and their families. There are 73 million children 0 to 18 years of age in the United States, comprising 25% of the population (Agency for Healthcare Research and Quality, 2008). The health status of children in the United States has improved in a number of areas, including increased immunization rates for all children, decreased adolescent birth rate, and improved child health outcomes. Unfortunately millions of children and their families have no health insurance, which results in a lack of access to care and health promotion services. In addition, disparities in pediatric health care are related to race, ethnicity, socioeconomic status, and geographic factors (see Research Focus box). Patterns of child health are shaped by medical progress and societal trends (Dougherty, Meikle, Owens, et al, 2005; Wise, 2004, 2005). The *Healthy People 2020* Leading Health Indicators (Box 1-1) provide a

---

BOX 1-1   *HEALTHY PEOPLE 2020*

Goals
Increase quality and length of healthy life
Eliminate health disparities

Leading Health Indicators
Physical activity
Overweight and obesity
Tobacco use
Substance abuse
Responsible sexual behavior
Mental health
Injury and violence
Environmental quality
Immunization
Access to health care

From US Department of Health and Human Service: *Healthy people 2020: understanding and improving health.*

---

framework for identifying essential components for child health promotion programs designed to prevent future health problems in our nation's children.

RESEARCH FOCUS

National Children's Study

The National Children's Study is the largest prospective, long-term study of children's health and development conducted in the United States. The study is designed to follow 100,000 children and their families from birth to age 21 years to understand the link between children's environments and their physical and emotional health and development (American Academy of Pediatrics, 2008). Researchers hoped that a study of this magnitude will provide information on innovative interventions for families, children, and health care providers to eradicate unhealthy diets, dental caries, and childhood obesity and to bring a significant reduction in violence, injury, substance abuse, and mental health disorders among the nation's children. This study supports the *Healthy People 2020* primary goals to increase the quality and years of healthy life and eliminate health disparities related to race, ethnicity, and socioeconomic status (US Department of Health and Human Services, 2009).

HEALTH PROMOTION

Many leading causes of disease, disability, and death in children (i.e., prematurity, nutritional deficiencies, injuries, chronic lung disease, obesity, cardiovascular disease, depression, violence, substance abuse, and human immunodeficiency virus/acquired immunodeficiency syndrome [HIV/AIDS]) can be significantly reduced or prevented in children and adolescents by addressing six categories of behavior (World Health Organization, 2007):

1. Tobacco use
2. Behavior that results in injury and violence
3. Alcohol and substance use
4. Dietary and hygienic practices that cause disease
5. Sedentary lifestyle
6. Sexual behavior that causes unintended pregnancy and disease

Child health promotion provides opportunities to reduce differences in current health status among members of different groups and ensure equal opportunities and resources to enable all children to achieve their fullest health potential.

Nutrition

Nutrition is an essential component for healthy growth and development. Human milk is the preferred form of nutrition for all infants. Breastfeeding provides the infant with micronutrients, immunologic properties, and several enzymes that enhance digestion and absorption of these nutrients. A recent resurgence in breastfeeding has occurred due to the education of mothers and fathers regarding its benefits and increased social support.

Children establish life-long eating habits during the first 3 years of life, and the nurse is instrumental in educating parents about the process of feeding and the importance of nutrition. Most eating preferences and attitudes related to food are established by family influences and culture. During adolescence, parental influence diminishes and the adolescent makes food choices related to peer acceptability and sociability. Occasionally these choices are detrimental to adolescents with chronic illnesses like diabetes, obesity, chronic lung disease, hypertension, cardiovascular risk factors, and renal disease.

Families that struggle with lower incomes, homelessness, and migrant status generally lack the resources to provide their children with adequate food intake, nutritious foods such as fresh fruits and vegetables, and appropriate protein intake. The result is nutritional deficiencies with subsequent growth and developmental delays, depression, and behavior problems.

Dental Care

Dental caries is the single most common chronic disease of childhood (Cheng, Han, and Gansky, 2008; Heuer, 2007). Nearly one in five children between the ages of 2 and 4 years has visible cavities (Kagihara, Niederhauser, and Stark, 2009). The most common form of early dental disease is early childhood caries, which may begin before the first birthday and progress to pain and infection within the first 2 years of life (Edelstein, 2005). Preschoolers of low-income families are twice as likely to develop tooth decay and only half as likely to visit the dentist as other children. Early childhood caries is a preventable disease, and nurses play an essential role in educating children and parents about practicing dental hygiene beginning with the first tooth eruption; drinking fluoridated water, including bottled water; and instituting early dental preventive care.

Immunizations

The two public health interventions that have had the greatest impact on world health are clean drinking water and childhood vaccination programs. Immunization rates differ depending on children's race and ethnicity, family income, the state in which they live, types of vaccinations, and their age (whether adolescent or younger children) (Dougherty, Meikle, Owens, et al, 2005). The nurse should review individual immunization records at every clinic visit, avoid missing opportunities to vaccinate, and encourage parents to keep immunizations current (US Department of Health and Human Services, 2009). Nurses are responsible for keeping up with changes in immunization schedules, recommendations, and research related to childhood vaccines.

CHILDHOOD HEALTH PROBLEMS

Changes in modern society, including advancing medical knowledge and technology, the proliferation of information systems, economically trouble times, and various changes and disruptive influences on the family, are leading to significant medical problems that affect the health of children (Lichter, 2005). Recent concern has focused on groups of children who are at highest risk, such as children born prematurely or with very low birth weight (VLBW) or low birth weight (LBW), children attending child care centers, children who live in poverty or are homeless, children of immigrant families, and children with chronic medical and psychiatric illness and disabilities. In addition, these children and their families face multiple barriers to adequate health, dental, and psychiatric care. The new morbidity, also known as *pediatric social illness*, refers to the behavior, social, and educational problems that children face. Problems that can negatively impact a child's development include poverty, violence, aggression, noncompliance, school failure, and adjustment to parental separation and divorce. In addition, mental health issues cause challenges in childhood and adolescence. One out of five adolescents has a mental health problem, and 1 out of 10 has a serious emotional problem that affects daily functioning (Coury, 2006).

Obesity and Type 2 Diabetes

Childhood obesity is the most common nutritional problem among American children, is increasing in epidemic proportions, and is associated with type 2 diabetes (Matyka, 2008; Cali and Caprio, 2008). Obesity in children and adolescents is defined as a body mass index at or greater than the 95th percentile for youth of the same age and gender (Schwartz and Chadha, 2008). The National Health and Nutrition Examination Survey reported that the prevalence of overweight children doubled and the prevalence of overweight adolescents tripled between 1980 and 2000 (American Dietetic Association, 2008).

Advancements in entertainment and technology such as television, computers, and video games have contributed to the growing childhood obesity problem in the United States. Approximately 63% of 8- to 18-years-olds have a television in their bedrooms and watch it an average of 4 hours a day (Robinson and Sargent, 2005). Minority populations, especially African-American and Hispanic children from low-income families, watch more than 4 hours of television daily, exacerbating the effects of sedentary activity and intake of high-caloric, fatty foods (Fitzgibbon and Stolley, 2004). Lack of physical activity related to limited resources, unsafe environments, and inconvenient play and exercise facilities, combined with easy access to television and video games, increases the incidence of obesity among low-income, minority children. Overweight youth, especially children of Hispanic, African-American, and Native American descent, have increased risk for developing hypercholesterolemia, insulin resistance, diabetes, hypertension, and heart disease (Schwartz and Chadha, 2008; Matyka, 2008) (Fig. 1-1). The U.S. Department of Health and Human Services (2009) suggests that nurses focus on prevention strategies to reduce the incidence of overweight children from the current 20% in all ethnic groups, to less than 6%.

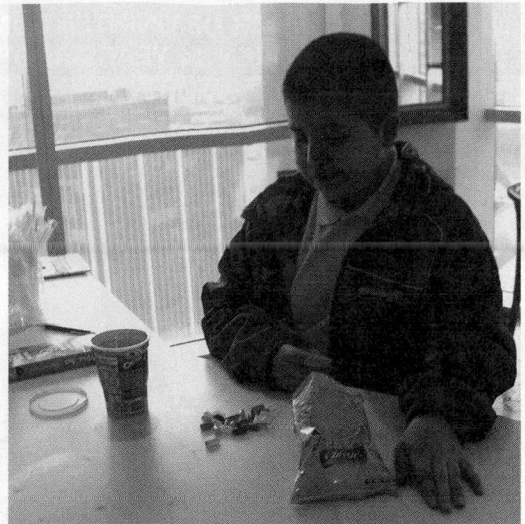

Fig. 1-1 The American culture's intake of high-caloric fatty foods contributes to obesity in children.

Childhood Injuries

Injuries are the most common cause of death and disability to children in the United States (Schnitzer, 2006) (Table 1-1). Motor vehicle accidents (MVAs) continue to be the most common cause of death in children older than 1 year of age. Other unintentional injuries (head injuries, drowning, burns, and firearm accidents) take the lives of children every day. Many childhood injuries and fatalities could be prevented by implementing programs of accident prevention and health promotion.

The type of injury and the circumstances surrounding it are closely related to normal growth and development (Box 1-2). As children develop, their innate curiosity compels them to investigate the environment and to mimic the behavior of others. This is essential to acquire competency as an adult, but can also predispose children to numerous hazards.

The child's developmental stage partially determines the types of injuries that are most likely to occur at a specific age and helps provide clues to preventive measures. For example, small infants are helpless in any environment. When they begin to roll over or propel themselves, they can fall from unprotected surfaces. The crawling infant, who has a natural tendency to place objects in the mouth, is at risk for aspiration or poisoning. The mobile toddler, with the instinct to explore and investigate and the ability to run and climb, may experience falls, burns, and collisions with objects. As children grow older, their absorption with play makes them oblivious to environmental hazards such as street traffic or water. The need to conform and gain acceptance compels older children and adolescents to accept challenges and dares. Although the rate of injuries is high in children less than 9 years of age, most fatal injuries occur in later childhood and adolescence.

The pattern of deaths caused by unintentional injuries, especially from MVAs, drowning, and burns, is remarkably consistent in most Western societies. The leading causes of death from injuries and their trends are presented in Table 1-1. The majority of deaths from injuries occur in boys. It is

TABLE 1-1 NUMBER OF UNINTENTIONAL INJURY DEATHS FOR LEADING CAUSES AMONG CHILDREN 14 YEARS AND YOUNGER

TYPE OF INCIDENT	NUMBER OF DEATHS IN 1987	NUMBER OF DEATHS IN 2004	PERCENT DECREASE/INCREASE
Motor vehicle crash	3587	2431	↓32%
Drowning	1363	761	↓44%
Pedestrian injury	1283	583	↓55%
Fire and/or burn injury	1233	512	↓58%
Suffocation	690	963	↑28%
Bike	389	132	↓66%
Falls	149	107	↓28%
Poisoning	100	86	↓14%
Firearm	247	63	↓74%

1987-2004 Unintentional Injury Deaths, Ages 0 to 14, United States

From Safe Kids USA: *Injury trends fact sheet,* Washington, DC, 2009, Safe Kids Worldwide, available at www.safekids.org/our-work/research/fact-sheets/injury-trends-fact-sheet.html (accessed June 21, 2010).

BOX 1-2 CHILDHOOD INJURIES: RISK FACTORS

Sex—Preponderance of males; difference mainly the result of behavioral characteristics, especially aggression

Temperament—Children with difficult temperament profile, especially persistence, high activity level, and negative reactions to new situations

Stress—Predisposes children to increased risk taking and self-destructive behavior; general lack of self-protection

Alcohol and drug use—Associated with higher incidence of motor vehicle injuries, drownings, homicides, and suicides

History of previous injury—Associated with increased likelihood of another injury, especially if initial injury required hospitalization

Developmental characteristics
- Mismatch between child's developmental level and skill required for activity (e.g., all-terrain vehicles)
- Natural curiosity to explore environment
- Desire to assert self and challenge rules
- In older child, desire for peer approval and acceptance

Cognitive characteristics (age specific)

Infant—Sensorimotor: explores environment through taste and touch

Young child
- Object permanence: actively searches for attractive object
- Cause and effect: lacks awareness of consequential dangers

- Transductive reasoning: may fail to learn from experiences (e.g., perceives falling from a step as a different type of danger from climbing a tree)
- Magical and egocentric thinking: is unable to comprehend danger to self or others

School-age child—Transitional cognitive processes: is unable to fully comprehend causal relationships; attempts dangerous acts without detailed planning regarding consequences

Adolescent—Formal operations: is preoccupied with abstract thinking and loses sight of reality; may lead to feeling of invulnerability

Anatomic characteristics (especially in young children)
- Large head—Predisposes to cranial injury
- Large spleen and liver with wide costal arch—Predisposes to direct trauma to these organs
- Small and light body—May be thrown easily, especially inside a moving vehicle

Other factors—Poverty, family stress (e.g., maternal illness, recent environmental change), substandard alternative child care, young maternal age, low maternal education, multiple siblings

important to note that accidents continue to account for more than three times as many teen deaths as any other cause (Annie E Casey Foundation, 2009). Fortunately, prevention strategies such as the use of car restraints, bicycle helmets, and smoke detectors have significantly decreased fatalities for children.

Nevertheless, the overwhelming causes of death in children are MVAs, including occupant, pedestrian, bicycle, and motorcycle deaths; these account for more than half of all injury deaths (Centers for Disease Control and Prevention, 2006). Children under 1 year of age have the highest rate of death from MVAs, primarily from a failure to properly use car restraints (Fig. 1-2).

Pedestrian accidents involving children account for significant numbers of motor vehicle–related deaths. Most of these accidents occur at midblock, at intersections, in driveways, and in parking lots. Driveway injuries typically involve small children and large vehicles backing up.

Bicycle-associated injuries also cause a number childhood deaths. Children ages 5 to 9 years are at greatest risk of bicycling fatalities. The majority of bicycling deaths are from head injuries. Helmets reduce the risk of head injury by 85%, but few children wear helmets (National Safety Council, 2000). Community-wide bicycle helmet campaigns and mandatory-use laws have resulted in significant increases in helmet use. Still, issues such as stylishness, comfort, and social acceptability remain important factors in noncompliance. Nurses can educate children and families about pedestrian and bicycle safety. In particular, school nurses can promote helmet wearing and encourage peer leaders to act as role models.

Drowning and burns are among the top three leading causes of deaths for males and females throughout childhood (Fig. 1-3). In addition, improper use of firearms is a major cause of death among males (Fig. 1-4). During infancy, more boys die from aspiration or suffocation than do girls (Fig. 1-5). Approximately 70% of all unintentional poisonings are reported in children under 2 years of age (Bronstein, Spyker, Cantilena, et al, 2008; Franklin and Rodgers, 2008) (Fig. 1-6). By ages 4 to 5 years, unintentional poisonings are uncommon. Intentional poisoning, associated with drug and alcohol abuse and suicide attempt, is the second leading cause of death in adolescent females and third leading cause in adolescent males.

Violence

Each day, 10 children in the United States are murdered by gunfire, equivalent to approximately one child every 2½ hours (Groves, 2005). Strikingly higher homicide rates are found among minority populations, especially African-American children. The causes of violence against children and self-inflicted violence are not fully understood. Violence seems to permeate American households through television programs, commercials, video games, and movies, all of which tend to desensitize the child toward violence. Violence also permeates the schools with the availability of guns, illicit drugs, and gangs. The problem of child homicide is extremely complex and involves numerous social, economic, and other influences. Prevention lies in better understanding of the social and psychologic factors that lead to the high rates of homicide and suicide. Nurses need to be especially aware of young people who harm animals or start fires, are depressed, are repeatedly in trouble with the criminal justice system, or are associated with groups known to be violent. Prevention requires early identification and rapid therapeutic intervention by qualified professionals.

Pediatric nurses can assess children and adolescents for risk factors related to violence. Families that own firearms must be educated about their safe use and storage. The presence of a gun in a household increases the risk of suicide by about five-fold and the risk of homicide by about threefold. Technologic changes such as childproof safety devices and loading indicators could improve the safety of firearms (see Community Focus box).

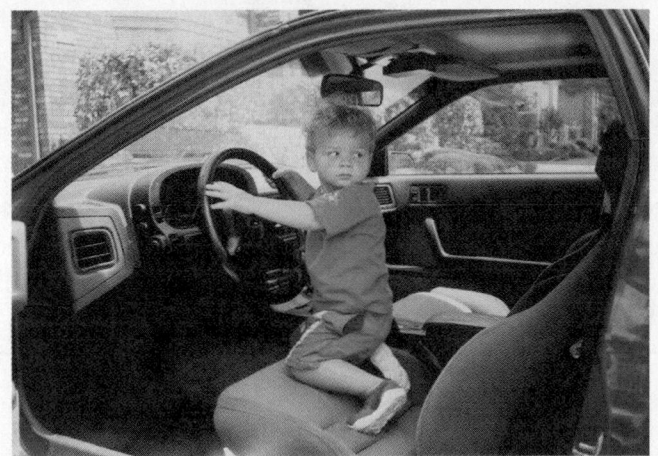

Fig. 1-2 Motor vehicle injuries are the leading cause of death in children older than 1 year of age. The majority of fatalities involve occupants who are unrestrained.

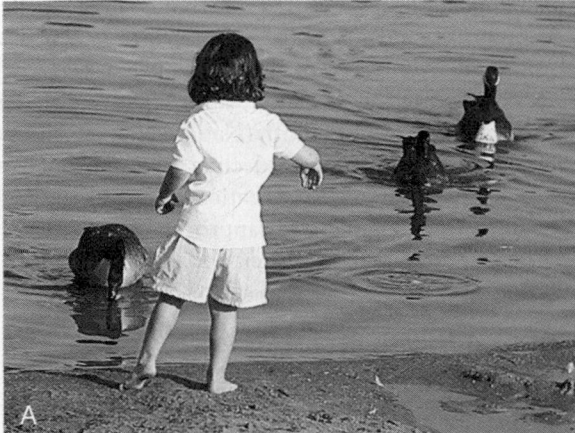 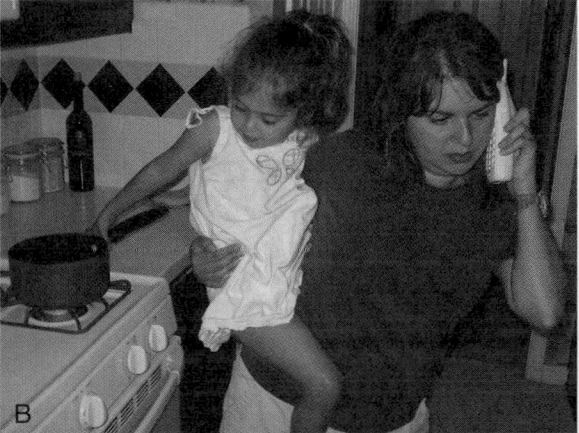

Fig. 1-3 A, Drowning is one of the leading causes of death. Children left unattended are unsafe even in shallow water. **B,** Burns are among the top three leading causes of death from injury in children ages 1 to 14 years.

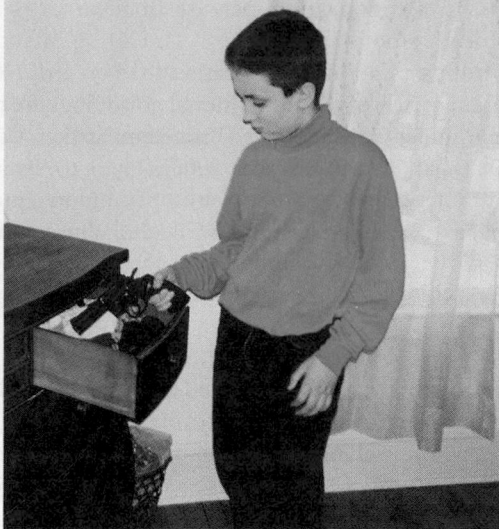

Fig. 1-4 Improper use of firearms is the fourth leading cause of death from injury in children 5 to 14 years of age.

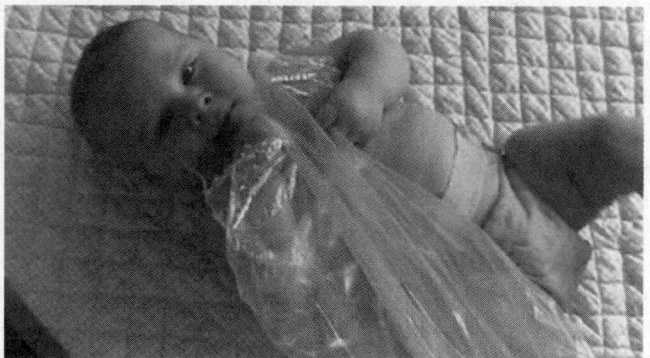

Fig. 1-5 Mechanical suffocation is the leading cause of death from injury in infants.

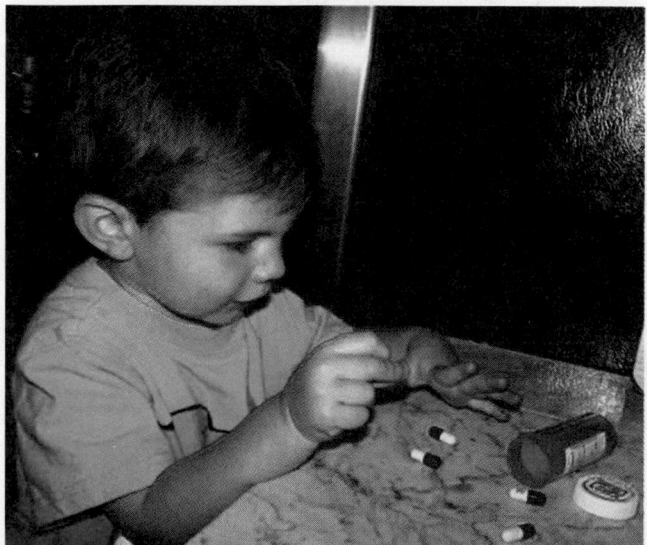

Fig. 1-6 Poisoning causes a considerable number of injuries in children under 4 years of age. Medications should never be left where young children can reach them.

COMMUNITY FOCUS
Violence in Children

Community violence has reached epidemic proportions in the United States. Recently, political leaders have recognized violence as a public health emergency and a preventable problem (Groves, 2005). The serious problem of community violence affects the lives of many children and expands throughout the family, schools, and the workplace. Nurses working with children, adolescents, and families have a critical role in reducing violence through early identification and symptom recognition of the mental-emotional stress that can result from these experiences.

Violent crimes continue to be a significant health issue for children, with homicide being the second leading cause of death in 15- to 19-year-olds (Annie E Casey Foundation, 2009). The multifaceted origins of violence include developmental factors, gang involvement, access to firearms, drugs, the media, poverty, and family conflict. Often the silent and underrecognized victims are the children who witness acts of community violence. Studies suggest that chronic exposure to violence has a negative effect on a child's cognitive, social, psychologic, and moral development. Also, multiple exposures to episodes of violence do not inoculate children against the negative effects; continued exposure can result in lasting symptoms of stress. Children living with chronic violence may exhibit behaviors such as difficulty concentrating in school, memory impairment, aggressive play, uncaring behaviors, and constricted activities and thinking for fear of reliving the traumatic event (Groves, 2005).

National concern about the increasing prevalence of violent crimes has prompted nurses to actively participate in ensuring that children grow up in safe environments. Pediatric nurses are positioned to assess children and adolescents for signs of exposure to violence and well-known risk factors; nurses also can provide nonviolent problem-solving strategies, counseling, and referrals. These activities affect community practice and expand the nurse's role in the future health environment. Professional resources include the following:

National Domestic Violence Hotline
PO Box 161810
Austin, TX 78716
800-799-SAFE
www.ndvh.org

Substance Abuse

Risk-taking behaviors, particularly in males, tend to begin in the first decade of life and continue into adolescence with drinking alcohol while driving, speeding, carrying a weapon, or using illicit drugs. Adolescent trends in cigarette smoking, alcohol use, and illicit drug abuse have declined since 2002. Approximately 9.8% of youth reported cigarette smoking, 15.9% reported alcohol use, and 9.5% reported illicit drug abuse within the past month (National Survey on Drug Use and Health, 2008). The slight decline in American youth's illicit drug use is attributed to education regarding the adverse effects of illicit drugs, parental disapproval, decreased availability of drugs, and consistent participation in church and organized activities such as scouts and sports.

Mental Health Problems

Mental health problems affect one out of five school-age children in the United States. Children and adolescents with mental health problems are more likely to drop out of school than those with other disabilities (Kelleher, 2005). One of the most common mental health problems is attention deficit hyperactivity disorder (ADHD) (Kelleher, 2005). ADHD is characterized by inattentiveness, impulsivity, and at times hyperactivity, and it may occur in children as early as 3 years of age (Medd, 2003). ADHD affects every aspect of the child's life, but is most obvious in the classroom. Medication, counseling, classroom interventions, behavior management strategies, and family education and counseling are all appropriate strategies to help children with mental health problems succeed.

Suicide is defined as a self-chosen death and is the third leading cause of death in children ages 10 to 19 (Doucette, 2005). The American Association of Suicidology (2009) estimates that there are 11.5 youth (15 to 24 years of age) suicides ever day. Suicide is preventable. Nurses should be alert to the symptoms of mental illness and potential suicidal ideation and be aware of potential resources for high-quality integrated mental health services (Coury, 2006).

MORTALITY

Mortality statistics describe the incidence or number of individuals who have died over a specific period. They are usually presented as rates per 100,000. Mortality rates are calculated from a sample of death certificates. In the United States the National Center for Health Statistics, under the Department of Health and Human Services, Public Health Service, is responsible for the collection, analysis, and dissemination of data on the health of the American people (Federal Interagency Forum on Child and Family Statistics, 2007).

The tabulation of race for live births (the denominator of infant mortality rates) has changed from race of child to race of mother. Formerly, for a child of mixed parentage in which one parent was Caucasian, the child was assigned the race of the other parent. In general, this change in assignment of race from child to mother has resulted in more Caucasian births and fewer non-Caucasian births. However, infant deaths are recorded by the decedent's race, resulting in a lower infant mortality rate for Caucasians than non-Caucasians. As a result of these changes in the early 1990s, figures for births, deaths, and infant mortality rates by race are not comparable to statistics reported before these changes were made.

Infant Mortality

The infant mortality rate is the number of deaths during the first year of life per 1000 live births. It may be further divided into neonatal mortality (<28 days of life) and postneonatal mortality (28 days to 11 months). In the United States infant mortality has decreased dramatically. At the beginning of the twentieth century the rate was approximately 200 infant deaths per 1000 live births. In 2006 the infant mortality rate was 6.69 deaths per 1000 live births (Heron, Hoyert, Murphy, et al, 2009).

From a worldwide perspective, however, the United States lags behind other nations in reducing infant mortality. In 2006 the United States ranked last among 29 nations that have a population of at least 2.5 million and had infant mortality rates equal to or lower than that of the United States. Hong Kong, Japan, Sweden, and Finland have the three lowest rates, with the United States ranked last behind Poland and Malaysia (Heron, Sutton, Xu, et al, 2010).

Birth weight is considered the major determinant of neonatal death in technologically developed countries. There is a relationship between LBW and infant morbidity and mortality (Heron, Sutton, Xu, et al, 2010). The lower the birth weight, the higher the mortality. The relatively high incidence of LBW (<2500 g [5.5 lb]) in the United States is considered a key factor in its higher neonatal mortality rate when compared with other countries. Access to and the use of high-quality prenatal care is a promising preventive strategy to decrease early delivery and infant mortality. Other factors that increase the risk of infant mortality include African-American race, male gender, short or long gestation, maternal age, and lower level of maternal education (Heron, Sutton, Xu, et al, 2010).

As Table 1-2 demonstrates, many of the leading causes of death during infancy continue to occur during the perinatal period. The first four causes—congenital anomalies, disorders relating to short gestation and unspecified LBW, sudden infant death syndrome, and newborn affected by maternal complications of pregnancy—accounted for about half of all deaths of infants under 1 year of age (Heron, Hoyert, Murphy, et al, 2009). LBW is a major indicator of infant health and a

RANK	CAUSE OF DEATH (BASED ON 10th REVISION, INTERNATIONAL CLASSIFICATION OF DISEASES)	PERCENT	RATE
	All races, all causes	100.00	677.3
1	Congenital anomalies	19.7	133.6
2	Disorders relating to short gestation and unspecified low birth weight	16.0	108.4
3	Sudden infant death syndrome	7.2	49.1
4	Newborn affected by maternal complications of pregnancy	6.1	41.0
5	Accidents (unintentional injuries)	4.2	28.7
6	Newborn affected by complications of placenta, cord, and membranes	3.9	26.4
7	Bacterial sepsis of newborn	2.7	18.3
8	Respiratory distress of newborn	2.5	17.0
9	Neonatal hemorrhage	2.1	14.2
10	Diseases of circulatory system	2.1	14.2

TABLE 1-2 INFANT MORTALITY RATE AND PERCENTAGE OF TOTAL DEATHS FOR 10 LEADING CAUSES OF INFANT DEATH IN 2007 (RATE PER 1000 LIVE BIRTHS)

Modified from Heron M, Hoyert DL, Murphy SL, et al: Deaths: final data for 2006, *Natl Vital Stat Rep* 57(14):1-134, 2009.

TABLE 1-3	FIVE LEADING CAUSES OF DEATH IN CHILDREN IN UNITED STATES: SELECTED AGE INTERVALS, 2007 (RATE PER 100,000 POPULATION)							
	AGES 1-4 YEARS		**AGES 5-9 YEARS**		**AGES 10-14 YEARS**		**AGES 15-19 YEARS**	
RANK	CAUSE	RATE	CAUSE	RATE	CAUSE	RATE	CAUSE	RATE
	All causes	28.2	All causes	13.6	All causes	16.7	All causes	61.6
1	Accidents	9.5	Accidents	4.8	Accidents	5.9	Accidents	29.7
2	Congenital anomalies	3.1	Cancer	2.4	Cancer	2.3	Homicide	9.6
3	Homicide	2.2	Congenital anomalies	1.0	Homicide	1.0	Suicide	6.8
4	Cancer	2.2	Homicide	0.7	Suicide	0.9	Cancer	3.0
5	Heart disease	1.0	Heart disease	0.5	Congenital anomalies	0.8	Heart disease	1.5

Modified from Heron M, Sutton PD, Xu J, et al: Annual summary of vital statistics—2007, *Pediatrics* 125(1):13, 2010.

significant predictor of infant mortality (Heron, Sutton, Xu, et al, 2010). Many birth defects are associated with LBW, and reducing the incidence of LBW will help prevent congenital anomalies. Infant mortality resulting from HIV infection decreased significantly during the 1990s. In 2003 HIV/AIDS accounted for less than 0.2% of all infant deaths (Heron, Sutton, Xu, et al, 2010).

When infant death rates are categorized according to race, a disturbing difference is seen. Infant mortality for Caucasians is considerably lower than for all other races in the United States, with African-Americans having twice the rate of Caucasians. Although the infant mortality of all racial groups increased slightly between 2001 and 2002, the gap has remained constant, with the infant mortality rate expressed as a ratio of African-American to Caucasian deaths being relatively unchanged for the past decade (Heron, Sutton, Xu, et al, 2010). The LBW rate is also much higher for African-American infants than for any other group. One encouraging note is that the gap in mortality rates between Caucasian and non-Caucasian races other than African-Americans has narrowed in recent years. Infant mortality rates for Hispanics and Asian–Pacific Islanders have decreased dramatically during the past 2 decades (Heron, Sutton, Xu, et al, 2010).

Childhood Mortality

Death rates for children older than 1 year of age have always been lower than those for infants. Children ages 5 to 14 years have the lowest rate of death. However, a sharp rise occurs during later adolescence, primarily from injuries, homicide, and suicide (Table 1-3). In 2007 these causes were responsible for approximately 75% of deaths in teenagers and young adults 15 to 19 years old (Heron, Sutton, Xu, et al, 2010). The trend in racial differences that occurs in infant mortality is also apparent in childhood deaths for all ages and for both sexes. Caucasians have fewer deaths for all ages, and male deaths outnumber female deaths.

After 1 year of age, the cause of death changes dramatically, with unintentional injuries (accidents) being the leading cause from the youngest ages to the adolescent years. Violent deaths have been steadily increasing among young people ages 10 through 25 years, especially African-Americans and males. Homicide is the second leading cause of death in the 15- to 19-year age-group (see Table 1-3). Children 12 years of age and older tend to be killed by nonfamily members (acquaintances and gangs, typically of the same race) and most frequently by firearms. Suicide, a form of self-violence, is the third leading cause of death among children and adolescents 15 to 19 years of age.

MORBIDITY

Measurements of the prevalence of a specific illness in the population at a particular time are known as morbidity statistics. Morbidity statistics are generally presented as rates per 1000 population. Unlike mortality, morbidity is difficult to define and may denote acute illness, chronic disease, or disability. The source of data also influences the statistics. Common sources include reasons for visits to physicians; diagnoses for hospital admission; or household interviews such as the National Health Interview Survey, Child Health Supplement. Unlike death rates, which are updated annually, morbidity statistics are revised less frequently and do not necessarily represent the general population.

Childhood Morbidity

Acute illness is defined as an illness with symptoms severe enough to limit activity or require medical attention. Respiratory illness accounts for approximately 50% of all acute conditions, 11% are caused by infections and parasitic disease, and 15% are caused by injuries. The chief illness of childhood is the common cold.

The types of diseases that children contract during childhood vary according to age. For example, upper respiratory tract infections and diarrhea decrease in frequency with age, whereas other disorders, such as acne and headaches, increase. Children who have had a particular type of problem are more likely to have that problem again. Morbidity is not distributed randomly in children. Children from poor families do not fare as well on health indicators compared with children from nonpoor families (Federal Interagency Forum on Child and Family Statistics, 2007). This finding suggests the need for heightened efforts to improve access to health care for low-income children.

Recent concern has focused on groups of children who have increased morbidity: homeless children, children living in poverty, LBW children, children with chronic illnesses, foreign-born adopted children, and children in daycare centers. A number of factors place these groups at risk for poor health. A major cause is barriers to health care, especially for the homeless, the poverty stricken, and those with chronic health problems. Other factors include improved survival of children with chronic health problems, particularly infants of VLBW.

EVOLUTION OF CHILD HEALTH CARE IN THE UNITED STATES

Children in Colonial America were born into a world with many hazards to their health and survival. Epidemics were common. Control or treatment was unknown. Physicians were few, and only a small number had any formal training. Midwives were untrained, basing their practice on experience. Books providing information on child care and feeding were scarce and, when available, were useful only to a minority of parents who were literate.

Medical care by physicians was limited to wealthy families who lived in or could travel to more developed cities. Children who lived on farms were mainly cared for by another family member or by a competent neighbor. Traveling medicine men, with their various forms of quackery, were common. Children who were bought as slaves or born to slaves had only as much care as their owner was able or willing to provide. Native American children were treated according to the tradition of each tribe, which was often a mixture of medicine, magic, and religion. With the colonization of America, Native Americans were exposed to many new, often fatal diseases.

Statistics on childhood mortality during the Colonial period are largely unavailable. Epidemic diseases included smallpox, measles, mumps, chickenpox, influenza, diphtheria, yellow fever, cholera, and whooping cough. However, the disease that surpassed all others as a cause of childhood death was dysentery. Sometimes entire families succumbed to this illness. Other diseases that contributed to childhood illness were the "slow epidemics" of tuberculosis, nutritional diseases, and injuries.

Although scientific knowledge was accumulating, especially from work done in Europe, there were no organized efforts in the United States to apply that knowledge to the care of the sick. It was not until the Industrial Revolution was well under way in the nineteenth century that the consequences of childhood illness and injury and the effects of child labor, poverty, and neglect became widely recognized. The end of the nineteenth century is often regarded as the dark ages of pediatrics, and the first half of the twentieth century is regarded as the dawn of improved health care for children.

The study of pediatrics began in the late 1800s, particularly under the influence of a Prussian-born physician, Abraham Jacobi (1830-1919), who is referred to as the Father of Pediatrics. With several other physicians he broke new ground in the scientific and clinical investigation of childhood diseases. One outstanding achievement was the establishment of "milk stations," where mothers could bring sick children for treatment and learn the importance of pure milk and its proper preparation.

The crusade for pure milk helped bring the dairy industry under legal control and led to the establishment of infant welfare stations. The remarkable decline in infant mortality since 1900 has been achieved through prevention and health-promoting measures such as improved sanitation and pasteurization of milk. Before these regulations existed, the unsanitary milk supply was a chief source of infantile diarrhea and tuberculosis. Cows were often kept in filthy stables and fed garbage and distillery wastes. Milk from cows that were fed distillery wastes was reported to make infants "tipsy."

At the same time, increasing concern developed for the social welfare of children, especially those who were homeless or employed as factory laborers. The work of one reformer, Lillian Wald (1867-1940), had far-reaching effects on child health and nursing. She founded the Henry Street Settlement in New York City, which eventually provided nursing services; social work; and an organized program of social, cultural, and educational activities. Wald is regarded as the founder of public health or community nursing. She was instrumental in establishing the role of the first full-time school nurse, Lina Rogers. Soon other nurses were employed to teach parents and children about the prevention or treatment of minor skin conditions, malnutrition, and other impairments or illnesses identified in the school. An outgrowth of nursing involvement in school health was the development of pediatric courses and specialized clinical experience in schools of nursing.

As more causes of disease were identified, health care workers emphasized isolation and asepsis. In the early 1900s children with contagious diseases were isolated from adult patients. Parents were prohibited from visiting because they might transmit disease to and from the home. Even toys and personal articles of clothing were kept from the child. It was not until the 1940s and the famous work of Spitz and Robertson on institutionalized children that the effects of isolation and maternal deprivation were recognized. This research brought forth a surge of interest in the psychologic health of children and resulted in changes for hospitalized children, such as rooming-in, sibling visitations, child life (play) programs, pre-hospitalization preparation, parent education, and hospital schooling.

Influenced by social reformers such as Lillian Wald, national leaders took action to improve children's living conditions. In 1909 President Theodore Roosevelt called the first White House Conference on Children, which focused on the care of dependent children and the deplorable working conditions of youngsters. As a result of this conference, the U.S. Children's Bureau was established in 1912 and placed under the Department of Health, Education and Welfare (now the Department of Health and Human Services).

The establishment of the Children's Bureau marked the beginning of a period of studies of economic and social factors related to infant mortality, maternal deaths, and maternal and infant care in rural areas, all of which created a stimulus for better standards of care for mothers and children. These studies led to the first Maternity and Infancy Act (Sheppard-Towner Act) in 1921, which provided grants to states to develop a Division of Maternal and Child Health (MCH) as a unit of the health department. This bill eventually lapsed because of opposition from those (especially the American Medical Association) who viewed it as a socialist movement. Nevertheless, the passage of the Maternity and Infancy Act was a turning point for the creation of the American Academy of Pediatrics in 1930.

With the passage of Title V of the Social Security Act (SSA) in 1935, a federal-state partnership was established under the administration of the Children's Bureau. Title V included federal grants-in-aid to states (matched by state funds) for three types of work: MCH, Crippled Children's Services (CCS), and child welfare services. The first programs provided by Title V were prenatal, postnatal, and child health clinics and training of personnel. The early emphasis of the CCS program was on orthopedic care. With the recognition that a child's ability to function could be limited by a chronic illness, state CCS programs became involved with children who had developmental, behavioral, and educational problems and, more recently, with home care of children with complex medical conditions. This broadened concept was reflected in 1985 by the passage of legislation that changed the name of the CCS to the Program for Children with Special Health Needs (CSHN).

Other federal programs that have had a major impact on maternal and child health include:

Medicaid—In 1965 Medicaid was created under Title XIX of the SSA to reduce financial barriers to health care for the poor. It is the largest maternal-child health program. A major project under Medicaid is the Child Health Assessment Program (CHAP), which provides services for a large number of pregnant women and children. Not all poor children are eligible for Medicaid; financial eligibility varies considerably from state to state.

Women, Infants, and Children (WIC)—In 1974 the WIC Special Supplemental Food Program was started. This program provides nutritious food and nutrition education to low-income, pregnant, postpartum, and lactating women and to infants and children up to age 5 years. Other nutrition programs include Food Stamps, National School Lunch Program, School Breakfast Program, and Child Care Food Program. The Child Care Food Program provides financial assistance for nutritious meals to children in daycare centers, family and group daycare homes, and Head Start centers.

Education for All Handicapped Children Act (P.L. 94-142)—In 1975 P.L. 94-142 was passed to provide free, appropriate public education to all handicapped children from ages 3 to 21 years and to provide for supportive services (such as speech and counseling) that ensure the benefit of special education.

Education of the Handicapped Act Amendments of 1986 (P.L. 99-457)—In 1986 P.L. 99-457 was passed to allow for the provision of federal funding to states to develop and implement a statewide, comprehensive, coordinated, and multidisciplinary program of early intervention services for handicapped infants and toddlers and their families.

Omnibus Budget Reconciliation Act of 1990—Passage of this act required states to extend Medicaid coverage to all children ages 6 to 18 years with family incomes below 133% of the poverty level.

Family and Medical Leave Act (FMLA)—Signed into law in 1993, FMLA allows eligible employees to take up to 12 weeks of unpaid leave from their jobs every year to care for newborn or newly adopted children; to care for children, parents, or spouses who have serious health conditions; or to recover from their own serious health conditions. After the leave, the law entitles employees to return to their previous jobs or to equivalent jobs with the same pay, benefits, and other conditions.

Health Insurance Portability and Accountability Act (HIPAA)—The first federal privacy standards to protect patients' medical records and other health information provided to health plans, doctors, hospitals, and other health care providers took effect on April 14, 2003. HIPAA, developed by the Department of Health and Human Services, sets new standards that provide patients with access to their medical records and more control over how their personal health information is used and disclosed. For further information, see the website www. hhs.gov/ocr/hipaa.

Despite the number of federal and state programs available to assist children and families, health care in the United States has serious barriers, including (1) financial barriers, such as not having insurance, having insurance that does not cover certain services, or being unable to pay for services; (2) system barriers, such as having to travel great distances for health care or state-to-state variations in Medicaid benefits; and (3) knowledge barriers, such as a lack of understanding about the need for or value of prenatal or child health supervision or a lack of awareness of the services that are available. The current thrust in health care is to improve children's and families' access to health care.

One of the major changes in health care delivery has been the establishment of a prospective payment system based on diagnosis-related groups (DRGs). The DRG categories define pretreatment (prospective) billing for almost all U.S. hospitals reimbursed by Medicaid. Because hospitals are financially responsible when Medicaid patients exceed the allotted admission stay, more patients are discharged early. This has created an immense need for home care and other community-based services. Health care cost containment remains a national priority, and some form of prospective payment affects almost everyone. Nurses need to be aware of changing trends in health care economics and be prepared to meet the challenges presented by managed care companies and health maintenance organizations (HMOs).

THE ART OF PEDIATRIC NURSING

PHILOSOPHY OF CARE

Nursing of infants, children, and adolescents is consistent with the definition of nursing as "the diagnosis and treatment of human responses to actual or potential health problems." This definition incorporates the four essential features of contemporary nursing practice (American Nurses Association, 2003):

1. Attention to the full range of human experiences and responses to health and illness without restriction to a problem-focused orientation
2. Integration of objective data with knowledge gained from an understanding of the patient or group's subjective experience
3. Application of scientific knowledge to the processes of diagnosis and treatment
4. Provision of a caring relationship that facilitates health and healing

Family-Centered Care

The philosophy of family-centered care recognizes the family as the constant in a child's life. Service systems and personnel must support, respect, encourage, and enhance the family's strength and competence by developing a partnership with parents (National Center for Cultural Competence, 2007). Nurses support families in their natural care-giving and decision-making roles by building on their unique strengths and acknowledging their expertise in caring for their child both within and outside the hospital setting (National Center for Cultural Competence, 2007). The nurse considers the needs of all family members in relation to the care of the child (Box 1-3). The philosophy acknowledges diversity among family structures and backgrounds; family goals, dreams, strategies, and actions; and family support, service, and information needs (Hooper, 2008).

Two basic concepts in family-centered care are enabling and empowerment. Professionals enable families by creating opportunities and means for all family members to display their current abilities and competencies and to acquire new ones to meet the needs of the child and family. Empowerment describes the interaction of professionals with families in such a way that families maintain or acquire a sense of control over their family lives and acknowledge positive changes that result from helping behaviors that foster their own strengths, abilities, and actions.

BOX 1-3   KEY ELEMENTS OF FAMILY-CENTERED CARE

Incorporating into policy and practice the recognition that the family is the constant in a child's life while the service systems and support personnel within those systems fluctuate

Facilitating family-professional collaboration at all levels of hospital, home, and community care:
- Care of an individual child
- Program development, implementation, and evaluation
- Policy formation

Exchanging complete and unbiased information between family members and professionals in a supportive manner at all times

Incorporating into policy and practice the recognition and honoring of cultural diversity, strengths, and individuality within and across all families, including ethnic, racial, spiritual, social, economic, educational, and geographic diversity

Recognizing and respecting different methods of coping and implementing comprehensive policies and programs that provide developmental, educational, emotional, environmental, and financial support to meet the diverse needs of families

Encouraging and facilitating family-to-family support and networking

Ensuring that home, hospital, and community service and support systems for children needing specialized health and developmental care and their families are flexible, accessible, and comprehensive in responding to diverse family-identified needs

Appreciating families as families and children as children, recognizing that they possess a wide range of strengths, concerns, emotions, and aspirations beyond their need for specialized health and developmental services and support

From Shelton TL, Stepanek JS: *Family-centered care for children needing specialized health and developmental services*, Bethesda, Md, 1994, Association for the Care of Children's Health.

Although caring for the family is strongly emphasized throughout this text, it is highlighted in features such as Cultural Competence and Family-Centered Care boxes (see p. 16).

Atraumatic Care

Atraumatic care is the provision of therapeutic care in settings, by personnel, and through the use of interventions that eliminate or minimize the psychologic and physical distress experienced by children and their families in the health care system. Therapeutic care encompasses the prevention, diagnosis, treatment, or palliation of acute or chronic conditions. Setting refers to the place in which that care is given—the home, the hospital, or any other health care setting. Personnel includes anyone directly involved in providing therapeutic care. Interventions range from psychologic approaches, such as preparing children for procedures, to physical interventions, such as providing space for a parent to room in with a child. Psychologic distress may include anxiety, fear, anger, disappointment, sadness, shame, or guilt. Physical distress may range from sleeplessness and immobilization to disturbances from sensory stimuli such as pain, temperature extremes, loud noises, bright lights, or darkness. Thus atraumatic care is concerned with the where, who, why, and how of any procedure performed on a child for the purpose of preventing or minimizing psychologic and physical stress (Wong, 1989).

The overriding goal in providing atraumatic care is: first, do no harm. Three principles provide the framework for achieving this goal: (1) prevent or minimize the child's separation from the family, (2) promote a sense of control, and (3) prevent or minimize bodily injury and pain. Examples of providing atraumatic care include fostering the parent-child relationship during hospitalization, preparing the child before any unfamiliar treatment or procedure, controlling pain, allowing the child privacy, providing play activities for expression of fear and aggression, providing choices to children, and respecting cultural differences.

ROLE OF THE PEDIATRIC NURSE

The pediatric nurse is responsible for promoting the health and well-being of the child and family. Nursing functions vary according to regional job structures, individual education and experience, and personal career goals. Just as patients (children and their families) have unique backgrounds, each nurse brings an individual set of variables that affect the nurse-patient relationship. No matter where pediatric nurses practice, their primary concern is the welfare of the child and family.

Therapeutic Relationship

The establishment of a therapeutic relationship is the essential foundation for providing high-quality nursing care. Pediatric nurses need to have meaningful relationships with children and their families and yet remain separate enough to distinguish their own feelings and needs. In a therapeutic relationship, caring, well-defined boundaries separate the nurse from the child and family. These boundaries are positive and professional and promote the family's control over the child's health care. These boundaries are essential for effective family advocacy (Jacobson, 2002). Both the nurse and the family are empowered and maintain open communication. In a nontherapeutic relationship these boundaries are blurred, and many of the nurse's actions may serve personal needs, such as a need to feel wanted and involved, rather than the family's needs.

Exploring whether relationships with patients are therapeutic or nontherapeutic helps nurses identify problem areas early in their interactions with children and families (see Nursing Care Guidelines box). Although questions regarding the nurse's involvement may label certain actions negative or positive, no one action makes a relationship therapeutic or nontherapeutic. For example, a nurse may spend additional time with the family but still recognize his or her own needs and maintain professional separateness. An important clue to nontherapeutic relationships is the staff's concerns about their peer's actions with the family.

Family Advocacy and Caring

Although nurses are responsible to themselves, the profession, and the institution of employment, their primary responsibility is to the consumer of nursing services: the child and family. The nurse must work with family members, identify their goals and needs, and plan interventions that best address the defined problems. As an advocate, the nurse assists the child and family in making informed choices and acting in the child's best interest. Advocacy involves ensuring that families are aware of all available health services, adequately informed of treatments and procedures involved in the child's care, and encouraged to change or support existing health care practices. The United Nations' Declaration of the Rights of the Child (Box 1-4) provides guidelines for nursing practice to ensure that every child receives optimum care.

As nurses care for children and families, they must demonstrate caring, compassion, and empathy for others. Aspects of caring embody the concept of atraumatic care and the development of a therapeutic relationship with patients. Parents perceive caring as a sign of quality in nursing care, which is often focused on the nontechnical needs of the child and family. Parents describe "personable" care as actions by the nurse that include acknowledging the parent's presence, listening, making the parent feel comfortable in the hospital environment, involv-

---

 NURSING CARE GUIDELINES

Exploring Your Relationships with Children and Families

To foster therapeutic relationships with children and families, you must first become aware of your caregiving style, including how effectively you take care of yourself. The following questions should help you understand the therapeutic quality of your professional relationships.

Negative Actions

Are you overinvolved with children and their families?
- Do you work overtime to care for the family?
- Do you spend off-duty time with children's families, either in or out of the hospital?
- Do you call frequently (either the hospital or home) to see how the family is doing?
- Do you show favoritism toward certain patients?
- Do you buy clothes, toys, food, or other items for the child and family?
- Do you compete with other staff members for the affection of certain patients and families?
- Do other staff members comment to you about your closeness to the family?
- Do you attempt to influence families' decisions rather than facilitate their informed decision making?

Are you underinvolved with children and families?
- Do you restrict parent or visitor access to children, using excuses such as the unit is too busy?
- Do you focus on the technical aspects of care and lose sight of the person who is the patient?

Are you overinvolved with children and underinvolved with their parents?
- Do you become critical when parents do not visit their children?
- Do you compete with parents for their children's affection?

Positive Actions

Do you strive to empower families?
- Do you explore families' strengths and needs in an effort to increase family involvement?
- Have you developed teaching skills to instruct families rather than doing everything for them?
- Do you work with families to find ways to decrease their dependence on health care providers?
- Can you separate families' needs from your own needs?

Do you strive to empower yourself?
- Are you aware of your emotional responses to different people and situations?
- Do you seek to understand how your own family experiences influence reactions to patients and families, especially as they affect tendencies toward overinvolvement or underinvolvement?
- Do you have a calming influence, not one that will amplify emotionality?
- Have you developed interpersonal skills in addition to technical skills?
- Have you learned about ethnic and religious family patterns?
- Do you communicate directly with persons with whom you are upset or take issue?
- Are you able to "step back" and withdraw emotionally, if not physically, when emotional overload occurs, yet remain committed?
- Do you take care of yourself and your needs?
- Do you periodically interview family members to determine their current issues (e.g., feelings, attitudes, responses, wishes), communicate these findings to peers, and update records?
- Do you avoid relying on initial interview data, assumptions, or gossip regarding families?
- Do you ask questions if families are not participating in care?
- Do you assess families for feelings of anxiety, fear, intimidation, worry about making a mistake, a perceived lack of competence to care for their child, or fear of health care professionals overstepping their boundaries into family territory, or vice versa?
- Do you explore these issues with family members and provide encouragement and support to enable families to help themselves?
- Do you keep communication channels open among self, family, physicians, and other care providers?
- Do you resolve conflicts and misunderstandings directly with those who are involved?
- Do you clarify information for families or seek the appropriate person to do so?

Do you recognize that from time to time a therapeutic relationship can change to a social relationship or an intimate friendship?
- Are you able to acknowledge the fact when it occurs and understand why it happened?
- Can you ensure that there is someone else who is more objective who can take your place in the therapeutic relationship?

BOX 1-4   UNITED NATIONS' DECLARATION OF THE RIGHTS OF THE CHILD

All children need:
- To be free from discrimination
- To develop physically and mentally in freedom and dignity
- To have a name and nationality
- To have adequate nutrition, housing, recreation, and medical services
- To receive special treatment if handicapped
- To receive love, understanding, and material security
- To receive an education and develop his or her abilities
- To be the first to receive protection in disaster
- To be protected from neglect, cruelty, and exploitation
- To be brought up in a spirit of friendship among people

---

ing the parent and child in the nursing care, showing interest in and concern for their welfare, showing affection and sensitivity to the parent and child, communicating with them, and individualizing the nursing care. Parents perceive personable nursing care as being integral to establishing a positive relationship.

Disease Prevention and Health Promotion

Every nurse involved in caring for children must understand the importance of disease prevention and health promotion. A nursing care plan must include a thorough assessment of all aspects of child growth and development, including nutrition, immunizations, safety, dental care, socialization, discipline, and education. If problems are identified, the nurse intervenes directly or refers the family to other health care providers or agencies.

The best approach to prevention is education and anticipatory guidance. In this text each chapter on health promotion includes sections on anticipatory guidance. An appreciation of the hazards or conflicts of each developmental period enables the nurse to guide parents regarding childrearing practices aimed at preventing potential problems. One significant example is safety. Because each age-group is at risk for special types of injuries, preventive teaching can significantly reduce injuries, lowering permanent disability and mortality rates.

Prevention also involves less obvious aspects of caring for children. The nurse is responsible for providing care that promotes mental well-being (e.g., enlisting the help of a child life specialist during a painful procedure such as an immunization).

Health Teaching

Health teaching is inseparable from family advocacy and prevention. Health teaching may be the nurse's direct goal, such as during parenting classes, or may be indirect, such as helping parents and children understand a diagnosis or medical treatment, encouraging children to ask questions about their bodies, referring families to health-related professional or lay groups, supplying patients with appropriate literature, and providing anticipatory guidance.

Health teaching is one area in which nurses often need preparation and practice with competent role models, since it involves transmitting information at the child's and family's level of understanding and desire for information. As an effective educator, the nurse focuses on providing the appropriate

health teaching with generous feedback and evaluation to promote learning.

Support and Counseling

Attention to emotional needs requires support and, sometimes, counseling. The role of child advocate or health teacher is supportive by virtue of the individualized approach. The nurse can offer support by listening, touching, and being physically present. Touching and physical presence are most helpful with children because they facilitate nonverbal communication. Counseling involves a mutual exchange of ideas and opinions that provides the basis for mutual problem solving. It involves support, teaching, techniques to foster the expression of feelings or thoughts, and approaches to help the family cope with stress. Optimally, counseling not only helps resolve a crisis or problem but also enables the family to attain a higher level of functioning, greater self-esteem, and closer relationships. Although counseling is often the role of nurses in specialized areas, counseling techniques are discussed in various sections of this text to help students and nurses cope with immediate crises and refer families for additional professional assistance.

Coordination and Collaboration

The nurse, as a member of the health care team, collaborates and coordinates nursing care with the care activities of other professionals. A nurse working in isolation rarely serves the child's best interests. The concept of holistic care can be realized through a unified, interdisciplinary approach by being aware of individual contributions and limitations and collaborating with other specialists to provide high-quality health services. Failure to recognize limitations can be nontherapeutic at best and destructive at worst. For example, the nurse who feels competent in counseling but who is really inadequate in this area may not only prevent the child from dealing with a crisis but also impede future success with a qualified professional.

Even nurses who practice in isolated geographic areas widely separated from other health professionals cannot be considered independent. Every nurse works interdependently with the child and family, collaborating on assessing needs and planning interventions so that the final care plan truly meets the child's needs. Numerous disciplines often work together to formulate a comprehensive approach without consulting patients regarding their ideas or preferences. The nurse is in a vital position to include patients in their care, either directly or indirectly, by communicating their thoughts to the health care team.

Ethical Decision Making

Ethical dilemmas arise when competing moral considerations underlie various alternatives. Parents, nurses, physicians, and other health care team members may reach different but morally defensible decisions by assigning different weights to competing moral values. These competing moral values may include **autonomy**, the patient's right to be self-governing; **nonmaleficence**, the obligation to minimize or prevent harm; **beneficence**, the obligation to promote the patient's well-being; and **justice**, the concept of fairness. Nurses must determine the most beneficial or least harmful action within the framework of societal mores, professional practice standards, the law, institutional rules, the family's value system and religious traditions, and the nurse's personal values.

Nurses must prepare themselves systematically for collaborative ethical decision making. They can accomplish this through formal course work, continuing education, contemporary literature, and work to establish an environment conducive to ethical discourse. Moreover, nurses must be educated on the mechanisms for dispute resolution, case review by ethics committees, procedural safeguards, state statutes, and case law (Woods, 2005).

The nurse also uses the professional code of ethics for guidance and as a means for professional self-regulation. The Code of Ethics for Nurses by the American Nurses Association focuses on the nurse's accountability and responsibility to the patient and emphasizes the nursing role as an independent professional, one that upholds its own legal liability.

Nurses may face ethical issues regarding patient care, such as the use of lifesaving measures for VLBW newborns or the terminally ill child's right to refuse treatment. They may struggle with questions regarding truthfulness, balancing their rights and responsibilities in caring for children with AIDS, whistleblowing, or allocating resources. Throughout the text such dilemmas are addressed in boxes titled Ethical Decision Making. Conflicting ethical arguments are presented to help nurses clarify their value judgments when confronted with sensitive issues.

RESEARCH AND EVIDENCE-BASED PRACTICE

Nurses should contribute to research because they are the individuals observing human responses to health and illness. The current emphasis on measurable outcomes to determine the efficacy of interventions (often in relation to the cost) demands that nurses know whether clinical interventions result in positive outcomes for their patients. This demand has influenced the current trend toward **evidence-based practice (EBP)**, which implies questioning why something is effective and whether a better approach exists. The concept of EBP also involves analyzing and translating published clinical research into the everyday practice of nursing. When nurses base their clinical practice on science and research and document their clinical outcomes, they will be able to validate their contributions to health, wellness, and cure, not only to their patients, third-party payers, and institutions but also to the nursing profession. Evaluation is essential to the nursing process, and research is one of the best ways to accomplish this.

EBP is the collection, interpretation, and integration of valid, important, and applicable patient-reported, nurse-observed, and research-derived information. Evidence-based nursing practice combines knowledge with clinical experience and intuition. It provides a rational approach to decision making that facilitates best practice (Scott and McSherry, 2009; van Achterberg, Schoonhoven, and Grol, 2008). EBP is an important tool that complements the nursing process by using critical thinking skills to make decisions based on existing knowledge. The traditional nursing process approach to patient care can be used to conceptualize the essential components of EBP nursing (Table 1-4). During the assessment and diagnostic phases of the nursing process, the nurse establishes important clinical questions and completes a critical review of existing knowledge. EBP also begins with identification of the problem. The nurse asks clinical questions in a concise, organized way that allows for clear answers. Once the specific questions are identified, extensive searching for the best information to answer the question begins. The nurse evaluates clinically relevant research, analyzes findings from the history and physical examinations, and reviews the specific pathophysiology of the defined problem. The third step in the nursing process is to develop a care plan. In evidence-based nursing practice, the care plan is established on completion of a critical appraisal of what is known and not known about the defined problem. Next, in the traditional nursing process, the nurse implements the care plan. By integrating evidence with clinical expertise, the nurse focuses care on the patient's unique needs. A template for organizing the evidence is found in Box 1-5. The final step in EBP is consistent with the final phase of the nursing process: to evaluate the effectiveness of the care plan.

Searching for evidence in this modern era of technology can be overwhelming. For nurses to implement EBP, they must have access to appropriate, recent resources such as online search engines and journals. In many institutions computer terminals are available on patient care units, with the Internet and online journals easily accessible. Another important resource for the implementation of EBP is time. The nursing shortage and ongoing changes in many institutions have compounded the issue of nursing time allocation for patient care, education, and training. In some institutions nurses are given paid time away from performing patient care to participate in activities that promote EBP. This requires an organizational environment that values EBP and its potential impact on patient care. As knowledge is generated regarding the significant impact of EBP on patient care outcomes, it is hoped that the organizational culture will change to support the staff nurse's participa-

TABLE 1-4	THE NURSING PROCESS AND EVIDENCE-BASED PRACTICE		
NURSING PROCESS	**ACTIONS**	**EVIDENCE-BASED PRACTICE**	**ACTIONS**
Assessment	Collect patient data	Ask the question	Clearly identifies specific patient problems and needs
Diagnosis	Analyze assessment data and determines diagnosis	Search for evidence	Collects information relevant to patient's identified problems and needs
Planning	Develop care plan	Analyze evidence	Critically appraises published literature
Implementation	Initiate interventions identified in care plan	Apply evidence to practice	Integrates evidence with clinical expertise and patient's unique needs
Evaluation	Evaluate patient's progress toward attainment of outcomes	Evaluate effectiveness	Evaluates effectiveness of integration of evidence

BOX 1-5 EVIDENCE-BASED PRACTICE TEMPLATE

Ask the Question

_____

_____

Search for the Evidence

Search strategies: _____

Databases used: _____

Critically Analyze the Evidence

GRADE criteria: _____

Apply the Evidence: Nursing Implications

_____

_____

_____

References

_____

_____

_____

TABLE 1-5 THE GRADE CRITERIA TO EVALUATE THE QUALITY OF THE EVIDENCE

QUALITY	TYPE OF EVIDENCE
High	Consistent evidence from well-performed randomized clinical trials (RCTs) or exceptionally strong evidence from unbiased observational studies
Moderate	Evidence from RCTs with important limitations (inconsistent results, methodologic flaws, indirect evidence, or imprecise results) or unusually strong evidence from unbiased observational studies
Low	Evidence for at least one critical outcome from observational studies, from RCTs with serious flaws, or from indirect evidence
Very Low	Evidence for at least one of the critical outcomes from unsystematic clinical observations or very indirect evidence

QUALITY	RECOMMENDATION
Strong	Desirable effects clearly outweigh undesirable effects, or vice versa
Weak	Desirable effects closely balanced with undesirable effects

Adapted from Guyatt GH, Oxman AD, Visit GE, et al: GRADE: an emerging consensus on rating quality of evidence and strength of recommendations, *BMJ* 336:924-926, 2008.

tion in EBP. As the amount of available evidence increases, so does our need to critically evaluate the evidence.

Throughout this book, EBP boxes summarize the existing evidence that promotes excellence in clinical care. The GRADE criteria are used to evaluate the quality of research articles used to develop practice guidelines (Guyatt, Oxman, Vist, et al, 2008). Table 1-5 defines how the nurse rates the quality of the evidence using the GRADE criteria and establishes a strong versus weak recommendation. Each EBP box rates the quality of existing evidence and the strength of the recommendation for practice change.

CRITICAL THINKING AND THE PROCESS OF PROVIDING NURSING CARE TO CHILDREN AND FAMILIES

CRITICAL THINKING

A systematic thought process is essential to a profession. It assists the professional in meeting the patient's needs. Critical thinking is purposeful, goal-directed thinking that assists individuals in making judgments based on evidence rather than guesswork (Walsh and Seldomridge, 2006; Alfaro-LeFevre, 2005). It is based on the scientific method of inquiry, which is also the basis for the nursing process. Critical thinking and the nursing process are considered crucial to professional nursing in that they constitute a holistic approach to problem solving.

Critical thinking is a complex developmental process based on rational and deliberate thought. Becoming a critical thinker provides a common denominator for knowledge that exemplifies disciplined and self-directed thinking. The knowledge is acquired, assessed, and organized by thinking through the clinical situation and developing an outcome focused on optimum

patient care. Critical thinking transforms the way in which individuals view themselves, understand the world, and make decisions. In recognition of the importance of this skill, Critical Thinking Exercises are included in this text. These exercises present a nursing practice situation that challenges the student to use the skills of critical thinking to come to the best conclusion. A series of questions lead the student to explore the evidence, assumptions underlying the problem, nursing priorities, and support for nursing interventions that allow the nurse to make a rational and deliberate response. These thinking exercises are designed to enhance nursing performance in clinical judgment.

NURSING PROCESS

The nursing process is a method of problem identification and problem solving that describes what the nurse actually does (Alfaro-LeFevre, 2005). The five-step nursing process model is assessment, diagnosis (problem identification), planning (with outcome development), implementation, and evaluation. The second step of the nursing process, nursing diagnosis, involves the naming the child's or family's problem in standardized nursing language. In the American Nurses Association (2003) Standards of Practice, the nursing diagnosis phase of the nursing process is separated into two steps: nursing diagnosis and outcome identification.

Assessment

Assessment is a continuous process that operates at all phases of problem solving and is the foundation for decision making. Assessment involves multiple nursing skills and consists of the purposeful collection, classification, and analysis of data from a variety of sources. To provide an accurate and comprehensive assessment, the nurse must consider information about the patient's biophysical, psychologic, sociocultural, and spiritual background.

Nursing Diagnosis

The second stage of the nursing process is problem identification and nursing diagnosis. At this point the nurse must interpret and make decisions about the data gathered. The nurse organizes or clusters these data into categories to identify significant areas and makes one of the following decisions:

- No dysfunctional health problems are evident; no interventions are indicated.
- Risk for dysfunctional health problems exists; interventions are needed for health promotion.
- Actual dysfunctional health problems are evident; interventions are needed for health promotion.

The nursing diagnosis is the naming of the cue clusters that are obtained during the assessment phase. According to NANDA International (formerly the North American Nursing Diagnosis Association), the currently accepted definition of the term **nursing diagnosis** is that it is a clinical judgment about individual, family, or community responses to actual and potential health problems and life processes. Nursing diagnoses provide the basis for selecting nursing interventions to achieve outcomes for which the nurse is accountable (Johnson, Bulechek, Dochterman, et al, 2001). The **Nursing Interventions Classification (NIC)** consists of a standardized list of more than 400 examples of care provided by nurses in clinical practice. The **Nursing Outcomes Classification (NOC)** is a comprehensive, standardized system of patient outcomes that can be used to evaluate the results of specific nursing interventions. Examples of NIC and NOC concepts are listed in each Nursing Care Plan in this text to provide an understanding of the standardized language and how it relates to the individualized plan.

Not all children have actual health problems; some have a potential health problem, which is a risk state that requires nursing intervention to prevent the development of an actual problem. Potential health problems may be indicated by risk factors, or signs, that predispose a child and family to a dysfunctional health pattern and are limited to individuals at greater risk than the population as a whole. Nursing intervention are directed toward reducing risk factors. To differentiate actual from potential health problems, the word *risk* is included in the nursing diagnosis statement (e.g., Risk for Infection).

Signs and symptoms refer to a cluster of cues and defining characteristics that are derived from patient assessment and indicate actual health problems. When a defining characteristic is essential for the diagnosis to be made, it is considered critical. These critical defining characteristics help differentiate between diagnostic categories. For example, in deciding between the diagnostic categories related to family function and coping, the nurse uses defining characteristics to choose the most appropriate nursing diagnosis (see Family-Centered Care box).

Planning

After identifying the nursing diagnoses, the nurse develops a care plan and establishes outcomes or goals. The **outcome** is the projected or expected change in a patient's health status, clinical condition, or behavior that occurs after nursing interventions have been instituted. The ultimate goal of nursing care

 FAMILY-CENTERED CARE

Using Defining Characteristics to Select an Appropriate Nursing Diagnosis

An 18-month-old only child is admitted with respiratory distress and a presumptive diagnosis of epiglottitis. Initial nursing actions focus on the child's physiologic status. As the condition stabilizes, the nurse gathers family assessment data. The child's immunizations are current, he is clean and well nourished, and his developmental age is appropriate. The parents are both present at admission. The mother is distraught about the sudden onset of respiratory distress. She states that earlier her child had only a "runny nose" and she thought it was just a cold. When the child suddenly began to have difficulty breathing, she felt helpless and unable to relieve her child's discomfort. She states: "Nothing I did made him any better. If I had known this could happen, I would have brought him to the hospital sooner. I feel like a bad mother." In the hospital, after explanations by the nurses, the mother understands that epiglottitis is a sudden illness that typically follows symptoms of a cold. She is cooperative and asks what she can do to make her child more comfortable. She implements all the suggestions of the health care team. The father supports both the child and mother, although he assumes a more passive, "listening" role.

Three nursing diagnoses that relate to family and parent situations may be relevant. The first step is to review the diagnoses and the defining characteristics and decide which one is most appropriate:

1. Parenting, Impaired—Inability of the primary caretaker to create, maintain, or regain an environment that nurtures the child's growth and development
   Selected defining characteristics:
   - Insecure (or lack of) attachment to infant
   - Poor or inappropriate caretaking skills
2. Conflict, Parental Role—Parent experience of role confusion and conflict in response to crisis
   Selected defining characteristics:
   - Parent expressing concerns about changes in parental role
   - A demonstrated disruption in care or caretaking routines
   - Parent expressing concerns or feelings of inadequacy to provide for the child's physical and emotional needs during hospitalization or in home
   - Parent verbalizing or demonstrating feelings of guilt, anger, fear, anxiety, or frustration about effect of child's illness on family process
3. Family Processes, Interrupted—A change in family relationships or functioning.
   Selected defining characteristics:
   - Expressions of conflict within the family
   - Changes in communication patterns among family members

Of these three diagnoses, the most relevant one is *Conflict, Parental Role.* The parents demonstrate attachment behavior to their child and are attentive to his needs. They appear to have appropriate parenting skills and are able to communicate effectively with each other. Neither parent expressed any conflict within the family. The sudden onset of this child's illness has interrupted the mother's usual role and caused her to feel inadequate, anxious, and guilty. However, the mother is able to adapt to this crisis. She demonstrates an ability to cope by learning and implementing new comforting skills for her child. The defining characteristics of the other two diagnoses require maladaptive characteristics that are clearly not demonstrated by these parents.

is to convert the nursing diagnoses into a desired health state. The care plan must be established before specific nursing interventions are developed and implemented.

Implementation

The implementation phase begins when the nurse puts the selected intervention into action and accumulates feedback data regarding its effects (or the patient's response to the intervention). The feedback returns in the form of observation and communication and provides a database on which to evaluate the outcome of the nursing intervention. It is imperative that continual assessment of the patient's status occur throughout all phases of the nursing process, thus making the process a dynamic rather than static problem-solving method. Throughout the implementation stage, the main concerns are the patient's physical safety and psychologic comfort in terms of atraumatic care.

Evaluation

Evaluation is the last step in the decision-making process. The nurse gathers, sorts, and analyzes data to determine whether (1) the established outcome has been met, (2) the nursing interventions were appropriate, (3) the plan requires modification, or (4) other alternatives should be considered. The evaluation phase either completes the nursing process (outcome is met) or serves as the basis for selecting alternative interventions to solve the specific problem.

With the current focus on patient outcomes in health care, the patient's care is evaluated not only at discharge but thereafter as well to ensure that the outcomes are met and there is adequate care for resolving existing or potential health problems. One federal agency that has developed clinical guidelines is the Agency for Healthcare Research and Quality.*

Documentation

Although documentation is not one of the five steps of the nursing process, it is essential for evaluation. The nurse can assess, diagnose and identify problems, plan, and implement without documentation; however, evaluation is best performed with written evidence of progress toward outcomes. The patient's medical record should include evidence of those elements listed in the Nursing Care Guidelines box.

📋 NURSING CARE GUIDELINES

Documentation of Nursing Care

- Initial assessments and reassessments
- Nursing diagnoses and/or patient care needs
- Interventions identified to meet the patient's nursing care needs
- Nursing care provided
- Patient's response to, and the outcomes of, the care provided
- Abilities of patient and/or, as appropriate, significant other(s) to manage continuing care needs after discharge

---

QUALITY OUTCOME MEASURES

Quality of care refers to the degree to which health services for individuals and populations increase the likelihood of desired health outcomes and are consistent with current professional knowledge (Institute of Medicine, 2000). Since nurses are the principal caregivers within health care institutions, high-quality nursing outcomes are used as an indicator of the ability to provide excellence in patient care. Nurse-sensitive indicators are chosen by using specific evaluation criteria (Box 1-6). Specific examples of patient-centered outcome measures estab-

---

BOX 1-6 QUALITY OUTCOME MEASURES: EVALUATION CRITERIA

Logical order for evaluating quality outcome measures:
1. Importance to measure and report
2. Scientific acceptability
3. Usability
4. Feasibility

BOX 1-7 NATIONAL QUALITY FORUM: PATIENT-CENTERED OUTCOME MEASURES*

Death among surgical inpatients with treatable serious complications (failure to rescue)—The percentage of major surgical inpatients who experience a hospital-acquired complication and die

Pressure ulcer prevalence—Percentage of inpatients who have a hospital-acquired pressure ulcer

Falls prevalence—Number of inpatient falls per inpatient days

Falls with injury—Number of inpatient falls with injuries per inpatient days

Restraint prevalence—Percentage of inpatients who have a vest or limb restraint

Urinary catheter–associated urinary tract infection for intensive care unit (ICU) patients—Rate of urinary tract infections associated with use of urinary catheters for ICU patients

Central line catheter–associated bloodstream infection rate for ICU and high-risk nursery patients—Rate of bloodstream infections associated with use of central line catheters for ICU and high-risk nursery patients

Ventilator-associated pneumonia for ICU and high-risk nursery patients—Rate of pneumonia associated with use of ventilators for ICU and high-risk nursery patients

Copyright © 2006 by the Joint Commission on Accreditation of Healthcare Organization, One Renaissance Boulevard, Oakbrook Terrace, IL 60181. NOTE: The Implementation Guide for the NQF Endorsed Nursing-Sensitive Care Performance Measures [Version 1.00, December 2005] is the intellectual property of and copyrighted by the Joint Commission on Accreditation of Healthcare Organizations, Oakbrook Terrace, Illinois. It is used in this text with the permission of The Joint Commission. Updates can be found at www.jointcommission.org/performancemeasurement/ measurereservelibrary/nqf_nursing.htm.
*Measures include only those related to the pediatric population.

---

lished by the National Quality Forum are found in Box 1-7. A comprehensive resource, the Quality and Safety Education for Nurses, is funded by the Robert Wood Johnson Foundation.†

Quality outcome evaluation criteria establish a framework for measuring nursing care performance. In addition to using the National Quality Forum's measurement evaluation criteria, nurses should evaluate each quality-nursing indicator to ensure it is an essential component of health care quality established by the Institute of Medicine (2000). These components include the following:
- Safe
- Effective
- Patient-centered
- Timely
- Efficient
- Equitable

---

*540 Gaither Road, Suite 2000, Rockville, MD 20850; 301-427-1364; info@ahrq.gov; www.ahrq.gov.

†University of North Carolina at Chapel Hill, School of Nursing, Carrington Hall, CB# 7460, Chapel Hill, North Carolina 27599; 919-843-9985; fax: 919-843-3884; e-mail: qsen@unc.edu; www.qsen.org.

Throughout the chapters that focus on serious health problems, we have developed examples of quality outcome measures for specific diseases that reflect patient-centered outcomes. Quality outcome measures promote interdisciplinary teamwork, and the boxes throughout this book exemplify measures of effective collaboration to improve care. Quality Patient Outcomes boxes throughout this book are developed to assist health care professionals in identifying appropriate measures that evaluate the quality of patient care.

KEY POINTS

- Although the infant mortality rate in the United States has declined over the past few decades, the United States lags significantly behind most other major countries, such as Canada.
- LBW, which is closely related to early gestational age, is considered the leading cause of neonatal death in the United States.
- Injuries are the leading cause of death in children over age 1 year, with the majority being MVA injuries.
- Childhood morbidity encompasses acute illness, chronic disease, and disability.
- Eighty percent of childhood illnesses are attributable to infections, with respiratory tract infections occurring two or three times more often than all other illnesses combined.
- The *new morbidity* refers to behavioral, social, and educational problems that can significantly alter a child's health.
- Developmental stage and environment are important determinants of the prevalence of injuries at a given age and thus help to direct preventive measures.
- The philosophy of family-centered care recognizes that the family is the constant in a child's life and that service systems and personnel must support, respect, and enhance the family's strength and competence.

- Atraumatic care is the provision of therapeutic care in settings, by personnel, and through the use of interventions that eliminate or minimize the psychologic and physical distress experienced by children and their families in the health care system.
- The pediatric nurse's roles include a therapeutic relationship, family advocacy, disease prevention and health promotion, health teaching, support and counseling, coordination and collaboration, ethical decision making, and research.
- EBP is the collection, interpretation, and integration of valid, important, and applicable patient-reported, nurse-observed, and research-derived information.
- The process of nursing children and families includes accurate and comprehensive assessment, analysis and synthesis of assessment data to arrive at a nursing diagnosis, planning of care, implementation of the plan, and evaluation of interventions.
- Since nurses are the principal caregivers within health care institutions, quality outcomes are used as a measure of the ability to provide excellence in patient care.

REFERENCES

Agency for Healthcare Research and Quality: *National healthcare disparities report,* Rockville, Md, 2008, US Department of Health and Human Services.

Alfaro-LeFevre R: *Applying nursing process: a tool for critical thinking,* ed 6, Philadelphia, 2005, Lippincott.

American Academy of Pediatrics: *The national children's study,* 2008, available at www.aap.org/family/natlchstudy.htm (accessed January 2, 2009).

American Association of Suicidology: *Youth suicide fact sheet,* 2009, available at www.suicidology.org (accessed December 2, 2009).

American Dietetic Association: Position of the American Dietetic Association: nutrition guidance for healthy children ages 2 to 11 years, *J Am Dietetic Assoc* 108(6):1038-1047, 2008.

American Nurses Association: *Nursing: scope and standards of practice,* Washington, DC, 2003, The Association.

Annie E Casey Foundation: *Kids count data book: state profiles of child well-being,* Baltimore, 2009, The Foundation.

Bronstein AC, Spyker DA, Cantilena LR, et al: 2007 Annual report of the American Association of Poison Control Centers' national poison data system: 25th annual report, *Clin Toxicol* 46(1):927-1057, 2008.

Cali AMG, Caprio S: Prediabetes and type 2 diabetes in youth: an emerging epidemic disease? *Curr Opin Endocrinol Diabetes Obes* 15:123-127, 2008.

Centers for Disease Control and Prevention: *CDC injury fact book,* Atlanta, 2006, National Center for Injury Prevention and Control.

Cheng NF, Han PZ, Gansky SA: Methods and software for estimating health disparities: the case of children's oral health, *Am J Epidemiol* 168(8):906-914, 2008.

Coury DL: Over the rainbow: advancing child health in the new millennium, *Ambul Pediatr* 6(3):134-137, 2006.

Doucette A: Youth suicide. In Cosby AG, Greenberg RE, Southward LH, et al, editors: *About children: an authoritative resource on the state of childhood today,* Elk Grove Village, Ill, 2005, American Academy of Pediatrics.

Dougherty D, Meikle SF, Owens P, et al: Children's health care in the First National Healthcare Quality Report and National Healthcare Disparities Report, *Med Care* 43(3 Suppl):I58-I63, 2005.

Edelstein BL: Tooth decay: the best of times, the worst of times. In Cosby AG, Greenberg RE, Southward LH, et al, editors: *About children: an authoritative resource on the state of childhood today,* Elk Grove Village, Ill, 2005, American Academy of Pediatrics.

Federal Interagency Forum on Child and Family Statistics: *America's children: key national indicators of well-being,* Washington, DC, 2007, US Government Printing Office.

Fitzgibbon ML, Stolley MR: Environmental changes may be needed for prevention of overweight in minority children, *Pediatr Ann* 33:45-49, 2004.

Franklin RL, Rodgers GB: Unintentional child poisoning treated in the United States hospital emergency departments: national estimates of incident cases, population-based poisoning rates, and product involvement, *Pediatrics* 122(6):1244-1251, 2008.

Groves BM: Violence in the lives of children. In Cosby AG, Greenberg RE, Southward LH, et al, editors: *About children: an authoritative resource on the state of childhood today,* Elk Grove Village, Ill, 2005, American Academy of Pediatrics.

Guyatt GH, Oxman AD, Vist GE, et al: GRADE: an emerging consensus on rating quality of evidence and strength of recommendations, *BMJ* 336:924-926, 2008.

Heuer S: Family-centered care, *J Spec Pediatr Nurs* 12(1):61-65, 2007.

Hooper VD: Patient-family centered care: are we there yet? *J Peri Anesthesia Nurs* 23(6):440-442, 2008.

Heron M, Hoyert DL, Murphy SL, et al: Deaths: final data for 2006, *Natl Vital Stat Rep* 57(14): 1-134, 2009.

Heron M, Sutton PD, Xu J, et al: Annual summary of vital statistics: 2007, *Pediatrics* 125(1):4-15, 2010.

Institute of Medicine: *Crossing the quality chasm,* Washington, DC, 2000, The Institute.

Jacobson GA: Maintaining professional boundaries: preparing nursing students for the challenge, *J Nurs Educ* 41(6):279-281, 2002.

Johnson M, Bulechek G, Dochterman J, et al: *Nursing diagnosis, outcomes and interventions,* St. Louis, 2001, Mosby.

Kagihara LE, Niederhauser VP, Stark M: Assessment, management, and prevention of early childhood caries, *J Am Acad Nurse Pract* 21(1):1-10, 2009.

Kelleher K: Mental health. In Cosby AG, Greenberg RE, Southward LH, et al, editors: *About children: an authoritative resource on the state of childhood today,* Elk Grove Village, Ill, 2005, American Academy of Pediatrics.

Lichter DT: Families: diversity and change. In Cosby AG, Greenberg RE, Southward LH, et al, editors: *About children: an authoritative resource on the state of childhood today,* Elk Grove Village, Ill, 2005, American Academy of Pediatrics.

Matyka KA: Type 2 diabetes in childhood: epidemiological and clinical aspects, *Br Med Bull* 86:59-75, 2008.

Medd SE: Children with ADHD need our advocacy, *J Pediatr Health Care* 17:102-104, 2003.

National Center for Cultural Competence: *A guide for advancing family-centered and culturally and linguistically competent care,* Washington, DC, 2007, Georgetown University Center for Child and Human Development.

National Safety Council: *Injury facts,* Itasca, Ill, 2000, The Council.

National Survey on Drug Use and Health: *Trends in substance use, dependence or abuse, and treatment among adolescents: 2002-2007,* Rockville, Md, December 4, 2008, Office of Applied Studies.

Robinson TN, Sargent JD: Children and media. In Cosby AG, Greenberg RE, Southward LH, et al, editors: *About children: an authoritative resource on the state of childhood today,* Elk Grove Village, Ill, 2005, American Academy of Pediatrics.

Schnitzer PG: Prevention of unintentional childhood injuries, *Am Fam Physician* 74(11):1864-1869, 2006.

Schwartz MS, Chadha A: Type 2 diabetes mellitus in childhood: obesity and insulin resistance, *J Am Osteopath Assoc* 108:518-524, 2008.

Scott K, McSherry R: Evidence-based nursing: clarifying the concepts for nurses in practice, *J Clin Nurs* 18(8):1085-1095, 2009.

US Department of Health and Human Services: *Healthy people 2020: the road ahead,* 2009, available at www.healthypeople.gov/hp2020/default.asp (accessed January 19, 2009).

van Achterberg T, Schoonhoven L, Grol R: Nursing implementation science: how evidence-based nursing requires evidence-based implementation, *J Nurs Scholar* 40(4):302-310, 2008.

Walsh CM, Seldomridge LA: Critical thinking: back to square two, *J Nurs Educ* 45(6):212-219, 2006.

Wise PH: Medical progress and inequalities in child health. In Cosby AG, Greenberg RE, Southward LH, et al, editors: *About children: an authoritative resource on the state of childhood today,* Elk Grove Village, Ill, 2005, American Academy of Pediatrics.

Wise PH: The transformation of child health in the United States, *Health Affairs* 23(5): 9-25, 2004.

Wong D: Principles of atraumatic care. In Feeg V, editor: *Pediatric nursing: forum on the future: looking toward the 21st century,* Pitman, NJ, 1989, Anthony J Jannetti.

Woods M: Nursing ethics education: are we really delivering the good(s)? *Nurs Ethics* 12(1):5-18, 2005.

World Health Organization: *School health and youth health promotion,* 2007, available at www.who.int/school_youth_health/en (accessed January 26, 2007).

Social, Cultural, and Religious Influences on Child Health Promotion

Annaka G. Thibodeaux and Kim Mooney-Doyle

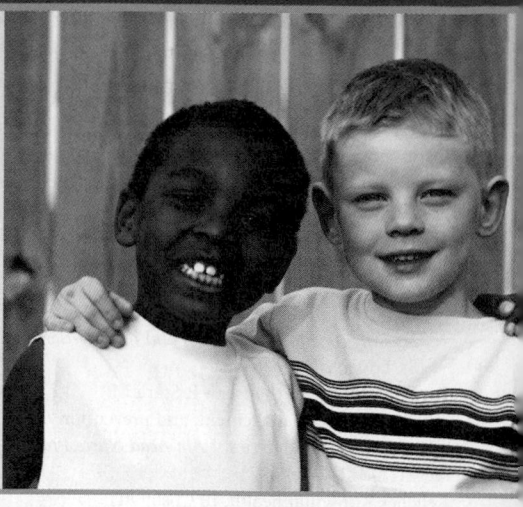

evolve WEBSITE

http://evolve.elsevier.com/wong/ncic
Case Study
    Cultural Considerations
Key Points Audio Summaries
NCLEX Review Questions
Skill
    Providing Culturally Sensitive Care
Spanish/English Translations
WebLinks

RELATED TOPICS

Communicating with Families Through an Interpreter, **Ch. 6**
Family Influences on Child Health Promotion, **Ch. 3**
Lactose Intolerance, **Ch. 13**
Nutritional Assessment, **Ch. 6**
Sickle Cell Anemia, **Ch. 35**
Skin, **Ch. 6**
Toddler, **Ch. 14;** Preschooler, **Ch. 15;** School-Age Child, **Ch. 17;**
    Adolescent, **Ch. 19**
Vegetarian Diets, **Ch. 13**

CHAPTER OUTLINE

CULTURE

Promoting the health of pediatric patients requires a nurse to understand social, cultural, and religious influences on children. This in turn depends on a purposeful awareness of the child's sociocultural context. A holistic view of care was first described by Madeleine Leininger, the recognized founder of transcultural nursing, in her culture care diversity and universality theory (Leininger, 2001). The theory provides an intellectual framework and a research methodology for providing culturally congruent patient care. As the ethnic, racial, and cultural diversity in the U.S. population increases, it is imperative that nurses become competent in transcultural nursing (Munoz and Luckmann, 2005). They must remain aware that every family, child, and health care provider comes to a clinical encounter with a cultural lens through which they see and interpret the world.

Transcultural nursing care is important considering the ever-changing population. The demographic profile of the United States 2000 census includes 69% non-Hispanic white,

13% Hispanic/Latino, 12% Black/African-American, and 4% Asian (US Census Bureau, 2001).

Nurses can become culturally competent by learning about and developing an understanding of cultures other than their own, being sensitive to the effects of culture on the nursing care of patients, and understanding how their own culture affects their ability to provide care to others (Dunn, 2002).

Culture is a rich context through which people view and respond to their world (see Cultural Competence box). It also provides the lens through which all facets of human behavior can be interpreted (Spector, 2009). Culture is composed of individuals who share a set of values, beliefs, practices (e.g., language, dress, diet, health care), social relationships, laws, politics, economics, and norms of behavior that are learned, integrative, social, and satisfying. Culture is an ingrained orientation to life that serves as a frame of reference for individual perception and judgment. Culture is, essentially, the way of life of a group of people that incorporates experiences of the past, influences thought and action in the present, and transmits these traditions to future group members. Families pass their culture on to children, and the children perceive the world through this cultural lens. Culture adapts to the ever-changing world as group members abandon, modify, or assume new patterns of living and behavior to meet the group's needs.

CULTURAL COMPETENCE

Cultural Definitions

> Culture characterizes a particular group with its values, beliefs, norms, patterns, and practices that are learned, shared, and transmitted from one generation to another (Leininger, 2001). Culture differs from both race and ethnicity. Race is a biologic term distinguishing variety in humans by physical traits. Ethnicity is the affiliation of a set of persons who share a unique cultural, social, and linguistic heritage. Socialization is the process by which society communicates its competencies, values, and expectations to children (Trawick-Smith, 2006). Culture is a complex whole in which each part is interrelated. It is an umbrella term that holds together many interrelated yet unique aspects of humanity like beliefs, tradition, life ways, and heritage. It is much more than a country of origin or a demographic designation such as African-American or Caucasian.

Material overt, or manifest, culture refers to the observable components of a culture, such as material objects (dress, art, utensils, and other artifacts) and actions. Nonmaterial covert culture refers to those aspects that cannot be observed directly, such as ideas, beliefs, customs, and feelings. Related to the large culture are many subcultures, each with an identity of its own. Children are socialized into a particular subculture rather than into the culture as a whole. Subcultural influences, such as ethnicity and social class, are discussed in more detail later in this chapter.

Cultures and subcultures contribute to the uniqueness of child members in such a subtle way and at such an early age that children grow up to think that their beliefs, attitudes, values, and practices are the "correct" or "normal" ones. By age 5 years, children can identify persons who belong to their own race or cultural background. During later primary years, children can identify those from different cultures (Trawick-Smith, 2006). A set of values learned in childhood is likely to characterize children's attitudes and behavior for life, influencing their long-range goals and their short-range, impulsive inclinations. Thus every ongoing society socializes each succeeding generation to its cultural heritage.

The manner and sequence of the growth and development phenomenon are universal and fundamental features of all children; however, children's varied behavioral responses to similar events are often determined by their culture. Culture plays a critical role in the parenting behaviors that facilitate children's development (Melendez, 2005). Children acquire the skills, knowledge, beliefs, and values important to their own family and culture. Cultural backgrounds can influence the pace of acquisition of cognitive and motor skills as well as the child's social and emotional development (Trawick-Smith, 2006).

Cultures may also differ in whether status in a group is based on age or on skill. Even children's play and their types of games are culturally determined. In some cultures children play in groups composed of members of the same sex; in others they play in mixed-sex groups. In some cultures team games predominate; in others most play is limited to individual games.

Standards and norms vary from culture to culture and from location to location; a practice that is accepted in one area may meet with disapproval or create tension in another. The extent to which cultures tolerate divergence from the established norm also varies among cultures and subcultural groups. Although conforming to cultural norms provides a degree of security, it is a decided deterrent to change.

THE CHILD AND FAMILY IN NORTH AMERICA

Context provides perspective for nursing care. The health and well-being of the child in the North American family is influenced by two distinct contexts: the context of family and the context of culture. Therefore understanding these layers of influence on pediatric health is integral to developing a family-centered and culturally competent nursing practice (Thibodeaux and Deatrick, 2007). America's orientation toward homogenization—"the great melting pot"—is changing to an orientation of complex cultural diversity. Increased awareness of the growing proportion of ethnic minorities that make up the U.S. population, coupled with a new appreciation for ethnic diversity, has resulted in a renewed interest in cultural variation.

The frontier background of the American culture has contributed to the overall orientation to life and childrearing. Americans have always had a basic optimistic view of the world, a belief that things can be better and that the children can and will be better off than their parents. With this hopeful outlook, a general future orientation, and the possibility of upward social mobility, American culture typically encourages development of self-confidence and autonomy in children. Children are generally permitted a greater degree of freedom than in more tradition-oriented cultures.

Family life in North America is characterized by increasing geographic and economic mobility. Families are less reliant on tradition, are fragmented, and have limited opportunity to transmit and acquire the traditional and accepted customs of a culture. Consequently, young adults rely to a greater extent on the professed experts, peers, and the mass media for acquisition of acceptable patterns of behavior, including childrearing practices. Conflicting information can be a source of confusion and frustration as parents attempt to determine the comparatively stable, essential components of the culture and transmit these to their children.

Children in North America grow up with a number of adults who differ from one another but who all provide input as role models, teachers, and standards for behavior. Most children live in some form of nuclear family located in sharply differentiated neighborhoods determined by income and ethnic status within a highly technical, largely urban society. Class differences in childrearing persist, but they are becoming less divergent.

Early in life children in minority cultures become aware of their cultural context and the discriminatory attitudes of the majority culture toward their racial or ethnic group. The direct effects of discrimination are anger and low self-esteem, which manifest in a variety of behaviors. Attitudes are slowly changing in some groups and in some places. With a relatively recent emergence of racial and ethnic pride along with a growing awareness, interest, and understanding of the majority, children in minority groups are becoming more secure and confident in their racial or ethnic identity. Individuals vary in their reactions to membership in a minority group, and much of this variation can be attributed to familial factors. The most important influences on development of a positive self-image are warm, understanding parents who actively foster their children's growth. Parents who accept their children and react positively and constructively rather than in a negative manner will help their children develop feelings of self-worth, self-esteem, and self-acceptance. The more adequate children feel, the more positive their attitudes toward peers in both the majority and minority groups and the greater their ability to withstand prejudice and intolerance and build lasting relationships.

SOCIAL ROLES

Much of children's self-concept comes from their ideas about their social roles. Roles are cultural creations; therefore the culture prescribes patterns of behavior for persons in a variety of social positions. All persons who hold similar social positions have an obligation to behave in a particular manner. A role prohibits some behaviors and allows others. Because culture outlines and clarifies roles, it is a significant influence on the development of children's self-concept (i.e., attitudes and beliefs they have about themselves).

A social group consists of a system of roles carried out in both primary and secondary groups. A **primary group** has intimate, continued, face-to-face contact; mutual support of members; and the ability to order or constrain a considerable proportion of individual members' behavior. Two such groups are the family and the peer group, both of which have a great deal of influence on the child.

Secondary groups are groups that have limited, intermittent contact and generally less concern for members' behavior. These groups offer little in terms of support or pressure toward conformity except in rigidly limited areas. Examples of secondary groups are professional associations and social organizations such as church groups.

A concept of social role also depends largely on whether a child is reared in a primary- or secondary-group community. Children are subjected to perceptibly different forms of parental training in these two types of environments.

Primary- and Secondary-Group Influences

Children are raised within a primary-group environment and within a secondary-group environment. The influences, strengths, and limitations of both groups are significant. In a primary-group community (e.g., family; peer group; some contemporary rural, religious, or ethnic communities), all members know each other, most belong to the same subgroups, and all are concerned about each member's behavior. Community members have a high degree of material and psychologic support and one traditional set of values that the entire group agrees on and supports; thus there is little conflict of values. In a stable community where the members remain within comparatively defined limits and relatives are likely to live close together, young members have ample opportunity to observe and absorb cultural practices and customs. Any member of the community feels justified in evaluating and censuring the conduct of another member.

Children reared in the relative isolation of secondary-group environmental influences tend to learn that there is only one acceptable way to respond to any given situation. The entire group agrees, and any tendency to deviate is met with collective disapproval. It is the parents' duty to see that the children learn and follow social roles and modes of behavior defined and strengthened by the views of the community.

The childrearing orientation in a secondary-group environment, such as urban communities, can differ considerably from that of a primary-group environment. The interaction between primary and secondary groups may reinforce values when both groups endorse that value, or create confusion or conflict when one group rejects a value accepted by the other. An urban community is dynamic. Many of the traditional behaviors and values may not meet the needs of the changing society. Consequently, parents are often uncertain about what to teach their children. They may wish to rear their children with values consistent with their own, but the differences in experience between the generations are too great. As a result, they often grant their children autonomy in some areas of decision making early in the developmental process, and other secondary groups assume a greater influence. None of the groups is highly dominant in its influence; therefore the children are exposed to an eclectic set of values and expectations, some in agreement and some in conflict. From these they must ultimately select those that they determine to be best for them and adopt them to form a consistent set of roles and behaviors to incorporate into the self-concept.

Self-Esteem and Culture

Culture influences a child's sense of self-esteem (Trawick-Smith, 2006). Some cultures are more collective in thought and action. A child from a collective culture will hold an inclusive view of self. Self-evaluation is related to the accomplishments or competencies of the entire family or community. School experiences that focus on personal achievement may promote positive self-esteem in some children but not in others who are more dependent on the success of a whole family or peer group.

Their sense of control may not come from individual self-reliance but rather from a feeling of worth in their family or community (Trawick-Smith, 2006).

Families and culture also influence the criteria children use to evaluate their own abilities. Additionally cultures vary in whether they instill an internal locus of control (a belief in the ability to regulate one's own life). Effects on self-esteem are minimal if those beliefs are directed by parents and are in accordance with cultural customs (Trawick-Smith, 2006). Ethnic pride can help children to maintain a positive self-image and counteract the effects of prejudice, which can have a negative impact on emotional health (Trawick-Smith, 2006).

CULTURAL SHOCK AND CULTURAL COMPETENCE

Cultural shock is characterized by the inability to respond to or function within a new or strange situation. It can occur when the values and beliefs of a new cultural setting are radically different from those of the person's native culture (Munoz and Luckmann, 2005). This state of shock or uneasiness can happen to a patient in a hospital or to a nurse caring for patients with different cultural backgrounds. Immigrants to a new country and persons from a subcultural group experience the same cultural shock when they must adjust to the ways of an unfamiliar subgroup or setting.

Numerous factors influence reactions to a new environment. Language barriers, including dialects and jargon specific to a subcultural group, inhibit effective communication. Habits and customs, such as different role behaviors or etiquette, and differences in attitudes and beliefs are puzzling to the newcomer in an unfamiliar environment. The child and family experiencing cultural shock can feel an intense sense of isolation, loneliness, and fear (Crom, 1995).

Nurses are challenged to overcome cultural shock and develop cultural sensitivity, an awareness of cultural similarities and differences. Doing so helps the nurse practice culturally competent care. This requires changing the way people think about, understand, and interact within the world around them (see Critical Thinking Exercise). The development of cultural competence is an ongoing, interactive process that involves six elements (Dunn, 2002):

1. Working on changing one's world view by examining one's own values and behaviors and working to reject racism and institutions that support it
2. Becoming familiar with core cultural issues by recognizing these issues and exploring them with patients
3. Becoming knowledgeable about the cultural groups one works with while learning about each individual patient's unique history
4. Becoming familiar with core cultural issues related to health and illness and communicating in a way that encourages patients to explain what an illness means to them
5. Developing a relationship of trust with patients and creating a welcoming atmosphere in the health care setting
6. Negotiating for mutually acceptable and understandable interventions of care

---

💡 CRITICAL THINKING EXERCISE
Reducing Cultural Shock

A woman from the Middle East is visiting her child who is hospitalized for a serious illness. Her husband left for home a short time ago to wash and change clothes. She speaks little English. You need to obtain her consent for an emergency procedure. She is hesitant and refuses to sign the consent form. What should you do?

1. Evidence—Are there sufficient data to draw any conclusions about this woman's actions?
2. Assumptions—Describe any underlying assumptions about each of the following:
   a. Arab culture
   b. Need for interpreter
   c. Approval for emergency procedures
   d. Documentation of the need for the emergency procedure
3. What priorities for nursing care should be established at this time?
4. Does the evidence support your nursing intervention(s)?

When minority groups immigrate to another country, a certain degree of cultural and ethnic blending occurs through the involuntary process of acculturation, those gradual changes produced in a culture by the influence of another culture that cause one or both cultures to be more similar to each other. However, the changes occur to various degrees in different families and groups. Many groups continue to identify with their traditional heritage while adapting to the ill-defined concept of the "American way." Acculturation may be referred to as assimilation, which is the process of developing a new cultural identity (Spector, 2009).

SUBCULTURAL INFLUENCES

Except in rare situations, children grow and develop in a blend of cultures and subcultures. In a large, complex society such as the United States, different groups have their own set of standards, values, and expectations within the collective ways of the large culture. Most subcultures were formed when groups of people clustered together by preference, by external pressures from the majority culture, or by geographic isolation. Although many cultural differences are related to geographic boundaries, subcultures are not always restricted by location. Some subcultures are even related to the stages of development and have traditions, games, loyalties, and rules. The behavior of school-age children and adolescents demonstrates age-related subcultures. The culture is handed down by word of mouth from one "generation" to the next, and its rituals and behavior standards are highly resistant to outside influence.

Children's membership in a cultural subgroup is, for the most part, involuntary. They are born into a family with a specific ethnic or racial heritage, socioeconomic level, and religious beliefs. Although the complex American society has countless subcultures and considerable variation in the way of life, those subcultures that seem to have the greatest influence on childrearing are ethnicity, social class, and occupational role. In addition, schools and peer-group subcultures are strong influences in the socialization of the child.

> **! NURSING ALERT**
>
> American cultures and subcultures can be so diverse, it is essential that nurses be aware of and knowledgeable about the predominant groups in their work community and apply this knowledge in their practice.

> **! NURSING ALERT**
>
> Any generalization made about an ethnic group may not apply to certain groups or individuals.

ETHNICITY

Ethnicity is the classification of or affiliation with any of the basic groups or divisions of humankind or any heterogeneous population differentiated by customs, characteristics, language, or similar distinguishing factors. Ethnic differences extend to many areas and include such manifestations as family structure, language, food preferences, moral codes, and expression of emotion. Some standards of behavior (e.g., the traditional role of the father) result from the cultural heritage of the specific ethnic group. Others reflect the interaction between subcultures, most notably between members of the majority culture and a minority subculture. The term *ethnic* has aroused strong negative feelings, and the general population often rejects this term (Spector, 2009).

To establish their place in the group, children learn to follow a mode of behavior that is in accordance with standards distinctive to the group and learn how they can expect others to behave toward them. They take their cues by observing and imitating those to whom they are exposed. For example, children of a racial minority form a perception of their role as a group member by observing how role models within the subgroup respond to treatment by people outside the subgroup. When they see group members display an attitude of inferiority, they assume this to be the appropriate behavior and incorporate these perceptions into their own self-concept.

In the United States the cross-cultural lines are becoming blurred as subcultures are assimilated and blended into the larger culture (Fig. 2-1). Although ethnic differences in child-rearing are probably diminishing, they remain important. It is particularly difficult for persons to attempt to maintain an identity within a subculture while living and conforming to the requirements of the larger culture.

Leavitt, Martinson, Liu, and colleagues (1999) found that immigrants from China who provided care for their children with cancer focused on dietary intake, whereas families that were of Caucasian descent focused on emotional support. The cultural framework directed the healing practices. Interestingly, the same study found that both groups shared the beliefs that mothers were the primary caregivers for the sick child. In this example one cultural behavior was unique to each cultural group while the other was similar. Consequently, children reared in this environment can become confused about roles and values of two or more cultures if they conflict. They usually adopt those of the more influential or higher-status culture. Youth, in particular, are influenced by the locally dominant group.

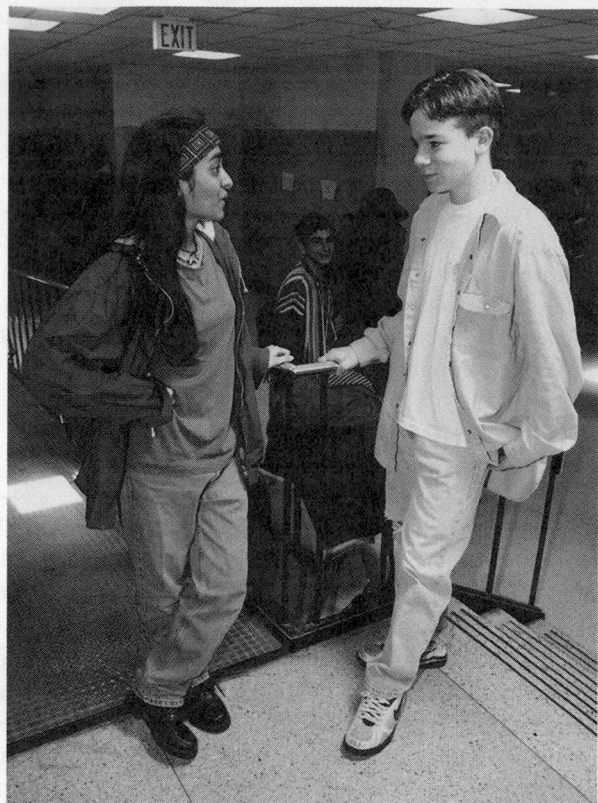

Fig. 2-1 Youngsters from different cultural backgrounds interact within the larger culture.

Ethnocentrism is the emotional attitude that one's own ethnic group is superior to others; that one's values, beliefs, and perceptions are the correct ones; and that the group's ways of living and behaving are the best way (Spector, 2009). Ethnic stereotyping or labeling stems from ethnocentric views. Ethnocentrism implies that all other groups are inferior and that their ways are not in the best interests of the group. It is a common attitude among a dominant ethnic group and strongly influences a person's ability to evaluate objectively the beliefs and behaviors of others. Nurses must overcome the natural tendency to have ethnocentric attitudes when caring for people from different cultures (Williams and Kruse, 1999). The culturally competent nurse has empathy for others, maintains an openness to feeling what the other feels, and remains curious and willing to ask questions to gain a better understanding. In addition, the nurse has a basic respect for self and others, and acknowledges the intrinsic value of all humans (Carrillo, Green, and Betancourt, 1999).

MINORITY-GROUP MEMBERSHIP

The United States has more racial, ethnic, and religious minority groups than any other country. Ethnic minority groups are becoming increasingly important because these groups are producing children at a faster rate than the majority Caucasian population. Consequently, the minority population is increasing. The rapidly emerging U.S. minority population will present special needs and require resources beyond what is currently available (Murdock, 2005).

The 2000 U.S. census revealed more than 280 million people in the United States, with 6.8 million reporting an ethnicity of more than two races. Blacks, or African-Americans, alone or in combination with another race, number more than 35 million, and Hispanics or Latinos of any race are more than 35 million. The Hispanic population increased 58%, or 13 million people, from 1990 to 2000 (US Census Bureau, 2001). Currently, Hispanics are the fastest growing minority in the United States and have many health needs that are not being met (Murdock, 2005; Warda, 2000). By the year 2010, Hispanics will surpass non-Hispanic blacks as the largest U.S. racial or ethnic group. In 2050 almost 30% of the U.S. population is expected to be Hispanic (Murdock, 2005) (see Cultural Competence box).

🌐 CULTURAL COMPETENCE

Overview of Race and Hispanic Origin in Census 2000

The federal government defines *race* and *Hispanic origin* as two separate and distinct concepts. In the 2000 U.S. Census, respondents were first asked if they are of Spanish/Hispanic/Latino origin. The second question asked respondents to report the race or races they considered themselves to be. The definitions of racial groups included (U.S. Census Bureau, 2001):

Whites—People having "origins in any of the original peoples of Europe, the Middle East, or North Africa"

African-Americans—Referred to as blacks and defined as "any persons whose lineage included ancestors who originated from any of the black racial groups of Africa"

Asians or Pacific Islanders—Any person with "origins in any of the original peoples of the Far East, Southeast Asia, the Indian subcontinent"

Native Hawaiian and Other Pacific Islanders—"People having origins in any of the original peoples of Hawaii, Guam, Samoa, or other Pacific Islands"

Native Americans—Referred to as American Indians and Alaskan Natives and defined as "persons having origins in the original peoples of North America and South America (including Central America), and who maintain cultural identification through tribal affiliations or community attachment"

SOCIOECONOMIC CLASS

Family relationships may be stronger in some ethnic or cultural groups than others. However, the influence of socioeconomic class cannot be overlooked. This relates to the family's economic and educational levels. Strong family relationships exist among those of lower socioeconomic class who have few resources and must rely on the support of a family network to meet physical and emotional needs. Middle- and upper-class people often have resources that reach beyond the extended family. They are able to access physical and emotional support in the community (Giger and Davidhizar, 1999). Do not confuse the term *socioeconomic class* with cultural or ethnic diversity. Children of a specific race are not necessarily of low socioeconomic status. Additionally, children of poverty do not automatically have developmental delays (Trawick-Smith, 2006).

Communication Skills

Any concept that occurs to a person can be expressed in language. However, ease of communication and use of language codes vary among the social classes. Language is much more restricted in the lower classes, and grammar usage differs more than pronunciation. Persons in the middle classes use different grammar from those in the lower classes and are able to express more complicated ideas; persons in the lower classes use very simple grammar and are less likely to offer explanations.

These communication differences are highly significant in relation to school achievement. School is constructed around the elaborate language codes of the middle class; therefore children from the lower class who lack an understanding of these language skills are placed at a decided disadvantage. This is particularly true for bilingual children and children from ethnic groups that have developed a unique dialect.

Historically, schools have participated in devaluing Native American languages, cultures, and traditional ways of learning and knowing (Robinson-Zanartu, 1996). Unfortunately, Native American children have been deficient in their preparation for school (Dykeman, Nelson, and Appleton, 1995). Also, children of Native American nations have been at risk for low achievement, overrepresentation in special education, and dropping out (Robinson-Zanartu, 1996). Many regional dialects and variations in language usage must be considered when communicating with persons from these groups. English words that sound like another word in a foreign language can cause considerable misunderstanding.

SCHOOLS

When children enter school, their radius of relationships extends to include a wider variety of peers and a new focus of authority. Although parents continue to exert the major influence on children, in the school environment teachers have the most significant psychologic impact on their development and socialization. The teachers' function is primarily limited to teaching, but, like parents, they are concerned about the children's emotional welfare. Both parents and teachers must constrain behavior and enforce standards of conduct.

Socialization

Next to the family, the schools exert the major force in providing continuity between generations by conveying a vast amount of culture from the older members to the young. This prepares children to carry out the traditional social roles they are expected to assume as adults in society. School is the center of cultural diffusion wherein the cultural standards of the larger group are disseminated to the local community. It governs what is taught and, to a large extent, how it is taught. School rules and regulations regarding attendance, authority relationships, and the system of penalties and rewards based on achievement transmit to the child the behavioral expectations of the adult world of employment and relationships. School is often the only institution in which children systematically learn about the negative consequences of behaviors that depart from social expectations. In addition, the school provides an opportunity for some children to participate in the larger society in rewarding ways and often provides avenues for social mobility for both students and teachers. Individuals in the lower classes are offered the opportunity for further education and the capacity to move up in the social strata.

Teachers are responsible for transmitting the knowledge and values of the dominant culture (i.e., those values on which there is broad consensus). They are expected to stimulate and guide children's intellectual development, sense of esthetics, and creative problem solving.

Traditionally the socialization process of school began when the child entered kindergarten or first grade. Today, with more than 60% of mothers of preschool children working outside the home, this socialization process begins much earlier for a significant number of children in a variety of childcare settings.

Children of some cultural groups fare less well in school. They come from underrepresented groups, including African-American, Mexican-American, Puerto-Rican, and Native-American children (Trawick-Smith, 2006). These cultural variations can be attributed to high rates of poverty, different cognitive styles, ineffective schools, and parents' views of schools as oppressive to cultural and traditional values (Trawick-Smith, 2006).

COMMUNITIES

Surveys of more than 1 million youth in the United States in grades 6 to 12 have shown that persons who experience a higher number of specific assets in their lives are more likely to make healthy choices and avoid high-risk behaviors. These assets offer a framework for positive child and adolescent development. The child or adolescent's community is made up of family, school, neighborhood, youth organization, and other members.

Four categories of external assets that youth receive from the community are (Search Institute, 2007):

1. Support—Young people need to feel support, care, and love from their families, neighbors, and others. They also need organizations and institutions that offer positive, supportive environments.
2. Empowerment—Young people need to feel valued by their community and be able to contribute to others. They need to feel safe and secure.
3. Boundaries and expectations—Young people need to know what is expected of them and what activities and behaviors are within the community boundaries and what are outside of them.
4. Constructive use of time—Young people need opportunities for growth through constructive, enriching opportunities and through quality time at home.

Internal assets must also be nurtured in the community's young members. These internal qualities guide choices and create a sense of centeredness, purpose, and focus. The four categories of internal assets are (Search Institute, 2007):

1. Commitment to learning—Young people need to develop a commitment to education and life-long learning.
2. Positive values—Youth need to have a strong sense of values that direct their choices.
3. Social competencies—Young people need competencies that help them make positive choices and build relationships.
4. Positive identity—Young people need a sense of their own power, purpose, worth, and promise.

Social Capital

Social capital is a health-related concept that provides a way for pediatric nurses to include a social context in their assessments. It considers where and how the children and families they care for live. Social capital is defined as the total sum of the social relationships within the family and the family's relationship with peers, with institutions (schools, clubs, faith-based organizations), and with communities that affect the health and well-being of children (Looman and Lindeke, 2005). It is the way people mobilize resources and allows them to turn relationships into resources. Families develop a sense of belonging and find strength in knowing others in the same situation (Looman, 2004). The focus is on the interaction rather than specific supports. Research shows that social capital is related to positive health outcomes (Looman and Lindeke, 2005). Pediatric nurses can include social capital in their practice by bringing families, community members, and professionals together for a common purpose. Nurses can also include social capital in practice by encouraging repeated contacts over time, encouraging storytelling, and advocating for community experiences that enhance health-promoting behaviors (Looman and Lindeke, 2005).

PEER CULTURES

Peer groups also have an impact on the socialization of children (Fig. 2-2). Peer relationships become increasingly important and influential as children proceed through school. In school, children have what can be regarded as a culture of their own. This is even more apparent in an unsupervised playgroup, since in school the culture is partly produced by adults.

During their lives children are exposed to value systems such as those of the family, ethnic group, and social class. In peer-group interaction they confront a variety of these sets of values. The values imposed by the peer group are especially compelling because children must accept and conform to them to be accepted as members of the group. When the peer values are not too different from those of family and teachers, the mild

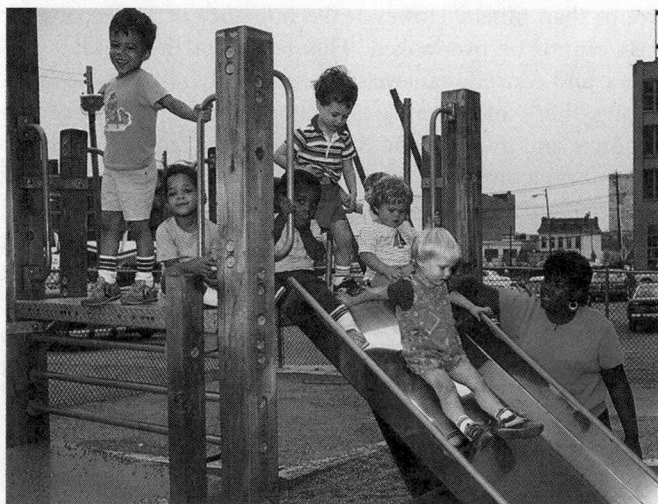

Fig. 2-2 Children from a variety of cultural and ethnic backgrounds begin to socialize in the child care setting.

conflict created by these small differences serves to separate children from the adults in their lives and to strengthen the feeling of belonging to the peer group.

The kind of socialization provided by the peer group depends on the subculture that develops from its members' background, interests, and capabilities. Some groups support school achievement, others focus on athletic prowess, and still others are decidedly against educative goals. Scholastic achievement is strongly related to the peer group's value system. Many conflicts between teachers and students and between parents and students can be attributed to fear of rejection by peers. What is expected from parents regarding academic achievement and what is expected from the peer culture often conflict, especially during high school. Chapter 19 discusses this in further detail.

Although the peer group has neither the traditional authority of the parents nor the legal authority of the schools for teaching information, it manages to convey a substantial amount of information to its members, especially on taboo subjects such as sex and drugs. Children's need for the friendship of their peers brings them into an increasingly complex social system. Through peer relationships, children learn to deal with dominance and hostility and to relate with persons in positions of leadership and authority. Other functions of the peer subculture are to relieve boredom and to provide recognition that individual members do not receive from teachers and other authority figures.

The peer-group culture has secrets, mores, and codes of ethics that promote group solidarity and detachment from adults. They have traditions and folkways, including age-related games and other activities, that are transferred from "generation to generation" of schoolchildren and that have a great influence over the behavior of all group members. As children move from one level to the next, they discard folkways of the younger group as they adopt those of the new group. For example, a school-age child rides a bicycle to school; the high school student prefers a car. As they advance, children are forward oriented only—they look forward with anticipation but may look backward with contempt.

BICULTURE

Some children are exposed to the values, role relationships, and lifestyles of two or more cultures. The virtual "straddling" of two cultures is referred to as **biculturation** and involves the ability to efficiently bridge the gap between an individual's culture of origin and the dominant culture (Rogers, 1995). This may occur because the child's parents are from two or more different cultures. In Hawaii, for example, it is common for children to be from four or more cultures. Other children straddle cultures as members of a minority culture within the dominant culture. This biculture is sometimes observed in the playgroup but usually is not a significant factor until children enter school. Then they must unlearn some of the established practices of one culture to become socialized in the other, especially in role relationships. For example, children from Hispanic and Asian cultures are taught to look away when scolded; in U.S. schools the teacher expects direct eye contact—"Look at me when I speak to you." Children learn new roles and social behavior more rapidly than their adult counterparts.

This biculture is particularly marked in language differences. The bilingual child is said to be at a disadvantage in school situations of the dominant culture, in which there is controversy over bilingual education. Those supporting bilingual education adhere to the principle that children will understand more readily and perform more realistically (especially in testing situations) if learning is directed in their own language; others contend that children living in a dominant culture should adopt the ways of that culture, including language. The child faces less conflict when the school supports his or her language and culture, even if the dominant language is used.

MASS MEDIA

The media provide children with a means for extending their knowledge about the world in which they live and have helped narrow the differences between social classes. However, many people are concerned about the enormous influence the media can have on the developing child and on health promotion behaviors (see Research Focus box). Children and adolescents in the United States spend more than 6 hours per day utilizing entertainment media (Council on Communications and Media, 2009). Increased use of entertainment media has been associated with the epidemic of obesity in children and adolescents and increased aggression in children (Jordan, 2004; Council on Communications and Media, 2009).

RESEARCH FOCUS

Entertainment Media and High-Risk Behaviors

Researchers have established links between mass media and an increase in the use of tobacco, alcohol, and violent behavior in adolescents (Council on Communications and Media, 2009; American Academy of Pediatrics, 2001; Strasburger and Donnerstein, 1999). The images of risky behavior presented by the media may serve to establish or reinforce teenagers' perceptions of their social environment. Also, media content may directly influence risk perception; media protagonists seldom suffer adverse consequences of their behaviors despite their grossly distorted experiences with violence, illness, or crime.

Children may identify closely with people or characters portrayed in reading materials, movies, videos, and television programs and commercials. Pediatric nurses can educate and support parents on the effects of mass media on their children through the following recommendations (Jordan, 2004):

- Be aware of the content of the child's media and amount of time spent looking at a screen.
- Help young children watching television to find educational programs.
- Remove television, Internet-accessible computers, and videogame systems from the bedroom to decrease the amount of time spent using these activities.
- Limit television viewing to 2 hours a day or less.
- Model good practices.
- Watch age-appropriate programs and play age-appropriate games with children.

Reading Materials

The oldest form of mass media—books, newspapers, and magazines—contributes to children's competence in almost every direction and provides enjoyment. Recognition of the impact that reading matter in schools has on value systems and the socialization process has prompted reevaluation of textbook content in several areas, such as stereotyped male and female role models, the sugar-coated view of life situations, and the biased history of minority groups.

Reading aloud to children is a vital activity in promoting success in reading. It provides cognitive and language stimulation, is a forum for quality parent-child interaction, and may reduce parent stress (Klass, Needlman, and Zuckerman, 2002).

Movies

Movies that are not closely bound to reality and often portray an assortment of socially approved behaviors perhaps make a contribution to children's value systems and do provide opportunities for desirable social learning. On the other hand, children, especially adolescents, flock to "macho" movies and those whose heroes resort to violent resolution of problems, such as karate and wild automobile chases. The carryover of these influences into daily life and relationships may account in part for the increase in violent behavior of young persons.

A recent concern is the violent and R-rated movies available to children and teenagers in theaters and through cable television and DVDs. The content of movies has changed markedly over the past few years, with mutilation being a major theme. To children who are unable to distinguish between reality and fantasy, these films play on their deepest fears and result in bedtime fears, nightmares, and a fearful view of the world.

Television

The medium that has the most impact on children in the United States today is television; it has become one of the most significant socializing agents in the lives of young children. The programs and commercials provide multiple sources for acquiring information, modeling behaviors, and observing value orientations. Besides producing a leveling effect on class differences in general information and vocabulary, TV exposes children to a wider variety of topics and events than they encounter in day-to-day life. Television always has time to talk to children and is a form of access to the adult world. Positive results occur only when viewing is relatively light, yet the average child in the United States over the age of 8 spends more time watching television or using a computer and video games (>6 hours/day) than in any other activity except sleeping (Fig. 2-3) (Council on Communications and Media, 2009).

Television can offer some beneficial effects on the growing child. In their follow-up study of adolescents who had participated as preschoolers in an investigation of television use, researchers found that children who viewed educational programs as preschoolers had higher grades, read more books, valued achievement, had greater creativity, and were less aggressive (Anderson, Huston, Schmitt, et al, 2001).

Most researchers have concluded, however, that protracted television viewing can have negative effects on children. Increased verbal and physical aggressiveness, reduced persistence at problem solving, greater sex-role stereotyping, and reduced creativity have been reported repeatedly. In fairness, no one has yet defined the long-term effects of other electronic factors such as stereo headphones versus conversation, com-

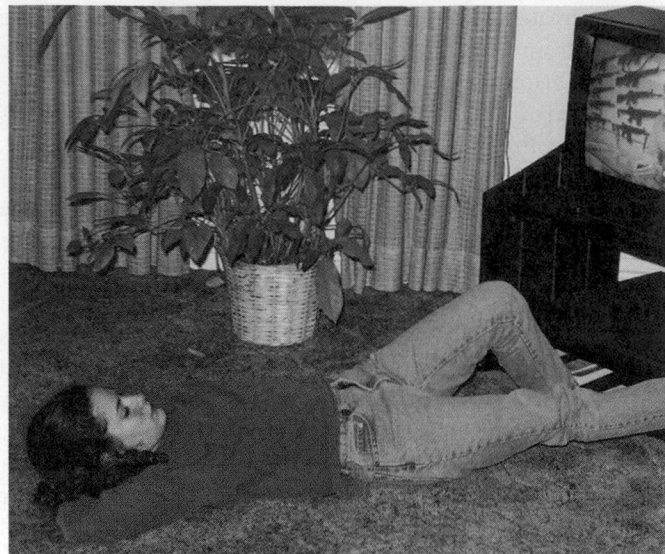

Fig. 2-3 The average child in the United States spends more time watching television than in any other activity except sleeping.

puter games or drills versus active social play, or DVDs versus books. However, clearly children in the modern electronic environment are constantly stimulated from the outside, which allows them little time to reflect and develop the inner speech that feeds brain development.

Most programs are designed to attract attention by visual jolts; the child establishes the habit of ignoring language in favor of hectic visual and auditory gimmicks. Like movies, television programs and commercials contain many implicit and explicit messages that promote alcohol consumption, smoking, violence, and promiscuous or unsafe sexual activity. An area of particular concern is unmonitored use of the Internet with videos sensationalizing violence, sex, suicide, and other destructive behaviors.

SOCIOECONOMIC INFLUENCES

POVERTY

A subcultural influence closely related to but different from social class is the condition known as **poverty**. It is a relative concept and is usually associated with the general standards of a population. The term *poverty* implies both visible and invisible impoverishment. It is a condition in which families live without adequate resources (Trawick-Smith, 2006). Visible poverty refers to lack of money or material resources, which includes poor nutrition, insufficient clothing, poor sanitation, and deteriorating housing. Invisible poverty refers to social and cultural deprivation such as limited employment opportunities, inferior educational opportunities, lack of or inferior medical services and health care facilities, and an absence of public services.

An **absolute standard** of poverty attempts to delimit a basic set of resources needed for adequate existence; a **relative standard** reflects the median standard of living in a society and is the term used in referring to childhood poverty in the United States; that is, what appears to be deprivation in one area may be a standard or norm in another.

An important development affecting the American family since the end of World War II is the widening disparity in income status among generations. Children from families with a single mother compose the largest group of children in poverty in the country (Wertheimer, 2005).

Growth in the number of poor children over the past decade has not been due to an increase in the number of welfare-dependent families, but to growth in the ranks of the working poor. Between 1994 and 2000, the poverty rate fell approximately 30%, but the trend has recently reversed, and the poverty rate rose 6% between 2000 and 2007. Approximately 18% of children in the United States live below the national poverty threshold, which is currently estimated at $21,027 for two adults and two children (Annie E Casey Foundation, 2009). In addition, approximately 20% of children live in neighborhoods where more than 20% of the population currently lives below the federal poverty threshold.

Such factors illustrate the growing inability of the American family to provide economic essentials for their children. Approximately 11.6% (about 8.5 million) of all children in the United States were uninsured in 2002 (Szilagyi, 2005). Uninsured children are more likely to miss school, jeopardizing their education as well as their health.

A high correlation between poverty and illness has long been observed. Impoverished families suffer from poor nutrition; without medical insurance, they have little if any preventive health care, inadequate health maintenance, and limited access to health services. One of the most significant health problems related to poverty is a high infant mortality rate. Although the rate of infant mortality has decreased in the United States, it still remains higher than that of most industrialized nations (Annie E Casey Foundation, 2009). Day-to-day needs of food, clothing, and lodging take precedence over health care as long as the ailing person feels able to perform activities of daily living.

Poor families may be denied access to some institutions for emergency or other hospital care. Frequently they must travel long distances to service centers that are willing to assume their care. In an emergency they must find money for taxi fare, borrow an automobile, or seek other means of transportation. They must find care for dependents, such as other infants and small children, or take them along when taking the ill child for care. Families tend to delay preventive care indefinitely unless health services are relatively accessible. They are more likely to consult folk practitioners or other persons within their community.

Poor nutrition accounts for many health problems in the lower classes. Lack of funds, education, and readily available healthy foods results in a diet that may be seriously lacking in essential food substances, especially protein, vitamins, and iron. This inadequate diet often leads to nutritional deficiency disorders and growth retardation in children. On the other hand, these issues may contribute to pediatric overweight and type 2 diabetes because nonnourishing foods are less expensive and are easier to access in some neighborhoods.

Dental problems are more prevalent because of deficient preventive care. Lack of standard immunizations together with reduced resistance from poor nutrition renders children in poor segments of the population vulnerable to communicable diseases. Poor sanitation and crowded living conditions also contribute to the higher incidence and perpetuation of illness. In general, poor people become ill more frequently and remain ill for longer periods than those in the general population.

HOMELESSNESS

One of the most pressing problems in the United States is the growing number of homeless families. Homeless individuals are those persons who lack resources and community ties necessary to provide for their own adequate shelter. In the past the homeless population traditionally included single adults, mostly men. Families with children make up 40% of the homeless population, compared with single men, who make up about 41% of the group (Redlener, 2005). Homeless children have increased in numbers as poverty has become feminized, minorities have become poorer, and low-income housing has become less accessible. Estimates of the number of homeless children in the United States may be as high as 1 million; about 10% of the children living in poverty were homeless (Redlener, 2005). Many homeless children are younger than 5 years and are from minority groups.

Most homelessness is a direct result of increasing number of people in poverty combined with a lack of decent, affordable housing. Other reasons include job layoffs, low incomes, parental mental illness, domestic conflict, and unexpected family or economic crises.

Another group of homeless children are the "runaway" and "throwaway" adolescents. Approximately 12% of the homeless population consists of adolescents (National Coalition to End Homelessness, 2009). Many runaways are victims of physical and sexual abuse and leave home because of long-term family or school problems. Poor parent-child relationships, extreme family conflict, feelings of alienation from parents, inconsistent supervision, and unpredictability in discipline are other factors often cited. These adolescents and young adults are at risk for violence, exploitation, substance abuse, and sexually transmitted infections (including HIV and AIDS).

Lack of a permanent housing deprives children of the most basic necessities for proper growth and development. Homelessness disrupts a child's friendships and schooling (Strehlow and Amos-Jones, 1999). Homeless children suffer from physical and mental disorders more often than do poor children who have a permanent residence. Homeless children lack basic health care, including routine immunization and screening for routine problems, and they suffer high rates of acute and chronic illnesses (Redlener, 2005).

MIGRANT FAMILIES

Children in migrant farm worker families are medically underserved. Their numbers are staggering; of the 2 million migrant farm workers who labor in the United States, 63% are accompanied by minor children (Gentry, Quandt, Davis, et al, 2007). These children face both acute and chronic health care issues as a result of poverty, parental occupation, and assimilation into American culture. They are often exposed to risks similar to those facing their parents, since they may accompany them into the fields. These children frequently live in substandard housing conditions, which are subject to overcrowding and transmission of communicable diseases.

Migrant farm worker families face many obstacles when attempting to interface with the U.S. health care system. Three of every five families live below the federally designated poverty line and may lack insurance. The family's use of health care may be affected by parental work schedules and access to transportation. Their own limited English proficiency is further exacerbated by a health care encounter that lacks cultural sensitivity, translation services, and language capability. Cultural expectations of the health care system may differ between the farm worker families and health care providers. This may ultimately have a negative effect on families' utilization of the health care system. In fact, many families living on the U.S.-Mexico border seek the majority of care for their children in Mexico, regardless of their insurance status. In addition, less than 20% of migrant farm worker families use the primary care and health promotion centers that are federally funded through the 1962 Migrant Health Act (Gentry, Quandt, Davis, et al, 2007). ⊖ These two statistics demonstrate the need for culturally sensitive care that is consistent with the perceived needs and expectations of the recipients of such care.

Nurses and other health care providers should be mindful of the persistence of various forms of child labor in the United States (Hindman, 2006). Approximately 50% of 12- to 15-year-olds participate in some sort of paid activity each year, and half of this population have jobs in which they are considered employees. Children, adolescents, and young adults may work in a variety of areas, including agriculture, construction, retail, or even street trades or scams. Youth who work on family farms often face the greatest risk of injury and death from handling dangerous or heavy machinery. Youth who work in street trades and scams or traveling sales crews may be subject to physical or verbal abuse or victimization (Hindman, 2006).

CULTURAL INFLUENCES

⊖ Nurses need to consider clients' cultural differences when providing health care. An understanding of the various beliefs regarding the causation of illness and disease, as well as traditional health practices, is essential to successful intervention. The more nurses know about the values, beliefs, and customs of other ethnic groups and how to elicit this information from families, the better they are able to meet the needs of these families and to gain their cooperation and compliance.

CULTURAL RELATIVITY

Although clinical characteristics of a disease or condition are essentially the same across cultures, how a child or family interprets or experiences the disease or condition varies. Culture as an influence is one obvious explanation for variance. **Cultural relativity** is the concept that any behavior must be judged first in the context of the culture in which it occurs. Cultural factors such as belief systems and view of the world influence the patient's and family's response to health care. These cultural beliefs and behaviors influence adherence to a treatment plan (Munoz and Luckmann, 2005). Some cultures, for example, may view a chronic illness or disability as affecting only particu-

lar aspects of a child's life, and the child as a whole is viewed as normal. In contrast, other families may describe the illness as having global effects on many aspects of the child's present and future life (Martinson, Armstrong, and Qiao, 1997). These contrasting views may result in parents having different goals and expectations for their children.

Culture influences the assignment of gender roles, perception of disease, and perception of the side effects of the disease and the treatment the child should receive. For example, the family may expect the mother to be the primary caregiver. This places her at risk for caregiver strain when she is caring for a sick child.

Nurses can often recognize a family's health-related cultural perceptions and interpretations through discussion and observation. They should explore and consider implications of these perceptions when planning culturally appropriate interventions. Nurses must be comfortable having discussions with families about their cultural beliefs and practices. The conversations can begin easily as, "I want to take the best care of your child and family as possible. Is there anything in particular about your beliefs [cultural, religious, family] that you think I should know?"

RELATIONSHIPS WITH HEALTH CARE PROVIDERS

The manner of relating with health care providers differs considerably among cultural groups. For some nurses, one area of conflict is the attitude toward time and waiting that is part of some cultures. The time orientation of Hispanic and African-American ethnic groups is in the present. For example, African-Americans are flexible in their time orientation; an African-American family may be late for or miss appointments because other issues take precedence, and they may not communicate this to the health agency. Hispanics, too, have a relaxed view of time. Whereas the dominant culture in the United States says that "time flies," the Hispanic says that "time walks."

The Japanese, on the other hand, consider time to be valuable and to be used wisely. They tend to be punctual for medical appointments and persistent in following prescribed regimens. A Vietnamese family will subordinate time to values considered to be more significant, such as propriety. They may be late for an appointment because of an overextended visit by a friend in their home. In general, Asian-Americans view the American focus on time as offensive. They spend hours getting to know people and view predetermined, abrupt endings as rude. Introductory small talk is considered good manners.

Navajo Indians view time on a continuum with no beginning and no end. The present-time orientation may cause a Navajo to eat two meals a day today, four meals tomorrow, no meals the next day, and three meals the day after. This becomes an important nursing consideration if a Navajo is told to take medication with meals to ensure three doses per day.

In many cultural groups the mother assumes the responsibility for health care; in others both parents are involved equally in relationships with health workers. A somewhat different approach is apparent in some of the Asian cultures. For example, a Vietnamese or Filipino father, as unquestioned head of the family, is traditionally the one who interacts with persons, including health care providers, outside the family unit. In the Hispanic family the father, as head of the house, makes decisions regarding illness and treatment of adult family members, but the grandmother in the extended family is consulted regarding child care. Usually the family confers with other members before reaching a decision regarding treatment or hospitalization of a child. The Arab family also relies on others to give advice and guidance in a time of crisis. A Japanese father may appear to be passive and uninvolved but actually is involved according to his own cultural standards.

> **⚠ NURSING ALERT**
>
> In working with families, it is essential for nurses to identify key members and decision makers; failure to include these significant individuals in teaching can seriously hinder adherence to the care plan.

Nurses should learn about any specific attitudes regarding the manner of approach to a child in a given culture. Navajo Indians do not like a stranger near their infants. They fear that the stranger may "witch" the child and cause the child harm. On the other hand, if a stranger, particularly a woman, lavishes attention on a Hispanic infant but fails to touch the child, some Hispanics believe the infant will develop symptoms of the "evil eye" (see p. 33). Vietnamese and Korean families may become upset if a newborn is admired at length for fear the evil spirits will overhear and desire the infant.

Some groups, such as the Amish, consider a child's admission to the hospital a family affair, with all members gathering to support and console the child and parents. In other groups the family is willing to relinquish the care of the child to the hospital authority without interference. Their visits with the child are short, although intense, but hospital staff may misinterpret this behavior as disinterest or abandonment.

All ethnic groups are entitled to be treated with dignity and respect. Family members should be addressed by their last names; many groups consider it an affront to be called by their first names. Stereotyping is to be condemned. People are individuals who are evaluated in relation to their cultural standards, needs, and preferences. For example, believing that fathers are never involved in the direct care of their child can result in wrong assumptions about a culture (Fig. 2-4).

Nurses who are members of a majority culture may encounter tension and distrust in a child from a minority culture as a result of the child's learned conceptions or relationships with other persons in the majority group. Based on these perceptions, minority children may suspect that nurses have hostile feelings toward them and fear ill treatment. When such children are hospitalized, this suspicion increases the feelings of loneliness and helplessness that accompany fearful events and separation from families. The reverse situation may be encountered by a nurse from a minority culture attempting to meet the needs of a child who has been conditioned to view the nurse's cultural or ethnic group as inferior. Either situation is more likely to occur if the nurse or the child has had little or no personal contact with the other's culture. For example, a child from a minority culture from the inner city who lives in a neighborhood and attends school only with children from his

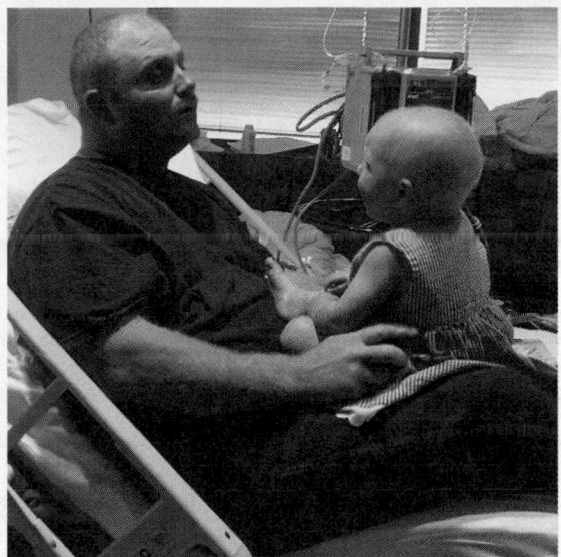

Fig. 2-4 Many fathers assume an active parenting role. (Courtesy E. Jacob, Texas Children's Hospital, Houston.)

or her minority culture may be more suspicious of a nurse from a different culture than would a child from the same minority group who lives in a culturally diverse neighborhood or attends an integrated school. Becoming familiar with cultures different from one's own and making an effort to know each other as individuals can shatter myths and, with time, build the trust needed to establish rewarding relationships between children, their families, and the nurse.

Communication

Communication is basic to all human relationships, but it may be a source of distress and misunderstanding between persons from different ethnic groups, especially if the languages are different. Prejudice is one of the biggest barriers to cross-cultural communication. The Office of Minority Health and Health Disparities of the U.S. Department of Health and Human Services has established national standards on culturally and linguistically appropriate services in health care. Health care organizations must ensure the competence of language assistance provided to person with limited English proficiency by interpreters and bilingual staff. Family and friends should not be used for interpretation services except on the patient's request (Shaw-Taylor, 2002). (See Communicating with Families Through an Interpreter, Chapter 6.)

Part of culturally sensitive communication is taking time to assess beliefs and values. In a study on childhood asthma, management researchers discovered that parents who believed asthma to be intermittent rather than a chronic condition provided suboptimal treatment to their child (Yoos, Kitzman, Henderson, et al, 2007). It is vital that the family members fully understand all implications of a child's care and management before they consent for special procedures or assume responsibility for the child's medication administration. Some persons with poor or limited language comprehension may simply smile and nod in agreement if they do not understand the questions or directives. It is not uncommon for an Asian family to indicate "yes" when in fact they mean "no" in order to avoid social disharmony. They tend to address issues indirectly rather than through confrontation and may become evasive when direct questioning makes them uncomfortable.

NURSING TIP Helpful communication tools include:

- Ask open-ended questions about cultural needs, health beliefs, and etiquette for communication.
- If a live interpreter is not available, use a language line telephone interpreter.
- Have legal consent forms and explanations of common diagnostic tests available in several languages.
- Keep cards with common greetings, phrases, and names of body parts in the family's language with the patient's chart (e.g., miseries [pain] and locked bowels [constipation] for African-Americans; and *caida de la mollera* [fallen fontanel from dehydration], *susto* [fright], *dolor, duels,* or *lele* [pain], and *la diarrhea* [diarrhea] for Hispanics).

Nonverbal communication is a practiced art in many Native American tribes, and the members are highly sensitive to body language. They emphasize periods of silence to formulate thoughts in preparation for speech and often remain silent after listening to others to properly assimilate what has been said. Interruption, interjection, or haste to arrive at a conclusion is perceived as immature behavior.

Different cultures view eye contact differently. Although Caucasians are advised to look people straight in the eye, persons in some ethnic groups avoid eye contact and become uncomfortable when conversing with health care workers. In non-Western cultures a patient may not look directly into the nurse's eyes as a sign of respect. Some Native Americans make eye contact during the initial greeting, but consider continued, unwavering eye contact insulting and disrespectful. Asians may consider eye contact a sign of hostility or impoliteness.

The level of comfort with body space or distance from others varies among cultures. Caucasians are generally comfortable at arm's length, Hispanics tend to get closer, and some Asians prefer a greater distance. Also, gestures may have different meanings. For example, some Asians consider pointing with a finger or foot disrespectful. Some Native Americans consider vigorous handshaking a sign of aggression, whereas to Caucasians the gesture is a sign of goodwill and strong character.

Families may be reluctant to question or otherwise initiate contact with health professionals. In Asian cultures, for example, it is considered a sign of disrespect to question persons of authority. A Japanese family may wait silently rather than ask or question. They believe the health professionals know best and will meet their needs without being asked. They also think it is important to avoid criticism. Criticism can cause the Japanese-American to "lose face," to feel ashamed, which is highly undesirable.

Language has been considered the biggest barrier to the use of health care services by many families, especially Southeast Asians (Mattson, 1995). Often, families may have poor language comprehension, so it is necessary to speak slowly and carefully, not loudly, when conversing with them. Many persons are able to read and write English better than they can speak or understand it. Also, people usually revert to their dominant language in anxiety-provoking situations, even if they are able to communicate satisfactorily under ordinary circumstances.

Terms of address and use of first and last names vary among cultures and can create confusion in institutions. For example,

in Asian cultures, the family name is given first in respect for the family and the given names follow. Therefore all siblings in a family have the same first name (or, in some families, the same middle name). The Mennonites refer to children as sons and daughters of a particular parent, such as "Josiah's son," rather than by the children's names.

Although all people share the basic emotions, there are decided ethnic variations in the ways emotions are expressed. People in some cultures (e.g., Italian, Latin, or Jewish background) express emotions openly and are accustomed to sharing their sorrows and joys with family and friends. Conversely, Nordic and Asian groups are more restrained in expressing emotion.

Health care providers generally ask questions and use handouts, booklets, and—particularly with children—dolls and pictures as communication aids. This is uncommon in some cultures. For example, Native American healers ask few questions and do not use forms. Nurses need to consider both verbal and nonverbal communication techniques to interact effectively with children and their families from different cultures (see Nursing Care Guidelines box).

FOOD CUSTOMS

Food customs and symbolism of various cultural, ethnic, and religious groups are an integral part of their lives. Although in a large country such as the United States most people have adopted the eclectic food habits that have evolved over generations, many still retain ethnic and geographic food traditions and preferences. Special holidays, ceremonies, and life experiences such as births, birthdays, weddings, and death are often marked by special food items or feasts. In many cultures specific food practices are followed during pregnancy in the belief that certain foods damage or benefit the developing fetus. The distinctive food customs of ethnic groups are a product of their native environment, determined by availability.

A number of restrictions are related to food items. Some have a physiologic origin, such as lack of dairy foods in the diets of some persons of African or Asian ancestry with lactose intolerance. Others are religious restrictions, such as kosher foods and food preparation of the Orthodox Jewish faith and the vegetarian diet of Seventh Day Adventists. (See Vegetarian Diets, Chapter 13.)

Children in a strange environment, such as the hospital, feel much more comfortable when they are served familiar foods. Hospital food often tastes strange and bland, especially to children who enjoy the highly seasoned foods of their culture. Also, the family may be concerned that the child is not receiving foods appropriate to their culture and beliefs. When possible, provide the children's ethnic foods or allow families to bring favorite foods that are not on the hospital menu. Concern for differences in food habits and patterns projects an attitude of respect for the family's ethnic or religious heritage (Ohio State University Extension, 2005).

It is also important for nurses and other health care providers to be mindful of the meaning of food and eating within a family or community. Feeding and food preparation are ways in which families nurture and care for one another. This is especially true in the parent-child relationship. Parents and

---

NURSING CARE GUIDELINES

Culturally Sensitive Interactions

Nonverbal Strategies

Invite family members to choose where they would like to sit or stand, allowing them to select a comfortable distance.

Observe interactions with others to determine which body gestures (e.g., shaking hands) are acceptable and appropriate. Ask when in doubt. Know when physical contact is prohibited.

Avoid appearing rushed.

Be an active listener.

Observe for cues regarding appropriate eye contact. Avoiding eye contact may be a sign of respect.

Learn appropriate use of pauses or interruptions for different cultures.

Ask for clarification if nonverbal meaning is unclear.

Learn if smiling indicates friendliness or if it is taboo (Spector, 2009).

Verbal Strategies

Learn proper terms of address.

Use a positive tone of voice to convey interest.

Speak concisely and thoughtfully, not loudly, when families have poor language comprehension.

Encourage questions.

Learn basic words and sentences of family's language, if possible.

Avoid professional terms.

When asking questions, tell family why the questions are being asked, the way in which the information they provide will be used, and how it might benefit their child.

Repeat important information more than once.

Always give the reason for a treatment or prescription.

Use information written in the family's language.

Arrange for the services of an interpreter when necessary (see Chapter 6).

Learn from families and representatives of their culture methods of communicating information without creating discomfort.

Address intergenerational needs (e.g., family's need to consult with others).

---

other family members may struggle with this desire to feed and nurture their child in circumstances when the child does not want to eat or cannot tolerate oral intake (i.e., a child receiving chemotherapy). Nurses can encourage families to nurture the sick child in other ways, such as touch, reading, or other enjoyable activities.

HEALTH BELIEFS AND PRACTICES

The nurse encounters people of many different racial and ethnic origins in the process of meeting the health needs of children and families. Some of these families have become so enculturated to the majority culture that their health beliefs and practices are consistent with those of the health care system. For many families, however, traditional practices and beliefs are an integral part of their daily lives. Health care workers should be aware that other people might live by different rules and priorities, which decisively influence health-related behavior.

A model for learning about health traditions that differ from the Western, or modern, health care system is based on three dimensions:

1. What are the physical aspects of caring for the body (e.g., are there special clothes, foods, medicines)?
2. What are the mental parts of caring for health (e.g., feelings, attitudes, rituals, actions)?
3. What are the spiritual aspects of health (who I am, spiritual customs, prayers, healers)?

For each of these dimensions, one must consider the cultural traditions used to maintain health, protect health, and restore health (Spector, 2009).

HEALTH BELIEFS

The beliefs related to the cause of illness and the maintenance of health are an integral part of a family's cultural heritage. Often inseparable from religious beliefs, they influence the way families cope with health problems and respond to health care providers. Predominant among most cultures are beliefs related

to natural forces, supernatural forces, and imbalance between forces.

Natural Forces

The most common natural forces held responsible for ill health if the body is not adequately protected include cold air entering the body and impurities in the air. For example, a Chinese parent may overdress the infant in an effort to keep cold wind from entering the child's body. The Chinese believe that cold weather, rain, or wind is responsible for "cold" conditions. They also believe that an innate energy called *chi* enters and leaves the body through the mouth, nose, and ears and flows through the body in definite pathways, or meridians, at specific times and locations. The Chinese believe that a lack of chi and blood causes fatigue, low energy, and a variety of ailments.

In the African-American culture, some individuals believe natural phenomena such as phases of the moon, seasons of the year, and planet positions affect the body and its processes; therefore health maintenance is strongly associated with the ability to read "the signs." Some cultures consider behaviors such as overeating, overwork, anxiety, and inadequate food and sleep to be natural causes of illness. Most Native Americans consider health to be a state of harmony with nature and the universe.

Supernatural Forces

High on the list of causes of illness are forces beyond comprehension and logical explanation. Some cultures view evil influences such as voodoo, witchcraft, or evil spirits as causes of illness, especially those illnesses that cannot be explained by other means.

A health belief that is common among people from Latin American, Mediterranean, some Asian, and some African societies is the concept of the "evil eye" (Spector, 2009). It is part of the concept of health as a state of balance and illness as a state of imbalance (see following section). Strength and power are associated with the evil eye; therefore, as long as an individual's strength and weakness remain in balance, he or she is unlikely to become a victim of the evil eye. Weaknesses are not necessarily physical. For example, an excess of some emotion, such as envy, can create weakness. Infants and small children, because of immature development of their internal strength-weakness states, are especially vulnerable to the gaze of the evil eye. Consequently, the evil eye serves to rationalize an inexplicable onset of illness in children who display symptoms such as restlessness, crying, diarrhea, vomiting, and fever.

Health Protection

Cultural traditions used in the protection of health may include protective objects, which may be worn, carried, or hung in the home or room. For example, amulets are objects or charms that are worn on a string or chain to protect the wearer from the evil eye or evil spirits. It is important to allow people to wear these objects in the health care setting. Another cultural practice is the inclusion of substances in the diet that protect health. For example, the ginseng root is used to "build the blood" in the Chinese culture. Religious practices, such as burning candles or prayer, are also traditions used to protect health (Spector, 2009).

Imbalance of Forces

The concept of balance or equilibrium is widespread throughout the world. One of the most common imbalances supported by the Hispanic, Filipino, Chinese, and Arab cultures is that which exists between "hot" and "cold." This belief is reputedly derived from the Hippocratic theory of humoral pathology, which states that illness is caused by an imbalance of the four humors: phlegm, blood, black bile, and yellow bile (Sekhon, 1996). "Hot" and "cold" describe certain properties and conditions completely unrelated to temperature. Diseases, areas of the body, foods, and illnesses are classified as either "hot" or "cold." In Chinese health belief the forces are termed *yin* (cold) and *yang* (hot) (Wang and Martinson, 1996). To maintain health and prevent illness, these forces must be kept in balance.

Illness is treated by restoring normal balance through the application of appropriate "hot" or "cold" remedies. A "cold" condition such as a respiratory disease is believed to be caused by exposure to cold weather, rain, or cold wind entering the body; it is treated by administration of "hot" foods, herbs, or drugs. Menstruation is considered a "hot" condition; therefore women are cautioned against ingesting "hot" foods, which might increase menstrual flow or produce cramping. Ingesting too much of either "hot" or "cold" foods can also be interpreted as a cause of illness.

Health care workers who are aware of this belief are better able to understand why some persons refuse to eat certain foods. It is often useful to discuss the diet with the family to determine their beliefs regarding food choices. It is possible to help families devise a diet that contains the necessary balance of basic food groups prescribed by the medical subculture while conforming to the beliefs of the ethnic subculture.

The "hot-cold" food classification may have adverse effects. For example, in some cultures newborn infants are often started on evaporated milk formulas. Evaporated milk is considered a "hot" food, whereas whole milk is viewed as a "cold" food. Infants tend to develop rashes, which are believed to be caused by "hot" foods; in such cases parents may decide to switch to whole milk. However, parents fear that it is dangerous to change too rapidly, so they often feed the child some type of neutralizing substance, which may create additional health problems. The nurse can help avoid such a problem by determining the family's preference before discharge from the hospital and prescribing a formula that is agreeable to both the family and the practitioner.

HEALTH PRACTICES

Cultures have numerous similarities regarding prevention and treatment of illness. All cultures have some types of home remedies that they apply before seeking help from other persons. Within the ethnic community, folk healers who are endowed with the ability to "cure" maladies are sought for special situations and when home remedies are unsuccessful. The *curandero* (male) or *curandera* (female) of the Mexican-American community is believed to have healing powers that are a gift from God. The Asian consults an herbalist, knowledgeable in medicines, or perhaps an ethnic practitioner in Asian therapies, including acupuncture (insertion of needles), acupressure (application of pressure), and moxibustion (application of heat). Native Americans consult a variety of healers with specific skills and knowledge. Specialized medicine persons diagnose illness, provide nonsacred treatments (usually by way of massage and herbs), and care for souls. Other specialists perform services or effect cures through the use of spiritual means. Native Hawaiians consult *kahunas* and practice *ho'oponopono* to heal family imbalance or disputes.

The folk healers are powerful persons in their community and can acquire information about an illness without resorting to probing questions. They "speak the language" of the family who seeks help and often combine their rituals and potions with prayer and entreaties to God. They also are able to create an atmosphere conducive to successful management. Furthermore, they exhibit a sincere interest in the family and their problem.

Some folk remedies are compatible with the medical regimen and are useful to reinforce the treatment plan. For example, aspirin (a "hot" medication) is an appropriate therapy for "cold" diseases such as the common cold and arthritis. It is not uncommon to discover that a folk prescription has a scientific basis. In any case, respect practices that do no harm patients.

In cultures that believe in the concept, overcoming the effect of the evil eye usually requires specialized rituals conducted by the appropriate practitioner. For example, the Chicano curandero ascertains that the condition is truly the result of the evil eye by performing an assessment ritual and then performs a curative ritual. Sometimes faith in the folk practitioner delays obtaining needed medical treatment, although the practitioner usually suggests medical care if his or her ministrations are unsuccessful.

Health practices of different cultures may also present problems of assessment and interpretation. For example, certain cultural practices or remedies can be misdiagnosed as evidence of child abuse by uninformed professionals (Box 2-1). It is important to explain why some of these and other familiar remedies may now be considered harmful. Families need to

BOX 2-1 CULTURAL PRACTICES POSSIBLY CONSIDERED ABUSIVE BY THE DOMINANT CULTURE

Coining—A Vietnamese practice that may produce weltlike lesions on the child's back when the edge of a coin is repeatedly rubbed lengthwise on the oiled skin to rid the body of disease.

Cupping—An Old World practice (also practiced by the Vietnamese) of placing a container (e.g., tumbler, bottle, jar) containing steam against the skin surface to "draw out the poison" or other evil element. When the heated air within the container cools, a vacuum is created that produces a bruiselike blemish on the skin directly beneath the mouth of the container.

Burning—A practice of some Southeast Asian groups whereby small areas of skin are burned to treat enuresis and temper tantrums.

Female genital mutilation (female circumcision)—Removal of or injury to any part of the female genital organ; practiced in Africa, the Middle East, Latin America, India, Asia, North America, Australia, and Western Europe.

Forced kneeling—A child discipline measure of some Caribbean groups in which a child is forced to kneel for a long time.

Topical garlic application—A practice of Yemenite Jews in which crushed garlic cloves or garlic–petroleum jelly plaster is applied to the wrists to treat infectious disease. The practice can result in blisters or garlic burns.

Traditional remedies that contain lead—Greta and azarcon (Mexico; used for digestive problems), paylooah (Southeast Asia; used for rash or fever), and surma (India; used as a cosmetic to improve eyesight).

FAMILY-CENTERED CARE
Cultural Awareness

I am a pediatric emergency nurse with a high regard for cultural diversity and a respect for healing practices and beliefs. I even made a manual for my emergency department that contains some of the information needed to help us understand and communicate with subcultures in the urban community we serve. Although I learned a great deal putting this manual together, it doesn't come close to the lesson I learned with the following experience.

A 15-month-old Bosnian girl in status epilepticus was carried in by her parents. They were frightened and spoke little English. I learned that the child had received a measles, mumps, and rubella (MMR) immunization the day before. As I proceeded to unwrap her from the blanket she was in, I quickly assessed the ABCs (airway, breathing, and circulation). I noticed that she was warm (probably a febrile seizure) and that a rag soaked in alcohol was tied around each thigh. Focusing on her potential airway compromise and trying to calm the parents, I proceeded to put an oxygen mask on her, undress her for a full assessment, and remove the alcohol rags. I spoke to the parents all the while in a calm, soothing voice. Once I had established an intravenous line and given her lorazepam (Ativan), the seizures stopped. So did the communication between her parents and me. I noticed that they would no longer give me eye contact, and the mother would not even speak to me after the seizures stopped. It wasn't until I was returning to the department from admitting her that I realized why they might have stopped communicating with me—I had removed the rags! Had I only thought to replace the rags or asked their permission to remove the rags, things may have been different.

Laura L. Kuensting, MSN(R), RN
Cardinal Glennon Children's Hospital
St. Louis, Missouri

! NURSING ALERT

Avoid attacking traditional health cultural beliefs and practices as wrong or harmful, or implying that biomedical measures are uniformly correct and effective and the only way to prevent illness or treat sickness. Such attacks usually result in rejection of biomedical health care practitioners and health teaching based on biomedicine or scientific facts.

understand how such practices can place them in jeopardy with child protective services, and they need to explore alternative measures that are more acceptable to the dominant culture (Hayes and Dreher, 1991).

Other cultural health remedies that are harmful include eating clay or excessive amounts of salt. A mercury compound, *azogue* (the Spanish name for quicksilver), is commonly used in Mexico and sometimes sold illegally to low-income Hispanic families in the United States as a remedy for diarrhea. Alert health care workers know that the drug can cause permanent central nervous system damage. A careful history can reveal these practices, but it may require the collaboration of a folk healer to convince a user to stop.

Faith healing and religious rituals are closely allied with many folk-healing practices. Wearing of amulets, medals, and other religious relics believed by the culture to protect the individual and facilitate healing is a common practice. It is important for health workers to recognize the value of this practice and keep the items where the family has placed them or nearby. It offers comfort and support and rarely impedes medical and nursing care. If an item must be removed during a procedure, it should be replaced, if possible, when the procedure is completed. The nurse should explain the reason for its temporary removal to the family to reassure them their wishes will be respected (see Family-Centered Care box).

Nurses can be most effective when operating from a multicultural perspective, which means using appropriate aspects of the culture in question to develop culturally acceptable health care interventions. When the folk practices do not interfere with the patient's welfare, they need not be discouraged. Often a compromise can be reached that accomplishes the nurse's goal while maintaining the patient's dignity and self-esteem.

IMPORTANCE OF CULTURAL COMPETENCE TO NURSES

A consensus exists among nurses that cultural competence of professional nursing practice should be raised (Lester, 1998). The challenge for nurses is to gain knowledge about cultural care values, beliefs, and practices and to use this knowledge in the care they provide (Leininger, 2001). To understand and deal effectively with families in a multicultural community, nurses must be aware of their own attitudes and values. Nurses, too, are a product of their own cultural background and education. They are part of the "nursing culture." Nurses function within the framework of a professional culture with its own values and traditions and, as such, become socialized into that culture by educational programs and later by the work environment and professional associations.

Frequently nurses and other health care workers are not aware of their own cultural values and how those values influence their thoughts and actions. A model for self-examination on cultural competence is the ASKED model (Box 2-2). Recognizing that a behavior may be characteristic of a culture rather than being an "abnormal" behavior places nurses at an advantage in their relationships with families. Ethnocentric

---

BOX 2-2   **ASKED MODEL OF CULTURAL COMPETENCE**

Awareness—Am I aware of my personal biases and prejudices toward cultural groups different from mine?

Skill—Do I have the skill to conduct a cultural assessment and perform a culturally based physical assessment in a sensitive manner?

Knowledge—Do I have knowledge of the patient's worldview and the field of bicultural ecology?

Encounters—How many face-to-face encounters have I had with patients from diverse cultural backgrounds?

Desire—Do I genuinely desire to be culturally competent?

From Campinha-Bacote J: Cultural competence in psychiatric nursing: have you "ASKED" the right questions? *J Am Psychiatr Nurses Assoc* 8(6):183-187, 2002, available at www.nursingworld.org/MainMenuCategories/ANAMarketplace/ANAPeriodicals/OJIN/TableofContents/Volume82003/No1Jan2003/AddressingDiversityinHealthCare.aspx (accessed November 19, 2009). © 2002 by J. Campinha-Bacote.

🌐 **CULTURAL COMPETENCE**

Five Components of Cultural Competence

Cultural competence includes following five components (Munoz and Luckmann, 2005):

1. Cultural awareness—A cognitive process through which the nurse appreciates and is sensitive to the cultural values of the patient and family
2. Cultural knowledge—The foundation the nurse builds through formal and informal education that includes world views of different cultures, values, beliefs, and perceptions about health and illness
3. Cultural skill—The ability to include cultural data in the nursing assessment through the collection of cultural data in the health interview and observations
4. Cultural encounter—The process through which the nurse seeks opportunities to engage in cross-cultural interactions directly or indirectly
5. Cultural desire—The genuine and sincere motivation to work effectively with minority clients; can only be achieved if the individual wants to engage in the process of acquiring cultural competence

---

approaches to nursing care are ineffective in meeting health and nursing needs of diverse cultural groups of patients (American Nurses Association, 1991). When nurses respect the cultural differences of a family, they are better able to determine whether the behavior is distinctive to the individual or a characteristic of the culture. What appears to be puzzling behavior may simply be the customary response in the culture (e.g., expression of emotion).

Cultural standards and values, the family structure and function, and past experiences with health care influence a family's feelings and attitudes toward health, their children, and health care delivery systems. It is often difficult for nurses to be nonjudgmental and objective in working with families whose behaviors and attitudes differ from or conflict with their own. The nurse needs to understand how his or her own cultural background influences the way care is delivered (American Nurses Association, 1991).

Relying only on one's own values and experiences for guidance can result in frustration and disappointment. It is one thing to know what is needed to deal with a health problem; it is often more difficult to implement a fruitful course of action unless nurses work within the cultural and socioeconomic framework of the family (see Critical Thinking Exercise, p. 23).

It is essential to make an effort to adapt ethnic practices to the family's health needs rather than attempt to change longstanding beliefs. To aid their efforts to understand and respect the cultural beliefs of families, nurses should have a readily available resource file containing pertinent information about the cultural and subcultural characteristics of the community in which they practice (e.g., traditional practices related to infant feeding practices and the time and manner of weaning and toilet training). Cultural competence is a process that is facilitated by recognizing cultural differences, integrating cultural knowledge, and acting in a culturally appropriate manner (Munoz and Luckmann, 2005) (see Cultural Competence box).

CULTURAL AWARENESS

Cultural and religious rituals are important practices among families from various cultures. An example is the Jewish *upsher-*

enish ceremony, which celebrates a boy's first haircut when he reaches 3 years of age. Any procedure requiring haircutting, such as placement of an intravenous line in a scalp vein, must be discussed with parents to obtain their permission.

Table 2-1 outlines some characteristics of selected cultures. Nurses must assess the cultural and religious practices of families to identify how these practices are similar to and different from those of their own cultural and religious backgrounds. Guidelines for culturally sensitive interactions are described on p. 33.

❗ **NURSING ALERT**

These generalizations are presented to help nurses learn the unique beliefs and practices of various groups and are not meant to be stereotypes of any group. It is critical to remember that no cultural group is homogeneous, every racial and ethnic group contains great diversity, and knowledge of a culture may not reflect an individual member's beliefs (Nance, 1995; Kleinman and Benson, 2006).

Concepts that come from medical anthropology can provide a framework for addressing health care issues. These concepts can have a direct impact on patient care. It leads the nurse away from an ethnocentric or medicocentric view of the health care encounter into the health care reality as constructed by the patient and family. This is relevant for addressing many of the problems that plague the American health care system: patient dissatisfaction with the health care they receive, unequal distribution of high-quality health care, and excessive cost (Kleinman, Eisenberg, and Good, 1978; Kleinman and Benson, 2006).

It is also important for nurses to recognize that disease and illness are distinct entities. Clinicians diagnose and treat diseases, "abnormalities in the structure and function of body organs and systems" (Kleinman, Eisenberg, and Good, 1978). Patients suffer from and deal with illnesses, "the human experience of sickness" (Kleinman, Eisenberg, and Good, 1978). Illness and disease are not interchangeable; illness may occur even when disease is not present, and the course of a disease may vary substantially from the experience of illness.

TABLE 2-1	BROAD CULTURAL CHARACTERISTICS RELATED TO HEALTH CARE OF CHILDREN AND FAMILIES		
HEALTH BELIEFS	**HEALTH PRACTICES**	**FAMILY RELATIONSHIPS**	**COMMUNICATION**
African			
Illness classified as:	Self-care and folk medicine prevalent	Strong kinship bonds in extended family; members come to aid of others in crisis	Alert to any evidence of discrimination
Natural—Affected by forces of nature without adequate protection (e.g., cold air, pollution, food and water)	Folk therapies usually religious in origin	Less likely to view illness as a burden	Place importance on nonverbal behavior
	Folk therapies often not shared with the medical provider	Place strong emphasis on work and ambition	Affection shown by touching and hugging
Unnatural—God's punishment for improper behavior	Prayer as common means for prevention and treatment	Elders cared for and respected	Silence may indicate lack of trust
May see illness as the "will of God"			Initial eye contact to show respect; maintaining eye contact can be viewed as aggressive
			Best to use direct but caring approach
Chinese			
A healthy body viewed as gift from parents and ancestors and must be cared for	Goal of therapy is to restore balance of yin and yang	Extended family pattern common	Open expression of emotions unacceptable
Health seen as one of the results of balance between the forces of **yin** (cold) and **yang** (hot)—energy forces that rule the world	Acupuncturist needles applied to appropriate meridians identified in terms of yin and yang	Strong concept of loyalty of young to old	Often smile when they do not comprehend
	Acupressure and **tai chi** replacing acupuncture in some areas	Respect for elders taught at early age—acceptance without questioning or talking back	Eye contact avoided as sign of respect
Illness caused by imbalance	**Moxibustion**—Application of heat to skin over specific meridians	Children's behavior a reflection on family	
Blood believed to be source of life and is not regenerated	Wide use of medicinal herbs procured and applied in prescribed ways	Family and individual honor and "face" important	
Chi is innate energy	Meals may or may not be planned to balance hot and cold	Self-reliance and self-esteem highly valued; self-expression repressed	
Haitian			
Illness seen as a punishment	Health a personal responsibility	Maintenance of family reputation paramount	Recent immigrants and older persons may speak only Haitian Creole
Natural cause (*maladi bone die*—disease of the Lord) caused by environmental factors, movement of blood within the body, changes between hot and cold, and bone displacement	Foods have properties of "hot"/"cold" and "light"/"heavy" and must be in harmony with one's life cycle and bodily states	Lineal authority supreme; children in a subordinate position in family hierarchy	Often smile and nod in agreement when do not understand
	Natural illnesses treated by home and folk remedies first	Children valued for parental security in old age and expected to contribute to family welfare at an early age	Quiet and gentle communication style and lack of assertiveness lead health care providers to falsely believe they comprehend health teaching and are compliant
Supernatural (*loa*—spirits' anger)	May use religious medallions, rosary beads, or figure of saint to pray with		
Good health seen as the maintenance of equilibrium			May not ask questions if health care provider is busy or rushed
Prayer and good spiritual habits important			
Japanese			
Shinto religious influence	Energy restored by means of acupuncture, acupressure, massage, and moxibustion along affected meridians	Close intergenerational relationships	Make significant use of nonverbal communication with subtle gestures and facial expression
Human inherently good		Generational categories:	
Evil caused by outside spirits		***Issei***—First generation to live in United States	Tend to suppress emotions
Illness caused by contact with polluting agents (e.g., blood, corpses, skin diseases)	***Kampō* medicine**—Use of natural herbs	***Nisei***—Second generation	Will often wait silently
	Believe in removal of diseased parts	***Sansei***—Third generation	
Health achieved through harmony and balance between self and society	Trend is to use both Western and Asian healing methods	***Yonsei***—Fourth generation	
	Care for disabled viewed as family's responsibility	Family tends to keep problems to self	
Disease caused by disharmony with society and not caring for body	Take pride in child's good health	Value self-control and self-sufficiency	
	Seek preventive care, medical care for illness	Concept of ***haji*** (shame) imposes strong control; unacceptable behavior of children reflects on family	

Continued

TABLE 2-1	BROAD CULTURAL CHARACTERISTICS RELATED TO HEALTH CARE OF CHILDREN AND FAMILIES—cont'd		
HEALTH BELIEFS	**HEALTH PRACTICES**	**FAMILY RELATIONSHIPS**	**COMMUNICATION**
Mexican-American			
Health controlled by environment, fate, and will of God	Seek help from *curandero* or *curandera*, especially in rural areas	Strong kinship—extended families include **compadres** (godparents) established by ritual kinship	Spanish speaking or bilingual
Certain illnesses considered "hot" and "cold" states and are treated with food that complements those states	**Curandero(a)** receives position by birth, apprenticeship, or a "calling" via dream or vision	Children valued highly and desired, taken everywhere with family	May have a strong preference for native language and revert to it in times of stress
Disease based on imbalance between individual and environment	Treatments involve use of herbs, rituals, and religious artifacts	Elderly treated with respect	May shake hands or engage in introductory embrace
	Practice for severe illness—make promises, visit shrines, offer medals and candles, offer prayers		Interpret prolonged eye contact as disrespectful
	Adhere to "hot" and "cold" food prescriptions and prohibitions for prevention and treatment of illness		Relaxed concept of time—may be late to appointments
Native American			
Believe health is state of harmony with nature and universe	Distinction made between indigenous health problem requiring native healer or practice and Western disease requiring other medical care	Cultures vary in kinship structure	Use anecdotes or metaphors to discuss a situation
Respect bodies through proper management		Extended family structure—usually includes relatives from both sides of family	Long pauses indicate careful consideration
Depend on individual belief in traditional culture	Health practices include self-sufficiency and harmonious living	Elder members assume leadership roles	Nonverbal communication
Traditional health beliefs holistic and wellness oriented	Participation in religious ceremonies and prayer promotes health		Respect indicated by avoiding eye contact
			Individuals usually speak for themselves
Puerto Rican			
Subscribe to the "hot-cold" theory of causation of illness	Infrequent use of health care system	Family usually large and home centered—the core of existence	Spanish speaking or bilingual
Believe some illness caused by evil forces	Seek folk healers (*espiritistas*)—use of herbs, rituals	Father has authority in family	Strong sense of family privacy—may view questions regarding family as impudent
Destiny (*Si Dios quiere*—if God wants) is in control of health	Treatment classified as "hot" or "cold"	Great respect for elders	
	Many varieties of herbal teas used to treat illness and promote healing	Children valued—seen as a gift from God	
		Children taught to obey and respect parents	
Vietnamese			
Good health considered to be balance between yin and yang	Family uses all means possible before using outside agencies for health care	Family is revered institution	May hesitate to ask questions
Concept of health based on harmony and balance	Regard health as family responsibility; outside aid sought when resources run out	Multigenerational families	Questioning authority is sign of disrespect; asking questions considered impolite
Rituals used to prevent illness	Use herbal medicine, spiritual practices, and acupuncture	Family is chief social network	May avoid eye contact with health professionals as a sign of respect
	May consider head sacred and feet profane; avoid touching head after feet	Children highly valued	
	May use cupping, coin rubbing, or pinching skin	Individual needs and interests subordinate to those of a family group	
	May inhale aromatic oils, take herbal teas, or wear strings tied on body	Father is main decision maker	
		Women taught submission to men	
		Parents expect respect and obedience from children	

Data from Galanti G: *Caring for patients from different cultures,* ed 3, Philadelphia, 2004, University of Pennsylvania Press; Lipson JG, Dibble SL, Minarik PA: *Culture and clinical care: a pocket guide,* San Francisco, 2005, UCSF Nursing Press; Purnell LD, Paulanka BJ: *Transcultural health care: a culturally competent approach,* Philadelphia, 2003, Davis; and Spector RE: *Cultural diversity in health and illness,* ed 6, Upper Saddle River, NJ, 2004, Pearson Prentice Hall.

Illness is culturally constructed; an individual's culture influences how a sickness is perceived, labeled, and explained. Culture also influences the meaning assigned to the illness, the role the individual with the sickness adopts, and the response of the family and community to the sickness.

Tension may arise when the perception of the illness and disease varies widely among the patient, family, and health care team. Failure of health care providers to recognize these disparities may be partially to blame in cases of noncompliance, delivery of inadequate care, and patient or family dissatisfaction. To begin addressing these issues, it is important for nurses to understand the various domains of health care in which individuals operate in American society: professional (health care providers and institutions), popular (family, community, and lay literature), and folk (nonprofessional healers) (Kleinman, Eisenberg, and Good, 1978). Each domain possesses a method for defining and explaining the sickness and what should be done to address it. The challenge for nurses and other health care providers is to address this disconnect with families and develop mutually agreed on goals. Nurses are in a prime position to assume this role, since understanding the human response to disease is central to their role. In addition, collaboration with the child and family is central to the role of the pediatric nurse.

Not all health care providers feel adequately prepared to care for culturally diverse populations. A study of 1700 resident physicians by Betancourt (2007) revealed that 25% to 30% of them did not feel prepared to deal with families who are mistrustful of the health care system, those with limited English proficiency, those whose health perspective differs from a Western-based model, those adults who incorporate other family into the decision-making process, or those who bring their spirituality into the health care environment. Unfortunately, the numbers may not be too different for nursing and other health care professionals. Such statistics are a wake-up call for anyone who strives for high-quality patient care.

One method of addressing this disconnect with families and beginning collaboration is by understanding the family's explanatory model of illness. The questions in Box 2-3, developed by Arthur Kleinman, a physician and anthropologist, aim to elicit an individual's beliefs about the disease or illness, the meaning attached to it, goals, and expectations of the outcome and role of the health care provider. The wording may need to be adapted depending on the child, family, setting, and clinical issue to be addressed. Nurses can then point out areas of discrepancy for further dialogue, negotiation, and collaboration. This discussion, when conducted with a genuine interest in the family and child's perspective, is a significant step in building trusting relationships, promoting adherence, decreasing disparities, and increasing health care satisfaction.

HEREDITARY FACTORS

Some groups of people are more susceptible or more resistant to certain illnesses than other groups. An innate susceptibility is acquired through generations of evolutionary changes that take place within constrained or segregated populations. The proximity to disease, environmental factors, and general physical status are significant factors associated with health problems.

Historically, the increased health risks associated with ethnicity have been explained in terms of genetic differences or related factors such as socioeconomic status (Scribner, 1996). The genetic constitution of individuals in groups is known to influence the degree to which they are susceptible to a specific disorder. It may be a result of an inherent lack of resistance to a disease organism; a trait that is an advantage in one environment but places the possessor at a disadvantage in another; or intermarriage within a relatively narrow range of geographic, ethnic, or religious restrictions.

A classic example of a geographic constraint is the common communicable disease rubeola. The rubeola virus, or the populations that were continually exposed to it, became altered in such a way that the disease was considered to be a universal disease of childhood from which the majority of children suffered without ill effects. When other populations (e.g., the inhabitants of the Hawaiian Islands) were exposed to the virus by explorers and missionaries, they experienced a violent response that resulted in high mortality.

Another communicable disease, tuberculosis, appears to be more prevalent in certain ethnic groups such as the Native Americans of the Southwest, Vietnamese immigrants, and Mexican-Americans. In many populations it is difficult to determine how much the increased incidence can be attributed to ethnic factors and how much is related to lifestyles in the lower social strata.

A number of diseases show ethnic or racial differences (Box 2-4). For example, Tay-Sachs disease, characterized by early neurologic deterioration and mental retardation, primarily affects Ashkenazi Jewish families, particularly those of northeastern European origin, whereas Sephardic Jewish families appear to be no more at risk for the disease than other populations. The incidence of cystic fibrosis is highest in Caucasians and almost nonexistent in Asians, and the rare affected African-Americans are usually in areas where there is likely to be mixed ancestry. A classic disorder of African-Americans is sickle cell disease (see Chapter 35); however, the incidence of cardiovascular disease, pneumonia, and diabetes is also high in this group. Native Americans have particularly high rates of diabetes, tuberculosis, diarrhea, alcoholism, and suicide. Consider

---

BOX 2-3	QUESTIONS THAT EXPLORE A FAMILY'S PERSPECTIVE ON CULTURE, ILLNESS, AND CARE

- What do you think caused your problem?
- Why do you think it started when it did?
- What do you think your sickness does to you? How does it work?
- How severe is your sickness? Will it have a short or long course?
- What kind of treatment do you think you should receive?
- What are the most important results you hope to receive from this treatment?
- What are the chief problems your sickness has caused for you?
- What do you fear most about your sickness?

Adapted from Kleinman A, Eisenberg L, Good B: Culture, illness, and care: clinical lessons from anthropologic and cross-cultural research, *Ann Intern Med* 88:251-258, 1978.

BOX 2-4	DISTRIBUTION OF SELECTED GENETIC TRAITS AND DISORDERS BY POPULATION OR ETHNIC GROUP

Åland Islanders (Finland)
Ocular albinism (Forsius-Eriksson type)

Alaskan Natives
Congenital adrenal hyperplasia
Pseudocholinesterase deficiency
Methemoglobinemia

Amish
Limb-girdle muscular dystrophy (Adams and Allen Counties, Indiana)
Ellis–van Creveld syndrome (Lancaster County, Pennsylvania)
Pyruvate kinase deficiency (Mifflin County, Ohio)
Hemophilia B (Holmes County, Pennsylvania)

Armenians
Familial Mediterranean fever

Blacks (African-Americans, Africans)
Sickle cell disease
Hemoglobin C disease
Hereditary persistence of hemoglobin F
Glucose-6-phosphate dehydrogenase (G6PD) deficiency, African type
Lactase deficiency, adult
β-Thalassemia

Burmese
Hemoglobin E disease

Chinese
α-Thalassemia
G6PD deficiency, Chinese type
Lactase deficiency, adult

Costa Rican
Malignant osteopetrosis

English
Cystic fibrosis
Hereditary amyloidosis, type III

Finns
Congenital nephrosis
Generalized amyloidosis syndrome, V
Polycystic liver disease
Retinoschisis
Aspartylglycosaminuria
Diastrophic dwarfism

French Canadians (Quebec)
Tyrosinemia
Morquio syndrome

Gypsies (Roma) (Czech Republic)
Congenital glaucoma

Hopi Indians
Tyrosinase-positive albinism

Icelanders
Phenylketonuria

Irish
Phenylketonuria
Neural tube defects

Japanese
Acatalasia
Cleft lip and palate
Oguchi disease

Jews
Ashkenazi
Tay-Sachs disease (infantile)
Niemann-Pick disease (infantile)
Gaucher disease (adult type)
Familial dysautonomia (Riley-Day syndrome)
Bloom syndrome
Torsion dystonia
Factor XI (plasma thromboplastin antecedent) deficiency

Sephardic
Familial Mediterranean fever
Ataxia-telangiectasia (Morocco)
Cystinuria (Libya)
Glycogen storage disease III (Morocco)

Lebanese
Dyggve-Melchior-Clausen syndrome

Mediterranean People (Italians, Greeks)
G6PD deficiency, Mediterranean type
β-Thalassemia
Familial Mediterranean fever

Middle Eastern People
Dubin-Johnson syndrome (Iran)
Ichthyosis vulgaris (Iraq)
Werdnig-Hoffmann disease (Karaite Jews)
G6PD deficiency, Mediterranean type
Phenylketonuria (Yemen)
Metachromatic leukodystrophy (Habbani Jews, Saudi Arabia)

Navajo Indians
Ear anomalies

Nova Scotia Acadians
Niemann-Pick disease, type D

Polish
Phenylketonuria

Polynesians
Clubfoot

Portuguese
Azorean disease (Joseph disease)

Scandinavians (Norway, Sweden, Denmark)
Cholestasis-lymphedema (Norway)
Sjögren-Larsson syndrome (Sweden)
Krabbe disease
Phenylketonuria

Scots
Phenylketonuria
Cystic fibrosis
Hereditary amyloidosis, type III

Thai
Lactase deficiency, adult
Hemoglobin E disease

Zuni Indians
Tyrosine-positive albinism

racial and ethnic differences in relation to diseases and defects as they are discussed throughout the book.

Common food items and drugs may cause health problems in certain ethnic groups. For example, people of Mediterranean, African, and Asian origin frequently have glucose-6-phosphate dehydrogenase (G6PD) deficiency. They may develop acute hemolytic anemia after they ingest fava (horse or broad) beans or certain drugs such as aspirin preparations, sulfonamides, or primaquine. Other groups, especially southern Europeans, Jews, Arabs, African-Americans, Asians, and Native Americans, have a deficiency of lactase, the enzyme needed to metabolize lactose. Ingestion of lactose can cause abdominal distention, flatus, and diarrhea. Unknowing but well-meaning health care workers may be responsible for these symptoms in their patients when they prescribe foods or food supplements containing lactose as sources of nutrients.

PHYSICAL CHARACTERISTICS

Members of different racial groups have observable differences in physical appearance. The most obvious are skin and hair coloring and texture. Skin color is determined by the amount of melanin in the skin. People from countries located near the equator have darkly pigmented skin, which protects the skin from the year-round exposure to the sun's rays; those from northern countries have light skin, which provides for maximum exposure to the sun's rays (necessary for vitamin D metabolism) during the short daylight hours. Skin color can show wide variations between these two extremes because of geographic origin or intermixing of persons with dark and light skin color.

As a consequence of the dark pigmentation, the detection of skin color changes can be difficult and requires modification of assessment techniques. For example, vasomotor alterations, cyanosis, and jaundice are not easily recognized in very dark skin. Variations in skin color can alter the appearance of the skin in a given circumstance (see Table 6-8).

In the newborn, variations are often related to racial or ethnic origin. For example, newborn infants of Asian and African-American parents are smaller than infants of Caucasian parents, and bluish pigmented areas (mongolian spots) on the sacral region are a common observation in Asian, African-American, Native American, and Mexican infants. It is important that health care providers be familiar with these birthmarks. They should be documented at newborn examinations and subsequent visits so they are not suddenly interpreted as bruises (Garwick and Auger, 2000).

Evaluation of stature and body build reveals some racial tendencies. Children from Asian countries are commonly smaller, falling below the 10th percentile on weight and height charts used for children in the United States. This difference in stature can lead to misinterpretation of health status and capabilities. A small child may appear intelligent for body size but be of average mental ability for age.

RELIGIOUS INFLUENCES

Probably the most influential factor shaping the U.S. culture is the Judeo-Christian faith. Many immigrants came to the United States for religious freedom and established a religious and moral atmosphere that persists today. However, individual differences are part of the general culture.

The family's religious orientation dictates a code of morality and influences the family's attitudes toward education, male and female role identity, and their ultimate destiny. It may also determine the school that the children attend, their companions, and often their mate selection. Religious beliefs are such an integral part of many cultures that it is difficult to distinguish the culture from the religion. In a few instances, such as in the Mennonite and Amish communities, religion is the basis for a common way of life that determines where the children are raised and their lifestyle.

RELIGIOUS BELIEFS

Religious and spiritual dimensions are among the most important influences in many people's lives (Fig. 2-5). The terms *religion* and *spirituality* are often used interchangeably; however, spirituality includes religion. Both religion and spirituality lend meaning in life and provide a source of love and relatedness between individuals and their God (Lukoff, Lu, and Turner, 1995). Nurses promote holistic nursing care through an integration of spiritual and psychosocial care. The care focuses on activities that support a person's system of beliefs and worship, such as praying, reading religious materials, and performing religious rituals. Meeting the spiritual needs of the child and family can provide strength, whereas unmet spiritual needs can result in spiritual distress and debilitation (Fulton and Moore, 1995). In practice, application of the nursing process for spiritual care (Box 2-5) can enhance the spiritual well-being of the child and family.

Religion influences the lifestyles of most cultures. Among many groups, illness, injury, or death is believed to be sent by God as a punishment for sin. Some may believe that health workers will be unable to help a person whom God is punishing and may express a fatalistic attitude toward treatment, stating that the illness is "the will of God." Others view it as a test of

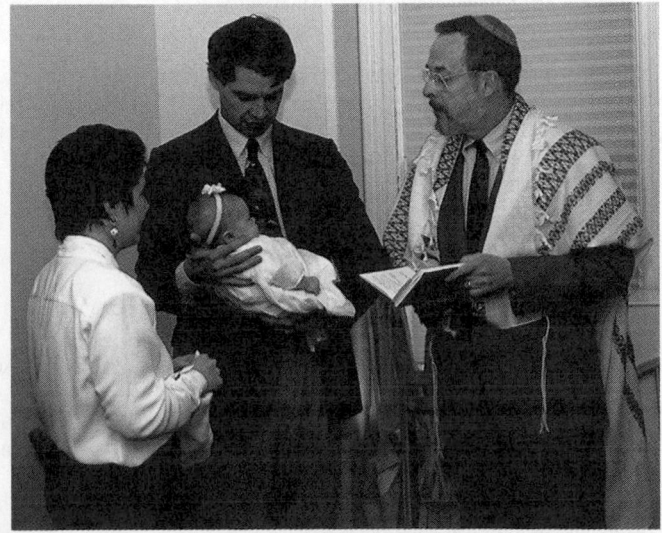

Fig. 2-5 Soon after an infant is born, many families have special religious ceremonies.

<table>
<tr><td>

BOX 2-5   **GUIDELINES FOR INTEGRATING SPIRITUAL CARE INTO PEDIATRIC NURSING PRACTICE**

- Demonstrate respect for the child and family's religious beliefs and practices.
- Support visitation and contact with family members, members of the patient's spiritual community, and spiritual leaders.
- Refer patients and families who have symptoms of spiritual distress or ask for religious or spiritual rituals to the institution's chaplaincy department.
- Use developmentally appropriate language when talking with children about spiritual concerns.
- Develop self-awareness of your own spiritual perspective.
- Familiarize yourself with the religious worldviews of cultural group in the population of patients you care for.
- Allow children and families to teach you about the specifics of their religious beliefs.
- Listen for understanding rather than agreement or disagreement.

</td></tr>
</table>

Data from Brooks B: Spirituality. In Kline N, editor: *Essentials of pediatric oncology nursing: a core curriculum,* ed 2, Glenview, Ill, 2004, Association of Pediatric Oncology Nurses; Barnes LL, Plotnikoff GA, Fox K, et al: Spirituality, religion, and pediatrics: intersecting worlds of healing, *Pediatrics* 106(4 Suppl):899-908, 2000.

child's health or therapy, the family's wishes are respected. The nurse should ask family members whether they want a clergy member present and whether they prefer hospital staff to call or prefer to do this on their own.

> **NURSING TIP** Children will rarely voice a need for spiritual support. Listen closely for indirect references.

It is important to determine the family's wishes regarding baptism, rites or practices related to death, and other religious rituals (such as circumcision, communion, or use of amulets or icons). Many religions have special clothing requirements, such as a cap (kippah) for the head (Orthodox Jews) or underclothes (Mormons). Respecting these rituals is especially important during a physical examination or preparation for surgery. An important role of the nurse is to be aware of families' spiritual needs and convey an attitude of concern for this important element of the child's care. Religion, which offers families understanding and spiritual support, is a valuable asset to health care. Table 2-2 outlines characteristics of selected religions with beliefs that affect health care.

strength, like the testing of Job in the Bible, and strive to remain faithful and overcome the conflicts.

The nurse clarifies dietary restrictions with the family, especially in denominations with many variations. Except when specific religious practices (such as fasting) interfere with the

In some instances the rights of the family and the responsibility of the state may be in conflict. For example, Jehovah's Witnesses refuse blood transfusions for themselves and for their children. Parents, by law, have the primary obligation to care for and make decisions about their minor children. However, the legal principle of *parens patriae* says that the state has an

TABLE 2-2   RELIGIOUS BELIEFS THAT MAY AFFECT NURSING CARE

BIRTH AND DEATH	DIET AND FOOD PRACTICES	MEDICAL CARE
Buddhist		
Birth—No baptism	Restrictions on some food combinations; extremes must be avoided.	Illness is believed to be a trial to aid development of soul; illness results from Karmic causes.
Infant presentation		
Death—Last rite chanting is often practiced at bedside soon after death; the deceased's family or Buddhist priest should be contacted.	Some sects are strictly vegetarian.	Surgery is permitted, but extremes must be avoided. Cleanliness is of great importance.
Organ donation/transplantation—Organ donation is a matter of individual conscience.	Discourage use of alcohol and drugs.	Family, community, and Buddhist priest are supportive visitors.
Church of Christ, Scientist (Christian Science)		
Birth—No baptism	Abstain from alcohol and some forms of tea and coffee.	Oppose human intervention with drugs or other therapies; however, accept legally required immunizations.
Death—No last rites; autopsy is not permitted except in cases of sudden death; individuals can choose burial or cremation.		Accept physical and moral healing.
Organ donation/transplantation—Church takes no specific position on transplantation as distinct from other medical or surgical procedures. Individuals decide on organ donation.		Family, friends, and members of spiritual community may visit.
Church of Jesus Christ of Latter Day Saints (Mormon)		
Birth—No baptism	Prohibit tea (except herbal), coffee, and alcohol.	Devout adherents believe in divine healing. Medical therapy is not prohibited.
Infant is blessed by church official at first opportunity after birth (in church).	Some individuals avoid chocolate and other products that contain caffeine.	Spiritual items—A "garment" (type of underwear) that is considered sacred; person may not want to remove it.
Baptism by immersion at 8 years.	Fasting for 24 hours each month.	Family, friends, and church members are supportive visitors.
Death—Believe that it is proper to bury the dead in the ground; cremation is discouraged.		
Organ donation/transplantation—Individuals can choose whether to will organs to be used in transplants.		

TABLE 2-2	RELIGIOUS BELIEFS THAT MAY AFFECT NURSING CARE—cont'd	
BIRTH AND DEATH	**DIET AND FOOD PRACTICES**	**MEDICAL CARE**
Hindu **Birth**—No baptism **Death**—Certain prescribed rites are followed after death; priest may tie thread around neck or wrist to signify blessing; family will wash the body; are particular about who touches their dead; bodies are to be cremated. **Organ donation/transplantation**—No religious laws prohibiting donation; individual decision.	Many dietary restrictions. Eating meat is forbidden.	With an amputation, loss of a limb is believed to represent sins committed in previous life. Accept most modern medical practices; some belief in faith healing. Spiritual item—Person may wear a thread around wrist or body; do not remove it. Family, community members, and priest are supportive visitors.
Islam (Muslim/Moslem) **Birth**—At birth, the first words said to the infant in his or her right ear are *Allah-o-Akbar* (Allah is great), and the remainder of the Call for Prayer is recited. An *Aqeeqa* (party) to celebrate the birth of the child is arranged by the parents. Male children are circumcised. **Death**—At the time of death, specific rituals (e.g., bathing, wrapping the body in cloth) must be done by same-sex Muslim. Before moving and handling the body, it is preferable to contact someone from the person's mosque or the local Islamic Society to perform these rituals. **Organ donation/transplantation**—Individual decides on organ donation/transplantation.	Prohibit all pork products and alcohol. Fasting is practiced during the ninth month of the Islamic year (Ramadan).	Believers are encouraged in the Qu'ran to seek treatment. It is taught that only Allah cures; however, Muslims are taught not to refuse treatment in the belief that Allah will take care of them because he also chooses at times to work through the efforts of humans. Other practices—Right hand is used for eating; left hand is for hygiene. Family and friends are supportive visitors.
Jehovah's Witnesses **Birth**—No baptism **Death**—No official last rites are practiced when death occurs. **Organ donation/transplantation**—Organ donation is forbidden.	No tobacco; moderate alcohol permissible.	Blood or blood products are not allowed; volume expanders are permissible if not derived from blood.
Judaism (Orthodox and Conservative) **Birth**—No baptism Ritual circumcision of male infants on eighth day; performed by mohel (ritual circumciser familiar with Jewish law and aseptic technique). **Death**—According to tradition, during last moments of life, relatives and close friends remain with the deceased. Amputated limbs or surgically removed tissues should be made available to family for burial. Cremation not allowed. **Organ donation/transplantation**—Organ transplantation/donation is complex issue; sometimes they are practiced.	Numerous dietary kosher laws exist; followers are allowed only meat from animals that are vegetable eaters and are ritually slaughtered; predatory fowl, shellfish, and pork are prohibited. Milk products served first can be followed by meat in a few minutes, but milk may not be consumed for several hours after eating meat. Fasting is part of Yom Kippur observance. Matzo replaces leavened bread during Passover week.	May resist surgical procedures during Sabbath, which extends from sundown Friday until sundown Saturday. Illness is grounds for violating dietary laws. Spiritual items—Men may wear prayer shawl, yarmulka (cap) while praying. Family, friends, and rabbi are supportive visitors.
Roman Catholic **Birth**—Infant baptism; especially urgent if poor prognosis, when it may be performed by anyone **Death**—Sacrament of the Sick is performed if prognosis is poor while patient is alive. **Organ donation/transplantation**—Transplantation of organs is viewed by Catholics as ethically and morally acceptable to Vatican; organ donation is viewed as an act of charity.	Abstaining from meat is practiced on Ash Wednesday, Good Friday, and Fridays during Lent (as a rule).	Encourage anointing of the sick Spiritual items—Rosary beads, crucifix Traditional church teaching does not approve of contraceptives or abortion.

Data from Galanti G: *Caring for patients from different cultures*, ed 3, Philadelphia, 2004, University of Pennsylvania Press; Lipson JG, Dibble SL, Minarik PA: *Culture and clinical care: a pocket guide*, San Francisco, 2005, UCSF Nursing Press; Purnell LD, Paulanka BJ: *Transcultural health care: a culturally competent approach*, Philadelphia, 2003, Davis; Spector RE: *Cultural diversity in health and illness*, ed 6, Upper Saddle River, NJ, 2004, Pearson Prentice Hall.

overriding interest in the health and welfare of its citizens. Parents' refusal of medical treatment for their child that is deemed essential can be interpreted as neglect. In addition to advocating for the child and family, the nurse's role may include assuming the role of consultant to the staff and family regarding new, alternative methods of transfusion and, if necessary, coordinating with officials to petition juvenile or family court for temporary guardianship of the child.

KEY POINTS

- Culture is the pattern of assumptions, beliefs, and practices, encompassing other products of human work and thoughts specific to members of an intergenerational group, community, or population.
- Nurses have a responsibility to understand the influence of culture, race, and ethnicity on the development of social and emotional relationships, childrearing practices, and attitudes toward health.
- A child's self-concept evolves from ideas about his or her social roles.
- Primary groups are characterized by intimate contact, mutual support, and behavior constraint among members.
- Secondary groups have limited, intermittent contact; little mutual support; and no pressure for conformity.
- Culture influences a child's self-esteem.
- Important subcultural influences on children include ethnicity, social class, occupation, schools, peers, biculture, and mass media.
- A trend that has significantly influenced the American family is increasing geographic and economic mobility.
- The minority group population is increasing in the United States, whereas the percentage of the Caucasian population is decreasing.
- Socioeconomic influences play a major role in opportunities for health promotion and wellness.

- Religious practices greatly influence health promotion beliefs in families.
- A child's physical characteristics and susceptibility to health problems are related to ethnic and cultural variations of hereditary and socioeconomic forces.
- Groups of children suffering from greater physical and mental health problems are those living in poverty, those who are homeless, or those who have migrant families.
- Drug response, food sensitivity, disease resistance, physical characteristics, and disease states may demonstrate ethnic or cultural variations.
- Because verbal and nonverbal communication is an important cultural consideration, nurses need to acknowledge and respect their patient's practices for productive interaction to occur.
- Cultural beliefs related to cause of illness and maintenance of health may focus on natural forces, supernatural forces, or imbalance of forces.
- The development of cultural competence is continual and an important concept in the nursing process. Nurses can facilitate this process by recognizing cultural differences, integrating cultural knowledge, and acting in a culturally appropriate manner.
- No cultural group is homogeneous; every racial and ethnic group contains great diversity.

ANSWERS TO CRITICAL THINKING EXERCISE

Reducing Cultural Shock

1. An understanding of the Arab culture provides insight into the woman's hesitancy to make decisions in her husband's absence.
2. a. Typically in the Arab culture men make the decisions and women are expected to support these decisions.
   b. The need for an interpreter is evident to make certain the mother understands the seriousness of the situation.
   c. Knowledge of the process for obtaining approval for emergency procedures without informed consent will facilitate the best care for the child.

d. Appropriate documentation of how approval was obtained without parental consent is essential.
3. The first priority is to make certain the child is receiving the best care possible and that the necessary procedure is performed as soon as possible. The next priority is to ensure the mother understands the urgency of the situation by using an interpreter.
4. The child's health status is most important at this time.

REFERENCES

American Academy of Pediatrics, Committee on Public Education: Children, adolescents, and television, *Pediatrics* 107(2):423-426, 2001.

American Nurses Association: *Position statement: cultural diversity in nursing practice*, 1991, available at www.nursingworld.org/EthicsHumanRights (accessed December 2, 2009).

Anderson DR, Huston AC, Schmitt KL, et al: Early childhood television viewing and adolescent behavior: the recontact study, *Monogr Soc Res Child Dev* 66(1):I-VIII, 1-147, 2001.

Annie E Casey Foundation: *2009 Kids count data book: state profiles of child well-being*, Baltimore, 2009, The Foundation.

Betancourt J: Commentary on "Current approaches to integrating elements of cultural competence in nursing education," *J Transcult Nurs* 18(25s):25s-27s, 2007.

Carrillo JE, Green AR, Betancourt JR: Cross-cultural primary care: a patient-based approach, *Ann Intern Med* 130(10):829-834, 1999.

Council on Communications and Media: Media violence—policy statement, *Pediatrics* 124(5):1495-1503, 2009.

Crom DB: The experience of South American mothers who have a child being treated for malignancy in the United States, *J Pediatr Oncol Nurs* 12(3):104-112, 1995.

Dunn AM: Culture competence and the primary care provider, *J Pediatr Health Care* 16(3):105-111, 2002.

Dykeman C, Nelson JR, Appleton V: Building strong working alliances with American Indian families, *Soc Work Educ* 17(3):148-157, 1995.

Fulton RA, Moore CM: Spiritual care of the school-age child with a chronic condition, *J Pediatr Nurs* 10(4):224-231, 1995.

Garwick A, Auger S: What do providers need to know about American Indian culture? Recommendations from urban Indian family caregivers, *Fam Systems Health* 18:177-189, 2000.

Gentry K, Quandt SA, Davis SW, et al: Child healthcare in two farmworker populations, *J Commun Health* 32(6):419-431, 2007.

Giger JN, Davidhizar RE: *Transcultural nursing: assessment and intervention*, ed 3, St Louis, 1999, Mosby.

Hayes J, Dreher C: Providing culturally sensitive care. In Smith D, editor: *Comprehensive child and family nursing skills*, St Louis, 1991, Mosby.

Hindman HD: Unfinished business: the persistence of child labor in the US, *Employee Responsibilities Rights J* 18(2):125-131, 2006.

Jordan A: The role of media in children's development: an ecological perspective, *J Dev Behav Pediatr* 25(3):196-206, 2004.

Klass P, Needlman R, Zuckerman B: Reach out and get your patients to read, *Contemp Pediatr* 19(1):51-58, 2002.

Kleinman A, Benson P: Anthropology in the clinic: the problem of cultural competency and how to fix it, *PLoS Medicine* 3(10):1673-1676, 2006.

Kleinman A, Eisenberg L, Good B: Culture, illness, and care: clinical lessons from anthropologic and cross-cultural research, *Ann Intern Med* 88:251-258, 1978.

Leavitt M, Martinson ID, Liu C, et al: Common themes and ethnic differences in family caregiving the first year after diagnosis of childhood cancer, part II, *J Pediatr Nurs* 14(2):110-122, 1999.

Leininger MM: The theory of culture care diversity and universality. In Leininger MM, editor: *Culture care diversity and universality: a theory of nursing*, Sudbury, Mass, 2001, Jones & Bartlett.

Lester N: Cultural competence: a nursing dialogue 2, *Am J Nurs* 98(9):36-42, quiz 43, 1998.

Looman WS: Defining social capital for nursing: experiences of family caregivers of children with chronic conditions, *J Fam Nurs* 10:412-428, 2004.

Looman WS, Lindeke LL: Health and social context: social capital's utility as a construct for nursing and health promotion, *J Pediatr Health Care* 19(2):90-94, 2005.

Lukoff D, Lu FG, Turner R: Cultural considerations in the assessment and treatment of religious and spiritual problems, *Psychiatr Clin North Am* 18(3):467-485, 1995.

Martinson IM, Armstrong V, Qiao J: The experience of the family of children with chronic illness at home in China, *Pediatr Nurs* 23(4):371-375, 1997.

Mattson S: Culturally sensitive perinatal care for Southeast Asians, *J Obstet Gynecol Neonat Nurs* 24(4):335-341, 1995.

Melendez L: Parental beliefs and practices around early self-regulation: the impact of culture and immigration, *Infants Young Child* 18(2):136-146, 2005.

Munoz CC, Luckmann J: *Transcultural communication in nursing*, Clifton Park, NY, 2005, Thomson Delmar Learning.

Murdock SH: Minority child population growth. In Cosby AG, Greenberg RE, Southward LH, et al, editors: *About children: an authoritative resource on the state of childhood today*, Elk Grove Village, Ill, 2005, American Academy of Pediatrics.

Nance TA: Intercultural communication: finding common ground, *J Obstet Gynecol Neonat Nurs* 24(3):249-255, 1995.

National Coalition to End Homelessness: Youth, 2009, available at www.endhomelessness.org/section/policy/focusareas/youth (accessed March 28, 2009).

Ohio State University Extension: Cultural diversity: eating in America, 2005, available at www.nal.usda.gov/fnic/etext/000010.html (accessed April 20, 2005).

Redlener I: Homelessness and its consequences. In Cosby AG, Greenberg RE, Southward LH, et al, editors: *About children: an authoritative resource on the state of childhood today*, Elk Grove Village, Ill, 2005, American Academy of Pediatrics.

Robinson-Zanartu C: Serving Native American children and families: considering cultural variables, *Lang Speech Hearing Serv Schools* 27:373-384, 1996.

Rogers G: Educating case managers for culturally competent practice, *J Case Manage* 4(2):60-65, 1995.

Scribner R: Paradox as paradigm: the health outcomes of Mexican Americans, *Am J Pub Health* 86(3):303-304, 1996.

Search Institute: *Developmental assets lists*, 2007, available at www.search-institute.org/developmental-assets/lists (accessed December 2, 2009).

Sekhon SK: Insights into South Asian culture: food and nutritional values, *Topics Clin Nutr* 11(4):47-56, 1996.

Shaw-Taylor Y: Culturally and linguistically appropriate health care for racial or ethnic minorities: analysis of the US Office of Minority Health's recommended standards, *Health Policy* 62:211-221, 2002.

Spector RE: *Cultural diversity in health and illness*, ed 7, Upper Saddle River, NJ, 2009, Prentice-Hall.

Strasburger VC, Donnerstein E: Children, adolescents, and the media: issues and solutions, *Pediatrics* 103(1):129-139, 1999.

Strehlow AJ, Amos-Jones T: The homeless as a vulnerable population, *Nurs Clin North Am* 34(2):261-274, 1999.

Szilagyi PG: Health insurance. In Cosby AG, Greenberg RE, Southward LH, et al, editors: *About children: an authoritative resource on the state of childhood today*, Elk Grove Village, Ill, 2005, American Academy of Pediatrics.

Trawick-Smith J: *Early childhood development: a multicultural perspective*, ed 4, Upper Saddle River, NJ, 2006, Prentice-Hall.

Thibodeaux AG, Deatrick JA: Cultural influence on family management of children with cancer, *J Pediatr Oncol Nurs* 24(4):227-233, 2007.

US Census Bureau: Overview of race and Hispanic origin: census 2000 brief, 2001, available at www.census.gov/prod/2001pubs/c2kbr01-1.pdf (accessed December 2, 2009).

Wang R, Martinson IM: Behavioral responses of healthy Chinese siblings to the stress of childhood cancer in the family, *J Pediatr Nurs* 11(6):383-391, 1996.

Warda MR: Mexican Americans' perceptions of culturally competent care, *West J Nurs Res* 22(2):203-224, 2000.

Wertheimer R: Poverty. In Cosby AG, Greenberg RE, Southward LH, et al, editors: *About children: an authoritative resource on the state of childhood today*, Elk Grove Village, Ill, 2005, American Academy of Pediatrics.

Williams LA, Kruse L: A culture fair: a creative, fun, and informative method of cultural awareness education, *J Staff Dev* 15(2):71-74, 1999.

Yoos HL, Kitzman H, Henderson C, et al: The impact of parental illness representation on disease management in childhood asthma, *Nurs Res* 56(3):167-174, 2007.

CHAPTER

3

Family Influences on Child Health Promotion

Marilyn J. Hockenberry

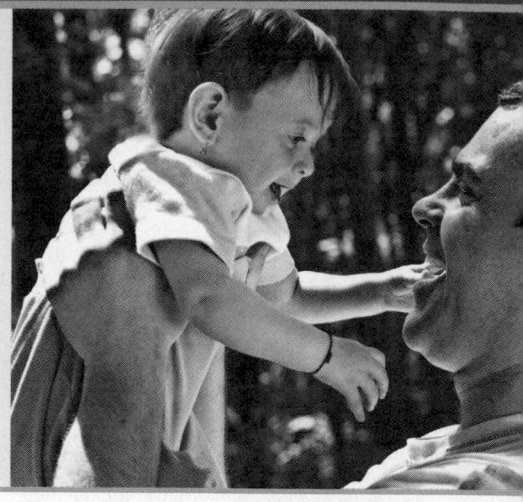

evolve WEBSITE

http://evolve.elsevier.com/Wong/NCIC
Case Study
   Family Functioning
Key Points Audio Summaries
NCLEX Review Questions
Spanish/English Translations
WebLinks

RELATED TOPICS

CHAPTER OUTLINE

GENERAL CONCEPTS

DEFINITION OF FAMILY

The term family has been defined in many different ways according to the individual's own frame of reference, values, or discipline. There is no universal definition of family; a family is what an individual considers it to be. Biology describes the family as fulfilling the biologic function of perpetuation of the species. Psychology emphasizes the interpersonal aspects of the family and its responsibility for personality development. Economics views the family as a productive unit providing for material needs. Sociology depicts the family as a social unit interacting with the larger society, creating the context within which cultural values and identity are formed. Others define family in terms of the relationships of the persons who make up the family unit. The most common type of relationships are consanguineous (blood relationships), affinal (marital relationships), and family of origin (family unit a person is born into).

Earlier definitions of family emphasized that family members were related by legal ties or genetic relationships and lived in the same household with specific roles. Later definitions have been broadened to reflect both structural and functional changes. A family can be defined as an institution where individuals, related through biology or enduring commitments, and representing similar or different generations and genders, participate in roles involving mutual socialization, nurturance, and emotional commitment (Hanson, Gedaly-Duff, and Kaakinen, 2005).

Considerable controversy has surrounded the newer concepts of family, such as communal families, single-parent families, and homosexual families. To accommodate these and other varieties of family styles, the descriptive term household is frequently used.

⚠ NURSING ALERT

The nurse's knowledge and the sensitivity with which he or she assesses a household will determine the types of interventions that are appropriate to support family members.

Nursing care of infants and children is intimately involved with care of the child *and* the family. Family structure and dynamics can have an enduring influence on a child, affecting the child's health and well-being (American Academy of Pediatrics, 2003). Consequently, nurses must be aware of the functions of the family, various types of family structures, and theories that provide a foundation for understanding the changes within a family and for directing family-oriented interventions.

FAMILY THEORIES

A family theory can be used to describe families and how the family unit responds to events both within and outside the family. Each family theory makes assumptions about the family and has inherent strengths and limitations (Hanson, Gedaly-Duff, and Kaakinen, 2005). Most nurses use a combination of theories in their work with children and families. Commonly used theories are family systems theory, family stress theory, and developmental theory (Table 3-1).

Family Systems Theory

Family systems theory is derived from general systems theory, a science of "wholeness" that is characterized by interaction among the components of the system and between the system and the environment (Bomar, 2004). General systems theory expanded scientific thought from a simplistic view of direct cause and effect (A causes B) to a more complex and interrelated theory (A influences B, but B also affects A). In family systems theory, the family is viewed as a system that continually interacts with its members and the environment. The emphasis is on the interaction between the members; a change in one family member creates a change in other members, which

in turn results in a new change in the original member. Consequently, a problem or dysfunction does not lie in any one member but rather in the type of interactions used by the family. Because the interactions, not the individual members, are viewed as the source of the problem, the family becomes the patient and the focus of care. Examples of the application of family systems theory to clinical problems are nonorganic failure to thrive and child abuse. According to family systems theory, the problem does not rest solely with the parent or child but with the type of interactions between the parent and the child and the factors that affect their relationship.

The family is viewed as a whole that is different from the sum of the individual members. For example, a household of parents and one child consists of not only three individuals, but also four interactive units. These units include three dyads (the marital relationship, the mother-child relationship, and the father-child relationship) and a triangle (the mother-father-child relationship). In this ecologic model, the family system functions within a larger system, with the family dyads in the center of a circle surrounded by the extended family, the subculture, and the culture, with the larger society at the periphery.

Bowen's family systems theory (Hanson, Gedaly-Duff, and Kaakinen, 2005) emphasizes that the key to healthy family function is the members' ability to distinguish themselves from each other both emotionally and intellectually. The family unit has a high level of adaptability. When problems arise within the family, change occurs by altering the interaction or feedback messages that perpetuate disruptive behavior. Feedback refers to processes in the family that help identify strengths and needs and determine how well goals are accomplished. Positive feedback initiates change; negative feedback resists change (Goldenberg and Goldenberg, 2008). When the family system is disrupted, change can occur at any point in the system.

A major factor that influences a family's adaptability is its boundary, an imaginary line that exists between the family and its environment (Hanson, Gedaly-Duff, and Kaakinen, 2005). Families have varying degrees of openness and closure in these boundaries. For example, one family has the capacity to reach out for help, whereas another considers help threatening. Knowledge of boundaries is critical when teaching or counseling families. Families with open boundaries may demonstrate a greater receptivity to interventions, whereas families demonstrating closed boundaries often require increased sensitivity and skill on the part of the nurse to gain their trust and acceptance. The nurse who uses family systems theory should assess the family's ability to accept new ideas, information, resources, and opportunities and to plan strategies.

Family Stress Theory

Family stress theory explains how families react to stressful events and suggests factors that promote adaptation to stress (Hanson, Gedaly-Duff, and Kaakinen, 2005). Families encounter stressors (events that cause stress and have the potential to effect a change in the family social system), including those that are predictable (e.g., parenthood) and those that are unpredictable (e.g., illness, unemployment). These stressors are cumulative, involving simultaneous demands from work, family, and community life. Too many stressful events occurring within a

TABLE 3-1	SUMMARY OF FAMILY THEORIES AND APPLICATIONS		
ASSUMPTIONS	**STRENGTHS**	**LIMITATIONS**	**APPLICATIONS**
Family Systems Theory			
A change in any one part of a family system affects all other parts of the family system (circular causality). Family systems are characterized by periods of rapid growth and change and periods of relative stability. Both too little change and too much change are dysfunctional for the family system; therefore a balance between morphogenesis (change) and morphostasis (no change) is necessary. Family systems can initiate change, as well as react to it.	Applicable for family in normal everyday life, as well as for family dysfunction and pathology Useful for families of varying structure and various stages of life cycle	More difficult to determine cause-and-effect relationships because of circular causality	Mate selection, courtship processes, family communication, boundary maintenance, power and control within family, parent-child relationships, adolescent pregnancy and parenthood
Family Stress Theory			
Stress is an inevitable part of family life, and any event, even if positive, can be stressful for family. Family encounters both normative expected stressors and unexpected situational stressors over life cycle. Stress has a cumulative effect on family. Families cope with and respond to stressors with a wide range of responses and effectiveness.	Potential to explain and predict family behavior in response to stressors and to develop effective interventions to promote family adaptation Focuses on positive contribution of resources, coping, and social support to adaptive outcomes Can be used by many disciplines in health field	Relationships between all variables in framework not yet adequately described Not yet known if certain combinations of resources and coping strategies are applicable to all stressful events	Transition to parenthood and other normative transitions, single-parent families, families experiencing work-related stressors (dual-earner family, unemployment), acute or chronic childhood illness or disability, infertility, death of a child, divorce, teenage pregnancy and parenthood
Developmental Theory			
Families develop and change over time in similar and consistent ways. Family and its members must perform certain time-specific tasks set by themselves and by persons in the broader society. Family role performance at one stage of family life cycle influences family's behavioral options at next stage. Family tends to be in stage of disequilibrium when entering a new life-cycle stage and strives toward homeostasis within stages.	Provides a dynamic, rather than static, view of family Addresses both changes within family and changes in family as a social system over its life history Anticipates potential stressors that normally accompany transitions to various stages and when problems may peak because of lack of resources	Traditional model more easily applied to two-parent families with children Use of age of oldest child and marital duration as marker of stage transition sometimes problematic (e.g., in stepfamilies, single-parent families)	Anticipatory guidance, educational strategies, and developing or strengthening family resources for management of transition to parenthood; family adjustment to children entering school, becoming adolescents, leaving home; management of "empty nest" years and retirement

relatively short period (usually 1 year) can overwhelm the family's ability to cope and place it at risk for breakdown or physical and emotional health problems among its members. When the family experiences too many stressors for it to cope adequately, a state of crisis ensues. For adaptation to occur, a change in family structure or interaction is necessary.

The **resiliency model of family stress, adjustment, and adaptation** emphasizes that the stressful situation is not necessarily pathologic or detrimental to the family but demonstrates that the family needs to make fundamental structural or systemic changes to adapt to the situation (McCubbin and McCubbin, 1994).

Developmental Theory

Developmental theory is an outgrowth of several theories of development. Duvall (1977) described eight developmental tasks of the family throughout its life span (Box 3-1). The family is described as a small group, a semiclosed system of personalities that interacts with the larger cultural social system. As an interrelated system, the family does not have changes in one part without a series of changes in other parts.

Developmental theory addresses family change over time using Duvall's family life cycle stages, based on the predictable changes in the family's structure, function, and roles, with the age of the oldest child as the marker for stage transition. The arrival of the first child marks the transition from stage I to stage II. As the first child grows and develops, the family enters subsequent stages. In every stage the family faces certain developmental tasks. At the same time, each family member must achieve individual developmental tasks as part of each family life cycle stage.

Developmental theory can be applied to nursing practice. For example, the nurse can assess how well new parents are accomplishing the individual and family developmental tasks associated with transition to parenthood. New applications should emerge as more is learned about developmental stages for nonnuclear and nontraditional families.

FAMILY NURSING INTERVENTIONS

In working with children, the nurse must include family members in their care plan. Research confirms parents' desire

---

BOX 3-1   DUVALL'S DEVELOPMENTAL STAGES OF THE FAMILY

Stage I—Marriage and an Independent Home: The Joining of Families
Reestablish couple identity.
Realign relationships with extended family.
Make decisions regarding parenthood.

Stage II—Families with Infants
Integrate infants into the family unit.
Accommodate to new parenting and grandparenting roles.
Maintain marital bond.

Stage III—Families with Preschoolers
Socialize children.
Parents and children adjust to separation.

Stage IV—Families with Schoolchildren
Children develop peer relations.
Parents adjust to their children's peer and school influences.

Stage V—Families with Teenagers
Adolescents develop increasing autonomy.
Parents refocus on midlife marital and career issues.
Parents begin a shift toward concern for the older generation.

Stage VI—Families as Launching Centers
Parents and young adults establish independent identities.
Parents renegotiate marital relationship.

Stage VII—Middle-Aged Families
Reinvest in couple identity with concurrent development of independent interests.
Realign relationships to include in-laws and grandchildren.
Deal with disabilities and death of older generation.

Stage VIII—Aging Families
Shift from work role to leisure and semiretirement or full retirement.
Maintain couple and individual functioning while adapting to the aging process.
Prepare for own death and dealing with the loss of spouse and/or siblings and other peers.

Modified from Wright LM, Leahey M: *Nurses and families: a guide to family assessment and intervention,* Philadelphia, 1984, Davis.

BOX 3-2   FAMILY NURSING INTERVENTIONS

- Behavior modification
- Case management and coordination
- Collaborative strategies
- Contracting
- Counseling, including support, cognitive reappraisal, and reframing
- Empowering families through active participation
- Environmental modification
- Family advocacy
- Family crisis intervention
- Networking, including use of self-help groups and social support
- Providing information and technical expertise
- Role modeling
- Role supplementation
- Teaching strategies, including stress management, lifestyle modifications, and anticipatory guidance

From Friedman MM, Bowden VR, Jones EG: *Family nursing: research theory and practice,* ed 5, Upper Saddle River, NJ, 2003, Prentice Hall.

---

and expectation to participate in their child's care (Power and Franck, 2008). To discover family dynamics, strengths, and weaknesses, a thorough family assessment is necessary (see Chapter 6). The nurse's choice of interventions depends on the theoretic family model that is used (Box 3-2). For example, in family systems theory, the focus is on the interaction of family members within the larger environment (Goldenberg and Goldenberg, 2008). In this case, using group dynamics to involve all members in the intervention process and being a skillful communicator are essential. Systems theory also presents excellent opportunities for anticipatory guidance. Because each family member reacts to every stress experienced by that system, nurses can intervene to help the family prepare for and cope with changes. In family stress theory the nurse employs crisis intervention strategies to help family members cope with the challenging event. In developmental theory the nurse provides anticipatory guidance to prepare members for transition to the next family stage. Nurses who think family involvement plays a key role in the care of a child are more likely to include families in the child's daily care (Fisher, Lindhorst, Matthews, et al, 2008).

FAMILY STRUCTURE AND FUNCTION

FAMILY STRUCTURE

The **family structure**, or **family composition**, consists of individuals, each with a socially recognized status and position, who interact with one another on a regular, recurring basis in socially sanctioned ways (Hanson, Gedaly-Duff, and Kaakinen, 2005). When members are gained or lost through events such as marriage, divorce, birth, death, abandonment, or incarceration, the family composition is altered and roles must be redefined or redistributed.

Traditionally, the family structure was either a nuclear or extended family. In recent years, family composition has assumed new configurations, with the single-parent family and blended family becoming prominent forms. The predominant structural pattern in any society depends on the mobility of families as they pursue economic goals and as relationships change. It is not uncommon for children to belong to several different family groups during their lifetime.

Nurses must be able to meet the needs of children from many diverse family structures and home situations. A family's particular structure affects the direction of nursing care. The U.S. Census Bureau uses four definitions for families: the traditional nuclear family, the nuclear family, the blended family or household, and the extended family or household.

Traditional Nuclear Family

A **traditional nuclear family** consists of a married couple and their biologic children. Children in this type of family live with both biologic parents and, if siblings are present, only full brothers and sisters (i.e., siblings who share the same two biologic parents). No other persons are present in the household (i.e., no steprelatives, foster or adopted children, half-siblings, other relatives, or nonrelatives).

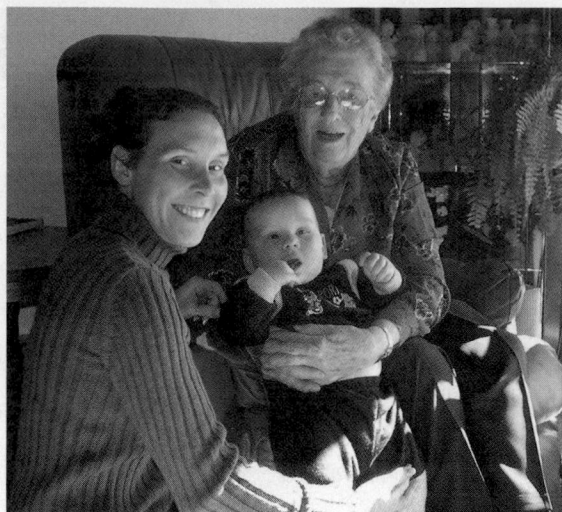

Fig. 3-1 Children benefit from interaction with grandparents, who sometimes assume the parenting role.

Nuclear Family

The nuclear family is composed of two parents and their children. The parent-child relationship may be biologic, step, adoptive, or foster. Sibling ties may be biologic, step, half, or adoptive. The parents are not necessarily married. No other relatives or nonrelatives are present in the household.

Blended Family

A blended family or household, also called a reconstituted family, includes at least one stepparent, stepsibling, or half-sibling. A stepparent is the spouse of a child's biologic parent but is not the child's biologic parent. Stepsiblings do not share a common biologic parent; the biologic parent of one child is the stepparent of the other. Half-siblings share only one biologic parent.

Extended Family

An extended family or household includes at least one parent, one or more children, and one or more members (related or unrelated) other than a parent or sibling. Parent-child and sibling relationships may be biologic, step, adoptive, or foster.

In many nations and among many ethnic and cultural groups, households with extended families are common. Within the extended family, grandparents often find themselves rearing their grandchildren (Fig. 3-1). Young parents are often considered too young or too inexperienced to make decisions independently. Often, the older relative holds the authority and makes decisions in consultation with the young parents. Sharing residence with relatives also assists with the management of scarce resources and provides child care for working families. A resource for extended families is the Grandparent Information Center.*

---

*For information, contact the local AARP representative or office; www.aarp.org/family/grandparenting.

Single-Parent Family

In the United States an estimated 21.7 million children live in single-parent families (Annie E Casey Foundation, 2009). The contemporary single-parent family has emerged partially as a consequence of the women's rights movement and also as a result of more women (and men) establishing separate households because of divorce, death, desertion, or single parenthood. In addition, a more liberal attitude in the courts has made it possible for single people, both male and female, to adopt children. Although mothers usually head single-parent families, it is becoming more common for fathers to be awarded custody of dependent children in divorce settlements. With women's increased psychologic and financial independence and the increased acceptability of single parents in society, more unmarried women are deliberately choosing mother-child families. Frequently, these mothers and children are absorbed into the extended family. The challenges of single-parent families are discussed on p. 63.

Binuclear Family

The term binuclear family refers to parents continuing the parenting role while terminating the spousal unit. The degree of cooperation between households and the time the child spends with each can vary. In joint custody the court assigns divorcing parents equal rights and responsibilities concerning the minor child or children. These alternate family forms are efforts to view divorce as a process of reorganization and redefinition of a family rather than as a family dissolution. Joint custody and coparenting are discussed further on p. 63.

Polygamous Family

Although it is not legally sanctioned in the United States, the conjugal unit is sometimes extended by the addition of spouses in polygamous matings. Polygamy refers to either multiple wives (polygyny) or, rarely, husbands (polyandry). Many societies practice polygyny that is further designated as sororal, in which the wives are sisters, or nonsororal, in which the wives are unrelated. Sororal polygyny is widespread throughout the world. Most often, mothers and their children share a husband and father, with each mother and her children living in the same or separate household.

Communal Family

The communal family emerged from disenchantment with most contemporary life choices. Although communal families may have divergent beliefs, practices, and organization, the basic impetus for formation is often dissatisfaction with the nuclear family structure, social systems, and goals of the larger community. Relatively uncommon today, communal groups share common ownership of property. In cooperatives, property ownership is private, but certain goods and services are shared and exchanged without monetary consideration. There is strong reliance on group members and material interdependence. Both provide collective security for nonproductive members, share homemaking and childrearing functions, and help overcome the problem of interpersonal isolation or loneliness.

Gay, Lesbian, Bisexual, and Transgender Families

A same-sex, homosexual, or gay/lesbian/bisexual/transgender (GLBT) family is one in which there is a legal or common-law tie between two persons of the same sex who have children (Blackwell, 2007). There are a growing number of families with same-sex parents in the United States, with an estimated one fourth of all same-sex couples raising children (Pawelski, Perrin, Foy, et al, 2006). Although some children in gay/lesbian households are biologic from a former marriage or relationship, children may be present in other circumstances. They may be foster or adoptive parents, lesbian mothers may conceive through artificial fertilization, or a gay male couple may become parents through use of a surrogate mother.

When children are brought up in GLBT families, the relationships seem as natural to them as heterosexual parents do to their offspring. In other cases, however, disclosure of parental homosexuality ("coming out") to children can be a concern for families. There are a number of factors to consider before disclosing this information to children. Parents should be comfortable with their own sexual preference and should discuss this with the children as they become old enough to understand relationships. Discussions should be planned and take place in a quiet setting where interruptions are unlikely.

Nurses need to be nonjudgmental and to learn to accept differences rather than demonstrate prejudice that can have a detrimental effect on the nurse-child-family relationship (Blackwell, 2007). Moreover, the more nurses know about the child's family and lifestyle, the more they can help the parents and the child.

FAMILY STRENGTHS AND FUNCTIONING STYLE

Family function refers to the interactions of family members, especially the quality of those relationships and interactions (Bomar, 2004). Researchers are interested in family characteristics that help families function effectively. Knowledge of these factors guides the nurse throughout the nursing process and helps the nurse to predict ways that families may cope and respond to a stressful event, to provide individualized support that builds on family strengths and unique functioning style, and to assist family members in obtaining resources.

Family strengths and unique functioning styles (Box 3-3) are significant resources that nurses can use to meet family needs. Building on qualities that make a family work well and strengthening family resources make the family unit even stronger. All families have strengths as well as vulnerabilities.

FAMILY ROLES AND RELATIONSHIPS

Each individual has a position, or status, in the family structure and plays culturally and socially defined roles in interactions within the family. Each family also has its own traditions and values and sets its own standards for interaction within and outside the group. Each determines the experiences the children should have, those they are to be shielded from, and how each of these experiences meets the needs of family members. When family ties are strong, social control is highly effective, and most

---

BOX 3-3   QUALITIES OF STRONG FAMILIES

- A belief and sense of **commitment** toward promoting the well-being and growth of individual family members, as well as the family unit
- **Appreciation** for the small and large things that individual family members do well and **encouragement** to do better
- Concentrated effort to spend **time** and do things together, no matter how formal or informal the activity or event
- A sense of **purpose** that permeates the reasons and basis for "going on" in both bad and good times
- A sense of **congruence** among family members regarding the value and importance of assigning time and energy to meet needs
- The ability to **communicate** with one another in a way that emphasizes positive interactions
- A clear set of **family rules, values,** and **beliefs** that establishes expectations about acceptable and desired behavior
- A varied repertoire of **coping strategies** that promote positive functioning in dealing with both normative and nonnormative life events
- The ability to engage in **problem-solving** activities designed to evaluate options for meeting needs and procuring resources
- The ability to be **positive** and see the positive in almost all aspects of their lives, including the ability to see crisis and problems as an opportunity to learn and grow
- **Flexibility** and **adaptability** in the roles necessary to procure resources to meet needs
- A **balance** between the use of internal and external family resources for coping and adapting to life events and planning for the future

From Dunst C, Trivette C, Deal A: *Enabling and empowering families: principles and guidelines for practice,* Cambridge, Mass, 1988, Brookline Books.

---

members conform to their roles willingly and with commitment. Conflicts arise when people do not fulfill their roles in ways that meet other family members' expectations, either because they are unaware of the expectations or because they choose not to meet them.

PARENTAL ROLES

In all family groups the socially recognized status of father and mother exists with socially sanctioned roles that prescribe appropriate sexual behavior and childrearing responsibilities. The guides for behavior in these roles serve to control sexual conflict in society and provide for prolonged care of children. The degree to which parents are committed and the way they play their roles are influenced by a number of variables and by the parents' unique socialization experience.

Parental role definitions have changed as a result of the changing economy and increased opportunities for women (Bomar, 2004). As the woman's role has changed, the complementary role of the man has also changed. Many fathers are more active in childrearing and household tasks. As the redefinition of sex roles continues in American families, role conflicts may arise in many families because of a cultural lag of the persisting traditional role definitions.

ROLE LEARNING

Roles are learned through the socialization process. During all stages of development children learn and practice, through interaction with others and in their play, a set of social roles and the characteristics of other roles. They behave in patterned and more or less predictable ways because they learn roles that define mutual expectations in typical social relationships. Although role definitions are changing, the basic determinants of parenting remain the same. Several determinants of parenting infants and young children are parental personality and mental well-being, systems of support, and child characteristics. These determinants have been used as consistent measurements to determine a person's success in fulfilling the parental role.

Parents, peers, authority figures, and other socializing agents who use positive and negative sanctions to ensure conformity to their norms transmit role conceptions. Role behaviors positively reinforced by rewards such as love, affection, friendship, and honors are strengthened. Negative reinforcement takes the form of ridicule, withdrawal of love, expressions of disapproval, or banishment.

In some cultures the role behavior expected of children conflicts with desirable adult behavior. One of the family's responsibilities is to develop culturally appropriate role behavior in children. Children learn to perform in expected ways consistent with their position in the family and culture. The observed behavior of each child is a single manifestation—a combination of social influences and individual psychologic processes. In this way the uniting of the child's intrapersonal system (the self) with the interpersonal system (the family) is simultaneously understood as the child's conduct.

Role structuring initially takes place within the family unit, in which the children fulfill a set of roles and respond to the roles of their parents and other family members (Hanson, Gedaly-Duff, and Kaakinen, 2005). Children's roles are shaped primarily by the parents, who apply direct or indirect pressures to induce or force children into the desired patterns of behavior or direct their efforts toward modification of the role responses of the child on a mutually acceptable basis. Parents have their own techniques and determine the course that the socialization process follows.

Children respond to life situations according to behaviors learned in reciprocal transactions. As they acquire important role-taking skills, their relationships with others change. For instance, when a teenager is also the mother but lives in a household with the grandmother, the teenager may be viewed more as an adolescent than as a mother. Children become proficient at understanding others as they acquire the ability to discriminate their own perspectives from those of others. Children who get along well with others and attain status in the peer group have well-developed role-taking skills.

Family Size and Configuration

Parenting practices differ between small and large families. Small families place more emphasis on the individual development of the children. Parenting is intensive rather than extensive, and there is constant pressure to measure up to family expectations. Children's development and achievement are measured against those of other children in the neighborhood and social class. In small families, children have more democratic participation than in larger families. Adolescents in small families identify more strongly with their parents and rely more on them for advice. They have well-developed, autonomous

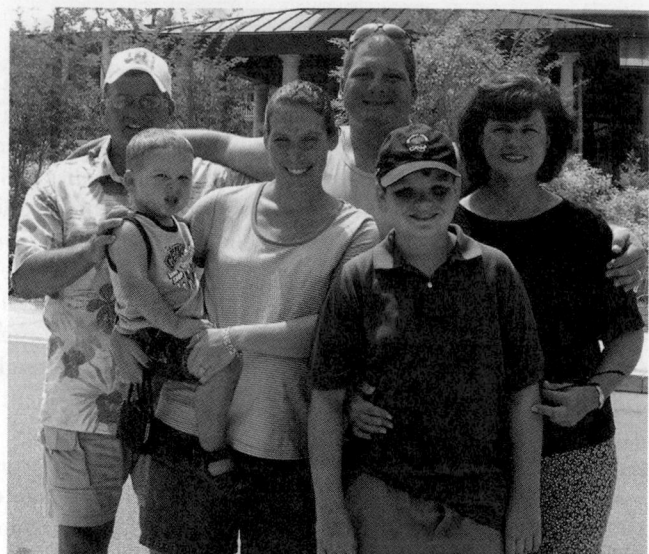

Fig. 3-2 Family structure and function promotes strong relationships among its members.

inner controls as contrasted with adolescents from larger families, who rely more on adult authority.

Children in a large family are able to adjust to a variety of changes and crises. There is more emphasis on the group and less on the individual (Fig. 3-2). Cooperation is essential, often because of economic necessity. The large number of people sharing a limited amount of space requires a greater degree of organization, administration, and authoritarian control. A dominant family member (a parent or older child) wields control. The number of children reduces the intimate, one-to-one contact between the parent and any individual child. Consequently, children turn to each other for what they cannot get from their parents. The reduced parent-child contact encourages individual children to adopt specialized roles to gain recognition in the family.

Older siblings in large families often administer discipline. Siblings are usually attuned to what constitutes misbehavior. Sibling disapproval or ostracism is frequently a more meaningful disciplinary measure than parental interventions. In situations such as death or illness of a parent, an older sibling often assumes responsibility for the family at considerable personal sacrifice. Large families generate a sense of security in the children that is fostered by sibling support and cooperation. However, adolescents from a large family are more peer oriented than family oriented.

Sibling Interactions
Spacing of Children

Age differences between siblings affect the childhood environment, but to a lesser extent than does the sex of the sibling. The arrival of a sibling is difficult for toddlers and preschool children, especially between the ages of 2 and 3 years old. At this age, they are still very attached to their parents and do not understand the concept of sharing. An older child is able to understand the situation and is likely to see the newcomer as a threat, although the child does feel the loss of the only-child status (Hanson, Gedaly-Duff, and Kaakinen, 2005). In general,

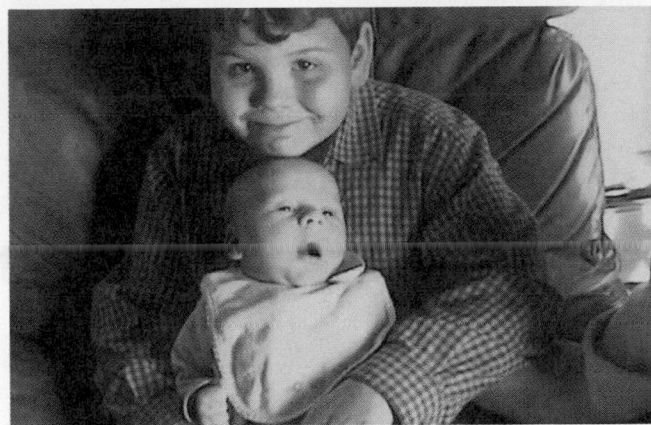

Fig. 3-3 Older school-age children often enjoy taking responsibility for the care of a younger sibling.

the narrower the spacing between siblings, the more the children influence one another, especially in emotional characteristics. The wider the spacing, the greater the influence of the parents.

Traditionally, sibling relationships were viewed from a Freudian perspective that emphasized the concept of sibling rivalry. Researchers have viewed siblings through developmental or ecologic frameworks that focus on interactions within family systems (Friedman, Bowden, and Jones, 2003). The results of these broader perspectives provide a picture of rich and varied sibling interactions (Fig. 3-3).

Sibling Functions

The sibling relationship's most unique feature is its duration. The longest relationship one will share with another human being is the sibling relationship, which lasts through a lifetime (often 50 to 80 years), compared with the child-parent relationship of approximately 30 to 50 years. Siblings spend long periods together and get to know each other at their best and worst.

Siblings exert power, exchange services, and express feelings in reciprocal ways that are often not revealed in the presence of the parents. They see themselves in their brother or sister, experience life vicariously through their sibling's behavior, and begin to expand on their own possibilities. Siblings can also be touchstones for what the other would *not* like to be, and they use each other as yardsticks for comparison. They provide a sounding board for each other and offer a safe forum for experimenting with new behaviors and roles. Brothers and sisters provide each other with tangible services (e.g., lending money, clothing, toys, or sports equipment; teaching a skill), help each other with childhood problems, provide support in dealing with parents or others outside the family, and provide introductions to new friendship groups. Children learn to negotiate and bargain, and sometimes to manipulate, from their siblings. Their interactions with each other provide opportunities for conflict and conflict resolution. They protect one another from parental-executive abuse of power and can form a coalition to deal with the issues of authority, power, and emotional support. Negotiating with parents is stronger when siblings act together rather than singly.

Tattling can be an important lever in sibling interactions. On the other hand, siblings often have a conspiracy of silence, leaving the parents feeling isolated and excluded. A willingness to maintain each other's privacy often forges a powerful bond of loyalty that distinguishes the relationship between siblings from that between friends.

More Active Sibling Relationships

Sibling relationships vary among cultures. Some factors may be giving the sibling relationship greater significance in American families than in the past. Shrinking family size, longer life spans, divorce and remarriage, geographic mobility, maternal employment, alternative sources of child care, competitive pressures, stress, and parental insufficiency may be propelling siblings into greater contact and emotional interdependence than ever before. Siblings often join forces to confront the trauma of divorce, and they frequently rely on each other for support when parents remarry. The large number of working mothers means that young siblings today have significant amounts of time when a personally committed adult does not monitor their relationship. Often an older sibling is required to baby-sit, resulting in children spending more and more time together unsupervised. In a worried, mobile, small-family, high-stress, fast-paced, parent-absent society, children often turn to a brother or sister to meet their needs for contact, constancy, and permanency.

Ordinal Position

Researchers have observed that the birth position of children affects their personalities. Parents treat children differently, and sibling interactions are different, depending on the child's position within the family. Power is unequally distributed among siblings. Older siblings attempt to dominate younger ones. Therefore younger siblings develop interpersonal skills, the ability to negotiate, and an ability to accept unfavorable outcomes to a greater extent than older siblings. Later-born children are obliged to interact with other siblings from birth and seem to be more outgoing and make friends more easily than firstborns. Children vary tremendously, and generalizations do not always apply to the individual. General characteristics of children in the various ordinal positions are presented in Box 3-4.

The Only Child

Being the only child in a family has traditionally been considered a disadvantage. Only children have been described as selfish, spoiled, dependent, and lonely. However, they do not demonstrate more evidence of maladjustment or self-centeredness than other children and tend to strongly resemble firstborn children in respects such as higher educational goals. Only children perform better on cognitive tests, are more mature, are more socially sensitive, and demonstrate superiority in language facility compared with other children.

Only children also enjoy the advantage of having parents who can devote more time to them, talk to them, and stimulate them in intellectual activities. However, parents also exert greater pressure for mature behavior at an early age and for achievement. Relative isolation from peers contributes to intellectual pursuits and encourages a rich fantasy life, independence, and originality.

BOX 3-4   INFLUENCE OF ORDINAL POSITION ON CHILDREN

Firstborn Children

Are more achievement oriented
Are more dominant
Receive more physical punishment
Are allowed to show more aggression to siblings
Have stronger consciences; are more self-disciplined and inner directed
Are more socially anxious
Are prone to feelings of guilt
Identify more with parents than with peers
Are more conservative
Are subject to greater parental expectations
Begin to speak earlier in life
Demonstrate higher intellectual achievement
Plan better and experience fewer frustrations
Are likely to be most wanted

Middle Children

Have more demands made on them for household help
Are praised less often
Receive less of the parents' time
Learn to compromise and be adaptable
Are less stimulated toward achievement
Are more difficult to characterize because of a variety of positions in the family

Youngest Children

Are less dependent than firstborn children
Are less tense, more affectionate, and more good natured
Tend to identify more with peer group than with parents
Are more flexible in their thinking
Are popular with classmates
Have fewer demands placed on them for household help

Only Children

Have many of the same characteristics as firstborn children
Are more mature and cultivated
Experience greater parental pressure for mature behavior and achievement
Demonstrate superiority in language facility
Rarely develop into stereotype of spoiled, selfish child
Often enjoy a rich fantasy life as a result of isolation

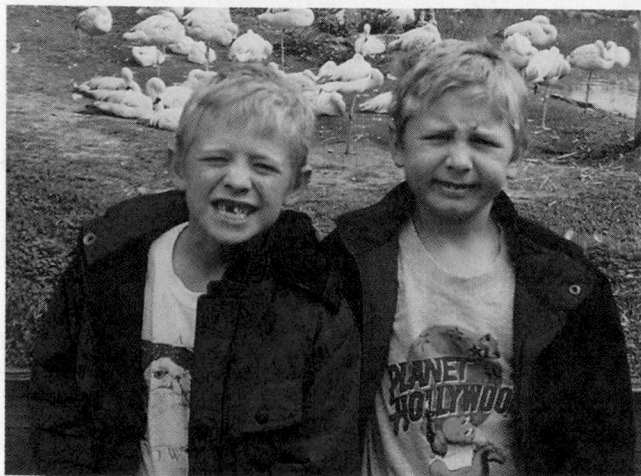

Fig. 3-4 Fraternal twins.

BOX 3-5   CHARACTERISTICS OF TWINS

MONOZYGOTIC (MZ) OR IDENTICAL TWINS	DIZYGOTIC (DZ) OR FRATERNAL TWINS
Result of one fertilized ovum that became separated early in development	Result of fertilization of two ova
Alike physically and genetically	Differ physically and genetically
Same sex	May be same or opposite sex
Frequency:	Frequency:
• Occurs uniformly in all populations	• Varies among races (highest in African-Americans, lowest in Asians, intermediate in Caucasians)
• Unaffected by maternal age	• More common with advancing maternal age (maximum at ages 35 to 39, then decreases rapidly)
Tendency unaffected by heredity	Marked familial tendency
	Expressed only in the female
	Fathers appear to transmit disposition toward double ovulation to daughters
Similar behavior	Dissimilar behavior; more sibling rivalry

Multiple Births

A deviation in early development that occurs with variable frequency is multiple births. Twins are not uncommon in the population, but triplets are rare and quadruplets or quintuplets are extremely unusual. In any of these situations, the offspring can be of the like or unlike sex (i.e., derived from a single ovum; from multiple ova; or from a combination of the two, which can involve one or more cell divisions). The cause of twinning is unknown, but the increase in the number of larger multiples (quintuplets, sextuplets) in recent years has been associated with fertility treatments such as ovulation-inducing drugs or in vitro fertilization. Because women in their thirties are almost 2.5 times as likely as women in their twenties to have higher-order plural births, increased childbearing among older women and the expanded use of fertility drugs have been associated with a rise in the multiple-birth ratio (Hamilton, Minino, Martin, et al, 2007).

Twins are of two distinct types: **identical**, or **monozygotic (MZ)**, and **fraternal** (Fig. 3-4), or **dizygotic (DZ)** (Box 3-5). In 2004 in the United States the overall rate of twin birth was 32.2 per 1000 births, a record high (Martin, Kung, Mathews, et al, 2008); one third are MZ twins, and two thirds are DZ twins.

A special kind of sibling relationship is observed in twins, although getting along with each other and quarreling are not much different from these behaviors in any other two siblings, especially if they are different-sex fraternal twins. Twins tend to work out a relationship that is reasonably satisfactory to both and demonstrate early independence from parental attention. They develop a remarkable capacity for cooperative play and considerable loyalty and generosity toward each other. It is not uncommon for them to evolve a private language between themselves that may interfere with the development of the family language.

In a twinship, one member of the pair, to a greater or lesser extent, is more dominant, outgoing, and assertive than the other, often to the consternation of their parents. However, the seemingly more passive twin is able to accomplish as much and get his or her way as frequently as the more assertive twin.

Researchers have also observed a difference in behavior between identical and fraternal twins. There is near-unison in the actions of identical twins (although they alternate in assuming the leadership), but fraternal twins, even of the same sex, do not display this quality. Sibling rivalry can be pronounced in fraternal twins, especially in different-sex twins.

Identical twins also differ in their response to the tendency of some parents to treat twins exactly alike. The present philosophy is to determine the degree to which the children demonstrate an inclination toward togetherness. Some twins thrive best when they are constantly in each other's company; others prefer more individuality and separateness. Early years of togetherness are often the basis of the children's security, and separating them too early may produce unnecessary stresses. Fostering individual differences as they become evident could ease the process of separation when it becomes advisable.

Parental Adjustment

The entrance of any new member into a household creates stress, but with multiple births two or more new members must be incorporated into the family at the same time. The problems are obvious. Two infants must be provided with physical care, including feeding, diapering, and all of the purchasing and preparation that accompanies the care of any infant. Scheduling becomes crucial, and advancement in development brings new problems and adjustments (e.g., space and sleeping arrangements, selection of a stroller and other equipment). Care must be observed in selecting toys. As play becomes a serious business, some toys that would be safe and appropriate for a single child become weapons when two infants share a playpen. It is a good idea to select different toys for each child as they grow older and encourage sharing.

It is especially important for parents to maintain relationships with each other and other family members. Parents need to arrange time together as often as possible. The National Organization of Mothers of Twins Clubs, Inc.,* has local chapters throughout the United States to offer information and support to parents of twins and is highly recommended as a resource. *Twins Magazine* (www.twinsmagazine.com) is a place to seek and give advice about parenting multiples.

PARENTING

MOTIVATION FOR PARENTHOOD

A dominant characteristic in all societies is that adults are expected to become parents and to be gratified by the experience. Pressures of tradition, sentiment regarding the state of parenthood, and religious beliefs influence decision making because conformity to social-role expectations is a strong influence in family planning.

Factors that influence family size are social class, religion, race, financial stability, type of conjugal-role relationships, and the social-psychologic aspects of sexual relations (Hanson, Gedaly-Duff, and Kaakinen, 2005). In the case of divorce and remarriage, an individual may decide to have more children with the new spouse.

PREPARATION FOR PARENTHOOD

The basic goals of parenting are to promote the physical survival and health of children, to foster the skills and abilities necessary to be self-sustaining adults, and to foster behavioral capabilities for optimizing cultural values and beliefs (Deave, Johnson, and Ingram, 2008). However, new parents often approach parenthood with limited experience and knowledge. Parents learn by trial and error, committing the same mistakes that have been committed by countless other parents, but they somehow manage to accomplish the task, becoming more skilled with each additional child.

Tradition, rather than rational planning, furnishes the chief norms for childrearing. Experience in having been nurtured as a child is an essential component of successful parenting. Their own parents are probably the only persons whom parents observe intimately in the parental role. This results in a generational continuity—parents rear their own children in much the same way that they themselves were reared. Other essential skills that parents need to feel comfortable in the parenting role include a basic understanding of childhood growth and development, bathing, feeding, use of play, and interpersonal communication skills.

TRANSITION TO PARENTHOOD

Although experts disagree as to whether the birth of the first child should be labeled a crisis, the early weeks of an infant's life call for parents to make drastic adjustments. A child's birth presents the challenge of providing total care 24 hours a day for a new member of the family (Deave, Johnson, and Ingram, 2008). A crisis may occur if the event is perceived as disturbing old habits and relationships and eliciting new responses. The birth requires role changes and significantly modifies former relationships. In addition to the roles of husband and wife, the couple must assume the roles of father and mother.

The advent of a new family member requires that the family cope with greater financial responsibilities, a possible loss of income, changes in sleeping habits, and less time for the parents to spend with each other (especially if it is a firstborn) and with other children. If these events are perceived as aversive, it can disrupt the couple's bond and reduce their intimacy and affection.

Parental Factors Affecting Transition to Parenthood

No amount of preparation can fully prepare prospective parents for an infant's constant and immediate needs. The importance of early parent-infant interactions is addressed in the discussion of the neonate, especially the attachment process (see Chapter 8). Factors affecting parenting are the age of the parents, the quality of the parental relationship, the amount of previous experience with childrearing, parental support systems, and the effects of stress on parental behavior (Deave, Johnson, and Ingram, 2008).

---

*NOMOTC Executive Office, 2000 Mallory Lane, Suite 130-600, Franklin, TN 37067; www.nomotc.org.

Parental Age

From a physiologic health perspective, the most satisfactory ages for childbearing are the years between 18 and 35. During this time, parents are considered to be in optimum health, with a predicted life span that allows sufficient time and vigor to raise a family. However, the age at which parents begin their families has changed over the past few decades in the United States, with a substantial increase in the birth rate for women 30 to 44 years of age and a decline for women ages 20 to 29 years.

Father Involvement

Current practices that encourage early father-infant interaction indicate that fathers are as intrigued with their newborns as mothers are (see discussion on paternal engrossment under Promote Parent-Infant Bonding [Attachment], Chapter 8). Even fathers who have little initial contact with their newborn become involved with them over the next few months (Fig. 3-5), although the type of interaction is different from that of the mother. For example, mothers are more likely to hold, soothe, care for, or play quietly with their infants, whereas fathers are more boisterous and engage in more physically stimulating activities. However, fathers are more than just playmates. They are often successful at soothing a distressed infant. A secure attachment to the father can help offset the consequences of an insecure attachment to the mother.

Parenting Education

First-time parents who have prepared themselves to be parents experience less stress adjusting to the birth of a new baby than those who have not. Programs designed to take place near the time of birth or soon after can be more helpful in easing transitional stress than earlier programs (Deave, Johnson, and Ingram, 2008).

Many parents are looking for ways to be a better parent. Nurses can offer a number of suggestions, including being an active listener, having an active role in education, keeping up with technology, keeping up with regular visits to the child's health care provider and vaccinations, ensuring safety in and out of the home, spending quality time with the child, and focusing on improving overall family communication (Fig. 3-6).

Other factors influencing the transition to the parental role include the following:

- Parents with previous experience, such as another child, appear to be more relaxed, have less conflict in disciplinary relationships, and are more aware of normal growth and development.
- The amount of stress experienced by one or both parents may interfere with their ability to be patient and understanding and to cope with their children's behavior.
- Special characteristics of the infant, such as being temperamentally difficult, can cause the parents to lose confidence and doubt their abilities. Infants with special care needs (such as those associated with a disability) can be a significant source of added stress.
- Stressed marital relationships can have a negative effect on parental transition because marital tension can alter caregiving routines and interfere with enjoyment of the infant. Conversely, parents' support and encouragement of one another serve as positive influences on establishing a satisfying parental role.

Support Systems

Successful adaptation to the stress of transition to parenthood involves at least two types of family resources (McCubbin and McCubbin, 1994). Internal resources such as adaptability and integration are the first type of resource. Changing from an orderly, predictable life to a relatively disordered, unpredictable one is a universal adaptation that families must make. Rigid schedules are impossible to maintain, and former activities must be curtailed or abandoned. Adaptation is reflected in learning to be patient, becoming better organized, and becoming more flexible. Integration refers to the couple's attempt to continue some activities they engaged in before they became parents. In this way couples are able to maintain a sense of continuity and appreciate the importance of the husband-wife relationship (McCubbin and McCubbin, 1994).

The second resource is the use of coping strategies that strengthen the family's organization and functioning. These

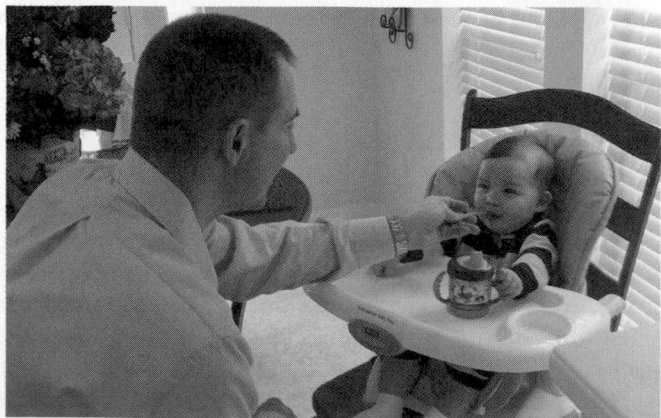

Fig. 3-5 Fathers who assume care of their children may feel more comfortable and successful in their parenting role.

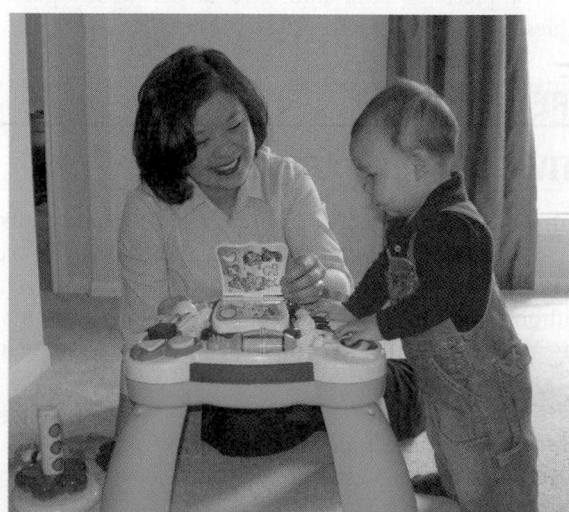

Fig. 3-6 Quality time spent with a child is essential to a family's health and well-being.

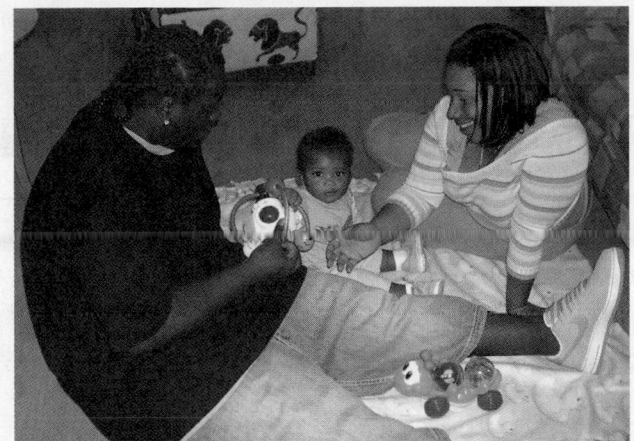

Fig. 3-7 Learning new roles together as a mother and father can enhance parenting relationships.

include the use of social support systems and community resources and the adoption of a future orientation. Interpersonal supports that provide information, advice, and caretaking can be derived from friends, relatives, and neighbors. Relationships with family, friends, and community are essential. For parents, positive, supportive work relationships are important. Equally important is time spent with friends. Arranging for time away from the child or children is also beneficial. One parent can assume care of the family to allow the other parent some time to himself or herself. Adoption of a future orientation reassures parents that things will get better, that they will cope, and that it is realistic to plan for the time when they will be able to engage in self-fulfilling activities.

It is also reassuring to know that others experience ambivalent feelings toward parenthood and share the same difficulties and frustrations. Exchanging ideas and experiences with other parents and each other provides an opportunity to voice concerns and to learn new ways to cope with multiple childrearing problems (Fig. 3-7).

PARENTING BEHAVIORS

Parental Styles of Control

Parenting styles have been described in many different ways. Within a social interactional learning model, parenting can be positive or coercive (Liddle, Santisteban, Levant, et al, 2002). A positive approach to parenting encourages skill development, whereas a coercive approach uses negative reinforcement and often causes a destructive effect on relationships.

Parenting styles are often classified as authoritarian, permissive, or authoritative (Hoeve, Dubas, Eichelsheim, et al, 2009; Hubbs-Tait, Kennedy, Page, et al, 2008). **Authoritarian** or **dictatorial** parents try to control their children's behavior and attitudes through unquestioned mandates. They establish rules and regulations or standards of conduct that they expect to be followed rigidly and unquestioningly. The message is: "Do it because I say so." Punishment need not be corporal but may be stern withdrawal of love and approval. Careful training often results in rigidly conforming behavior in the children, who tend to be sensitive, shy, self-conscious, retiring, and submissive. They are more likely to be courteous, loyal, honest, and dependable but docile. These behaviors are more typically observed when close supervision and affection accompany parental authority. If not, this style of parenting may be associated with both defiant and antisocial behavior.

Permissive parents exert little or no control over their children's actions. They avoid imposing their own standards of conduct and allow their children to regulate their own activity as much as possible. These parents consider themselves to be resources for the children, not role models. If rules do exist, the parents explain the underlying reason, elicit the children's opinions, and consult them in decision-making processes. They employ lax, inconsistent discipline; do not set sensible limits; and do not prevent the children from upsetting the home routine. These parents rarely punish the children.

Authoritative or **democratic** parents combine practices from both of the previously described parenting styles. They direct their children's behavior and attitudes by emphasizing the reason for rules and negatively reinforcing deviations. They respect the individuality of each child and allow the child to voice objections to family standards or regulations. Parental control is firm and consistent but tempered with encouragement, understanding, and security. Control is focused on the issue, not on withdrawal of love or the fear of punishment. These parents foster "inner-directedness," a conscience that regulates behavior based on feelings of guilt or shame for wrongdoing, not on fear of being caught or punished. Parents' realistic standards and reasonable expectations produce children with high self-esteem who are self-reliant, assertive, inquisitive, content, and highly interactive with other children.

There are differing philosophies in regard to parenting. Childrearing is a culturally bound phenomenon, and children are socialized to behave in ways that are important to their family. In the authoritative style, authority is shared and children are included in discussions, fostering an independent and assertive style of participation in family life. When working with individual families, nurses should give these differing styles equal respect.

LIMIT SETTING AND DISCIPLINE

In its broadest sense, **discipline** means *to teach* or refers to a set of rules governing conduct. In a narrower sense, it refers to the action taken to enforce the rules after noncompliance. **Limit setting** refers to establishing the rules or guidelines for behavior. For example, parents can place limits on the amount of time children spend watching television or chatting online. The clearer the limits that are set and the more consistently they are enforced, the less need there is for disciplinary action.

Nurses can help parents establish realistic and concrete "rules." Limit setting and discipline are positive, necessary components of childrearing and serve several useful functions as they help children:

- Test their limits of control
- Achieve in areas appropriate for mastery at their level
- Channel undesirable feelings into constructive activity
- Protect themselves from danger
- Learn socially acceptable behavior

Children want and need limits. Unrestricted freedom is a threat to their security and safety. By testing the limits imposed on them, children learn the extent to which they can manipulate their environment and gain reassurance from knowing that others are there to protect them from potential harm.

Minimizing Misbehavior

The reasons for misbehavior may include attention, power, defiance, and a display of inadequacy (e.g., the child misses classes because of a fear that he or she is unable to do the work). Children may also misbehave because the rules are not clear or consistently applied. Acting-out behavior, such as a temper tantrum, may represent uncontrolled frustration, anger, depression, or pain. The best approach is to structure interactions with children to prevent or minimize unacceptable behavior (see Family-Centered Care box).

FAMILY-CENTERED CARE
Minimizing Misbehavior

- Set realistic goals for acceptable behavior and expected achievements.
- Structure opportunities for small successes to lessen feelings of inadequacy.
- Praise children for desirable behavior with attention and verbal approval.
- Structure the environment to prevent unnecessary difficulties (e.g., place fragile objects in inaccessible area).
- Set clear and reasonable rules; expect the same behavior regardless of the circumstances; if exceptions are made, clarify that the change is for one time only.
- Teach desirable behavior through own example, such as using a quiet, calm voice rather than screaming.
- Review expected behavior before special or unusual events, such as visiting a relative or having dinner in a restaurant.
- Phrase requests for appropriate behavior positively, such as "Put the book down," rather than "Don't touch the book."
- Call attention to unacceptable behavior as soon as it begins; use distraction to change the behavior or offer alternatives to annoying actions, such as exchanging a quiet toy for one that is too noisy.
- Give advance notice or "friendly reminders," such as "When the TV program is over, it is time for dinner" or "I'll give you to the count of three and then we have to go."
- Be attentive to situations that increase the likelihood of misbehaving, such as overexcitement or fatigue, or decreased personal tolerance to minor infractions.
- Offer sympathetic explanations for not granting a request, such as "I am sorry I can't read you a story now, but I have to finish dinner. Then we can spend time together."
- Keep any promises made to children.
- Avoid outright conflicts; temper discussions with statements such as "Let's talk about it and see what we can decide together" or "I have to think about it first."
- Provide children with opportunities for power and control.

General Guidelines for Implementing Discipline

Regardless of the type of discipline used, certain principles are essential to ensure the efficacy of the approach (see Family-Centered Care box). Many strategies, such as behavior modification, can only be implemented effectively when principles of consistency and timing are followed. A pattern of intermittent or occasional enforcement of limits actually prolongs the undesired behavior because children learn that if they are persistent, the behavior is permitted eventually. Delaying punishment weakens its intent, and practices such as telling the child, "Wait

until your father comes home," are not only ineffectual, but also convey negative messages about the other parent.*

FAMILY-CENTERED CARE
Implementing Discipline

Consistency—Implement disciplinary action exactly as agreed on and for each infraction.

Timing—Initiate discipline as soon as child misbehaves; if delays are necessary, such as to avoid embarrassment, verbally disapprove of the behavior and state that disciplinary action will be implemented.

Commitment—Follow through with the details of the discipline, such as timing of minutes; avoid distractions that may interfere with the plan, such as telephone calls.

Unity—Make certain that all caregivers agree on the plan and are familiar with the details to prevent confusion and alliances between child and one parent.

Flexibility—Choose disciplinary strategies that are appropriate to child's age and temperament and the severity of the misbehavior.

Planning—Plan disciplinary strategies in advance and prepare child if feasible (e.g., explain use of time-out); for unexpected misbehavior, try to discipline when you are calm.

Behavior orientation—Always disapprove of the behavior, not the child, with such statements as "That was a wrong thing to do. I am unhappy when I see behavior like that."

Privacy—Administer discipline in private, especially with older children, who may feel ashamed in front of others.

Termination—After the discipline is administered, consider child as having a "clean slate," and avoid bringing up the incident or lecturing.

Types of Discipline

To deal with misbehavior, parents need to implement appropriate disciplinary action. Many approaches are available. **Reasoning** involves explaining why an act is wrong and is usually appropriate for older children, especially when moral issues are involved. However, young children cannot be expected to "see the other side" because of their egocentrism. Children in the preoperative stage of cognitive development (toddlers and preschoolers) have a limited ability to distinguish between their point of view and that of others. Sometimes children use "reasoning" as a way of gaining attention. For example, they may misbehave thinking the parents will give them a lengthy explanation of the wrongdoing and knowing that negative attention is better than no attention. When children use this technique, parents should end the explanation by stating, "This is the rule, and this is how I expect you to behave. I won't explain it any further."

Unfortunately, reasoning is often combined with **scolding**, which sometimes takes the form of shame or criticism. For example, the parent may state, "You are a bad boy for hitting your brother." Children take such remarks seriously and personally, believing that they *are* bad.

Positive and negative reinforcement is the basis of **behavior modification** theory—behavior that is rewarded will be repeated; behavior that is not rewarded will be extinguished. Using **rewards** is a positive approach. By encouraging children to behave in specified ways, the parents can decrease the ten-

---

*For parenting of kindergarten through sixth grade children, see http://childparenting.about.com and www.kidshealth.org.

dency to misbehave. With young children, using paper stars is an effective method. For older children, the "token system" is appropriate, especially if a certain number of stars or tokens yields a special reward, such as a trip to the movies or a new book. In planning a reward system, the parents must explain expected behaviors to the child and establish rewards that are reinforcing. They should use a chart to record the stars or tokens and always give an earned reward promptly. Verbal approval should always accompany extrinsic rewards.

Consistently **ignoring** behavior will eventually extinguish or minimize the act. Although this approach sounds simple, it is difficult to implement consistently. Parents frequently "give in" and resort to previous patterns of discipline. Consequently, the behavior is actually reinforced because the child learns that persistence gains parental attention. For ignoring to be effective, parents should (1) understand the process, (2) record the undesired behavior before using ignoring to determine whether a problem exists and to compare results after ignoring is begun, (3) determine whether parental attention acts as a reinforcer, and (4) be aware of "response burst." Response burst is a phenomenon that occurs when the undesired behavior increases after ignoring is initiated because the child is "testing" the parents to see if they are serious about the plan.

The strategy of **consequences** involves allowing children to experience the results of their misbehavior. It includes three types:

1. Natural—Those that occur without any intervention, such as being late and having to clean up the dinner table
2. Logical—Those that are directly related to the rule, such as not being allowed to play with another toy until the used ones are put away
3. Unrelated—Those that are imposed deliberately, such as no playing until homework is completed or the use of time-out

Natural or logical consequences are preferred and effective if they are meaningful to children. For example, the natural consequence of living in a messy room may do little to encourage cleaning up, but allowing no friends over until the room is neat can be motivating! Withdrawing privileges is often an unrelated consequence. After the child experiences the consequence, the parent should refrain from any comment, because the usual tendency is for the child to try to place blame for imposing the rule.

Time-out is a refinement of the common practice of sending the child to his or her room and is a type of unrelated consequence. It is based on the premise of removing the reinforcer (i.e., the satisfaction or attention the child is receiving from the activity). When placed in an unstimulating and isolated place, children become bored and consequently agree to behave in order to reenter the family group (Fig. 3-8). Time-out avoids many of the problems of other disciplinary approaches. No

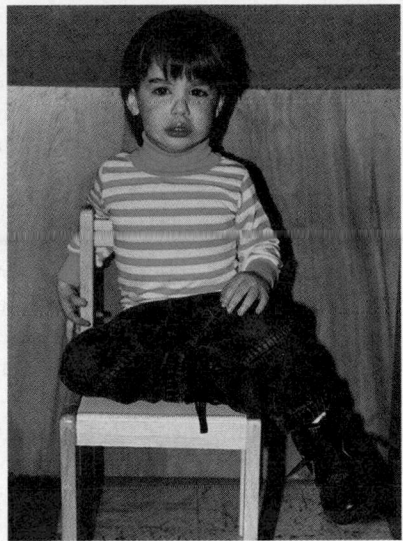

Fig. 3-8 Time-out is an excellent disciplinary strategy for young children.

physical punishment is involved; no reasoning or scolding is given; and the parent does not need to be present for all of the time-out, thus facilitating consistent application of this type of discipline. Time-out offers both the child and the parent a "cooling off" time. To be effective, however, time-out must be planned in advance (see Family-Centered Care box).

FAMILY-CENTERED CARE

Using Time-Out

Select an area for time-out that is safe, convenient, and unstimulating, but where the child can be monitored, such as the bathroom, hallway, or laundry room.
Determine what behaviors warrant a time-out.
Make certain children understand the "rules" and how they are expected to behave.
Explain to children the process of time-out:
- When they misbehave, they will be given *one* warning.
- If they do not obey, they will be sent to the place designated for time-out.
- They are to sit there for a specified period.
- If they cry, refuse, or display any disruptive behavior, the time-out period will begin *after* they quiet down.
- When they are quiet for the duration of the time, they can then leave the room.
A rule for the length of time-out is *1 minute per year of age;* use a kitchen timer with an audible bell to record the time rather than a watch.
Implement time-out in a public place by selecting a suitable area, or explain to children that time-out will be spent immediately on returning home.

Corporal or **physical punishment** most often takes the form of spanking (Larzelere, 2008). Based on the principles of aversive therapy, inflicting pain through spanking causes a dramatic short-term decrease in the behavior. However, this approach has serious flaws: (1) it teaches children that violence is acceptable; (2) it may physically harm the child if it is the result of parental rage; and (3) children become "accustomed" to spanking, requiring more severe corporal punishment over time. Spanking can result in severe physical and psychologic injury, and it interferes with effective parent-child interaction (Cain, 2008). In addition, when the parents are not around, children are likely to misbehave, since they have not learned to behave well for their own sake. Parental use of corporal punishment may also interfere with the child's development of moral reasoning.

SPECIAL PARENTING SITUATIONS

Parenting is a demanding task under ideal circumstances, but when parents and children face situations that deviate from "the norm," the potential for family disruption is increased. Situations that are encountered frequently are divorce, single parenthood, blended families, adoption, and dual-career families. In addition, as cultural diversity increases in our communities, many immigrants are making the transition to parenthood and a new country, culture, and language simultaneously. Other situations that create unique parenting challenges are parental alcoholism, homelessness, and incarceration. Although these topics are not addressed here, the reader may wish to investigate them further.

PARENTING THE ADOPTED CHILD

Adoption establishes a legal relationship between a child and parents who are not related by birth, but who have the same rights and obligations that exist between children and their biologic parents. In the past the biologic mother alone made the decision to relinquish the rights to her child. In recent years the courts have acknowledged the legal rights of the biologic father regarding this decision. Concerned child advocates have questioned whether decisions that honor the father's rights are in the best interests of the child. As the child's rights have become recognized, older children have successfully dissolved their legal bond with their biologic parents to pursue adoption by adults of their choice. Furthermore, there is a growing interest and demand within the gay and lesbian (GLBT) community to adopt.

Unlike biologic parents, who prepare for their child's birth with prenatal classes and the support of friends and relatives, adoptive parents have fewer sources of support and preparation for the new addition to their family. Nurses can provide the information, support, and reassurance needed to reduce parental anxiety regarding the adoptive process and refer adoptive parents to state parental support groups. Such sources can be contacted through a state or county welfare office.

The sooner infants enter their adoptive home, the better the chances of parent-infant attachment. However, the more caregivers the infant had before adoption, the greater the risk for attachment problems. The infant must break the bond with the previous caregiver and form a new bond with the adoptive parents. Difficulties in forming an attachment depend on the amount of time he or she has spent with caregivers early in life as well as the number of caregivers (e.g., the birth mother, nurse, adoption agency personnel).

Siblings, adopted or biologic, who are old enough to understand should be included in decisions regarding the commitment to adopt, with reassurance that they are not being replaced. Ways that the siblings can interact with the adopted child should be stressed (Fig. 3-9).

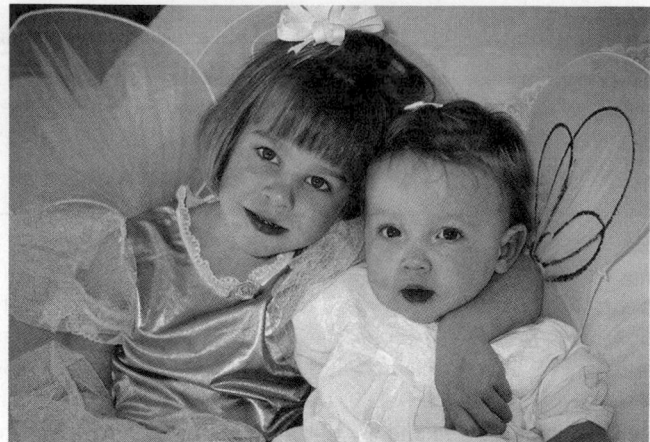

Fig. 3-9 An older sister lovingly embraces her adopted sister.

Issues of Origin

The task of telling children that they are adopted can be a cause of deep concern and anxiety. There are no clear-cut guidelines for parents to follow in determining when and at what age children are ready for the information. Parents are naturally reluctant to present such potentially unsettling news. However, it is important that parents not withhold the adoption from the child, since it is an essential component of the child's identity (see Critical Thinking Exercise).

❓ CRITICAL THINKING EXERCISE

Parenting the Adopted Child

Twelve-month-old Justin was adopted at birth. His parents tell you that they wonder when they should tell Justin that he is adopted. As the nurse, what counseling and advice should you give Justin's parents?

Questions
1. Evidence—Is there sufficient information to draw any conclusions about this situation?
2. Assumptions—Describe some underlying assumptions about the following:
   a. The best time to tell children that they are adopted
   b. The manner in which parents should tell their child about adoption
   c. Children's reactions to being told they are adopted
3. What implications for nursing care can be drawn at this time?
4. Does the evidence support your conclusion?

The timing arises naturally as parents become aware of the child's readiness. Most authorities believe that children should be informed at an age young enough so that, as they grow older, they do not remember a time when they did not know they were adopted. The time is highly individual, but must be right for both the parents and the child. It may be when children ask where babies come from, at which time children can also be told the facts of their adoption. If they are told in a way that conveys the idea that they were active participants in the selection process, they will be less likely to feel that they were abandoned victims in a helpless situation. For example, parents can tell children that their personal qualities drew the parents to them. It is wise for parents who have not previously discussed adoption to tell children that they are adopted before the children enter school to avoid having them learn it from third parties. Complete honesty between parents and children strengthens the relationship.

Parents should anticipate behavior changes after the disclosure, especially in older children. Children who are struggling with the revelation that they are adopted may benefit from individual and family counseling. Children may use the fact of their adoption as a weapon to manipulate and threaten parents. Statements such as "My real mother would not treat me like this" or "You don't love me as much because I'm adopted" hurt parents and increase their feelings of insecurity. Such statements may also cause parents to become overpermissive. Adopted children need the same undemanding love, combined with firm discipline and limit setting, as any other child.

Adolescence

Adolescence may be an especially trying time for parents of adopted children. The normal confrontations of adolescents and parents assume more painful aspects in adoptive families. Adolescents may use their adoption to defy parental authority or as a justification for aberrant behavior. As they attempt to master the task of identity formation, they may begin to have feelings of abandonment by their biologic parents. Gender differences in reacting to adoption may surface.

Adopted children fantasize about their biologic parents and may feel the need to discover their parents' identity to define themselves and their own identity. It is important for parents to keep the lines of communication open and to reassure their child that they understand the need to search for their identity. In some states, birth certificates are made legally available to adopted children when they come of age. Parents should be honest with questioning adolescents and tell them of this possibility (the parents themselves are unable to obtain the birth certificate; it is the children's responsibility if they desire it).

Cross-Racial and International Adoption

Adoption of children from racial backgrounds different from that of the family is commonplace. In addition to the problems faced by adopted children in general, children of a cross-racial adoption must deal with physical and sometimes cultural differences. It is advised that parents who adopt children with different ethnic background do everything to preserve the adopted children's racial heritage.

! **NURSING ALERT**

As a health care provider, it is important not to ask the wrong questions, such as "Is she yours, or is she adopted?" "What do you know about the 'real' mother?" "Do they have the same father?" or "How much did it cost to adopt him?"

Although the children are full-fledged members of an adopting family and citizens of the adopted country, if they have a strikingly different appearance from other family members or exhibit distinct racial or ethnic characteristics, challenges may be encountered outside the family. Bigotry may appear among relatives and friends. Strangers may make thoughtless comments and talk about the children as though they were not members of the family. It is vital that family members declare

to others that this is their child and a cherished member of the family.

In international adoptions the medical information the parents receive may be incomplete or sketchy; weight, height, and head circumference are often the only objective information present in the child's medical record. Many internationally adopted children were born prematurely, and common health problems such as infant diarrhea and malnutrition delay growth and development. Some children have serious or multiple health problems that can be stressful for the parents.

PARENTING AND DIVORCE

Since the mid-1960s, a marked change in the stability of families has been reflected in increased rates of divorce, single parenthood, and remarriage. In 2008 the divorce rate for the United States was 3.6 per 1000 total population (Centers for Disease Control and Prevention, 2008). The divorce rate has changed little since 1987. In the decade before that, the rate increased yearly, with a peak in 1979. Although almost half of all divorcing couples are childless, it is estimated that more than 1 million children experience divorce each year.

The process of divorce begins with a period of marital conflict of varying length and intensity, followed by a separation, the actual legal divorce, and the reestablishment of different living arrangements (Box 3-6). Because a function of parenthood is to provide for the security and emotional welfare of children, disruption of the family structure often engenders strong feelings of guilt in the divorcing parents.

During a divorce, parents' coping abilities may be compromised. The parents may be preoccupied with their own feelings, needs, and life changes and be unavailable to support their children. Newly employed parents, usually mothers, are likely to leave children with new caregivers, in strange settings, or alone after school. The parent may also spend more time away from

---

BOX 3-6 **STAGES OF THE DIVORCE PROCESS**

Acute Phase
The married couple makes the decision to separate.
This phase includes the legal steps of filing for dissolution of the marriage and, usually, the departure of the father from the home.
This phase lasts from several months to more than a year and is accompanied by familial stress and a chaotic atmosphere.

Transitional Phase
The adults and children assume unfamiliar roles and relationships within a new family structure.
This phase is often accompanied by a change of residence, a reduced standard of living and altered lifestyle, a larger share of the economic responsibility being shouldered by the mother, and radically altered parent-child relationships.

Stabilizing Phase
The postdivorce family reestablishes a stable, functioning family unit.
Remarriage frequently occurs, with concomitant changes in all areas of family life.

Modified from Wallerstein JS: Children of divorce: stress and developmental tasks. In Garmezy N, Rutter M, editors: *Stress, coping, and development in children*, New York, 1988, McGraw-Hill.

home, searching for or establishing new relationships. Sometimes, however, the adult feels frightened and alone and begins to depend on the child as a substitute for the absent parent. This dependence places an enormous burden on the child.

Common characteristics in the custodial household after separation and divorce include disorder, coercive types of control, inflammable tempers in both parents and children, reduced parental competence, a greater sense of parental helplessness, poorly enforced discipline, and diminished regularity in household routines. Noncustodial parents are seldom prepared for the role of visitor, may assume the role of recreational and "fun" parent, and may not have a residence suitable for children's visits. They may also be concerned about maintaining the arrangement over the years to follow.

Impact of Divorce on Children

Parental divorce is an additional childhood adversity that contributes to poor mental health outcomes, especially when combined with child abuse. Parental psychopathology may be one possible mechanism to explain the relationships between child abuse, parental divorce, and psychiatric disorders and suicide attempts (Afifi, Boman, Fleisher, et al, 2009). Even when a divorce is amicable and open, children recall parental separation with the same emotions felt by victims of a natural disaster: loss, grief, and vulnerability to forces beyond their control.

The impact of divorce on children depends on several factors, including the age and sex of the children, the outcome of the divorce, and the quality of the parent-child relationship and parental care during the years following the divorce. Family characteristics are more crucial to the child's well-being than specific child characteristics, such as age or sex. High levels of ongoing family conflict are related to problems of social development, emotional stability, and cognitive skills for the child (see Research Focus box).

⬛ RESEARCH FOCUS

Impact of Divorce

Children who reported that their divorced parents were cooperative had better relationships with their parents, grandparents, stepparents, and siblings (Ahrons, 2007). Complications associated with divorce include efforts on the part of one parent to subvert the child's loyalties to the other, abandonment to other caregivers, and adjustment to a stepparent.

A major problem occurs when children are "caught in the middle" between the divorced parents. They become the message bearer between the parents, are often quizzed about the other parent's activities, and have to listen to one parent criticize the other. A nurse may be able to help the child get out of the middle by stating "I messages" based on the formula of "I feel (state the feeling) when you (state the source). I would like it if you . . . ." An example of an "I message" is: "I do not feel comfortable when you ask me questions about mom; maybe you could ask her yourself." This approach enables the child to feel in control.

Feelings of children toward divorce vary with age (Box 3-7). Previously, researchers believed that divorce had a greater impact on younger children, but recent observations indicate that divorce constitutes a major disruption for children of all

ages. The feelings and behaviors of children may be different for various ages and gender, but all children suffer stress second only to the stress produced by the death of a parent. Although considerable research has looked at sex differences in children's adjustments to divorce, the findings are not conclusive.

Some children feel a sense of shame and embarrassment concerning the family situation. Sometimes children see themselves as different, inferior, or unworthy of love, especially if they feel responsible for the family dissolution. Although the social stigma attached to divorce no longer produces the emotions it did in the past, such feelings may still exist in small towns or in some cultural groups and can reinforce children's negative self-image. The lasting effects of divorce depend on the children's and the parents' adjustment to the transition from an intact family to a single-parent family and, often, to a reconstituted family.

Although most studies have concentrated on the negative effects of divorce on youngsters, some positive outcomes of divorce have been reported. A successful postdivorce family, either a single-parent or a reconstituted family, can improve the quality of life for both adults and children. If conflict is resolved, a better relationship with one or both parents may result, and some children may have less contact with a disturbed parent. Greater stability in the home setting and the removal of arguing parents can be a positive outcome for the child's long term well-being.

Telling the Children

Parents are understandably hesitant to tell children about their decision to divorce. Most parents neglect to discuss either the divorce or its inevitable changes with their preschool child. Without preparation, even children who remain in the family home are confused by the parental separation. Frequently, children are already experiencing vague, uneasy feelings that are more difficult to cope with than being told the truth about the situation.

If possible, the initial disclosure should include both parents and siblings, followed by individual discussions with each child. Sufficient time should be set aside for these discussions, and they should take place during a period of calm, not after an argument. Parents who physically hold or touch their children provide them with a feeling of warmth and reassurance. The discussions should include the reason for the divorce, if age appropriate, and reassurance that the divorce is not the fault of the children.

Parents should not fear crying in front of the children, because their crying gives the children permission to cry also. Children need to ventilate their feelings. Children may feel guilt, a sense of failure, or that they are being punished for misbehavior. They normally feel anger and resentment and should be allowed to communicate these feelings without punishment. They also have feelings of terror and abandonment. They need consistency and order in their lives. They want to know where they will live, who will take care of them, if they will be with their siblings, and if there will be enough money to live on. Children may also wonder what will happen on special days such as birthdays and holidays, whether both parents will come to school events, and whether they will still have the same friends. Children fear that if their parents stopped loving each

BOX 3-7 FEELINGS AND BEHAVIORS OF CHILDREN RELATED TO DIVORCE

Infancy
Effects of reduced mothering or lack of mothering
Increased irritability
Disturbance in eating, sleeping, and elimination
Interference with attachment process

Early Preschool Children (Ages 2 to 3 Years)
Frightened and confused
Blame themselves for the divorce
Fear of abandonment
Increased irritability, whining, tantrums
Regressive behaviors (e.g., thumb sucking, loss of elimination control)
Separation anxiety

Later Preschool Children (Ages 3 to 5 Years)
Fear of abandonment
Blame themselves for the divorce; decreased self-esteem
Bewilderment regarding all human relationships
Become more aggressive in relationships with others (e.g., siblings, peers)
Engage in fantasy to seek understanding of the divorce

Early School-Age Children (Ages 5 to 6 Years)
Depression and immature behavior
Loss of appetite and sleep disorders
May be able to verbalize some feelings and understand some divorce-related changes
Increased anxiety and aggression
Feelings of abandonment by departing parent

Middle School-Age Children (Ages 6 to 8 Years)
Panic reactions
Feelings of deprivation—loss of parent, attention, money, and secure future
Profound sadness, depression, fear, and insecurity
Feelings of abandonment and rejection
Fear regarding the future

Difficulty expressing anger at parents
Intense desire for reconciliation of parents
Impaired capacity to play and enjoy outside activities
Decline in school performance
Altered peer relationships—become bossy, irritable, demanding, and manipulative
Frequent crying, loss of appetite, sleep disorders
Disturbed routine, forgetfulness

Later School-Age Children (Ages 9 to 12 Years)
More realistic understanding of divorce
Intense anger directed at one or both parents
Divided loyalties
Ability to express feelings of anger
Ashamed of parental behavior
Desire for revenge; may wish to punish the parent they hold responsible
Feelings of loneliness, rejection, and abandonment
Altered peer relationships
Decline in school performance
May develop somatic complaints
May engage in aberrant behavior such as lying, stealing
Temper tantrums
Dictatorial attitude

Adolescents (Ages 12 to 18 Years)
Able to disengage themselves from parental conflict
Feelings of a profound sense of loss—of family, childhood
Feelings of anxiety
Worry about themselves, parents, siblings
Expression of anger, sadness, shame, embarrassment
May withdraw from family and friends
Disturbed concept of sexuality
May engage in acting-out behaviors

other, they could stop loving them. Their need for love and reassurance is tremendous at this time.

Custody and Parenting Partnerships

In the past, when parents separated, the mother was given custody of the children with visitation agreements for the father. Now both parents and the courts are seeking alternatives. Current belief is that neither fathers nor mothers should be awarded custody automatically. Custody should be awarded to the parent who is best able to provide for the children's welfare. In some cases, children experience severe stress when living or spending time with a parent. Many fathers have demonstrated both their competence and their commitment to care for their children.

Often overlooked are the changes that may occur in the children's relationships with other relatives, especially grandparents. Grandparents are increasingly involved in the care of young children (Fergusson, Maughan, and Golding, 2008). Grandparents on the noncustodial side are often kept from their grandchildren, whereas those on the custodial side may be overwhelmed by their adult child's return to the household with grandchildren.

Two other types of custody arrangements are divided custody and joint custody. **Divided custody**, or **split custody**, means that each parent is awarded custody of one or more of the

children, thereby separating siblings. For example, sons might live with the father and daughters with the mother.

Joint custody takes one of two forms. In **joint physical custody**, the parents alternate the physical care and control of the children on an agreed-on basis while maintaining shared parenting responsibilities legally. This custody arrangement works well for families who live close to each other and whose occupations permit an active role in the care and rearing of the children. In **joint legal custody**, the children reside with one parent but both parents are the children's legal guardians, and both participate in childrearing.

Coparenting offers substantial benefits for the family: children can be close to both parents, and life with each parent can be more normal (as opposed to having a disciplinarian mother and a recreational father). To be successful, parents in these arrangements must be highly committed to provide normal parenting and to separate their marital conflicts from their parenting roles. No matter what type of custody arrangement is awarded, the primary consideration is the welfare of the children.

SINGLE PARENTING

An individual may acquire single-parent status as a result of divorce, separation, death of a spouse, or birth or adoption of a child. Although divorce rates have stabilized, the number of single-parent households continues to rise. In 2007, 32% of children younger than 18 years of age lived in single-parent families, and the majority of single parents were women (Kreider and Elliott, 2009; Annie E Casey Foundation, 2009). Although some women are single parents by choice, most never planned on being single parents, and many feel pressure to marry or remarry.

Managing shortages of money, time, and energy is often a concern for single parents. Studies repeatedly confirm the financial difficulties of single-parent families, particularly single mothers. In 2004 only one third of mother-headed households received any child support or alimony (Annie E Casey Foundation, 2009). In fact, the stigma of poverty may be more keenly felt than the discrimination associated with being a single parent. These families are often forced by their financial status to live in communities with inadequate housing and personal safety concerns. Single parents often feel guilty about the time spent away from their children. Divorced mothers, from marriages in which the father assumed the role of bread-winner and the mother the household maintenance and parenting roles, have considerable difficulty adjusting to their new role of breadwinner. Many single parents have trouble arranging for adequate child care, particularly for a sick child.

Being a teenage parent adds to the financial burden of being a single parent and can have long-term consequences for the mother and child. Poverty is a well-known predictor of adverse effects on a child's health and well-being. Approximately 78% of children born to a teenage mother who did not marry or graduate high school live in poverty. In contrast, only 9% of children born to women over 20 who marry and finish high school live in poverty (Annie E Casey Foundation, 2009).

Social supports and community resources needed by single-parent families include health care services that are open on evenings and weekends; high-quality child care; respite child care to relieve parental exhaustion and prevent burnout; and parent enhancement centers for advancing education and job skills, providing recreational activities, and offering parenting education. Single parents need social contacts separate from their children for their own emotional growth and that of their children. Parents Without Partners, Inc.,* is an organization designed to meet the needs of single parents.

Single Fathers

Fathers who have custody of their children have many of the same problems as divorced mothers. They feel overburdened by the responsibility; depressed; and concerned about their ability to cope with the emotional needs of the children, especially girls. Some fathers lack home-making skills. They may find it difficult at first to coordinate household tasks, school visits, and other activities associated with managing a household alone.

PARENTING IN RECONSTITUTED FAMILIES

In the United States, many of the children living in homes where parents have divorced will experience another major

change in their lives such as the addition of a stepparent or new siblings (Hanson, Gedaly-Duff, and Kaakinen, 2005). The entry of a stepparent into a ready-made family requires adjustments for all family members. Some obstacles to the role adjustments and family problem solving include disruption of previous life-styles and interaction patterns, complexity in the formation of new ones, and lack of social supports. Despite these problems, most children from divorced families want to live in a two-parent home.

Cooperative parenting relationships can allow more time for each set of parents to be alone to establish their own relationship with the children. Under ideal circumstances, power conflicts between the two households can be reduced, and tension and anxiety can be lessened for all family members. In addition, the children's self-esteem can be increased, and there is a greater likelihood of continued contact with grandparents. Flexibility, mutual support, and open communication are critical in successful relationships in stepfamilies and stepparenting situations.

PARENTING IN DUAL-EARNER FAMILIES

No change in family lifestyle has had more impact than the large numbers of women moving away from the traditional home-maker role and entering the workplace (Hanson, Gedaly-Duff, and Kaakinen, 2005). The trend toward increased numbers of dual-earner families is unlikely to diminish significantly. As a result, the family is subject to considerable stress as members attempt to meet often competing demands of occupational needs and those regarded as necessary for a rich family life.

Role definitions are frequently altered to arrange a more equitable division of time and labor, as well as to resolve conflict, especially conflict related to traditional cultural norms. Overload is a common source of stress in a dual-earner family, and social activities are significantly curtailed. Time demands and scheduling are major problems for all individuals who work. When the individuals are parents, the demands can be even more intense. Dual-earner couples may increase the strain on themselves to avoid creating stress for their children. Although there is no evidence to indicate that the dual-earner lifestyle is stressful to children, the stress experienced by the parents may affect the children indirectly.

Working Mothers

Working mothers have become the norm in the United States. Maternal employment may have variable effects on preschool children's health (Mindlin, Jenkins, and Law, 2009). The quality of child care is a persistent concern for all working parents (see Evidence-Based Practice box). Determinants of child care quality are based on health and safety requirements, responsive and warm interaction between staff and children, developmentally appropriate activities, trained staff, limited group size, age-appropriate caregivers, adequate staff-to-child ratios, and adequate indoor and outdoor space. Nurses play an important role in helping families find suitable sources of child care and prepare children for this experience (see Alternate Child Care Arrangements, Chapter 10).

---

*1650 South Dixie Hwy, Suite 402, Boca Raton, FL 33432; 800-637-7974; http://parentswithoutpartners.org.

Daycare for Preschool Children

ASK THE QUESTION

Does daycare have an effect on preschool education, health, and welfare?

SEARCH FOR THE EVIDENCE

Search strategies

Randomized controlled trials of daycare for preschool children were identified using electronic databases, hand searches of relevant literature, and contact with authors.

Databases used

MEDLINE, EMBASE, Cochrane Controlled Trials Register, Social Science Citation Index, PsycLIT, ERIC

CRITICALLY ANALYZE THE EVIDENCE

GRADE criteria: Evidence quality high; recommendation strong (Guyatt, Oxman, Vist, et al, 2008)

A Cochrane Library systematic review found seven randomized control trials and one quasi-randomized study after examining 920 abstracts and 19 books (Zortich, Roberts, and Oakley, 2005). All of the eight studies were conducted in the United States. In these eight studies, a total of 2203 children were randomized to daycare or a control group. All subjects were less than 4 years old at enrollment. Daycare ranged from 2 hr/wk for 8 months to 7 hr/day, 5 day/wk, for 7 years. All studies examined cognitive development, six studies examined school performance, four studies evaluated behavior, and one study assessed children's health.

The NICHD Early Child Care Research Network (Belsky, Vandell, Burchinal, et al, 2007) followed more than 1300 children receiving early child care and found that, although parenting was a stronger and more consistent predictor of children's development than early child care experiences, higher-quality care predicted higher vocabulary scores, and higher daycare exposure predicted more teacher-reported problem behaviors through sixth grade.

Bradley and Vandell (2007) evaluated studies of early child care with specific attention to the impact of the child's age, the time spent in child care, and quality and type of care facility on adaptive functioning. Children who were younger when child care began and were cared for 30 or more hours a week experienced stress-related behaviors. These children had higher language scores. The likelihood of communicable illness and ear infections was increased when six or more children were together.

APPLY THE EVIDENCE: NURSING IMPLICATIONS

- Parenting is a stronger and more consistent predictor of child development than the early child care experience.
- Studies revealed out-of-home daycare has beneficial effects for children, enhancing cognitive development and preventing later school failures.
- Observational studies have reported that daycare can negatively affect child development.
- Evidence suggests that out-of-home daycare can have a positive effect on social outcomes for children and their families.

References

Belsky J, Vandell DL, Burchinal M, et al: Are there long-term effects of early child care? *Child Development* 78(2):681-701, 2007.

Bradley RH, Vandell DL: Child care and the well-being of children, *Arch Pediatr Adolesc Med* 161(7):669-676, 2007.

Guyatt GH, Oxman AD, Vist GE, et al: GRADE: an emerging consensus on rating quality of evidence and strength of recommendations, *BMJ* 336:924-926, 2008.

Zortich B, Roberts I, Oakley A: Day care for pre-school children, *Cochrane Database Syst Rev* (2):CD000564, 2000. In *The Cochrane Library*, issue 3, 2005.

FOSTER PARENTING

The term **foster care** is defined as placement in an approved living situation away from the family of origin (Annie E Casey Foundation, 2009; American Academy of Pediatrics, 2000). The living situation may be an approved foster home, possibly with other children, or a preadoptive home. Each state provides a standard for the role of foster parent and a process by which to become one. These "parents" contract with the state to provide a home for children for a limited duration. Most states require about 27 hours of training before being on contract and at least 12 hours of continuing education a year. Foster parents may be required to attend a foster parent support group that is often separate from a state agency. Each state has guidelines regarding the relative health of the prospective foster parents and their families, background checks regarding legal issues for the adults, personal interviews, and a safety inspection of the residence and surroundings (Chamberlain, Price, Leve, et al, 2008).

Foster homes include both kinship and nonrelative placements. Since the 1980s, the proportion of children in out-of-home care placed with relatives has increased rapidly and been accompanied by a decrease in the number of foster families. As with their nonfoster counterparts, much of the child's adjust-ment depends on the family's stability and available resources. Even though foster homes are designed to provide short-term care, it is not unusual for children to stay for many years.

Nurses should be aware that nearly 700,000 children spend time living in foster care in a given year, many of them facing developmental concerns (Annie E Casey Foundation, 2009; American Academy of Pediatrics, 2000). Children from lower-income, single-mother, and mother-partner families are considerably more likely to be living in foster care (Berger and Waldfogel, 2004). Children in foster care tend to have a higher than normal incidence of acute and chronic health problems and may experience feelings of isolation or confusion (Annie E Casey Foundation, 2009). Foster children are often at risk because of their previous caretaking environment. Nurses should strive to implement strategies to improve the health care for this group of children. In particular, assessment and case management skills are required to involve other disciplines in meeting their needs.

ACCOMMODATING CONTEMPORARY PARENTING SITUATIONS

During recent years, both the private and government sectors have identified specific problems of contemporary families.

Many of these issues involve working parents. One significant stressor for the working single parent or for dual-earner families is when a child becomes ill. The frequency of childhood illness, exclusion practices of most licensed child care programs, and employer's limited sick-leave policies are other contributing factors. Most authorities agree that a familiar face and place are important components of sick-child care, and some argue that the only place for an ill child is at home with a parent or other relative.

Some employers have become more family focused and provide time off for parents to be with sick children. Increasing numbers are becoming more generous in the amount of time they allow parents (fathers as well as mothers) to remain at home after the birth or adoption of a child. Flexible work schedules and family-oriented legislation can ease the burden of managing family and work responsibilities. The passage of the Family and Medical Leave Act (FMLA) in 1993 set the stage for a greater focus on the issues of contemporary families. FMLA allows eligible employees to take up to 12 weeks of unpaid leave each year to care for newborn or newly adopted children, parents, or spouses who have serious health conditions, or to recover from their own serious health condition.

KEY POINTS

- Because there is no agreement about the definition of family, a family is what an individual considers it to be.
- Three theories that have significant application to pediatric nursing are family systems theory, family stress theory, and developmental theory.
- Although the traditional family structure is nuclear or extended, in recent years other forms, such as the single-parent family, have become more prominent.
- Family size and position within the family structure have a strong impact on a child's development.
- Interpersonal skills and a basic understanding of childhood growth and development are two essential areas of focus for parents.
- Parental control tends to be predominantly one of three types: authoritarian, permissive, or authoritative.

- Three areas of special concern to adoptive families include the initial attachment process, the task of telling the children they are adopted, and identity formation during adolescence.
- Marital factors within the home significantly influence a child's development. The impact of divorce on a child depends on the child's age, the outcome, and the quality of the parent-child relationship and parental care following the divorce.
- Single parenting and stepparenting create adjustment difficulties and add stress to the already demanding parental role. Significant numbers of children will live in a single-parent or reconstituted family at some point.

ANSWERS TO CRITICAL THINKING EXERCISE

Parenting the Adopted Child

1. Yes. Although there is no one best time to tell children they are adopted, most authorities believe that children should be informed before they enter school to avoid learning about it from third parties. In addition, authorities agree that children should be told at an age young enough so that, as they grow older, they do not remember a time when they did not know they were adopted.

2. **a.** The best time is highly individualized and based on the child's readiness. For some children, this may be when they ask about where babies come from. Children have a more difficult adjustment if disclosure occurs when they are older, and waiting until adolescence is too late.
   b. Parents should be completely honest with the child and provide information about the adoption in a matter-of-fact way. Sharing the story of adoption is an important parental responsibility and can be handled much like a parent shares birth experiences with a biologic child.
   c. Parents should anticipate that children may act out after being told that they are adopted. Some children use the fact of their adoption as a weapon to manipulate and threaten their parents. Allowing children to express their feelings and emotions after they have been told about their adoption is important.

3. Because Justin's parents have requested guidance, it is appropriate for you, as the nurse, to provide information about how and when they should tell Justin he is adopted. However, the nurse's first priority is to be certain that Justin's parents are comfortable with this information, and that they feel free to ask any further questions and to obtain additional information. Because Justin is only 12 months old, his parents have time to think about how they will present this information to Justin and to prepare for the disclosure. They also have time to discuss how they will react to the feelings, emotions, and behaviors that Justin may demonstrate after he learns he is adopted.

4. Yes, at the present time, most authorities agree that children should be told about the fact that they are adopted, and that disclosure of this information should occur before the school-age years.

REFERENCES

Afifi TO, Boman J, Fleisher W, et al: The relationship between child abuse, parental divorce, and lifetime mental disorders and suicidality in a nationally representative adult sample, *Child Abuse Negl* 33(3):139-147, 2009.

Ahrons CR: Family ties after divorce: long-term implications for children, *Family Process* 46(1):53-65, 2007.

American Academy of Pediatrics: Family pediatrics: report of the Task Force on the Family, *Pediatrics* 111(6):1541-1571, 2003.

American Academy of Pediatrics, Committee on Early Childhood, Adoption, and Dependent Care: Development issues for young children in foster care (RE0012), *Pediatrics* 106(5): 1145-1150, 2000.

Annie E Casey Foundation: *2009 Kids count data book: state profiles of child well-being,* Baltimore, 2009, The Foundation.

Berger L, Waldfogel J: Out-of-home placement of children and economic factors: an empirical analysis, *Rev Econo Household* 2(4):387-411, 2004.

Blackwell CW: Belief in the "free choice" model of homosexuality: a correlate of homophobia in registered nurses, *J LGBT Health Res* 3(3):31-40, 2007.

Bomar PJ: *Promoting health in families,* ed 3, Philadelphia, 2004, Saunders.

Cain DS: Parenting online and lay literature on infant spanking: information readily available to parents, *Soc Work Health Care* 47(2):174-184, 2008.

Centers for Disease Control and Prevention: Births marriages, divorces, and deaths: provisional date for February 2008, *Natl Vital Stat Rep* 57(5):1-6, 2008.

Chamberlain P, Price J, Leve LD, et al: Prevention of behavior problems for children in foster care: outcomes and mediation effects, *Prev Sci* 9(1):17-27, 2008.

Deave T, Johnson D, Ingram J: Transition to parenthood: the needs of parents in pregnancy and early parenthood, *BMC Pregnancy Childbirth* 29(8):30, 2008.

Duvall ER: *Family development,* ed 5, Philadelphia, 1977, Lippincott.

Fergusson E, Maughan B, Golding J: Which children receive grandparental care and what effect does it have? *Child Psychol Psychiatry* 49(2):161-169, 2008.

Fisher C, Lindhorst H, Matthews T, et al: Nursing staff attitudes and behaviors regarding family presence in the hospital setting, *J Adv Nurs* 64(6):615-624, 2008.

Friedman MM, Bowden VR, Jones EG: *Family nursing: research theory and practice,* ed 5, Upper Saddle River, NJ, 2003, Prentice Hall.

Goldenberg I, Goldenberg H: *Family theory: an overview,* ed 7, Pacific Grove, Calif, 2008, Brooks-Cole Cengage Learning.

Hamilton BE, Minino AM, Martin JA, et al: Annual summary of vital statistics: 2005, *Pediatrics* 119(2):345-360, 2007.

Hanson SMH, Gedaly-Duff V, Kaakinen JR: *Family health care nursing,* ed 3, Philadelphia, 2005, Davis.

Hoeve M, Dubas JS, Eichelsheim VI, et al: The relationship between parenting and delinquency: a meta-analysis, *J Abnorm Child Psychol* 37(6):749-775, 2009.

Hubbs-Tait L, Kennedy TS, Page MC, et al: Parental feeding practices predict authoritative, authoritarian, and permissive parenting styles, *J Am Diet Assoc* 108(7):1154-1161, 2008.

Kreider RM, Elliott DB: America's families and living arrangements: 2007. In *US Census Bureau: Current population reports,* Washington, DC, 2009, The Bureau.

Larzelere RE: Disciplinary spanking: the scientific evidence, *J Dev Behav Pediatr* 29(4):334-335, 2008.

Liddle HA, Santisteban DA, Levant RF, et al: *Family psychology,* Washington, DC, 2002, American Psychological Association.

Martin JA, Kung KC, Mathews TJ, et al: Annual summary of vital statistics: 2006, *Pediatrics* 121(4):788-801, 2008.

McCubbin MA, McCubbin HI: Families coping with illness: the resiliency model of family stress, adjustment, and adaptation. In Danielson CB, Bissel BH, Winstead-Fry P, editors: *Families, health, and illness,* St. Louis, 1994, Mosby.

Mindlin M, Jenkins R, Law C: Maternal employment and indicators of child health: a systemic review in pre-school children in OECD countries, *J Epidemiol Commun Health* 63(5):340-350, 2009.

Pawelski JG, Perrin EC, Foy JM, et al: The effects of marriage, civil union, and domestic partnership laws on the health and well-being of children, *Pediatrics* 118(1):349-364, 2006.

Power N, Franck L: Parent participation in the care of hospitalized children: a systematic review, *J Adv Nurs* 62(6):622-641, 2008.

Community-Based Nursing Care of the Child and Family

Christine A. Brosnan and Sandra L. Upchurch

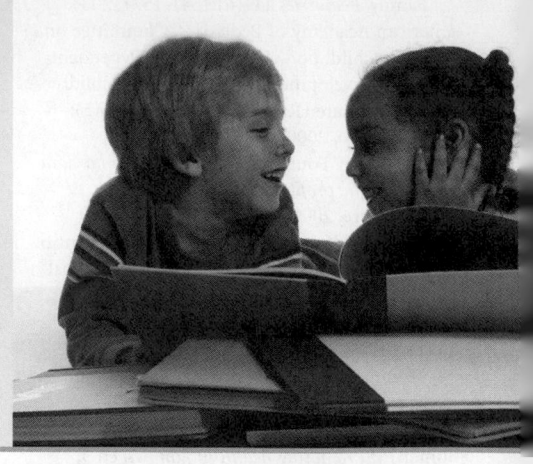

evolve WEBSITE

RELATED TOPICS

CHAPTER OUTLINE

COMMUNITY HEALTH CONCEPTS

COMMUNITY

Healthy communities provide children not only with high-quality medical care, but also with a nurturing, safe place to live and grow. They provide a good infrastructure, which includes such structures as roads, sidewalks, schools, and playgrounds. Healthy communities address concerns through collaboration between and among citizens, businesses, and governmental and private agencies. They address the concerns using problem-solving strategies within the confines of the community's value system, thus increasing the community's own capacity to meet its needs (Flynn and Ivanov, 2004). The health of children and their families is greatly influenced by their community, and nurses can make a significant contribution by working with the community to promote children's health. Nurses working with pediatric populations need to understand the concepts and processes critical to addressing pediatric concerns from a community health perspective.

This chapter focuses on community health nursing as it relates to children. First, it outlines and defines the concepts that serve as the basis of the community health nursing process.

Next, it describes the process step by step. It illustrates the use of the process in addressing a very real child health concern: bicycle safety.

> **NURSING TIP** Knowing the characteristics of a healthy community will help the nurse develop a care plan. A healthy community shapes its own future by embracing diversity and connecting its people and resources. Members of organizations in healthy communities are being asked to show their impact, that is, the actual costs and benefits of their work.

A **community** can be defined as a group of individuals with shared characteristics or interests who relate to each other (Allender and Spradley, 2005a). A community includes children and families, the physical environment, educational facilities, safety and transportation resources, political and governmental agencies, health and social services, communication resources, economic resources, and recreational facilities (Anderson and McFarlane, 2008b). Community health initiatives are directed at either the health of the community as a whole or at specific populations within the community that have unique needs. In this context, **populations** can be described as groups of people who live in a community, such as school-age children. Common values often guide behaviors of populations in relation to health promotion and disease prevention activities. Subpopulations, or aggregates, are more narrowly defined groups (e.g., obese middle-school children) toward whom nurses direct activities to improve the health status of individuals in the group (McEwen and Nies, 2007). A geographic community is one that is delineated by its geographic boundaries. These boundaries may be defined, for example, by zip codes, census tracts, or city limits. Individuals in a community who collaborate to solve a problem that affects them, whether it be a health problem, a financial problem, or a social problem, are often called a community of solution (Allender and Spradley, 2005a).

Community care involves a collaboration of individuals and groups, including health care providers, advocates, governments, managed care organizations, businesses, children, and families, within a specific community. The goal of the collaborative effort is to provide services that promote the child health initiatives of *Healthy People 2020* (www.healthypeople.gov) (US Department of Health and Human Services, 2009). Community care is "without walls" in that the services of the health care system are frequently redesigned to meet the community's changing needs. Those involved in community care collaborate with the community to identify, plan, intervene, and evaluate activities that improve the community's health (Anderson and McFarlane, 2008b). Stakeholders in the process are individuals in the community who contribute resources, services, and financial support; implement interventions; or are the recipients of services (Smith and Maurer, 2005).

Community health nursing focuses on promoting and maintaining the health of individuals, families, and groups in the community setting. It is a synthesis of nursing and public health, emphasizing personal responsibility for health and self-care. At its best, community health nursing empowers communities by enabling members to gain the knowledge and skills needed to fulfill their own needs.

Community health concepts are useful in addressing health concerns in many different settings (Box 4-1). These health concerns are addressed by the American Nurses Association (2007) *Public Health Nursing's Scope and Standards of Practice,* which incorporate both standards of care (assessment, diagnosis, outcome identification, planning, implementation, and evaluation) and standards of professional performance (quality of care, performance appraisal, education, collegiality, collaboration, research, and resource utilization). The Quad Council of Public Health Nursing Organizations (2003), an alliance of the four national nursing organizations that addresses public health nursing issues, finalized core competencies to be used in conjunction with these documents (Box 4-2).

The roles and functions of the community health nurse continue to evolve. In the future, more pediatric nurses will be working in community settings. The Health Resources and Services Administration (2004) reported that 22.7% of the total registered nurse workforce was employed in a community or public health setting or in ambulatory care. Only 57.4% of registered nurses practiced in hospital settings, and a slight trend is developing away from hospitals as the major employer of nurses.

Traditionally, the roles and functions of community health nurses included caregiver, advocate, case manager, case finder, counselor, educator, epidemiologist, group process leader, health planner, and manager (Clark, 2008). For example, the nurse employed in a pediatric outpatient clinic functions in a number of roles to provide care to a child with type 2 diabetes. The nurse provides case management by coordinating care among the disciplines, counseling by supporting the child and family through a developmental crisis, and case finding by identifying risk factors in the child's siblings. New roles are always emerging for the nurse who works with pediatric populations in the community. The work involved during times of natural disasters, public health threats, and terrorism attacks is one example (Box 4-3).

The Institute of Medicine developed a list of core functions to guide the work of public health professionals, including nurses. The core functions are directed at providing population-wide services and personal and home services for people at risk (Institute of Medicine, 1988; Allender and Spradley, 2005b). The population-wide services are based on assessment of health status monitoring and on disease surveillance, policy development, and assurance that can be translated into service. The skill set important for the nurse in a public health setting includes the ability to analyze data, measure health status, connect people to organizations, bring about change in organizations, build strength in diversity, build coalitions, develop interdisciplinary teams, and devise approaches to quality improvement (Gebbie and Hwang, 2000). For example, the pediatric nurse employed in a managed care environment may be asked to develop a creative approach to teaching children with asthma about peak flow meters during emergency department visits. Included in the request may be a mechanism for

---

BOX 4-1   COMMUNITY HEALTH CARE SETTINGS

- Home health agencies
- Schools
- Physicians' offices
- Ambulatory health clinics
- Emergency departments
- Triage call centers
- Insurance agencies
- Health departments
- International relief agencies
- Health education agencies
- Juvenile detention facilities
- Camps
- Daycare centers
- Foster care facilities
- Parishes
- Hospices
- Occupational health sites
- Rehabilitation agencies

BOX 4-2   PUBLIC HEALTH NURSING COMPETENCIES

Domain #1—Analytic Assessment Skills
Domain #2—Policy Development/Program Planning Skills
Domain #3—Communication Skills
Domain #4—Cultural Competency Skills
Domain #5—Community Dimensions of Practice Skills
Domain #6—Basic Public Health Sciences Skills
Domain #7—Financial Planning and Management Skills
Domain #8—Leadership and Systems Thinking Skills

Quad Council of Public Health Nursing Organizations: *Quad council PHN competencies,* 2003, available at www.astdn.org/publication_quad_council_phn_competencies.htm (accessed April 14, 2009).

BOX 4-3	EVOLVING ROLE OF THE PEDIATRIC NURSE: NATURAL AND MAN-MADE DISASTERS

Communities are affected by disasters, either natural disasters like hurricanes and wildfires or man-made disasters like terrorist attacks. During disasters, communities may not have the resources to respond and recover on their own. Pediatric nurses in all settings need to know disaster management stages, which include:

1. **Prevention**—Identification of disaster risks, education about what actions to take
2. **Preparedness and planning**
   A. For **individuals and families**—Training in first aid, an emergency disaster kit, a predetermined place to meet, and a communication plan
   B. For **communities and agencies**—Determination of the lines of authority and communication; coordination of personnel, supplies, and equipment; evacuation; rescue; and care of the dead
3. **Response**—Begins after the disaster; implementation of plans, which may include shelter in place for individuals, evacuation, or search and rescue; calmness and patience essential characteristics for all individuals involved

An important question for nurses to consider is, Will nurses care for patients in the community during the disaster or will they stay with their own family? (See Internet Resources.)

Adapted from Mendias EP, Grimes DE: Preventing and managing community emergencies: disasters and infectious diseases. In Anderson ET, McFarlane J, editors: *Community as partner*, Philadelphia, 2008, WoltersKluwer/Lippincott Williams & Wilkins; and Summerlin EB: Natural and man-made disasters. In Nies MA, McEwen M, editors: *Community/public health nursing: promoting the health of populations*, Philadelphia, 2007, Saunders.

evaluating the cost of the approach and the occurrence of repeated emergency department visits.

NURSING TIP To study improvement in patient care, the Institute of Medicine convened the First Annual Crossing the Quality Chasm Summit: a Focus on Communities. Members of the group realized that "communities could serve as 'laboratories of innovation' to assess what does or doesn't work before a policy is adopted." A community-level perspective is important for a realistic health care system (Adams, Greiner, and Corrigan, 2004).

DEMOGRAPHY

Demography is the study of population characteristics. Demographic characteristics include age, gender, race and ethnicity, socioeconomic status, and education. Individuals, families, and communities have demographic characteristics that may affect their health risks (Cashaw, 2008). **Risk** is the probability of developing a disease, injury, or illness. Age is one of the most important risk factors to consider for disease prevention and the development of certain health conditions. For example, all children under age 5 years and especially those under 6 months of age are at higher risk for respiratory syncytial virus than older children (Hall, Weinberg, and Iwane, 2009). Gender also plays an important role. Males are at much greater risk of hemophilia A and B than females. Certain races and ethnic groups have long been associated with increased risk for certain diseases and disorders, but it is now thought that, aside from genetic predisposition, there is a complicated relationship between minority status and socioeconomic status that increases

the risk for disease and disability (Smith, 2000). Low socioeconomic status predisposes children to a variety of problems. Poor children are more likely to be hospitalized for pneumonia, asthma, dehydration, and gastroenteritis than children from affluent families (Institute of Medicine, 1998; Committee on Evaluation of Children's Health, 2004). Preschool children without health insurance are also less likely to be immunized against childhood illnesses than children who have private insurance (Santoli, Huet, Smith, et al, 2004).

NURSING TIP Nurses should recognize the importance of social capital in the populations where they work. Social capital is similar to social support at the individual level. It is a sociocultural aspect of health that permits access to and participation in relationships that provide resources required for the necessities of life (Clark, 2008).

EPIDEMIOLOGY

Epidemiology is the science of population health applied to the detection of morbidity and mortality in a population. The **epidemiologic process** identifies the distribution and causes of disease or injury across a population (Cashaw, 2008). It also serves as an important component in developing health programs. For example, *Healthy People 2020* incorporates a process to develop a set of health objectives for the United States (US Department of Health and Human Services, 2009). Health professionals in community, state, and health care organizations use the objectives as a guide to develop programs that have the greatest impact on children's health.

Distribution of Disease, Injury, or Illness

Morbidity rates are used to measure disease and injury, and, along with natality (ratio of live births in an area to the population of that area) and mortality rates, they present an objective picture of a community's health status. There are two types of morbidity rates: incidence and prevalence. **Incidence** measures the occurrence of new events in a population during a time period. **Prevalence** measures existing events in a population during a time period (Hennekens and Buring, 1987). For example, the incidence of type 1 diabetes in a community is estimated by counting the new cases in a population and dividing that figure by the number of people at risk. The prevalence is estimated by counting the existing cases of type 1 diabetes in a population and dividing that figure by the number of people at risk. Both incidence and prevalence are usually given as rates per 1000, 10,000, or 100,000 population, depending on their frequency. Box 4-4 presents frequently used rates.

Epidemiologic Triangle

Three factors form the **epidemiologic triangle**, and their interrelationship alters the risk of acquiring a disease or condition (McKeown and Messias, 2006). These factors are agent, host, and environment. An **agent** is responsible for causing a disease and may be an infectious agent such as *Mycobacterium tuberculosis*, a chemical agent such as lead in paint, or a physical agent such as fire. **Host** factors are those that are specific to an individual or group. These can be genetic factors that cannot be controlled, or they can be lifestyle factors, such as food selection or exercise patterns. **Environmental** factors provide a

BOX 4-4	FREQUENTLY USED MORTALITY AND MORBIDITY RATES

$$\text{Crude birth rate} = \frac{\text{Number of births in a population within a time period} \times 1000}{\text{Total population}}$$

$$\text{Crude death rate} = \frac{\text{Number of deaths in a population within a time period} \times 1000}{\text{Total population}}$$

$$\text{Cause-specific death rate} = \frac{\text{Number of deaths in a population due to a certain disease within a time period} \times 1000}{\text{Total population}}$$

$$\text{Age-specific death rate} = \frac{\text{Number of deaths in a population in a certain age-group within a time period} \times 1000}{\text{Total population in that age-group}}$$

$$\text{Incidence of disease} = \frac{\text{Number of new events in a population within a time period} \times 1000}{\text{Total at-risk population}}$$

$$\text{Prevalence of disease} = \frac{\text{Number of existing events in a population within a time period} \times 1000}{\text{Total at-risk population}}$$

setting and include the climatic conditions in which the host lives and factors related to the home, neighborhood, and school.

Levels of Prevention

Community health programs are based on three classic levels of prevention (Leavell and Clark, 1965). **Primary prevention** focuses on health promotion and prevention of disease or injury. Examples of primary prevention activities include well-child care clinics, immunization programs, safety programs (bike helmets, car seats, seat belts, childproof containers), nutrition programs, environmental efforts (clean air programs), sanitation measures (chlorinated water, garbage removal, sewage treatment), and community parenting classes. **Secondary prevention** focuses on screening and early diagnosis of disease. Examples of secondary interventions include tuberculosis and lead screening programs and mental health counseling for stressful events such as separation, divorce, death, or community natural disasters (e.g., earthquakes, floods, and hurricanes). **Tertiary prevention** focuses on optimizing function for children with disabilities or chronic diseases. Tertiary interventions include rehabilitation and disease management programs for asthma, sickle cell disease, cancer, and anorexia and special education programs for children.

Screening

Community health nurses are frequently involved in screening, a secondary prevention activity. The purpose of screening is to detect and treat disease early in its pathogenesis to prevent the spread and progression of the disease (Wilson and Jungner, 1968). However, screening is not appropriate for every condition. In a seminal article, Wilson and Jungner (1968) described 10 principles for assessment tools that should be used when developing screening programs (Box 4-5). Although screening may bring benefits, a certain amount of risk is associated with any intervention. Screening poses the psychologic risk associated with false-positive results. There is the danger that a parent may continue to worry and perhaps treat a child with a positive screen differently even after further diagnostic testing determines the child is normal (Moran, Quirk, Duff, et al, 2007; van der Ploeg, Lanting, Kauffman-de Boer, et al, 2008). It is essen-

BOX 4-5	PRINCIPLES OF EARLY DISEASE DETECTION

1. The condition sought should be an important health problem.
2. There should be an accepted treatment for patients with recognized disease.
3. Facilities for diagnosis and treatment should be available.
4. There should be a recognizable latent or early symptomatic stage.
5. There should be a suitable test or examination.
6. The test should be acceptable to the population.
7. The natural history of the condition, including development from latent to declared disease, should be adequately understood.
8. There should be an agreed policy on whom to treat.
9. The cost of case finding (including diagnosis and treatment of patients diagnosed) should be economically balanced in relation to possible expenditures on medical care as a whole.
10. Case finding should be a continuing process and not a "once and for all" project.

From Wilson JMG, Jungner G: *Principles and practice of screening for disease,* Public Health Papers 34, Geneva, 1968, World Health Organization.

tial to determine the evidence for a proposed screening program before beginning the program to ensure the benefits exceed the risks and cost (see Evidence-Based Practice box).

ECONOMICS

A basic understanding of the economics of health care is essential because it enables the nurse to participate in decision making about the value of children's health programs. Economists theorize that individuals and societies view health as a basic utility, that is, something that is perceived as important and valuable (Gold, 1996). Other basic utilities are food, shelter, and clothing. People are willing to trade resources, such as money and time, for a program or intervention that will improve their health. Economists measure the amount of resources individuals and communities are willing to pay for good health. They also examine how different groups prioritize health care needs and allocate health care dollars. Methods for defining and estimating cost have been well described, as has

EVIDENCE-BASED PRACTICE

Acanthosis Nigricans and the Risk of Type 2 Diabetes in Children

ASK THE QUESTION

In a school-aged population, is acanthosis nigricans (AN) screening effective in detecting insulin resistance?

SEARCH FOR THE EVIDENCE

Search strategies

Keywords *acanthosis nigricans, screening,* and *insulin resistance* were used to find articles published in English between 1996 and 2009. Studies were limited to children who were 0 to 18 years of age.

Databases used

PubMed, CINAHL, Cochrane Database of Systematic Reviews, Centers for Disease Control and Prevention (CDC)

CRITICALLY ANALYZE THE EVIDENCE

GRADE criteria: Evidence quality low; recommendation weak (Guyatt, Oxman, Vist, et al, 2008)

Seven correlational studies were reviewed. Five of the studies screened community or school populations, and two studies screened clinic populations. In six of the studies, the prevalence of AN ranged from 5% in a general pediatric population (Drobac, Brickman, Smith, et al, 2004) to 73% in a sample of overweight children (Kobaissi, Weigensberg, Ball, et al, 2004). In the seventh study, Ice, Murphy, Minor, and colleagues (2009) screened 40,361 children to determine risk factors associated with metabolic syndrome. They reported that, in a sample of 676 children with AN, 60.8% were also insulin resistant. A limitation of the study was that the researchers did not measure insulin resistance in children without AN, making it impossible to compare the two groups. In general, obesity was found to be a more effective predictor of insulin resistance than AN (Kobaissi, Weigensberg, Ball, et al, 2004; Mukhtar, Cleverley, Voorhees, et al, 2001; Nguyen, Keil, Russell, et al, 2001). The CDC discourages community and school screening for AN because there is insufficient evidence that it predicts diabetes development (Centers for Disease Control and Prevention, 2005).

APPLY THE EVIDENCE: NURSING IMPLICATIONS

- AN screening should not be adopted as part of a community or schoolwide screening program.
- Further research is needed to determine the most predictive indicator of diabetes development.

References

Centers for Disease Control and Prevention: CDC statement on screening children for acanthosis nigricans in schools and communities, *News and Information—CDC Statements on Diabetes Issues,* 2005, available at www.cdc.gov/diabetes/news (accessed April 3, 2009).

Drobac S, Brickman W, Smith T, et al: Evaluation of a type 2 diabetes screening protocol in an urban pediatric clinic, *Pediatrics* 114(1):141-148, 2004.

Guyatt GH, Oxman AD, Vist GE, et al: GRADE: an emerging consensus on rating quality of evidence and strength of recommendations, *BMJ* 336:924-926, 2008.

Ice CL, Murphy E, Minor VE, et al: Metabolic syndrome in fifth grade children with acanthosis nigricans: results from the CARDIAC project, *World J Pediatr* 5(1), 2009, available at www.wjpch.com (accessed February 15, 2009).

Kobaissi HA, Weigensberg MJ, Ball GD, et al: Relation between acanthosis nigricans and insulin sensitivity in overweight Hispanic children at risk for type 2 diabetes, *Diabetes Care* 27(6):1412-1416, 2004.

Mukhtar Q, Cleverley G, Voorhees RE, et al: Prevalence of acanthosis nigricans and its association with hyperinsulinemia in New Mexico adolescents, *J Adolesc Health* 28(5):372-376, 2001.

Nguyen TT, Keil MF, Russell DL, et al: Relation of acanthosis nigricans to hyperinsulinemia and insulin sensitivity in overweight African American and white children, *J Pediatr* 138(4):474-480, 2001.

---

the need for a standardized approach to the measurement of cost and effects (Brosnan and Swint, 2001; Drummond, Sculpher, Torrance, et al, 2005).

Economic evaluation provides objective information to establish a program's value to the community. An example is the use of ambulatory blood pressure monitoring to evaluate the presence of continuous stage 1 hypertension versus white coat hypertension in children. Swartz, Srivaths, Croix, and colleagues (2008) reviewed the records of 267 children who were referred for diagnosis of stage 1 hypertension because of initial readings of increased blood pressure. They determined that the use of 24-hour ambulatory monitoring before initiating more expensive diagnostic tests would have identified children with benign white coat hypertension who did not need treatment. The authors reported that the potential savings of ambulatory blood pressure monitoring were in excess of $2 million for every 1000 children referred.

> **NURSING TIP** In today's health care climate of interdisciplinary practice and managed care, nurses are expected to understand basic economic concepts and collaborate with others in applying the methods of cost analysis to their practice. Nurses who are unable to do this risk loss of decision-making responsibilities for themselves and their patients.

A **cost-effectiveness analysis,** the most common type of economic evaluation, requires a comparison of one program with an alternative. In this type of analysis the costs of nursing interventions are calculated in dollars, and end points are calculated in health units (such as lives saved or hospital days avoided). The results are presented in a ratio with costs in the numerator and health units in the denominator. For example, Caviness, Cantor, Allen, and colleagues (2004) analyzed the impact of providing antibodies to prevent bacterial endocarditis in children with fever and a history of cardiac pathologic conditions who were scheduled for urinary catheterization. They found the cost ranged from $70 million to $95 million per case of bacterial endocarditis prevented. They concluded that preventive antibody treatment was not cost-effective.

COMMUNITY NURSING PROCESS

In community nursing the focus of the nursing process shifts from the individual child and family to the community or target population. The stages of the process (assessment, diagnosis, planning, intervention, and evaluation) are similar whether the client is one child or a population of children. Only the types of interventions and indicators of wellness and illness differ

(Anderson and McFarlane, 2008a). Assessment is focused on collecting subjective and objective information about the target population to diagnose problems based on community needs. Planning involves the development of community-centered interventions. The nurse works with the community to implement a program that enables members to reach their goals and to evaluate whether the goals were met. Community nursing is collaborative, and the nurse is one member of a community team that includes other health professionals, educators, politicians, religious leaders, members of public and voluntary organizations, and consumers. The nurse's role depends on the project's scope, the target population, and the team members' expertise. For instance, the school nurse may assume a leadership role in planning for the health needs of elementary schoolchildren and serve as a panel member on a citywide committee assessing environmental pollution.

COMMUNITY NEEDS ASSESSMENT

The assessment phase of the community nursing process is called a community needs assessment. Assessment involves the collection of subjective and objective information about a community. Subjective information indicates what community members say are their most important needs and can be determined in a number of ways. One way is to distribute questionnaires to a sample of people living in the community. Another way is to interview community members directly by telephoning or meeting with individuals, such as community leaders, who represent the group or who have a special role in the group. The needs community stakeholders express, or their felt needs, must be considered in planning interventions.

The nurse collects objective information, or data, either by direct observation or through written sources. A windshield tour is one method of direct observation. Nurses drive through a neighborhood and take notes about the environment, including the appearance of houses, the presence of sidewalks and gutters, and the number of public areas. Objective information about the community's health status can also be obtained from such sources as the chamber of commerce, census bureaus, libraries, state health departments, and the Internet sites of voluntary health organizations and government agencies. Information about community resources can be found in service directories compiled by organizations such as the United Way and population-specific books provided by public and voluntary agencies.

One way to organize an assessment is to use a guide that lists community systems that need to be examined. This process is similar to using a physical assessment guide to examine the different body systems in an individual patient. Anderson (2008) described eight community systems that the nurse should examine: health and social services, communication, recreation, physical environment, education, safety and transportation, politics and government, and economics. During the assessment the nurse studies how well each component in the community functions and interacts to meet the health needs of children. The nurse also identifies the community's strengths and determines whether any barriers prevent access to care for children and their families (see Critical Thinking Exercise).

Once the assessment is completed, the community nurse collaborates with team members to analyze the results of surveys

---

❓ CRITICAL THINKING EXERCISE
Development of an After-School Program

Mary Jones is the school nurse at Ivy Elementary School. She has been in the position for 5 years and knows many of the teachers and staff members well. She eats lunch with a group of teachers daily and attends the children's choral programs. In the past, the principal at Ivy supported Ms. Jones's idea to teach a group of children with multiple dental caries about brushing their teeth. The staff and principal visit her office often, asking health-related questions and seeking information about students', their own, and their families' health. One concern is repeatedly discussed. A number of the children go home to limited adult supervision after school. Many teachers think an after-school program with activities would help students.

Ivy Elementary School: The school houses grades K-5, has 400 students, and serves a geographic area of three census tracts. The school has been in the neighborhood for 20 years and has an active parent-teacher association. Most children are bused to and from the school. The school has a race/ethnicity mix of 45% Hispanic, 35% African-American, 15% non-Hispanic Caucasian, and 5% other. Almost 50% of the students are eligible for the free school lunch program; more than 30% of the children are overweight or at risk for overweight.

1. Evidence—Is there sufficient evidence to develop an after-school program?
2. Assumptions—Describe some underlying assumptions about the following:
   a. Completing the needs assessment for the after-school program
   b. Obtaining objective data
   c. Obtaining subjective data
   d. Finding out about components of successful after-school programs
   e. After-school program's cultural acceptability to families
3. What implications and priorities can be drawn?
4. Does the evidence objectively support your conclusion?

---

and questionnaires, determines whether the needs described by community members can be met by existing community agencies, and identifies individuals at highest risk. During the analysis the demographic characteristics and the morbidity and mortality rates in the community are compared with a standard. Comparisons can be made on the basis of time or place. In time comparisons, the nurse contrasts the rates in the current year with the rates during an earlier period. In place comparisons, the nurse contrasts the rates in the community with those of a standard population. Standard rates may come from another community or from city, state, or national studies. For example, the rate of tuberculosis in a group of preschool children in the community in 2002 could be compared with the rate of tuberculosis in preschool children in the state in 2002.

A community health diagnosis is the reflection of health status, risks, or needs in relation to a causative agent. The format of a community diagnosis is similar to that of an individual nursing diagnosis in that it identifies a problem (need) and the etiology related to that problem (causative agent). An example of a community nursing diagnosis is "Increase in body mass index (BMI) among elementary school students compared with the national standard related to high intake of calories and sedentary lifestyle" (Anderson and McFarlane, 2008a).

COMMUNITY PLANNING

The nurse collaborates with community members in developing a plan that addresses the needs and problems of the target population. To maximize the use of community resources, problems should first be prioritized on the basis of their severity, the community's felt needs, and the community nurse's ability to bring about change. The nurse should also conduct a literature search for approaches that have proved effective in addressing the problem. Once the problems are prioritized, the nurse works with community members to develop at least one goal for each problem the members will address. Goals are outcomes that give direction to interventions and provide a measure of the change the interventions produced. Community interventions frequently take the form of health programs for improving the health status of the target population. Community

health programs are based on three levels of prevention: primary, secondary, and tertiary. For example, a goal for the community diagnosis of increased BMI among elementary schoolchildren is "Within 2 years the number of students with BMIs above the 95th percentile for age and sex will decrease by 20%." The nurse and community members then begin to plan a health program that includes a number of interventions to address this serious problem.

The planning group considers the resources that are already available in the community and those that will be needed for implementing a health program, including personnel, supplies

---

BOX 4-6   EXAMPLE OF COMMUNITY ASSESSMENT AND PLANNING

Lakewood is an elementary school with 500 prekindergarten to sixth-grade children. The school nurse was asked to conduct a needs assessment of the school community and to develop a care plan. The schoolchildren and their families were the target population.

Community Needs Assessment

The school nurse formed a team of community members that included parents of students who attend Lakewood Elementary School, faculty and staff, health care professionals, local religious leaders, and politicians. The group met at regular intervals. Their first task was to complete the community assessment. Team members mailed questionnaires to a random sample of families who had children attending Lakewood. They held focus groups with community members to obtain subjective information about the needs of the school community. Team members obtained objective data from the local health department, school records, and the U.S. Census Bureau. The nurse also conducted a windshield tour of the neighborhood surrounding the school. The following information was collected:

People—Lakewood is located in an ethnically diverse area composed of 20% Hispanics, 40% African-Americans, 30% non-Hispanic Caucasians, and 10% Asians. The ethnicity of students in the school is representative of the surrounding area. Lakewood is located in a large southwestern city.

Safety and transportation—School bus service was rated excellent by a majority of those surveyed. The last school bus accident occurred 10 years ago. There were no fatalities, but a few children had minor injuries. Many children bicycle to school. Over the past 5 years there were 10 bicycle accidents involving children from Lakewood. One of these accidents resulted in a fatality. In the 5 years before that three bicycle accidents occurred, and none involved a fatality. Teachers noted that many of the children do not wear bicycle helmets and that the bicycles appear old and in need of repair. Parents complained that neighborhood streets are narrow and few have curbs and sidewalks. In fact, most streets are bordered by ditches.

Economics—Although 94% of families had at least one fully employed member, 45% of the families lived below the poverty level. The number below poverty level had not changed in 10 years.

Education—Sixty percent of the adult population had a high school diploma, and 10% of this group had completed at least 1 year of college. School attendance at Lakewood was higher than overall state attendance rates.

Communication—Ninety-five percent of homes had telephones, compared with 85% 10 years ago. An estimated 10% of the target population did not speak English; Spanish was the primary language spoken in this group.

Recreation—Few places were available for small children to play. The focus groups recommended more parks and playgrounds.

Politics and government—The school system was strongly centralized and headed by a school superintendent. The city had a mayor and city council.

Social—Of those families living below the poverty level, 60% received some type of welfare assistance, including food stamps. The school lunch program served 95% of the children attending the school.

Health—Childhood immunization rates for all recommended diseases among kindergarten children in the community was 96%. This rate compared favorably to a report indicating that only 75% of states have attained

the goal of having at least 95% of kindergarten children immunized (Centers for Disease Control and Prevention, 2007). Vision and hearing screening programs at Lakewood resulted in the referral of 5% of the students for vision problems and 2% of the students for hearing problems. Review of student records indicated that all those children referred received diagnostic follow-up and treatment when indicated. Heights and weights were obtained on all students annually, and the body mass index (BMI) was determined for each student. BMI is calculated by dividing the weight in kilograms by the square of the height in meters (Flegal, Carroll, Kuzmarski, et al, 1998). Results indicated that 19% of students were above the 95th percentile for age and sex, compared with 17% nationally (Ogden, Carroll, Curtin, et al, 2006). In focus groups, students and teachers noted that school breakfasts and lunches were high in carbohydrates and fats. They also observed that decreased recess time resulted in decreased student activity during school hours.

Based on the above assessment, the following community diagnoses were made:

- Increase in injuries related to bicycle accidents
- Increase in weight among students compared with the national standard related to high intake of calories and sedentary lifestyle

Planning

Team members agreed that the increase in weight among the children should be closely monitored over the next 5 years. They also agreed that increased frequency of bicycle accidents among students was the highest priority problem, and the team developed the following goals: (1) within 6 months all children will wear helmets when bicycling, (2) within 1 year all students' bikes will be well-maintained, and (3) within 2 years no child going to or returning from school will be involved in a bicycle accident.

Team members reviewed the literature for examples of communities that had experienced similar problems, contacted school and health department officials in other areas of the country, examined the results of successful programs, and planned a health program that addressed the unique needs of the target population. The program was titled "Lakewood Bikes Safely." Program activities were the following:

1. Each September the school nurse will address the school's parent association about the importance of bicycle safety, including the need to wear a helmet and to maintain bicycle equipment. As part of the presentation, a community policeman will discuss safety guidelines.
2. The school nurse will work with parents who have a financial need to help them obtain bicycle helmets for their children and funding for bike maintenance.
3. Within 6 months school administrators and community members will petition the city to provide identified bicycle trails.

Team members determined the resources needed to implement the program, including personnel, supplies, and equipment. They estimated the total cost of setting up the program and maintaining it for 5 years and applied for funding to the school district and to the city and state health departments. The school nurse and other team members assumed responsibility for the timely implementation and evaluation of the Lakewood Bikes Safely program.

and equipment, office space, phones, and computers. The group makes decisions about the program's timeline, budget, and strategies to obtain funding. The nurse may also contact health professionals who have implemented successful programs in other communities; they can provide valuable time-saving tips and suggestions. Program descriptions are found through professional contacts, online resources, and literature reviews. An example of a community assessment and planning project is presented in Box 4-6.

COMMUNITY IMPLEMENTATION

During program implementation the nurse and community members carry out the interventions. Whether the program is simple or complex, oversight is needed to ensure that everyone involved is communicating with each other, following the plan's guidelines, keeping within the timeline, and documenting daily activities and expenses. The documentation proves invaluable during the evaluation phase of the process.

COMMUNITY EVALUATION

Evaluation identifies whether the goals and program objectives are met. Various models of program evaluation exist. A structure, process, and outcome method is commonly used by health care organizations. Donabedian (1980) described this approach as:

Structure—Where and by whom is the care delivered in a program?

Process—Was the care delivered using operational standards and within the financial guidelines of the program?

Outcome—What was the impact on health status? Was there an improvement?

Structure focuses on the qualifications of personnel; the adequacy of buildings, offices, supplies, and equipment; and the characteristics of the target population. Process focuses on the interaction of patients and providers. Process indicators include the number of people who attend a health education program, the number of pamphlets distributed, and the efficiency of the program. Outcome focuses on whether program objectives and community goals were met. Program evaluation should be ongoing to monitor performance improvement initiatives, improve the way health care is delivered, and hence improve the health status of the target population.

Another approach to evaluation can involve the two components of formative and summative evaluation. Formative evaluation occurs all along the nursing process—assessment, planning, and implementation. Continuous formative evaluation can prevent problems that could affect outcomes, since modifications can be made immediately to adjust or improve the program. The modifications can involve such areas as educational materials, facilities, personnel assignments, or attitudes. Summative evaluation involves measuring the extent to which the goals were met. It is the end point or the sum of the results of the intervention (Smith and Maurer, 2005; Worral, 2008). The terms *formative* and *summative evaluation* are sometimes used as synonyms for process and outcome evaluation, respectively.

> **NURSING TIP** Too often nurses focus most of their attention on assessment, planning, and implementation. Evaluation, which would delineate the outcomes, costs, and benefits of their work, is an integral component of the nursing process that should not be overlooked.

▐ KEY POINTS

- Caring for children within a community requires a multidisciplinary approach.
- Healthy communities provide children with not only high-quality medical care but also a nurturing, safe place to live and grow.
- Community health nursing focuses on promoting and maintaining the health of individuals, families, and groups in the community setting.
- Individuals, families, and communities have demographic characteristics that may affect their risk for disease or injury.
- Epidemiology is the science of population health applied to the detection of morbidity and mortality in a population.
- Community health programs are based on three levels of intervention: primary, secondary, and tertiary.
- Economic evaluations provide objective information to establish a program's value to society.
- A community needs assessment involves collection of subjective and objective information about the community.
- A community health diagnosis is similar to a nursing diagnosis, with an identified problem and a defined cause.
- Program planning and implementation in the community require collaboration between the nurse and community members who are in positions to promote change.
- Evaluation of effective community programs includes consideration of the program's structure, process, and outcomes.

▐ ANSWERS TO CRITICAL THINKING EXERCISE

Development of an After-School Program

1. **No**, there are not sufficient data to develop a program.
2. **a.** There are sufficient data to warrant Ms. Jones conducting a needs assessment to see whether stakeholders (e.g., parents, teachers, the principal, the parent-teacher organization

[PTO]) would see starting an after school program as a priority.

b. Objective data for the assessment could be obtained through such methods as a mail-out survey to the parents. Additionally, Ms. Jones may need to assess what after-school programs (i.e., resources) are currently available in the area, including the cost per child for care. A windshield survey could be conducted.

c. Subjective data could be obtained from the teachers during a focus group or from the parents during a parent-teacher organization (PTO) meeting.

d. The nurse could perform a literature search to learn about successful components of after-school programs and research-based evaluations of the programs.

e. Objective and subjective data could be gathered from parents to determine whether an after-school program would be considered acceptable to them.

3. With the present information, Ms. Jones should continue to informally collect data about the need for an after-school program in her conversations with the staff, principal, stu-

dents, and parents. She could consider convening a group of stakeholders to explore whether and how to proceed with the assessment. The nurse would be alert to other areas of health concerns that might take priority, such as out breaks of head lice or an increase in the number of bicycle accidents.

4. Ms. Jones conducted a literature search about research on after-school programs. She searched PubMed using the terms *after-school programs* and *children*. She found a number of relevant articles with three that caught her attention: "After School Program Impact on Physical Activity and Fitness: A Meta-Analysis" (Beets, Beighle, Erwin, et al, 2009), "After-School Youth Development Programs: A Developmental-Ecological Model of Current Research" (Riggs and Greenberg, 2004), and "Management Matters: Sustaining Funds for Youth Development Programs" (Walker, 2006).

REFERENCES

Adams K, Greiner AC, Corrigan JM, editors: *First annual Crossing the Quality Chasm Summit: a focus on communities,* Washington, DC, 2004, Institute of Medicine, National Academies Press.

Allender JA, Spradley BW: Opportunities and challenges of community health nursing. In Allender JA, Spradley BW, editors: *Community health nursing: promoting and protecting the public's health,* Philadelphia, 2005a, Lippincott Williams & Wilkins.

Allender JA, Spradley BW: Roles and settings for community health nursing practice. In Allender JA, Spradley BW, editors: *Community health nursing: promoting and protecting the public's health,* Philadelphia, 2005b, Lippincott Williams & Wilkins.

American Nurses Association: *Public health nursing's scope and standards of practice,* Washington, DC, 2007, American Nurses Publishing.

Anderson ET: A model to guide practice. In Anderson ET, McFarlane J, editors: *Community as partner,* Philadelphia, 2008, Lippincott Williams & Wilkins.

Anderson ET, McFarlane J: Community analysis and nursing diagnosis. In Anderson ET, McFarlane J, editors: *Community as partner,* Philadelphia, 2008a, Lippincott Williams & Wilkins.

Anderson ET, McFarlane J: Community assessment. In Anderson ET, McFarlane J, editors: *Community as partner,* Philadelphia, 2008b, Lippincott Williams & Wilkins.

Beets MW, Beighle A, Erwin HE, et al: After school program impact on physical activity and fitness: a meta-analysis, *Am J Prev Med* 36(6):527-537, 2009.

Brosnan CA, Swint JM: Cost analysis: concepts and application, *Public Health Nurs* 18(1):13-18, 2001.

Cashaw SA: Epidemiology, demography, and community health. In Anderson ET, McFarlane J, editors: *Community as partner,* Philadelphia, 2008, Lippincott Williams & Wilkins.

Caviness AC, Cantor SB, Allen CH, et al: A cost-effectiveness analysis of bacterial

endocarditis prophylaxis for febrile children who have cardiac lesions and undergo urinary catheterization in the emergency department, *Pediatrics* 113(5):1291-1296, 2004.

Centers for Disease Control and Prevention: Vaccination coverage among children in kindergarten—United States, 2006-07 School Year, *MMWR* 56(32):819-821, 2007.

Clark MJ: Community health nursing. In Clark MJ, editor: *Community health nursing: advocacy for population health,* Upper Saddle River, NJ, 2008, Pearson Education.

Committee on Evaluation of Children's Health: *Children's health, the nation's wealth,* Washington, DC, 2004, Institute of Medicine, National Academies Press.

Donabedian A: *The definition of quality and approaches to its assessment,* Ann Arbor, Mich, 1980, Health Administration Press.

Drummond MF, Sculpher MJ, Torrance GW, et al: *Methods for the economic evaluation of health care programmes,* ed 3, New York, 2005, Oxford University Press.

Flegal KM, Carroll MD, Kuzmarski RJ, et al: Overweight and obesity in the United States: prevalence and trends, *Int J Obes Relat Metab Disord* 22(1):39-47, 1998.

Flynn BC, Ivanov LL: Health promotion through healthy cities. In Stanhope M, Lancaster J: *Community and public health nursing,* St. Louis, 2004, Mosby.

Gebbie KM, Hwang I: Preparing currently employed public health nurses for changes in the health system, *Am J Public Health* 90(5):716-721, 2000.

Gold MR: Identifying and valuing outcomes. In Gold MR, Siegel JE, Russell LB, et al, editors: *Costeffectiveness in health and medicine,* New York, 1996, Oxford University Press.

Hall CB, Weinberg GA, Iwane MK: The burden of respiratory syncytial virus infection in young children, *N Engl J Med* 360(6):588-598, 2009.

Health Resources and Services Administration: *Findings from the national sample of RN's,* Rockville, Md, 2004, US Department of Health and Human Services, available at

http://bhpr.hrsa.gov/healthworkforce/rnsurvey04/2.htm (accessed April 15, 2009).

Hennekens CH, Buring JE: *Epidemiology in medicine,* Boston, 1987, Little Brown.

Institute of Medicine: *America's children: health insurance and access to care,* Washington, DC, 1998, National Academy Press.

Institute of Medicine: *The future of public health,* Washington, DC, 1988, National Academy Press.

Leavell HR, Clark EG: *Preventive medicine for the doctor in his community: an epidemiologic approach,* ed 3, New York, 1965, McGraw-Hill.

McEwen M, Nies AM: Health: a community view. In Nies AM, McEwen M: *Community/public health nursing,* ed 4, St Louis, 2007, Mosby.

McKeown RE, Messias DK: Epidemiologic applications. In Stanhope M, Lancaster J, editors: *Foundations of nursing in the community,* ed 2, St. Louis, 2006, Mosby.

Moran J, Quirk K, Duff A, et al: Newborn screening for CF in a regional paediatric centre: the psychosocial effects of false-positive IRT results on parents, *J Cystic Fibrosis* 6:250-254, 2007.

Ogden CL, Carroll MD, Curtin LR, et al: Prevalence of overweight and obesity in the United States, 1999-2004, *JAMA* 295(13):1549-1555, 2006.

Quad Council of Public Health Nursing Organizations: *Quad council PHN competencies,* 2003, available at www.astdn.org/publication_quad_council_phn_competencies.htm (accessed April 14, 2009).

Riggs NR, Greenberg MT: After-school youth development programs: a developmental-ecological model of current research, *Clin Child Fam Psychol Rev* 7(3):177-190, 2004.

Santoli JM, Huet NJ, Smith PJ, et al: Insurance status and vaccination coverage among US preschool children, *Pediatrics* 113(6 Suppl): 1959-1964, 2004.

Smith GD: Learning to live with complexity: ethnicity, socioeconomic position, and health in Britain and the United States, *Am J Public Health* 90:1694-1698, 2000.

Smith CM, Maurer FA: Evaluation of nursing care with communities. In Maurer FA, Smith CM, editors: *Community/public health nursing practice,* St. Louis, 2005, Mosby.

Swartz SJ, Srivaths PR, Croix B, et al: Cost-effectiveness of ambulatory blood pressure monitoring in the initial evaluation of hypertension in children, *Pediatrics* 122(6):1177-1181, 2008.

US Department of Health and Human Services: *Healthy people 2020: the road ahead, 2009,* available at www.healthypeople.gov/hp2020/default.asp (accessed Jan 19, 2009).

van der Ploeg CPB, Lanting CI, Kauffman-de Boer MA, et al: Examination of long-lasting parental concern after false-positive results of neonatal hearing screening, *Arch Dis Child* 93:508-511, 2008.

Walker KE, Management matters: sustaining funds for youth development programs,

J Public Health Manage Pract (Suppl): S17-S22, 2006.

Wilson JMG, Jungner G: *Principles and practice of screening for disease,* Public Health Papers 34, Geneva, 1968, World Health Organization.

Worral PS: Evaluation in healthcare education. In Bastable SB: *Nurse as educator: principles of teaching and learning for nursing practice,* Boston, 2008, Jones & Bartlett.

INTERNET RESOURCES

American Public Health Association—www.apha.org

Children Now—www.childrennow.org

Health Resources and Services Administration—www.hrsa.gov

Healthy People 2020—www.healthypeople.gov

Institute of Medicine—www.iom.edu

Kids Count Data, Annie E. Casey Foundation—www.kidscount.org

National Institute of Environmental Health Sciences—www.niehs.nih.gov

National Safety Council—www.nsc.org

Office of Disease Prevention and Health Promotion—http://odphp.osophs.dhhs.gov

Safe Kids Worldwide—www.safekids.org

U.S. Census Bureau, national and state census information—www.census.gov

U.S. Department of Education—www.ed.gov

U.S. Department of Health and Human Services—www.os.dhhs.gov

World Health Organization—www.who.int

CHAPTER

5

Hereditary Influences on Health Promotion of the Child and Family

Cynthia A. Prows

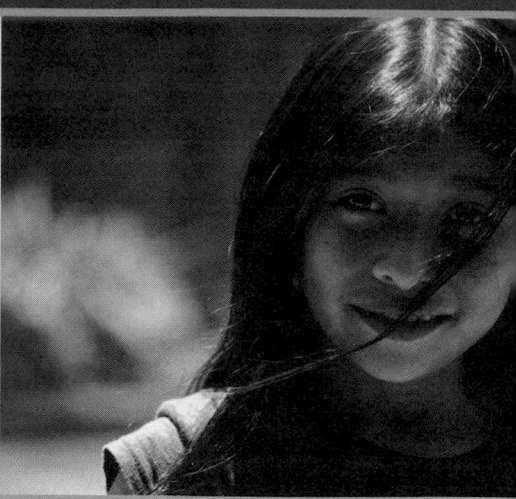

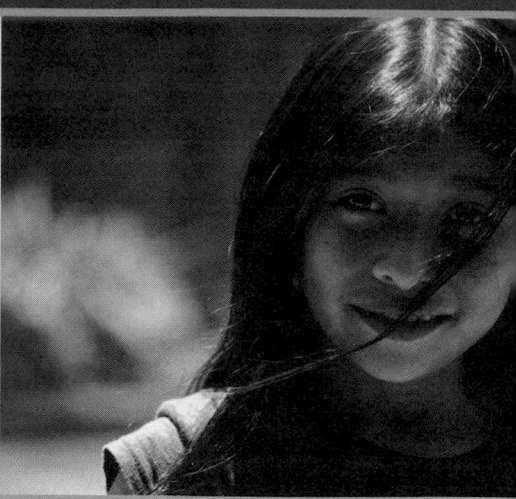 WEBSITE

RELATED TOPICS

CHAPTER OUTLINE

GENETIC INFLUENCES ON HEALTH

The twentieth century was a time of intense work and discovery in the field of medical genetics (McKusick, 2002), or the study of human hereditary disease. The modern era of medical genetics began with the discovery of inborn errors of metabolism, launched by the work of Archibald Garrod when, in 1902, he discovered alkaptonuria. This would be the precursor of modern biochemical genetics. In the second half of the twentieth century, pioneers Beadle and Tatum laid the foundation of molecular genetics when they discovered the pathway of genetic information from deoxyribonucleic acid (DNA) to ribonucleic acid (RNA) to protein. In 1956, Ingram discovered the molecular defect responsible for sickle cell disease. From that point forward, research in medical genetics focused on identifying the protein (enzyme) products of specific genes and relating them to disease processes. Cytogenetics, the study of chromosome disorders, started in 1952 with Lejeune's discovery of the genetic basis of Down syndrome. In recent times, molecular-based knowledge and technologies have been greatly accelerated by the Human Genome Project (HGP), which is rapidly identifying genes and DNA variations associated with disease.

The HGP, an international collaborative research program that spanned 13 years, accomplished its end objective in 2003 when researchers uncovered the sequence of the gene-rich areas of the genome. The genetic information obtained through the HGP represented a major step toward understanding human genes and opened new horizons in every aspect of medicine and biology with a major impact on health promotion, disease prevention, and treatment (Collins, Green, Guttmacher, et al, 2003).

Much effort has focused on identifying gene variations. As a human species, we are 99.9% alike; however, it may be the 0.1% variation that will help us understand the genetic risk for illnesses. Researchers hope to devise treatment strategies that are specific to an individual's genetic predisposition or molecular mechanism of disease. Another outcome of the HGP is the study of how inheritance affects the body's response to medications, a field called pharmacogenetics or pharmacogenomics. The clinical application of this allows for individualized medication selection and dosing to improve efficacy and safety. In addition, drugs can be developed that target specific molecular and cellular disease mechanisms.

The information garnered from the HGP has affected areas beyond the realm of science, as it began to affect human life and ethical decision making. It is not surprising that part of the total budget for the project was allotted to the Ethical, Legal, and Social Implications (ELSI) program to deal with the new genetic information. Research by the ELSI program has focused on issues such as genetic discrimination, privacy, education, informed consent, and DNA banking. It will continue to look at new issues generated by increasing knowledge of the human genome.

Nurses and other health care providers are increasingly faced with incorporating genetic-genomic information into their practice. In response to this need, the Consensus Panel on Genetic/Genomic Nursing Competencies was established in 2006. This independent panel of nurse leaders from clinical, research, and academic settings established essential minimal competencies necessary for nurses to deliver competent genetic- and genomic-focused nursing care. The American Association of Colleges of Nursing overwhelmingly endorsed the revised baccalaureate essentials document, which identified genetics and genomics as strong forces influencing the role of nurses in patient care. This chapter provides foundational information to help nurses begin using genetics and genomics information and technology when caring for children and families (Box 5-1).

HEREDITY AND ENVIRONMENT IN HUMAN DISEASE

Before the discoveries of the HGP, the total number of human genes had been estimated at approximately 50,000 to 100,000. It is now known that the human genome consists of 20,000 to 25,000 genes, a surprisingly low number for a sophisticated species (International Human Genome Sequencing Consortium, 2004).

Genes are segments of DNA that contain genetic information necessary to control a certain physiologic function or characteristic. These segments are often referred to as *sites,* or *loci,* indicating a physical or "geographic" location on a chromosome. Genetic disorders may result from gene mutations (single-gene, polygenic, or mitochondrial disorders) or chromosome abnormalities. Genes that encode proteins are termed structural genes. Mutations in structural genes may have significant qualitative and quantitative effects on the synthesis of the corresponding protein, with potential clinical consequences. Proteins can be classified as structural (or constitutive) proteins, and those that affect the metabolism of other molecules or substrates (enzymes). Table 5-1 summarizes the effects of protein disorders on selected genetic diseases. Such alterations in an individual genome may have been inherited from a parent or may represent an event that is new to that person and may be the first case in that family (new mutation). It is therefore erroneous to consider all genetic disorders as having a positive family history.

In earlier times, human diseases were thought to be either clearly genetic or typically environmental. However, the observation that some genetic disorders are congenital (present at birth) whereas others are expressed later in life has led scientists to conclude that many, if not most, diseases are caused by a genetic predisposition that can be activated by an environmental trigger. The concept of complex (or multifactorial) diseases emerged from this thought. Examples of such interactions are found in single-gene disorders, such as phenylketonuria (PKU) and sickle cell disease, and multifactorial conditions, such as cancer and neural tube defects (NTDs). PKU is a disorder resulting from the (genetically determined) absence of an enzyme that metabolizes the amino acid phenylalanine. However, the deleterious effects in the infant are expressed only after sufficient ingestion of phenylalanine-containing substances, such as milk (environmental trigger). Even in the case of a "classic" genetic condition, such as sickle cell disease, its acute symptoms are precipitated by certain conditions such as lowered oxygen tension, infection, or dehydration.

Cancer is another example of genetic-environment interplay and explains the difference between inherited conditions and

BOX 5-1   KEY GENETIC TERMS

AFP—Abbreviation of alpha-fetoprotein, a protein produced by the developing fetus. Alterations in AFP can be used as a marker suggestive of neural tube defect (increased AFP) and Down syndrome (decreased AFP).

Alleles—One version of a gene at a given location (locus) along a chromosome. The most common version of a gene in a population is called the **wild type allele**.

Amniocentesis—Prenatal diagnostic procedure that consists of transabdominally withdrawing a small sample of amniotic fluid for genetic analysis of embryonic cells. Biochemical analysis and chromosome studies can be performed in such cells. This procedure is usually performed 14 to 20 weeks.

Aneuploidy—An abnormal chromosome pattern in which the total number of chromosomes is not a multiple of the haploid number (n = 23) (e.g., persons with 45 or 47 chromosomes, as in Turner or Down syndrome, respectively). Such monosomies and trisomies are examples of aneuploidy.

Association—Nonrandom cluster of malformations, the cause of which varies from person to person (e.g., VATER association).

Autosomes—The 22 pairs of chromosomes in somatic cells that do not greatly influence sex determination at conception. This does not include the sex chromosomes, X and Y.

Carrier—A clinically normal (asymptomatic) person who possesses a genetic alteration, either in the form of a gene or chromosome change. A carrier has the potential of transmitting that abnormality to an offspring who will then express the abnormal phenotype. Examples of carrier states include a sickle cell disease carrier ("trait") and a balanced carrier of a chromosome translocation.

Centromere—Chromosomal region that separates the chromosome arms and unites the chromatids. Centromeres attach to spindle fibers during cell division, ensuring through disjunction an equal distribution of chromosomes or chromatids.

Chromosome—Filament-like nuclear structure that consists of chromatin, stores genetic information as base sequences in DNA, and has a constant number for each species. Chromosomes are found in pairs in somatic cells (homologous chromosomes) and in single copies in germ cells. One member of a homologous pair is of paternal origin, the other of maternal origin. Homologous chromosomes have identical number and arrangement of genes.

Chromosome aberrations—Genetic disorders that result from variation in number or structure of chromosomes.

Chromosomes, acrocentric—Chromosomes in which the centromere is distally placed. Human chromosomes in groups D and G are acrocentric.

Chromosomes, metacentric—Chromosomes in which the centromere is located approximately in the midpoint of the chromosome, resulting in arms of approximately equal length. Human chromosomes A(1), A(3), and E(16) are metacentric.

Chromosomes, submetacentric—Chromosomes in which the centromere is located closer to one telomere than to the other. Human B group chromosomes are submetacentric.

Concordant—A condition in which two individuals have the same genetic trait; usually applied to monozygotic twin concordance studies.

Congenital—Present at birth. A congenital disease may or may not be genetic. Likewise, a genetic disease may or may not be congenital, although the causative genes are present at birth.

Crossing-over—The genetic event that results in exchange of genetic material between homologous chromosomes during prophase I of meiosis.

CVS—Abbreviation of chorionic villi sampling, a prenatal diagnostic procedure in which a small amount of chorionic villi material (embryonic tissue) is aspirated for genetic analysis of the developing embryo. This procedure is usually performed during the first trimester of pregnancy.

Cytogenetics—Study of chromosomes, with special focus on chromosome abnormalities.

Deformation—Fetal abnormality caused by extrinsic factors (e.g., uterine position).

Diploid—A cell that contains two copies of each chromosome. The term is often extended to include an individual carrying such cells. The diploid number (2n) in humans is 46.

Deletion—The loss of chromosomal material. An example of a terminal deletion is found in cri du chat (cat's cry) syndrome, in which there is loss of a portion of the short arm of chromosome B(5). Deleted fragments may attach to another chromosome (see Translocation).

DNA—Abbreviation of deoxyribonucleic acid, a double-helix molecule consisting of an assembly of nucleotides (phosphate–sugar [deoxyribose]–nitrogenous base). DNA bases (cytosine, guanine, thymine, adenine) encode genetic information, which is *transcribed* into messenger RNA and further *translated* into proteins.

DNA, mitochondrial (mtDNA)—DNA located in the mitochondria of cells. Inheritance of mtDNA is independent from paternal genetics.

DNA, nuclear (nDNA)—DNA located in the nucleus of cells.

Dominant—An allele that is phenotypically expressed in single copy (heterozygote) and in double copy (homozygote). Example: polydactyly.

FISH analysis—Fluorescent in situ hybridization, a process by which chromosomes or portions of chromosomes are "painted" with fluorescent molecules. This technique is useful for identifying chromosomal microdeletions.

Gamete (germ cell)—A mature reproductive cell containing the haploid number of chromosomes (n = 23); in males, the spermatozoon; in females, the ovum. The union of gametes in sexual reproduction initiates the development of a new individual.

Gametogenesis—A series of mitotic and meiotic cell divisions occurring in the gonads that lead to the production of gametes; in males, spermatogenesis; in females, oogenesis. Reduction in the number of chromosomes (2n → n) during gametogenesis occurs in the first meiotic division (meiosis I).

Gene—A segment of nucleic acid that contains genetic information necessary to control a certain function, such as the synthesis of a polypeptide (structural gene). This segment is often referred to as a site, or locus, on a chromosome.

Genetic counseling—The process by which genetic information is given to patients and their families. Information about a genetic disease may include its natural history, recurrence risk, and management.

Genetics—Study of individual genes and their impact on relatively rare single-gene disorders.

Genome—Complete genetic information of an organism, usually described as total number of base pairs. The human genome contains approximately 3 billion base pairs.

Genomics—Study of all the genes in the human genome together, including their interactions with each other and the environment, and the influence of other psychosocial and cultural factors.

Genotype—Genetic constitution that determines the physical and chemical characteristics of an individual.

Haploid—The number of chromosomes present in a gamete. Also, a cell that contains one copy of each chromosome. The haploid number (n) in humans is 23. The diploid number of chromosomes (46) is reconstituted in the zygote on fertilization of two haploid gametes.

Hemizygote—A condition in which an allele is present in a single copy. Males are hemizygous for all markers (genes) located on the X chromosome.

Heterozygote—An individual who has two different alleles at a given locus on a pair of homologous chromosomes; for example, in the case of the *HexA* gene, Hh (or +/−).

Homologous—Referring to chromosomes with matching genes, or to those genes individually.

Homozygote—An individual possessing a pair of identical alleles at a given locus; for example, in the case of the *HexA* gene, above, HH (or +/+) and hh (or −/−).

Human Genome Project—International research project to map each human gene and sequence the human genome.

Imprinting—Phenomenon in which an allele at a given locus is altered or inactivated, depending on whether it is inherited from mother or father; implies a functional difference in genes inherited from the two parents and explains some variation in expression.

Karyotype—The chromosome constitution of an individual represented by a laboratory-made display in which chromosomes are arranged by size and centromere position.

BOX 5-1   **KEY GENETIC TERMS—cont'd**

Locus—The chromosome location of a specific gene (or site). Plural: loci.

Malformation—A primary morphologic defect occurring as a result of abnormal morphogenesis.

Malformation, major—Structural abnormality with serious medical, surgical, or cosmetic consequences.

Malformation, minor—Structural abnormality that has no serious consequences or is a normal variation (e.g., extra nipple or umbilical hernia).

Meiosis—A reductional type of cell division, in which the chromosome number is halved. In humans, meiosis is one of the processes that lead to the formation of haploid gametes (n = 23).

Mendelian inheritance—The mode of inheritance of single-gene traits. The term is derived from Gregor Mendel, the pioneer of genetics.

Microdeletion—Chromosome deletion too small to be detected by standard cytogenetic techniques; can be detected by FISH analysis, which is a molecular cytogenetic technique.

Mitochondrion—Cellular organelle responsible for converting nutrients into energy and for many other specialized tasks. Mitochondria are the only part of the body known to have their own separate and unique DNA; mitochondrial DNA (mtDNA) is inherited exclusively from the mother. Plural: mitochondria.

Mitosis—Type of equational cell division in which the resulting daughter cells have the same number of chromosomes as each other and the mother cell.

Monosomy—The aneuploid condition of having a chromosome represented by a single copy in a somatic cell, that is, the absence of a chromosome from a given pair. Generally, monosomies are not compatible with life, except in the case of a missing X chromosome in Turner syndrome (45,XO).

Mosaicism—Condition in which an individual harbors two or more genetically distinct cell lines. Generally, one cell line is normal and one is abnormal; it results from mitotic nondisjunction, a postzygotic event.

Multifactorial—Complex interaction of both genetic and environmental factors that produces an effect on an individual. Disease processes resulting from multifactorial inheritance are referred to as *complex diseases.*

Mutation—Structural or chemical alteration in genetic material that persists and is transmitted to future generations. Mutations can occur naturally *(spontaneous)* or can be induced by a variety of physical (temperature, radiation), chemical (various substances such as nitrogen mustard), or biologic (certain viruses) mutagens.

Nondisjunction—Failure of homologous chromosomes or chromatids to separate properly during anaphase meiosis I and II, or mitosis, resulting in daughter cells with unequal chromosome numbers. Meiotic nondisjunction may result in gametes with abnormal chromosome number, which on fertilization may produce aneuploidy. Mitotic nondisjunction in a developing embryo may result in mosaicism.

Oncogene—A gene or group of genes, usually involved in cell division, whose malfunction (e.g., a mutation) will result in malignant transformation.

Pedigree chart (family tree, genogram)—A diagram that describes family relationships, gender, disease status, or other relevant information about a family, illustrating the genetic variation within a family.

Penetrance—Frequency with which a heritable trait is manifested in individuals possessing the gene.

Phenotype—Any observable or measurable expression of gene function in an individual. For instance, eye color and hemoglobin type are phenotypic expressions of specific genes. Phenotypes may result from interaction of genotype and environment.

Polygenic—Inheritance involving many genes at separate loci whose combined, additive effects produce a given phenotype.

Polyploidy—Chromosome condition in which the diploid chromosome number of a cell varies by increments of 23. For example, a triploid cell or individual would have 69 chromosomes (46 + 23); a tetraploid, 92 (46 + 23 + 23).

Proband (index case)—The clinically identified person who displays the characteristics of features of the disease in question; also referred to as propositus (feminine: proposita).

Recessive—Refers to an allele whose phenotypic expression occurs in homozygous or hemizygous conditions. In heterozygosity, a recessive allele is masked by its dominant homologous counterpart. Example: cystic fibrosis.

Recombination—The occurrence among the offspring of new combinations of alleles as a result of genetic material exchange following crossovers during parental gametogenesis.

RNA—Abbreviation of ribonucleic acid, a single-stranded molecule consisting of an assembly of nucleotides (phosphate–sugar [ribose]–nitrogenous base). RNA bases (cytosine, guanine, uracil, adenine) encode genetic information, which is *translated* into proteins.

Sex-linked—The transmission of a trait whose causative gene is located on a sex chromosome (X or Y). Most sex-linked genes in humans are located on the X chromosome (X-linked).

Somatic cell—Body tissue cells with diploid complement of 46 chromosomes.

Sporadic—A descriptor for birth defects or disorders occurring as a new case in a family and not inherited.

Syndrome—A collection of multiple primary malformations or defects all due to a single underlying cause. Examples: Down syndrome (chromosome abnormality), Marfan syndrome (single-gene disorder).

Telomere—The distal portion of a chromosome.

Teratogen—An environmental agent capable of producing a birth defect.

Transcription—The process by which genetic information is copied from DNA to RNA.

Translation—The step in protein synthesis during which an amino acid sequence is assembled according to the genetic information contained in messenger RNA (mRNA).

Translocation—Transfer of all or part of a chromosome to a different chromosome after chromosome breakage; can be balanced, producing no phenotypic effects, or unbalanced, producing severe or lethal effects.

Trisomy—An aneuploid condition caused by the presence of an extra chromosome, which is added to a given chromosome pair and results in a total number of 47 chromosomes per cell. Down syndrome is the most common human autosomal trisomy.

X inactivation (lyonization)—The process by which, in a normal female, most of genes on one of the X chromosomes are inactivated during early embryonic development, so that alleles on active chromosome are allowed full expression.

X-linked inheritance—Transmission of a trait whose causative gene is located on the X chromosome.

Zygote—Cell resulting from the fusion of male and female gametes.

---

somatic cell genetic disorders. A normal somatic cell (any body cell other than the ova and sperm) may become a cancer cell after acquiring a series of gene changes. This process is the typical "genetic" cause of cancer. In a small subset of families, a mutation in a gene normally involved in regulation of cell growth, DNA repair, or cell death (apoptosis) is transmitted through the germ cells (ova and sperm). Children who inherit the genetic mutation will have it in all of their somatic cells, making them more susceptible to subsequent genetic changes in one or more cells that may transform into cancer cells. An increasing number of tests are available to identify at-risk family members who have inherited a cancer-susceptibility genetic mutation. However, this type of testing in children is controversial. Beyond the genetic component of cancer, there is little dispute that environmental insult, such as tobacco smoking, sun exposure, and radiation, can be carcinogenic. Such environmental triggers are capable of spontaneously creating noninherited mutations in genes that regulate cell growth and cell response to cell abnormalities that can eventually lead to malignant transformation.

TABLE 5-1	SELECTED PROTEINS INVOLVED IN GENETIC DISEASE	
PROTEIN INVOLVED	**ALTERED MECHANISM OF ACTION DUE TO MUTATIONS**	**RESULTING DISORDER**
Constitutive Proteins		
Globins	Altered oxygen transport	Hemoglobinopathies: • Sickle cell disease • Thalassemias
Dystrophin	Muscle cell defect	Muscular dystrophies
Coagulation factors VIII and IX	Abnormal clotting activity	Hemophilia A and B
Enzymes		
Phenylalanine hydroxylase	Interrupted metabolism of phenylalanine and accumulation of toxic precursors (phenylalanine and phenylketones)	Phenylketonuria
Hexosaminidase A (HexA)	Interrupted metabolism and accumulation of precursors (GM_2 ganglioside)	Tay-Sachs disease
Hypoxanthine-guanine phosphoribosyltransferase (HGPRT)	Disruption of metabolic feedback mechanism and accumulation of end product (uric acid)	Lesch-Nyhan syndrome
3-Hydroxy-3-methylglutaryl coenzyme A (HMG-CoA) reductase	Disruption of metabolic feedback mechanism and accumulation of end product (cholesterol)	Familial hypercholesterolemia

Evidence is growing that genes play an important role in human susceptibility and resistance to infection even in cases with a clear environmental cause of the infectious disease. Evidence for this genetic element in resistance gained heightened recognition during the first decade of the acquired immunodeficiency (AIDS) epidemic. Researchers discovered that adults with a specific deletion in both copies of their *CCR5* genes did not become infected with human immunodeficiency virus (HIV) despite repeated exposure. Later it was found that children exposed in utero to HIV typically had a significantly delayed onset of disease if at least one of their *CCR5* genes had the specific mutation (Romiti, Colognesi, Cancrini, et al, 2000). Understanding the mechanism of resistance associated with *CCR5* mutation led to a novel molecular therapy (Wilkin, Su, Kuritzkes, et al, 2007).

CONGENITAL ANOMALIES

Embryogenesis and fetal development are an intricate and precisely timed series of events in which all parts must be properly integrated to ensure a coordinated whole. Insults during development or abnormalities in differentiation or in the proper timing of organogenesis may result in a variety of congenital anomalies. Congenital anomalies, or birth defects, occur in 2% to 4% of all live-born children and are often classified as deformations, disruptions, dysplasias, or malformations. Deformations are often caused by extrinsic mechanical forces on normally developing tissue. Club foot is an example of a deformation often caused by uterine constraint. Disruptions result from the breakdown of previously normal tissue. Congenital amputations caused by amniotic bands (fibrous strands of amnion that wrap around different body parts during development) are examples of disruption anomalies (Zieve, Juhn, and Eltz, 2009). Dysplasias result from abnormal organization of cells into a particular tissue type. Congenital abnormalities of the teeth, hair, nails, or sweat glands may be manifestations of one of the more than 100 different ectodermal dysplasia syndromes (National Foundation for Ectodermal Dysplasia, 2009). Malformations are abnormal formations of organs or body parts resulting from an abnormal developmental process. Most malformations occur before 12 weeks of gestation. Cleft lip, an example of a malformation, occurs at approximately 5 weeks of gestation when the developing embryo naturally has two clefts in the area. Normally between 5 and 7 weeks, cells rapidly divide and migrate to fill in those clefts. If there is an abnormality in this developmental process, the embryo is left with either a unilateral or bilateral cleft lip that may also involve the palate.

The types of anomalies that can result from genetic or prenatal environmental causes can be major structural abnormalities with serious medical, surgical, or quality-of-life consequences, or they can be minor anomalies or normal variants with no serious consequences, such as a sacral dimple, an extra nipple, or a café-au-lait spot. Congenital anomalies can occur in isolation, such as congenital heart defect, or multiple anomalies may be present. A recognized pattern of anomalies resulting from a single specific cause is called a syndrome (e.g., Down syndrome or fetal alcohol syndrome). A nonrandom pattern of malformations for which a cause has not been determined is called an association (e.g., VACTERL [vertebral defects, anal atresia, cardiac defect, tracheoesophageal fistula, and renal and limb defects] association). When a single anomaly leads to a cascade of additional anomalies, the pattern of defects is referred to as a sequence. Pierre Robin sequence begins with the abnormal development of the mandible, resulting in abnormal placement of the tongue during development. The normal developmental process for the palate is prevented because the tongue obstructs the migration of the palatal shelves toward the midline and a cleft palate remains. Consequently, infants born with Pierre Robin sequence have a recessed mandible and an abnormally placed tongue and are at risk for obstructive apnea. NTDs, cleft lip and palate, deafness, congenital heart defects, and cognitive impairment are examples of congenital malformations that can occur in isolation or as part of a syndrome, association, or sequence and can have different causes, such as single-gene or chromosome abnormalities, prenatal exposures, or multifactorial causes.

GENETIC DISORDERS

Genetic disorders can be caused by chromosome abnormalities as seen in Turner syndrome, Down syndrome, or velo-cardio-facial syndrome (VCFS); single-gene mutations as seen in sickle cell anemia, neurofibromatosis, or Duchenne muscular dystrophy; a combination of genetic and environmental factors as seen in NTDs or maturity onset diabetes in the young; and mitochondrial DNA (mtDNA) mutations as seen in nonsyndromic deafness susceptibility due to aminoglycoside sensitivity. Whereas numeric or structural chromosome aberrations automatically involve large groups of genes, a small gene mutation does not alter chromosome structure and number. Alterations in single genes (single-gene disorders) or in many genes (polygenic disorders) may represent too small a lesion to cause an identifiable alteration in chromosomal structure. Human nucleated somatic cells contain approximately 25,000 genes distributed, in the form of tightly coiled DNA molecules, along 46 chromosomes. Since human chromosomes vary in size, the larger the chromosome, the greater the number of genes carried.

Both numeric and structural abnormalities of autosomes (all chromosomes except the X and Y chromosomes) account for a variety of syndromes usually characterized by cognitive deficiencies. A few are associated with a group of characteristics that clearly indicate the precise chromosome anomaly. Nurses often note dysmorphic facial features, behavioral characteristics such as an unusual cry and poor feeding behavior, and other neurologic manifestations such as hypotonia or abnormal reflex responses, which may alert them to these and other chromosome abnormalities.

Numeric Chromosome Abnormalities

With the exception of brief periods of gametogenesis, human beings are diploid individuals, and human somatic cells are diploid (a cell that contains two copies of each chromosome). A diploid chromosome number in humans is represented by the notation 2n = 46. A haploid chromosome constitution (n = 23) is found in germ cells, the male and female gametes (sperm and ova). Somatic cells contain 44 autosomes (the 22 pairs of chromosomes that do not greatly influence sex determination at conception) and two sex chromosomes, XX in females and XY in males. For the purpose of cytogenetic studies, chromosomes are usually displayed in a karyotype, the laboratory-made arrangement of specially prepared chromosomes according to their size and centromere position. The location of the centromere allows the classification of human chromosomes as acrocentric, submetacentric, and metacentric chromosomes (Fig. 5-1).

Numeric chromosome abnormalities occur whenever entire chromosomes are added or deleted. The addition of one or more chromosomes to each pair (increments of the haploid number, 23) will result in triploid cells with 69 chromosomes (46 + 23), or tetraploid cells with 92 chromosomes (46 + 23 + 23), and so on. The product of this uniform addition of chromosomes to all the original pairs is termed euploidy, a euploid cell being one whose chromosome number is a multiple of 23.

Individuals who are triploid (3n = 69) have a genetic imbalance of such magnitude that the few who are carried to term

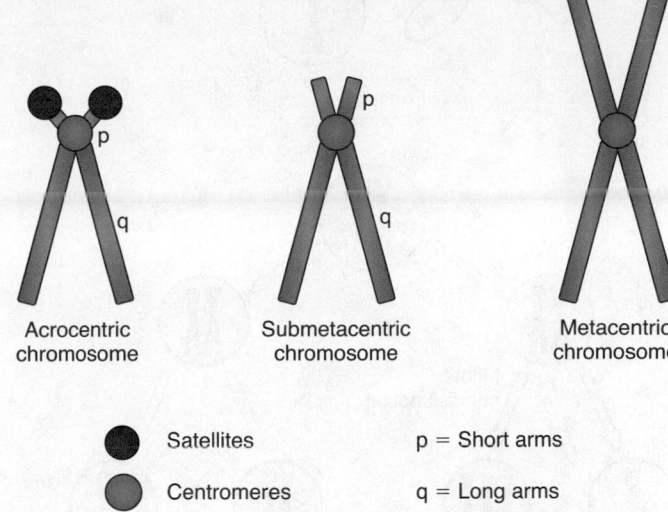

| Satellites | p = Short arms |
| Centromeres | q = Long arms |

Fig. 5-1 Chromosome classification by centromere position. Positioning of centromeres results in chromosomes with extremely short arms (acrocentric chromosomes), relatively short arms (submetacentric chromosomes), or arms of equal length (metacentric chromosomes).

have severe multiple abnormalities that limit their life span to a few hours or days. On the other hand, one chromosome may be added to or lost from one of the pairs, creating a condition of aneuploidy. When one chromosome is added to a pair, the embryo, fetus, or child is described as having a trisomy, and the total chromosome number is 47. Most fetuses that have an autosomal trisomy are not live born. Fetuses with trisomy 21, trisomy 18, and trisomy 13 may be live born. When one chromosome is lost from the pair, the fetus is described as having a monosomy, and the total chromosome number in somatic cells is 45. The loss of a chromosome and its related complement of genes is overall more detrimental than the addition of a chromosome. The only monosomy compatible with life is monosomy X (Turner syndrome); yet most 45,X pregnancies spontaneously miscarry (Sybert and McCauley, 2004).

The most common cause of alteration in the number of chromosomes is a misdistribution of chromosomes during mitosis or meiosis. As somatic cells multiply by mitosis, each daughter cell receives the same chromosome number as the mother cell. This equitable chromosome sharing in anaphase is due to a phenomenon termed disjunction, by which chromatids of each chromosome separate and migrate to opposite poles of the cell. Disruption of this orderly chromosome distribution occurs in nondisjunction, which can occur during both mitosis and meiosis. In mitosis, failure of chromatids to separate properly during anaphase will result in daughter cells with different chromosome numbers (e.g., 45 and 47, instead of 46 and 46). Of those, the 45-chromosome monosomic cells will tend to degenerate and die, but those with the extra chromosome (trisomic) will continue to divide and generate a complete line of trisomic cells.

When mitotic nondisjunction occurs during embryonic development (Fig. 5-2), the trisomic cell line proliferates concomitantly with the normal cell line, and an individual with mosaicism for that particular chromosome result. Mosaicism,

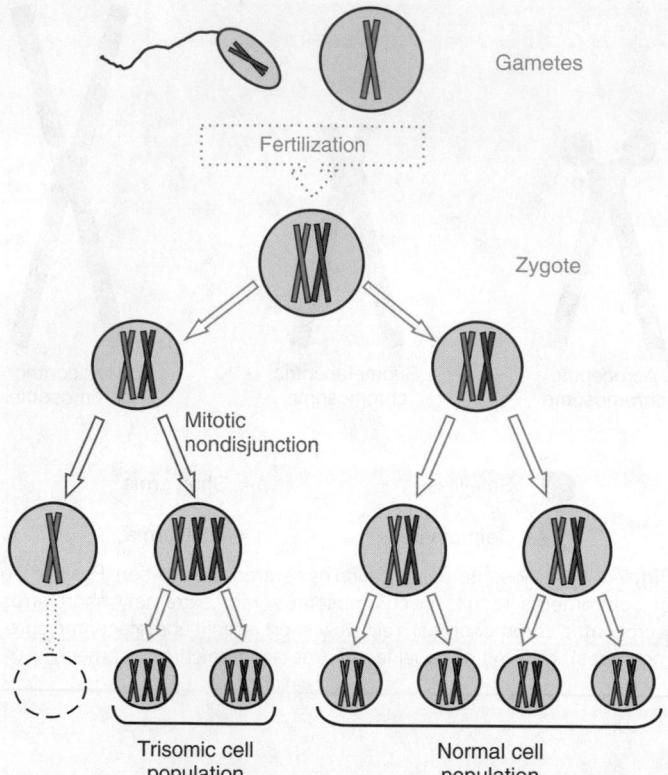

Fig. 5-2 Mitotic nondisjunction resulting in individual with different cell populations (mosaicism). This event occurs during embryonic development, after normal zygote was formed by fertilization of two normal gametes. Only one chromosome pair is represented. As represented here, mitotic nondisjunction and uneven chromosome distribution result in some cell populations with the extra chromosome, whereas other cell lines have the normal chromosome complement.

therefore, results in an individual (mosaic) with two or more genetically different cell populations. The chromosomal notation for a male with mosaic type of Down syndrome, for example, is 46,XY/47,XY,+21). The slash (/) indicates a dual cell population in which one has the normal chromosomal constitution (46,XY), while the other carries an extra chromosome 21 and has a total chromosome number of 47. The percentage, or level, of mosaicism depends on the stage of embryonic development in which the cell division error occurs. If it occurs at the first cell division after fertilization, the level of mosaicism may be as high as 50%. If the cell division error occurs in later development, the abnormal cells may be localized to one cell type, such as the brain tissue or germ cell line (ovaries or testes). The extent of clinical manifestations is determined by the type of tissues that contain cells with abnormal chromosome numbers and the percentage of affected cells, and may vary from near normal to a fully manifested syndrome.

Meiotic nondisjunction (Fig. 5-3) is a major cause of aneuploidy, an abnormal chromosome pattern in which the total number of chromosomes is not a multiple of the haploid number, 23. Nondisjunction can occur during meiosis I and II, during both oogenesis and spermatogenesis, resulting in gametes with aneuploid chromosome number (e.g., 22 or 24, instead of 23). As in the case of somatic cells, gametes lacking a chromosome are not likely to survive, but gametes with an

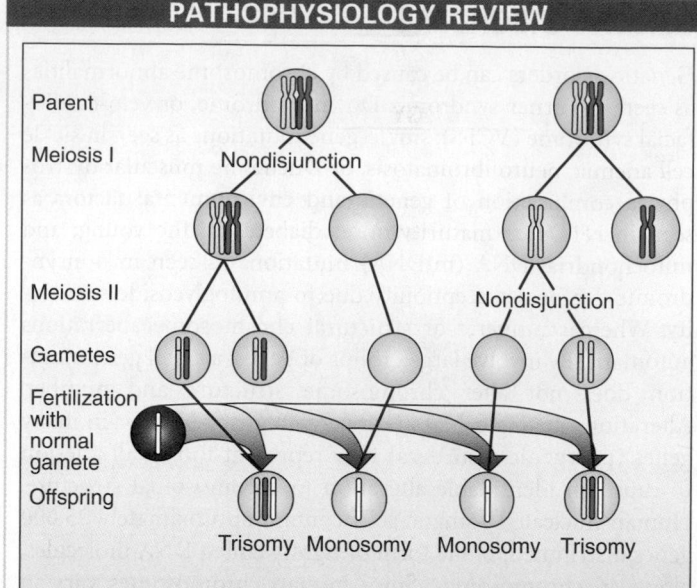

Fig. 5-3 Nondisjunction causes aneuploidy when chromosomes or sister chromatids fail to divide properly. (From Jorde LB, Carey JC, Bamshad MJ, et al: *Medical genetics*, ed 3, St Louis, 2003, Mosby.)

extra chromosome are more often viable. Fertilization of an aneuploid gamete with a normal gamete will produce an aneuploid zygote. The most common aneuploidies in humans are trisomies.

Autosome Aneuploidies

Examples of numeric alterations affecting the autosomes include some of the most common trisomies found in humans: trisomy 21 (Down syndrome), trisomy 18 (Edwards syndrome), and trisomy 13 (Patau syndrome) (Table 5-2).

Trisomy 21

Down syndrome affects 1 in 800 to 1 in 1000 live births and is the most common aneuploidy compatible with life expectancy into adulthood. Physical and cognitive abnormalities vary. Intelligence quotient (IQ) range is typically mild to moderate impairment. In spite of modern medical developments, life expectancy is still shortened, with 20% dying in the first decade, and 50% by age 60 years. Adults with Down syndrome are also more likely to develop Alzheimer disease; more than 75% of those over age 60 are affected with the disease (Rimoin, Connor, Pyeritz, et al, 2002).

The chromosomal constitution of Down syndrome is variable, with three possible configurations (Lashley, 2005):

1. **Trisomy**—The nomenclature for a female with trisomy is 47,XX+21 and for a male with trisomy is 47,XY,+21. Trisomy encompasses 92% of all cases of Down syndrome. The extra chromosome 21 is unattached and segregates freely during meiosis. The risk for this type of Down syndrome increases linearly with increasing maternal age (from 1:1500 live births for mothers age 20 years, to 1:50 live births for mothers over age 45) (Jones, 2006); however, because young women have more babies, about 75% of babies with trisomy 21 are born to younger mothers.

TABLE 5-2   PARTIAL LIST OF CHROMOSOMAL GENETIC DISORDERS

DISORDER	GENETIC ETIOLOGY	POSSIBLE PERIODS OF RECOGNITION	MAJOR FINDINGS	RESOURCES*
Angelman syndrome	Chr—Deletion, uniparental disomy, or abnormal methylation of chromosome 15	Prenatal to early childhood	Significant motor, cognitive, and speech delays; microcephaly; ataxia	www.geneclinics.org/profiles/angelman/details.html http://ghr.nlm.nih.gov/condition=angelmansyndrome www.angelman.org
Beckwith-Wiedemann syndrome	AD or Chr—Abnormal methylation of chromosome 11, uniparental disomy of paternal chromosome 11, or structural abnormality in critical region	Prenatal to newborn	Overgrowth syndrome; often recognized in newborn period due to abnormally large tongue; abdominal wall defects; hypoglycemia in infancy	www.ncbi.nlm.nih.gov/bookshelf/br. fcgi?book=gene&part=bws http://ghr.nlm.nih.gov/condition= beckwithwiedemannsyndrome www.beckwith-wiedemann.info
Cri du chat syndrome	Chr—46,XX,del(5p) or 46,XY,del(5p)	Prenatal to newborn	Microcephaly; high-pitched, catlike cry; significant motor and cognitive delays	http://ghr.nlm.nih.gov/condition=criduchatsyndrome www.fivepminus.org
Down syndrome (trisomy 21)	Chr—47,XX,+21 or 47,XY,+21	Prenatal to newborn	Mild to moderate cognitive impairment, characteristic facial features, hypotonia	http://ghr.nlm.nih.gov/condition=downsyndrome http://aappolicy.aappublications.org/cgi/content/full/ pediatrics;107/2/442 www.ndss.org www.nads.org
Edwards syndrome (trisomy 18)	Chr—47,XX,+18 or 47,XY,+18	Prenatal to newborn	Multiple congenital anomalies; significantly shortened life span; if survival beyond 1 yr, severe cognitive impairment	http://ghr.nlm.nih.gov/condition=trisomy18 www.trisomy18.org
Klinefelter syndrome	Chr—47,XXY	Prenatal; adolescence to adulthood	Gynecomastia, small testes, normal sex drive and function but infertility common	http://ghr.nlm.nih.gov/condition=klinefeltersyndrome
Patau syndrome (trisomy 13)	Chr—47,XX,+13 or 47,XY,+13	Prenatal to newborn	Multiple congenital anomalies; significantly shortened life span; if survival beyond 1 yr, severe cognitive impairment	http://ghr.nlm.nih.gov/condition=trisomy13 www.livingwithtrisomy13.org/index.htm
Prader-Willi syndrome	Chr—Absence of paternally derived region of chromosome 15 or abnormally methylated critical region of chromosome 15	Prenatal; infancy to early childhood	Severe hypotonia, failure to thrive in early infancy; after 1-2 yr of age, excessive eating—including nonfood items; morbid obesity; cognitive impairment; distinctive behavioral problems; hypogonadism	www.ncbi.nlm.nih.gov/bookshelf/br. fcgi?book=gene&part=pws http://ghr.nlm.nih.gov/condition=praderwillisyndro me
Turner syndrome	Chr—45,XO	Prenatal to adolescence	Lymphedema at birth, coarctation, short stature, ovarian dysgenesis, lack of secondary sex characteristics during adolescence	http://ghr.nlm.nih.gov/condition=turnersyndrome http://pediatrics.aappublications.org/cgi/content/ full/111/3/692

AD, Autosomal dominant; *Chr,* chromosomal.

*Support groups are listed on most websites. However, before referring families to support groups, particularly for families that discovered the diagnosis prenatally, carefully review the support group and describe its focus to the couple so they can make an informed decision about whether to visit it.

2. **Translocation Down syndrome**—The accepted nomenclature for a male with Down syndrome due to robertsonian translocation between acrocentric chromosomes 14 and 21 is 46,XY,t(14;21). Translocation (discussed later) accounts for approximately 4% of all male and female Down syndrome cases. The majority of cases are sporadic (without family history), but about 25% have one balanced translocation carrier parent. When one such carrier and a partner with normal chromosomes reproduce, their theoretical chances of producing a live-born child with Down syndrome are 33%, but the actual observed risk is approximately 15% if the mother is the carrier and less than 10% if the father is the carrier. The observed chance of producing a live-born child who is a balanced translocation carrier approaches 50%. Because chromosome 21 is an acrocentric chromosome, it is possible for the translocation to be with both chromosome 21s. A carrier mother [45,XX,t(21;21)] or father [45,XY,t(21;21)] of the translocation would have a 100% chance of producing a child with Down syndrome, since the other

parent would normally contribute one chromosome 21. This latter situation is one of the rare examples in genetics where an abnormality is passed on to *all* living progeny.

3. **Mosaic Down syndrome**—The nomenclature for a female with mosaic Down syndrome is 46,XX/47,XX+21. This rarer type of Down syndrome can occur in males and females. It results from mitotic nondisjunction during early embryonic development of a normal zygote. Children with this type have mixed cell populations, some with the normal karyotype, others with the extra chromosome. Contrary to what one might expect, children with mosaic Down syndrome do not necessarily have a better developmental outcome than those with free trisomy type. The proportion of trisomic cells in various tissues and organs play a role in the child's developmental potential and syndrome-associated potential health problems.

Trisomy 18

Edwards syndrome is a fairly common trisomy in fetuses. Those who are live born have severe cognitive impairment and physical abnormalities that contribute to a limited life span.

Trisomy 13

Patau syndrome carries more severe malformations than the previous two trisomies discussed, consistent with the increased size of the extra chromosome and greater gene imbalance. Life span is significantly shortened.

Sex Chromosome Aneuploidies

Alterations in number may also involve the sex chromosomes (see Table 5-2). The possible mechanisms by which sex chromosome abnormalities may occur are the same as those previously described (i.e., prefertilization nondisjunction during one of the meiotic divisions of gametogenesis in either parent or in the early postfertilization divisions of the zygote). An alteration in the number of sex chromosomes usually does not produce the profound effects that are associated with the autosomal trisomies. Intelligence may be normal or low normal, or the child may have some learning disabilities, but moderate or severe cognitive impairment is less common. Some of the most common genetic disorders caused by sex chromosome aneuploidies are Klinefelter, XYY, triple-X female, and Turner syndromes.

47,XXY

Klinefelter syndrome is the most common of all sex chromosome aneuploidies. Physical abnormalities include elements of decreased masculinization, such as gynecomastia; hypogonadism (with sterility resulting from degeneration of seminiferous tubules); and increased pubis-to-sole length, reflecting elongated lower limbs (Fig. 5-4). Mental development is normal in most cases, with a mean full-scale IQ between 85 and 90. Cognitive difficulties tend to be in expressive language, auditory processing, and auditory memory. Chromosome mosaicism (46,XY/47,XXY) rarely occurs and results in individuals with milder manifestations than their trisomic counterparts. Overall, the phenotype of Klinefelter syndrome is highly variable,

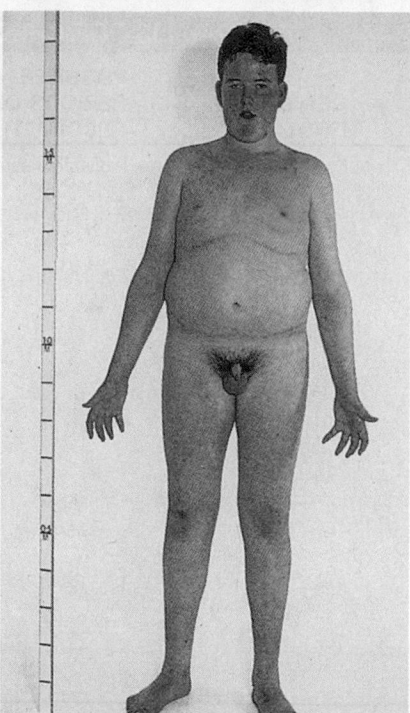

Fig. 5-4 Klinefelter syndrome. This young man exhibits many characteristics of Klinefelter syndrome: small testes, some development of the breasts, sparse body hair, and long limbs. This syndrome results from the presence of two or more X chromosomes with one Y chromosome (genotypes XXY or XXXY, for example). (From Patton KT, Thibodeau GA: *Anatomy and physiology,* ed 7, St Louis, 2010, Mosby.)

making it difficult, in the absence of chromosome studies, to make a prepubertal clinical diagnosis.

47,XYY

This genotype was reported in the early 1960s by Patricia Jacobs, a Scottish cytogeneticist who detected an increased frequency of double-Y men among inmates of penal institutions in Great Britain. In early reports an extra Y chromosome was reported as being responsible for an individual's increased tendency toward aggression against property (as opposed to aggression against humans). A detailed statistical analysis by Digamber Borgaonkar (Johns Hopkins University) of more than 200 cases later revealed that the only correlates with an extra Y chromosome were tall stature (>6 feet) and skin disorders, such as persistent adulthood acne. That large study found no significant correlations between XYY and cognitive impairment and aggressive tendencies, and the syndrome remains today a scientific curiosity. A majority of children produced by XYY fathers have normal chromosomal constitution, probably reflecting a selective advantage of normal haploid gametes over aneuploid ones.

45,XO

Turner syndrome, originally described clinically as ovarian dysgenesis (with gonads consisting of streaks of connective tissue and devoid of germ cells), is an example of a monosomy that is compatible with life. Clinical manifestations are variable in expression. Intellectually, verbal IQ exceeds performance IQ.

There is no prepubertal growth spurt, and girls with Turner syndrome are generally infertile. It is common practice to administer female hormones around the time that puberty would occur to provide the girl with Turner syndrome some secondary sex characteristics; however, the female hormones may further stunt growth and must be used judiciously. The child's growth is usually normal until 3 years of age and then slows, gradually drifting away from the normal growth curve. Treatment for the decreased growth velocity includes growth hormone and anabolic steroids. Mosaicism also occurs in Turner syndrome (e.g., 46,XX/45,XO), resulting in milder expression of the phenotype. Girls with Turner syndrome may have difficulty with peer relationships and with understanding social cues. They may exhibit behavioral problems, especially immature, socially isolated behavior. Most, however, lead productive lives and function as independent adults.

47,XXX

A relatively common condition (1:1000 live female births), females with triple-X display a normal phenotype, with an increased risk of learning disabilities when compared with their euploid sisters. Gynecologic complications include delayed menarche and premature menopause. As with XXY men, the offspring of XXX women is largely normal, indicative of a selective advantage of euploid gametes.

Structural Chromosome Abnormalities

Chromosomes are subject to structural alterations resulting from breakage and rearrangement. Chromosome breakage has long been recognized as a significant source of genetic abnormalities. Many clastogens (chromosome-breaking agents) have been identified, including physical (e.g., ionizing radiation), chemical (e.g., chlorpromazine), and biologic (e.g., viral infections) agents. Chromosome breakage can also result from many nonspecific causes, such as influenza. These breaks are usually restricted to somatic cells and are temporary. Chromosome breakage becomes significant when it is permanent (or long lasting) and when these permanent changes, in addition to appearing in somatic cells, are also present in germ cells and thus have the potential of being transmitted to the offspring.

A chromosome deletion occurs when chromosome breakage results in loss of the broken fragment at a chromosome's terminal end or within the chromosome. Chromosome deletions often have significant clinical impact, as in a chromosome 5 terminal deletion that results in cri du chat syndrome. Chromosome breakage can create unstable end points ("sticky ends"), which predispose the chromosomes to a variety of rearrangements of the fragments. A relatively rare structural abnormality that can occur as a result of chromosomal "sticky ends" is a ring chromosome. If a break occurs in the terminal end of both arms of a chromosome, the ends may fuse together, forming a circle. Like any structural alteration of a chromosome, the clinical manifestations depend on which genes are lost.

A more common rearrangement resulting from chromosome breakage is a translocation, which occurs when a chromosomal fragment reunites with another, nonhomologous chromosome. Two types of translocations have clinical significance: reciprocal translocations and robertsonian transloca-

tions. In a reciprocal translocation, breaks occur in two different chromosomes and the fragments are mutually exchanged, resulting in derivative chromosomes. Robertsonian translocations occur when the short arms of two acrocentric chromosomes (pairs 13 to 15 and pairs 21 and 22) break off and the remaining long arms fuse at the centromere, forming a "single chromosome" (Fig. 5-5). Both types result in individuals who have the correct amount of genetic information (although "rearranged"), and therefore no clinical manifestations are expected. These persons are termed balanced translocation carriers. These asymptomatic, balanced translocation carriers (either male or female) may pass the translocation to their offspring in a balanced or unbalanced form, depending on how the chromosomes segregate to the gametes. If it is passed in the unbalanced form, the combination is often lethal, and an early spontaneous abortion occurs. The chance of having a liveborn child with birth defects associated with the unbalanced translocation depends on the quantity and role of the missing or additional genetic material. Approximately 5% of cases of repeated spontaneous abortion (two or more) can be attributed to a balanced translocation carrier parent.

Some structural chromosome abnormalities are too small to reliably visualize under a light microscope but are still clinically relevant. Fragile, or weak, sites associated with expanded triplet

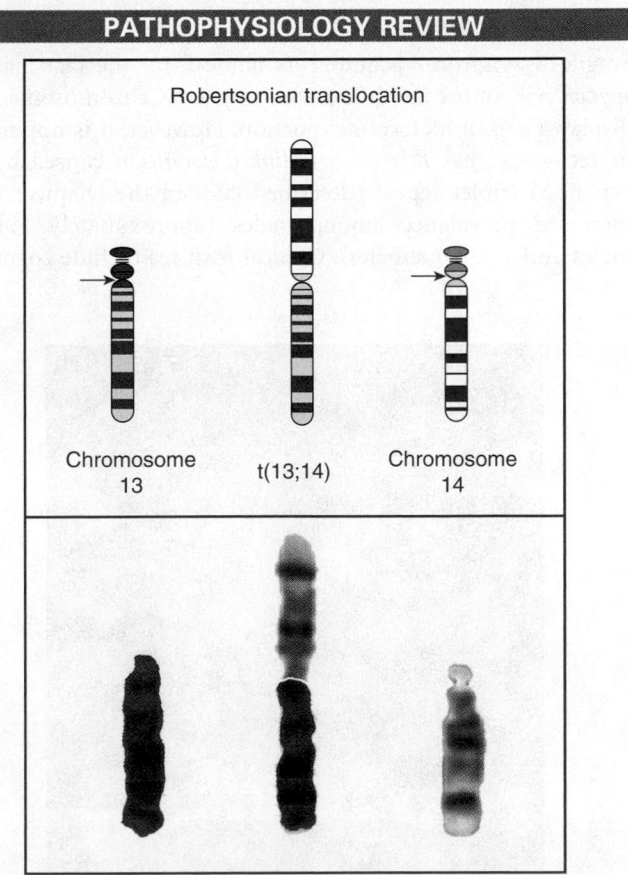

PATHOPHYSIOLOGY REVIEW

Robertsonian translocation

Chromosome 13   t(13;14)   Chromosome 14

Chromosomes in parent who carries a 14/21 Robertsonian translocation

Fig. 5-5 Translocation. In a robertsonian translocation the long arms of two acrocentric chromosomes (13 and 14) fuse, forming a single chromosome. (From Jorde LB, Carey JC, Bamshad MJ, et al: *Medical genetics*, ed 3, St Louis, 2003, Mosby.)

repeats (described later in the chapter) have been identified on both the autosomes and the X chromosome. A classic example is fragile X syndrome. **Contiguous gene syndromes** are disorders characterized by a microdeletion or microduplication of smaller chromosome segments, which may require special analysis techniques or molecular testing to detect (Brown, 2003). **Microdeletion syndromes**, such as VCFS, are more common than microduplication syndromes.

46,XX,del(5p) or 46,XY,del(5p)

Cri du chat, or cat's cry, syndrome is a rare (1:50,000 live births) (Jorde, Carey, Bamshad, et al, 2003) chromosome deletion syndrome resulting from loss of the small arm of chromosome 5. In early infancy this syndrome manifests with a typical but nondistinctive facial appearance, often a "moon-shaped" face with wide-spaced eyes (hypertelorism) (Fig. 5-6). As the child grows, this feature is progressively diluted, and by age 2 years the child is indistinguishable from age-matched controls. Profound cognitive impairment persists throughout their short life; many die in infancy. Typical of this disease is a crying pattern that is abnormal and catlike. At times it sounds like an angry cat, at others like a soft mewing sound. This is a result of a laryngeal atrophy that improves with age. By age 3 years the crying pattern is still abnormal, but it acquires a normal pitch and loses its catlike quality.

Fragile X Syndrome

Fragile X syndrome acquired its name from the fact that, in special cell culture conditions, the affected X chromosome may display a gap in its terminal portion. However, it is important to recognize that *this is an X-linked condition* caused by an expanded triplet repeat (described later in the chapter) with increased prevalence among males (approximately 1:4000 males and 1:6000 females). Clinical features include cognitive

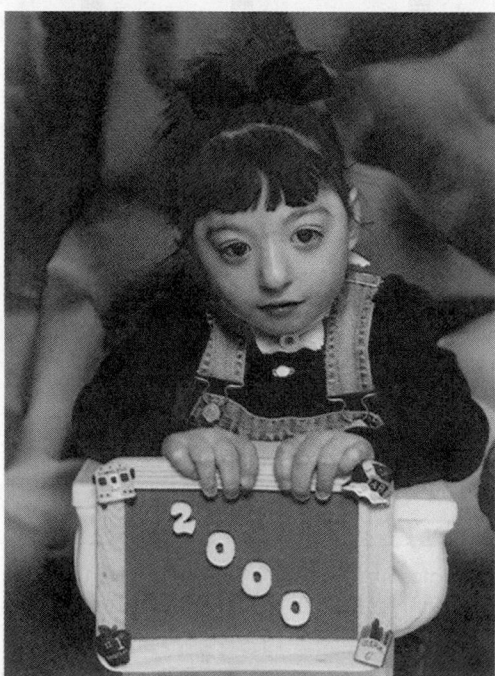

Fig. 5-6 Eight-year-old child with cri du chat (cat's cry) syndrome. Notice the wide-spaced eyes (hypertelorism) and "moon face."

impairment and a typical facial appearance, with an elongated face and large ears (Gardner and Sutherland, 2004).

Velo-Cardio-Facial Syndrome

VCFS, sometimes called DiGeorge syndrome, is the most common (1:2000) microdeletion syndrome. It is caused by a specific microdeletion within the long arm of chromosome 22 (22q11.2 deletion) (Shprintzen, 2008). Manifestations of this condition are variable, with approximately 180 different possible clinical features described. Although no one feature is found in every patient, cognitive impairment is common and can range from full-scale measured IQ in the borderline low-normal range with characteristic learning disabilities to mild cognitive impairment (Antshel, Fremont, Kates, et al, 2008). Although most patients' deletion is caused by a sporadic event, those with the condition can transmit the microdeletion in an autosomal dominant manner. Therefore their chances of producing a child with VCFS are 50% with each pregnancy.

Chromosome Instability Syndromes

Chromosome instability syndromes are a heterogeneous group of genetic disorders characterized by a high frequency of chromosome breakage observed in vitro. They include ataxia telangiectasia, Fanconi anemia, and xeroderma pigmentosum. These syndromes are associated with decreased immune function and an increased incidence of cancer.

SINGLE-GENE DISORDERS

Chromosome anomalies typically affect large numbers of genes; however, a **single-gene disorder** is caused by an abnormality within a gene or in a gene's regulatory region. Single-gene disorders display a mendelian pattern of dominant or recessive inheritance that was first delineated in the mid-nineteenth century by Gregor Mendel's experiments with plants. Single-gene disorders can affect all body systems and may have mild to severe expressions. Since single-gene disease involves very short DNA segments within a chromosome, they cannot be detected by chromosome analysis and demand specific and sophisticated molecular detection methods, such as DNA-based techniques (Table 5-3).

Mendelian inheritance laws allow for risk prediction in single-gene disorders; however, phenotypic expression may be altered by incomplete penetrance or variable expressivity of the responsible allele. An allele is said to have **reduced** or **incomplete penetrance** in a population when a proportion of persons who possess that allele do not express the phenotype. An allele is said to have **variable expressivity** when individuals possessing that allele display the features of the syndrome in various degrees, from mild to severe. If a person expresses even the mildest possible phenotype, the allele is penetrant in that individual.

Autosomal Inheritance Patterns
Autosomal Dominant Inheritance

General characteristics of **autosomal dominant inheritance** are presented in Box 5-2. A clear understanding of transmission of autosomal inheritance patterns requires the understanding of a few basic facts. First, most genetic diseases are rare. The prob-

TABLE 5-3 SELECT TECHNIQUES OF DNA ANALYSIS AND DISEASE DETECTION

TECHNIQUE	PURPOSE AND METHODOLOGY	APPLICATION
Basic Techniques		
DNA extraction	Extracted DNA can be immediately analyzed or stored for future use.	DNA extracted from variety of cells (amniocytes, lymphoblasts, single cell from eight-cell stage embryo) and tissues (skin, cheek cells, hair root, chorionic villi, archived pathology specimens)
Polymerase chain reaction (PCR)	Rapid amplification of small quantities of genetic material (DNA or RNA). Short lengths of DNA (primers) bind to specific DNA regions and initiate their replication. Several repetitions of this process can amplify a desired DNA region (and only this region) several thousand fold.	Essential technique for many molecular genetic diagnostic tests, but limited to already sequenced DNA genes or regions
Post-PCR Analysis		
Sequence of all exons and intron-exon boundaries of a gene	As cost decreases, this is becoming preferred test for genes that have many possible disease-associated mutations throughout the gene.	*BRCA1, BRCA2*, familial adenomatous polyposis Picks up all mutations except large gene deletions, but may pick up a mutation not previously described and may not be able to tell if it has any pathologic significance.
Sequence-specific amplification and amplification refractory mutation system (ARMS)	Detection of already sequenced mutations by means of sequence-specific primers. ARMS detects presence or absence of specific mutation.	Cystic fibrosis Hemoglobinopathies (sickle cell disease, thalassemias)
Oligonucleotide ligation assay (OLA)	Two complementing small nucleotide probes reciprocally bind to DNA. Mutation is detected, since it prevents appropriate binding of probes to DNA.	Cystic fibrosis Familial hypercholesterolemia
Restriction enzyme analysis of PCR products	Commercially available bacterial endonucleases bind to specific DNA sequences and cut molecule at that point.	Charcot-Marie-Tooth disease Duchenne and Becker muscular dystrophies
Single-stranded conformation polymorphism analysis (SSCP)	Some mutations resulting from base substitutions cause changes in secondary structure of DNA. SSCP detects such conformational changes indicative of occurring mutations.	
Heteroduplex analysis	The conformational properties of the double-stranded molecules are used to distinguish different base pairing (i.e., mutations).	
Non-PCR–Based Analysis		
Southern blotting	After cutting DNA with restriction enzymes, fragments are analyzed for mutations or repeated base sequences.	Fragile X syndrome (CGG repeats) Huntington disease (CAG repeats) Some thalassemias (e.g., Bart thalassemia)

CAG, Cytosine-adenine-guanine; *CGG*, cytosine-guanine-guanine; *DNA*, deoxyribonucleic acid; *RNA*, ribonucleic acid.

ability that two affected persons will mate is very low for most genetic disorders (with the exception of societal selection, as in the case of achondroplasia). Second, depending on the disease, if one parent is affected, he or she is much more likely to be heterozygous (have one mutant allele) than homozygous (have two mutant alleles). Usually, an individual with two dominant mutant alleles will experience physical or mental abnormalities at a much more severe level.

Those assumptions being accepted, two questions remain: (1) what are the chances of transmitting the mutant allele to the offspring? and (2) what are the risks of the offspring being affected? If a gene has only two alleles, one normal and one mutant, then three possible allele combinations exist: normal/normal, normal/mutant, and mutant/mutant. In autosomal dominant conditions, only persons with normal/normal combination will be disease free, assuming that the mutant allele is 100% penetrant. Fig. 5-7 shows the relationships between genotypes and phenotypes for an autosomal dominant trait. Considering that genetic diseases are rare and that persons who

are homozygous for the mutated allele are more severely affected, it is most likely that an affected individual who is heterozygous for the mutant allele will mate with a genotypically normal partner (Fig. 5-8, *A*). The outcomes of these matings are best expressed by the use of **Punnett squares**. Also depicted (Fig. 5-8, *B*) is the mating of a homozygote for the mutated gene with a genotypically normal partner. The result of these matings is one of the few instances in medical genetics in which *all* progeny have a 100% chance of being affected, assuming that the mutant allele they receive is 100% penetrant. These matings, however, are extremely rare.

Many children diagnosed with an autosomal dominant disorder have a positive family history of the disease. In other instances, that child may represent the first occurrence of that condition in the family. In the latter case, the event may be due to a new mutation (**fresh mutation**) in that child or to the presence of the mutation only in the germ cells of a healthy parent. The birth of other affected children indicates the second possibility. The range of expression of autosomal dominant genes is highly variable, from minor manifestations (e.g., poly-dactyly), to severe, debilitating, and life-threatening disease (e.g., neurofibromatosis). Depending on the degree of disability the condition imposes on the individual and the ability to procreate, the mutated gene either will be eliminated or will continue to be passed on through several generations. In addition, in diseases that have a late age of onset (e.g., Huntington disease), a person with a disease-associated mutation may be healthy and asymptomatic during childbearing years and be unaware of the risk of passing on the mutant allele to offspring. Consequently, the mutant allele continues to be passed on through several generations.

Other examples of autosomal dominant disorders include achondroplasia, neurofibromatosis, and Marfan syndrome. An idealized pedigree for autosomal dominant inheritance is found in Fig. 5-9 and discussed in the Nursing Care Guidelines box (p. 111). The gene mutation associated with achondroplasia is considered 100% penetrant. The pedigree in the figure demonstrates that although an affected parent has a 50% chance with each pregnancy of transmitting the gene mutation associated with achondroplasia, 50% of offspring do not necessarily inherit the gene mutation. Selected examples of autosomal dominant disorders are found in Table 5-4.

Autosomal Recessive Inheritance

General characteristics of autosomal recessive inheritance are presented in Box 5-3. Children who display an autosomal recessive disorder are always homozygous for that trait (both the maternally and paternally inherited alleles contain disease-associated mutations). This is due to the fact that a recessive

Text continued on p. 95.

BOX 5-2 AUTOSOMAL DOMINANT INHERITANCE: CHARACTERISTICS*

- Males and females are equally likely to be affected.
- A single copy of the mutant allele is typically sufficient to cause the phenotype to express, and therefore a carrier state does not exist. However, if the mutant allele is not fully penetrant (some individuals in a population with the same mutant allele do not express the trait), then the unaffected person with the mutant allele may be referred to as a carrier of the reduced penetrant allele.
- The homozygote for the mutant allele is usually more severely affected than the heterozygote.
- The phenotype appears in consecutive generations unless the condition was due to a new dominant mutation.
- Children of an affected parent have a 50% chance of inheriting the mutant allele and being affected.
- If the mutant allele is 100% penetrant, then phenotypically normal persons in a family pedigree are free of the mutant allele and do not transmit the phenotype to their offspring. However, due to variable expressivity, careful clinical examination and laboratory studies may be necessary before concluding that a person is truly "phenotypically normal."

*All partners of affected persons here are considered genotypically normal.

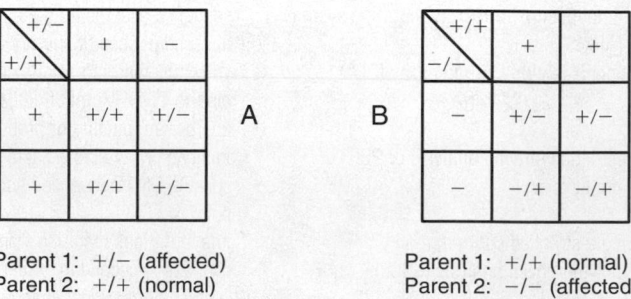

Parent 1: +/− (affected)
Parent 2: +/+ (normal)

Outcomes per pregnancy:
50% +/− (affected)
50% +/+ (normal)

Parent 1: +/+ (normal)
Parent 2: −/− (affected)

Outcomes per pregnancy:
100% +/− (affected)

+ Normal ("wild-type") allele
− Mutant allele

Fig. 5-8 Determination of mating outcomes in autosomal dominant inheritance obtained with Punnett squares. **A,** Possible outcomes of the mating of an affected heterozygous individual (+/−) with a normal partner (+/+). **B,** Mating of an affected homozygous individual (−/−) and a normal partner (+/+).

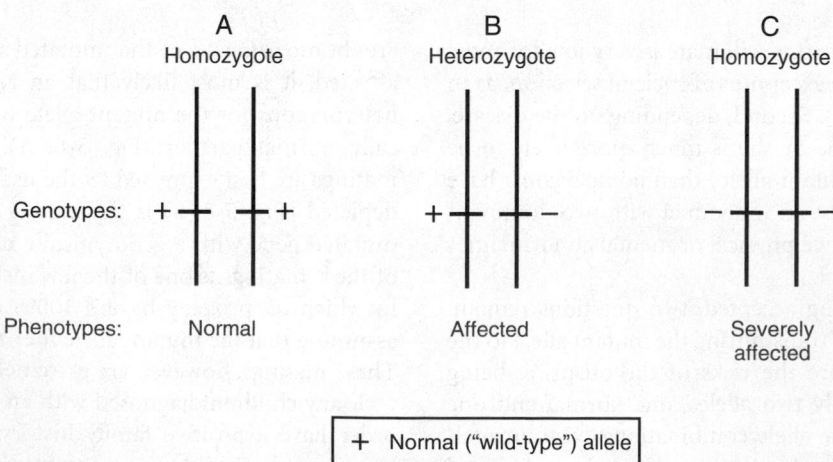

+ Normal ("wild-type") allele
− Mutant allele

Fig. 5-7 Dominant inheritance pattern. Schematic representation of the three possible allelic arrangements of a gene with two alleles. Depicted here are genotypes and possible phenotypes for a trait transmitted by a dominant gene. The presence of a single copy of the mutant allele in heterozygous person **(B)** is sufficient to express the phenotype in question. Double dose of the mutated allele, in homozygous person **(C)**, results in more severe expression of the phenotype.

PATHOPHYSIOLOGY REVIEW

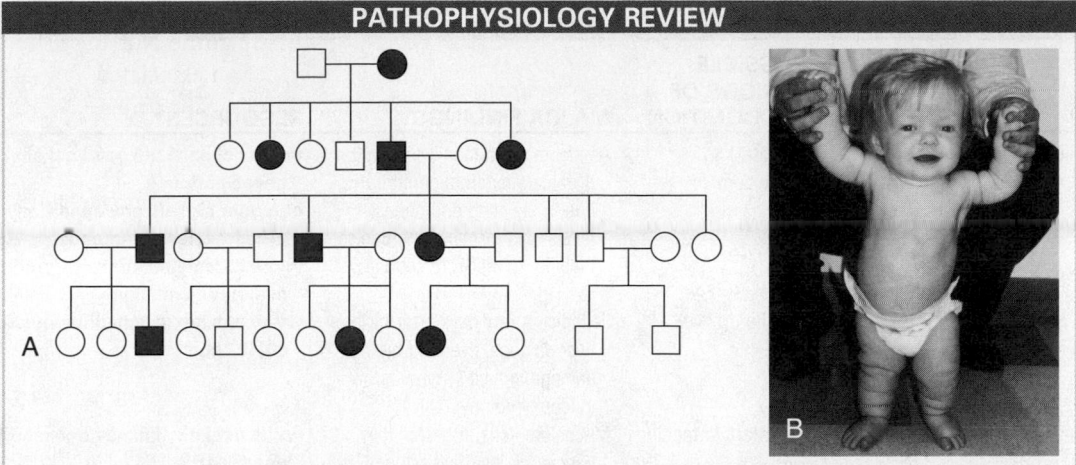

Fig. 5-9 Pedigree for achondroplasia. **A,** Pedigree showing the transmission of an autosomal dominant disease. **B,** Achondroplasia. This girl has short limbs relative to trunk length. She also has a prominent forehead, low nasal root, and redundant skin folds in the arms and legs. (**B,** From Jorde LB, Carey JC, Bamshad MJ, et al: *Medical genetics,* ed 3, St Louis, 2003, Mosby.)

TABLE 5-4	PARTIAL LIST OF MENDELIAN INHERITED GENETIC DISORDERS			
DISORDER	**GENETIC ETIOLOGY**	**POSSIBLE PERIODS OF RECOGNITION**	**MAJOR FINDINGS**	**RESOURCES***
Achondroplasia	AD	Prenatal to newborn	Dwarfism with legs and arms significantly shorter than torso; characteristic facial features	www.geneclinics.org/profiles/achondroplasia/details.html http://ghr.nlm.nih.gov/condition=achondroplasia www.lpaonline.org/mc/page.do
Adenosine deaminase deficiency	AR	Prenatal†; infant period most common; onset can be delayed until adulthood	Enzyme deficiency that results in severe combined immunodeficiency	www.ncbi.nlm.nih.gov/bookshelf/br.fcgi?book=gene&part=ada http://ghr.nlm.nih.gov/condition=adenosinedeaminasedeficiency www.primaryimmune.org
Ataxia telangiectasia	AR	Prenatal† to early childhood	Immunodeficiency, neurodegenerative, acute sensitivity to ionizing radiation that increases risk for cancer	www.ninds.nih.gov/disorders/a_t/a-t.htm www.cancer.gov/cancertopics/factsheet/risk/ataxia http://ghr.nlm.nih.gov/condition=ataxiatelangiectasia www.atcp.org
Beckwith-Wiedemann syndrome	AD or Chr—Abnormal methylation of chromosome 11, uniparental disomy of paternal chromosome 11, or structural abnormality in critical region	Prenatal to newborn	Overgrowth syndrome; often recognized in newborn period due to abnormally large tongue; abdominal wall defects; hypoglycemia in infancy	www.ncbi.nlm.nih.gov/bookshelf/br.fcgi?book=gene&part=bws http://ghr.nlm.nih.gov/condition=beckwithwiedemannsyndrome www.beckwith-wiedemann.info
Bloom syndrome	AR	Prenatal† to early childhood	Prenatal and postnatal growth retardation; chromosome instability leading to sun sensitivity, high cancer risk, immunodeficiency	www.ncbi.nlm.nih.gov/bookshelf/br.fcgi?book=gene&part=bloom http://ghr.nlm.nih.gov/condition=bloomsyndrome

AD, Autosomal dominant; *AR,* autosomal recessive; *Chr,* chromosomal; *DNA,* deoxyribonucleic acid; *XL,* X-linked.

*Support groups are listed on most websites. However, before referring families to support groups, particularly for families that discovered the diagnosis prenatally, carefully review the support group and describe its focus to the couple so they can make an informed decision about whether to visit it.

†Mutation(s) in affected family member or in carrier parents need to be known before prenatal testing can be informative.

Continued

TABLE 5-4   PARTIAL LIST OF MENDELIAN INHERITED GENETIC DISORDERS—cont'd

DISORDER	GENETIC ETIOLOGY	POSSIBLE PERIODS OF RECOGNITION	MAJOR FINDINGS	RESOURCES*
Congenital adrenal hyperplasia	AR	Prenatal† to newborn	Ambiguous genitalia—virilization of female external genitalia due to elevated androgen levels; salt loss in some due to inability to reabsorb sodium	www.ncbi.nlm.nih.gov/bookshelf/br.fcgi?book=gene&part=cah http://ghr.nlm.nih.gov/condition=21hydroxylasedeficiency www.caresfoundation.org/productcart/pc/overview_cah.html
Crigler-Najjar syndrome	AR	Newborn	Jaundice a few days after birth, liver damage, eventual brain damage in type 1; type 2 milder symptoms	www.nlm.nih.gov/medlineplus/ency/article/001127.htm
Cystic fibrosis	AR	Prenatal† to toddler	Meconium ileus at birth; pancreatic insufficiency and malabsorption; chronic pulmonary inflammation and infection	www.ncbi.nlm.nih.gov/bookshelf/br.fcgi?book=gene&part=cf http://ghr.nlm.nih.gov/condition=cysticfibrosis www.cff.org
Duchenne muscular dystrophy	XL recessive	Prenatal† to early childhood	Delayed milestones, progressive skeletal muscle disease, dilated cardiomyopathy	www.ncbi.nlm.nih.gov/bookshelf/br.fcgi?book=gene&part=dbmd http://ghr.nlm.nih.gov/condition=duchenneandbeckermusculardystrophy www.mda.org/disease/DMD.html
Familial adenomatous polyposis (Gardner syndrome, Turcot syndrome)	AD—Mutation in APC gene	Childhood to adulthood	Hundreds to thousands of adenomatous polyps in the distal portion of colon; colon cancer; extra colonic polyps and tumors	www.ncbi.nlm.nih.gov/bookshelf/br.fcgi?book=gene&part=fap http://ghr.nlm.nih.gov/condition=familialadenomatouspolyposis
Fanconi anemia	Most forms AR; at least one form XL	Prenatal† to childhood	Multiple malformations, progressive bone marrow failure, chromosome breakage in cell culture	www.ncbi.nlm.nih.gov/bookshelf/br.fcgi?book=gene&part=fa#fa http://marrowfailure.cancer.gov/FA.html
Fragile X syndrome	XL—Expanded triplet repeat	Prenatal; childhood to adolescent	Moderate cognitive impairment in males, mild cognitive impairment in females	www.ncbi.nlm.nih.gov/bookshelf/br.fcgi?book=gene&part=fragilex http://ghr.nlm.nih.gov/condition=fragilexsyndrome
Friedreich ataxia	AR (most have expanded triplet repeat in one or both genes)	Prenatal† to childhood	Slowly progressive ataxia, cardiomyopathy	www.ncbi.nlm.nih.gov/bookshelf/br.fcgi?book=gene&part=friedreich http://ghr.nlm.nih.gov/condition=friedreichataxia
Galactosemia	AR	Prenatal† to neonatal	Failure to thrive, hepatocellular damage, sepsis, bleeding, cognitive impairment, death if untreated	www.ncbi.nlm.nih.gov/bookshelf/br.fcgi?book=gene&part=galactosemia http://ghr.nlm.nih.gov/condition=galactosemia
Gaucher disease	AR	Prenatal† to adulthood	Three major types: • Type 1 most common; hepatosplenomegaly, bone disease, sometimes lung disease • Type 2 neurodegenerative, lethal by 4 yr • Type 3 neurodegenerative disease, can live to adulthood	www.ncbi.nlm.nih.gov/bookshelf/br.fcgi?book=gene&part=gaucher http://ghr.nlm.nih.gov/condition=gaucherdisease

AD, Autosomal dominant; *AR,* autosomal recessive; *Chr,* chromosomal; *DNA,* deoxyribonucleic acid; *XL,* X-linked.

*Support groups are listed on most websites. However, before referring families to support groups, particularly for families that discovered the diagnosis prenatally, carefully review the support group and describe its focus to the couple so they can make an informed decision about whether to visit it.

†Mutation(s) in affected family member or in carrier parents need to be known before prenatal testing can be informative.

TABLE 5-4		PARTIAL LIST OF MENDELIAN INHERITED GENETIC DISORDERS—cont'd		
DISORDER	**GENETIC ETIOLOGY**	**POSSIBLE PERIODS OF RECOGNITION**	**MAJOR FINDINGS**	**RESOURCES***
Glucose-6-phosphate dehydrogenase (G6PD) deficiency	XL recessive	Infant to adulthood	Hemolytic anemia; expression dependent on exposure to environmental triggers (eating fava beans, certain infections, and certain drugs)	www.nlm.nih.gov/medlineplus/ency/article/000528.htm http://ghr.nlm.nih.gov/condition=glucose6phosphatedehydrogenasedeficiency
Hemophilia A, hemophilia B	XL recessive	Prenatal† to adulthood depending on extent of deficient clotting activity	Hemophilia A—Factor VIII deficiency; hemophilia B—Factor IX deficiency Both diagnosed in infancy period in those with severe deficiency; brought to attention by spontaneous joint or deep muscle bleeds	www.ncbi.nlm.nih.gov/bookshelf/br.fcgi?book=gene&part=hemo-a www.ncbi.nlm.nih.gov/bookshelf/br.fcgi?book=gene&part=hemo-b http://ghr.nlm.nih.gov/condition=hemophilia
Huntington disease	AD expanded triplet repeat	Prenatal for couples with family history; most often diagnosed in adulthood	Progressive neurodegenerative disease with mean age of onset in third to fourth decade of life; death typically within 20 yr of symptom onset	www.ncbi.nlm.nih.gov/bookshelf/br.fcgi?book=gene&part=huntington http://ghr.nlm.nih.gov/condition=huntingtondisease
Hurler syndrome	AR	Prenatal†; infant to childhood	Progressive lysosomal storage disease; death by 10 yr of age in severely affected; mildly affected can live into adulthood	www.ncbi.nlm.nih.gov/bookshelf/br.fcgi?book=gene&part=mps1 http://ghr.nlm.nih.gov/condition=mucopolysaccharidosistypei
Hypophosphatemic vitamin D–resistant rickets	XL dominant	Infant to childhood	Kidney abnormality resulting in overexcretion of phosphate in urine; secondary bone defects result	www.merck.com/mmhe/print/sec11/ch146/ch146g.html
Incontinentia pigmenti	XL dominant	Prenatal†; newborn to infant	Often prenatally lethal in males; those who survive should have chromosome testing; blistering of skin, later linear hypopigmentation of skin; small, missing teeth; sparse, wiry hair; vascular retinal abnormalities	www.ncbi.nlm.nih.gov/bookshelf/br.fcgi?book=gene&part=i-p http://ghr.nlm.nih.gov/condition=incontinentiapigmenti
Li-Fraumeni syndrome	AD	Prenatal†; 50% have first cancer by age 40	Predisposition to multiple primary cancers at various body sites	www.ncbi.nlm.nih.gov/bookshelf/br.fcgi?book=gene&part=li-fraumeni http://ghr.nlm.nih.gov/condition=lifraumenisyndrome
Malignant hyperthermia	AD	Prenatal† or before drug exposure (if family history and family mutation known)	Susceptibility to uncontrolled skeletal muscle hypermetabolism when exposed to certain anesthetics and succinylcholine; first symptoms tachycardia, tachypnea, then progressive symptoms and death if not quickly treated	www.ncbi.nlm.nih.gov/bookshelf/br.fcgi?book=gene&part=mhs http://ghr.nlm.nih.gov/condition=malignanthyperthermia www.mhaus.org
Marfan syndrome	AD	Prenatal†; neonatal to adulthood depending on number and severity of features and presence or absence of family history	Connective tissue disorder primarily affecting cardiovascular, skeletal, and ocular systems	www.ncbi.nlm.nih.gov/bookshelf/br.fcgi?book=gene&part=marfan http://ghr.nlm.nih.gov/condition=marfansyndrome

Continued

TABLE 5-4   PARTIAL LIST OF MENDELIAN INHERITED GENETIC DISORDERS—cont'd

DISORDER	GENETIC ETIOLOGY	POSSIBLE PERIODS OF RECOGNITION	MAJOR FINDINGS	RESOURCES*
Myotonic dystrophy	AD expansion mutation; *DMPK* for type 1; *CNBP* for type 2	Prenatal if gene expansion mutation identified in affected parent Type 1—Birth in congenital form; child to adulthood for other forms Type 2—Onset typically in third decade	Variable presentation Classic type 1—Affects skeletal and smooth muscle characterized by muscle weakness, wasting, myotonia, cardiac conduction abnormalities Type 2—Muscle weakness, myotonia, posterior subcapsular cataracts, insulin insensitivity (increasingly common with age)	www.ncbi.nlm.nih.gov/bookshelf/br.fcgi?book=gene&part=myotonic-d www.ncbi.nlm.nih.gov/bookshelf/br.fcgi?book=gene&part=myotonic-d2 http://ghr.nlm.nih.gov/condition=myotonicdystrophy
Neurofibromatosis	AD	Type 1—Childhood to adulthood Type 2—Adolescence to adulthood	Type 1—Six or more café-au-lait spots, axillary and inguinal freckling, neurofibromas, iris Lisch nodules; learning disabilities common. Type 2—Vestibular schwannomas	www.ncbi.nlm.nih.gov/bookshelf/br.fcgi?book=gene&part=nf1 http://ghr.nlm.nih.gov/condition=neurofibromatosistype1 www.ncbi.nlm.nih.gov/bookshelf/br.fcgi?book=gene&part=nf2 http://ghr.nlm.nih.gov/condition=neurofibromatosistype2
Oculocutaneous albinism type 1	AR	Prenatal†; birth to childhood	Hypopigmentation of skin and hair due to reduced melanin production; nystagmus, iris translucency; significant vision impairment	www.ncbi.nlm.nih.gov/bookshelf/br.fcgi?book=gene&part=oca1 http://ghr.nlm.nih.gov/condition=oculocutaneousalbinism
Phenylketonuria	AR	Prenatal†; newborn	Minimal or absent phenylalanine hydroxylase activity resulting in profound cognitive impairment if not treated early with dietary restriction of phenylalanine	www.ncbi.nlm.nih.gov/bookshelf/br.fcgi?book=gene&part=pku http://ghr.nlm.nih.gov/condition=phenylketonuria
Pompe disease (glycogen storage disease type II)	AR	Prenatal†; newborn to infant	Hypotonia, cardiomegaly, and hypertrophic cardiomyopathy, failure to thrive; death within first yr of life; early enzyme therapy may prevent or delay symptoms	www.ncbi.nlm.nih.gov/bookshelf/br.fcgi?book=gene&part=gsd2 http://ghr.nlm.nih.gov/condition=pompedisease
Porphyria, acute intermittent	AD (low penetrance)	Adolescence to adulthood	Acute attacks include abdominal pain; peripheral neuropathy; neuropsychiatric symptoms	www.ncbi.nlm.nih.gov/bookshelf/br.fcgi?book=gene&part=aip http://ghr.nlm.nih.gov/condition=porphyria
Sickle cell disorder (sickle cell anemia; sickle-hemoglobin C disease; sickle β-thalassemia)	AR	Prenatal to newborn; if missed on newborn screen, childhood	Severe pain at site of vascular occlusion leading to tissue ischemia; organ dysfunction possible at site of vascular occlusion	www.ncbi.nlm.nih.gov/bookshelf/br.fcgi?book=gene&part=sickle http://ghr.nlm.nih.gov/condition=sicklecelldisease
Tay-Sachs disease (hexosaminidase A deficiency)	AR	Prenatal to infant	Neurodegenerative disease Acute type—Progressive weakness, loss of motor skills, seizures, blindness, spasticity, death by about 4 yr Subacute type—May have onset in childhood or adulthood with variable progressive neurologic findings	www.ncbi.nlm.nih.gov/bookshelf/br.fcgi?book=gene&part=tay-sachs http://ghr.nlm.nih.gov/condition=taysachsdisease

AD, Autosomal dominant; *AR,* autosomal recessive; *Chr,* chromosomal; *DNA,* deoxyribonucleic acid; *XL,* X-linked.

*Support groups are listed on most websites. However, before referring families to support groups, particularly for families that discovered the diagnosis prenatally, carefully review the support group and describe its focus to the couple so they can make an informed decision about whether to visit it.

†Mutation(s) in affected family member or in carrier parents need to be known before prenatal testing can be informative.

TABLE 5-4	PARTIAL LIST OF MENDELIAN INHERITED GENETIC DISORDERS—cont'd			
DISORDER	**GENETIC ETIOLOGY**	**POSSIBLE PERIODS OF RECOGNITION**	**MAJOR FINDINGS**	**RESOURCES***
β-Thalassemia	AR	Prenatal†; newborn screening; by 2 yr of age if missed on screen	Microcytic hypochromic anemia, absent or reduced β-hemoglobin; severe anemia and secondary hepatosplenomegaly	www.ncbi.nlm.nih.gov/bookshelf/br.fcgi?book=gene&part=b-thal http://ghr.nlm.nih.gov/condition=betathalassemia
Velo-cardio-facial syndrome	AD and Chr—46,XX,del(22.11.2) or 46,XY,del(22.11.2)	Prenatal to adulthood	Extremely variable condition; nearly 200 possible features described; most common are cognitive impairment, palatal structural or functional abnormalities, conotruncal heart defects, mild immunodeficiencies	www.ncbi.nlm.nih.gov/bookshelf/br.fcgi?book=gene&part=gr_22q11deletion http://ghr.nlm.nih.gov/condition=22q112deletionsyndrome
Xeroderma pigmentosum	AR (abnormalities in genes responsible for DNA repair)	Prenatal† to 2 yr	Acute sun sensitivity (severe sunburns and blistering with minimal exposure) and over 1000 fold increased risk of cutaneous and ocular neoplasms; in some cases, sensitivity to x rays	www.ncbi.nlm.nih.gov/bookshelf/br.fcgi?book=gene&part=xp www.cc.nih.gov/ccc/patient_education/pepubs/xp7_17.pdf

---

BOX 5-3   AUTOSOMAL RECESSIVE INHERITANCE: CHARACTERISTICS

- Males and females are equally likely to be affected.
- A carrier state exists. Both males and females can be carriers.
- The disease rarely appears in multiple generations unless there is consanguinity in the family or the family is part of a racial, ethnic, or cultural group in which the frequency of the mutated allele is high. Members of the generation who have affected children are usually asymptomatic (heterozygous) carriers.
- Carrier parents have a 25% chance of producing an affected child and a 50% chance of producing a carrier child in each and every pregnancy.
- Parent consanguinity may be a factor when a child is affected with a rare recessive disease.

---

allele is one whose phenotypic expression occurs only when both genes have disease-associated mutations. Although this makes the alleles homozygous because both alleles are recessive, the disease-associated mutation may be different in each allele. When this is the case, the pair of alleles is more accurately referred to as compound heterozygous for the recessive trait. In the heterozygote, a recessive allele is "masked" by the wild type (normal) allele, which is dominant (Fig. 5-10). Whereas the possible pregnancy outcomes in autosomal dominant pattern (see Fig. 5-7) are children who are either affected (if the gene mutation is fully penetrant) or unaffected when completely free of the gene mutation, in autosomal recessive inheritance a third possibility arises, that of a heterozygous carrier (see Fig. 5-10, B). These are individuals who are clinically normal (or nearly normal), but who are at risk of having offspring who are affected.

Identification of such carriers is of paramount importance for genetic counseling. In the case of an unaffected couple who produces a child with a recessive disease, identification is easy; since they each must contribute a mutant allele, they must be considered obligate carriers, even in the absence of specific carrier testing for that gene. Specific tests to detect heterozygous carriers of a variety of genetic diseases are available, but it would be impractical and certainly not cost-effective to use all available tests to screen all prospective parents without specific risk factors. Genetic screening for carriers is usually limited to populations at risk, either because they belong to a high-risk group for a certain disorder (e.g., Ashkenazi Jews and Tay-Sachs disease) or because of positive family history. Carriers for some specific disorders can be identified by specific tests before conception, by means of routine screening, or after conception by means of prenatal diagnosis (e.g., Tay-Sachs disease, cystic fibrosis [CF], sickle cell disorder). It is estimated that each person carries from three to eight mutated genes for a severe recessive disease. For example, 1 in 25 persons in the United States and Northern European populations carries a recessive gene mutation for CF. In the African-American population, 1 in 10 persons is a carrier for the sickle cell gene mutation. For PKU, the carrier rate in the general population is 1 in 50.

However, since genetic diseases are rare, the probability of the mating of two persons who carry the same gene in the same allelic configuration is very small. The chances are increased if mating occurs among persons who select a mate because of geographic, ethnic, or religious restrictions or blood relationship (consanguinity). For example, 1 in 30 Ashkenazi Jews is a carrier of a gene mutation associated with Tay-Sachs disease, and 1 in 3600 live births would be affected without preconception screening. For comparison, the frequency of Tay-Sachs

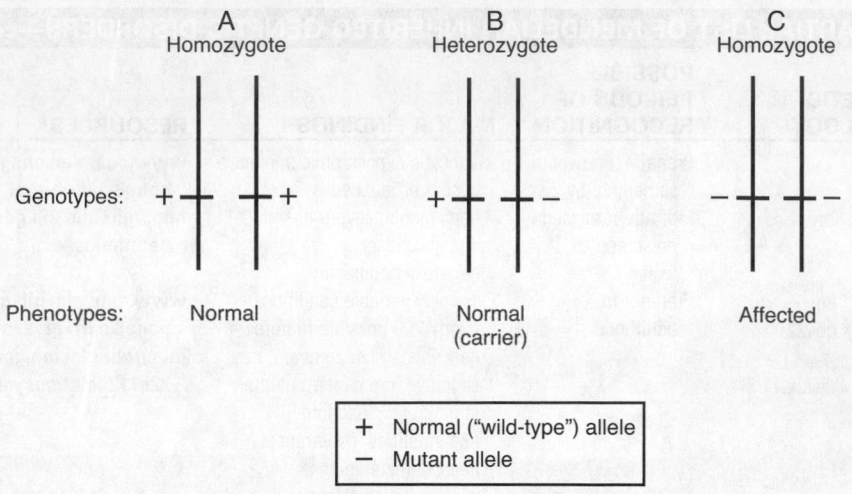

Fig. 5-10 Recessive inheritance pattern. Schematic representation of the three possible allelic arrangements of a gene with two alleles. Depicted here are genotypes and possible phenotypes for a trait transmitted by a recessive gene. The presence of a single copy of the mutant allele in the heterozygous person **(B)** results in a phenotypically normal individual who carries the mutant allele. The affected phenotype is only expressed in presence of a double dose of the mutated allele **(C)**.

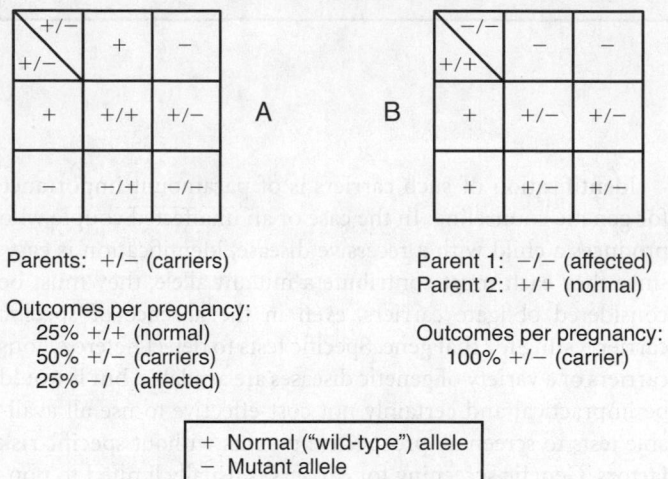

Parents: +/− (carriers)

Outcomes per pregnancy:
 25% +/+ (normal)
 50% +/− (carriers)
 25% −/− (affected)

Parent 1: −/− (affected)
Parent 2: +/+ (normal)

Outcomes per pregnancy:
 100% +/− (carrier)

+ Normal ("wild-type") allele
− Mutant allele

Fig. 5-11 Autosomal recessive inheritance: Punnett squares. **A,** Possible outcomes of mating of two heterozygous carriers (+/−). **B,** Mating of affected homozygous individual (−/−) and normal partner (+/+). Percentages shown refer to outcome possibilities in each pregnancy.

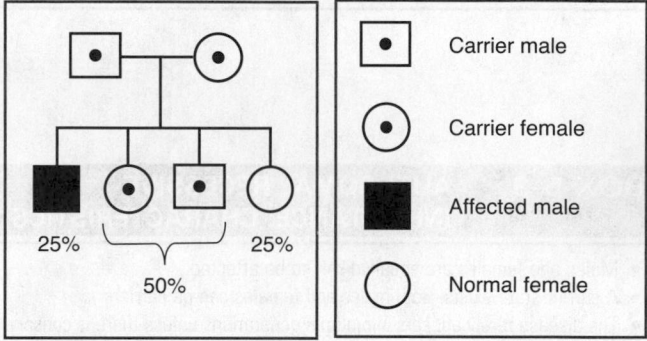

Fig. 5-12 Autosomal recessive inheritance: typical pedigree. The idealized pedigree on the left represents possible outcomes of the mating of two heterozygous carriers (+/−). Percentages express risks for each pregnancy resulting from this mating.

disease outside this population is 100 times smaller (i.e., 1 in 360,000 live births).

Other examples of autosomal recessive disorders include the thalassemias, congenital adrenal hyperplasia, and galactosemia. Fig. 5-11 illustrates two situations involving autosomal recessive traits. Fig. 5-11, *A,* depicts the most common occurrence in autosomal recessive disorders: the mating of two carrier parents with each pregnancy carrying a 25% chance of producing an affected child. Fig. 5-11, *B,* reflects the mating of an affected parent with a genotypically normal partner, in which 100% of the offspring will be carriers. An idealized pedigree representing the mating of two heterozygous (asymptomatic) carriers and its possible outcomes in each and every pregnancy is shown in Fig. 5-12. Selected examples of autosomal recessive disorders are found in Table 5-4.

Sex-Linked Inheritance Patterns

The transmission of genes located on one of the sex chromosomes (either X or Y) is termed sex-linked inheritance. However, few genes have been found on the Y chromosome, so frequently the terms *sex-linked* and *X-linked* are interchangeably (and incorrectly) used. The testicular organizing region of the Y chromosome determines the formation of testes and the development of male sexual structures during embryonic growth. A gene for hairy ears, with high prevalence in southern Asia, has also been located on the Y chromosome. Inheritance of Y-linked genes follows a father-to-son, or male-to-male, pattern. It is important to remember that men give their X chromosomes to their daughters (and their Y to their sons), so in analyzing a family pedigree, male-to-male transmission of a gene rules out X-linked inheritance.

Women have two homologous X chromosomes; therefore inheritance of genes located on the X chromosome (X-linked inheritance) follows the same pattern as that for autosomal genes. However, in the case of males, the X and Y chromosomes have small areas of homology and therefore do not pair side-

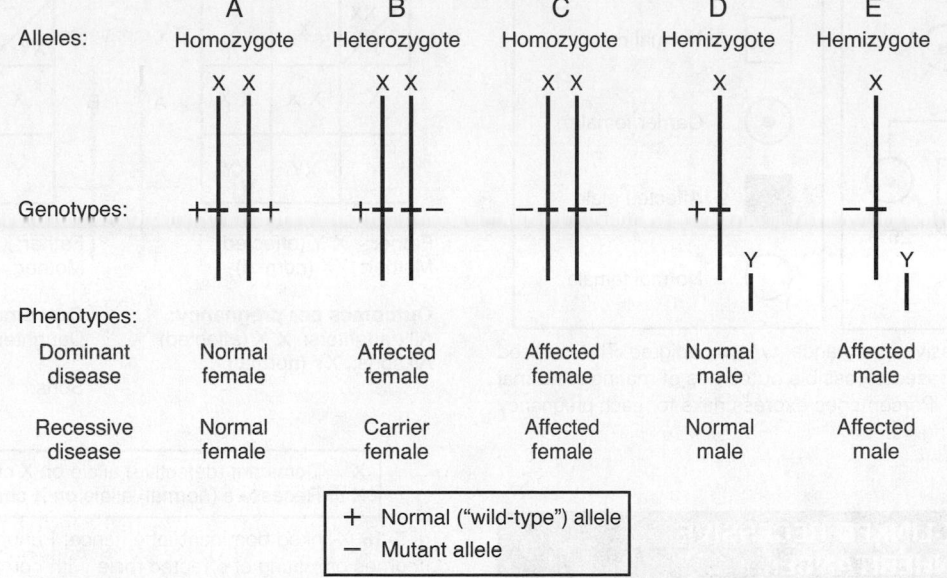

Fig. 5-13 X-linked inheritance pattern. **A to C,** Possible allelic arrangements of an X-linked gene in females. Note that phenotypic expression of an X-linked gene in women is typically similar to that of an autosomal gene. However, unequal X inactivation could result in more active X chromosomes with the mutation and could result in symptoms. **D** and **E,** Uneven pairing of X and Y chromosomes in males, and its phenotypic expressions. Note that there are no carrier males, since the phenotype is determined solely by the characteristic of X-linked allele. Hemizygous males are either normal or affected.

by-side during meiosis. Because of this, men are hemizygous for all genes on the X chromosome that do not have a homologous site on the Y chromosome, and their alleles are represented as single copies. Therefore, in the inheritance of an X-linked gene, the single-copy presence of its normal, or its mutant, allele will result in the expression of the normal or mutant phenotype, respectively. This is true for both dominant and recessive X-linked diseases in males (Fig. 5-13).

X-Linked Recessive Inheritance

In females the alleles of an X-linked recessive gene behave as the alleles of any autosomal recessive gene: the effect of the abnormal allele is "hidden" by the normal (dominant) allele. Therefore females who have a disease-associated mutation in both members of the gene pair will express the phenotype. Although it is rare for females to express the phenotype if only one member of the gene pair carries a disease-associated mutation, it is possible due to X inactivation.

Soon after fertilization, it is normal for one X chromosome in females to be inactivated through a natural process called **methylation.** This occurs in each cell in the early blasotcyst stage, and whether the paternal or maternal X is inactivated is random in each cell. At the time this occurs, the X that has been inactivated will remain so through all subsequent cell divisions. Females who express a phenotype may do so due to the inactivation of a greater proportion of X chromosomes carrying the normal allele in the tissues or organs associated with the disorder. Examples of X-linked recessive disorders include hemophilia types A and B and Duchenne muscular dystrophy. Fig. 5-14 illustrates the outcomes of each pregnancy between an affected man and a normal woman (see Fig. 5-14, *A*), and between a normal man and a carrier woman (see Fig. 5-14, *B*). An idealized pedigree depicting the mating between a genetically

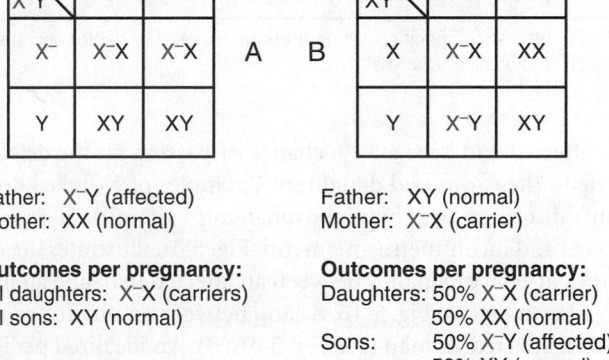

Father: X⁻Y (affected)   Father: XY (normal)
Mother: XX (normal)   Mother: X⁻X (carrier)

Outcomes per pregnancy: **Outcomes per pregnancy:**
All daughters: X⁻X (carriers)   Daughters: 50% X⁻X (carrier)
All sons: XY (normal)   50% XX (normal)
                                             Sons: 50% X⁻Y (affected)
                                                        50% XY (normal)

X⁻ = Recessive (defective) allele on X chromosome
X = Dominant (normal) allele on X chromosome

Fig. 5-14 X-linked recessive inheritance: Punnett squares. **A,** Possible outcomes of mating of affected male with normal female. **B,** Mating of normal male and carrier female. Percentages refer to outcome possibilities in each pregnancy.

normal man and a carrier woman, and its possible outcomes per pregnancy, is shown in Fig. 5-15. The primary characteristics of X-linked recessive inheritance are listed in Box 5-4.

X-Linked Dominant Inheritance

X-linked dominant inheritance (see Fig. 5-13) is rare. The main characteristics of X-linked dominant inheritance are (1) both males and females can be affected, but females, because of the random nature of X inactivation, are usually less severely affected than males; (2) affected men do not transmit the defective allele to their sons; and (3) all daughters of an affected man

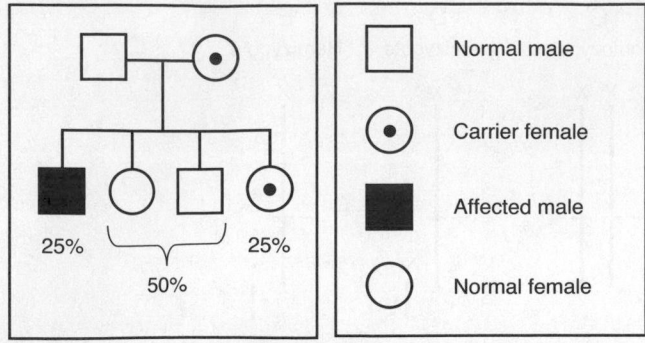

Fig. 5-15 X-linked recessive inheritance: typical pedigree. The idealized pedigree on the left represents possible outcomes of mating of normal male and carrier female. Percentages express risks for each pregnancy resulting from this mating.

BOX 5-4   X-LINKED RECESSIVE INHERITANCE: CHARACTERISTICS*

- Most affected persons are male. Affected females are extremely rare.
- Males transmit their Y chromosome to their sons; therefore father-to-son transmission of X-linked traits is not possible except in the rare instance of nondisjunction when a sperm carries both an X and Y chromosome.
- All daughters of an affected male are (heterozygous) carriers; none is affected (homozygous).
- Sons of carrier females have a 50% chance of inheriting the mutant allele and being affected (hemizygous). Daughters have a 50% risk of inheriting the mutant allele and being (heterozygous) carriers.

*Unless otherwise specified, all partners of affected or carrier persons here are genotypically normal.

are affected and have a 50% chance of passing on the defective allele to their sons and daughters. Examples of X-linked dominant disorders are hypophosphatemic vitamin D–resistant rickets and incontinentia pigmenti. Fig. 5-16 illustrates the outcomes of each pregnancy between an affected man and an unaffected woman (see Fig. 5-16, *A*) and between an unaffected man and an affected woman (see Fig. 5-16, *B*). An idealized pedigree representing the mating of an affected man with a genetically normal woman is shown in Fig. 5-17.

VARIABLE PATTERNS OF GENE EXPRESSION AND INHERITANCE

A number of variables have been observed that explain or modify basic inheritance patterns and the effects of chromosome abnormalities. Some of these variations have been recognized for some time; others are newly discovered phenomena that explain some apparent contradictions in the established patterns of inheritance. Also, some disorders have been reported to follow more than one inheritance pattern in different families (e.g., a classically recessive disorder may occasionally be reported to be following a dominant or X-linked pattern in other families). This phenomenon is known as locus heterogeneity (King, Rotter, and Motulsky, 2002).

The most notable of these gene variations is mutation. As discussed above, mutations are heritable changes in the DNA sequence of a gene. Mutations can result from a substitution of

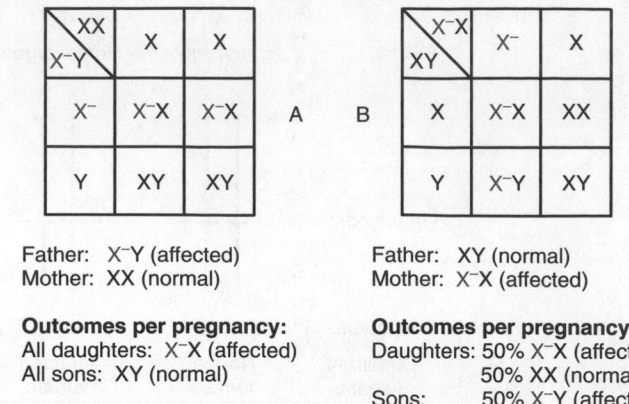

Father: X⁻Y (affected)
Mother: XX (normal)

Outcomes per pregnancy:
All daughters: X⁻X (affected)
All sons: XY (normal)

Father: XY (normal)
Mother: X⁻X (affected)

Outcomes per pregnancy:
Daughters: 50% X⁻X (affected)
          50% XX (normal)
Sons: 50% X⁻Y (affected)
         50% XY (normal)

X⁻ = Dominant (defective) allele on X chromosome
X = Recessive (normal) allele on X chromosome

Fig. 5-16 X-linked dominant inheritance: Punnett squares. **A,** Possible outcomes of mating of affected male with normal female. **B,** Mating of normal male and affected female. Percentages shown refer to outcome possibilities in each pregnancy.

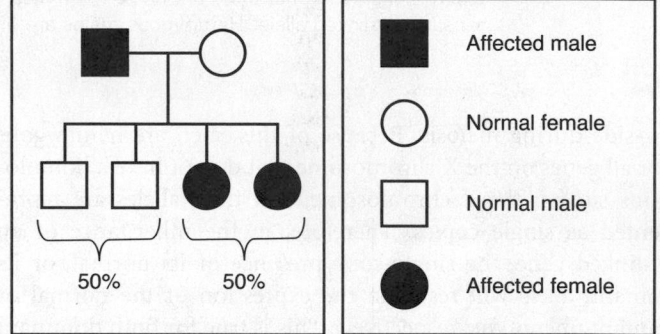

Affected male

Normal female

Normal male

Affected female

Fig. 5-17 X-linked dominant inheritance: typical pedigree. The idealized pedigree on the left represents possible outcomes of mating of affected male and normal female. Percentages depicted express risks for each pregnancy resulting from this mating. Since the mutant allele is carried in the X chromosome, an affected male will transfer it to 100% of his daughters.

bases (**point mutations**) or the insertion or deletion of bases (Korf, 2000). Some genes have a high mutation rate, and various forms of the resulting disease may have varying expression. One example is the *CFTR* gene, in which more than 1000 different CF-associated mutations have been identified (the vast majority being point mutations or small deletions). Mutations can occur in somatic cells or in germ cells. Somatic cell mutations are passed on to the daughter cells of the mutated cell, but are not transmitted to the offspring. Germ cells mutations affect the gametes and are hereditary. Mutation rates are not constant for all genes, so some diseases may occur with much greater frequency than others.

Variable expression is an important concept that describes differences in the extent and severity of phenotype. There is a continuum of expression for any affected person from very mild to severe clinical manifestations. For those with very mild manifestations, it may take an expert clinician to identify the condition. For example, a parent of a child with classic neurofibromatosis may exhibit only a few "birth marks" that a medical geneticist, genetics advanced practice nurse, or genetic counselor would recognize as café-au-lait spots, one of the manifestations of neurofibromatosis.

The discovery of expansion mutations in some genetic disorders has helped explain their variation in inheritance patterns and clinical expression (Nelson, 1996). Within genes are sequences of DNA nucleotide repeats. A normal gene has a certain number of these repeats, for example, the *FMR1* gene on the X chromosome usually has about 5 to 40 repeats. When *FMR1* has 59 to 200 repeats, that area of the gene can become unstable and gain further repeats during meiosis. Females who have this number of repeats are considered carriers of a premutation for fragile X syndrome. A person with fragile X has a full mutation allele with hundreds to thousands of repeats. Because fragile X syndrome is an X-linked disorder, females are less likely to be affected because of the presence of a normal allele on the homologous X chromosome. These expanding repeats have also been found to occur in autosomal dominant disorders such as myotonic dystrophy and in autosomal recessive disorders such as Friedreich ataxia (Chamberlain, 1996). Expansion mutations that have a tendency to further expand when transmitted from one generation to the next can display phenotypic anticipation. Pedigrees display anticipation when individuals in successive generations develop the disorder at an earlier age and/or with more severe manifestations.

Genomic imprinting and uniparental disomy are two genetic phenomena that consider the parental origin of genetic information (i.e., maternally or paternally derived). The concept of genomic imprinting refers to modification, in some instances, of genetic material, resulting in phenotypic differences based on whether the genes and chromosomes were derived from the mother or the father. Genomic imprinting is exhibited during pregnancy, when paternally derived chromosomes seem to positively influence placental development and maternally derived chromosomes seem to positively influence fetal development. This phenomenon also occurs in some genetic disorders, such as Prader-Willi and Angelman syndromes. In both these disorders about two thirds of affected individuals have a deletion of the same segment of chromosome 15. However, the clinical manifestations of Prader-Willi and Angelman syndromes are markedly different. If the deletion occurs on the paternally derived chromosome 15, the child exhibits Prader-Willi syndrome; if the deletion occurs on the maternally derived chromosome 15, the child manifests Angelman syndrome (Jorde, Carey, Bamshad, et al, 2003). Prader-Willi syndrome is characterized by failure to thrive and central hypotonia in the newborn and infancy period with later insatiable hunger that can lead to morbid obesity during childhood. Children with Prader-Willi syndrome also have cognitive dysfunction, typical dysmorphic features, behavioral disturbances, hypothalamic hypogonadism, and short stature. In contrast, Angelman syndrome includes severe cognitive impairment, characteristic facies, abnormal (puppetlike) gait, and paroxysms of inappropriate laughter. Children with Angelman syndrome are usually nonverbal, although they may vocalize (Fridman, Varela, Kok, et al, 2000).

In some cases both copies of a chromosome pair are determined to have come from one parent, either the mother or the father, instead of one from each; this phenomenon is called uniparental disomy (Fridman, Varela, Kok, et al, 2000). An example of uniparental disomy was reported with CF, in which both chromosomes, each with a mutant recessive gene, came from the carrier mother; the father was not a carrier. In cases that appear to be nonpaternal, uniparental disomy may be a factor. One of several theories about uniparental disomy is that the chromosome pair was originally a trisomy and the father's chromosome was randomly eliminated, leaving two copies of the mother's chromosome. Because the chromosomes appear as a normal "pair," diagnosis of this situation is only possible with molecular (DNA) techniques. Uniparental disomy has also been reported with Beckwith-Wiedemann syndrome, which is characterized by overgrowth and hypoglycemia at birth (see Table 5-2).

MITOCHONDRIAL DISORDERS

The nucleus is not the only site of genetic information. Extranuclear DNA is found in a cytoplasmic cellular organelle, the mitochondrion, whose primary function in cellular metabolism is the production of energy. Mutations in mtDNA also account for nonmendelian inheritance patterns. Inheritance of traits contained in mtDNA is exclusively maternal, since only the mitochondria from the ovum are transmitted to the zygote. Mitochondria are not contained within the sperm head.

An additional complexity in mitochondrial inheritance results from the fact that, during mitosis, mitochondria are randomly distributed among the daughter cells, so that both normal and mutated mitochondria may be found in the same cell, a phenomenon known as heteroplasmy (Korf, 2000). This leads to variable dosages of mutated mtDNA between tissues and organs. This variation in mutation load leads to a highly variable spectrum of clinical manifestations, and individuals with the same mtDNA mutation may range from symptom free, to mildly affected, to severely impaired. Symptoms may include seizures, pancreatitis, and metabolic disease. Different manifestations may be seen in different members of the same family. Heteroplasmy complicates the use of prenatal diagnosis. Once the mtDNA mutation is identified in the mother, her pregnancies can be tested for the same mutation. However, the mutation load identified in sampled fetal tissue (chorionic villi or amniocytes) may not correspond to other fetal tissues, the mutational load of which will continue to change during development due to random mitotic segregation of cytoplasmic organelles. Consequently, it is not possible to predict the unborn child's phenotype based on prenatal test results.

mtDNA mutations are responsible for various childhood diseases (Table 5-5), such as Leigh syndrome (movement disorder, respiratory dyskinesia, regression, hypotonia, seizures, and failure to thrive). Because mitochondrial disorders have such variability of expression, determining the diagnosis can be confusing. However, when a child has an unexplained constellation of symptoms, a mitochondrial disorder should be considered. Examples of mitochondrial syndromes include Kearns-Sayre syndrome (external ophthalmoplegia, pigmentary retinopathy, heart block, ataxia, increased cerebrospinal fluid protein); myoclonic epilepsy with ragged red fibers, or MERRF (myoclonic epilepsy, myopathy, dementia); and MELAS (mitochondrial encephalomyopathy, lactic acidosis,

TABLE 5-5   **PARTIAL LIST OF MITOCHONDRIAL GENETIC DISORDERS**

DISORDER	GENETIC ETIOLOGY	POSSIBLE PERIODS OF RECOGNITION	MAJOR FINDINGS	RESOURCES*
Kearns-Sayre syndrome	Mit—Maternal inheritance but affected women only have approximately 1 in 24 risk of having affected offspring; maternal transmission to more than one child has not been reported	Infancy; before 20 yr of age	Three overlapping phenotypes that can be seen in same family and used to be distinguished as three different diseases; multisystem disease primarily affecting CNS, endocrine system, skeletal muscles, heart, retina	www.ncbi.nlm.nih.gov/bookshelf/br. fcgi?book=gene&part=kss
Leigh syndrome; NARP (neurogenic muscle weakness, ataxia, retinitis pigmentosa)	Mit—Many different mitochondrial genes implicated	Leigh—Infancy NARP—Childhood	Symptoms depend on mutation load and tissue distribution of disease causing mtDNA mutation; progressive, neurodegenerative disorder Leigh onset typically after viral infection; 75% die by 3 yr of age NARP onset typically in childhood; ataxia, learning difficulties, episodic deterioration possible following viral infections	www.ncbi.nlm.nih.gov/bookshelf/br. fcgi?book=gene&part=narp
MELAS (mitochondrial encephalomyopathy, lactic acidosis, and strokelike episodes)	Mit	Early childhood	Encephalopathy, seizures, recurrent vomiting, recurrent headaches, exercise intolerance, strokelike episodes	www.ncbi.nlm.nih.gov/bookshelf/br.fcgi? book=gene&part=melas http://ghr.nlm.nih.gov/condition= mitochondrialencephalomyopathylactic acidosisandstrokelikeepisodes
MERRF (myoclonic epilepsy associated with ragged red fibers)	Mit	Childhood	Myoclonus, generalized epilepsy, ataxia, dementia	www.ncbi.nlm.nih.gov/bookshelf/br. fcgi?book=gene&part=merrf

CNS, Central nervous system; *Mit,* mitochondrial; *mtDNA,* mitochondrial deoxyribonucleic acid.
*Support groups are listed on most websites. However, before referring families to support groups, particularly for families that discovered the diagnosis prenatally, carefully review the support group and describe its focus to the couple so they can make an informed decision about whether to visit it.

strokelike episodes) (Korf, 2000). Nuclear DNA (nDNA) mutations can also cause disorders of the mitochondria, so not all "mitochondrial disorders" are caused by mutations in mtDNA.

HEREDITARY CANCER PREDISPOSITION GENES

The process of carcinogenesis implies permanent changes in the DNA of the targeted cell. Early observations recognized genetic influences in cancer: (1) certain types of cancer occur more frequently within certain families (breast, colon, ovarian, some leukemias); (2) some well-defined genetic disorders show a predisposition to various malignancies (familial adenomatous polyposis and colon cancer, Bloom syndrome and lymphomas); (3) many chromosome abnormalities occur frequently with malignancies (Philadelphia chromosome in chronic myelogenous leukemia); and (4) certain chromosome aneuploidies predispose the person to cancer (Down syndrome and acute leukemias).

The discovery of oncogenes in the early 1970s marked the beginning of a new era in the field of cancer genetics (Box 5-5). Initially thought to be carried exclusively by retroviruses, oncogenes were later identified as natural genes that existed in all mammals. Early investigations suggested that oncogenes were found in inactive form (i.e., no correlation with cancer could be identified in this state). In reality, oncogenes are normally involved in cell growth and division. A mutation in an oncogene can disrupt this normal process and transform a normal cell into one that has uncontrolled cell growth or division, predisposing the cell to further mutations that eventually transform the cell into one that is malignant.

Since the discovery of oncogenes, two other classes of genes associated with cancer development have been identified: tumor suppressor genes and mismatch repair genes. Tumor suppressor genes normally inhibit cell growth and division. A mutation in these genes can interfere with this normal function and lead to uninhibited cell growth and division. Among this group is *p53* (sometimes called *TP53*), whose germ cell (or hereditary) mutations are associated with Li-Fraumeni syndrome and whose somatic cell mutations (sporadic) result in various malignancies, such as bladder cancer. Li-Fraumeni syndrome is inherited as an autosomal dominant trait that predisposes children and young adults to the development of various tumors, including osteosarcoma; soft tissue sarcomas; breast, brain, and adrenocortical carcinomas; and leukemia.

Mismatch repair genes normally function by recognizing and repairing DNA errors that occur during replication or mutations that are caused by external agents such as ultraviolet light or chemical exposure. Xeroderma pigmentosum is a classic example of inherited predisposition to cancers caused by a germline mutation in one of several possible mismatch repair genes. Infants and children with xeroderma pigmentosum are at considerable risk for skin cancers triggered by sun and ultraviolet light exposure.

MULTIFACTORIAL (COMPLEX) DISORDERS

A number of frequently encountered diseases and defects show an increased incidence in some families but have no clear-cut affected-unaffected classification. Although the incidence is higher than would be expected by chance, no specific mode of inheritance can be identified. In some, environmental factors, including the prenatal environment, appear to play an important role. These conditions are classified as multifactorial disorders, in which a genetic susceptibility and specific environmental agents interact to produce a disease state. Multifactorial disorders include NTDs, cleft lip and cleft palate, many congenital heart defects, congenital hip dislocation, and pyloric stenosis.

Recurrence risks for multifactorial conditions are empirically based on observed recurrence within a population. In general, recurrence risk is usually low (<10%). For example, NTDs occur in 1 out of 1000 births in the general population. The recurrence risk after the first affected child is 2 or 3 out of 100 births (American Academy of Pediatrics, 1999). Advances in genetics are enhancing knowledge of multifactorial inheritance and familial risks (King, Rotter, and Motulsky, 2002).

DISORDERS OF THE INTRAUTERINE ENVIRONMENT

The intrauterine environment can have a profound and permanent effect on the developing fetus, with or without chromosome or single-gene abnormalities. Intrauterine growth retardation, for example, can occur with many genetic syndromes, such as Down, Russell-Silver, Prader-Willi, and Turner syndromes (Rimoin, Connor, Pyeritz, et al, 2002), or it can be caused by nongenetic factors such as maternal alcohol ingestion. Placental abnormalities are increasingly being found to be the etiologic factor in neurodevelopmental disorders (such as cerebral palsy and cognitive impairment) that were previously attributed to asphyxia during delivery (Bos, Einspieler, and Prechtl, 2001).

Teratogens, agents that cause birth defects when present in the prenatal environment, account for the majority of adverse intrauterine effects not attributable to genetic factors. Types of teratogens include drugs (phenytoin [Dilantin], warfarin [Coumadin], isotretinoin [Accutane]), chemicals (ethyl alcohol, cocaine, lead), infectious agents (rubella, cytomegalovirus), physical agents (maternal ionizing radiation, hyperthermia), and metabolic agents (maternal PKU). Many of these teratogenic exposures and the resulting effects are completely preventable, such as ingestion of alcohol resulting in fetal alcohol syndrome or fetal alcohol effects, which causes severe birth defects, including cognitive impairment. The incidence of fetal alcohol syndrome is estimated at 5.2 per 10,000 live births (American Academy of Pediatrics, 2000). (See Chapter 11.)

CYTOGENETIC DIAGNOSTIC TECHNIQUES

Chromosomes are usually studied under light microscopy. After a significant number of cells are prepared so the chromosomes can be visualized during mitotic metaphase under a light microscope and imaged through a computer, their chromosomes are displayed in a karyotype, arranged according to their size, position of their centromeres, and banding patterns. A relatively recent advance called chromosome painting uses DNA probes attached to different colored fluorescent dyes to identify chromosomes by their color (Fig. 5-18). Robotic cell harvesters and computerized imaging systems have drastically cut down on manual labor; however, expert technicians and cytogeneticists are still necessary to analyze and interpret karyotypes whether they are traditionally stained or fluorescently colored. The most common human cells used for chromosomes studies are peripheral blood leukocytes obtained by venipuncture and cells obtained by biopsy from a variety of tissues, such as skin (including fetal skin cells), chorionic villi, and bone marrow.

Numeric abnormalities such as trisomies and gross structural anomalies such as deletions, duplications, and translocations of larger segments of genetic material may be detectable by karyotype analysis. Large chromosome structural anomalies may be visualized with the help of basic staining techniques, and various types of banding procedures (e.g., Giemsa, or G, banding; centromeric, or C, banding; replication banding). Very small changes, such as microdeletions, microduplications,

PATHOPHYSIOLOGY REVIEW

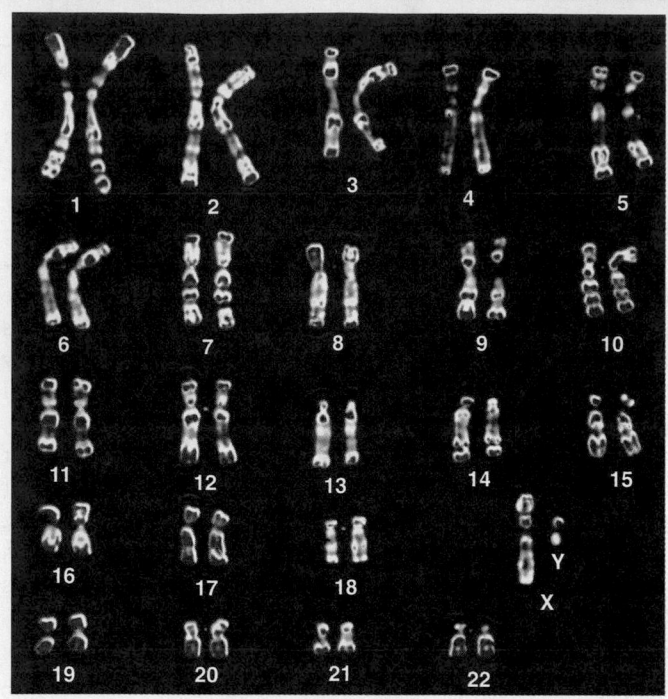

9.2 µm

Fig. 5-18 Human karyotype. (From Raven PH, Johnson G, Singer S, et al: *Biology*, ed 8, New York, 2008, McGraw-Hill.)

and fragile sites, usually require special molecular techniques such as fluorescent in situ hybridization (FISH) which uses fluorescent-labeled single-stranded DNA probes designed to attach to specific areas of chromosomes. For example, the FISH test used to diagnose VCFS contains probes that adhere to 22q11.2. Although persons with VCFS have two chromosome 22s, the FISH probe attaches to the specific region on only one of the chromosomes, since on the other the region of interest is deleted. A more recent test done in some cytogenetics laboratories, comparative genomic hybridization, uses molecular probes to detect up to thousands of submicroscopic imbalances throughout the genome (Edelmann and Hirschhorn, 2009).

MOLECULAR DIAGNOSTIC TECHNIQUES

Information derived from the HGP has led to significant advances in the diagnosis of genetic disease. Identification of single-gene mutations responsible for some genetic disorders is now possible as increasing numbers of genes are being mapped (located on a specific chromosome or segment of a chromosome). In some conditions, such as CF, sickle cell disease, Huntington disease, and fragile X syndrome, the specific gene is known and tests are available to detect many of the specific disease-associated mutations. For some disorders, such as familial adenomatous polyposis, sequencing of the related gene may be necessary because mutations can be found anywhere in the gene and there are not any particular common mutations to target. Gene sequencing is more labor intensive and expensive than targeted DNA mutation testing. A regularly updated Internet source for available genetic tests can be found at

GeneTests at the University of Washington, Seattle (www.gene-tests.org). At the time of this writing, GeneTests listed nearly 600 laboratories that provided clinical genetic testing for more than 1400 different genetic disorders.

PREDISPOSITION GENETIC TESTING

Molecular diagnostic techniques have enabled **predisposition testing**, which is the identification of gene mutations associated with genetic disorders in asymptomatic individuals. Depending on the penetrance of the allele(s), these may be considered presymptomatic or susceptibility tests.

Familial adenomatous polyposis is one of several overlapping conditions associated with mutation in the *APC* gene. These mutations are considered virtually 100% penetrant, resulting in hundreds to thousands of adenomatous polyps and eventual colon cancer. Once the *APC* mutation has been identified in an affected family member, at-risk family members can be tested for the same mutation. Because of the high penetrance, such testing in asymptomatic individuals would be considered presymptomatic testing. *APC* mutation testing in at-risk children is done to identify those who need colon screening and to identify polyp formation early so cancer-preventive surgical decisions can be made (Lynch, Lynch, Lynch, et al, 2008).

Hereditary breast and ovarian cancer has primarily been associated with mutations in either *BRCA1* or *BRCA2*. Penetrance of mutations in these genes has been reported to be as high as 85% for breast cancer and lower for other associated cancers (ovarian, prostate, pancreatic, gastrointestinal, and melanoma). Once the *BRCA1* or *BRCA2* mutation has been identified in an affected family member, asymptomatic at-risk family members can be tested for the same mutation. Onset and type of cancer varies between members of a family identified with a mutation. In addition, although some members may develop one or more of the associated cancers, other mutation-carrying members may die in their eighties without ever developing cancer (Nusbaum and Isaacs, 2007; Fossland, Stroop, Schwartz, et al, 2009). Therefore testing for mutations in *BRCA1* and *BRCA2* in an asymptomatic family member is considered susceptibility testing. This type of testing is discouraged in at-risk children until they are cognitively and emotionally able to make an informed decision about testing for themselves (American Academy of Pediatrics, 2001).

THERAPEUTIC MANAGEMENT OF GENETIC DISEASE

Therapy for genetic disease is currently aimed at correcting the phenotypic expression of gene abnormalities, and therefore the major goal of therapy is modification of the internal or external environment to correct or minimize the effects of the genetic defect. However, the HGP has opened doors to genotype intervention, and clinical applications of gene manipulation techniques are currently being tested.

Phenotype Modification

Examples of currently used intervention aimed at modifying the phenotypic expression of genetic disorders follow.

Surgical Management

Surgical repair of structural defects has made it possible to prolong life in a number of multifactorial disorders, such as congenital heart disease and NTDs. Numerous facial and limb deformities can be corrected by plastic and reconstructive techniques. In the case of familial adenomatous polyposis, the colon is surgically removed to prevent colon cancer that would eventually develop in one or more of the countless polyps that line the colon. The use of splenectomy in several hereditary disorders of blood cells prevents the trapping and destruction of abnormal blood cells in that organ. Early diagnosis and enucleation in retinoblastoma have reduced the mortality from this malignant eye tumor. Fetal surgery may also be performed for some life-threatening anomalies such a diaphragmatic hernia. Corrective surgery for children born with ambiguous genitalia (e.g., girls with congenital adrenal hyperplasia), although widely used, has been recently the focus of controversy that involves the issue of parental versus affected individual (future) preferences.

Diet Modification

For disorders in which an enzyme deficiency causes a toxic accumulation of a substance or its by-products, restricting the intake of foods containing that substance may prevent irreversible damage from the improper metabolism of these compounds. This dietary control is lifelong and requires a high level of adherence. Examples in infants and children include the low-phenylalanine diet prescribed for PKU, elimination of dairy products containing lactose for hereditary lactase deficiency, avoidance of foods containing or producing galactose for galactosemia, and a diet low in branched-chain amino acids for maple syrup urine disease. Women with PKU who have not maintained dietary control must reinstitute a strict low-phenylalanine diet before conception and maintain it throughout pregnancy to prevent a high risk of adverse fetal effects (see Chapter 9).

Preconception and prenatal folic acid supplementation has been shown to reduce the incidence or recurrence of NTDs (see Chapter 11). Therefore in 1992 the U.S. Public Health Service recommended that all women capable of becoming pregnant should consume 0.4 mg of folic acid per day. This recommendation was added to the existing mandate by the U.S. Food and Drug Administration that, as of 1998, folic acid would be added to enriched grain products. This would add 0.1 mg folic acid to the daily diet of the average person. Since that time, the incidence of NTDs has declined by 19% (Honein, Paulozzi, Mathews, et al, 2001). Women who have previously had a pregnancy affected by an NTD are advised to take 4.0 mg of folic acid per day beginning 1 month before conception and continuing throughout the first trimester of pregnancy. The risk of recurrence of an NTD in another pregnancy is reduced by 72% in women following this regimen.

Metabolic Manipulation

In some deficiency diseases, supplying the missing product that cannot be synthesized prevents undesirable effects. For example, thyroid hormone is prescribed to prevent the damaging effects of hypothyroidism, and providing the missing blood factors prevents life-threatening and debilitating hemorrhages in persons with different types of hemophilia. Other examples are insulin for diabetes mellitus, growth hormone for growth hormone deficiency, and corticosteroids for adrenogenital syndrome.

Removal of toxic substances that accumulate in vital tissues as a result of a hereditary disease can prevent disabling complications. Some of the deleterious effects of hemochromatosis, a hereditary disorder characterized by an excess accumulation of iron in the liver, heart, and pancreas, can be reduced with the removal of iron by administration of chelating agents or periodic therapeutic phlebotomies.

Diet supplements can be given when the individual is unable to synthesize or effectively utilize substances needed as cofactors in metabolism. This includes the use of vitamin B_{12} in persons with pernicious anemia, whose absorption of this vitamin is impaired. Vitamin and cofactor supplementation may be used to treat mitochondrial disease. Phenobarbitone can be used to enhance hepatic metabolism of unconjugated bilirubin in children with Crigler-Najjar syndrome type 2, thus helping prevent brain damage (kernicterus) and jaundice (Scriver, Beaudet, Sly, et al, 2001).

Avoidance of Drugs or Other Harmful Substances

In drug-induced disease, such as glucose-6-phosphate dehydrogenase (G6PD) deficiency and the porphyrias, avoidance of the drugs that precipitate a reaction is a simple preventive measure. These include aspirin and quinine-based antimalarial medications in the case of G6PD deficiency, and ethanol, barbiturates, anticonvulsants, sulfonamides, and oral contraceptives in the case of acute intermittent porphyria (Scriver, Beaudet, Sly, et al, 2001). Some anesthetic agents may precipitate symptoms of malignant hyperthermia and myotonic dystrophy.

Immunologic Prevention

The administration of immunoglobulin to Rh-negative mothers after the birth of an Rh-positive infant is effective in preventing Rh-antibody formation, which causes hemolytic disease of the newborn in subsequent births.

Transplantation

Better control of tissue incompatibility problems is improving the survival of children undergoing replacement of nonfunctioning organs with normal organs. Transplanted organs include the kidneys in hereditary polycystic kidneys, the heart in severe cardiac myopathy, the liver in hepatic atresia, and bone marrow.

Gene Product Replacement

Recombinant DNA technology makes it possible to produce large quantities of certain gene products. Such technology avoids the infectious contamination risk that accompanied extraction of gene products from mass quantities of human blood or tissue.

The administration of gene products is especially applicable when the missing product is a circulatory peptide or protein, as in coagulation factor VIII or IX in hemophilia type A and type B, respectively (Saenko and Pipe, 2006). If the gene product is membrane bound, as is the case for enzymes deficient in various lysosomal storage diseases, the natural enzyme product may need to be purposefully altered so that it can enter the cell through a naturally occurring cell receptor. Gaucher disease was the first lysosomal disorder to be successfully treated in this manner, and lessons learned in the process have led to more recent enzyme replacement therapies for disorders such as Pompe disease and Hurler syndrome (Bailey, 2008). If the missing gene product is a substance that acts within a metabolic pathway of a specific organ protected by a barrier, such as the enzyme hexosaminidase A in Tay-Sachs disease (blood-brain barrier), injectable products become ineffective and replacement is more problematic. The introduction of a foreign gene product may eventually trigger an immune reaction, as has been observed in hemophilia when the recipient develops antibody against the clotting factor, greatly reducing the efficiency of an otherwise successful therapy.

Gene Transfer

Gene transfer can be achieved through introduction of a normal gene by a harmless virus vector. For example, introduction of a normally functioning gene may correct an abnormal phenotype resulting from the absence of that gene. Introduction of a toxic gene may cause apoptosis of a cancer cell. Introduction of antigen or cytokine gene can stimulate the immune system to eliminate malignant cells. This approach has been attempted in humans with the transfer of normal gene copies of β-hemoglobin into bone marrow cells in an effort to treat a form of β-thalassemia; it has also been used in sickle cell disease and in adenosine deaminase deficiency. Gene therapy research has suffered a number of setbacks in clinical research, and the search for safer, more effective ways to transfer genes into human cells continues.

Environmental Modification

Inherited diseases or defects with no therapeutic modality can be modified to enhance the quality of life for the affected individual. Some examples of environmental manipulation include hearing aids for children with congenital hearing loss, glasses or vision enhancers such as books in enlarged print or Braille for the visually impaired, mobilizing devices such as braces and wheelchairs for persons with muscle and bone impairment, prosthetic devices for those with limb deficiencies, and infant stimulation programs to maximize the potential of children who are developmentally delayed. Environmental manipulation also includes protection from the damaging effects of the environment, such as exposure to sunlight, which can cause skin fragility and blistering in persons with porphyrias and increases the risk of skin cancers in patients with xeroderma pigmentosum and oculocutaneous albinism (Kingston, 2002).

IMPACT OF HEREDITARY DISORDERS ON THE FAMILY

GENETIC TESTING

Genetic testing can be broadly divided into two categories: diagnostic testing and screening. Tests to detect a disease-associated genetic mutation in symptomatic individuals are rapidly assuming greater importance in management of genetic disorders as more genes and mutations are identified and techniques are developed for easy application of the tests. Dramatic improvements in testing capabilities also provide opportunities to identify disease-associated mutations in people before they become symptomatic. With improved technology, mass screening for numerous genetic disorders will probably become routine. However, to be truly effective, screening programs depend on thorough education of both health professionals and the public regarding these programs and the limitations and implications of testing. The religious, moral, ethical, and legal issues revolving around screening and prenatal diagnosis are extensive and change over time (Farrell, Certain, and Farrell, 2001).

Purposes of Screening

Genetic screening is presumptive identification of an unrecognized genetic predisposition for future disease in individuals or their progeny for which preventive or disease course–altering interventions exist. In general, genetic screening targets populations, whereas genetic diagnostic testing targets individuals. The first corollaries of any genetic screening intervention must be *voluntary participation, equal access to all,* and *confidentiality* (both in conducting the tests and in handling records and results). In addition, education and counseling about tests and procedures must be an integral part of any screening program. Attention must be paid to quality control of all aspects of testing and laboratory procedures.

Genetic screening has three purposes: (1) to provide for early recognition of a disease, before symptoms occur, for which effective intervention and therapy exist (e.g., PKU); (2) to identify carriers of a genetic disease for the purpose of maximizing parenthood planning options (e.g., Tay-Sachs disease); and (3) to obtain population data on frequency, spectrum, and natural history of genetic variations not currently known to be associated with disease.

Screening for genetic disorders can occur during various times in a person's life: (1) preconception screening of selected populations for heterozygous carriers (e.g., Ashkenazi Jewish carrier screening panel) (Gross, Pletcher, Monaghan, et al, 2008); (2) screening of relatives of known carrier or affected individuals within a family, for the purpose of reproductive decision making; (3) postconceptional (prenatal) screening (e.g., maternal serum screen for identifying risks for NTDs and chromosome abnormalities); and (4) newborn screening (e.g., panel for PKU in all newborns, as mandated by law in all U.S. states).

Newborn Screening

Newborn screening began in the 1960s when Guthrie devised the blood spot test to screen for PKU. Newborn screening for PKU was begun in all states, and currently each state offers screening for a growing number of disorders such as hemoglobinopathies, galactosemia, hypothyroidism, and congenital adrenal hypoplasia. In the past, decisions about which disorder to include were based on the following criteria:

- The disease occurs with a significant frequency.
- An inexpensive and reliable method of testing exists.
- There is effective treatment and intervention.
- If untreated, the baby will die or be severely developmentally impaired.
- An affected newborn may appear normal at birth.

Because the actual disorders screened by individual states varied considerably, the American College of Medical Genetics (ACMG) was commissioned by the Maternal Child Health Bureau of the Health Resources and Services Administration to develop a uniform screening panel. The ACMG task force used the following minimum criteria when considering which disorders to include (American College of Medical Genetics Newborn Screening Expert Group, 2006):

- It can be identified at a phase (24 to 48 hours after birth) at which it would not ordinarily be clinically detected.
- A test with appropriate sensitivity and specificity is available for it.
- There are demonstrated benefits of early detection, timely intervention, and efficacious treatment of the condition being tested.

A panel of 29 core conditions and 25 secondary conditions was recommended by ACMG in its 2006 report (Sweetman, Millington, Therrell, et al, 2006). With advancing technology the number of conditions screened by individual states can be expected to change. A regularly updated list of conditions offered in each state's newborn screening panel can be found at the National Newborn Screening and Genetics Resource Center website (http://genes-r-us.uthscsa.edu).

Because many of the conditions tested for are metabolic disorders, it is important that the first newborn screening blood sample be obtained at least 24 hours after the first protein feeding or within the first 72 hours of life. Infants found to be screen positive (thus at high risk) for a metabolic condition such as PKU or galactosemia are immediately referred to a medical center for testing to confirm the diagnosis and initiate treatment. Of course, this relies on a coordinated follow-up program that includes well-informed primary care providers and nurses who can locate newborns with abnormal screening results and facilitate the necessary follow-up visits.

Screening for Reproductive Information

Screening for heterozygotes (carriers) can detect unaffected persons with certain variant genes who, when they mate with an individual who carries a similar variant gene, are at high risk of producing an affected offspring. These individuals are thus provided with the information they need for making decisions about family planning. Carriers of a number of diseases can be detected by laboratory tests, but, because of the rarity of these diseases, mass screening is not feasible except in persons or populations known to be at risk. Persons at risk include close relatives of those with an inborn error of metabolism or other detectable disorder, and certain ethnic populations known to have a high incidence of a specific disease, such as sickle cell anemia in African-Americans, Tay-Sachs disease in Ashkenazi Jews, and thalassemia in people of Mediterranean ancestry.

This type of screening is sometimes controversial. Screening for carrier status for CF is one such situation that has the potential to create ethical dilemmas. Children with CF have a disease-associated mutation in each of their *CFTR* genes. More than 1000 different *CFTR* mutations have been identified, yet carrier testing for CF typically analyzes less than 100 of the possible *CFTR* mutations. Therefore, after screening, a couple may feel safe to proceed with pregnancy yet still have a child with CF.

Carrier status screening has influenced marriage partner selection. Some carriers have made life choices based on inaccurate understanding of the implications of carrier status (e.g., thinking they would get the disease or that they were at high risk for having an affected child regardless of whether the partner is also a carrier). These misunderstandings and their consequences underscore the importance of careful education before decision making regarding carrier screening.

Carrier testing for children is generally not recommended, since the information is for reproductive purposes. Instead, parents are counseled that the child should make a decision about carrier testing when she or he is old enough to make an informed choice. Yet newborn screening tests reveal carrier status for certain conditions such as CF and sickle cell. Careful counseling is necessary with carrier screening to ensure that individuals understand the limitations of testing and the implications of results. Even with careful counseling, there may be significant misunderstanding or misuse of information (Ciske, Haavisto, Laxova, et al, 2001; Farrell, Kosorok, Rock, et al, 2001).

Screening for Epidemiologic Information

Public health officials may use screening as a method for monitoring the incidence of diseases or malformations in a population to detect environmental or other causes that might significantly influence the incidence of the disorders. For example, geographic and socioeconomic variations in the incidence of NTDs eventually led to research that determined that folic acid supplementation of 0.4 mg/day in women of childbearing age reduces NTD occurrence by as much as 50% (Mills and Signore, 2004).

Significance of Screening to Families

Mass screening programs have received mixed acceptance from health professionals and the general public. Various groups have raised objections concerning the accuracy of the screening tests. An ideal genetic screening test must have high sensitivity (ability to detect true positives) and specificity (ability to detect true negatives); it must yield rapid results, be safe, and be cost-effective; it should cause minimum physical and emotional discomfort to all involved. Other reasons for controversy include health professionals' lack of knowledge about the testing purposes and implications of results, the public cost of testing (if government funded), and the psychologic implications of learning about carrier status. However, with several well-organized or legislated programs proving their value in preventing disease or of the damaging effects of disease, an increasing number of programs are gaining acceptance and support.

Potential benefits of carrier screening include facilitating genetic counseling and reproductive planning and providing useful information to other at-risk family members. Newborn screening provides for early detection and treatment initiation, maximizing quality of life. Yet realizing these benefits requires that couples and parents be given adequate information to make informed decisions about whether to pursue screening. For newborn screening, parent choice about testing may be limited by state regulations. Some states allow exemptions from newborn screening in certain situations, such as objections on religious grounds if there is a conflict with religious practices and beliefs of an established church. Regardless, parents need to be educated about the purpose; benefits, risks, and limitations of newborn screening; and the implications of abnormal results (Spahis and Bowers, 2006). Focus groups with parents have indicated that this type of education is preferred during the prenatal period (Campbell and Ross, 2003).

The social stigma of being the carrier of a "defective" gene may be a side effect of screening. In some families such knowledge is embarrassing and damaging to self-esteem. Teenagers may be especially vulnerable to the effects of knowing they carry a specific disease-associated gene mutation at a time when identity formation and peer approval are extremely important. Cultural views regarding this knowledge can have profound effects on the members of some ethnic groups. In some cases, social status within the cultural group can be impaired.

Probably the most important area for nursing practice is teaching, or the ability to convey clear, precise, and unambiguous information to clients. Families need to understand why the screening is proposed, what the results mean, and how the family can interpret false-positive and false-negative results (Baroni, Anderson, and Mischler, 1997). Anxiety is greater when families have not received sufficient information about the screening or testing process and its significance for their health. Families also have a right to know who assumes the cost of additional testing or retesting—the family or the state. The nurse is a valuable resource in ensuring that families are aware of alternatives and in helping them make the best decision (Spahis and Bowers, 2006).

PRENATAL TESTING

Pediatric nurses may encounter couples who had prenatal testing and are preparing for the anticipated care of their unborn child. Such couples may be making primary care arrangements; meeting professionals in the newborn intensive care unit; meeting with surgeons to learn about the surgeries their newborn will need in the first few days, weeks, or months of life; and talking with other parents who have children with the same condition. Thus it is important that pediatric nurses have a general understanding of the capabilities, limitations, and risks of prenatal testing.

Advances in technology have greatly increased the spectrum of available prenatal screening and diagnostic options. Although screening options are available for all pregnant women, prenatal diagnostic testing is reserved for pregnancies considered at increased risk for less than healthy outcomes. The purposes of prenatal testing include identifying congenital anomalies and genetic disorders that may need intervention during pregnancy or soon after delivery; enabling parents to prepare for the birth of a child who will require long-term medical or developmental interventions; and enabling parents to make decisions about placing their child for adoption or terminating the pregnancy. However, even normal prenatal test results do not guarantee the birth of a healthy baby. When referring a family for prenatal testing, the nurse can benefit from general guidelines, some of which are delineated in Box 5-6.

Prenatal Screening Tests

Biochemical maternal serum screening is used to detect pregnancies at increased risk for certain congenital anomalies and

---

BOX 5-6	INDICATIONS FOR PRENATAL TESTING

General Risk Factors
Maternal age of at least 35 years at time of delivery or at least 31 years if twin gestation
Elevated or low trisomy profile screen results

Specific Risk Factors
Previous child with a structural defect or chromosome abnormality
Previous stillbirth or neonatal death
Structural abnormality in mother or father
Balanced translocation in mother or father
Inherited disorders—Cystic fibrosis, metabolic disorders, sex-linked recessive disorders
Medical disease in mother—Diabetes mellitus, phenylketonuria
Exposure to a teratogen—Ionizing radiation, anticonvulsant medicines, lithium, isotretinoin, alcohol
Infection—Rubella, toxoplasmosis, cytomegalovirus
Abnormal ultrasound findings

Ethnic Risk Factors
Disorder—Ethnic or racial group
Tay-Sachs disease—Ashkenazi Jewish, French Canadian
Sickle cell anemia—Black African, Mediterranean, Arab, Indian, Pakistani
α- and β-Thalassemia—Mediterranean, Southern and Southeast Asian, Chinese

Modified from D'Alton ME, DeCherney AH: Prenatal diagnosis, *N Engl J Med* 328(2):114-120, 1993.

---

chromosome disorders. In the first trimester, maternal serum can be analyzed for free β-human chorionic gonadotropin (hCG) and pregnancy-associated plasma protein A. These values, in combination with nuchal fold translucency measurement, can be used to identify pregnancies at high risk for chromosome anomalies, particularly aneuploidy. In such situations, the couple is offered diagnostic testing, which may include chorionic villi sampling (CVS) or amniocentesis, depending on the fetus's gestational age. Risk for neural tube and abdominal wall defects is screened during the second trimester when alpha-fetoprotein (AFP) is detectable in maternal serum. Also during the second trimester, hCG, unconjugated estriol, and inhibin A can be measured to screen for aneuploidies. High-risk pregnancies can be further evaluated with diagnostic ultrasound, amniocentesis, or fetal cord blood sampling (American College of Obstetrics and Gynecology, 2007).

Prenatal Diagnostic Procedures

Recommendations for diagnostic testing may be triggered by preexisting risks (e.g., previous child with a genetic disorder), personal characteristics (e.g., member of subpopulation at risk for certain genetic diseases), or a newly identified risk following prenatal screening for the current pregnancy (see Box 5-6). Specific risk factors are usually identified in the family history, previous pregnancy outcomes, or the mother's medical history. Ethnic risk factors are based on a higher carrier frequency for certain genetic diseases in selected populations. Indications for prenatal diagnosis when any of these risk factors is present are based on a greater than general population risk that a congenital anomaly or genetic disorder will occur in the pregnancy. The specific risk is, of course, different for each situation.

Invasive prenatal diagnostic tests include CVS, amniocentesis, and fetal blood sampling. CVS can be performed between 10 and 12 weeks of gestation. Using either a transcervical or transabdominal approach guided by ultrasound, the clinician obtains a small biopsy of the chorionic villi. Cells from the sample can be grown for chromosome and single-gene disorder studies. Contamination of the sample with maternal cells can compromise the accuracy of test results. Amniocentesis is usually performed at 14 to 18 weeks of gestation under ultrasound guidance. Fetal skin cells that have sloughed off and are present in the amniotic fluid can be isolated and cultured for chromosome or single-gene analyses. AFP can be measured in the amniotic fluid and is a much more reliable indicator of an NTD or abdominal wall defect than maternal serum AFP. An additional test for an enzyme specific to neural tissue, acetylcholinesterase, may be done; if this test is positive in the presence of an elevated AFP level, it is diagnostic of an open NTD. A diagnostic ultrasound clarifies the extent and location of the NTD or abdominal wall defect. A less frequently used test is fetal blood sampling, in which blood is drawn from the umbilical vein. This procedure can be performed after 18 weeks of gestation and is usually done for prenatal evaluation of fetal hematologic abnormalities, inborn errors of metabolism, fetal infection, and rapid chromosome analysis (Rodeck, 2004).

A few additional diagnostic tests are infrequently used. Fetal biopsy is sometimes used to diagnose certain genetic skin disorders and metabolic disorders when DNA studies are unavailable or are uninformative. Fetal echocardiography may be performed for further diagnosis when a cardiac defect is noted on ultrasound. Research is under way to improve prenatal diagnostic testing.

A relatively new option for parents at risk for having a child with a genetic disorder is preimplantation genetic diagnosis. Through in vitro (test tube) fertilization, the embryo can be tested at the six- to eight-cell stage for specific genetic disorder. Normal or an unaffected carrier embryo or embryos are implanted. This technique has been used for Tay-Sachs disease, CF, and some X-linked disorders (Kent-First, 2000). It has been used by a couple who wished not only to avoid the birth of another child affected with Fanconi anemia, but also to have a healthy sibling who could provide a human lymphocyte antigen match for an affected sibling who needed stem cell transplantation (Verlinsky, Rechitsky, Schoolcraft, et al, 2001).

GENETIC EVALUATION AND COUNSELING

In recent years the role of genetics as an etiologic agent in disease and disability has assumed a more prominent place in the nursing care of infants and children. The expanded recognition of genetic diseases and disorders and an increasingly well-informed public are creating a justified demand for genetic evaluation, diagnosis, information regarding risks to present and future generations, and access to available therapies. Unfortunately, however, persons who need expert genetic counseling often make uninformed decisions on their own or are the victims of well-meaning but equally uninformed relatives, acquaintances, or paraprofessionals. Nurses involved in infant and child care continually encounter families that have a risk of transmitting a disorder to an offspring, as well as children who may have an undiagnosed genetic disorder that needs expert evaluation.

It is a nurse's responsibility to learn basic genetic principles, to be alert to situations in which families could benefit from genetic evaluation and counseling, to know about special services that can help manage and support affected children, and to be familiar with facilities in their areas where these services are available. In this way, nurses will be able to direct individuals and families to needed services and be active participants in the genetic evaluation and counseling process. Early identification of a genetic disorder allows anticipation of associated conditions and implementation of available preventive measures and therapy to avoid potential complications and to enhance the child's health. It may also prevent the unexpected birth of another affected child in the immediate or extended family.

Pediatric Indications for Genetic Consultation

The ACMG has produced guidelines for genetics consultation (Pletcher, Toriello, Noblin, et al, 2007). The indications can be broadly divided into preconception-prenatal, pediatric, and adult. The indications that are relevant for newborns through adolescents are:

- Family history of hereditary diseases, birth defects, or developmental problems
- Family history of sudden cardiac death or early-onset cancer
- Family history of mental illness
- Abnormal newborn screen
- Abnormal genetic test result ordered by a nongenetics professional who lacks the knowledge and experience to discuss implications of results
- Progressive neurologic condition
- Major congenital anomaly (e.g., cleft lip, congenital heart defect, limb abnormality, spina bifida)
- Pattern of major or minor anomalies suggestive of genetic disorder
- Congenital or early-onset hearing loss or vision loss
- Cognitive impairment or autism
- Abnormal sexual maturation or delayed puberty
- Abnormally tall or short stature when compared with other family members
- Excessive bleeding or excessive clotting
- Parental requests that child be evaluated by a genetics professional

Genetic evaluation for diagnostic purposes may occur at any point in the life span. In the newborn period, birth defects and abnormal newborn screen results are obvious reasons for referral. Beyond the newborn period, indicators for referral include metabolic disorders, developmental delays, growth delays, behavioral problems, cognitive delays, abnormal or delayed sexual development, and medical problems known to be associated with genetic diseases. For example, a preschooler with hyperactivity and autistic-like behaviors may need evaluation for fragile X syndrome, and a 17-year-old girl with primary amenorrhea and short stature should be evaluated for Turner syndrome (Gardner and Sutherland, 2004).

With so many recent advances in genetic testing, it is not unusual for a child or adult with longstanding medical problems, including cognitive impairment, to be referred for reevaluation of his or her condition as a possible genetic disorder that might not have been diagnosable a few years earlier, such as microdeletion disorders or single-gene mutations. If a genetic diagnosis is made, the patient is usually referred back to the primary care physician with recommendations for routine management.

Persons may not be affected themselves but may request genetic counseling about the heritability of a trait. A young couple contemplating childbearing may be concerned about a disorder in one of their families or may seek advice because they are related. A couple who are both members of a population at risk for certain genetic diseases may wish to determine whether they carry an associated gene mutation (e.g., African-Americans and sickle cell anemia, Ashkenazi Jews and Tay-Sachs disease, or persons of Mediterranean ancestry and thalassemia). A couple planning adoption might seek genetic evaluation and counseling regarding a prospective child.

More often, persons who inquire about the possibility of recurrence of a disease or disorder have a child, or had a child who died, with a genetic disease or disorder. They are concerned about the likelihood of having another, similarly affected child and may want to know what reproductive choices are available. They might seek this advice before initiating another pregnancy or after the mother is already pregnant. If prenatal diagnostic testing is not done, the history of a condition in an older sibling, such as galactosemia, alerts health personnel to initiate specific and thorough testing for the condition in a newborn. In this way, early therapy can be initiated, thus minimizing or eliminating the effects of the disease or defect.

Parents need to know the risk in their particular situation and how it relates to the random risk for any prospective parents. When families understand the risks involved, they can make informed decisions regarding family planning and available prenatal testing. Additional counseling is necessary if abnormal results are obtained so the couple can decide to continue or terminate the pregnancy. They need considerable support for either decision (Veach, LeRoy, and Bartels, 2003). Parents may also have concerns about risks to unaffected siblings and about reproductive implications for their affected and unaffected offspring.

Genetic Services

Comprehensive genetic services consist of a group of specialists, which may include clinical geneticists, advanced practice nurses in genetics, genetic counselors, psychologists, biochemical geneticists, cytogeneticists, molecular geneticists, nurses, social workers, and other auxiliary personnel. The services are most often under the leadership of a physician trained in medical genetics, who assumes responsibility for the medical aspects of the problem. Although genetic centers were typically considered a resource for genetic evaluation, diagnosis, and counseling, a growing number of centers are managing the health care needs of patients with complex, rare genetic disorders. Some centers specialize in treatment of genetic disorders (e.g., enzyme replacement therapy for lysosomal storage disorders). Most centers are associated with a large medical center, which may have extensive outreach programs with satellite

clinics throughout adjacent urban and rural areas. Numerous specialty clinics also deal with specific genetic disorders (such as CF, muscular dystrophy, hemophilia, or craniofacial anomalies) and provide their own genetic counseling services. Unfortunately, these units are concentrated in and around large metropolitan areas. As a result, counseling is not always accessible to a large number of people who could benefit from the service.

Unlike a medical prognosis, which predicts the outcome of a disease for an individual, a genetic prognosis may have implications for others as well, including members of the immediate family, other relatives, and future offspring. During a genetic evaluation or follow-up visit, a genetics professional obtains or updates the patient's family history and pedigree, developmental history, and medical history (including pregnancy, labor, and delivery information); performs a physical examination, including dysmorphic features; and orders appropriate testing such as biochemical, cytogenetic, or molecular procedures. A genetic diagnosis may or may not be made initially. Genetic evaluation and counseling are time consuming and labor intensive. The pediatric nurse can facilitate the referral and help the family understand the sometimes lengthy process in arriving at a diagnosis. Nurses can also collect preliminary histories, including family history, and help parents prepare questions for the counseling session (Consensus Panel on Genetic/Genomic Nursing Competencies, 2006).

Genetic counseling is a communication process that deals with the human problems associated with the occurrence, or risk of occurrence, of a genetic disorder in a family. This process involves an attempt by one or more appropriately trained persons to help the individual or family:

- Comprehend the medical facts, including the diagnosis, the probable course of the disorder, and the available management
- Appreciate the way heredity contributes to the disorder and the risk of recurrence in specified relatives
- Understand the options for dealing with the risk of recurrence
- Choose the course of action that seems appropriate to them in view of their risk and family goals and act in accordance with that decision
- Make the best possible adjustment to the disorder in an affected family member and to the risk of recurrence of that disorder

Estimation of Risks

Effective genetic counseling based on a diagnosis or known risk factors requires a thorough evaluation of each situation. The genetics nurse or counselor derives risks of occurrence or recurrence from information acquired through a thorough family history, including known genetic information. A careful, detailed family history not only provides a picture of the proband (the affected person, or index case) in relation to other family members, but also may identify others who are similarly affected or who might be presymptomatic or at risk of producing affected children. Analyzing the pattern of affected family members can assist in confirming a tentative diagnosis or in determining the level of risk in multifactorial inheritance.

An accurate diagnosis is essential to provide specific risk figures. There are more than 10,000 known inherited disorders, many of which have similar clinical manifestations but different modes of inheritance. For example, symptoms in the early stages of severe X-linked muscular dystrophy appear much like those of the milder autosomal recessive and autosomal dominant varieties, autosomal recessive neurogenic muscular atrophies, and nongenetic poliomyelitis. The significance of the risks related to each type of disorder is readily apparent. For disorders with an unknown or multifactorial cause, recurrence risks are termed *empiric*, meaning they are based on observations of recurrence in similar situations, rather than *theoretic*, meaning they are based on mendelian inheritance patterns.

Communicating Risks

When explaining reproductive risk estimates, the genetics nurse or counselor does not attempt to make recommendations or decisions for patients. The nurse or counselor communicates comprehensive and current information about the nature of the disorder, the extent of risk involved, the probable consequences, and alternative solutions. The nurse then supports the informed patients regarding their decisions about whether to pursue preconception or prenatal testing and what to do in response to test results. However, genetics professionals recognize that recommendations do have a place when genetic testing is used to identify risk for diseases or disorders that have available treatments that can prevent, delay, or improve symptoms. Children who test positive for a mutation in the *APC* gene associated with familial adenomatous polyposis will eventually develop colon polyps, and eventually one or more will become cancerous. Therefore genetics professionals recommend specific screening measures for these children; when polyps are discovered, the professionals recommend a surgical consult to discuss colectomy options. As with any health care encounter, shared decision making with parents is the goal.

It is helpful to explain risks in different ways and to use examples to aid in understanding the meaning of probabilities. Most people do not have an adequate knowledge of genetics and human biology to fully comprehend these complex concepts. Words and concepts that can be used include *percentages*, *chance*, *odds*, and *likelihood*. For example, if a 40-year-old woman has a 1:112 risk of having a child with Down syndrome, other ways to explain it include, "You have about a 1% chance of having a baby with Down syndrome," or "Out of 112 women your age having a baby, odds are that one of them will have a child with Down syndrome." Games of probability can also be used, such as flipping coins, baseball pools, and lotteries.

Nurses can contact a family before genetic consultation to assess the family's needs and attempt to reduce their anxiety. The telephone contact can also be used to obtain a family history and explain the clinic procedures. Many families are concerned about such things as whether they will be required to undress, whether blood is to be drawn, whether they can accompany the child during the visit, or whether they will be told what to do about reproduction. Families who know what to expect are able to gain more from a genetics consultation.

> **! NURSING ALERT**
>
> Families may misunderstand probability, even when it is fully explained. The nurse should impress on them that each pregnancy is an independent event. Often parents who are told that a recessive disorder carries a 1:4 risk of recurrence incorrectly reason that because they already have one affected child, the next three will be unaffected. Chance has no memory; the risk is 1:4 for each and every pregnancy.

ROLE OF NURSES IN GENETICS

All nurses need to be prepared to use genetic and genomic information and technology when providing care. Nearly 50 nursing organizations endorsed essential minimum competencies necessary for nurses to deliver competent genetic and genomic focused nursing care (Consensus Panel on Genetic/Genomic Nursing Competencies, 2006). The professional practice domains include applying/integrating genetic knowledge into nursing assessment; identifying and referring clients who may benefit from genetic information or services; identifying genetics resources and services to meet clients' needs; and providing care and support before, during, and after providing genetic information and/or services. Often a nurse is the first one to recognize the need for genetic evaluation by identifying an inherited disorder in a family history or by noting physical, cognitive, or behavioral abnormalities when performing a nursing assessment (Box 5-7).

Nurses who specialize in genetics are guided by the Genetics/Genomics Nursing Scope and Standards of Practice (International Society of Nurses in Genetics, 2006). Genetics

> **BOX 5-7   ASSESSMENT CLUES TO GENETIC DISORDERS***
>
> **Major or minor birth defects (anomalies) and dysmorphic features**—Cardiac defect, ear or eye abnormalities, micrognathia, forehead prominence, hairline low set on forehead or nape of neck, wide-set eyes (hypertelorism), epicanthal folds, low-set or abnormal ears.
> **Growth abnormalities**—Short stature, overgrowth, asymmetric growth, intrauterine growth retardation
> **Skeletal abnormalities**—Limb abnormalities, asymmetry, scoliosis, hyperextensible joints, hypotonic or hypertonic muscle tone, pectus excavatum, finger or joint abnormalities
> **Visual or hearing problems**—Coloboma of the iris, hearing loss, congenital or early-onset cataracts
> **Metabolic disorders**—Unusual odor of breath, urine, or stool
> **Sexual development abnormalities**—Ambiguous genitalia, micropenis, delayed onset of puberty, primary amenorrhea, precocious sexual development, large testicles
> **Skin disorders**—Unusual pigmentation patterns (e.g., café-au-lait spots, vitiligo), dry and scaly skin, skin tumors, hyperextensible skin
> **Recurrent infection or immunodeficiency**—Ear infection, pneumonia, poor healing of umbilicus
> **Development and speech delays or loss of developmental milestones**
> **Cognitive delays**—Learning disabilities, mild to severe cognitive impairment
> **Behavioral disorders**—Attention deficit disorders with or without hyperactivity, autistic behavior, aggressive behavior
>
> *Increased concern for genetic etiology if two or more findings are present.

nurses at the basic level tend to work in clinics that focus on services for patients with specific single-gene disorders such as CF, sickle cell disease, muscular dystrophy, and hemophilia. They may also work in genetics clinics. Genetics nurses in advanced practice work in a variety of specialty clinics or genetics centers. These nurses evaluate a patient's medical, developmental, prenatal, birth, and family histories; perform physical examinations, including dysmorphology examination; order tests and diagnostic procedures and evaluate their results; prescribe therapies that are within their scope of practice; and evaluate patient outcomes. Genetics nurses collaborate with teams that include medical geneticists and genetic counselors.

This chapter highlights the role of all nurses who care for children and their families. The *Essential Nursing Competencies and Curricula Guidelines for Genetics and Genomics* (Consensus Panel on Genetic/Genomic Nursing Competencies, 2006) is used as a framework for discussion (Box 5-8).

Nursing Assessment: Applying and Integrating Genetic and Genomic Knowledge

Family health history is an important tool to identify individuals and families at increased risk for disease, risk factors for disease (such as obesity), and inheritance patterns of diseases. Because of its importance, all nurses need to be able to elicit family history information and document the collected information in pedigree format.

When eliciting a family health history, nurses should collect information about all family members within a minimum of three generations. This process usually takes 20 to 30 minutes. When possible, it is best to include both parents in the interview to elicit information about relatives on both sides of the family. Medical records, birth and death records, family Bibles, and photograph albums are helpful resources, and persons being interviewed should be instructed to bring such items if they are available. It may be necessary to consult other members of the family. The level of education and the degree of understanding vary widely among informants and influence their reliability. The informants may be reticent, particularly if they view the disorder as something to be ashamed of or in some way threatening. Sometimes true relationships may be concealed, such as adoption or misattributed paternity.

Skillful interviewing is necessary to obtain essential, but often embarrassing or private information. Since the parents may not be married, they should be addressed as couples or

---

BOX 5-8   ESSENTIAL NURSING COMPETENCIES FOR GENETICS AND GENOMICS: PROFESSIONAL PRACTICE DOMAIN

Nursing Assessment: Applying/Integrating Genetic and Genomic Knowledge
The registered nurse:
- Demonstrates an understanding of the relationship of genetics and genomics to health, prevention, screening, diagnostics, prognostics, selection of treatment, and monitoring of treatment effectiveness
- Demonstrates ability to elicit a minimum of three-generation family health history information
- Constructs a pedigree from collected family history information using standardized symbols and terminology
- Collects personal, health, and developmental histories that consider genetic, environmental, and genomic influences and risks
- Conducts comprehensive health and physical assessments which incorporate knowledge about genetic, environmental, and genomic influences and risk factors
- Critically analyzes the history and physical assessment findings for genetic, environmental, and genomic influences and risk factors
- Assesses clients'* knowledge, perceptions, and responses to genetic and genomic information
- Develops a plan of care that incorporates genetic and genomic assessment information

Identification
The registered nurse:
- Identifies clients who may benefit from specific genetic and genomic information and/or services based on assessment data
- Identifies credible, accurate, appropriate, and current genetic and genomic information, resources, services, and/or technologies specific to given clients
- Identifies ethical, ethnic/ancestral, cultural, religious, legal, fiscal, and societal issues related to genetic and genomic information and technologies

- Defines issues that undermine the rights of all clients for autonomous, informed genetic- and genomic-related decision making and voluntary action

Referral Activities
The registered nurse:
- Facilitates referrals for specialized genetic and genomic services for clients as needed

Provision of Education, Care, and Support
The registered nurse:
- Provides clients with interpretation of selective genetic and genomic information or services
- Provides clients with credible, accurate, appropriate, and current genetic and genomic information, resources, services, and/or technologies that facilitate decision making
- Uses health promotion/disease prevention practices that (1) consider genetic and genomic influences on personal and environmental risk factors; and (2) incorporate knowledge of genetic and/or genomic risk factors (e.g., a client with a genetic predisposition for high cholesterol who can benefit from a change in lifestyle that will decrease the likelihood that the genetic risk will be expressed)
- Uses genetic- and genomic-based interventions and information to improve clients' outcomes
- Collaborates with health care providers in providing genetic and genomic health care
- Collaborates with insurance providers/payers to facilitate reimbursement for genetic and genomic health care services
- Performs interventions/treatments appropriate to clients' genetic and genomic health care needs
- Evaluates impact and effectiveness of genetic and genomic technology, information, interventions, and treatments on clients' outcome

From Consensus Panel on Genetic/Genomic Nursing Competencies: *Essentials of genetic and genomic nursing: competencies, curricula guidelines, and outcome indicators,* ed 2, Silver Spring, Md, 2009, American Nurses Association.
*Clients as defined by document are recipients of health care; this may include persons, families, communities, and/or populations from any race, ethnicity or ancestry, culture, or religious background.

partners and asked about other unions that may have produced a pregnancy. In eliciting a birth history from the mother and father, the nurse should specifically ask about abortions, miscarriages, and stillbirths in addition to live births. To identify all members of the family tree, it is best to ask about pregnancies even of young teenagers. When inquiring about family diseases, the nurse might ask the question in different ways. For example, if a person denies any cognitive impairment in the family, asking other questions, such as about learning problems, being in special education classes, and failing or not completing school, may uncover a family history.

The family history is recorded in the form of a **pedigree chart** or family tree (in some disciplines termed a **genogram**), using standard symbols to indicate persons, relationships, and significant details related to them (Bennett, Steinhaus, Uhrich, et al, 1995) (Fig. 5-19). Construction of a pedigree begins with the affected child (proband, index case, or original patient) and all of the mother's pregnancies (Fig. 5-20, *A*). Next, the maternal family history is explored in a similar manner (Fig. 5-20, *B*); then information is gathered about relatives on the father's side, as well as any children or pregnancies that may have occurred through the father's previous unions (Fig. 5-20, *C*) (see Nursing Care Guidelines box). It is important at this point to determine whether the couple might be related in any way, although contrary to popular belief, this is usually a concern only for first cousins or closer relatives. The first-cousin risk for birth defects is about 5% compared with the general population risk of 2% to 3%. The primary risk increase is for autosomal recessive disorders, in which the chance that two individuals carry the same rare, deleterious gene is increased if they are related.

The nurse solicits information not only about other affected family members but also about (1) births (live birth, stillbirths, and abortions [especially spontaneous abortions], including gestational age of pregnancy); (2) infertility problems; (3) matings (legally sanctioned, consanguineous, multiple, unwed, and other complex relationships); (4) health of family members, including any other genetic diseases or disorders or birth defects; and (5) death and causes of death, including early

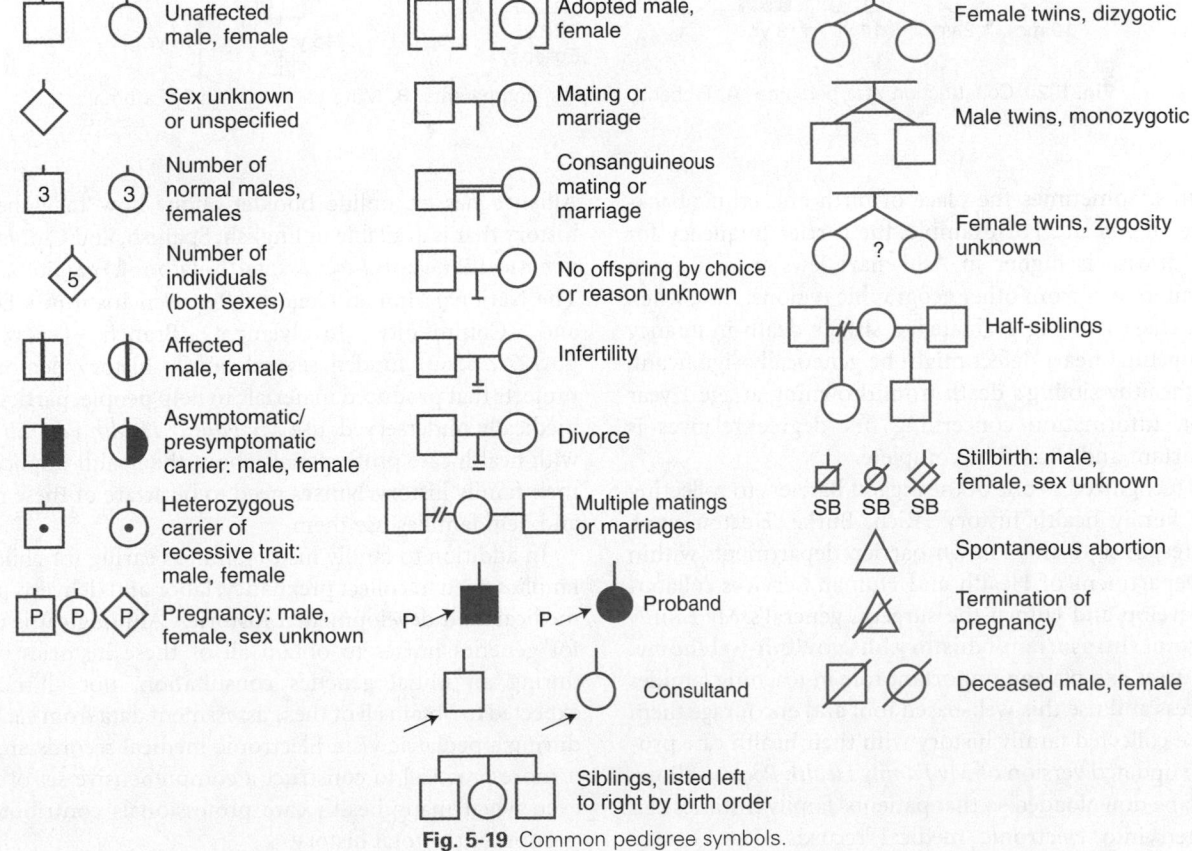

Fig. 5-19 Common pedigree symbols.

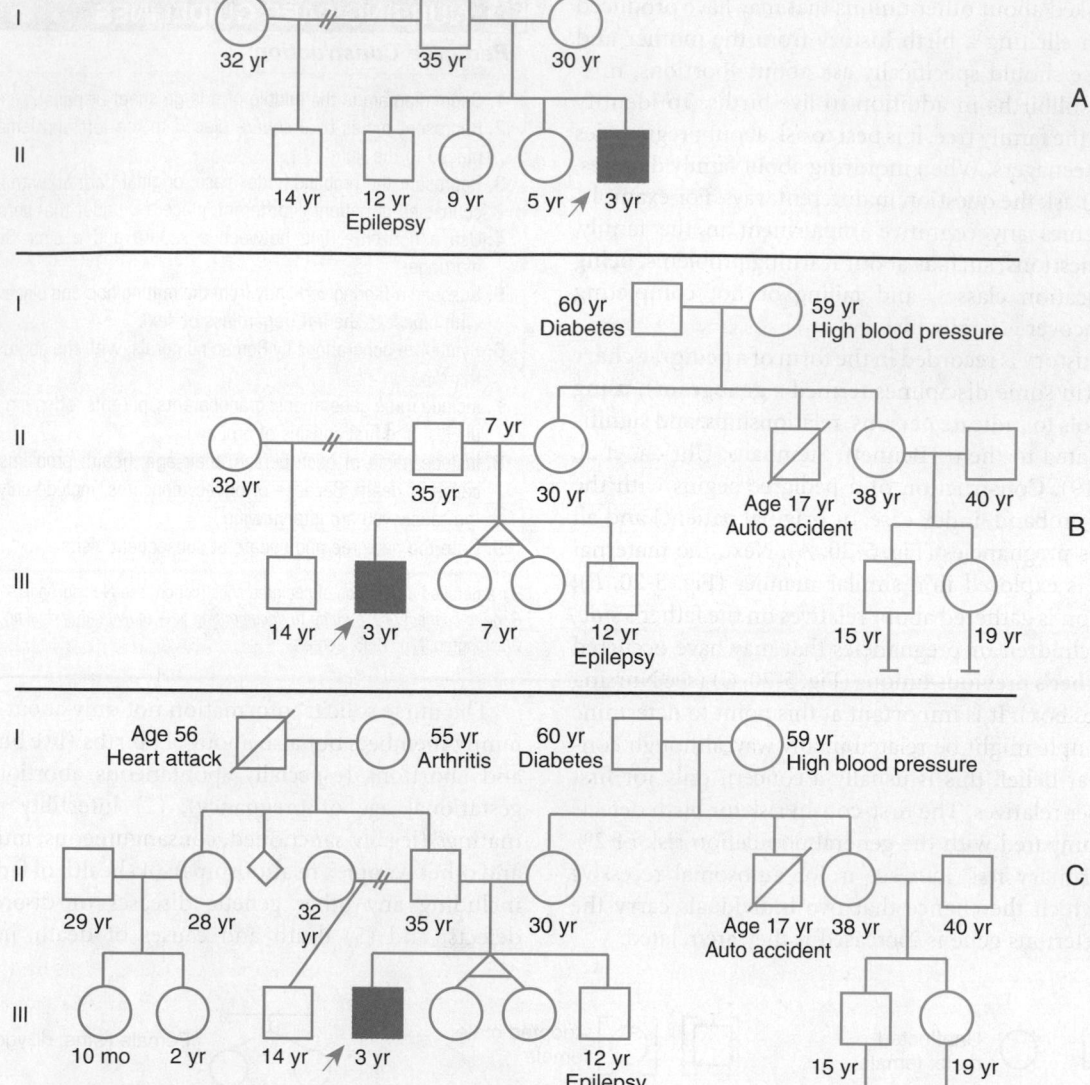

Fig. 5-20 Construction of a pedigree. **A,** Proband, siblings, and parents. **B,** Maternal relatives. **C,** Paternal relatives added.

infant deaths. Sometimes the place of birth and ethnic background are significant. For example, the carrier frequency for Tay-Sachs disease is higher in Ashkenazi Jews from Eastern Europe than in Jews from other geographic regions. Also, when a pedigree chart is being evaluated, a sister's death in infancy from a congenital heart defect might be genetically significant, whereas a healthy sibling's death from drowning at age 1 year would not. Information concerning first-degree relatives is most important and should be complete.

Time is recognized as one of the biggest barriers to collecting a detailed family health history (Rich, Burke, Heaton, et al, 2004). In response to this known barrier, departments within the U.S. Department of Health and Human Services collaborated to develop and launch the surgeon general's *My Family Health Portrait* (https://familyhistory.hhs.gov/fhh-web/home.action). Nurses can play an important role in teaching families how to access and use this web-based tool and encourage them to share the collected family history with their health care providers. The updated version of *My Family Health Portrait* allows the code to be downloaded so that patients' family histories can be imported into electronic medical records. The Genetic

Alliance has an online booklet about how to gather family history that is available in English, Spanish, and Chinese (www.geneticalliance.org/ksc_assets/tools/book1ga_ll022309.pdf). The National Human Genome Research Institute's Education and Community Involvement Branch (www.genome.gov/27026369) funded several family history demonstration projects that produced materials to help people, particularly the medically underserved, use *My Family Health Portrait* and talk with health care professionals about the health implications of their family history. Nurses need to be aware of these resources and help families use them.

In addition to family history, nurses caring for children and families need to collect pregnancy, labor and delivery, perinatal, medical, and developmental histories. Although it is common for genetics nurses to obtain all of these histories before or during an initial genetics consultation, not all nurses are expected to obtain all of these assessment data from each patient during a pediatric visit. Electronic medical records are making it more practical to construct a comprehensive set of histories even when many health care professionals contribute only a portion of the total history.

All nurses are taught to perform physical assessments, but they are seldom taught to recognize minor anomalies and dysmorphology that may suggest a genetic disorder. Yet nurses are keen in recognizing delays in development, behavior differences, and global appearances that raise concern that a newborn, infant, child, or adolescent needs further evaluation. Although dysmorphology is beyond the scope of this chapter, readers are encouraged to review the January 2009 issue of *American Journal of Medical Genetics* (Carey, 2009). Drawings and photographs of normal and abnormal morphologic characteristics are provided for the head, face, and extremities, together with accepted dysmorphology terminology. Nurses knowledgeable in dysmorphology are able to articulate specific concerns about a child's appearance rather than relying on the outdated and offensive phrase, "funny looking kid." When a major anomaly is identified, nurses should raise suspicion that the child could have additional congenital anomalies. When three or more minor anomalies are identified, nurses should suspect the possibility of an underlying syndrome. However, it is important to consider the biologic parents' physical appearance, development, and behavior when considering the relevance of the child's combination of minor anomalies.

Identification and Referral

Nurses have an important role in identifying patients and families who have, or are at risk for developing or transmitting, a genetic condition (see Box 5-7 for assessment clues to genetic disorders). Once family and patients concerns are identified, they may need help identifying and accessing necessary services. Nurses need to become familiar with the genetic services in their areas. As mentioned before, many services tend to be in large metropolitan areas. A regularly updated resource for locating genetics clinics can be found at www.genetests.org (click on Clinic Directory tab). Contact information for specific genetics professionals can be found at the following websites: geneticists, www.acmg.net (click on Find a Geneticist); genetics nurses, www.isong.org (call or e-mail office); and genetic counselors, www.nsgc.org (click on Find a Counselor). In addition, state health departments either offer services or can help identify health professionals with specialty training in genetics.

When facilitating genetics consultations, nurses should share with the genetics professional the findings in the histories they collected that triggered the consultation. Nurses can also help the referral process by determining and communicating the family's initial concerns, their state of knowledge about the reason for referral, and their attitudes and beliefs concerning genetics.

Providing Education, Care, and Support

Maintaining contact with the family or making a referral to a health care practice or an agency that can provide a sustained relationship is critical. As mentioned, it is becoming more common for genetics health care professionals to provide regular follow up and management, particularly for children with rare genetic disorders. However, some families choose not to have follow-up visits with genetic experts.

Regardless of whether families choose to receive continued care with a genetics center, clinic, or professional, nurses can help patients and families process and clarify the information they receive during a genetics visit. Misunderstanding of this information can have many causes, including cultural differences, the disparity of knowledge between the counselor and the family, and the heightened emotion surrounding genetic counseling. Family members have difficulty absorbing all the information presented during a genetics evaluation and counseling session. Knowing this, genetics professionals write and send clinic summary letters to families. The nurse may need to help the family understand terminology in the letter, help them identify and articulate remaining questions or areas of clarification, and coach them through the process of accessing genetics health professionals to get remaining questions and concerns answered. Information often needs to be repeated several times before the family understands the content and its implications.

Nurses must assess for and address parents' feelings of guilt about carrying "bad genes" or having "made my child sick." Depending on the type of cytogenetic disorder, the nurse may be able to absolve the parents of guilt by explaining the random nature of segregation during both gamete formation and fertilization and that errors in cell division unique to the pregnancy in question are not likely to happen again and are not inherited. If the condition is a mendelian-inherited or mitochondrial disorder, it is important to assess parents' understanding of recurrence risk, help them understand the chances that a subsequent pregnancy will not be affected, and ensure they have been given information about their options for future children (preimplantation diagnosis, use of donor egg or sperm, prenatal diagnosis, or adoption). Families often try to reason that some unrelated event caused the abnormality (e.g., a fall, a urinary tract infection, or "one glass of wine") before the mother was aware that she was pregnant. These misconceptions need to be assessed and dispelled.

After a genetics visit, and sometimes before the visit, parents often use the Internet to find answers to their questions. During the initial genetics evaluation, a diagnosis may not be possible. Instead, findings in medical, developmental, and family histories lead the professional to order genetic tests and other diagnostic procedures. Diagnoses under consideration are discussed briefly with the parents. Some parents are satisfied with the brief information and do not care to find out more until the actual diagnosis is established. Other parents go home and seek as much information as they can about the diagnoses under consideration. The information they find can be terrifying and overwhelming and inaccurate or misleading. Nurses can play an important role in helping parents identify reliable, accurate resources for information at whatever time they desire it. It is also important to stress that everything that is described for a genetic condition may not be relevant to their child. Before the follow-up genetics visit when test and procedure results are discussed, nurses can help parents identify and write down the questions and concerns they need addressed before leaving the clinic.

Once a genetics diagnosis is made or a genetic predisposition to a delayed-onset disorder is identified, nurses need to have frequent contact with patients and families as they attempt to incorporate recommended therapies or disease-prevention strategies into their daily lives. For example, a disorder such as PKU requires conscientious diet management; therefore it is important to make certain that the family understands and follows instructions and is able to navigate the health care system to access the essential formula and low-phenylalanine food products. An infant evaluated for cleft palate and cardiac defect and subsequently found to have VCFS requires surgical intervention for the congenital malformations. The infant also benefits from early intervention services and eventually an individualized education plan in school, since developmental delay and eventual learning problems are common.

Initial and ongoing assessment of the family's coping abilities, resources, and support systems is vital to determine their need for additional assistance and support. As with any family who has a child with chronic health care needs, nurses must teach the family to become the child's advocate. Nurses can help families locate agencies and clinics specializing in a specific disorder or its consequences that can provide services (e.g., equipment, medication, and rehabilitation), educational programs, and parent support groups. Referral to local and national support groups or contact with a local family that has a child with the same condition can be helpful for new parents. Privacy and confidentiality are imperative, and both families must give permission before their contact information is given (International Society of Nurses in Genetics, 2006). Nurses can also be instrumental in helping parents start a support group when none is available.

Parental attachment and adjustment to the baby can be supported and facilitated by nursing interventions. Assessing the parents' understanding of the child's disorder and providing simple and truthful explanations can help them begin to understand their child's health issues. Guiding the parents in recognizing their child's cues, responses, and strengths can be helpful even for experienced parents. A caring attitude conveys the value of their child and, by extension, their value as parents. The nurse can help the parents identify their strengths as a family and identify support that is available to them.

Giving birth to and raising a child with a genetic disorder is not necessarily a lifetime burden. It is important for nurses to ask parents to describe their experience raising their child with a particular genetic condition. What has been the impact on their family? While parents may initially experience negative outcomes, such as shock, emotional distress, and grief, families can adapt and thrive. Resources for managing stress and restoring balance in the lives of families affected by a genetic condition can help. Van Riper's (2007) research has identified nursing interventions that can promote resilience and adaptation in families of children with Down syndrome. Van Riper's recommendations are useful for families of children with any type of genetic disorder:

- Recognize multiple stressors, strains, and transitions in their lives (e.g., unmet family needs).
- Discuss and implement strategies for reducing family demands (e.g., setting priorities and reducing the number of outside activities family members are involved in).
- Identify and use individual, family, and community resources (e.g., humor, family flexibility, supportive extended family, respite care, local support groups, and Internet resources).
- Expand the range and efficacy of their coping strategies (e.g., increase the use of active strategies such as reframing, mobilize their ability to acquire and accept help, and decrease the use of passive appraisal).
- Encourage the use of an affirming style of family problem-solving communication (e.g., one that conveys support and caring and exerts a calming influence).

Some families do struggle after learning their child has a genetic disorder. Families may feel ashamed of a hereditary disorder and seek to blame their partner for transmitting a faulty gene or chromosome. Intrafamilial strife, hostility, and marital or couple disharmony, sometimes to the point of family disintegration, can occur. Nurses should be alert for evidence of risk factors that indicate poor adjustment (e.g., child abuse, divorce, or other maladaptive behaviors). Referral to psychosocial professionals for crisis intervention may be necessary.

KEY POINTS

- Most if not all disease processes have a genetic component.
- Genetic diseases may be caused by chromosome abnormalities, gene mutations, or mtDNA mutations. In addition, expression of a genetic disease are often influenced by environmental factors.
- Congenital anomalies—errors of morphogenic development—may arise at any stage of development and demonstrate wide variability in causative factors. Environmental teratogens and maternal disease may also disrupt fetal development, leading to birth defects.
- Chromosome disorders are caused by abnormalities in either chromosome structure or number.
- Alterations in chromosome number occur as a result of unequal distribution of genetic material during gamete formation (meiotic nondisjunction) or early cell division of the zygote (mitotic nondisjunction).
- Genes can be located on an autosome or a sex chromosome. Their mode of expression can be dominant or recessive.
- Disorders caused by single-gene mutations are distributed in families according to predictable mendelian principles of inheritance, but recognition of the pattern may be influenced by variable expressivity and penetrance (frequency of expression). In addition, a genetic disorder can be phenotypically expressed by seemingly unrelated manifestations.
- Most current interventions for genetic disease aim at correcting or modifying the phenotypic expression.
- The objectives of genetic testing are to detect the presence of disease in individuals, detect unaffected carriers of a disease, and monitor the incidence of disease or malformations in a population.
- Prenatal testing is aimed at both screening (ultrasound and maternal biochemical marker testing) and diagnosis (amniocentesis, ultrasound, CVS, and fetal cord blood sampling).
- A genetic counseling goal is to provide individuals and families with information needed to make informed decisions about a course of action that is most appropriate to them.
- Competent nursing practice includes applying and integrating genetic and genomic knowledge during nursing assessment; when identifying and referring patients and families who may benefit from genetic services; when identifying resources for patients and families; and when providing education, care, and support.

REFERENCES

American Academy of Pediatrics: Ethical issues with genetic testing in pediatrics, *Pediatrics* 107(6):1451-1455, 2001.

American Academy of Pediatrics, Committee on Substance Abuse and Committee on Children with Disabilities: Fetal alcohol syndrome and alcohol-related neurodevelopmental disorders, *Pediatrics* 106(2 Pt 1):358-361, 2000.

American Academy of Pediatrics: Folic acid for the prevention of neural tube defects, *Pediatrics* 104(2):325-327, 1999.

American College of Medical Genetics Newborn Screening Expert Group: Newborn screening: toward a uniform screening panel and system—executive summary, *Genet Med* 8(5 Suppl):1S-11S, 2006.

American College of Obstetrics and Gynecology: Screening for fetal chromosomal abnormalities: clinical management guidelines for obstetrician-gynecologists, *Obstet Gynecol* 109(1):217-227, 2007.

Antshel KM, Fremont W, Kates WR, et al: The neurocognitive phenotype in velo-cardio-facial syndrome: a developmental perspective, *Dev Disabil Res Rev* 14(1):43-51, 2008.

Bailey L: An overview of enzyme replacement therapy for lysosomal storage diseases, *Online J Issues Nursing* 13(1):Manuscript 3, 2008.

Baroni MA, Anderson YE, Mischler E: Cystic fibrosis newborn screening: impact of early screening results on parenting stress, *Pediatr Nurs* 23(2):143-151, 1997.

Bennett RL, Steinhaus KA, Uhrich SB, et al: Recommendations for standardized human pedigree nomenclature, *Am J Med Genet* 56:745-752, 1995.

Bos AF, Einspieler C, Prechtl HF: Intrauterine growth retardation, general movements, and neurodevelopmental outcome: a review, *Dev Med Child Neurol* 43(1):61-68, 2001.

Brown SM: *Essentials of medical genomic,* Hoboken, NJ, 2003, Wiley-Liss.

Campbell E, Ross LF: Parental attitudes regarding newborn screening of PKU and DMD, *Am J Med Genet* 120A(2):209-214, 2003.

Carey JC, editor: Elements of morphology: standard terminology, *Am J Med Genet A* 149A(1):1-127, 2009.

Chamberlain S: Friedreich's in relief, *Nat Genet* 12(4):344-345, 1996.

Ciske D, Haavisto A, Laxova A, et al: Genetic counseling and neonatal screening for cystic fibrosis: an assessment of the communication process, *Pediatrics* 107(4):699-705, 2001.

Collins FS, Green ED, Guttmacher AE, et al: A vision for the future of genomics research: a blueprint for the genomic era, *Nature* 422:1-13, 2003.

Consensus Panel on Genetic/Genomic Nursing Competencies: *Essential nursing competencies and curricula guidelines for genetics and genomics,* Silver Spring, Md, 2006, American Nurses Association.

Edelmann L, Hirschhorn K: Clinical utility of array CGH for the detection of chromosomal imbalances associated with mental retardation and multiple congenital anomalies, *Ann N Y Acad Sci* 1151:157-166, 2009.

Farrell M, Certain I, Farrell P: Genetic counseling and risk communication services of newborn screening programs, *Arch Pediatr Adolesc Med* 155(2):120-126, 2001.

Farrell P, Kosorok MR, Rock MJ, et al: Early diagnosis of cystic fibrosis through neonatal screening prevents severe malnutrition and improves long-term growth: Wisconsin Cystic Fibrosis Neonatal Screening Study Group, *Pediatrics* 107(1):1-13, 2001.

Fossland VS, Stroop JB, Schwartz RC, et al: Genetic issues in patients with breast cancer, *Surg Oncol Clin North Am* 18(1):53-71, viii, 2009.

Fridman C, Varela MC, Kok F, et al: Paternal UPD15: further genetic and clinical studies in four Angelman syndrome patients, *Am J Med Genet* 92(5):322-327, 2000.

Gardner RJ, Sutherland GR: *Chromosome abnormalities and genetic counseling,* ed 3, New York, 2004, Oxford University Press.

Gross SJ, Pletcher BA, Monaghan KG, et al: Carrier screening in individuals of Ashkenazi Jewish descent, *Genet Med* 10(1):54-56, 2008.

Honein M, Paulozzi LJ, Mathews TJ, et al: Impact of folic acid fortification of the US food supply on the occurrence of neural tube defects, *JAMA* 285(23):2981-2986, 2001.

International Human Genome Sequencing Consortium: Finishing the euchromatic sequence of the human genome, *Nature* 431:931-945, 2004.

International Society of Nurses in Genetics: *Genetics/genomics nursing: scope and standards of practice,* Silver Springs, Md, 2006, American Nurses Association.

Jones KL: *Smith's recognizable patterns of human malformation,* Philadelphia, 2006, Saunders.

Jorde LB, Carey JC, Bamshad MJ, et al: *Medical genetics,* ed 3, St. Louis, 2003, Mosby.

Kent-First M: The critical and expanding role of genetics in assisted reproduction, *Prenatal Diagnosis* 20(7):536-551, 2000.

King RA, Rotter JI, Motulsky AG: Approach to genetic basis of common diseases. In King RA, Rotter JI, Motulsky AG, editors: *The genetic basis of common diseases,* ed 2, New York, 2002, Oxford.

Kingston HM: *ABC of clinical genetics,* ed 3, London, 2002, BMJ Books.

Korf BR: *Human genetics: a problem-based approach,* ed 2, Cambridge, Mass, 2000, Blackwell Science.

Lashley FR: *Clinical genetics in nursing practice,* New York, 2005, Springer.

Lynch HT, Lynch JF, Lynch PM, et al: Hereditary colorectal cancer syndromes: molecular genetics, genetic counseling, diagnosis and management, *Fam Cancer* 7(1):27-39, 2008.

McKusick VA: History of medical genetics. In Rimoin DL, Connor MJ, Pyeritz RE, et al, editors: *Principles and practice of medical genetics,* New York, 2002, Churchill Livingstone.

Mills JL, Signore C: Neural tube defect rates before and after food fortification with folic acid, *Birth Defects Res A Clin Mol Teratol* 70:844-845, 2004.

National Foundation for Ectodermal Dysplasia: What is ED? Mascoutah, Ill, 2009, The Foundation, available at http://nfed.org/about_ed_faq.asp (accessed December 15, 2009).

Nelson DL: Allelic expansion underlies many genetic diseases, *Growth Genet Horm* 12(1):1-4, 1996.

Nusbaum R, Isaacs C: Management updates for women with a BRCA1 or BRCA2 mutation, *Molec Diagn Ther* 11(3):133-144, 2007.

Pletcher BA, Toriello HV, Noblin SJ, et al: Indications for genetic referral: a guide for healthcare providers, *Genet Med* 9(6):385-389, 2007.

Rich EC, Burke W, Heaton CJ, et al: Reconsidering the family history in primary care, *J Gen Intern Med* 19(3):273-280, 2004.

Rimoin DL, Connor MJ, Pyeritz RE, et al, editors: *Emery and Rimoin's principles and practice of medical genetics,* London, 2002, Churchill Livingstone.

Rodeck CH: Fetal blood sampling: historical perspectives, *NeoReviews* 5(6):e229-e231, 2004.

Romiti ML, Colognesi C, Cancrini C, et al: Prognostic value of a CCR5 defective allele in pediatric HIV-1 infection, *Mol Med* 6(1):28-36, 2000.

Saenko EL, Pipe SW: Strategies towards a longer acting factor VIII, *Haemophilia* 12(Suppl 3):42-51, 2006.

Scriver CR, Beaudet AL, Sly WS, et al, editors: *The metabolic and molecular bases of inherited disease,* New York, 2001, McGraw-Hill.

Shprintzen RJ: Velo-cardio-facial syndrome: 30 years of study, *Dev Disabil Res Rev* 14(1):3-10, 2008.

Spahis JK, Bowers NR: Navigating the maze of newborn screening, *MCN Am J Matern Child Nurs* 31(3):190-196, 2006.

Sweetman L, Millington DS, Therrell BL, et al: Naming and counting disorders (conditions) included in newborn screening panels, *Pediatrics* 117(5 Pt 2):S308-S314, 2006.

Sybert VP, McCauley E: Turner's syndrome, *N Engl J Med* 351:1227-1238, 2004.

Van Riper M: Families of children with Down syndrome: responding to "a change in plans" with resilience, *J Pediatr Nurs* 22(2):116-128, 2007.

Veach PM, LeRoy BS, Bartels DM: *Facilitating the genetic counseling process: a practice manual,* New York, 2003, Springer.

Verlinsky Y, Rechitsky S, Schoolcraft W, et al: Preimplantation diagnosis for Fanconi anemia combined with HLA matching, *JAMA* 285(24):3130-3133, 2001.

Wilkin JZ, Su Z, Kuritzkes DR, et al: HIV type 1 chemokine coreceptor use among antiretroviral-experienced patients screened for a clinical trial of a CCR5 inhibitor: AIDS Clinical Trial Group A5211, *Clin Infect Dis* 44(4):591-595, 2007.

Zieve D, Juhn G, Eltz DR: *Amniotic constriction bands,* 2009, available at www.nlm.nih.gov/medlineplus/ency/article/001579.htm (accessed June 9, 2009).

INTERNET RESOURCES

Ethical, Legal, and Social Issues (ELSI)—www.
genome.gov/PolicyEthics (NIH site) and
www.ornl.gov/hgmis/elsi/elsi.html
(Department of Energy site) (program
developed to study the issues surrounding the
availability of genetic information)

Family Village—www.familyvillage.wisc.edu
(information and resources for families with
disabilities and persons who provide services
for them)

GeneTests—www.genetests.org (genetic testing
resource; requires password to enter the site;
easy to obtain)

Genetic Alliance—www.geneticalliance.org
(international coalition of individuals,
professionals, and genetic support
organizations)

Genetic Home Reference—http://ghr.nlm.nih.
gov (handbook on basic human and
clinical genetics concepts, summaries

of a variety of genetic conditions, excellent
glossary)

Health on the Net Code of Conduct—www.hon.
ch/HONcode/Conduct.html (describes the
Health on the Net Foundation code of
conduct for medical and health websites,
which addresses the reliability and credibility
of information)

International Society of Nurses in Genetics—
www.isong.org (provides information about
various genetics education programs,
instructional resources, conferences targeting
nurses)

National Cancer Institute—www.cancer.gov
(provides accurate and up-to-date cancer
information)

National Coalition for Health Professional
Education in Genetics—www.nchpeg.org
(promotes access to human genetics
education resources for health

professionals in a variety of specialties and
disciplines)

National Human Genome Research Institute—
http://genome.gov (information on genome
research and its ethical, legal, and social
implications)

National Organization for Rare Disorders—
www.rarediseases.org (a federation
of voluntary health organizations
dedicated to helping people with rare
"orphan" diseases)

OMIM, Online Mendelian Inheritance in
Man—www.ncbi.nlm.nih.gov/Omim
(up-to-date summaries of human genes and
genetic disorders)

United Mitochondrial Disease Foundation—
www.umdf.org (provides information about
mitochondrial defects, including professional
and lay materials)

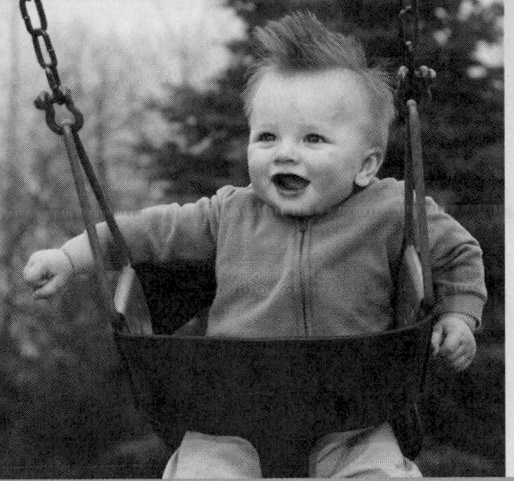

Communication and Physical Assessment of the Child

Marilyn J. Hockenberry

CHAPTER OUTLINE

GUIDELINES FOR COMMUNICATION AND INTERVIEWING

The most widely used method of communicating with parents on a professional basis is the interview process. Unlike social conversation, interviewing is a specific form of goal-directed communication. As nurses converse with children and adults, they focus on the individuals to determine the kind of persons they are, their usual mode of handling problems, whether they need help, and the way they react to counseling. Developing interviewing skills requires time and practice, but following some guiding principles can facilitate this process. An organized approach is most effective when using interviewing skills in patient teaching.

ESTABLISHING A SETTING FOR COMMUNICATION

Appropriate Introduction

Introduce yourself and ask the name of each family member who is present. Address parents or other adults by their appropriate titles, such as "Mr." and "Mrs.," unless they specify a preferred name. Record the preferred name on the medical record. Using formal address or their preferred names, rather than using first names or "mother" or "father," conveys respect and regard for the parents or other caregivers (Seidel, Ball, Dains, et al, 2007).

At the beginning of the visit, include children in the interaction by asking them their name, age, and other information. Nurses often direct all questions to adults, even when children are old enough to speak for themselves. This only terminates one extremely valuable source of information: the patient. When including the child, follow the general rules for communicating with children given in the Nursing Care Guidelines box on p. 122.

Assurance of Privacy and Confidentiality

The place where the nurse conducts the interview is almost as important as the interview itself. The physical environment should allow for as much privacy as possible, with distractions, such as interruptions, noise, or other visible activity, kept to a minimum. At times it is necessary to turn off a television, radio, or cellular telephone. The environment should also have some play provision for young children to keep them occupied during the parent-nurse interview (Fig. 6-1). Parents who are constantly interrupted by their children are unable to concentrate fully and tend to give brief answers to finish the interview as quickly as possible.

Confidentiality is another essential component of the initial phase of the interview. Since the interview is usually shared with other members of the health team care or the teacher (in the case of students), be certain to inform the family of the limits regarding confidentiality. If confidentiality is a concern in a particular situation, such as when talking to a parent suspected of child abuse or a teenager contemplating suicide, deal with

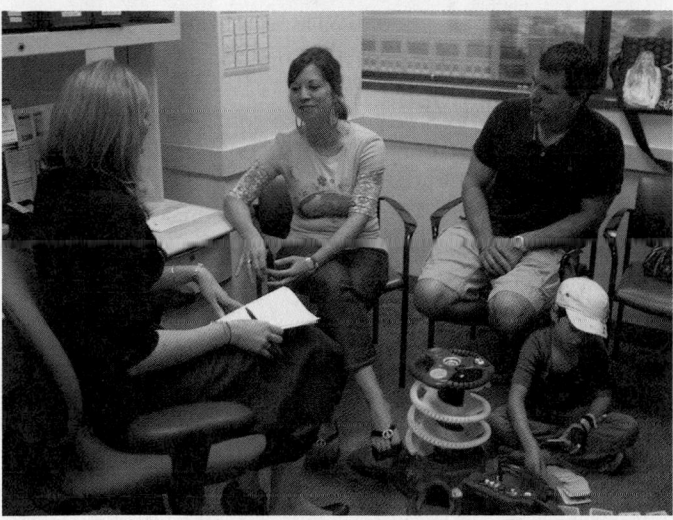

Fig. 6-1 Child plays while nurse interviews parent.

BOX 6-1   TELEPHONE TRIAGE GUIDELINES

Date and time
Background
- Name, age, sex
- Chronic illness
- Allergies, current medications, treatments, or recent immunizations

Chief complaint
General symptoms
- Severity
- Duration
- Other symptoms
- Pain

Systems review
Steps taken
- Advised to call emergency medical services (911)
- Advised to see practitioner
- Advised regarding home care
- Advised to call back if symptoms worsen or fail to improve

Resources for Telephone Triage Protocols

Beaulieu R, Jumphreys J: Evaluation of a telephone advice nurse in a nursing faculty managed pediatric community clinic, *J Pediatr Health Care* 22(3):175-181, 2008.

Marklund B, Ström M, Månsson J, et al: Computer-supported telephone nurse triage: an evaluation of medical quality and costs, *J Nurs Manage* 15:180-187, 2007.

Simonsen SM: *Telephone assessment: guidelines for practice*, ed 2, St Louis, 2001, Mosby.

---

this directly and inform the person that in such instances confidentiality cannot be ensured. However, the nurse judiciously protects information of a confidential nature.

COMPUTER PRIVACY AND APPLICATIONS IN NURSING

The use of computer technology to store and retrieve health information has become widespread. The health care community is increasingly concerned about the privacy and security of this health information. Any person accessing confidential health information is charged with managing safeguards for disclosure, since violations might incur civil damages.

Many institutions use computer and information applications in nursing (**nursing informatics**), such as electronic medical records, to record care and access information. Two important health care applications are record transmission, including facsimile (fax), electronic mail (e-mail), and telemedicine. The telemedicine application is capable of two-way video conferencing, transmission of radiographs, and clinical consultation between remote sites and centralized resources.*

TELEPHONE TRIAGE AND COUNSELING

Nurses are increasingly responsible for assessing children's symptoms and applying clinical judgment for further medical care (**triage**) via telephone report. Most often, health problems are assessed and prioritized according to urgency, and nurses provide treatment via telephone services. A well-designed telephone triage program is essential for safe, prompt, and consistent-quality health care (Beaulieu and Humphreys, 2008; Marklund, Ström, Månsson, et al, 2007). Telephone triage is more than "just a phone call," since a child's life is a high price to pay for poorly managed or incompetent telephone assessment skills. Typically, guidelines for telephone triage include asking screening questions; determining when to immediately refer to emergency medical services (dial 911); and determining when to refer to same-day appointments, appointments in 24 to 72 hours, appointments in 4 days or more, or home care (Box 6-1). Successful outcomes are based on the consistency and accuracy of the information provided. Telephone triage care management has increased access to high-quality health care services and empowered parents to participate in their child's medical care. Consequently patient satisfaction has significantly improved. Unnecessary emergency department and clinic visits have decreased, saving medical costs and time (with less absence from work) for families in need of health care.

! NURSING ALERT

Legal issues can emerge from errors in telephone triage care management. Always advise the parent that the child should see their health care provider if there is any doubt as to the seriousness of the illness.

COMMUNICATING WITH FAMILIES

COMMUNICATING WITH PARENTS

Although the parent and the child are separate and distinct individuals, the nurse's relationship with the child is frequently mediated by the parent, particularly with younger children. For the most part, nurses acquire information about the child by direct observation or through communication with the parents. Usually it can be assumed that, because of the close contact with the child, the parent gives reliable information. Assessing the

---

*Resources: Nicoll LH: *Nurses' guide to the Internet*, ed 3, Philadelphia, 2001, Lippincott. Also available is a bimonthly publication, *CIN: Computers, Informatics, Nursing*. To order, call 800-638-3030; fax: 301-714-2300; e-mail: CustomerService@LWW.com; www.cinjournal.com.

child requires input from the child (verbal and nonverbal), information from the parent, and the nurse's own observations of the child and interpretation of the relationship between the child and the parent. When children are old enough to be active participants in their own health maintenance, the parent becomes a collaborator in health care.

Encouraging the Parents to Talk

Interviewing parents not only offers the opportunity to determine the child's health and developmental status, but also offers information about factors that influence the child's life. Whatever the parent sees as a problem should be a concern of the nurse. These problems are not always easy to identify. Nurses need to be alert for clues and signals by which a parent communicates worries and anxieties. Careful phrasing with broad, open-ended questions such as "What is Jimmy eating now?" provides more information than several single-answer questions, such as "Is Jimmy eating what the rest of the family eats?"

Sometimes the parent will take the lead without prompting. At other times it may be necessary to direct another question on the basis of an observation, such as "Connie seems unhappy today" or "How do you feel when David cries?" If the parent appears to be tired or distraught, consider asking, "What do you do to relax?" or "What help do you have with the children?" A comment such as "You handle the baby very well. What kind of experience have you had with babies?" to new parents who appear comfortable with their first child gives positive reinforcement and provides an opening for questions they might have on the infant's care. Often all that is required to keep parents talking is a nod or saying "yes" or "uh-huh."

When attempting to elicit feelings and probe covert problems, avoid closed-ended questions that begin with "Does ...," "Did ...," or "Is ...," which usually require only a single response. In addition, asking questions such as "Does your son have any problems at school?" subtly implies a lack of parental skills and may make the parent defensive. Instead, say, "What ...," "How ...," "Tell me about ..." and encourage elaboration with "You were saying ..." or "You say that ...," or by reflecting back a key word. Open-ended questions are nonthreatening and encourage description.

Directing the Focus

Directing the focus of the interview while allowing maximum freedom of expression is one of the most difficult goals in effective communication. One approach is the use of open-ended or broad questions, followed by guiding statements. For example, if the parent proceeds to list the other children by name, say, "Tell me their ages, too." If the parent continues to describe each child in depth, which is not the purpose of the interview, redirect the focus by stating, "Let's talk about the other children later. You were beginning to tell me about Paul's activities at school." This approach conveys interest in the other children but focuses the assessment on the patient.

Listening and Cultural Awareness

Listening is the most important component of effective communication. When the purpose of listening is to understand the person being interviewed, it is an active process that requires

concentration and attention to all aspects of the conversation—verbal, nonverbal, and abstract. Major blocks to listening are environmental distraction and premature judgment.

Although it is necessary to make some preliminary judgments, listen with as much objectivity as possible by clarifying meanings and attempting to see the situation from the parent's point of view. Effective interviewers consciously control their reactions, responses, and the techniques they use (see Cultural Competence box).

⊕ CULTURAL COMPETENCE
Interviewing Without Judgment

It is easy to inject one's own attitudes and feelings into an interview. Often nurses' own prejudices and assumptions, which may include racial, religious, and cultural stereotypes, influence their perceptions of a parent's behavior. What the nurse may interpret as a parent's passive hostility or lack of interest may be shyness or an expression of anxiety. For example, in Western cultures eye contact and directness are signs of paying attention. However, in many non-Western cultures, including that of Native Americans, directness (such as looking someone in the eye) is considered rude. Children are taught to avert their gaze and to look down when being addressed by an adult, especially one with authority (Seidel, Ball, Dains, et al, 2007). Therefore nurses must make judgments about "listening," as well as verbal interactions, with an appreciation of cultural differences (see Nursing Care Guidelines box, p. 33, and Chapter 2).

Minimum verbal activity with active listening facilitates parent involvement. It is tempting to spend time explaining, describing, and interpreting health information when the opportunity presents itself. However, it is possible to provide effective health education by timing the information properly and presenting only as much as is necessary at the moment.

Careful listening relies on the use of clues, verbal leads, or signals from the interviewee to move the interview along. Frequent references to an area of concern, repetition of certain key words, or a special emphasis on something or someone serve as cues to the interviewer for the direction of inquiry. Concerns and anxieties are often mentioned in a casual, offhand manner. Even though they are casual, they are important and deserve careful scrutiny to identify problem areas. For example, a parent who is concerned about a child's habit of bed-wetting may casually mention that the child's bed was "wet this morning."

Using Silence

Silence as a response is often one of the most difficult interviewing techniques to learn. The interviewer requires a sense of confidence and comfort to allow the interviewee space in which to think without interruptions. Silence permits the interviewee to sort out thoughts and feelings and search for responses to questions. Silence can also be a cue for the interviewer to go more slowly, reexamine the approach, and not push too hard (Seidel, Ball, Dains, et al, 2007).

Sometimes it is necessary to break the silence and reopen communication. Do this in a way that encourages the person to continue talking about what is considered important. Breaking a silence by introducing a new topic or by prolonged talking essentially terminates the interviewee's opportunity to use the silence. Suggestions for breaking the silence include statements such as "Is there anything else you wish to say?"

"I see you find it difficult to continue; how may I help?" or "I don't know what this silence means. Perhaps there is something you would like to put into words but find difficult to say."

Being Empathic

Empathy is the capacity to understand what another person is experiencing from within that person's frame of reference; it is often described as the ability to put oneself in another's shoes. The essence of empathic interaction is accurate understanding of another's feelings (Mathiasen, 2006). Empathy differs from sympathy, which is *having* feelings or emotions similar to those of another person, rather than *understanding* those feelings (Mathiasen, 2006).

Providing Anticipatory Guidance

The ideal way to handle a situation is to deal with it *before* it becomes a problem. The best preventive measure is anticipatory guidance. Traditionally, anticipatory guidance focused on providing families information on normal growth and development and nurturing childrearing practices. For example, one of the most significant areas in pediatrics is injury prevention. Beginning prenatally, parents need specific instructions on home safety. Because of the child's maturing developmental skills, parents must implement home safety changes early to minimize risks to the child.

Unprepared parents can be disturbed by many normal developmental changes, such as a toddler's diminished appetite, negativism, altered sleeping patterns, and anxiety toward strangers. The chapters on health promotion provide the nurse information for counseling parents. However, anticipatory guidance should extend beyond giving general information during brief visits to empowering families to use the information as a means of building competence in their parenting abilities (Magar, Dabova-Missova, and Gjerdingen, 2006). To achieve this level of anticipatory guidance, the nurse should:

- Base interventions on needs identified by the family, not by the professional
- View the family as competent or as having the ability to be competent
- Provide opportunities for the family to achieve competence

Avoiding Blocks to Communication

A number of blocks to communication can adversely affect the quality of the helping relationship. The interviewer introduces many of these blocks, such as giving unrestricted advice or forming prejudged conclusions. Another type of block occurs primarily with the interviewees and concerns information overload. When individuals receive too much information or information that is overwhelming, they often demonstrate signs of increasing anxiety or decreasing attention. Such signals should alert the interviewer to give less information or to clarify what has been said. Box 6-2 lists some of the more common blocks to communication, including signs of information overload.

The nurse can correct communication blocks by careful analysis of the interview process. One of the best methods for improving interviewing skills is audiotape or videotape feedback. With supervision and guidance, the interviewer can recognize the blocks and consciously avoid them.

BOX 6-2 BLOCKS TO COMMUNICATION

Communication Barriers (Nurse)
Socializing
Giving unrestricted and sometimes unasked for advice
Offering premature or inappropriate reassurance
Giving overready encouragement
Defending a situation or opinion
Using stereotyped comments or clichés
Limiting expression of emotion by asking directed, closed-ended questions
Interrupting and finishing the person's sentence
Talking more than the interviewee
Forming prejudged conclusions
Deliberately changing the focus

Signs of Information Overload (Patient)
Long periods of silence
Wide eyes and fixed facial expression
Constant fidgeting or attempting to move away
Nervous habits (e.g., tapping, playing with hair)
Sudden interruptions (e.g., asking to go to the bathroom)
Looking around
Yawning, eyes drooping
Frequently looking at a watch or clock
Attempting to change topic of discussion

Communicating with Families Through an Interpreter

Sometimes communication is impossible because two people speak different languages. In this case it is necessary to obtain information through a third party, the interpreter. When using an interpreter, the nurse follows the same interviewing guidelines. Specific guidelines for using an adult interpreter are given in the Nursing Care Guidelines box.

NURSING CARE GUIDELINES

Using an Interpreter

- Explain to interpreter the reason for the interview and the type of questions that will be asked.
- Clarify whether a detailed or brief answer is required and whether the translated response can be general or literal.
- Introduce the interpreter to family and allow some time before the interview for them to become acquainted.
- Communicate directly with family members when asking questions to reinforce interest in them and to observe nonverbal expressions, but do not ignore interpreter.
- Pose questions to elicit only one answer at a time, such as "Do you have pain?" rather than "Do you have any pain, tiredness, or loss of appetite?"
- Refrain from interrupting family member and interpreter while they are conversing.
- Avoid commenting to interpreter about family members, since they may understand some English.
- Be aware that some medical words, such as *allergy*, may have no similar word in another language; avoid medical jargon whenever possible.
- Be aware that cultural differences may exist regarding views on sex, marriage, or pregnancy.
- Allow time after the interview for interpreter to share something that he or she thought could not be said earlier; ask about the interpreter's impression of nonverbal clues to communication and family members' reliability or ease in revealing information.
- Arrange for family to speak with the same interpreter on subsequent visits whenever possible.

Communicating with families through an interpreter requires sensitivity to cultural, legal, and ethical considerations (see Cultural Competence box). For example, in some cultures using a child as an interpreter is considered an insult to an adult because children are expected to show respect by not questioning their elders. In some cultures class differences between the interpreter and the family may cause the family to feel intimidated and less inclined to offer information. Therefore it is important to choose the translator carefully and provide time for the interpreter and family to establish rapport.

🌐 **CULTURAL COMPETENCE**

Using Children as Translators

When no one else is available to translate, children within the family are often asked to assume this role. In this situation it is important to stress *literal* translation of parent responses. To ensure correct translations, it may be necessary to interrupt the parent and ask the child to translate every few sentences. When using children as interpreters, ask questions directed at specific answers and assess the interpreted translation in terms of nonverbal expressions of communication. Note that some institutions prohibit or discourage the use of children as interpreters; check institutional policy for compliance.

Legal and ethical concerns may also arise. For example, in obtaining informed consent through an interpreter, the nurse should fully inform the family of all aspects of the particular procedure to which they are consenting. Issues of confidentiality may arise when family members related to another patient are asked to interpret for the family, thus revealing sensitive information that may be shared with other families on the unit. With increased sensitivity toward patient rights and confidentiality, many institutions now require consent forms produced in the patient's primary language.

❗ **NURSING ALERT**

When using translated materials, such as a health history form, be certain the informant is literate in the foreign language.

COMMUNICATING WITH CHILDREN

 Although the greatest amount of verbal communication is usually carried out with the parent, do not exclude the child during the interview. Pay attention to infants and younger children through play or by occasionally directing questions or remarks to them. Include older children as active participants.

In communication with children of all ages, the nonverbal components of the communication process convey the most significant messages. It is difficult to disguise feelings, attitudes, and anxiety when relating to children. They are alert to surroundings and attach meaning to every gesture and move that is made; this is particularly true of very young children.

Active attempts to make friends with children before they have had an opportunity to evaluate an unfamiliar person tend to increase their anxiety. Continue to talk to the child and parent but go about activities that do not involve the child directly, thus allowing the child to observe from a safe position. If the child has a special toy or doll, "talk" to the doll first. Ask simple questions such as "Does your teddy bear have a name?"

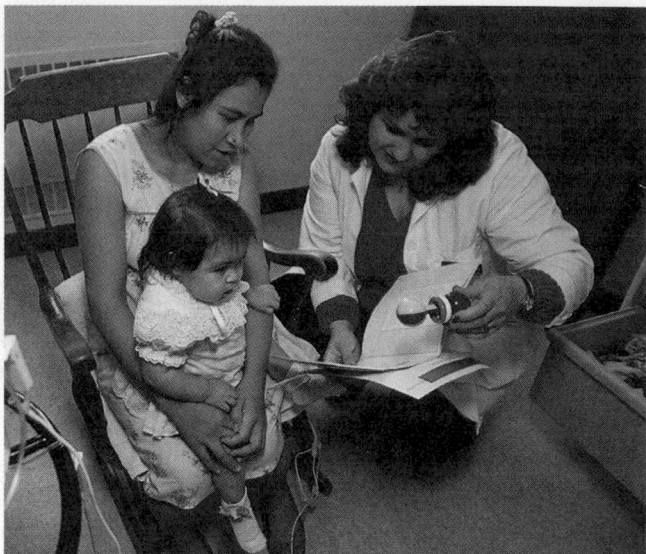
Fig. 6-2 Nurse assumes position at child's level.

📋 **NURSING CARE GUIDELINES**

Communicating with Children

- Allow children time to feel comfortable.
- Avoid sudden or rapid advances, broad smiles, extended eye contact, or other gestures that may be seen as threatening.
- Talk to the parent if child is initially shy.
- Communicate through transition objects such as dolls, puppets, and stuffed animals before questioning a young child directly.
- Give older children the opportunity to talk without the parents present.
- Assume a position that is at eye level with child (Fig. 6-2).
- Speak in a quiet, unhurried, and confident voice.
- Speak clearly, be specific, and use simple words and short sentences.
- State directions and suggestions positively.
- Offer a choice only when one exists.
- Be honest with children.
- Allow them to express their concerns and fears.
- Use a variety of communication techniques.

---

to ease the child into conversation. Other guidelines for communicating with children are in the Nursing Care Guidelines box. Specific guidelines for preparing children for procedures, a common nursing function, are in Chapter 27.

Communication Related to Development of Thought Processes

The normal development of language and thought offers a frame of reference for communicating with children. Thought processes progress from sensorimotor to perceptual to concrete and finally to abstract, formal operations. An understanding of the typical characteristics of these stages provides the nurse with a framework to facilitate social communication (Box 6-3).

Infancy

Because they are unable to use words, infants primarily use and understand nonverbal communication. Infants communicate their needs and feelings through nonverbal behaviors and vocalizations that can be interpreted by someone who is around them for a sufficient time. Infants smile and coo when content and cry when distressed. Crying is provoked by unpleasant

| BOX 6-3 | CHARACTERISTICS OF COMMUNICATIVE DEVELOPMENT IN YOUNG CHILDREN |

Perlocutionary Stage (0 to 8-9 Months)
Child is reflexive to stimuli.
Child shows increasing purpose in action.

Emerging Illocutionary Stage (8-9 to 12-15 Months)
Child communicates intentionally with signals and gestures.

Conventional Illocutionary–Emerging Locutionary Stage (12-15 to 18-24 Months)
Child communicates intentionally with gestures, vocalizations, and verbalizations.

Modified from Hoge DR, Parette HP: Facilitating communicative development in young children with disabilities, *Transdisc J* 5(2):113-130, 1995.

stimuli from inside or outside, such as hunger, pain, body restraint, or loneliness. Adults interpret this to mean that an infant needs something and consequently try to alleviate the discomfort and reduce tension. Crying (or the desire to cry) persists as a part of everyone's communication repertoire.

Infants respond to adults' nonverbal behaviors. They become quiet when they are cuddled, patted, or receive other forms of gentle physical contact. They receive comfort from the sound of a voice, even though they do not understand the words that are spoken. Until infants reach the age at which they experience stranger anxiety, they readily respond to any firm, gentle handling and quiet, calm speech. Loud, harsh sounds and sudden movements are frightening.

Older infants' attention is centered on themselves and their parents; therefore any stranger is a potential threat until proved otherwise. Holding out the hands and asking the child to "come" is seldom successful, especially if the infant is with the parent. If infants must be handled, simply pick them up firmly without gestures. Observe the position in which the parent holds the infant. Most infants learn to prefer a particular position and manner of handling. In general, infants are more at ease upright than horizontal. Also, hold infants so they can see their parents. Until they develop the understanding that an object (in this case the parent) removed from sight can still be present, they have no way of knowing the object is still there.

Early Childhood

Children younger than 5 years of age are egocentric. They see things only in relation to themselves and from their point of view. Therefore focus communication on them. Tell them what they can do or how they will feel. Experiences of others are of no interest to them. It is futile to use another child's experience in an attempt to gain the cooperation of small children. Allow them to touch and examine articles they will come in contact with. A stethoscope bell will feel cold; palpating a neck might tickle. Although they have not yet acquired sufficient language skills to express their feelings and wants, toddlers can effectively use their hands to communicate ideas without words. They push an unwanted object away, pull another person to show them something, point, and cover the mouth that is saying something they do not wish to hear.

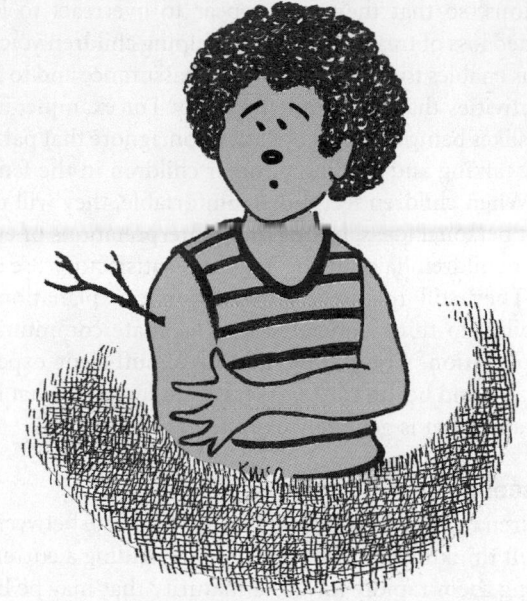

Fig. 6-3 A young child may take the expression "a little stick in the arm" literally.

Everything is direct and concrete to small children. They are unable to work with abstractions and interpret words literally. Analogies escape them because they are unable to separate fact from fantasy. For example, they attach literal meaning to such common phrases as "two-faced," "sticky fingers," or "coughing your head off." Children who are told they will get "a little stick in the arm" may not be able to envision an injection (Fig. 6-3). Therefore avoid using a phrase that might be misinterpreted by a small child (see Nursing Care Guidelines box, Chapter 27, p. 1004).

Young children assign human attributes to inanimate objects. Consequently they fear that objects may jump, bite, cut, or pinch all by themselves. Children do not know that these devices are unable to perform without human direction. To minimize their fear, keep unfamiliar equipment out of view until it is necessary.

School-Age Years

Younger school-age children rely less on what they see and more on what they know when faced with new problems. They want explanations and reasons for everything but require no verification beyond that. They are interested in the functional aspect of all procedures, objects, and activities. They want to know why an object exists, why it is used, how it works, and the intent and purpose of its user. They need to know what is going to take place and why it is being done to them specifically. For example, to explain a procedure such as taking blood pressure, show the child how squeezing the bulb pushes air into the cuff and makes the "silver" in the tube go up. Let the child operate the bulb. An explanation for the procedure might be as simple as, "I want to see how far the silver goes up when the cuff squeezes your arm." Consequently, the child becomes an enthusiastic participant.

School-age children have a heightened concern about body integrity. Because of the special importance they place on their body, they are sensitive to anything that constitutes a threat or suggestion of injury to it. This concern extends to their possessions, so that they may appear to overreact to loss or threatened loss of treasured objects. Helping children voice their concerns enables the nurse to provide reassurance and to implement activities that reduce their anxiety. For example, if a shy child dislikes being the center of attention, ignore that particular child by talking and relating to other children in the family or group. When children feel more comfortable, they will usually interject personal ideas, feelings, and interpretations of events.

Older children have an adequate and satisfactory use of language. They still require relatively simple explanations, but their ability to think concretely can facilitate communication and explanation. Commonly, they have sufficient experience with health and health care workers to understand what is happening and what is generally expected of them.

Adolescence

As children move into adolescence, they fluctuate between child and adult thinking and behavior. They are riding a current that is moving them rapidly toward a maturity that may be beyond their coping ability. Therefore, when tensions rise, they may seek the security of the more familiar and comfortable expectations of childhood. Anticipating these shifts in identity allows the nurse to adjust the course of interaction to meet the needs of the moment. No single approach can be relied on consistently, and encountering cooperation, hostility, anger, bravado, and a variety of other behaviors and attitudes is common. It is as much a mistake to regard the adolescent as an adult with an adult's wisdom and control as it is to assume that the teenager has the concerns and expectations of a child.

Frequently adolescents are more willing to discuss their concerns with an adult outside the family, and they often welcome the opportunity to interact with a nurse outside the presence of their parents. They accept anyone who displays a genuine interest in them. However, adolescents are quick to reject persons who attempt to impose their values on them, whose interest is feigned, or who appear to have little respect for who they are and what they think or say.

Interviewing the adolescent presents some special issues. The first may be whether to talk with the adolescent alone or with the adolescent and parents together. Of course, if the parent is not there, the only question is whether to suggest to the teenager that the parents be interviewed at another time. If the parents and teenager are together, talking with the adolescent first has the advantage of immediately identifying with the young person, thus fostering the interpersonal relationship. However, talking with the parents initially may provide insight into the family relationship. In either case, give both parties an opportunity to be included in the interview. If time is limited, such as during history taking, clarify this at the onset to avoid appearing to "take sides" by talking more with one person than with the other.

Confidentiality is of great importance when interviewing adolescents. Explain to parents and teenagers the limits of confidentiality, specifically that young persons' disclosures will not be shared unless they indicate a need for intervention, as in the case of suicidal behavior.

Another dilemma in interviewing adolescents is that two views of a problem frequently exist—the teenager's and the parents'. Clarification of the problem is a major task. However, providing both parties an opportunity to discuss their perceptions in an open and unbiased atmosphere can, by itself, be therapeutic. Demonstrating positive communication skills can help families communicate more effectively (see Nursing Care Guidelines box).

 NURSING CARE GUIDELINES
Communicating with Adolescents

Build a Foundation
Spend time together.
Encourage expression of ideas and feelings.
Respect their views.
Tolerate differences.
Praise good points.
Respect their privacy.
Set a good example.

Communicate Effectively
Give undivided attention.
Listen, listen, listen.
Be courteous, calm, and open minded.
Try not to overreact. If you do, take a break.
Avoid judging or criticizing.
Avoid the "third degree" of continuous questioning.
Choose important issues when taking a stand.
After taking a stand:
• Think through all options.
• Make expectations clear.

COMMUNICATION TECHNIQUES

In addition to such conventional interviewing methods as reflection and open-ended questions, a number of techniques encourage family members to express their thoughts and feelings in a less directive and confrontational manner. Several approaches are projective—they present nonspecific material that enables individuals to externalize or project inner aspects of themselves to others.

Nurses use a variety of verbal techniques to encourage communication. Some of these techniques are useful to pose questions or explore concerns in a less threatening manner. Others can be presented as word games, which are often well received by children. However, for many children and adults, talking about feelings is difficult, and verbal communication may be more stressful than supportive. In such instances, use several nonverbal techniques to encourage communication.

Box 6-4 describes both verbal and nonverbal techniques. Because of the importance of play in communicating with children, play is discussed more extensively below. Any of the verbal or nonverbal techniques can give rise to strong feelings that surface unexpectedly. Be prepared to handle them or to recognize when issues go beyond your ability to deal with them. At that point, consider an appropriate referral.

Play

Play is a universal language of children. It is one of the most important forms of communication and can be an effective technique in relating to them. The nurse can often pick up on clues about physical, intellectual, and social developmental progress from the form and complexity of a child's play

BOX 6-4   CREATIVE COMMUNICATION TECHNIQUES WITH CHILDREN

Verbal Techniques
"I" Messages
Relate a feeling about a behavior in terms of "I."
Describe effect behavior had on the person.
Avoid use of "you."
"You" messages are judgmental and provoke defensiveness.
Example—"You" message: "You are being uncooperative about doing your treatments."
Example—"I" message: "I am concerned about how the treatments are going because I want to see you get better."

Third-Person Technique
Express a feeling in terms of a third person ("he," "she," "they"). This is less threatening than directly asking children how they feel because it gives them an opportunity to agree or disagree without being defensive.
Example—"Sometimes when a person is sick a lot, he feels angry and sad because he cannot do what others can." Either wait silently for a response or encourage a reply with a statement such as "Did you ever feel that way?"
This approach allows children three choices: (1) to agree and, one hopes, express how they feel; (2) to disagree; or (3) to remain silent, which means they probably have such feelings but are unable to express them at this time.

Facilitative Response
Listen carefully and reflect back to patients the feelings and content of their statements.
Responses are empathic and nonjudgmental and legitimize the person's feelings.
Formula for facilitative responses: "You feel _____ because _____."
Example—If child states, "I hate coming to the hospital and getting needles," a facilitative response is, "You feel unhappy because of all the things that are done to you."

Storytelling
Use the language of children to probe into areas of their thinking while bypassing conscious inhibitions or fears.
The simplest technique is asking children to relate a story about an event, such as "being in the hospital."
Other approaches:
- Show children a picture of a particular event, such as a child in a hospital with other people in the room, and ask them to describe the scene.
- Cut out comic strips, remove words, and have child add statements for scenes.

Mutual Storytelling
Reveal child's thinking and attempt to change child's perceptions or fears by retelling a somewhat different story (more therapeutic approach than storytelling).
Begin by asking child to tell a story about something, then tell another story that is similar to child's tale but with differences that help child in problem areas.
Example—Child's story is about going to the hospital and never seeing his or her parents again. Nurse's story is also about a child (using different names but similar circumstances) in a hospital whose parents visit every day, but in the evening after work, until the child is better and goes home with them.

Bibliotherapy
Use books in a therapeutic and supportive process.
Provide children with an opportunity to explore an event that is similar to their own but sufficiently different to allow them to distance themselves from it and remain in control.
General guidelines for using bibliotherapy are:
1. Assess child's emotional and cognitive development in terms of readiness to understand the book's message.
2. Be familiar with the book's content (intended message or purpose) and the age for which it is written.

3. Read the book to the child if child is unable to read.
4. Explore the meaning of the book with the child by having child:
   - Retell the story
   - Read a special section with the nurse or parent
   - Draw a picture related to the story and discuss the drawing
   - Talk about the characters
   - Summarize the moral or meaning of the story

Dreams
Dreams often reveal unconscious and repressed thoughts and feelings.
Ask child to talk about a dream or nightmare.
Explore with child what meaning the dream could have.

"What If" Questions
Encourage child to explore potential situations and to consider different problem-solving options.
Example—"What if you got sick and had to go the hospital?" Children's responses reveal what they know already and what they are curious about, providing an opportunity for them to learn coping skills, especially in potentially dangerous situations.

Three Wishes
Ask, "If you could have any three things in the world, what would they be?"
If child answers, "That all my wishes come true," ask child for specific wishes.

Rating Game
Use some type of rating scale (numbers, sad to happy faces) to have child rate an event or feeling.
Example—Instead of asking youngsters how they feel, ask how their day has been "on a scale of 1 to 10, with 10 being the best."

Word Association Game
State key words and ask children to say the first word they think of when they hear the word.
Start with neutral words and then introduce more anxiety-producing words, such as "illness," "needles," "hospitals," and "operation."
Select key words that relate to some relevant event in the child's life.

Sentence Completion
Present a partial statement and have the child complete it. Some sample statements are:
- The thing I like best (least) about school is _____.
- The best (worst) age to be is _____.
- The most (least) fun thing I ever did was _____.
- The thing I like most (least) about my parents is _____.
- The one thing I would change about my family is _____.
- If I could be anything I wanted, I would be _____.
- The thing I like most (least) about myself is _____.

Pros and Cons
Select a topic, such as "being in the hospital," and have child list "five good things and five bad things" about it.
This is an exceptionally valuable technique when applied to relationships, such as things family members like and dislike about each other.

Nonverbal Techniques
Writing
Writing is an alternative communication approach for older children and adults.
Specific suggestions include:
- Keep a journal or diary.
- Write down feelings or thoughts that are difficult to express.
- Write "letters" that are never mailed (a variation is making up a "pen pal" to write to).
Keep an account of child's progress from both a physical and an emotional viewpoint.

Drawing
Drawing is one of the most valuable forms of communication—both nonverbal (from looking at the drawing) and verbal (from child's story of the picture).

Continued

BOX 6-4   CREATIVE COMMUNICATION TECHNIQUES WITH CHILDREN—cont'd

Nonverbal Techniques—cont'd
Drawing—cont'd
Children's drawings tell a great deal about them because they are projections of their inner selves.
Spontaneous drawing involves giving child a variety of art supplies and providing the opportunity to draw.
Directed drawing involves a more specific direction, such as "draw a person" or the "three themes" approach (state three things about child and ask child to choose one and draw a picture).

Guidelines for Evaluating Drawings
Use spontaneous drawings and evaluate more than one drawing whenever possible.
Interpret drawings in light of other available information about child and family, including the child's age and stage of development.
Interpret drawings as a whole rather than focusing on specific details of the drawing.
Consider individual elements of the drawing that may be significant:
- Sex of figure drawn first—Usually relates to child's perception of own sex role
- Size of individual figures—Expresses importance, power, or authority.
- Order in which figures are drawn—Expresses priority in terms of importance
- Child's position in relation to other family members—Expresses feelings of status or alliance
- Exclusion of a member—May denote feeling of not belonging or desire to eliminate

- Accentuated parts—Usually express concern for areas of special importance (e.g., large hands may be a sign of aggression)
- Absence of or rudimentary arms and hands—Suggest timidity, passivity, or intellectual immaturity; tiny, unstable feet may express insecurity, and hidden hands may mean guilt feelings
- Placement of drawing on the page and type of stroke—Free use of paper and firm, continuous strokes express security, whereas drawings restricted to a small area and lightly drawn in broken or wavering lines may be a sign of insecurity
- Erasures, shading, or cross-hatching—Expresses ambivalence, concern, or anxiety with a particular area

Magic
Use simple magic tricks to help establish rapport with child, encourage compliance with health interventions, and provide effective distraction during painful procedures.
Although the "magician" talks, no verbal response from child is required.

Play
Play is the universal language and "work" of children.
It tells a great deal about children because they project their inner selves through the activity.
Spontaneous play involves giving child a variety of play materials and providing the opportunity to play.
Directed play involves a more specific direction, such as providing medical equipment or a dollhouse for focused reasons, such as exploring child's fear of injections or exploring family relationships.

---

behaviors. Play requires minimum equipment or none at all. Many providers use therapeutic play to reduce the trauma of illness and hospitalization (see Chapter 27) and to prepare children for therapeutic procedures (see Chapter 27).

Because their ability to perceive precedes their ability to transmit, infants respond to activities that register on their physical senses. Patting, stroking, and other skin play conveys messages. Repetitive actions, such as stretching infants' arms out to the side while they are lying on their back and then folding the arms across the chest or raising and revolving the legs in a bicycling motion, will elicit pleasurable sounds. Colorful items to catch the eye or interesting sounds, such as a ticking clock, chimes, bells, or singing, can be used to attract children's attention.

Older infants respond to simple games. The old game of peek-a-boo is an excellent means of initiating communication with infants while maintaining a "safe," nonthreatening distance. After this intermittent eye contact, the nurse is no longer viewed as a stranger but as a friend. This can be followed by touch games. Clapping an infant's hands together for pat-a-cake or wiggling the toes for "this little piggy" delights an infant or small child. Talking to a foot or other part of the child's body is another effective tactic. Much of the nursing assessment can be carried out with the use of games and simple play equipment while the infant remains in the safety of the parent's arms or lap.

The nurse can capitalize on the natural curiosity of small children by playing games such as "Which hand do you take?" and "Guess what I have in my hand" or by manipulating items such as a flashlight or stethoscope. Finger games are useful. More elaborate materials, such as puppets and replicas of familiar or unfamiliar items, serve as excellent means of communi-

cating with small children. The variety and extent are limited only by the nurse's imagination.

Through play, children reveal their perceptions of interpersonal relationships with their family, friends, or hospital personnel. Children may also reveal the wide scope of knowledge they have acquired from listening to others around them. For example, through needle play, children may reveal how carefully they have watched each procedure by precisely duplicating the technical skills. They may also reveal how well they remember those who performed procedures. In one example, a child painstakingly reenacted every detail of a tedious medical procedure, including the role of the physician who had repeatedly shouted at her to be still for the long ordeal. Her anger at him was most evident during the play session and revealed the cause for her abrupt withdrawal and passive hostility toward the medical and nursing staff after the test.

Play sessions serve not only as assessment tools for determining children's awareness and perception of their illness, but also as methods of intervention and evaluation. In the previous example, when the child revealed anger toward the physician, the nurse acted the part of the patient but this time did not accept the physician's harsh commands to stay still. Instead, the nurse said to the physician all the things the child had wished she could say.

HISTORY TAKING

PERFORMING A HEALTH HISTORY

The format used for history taking may be (1) **direct**, where the nurse asks for information via direct interview with the informant; or (2) **indirect**, where the informant supplies the information by completing some type of questionnaire. The direct method is superior to the indirect approach or a combination of both. However, because time is limited, the direct approach is not always practical. If the nurse cannot use the direct approach, he or she should review parents' written responses and question them regarding any unusual answers. The categories listed in Box 6-5 encompass children's current and past health status and information about their psychosocial environment.

Identifying Information

Much of the identifying information may already be available from other recorded sources. However, if the parent and youngster seem anxious, use this opportunity to ask about such information to help them feel more comfortable.

Informant

One of the important elements of identifying information is the **informant**, the person(s) who furnishes the information. Record (1) who the person is (child, parent, or other), (2) an impression of reliability and willingness to communicate, and (3) any special circumstances such as the use of an interpreter or conflicting answers by more than one person.

Chief Complaint

The **chief complaint** is the specific reason for the child's visit to the clinic, office, or hospital. It may be the theme, with the present illness viewed as the description of the problem. Elicit the chief complaint by asking open-ended, neutral questions such as "What seems to be the matter?" "How may I help you?" or "Why did you come here today?" Avoid labeling-type questions such as "How are you sick?" or "What is the problem?" It is possible that the reason for the visit is not an illness or problem.

Occasionally, it is difficult to isolate one symptom or problem as the chief complaint because the parent may identify many. In this situation be as specific as possible when asking questions. For example, asking informants to state which *one* problem or symptom prompted them to seek help now may help them focus on the most immediate concern.

Present Illness

The history of the present illness* is a narrative of the chief complaint from its earliest onset through its progression to the present. Its four major components are (1) the details of **onset**, (2) a complete **interval** history, (3) the **present** status, and (4) the reason for seeking help **now**. The focus of the present illness is on all factors relevant to the main problem, even if they have disappeared or changed during the onset, interval, and present.

Analyzing a Symptom

Because pain is often the most characteristic symptom denoting the onset of a physical problem, it is used as an example for analysis of a symptom. Assessment includes (1) type, (2)

---

*The term *illness* is used in its broadest sense to denote any problem of a physical, emotional, or psychosocial nature. It is actually a history of the chief complaint.

| BOX 6-5 | OUTLINE OF A PEDIATRIC HEALTH HISTORY |

Identifying information

1. Name	6. Sex
2. Address	7. Religion
3. Telephone	8. Date of interview
4. Birth date and place	9. Informant
5. Race or ethnic group	

Chief complaint (CC)—To establish the major specific reason for the child's and parents' seeking professional health attention

Present illness (PI)—To obtain all details related to the chief complaint

Past history (PH)—To elicit a profile of the child's previous illnesses, injuries, or operations

1. Birth history (pregnancy, labor and delivery, perinatal history)	4. Current medications
2. Previous illnesses, injuries, or operations	5. Immunizations
3. Allergies	6. Growth and development
	7. Habits

Review of systems (ROS)—To elicit information concerning any potential health problem

1. General	10. Chest
2. Integument	11. Respiratory
3. Head	12. Cardiovascular
4. Eyes	13. Gastrointestinal
5. Ears	14. Genitourinary
6. Nose	15. Gynecologic
7. Mouth	16. Musculoskeletal
8. Throat	17. Neurologic
9. Neck	18. Endocrine

Family medical history—To identify genetic traits or diseases that have familial tendencies and to assess exposure to a communicable disease in a family member and family habits that may affect the child's health, such as smoking and chemical use

Psychosocial history—To elicit information about the child's self-concept

Sexual history—To elicit information concerning the child's sexual concerns or activities and any pertinent data regarding adults' sexual activity that influences the child

Family history—To develop an understanding of the child as an individual and as a member of a family and a community
1. Family composition
2. Home and community environment
3. Occupation and education of family members
4. Cultural and religious traditions
5. Family function and relationships

Nutritional assessment—To elicit information on the adequacy of the child's nutritional intake and needs
1. Dietary intake
2. Clinical examination

location, (3) severity, (4) duration, and (5) influencing factors (see Nursing Care Guidelines box; see also Pain Assessment, Chapter 7).

History

The history contains information relating to all previous aspects of the child's health status and concentrates on several areas that are ordinarily passed over in the history of an adult, such as birth history, detailed feeding history, immunizations, and growth and development. Since this section includes a great deal of information, use a combination of open-ended and fact-finding questions. For example, begin interviewing for each section with an open-ended statement such as "Tell me about your child's birth" to provide the informants the opportunity

NURSING CARE GUIDELINES
Analyzing the Symptom: Pain

Type
Be as specific as possible. With young children, asking the parents how they know the child is in pain may help describe its type, location, and severity. For example, a parent may state, "My child must have a severe earache because she pulls at her ears, rolls her head on the floor, and screams. Nothing seems to help." Help older children describe the "hurt" by asking them if it is sharp, throbbing, dull, or stabbing. Record whatever words they use in quotes.

Location
Be specific. "Stomach pains" is too general a description. Children can better localize the pain if they are asked to "point with one finger to where it hurts" or to "point to where Mommy or Daddy would put a Band-Aid." Determine if the pain radiates by asking, "Does the pain stay there or move? Show me with your finger where the pain goes."

Severity
Severity is best determined by finding out how it affects the child's usual behavior. Pain that prevents a child from playing, interacting with others, sleeping, and eating is most often severe. Assess pain intensity using a rating scale, such as a numeric or FACES scale (see Chapter 7).

Duration
Include the duration, onset, and frequency. Describe this in terms of activity and behavior, such as "pain reported to last all night, child refused to sleep and cried intermittently."

Influencing Factors
Include anything that causes a change in the type, location, severity, or duration of the pain: (1) precipitating events (those that cause or increase the pain), (2) relieving events (those that lessen the pain, such as medications), (3) temporal events (times when the pain is relieved or increased), (4) positional events (standing, sitting, lying down), and (5) associated events (meals, stress, coughing).

to relate what they think is most important. Ask fact-finding questions related to specific details whenever necessary to focus the interview on certain topics.

Birth History

The **birth history** includes all data concerning (1) the mother's health during pregnancy, (2) the labor and delivery, and (3) the infant's condition immediately after birth. Since prenatal influences have significant effects on a child's physical and emotional development, a thorough investigation of the birth history is essential. Because parents may question what relevance pregnancy and birth have on the child's present condition, particularly if the child is past infancy, explain why such questions are included. An appropriate statement may be, "I will be asking you some questions about your pregnancy and _____'s [refer to child by name] birth. Your answers will give me a more complete picture of his [or her] overall health."

Because emotional factors also affect the outcome of pregnancy and the subsequent parent-child relationship, investigate (1) concurrent crises during pregnancy and (2) prenatal attitudes toward the fetus. It is best to approach the topic of parental acceptance of pregnancy through indirect questioning. Asking parents if the pregnancy was planned is a leading statement because they may respond affirmatively for fear of criticism if the pregnancy was unexpected. Rather, encourage

parents to state their true reactions by referring to specific facts relating to the pregnancy, such as the spacing between offspring, an extended or short interval between marriage and conception, or a pregnancy during adolescence. The parent can choose to explore such statements with further explanations or, for the moment, may not be able to reveal such feelings. If the parent remains silent, return to this topic later in the interview.

Dietary History

Because parental concerns are common and nursing interventions are important in ensuring optimum nutrition, the dietary history is discussed in detail later in this chapter under Nutritional Assessment.

Previous Illnesses, Injuries, and Operations

When inquiring about past illnesses, begin with a general statement such as "What other illnesses has your child had?" Since parents are most likely to recall serious health problems, ask specifically about colds; earaches; and childhood diseases such as measles, rubella (German measles), chickenpox, mumps, pertussis (whooping cough), diphtheria, tuberculosis, scarlet fever, strep throat, recurrent ear infections, gastroesophageal reflux, tonsillitis, or allergic manifestations.

In addition to illnesses, ask about injuries that required medical intervention, operations, and any other reason for hospitalization, including the dates of each incident. Focus on injuries such as accidental falls, poisoning, choking, or burns, since these may be potential areas for parental guidance.

Allergies

Ask about commonly known allergic disorders such as hay fever and asthma; unusual reactions to drugs, food, or latex products; and reactions to other contact agents such as poisonous plants, animals, household products, or fabrics. If asked appropriate questions, most people can give reliable information about drug reactions (see Nursing Care Guidelines box).

NURSING CARE GUIDELINES
Taking an Allergy History

- Has your child ever taken any drugs or tablets that have disagreed with him or her or caused an allergic reaction? If yes, can you remember the name(s) of these drugs?
- Can you describe the reaction?
- Was the drug taken by mouth (as a tablet or syrup), or was it an injection?
- How soon after starting the drug did the reaction happen?
- How long ago did this happen?
- Did anyone tell you it was an allergic reaction, or did you decide for yourself?
- Has your child ever taken this drug, or a similar one, again? If yes, did your child experience the same problems?
- Have you told the doctors or nurses about your child's reaction or allergy?

! NURSING ALERT

Information about allergic reactions to drugs or other products is essential. Failure to document a serious reaction places the child at risk if the agent is given.

Current Medications

Inquire about current drug regimens, including vitamins, antipyretics (especially aspirin), antibiotics, antihistamines, decongestants, or herbs and homeopathic medications. List all medications, including name, dose, schedule, duration, and reason for administration. Often parents are unaware of the drug's actual name. Whenever possible, ask parents to bring the containers with them to the next visit, or ask for the name of the pharmacy and call for a list of all the child's recent prescription medications. However, this list will not include over-the-counter medications, which are important to know.

Immunizations

A record of all immunizations is essential. Since many parents are unaware of the exact name and date of each immunization, the most reliable source of information is a hospital, clinic, or private practitioner's record. All immunizations and "boosters" are listed, stating (1) the name of the specific disease, (2) the number of injections, (3) the dosage (sometimes lesser amounts are given if a reaction is anticipated), (4) the ages when administered, and (5) the occurrence of any reaction following the immunization.

! NURSING ALERT

Inquire about previous administration of any horse or other foreign serum. Inquire about recent administration of immune gamma globulin or blood transfusion because these necessitate a delay in giving live vaccines. And ask about anaphylactic reactions to neomycin, eggs, or any other component of a vaccine.

Growth and Development

The most important previous growth patterns to record are:
- Approximate weight at 6 months, 1 year, 2 years, and 5 years of age
- Approximate length at ages 1 and 4 years
- Dentition, including age of onset, number of teeth, and symptoms during teething

Developmental milestones include:
- Age of holding up head steadily
- Age of sitting alone without support
- Age of walking without assistance
- Age of saying first words with meaning
- Present grade in school
- Scholastic performance
- If the child has a best friend
- Interactions with other children, peers, and adults

Use specific and detailed questions when inquiring about each developmental milestone. For example, "sitting up" can mean many different activities, such as sitting propped up, sitting in someone's lap, sitting with support, sitting up alone but in a hyperflexed position for assisted balance, or sitting up unsupported with the back slightly rounded. A clue to misunderstanding of the requested activity may be an unusually early age of achievement.

Habits

Habits are an important area to explore (Box 6-6). Parents frequently express concerns during this part of the history.

BOX 6-6   HABITS TO EXPLORE DURING A HEALTH INTERVIEW

- Behavior patterns such as nail biting, thumb sucking, pica (habitual ingestion of nonfood substances), rituals ("security" blanket or toy), and unusual movements (head banging, rocking, overt masturbation, walking on toes)
- Activities of daily living, such as hour of sleep and arising, duration of nighttime sleep and naps, type and duration of exercise, regularity of stools and urination, age of toilet training, and daytime or nighttime bed-wetting
- Unusual disposition; response to frustration
- Use or abuse of alcohol, drugs, coffee, or tobacco

Encourage their input by saying, "Please tell me any concerns you have about your child's habits, activities, or development." Investigate further any concerns that parents express.

One of the most common concerns relates to sleep. Many children develop a normal sleep pattern, and all that is required during the assessment is a general overview of nighttime sleep and nap schedules. However, a number of children develop sleep problems (see Sleep Problems, Chapters 10 and 13). When sleep problems occur, the nurse needs a more detailed sleep history to guide appropriate interventions.*

Habits related to use of chemicals apply primarily to older children and adolescents. If a youngster admits to smoking, drinking, or using drugs, ask about the quantity and frequency. Questions such as "Many kids your age are experimenting with drugs and alcohol; have you ever had any drugs or alcohol?" may give more reliable data than questions such as "How much do you drink?" or "How often do you drink or take drugs?" Clarify that "drinking" includes all types of alcohol, including beer and wine. When quantities such as a "glass" of wine or a "can" of beer are given, ask about the size of the container.

If older children deny use of chemical substances, inquire about past experimentation. Asking, "You mean you never tried to smoke or drink?" implies that the nurse expects some such activity, and the youngster may be more inclined to answer truthfully. Be aware of the confidential nature of such questioning, the adverse effect that the parents' presence may have on the adolescent's willingness to answer, and the fact that self-reporting may not be an accurate account of chemical abuse.

Sexual History

The sexual history is an essential component of adolescents' health assessment. The history uncovers areas of concern related to sexual activity; alerts the nurse to circumstances that may indicate screening for sexually transmitted infections or testing for pregnancy; and provides information related to the need for sexual counseling, such as safer sex practices. Box 6-7 gives guidelines for anticipatory guidance topics for parents and adolescents.

One approach to initiating a conversation about sexual concerns is to begin with a history of peer interactions. Open-ended

---

*A sleep history and a sleep chart for the family to record the child's daily sleep and wake activities is available in Wilson D, Hockenberry M: *Wong's clinical manual of pediatric nursing*, ed 7, St Louis, 2008, Mosby.

BOX 6-7   ANTICIPATORY GUIDANCE— SEXUALITY

Ages 12 to 14 Years

Have adolescent identify supportive adult to discuss sexuality issues and concerns with.

Discuss advantages of delaying sexual activity.

Discuss making responsible decisions regarding normal sexual feelings.

Discuss role of gender, peer pressure, and the media in sexual decision making.

Discuss contraceptive options (advantages and disadvantages).

Provide education regarding sexually transmitted infections (STIs), including human immunodeficiency virus (HIV) infection; clarify risks and discuss condoms.

Discuss abuse prevention: avoiding dangerous situations, role of drugs and alcohol, and use of self-defense.

Have adolescent clarify values, needs, and ability to be assertive.

If adolescent is sexually active, discuss limiting partners, use of condoms, and contraceptive options.

Have confidential interview with adolescent (including a sexual history).

Discuss the evolution of sexual identity and expression.

Discuss breast examination or testicular examination.

Ages 15 to 18 Years

Support delaying sexual activity.

Discuss alternatives to intercourse.

Discuss "When are you ready for sex?"

Clarify values; encourage responsible decision making.

Discuss consequences of unprotected sex: early pregnancy, STIs, including HIV infection.

Discuss negotiating with partner and barriers to safer sex.

If adolescent is sexually active, discuss limiting partners, use of condoms, and contraceptive options.

Emphasize that sex should be safe and pleasurable for both partners.

Have confidential interview with adolescent.

Discuss concerns about sexual expression and identity.

Data from Wright K: Anticipatory guidance: developing a healthy sexuality, *Pediatr Ann* 26(2 Suppl):S142-S144, C3, 1997; and Fonseca H, Greydanus D: Sexuality in the child, teen and young adult: concepts for the clinician, *Prim Care Clin Office Pract* 34:275-292, 2007.

statements such as "Tell me about your social life" or "Who are your closest friends?" generally lead into a discussion of dating and sexual issues. To probe further, include questions about the adolescent's attitudes on such topics as sex education, "going steady," "living together," and premarital sex. Phrase questions to reflect concern rather than judgment or criticism of sexual practices.

In any conversation regarding sexual history, be aware of the language that is used in either eliciting or conveying sexual information. For example, avoid asking whether the adolescent is "sexually active," since this term is broadly defined. "Are you having sex with anyone?" is probably the most direct and best understood question. Since same-sex experimentation may occur, refer to all sexual contacts in nongender terms, such as "anyone" or "partners," rather than "girlfriends" or "boyfriends."

A detailed account of sexual partners is necessary if the patient has a history of, displays any symptoms of, or asks for treatment of a sexually transmitted infection. A difficult but necessary part of the interview is to determine the sites of possible infection. Since sexual diseases can be contracted in any

of the body orifices, inform the adolescent that a sexually transmitted infection can be acquired without visible signs of disease at nongenital sites.

Family Medical History

The family medical history is used primarily to discover any hereditary or familial diseases in the parents and child. In general, it is confined to **first-degree relatives** (parents, siblings, grandparents, and immediate aunts and uncles). Information for each family member includes age; marital status; state of health if living; cause of death if deceased; and any evidence of conditions such as early heart disease, sudden death from unknown cause, hypercholesterolemia, hypertension, cancer, diabetes mellitus, obesity, congenital anomalies, allergies, asthma, seizures, tuberculosis, sickle cell disease, cognitive impairment, hearing or visual deficits, psychiatric disorders such as depression or psychosis, and emotional problems. Confirm the accuracy of the reported disorders by inquiring about the symptoms, course, treatment, and sequelae of each diagnosis.

Geographic Location

One of the important areas to explore when assessing the family health history is geographic location, including the birthplace and travel to different areas in or outside of the country, for identification of possible exposure to endemic diseases. Although the primary interest is the child's temporary residence in various localities, also inquire about close family members' travel, especially during tours of military service or business trips. Children are especially susceptible to parasitic infestation in areas of poor sanitary conditions and to vector-borne diseases, such as those from mosquitoes or ticks in warm and humid or heavily wooded regions.

Family Structure

Assessment of the family, both its structure and function, is an important component of the history-taking process. Because the quality of the functional relationship between the child and family members is a major factor in emotional and physical health, family assessment is discussed separately and in greater detail apart from the more traditional health history.

Family assessment is the collection of data about the composition of the family and the relationships among its members. In its broadest sense, family refers to all those individuals who are considered by the family member to be significant to the nuclear unit, including relatives, friends, and social groups such as the school and church. Although family assessment is not family therapy, it can and frequently is therapeutic. Involving family members in discussing family characteristics and activities can provide insight into family dynamics and relationships.

Because of the time involved in performing an in-depth family assessment as presented here, be selective in deciding when knowledge of family function may facilitate nursing care (see Nursing Care Guidelines box). During brief contacts with families, a full assessment is not appropriate, and screening with one or two questions from each category may reflect the health of the family system or the need for additional assessment.

NURSING CARE GUIDELINES

Initiating a Comprehensive Family Assessment

Perform a comprehensive assessment on:
- Children receiving comprehensive well-child care
- Children experiencing major stressful life events (e.g., chronic illness, disability, parental divorce, death of a family member)
- Children requiring extensive home care
- Children with developmental delays
- Children with repeated accidental injuries and those with suspected child abuse
- Children with behavioral or physical problems that could be caused by family dysfunction

---

! NURSING ALERT

In assessing family composition, it is sometimes difficult to establish the status of the adult relationships. If the parent fails to mention the other parent, ask, "Where is the child's father [or mother]?" Avoid saying "husband" or "wife" because this assumes that only marital relationships exist.

Family structure refers to the composition of the family—who lives in the home and those social, cultural, religious, and economic characteristics that influence the child's and family's overall psychobiologic health (see also Chapters 2 and 3). Since the information elicited in this part of the history is often the most personal and confidential, include it toward the end of the interview when rapport is well established.

The most common method of eliciting information on the family structure is to interview family members. The principal areas of concern are (1) family composition, (2) home and community environment, (3) occupation and education of family members, and (4) cultural and religious traditions (Box 6-8).

Psychosocial History

The traditional medical history includes a personal and social section that concentrates on children's personal status, such as school adjustment and any unusual habits, and the family and home environment. Since several personal aspects are covered under development and habits, only those issues related to children's ability to cope and their self-concept are presented here.

Through observation, obtain a general idea of how children handle themselves in terms of confidence in dealing with others, answering questions, and coping with new situations. Observe the parent-child relationship for the types of messages sent to children about their coping skills and self-worth. Do the parents treat the child with respect, focusing on strengths, or is the interaction one of constant reprimands, with emphasis on weaknesses and faults? Do the parents help the child learn new coping strategies or support the ones the child uses?

BOX 6-8　　FAMILY ASSESSMENT INTERVIEW

General Guidelines

Schedule the interview with the family at a time that is most convenient for all parties; include as many family members as possible; clearly state the purpose of the interview.

Begin the interview by asking each person's name and their relationship to one another.

Restate the purpose of the interview and the objective.

Keep the initial conversation general to put members at ease and to learn the "big picture" of the family.

Identify major concerns and reflect these back to the family to be certain that all parties receive the same message.

Terminate the interview with a summary of what was discussed and a plan for additional sessions if needed.

Structural Assessment Areas
Family Composition

Immediate members of the household (names, ages, and relationships)

Significant extended family members

Previous marriages, separations, death of spouses, or divorces

Home and Community Environment

Type of dwelling, number of rooms, occupants

Sleeping arrangements

Number of floors, accessibility of stairs and elevators

Adequacy of utilities

Safety features (fire escape, smoke and carbon monoxide detectors, guardrails on windows, use of car restraint)

Environmental hazards (e.g., chipped paint, poor sanitation, pollution, heavy street traffic)

Availability and location of health care facilities, schools, play areas

Relationship with neighbors

Recent crises or changes in home

Child's reaction and adjustment to recent stresses

Occupation and Education of Family Members

Types of employment

Work schedules

Work satisfaction

Exposure to environmental or industrial hazards

Sources of income and adequacy

Effect of illness on financial status

Highest degree or grade level attained

Cultural and Religious Traditions

Religious beliefs and practices

Cultural and ethnic beliefs and practices

Language spoken in home

Assessment questions include:
- Does the family identify with a particular religious or ethnic group? Are both parents from that group?
- How is religious or ethnic background part of family life?
- What special religious or cultural traditions are practiced in the home (e.g., food choices and preparation)?
- Where were family members born, and how long have they lived in this country?
- What language does the family speak most frequently?
- Do they speak and understand English?
- What do they believe causes health or illness?
- What religious or ethnic beliefs influence the family's perception of illness and its treatment?
- What methods are used to prevent or treat illness?
- How does the family know when a health problem needs medical attention?
- Whom does the family contact when a member is ill?
- Does the family rely on cultural or religious healers or remedies? If so, ask them to describe the type of healer or remedy.
- Whom does the family go to for support (clergy, medical healer, relatives)?

Continued

BOX 6-8 FAMILY ASSESSMENT INTERVIEW—cont'd

Structural Assessment Areas—cont'd
Cultural and Religious Traditions—cont'd
- Does the family experience discrimination because of their race, beliefs, or practices? Ask them to describe.

Functional Assessment Areas
Family Interactions and Roles
Interactions refer to ways family members relate to each other. Chief concern is the amount of intimacy and closeness among the members, especially spouses.
Roles refer to behaviors of people as they assume a different status or position.
Observations include:
- Family members' responses to each other (cordial, hostile, cool, loving, patient, short tempered)
- Obvious roles of leadership versus submission
- Support and attention shown to various members
Assessment questions include:
- What activities does the family perform together?
- Whom do family members talk to when something is bothering them?
- What are members' household chores?
- Who usually oversees what is happening with the children, such as at school or health care?
- How easy or difficult is it for the family to change or accept new responsibilities for household tasks?

Power, Decision Making, and Problem Solving
Power refers to individual member's control over others in family; it is manifested through family decision making and problem solving.
Chief concern is clarity of boundaries of power between parents and children.
One method of assessment involves offering a hypothetical conflict or problem, such as a child failing school, and asking family how they would handle this situation.
Assessment questions include:
- Who usually makes the decisions in the family?

- If one parent makes a decision, can the child appeal to the other parent to change it?
- What input do children have in making decisions or discussing rules?
- Who makes and enforces the rules?
- What happens when a rule is broken?

Communication
Communication is concerned with clarity and directness of communication patterns.
Further assessment includes periodically asking family members if they understood what was just said and to repeat the message.
Observations include:
- Who speaks to whom
- If one person speaks for another or interrupts
- If members appear uninterested when certain individuals speak
- If there is agreement between verbal and nonverbal messages
Assessment questions include:
- How often do family members wait until others are through talking before "having their say"?
- Do parents or older siblings tend to lecture and preach?
- Do parents tend to "talk down" to the children?

Expression of Feelings and Individuality
Expressions are concerned with personal space and freedom to grow, with limits and structure needed for guidance.
Observing patterns of communication offers clues to how freely feelings are expressed.
Assessment questions include:
- Is it OK for family members to get angry or sad?
- Who gets angry most of the time? What do they do?
- If someone is upset, how do other family members try to comfort this person?
- Who comforts specific family members?
- When someone wants to do something, such as try out for a new sport or get a job, what is the family's response (offer assistance, discouragement, or no advice)?

Parent-child interactions also convey messages about body image. Do the parents label the child and body parts, such as "bad boy," "skinny legs," or "ugly scar"? Do the parents handle the child gently, using soothing touch to calm an anxious child, or do they treat the child roughly, using slaps or restraint to make the child obey? If the child touches certain parts of the body, such as the genitalia, do the parents make comments that suggest a negative connotation?

With older children many of the communication strategies discussed earlier in the chapter are useful in eliciting more definitive information about their coping and self-concept. Children can write down five things they like and dislike about themselves. The nurse can use sentence completion statements, such as "The thing I like best (or worst) about myself is _____"; "If I could change one thing about myself, it would be _____"; or "When I am scared, I _____."

Review of Systems

The review of systems is a specific review of each body system, following an order similar to that of the physical exami-

nation (see Nursing Care Guidelines box). Often the history of the present illness provides a complete review of the system involved in the chief complaint. Since asking questions about other body systems may appear irrelevant to the parents or child, precede the questioning with an explanation of why the data are necessary (similar to the explanation concerning the relevance of the birth history) and reassure the parents that the child's main problem has not been forgotten.

Begin the review of a specific system with a broad statement such as "How has your child's general health been?" or "Has your child had any problems with his eyes?" If the parent states that the child has had problems with some body function, pursue this with an encouraging statement such as "Tell me more about that." If the parent denies any problems, query for specific symptoms (e.g., "No headaches, bumping into objects, or squinting?"). If the parent reconfirms the absence of such symptoms, record positive statements in the history, such as "Mother denies headaches, bumping into objects, or squinting." In this way, anyone who reviews the health history is aware of exactly what symptoms were investigated.

NURSING CARE GUIDELINES

Review of Systems

General—Overall state of health, fatigue, recent or unexplained weight gain or loss (period of time for either), contributing factors (change of diet, illness, altered appetite), exercise tolerance, fevers (time of day), chills, night sweats (unrelated to climatic conditions), frequent infections, general ability to carry out activities of daily living

Integument—Pruritus, pigment or other color changes, acne, eruptions, rashes (location), tendency for bruising, petechiae, excessive dryness, general texture, disorders or deformities of nails, hair growth or loss, hair color change (for adolescent, use of hair dyes or other potentially toxic substances, such as hair straighteners)

Head—Headaches, dizziness, injury (specific details)

Eyes—Visual problems (behaviors indicative of blurred vision, such as bumping into objects, clumsiness, sitting close to television, holding a book close to face, writing with head near desk, squinting, rubbing the eyes, bending head in an awkward position), cross-eyes (strabismus), eye infections, edema of lids, excessive tearing, use of glasses or contact lenses, date of last optic examination

Ears—Earaches, discharge, evidence of hearing loss (ask about behaviors, such as need to repeat requests, loud speech, inattentive behavior), results of any previous auditory testing

Nose—Nosebleeds (epistaxis), constant or frequent runny or stuffy nose, nasal obstruction (difficulty breathing), alteration or loss of sense of smell

Mouth—Mouth breathing, gum bleeding, toothaches, toothbrushing, use of fluoride, difficulty with teething (symptoms), last visit to dentist (especially if temporary dentition is complete), response to dentist

Throat—Sore throats, difficulty swallowing, choking (especially when chewing food; may be from poor chewing habits), hoarseness or other voice irregularities

Neck—Pain, limitation of movement, stiffness, difficulty holding head straight (torticollis), thyroid enlargement, enlarged nodes or other masses

Chest—Breast enlargement, discharge, masses, enlarged axillary nodes (for adolescent girl, ask about breast self-examination)

Respiratory—Chronic cough, frequent colds (number per year), wheezing, shortness of breath at rest or on exertion, difficulty breathing, sputum production, infections (pneumonia, tuberculosis), date of last chest x-ray examination, skin reaction from tuberculin testing

Cardiovascular—Cyanosis or fatigue on exertion, history of heart murmur or rheumatic fever, anemia, date of last blood count, blood type, recent transfusion

Gastrointestinal (questions in regard to appetite, food tolerance, and elimination habits are asked elsewhere)—Nausea, vomiting (not associated with eating, may be indicative of brain tumor or increased intracranial pressure), jaundice or yellowing skin or sclera, belching, flatulence, recent change in bowel habits (blood in stools, change of color, diarrhea or constipation)

Genitourinary—Pain on urination, frequency, hesitancy, urgency, hematuria, nocturia, polyuria, unpleasant odor to urine, force of stream, discharge, change in size of scrotum, date of last urinalysis (for adolescent, sexually transmitted infection, type of treatment; for male adolescent, ask about testicular self-examination)

Gynecologic—Menarche, date of last menstrual period, regularity or problems with menstruation, vaginal discharge, pruritus, date and result of last Papanicolaou (Pap) smear (include obstetric history, as discussed under birth history, when applicable); if sexually active, type of contraception, sexually transmitted infection and type of treatment

Musculoskeletal—Weakness, clumsiness, lack of coordination, unusual movements, back or joint stiffness, muscle pains or cramps, abnormal gait, deformity, fractures, serious sprains, activity level

Neurologic—Seizures, tremors, dizziness, loss of memory, general affect, fears, nightmares, speech problems, any unusual habits

Endocrine—Intolerance to weather changes, excessive thirst or urination, excessive sweating, salty taste to skin, signs of early puberty

NUTRITIONAL ASSESSMENT

DIETARY INTAKE

Food consumption patterns of children have changed over the past 30 years (Nicklas, Demory-Luce, Yang, et al, 2004). The prevalence of overweight and obesity among children and adolescents has significantly increased (Hedley, Ogden, Johnson, et al, 2004). Knowledge of the child's dietary intake is an essential component of a nutritional assessment. However, it is also one of the most difficult factors to assess. Individuals' recall of food consumption, especially amounts eaten, is frequently unreliable. The food intake history of children and adolescents is prone to reporting error, mostly in the form of underreporting (Livingstone, Robson, and Wallace, 2004). People from different cultures may have difficulty adequately describing the types of food they eat. Despite these obstacles, a dietary evaluation is an important component of the child's assessment.

The **dietary reference intakes (DRIs)** are a set of four nutrient-based reference values that provide quantitative estimates of nutrient intake for use in assessing and planning dietary intake (American Academy of Pediatrics, 2004; Murphy and Poos, 2002). The specific DRIs are:

Estimated average requirement (EAR)—Nutrient intake estimated to meet the requirement of half the healthy individuals (50%) for a specific age and gender group.

Recommended dietary allowance (RDA)—Average daily dietary intake sufficient to meet the nutrient requirement of nearly all (97% to 98%) of healthy individuals for a specific age and gender group.

Adequate intake (AI)—Recommended intake level based on estimates of nutrient intake by healthy groups of individuals.

Tolerable upper intake level (UL)—Highest average daily nutrient intake level likely to pose no risk of adverse health effects. As intake increases above the UL, risk of adverse effects increases.

Fig. 6-4 contains MyPlate, which describes dietary intake in children. Specific questions used to conduct a nutritional assessment are given in Box 6-9. Every nutritional assessment should begin with a **dietary history**. The exact questions used to elicit a dietary history vary with the child's age. In general, the younger the child, the more specific and detailed the history should be. The overview elicited from the dietary history can be helpful in evaluating food frequency records. The history is also concerned with financial and cultural factors

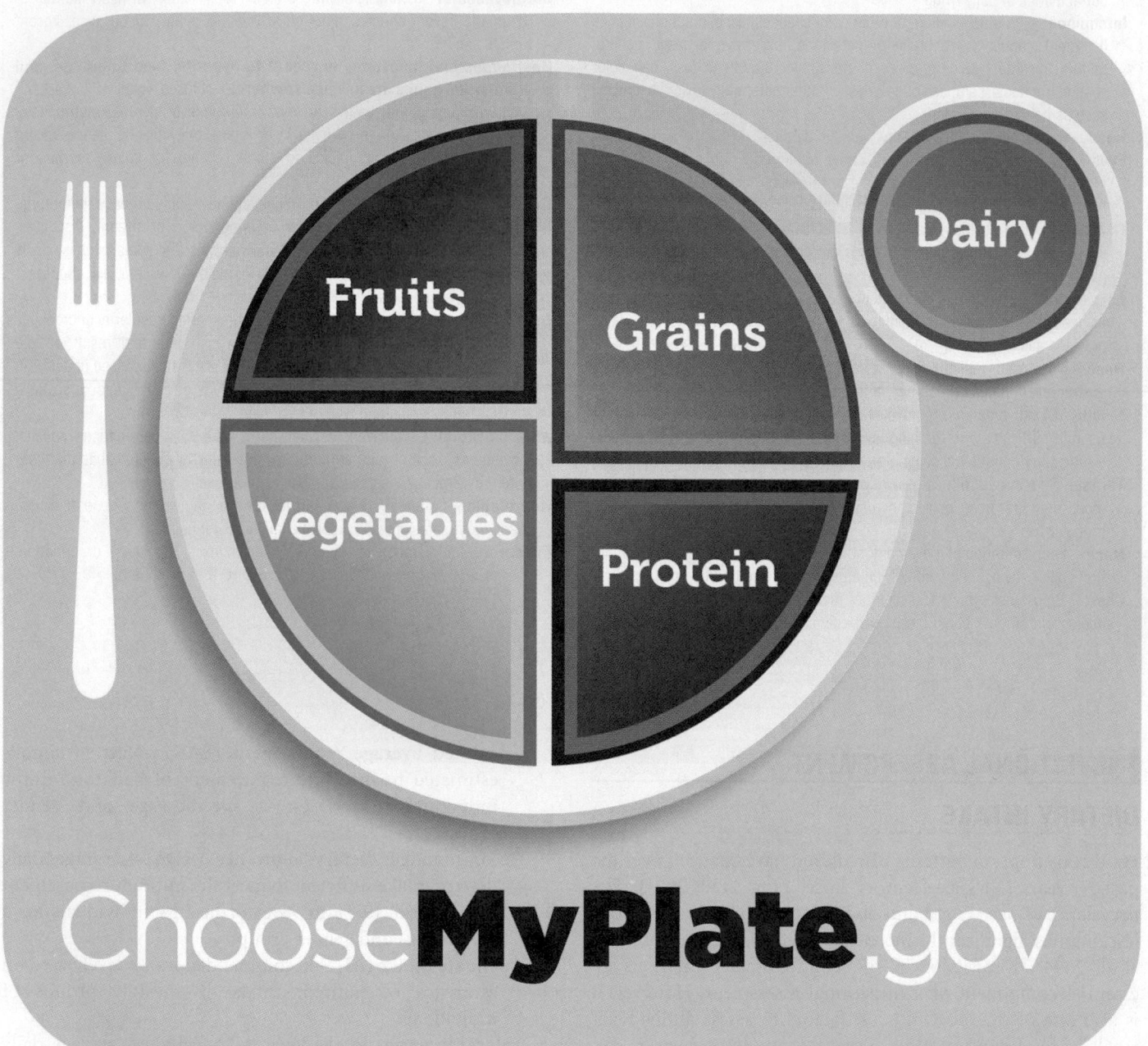

Fig. 6-4 MyPlate. MyPlate advocates building a healthy plate by making half of your plate fruits and vegetables and the other half grains and protein. Avoiding oversized portions, making half your grains whole grains, and drinking fat-free or low-fat (1%) milk are additional recommendations for a healthy diet. (From U.S. Department of Agriculture: *MyPlate*, Washington, DC, June 2011, The Service, available online at www.choosemyplate.gov.)

BOX 6-9   DIETARY REFERENCE INTAKES FOR AN INDIVIDUAL

Estimated average requirement (EAR)—Used to examine the possibility of inadequacy.

Recommended dietary allowance (RDA)—Dietary intake at or above this level usually has a low probability of inadequacy.

Adequate intake (AI)—Dietary intake at or above this level usually has a low probability of inadequacy.

Tolerable upper intake level (UL)—Dietary intake above this level usually places an individual at risk of adverse effects from excessive nutrient intake.

Dietary History

What are the family's usual mealtimes?

Do family members eat together or at separate times?

Who does the family grocery shopping and meal preparation?

How much money is spent to buy food each week?

How are most foods prepared—baked, broiled, fried, other?

How often does the family or your child eat out?
- What kinds of restaurants do you go to?
- What kinds of food does your child typically eat at restaurants?

Does your child eat breakfast regularly?

Where does your child eat lunch?

What are your child's favorite foods, beverages, and snacks?
- What are the average amounts eaten per day?
- What foods are artificially sweetened?
- What are your child's snacking habits?
- When are sweet foods usually eaten?
- What are your child's toothbrushing habits?

What special cultural practices are followed? What ethnic foods are eaten?

What foods and beverages does your child dislike?

How would you describe your child's usual appetite (hearty eater, picky eater)?

What are your child's feeding habits (breast, bottle, cup, spoon, eats by self, needs assistance, any special devices)?

Does your child take vitamins or other supplements? Do they contain iron or fluoride?

Does your child have any known or suspected food allergies? Is your child on a special diet?

Has your child lost or gained weight recently?

Are there any feeding problems (excessive fussiness, spitting up, colic, difficulty sucking or swallowing)? Are there any dental problems or appliances, such as braces, that affect eating?

What types of exercise does your child do regularly?

Is there a family history of cancer, diabetes, heart disease, high blood pressure, or obesity?

Additional Questions for Infants

What was the infant's birth weight? When did it double? Triple?

Was the infant premature?

Are you breast-feeding or have you breast-fed your infant? For how long?

If you use a formula, what is the brand?
- How long has the infant been taking it?
- How many ounces does the infant drink a day?

Are you giving the infant cow's milk (whole, low fat, skim)?
- When did you start?
- How many ounces does the infant drink a day?

Do you give your infant extra fluids (water, juice)?

If the infant takes a bottle to bed at nap or nighttime, what is in the bottle?

At what age did the child start on cereal, vegetables, meat or other protein sources, fruit or juice, finger food, table food?

Do you make your own baby food or use commercial foods, such as infant cereal?

Does the infant take a vitamin or mineral supplement? If so, what type?

Has the infant had an allergic reaction to any food(s)? If so, list the foods and describe the reaction.

Does the infant spit up frequently; have unusually loose stools; or have hard, dry stools? If so, how often?

How often do you feed your infant?

How would you describe your infant's appetite?

Modified from Murphy SP, Poos MI: Dietary reference intakes: summary of applications in dietary assessment, *Pub Health Nutr* 5(6A):843-849, 2002.

---

that influence food selection and preparation (see Cultural Competence box).

 CULTURAL COMPETENCE

Food Practices

Because cultural practices are prevalent in food preparation, consider carefully the kinds of questions that are asked and the judgments made during counseling. For example, some cultures, such as Hispanic, African-American, and Native American, include many vegetables, legumes, and starches in their diet that together provide sufficient essential amino acids, even though the actual amount of meat or dairy protein is low. (See Food Customs, Chapter 2.)

The most common and probably easiest method of assessing daily intake is the 24-hour recall. The child or parent recalls every item eaten in the past 24 hours and the approximate amounts. The 24-hour recall is most beneficial when it represents a typical day's intake. Some of the difficulties with a daily recall are the family's inability to remember exactly what was eaten and inaccurate estimation of portion size. To increase accuracy of reporting portion sizes, the use of food models and additional questions are recommended. In general, this method is most useful in providing *qualitative* information about the child's diet.

To improve the reliability of the daily recall, the family can complete a food diary by recording every food and liquid consumed for a certain number of days. A 3-day record consisting of 2 weekdays and 1 weekend day is representative for most people. Providing specific charts to record intake can improve compliance. The family should record items immediately after eating.

A food frequency questionnaire or record provides information about the number of times in a day, week, or month a child consumes items from the different food groups. In general, it provides a qualitative overview but has the advantage of avoiding recall based on a "typical" day. It can be especially useful when verifying a food history or diary.

CLINICAL EXAMINATION OF NUTRITION

A significant amount of information regarding nutritional deficiencies comes from a clinical examination, especially from assessing the skin, hair, teeth, gums, lips, tongue, and eyes. Hair, skin, and mouth are vulnerable because of the rapid turnover of epithelial and mucosal tissue. Table 6-1 summarizes clinical signs of possible nutritional deficiency or excess. Few are diagnostic for a specific nutrient, and if suspicious signs are found, they must be confirmed with dietary and biochemical data.

TABLE 6-1   CLINICAL ASSESSMENT OF NUTRITIONAL STATUS

EVIDENCE OF ADEQUATE NUTRITION	EVIDENCE OF DEFICIENT OR EXCESS NUTRITION	DEFICIENCY OR EXCESS*
General Growth		
Between 5th and 95th percentiles for height, weight, and head circumference	<5th or >95th percentile for growth	Protein, calories, fats, and other essential nutrients, especially vitamin A, pyridoxine, niacin, calcium, iodine, manganese, zinc
Steady gain with expected growth spurts during infancy and adolescence	Absence of or delayed growth spurts; poor weight gain	
Sexual development appropriate for age	Delayed sexual development	Excess vitamins A, D
Skin		
Smooth, slightly dry to touch	Hardening and scaling	Vitamin A
Elastic and firm	Seborrheic dermatitis	Excess niacin
Absence of lesions	Dry, rough, petechiae	Riboflavin
Color appropriate to genetic background	Delayed wound healing	Vitamin C
	Scaly dermatitis on exposed surfaces	Riboflavin, vitamin C, zinc
	Wrinkled, flabby	Niacin
	Crusted lesions around orifices, especially nares	Protein, calories, zinc
	Pruritus	Excess vitamin A, riboflavin, niacin
	Poor turgor	Water, sodium
	Edema	Protein, thiamine
		Excess sodium
	Yellow tinge (jaundice)	Vitamin B$_{12}$
		Excess vitamin A, niacin
	Depigmentation	Protein, calories
	Pallor (anemia)	Pyridoxine, folic acid, vitamins B$_{12}$, C, E (in premature infants), iron
		Excess vitamin C, zinc
	Paresthesia	Excess riboflavin
Hair		
Lustrous, silky, strong, elastic	Stringy, friable, dull, dry, thin	Protein, calories
	Alopecia	Protein, calories, zinc
	Depigmentation	Protein, calories, copper
	Raised areas around hair follicles	Vitamin C
Head		
Even molding, occipital prominence, symmetric facial features	Softening of cranial bones, prominence of frontal bones, skull flat and depressed toward middle	Vitamin D
Fused sutures after 18 months	Delayed fusion of sutures	Vitamin D
	Hard, tender lumps in occiput	Excess vitamin A
	Headache	Excess thiamine
Neck		
Thyroid not visible, palpable in midline	Thyroid enlarged, may be grossly visible	Iodine
Eyes		
Clear, bright	Hardening and scaling of cornea and conjunctiva	Vitamin A
Good night vision	Night blindness	Vitamin A
Conjunctiva—Pink, glossy	Burning, itching, photophobia, cataracts, corneal vascularization	Riboflavin
Ears		
Tympanic membrane—Pliable	Calcified (hearing loss)	Excess vitamin D
Nose		
Smooth, intact nasal angle	Irritation and cracks at nasal angle	Riboflavin
		Excess vitamin A
Mouth		
Lips—Smooth, moist, darker color than skin	Fissures and inflammation at corners	Riboflavin
		Excess vitamin A
Gums—Firm, coral pink, stippled	Spongy, friable, swollen, bluish red or black, bleed easily	Vitamin C
Mucous membranes—Bright pink, smooth, moist	Stomatitis	Niacin
Tongue—Rough texture, no lesions, taste sensation	Glossitis	Niacin, riboflavin, folic acid
	Diminished taste sensation	Zinc

TABLE 6-1   CLINICAL ASSESSMENT OF NUTRITIONAL STATUS—cont'd

EVIDENCE OF ADEQUATE NUTRITION	EVIDENCE OF DEFICIENT OR EXCESS NUTRITION	DEFICIENCY OR EXCESS*
Mouth—cont'd		
Teeth—Uniform white color, smooth, intact	Brown mottling, pits, fissures	Excess fluoride
	Defective enamel	Vitamins A, C, D, calcium, phosphorus
	Caries	Excess carbohydrates
Chest		
In infants, shape almost circular	Depressed lower portion of rib cage	Vitamin D
In children, lateral diameter increased in proportion to anteroposterior diameter	Sharp protrusion of sternum	Vitamin D
Smooth costochondral junctions	Enlarged costochondral junctions	Vitamins C, D
Breast development—Normal for age	Delayed development	See under General Growth; especially zinc
Cardiovascular System		
Pulse and blood pressure (BP) within normal limits	Palpitations	Thiamine
	Rapid pulse	Potassium
		Excess thiamine
	Arrhythmias	Magnesium, potassium
		Excess niacin, potassium
	Increased BP	Excess sodium
	Decreased BP	Thiamine
		Excess niacin
Abdomen		
In young children, cylindric and prominent	Distended, flabby, poor musculature	Protein, calories
	Prominent, large	Excess calories
In older children, flat	Potbelly, constipation	Vitamin D
Normal bowel habits	Diarrhea	Niacin
		Excess vitamin C
	Constipation	Excess calcium, potassium
Musculoskeletal System		
Muscles—Firm, well-developed, equal strength bilaterally	Flabby, weak, generalized wasting	Protein, calories
	Weakness, pain, cramps	Thiamine, sodium, chloride, potassium, phosphorus, magnesium
		Excess thiamine
	Muscle twitching, tremors	Magnesium
	Muscular paralysis	Excess potassium
Spine—Cervical and lumbar curves (double S curve)	Kyphosis, lordosis, scoliosis	Vitamin D
Extremities—Symmetric; legs straight with minimum bowing	Bowing of extremities, knock-knees	Vitamin D, calcium, phosphorus
	Epiphyseal enlargement	Vitamins A, D
	Bleeding into joints and muscles, joint swelling, pain	Vitamin C
Joints—Flexible, full range of motion, no pain or stiffness	Thickening of cortex of long bones with pain and fragility, hard tender lumps in extremities	Excess vitamin A
	Osteoporosis of long bones	Calcium
		Excess vitamin D
Neurologic System		
Behavior—Alert, responsive, emotionally stable	Listless, irritable, lethargic, apathetic (sometimes apprehensive, anxious, drowsy, mentally slow, confused)	Thiamine, niacin, pyridoxine, vitamin C, potassium, magnesium, iron, protein, calories
		Excess vitamins A, D, thiamine, folic acid, calcium
Absence of tetany, convulsions	Masklike facial expression, blurred speech, involuntary laughing	Excess manganese
	Convulsions	Thiamine, pyridoxine, vitamin D, calcium, magnesium
		Excess phosphorus (in relation to calcium)
Intact peripheral nervous system	Peripheral nervous system toxicity (unsteady gait, numb feet and hands, fine motor clumsiness)	Excess pyridoxine
Intact reflexes	Diminished or absent tendon reflexes	Thiamine, vitamin E

*Nutrients listed are deficient unless specified as excess.

Generally, the clinical examination does not reveal children *at risk* for a deficiency or excess.

Anthropometry, an essential parameter of nutritional status, is the measurement of height, weight, head circumference, proportions, skinfold thickness, and arm circumference in young children. Height and head circumference reflect past nutrition, whereas weight, skinfold thickness, and arm circumference reflect present nutritional status, especially of protein and fat reserves. Skinfold thickness is a measurement of the body's fat content because approximately half the body's total fat stores are directly beneath the skin. The upper arm muscle circumference is correlated with measurements of total muscle mass. Since muscle serves as the body's major protein reserve, this measurement is considered an index of the body's protein stores. Ideally, growth measurements are recorded over time, and comparisons are made regarding the *velocity* of growth based on previous and present values.

Numerous biochemical tests are available for assessing nutritional status and include analysis of plasma; blood cells; urine; and tissues from liver, bone, hair, and fingernails. Many of these tests are complicated and are not performed routinely. Common laboratory procedures for nutritional status include measurement of hemoglobin, hematocrit, transferrin, albumin, creatinine, and nitrogen. Appendix C provides laboratory values for these tests and more specific nutrient measurements.

EVALUATION OF NUTRITIONAL ASSESSMENT

After collecting the data needed for a thorough nutritional assessment, evaluate the findings to plan appropriate counseling. From the data, assess whether the child is (1) malnourished, (2) at risk for becoming malnourished, (3) well nourished with adequate reserves, or (4) overweight or obese.

Analyze the daily food diary for the variety and amounts of foods suggested in MyPlate (see Fig. 6-4). For example, if the list includes no vegetables, inquire about this rather than assuming that the child dislikes vegetables, since it is possible that none were served that day. Also, evaluate the information in terms of the family's ethnic practices and financial resources. Encouraging increased protein intake with additional meat is not always feasible for families on a limited budget and may conflict with food practices that use meat sparingly, such as in Asian meal preparation.

GENERAL APPROACHES TOWARD EXAMINING THE CHILD

SEQUENCE OF THE EXAMINATION

Ordinarily, the sequence for examining patients follows a head-to-toe direction. The main function of such a systematic approach is to provide a general guideline for assessment of each body area to avoid omitting segments of the examination. The standard recording of data also facilitates exchange of information among different professionals. The typical organization of a physical examination is in the chapter outline. In examining children, this orderly sequence is frequently altered to accommodate the child's developmental needs, although the

examination is recorded following the head-to-toe model. Using developmental and chronologic age as the main criteria for assessing each body system accomplishes several goals:

- Minimizes stress and anxiety associated with assessment of various body parts
- Fosters a trusting nurse-child-parent relationship
- Allows for maximum preparation of the child
- Preserves the essential security of the parent-child relationship, especially with young children
- Maximizes the accuracy and reliability of assessment findings

PREPARATION OF THE CHILD

Although the physical examination consists of painless procedures, for some children the use of a tight arm cuff, probes in the ears and mouth, pressure on the abdomen, and a cold piece of metal to listen to the chest are stressful. Therefore the nurse should use the same considerations discussed in Chapter 27 for preparing children for procedures. In addition to that discussion, general guidelines related to the examining process are given in the Nursing Care Guidelines box.

The physical examination should be as pleasant as possible, as well as educational. For example, use of a detailed drawing or anatomically correct doll can help preschoolers and older children learn about their bodies (Vessey, 1995). The paper-doll technique is a useful approach to teaching children about the body part that is being examined (Fig. 6-5). At the conclusion of the visit, the child can bring home the paper doll as a memento.

Table 6-2 summarizes guidelines for positioning, preparing, and examining children at various ages. Because no child fits precisely into one age category, it may be necessary to vary the approach after a preliminary assessment of the child's developmental achievements and needs. Even with the best approach, many toddlers are uncooperative and inconsolable for much of the physical examination. However, some seem intrigued by the new surroundings and unusual equipment and respond more like preschoolers than toddlers. Likewise, some early preschool-

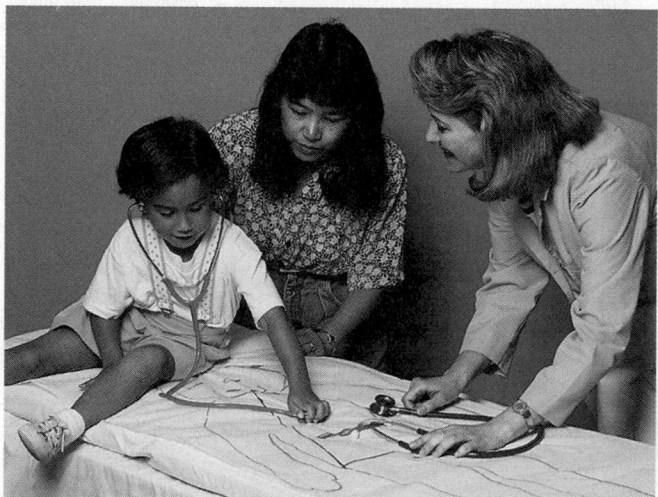

Fig. 6-5 Using paper-doll technique to prepare child for physical examination.

NURSING CARE GUIDELINES

Performing Pediatric Physical Examination

Perform the examination in an appropriate, nonthreatening area:
- Have room well lit and decorated with neutral colors.
- Have room temperature comfortably warm.
- Place all strange and potentially frightening equipment out of sight.
- Have some toys, dolls, stuffed animals, and games available for child.
- If possible, have rooms decorated and equipped for different-age children.
- Provide privacy, especially for school-age children and adolescents.

Provide time for play and becoming acquainted.

Observe behaviors that signal child's readiness to cooperate:
- Talking to the nurse
- Making eye contact
- Accepting the offered equipment
- Allowing physical touching
- Choosing to sit on examining table rather than parent's lap

If signs of readiness are not observed, use the following techniques:
- Talk to parent while essentially "ignoring" child; gradually focus on child or a favorite object, such as a doll.
- Make complimentary remarks about child, such as appearance, dress, or a favorite object.
- Tell a funny story or play a simple magic trick.
- Have a nonthreatening "friend" available, such as a hand puppet to "talk" to child for the nurse (see Fig. 6-26, *A*).

If child refuses to cooperate, use the following techniques:
- Assess reason for uncooperative behavior; consider that a child who is unduly afraid may have had a traumatic experience.
- Try to involve child and parent in process.
- Avoid prolonged explanations about examining procedure.
- Use a firm, direct approach regarding expected behavior.
- Perform examination as quickly as possible.
- Have attendant gently restrain child.
- Minimize any disruptions or stimulation.
- Limit number of people in room.
- Use isolated room.
- Use quiet, calm, confident voice.

Begin examination in a nonthreatening manner for young children or children who are fearful:
- Use activities that can be presented as games, such as test for cranial nerves (see Table 6-13) or parts of developmental screening tests (see Appendix A).
- Use approaches such as Simon Says to encourage child to make a face, squeeze a hand, stand on one foot, and so on.
- Use paper-doll technique:
  1. Lay child supine on an examining table or floor that is covered with a large sheet of paper.
  2. Trace around child's body outline.
  3. Use body outline to demonstrate what will be examined, such as drawing a heart and listening with stethoscope before performing activity on child.

If several children in the family will be examined, begin with most cooperative child to model desired behavior.

Involve child in examination process:
- Provide choices, such as sitting on table or in parent's lap.
- Allow child to handle or hold equipment.
- Encourage child to use equipment on a doll, family member, or examiner.
- Explain each step of the procedure in simple language.

Examine child in a comfortable and secure position:
- Sitting in parent's lap
- Sitting upright if in respiratory distress

Proceed to examine the body in an organized sequence (usually head to toe) with the following exceptions:
- Alter sequence to accommodate needs of different-age children (see Table 6-2).
- Examine painful areas last.
- In emergency situation, examine vital functions (airway, breathing, and circulation) and injured area first.

Reassure child throughout the examination, especially about bodily concerns that arise during puberty.

Discuss findings with family at the end of the examination.

Praise child for cooperation during the examination; give a reward such as a small toy or sticker.

---

ers may require more of the "security measures" employed with younger children, such as continued parent-child contact, and less of the preparatory measures used with preschoolers, such as playing with the equipment before and during the actual examination (Fig. 6-6).

Despite numerous variations in the general approaches, some common ones are detailed here. For example, the suggested sequence may change considerably when the child is in pain or when obvious physical defects are present. In either situation, examine the affected area last to minimize distress early in the examination and to focus on normal, healthy, functioning body parts.

PHYSICAL EXAMINATION

Although the approach to and sequence of the physical examination differ according to the child's age, the following discussion outlines the traditional model for physical assessment. The focus includes all pediatric age-groups; however, see Chapter 8 for a detailed discussion of a newborn assessment. Because the physical examination is a vital part of preventive pediatric care, Fig. 6-7 gives a schedule for periodic health visits.

GROWTH MEASUREMENTS

Measurement of physical growth in children is a key element in evaluating their health status. Physical growth parameters include weight, height (length), skinfold thickness, arm circumference, and head circumference. Values for these growth parameters are plotted on percentile charts, and the child's measurements in percentiles are compared with those of the general population.

Growth Charts

The most commonly used growth charts in the United States are from the National Center for Health Statistics (NCHS) (Ogden, Kuczmarski, Flegal, et al, 2002). The growth charts have been revised to include the body mass index–for-age (BMI-for-age) charts, 3rd and 97th smoothed percentiles for all charts, and the 85th percentile for the weight-for-stature and BMI-for-age charts (see Appendix B). The data were collected from five national surveys between 1963 and 1994. The revised charts have eliminated the disjunctions between the curves for infants and other children and have been extended for children and adolescents to 20 years.

Skill—Measuring Physical Growth

TABLE 6-2   AGE-SPECIFIC APPROACHES TO PHYSICAL EXAMINATION DURING CHILDHOOD

POSITION	PREPARATION	SEQUENCE
Infant Before able to sit alone—Supine or prone, preferably in parent's lap; before 4-6 months, can place on examining table After able to sit alone—Sitting in parent's lap whenever possible; if on table, place with parent in full view	Completely undress if room temperature permits. Leave diaper on male infant. Gain cooperation with distraction, bright objects, rattles, talking. Smile at infant; use soft, gentle voice. Pacify with bottle of sugar water or feeding. Enlist parent's aid for restraining to examine ears, mouth. Avoid abrupt, jerky movements.	If quiet, auscultate heart, lungs, abdomen. Record heart and respiratory rates. Palpate and percuss same areas. Proceed in usual head-to-toe direction. Perform traumatic procedures last (eyes, ears, mouth [while crying]). Elicit reflexes as body part is examined. Elicit Moro reflex last.
Toddler Sitting or standing on or by parent Prone or supine in parent's lap	Have parent remove outer clothing. Remove underwear as body part is examined. Allow to inspect equipment; demonstrating use of equipment is usually ineffective. If uncooperative, perform procedures quickly. Use restraint when appropriate; request parent's assistance. Talk about examination if cooperative; use short phrases. Praise for cooperative behavior.	Inspect body area through play: "count fingers," "tickle toes." Use minimum physical contact initially. Introduce equipment slowly. Auscultate, percuss, palpate whenever quiet. Perform traumatic procedures last (same as for infant).
Preschool Child Prefer standing or sitting Usually cooperative prone or supine Prefer parent's closeness	Request self-undressing. Allow to wear underpants if shy. Offer equipment for inspection; briefly demonstrate use. Make up story about procedure (e.g., "I'm seeing how strong your muscles are" [blood pressure]). Use paper-doll technique. Give choices when possible. Expect cooperation; use positive statements (e.g., "Open your mouth").	If cooperative, proceed in head-to-toe direction. If uncooperative, proceed as with toddler.
School-Age Child Prefer sitting Cooperative in most positions Younger child prefers parent's presence Older child may prefer privacy	Respect need for privacy. Request self-undressing. Allow to wear underpants. Give gown to wear. Explain purpose of equipment and significance of procedure, such as otoscope to see eardrum, which is necessary for hearing. Teach about body function and care.	Proceed in head-to-toe direction. May examine genitalia last in older child.
Adolescent Same as for school-age child Offer option of parent's presence	Allow to undress in private. Give gown. Expose only area to be examined. Respect need for privacy. Explain findings during examination: "Your muscles are firm and strong." Matter-of-factly comment about sexual development: "Your breasts are developing as they should be." Emphasize normalcy of development. Examine genitalia as any other body part; may leave to end.	Same as older school-age child. May examine genitalia last.

The weight-for-age percentile distributions are now continuous between the infant and the older child charts at 24 to 36 months. The length-for-age to stature-for-age and weight-for-length to weight-for-stature curves are parallel in the overlapping ages of 24 to 36 months. The revised weight-for-stature charts provide a smoother transition from the weight-for-length charts for preschool-age children.

The most prominent change to the complement of growth charts for older children and adolescents is the addition of the BMI-for-age growth curves. The BMI-for-age charts were developed with national survey data (1963 to 1994), excluding data from the 1988 to 1994 National Health and Nutrition Examination Surveys III (NHANES III) for children older than 6 years because an increase in body weight and BMI occurred between NHANES III and previous national surveys. Without this exclusion, the 85th and 95th percentile curves would have been higher, and fewer children and adolescents would have been classified as at risk of or overweight. Therefore the BMI-for-age growth curves do not represent the current population of children older than 6 years of age.

> **! NURSING ALERT**
>
> The sex-specific BMI-for-age charts for ages 2 to 20 years replace the 1977 NCHS weight-for-stature charts that were limited to prepubescent boys younger than 11½ years and with statures less than 145 cm (4 feet, 9 inches), and to prepubescent girls younger than 19 years and with statures less than 137 cm (4 feet, 6 inches).

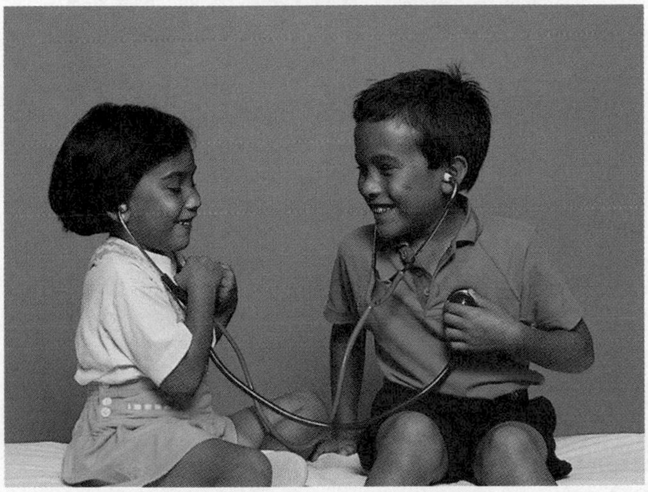

Fig. 6-6 Preparing children for physical examination.

Breast- and Formula-Fed Infants

The national survey data better represent the combined size and growth patterns of the general U.S. population (1971 to 1994). Over the past 30 years in the United States, approximately half of all infants were reported to have been breast-fed, and approximately one third were breast-fed for 3 months or more. Therefore, compared with the 1977 NCHS growth charts, the nationally representative data on which the revised infant growth charts are based better represent the combined growth patterns of breast-fed and formula-fed infants in the U.S. population (Ogden, Kuczmarski, Flegal, et al, 2002).

Special Groups

Although differences in size and growth occur among the major racial and ethnic groups in the United States, these appear to be small and inconsistent. Therefore the revised

	Infancy							Early Childhood							Middle Childhood						Adolescence							
Age	Newborn	3-5 d	By1mo	2 mo	4 mo	6 mo	9 mo	12mo	15mo	18mo	24mo	30mo	3 y	4 y	5 y	6 y	7 y	8 y	9 y	10 y	11 y	12 y	13 y	14 y	15 y	16 y	17 y	18 y
History Initial/Interval	•	•	•	•	•	•	•	•	•	•	•	•	•	•	•	•	•	•	•	•	•	•	•	•	•	•	•	•
Measurements																												
Length/Height and Weight	•	•	•	•	•	•	•	•	•	•	•	•	•	•	•	•	•	•	•	•	•	•	•	•	•	•	•	•
Head Circumference	•	•	•	•	•	•	•	•	•	•	•																	
Weight for Length	•	•	•	•	•	•	•	•	•	•																		
Body Mass Index											•	•	•	•	•	•	•	•	•	•	•	•	•	•	•	•	•	•
Blood Pressure	★	★	★	★	★	★	★	★	★	★	★	★	★	★	•	•	•	•	•	•	•	•	•	•	•	•	•	•
Sensory Screening																												
Vision	★	★	★	★	★	★	★	★	★	★	★	★	•	•	•	•	★	•	★	•	★	•	★	★	•	★	★	•
Hearing	•	★	★	★	★	★	★	★	★	★	★	★	★	•	•	•	★	•	★	•	★	★	★	★	★	★	★	★
Developmental/ Behavioral Assessment																												
Developmental Screening							•			•		•																
Autism Screening										•	•																	
Developmental Surveillance	•	•	•	•	•	•		•	•		•		•	•	•	•	•	•	•	•	•	•	•	•	•	•	•	•
Psychosocial/ Behavioral Assessment	•	•	•	•	•	•	•	•	•	•	•	•	•	•	•	•	•	•	•	•	•	•	•	•	•	•	•	•
Alcohol and Drug Use Assessment																					★	★	★	★	★	★	★	★
Physical Examination	•	•	•	•	•	•	•	•	•	•	•	•	•	•	•	•	•	•	•	•	•	•	•	•	•	•	•	•
Procedures																												
Newborn Metabolic/ Hemoglobin Screening	←——	•	——→																									
Immunization	•	•	•	•	•	•	•	•	•	•	•	•	•	•	•	•	•	•	•	•	•	•	•	•	•	•	•	•
Hematocrit or Hemoglobin					★			•			★	★		★	★	★	★	★	★	★	★	★	★	★	★	★	★	★
Lead Screening						★	★	• or ★		★	• or ★		★	★	★	★												
Tuberculin Test		★				★		★		★	★		★	★	★	★	★	★	★	★	★	★	★	★	★	★	★	★
Dyslipidemia Screening											★			★		★		★		★	★	★	★	★	★	★	★	•
STI Screening																					★	★	★	★	★	★	★	★
Cervical Dysplasia Screening																					★	★	★	★	★	★	★	★
Oral Health						★	★	• or ★		• or ★	• or ★	• or ★	•			•												
Anticipatory Guidance	•	•	•	•	•	•	•	•	•	•	•	•	•	•	•	•	•	•	•	•	•	•	•	•	•	•	•	•

Key: • = To be performed; ★ = risk assessment to be performed, with appropriate action to follow, if positive; ←—•—→ = range during which a service may be provided, with the symbol indicating the preferred age.

Fig. 6-7 Preventive health care chart. *STI,* Sexually transmitted infection. (Modified from American Academy of Pediatrics Committee on Practice and Ambulatory Medicine and Bright Futures Steering Committee: Recommendations for preventive pediatric health care, *Pediatrics* 120(6):1376, 2007.)

growth charts include all infants and children whatever their race or ethnicity. Because the growth patterns of preterm, very low–birth-weight (VLBW) (<1500 g [3.3 lb]) infants are considerably different from those of higher birth-weight, full-term infants and specialized growth charts exist to track the growth of VLBW infants, data for VLBW infants were excluded from the revised charts.

Version of the Growth Charts

Three different versions of the charts are available (**www.cdc. gov/growthcharts**). The first set contains all nine smoothed percentile lines (3rd, 5th, 10th, 25th, 50th, 75th, 90th, 95th, 97th), and the second and third sets contain seven smoothed percentile lines. The second set contains the 5th and 95th percentile lines, and the third set contains the 3rd and 97th percentile lines at the extreme ends of the distribution. In addition, the charts for weight-for-stature and BMI-for-age contain the 85th percentile. In all the growth charts, age is truncated to the nearest full month, for example, 1 month (1.0 to 1.9 months), 11 months (11.0 to 11.9 months), and 23 months (23.0 to 23.9 months).

The three sets of charts are provided to meet the needs of various users. Set 1 shows all the major percentile curves but may have limitations when the curves are close together, especially at the youngest ages. Most users in the United States may wish to use the format shown in set 2 for the majority of routine clinical applications (see Appendix C). Pediatric endocrinologists and others dealing with special populations, such as children with failure to thrive, may wish to use the format in set 3.

Nurses are often responsible for measuring growth in children, so it is essential that they understand the revised growth charts. Several important differences exist between the 1977 and the revised charts with significant implications for classifying children as underweight or overweight. Nurses need to become familiar with determining BMI, which only requires information about the child's weight and height.* With the increasing number of overweight children in the United States, the BMI charts are a critical component of children's physical assessment.

> **! NURSING ALERT**
>
> BMI-for-age may be used to identify children and adolescents at the upper end of the distribution who are either overweight (≥95th percentile) or at risk for being overweight (≥85th and <95th percentile) (Ogden, Carroll, and Flegal, 2008). Formulas for determining BMI are available at www.cdc.gov/nccdphp/dnpa/bmi and in Appendix B.

Children whose growth may be questionable include:
- Children whose height and weight percentiles are widely disparate (e.g., height in the 10th percentile and weight in the 90th percentile, especially with above-average skinfold thickness)

---

*BMI (English) = [Weight in pounds ÷ (Height in inches × Height in inches)] × 703. BMI (metric) = Weight in kilograms ÷ [Height in meters]². NOTE: This formula is the BMI calculation for adults, used in some pediatric settings; for child and adolescent BMI table and plotting, see Appendix B.

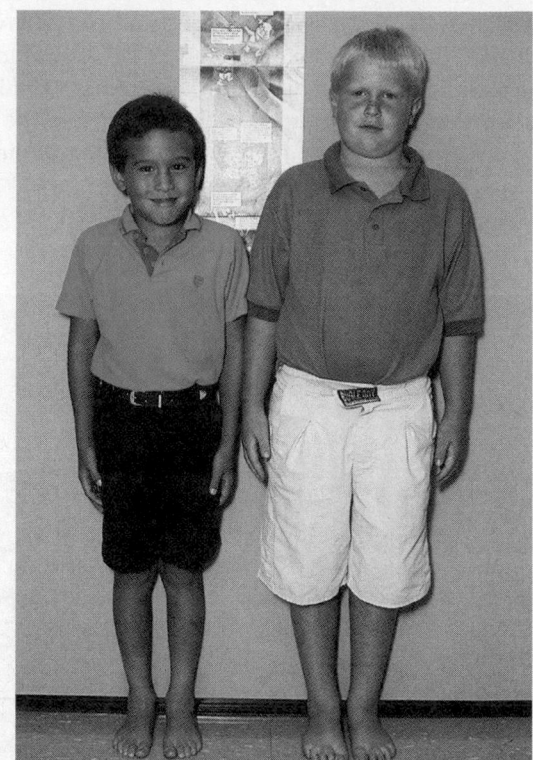

Fig. 6-8 These children of identical age (8 years) are markedly different in size. Child on left, of Asian descent, is at 5th percentile for height and weight. Child on right is above 95th percentile for height and weight. However, both children demonstrate normal growth patterns.

- Children who fail to follow the expected growth velocity in height and weight, especially during the rapid growth periods of infancy and adolescence
- Children who show a sudden increase (except during puberty), decrease, or no change in a previously steady growth pattern.

Because growth is a continuous but uneven process, the most reliable evaluation lies in comparing growth measurements over time. It is important to remember that normal growth patterns vary among children the same age (Fig. 6-8).

Ethnic Differences in Growth

A potential concern with the U.S. growth charts is their accuracy in evaluating the growth of children from different ethnic and socioeconomic backgrounds. These growth charts can serve as a reference guide for all racial or ethnic groups if used from the perspective that different groups of children have varying normal distributions on the growth curves.

Length

The term **length** refers to measurements taken when children are supine (also referred to as **recumbent length**). Until children are 24 months old (or 36 months if using the chart for birth to 36 months), measure recumbent length. Because of the normally flexed position during infancy, fully extend the body by (1) holding the head in midline, (2) grasping the knees together gently, and (3) pushing down on the knees until the legs are fully extended and flat against the table. If using a measuring board, place the head firmly at the top of the board and the heels of the feet firmly against the footboard.

If such a measuring device is not available, measure length by placing the child on a paper-covered surface, marking the end points of the top of the head and the heels of the feet, and measuring between these two points (Fig. 6-9). For accurate measurement, hold the writing utensil at a right angle to the table when marking the cephalic point; position the feet with the toes pointing directly to the ceiling when marking the heel point. Regardless of the method used, have someone assist in holding the child's head in midline while you extend the legs and take the measurements.

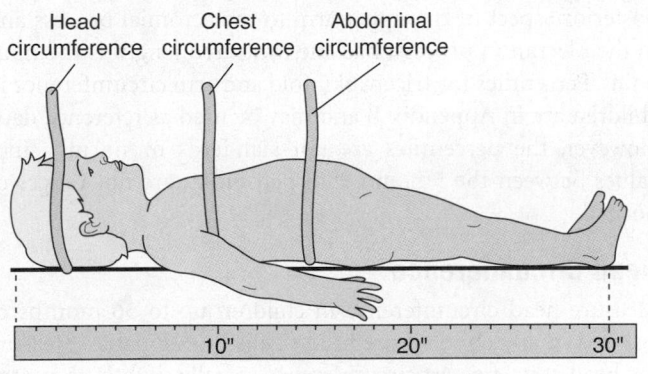

Fig. 6-9 Measurement of head, chest, and abdominal circumference and crown-to-heel (recumbent) length. (From Price DL: *Pediatric nursing: an introductory text,* ed 10, St Louis, 2007, Saunders.)

Height

The term **height** (or **stature**) refers to the measurement taken when a child is standing upright. Measure height by having the child, with shoes removed, stand as tall and straight as possible, with the head in midline and the line of vision parallel to the ceiling and floor. Be certain the child's back is to the wall or other vertical flat surface, with the heels, buttocks, and back of the shoulders touching the wall and the medial malleoli touching if possible (Fig. 6-10). Check for and correct bending of the knees, slumping of the shoulders, or raising of the heels.

> **NURSING TIP** Normally, height is less if measured in the afternoon than in the morning. To minimize this variation, apply modest upward pressure under the jaw or the mastoid processes behind the ears.

For the most accurate measurement, use a wall-mounted unit (**stadiometer**; see Fig. 6-10). The movable measuring rod of platform scales is accurate only if it remains parallel to the floor and rests securely on the topmost part of the head. To improvise a flat surface for measuring length, attach a paper or metal tape or yardstick to the wall, position the child adjacent to the tape, and place a three-dimensional object, such as a thick book or box, on top of the head. Rest the side of the object firmly against the wall to form a right angle. Measure length or stature to the nearest 1 mm or ⅛ inch.

Weight

Weight is measured with an appropriately sized balance beam scale, which measures weight to the nearest 10 g (0.35 oz) for

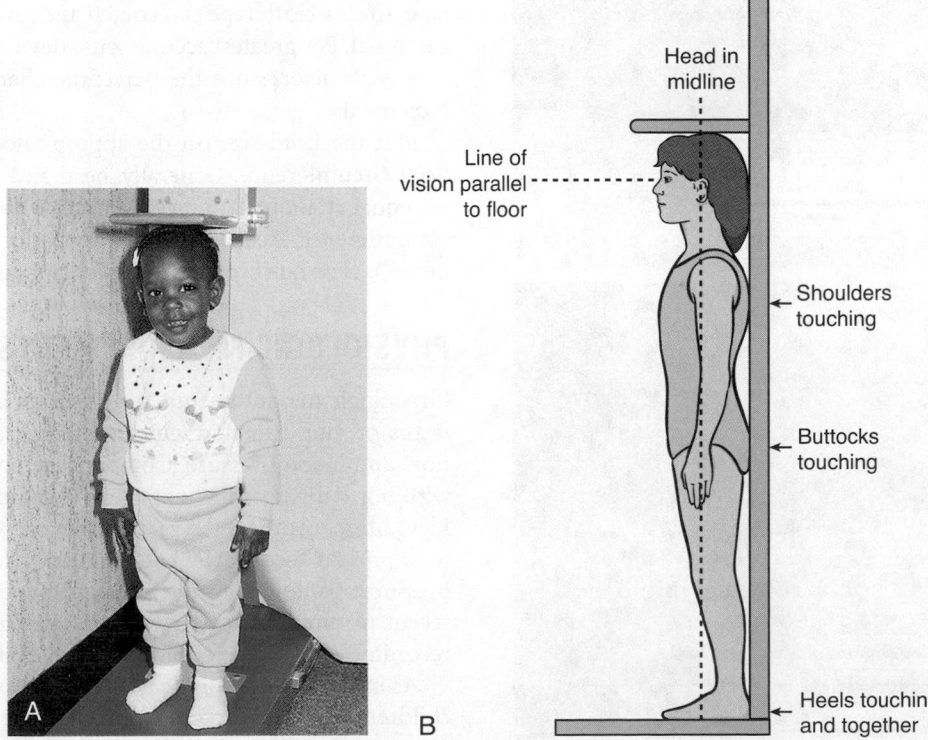

Fig. 6-10 **A** and **B,** Measurement of height. (**A,** From Seidel HM, Ball JW, Dains JE, et al: *Mosby's guide to physical examination,* ed 6, St Louis, 2007, Mosby. **B,** From Wilson S: *Health assessment for nursing practice,* ed 4, St Louis, 2009, Mosby.)

infants and 100 g (0.22 lb) for children. Before weighing the child, balance the scale by setting it at 0 and noting if the balance registers exactly in the middle of the mark. If the end of the balance beam rises to the top or bottom of the mark, more or less weight, respectively, is needed. Some scales are designed to self-correct, but others need to be recalibrated by the manufacturer. Scales vary in their accuracy; infant scales tend to be more accurate than adult platform scales, and newer scales tend to be more accurate than older ones, especially at the upper levels of weight measurement. When precise measurements are necessary, two nurses should take the weight independently; if there is a discrepancy, take a third reading.

Take measurements in a comfortably warm room. When the birth to 36-month growth charts are used, children should be weighed nude. Older children are usually weighed while wearing their underpants or a light gown. However, always respect the privacy of all children. If the child must be weighed wearing some article of clothing or some type of special device, such as a prosthesis or an armboard for an intravenous device, note this when recording the weight. Children who are measured for recumbent length are usually weighed on an infant platform scale and placed in a lying or sitting position. When weighing a child, place your hand lightly above the infant to prevent him or her from accidentally falling off the scale (Fig. 6-11, *A*) or stand close to the toddler, ready to prevent a fall (Fig. 6-11, *B*). For maximum asepsis, cover the scale with a clean sheet of paper between each child's measurement.

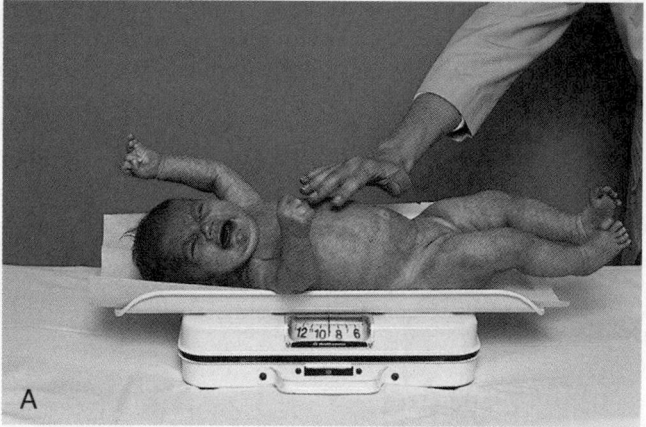

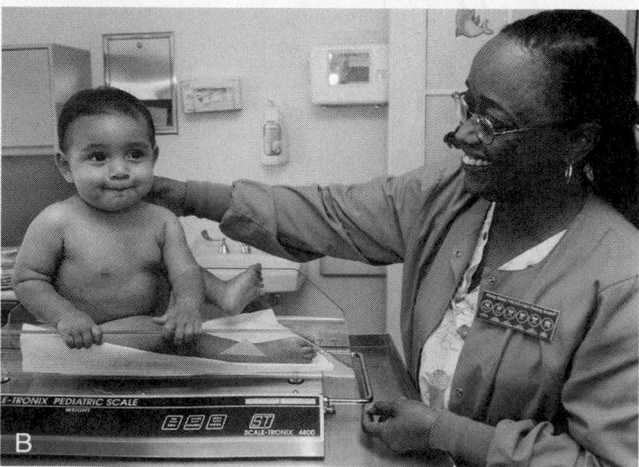

Fig. 6-11 A, Infant on scale. **B,** Toddler on scale. Note presence of nurse to prevent falls. (**B,** Courtesy Paul Vincent Kuntz, Texas Children's Hospital, Houston.)

Skinfold Thickness and Arm Circumference

Measures of relative weight and stature cannot distinguish between adipose (fat) tissue and muscle. One convenient measure of body fat is skinfold thickness, which is increasingly recommended as a routine measurement. Measure skinfold thickness with special calipers, such as the Lange calipers. The most common sites for measuring skinfold thickness are the triceps (most practical for routine clinical use), subscapula, suprailiac, abdomen, and upper thigh. For greatest reliability, follow the exact procedure for measurement and record the average of at least two measurements of one site.

Arm circumference is an indirect measure of muscle mass. Measurement of arm circumference follows the same procedure as for skinfold thickness except the midpoint is measured with a paper or steel tape. Place the tape vertically, along the posterior aspect of the upper arm to the acromial process and to the olecranon process; half the measured length is the midpoint. Percentiles for triceps skinfold and arm circumference in children are in Appendix B and may be used as reference data. However, the percentiles are not standards or norms, since values between the 5th and 95th percentiles are not ranges of normal.

Head Circumference

Measure head circumference in children up to 36 months of age and in any child whose head size is questionable. Measure the head at its greatest circumference, usually slightly above the eyebrows and pinna of the ears and around the occipital prominence at the back of the skull (see Fig. 6-9). Because head shape can affect the location of the maximum circumference, more than one measurement at points above the eyebrows is necessary to obtain the most accurate measure. Use a paper or metal tape, since a cloth tape can stretch and give a falsely small measurement. For greatest accuracy, use devices marked with tenths of a centimeter, since the percentile charts have only 0.5-cm increments.

Plot the head size on the appropriate growth chart under head circumference. Generally, head and chest circumferences are equal at about 1 to 2 years of age. During childhood, chest circumference exceeds head size by about 5 to 7 cm (2 to 2.75 inches). (For newborns see Physical Assessment, Chapter 8.)

PHYSIOLOGIC MEASUREMENTS

Physiologic measurements, key elements in evaluating physical status of vital functions, include temperature, pulse, respiration, and blood pressure. Compare each physiologic recording with normal values for that age-group (see inside back cover). In addition, compare the values taken on preceding health visits with present recordings. For example, a falsely elevated blood pressure reading may not indicate hypertension if previous recent readings have been within normal limits. The isolated recording may indicate some stressful event in the child's life.

As in most procedures carried out with children, treat older children and adolescents much the same as adults. However, give special consideration to preschool children (see Atraumatic Care box). For best results in taking vital signs of infants, count respirations first (before the infant is disturbed), take the pulse next, and measure temperature last. If vital signs cannot be taken without disturbing the child, record the child's behavior (e.g., crying) along with the measurement.

ATRAUMATIC CARE

Reducing Young Children's Fears

Young children, especially preschoolers, fear intrusive procedures because of their poorly defined body boundaries. Therefore avoid invasive procedures, such as measuring rectal temperature, whenever possible. Also, avoid using the word "take" when measuring vital signs, since young children interpret words literally and may think that their temperature or other function will be taken away. Instead, say, "I want to know how warm you are."

Temperature

Temperature is the measure of heat content within an individual's body. The core temperature most closely reflects the temperature of the blood flow through the carotid arteries to the hypothalamus. Core temperature is relatively constant despite wide fluctuations in the external environment. When a child's temperature is altered, receptors in the skin, spinal cord, and brain respond in an attempt to achieve normothermia, a normal temperature state. In pediatrics, there is a lack of consensus regarding what temperature constitutes normothermia for every child. For rectal temperatures in children, a value of 37° to 37.5° C (98.6° to 99.5° F) is an acceptable range, where heat loss and heat production are balanced. For neonates, a core body temperature between 36.5° and 37.6° C (97.7° and 99.7° F) is a desirable range. In the neonate, obtain temperature measurements for monitoring adequacy of thermoregulation, not fever; therefore temperature measurements in each infant should be carefully considered in the context of the *purpose* and the environment.

The nurse can measure temperature in healthy children at several body sites via oral, rectal, axillary, ear canal, tympanic membrane, temporal artery, or skin route (Box 6-10). For the ill child other sites for temperature measurement that have been investigated include the urinary bladder, pulmonary artery, and esophageal and nasopharyngeal sites (Martin and Kline, 2004) (Box 6-11). One of the most important influences on the accuracy of temperature is improper temperature-taking technique. Detailed discussion of temperature-taking methods and visual examples of proper techniques are given in Table 6-3. For a critical review of the evidence on temperature taking methods, see the Evidence-Based Practice box.

The most frequently used temperature measurement devices in infants and children are as follows (Healthcare Product Comparison System, 2004a, 2004b):

Electronic intermittent thermometers—Measure the patient's temperature at oral, rectal, and axillary sites and are used as primary diagnostic indicators

Infrared thermometers—Measure the patient's temperature by collecting emitted thermal radiation from a particular site (e.g., ear canal)

Electronic continuous thermometers—Measure the patient's temperature during the administration of

Text continued on p. 148.

BOX 6-10   RECOMMENDED TEMPERATURE SCREENING ROUTES IN INFANTS AND CHILDREN

Birth to 2 Years
Axillary
Rectal—if definitive temperature reading is needed for infants over 1 month of age

2 to 5 Years
Axillary
Tympanic
Oral—when child can hold thermometer under tongue
Rectal—if definitive temperature reading is needed

Over 5 Years
Oral
Axillary
Tympanic

BOX 6-11   ALTERNATIVE TEMPERATURE MEASUREMENT SITES FOR THE ILL CHILD

Skin
Probe is placed on the skin to determine heat output in response to changes in the patient's skin temperature.
Skin temperature sensors are most often used for neonates and infants placed in radiant heat warmers or isolettes (using servocontrol feature of the apparatus). In turn, the heater unit warms to a set point to maintain the infant's temperature within a specified range.
ThermoSpot is an example of a device allowing continuous thermal monitoring in neonates.

Urinary Bladder
A thermistor or thermocouple is placed within the indwelling bladder catheter. The catheter tip immersed in the bladder provides a continuous temperature read-out on the bedside monitor.
This is not a true measure of core temperature but responds better than rectal and skin temperatures to core body changes.
Because of thermistor sizes, this method is unusable with neonates and small infants.

Pulmonary Artery
A catheter is placed into the heart to obtain a reading in the pulmonary artery.
It is used in critical care settings or operating rooms only in patients requiring aggressive monitoring.
Catheter is not available in sizes for neonates or small infants.

Esophageal Site
Probe is inserted into the lower third of the esophagus at the level of the heart.
This is used in critical care settings or operating rooms.
Several companies have esophageal stethoscopes with temperature probe monitors for patients in the operating room that show a continuous temperature reading.

Nasopharyngeal Site
Probe is inserted into the nasopharynx, posterior to the soft palate, and provides an estimate of hypothalamic temperature.
This is used in critical care settings or operating rooms.

Data from Kumar PR, Nisarga R, Gowda B: Temperature monitoring in newborns using ThermoSpot, *Indian J Pediatr* 71(9):795-796, 2004; Martin SA, Kline AM: Can there be a standard for temperature measurement in the pediatric intensive care unit? *AACN Clin Issues* 15(2):254-266, 2004; and Maxton FJC, Justin L, Gilles D: Estimating core temperature in infants and children after cardiac surgery: a comparison of six methods, *J Adv Nurs* 45(2):214-222, 2004.

| TABLE 6-3 | TEMPERATURE MEASUREMENT LOCATIONS FOR INFANTS AND CHILDREN |

TEMPERATURE SITE

Oral

Place tip under tongue in right or left posterior sublingual pocket, not in front of tongue. Have child keep mouth closed, without biting on thermometer.

Pacifier thermometers measure intraoral or supralingual temperature and are available but lack support in the literature.

Several factors affect mouth temperature: eating and mastication, hot or cold beverages, open-mouth breathing, ambient temperature.

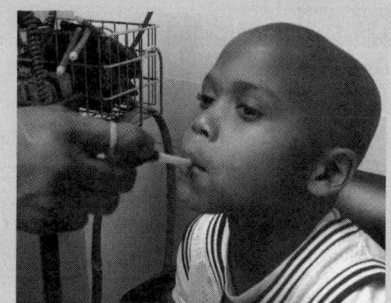

Axillary

Place tip under arm in center of axilla and keep close to skin, not clothing. Hold child's arm firmly against side. Temperature may be affected by poor peripheral perfusion (results in lower value), clothing or swaddling, use of radiant warmer, or amount of brown fat in cold-stressed neonate (results in higher value).

Advantage—Avoids intrusive procedure and eliminates risk of rectal perforation.

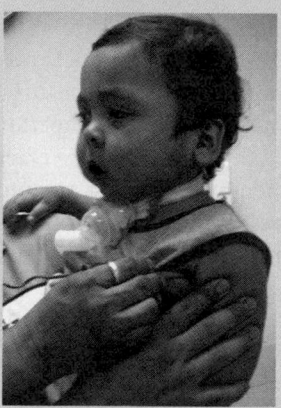

Ear Based (Aural)

Insert small infrared probe deeply into canal to allow sensor to obtain measurement. Size of probe (most are 8 mm) may influence accuracy of result. In young children this may be a problem because of small diameter of canal. Proper placement of ear is controversial related to whether the pinna should be pulled in manner similar to that used during otoscopy (see p. 160).

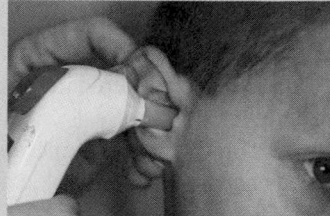

Rectal

Place well-lubricated tip at maximum 2.5 cm (1 inch) into rectum for children and 1.5 cm (0.6 inch) for infants; securely hold thermometer close to anus.

Child may be placed in side-lying, supine, or prone position (i.e., supine with knees flexed toward abdomen); cover penis, since procedure may stimulate urination. A small child may be placed prone across parent's lap.

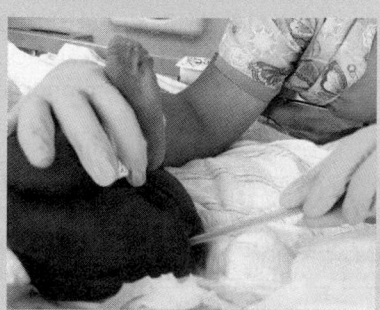

Temporal Artery

An infrared sensor probe scans across forehead, capturing heat from arterial blood flow. Temporal artery is only artery close enough to skin's surface to provide access for accurate temperature measurement.

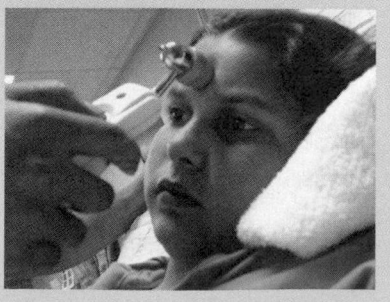

Data from Martin SA, Kline AM: Can there be a standard for temperature measurement in the pediatric intensive care unit? *AACN Clin Issues* 15(2):254-266, 2004; and Falzon A, Grech V, Caruana B, et al: How reliable is axillary temperature measurement? *Acta Paediatr* 92(3):309-313, 2003. Oral, axillary, rectal, and temporal artery images courtesy Paul Vincent Kuntz, Texas Children's Hospital, Houston.

EVIDENCE-BASED PRACTICE

Temperature Measurement in Pediatrics

ASK THE QUESTION

In infants and children, what is the most accurate method for measuring temperature?

SEARCH FOR THE EVIDENCE

Search strategies

Clinical research studies related to this issue were identified by searching for English publications within past 10 years, research-based articles (level 3 or lower), infant and child populations, comparisons to gold standard: rectal thermometry.

Databases used

PubMed, Cochrane Collaboration, MD Consult, Joanna Briggs Institute, National Guideline Clearinghouse (AHRQ), TRIP Database Plus, PedsCCM, BestBETs

CRITICALLY ANALYZE THE EVIDENCE

GRADE criteria: Evidence quality moderate; recommendation strong (Guyatt, Oxman, Vist, et al, 2008)

Rectal temperature—Rectal measurement remains the clinical gold standard for the precise diagnosis of fever in infants and children (Greenes and Fleisher, 2004; Riddell and Eppich, 2003; University of Michigan, 2003). However, this procedure is more invasive and is contraindicated for infants less than 1 month old, children with recent rectal surgery, children with diarrhea or anorectal lesions, and children receiving chemotherapy (cancer treatment usually affects mucosa and causes neutropenia). Findings are affected by depth of insertion and presence of stool. Rectal temperatures are slow to change in relation to changing core temperature. Many parents are uncomfortable with this method, and children may resent it. It has capacity to spread contaminants found in stool.

Oral temperature (OTs)—OT indicates rapid changes in core body temperature, but accuracy may be an issue when compared with the rectal site (Jensen, Jensen, Madsen, et al, 2000). OTs are considered the standard for temperature measurement (Gilbert, Barton, and Counsell, 2002), but are contraindicated in children who have an altered level of consciousness, are receiving oxygen, are mouth breathing, are experiencing mucositis, had recent oral surgery or trauma, or are under 5 years of age (Carroll, 2000; El-Radhi and Barry, 2006). Limitations of OTs include the effects of ambient room temperature and recent oral intake (Carroll, 2000; Martin and Kline, 2004). Even patients with no obvious mouth breathing were found to have OTs in the normal range despite the presence of clinical fever (Tandberg and Sklar, 1983). O'Brien, Rogers, Holden, and colleagues (2000) found OT-predictive thermometers to read significantly lower than other core temperature measurements and miss one out of seven fevers.

Axillary temperature—This is inconsistent and insensitive in infants and children over 1 month old (Jean-Mary, Dicanzio, Shaw, et al, 2002; Falzon, Grech, Caruana, et al, 2003). In neonates with fever the axillary temperature cannot be used interchangeably with rectal measurement (Muller, van Berkel, and de Beaufort, 2008). Despite its low sensitivity and specificity in detecting fever, the axillary site is recommended by the American Academy of Pediatrics (2001) as a screening test for fever in infants 1 month of age.

Ear (aural) temperature—This is not a precise measurement of body temperature. Meta-analysis of 101 studies comparing tympanic membrane temperatures with rectal temperatures in children concluded that the tympanic method demonstrated a wide range of variability, limiting its application in a pediatric setting (Craig, Lancaster, Taylor, et al, 2002). More recently published reviews continue to find poor sensitivity using infrared ear thermometry (Dodd, Lancaster, Craig, et al, 2006). Diagnosis of fever without a focus should not be made based on tympanic thermometry, since it is not an accurate measure of core temperature (Dodd, Lancaster, Craig, et al, 2006; Craig, Lancaster, Taylor, et al, 2002; Riddell and Eppich, 2003).

Temporal artery temperature (TAT)—TAT was not predictable for fever in children under 3 months but could be used as a screening tool for detecting fever less than 38° C (100.4° F) in children 3 to 24 months old (Schuh, Komar, Stephens, et al, 2004). Temporal temperature can be used as a rapid assessment screening tool to identify rectal fever over 39° C (102.2° F) in children 3 to 24 months old, but is unreliable as a screening tool for infants under 3 months (Siberry, Diener-West, Schappell, et al, 2002). These published studies examining the accuracy and precision of TATs in infants and children are limited by small sample sizes. Previous samples included subjects primarily under the age of 36 months, although one abstract was found of a study that examined 75 TATs in children 6 to 12 years old (Pidwell, Heavrin, Santen, et al, 2000). Settings that have been used to study TATs in pediatric patients include the emergency center (Greenes and Fleisher, 2001; Pidwell, Heavrin, Santen, et al, 2000; Schuh, Komar, Stephens, et al, 2004; Siberry, Diener-West, Schappell, et al, 2002), physician's office (Callanan, 2003), pediatric intensive care unit (Hebbar, Fortenberry, Rogers, et al, 2005), and operating room (Al-Mukhaizeem, Allen, Komar, et al, 2004).

APPLY THE EVIDENCE: NURSING IMPLICATIONS

- No single site used for temperature assessment provides unequivocal estimates of core body temperature.
- Studies show that the axillary and tympanic measures demonstrate poor agreement when these modes are compared with more accurate core temperature methods. The differences are more evident as temperature increases, regardless of age.
- When an accurate method for obtaining a correct reflection of core temperature is needed, the rectal temperature is recommended in younger children and the oral route in older children.
- For infants less than 1 month of age, the American Academy of Pediatrics (2001) recommends axillary temperatures.

References

Al-Mukhaizeem F, Allen U, Komar L, et al: Comparison of temporal artery, rectal and esophageal core temperatures in children: results of a pilot study, *Paediatr Child Health* 9(7):461-465, 2004.

American Academy of Pediatrics, Committee on Environmental Health: Technical report: mercury in the environment: implications for pediatricians, *Pediatrics* 108(1):197-205, 2001.

Callanan D: Detecting fever in young infants: reliability of perceived, pacifier, and temporal artery temperatures in infants younger than 3 months of age, *Pediatr Emerg Care* 19(4):240-243, 2003.

Carroll M: An evaluation of temperature measurement, *Nurs Stand* 14(44):39-43, 2000.

Craig JV, Lancaster GA, Taylor S, et al: Infrared ear thermometry compared with rectal thermometry in children: a systemic review, *Lancet* 360:603-609, 2002.

Dodd SR, Lancaster GA, Craig JV, et al: In a systematic review, infrared ear thermometry for fever diagnosis in children finds poor sensitivity, *J Clin Epidemiol* 59:354-357, 2006.

El-Radhi AS, Barry W: Thermometry in paediatric practice, *Arch Dis Child* 91(4):351-356, 2006.

Falzon A, Grech V, Caruana B, et al: How reliable is axillary temperature measurement? *Acta Paediatr* 92(3):309-313, 2003.

Gilbert M, Barton AJ, Counsell CM: Comparison of oral and tympanic temperatures in adult surgical patients, *Appl Nurs Res* 15(1):42-47, 2002.

Greenes DS, Fleisher GR: When body temperature changes, does rectal temperature lag? *J Pediatr* 144(6):824-826, 2004.

Greenes DS, Fleisher GR: Accuracy of a noninvasive temporal artery thermometer for use in infants, *Arch Pediatr Adolesc Med* 155(3):376-381, 2001.

Continued

EVIDENCE-BASED PRACTICE—cont'd

Temperature Measurement in Pediatrics

References—cont'd

Guyatt GH, Oxman AD, Vist GE, et al: GRADE: an emerging consensus on rating quality of evidence and strength of recommendations, *BMJ* 336: 924-926, 2008.

Hebbar K, Fortenberry JD, Rogers K, et al: Comparison of temporal artery thermometer to standard temperature measurement in pediatric intensive care unit patients, *Pediatr Crit Care Med* 6(5):557-561, 2005.

Jean-Mary MB, Dicanzio J, Shaw J, et al: Limited accuracy and reliability of infrared axillary and aural thermometers in a pediatric outpatient population, *J Pediatr* 141(5):671-676, 2002.

Jensen BN, Jensen FS, Madsen SN, et al: Accuracy of digital tympanic, oral, axillary, and rectal thermometers compared with standard rectal mercury thermometers, *Eur J Surg* 166(11):848-851, 2000.

Martin SA, Kline AM: Can there be a standard for temperature measurement in the pediatric intensive care unit? *AACN Clin Issues* 15(2):254-266, 2004.

Muller PCE, van Berkel LH, de Beaufort AJ: Axillary and rectal temperature measurements poorly agree in newborn infants, *Neonatology* 94:31-34, 2008.

O'Brien DL, Rogers IR, Holden W, et al: The accuracy of oral predictive and infrared emission detection tympanic thermometers in an emergency department setting, *Acad Emerg Med* 7(9):1061-1064, 2000.

Pidwell WB, Heavrin BS, Santen SA, et al: Accuracy of temporal artery thermometer (abstract), *Ann Emerg Med* 36(4):S5, 2000.

Riddell A, Eppich W: Should tympanic temperature measurement be trusted? BestBETs, 2003, available at www.bestbets.org/cgi-bin/bets.pl?record=00340 (accessed April 2005).

Schuh S, Komar L, Stephens D, et al: Comparison of the temporal artery and rectal thermometry in children in the emergency department, *Pediatr Emerg Care* 20(11):736-741, 2004.

Siberry GK, Diener-West M, Schappell E, et al: Comparison of temple temperatures with rectal temperatures in children under 2 years of age, *Clin Pediatr* 41(6):405-414, 2002.

Tandberg D, Sklar D: Effect of tachypnea on the estimation of body temperature by an oral thermometer, *N Engl J Med* 308(16):945-946, 1983.

University of Michigan: Rectal temperature is still the gold standard for determining the presence or absence of fever, Evidence-Based Pediatrics Web Site, 2003, available at www.med.umich.edu/pediatrics/ebm/cats/fever.htm (accessed April 2005).

BOX 6-12 **TYPES OF THERMOMETERS USED TO MEASURE TEMPERATURE IN INFANTS AND CHILDREN**

Electronic Thermometer

Temperature is sensed with an electronic component called thermistor mounted at the tip of a plastic and stainless steel probe, which is connected to an electronic recorder. A disposable plastic cover is used for infection control.

Temperature measurement appears on digital display within 60 seconds.

Probe can be placed in mouth, axilla, or rectum.

Infrared Thermometer

Thermal radiation is measured from axilla, ear canal, or tympanic membrane.

Temperature measurement appears on digital display in approximately 1 second.

Three types are available for ear-based use: tympanic, ear canal, and arterial heat balance via the ear canal (AHBE).

Often these devices are all inappropriately referred to as *tympanic thermometers*.

Temperatures measured in this way reflect arterial (bloodstream) temperature.

Ear-Based Temperature Sensor

Although this is frequently used in pediatric settings (especially ambulatory clinics), debate continues on the reliability of ear-based thermometry in screening febrile children.

Most models use "offsets" for internal calculations that transform ear temperature into supposedly equivalent oral or rectal temperatures.

Ear Sensor (LighTouch LTX)

This measures the infrared heat energy radiating from canal opening, scans canal for highest temperature reading, and then calculates arterial temperature (correlates highly with core or internal body temperature).

It is available in two sizes; smaller size of LighTouch Pedi-Q is for infants and toddlers.

Axillary Sensor (LighTouch LTN)

This measures the infrared heat energy radiating from the axilla.

It can be used on wet skin; in incubators; or under radiant heaters, warming pads, or other heat sources.

Digital Thermometer

A probe is connected to a microprocessor chip, which translates signals into degrees and sends temperature measurement to digital display.

It is used like an oral electronic thermometer and can be used for measuring oral, rectal, and axillary temperature.

It is more accurate and easier to read, but somewhat more expensive, than plastic strip thermometer.

Liquid Crystal Skin Contact Thermometer (Chemical Dot Thermometer)

This single-use, disposable, flexible thermometer has a specific chemical mixture in each circle that changes color to measure temperature increments of $\frac{2}{10}$ of a degree.

There are two types:

1. Kept in mouth (1 minute), axilla (3 minutes), or rectum (3 minutes); color change is read 10 to 15 seconds after removing thermometer
2. Wearable, continuous-use thermometer, which is placed under axilla; may be read within 2 to 3 minutes after placement and continuously thereafter; discard and replace every 48 hours

---

general anesthesia, treatment of hypothermia or hyperthermia, and other situations that require continuous monitoring

Box 6-12 provides a detailed description of these devices.

! **NURSING ALERT**

The belief that core temperature can be estimated by adding 1° C to the temperature taken in the axilla is incorrect. Do not add a degree to the finding obtained by taking a temperature by the axillary route (Craig, Lancaster, Williamson, et al, 2000).

Pulse

A satisfactory pulse can be taken radially in children older than 2 years of age. However, in infants and young children, the apical impulse (heard through a stethoscope held to the chest at the apex of the heart) is more reliable (see Fig. 6-33 for location of pulses). Count the pulse for 1 full minute in infants and young children because of possible irregularities in rhythm. However, when frequent apical rates are necessary, use shorter counting times (e.g., 15- or 30-second intervals). For greater accuracy, measure the apical rate while the child is asleep; record the child's behavior along with the rate. Grade pulses

TABLE 6-4	GRADING OF PULSES
GRADE	**DESCRIPTION**
0	Not palpable
+1	Difficult to palpate, thready, weak, easily obliterated with pressure
+2	Difficult to palpate, may be obliterated with pressure
+3	Easy to palpate, not easily obliterated with pressure (normal)
+4	Strong, bounding, not obliterated with pressure

TABLE 6-5	NORMATIVE DINAMAP BLOOD PRESSURE VALUES (SYSTOLIC/ DIASTOLIC; MEAN ARTERIAL PRESSURE IN PARENTHESES)		
AGE-GROUP	**MEAN**	**90th PERCENTILE**	**95th PERCENTILE**
Newborn (1-3 days)	65/41 (50)	75/49 (59)	78/52 (62)
1 month-2 years	95/58 (72)	106/68 (83)	110/71 (86)
2-5 years	101/57 (74)	112/66 (82)	115/68 (85)

From Park M, Menard S: Normative oscillometric blood pressure values in the first 5 years in an office setting, *Am J Dis Child* 143(7):860-864, 1989.

according to the criteria in Table 6-4. Compare radial and femoral pulses at least once during infancy to detect the presence of circulatory impairment, such as coarctation of the aorta. (See inside back cover for normal rates for pediatric age-groups.)

Respiration

Count the respiratory rate in children in the same manner as for the adult patient. However, in infants observe abdominal movements, since respirations are primarily diaphragmatic. Because the movements are irregular, count them for 1 full minute for accuracy (see also p. 164). (See inside back cover for normal respiratory rates in children.)

Blood Pressure

Blood pressure (BP) measurement by noninvasive methods is part of a routine vital sign determination. Measure BP annually in children 3 years of age through adolescence and in children with symptoms of hypertension, children in emergency departments and intensive care units, and high-risk infants (National High Blood Pressure Education Program Working Group on High Blood Pressure in Children and Adolescents, 2004).

Measurement Devices

Ambulatory BP monitoring in children and adolescents is a valuable method for assessing and managing suspected hypertension (Bald, 2002). Also measure BP using electronic devices that employ oscillometric or Doppler techniques. In oscillometry, pressure changes are transmitted through the arterial wall to the pressure cuff, and the oscillations are detected by a pressure-sensitive indicator. Oscillometers have digital read-outs for systolic, diastolic, and mean arterial pressures (MAP) and for pulse. The MAP is not the same as the mean BP (arithmetic average of systolic and diastolic pressures). Rather, it is a value somewhat lower than the arithmetic mean. BP readings using oscillometry, such as Dinamap, are generally higher (10 mm Hg higher) than measurements using auscultation (Park, Menard, and Schoolfield, 2005) (Table 6-5). Differences between Dinamap and auscultatory readings prevent the interchange of the readings by the two methods. The oscillometric BP monitoring method is a reliable screening tool used in a variety of age-groups (Mattu, Heran, and Wright, 2004a, 2004b).

Doppler ultrasound translates changes in ultrasound frequency caused by blood movement within the artery to audible sound by means of a transducer in the cuff. This technique is useful for systolic pressure measurement but is unreliable for diastolic pressure measurement. Oscillometric and Doppler instruments are useful in measuring BP in infants and have largely replaced the flush method, which reflects only the mean BP, and the auscultatory method.

Selection of Cuff

No matter what type of noninvasive technique is used, the most important factor in accurately measuring BP is the use of an appropriately sized cuff (cuff size refers only to the inner inflatable bladder, not the cloth covering). A technique to establish an appropriate cuff size is to choose a cuff with a bladder width that is approximately 40% of the arm circumference midway between the olecranon and the acromion (see Research Focus box). This will usually be a cuff bladder that covers 80% to 100% of the circumference of the arm (Fig. 6-12) (Beevers, Lip, and O'Brien, 2001; National Institutes of Health, National Heart, Lung, and Blood Institute, 1996). Cuffs that are either too narrow or too wide affect the accuracy of BP measurements. If the cuff size is too small, the reading on the device is falsely high. If the cuff size is too large, the reading is falsely low (Clark, Kieh-Lai, Sarnaik, et al, 2002).

RESEARCH FOCUS

Selection of a Blood Pressure Cuff

Researchers have found that selection of a cuff with a bladder width equal to 40% of the upper arm circumference most accurately reflects directly measured radial arterial pressure (Clark, Kieh-Lai, Sarnaik, et al, 2002).

Using limb circumference for selecting cuff width more accurately reflects direct arterial BP than using limb length, since this method takes into account variations in arm thickness and the amount of pressure required to compress the artery. For measurement on sites other than the upper arms, use the limb circumference, although the shape of the limb (e.g., conical shape of the thigh) may prevent appropriate placement of the cuff and inaccurately reflect intraarterial BP (Table 6-6).

When using a site other than the arm, BP measurements using noninvasive techniques may differ. Generally, systolic pressure in the lower extremities (thigh or calf) is greater than pressure in the upper extremities, and systolic BP in the calf is higher than that in the thigh (Fig. 6-13). Table 6-7 lists these differences that are applied to oscillometric measurements taken on the right extremities with the child supine and the cuff size based on the circumference method.

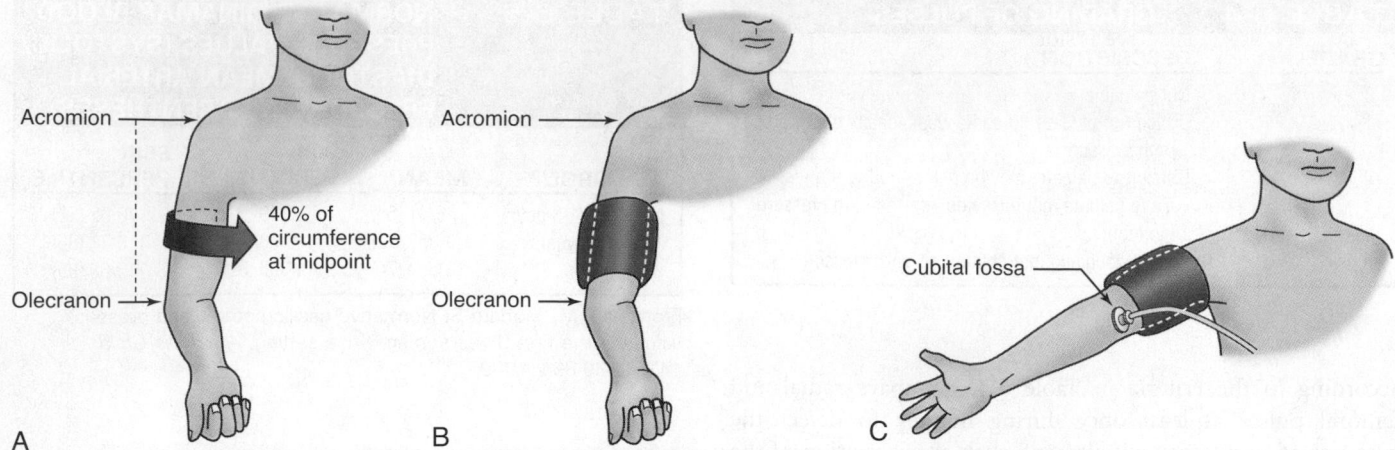

Fig. 6-12 Determination of proper cuff size. **A,** Cuff bladder width should be approximately 40% of circumference of arm measured at a point midway between olecranon and acromion. **B,** Cuff bladder length should cover 80% to 100% of circumference of arm. **C,** Blood pressure should be measured with cubital fossa at heart level. Arm should be supported. Stethoscope bell is placed over brachial artery pulse, proximal and medial to cubital fossa and below bottom edge of cuff. (From National Institutes of Health, National Heart, Lung, and Blood Institute: *Update on the Task Force Report [1987] on high blood pressure in children and adolescents: a working group report from the National High Blood Pressure Education Program*, NIH Pub No 96-3790, Bethesda, Md, September 1996, The Institutes.)

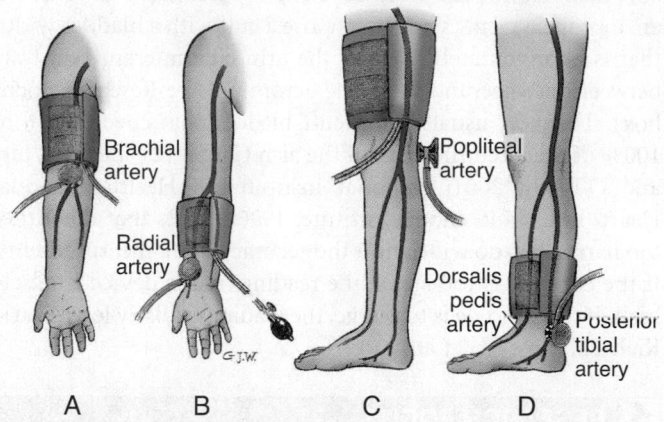

Fig. 6-13 Sites for measuring blood pressure. **A,** Upper arm. **B,** Lower arm or forearm. **C,** Thigh. **D,** Calf or ankle.

TABLE 6-7	DIFFERENCES IN OSCILLOMETRIC SYSTOLIC BLOOD PRESSURE BETWEEN ARM AND LOWER EXTREMITY SITES IN NORMAL CHILDREN	
AGE-GROUP (yr)	**SYSTOLIC BLOOD PRESSURE × (MEAN ± SD)**	
	ARM-THIGH	**ARM-CALF**
4-8	−7.1 ± 6.8	−9.3 ± 7.4
9-16	−2.4 ± 7.7	−5.0 ± 26.9

From Park M, Lee D, Johnson GA: Oscillometric blood pressures in the arm, thigh, and calf in healthy children and those with aortic coarctation, *Pediatrics* 91(4):761-765, 1993.

! NURSING ALERT

When taking BP, use an appropriately sized cuff. When the correct size is not available, use an oversized cuff rather than an undersized one or use another site that more appropriately fits the cuff size. Do not choose a cuff based on the name of the cuff (e.g., an "infant" cuff may be too small for some infants).

TABLE 6-6	RECOMMENDED DIMENSIONS FOR BLOOD PRESSURE CUFF BLADDERS		
AGE	**WIDTH (cm)**	**LENGTH (cm)**	**MAXIMUM ARM CIRCUMFERENCE (cm)***
Newborn	4	8	10
Infant	6	12	15
Child	9	18	22
Small adult	10	24	26
Adult	13	30	34
Large adult	16	38	44
Thigh	20	42	52

From National High Blood Pressure Education Program Working Group on High Blood Pressure in Children and Adolescents: The fourth report on the diagnosis, evaluation, and treatment of high blood pressure in children and adolescents, *Pediatrics* 114(2 Suppl 4th Rep):555-576, 2004.
*Calculated so that largest arm would still allow bladder to encircle arm by at least 80%.

Measurement and Interpretation

Measuring and interpreting BP in infants and children require attention to correct procedure because (1) limb sizes vary and cuff selection must accommodate the circumference; (2) excessive pressure on the antecubital fossa affects the Korotkoff sounds; (3) children easily become anxious, which can elevate BP; and (4) BP values change with age and growth. In children and adolescents, determine the normal range of BP by body size and age. BP standards that are based on gender, age, and height provide a more precise classification of BP according to body size. This approach avoids misclassifying children who are very tall or very short. The revised BP tables now include the 50th,

90th, 95th, and 99th percentiles (with standard deviations) by gender, age, and height (see inside back cover).

> **! NURSING ALERT**
>
> Compare BP in the upper and lower extremities to detect abnormalities, such as coarctation of the aorta, in which the lower extremity pressure is less than the upper extremity pressure.

To use the tables in a clinical setting, determine the height percentile by using the newly revised Centers for Disease Control and Prevention growth charts (www.cdc.gov/growthcharts). The child's measured systolic BP and diastolic BP are compared with the numbers provided in the table (boys or girls) according to the child's age and height percentile. The child is normotensive if the BP is below the 90th percentile. If the BP is at or above the 90th percentile, repeat the BP measurement at that visit to verify an elevated BP. BP measurements between the 90th and 95th percentiles indicate prehypertension and necessitate reassessment and consideration of other risk factors. In addition, if an adolescent's BP is more than 120/80 mm Hg, consider the patient prehypertensive even if this value is below the 90th percentile. This BP level typically occurs for systolic BP at 12 years old and for diastolic BP at 16 years old. If the child's BP (systolic or diastolic) is at or above the 95th percentile, the child may be hypertensive, and the measurement must be repeated on at least two occasions to confirm diagnosis (National High Blood Pressure Education Program Working Group on High Blood Pressure in Children and Adolescents, 2004) (see Nursing Care Guidelines box).

> **📋 NURSING CARE GUIDELINES**
>
> ***Using the Blood Pressure Tables***
>
> 1. Use the standard height charts to determine the height percentile.
> 2. Measure and record the child's systolic blood pressure (SBP) and diastolic blood pressure (DBP).
> 3. Use the correct gender table for SBP and DBP.
> 4. Find the child's age on the left side of the table. Follow the age row horizontally across the table to the intersection of the line for the height percentile (vertical column).
> 5. There, find the 50th, 90th, 95th, and 99th percentiles for SBP in the left columns and for DBP in the right columns.
>   - BP less than 90th percentile is normal.
>   - BP between the 90th and 95th percentiles is prehypertension. In adolescents, BP of 120/80 mm Hg or greater is prehypertension, even if this figure is less than the 90th percentile.
>   - BP over the 95th percentile may be hypertension.
> 6. If the BP is over the 90th percentile, the BP should be repeated twice at the same office visit, and an average SBP and DBP should be used.
> 7. If the BP is over the 95th percentile, BP should be staged. If BP is stage 1 (95th to 99th percentile plus 5 mm Hg), BP measurements should be repeated on two more occasions. If hypertension is confirmed, evaluation should proceed. If BP is stage 2 (>99th percentile plus 5 mm Hg), prompt referral should be made for evaluation and therapy. If the patient is symptomatic, immediate referral and treatment are indicated.
>
> From National High Blood Pressure Education Program Working Group on High Blood Pressure in Children and Adolescents: The fourth report on the diagnosis, evaluation, and treatment of high blood pressure in children and adolescents, *Pediatrics* 114(2 Suppl 4th Rep):555-576, 2004.

Orthostatic Hypotension

Orthostatic hypotension (OH), also called postural hypotension or orthostatic intolerance, often manifests as syncope (fainting), vertigo (dizziness), or lightheadedness and is caused by decreased blood flow to the brain (cerebral hypoperfusion). Normally blood flow to the brain is maintained at a constant level by a number of compensating mechanisms that regulate systemic BP. When one assumes a sitting or standing position from a supine or recumbent position, peripheral capillary vasoconstriction occurs, and blood that was pooling in the lower vasculature is returned to the heart for redistribution to the head and remainder of the body. When this mechanism fails or is slow to respond, the person may experience vertigo or syncope. One of the most common causes of OH is hypovolemia, which may be induced by medications such as diuretics, vasodilator medications, and prolonged immobility or bed rest. Other causes of OH include dehydration, diarrhea, emesis, fluid loss from sweating and exertion, alcohol intake, dysrhythmias, diabetes mellitus, sepsis, and hemorrhage.

BP measurements taken with the child supine then standing (at least 2 minutes in each position) may demonstrate variability and assist in the diagnosis of OH. The child with a sustained drop in systolic pressure of more than 20 mm Hg or in diastolic pressure of more than 10 mm Hg after standing for 2 minutes without an increase in heart rate of more than 15 beats/min most likely has an autonomic deficit. Nonneurogenic causes of OH have a compensatory increase in pulse of more than 15 beats/min as well as a drop in BP, as noted previously. For the child or adolescent with vertigo, lightheadedness, nausea, syncope, diaphoresis, and pallor, it is important to monitor BP and heart rate to determine the original cause. BP is an important diagnostic measurement in children and adolescents and must be a part of the routine monitoring of vital signs.

> **! NURSING ALERT**
>
> Published norms for BP, such as those on the inside back cover, are valid only if you use the same method of measurement (auscultation and cuff size determination) in clinical practice.

GENERAL APPEARANCE

The child's general appearance is a cumulative, subjective impression of the child's physical appearance, state of nutrition, behavior, personality, interactions with parents and nurse (also siblings if present), posture, development, and speech. Although the nurse records general appearance at the beginning of the physical examination, it encompasses all the observations of the child during the interview and physical assessment.

Note the facies, the child's facial expression and appearance. For example, the facies may give clues to children who are in pain; have difficulty breathing; feel frightened, discontented, or unhappy; are mentally delayed; or are acutely ill.

Observe the posture, position, and types of body movement. The child with hearing or vision loss may characteristically tilt the head in an awkward position to hear or see better. The child in pain may favor a body part. The child with low self-esteem or a feeling of rejection may assume a slumped, careless, and apathetic pose. Likewise, a child with confidence, a feeling of self-worth, and a sense of security usually demonstrates a tall, straight, well-balanced posture. While observing such body language, do not interpret too freely but rather record objectively.

Note the child's hygiene in terms of cleanliness; unusual body odor; the condition of the hair, neck, nails, teeth, and feet; and the condition of the clothing. Such observations are excellent clues to possible instances of neglect, inadequate financial resources, housing difficulties (e.g., no running water), or lack of knowledge concerning children's needs.

Behavior includes the child's personality, activity level, reaction to stress, requests, frustration, interactions with others (primarily the parent and nurse), degree of alertness, and response to stimuli. Some mental questions that serve as reminders for observing behavior include: What is the child's overall personality? Does the child have a long attention span, or is he or she easily distracted? Can the child follow two or three commands in succession without the need for repetition? What is the youngster's response to delayed gratification or frustration? Does the child use eye contact during conversation? What is the child's reaction to the nurse and family members? Is the child quick or slow to grasp explanations?

Development can be assessed by carefully observing the child, but verify your impressions with screening tests. This chapter and Chapter 24 discuss various tests for assessing development, speech, vision, and hearing.

Under general appearance, record an overall estimate of the child's speech development, motor skills, coordination, and recent area of achievement. For example, the following statement may apply to an 18-month-old child: "Motor development advanced for age; climbs, runs, jumps (most recent motor skill), manipulates small objects with ease; excellent coordination and balance; beginning to name many objects; uses two-word phrases; and enjoys 'talking' to self and others."

SKIN

Assess skin for color, texture, temperature, moisture, turgor, lesions, and rashes. Examination of the skin and its accessory organs primarily involves inspection and palpation. Touch allows the nurse to assess the texture, turgor, and temperature of the skin (Turnbull, 2000). The normal color in light-skinned children varies from a milky white and rose to a deeply hued pink. Dark-skinned children, such as those of Native American, Hispanic, or African descent, have inherited various brown, red, yellow, olive green, and bluish tones in their skin. Asian persons have skin that is normally of a yellow tone. Several variations in skin color can occur, some of which warrant further investigation. The types of color change and their appearance in children with light or dark skin are summarized in Table 6-8.

Normally the skin texture of young children is smooth, slightly dry, and not oily or clammy. Evaluate skin temperature by symmetrically feeling each part of the body and comparing upper areas with lower ones. Note any difference in temperature.

Determine tissue turgor, or elasticity in the skin, by grasping the skin on the abdomen between the thumb and index finger, pulling it taut, and quickly releasing it. Elastic tissue immediately resumes its normal position without residual marks or creases. In children with poor skin turgor, the skin remains suspended or tented for a few seconds before slowly falling back on the abdomen. Skin turgor is one of the best estimates of adequate hydration and nutrition.

Accessory Structures

Inspection of the accessory structures of the skin may be performed while examining the skin, scalp, or extremities.

Inspect the hair for color, texture, quality, distribution, and elasticity. Children's scalp hair is usually lustrous, silky, strong,

TABLE 6-8	DIFFERENCES IN COLOR CHANGES OF RACIAL GROUPS	
DESCRIPTION	**APPEARANCE IN LIGHT SKIN**	**APPEARANCE IN DARK SKIN**
Cyanosis—Bluish tone through skin; reflects reduced (deoxygenated) hemoglobin	Bluish tinge, especially in palpebral conjunctiva (lower eyelid), nail beds, earlobes, lips, oral membranes, soles, and palms	Ashen gray lips and tongue
Pallor—Paleness; may be sign of anemia, chronic disease, edema, or shock	Loss of rosy glow in skin, especially face	Ashen gray appearance in black skin; More yellowish brown color in brown skin
Erythema—Redness; may be result of increased blood flow from climatic conditions, local inflammation, infection, skin irritation, allergy, or other dermatoses, or may be caused by increased numbers of red blood cells as compensatory response to chronic hypoxia	Redness easily seen anywhere on body	Much more difficult to assess; rely on palpation for warmth or edema
Ecchymosis—Large, diffuse areas, usually black and blue, caused by hemorrhage of blood into skin; typically result of injuries	Purplish to yellow-green areas; may be seen anywhere on skin	Very difficult to see unless in mouth or conjunctiva
Petechiae—Same as ecchymosis except for size: small, distinct, pinpoint hemorrhages ≤2 mm in size; can denote some type of blood disorder, such as leukemia	Purplish pinpoints most easily seen on buttocks, abdomen, and inner surfaces of arms or legs	Usually invisible except in oral mucosa, conjunctiva of eyelids, and conjunctiva covering eyeball
Jaundice—Yellow staining of skin usually caused by bile pigments	Yellow staining seen in sclerae of eyes, skin, fingernails, soles, palms, and oral mucosa	Most reliably assessed in sclerae, hard palate, palms, and soles

and elastic. Genetic factors affect the appearance of hair. For example, the hair of African-American children is usually curlier and coarser than that of Caucasian children. Hair that is stringy, dull, brittle, dry, friable, and depigmented may suggest poor nutrition. Record any bald or thinning spots. Loss of hair in infants may indicate lying in the same position and may be a cue to counsel parents concerning the child's stimulation needs.

Inspect the hair and scalp for general cleanliness. Persons in some ethnic groups condition their hair with oils or lubricants that, if not thoroughly washed from the scalp, clog the sebaceous glands, causing scalp infections. Also examine the area for lesions; scaliness; evidence of infestation, such as lice or ticks; and signs of trauma, such as ecchymosis, masses, or scars.

In children who are approaching puberty, look for growth of secondary hair as a sign of normally progressing pubertal changes. Note precocious or delayed appearance of hair growth because, although not always suggestive of hormonal dysfunction, it may be of great concern to the early- or late-maturing adolescent.

Inspect the nails for color, shape, texture, and quality. Normally the nails are pink, convex, smooth, and hard but flexible (not brittle). The edges, which are usually white, should extend over the fingers. Dark-skinned individuals may have more deeply pigmented nail beds. Short, ragged nails are typical of habitual biting. Uncut, dirty nails are a sign of poor hygiene.

The palm normally shows three flexion creases (Fig. 6-14, *A*). In some situations such as Down syndrome, the two distal horizontal creases are fused to form a single horizontal crease (the **single palmar crease**, or **transpalmar crease**) (Fig. 6-14, *B*). If grossly abnormal lines or folds are observed, sketch a picture to describe them and refer the finding to a specialist for further investigation.

LYMPH NODES

Lymph nodes are usually assessed during examination of the part of the body in which they are located. The body's lymphatic drainage system is extensive. Fig. 6-15 shows the usual sites for palpating accessible lymph nodes.

Palpate nodes using the distal portion of the fingers and gently but firmly pressing in a circular motion along the regions where nodes are normally present. During assessment of the nodes in the head and neck, tilt the child's head upward slightly but without tensing the sternocleidomastoid or trapezius muscles. This position facilitates palpation of the **submental, submandibular, tonsillar,** and **cervical nodes.** Palpate the **axillary nodes** with the child's arms relaxed at the sides but slightly abducted. Assess the **inguinal nodes** with the child in the supine position.

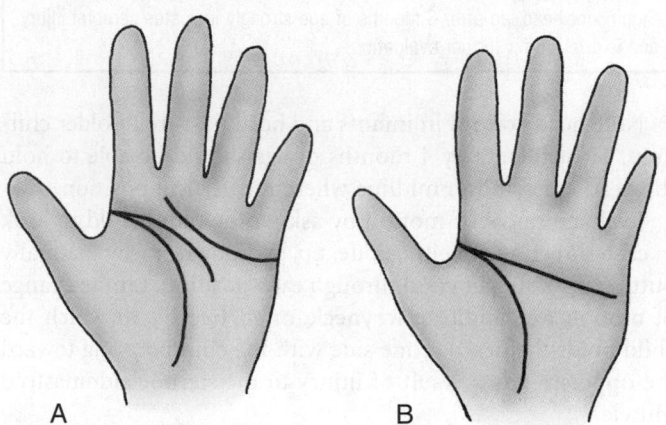

Fig. 6-14 Examples of flexion creases on palm. **A,** Normal. **B,** Transpalmar crease.

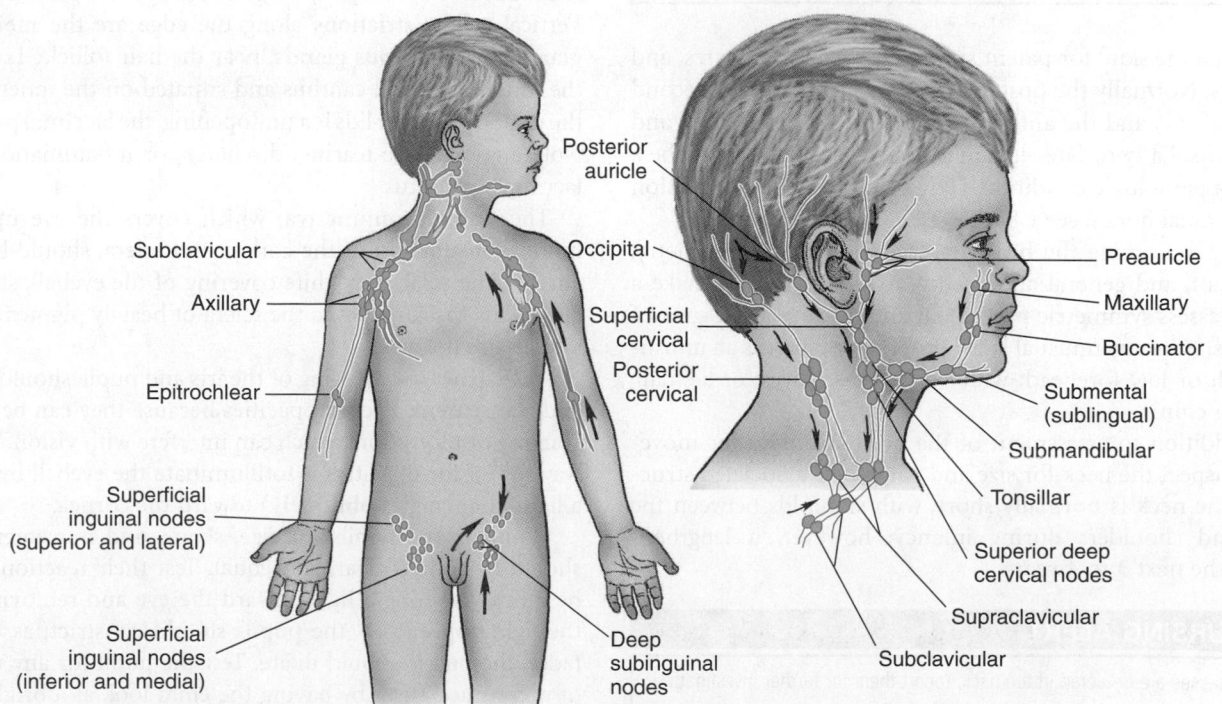

Fig. 6-15 Location of superficial lymph nodes. *Arrows* indicate directional flow of lymph.

Note size, mobility, temperature, and tenderness, as well as reports by the parents regarding any visible change of enlarged nodes. In children, small, nontender, movable nodes are usually normal. Tender, enlarged, warm, erythematous lymph nodes generally indicate infection or inflammation close to their location. Report such findings for further investigation.

HEAD AND NECK

⊖ Observe the head for general shape and symmetry. A flattening of one part of the head, such as the occiput, may indicate that the child continually lies in this position. Marked asymmetry is usually abnormal and may indicate premature closure of the sutures (**craniosynostosis**).

> **! NURSING ALERT**
>
> Significant head lag after 6 months of age strongly indicates cerebral injury and is referred for further evaluation.

Note head control in infants and head posture in older children. Most infants by 4 months of age should be able to hold the head erect and in midline when in a vertical position.

Evaluate range of motion by asking the older child to look in each direction (to either side, up, and down) or by manually putting the younger child through each position. Limited range of motion may indicate **wryneck**, or **torticollis**, in which the child holds the head to one side with the chin pointing toward the opposite side a result of injury to the sternocleidomastoid muscle.

> **! NURSING ALERT**
>
> Hyperextension of the head (opisthotonos) with pain on flexion is a serious indication of meningeal irritation and is referred for immediate medical evaluation.

Palpate the skull for patent sutures, fontanels, fractures, and swellings. Normally the posterior fontanel closes by the second month of life, and the anterior fontanel fuses between 12 and 18 months. Early or late closure is noted, since either may be a sign of a pathologic condition. (For a more detailed discussion of the cranial bones, see Chapter 8.)

While examining the head, observe the face for symmetry, movement, and general appearance. Ask the child to "make a face" to assess symmetric movement and disclose any degree of paralysis. Note any unusual facial proportion, such as an unusually high or low forehead; wide- or close-set eyes; or a small, receding chin.

In addition to assessment of the head and neck for movement, inspect the neck for size and palpate its associated structures. The neck is normally short, with skinfolds between the head and shoulders during infancy; however, it lengthens during the next 3 to 4 years.

> **! NURSING ALERT**
>
> If any masses are detected in the neck, report them for further investigation. Large masses can block the airway.

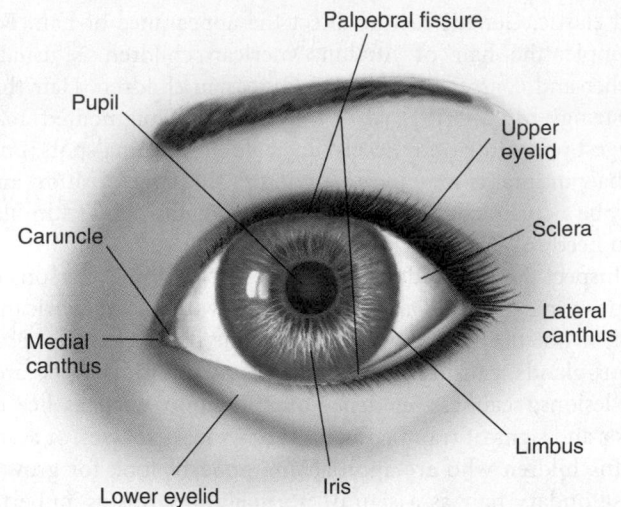

Fig. 6-16 External structures of eye.

EYES

Inspection of External Structures

⊖ Inspect the lids for proper placement on the eye. When the eye is open, the upper lid should fall near the upper iris. When the eyes are closed, the lids should completely cover the cornea and sclera (Fig. 6-16).

Determine the general slant of the **palpebral fissures** or lids by drawing an imaginary line through the two points of the medial canthus and across the outer orbit of the eyes and aligning each eye on the line. Usually the palpebral fissures lie horizontally. However, in Asians the slant is normally upward.

Also inspect the inside lining of the lids, the **palpebral conjunctivae**. To examine the lower conjunctival sac, pull the lid down while the patient looks up. To evert the upper lid, hold the upper lashes and gently pull *down* and *forward* as the child looks down. Normally the conjunctiva appears pink and glossy. Vertical yellow striations along the edge are the **meibomian glands**, or **sebaceous glands**, near the hair follicle. Located in the inner or medial canthus and situated on the inner edge of the upper and lower lids is a tiny opening, the **lacrimal punctum**. Note any excessive tearing, discharge, or inflammation of the lacrimal apparatus.

The **bulbar conjunctiva**, which covers the eye up to the limbus, or junction of the cornea and sclera, should be transparent. The **sclera**, or white covering of the eyeball, should be clear. Tiny black marks in the sclera of heavily pigmented individuals are normal.

The **cornea**, or covering of the iris and pupil, should be clear and transparent. Record opacities because they can be signs of scarring or ulceration, which can interfere with vision. The best way to test for opacities is to illuminate the eyeball by shining a light at an angle (**obliquely**) toward the cornea.

Compare the pupils for size, shape, and movement. They should be round, clear, and equal. Test their reaction to light by quickly shining a light toward the eye and removing it. As the light approaches, the pupils should constrict; as the light fades, the pupils should dilate. Test the pupil for any response of **accommodation** by having the child look at a bright, shiny object at a distance and quickly moving the object toward the face. The pupils should constrict as the object is brought near the eye. Record normal findings on examination of the pupils as PERRLA, which stands for "*P*upils *E*qual, *R*ound, *R*eact to *L*ight, and *A*ccommodation."

Inspect the iris and pupil for color, size, shape, and clarity. Permanent eye color is usually established by 6 to 12 months of age. While inspecting the iris and pupil, look for the lens. Normally the lens is not visible through the pupil.

Inspection of Internal Structures

The ophthalmoscope permits visualization of the interior of the eyeball with a system of lenses and a high-intensity light. The lenses permit clear visualization of eye structures at different distances from the nurse's eye and correct visual acuity differences in the examiner and child. Use of the ophthalmoscope requires practice to know which lens setting produces the clearest image.

The ophthalmic and otic heads are usually interchangeable on one "body" or handle, which encloses the power source, either disposable or rechargeable batteries. The nurse should practice changing the heads, which snap on and are secured with a quarter turn, and replacing the batteries and light bulbs. Nurses who are not directly involved in physical assessment are often responsible for ensuring that the equipment functions properly.

Preparing the Child

The nurse can prepare the child for the ophthalmoscopic examination by showing the child the instrument, demonstrating the light source and how it shines in the eye, and explaining the reason for darkening the room. For infants and young children who do not respond to such explanations, it is best to use distraction to encourage them to keep their eyes open. Forcibly parting the lids results in an uncooperative, watery eyed child and a frustrated nurse. Usually, with some practice, the nurse can elicit a red reflex almost instantly while approaching the child and may also gain a momentary inspection of the blood vessels, macula, or optic disc.

Funduscopic Examination

Fig. 6-17 shows the structures of the back of the eyeball, or the fundus. The fundus is immediately apparent as the red reflex.

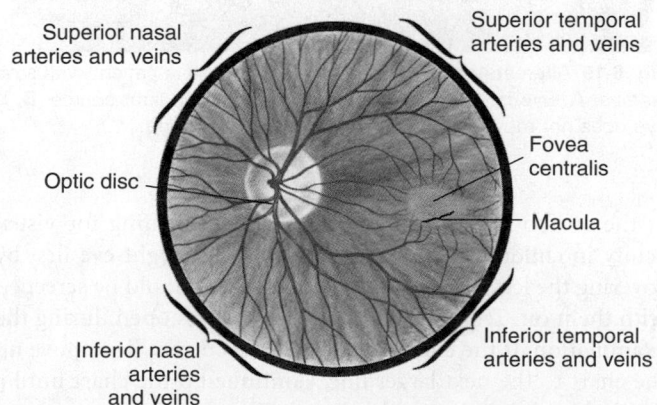

Fig. 6-17 Structures of fundus. (From Seidel HM, Ball JW, Dains JE, et al: *Mosby's guide to physical examination,* ed 6, St Louis, 2007, Mosby.)

The intensity of the color increases in darkly pigmented individuals.

> ### ! NURSING ALERT
>
> A brilliant, uniform red reflex is an important sign because it rules out many serious defects of the cornea, aqueous chamber, lens, and vitreous chamber. Any dark shadows or opacities are recorded because they indicate some abnormality in any of these structures.

As the ophthalmoscope is brought closer to the eye, the most conspicuous feature of the fundus is the optic disc, the area where the blood vessels and optic nerve fibers enter and exit the eye. The disc is creamy pink and lighter in color than the surrounding fundus. Normally it is round or vertically oval.

After locating the optic disc, inspect the area for blood vessels. The central retinal artery and vein appear in the depths of the disc and emanate outward with visible branching. The veins are darker and about one fourth larger than the arteries. Normally the branches of the arteries and veins cross each other.

Other structures that are common are the macula, the area of the fundus with the greatest concentration of visual receptors, and, in the center of the macula, a minute glistening spot of reflected light called the fovea centralis; this is the area of most perfect vision.

Vision Testing

Several tests are available for assessing vision. This discussion focuses on four areas: (1) ocular alignment, (2) visual acuity, (3) peripheral vision, and (4) color vision. Vision screening should be performed by age 3 and annually after that or more often if there are concerns (American Academy of Pediatrics, 2003a; Wall, Marsh-Tootle, Evans, et al, 2002). Chapter 24 discusses behavioral and physical signs of visual impairment.

Ocular Alignment

Normally, by the age of 3 to 4 months, children are able to fixate on one visual field with both eyes simultaneously (binocularity). One of the most important tests for binocularity is alignment of the eyes to detect nonbinocular vision, or strabismus (Halle, 2002). In strabismus, or cross-eye, one eye deviates from the point of fixation. If the misalignment is constant, the weak eye becomes "lazy," and the brain eventually suppresses the image produced by that eye. If strabismus is not detected and corrected by ages 4 to 6 years, blindness from disuse, known as amblyopia, may result.

Tests commonly used to detect misalignment are the corneal light reflex and the cover tests. To perform the corneal light reflex test, or Hirschberg test, shine a flashlight or the light of the ophthalmoscope directly into the patient's eyes from a distance of about 40.5 cm (16 inches). If the eyes are orthophoric, or normal, the light falls symmetrically within each pupil (Fig. 6-18, *A*). If the light falls off center in one eye, the eyes are misaligned. Epicanthal folds, excess folds of skin that extend from the roof of the nose to the inner termination of the eyebrow and that partially or completely overlap the inner canthus of the eye, may give a false impression of misalignment (pseudostrabismus) (Fig. 6-18, *B*). Epicanthal folds are often found in Asian children.

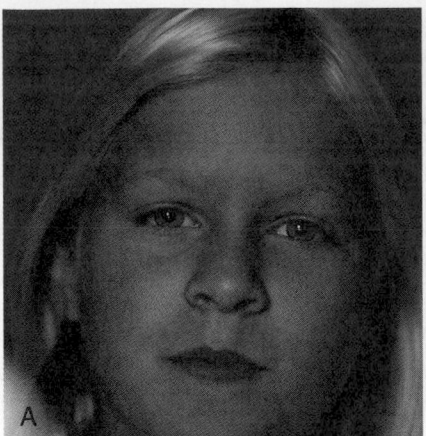
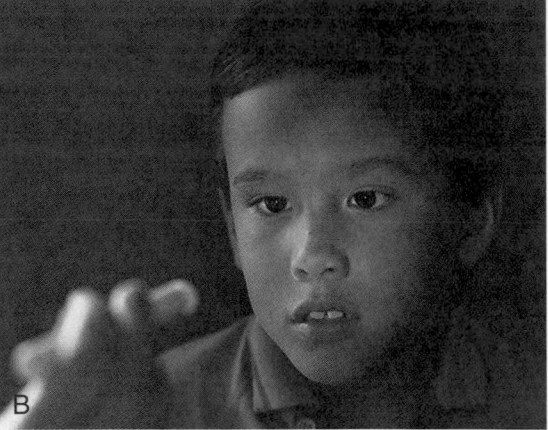

Fig. 6-18 A, Corneal light reflex test demonstrating orthophoric eyes. **B,** Pseudostrabismus. Inner epicanthal folds cause eyes to appear misaligned; however, corneal light reflexes fall perfectly symmetrically.

In the **cover test**, one eye is covered, and the movement of the *uncovered* eye is observed while the child looks at a near (33 cm [13 inches]) or distant (6 m [20 feet]) object. If the uncovered eye does not move, it is aligned. If the uncovered eye moves, a misalignment is present because, when the stronger eye is temporarily covered, the misaligned eye attempts to fixate on the object.

In the **alternate cover test**, occlusion shifts back and forth from one eye to the other, and movement of the eye that was *covered* is observed as soon as the occluder is removed while the child focuses on a point in front of him or her (Fig. 6-19). If normal alignment is present, shifting the cover from one eye to the other will not cause the eye to move. If misalignment is present, eye movement will occur when the cover is moved. This test takes more practice than the other cover test because the occluder must be moved back and forth quickly and accurately to see the eye move. Because deviations can occur at different ranges, it is important to perform the cover tests at both close and far distances.

> ### ! NURSING ALERT
>
> The cover test is usually easier to perform if the examiner uses his or her hand rather than a card-type occluder (see Fig. 6-19). Attractive occluders fashioned like an ice cream cone or happy-face lollipop cut from cardboard are also well received by young children.

Photoscreening is a technique used to screen for amblyopia, refractive disorders, and media opacities (American Academy of Pediatrics, 2003a; Berry, Simons, Siatkowski, et al, 2001). Using a camera, the nurse obtains images of the pupillary reflexes (reflections) and red reflexes (Bruckner test) (American Academy of Pediatrics, 2003a). Photoscreening offers an effective way to screen infants, preverbal children, and those with developmental delays who are difficult to screen.

Visual Acuity Testing in Children Beyond Infancy

The most common test for measuring visual acuity is the **Snellen letter chart**, which consists of lines of letters of decreasing size. The American Academy of Pediatrics (2003a) recommends that children stand 10 feet from the chart with their heels

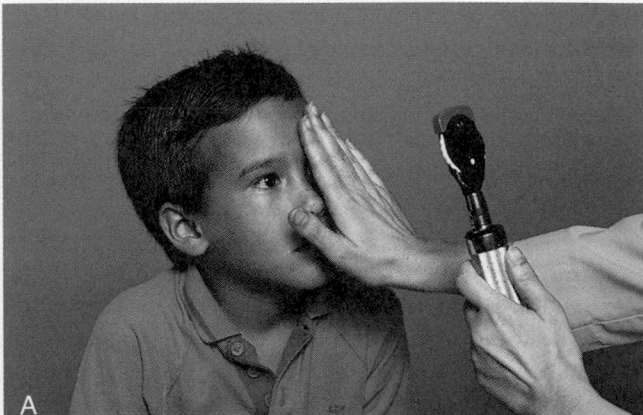
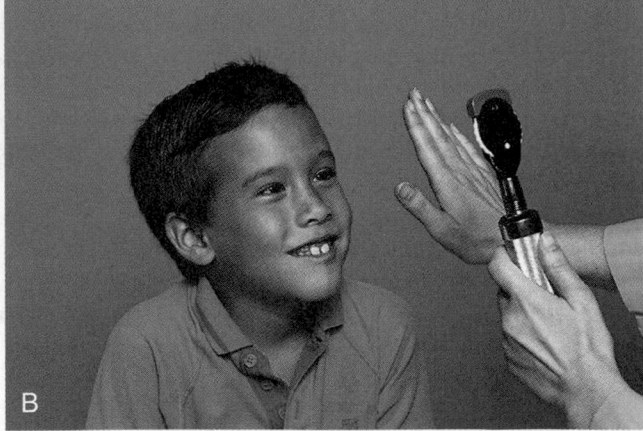

Fig. 6-19 Alternate cover test to detect amblyopia in patient with strabismus. **A,** Eye is occluded, and child is fixating on light source. **B,** If eye does not move when uncovered, eyes are aligned.

at the 10-foot line during testing. When screening for visual acuity in children, the nurse tests the child's right eye first by covering the left. Children who wear glasses should be screened with them on. Tell the child to keep both eyes open during the examination. If the child fails to read the current line, move up the chart to the next larger line. Continue up the chart until a line is found that the child can pass. Then begin moving down the chart again until the child fails to read the line. To pass each line, the child must correctly identify four of six symbols on the line. Repeat the procedure, covering the right eye. Table 6-9 provides a list of visual screening tests for children and guidelines for referral recommended by the American Academy of Pediatrics (2003a).

For children unable to read letters and numbers, the **tumbling E** or **HOTV** test is useful (Coats and Jenkins, 1997). The tumbling E test uses the capital letter E pointing in four different directions. The child is asked to point in the direction the E is facing. The HOTV test consists of a wall chart composed of the letters H, O, T, and V. The child is given a board containing a large H, O, T, and V. The examiner points to a letter on the wall chart, and the child matches the correct letter on the board held in his or her hand. The tumbling E and HOTV are excellent tests for preschool-age children.

If a child is unable to perform the tumbling E or HOTV test, use the Allen card test. The **Allen card test** uses common figures to test the child's vision. It is important to assess whether the child is able to identify the pictures before actual vision testing. The examiner walks backward slowly, flipping through the cards and presenting different pictures to the child. The examiner continues to move backward as the child correctly calls out the figures. When the child begins to miss the figure on the cards, the examiner moves forward to confirm that the child is able to identify the figures at that point. All Allen card figures are 20/30 in size. The farthest distance at which the child is able to accurately identify the pictures becomes the numerator, and 30 becomes the denominator. For example, if the child is able to identify the pictures accurately at 15 feet, record the visual acuity as 15/30. This is equivalent to 20/40 or 10/20 visual acuity.

Visual Acuity Testing in Infants and Difficult-to-Test Children

In newborns, vision is tested mainly by checking for **light perception** by shining a light into the eyes and noting responses such as pupillary constriction, blinking, following the light to midline, increased alertness, or refusal to open the eyes after exposure to the light. Although the simple maneuver of checking light perception and eliciting the pupillary light reflex indicates that the anterior half of the visual apparatus is intact, it does not confirm that the infant can see. In other words, this test does not assess whether the brain receives the visual message and interprets the signals.

Another test of visual acuity is the infant's ability to fix on and follow a target. Although any brightly colored or patterned object can be used, the human face is excellent. Hold the infant upright while moving your face slowly from side to side.

> **! NURSING ALERT**
>
> If visual fixation and following are not present by 3 to 4 months of age, further ophthalmologic evaluation is necessary.

Other signs that may indicate visual loss or other serious eye problems include fixed pupils, strabismus, constant nystagmus, the setting-sun sign, and slow lateral movements. Unfortunately, it is difficult to test each eye separately; the presence of such signs in one eye could indicate unilateral blindness.

Special tests are available for testing infants and other difficult-to-test children to assess acuity or confirm blindness. For example, in **visually evoked potentials**, the eyes are stimulated with a bright light or pattern, and electrical activity to the visual cortex is recorded through scalp electrodes. Acuity is assessed by using progressively smaller patterns.

Peripheral Vision

In children who are old enough to cooperate, estimate **peripheral vision**, or the visual field of each eye, by having the children fixate on a specific point directly in front of them while an object, such as a finger or a pencil, is moved from beyond the field of vision into the range of peripheral vision. As soon as children see the object, have them say "stop." At that point measure the angle from the anteroposterior axis of the eye (straight line of vision) to the peripheral axis (point at which the object is first seen). Check each eye separately and for each quadrant of vision. Normally children see about 50 degrees upward, 70 degrees downward, 60 degrees nasalward, and 90 degrees temporally. Limitations in peripheral vision may indicate blindness from damage to structures within the eye or to any of the visual pathways.

Color Vision

Another important test is for color vision. It is estimated that 8% to 10% of Caucasian males and less than half that percentage of African-American males inherit the X-linked disorder known as **color vision deficit** (also known as **color blindness**, a less acceptable term). From 0.5% to 1% of Caucasian females are affected. Although the severity of impaired perception of color varies considerably, the two most common types are **protanomaly**, in which the child confuses gray with pink or pale blue with green, and **deuteranomaly**, in which the child confuses gray with pale purple or green. In most of these individuals the color vision deficit causes no major problems. However, some individuals with more severe deficits may be unable to distinguish amber or red traffic lights, fail to see a red brake light on the rear of a car, have difficulty distinguishing green traffic lights from incandescent street lamps, and have a poor sense of color coordination of clothing. For school-age children the greatest difficulty lies in performance of academic skills that use color as a visual aid. Adolescents may be ineligible for certain vocational opportunities, such as electronics, photography, printing, interior decorating, pharmaceuticals, textiles, police work, and several types of military service.

The tests available for color vision include the **Ishihara test** and the **Hardy-Rand-Rittler test**. Each consists of a series of cards (pseudoisochromatic) that contain a color field composed of spots of a certain "confusion" color. Against the field is a number or symbol similarly printed in dots but of a color likely to be confused with the field color by the person with a color vision deficit. As a result, the figure or letter is invisible to an affected individual but is clearly seen by a person with normal vision.

EARS

Inspection of External Structures

The entire external earlobe is called the **pinna**, or **auricle**; one is located on each side of the head. Measure the height alignment of the pinna by drawing an imaginary line from the

TABLE 6-9	EYE EXAMINATION GUIDELINES*		
FUNCTION	**RECOMMENDED TESTS**	**REFERRAL CRITERIA**	**COMMENTS**
Ages 3-5 Yr			
Distance visual acuity	Snellen letters Snellen numbers Tumbling E HOTV Picture test: • Allen figures • LEA symbols	1. <4 of 6 correct on 20-foot (6-m) line with either eye tested at 10 foot (3 m) monocularly (i.e., <10/20 or 20/40) or 2. Two-line difference between eyes, even within passing range (i.e., 10/12.5 and 10/20 or 20/25 and 20/40)	1. Tests are listed in decreasing order of cognitive difficulty; highest test that child is capable of performing should be used; in general, tumbling E or HOTV test should be used for children 3-5 yr of age and Snellen letters or numbers for children 6 yr and older. 2. Testing distance of 10 feet (3 m) is recommended for all visual acuity tests. 3. Line of figures is preferred over single figures. 4. Nontested eye should be covered by occluder held by examiner or by adhesive occluder patch applied to eye; examiner must ensure that it is not possible to peek with nontested eye.
Ocular alignment	Cross cover test at 10 feet (3 m) Random dot E stereo test at 18 inches (40 cm) Simultaneous red reflex test (Bruckner test)	Any eye movement <4 of 6 correct Any asymmetry of pupil color, size, brightness	Child must be fixing on a target while cross cover test is performed. Use direct ophthalmoscope to view both red reflexes simultaneously in a darkened room from 2-3 feet (0.6-0.9 m) away; detects asymmetric refractive errors as well.
Ocular media clarity (cataracts, tumors, etc.)	Red reflex	White pupil, dark spots, absent reflex	Use direct ophthalmoscope in a darkened room. View eyes separately at 12-18 inches (30-45 cm); white reflex indicates possible retinoblastoma.
≥6 Years			
Distance visual acuity	Snellen letters Snellen numbers Tumbling E HOTV Picture test: • Allen figures • LEA symbols	1. <4 of 6 correct on 15-foot (4.5-m) line with either eye tested at 10 feet (3 m) monocularly (i.e., <10/15 or 20/30) or 2. Two-line difference between eyes, even within the passing range (i.e., 10/10 and 10/15 or 20/20 and 20/30)	1. Tests are listed in decreasing order of cognitive difficulty; highest test that child is capable of performing should be used; in general, tumbling E or HOTV test should be used for children 3-5 yr of age and Snellen letters or numbers for children 6 yr and older. 2. Testing distance of 10 feet (3 m) is recommended for all visual acuity tests. 3. Line of figures is preferred over single figures. 4. Nontested eye should be covered by occluder held by examiner or by adhesive occluder patch applied to eye; examiner must ensure that it is not possible to peek with nontested eye.
Ocular alignment	Cross cover test at 10 feet (3 m) Random dot E stereo test at 18 inches (40 cm) Simultaneous red reflex test (Bruckner test)	Any eye movement <4 of 6 correct Any asymmetry of pupil color, size, brightness	Child must be fixing on target while cross cover test is performed. Use direct ophthalmoscope to view both red reflexes simultaneously in a darkened room from 2-3 feet (0.6-0.9 m) away; detects asymmetric refractive errors as well.
Ocular media clarity (cataracts, tumors, etc.)	Red reflex	White pupil, dark spots, absent reflex	Use direct ophthalmoscope in a darkened room. View eyes separately at 12-18 inches (30-45 cm); white reflex indicates possible retinoblastoma.

From American Academy of Pediatrics, Committee on Practice and Ambulatory Medicine, Section on Ophthalmology: Eye examination in infants, children, and young adults by pediatricians, *Pediatrics* 111(4):902-907, 2003.
*Assessing visual acuity (vision screening) is one of the most sensitive techniques for detection of eye abnormalities in children. The American Academy of Pediatrics Section on Ophthalmology, in cooperation with American Association for Pediatric Ophthalmology and Strabismus and American Academy of Ophthalmology, has developed these guidelines to be used by physicians, nurses, educational institutions, public health departments, and other professionals who perform vision evaluation services.

outer orbit of the eye to the occiput, or most prominent protuberance of the skull. The top of the pinna should meet or cross this line. Low-set ears are commonly associated with renal anomalies or cognitive impairment. Measure the angle of the pinna by drawing a perpendicular line from the imaginary horizontal line and aligning the pinna next to this mark. Normally the pinna lies within a 10-degree angle of the vertical line (Fig. 6-20). If it falls outside this area, record the deviation and look for other anomalies.

Normally the pinna extends slightly outward from the skull. Except in newborn infants, ears that are flat against the head or protruding away from the scalp may indicate problems. Flattened ears in an infant may suggest a frequent side-lying position and, just as with isolated areas of hair loss, may be a clue to investigate parents' understanding of the child's stimulation needs.

Inspect the skin surface around the ear for small openings, extra tags of skin, or sinuses. If a sinus is found, note this

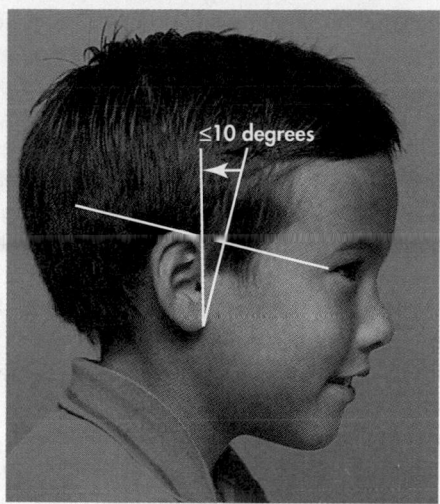

Fig. 6-20 Ear alignment.

because it may represent a fistula that drains into some area of the neck or ear. Cutaneous tags represent no pathologic process but may cause parents concern in terms of the child's appearance.

Also assess the ear for hygiene. An otoscope is not necessary for looking into the external canal to note the presence of **cerumen**, a waxy substance produced by the ceruminous glands in the outer portion of the canal. Cerumen is usually yellow-brown and soft. If an otoscope is used and any discharge is visible, note its color and odor. Avoid transmitting potentially infectious material to the other ear or to another child through hand washing and using disposable specula or sterilizing reusable specula between each examination.

Inspection of Internal Structures

The head of the otoscope permits visualization of the tympanic membrane by use of a bright light, a magnifying glass, and a speculum. Some otoscopes have an attachment for a pneumonic device to insert air into the canal to determine membrane compliance (movement). The speculum, which is inserted into the external canal, comes in a variety of sizes to accommodate different canal widths. The largest speculum that fits comfortably into the ear is used to achieve the greatest area of visualization. The lens, or magnifying glass, is movable, allowing the examiner to insert an object, such as a curette, into the ear canal through the speculum while still viewing the structures through the lens.

Positioning the Child

Before beginning the otoscopic examination, position the child properly and gently restrain (sit on parents lap and hold parents hands) if necessary. Older children usually cooperate and do not need restraint. However, prepare them for the procedure by allowing them to play with the instrument, demonstrating how it works, and stressing the importance of remaining still. A helpful suggestion is to let them observe you examining the parent's ear. Restraint is needed for younger children because the ear examination upsets them (see Atraumatic Care box).

As you insert the speculum into the meatus, move it around the outer rim to accustom the child to the feel of something entering the ear. If examining a painful ear, touch a nonpainful

part of the affected ear, then examine the unaffected ear, and finally return to the painful ear. By this time the child is usually less fearful of anything causing discomfort to the ear and will cooperate more.

For their protection and safety, restrain infants and toddlers for the otoscopic examination. There are two general positions of restraint. In one the child is seated sideways in the parent's lap with one arm hugging the parent and the other arm at the side. The ear to be examined is toward the nurse. With one arm the parent holds the child's head firmly against his or her chest, and with the other arm hugs the child, thereby securing the child's free arm (Fig. 6-21, *A*). Examine the ear using the same procedure for holding the otoscope as described later.

The other position involves placing the child on the side, back, or abdomen with the arms at the side and the head turned

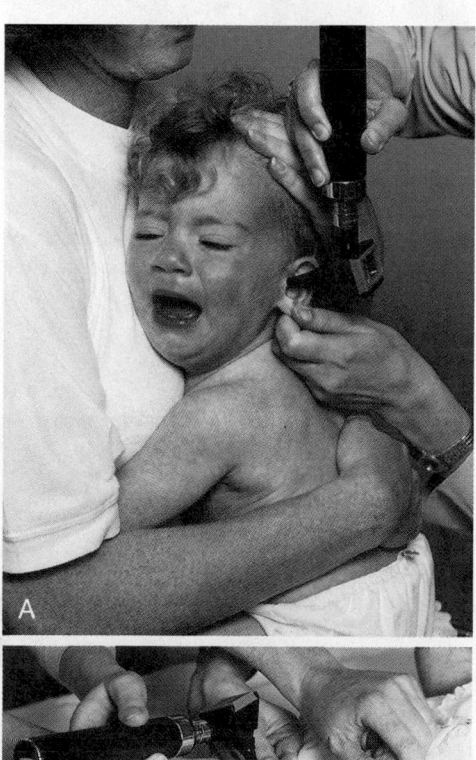

Fig. 6-21 Position for restraining child (**A**) and infant (**B**) during otoscopic examination.

so that the ear to be examined points toward the ceiling. Lean over the child, use the upper part of the body to restrain the arms and upper trunk movements, and use the examining hand to stabilize the head. This position is practical for young infants or for older children who need minimum restraint, but it may not be feasible for other children who protest vigorously. For safety, enlist the parent's or an assistant's help in immobilizing the head by firmly placing one hand above the ear and the other on the child's side, abdomen, or back (Fig. 6-21, *B*).

With cooperative children, examine the ear with the child in a side-lying, sitting, or standing position. One disadvantage to standing is that the child may "walk away" as the otoscope enters the canal. If the child is standing or sitting, tilt the head slightly toward the child's opposite shoulder to achieve a better view of the drum (Fig. 6-22).

With the thumb and forefinger of the free (usually non-dominant) hand, grasp the auricle. For the two positions of

restraint, hold the otoscope upside down at the junction of its head and handle with the thumb and index finger. Place the other fingers against the skull to allow the otoscope to move with the child in case of sudden movement. In examining a cooperative child, hold the handle with the otic head upright or upside down. Use the dominant hand to examine both ears or reverse hands for each ear, whichever is more comfortable.

Before using the otoscope, visualize the external ear and the tympanic membrane as being superimposed on a clock (Fig. 6-23). The numbers are important geographic landmarks. Introduce the speculum into the meatus between the 3 and 9 o'clock positions in a *downward* and *forward* position. Because the canal is curved, the speculum does not permit a panoramic view of the tympanic membrane unless the canal is straightened. In infants the canal curves upward. Therefore pull the pinna *down* and *back* to the 6 to 9 o'clock range to straighten the canal (Fig. 6-24, *A*). With older children, usually those older

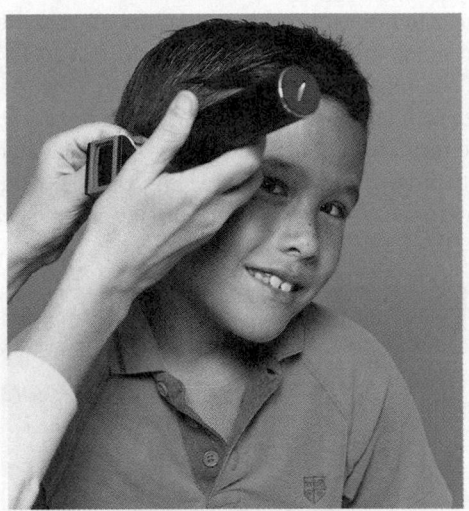

Fig. 6-22 Positioning head by tilting it toward opposite shoulder for full view of tympanic membrane.

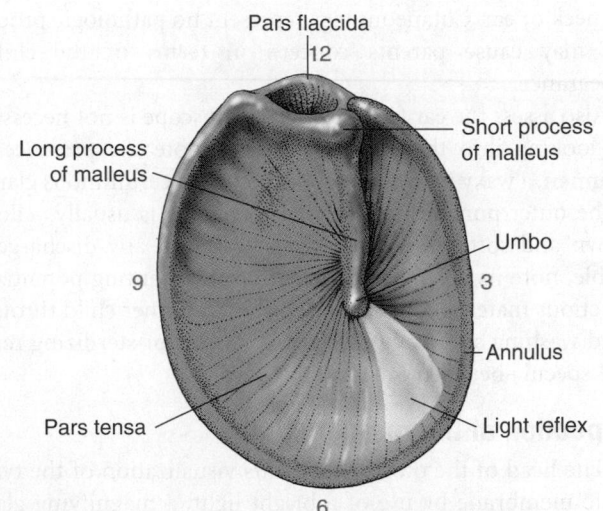

Fig. 6-23 Landmarks of tympanic membrane. (From Rothrock JC: *Alexander's care of the patient in surgery*, ed 13, St Louis, 2006, Mosby.)

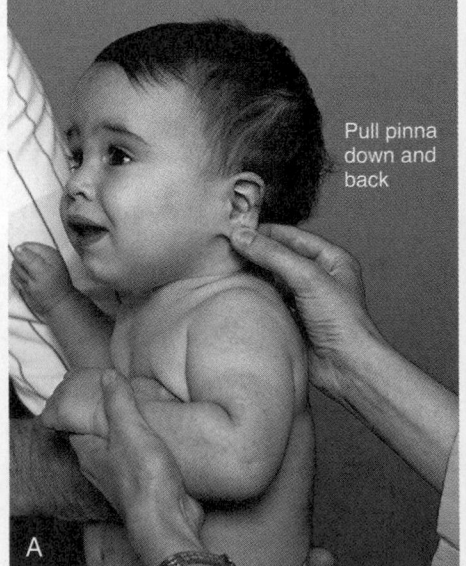

Pull pinna down and back

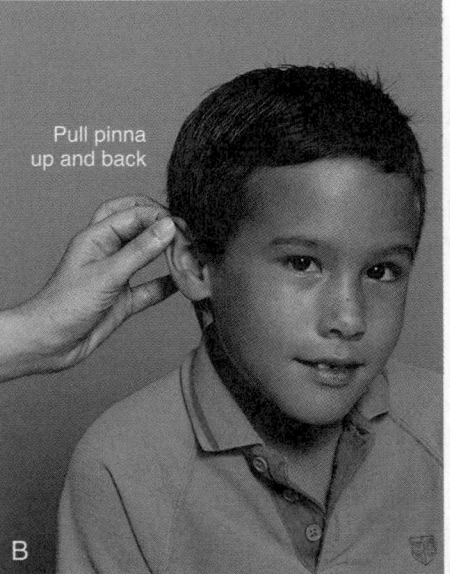

Pull pinna up and back

Fig. 6-24 Positioning for visualizing eardrum in infant (**A**) and in child older than 3 years of age (**B**).

than 3 years of age, the canal curves downward and forward. Therefore pull the pinna *up* and *back* toward a 10 o'clock position (Fig. 6-24, *B*). If you have difficulty visualizing the membrane, try repositioning the head, introducing the speculum at a different angle, and pulling the pinna in a slightly different direction. Do not insert the speculum past the cartilaginous (outermost) portion of the canal, usually a distance of 0.60 to 1.25 cm (0.25 to 0.5 inch) in older children. Insertion of the speculum into the posterior or bony portion of the canal causes pain.

In neonates and young infants the walls of the canal are pliable and floppy because of the underdeveloped cartilaginous and bony structures. Therefore the very small 2-mm speculum usually needs to be inserted deeper into the canal than in older children. Exercise great care not to damage the walls or drum. For this reason, only an experienced examiner should insert an otoscope into the ears of very young infants.

Otoscopic Examination

As you introduce the speculum into the external canal, inspect the walls of the canal, the color of the tympanic membrane, the light reflex, and the usual landmarks of the bony prominences of the middle ear. The walls of the external auditory canal are pink, although they are more pigmented in dark-skinned children. Minute hairs are evident in the outermost portion, where cerumen is produced. Note signs of irritation, foreign bodies, or infection.

Foreign bodies in the ear are not uncommon in children and range from erasers to beans. Symptoms may include pain, discharge, and affected hearing. Remove soft objects, such as paper or insects, with forceps. Remove small, hard objects, such as pebbles, with a suction tip, a hook, or irrigation. However, irrigation is contraindicated if the object is vegetative matter, such as beans or pasta, which swells when in contact with fluid.

> **! NURSING ALERT**
>
> If there is any doubt about the type of object in the ear and the appropriate method to remove it, refer the child to the appropriate practitioner.

The **tympanic membrane** is a translucent, light pearly pink or gray. Note marked erythema (which may indicate suppurative otitis media); a dull, nontransparent grayish color (some-times suggestive of serous otitis media); or ashen gray areas (signs of scarring from a previous perforation). A black area usually suggests a perforation of the membrane that has not healed.

The characteristic tenseness and slope of the tympanic membrane cause the light of the otoscope to reflect at about the 5 or 7 o'clock position. The **light reflex** is a fairly well-defined, cone-shaped reflection, which normally points away from the face.

The **bony landmarks** of the drum are formed by the **umbo**, or tip of the malleus. It appears as a small, round, opaque, concave spot near the center of the drum. The **manubrium** (long process or handle) of the malleus appears to be a whitish line extending from the umbo upward to the margin of the membrane. At the upper end of the long process near the 1 o'clock position (in the right ear) is a sharp, knoblike protuberance, representing the short process of the malleus. Note the absence of the light reflex or loss or abnormal prominence of any of these landmarks.

Auditory Testing

Several types of hearing tests are available and recommended for screening in infants and children (American Academy of Pediatrics, 2003b) (Table 6-10). Universal newborn hearing screening is available in almost every state in the United States. The nurse must operate under a high index of suspicion for those children who may have conditions associated with hearing loss, whose parents are concerned about hearing loss, and who may have developed behaviors that indicate auditory impairment (Cunningham and Cox, 2003). Chapter 24 discusses types of hearing loss, causes, clinical manifestations, and appropriate treatment.

NOSE

Inspection of External Structures

The nose is located in the middle of the face just below the eyes and above the lips. Compare its placement and alignment by drawing an imaginary vertical line from the center point between the eyes down to the notch of the upper lip. The nose should lie exactly vertical to this line, with each side exactly symmetric. Note its location, any deviation to one side, and asymmetry in overall size and in diameter of the nares (nostrils). The bridge of the nose is sometimes flat in Asian and

(Anatomy Review—External and Internal Structures of the Nose)

TABLE 6-10	AUDITORY TESTS FOR INFANTS AND CHILDREN		
AGE	**AUDITORY TEST AND AVERAGE TIME**	**TYPE OF MEASUREMENT**	**PROCEDURE**
All ages	Evoked otoacoustic emissions, 10-min test	Physiologic test specifically measuring cochlear (outer hair cell) response to presentation of stimulus	Small probe containing sensitive microphone is placed in ear canal for stimulus delivery and response detection.
Birth-9 months	Auditory brainstem response, 15-min test	Electrophysiologic measurement of activity in auditory nerve and brainstem pathways	Placement of electrodes on child's head detects auditory stimuli presented though earphones one ear at a time.
9 months-2½ yr	Conditioned oriented responses or visual reinforced audiometry, 30-min test	Behavioral tests measuring child's responses to speech and frequency-specific stimuli presented through speakers	Both techniques condition child to associate speech or frequency-specific sound with reinforcement stimulus, such as lighted toy.

Modified with permission from Bachmann KR, Arvedson JC: Early identification and intervention for children who are hearing impaired, *Pediatr Rev* 19:155-165, 1998.

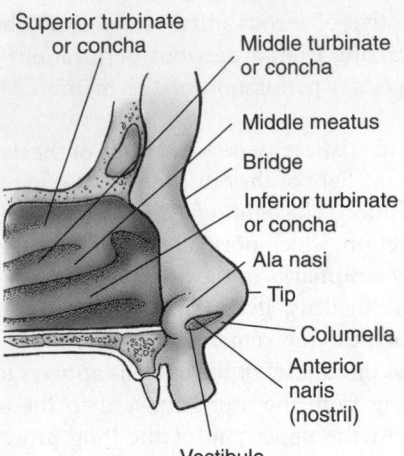

Superior turbinate or concha
Middle turbinate or concha
Middle meatus
Bridge
Inferior turbinate or concha
Ala nasi
Tip
Columella
Anterior naris (nostril)
Vestibule

Fig. 6-25 External landmarks and internal structures of nose.

African-American children. Observe the alae nasi for any sign of flaring, which indicates respiratory difficulty. Always report any flaring of the alae nasi. Fig. 6-25 illustrates the landmarks used in describing the external structures of the nose.

Inspection of Internal Structures

Inspect the anterior vestibule of the nose by pushing the tip upward, tilting the head backward, and illuminating the cavity with a flashlight or otoscope without the attached ear speculum. Note the color of the mucosal lining, which is normally redder than the oral membranes, as well as any swelling, discharge, dryness, or bleeding. There should be no discharge from the nose.

On looking deeper into the nose, inspect the turbinates, or concha, plates of bone that jut into the nasal cavity and are enveloped by mucous membrane. The turbinates greatly increase the surface area of the nasal cavity as air is inhaled. The spaces or channels between the turbinates are called the meatus and correspond to each of the three turbinates. Normally the front end of the inferior and middle turbinate and the middle meatus are seen. They should be the same color as the lining of the vestibule.

Inspect the septum, which should divide the vestibules equally. Note any deviation, especially if it causes an occlusion of one side of the nose. A perforation may be evident within the septum. If this is suspected, shine the light of the otoscope into one naris and look for admittance of light to the other. Because olfaction is an important function of the nose, testing for smell may be done at this point or as part of cranial nerve assessment (see Table 6-13).

MOUTH AND THROAT

With a cooperative child, the nurse can accomplish almost the entire examination of the mouth and throat without the use of a tongue blade. Ask the child to open the mouth wide; to move the tongue in different directions for full visualization; and to say "ahh," which depresses the tongue for full view of the back of the mouth (tonsils, uvula, and oropharynx). For a closer look at the buccal mucosa, or lining of the cheeks, ask

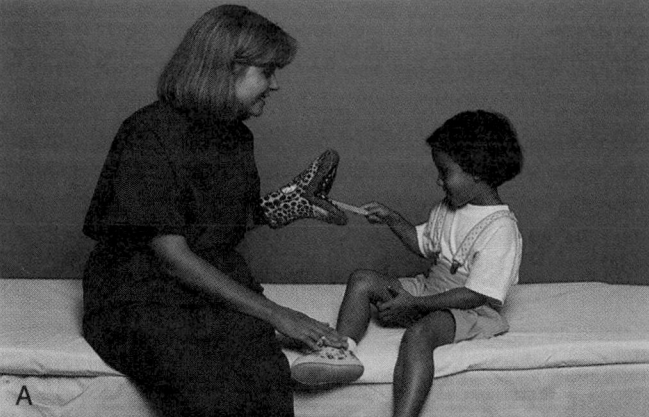

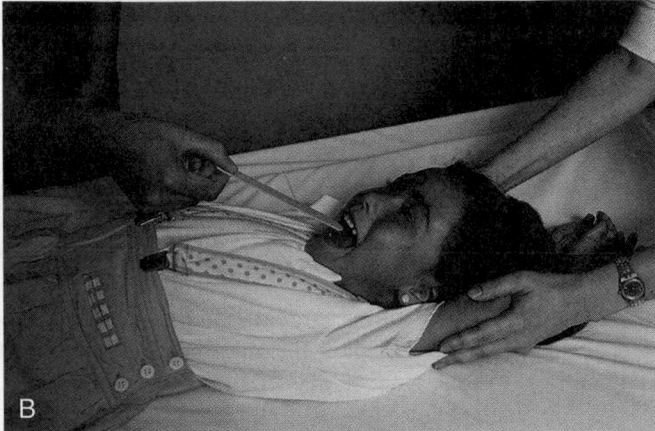

Fig. 6-26 A, Encouraging child to cooperate. **B,** Positioning child for examination of mouth.

children to use their fingers to move the outer lip and cheek to one side (see Atraumatic Care box).

ATRAUMATIC CARE

Encouraging Opening the Mouth for Examination

- Perform the examination in front of a mirror.
- Let child first examine someone else's mouth, such as the parent, the nurse, or a puppet (Fig. 6-26, A), and then examine child's mouth.
- Instruct child to tilt the head back slightly, breathe deeply through the mouth, and hold the breath; this action lowers the tongue to the floor of the mouth without the use of a tongue blade.
- Lightly brushing the palate with a cotton swab also may open the mouth for assessment.

Infants and toddlers usually resist attempts to keep the mouth open. Because inspecting the mouth is upsetting, leave it for the end of the physical examination (along with examination of the ears) or do it during episodes of crying. However, the use of a tongue blade (preferably flavored) to depress the tongue may be needed. Place the tongue blade along the *side* of the tongue, not in the center back area where the gag reflex is elicited. Fig. 6-26, *B*, illustrates proper positioning of the child for the oral examination.

The major structure of the exterior of the mouth is the lips. The lips should be moist, soft, smooth, and pink, or a deeper hue than the surrounding skin. The lips should be symmetric when relaxed or tensed. Assess symmetry when the child talks or cries.

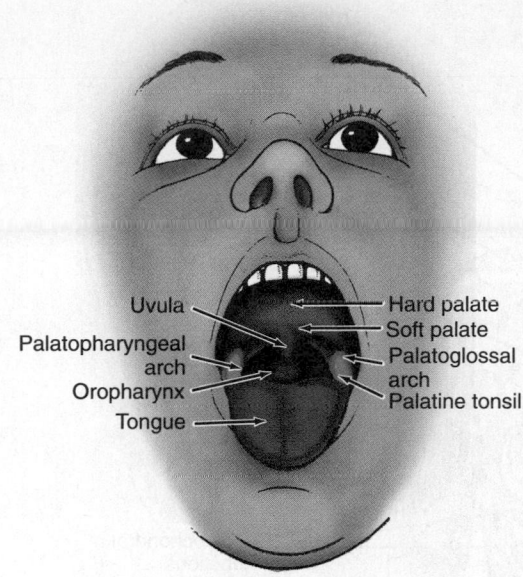

Uvula
Palatopharyngeal arch
Oropharynx
Tongue
Hard palate
Soft palate
Palatoglossal arch
Palatine tonsil

Fig. 6-27 Interior structures of mouth.

Inspection of Internal Structures

The major structures that are visible within the oral cavity and oropharynx are the mucosal lining of the lips and cheeks, gums (or gingiva), teeth, tongue, palate, uvula, tonsils, and posterior oropharynx (Fig. 6-27). Inspect all areas lined with mucous membranes (inside the lips and cheeks, gingiva, underside of the tongue, palate, and back of the pharynx) for color, any areas of white patches or ulceration, bleeding, sensitivity, and moisture. The membranes should be bright pink, smooth, glistening, uniform, and moist.

Inspect the teeth for number in each dental arch, for hygiene, and for occlusion or bite (see also Teething, Chapter 12). Discoloration of tooth enamel with obvious plaque (whitish coating on the surface of the teeth) is a sign of poor dental hygiene and indicates a need for counseling. Brown spots in the crevices of the crown of the tooth or between the teeth may be caries (cavities). Chalky white to yellow or brown areas on the enamel may indicate fluorosis (excessive fluoride ingestion). Teeth that appear greenish black may be stained temporarily from ingestion of supplemental iron.

Examine the gums (gingiva) surrounding the teeth. The color is normally coral pink, and the surface texture is stippled, similar to the appearance of an orange peel. In dark-skinned children the gums are more deeply colored, and a brownish area is often observed along the gum line.

Inspect the tongue for papillae, small projections that contain several taste buds and give the tongue its characteristic rough appearance. Note the size and mobility of the tongue. Normally the tip of the tongue should extend to the lips or beyond.

The roof of the mouth consists of the hard palate, which is located near the front of the oral cavity, and the soft palate, which is located toward the back of the pharynx and has a small midline protrusion called the uvula. Carefully inspect the palates to ensure they are intact. The arch of the palate should be dome shaped. A narrow, flat roof or a high, arched palate affects the placement of the tongue and can cause feeding and speech problems. Test movement of the uvula by eliciting a gag reflex. It should move upward to close off the nasopharynx from the oropharynx.

Examine the oropharynx and note the size and color of the palatine tonsils. They are normally the same color as the surrounding mucosa; glandular, rather than smooth in appearance; and barely visible over the edge of the palatoglossal arches. The size of the tonsils varies considerably during childhood. However, report any swelling, redness, or white areas on the tonsils.

CHEST

Inspect the chest for size, shape, symmetry, movement, breast development, and the bony landmarks formed by the ribs and sternum. The rib cage consists of 12 ribs on each side and the sternum, or breast bone, located in the midline of the trunk (Fig. 6-28). The sternum is composed of three main parts. The manubrium, the uppermost portion, can be felt at the base of the neck at the suprasternal notch. The largest segment of the sternum is the body, which forms the sternal angle (angle of Louis) as it articulates with the manubrium. At the end of the body is a small, movable process called the xiphoid. The angle of the costal margin as it attaches to the sternum is called the costal angle and is normally about 45 to 50 degrees. These bony structures are important landmarks in the location of ribs and intercostal spaces (ICSs), which are the spaces between the ribs. They are numbered according to the rib directly *above* the space. For example, the space immediately below the second rib is the second ICS.

The thoracic cavity is also divided into segments by drawing imaginary lines on the chest and back. Fig. 6-29 illustrates the anterior, lateral, and posterior divisions.

Measure the size of the chest by placing the measuring tape around the rib cage at the nipple line (see Fig. 6-9). For greatest accuracy, take two measurements—one during inspiration and the other during expiration—and record the average. Chest size is important mainly in relation to head circumference (see p. 144). Always report marked disproportions because most are caused by abnormal head growth, although some may be a result of altered chest shape, such as barrel chest (chest is round) or pigeon chest (sternum protrudes outward).

During infancy the chest's shape is almost circular, with the anteroposterior (front-to-back) diameter equaling the transverse, or lateral (side-to-side), diameter. As the child grows, the chest normally increases in the transverse direction, causing the anteroposterior diameter to be less than the lateral diameter. Note the angle made by the lower costal margin and the sternum, and palpate the junction of the ribs with the costal cartilage (costochondral junction) and sternum, which should be fairly smooth.

Movement of the chest wall should be symmetric bilaterally and coordinated with breathing. During inspiration the chest rises and expands, the diaphragm descends, and the costal angle increases. During expiration the chest falls and decreases in size, the diaphragm rises, and the costal angle narrows (Fig. 6-30). In children younger than 6 or 7 years of age, respiratory movement is principally abdominal or diaphragmatic. In older children, particularly girls, respirations are chiefly thoracic. In

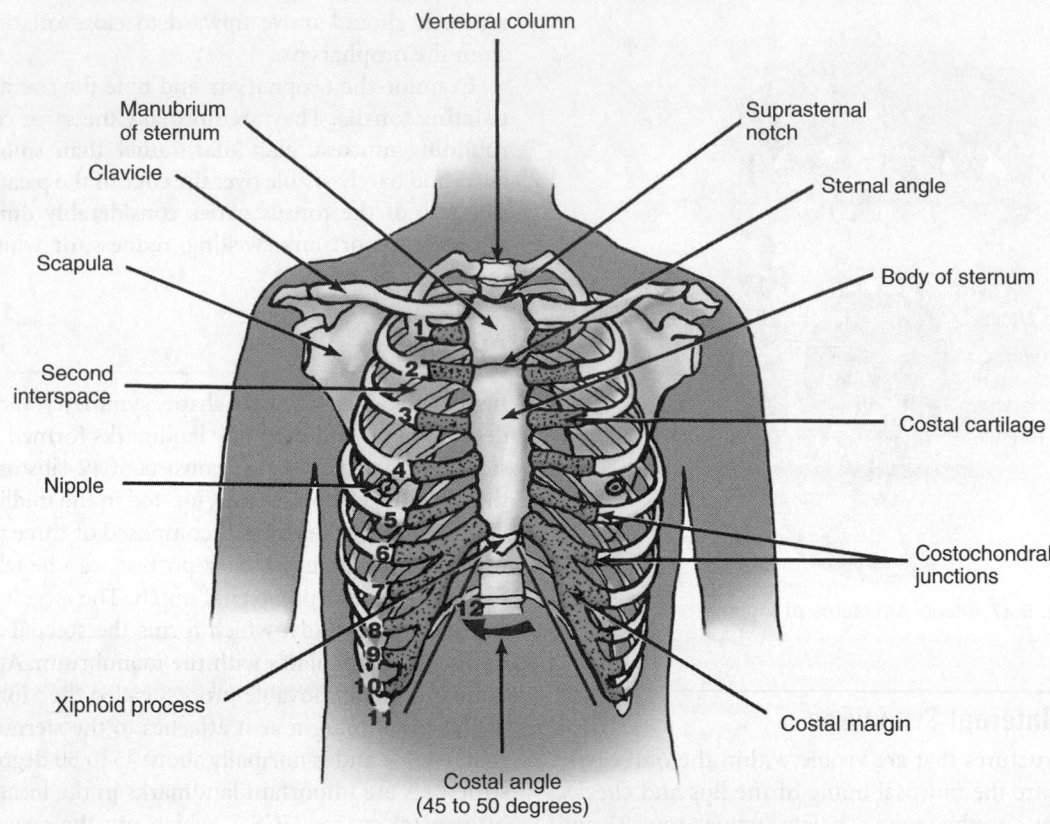

Fig. 6-28 Rib cage.

either case the chest and abdomen should rise and fall together. Always report any asymmetry of movement.

While inspecting the skin surface of the chest, observe the position of the nipples and any evidence of breast development. Normally the nipples are located slightly lateral to the midclavicular line between the fourth and fifth ribs. Note symmetry of nipple placement and normal configuration of a darker pigmented areola surrounding a flat nipple in the prepubertal child.

Pubertal breast development usually begins in girls between 10 and 14 years of age (see Chapter 19. Record early (precocious) or delayed breast development, as well as evidence of any other secondary sexual characteristics. In males breast enlargement (**gynecomastia**) may be caused by hormonal or systemic disorders, but more commonly it is a result of adipose tissue from obesity or a transitory body change during early puberty. In either situation investigate the child's feelings regarding breast enlargement.

In adolescent girls who have achieved sexual maturity, palpate the breasts for evidence of any masses or hard nodules. Use this opportunity to discuss the importance of routine breast self-examination. Emphasize that most palpable masses are benign to decrease any fear or concern that results when a mass is felt.

LUNGS

The lungs are situated inside the thoracic cavity, with one lung on each side of the sternum. Each lung is divided into an **apex**, which is slightly pointed and rises above the first rib; a **base**, which is wide and concave and rides on the dome-shaped diaphragm; and a **body**, which is divided into lobes. The right lung has three lobes: the upper, middle, and lower. The left lung has only two lobes, the upper and lower, because of the space occupied by the heart (Fig. 6-31).

Inspection of the lungs primarily involves observation of respiratory movements. Evaluate respirations for (1) rate (number per minute), (2) rhythm (regular, irregular, or periodic), (3) depth (deep or shallow), and (4) quality (effortless, automatic, difficult, or labored). Note the character of breath sounds, such as noisy, grunting, snoring, or heavy.

Evaluate respiratory movements by placing each hand flat against the back or chest with the thumbs in midline along the lower costal margin of the lungs. The child should be sitting during this procedure and, if cooperative, should take several deep breaths. During respiration your hands will move with the chest wall. Assess the amount and speed of respiratory excursion and note any asymmetry of movement.

Experienced examiners may percuss the lungs. Percuss the anterior lung from apex to base, usually with the child in the supine or sitting position. Percuss each side of the chest in sequence to compare the sounds. When percussing the posterior lung, the procedure and sequence are the same, although the child should be sitting. Resonance is heard over all the lobes of the lungs that are not adjacent to other organs. Record and report any deviation from the expected sound.

Auscultation

Auscultation involves using the stethoscope to evaluate breath sounds (see Nursing Care Guidelines box). Breath sounds are best heard if the child inspires deeply (see Atraumatic Care box). In the lungs breath sounds are classified as vesicular, bronchovesicular, or bronchial (Box 6-13).

Absent or diminished breath sounds are always an abnormal finding warranting investigation. Fluid, air, or solid masses in the pleural space all interfere with the conduction of breath sounds. Diminished breath sounds in certain segments of the lung can alert the nurse to pulmonary areas that may benefit from chest physiotherapy. Increased breath sounds after pulmonary therapy indicate improved passage of air through the respiratory tract. Box 6-14 lists terms used to describe various respiration patterns.

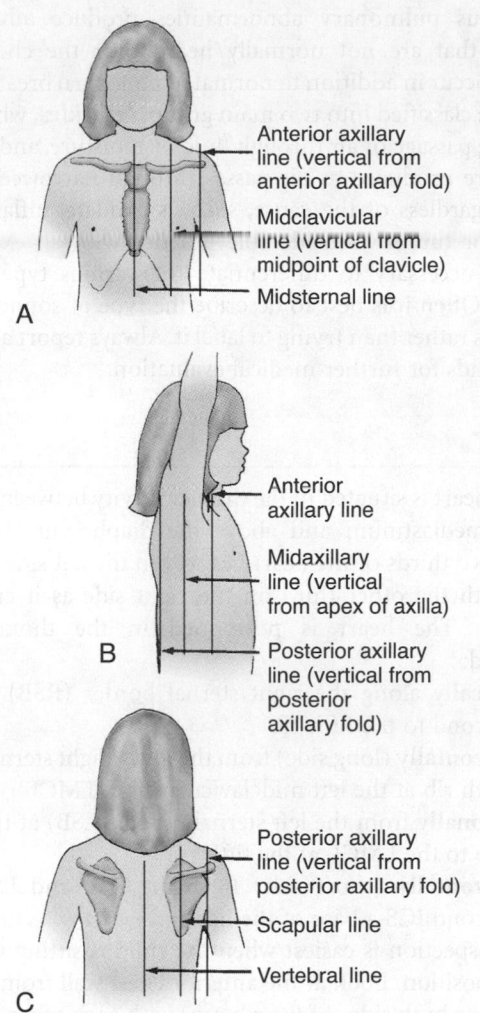

Fig. 6-29 Imaginary landmarks of chest. **A,** Anterior. **B,** Right lateral. **C,** Posterior.

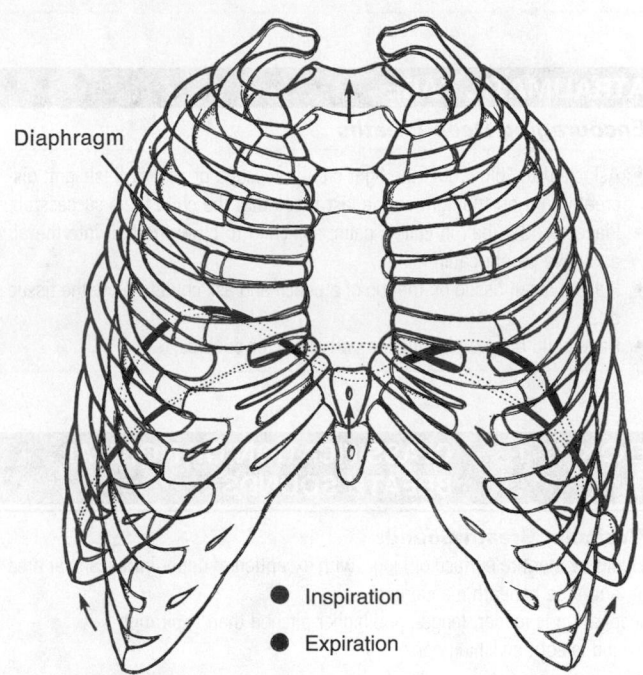

Fig. 6-30 Movement of chest during respiration.

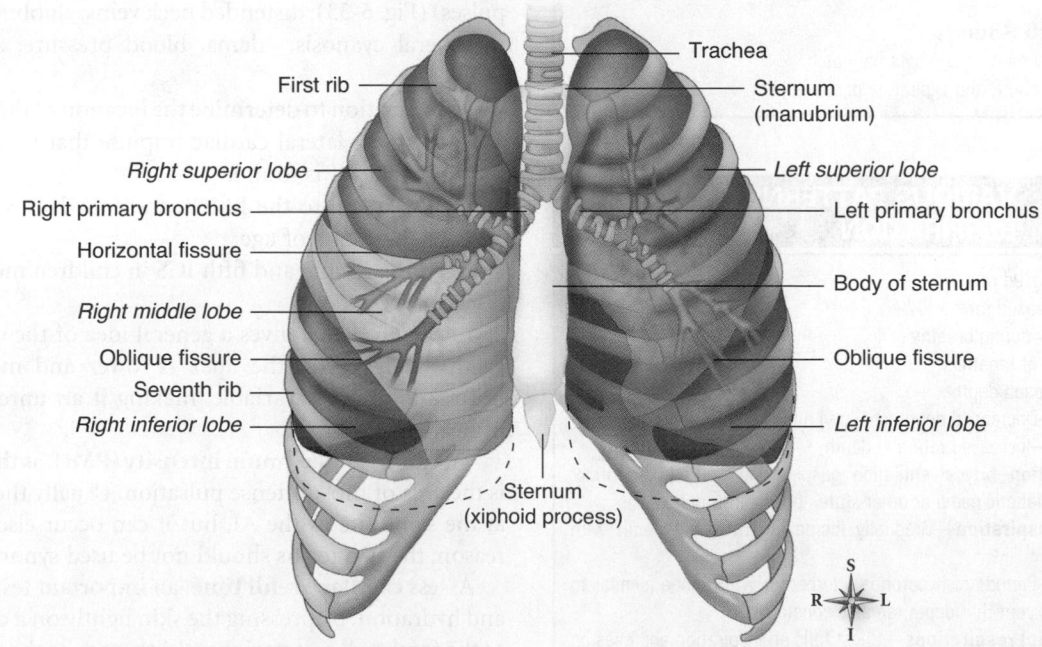

Fig. 6-31 Location of lobes of lungs within thoracic cavity. (From Patton KT, Thibodeau GA: *Anatomy and physiology,* ed 7, St Louis, 2010, Mosby.)

NURSING CARE GUIDELINES

Effective Auscultation

- Make certain child is relaxed and not crying, talking, or laughing. Record if child is crying.
- Check that room is comfortable and quiet.
- Warm stethoscope before placing it against skin.
- Apply firm pressure on chest piece but not enough to prevent vibrations and transmission of sound.
- Avoid placing stethoscope over hair or clothing, moving it against skin, breathing on tubing, or sliding fingers over chest piece, which may cause sounds that falsely resemble pathologic findings.
- Use a symmetric and orderly approach to compare sounds.

ATRAUMATIC CARE

Encouraging Deep Breaths

- Ask child to "blow out" the light on an otoscope or pocket flashlight; discreetly turn off the light on the last try so that the child feels successful.
- Place a cotton ball in child's palm; ask child to blow the ball into the air and have parent catch it.
- Place a small tissue on the top of a pencil and ask child to blow the tissue off.
- Have child blow a pinwheel, a party horn, or bubbles.

BOX 6-13   CLASSIFICATION OF NORMAL BREATH SOUNDS

Vesicular Breath Sounds
Heard over entire surface of lungs, with exception of upper intrascapular area and area beneath manubrium.
Inspiration is louder, longer, and higher pitched than expiration.
Sound is soft, swishing noise.

Bronchovesicular Breath Sounds
Heard over manubrium and in upper intrascapular regions where trachea and bronchi bifurcate.
Inspiration is louder and higher pitched than in vesicular breathing.

Bronchial Breath Sounds
Heard only over trachea near suprasternal notch.
Inspiratory phase is short, and expiratory phase is long.

BOX 6-14   VARIOUS PATTERNS OF RESPIRATION

Tachypnea—Increased rate
Bradypnea—Decreased rate
Dyspnea—Distress during breathing
Apnea—Cessation of breathing
Hyperpnea—Increased depth
Hypoventilation—Decreased depth (shallow) and irregular rhythm
Hyperventilation—Increased rate and depth
Kussmaul respiration—Hyperventilation, gasping and labored respiration; usually seen in diabetic coma or other states of respiratory acidosis
Cheyne-Stokes respiration—Gradually increasing rate and depth with periods of apnea
Biot respiration—Periods of hyperpnea alternating with apnea (similar to Cheyne-Stokes except that depth remains constant)
Seesaw (paradoxic) respirations—Chest falls on inspiration and rises on expiration
Agonal—Last gasping breaths before death

Various pulmonary abnormalities produce **adventitious sounds** that are not normally heard over the chest. These sounds occur in addition to normal or abnormal breath sounds. They are classified into two main groups: **crackles**, which result from the passage of air through fluid or moisture, and **wheezes**, which are produced as air passes through narrowed passageways, regardless of the cause, such as exudate, inflammation, spasm, or tumor. Considerable practice with an experienced tutor is necessary to differentiate the various types of lung sounds. Often it is best to describe the type of sound heard in the lungs rather than trying to label it. Always report any abnormal sounds for further medical evaluation.

HEART

The heart is situated in the thoracic cavity between the lungs in the mediastinum and above the diaphragm (Fig. 6-32). About two thirds of the heart lies within the left side of the rib cage, with the other third on the right side as it crosses the sternum. The heart is positioned in the thorax like a trapezoid:

> **Vertically** along the right sternal border (RSB) from the second to the fifth rib
> **Horizontally** (long side) from the lower right sternum to the fifth rib at the left midclavicular line (LMCL)
> **Diagonally** from the left sternal border (LSB) at the second rib to the LMCL at the fifth rib
> **Horizontally** (short side) from the RSB and LSB at the second ICS—base of the heart

Inspection is easiest when the child is sitting in a semi-Fowler position. Look at the anterior chest wall from an angle, comparing both sides of the rib cage with each other. Normally they should be symmetric. In children with thin chest walls, a pulsation may be visible. Because comprehensive evaluation of cardiac function is not limited to the heart, also consider other findings such as the presence of all pulses (especially the femoral pulses) (Fig. 6-33), distended neck veins, clubbing of the fingers, peripheral cyanosis, edema, blood pressure, and respiratory status.

Use palpation to determine the location of the **apical impulse (AI)**, the most lateral cardiac impulse that may correspond to the apex. The AI is found:

- Just lateral to the LMCL and fourth ICS in children less than 7 years of age
- At the LMCL and fifth ICS in children more than 7 years of age

Although the AI gives a general idea of the size of the heart (with enlargement, the apex is lower and more lateral), its normal location is variable, making it an unreliable indicator of heart size.

The **point of maximum intensity (PMI)**, as the name implies, is the area of most intense pulsation. Usually the PMI is located at the same site as the AI, but it can occur elsewhere. For this reason, the two terms should not be used synonymously.

Assess **capillary refill time**, an important test for circulation and hydration, by pressing the skin lightly on a central site, such as the forehead, or a peripheral site, such as the top of the hand, to produce a slight blanching. The time it takes for the blanched area to return to its original color is the capillary refill time.

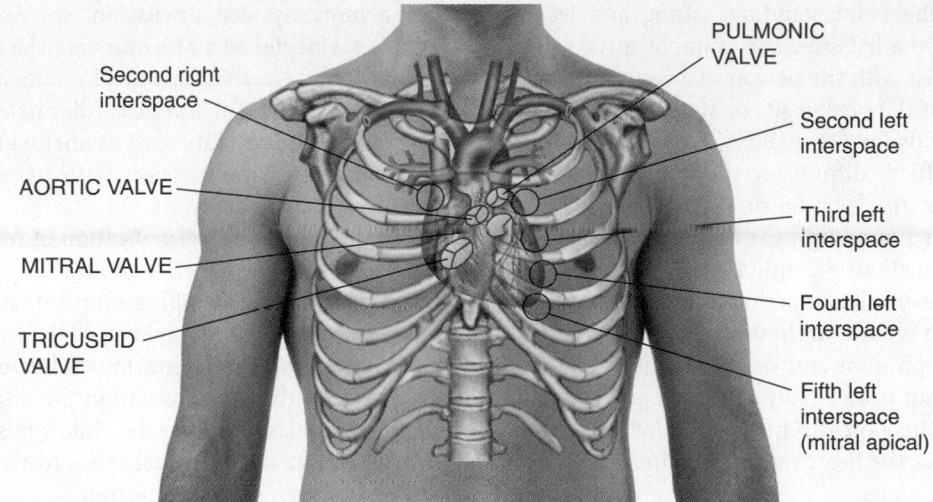

Fig. 6-32 Position of heart within thorax. (From Seidel HM, Ball JW, Dains JE, et al: *Mosby's guide to physical examination*, ed 5, 2003, St Louis, Mosby.)

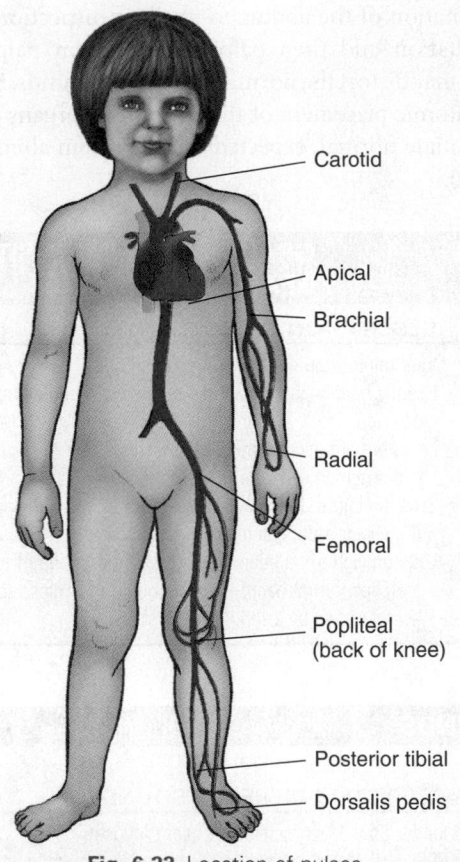

Fig. 6-33 Location of pulses.

> **! NURSING ALERT**
>
> Capillary refill should be brisk—less than 2 seconds. Prolonged refill may be associated with poor systemic perfusion or a cool ambient temperature.

Auscultation

Origin of Heart Sounds

The heart sounds are produced by the opening and closing of the valves and the vibration of blood against the walls of the heart and vessels. Normally two sounds—S_1 and S_2—are heard,

which correspond, respectively, to the familiar "lub dub" often used to describe the sounds. S_1 is caused by closure of the **tricuspid** and **mitral valves** (sometimes called the **atrioventricular valves**). S_2 is the result of closure of the **pulmonic** and **aortic valves** (sometimes called **semilunar valves**). Normally the split of the two sounds in S_2 is distinguishable and widens during inspiration. **Physiologic splitting** is a significant normal finding.

> **! NURSING ALERT**
>
> Fixed splitting, in which the split in S_2 does not change during inspiration, is an important diagnostic sign of atrial septal defect.

Two other heart sounds, S_3 and S_4, may be produced. S_3 is normally heard in some children; S_4 is rarely heard as a normal heart sound; it usually indicates the need for further cardiac evaluation.

Differentiating Normal Heart Sounds

Fig. 6-34 illustrates the approximate anatomic position of the valves within the heart chambers. Note that the anatomic location of valves does not correspond to the area where the sounds are heard best. The auscultatory sites are located in the direction of the blood flow through the valves.

Normally S_1 is louder at the apex of the heart in the mitral and tricuspid area, and S_2 is louder near the base of the heart in the pulmonic and aortic area (Table 6-11). Listen to each sound by inching down the chest. Auscultate the following areas for sounds, such as murmurs, which may radiate to these sites: sternoclavicular area above the clavicles and manubrium, area along the sternal border, area along the left midaxillary line, and area below the scapulae.

> **NURSING TIP** To distinguish between S_1 and S_2 heart sounds, simultaneously palpate the carotid pulse with the index and middle fingers and listen to the heart sounds; S_1 is synchronous with the carotid pulse.

Auscultate the heart with the child in at least two positions: sitting and reclining. If adventitious sounds are detected, further evaluate them with the child standing, sitting and leaning forward, and lying on the left side. For example, atrial sounds such as S₄ are heard best with the person in a recumbent position and usually fade if the person sits or stands.

Evaluate heart sounds for (1) quality (they should be clear and distinct, not muffled, diffuse, or distant); (2) intensity, especially in relation to the location or auscultatory site (they should not be weak or pounding); (3) rate (they should have the same rate as the radial pulse); and (4) rhythm (they should be regular and even). A particular arrhythmia that occurs normally in many children is **sinus arrhythmia**, in which the heart rate increases with inspiration and decreases with expiration. Differentiate this rhythm from a truly abnormal arrhythmia by having children hold their breath. In sinus arrhythmia, cessation of breathing causes the heart rate to remain steady.

Heart Murmurs

Another important category of the heart sounds is **murmurs**, which are produced by vibrations within the heart chambers or in the major arteries from the back-and-forth flow of blood.

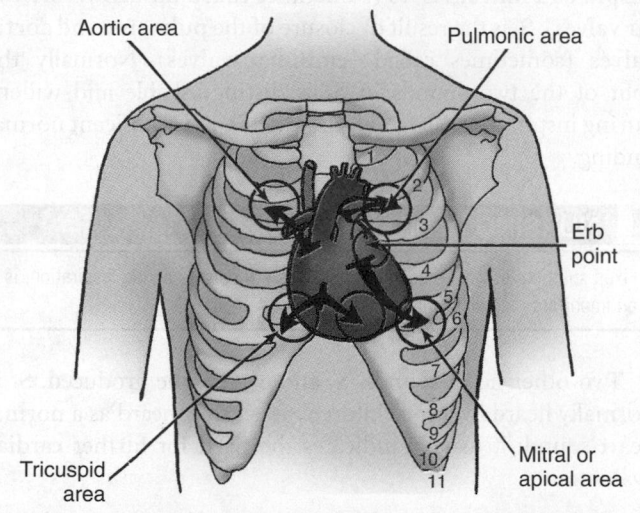

Fig. 6-34 Direction of heart sounds for anatomic valve sites and areas *(circled)* for auscultation.

(For a more detailed discussion, see Assessment of Cardiac Function, Chapter 34.) Murmurs are classified as:

Innocent—No anatomic or physiologic abnormality exists.

Functional—No anatomic cardiac defect exists, but a physiologic abnormality such as anemia is present.

Organic—A cardiac defect with or without a physiologic abnormality exists.

The description and classification of murmurs are skills that require considerable practice and training. In general, recognize murmurs as distinct swishing sounds that occur in addition to the normal heart sounds and record the (1) location, or the area of the heart in which the murmur is heard best; (2) time of the occurrence of the murmur within the S₁-S₂ cycle; (3) intensity (evaluate in relationship to the child's position); and (4) loudness. Table 6-12 lists the usual subjective method of grading the loudness or intensity of a murmur.

ABDOMEN

Examination of the abdomen involves inspection, followed by auscultation and then palpation. Perform palpation last because it may distort the normal abdominal sounds. Knowledge of the anatomic placement of the abdominal organs is essential to differentiate normal, expected findings from abnormal ones (Fig. 6-35).

TABLE 6-12	GRADING THE INTENSITY OF HEART MURMURS	
GRADE	**DESCRIPTION**	
I	Very faint; often not heard if child sits up	
II	Usually readily heard; slightly louder than grade I; audible in all positions	
III	Loud, but not accompanied by a thrill	
IV	Loud, accompanied by a thrill	
V	Loud enough to be heard with a stethoscope barely touching the chest; accompanied by a thrill	
VI	Loud enough to be heard with the stethoscope not touching the chest; often heard with the human ear close to the chest; accompanied by a thrill	

TABLE 6-11	SEQUENCE OF AUSCULTATING HEART SOUNDS*	
AUSCULTATORY SITE	**CHEST LOCATION**	**CHARACTERISTICS OF HEART SOUNDS**
Aortic area	Second right intercostal space close to sternum	S₂ heard louder than S₁; aortic closure heard loudest
Pulmonic area	Second left intercostal space close to sternum	Splitting of S₂ heard best, normally widens on inspiration; pulmonic closure heard best
Erb point	Second and third left intercostal spaces close to sternum	Frequent site of innocent murmurs and those of aortic or pulmonic origin
Tricuspid area	Fifth right and left intercostal spaces close to sternum	S₁ heard as louder sound preceding S₂ (S₁ synchronous with carotid pulse)
Mitral or apical area	Fifth intercostal space, left midclavicular line (third to fourth intercostal space and lateral to left midclavicular line in infants)	S₁ heard loudest; splitting of S₁ may be audible because mitral closure is louder than tricuspid closure
		S₁ heard best at beginning of expiration with child in recumbent or left side-lying position; occurs immediately after S₂; sounds like word S₁ S₂ S₃: "Ken-tuc-ky"
		S₄ heard best during expiration with child in recumbent position (left side-lying position decreases sound); occurs immediately before S₁; sounds like word S₄ S₁ S₂: "Ten-nes-see"

*Use both diaphragm and bell chest pieces when auscultating heart sounds. Bell chest piece is necessary for low-pitched sounds of murmurs, S₃, and S₄.

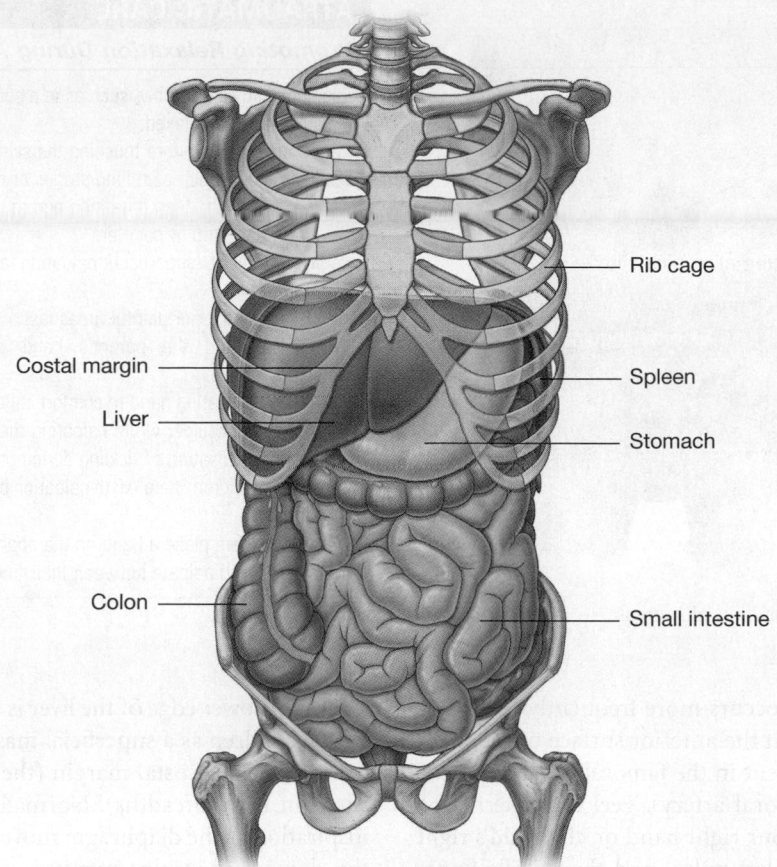

Fig. 6-35 Location of structures in abdomen. (From Drake RL, Vogl W, Mitchell AWM: *Gray's anatomy for students*, 2005, New York: Churchill Livingstone.)

For descriptive purposes, the abdominal cavity is divided into four quadrants by drawing a vertical line midway from the sternum to the symphysis pubis and a horizontal line across the abdomen through the umbilicus. The sections are named:

- Left upper quadrant
- Left lower quadrant
- Right upper quadrant
- Right lower quadrant

Inspection

Inspect the contour of the abdomen with the child erect and supine. Normally the abdomen of infants and young children is cylindric and, in the erect position, fairly prominent because of the physiologic lordosis of the spine. In the supine position the abdomen appears flat. A midline protrusion from the xiphoid to the umbilicus or symphysis pubis is usually **diastasis recti**, or failure of the rectus abdominis muscles to join in utero. In a healthy child a midline protrusion is usually a variation of normal muscular development.

> **! NURSING ALERT**
>
> A tense, boardlike abdomen is a serious sign of paralytic ileus and intestinal obstruction.

The skin covering the abdomen should be uniformly taut, without wrinkles or creases. Sometimes silvery, whitish striae ("stretch marks") are seen, especially if the skin has been stretched as in obesity. Superficial veins are usually visible in light-skinned, thin infants, but distended veins are an abnormal finding.

Observe movement of the abdomen. Normally chest and abdominal movements are synchronous. In infants and thin children **peristaltic waves** may be visible through the abdominal wall; they are best observed by standing at eye level to and across from the abdomen. Always report this finding.

🖲 Examine the umbilicus for size, hygiene, and evidence of any abnormalities, such as hernias. The umbilicus should be flat or only slightly protruding. If a herniation is present, palpate the sac for abdominal contents and estimate the approximate size of the opening. **Umbilical hernias** are common in infants, especially in African-American children.

Hernias may exist elsewhere on the abdominal wall (Fig. 6-36). An **inguinal hernia** is a protrusion of peritoneum through the abdominal wall in the inguinal canal. It occurs mostly in males, is frequently bilateral, and may be visible as a mass in the scrotum. To locate a hernia, slide the little finger into the external inguinal ring at the base of the scrotum and ask the child to cough. If a hernia is present, it will hit the tip of the finger.

> **NURSING TIP** If the child is too young to cough, have the child blow up a balloon or laugh to raise the intraabdominal pressure sufficiently to demonstrate the presence of an inguinal hernia.

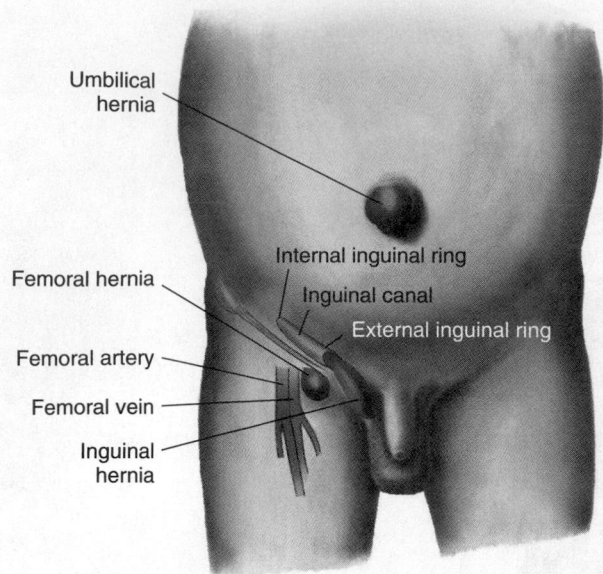

Umbilical hernia

Internal inguinal ring

Inguinal canal

External inguinal ring

Femoral hernia

Femoral artery

Femoral vein

Inguinal hernia

Fig. 6-36 Location of hernias.

ATRAUMATIC CARE

Promoting Relaxation During Abdominal Palpation

Position child comfortably, such as in a semireclining position in the parent's lap, with knees flexed.

Warm your hands before touching the skin.

Use distraction, such as telling stories or talking to child.

Teach child to use deep breathing and to concentrate on an object.

Give infant a bottle or pacifier.

Begin with light, superficial palpation and gradually progress to deeper palpation.

Palpate any tender or painful areas last.

Have child hold the parent's hand and squeeze it if palpation is uncomfortable.

Use the nonpalpating hand to comfort child, such as placing the free hand on the child's shoulder while palpating the abdomen.

To minimize sensation of tickling during palpation:
- Have children "help" with palpation by placing a hand over the palpating hand.
- Have them place a hand on the abdomen with the fingers spread wide apart, and palpate between their fingers.

A **femoral hernia**, which occurs more frequently in girls, is felt or seen as a small mass on the anterior surface of the thigh just below the inguinal ligament in the femoral canal (a potential space medial to the femoral artery). Feel for a hernia by placing the index finger of your right hand on the child's right femoral pulse (left hand for left pulse) and the middle finger flat against the skin toward the midline. The ring finger lies over the femoral canal, where the herniation occurs. Palpation of hernias in the pelvic region is often part of the genital examination.

Auscultation

The most important finding to listen for is **peristalsis**, or **bowel sounds**, which sound like short metallic clicks and gurgles. Record their frequency per minute (e.g., 5 sounds/min). Stimulate bowel sounds by stroking the abdominal surface with a fingernail. Report absence of bowel sounds or hyperperistalsis, since either usually denotes an abdominal disorder.

Palpation

There are two types of palpation: superficial and deep. For **superficial palpation**, lightly place your hand against the skin and feel each quadrant, noting any areas of tenderness, muscle tone, and superficial lesions such as cysts. Because superficial palpation is often perceived as tickling, use several techniques to minimize this sensation and relax the child (see Atraumatic Care box). Admonishing the child to stop laughing only draws attention to the sensation and decreases cooperation.

Deep palpation is for palpating organs and large blood vessels and for detecting masses and tenderness that were not discovered during superficial palpation. Palpation usually begins in the lower quadrants and proceeds upward to avoid missing the edge of an enlarged liver or spleen. Except for palpating the liver, successful identification of other organs, such as the spleen, kidney, and part of the colon, requires considerable practice with tutored supervision. Report any questionable mass. The lower edge of the liver is sometimes felt in infants and young children as a superficial mass 1 to 2 cm (0.4 to 0.8 inch) below the right costal margin (the distance is sometimes measured in fingerbreadths). Normally, the liver descends during inspiration as the diaphragm moves downward. Do not mistake this downward displacement as a sign of liver enlargement.

❗ NURSING ALERT

If the liver is palpable 3 cm (1.2 inch) below the right costal margin or the spleen is palpable more than 2 cm (0.8 inch) below the left costal margin, these organs are enlarged—a finding that is always reported for further medical investigation.

Palpate the **femoral pulses** by placing the tips of two or three fingers (index, middle, or ring) along the inguinal ligament about midway between the iliac crest and symphysis pubis. Feel both pulses simultaneously to make certain that they are equal and strong (Fig. 6-37).

❗ NURSING ALERT

Absence of femoral pulses is a significant sign of coarctation of the aorta and is referred for medical evaluation.

GENITALIA

Examination of genitalia conveniently follows assessment of the abdomen while the child is still supine. In adolescents inspection of the genitalia may be left to the end of the examination. The best approach is to examine the genitalia matter-of-factly, placing no more emphasis on this part of the assessment than on any other segment. It helps to relieve children's and parents' anxiety by telling them the results of the findings; for example, the nurse might say, "Everything looks fine here."

If it is necessary to ask questions, such as about discharge or difficulty urinating, respect the child's privacy by covering

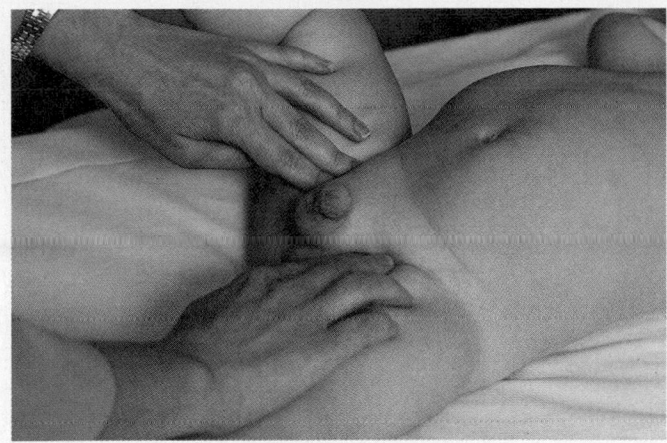

Fig. 6-37 Palpating for femoral pulses.

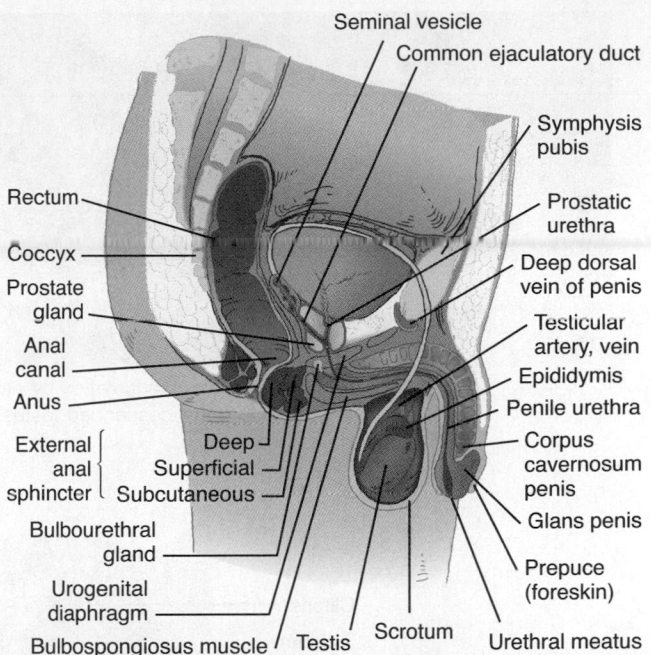

Fig. 6-38 Major structures of genitalia in uncircumcised postpubertal male. (From Black JM: *Medical-surgical nursing: clinical management for positive outcomes*, ed 8, St Louis, 2008, Saunders.)

the lower abdomen with the gown or underpants. To prevent embarrassing interruptions, keep the door or curtain closed and post a "do not disturb" sign. Have a drape ready to cover the genitalia if someone enters the room.

In examining the genitalia, wear gloves to avoid contact with body substances. It might be helpful for the adolescent to know that wearing gloves also prevents skin-to-skin contact.

The genital examination is an excellent time for eliciting questions or concern about body function or sexual activity. Also use this opportunity to increase or reinforce the child's knowledge of reproductive anatomy by naming each body part and explaining its function. This part of the health assessment is an opportune time to teach testicular self-examination to boys.

Male Genitalia

Note the external appearance of the glans and shaft of the penis, the prepuce, the urethral meatus, and the scrotum (Fig. 6-38). The penis is generally small in infants and young boys until puberty, when it begins to increase in both length and width. In an obese child the penis often looks abnormally small because of the folds of skin partially covering it at the base. Be familiar with normal pubertal growth of the external male genitalia to compare the findings with the expected sequence of maturation (see Chapter 16).

Examine the **glans** (head of the penis) and **shaft** (portion between the perineum and prepuce) for signs of swelling, skin lesions, inflammation, or other irregularities. Any of these signs may indicate underlying disorders, especially sexually transmitted infections.

Carefully inspect the **urethral meatus** for location and evidence of discharge. Normally it is centered at the tip of the glans. Also note hair distribution. Normally, before puberty, no pubic hair is present. Soft, downy hair at the base of the penis is an early sign of pubertal maturation. In older adolescents hair distribution is diamond-shaped from the umbilicus to the anus.

Note the location and size of the **scrotum**. The scrota hang freely from the perineum behind the penis, and the left scrotum normally hangs lower than the right. In infants the scrota appear large in relation to the rest of the genitalia. The skin of the scrotum is loose and highly rugated (wrinkled). During early adolescence the skin normally becomes redder and coarser.

In dark-skinned children the scrota are usually more deeply pigmented.

Palpation of the scrotum includes identification of the testes, epididymis, and, if present, inguinal hernias. The two **testes** are felt as small, ovoid bodies about 1.5 to 2 cm (0.6 to 0.8 inch) long—one in each scrotal sac. They do not enlarge until puberty, when they approximately double in size.

When palpating for the presence of the testes, avoid stimulating the **cremasteric reflex**, which is stimulated by cold, touch, emotional excitement, or exercise. This reflex pulls the testes higher into the pelvic cavity. Several measures are useful in preventing the cremasteric reflex during palpation of the scrotum. First, warm the hands. Second, if the child is old enough, examine him in a tailor or "Indian" position, which stretches the muscle, preventing its contraction (Fig. 6-39, *A*). Third, block the normal pathway of ascent of the testes by placing the thumb and index finger over the upper part of the scrotal sac along the inguinal canal (Fig. 6-39, *B*). If there is any question concerning the existence of two testes, place the index and middle fingers in a scissors fashion to separate the right and left scrota. If, after using these techniques, you have not palpated the testes, feel along the inguinal canal and perineum to locate masses that may be undescended testes. Although undescended testes may descend at any time during childhood and are checked at each visit, report any failure to palpate the testes.

Female Genitalia

The examination of female genitalia is limited to inspection and palpation of external structures. If a vaginal examination is required, the nurse should make an appropriate referral unless he or she is qualified to perform the procedure.

A convenient position for examination of the genitalia involves placing the young child supine on the examining table or in a semireclining position on the parent's lap with the feet

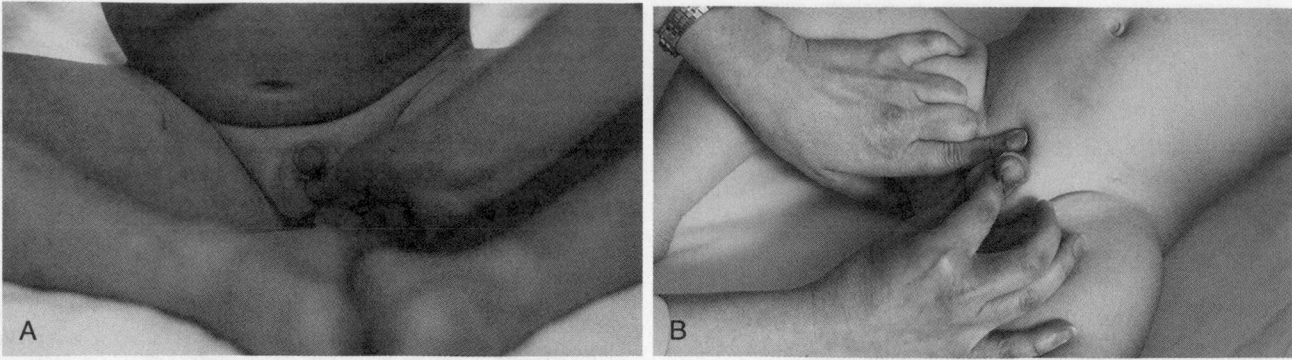

Fig. 6-39 A, Preventing cremasteric reflex by having child sit in tailor position. **B,** Blocking inguinal canal during palpation of scrotum for descended testes.

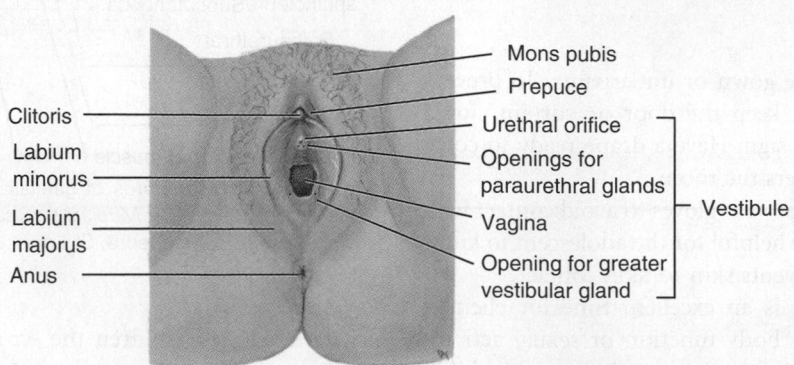

Clitoris
Labium minorus
Labium majorus
Anus

Mons pubis
Prepuce
Urethral orifice
Openings for paraurethral glands
Vagina
Opening for greater vestibular gland

Vestibule

Fig. 6-40 External structures of genitalia in postpubertal female. Labia are spread to reveal deeper structures. (From Applegate E: *The anatomy and physiology learning system,* ed 3, St Louis, 2006, Saunders.)

supported on your knees as you sit facing the child. Divert the child's attention from the examination by instructing her to try to keep the soles of her feet pressed against each other. Separate the labia majora with the thumb and index finger and retract outward to expose the labia minora, urethral meatus, and vaginal orifice.

Examine the female genitalia for size and location of the structures of the **vulva,** or **pudendum** (Fig. 6-40). The **mons pubis** is a pad of adipose tissue over the symphysis pubis. At puberty the mons is covered with hair, which extends along the labia. The usual pattern of female hair distribution is an inverted triangle. The appearance of soft, downy hair along the labia majora is an early sign of sexual maturation. Note the size and location of the **clitoris,** a small, erectile organ located at the anterior end of the labia minora. It is covered by a small flap of skin, the **prepuce.**

The **labia majora** are two thick folds of skin running posteriorly from the mons to the posterior commissure of the vagina. Internal to the labia majora are two folds of skin called the **labia minora.** Although the labia minora are usually prominent in the newborn, they gradually atrophy, which makes them almost invisible until their enlargement during puberty. The inner surface of the labia should be pink and moist. Note the size of the labia and any evidence of fusion, which may suggest male scrota. Normally no masses are palpable within the labia.

The **urethral meatus** is located posterior to the clitoris and is surrounded by the Skene glands and ducts. Although not a prominent structure, the meatus appears as a small V-shaped slit. Note its location, especially if it opens from the clitoris or inside the vagina. Gently palpate the glands, which are common sites of cysts and sexually transmitted lesions.

The **vaginal orifice** is located posterior to the urethral meatus. Its appearance varies depending on individual anatomy and sexual activity. Ordinarily, examination of the vagina is limited to inspection. In virgins a thin crescent-shaped or circular membrane, called the **hymen,** may cover part of the vaginal opening. In some instances it completely occludes the orifice. After rupture, small rounded pieces of tissue called **caruncles** remain. Although an imperforate hymen denotes lack of penile intercourse, a perforate one does not necessarily indicate sexual activity (see also Sexual Abuse, Chapter 16).

> **❗ NURSING ALERT**
>
> In girls who have been circumcised, the genitalia will appear different. Do not show surprise or disgust, but note the appearance and discuss the procedure with the young woman (see also Cultural Competence box, p. 120).

Surrounding the vaginal opening are **Bartholin glands,** which secrete a clear, mucoid fluid into the vagina for lubrication during intercourse. Palpate the ducts for cysts. Also note the discharge from the vagina, which is usually clear or white.

ANUS

After examination of the genitalia, it is easy to identify the anal area, although the child should be placed on the abdomen. Note the general firmness of the buttocks and symmetry of the **gluteal folds**. Assess the tone of the anal sphincter by eliciting the **anal reflex (anal wink)**. Gently scratching the anal area results in an obvious quick contraction of the external anal sphincter.

BACK AND EXTREMITIES

Spine

Note the general **curvature** of the spine. Normally the back of a newborn is rounded or **C** shaped from the thoracic and pelvic curves. The development of the cervical and lumbar curves approximates development of various motor skills, such as cervical curvature with head control, and gives the older child the typical double **S** curve.

Marked curvatures in posture are abnormal. **Scoliosis**, lateral curvature of the spine, is an important childhood problem, especially in girls. Although scoliosis may be identified by observing and palpating the spine and noting a sideways displacement, more objective tests include:

- With the child standing erect, clothed only in underpants (and bra if older girl), observe from behind, noting asymmetry of the shoulders and hips.
- With the child bending forward so that the back is parallel to the floor, observe from the side, noting asymmetry or prominence of the rib cage.

A slight limp, a crooked hemline, or complaints of a sore back are other signs and symptoms of scoliosis.

Inspect the back, especially along the spine, for any tufts of hair, dimples, or discoloration. Mobility of the vertebral column is easy to assess in most children because of their tendency to be in constant motion during the examination. However, you can test mobility by asking the child to sit up from a prone position or to do a modified sit-up exercise.

Movement of the cervical spine is an important diagnostic sign of neurologic problems, such as meningitis. Normally movement of the head in all directions is effortless.

❗ NURSING ALERT

Hyperextension of the neck and spine, or opisthotonos, which is accompanied by pain when the head is flexed, is always referred for immediate medical evaluation.

Extremities

Inspect each extremity for symmetry of length and size; refer any deviation for orthopedic evaluation. Count the fingers and toes to be certain of the normal number. This is so often taken for granted that an extra digit (**polydactyly**) or fusion of digits (**syndactyly**) may go unnoticed.

Inspect the arms and legs for temperature and color, which should be equal in each extremity, although the feet may normally be colder than the hands.

Assess the shape of bones. There are several variations of bone shape in children. Although many of them cause parents concern, most are benign and require no treatment. **Bowleg**, or **genu varum**, is lateral bowing of the tibia. It is clinically present when the child stands with an outward bowing of the legs, giving the appearance of a bow. Usually there is an outward

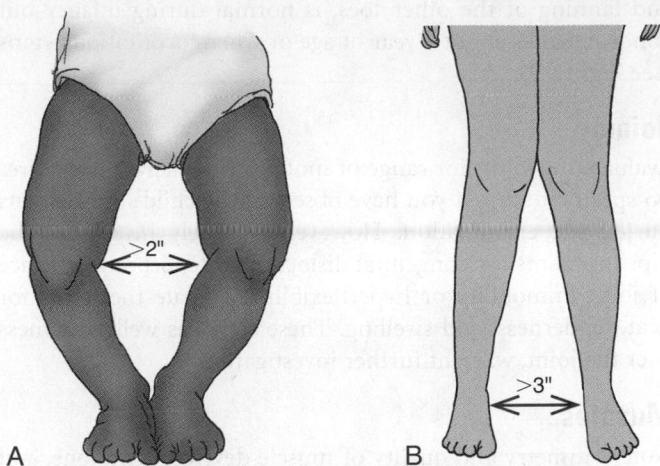

Fig. 6-41 A, Bowleg. **B**, Knock-knee.

curvature of both femur and tibia (Fig. 6-41, *A*). Toddlers are usually bowlegged after beginning to walk until all their lower back and leg muscles are well developed. Unilateral or asymmetric bowlegs that are present beyond the age of 2 to 3 years, particularly in African-American children, may represent pathologic conditions requiring further investigation.

Knock-knee, or **genu valgum**, appears as the opposite of bowleg, in that the knees are close together but the feet are spread apart. It is determined clinically by using the same method as for genu varum but by measuring the distance between the malleoli, which normally should be less than 7.5 cm (3 inches) (Fig. 6-41, *B*). Knock-knee is normally present in children from about 2 to 7 years of age. Knock-knee that is excessive, asymmetric, accompanied by short stature, or evident in a child nearing puberty requires further evaluation.

Next inspect the feet. Infants' and toddlers' feet appear flat because the foot is normally wide and the arch is covered by a fat pad. Development of the arch occurs naturally from the action of walking. Normally, at birth the feet are held in a valgus (outward) or varus (inward) position. To determine whether a foot deformity at birth is a result of intrauterine position or development, scratch the outer, then inner, side of the sole. If the foot position is self-correctable, it will assume a right angle to the leg. As the child begins to walk, the feet turn outward less than 30 degrees and inward less than 10 degrees.

Toddlers have a "toddling" or broad-based gait, which facilitates walking by lowering the center of gravity. As the child reaches preschool age, the legs are brought closer together. By school age the walking posture is much more graceful and balanced.

The most common gait problem in young children is **pigeon toe**, or **toeing in**, which usually results from torsional deformities, such as internal tibial torsion (abnormal rotation or bowing of the tibia). Tests for tibial torsion include measuring the thigh-foot angle, which requires considerable practice for accuracy.

Elicit the **plantar** or **grasp reflex** by exerting firm but gentle pressure with the tip of the thumb against the lateral sole of the foot from the heel upward to the little toe and then across to the big toe. The normal response in children who are walking is flexion of the toes. **Babinski sign**, dorsiflexion of the big toe and fanning of the other toes, is normal during infancy but abnormal after about 1 year of age or when locomotion begins (see Fig. 12-9).

Joints

Evaluate the joints for range of motion. Normally this requires no specific testing if you have observed the child's movements during the examination. However, routinely investigate the hips in infants for congenital dislocation. Report any evidence of joint immobility or hyperflexibility. Palpate the joints for heat, tenderness, and swelling. These signs, as well as redness over the joint, warrant further investigation.

Muscles

Note symmetry and quality of muscle development, tone, and strength. Observe development by looking at the shape and contour of the body in both a relaxed and a tensed state. Estimate tone by grasping the muscle and feeling its firmness when it is relaxed and contracted. A common site for testing tone is the biceps muscle of the arm. Children are usually willing to "make a muscle" by clenching their fist.

Estimate strength by having the child use an extremity to push or pull against resistance, as in the following examples:

Arm strength—Child holds the arms outstretched in front of the body and tries to raise the arms while downward pressure is applied.

Hand strength—Child shakes hands with nurse and squeezes one or two fingers of the nurse's hand.

Leg strength—Child sits on a table or chair with the legs dangling and tries to raise the legs while downward pressure is applied.

Note symmetry of strength in the extremities, hands, and fingers, and report evidence of **paresis**, or weakness.

NEUROLOGIC ASSESSMENT

The assessment of the nervous system is the broadest and most diverse part of the examination process, since every human function, both physical and emotional, is controlled by neurologic impulses. Much of the neurologic examination has already been discussed, such as assessment of behavior, sensory testing, and motor function. The following focuses on a general appraisal of cerebellar function, deep tendon reflexes, and the cranial nerves.

Cerebellar Function

The cerebellum controls balance and coordination. Much of the assessment of cerebellar function is included in observing the child's posture, body movements, gait, and development of fine and gross motor skills. Tests such as balancing on one foot and the heel-to-toe walk assess balance. Test coordination by asking the child to reach for a toy, button clothes, tie shoes, or draw a straight line on a piece of paper (provided the child is old enough to do these activities). Coordination can also be tested by any sequence of rapid, successive movements, such as quickly touching each finger with the thumb of the same hand.

Several tests for cerebellar function can be performed as games (Box 6-15). When a Romberg test is done, stay beside the child if there is a possibility that he or she might fall. School-

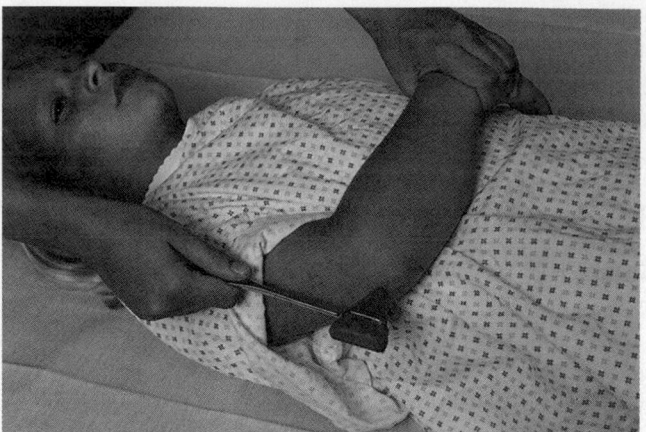

Fig. 6-42 Testing for triceps reflex. Child is placed supine, with forearm resting over chest, and triceps tendon is struck. Alternate procedure: child's arm is abducted, with upper arm supported and forearm allowed to hang freely. Triceps tendon is struck. Normal response is partial extension of forearm.

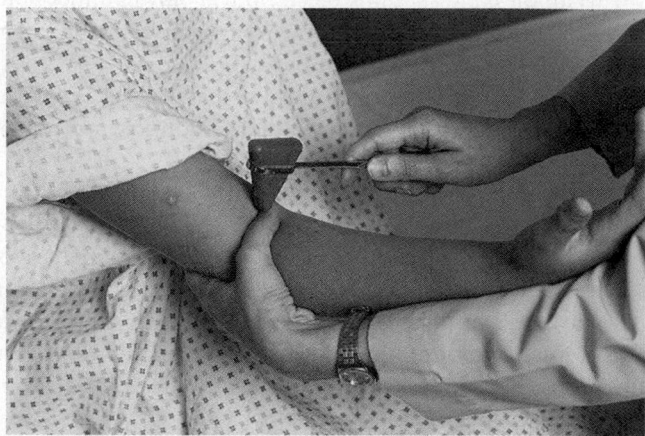

Fig. 6-43 Testing for biceps reflex. Child's arm is held by placing partially flexed elbow in examiner's hand with thumb over antecubital space. Examiner's thumbnail is struck with hammer. Normal response is partial flexion of forearm.

BOX 6-15   TESTS FOR CEREBELLAR FUNCTION

Finger-to-nose test—With child's arm extended, ask child to touch the nose with the index finger with eyes open and then closed.

Heel-to-shin test—Have child stand and run the heel of one foot down the shin or anterior aspect of the tibia of the other leg, both with eyes opened and then closed.

Romberg test—Have child stand with eyes closed and heels together; falling or leaning to one side is abnormal and is called Romberg sign.

---

age children should be able to perform these tests, although in the finger-to-nose test preschoolers normally can only bring the finger within 5 to 7.5 cm (2 to 3 inches) of the nose. Difficulty in performing these exercises indicates poor sense of position (especially with the eyes closed) and incoordination (especially with the eyes opened).

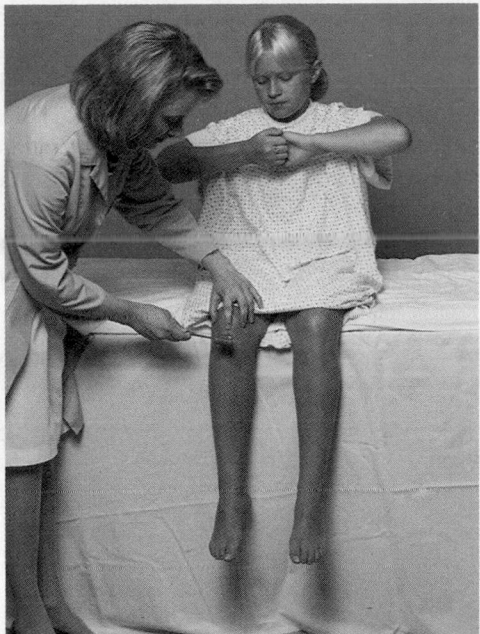

Fig. 6-44 Testing for patellar, or knee jerk, reflex, using distraction. Child sits on edge of examining table (or on parent's lap) with lower legs flexed at knee and dangling freely. Patellar tendon is tapped just below kneecap. Normal response is partial extension of lower leg.

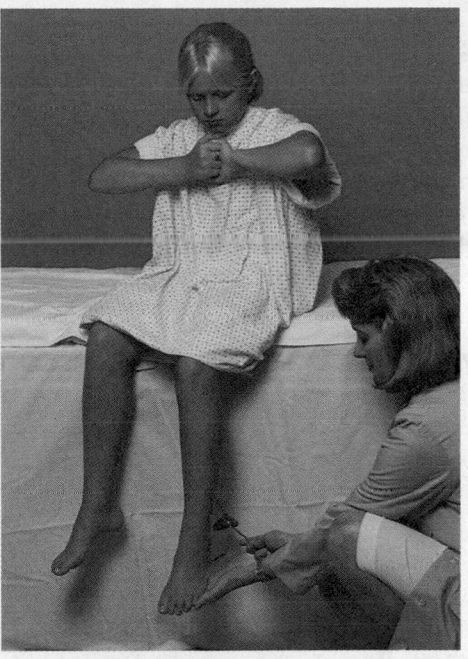

Fig. 6-45 Testing for Achilles reflex. Child should be in same position as for knee jerk reflex. Foot is supported lightly in examiner's hand, and Achilles tendon is struck. Normal response is plantar flexion of foot (foot pointing downward).

PATHOPHYSIOLOGY REVIEW

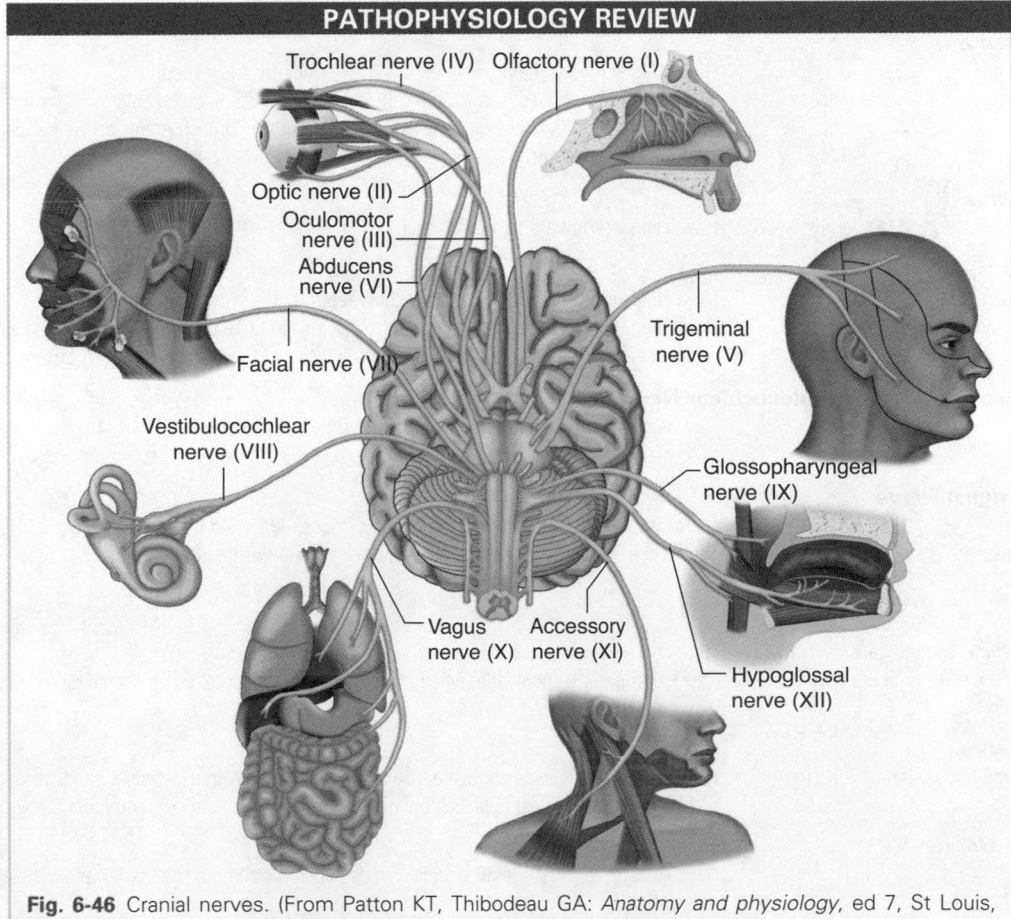

Fig. 6-46 Cranial nerves. (From Patton KT, Thibodeau GA: *Anatomy and physiology*, ed 7, St Louis, 2009, Mosby.)

Reflexes

Testing reflexes is an important part of the neurologic examination. Persistence of primitive reflexes (see Chapter 8), loss of reflexes, or hyperactivity of deep tendon reflexes is usually a result of a cerebral insult.

Elicit reflexes by using the rubber head of the reflex hammer, flat of the finger, or side of the hand. If the child is easily frightened by equipment, use your hand or finger. Although testing reflexes is a simple procedure, the child may inhibit the reflex by unconsciously tensing the muscle. To avoid tensing, distract younger children with toys or talk to them. Older children can concentrate on the exercise of grasping their two hands in front of them and trying to pull them apart. This diverts their attention from the testing and causes involuntary relaxation of the muscles.

Deep tendon reflexes are stretch reflexes of a muscle. The most common deep tendon reflex is the **knee jerk reflex**, or

TABLE 6-13 ASSESSMENT OF CRANIAL NERVES	
DESCRIPTION AND FUNCTION	**TESTS**
I—Olfactory Nerve Olfactory mucosa of nasal cavity Smell	With eyes closed, have child identify odors such as coffee, alcohol from a swab, or other smells; test each nostril separately.
II—Optic Nerve Rods and cones of retina, optic nerve Vision	Check for perception of light, visual acuity, peripheral vision, color vision, and normal optic disc.
III—Oculomotor Nerve Extraocular muscles of eye: • Superior rectus—moves eyeball up and in • Inferior rectus—moves eyeball down and in • Medial rectus—moves eyeball nasally • Inferior oblique—moves eyeball up and out Pupil constriction and accommodation Eyelid closing	Have child follow an object (toy) or light in six cardinal positions of gaze (see Fig. 6-47). Perform *PERRLA* (*P*upils *E*qual, *R*ound, *R*eact to *L*ight, and *A*ccommodation). Check for proper placement of lid.
IV—Trochlear Nerve Superior oblique muscle—moves eye down and out	Have child look down and in (see Fig. 6-47).
V—Trigeminal Nerve Muscles of mastication Sensory—face, scalp, nasal and buccal mucosa	Have child bite down hard and open jaw; test symmetry and strength. With child's eyes closed, see if child can detect light touch in mandibular and maxillary regions. Test corneal and blink reflex by touching cornea lightly (approach from side so that child does not blink before cornea is touched).
VI—Abducens Nerve Lateral rectus muscle—moves eye temporally	Have child look toward temporal side (see Fig. 6-47).
VII—Facial Nerve Muscles for facial expression Anterior two thirds of tongue (sensory)	Have child smile, make funny face, or show teeth to see symmetry of expression. Have child identify sweet or salty solution; place each taste on anterior section and sides of protruding tongue; if child retracts tongue, solution will dissolve toward posterior part of tongue.
VIII—Auditory, Acoustic, or Vestibulocochlear Nerve Internal ear Hearing and balance	Test hearing; note any loss of equilibrium or presence of vertigo.
IX—Glossopharyngeal Nerve Pharynx, tongue Posterior third of tongue Sensory	Stimulate posterior pharynx with a tongue blade; child should gag. Test sense of sour or bitter taste on posterior segment of tongue.
X—Vagus Nerve Muscles of larynx, pharynx, some organs of gastrointestinal system, sensory fibers of root of tongue, heart, and lung	Note hoarseness of voice, gag reflex, and ability to swallow. Check that uvula is in midline; when stimulated with tongue blade, it should deviate upward and to stimulated side.
XI—Accessory Nerve Sternocleidomastoid and trapezius muscles of shoulder	Have child shrug shoulders while applying mild pressure; with examiner's hands placed on shoulders, have child turn head against opposing pressure on either side; note symmetry and strength.
XII—Hypoglossal Nerve Muscles of tongue	Have child move tongue in all directions; have child protrude tongue as far as possible; note any midline deviation. Test strength by placing tongue blade on one side of tongue and having child move it away.

patellar reflex (sometimes called the quadriceps reflex). Figs. 6-42 to 6-45 illustrate the reflexes normally elicited. Report any diminished or hyperreflexive response for further evaluation.

Cranial Nerves

Assessment of the cranial nerves is an important area of neurologic assessment (Fig. 6-46; Table 6-13). With young children, present the tests as games to foster trust and security at the beginning of the examination. Also include the cranial nerve test when examining each system, such as tongue movement and strength, gag reflex, swallowing, cardinal positions of gaze (Fig. 6-47), and position of the uvula during examination of the mouth.

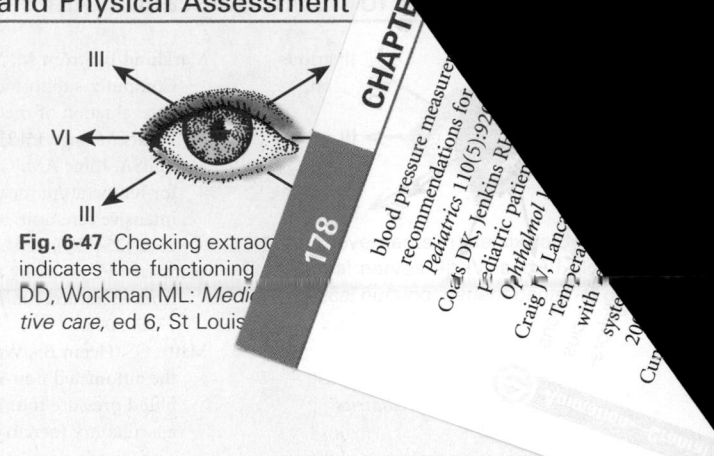

Fig. 6-47 Checking extraoc... indicates the functioning... DD, Workman ML: *Medi... tive care*, ed 6, St Louis...

KEY POINTS

- To effectively establish a setting for communication, nurses must make an appropriate introduction and ensure privacy and confidentiality.
- When communicating with parents, nurses need to encourage parental involvement, listen carefully, use silence, and be empathic.
- Communication with children must reflect their developmental stage.
- Nonverbal communication with children may take the form of writing, drawing, and play.
- The objectives of performing a health history are to identify pertinent information, determine the chief complaint, analyze the present illness, secure the patient's health history, review biologic systems, and record a family medical history and child psychosocial and sexual history.
- Family assessment is the collection of data about family composition and relationships among its members; it also focuses on home and community environment, parents' occupation and education, and cultural and religious traditions.
- The family function interview examines interaction and roles, power, decision making, problem solving, communication, and expression of feelings and individuality.
- Nutritional assessment is performed by determination of dietary intake, clinical examination, and biochemical analysis.
- Growth measurements during the physical examination focus on length or height, weight, skinfold thickness, and arm and head circumference. Assessment of growth is measured against standard growth charts to determine a child's status in comparison with other children of the same age.

- Measurements of temperature, pulse, respiration, and BP constitute the physiologic approach to assessment.
- The child's general appearance is a cumulative, subjective impression of physical appearance, state of nutrition, behavior, personality, interactions with parents and nurse, posture, development, and speech.
- Assessment of the skin, which primarily involves inspection and palpation, focuses on color, texture, temperature, moisture, and turgor. The nurse needs to be aware of both physiologic and ethnic factors that may affect these areas.
- In assessment of the lymph nodes, the nurse examines, by palpation, the part of the body in which the glands are located.
- The head is inspected for shape, symmetry, mobility, and muscle control.
- Examination of the eyes includes placement and alignment, inspection of external and internal structures, and vision testing.
- The ear examination encompasses placement and alignment, external and internal structures, and auditory testing.
- The lungs are examined by inspection, palpation, percussion, and auscultation.
- Auscultation is the most important procedure for examining the heart.
- Abdominal assessment follows an orderly sequence of inspection, auscultation, and palpation, since palpation may distort normal abdominal sounds.
- Examination of the genitalia may provoke anxiety in the child, and the nurse must avoid any transference of anxiety.
- Neurologic assessment addresses behavior; motor, sensory, and cerebellar function; reflexes; and cranial nerves.

REFERENCES

American Academy of Pediatrics: *Pediatric nutrition handbook*, ed 5, Elk Grove Village, Ill, 2004, The Academy.

American Academy of Pediatrics, Committee on Practice and Ambulatory Medicine, Section on Ophthalmology: Eye examination in infants, children, and young adults by pediatricians, *Pediatrics* 111(4):902-907, 2003a.

American Academy of Pediatrics, Committee on Practice and Ambulatory Medicine, Section

on Otolaryngology and Bronchoesophagology: Hearing assessment in infants and children: recommendations beyond neonatal screening, *Pediatrics* 111(2):436-440, 2003b.

Bald M: Ambulatory blood pressure monitoring in children and adolescents, *Minerva Paediatr* 54(1):13-24, 2002.

Beaulieu R, Humphreys J: Evaluation of a telephone advice nurse in a nursing faculty managed pediatric community clinic, *J Pediatr Health Care* 22(3):175-181, 2008.

Beevers G, Lip GYH, O'Brien E: ABC of hypertension blood pressure measurement, part I, Sphygmomanometry: factors common to all techniques, *BMJ* 322(7292):981-985, 2001.

Berry BE, Simons BD, Siatkowski RM, et al: Preschool vision screening using the MTI-Photoscreener, *Pediatr Nurs* 27(1):27-34, 2001.

Clark JA, Kieh-Lai MW, Sarnaik A, et al: Discrepancies between direct and indirect

ments using various
arm cuff selection,
0-923, 2002.
: Vision assessment of the
: refinements, *Am Acad*
(1):1-12, 1997.
ster GA, Williamson PR, et al:
re measured at the axilla compared
ctum in children and young people:
matic review, *BMJ* 320(7243):1174-1178,
00.
ningham M, Cox EO: Hearing assessment in
infants and children: recommendations
beyond neonatal screening, *Pediatrics*
111(2):436-440, 2003.

Halle C: Achieve new vision screening objectives,
Nurse Pract 27(3):15-35, 2002.

Healthcare Product Comparison System:
Thermometers, electronic, infrared, Plymouth
Meeting, Penn, July 2004a, ECRI.

Healthcare Product Comparison System:
*Thermometers, electronic, thermistor/
thermocouple, patient,* Plymouth Meeting,
Penn, July 2004b, ECRI.

Hedley AA, Ogden CL, Johnson CL, et al:
Prevalence of overweight and obesity among
US children, adolescents, and adults,
1999-2002, *JAMA* 291(23):2847-2850, 2004.

Livingstone MBE, Robson PJ, Wallace MW:
Issues in dietary intake assessment of children
and adolescents, *Br J Nutr* 92(Suppl 2):
S213-S222, 2004.

Magar NA, Dabova-Missova S, Gjerdingen DK:
Effectiveness of targeted anticipatory guidance
during well-child visits: a pilot trial, *J Am
Board Fam Med* 19(5):450-458, 2006.

Marklund B, Ström M, Månsson J, et al:
Computer-supported telephone nurse triage:
an evaluation of medical quality and costs,
J Nurs Manage 15(2):180-187, 2007.

Martin SA, Kline AM: Can there be a standard
for temperature measurement in the pediatric
intensive care unit? *AACN Clin Issues*
15(2):254-266, 2004.

Mathiasen H: Empathy and sympathy: voices
from literature, *Am J Cardiol* 97(12):1789-
1790, 2006.

Mattu GS, Heran BS, Wright JM: Comparison of
the automated non-invasive oscillometric
blood pressure monitor (BpTRU™) with the
auscultatory mercury sphygmomanometer in
a paediatric population, *Blood Pressure Monit*
9(1):39-45, 2004a.

Mattu GS, Heran BS, Wright JM: Overall
accuracy of the BpTRU™—an automated
electronic blood pressure device, *Blood Press
Monit* 9(1):47-52, 2004b.

Murphy SP, Poos MI: Dietary reference intakes:
summary of applications in dietary
assessment, *Public Health Nutr* 5(6A):843-849,
2002.

National High Blood Pressure Education
Program Working Group on High Blood
Pressure in Children and Adolescents: The
fourth report on the diagnosis, evaluation,
and treatment of high blood pressure in
children and adolescents, *Pediatrics* 114(2
Suppl 4th Rep):555-576, 2004.

National Institutes of Health, National Heart,
Lung, and Blood Institute: *Update on the Task
Force Report (1987) on high blood pressure in
children and adolescents: a working group*

*report from the National High Blood Pressure
Education Program,* NIH Pub No 96-3790,
Bethesda, Md, September 1996, The
Institutes.

Nicklas TA, Demory-Luce D, Yang SJ, et al:
Children's food consumption patterns have
changed over 2 decades (1973-1994): the
Bogalusa heart study, *J Am Diet Assoc*
104(7):1127-1140, 2004.

Ogden CL, Carroll MD, Flegal KM: High body
mass index for age among US children and
adolescents, 2003-2006, *JAMA* 299(20):2401-
2405, 2008.

Ogden CL, Kuczmarski RJ, Flegal KM, et al:
Centers for Disease Control and Prevention
2000 growth charts for the United States:
improvements to the 1977 National Center
for Health Statistics version, *Pediatrics*
109(1):45-60, 2002.

Park MK, Menard SW, Schoolfield J:
Oscillometric blood pressure standards for
children, *Pediatr Cardiol* 26(5):601-607,
2005.

Seidel HM, Ball JW, Dains JE, et al: *Mosby's guide
to physical examination,* ed 6, St. Louis, 2007,
Mosby.

Turnbull R: Skin assessment in children: a
methodical approach, *Nurs Times* 96(41):33-
34, 2000.

Vessey JA: Developmental approaches to
examining young children, *Pediatr Nurs*
21(1):53-56, 1995.

Wall TC, Marsh-Tootle W, Evans HH, et al:
Compliance with vision-screening guidelines
among a national sample of pediatricians,
Ambul Pediatr 2(6):449-455, 2002.

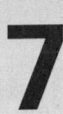

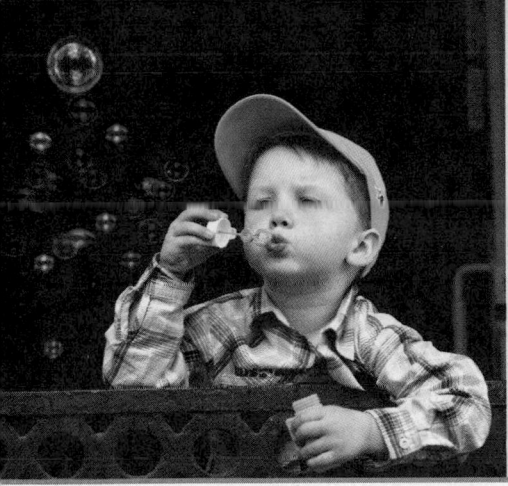

Pain Assessment and Management in Children

Eufemia Jacob

CHAPTER OUTLINE

The evidence-based literature on pediatric pain assessment and management grows considerably each year. Pain measurement tools that were developed more than 20 years ago continue to be refined and are becoming available electronically. Available treatment options for pediatric acute and chronic pain are continually being evaluated, and new technologies and administration options become available every day. Unfortunately, despite the advances in acute and chronic pediatric pain management over the past 15 to 20 years, many children and adolescents continue to suffer from inadequately treated pain of all types (Perquin, Hazebroek-Kampschreur, Hunfeld, et al, 2000a, 2000b). Several research studies suggest that the undertreatment of pain in children is related to inconsistent practices in pain assessment, administration of analgesics at subtherapeutic levels, prolonged intervals in between medications, and lack of systematic monitoring and evaluation of relief (Jacob and

Nursing Care Plan—The Child in Pain

Puntillo, 2000; Jacob, Miaskowski, and Savedra, et al, 2003a, 2003b; Jacob and Mueller, 2008).

PAIN ASSESSMENT

The pain experience in children is influenced by the child's age and developmental level, the cause of the pain, the nature of the pain, and the child's ability to express the pain in a meaningful way (Box 7-1). Pediatric pain assessment tools need to reflect the variations in children's cognitive, emotional, and physical capabilities. The family plays an important role in pain assessment. The Pediatric Initiative on Methods, Measurement, and Pain Assessment in Clinical Trials (PedIMMPACT) group recommended six core domains and specific measures to assess and measure pain in children (McGrath, Walco, Turk, et al, 2008). These domains include pain intensity, global judgment

---

BOX 7-1 DEVELOPMENTAL CHARACTERISTICS OF CHILDREN'S RESPONSES TO PAIN

Young Infant

Generalized body response of rigidity or thrashing, possibly with local reflex withdrawal of stimulated area

Loud crying

Facial expression of pain (brows lowered and drawn together, eyes tightly closed, and mouth open and squarish)

No association demonstrated between approaching stimulus and subsequent pain

Older Infant

Localized body response with deliberate withdrawal of stimulated area

Loud crying

Facial expression of pain or anger

Physical resistance, especially pushing the stimulus away after it is applied

Young Child

Loud crying, screaming

Verbal expressions such as "Ow," "Ouch," "It hurts"

Thrashing of arms and legs

Attempts to push stimulus away before it is applied

Lack of cooperation; need for physical restraint

Requests termination of procedure

Clings to parent, nurse, or other significant person

Requests emotional support, such as hugs or other forms of physical comfort

May become restless and irritable with continuing pain

Behaviors occurring in anticipation of actual painful procedure

School-Age Child

May see all behaviors of young child, especially during actual painful procedure, but less in anticipatory period

Stalling behavior, such as "Wait a minute" or "I'm not ready"

Muscular rigidity, such as clenched fists, white knuckles, gritted teeth, contracted limbs, body stiffness, closed eyes, wrinkled forehead

Adolescent

Less vocal protest

Less motor activity

More verbal expressions, such as "It hurts" or "You're hurting me"

Increased muscle tension and body control

Data from Craig KD, McMahon, Morison, et al: Developmental changes in infant pain expression during immunization injections, *Soc Sci Med* 19(12):1331-1337, 1984; and Katz ER, Kellerman J, Siegel SE: Behavioral distress in children with cancer undergoing medical procedures: developmental considerations, *J Consult Clin Psychol* 48(3):356-365, 1980.

---

of satisfaction with treatment, symptoms and adverse events, physical recovery, emotional response, and economic factors. These domains are discussed for assessment of both acute pain and chronic and recurrent pain.

ASSESSMENT OF ACUTE PAIN

Acute pain may be related to medical treatments, surgical procedures, injury, infection, or exacerbations of underlying disease.

Pain Intensity

Traditionally, pediatric pain assessment tools are described as being behavioral, physiologic, or self-report and are used predominantly to measure pain intensity. Many pediatric pain assessment tools have been validated and are widely used. Behavioral measures of pain are generally used for children from infancy to age 4 years (Table 7-1), and self-report measures are used for children over 4 years of age (Table 7-2). Self-report measures are not valid for children under 4 years of age because most children under 4 cannot accurately report the intensity of their pain. Distress behaviors, such as vocalization of sounds associated with pain, changes in facial expression, and unexpected or unusual body movements, have been associated with pain (Figs. 7-1 and 7-2). Understanding that these behaviors are associated with pain makes assessing pain in small children with limited communication skills a little easier. However, discriminating between pain behaviors and reactions to other sources of distress, such as hunger, anxiety, or other types of discomfort, is not always easy. These factors decrease the specificity and sensitivity of behavioral measures (see Table 7-1).

Behavioral pain assessment may provide a more complete picture of the total pain experience when administered in conjunction with a subjective self-report measure. Behavioral pain measurement tools may be more time consuming than self-reports because they depend on a trained observer to watch and record children's behaviors such as vocalization, facial expression, and body movements that suggest discomfort. In addition, they are most reliable when used to measure short, sharp procedural pain, such as during injections or lumbar punctures, or when assessing pain in infants. They are less reliable when measuring recurrent or chronic pain and when assessing pain in older children, where pain scores on behavioral measures do not always correlate with the children's own reports of pain intensity.

The four most commonly used behavioral pain measurement tools are the FLACC, CHEOPS, TPPPS, and PPPRS (see Table 7-1). The FLACC Pain Assessment Tool is an interval scale that includes the five categories of behavior: facial expression (F), leg movement (L), activity (A), cry (C), and consolability (C) (Manworren and Hynan, 2003; Merkel, Voepel-Lewis, Shayevitz, et al, 1997). It measures each behavior on a 0 to 10 scale, with total scores ranging from 0 (no pain behaviors) to 10 (most possible pain behaviors).

The Children's Hospital of Eastern Ontario Pain Scale (CHEOPS) was developed in collaboration with experienced recovery room nurses who were queried as to what behaviors

Text continued on p. 185.

TABLE 7-1 SUMMARY OF SELECTED BEHAVIORAL PAIN ASSESSMENT SCALES FOR YOUNG CHILDREN

AGES OF USE	RELIABILITY AND VALIDITY	VARIABLES	SCORING RANGE
Objective Pain Score (OPS) (Hannallah, Broadman, Belman, et al, 1987)			
4 mo–18 yr	Concurrent validity with linear analog pain scale, Spearman's r: 0.721 with scores ≥6 and 0.419 with scores <6 Interrater agreement, coefficient alpha: 0.986 for one rater and 0.983 for the other Concurrent validity with CHEOPS, Pearson correlation coefficient: 0.88 and 0.94	Blood pressure (0-2) Crying (0-2) Moving (0-2) Agitation (0-2) Verbal evaluation/body language (0-2)	0 = no pain; 10 = worst pain
Children's Hospital of Eastern Ontario Pain Scale (CHEOPS) (McGrath, Johnson, Goodman, et al, 1985)			
1-5 yr	Interrater reliability: 90%-99.5% Internal correlation: significant correlations between pairs of items Concurrent validity between CHEOPS and visual analog scale (VAS): 0.91; between individual and total scores of CHEOPS and VAS: 0.50-0.86 Construct validity with preanalgesia and postanalgesia scores: 9.9-6.3	Cry (1-3) Facial (0-2) Child verbal (0-2) Torso (1-2) Touch (1-2) Legs (1-2)	4 = no pain; 13 = worst pain
Nurses Assessment of Pain Inventory (NAPI) (Stevens, 1990)			
Newborn–16 yr	Not tested by original author. Later tested by Joyce, Schade, Keck, et al (1994) Interrater agreement: weighted kappa 0.37-0.80 Discriminant validity: statistically significant differences between preanalgesia and postanalgesia scores ($p < 0.0001$) Reliability: Cronbach alpha: 0.35-0.69	Body movement (0-2) Facial (0-3) Touching (0-2)	0 = no pain; 7 = worst pain
Behavioral Pain Score (BPS) (Robieux, Kumar, Radhakrishnan, et al, 1991)			
3-36 mo	Original article stated, "Reliability of the VAS and BPS scores was tested by a k test"; no further testing of reliability or validity mentioned	Facial expression (0-2) Cry (0-3) Movements (0-3)	0 = no pain; 8 = worst pain
Modified Behavioral Pain Scale (MBPS) (Taddio, Nulman, Koren, et al, 1995)			
4-6 mo	Concurrent validity between MBPS and VAS scores: correlation coefficient 0.68 ($p < 0.001$) and 0.74 ($p < 0.001$) Construct validity using prevaccination and postvaccination scores with EMLA (lidocaine-prilocaine) versus placebo: significantly lower scores with EMLA ($p < 0.01$) Internal consistency of items: significant correlations between items Interrater agreement ICC: 0.95, $p < 0.001$ Test-retest reliability: 0.95, $p < 0.001$	Facial expression (0-3) Cry (0-4) Movements (0, 2, 3)	0 = no pain; 10 = worst pain
Riley Infant Pain Scale (RIPS) (Schade, Joyce, Gerkensmeyer, et al, 1996)			
<36 mo and for children with cerebral palsy	Interrater agreement using intraclass correlation coefficient: 0.53-0.83, $p < 0.0001$ Discriminant validity using Mann-Whitney U test with preanalgesia and postanalgesia scores: statistically significant ($p < 0.001$) Sensitivity: 0.31-0.23 Specificity: 0.86-0.90 Interrater reliability using 2-way cross tabulations and kappa statistics (r[87] = 0.94; $p < 0.001$) and kappa values above 0.50 for each category	**0** Neutral face/smiling, calm, sleeping quietly, no cry, consolable, moves easily **1** Frowning/grimace, restless body movements, restless sleep, whimpering, winces with touch **2** Clenched teeth, moderate agitation, sleeps intermittently, difficult to console, cries with touch **3** Full cry expression, thrashing/flailing, sleeping prolonged periods interrupted by jerking or no sleep, screaming/high-pitched cry, inconsolable, screams when touched/moved	0 = no pain; 3 = worst pain

Continued

TABLE 7-1 SUMMARY OF SELECTED BEHAVIORAL PAIN ASSESSMENT SCALES FOR YOUNG CHILDREN—cont'd

AGES OF USE	RELIABILITY AND VALIDITY	VARIABLES	SCORING RANGE
FLACC Postoperative Pain Tool (Merkel, Voepel-Lewis, Shayevitz, et al, 1997)			
2 mo–7 yr	Validity using analysis of variance for repeated measures to compare FLACC scores before and after analgesia; preanalgesia FLACC scores significantly higher than postanalgesia scores at 10, 30, and 60 min ($p < 0.001$ for each time)	Face (0-2) Legs (0-2) Activity (0-2) Cry (0-2) Consolability (0-2)	0 = no pain; 10 = worst pain
	Correlation coefficients used to compare FLACC pain scores and OPS pain scores; significant positive correlation between FLACC and OPS scores ($r = 0.80$; $p < 0.001$); positive correlation also found between FLACC scores and nurses' global ratings of pain ($r[47] = 0.41$; $p < 0.005$)		

FLACC Scale*

	0	1	2
Face	No particular expression or smile	Occasional grimace or frown, withdrawn, disinterested	Frequent to constant frown, clenched jaw, quivering chin
Legs	Normal position or relaxed	Uneasy, restless, tense	Kicking, or legs drawn up
Activity	Lying quietly, normal position, moves easily	Squirming, shifting back and forth, tense	Arched, rigid, or jerking
Cry	No cry (awake or asleep)	Moans or whimpers, occasional complaint	Crying steadily, screams or sobs, frequent complaints
Consolability	Content, relaxed	Reassured by occasional touching, hugging, or talking to; distractible	Difficult to console or comfort

*From Merkel SI, Voepel-Lewis T, Shayevitz JR, et al: The FLACC: a behavioral scale for scoring postoperative pain in young children, *Pediatr Nurs* 23(3):293-297, 1997. Used with permission of Jannetti Publications, Inc., and the University of Michigan Health System. Can be reproduced for clinical and research use.

TABLE 7-2 PAIN RATING SCALES FOR CHILDREN

PAIN SCALE, DESCRIPTION	INSTRUCTIONS	RECOMMENDED AGE, COMMENTS
FACES Pain Rating Scale* Consists of six cartoon faces ranging from smiling face for "no pain" to tearful face for "worst pain"	*Original instructions:* Explain to child that each face is for a person who feels happy because there is no pain (hurt) or sad because there is some or a lot of pain. FACE 0 is very happy because there is no hurt. FACE 1 hurts just a little bit. FACE 2 hurts a little more. FACE 3 hurts even more. FACE 4 hurts a whole lot, but FACE 5 hurts as much as you can imagine, although you don't have to be crying to feel this bad. Ask child to choose face that best describes own pain. Record number under chosen face on pain assessment record. *Brief word instructions:* Point to each face using the words to describe the pain intensity. Ask child to choose face that best describes own pain, and record appropriate number.	For children as young as 3 yr. Using original instructions without affect words, such as happy or sad, or brief words resulted in same range of pain rating, probably reflecting child's rating of pain intensity. For coding purposes, numbers 0, 2, 4, 6, 8, 10 can be substituted for 0-5 system to accommodate 0-10 system. The FACES provides three scales in one: facial expressions, numbers, and words. Research supports cultural sensitivity of FACES for Caucasian, African-American, Hispanic, Thai, Chinese, and Japanese children.

| 0 No hurt | 1 or 2 Hurts little bit | 2 or 4 Hurts little more | 3 or 6 Hurts even more | 4 or 8 Hurts whole lot | 5 or 10 Hurts worst |

*See footnote on p. 184.

TABLE 7-2	PAIN RATING SCALES FOR CHILDREN—cont'd	
PAIN SCALE, DESCRIPTION	**INSTRUCTIONS**	**RECOMMENDED AGE, COMMENTS**
Oucher (Beyer, Denyes, and Villarruel, 1992)		

Consists of six photographs of Caucasian child's face representing "no hurt" to "biggest hurt you could ever have"; also includes vertical scale with numbers from 0 to 100; scales for African-American and Hispanic children have been developed (Villarruel and Denyes, 1991)	*Numeric scale:*
	   Point to each section of scale to explain variations in pain intensity: "0 means no hurt."
	   "This means little hurts" (pointing to lower part of scale, 1-29).
	   "This means middle hurts" (pointing to middle part of scale, 30-69).
	   "This means big hurts" (pointing to upper part of scale, 70-99).
	   "100 means the biggest hurt you could ever have."
	   Score is actual number stated by child.
	Photographic scale:
	   Point to each photograph and explain variations in pain intensity using following language: 1st picture from the bottom is "no hurt," 2nd is "a little hurt," 3rd is "a little more hurt," 4th is "even more hurt than that," 5th is "pretty much or a lot of hurt," and 6th is "biggest hurt you could ever have."
	   Score pictures from 0 to 5, with bottom picture scored as 0.
	General:
	   Practice using Oucher by recalling and rating previous pain experiences (e.g., falling off bike). Child points to number or photograph that describes pain intensity associated with experience. Obtain current pain score from child by asking, "How much hurt do you have right now?"
		Children 3-13 yr
		Use numeric scale if child can count to 100 by ones and identify the larger of any 2 numbers, or by tens (Jordan-Marsh, Yoder, Hall, et al, 1994).
		Determine whether child has cognitive ability to use photographic scale; child should be able to rank six geometric shapes from largest to smallest.
		Determine which ethnic version of Oucher to use. Allow child to select version of Oucher, or use version that most closely matches physical characteristics of child.
		NOTE: Ethnically similar scale may not be preferred by child when given choice of ethnically neutral cartoon scale (Luffy and Grove, 2003).

Poker Chip Tool (Hester, Foster, Jordan-Marsh, et al, 1998)		
Uses four red poker chips placed horizontally in front of child	Say to child: "I want to talk with you about the hurt you may be having right now." Align chips horizontally in front of child on bedside table, clipboard, or other firm surface. Tell child, "These are pieces of hurt." Beginning at chip nearest child's left side and ending at one nearest right side, point to chips and say, "This (1st chip) is a little bit of hurt and this (4th chip) is the most hurt you could ever have." For a young child or for any child who may not fully comprehend the instructions, clarify by saying, "That means this (1) is just a little hurt, this (2) is a little more hurt, this (3) is more yet, and this (4) is the most hurt you could ever have." Do not give children an option for 0 hurt. Research with Poker Chip Tool has verified that children without pain will so indicate by responses such as, "I don't have any." Ask child, "How many pieces of hurt do you have right now?" After initial use of Poker Chip Tool, some children internalize the concept "pieces of hurt." If child gives response such as "I have one right now," before you ask or before you lay out poker chips, record number of chips on Pain Flow Sheet. Clarify child's answer by statements such as "Oh, you have a little hurt? Tell me about the hurt."	Children as young as 4 yr Determine whether child has cognitive ability to use numbers by identifying larger of any 2 numbers.
Word-Graphic Rating Scale† (Tesler, Savedra, Holzemer, et al, 1991)		
Uses descriptive words (may vary in other scales) to denote varying intensities of pain	Explain to child, "This is a line with words to describe how much pain you may have. This side of the line means no pain, and over here the line means worst possible pain." (Point with your finger where "no pain" is, and run your finger along the line to "worst possible pain," as you say it.) "If you have no pain, you would mark like this." (Show example.) "If you have some pain, you would mark somewhere along the line, depending on how much pain you have." (Show example.) "The more pain you have, the closer to worst pain you would mark. The worst pain possible is marked like this." (Show example.) "Show me how much pain you have right now by marking with a straight, up-and-down line anywhere along the line to show how much pain you have right now." With millimeter rule, measure from the "no pain" end to mark and record this measurement as pain score.	Children 4-17 yr

No pain	Little pain	Medium pain	Large pain	Worst possible pain

†See footnote on p. 184.

Continued

TABLE 7-2	PAIN RATING SCALES FOR CHILDREN—cont'd	
PAIN SCALE, DESCRIPTION	**INSTRUCTIONS**	**RECOMMENDED AGE, COMMENTS**
Numeric Scale Uses straight line with end points identified as "no pain" and "worst pain" and sometimes "medium pain" in the middle; divisions along line marked in units from 0-10 (high number may vary)	Explain to child that at one end of line is 0, which means that person feels no pain (hurt). At other end is usually 5 or 10, which means the person feels worst pain imaginable. The numbers 1-5 or 1-10 are for very little pain to a whole lot of pain. Ask child to choose number that best describes own pain.	Children as young as 5 yr, as long as they can count and have some concept of numbers and their values in relation to other numbers Scale may be used horizontally or vertically. Number coding should be same as other scales used in facility.

No pain   Worst pain

| 0 | 1 | 2 | 3 | 4 | 5 | 6 | 7 | 8 | 9 | 10 |

| **Visual Analog Scale (VAS) (Cline, Herman, Shaw, et al, 1992)**
Defined as vertical or horizontal line that is drawn to certain length, such as 10 cm (4 inches), and anchored by items that represent extremes of the subjective phenomenon being measured, such as pain | Ask child to place mark on line that best describes amount of own pain. With centimeter ruler, measure from "no pain" end to the mark, and record this measurement as the pain score. | Children as young as 4½ yr, preferably 7 yr Vertical or horizontal scale may be used. Research shows that children ages 3-18 yr least prefer VAS compared with other scales (Luffy and Grove, 2003; Wong and Baker, 1988). |

No pain   Worst pain

| **Color Tool (Eland and Banner, 1999)**
Uses markers for child to construct own scale that is used with body outline | Present eight markers to child in random order. Ask child, "Of these colors, which color is like _____?" (the event identified by child as having hurt the most). Place the marker (represents severe pain) away from other markers. Ask child, "Which color is like a hurt, but not quite as much as _____?" (the event identified by child as having hurt the most). Place this marker with the marker chosen to represent severe pain. Ask child, "Which color is like something that hurts just a little?" Place the marker with the other colors. Ask child, "Which color is like no hurt at all?" Show the four marker choices to the child in order from worst to no-hurt color. Ask child to show on body outlines where he or she hurts, using markers chosen. After child has colored hurts, ask if they are current hurts or hurts from the past. Ask if child knows why the area hurts if it is not clear to you why it does. | Children as young as 4 yr, provided they know their colors, are not color blind, and are able to construct the scale if in pain |

*Wong-Baker FACES Pain Rating Scale reference manual describing development and research of the scale is available from City of Hope Pain/Palliative Care Resource Center, 1500 East Duarte Road, Duarte, CA 91010; 626-359-8111, ext. 3829; fax: 626-301-8941; **www1.us.elsevierhealth.com/FACES**.

†Instructions for Word-Graphic Rating Scale from Acute Pain Management Guideline Panel: *Acute pain management in infants, children, and adolescents: operative and medical procedures; quick reference guide for clinicians,* ACHPR Pub. No. 92-0020, Rockville, Md, 1992, Agency for Health Care Research and Quality, US Department of Health and Human Services. Word-Graphic Rating Scale is part of the Adolescent Pediatric Pain Tool and is available from Pediatric Pain Study, University of California, School of Nursing, Department of Family Health Care Nursing, San Francisco, CA 94143-0606; 415-476-4040.

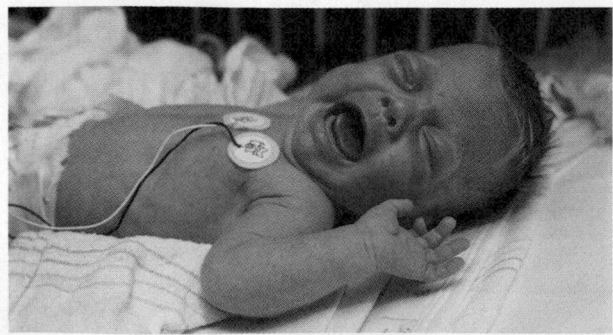

Fig. 7-1 Full, robust crying of preterm infant after heel stick. (Courtesy Halbouty Premature Nursery, Texas Children's Hospital, Houston; photo by Paul Vincent Kuntz.)

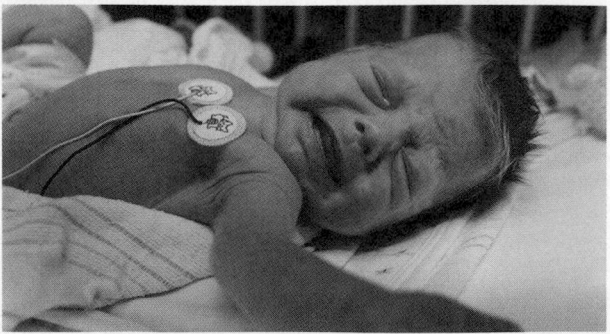

Fig. 7-2 The face of pain after heel stick. Note eye squeeze, brow bulge, nasolabial furrow, and wide-spread mouth. (Courtesy Halbouty Premature Nursery, Texas Children's Hospital, Houston; photo by Paul Vincent Kuntz.)

they most frequently observed to determine whether a child is in pain (McGrath, Johnson, Goodman, et al 1985; Suraseranivongse, Montapaneewat, Manon, et al, 2005). Six categories of behaviors are identified: cry, facial, verbal, torso, touch, and legs. Scoring was devised so that 0 equals behavior that is the antithesis of pain, 1 means the behavior is not indicative of pain and is not the antithesis of pain, 2 indicates behavior consistent with mild or moderate pain, and 3 means the behavior is indicative of severe pain. The range of the total score is 4 to 13.

The Toddler-Preschooler Postoperative Pain Scale (TPPPS) is an observational scale developed for measuring postoperative pain in children ages 1 to 5 years (Suraseranivongse, Montapaneewat, Manon, et al, 2005; Tarbell, Cohen, and Marsh, 1992). It consists of three pain behavior categories: vocal pain expression, facial pain expression, and bodily pain expression. Vocal pain expression includes verbal pain complaints such as crying, screaming, groaning, moaning, and grunting. Facial pain expression includes open mouth with lips pulled back at corners, squinting or closed eyes, furrowed forehead, and brow bulge. Bodily pain is indicated by restless motor behavior when touched in a painful area.

The Parent's Postoperative Pain Rating Scale (PPPRS) is a scale that parents may use to rate their children's pain by noting changes in the frequency of a number of behaviors (Chambers, 2003; Chambers and Craig, 1998; Finley, Chambers, McGrath, et al, 2003). The Parents' Postoperative Pain Measure (PPPM), for use by parents, was developed based on cues parents reported observing in their children after surgery such as changes in appetite and activity level.

The only pain measurement tool recommended for use with children in critical care settings is the COMFORT scale (Ambuel, Hamlett, Marx, et al, 1992). The COMFORT scale is a behavioral, unobtrusive method of measuring distress in unconscious and ventilated infants, children, and adolescents. This scale has eight indicators: alertness, calmness/agitation, respiratory response, physical movement, blood pressure, heart rate, muscle tone, and facial tension. Each indicator is scored between 1 and 5 based on the behaviors exhibited by the patient. The provider observes the patient unobtrusively for 2 minutes and derives the total score by adding the scores of each indicator. The total scores can range between 8 and 40. A score of 17 to 26 generally indicates adequate sedation and pain control.

The PedIMMPACT statement recommends the Poker Chips Tool for children 3 to 4 years of age (Hester, Foster, and Kristensen, 1990), the Faces Pain Scale–Revised for children 4 to 12 years of age (Hicks, von Baeyer, Spafford, et al, 2001) the Visual Analog Scale (VAS) for children 8 years and older (Scott, Ansell, and Huskisson, 1977).

The Poker Chip Tool consists of a set of four red plastic poker chips. Each chip is used to denote a "piece of hurt," and the child is asked to choose "how many pieces of hurt do you have right now?" The child responds that he or she does not have any pieces of hurt, or one chip corresponds to "a little hurt," the second chip indicates "a little more hurt," the third chip means "more hurt," and the fourth chip equals the "most hurt you could ever have." The scores range from 0 to 4. The Poker Chip Tool has undergone extensive psychometric testing by various teams of investigators (Gharaibeh and

Abu-Saad 2002; Goodenough, Addicoat, Champion, et al, 1997; Suraseranivongse, Montapaneewat, Manon, et al, 2005).

There are many different "faces" scales for the measurement of pain intensity. Although children who are 4 or 5 years old are able to use self-report measures, cognitive characteristics of the preoperational stage influence their ability to use these scales. Simple, concrete anchor words, such as "no hurt" to "biggest hurt," are more appropriate than "least pain sensation to worst intense pain imaginable." The ability to discriminate degrees of pain in facial expressions appears to be reasonably established by 3 years of age (see Table 7-2). Faces scales provide a series of facial expressions depicting gradations of pain. The faces are appealing because children can simply point to the face that represents how they feel.

The Bieri Faces Pain Scale–Revised (Hicks, von Baeyer, Spafford, et al, 2001) and the WB FACES Pain Scale (Wong and Baker, 1988) are the most widely used faces pain measurement tools. The Bieri scale consists of six faces depicting increasing gradation of pain severity from 0 = "no pain" on the left face to 5 = "most pain possible" on the right face. In developing this scale, the authors did not include a smiling face at the "no pain" end or tears at the "most pain" end and validated it so that it is equivalent to a 0 to 10 metric system. The WB FACES Pain Scale consists of six cartoon faces ranging from a smiling face for "no pain" to a tearful face for "worst pain." The child is asked to choose a face that describes his or her pain. Although the PedIMMPACT group recommended the Faces Pain Scale–Revised, most children prefer the WB FACES Pain Scale (Chambers, Giesbrecht, Craig, et al, 1999; Keck, Gerkensmeyer, Joyce, et al, 1996; Luffy and Grove, 2003; West, Oakes, Hinds, et al, 1994). The WB FACES pain scale is widely used in children's hospitals across the United States.

For children 8 years and older, the Numeric Rating Scale (NRS), specifically the 0 to 10 scale, is most widely used in clinical practice because it is easy to use. However, there is little research to support the reliability and validity of the NRS, except in the context of the Oucher Pain Scale (Beyer, Turner, Jones, et al, 2005) (see Table 7-2). Although the VAS requires a higher degree of abstraction than the NRS, the PedIMMPACT group recommends the VAS because of the lack of supportive evidence through psychometric studies with the NRS in children and adolescents.

Global Judgment of Improvement and of Satisfaction with Treatment

Patients or patient surrogates may provide a collection of their perspective of all aspects of the treatment experience by allowing them to rate a global judgment of satisfaction with treatment. Patient or parent global judgments focus on the patient's experience. The ratings will mean something different from one patient or surrogate to another. Although some may focus on the relief of pain, others may consider side effects of the treatment. The global question should be specific so the patient is able to give a focused response in the answer. For example, a focused global question would read, "Considering pain relief, side effects, physical recovery, and emotional recovery, how satisfied were you with the intervention your child received for pain?"

Adverse Events and Symptoms

Treatment-emergent adverse events refer to signs, symptoms, laboratory findings, or diseases that occur after medications for pain are initiated. Constipation is the most common adverse event associated with prolonged opioid use, yet is not commonly screened for in children with pain. There is no particular strategy to measure either the occurrence or severity of treatment-emergent adverse events. Children older than 10 years may be able to provide this information. In younger children the nurse must be extra vigilant and should ask parents or caregivers about any perceived adverse events and symptoms.

Physical Recovery

The domain of physical recovery includes those aspects of physical functioning that are influenced by the procedure or injury causing acute pain. Assessments of the physical recovery would include time to ambulation, time to resume swallowing, time to normal spirometry, return to normal nutritional intake, and time out of bed. However, measures such as tolerance of physical therapy may be inconsistent. One child may be intolerant of physical therapy because he or she did not want to participate, whereas another child might be considered intolerant of physical therapy if the therapy was associated with pain, profuse crying, and refusal to do the work. The PedIMMPACT group recommends assessing existing measures of physical recovery for the purposes of evaluating interventions to control pain following procedures and injuries that have specific effects on physical functioning.

Emotional Response

The domain of emotional response includes all aspects of negative affect or distress secondary to pain such as anxiety, depression, fear, distress, dysphoria, or unhappiness. Behaviors indicating avoidance, withdrawal, or resistance need to be assessed. In children 8 years and older, the PedIMMPACT group recommends the use of the Adolescent Pediatric Pain Tool (APPT) (Savedra, Holzemer, Tesler, et al, 1993), which allows children to describe the quality of the pain using a word list. The 56 words are grouped according to sensory, affective, and evaluative qualities of pain. This measurement tool has been validated.

ASSESSMENT OF CHRONIC AND RECURRENT PAIN

Pain that persists for 3 months or more or beyond the expected period of healing is defined as chronic pain. Complex regional pain syndrome and chronic daily headache are the most common types of chronic pain conditions in children. Pain that is episodic and recurs is defined as recurrent pain. The time frame within which episodes of pain recur is at least 3 months. Recurrent pain syndromes in children include migraine headache, episodic sickle cell pain, recurrent abdominal pain, and recurrent limb pain (see Research Focus box).

Chronic or recurrent pain adversely affects the psychosocial and physical well-being of children. The domains for the assessment of chronic or recurrent pain are the same for acute pain (pain intensity, global judgment of satisfaction with treatment,

RESEARCH FOCUS
Pain in School-Age Children

Van Dijk, McGrath, Pickett, and colleagues (2006) reported that 57% of school-age children have at least one recurrent pain (headaches, stomach pains, growing pains), and at least 6% have one or more chronic pain episodes (disease related, back pain).

symptoms and adverse events, physical functioning, emotional functioning, economic factors), plus two additional domains: role functioning and sleep. Because the time course of chronic or recurrent pain is different from that of acute pain, measures used to assess chronic pain often evaluate the symptom over time.

Pain diaries are commonly used to assess pain symptoms and response to treatment in children and adolescents with recurrent or chronic pain (Ely, Dampier, Gilday, et al, 2002; Dampier, Ely, Brodecki, et al, 2002a, 2002b; Stinson, Stevens, Feldman, et al, 2008; Palermo and Valenzuela, 2003; Palermo, Valenzuela, and Stork, 2004; Stone, Broderick, Schwartz, et al, 2003). Most pain diaries use NRS or VAS with varying anchors such as faces scales or words. Diary studies have included children as young as 6 years. Conventional paper-and-pencil measures have been associated with several limitations such as poor compliance, missing data, hoarding of responses, and back and forward filling (Palermo and Valenzuela, 2003; Stone, Broderick, Schwartz, et al, 2003) (see Research Focus box).

RESEARCH FOCUS
Electronic Diaries

An increasing number of studies are converting paper diaries into electronic diaries for use in school-age children and adolescents with recurrent or chronic pain (Palermo, Valenzuela, and Stork, 2004; Stinson, Stevens, Feldman, et al, 2008; Stone, Broderick, Schwartz, et al, 2003). Electronic diaries were found to show higher accuracy of children's diary responses and higher compliance rates when compared with the paper format. However, electronic diaries are more expensive and may have a number of logistical issues left to resolve.

The PedIMMPACT group recommends the same approach for measuring global judgment of satisfaction with treatment of symptoms and adverse events. The physical functioning domain in chronic or recurrent pain is focused on activities of everyday life, such as sitting or walking, or on more vigorous activities such as running and other sports. The recommendation is to use a measure such as the functional disability inventory (FDI) (Walker and Greene, 1991) for assessing physical functioning in school-age children and adolescents. The FDI assesses the child's ability to perform everyday physical activities and has established psychometric properties with different populations (Claar and Walker, 2006; Reid, Lang, and McGrath, 1997; Vervoort, Goubert, Eccleston, et al, 2006). For children less than 7 years of age the Pediatric Quality of Life Scale (PedsQL), developed by Varni, Seid, and Rode (1999), is a multidimensional scale with both parent and child versions that is recommended for assessing physical, emotional, social, and academic functioning as they relate to the child's pain. The PedsQL and the PedMIDAS (Hershey, Powers, Vockell, et al,

2001, 2004) have been validated for measurement of role functioning in children with chronic or recurrent pain.

The emotional functioning domain most often refers to the presence of depression or anxiety, which may be more prevalent in children with chronic or recurrent pain (Palermo, 2000). The Children's Depression Inventory (Kovacs, 1981) and the Revised Child Anxiety and Depression Scale (Chorpita, Yim, Moffitt, et al, 2000) have been used to assess anxiety and depression in children and adolescents with chronic or recurrent pain. Fortunately, most children with chronic or recurrent pain do not experience clinical levels of anxiety or depression.

Sleep disruption is also common in those with chronic or recurrent pain. More than half of children with pain-related conditions report difficulties sleeping (Walters and Williamson, 1999; Palermo and Kiska, 2005). A sleep diary can be useful in keeping a record of activities surrounding sleep, including bed time, time to fall asleep, number of night awakenings, waking in the morning, and especially any pain or other circumstance that interfered with sleeping. The sleep diary was validated using sleep actigraphy in healthy children ages 13 and 14 years (Gaina, Sekine, Chen, et al, 2004). The Sleep Habits Questionnaire (Owens, Spirito, and McGuinn, 2000) may be useful for assessing sleep behaviors in school-age children with chronic or recurrent pain.

MULTIDIMENSIONAL MEASURES

The number of pain measures available for use in infants, young children, and adolescents has increased dramatically and adds a layer of complexity to the assessment of pain in children. The current trend supports a common metric for measurement of pain in children (von Baeyer and Hicks, 2000). Most instruments consist of 0 for no pain to a range of 4 to 160 for the top anchors in pain measures. A pain score of 5 may mean a lot of pain (if a 0 to 5 scale is used) or very little (if a 0 to 100 scale is used), and it may not be clearly specified which score corresponds to which scale. Other health care providers who do not specialize in pediatric pain may be confused by the available instruments and scoring methods and may not be able to determine the effectiveness of interventions by the pain score documented. An advantage to using a common metric is that a certain score may be considered as the point at which an intervention is required, or a point at which relief may be considered adequate (von Baeyer and Hicks, 2000). The 0 to 10 system was reported to be preferred by health care providers and would make pain scores easier to read, interpret, and integrate into research and practice.

Several cognitive skills, such as measurement, classification, and seriation (the ability to accurately place in ascending or descending order), become apparent between 7 and 10 years of age. Older children are able to use a 0 to 10 NRS used by adolescents and adults. However, the use of the 0 to 10 NRS is only an assessment of pain intensity, which may not change in some pain states (Jacob, Miaskowski, Savedra, et al, 2003a, 2003b). Other dimensions such as pain quality, pain location, and spatial distribution of pain may change without a change in pain intensity.

Two multidimensional assessment tools have been well validated for children 8 years and older. The APPT, modeled after

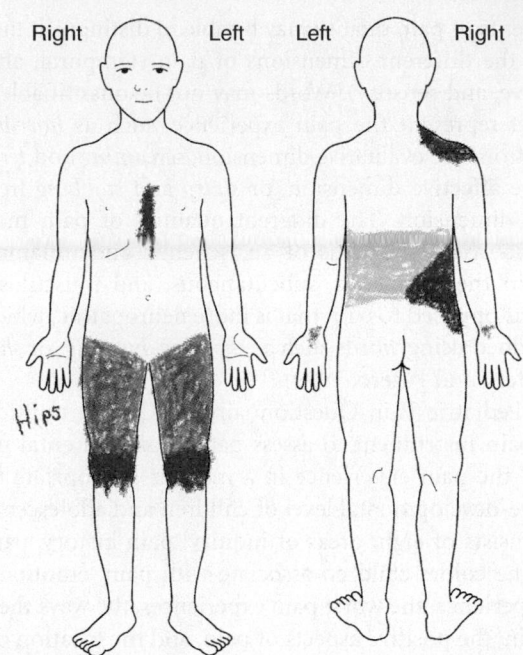

Fig. 7-3 Adolescent Pediatric Pain Tool: body outlines for pain assessment. Instructions: "Color in the areas on these drawings to show where you have pain. Make the marks as big or as small as the place where the pain is." Tool has been completed by a child with sickle cell disease. (From Savedra MC, Tesler MD, Holzemer WL, Ward JA, School of Nursing, University of California–San Francisco; copyright 1989, 1992.)

the McGill Pain Questionnaire (Melzack, 1975), is a multidimensional pain measurement instrument used with children and adolescents to assess pain location, intensity, and quality (Fig. 7-3). The APPT is an instrument with an anterior and posterior body outline on one side and a 100-mm word-graphing rating scale with a pain descriptor on the other side (Savedra, Tesler, Holzemer, et al, 1989; Wilkie, Holzemer, Tesler, et al, 1990; Tesler, Savedra, Holzemer, et al, 1991; Savedra, Holzemer, Tesler, et al, 1993). Each of the three components of the APPT is scored separately. The body outline is scored by placing a clear plastic template overlay with 43 body areas on the body outline diagram. An estimate of the pervasiveness of the pain is made by counting the number of body areas marked. A ruler or micrometer preprinted on the APPT is used to score the word-graphic rating scale. The number of millimeters from the left side of the scale to the point marked by the child is measured; and the numeric value provides an overall evaluation of the amount of pain the child is experiencing. The total number of words on the descriptor list is counted, and scores range from 0 to 56. The clinician then counts the number of words selected in each of three categories—evaluative (0-8), sensory (0-37), and affective (0-11)—and calculates a percentage score for each one (Savedra, Holzemer, Tesler, et al, 1993).

An advantage to using the APPT is that, in some pain states, pain intensity ratings do not change, but pain location and spatial distribution of pain may decrease over time (Jacob, Miaskowski, Savedra, et al, 2003a, 2003b). The total surface area may decrease, but some children may perceive the remaining sites as equal in pain intensity. In addition to pain location, assessments of pain quality may be able to distinguish the presence of the different dimensions of pain (temporal, affective, evaluative, and sensory). Words may not be quantifiable on an NRS, yet represent the pain experience, such as *horrible* and *terrible* from the evaluative dimension, *screaming* and *terrifying* from the affective dimension, or *sharp* and *stabbing* from the sensory dimension. The different qualities of pain may also represent whether pain is of an ischemic and inflammatory nature in the cutaneous, subcutaneous, and musculoskeletal tissues, as opposed to pain that is more neuropathic, which may be described using words such as *shooting, burning,* or *shocklike* (McCaffery and Pasero, 1999).

The Pediatric Pain Questionnaire (PPQ) is a multidimensional pain instrument to assess patient and parental perceptions of the pain experience in a manner appropriate for the cognitive-developmental level of children and adolescents. The PPQ consists of eight areas of inquiry: pain history, pain language, the colors children associate with pain, emotions children experience, the worst pain experiences, the ways they cope with pain, the positive aspects of pain, and the location of their current pain. The three components of the PPQ include VASs; color-coded rating scales; and verbal descriptors to provide information about the sensory, affective, and evaluative dimensions of chronic pain (Varni, Thompson, and Hanson, 1987). There is also information about the child and family's pain history, symptoms, pain relief interventions, and socioenvironmental situations that may influence pain. The child, parent, and physician each complete the form separately.

ASSESSMENT OF PAIN IN SPECIFIC POPULATIONS

PAIN IN NEONATES

Assessment of pain in the preverbal child is difficult, especially in the neonate, since the most reliable indicator of pain, self-report, is not possible. Evaluation must be based on physiologic changes and behavioral observations (Box 7-2). Although behaviors such as vocalizations, facial expressions, body movements, and general relaxation state are common to all infants, they vary with different situations. Crying associated with pain is more intense and sustained (see Fig. 7-1). Facial expression is the most consistent and specific characteristic; scales are available to systematically evaluate facial features, such as eye squeeze, brow bulge, open mouth, and taut tongue (Hadjistavropoulos, Craig, Grunau, et al, 1997). Most infants respond with increased body movements, but the infant may be experiencing pain even when lying quietly with eyes closed. The preterm infant's response to pain may be behaviorally blunted or absent; however, there is ample evidence that such infants are neurologically capable of feeling pain. In addition, infants in awake or alert states demonstrate a more robust reaction to painful stimuli than infants in sleep states. Also, an infant receiving a muscle-paralyzing agent (vecuronium) is incapable of a behavioral or visible pain response.

Although regular use of pain assessment tools can assist caregivers in determining whether the infant is in pain, caregivers must consider the infant's maturity, behavioral state, energy

---

BOX 7-2   MANIFESTATIONS OF ACUTE PAIN IN THE NEONATE

Physiologic Responses

Vital signs—Observe for variations.
- Increased heart rate
- Increased blood pressure
- Rapid, shallow respirations

Oxygenation
- Decreased transcutaneous oxygen saturation (tcPo₂)
- Decreased arterial oxygen saturation (Sao₂)

Skin—Observe color and character.
- Pallor or flushing
- Diaphoresis
- Palmar sweating

Other observations
- Increased muscle tone
- Dilated pupils
- Decreased vagal nerve tone
- Increased intracranial pressure
- Laboratory evidence of metabolic or endocrine changes: hyperglycemia, lowered pH, elevated corticosteroids

Behavioral Responses

Vocalizations—Observe quality, timing, and duration.
- Crying
- Whimpering
- Groaning

Facial expression—Observe characteristics, timing, orientation of eyes and mouth.
- Grimaces
- Brow furrowed
- Chin quivering
- Eyes tightly closed
- Mouth open and squarish

Body movements and posture—Observe type, quality, and amount of movement or lack of movement; relationship to other factors.
- Limb withdrawal
- Thrashing
- Rigidity
- Flaccidity
- Fist clenching

Changes in state—Observe sleep, appetite, activity level.
- Changes in sleep-wake cycles
- Changes in feeding behavior
- Changes in activity level
- Fussiness, irritability
- Listlessness

---

resources available to respond, and risk factors for pain. In infants with diminished ability to respond robustly to pain, it is imperative to presume that pain exists in all situations that are usually considered painful for adults and children, even in the absence of behavioral or physiologic signs (Sweet and McGrath, 1998).

Several pain assessment tools for neonates have been developed (Table 7-3). One tool used by nurses who work with premature and full-term infants in the neonatal intensive care setting is called CRIES, which is an acronym for the tool's physiologic and behavioral indicators of pain: *C*rying, *R*equiring increased oxygen, *I*ncreased vital signs, *E*xpression, and *S*leeplessness. Each indicator is scored from 0 to 2, with a total possible pain score, representing the worst pain, of 10. A pain

TABLE 7-3   SUMMARY OF PAIN ASSESSMENT SCALES FOR INFANTS

AGES OF USE	RELIABILITY AND VALIDITY	VARIABLES	SCORING RANGE
Postoperative Pain Score (POPS) (Barrier, Attia, Mayer, et al, 1987)			
1-7 mo	Not tested by original authors Later tested by Joyce, Schade, Keck, et al (1994); high interrater agreement (reliability); discriminant validity (p <0.0001); reliability with high Cronbach alpha ranging from 0.79-0.88	Sleep (0-2) Flexion fingers/toes (0-2) Facial expression (0-2) Sucking (0-2) Quality of cry (0-2) Tone (0-2) Spontaneous motor activity (0-2) Consolability (0-2) Spontaneous excitability (0-2) Sociability (0-2)	0 = worst pain; 20 = no pain
Neonatal Infant Pain Scale (NIPS) (Lawrence, Alcock, McGrath, et al, 1993)			
Average gestational age 33.5 wk	Interrater reliability: 0.92 and 0.97 Construct validity using analysis of variance between scores before, during, and after procedure: F = 18.97, df = 2.42, p <0.001 Concurrent validity between NIPS and visual analog scale (VAS) using Pearson correlations: 0.53-0.84 Internal consistency using Cronbach alpha: 0.95, 0.87, and 0.88 for before, during, and after procedure scores	Facial expression (0-1) Arms (0-1) Cry (0-2) Legs (0-1) Breathing patterns (0-1) State of arousal (0-1)	0 = no pain; 7 = worst pain
Pain Assessment Tool (PAT) (Hodgkinson, Bear, Thorn, et al, 1994)			
27 wk of gestational age—full term	No reliability or validity discussed by original authors	Posture/tone (1-2) Respirations (1-2) Sleep pattern (0-2) Heart rate (1-2) Expression (1-2) Saturations (0-2) Color (0-2) Blood pressure (0-2) Cry (0-2) Nurse's perception (0-2)	4 = no pain; 20 = worst pain
Pain Rating Scale (PRS) (Joyce, Schade, Keck, et al, 1994)			
1-36 mo	Interrater agreement: r = 0.65-0.84, p <0.0001 Discriminant validity: statistically significant t-tests (p <0.0001)	**0** Smiling, sleeping, no change when moved/touched **1** Takes small amount orally, restless, moving, cries **2** Not drinking/eating, short periods of cries, distracted with rocking or pacifier **3** Change in behavior, irritable, arms/legs shake/jerk, facial grimace **4** Flailing, high-pitched wailing, parents request pain medication, unable to distract **5** Sleeping prolonged periods interrupted by jerking, continuous crying, rapid and shallow respirations	0 = no pain; 5 = worst pain
CRIES (Krechel and Bildner, 1995)			
32-60 wk of gestational age	Concurrent validity between CRIES and POPS: 0.73 (p <0.0001, n = 1382); Spearman correlation between subjective report and POPS and CRIES: 0.49 (p <0.0001, n >1300) Discriminant validity using before and after analgesia scores: Wilcoxon sign rank test: mean decline of 3.0 units (p <0.0001, n = 74) Interrater reliability using Spearman correlation coefficient: r = 0.72 (p <0.0001, n = 680)	Crying (0-2) Requires increased oxygen (0-2) Increased vital signs (0-2) Expression (0-2) Sleepless (0-2)	0 = no pain; 10 = worst pain

Continued

TABLE 7-3	SUMMARY OF PAIN ASSESSMENT SCALES FOR INFANTS—cont'd		
AGES OF USE	**RELIABILITY AND VALIDITY**	**VARIABLES**	**SCORING RANGE**

Premature Infant Pain Profile (PIPP) (Stevens, Johnston, Petryshen, et al, 1996)

28-40 wk of gestational age	Internal consistency using Cronbach alpha: 0.75-0.59; standardized item alpha for six items: 0.71 Construct validity using handling versus painful situations: statistically significant differences (paired $t = 12.24$, two-tailed $p < 0.0001$, and Mann-Whitney U = 765.5, $p < 0.00001$) and using real versus sham heel stick procedures with infants ages 28-30 wk of gestational age ($t = 2.4$, two-tailed $p < 0.02$, and Mann-Whitney U = 132, $p < 0.016$) and with full-term boys undergoing circumcision with topical anesthetic versus. placebo ($t = 2.6$, two-tailed $p < 0.02$, or nonparametric equivalent Mann-Whitney U test, U = 145.7, two-tailed $p < 0.02$)	Gestational age (0-3) Eye squeeze (0-3) Behavioral state (0-3) Nasolabial furrow (0-3) Heart rate (0-3) Oxygen saturation (0-3) Brow bulge (0-3)	0 = no pain; 21 = worst pain

Scale for Use in Newborns (SUN) (Blauer and Gerstmann, 1998)

0-28 days	No reliability; face validity, content validity, construct validity using extreme groups	Central nervous system state (0-4) Movement (0-4) Breathing (0-4) Tone (0-4) Heart rate (0-4) Face (0-4) Mean blood pressure (0-4)	0 = no pain; 28 = worst pain Average baseline score 10-14 A 2 represents normal or baseline value

Neonatal Pain, Agitation, and Sedation Scale (NPASS) (Puchalski and Hummel, 2002)

Birth (23 wk of gestational age) and full-term newborns up to 100 days	Interrater reliability using ICC: 0.95 CI for preintervention and postintervention pain scale; 0.95 CI for preintervention and postintervention sedation scale
	Internal consistency (Cronbach alpha):
	  Preintervention pain scale, 0.75 and 0.71 raters 1 and 2
	  Postintervention pain scale, 0.25 and 0.27 raters 1 and 2
	  Preintervention sedation scale, 0.88 and 0.81 raters 1 and 2
	  Postintervention sedation scale, 0.86 and 0.89 raters 1 and 2
		Cry/irritability (0-2)
		Behavior/state (0-2)
		Facial expression (0-2)
		Extremities/tone (0-2)
		Vital signs—heart rate, respiratory rate, blood pressure, SaO$_2$ (0-2)
			Pain score: 0 = no pain; 10 = intense pain
			Sedation score: 0 = no sedation; 10 = deep sedation

CRIES Neonatal Postoperative Pain Scale

	0	1	2
Crying	No	High pitched	Inconsolable
Requires oxygen for saturation >95%	No	<30%	>30%
Increased vital signs	Heart rate and blood pressure ≤ preoperative state	Heart rate and blood pressure increase <20% of preoperative state	Heart rate and blood pressure increase >20% of preoperative state
Expression	None	Grimace	Grimace, grunt
Sleepless	No	Wakes at frequent intervals	Constantly awake

score greater than 4 is considered significant. This tool has been tested for reliability and validity for postoperative pain in infants between the ages of 32 weeks of gestation up to 20 weeks postterm (60 weeks) (Sweet and McGrath, 1998).

The Premature Infant Pain Profile (PIPP) was developed specifically for preterm infants (Sweet and McGrath, 1998). The category "gestational age at time of observation" gives a higher pain score to infants with lower gestational age. Infants who are asleep 15 seconds before the painful procedure also receive additional points for their blunted behavioral responses to painful stimuli.

The Neonatal Pain, Agitation, and Sedation Scale (NPASS) was originally developed to measure pain or sedation in preterm infants after surgery. It measures five criteria (see Table 7-3) in two dimensions (pain and sedation) and is used in neonates as young as 23 weeks of gestation up to infants 100 days old. Extra points are added in the pain scale dimension for preterm infants based on gestational age.

CHILDREN WITH COMMUNICATION AND COGNITIVE IMPAIRMENT

The assessment of pain in children with communication and cognitive impairment can be challenging. Children who have significant difficulties in communicating with others about their pain include those who have significant neurologic impairments (e.g., cerebral palsy), cognitive impairment, metabolic disorders, autism, severe brain injury, and communication barriers (e.g., critically ill children who are on ventilators or heavily sedated or have neuromuscular disorders, loss of hearing, or loss of vision) and consequently are at greater risk for undertreatment of pain. Children with communication and cognitive deficits often experience spasticity, contractures, injury, infection, and orthopedic surgical treatment that may be painful. Behaviors include moaning, inconsistent patterns of play and sleep, changes in facial expression, and other physical problems that may mask expression of pain and be difficult to interpret (Hadden and von Baeyer, 2002).

The mother or primary caregiver may be the most important source of information when assessing pain in children with developmental delays (Breau, MacLaren, McGrath, et al, 2003). Stallard, Williams, Lenton, and colleagues (2001) asked the parents of cognitively impaired and noncommunicative children to assess the presence, severity, and duration of their pain during a 2-week observation period. Parents reported that 84% experienced pain on 5 or more separate days, with 32% experiencing pain on 12 or more days. Of the 74 episodes that lasted longer than 30 minutes, 33.8% occurred at night. Most pain episodes lasted longer than 10 minutes, with 48% of the children having episodes lasting longer than 10 minutes on 5 or more days. Although the experience of pain was common among this group of children, none was receiving treatment for relief or management of pain (see Research Focus box).

RESEARCH FOCUS

Pain Reporting in Cognitively Impaired Children

Up to 60% of parents of children with severe cognitive impairment reported that their child experienced pain or severe discomfort that was not being effectively managed (Lenton, Stallard, Lewis, et al, 2001; Stallard, Williams, Velleman, et al, 2002). The most frequently reported pain behaviors are crying; being less active; seeking comfort; moaning; not cooperating; being irritable; being stiff, spastic, tense, or rigid; sleeping less; being difficult to satisfy or pacify; flinching or moving body part away; and being agitated or fidgety (Hadden and von Baeyer, 2002). Parents also reported that some daily living activities were painful such as assisted stretching and walking, independent standing, toileting, putting on splints, occupational therapy, range of motion, and physical therapy.

The Non-communicating Children's Pain Checklist (NCCPC) is a pain measurement tool specifically designed for children with cognitive impairments (Breau, McGrath, Camfield, et al, 2002). The scale discriminates between periods of pain and calm and can predict behavior during subsequent episodes of pain (Fig. 7-4). The scale consists of six subscales (vocal, social, facial, activity, body and limbs, physiologic signs), which are scored based on the number of times the items are observed over a 10-minute period (0 = not at all; 1 = just a little; 2 = fairly often; 3 = very often).

The Pain Indicator for Communicatively Impaired Children (PICIC) distinguishes between pain and nonpain in children with life-threatening illness who have communication challenges (Stallard, Williams, Velleman, et al, 2002). The PICIC has six core pain cues: crying with or without tears; screaming, yelling, groaning, or moaning; screwed up or distressed looking face; body appearing stiff or tense; difficulty in comforting or consoling; and flinching or moving away if touched. The items are rated using a 4-point Likert scale (1 = not at all, 2 = a little, 3 = often, 4 = all the time).

CULTURAL DIFFERENCES

A major challenge in the assessment and management of pain in children is the cultural appropriateness of pain assessment tools that have been validated only in Caucasian and English-speaking children (see Cultural Competence box). Cultural background may influence the validity and reliability of pain assessment tools developed in a single cultural context (Bernstein and Pachter, 2003).

CULTURAL COMPETENCE

Pain Scales

Observational scales and interview questionnaires for pain may not be as reliable for pain assessment as self-report scales in children of Hispanic origin. Children of Asian descent, who may learn to read Chinese characters vertically downward and from right to left, may have difficulty using horizontally oriented scales.

The Oucher Pain Scale (see Table 7-2), originally developed and validated as a self-report of pain intensity for Caucasian children 3 to 12 years old, now features photographs of children who more closely match the physical characteristics of African-American and Hispanic children (Beyer and Knott, 1998). The Oucher Faces Pain Scale consists of six photographs on the right side and a 0 to 100 scale on the left side. The photographs show the face of one child with the pictures arranged to show increasing levels of discomfort. Each version has been tested primarily with children in each ethnic group. Children use the Oucher by selecting a photograph or number that most closely represents the level of pain intensity they are experiencing (Beyer and Knott, 1998). These tools address cultural issues in accuracy of pain assessment and were designed to promote cultural sensitivity and self-esteem for minority, non-Caucasian children.

A comparison of surgery-related experiences in 25 African-American and 30 Caucasian children showed no significant difference in self-report of pain (Bohannon, 1995). However, physiologic parameters were found to be higher and behavioral distress scores lower in African-American children. Lower levels of analgesia and higher pain tolerance were also reported in a sample of Chinese pediatric burn and surgical (herniorrhaphy and appendectomy) patients compared with levels common for children in Western countries with comparable injuries or procedures (Hu, Zhang, and Chen, 1991a, 1991b).

The APPT also has a Spanish version (Van Cleve, Muñoz, Bossert, et al, 2001) that has been used in children and adolescents with cancer (Jacob and Mueller, 2008; Van Cleve, Bossert, Beecroft, et al, 2004).

Non-communicating Children's Pain Checklist — Postoperative Version (NCCPC-PV)

NAME:_____   UNIT/FILE #: _____   DATE:_____ (dd/mm/yy)

OBSERVER:_____ START TIME:_____ AM/PM   STOP TIME:_____ AM/PM

How often has this child shown these behaviours in the last 10 minutes? Please circle a number for each behaviour. If an item does not apply to this child (for example, this child cannot reach with his/her hands), then indicate "not applicable" for that item.

0 = NOT AT ALL   1 = JUST A LITTLE   2 = FAIRLY OFTEN   3 = VERY OFTEN   NA = NOT APPLICABLE

I. Vocal

1. Moaning, whining, whimpering (fairly soft)..	0	1	2	3	NA
2. Crying (moderately loud)..	0	1	2	3	NA
3. Screaming/yelling (very loud)...	0	1	2	3	NA
4. A specific sound or word for pain (e.g., a word, cry, or type of laugh)..........	0	1	2	3	NA

II. Social

5. Not cooperating, cranky, irritable, unhappy..	0	1	2	3	NA
6. Less interaction with others, withdrawn..	0	1	2	3	NA
7. Seeking comfort or physical closeness...	0	1	2	3	NA
8. Being difficult to distract, not able to satisfy or pacify..............................	0	1	2	3	NA

III. Facial

9. A furrowed brow...	0	1	2	3	NA
10. A change in eyes, including: squinching of eyes, eyes opened wide, eyes frowning	0	1	2	3	NA
11. Turning down of mouth, not smiling...	0	1	2	3	NA
12. Lips puckering up, tight, pouting, or quivering...	0	1	2	3	NA
13. Clenching or grinding teeth, chewing, or thrusting tongue out	0	1	2	3	NA

IV. Activity

14. Not moving, less active, quiet...	0	1	2	3	NA
15. Jumping around, agitated, fidgety..	0	1	2	3	NA

V. Body and Limbs

16. Floppy..	0	1	2	3	NA
17. Stiff, spastic, tense, rigid	0	1	2	3	NA
18. Gesturing to or touching part of the body that hurts	0	1	2	3	NA
19. Protecting, favoring, or guarding part of the body that hurts	0	1	2	3	NA
20. Flinching or moving the body part away, being sensitive to touch...............	0	1	2	3	NA
21. Moving the body in a specific way to show pain (e.g., head back, arms down, curls up, etc.)	0	1	2	3	NA

VI. Physiological

22. Shivering..	0	1	2	3	NA
23. Change in color, pallor..	0	1	2	3	NA
24. Sweating, perspiring..	0	1	2	3	NA
25. Tears..	0	1	2	3	NA
26. Sharp intake of breath, gasping..	0	1	2	3	NA
27. Breath holding..	0	1	2	3	NA

SCORE SUMMARY

Category	I	II	III	IV	V	VI	TOTAL
Score							

Fig. 7-4 Non-communicating Children's Pain Checklist. (Copyright 2004, Lynn Breau, Patrick McGrath, Allen Finley, and Carol Camfield. Reprinted with permission.)

There are several documented barriers to effective pain treatment in non–English speaking patients, including inadequate assessment of pain, concern about side effects of and tolerance to analgesics, patient and family reluctance to report pain, fear that pain means worse disease, reluctance to take pain medications, and lack of adherence to prescribed analgesics (Abbe, Simon, Angiolillo, et al, 2006; Bruera, Willey, Ewert-Flannagan, et al, 2005; Flores and Vega, 1998; Flores, Abreu, Olivar, et al, 1998). Non–English speaking patients pose additional language and cultural barriers that make pain assessment and treatments

USING THE NCCPC-PV

The NCCPC-PV was designed to be used for children, aged 3 to 18 years, who are unable to speak because of cognitive (mental/intellectual) impairments or disabilities. It can be used *whether or not* a child has physical impairments or disabilities. Descriptions of the types of children used to validate the NCCPC-PV can be found in: Breau, L.M., Finley, G.A., McGrath, P.J. & Camfield, C.S. (2002). Validation of the Non-communicating Children's Pain Checklist — Postoperative Version. *Anesthesiology, 96* (3), 528-535. The NCCPC-PV was designed to be used without training by parents and caregivers (carers), or by other adults who are not familiar with a specific child (do not know them well).

The NCCPC-PV may be freely copied for clinical use or use in research funded by not-for-profit agencies. For-profit agencies should contact Lynn Breau: Pediatric Pain Research, IWK Health Centre, 5850 University Avenue, Halifax, Nova Scotia, Canada, B3J 3G9 (lbreau@ns.sympatico.ca).

The NCCPC-PV was intended for use for pain after surgery or due to other procedures conducted in hospital. If short- or long-term pain is suspected for a child at home or in a long-term residential setting, the **Non-communicating Children's Pain Checklist — Revised** may be used. It can be obtained by contacting Lynn Breau. Information regarding the NCCPC-R can be found in: Breau, L.M., McGrath, P.J., Camfield, C.S. & Finley, G.A. (2002). Psychometric Properties of the Non-communicating Children's Pain Checklist—Revised. *Pain, 99,* 349-357.

ADMINISTRATION

To complete the NCCPC-R, base your observations on the child's behavior over **10 minutes**. *It is not necessary to watch the child continuously for this period.* However, it is recommended that the observer be in the child's presence for the majority of this time (e.g., be in the same room with the child). Although shorter observation periods may be used, the cut-off scores described below may not apply.

At the end of the observation time, indicate how frequently (how often) each item was seen or heard. This should not be based on the child's typical behavior or in relation to what he or she usually does. A guide for deciding the frequency of items is below:

> 0 = Not present at all during the observation period. (Note: If the item is not present because the child is not capable of performing that act, it should be scored as "NA").
> 1 = Seen or heard rarely (hardly at all), but is present.
> 2 = Seen or heard a number of times, but not continuous (not all the time).
> 3 = Seen or heard often, almost continuous (almost all the time); anyone would easily notice this if they saw the child for a few moments during the observation time.
> NA = Not applicable. This child is not capable of performing this action.

SCORING

1. Add up the scores for each subscale and enter below that subscale number in the Score Summary at the bottom of the sheet. Items marked "NA" are scored as "0" (zero).
2. Add up all subscale scores for Total Score.
3. Check whether the child's score is greater than the cut-off score.

CUT-OFF SCORE

Based on the scores of 24 children aged 3 to 18 (Breau, Finley, McGrath & Camfield, 2002), a **Total Score of 11 or more** indicates a child has **moderate to severe pain**. Based on unpublished data from this same sample, a *Total score of 6-10* indicates a child has **mild pain**. When parents and caregivers completed the NCCPC-PV in hospital for the study group, this was accurate 88% of the time. When other observers completed the NCCPC-PV, this was accurate 75% of the time. A Total Score of 10 or less indicates less than moderate/severe pain. This was correct in the study group for parents and caregivers 81% of the time, and for other observers 63% of the time.

USE OF CUT-OFF SCORES

As with all observational tools, caution should be taken in using cut-off scores, because they may not be 100% accurate. They should not be used as the only basis for deciding whether a child should be treated for pain. In some cases children may have lower scores when pain is present. For more detailed instructions for use of the NCCPC-PV in such situations, please refer to the full manual, available from Lynn Breau: Pediatric Pain Research, IWK Health Centre, 5850 University Avenue, Halifax, Nova Scotia, Canada, B3J 3G9 (lbreau@ns.sympatico.ca).

Fig. 7-4, cont'd.

more challenging (see Research Focus box). To minimize the risk of undertreatment of pain, clinicians may give non–English speaking children and adolescents the body outline diagram of the APPT and encourage them to use the diagram for communicating the location and extensiveness of pain (Jacob and Mueller, 2008).

CHILDREN WITH CHRONIC ILLNESS AND COMPLEX PAIN

Questionnaires and pain assessment scales do not always provide the most meaningful means of assessing pain in children, particularly for those with complex pain. Some children

RESEARCH FOCUS
Pain Reporting in Non–English-Speaking Children

Jacob, McCarthy, Sambuco, and colleagues (2008) examined the pain experience of Spanish-speaking children with cancer who were asked about their pain during the week before a scheduled oncology clinic appointment. They found that 41% of the patients were experiencing pain. Some were experiencing moderate to severe pain and did not receive medications because they did not report their pain.

cannot relate to a face or a number that describes their pain. Other children, such as those with cancer, are experiencing multiple symptoms and may find it difficult to isolate the pain from other symptoms. Rating the pain does not always accurately convey to others how they really feel (Woodgate and Yanofsky, 2004).

The most important aspect of pain assessment for children with chronic illness, particularly those with complex pain, is the relationship that develops between the child and the family. This relationship offers health care providers a sense of what the pain experience means to the child and family. The pain experience can interfere with the child's ability to eat, sleep, and perform daily activities and routines (Miaskowski and Lee, 1999; Morin, Gibson, and Wade, 1998) and may be complicated by pain processes that occur in the central nervous system, side effects of medical treatments, and complications associated with disease management.

Other important components of assessment include the onset of pain; pain duration or pattern; the effectiveness of the current treatment; factors that aggravate or relieve the pain; other symptoms and complications concurrently felt; and interference with the child's mood, function, and interactions with family (McCaffery and Pasero, 1999). In addition to asking the child or parent when the pain started and how long the pain lasts, the nurse can assess variations and rhythms by asking whether the pain is better or worse at certain times of the day or night. If the child has had pain for a while, the child or parent may know which medications and doses are helpful. They may also have found some nonpharmacologic methods that have helped. The nurse may ask the child or parent if there are activities, positions, and other events that may increase the pain. Pain may be accompanied by other symptoms such as nausea and poor appetite, and it may interfere with sleep and other activities.

Other aspects warranting careful assessment that may pose barriers to effective management include family issues and relationships, fears and concerns about addictions (see Community Focus box, p. 211), the clinician's and family's lack of knowledge about pain, inappropriate use of pain medications, ineffective management of adverse effects from medications, and the use of different modalities (McCaffery and Pasero, 1999).

PAIN MANAGEMENT

Children may experience pain as a result of surgery, injuries, acute and chronic illnesses, and medical or surgical procedures. Unrelieved pain may lead to potential long-term physiologic, psychosocial, and behavioral consequences (Goldschneider and

Anand, 2003; Weisman, Bernstein, and Schechter, 1998). Management of pain should be a priority for all pediatric health care providers.

NONPHARMACOLOGIC MANAGEMENT

Pain is often associated with fear, anxiety, and stress. A number of nonpharmacologic techniques, such as distraction, relaxation, guided imagery, and cutaneous stimulation, can help with pain control (see Nursing Care Guidelines box). It is also important to provide coping strategies that help reduce pain perception, make pain more tolerable, decrease anxiety, and enhance the effectiveness of analgesics or reduce the dosage required (Rusy and Weisman, 2000). Techniques decrease the perceived threat of pain, provide a sense of control, enhance comfort, and promote rest and sleep (McCaffery and Pasero, 1999). Despite a paucity of research on the effectiveness of many of these interventions, the strategies are safe, noninvasive, and inexpensive, and most are independent nursing functions. Environmental and psychologic factors may exert a powerful influence on children's pain perceptions and may be modified by using psychosocial strategies, education, parental support, and cognitive-behavioral interventions. For children undergoing repeated painful procedures, cognitive-behavioral interventions are effective for decreasing anxiety and distress (McGrath and Hillier, 2003).

If the child cannot identify a familiar coping technique, the nurse can describe several strategies and let the child select the most appealing one. Experimentation with several strategies that are suitable to the child's age, pain intensity, and abilities is often necessary to determine the most effective approach. Parents should be involved in the selection process; they may be familiar with the child's usual coping skills and can help identify potentially successful strategies. Involving parents also encourages their participation in learning the skill with the child and acting as coach. If the parent cannot assist the child, other appropriate persons may include a grandparent, older sibling, nurse, or child-life specialist (McGrath and Hillier, 2003).

Children should learn to use a specific strategy before pain occurs or before it becomes severe. To reduce the child's effort, instructions for a strategy, such as distraction or relaxation, can be audiotaped and played during a period of comfort. However, even after they have learned an intervention, children often need help using it during a painful procedure. The intervention can also be used after the procedure. This gives the child a chance to recover, feel mastery, and cope more effectively (McGrath and Hillier, 2003).

Several studies have documented the effectiveness of nonpharmacologic analgesia, such as containment, positioning, nonnutritive sucking, and kangaroo holding, in neonates during painful procedures. Containment is achieved through positioning and blanket rolls (Cole and Jorgensen, 1997). It provides a "nest" that enhances the infant's feelings of security and decreases stress. Comforting measures and swaddling reduce crying and heart rate after procedures such as heel punctures and injections (see Research Focus box).

Nonnutritive sucking (pacifier) (Fig. 7-5) reduces behavioral, physiologic, and hormonal responses to pain from procedures, such as heel punctures, venipuncture, and immunization

NURSING CARE GUIDELINES
Nonpharmacologic Strategies for Pain Management

General Strategies

Consult child-life specialist.

Use nonpharmacologic interventions to supplement, not replace, pharmacologic interventions, and use for mild pain and pain that is reasonably well controlled with analgesics.

Form a trusting relationship with child and family.

Express concern regarding their reports of pain and intervene appropriately.

Take an active role in seeking effective pain management strategies.

Use general guidelines to prepare child for procedure.

Prepare child before potentially painful procedures, but avoid "planting" the idea of pain.

- For example, instead of saying, "This is going to (or may) hurt," say, "Sometimes this feels like pushing, sticking, or pinching, and sometimes it doesn't bother people. Tell me what it feels like to you."
- Use "nonpain" descriptors when possible (e.g., "It feels like heat" rather than "It's a burning pain"). This allows for variation in sensory perception, avoids suggesting pain, and gives the child control in describing reactions.
- Avoid evaluative statements or descriptions (e.g., "This is a terrible procedure" or "It really will hurt a lot").

Stay with child during a painful procedure.

Allow parents to stay with child if child and parent desire; encourage parent to talk softly to child and to remain near child's head.

Involve parents in learning specific nonpharmacologic strategies and in assisting child with their use.

Educate child about the pain, especially when explanation may lessen anxiety (e.g., that pain may occur after surgery and does not indicate something is wrong); reassure the child that he or she is not responsible for the pain.

For long-term pain control, offer the child a doll, which represents "the patient," and allow child to do everything to the doll that is done to them; emphasize pain control through the doll by stating, "Dolly feels better after the medicine."

Teach procedures to child and family for later use.

Specific Strategies
Distraction

Involve parent and child in identifying strong distractors.

Involve child in play; use radio, tape recorder, CD player, or computer game; have child sing or use rhythmic breathing.

Have child take a deep breath and blow it out until told to stop.

Have child blow bubbles to "blow the hurt away."

Have child concentrate on yelling or saying "ouch," with instructions to "yell as loud or soft as you feel it hurt; that way I know what's happening."

Have child look through kaleidoscope (type with glitter suspended in fluid-filled tube) and encourage him or her to concentrate by asking, "Do you see the different designs?"

Use humor, such as watching cartoons, telling jokes or funny stories, or acting silly with child.

Have child read, play games, or visit with friends.

Relaxation

With an infant or young child:

- Hold in a comfortable, well-supported position, such as vertically against the chest and shoulder.

- Rock in a wide, rhythmic arc in a rocking chair or sway back and forth, rather than bouncing child.
- Repeat one or two words softly, such as "Mommy's here."

With a slightly older child:

- Ask child to take a deep breath and "go limp as a rag doll" while exhaling slowly; then ask child to yawn (demonstrate if needed).
- Help child assume a comfortable position (e.g., pillow under neck and knees).
- Begin progressive relaxation: starting with the toes, systematically instruct child to let each body part "go limp" or "feel heavy"; if child has difficulty relaxing, instruct child to tense or tighten each body part and then relax it.
- Allow child to keep eyes open, since children may respond better if eyes are open rather than closed during relaxation.

Guided Imagery

Have child identify some highly pleasurable real or imaginary experience.

Have child describe details of the event, including as many senses as possible (e.g., "feel the cool breezes," "see the beautiful colors," "hear the pleasant music").

Have child write down or tape record script.

Encourage child to concentrate only on the pleasurable event during the painful time; enhance the image by recalling specific details by reading the script or playing the tape.

Combine with relaxation and rhythmic breathing.

Positive Self-Talk

Teach child positive statements to say when in pain (e.g., "I will be feeling better soon," "When I go home, I will feel better, and we will eat ice cream").

Thought Stopping

Identify positive facts about the painful event (e.g., "It does not last long").

Identify reassuring information (e.g., "If I think about something else, it does not hurt as much").

Condense positive and reassuring facts into a set of brief statements and have child memorize them (e.g., "Short procedure, good veins, little hurt, nice nurse, go home").

Have child repeat the memorized statements whenever thinking about or experiencing the painful event.

Behavioral Contracting

Informal—May be used with children as young as 4 or 5 years of age:

- Use stars, tokens, or cartoon character stickers as rewards.
- Give a child who is uncooperative or procrastinating during a procedure a limited time (measured by a visible timer) to complete the procedure.
- Proceed as needed if child is unable to comply.
- Reinforce cooperation with a reward if the procedure is accomplished within specified time.

Formal—Use written contract, which includes:

- Realistic (seems possible) goal or desired behavior
- Measurable behavior (e.g., agrees not to hit anyone during procedures)
- Contract written, dated, and signed by all persons involved in any of the agreements
- Identified rewards or consequences that are reinforcing
- Goals that can be evaluated
- Commitment and compromise requirements for both parties (e.g., while timer is used, nurse will not nag or prod child to complete procedure)

---

injections. The administration of concentrated sucrose with or without nonnutritive sucking has calming and pain-relieving effects for invasive procedures in neonates (see Evidence-Based Practice box). In one study the amount of time crying was decreased with 0.24 to 0.48 g (0.008 to 0.17 oz) (2 ml of a 12% to 24% sucrose solution) administered orally 2 minutes before a heel lance or venipuncture (Stevens, Yamada, and Ohlsson, 2005).

Kangaroo care is a skin-to-skin holding of infants dressed only in diapers against their mother's or father's chest (Gray,

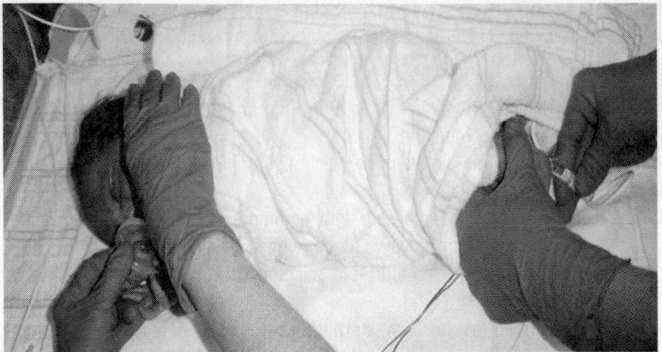

Fig. 7-5 Sucking following oral sucrose can enhance analgesia before a heel stick in a preterm infant.

RESEARCH FOCUS

Nonpharmacologic Methods of Pain Management

In infants between 27 and 34 weeks of gestational age, those infants who were swaddled after a routine heel stick procedure were able to calm crying immediately, decrease heart rate, and return to a sleep state; in comparison, infants who were not swaddled took a minimum of 10 minutes to return to baseline physiologic and behavioral levels (Fearon, Kisilevsky, Hains, et al, 1997). Proper positioning with the infant held in a midline orientation, hand to mouth activity, and proper flexion can promote self-soothing behaviors. "Facilitated tucking," which is holding the infant's extremities flexed and contained close to the trunk, during heel lance procedures decreases heart rate and crying time and promotes stability in the sleep-wake cycles after the lance.

EVIDENCE-BASED PRACTICE
Carol Turnage Carrier

Reduction of Minor Procedural Pain in Infants

ASK THE QUESTION

In newborns and infants, does sucrose provide adequate analgesia during minor painful procedures? Are the effects age dependent?

SEARCH FOR THE EVIDENCE

Search strategies

Search selection criteria included English publications within past 10 years, research-based articles (level 1 or lower) on neonates or infants undergoing venipuncture or immunizations.

Databases used

PubMed, Cochrane Collaboration, MD Consult, Joanna Briggs Institute, National Guideline Clearinghouse (AHQR), TRIP Database Plus, PedsCCM, BestBETs

CRITICALLY ANALYZE THE EVIDENCE

GRADE criteria: Evidence quality high; recommendation strong (Guyatt, Oxman, Vist, et al, 2008)

Venipuncture versus heel lance for blood sampling

- Four randomized controlled trials reviewed by the Cochrane Collaboration (Shah and Ohlsson, 2004) compared the efficacy and painfulness of blood sampling by venipuncture or heel lance in full-term neonates. The researchers concluded that venipuncture performed by skilled phlebotomists results in less pain than heel stick for blood sampling. Decreased pain scores, cry duration, and mother's rating of infant's pain demonstrated venipuncture as the preferred method of blood collection. The researchers noted that infants receiving heel stick may also require more than one stick to get enough for the sample, whereas venipuncture reduces the risk of additional sticks.

Glucose versus EMLA cream for venipuncture in neonates

- In a randomized control, double-blind study of 201 newborn infants (Gradin, Lenclen, Gajdos, et al, 2002), 99 received EMLA (lidocaine and prilocaine) and oral placebo, and 102 were given 30% oral glucose and placebo on the skin. The 30% glucose group had significantly lower Premature Infant Pain Profile (PIPP) scores and duration of crying than the EMLA group. Significantly fewer patients in the glucose group were scored on the PIPP as having pain or a score above 6 (19.3% compared with 41.7%).

Glucose compared with EMLA for venipuncture pain

- In a randomized control, double-blind study, Lindh, Wiklund, Blomquist, and colleagues (2003) compared the pain response of 90 infants divided equally into EMLA plus 1 ml water by mouth as control placebo with a treatment group given occlusive dressing plus 1 ml oral glucose (300 mg/ml). The combination of EMLA and oral glucose significantly reduced pain response associated with diphtheria-pertussis-tetanus immunizations in 3-month-old infants.

Sucrose for minor painful procedures (heel lance and venipuncture)

- One hundred fifty full-term newborns were randomly assigned to one of six treatment groups: (1) no treatment, (2) 2 ml sterile water placebo, (3) 2 ml 30% glucose, (4) 2 ml 30% sucrose, (5) 2 ml 30% sucrose with pacifier, and (6) pacifier alone. Results: The pacifier alone was more effective than sweet solutions, sweet solutions and pacifier were significantly more effective than the placebo, and sucrose and glucose were equally effective in lowering pain scores (Carbajal, Chauvet, Couderc, et al, 1999).

- Acharya, Annamali, Taub, and colleagues (2004) studied 28 infants (mean gestation at birth of 30.5 weeks and postnatal age of 27.2 days) who received either 2 ml of a placebo of sterile water or 25% sucrose slowly over 2 minutes into the mouth by syringe 4 minutes before two routine venipunctures. Results: Behavioral state and difficulty and duration of venipuncture were not significantly different between the two liquids. Heart rate, crying times, and neonatal facial coding system scores were significantly lower in the treatment group.

- Abad, Diaz-Gomez, Domenech, and colleagues (2001) compared oral sucrose with EMLA in a prospective randomized trial of 51 full-term newborn infants less than 4 days old receiving venipuncture. The 2 ml of 24% sucrose solution alone was the most effective analgesic compared with placebo (spring water), EMLA, or EMLA combined with 2 ml sucrose. The combination of EMLA and sucrose did not enhance the analgesic effects.

- In the Stevens, Yamada, and Ohlsson (2005) review, 21 randomized control trials met criteria for review, 11 with full-term infants and nine with preterm infants, with one study including both populations (1616 infants; maximum postnatal age of 28 days after reaching 40 weeks corrected age). Heel lance was the most common procedure observed as the painful stimulus; three studies used venipuncture. Sucrose in a wide variety of dosages delivered by syringe or pacifier was found to decrease crying time, heart rate, facial action, and composite pain scores during venipuncture and heel lance. These reviewers recommend the use of sucrose in a range of 0.012 to 0.12 g (0.05 to 0.5 ml) of a 24% solution 2 minutes before a single heel lance or venipuncture for safe and effective pain relief. They also recommend concomitant use of other methods of pain relief, since some studies included use of pacifier, rocking, kangaroo care, or holding along with sucrose intervention.

Reduction of Minor Procedural Pain in Infants

APPLY THE EVIDENCE AND NURSING IMPLICATIONS

Sucrose

- Sucrose is effective in reducing pain response in infants 6 months and less undergoing minor acute painful procedures.
- Adverse effects such as hyperglycemia, aspiration, or necrotizing enterocolitis have not been reported with sucrose administered without additives.
- The most effective dose has been 24% solution given at least 2 minutes before a procedure.
- Doses of 50% to 75% have been effective for relieving pain during immunizations in infants up to 6 months of age, suggesting that higher concentrations may be required for older infants.
- Effective dose volumes range from 0.05 to 2 ml, with lower volumes used for low-birth-weight infants and larger volumes used for older infants.
- The analgesic effect of sucrose in combination with sucking a bottle or pacifier appears to be enhanced.
- Studies of older infants have used both increased volume and concentration of sucrose.
- Sucrose in combination with nonpharmacologic support during a procedure may increase the analgesic response for older infants (2 months) even with lower concentrations of sucrose. Interventions include pacifier, holding, swaddling, skin-to-skin contact, and rocking.
- Administration can be by labeled oral syringe, dipped pacifier, or bottle, depending on the infant's ability and age.
- The advantages of minimum wait time, low cost, and decreased risk of adverse effects were significant.
- Effects of repeated dosing over time and dosing of infants less than 27 weeks are not known.

Glucose

- Glucose 30% 1 ml given orally by syringe is more effective than EMLA for venipuncture pain.
- Comparisons between sucrose and glucose have been inconclusive.

References

Abad F, Diaz-Gomez NM, Domenech E, et al: Oral sucrose compares favorably with lidocaine-prilocaine cream for pain relief during venepuncture in neonates, *Acta Paediatr* 90:160-165, 2001.

Acharya AB, Annamali S, Taub NA, et al: Oral sucrose analgesia for preterm infant venepuncture, *Arch Dis Child Fetal Neonatal Educ* 89:F17-F18, 2004.

Carbajal R, Chauvet X, Couderc S, et al: Randomised trial of analgesic effects of sucrose, glucose, and pacifiers in term neonates, *BMJ* 319(7222):1393-1397, 1999.

Gradin M, Lenclen R, Gajdos V, et al: Crossover trial of analgesic efficacy of glucose and pacifier in very preterm neonates during subcutaneous injections, *Pediatrics* 110(6):1053-1057, 2002.

Guyatt GH, Oxman AD, Vist GE, et al: GRADE: an emerging consensus on rating quality of evidence and strength of recommendations, *BMJ* 336: 924-926, 2008.

Lindh V, Wiklund U, Blomquist HK, et al: EMLA cream and oral glucose for immunization pain in 3-month old infants, *Pain* 104(1-2):381-388, 2003.

Shah V, Ohlsson A: Venepuncture versus heel lance for blood sampling in term neonates, *Cochrane Database Syst Rev* (4):CD001452.pub2; DOI: 10.1002/14651858.CD001452.pub2, 2004.

Stevens B, Yamada J, Ohlsson A: *Sucrose for analgesia in newborn infants undergoing painful procedures* (review), 2005. In Cochrane Neonatal Collaboration, available at www.thecochranelibrary.com (accessed April 16, 2009).

Watt, and Blass, 2000; Johnston, Stevens, Pinelli, et al, 2003). Infants who spent 1 to 3 hours in kangaroo care showed increased frequency in quiet sleep, longer duration of quiet sleep, and decreased crying in the neonatal intensive care unit (NICU), and they cried less at the age of 6 months when compared with neonates who did not receive skin-to-skin contact (see Research Focus box).

RESEARCH FOCUS

Kangaroo Care

Significant differences were found in pain responses during heel lancing between infants who were kangaroo held and those who were not. In the study by Gray, Watt, and Blass (2000), heart rate increased by 8 to 10 beats/min in the kangaroo care group versus 36 to 38 beats/min in the control group of neonates who were swaddled in bassinets; grimacing was 64% less and crying was 82% less in the kangaroo-held infants.

In another study, infant responses to pain during heel lance procedures were studied using kangaroo holding (Fig. 7-6), with the neonate held upright at a 60-degree angle between the mother's breasts for maximal skin-to-skin contact (Johnston, Stevens, Pinelli, et al, 2003). A blanket was placed over the neonate's back, and the mother's clothes were wrapped around the neonate for 30 minutes before the lancing procedure,

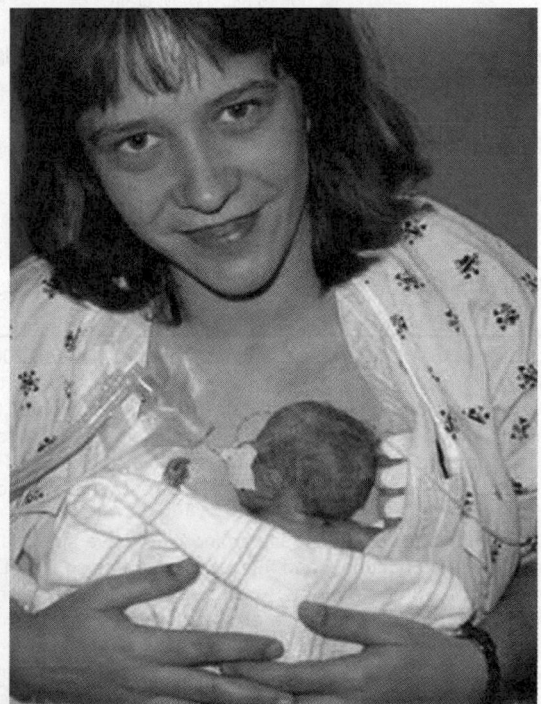

Fig. 7-6 Mother using kangaroo hold with her newborn infant. Note placement of the infant directly on the mother's skin.

during, and at least 30 minutes after the heel stick. Another group remained in the isolette in a prone position, swaddled with a blanket and the heel accessible, for 30 minutes before the heel lancing procedure. Pain scores were significantly lower in kangaroo-held infants.

COMPLEMENTARY PAIN MEDICINE

Many terms are used to describe approaches to health care that are outside the realm of conventional medicine as practiced in the United States. Complementary and alternative medicine (CAM), as defined by the National Center for Complementary and Alternative Medicine, is a group of diverse medical and health care systems, practices, and products that are not currently considered part of conventional medicine (Myers, Stuber, Bonamer-Rheingans, et al, 2005) (see Complementary and Alternative Therapy box). Although some scientific evidence exists regarding some CAM therapies, for most, key questions are yet to be answered through well-designed scientific studies—questions such as whether these therapies are safe and whether they work for the diseases or medical conditions for which they are used.

Current estimates of pediatric CAM use range from 10% to 15%, derived from children sampled at health care facilities, children with chronic conditions, and/or use in countries other than the United States. For the U.S. population, pediatric CAM use was estimated to be 31% to 84% (Myers, Stuber, Bonamer-Rheingans, et al, 2005; Rusy and Weisman, 2000). Those who used CAM were found in each age-group, and the mean age was 10.3 years. The majority used unconventional therapy for

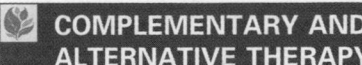

COMPLEMENTARY AND ALTERNATIVE THERAPY

Five Classifications of Complementary and Alternative Medicine

Complementary and alternative medicine therapies are grouped into five classes: biologically based (foods, special diets, herbal or plant preparations, vitamins, other supplements); manipulative treatments (chiropractic, osteopathy, massage); energy based (Reiki, bioelectric or magnetic treatments, pulsed fields, alternating and direct currents); mind-body techniques (mental healing, expressive treatments, spiritual healing, hypnosis, relaxation); and alternative medical systems (homeopathy; naturopathy; ayurvedic; traditional Chinese medicine, including acupuncture and moxibustion).

chronic, as opposed to life-threatening, medical conditions. The therapies that are increasingly used include herbal medicine, massage, megavitamins, self-help groups, folk remedies, energy healing, and homeopathy (Myers, Stuber, Bonamer-Rheingans, et al, 2005; Rusy and Weisman, 2000).

PHARMACOLOGIC MANAGEMENT

Nonopioids, including acetaminophen (Tylenol, Paracetamol) and nonsteroidal antiinflammatory drugs (NSAIDs), are suitable for mild to moderate pain (Table 7-4). Opioids are needed for moderate to severe pain (Table 7-5). A combination of the two analgesics acts on the pain system on two levels: nonopioids primarily act at the peripheral nervous system and opioids primarily act at the central nervous system. This approach provides increased analgesia without increased side

Skill—Calculating Safe Dosages for Children

Pediatric Drug Dosage Calculations

TABLE 7-4	NONSTEROIDAL ANTIINFLAMMATORY DRUGS (NSAIDs) APPROVED FOR CHILDREN*	
DRUG	**DOSAGE**	**COMMENTS**
Acetaminophen (Tylenol)	10-15 mg/kg/dose q 4-6 hr not to exceed 5 doses in 24 hr or 75 mg/kg/day, orally	Available in numerous preparations Nonprescription Higher dosage range may provide increased analgesia
Choline magnesium trisalicylate (Trilisate)	Children <37 kg (81.5 lb): 50 mg/kg/day divided into 2 doses Children >37 kg (81.5 lb): 2250 mg/day divided into 2 doses	Available in suspension, 500 mg/5 ml Prescription
Ibuprofen (children's Motrin, children's Advil)	Children >6 mo: 5-10 mg/kg/dose q 6-8 hr not to exceed 40 mg/kg/day	Available in numerous preparations Available in suspension, 100 mg/5 ml, and drops, 100 mg/2.5 ml Nonprescription
Naproxen (Naprosyn)	Children >2 yr: 5-7 mg/kg/dose every 8-12 hr	Available in suspension, 125 mg/5 ml, and several different dosages for tablets Prescription
Tolmetin (Tolectin)	Children >2 yr: 5-7 mg/kg/dose every 6-8 hr	Available in 200-mg, 400-mg, and 600-mg tablets Prescription

Data from Lacy CF: Lexi-Comp's drug information handbook 2009-2010, ed 18, Hudson, Ohio, 2009, Lexi-Comp, Inc.

NOTE: Newer formulations of NSAIDs selectively inhibit one of the enzymes of cyclooxygenase (COX-2, which is responsible for pain transmission) but do not inhibit the other (COX-1). Inhibition of COX-1 decreases prostaglandin production, which is necessary for normal organ function. For example, prostaglandins help maintain gastric mucosal blood flow and barrier protection, regulate blood flow to the liver and kidneys, and facilitate platelet aggregation and clot formation. Theoretically, the COX-2 NSAIDs provide similar analgesic and antiinflammatory benefits with fewer gastric and platelet side effects than the nonselective agents. COX-2 NSAIDs are approved for use in patients >18 years of age.

*All NSAIDs in this table (except acetaminophen) have significant antiinflammatory, antipyretic, and analgesic actions. Acetaminophen has a weak antiinflammatory action, and its classification as an NSAID is controversial. Patients respond differently to various NSAIDs; therefore changing from one drug to another may be necessary for maximum benefit. Acetylsalicylic acid (aspirin) is also an NSAID but is not recommended for children because of its possible association with Reye syndrome. The NSAIDs in this table have no known association with Reye syndrome. However, caution should be exercised in prescribing any salicylate-containing drug (e.g., choline magnesium trisalicylate) for children with known or suspected viral infection. Side effects of ibuprofen, naproxen, and tolmetin include nausea, vomiting, diarrhea, constipation, gastric ulceration, bleeding nephritis, and fluid retention. Acetaminophen and choline magnesium trisalicylate are well tolerated in the gastrointestinal tract and do not interfere with platelet function. NSAIDs (except acetaminophen) should not be given to patients with allergic reactions to salicylates. All the NSAIDs should be used cautiously in patients with renal impairment.

TABLE 7-5 DOSAGE OF SELECTED OPIOIDS FOR CHILDREN

DRUG	APPROPRIATE EQUIANALGESIC	APPROXIMATE EQUIANALGESIC PARENTERAL DOSE	RECOMMENDED STARTING DOSE (CHILDREN <50 kg (110 lb) BODY WEIGHT)*	
			ORAL	PARENTERAL
Morphine	30 mg q 3-4 hr	10 mg q 3-4 hr	0.2-0.4 mg/kg q 3-4 hr 0.3-0.6 mg/kg time released q 12 hr	0.1-0.2 mg/kg IM q 3-4 hr 0.02-0.1 mg/kg IV bolus q 2 hr 0.015 mg/kg q 8 min PCA 0.01-0.02 mg/kg/hr IV infusion (neonates) 0.01-0.06 mg/kg/hr IV infusion (child)
Fentanyl (Sublimaze) (oral mucosal form [Actiq])†	Not available	0.1 mg IV	5-15 mcg/kg; maximum dose 400 mcg	0.5-1.5 mcg/kg IV bolus q 30 min 1-2 mcg/hr IV infusion
Codeine‡	200 mg q 3-4 hr	130 mg q 3-4 hr	1 mg/kg q 3-4 hr	Not recommended
Hydromorphone§ (Dilaudid)	7.5 mg q 3-4 hr	1.5 mg q 3-4 hr	0.04-0.1 mg/kg q 3-4 hr	0.02-0.1 mg/kg q 3-4 hr 0.005-0.2 mg/kg IV bolus q 2 hr
Hydrocodone and acetaminophen (Lorcet, Lortab, Vicodin, others)	30 mg q 3-4 hr	Not available	0.2 mg/kg q 3-4 hr	Not available
Levorphanol (Levo-Dromoran)	4 mg q 6-8 hr	2 mg q 6-8 hr	0.04 mg/kg q 6-8 hr	0.02 mg/kg q 6-8 hr
Meperidine (Demerol)‖	300 mg q 2-3 hr	100 mg q 3 hr	Not recommended	0.75 mg/kg q 2-3 hr
Methadone (Dolophine, others)¶	20 mg q 6-8 hr	10 mg q 6-8 hr	0.2 mg/kg q 6-8 hr	0.1 mg/kg q 6-8 hr
Oxycodone (Roxicodone, OxyContin; also in Percocet, Percodan, Tylox, others)	20 mg q 3-4 hr	Not available	2 mg/kg q 3-4 hr**	Not available

Data from Acute Pain Management Guideline Panel: *Acute pain management: operative or medical procedures and trauma: clinical practice guideline,* AHCPR Pub. No. 92-0032, Rockville, Md, 1992, Agency for Health Care Policy and Research, Public Health Service, US Department of Health and Human Services; Berde C, Ablin A, Glazer J, et al: American Academy of Pediatrics Report of the Subcommittee on Disease-Related Pain in Childhood Cancer, *Pediatrics* 86(5 pt 2):820, 1990.

IM, Intramuscular; *IV,* intravenous; *PCA,* patient-controlled analgesia.

NOTE: Published tables vary in suggested doses that are equianalgesic to morphine. Clinical response is criterion that must be applied for each patient; titration to clinical response is necessary. Because there is not complete cross-tolerance among these drugs, it is usually necessary to use a lower than equianalgesic dose when changing drugs and to retitrate to response.

CAUTION: Recommended doses do not apply to patients with renal or hepatic insufficiency or other conditions affecting drug metabolism and kinetics.

*CAUTION: Doses listed for patients with body weight <50 kg (110 lb) cannot be used as initial starting doses in infants <6 months of age. For nonventilated infants <6 months, the initial opioid dose should be about ¼ to ⅓ of the dose recommended for older infants and children. For example, morphine could be used at a dose of 0.03 mg/kg instead of the traditional 0.1 mg/kg.

†Actiq is indicated only for management of breakthrough cancer pain in patients with malignancies who are already receiving and are tolerant to opioid therapy, but it can be used for preoperative or preprocedural sedation and analgesia.

‡CAUTION: Codeine doses above 65 mg often are not appropriate because of diminishing incremental analgesia with increasing doses but continually increasing constipation and other side effects. Dosages are from McCaffery M, Pasero C: *Pain: a clinical manual,* ed. 2, St. Louis, 1999, Mosby.

§For morphine, hydromorphone, and oxymorphone, rectal administration is an alternate route for patients unable to take oral medications, but equianalgesic doses may differ from oral and parenteral doses because of pharmacokinetic differences.

‖Meperidine is not recommended for continuous pain control (e.g., postoperatively) because of risk of normeperidine toxicity.

¶Initial dose is 10%-25% of equianalgesic morphine dose. Parenteral Dolophine is no longer available in the United States.

**CAUTION: Doses of aspirin and acetaminophen in combination with opioid or nonsteroidal antiinflammatory drug preparations must also be adjusted to patient's body weight. Daily dose of acetaminophen should not exceed 75 mg/kg, or 4000 mg.

effects. Several combinations, such as acetaminophen with codeine, may have increasing doses of the opioid but a constant dose of the nonopioid (Table 7-6). Before increasing the opioid, it may be preferable to increase the nonopioid component, for example, adding one regular-strength acetaminophen tablet (325 mg) to acetaminophen 300 mg with codeine 15 mg (Tylenol No. 2) before advancing to acetaminophen 300 mg with codeine 30 mg (Tylenol No. 3) or codeine 60 mg (Tylenol No. 4). However, if this approach is not successful, pain management will require a stronger opioid (see Table 7-5).

Oxycodone is available without a nonopioid in an immediate release and a controlled release preparation (OxyContin). The oxycodone dose can be safely increased without the risk of toxicity from excessive acetaminophen use. Actions of various opioids differ. Morphine is considered the gold standard for the management of severe pain. When morphine is not a suitable

TABLE 7-6   COANALGESIC ADJUVANT DRUGS

DRUG	DOSAGE	INDICATIONS	COMMENTS
Antidepressants			
Amitriptyline	0.2-0.5 mg/kg PO hs Titrate upward by 0.25 mg/kg q 5-7 days prn Available in 10- and 25-mg tablets Usual starting dose: 10-25 mg	Continuous neuropathic pain with burning, aching, dysthesia with insomnia	Provides analgesia by blocking reuptake of serotonin and norepinephrine, possibly slowing transmission of pain signals Helps with pain related to insomnia and depression (use nortriptyline if patient is oversedated) Analgesic effects seen earlier than antidepressant effects
Nortriptyline	0.2-1.0 mg/kg PO AM or bid Titrate up by 0.5 mg q 5-7 days Maximum: 25 mg/dose	Neuropathic pain as above without insomnia	Side effects include dry mouth, constipation, urinary retention
Anticonvulsants			
Gabapentin	5 mg/kg PO hs Increase to bid on day 2, tid on day 3 Maximum: 300 mg/day	Neuropathic pain	Mechanism of action unknown Side effects include sedation, ataxia, nystagmus, dizziness
Carbamazepine	<6 yr—2.5-5 mg/kg PO bid initially Increase 20 mg/kg/24 hr, divide bid every week prn Maximum: 100 mg bid 6-12 yr—5 mg/kg PO bid initially Increase 10 mg/kg/24 hr; divide bid every week prn to usual max: 100 mg/dose bid >12 yr—200 mg PO bid initially Increase 200 mg/24 hr, divide bid every week prn to max: 1.6-2.4 g/24 hr	Sharp, lancinating neuropathic pain Peripheral neuropathies Phantom limb pain	Similar analgesic effect to amitriptyline Monitor blood levels for toxicity only Side effects include decreased blood counts, ataxia, gastrointestinal irritation
Anxiolytics			
Lorazepam	0.03-0.1 mg/kg q 4-6 hr PO or IV Maximum: 2 mg/dose	Muscle spasm Anxiety	May increase sedation in combination with opioids Can cause depression with prolonged use
Diazepam	0.1-0.3 mg/kg q 4-6 hr PO or IV Maximum: 10 mg/dose		
Corticosteroids			
Dexamethasone	Dose dependent on clinical situation; higher bolus doses in cord compression, then lower daily dose Try to wean to NSAIDs if pain allows Cerebral edema: 1-2 mg/kg load then 1-1.5 mg/kg/day divided q 6 hr Maximum: 4 mg/dose Antiinflammatory: 0.08-0.3 mg/kg/day divided q 6-12 hr	Pain from increased intracranial pressure Bony metastasis Spinal or nerve compression	Side effects include edema, gastrointestinal irritation, increased weight, acne Use gastroprotectants such as H$_2$-blockers (ranitidine) or proton pump inhibitors such as omeprazole for long-term administration of steroids or NSAIDs in end-stage cancer with bony pain
Others			
Clonidine	2-4 mcg/kg PO q 4-6 hr May also use a 100 mcg transdermal patch q 7 days for patients >40 kg (88 lb)	Neuropathic pain Lancinating, sharp, electrical, shooting pain Phantom limb pain	α_2-Adenoreceptor agonist modulates ascending pain sensations Routes of administration: oral, transdermal, and spinal Management of withdrawal symptoms Monitor for orthostatic hypertension, decreased heart rate Sedation common
Mexiletine	2-3 mg/kg/dose PO tid, may titrate 0.5 mg/kg q 2-3 wk prn Maximum: 300 mg/dose		Similar to lidocaine, longer acting Stabilizes sodium conduction in nerve cells, reduces neuronal firing Can enhance action of opioids, antidepressants, anticonvulsants Side effects include dizziness, ataxia, nausea, vomiting May measure blood levels for toxicity

bid, Twice a day; *hs,* at bedtime; *IV,* intravenous; *NSAIDs,* nonsteroidal antiinflammatory drugs; *PO,* by mouth; *prn,* as needed; *q,* every; *tid,* three times a day.

opioid, drugs such as hydromorphone (Dilaudid) and fentanyl (Sublimaze) are effective substitutes. Although fentanyl is used as an anesthetic in the operating room, it is classified as an analgesic. It can be safely administered by nurses by the intravenous (IV), intramuscular (IM), transmucosal, and transdermal routes (Algren, Gursoy, Johnson, et al, 1998; Golianu, Krane, Galloway, et al, 2000).

! NURSING ALERT

The optimum dosage of an analgesic is one that controls pain without causing undesirable side effects. This usually requires **titration**, the gradual adjustment of drug dosage (usually by increasing the dose) until optimum pain relief without excessive sedation is achieved. Dosage recommendations are only safe initial dosages (see Tables 7-5 and 7-6), not optimum dosages.

Several drugs, known as coanalgesics or adjuvant analgesics, may be used alone or with opioids to control pain symptoms and opioid side effects. Drugs frequently used to relieve anxiety, cause sedation, and provide amnesia are diazepam (Valium) and midazolam (Versed); however, these drugs are not analgesics and should be used to enhance the effects of analgesics, not as a substitute for analgesics. Other adjuvants include tricyclic antidepressants (e.g., amitriptyline, imipramine) and antiepileptics (e.g., gabapentin, carbamazepine, clonazepam) for neuropathic pain (see Table 7-6), stool softeners and laxatives for constipation, antiemetics for nausea and vomiting, diphenhydramine for itching, steroids for inflammation and bone pain, and dextroamphetamine and caffeine for possible increased pain and sedation (Table 7-7) (McCaffery and Pasero, 1999).

The use of placebos to determine whether the patient is having pain is unjustified and unethical; a positive response to a placebo, such as a saline injection, is common in patients who have a documented organic basis for pain. Therefore the deceptive use of placebos does not provide useful information about the presence or severity of pain. The use of placebos can cause side effects similar to those of opioids, can destroy the patient's trust in the health care staff, and raises serious ethical and legal questions. The American Society of Pain Management Nursing has issued a position statement against the use of placebos to treat pain (McCaffery and Pasero, 1999).

TABLE 7-7 MANAGEMENT OF OPIOID SIDE EFFECTS

SIDE EFFECT	ADJUVANT DRUGS	NONPHARMACOLOGIC TECHNIQUES
Constipation	**Senna and docusate sodium** *Tablet:* 2-6 yr: Start with $\frac{1}{2}$ tablet once a day; maximum: 1 tablet twice a day 6-12 yr: Start with 1 tablet once a day; maximum: 2 tablets twice a day >12 yr: Start with 2 tablets once a day; maximum: 4 tablets twice a day *Liquid:* 1 mo–1 yr: 1.25-5 ml q hs 1-5 yr: 2.5-5 ml q hs 5-15 yr: 5-10 ml q hs >15 yr: 10-25 ml q hs **Casanthranol and docusate sodium** *Liquid:* 5-15 ml q hs *Capsules:* 1 cap PO q hs **Bisacodyl:** PO or PR 3-12 yr: 5 mg/dose/day >12 yr: 10-15 mg/dose/day **Lactulose** 7.5 ml/day after breakfast Adult: 15-30 ml/day PO **Mineral oil:** 1-2 tsp/day PO **Magnesium citrate** <6 yr: 2-4 ml/kg PO once 6-12 yr: 100-150 ml PO once >12 yr: 150-300 ml PO once **Milk of Magnesia** <2 yr: 0.5 ml/kg/dose PO once 2-5 yr: 5-15 ml/day PO 6-12 yr: 15-30 ml PO once >12 yr: 30-60 ml PO once	Increase water intake Prune juice, bran cereal, vegetables Exercise
Sedation	**Caffeine:** single dose of 1-1.5 mg PO **Dextroamphetamine:** 2.5-5 mg PO in AM and early afternoon **Methylphenidate:** 2.5-5 mg PO in AM and early afternoon Consider opioid switch if sedation persists	Caffeinated drinks (e.g., Mountain Dew, cola drinks)
Nausea, vomiting	**Promethazine:** 0.5 mg/kg q 4-6 hr; maximum: 25 mg/dose **Ondansetron:** 0.1-0.15 mg/kg IV or PO q 4 hr; maximum: 8 mg/dose **Granisetron:** 10-40 mcg/kg q 2-4 hr; maximum: 1 mg/dose **Droperidol:** 0.05-0.06 mg/kg IV q 4-6 hr; can be very sedating	Imagery, relaxation Deep, slow breathing
Pruritus	**Diphenhydramine:** 1 mg/kg IV or PO q 4-6 hr prn; max: 25 mg/dose **Hydroxyzine:** 0.6 mg/kg/dose PO q 6 hr; maximum: 50 mg/dose **Naloxone:** 0.5 mcg/kg q 2 min until pruritus improves (diluted in solution of 0.1 mg of naloxone per 10 ml of saline) **Butorphanol:** 0.3-0.5 mg/kg IV (use cautiously in opioid-tolerant children; may cause withdrawal symptoms); maximum: 2 mg/dose because mixed agonist-antagonist	Oatmeal baths, good hygiene Exclude other causes of itching Change opioids
Respiratory depression: mild to moderate	Hold dose of opioid Reduce subsequent doses by 25%	Arouse gently, give oxygen, encourage to deep breathe

Continued

TABLE 7-7	MANAGEMENT OF OPIOID SIDE EFFECTS—cont'd	
SIDE EFFECT	**ADJUVANT DRUGS**	**NONPHARMACOLOGIC TECHNIQUES**
Respiratory depression: severe	**Naloxone** *During disease pain management:* 0.5 mcg/kg in 2 min increments until breathing improves (American Pain Society, 1999; McCaffery and Pasero, 1999) Reduce opioid dose if possible Consider opioid switch *During sedation for procedures:* 5-10 mcg/kg until breathing improves (Yaster, Krance, Kaplan, et al, 1997) Reduce opioid dose if possible Consider opioid switch	Oxygen, bag and mask if indicated
Dysphoria, confusion, hallucinations	Evaluate medications, eliminate adjuvant medications with central nervous system effects as symptoms allow Consider opioid switch if possible **Haloperidol** (Haldol): 0.05-0.15 mg/kg/day divided in 2-3 doses; maximum: 2-4 mg/day	Rule out other physiologic causes
Urinary retention	Evaluate medications, eliminate adjuvant medications with anticholinergic effects (e.g., antihistamines, tricyclic antidepressants) Occurs more frequently with spinal analgesia than with systemic opioid use **Oxybutynin** 1 yr: 1 mg tid 1-2 yr: 2 mg tid 2-3 yr: 3 mg tid 4-5 yr: 4 mg tid >5 yr: 5 mg tid	Rule out other physiologic causes In/out or indwelling urinary catheter

hs, At bedtime; *IV,* intravenous; *PO,* by mouth; *PR,* by rectum; *prn,* as needed; *q,* every; *tid,* three times a day.

Children (except infants younger than about 3 to 6 months) metabolize drugs more rapidly than adults. Younger children may require higher doses of opioids to achieve the same analgesic effect. Therefore the therapeutic effect and duration of analgesia vary. Children's dosages are usually calculated according to body weight, except in children with a weight greater than 50 kg (110 lb), where the weight formula may exceed the average adult dose. In this case the adult dose is used.

A reasonable starting dose of opioid for infants under 6 months who are not mechanically ventilated is one fourth to one third of the recommended starting dose for older children. The infant is monitored closely for signs of pain relief and respiratory depression. The dose is titrated to effect. Because tolerance can develop rapidly, large doses may be needed for continued severe pain (McCaffery and Pasero, 1999). If pain relief is inadequate, the initial dose is increased (usually by 25% to 50% if pain is moderate, or by 50% to 100% if pain is severe) to provide greater analgesic effectiveness. Decreasing the interval between doses may also provide more continuous pain relief. A major difference between opioids and nonopioids is that nonopioids have a ceiling effect, which means that doses higher than the recommended dose will not produce greater pain relief. Opioids do not have a ceiling effect other than that imposed by side effects; therefore larger dosages can be safely given for increasing severity of pain.

Parenteral and oral dosages of opioids are not the same. Because of the first-pass effect, an oral opioid is rapidly absorbed from the gastrointestinal tract and is partially metabolized in the liver before reaching the central circulation. Therefore oral dosages must be larger to compensate for the partial loss of analgesic potency to achieve equianalgesia (equal analgesic effect). Conversion factors (Table 7-8) for selected opioids must

be used when a change is made from IV (preferred) or IM to oral. Immediate conversion from IM or IV to the suggested equianalgesic oral dose may result in a substantial error. For example, the dose may be significantly more or less than what the child requires. Small changes ensure small errors. Several routes of analgesic administration can be used (Box 7-3), and the most effective and least traumatic route of administration should be selected.

Preventive pain control is best provided through continuous IV infusion rather than intermittent boluses. If intermittent boluses are given, make certain the intervals between doses do not exceed the drug's expected duration of effectiveness. For extended pain control with fewer administration times, drugs that provide longer duration of action (e.g., some NSAIDs, time-released morphine or oxycodone, methadone, levorphanol) can be used.

Continuous analgesia is not always appropriate, since not all pain is continuous. Frequently, temporary pain control or conscious sedation is needed to provide analgesia before a scheduled procedure. When pain can be predicted, the drug's peak effect should be timed to coincide with the painful event. For example, with opioids the peak effect is approximately a half hour for the IV route; with nonopioids the peak effect occurs about 2 hours after oral administration. For rapid onset and peak of action, opioids that quickly penetrate the blood-brain barrier (e.g., IV fentanyl) provide excellent pain control.

Patient-Controlled Analgesia

A significant advance in the administration of IV, epidural, or subcutaneous analgesics is the use of patient-controlled analgesia (PCA). As the name implies, the patient controls the

TABLE 7-8	EQUIANALGESIA OF SELECTED ANALGESICS		
DRUG*		**EQUAL TO ORAL MORPHINE (mg)**	**EQUAL TO INTRAMUSCULAR OR INTRAVENOUS MORPHINE (mg)**
Hydromorphone (Dilaudid), 1 mg		4	1.3
Codeine, 30 mg		4.5	1.5
Meperidine (Demerol), 50 mg		4.8	1.6
Codeine, 30 mg; acetaminophen, 300 mg (Tylenol No. 3)		7.2	2.4
Oxycodone, 5 mg; aspirin, 325 mg (Percodan)		7.2	2.4
Oxycodone, 5 mg; aspirin, 325 mg (Percodan)		7.2	2.4
Hydrocodone, 5 mg; acetaminophen, 500 mg (Vicodin, Lortab)		9	3
Oxycodone, 5 mg; acetaminophen, 500 mg (Tylox)		9	3
Methadone (Dolophine), 10 mg		15	7.5
Acetaminophen, 325 mg (Tylenol)		2.7	0.9
Aspirin, 325 mg		2.7	0.9
Acetaminophen, 500 mg (Tylenol Extra Strength)		4	1.3
Codeine, 60 mg; acetaminophen, 300 mg (Tylenol No. 4)		11.7	3.9
Fentanyl, transdermal patch (Duragesic) (based on 25 mcg/hr patch applied q 3 days = 50 mg oral morphine q 24 hr or divided into 6 doses = 8.3 mg) or use:		8.3	2.77

Recommended Initial Duragesic Dose Based on Daily Oral Morphine Dose†

ORAL 24-HOUR MORPHINE (mg/day)	**DURAGESIC DOSE (mg/hr)**
45-134	25
135-224	50
225-314	75
315-404	100
405-494	125
495-584	150
585-674	175
675-764	200
765-854	225
855-944	250
945-1034	275
1035-1124	300

Courtesy Betty R. Ferrell, PhD FAAN, 1999. Used with permission.
NOTE: When converting to oral oxycodone from oral morphine, an appropriate conservative estimate is 15-20 mg of oxycodone per 30 mg of morphine; however, when converting to oral morphine from oral oxycodone, an appropriate conservative estimate is 30 mg of morphine per 30 mg of oxycodone (McCaffery M, Pasero C: *Pain: a clinical manual,* ed. 2, St. Louis, 1999, Mosby).
*Oral medication with exception of fentanyl.
†Data from Duragesic package insert, Janssen Pharmaceutical Products, Titusville, NJ, 2001.

amount and frequency of the analgesic, which is typically delivered through a special infusion device. Children who are physically able to "push a button" (i.e., 5 to 6 years of age) and who can understand the concept of pushing a button to obtain pain relief can use PCA (Maxwell and Yaster, 2000). Although it is controversial, parents and nurses have used the IV PCA system for the child. Nurses can efficiently use the infusion device on a child of any age to administer analgesics to avoid signing for and preparing opioid injections every time one is needed (Fig. 7-7). When PCA is used as "nurse- or parent-controlled" analgesia, the concept of patient control is negated, and the inherent safety of PCA needs to be monitored. Research has reported safe and effective analgesia in children when the patient, parent, or nurse controlled the PCA (Algren, Gursoy, Johnson, et al, 1998; Maxwell and Yaster, 2000).

PCA infusion devices typically allow for three methods or modes of drug administration to be used alone or in combination:

1. Patient-administered boluses that can be infused only according to the preset amount and lockout interval (time between doses). More frequent attempts at self-administration may mean the patient needs the dose and time adjusted for better pain control.
2. Nurse-administered boluses that are typically used to give an initial loading dose to increase blood levels rapidly and to relieve breakthrough pain (pain not relieved with the usual programmed dose).
3. Continuous basal rate infusion that delivers a constant amount of analgesic and prevents pain from returning during those times, such as sleep, when the patient cannot control the infusion.

As with any type of analgesic management plan, continued assessment of the child's pain relief is essential for the greatest benefit from PCA. Typical uses of PCA are for controlling pain from surgery, sickle cell crisis, trauma, and cancer. Morphine is the drug of choice for PCA and usually comes in

BOX 7-3   ROUTES AND METHODS OF ANALGESIC DRUG ADMINISTRATION

Oral

Oral route preferred because of convenience, cost, and relatively steady blood levels

Higher dosages of oral form of opioids required for equivalent parenteral analgesia

Peak drug effect occurring after 1 to 2 hours for most analgesics

Delay in onset a disadvantage when rapid control of severe or fluctuating pain is desired

Sublingual, Buccal, or Transmucosal

Tablet or liquid placed between cheek and gum (buccal) or under tongue (sublingual)

Highly desirable because more rapid onset than oral route

- Produces less first-pass effect through liver than oral route, which normally reduces analgesia from oral opioids (unless sublingual or buccal form is swallowed, which occurs often in children)

Few drugs commercially available in this form

Many drugs can be compounded into sublingual troche or lozenge.*

- Actiq—Oral transmucosal fentanyl citrate in hard confection base on a plastic holder; indicated only for management of breakthrough cancer pain in patients with malignancies who are already receiving and are tolerant to opioid therapy, but can be used for preoperative or preprocedural sedation and analgesia

Intravenous (IV) (Bolus)

Preferred for rapid control of severe pain

Provides most rapid onset of effect, usually in about 5 minutes

Advantage for acute pain, procedural pain, and breakthrough pain

Needs to be repeated hourly for continuous pain control

Drugs with short half-life (morphine, fentanyl, hydromorphone) preferable to avoid toxic accumulation of drug

IV (Continuous)

Preferred over bolus and intramuscular injection for maintaining control of pain

Provides steady blood levels

Easy to titrate dosage

Subcutaneous (SC) (Continuous)

Used when oral and IV routes not available

Provides equivalent blood levels to continuous IV infusion

Suggested initial bolus dose to equal 2-hour IV dose; total 24-hour dose usually requires concentrated opioid solution to minimize infused volume; use smallest gauge needle that accommodates infusion rate

Patient-Controlled Analgesia (PCA)

Generally refers to self-administration of drugs, regardless of route

Typically uses programmable infusion pump (IV, epidural, SC) that permits self-administration of boluses of medication at preset dose and time interval (lockout interval is time between doses)

PCA bolus administration often combined with initial bolus and continuous (basal or background) infusion of opioid

Optimum lockout interval not known but must be at least as long as time needed for onset of drug

- Should effectively control pain during movement or procedures
- Longer lockout provides larger dose

Family-Controlled Analgesia

One family member (usually a parent) or other caregiver designated as child's primary pain manager with responsibility for pressing PCA button

Guidelines for selecting a primary pain manager for family-controlled analgesia:

- Spends a significant amount of time with the patient
- Is willing to assume responsibility of being primary pain manager
- Is willing to accept and respect patient's reports of pain (if able to provide) as best indicator of how much pain the patient is experiencing; knows how to use and interpret a pain rating scale
- Understands the purpose and goals of patient's pain management plan

- Understands concept of maintaining a steady analgesic blood level
- Recognizes signs of pain and side effects and adverse reactions to opioid

Nurse-Activated Analgesia

Child's primary nurse designated as primary pain manager and is only person who presses PCA button during that nurse's shift

Guidelines for selecting primary pain manager for family-controlled analgesia also applicable to nurse-activated analgesia

May be used in addition to basal rate to treat breakthrough pain with bolus doses; patient assessed every 30 minutes for need for bolus dose

May be used without a basal rate as a means of maintaining analgesia with around-the-clock bolus doses

Intramuscular

NOTE: Not recommended for pain control; not current standard of care

Painful administration (hated by children)

Tissue and nerve damage caused by some drugs

Wide fluctuation in absorption of drug from muscle

Faster absorption from deltoid than from gluteal sites

Shorter duration and more expensive than oral drugs

Time consuming for staff and unnecessary delay for child

Intranasal

Available commercially as butorphanol (Stadol NS); approved for those older than 18 years of age

Should not be used in patient receiving morphinelike drugs because butorphanol is partial antagonist that will reduce analgesia and may cause withdrawal

Intradermal

Used primarily for skin anesthesia (e.g., before lumbar puncture, bone marrow aspiration, arterial puncture, skin biopsy)

Local anesthetics (e.g., lidocaine) cause stinging, burning sensation

Duration of stinging dependent on type of "caine" used

To avoid stinging sensation associated with lidocaine:

- Buffer the solution by adding 1 part sodium bicarbonate (1 mEq/ml) to 9 to 10 parts 1% or 2% lidocaine with or without epinephrine (see Evidence-Based Practice box, p. 210)

Normal saline with preservative, benzyl alcohol, anesthetizes venipuncture site

Same dose used as for buffered lidocaine (see Evidence-Based Practice box, p. 210)

Topical or Transdermal

EMLA (eutectic mixture of local anesthetics [lidocaine and prilocaine]) cream and anesthetic disk or LMX4 (4% lidocaine cream)

- Eliminates or reduces pain from most procedures involving skin puncture
- Must be placed on intact skin over puncture site and covered by occlusive dressing or applied as anesthetic disc for 1 hour or more before procedure (see Evidence-Based Practice box, p. 207)

Lidocaine-tetracaine (Synera, S-Caine)

- Apply for 20 to 30 minutes
- Do not apply to broken skin

LAT (lidocaine-adrenaline-tetracaine), tetracaine-phenylephrine (tetraphen)

- Provides skin anesthesia about 15 minutes after application on nonintact skin
- Gel (preferable) or liquid placed on wounds for suturing
- Adrenaline not for use on end arterioles (fingers, toes, tip of nose, penis, earlobes) because of vasoconstriction

Transdermal fentanyl (Duragesic)

- Available as patch for continuous pain control
- Safety and efficacy not established in children younger than 12 years of age
- Not appropriate for initial relief of acute pain because of long interval to peak effect (12 to 24 hours); for rapid onset of pain relief, give an immediate-release opioid
- Orders for "rescue doses" of an immediate-release opioid recommended for breakthrough pain, a flare of severe pain that breaks through the medication being administered at regular intervals for persistent pain

BOX 7-3   ROUTES AND METHODS OF ANALGESIC DRUG ADMINISTRATION—cont'd

Topical or Transdermal—cont'd

- Has duration of up to 72 hours for prolonged pain relief
- If respiratory depression occurs, possible need for several doses of naloxone

Vapocoolant

- Use of prescription spray coolant, such as Fluori-Methane or ethyl chloride (Pain-Ease); applied to the skin for 10 to 15 seconds immediately before the needle puncture; anesthesia lasts about 15 seconds
- Some children dislike cold; may be more comfortable to spray coolant on a cotton ball and then apply this to the skin
- Application of ice to the skin for 30 seconds found to be ineffective

Rectal

Alternative to oral or parenteral routes

Variable absorption rate

Generally disliked by children

Many drugs able to be compounded into rectal suppositories*

Regional Nerve Block

Use of long-acting local anesthetic (bupivacaine or ropivacaine) injected into nerves to block pain at site

Provides prolonged analgesia postoperatively, such as after inguinal herniorrhaphy

May be used to provide local anesthesia for surgery, such as dorsal penile nerve block for circumcision or for reduction of fractures

Inhalation

Use of anesthetics, such as nitrous oxide, to produce partial or complete analgesia for painful procedures

Side effects (e.g., headache) possible from occupational exposure to high levels of nitrous oxide

Epidural or Intrathecal

Involves catheter placed into epidural, caudal, or intrathecal space for continuous infusion or single or intermittent administration of opioid with or without a long-acting local anesthetic (e.g., bupivacaine, ropivacaine)

Analgesia primarily from drug's direct effect on opioid receptors in spinal cord

Respiratory depression rare but may have slow and delayed onset; can be prevented by checking level of sedation and respiratory rate and depth hourly for initial 24 hours and decreasing dose when excessive sedation is detected

Nausea, itching, and urinary retention common dose-related side effects from the epidural opioid

Mild hypotension, urinary retention, and temporary motor or sensory deficits common unwanted effects of epidural local anesthetic

Catheter for urinary retention inserted during surgery to decrease trauma to child; if inserted when child is awake, anesthetize urethra with lidocaine

Data primarily from American Pain Society: *Principles of analgesic use in the treatment of acute pain and chronic cancer pain*, ed 4, Glenview, Ill, 1999, The Society; and McCaffery M, Pasero C: *Pain: a clinical manual*, ed 2, St Louis, 1999, Mosby.

*For further information about compounding drugs in troche or suppository form, contact Professional Compounding Centers of America (PCCA), 9901 S. Wilcrest Drive, Houston, TX 77009; 800-331-2498; **www.pccarx.com**.

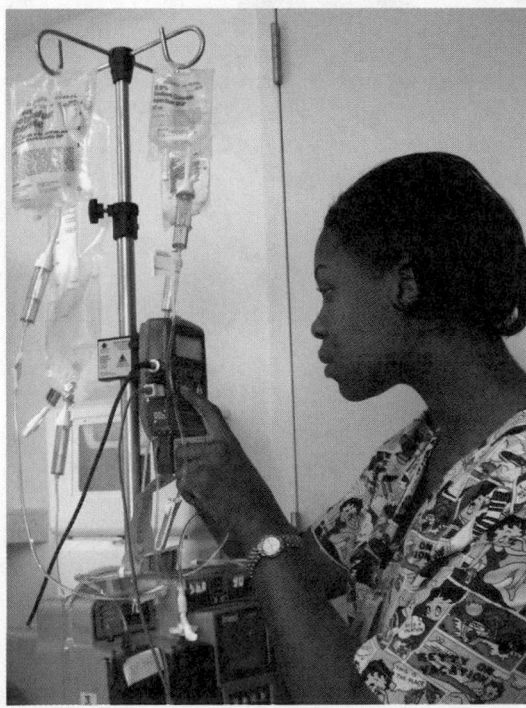

Fig. 7-7 Nurse programming a patient-controlled analgesia pump to administer analgesia.

a concentration of 1 mg/ml (Table 7-9). Other options are hydromorphone (0.2 mg/ml) and fentanyl (0.01 mg/ml).

Hydromorphone is often used when patients are not able to tolerate side effects such as pruritus and nausea from the morphine PCA (Algren, Gursoy, Johnson, et al, 1998; Maxwell and

Yaster, 2000). Some physicians may still prescribe meperidine. However, meperidine is the least potent and shortest-acting of the synthetic opioids and the least effective in providing analgesia for severe pain. More important, it may increase the risk of seizures when administered chronically because of the excitatory effects on the nervous system of its metabolite, normeperidine. Some authors (Nadvi, Sarnaik, and Ravindranath, 1999) have argued that the incidence of meperidine-associated seizures is extremely small (0.4% of patients; 0.06% of admissions) and the risk of seizures should not dissuade clinicians from using this drug. However, the American Pain Society recommends that meperidine be reserved for brief treatment courses for patients who have reported and demonstrated its effectiveness, or who have allergies or uncorrectable intolerances to other opioids. Meperidine should not be used for longer than 48 hours or in dosages greater than 600 mg/24 hr (Max, Payne, Edwards, et al, 1999).

Epidural Analgesia

Epidural analgesia is used to manage pain in selected cases. Although an epidural catheter can be inserted at any vertebral level, it is usually placed into the epidural space of the spinal column at the lumbar or caudal level (Fig. 7-8). The thoracic level is usually reserved for older children or adolescents who have had an upper abdominal or thoracic procedure, such as a lung transplant. An opioid (usually fentanyl, hydromorphone, or preservative-free morphine, which is often combined with a long-acting local anesthetic such as bupivacaine or ropivacaine) is instilled via single or intermittent bolus, continuous infusion, or patient-controlled epidural analgesia. Analgesia results from the drug's effect on opiate receptors in the dorsal horn of the

TABLE 7-9	SUGGESTED INTRAVENOUS PATIENT-CONTROLLED ANALGESIA OPIOID INFUSION ORDERS			
DRUG	BASAL RATE (mcg/kg/hr)	BOLUS RATE (mcg/kg/dose)	LOCKOUT PERIOD (min)	MAXIMUM DOSE (mg/kg/hr)
Morphine	10-30	10-30	6-10	0.1-0.15
Hydromorphone	3-5	6-10	0.015-0.02	3-5
Fentanyl	0.5-1.00	0.5-1.0	6-10	0.002-0.004

From Yaster M, Krance EJ, Kaplan RF, et al: *Pediatric pain management and sedation handbook,* St. Louis, 1997, Mosby.

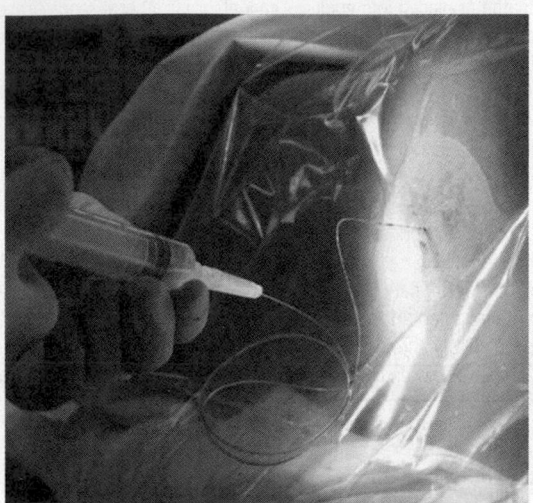

Fig. 7-8 Epidural analgesia catheter placement.

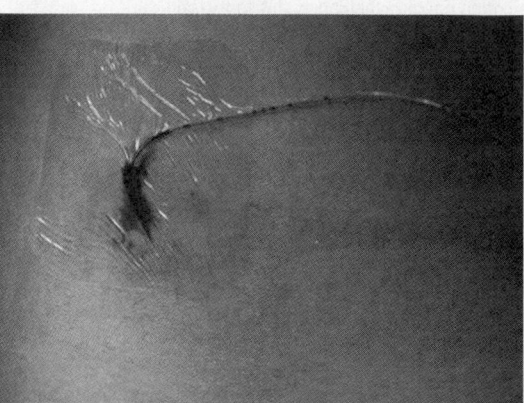

Fig. 7-9 Dressing covering site of epidural catheter.

spinal cord, rather than the brain. As a result, respiratory depression is rare, but if it occurs, it develops slowly, typically 6 to 8 hours after administration (Golianu, Krane, Galloway, et al, 2000). Properly securing the epidural catheter with an occlusive dressing decreases the possibility of soiling or inadvertently displacing the catheter (Fig. 7-9). Careful monitoring of sedation level and respiratory status is critical to prevent opioid-induced respiratory depression. Assessment of pain and the skin condition around the catheter site are important aspects of nursing care (Golianu, Krane, Galloway, et al, 2000).

Transmucosal and Transdermal Analgesia

Oral transmucosal fentanyl (Oralet) provides nontraumatic preoperative and preprocedural analgesia and sedation (Golianu, Krane, Galloway, et al, 2000). Fentanyl is also available as a transdermal patch (Duragesic). Although contraindicated for acute pain management, it may be used for older children and adolescents who have cancer pain or sickle cell pain or for patients who are opioid tolerant.

One of the most significant improvements in the ability to provide atraumatic care to children is the anesthetic cream LMX4 (a 4% liposomal lidocaine cream) or EMLA (a eutectic mixture of local anesthetics) (Abdelkefi, Abdennebi, Mellouli, et al, 2004; Choi, Irwin, Hui, et al, 2003; Egekvist and Bjerring, 2000; Gad, Olsen, Lysgaard, et al, 2005; Rogers and Ostrow, 2004; Santiago, Abad, Fernandez, et al, 2000; Uziel, Berkovitch, Gazarian, et al, 2003). The eutectic mixture (lidocaine 2.5% and prilocaine 2.5%), whose melting point is lower than that of the two anesthetics alone, permits effective concentrations of the

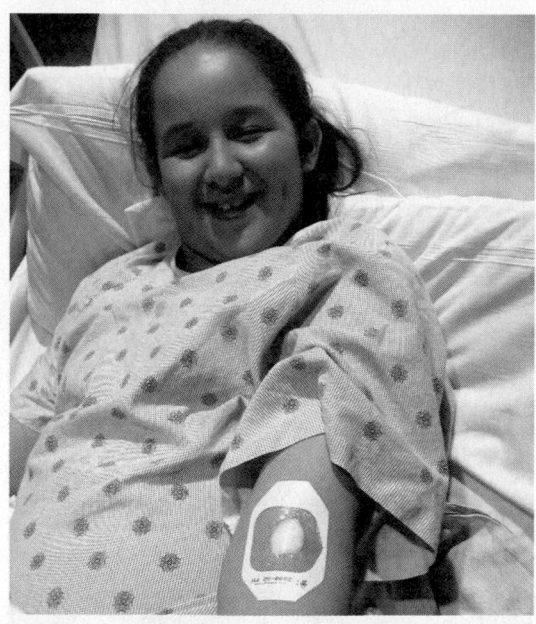

Fig. 7-10 LMX is an effective analgesic before intravenous insertion or blood draw.

drug to penetrate intact skin (see Evidence-Based Practice box, p. 207, and Fig. 7-10). Transdermal patches such as Synera are effective methods to administer topical analgesia before painful procedures. A recent review of the evidence comparing these patches to EMLA is found in the Evidence-Based Practice box (p. 208).

In some situations there is not enough time for topical preparations like LMX or EMLA to take effect, and refrigerant sprays such as ethyl chloride and fluorimethane can be used (Reis and Holubkov, 1997). When sprayed on the skin, these

EVIDENCE-BASED PRACTICE

EMLA Versus LMX for Pain Reduction of Peripheral Intravenous Access in Children

ASK THE QUESTION

In children is EMLA (lidocaine and prilocaine) a better anesthetic cream than LMX (lidocaine) in reducing pain from peripheral intravenous (PIV) access?

SEARCH FOR THE EVIDENCE

Search strategies
Search selection criteria included English language publications within past 5 years, research-based articles on children undergoing PIV access.

Databases used
PubMed, Cochrane Collaboration, MD Consult, Joanna Briggs Institute, National Guideline Clearinghouse (AHQR), TRIP Database Plus, PedsCCM, BestBETs

CRITICALLY ANALYZE THE EVIDENCE

GRADE criteria: Evidence quality moderate; recommendation strong (Guyatt, Oxman, Vist, et al, 2008)

Three studies were found that evaluated the two anesthetics for PIV access. All three were randomized control trials (level 1). All three studies found that a 30-minute application of LMX is as effective as a 60-minute application of EMLA for producing topical anesthesia for PIV access in children. None of the studies found PIV access difficulty was influenced by EMLA or LMX.

1. The two local anesthetics (EMLA versus LMX) were compared in a group of 120 children 5 to 17 years of age scheduled for venipuncture in two sites. No differences were found in patients' perception of pain or parental and nurse observation scores (Eichenfield, Funk, Fallon-Friedlander, et al, 2002).
2. EMLA and LMX were compared in a group of 30 healthy children 7 to 13 years of age. Self-report measures showed no difference in reported pain when examining the two anesthetics (Kleiber, Sorenson, Whiteside, et al, 2002).
3. EMLA and LMX were compared in 60 children, 8 to 17 years of age, randomized to either LMX or EMLA. No differences were found between the groups. LMX caused less blanching (Koh, Harrison, Myers, et al, 2004).

APPLY THE EVIDENCE: NURSING IMPLICATIONS

LMX offers several advantages: rapid onset of action, lower cost, and no risk of methemoglobinemia in children of all ages. Apply LMX for 30 minutes before establishing PIV access.

Nursing implications include the following:
- Age—More than 34 weeks of gestation
- Time of onset—30 minutes
- Duration—1 hour
- Removal—No more than 2 hours after application
- Multiple sites—Yes
- Use with abraded skin—No
- Impact on PIV access difficulty—None
- Do not use within 2 hours before vesicants
- Maximum area/dose—For children weighing less than 20 kg (44 lb), apply to area less than 100 cm^2
- Cover with occlusive dressing

References

Eichenfield LF, Funk A, Fallon-Friedlander S, et al: A clinical study to evaluate the efficacy of Ela-Max as compared with eutectic mixture of local anesthetics cream for pain reduction of venipuncture in children, *Pediatrics* 109(6):1092-1099, 2002.

Guyatt GH, Oxman AD, Vist GE, et al: GRADE: an emerging consensus on rating quality of evidence and strength of recommendations, *BMJ* 336:924-926, 2008.

Kleiber C, Sorenson M, Whiteside K, et al: Topical anesthetics for intravenous insertion in children: a randomized equivalency study, *Pediatrics* 110:758-761, 2002.

Koh JL, Harrison D, Myers R, et al: A randomized, double-blind comparison study of EMLA and ELA-Max for topical anesthesia in children undergoing intravenous insertion, *Pediatr Anesthesiol* 14:977-982, 2004.

---

sprays vaporize, rapidly cool the area, and provide superficial anesthesia. Hospital formularies may have other products with lidocaine, prilocaine, or amethocaine topical preparations that require less time for application.

The intradermal route is sometimes used to inject a local anesthetic, typically lidocaine, into the skin to reduce the pain from a lumbar puncture, bone marrow aspiration, or venous or arterial access. One problem with the use of lidocaine is the stinging and burning that initially occur. However, the use of buffered lidocaine with sodium bicarbonate (see Evidence-Based Practice box, p. 210) reduces the stinging sensation (Wong and Pasero, 1997a, 1997b). Warming the lidocaine to 37° C (98.6° F) may accomplish the same effect (McCaffery and Pasero, 1999). A needle-free injection system also be can used to provide intradermal anesthesia (see Evidence-Based Practice box, p. 209).

Timing of Analgesia

The right timing for administering analgesics depends on the type of pain. For continuous pain control, such as for postoperative or cancer pain, a preventive schedule of medication around the clock (ATC) is effective. The ATC schedule avoids the low plasma concentrations that permit breakthrough pain. If analgesics are administered only when pain returns (a typical use of the prn, or "as needed," order), pain relief may take several hours. This may require higher doses, leading to a cycle of undermedication of pain alternating with periods of overmedication and drug toxicity. This cycle of erratic pain control also promotes "clock watching," which may be erroneously equated with addiction. Nurses can effectively use prn orders by giving the drug at regular intervals, since "as needed" should be interpreted as "as needed to prevent pain," not "as little as possible."

EVIDENCE-BASED PRACTICE   *Terri L. Brown*

Analgesic Patches: Synera to Decrease Pain During Painful Procedures

ASK THE QUESTION

Do topical analgesic patches (e.g., lidocaine-tetracaine [Synera, S-Caine]) offer additional advantages (less time, ease of use, lower cost, higher effectiveness, decreased anxiety) in relieving pain during peripheral intravenous (PIV) cannulation in children compared with LMX (lidocaine) cream and buffered lidocaine via injection?

SEARCH FOR THE EVIDENCE

Search strategies

English research-based publications on lidocaine-tetracaine patches for venipuncture without time limitation were included. Exclusions included epidural use, dermatologic procedures, and S-Caine Peel

Databases used

Cochrane Collaboration Database, Joanna Briggs Institute, National Guideline Clearinghouse (AHRQ), PubMed, SUMSearch, CINAHL, Scopus, Micromedex, UpToDate, BestBETs, manufacturer's websites (Endo Pharmaceuticals, ZARS Pharma)

CRITICALLY ANALYZE THE EVIDENCE

GRADE criteria: Evidence quality strong; recommendation strong (Guyatt, Oxman, Vist, et al, 2008)

Two randomized controlled trials (RCTs) in children and two RCTs in adults have demonstrated that Synera is effective in inducing local anesthesia before PIV access. One RCT in adults concluded that Synera was as effective as EMLA in a much shorter timeframe with fewer adverse reactions (Sawyer, Febbraro, Masud, et al, 2009). The manufacturer reports 23 additional clinical trials (including one demonstrating safety in infants as young as 4 months), but these were not found in the search of published literature.

Pediatric studies

Synera reduced PIV cannulation pain and did not alter the success rate in a double-blind, placebo-controlled RCT of 45 children 3 to 17 years old in a suburban emergency center (Singer, Taira, Chisena, et al, 2008). Synera or a placebo patch was placed over the antecubital or hand vein. The median self-reported pain using a visual analog scale (VAS) or Wong-Baker faces scale in the Synera group was significantly lower than in the placebo group ($p = 0.04$). PIV cannulation success on the first attempt was similar in both groups (90% versus 85%).

In a double-blind, placebo-controlled RCT, a 20-minute application of the S-Caine Patch was effective in lessening pain in 64 children scheduled for vascular access at two centers (Sethna, Verghese, Hannallah, et al, 2005). Synera was developed under the name of S-Caine Patch and renamed at time of U.S. Food and Drug Administration approval. The pain patch significantly reduced pain compared with placebo (median Oucher scores of 0 versus 60; $p < 0.001$); 59% of children in the pain patch group reported no pain compared with 20% in the placebo group. Investigator estimations of pain and independent observer ratings also favored the S-Caine Patch ($p < 0.001$). Mild skin erythema (<38%) and edema (<2%) occurred with similar frequencies between the groups.

Cost-effectiveness

In a decision model on cost-effectiveness of topical and inhalation analgesics during PIV cannulation in the pediatric emergency setting, Pershad, Steinberg, and Waters (2008) concluded that the lidocaine-tetracaine (S-Caine) patch ranked fifth out of eight agents. Costs included the cost of the agent plus costs associated with time in the emergency department. Additional variables considered were peak onset time, PIV cannulation success rate, and mean reduction in VAS scores. Seventeen RCTs involving 1287 children were included in the cost analysis. Researchers found "the needle-free jet injection of lidocaine device [J-Tip®] had the lowest incremental cost-effectiveness ratio, followed by intradermal injection of buffered lidocaine; lidocaine iontophoresis; nitrous oxide inhalation analgesia; a heated lidocaine and tetracaine patch; sonophoresis with lidocaine cream, 4%; lidocaine cream alone, 4% [LMX®]; and use of a eutectic mixture of lidocaine and prilocaine cream [EMLA®]" (Pershad, Steinberg, and Waters, 2008).

APPLY THE EVIDENCE: NURSING IMPLICATIONS

- Synera use during PIV cannulation in children 3 years and older decreases pain.
- Do not use in children with a sensitivity to lidocaine, tetracaine, para-aminobenzoic acid (PABA), or amide or ester-type anesthetics. Use with caution in patients with hepatic impairment or receiving class I antiarrhythmic drugs (such as tocainide and mexiletine). Do not apply to broken skin.
- Use immediately after opening pouch, since patch begins to heat once removed from pouch. To ensure proper heating without thermal injury, do not cut the patch or remove any layers of the patch and ensure the holes on the patch are not covered by clothing.
- Do not keep the patch on longer than 20 to 30 minutes.
- There are limited data to support the safety of applying multiple patches simultaneously or sequentially. Follow the distributor's recommendations to *not* apply multiple patches.
- As with all transdermal patches containing medication, after use fold adhesive together and dispose of used patches in a location out of the reach of children.
- Do not use in magnetic resonance imaging suite.

References

Guyatt GH, Oxman AD, Vist GE, et al: GRADE: an emerging consensus on rating quality of evidence and strength of recommendations, *BMJ* 336:924-926, 2008.

Pershad J, Steinberg S, Waters T: Cost-effectiveness analysis of anesthetic agents during peripheral intravenous cannulation in the pediatric emergency department, *Arch Pediatr Adolesc Med* 162(20):952-961, 2008.

Sawyer J, Febbraro S, Masud S, et al: Heated lidocaine/tetracaine patch (Synera™, Rapydan™) compared with lidocaine/prilocaine cream (EMLA®) for topical anaesthesia before vascular access, *Br J Anaesthesia* 102(2):210-215, 2009.

Sethna NF, Verghese ST, Hannallah RS, et al: A randomized controlled trial to evaluate S-Caine Patch™ for reducing pain associated with vascular access in children, *Anesthesiology* 102(2):403-408, 2005.

Singer AJ, Taira BR, Chisena EN, et al: Warm lidocaine/tetracaine patch versus placebo before pediatric intravenous cannulation: a randomized controlled trial, *Ann Emerg Med* 52(1):41-47, 2008.

Terri L. Brown

EVIDENCE-BASED PRACTICE

Needle-Free Injection System: J-Tip to Administer Buffered Lidocaine

ASK THE QUESTION

In pediatrics, are needle-free injection systems (e.g., J-Tip) effective and safe in relieving pain during peripheral intravenous (PIV) cannulation?

SEARCH FOR THE EVIDENCE

Search strategies

English language research-based publications on jet injectors for delivery of lidocaine during PIV cannulation without time limitation were included. Exclusions included dental products, insulin, growth factor, and medications other than lidocaine.

Databases used

Cochrane Collaboration Database, Joanna Briggs Institute, National Guideline Clearinghouse (AHRQ), PubMed, SUMSearch, CINAHL, Scopus, UpToDate, BestBETs, manufacturers' or distributors' websites (National Medical Products, Bioject, and Injex)

CRITICALLY ANALYZE THE EVIDENCE

GRADE criteria: Evidence quality strong; recommendation strong (Guyatt, Oxman, Vist, et al, 2008)

Three randomized controlled trials (RCTs) conducted in children reached favorable conclusions using J-Tip to administer buffered lidocaine for pain prevention during PIV cannulation. Two of the studies found J-Tip superior in pain prevention to LMX (lidocaine cream) or EMLA (a eutectic mix of lidocaine and prilocaine) and no different in the success rate of PIV access on first attempt.

J-Tip with 0.2 ml 1% buffered lidocaine provided greater anesthesia than a 30-minute application of LMX in children ages 8 to 15 years undergoing 22-gauge or 24-gauge PIV catheter insertion (Spanos, Booth, Koenig, et al, 2008). Seventy children in a tertiary care pediatric emergency department self-reported pain using a visual analog scale (VAS) before and after PIV cannulation. Blinded observer VAS scores from videotapes were also assigned for pain at jet injection and PIV catheter insertion. Subject VAS scores were significantly different immediately after PIV catheter insertion (17.3 for J-Tip versus 44.6 for LMX, p <0.001). Blinded reviewer VAS scores were not statistically significant (21.7 for J-Tip versus 31.9 for LMX, p = 0.23). Researchers also concluded that J-Tip did not alter the insertion site or affect the success of PIV success on first attempt and that multiple injections could be performed if necessary without causing lidocaine toxicity.

J-Tip with 0.25 ml of 1% buffered lidocaine provided greater anesthesia than application of 2.5 g of EMLA in a study of 116 children ages 7 to 19 years undergoing PIV catheter insertion (Jimenez, Bradford, Seidel, et al, 2006). The subjects' self-report median pain ratings of PIV cannulation using a 0 to 10 VAS were 0 for J-Tip and 3 for EMLA (p = 0.0001 for patients receiving EMLA ≥60 minutes before cannulation; and p = 0.0013 for those receiving EMLA <60 minutes before). Additionally, more scores were favorable for the J-Tip application (84% reported no pain at the time of injection) compared with EMLA application (61% reported pain at time of Tegaderm dressing removal; p = 0.004). No significant differences were found in the number of PIV attempts. The cost of the J-Tip ($2.10) was less than the cost of EMLA ($2.80) at the study facility. J-Tip makes a popping sound when activated, and investigators provided an additional J-Tip for each subject to see and hear how it worked before actual use, if desired.

J-Tip with 0.2 ml of 1% buffered lidocaine was no more effective than jet-delivered placebo (preservative-free normal saline) during PIV cannulation, but may provide superior analgesia compared with no local anesthetic pretreatment (Auerbach, Tunik, and Mojica, 2009). In phase I, 150 children 5 to 18 years of age received either J-Tip (0.2 ml of buffered 1% lidocaine) or jet-delivered placebo (0.2 ml of preservative-free normal saline) 60 seconds before PIV cannulation in an emergency department. Subjects reported pain on injection and on PIV cannulation using a 100-mm color analog scale. In phase II, 47 children described the effect of using the jet device. The mean needle insertion pain score for jet lidocaine, 28 mm, was similar to the mean score for placebo, 34 mm, and lower than the no device group, 52 mm. Most patients reported they would request this device for future PIV access. Providers' ratings of their ability to visualize veins and the patient cooperation were similar in all three groups.

Cost-effectiveness

In a decision model on cost-effectiveness of topical and inhalation analgesics during PIV cannulation in the pediatric emergency setting, Pershad, Steinberg, and Waters (2008) concluded that J-Tip had the lowest incremental cost-effectiveness ratio of eight agents. Costs included the cost of the agent plus costs associated with time in the emergency department. Additional variables considered were peak onset time, PIV cannulation success rate, and mean reduction in VAS scores. Additional agents included were intradermal injection of buffered lidocaine, lidocaine iontophoresis, nitrous oxide inhalation analgesia, Synera (lidocaine-tetracaine patch), Sonosite (sonophoresis with lidocaine cream), LMX, and EMLA. Seventeen RCTs involving 1287 children were included in the cost analysis.

APPLY THE EVIDENCE: NURSING IMPLICATIONS

- J-Tip with 0.2 ml of buffered lidocaine 1% decreases pain during PIV insertion.
- Wait 1 minute after administration before attempting PIV insertion.
- Do not use in children with a known hypersensitivity to lidocaine or other amide-type local anesthetics such as prilocaine, mepivacaine, bupivacaine, or etidocaine.

References

Auerbach M, Tunik M, Mojica M: A randomized, double-blind controlled study of jet lidocaine compared to jet placebo for pain relief in children undergoing needle insertion in the emergency department, *Acad Emerg Med* 16(1):1-6, 2009.

Guyatt GH, Oxman AD, Vist GE, et al: GRADE: an emerging consensus on rating quality of evidence and strength of recommendations, *BMJ* 336:924-926, 2008.

Jimenez N, Bradford H, Seidel KD, et al: A comparison of a needle-free injection system for local anesthesia versus EMLA® for intravenous catheter insertion in the pediatric patient, *Anesth Analgesia* 102(2):411-414, 2006.

Pershad J, Steinberg S, Waters T: Cost-effectiveness analysis of anesthetic agents during peripheral intravenous cannulation in the pediatric emergency department, *Arch Pediatr Adolesc Med* 162(20):952-961, 2008.

Spanos S, Booth R, Koenig H, et al: Jet injection of 1% buffered lidocaine versus topical ELA-Max for anesthesia before peripheral intravenous catheterization in children: a randomized controlled trial, *Pediatr Emerg Care* 24(8):511-515, 2008.

Angela Morgan

EVIDENCED-BASED PRACTICE

Buffered Lidocaine for Pain Reduction During Peripheral Intravenous Access in Children

ASK THE QUESTION

In children is buffered lidocaine an appropriate anesthetic for reducing pain during peripheral intravenous (PIV) access?

SEARCH FOR THE EVIDENCE

Search strategies

Search criteria included English publications within the past 5 years, research-based articles (level 3 or lower) on children undergoing PIV access. Two of the articles reviewed were more than 5 years old but were included based on the limited literature in this area.

Databases used

PubMed, Cochrane Collaboration, MD Consult, Joanna Briggs Institute, National Guideline Clearinghouse (AHQR), TRIP Database, PedsCCM, BestBETs

CRITICALLY ANALYZE THE EVIDENCE

GRADE criteria: Evidence quality strong; recommendation strong (Guyatt, Oxman, Vist, et al, 2008)

A review of the literature revealed 10 studies evaluating buffered lidocaine given before PIV access from 1991 through 1999 (Murphy, 2000). Four of the studies were specific to pediatrics. Findings from the pediatric studies support buffered lidocaine as a pain reduction measure in children before PIV access.

- A randomized trial consisting of 69 subjects ranging from 4 to 17 years of age (61% female) evaluated buffered lidocaine versus LMX (liposomal lidocaine cream) before PIV access. Results showed both interventions decreased pain and no significant differences in pain levels between the buffered lidocaine and LMX groups. The LMX group stated that the pain came with the removal of the occlusive dressing from the site (Luhmann, Hurt, Shootman, et al, 2004).
- Fein, Boardman, Stevenson, and colleagues (1998) evaluated buffered lidocaine versus no pain control measures in a group of 99 children requiring PIV access in the emergency department (ED). PIV access without buffered lidocaine was significantly more painful than PIV access with buffered lidocaine.
- Sacchetti and Carraccio (1996) evaluated subcutaneous lidocaine versus no pain control measures in 110 children under 2 years of age before PIV access in the ED. No significant differences in pain levels were found in the groups. A weakness to this trial was that it was not blinded or randomized.
- A clinical trial of 59 children requiring PIV access in the ED evaluated the use and nonuse of subcutaneous lidocaine before PIV access. PIV access without lidocaine was significantly more painful than PIV access with lidocaine regardless of catheter size. Trial weaknesses included a small sample size with wide confidence levels and no randomization (Klein, Shugerman, Leigh-Taylor, et al, 1995).

APPLY THE EVIDENCE: NURSING IMPLICATIONS

Buffered lidocaine

- Age—More than 2 years
- Time of onset—Immediate
- Duration—1 hour
- Multiple sites—Yes
- Use with abraded skin—No
- Impact on PIV access difficulty—Possibility of some vasoconstriction
- Do not use within 2 hours before vesicants
- Dose—0.1 to 0.5 ml buffered 1% lidocaine, to a maximum of 0.45 ml/kg/dose; can repeat dose after 2 hours
- Consideration—An "extra stick" and ineffective buffered lidocaine administration may result in pain during both local administration and PIV access. Expertise in administering buffered lidocaine is an important factor related to its effectiveness.

References

Fein JA, Boardman CR, Stevenson S, et al: Saline with benzyl alcohol as intradermal anesthesia for intravenous line placement in children, *Pediatr Emerg Care* 14(2):119-122, 1998.

Guyatt GH, Oxman AD, Vist GE, et al: GRADE: an emerging consensus on rating quality of evidence and strength of recommendations, *BMJ* 336:924-926, 2008.

Klein EJ, Shugerman RP, Leigh-Taylor K, et al: Buffered lidocaine: analgesia for intravenous line placement in children, *Pediatrics* 95(5):709-712, 1995.

Luhmann J, Hurt S, Shootman M, et al: A comparison of buffered lidocaine versus ELA-Max before peripheral intravenous catheter insertions in children, *Pediatrics* 113(3 Pt 1):217-220, 2004.

Murphy R: *Prior injection of local anaesthetic and the pain and success of intravenous cannulation,* 2000, available at www.bestbets.org (accessed March 2005).

Sacchetti AD, Carraccio C: Subcutaneous lidocaine does not affect the success rate of intravenous access in children less than 24 months of age, *Acad Emerg Med* 3(11):1016-1019, 1996.

Monitoring Side Effects

Both NSAIDs and opioids have side effects, although the major concern is with those from opioids (Box 7-4). Respiratory depression is the most serious complication and is most likely to occur in sedated patients. The respiratory rate may decrease gradually or respirations may cease abruptly; lower limits of normal are not established for children, but any significant change from a previous rate calls for increased vigilance. A slower respiratory rate does not necessarily reflect decreased arterial oxygenation; an increased depth of ventilation may compensate for the altered rate. If respiratory depression or arrest occurs, be prepared to intervene quickly (see Nursing Care Guidelines box).

Although respiratory depression is the most dangerous side effect, constipation is a common, and sometimes serious, side effect of opioids, which decrease peristalsis and increase anal sphincter tone. Prevention with stool softeners and laxatives is more effective than treatment once constipation occurs. Dietary treatment, such as increased fiber, is usually not sufficient to promote regular bowel evacuation. However, dietary measures, such as increased fluid and fruit intake, and physical activity are encouraged. Pruritus from epidural or IV infusion is treated with low doses of IV naloxone, nalbuphine, or diphenhydramine. Nausea, vomiting, and sedation usually subside after 2 days of opioid administration, although oral or rectal antiemetics are sometimes necessary.

BOX 7-4   SIDE EFFECTS OF OPIOIDS

General
Constipation (possibly severe)
Respiratory depression
Sedation
Nausea and vomiting
Agitation, euphoria
Mental clouding
Hallucinations
Orthostatic hypotension
Pruritus
Urticaria
Sweating
Miosis (may be sign of toxicity)
Anaphylaxis (rare)

Signs of Tolerance
Decreasing pain relief
Decreasing duration of pain relief

Signs of Withdrawal Syndrome in Patients with Physical Dependence
Initial Signs of Withdrawal
Lacrimation
Rhinorrhea
Yawning
Sweating

Later Signs of Withdrawal
Restlessness
Irritability
Tremors
Anorexia
Dilated pupils
Gooseflesh
Nausea, vomiting

NURSING CARE GUIDELINES
Managing Opioid-Induced Respiratory Depression

If Respirations Are Depressed
Assess sedation level.
Reduce infusion by 25% when possible.
Stimulate patient (shake shoulder gently, call by name, ask to breathe).
Administer oxygen.

If Patient Cannot Be Aroused or Is Apneic
Initiate resuscitation efforts as appropriate.
Administer naloxone (Narcan):
- For children weighing less than 40 kg (88 lb), dilute 0.1 mg naloxone in 10 ml sterile saline to make 10 mcg/ml solution and give 0.5 mcg/kg.
- For children weighing more than 40 kg (88 lb), dilute 0.4-mg ampule in 10 ml sterile saline and give 0.5 ml.

Administer bolus by slow intravenous push every 2 minutes until effect is obtained.
Closely monitor patient. Naloxone's duration of antagonist action may be shorter than that of the opioid, requiring repeated doses of naloxone.
NOTE: Respiratory depression caused by benzodiazepines (e.g., diazepam [Valium] or midazolam [Versed]) can be reversed with flumazenil (Romazicon). Pediatric dosing experience suggests 0.01 mg/kg (0.1 ml/kg); if no (or inadequate) response after 1 to 2 minutes, administer same dose and repeat as needed at 60-second intervals for maximum dose of 1 mg (10 ml) (Yaster, Krance, Kaplan, et al, 1997).

Both tolerance and physical dependence can occur with prolonged use of opioids (see Community Focus box). **Physical dependence** is a normal, natural, physiologic state of "neuroadaptation." When opioids are abruptly discontinued without weaning, withdrawal symptoms occur 24 hours later and reach a peak within 72 hours. Symptoms of withdrawal include signs of neurologic excitability (irritability, tremors, seizures, increased motor tone, insomnia), gastrointestinal dysfunction (nausea, vomiting, diarrhea, abdominal cramps), and autonomic dysfunction (sweating, fever, chills, tachypnea, nasal congestion, rhinitis). Withdrawal symptoms can be anticipated and prevented by weaning patients from opioids that were administered for more than 5 to 10 days. Adherence to a weaning protocol to prevent or minimize withdrawal symptoms from opioids is required. A weaning flowsheet (Fig. 7-11, *A*) may be used to assess the efficacy of opioid weaning in

COMMUNITY FOCUS
Fear of Opioid Addiction

One of the reasons for the unfounded but prevalent fear of addiction from opioids used to relieve pain is a misunderstanding of the differences between physical dependence, tolerance, and addiction. Health care professionals and the community often confuse addiction with the physiologic effects of opioids, when in reality these three events are unrelated.

The American Society of Addiction Medicine defines these three terms as follows:

Physical dependence on an opioid is a physiologic state in which abrupt cessation of the opioid, or administration of an opioid antagonist, results in a withdrawal syndrome. Physical dependence on opioids is an expected occurrence in all individuals who continuously use opioids for therapeutic or nontherapeutic purposes. It does not, in and of itself, imply addiction.

Tolerance is a form of neuroadaptation to the effects of chronically administered opioids (or other medications) that is indicated by the need for increasing or more frequent doses of the medication to achieve the initial effects of the drug. A person may develop tolerance both to the analgesic effects of opioids and to some of the unwanted side effects, such as respiratory depression, sedation, or nausea. Tolerance is variable in occurrence, but it does not, in and of itself, imply addiction.

Addiction in the context of pain treatment with opioids is characterized by a persistent pattern of dysfunctional opioid use that may involve any or all of the following:
- Adverse consequences associated with the use of opioids
- Loss of control over the use of opioids
- Preoccupation with obtaining opioids, despite the presence of adequate analgesia

Unfortunately, individuals who have severe, unrelieved pain may become intensely focused on finding relief. Sometimes behaviors such as "clock watching" make patients appear to others to be preoccupied with obtaining opioids. However, this preoccupation focuses on finding relief of pain, not on using opioids for reasons other than pain control. This phenomenon has been termed *pseudoaddiction* and must not be confused with real addiction.

Nurses must educate older children, parents, and health professionals about the extremely low risk of real addiction (<1%) from the use of opioids to treat pain. Infants, young children, and comatose or terminally ill children simply cannot become addicted because they are incapable of a consistent pattern of drug-seeking behavior, such as stealing, drug dealing, prostitution, and use of family income, to obtain opioids for nonanalgesic reasons.

Data from American Society of Addiction Medicine: *Public policy statement on definitions related to the use of opioids for pain treatment,* February 2001, available at www.asam.org/Pain.html (accessed December 8, 2009).

Children's Hospital Oakland Opioid Weaning Flowsheet and Guidelines for Use of the Form

Analgesia/sedation orders (drug/dose/frequency)

Date			
Drug			
Administration time			
Dose ↑ or ↓ or freq change			

		Time:		
Choose one: Crying/agitated 25%-50% of interval Crying/agitated >50% of interval	2 3			
Choose one: Sleeps ≤25% of interval Sleeps 26%-75% of interval Sleeps >75% of interval	3 2 1			
Choose one: Hyperactive Moro Markedly hyperactive Moro	2 3			
Choose one: Mild tremors, disturbed Moderate/severe tremors, disturbed	1 2			
Increased muscle tone	2			
Temperature 37.2°-38.4°C	1			
Temperature >38.4°C	2			
Respiratory rate >60 (extubated)	2			
Suction >twice/interval (intubated)	2			
Sweating	1			
Frequent yawning (>3-4/interval)	1			
Sneezing (>3-4/interval)	1			
Nasal stuffiness	1			
Emesis	2			
Projectile vomiting	3			
Loose stools	2			
Watery stools	3			
TOTAL SCORE				
ADJUSTED SCORE				
INITIALS OF PERSON SCORING				

Directions: Score every 2-4 hours per guideline
Score greater than 8-12 may indicate withdrawal

Guidelines for use of the flow sheet

Use of form

Use the flowsheet for all infants who have received continuous or around-the-clock opioid medication for 3 days or more, or more than 3 doses per day for more than 5 days. This patient population will most often include postoperative patients, agitated intubated infants, and all post-ECMO patients.

Instructions
1. Write drug, dose, and frequency of analgesics and sedatives ordered.
2. Enter date, name of drug (abbreviated MS=morphine sulfate or FENT=fentanyl), and administration time of drugs given in the appropriate boxes; indicate if dose frequency given is an increase or decrease from the ordered dose.
3. Scoring must be performed every 4 hours during weaning of opioids, every 2 hours if score is 8 or greater. The score for each item indicates the presence of the sign during the previous 2-4 hours (depending on the scoring interval). Every 4-hour scoring should continue until the patient is off all opioids for 48-72 hours. Place a "0" in the column after the sign if it is not seen during the scoring period.

Central nervous system
Crying behavior: Score 2 points if patient exhibits crying or cry behavior for a duration of ≤50% of the scoring interval. Score 3 points if cumulative crying behavior totals >50% of the scoring interval.
NOTE: Crying behavior is accompanied by the facial expressions associated with crying, but without audible sounds because of endotracheal intubation.
Sleeping: Score 3 points if patient sleeps for ≤25% of the scoring interval. Score 2 points if patient sleeps for 26%-75% of the scoring interval. Score 1 point if patient sleeps for >75% of the scoring interval.
Moro (startle) reflex: Score 2 points if patient has some arm and/or leg extension when touched or when disturbed by loud noises. Score 3 points if patient has marked arm and/or leg extension that is accompanied by crying behavior, hyperalert state, or continued arm and/or leg tremors after being startled.
Tremors—disturbed: Score 1 point if patient has mild tremors when disturbed. Score 2 points if patient has moderate to severe tremors when disturbed. NOTE: Tremors are alternating movements that are rhythmic, of equal rate and amplitude, and can usually be stopped by flexion of the limb.
Increased muscle tone: Score 2 points if patient exhibits fisting or tight flexion of extremities that are difficult to extend.

Metabolic
Temperature: Score 1 point if patient's temperature is 37.2°-38.4°C. Score 2 points if patient's temperature is >38.4°C.
Respiratory rate: Score 1 point if patient's spontaneous respiratory rate is >60/minute. Score 2 points if patient's spontaneous respiratory rate is >60/minute and accompanied by retractions.
Suction: Score 2 points if patient is suctioned more than twice during a 4-hour period.
Sweating: Score 1 point if patient exhibits any type of sweating, including beads of sweat, or if skin is moist to touch.
Yawning: Score 1 point if patient yawns >3-4 times in succession or yawns 1-2 times often during a 4-hour period.
Sneezing: Score 1 point if patient sneezes >3-4 times in succession or sneezes 1-2 times during a 4-hour period.
Nasal stuffiness: Score 1 point for nasal stuffiness.

Gastrointestinal
Emesis of formula/stomach contents: Score 2 points if patient has 1 or more episodes of emesis during a 4-hour period.
Projectile vomiting: Score 3 points if patient has 1 or more episodes of projectile vomiting.
Loose stools: Score 2 points if patient has loose stools characterized by a water ring around some solid stool. The stools will often be frequent. NOTE: Do not score for "breast milk" stools: frequent, small, seedy, yellow stools.
Watery stools: Score 3 points if patient has stools that consist of only liquid. The stools will often be frequent.

Total score: Add up all the scores in the column and place the total score in this box. Clinical signs that appear continuously, such as respiratory rate >60 or regular poor feeding, should be included in the total score.
Adjusted score: The adjusted score is used when a sign is detected that is expected to occur independently of withdrawal, due to a preexisting condition (high respiratory rate in infant with bronchopulmonary dysplasia). The decision to adjust the score should be made after discussion with the healthcare team during rounds, and the rationale should be recorded in a problem-oriented note. Circle the signs to be excluded and deduct the points from the total score to obtain the adjusted score.
Initials of person scoring: The person scoring should write his/her initials in this space.

A

Fig. 7-11 A, Weaning flowsheet to monitor opioid weaning in neonates.

neonates (Franck and Vilardi, 1995; Franck, Vilardi, Durand, et al, 1998). In older infants and young children (7 months to 10 years) the Withdrawal Assessment Tool–1 (Fig. 7-11, *B*) may be use to assess and monitor withdrawal symptoms in pediatric critically ill children who are exposed to opioids and benzodiazepines for prolonged periods (Franck, Harris, Soetenga, et al, 2008).

Tolerance occurs when the dose of an opioid needs to be increased to achieve the same analgesic effects that was previously achieved at a lower dose (see Community Focus box). Tolerance may develop after 10 to 21 days of morphine administration. Treatment of tolerance involves increasing the dose or decreasing the duration between doses. Treatment of physical dependence involves gradually reducing the dose over

several days to prevent withdrawal symptoms, as follows (Max, Payne, Edwards, et al, 1999):
- Gradually reduce dose (similar to tapering of steroids).
- Give half of previous daily dose every 6 hours for first 2 days.
- Then reduce dose by 25% every 2 days. Continue this schedule until the patient reaches a total daily dose of 0.6 mg/kg of morphine (or equivalent). After 2 days on this dose, discontinue opioid.
- You may also switch to oral methadone, using one fourth of equianalgesic dose as initial weaning dose and proceeding as described above.

Parents and older children may fear addiction when opioids are prescribed. The nurse should address these concerns with

WITHDRAWAL ASSESSMENT TOOL – 1 (WAT–1)

Patient Identifier												
	Date:											
	Time:											
Information from patient record, previous 12 hours												
Any loose /watery stools	No = 0 Yes = 1											
Any vomiting/wretching/gagging	No = 0 Yes = 1											
Temperature > 37.8°C	No = 0 Yes = 1											
2 minute pre-stimulus observation												
State	SBS* ≤ 0 or asleep/awake/calm = 0 SBS* ≥ +1 or awake/distressed = 1											
Tremor	None/mild = 0 Moderate/severe = 1											
Any sweating	No = 0 Yes = 1											
Uncoordinated/repetitive movement	None/mild = 0 Moderate/severe = 1											
Yawning or sneezing	None or 1 = 0 ≥2 = 1											
1 minute stimulus observation												
Startle to touch	None/mild = 0 Moderate/severe = 1											
Muscle tone	Normal = 0 Increased = 1											
Post-stimulus recovery												
Time to gain calm state (SBS* ≤ 0)	< 2min = 0 2 - 5min = 1 > 5 min = 2											
Total Score (0-12)												

WITHDRAWAL ASSESSMENT TOOL (WAT–1) INSTRUCTIONS

- Start WAT-1 scoring from the **first day of weaning** in patients who have received opioids +/or benzodiazepines by infusion or regular dosing for prolonged periods (e.g., > 5 days). Continue twice daily scoring until 72 hours after the last dose.
- The Withdrawal Assessment Tool (WAT-1) should be completed along with the SBS[1] at least once per 12 hour shift (e.g., at 08:00 and 20:00 ± 2 hours). The progressive stimulus used in the SBS[1] assessment provides a standard stimulus for observing signs of withdrawal.

Obtain information from patient record (this can be done before or after the stimulus):
  ✓ **Loose/watery stools**: Score 1 if any loose or watery stools were documented in the past 12 hours; score 0 if none were noted.
  ✓ **Vomiting/wretching/gagging**: Score 1 if any vomiting or spontaneous wretching or gagging were documented in the past 12 hours; score 0 if none were noted
  ✓ **Temperature > 37.8°C**: Score 1 if the modal (most frequently occurring) temperature documented was greater than 37.8°C in the past 12 hours; score 0 if this was not the case.

2 minute pre-stimulus observation:
  ✓ **State**: Score 1 if awake and distress (SBS[1]: ≥ +1) observed during the 2 minutes prior to the stimulus; score 0 if asleep or awake and calm/cooperative (SBS[1] ≤ 0).
  ✓ **Tremor**: Score 1 if moderate to severe tremor observed during the 2 minutes prior to the stimulus; score 0 if no tremor (or only minor, intermittent tremor).
  ✓ **Sweating**: Score 1 if any sweating during the 2 minutes prior to the stimulus; score 0 if no sweating noted.
  ✓ **Uncoordinated/repetitive movements**: Score 1 if moderate to severe uncoordinated or repetitive movements such as head turning, leg or arm flailing or torso arching observed during the 2 minutes prior to the stimulus; score 0 if no (or only mild) uncoordinated or repetitive movements.
  ✓ **Yawning or sneezing > 1**: Score 1 if more than 1 yawn or sneeze observed during the 2 minutes prior to the stimulus; score 0 if 0 to 1 yawn or sneeze.

1 minute stimulus observation:
  ✓ **Startle to touch**: Score 1 if moderate to severe startle occurs when touched during the stimulus; score 0 if none (or mild).
  ✓ **Muscle tone**: Score 1 if tone increased during the stimulus; score 0 if normal.

Post-stimulus recovery:
  ✓ **Time to gain calm state (SBS[1] ≤ 0)**: Score 2 if it takes greater than 5 minutes following stimulus; score 1 if achieved within 2 to 5 minutes; score 0 if achieved in less than 2 minutes.
  Sum the 11 numbers in the column for the total WAT-1 score (0-12).

B

Fig. 7-11, cont'd. B, Withdrawal assessment tool for infants and children. *SBS,* State behavioral scale. (**A,** Modified from Franck L, Vilardi J: Assessment and management of opioid withdrawal in ill neonates, *Neonatal Netw* 14[2]:39-48, 1995; **B,** © 2007 LS Franck and MAQ Curley. All rights reserved. Reprinted in Franck LS, Harris SK, Soetenga DJ, et al: The Withdrawal Assessment Tool–1 (WAT–1): an assessment instrument for monitoring opioid and benzodiazepine withdrawal symptoms in pediatric patients, *Pediatr Crit Care Med* 9[6]:577, 2008. *From Curley MQ, Harris SK, Fraser KA, et al: State behavioral scale: a sedation assessment instrument for infants and young children supported on mechanical ventilation, *Pediatr Crit Care Med* 7(2):107-114, 2008.)

assurance that any such risk is extremely low. It may be helpful to ask the question, "If you did not have this pain, would you want to take this medicine?" The answer is invariably no, which reinforces the solely therapeutic nature of the drug. It is also important to avoid making statements to the family such as "We don't want you to get used to this medicine," or "By now you shouldn't need this medicine," which may reinforce the fear of becoming addicted. Whereas both physical dependence and tolerance are physiologic states, addiction or psychologic dependence is a psychologic state and implies a "cause-effect" mode of thinking, such as "I need the drug because it makes me feel better." Infants and children do not have the cognitive ability to make the cause-effect association and therefore cannot become addicted. The use of opioid analgesics early in life has not been demonstrated to increase the risk for addiction later in life. Nurses need to explain to parents the differences among physical dependence, tolerance, and addiction and allow them to express concerns about the use and duration of use of opioids. Infants and children, when treated appropriately with opioids, may be at risk for physical tolerance and physical dependence, but not psychologic dependence or addiction (McCaffery and Pasero, 1999).

Evaluation of Effectiveness of Pain Regimen

The response to therapy should be evaluated 15 to 30 minutes after each dose, and titration should continue to the highest achievable amount of relief (Max, Payne, Edwards, et al, 1999). In a retrospective study that examined the pain experience of children with sickle cell disease, evidence of pain relief from medications was documented for less than half (44.8%) of the patients in the emergency department (ED) (Jacob and Mueller, 2008). Even though The Joint Commission required documentation of pain assessments with vital signs, evidence of pain relief was not documented in 41.4% of the episodes. Titration methods in the ED or during the course of hospitalization, if used, were not reflected in the amount of medications received by the children (Jacob and Mueller, 2008; Jacob, Miaskowski, Savedra, et al, 2003a, 2003b).

In a study of nursing practice related to pain assessment and management in different pediatric specialty units, nurses noted complaints of pain, but seldom documented specific pain scores or responses to analgesics after administration (Jacob and Puntillo, 2000). Pain scores were not available before and after analgesics, and it was therefore not possible to conclude whether analgesics were effective. Nurses therefore need to evaluate and monitor pain in a timely fashion after administration of analgesic and titrate dosage to effect. Nurses also need to make recommendations for an alternate analgesic; for addition of another analgesic; or for a combination of analgesics, adjuvants, and nonpharmacologic strategies.

CONSEQUENCES OF UNTREATED PAIN IN INFANTS

Despite current research on the neonate's experience of pain, infant pain often remains inadequately managed. The mismanagement of infant pain is partially the result of misconceptions regarding the effects of pain on the neonate and the lack of knowledge of immediate and long-term consequences of untreated pain. Infants respond to noxious stimuli through physiologic indicators (increased heart rate and blood pressure, variability in heart rate and intracranial pressure, and decreases in Sao_2 and skin blood flow) and behavioral indicators (muscle rigidity, facial expression, crying, withdrawal, and sleeplessness) (Anand, Grunau, and Oberlander, 1997; Bildner and Krechel, 1996). The physiologic and behavioral changes, as well as a variety of neurophysiologic responses to noxious stimulation, are responsible for acute and long-term consequences of pain.

Several harmful effects occur with unrelieved pain, particularly when pain is prolonged. Pain triggers a number of physiologic stress responses in the body, and they lead to negative consequences that involve multiple systems. Unrelieved pain may prolong the stress response and adversely affect an infant's or child's recovery, whether it is from trauma, surgery, or disease. (See Research Focus box.)

🔍 RESEARCH FOCUS

Deep Intraoperative Anesthesia

In a landmark study by Anand and Hickey (1992), 30 neonates received deep intraoperative anesthesia with high doses of the opioid sufentanil, followed postoperatively by an infusion of opioids for 24 hours, and 15 neonates received lighter anesthesia with halothane and morphine followed postoperatively by intermittent morphine and diazepam. The 15 neonates who received the lighter anesthesia and intermittent postoperative opioids had more severe hyperglycemia and lactic acidemia, and 4 postoperative deaths occurred in the group. The 30 neonates who received deep anesthesia had a lower incidence of complications (sepsis, metabolic acidosis, disseminated intravascular coagulation) and no deaths.

Poorly controlled acute pain can predispose patients to chronic pain syndromes. See Box 7-5 for a list of numerous complications of untreated pain in infants. A guiding principle in pain management is that prevention of pain is always better than treatment (Benjamin, Swinson, and Nagel, 2000). Pain that is established and severe is often more difficult to control. When pain is unrelieved, sensory input from injured tissues reaches spinal cord neurons and may enhance subsequent responses. Long-lasting changes in cells within spinal cord pain pathways may occur after a brief painful stimulus and may lead to the development of chronic pain conditions. Basbaum (1999a, 1999b) reported a series of studies that emphasize a distinct neurochemistry of acute and persistent pain and concluded that persistent pain is not merely a prolonged acute pain symptom of some other disease. Underlying physiologic mechanisms lead to the persistence of pain (Marx, 2004; Woolf and Salter, 2000).

Anand and Hickey (1987) described additional responses of infants to painful stimuli from their own unpublished and other scientific studies. Chemical and hormonal responses were observed following noxious stimuli without the use of an anesthetic or analgesic. Such responses included increases in β-endorphin secretion (an endogenous opioid), plasma renin activity, plasma epinephrine and norepinephrine, catecholamines, growth hormone, glucagon, aldosterone, and other corticosteroids. The result of these chemical and hormonal increases includes the breakdown of fat and carbohydrate stores; prolonged hyperglycemia; and increased serum lactate,

BOX 7-5 CONSEQUENCES OF UNTREATED PAIN IN INFANTS

Acute Consequences
Periventricular-intraventricular hemorrhage
Increased chemical and hormone release
Breakdown of fat and carbohydrate stores
Prolonged hyperglycemia
Higher morbidity for neonatal intensive care unit patients
Memory of painful events
Hypersensitivity to pain
Prolonged response to pain
Inappropriate innervation of the spinal cord
Inappropriate response to nonnoxious stimuli
Lower pain threshold

Potential Long-Term Consequences
Higher somatic complaints of unknown origin
Greater physiologic and behavioral responses to pain
Increased prevalence of neurologic deficits
Psychosocial problems
Neurobehavioral disorders
Cognitive deficits
Learning disorders
Poor motor performance
Behavioral problems
Attention deficits
Poor adaptive behavior
Inability to cope with novel situations
Problems with impulsivity and social control
Learning deficits
Emotional temperament changes in infancy or childhood
Accentuated hormonal stress responses in adult life

pyruvate, total ketone bodies, and nonesterified fatty acids. Such consequences can lead to a greater morbidity for neonates in the NICU. Several experimental studies revealed a significant decrease in these responses when adequate analgesia was used before the painful procedure. One study showed that the standardization of postoperative pain management strategies for infants in the NICU led to the following improvements: (1) decreased length of time to extubation, (2) decreased length of stay, (3) better fluid management, and (4) reduced side effects of opioids. The authors also noted improved pain management documentation, decreased cost, and decreased nursing time (Furdon, Eastman, Benjamin, et al, 1998) (see Atraumatic Care box).

ATRAUMATIC CARE

Use of Opioids and Extubation Practice

Traditional belief holds that the continued use of opioids for neonates in the postoperative period results in prolonged intubation. Consequently, traditional practice is to discontinue all opioids several hours before and after extubation, thus preventing pain relief. Furdon, Eastman, Benjamin, and colleagues (1998) found that continuous opioid infusion in infants without an underlying pulmonary or neurologic pathologic condition actually shortened the time to extubation and caused no problems of respiratory depression that required reintubation. Preliminary evidence suggests that the use of preemptive analgesia with a continuous infusion of low-dose morphine reduces the incidence of poor neurologic outcomes in preterm neonates who require ventilatory support.

An experience known as the windup phenomenon has been attributed to a decreased pain threshold and chronic pain. Central and peripheral mechanisms that occur in response to noxious tissue injury have been studied in an attempt to explain a prolonged neonatal response to pain characteristic of the windup phenomenon. After exposure to noxious stimuli, multiple levels of the spinal cord experience an altered excitability. This altered excitability may cause nonnoxious stimuli, such as routine nursing care and handling, to be perceived as noxious stimuli. The nonnoxious stimuli produce the same physiologic response to stress that noxious stimuli would produce, leading to chronic pain. Long-term exposure to chronic pain may be responsible for more biologic and clinical consequences in critically ill premature infants than acute pain (Anand, Grunau, and Oberlander, 1997).

Researchers have found that nerve damage resulting from tissue injury stimulates collateral nerve growth by surrounding undamaged nerves. This collateral growth is responsible for inappropriate innervation in the spinal cord, which processes information from the surrounding undamaged nerves (Anand, Grunau, and Oberlander, 1997). Based on evidence from a study of human infants and adult rats exposed to neonatal pain, additional long-term consequences of neonatal pain include potential emotional temperament changes in infancy or childhood, accentuated hormonal stress responses in adult life, a preference for alcohol, and decreased exploratory behaviors (Anand, Grunau, and Oberlander, 1997).

Consequences of a history of extremely low birth weight and early pain exposure that may be attributed to pain and environmental stress include increased prevalence of neurologic deficits, psychosocial problems, and neurobehavioral disorders. Additional sequelae include cognitive deficits, learning disorders, poor motor performance, behavioral problems, attention deficits, poor adaptive behavior, inability to cope with novel situations, problems with impulsivity and social control, and learning deficits (Anand, Grunau, and Oberlander, 1997).

The limited available knowledge with respect to the consequences of infant pain suggests serious potential deleterious effects of untreated pain (see Box 7-5). Prevention of acute pain and treatment of chronic pain have been documented as beneficial in reducing the morbidity and mortality associated with frequent exposure to pain in premature infants (Anand and Carr, 1989; Anand and Hickey, 1987, 1992). Nurses who care for infants and children should consider the potential acute and long-term effects of pain on their young patients and be advocates in treating and preventing pain.

COMMON PAIN STATES IN CHILDREN

PAINFUL AND INVASIVE PROCEDURES

Several painful and invasive procedures require the administration of anesthetics and analgesics. For circumcision pain, caudal or penile blocks are employed before the procedure, then parents are instructed how to apply lidocaine gels for the first 24 to 36 hours after the circumcision. For open wounds, bupivacaine may be instilled with or without epinephrine onto the dressing applied to skin to minimize pain for up to 48 hours after the procedure. For graft donor sites, analgesia is maintained by using a foam dressing soaked with bupivacaine (0.25%, 2 mg/kg; 0.8 ml/kg) and applying it to the donor surface. A continuous infusion of 0.25% bupivacaine at 1 to 3 ml/hr via a standard 18-gauge epidural catheter is then curled on the outer or inner surface of the foam (Cousins and Power, 2003). Wound perfusion of bupivacaine is useful for iliac crest bone graft donor sites (used for alveolar bone grafting in some techniques of cleft palate repair). A standard 18-gauge epidural catheter is also used with a very low infusion rate (1 to 3 ml/hr) of bupivacaine. For minor and some intermediate procedures, the local anesthetic infiltration with bupivacaine is commonly used. Some examples of these procedures include surface wounds and tunneling procedures in the anesthetized child requiring inguinal surgery; insertion of ventriculoperitoneal shunts, central venous lines, or central venous catheter-reservoir systems; and similar procedures.

Procedural Sedation and Analgesia

Severe pain associated with invasive procedures and anxiety associated with diagnostic imaging can be managed with sedation and analgesia (Meredith, O'Keefe, and Galwankar, 2008). Sedation involves a wide range of levels of consciousness (Box 7-6). A thorough patient assessment is essential before procedural sedation. Key components to include in the patient history include:

Past medical history—Major illnesses such as asthma, psychiatric disorders, cardiac disease, hepatic or renal impairment; previous hospitalizations or surgeries; history of previous anesthesia or sedation.

Allergies—Opiates, benzodiazepines, barbiturates, local anesthetics, or others.

Current medications—Cardiovascular medications, central nervous system depressants. Use caution with chronic benzodiazepine and opiate users; administration of reversal agents may induce withdrawal or seizures.

Drug use—Narcotics, benzodiazepines, barbiturates, cocaine, and alcohol.

Last oral intake—For nonemergent cases, some guidelines recommend more than 6 hours for solid food and more than 2 hours for clear liquid.

Volume status—Vomiting, diarrhea, fluid restriction, urinary output, making tears.

A physical status evaluation using the ASA Physical Status Classification (Meredith, O'Keefe, and Galwankar, 2008) is documented before administering analgesia and sedation:

Class I—A normally health patient

Class II—A patient with mild systemic disease

Class III—A patient with severe systemic disease

Class IV—A patient with severe systemic disease that is a constant threat to life

Class V—A moribund patient who is not expected to survive without the operation

To provide a safe environment for procedural sedation and analgesia (PSA), equipment should be readily available to prevent or manage adverse events and complications (Box 7-7). The patient should have an IV access for titration of sedation and analgesic medications and for administration of possible antagonists and fluids. Trained personnel (physician, registered nurse, respiratory therapist) whose sole responsibility is to monitor the patient (rather than performing or assisting with the procedure) should be present to monitor for adverse events and complications. Common medications used for PSA are found in Table 7-10.

POSTOPERATIVE PAIN

Surgery and traumatic injuries (fractures, dislocations, strains, sprains, lacerations, burns) generate a catabolic state as a result of increased secretion of catabolic hormones and lead to alterations in blood flow, coagulation, fibrinolysis, substrate metabolism, and water and electrolyte balance and increase the demands on the cardiovascular and respiratory systems (Cousins and Power, 2003). The major endocrine and metabolic changes occur during the first 48 hours after surgery or trauma. Local anesthetics and opioid neural blockade may effectively mitigate the physiologic responses to surgical injury.

Pain associated with surgery to the chest (e.g., repair of congenital heart defects, chest trauma) or abdominal regions (e.g., appendectomy, cholecystectomy, splenectomy) may result in pulmonary complications. Pain leads to decreased muscle movement in the thorax and abdominal area and leads to

---

BOX 7-6   LEVELS OF SEDATION

Minimal Sedation (Anxiolysis)
Patient responds to verbal commands.
Cognitive function may be impaired.
Respiratory and cardiovascular systems are unaffected.

Moderate Sedation (Previously Conscious Sedation)
Patient responds to verbal commands but may not respond to light tactile stimulation.
Cognitive function is impaired.
Respiratory function is adequate; cardiovascular system is unaffected.

Deep Sedation
Patient cannot be easily aroused except with repeated or painful stimuli.
Ability to maintain airway may be impaired.
Spontaneous ventilation may be impaired; cardiovascular function is maintained.

General Anesthesia
Loss of consciousness, patient cannot be aroused with painful stimuli.
Airway cannot be maintained adequately and ventilation is impaired.
Cardiovascular function may be impaired.

From Meredith JR, O'Keefe KP, Galwankar S: Pediatric procedural sedation and analgesia, *J Emerg Trauma Shock* 1(2):88-96, 2008.

BOX 7-7   PROCEDURAL SEDATION AND ANALGESIA EQUIPMENT NEEDS

- High-flow oxygen and delivery method
- Airway management materials: endotracheal tubes, bag valve masks, and laryngoscopes
- Pulse oximetry, blood pressure monitor, electrocardiography,* capnography*
- Suction and large-bore catheters
- Vascular access supplies
- Resuscitation drugs, intravenous fluids
- Reversal agents, including flumazenil and naloxone

*May be optional devices.

TABLE 7-10   PROCEDURAL SEDATION AND ANALGESIA AGENTS

CLASSIFICATION	NAME	DOSE AND ROUTE	PEAK EFFECT	SIDE EFFECTS
Opiates				
Natural	Morphine	0.1-0.2 mg/kg IV	15 min	Sedation, somnolence, respiratory distress or depression, pruritus
Synthetic	Fentanyl	1-2 mcg/kg IV	10 min	Respiratory distress or depression, apnea, seizures, shock, chest wall rigidity (most rapid infusion or high doses)
Sedatives				
Benzodiazepines	Midazolam	0.02-0.1 mg/kg IV	5 min	Respiratory distress or depression, apnea, premature
		0.2-0.5 mg/kg IN	20-30 min	ventricular contractions, amnesia, blurred vision, or
		0.5-0.75 mg/kg PO	20-30 min	hyperexcitability
Barbiturates	Pentobarbital	2-5 mg/kg PR; maximum: 150 mg	15-60 min	Hypoventilation, apnea, bradycardia, hypotension,
		1-3 mg/kg IV; maximum: 150 mg	1 min	syncope, nausea
Hypnotics	Propofol	1 mg/kg IV, then 0.5 mg/kg IV over 30-60 min	6-7 min	Pain on injection, involuntary movements, hypotension, apnea
	Etomidate	0.1-0.2 mg/kg IV	30 sec	Pain on injection, involuntary movements
Dissociative				
Injected	Ketamine	1-2 mg/kg IV	5 min	Laryngospasm, severe hypotension or hypertension,
		3-5 mg/kg IM	10 min	respiratory depression, apnea, excessive salivation
Adjuvants for ketamine	Atropine	1 mg/kg IM or IV; minimum: 0.1 mg; maximum: 0.5 mg		Tachycardia, dizziness, blurred vision, photophobia
	Midazolam	0.05 mg/kg IV	5 min	See above
Inhaled	Nitrous oxide	30%-50% nitrous oxide, mixed with oxygen	3-5 min	Hypotension, vertigo
Reversal Agents				
Opioid reversal	Naloxone	<5 yr or <9 kg (20 lb): 0.1 mg/kg IV, IM, SC, or ET q 2-3 min	1-2 hr	May precipitate withdrawal in patients receiving opiates
		>5 yr or >9 kg (20 lb): 2 mg IV, IM, SC, or ET q 2-3 min	1-2 hr	Injection site pain
Benzodiazepine reversal	Flumazenil	0.02 mg/kg IV q 1 min; maximum: 1 mg		

ET, Endotracheal tube; *IM,* intramuscular; *IN,* intranasal; *IV,* intravenous; *PR,* per rectum; *q,* every; *SC,* subcutaneous.

decreased tidal volume, vital capacity, functional residual capacity, and alveolar ventilation. The patient is unable to cough and clear secretions, and the risk for complications such as pneumonia and atelectasis is high. Severe postoperative pain also results in sympathetic overactivity, which leads to increases in heart rate, peripheral resistance, blood pressure, and cardiac output. The patient eventually experiences an increase in cardiac demand and myocardial oxygen consumption and a decrease in oxygen delivery to the tissues.

The basis for good postoperative pain control in children is preemptive analgesia. **Preemptive analgesia** involves administration of medications (e.g., local and regional anesthetics, analgesics) before the child experiences the pain or before surgery is performed so that the sensory activation and changes in the pain pathways of the peripheral and central nervous system can be controlled. Preemptive analgesia lowers postoperative pain, lowers analgesic requirement, lowers hospital stay, lowers complications after surgery, and minimizes the risks for peripheral and central nervous system sensitization that can lead to persistent pain (Cousins and Power, 2003).

A combination of medications (**multimodal** or **balanced analgesia**) is used for postoperative pain and may include NSAIDs, local anesthetics, nonopioids, and opioid analgesics to achieve optimum relief and minimize side effects. Opioids (see Table 7-5) administered ATC during the first 48 hours or administered via PCA (see Table 7-9) are commonly prescribed

postoperatively. The duration of use is frequently limited to days, since the cause of pain usually resolves. The combination of the IV NSAID ketorolac and morphine using a PCA device is frequently prescribed after thoracic surgery. Morphine delivered by PCA leads to a lower total dosage of opioid analgesia when compared with the administration of intermittent doses of analgesic as required. After bowel surgery, a mixture of a local anesthetic (bupivacaine) and a low-dose opioid (fentanyl) delivered by epidural route improves the rate of recovery and minimizes the gastrointestinal effects (e.g., bowel stasis, nausea, vomiting). Once bowel function has been restored, oral opioids such as immediate release and controlled release preparations are preferred in older children. Controlled release opioids facilitate ATC dosing and improve sleep. They are also associated with a lower incidence of nausea, sedation, and breakthrough pain.

BURN PAIN

Because burn pain has multiple components, involves repeated manipulations over the injured painful sites, and has changing pattern over time, it is difficult and challenging to control. Burn pain includes a constant background pain that is felt at the wound sites and surrounding areas. Burn pain is exacerbated (breakthrough pain) by movements such as changing position, turning in bed, walking, or even breathing. Areas of normal skin that have been harvested for skin grafts (donor sites) also are painful. Pain is commonly experienced with intense tingling or itching sensations when skin grafting is required. During the healing process, when the tissue and nerve regenerate, the necrotic tissue (eschar) is excised until viable tissue is reached. The healing process may last for months to years. Pain or paresthetic sensations (itching, tingling, cold sensations, etc.) may persist. In addition, discomfort may be associated with immobilization of limbs in splints or garments, as well as multiple surgical interventions such as skin grafting and reconstructive surgery (Choiniere, 2003).

Multiple therapeutic procedures are carried out during the course of treatment. These procedures (dressing changes, wound débridement and cleansing, physical therapy sessions) occur daily or even several times a day (see Chapter 27). Providing proper analgesia without interfering with the patient's awareness during and after the procedure is the biggest challenge in the management of burn pain. Fentanyl or alfentanil has a major advantage over morphine because of the short duration. Fentanyl can prevent oversedation after the procedure. For less painful procedures, premedication with oral morphine, oral ketamine, or milder opioids 15 minutes before the procedure may be sufficient. Depending on the patient's anxiety level, a benzodiazepine (e.g., lorazepam) before the procedure may be beneficial. For longer procedures, morphine is the mainstay of treatment. Some patients may require moderate to deep sedation and analgesia. Oral oxycodone with midazolam and acetaminophen, in addition to nitrous oxide, may be needed. IV ketamine administered at subtherapeutic doses has been one of the most extensively used anesthetics for burn patients. The dysphoria and unpleasant reactions associated with ketamine administration may be minimized with premedication with a benzodiazepine. If ketamine is used with either morphine or fentanyl, the regimen could have opioid-sparing actions and reduce the opioid-related side effects.

Psychologic interventions are helpful in the treatment of burn pain. These interventions include hypnosis, relaxation training (breathing exercises, progressive muscle relaxation), biofeedback, stress inoculation training, cognitive-behavioral strategies (guided imagery, distraction, coping skills), and group and individual psychotherapy. They can be used alone or in combination. All these techniques can help the patient relax and maintain a sense of control (Choiniere, 2003). A major disadvantage of these interventions is they require time and discipline and often patients are too stressed, fatigued, disoriented, or sick to engage in them.

RECURRENT HEADACHES IN CHILDREN

Recurrent headaches in children can be caused by several factors, including tension, dental braces, imbalance or weakness of eye muscles causing deviation in alignment and refractive errors, sequelae to accidents, sinusitis and other cranial infection or inflammation, increased intracranial pressure, epileptic attacks, drugs, obstructive sleep apnea, and rarely hypertension (see Chapter 37). Other causes may include arteriovenous malformations, disturbances in cerebrospinal fluid flow or absorption, intracranial hemorrhages, ocular and dental diseases, bacterial infections, and brain tumors.

Severe pain is the most disturbing symptom in migraine. Tension-type headache is usually mild or moderate, often producing a pressing feeling in the temples, like a "tight band around the head." Continuous, daily, or near-daily headache with no specific cause occurs in a small subgroup of children. In epilepsy, headaches commonly occur immediately before, during, or after a seizure attack.

Treatment of recurrent headaches requires an understanding of the antecedents and consequences of headache pain. A headache diary can allow the child to record the time of onset, activities before the onset, any worries or concerns as far back as 24 hours before the onset, severity and duration of pain, pain medications taken, and activity pattern during headache episodes. The headache diary allows ongoing monitoring of headache activity, indicates the effects of interventions, and guides treatment planning.

Headache management involves two main behavioral approaches: (1) teaching patients self-control skills to prevent headache (biofeedback techniques and relaxation training), and (2) modifying behavior patterns that increase the risk of headache occurrence or reinforce headache activity (cognitive-behavioral stress management techniques). Biofeedback is a technology-based form of relaxation therapy and can be useful in assessing and reinforcing learning of relaxation skills such as progressive muscle relaxation, deep breathing, and imagery. Children as young as 7 years of age are able to learn these skills and with 2 to 3 weeks of practice are able to decrease the time needed to achieve relaxation.

To modify behavior patterns that increase the risk of headache or reinforce headache activity, the nurse instructs parents to avoid giving excessive attention to their child's headache and to respond matter-of-factly to pain behavior and requests for special attention (Holden, Deichmann, and Levy, 1999). Parents learn to assess whether the child is avoiding school or social performance demands because of headache. Parents are taught to focus attention on adaptive coping such as the use of relaxation techniques and maintenance of normal activity patterns. When using cognitive-behavioral stress management techniques, the parents identify negative thoughts and situations that may be associated with increased risk for headache. The parent teaches the child to activate positive thoughts and engage in adaptive behavior appropriate to the situation.

RECURRENT ABDOMINAL PAIN IN CHILDREN

Recurrent abdominal pain (RAP) or functional abdominal pain is defined as pain that occurs at least once per month for 3 consecutive months, accompanied by pain-free periods, and is severe enough that it interferes with a child's normal activities (see Chapter 18). Management of RAP is highly individualized to reflect the causes of the pain and the psychosocial needs of the child and family. A clear understanding of the child's characteristics (anxiety, physical health, temperament, coping skills, experience, learned response, depression), child's disability (school attendance, activities with family, social interactions, pain behaviors), environmental factors (family attitudes and behavioral patterns, school environment, community, friendships), and the pain stimulus (disease, injury, stress) is important in planning management strategies (Collins and Weisman, 2003).

Before any workup of the pain, the nurse informs the family that RAP is common in children and only 10% of children with RAP have an identifiable organic cause for their pain symptom. Medical workup is dictated by the child's symptoms and signs in combination with knowledge about common organic causes of RAP. If an organic cause is found, it will be treated appropriately. Even if no organic cause is found, the nurse needs to communicate to the child and family a belief that the pain is real. Usually the abdominal pain goes away, but even if problems are identified, they may not be the actual cause and pain may persist, may be replaced by another symptom, or may go away on its own. The management plan includes regular follow-up at a 3- to 4-month intervals, a list of symptoms that call for earlier contact, and biobehavioral pain management techniques. The goal is to minimize the impact of the pain on the child's activities and the family's life (Collins and Weisman, 2003).

Case reports have demonstrated the effectiveness of implementing a time-out procedure, token systems, and positive reinforcement based on operant theory treatment modalities. Stress management and cognitive-behavioral strategies have also been successful. Parent training in how to avoid positive reinforcement of sick behaviors and focus on rewarding healthy behaviors is important. Over the course of several sessions, parents are educated about RAP, how to distinguish between sick and well behaviors, a reward system for well behaviors, and the importance of reinforcing relaxation and coping skills taught to children for pain management. Treatment may consist of a varying number of sessions over 1 to 6 months and may include various components such as monitoring symptoms, limiting parent attention, relaxation training, increasing dietary fiber, and requiring school attendance. Response rates are 25% without abdominal pain and 56% to 75% improvements in symptoms (Collins and Weisman, 2003). The use of cognitive-behavioral therapy has been documented to reduce or eliminate pain in children with RAP and highlights the involvement of parents in supporting their child's self-management behavior. No negative side effects of symptom substitution occurred with the interventions. (See Research Focus box.)

RESEARCH FOCUS

Recurrent Abdominal Pain

One study demonstrated that the combination of self-regulation and cognitive-behavioral interventions along with fiber intervention is more effective for treating recurrent abdominal pain (RAP) than using fiber alone (Weydert, Ball, and Davis, 2003).

Two studies evaluated the use of famotidine (See, Birnbaum, Schechter, et al, 2001) and pizotifen (Symon and Russell, 1995) for the treatment of abdominal pain. Famotidine is an H_2-receptor antagonist that was given twice daily (0.5 mg/kg/dose). It was demonstrated to improve pain in 68% of children and decreased the peptic index score (composite score for nausea, vomiting, appetite loss, epigastric pain, weight loss, and nocturnal awakening). Pizotifen is a serotonin antagonist that was tested in 14 children given at 5 ml (0.25 mg) twice daily for 1 month. Patients who received pizotifen had fewer days of abdominal pain, a lower index of severity, and a lower index of misery when compared with those receiving a placebo. The only side effects noted were slight drowsiness and slight weight gain. Pizotifen is available worldwide but not approved for use in the United States.

PAIN IN CHILDREN WITH SICKLE CELL DISEASE

A painful episode is the most frequent cause for ED visits and hospital admissions among children with sickle cell disease (see Chapter 35). The acute painful episode in sickle cell disease is the only pain syndrome in which opioids are considered the major therapy and are started in early childhood and continued throughout adult life. A source of frustration for patients and clinicians is that most current analgesic regimens are inadequate in controlling some of the most severe painful episodes. A multidisciplinary approach that involves both pharmacologic and nonpharmacologic modalities (cognitive-behavioral intervention, heat, massage, physical therapy) is needed, but not often implemented. The goals of treatment of the acute episode may not be to take all the pain away, which is usually impossible, but to make the pain tolerable to the patient until the episode resolves and to increase function and patient participation in activities of daily living (Benjamin, Dampier, Jacox, et al, 1999; Max, Payne, Edwards, et al, 1999).

Patients coming to an ED for acute painful episodes usually have exhausted all home care options or outpatient therapy (Benjamin, Dampier, Jacox, et al, 1999; Max, Payne, Edwards, et al, 1999). The nurse should ask patients what the usual medication, dosage, and side effects were in the past; the usual medication taken at home; and medication taken since the onset of present pain. The patient may be on long-term opioid therapy at home and therefore may have developed some degree of tolerance. A different potent opioid or a larger dose of the same medication may be indicated. Because mixed opioid-agonist-antagonists (e.g., pentazocine, nalbuphine, butorphanol) may precipitate withdrawal syndromes, avoid these if patients were taking long-term opioids at home. A "passport" card with patient information about the diagnosis, previous complications, suggested pain management regimen, and name and contact information of the primary hematologist is helpful for parents and facilitates management of pain in the ED.

The patient is admitted for inpatient management of severe pain if adequate relief is not achieved in the ED (Benjamin, Dampier, Jacox, et al, 1999; Max, Payne, Edwards, et al, 1999). For severe pain, IV administration with bolus dosing and continuous infusion using a PCA device may be necessary. Patients requiring more than 5 to 7 days of opioids should have tapering doses to avoid the physiologic symptoms of withdrawal (dysphoria, nasal congestion, diarrhea, nausea and vomiting, sweating, and seizures). Appropriate weaning of the PCA schedules start with reduction of the continuous infusion rate before discontinuation, while the patient continues to use demand doses for analgesia. Morphine-equivalent equianalgesic conversions may be used to convert continuous infusion rates to equivalent oral analgesics (see Table 7-8). Doses of long-acting oral analgesics, such as sustained release oral morphine, may also be used to replace continuous infusion dosing. The demand doses can be subsequently reduced if analgesia remains adequate.

Patients who are administered doses of opioids that are inadequate to relieve their pain, or whose doses are not tapered after a course of treatment, may develop iatrogenic **pseudoaddiction**, which resembles addiction (Elander, Lusher, Bevan, et al,

2004). Pseudoaddiction or clock-watching behavior may be resolved by communicating with patients to ensure accurate assessment, involving them in decisions about their pain management, and administering adequate opioid doses (Elander, Lusher, Bevan, et al, 2004).

CANCER PAIN IN CHILDREN

Pain in children with cancer is present before diagnosis and treatment and may resolve after initiation of anticancer therapy. However, treatment-related pain is common (see Table 7-11 and Research Focus box). Pain may be related to an operation, mucositis, a phantom limb, or infection. Pain can also be related to chemotherapy and procedures such as bone marrow aspiration, needle puncture, and lumbar puncture (Collins, Byrnes, Dunkel, et al, 2000). Tumor-related pain frequently occurs when the child relapses or when tumors become resistant to treatment. Intractable pain may occur in patients with solid tumors that metastasize to the central or peripheral nervous system. In young adult survivors of childhood cancer, chronic pain conditions may develop, including complex regional pain syndrome of the lower extremity, phantom limb pain, avascular necrosis, mechanical pain related to bone that failed to unite after tumor resection, and postherpetic neuralgia.

Oral mucositis (ulceration of the oral cavity and throat) may occur in 40% of patients undergoing chemotherapy or radio-

RESEARCH FOCUS

Cancer-Related Pain

In one study of children with cancer, pain was the most prevalent symptom (84.4%) and was rated as moderate to severe (86.6%) and highly distressing (52.8%) (Collins, Byrnes, Dunkel, et al, 2000).

therapy and in 76% of patients undergoing bone marrow transplant (Berger, Henderson, Nadoolman, et al, 1995). No present therapy adequately relieves the pain of these lesions. Antihistamines, local anesthetics, and opioids provide only temporary relief, may block taste perception, or may produce additional side effects such as lethargy and constipation. Initial treatment includes single agents (saline, opioids, sodium bicarbonate, hydrogen peroxide, sucralfate suspension, clotrimazole, nystatin, viscous lidocaine, amphotericin B, dyclonine) or mouthwash mixtures using a combination of agents (lidocaine, diphenhydramine, Maalox or Mylanta, nystatin). The mucositis after bone marrow transplantation may be prolonged, continuously intense, exacerbated by mouth care and swallowing, or worse during waking hours. The patient may be unable to eat or swallow. Morphine administered as a continuous infusion or delivered by PCA device may be required until mucositis is resolved (Collins and Weisman, 2003).

Other treatment-related pain includes (1) abdominal pain after allogeneic bone marrow transplantation, which may be

TABLE 7-11	CANCER PAIN IN CHILDREN	
TYPE	**CLINICAL PRESENTATION**	**CAUSES**
Bone		
Skull	Aching to sharp, severe pain generally more pronounced with	Infiltration of bone
Vertebrae	movement; point tenderness common	Skeletal metastases—Irritation and stretching of pain
Pelvis and femur	Skull—Headaches, blurred vision	receptors in periosteum and endosteum
	Spine—Tenderness over spinous process	Prostaglandins released from bone destruction
	Extremities—Pain associated with movement or lifting	
	Pelvis and femur—Pain associated with movement; pain with	
	weight bearing and walking	
Neuropathic		
Peripheral	Complaints of pain without any detectable tissue damage	Nerve injury caused by tumor infiltration; can also be
Plexus	Abnormal or unpleasant sensations, generally described as	caused by injury from treatment (e.g., vincristine toxicity)
Epidural	tingling, burning, or stabbing	Infiltration or compression of peripheral nerves
Cord compression	Often a delay in onset	Surgical interruption of nerves (phantom pain after
	Brief, shooting pain	amputation)
	Increased intensity of pain with receptive stimuli	
Visceral		
Soft tissue	Poorly localized	Obstruction—Bowel, urinary tract, biliary tract
Tumors of bowel	Varies in intensity	Mucosal ulceration
Retroperitoneum	Pressure, deep or aching	Metabolic alteration
		Nociceptor activation, generally from distention or
		inflammation of visceral organs
Treatment Related		
Mucositis	Difficulty swallowing, pain from lesions in oropharynx; may	Direct side effects of treatment for cancer:
Infection	extend throughout entire gastrointestinal tract	Chemotherapy
Postlumbar puncture	Infection may be localized pain from focused infection or	Radiation
headaches	generalized (i.e., tissue infection versus septicemia)	Surgery
Radiation dermatitis	Severe headache after lumbar puncture	
Postsurgical	Skin inflammation causing redness and breakdown	
	Pain related to tissue trauma secondary to surgery	

associated with acute graft-versus-host disease; (2) abdominal pain associated with typhlitis (infection of the cecum), which occurs when the patient is immunocompromised; (3) phantom sensations and phantom limb pain after an amputation; (4) peripheral neuropathy after administration of vincristine; and (5) medullary bone pain, which may be associated with administration of granulocyte colony–stimulating factor (Collins and Weisman, 2003) (see Research Focus box).

RESEARCH FOCUS

Procedure-Related Cancer Pain

Almost 40% of all pain episodes in children with cancer may be attributed to procedures (Ljungman, Gordh, Sorensen, et al, 1999, 2000, 2001; Ljungman, Kreuger, Andreasson, et al, 2000).

Survivors of childhood cancer describe vivid memories of their experience with repeated painful procedures during treatment. These procedures include needle puncture for IM chemotherapy (L-asparaginase), IV lines, port access and blood draws, lumbar puncture, bone marrow aspiration and biopsy, removal of central venous catheters, and other invasive diagnostic procedures. Fear and anxiety related to these procedures may be minimized with parent and child preparation. The preparation starts with obtaining information from the parent about the child's coping styles, explaining the procedure, and enlisting their support, followed by an age-appropriate explanation to the child. Topical analgesics (cold sprays, EMLA, amethocaine gels), as discussed previously, are effective in providing analgesia before needle procedures.

Lumbar puncture for administration of chemotherapy (cytarabine, methotrexate) and collection of cerebrospinal fluid may lead to a leak at the puncture site and low intracranial pressure (Collins and Weisman, 2003). Some children may experience postdural puncture headache, which may be treated by administering nonopioid analgesics and placing the patient in the supine position for 1 hour after the procedure. The pain related to bone marrow aspiration is due to the insertion of a large needle into the posterior iliac space and the unpleasant sensation experienced at the time of marrow aspiration. Cognitive-behavioral therapy (guided imagery, relaxation, music therapy, hypnosis), conscious sedation, and general anesthesia have been effective in decreasing pain and distress during the procedure.

If the patient is neutropenic (absolute neutrophil count <500/mm^3), the antipyretic action of acetaminophen may mask a fever. In patients with thrombocytopenia (platelet count <50,000/mm^3), who may be at risk for bleeding, NSAIDs are contraindicated. Morphine is the most widely used opioid for moderate to severe pain and may be administered via the oral (including sustained release formulations such as MS Contin and Kadian), IV, subcutaneous, epidural, and intrathecal routes. When dose-limiting side effects of morphine develop, hydromorphone has been reported to be effective in several studies of children with cancer (Drake, Longworth, and Collins, 2004) (see Research Focus box).

The most common clinical syndrome of neuropathic pain is painful peripheral neuropathy caused by chemotherapeutic

RESEARCH FOCUS

Morphine Versus Hydromorphone

In a study of children and adolescents with mucositis after bone marrow transplantation, which compared morphine to hydromorphone using patient-controlled analgesia, hydromorphone was well tolerated and had a potency ratio of approximately 6:1 relative to morphine (Drake, Longworth, and Collins, 2004).

agents, particularly vincristine and cisplatin, and rarely cytarabine (Collins and Weisman, 2003). After withdrawal of the chemotherapy, the neuropathy may resolve over weeks to months, or it may persist even after withdrawal. Neuropathic pain is associated with at least one of the following: (1) pain that is described as electric or shocklike, stabbing, or burning; (2) signs of neurologic involvement (paralysis, neuralgia, pain hypersensitivity) other than those associated with the progression of the tumor; and (3) the location of the solid organ cancer consistent with neurologic damage that could give rise to neuropathic pain. Dying children with cancer who experience neuropathic pain have higher baseline requirements of morphine and require more rapid increases of morphine than dying children without neuropathic pain (Dougherty and DeBaun, 2003). Children with neuropathic pain often require massive opioid infusion (>3 mg/kg/hr of IV morphine dose equivalent, or approximately 100-fold greater than standard starting infusion rates). An epidural or subarachnoid infusion may be initiated if the patient experiences dose-limiting side effects of opioids or if pain is resistant to opioids.

Tricyclic antidepressants (amitriptyline, desipramine) and anticonvulsants (gabapentin, carbamazepine) have demonstrated effectiveness in neuropathic cancer pain (see Research Focus box). The tricyclic antidepressants have many actions that could be involved in their pain-relieving effect and have been considered the mainstay of therapy for neuropathic pain (Sindrup, Otto, Finnerup, et al, 2005).

RESEARCH FOCUS

Tricyclic Antidepressants to Treat Neuropathic Pain

Randomized controlled trials showed that 60% to 70% of patients with neuropathic pain achieve relief with tricyclic antidepressants (Sindrup, Otto, Finnerup, et al, 2005).

Klepstad, Borchgrevink, Hval, and colleagues (2001) reported the pain experience of a 12-year-old girl with severe neuropathic pain caused by a cervical spinal tumor. Two weeks after resection of the tumor, the child experienced increased pain in her neck, which was superficial and distributed in the dermatomes below the cervical medullary lesion. Touch provoked pain, and it did not decrease in intensity despite a subcutaneous infusion of morphine at 160 mg/24 hr. The child screamed from increased pain when her parents or siblings tried to comfort her with bodily contact. Pain was relieved after administration of 7.5 to 10 mg IV ketamine. Ketamine is an N-methyl-d-aspartate (NMDA) antagonist, which has undesirable side effects (sedation, nausea, dissociative reactions, muteness, dizziness, and visual distortions) and short duration of action (Sang, 2000). After administration of ketamine, the child was able to tolerate touch without pain paroxysms. A continuous IV infusion was eventually initiated for convenience, and benzodiazepines were added to avoid the psychomimetic effects associated with ketamine.

More recently Finkel, Pestieau, and Quezado (2007) used subanesthetic doses of ketamine to treat 11 children and adolescents who were on high doses of opioids and had uncontrolled cancer pain. Ketamine appeared to improve pain control and to have an opioid-sparing effect. Members of a pain management consulting service directed and titrated the ketamine to address symptoms. The ketamine dosage range used (0.1 to 1 mg/kg/hr) was lower than that used for anesthetic purposes. Lorazepam (0.025 mg/kg/12 hr) was administered concurrently during ketamine treatment. Continuous monitoring included heart rate, noninvasive blood pressure, respiratory rate, and oxygen saturation.

Although ketamine is frequently used to ensure analgesia and sedation during painful procedures in children, the long-term use of ketamine for the treatment of neuropathic pain in children has not been systematically studied and is not of clinical benefit for all patients (Klepstad, Borchgrevink, Hval, et al, 2001). In randomized studies of patients with chronic neuropathic pain, only some patients had a beneficial response to ketamine (Haines and Gaines, 1999; Max, Byas-Smith, Gracely, et al, 1995; Mitchell, 2001). Other N-methyl-D-aspartate (NMDA) antagonists (dextromethorphan, memantine) are available for clinical use, but no reports on their use in children with neuropathic pain related to cancer have been documented.

PAIN AND SEDATION IN END-OF-LIFE CARE

Many patients at the end of life require doses of opioids that make them sedated but arousable as their disease progresses (cancer, human immunodeficiency virus, cystic fibrosis, neurodegenerative disease). Patients achieve comfort with a combination of opioids and adjuvant analgesics in most situations. Parents need reassurance that the opioids are treating pain but not causing the child's death and that the child's advancing disease is the cause of death.

A small group of patients have intolerable side effects or inadequate analgesia despite extremely aggressive use of medications to relieve pain and side effects. Continuous sedation may be a means of relieving suffering when there is no feasible or acceptable means of providing analgesia that preserves alertness. A continuing high-dose infusion of opioids along with sedation is prescribed to reduce the possibility that a child might experience unrelieved pain but be too sedated to report it. Sedation in these situations is widely regarded as providing comfort, not euthanasia. Clinicians and ethicists have a range of views regarding assisted suicide and euthanasia, but they all agree that no child or parent should choose death because of inadequate efforts to relieve pain and suffering (Berde and Collins, 2003).

▮ KEY POINTS

- Although the ability to measure pain in children has improved dramatically in recent years, assessment of pain in children continues to be complex and challenging.
- Behavioral assessment is useful for measuring pain in infants and preverbal children who do not have the language skills to communicate that they are in pain, or when mental clouding and confusion limit a child's ability to communicate.
- Physiologic measures are not able to distinguish between physical responses to pain and other forms of stress to the body.
- The number of pain measurement tools that are available for use in infants and young children has increased dramatically and adds a layer of complexity to the assessment of pain in children.
- Important components of assessment include the onset of pain; pain duration or pattern; effectiveness of the current treatment; factors that aggravate or relieve the pain; other symptoms and complications concurrently felt; and interference with the child's mood, function, and interactions with family.
- The administration of sucrose with and without nonnutritive sucking has a calming and pain-relieving effects for invasive procedures in neonates.
- One of the most significant improvements in the ability to provide atraumatic care to children is the anesthetic creams LMX or EMLA.
- Nonopioids, including acetaminophen (Tylenol, Paracetamol) and NSAIDs, are suitable for mild to moderate pain; opioids are needed for moderate to severe pain.
- Several drugs, known as coanalgesics or adjuvant analgesics, may be used alone or with opioids to control pain symptoms and opioid side effects.

- A significant advance in the administration of IV, epidural, or subcutaneous analgesics is the use of PCA.
- Although respiratory depression is the most feared side effect of opioids, constipation is a common, and sometimes serious, side effect, which decrease peristalsis and increase anal sphincter tone.
- Several harmful effects occur with unrelieved pain, particularly when pain is prolonged.
- Surgery and traumatic injuries (fractures, dislocations, strains, sprains, lacerations, burns) generate a catabolic state as a result of increased secretion of catabolic hormones and lead to alterations in blood flow, coagulation, fibrinolysis, substrate metabolism, and water and electrolyte balance, and increase the demands on the cardiovascular and respiratory systems.
- Because burn pain has multiple components, involves repeated manipulations over the injured painful sites, and has changing patterns over time, it is difficult and challenging to control.
- Treatment of recurrent headaches requires an understanding of the antecedents and consequences of headache pain.
- RAP or functional abdominal pain is defined as pain that occurs at least once per month for 3 consecutive months, accompanied by pain-free periods, and is severe enough that it interferes with a child's normal activities.
- A painful episode is the most frequent cause for ED visits and hospital admissions among children with sickle cell disease.
- Pain is the most prevalent symptom reported by children with cancer.

- Injections from immunizations, IM antibiotics in the ED or physician's office, and blood draws are common sources of pain in children.
- For nonpainful procedures such as radiologic imaging studies, several medications are used to sedate, minimize anxiety, and induce amnesia.

- Several painful and invasive procedures require the administration of anesthetics and analgesics.

REFERENCES

Abbe M, Simon C, Angiolillo A, et al: A survey of language barriers from the perspective of pediatric oncologists, interpreters, and parents, *Pediatr Blood Cancer* 47(6):819-824, 2006.

Abdelkefi A, Abdennebi YB, Mellouli F, et al: Effectiveness of fixed 50% nitrous oxide oxygen mixture and EMLA cream for insertion of central venous catheters in children, *Pediatr Blood Cancer* 43(7):777-779, 2004.

Algren JT, Gursoy F, Johnson TD, et al: The effect of nitrous oxide diffusion on laryngeal mask airway cuff inflation in children, *Paediatr Anaesth* 8(1):31-36, 1998.

Ambuel B, Hamlett KW, Marx CM, et al: Assessing distress in pediatric intensive care environments: the COMFORT scale, *J Pediatr Psychol* 17(1):95-109, 1992.

American Pain Society: *Principles of analgesic use in the treatment of acute pain and chronic cancer pain,* ed 4, Glenview, Ill, 1999, The Society.

Anand KJ, Carr DB: The neuroanatomy, neurophysiology, and neurochemistry of pain, stress, and analgesia in newborns and children, *Pediatr Clin North Am* 36(4):795-822, 1989.

Anand KJ, Grunau RE, Oberlander TF: Developmental character and long-term consequences of pain in infants and children, *Child Adolesc Psychiatr Clin North Am* 6(4):703-724, 1997.

Anand KJ, Hickey PR: Halothane-morphine compared with high-dose sufentanil for anesthesia and postoperative analgesia in neonatal cardiac surgery, *N Engl J Med* 326(1):1-9, 1992.

Anand KJ, Hickey PR: Pain and its effects in the human neonate and fetus, *N Engl J Med* 317(21):1321-1329, 1987.

Barrier G, Attia J, Mayer MN, et al: Measurement of postoperative pain and narcotic administration in infants using a new clinical scoring system, *Anesthesiology* 67(3A):A532, 1987.

Basbaum AI: Distinct neurochemical features of acute and persistent pain, *Proc Natl Acad Sci USA* 96(14):7739-7743, 1999a.

Basbaum AI: Spinal mechanisms of acute and persistent pain, *Reg Anesth Pain Med* 24(1):59-67, 1999b.

Benjamin LJ, Dampier CD, Jacox AK, et al: *Guideline for the management of acute and chronic pain in sickle cell disease,* Glenview, Ill, 1999, American Pain Society.

Benjamin L, Swinson G, Nagel R: Sickle cell anemia day hospital: an approach for the management of uncomplicated painful crises, *Blood* 95:1130-1137, 2000.

Berde C, Collins J: Cancer pain and palliative care in children. In Melzack R, Wall P, editors: *Handbook of pain management,* St. Louis, 2003, Churchill Livingstone.

Berger A, Henderson M, Nadoolman W, et al: Oral capsaicin provides temporary relief for oral mucositis pain secondary to chemotherapy/radiation therapy, *J Pain Symptom Manage* 10(3):243-248, 1995.

Bernstein B, Pachter L: Cultural considerations in children's pain. In Schechter N, Berde C, Yaster M, editors: *Pain in infants, children, and adolescents,* Philadelphia, 2003, Lippincott Williams & Wilkins.

Beyer JE, Denyes MJ, Villarruel AM: The creation, validation and continuing development of the Oucher: a measure of pain intensity in children, *J Pediatr Nurs* 7(5):335-346, 1992.

Beyer JE, Knott CB: Construct validity estimation for the African-American and Hispanic versions of the Oucher scale, *J Pediatr Nurs* 13(1):20-31, 1998.

Beyer JE, Turner SB, Jones L, et al: The alternate forms reliability of the Oucher pain scale, *Pain Manage Nurs* 6(1):10-17, 2005.

Bildner J, Krechel SW: Increasing staff nurse awareness of postoperative pain management in the NICU, *Neonat Netw* 15(1):11-16, 1996.

Blauer T, Gerstmann D: A simultaneous comparison of three neonatal pain scales during common NICU procedures, *Clin J Pain* 14(1):39-47, 1998.

Bohannon A: *Physiological, self-report, and behavioral ratings of pain in 3 to 7 year old African-American and Anglo-American children,* Miami, 1995, University of Miami.

Breau LM, MacLaren J, McGrath PJ, et al: Caregivers' beliefs regarding pain in children with cognitive impairment: relation between pain sensation and reaction increases with severity of impairment, *Clin J Pain* 19(6):335-344, 2003.

Breau LM, McGrath PJ, Camfield CS, et al: Psychometric properties of the Non-communicating Children's Pain Checklist–Revised, *Pain* 99:349-357, 2002.

Bruera E, Willey JS, Ewert-Flannagan PA, et al: Pain intensity assessment by bedside nurses and palliative care consultants: a retrospective study, *Support Care Cancer* 13(4):228-231, 2005.

Chambers C: The role of family factors in pediatric pain. In Finley GA, McGrath PJ, editors: *Pediatric pain: biological and social context,* Seattle, 2003, IASP Press.

Chambers C, Craig K: An intrusive impact of anchors in children's faces pain scales, *Pain* 78:27-37, 1998.

Chambers CT, Giesbrecht K, Craig KD, et al: A comparison of faces scales for the measurement of pediatric pain: children's and parents' ratings, *Pain* 83:25-35, 1999.

Choi WY, Irwin MG, Hui TW, et al: EMLA cream versus dorsal penile nerve block for postcircumcision analgesia in children, *Anesth Analg* 96(2):396-399, 2003.

Choiniere M: Pain of burns. In Melzack R, Wall P, editors: *Handbook of pain management,* St. Louis, 2003, Churchill Livingstone.

Chorpita BF, Yim L, Moffitt C, et al: Assessment of symptoms of DSM-IV anxiety and depression in children: a revised child anxiety and depression scale, *Behav Res Ther* 38(8):835-855, 2000.

Claar RL, Walker LS: Functional assessment of pediatric pain patients: psychometric properties of the functional disability inventory, *Pain* 121(1-2):77-84, 2006.

Cline ME, Herman J, Shaw ER, et al: Standardization of the visual analogue scale, *Nurs Res* 41(6):378-380, 1992.

Cole J, Jorgensen K: Medical, developmental, and pharmacologic intervention: the essence of collaboration, *Neonat Netw* 16:56-58, 1997.

Collins JJ, Byrnes ME, Dunkel IJ, et al: The measurement of symptoms in children with cancer, *J Pain Symptom Manage* 19(5):363-377, 2000.

Collins J, Weisman S: Management of pain in childhood cancer. In Schechter N, Berde C, Yaster M, editors: *Pain in infants, children, and adolescents,* Philadelphia, 2003, Lippincott Williams & Wilkins.

Cousins M, Power I: Acute and postoperative pain. In Melzack R, Wall P, editors: *Handbook of pain management,* St. Louis, 2003, Churchill Livingstone.

Dampier C, Ely B, Brodecki D, et al: Characteristics of pain managed at home in children and adolescents with sickle cell disease by using diary self-reports, *J Pain* 3(6):461-470, 2002a.

Dampier C, Ely B, Brodecki D, et al: Home management of pain in sickle cell disease: a daily diary study in children and adolescents, *J Pediatr Hematol Oncol* 24(8):643-647, 2002b.

Dougherty M, DeBaun MR: Rapid increase of morphine and benzodiazepine usage in the last 3 days of life in children with cancer is related to neuropathic pain, *J Pediatr* 142(4):373-376, 2003.

Drake R, Longworth J, Collins JJ: Opioid rotation in children with cancer, *J Palliat Med* 7(3):419-422, 2004.

Egekvist H, Bjerring P: Effect of EMLA cream on skin thickness and subcutaneous venous diameter: a randomized, placebo-controlled study in children, *Acta Dermatol Venereol* 80(5):340-343, 2000.

Eland JA, Banner W: Analgesia, sedation, and neuromuscular blockage in pediatric critical care. In Hazinski ME, editor: *Manual of pediatric critical care*, St. Louis, 1999, Mosby.

Elander J, Lusher J, Bevan D, et al: Understanding the causes of problematic pain management in sickle cell disease: evidence that pseudoaddiction plays a more important role than genuine analgesic dependence, *J Pain Symptom Manage* 27(2):156-169, 2004.

Ely B, Dampier C, Gilday M, et al: Caregiver report of pain in infants and toddlers with sickle cell disease: reliability and validity of a daily diary, *J Pain* 3(1):50-57, 2002.

Fearon I, Kisilevsky BS, Hains SM, et al: Swaddling after heel lance: age-specific effects on behavioral recovery in preterm infants, *Develop Behav Pediatr* 18:222-232, 1997.

Finkel JC, Pestieau SR, Quezado ZM: Ketamine as an adjuvant for treatment of cancer pain in children and adolescents, *J Pain* 8(6):515-521, 2007.

Finley GA, Chambers CT, McGrath PJ, et al: Construct validity of the parents' postoperative pain measure, *Clin J Pain* 19(5):329-334, 2003.

Flores G, Vega LR: Barriers to health care access for Latino children: a review, *Fam Med* 30(3):196-205, 1998.

Flores G, Abreu M, Olivar MA, et al: Access barriers to health care for Latino children, *Arch Pediatr Adolesc Med* 152(11):1119-1125, 1998.

Franck LS, Harris SK, Soetenga DJ, et al: The Withdrawal Assessment Tool–1 (WAT-1): an assessment instrument for monitoring opioid and benzodiazepine withdrawal symptoms in pediatric patients, *Pediatr Crit Care Med* 9(6):573-580, 2008.

Franck LS, Vilardi J: Assessment and management of opioid withdrawal in ill neonates, *Neonat Netw* 14(2):39-48, 1995.

Franck LS, Vilardi J, Durand D, et al: Opioid withdrawal in neonates after continuous infusions of morphine or fentanyl during extracorporeal membrane oxygenation, *Am J Crit Care* 7(5):364-369, 1998.

Furdon SA, Eastman M, Benjamin K, et al: Outcome measures after standardized pain management strategies in postoperative patients in the neonatal intensive care unit, *J Perinat Neonatal Nurs* 12(1):58-69, 1998.

Gad LN, Olsen KS, Lysgaard AB, et al: Optimized use of EMLA cream in children—secondary publication: a randomized, prospective, controlled comparison of two application regimes, *Ugeskr Laeger* 167(4):404-407, 2005.

Gaina A, Sekine M, Chen X, et al: Validity of child sleep diary questionnaire among junior high school children, *J Epidemiol* 14(1):1-4, 2004.

Gharaibeh M, Abu-Saad H: Cultural validation of pediatric pain assessment tools: Jordanian perspective, *J Transcult Nurs* 13(1):12-18, 2002.

Goldschneider K, Anand K: Long-term consequences of pain in neonates. In Schechter N, Berde C, Yaster M, editors: *Pain in infants, children, and adolescents*, Philadelphia, 2003, Lippincott Williams & Wilkins.

Golianu B, Krane EJ, Galloway KS, et al: Pediatric acute pain management, *Pediatr Clin North Am* 47(3):559-587, 2000.

Goodenough B, Addicoat L, Champion GD, et al: Pain in 4- to 6-year-old children receiving intramuscular injections: a comparison of the Faces Pain Scale with other self-report and behavioral measures, *Clin J Pain* 13(1):60-73, 1997.

Gray L, Watt L, Blass E: Skin-to-skin contact is analgesic in healthy newborns, *Pediatrics* 105(1):110-111, 2000.

Hadden KL, von Baeyer CL: Pain in children with cerebral palsy: common triggers and expressive behaviors, *Pain* 99(1-2):281-288, 2002.

Hadjistavropoulos HD, Craig KD, Grunau RE, et al: Judging pain in infants: behavioural, contextual, and developmental determinants, *Pain* 73(3):319-324, 1997.

Haines DR, Gaines SP: N of 1 randomised controlled trials of oral ketamine in patients with chronic pain, *Pain* 83(2):283-287, 1999.

Hannallah RS, Broadman LM, Belman AB, et al: Comparison of caudal and ilioinguinal/iliohypogastric nerve blocks for control of post-orchiopexy pain in pediatric ambulatory surgery, *Anesthesiology* 66:832-834, 1987.

Hershey AD, Powers SW, Vockell AL, et al: Development of a patient-based grading scale for PedMIDAS. *Cephalalgia* 24(10):844-849, 2004.

Hershey AD, Powers SW, Vockell AL, et al: PedMIDAS: development of a questionnaire to assess disability of migraines in children, *Neurology* 57(11):2034-2039, 2001.

Hester NO, Foster RL, Jordan-Marsh M, et al: Putting pain measurement into clinical practice. In Finley GA, McGrath PJ, editors: *Measurement of pain in infants and children*, vol. 10, Seattle, 1998, International Association for the Study of Pain Press.

Hester N, Foster R, Kristensen K: Measurement of pain in children: generalizability and validity of the pain ladder and poker chip tool, *Adv Pain Res Ther* 15:79-84, 1990.

Hicks CL, von Baeyer CL, Spafford PA, et al: The Faces Pain Scale—Revised: toward a common metric in pediatric pain measurement, *Pain* 93(2):173-183, 2001.

Hodgkinson K, Bear M, Thorn J, et al: Measuring pain in neonates: evaluating an instrument and developing a common language, *Austral J Adv Nurs* 12(1):17-22, 1994.

Holden E, Deichmann M, Levy J: Empirically supported treatments in pediatric psychology: recurrent pediatric headache, *J Pediatr Psychol* 24:91-100, 1999.

Hu Y, Zhang G, Chen Z: Evaluation of pain tolerance of children in Xinjiang, China, from analgesic measures for surgery (abstract), *J Pain Symptom Manage* 6:205, 1991a.

Hu Y, Zhang G, Chen Z: Pain after burn injuries among Chinese children: a further study on transcultural and ethnic differences of pain (abstract), *J Pain Symptom Manage* 6:155, 1991b.

Jacob E, McCarthy KS, Sambuco G, et al: Intensity, location, and quality of pain in Spanish-speaking children with cancer, *Pediatr Nurs* 34(1):45-52, 2008.

Jacob E, Miaskowski C, Savedra M, et al: Changes in intensity, location, and quality of vaso-occlusive pain in children with sickle cell disease, *Pain* 102(1-2):187-193, 2003a.

Jacob E, Miaskowski C, Savedra M, et al: Management of vaso-occlusive pain in children with sickle cell disease, *J Pediatr Hematol Oncol* 25(4):307-311, 2003b.

Jacob E, Mueller BU: Pain experience of children with sickle cell disease who had prolonged hospitalizations for acute painful episodes, *Pain Med* 9(1):13-21, 2008.

Jacob E, Puntillo KA: Variability of analgesic practices for hospitalized children on different pediatric specialty units, *J Pain Symptom Manage* 20(1):59-67, 2000.

Johnston CC, Stevens B, Pinelli J, et al: Kangaroo care is effective in diminishing pain response in preterm neonates, *Arch Pediatr Adolesc Med* 157(11):1084-1088, 2003.

Jordan-Marsh M, Yoder L, Hall D, et al: Alternate Oucher form testing gender, ethnicity and age variations, *Res Nurs Health* 17:111-118, 1994.

Joyce BA, Schade JG, Keck JF, et al: Reliability and validity of preverbal pain assessment tools, *Issues Comp Pediatr Nurs* 17:121-135, 1994.

Keck JF, Gerkensmeyer JE, Joyce BA, et al: Reliability and validity of the Faces and Word Descriptor Scales to measure procedural pain, *J Pediatr Nurs* 11(6):368-374, 1996.

Kovacs M: Rating scales to assess depression in school-aged children, *Acta Paedopsychiatr* 46(5-6):305-315, 1981.

Klepstad P, Borchgrevink P, Hval B, et al: Long-term treatment with ketamine in a 12-year-old girl with severe neuropathic pain caused by a cervical spinal tumor, *J Pediatr Hematol Oncol* 23(9):616-619, 2001.

Krechel SW, Bildner J: CRIES: a new neonatal postoperative pain measurement score: initial testing of validity and reliability, *Pediatr Anaesth* 5:53-61, 1995.

Lawrence J, Alcock D, McGrath P, et al: The development of a tool to assess neonatal pain, *Neonat Netw* 12(6):59-66, 1993.

Lenton S, Stallard P, Lewis M, et al: Prevalence and morbidity associated with non-malignant, life-threatening conditions in childhood, *Child Care Health Devel* 27(5):389-398, 2001.

Ljungman G, Gordh T, Sorensen S, et al: Lumbar puncture in pediatric oncology: conscious sedation vs. general anesthesia, *Med Pediatr Oncol* 36(3):372-379, 2001.

Ljungman G, Gordh T, Sorensen S, et al: Pain variations during cancer treatment in children: a descriptive survey, *Pediatr Hematol Oncol* 17(3):211-221, 2000.

Ljungman G, Gordh T, Sorensen S, et al: Pain in paediatric oncology: interviews with children, adolescents and their parents, *Acta Paediatr* 88(6):623-630, 1999.

Ljungman G, Kreuger A, Andreasson S, et al: Midazolam nasal spray reduces procedural anxiety in children. *Pediatrics* 105(1 Pt 1):73-78, 2000.

Luffy R, Grove SK: Examining the validity, reliability, and preference of three pediatric pain measurement tools in African-American children, *Pediatr Nurs* 29(1):54-60, 2003.

Manworren R, Hynan L: Clinical validation of FLACC: Preverbal Patient Pain Scale, *Pediatr Nurs* 29(2):140-146, 2003.

Marx J: Pain research: prolonging the agony, *Science* 305(5682):326-329, 2004.

Max MB, Byas-Smith MG, Gracely RH, et al: Intravenous infusion of the NMDA antagonist, ketamine, in chronic posttraumatic pain with allodynia: a double-blind comparison to alfentanil and placebo, *Clin Neuropharmacol* 18(4):360-368, 1995.

Max MB, Payne R, Edwards WT, et al: *Principles of analgesic use in the treatment of acute pain and cancer pain*, Glenview, Ill, 1999, American Pain Society.

Maxwell L, Yaster M: Perioperative management issues in pediatric patients, *Anesthesiol Clin North Am* 18(3):601-632, 2000.

McCaffery M, Pasero C: *Pain clinical manual*, St. Louis, 1999, Mosby.

McGrath P, Hillier L, editors: *Modifying the psychologic factors that intensify children's pain and prolong disability*, Philadelphia, 2003, Lippincott Williams & Wilkins.

McGrath PJ, Johnson G, Goodman JT, et al: The CHEOPS: a behavioral scale to measure postoperative pain in children. In Fields H, Dubner R, Cervero F, editors: *Advances in pain research and therapy*, New York, 1985, Raven Press.

McGrath PJ, Walco GA, Turk DC, et al: Core outcome domains and measures for pediatric acute and chronic/recurrent pain clinical trials: PedIMMPACT recommendations, *J Pain* 9(9):771-783, 2008.

Melzack R: The McGill pain questionnaire: major properties and scoring methods, *Pain* 1:277-299, 1975.

Meredith JR, O'Keefe KP, Galwankar S: Pediatric procedural sedation and analgesia, *J Emerg Trauma Shock* 1(2):88-96, 2008.

Merkel SI, Voepel-Lewis T, Shayevitz JR, et al: The FLACC: a behavioral scale for scoring postoperative pain in young children, *Pediatr Nurs* 23(3):293-297, 1997.

Miaskowski C, Lee K: Pain, fatigue, and sleep disturbances in oncology outpatients receiving radiation therapy for bone metastasis: a pilot study, *J Pain Symptom Manage* 17(5):320-332, 1999.

Mitchell AC: An unusual case of chronic neuropathic pain responds to an optimum frequency of intravenous ketamine infusions, *J Pain Symptom Manage* 21(5):443-446, 2001.

Morin C, Gibson D, Wade J: Self-reported sleep and mood disturbance in chronic pain patients, *Clin J Pain* 14(4):311-314, 1998.

Myers C, Stuber ML, Bonamer-Rheingans JI, et al: Complementary therapies and childhood cancer, *Cancer Control* 12(3):172-180, 2005.

Nadvi SZ, Sarnaik S, Ravindranath Y: Low frequency of meperidine-associated seizures in sickle cell disease, *Clin Pediatr (Phila)* 38(8):459-462, 1999.

Owens JA, Spirito A, McGuinn M: The Children's Sleep Habits Questionnaire (CSHQ): psychometric properties of a survey instrument for school-aged children, *Sleep* 23(8):1043-1051, 2000.

Palermo TM: Impact of recurrent and chronic pain on child and family daily functioning: a critical review of the literature, *J Dev Behav Pediatr* 21(1):58-69, 2000.

Palermo TM, Kiska R: Subjective sleep disturbances in adolescents with chronic pain: relationship to daily functioning and quality of life, *J Pain* 6(3):201-207, 2005.

Palermo T, Valenzuela D: Use of pain diaries to assess recurrent and chronic pain in children, *Suffer Child* 3:1-14, 2003.

Palermo TM, Valenzuela D, Stork PP: A randomized trial of electronic versus paper pain diaries in children: impact on compliance, accuracy, and acceptability, *Pain* 107(3):213-219, 2004.

Perquin CW, Hazebroek-Kampschreur AA, Hunfeld JA, et al: Chronic pain among children and adolescents: physician consultation and medication use, *Clin J Pain* 16(3):229-235, 2000a.

Perquin CW, Hazebroek-Kampschreur AA, Hunfeld JA, et al: Pain in children and adolescents: a common experience, *Pain* 87(1):51-58, 2000b.

Puchalski M, Hummel P: The reality of neonatal pain, *Adv Neonatal Care* 2(5):233-244, 2002.

Reid GJ, Lang BA, McGrath PJ: Primary juvenile fibromyalgia: psychological adjustment, family functioning, coping, and functional disability, *Arthritis Rheum* 40(4):752-760, 1997.

Reis E, Holubkov R: Vapocoolant spray is equally effective as EMLA cream in reducing immunization pain in school-aged children, *Pediatrics* 100(6):e5, 1997.

Robieux I, Kumar R, Radhakrishnan S, et al: Assessing pain and analgesia with a lidocaine-prilocaine emulsion in infants and toddlers during venipuncture, *J Pediatr* 118(6):971-973, 1991.

Rogers TL, Ostrow CL: The use of EMLA cream to decrease venipuncture pain in children, *J Pediatr Nurs* 19(1):33-39, 2004.

Rusy L, Weisman S: Complementary therapies for acute pediatric pain management, *Pediatr Clin North Am* 47(3):589-599, 2000.

Sang CN: NMDA-receptor antagonists in neuropathic pain: experimental methods to clinical trials, *J Pain Symptom Manage* 19(1 Suppl):S21-S25, 2000.

Santiago A, Abad P, Fernandez C, et al: Premedication with EMLA cream for ambulatory surgery in children, *Ambu Surg* 8(3):157, 2000.

Savedra MC, Holzemer WL, Tesler MD, et al: Assessment of postoperation pain in children and adolescents using the adolescent pediatric pain tool, *Nurs Res* 42(1):5-9, 1993.

Savedra MC, Tesler MD, Holzemer WL, et al: Pain location: validity and reliability of body outline markings by hospitalized children and adolescents, *Res Nurs Health* 12:307-314, 1989.

Schade JG, Joyce BA, Gerkensmeyer J, et al: Comparison of three preverbal scales for postoperative pain assessment in a diverse pediatric sample, *J Pain Symptom Manage* 12(6):348-359, 1996.

Scott PJ, Ansell BM, Huskisson EC: Measurement of pain in juvenile chronic polyarthritis, *Ann Rheum Dis* 36(2):186-187, 1977.

See MC, Birnbaum AH, Schechter CB, et al: Double-blind, placebo-controlled trial of famotidine in children with abdominal pain and dyspepsia, *Dig Dis Sci* 46:985-992, 2001.

Sindrup SH, Otto M, Finnerup NB, et al: Antidepressants in the treatment of neuropathic pain, *Basic Clin Pharmacol Toxicol* 96(6):399-409, 2005.

Stallard P, Williams L, Lenton S, et al: Pain in cognitively impaired, non-communicating children, *Arch Dis Child* 85(6):460-462, 2001.

Stallard P, Williams L, Velleman R, et al: The development and evaluation of the pain indicator for communicatively impaired children (PICIC), *Pain* 98(1-2):145-149, 2002.

Stevens B: Development and testing of a pediatric pain management sheet, *Pediatr Nurs* 16(6):543-548, 1990.

Stevens B, Johnston C, Petryshen P, et al: Premature Infant Pain Profile: development and initial validation, *Clin J Pain* 12:13-22, 1996.

Stevens B, Yamada J, Ohlsson A: *Sucrose for analgesia in newborn infants undergoing painful procedures* (review), 2005. In Cochrane Neonatal Collaboration, available at www.thecochranelibrary.com (accessed November 30, 2009).

Stinson JN, Stevens BJ, Feldman BM, et al: Construct validity of a multidimensional electronic pain diary for adolescents with arthritis, *Pain* 136(3):281-292, 2008.

Stone AA, Broderick JE, Schwartz JE, et al: Intensive momentary reporting of pain with an electronic diary: reactivity, compliance, and patient satisfaction, *Pain* 104(1-2):343-351, 2003.

Suraseranivongse S, Montapaneewat T, Manon J, et al: Cross-validation of a self-report scale for postoperative pain in school-aged children, *J Med Assoc Thai* 88:412-418, 2005.

Sweet S, McGrath P: Physiological measures of pain. In Finley GA, McGrath PJ, editors: *Measurement of pain in infants and children*, Seattle, 1998, IASP Press.

Symon DN, Russell G: Double blind placebo controlled trial of pizotifen syrup in the treatment of abdominal migraine, *Arch Dis Child* 72(1):48-50, 1995.

Taddio A, Nulman I, Koren BS, et al: A revised measure of acute pain in infants, *J Pain Symptom Manage* 10(6):456-463, 1995.

Tarbell SE, Cohen IT, Marsh JL: The Toddler-Preschooler Postoperative Pain Scale: an observational scale for measuring postoperative pain in children aged 1-5: preliminary report, *Pain* 50(3):273-280, 1992.

Tesler MD, Savedra MC, Holzemer WL, et al: The word-graphic rating scale as a measure of children's and adolescents' pain intensity, *Res Nurs Health* 14:361-371, 1991.

Uziel Y, Berkovitch M, Gazarian M, et al: Evaluation of eutectic lidocaine/prilocaine cream (EMLA) for steroid joint injection in children with juvenile rheumatoid arthritis: a double blind, randomized, placebo controlled trial, *J Rheumatol* 30(3):594-596, 2003.

Van Cleve L, Bossert E, Beecroft P, et al: The pain experience of children with leukemia during the first year after diagnosis, *Nurs Res* 53(1):1-10, 2004.

Van Cleve L, Muñoz C, Bossert EA, et al: Children's and adolescents' pain language in Spanish: translation of a measure, *Pain Manage Nurs* 2(3):110-118, 2001.

Van Dijk A, McGrath PA, Pickett W, et al: Pain prevalence in 9- to 13-year-old schoolchildren, *Pain Res Manage* 11(4):234-240, 2006.

Varni JW, Seid M, Rode CA: The PedsQL: measurement model for the pediatric quality of life inventory, *Med Care* 37(2):126-139, 1999.

Varni JW, Thompson KL, Hanson V: The Varni/Thompson Pediatric Pain Questionnaire, part I, Chronic musculoskeletal pain in juvenile rheumatoid arthritis, *Pain* 28:27-38, 1987.

Vervoort T, Goubert L, Eccleston C, et al: Catastrophic thinking about pain is independently associated with pain severity, disability, and somatic complaints in school children and children with chronic pain, *J Pediatr Psychol* 31(7):674-683, 2006.

Villarruel AM, Denyes MJ: Pain assessment in children: theoretical and empirical validity, *Adv Nurs Sci* 14(2):32-41, 1991.

von Baeyer C, Hicks C: Support for a common metric for pediatric pain intensity scales, *Pain Res Manage* 4(2):157-160, 2000.

Walker LS, Greene JW: The functional disability inventory: measuring a neglected dimension of child health status, *J Pediatr Psychol* 16(1):39-58, 1991.

Walters A, Williamson G: The role of activity restriction in the association between pain and depression: a study of pediatric patients with chronic pain, *Child Health Care* 28:33-50, 1999.

Weisman S, Bernstein B, Schechter N: Consequences of inadequate analgesia during painful procedures in children, *Arch Pediatr Adolesc Med* 152:147-149, 1998.

West N, Oakes L, Hinds PS, et al: Measuring pain in pediatric oncology ICU patients, *J Pediatr Oncol Nurs* 11(2):64-70, 1994.

Weydert J, Ball T, Davis M: Systematic review of treatments for recurrent abdominal pain, *Pediatrics* 111(1):1-3, 2003.

Wilkie DJ, Holzemer WL, Tesler MD, et al: Measuring pain quality: validity and reliability of children's and adolescents' pain language, *Pain* 41(2):151-159, 1990.

Wong DL, Baker CM: Pain in children: comparison of assessment scales, *Pediatr Nurs* 14(1):9-17, 1988.

Wong D, Pasero CL: Reducing the pain of lidocaine, *Am J Nurs* 97(1):17-18, 1997a.

Wong D, Pasero CL: Using local anesthetics to control procedural pain, *Am J Nurs* 97(1):17, 1997b.

Woodgate R, Yanofsky R: A different perspective to approaching cancer symptoms in children, *J Pain Symptom Manage* 26(3):800-817, 2004.

Woolf CJ, Salter MW: Neuronal plasticity: increasing the gain in pain, *Science* 288(5472):1765-1769, 2000.

Yaster M, Krance EJ, Kaplan RF, et al: *Pediatric pain management and sedation handbook*, St. Louis, 1997, Mosby.

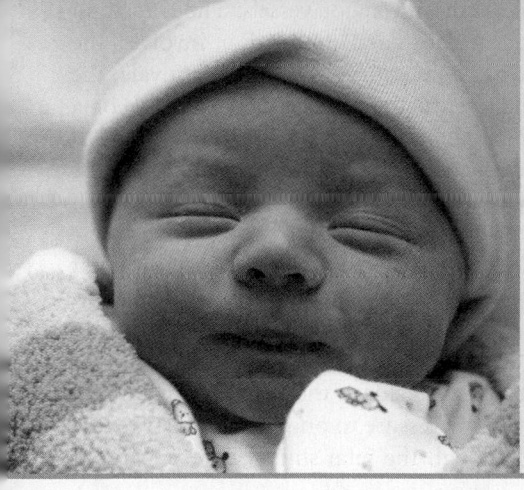

Health Promotion of the Newborn and Family

Barbara J. Wheeler

Evolve WEBSITE

http://evolve.elsevier.com/wong/ncic

Anatomy Review
  Location of Sutures and Fontanels
Animations
  Bradycardia
  Fetal Circulation
Case Studies
  Breast-Feeding
  The Normal Newborn
Critical Thinking Exercises
  Circumcision
  Formula Preparation
Key Points Audio Summaries
NCLEX Review Questions
Pediatric Assessment Video Clips
Skill
  Infant Feeding
Spanish/English Translations
WebLinks

RELATED TOPICS

Administration of Medication, **Ch. 27**
Ambiguous Genitalia, **Ch. 11**
Birth Injuries, **Ch. 9**
Blood Specimens, **Ch. 27**
Cardiac Development and Function: Embryologic
  Development, **Ch. 34**
Changes in Fluid Volume Related to Growth, **Ch. 28**
Congenital Heart Disease, **Ch. 34**
Dermatologic Problems in the Newborn, **Ch. 9**
Diaper Dermatitis, **Ch. 13**
Fluoride, **Ch. 14**
The High-Risk Newborn and Family, **Ch. 10**
Motor Vehicle Injuries, **Chs. 12 and 14**
Multiple Births, **Ch. 3**
Neonatal Pain, **Ch. 7**
Nutrition, **Ch. 12**
Physical Examination, **Ch. 6**
Sibling Rivalry, **Ch. 14**
The Skin, **Ch. 18**

CHAPTER OUTLINE

ADJUSTMENT TO EXTRAUTERINE LIFE

The most profound physiologic change required of the newborn is transition from fetal or placental circulation to independent respiration. The loss of the placental connection means the loss of complete metabolic support, particularly the supply of oxygen and the removal of carbon dioxide. The normal stresses of labor and delivery cause alterations in placental gas exchange patterns, acid-base balance in the blood, and cardiovascular activity in the neonate. Factors that interfere with normal transition or increase fetal hypoxia, hypercapnia, and acidosis will affect the fetus's adjustment to extrauterine life.

IMMEDIATE ADJUSTMENTS

Respiratory System

The most critical and immediate physiologic change required of the newborn is the onset of breathing. The stimuli that help initiate respiration are primarily chemical and thermal. Chemical factors in the blood (low oxygen, high carbon dioxide, and low pH) initiate impulses that excite the respiratory center in the medulla. The primary thermal stimulus is the sudden chilling of the infant, who leaves a warm environment and enters a relatively cooler atmosphere. This abrupt change in temperature excites sensory impulses in the skin that are transmitted to the respiratory center. Tactile stimulation may assist in initiating respiration. Descent through the birth canal and normal handling during delivery, such as drying the skin, help stimulate respiration in uncompromised infants. Acceptable methods of tactile stimulation include slapping or flicking the soles of the feet or gently rubbing the newborn's back, trunk, or extremities (American Academy of Pediatrics, 2006a). Slapping the newborn's buttocks or back is a harmful technique and should not be done. Prolonged tactile stimulation, beyond one or two slaps or flicks to the soles of the feet or rubbing the back once or twice, can waste precious time in the event of respiratory difficulty and can cause additional damage in infants who have become hypoxemic before or during the birth process.

The initial entry of air into the lungs is opposed by the surface tension of the fluid that filled the fetal lungs and alveoli. Some fetal lung fluid is removed during the normal forces of labor and delivery. As the chest emerges from the birth canal, fluid is squeezed from the lungs through the nose and mouth. After complete emergence of the neonate's chest, a brisk recoil of the thorax occurs. Air enters the upper airway to replace the lost fluid. In cesarean birth the chest is not compressed, and the newborn may need additional respiratory support or monitoring until remaining fetal lung fluid is absorbed by the pulmonary capillaries and lymphatic vessels.

In the alveoli the fluid's surface tension is reduced by **surfactant**, a substance produced by the alveolar epithelium that coats the alveolar surface. Chapter 10 discusses the effect of surfactant in facilitating breathing in relation to respiratory distress syndrome.

Circulatory System

As important as the initiation of respiration are the circulatory changes that allow blood to flow through the lungs. These changes occur more gradually and are the result of pressure changes in the lungs, heart, and major vessels. The transition from fetal circulation to postnatal circulation involves the functional closure of the **fetal shunts**: the foramen ovale, the ductus arteriosus, and eventually the ductus venosus. (For a brief review of fetal circulation, see Chapter 34.)

Once the lungs are expanded, the inspired oxygen dilates the pulmonary vessels, which decreases pulmonary vascular resistance and consequently increases pulmonary blood flow. As the lungs receive blood, the pressure in the right atrium, right ventricle, and pulmonary arteries decreases. At the same time, there is a progressive rise in systemic vascular resistance and an increased volume of blood as a result of cord clamping. This increases the pressure in the left side of the heart. Because blood flows from an area of high pressure to one of low pressure, the circulation of blood through the fetal shunts is reversed (see Fig. 34-2).

The most important factor controlling ductal closure is the increased oxygen concentration of the blood. Secondary factors are the fall in endogenous prostaglandins and acidosis. The foramen ovale closes functionally at or soon after birth from compression of the two portions of the atrial septum. The ductus arteriosus is closed functionally by the fourth day in well neonates, but closure may be delayed in ill or preterm infants. Anatomic closure from deposition of fibrin and cell products takes considerably longer. Because of the reversible flow of blood through the ductus arteriosus during the early neonatal period, a functional murmur is occasionally heard.

PHYSIOLOGIC STATUS OF OTHER SYSTEMS

Thermoregulation

Next to establishing respiration, heat regulation is most critical to the newborn's survival. Although the newborn's capacity for heat production is adequate, several factors predispose the newborn to excessive heat loss. First, the newborn's large surface area relative to his or her weight facilitates heat loss to the environment. The newborn's large body surface is partially compensated for by a usual position of flexion, which decreases the amount of surface area exposed to the environment.

The second factor that contributes to loss of body heat is the newborn's thin layer of subcutaneous fat. Since core body temperature is approximately 1°F (~0.5°C) higher than surface body temperature, this temperature gradient (difference) causes a heat transfer from a higher to lower temperature.

A third factor is the newborn's mechanism for producing heat. Unlike the child or adult, who can increase heat production through shivering, the chilled neonate cannot shiver but produces heat through **nonshivering thermogenesis (NST)**. NST (or chemical thermogenesis) is produced by stimulating cellular respiration, resulting in increased need for oxygen and glucose (see Thermoregulation, Chapter 10). A thermogenic source unique to the full-term newborn is **brown adipose tissue (BAT)**, or brown fat, which owes its name to its larger content of mitochondrial cytochromes. BAT has a greater capacity for heat production through intensified metabolic activity than does ordinary adipose tissue. Heat generated in the brown fat is distributed to other parts of the body by the blood, which is warmed as it flows through the layers of this tissue.

Superficial deposits of brown fat are located between the scapulae, around the neck, in the axillae, and behind the sternum. Deeper layers surround the kidneys, trachea, esophagus, some major arteries, and adrenals. The location of the brown fat may explain why the nape of the neck often feels warmer than the rest of the body. Brown fat can affect the accuracy of axillary temperature measurement (see p. 242).

Because of these factors predisposing infants to loss of body heat, it is essential that newly born infants are quickly dried and either provided with warm, dry blankets or placed skin-to-skin with their mothers after delivery.

Although concern is usually for newborns' ability to conserve heat, they also can have difficulty dissipating heat in an overheated environment, increasing the risk of hyperthermia.

Hematopoietic System

The blood volume of the newborn depends largely on the amount of blood transferred via the placenta before clamping of the cord. The blood volume of the full-term infant is about 80 to 85 ml/kg of body weight. Immediately after birth the total blood volume averages 300 ml, but, depending on how long the infant is attached to the placenta, as much as 100 ml can be added to the blood volume. Common laboratory test blood values for the newborn are listed in Appendix C.

Fluid and Electrolyte Balance

Changes occur in the total body water volume, extracellular fluid volume, and intracellular fluid volume during the transition from fetal to postnatal life. The fetus is composed almost entirely of water early in gestation and at term is 73% fluid, compared with 58% in the adult. The fetus has more extracellular fluid than intracellular fluid, but this shifts progressively throughout postnatal life, probably because of the growth of cells at the expense of extracellular fluid. The infant has a proportionately higher ratio of extracellular fluid than the adult and consequently has a higher level of total body sodium and chloride and a lower level of potassium, magnesium, and phosphate (see Chapter 28).

An important aspect of fluid balance is its relationship to other systems. The rate of fluid exchange is seven times greater in the infant than in the adult, and the infant's rate of metabolism is twice as great in relation to body weight. As a result, twice as much acid is formed, leading to more rapid development of acidemia. In addition, the immature kidneys cannot sufficiently concentrate urine to conserve body water. These three factors make the infant more prone to dehydration, acidosis, and overhydration.

Gastrointestinal System

The newborn's ability to digest, absorb, and metabolize food is adequate but limited in certain functions. Enzymes are available to catalyze proteins and simple carbohydrates (monosaccharides and disaccharides), but deficient production of pancreatic amylase impairs utilization of complex carbohydrates (polysaccharides). A deficiency of pancreatic lipase limits the absorption of fats, especially with ingestion of foods that have high saturated fatty acid content, such as cow's milk. Human milk, despite its high fat content, is easy to digest and absorb because it contains enzymes such as lipase, which assist in digestion.

The liver is the most immature of the gastrointestinal organs. The activity of the enzyme glucuronyl transferase is reduced, affecting the conjugation of bilirubin with glucuronic acid, which contributes to physiologic jaundice of the newborn. The liver is also deficient in forming plasma proteins, which likely plays a role in the edema usually seen at birth. Prothrombin and other coagulation factors are also low. The liver stores less glycogen at birth than later in life. Consequently, the newborn is prone to hypoglycemia, which may be prevented by early and effective feeding, especially breast-feeding.

Some salivary glands are functioning at birth, but the majority do not begin to secrete saliva until about age 2 to 3 months, when drooling is common. The stomach capacity is limited to about 90 ml in an average-sized full-term infant (3.4 kg [7.5 lb]); thus the infant requires frequent small feedings. Newborns who breast-feed usually have more frequent feedings and more frequent stools than infants who receive formula.

The infant's intestine is longer in relation to body size than that in the adult. Therefore it has a proportionately larger number of secretory glands and a larger surface area for absorption compared with the adult's intestine. Rapid peristaltic waves and simultaneous nonperistaltic waves occur along the entire intestine. These waves, called the **migrating motor complex (MMC)**, propel nutrients forward. The relative immaturity of the MMC, combined with decreased lower esophageal sphincter (LES) pressure, inappropriate relaxation of the LES, and delayed gastric emptying, makes regurgitation a common occurrence. Progressive changes in the stooling pattern indicate a properly functioning gastrointestinal tract (Box 8-1).

Renal System

All structural components are present in the renal system, but the kidney has a functional deficiency in its ability to concentrate urine and to cope with fluid and electrolyte fluctuations, such as dehydration or a concentrated solute load.

Total volume of urinary output per 24 hours is about 200 to 300 ml by the end of the first week. The bladder involuntarily empties when stretched by a volume of 15 ml, resulting in as

---

BOX 8-1 CHANGE IN STOOLING PATTERNS OF NEWBORNS

Meconium
This is the infant's first stool, composed of amniotic fluid and its constituents, intestinal secretions, shed mucosal cells, and possibly blood (ingested maternal blood or minor bleeding of alimentary tract vessels).
Passage of meconium occurs within the first 24 hours for the vast majority of newborns, although it is delayed in premature infants (Metaj, Laroia, Lawrence, et al, 2003).

Transitional Stools
These usually appear by the third day after initiation of feeding.
They are greenish brown to yellowish brown, thin, and less sticky than meconium and may contain some milk curds.

Milk Stools
These usually appear by the fourth day.
In breast-fed infants stools are yellow to golden, are pasty in consistency, and have an odor similar to that of sour milk.
In formula-fed infants stools are pale yellow to light brown, are firmer in consistency, and have a more offensive odor.

many as 20 voidings per day. The first voiding should occur within 24 hours. The urine is colorless and odorless and has a specific gravity of approximately 1.020.

Integumentary System

At birth all the structures within the skin are present, but many of the functions of the integument are immature. The two layers of the skin, the epidermis and dermis, are loosely bound to each other and are very thin. Rete pegs, which later in life anchor the epidermis to the dermis, are not developed. Slight friction across the epidermis, such as from rapid removal of tape, can cause separation of these layers and blister formation or loss of the epidermis. In full-term infants the transitional zone between the cornified and living layers of the epidermis is effective in preventing fluid from reaching the skin surface.

The sebaceous glands are active late in fetal life and in early infancy because of high levels of maternal androgens. They are most densely located on the scalp, face, and genitalia and produce the grayish white, greasy vernix caseosa that covers the infant at birth. Plugging of the sebaceous glands causes milia.

The eccrine glands, which produce sweat in response to heat or emotional stimuli, are functional at birth, and by 3 weeks of age palmar sweating on crying reaches levels equivalent to those of anxious adults. Observing palmar sweating is helpful in assessing pain. The eccrine glands produce sweat in response to higher temperatures than those required in adults, and the retention of sweat may result in milia. The apocrine glands, sweat glands that develop as attachments to hair follicles, remain small and nonfunctional until puberty.

The growth phases of hair follicles usually occur simultaneously at birth. During the first few months the synchrony between hair loss and regrowth is disrupted, and there may be overgrowth of hair or temporary alopecia. Boys' hair grows faster than girls' hair, and in both sexes scalp hair growth is slower at the crown.

Because the amount of melanin is low at birth, newborns are lighter skinned than they will be as children. Consequently, infants are more susceptible to the harmful effects of ultraviolet light such as the sun.

Musculoskeletal System

At birth the skeletal system contains larger amounts of cartilage than ossified bone, although the process of ossification is fairly rapid during the first year. The nose, for example, is predominantly cartilage at birth and is frequently flattened by the force of delivery. The six skull bones are relatively soft and not yet joined. The sinuses are incompletely formed as well.

Unlike the skeletal system, the muscular system is almost completely formed at birth. Hypertrophy, rather than hyperplasia, of cells causes the growth in the size of muscular tissue.

Defenses Against Infection

The infant is born with several defenses against infection. The first line of defense is the skin and mucous membranes, which protect the body from invading organisms. The second line of defense is the cellular elements of the immunologic system, which produces several types of cells capable of attacking a pathogen. The neutrophils and monocytes are phagocytes, cells that engulf, ingest, and destroy foreign agents. Eosinophils also probably have a phagocytic property because in the presence of foreign protein they increase in number. The lymphocytes (T and B cells) are capable of being converted to other cell types, such as monocytes and antibodies. Although the phagocytic properties of the blood are present in the infant, the tissues' inflammatory response to localize an infection is immature.

The third line of defense is the formation of specific antibodies to an antigen. This process requires exposure to various foreign agents for antibody production to occur. Infants are generally not capable of producing their own immunoglobulins until the beginning of the second month of life, but they receive considerable passive immunity in the form of immunoglobulin G (IgG) from the maternal circulation and from human milk (see p. 260). They are protected against most major childhood diseases, including diphtheria, measles, poliomyelitis, and rubella, for about 3 months, provided that the mother has developed antibodies to these illnesses.

Endocrine System

Ordinarily, the newborn's endocrine system is adequately developed, but its functions are immature. For example, the posterior lobe of the pituitary gland produces limited quantities of antidiuretic hormone, or vasopressin, which inhibits diuresis. This renders the newborn highly susceptible to dehydration.

The effect of maternal sex hormones is particularly evident in the newborn. The labia are hypertrophied, and the breasts in both sexes may be engorged and secrete milk (witch's milk) during the first few days of life to as long as 2 months of age. Female newborns may have pseudomenstruation (more often seen as a milky secretion rather than actual blood) from a sudden drop in progesterone and estrogen levels.

Neurologic System

At birth the nervous system is incompletely integrated but sufficiently developed to sustain extrauterine life. Most neurologic functions are primitive reflexes. The autonomic nervous system is crucial during transition because it stimulates initial respirations, helps maintain acid-base balance, and partially regulates temperature control.

Myelination of the nervous system follows the cephalocaudal-proximodistal (head-to-toe–center-to-periphery) laws of development and is closely related to the observed mastery of fine and gross motor skills. Myelin is necessary for rapid and efficient transmission of some, but not all, nerve impulses along the neural pathway. Tracts that develop myelin earliest are the sensory, cerebellar, and extrapyramidal. This accounts for the acute senses of taste, smell, and hearing and the perception of pain in the newborn. All cranial nerves are myelinated except the optic and olfactory nerves.

Sensory Functions

The newborn's sensory functions are remarkably well developed and have a significant effect on growth and development, including the attachment process.

Vision

At birth the eye is structurally incomplete. The fovea centralis is not yet completely differentiated from the macula. The ciliary muscles are also immature, limiting the eyes' ability to accommodate and fixate on an object for any length of time. The pupils react to light, the blink reflex is responsive to minimum stimulus, and the corneal reflex is activated by a light touch. Tear glands usually do not begin to function until 2 to 4 weeks of age.

The newborn has the ability to momentarily fixate on a bright or moving object that is within 20 cm (8 inches) and in the midline of the visual field. In fact, the infant's ability to fixate or coordinate movement is greater during the first hour of life than during the succeeding several days. Visual acuity is reported to be between 20/100 and 20/400, depending on the vision measurement techniques (see Table 6-9).

The infant also demonstrates visual preferences: medium colors (yellow, green, pink) over dim or bright colors (red, orange, blue); black-and-white contrasting patterns, especially geometric shapes and checkerboards; large objects with medium complexity rather than small, complex objects; and reflecting objects over dull ones.

Hearing

Once the amniotic fluid has drained from the ears, the infant probably has auditory acuity similar to that of an adult. The newborn is able to detect a loud sound of about 90 dB and reacts with a startle (Moro) reflex. The newborn's response to sounds of low frequency and high frequency differs; the former, such as a heartbeat, metronome, or lullaby, tends to decrease an infant's motor activity and crying, whereas the latter elicits an alerting reaction.

Infants have an early sensitivity to the sound of human voices and to specific speech sounds. For example, infants younger than 3 days of age can distinguish their mother's voice from that of other females. As early as 5 days, newborns can differentiate between stories read by their mother's voice (in utero) versus stories read by another woman's voice after birth.

The internal and middle ear structures are large at birth, but the external canal is small. The mastoid process and the bony part of the external canal have not yet developed. Consequently, the tympanic membrane and facial nerve are close to the surface and can be easily damaged.

Smell

Newborns react to strong odors such as alcohol or vinegar by turning their heads away. Breast-fed infants are able to smell breast milk and will cry for their mothers when the breasts are leaking. Infants are also able to differentiate their mother's breast milk from that of other women by scent alone. Many believe maternal odors influence the attachment process and successful breast-feeding. Unnecessary routine washing of the breasts may interfere with establishment of early breast-feeding.

Taste

The newborn can distinguish between tastes, and various types of solutions elicit differing facial reflexes. A tasteless solution elicits no facial expression; a sweet solution elicits an eager suck and a look of satisfaction; a sour solution causes the usual puckering of the lips; and a bitter liquid produces an angry, upset expression.

Touch

The newborn perceives tactile sensation in any part of the body, although the face (especially the mouth), hands, and soles of the feet seem to be most sensitive. Sufficient evidence now shows that touch and motion are essential components in the attachment process and in normal growth and development. Gentle patting of the back or rubbing of the abdomen usually elicits a calming response from the infant. However, painful stimuli, such as a pinprick, elicit an upset response.

NURSING CARE OF THE NEWBORN AND FAMILY

ASSESSMENT

The newborn requires thorough, skilled observation to ensure a satisfactory adjustment to extrauterine life. Physical assessment after delivery is divided into four phases: (1) the initial assessment, which includes the Apgar scoring system; (2) transitional assessment during periods of reactivity; (3) assessment of gestational age; and (4) a comprehensive, systematic physical examination. In addition, the nurse must be aware of those behaviors that signal successful attachment between the infant and parents. Awareness of the expected normal findings during each assessment process helps the nurse recognize any deviation that may prevent the infant from progressing unevenfully through the early postnatal period. With shorter hospital stays, accomplishing a thorough newborn assessment and comprehensive parent teaching may be a challenge (see p. 271).

Initial Assessment: Apgar Scoring

The most frequently used method to assess the newborn's immediate adjustment to extrauterine life is the Apgar scoring system (Stoll, 2007). The score is based on observation of heart rate, respiratory effort, muscle tone, reflex irritability, and color (Table 8-1). Each item is given a score of 0, 1, or 2. Evaluations of all five categories are made 1 and 5 minutes after birth and are repeated every 5 minutes until the infant's condition stabilizes. Total scores of 0 to 3 represent severe distress, scores of 4 to 6 signify moderate difficulty, and scores of 7 to 10 indicate absence of difficulty in adjusting to extrauterine life. Many healthy newborns do not achieve a score of 10 because the body is not completely pink. The degree of physiologic immaturity

TABLE 8-1	INFANT EVALUATION AT BIRTH: APGAR SCORING SYSTEM		
SIGN	**0**	**1**	**2**
Heart rate	Absent	Slow, <100 beats/min	>100 beats/min
Respiratory effort	Absent	Irregular, slow, weak cry	Good, strong cry
Muscle tone	Limp	Some flexion of extremities	Well flexed
Reflex irritability	No response	Grimace	Cry, sneeze
Color	Blue, pale	Body pink, extremities blue	Completely pink

affects the Apgar score. For example, a healthy preterm infant may receive a low score due to low tone and reduced reflex irritability. Infection, congenital anomalies, maternal sedation or analgesia, hypovolemia, and neuromuscular disorders also affect the Apgar score.

The Apgar score reflects the infant's general condition at 1 and 5 minutes based on the five parameters described above. The Apgar score is not a tool, however, that stands on its own to either interpret past events or predict future events linked to the infant's neurologic or physical status. The Apgar score is not used to determine the newborn's need for resuscitation at birth; when necessary, resuscitative efforts should begin before the 1-minute Apgar score is obtained (American Academy of Pediatrics, 2006b).

Transitional Assessment: Periods of Reactivity

The newborn exhibits behavioral and physiologic characteristics that can at first appear to be signs of stress. During a newborn's initial 24 hours, changes in heart rate, respiration, motor activity, color, mucus production, and bowel activity occur in an orderly, predictable sequence, which is normal and indicates lack of stress. Distressed infants also progress through these stages but at a slower rate.

For 6 to 8 hours after birth the newborn is in the first period of reactivity. During the first 30 minutes the infant is alert, cries vigorously, may suck his or her fingers or fist, and appears interested in the environment. At this time the neonate's eyes are usually open; thus this is an excellent opportunity for mother, father, and child to see each other. Because the healthy, full-term newborn has a vigorous suck reflex, this is an opportune time to begin breast-feeding. The newborn usually grasps the nipple quickly, satisfying both mother and child. This is particularly important to remember, because it is likely that after this initial highly active state the infant may be sleepy and uninterested in sucking. Physiologically the respiratory rate can be as high as 80 breaths/min, crackles may be heard, heart rate may reach 180 beats/min, bowel sounds are active, mucus secretions are increased, and temperature may decrease slightly.

After this initial stage of alertness and activity, the infant enters the second stage of the first reactive period, which generally lasts 2 to 4 hours. Heart and respiratory rates decrease, temperature continues to fall, mucus production decreases, and urine or stool is usually not passed. The infant is in a state of sleep and relative calm. Any attempt at stimulation usually elicits a minimal response. Because of the decrease in body temperature, avoid undressing or bathing the infant during this time.

The second period of reactivity begins when the infant wakes from this deep sleep; it lasts about 2 to 5 hours and provides another excellent opportunity for child and parents to interact. The infant is again alert and responsive, heart and respiratory rates increase, the gag reflex is active, gastric and respiratory secretions are increased, and passage of meconium commonly occurs. This period is usually over when the amount of respiratory mucus has decreased. After this stage is a period of stabilization of physiologic systems and a vacillating pattern of sleep and activity.

Behavioral Assessment

An important area of assessment is observation of behavior. Infants' behavior helps shape their environment, and their

---

> **BOX 8-2   CLUSTERS OF NEONATAL BEHAVIORS IN BRAZELTON NEONATAL BEHAVIORAL ASSESSMENT SCALE**
>
> **Habituation**—Ability to respond to and then inhibit response to discrete stimulus (light, rattle, bell, pinprick) while asleep
> **Orientation**—Quality of alert states and ability to attend to visual and auditory stimuli while alert
> **Motor performance**—Quality of movement and tone
> **Range of state**—Measure of general arousal level or arousability of infant
> **Regulation of state**—How infant responds when aroused
> **Autonomic stability**—Signs of stress (tremors, startles, skin color) related to homeostatic (self-regulating) adjustment of the nervous system
> **Reflexes**—Assessment of several neonatal reflexes

Data from Brazelton TB, Nugent JK: *Neonatal behavioural assessment scale*, London, 1996, MacKeith Press.

---

ability to react to various stimuli affects how others relate to them. The principal areas of behavior for newborns are sleep, wakefulness, and activity such as crying.

One method of systematically assessing the infant's behavior is use of the Brazelton Neonatal Behavioral Assessment Scale (BNBAS) (Brazelton and Nugent, 1996). The BNBAS is an interactive examination that assesses the infant's response to 28 items organized in clusters (Box 8-2). It is generally used as a research or diagnostic tool and requires special training.

In addition to its use as an initial and ongoing tool to assess neurologic and behavioral responses, the scale can be used to assess initial parent-child relationships; to help identify caregivers who may benefit from a role model; and to guide parents, helping them focus on their infant's individuality and develop a deeper attachment. Studies have demonstrated that, by showing parents the unique characteristics of their infant, health care providers can enable them to develop a more positive perception of the infant, with increased interaction between infant and parents.

Patterns of Sleep and Activity

Newborns begin life with a systematic schedule of sleep and activity that is initially evident during the periods of reactivity. For the next 2 or 3 days most infants sleep almost constantly to recover from the exhausting birth process.

Infants have six distinct sleep-wake states, which represent a particular form of neural control (Table 8-2). As gestational and postconceptional maturity increases, each state becomes more precisely defined according to the behaviors observed. State is defined as a "group of characteristics that regularly occur together" (Blackburn, 2007); these include body activity, eye and facial movements, respiratory pattern, and response to internal and external stimuli. The six sleep-wake states are quiet (deep) sleep, active (light) sleep, drowsy, awake (quiet), active alert, and crying. Infants respond to internal and external environmental factors by controlling sensory input and regulating the sleep-wake states; the ability to make smooth transitions between states is called state modulation. The ability to regulate sleep-wake states is essential in the infant's neurobehavioral development. The more immature the infant, the less he or she is able to cope with factors, external or internal, that affect the sleep-wake patterns.

TABLE 8-2	STATES OF SLEEP AND ACTIVITY
STATE AND BEHAVIOR	**IMPLICATIONS FOR PARENTS**
Deep Sleep (Quiet) Closed eyes Regular breathing No movement except for occasional sudden bodily twitch No eye movement	Continue usual household noises because external stimuli do not arouse infant. Leave infant alone if sudden loud noise awakens infant and child cries. Do not attempt to feed.
Light Sleep (Active) Closed eyes Irregular breathing Slight muscular twitching of body Rapid eye movements under closed eyelids May smile	External stimuli that did not arouse infant during regular sleep may minimally arouse child. Periodic groaning or crying is usual; do not interpret as indication of pain or discomfort.
Drowsy Eyes may be open Irregular breathing Active body movement variable, with occasional mild startles	Most stimuli arouse infant, but infant may return to sleep state. Pick infant up during this time rather than leaving in crib. Provide mild stimulus to awaken. Infant may enjoy nonnutritive sucking.
Quiet Alert Eyes wide open and bright Responds to environment by active body movement and staring at close-range objects Minimum body activity Regular breathing Focuses attention on stimuli	Satisfy infant's needs such as hunger or nonnutritive sucking. Place infant in area of home where activity is continuous. Place toys in crib or playpen. Place objects within 17.5-20 cm (7-8 inches) of infant's view. Intervene to console.
Active Alert May begin with whimpering and slight body movement Eyes open Irregular breathing	Remove intense internal or external stimuli because of increased sensitivity to stimuli.
Crying Progresses to strong, angry crying and uncoordinated thrashing of extremities Eyes open or tightly closed Grimaces Irregular breathing	Comforting measures that were effective during alert state are usually ineffective. Rock and swaddle to decrease crying. Intervene to reduce fatigue, hunger, or discomfort.

Portions adapted from Blackburn S, Loper DL: *Maternal, fetal, and neonatal physiology: a clinical perspective*, Philadelphia, 1992, Saunders.

Recognition and knowledge of sleep-wake states are important in planning nursing care. It is also important for nurses to help parents and caregivers understand the significance of the infant's behavioral responses to daily caregiving and how these states can be altered. A classic example is the newborn who feeds vigorously in the active alert state but not in the deep sleep state. The neurologic assessment of a newborn will differ significantly in these two states. Newborns typically spend as much as 16 to 18 hours a day sleeping and do not necessarily follow a pattern of light-dark diurnal rhythm. With increasing age, sleep-wake states change, with increasing amounts of time spent in awake alert states and decreasing amounts in sleep time. Approximately 50% of total sleep time is spent in irregular or rapid eye movement sleep.

Cry

The newborn should begin extrauterine life with a strong, lusty cry. The sounds produced by crying can be described as hunger, anger, pain, and "bid for attention" cries. Discomfort (pain) sounds initially consist of gasps and cries in which the consonant *H* is clearly distinguishable. The duration of crying in each infant varies as much as the duration of sleep. Some newborns may cry for as little as 5 minutes or as much as 2 hours or more per day.

Variations in the initial cry can indicate underlying abnormalities. A weak, groaning cry or grunting during expiration usually indicates a respiratory disturbance. Absent, weak, or constant crying may suggest a pathologic state such as tension pneumothorax or perinatal asphyxia. Crying status alone, however, is not a diagnostic tool.

Assessment of Attachment Behaviors

One of the most important areas of assessment is careful observation of those behaviors thought to indicate the formation of emotional bonds between the newborn and family, especially the mother. Although bonding and attachment are sometimes referred to as separate phenomena, with bonding representing the development of emotional ties from parent to infant and attachment representing the emotional ties from infant to parent, in this discussion and the one on p. 268, the terms are used interchangeably to denote both processes.

Unlike physical assessment of the neonate, which follows concrete guidelines, assessment of parent-child attachment requires much more skill in terms of observation and interviewing. The assessment process is even more challenging with short hospital stays for mothers and their newborn infants. Rooming-in of mother and infant and visits by father, siblings, and grandparents facilitate recognition of behaviors that demonstrate positive or negative attachment. Guidelines for assessment of bonding behaviors are in the Nursing Care Guidelines box.

📋 NURSING CARE GUIDELINES

Assessing Attachment Behavior

- When you bring the infant to the parents, do they reach out for the child and call the child by name?
- Do the parents speak about the child in terms of identification (e.g., whom the infant looks like; what appears special about their child compared with other infants)?
- When parents are holding the infant, what kind of body contact is there? Do parents feel at ease in changing the infant's position; are fingertips or whole hands used; are there parts of the body they avoid touching or parts of the body they investigate and scrutinize?
- When the infant is awake, what kinds of stimulation do the parents provide? Do they talk to the infant, to each other, or to no one? How do they look at the infant—direct visual contact, avoidance of eye contact, or looking at other people or objects?
- How comfortable do the parents appear in terms of caring for the infant? Do they express any concern regarding their ability or disgust for certain activities, such as changing diapers?
- What type of affection do they demonstrate to the newborn, such as smiling, stroking, kissing, or rocking?
- If the infant is fussy, what kinds of comforting techniques do the parents use, such as rocking, swaddling, talking, or stroking?

Talking to the parents uncovers many variables that can affect the development of attachment and parenting. (See also Child Maltreatment, Chapter 16.) What expectations do they have for this child? In other words, how similar are their predictions of the fantasy child and their realizations about the real child? Encourage them to talk about their relationship with their own parents, since the type of parenting that parents received as children influences their childrearing practices. Is this a planned birth? How do they see the addition of a dependent family member affecting their lifestyle? What arrangements have they made for such changes in lifestyle? What support system or significant others are available for assistance? What are their views regarding childrearing?

The labor process significantly affects the immediate attachment of mothers to their newborn children. Factors such as a long labor, feeling tired or "drugged" after delivery, and problems with breast-feeding may delay the development of initial positive feelings toward the newborn.

During pregnancy, and often even before conception, parents develop an image of the "ideal or fantasy infant." The unborn child has an imagined appearance, pattern of behavior, expected accomplishments, and predetermined effect on the family's lifestyle. At birth the fantasy infant becomes the real infant. How closely the dream child resembles the real child influences the bonding process. Assessing such expectations during pregnancy and at the time of the infant's birth allows identification of discrepancies in the parents' fantasy versus the real child.

The Neonatal Perception Inventories (NPI) (Broussard, 1979) assess the mother's perception of her real infant compared with her image of an "average" infant. It has been hypothesized that, for optimum mothering to occur, the mother needs to see her infant as better than an "average" baby. Mothers who do not rate their infants as better than average may be at risk for developing parenting abilities that fail to meet the infant's needs. The NPI II (completed 4 weeks after delivery) accurately predicted later childhood adjustment problems, whereas the NPI I (completed 1 or 2 days after the infant's birth) did not (Broussard, 1976). In follow-up studies over a 19-year period, infants who were negatively perceived had the greatest risk for developing behavioral and emotional disorders (Broussard, 1984).

Because attachment involves a mutually reciprocal interchange, observing the interaction between parent and infant is important. An excellent opportunity exists during feeding. A useful instrument for systematically describing the parent's and infant's behaviors is the Feeding Scale developed by the Nursing Child Assessment Satellite Training (NCAST) program (Barnard, 1994). It consists of 76 behavioral items; 50 items describe the parent's behavior regarding (1) sensitivity to cues, (2) response to child's distress, (3) social-emotional growth fostering, and (4) cognitive growth fostering. Twenty-six items focus on the child's behavior in terms of (1) clarity of cues and (2) responsiveness to parent. The results can be shared with parents to encourage discussion of feelings about the infant and to highlight behaviors of the couple that foster successful interaction. The Feeding Scale is appropriate for use with infants during the first year. Training to become a certified tester is available through the NCAST program.*

Clinical Assessment of Gestational Age

Assessment of gestational age is important because perinatal morbidity and mortality are related to gestational age and birth weight. A frequently used method is the Simplified Assessment of Gestational Age by Ballard, Novack, and Driver (1979) (Fig. 8-1, *A*). The Ballard scale, an abbreviated version of the Dubowitz scale (Dubowitz and Dubowitz, 1977), measures gestational ages of infants between 35 and 42 weeks. It assesses six external physical and six neuromuscular signs. Each sign has a number score, and the cumulative score correlates with a maturity rating of 26 to 44 weeks of gestation.

The New Ballard Scale, a revision of the original scale, can be used with newborns as young as 20 weeks of gestation (Ballard, Khoury, Wedig, et al, 1991). The tool has the same physical and neuromuscular sections but includes scores that reflect signs of extremely premature infants, such as fused eyelids; imperceptible breast tissue; sticky, friable, transparent skin; no lanugo; and square-window (flexion of wrist) angle of greater than 90 degrees (see Fig. 8-1, *A*, and a description of the tests in Box 8-3). The examination of infants with a gestational age of 26 weeks or less should be performed at a postnatal age of less than 12 hours. For infants with a gestational age of at least 26 weeks, the examination can be performed up to 96

---

*For information contact NCAST-AVENUW, University of Washington, PO Box 357920, Seattle, WA 98195-7920; 206-543-8528, fax: 206-685-3284; e-mail: ncast@u.washington.edu; **www.ncast.org**.

ESTIMATION OF GESTATIONAL AGE BY MATURITY RATING

NEUROMUSCULAR MATURITY

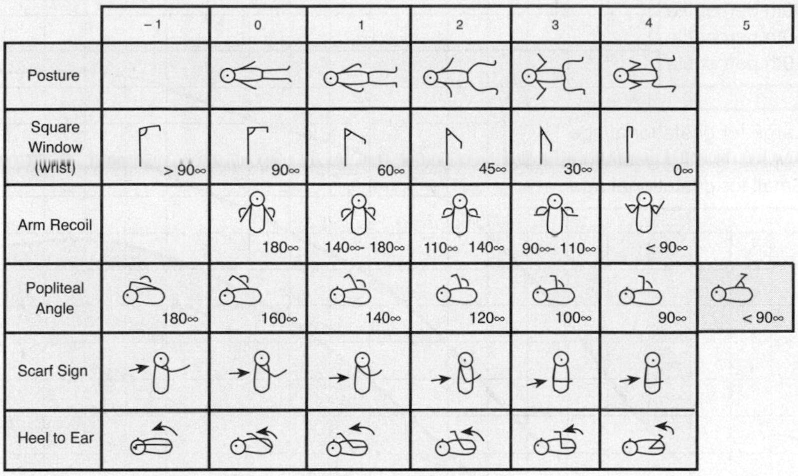

	−1	0	1	2	3	4	5
Posture							
Square Window (wrist)	> 90°	90°	60°	45°	30°	0°	
Arm Recoil		180°	140°–180°	110°–140°	90°–110°	< 90°	
Popliteal Angle	180°	160°	140°	120°	100°	90°	< 90°
Scarf Sign							
Heel to Ear							

PHYSICAL MATURITY

Skin	sticky friable transparent	gelatinous red, translucent	smooth pink, visible veins	superficial peeling &/or rash, few veins	cracking pale areas rare veins	parchment deep cracking no vessels	leathery cracked wrinkled
Lanugo	none	sparse	abundant	thinning	bald areas	mostly bald	
Plantar Surface	heel-toe 40-50 mm: -1 <40 mm: -2	>50 mm no crease	faint red marks	anterior transverse crease only	creases ant. 2/3	creases over entire sole	
Breast	imperceptible	barely perceptible	flat areola no bud	stippled areola 1-2 mm bud	raised areola 3-4 mm bud	full areola 5-10 mm bud	
Eye/Ear	lids fused loosely: -1 tightly: -2	lids open pinna flat stays folded	slightly curved pinna; soft; slow recoil	well-curved pinna; soft but ready recoil	formed & firm instant recoil	thick cartilage ear stiff	
Genitals (male)	scrotum flat, smooth	scrotum empty faint rugae	testes in upper canal rare rugae	testes descending few rugae	testes down good rugae	testes pendulous deep rugae	
Genitals (female)	clitoris prominent labia flat	prominent clitoris small labia minora	prominent clitoris enlarging minora	majora & minora equally prominent	majora large minora small	majora cover clitoris & minora	

MATURITY RATING

score	weeks
-10	20
-5	22
0	24
5	26
10	28
15	30
20	32
25	34
30	36
35	38
40	40
45	42
50	44

A

Fig. 8-1 **A,** Ballard scale for newborn maturity rating. Expanded scale includes extremely premature infants and has been refined to improve accuracy in more mature infants. (**A,** From Ballard JL, Khoury JC, Wedig K, et al: New Ballard score expanded to include extremely premature infants, *J Pediatr* 119:417, 1991.)

Continued

hours after birth. To ensure accuracy, it is recommended that the initial examination be performed within the first 48 hours of life. In a study of preterm infants ranging from 29 to 35 weeks at birth, Ballard scores completed 7 days after birth were found to either overestimate or underestimate gestational age by up to 2 weeks (Sasidharan, Dutta, and Narang, 2009).

The New Ballard Scale overestimates gestational age by 2 to 4 days in infants younger than 37 weeks of gestation, especially at gestational ages of 32 to 37 weeks (Ballard, Khoury, Wedig, et al, 1991). In one study, the Ballard scale was shown to overestimate gestational age of infants less than 28 weeks by as much as 1.3 to 3.3 weeks (Donovan, Tyson, Ehrenkranz, et al, 1999), so other indices of gestational age must also be used in this age-group.

Trotter (2009) indicates that the optimal timing for gestational age assessment in extremely preterm neonates has not been determined primarily because of neuromuscular adjust- ments following birth; in addition, conditions such as asphyxia or maternal medications administered during delivery may alter neuromuscular function. One suggested alternative to an inconclusive neuromuscular evaluation is to assess the physical criteria, multiply by a factor of 2, and assign a gestational age based on the score obtained with this method (Trotter, 2009).

Weight Related to Gestational Age

The infant's weight at birth also correlates with the incidence of perinatal morbidity and mortality. Birth weight alone, however, is a poor indicator of gestational age and fetal maturity. Maturity implies functional capacity—the degree to which the neonate's organ systems are able to adapt to the requirements of extrauterine life. Therefore gestational age is more closely related to fetal maturity than is birth weight. Because heredity influences size at birth, it is important to note the sizes of other family members as part of the assessment process.

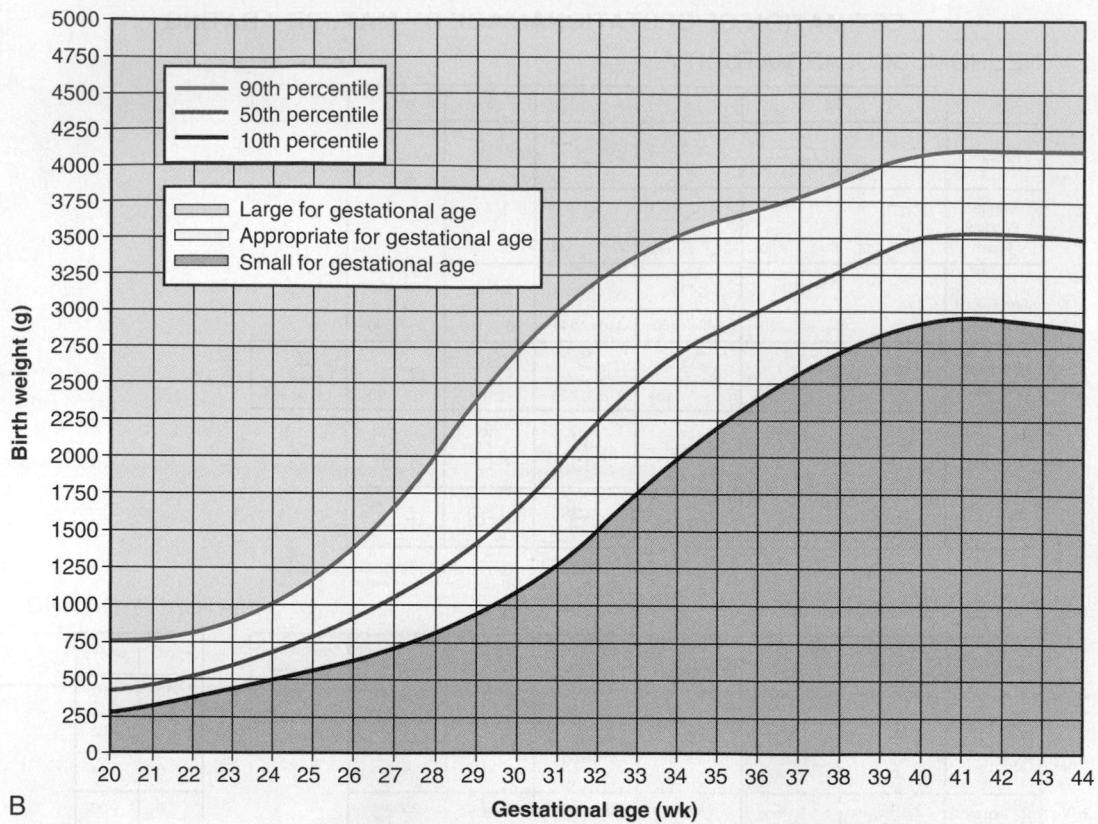

B

Fig. 8-1, cont'd. B, Intrauterine growth: birth weight percentiles based on live single births at gestational ages 20 to 44 weeks. (**B,** Data from Alexander GR, Himes JH, Kaufman RB, et al: A United States national reference for fetal growth, *Obstet Gynecol* 87(2):163-168, 1996.)

BOX 8-3	TESTS USED IN ASSESSING GESTATIONAL AGE

See Fig. 8-1, *A,* for score categories and maneuvers.

Posture—With infant quiet and in a supine position, observe degree of flexion in arms and legs. Muscle tone and degree of flexion increase with maturity. *Score:* Full flexion of the arms and legs = 4.

Square window—With thumb supporting back of arm below wrist, apply gentle pressure with index and third fingers on dorsum of hand without rotating infant's wrist. Measure angle between base of thumb and forearm. *Score:* Full flexion (hand lies flat on ventral surface of forearm) = 4.

Arm recoil—With infant supine, fully flex both forearms on upper arms, hold for 5 seconds; pull down on hands to fully extend and rapidly release arms. Observe rapidity and intensity of recoil to a state of flexion. *Score:* A brisk return to full flexion = 4.

Popliteal angle—With infant supine and pelvis flat on a firm surface, flex lower leg on thigh and then flex thigh on abdomen. While holding knee with thumb and index finger, extend lower leg with index finger of other hand. Measure degree of angle behind knee (popliteal angle). *Score:* An angle of less than 90 degrees = 5.

Scarf sign—With infant supine, support head in midline with one hand; use other hand to pull infant's arm across the shoulder so that infant's hand touches shoulder. Determine location of elbow in relation to midline. *Score:* Elbow does not reach midline = 4.

Heel to ear—With infant supine and pelvis flat on a firm surface, pull foot as far as possible up toward ear on same side. Measure distance of foot from ear and degree of knee flexion (same as popliteal angle). *Score:* Knees flexed with a popliteal angle of less than 10 degrees = 4.

Intrauterine growth curves developed by Battaglia and Lubchenco (1967) have been used to classify infants according to birth weight and gestational age. Since that time, other intrauterine growth charts have emerged to reflect a more heterogeneous sample population than previously described (Cunningham, Gant, Leveno, et al, 2001). The primary intrauterine growth charts that provide national reference data include the work of Alexander, Himes, Kaufman, and colleagues (1996), which represents more than 3.1 million live births in the United States (see Fig. 8-1, *B*); Thomas, Peabody, Turnier, and colleagues (2000); and Arbuckle, Wilkins, and Sherman (1993) and Kramer, Platt, Wen, and colleagues (2001), which represent intrauterine growth among the Canadian population. Thomas, Peabody, Turnier, and colleagues (2000) concluded that intrauterine growth measured by head circumference, birth weight, and length varies according to race and gender. These researchers also found that altitude did not seem to significantly affect birth weight as other authors have suggested. It is recommended that the reader access and use the most current intrauterine growth chart specific to the population being evaluated. Classification of infants at birth by both weight and gestational age provides a satisfactory method for predicting mortality risks and providing guidelines for management of the neonate.

The infant's birth weight, length, and head circumference are plotted on standardized graphs that identify normal values for gestational age. The infant whose weight is **appropriate for**

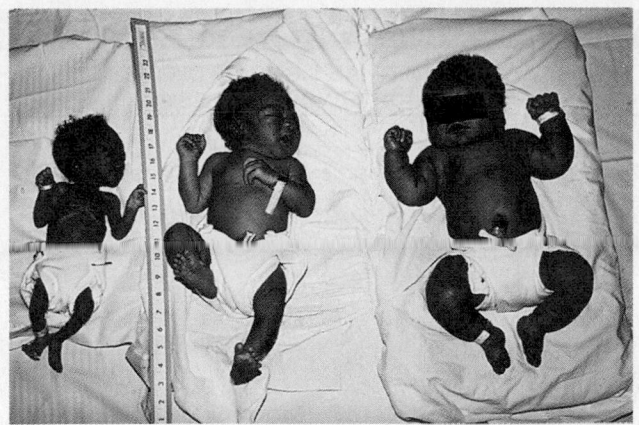

Fig. 8-2 Three infants, same gestational age, weighing 600, 1400, and 2750 g (1.3, 3, and 6 lb), respectively, from left to right. (From *Perinatal assessment of maturation,* National Audiovisual Center, Washington, DC.)

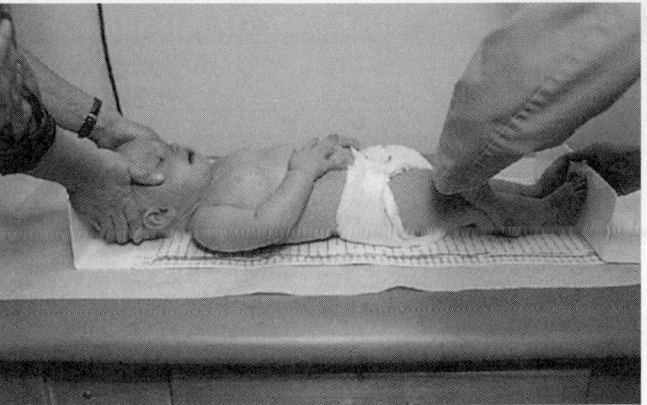

Fig. 8-3 Measurement of infant length.

gestational age (AGA) (between the 10th and 90th percentiles) can be presumed to have grown at a normal rate regardless of the length of gestation—preterm, term, or postterm. The infant who is **large for gestational age (LGA)** (>90th percentile) can be presumed to have grown at an accelerated rate during fetal life; the **small-for-gestational-age (SGA)** infant (<10th percentile) can be presumed to have grown at a restricted rate during intrauterine life. When gestational age is determined according to the Ballard scale, the newborn will fall into one of the following nine possible categories for birth weight and gestational age: AGA—term, preterm, postterm; SGA—term, preterm, postterm; or LGA—term, preterm, postterm. Fig. 8-2 illustrates the disparity between birth weights of three preterm infants of the same gestational age. Birth weight influences mortality: the lower the birth weight, the higher the mortality. The same is true for gestational age: the lower the gestational age, the higher the mortality.

Physical Assessment

The discussion of physical examination focuses on normal findings, variations from the norm that require little or no intervention, and specific potential danger signs that require more careful observation. General guidelines for conducting a physical examination are in the Nursing Care Guidelines box. Table 8-3 summarizes the physical examination of the newborn. (See Chapter 6 for further discussion of examination techniques.)

General Measurements

Several important measurements of the newborn are significant when compared with each other, as well as when recorded over time on a graph. For the full-term infant, average head circumference is between 33 and 35 cm (13 and 14 inches). Head circumference may be somewhat less than that immediately after birth because of the molding process that occurs during vaginal delivery. Usually by the second or third day the normal size and contour of the skull have replaced the molded one.

Chest circumference is 30.5 to 33 cm (12 to 13 inches). Head circumference is usually about 2 to 3 cm (about 1 inch) greater than chest circumference. Because of the molding of the head during delivery, these measurements may initially appear equal. However, if the head is significantly smaller than the chest,

---

NURSING CARE GUIDELINES

Physical Examination of the Newborn

Provide a normothermic and nonstimulating examination area.
Check that equipment and supplies are working properly and are accessible.
Proceed quickly to avoid stressing infant.
Undress only body area examined to prevent heat loss.
Proceed in an orderly sequence (usually head to toe) with the following exceptions:
- Perform all procedures that require quiet first, such as auscultating the lungs, heart, and abdomen.
- Perform disturbing procedures, such as testing reflexes, last.
- Measure head, chest, and length at same time to compare results.

Comfort infant during and after examination; involve parent in:
- Talking softly
- Holding the infant's hands against the chest
- Swaddling and holding
- Giving a pacifier or gloved finger to suck

---

microcephaly or premature closure of the sutures (**craniosynostosis**) is a possibility. If the head is more than 4 cm (1.6 inches) larger than the chest in circumference and this relationship remains constant or increases over several days, then hydrocephalus must be considered. Other causes of increased head circumference are caput succedaneum, cephalhematoma, subgaleal hemorrhage, and subdural hematoma. Prematurity and intrauterine malnutrition also can cause the head measurement to be significantly larger than the chest circumference, but this is because of decreased chest size, not increased head circumference.

Head circumference may also be compared with crown-to-rump length, or sitting height. Crown-to-rump measurements are usually 31 to 35 cm (12.5 to 14 inches) and are approximately equal to head circumference. The relationship of the head and crown-to-rump measurements is more reliable than that of the head and chest. Severn (1994) noted that neonatal head circumference and crown-to-rump length provide a more accurate means for identifying infants at risk; head circumference was shown to be equal to or up to 1 cm (0.4 inch) more than crown-to-rump length in 62% of the infants examined and determined to be normocephalic.

Head-to-heel length is also measured. It is important to extend the legs completely when measuring total body length (Fig. 8-3). The average length of the newborn is 48 to 53 cm (19 to 21 inches).

TABLE 8-3   SUMMARY OF PHYSICAL ASSESSMENT OF THE NEWBORN

Animation—Bradycardia

USUAL FINDINGS	COMMON VARIATIONS, MINOR ABNORMALITIES	POTENTIAL SIGNS OF DISTRESS, MAJOR ABNORMALITIES
General Measurements		
Head circumference—33-35 cm (13-14 inches); about 2-3 cm (1 inch) larger than chest circumference	Molding after birth altering head circumference	Head circumference <10th or >90th percentile
Chest circumference—30.5-33 cm (12-13 inches)	Head and chest circumferences equal for first 1-2 days after birth	
Crown-to-rump length—31-35 cm (12.2-14 inches); approximately equal to head circumference		
Head-to-heel length—48-53 cm (19-21 inches)		
Birth weight—2700-4000 g (6-9 lb)	Loss of 10% of birth weight in first week; regained in 10-14 days, depending on feeding method	Birth weight <10th or >90th percentile
Vital Signs		
Temperature, axillary—36.5°-37° C (97.7°-98° F)	Crying increasing body temperature slightly	Hypothermia
	Radiant warmer falsely increasing axillary temperature	Hyperthermia
Heart rate, apical—120-140 beats/min	Crying increasing heart rate; sleep decreasing heart rate	⊖ Bradycardia—Resting rate <80-100 beats/min
	During 1st period of reactivity (6-8 hr), rate ≤180 beats/min	Tachycardia—Rate >160-180 beats/min
		Irregular rhythm
Respirations—30-60 breaths/min	Crying increasing respiratory rate; sleep decreasing respiratory rate	Tachypnea—Rate >60 breaths/min
	During 1st period of reactivity (6-8 hr), rate up to 80 breaths/min	Apnea—20 sec or more
Blood pressure (BP), oscillometric: 65/41 mm Hg in arm and calf	Crying and activity increasing BP	Oscillometric systolic pressure in calf 6-9 mm Hg less than in upper extremity (sign of coarctation of aorta)
		Systolic pressure >90 mm Hg is considered hypertension (Falkner, 2007)
General Appearance		
Posture—Flexion of head and extremities, which rest on chest and abdomen	Frank breech—Extended legs, abducted and fully rotated thighs, flattened occiput, extended neck	Limp posture—Extension of extremities
Skin		
At birth, bright red, puffy, smooth	Neonatal jaundice after first 24 hr	Progressive jaundice, especially in first 24 hr
2nd-3rd day, pink, flaky, dry	Ecchymoses or petechiae caused by birth trauma	Generalized cyanosis
Vernix caseosa	Milia—Distended sebaceous glands that appear as tiny white papules on cheeks, chin, and nose	Pallor
Lanugo		Mottling
Edema around eyes, face, legs, dorsa of hands, feet, and scrotum or labia	Miliaria or sudamina—Distended sweat (eccrine) glands that appear as minute vesicles, especially on face	Grayness
Acrocyanosis—Cyanosis of hands and feet	Erythema toxicum—Pink papular rash with vesicles superimposed on thorax, back, buttocks, and abdomen; may appear in 24-48 hr and resolve after several days	Plethora
Cutis marmorata—Transient mottling when infant is exposed to decreased temperature	Harlequin color change—Clearly outlined color change as infant lies on side; lower half of body becomes pink, and upper half is pale	Hemorrhage, ecchymoses, or petechiae that persist
		Sclerema—Hard and stiff skin
		Poor skin turgor
	Mongolian spots—Irregular areas of deep blue pigmentation, usually in sacral and gluteal regions; seen predominantly in newborns of African, Native American, Asian, or Hispanic descent (see figure at right)	Rashes, pustules, or blisters
		Café-au-lait spots—Light brown spots
		Nevus flammeus—Port-wine stain
	Telangiectatic nevi ("stork bites")—Flat, deep pink, localized areas usually seen on back of neck	

TABLE 8-3	SUMMARY OF PHYSICAL ASSESSMENT OF THE NEWBORN—cont'd	
USUAL FINDINGS	**COMMON VARIATIONS, MINOR ABNORMALITIES**	**POTENTIAL SIGNS OF DISTRESS, MAJOR ABNORMALITIES**
Head		
Anterior fontanel—Diamond shaped; size varies from barely palpable to 4-5 cm (0.5-2 inches) (see Fig. 8-7) Posterior fontanel—Triangular, 0.5-1 cm (0.2-0.4 inches) Fontanels flat, soft, and firm Widest part of fontanel measured from bone to bone, not suture to suture	Molding after vaginal delivery Third sagittal (parietal) fontanel Bulging fontanel because of crying or coughing Caput succedaneum—Edema of soft scalp tissue Cephalhematoma (uncomplicated)—Hematoma between periosteum and skull bone	Fused sutures Bulging or depressed fontanels when quiet Widened sutures and fontanels Craniotabes—Snapping sensation along lambdoid suture that resembles indentation of Ping-Pong ball
Eyes		
Lids usually edematous Color—Slate gray, dark blue, brown Absence of tears Red reflex Corneal reflex in response to touch Pupillary reflex in response to light Blink reflex in response to light or touch Rudimentary fixation on objects and ability to follow to midline	Epicanthal folds in Asian infants Searching nystagmus or strabismus Subconjunctival (scleral) hemorrhages: ruptured capillaries, usually at limbus	Pink color of iris Purulent discharge Upward slant in non-Asians Hypertelorism (≥3 cm [1.8 inches]) Hypotelorism Congenital cataracts Constricted or dilated fixed pupil Absence of red reflex Absence of pupillary or corneal reflex Inability to follow object or bright light to midline Yellow sclera
Ears		
Position—Top of pinna on horizontal line with outer canthus of eye Startle (Moro) reflex elicited by loud, sudden noise Pinna flexible, cartilage present	Inability to visualize tympanic membrane because of filled aural canals Pinna flat against head Irregular shape or size Pits or skin tags	Low placement of ears Absence of startle (Moro) reflex in response to loud noise Minor abnormalities possible signs of various syndromes, especially renal
Nose		
Nasal patency Nasal discharge—Thin white mucus Sneezing	Flattened and bruised	Nonpatent canals Thick, bloody nasal discharge Flaring of nares (alae nasi) Single nasal canal Copious nasal secretions or stuffiness (may be minor)
Mouth and Throat		
Intact, high-arched palate Uvula in midline Frenulum of tongue Frenulum of upper lip Sucking reflex—Strong and coordinated Rooting reflex Gag reflex Extrusion reflex Absent or minimum salivation Vigorous cry	Natal teeth—Teeth present at birth; benign but may be associated with congenital defects Epstein pearls—Small, white epithelial cysts along midline of hard palate	Cleft lip Cleft palate Large, protruding tongue or posterior displacement of tongue Profuse salivation or drooling Candidiasis (thrush)—White, adherent patches on tongue, palate, and buccal surfaces Inability to pass nasogastric tube Hoarse, high-pitched, weak, absent, or other abnormal cry Stridor
Neck		
Short, thick, usually surrounded by skinfolds Tonic neck reflex	Torticollis (wry neck)—Head held to one side with chin pointing to opposite side	Excessive skinfolds or webbing Resistance to flexion Absence of tonic neck reflex Fractured clavicle; crepitus
Chest		
Anteroposterior and lateral diameters equal Slight sternal retractions evident during inspiration Xiphoid process evident Breast enlargement	Funnel chest (pectus excavatum) Pigeon chest (pectus carinatum) Supernumerary nipples Secretion of milky substance from breasts ("witch's milk")	Depressed sternum Marked retractions of chest and intercostal spaces during respiration Asymmetric chest expansion Redness and firmness around nipples Wide-spaced nipples

Continued

TABLE 8-3   **SUMMARY OF PHYSICAL ASSESSMENT OF THE NEWBORN—cont'd**

USUAL FINDINGS	COMMON VARIATIONS, MINOR ABNORMALITIES	POTENTIAL SIGNS OF DISTRESS, MAJOR ABNORMALITIES
Lungs Respirations chiefly abdominal Cough reflex absent at birth, present by 1-2 days Bilateral equal bronchial breath sounds	Rate and depth of respirations may be irregular; periodic breathing Crackles shortly after birth	Inspiratory stridor Expiratory grunting Retractions Persistent irregular breathing Periodic breathing with repeated apneic spells Seesaw respirations (paradoxic) Apnea Unequal breath sounds Persistent fine, medium, or coarse crackles Wheezing Diminished breath sounds Peristaltic bowel sounds on one side, with diminished breath sounds on same side
Heart Apex—4th-5th intercostal space, lateral to left sternal border S_2 slightly sharper and higher in pitch than S_1	Sinus arrhythmia—Heart rate increasing with inspiration and decreasing with expiration Transient cyanosis on crying or straining	Dextrocardia—Heart on right side Displacement of apex, muffled heart sound Cardiomegaly Abdominal shunts Murmur Thrill Persistent central cyanosis Hyperactive precordium
Abdomen Cylindric in shape Liver—Palpable 2-3 cm (0.8-1.8 inches) below right costal margin Spleen—Tip palpable at end of 1st week of age Kidneys—Palpable 1-2 cm (0.4-0.8 inches) above umbilicus Umbilical cord—Bluish white at birth with 2 arteries and 1 vein Femoral pulses—Equal bilaterally	Umbilical hernia Diastasis recti—Midline gap between recti muscles Wharton jelly—Unusually thick umbilical cord	Abdominal distention Localized bulging Distended veins Absent bowel sounds Enlarged liver and spleen Ascites Visible peristaltic waves Scaphoid or concave abdomen Moist umbilical cord Presence of only 1 artery in cord Urine, stool, or pus leaking from cord or cord insertion site Periumbilical erythema Palpable bladder distention after scant voiding Absent femoral pulses Cord bleeding or hematoma Omphalocele or gastroschisis—Protrusion of abdominal contents through umbilical cord or abdominal wall Bladder exstrophy
Female Genitalia Labia and clitoris usually edematous Urethral meatus behind clitoris Vernix caseosa between labia Urination within 24 hr	Pseudomenstruation—Blood-tinged or mucoid discharge Hymenal tag	Enlarged clitoris with urethral meatus at tip Fused labia Absence of vaginal opening Meconium from vaginal opening No urination within 24 hr Masses in labia Ambiguous genitalia Bladder exstrophy

Abdominal circumference need not be routinely measured in the newborn, but should be done in the event of abdominal distention to determine changes in girth over time. Abdominal circumference is measured just above the level of the umbilicus. Because the umbilical cord is still attached, making measurements across the umbilicus (see Fig. 6-9) is too variable in

newborns. Measuring the abdominal circumference below the umbilical region is also unsuitable because bladder status may affect the reading.

Measure body weight soon after birth because weight loss occurs fairly rapidly. Normally the newborn loses up to 10% of the birth weight by 3 to 4 days of age because of loss of exces-

TABLE 8-3   SUMMARY OF PHYSICAL ASSESSMENT OF THE NEWBORN—cont'd

USUAL FINDINGS	COMMON VARIATIONS, MINOR ABNORMALITIES	POTENTIAL SIGNS OF DISTRESS, MAJOR ABNORMALITIES
Male Genitalia		
Urethral opening at tip of glans penis	Urethral opening covered by prepuce	Hypospadias—Urethral opening on ventral surface of penis
Testes palpable in each scrotum	Inability to retract foreskin	
Scrotum usually large, edematous, pendulous, and covered with rugae; usually deeply pigmented in dark-skinned ethnic groups	Epithelial pearls—Small, firm, white lesions at tip of prepuce	Epispadias—Urethral opening on dorsal surface of penis
Smegma	Erection or priapism	Chordee—Ventral curvature of penis
Urination within 24 hr	Testes palpable in inguinal canal	Testes not palpable in scrotum or inguinal canal
	Scrotum small	No urination within 24 hr
		Inguinal hernia
		Hypoplastic scrotum
		Hydrocele—Fluid in scrotum
		Masses in scrotum
		Meconium from scrotum
		Discoloration of testes
		Ambiguous genitalia
		Bladder exstrophy
Back and Rectum		
Spine intact, no openings, masses, or prominent curves	Green liquid stools in infant under phototherapy	Anal fissures or fistulas
Trunk incurvation reflex	Delayed passage of meconium in very low–birth-weight neonates	Imperforate anus
Anal reflex		Absence of anal reflex
Patent anal opening		No meconium within 36-48 hr
Passage of meconium within 48 hr		Pilonidal cyst or sinus
		Tuft of hair along spine
		Spina bifida (any degree)
Extremities		
10 fingers and toes	Partial syndactyly between 2nd and 3rd toes	Polydactyly—Extra digits
Full range of motion	2nd toe overlapping 3rd toe	Syndactyly—Fused or webbed digits
Nail beds pink, with transient cyanosis immediately after birth	Wide gap between 1st (hallux) and 2nd toes	Phocomelia—Hands or feet attached close to trunk
Creases on anterior ⅔ of sole	Deep crease on plantar surface of foot between 1st and 2nd toes	Hemimelia—Absence of distal part of extremity
Sole usually flat	Asymmetric length of toes	Hyperflexibility of joints
Symmetry of extremities	Dorsiflexion and shortness of hallux	Persistent cyanosis of nail beds
Equal muscle tone bilaterally, especially resistance to opposing flexion		Yellowing of nail beds
Equal bilateral brachial pulses		Sole covered with creases
		Transverse palmar (simian) crease
		Fractures
		Decreased or absent range of motion
		Dislocated or subluxated hip
		Limitation in hip abduction
		Unequal gluteal or leg folds
		Unequal knee height (Allis or Galeazzi sign)
		Audible clunk on abduction (Ortolani sign)
		Asymmetry of extremities
		Unequal muscle tone or range of motion
Neuromuscular System		
Extremities usually in some degree of flexion	Quivering or momentary tremors	Hypotonia—Floppy, poor head control, extremities limp
Extension of extremity followed by previous position of flexion		Hypertonia—Jittery, arms and hands tightly flexed, legs stiffly extended, startles easily
Head lag while sitting, but momentary ability to hold head erect		Asymmetric posturing (except tonic neck reflex)
Ability to turn head from side to side when prone		Opisthotonic posturing—Arched back
Ability to hold head in horizontal line with back when held prone		Signs of paralysis
		Tremors, twitches, and myoclonic jerks
		Marked head lag in all positions

sive extracellular fluid and meconium, as well as limited food intake, especially in breast-fed infants. The birth weight is usually regained by the tenth to fourteenth day of life, depending on method of feeding. Most newborns weigh 2700 to 4000 g (6 to 9 lb), the average weight being about 3400 g (7.5 lb). Accurate birth weights and lengths are important because

they provide a baseline for assessment of risk status and future growth.

Vital Signs

Another category of measurements is vital signs. Axillary temperatures are taken because insertion of a thermometer into the

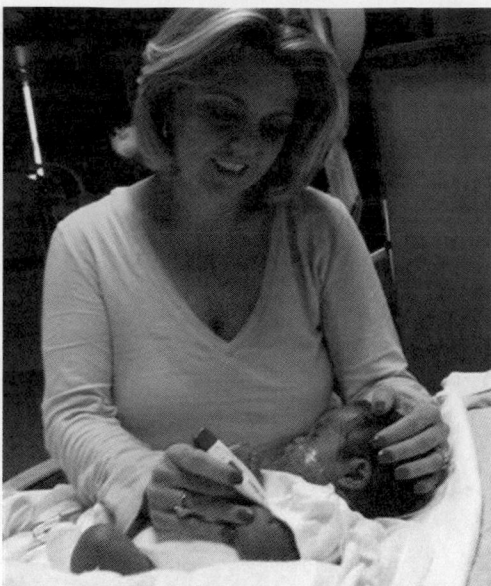

Fig. 8-4 Mother taking axillary temperature with digital thermometer. (Courtesy E. Jacob, Texas Children's Hospital, Houston.)

rectum can cause perforation of the mucosa. (See Table 6-3 and Fig. 8-4.) Core (internal) body temperature varies according to the period of reactivity but is normally 36.5° to 37.6°C (97.7° to 99.7°F). Skin temperature is slightly lower than core body temperature. Therefore axillary temperature is generally less than rectal temperature, measuring about 0.2°C lower (Hussink Muller, van Berkel, and de Beaufort, 2008).

Because BAT is located in the axillary pocket, axillary readings may be elevated whenever NST occurs (see p. 228). However, axillary readings are normal in cold-stressed infants when NST is not triggered or is overwhelmed. The single best method for determining the newborn infant's temperature in any given situation remains elusive when considering the available studies. Controversy exists regarding the accuracy of tympanic membrane sensors. Bliss-Holtz (1993) compared axillary and tympanic membrane temperatures in neonates and found that tympanic membrane temperature measurements were helpful in determining the infant's thermal state. However, other studies have found tympanic membrane temperatures to have high variability according to neonatal environment (bassinet or open crib, radiant warmer, and incubator) (Hicks, 1996; Leick-Rude and Bloom, 1998) and limited usefulness in critically ill neonates (Weiss, Poeltler, and Gocka, 1993; Wilshaw, Beckstrand, Waid, et al, 1999). One study concluded that tympanic membrane temperatures were unacceptable for detecting fever in children under 6 years of age (Lanham, Walker, Klocke, et al, 1999). A meta-analysis of 101 studies comparing tympanic membrane temperatures with rectal temperatures in children concluded that the tympanic method demonstrated a wide range of variability, limiting its application in a pediatric setting (Craig, Lancaster, Taylor, et al, 2002).

The Canadian Paediatric Society (2009) outlines concerns regarding safety and accuracy of tympanic temperature measurement in newborns because of the size of a newborn's external ear canal relative to the size of the thermometer probe. To ensure accuracy, the probe, which may be up to 8 mm (0.3 inch) in diameter, must be deeply inserted into the ear canal to

allow orientation of the sensor near or against the tympanic membrane. At birth, the average diameter of the canal is just 4 mm (0.16 inch); at 2 years of age it is just 5 mm (0.2 inch). The Canadian Paediatric Society concurs with earlier writers Bliss-Holtz (1995) and Yetman, Coody, West, and colleagues (1993) in their conclusion that infrared tympanic membrane technology has yet to meet clinical needs for use in newborn infants. Infrared axillary and digital thermometers are used in many neonatal units because they give rapid readings and are easy to clean. Studies demonstrate their usefulness in well, full-term newborns (Sganga, Wallace, Kiehl, et al, 2000), but accuracy with critically ill neonates is less predictable (Seguin and Terry, 1999; Wilshaw, Beckstrand, Waid, et al, 1999). Bailey and Rose (2001) concluded that tympanic membrane temperatures (versus axillary) in healthy preterm infants were reliable, were cost-effective, and decreased the amount of handling required for monitoring. Skin temperature readings have also been found to vary with probe site placement; bed type; environmental temperature; and the use of blankets, clothing, and nesting devices (Leick-Rude and Bloom, 1998). Jones, Kleber, Eckert, and colleagues (2003) compared rectal temperatures of infants under 2 months of age with calibrated digital thermometers and mercury glass thermometers. The study of 120 infants found that the digital thermometers measured a higher temperature (mean average of 0.7°F; range 0° to 1.6°F) than the mercury glass thermometers. The researchers concluded that the error in measurement was attributable to the digital thermometer used.

Advantages of digital thermometers in neonatal care include relatively easy readability by parents and caretakers in the home, improvement of discharge planning effectiveness, and decreased risk of breakage and associated complications compared with glass thermometers. Both the American Academy of Pediatrics (2003b) and the Canadian Paediatric Society (2009) have advised that mercury thermometers no longer be used in hospitals, clinics, and homes to decrease mercury exposure hazard.

Temporal artery thermometers (TATs) are available for use in the general pediatric population, and parents often report ease of use and less discomfort with such methods. Greenes and Fleisher (2001) concluded that the TAT had limited sensitivity in infants for detecting rectal fever, yet the TAT was more accurate than the tympanic thermometer. Siberry, Diener-West, Schappell, and colleagues (2002) compared the infrared TAT (using an infrared device [Exergen, Watertown, Massachusetts]) with the rectal temperature measurement (digital thermometer) and found poor predictability for fever in children 0 to 3 months old. The authors concluded that the TAT could be used as a rapid assessment screening tool to identify rectal fever in children 3 to 24 months old, but TAT was unreliable as a screening tool for infants under 3 months. Schuh, Komar, Stephens, and colleagues (2004) compared rectal temperatures with TAT measurements in an emergency department population of children under 24 months and concluded that the TAT was not predictable for fever in children under 3 months but could be used as a screening tool for detecting fever of at least 38.3°C (100.9°F) in children 3 to 24 months. Holzhauer, Reith, Sawin, and colleagues (2009) determined that TAT did not accurately detect rectal fever in infants and children aged 3 to 36 months; the researchers did find that TAT was less traumatic for small children than rectal temperature measurement.

In most studies regarding newborn temperature, the glass mercury thermometer is the gold standard against which other methods are compared. Nurses must be cognizant of the many variables involved and be able to make clear clinical decisions based on accurate and objective data. Some examples of variables include:

Site—Axillary, rectal, tympanic, skin

Environment—Radiant warmer, open crib, incubator, clothing, or nesting

Purpose—Fever, possible sepsis (in which case the temperature may be lower than normal in newborns), and thermoregulation in the transition phase

Instrument—Electronic, digital, or infrared

Nurses must also consider cost-effectiveness (nursing care time and instrument operation cost) and potential cross-contamination risks when evaluating neonatal temperature measurement (Sganga, Wallace, Kiehl, et al, 2000). Ease of use and infant comfort are important factors to consider when teaching parents about taking the newborn's temperature at home. Further research is needed to perfect thermometers that accurately reflect the infant's core temperature to effectively plan nursing care and maintain a stable temperature.

Pulse and respirations vary according to the periods of reactivity and to the infant's behavior but are usually 120 to 140 beats/min and 30 to 60 breaths/min. Both are counted for a full 60 seconds to detect irregularities in rate, rhythm, and quality. The heart rate is taken apically with a stethoscope, and the brachial and femoral arteries are palpated for equality of strength or fullness.

Measurement of blood pressure (BP) provides baseline data and may indicate cardiovascular problems. BP is affected by gestational age and birth weight. During the first postnatal week BP increases by 1 to 2 mm Hg/day; during the first 6 weeks of life it increases by approximately 1 mm Hg/wk (Tulassy, Ramanathan, Evans, et al, 2005). Falkner (2007) suggests that the upper 95% confidence limit for a 40-week term infant is 90 mm Hg (systolic) and that a term infant with a systolic blood pressure exceeding this limit is considered hypertensive. For infants with murmurs, suspicion of congenital heart disease, or any concerns regarding tissue perfusion or fluid volume, BP is most easily and accurately assessed using oscillometry (Dinamap), although the device is less reliable when the mean arterial BP is below 35 mm Hg (Fig. 8-5). Oscillometric BP is more accurate when the newborn is in quiet or sleep state and an appropriate cuff width–to-arm or calf ratio of 0.45 to 0.70 (approximately ½ to ¾) is used (Nuntnarumit, Yang, and Bada-Ellzey, 1999). It is also recommended that two or three BP measurements be taken in sick infants and that the mean BP be used because there is less error than when using systolic and diastolic readings. For healthy term infants, the average oscillometric systolic/diastolic BP is 65/45 mm Hg on day 1 of life, changing to 69.5/44.5 by day 3 (Kent, Kecskes, Shadbolt, et al, 2007). Compare BP in the upper and lower extremities, which should be equal.

Calf BP measurements are comparable to brachial pressures in newborns and infants less than 1 year of age and are often

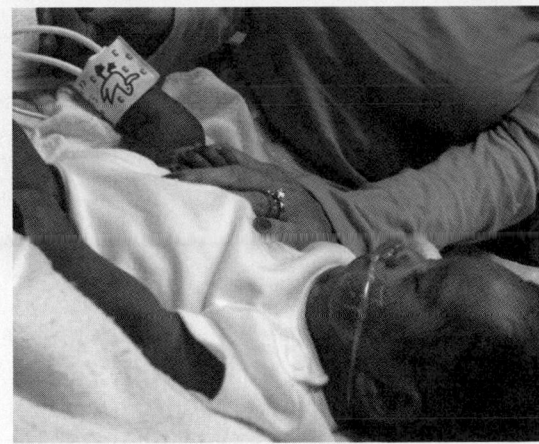

Fig. 8-5 Measurement of blood pressure using oscillometry. (Courtesy E. Jacob, Texas Children's Hospital, Houston.)

more accessible. For consistency, some recommend that baseline calf and brachial pressures be taken initially and the site documented (Axton, Smith, Bertrand, et al, 1995). Although recent normative BP values are for healthy term infants (Kent, Kecskes, Shadbolt, et al, 2007), there remains a distinct need for further studies to clarify the norms for preterm newborns (Tulassy, Ramanathan, Evans, et al, 2005; Nuntnarumit, Yang, and Bada-Ellzey, 1999).

A suggested schedule for monitoring heart and respiratory rates and temperature is within the first hour of life, then once every 8 hours until discharge. This schedule may vary according to institutional policy. Any change in the infant's color, breathing, muscle tone, or behavior necessitates more frequent monitoring.

Although uncommon, neonatal hypertension may be a sign of a significant underlying problem such as renal, cardiac, or thromboembolic pathologic condition, or it may be associated with a medication treatment regimen. The nurse should bring neonatal hypertension to the primary practitioner's attention for further evaluation.

General Appearance

In the full-term newborn the posture is one of flexion, a result of in utero position (Fig. 8-6). Most infants are born in a vertex (head first) presentation and keep the head flexed, with the chin resting on the upper chest. The arms are flexed at the elbows and rest, folded, on the chest with hands clenched or fisted. The legs are flexed at the knees, the hips are flexed with thighs resting on the abdomen, and the feet are dorsiflexed against the anterior aspect of the legs. The vertebral column is also flexed.

Note any deviation from this characteristic fetal position. For example, preterm and hypoxic infants do not assume an attitude of total flexion but rather one of limp or hypotonic extension. Nonvertex presentations also result in variations in posture. In breech presentations the posture depends on the presenting part; a frank breech presentation results in extended legs, abducted and fully rotated thighs, a flattened head on top, and a neck that appears elongated.

Observe the infant's behavior, especially the degree of alertness, drowsiness, and irritability, which are common signs of

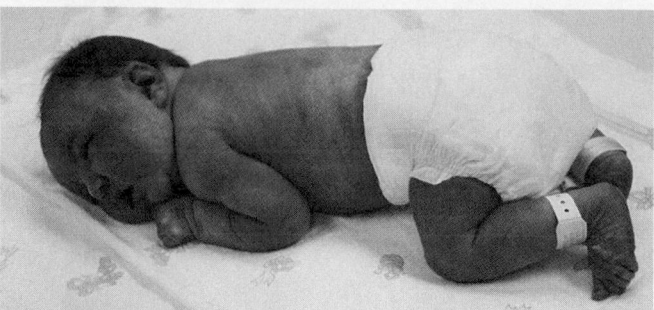

Fig. 8-6 Flexion position of neonate. NOTE: Prone position is avoided for infant sleeping.

neurologic problems. Ask the following questions when assessing behavior:

- Is the infant easily awakened by a loud noise?
- Is the infant comforted by rocking, sucking, or cuddling?
- Does the infant seem to have periods of deep and light sleep?
- When awake, does the infant seem satisfied after a feeding?
- What stimuli elicit responses from the infant?

Skin

The texture of the newborn's skin is velvety smooth and puffy, especially about the eyes, the legs, the dorsal aspect of the hands and feet, and the scrotum or labia.

Skin color depends on racial and familial background and varies greatly among newborns. In general, the Caucasian infant is usually pink to red; the African-American newborn may appear a pinkish or yellowish brown; infants of Hispanic descent may have an olive tint or a slight yellow cast to the skin; infants of Asian descent may be a rosy or yellowish tan; and the color of Native American newborns depends on the tribe and can vary from light pink to dark reddish brown. By the second or third day the skin turns to its more natural tone and is drier and flakier.

Observe the color of the skin in relation to activity, position, and temperature changes. In general, the infant becomes redder when crying and may demonstrate transient periods of cyanosis during the first few hours of life (not associated with apnea or bradycardia). Table 8-3 describes several other color changes and minor skin blemishes.

At birth the skin may be covered with a grayish white, cheeselike substance called **vernix caseosa**, a mixture of sebum and desquamating cells. If it is not removed during the bath, it will be absorbed by about 24 to 48 hours. A fine, downy hair called **lanugo** may be present on the skin, especially on the forehead, cheeks, shoulders, and back.

Head

General observation of the head's contour is important because molding occurs in almost all vaginal deliveries. In a vertex delivery the head is usually flattened at the forehead, with the apex rising and forming a point at the end of the parietal bones, and the posterior skull or occiput dropping abruptly. The usual, more oval contour of the head is apparent by 1 or 2 days after

birth. The change in shape occurs because the bones of the cranium are not fused, allowing for overlapping of the edges of these bones to accommodate to the size of the birth canal during delivery. Such molding does not occur in infants born by cesarean section unless there has been prolonged labor or the head has been engaged in the pelvis.

Six bones—the frontal, occipital, two parietals, and two temporals—constitute the cranium. Between the junctions of these bones are bands of connective tissue called **sutures**. At the junction of the suture are wider spaces of unossified membranous tissue called **fontanels**. ⊖ The two most prominent fontanels are the anterior fontanel, formed by the junction of the sagittal, coronal, and frontal sutures, and the posterior fontanel, formed by the junction of the sagittal and lambdoid sutures (Fig. 8-7, *A*).

Two other fontanels—the sphenoidal and mastoid—are normally present but are not usually palpable. An additional fontanel located between the anterior and posterior fontanels along the sagittal suture is found in some neonates but is also found in some infants with Down syndrome. Note and record the presence of this sagittal or parietal fontanel.

> **NURSING TIP** The location of the sutures is easily remembered because the coronal suture "crowns" the head, and the sagittal suture "separates" the head.

Palpate the skull for all sutures and fontanels by using the tip of the index finger and running it along the ends of the bones (Fig. 8-7, *B*). Sutures feel like cracks between the skull bones; fontanels feel like wider "soft spots" at the junction of sutures. Note their size, shape, molding, and any abnormal closure.

The anterior fontanel is diamond shaped and measures 4 to 5 cm (about 2 inches) at its widest point (from bone to bone, rather than from suture to suture). The posterior fontanel is triangular, measuring between 0.5 and 1 cm (<0.5 inch) at its widest part. It is easily located by following the sagittal suture toward the occiput. The posterior fontanel may not be palpable after birth because of edema (caput) or other cranial molding.

The fontanels should feel flat, firm, and well demarcated against the bony edges of the skull. Frequently pulsations are visible at the anterior fontanel. Coughing, crying, or lying down may temporarily cause the fontanels to bulge and become more taut.

Palpate the skull for any unusual masses or prominences, particularly those resulting from birth trauma, such as caput succedaneum or cephalhematoma. (See Chapter 9.) Because of the pliability of the skull, exerting pressure at the margin of the parietal and occipital bones along the lambdoid suture may produce a snapping sensation similar to the indentation of a Ping-Pong ball. This phenomenon, known as physiologic **craniotabes**, may be found normally, especially in newborns of breech birth, but also may be associated with hydrocephalus, congenital syphilis, or rickets.

Assess the degree of head control. Although head lag is normal, the full-term newborn has some ability to control the head in certain positions. If the supine infant is pulled by the arms into a semi-Fowler position, head lag and hyperextension

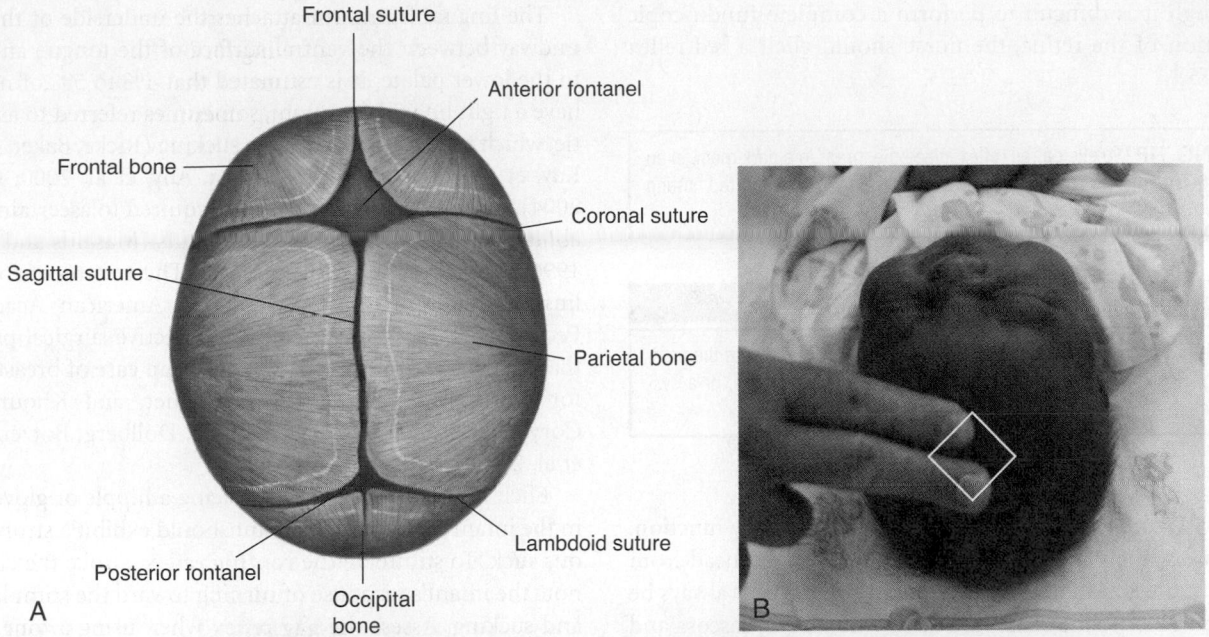

Fig. 8-7 A, Location of sutures and fontanels. **B,** Palpating anterior fontanel.

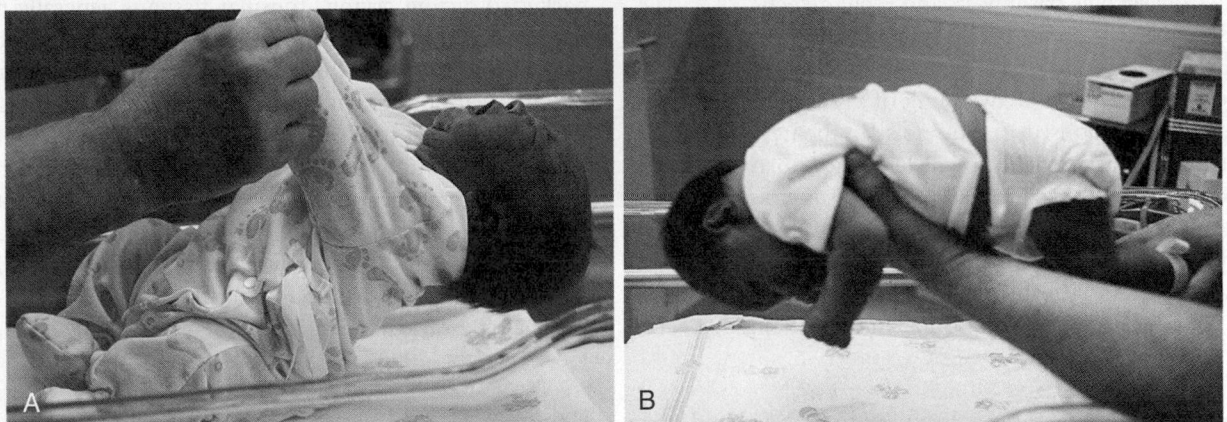

Fig. 8-8 Head control in infant. **A,** Inability to hold head erect when pulled to sitting position. **B,** Ability to hold head erect when placed in ventral suspension.

occur (Fig. 8-8, *A*). However, as infants are brought forward into a sitting position, they attempt to control their heads in an upright position. As the head falls forward onto the chest, many infants attempt to right it into the erect position. If they are held in ventral suspension (i.e., held prone above and parallel to the examining surface), the head is held in a straight line with the spinal column (Fig. 8-8, *B*). When lying on the abdomen, newborns have the ability to lift the head slightly, turning it from side to side. Marked head lag is seen in neonates with Down syndrome, prematurity, hypoxia, and metabolic and neurologic disorders.

Eyes

Because newborns tend to keep their eyes tightly closed, begin the examination of the eyes by observing the lids for edema, which is normally present for 2 days after delivery. Observe the eyes for symmetry and for hypertelorism (wide spacing between the eyes), but do not measure the distance between the inner canthi unless there is cause for further investigation. Tears may be present at birth, but purulent discharge from the eyes shortly after birth is abnormal.

To visualize the surface structures of the eye, hold the infant supine and gently lower the head. The eyes will usually open, similar to the mechanism of a doll's eyes. The sclera should be white and clear.

Examine the cornea for any opacities or haziness. The corneal reflex is present at birth but is generally not elicited unless cerebral or eye damage is suspected. The pupil usually responds to light by constricting. Absence of the pupillary reflex, particularly by 3 weeks of age, suggests blindness. A fixed, dilated, or constricted pupil may indicate central nervous system damage. A searching nystagmus is common after birth. Strabismus is a normal finding because of the lack of binocularity.

Note the color of the iris. Most light-skinned newborns have slate gray or dark blue eyes, whereas dark-skinned infants have brown eyes. Absence of color is characteristic of albinism.

Although it is difficult to perform a complete funduscopic examination of the retina, the nurse should elicit a red reflex (see p. 155).

> **NURSING TIP** To elicit a red reflex, place the infant in a dark room. In an alert state many newborns will open the eyes in a supported sitting position.

> **! NURSING ALERT**
>
> Always record and report absence of the red reflex. It may indicate the presence of glaucoma, retinal abnormality, retinoblastoma, cataracts, or a systemic disease (American Academy of Pediatrics, 2008d).

Ears

Examine the ears for position, structure, and auditory function. The pinna is often flattened against the side of the head from pressure in utero. An otoscopic examination may not always be performed because the canals are filled with vernix caseosa and amniotic fluid, making visualization of the tympanic membrane difficult. Periauricular skin tags, sinuses, and misshapen or low-set ears may be familial or associated with other congenital defects such as trisomy 18 and renal defects.

One way to assess auditory ability is by making a sharp, loud noise close to the infant's head and noting the presence of the startle reflex (Table 8-4) or twitching of the eyelids. However, the absence of a response to a loud noise in the newborn is not diagnostic for hearing deficit. Full-term newborns have the ability to habituate to noxious stimuli such as noise and may not react every time. Also, be aware of newborns considered at risk for hearing loss so that early testing can be performed (see Universal Newborn Hearing Screening, p. 254). (See Auditory Testing, Chapter 6, and Hearing Impairment, Chapter 24.)

Nose

Assess patency of the nasal canals by holding your hand over the infant's mouth and one canal and noting the passage of air through the unobstructed opening. If nasal patency is questionable, report it, since most newborns are obligatory nose breathers and are unable to breathe orally in response to nasal occlusion.

The nose is usually flattened after birth, and bruises are common, especially if forceps were used. Thin, white mucus is common in the newborn, but a thick, bloody nasal discharge should be evaluated. Sneezing is common.

Mouth and Throat

Inspect the mouth's existing structures. The palate is normally high arched and somewhat narrow. Inspect the hard and soft palates for any clefts, which warrant further investigation. A common finding is Epstein pearls—small, white, epithelial cysts along both sides of the midline of the hard palate. They are insignificant and disappear in several weeks.

The frenulum of the upper lip is a band of thick, pink tissue that lies under the inner surface of the upper lip and extends to the maxillary alveolar ridge. It usually disappears as the maxilla grows. It is particularly evident when the infant yawns or smiles.

The lingual frenulum attaches the underside of the tongue midway between the ventral surface of the tongue and the tip to the lower palate. It is estimated that 4% to 5% of newborns have a tight lingual frenulum, sometimes referred to as tongue-tie, which may restrict adequate sucking (Ricke, Baker, Madlon-Kay, et al, 2005; Messner, Lalakea, Aby, et al, 2000; Griffiths, 2004). Further evaluation may be required to ascertain sucking ability, particularly in breast-fed infants (Masaitis and Kaempf, 1996; Wiessinger and Miller, 1995). The treatment for a tight lingual frenulum advocated by the American Academy of Pediatrics is frenotomy, a safe and effective surgical procedure that improves comfort, effectiveness, and ease of breast-feeding for mother and infant (Ballard, Auer, and Khoury, 2002; Coryllos, Genna, and Salloum, 2004; Dollberg, Botzer, Grunis, et al, 2006).

Elicit the sucking reflex by placing a nipple or gloved finger in the infant's mouth. The infant should exhibit a strong, vigorous suck. To stimulate the rooting reflex, stroke the cheek and note the infant's response of turning toward the stimulated side and sucking. Assess the gag reflex when using a tongue blade to visualize the oropharynx.

Inspect the uvula while the infant is crying and the chin is depressed. However, the uvula may be retracted upward and backward during crying. Tonsillar tissue is generally not seen in the newborn. Natal teeth (teeth present at birth as opposed to neonatal teeth—teeth that erupt during the first month of life) are seen infrequently and erupt chiefly at the position of the lower central incisors. They are reported because they are sometimes found in infants with developmental abnormalities and syndromes, including cleft lip and palate. Most natal teeth are loosely attached. However, current research suggests preserving them until they exfoliate naturally (Leung and Robson, 2006; McDonald, Avery, and Dean, 2004), unless breast-feeding is impaired by the neonate biting the breast or the teeth are very loose (Wright, 2000).

Neck

Because the newborn's neck is short and covered with folds of tissue, for adequate assessment allow the head to fall gently backward in slight hyperextension while supporting the back in a slightly raised position. Observe for range of motion, shape, and any abnormal masses, and palpate each clavicle for possible fractures. (See Fractures, Chapter 9.)

Chest

The shape of the newborn's chest is almost circular, with equal anteroposterior and lateral diameters. The ribs are flexible, and slight intercostal retractions are normal on inspiration. The xiphoid process is commonly visible as a small protrusion at the end of the sternum. The sternum is raised and slightly curved.

Inspect the breasts for size; shape; and nipple formation, location, and number. Maternal hormones cause breast enlargement that appears in many newborns of either gender by the second or third day. Occasionally the infant's breasts will secrete a milky substance (sometimes called witch's milk). Infrequently, more than two nipples are present; if these are found, evaluate the kidneys because of the association of extra nipples with renal anomalies.

TABLE 8-4	ASSESSMENT OF REFLEXES IN THE NEWBORN
REFLEXES	**EXPECTED BEHAVIORAL RESPONSES**

Localized

Eyes

Blinking or corneal reflex	Infant blinks at sudden appearance of bright light or at approach of object toward cornea; persists throughout life.
Pupillary	Pupil constricts when bright light shines toward it; persists throughout life.
Doll's eye	As head is moved slowly to right or left, eyes lag behind and do not immediately adjust to new position of head; disappears as fixation develops; if persists, indicates neurologic damage.

Nose

Sneeze	Nasal passages respond spontaneously to irritation or obstruction; persists throughout life.
Glabellar	Tapping briskly on glabella (bridge of nose) causes eyes to close tightly; usually disappears in infancy.

Mouth and Throat

Sucking	Infant begins strong sucking movements of circumoral area in response to stimulation; persists throughout infancy, even without stimulation, such as during sleep.
Gag	Stimulation of posterior pharynx by food, suction, or passage of tube causes infant to gag; persists throughout life.
Rooting	Touching or stroking cheek along side of mouth causes infant to turn head toward that side and begin to suck; should disappear at about age 3-4 mo, but may persist for up to 12 mo.
Extrusion	When tongue is touched or depressed, infant responds by forcing it outward; disappears by age 4 mo.
Yawn	Infant has spontaneous response to decreased oxygen by increasing amount of inspired air; persists throughout life.
Cough	Irritation of mucous membranes of larynx or tracheobronchial tree causes coughing; persists throughout life; usually present after 1st day of birth.

Extremities

Grasp	Touching palms or soles near base of digits causes flexion of hands and toes (see Fig. 8-10, *A*); palmar grasp lessens after age 3 mo, to be replaced by voluntary movement; plantar grasp lessens by 8 mo of age.
Babinski	Stroking outer sole of foot upward from heel and across ball of foot causes toes to hyperextend and hallux to dorsiflex (see Fig. 8-10, *B*); disappears after age 1 yr.
Ankle clonus	Briskly dorsiflexing foot while supporting knee in partially flexed position results in 1-2 oscillating movements ("beats"); eventually no beats should be felt.

Mass

Moro	Sudden jarring or change in equilibrium causes sudden extension and abduction of extremities and fanning of fingers, with index finger and thumb forming a C shape, followed by flexion and adduction of extremities; legs may weakly flex; infant may cry (Fig. 8-9, *A*); disappears after age 3-4 mo, usually strongest during first 2 mo.
Startle	Sudden loud noise causes abduction of arms with flexion of elbows; hands remain clenched; disappears by age 4 mo.
Perez	While infant is prone on firm surface, thumb is pressed along spine from sacrum to neck; infant responds by crying, flexing extremities, and elevating pelvis and head; lordosis of spine, defecation, and urination may occur; disappears by age 4-6 mo.
Asymmetric tonic neck	When infant's head is turned to one side, arm and leg extend on that side, and opposite arm and leg flex (Fig. 8-9, *B*); disappears by age 3-4 mo, to be replaced by symmetric positioning of both sides of body.
Trunk incurvation (Galant) reflex	Stroking infant's back alongside spine causes hips to move toward stimulated side; disappears by age 4 wk.
Dance or step	If infant is held so that sole of foot touches hard surface, there is reciprocal flexion and extension of leg, simulating walking (Fig. 8-9, *C*); disappears after age 3-4 wk, to be replaced by deliberate movement.
Crawl	When placed on abdomen, infant makes crawling movements with arms and legs; disappears at about age 6 wk (Fig. 8-9, *D*).
Placing	When infant is held upright under arms and dorsal side of foot is briskly placed against hard object, such as table, leg lifts as if foot is stepping on table; age of disappearance varies.

Lungs

The newborn's normal respirations are irregular and abdominal, and the rate is between 30 and 60 breaths/min. Periods of **apnea** lasting more than 20 seconds are abnormal and may be accompanied by **bradycardia**. After the first forceful breaths required to initiate respiration, subsequent breaths should be easy and fairly regular in rhythm. Occasional irregularities occur in relation to crying, sleeping, and feeding. **Periodic breathing** is common in full-term newborns and consists of rapid nonlabored respirations followed by pauses of less than 20 seconds; periodic breathing may be more prominent during sleep and is not accompanied by status changes such as cyanosis or bradycardia.

Perform auscultation when the infant is quiet. Bronchial breath sounds should be equal bilaterally. Report any differ-ences in auscultatory findings between symmetric sites. Crackles soon after birth may indicate areas of atelectasis or the presence of fluid, which represents the normal transition of the lungs to extrauterine life. However, wheezes, persistence of crackles, and stridor should be reported.

> ### ! NURSING ALERT
>
> Signs of respiratory distress include tachypnea, grunting, nasal flaring, intercostal retractions, stridor, abnormal breath sounds, cyanosis, and pallor.

Heart

Heart rate may range from 100 to 180 beats/min shortly after birth and, when the infant's condition has stabilized, from 120 to 140 beats/min. Palpate to find the **point of maximum**

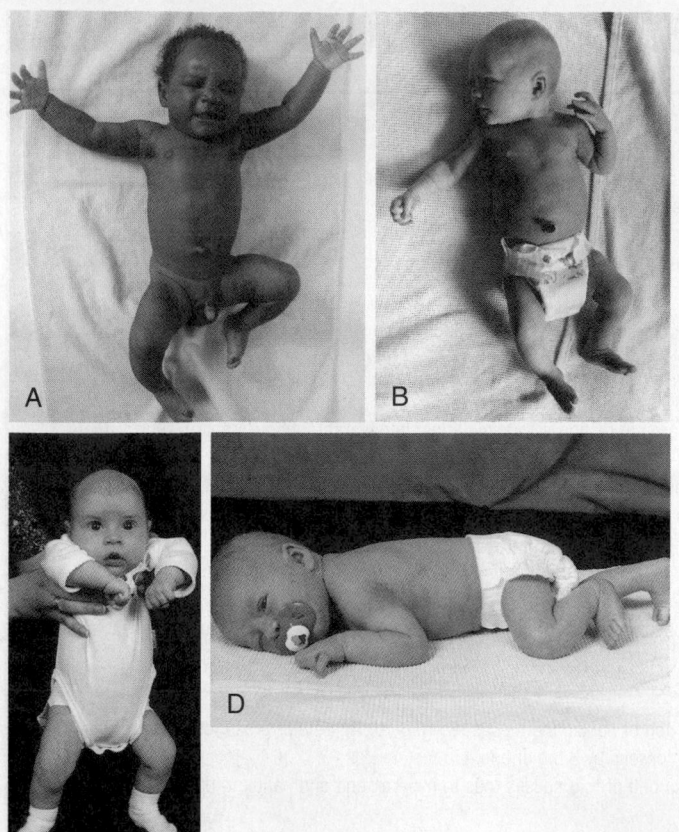

Fig. 8-9 A, Moro reflex. **B,** Tonic neck reflex. **C,** Dance reflex. **D,** Crawl reflex. (Courtesy Paul Vincent Kuntz, Texas Children's Hospital, Houston.)

intensity (PMI), which is usually in the fourth to fifth intercostal space, medial to the left midclavicular line. The PMI gives some indication of the location of the heart, which may be displaced in conditions such as congenital diaphragmatic hernia or pneumothorax. **Dextrocardia**, an anomaly wherein the heart is on the right side of the body, should be reported (the abdominal organs may also be reversed), along with associated circulatory abnormalities.

> **NURSING TIP** Because auscultation of neonatal breath sounds and heart tones is often difficult for the untrained ear, practice auscultating one parameter at a time. Close your eyes and mentally block out the extraneous sounds heard, such as room noise or neonatal movement; offer the newborn a pacifier or gloved finger. Auscultation of a murmur and decreased air movement in specific lung fields requires patience and practice; it may require auscultating the heart tones or breath sounds for 1 to 3 minutes each.

Auscultation of the specific components of the heart sounds is difficult because of the rapid rate and effective transmission of respiratory sounds. However, the first (S_1) and second (S_2) sounds should be clear and well defined; the second sound is somewhat higher in pitch and sharper than the first. Murmurs are frequently heard in the newborn, especially over the base of the heart or at the left sternal border in the third or fourth interspace. Ordinarily they are not associated with specific cardiac defects but frequently represent the

incomplete functional closure of fetal shunts (Fuloria and Kreiter, 2002). (Chapter 6 discusses grading of heart murmurs.) However, always record and report any murmur or other unusual sounds.

Abdomen

The normal contour of the abdomen is cylindric and prominent with visible veins. Bowel sounds are audible within the first 15 to 20 minutes after birth. Visible peristaltic waves may be observed in thin newborns but should not be seen in well-nourished infants.

Inspect the umbilical cord to determine the presence of two arteries, which look like papular structures, and one vein, which has a larger lumen than the arteries and a thinner vessel wall. At birth the cord appears bluish white and moist. After clamping, it begins to dry and appears a dull, yellowish brown. It progressively shrivels and turns greenish black. If the umbilical cord appears unusually large in diameter at the base, inspect for the presence of a hematoma or small omphalocele. The cord must not be clamped over an omphalocele, since part of the intestine will be clamped, causing tissue necrosis. One practical rule of thumb is to cut the cord distally 10 to 12 cm (4 to 5 inches) from a questionable enlargement until further examination is carried out by a practitioner. The extra length can be cut once normal anatomy has been identified.

A cord that is draining and erythematous at the base should be investigated by the primary practitioner. The cord undergoes a process of dry gangrene decay, which has an odor; therefore odor alone may not be a reliable index of suspicion for **omphalitis**.

Palpate after inspecting the abdomen. The liver is normally palpable 1 to 3 cm (about 0.5 to 1 inch) below the right costal margin. The tip of the spleen can sometimes be felt, but a palpable spleen more than 1 cm below the left costal margin suggests enlargement and warrants further investigation. Although the nurse should palpate both kidneys, this maneuver requires considerable practice. When felt, the lower half of the right kidney and the tip of the left kidney are 1 to 2 cm (about 0.5 to 1 inch) above the umbilicus. During examination of the lower abdomen, palpate for femoral pulses, which should be strong and equal bilaterally.

Female Genitalia

Normally the labia majora and minora (the minora may be more prominent) and clitoris are edematous, especially after a breech delivery. However, carefully inspect the labia and clitoris to identify any evidence of ambiguous genitalia or other abnormalities. Normally in a girl the urethral opening is located behind the clitoris. Any deviation from this may mistakenly suggest that the clitoris is a small penis, which can occur in conditions such as congenital adrenal hyperplasia.

A **hymenal tag** is occasionally visible from the posterior opening of the vagina. It is composed of tissue from the hymen and the labia minora and usually disappears in several weeks. Generally, the vaginal vault is not inspected.

Vaginal discharge may be noted during the first week of life. This **pseudomenstruation** is a manifestation of the abrupt decrease in maternal hormones and usually disappears by 2 to 4 weeks of age. Fecal discharge from the vaginal opening indicates a rectovaginal fistula and must be reported. Vernix caseosa may be present in large amounts between the labia. Vigorous attempts to remove all the vernix through bathing are avoided to prevent tissue damage. With routine bathing and care, vernix will disappear after several days.

Male Genitalia

Inspect the penis for the urethral opening, which is located at the tip. However, the opening may be totally covered by the prepuce, or foreskin, which covers the glans penis. A tight prepuce is a common finding in newborns and does not indicate phimosis. It should not be forcefully retracted; locating the urinary meatus is usually possible without retracting the foreskin (Cavaliere, 2009). Smegma, a white cheesy substance, is commonly found around the glans penis, under the foreskin. An erection is common in the newborn. Small, white, firm lesions called epithelial pearls may be seen at the tip of the prepuce.

The scrotum may be large, edematous, and pendulous in the full-term neonate, especially in the infant born in breech position. It is more deeply pigmented in dark-skinned infants. A noncommunicating hydrocele commonly occurs unilaterally and disappears within a few months. Palpate the scrotum for the presence of testes. (See Chapter 6.)

In small newborns, particularly premature infants, the undescended testes may be palpable within the inguinal canal. Absence of the testes may also be a sign of ambiguous genitalia, especially when accompanied by a small scrotum and penis. Inguinal hernias may or may not be manifested immediately after birth. A hernia is easier to detect when the infant is crying. Palpable lymph nodes are most commonly found in the inguinal area. Report a discolored or dusky scrotum, scrotal edema, or palpation of a small mass to the practitioner because these may be a sign of testicular torsion (Juretschke, 2000).

Back and Anus

Inspect the spine with the infant prone. The shape of the spine is gently rounded, with none of the characteristic S-shaped curves seen later in life. Any abnormal openings or sinuses, masses, dimples, or soft areas are noted. A protruding sac anywhere along the spine, but most commonly in the sacral area, indicates some type of spina bifida. A small sinus, which may or may not be communicating with the spine, is a pilonidal sinus. It is frequently covered with a tuft of hair. Although it may have no pathologic significance, a pilonidal cyst may indicate the existence of spina bifida occulta or be a portal of entry into the spinal column. With the infant still prone, note symmetry of the gluteal folds. Report any evidence of asymmetry. Skilled examiners test for developmental dysplasia of the hip. (See Chapter 11.)

The presence of an anal orifice and passage of meconium through the orifice during the first 24 to 48 hours of life indicates anal patency. If the nurse suspects an imperforate anus, report this to the practitioner for further evaluation. The presence of meconium or stool on the perineum is not an indication of rectal patency; a fistula may exist wherein stool is evacuated via the vagina, scrotum, or raphe. Therefore it is imperative to check anal patency with a small rubber catheter should any doubt regarding patency exist.

Extremities

Examine the extremities for symmetry, range of motion, and signs of malformation or trauma. Count the fingers and toes, and note supernumerary digits (polydactyly) or fusion of digits (syndactyly). A partial syndactyly between the second and third toes is a common variation seen in otherwise normal infants. More extensive fusion is abnormal, and the nurse should report this to the practitioner.

Observe range of motion of the extremities throughout the entire examination. The newborn will demonstrate full range of motion in the elbow, hip, shoulder, and knee joints. Movements should be symmetric, smooth, and unrestricted. The absence of arm movement signals a potential birth injury paralysis such as Klumpke or Erb-Duchenne paralysis. (See Birth Injuries, Chapter 9.) An asymmetric or partial Moro reflex should alert the practitioner to further evaluate upper extremity mobility. Examine the lower extremities for limb length, symmetry, and hip abduction and flexion.

Examine the nails; the nail beds should be pink, although slight blueness is evident in acrocyanosis. Persistent cyanosis of the nail beds may indicate hypoxia or vasoconstriction. Yellowing of the nail beds may indicate intrauterine distress, postterm birth, or hemolytic disease. Short or absent nails are seen in preterm infants, whereas long nails, extending over the ends of the fingers, are characteristic of postterm newborns.

The palms of the hands should have the usual creases (see Fig. 6-14). A transverse palmar crease (simian crease) suggests Down syndrome but may also be a normal finding. The full-term newborn usually has creases covering the entire sole of the foot. In postterm infants the sole is covered with deep creases, and in preterm infants the creases may partially cover the sole or may be absent. The soles are flat with prominent fat pads. Note any foot abnormalities.

Two reflexes are elicited. The first is the grasp reflex. Touching the palms or soles near the base of the digits causes flexion or grasping (Fig. 8-10, *A*). The other is Babinski reflex. Stroking the outer sole of the foot upward from the heel across the ball of the foot causes the big toe to dorsiflex and the other toes to hyperextend (Fig. 8-10, *B*, and Table 8-4).

Inspect the extremities for evidence of fractures from birth trauma. The clavicle, humerus, and femur are most commonly involved. Limitation of movement, crepitus, visible deformity, asymmetry of reflexes, and malposition of the site suggest a fracture.

It is important to assess neonatal muscle tone. By attempting to extend a flexed extremity, determine whether tone is equal bilaterally. Extension of any extremity is usually met with resistance, and when released, the extremity returns to its previous flexed position. Hypotonia suggests some degree of hypoxia, neurologic or muscular disorder, or Down syndrome. Asymmetry of muscle tone may indicate a degree of paralysis from damage to the central nervous system. Failure to move the lower limbs suggests a spinal cord lesion or injury. Sustained rhythmic tremors, twitches, and myoclonic jerks characterize neonatal seizures or may indicate neonatal abstinence syndrome. (See Neonatal Seizures and Drug-Exposed Infants, Chapter 10.) Sudden asynchronous jerking movements, quivering, or momentary tremors are usually normal.

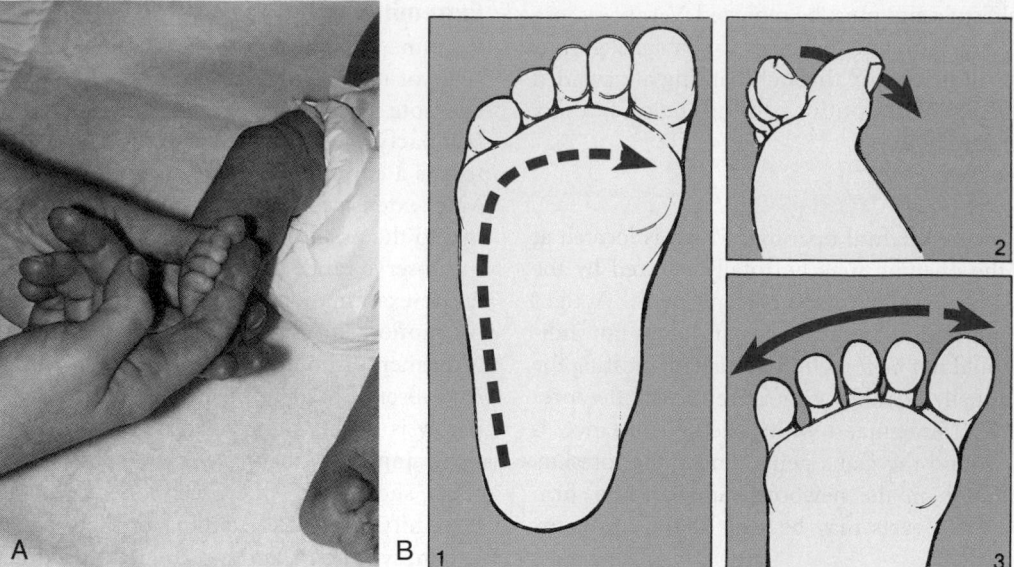

Fig. 8-10 A, Plantar or grasp reflex. **B,** Babinski reflex. *1,* Direction of stroke. *2,* Dorsiflexion of big toe. *3,* Fanning of toes. (**A** from Zitelli BJ, Davis HW: *Atlas of pediatric physical diagnosis,* ed 4, St Louis, 2002, Mosby.)

Neurologic System

Assessing neurologic status is a critical part of the physical examination of the newborn. Much of the neurologic testing takes place during evaluation of body systems, such as eliciting localized reflexes and observing posture, muscle tone, head control, and movement. However, several important mass (total body) reflexes also need to be elicited. Test these at the end of the examination, since they may disturb the infant and interfere with auscultation. Table 8-4 describes these reflexes and several local reflexes. Record and report the absence, asymmetry, persistence, or weakness of a reflex.

The nursing process in the care of the healthy newborn is outlined in Box 8-4.

MAINTAIN A PATENT AIRWAY

Establishing a patent airway is the primary objective in the delivery room. When the newborn is supine, a neutral neck position (avoiding neck flexion or hyperextension) is critical to achieving and maintaining a patent airway. After feeding, position the infant to facilitate drainage of secretions.

The American Academy of Pediatrics (2005a) recommends the supine position during sleep for all newborns. This recommendation is based on the association between sleeping prone and sudden infant death syndrome. (See Chapter 13.) Since the initial recommendation in 1992 that all infants be placed in the supine position to sleep, there has been no evidence of an increased number of complications, such as choking or vomiting, when infants are placed in a supine sleep position (Malloy, 2002). There has, however, been an increase in the number of infants with cranial asymmetry, particularly unilateral flattening of the occiput (American Academy of Pediatrics, 2003a). Health care professionals must educate parents on prevention of deformational plagiocephaly by encouraging alternate positions when baby is awake. (See also Positional Plagiocephaly, Chapter 11.)

Suctioning, if needed, may be done with a bulb syringe. Used bulb syringes should be replaced every 24 hours in the hospital and boiled for 10 minutes after use in the home to prevent bacterial contamination. If more forceful removal of secretions is required, mechanical suction is used. Use of the proper-sized catheter and correct suctioning technique are essential to prevent mucosal damage and edema. Gentle suctioning is necessary to prevent laryngospasm, reflex bradycardia, and other cardiac arrhythmias from vagal stimulation. Oropharyngeal suctioning is performed for up to 5 seconds with sufficient time between each attempt to allow the infant to reoxygenate. If nasal suctioning is necessary, it must be done *after* oral suctioning to minimize the possibility of aspiration of oropharyngeal contents (American Academy of Pediatrics, 2006a).

The stomach may be emptied (aspirated) to remove the contents; passing a catheter to the stomach may also rule out esophageal atresia. Closely monitor vital signs, and report immediately any indication of respiratory distress.

To avoid aspiration of amniotic fluid or mucus, clear the mouth and pharynx first, then the nasal passages (remember m *before* n), to prevent a gasp and inspiration of large amounts of oropharyngeal secretions. Compress the bulb syringe before insertion to avoid forcing secretions into the bronchi.

MAINTAIN A STABLE BODY TEMPERATURE

Conserving the newborn's body heat is an essential nursing goal. At birth a major cause of heat loss is evaporation, the loss of heat through moisture. The amniotic fluid that bathes the infant's skin favors evaporation, especially when combined with the cool atmosphere of the delivery room. Rapidly drying the skin and hair with a warmed towel and placing the infant in a heated environment will minimize heat loss through evaporation.

Another source of heat loss is radiation, the loss of heat to cooler solid objects in the environment that are not in direct

BOX 8-4   NURSING PROCESS: THE HEALTHY NEWBORN AND FAMILY

Assessment

A brief initial assessment is performed to detect any problems that may impair an effective newborn transition. Once the infant has stabilized and maternal-infant contact has occurred, a more thorough examination may take place, including the gestational age assessment.

Nursing Diagnoses

Nursing diagnoses are established after analysis of the findings of the physical assessment. Nursing diagnoses for the newborn include the following:

- Ineffective Airway Clearance related to airway obstruction with mucus, blood, and amniotic fluid; and inability to clear mucus by cough and expectoration
- Risk for Imbalanced Body Temperature related to imbalance between body heat loss and heat production
- Pain related to heel stick, circumcision, venipuncture
- Readiness for Enhanced Parenting related to knowledge of newborn's social capabilities, knowledge of newborn's dependency needs, and knowledge of biologic characteristics of the newborn
- Ineffective Role Performance related to misinterpretation of newborn's behavioral cues and inadequate knowledge about newborn's basic care needs (feeding, bathing, sleep-wake patterns, stooling and voiding patterns)
- Risk for Unstable Glucose Level related to increased glucose utilization at birth and decreased endogenous glucose supply
- Neonatal Jaundice related to increasing serum bilirubin levels, inability to metabolize and excrete bilirubin, and increased hemolysis

Planning

Expected outcomes can apply both to the infant and the parents. Expected outcomes for the newborn during the immediate recovery period include that the infant will:

- Maintain effective breathing pattern
- Maintain effective thermoregulation
- Maintain adequate cardiac output, circulation, and tissue perfusion
- Remain free from infection
- Receive necessary nutrition for growth
- Receive bilirubin assessment and screening within the first week of life to determine risk for increasing levels of serum bilirubin

Expected outcomes for the parents include that they will:

- Attain knowledge, skill, and confidence relevant to infant care activities
- State understanding of biologic and behavioral characteristics of the newborn
- Begin to integrate the newborn into the family

Implementation and Interventions

A number of intervention strategies for the newborn infant are discussed on pp. 250-273.

Evaluation

The effectiveness of the established outcomes and nursing interventions for the newborn and family is determined by continual assessment and evaluation of the infant's response to the extrauterine environment and the family's willingness to integrate the newborn into the existing family matrix. The nurse can be reasonably assured that care was effective to the extent that the stated outcomes for care were achieved.

---

contact with the infant. Loss of heat through radiation increases as these solid objects become colder and closer to the infant. The temperature of ambient (surrounding) air in the incubator essentially has no effect on loss of heat through radiation. This is a critical point to remember when attempting to maintain a constant temperature for the infant, because even when the temperature of the ambient air is optimum, the infant can become hypothermic. The use of a radiant heating device, such as a heat lamp, with an incubator may cause the infant to overheat because the neonate cannot effectively dissipate radiant heat through the Plexiglas wall of the incubator. For this same reason, do not expose an incubator to direct sunlight.

An example of radiant heat loss is the placement of the incubator close to a cold window or air conditioning unit. The cold from either source will cool the incubator walls and subsequently the neonate's body. To prevent this, the incubator is placed as far away as possible from walls, windows, or ventilating units.

Heat loss can also occur through conduction and convection. **Conduction** involves loss of body heat from direct skin contact with a cooler solid object. The nurse can minimize this by placing the infant on a padded, covered surface rather than directly on a cool hard table and by providing insulation with clothes and blankets. Placing the newborn nestled close to the mother, such as in her arms or on her abdomen immediately after delivery in **skin-to-skin** (kangaroo care) contact, is beneficial in terms of conserving newborn heat and fostering maternal attachment and breast-feeding.

Convection is similar to conduction, except that heat loss is aided by surrounding air currents. For example, placing the infant in the direct flow of air from a fan or air conditioner vent causes rapid heat loss through convection. Transporting the neonate in a crib with solid sides reduces airflow around the infant.

PROTECT FROM INFECTION AND INJURY

The most important practice for preventing cross-infection is thorough hand washing by all individuals involved in the infant's care. Other procedures to prevent infection include eye care, umbilical care, bathing, and care of the circumcision. Artificial and long fingernails are discouraged for those working in neonatal care because the former have been implicated in the transmission of *Pseudomonas* organisms (Moolenaar, Crutcher, San Joaquin, et al, 2000; Foca, Jacob, Whittier, et al, 2000); contaminated hand soaps have been identified in one neonatal *Serratia marcescens* outbreak (Rabier, Bataillon, Jolivet-Gougeon, et al, 2008). Vitamin K is administered to protect against hemorrhage.

Identification

Proper identification of the newborn is essential. The nurse must verify that identifying bands are securely fastened on the newborn and verify the information (name, sex, mother's admission number, date, and time of birth) against the birth records and the child's gender. Some institutions use methods of infant identification such as a color photograph kept in the medical record, storage of blood for DNA genotyping, and electronic surveillance systems for infant security. Footprinting or fingerprinting alone is not currently recommended for newborn identification (American Academy of Pediatrics and American College of Obstetricians and Gynecologists, 2007); however, many institutions continue to practice footprinting. Electronic tags that give off a radio frequency are also being used to prevent newborn abductions (Shogan, 2002). Another measure to decrease infant abduction is to discontinue the publication of birth announcements in the local newspaper.

A proactive hospital emergency plan should be implemented to prevent infant abduction and to respond promptly and effectively if one occurs (Geller, 2000). A mock newborn abduction drill is an effective method to evaluate staff competence and response to the incident (Shogan, 2002). *All* hospital personnel should be educated regarding newborn abduction, preventive strategies, and methods to identify the potential risk of such an occurrence.

The nurse needs to discuss safety issues with the mother before and after delivery of the newborn to ensure adequate understanding of safety measures to prevent newborn abduction. Thirty-two percent of infant abductions occur from health care facilities (Burgess, Carr, Nahirny, et al, 2008). A written copy of safety instructions should also be given to the parent. Instruct parents to look at identification badges of nurses and any hospital personnel who come in contact with the infant and not to relinquish their infants to anyone without proper identification. Some hospital employees in newborn and maternity areas wear color-coded badges or symbols that are changed frequently to decrease the likelihood of infant abduction. Mothers are also advised not to leave the infant alone in the crib while they shower or use the bathroom; rather, they should ask to have the infant returned to the nursery if a family member is not present in the room. Encourage parents and staff to use a password system when the newborn is taken from the room as a routine security measure. The nurse should document in the chart that these instructions were given and that appropriate identification band checks are routinely made throughout each shift.

Nursing staff are also educated regarding the "typical" abductor profile and to be constantly aware of visitors with unusual behavior. The typical abductor is a female between the ages of 15 and 44 who often has a large build and low self-esteem. She may be emotionally disturbed because of the loss of her own child or inability to conceive and may have a strained relationship with her husband or partner. The typical abductor may also be seen visiting the newborn nursery or neonatal intensive care unit (NICU) before the abduction and may ask questions about the care of or the health of a specific newborn. The abductor may familiarize herself with the hospital routine and may also impersonate a health care worker.

The nurse should advise parents that infant safety measures must be implemented after discharge from hospital as well, since home abductions have nearly doubled in recent years, and make up 49% of all infant abductions; those from public places have tripled to 9% of abductions (Burgess, Carr, Nahirny, et al, 2008). Instruct parents to be cautious of anyone they do not know well, particularly persons they met during the pregnancy who show excessive interest or who show up at their home unannounced (Burgess, Carr, Nahirny, et al, 2008).

Eye Care

Prophylactic eye treatment against ophthalmia neonatorum, infectious conjunctivitis of the newborn, includes the use of (1) silver nitrate (1%) solution, (2) erythromycin (0.5%) ophthalmic ointment or drops, or (3) tetracycline (1%) ophthalmic ointment or drops (preferably in single-dose ampules or tubes)

(see Nursing Care Guidelines box). *Chlamydia trachomatis* is the major cause of ophthalmia neonatorum in the United States. Silver nitrate is effective against gonococcal conjunctivitis. Topical antibiotics (tetracycline and erythromycin) and silver nitrate have not proved to be effective in the prevention and treatment of chlamydial conjunctivitis. A 14-day course of oral erythromycin or ethylsuccinate may be given for chlamydial conjunctivitis (American Academy of Pediatrics, 2009b). The administration of oral erythromycin to infants less than 6 weeks old has been associated with the development of infantile hypertrophic pyloric stenosis; therefore parents should be informed of the potential risks and signs of the illness (American Academy of Pediatrics, 2009b).

📋 NURSING CARE GUIDELINES

Ophthalmia Neonatorum Prophylaxis

- Clean the eyelids with cotton and sterile water if needed.
- Separate lids and apply 2 drops or a 1 to 2 cm (0.5 inch) ribbon of ointment in each conjunctival sac.
- Massage lids to ensure spread of the medication.
- Wipe excess medication from eye with cotton 1 minute after application.
- Do not rinse eyes.

Although eye prophylaxis is mandatory in the United States, health care facilities are free to choose specific drugs. Effective prophylaxis may be better directed at treating maternal chlamydial infection in areas where that organism is prevalent.

NURSING TIP A chemical conjunctivitis may occur within 24 hours of instillation of ophthalmic prophylaxis. The clinical features include mild lid edema and a sterile, nonpurulent eye discharge (Fuloria and Kreiter, 2002). Report purulent eye discharge to the primary practitioner for further investigation.

Studies on maternal attachment suggest that in the first hour of life a newborn has a greater ability to focus on coordinated movement than at any other time during the next several days. Because eye contact is important in the development of maternal-infant bonding, routine administration of silver nitrate or antibiotics can be postponed for up to 1 hour after birth. However, practitioners must ensure that the drug is given by 1 hour of age.

Vitamin K Administration

Shortly after birth, vitamin K is administered to prevent hemorrhagic disease of the newborn. (See Chapter 9.) Normally, the intestinal flora synthesizes vitamin K. However, because the infant's intestine is presumably sterile at birth and because breast milk contains low levels of vitamin K, the supply is inadequate for at least the first 3 to 4 days. The major function of vitamin K is to catalyze the synthesis of prothrombin in the liver, which is needed for blood clotting. The vastus lateralis muscle is the traditionally recommended injection site, but the ventrogluteal (not dorsogluteal) muscle can be used.

Several countries have noted a resurgence in later onset of vitamin K deficiency bleeding (VKDB) after practicing orally administered prophylaxis (American Academy of Pediatrics, 2003c). Current recommendations are that vitamin K be given to all newborns as a single intramuscular dose of 0.5 to 1.0 mg (American Academy of Pediatrics and American College of Obstetricians and Gynecologists, 2007). Additional study is needed on the efficacy, safety, and bioavailability of oral preparations and on the most effective dosing regimens to prevent VKDB (see Research Focus box).

RESEARCH FOCUS

Infant Pain Response and Maternal Hypertension

France, Taddio, Shah, and colleagues (2009) recently found that, when given an intramuscular injection of vitamin K, infants of mothers with a family history of hypertension had significantly shorter crying times and marginally lower facial grimacing scores than infants without maternal history of hypertension. The researchers concluded that reduced pain responses in infants at risk for hypertension is not a learned response but rather a product of genetic or prenatal influences.

Hepatitis B Vaccine Administration

To decrease the incidence of hepatitis B virus (HBV) in children and its serious consequences (cirrhosis and liver cancer) in adulthood, the first of three doses of HBV vaccine is recommended between birth and 2 months of age for all newborns born to hepatitis B surface antigen (HBsAg)–negative mothers. The injection is given in the vastus lateralis muscle, since this site is associated with a better immune response than the dorsogluteal area (although the dorsogluteal muscle typically is not used in infants in the United States) (American Academy of Pediatrics, 2009b). (See Immunizations, Chapter 12.) Giving the infant concentrated oral sucrose can reduce the pain of the injection (Stevens, Yamada, and Ohlsson, 2004). Preterm infants born to HBsAg-negative mothers should be vaccinated as early as 30 days of age regardless of gestational age or birth weight. Preterm infants weighing less than 2000 g (4.4 lb) who are ready to be released from hospital should receive hepatitis B vaccine just before hospital discharge. Infants born to HBsAg-positive mothers should be immunized within 12 hours after birth with HBV vaccine and hepatitis B immune globulin at separate sites, regardless of gestational age or birth weight (American Academy of Pediatrics, 2009b).

Newborn Screening for Disease

Blood sampling can detect a large number of congenital disorders in the newborn period so that early intervention can take place to decrease the long-term effects and cost of not treating such conditions. Currently no national policy regulates newborn screening; therefore the extent of screening has been largely determined by state laws and individual practice. All states now mandate screening tests for phenylketonuria (PKU) and congenital hypothyroidism (see Chapters 9 and 35); many states also have programs that include screening for sickle cell disease and galactosemia. Because of concern regarding the inconsistency among states in screening for such conditions based on cost, population demographics, resource availability, and political environment, the Task Force on Newborn Screening was formed by the American Academy of Pediatrics and other federal health care agencies and has developed a number of resolutions and policies to better address the issue of newborn screening (American Academy of Pediatrics, 2008b).

The advent of tandem mass spectrometry has expanded newborn screening to include detection of disorders of fatty acid oxidation, amino acids, and organic acids. This technology uses a minimum amount of blood and can identify more than 40 different disorders in 2 minutes (Bryant, Horns, Longo, et al, 2004). Tandem mass spectrometry has improved sensitivity and specificity for the detection of such conditions as hyperphenylalaninemia (PKU) and has a lower rate of false-positive results than other standardized testing methods.

The nurse's responsibility is to educate parents regarding the importance of screening and to collect appropriate specimens at the recommended time (after 24 hours of age or after the introduction of feedings; hospitalized infants must be screened before 7 days of age). With early newborn discharge before 24 hours, adequate screening for PKU requires a follow-up test within 2 weeks (Kaye and American Academy of Pediatrics, 2006). Accurate screening depends on high-quality blood spots on approved filter paper forms. The blood should completely saturate the filter paper spot on one side only. The paper should not be handled, placed on wet surfaces, or contaminated with any substance (see Atraumatic Care box). The American Academy of Pediatrics (2008a) recommends routine prenatal and perinatal human immunodeficiency virus (HIV) counseling and testing for all pregnant women. Benefits of early identification of HIV-infected infants include:

- Early antiretroviral therapy and aggressive nutritional supplementation
- Appropriate changes in their immunization schedule
- Monitoring and evaluation of immunologic, neurologic, and neuropsychologic functions for possible changes caused by antiretroviral therapy
- Initiation of special educational services
- Evaluation of the need for other therapies, such as immunoglobulin for the prevention of bacterial infections
- Tuberculosis screening and treatment
- Management of communicable disease exposures

Cesarean section, performed before the rupture of membranes or the onset of labor, may prevent mother-to-child transmission of HIV in optimally treated women and is associated with a 50% or more reduction in the risk of mother-to-child transmission among HIV-infected women who are either not receiving antiretroviral therapy or are receiving minimal therapy. For infants whose mother's HIV status is unknown, rapid HIV antibody testing provides information within 12 hours of the infant's birth. Antiretroviral prophylaxis is started as soon as possible, pending completion of confirmatory HIV testing. Breast-feeding is delayed until confirmatory testing is done. If the test is negative, prophylaxis is stopped and breast-feeding may start. If the test is positive, infants should be treated with antiretroviral prophylaxis for 6 weeks, and the mother should not breast-feed (American Academy of Pediatrics, 2008a). HIV-exposed infants who test negative initially should undergo further testing at 1 to 2 months and at 4 to 6 months of age to exclude or identify HIV infection (Havens, Mofenson, and Committee on Pediatric AIDS, 2009). For information on several diseases that may be included in newborn screening, see American Academy of Pediatrics' Introduction to the Newborn Screening Fact Sheets (Kaye and American Academy of Pediatrics, 2006).

ATRAUMATIC CARE

Heel Punctures

Repeated heel lancing is often necessary to obtain sufficient blood for a number of newborn blood tests, including newborn screening. It has been anecdotally observed that newborns appear to withdraw the heel when touched for subsequent heel punctures. Taddio, Shah, Gilbert-MacLeod, and colleagues (2002) found that infants of diabetic mothers exposed to multiple heel punctures in the first 24 to 36 hours of life learned to anticipate pain and exhibited more intense pain responses. The use of automated lancet devices such as Tenderfoot cause less pain and require fewer punctures than manual lance blades (Blain-Lewis, 1992; Paes, Janes, Vegh, et al, 1993). Additional studies have shown that venipuncture performed by an experienced phlebotomist elicited fewer pain responses (as measured by the Premature Infant Pain Profile [PIPP]) from full-term newborns than did heel punctures (Shah and Ohlsson, 2001). In addition, the need for additional skin punctures was reduced with venipuncture. Although maternal anxiety was initially higher in the venipuncture group, mothers who observed the venipuncture reported observing less pain response than mothers who observed heel punctures.

Oral sucrose and nonnutritive sucking have proved effective in decreasing the pain associated with heel punctures in preterm and full-term infants during the first week of life (Taddio, Shah, and Katz, 2009; Stevens, Yamada, and Ohlsson, 2004; Gibbins, Stevens, Hodnett, et al, 2002; Harrison, Johnston, and Loughnan, 2003); however, the exact dose range that proves effective varies among several studies (Stevens, Yamada, and Ohlsson, 2004). In one study, infants experiencing venipuncture were given either oral sucrose (30%) and a skin placebo or the eutectic mixture of local anesthetic (EMLA). Pain scores were measured with the PIPP, and infants receiving the oral sucrose solution exhibited fewer pain symptoms than those in the EMLA group (Gradin, Eriksson, Holmqvist, et al, 2002). Newborns given 2 ml of concentrated oral sucrose solution showed a significant reduction in crying time and heart rate in comparison with controls (given sterile water) during heel stick sampling and other painful stimuli (Stevens, Yamada, and Ohlsson, 2004).

Evidence indicates that as little as 2 ml of a 24% oral sucrose solution is effective in decreasing pain in full-term and preterm infants. In addition, the best analgesic effect is achieved when sucrose is administered 2 minutes before the painful procedure with a pacifier or syringe. In one study protocol where oral sucrose was effective, 0.5 ml of 24% oral sucrose solution was administered 2 minutes before the heel puncture, during, and 5 minutes after the heel puncture (Gibbins, Stevens, Hodnett, et al, 2002). Eriksson and Finnstrom (2004) found

that repeated administration of a 30% sucrose solution before heel lance in healthy full-term infants did not decrease the pain-relieving effect of the glucose solution; the study's aim was to determine whether multiple oral glucose administration would cause tolerance to glucose.

The mother's holding the infant in skin-to-skin contact has also been shown to significantly reduce the child's distress during the procedure (Johnston, Filion, Campbell-Yeo, et al, 2009; Blass and Watt, 1999; Gray, Watt, Blass, 2000; Johnston, Stevens, Pinelli, et al, 2003). Breast-feeding during heel puncture in full-term newborns has been shown to be effective in decreasing pain scores when compared with placebo or an oral sucrose solution (Carbajal, Veerapen, Couderc, et al, 2003; Codipietro, Ceccarelli, and Ponzone, 2008).

After a review of several published studies examining the benefit of applying the topical anesthetic EMLA to reduce the pain of heel lance in full-term and preterm infants, Weise and Nahata (2005) report no differences in pain response between the use of EMLA versus placebo. Thus this product appears to confer no benefit on newborns undergoing heel lance procedures.

Music was found to decrease the pain response to heel stick in a small group of preterm infants (Butt and Kisilevsky, 2000). A study comparing the effects of swaddling and containment on preterm infants undergoing heel stick failed to demonstrate significant differences between the two interventions (Huang, Tung, Kuo, et al, 2004).

These studies provide evidence of a number of effective ways to decrease the pain associated with heel puncture in full-term and preterm newborns. It is essential that nurses use *all* available resources to advocate for the prevention and management of neonatal pain during such procedures as heel puncture. Because the overall goal is to decrease the effect of painful interventions such as heel stick on infants, a combination of pharmacologic and nonpharmacologic interventions is recommended (Yamada, Stinson, Lamda, et al, 2008). (See also Atraumatic Care box, p. 257.)

A number of commercially available oral sucrose solutions now exist, including Toot-Sweet, a 24% sucrose solution from Hawaii Medical, LLL, and Sweet-Ease, 24% sucrose solution, from Children's Medical Ventures, Norwell, Massachusetts. When these are not available, the pharmacy may mix an oral sucrose solution to ensure a clean product. An approximate 25% sucrose solution is made by mixing 1 tsp of granulated (table) sugar with 4 tsp of sterile water; however, this method is the least desirable to prevent contamination of the solution and subsequent problems.

Universal Newborn Hearing Screening

It has been estimated that screening children for hearing loss by risk factors alone fails to identify approximately 50% of all newborns with a congenital hearing loss. Furthermore, infants who are hard of hearing or deaf, yet receive intervention before the age of 6 months, maintain appropriate language development matching their cognitive abilities through the age of 5 years (Yoshinaga-Itano, Sedey, Coulter, et al, 1998). For these reasons the American Academy of Pediatrics Joint Committee on Infant Hearing (2007b) recommends universal hearing screening of all newborns before discharge from the birthing hospital. Infants may be screened for hearing loss by auditory brainstem response or evoked otoacoustic emissions. Newborns who fail the initial screening require referral for outpatient retesting and intervention by 1 month of age; newborns who do not receive initial screening before discharge should also be tested by 1 month (American Academy of Pediatrics, 2007b; Connolly, Carron, and Roark, 2005). A subsequent audiologic assessment should be performed at least once by 24 to 36 months of age if the infant has any hearing risk factors despite passing the newborn hearing screening (American Academy of Pediatrics, 2009c).

Bathing

Bath time is an opportunity for the nurse to accomplish much more than general hygiene. It is an excellent time for observing the infant's behavior, state of arousal, alertness, and muscular activity. Bathing is usually performed after the vital signs, especially the temperature, have stabilized.

With the possibility of transmission of HBV and HIV via maternal blood and blood-stained amniotic fluid, the traditional timing of the newborn's bath has been questioned. Studies indicate that healthy full-term newborns with a stable body temperature can be bathed as early as 1 hour of age without experiencing problems, provided that effective thermoregulation measures are taken after the bath (Penny-MacGillivray, 1996; Behring, Vezeau, and Fink, 2003; Varda and Behnke, 2000; Medves and O'Brien, 2004). Take caution, however, to avoid instituting routine newborn bathing according to a rigid schedule; nursing interventions such as bathing should instead be based on individualized assessment and family interaction needs.

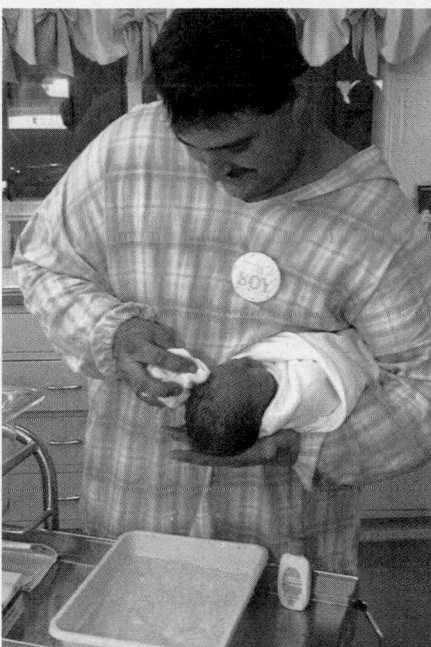

Fig. 8-11 Bath time is an excellent opportunity for parents to learn about their newborn.

Because of the possibility of blood and body fluid contagions, as part of Standard Precautions, nurses should wear gloves when handling the newborn until blood and amniotic fluid are removed by bathing.

The bath time provides an opportunity for the nurse to involve the parents in the care of their child, to teach correct hygiene procedures, and to help them learn about their infant's individual characteristics (Fig. 8-11). The bath may also be used to help parents learn and better understand their newborn's behavioral characteristics using the BNBAS. The nurse stresses appropriate bathing supplies and the need for safety in terms of water temperature and supervision of the infant at all times during the bath.

Encourage parents to examine every finger and toe of their infant during bathing. Frequently normal variations such as milia, **erythema toxicum** (rash), or "stork bites" worry parents who are unaware of the insignificance of such findings. Minor birth injuries may appear as major defects to them. Explaining how these occurred and when they will disappear reassures parents of their infant's normalcy. Chapter 9 discusses common variations.

One of the most important considerations in skin cleansing is preservation of the skin's "acid mantle," which is formed by the uppermost horny layer of the epidermis; sweat; superficial fat; metabolic products; and external substances such as amniotic fluid, microorganisms, and chemicals. The infant's skin surface has a pH of about 5 soon after birth, and the bacteriostatic effects of this pH are significant. In addition, newborn skin is covered with host-defense proteins, such as lysozyme and lactoferrin, which contribute importantly to a newborn's defense against bacterial infections (Walker, Akinbi, Meinzen-Derr, et al, 2008). Consequently, use only plain warm water for routine bathing. If a cleanser is needed, Dove (fragrance free) has a neutral pH and is mild. Alkaline soaps, oils, powder, and lotions are not used because they alter the acid mantle, thus providing a medium for bacterial growth. Talcum powder has the added risk of aspiration if it is applied close to the infant's face. Corn starch powder may also cause respiratory problems and aspiration. (See Diaper Dermatitis, Chapter 13.)

Parents should be involved in a discussion regarding the newborn's bath at home. It is recommended that for the first 2 to 4 weeks the infant be bathed no more than two or three times per week with a plain warm sponge bath. This practice will help maintain the integrity of the newborn's skin and allow time for the umbilical cord to dry completely. Routine daily bathing for newborns is no longer recommended.

Cleansing should proceed in the cephalocaudal (head-to-toe) direction. Vigorous rubbing to remove vernix is unnecessary and may cause more harm than good. A diaper is applied after the bath, and the infant is clothed appropriately to prevent heat loss.

The nurse should discuss the choice of cloth or disposable diapers with parents. Disposable diapers are the most convenient, although a diaper service eliminates the need to shop for replacement diapers. Disposable diapers with absorbent gelling material have benefits related to preserving healthy skin; preventing diaper dermatitis, especially beyond the neonatal period (see Chapter 13); and controlling contamination of the environment because of their better containment of urine and feces.

Care of the Umbilicus

Because the umbilical stump is an excellent medium for bacterial growth, various methods of cord care have been practiced to prevent infection. Some methods popular in the past include the use of an antimicrobial agent such as bacitracin or triple dye, or agents such as alcohol or povidone. Many studies report that the use of antiseptic agents prolongs cord drying and separation (Zupan, Garner, and Omari, 2004; Dore, Buchan, Coulas, et al, 1998). Although studies regarding bacterial growth and colonization according to the cleansing method used have produced varied results (Janssen, Selwood, Dobson, et al, 2003; Golombek, Brill, and Salice, 2002; Dore, Buchan, Coulas, et al, 1998), a Cochrane Review of 21 studies found no significant difference between cords treated with antiseptics compared with dry cord care or placebo; there were no reported systemic infections or deaths, and a trend towards reduced colonization was found in cords treated with antiseptics (Zupan, Garner, and Omari, 2004). Current recommendations for cord care by the Association of Women's Health, Obstetric and Neonatal Nurses (2007) includes cleaning the cord initially with sterile water or a neutral pH cleanser, then subsequently cleaning the cord with water.

Nurses working in neonatal care must carefully evaluate the available studies and compare the risks and benefits regarding the method of cord care within their own population of newborns and families. Particularly in the developing world, infants may encounter increased risk of potentially life-threatening sepsis; thus antimicrobial treatment may be appropriate in some settings (Mullany, Darmstadt, Katz, et al, 2009). A recent randomized controlled study showed that use of a newer antimicrobial for cord care, chlorhexidine powder, resulted in faster cord separation time and fewer complications than dry cord care (Kapellen, Gebauer, Brosteanu, et al, 2009). Regardless of the method used, nurses must teach parents about the importance of observation and monitoring of the cord, in addition to cord care methods, in discharge planning.

The diaper is placed below the cord to avoid irritation and wetness on the site. Parents are instructed regarding stump deterioration and proper umbilical care. The stump deteriorates through the process of dry gangrene. Cord separation time is influenced by a number of factors, including type of cord care, type of delivery, and other perinatal events. The average cord separation time is 5 to 15 days. It takes a few more weeks for the cord base to heal completely after cord separation. During this time, care consists of keeping the base clean and dry and observing for any signs of infection.

With early hospital discharge, newborns may be discharged before it is safe to remove the cord clamp. Teach the parent how to safely remove the clamp once the newborn is at least 24 hours old and no oozing from the cord is evident.

Circumcision

Circumcision, the surgical removal of the foreskin on the glans penis, is usually done in the hospital, although it is not a common practice in most countries. In the United States, however, circumcision rates have increased significantly over time: 61.1% of U.S. boys born from 1997 to 2000 were circumcised, compared with 48.3% of U.S. boys born from 1988 to 1991 (Nelson, Dunn, Wan, et al, 2005). Despite the frequency of the procedure in the United States, there is still much controversy regarding the benefits and risks (Box 8-5). One study that received considerable criticism demonstrated a ninefold increase in urinary tract infections in uncircumcised boys during the first year of life (Bartman, 2001; Schoen, Colby, and Ray, 2000). Other researchers have responded that such infections are best prevented by practicing good hygiene, rather than advocating an invasive procedure such as circumcision (Kinkade, Meadows, and Gracia-Trujillo, 2005).

Recently, research has explored the possible link between circumcision and reduced transmission of communicable illnesses such as human papillomavirus (HPV) and HIV in later life. Several researchers report that circumcision is associated with reduced likelihood of transmission of HPV in men known to be exposed (Lu, Wu, Nielson, et al, 2009; Nielson, Schiaffino, Dunne, et al, 2009). Warner, Ghanem, Newman, and colleagues (2009) report that circumcision is associated with substantially reduced transmission of HIV in men known to be exposed. There is concern, however, regarding findings from such observational studies, since there is no opportunity for control of confounding variables (factors other than circumcision that explain the results). A Cochrane Review cautioned against adoption of circumcision as a public health measure until stronger prospective studies demonstrate a clear link between lack of circumcision and disease transmission (Siegfried, Muller, Volmink, et al, 2003). Since that caution, some prospective studies have reported reduced risk of HIV transmission after adult circumcision in high-risk groups (Bailey, Moses, Parker, et al, 2007; Gray, Kigozi, Serwadda, et al, 2007). More research is needed to better understand any possible link between neonatal circumcision and subsequent risk of sexually transmitted infection.

The American Academy of Pediatrics (1999) issued a circumcision policy statement stating that the medical benefits of male newborn circumcision are not sufficiently significant to recommend it as a routine procedure. The academy statement emphasizes parental autonomy to determine what is in the best interest of their newborn boy. The policy encourages the physician to ensure that parents have been given accurate and unbiased information about the risks, benefits, and alternatives before making an informed choice and that they understand that circumcision is an elective procedure. In addition to examining the medical benefits of newborn circumcision, the academy recommended that if parents decide to have their male infant circumcised, procedural analgesia should be provided.

This policy statement has direct implications for nurses caring for newborns and their families. First, because nurses are in a unique position to educate parents regarding the care of their newborns, they must take responsibility for ensuring that each parent has accurate and unbiased information on which to make an informed decision. Parents need to know the options for pain control, especially the choice of topical or injected anesthesia, and their option of observing the procedure.*

Second, the nurse should use nonpharmacologic interventions as an adjunct to reduce the pain of this operative procedure (see Atraumatic Care box). Despite adequate scientific evidence that newborns feel and respond to pain, circumcisions are still performed in the United States with either insufficient analgesia or no analgesia at all. Nurses can use the academy's policy statement to advocate more effectively for the use of optimum pain relief during circumcision.

Four types of anesthesia and analgesia are used in newborns undergoing circumcision: ring block, dorsal penile nerve block

Critical Thinking Exercise—Circumcision (margin tab)

BOX 8-5   RISKS AND BENEFITS OF NEONATAL CIRCUMCISION

Risks (Complications)

Hemorrhage

Infection

Dehiscence (separation of approximated edges of skin)

Meatitis (from loss of protective foreskin)

Adhesions

Concealed penis

Urethral fistula

Meatal stenosis

Pain in unanesthetized infants (long-term consequences unknown, but short-term stresses include increased heart rate, behavior changes, prolonged crying, increased cortisol levels, and decreased blood oxygenation)

Benefits

Prevention of penile cancer and posthitis (inflammation of prepuce)

Decreased incidence of balanitis (inflammation of glans) and possibly urinary tract infection in infants

Reduction or prevention of acquisition and transmission of sexually transmitted infections

Prevention of complications associated with later circumcision

Preservation of male's body image that is consistent with peers (in countries where procedure is common)

Should we have our son circumcised? is available from the American Academy of Pediatrics, 141 Northwest Point Blvd., Elk Grove Village, IL 60009-1098; 847-434-4000; fax: 847-434-8000; www.aap.org.

ATRAUMATIC CARE

Guidelines for Pain Management During Neonatal Circumcision*

Pharmacologic Interventions

Use of Topical Anesthetic Only

1. One hour before the procedure, administer acetaminophen (e.g., Tylenol 15 mg/kg) as ordered by the practitioner.
2. Place a thick layer (1 g) of EMLA† or LMX4‡ cream around the penis where the prepuce (foreskin) attaches to the glans. Avoid placing cream on the tip of the penis where it may come in contact with urethral opening.
3. Cover the penis with a "finger cot" that is cut from a vinyl or latex glove, or a piece of plastic wrap, and secure bottom of covering with tape. Avoid using Tegaderm or large amounts of tape on the skin because removing the adhesive causes pain and can irritate the fragile skin.
4. If the infant urinates during the time EMLA is applied (1 hour) and a significant amount of EMLA is removed, reapply the cream and covering. The total application of EMLA should not exceed a surface area of 10 cm² (1.25 × 1.25 inches).
5. Remove cream with clean cloth or tissue. Blanching of skin is an expected reaction to EMLA's application under an occlusive dressing; erythema and some edema may occur also.
6. Two minutes before starting the procedure, give the infant a sucrose solution; 24% (weight/volume) sucrose solution is available commercially from Children's Medical Ventures (800-345-6443), or may be easily made by a hospital pharmacy. Use this solution to coat the pacifier (recoat several times before and during the procedure).
7. After the procedure, apply petrolatum or A&D ointment on a 2 × 2 inch dressing before diapering infant to prevent the wound from adhering to the dressing or diaper.
8. Administer acetaminophen as ordered by the practitioner 4 hours after the initial dose; give additional doses as needed but not to exceed five doses in 24 hours or a maximum dose of 75 mg/kg/day.

Use of Dorsal Penile Nerve Block (DPNB) or Ring Block

1. One hour before the procedure administer acetaminophen as ordered by the practitioner.
2. One hour before procedure, apply EMLA. For the DPNB apply EMLA to the prepuce as described previously and at the penile base. For the ring block

apply EMLA to the prepuce as described previously and to the shaft of the penis. Use a topical anesthetic in conjunction with the DPNB or ring block to avoid the pain of injecting the anesthetic.

3. Use a 30-gauge needle to administer the lidocaine.§ For the DPNB, 0.4 ml of the lidocaine is infiltrated at the 10:30 and 1:30 o'clock positions in Buck fascia at the penile base. For the ring block, 0.4 ml of lidocaine is infiltrated subcutaneously on each side of the shaft of the penis below the prepuce.
4. For maximum anesthesia, wait 5 minutes after injection of lidocaine. An alternative anesthetic agent is chloroprocaine, which is as effective as lidocaine after 3 minutes.
5. Approximately 2 minutes before the circumcision, administer concentrated oral sucrose solution as described previously.
6. After the procedure, apply A&D ointment or petrolatum and administer acetaminophen as described previously.

Nonpharmacologic Interventions

In addition to the preceding pharmacologic interventions:

- If using a Circumstraint board, pad with blankets or other thick, soft material such as "lamb's wool." A more comfortable, padded, and physiologic restraint that places the infant semireclining can also decrease distress‖ (Stang, Snellman, Condon, et al, 1997).
- Provide the parents, caregiver, or another staff member with the option to hold the infant during the procedure or to be present during the circumcision.
- Swaddle the upper body and legs to provide warmth and containment and to reduce movement.
- If the patient is not swaddled and is unclothed, use a radiant warmer to prevent hypothermia. Shield infant's eyes from overhead lights.
- Prewarm any topical solutions to be used in sterile preparation of the surgical site by placing in a warm blanket or towel.
- Play infant relaxation music¶ before, during, and after procedure; allow parents or other caregiver the option of choosing the music.
- After the procedure, remove restraints and swaddle. Immediately have the parent, other caregiver, or nursing staff hold the infant. Continue to have the infant suck on pacifier or offer feeding.

Data from Broadman LM, Hannallah RS, Belman AB, et al: Post-circumcision analgesia: a prospective evaluation of subcutaneous ring block of the penis, *Anesthesiology* 67:339-402, 1987; Howard CR, Howard FM, Weitzman ML: Acetaminophen analgesia in neonatal circumcision: the effect on pain, *Pediatrics* 93(4):641-646, 1994; Lander J, Brady-Fryer B, Metcalfe JB, et al: Comparison of ring block, dorsal penile nerve block, and topical anesthesia for neonatal circumcision, *JAMA* 278:2157-2162, 1997; Mintz MR, Grillo R: Dorsal penile nerve block for circumcision, *Clin Pediatr* 28:590-591, 1989; Serour F, Mandelberg A, Mori J: Slow injection of local anesthetic will decrease pain during dorsal penile nerve block, *Acta Anesthesiol Scand* 42:926-928, 1998; Spencer DM, Miller KA, O'Quinn M, et al: Dorsal penile nerve block in neonatal circumcision: chloroprocaine versus lidocaine, *Am J Perinatol* 9(3):214-218, 1992; Stang H, Snellman LW, Condon LM, et al: Beyond dorsal penile nerve block: a more humane circumcision, *Pediatrics* 100(2):E3, 1997, available at www.pediatrics.org/cgi/content/full/100/2/e3 (accessed November 25, 2009); Stevens B, Yamada J, Ohlsson A: Sucrose for analgesia in newborn infants undergoing painful procedures, *Cochrane Database Syst Rev* (3):CD001069, 2004; Taddio A, Stevens B, Craig K, et al: Efficacy and safety of lidocaine-prilocaine cream (EMLA) for pain during circumcision, *N Engl J Med* 336(17):1197-1201, 1997.

*There is sufficient evidence and support for use of a combination of pharmacologic and nonpharmacologic interventions to holistically manage neonatal circumcision pain. Combined analgesia, nonpharmacologic interventions (such as swaddling), and local anesthesia may be used during the procedure to provide holistic pain management (Taddio, Pollock, Gilbert-MacLeod, et al, 2000; Anand and International Evidence-Based Group for Neonatal Pain, 2001; Geyer, Ellsbury, Kleiber, et al, 2002; Razmus, Dalton, and Wilson, 2004).

†On March 11, 1999, the US Food and Drug Administration approved use of EMLA in infants age 37 weeks of gestation, provided practitioners followed recommendations regarding maximal dose and limits for exposure time to the medication. In addition, practitioners are advised not to use EMLA with infants who are receiving methemoglobinemia-inducing medications such as acetaminophen or phenobarbital. Although the package insert warns that patients taking acetaminophen are at greater risk for developing methemoglobinemia, there have been no reported cases of this complication in children taking acetaminophen and using EMLA.

‡LMX4 (previously Ela-Max) is a 4% lidocaine cream reported to be effective within 30 minutes of application for venipuncture. There is no need to apply an occlusive dressing over LMX4 cream as recommended for EMLA (Wong, 2003). Use of LMX4 for pain relief of pediatric meatotomy has been reported previously (Smith and Gjellum, 2004). Despite anecdotal reports of its use in neonatal circumcision, at this time no studies are available regarding the use or effectiveness of LMX4 for neonatal circumcision analgesia.

§In one study the use of buffered lidocaine, which normally reduces stinging sensation of lidocaine, did not provide effective anesthesia for DPNB (Stang, Snellman, Condon, et al, 1997). The study on slow injection of the anesthetics lidocaine and bupivacaine compared 40 versus 80 seconds in patients ages 15 to 53 years (Serour, Mandelberg, and Mori, 1998).

‖For information on Stang Circ Chair, contact Pedicraft, 4134 Saint Augustine Rd, Jacksonville, FL 32207, 800-223-7649; e-mail: info@pedicraft.com; www.pedicraft.com.

¶Suggested infant relaxation music: Heartbeat Lullabies by Terry Woodford. Available from Baby-Go-To-Sleep Center, Audio-Therapy Innovations, Inc., PO Box 550, Colorado Springs, CO 80901, 800-537-7748.

(DPNB), topical anesthetic such as EMLA (prilocaine-lidocaine), and oral sucrose. Oral acetaminophen and comfort measures such as music, sucking on a pacifier, and soothing voices have not proved to be effective in reducing the pain of circumcision when used alone (Williamson, 1997).

A Cochrane Review (Brady-Fryer, Wiebe, and Lander, 2004) reports that DPNB is the most frequently studied intervention and the most effective method of preventing circumcision pain. Ring block is also effective in reducing pain and is reported to be technically easier and potentially safer because it eliminates the risk of injecting lidocaine into the dorsal vessels. The topical application of EMLA to the penis before circumcision has also been helpful in reducing operative pain (Taddio, Ohlsson, and Ohlsson, 2000). An occlusive dressing must be placed over the cream, which must be applied approximately 1 hour before the procedure. Although this preparation may be perceived as complicated and requiring too much advance notice, it is important to remember that most newborns are kept NPO (nothing by mouth) for 1 to 2 hours before the procedure to prevent aspiration. In clinical practice, however, the issues of difficulty in application and time required to reach maximum effect may result in EMLA being used less often as an anesthetic (Brady-Fryer, Wiebe, and Lander, 2004). The use of EMLA cream for neonatal circumcision has not been associated with methemoglobinemia, a serious but rare complication associated with prilocaine. A localized rash has been associated with EMLA when used for circumcision.

A nonpharmacologic strategy for providing pain relief for circumcision is the use of intraoral sucrose. The administration of a concentrated dose of oral sucrose and nonnutritive sucking have proved more effective than no treatment in decreasing procedural pain (venipuncture, heel stick, circumcision) in full-term and preterm infants in many studies (Herschel, Khoshnood, Ellman, et al, 1998; Stevens, Taddio, Ohlsson, et al, 1997; Stevens, Johnston, Franck, et al, 1999). A Cochrane Review (Stevens, Yamada, and Ohlsson, 2004) concludes that oral sucrose is safe and effective for reducing procedural pain for single painful events, although the optimum dose for maximum pain relief is not yet known. Research addressing the use of sucrose as an adjunct to other nonpharmacologic and pharmacologic pain management methods is needed. Many nurses use intraoral sucrose to reduce the pain associated with procedures such as circumcision, venipuncture, and heel stick.

The Cochrane group exploring pain relief for neonatal circumcision (Brady-Fryer, Wiebe, and Lander, 2004) recommends that future research focus on benefits of infants receiving two or more active interventions for pain relief, and states that a placebo or no-treatment group is no longer acceptable. Studies exploring the use of several strategies concurrently, such as that conducted by Razmus, Dalton, and Wilson (2004), which included groups receiving both sucrose and ring block compared with ring block alone, have the most potential to clarify optimum strategies.

A recent Cochrane Review on pain relief for boys undergoing circumcision emphasized the need for postoperative pain relief (Cyna and Middleton, 2008). The authors advocate anticipating and controlling postoperative pain both to enhance patient comfort and to decrease crying and agitation that may increase the risk of postoperative bleeding.

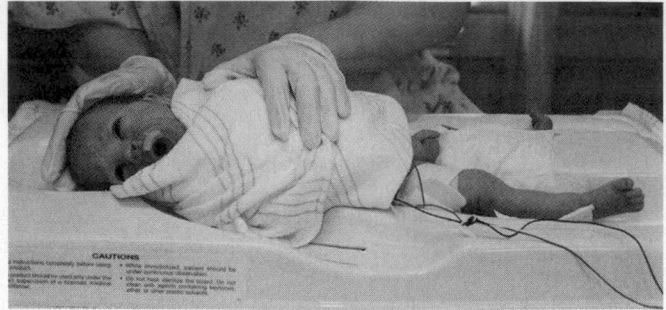

Fig. 8-12 Proper positioning of infant in Circumstraint. (Courtesy Paul Vincent Kuntz, Texas Children's Hospital, Houston.)

Circumcision is usually performed in the nursery. It should not be performed immediately after delivery because of the neonate's unstable physiologic status and increased susceptibility to stress. Preoperative nursing care includes allowing the infant nothing by mouth before the procedure to prevent aspiration of vomitus (about 1 to 2 hours); however, the necessity of this practice has been challenged (Kraft, 2003). Additional measures include the surgical time-out, checking for a signed consent form, and adequately restraining the infant, usually on a special board (Fig. 8-12) or physiologic circumcision restraint chair. The circumcision chair is padded and allows free movement of the newborn's extremities without compromising the surgical field. In addition, the chair allows the infant to sit at a 30- to 45-degree angle, and it is adjustable to accommodate smaller newborns (Stang, Snellman, Condon, et al, 1997). All the equipment used for the procedure, such as gloves, instruments, dressings, and draping towels, must be sterile.

The procedure involves freeing the foreskin from the glans penis by using a scalpel, Gomco or Mogen clamp (see Cultural Competence box), or Plastibell. In the Gomco technique the foreskin is clamped, cut with a scalpel, and removed; the clamp crushes the nerve endings and blood vessels, promoting hemostasis. In the Plastibell procedure the foreskin is removed using a plastic ring and a string tied around the foreskin like a tourniquet. The excess foreskin is trimmed. In about 5 to 8 days the plastic ring separates and falls off.

Once the procedure is completed, the infant is released from the restraints and comforted. If the parents were not present during the procedure, they are informed of the infant's status and reunited with their son.

Care of the circumcision depends on the type of procedure. If a clamp (Gomco or Mogen) was used, a petrolatum gauze dressing may be applied loosely to prevent adherence to the diaper. If the Plastibell was applied, no special dressing is required. Because the area is tender, the diaper is applied loosely to prevent friction against the penis. The circumcision is evaluated for excessive bleeding in the first few hours after the procedure, and the first void is recorded. A recommended standard is to evaluate the site every 30 minutes for at least 2 hours and then at least every 2 hours thereafter (Williamson, 1997).

NURSING TIP To check for the first void in disposable diapers made of absorbent gelling material, pinch the crotch of the diaper for a "clumpy, doughy" feeling, since these diapers will feel dry despite voiding.

CULTURAL COMPETENCE
Circumcision

In the Jewish culture circumcision is performed during a ceremony called a berith, or brit, which takes place on the eighth day of life. A specially trained professional known as a mohel stretches the prepuce over the glans, pulling it through a slit in a shield (usually a Mogen clamp) and cutting it with a knife. The traditional technique is not sterile, and bleeding is controlled by tight bandaging around the penis (Cohen, Drucker, Vainer, et al, 1992). The infant may be given some sweet wine before the procedure. Blankets instead of straps are usually used to restrain the infant to a board, and the parents are present (Trochtenberg, 1990).

Female circumcision (mutilation) is practiced in some parts of Africa, the Middle East, and Southeast Asia—and in immigrants from these countries to the United States, Australia, Canada, and Europe. In the most extensive operation (excision or infibulation) the clitoris, labia minora, and medial aspects of the labia majora are removed. The remainder of the labia majora is sewn closed, except for a small opening for urine and menses (American Academy of Pediatrics, 1998; McCleary, 1994; Abubakar, Iliyasu, Kabir, et al, 2004). Anesthesia is rarely used. In African and Asian cultures, female circumcision is used to prove virginity and to reduce sexual pleasure, thus promoting fidelity. The World Health Organization (2008) condemns all forms of female genital mutilation.

BOX 8-6   ADVANTAGES OF HUMAN MILK COMPARED WITH FORMULA

- Contains adequate (not excessive) protein; has greater quantities of certain amino acids, including cystine and taurine
- Contains more lactalbumin (produces easily digested curds) than casein (produces large, hard curds)
- Contains more lactose, which in the gut stimulates growth of microorganisms, which synthesize some B vitamins and produce organic acids that may restrict or prevent the growth of harmful bacteria
- Contains more monounsaturated fatty acids, which enhance absorption of fat and calcium
- Contains adequate (not excessive) minerals, with exception of fluoride (low)
- Contains low amounts of iron and zinc, but these are more readily absorbed
- Contains less calcium and phosphorus but a more favorable ratio of the minerals, which prevents excessive calcium excretion
- Contains adequate amounts of vitamins A, B complex, and E; vitamin C content depends on maternal intake; vitamin D is low but more readily absorbed
- Contains growth modulators that modify growth or maturation
- Offers several immunologic benefits: contains various immunoglobulins, especially immunoglobulin A; macrophages, granulocytes, T- and B-cell lymphocytes; and other factors that inhibit bacterial growth
- Has laxative effect
- Is economical, readily available, and sanitary
- Has psychologic benefits of a close bond between infant and mother during feeding

---

Normally, on the second day a yellowish white exudate forms as part of the granulation process. This is not a sign of infection and is not forcibly removed. As healing progresses, the exudate disappears. Parents are educated to report any evidence of bleeding, unusual swelling, or absence of voiding to the practitioner.

PROVIDE OPTIMUM NUTRITION

Selection of a feeding method is one of the major decisions parents face. It is best to explore feeding options before the infant is born when parents are better able to understand the importance of infant nutrition and the choices available. Nurses should be at the forefront in providing parent(s) with accurate and unbiased information needed to make a conscientious, informed decision regarding feeding method. In general, there are two primary choices: human milk and commercially prepared cow's milk–based formula. These two methods have significant nutritional, economic, and psychologic differences (Box 8-6).

Cultural Influences on Infant Feeding

Cultural beliefs and practices are significant influences on infant feeding methods. As many as 50 of 120 cultures studied typically do not give colostrum to newborns and only begin breast-feeding after the milk has "come in." These groups include some Filipinos, Hispanics, Vietnamese, Hmong, Koreans, and Nigerians. When breast-feeding is delayed until the milk is in, babies are given prelacteal food. In India, infants may be fed liquids such as honey, tea, water, or sugar water before the initiation of breast-feeding (Choudhry, 1997). Other cultures begin breast-feeding immediately and offer the breast each time the infant cries. Cultural attitudes regarding modesty and breast-feeding are important considerations. Language barriers may also prevent successful breast-feeding and counseling in some situations. Even among Hispanic Spanish-speaking people, terminology used in one country for the act of breast-feeding or describing the breasts may be offensive in another Spanish-speaking country.

Hernandez (2006) suggests that knowledge of the Hispanic woman's immigration status is important when discussing breast-feeding; U.S.-born Hispanic women are less likely to initiate breast-feeding, whereas those recently immigrated are more likely to continue the social norm of breast-feeding. Breast-feeding classes in Spanish for the new mother and grandmother may enhance discussion of practices related to exclusive breast-feeding in the first few months (Hernandez, 2006). Mexican women have a custom called *la cuarentena*, which means the woman has 40 days of rest after giving birth; during this time the mother is relieved of housekeeping duties and may focus on the new infant. The maternal grandmother traditionally assists the mother during this time. Other Hispanic customs related to infant feeding include the belief in herbal teas consumed by the breast-feeding mother to settle the infant's stomach; commonly given teas include *manzanilla* (chamomile) and anise. In Hispanic families the breast-feeding mother commonly consumes traditional cultural foods to acculturate the infant to such foods (Hernandez, 2006).

The Muslim and Jewish cultures value breast-feeding of infants. Muslim women also have the tradition of the 40-day rest period in which the woman is relieved of housekeeping duties and other women help care for her. During this time the mother may exclusively breast-feed; however, Muslim women typically terminate exclusive breast-feeding early in infancy (Chertok, Shoham-Vardi, and Hallak, 2004). Breast-feeding for Jewish women is perceived as being important but is highly influenced by maternal education level, assimilated cultural values depending on geographic region of origin, and previous breast-feeding experience (Chertok, Shoham-Vardi, and Hallak, 2004).

With the large percentage of immigrants in the United States, it is incumbent on nurses to discuss cultural values related to breast-feeding and the benefits of breast-feeding so the mother can make an informed decision. Hernandez (2006) relates the story of a young Mexican woman who delivered an infant in the United States but started bottle-feeding instead of breast-feeding. When asked about this, she told the nurse that since there was a packet of formula in the infant's crib at discharge, she interpreted this as the cultural norm in the United States and did not breast-feed. The nursing implications are clear: clarify with the mother what her expectations are regarding infant feeding and assist her in meeting those goals.

Sociocultural values may preclude the mother receiving adequate information regarding breast-feeding; for example, if the family is strongly patriarchal and the father is the only English-speaking person in the family, the necessary information being conveyed to the mother by the health care provider may not be correctly translated. Persons immigrating to the United States often tend to acquire the local customs, and, although breast-feeding may have been common in their own country, they may abandon the practice in the United States, considering it "outdated" (Riordan and Gill-Hopple, 2001) (see Cultural Competence box).

⊕ CULTURAL COMPETENCE

Acculturation

Acculturation is a process whereby members of one cultural group adopt the beliefs and behaviors of another group. Singh, Kogan, and Dee (2007) identified the effects of immigration on breast-feeding rates in the United States based on the 2003 National Survey of Children's Health. In this study women who immigrated from other countries to the United States and had a native-born infant were significantly more likely to initiate and maintain breast-feeding for 6 to 12 months compared with women who had immigrant parents and a native-born infant. Acculturation in this study was associated with lower breast-feeding rates among Hispanic and non-Hispanic women.

Human Milk

Human milk is the best option for infant nutrition up to 1 year of age. Breast milk consists of a number of micronutrients that are bioavailable, meaning these nutrients are available in quantities and qualities that make them easily digestible by the newborn and absorbed for energy and growth. A variety of immunologic properties are found exclusively in human milk. Human milk has been shown to be effective in protecting the newborn against respiratory tract infections and decreasing the incidence of hospital admissions for respiratory tract illnesses in generally healthy infants (Bachrach, Schwarz, and Bachrach, 2003); gastrointestinal infections caused by enterococci; otitis media, numerous allergies, and atopy; and type 2 diabetes (Beaudry, Dufour, and Marcoux, 1995; Dewey, Heinig, and Nommsen-Rivers, 1995; Scariati, Grummer-Strawn, and Fein, 1997; Young, Martens, Taback, et al, 2002). Some studies have demonstrated that breast-feeding has an analgesic effect on newborns during painful procedures such as heel puncture (Gray, Miller, Phillip, et al, 2002; Carbajal, Veerapen, Couderc, et al, 2003).

The fat content of human milk is composed of lipids, triglycerides, and cholesterol; cholesterol is an essential element for brain growth. The function of these lipids is to allow optimum intestinal absorption of fatty acids and provide essential fatty acids and polyunsaturated fatty acids. Furthermore lipids contribute approximately 50% of the total calories in human milk (Lawrence and Lawrence, 2005). Although the overall fat content in human milk is higher than that of cow's milk–based formula, it is used more efficiently by the infant.

The primary source of carbohydrate in human milk is lactose, which is present in higher concentrations (6.8 g/dl) than in cow's milk–based formula (4.9 g/dl). Other carbohydrates found in human milk include glucose, galactose, and glucosamine. The carbohydrates serve not only as a large percentage of the total calories in human milk, but also have a protective function; the oligosaccharides (prebiotic) in human milk stimulate the growth of *Lactobacillus bifidus* (a probiotic) and prevent bacteria from adhering to epithelial surfaces (Lawrence and Lawrence, 2005).

Human milk contains the two proteins, whey (lactalbumin) and casein (curd), in a ratio of approximately 60:40 (versus 20:80 to 100% whey in different brands of cow's milk–based formula). This ratio in human milk makes it more digestible and produces the soft stools seen in infants who breast-feed. Thus human milk has a laxative effect and constipation is uncommon. The whey protein, lactoferrin, in human milk has iron-binding characteristics with bacteriostatic capabilities, particularly against gram-positive and gram-negative aerobes, anaerobes, and yeasts (Lawrence and Lawrence, 2005).

Lysozyme is found in large quantities in human milk with bacteriostatic functions against gram-positive bacteria and *Enterobacteriaceae* organisms. Human milk also contains numerous other host defense factors such as macrophages, granulocytes, and T and B lymphocytes. Casein in human milk greatly enhances the absorption of iron, thus preventing iron-dependent bacteria from proliferating in the gastrointestinal tract (Biancuzzo, 2003). Secretory immunoglobulin A (IgA) is found in high levels in colostrum, but levels gradually decrease over the first 14 days of life. Secretory IgA is an immunoglobulin that prevents viruses and bacteria from invading the intestinal mucosa in breast-fed newborns, thus protecting them from infection (Hanson and Korotkova, 2002). This whey protein is also believed to play an important role in preventing the development of allergies (Biancuzzo, 2003).

Several digestive enzymes also present in human milk include amylases, lipases, proteases, and ribonucleases, which enhance digestion and absorption of various nutrients (Lawrence and Lawrence, 2005). The amounts of lipid- and water-soluble vitamins, as well as electrolytes, minerals, and trace elements, in human milk are sufficient for infant growth, development, and energy needs during the first 6 months of life. The one possible exception is vitamin D, which is found in varying amounts depending on the mother's intake of vitamin D–fortified food and exposure to ultraviolet light. Therefore, to prevent vitamin D deficiency rickets, the American Academy of Pediatrics (Wagner, Greer, and American Academy of Pediatrics, 2008) now recommends that infants who are exclusively breast-fed, who are breast-fed and consuming less than 1000 ml of vitamin D–fortified formula or milk per day, or who are ingesting less than 1000 ml/day of vitamin D–fortified formula or milk be supplemented with 400 international units of vitamin D (oral) per day. In addition, older children who do not consume at least 400 international units of vitamin D–fortified milk or vitamin D–fortified foods should receive a supplement of 400 international units of vitamin D daily. The Canadian Paediatric Society (2007) suggests that for children living in its northernmost climates, it may be reasonable to double this recommendation to 800 international units per day, to compensate for extremely limited exposure to sunlight.

Studies have also shown that feeding infants human milk produces children with higher intelligence than their counterparts fed on cow's milk–based formula (Anderson, Johnstone, and Remley, 1999; Lanting, Fidler, Huisman, et al, 1994). Additional beneficial components of human milk include prostaglandins; epidermal growth factor; docosahexaenoic acid (DHA); arachidonic acid (AA); taurine; carnitine; cytokine; interleukins; and natural hormones such as thyroid-releasing hormone, gonadotropin-releasing hormone, and prolactin.

Human milk also has variations related to the timing of the lactation cycle. Colostrum, for example, is rich in immunoglobulins and vitamin K and has a higher protein content than mature milk; however, it has a lower fat content. Transitional milk replaces colostrum when the mother's milk supply starts increasing, and eventually mature milk becomes the primary milk source. There is also diurnal variation in the biochemistry of mature human milk. Human milk also varies with respect to gestational age; preterm human milk differs from mature milk in its biochemical composition (Lawrence and Lawrence, 2005). Nonphysiologic advantages of human milk are discussed in the next section.

Breast-Feeding

Human milk is the preferred form of nutrition for the full-term infant. *Healthy People 2020* has a goal to increase breast-feeding rates in the United States to 75% in early postpartum and to 50% for mothers who continue to breast-feed for at least 6 months US Department of Health and Human Services, 2009). Data from the 2003 Ross Mothers Survey indicate that the overall rate of breast-feeding in the hospital was 66%, down four points from 2002 (70.1%); breast-feeding at 6 months of age in 2003 was reported to be 32.8%, down slightly from the previous year (33.2%) (Ross Mothers Survey, 2003). The Centers for Disease Control and Prevention (2007) analyzed data from the National Immunization Survey and found that, among infants born in 2004, 30.5% and 11.3% were exclusively breast-feeding at 3 and 6 months, respectively. Both surveys found similar disparities in breast-feeding rates: lower breast-feeding rates at 6 months occurred in African-American women and in women without a college degree. Full-time employment at 6 months was a strong contributing factor to the decrease in breast-feeding, and enrollment in the Women, Infants, and Children (WIC) program was also found to have a negative impact on the initiation of breast-feeding in the hospital (55.2% for non-WIC versus 32.3% for WIC participants) (Ross Mothers Survey, 2003).

In a survey breast-feeding mothers indicated that the determining factors for changing to bottle-feeding included the mother's perception of the father's attitude toward breast-feeding and the mother's uncertainty regarding the amount of milk the infant would receive (Arora, McJunkin, Wehrer, et al, 2000). These findings have important implications for involving fathers in education and discussion regarding breast-feeding before and during the pregnancy. Fathers may feel left out during the newborn period if they have little involvement other than diapering and holding the infant. Encouraging fathers regarding their positive role in supporting the mother in her breast-feeding may help decrease feelings of isolation, benefit mother-infant interaction, and decrease a sense of helplessness and isolation.

The American Academy of Pediatrics (2005b) has reaffirmed its position recommending exclusive breast-feeding until 6 months of age, with continued breast-feeding to at least 1 year of age and beyond as long as is mutually desirable by mother and infant. The academy also supports programs that enable women to continue breast-feeding after returning to work. In its support of breast-feeding practices, the academy further discourages the advertisement of infant formula to breast-feeding mothers and distribution of formula discharge packs without the advice of a health care provider.

The Baby-Friendly Hospital Initiative (BFHI) is a joint effort of the World Health Organization and UNICEF to promote and support breast-feeding as the model for optimum infant nutrition. BFHI developed 10 research-supported practices as guidelines for maternity facilities worldwide to promote breast-feeding (Kyenkya-Isabirye, 1992; Wright, Rice, and Wells, 1996) (Box 8-7).

In addition to the physiologic qualities of human milk, the most outstanding psychologic benefit of breast-feeding is the close maternal-child relationship. The infant is nestled close to the mother's skin, can hear the rhythm of her heartbeat, can feel the warmth of her body, and has a sense of peaceful security. The mother has a close feeling of union with her child and

---

BOX 8-7   TEN STEPS TO SUCCESSFUL BREAST-FEEDING

Every facility providing maternity services and care for newborn infants should:

1. Have a written breast-feeding policy that is routinely communicated to all health care staff.
2. Train all health care staff in skills necessary to implement this policy.
3. Inform all pregnant women about the benefits and management of breast-feeding.
4. Help mothers initiate breast-feeding within a half hour of birth.
5. Show mothers how to breast-feed and how to maintain lactation even if they are separated from their infants.
6. Give newborn infants no food or drink other than breast milk, unless medically indicated.
7. Practice rooming-in—allow mothers and infants to remain together—24 hours a day.
8. Encourage breast-feeding on demand.
9. Give no artificial teats or pacifiers (also called dummies or soothers) to breast-feeding infants.
10. Foster the establishment of breast-feeding support groups and refer mothers to them on discharge from the hospital or clinic.

From Kyenkya-Isabirye M: UNICEF launches the Baby-Friendly Hospital Initiative, *MCN* 17(4):177-179, 1992; and Wright A, Rice S, Wells S: Changing hospital practices to increase the duration of breastfeeding, *Pediatrics* 97(5):669-676, 1996.

Case Study—Breast-Feeding

feels a sense of accomplishment and satisfaction as the infant suckles milk from her.

Human milk is the most economical form of feeding. It is always available, ready to serve at room temperature, and free of contamination. The projected monetary savings for a population of breast-feeding infants in relation to preventive medicine are considered significant (Ball and Wright, 1999; Montgomery and Splett, 1997). Although human milk is not sterile, healthy full-term infants can tolerate varying amounts of nonpathogenic and pathogenic organisms. The protection against infection can provide additional cost savings in terms of fewer medical visits and less time lost from work for the employed mother.

Breast-fed infants, especially beyond 2 to 3 months of age, tend to grow at a satisfactory but slower rate than bottle-fed infants (Dewey, Heinig, Nommsen, et al, 1991; de Onis and Onyango, 2003). Infants who are exclusively breast-fed have decreased amount of free fat and thus tend to appear leaner than their formula-fed counterparts (Butte, Wong, Hopkinson, et al, 2000; Dewey, Heinig, Nommsen, et al, 1993). The National Center for Health Statistics' growth charts (see Appendix B) have been adjusted to reflect exclusively breast-fed infants, who have a slower growth rate during the first several months of life. By the age of 12 to 15 months breast-fed infants weigh approximately the same as their bottle-fed counterparts.

Contraindications to breast-feeding include (Lawrence and Lawrence, 2005; American Academy of Pediatrics, 2005b):

- Maternal chemotherapy-antimetabolites and certain antineoplastic drugs
- Active tuberculosis not under treatment in mother
- HIV in mother
- Galactosemia in infant
- Maternal herpes simplex lesion on a breast
- Cytomegalovirus (CMV); may be a risk to preterm infants receiving CMV-infected donor milk, not to infected mother's infant, who already has CMV
- Maternal substance abuse (e.g., cocaine, methamphetamines, marijuana) (NOTE: Maternal methadone treatment for substance abuse is not a contraindication to breast-feeding.)
- Human T-cell leukemia virus type 1
- Mothers receiving diagnostic or radioactive isotopes or who have had exposure to radioactive materials (for as long as there is radioactivity in milk)

A small number of medications are contraindicated for breast-feeding mothers. Consult a reference text such as Hale (2008). Mastitis is usually not a contraindication if the discomfort is tolerable.

Some herbal products are presented as safe and effective alternatives to prescription or over-the-counter medications. Certain herbal agents, namely the galactogogues, are reported to increase breast milk production. Data are still insufficient to confirm or deny the assertion of increased milk production using galactogogues, and nurses should caution mothers to seek advice from a practitioner to ensure that the herbal preparations will not harm the breast-feeding infant (Conover and Buehler, 2004).

Breast-feeding can be done with twin births and other multiples. If the infants are full term, they can begin feedings imme-

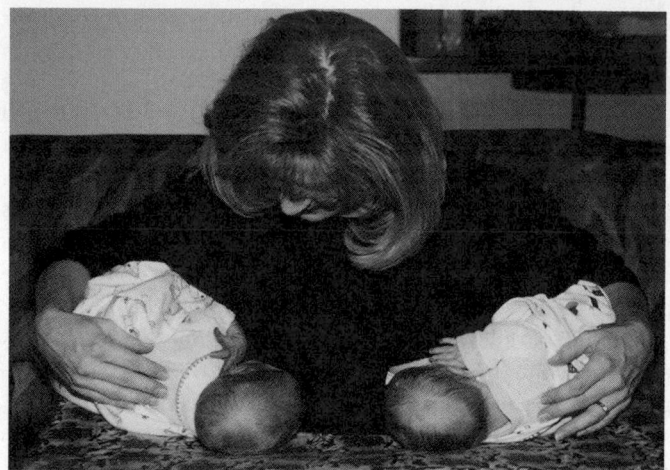

Fig. 8-13 Simultaneous breast-feeding of twins.

diately after birth (Fig. 8-13). Simultaneous feeding promotes the rapid production of milk needed for both infants and makes the milk that would normally be lost in the let-down reflex available to one of the twins. When only one infant is hungry, the mother should feed singly. She should also alternate breasts when feeding each infant and avoid favoring one breast for one infant. The sucking patterns of infants vary, and each infant needs the visual stimulation and exercise that alternating breasts provides.

> **! NURSING ALERT**
>
> Do not use microwaves to defrost frozen human milk. High-temperature microwaving (72° to 98° C [162° to 208° F]) significantly destroys the antiinfective factors and vitamin C content (Quan, Yang, Rubinstein, et al, 1992). The safety of low-temperature microwaving (20° to 53° C [68° to 127° F]) remains questionable. One of the best ways to thaw frozen human milk is to place it under a warm flow of tap water. Several commercial bottle warmers are now available to thaw or warm up breast milk. Test the temperature of the milk before feeding.

A concern many mothers have is the perceived inconvenience of loss of freedom and independence. Being committed to feeding the infant every 2 to 3 hours can be overwhelming, especially to women with multiple responsibilities. Many women resume their careers shortly after their pregnancy and prefer to bottle-feed. Combining breast-feeding and employment is possible, and Chapter 12 discusses suggestions for the mother. Although breast-feeding is the preferred form of infant feeding, mothers' decisions regarding their preferences must be supported and respected.

Successful breast-feeding probably depends more on the mother's desire to breast-feed, satisfaction with breast-feeding, and available support systems than on any other factors. Mothers need support, encouragement, and assistance during their postpartum hospital stay and at home to enhance their opportunities for success and satisfaction.

Three main criteria have been proposed as essential in promoting breast-feeding: absence of a rigid feeding schedule, correct positioning of the infant at the breast to achieve a deep alveolar latch, and correct suckling technique. Correct suckling for breast-feeding is defined as a wide-open mouth, tongue

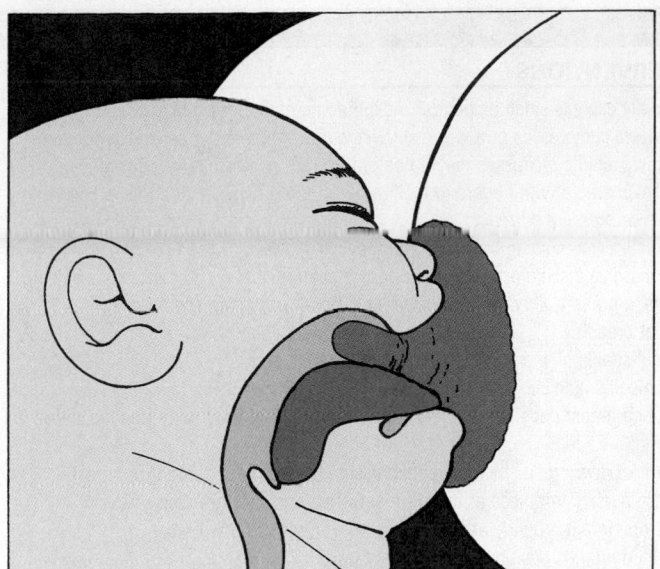

Fig. 8-14 The tongue is under the areola, with tip of the nipple at back of the wide-open mouth.

under the areola, and expression of milk by effective alveolar compression (Fig. 8-14).

The following interventions promote breast-feeding:

- Frequent and early breast-feeding, especially during the first hour of life; immediate skin-to-skin contact; rooming-in; and feeding on demand
- Direct modeling of the importance of breast-feeding by health care providers, such as implementing demand nursing with no formula supplementation and decreased emphasis on infant formula products
- Increased information and support to mothers after discharge, especially follow-up telephone calls
- Early breast pumping every 2 to 3 hours for 20 minutes bilaterally if the newborn is unable to nurse immediately (increases oxytocin production and thus milk production)

Nurses play a significant role in the breast-feeding decision and must make themselves available to families for guidance and support. Several excellent books and organizations, such as La Leche League International,* are available as resources for professionals and breast-feeding mothers.

Breast-Feeding Problems

Many mothers have concerns regarding breast-feeding, and, with earlier discharge from postpartum units, problems such as engorgement and painful nipples may occur after the mother is home. New mothers are often concerned about their milk supply, and excessive anxiety can affect successful lactation (see Family-Centered Care box).

Table 8-5 summarizes the more common breast-feeding problems and the interventions to correct them. Most of these problems are easily prevented or easily remedied, provided the mother receives education and guidance. Assessment should include a detailed history, examination of the breasts, and observation of the breast-feeding (see Nursing Care Guidelines box).

*PO Box 4079, Schaumburg, IL 60168-4079; 800-LA-LECHE or 847-519-7730; www.llli.org.

In Canada: PO Box 700, Winchester, ON K0C 2K0; 613-774-4900 or 800-665-4324; www.lllc.ca.

FAMILY-CENTERED CARE
Breast-Feeding and Infant Weight Gain

Mothers whose breast-fed infants fail to gain weight according to standard growth curves published before 2000 may be told that their milk, although nutritionally good for the baby from an immunologic standpoint, lacks fat for adequate growth. The Centers for Disease Control and Prevention (2010) now recommends the WHO growth charts be used for children less than 24 months of age instead of the CDC growth charts. The basis for this recommendation is that the healthy breastfed infant is the standard against which all other infants of this age are compared in the WHO growth charts. The CDC growth charts continue to be recommended for children over 24 months. In addition, mothers may be told by relatives to stop breast-feeding the infant because he or she does not weigh as much as the same-age infant who is being bottle-fed. However, evidence indicates that the older standard growth charts may not reflect normal growth patterns of infants who are breast-fed. Infants who are breast-fed grow more rapidly during the first 2 months of life, but growth is slower from 3 to 12 months when compared with the previous National Center for Health Statistics (NCHS) growth reference data charts. In the second year of life, breast-fed infants gain weight faster than is reflected by reference charts, and by 24 months their average weight approximates current growth charts (Dewey, Peerson, Brown, et al, 1995; de Onis and Onyango, 2003). Breast-fed infants are leaner and have less body fat than formula-fed infants, but growth in head circumference is greater in the breast-fed group. The American Academy of Pediatrics (2009a) suggests that weight gain in formula-fed infants is excessive and that there are no detrimental effects to the slower weight gain of breast-fed infants. There is evidence that breast-fed infants regulate their energy intake, thus decreasing the propensity toward obesity in later life.

The World Health Organization (2006) has also published new growth standards for children that are based on the growth of healthy breast-fed infants throughout the first year of life (www.who.int/childgrowth/standards/en).

An important factor in the development of the dietary reference intakes by the Institute of Medicine (see p. 524, Chapter 13) that affects children, particularly infants 0 to 6 months, is that the adequate intakes are based on the nutrient intake of full-term, healthy, breast-fed infants (by well-nourished mothers), which now represents the gold standard for infant nutrition in this age-group

In recent years there has been increased concern about the long-term effects of obesity among Americans, with acknowledgment that early childhood nutrition may play an important role in feeding habits that affect health throughout adulthood. Rapid weight gain during infancy has been correlated with overweight toddlers and preschoolers (Dennison, Edmunds, Stratton, et al, 2006; Goodell, Wakefield, and Ferris, 2009; Taveras, Rifas-Shiman, Belfort, et al, 2009). Kramer, Guo, Platt, and colleagues (2004) found that infants who were fed formula or other milk and breast milk (versus exclusive breast milk intake) had significantly higher growth velocity (in weight and length) than breast-fed counterparts, especially at 3 to 6 months of age. Grummer-Strawn, Mei, and the Centers for Disease Control and Prevention Pediatric Nutrition Surveillance System (2004) found that prolonged breast-feeding (≥6 months) provided a dose-response, protective relationship against the risk of being overweight (body mass index for age ≥95th percentile by 2000 National Health and Nutrition Examination Survey growth charts) in 4-year-old non-Hispanic Caucasian children. The authors concluded that breast-feeding longer than 6 months provides health benefits that extend well beyond the period of breast-feeding. In 2000 NCHS revised the growth charts to reflect differences in growth in infants who are breast- and bottle-fed. The new growth charts can be downloaded from the Centers for Disease Control and Prevention website, www.cdc.gov/growthcharts.

Nurses can share these findings with parents to allay fears of an inadequate milk supply, which can discourage mothers from continuing to breast-feed. Also, an evaluation of growth, especially if weight-for-length is less than 2 standard deviations below the mean, must be viewed carefully to avoid the diagnosis of growth failure in infants with no other evidence of inadequate nutrition (see Chapter 13).

TABLE 8-5	BREAST-FEEDING PROBLEMS	
PROBLEM	**COMMENTS**	**INTERVENTIONS**
Engorgement	Best intervention is *prevention* with proper deep areolar latch-on and frequent nursing on both breasts for complete emptying of ducts. If engorgement occurs, infant may be unable to properly grasp distended areola.	Manually express small amount of milk; electric pump may be beneficial for some. Use warm compresses or a warm shower *before feeding;* for severely engorged breasts, cold compresses may be helpful to reduce vascularity *after feeding.* Compress areola with fingers to facilitate infant's grasp (C-hold); this is known as *reverse pressure softening.* Use well-fitting nursing brassiere and wear 24 hr/day. For excessive discomfort, take ibuprofen or acetaminophen 30 min before feeding.

Painful nipples	Most common causes are poor feeding technique, improper care of breasts, or poor hygiene with bacterial or fungal infection.
	If left untreated, discomfort may cause mother to terminate breast-feeding.
		Massage breasts; vary position of infant's mouth on nipple and areola.
		Care of breasts:
		  Avoid soaps, oils, or self-prescribed treatments.
		  Air nipples as much as possible.
		  Change breast pads frequently; avoid plastic-backed pads (may trap moisture).
		Feeding:
		  Start let-down reflex by manual expression before putting infant to breast.
		  Begin nursing with less affected breast, then nurse on affected side.
		  Position infant properly at breast to achieve deep areolar grasp.
		  Change infant's position.
		  For excessive discomfort, take analgesics 30 min before feeding; apply cool compresses to nipples after feeding.

Delayed let-down reflex	Reflex essential to delivery of milk from alveoli and smaller milk ducts into larger lactiferous ducts; controlled primarily by release of prolactin and oxytocin. Pain, stress, and anxiety can interfere with reflex.	Provide quiet, relaxing atmosphere for nursing (e.g., soothing music, privacy, pillows for positioning, decreased distractions). Stroke breast gently. Apply warmth to breast. May need to use oxytocin nasal spray (compounded prescription) to induce reflex (use only in newborn period).
Inadequate milk supply	Production of milk depends on supply and demand. Inadequate supply rarely is related to organic causes, such as decreased glandular tissue, but may occur after breast augmentation or reduction surgery, or as a result of a hormonal imbalance such as polycystic ovarian syndrome.	Continue breast-feeding every 2-3 hr. Massage breasts before feeding. Apply warm compresses before pumping or feeding. Avoid use of supplemental formula before breast-feeding is well established to prevent nipple preference and satiation (infant will not be hungry enough to breast-feed). Reassure mother that her milk supply will likely be adequate and it depends on frequent nursing. Encourage more frequent nursing (at least 6-10 times daily, initially at both breasts). Encourage adequate rest, nutrition, and fluids. Monitor infant's growth; in some cases formula supplementation may be indicated. An alternative to bottle-feeding is use of a supplemental feeding device consisting of a plastic bag or syringe for formula and a thin feeding tube placed next to mother's nipple during nursing.
Plugged ducts	This may occur at any time, especially during first 6 wk.	Continue breast-feeding every 2-3 hr. Massage breasts before feeding. Apply warm compresses before pumping or feeding. Alternate feeding positions, positioning infant's chin toward obstructed area.
Mastitis	Inflammation or infection in mammary gland or tissue by *Staphylococcus aureus;* results from inadequate emptying of ducts or from cracks in nipple skin; may be associated with fever and flulike symptoms. Prevention: see Interventions for Plugged ducts, above. If mastitis occurs, current treatment is 10 days of antibiotics (usually amoxicillin or cephalexin, started with onset of symptoms). If symptoms of intense "burning" in breasts with erythema of nipples, consider *Candida* infection of ducts (oral fluconazole [Diflucan] is treatment).	Continue breast-feeding during this time to keep breast well drained (unless contraindicated for medical reasons such as systemic illness).
Unsuccessful latch-on	Improper positioning of infant at breast, inability to achieve deep areolar grasp, sleepiness, or improper suckling technique may cause this common problem; flat, large, or inverted nipples may also be a factor.	Mother and newborn must be anatomically positioned so that infant's mouth is in full contact with breast; mother should use C-hold; newborn's mouth is opened wide, and most of areola is grasped (see Fig. 8-14), especially with lower lip; frequent swallowing should be heard as evidence of spontaneous and successful suckling. Anatomic problems such as flat or inverted nipples may be managed by mother wearing nipple shields to elongate or make nipples more accessible. Additional pumping may be necessary after nursing when shield is used.

NURSING CARE GUIDELINES

Observing the Breast-Feeding Pair

- Position of mother, her body language, and any possible tension.
- Position of infant. Child's ventral (front) surface is next to mother's ventral surface with the face directly in front of the breast ("tummy to tummy"). The infant cannot swallow if the head has to turn to the breast.
- Position of mother's hand on the breast. Using the thumb on top and fingers supporting the breast encircling the areola (the C-hold) facilitates infant's ability to grasp the areola properly.
- Flanged position of infant's lips on the areola. The lips should gently grasp most of the areola, with the lower lip covering more of the areola than the upper lip.
- Baby's chin, not the nose, touching mother's breast (Newman and Pitman, 2000).
- Use of alternate breasts and feeding time on each breast.
- Technique to break suction. The mother should release suction using fingers between the areola and lips, not pulling infant from the breast abruptly.

Encourage frequent feedings to increase milk production; use of supplemental formula, water, glucose water, or solid foods will result in decreased breast milk intake and ultimately decreased production.

Many breast-feeding problems respond rapidly to simple interventions, such as correcting the infant's feeding position. However, the mother needs continual reassurance of success and the support that allows her the needed rest and relaxation to nurse her infant. Referral to supportive agencies, such as local groups of La Leche League International, or to a lactation specialist may be beneficial.

Bottle-Feeding

Bottle-feeding generally refers to the use of bottles for feeding commercial or evaporated milk formula rather than using the breast, although in some instances human milk may be expressed and fed with a bottle. Bottle-feeding is an acceptable method of feeding. However, nurses should not assume that new parents automatically know how to bottle-feed their infant. Parents who choose bottle-feeding also need support and assistance in meeting their infant's needs.

Providing newborns with nutrition is only one aspect of the feeding. Holding them close to the body while rocking or cuddling them helps ensure the emotional component of feeding. Like breast-fed infants, bottle-fed infants need to be held on alternate sides of the lap to expose them to different stimuli. The feeding should not be hurried. Even though they may suck vigorously for the first 5 minutes and seem to be satisfied, they should be allowed to continue sucking. Infants need at least 2 hours of sucking a day. If there are six feedings per day, then about 20 minutes of sucking at each feeding provides for oral gratification.

Propping the bottle is discouraged because:
- It denies the infant the important component of close human contact.
- The infant may aspirate formula into the trachea and lungs while sleeping.
- It may facilitate the development of middle ear infections. As the infant lies flat and sucks, milk that has pooled in

the pharynx becomes a suitable medium for bacterial growth. Bacteria then enter the eustachian tube, which leads to the middle ear, causing acute otitis media.
- It encourages continuous pooling of formula in the mouth, which can lead to caries when the teeth erupt. (See Chapter 14.)

! NURSING ALERT

Warming bottles in the microwave oven is not recommended because of the risk of burns from excessively hot temperatures of the milk or bottles exploding. When milk is warmed in the microwave, it is not warmed evenly and may be too hot in places, causing mouth burns. If mother's milk is warmed in the microwave, there is significant loss of antiinfective cells and properties within the milk (Quan, Yang, Rubinstein, et al, 1992).

Preparation of Formula

The two traditional ways of preparing formula are the terminal heat method (all the utensils and formula are boiled together for 25 minutes) and the aseptic method (the equipment is boiled separately, after which the formula is poured into the bottles). Because of improved sanitary conditions in developed countries, neither of these methods is essential. The clean technique is satisfactory, including using a dishwasher. Persons preparing the formula wash their hands well and then wash all the equipment used to prepare the formula, including the cans of formula or evaporated milk. The formula is prepared and bottled and refrigerated if not used for feeding immediately. Warming the formula is optional. Any milk remaining in the bottle after the feeding is discarded because it is an excellent medium for bacterial growth. Opened cans of formula are covered and refrigerated until the next feeding.

Stress to families that the proportions must not be altered—neither diluted to extend the amount of formula nor concentrated to provide more calories, unless directed by the practitioner to increase caloric content. Recommendations for labeling infant formulas require that the directions for preparation and use of the formula include pictures and symbols for nonreading individuals. In addition, manufacturers are translating the directions into foreign languages, such as Spanish and Vietnamese, to prevent misunderstanding and errors in formula preparation.

Although low-iron infant formula is available, it is not recommended for use in infants less than 1 year of age. Currently no evidence exists that iron-fortified formula (containing ≥4 mg/L iron) increases gastrointestinal symptoms such as constipation (American Academy of Pediatrics, 2009a).

Feeding Schedules

Ideally, feeding schedules should be determined by the infant's hunger. Demand feedings are given when the infant signals readiness. Scheduled feedings are arranged at predetermined intervals. Some hospitals routinely feed infants every 3 to 4 hours. Although this may be satisfactory for bottle-fed infants, it hinders the breast-feeding process. Since breast-fed infants tend to be hungry every 2 to 3 hours because of the easy digestibility of the milk, they should be fed on demand.

Supplemental feedings should not be offered to breast-fed infants before lactation is well established because they may

Critical Thinking Exercise—Formula Preparation

satiate the infant and may cause nipple preference. Supplemental water is not needed by breast- or bottle-fed infants, even in hot climates (American Academy of Pediatrics, 2009a). Satiated infants suck less vigorously at the breast, and milk production depends on the breast being emptied at each feeding. If milk is allowed to accumulate in the ducts, causing breast engorgement, ischemia results, suppressing the activity of the acini, or milk-secreting cells. Consequently, milk production is reduced. In addition, the process of sucking from a bottle is different from breast nipple compression. The relatively inflexible rubber nipple prevents the tongue from its usual rhythmic action. Infants learn to put the tongue against the nipple holes to slow down the more rapid flow of fluid. When infants use these same tongue movements during breast-feeding, they may push the human nipple out of the mouth and may not grasp the areola properly.

Usually by 3 weeks of age, lactation is well established. Bottle-fed infants consume about 2 to 3 oz of formula at each feeding and are fed approximately six times a day. The quantity of formula consumed is based on the caloric need of 108 kcal/kg/day; therefore a newborn who weighs 3 kg (6.6 lb) requires 324 kcal/day. Because commercial formula for full-term infants has 20 kcal/oz, about 480 ml (16 oz) will provide the daily caloric requirement. Breast-fed infants may feed as frequently as 10 to 12 times a day.

Feeding Behavior

Five behavioral stages occur during successful feeding. Recognizing these steps can assist nurses in identifying potential feeding problems caused by improper feeding techniques (see discussion of NCAST Feeding Scale, p. 234). Prefeeding behavior, such as crying or fussing, demonstrates the infant's level of arousal and degree of hunger. To encourage the infant to grasp the breast properly, it is preferable to begin feeding during the quiet alert state, before the infant becomes upset. Approach behavior is indicated by sucking movements or the rooting reflex.

Attachment behavior includes those activities that occur from the time the infant receives the nipple and sucks (sometimes more pronounced during initial attempts at breast-feeding). Consummatory behavior consists of coordinated sucking and swallowing. Persistent gagging might indicate unsuccessful consummatory behavior. Satiety behavior is observed when infants let the parent know that they are satisfied, usually by falling asleep.

Commercially Prepared Formulas

The analysis of human and whole cow's milk indicates that the latter is unsuitable for infant nutrition. Whole cow's milk has a high protein content, has low fat and lipid content, and may cause intestinal bleeding and lead to iron deficiency anemia in infants. There has also been some question regarding the unmodified protein content of whole cow's milk, which may trigger an undesired immune response and thus increase the incidence of allergies in children at an early age.

Commercially prepared formulas are cow's milk–based formulas that have been modified to resemble the nutritional content of human milk. These formulas are altered from cow's milk by removing butterfat, decreasing the protein content, and adding vegetable oil and carbohydrate. Some cow's milk–based

formulas have demineralized whey added to yield a whey/casein ratio of 60:40. The standard cow's milk–based formulas, regardless of the commercial brand, have similar compositions of vitamins, minerals, protein, carbohydrates, and essential amino acids, with minor variations such as the source of carbohydrate (Akers and Groh-Wargo, 2005), nucleotides to enhance immune function, and long-chain polyunsaturated fatty acids (LCPUFAs) DHA and AA, which are thought to improve brain function (Georgieff, 2001; Gil, Ramirez, and Gil, 2003). DHA and AA are both found in large quantities in human milk but until recently were not present in most infant formulas. Studies in full-term infants receiving supplements with DHA and AA have produced mixed results regarding brain function and visual acuity. Many studies report a variety of sources for LCPUFAs, including egg yolk lipid, phospholipids, and triglyceride. The evidence for supplementation of formula for preterm infants with LCPUFAs, however, has been more convincing; it produces some transient improvement in visual acuity and general development (American Academy of Pediatrics, 2009a). There do not appear to be any adverse effects associated with LCPUFA supplementation in preterm infants with respect to the incidence of bronchopulmonary disease, necrotizing enterocolitis, or other conditions of prematurity (American Academy of Pediatrics, 2009a). Standard cow's milk–based formulas are also sold as low iron and iron fortified; however, only the iron-fortified formulas meet the iron requirements of infants (American Academy of Pediatrics, 2009a).

The presence of the probiotics *Lactobacillus rhamnosus GG* and *Bifidobacterium lactis* in breast milk has led to the addition of prebiotic components to cow's milk–based formula. Prebiotic oligosaccharides are food ingredients that promote the growth and activity of bacteria such as *Lactobacillus* and *Bifidobacterium*, which benefit the host (Douglas and Sanders, 2008; Vandenplas, 2002). Some of the reported advantages include a decreased number of intestinal infections, otitis media, and acute respiratory tract infections (Rautava, Salminen, and Isolauri, 2009). The addition of a prebiotic oligosaccharide was reported to have modified formula-fed infants' intestinal flora and aided in decreasing upper respiratory tract and gastrointestinal infections (Arslanoglu, Moro, and Boehm, 2007).

Commercially prepared infant formulas fall into four main categories: (1) cow's milk–based formulas, available in 20 kcal/fl oz as liquid (ready to feed), as powder (requires dilution with water), or as a concentrated liquid (requires dilution with water); (2) soy-based formulas, available commercially in ready-to-feed 20 kcal/fl oz powder and concentrated liquid forms, commonly used for children who are lactose or cow's milk protein intolerant; (3) casein- or whey-hydrolysate formulas, commercially available in ready-to-feed and powder forms and used primarily for children who cannot tolerate or digest cow's milk or soy-based formulas; and (4) amino acid formulas.

The American Academy of Pediatrics Committee on Nutrition (2008c) recommends the use of soy protein–based formulas for infants with galactosemia and hereditary lactase deficiency, and in situations where a vegetarian diet is preferred. For infants with documented allergies caused by cow's milk, extensively hydrolyzed protein formula should be considered, since up to 14% of these infants will also have a soy protein allergy. Some researchers have speculated that exclusive use of soy formula in infants may adversely affect their endocrine, reproductive, and immune systems. This concern is related to isoflavones in soy and possible alteration in sexual maturity, immune response, and thyroid function (Greim, 2004; Chen and Rogan, 2004). Chen and Rogan (2004) note an urgent need to evaluate the effects of isoflavones in soy infant formula clinically, prospectively, and longitudinally. Others report no long-term untoward effects from the ingestion of isoflavones in soy formula (Merritt and Jenks, 2004; Giampietro, Bruno, Furcolo, et al, 2004). The American Academy of Pediatrics (2008c) states that there is currently no conclusive evidence that dietary soy products adversely affect human development, reproduction, or endocrine function.

The casein- or whey-hydrolysate formulas are considered to be less antigenic than either cow's milk– or soy-based formulas. The protein hydrolysate formulas (casein and whey) are derived from cow's milk–based formula by a process of heat, filtration, and enzyme treatment designed to break the peptide chains into more digestible proteins. The hydrolysate formulas have the reported disadvantage of tasting bad; some have commercially added flavoring. Neocate and EleCare are amino acid formulas, designed for infants who are extremely sensitive to cow's milk–based, soy-based, and partially or extensively hydrolyzed casein- and whey-based formulas. Both Neocate and EleCare are available in powder form. A variety of formulas are manufactured for infants and children with special needs (Table 8-6).

Follow-up formulas are marketed as a transitional formula for infants older than 6 months who are also eating solid foods. These generally contain a higher percentage of calories from protein and carbohydrate sources, a higher amount of iron and vitamins, and a lower amount of fat than standard cow's milk–based formulas. Many nutrition experts and the American Academy of Pediatrics (2009c), however, discount the necessity of follow-up formulas if the infant is receiving an adequate amount of solid food containing sufficient iron, vitamins, and minerals.

Alternate Milk Products

In the United States few infants are fed evaporated milk formula, and its use is not recommended by the American Academy of Pediatrics (2009c). However, it has many advantages over

TABLE 8-6	NORMAL AND SPECIAL INFANT FORMULAS*†
FORMULA (MANUFACTURER)	**COMMENTS AND NUTRITIONAL CONSIDERATIONS‡**
Full-Term Infant Nutrition	
Similac Advance EarlyShield (Abbott)	Contains prebiotics (galactooligosaccharides), antioxidant, DHA, AA, and nucleotides
Enfamil Premium Lipil with Triple Health Guard (Mead Johnson)	Contains sources of DHA and AA; iron fortified; prebiotics added
Enfamil AR and Enfamil AR Lipil (contains AA and DHA) (Mead Johnson)	For mild gastroesophageal reflux; contains rice starch; iron fortified
Good Start Gentle Plus (Nestlé) and Good Start Protect Plus	Contains sources of DHA and AA; Protect Plus contains *Bifidus* BL
Similac PM 60/40 (Abbott)	Powder only; low solute load; for infants with impaired renal, digestive, and cardiovascular function; lower calcium, potassium, and phosphorus content
Enfamil Gentlease Lipil (Mead Johnson)	Added DHA, ARA; decreased lactose content
Formulas for Cow's Milk Protein–Sensitive and Lactose-Intolerant Infants*	
Similac Isomil and Similac Isomil Advance (contains AA and DHA) (Abbott)	Soy protein; for lactose intolerance and galactosemia
Enfamil ProSobee and Enfamil ProSobee Lipil (contains AA and DHA) (Mead Johnson)	Soy protein; for lactose intolerance and galactosemia
Similac Isomil DF (Abbott)	Partially hydrolyzed (corn starch); contains fiber; for diarrhea in infants >6 mo; lessens amount and duration of watery stools
Nestlé Alsoy (Nestlé)	Soy protein, with DHA and AA
Similac Sensitive Lactose Free and Lactose Free Advance (contains AA and DHA) (Abbott)	Corn syrup solids and sucrose; for lactose malabsorption; iron fortified
Enfamil LactoFree and LactoFree Lipil (contains AA and DHA) (Mead Johnson)	Corn syrup solids; lactose intolerance
Protein Hydrolysate–Based and Amino Acid–Based Formulas	
Similac Alimentum and Alimentum Advance (contains AA and DHA) (Abbott)	Liquid; hydrolyzed casein; hypoallergenic; lactose free; nutritionally complete; gastrointestinal malabsorption
Enfamil Nutramigen and Nutramigen Lipil (contains AA and DHA) (Mead Johnson)	Powder; hydrolyzed casein; hypoallergenic; lactose and sucrose free; nutritionally complete; for galactosemia
Enfamil Pregestimil (Mead Johnson)	Powder; hydrolyzed casein; lactose and sucrose free; easily digestible; used for postoperative bowel resection and malabsorption conditions
Neocate (Nutricia North America)	Powder; amino acid based; for children sensitive to soy, cow's milk protein, and hydrolyzed formula; nutritionally complete; high cost is factor
EleCare (Abbott)	Powder; amino acid–based formula; hypoallergenic; nutritionally complete; iron fortified; for children sensitive to soy, cow's milk protein, and hydrolyzed formula; high cost is a factor

AA, Arachidonic acid; *DHA*, docosahexaenoic acid.
*Major retail companies manufacture their own brands of term infant formulas that comply with the Food and Drug Administration guidelines for infant formula composition; these are often less expensive than brand name formulas and contain the same ingredients.
†This is not an exhaustive list of infant formulas. Other formulas with special additives and uses are available, and information may be obtained from formula company representative.
‡All formulas in this table provide 20 kcal/oz.

whole milk. It is readily available in cans; needs no refrigeration if unopened; is less expensive than commercial formula; provides a softer, more digestible curd; and contains more lactalbumin and a higher calcium/phosphorus ratio. Disadvantages of evaporated milk for infant nutrition include low iron and vitamin C concentrations, excessive sodium and phosphorus, decreased vitamin A and D (except in fortified forms), and poorly digested fat (Akers and Groh-Wargo, 2005). A common method for preparing evaporated milk formula is diluting the 13-oz can of milk with 19½ oz of water and adding 3 tbsp of sugar or commercially processed corn syrup.

Evaporated milk must not be confused with condensed milk, which is a form of evaporated milk with 45% more sugar. Because of its high carbohydrate concentration and disproportionately low fat and protein content, condensed milk is not used for infant feeding. Likewise, skim milk and low-fat milk must not be used because they are deficient in caloric concentration, significantly increase the renal solute load and water demands, and deprive the body of essential fatty acids.

Goat's milk is a poor source of iron and folic acid. It has an excessively high renal solute load as a result of its high protein content and can cause metabolic acidosis, making it unsuitable for infant nutrition (American Academy of Pediatrics, 2009c; Hendriksz and Walter, 2004). Some parents believe that goat's milk is less allergenic than other available milk sources and may feed it to their infants to reduce allergic milk reactions. However, infants allergic to cow's milk have experienced anaphylaxis with their first exposure to goat's milk (Pessler and Nejat, 2004).

Raw, unpasteurized milk from any animal source is unacceptable for infant nutrition.

PROMOTE PARENT-INFANT BONDING (ATTACHMENT)

The process of parenting is based on a relationship between parent and infant. As more is learned of the complexity of neonates and their potential for influencing and shaping their environments, particularly their interaction with significant others, it is apparent that promoting positive parent-child relationships necessitates an understanding of behavioral steps in attachment, including variables that enhance or hinder this process. Nurses also must be skilled in methods of teaching parents to develop a stronger relationship with their children, especially by recognizing potential problems (see Assessment of Attachment Behaviors, p. 233).

Infant Behavior

Nurses must appreciate the individuality and uniqueness of each infant. According to the individual temperament, the infant will change and shape the environment, which will undoubtedly influence future development. An infant who sleeps 20 hours a day will be exposed to fewer stimuli than one who sleeps 16 hours a day. In turn, each infant will likely elicit a different response from parents. The infant who is quiet, undemanding, and passive may receive much less attention than the infant who is responsive, alert, and active. Behavioral characteristics such as irritability and consolability can influence the ease of transition to parenthood and the parent's perception of the infant.

> ### BOX 8-8　HOW TO MAKE THE INFANT'S WORLD MORE EXCITING
>
> - Infant prefers animated and auditory objects.
> - Objects should be placed about 20 cm (8 inches) away from infant.
> - Infant enjoys novelty and quickly tires of seeing same objects; mobile should be changed frequently.
> - Infant prefers to look at medium-intensity colors and contrasting colors, such as black and white.
> - Infant likes geometric shapes and checkerboards; prefers patterns over straight lines.
> - Contrasting lights and reflective surfaces such as mirrors are especially interesting.
> - But most of all, nothing is as fascinating as the human face and voice!

Nurses can positively influence the attachment of parent and child. The first step is recognizing individual differences and explaining to parents that such characteristics are normal. For example, some people believe that infants sleep throughout the day, except for feedings. For some newborns this may be true, but for many it is not. Understanding that the infant's wakefulness is part of biologic rhythm and not a reflection of inadequate parenting can be crucial in promoting healthy parent-child relationships. Another aspect of helping parents involves supplying guidelines on how to enhance the infant's development during awake periods. Placing the child in a crib to stare at the same mobile every day is not exciting, but carrying the infant into each room as one does daily chores can be fascinating. A few suggestions can make life more stimulating for the infant and gratifying for the parents (Box 8-8).

Maternal Attachment

Research has suggested that there is a maternal sensitive period immediately and for a short time after birth when mothers have a unique ability to attach to their infants (Klaus, Kennell, and Klaus, 1995). Mothers demonstrate a predictable and orderly pattern of behavior during the attachment process. When mothers are presented with their nude infants, they begin to examine the infant with their fingertips, concentrating on touching the extremities, and then proceed to massage and encompass the trunk with their entire hands. Assuming the **en face position**, in which the mother's and infant's eyes meet in visual contact in the same vertical plane, is significant in the formation of affectional ties (Fig. 8-15). Although similar patterns of touching have been observed, additional studies demonstrate different patterns for mothers, as well as the same pattern for nonmaternal persons, such as male and female nurses. Consequently, nurses must exercise caution in interpreting behaviors such as touching.

Several studies have attempted to substantiate the long-term benefits of providing parents with opportunities to optimally bond with their infant during the initial postpartum period. Although there is some evidence that increased parent-child contact encourages prolonged breast-feeding and may minimize the risks of parenting disorders, conclusions about the long-term effects of such early intervention on parenting and child development must be viewed cautiously. In addition, some authorities claim that the emphasis on bonding has been unjustified and may lead to guilt and fear in parents who did not have early contact with their infant. There is concern that literal interpretation of "sensitive" or "critical" might imply

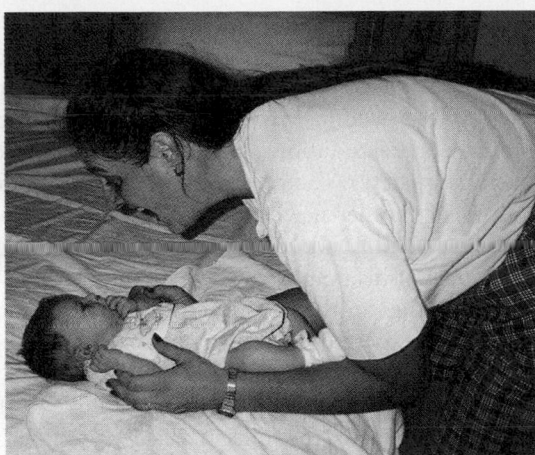

Fig. 8-15 En face position between parent and infant can be significant in attachment process.

that, without early contact, optimum bonding cannot occur or, conversely, that early contact alone is sufficient to ensure competent parenting.

The nurse should stress to parents that, although early bonding may be valuable, it does not represent an "all or none" phenomenon. Throughout the child's life there will be multiple opportunities for the development of parent-child attachment. Bonding is a complex process that develops gradually and is influenced by numerous factors, only one of which is the type of initial contact between the newborn and parent. In a concept analysis of parent-infant attachment, Goulet, Bell, St-Cyr, and colleagues (1998) describe attributes of parent-infant attachment as proximity, reciprocity, and commitment. Within these attributes are further dimensions, which include contact, emotional state, individualization, complementarity, sensitivity, centrality, and parent role exploration. The researchers describe the parent-infant attachment process as one that is complex and therefore cannot be evaluated simply by the observations of attitudes and behaviors of parents toward their infants. Further research into the reciprocal relationships between infant and parent and the situational factors that influence such relationships are recommended.

One component of successful maternal attachment is *reciprocity* (Brazelton, 1974). As the mother responds to the infant, the infant must respond to the mother by some signal, such as sucking, cooing, eye contact, grasping, or *molding* (conforming to other's body during close physical contact). The first step is *initiation,* in which interaction between infant and parent begins. Next is *orientation,* which establishes the partners' expectations of each other during the interaction. Following orientation is *acceleration* of the attention cycle to a peak of excitement. The infant reaches out and coos, both arms jerk forward, the head moves backward, the eyes dilate, and the face brightens. After a short time, *deceleration* of the excitement and *turning away* occur, in which the infant's eyes shift away from the mother's and the child may grasp his or her own shirt. During this cycle of nonattention, repeated verbal or visual attempts to reinitiate the infant's attention are ineffective. This deceleration and turning away probably prevent the infant from being overwhelmed by excessive stimuli. In a good interaction both partners have synchronized their attention-nonattention cycles. Parents or other caregivers who do not allow the infant

to turn away and who continually attempt to maintain visual contact may encourage the infant to turn off the attention cycle and thus prolong the nonattention phase.

Although this description of reciprocal interacting behavior is usually observed in the infant by 2 to 3 weeks of age, nurses can use this information to teach parents how to interact with their infant. Recognizing the attention versus nonattention cycles and understanding that the latter is not a rejection of the parent helps parents develop competence in parenting. A recent study reported that co-regulation, where mothers and infants understood and responded appropriately to such cues as attention and inattention, was linked with increased attachment and better infant mental and psychomotor development (Evans and Porter, 2009). There are reports that maternal postpartum depression negatively affects attachment to the infant unless specific interventions are implemented. In one study mothers who were depressed showed a decreased sensitivity to the infants' needs and expressed fewer affirmations of their infants' behaviors and more negations when compared with nondepressed mothers (Murray, Fiori-Cowley, Hopper, et al, 1996). Insecure infant attachments were more likely to occur in depressed mothers when measured at 18 months postpartum. Overall, infants of depressed mothers showed no more pervasive distress or avoidance than the nondepressed control group, but did demonstrate more instances of disruptive behavior, which were precipitated by maternal negating. Conversely, a recent study of pregnant women demonstrated that concerns about attachment prenatally contribute to an increased risk for postpartum depression (Monk, Leight, and Fang, 2008).

Paternal Engrossment

Fathers also show specific attachment behaviors to the newborn. This process of paternal **engrossment**, forming a sense of absorption, preoccupation, and interest in the infant, includes (1) visual awareness of the newborn, especially focusing on the child's beauty; (2) tactile awareness, often expressed in a desire to hold the infant; (3) awareness of distinct characteristics with emphasis on those features of the infant that resemble the father; (4) perception of the infant as perfect; (5) development of a strong feeling of attraction to the child that leads to intense focusing of attention on the infant; (6) extreme elation; and (7) a sense of deep self-esteem and satisfaction. These responses are greatest during the early contacts with the infant and are intensified by the neonate's normal reflex activity, especially the grasp reflex and visual alertness. In addition to behavioral reactions, fathers also demonstrate physiologic responses such as increased heart rate and blood pressure during interactions with their newborns. In one study the attachment scores of inexperienced or first-time fathers were not significantly different from the attachment scores of experienced fathers. The researchers found support for the concept that the love relationship a father develops for a second or subsequent child is as strong and unique as for the first child (Ferketich and Mercer, 1995).

Fathers of preterm infants reported they first felt a bond or love with their high-risk newborn when they held the infant for the first time; the earlier the father was able to hold his infant, the earlier the father reported feelings of warmth and love for the newborn (Sullivan, 1999).

The process of engrossment has significant implications for nurses. It is imperative to recognize the importance of early father-infant contact in this process. Fathers need to be encouraged to express their positive feelings, especially if such emotions are contrary to any belief that fathers should remain stoic. If this is not clarified, fathers may feel confused and attempt to suppress the natural sensations of absorption, preoccupation, and interest to conform with societal expectations.

Mothers also need to be aware of the responses of the father toward the newborn, since one of the consequences of paternal preoccupation with the infant is less overt attention toward the mother. If both parents are able to share their feelings, each can appreciate the process of attachment toward their child and will avoid the unfortunate conflict of being insensitive and unaware of the other's needs. In addition, a father who is encouraged to form a relationship with his newborn is less likely to feel excluded and abandoned once the family returns home and the mother directs her attention toward caring for the infant.

Ideally, the process of engrossment should be discussed with parents before the delivery, such as in prenatal classes, to reinforce the father's awareness of his natural feelings toward the expected child. Focusing on the future experience of seeing, touching, and holding one's newborn may also help expectant fathers become more comfortable in accepting their paternal feelings. This in turn can assist them in being more supportive toward the mother, especially as labor and delivery draw near.

At the infant's birth the nurse can play a vital role in helping the father express engrossment by assessing the neonate in front of the couple; pointing out normal characteristics; encouraging identification through consistent referral to the child by name; encouraging the father to cuddle, hold, and talk to the infant; and demonstrating whenever necessary the soothing powers of caressing, stroking, and rocking the child (Fig. 8-16).

The father's role in supporting the mother during this period cannot be overemphasized. Once the mother has held the newborn skin-to-skin the father may also be encouraged to hold the newborn skin-to-skin while the mother rests. Fathers are encouraged to be with the mother during labor and delivery, to spend time alone with the mother and newborn after delivery, and to "room in" with the mother and infant. Education programs should be made available to new fathers and include information on holding the newborn, bathing, assisting the mother with breast-feeding, problems associated with breast-feeding and potential solutions, and care of the newborn at home (including safety). The integration of the father into the existing dyad of mother-newborn to form a new family—a triad—will help solidify his role as parent and partner in the care and support of his family.

The nurse watches for the same indications of affection from the father as those expected in the mother, such as visual contact in the en face position and embracing the infant close to the body. When present, such behaviors are reinforced. If such responses are not obvious, the nurse needs to assess the father's feelings regarding this birth, cultural beliefs that may prevent his expression of emotions, and other factors to facilitate his positive attachment during this critical period.

Siblings

Although the attachment process has been discussed almost exclusively in terms of the parents and infants, it is essential that nurses be aware of other family members, such as siblings, grandparents, and members of the extended family, who need preparation for the acceptance of this new child. Young children in particular need sensitive preparation for the birth to minimize sibling jealousy.

In support of family-centered care, there is an increasing trend to encourage siblings to visit the mother on the postpartum unit and to hold the newborn (Fig. 8-17). Another trend has been the presence of siblings at childbirth. Unlike sibling visitation, this practice has been controversial, yet truly family-centered care encompasses siblings, grandparents, and other significant persons from the extended family unit (Tomlinson, Bryan, and Esau, 1996). The American Academy of Pediatrics and American College of Obstetricians and Gynecologists (2007) support the presence of siblings at childbirth and visitation of the newborn and mother; basic guidelines for infection control and adult supervision are also recommended. Children exhibit different degrees of involvement in the birth process. Young children may fall asleep toward the end of delivery. Some reported benefits include children's increased knowledge of the birth process, less regressive behavior after the birth, and more mothering and caregiving behavior toward the infant. Some practitioners add facilitated family bonding and assimilation of the newborn into the family as positive outcomes. Parents whose children attended the birth have echoed these same benefits and have expressed their desire to repeat the experience should another pregnancy occur. Despite these positive findings, opponents believe that allowing children to observe a delivery could lead to emotional difficulties, although no research supports this contention. As research mounts, birthing centers that allow siblings at the birth are developing more definitive guidelines, such as an age requirement of at least 4 to 5 years, the presence of a supportive person for the sibling only, and an adequate sequence of preparation in which parents explore all options for preparing their other children.

From observations during sibling visitation, there is evidence that sibling attachment occurs. However, the en face

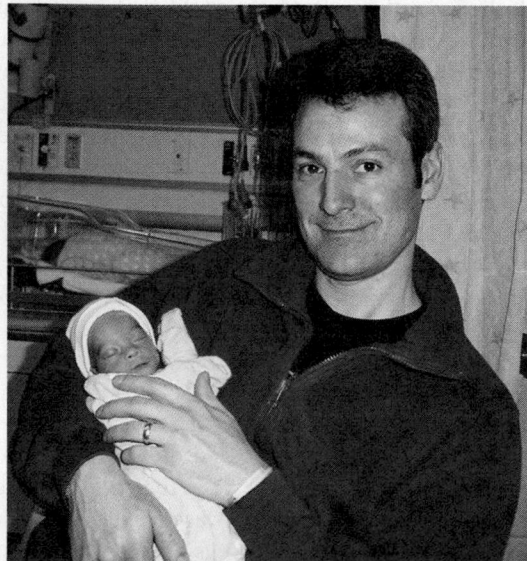

Fig. 8-16 A desire to hold the infant and participate in caregiving activities is an important step in the paternal attachment process.

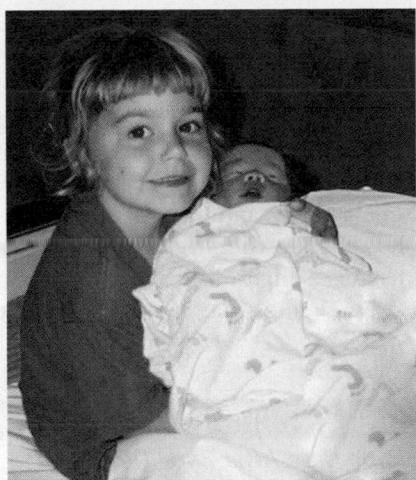

Fig. 8-17 Sibling visitation shortly after birth can be significant in the attachment process.

position is assumed much less often among the newborn and siblings than between mother and newborn, and when this position is used, it is brief. Siblings focus more on the head or face than on touching or talking to the infant. The siblings' verbalizations are focused less on attracting the infant's attention and more on addressing the mother about the newborn. Children who have established a prenatal relationship with the fetus have demonstrated more attachment behaviors, supporting the suggestion of encouraging prenatal acquaintance. Additional research is needed to establish theories on sibling bonding like those that have been constructed for parental bonding.

Multiple Births and Subsequent Children

A component of attachment that has special meaning for families with multiple births, monotropy refers to the principle that a person can become optimally attached to only one individual at a time. If a parent can form only one attachment at a time, how can all the siblings of a multiple birth receive optimum emotional care? Until recently a paucity of research had been done on bonding and multiple births, and even less is known about paternal engrossment and sibling attachment. In regard to maternal-twin bonding, the conclusions of different authors vary. Some report that mothers bond equally to each twin at the time of birth, even if one twin is ill. Others suggest that mothers of twins may take months or even years to form individual attachments and even longer if the twins are identical. Damato (2004) studied mothers of twins and found that postpartum depression had a negative impact on the maternal-infant relationship; when either one or both newborns (of twins) were admitted to the NICU, the mother's feelings of attachment were decreased at the time of the admission and up to 9 weeks postpartum. The author highlights the need for mothers of twins to have multiple opportunities to interact with twins shortly after birth through breast-feeding, skin-to-skin contact, and complete access to and care of the infants.

In a qualitative metasynthesis, Beck (2002) reported that mothers of multiples have unique needs related to the following themes: the impact of the burden of constant care for the infants, the myriad emotions experienced in the process of childbirth and childrearing, support by the children's father and mother's close friends, provision of equal attention to each infant, and acknowledgment of each infant's individuality.

Nurses can be instrumental in promoting bonding at multiple births. The most important principle is to assist the parents in recognizing the individuality of the children, especially monozygotic (identical) twins. The mother should visit with each newborn, including a sick infant, as much as possible after birth. Rooming-in and breast-feeding are encouraged. The nurse emphasizes any characteristics that are unique to each child and calls each infant by name, rather than calling them "the twins." Asking the family questions such as "How do you tell Sally and Amy apart?" and "In what ways are Sally and Amy different and similar?" helps point out their individual characteristics. Behaviors on the BNBAS can be used to illustrate these differences and to stress effective strategies for dealing with multiple personalities at the same time. (Other strategies for promoting individualism are discussed under Multiple Births in Chapter 3.)

Cobedding of twins or other multiples may be done in the hospital to maintain the bond between siblings that was formed in utero (Della Porta, Aforismo, and Butler-O'Hara, 1998). However, the American Academy of Pediatrics (2007a) has recommended against families cobedding at home. Because neither the safety nor the benefits of cobedding for newborns has been documented in the literature, the academy recommends families be counseled to follow safe sleeping practices, which currently dictate that infants sleep alone for optimal safety.

Another area of attachment that has received minimum attention is maternal bonding of multiparous mothers. Research suggests that "taking on" a second child has several additional tasks:

- Promoting acceptance and approval of the second child
- Grieving and resolving the loss of an exclusive dyadic relationship with the first child
- Planning and coordinating family life to include a second child
- Reformulating a relationship with the first child
- Identifying with the second child by comparing this child with the first child in terms of physical and psychologic characteristics
- Assessing one's affective capabilities in providing sufficient emotional support and nurturance simultaneously to two children

Employed mothers who have a second child report fewer concerns than unemployed mothers regarding general aspects of separation from their child and the effect of separation on the child, but they have similar concerns regarding separation because of employment as they had with the first child. It appears that although experience may decrease some concerns, it may not minimize others.

PREPARE FOR DISCHARGE AND HOME CARE

With shorter postpartum stays, as well as a trend toward mother-infant care, also called dyad or couplet care, discharge planning, referral, and home visiting have become important components of comprehensive newborn care. First-time, as well as experienced, parents benefit from guidance and assistance with the infant's care, such as breast- or bottle-feeding, and with the family's integration of a new member, particularly sibling adjustment.

To assess and meet these needs, teaching must begin early, ideally before the birth. Not only is the postpartum stay short (as little as 12 to 24 hours), but mothers are also in the taking-in phase, where they demonstrate passive and dependent behaviors. On the first postpartum day, because of fatigue and excitement about the newborn, women may not be able to absorb large amounts of information. This time may need to be spent highlighting essential aspects of care, such as infant safety and feeding. Parents may also be given a list of mother and infant care topics as part of the nursing admission history to choose issues they wish to review before going home. Teaching before discharge should focus on newborn feeding patterns, monitoring diapers for stools and voiding, jaundice, and infant crying (see Family-Centered Care box).

FAMILY-CENTERED CARE

Early Newborn Discharge Criteria

- It was a singleton birth between 38 and 42 weeks of gestation.
- Baby was delivered by uncomplicated vaginal delivery.
- Birth weight is appropriate for gestational age.
- Physical examination was normal.
- Vital signs are normal and stable as measured in an open crib with adequate clothing.
- Infant has urinated and passed at least one stool.
- Infant has completed at least two successful feedings.
- Clinical significance of jaundice, if present, has been determined and appropriate management or follow-up plans put in place.
- Appropriate maternal and infant blood tests have been performed.
- Appropriate neonatal immunizations have been administered.
- Newborn hearing screening has been completed per hospital protocol and state regulations.
- Family, environmental, and social risk factors have been assessed.
- Documentation is in place that mother has received usual infant care training and has demonstrated competency.
- Support persons are available to assist mother and her infant after discharge.
- Continuing medical care is planned, including that infants discharged sooner than 48 hours be examined within 48 hours of discharge from hospital.

Data from American Academy of Pediatrics: Policy statement: hospital stay for healthy terms newborns, *Pediatrics* 113(5):1434-1436, 2004.

Although legislation has been enacted guaranteeing most mothers a minimum of 48 hours' hospitalization, studies indicate that many mothers are leaving the hospital as early as 8 to 12 hours after vaginal delivery. The American Academy of Pediatrics (2004) has established guidelines for postpartum discharge before 48 hours of age. The academy emphasizes that the primary care physician rather than an insurance company should make the determination of appropriate discharge time. Nurses must continue to work within the confines of available resources and time to maintain adequate quality of care for mothers and infants.

Although many mothers and newborns may be safely discharged within 12 to 24 hours without detriment to their health, others may require a longer stay. Follow-up home care within days (or even hours after discharge when minor problems are

anticipated) is important to curtail hospital costs and provide adequate maternal-newborn care with minimum complications. Despite the changing spectrum of well-newborn health care, the nurse's role continues to be that of providing ongoing assessments of each mother-newborn dyad to ensure a safe transition to home and a successful adaptation into the family unit. The ultimate safety and success of early newborn discharge from hospital are contingent on using clear discharge criteria and having a high-quality early follow-up program (Radmacher, Massey, and Adamkin, 2002) (see Community Focus box).

COMMUNITY FOCUS

Newborn Home Care After Early Discharge*

Wet diapers—Minimum of one for each day of life (day 2 = 2 wets; day 3 = 3 wets) until fifth or sixth day, at which time 5 or 6 per day to 14 days, then 6 to 10 per day.

Breast-feeding—Successful latch-on and feeding every $1\frac{1}{2}$ to 3 hours daily. Swallowing should be audible.

Formula feeding—Successful, voiding as above, taking 1 to 3 oz (approximately) on demand or at least every 3 to 4 hours. Should be easily aroused for feeding.

Circumcision—Wash with warm water only; yellow exudate forming, non-bleeding, Plastibell intact for 48 hours.

Stools—At least one soft stool every 48 to 72 hours (bottle-feeding), or two or three per day (breast-feeding).

Color—Pink to ruddy when crying; pink centrally when at rest or asleep.

Activity—Four or five wakeful periods per day; alerts to environmental sounds and voices.

Jaundice—Physiologic jaundice (not appearing in first 24 hours), feeding, voiding, and stooling as noted above. Notify practitioner of suspicion of pathologic jaundice (if it appears within 24 hours of birth, ABO or Rh problems are suspected), decreased activity, poor feeding, dark orange skin color persisting after the fifth day in light-skinned newborn. Obtain transcutaneous bilirubin before discharge and identify risk per hour-specific risk nomogram; follow up with practitioner within 48 hours after discharge if discharged home before 24 hours old (see Hyperbilirubinemia, Chapter 9).

Cord—Kept above diaper line; drying.

Vital signs—Heart rate 120 to 140 beats/min at rest; respiratory rate 30 to 55 breath/min at rest without evidence of sternal retractions, grunting, or nasal flaring; temperature 36.3° to 37° C (97.3° to 98.6° F) axillary.

Position of sleep—On back.

*Any deviation from the above or suspicion of poor newborn adaptation should be reported to the practitioner at once.

With family structures changing, it is essential that nurses identify the primary caregiver, which may not always be the mother but may be a father, grandparent, or baby-sitter. Depending on the family composition, the mother's primary support system in the care of the newborn may not always be the traditional husband or male companion.

Nurses should not assume that terminology associated with mother-infant care is understood. Words relating to the anatomy (e.g., *meconium, labia, edema,* and *genitalia*) and to breast-feeding (e.g., *areola, colostrum,* and *let-down reflex*) may be unfamiliar to mothers. Mothers with other children do not necessarily understand more words, and young age and less education decrease comprehension.

An essential area of discharge counseling is the safe transport of the newborn home from the hospital. Ideally this information should be provided before delivery to allow parents to purchase a federally approved infant car safety seat restraint. An emerging trend is to hold the birthing center or hospital liable for any harm incurred as result of discharging a newborn without ensuring that the child is safely secured in an appropriate car safety seat restraint.

When purchasing a car safety seat restraint, parents should consider cost and convenience. The convertible-type seats are more expensive initially but cost less than two separate car restraint systems (infant-only model or infant-toddler convertible model). (See Chapter 12.) Convenience is a major factor, since a cumbersome restraint may be used less and improperly. Before buying a car safety seat restraint, it is best to try out different models. For example, some types are too large for subcompact cars. Asking friends about the advantages and disadvantages of their restraints is helpful, but borrowing their car seat or purchasing a used one can be dangerous. Parents should use only a restraint that has directions for use and a certification label stating that it complies with federal motor vehicle safety standards (both should be on the seat). They should not use a restraint that has been involved in a crash. Some service clubs and hospitals have loan programs for vehicle safety restraints. Information about approved models and other aspects of car safety seat restrains is available from several sources.*

---

*American Academy of Pediatrics, 141 Northwest Point Blvd., Elk Grove Village, IL 60007; 847-434-4000, fax: 847-434-8000; *Car safety seats: a guide for families 2009* is available at www.aap.org/family/carseatguide.htm. National Highway Traffic Safety Administration Auto Safety Hotline, 888-327-4236; www.nhtsa.dot.gov. For children with special needs, contact the National Easter Seal Society, 800-221-6827, and ask about Special KARS (Kids Are Riding Safe; www.easterseals.com. Riley Hospital for Children National Center for Safe Transportation of Children with Special Healthcare Needs, 800-755-0912; www.preventinjury.org.

Parents are cautioned against placing an infant in the front seat of a car with a passenger-side air bag. Infants weighing less than 9 kg (20 lb) or younger than 1 year should always be placed in a rear-facing child safety seat in the back seat of the car.

In the United States and Canada, all states and provinces have mandated the use of child restraints. Therefore hospitals and birthing centers should have policies regarding the safe discharge of a newborn in a car safety seat and provisions for parents to learn to use the device correctly. Parents are more likely to use a restraint correctly and consistently if the proper use of one is demonstrated and its necessity is stressed.

Although federal safety standards do not specify the minimum weight of an infant and the appropriate type of restraint, newborns weighing 2000 g (4.4 lb) receive relatively good support in convertible seats with a seat back–to-crotch strap height of 14 cm (5.5 inches) or less. Rolled blankets and towels may be needed between the crotch and legs to prevent slouching and can be placed along the sides to minimize lateral movements. Seats with shields (large padded surfaces in front of the child) and armrests (found on some older models) are unacceptable because of their proximity to the infant's face and neck. (For a discussion of appropriate car restraints for preterm infants, see p. 341, and for infants, see Motor Vehicle Injuries in Chapters 12 and 14.) Padding is never placed underneath or behind the infant because it creates slack in the harness, leading to the possibility of the child's ejection from the seat in the event of a crash.

The use of an appropriate car safety seat restraint is also encouraged to prevent injuries to children riding in airplanes. The Federal Aviation Administration recommends that children less than 4 years old ride in an approved safety restraint seat to prevent harm during turbulent weather, landing, and takeoff (American Academy of Pediatrics, 2002).

KEY POINTS

- Transition from fetal or placental circulation to independent respiration is the most important physiologic change required of the newborn.
- Chemical and thermal factors help initiate the neonate's first breaths.
- Circulatory changes in the neonate result from shifts in pressure in the heart and major vessels and from functional closures of the fetal shunts.
- The newborn's relatively large surface area, thin layer of subcutaneous fat, and unique mechanism for producing heat predispose the newborn to excessive heat loss.
- The infant's high rate of metabolism is closely correlated with the rate of fluid exchange, which is seven times greater in the infant than in the adult.
- The skin and mucous membranes and antibodies are the first and second lines of defense against infection.
- Apgar scoring, the initial assessment of the newborn, focuses on heart rate, respiratory effort, muscle tone, reflex irritability, and color.
- Physical assessment of the newborn includes clinical assessment of gestational age, general measurements, general appearance, head-to-toe assessment, and parent-infant attachment or bonding.

- Neurologic assessment focuses on reflexes and posture, muscle tone, head control, and movement and is best accomplished during the general physical examination.
- Behavioral assessment of newborns with the BNBAS examines responses to seven categories: habituation, orientation, motor performance, range of state, regulation of state, autonomic stability, and reflexes.
- An instrument for assessing the reciprocal interchange between parent and infant is the NCAST Feeding Scale.
- Physical care for the newborn includes maintaining a patent airway, maintaining a stable body temperature, protecting from infection and injury, and providing optimum nutrition.
- Although the attachment, or bonding, process primarily affects infants and parents, siblings and other family members also play an important role.
- With short postpartum stays, teaching should begin before birth and continue after discharge with telephone or home visit follow-up.
- An essential aspect of discharge teaching is ensuring the newborn's safe transportation home in a federally approved, backward-facing car safety seat restraint.

REFERENCES

Abubakar I, Iliyasu Z, Kabir M, et al: Knowledge, attitude and practice of female genital cutting among antenatal patients in Aminu Kano Teaching Hospital, *Nigerian J Med* 13(3):254-258, 2004.

Akers SM, Groh-Wargo SL: Normal nutrition during infancy. In Samour PQ, Helm KK, Lang CE, editors: *Handbook of pediatric nutrition,* ed 3, Sudbury, Mass, 2005, Jones & Bartlett.

Alexander GR, Himes JH, Kaufman RB, et al: A United States national reference for fetal growth, *Obstet Gynecol* 87(2):163-168, 1996.

American Academy of Pediatrics, Committee on Nutrition: *Pediatric nutrition handbook,* ed 6, Elk Grove Village, Ill, 2009a, The Academy.

American Academy of Pediatrics, Committee on Infectious Diseases: *Red book: 2009 report of the Committee on Infectious Diseases,* ed 28, Elk Grove Village, IL, 2009b, The Academy.

American Academy of Pediatrics: Clinical report—hearing assessment in infants and children: recommendations beyond neonatal screening, *Pediatrics* 124(4):1252-1263, 2009c.

American Academy of Pediatrics, Committee on Pediatric AIDS: HIV testing and prophylaxis to prevent mother-to-child transmission in the United States, *Pediatrics* 122(5):1127-1134, 2008a.

American Academy of Pediatrics, Newborn Screening Authoring Committee: Newborn screening expands: recommendations for pediatricians and medical homes— implications for the system, *Pediatrics* 121(1):192-217, 2008b.

American Academy of Pediatrics, Committee on Nutrition: Use of soy protein-based formulas in infant feeding, *Pediatrics* 121(5):1062-1068, 2008c.

American Academy of Pediatrics, Section on Ophthalmology: Red reflex examination in neonates, infants, and children, *Pediatrics* 122(6):1401-1404, 2008d.

American Academy of Pediatrics: Committee on Fetus and Newborn: Cobedding twins and higher-order multiples in a hospital setting, *Pediatrics* 120(6):1359-1366, 2007a.

American Academy of Pediatrics, Joint Committee on Infant Hearing: Year 2007 position statement: principles and guidelines for early hearing detection and intervention programs, *Pediatrics* 120:898-921, 2007b.

American Academy of Pediatrics: *Neonatal resuscitation textbook,* 5th edition, Dallas, 2006a, American Heart Association.

American Academy of Pediatrics: Policy statement: the Apgar score, *Pediatrics* 117(4):1444-1447, 2006b.

American Academy of Pediatrics: The changing concept of sudden infant death syndrome: diagnostic coding shifts, controversies regarding the sleeping environment, and new variables to consider in reducing risk, *Pediatrics* 116(5):1245-1255, 2005a (reaffirmed January 2009).

American Academy of Pediatrics: Policy statement: breastfeeding and the use of human milk, *Pediatrics* 115(2):496-506, 2005b.

American Academy of Pediatrics: Policy statement: hospital stay for healthy terms newborns, *Pediatrics* 113(5):1434-1436, 2004.

American Academy of Pediatrics: Clinical report: prevention and management of positional skull deformities in infants, *Pediatrics* 112(1):199-202, 2003a.

American Academy of Pediatrics: Facilities and equipment for the care of pediatric patients in a community hospital, *Pediatrics* 111(5):1120-1122, 2003b (reaffirmed September 1, 2007).

American Academy of Pediatrics: Policy statement: controversies concerning vitamin K and the newborn, *Pediatrics* 112(1):191-192, 2003c.

American Academy of Pediatrics, Committee on Injury and Poison Prevention: Selecting and using the most appropriate car safety seats for growing children: guidelines for counseling parents, *Pediatrics* 109(3):550-553, 2002.

American Academy of Pediatrics, Task Force on Circumcision: Circumcision policy statement, *Pediatrics* 103(3):686-693, 1999.

American Academy of Pediatrics, Committee on Bioethics: Female genital mutilation, *Pediatrics* 102(1):153-156, 1998.

American Academy of Pediatrics, American College of Obstetricians and Gynecologists: *Guidelines for perinatal care,* ed 6, Elk Grove Village, Ill, 2007, The Academy.

Anand KJS, International Evidence-Based Group for Neonatal Pain: Consensus statement for the prevention and management of pain in the newborn, *Arch Pediatr Adolesc Med* 155(2):173-179, 2001.

Anderson JW, Johnstone BM, Remley DT: Breastfeeding and cognitive development: a meta-analysis, *Am J Clin Nutr* 70(4):525-535, 1999.

Arbuckle T, Wilkins R, Sherman G: Birth weight percentiles by gestational age in Canada, *Obstet Gynecol* 81(1):39-48, 1993.

Arora S, McJunkin C, Wehrer J, et al: Major factors influencing breastfeeding rates: mother's perception of father's attitude and milk supply, *Pediatrics* 106(5):e67, 2000.

Arslanoglu S, Moro GE, Boehm G: Early supplementation of probiotic oligosaccharides protects formula-fed infants against infections during the first 6 months of life, *J Nutr* 137(11):2420-2424, 2007.

Association of Women's Health, Obstetric and Neonatal Nurses: *Evidence-based clinical practice guideline: neonatal skin care,* 2nd edition, Washington, DC, 2007, The Association.

Axton SE, Smith LF, Bertrand S, et al: Comparison of brachial and calf blood pressures in infants, *Pediatr Nurs* 21(4):323-326, 1995.

Bachrach VR, Schwarz E, Bachrach LR: Breastfeeding and the risk of hospitalization for respiratory disease in infancy, *Arch Pediatr Adolesc Med* 157(3):237-243, 2003.

Bailey J, Rose P: Axillary and tympanic temperature recording in the preterm neonate: a comparative study, *J Adv Nurs* 34(4):465-474, 2001.

Bailey RC, Moses S, Parker CB, et al: Male circumcision for HIV prevention in young men in Kisumu, Kenya: a randomized controlled trial, *Lancet* 369(9562):643-656, 2007.

Ball TM, Wright AL: Health care costs of formula-feeding in the first year of life, *Pediatrics* 103(Suppl 4):S870-S876, 1999.

Ballard JL, Auer CE, Khoury JC: Ankyloglossia: assessment, incidence, and effect of frenuloplasty on the breastfeeding dyad, *Pediatrics* 110(5):e63, 1001, 2002.

Ballard JL, Khoury JC, Wedig K, et al: New Ballard score expanded to include extremely premature infants, *J Pediatr* 119:417-423, 1991.

Ballard JL, Novak KK, Driver M: A simplified score for assessment of fetal maturation of newly born infants, *J Pediatr* 95(5):769-774, 1979.

Barnard K: *NCAST feeding manual,* Seattle, 1994, University of Washington.

Bartman T: Newborn circumcision and urinary tract infections (letter), *Pediatrics* 107(1):210-214, 2001.

Battaglia FC, Lubchenco LO: A practical classification of newborn infants by weight and gestational age, *J Pediatr* 71(2):159-161, 1967.

Beaudry M, Dufour R, Marcoux S: Relation between infant feeding and infections during the first 6 months of life, *J Pediatr* 126(2):191-197, 1995.

Beck CT: Mothering multiples, *MCN* 27(4):214-221, 2002.

Behring A, Vezeau TM, Fink R: Timing of the newborn first bath: a replication, *Neonat Netw* 22(1):39-46, 2003.

Biancuzzo M: *Breastfeeding the newborn: clinical strategies for nurses,* ed 2, St Louis, 2003, Mosby.

Blackburn ST: *Maternal, fetal, and neonatal physiology: a clinical perspective,* ed 3, St Louis, 2007, Saunders.

Blain-Lewis N: Comparative studies of bruising and healing after heelstick, *Neonat Intensive Care* 5(5):18-21, 1992.

Blass EM, Watt LB: Suckling- and sucrose-induced analgesia in human newborns, *Pain* 83(3):611-623, 1999.

Bliss-Holtz J: Methods of newborn infant temperature monitoring: a research review, *Issues Compr Pediatr Nurs* 18(4):287-298, 1995.

Bliss-Holtz J: Determination of thermoregulatory state in full-term infants, *Nurs Res* 42(4):204-207, 1993.

Brady-Fryer B, Wiebe N, Lander JA: Pain relief for neonatal circumcision. In *Cochrane Database Syst Rev* 18(4):CD004217, 2004.

Brazelton TB: Mother-infant reciprocity. In Klaus MH, Leger T, Trause MA, editors: *Maternal attachment and mothering disorders: a round table,* Sausalito, Calif, 1974, Johnson & Johnson Baby Products.

Brazelton TB, Nugent JK: *Neonatal behavioral assessment scale,* London, 1996, MacKeith Press.

Broussard ER: The Pittsburgh firstborns at age 19 years. In Call J, Calerson E, Tyson R, editors:

Frontiers of infant psychiatry, vol 2, New York, 1984, Basic Books.

Broussard ER: Assessment of the adaptive potential of the mother infant system: the Neonatal Perception Inventories, *Semin Perinatol* 3(1):91-100, 1979.

Broussard ER: Neonatal prediction and outcome at 10/11 years, *Child Psychiatr Hum Dev* 7(2):85-93, 1976.

Bryant KG, Horns KM, Longo N, et al: A primer on newborn screening, *Adv Neonat Care* 4(5):306-317, 2004.

Burgess AW, Carr KE, Nahirny C, et al: Nonfamily infant abductions, 1983-2006, *Am J Nurs* 108(9):32-38, 2008.

Butt ML, Kisilevsky BS: Music modulates behavior of premature infants following heel lance, *Can J Nurs Res* 31(4):17-39, 2000.

Butte NF, Wong WW, Hopkinson JM, et al: Infant feeding mode affects early growth and body composition, *Pediatrics* 106(6):1355-1366, 2000.

Canadian Paediatric Society, Community Paediatrics Committee: *Temperature measurement in paediatrics*, reaffirmed February 2009, available at www.cps.ca/english/statements (accessed March 12, 2009).

Canadian Paediatric Society, First Nations, Inuit and Métis Health Committee: Vitamin D supplementation: recommendations for Canadian mothers and infants, *Paediatr Child Health* 12(7):583-589, 2007.

Carbajal R, Veerapen S, Couderc S, et al: Analgesic effect of breast feeding in term neonates: randomized controlled trial, *Br Med J* 326(7379):13, 2003.

Cavaliere T: Genitourinary assessment. In Tappero E, Honeyfield M, editors: *Physical assessment of the newborn: a comprehensive approach to the art of physical examination*, ed 4, Petaluma, Calif, 2009, NICU Ink.

Centers for Disease Control and Prevention: Use of World Health Organization and CDC growth charts for children aged 0-59 months in the United states, *MMWR Weekly* 59(rr09):1-15, 2010.

Centers for Disease Control and Prevention: Breastfeeding trends and updated national health objectives for exclusive breastfeeding—United States, birth years 2000-2004, *MMWR* 56(30):760-763, 2007.

Chen A, Rogan W: Isoflavones in soy infant formula: a review of evidence for endocrine and other activity in infants, *Ann Rev Nutr* 24:33-54, 2004.

Chertok IR, Shoham-Vardi I, Hallak M: Four-month breastfeeding duration in postcesarean women of different cultures in the Israeli Negev, *J Perinat Neonatal Nurs* 18(2):145-160, 2004.

Choudhry UK: Traditional practices of women from India: pregnancy, childbirth, and newborn care, *J Obstet Gynecol Neonatal Nurs* 26(5):533-539, 1997.

Codipietro L, Ceccarelli M, Ponzone A: Breastfeeding or oral sucrose solution in term neonates receiving heel lance: a randomized, controlled trial, *Pediatrics* 122(3):e716-721, 2008.

Cohen HA, Drucker MM, Vainer S, et al: Postcircumcision urinary tract infection, *Clin Pediatr* 31(6):322-324, 1992.

Connolly JL, Carron JD, Roark SD: Universal newborn hearing screening: are we achieving the Joint Committee on Infant Hearing (JCIH) objectives? *Laryngoscope* 115(2):232-236, 2005.

Conover E, Buehler BA: Use of herbal agents by breastfeeding women may affect infants, *Pediatr Ann* 33(4):235-240, 2004.

Coryllos A, Genna C, Salloum A. Congenital tongue-tie and its impact on breastfeeding. In American Academy of Pediatrics, Section on Breastfeeding: *Breastfeeding: best for baby and mother*, Elk Grove Village, Ill, 2004, The Academy.

Craig JV, Lancaster GA, Taylor S, et al: Infrared ear thermometry compared with rectal thermometry in children: a systematic review, *Lancet* 360(9333):603-609, 2002.

Cunningham FG, Gant NF, Leveno KJ, et al, editors: *Williams obstetrics*, ed 21, New York, 2001, McGraw Hill.

Cyna AM, Middleton P: Caudal epidural block versus other methods of postoperative pain relief for circumcision in boys, *Cochrane Database Syst Rev* 8(4):CD003005, 2008.

Damato EG: Prenatal attachment and other correlates of postnatal attachment to twins, *Adv Neonat Care* 4(5):274-291, 2004.

de Onis M, Onyango AW: The Centers for Disease Control and Prevention 2000 growth charts and the growth of breastfed infants, *Acta Paediatr* 92:413-419, 2003.

Della Porta K, Aforismo D, Butler-O'Hara M: Co-bedding of twins in the neonatal intensive care, *Pediatr Nurs* 24(6):529-531, 1998.

Dennison BA, Edmunds LS, Stratton HH, et al: Rapid infant weight gain predicts childhood overweight, *Obesity (Silver Spring)* 14(3):491-499, 2006.

Dewey KG, Heinig MJ, Nommsen LA, et al: Breastfed infants are leaner than formula-fed infants at 1 year of age: the DARLING study, *Am J Clin Nutr* 57(2):140-145, 1993.

Dewey K, Heinig MJ, Nommsen LA, et al: Adequacy of energy intake among breastfed infants in the DARLING study: relationships to growth velocity, morbidity, and activity levels, *J Pediatr* 119(4):538-547, 1991.

Dewey KG, Heinig MJ, Nommsen-Rivers LA: Differences in morbidity between breast-fed and formula-fed infants, *J Pediatr* 126(5 pt 1):696-702, 1995.

Dewey KG, Peerson JM, Brown KH, et al: Growth of breast-fed infants deviates from current reference data: a pooled analysis of US, Canadian and European data sets, *Pediatrics* 96(3 Pt 1):495-503, 1995.

Dollberg S, Botzer E, Grunis E, et al: Immediate nipple pain relief after frenotomy in breastfed infants with ankyloglossia: a randomized, prospective study, *J Pediatr Surg* 41(9):1598-1600, 2006.

Donovan EF, Tyson JE, Ehrenkranz RA, et al: Inaccuracy of Ballard scores before 28 weeks' gestation, *J Pediatr* 135(2 Pt 1):147-152, 1999.

Dore S, Buchan D, Coulas S, et al: Alcohol versus natural drying for newborn cord care, *J Obstet Gynecol Neonatal Nurs* 27(6):621-627, 1998.

Douglas LC, Sanders ME: Probiotics and prebiotics in dietetics practice, *J Am Diet Assoc* 108(3):510-521, 2008.

Dubowitz LMS, Dubowitz V: *Gestational age of the newborn*, Menlo Park, Calif, 1977, Addison-Wesley.

Eriksson M, Finnstrom O: Can daily repeated doses of orally administered glucose induce tolerance when given for neonatal pain relief? *Acta Paediatr* 93(2):246-249, 2004.

Evans CA, Porter CL: The emergence of mother-infant co-regulation during the first year: links to infants' developmental status and attachment, *Infant Behav Devel* 32(2):147-158, 2009.

Falkner B: Hypertension in children and adolescents. In Black HR, Elliott WJ, editors, *Hypertension*, Philadelphia, 2007, Saunders.

Ferketich SL, Mercer RT: Paternal-infant attachment of experienced and inexperienced fathers during infancy, *Nur Res* 44(1):31-37, 1995.

Foca M, Jacob K, Whittier S, et al: Endemic *Pseudomonas aeruginosa* infection in a neonatal intensive care unit, *N Engl J Med* 343(10):695-700, 2000.

France CR, Taddio A, Shah VS, et al: Maternal family history of hypertension attenuates neonatal pain response, *Pain* 142(3):189-193, 2009.

Fuloria M, Kreiter S: The newborn examination, part 1, Emergencies and common abnormalities involving the skin, head, neck, chest, and respiratory and cardiovascular systems, *Am Fam Physician* 65(1):61-68, 2002.

Geller M: Infant abduction in the hospital setting, *QRC Advisor* 16(5):1-4, 2000.

Georgieff MK: Taking a rational approach to the choice of formula, *Contemp Pediatr* 18(8):112-130, 2001.

Geyer J, Ellsbury D, Kleiber C, et al: An evidence-based multidisciplinary protocol for neonatal circumcision pain management, *J Obstet Gynecol Neonatal Nurs* 31(4):403-410, 2002.

Giampietro PG, Bruno G, Furcolo G, et al: Soy protein formulas in children: no hormonal effects in long-term feeding, *J Pediatr Endocrinol Metab* 17(2):191-196, 2004.

Gibbins S, Stevens B, Hodnett E, et al: Efficacy and safety of sucrose for procedural pain relief in preterm and term neonates, *Nurs Res* 51(6):375-382, 2002.

Gil A, Ramirez M, Gil M: Role of long-chain polyunsaturated fatty acids in infant nutrition, *Eur J Clin Nutr* 57(Suppl 1):S31-S34, 2003.

Golombek SG, Brill PE, Salice AL: Randomized trial of alcohol versus triple dye for umbilical cord care, *Clin Pediatr* 41(6):419-423, 2002.

Goodell LS, Wakefield DB, Ferris AM: Rapid weight gain during the first year of life predicts obesity in 2-3 year olds from a low-income, minority population, *J Community Health* 34(5):370-375, 2009.

Goulet C, Bell L, St-Cyr D, et al: A concept analysis of parent-infant attachment, *J Adv Nurs* 28(5):1071-1081, 1998.

Gradin M, Eriksson M, Holmqvist G, et al: Pain reduction at venipuncture in newborns: oral glucose compared with local anesthetic cream, *Pediatrics* 110(6):1053-1057, 2002.

Gray L, Miller LW, Phillip BL, et al: Breastfeeding is analgesic in healthy newborns, *Pediatrics* 109(4):590-593, 2002.

Gray L, Watt L, Blass EM: Skin-to-skin contact is analgesic in healthy newborns, *Pediatrics* 105(1):110-111, 2000, available at www.pediatrics.org/cgi/content/full/105/1/e14 (accessed November 25, 2009).

Gray RH, Kigozi G, Serwadda D, et al: Male circumcision for HIV prevention in men in Rakai, Uganda: a randomized trial, *Lancet* 369(9562):657-666, 2007.

Greenes DS, Fleisher GR: Accuracy of a noninvasive temporal artery thermometer for use in infants, *Arch Pediatr Adolesc Med* 155(3):376-381, 2001.

Greim HA: The endocrine and reproductive system: adverse effects of hormonally active substances? *Pediatrics* 113(4):1070-1075, 2004.

Griffiths DM: Do tongue-ties affect breastfeeding? *J Hum Lact* 20(4):409-414, 2004.

Grummer-Strawn LM, Mei Z, Centers for Disease Control and Prevention Pediatric Nutrition Surveillance System: Does breastfeeding protect against pediatric overweight? Analysis of longitudinal data from the Centers for Disease Control and Prevention Pediatric Nutrition Surveillance System, *Pediatrics* 113(2):e81-e86, 2004.

Hale T: *Medications and mothers' milk,* Amarillo, Tex, 2008, Pharmasoft.

Hanson LA, Korotkova M: The role of breastfeeding in prevention of neonatal infection, *Semin Neonatol* 7(4):275-281, 2002.

Harrison D, Johnston L, Loughnan P: Oral sucrose for procedural pain in sick hospitalized infants: a randomized-controlled trial, *J Paediatr Child Health* 39(8):591-597, 2003.

Havens PL, Mofenson LM, Committee on Pediatric AIDS: Evaluation and management of the infant exposed to HIV-1 in the United States, *Pediatrics* 123(1):175-187, 2009.

Hendriksz CJ, Walter JH: Feeding infants with undiluted goat's milk can mimic tryosinaemia type 1, *Acta Paediatr* 93(4):552-553, 2004.

Hernandez IF: Promoting exclusive breastfeeding for Hispanic women, *MCN* 31(5):318-324, 2006.

Herschel M, Khoshnood B, Ellman C, et al: Neonatal circumcision: randomized trial of a sucrose pacifier for pain control, *Arch Pediatr Adolesc Med* 152(3):279-284, 1998.

Hicks MA: A comparison of the tympanic and axillary temperatures of the preterm and term infant, *J Perinatol* 16(4):261-267, 1996.

Holzhauer JK, Reith V, Sawin KJ, et al: Evaluation of temporal artery thermometry in children 3-36 months old, *J Soc Pediatr Nurs* 14(4):239-244, 2009.

Huang CM, Tung WS, Kuo LL, et al: Comparison of pain responses of premature infants to the heelstick between containment and swaddling, *J Nurs Res* 12(1):31-40, 2004.

Hussink Muller PC, van Berkel LH, de Beaufort AJ: Axillary and rectal temperature measurements poorly agree in newborn infants, *Neonatology* 94(1):31-34, 2008.

Janssen PA, Selwood BL, Dobson SR, et al: To dye or not to dye: a randomized, clinical trial of a triple dye/alcohol regime versus dry cord care, *Pediatrics* 111(1):15-20, 2003.

Johnston CC, Filion F, Campbell-Yeo M, et al: Enhanced kangaroo mother care for heel lance in preterm infants: a crossover trial, *J Perinatol* 29(1):51-56, 2009.

Johnston CC, Stevens B, Pinelli J, et al: Kangaroo care is effective in diminishing pain response in preterm neonates, *Arch Pediatr Adolesc Med* 157(11):1084-1088, 2003.

Jones HL, Kleber CB, Eckert GJ, et al: Comparison of rectal temperature measured by digital vs. mercury glass thermometer in infants under 2 months old, *Clin Pediatr* 42(4):357-359, 2003.

Juretschke LJ: Unilateral neonatal testicular torsion, *J Obstet Gynecol Neonatal Nurs* 29(5):451-456, 2000.

Kapellen TM, Gebauer CM, Brosteanu O, et al: Higher rate of cord-related adverse events in neonates with dry umbilical cord care compared to chlorhexidine powder: results of a randomized controlled study to compare efficacy and safety of chlorhexidine powder versus dry care in umbilical cord care of the newborn, *Neonatology* 96(1):13-18, 2009.

Kaye CI, American Academy of Pediatrics, Committee on Genetics: Newborn Screening Fact Sheets, *Pediatrics* 118(3):e934-e963, 2006.

Kent AL, Kecskes Z, Shadbolt B, et al: Blood pressure in the first year of life in healthy infants born at term, *Pediatr Nephrol* 22(10):1743-1749, 2007.

Kinkade S, Meadows S, Gracia-Trujillo J: Does neonatal circumcision decrease morbidity? *J Fam Pract* 54(1):81-82, 2005.

Klaus MH, Kennell JH, Klaus PH: *Bonding: building the foundations of secure attachment and independence,* Menlo Park, Calif, 1995, Addison-Wesley.

Kraft NL: A pictorial and video guide to circumcision without pain, *Adv Neonat Care* 3(2):50-64, 2003.

Kramer MS, Guo T, Platt RW, et al: Feeding effects on growth during infancy, *J Pediatr* 145(5):600-605, 2004.

Kramer MS, Platt RW, Wen SW, et al: A new and improved population-based Canadian reference for birth weight for gestational age, *Pediatrics* 108(2):e35, 462, 2001.

Kyenkya-Isabirye M: UNICEF launches the Baby-Friendly Hospital Initiative, *MCN* 17(4):177-179, 1992.

Lanham DM, Walker B, Klocke E, et al: Accuracy of tympanic temperature readings in children under 6 years of age, *Pediatr Nurs* 25(1):39-42, 1999.

Lanting CI, Fidler V, Huisman M, et al: Neurological differences between 9-year-old children fed breast-milk or formula-milk as babies, *Lancet* 344(8933):1319-1322, 1994.

Lawrence RA, Lawrence RM: *Breastfeeding: a guide for the medical profession,* ed 6, St Louis, 2005, Mosby.

Leick-Rude MK, Bloom LF: A comparison of temperature-taking methods in neonates, *Neonat Netw* 17(5):21-37, 1998.

Leung AKC, Robson, WLM: Natal teeth: a review, *J Natl Med Assoc* 98(2):226-228, 2006.

Lu B, Wu Y, Nielson CM, et al: Factors associated with acquisition and clearance of human papillomavirus infection in a cohort of US men: a prospective study, *J Infect Dis* 199(3):363-371, 2009.

Malloy MH: Trends in postneonatal aspiration deaths and reclassification of sudden infant death syndrome: impact of the "Back to Sleep" program, *Pediatrics* 109(4):661-665, 2002.

Masaitis NS, Kaempf JW: Developing a frenotomy policy at one medical center: a case study approach, *J Hum Lact* 12(3):229-232, 1996.

McCleary PH: Female genital mutilation and childbirth: a case report, *Birth* 21(4):221-223, 1994.

McDonald RE, Avery DR, Dean JA: *Dentistry for the child and adolescent,* ed 8, St Louis, 2004, Mosby.

Medves M, O'Brien B: The effect of bather and location of first bath on maintaining thermal stability in newborns, *J Obstet Gynecol Neonatal Nurs* 33(2):175-182, 2004.

Merritt RJ, Jenks BH: Safety of soy-based formulas containing isoflavones: the clinical evidence, *J Nutr* 134(5):1220S-1224S, 2004.

Messner AH, Lalakea M, Aby J, et al: Ankyloglossia: incidence and affected feeding difficulties, *Arch Otolaryngol Head Neck Surg* 126(1):36-39, 2000.

Metaj M, Laroia N, Lawrence RA, et al: Comparison of breast-and formula-fed normal newborns in time to first stool and urine. *J Perinatol* 23:624-628, 2003.

Monk C, Leight KL, Fang Y: The relationship between women's attachment style and perinatal mood disturbance: implications for screening and treatment. *Arch Women's Mental Health* 11(2):117-129, 2008.

Montgomery DL, Splett PL: Economic benefit of breast-feeding infants enrolled in WIC, *J Am Diet Assoc* 97(4):379-385, 1997.

Moolenaar RL, Crutcher JM, San Joaquin VH, et al: A prolonged outbreak of *Pseudomonas aeruginosa* in a neonatal intensive care unit: did staff fingernails play a role in disease transmission? *Infect Control Hosp Epidemiol* 21(2):80-85, 2000.

Mullany LC, Darmstadt GL, Katz J, et al: Risk of mortality subsequent to umbilical cord infection among newborns of southern Nepal: cord infection and mortality, *Pediatr Infect Dis J* 28(1):17-20, 2009.

Murray L, Fiori-Cowley A, Hopper R, et al: The impact of postnatal depression and associated adversity on early mother-infant interactions and later infant outcomes, *Child Dev* 67(5):2512-2526, 1996.

Nelson CP, Dunn R, Wan J, et al: The increased incidence of newborn circumcision: data from the nationwide inpatient sample, *J Urology* 173(3):978-981, 2005.

Newman J, Pitman T: *The ultimate breastfeeding book of answers,* Roseville, Calif, 2000, Prima.

Nielson CM, Schiaffino MK, Dunne EF, et al: Associations between male anogenital human papillomavirus infection and circumcision by anatomic site sampled and lifetime number of female sex partners, *J Infect Dis* 199(1):7-13, 2009.

Nuntnarumit P, Yang W, Bada-Ellzey HS: Blood pressure measurements in the newborn, *Clin Perinatol* 26(4):981-996, 1999.

Paes B, Janes M, Vegh P, et al: A comparative study of heel-stick devices for infant blood collection, *Am J Dis Child* 147(3):346-348, 1993.

Penny-MacGillivray T: A newborn's first bath: when? *J Obstet Gynecol Neonatal Nurs* 25(6):481-487, 1996.

Pessler F, Nejat M: Anaphylactic reactions to goat's milk in a cow's milk allergic infant, *Pediatric Allergy Immunol* 15(2):183-185, 2004.

Quan R, Yang C, Rubinstein S, et al: Effects of microwave radiation on anti-infective factors in human milk, *Pediatrics* 89(4 Pt 1):667-669, 1992.

Rabier V, Bataillon S, Jolivet-Gougeon A, et al: Hand washing soap as a source of neonatal *Serratia marcescens* outbreak, *Acta Paediatrica* 97(10):1381-1385, 2008.

Radmacher P, Massey C, Adamkin D: Hidden morbidity with "successful" early discharge, *J Perinatol* 22:15-20, 2002.

Rautava S, Salminen S, Isolauri E: Specific probiotics in reducing the risk of acute infections in infancy: a randomized, double-blind, placebo-controlled study, *Br J Nutr* 101(11):1722-1726, 2009.

Razmus I, Dalton M, Wilson D: Pain management for newborn circumcision, *Pediatr Nurs* 20(5):414-417, 427, 2004.

Ricke LA, Baker NJ, Madlon-Kay DJ, et al: Newborn tongue-tie: prevalence and effect on breastfeeding, *J Am Board Fam Pract* 18(1):1-7, 2005.

Riordan J, Gill-Hopple K: Breastfeeding care in multicultural populations, *J Obstet Gynecol Neonatal Nurs* 30(2):216-223, 2001.

Ross Mothers Survey: Breastfeeding trends—2003, Columbus, OH, 2003, Ross Products Division, Abbott Laboratories. Available at http://abbottnutrition.com/resources/en_US/home/breastfeeding/BF_Trends_2003.pdf (accessed June 16, 2008).

Sasidharan K, Dutta S, Narang A: Validity of New Ballard score until 7th day of postnatal life in moderately preterm neonates, *Arch Dis Childhood Fetal Neonat* 94:F39-F44, 2009.

Scariati PD, Grummer-Strawn LM, Fein SB: A longitudinal analysis of infant morbidity and the extent of breastfeeding in the United States, *Pediatrics* 99(6):e5, 1997.

Schoen EJ, Colby CJ, Ray GT: Newborn circumcision decreases incidence and costs of urinary tract infections during first year of life, *Pediatrics* 105(4):789-793, 2000.

Schuh S, Komar L, Stephens D, et al: Comparison of the temporal artery and rectal thermometry in children in the emergency department, *Pediatr Emerg Care* 20(11):736-741, 2004.

Seguin J, Terry K: Neonatal infrared axillary thermometry, *Clin Pediatr* 38(1):35-40, 1999.

Serour F, Mandelberg A, Mori J: Slow injection of local anesthetic will decrease pain during dorsal penile nerve block, *Acta Anaesthesiol Scand* 42(8):926-928, 1998.

Severn CB: Head circumference–crown rump length: practical measurements for neonatal screening, *Neonat Intensive Care* 7(4):52-57, 1994.

Sganga A, Wallace R, Kiehl E, et al: A comparison of four methods of normal newborn temperature measurement, *MCN* 25(2):76-79, 2000.

Shah V, Ohlsson A: Venepuncture versus heel lance for blood sampling in term neonates. In *Cochrane Database Syst Rev* (2):CD001452, 2001.

Shogan MG: Emergency management plan for newborn abduction, *J Obstet Gynecol Neonatal Nurs* 31(3):340-346, 2002.

Siberry GK, Diener-West M, Schappell E, et al: Comparison of temple temperatures with rectal temperatures in children under 2 years of age, *Clin Pediatr* 41(6):405-414, 2002.

Siegfried N, Muller M, Volmink J, et al: Male circumcision for prevention of heterosexual acquisition of HIV in men, *Cochrane Database Syst Rev* (3):CD003362, 2003.

Singh GK, Kogan MD, Dee DL: Nativity/immigrant status, race/ethnicity, and socioeconomic determinants of breastfeeding initiation and duration in the United States, 2003, *Pediatrics* 119(Suppl 1):S38-S46, 2007.

Smith DP, Gjellum M: The efficacy of LMX versus EMLA for pain relief in boys undergoing office meatotomy, *J Urol* 172 (4 Pt 2):1760-1761, 2004.

Stang HJ, Snellman LW, Condon LM, et al: Beyond dorsal penile nerve block: a more humane circumcision, *Pediatrics* 100(2):e3, 1997, available at www.pediatrics.org/cgi/content/full/100/2/e3 (accessed November 25, 2009).

Stevens B, Johnston C, Franck L, et al: The efficacy of developmentally sensitive interventions and sucrose for relieving procedural pain in very low birth weight infants, *Nurs Res* 48(1):35-43, 1999.

Stevens B, Taddio A, Ohlsson A, et al: The efficacy of sucrose for relieving procedural pain in neonates: a systematic review and meta-analysis, *Acta Paediatr* 86(8):837-842, 1997.

Stevens B, Yamada J, Ohlsson A: Sucrose for analgesia in newborn infants undergoing painful procedures, *Cochrane Database Syst Rev* (3):CD001069, 2004.

Stoll B: Routine delivery room care. In Behrman RE, Kliegman RM, Jenson HB, et al, editors: *Nelson textbook of pediatrics*, ed 18, Philadelphia, 2007, Saunders.

Sullivan JR: Development of father-infant attachment in fathers of preterm infants, *Neonat Netw* 18(7):33-39, 1999.

Taddio A, Ohlsson K, Ohlsson A: Lidocaine-prilocaine cream for analgesia during circumcision in newborn boys, *Cochrane Database Syst Rev* (2):CD000494, 2000.

Taddio A, Pollock N, Gilbert-MacLeod C, et al: Combined analgesia and local anesthesia to minimize pain during circumcision, *Arch Pediatr Adolesc Med* 154(5):620-623, 2000.

Taddio A, Shah V, Gilbert-MacLeod C, et al: Conditioning and hyperalgesia in newborns exposed to repeated heel lances, *JAMA* 288(7):857-861, 2002.

Taddio A, Shah V, Katz J: Reduced infant response to a routine care procedure after sucrose analgesia, *Pediatrics* 123(3):e425-e429, 2009.

Taveras EM, Rifas-Shiman MB, Belfort MB, et al: Weight status in the first 6 months of life and obesity at 3 years of age, *Pediatrics* 123(4):1177-1183, 2009.

Thomas P, Peabody J, Turnier V, et al: A new look at intrauterine growth and the impact of race, altitude, and gender, *Pediatrics* 106(2):e21, 2000.

Tomlinson PS, Bryan AA, Esau AL: Family centered intrapartum care: revisiting an old concept, *J Obstet Gynecol Neonatal Nurs* 25(4):331-337, 1996.

Trochtenberg DS: Neonatal circumcision (letter to the editor), *N Engl J Med* 323(17):1206, 1990.

Trotter CW: Gestational age assessment. In Tappero EP, Honeyfield ME, editors: *Physical assessment of the newborn: a comprehensive approach to the art of physical examination*, ed 4, Santa Rosa, Calif, 2009, NICU Ink.

Tulassy T, Ramanathan R, Evans JR, et al: Renal vascular disease in the newborn. In Taeusch HW, Ballard RA, Gleason CA, editors: *Avery's diseases of the newborn*, ed 8, Philadelphia, 2005, Saunders.

US Department of Health and Human Services: Healthy people 2020 public meetings, Washington, DC, 2009, The Department, available at www.healthypeople.gov/hp2020/Objectives/ViewObjective.aspx?Id=177&TopicArea=Maternal%2c+Infant+and+Child+Health&Objective=MICH+HP2020%e2%80%9312&TopicAreaId=32 (accessed November 25, 2009).

Vandenplas Y: Oligosaccharides in infant formula, *Br J Nutr* 87(Suppl 2): S293-S296, 2002.

Varda KE, Behnke RS: The effect of timing the initial bath on newborn's temperature, *J Obstet Gynecol Neonatal Nurs* 29(1):27-32, 2000.

Wagner CL, Greer FR, American Academy of Pediatrics Section on Breastfeeding: Prevention of rickets and vitamin D deficiency in infants, children, and adolescents, *Pediatrics* 122(5):1142-1150, 2008.

Walker VP, Akinbi HT, Meinzen-Derr J, et al: Host defense proteins on the surface of neonatal skin: implications for innate immunity, *J Pediatrics* 152(6):777-781, 2008.

Warner L, Ghanem KG, Newman DR, et al: Male circumcision and risk of HIV infection among heterosexual African American men attending Baltimore sexually transmitted disease clinics, *J Infect Dis* 199(1):59-65, 2009.

Weise KL, Nahata MC: EMLA for painful procedures in infants, *J Pediatr Health Care* 19(1):42-47, 2005.

Weiss ME, Poeltler D, Gocka I: Infrared tympanic thermometry for neonatal temperature assessment, *J Obstet Gynecol Neonatal Nurs* 23(9):798-803, 1993.

Wiessinger D, Miller M: Breastfeeding difficulties as a result of tight lingual and labial frena: a case report, *J Hum Lact* 11(4):313-316, 1995.

Williamson ML: Circumcision anesthesia: a study of nursing implications for dorsal penile nerve block, *Pediatr Nurs* 23(10):59-63, 1997.

Wilshaw R, Beckstrand R, Waid D, et al: A comparison of the use tympanic, axillary, and rectal thermometers in infants, *J Pediatr Nurs* 14(2):88-93, 1999.

Wong D: Topical local anesthetics: two products for pain relief during minor procedures, *AJN* 103(6):42-45, 2003.

World Health Organization: WHO child growth standards, World Health Organization, Geneva, Switzerland, 2006, available at www.who.int/childgrowth/en (accessed July 2, 2009).

World Health Organization: *Eliminating female genital mutilation: an interagency statement*

UNAIDS, UNDP, UNECA, UNESCO, UNFPA, UNHCHR, UNHCR, UNICEF, UNIFEM, WHO, Geneva, 2008, The Organization.

Wright A, Rice S, Wells S: Changing hospital practices to increase the duration of breastfeeding, *Pediatrics* 97(5):669-676, 1996.

Wright JT: Normal formation and development defects of human dentition, *Pediatr Clin North Am* 47(5):975-1000, 2000.

Yamada J, Stinson J, Lamda J, et al: A review of systematic reviews on pain interventions in hospitalized infants, *Pain Res Manage* 13(5):413-420, 2008.

Yetman RJ, Coody DK, West MS, et al: Comparison of temperature measurements

by an aural infrared thermometer with measurements by traditional rectal and axillary techniques, *J Pediatr* 122(5):769-773, 1993.

Yoshinaga-Itano C, Sedey SL, Coulter DK, et al: Language of early- and late-identified children with hearing loss, *Pediatrics* 102(5):1161-1171, 1998.

Young TK, Martens PJ, Taback SP, et al: Type 2 diabetes mellitus in children: prenatal and early infancy risk factors among native Canadians, *Arch Pediatr Adolesc Med* 156(7):651-655, 2002.

Zupan J, Garner P, Omari AA: Topical umbilical cord care at birth, *Cochrane Database Syst Rev* (3):CD001057, 2004.

Health Problems of the Newborn

David Wilson

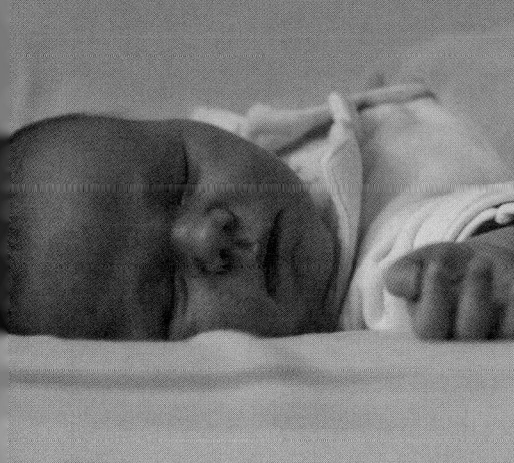

CHAPTER OUTLINE

▌BIRTH INJURIES

ⓔ Several factors predispose an infant to birth injuries. Maternal factors include uterine dysfunction that leads to prolonged or precipitous labor, preterm or postterm labor, and cephalopelvic disproportion. Injury may result from dystocia caused by fetal macrosomia, multifetal gestation, abnormal or difficult presentation (not caused by maternal uterine or pelvic conditions), and congenital anomalies. Intrapartum events that can result in scalp injury include the use of intrapartum monitoring of fetal heart rate and collection of fetal scalp blood for acid-base assessment. Obstetric birth techniques can cause injury. Forceps birth, vacuum extraction, version and extraction, and cesarean birth are potential contributory factors. Often more than one factor is present, and multiple predisposing factors may be related to a single maternal condition.

BOX 9-1	TYPES OF PHYSICAL INJURIES AT BIRTH

Soft Tissue Injury
Erythema
Abrasion
Petechiae
Ecchymoses
Subcutaneous fat necrosis
Subconjunctival (scleral) hemorrhage
Retinal hemorrhage
Hemorrhage into abdominal organ(s)

Head Injury
Caput succedaneum
Subgaleal hemorrhage
Cephalhematoma
Fracture (depressed or linear)
Intracranial hemorrhage

Neurologic Injury
Subdural or epidural hematoma
Facial paralysis
Brachial palsy (Erb-Duchenne paralysis, Klumpke palsy)
Phrenic nerve palsy (diaphragmatic paralysis)
Spinal cord injury

BOX 9-2	COMMON TYPES OF SOFT TISSUE INJURY

Erythema and abrasions—Usually the result of the application of forceps; discoloration the same configuration as the instrument
Petechiae—Nonraised, pinpoint hemorrhages caused by a sudden increase and then release of pressure during passage through the birth canal; may be seen on the chest, face, and head
Ecchymoses—Small hemorrhagic areas (larger than petechiae) that may occur after traumatic, precipitous, or breech delivery
Subcutaneous fat necrosis—Clearly outlined masses located in the subcutaneous tissues that are firm to the overlying skin but movable over the underlying tissue; most likely caused by traumatic manipulation during delivery
Subconjunctival (scleral) hemorrhages—The result of rupture of capillaries in the sclera from pressure on the fetal head during delivery; most commonly located in the limbus of the iris
Retinal hemorrhages—Flame-shaped, irregular, or round areas of bleeding in the retina from excessive pressure on the fetal head during delivery; extensive areas possibly indicative of subdural hematoma or brain trauma

Many injuries are minor and resolve spontaneously in a few days; others, although minor, require some degree of intervention. Still others can be serious or even fatal. Part of the nurse's responsibility is to identify such injuries so that appropriate interventions can be initiated as soon as possible. Birth injuries are classified according to the type of body structure involved (Box 9-1).

SOFT TISSUE INJURY

Infants may sustain various types of soft tissue injury during birth, primarily in the form of bruises and abrasions secondary to dystocia. Soft tissue injury usually occurs when there is some degree of disproportion between the presenting part and the maternal pelvis (**cephalopelvic disproportion**). Box 9-2 lists common types of soft tissue injury. The use of forceps to facilitate a difficult vertex delivery may produce discoloration or abrasions with the same configuration as the forceps on the sides of the neonate's face. Petechiae or ecchymoses may be observed on the presenting part after a breech or brow delivery. After a difficult or precipitous delivery, the sudden release of pressure on the head can produce scleral hemorrhages or generalized petechiae over the face and head. Petechiae and ecchymoses may also appear on the head, neck, and face of an infant born with a **nuchal cord**, giving the infant's face a cyanotic appearance. A well-defined circle of petechiae and ecchymoses may also appear on the occipital region of the newborn's head when a vacuum suction cup is applied during delivery. Rarely, lacerations occur during cesarean section.

These traumatic lesions generally fade spontaneously and without treatment within a few days. However, petechiae may be a manifestation of an underlying bleeding disorder and are evaluated.

Nursing Care Management

Nursing care is directed primarily toward assessing the injury, maintaining asepsis of the area to prevent breakdown and infection, and providing an explanation and reassurance to the parents. The nurse records an accurate description of the injury (e.g., extent of petechiae) to facilitate subsequent comparative nursing evaluations.

Regardless of how benign the injury, parents may be concerned and mourn the loss of the expected "perfect" infant. Explanations of the cause and treatment, if any, need to be thorough and repeated frequently. If the injury is temporarily disfiguring, such as extensive facial bruising, nurses can demonstrate acceptance of the child through their example of sensitive, personal care.

HEAD TRAUMA

Head trauma that occurs during the birth process is usually benign but occasionally results in more serious injury. The injuries that produce serious trauma, such as intracranial hemorrhage and subdural hematoma, are discussed in relation to neurologic disorders in the newborn. (See Chapters 10 and 37.) Skull fractures are discussed with other fractures sustained during the birth process. The three most common types of extracranial hemorrhagic injury are caput succedaneum, subgaleal hemorrhage, and cephalhematoma.

Caput Succedaneum

The most commonly observed scalp lesion is **caput succedaneum**, a vaguely outlined area of edematous tissue situated over the portion of the scalp that presents in a vertex delivery (Fig. 9-1, *A*). The swelling consists of serum and/or blood that has accumulated in the tissues above the bone. Typically the swelling extends beyond the bone margins (or sutures) and may be associated with overlying petechiae or ecchymosis. It is present at or shortly after birth. No specific treatment is necessary, and the swelling subsides within a few days.

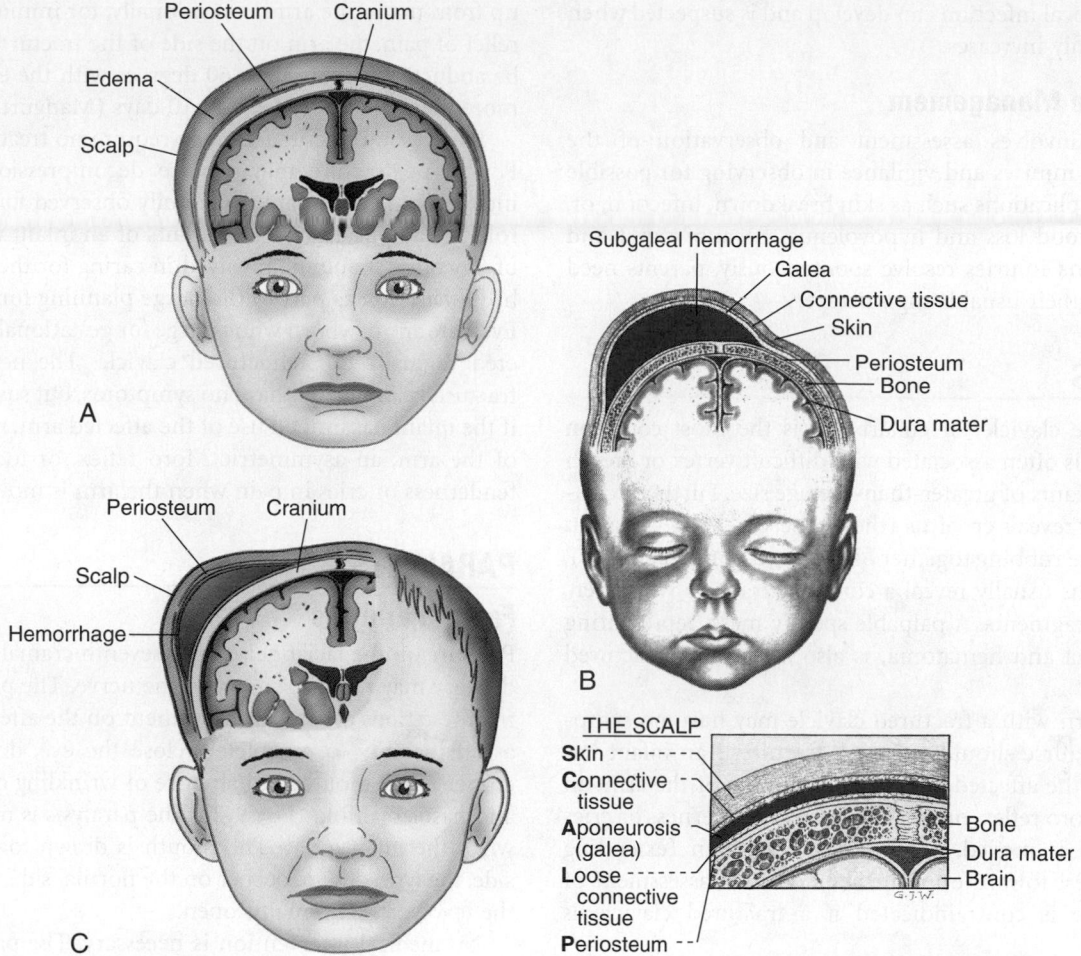

Fig. 9-1 A, Caput succedaneum. **B,** Subgaleal hemorrhage. **C,** Cephalhematoma. (**A** and **C,** From Seidel HM, Ball JW, Dains JE, et al: *Mosby's guide to physical examination,* ed 6, St Louis, 2006, Mosby.)

Subgaleal Hemorrhage

Subgaleal hemorrhage is bleeding into the subgaleal compartment (Fig. 9-1, *B*). The subgaleal compartment is a potential space that contains loosely arranged connective tissue. It is located beneath the galea aponeurosis, the tendinous sheath that connects the frontal and occipital muscles and forms the inner surface of the scalp. The injury occurs as a result of forces that compress and then drag the head through the pelvic outlet. The bleeding extends beyond bone, often posterior into the neck, and continues after birth, with the potential for serious complications and morbidity.

Early detection of the hemorrhage is vital; serial head circumference measurements and inspection of the back of the neck for increasing edema and a firm mass are essential. A boggy fluctuant mass over the scalp that crosses the suture line and moves as the baby is repositioned is an early sign of subgaleal hemorrhage (Doumouchtsis and Arulkumaran, 2006). Other signs include pallor, tachycardia, a forward and lateral positioning of the newborn's ears as the hematoma extends posteriorly, and increasing head circumference (Mangurten, 2006). Computed tomography (CT) or magnetic resonance imaging is useful in confirming the diagnosis. Replacement of lost blood and clotting factors is required in acute cases of

hemorrhage. Monitoring the infant for changes in level of consciousness and a decrease in the hematocrit is also key to early recognition and management. An increase in serum bilirubin levels may occur as a result of the degrading blood cells within the hematoma.

Cephalhematoma

A cephalhematoma forms when blood vessels rupture during labor or delivery to produce bleeding into the area between the bone and its periosteum. The injury occurs most often with primiparous women and is often associated with forceps delivery and vacuum extraction. Unlike caput succedaneum, the boundaries of the cephalhematoma are distinguishable and do not extend beyond the limits of the bone (Fig. 9-1, *C*). The cephalhematoma may involve one or both parietal bones but rarely affects the occipital and frontal bones. The swelling is usually minimum or absent at birth and increases in size on the second or third day. Blood loss is usually not significant.

No treatment is indicated for uncomplicated cephalhematoma. Most lesions are absorbed within 2 weeks to 3 months. Lesions that result in severe blood loss to the area or that involve an underlying fracture require further evaluation. Hyperbilirubinemia may result during resolution of the hematoma. A local infection can develop and is suspected when swelling suddenly increases.

Nursing Care Management

Nursing care involves assessment and observation of the common scalp injuries and vigilance in observing for possible associated complications such as skin breakdown, infection, or, rarely, acute blood loss and hypovolemia. Because caput and cephalhematoma injuries resolve spontaneously, parents need reassurance of their usual benign nature.

FRACTURES

Fracture of the clavicle, or collarbone, is the most common birth injury. It is often associated with difficult vertex or breech deliveries of infants of greater-than-average size. Further examination usually reveals crepitus (the coarse, crackling sensation produced by the rubbing together of fractured bone fragments), and radiographs usually reveal a complete fracture with overriding of the fragments. A palpable spongy mass, representing localized edema and hematoma, is also a sign of a fractured clavicle.

The newborn with a fractured clavicle may have no symptoms, but the nurse should suspect a fracture if an infant has limited use of the affected arm, malpositioning of the arm, an asymmetric Moro reflex, or focal swelling or tenderness or cries when the arm is moved. Eliciting the scarf sign (extending arm across chest toward opposite shoulder) for assessment of gestational age is contraindicated if a fractured clavicle is suspected.

In neonates, fractures of long bones, such as the femur or the humerus, are difficult to detect by radiographic examination. Although osteogenesis imperfecta is a rare finding, assess a newborn infant with a fracture for other evidence of this congenital disorder.

Fractures of the neonatal skull are uncommon. The bones, which are less mineralized and more compressible than bones in older infants and children, are separated by membranous seams that allow the head contour to adjust to the birth canal during delivery. Skull fractures usually follow a prolonged, difficult delivery or forceps extraction. Most fractures are linear, but some may be visible as depressed indentations that compress or decompress like a Ping-Pong ball. Management of depressed skull fractures is controversial; many resolve without intervention. Nonsurgical elevation of the indentation using a hand breast pump or vacuum extractor has been reported (Mangurten, 2006). Surgery may be required in the presence of bone fragments or signs of increased intracranial pressure. A similar finding in neonates is craniotabes, which is usually benign or may be associated with prematurity, rickets, or hydrocephalus. In this condition the cranial bone(s) moves freely on palpation and may be easily compressed.

Nursing Care Management

Often no intervention is prescribed other than proper body alignment, careful dressing and undressing of the infant, and handling and carrying techniques that support the affected bone. If the infant has a fractured clavicle, it is important to support the upper and lower back rather than pull the infant

up from under the arms. Occasionally, for immobilization and relief of pain, the arm on the side of the fractured clavicle may be abducted at more than 60 degrees with the elbow flexed at more than 90 degrees for 7 to 10 days (Mangurten, 2006).

Linear skull fractures usually require no treatment. A Ping-Pong–type fracture may require decompression by surgical intervention. The infant is carefully observed for signs of neurologic complications. The parents of an infant with a fracture of any bone should be involved in caring for the infant during hospitalization as part of discharge planning for care at home. Evaluate any newborn who is large for gestational age and delivered vaginally for a fractured clavicle. The newborn with a fractured clavicle may have no symptoms, but suspect a fracture if the infant has limited use of the affected arm, malpositioning of the arm, an asymmetric Moro reflex, or focal swelling or tenderness or cries in pain when the arm is moved.

PARALYSES

Facial Paralysis

Pressure on the facial nerve (the seventh cranial nerve) during delivery may result in injury to the nerve. The primary clinical manifestations are loss of movement on the affected side, such as an inability to completely close the eye, drooping of the corner of the mouth, and absence of wrinkling of the forehead and nasolabial fold (Fig. 9-2). The paralysis is most noticeable when the infant cries. The mouth is drawn to the unaffected side, the wrinkles are deeper on the normal side, and the eye on the involved side remains open.

No medical intervention is necessary. The paralysis usually disappears spontaneously in a few days but may take as long as several months.

Brachial Palsy

Brachial plexus injury results from forces that alter the normal position and relationship of the arm, shoulder, and

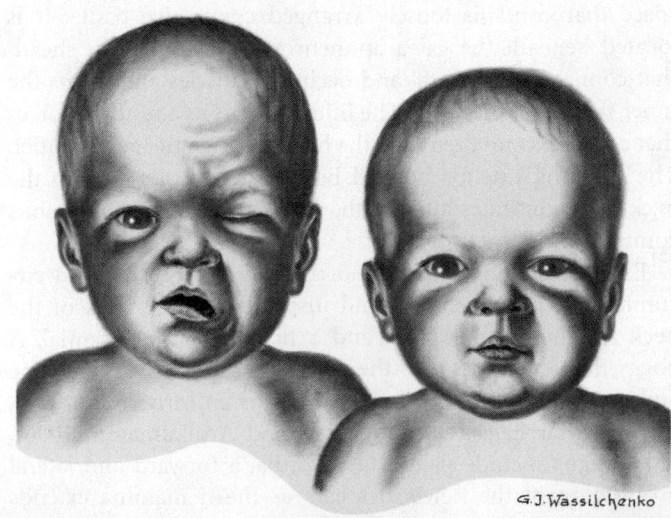

Fig. 9-2 A, Paralysis of right side of face 15 minutes after forceps delivery. Absence of movement on affected side is especially noticeable when infant cries. **B,** Same infant 24 hours later.

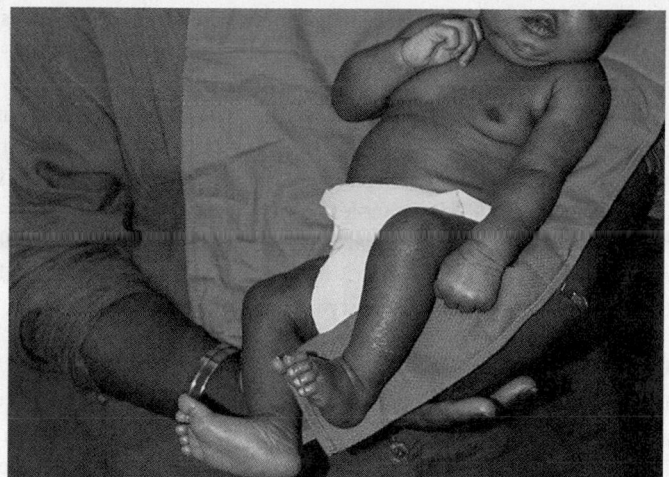

Fig. 9-3 Left-sided brachial plexus (Erb-Duchenne) palsy. Note extended, internally rotated arm and pronated wrist on affected side.

neck. **Erb palsy** (Erb-Duchenne paralysis) is caused by damage to the upper plexus and usually results from stretching or pulling away of the shoulder from the head, as might occur with shoulder dystocia or with a difficult vertex or breech delivery. Other identified risk factors include an infant with birth weight of over 4000 g (8.8 lb), a second stage of labor of less than 15 minutes, maternal body mass index greater than 29, and a vacuum-assisted extraction (Hudic, Fatusic, Sinanovic, et al, 2006). The less common lower plexus palsy, or Klumpke palsy, results from severe stretching of the upper extremity while the trunk is relatively less mobile.

The clinical manifestations of Erb palsy are related to the paralysis of the affected upper extremity and muscles. The arm hangs limp alongside the body. The shoulder and arm are adducted and internally rotated. The elbow is extended, and the forearm is pronated, with the wrist and fingers flexed; a grasp reflex may be present because finger and wrist movement remain normal, but the Moro reflex is absent (Tappero, 2009) (Fig. 9-3). In lower plexus palsy the muscles of the hand are paralyzed, with consequent wrist drop and relaxed fingers. In a third and more severe form of brachial palsy, total plexus injury, the entire arm and hand are paralyzed and hang limp and motionless at the side. The Moro reflex is absent on the affected side for all forms of brachial palsy.

Treatment of the affected arm is aimed at preventing contractures of the paralyzed muscles and maintaining correct placement of the humeral head within the glenoid fossa of the scapula. Complete recovery from stretched nerves usually takes 3 to 6 months. Full recovery is expected in 88% to 92% of infants (Paige and Moe, 2006). However, avulsion of the nerves (complete disconnection of the ganglia from the spinal cord that involves both anterior and posterior roots) results in permanent damage. For those injuries that do not improve spontaneously by 3 months, surgical intervention may be needed to relieve pressure on the nerves or to repair the nerves with grafting (Joyner, Soto, and Adam, 2006). In some cases injection of botulinum toxin A into the pectoralis major muscle may be effective in reducing muscle contractures after birth-related brachial plexus injuries (Price, Ditaranto, Yaylali, et al, 2007).

Phrenic Nerve Paralysis

Phrenic nerve paralysis results in diaphragmatic paralysis as demonstrated by ultrasonography, which shows paradoxic chest movement and an elevated diaphragm. Initially, chest radiography may not demonstrate an elevated diaphragm if the neonate is receiving positive pressure ventilation. The injury sometimes occurs in conjunction with brachial palsy. Respiratory distress is the most common and important sign of injury. Because injury to the phrenic nerve is usually unilateral, the lung on the affected side does not expand and respiratory efforts are ineffectual. Breathing is primarily thoracic, and cyanosis, tachypnea, or complete respiratory failure may be seen. Pneumonia and atelectasis on the affected side may also occur.

Nursing Care Management

Nursing care of the infant with facial nerve paralysis involves aiding the infant in sucking and helping the mother with feeding techniques. A comprehensive evaluation of the infant's oral motor skills by an infant feeding specialist is recommended to develop an effective multidisciplinary feeding regimen. Because part of the mouth cannot close tightly around the nipple, the use of a soft rubber nipple with a large hole may be helpful but should be used carefully to prevent choking. The infant may require partial gavage feeding and supplemental oral stimulation with a minimum amount of formula to prevent aspiration. Breast-feeding is not contraindicated, but the mother will need assistance in helping the infant grasp and compress the areolar area.

If the lid of the eye on the affected side does not close completely, instill artificial tears as needed to prevent drying of the conjunctiva, sclera, and cornea. The lid is often taped shut to prevent injury. If the infant requires eye care at home, teach the parents the procedure for administering eye drops before the infant is discharged from the nursery. (See Chapter 27.)

Nursing care of the newborn with brachial palsy is concerned primarily with proper positioning of the affected arm. The affected arm should be gently immobilized on the upper abdomen; passive range-of-motion exercises of the shoulder, wrist, elbow, and fingers are initiated at 7 to 10 days of age (Joyner, Soto, and Adam, 2006). Wrist flexion contractures may be prevented with the use of supportive splints. In dressing the infant, give preference to the affected arm. Undressing begins with the unaffected arm, and redressing begins with the affected arm to prevent unnecessary manipulation and stress on the paralyzed muscles. Teach parents to use the "football" position when holding the infant and to avoid picking the child up from under the axillae or by pulling on the arms.

The infant with phrenic nerve paralysis requires the same nursing care as any infant with respiratory distress. The family's emotional needs are also an important part of nursing care; the family needs reassurance regarding the neonate's progress toward an optimal outcome. Follow-up care is also essential because of the extended length of recovery. Parents may wish to contact the Brachial Plexus Palsy Foundation and visit the website for further information.*

*210 Spring Haven Circle, Royersford, PA 19468; www.brachialplexuspalsyfoundation.org.

Animation—Paralyzed Diaphragm

DERMATOLOGIC PROBLEMS IN THE NEWBORN

ERYTHEMA TOXICUM NEONATORUM

Erythema toxicum neonatorum, also known as *flea bite dermatitis* or *newborn rash,* is a benign, self-limiting eruption that usually appears within the first 2 days of life. The 1- to 3-mm lesions are firm, pale yellow or white papules or pustules on an erythematous base, which resemble flea bites. Erythema toxicum may appear as one or two isolated "flea bites" or as multiple lesions; the rash commonly disappears from one location and reappears elsewhere hours later. The rash appears most commonly on the face, proximal extremities, trunk, and buttocks, but it may be located anywhere on the body except the palms and soles. The rash may be more obvious during crying episodes. There are no systemic manifestations, and successive crops of lesions heal without pigmentation changes. The rash usually lasts approximately 5 to 7 days.

The cause is unknown. However, a smear of the pustule shows numerous eosinophils and a relative absence of neutrophils. Obtain bacterial, fungal, or viral cultures when the diagnosis is questionable. Although no treatment is necessary, parents are usually concerned about the rash and need to be reassured of its benign and transient nature.

CANDIDIASIS

Candidiasis, also known as moniliasis, is not uncommon in the newborn. *Candida albicans,* the organism usually responsible, may cause disease in any organ system. It is a yeastlike fungus (produces yeast cells and spores) that can be acquired from a maternal vaginal infection during delivery; by person-to-person transmission (especially from poor hand-washing technique); or from contaminated hands, bottles, nipples, or other articles. Mucocutaneous, cutaneous, and disseminated candidiasis are observed in this age-group. It is usually a benign disorder in the neonate and is often confined to the oral and diaper regions. (See Diaper Dermatitis, Chapter 13.)

Oral candidiasis (thrush) is characterized by white adherent patches on the tongue, palate, and inner aspects of the cheeks. Oral candidiasis can be distinguished from coagulated milk when attempts to remove the patches with a tongue blade are unsuccessful. The infant may refuse to suck or may feed poorly because of pain in the mouth. This condition tends to be acute in the newborn (rarely appears in first week of life) and chronic in older infants and young children. Thrush appears when the oral flora is altered as a result of antibiotic therapy or poor hand washing by the infant's caregiver. Although the disorder is usually self-limiting, spontaneous resolution may take as long as 2 months, during which time lesions may spread to the larynx, trachea, bronchi, and lungs and along the gastrointestinal tract.

The disease is treated with good hygiene, application of a fungicide, and correction of any underlying disturbance. The source of infection, usually the mother, should be treated to prevent reinfection. Topical application of 1 ml of nystatin (Mycostatin) over the surfaces of the oral cavity four times a day or every 6 hours is usually sufficient to prevent spread of the disease or prolongation of its course. Several other drugs may be used, including amphotericin B (Fungizone), clotrimazole (Lotrimin, Mycelex), fluconazole (Diflucan), or miconazole (Monistat, Micatin) given intravenously, orally, or topically. To prevent relapse, therapy should be continued for at least 2 days after the lesions disappear (Lawrence and Lawrence, 2005). Gentian violet solution may be used in addition to one of the antifungal drugs in chronic cases of oral thrush; however, the former does not treat gastrointestinal *Candida* organisms and may irritate the oral mucosa.

Nursing Care Management

Direct nursing care toward preventing spread of the infection and correct application of the prescribed topical medication. For candidiasis in the diaper area, teach the caregiver to keep the diaper area clean and to apply the medication to affected areas as prescribed. (See Diaper Dermatitis, Chapter 13.) Older infants can introduce *Candida* organisms into their mouths with hands contaminated by contact with diaper dermatitis.

In cases of oral thrush, administer nystatin after feedings. Distribute the medication over the surface of the oral mucosa and tongue with an applicator or syringe; the remainder of the dose is deposited in the mouth to be swallowed by the infant to treat any gastrointestinal lesions. In addition to good hygienic care, other measures to control thrush include rinsing the infant's mouth with plain water after each feeding before applying the medication and boiling reusable nipples and bottles for at least 20 minutes after a thorough washing (spores are heat resistant). Boil pacifiers for at least 20 minutes once daily, and treat the nipples of breast-feeding mothers to prevent reinfection. If the mother is breast-feeding, simultaneous treatment of the infant and mother is recommended if either is infected (Lawrence and Lawrence, 2005).

HERPES

Neonatal herpes is one of the most serious viral infections in the newborn, with a mortality rate of up to 60% in infants with disseminated disease. The disease may be classified according to the following types: (1) skin, eye, and mouth; (2) localized central nervous system (CNS) disease; or (3) disseminated infection involving multiple sites such as the lungs, liver, adrenal glands, CNS, skin, eyes, and mouth. Approximately 86% to 90% of herpes simplex virus (HSV) transmission occurs during delivery. The rash appears as vesicles or pustules on an erythematous base. Clusters of lesions are common. The lesions ulcerate and crust over rapidly. Fetal scalp monitoring sites are commonly the primary site of infection. The risk of infection during vaginal birth in the presence of genital herpes is estimated to be as high as 57% with active primary infection at term (Brown, Wald, Morrow, et al, 2003). However, in up to 80% of cases of neonatal HSV infection, the mother has no history or symptoms of infection at the time of birth, but serologic testing reveals evidence of the herpes virus (Kimberlin, 2005).

Most infants with neonatal herpes eventually develop this characteristic rash, but up to 20% of neonates with disseminated disease do not develop a skin rash (Kimberlin, 2007). Ophthalmologic clinical findings include chorioretinitis and microphthalmia; neurologic involvement such as microcephaly and encephalomalacia may also develop (Kimberlin, 2007). Disseminated infections may involve virtually every organ system, but the liver, adrenal glands, and lungs are most commonly affected. In HSV meningitis infants develop multiple lesions of cortical hemorrhagic necrosis. It can occur alone or with oral, eye, or skin lesions. The presenting symptoms, which may occur in the second to fourth week of life, include lethargy, poor feeding, irritability, and local or generalized seizures.

Infants with CNS and disseminated disease have a much higher mortality rate than those initially seen with skin, eye, or mouth disease. Neonatal HSV may be difficult to detect in the early newborn period, and nonspecific signs such as irritability, fever, poor feeding, or lethargy may be seen. When the diagnosis is delayed, mortality may be high even with antiviral therapy, and long-term irreversible complications such as seizures, blindness, and psychomotor and learning delays are not uncommon.

Nursing Care Management

Neonates with herpes virus or suspected infection (as a result of exposure) should be carefully evaluated for clinical manifestations. The absence of skin lesions in the neonate exposed to maternal herpes virus does not indicate absence of disease. Institute Contact Precautions (in addition to Standard Precautions) according to American Academy of Pediatrics and American College of Obstetricians and Gynecologists (2007) guidelines or hospital protocol. It is recommended that swabs of the mouth, nasopharynx, conjunctivae, rectum, and any skin vesicles be obtained from the exposed neonate. In addition, obtain urine, stool, blood, and cerebrospinal fluid specimens for culture. Antiviral therapy with acyclovir is initiated if the cultures are positive or if there is strong suspicion of herpes infection (American Academy of Pediatrics, 2009b).

Early recognition and treatment with antiviral therapy are key to the prevention of serious and often fatal complications. Closely evaluate for the disease infants who are seen in the first 5 or 6 weeks of life with the nonspecific signs of poor feeding, lethargy, fever, and irritability, with or without the characteristic rash.

BULLOUS IMPETIGO

Bullous impetigo is an infectious superficial skin condition most often caused by various strains of *Staphylococcus aureus*. Bullous vesicular lesions erupt on previously untraumatized or intact skin. The lesions may appear on any body surface and sometimes become widespread, but the usual distribution involves the buttocks, perineum, trunk, face, and extremities. The neonatal form may appear first in the diaper region (Morelli, 2007). They vary in size from a few millimeters to several centimeters, contain turbid fluid, and are easily ruptured (Morelli, 2007). The bullae rupture in 1 or 2 days, leaving a superficial red, moist, denuded area with little crusting. In some cases the condition may be mistaken for thermal injury or staphylococcal scalded skin syndrome (SSSS). Bullous impetigo lesions develop on intact skin, whereas lesions of SSSS spread systemically from an original infection site. There is no cutaneous sensitivity with bullous impetigo, and the Gram stain and blister cultures are positive for staphylococci.

Treatment usually involves the administration of oral antibiotics and topical application of mupirocin (Bactroban). Systemic treatment with erythromycin may be required if the lesions are near the mouth or in the event of abscess formation. Recovery is usually rapid and uneventful.

Nursing Care Management

Once the diagnosis is suspected, the infant is isolated until therapy is instituted to prevent spread of the infection to other infants. Persons who have come in contact with the infant are investigated to determine a possible source of the infecting organism. Scrutinize other infants who have mutual contacts for early detection of any infection. Instruct parents and other visitors regarding precautions for the prevention of infection, especially through hand washing and Standard Precautions. (See Infection Control, Chapter 27.)

To prevent older infants from scratching the lesions, the arms may need to be confined by using elbow restraints, by pulling the undershirt sleeves over the hands and securing the openings with tape, or by applying mittens. If restraints of any kind are used, the infant is allowed freedom of movement at supervised times. Rocking, cuddling, and holding during feeding are essential components of care.

BIRTHMARKS

Discolorations of the skin are common findings in the newborn infant. (See discussion on skin assessment under Physical Assessment, Chapter 8.) Most, such as mongolian spots or telangiectatic nevi, involve no therapy other than reassuring parents of the benign nature of these discolorations. However, some can be the manifestation of a disease that suggests further examination of the child and other family members (e.g., multiple flat, light brown café-au-lait spots often characterize the autosomal dominant hereditary disorder neurofibromatosis and are common findings in Albright syndrome).

Darker or more extensive lesions demand further inspection. Excision of the lesion is recommended when feasible or for biopsy. Such lesions include the reddish brown solitary nodule that appears on the face or upper arm and usually represents a spindle and epithelioid cell nevus (juvenile melanoma); a giant pigmented nevus (bathing trunk nevus), a dark brown to black irregular plaque that is at risk of transformation to malignant melanoma; and the dark brown or black macules that become more numerous with age (junctional or compound nevi).

Vascular birthmarks may be divided into vascular malformations and vascular tumors (hemangiomas). Experts now recommend labeling vascular tumors as **hemangiomas of infancy** or **infantile hemangiomas** to differentiate them from other vascular tumors and malformations. Hemangiomas may be further classified as localized, segmental, or multifocal (Miller and Frieden, 2005). Localized superficial hemangiomas tend to appear early in infancy and spontaneously resolve without therapy within several years, whereas the segmental variety is more likely to cause complications such as ulceration and vital organ compromise and to involve developmental defects. Multifocal hemangiomas are less likely to be associated with the complications seen with the segmental variety (Miller

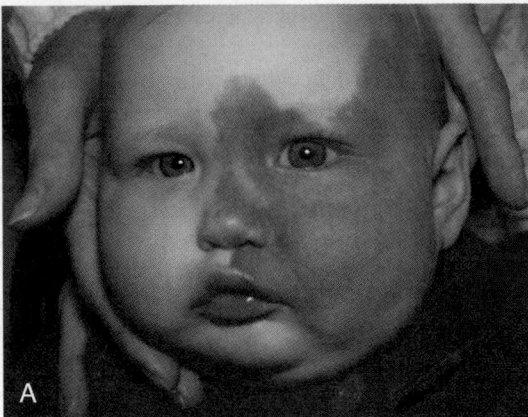 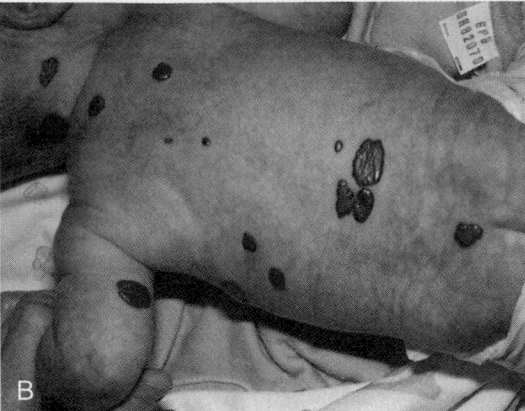

Fig. 9-4 A, Port-wine stain. **B,** Strawberry hemangioma. (From Zitelli BJ, Davis HW: *Atlas of pediatric physical diagnosis,* ed 4, St Louis, 2002, Mosby.)

and Frieden, 2005). This discussion focuses only on the more common hemangiomas of infancy.

Vascular stains (malformations) are permanent lesions that are present at birth and are initially flat and erythematous. Any vascular structure—capillary, vein, artery, or lymphatic—may be involved. The two most common vascular stains are port-wine stains (nevus flammeus) and transient macular stains such as the stork bite or salmon patch, usually located on the glabella or nape of the neck. Port-wine lesions are pink, red, or, rarely, purple stains of the skin that thicken, darken, and proportionately enlarge as the child grows (Fig. 9-4, *A*).

Port-wine stains may also be associated with structural malformations, such as glaucoma or leptomeningeal angiomatosis (tumor of blood or lymph vessels in the pia arachnoid, or Sturge-Weber syndrome) or bony or muscular overgrowth (Klippel-Trénaunay-Weber syndrome). Monitor children with port-wine stains on the eyelids, forehead, cheeks, or extremities for these syndromes with periodic ophthalmologic examination, neurologic imaging, and measurement of extremities.

The treatment of choice for port-wine stains is the flashlamp pulsed dye laser. The child's skin is reported to respond to therapy and have fewer side effects than in adults (Stier, Glick, and Hirsch, 2008). A series of treatments is usually needed (see Atraumatic Care box). The treatments can significantly lighten or completely clear the lesions with almost no scarring or pigment change.

ATRAUMATIC CARE

Laser Therapy

The laser pulse feels like the sharp snap of a rubber band on the skin, and each treatment may involve from 15 to 100 pulses. Therefore children should be given a general anesthetic, sedation, or a topical anesthetic, such as EMLA (eutectic mixture of local anesthetics [prilocaine 2.5% and lidocaine 2.5%]) or LMX4 (4% liposomal prilocaine).

Infantile hemangiomas, also sometimes referred to as strawberry or capillary hemangiomas, are benign cutaneous tumors that involve only capillaries. These are often not apparent at birth but may appear within a few weeks as an erythematous patch, enlarge considerably during the first year of life and then begin to involute spontaneously. It may take 5 to 12 years for complete resolution. As many as 50% of patients may be left with residual findings such as telangiectasia, redundant fatty tissue, or skin atrophy (Alster and Railan, 2006). These hemangiomas are bright red, rubbery nodules with a rough surface and a well-defined margin (Fig. 9-4, *B*). A relationship has been established between infantile hemangiomas and placental tissue (Metry, 2004). One study demonstrated that low birth weight was the most significant risk factor for infantile hemangioma (Drolet, Swanson, Frieden, et al, 2008).

Cavernous venous hemangiomas involve deeper vessels in the dermis and have a bluish red color and poorly defined margins. These latter forms may be associated with the trapping of platelets (Kasabach-Merritt syndrome) and subsequent thrombocytopenia.

Hemangiomas may also occur as part of the PHACE syndrome:

P—Posterior fossa brain malformation

H—Hemangiomas (segmental cervicofacial)

A—Arterial anomalies

C—Cardiac defects, including coarctation of the aorta

E—Eye anomalies

Most cavernous venous hemangiomas are large defects and are located on the face (Miller and Frieden, 2005). This neurocutaneous syndrome is diagnosed by the presence of a facial hemangioma in addition to either one or several of the other associated conditions; clinical outcomes vary according to the organs involved.

Although many localized superficial hemangiomas require no treatment because of their high rate of spontaneous involution, some vision and airway obstruction may necessitate therapy. Ulceration is a common complication, especially when the hemangioma is perineal or perioral. This may result in pain, bleeding, infection, and scarring. The pulsed dye laser can effectively reduce some hemangiomas; systemic prednisone administered for 2 to 3 weeks or longer may also deter further growth. Optional treatments may include interferon alfa, imiquimod, vincristine, bleomycin, cyclophosphamide, becaplermin, debulking surgery, and no treatment (Pandey, Gangopadhyay, and Upadhyay, 2008; Stier, Glick, and Hirsch, 2008).

Nursing Care Management

Birthmarks, especially those on the face, are upsetting to parents. Families need an explanation of the type of lesion, its significance, and possible treatment.* They can benefit from seeing photographs of other infants before and after treatment for port-wine stains or after the passage of time for hemangiomas. Pictures taken to follow the involution process may further help parents gain confidence that progress is taking place.

If laser therapy is performed, the lesion will have a purplish black appearance for 7 to 10 days, after which the blackness will fade and give way to redness with an eventual lightening of the treated area. During the treatment phase caution parents to avoid any trauma to the lesion or picking at the scab. Trim the infant's fingernails as an added precaution. Washing the area gently with water and dabbing it dry is adequate, although in some cases a topical antibiotic ointment may be used. Do not give any salicylates during the treatment phase because they decrease the effects of the therapy. Keep the infant out of the sun for several weeks and then protected with a sunscreen of at least SPF 15. Complications associated with laser treatment include possible secondary infection, keloid or pyogenic granuloma formation, localized dermatitis, and hyperpigmentation or hypopigmentation.

PROBLEMS RELATED TO PHYSIOLOGIC FACTORS

HYPERBILIRUBINEMIA

The term **hyperbilirubinemia** refers to an excessive level of accumulated bilirubin in the blood and is characterized by **jaundice**, or **icterus**, a yellowish discoloration of the skin and other organs. Hyperbilirubinemia is a common finding in the newborn and in most instances is relatively benign. However, in extreme cases, it can indicate a pathologic state.

Hyperbilirubinemia may result from increased unconjugated or conjugated bilirubin. The unconjugated form (Table 9-1) is the type most commonly seen in newborns. The following discussion of hyperbilirubinemia is limited to unconjugated hyperbilirubinemia.

Pathophysiology

Bilirubin is one of the breakdown products of hemoglobin that results from red blood cell (RBC) destruction. When RBCs are destroyed, the breakdown products are released into the circulation, where the hemoglobin splits into two fractions: heme and globin. The globin (protein) portion is used by the body, and the heme portion is converted to unconjugated bilirubin, an insoluble substance bound to albumin.

In the liver the bilirubin is detached from the albumin molecule and, in the presence of the enzyme glucuronyl transferase, is conjugated with glucuronic acid to produce a highly soluble substance, conjugated bilirubin glucuronide, which is then excreted into the bile. In the intestine, bacterial action reduces the conjugated bilirubin to urobilinogen, the pigment that gives stool its characteristic color. Most of the reduced bilirubin is excreted through the feces; a small amount is eliminated in the urine (Fig. 9-5).

Normally the body is able to maintain a balance between the destruction of RBCs and the use or excretion of by-products. However, when developmental limitations or a pathologic process interferes with this balance, bilirubin accumulates in the tissues to produce jaundice. Possible causes of hyperbilirubinemia in the newborn are:

- Physiologic (developmental) factors (prematurity)
- An association with breast-feeding or breast milk
- Excess production of bilirubin (e.g., hemolytic disease, biochemical defects, bruises)
- Disturbed capacity of the liver to secrete conjugated bilirubin (e.g., enzyme deficiency, bile duct obstruction)
- Combined overproduction and underexcretion (increased hemolytic process)
- Some conditions or disease states (e.g., glucose-6-phosphate dehydrogenase [G6PD] deficiency, hypothyroidism, galactosemia, infant of a diabetic mother)
- Genetic predisposition to increased production (Native Americans, Asians)

The first two causes, physiologic factors and an association with breast-feeding, are discussed in the following sections; the third major cause, hemolytic disease, is presented on p. 295.

Complications

Unconjugated bilirubin is highly toxic to neurons; therefore an infant with severe hyperbilirubinemia is at risk of developing **bilirubin encephalopathy**, a term that describes varying degrees of CNS damage resulting from the deposition of unconjugated bilirubin in brain cells. **Kernicterus** describes the yellow staining of the brain cells that may result in bilirubin encephalopathy. The damage occurs when the serum concentration reaches toxic levels, regardless of cause. There is evidence that a fraction of unconjugated bilirubin crosses the blood-brain barrier in neonates with physiologic hyperbilirubinemia. When certain pathologic conditions exist in addition to elevated bilirubin levels, the infant has an increased permeability of the blood-brain barrier to unconjugated bilirubin and, thus, potential irreversible damage. The exact level of serum bilirubin required to cause damage is not yet known.

Multiple factors contribute to bilirubin neurotoxicity; therefore serum bilirubin levels alone do not predict the risk of CNS injury. Factors that enhance the development of bilirubin encephalopathy include acidosis, lowered serum albumin levels, intracranial infections such as meningitis, and abrupt fluctuations in blood pressure. In addition, any condition that increases the metabolic demands for oxygen or glucose (e.g., fetal distress, hypoxia, hypothermia, or hypoglycemia) also increases the risk of CNS damage despite lower serum levels of bilirubin. The administration of hypertonic solutions such as glucose and sodium bicarbonate in acutely ill infants, which causes a sudden rise in serum osmolality, has also been a contributing factor in the development of bilirubin encephalopathy.

*Information is available from Birthmarks and Hemangiomas InterNETwork Support Group, http://members.tripod.com/~Michelle_G/SPTGP.html; and Vascular Birthmarks Foundation, 877-VBF-4646; www.birthmark.org.

TABLE 9-1   COMPARISON OF MAJOR TYPES OF UNCONJUGATED HYPERBILIRUBINEMIA*

PHYSIOLOGIC JAUNDICE	BREAST-FEEDING–ASSOCIATED JAUNDICE (EARLY ONSET)	BREAST MILK JAUNDICE (LATE ONSET)	HEMOLYTIC DISEASE
Cause			
Immature hepatic function plus increased bilirubin load from red blood cell (RBC) hemolysis	Decreased milk intake related to fewer calories consumed by infant before mother's milk is well established; enterohepatic shunting	Possible factors in breast milk that prevent bilirubin conjugation Less frequent stooling	Blood antigen incompatibility causing hemolysis of large numbers of RBCs Liver's inability to conjugate and excrete excess bilirubin from hemolysis
Onset			
After 24 hr (preterm infants, prolonged)	2nd-4th day	4th day	During first 24 hr (levels increase >5 mg/dl/day)
Peak			
3rd-4th day	3rd-5th day	10th-15th day	Variable
Duration			
Declines on 5th-7th day	Variable	May remain jaundiced for 3-12 wk or more	Depends on severity and treatment
Therapy			
Increase frequency of feedings and avoid supplements. Evaluate stooling pattern. Monitor transcutaneous bilirubin (TcB) or total serum bilirubin (TSB) level. Perform risk assessment (see Fig. 9-6, *A*). Use phototherapy if bilirubin levels increase significantly or significant hemolysis is present (see Fig. 9-6, *B*).	Breast-feed frequently (10-12 times/day); avoid supplements such as water, dextrose water, or formula. Evaluate stooling pattern; stimulate as needed. Perform risk assessment (see Fig. 9-6, *A*). Use phototherapy if bilirubin levels increase significantly or significant hemolysis is present (see Fig. 9-6, *B*). If phototherapy is instituted, evaluate benefits and harm of temporarily discontinuing breast-feeding; additional assessments may be required. Assist mother with maintaining milk supply; feed expressed milk as appropriate. After discharge, follow up according to hour of discharge (see p. 290).	Increase frequency of breast-feeding; use no supplementation such as glucose water; cessation of breast-feeding is not recommended. Perform risk assessment (see Fig. 9-6, *A*). Consider performing additional evaluations: glucose-6-phosphate dehydrogenase, direct and indirect serum bilirubin, family history, and others as necessary. May include home phototherapy with a temporary (10-12 hr) discontinuation of breast-feeding; a subsequent TSB may be drawn to evaluate a drop in serum levels. Assist mother with maintenance of milk supply and reassurance regarding her milk supply and therapy. Use formula supplements only at practitioner's discretion.	Monitor TcB or TSB level. Perform risk assessment (see Fig. 9-6, *A*). Postnatal—Use phototherapy; administer intravenous immunoglobulin per protocol; if severe, perform exchange transfusion. Prenatal—Perform transfusion (fetus). Prevent sensitization (Rh incompatibility) of Rh-negative mother with Rh₀(D) immune globulin (RhIg). If mother is breast-feeding, assist with maintenance and storage of milk; may bottle feed expressed milk as appropriate to therapy. Minimize maternal-infant separation, and encourage contact as appropriate.

*Table depicts patterns of jaundice in term infants; patterns in preterm infants will vary according to factors such as gestational age, birth weight, and illness.

The signs of bilirubin encephalopathy are those of CNS depression or excitation. Prodromal symptoms consist of decreased activity, lethargy, irritability, hypotonia, and seizures. Later these subtle findings are followed by development of athetoid cerebral palsy, cognitive delay, and deafness (Sgro, Shah, and Campbell, 2005). Long-term effects include evidence of neurologic damage, such as cognitive impairment, attention deficit hyperactivity disorder, delayed or abnormal motor movement (especially ataxia or athetosis), behavior disorders, perceptual problems, or sensorineural hearing loss.

Physiologic Jaundice

The most common cause of hyperbilirubinemia is the relatively mild and self-limited physiologic jaundice, or icterus neonatorum. Unlike hemolytic disease of the newborn (HDN) (see p. 295), physiologic jaundice is not associated with any pathologic process. Although almost all newborns experience elevated bilirubin levels, only about half demonstrate observable signs of jaundice.

Two phases of physiologic jaundice have been identified in full-term infants. In the first phase, bilirubin levels of formula-fed Caucasian and African-American infants gradually increase to approximately 5 to 6 mg/dl by 3 to 4 days of life, then decrease to a plateau of 2 to 3 mg/dl by the fifth day (Blackburn, 2007). Bilirubin levels maintain a steady plateau state in the second phase without increasing or decreasing until approximately 12 to 14 days, at which time levels decrease to the normal value of 1 mg/dl (Blackburn, 2007). This pattern varies according to racial group, method of feeding (breast versus bottle), and gestational age. In preterm formula-fed infants, serum bilirubin levels may peak as high as 10 to 12 mg/dl at 5 or 6 days of life and decrease slowly over a period of 2 to 4 weeks (Blackburn, 2007).

As noted above, infants of Asian descent (as well as Native Americans) have mean bilirubin levels almost twice those

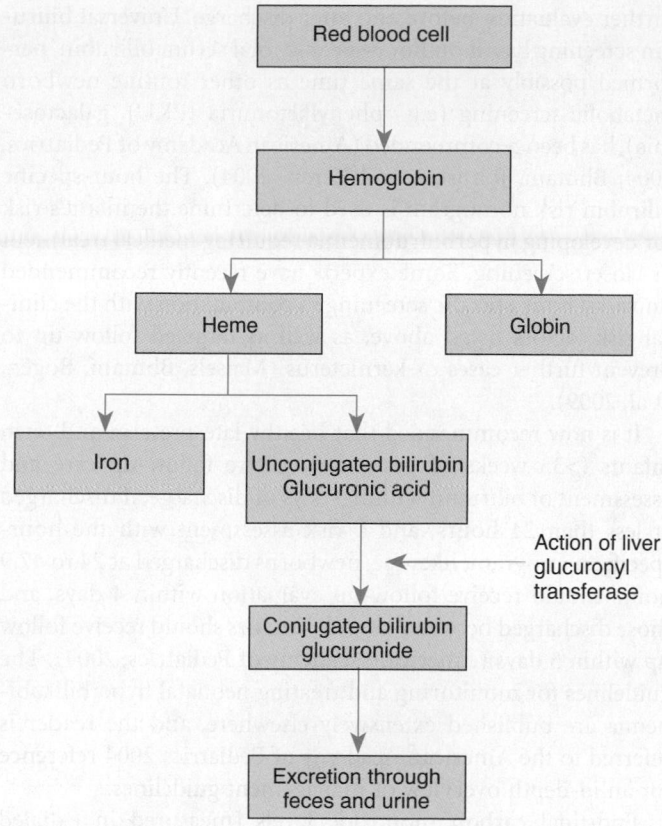

Fig. 9-5 Formation and excretion of bilirubin.

seen in Caucasians or African-Americans. An increased incidence of hyperbilirubinemia occurs in newborns from certain geographic areas, particularly areas around Greece (see Cultural Competence box). These populations may have G6PD deficiency, which can cause acute hemolytic anemia. Hyperbilirubinemia also develops in a small number of newborns with Crigler-Najjar syndrome, an inherited disorder in which there is an absence of glucuronyl transferase. Infants with metabolic disorders such as galactosemia or hypothyroidism may also develop hyperbilirubinemia.

🌐 CULTURAL COMPETENCE

Risk Factors for Hyperbilirubinemia

Neonates of East Asian ethnicity (China, Taiwan, Macao, Hong Kong, Japan, and Korea) are at higher risk for high mean serum bilirubin levels than neonates of any different ethnic origin. The apparent reason for this is the increased presence of certain genes in the East Asian population that modulate bilirubin metabolism in the liver (Watchko, 2009). Exclusive breast-feeding is another risk factor for neonatal hyperbilirubinemia. Watchko (2009) stresses that a combination of risk factors increases the newborn's likelihood of developing hyperbilirubinemia. Therefore infants of East Asian mothers who are breast-feeding should be carefully evaluated during the early neonatal period (first week of life) for elevated serum bilirubin levels.

Mechanisms Involved in Physiologic Jaundice

On average, newborns produce twice as much bilirubin as do adults because of higher concentrations of circulating erythrocytes and a shorter life span of RBCs (only 70 to 90 days, in contrast to 120 days in older children and adults). In addition, the liver's ability to conjugate bilirubin is reduced because of

limited production of glucuronyl transferase. Newborns also have a lower plasma-binding capacity for bilirubin because of lower albumin concentrations than older children. Normal changes in hepatic circulation following birth may contribute to excessive demands on liver function.

Normally, conjugated bilirubin is reduced to urobilinogen by the intestinal flora and excreted in feces. However, the relatively sterile and less motile newborn bowel is initially less effective in excreting urobilinogen. In the newborn intestine the enzyme β-glucuronidase is able to convert conjugated bilirubin into the unconjugated form, which is subsequently reabsorbed by the intestinal mucosa and transported to the liver. This process, known as enterohepatic circulation or enterohepatic shunting, is accentuated in the newborn and is thought to be a primary mechanism in physiologic jaundice (Blackburn, 2007). Feeding (1) stimulates peristalsis and produces more rapid passage of meconium, thus diminishing the amount of reabsorption of unconjugated bilirubin; and (2) introduces bacteria to aid in the reduction of bilirubin to urobilinogen. Colostrum, a natural cathartic, facilitates meconium evacuation.

Jaundice in Breast-Feeding Infants

Breast-feeding is associated with an increased incidence of jaundice. Two types have been identified. Breast-feeding–associated jaundice (early-onset jaundice) begins at 2 to 4 days of age and occurs in approximately 12% to 35% of breast-fed newborns (Blackburn, 2007). The jaundice is related to the process of breast-feeding and probably results from decreased caloric and fluid intake by breast-fed infants before the milk supply is well established, since fasting is associated with decreased hepatic clearance of bilirubin. A decrease in milk (fluid) intake may result in dehydration, which also concentrates the circulating bilirubin in the blood; however, supplemental fluids such as glucose water or water do not enhance bilirubin excretion and may delay the excretion process.

Breast milk jaundice (late-onset jaundice) begins around the fourth day and occurs in 2% to 4% of breast-fed infants (Blackburn, 2007). Rising levels of bilirubin peak during the second week and gradually diminish. Despite high levels of bilirubin that may persist for 3 to 12 weeks, these infants are well. The jaundice may be caused by factors in the breast milk (pregnanediol, fatty acids, and β-glucuronidase) that either inhibit the conjugation or decrease the excretion of bilirubin. Less frequent stooling by breast-fed infants may allow extended time for reabsorption of bilirubin from the intestine via the enterohepatic route described above (see Table 9-1).

Clinical Manifestations

The most obvious sign of hyperbilirubinemia is jaundice, the yellowish discoloration primarily of the sclera, nails, or skin. As a rule, jaundice that appears within the first 24 hours is caused by HDN, sepsis, or one of the maternally derived diseases such as diabetes mellitus or infections. Jaundice that appears on the second or third day, peaks on the third to fifth day, and declines on the fifth to seventh day is usually the result of physiologic jaundice; as noted above, this pattern may vary according to ethnic origin. The intensity of the jaundice is not always related to the degree of hyperbilirubinemia; therefore serum bilirubin levels are necessary.

Diagnostic Evaluation

Total serum bilirubin is measured to determine the degree of hyperbilirubinemia. Normal values of unconjugated bilirubin are 0.2 to 1.4 mg/dl. In the newborn, levels must exceed 5 mg/dl before jaundice (icterus) is observable. However, evaluation of jaundice is not based solely on serum bilirubin levels, but also on the timing of the appearance of clinical jaundice; gestational age at birth; age in days since birth; family history, including maternal Rh factor; evidence of hemolysis; feeding method; infant's physiologic status; and progression of serial serum bilirubin levels. The following criteria are indicators of pathologic jaundice that warrant further investigation as to the cause. It is not an all-inclusive list; other factors are also evaluated:

- Appearance of clinical jaundice within 24 hours of birth
- Persistent clinical jaundice over 2 weeks in full-term, formula-fed infant
- Total serum bilirubin levels over 12.9 mg/dl (term infant) or over 15 mg/dl (preterm infant); upper limit for breast-fed infant: 15 mg/dl
- Increase in serum bilirubin by 5 mg/dl/day
- Direct bilirubin exceeding 1.5 to 2 mg/dl
- Total serum bilirubin level over 95th percentile for age (in hours) on hour-specific risk nomogram (Fig. 9-6, *A*)

Following are risk factors that may place the term infant at high risk for hyperbilirubinemia: maternal race (e.g., Asian or Asian American), gestational age 35 to 36 weeks, significant bruising, cephalhematoma or significant bruising, exclusive breastfeeding, blood group incompatibility or hemolytic disease such as G6PD, and history of sibling with hyperbilirubinemia (Watchko, 2009).

Noninvasive monitoring of bilirubin via cutaneous reflectance measurements (transcutaneous bilirubinometry, or TcB) allows for repetitive estimations of total serum bilirubin and, when used correctly, may decrease the need for invasive monitoring. With shorter maternity stays, the value of transcutaneous bilirubin measurements as a screening tool for evaluating the need for obtaining serum bilirubin levels or closely monitoring the infant has received considerable attention. Some TcB monitors provide accurate measurements within 2 to 3 mg/dl in most neonatal populations at serum levels below 15 mg/dl (American Academy of Pediatrics, 2004). Regardless of the screening instrument chosen, it is important to note that, to date, no transcutaneous bilirubin meter measures the total serum bilirubin level, and they must be used according to published guidelines as screening tools, not as predictors of need for therapy. Multiple readings over time at a consistent site (e.g., sternum, forehead) are more valuable than a single reading. Once phototherapy has been initiated, TcB is no longer useful as a screening tool.

The use of hour-specific serum bilirubin levels to predict newborns at risk for rapidly rising levels has now become an official recommendation by the Academy of Pediatrics (2004) for monitoring healthy neonates at more than 35 weeks of gestation before discharge from the hospital. Using a nomogram (see Fig. 9-6, *A*) with three designated risk levels (high, intermediate, or low risk) of hour-specific total serum bilirubin values assists in determining which newborns might need further evaluation before and after discharge. Universal bilirubin screening based on hour-specific total serum bilirubin, performed possibly at the same time as other routine newborn metabolic screening (e.g., phenylketonuria [PKU], galactosemia), has been recommended (American Academy of Pediatrics, 2004; Bhutani, Johnson, and Keren, 2004). The hour-specific bilirubin risk nomogram is used to determine the infant's risk for developing hyperbilirubinemia requiring medical treatment or closer screening. Some experts have recently recommended universal hour-specific screening in combination with the clinical risk factors listed above, as well as targeted follow-up to prevent further cases of kernicterus (Maisels, Bhutani, Bogen, et al, 2009).

It is now recommended that healthy late-preterm and term infants (>35 weeks of gestation) receive follow-up care and assessment of bilirubin within 3 days of discharge, if discharged at less than 24 hours, and a risk assessment with the hour-specific nomogram; likewise, newborns discharged at 24 to 47.9 hours should receive follow-up evaluation within 4 days, and those discharged between 48 and 72 hours should receive follow up within 5 days (American Academy of Pediatrics, 2004). The guidelines for monitoring and treating neonatal hyperbilirubinemia are published extensively elsewhere, and the reader is referred to the American Academy of Pediatrics 2004 reference for an in-depth overview of management guidelines.

End-tidal carbon monoxide levels (measured in exhaled breath) may be of value in determining the presence of hemolysis and the rate of heme degradation and bilirubin production in some infants. These determinations are often useful in determining the need for surveillance during the first week of life (American Academy of Pediatrics, 2004).

Therapeutic Management

The primary goals in the treatment of hyperbilirubinemia are to prevent bilirubin encephalopathy and, as in any blood group incompatibility, to reverse the hemolytic process (see p. 288). The main form of treatment involves the use of phototherapy. Exchange transfusion is generally used for reducing dangerously high bilirubin levels that occur with hemolytic disease.

The pharmacologic management of hyperbilirubinemia with phenobarbital has centered primarily on the infant with hemolytic disease and is most effective when given to the mother several days before delivery. Phenobarbital promotes (1) hepatic glucuronyl transferase synthesis, which increases bilirubin conjugation and hepatic clearance of the pigment in bile; and (2) protein synthesis, which may increase albumin for more bilirubin binding sites. However, the use of phenobarbital in either the antenatal or the postnatal period has not proved to be as effective as other treatments in reducing bilirubin. Bilirubin production in the newborn can be decreased by inhibiting heme oxygenase—an enzyme needed for heme breakdown (to biliverdin)—with metalloporphyrins, especially tin protoporphyrin and tin mesoporphyrin. The use of heme-oxygenase inhibitors provides a preventive approach to hyperbilirubinemia (Dennery, 2005).

Healthy late-preterm and full-term infants with jaundice may also benefit from early initiation of feedings and frequent breast-feeding. These preventive measures are aimed at promoting increased intestinal motility, decreased enterohepatic

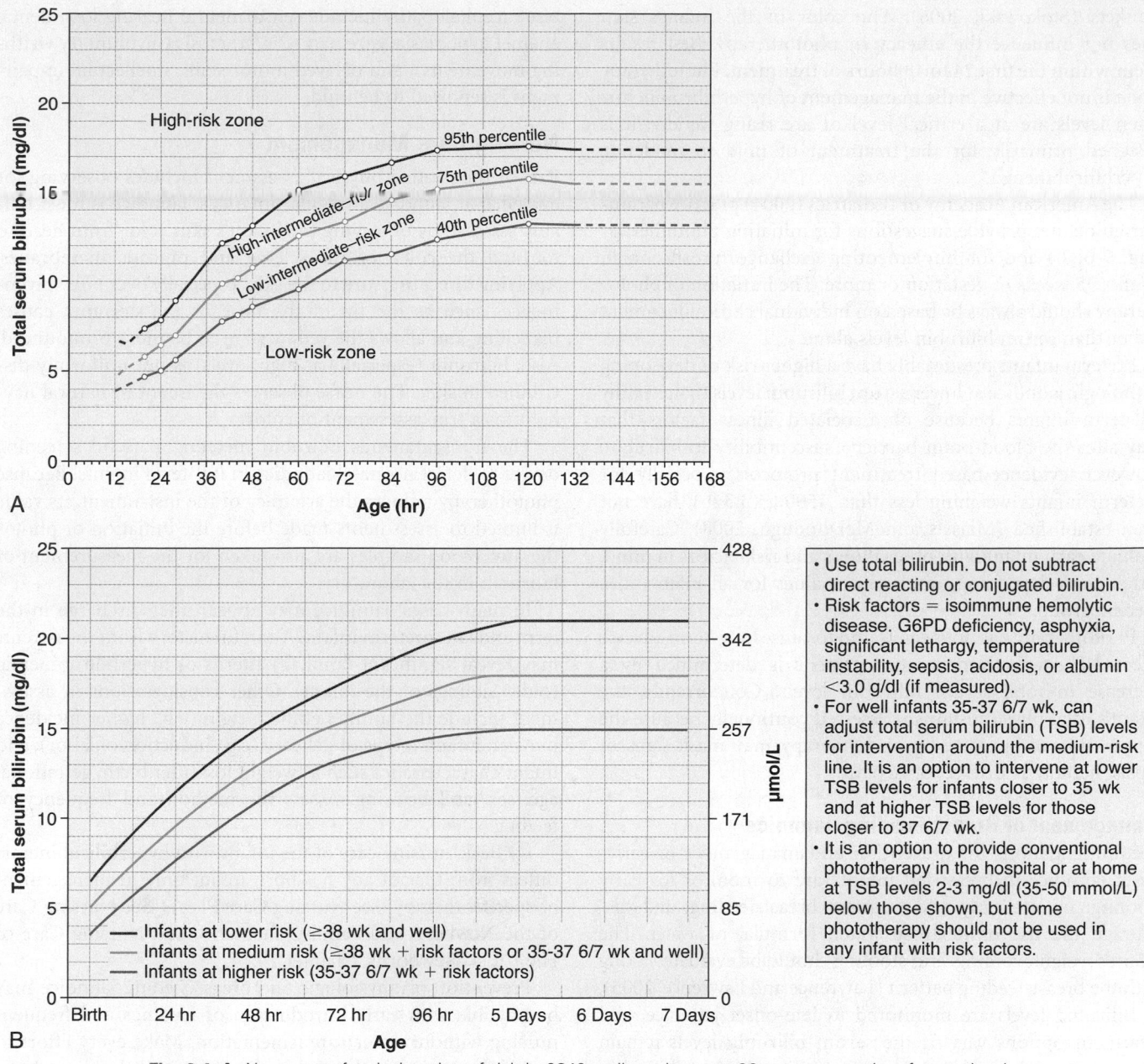

Fig. 9-6 A, Nomogram for designation of risk in 2840 well newborns at 36 or more weeks of gestational age with birth weight of 2000 g (4.4 lb) or more, or 35 or more weeks of gestational age and birth weight of 2500 g (5.5 lb) or more, based on the hour-specific serum bilirubin values. (This nomogram should not be used to represent the natural history of neonatal hyperbilirubinemia.) **B,** Guidelines for phototherapy in hospitalized infants of 35 or more weeks of gestation. (**A,** From Bhutani VK, Johnson L, Sivieri EM: Predictive ability of a predischarge hour-specific serum bilirubin for subsequent significant hyperbilirubinemia in healthy term and near-term newborns, *Pediatrics* 103(1):6-14, 1999. **B,** From American Academy of Pediatrics, Subcommittee on Hyperbilirubinemia: Management of hyperbilirubinemia in the newborn infant 35 or more weeks of gestation, *Pediatrics* 114(1):297-316, 2004.)

shunting, and normal bacterial flora in the bowel to effectively enhance the excretion of unconjugated bilirubin.

Phototherapy

Phototherapy consists of exposing the infant's skin to an appropriate light source. Light promotes bilirubin excretion by photoisomerization, which alters the structure of bilirubin to a soluble form (lumirubin).

For phototherapy to be effective, the infant's skin must be fully exposed to an adequate amount of light or irradiance.

When serum bilirubin levels are rapidly increasing or approximating critical levels, double or intensive phototherapy is recommended. This technique often involves the application of phototherapy with lights above the infant and another source of light (e.g., fiberoptic mattress) under the infant (Stokowski, 2006). The goal is to increase irradiance to the 430 to 490 nm band, which provides best results (American Academy of Pediatrics, 2004). Available commercial phototherapy delivery systems are numerous and include halogen spotlights, light-emitting diodes, fluorescent tubes or bank lights, and fiberoptic blankets (Stokowski, 2006). The color of the infant's skin does not influence the efficacy of phototherapy. Best results occur within the first 24 to 48 hours of treatment. Phototherapy alone is not effective in the management of hyperbilirubinemia when levels are at a critical level or are rising rapidly; it is designed primarily for the treatment of mild to moderate hyperbilirubinemia.

The American Academy of Pediatrics (2004) practice parameter guidelines provide suggestions for initiating phototherapy (Fig. 9-6, B) and for implementing exchange transfusion in infants 35 weeks of gestation or more. The initiation of phototherapy should always be based on individual clinical judgment rather than serum bilirubin levels alone.

Preterm infants presumably have a higher risk of developing pathologic jaundice at lower serum bilirubin levels than healthy full-term infants because of associated illness factors that may alter the blood-brain barrier's susceptibility to bilirubin. However, evidence-based treatment protocols, especially for preterm infants weighing less than 1500 g (3.3 lb), have not been established (Maisels and McDonough, 2008). Carefully evaluate each infant with other illness and risk factors in mind, rather than depending on absolute values for all infants in a specific group.

Phototherapy has not been found to cause long-term adverse effects. The effectiveness of treatment is determined by a decrease in total serum bilirubin levels. Concurrently, the infant's total physical status is assessed continually because the suppression of jaundice by phototherapy may mask signs of sepsis, hemolytic disease, or hepatitis.

Management of Breast-Feeding Jaundice

Recommendations for prevention and management of early-onset jaundice in breast-fed infants are to monitor for early stooling; initiate early and frequent breast-feeding; and discourage the use of dextrose water, formula, or water. The infant's weight, voiding, and stooling should be evaluated along with the breast-feeding pattern (Lawrence and Lawrence, 2005).

Bilirubin levels are monitored in late-onset jaundice, and treatment options vary. If the serum bilirubin levels remain above 16 mg/dl for more than 24 hours, obtain a bilirubin reading 2 hours after breast-feeding, which may then be interrupted for 10 to 12 hours (provide fluid and calories during this time) and repeat levels drawn; with a serum bilirubin level decrease of 2 mg/dl or more and levels below 15 mg/dl, the infant may resume breast-feeding. If levels do not drop significantly, further evaluation is necessary (Lawrence and Lawrence, 2005). It is not within the scope of this text to discuss the full spectrum of treatment possibilities; therefore consult other sources. Whenever possible, offer parents the option of continuing breast-feeding, provided that the jaundiced infant is closely monitored for additional contributing factors. Home phototherapy and continued breast-feeding are options for the family with a jaundiced newborn.

Prognosis

Early recognition and treatment of neonatal hyperbilirubinemia prevent unnecessary medical therapies, parent-infant separation, breast-feeding disruption and possibly failure, and bilirubin encephalopathy. The characteristic features of bilirubin encephalopathy include sensorineural hearing loss, dental enamel hypoplasia, gaze paralysis, athetosis (involuntary writhing movements), and delayed motor skills; intellectual impairment is reported to be mild.

Nursing Care Management

Part of the routine physical assessment includes observing for evidence of jaundice at regular intervals. Jaundice is most reliably assessed by observing the infant's skin color from head to toe and the color of the sclerae and mucous membranes. Applying direct pressure to the skin, especially over bony prominences such as the tip of the nose or the sternum, causes blanching and allows the yellow stain to be more pronounced. Also, bilirubin (especially at high levels) is not uniformly distributed in skin. The nurse observes the infant in natural daylight for a true assessment of color.

The transcutaneous bilirubin meter is a useful screening device to detect neonatal jaundice in full-term infants. Because phototherapy reduces the accuracy of the instrument, its value is limited to assessments made before the initiation of phototherapy. Blood samples are also taken for the measurement of bilirubin in the laboratory.

In many cases, jaundice may appear after discharge in the term and late-preterm infant. A careful history from the parents may reveal significant familial patterns of hyperbilirubinemia (older siblings of the infant). Other considerations in assessment include the family's ethnic origin (e.g., higher incidence in Asian infants); type of delivery (e.g., induction of labor); and infant characteristics such as weight loss after birth, gestational age, sex, and bruising. Assess the method and frequency of feeding.

ⓔ Basic nursing care of the infant with hyperbilirubinemia differs from that of any newborn infant only in management of specific therapy (see Nursing Care Plan). (See Nursing Care of the Newborn and Family, Chapter 8, and Nursing Care of High-Risk Newborns, Chapter 10.)

Prevention of physiologic and breast-feeding jaundice may be possible with early introduction of feedings and frequent nursing without water supplementation. Make every effort to provide an optimum thermal environment to reduce metabolic needs.

> **QUALITY PATIENT OUTCOMES: Neonatal Hyperbilirubinemia**
> Total serum bilirubin level will be maintained below high-risk critical value (as determined on the hour-specific total serum bilirubin nomogram).

Phototherapy

The infant who receives phototherapy is placed under the light source, exposing as much skin surface as possible, and repositioned frequently to expose all body surface areas to the light. Once phototherapy has been initiated, frequent (every 6 to 12 hours) serum bilirubin levels are necessary because visual and transcutaneous assessments of jaundice are no longer considered valid.

The nurse institutes several precautions to protect the infant during phototherapy. An opaque mask shields the infant's eyes to prevent exposure to the light (Fig. 9-7). The eye shield should be properly sized and positioned to cover the eyes completely

NURSING CARE PLAN

The Newborn with Jaundice

NURSING DIAGNOSIS	EXPECTED PATIENT OUTCOMES	NURSING INTERVENTIONS	RATIONALE
Neonatal jaundice related to abnormal blood profile (increased breakdown of products of red blood cells), developmental age (immature blood-brain barrier and immature liver function)	Newborn will receive appropriate therapy to enhance bilirubin excretion. Newborn total serum bilirubin levels will remain below high risk or high-intermediate risk zone.	Initiate breast-feeding within 1st hour of life in delivery room.	To promote breast milk intake and stooling To enhance parent-infant interaction and acquaintance with newborn
		If formula feeding, assist parents in initiation of early feeding.	To promote milk intake and stooling
Child's/Family's Defining Characteristics (Subjective and Objective Data)	**The Following NOC Concepts Apply to These Outcomes** Risk Control Newborn Adaptation	Assess skin for jaundice every 4 hr.	To detect evidence of clinical jaundice and rising bilirubin levels
Clinical jaundice evident within 24 hr of birth.		Monitor transcutaneous bilirubin levels per institution protocol or at least every 6-8 hr. Obtain serum bilirubin (collaborative intervention).	To detect rising levels of bilirubin for institution of appropriate therapy
Altered breast-feeding (ineffective latch-on, nurses <6-8 times in 24-hr period) Altered stooling pattern (<1 stool in 24 hr)		Monitor intake and output with each occurrence.	To evaluate effectiveness of breast-feeding or formula intake by measuring urinary and stool output To provide accurate record of output to evaluate effectiveness of feedings
		Maintain accurate record of urinary and stool output and assist parents in same.	To evaluate effectiveness of feedings
		Monitor vital signs per unit protocol or at least every 8 hr. Report signs of poor transition to extrauterine life.	To evaluate transitional events and ensure infant is making an effective transition without cardiorespiratory, metabolic, thermoregulatory, or other physiologic problems
		Instruct parents regarding newborn care, including jaundice—appearance, significance, importance of follow-up visit to practitioner within 2-3 days of discharge, feeding methods, and stooling and voiding patterns.	To promote physical care of newborn and decrease parents' anxiety related to home care
		The Following NIC Concepts Apply to These Interventions Risk Identification Nutrition Management Breastfeeding Assistance Lactation Counseling Newborn Monitoring Newborn Care Fluid Monitoring	

NURSING DIAGNOSIS	EXPECTED PATIENT OUTCOMES	NURSING INTERVENTIONS	RATIONALE
Readiness for Enhanced Parenting related to birth of a new family member	Parent(s) of newborn will assume responsibility for emotional and physical care and well-being of the new family member.	Initiate skin-to-skin contact between mother and newborn and father and newborn in delivery room within 1st hr of birth.	To enhance breast-feeding and parent-infant interaction and to promote early stooling and bilirubin clearance
Child's/Family's Defining Characteristics (Subjective and Objective Data)	**The Following NOC Concepts Apply to These Outcomes** Parent-Infant Attachment Parenting: Social Safety Caregiver Home Care Readiness	Encourage early breast-feeding in 1st hr of birth. Perform physical assessment with parents present and show typical newborn characteristics. Point out state traits such as quiet awake and cues to feeding readiness.	To promote parents' knowledge of infant physical characteristics and behavior
Parent(s) express willingness to enhance parenting. Emotional support of child is evident; bonding or attachment is evident.		Encourage parent participation in care behaviors such as diapering, formula feeding (as applicable), and bathing.	To enhance parental feeling of contribution as newborn's primary caretakers To promote familiarity with behaviors and decrease parental anxiety
		Encourage sibling visitation and participation in care and holding of newborn as age-appropriate.	To promote sibling participation in care and acceptance of new family member
		The Following NIC Concepts Apply to These Interventions Anxiety Reduction Family Support Family Process Maintenance Parent Education: Infant	

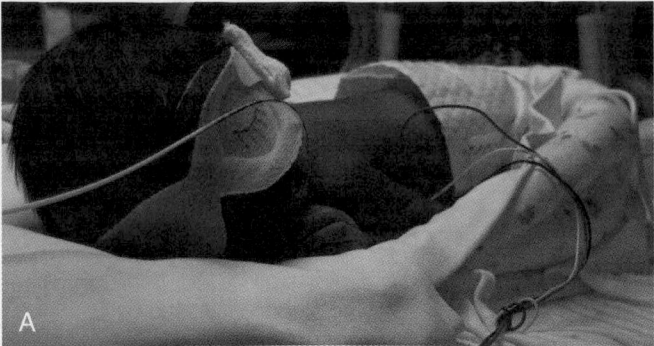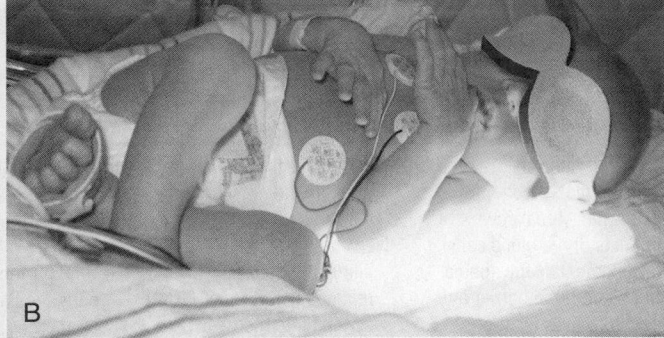

Fig. 9-7 A, Infant receiving phototherapy; note nested boundaries for comfort and eye protection. **B,** Newborn laying on phototherapy light source, which may be used with overhead lights to provide intensive phototherapy. (Courtesy E. Jacobs, Texas Children's Hospital, Houston.)

but prevent any occlusion of the nares. The infant's eyelids are closed before the mask is applied because the corneas may become excoriated if they come in contact with the dressing. The nurse checks the newborn's eyes at least every 4 to 6 hours for evidence of discharge, excessive pressure on the lids, or corneal irritation. Remove eye shields during feedings, which provide the opportunity for visual and sensory stimulation.

Monitor infants who are in an open crib receiving phototherapy for temperature instability, since phototherapy may cause an increase in the body temperature. The distance between the phototherapy light source and the infant must be maintained as outlined by the manufacturer's guidelines; halogen lights placed too close to the infant's skin may cause burns (Stokowski, 2006). Maintaining the infant in a flexed position with rolled blankets along the sides of the body helps maintain heat and provides comfort.

Accurate charting is another important nursing responsibility and includes (1) times that phototherapy is started and stopped, (2) proper shielding of the eyes, (3) type of phototherapy unit (by manufacturer), (4) number of lamps, (5) distance between surface of lamps and infant, (6) use of phototherapy in combination with an incubator or open bassinet, (7) photometer measurement of light intensity (microwatts), and (8) side effects.

Side Effects of Phototherapy

Minor side effects for which the nurse should be alert include loose, greenish stools; transient skin rashes; mild hyperthermia; increased metabolic rate; and priapism. Dehydration and electrolyte disturbances, such as hypocalcemia, are uncommon yet may occur. To prevent or minimize these effects, the nurse monitors the temperature to detect early signs of hypothermia or hyperthermia, and observes the skin for evidence of dehydration and drying, which can lead to excoriation and breakdown. Oily lubricants or lotions are not used on the skin to prevent increased tanning. Full-term and late-preterm infants receiving phototherapy may require additional fluid volume or feedings to compensate for insensible and intestinal fluid loss. Because phototherapy enhances the excretion of unconjugated bilirubin through the bowel, loose stools may indicate accelerated bilirubin excretion. Frequent stooling can cause perianal irritation; therefore meticulous skin care, especially keeping the skin clean and dry, is essential.

Once phototherapy is permanently discontinued, there is often a subsequent increase in the serum bilirubin level, often called the "rebound effect." This is usually transient and resolves without resuming therapy.

Another reaction to phototherapy is the **bronze-baby syndrome,** in which the serum, urine, and skin turn grayish brown several hours after the infant is placed under the light. This reaction is probably caused by retention of a bilirubin breakdown product of phototherapy, possibly copper porphyrin. The syndrome almost always occurs in infants who have elevated conjugated hyperbilirubinemia and some degree of cholestasis. The browning generally resolves after discontinuation of phototherapy.

Family Support

Parents need reassurance concerning their infant's progress. The nurse explains all the procedures to familiarize them with the benefits and risks. Reassure parents that the naked infant under the bilirubin light is warm and comfortable. Remove eye shields and turn off phototherapy when the parents are visiting to facilitate the attachment process. Also reassure parents that the neonate is accustomed to darkness after months of intrauterine existence and benefits a great deal from auditory and tactile stimulation (see Family-Centered Care box).

⚙ FAMILY-CENTERED CARE
Phototherapy and Parent-Infant Interaction

The traditional use of phototherapy has evoked concerns regarding a number of psychobehavioral issues, including parent-infant separation, potential social isolation, decreased sensorineural stimulation, altered biologic rhythms, altered feeding patterns, and activity changes. Parental anxiety is greatly increased, particularly at the sight of the newborn blindfolded and under special lights. The interruption of breast-feeding for phototherapy is a potential deterrent to successful maternal-infant attachment and interaction.

Because research has demonstrated that bilirubin catabolism occurs primarily within the first few hours of the initiation of phototherapy, there is increased support for the removal of the infant from treatment for feeding and holding. The benefits of stopping phototherapy for parental feeding and holding outweigh concerns related to the clearance of bilirubin in the healthy full-term newborn with mild to moderate hyperbilirubinemia. Home phototherapy offers an additional opportunity to foster parent-infant attachment.

The initiation of any treatment requires informed consent by the parents; however, in the case of phototherapy, parents may feel considerable anxiety when nurses use such words as "kernicterus" and "possible harm to the brain" to describe possible effects of hyperbilirubinemia. It is imperative that nurses remain sensitive to parents' feelings and information needs during this process. An important nursing intervention is the assessment of the parents' understanding of the treatment involved and clarification of the nature of the therapy.

One of the most important nursing interventions is recognition of breast-feeding jaundice. Lack of familiarity among health professionals has caused many newborns prolonged hospitalization, termination of breast-feeding, and unnecessary phototherapy. Care of the new mother may include supporting successful and frequent breast-feeding. Parents also need reassurance of the benign nature of the jaundice and encouragement to resume breast-feeding if temporary cessation is prescribed. Unfortunately, jaundice increases the risk of breast-feeding being discontinued and development of the **vulnerable child syndrome**—the parents' belief that their child has suffered a "close call" and is vulnerable to serious injury.

Discharge Planning and Home Care

With short hospital stays, mothers and infants may be discharged before evidence of jaundice is present. It is imperative that the nurse discuss signs of jaundice with the mother because any clinical symptoms will probably appear at home. Teach parents to evaluate the number of voids and evidence of adequate breast-feeding once the infant is home and encourage them to bring the newborn to the hospital, clinic, or primary care practitioner if there are indications of hyperbilirubinemia. Breast-feeding mother-infant dyads must receive appropriate guidance and assistance with breast-feeding to ensure the infant is receiving an adequate amount of breast milk and that stooling is occurring. A follow-up visit to the health care practitioner within 2 or 3 days after discharge to evaluate feeding and elimination patterns and jaundice is important in the posthospital care of the full-term newborn (see Diagnostic Evaluation, p. 290, for follow-up recommendations).

If home phototherapy is instituted, the hospital, durable medical equipment company representative, or home health care nurse is usually responsible for teaching family members and assessing their abilities to implement the treatment safely and in a timely manner. General guidelines for home care preparation and education are discussed in Chapters 8, 25, and 26. Written instructions and supervision of care—especially the application of eye shields, if needed—are essential. The minor side effects of phototherapy are reviewed, and parents may need instruction in taking axillary temperatures and recording times and amounts of feedings and the number of wet diapers and stools.

Regardless of how benign the disorder or the therapy, parents need support and understanding. In jaundice associated with breast-feeding, follow-up blood studies are usually required to assess the progress of the jaundice. If temporary cessation of breast-feeding is prescribed, teach mothers to pump the breasts every 2 to 3 hours to maintain lactation; the expressed milk is properly stored for use after breast-feeding is resumed. Nurses should take measures to help the mother achieve successful breast-feeding, including consultation with a lactation specialist on an outpatient basis.

HEMOLYTIC DISEASE OF THE NEWBORN

Hyperbilirubinemia in the first 24 hours of life is most often the result of **hemolytic disease of the newborn (HDN)**, an abnormally rapid rate of RBC destruction. Anemia caused by this destruction stimulates the production of RBCs, which in turn provides increasing numbers of cells for hemolysis. Major causes of increased erythrocyte destruction are isoimmunization (primarily RhD) and ABO incompatibility.

Blood Incompatibility

The membranes of human blood cells contain a variety of **antigens**, also known as agglutinogens, substances capable of producing an immune response if recognized by the body as foreign. The reciprocal relationship between antigens on RBCs and antibodies in the plasma causes **agglutination** (clumping). In other words, antibodies in the plasma of one blood group (except the AB group, which contains no antibodies) produce agglutination when mixed with antigens of a different blood group. In the ABO blood group system the antibodies occur naturally. In the Rh system the person must be exposed to the Rh antigen before significant antibody formation takes place and causes a sensitivity response known as **isoimmunization**.

Rh Incompatibility (Isoimmunization)

The Rh blood group consists of several antigens (with D being the most prevalent). For simplicity, only the terms **Rh positive** (presence of antigen) and **Rh negative** (absence of antigen) are used in this discussion. (See Autosomal Inheritance Patterns, Chapter 5.) The presence or absence of the naturally occurring Rh factor determines the blood type.

Ordinarily, no problems are anticipated when the Rh blood types are the same in both mother and fetus or when the mother is Rh positive and the infant is Rh negative. Difficulty may arise when the mother is Rh negative and the infant is Rh positive. Although the maternal and fetal circulations are separate, there is evidence of a bidirectional trafficking of fetal RBCs and cell-free DNA to the maternal circulation (Moise, 2007). More commonly, however, fetal RBCs enter into the maternal circulation at the time of delivery. The mother's natural defense mechanism responds to these alien cells by producing anti-Rh antibodies.

Under normal circumstances, this process of isoimmunization has no effect on the fetus during the first pregnancy with an Rh-positive fetus, since the initial sensitization to Rh antigens rarely occurs before the onset of labor. However, with the increased risk of fetal blood being transferred to the maternal circulation during placental separation, maternal antibody production is stimulated. During a subsequent pregnancy with an Rh-positive fetus, these previously formed maternal antibodies to Rh-positive blood cells enter the fetal circulation, where they attach to and destroy fetal erythrocytes (Fig. 9-8). Multiple gestations, abruptio placentae, placenta previa, manual removal of the placenta, and cesarean delivery increase the incidence of transplacental hemorrhage and subsequent isoimmunization (Moise, 2008).

Because the condition begins in utero, the fetus attempts to compensate for the progressive hemolysis by accelerating the rate of erythropoiesis. As a result, immature RBCs

PATHOPHYSIOLOGY REVIEW

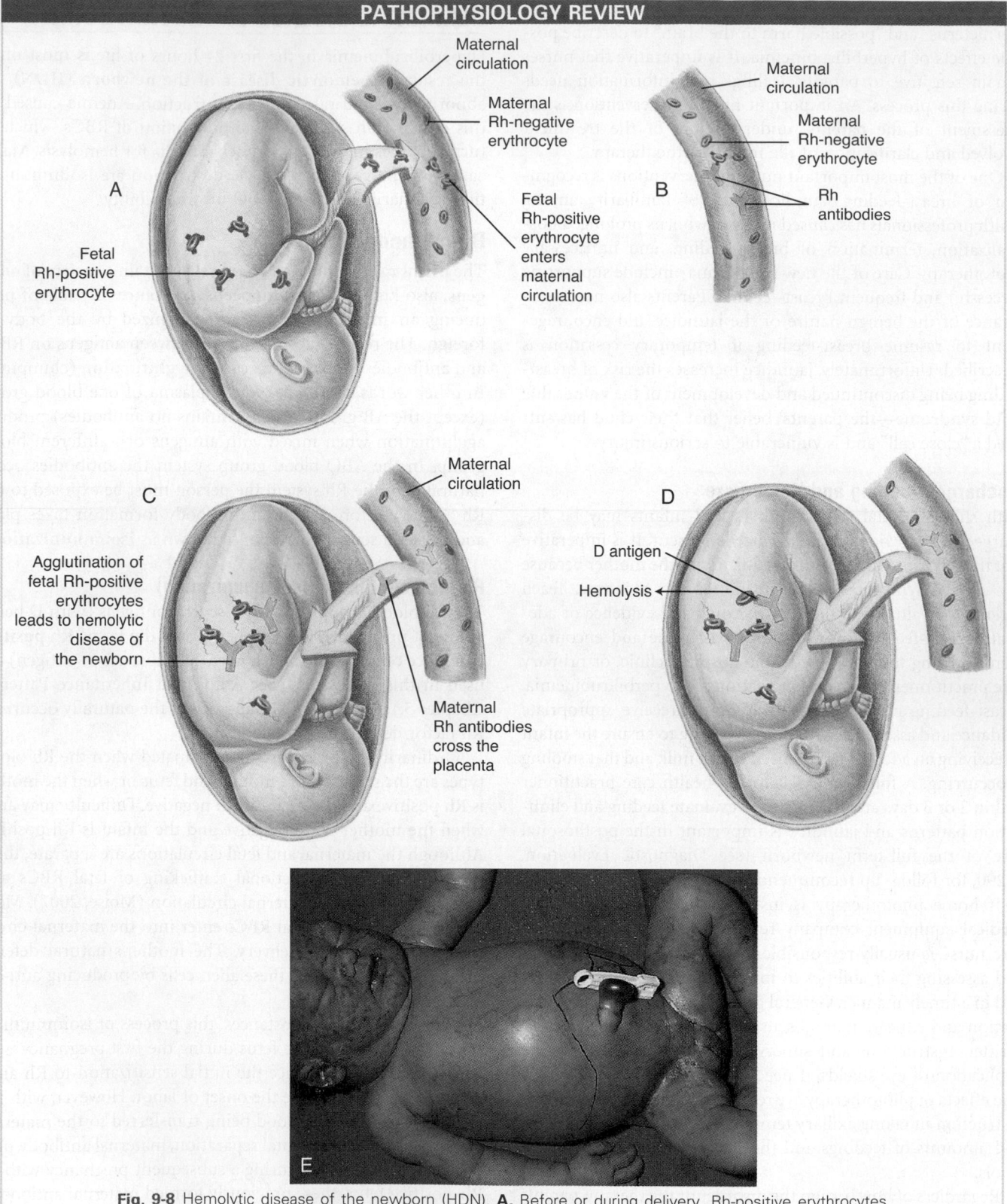

Fig. 9-8 Hemolytic disease of the newborn (HDN). **A,** Before or during delivery, Rh-positive erythrocytes from the fetus enter the blood of an Rh-negative woman through a tear in the placenta. **B,** The mother is sensitized to the Rh antigen and produces Rh antibodies. Because this usually happens after delivery, there is no effect on the fetus in the first pregnancy. **C,** During a subsequent pregnancy with an Rh-positive fetus, Rh-positive erythrocytes cross the placenta, enter the maternal circulation, and **(D)** stimulate the mother to produce antibodies against the Rh antigen. The Rh antibodies from the mother cross the placenta, causing agglutination and hemolysis of fetal erythrocytes, and HDN develops **(E).** (From McCance K, Huether S: *Pathophysiology: the biological basis for disease in adults and children,* ed 6, St Louis, 2010, Mosby.)

(erythroblasts) appear in the fetal circulation; hence the term erythroblastosis fetalis.

The development of maternal sensitization to Rh-positive antigens exhibits wide variability. Sensitization may occur during the first pregnancy if the woman previously received an Rh-positive blood transfusion. No sensitization may occur in situations in which a strong placental barrier prevents transfer of fetal blood into the maternal circulation. Approximately 10% to 15% of sensitized mothers have no hemolytic reaction in the newborn. In addition, some Rh-negative women, even though exposed to Rh-positive fetal blood, are immunologically unable to produce antibodies to the foreign antigen.

In the most severe form of erythroblastosis fetalis (hydrops fetalis), the progressive hemolysis causes fetal hypoxia; cardiac failure; generalized edema (anasarca); and fluid effusions into the pericardial, pleural, and peritoneal spaces (hydrops). The fetus may be delivered stillborn or in severe respiratory distress. Maternal Rh immunoglobulin (RhIg) administration, early intrauterine detection of fetal anemia by ultrasonography (serial Doppler assessment of the peak velocity in the fetal middle cerebral artery), and subsequent treatment by fetal blood transfusions or high-dose intravenous immunoglobulin (IVIG) have dramatically improved the outcome of affected fetuses (Moise, 2008).

ABO Incompatibility

Hemolytic disease can also occur when the major blood group antigens of the fetus are different from those of the mother. The major blood groups are A, B, AB, and O. The incidence of these blood groups varies according to race and geographic location. In the North American Caucasian population, 46% have type O blood, 42% have type A blood, 9% have type B blood, and 3% have type AB blood.

The presence or absence of antibodies and antigens determines whether agglutination will occur. Antibodies in the plasma of one blood group (except the AB group, which contains no antibodies) will produce agglutination (clumping) when mixed with antigens of a different blood group. Naturally occurring antibodies in the recipient's blood cause agglutination of a donor's RBCs. The agglutinated donor cells become trapped in peripheral blood vessels, where they hemolyze, releasing large amounts of bilirubin into the circulation.

The most common blood group incompatibility in the neonate is between a mother with O blood group and an infant with A or B blood group. Hemolysis due to anti-A is more common than for anti-B (see Table 9-2 for possible ABO incompatibilities). Naturally occurring anti-A or anti-B antibodies already present in the maternal circulation cross the placenta and attach to fetal RBCs, causing hemolysis. Usually

the hemolytic reaction is less severe than in Rh incompatibility; however, rare cases of hydrops have been reported (Black and Maheshwari, 2009). Unlike the Rh reaction, ABO incompatibility may occur in the first pregnancy. The risk of significant hemolysis in subsequent pregnancies is thought to be unchanged from the first.

Clinical Manifestations

Jaundice appears shortly after birth (during the first 24 hours), and serum levels of unconjugated bilirubin rise rapidly. Anemia results from the hemolysis of large numbers of erythrocytes, and hyperbilirubinemia and jaundice result from the liver's inability to conjugate and excrete the excess bilirubin. Most newborns with HDN are not jaundiced at birth. However, hepatosplenomegaly and varying degrees of hydrops may be evident. If the infant is severely affected, hydrops, anemia, and hypovolemic shock are apparent. Hypoglycemia may occur as a result of pancreatic cell hyperplasia.

Diagnostic Evaluation

Early identification and diagnosis of RhD sensitization is important in the management and prevention of fetal complications. A maternal antibody titer (indirect Coombs test) should be drawn at the first prenatal visit. Genetic testing allows early identification of paternal zygosity at the RhD gene locus, thus allowing earlier detection of the potential for isoimmunization and avoiding further maternal or fetal testing (Moise, 2008). Amniocentesis can be used to test the fetal blood type of a woman whose antibody screen is positive; the use of polymerase chain reaction may determine the fetal blood type, hemoglobin, hematocrit, and presence of maternal antibodies. Chorionic villus sampling has drawbacks that preclude its use, including possible spontaneous abortion of the fetus and fetomaternal hemorrhage, which would make the situation worse. With either method the determination of an Rh-negative fetus requires no further treatment. The detection of cell-free fetal DNA in the maternal plasma of RhD–negative women to detect an RhD-positive fetus has been used successfully in the United Kingdom; however, this technology is not yet available in the United States (Finning, Martin, and Daniels, 2009; Moise, 2008). Such testing would negate the necessity of amniocentesis for fetal blood type.

Ultrasonography is an important adjunct in the detection of isoimmunization. Alterations in the placenta, umbilical cord, and amniotic fluid volume, as well as the presence of fetal hydrops, can be detected with high-resolution ultrasonography, allowing early, noninvasive treatment before the development of erythroblastosis. Serial Doppler ultrasonography of fetal middle cerebral artery peak velocity is often used to detect and measure fetal hemoglobin and, subsequently, fetal anemia (Moise, 2008). Erythroblastosis fetalis caused by Rh incompatibility can also be assessed by evaluating rising anti-Rh antibody titers in the maternal circulation (indirect Coombs test) or by testing the optical density of amniotic fluid (delta OD 450 test), because bilirubin discolors the fluid. The disease in the newborn is suspected on the basis of the timing and appearance of jaundice (see Table 9-1) and can be confirmed postnatally by detecting antibodies attached to the circulating erythrocytes of affected infants (direct Coombs test, or direct antiglobulin test).

TABLE 9-2	POTENTIAL MATERNAL-FETAL ABO INCOMPATIBILITIES	
MATERNAL BLOOD GROUP	**INCOMPATIBLE FETAL BLOOD GROUP**
O	A or B
B	A or AB
A	B or AB

The Coombs test is routinely performed on cord blood samples from infants born to Rh-negative mothers.

Therapeutic Management

The primary aim of therapeutic management of isoimmunization is prevention. Postnatal therapy usually entails phototherapy for mild cases and exchange transfusion for more severe forms. In severe cases of hydrops, aggressive interventions such as pericardial and pleural fluid aspiration, mechanical ventilatory support, and inotrope therapy may be required for stabilization. Although phototherapy may control bilirubin levels in mild cases, the hemolytic process may continue, causing severe anemia (if untreated) between 7 and 21 days of life.

Prevention of Rh Isoimmunization

The administration of RhIg, a human gamma-globulin concentrate of anti-D, to all unsensitized Rh-negative mothers after delivery or abortion of an Rh-positive infant or fetus prevents the development of maternal sensitization to the Rh factor. The injected anti-Rh antibodies destroy (by subsequent phagocytosis and agglutination) fetal RBCs passing into the maternal circulation before the mother's immune system can recognize them. Because the immune response is blocked, anti-D antibodies and memory cells (which produce the primary and secondary immune responses, respectively) are not formed. The inhibition of memory cell formation is especially important because memory cells provide long-term immunity by initiating a rapid immune response once the antigen is reintroduced (McCance and Huether, 2010).

To be effective, RhIg (such as RhoGAM) must be administered to unsensitized mothers within 72 hours (but possibly as long as 3 to 4 weeks) after the first delivery, miscarriage, or abortion, and repeated after subsequent pregnancies. The administration of RhIg at 26 to 28 weeks of gestation further reduces the risk of Rh isoimmunization. RhIg is not effective against existing Rh-positive antibodies in the maternal circulation. RhIg is administered intramuscularly, not intravenously, and only to Rh-negative women with a negative Coombs test—never to the infant or father.

The use of a heme-oxygenase inhibitor, such as tin mesoporphyrin (given intramuscularly to the newborn), has proved effective in preventing neonatal hyperbilirubinemia.

Maternal administration of high-dose IVIG, alone or in combination with plasmapheresis, decreases the fetal effects of RhD isoimmunization (Moise, 2002; Urbaniak, 2008).

Studies have also demonstrated the effectiveness of neonatal IVIG at decreasing the severity of RBC destruction (hemolysis) in HDN and subsequent development of jaundice; IVIG administered to the neonate attacks the maternal cells that destroy neonatal RBCs, slowing the progression of bilirubin production (Mundy, 2005). This therapy, often used in conjunction with phototherapy, may decrease the necessity for exchange transfusion (Gottstein and Cooke, 2003).

Intrauterine Transfusion

Infants of mothers already sensitized may be treated by intrauterine transfusion, which consists of infusing blood into the fetus's umbilical vein. The need for therapy is based on the antenatal diagnosis of isoimmunization by determining the optical density of amniotic fluid (by amniocentesis) as an index of fetal hemolysis, or by serial ultrasonography, which may detect the presence of fetal hydrops and anemia as early as 16 weeks of gestation. With ultrasound technology fetal transfusion may be accomplished directly via the umbilical vein, infusing Rh O-negative packed RBCs to raise the fetal hematocrit to 40% to 50%; fetal movement and transfusion risks are minimized by administering a muscle-paralyzing drug for temporary fetal paralysis. The frequency of intrauterine transfusions may vary according to institution yet may be as often as every 2 weeks until the fetus reaches pulmonary maturity at approximately 37 to 38 weeks of gestation (Moise, 2002, 2008).

Exchange Transfusion

Exchange transfusion, in which the infant's blood is removed in small amounts (usually 5 to 10 ml at a time) and replaced with compatible blood (Rh-negative blood), is a standard mode of therapy for treatment of severe hyperbilirubinemia that is unresponsive to phototherapy, and it is the treatment of choice for severe hyperbilirubinemia and hydrops caused by Rh incompatibility. Exchange transfusion removes the sensitized erythrocytes, lowers the serum bilirubin level to prevent bilirubin encephalopathy, corrects the anemia, and prevents cardiac failure. Indications for exchange transfusion include rapidly increasing serum bilirubin levels and hemolysis despite aggressive phototherapy. The criteria for exchange transfusion in preterm infants vary according to associated illness factors. The American Academy of Pediatrics (2004) practice parameter guidelines provide suggestions for initiating phototherapy and exchange transfusion in infants 35 weeks of gestation or more. An infant born with hydrops fetalis or signs of cardiac failure is a candidate for immediate exchange transfusion with fresh whole blood.

For exchange transfusion, fresh whole blood is typed and cross-matched to the mother's serum. The amount of donor blood used is usually double the infant's blood volume, which is approximately 85 ml/kg body weight. The double-volume exchange transfusion replaces approximately 85% of the neonate's blood.

An exchange transfusion is a sterile surgical procedure. A catheter is inserted into the umbilical vein and threaded into the inferior vena cava. Depending on the infant's weight, 5 to 10 ml of blood is withdrawn within 15 to 20 seconds, and the same volume of donor blood is infused until the targeted volume (double the estimated blood volume) is reached. If the donor blood has been citrated (addition of citrate phosphate dextrose adenine to prevent coagulation), calcium gluconate may be given after the infusion of each 100 ml of donor's blood to prevent hypocalcemia.

ABO Incompatibility

The treatment for ABO hemolytic disease is early detection and implementation of phototherapy for the reduction of hyperbilirubinemia. The initial diagnosis is often more difficult because the direct Coombs test may be negative or weakly reactive. The presence of jaundice within the first 24 hours, elevated serum bilirubin levels, RBC spherocytosis, and increased erythrocyte production is diagnostic of ABO incompatibility. In some centers IVIG transfusions are used in combination with phototherapy to treat ABO incompatibility. Exchange transfusion is not commonly required for ABO incompatibility except when phototherapy fails to decrease bilirubin concentrations.

Prognosis

The severe anemia of isoimmunization may result in stillbirth, shock, congestive heart failure, poor feeding, or poor weight gain. Perinatal survival rates for HDN are reported to be above 90% as a result of early prenatal detection and intrauterine management (Moise, 2008). Complications from exchange transfusion are uncommon; however, close monitoring is imperative.

Nursing Care Management

The initial nursing responsibility is recognizing jaundice. The possibility of hemolytic disease can be anticipated from the prenatal and perinatal history. Prenatal evidence of incompatibility, maternal blood type O, and a positive Coombs test are cause for increased vigilance for early signs of jaundice in an infant.

If an exchange transfusion is required, the nurse prepares the infant and the family and assists the practitioner with the procedure. The infant must remain NPO ("nothing by mouth") during the procedure; therefore a peripheral infusion of dextrose and electrolytes is established. The nurse documents blood volumes exchanged, including the amount of blood withdrawn and infused, the time of each procedure, and the cumulative record of the total volume exchanged. The nurse also evaluates vital signs frequently (monitored electronically during the procedure) and correlates them with the removal and infusion of blood. If signs of cardiac or respiratory problems occur, the procedure is stopped temporarily and resumed once the infant's cardiorespiratory function stabilizes. The nurse also observes for signs of transfusion reaction (temperature instability, hypotension, tachycardia, bradycardia, rash) and maintains adequate neonatal thermoregulation, blood glucose levels, and fluid balance.

Family Support

Parents often feel guilty because they think they have caused the blood incompatibility. Parents should never be made to feel responsible or negligent. The nurse encourages them to express their thoughts. The nurse should praise parents for actions they took to prevent any problems, such as frequent antepartum examinations and blood tests.

HYPOGLYCEMIA

Neonatal hypoglycemia has many recognized causes; the following discussion primarily focuses on transient neonatal hypoglycemia.

Hypoglycemia is present when the newborn's blood glucose concentration is lower than the body's requirement for cellular energy and metabolism. However, the precise definition of hypoglycemia for every newborn in regard to gestational age, birth weight, metabolic needs, and illness or wellness state remains unknown. Cornblath, Hawdon, Williams, and colleagues (2000) have suggested an operational threshold at which interventions to increase serum glucose levels should be insti-

tuted to prevent serious effects. For the healthy full-term infant, born after an uneventful pregnancy and delivery, recommendations are to monitor glucose levels only in the presence of risk factors (see following) or clinical manifestations of hypoglycemia; in these infants a plasma glucose of less than 45 mg/dl (2.5 mmol/L) requires intervention. Healthy full-term, breast-fed newborns may not fit into this category because human milk appears to provide adequate substrate (Cornblath, Hawdon, Williams, et al, 2000). Hoseth, Joergensen, Ebbesen, and colleagues (2000) evaluated blood glucose levels in healthy full-term, breast-fed infants and found significant hypoglycemia in only 2 of the 223 infants during the first 4 days of life (see Research Focus box). Maternal tobacco use, method of delivery, and anesthetics did not affect the infants' glucose levels.

> ### RESEARCH FOCUS
>
> ### *Early Breast-Feeding in Infants of Women with Gestational Diabetes*
>
> Chertok, Raz, Shoham, and colleagues (2009) reported on a study of 84 infants of women with gestational diabetes who were breast-fed in the delivery room; these infants had higher mean blood glucose levels than those who were not breast-fed in the delivery room and also in comparison to infants fed formula for the first feeding. The researchers postulated that early breast-feeding may facilitate glycemic stability in infants born to women with gestational diabetes.

In infants who are at risk for altered metabolism as a result of maternal illness factors (diabetes [gestational or otherwise], pregnancy-induced hypertension, terbutaline administration) or newborn factors (perinatal hypoxia, infection, hypothermia, polycythemia, congenital malformations, hyperinsulinism, smallness for gestational age, fetal hydrops, late-preterm birth), close observation and monitoring of blood glucose levels within 2 to 3 hours of birth are recommended. If the newborn has a blood glucose below 36 mg/dl (2.0 mmol/L), intervention such as breast- or bottle-feeding should be instituted; if levels remain low despite feeding, intravenous dextrose is warranted. In such infants the treatment should be aimed at maintaining the blood glucose levels above 45 mg/dl (2.5 mmol/L) (Cornblath, Hawdon, Williams, et al, 2000). Blood glucose levels for infants with severe hyperinsulinism may need to be higher (60 mg/dl [3.3 mmol/L]) to prevent serious effects. Hypoglycemia in preterm infants requires further study, but it has been suggested that values be maintained above 47 mg/dl (2.6 mmol/L) (Cornblath, Hawdon, Williams, et al, 2000). Cowett and Loughead (2002) concluded that plasma glucose levels below 45 mg/dl (2.5 mmol/L) are suboptimal for either the term or preterm infant and appropriate therapy should be implemented in such infants.

The decision of when to treat the hypoglycemic newborn is not based on a single plasma glucose value but on a number of clinical factors (Rozance and Hay, 2006; Sperling and Menon, 2004).

Pathophysiology

After birth the infant must supply nutrients to meet energy requirements for maintaining body temperature, respiration, muscular activity, and regulation of blood glucose. Glucose comes primarily from glycogen stores deposited in the liver, heart, and skeletal muscles during the last trimester of pregnancy.

The brain is especially dependent on adequate glucose supply for appropriate function. There is evidence of a major shift in energy metabolism from glucose to carbohydrate in newborns during the first several hours of life; hence the importance of providing adequate energy substrate. Although newborns demonstrate the ability to use ketones and amino acids as energy substrate, there are certain limitations. Infants with severe hyperinsulinism are unable to compensate metabolically and require more glucose than normal. Conditions that decrease the availability of substrate or prevent appropriate metabolism of available substrate place the infant at risk for hypoglycemia. These include intrauterine growth failure, prematurity, maternal diabetes, maternal use of hypoglycemic drugs, maternal administration of tocolytics such as terbutaline and ritodrine, intrapartum administration of glucose, perinatal hypoxia, infection, hypothermia, polycythemia, fetal hydrops, inborn errors of metabolism (IEMs) such as galactosemia, certain congenital malformations, endocrine disorders, abnormal extrauterine transition, and failure to receive adequate perinatal nutrition.

Both transient neonatal hypoglycemia and recurrent hypoglycemia are based on conditions with decreased hepatic glucose production. Transient neonatal hypoglycemia is associated with intrapartum glucose administration, terbutaline administration, gestational diabetes, intrauterine growth restriction, perinatal stress or asphyxia, prematurity, cold stress, polycythemia, and size that is large for gestational age. Recurrent hypoglycemia is observed in neonates with excessive insulin production or hyperinsulinism and includes infants with IEMs, Beckwith-Wiedmann syndrome, nesidioblastosis, Rh isoimmunization, and certain rare endocrine disorders (Cowett and Loughead, 2002; Miclic, 2008; Sperling, 2007).

Clinical Manifestations

The signs of hypoglycemia are usually vague and often indistinguishable from those observed in other newborn conditions, such as hypocalcemia, septicemia, CNS disorders, or cardiorespiratory problems. Because the brain depends on glucose for energy, cerebral signs such as jitteriness, tremors, twitching, weak or high-pitched cry, lethargy, hypotonia, limpness, seizures, and coma are prominent. Other clinical manifestations are cyanosis, apnea, rapid and irregular respirations, sweating, eye rolling, and refusal to feed. The symptoms often are transient but recurrent.

Diagnostic Evaluation

Diagnosis is confirmed by direct analysis of blood glucose concentration. Two consecutive specimens of blood should be analyzed because of the many factors that can affect readings.

Point-of-care blood glucose monitors in neonatal care must be accurate, rapid, and inexpensive; must demonstrate reliability with neonatal hematocrit ranges; must accept small blood volumes; and must provide reliable data for diagnosing neonatal hypoglycemia and hyperglycemia (Desphande and Platt, 2005; Sirkin, Jalloh, and Lee, 2002). Blood glucose measurements with a reagent strip such as Dextrostix or Chemstrip bG,

read manually or with a glucose reflectance meter, are considered inaccurate and unreliable (Desphande and Platt, 2005).

Strict quality monitoring, regular calibration, and adherence to strict protocols are necessary to ensure accuracy. The most accurate method is the laboratory analysis of serum glucose. Blood specimens may be obtained from heel, arterial, or venous punctures. (See Atraumatic Care box, p. 254 [Chapter 8].)

Proper handling of the specimen is essential because storage at room temperature increases glycolysis. Accurate readings can be facilitated by storing the blood sample on ice to slow cellular metabolism or by removing the RBCs through centrifugation.

Therapeutic Management

Intravenous infusion of glucose is one method of treating hypoglycemia. In full-term infants who are borderline hypoglycemic and *clinically asymptomatic*, the early institution of milk feeding (breast or formula) may reestablish normoglycemia, thus avoiding the need for intravenous glucose. Milk feeding likely stimulates ketogenesis and facilitates gluconeogenesis (Sperling and Menon, 2004). Infants who are at increased risk for developing hypoglycemia should have their blood glucose measured within 1 hour after birth. The procedure should be repeated every 1 to 2 hours for the first 6 to 8 hours, then every 4 to 6 hours for 2 days.

Oral glucose feedings are often used as a treatment for hypoglycemia in healthy newborns. However, formula and breast milk are just as effective. Hypoglycemia is preventable in most instances by the initiation of early feeding in healthy, asymptomatic term newborns (Cowett and Loughead, 2002). Breast-fed infants should be put to breast as soon as possible after delivery. (See Infants of Diabetic Mothers, Chapter 10, for management of hypoglycemia related to transient hyperinsulinemia.)

A systematic review by the Joanna Briggs Institute (2007) concluded that early and exclusive breast-feeding is safe and adequate to meet the metabolic needs of healthy term infants; such infants do not require glucose monitoring, nor do they require supplemental feeding with dextrose water or other milk substitutes. The study further stressed the importance of maintaining newborn thermoregulation to prevent hypoglycemia.

QUALITY PATIENT OUTCOMES: Neonatal Hypoglycemia
- Maintains blood glucose level above 45 mg/dl
- No clinical evidence of hypoglycemia
- Receives adequate carbohydrate intake

Nursing Care Management

Much of the nursing responsibility for the infant with hypoglycemia involves identification of the problem through careful observation of physical status. Another concern is to reduce environmental factors, such as cold stress and respiratory difficulty, which predispose the infant to the development of a decreased blood glucose level.

An intravenous glucose infusion is required for infants with symptomatic hypoglycemia who are unable to tolerate oral feedings, infants who are unable to maintain adequate glucose levels with oral feedings, and infants with profound hypoglycemia. An initial bolus infusion of 2 ml/kg of 10% dextrose over 1 minute followed by a continuous dextrose infusion of 6 to

8 mg/kg is appropriate therapy for the hypoglycemic infant (Miclic, 2008). Major nursing objectives include preventing, anticipating, and recognizing potential dangers of concentrated dextrose infusion. Too-rapid infusion of the hypertonic solution can cause circulatory overload, hyperglycemia, and intracellular dehydration. Maintaining the ordered flow rate with an intravenous pump and checking and charting hourly intake decrease the chance of such problems.

The infusion is administered through a peripheral vein to increase hemodilution of the concentrated solution and prevent irritation of the vessel walls. Extravasation of the fluid into the surrounding area can cause tissue sloughing. Termination of the glucose solution must be gradual to prevent hypoglycemia caused by hyperinsulinism.

Because hypoglycemia may be a symptom of some other underlying pathophysiologic process, parents are usually concerned about their infant's progress, particularly because these infants do not feed well or demonstrate behaviors that are typical of healthy infants. Nurses need to be aware of parents' thoughts, allow them to express their feelings, and update them on the infant's progress.

HYPERGLYCEMIA

Hyperglycemia in the newborn is usually defined as a blood glucose concentration greater than 125 mg/dl in the full-term infant or greater than 150 mg/dl in the preterm infant. Those affected are usually low-birth-weight infants who are unable to tolerate intravenous glucose infusions at the usual rate. The glucose intolerance is probably related to general immaturity of the usual regulatory mechanisms. Increased blood glucose levels may also occur in infants with sepsis or decreased insulin sensitivity (such as infants with transient diabetes mellitus), infants receiving methylxanthines, and infants who are stressed (e.g., infants with respiratory distress syndrome, infants undergoing surgical procedures).

Hyperglycemia is usually asymptomatic but detected on routine screening. Most often, hyperglycemia is treated by reducing the infant's glucose intake. Untreated hyperglycemia may result in an osmotic diuresis with subsequent fluid volume loss and dehydration; if severe, it may result in an intraventricular hemorrhage as a result of fluid shifts in the CNS (Blackburn, 2007). Insulin infusion is sometimes administered to very low–birth-weight infants who require but are unable to tolerate intravenous dextrose solutions with concentrations greater than 5 g/dl.

Nursing Care Management

Monitor blood glucose frequently, especially in the infant receiving insulin. This requires numerous heel sticks, and sites should be rotated to minimize tissue damage. (See Blood Specimens, Chapter 27, and the Atraumatic Care box titled "Heel Punctures" in Chapter 8.) Carefully measure urinary output to detect any evidence of glycosuria and possible osmotic diuresis.

As in the care of all infants, give parents a careful explanation of the therapy, provide frequent progress reports, and support them to reduce anxiety. (See Nursing Care of High-Risk Newborns, Chapter 10.)

HYPOCALCEMIA

As with many conditions in the neonate, hypocalcemia is difficult to differentiate from other disorders (sepsis, meningitis, narcotic withdrawal, hypoglycemia), and the etiology may be ill defined. The incidence is highest at two times during the neonatal period. Early-onset hypocalcemia, which appears within the first 24 to 48 hours, is the more common form and typically affects the preterm or small-for-gestational-age infant and any infant who has experienced perinatal asphyxia. Preterm infants may have hypocalcemia as a result of inadequate calcium intake, increased calcitonin levels, possibly resistance to parathyroid hormone activation preventing calcium removal from bones, acidosis, and decreased vitamin D intake and absorption (Blackburn, 2007). An infant born to a diabetic mother may also experience early hypocalcemia, possibly as a result of relative maternal hyperparathyroidism and transient neonatal hypoparathyroidism. Symptoms include jitteriness, prolonged QT interval, apnea, cyanotic episodes, a high-pitched cry, and abdominal distention.

Late-onset hypocalcemia, which is not apparent until after the first 3 or 4 days of life, is referred to as cow's milk–induced hypocalcemia or neonatal tetany. Although uncommon in developed countries, it may be observed in well-nourished infants who are fed modified cow's milk, such as evaporated milk formula. Cow's milk, which has a high phosphorus content, produces hyperphosphatemia and a resultant hypocalcemia by increasing calcium deposition in the bone and soft tissues. Late hypocalcemia may also be seen in infants with intestinal malabsorption, hyperinsulinemia, hypoparathyroidism, or hypomagnesemia.

The manifestations of neonatal tetany reflect neuromuscular irritation: twitching, tremors, irritability, high-pitched cry, tachycardia, and rarely seizures (Blackburn, 2007). The preterm neonate with hypocalcemia may be asymptomatic. Neonatal tetany is rarely seen in industrialized countries because of the prevalent use of commercial formula or human milk as the newborn's primary source of nutrition.

In some preterm neonates, rickets and osteopenia may occur as a result of calcium or phosphorus deficiency in association with vitamin D deficiency, which prevents adequate intestinal absorption of minerals (Blackburn, 2007). Very low–birth-weight infants, infants with chronic conditions such as chronic lung disease (bronchopulmonary dysplasia), and infants on prolonged diuretic management are at particular risk for developing rickets and osteopenia (Blackburn, 2007). There have been reported cases of vitamin D deficiency in healthy breast-fed infants who received minimal ultraviolet light exposure or whose breast-feeding mother had a diet deficient in vitamin D; hence the American Academy of Pediatrics' (2008a) recommendation for vitamin D supplementation (400 international units/day, oral) in all newborns exclusively breast-fed.

Diagnostic Evaluation

Diagnosis of hypocalcemia is confirmed with serum electrolyte determinations. Normal infant serum calcium values are usually in the range of 7.0 to 8.0 mg/dl (1.75 to 2.0 mmol/L) (Blackburn, 2007).

In full-term infants hypocalcemia is indicated at total serum calcium levels below 7.8 to 8 mg/dl (1.95 to 2.0 mmol/L) or ionized calcium levels (the biologically important fraction of calcium) below 3.0 to 4.4 mg/dl (1.1 mmol/L). In preterm infants a lower limit of 7.0 mg/dl (1.8 mmol/L) is considered hypocalcemic (Blackburn, 2007). Most clinicians consider the serum ionized calcium to be the best standard for monitoring blood calcium activity.

Therapeutic Management

In most instances early-onset hypocalcemia is temporary and resolves in 1 to 3 days. Restoration of a normal calcium level is facilitated by early feedings, physiologic correction of hypoparathyroidism, and, sometimes, administration of calcium supplements.

Treatment of hypocalcemia involves intravenous administration of 10% calcium gluconate. The drug is administered slowly over 10 to 30 minutes or as a continuous infusion; intravenous administration should not exceed 100 mg/min (Custer and Rau, 2009). Rapid intravenous calcium administration may cause cardiac dysrhythmias and circulatory collapse. The heart rate and blood pressure should be electronically monitored. Take care to ascertain that the infusion device is positioned within the vein because extravasation into surrounding tissue causes local necrosis, calcification, and sloughing. *Intramuscular* administration of calcium gluconate is *contraindicated* because it precipitates in the tissue, causing necrosis. If the infant can tolerate oral fluids, oral doses of calcium are given with formula. Adequate intake of vitamin D and phosphorus is imperative, especially in extremely low– and very low–birth-weight infants. Exercise caution in the use of oral calcium salts because of their hypertonicity and subsequent effects on the bowel of at-risk infants.

Nursing Care Management

Nursing care of the infant with hypocalcemia is directed toward identifying infants at risk for early hypocalcemia, observing for clinical manifestations in such infants, and administering supplemental calcium, vitamin D, and phosphorus. Monitor the infant continuously during intravenous infusions. Calcium gluconate can cause tissue necrosis and scar formation; therefore it is recommended that superficial veins such as those on the scalp be avoided. To prevent tissue necrosis, carefully observe the infusion site and changes it as needed. Calcium gluconate is also incompatible with a number of drugs, most notably sodium bicarbonate.

The nurse also observes for signs of acute hypercalcemia (vomiting, bradycardia). If such symptoms occur, discontinue the injection or infusion and notify the practitioner. Institute seizure precautions because seizures are common.

To prevent late-onset hypocalcemia, the nurse provides preventive care and anticipatory guidance regarding the correct use of an infant formula containing the appropriate balance of calcium and phosphorus and assists the parent in planning for meeting the growing infant's nutritional needs through an affordable commercial infant formula.

If the infant is discharged on formula feedings supplemented with calcium, teach the parents the correct procedure for diluting the mineral in the formula and advise them to use only the prescribed formula. Also teach parents to observe for any signs of hypocalcemia or hypercalcemia in the infant receiving supplemental calcium.

HEMORRHAGIC DISEASE OF THE NEWBORN

Hemorrhagic disease of the newborn, or vitamin K deficiency bleeding, is a bleeding disorder that occurs as a result of a vitamin K deficiency. Hemorrhagic disease may be classified according to appearance as early, classic, or late onset. Newborns' vitamin K stores are virtually absent and prothrombin activity is moderately deficient, decreases until approximately 72 hours after birth, and then begins to increase. Consequently, vitamin K–dependent coagulation factors (II, VII, IX, X) are significantly reduced. In addition, the newborn's relatively sterile intestinal tract is unable to synthesize the vitamin until feedings have begun.

Signs and symptoms of hemorrhagic disease typically appear within hours of birth and can include oozing from the umbilicus or circumcision site, bloody or black stools, hematuria, ecchymoses on the skin and scalp, epistaxis, or bleeding from punctures. Classic hemorrhagic disease usually occurs 1 to 7 days after birth. Signs and symptoms are the same as those seen with early-onset disease. Diagnosis is confirmed by findings of prolonged prothrombin time and partial thromboplastin time accompanied by normal platelet count and fibrinogen level.

Infants born to mothers who are taking antiepileptic drugs phenytoin and phenobarbital may have a severe form of hemorrhagic disease of the newborn and should be carefully evaluated and treated accordingly. The bleeding is most severe within the first 24 hours of life and may require treatment with intravenous vitamin K and fresh frozen plasma (Stoll, 2007).

A late form of hemorrhagic disease (late onset) appears at approximately 2 to 12 weeks of age. This form occurs in totally or predominantly breast-fed infants who did not receive adequate vitamin K prophylaxis at birth. Although vitamin K levels in breast milk appear to be lower than in cow's milk–based formulas, previous studies indicate that hemorrhagic disease occurred in infants who were exclusively breast-fed and who did not receive the standard prophylaxis at birth or were given a single dose of oral vitamin K (Lawrence and Lawrence, 2005). Manifestations of late-onset disease include evidence of intracranial hemorrhage; deep ecchymoses; and bleeding from the gastrointestinal tract, mucous membranes, skin punctures, or surgical incisions.

Therapeutic Management

The goal of management is prevention of hemorrhagic disease of the newborn with prophylactic administration of vitamin K. In the United States, intramuscular administration of vitamin K (phytonadione [AquaMEPHYTON, Mephyton]) in a dose of 0.5 to 1 mg once during the first few hours after birth is standard practice. The current recommendation to prevent hemorrhagic disease in infants who are breast-fed is to provide intramuscular vitamin K at birth and for the mother to have a well-balanced diet (American Academy of Pediatrics, 2009a). The administration of oral vitamin K is currently not recommended to prevent neonatal hemorrhagic disease (Stoll, 2007).

In newborns with hemorrhagic disease, treatment is the same as the preventive measures except that the vitamin may be given intravenously to prevent a hematoma at an intramuscular site. Bleeding usually ceases within 2 to 4 hours of vitamin K administration.

Nursing Care Management

Nursing care primarily involves prevention through careful administration of the vitamin into the vastus lateralis or ventrogluteal (not dorsogluteal) muscle. In instances in which this procedure is not routinely carried out (e.g., home births or emergency deliveries), the nurse observes for signs of the bleeding disorder and notifies the practitioner for appropriate diagnosis and treatment. Encourage breast-feeding mothers to increase their intake of foods containing vitamin K; the best sources are green vegetables, especially broccoli.

INBORN ERRORS OF METABOLISM

IEMs include a large number of inherited diseases caused by interruptions in the various pathways involved in the metabolism of protein, carbohydrates, or lipids. Fig. 9-9 is a conceptual model representing the multiple interactions in a metabolic pathway in health and disease. **Metabolic pathways** are series of biochemical reactions by which substrates are sequentially converted into other by-products, aiming at a final end-product that can be successfully used or eliminated by the body. Each of these transformations is mediated by an enzyme, which is under the control of a specific structural gene. Fig. 9-9, *A*, represents the normal metabolic conversion of substance **A** into end-product **K**, via by-products **B, C, D**, etc. Enzymes **b** and **c**, whose synthesis is controlled by genes β and δ, catalyze steps **B** → **C** and **C** → **D**, respectively. A feedback loop ensures physiologic levels of **K**. A gene mutation may result in qualitative or quantitative changes in the enzyme, resulting in a different (and therefore ineffective) enzyme, or in the decreased synthesis of the enzyme, including its total absence. This ineffective (or missing) enzyme will interrupt the pathway, resulting in accumulation of the by-product that immediately precedes the blockage, as well as lack of the by-products beyond the blockage. IEMs can occur as a result of such accumulations or absences of an essential by-product.

In Fig. 9-9, *B*, a mutation in gene β prevents normal synthesis of enzyme **b**, creating an interruption of the pathway between **B** and **C**. Assuming a continuous uptake of **A**, two outcomes ensue: accumulation of **B**, and depletion of all products beyond the block (**C, D, ... K**). An example of this situation is Tay-Sachs disease (or GM₂ gangliosidosis). In this disease, a mutation in the *HexA* gene (here exemplified by β) causes the lack of the enzyme hexosaminidase A (HexA), represented by **b**. Absence of **b** creates an accumulation of ganglioside GM₂ (**B**)—lipids, in nerve cells, resulting in the clinical manifestations of this progressive neurologic disorder because the lipids are not broken down by the cellular liposomes.

Fig. 9-9, *C*, depicts a mutation in gene δ, which causes depletion of enzyme **c** and interrupts the metabolic conversion of **C** into **D**. In this instance, an alternative pathway **C** → **E** → **F** is opened. This event may have two outcomes: product **F** may eventually be converted into **K**, with no significant clinical con-

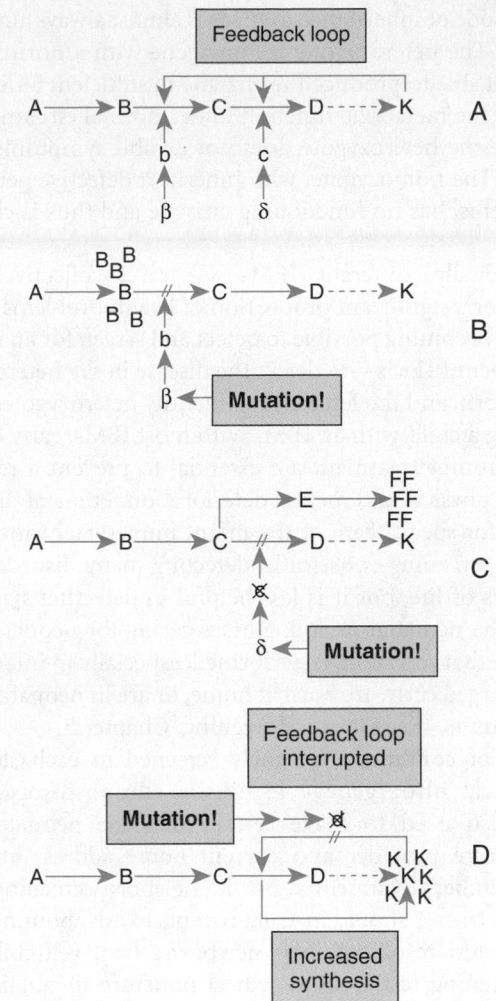

Fig. 9-9 Metabolic pathway. **A,** Normal metabolic pathway. **B,** Mutation of gene β. **C,** Mutation of gene δ. **D,** Genetic alteration of enzyme d. *A,* Substance; *B-F,* by-products; *K,* end-product; *b, c,* and, *d,* enzymes; β and δ, genes. (Adapted from da Cunha MF: Genetic basis of human disease. In Bullock BA, Henze RL, editors: *Focus on physiology,* Philadelphia, 2000, Lippincott.)

sequences; or **F** may represent the end-point to the alternative pathway. If accumulation of **F** reaches toxic levels, a disease process may occur. Such is the case with PKU, an IEM that creates an intolerance to the amino acid phenylalanine. The missing enzyme (**c**, in this case), which results from mutation in the phenylalanine hydroxylase (*PAH*) gene (δ), is phenylalanine hydroxylase. The alternative pathway leads to the formation and accumulation of phenylketones (**F**). In combination with phenylalanine deficiency, an excessive amount of phenylketones contributes to the postnatal completion of myelination of nerves, resulting in profound cognitive impairment.

Fig. 9-9, *D*, represents a genetic alteration of the enzyme **d**, which is involved in the feedback control of synthesis of **K**. As a result, **K** may accumulate to toxic levels. The prototype genetic disease here is Lesch-Nyhan syndrome, in which **d** is the enzyme hypoxanthine-guanine phosphoribosyltransferase (HGPRT) and **K** is uric acid. A deficiency in HGPRT and accumulation of uric acid to extremely high levels will result in the development of cognitive impairment and self-mutilation tendency.

The mode of inheritance in IEMs is almost always autosomal recessive. The heterozygote has one gene with a normal effect and is still able to produce the enzyme in sufficient amounts to carry out the metabolic function under normal circumstances. Therefore the heterozygote does not exhibit symptoms of the disorder. The homozygote, who inherits a defective gene from both parents, has no functioning enzyme and thus is clinically affected.

Individually, different IEMs are rare; collectively they account for a significant proportion of health problems in children. It is becoming possible to detect and screen for an increasing number of IEMs—to detect the disease in the heterozygote, the newborn, and the fetus and to identify heterozygotes at risk for having a child with an IEM. With most IEMs, early diagnosis and prompt treatment are essential to prevent a relentless course of physical and mental deterioration. Prenatal diagnosis provides for special care of the infant immediately after birth. Neonatal screening is useful in detecting many disorders after a few days of life, but it is less helpful in detecting symptoms early in the neonatal period. Nurses caring for neonates must be certain that screening is performed, especially in infants who are discharged early, are born at home, or are in neonatal intensive care units. (See Genetic Screening, Chapter 5.)

A list of conditions routinely screened in each state can be found at http://genes-r-us.uthscsa.edu/nbsdisorders.pdf. Nurses also need to make certain that the neonate has a primary care provider and current home address and telephone number documented on the newborn screening blood spot card. Nurses should instruct parents to ask about newborn screening test results at their newborn's first well-child visit. Most screening tests require a heel puncture to obtain sufficient blood to completely cover circles on special blotting paper. A new screening test, tandem mass spectrometry, has the potential to identify up to 40 IEMs. With tandem mass spectrometry, earlier identification of IEMs may prevent further developmental delays and morbidities in affected children. (See Atraumatic Care box, p. 254, for measures to reduce the pain of lancing and squeezing the heel, and see Newborn Screening for Disease, Chapter 8.)

Some nonspecific manifestations—including lethargy, poor feeding, vomiting, diarrhea, hypoglycemia, metabolic acidosis, respiratory distress, apnea, hypothermia, coma, and seizures—occur in a wide variety of genetic and acquired disorders. The time of onset may be important. Most IEMs produce no symptoms during the first 24 hours of life. Other manifestations that may indicate an IEM include jaundice, hepatomegaly, unusual odor (sweat, urine, feces), abnormal eating patterns (food aversions, vomiting after eating certain foods), coarse facial features, macroglossia (enlarged tongue), abnormal hair, dysmorphic features, and abnormal eye findings (e.g., cataracts, retinal changes). A family history of neonatal deaths (within the same sibling group, or among family members) alerts the observer to the possibility of an IEM. The initial recognition of signs that might indicate an IEM is the responsibility of health professionals, including nurses.

Although there are many categories of IEMs, only three are discussed here because they can be identified in the neonatal period and because treatment has been reasonably successful. They are examples of (1) disorders of protein metabolism (PKU), (2) disorders of carbohydrate metabolism (galactosemia), and (3) disorders of hormone synthesis (congenital hypothyroidism). (Table 5-4 outlines other IEMs.)

PHENYLKETONURIA

PKU, a genetic disease inherited as an autosomal recessive trait, is caused by an absence of the enzyme phenylalanine hydroxylase needed to metabolize the essential amino acid phenylalanine. The prevalence of PKU varies widely in the United States because different states have different definition criteria for what constitutes hyperphenylalaninemia and PKU. The reported figures for PKU range from 1 per 19,000 to 1 per 13,500 live births. The disease has a wide variation of incidence by ethnic groups. The disease is most prevalent among individuals of Northern European ancestry, American Indians, and Alaskan Natives, whereas African-American, Hispanic, Jewish, and Asian individuals account for the lowest frequencies (Hellekson, 2001). Among African-Americans, for instance, the incidence of PKU is 1 per 50,000 live births (McPhee and Ganong, 2006).

Classic PKU is at one end of a spectrum of conditions that involve defects of amino acids phenylalanine and tyrosine metabolism known as hyperphenylalaninemia. Within the spectrum of hyperphenylalaninemia are conditions with varying degrees of severity depending on the degree of enzyme deficiency (Rezvani, 2007). Because other forms are the result of a deficiency of other enzymes and are diagnosed and treated differently, the following discussion of PKU is limited to the severe, classic form.

Pathophysiology

In PKU the hepatic enzyme phenylalanine hydroxylase, which controls the conversion of phenylalanine to tyrosine, is absent. This results in the accumulation of phenylalanine in the bloodstream and urinary excretion of abnormal amounts of its metabolites, the phenyl acids (Fig. 9-10). One of these phenyl ketones, phenylpyruvic acid, gives urine the characteristic musty odor associated with this disease and is responsible for the term *phenylketonuria*.

Amino acids produced by the metabolism of phenylalanine are absent in PKU. One of these, tyrosine, is needed to form the pigment melanin and the hormones epinephrine and thyroxine. Decreased melanin production results in similar phenotypes of most children with PKU: blond hair, blue eyes, and fair skin that is particularly susceptible to eczema and other dermatologic problems. Children with a genetically darker skin color may be red haired or brunette.

Severe hyperphenylalaninemia (>360 to 600 mmol/L) causes progressive damage to the developing brain with severe consequences: defective myelination, cystic degeneration of the gray and white matter, and disturbances in cortical lamination. Cognitive impairment occurs before the metabolites are detected in the urine and will progress if ingested phenylalanine levels are not lowered.

Clinical Manifestations

Clinical manifestations of PKU include growth failure (failure to thrive); frequent vomiting; irritability; hyperactivity; and

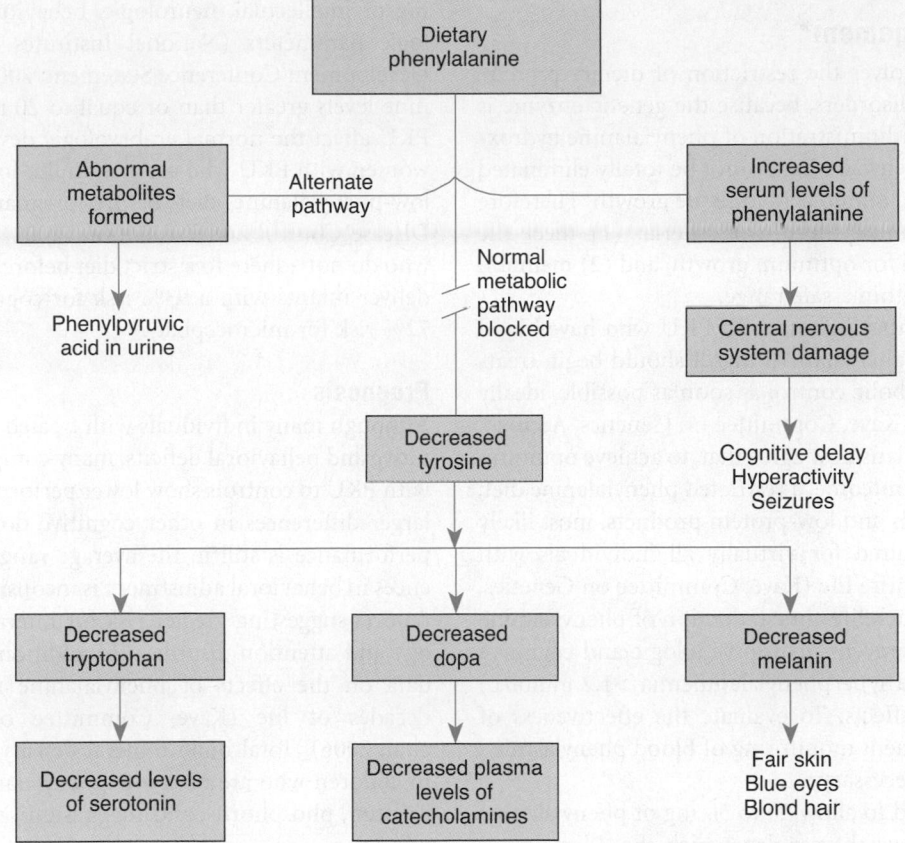

Fig. 9-10 Metabolic errors and consequences in phenylketonuria.

unpredictable, erratic behavior. Older children commonly display bizarre or schizoid behavior patterns such as fright reactions, screaming episodes, head banging, arm biting, disorientation, failure to respond to strong stimuli, and spasticity or catatonia-like positions. Many of the severely cognitively impaired children have seizures, and approximately 80% of untreated persons with PKU demonstrate abnormal electroencephalographs, regardless of whether overt seizures occur.

Diagnostic Evaluation*

The objective in diagnosing or treating the disorder is to prevent cognitive impairment. The most commonly used test for screening newborns is the Guthrie bacterial inhibition assay for phenylalanine in the blood. *Bacillus subtilis*, present in the culture medium, grows if the blood contains an excessive amount of phenylalanine. The normal range of blood phenylalanine concentration in newborns is 0.5 to 1 mg/dl. The Guthrie test detects serum phenylalanine levels greater than 4 mg/dl (normal value is 1.6 mg/dl). Only fresh heel blood, not cord blood, can be used for the test.

Newborn screening tests are mandatory in all 50 U.S. states. The screening test is most reliable if the blood sample is taken after the infant has ingested a source of protein. Because of early

discharge of newborns, recommendations for screening include (1) collecting the initial specimen as close as possible to discharge and no later than 7 days after birth, (2) obtaining a subsequent sample by 2 weeks of age if the initial specimen is collected before the newborn is 24 hours old, and (3) designating a primary care provider to all newborns before discharge for adequate newborn follow-up screening (Kaye, Committee on Genetics, Accurso, et al, 2006). In several states a second newborn screening is performed when the infant is 1 to 2 weeks old, on the basis that a maximum number of children with genetic disorders will be identified (American Academy of Pediatrics, 2008b). After a positive screen, diagnostic testing must be performed promptly (Kaye, Committee on Genetics, Accurso, et al, 2006).

When collecting the specimen, avoid "layering" the blood specimen on the special Guthrie paper. Layering is placing one drop of blood on top of the other or overlapping the specimen. Best results are obtained by collecting the specimen with a pipette from the heel stick and spreading the blood uniformly over the blot paper.

A major concern is that a significant number of infants are not rescreened for PKU after early discharge and are at risk for a missed or delayed diagnosis. Give special consideration to screening infants born at home who have no hospital contact, as well as infants adopted internationally.

Because of the possibility of variant forms of hyperphenylalaninemia, a natural dietary protein challenge test is recommended after approximately 3 months of dietary treatment to confirm the diagnosis of classic PKU.

*Always refer patient to a genetic metabolic specialist. For a reference list, visit the American Society of Human Genetics website, **www.ashg.org**.

Therapeutic Management*

Treatment of PKU involves the restriction of dietary protein. As with most genetic disorders, because the genetic enzyme is intracellular, systemic administration of phenylalanine hydroxylase is of no value. Phenylalanine cannot be totally eliminated because it is an essential amino acid in tissue growth. Therefore dietary management must meet two criteria: (1) meet the child's nutritional need for optimum growth, and (2) maintain phenylalanine levels within a safe range.

Professionals agree that infants with PKU who have blood phenylalanine levels higher than 10 mg/dl should begin treatment to establish metabolic control as soon as possible, ideally by 7 to 10 days of age (Kaye, Committee on Genetics, Accurso, et al, 2006). Most clinicians now agree that, to achieve optimum metabolic control and outcome, a restricted phenylalanine diet, including medical foods and low-protein products, most likely will be medically required for virtually all individuals with classic PKU for their entire life (Kaye, Committee on Genetics, Accurso, et al, 2006). Such life-time reduction of phenylalanine intake is necessary to prevent neuropsychologic and cognitive deficits, since even a mild hyperphenylalaninemia (>1.2 mmol/L) would produce such effects. To evaluate the effectiveness of dietary treatment, frequent monitoring of blood phenylalanine and tyrosine levels is necessary.

The diet is calculated to allow 20 to 30 mg of phenylalanine per kilogram of body weight per day, which should maintain serum phenylalanine levels between 2 and 8 mg/dl. Significant brain damage is likely to occur when levels are greater than 11 to 15 mg/dl. In the United States a level of 2 to 6 mg/dl is recommended for children 12 years and younger and 2 to 10 mg/dl for older persons (Kaye, Committee on Genetics, Accurso, et al, 2006). For optimum growth to occur, the diet begins no later than 3 weeks of age.

Because all natural food proteins contain approximately 15% phenylalanine, specially prepared milk substitutes are prescribed for the infant (Table 9-3). Some of these products are made from specially treated enzymatic casein hydrolysate, which provides only 0.4% phenylalanine (28.5 mg/8 oz). They also contain minerals and vitamins to provide a balanced nutritional formula. Tyrosine and several other amino acids are supplied in the formula. Because of the low phenylalanine content of breast milk, total or partial breast-feeding may be possible with close monitoring of phenylalanine levels (Lawrence and Lawrence, 2005). Diet substitutes for older children, such as Phenyl-Free 2 (Mead Johnson) and Phenex-2 (Ross), contain no phenylalanine and allow for greater exchanges with natural low-phenylalanine foods in the diet, leading to a more normal diet.

A low-phenylalanine diet begins as soon as possible after birth and continues throughout life. Adherence to this diet can be especially challenging in adolescence and adulthood. To evaluate the effectiveness of dietary treatment, frequent monitoring of blood phenylalanine and tyrosine levels is necessary. Achieving optimum outcomes also relies on periodic monitoring of intellectual, neurologic, behavioral, and neuropsychologic parameters (National Institutes of Health Consensus Development Conference Statement, 2001). Because phenylalanine levels greater than or equal to 20 mg/dl in mothers with PKU affect the normal embryologic development of the fetus, women with PKU who are not on life-long diet must resume a low-phenylalanine diet before pregnancy. The Centers for Disease Control and Prevention (2002) reported that women who do not adhere to a strict diet before and during pregnancy deliver infants with a 93% risk for cognitive impairment and 72% risk for microcephaly.†

Prognosis

Although many individuals with treated PKU manifest no cognitive and behavioral deficits, many comparisons of individuals with PKU to controls show lower performance on IQ tests, with larger differences in other cognitive domains. However, their performance is still in the average range. Evidence for differences in behavioral adjustment is inconsistent despite anecdotal reports suggesting greater risk for internalizing psychopathology and attention disorders. In addition, there are insufficient data on the effects of phenylalanine restriction over many decades of life (Kaye, Committee on Genetics, Accurso, et al, 2006). Total bone mineral density is considerably lower in children who are on a low-phenylalanine diet, even though calcium, phosphorus, and magnesium intakes are higher than normal.

Currently, treatment for many genetic diseases aims at modifying the phenotypical expression of those conditions. In the case of PKU, early childhood treatment with a reduced phenylalanine diet is highly successful at removing the possibility of cognitive impairment. However, PKU-rescued adults (i.e., those treated with reduction of phenylalanine in early childhood) remain unable to metabolize the amino acid and will always exhibit phenylalaninemia. For this reason, life-long low-phenylalanine diet is recommended (Moyle, Fox, Bynevelt, et al, 2007). PKU-rescued women who do not maintain low phenylalanine levels tend to produce children with cognitive and developmental impairments. Although indirectly related to the maternal PKU genotype, this is due to the fact that embryos are developing in a uterine environment with excessive concentrations of blood phenylalanine. To avoid this possibility, PKU-rescued women contemplating motherhood need to be placed again on low-phenylalanine diet for the duration of the pregnancy.

Recently sapropterin dihydrochloride, or BH4, has been used successfully in persons with hyperphenylalaninemia to decrease circulating phenylalanine levels. BH4 was given in weight-based daily oral doses of 5 to 20 mg/kg/day and was shown to effectively reduce phenylalanine levels in persons 8 years old and older (Lee, Treacy, Crombez, et al, 2008). Additional data indicate that BH4 may be safely tolerated by children as young as 4 years of age; in this study children were able to increase phenylalanine daily intake slightly because of the blood level reductions caused by the drug (Trefz, Burton, Longo, et al, 2009). It

---

*A resource for dietary management is Acosta PB, Yannicelli S: *The Ross metabolic formula system nutrition support protocols,* ed 4, Columbus, Ohio, 2001, Abbott Nutrition; 800-227-5767; http://abbottnutrition.com.

†For more information, contact American Society of Human Genetics, 9650 Rockville Pike, Bethesda, MD 20814; 301-634-7300, 866-HUM-GENE; www.ashg.org.

TABLE 9-3   FORMULAS FOR INFANTS AND TODDLERS WITH METABOLIC CONDITIONS*†

FORMULA (MANUFACTURER)	COMMENTS AND NUTRITIONAL CONSIDERATIONS
Phenyl-Free 1 (Mead Johnson)	Phenylalanine free; use for infants and toddlers with PKU; iron fortified; powder; phenylalanine from breast milk, infant formula, or other foods required to support growth; lactose free
Phenyl-Free 2 (Mead Johnson)	Phenylalanine free; use for children >1 yr of age and adults with PKU; iron fortified; powder; permits increased supplementation with normal foods; higher protein content than Phenyl-Free 1
Phenex-1 (Ross)	Phenylalanine free; powder; use for infants and toddlers with PKU
Phenex-2 (Ross)	Phenylalanine free; powder; use for children and adults with PKU
Phenyl-Free 2 HP (Mead Johnson)	Phenylalanine free; powder; use for children and adults with PKU; permits increased supplementation with normal foods
Similac Isomil Advance	Lactose-free, soy-based formula for infants with galactosemia; Similac Go & Grow for children 9-24 mo of age
RCF (Ross)	Carbohydrate-free soy formula with iron; may be used in children with carbohydrate intolerance or galactosemia
Enfamil ProSobee Lipil (Mead Johnson)	Soy-based, lactose-free formula for infants with galactosemia; contains AA and DHA (LCPUFAs) (see also Chapter 8, Infant Formulas)
Enfamil Next Step ProSobee Lipil (Mead Johnson)	Soy-based, lactose-free formula for infants with galactosemia; contains AA and DHA (for infants ≥9 mo old)

AA, Arachidonic acid; *DHA,* docosahexaenoic acid; *LCPUFAs,* long-chain polyunsaturated fatty acids; *PKU,* phenylketonuria.
*Ross Laboratories and Mead Johnson manufacture several specialty formulas for metabolic disorders for infants. For a comprehensive list of metabolic disease formulas, contact the manufacturers.
†This is not an exhaustive list of metabolic formulas or companies that offer such products. Reader is advised to consult primary care practitioner for additional information and specific guidelines for feeding children with special dietary needs.

is important to note that those taking BH4 in these studies remained on a phenylalanine diet restriction.

Nursing Care Management

The principal nursing considerations involve teaching the family regarding the dietary restrictions. Although the treatment may sound simple, the task of maintaining such a strict dietary regimen is demanding, especially for older children and adolescents. Foods with low phenylalanine levels (e.g., some vegetables [except legumes]; fruits; juices; and some cereals, breads, and starches) must be measured to provide the prescribed amount of phenylalanine. Most high-protein foods, such as meat and dairy products, are either eliminated or restricted to small amounts.

Maintaining the diet during infancy presents few problems. Parents can introduce solid foods such as cereal, fruits, and vegetables as usual to the infant. Difficulties arise as the child gets older. A decreased appetite and refusal to eat may reduce intake of the calculated phenylalanine requirement. The child's increasing independence may inhibit absolute control of what he or she eats. Either factor can result in decreased or increased phenylalanine levels. During the school years, peer pressure becomes a major force in deterring the child from eating the prescribed foods or abstaining from high-protein foods such as milkshakes or ice cream. Limitations of this diet are best illustrated by an example: a $\frac{1}{4}$-lb hamburger may provide a 2-day phenylalanine allowance for a school-age child. Illness and growth spurts increase the body's need for this essential amino acid. Adolescence is a particularly difficult period, and limiting foods containing phenylalanine in adolescents with PKU is challenging. Special camps to educate adolescent girls with PKU regarding appropriate food intake demonstrated short-term effects in decreasing blood phenylalanine levels (Singh, Kable, Guerrero, et al, 2000). However, studies show a gradual decline in diet compliance with consequent increases in blood phenylalanine levels during early adolescence and young adulthood (Walter and White, 2004).

The assistance of a registered dietitian is essential. Parents need a basic understanding of the disorder and practical suggestions regarding food selection and preparation.* A number of support groups for parents of children with PKU are available nationwide. Many Internet resources also contain valuable information regarding dietary counseling and food options. Meal planning is based on an exchange list. As soon as children are old enough, usually by early preschool, they should be involved in the daily calculation, menu planning, and formula preparation. A computer voice-activated calculator, cards, or colored beads can help children keep track of the daily allowance of phenylalanine foods. A system of goal setting, self-monitoring, contracts, and rewards can promote compliance in adolescents.

Family Support†

In addition to the problems related to a child with a chronic disorder (see Chapter 22), the parents have the burden of knowing they are carriers of the defect and must make serious decisions regarding future children. Prenatal testing is now available to detect the *PAH* mutation in heterozygotes. Genetic counseling is especially important to ensure that the heterozygote couple understands their recurrence risk. Genetic counseling is needed for the person with PKU when he or she is of reproductive age to learn about the chances of having a child with PKU or a child affected by a high phenylalanine in-utero environment. (See Role of Nurses in Genetic Counseling and Referral, Chapter 5.)

---

*A helpful resource is Schuett V, editor: *Low protein cookery for phenylketonuria,* ed 3, Madison, Wis, 1997, University of Wisconsin Press.
†National support groups include the Children's PKU Network, which offers a variety of support services: 3790 Via de la Valle, Suite 120, Del Mar, CA 92014; 800-377-6677; e-mail: PKUnetwork@aol.com; www.pkunetwork.org; and the National PKU Alliance, Christine Brown, Executive Director, PO Box 501, Tomahawk, WI 54487; 715-437-0477; www.npkua.org.

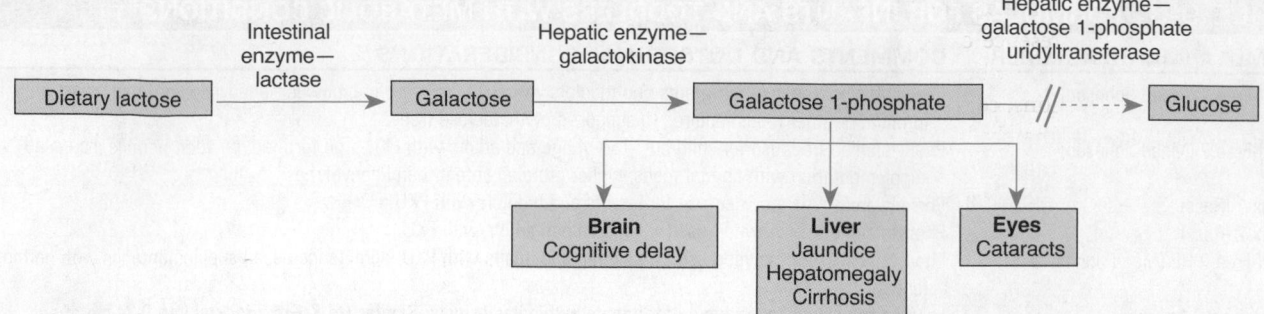

Fig. 9-11 Metabolic errors and consequences in galactosemia.

GALACTOSEMIA

Galactosemia is a rare autosomal recessive disorder that results from various gene mutations leading to three distinct enzymatic deficiencies. The most common type of galactosemia (classic galactosemia) results from a deficiency of a hepatic enzyme, galactose 1-phosphate uridyltransferase (GALT), and affects approximately 1 of 47,000 births. The other two varieties of galactosemia involve deficiencies in the enzymes galactokinase (GALK) and galactose 4'-epimerase (GALE); these are extremely rare disorders (Kaye, Committee on Genetics, Accurso, et al, 2006). All three enzymes (GALT, GALK, and GALE) are involved in the conversion of galactose into glucose (Fig. 9-11).

Accumulation of activated 1-phosphate metabolites of galactose (and fructose) is extremely toxic to various tissues, especially in the kidneys, liver, and nervous system. As galactose 1-phosphate accumulates in the blood, a series of abnormalities develop. Hepatic dysfunction leads to cirrhosis, resulting in jaundice in the infant by the second week of life. The spleen subsequently becomes enlarged as a result of portal hypertension. Cataracts are usually recognizable by 1 or 2 months of age; cerebral damage, manifested by the symptoms of lethargy and hypotonia, is evident soon afterward. Infants with galactosemia appear normal at birth, but on ingestion of milk (which has a high lactose content) they begin to show progressive symptoms, including vomiting, diarrhea, and weight loss (Askin and Diehl-Jones, 2003). *Escherichia coli* sepsis is another common initial clinical sign (Kaye, Committee on Genetics, Accurso, et al, 2006; Kishnani and Chen, 2007). Death during the first month of life is frequent in untreated infants.

Diagnostic Evaluation*

Diagnosis is made on the basis of the infant's history, physical examination, galactosuria, increased levels of galactose in the blood, or decreased levels of uridine diphosphate–galactose transferase activity in erythrocytes. The infant may display characteristics of malnutrition and dehydration; decreased muscle mass and body fat may be evident. Newborn screening for this disease is required in all states (http://genes-r-us.uthscsa.edu/nbsdisorders.pdf). Heterozygotes can also be identified, since they have significantly lower levels of the essential enzyme. Although asymptomatic, such individuals have been noted to spontaneously dislike and therefore limit the ingestion of galactose-containing foods.

Therapeutic Management

During infancy, treatment consists of eliminating all milk and lactose-containing formula, including breast milk. Traditionally, lactose-free formulas are used, with soy-protein formula being the feeding of choice (see Table 9-3). However, recent research suggests that elemental formula (galactose-free) may be more beneficial than soy formulas (Zlatunich and Packman, 2005). The American Academy of Pediatrics (2009a) recommends the use of soy formula for infants diagnosed with galactosemia. As the infant progresses to solids, only foods low in galactose should be consumed. Certain fruits are high in galactose, and some dietitians recommend that they be avoided. Nurses should give food lists to the family to ensure appropriate foods are chosen.

If galactosemia is suspected, implement supportive treatment and care, including monitoring for hypoglycemia, liver failure, bleeding disorders, and *E. coli* sepsis (Kaye, Committee on Genetics, Accurso, et al, 2006).

Prognosis

Follow-up studies of children treated from birth or within the first 2 months of life after symptoms appear have found long-term complications, such as ovarian dysfunction, cataracts, abnormal speech, cognitive impairment, growth restriction, and motor delay (Kaye, Committee on Genetics, Accurso, et al, 2006; Lashley, 2002). These findings have revealed that eliminating sources of galactose does not significantly improve the outcome. New therapeutic strategies, such as enhancing residual transferase activity, replacing depleted metabolites, or using gene replacement therapy, are needed to improve the prognosis for these children.

Nursing Care Management†

Nursing interventions are similar to those for PKU and other IEMs, except that dietary restrictions are easier to maintain

---

*Always refer patients to a genetic metabolic specialist. For a reference list visit the American Society of Human Genetics website, www.ashg.org.

†Information and support for parents can be found at the American Liver Foundation, www.liverfoundation.org; and at Parents of Galactosemic Children, Inc., PO Box 2401, Mandeville, LA 74070-2401; 866-900-PGC1; www.galactosemia.org.

because many more foods are allowed. However, reading food labels carefully for the presence of any form of lactose, especially dairy products, is mandatory. Many drugs, such as some of the penicillin preparations, contain lactose as filler and also must be avoided. Unfortunately, lactose is an unlabeled ingredient in many pharmaceuticals. Therefore instruct parents to ask their local pharmacist about galactose content of any over-the-counter or prescription medication.

CONGENITAL HYPOTHYROIDISM

Congenital hypothyroidism (CH) (formerly called by the undesirable term *cretinism*), an inborn error of thyroid metabolism, occurs in neonates who are born without the ability to synthesize adequate amounts of thyroid hormone. Results of screening tests in the United States indicate that CH occurs in approximately 1 of every 4000 to 1 of every 3000 newborns (Kaye, Committee on Genetics, Accurso, et al, 2006). Infants with Down syndrome have a much higher rate (1 in 140 newborns) of either permanent or transient forms of the disorder. Also, a higher incidence of other congenital abnormalities has been observed in infants with CH.

A number of etiologic factors are implicated in CH, and the condition may be permanent or transient. Permanent CH can result from defective thyroid gland development, an enzymatic defect in thyroxine synthesis (primary disease), or (rarely) pituitary dysfunction (secondary disease). Transient hypothyroidism results from intrauterine transfer of goiter-inducing substances (such as the antithyroid drugs), which inhibit thyroid hormone secretion. Although self-limiting, this type is potentially fatal because the infant's thyroid is unable to produce its own hormones once the maternal supply is terminated. In addition, regardless of etiology, a large goiter in a neonate may cause total obstruction of the airway. Many preterm infants have hypothyroidism (hypothyroxinemia) at birth as a result of hypothalamic and pituitary immaturity. However, this type is considered transient and often requires no treatment. Infants born prior to 28 weeks gestation may require temporary thyroid hormone replacement.

Clinical Manifestations

The severity of the disorder depends on the amount of thyroid tissue present and able to produce the necessary levels of thyroid hormones. Usually the newborn does not exhibit obvious signs of hypothyroidism immediately after birth because of the exogenous source of prenatal thyroid hormone supplied by the maternal circulation. However, subtle signs such as poor feeding, lethargy, prolonged neonatal jaundice, respiratory difficulty, cyanosis, constipation, hoarse cry, large fontanels, and bradycardia may be seen within the first few weeks of life. In addition, infants with CH may be born postterm (42 weeks). Clinical manifestations may be delayed in infants with a functional remnant of thyroid gland; infants with some types of familial hypothyroidism; and breast-fed infants, who may not display symptoms until weaned.

Classic features of untreated CH usually appear after approximately 6 weeks of life and include typical facial features (depressed nasal bridge, short forehead, puffy eyelids, and large tongue); thick, dry, mottled skin that feels cold to the touch; coarse, dry, lusterless hair; abdominal distention; umbilical hernia; hyporeflexia; bradycardia; hypothermia; hypotension with narrow pulse pressure; anemia; and widely patent cranial sutures. Bone age is greatly delayed from birth. The most serious consequence is delayed development of the nervous system, which leads to severe cognitive impairment. The severity of the intellectual deficit is related to the degree of hypothyroidism and the duration of the condition before treatment. Other nervous system manifestations include slow, awkward movements and abnormal deep tendon reflexes (often referred to as being "hung-up" because the relaxation phase after the contraction is slow), hypotonia, spasticity, speech disorders, fine motor incoordination, and strabismus.

Diagnostic Evaluation

Diagnosis is aimed at early identification of the disorder to prevent the serious impact on mental development and stunted physical growth as a result of delayed treatment. Mean IQ is reported to be proportional to the age when treatment is initiated (Kaye, Committee on Genetics, Accurso, et al, 2006). Neonatal screening consists of an initial filter-paper blood-spot thyroxine (T_4) measurement followed by measurement of thyroid-stimulating hormone (TSH) in infants with low T_4 values. Newborn screening is mandatory in all 50 U.S. states. Although it is best to obtain a heel stick blood sample for the test between 2 and 4 days of age, specimens are usually taken within the first 24 to 48 hours or before discharge as part of concurrent screening for other metabolic defects. Early screening can result in overdiagnosis (false positives), but this is preferable to missing the diagnosis.

For screening results that show a low level of T_4 (<10%), obtain TSH levels, and if these are elevated (>40 mU/L), further tests to determine the cause of the disease should be carried out (American Academy of Pediatrics and American Thyroid Association, 2006). Additional tests include serum measurement of T_4, triiodothyronine (T_3) resin uptake, free T_4, and thyroid-bound globulin. Tests of thyroid gland function (thyroid scan and uptake) usually involve oral administration of a radioactive isotope of iodine (^{131}I) and measurement of iodine uptake by the thyroid, usually within 24 hours. Patients with CH have low T_4, T_3, and free T_4 levels and decreased thyroid uptake of ^{131}I. Skeletal radiography is employed to assess bone age.

In the newborn, thyroid function studies are elevated in comparison with values in older children. Thus it is important to document the timing of the tests. In preterm and sick full-term infants, thyroid function tests are usually lower than in healthy full-term infants; a repeat T_4 and TSH may be evaluated after 30 weeks (corrected age) in newborns born before that time and after resolution of the acute illness in the sick full-term infant.

Therapeutic Management

Treatment involves life-long thyroid hormone replacement therapy that begins as soon as possible after diagnosis to abolish all signs of hypothyroidism and to reestablish normal physical and mental development. The drug of choice is synthetic levothyroxine sodium (Synthroid or Levothroid). Regular measurement of T_3, T_4, and TSH levels is important in ensuring optimum treatment. Optimum dosage of L-thyroxine should be able to maintain blood TSH concentration between 0.5 and 2.0 mU/L during the first 3 years of life (American Academy of Pediatrics and American Thyroid Association, 2006). Bone age surveys are also performed to ensure optimum growth.

Prognosis

If treatment begins shortly after birth (by 2 weeks of age) and is consistently maintained, normal physical growth and intelligence are possible. The most significant factor adversely affecting eventual intelligence appears to be inadequate treatment, which may be related to nonadherence.

Nursing Care Management

The most important nursing objectives include collecting an adequate specimen and identifying the disorder early. The integrity of the blood specimen must be maintained for the test to be accurate; overlaying of blood on the designated spot may produce inaccurate results. Blood is applied to only one side of the paper so that complete saturation is obtained. Keep the specimen paper dry and avoid excessive heat exposure.

Nurses caring for neonates must be certain that screening is performed, especially in infants who are preterm, discharged early, or born at home. Although the screening test is specific, some children may not be identified, and nurses in community health need to be aware of the earliest signs of the disorder. Parental remarks about an unusually "quiet and good" baby together with any of the early physical manifestations should lead to a suspicion of hypothyroidism, which requires a referral for specific tests.

Once the diagnosis is confirmed, parents need an explanation of the disorder and the necessity of life-long treatment. The nurse must stress the importance of compliance with the drug regimen for the child to achieve normal growth and development. Because the drug is tasteless, it can be crushed and added to formula, breast milk, water, or food. However, do not administer soy, fiber, or iron with the medication. If a dose is missed, twice the dose should be given the next day. Unless there are maternal contraindicative factors, breast-feeding is acceptable in infants with hypothyroidism (Lawrence and Lawrence, 2005). Parents also need to be aware of signs indicating overdose, such as rapid pulse, dyspnea, irritability, insomnia, fever, sweating, and weight loss. Ideally they should know how to count the pulse and be instructed to withhold a dose and consult their practitioner if the pulse rate is above a certain value. Signs of inadequate treatment are fatigue, sleepiness, decreased appetite, and constipation.

If the diagnosis was delayed past early infancy, the chance of permanent cognitive impairment is great. Parents need the same guidance in caring for their child as do others who have an offspring with cognitive impairment. (See Chapter 24.) They need an opportunity to discuss their feelings regarding late recognition of the disorder. Although treatment will not reverse the intellectual deficit, it may prevent further damage. Genetic counseling is important, especially if the disorder is caused by an inborn error of thyroid hormone synthesis, which is autosomal recessive. (See Chapter 5 for a discussion of genetic counseling.)

PROBLEMS CAUSED BY PERINATAL ENVIRONMENTAL FACTORS

CHEMICAL AGENTS

Prenatal environmental effects from chemicals such as alcohol, medications, or drugs; infectious disease; or radiation or other environmental factors may be regarded as nongenetic causes of congenital anomalies because these substances can produce congenital structural, functional, or growth defects. An agent that produces congenital malformations or increases their incidence is called a **teratogen**.

The relationship of the fetal and maternal circulations allows for the interchange of chemical substances across the placental membrane. Many drugs have been suspected of producing congenital malformations, and some have been definitely implicated. Some of the most recognized teratogenic drugs include alcohol, tobacco, antiepileptic medications (valproic acid, phenytoin), isotretinoin (Accutane), lithium, methotrexate, cocaine, and diethylstilbestrol. (See Chapter 10, Drug-Exposed Infants and Fetal Alcohol Syndrome or Alcohol-Related Birth Defects.) The limited metabolic capabilities of the fetal liver and its immature enzyme and transport systems render the unborn child ill equipped for maintaining homeostasis when chemical disturbances are imposed by the mother or the environment. This includes both substances produced by the mother in response to a disease state (such as diabetes) and exogenous substances ingested or inhaled by the mother.

The teratogenic effect of drugs is not believed to affect developing tissue until day 15 of gestation, when tissue differentiation begins to take place. Before that time, drugs usually have little effect because they are believed to have an insignificant affinity for undifferentiated tissue. Also, until implantation takes place, at approximately 7 days after conception, the embryo is not exposed to maternal blood that contains the drug. However, some drugs may affect the uterine lining, making it unsuitable for implantation. Drugs administered between days 15 and 90 may produce an effect if the tissue for which the drug has an affinity is in the process of differentiation at that time. After 90 days, when differentiation is complete, most fetal tissues are relatively resistant to teratogenic effects of drugs. However, the impact on ongoing neurologic development is not known.

Nursing Care Management

Caution expectant mothers against ingesting any medication without first consulting a practitioner. To help ensure that fewer women will inadvertently take some chemical that might harm the fetus, medication labels are now required to include information regarding the possible teratogenic effects. Excessive use of some commonplace drugs, such as alcohol, valproic acid, and isotretinoin, produces characteristic malformations in the fetus.

Nurses should be aware of Birth Defect Research for Children, Inc.,* which offers help and information to families with children with defects caused by maternal exposure to drugs, chemicals, radiation, or other environmental agents.

---

*800 Celebration Ave., Suite 225, Celebration, FL 34747; 407-466-8304; www.birthdefects.org.

RADIATION

Ionizing radiation in large doses has been shown to be both mutagenic and teratogenic in humans. Pelvic irradiation of pregnant women—from natural background radiation that is present everywhere in varying degrees, from occupational exposure, or from diagnostic or therapeutic procedures—is believed to be hazardous to the embryo, although the extent of teratogenicity and the exact dosage required to induce somatic change is not yet known. The risk of untoward effects to an irradiated fetus whose mother is undergoing diagnostic radiation by CT is reported to be the same as that of the general population, or 1% to 3% (Ratnapalan, Bona, and Koren, 2003). Patel, Reede, Katz, and colleagues (2007) affirm that, although there is a theoretical risk of carcinogenesis when the fetus is exposed to diagnostic radiation, with the radiation levels currently used there are no known risks for congenital malformations or cognitive impairment. These authors present an extensive review of diagnostic radiation methods used for pregnant and lactating mothers. Radiation may damage the conceptus at any time during its prenatal existence, and it is known that rapidly dividing and differentiating cells, such as those of the embryo, have increased radiosensitivity. As with other teratogens, the type of effect produced is closely correlated with the stage of development at which the radiation exposure occurs.

To help prevent the possibility of radiation damage, it is advisable (1) to avoid unnecessary radiation exposure, such as elective radiographs to the pelvis and abdomen, in women of childbearing age except during the 2 weeks immediately after menstruation; (2) to ascertain whether pregnancy is a possibility; and (3) to advise both men and women who have lower abdominal or pelvic radiographs to avoid conception for several months. Pregnant women should avoid radioactive iodine exposure, since iodine has an affinity for fetal thyroid tissue and can lead to developmental problems such as fetal goiter, microcephaly, intrauterine growth restriction, malignancy, and death. Women should also avoid the use of nonradioactive iodides in vaginal douche solutions, vaginal suppositories containing povidone-iodine (Betadine), and iodinized drugs for asthmatics during pregnancy (Blackburn, 2007).

The occurrence of childhood cancer as a result of prenatal or preconceptual radiation exposure has been reported to be unfounded (Mettler and Stazzone, 2007).

KEY POINTS

- Problems of the newborn may be attributed to birth injuries, transient metabolic illnesses, and IEMs.
- The forces of labor and delivery may cause soft tissue injury, head trauma, fractures, and paralysis.
- The most common forms of paralysis in the newborn are facial nerve, brachial plexus, and phrenic nerve palsies.
- Common skin problems of the newborn include erythema toxicum; candidiasis; bullous impetigo; and birthmarks, especially port-wine stains and hemangiomas.
- Because of their immature physiologic status, infants may be predisposed to hyperbilirubinemia, hypoglycemia, hyperglycemia, and hypocalcemia.
- In the newborn hyperbilirubinemia may result from excess production of bilirubin, decreased capacity of the liver to conjugate bilirubin, and/or deconjugation of bilirubin in the neonatal intestine (enterohepatic shunting).
- The primary treatment of hyperbilirubinemia is phototherapy.
- HDN is characterized by abnormally rapid destruction of RBCs as a result of blood incompatibility between mother and fetus.
- Hypoglycemia can often be prevented by initiating early feedings in the healthy asymptomatic newborn.
- Hemorrhagic disease of the newborn is characterized by oozing from the umbilicus or circumcision site, bloody or black stools, hematuria, ecchymoses, and epistaxis.
- The most significant IEMs are CH, PKU, and galactosemia.
- Thyroid replacement medication is required to treat CH.
- Life-long dietary control is the treatment of choice for PKU and galactosemia to prevent serious neurobehavioral deficits.
- Perinatal environmental factors such as chemicals, drugs ingested in pregnancy, and radiation may have fetal teratogenic effects.

REFERENCES

Alster TS, Railan D: Laser treatment of vascular birthmarks, *J Craniofac Surg* 17(4):720-723, 2006.

American Academy of Pediatrics: *Pediatric nutrition handbook,* ed 6, Elk Grove Village, Ill, 2009a, The Academy.

American Academy of Pediatrics: *Red book: 2009 report of the Committee on Infectious Diseases,* ed 28, Elk Grove, Ill, 2009b, The Academy.

American Academy of Pediatrics: Prevention of rickets and vitamin D deficiency in infants, children, and adolescents, *Pediatrics* 122(5):1142-1148, 2008a.

American Academy of Pediatrics, Newborn Screening Authoring Committee: Newborn screening expands: recommendations for pediatricians and medical homes—implications for the system, *Pediatrics* 121(2):192-217, 2008b.

American Academy of Pediatrics, Subcommittee on Hyperbilirubinemia: Clinical practice guideline: management of hyperbilirubinemia in the newborn infant 35 or more weeks of gestation, *Pediatrics* 114(1):297-316, 2004.

American Academy of Pediatrics, American College of Obstetricians and Gynecologists: *Guidelines for perinatal care,* ed 6, Elk Grove Village, Ill, 2007, The Academy.

American Academy of Pediatrics, American Thyroid Association: Update of newborn screening and therapy for congenital hypothyroidism, *Pediatrics* 117(6):2290-2303, 2006.

Askin DF, Diehl-Jones B: Liver, part 3, Pathophysiology of liver dysfunction, *Neonat Netw* 22(3):5-15, 2003.

Bhutani VK, Johnson LH, Keren R: Diagnosis and management of hyperbilirubinemia in the term neonate: for a safer first week, *Pediatr Clin North Am* 51(4):843-861, 2004.

Black LV, Maheshwari A: Disorders of the fetomaternal unit: hematologic manifestations in the fetus and neonate, *Semin Perinatol* 33(1):12-19, 2009.

Blackburn S: *Maternal, fetal, and neonatal physiology: a clinical perspective,* ed 3, St Louis, 2007, Saunders.

Brown ZA, Wald A, Morrow RA, et al: Effect of serologic status and cesarean delivery on transmission rates of herpes simplex virus from mother to infant, *JAMA* 289:203-209, 2003.

Centers for Disease Control and Prevention: Barriers to dietary control among pregnant women with phenylketonuria—United States, 1998-2000, *MMWR* 51(5):117-120, 2002.

Chertok IR, Raz I, Shoham I, et al: Effects of early breastfeeding on neonatal glucose levels of term infants born to women with gestational diabetes, *J Hum Nutr Diet* 22(2):166-169, 2009.

Cornblath M, Hawdon JM, Williams AF, et al: Controversies regarding definition of neonatal hypoglycemia: suggested operational thresholds, *Pediatrics* 105(5):1141-1145, 2000.

Cowett RM, Loughead JL: Neonatal glucose metabolism: differential diagnoses, evaluation, and treatment of hypoglycemia, *Neonat Netw* 21(4):9-18, 2002.

Custer JW, Rau RE, editors: *Harriet Lane handbook,* 18 edition, St. Louis, 2009, Mosby.

Dennery PA: Metalloporphyrins for the treatment of neonatal jaundice, *Curr Opin Pediatr* 17(2):167-169, 2005.

Desphande S, Platt MW: The investigation and management of neonatal hypoglycaemia, *Semin Fetal Neonat Med* 10(4):351-361, 2005.

Doumouchtsis SK, Arulkumaran S: Head injuries after instrumental vaginal deliveries, *Curr Opin Obstet Gynecol* 18(2):129-134, 2006.

Drolet BA, Swanson EA, Frieden IJ, et al: Infantile hemangiomas: an emerging health issue linked to an increased rate of low birth weight infants, *J Pediatr* 153(5):712-715, 2008.

Finning K, Martin P, Daniels G: The use of maternal plasma for prenatal RhD blood group genotyping, *Methods Mol Biol* 496:143-157, 2009.

Gottstein R, Cooke RW: Systematic review of intravenous immunoglobulin in haemolytic disease of the newborn, *Arch Dis Child Fetal Neonatal Ed* 88(1):F6-F10, 2003.

Hellekson KL: Practice guidelines: NIH consensus statement on phenylketonuria, *Am Fam Physician* 63(7):1430-1432, 2001.

Hoseth E, Joergensen A, Ebbesen F, et al: Blood glucose levels in a population of healthy, breast fed, term infants of appropriate size for gestational age, *Arch Dis Child Fetal Neonatal Educ* 83(2):F117-F119, 2000.

Hudic I, Fatusic Z, Sinanovic O, et al: Etiological risk factors for brachial plexus palsy, *J Matern Fetal Neonatal Med* 19(10):655-661, 2006.

Joanna Briggs Institute: Management of asymptomatic hypoglycaemia in healthy term neonates for nurses and midwives, *Nurs Standard* 22(8):35-38, 2007.

Joyner B, Soto MA, Adam HM: Brachial plexus injury, *Pediatr Rev* 27(6):238-239, 2006.

Kaye CI, Committee on Genetics, Accurso F, et al: Newborn screening fact sheets, *Pediatrics* 118(3):e934-e963, 2006.

Kimberlin DW: Herpes simplex virus infections of the newborn, *Semin Perinatol* 31(1):19-25, 2007.

Kimberlin DW: Herpes simplex virus infections in neonates and early childhood, *Semin Pediatr Infect Dis* 16:271-281, 2005.

Kishnani PS, Chen YT: Defects in galactose metabolism. In Kliegman RM, Behrman RE, Jenson HB, et al, editors: *Nelson textbook of pediatrics,* ed 18, Philadelphia, 2007, Saunders.

Lashley FR: Newborn screening: new opportunities and new challenges, *Newborn Infant Nurs Rev* 2(4):228-242, 2002.

Lawrence RA, Lawrence RM: *Breastfeeding: a guide for the medical profession,* ed 6, St Louis, 2005, Mosby.

Lee P, Treacy EP, Crombez E, et al: Safety and efficacy of 22 weeks of treatment with sapropterin dihydrochloride in patients with phenylketonuria, *Am J Med Genet A* 146A(22):2851-2859, 2008.

Maisels MJ, Bhutani VK, Bogen D, et al: Hyperbilirubinemia in the newborn infant ≥35 weeks' gestation: an update with clarifications, *Pediatrics* 124(4):1193-1198, 2009.

Maisels MJ, McDonough AF: Phototherapy for neonatal jaundice, *N Engl J Med* 358(9):920-928, 2008.

Mangurten HH: Birth injuries. In Fanaroff AA, Martin RJ, editors: *Neonatal-perinatal medicine: diseases of the fetus and infant,* ed 8, St Louis, 2006, Mosby.

McCance K, Huether S: *Pathophysiology: the biological basis for disease in adults and children,* ed 6, St Louis, 2010, Mosby.

McPhee SJ, Ganong WF: *Pathophysiology of disease: an introduction to clinical medicine,* ed 5, New York, 2006, Lang Medical Books.

Metry D: Update on hemangiomas of infancy, *Curr Opin Pediatr* 16(4):373-377, 2004.

Mettler FA, Stazzone MM: Environmental health hazards: pediatric radiation injuries. In Kliegman RM, Behrman RE, Jenson HB, et al, editors: *Nelson textbook of pediatrics,* ed 18, Philadelphia, 2007, Saunders.

Miclic TL: Neonatal glucose homeostasis, *Neonat Netw* 27(3):203-207, 2008.

Miller T, Frieden IJ: Hemangioma: new insights and classification, *Pediatr Ann* 34(3):179-187, 2005.

Moise KJ: Management of rhesus alloimmunization in pregnancy, *Obstet Gynecol* 112(1):164-176, 2008.

Moise KJ: Red cell alloimmunization. In Gabbe SG, Niebyl JR, Simpson KL, editors: *Obstetrics: normal and problem pregnancies,* ed 5, London, 2007, Churchill Livingstone.

Moise KJ: Management of rhesus alloimmunization in pregnancy, *Obstet Gynecol* 100(3):600-611, 2002.

Morelli JG: Cutaneous bacterial infections. In Kliegman RM, Behrman RE, Jenson HB, et al, editors: *Nelson textbook of pediatrics,* ed 18, Philadelphia, 2007, Saunders.

Moyle JJ, Fox AM, Bynevelt M, et al: A neuropsychological profile of off-diet adults with phenylketonuria, *J Clin Exp Neuropsychol* 29(4):436-441, 2007.

Mundy CA: Intravenous immunoglobulin in the management of hemolytic disease of the newborn, *Neonat Netw* 24(6):17-24, 2005.

National Institutes of Health Consensus Development Conference Statement: Phenylketonuria: screening and management, Oct 16-18, 2000, *Pediatrics* 108(4):972-982, 2001.

Paige PL, Moe PC: Neurologic disorders. In Merenstein GB, Gardner SL, editors: *Handbook of neonatal intensive care,* ed 6, St Louis, 2006, Mosby.

Pandey A, Gangopadhyay An, Upadhyay VD: Evaluation and management of infantile hemangioma: an overview, *Ostomy Wound Manage* 54(5):16-18, 20, 22-26, 28-29, 2008.

Patel SJ, Reede DL, Katz DS, et al: Imaging the pregnant patient for nonobstetric conditions: algorithms and radiation dose considerations, *Radiographics* 27(6):1705-1722, 2007.

Price AE, Ditaranto P, Yaylali I, et al: Botulinum toxin type A as an adjunct to the surgical treatment of the medial rotation deformity of the shoulder in birth injuries of the brachial plexus, *J Bone Joint Surg Br* 89(3):327-329, 2007.

Ratnapalan S, Bona N, Koren G: Ionizing radiation during pregnancy, *Can Fam Physician* 49:873-874, 2003.

Rezvani I: Defects in metabolism of amino acids. In Kliegman RM, Behrman RE, Jenson HB, et al, editors, *Nelson textbook of pediatrics,* ed 18, Philadelphia, 2007, Saunders.

Rozance PJ, Hay WH: Hypoglycemia in newborn infants: features associated with adverse outcomes, *Biol Neon* 90(2):74-86, 2006.

Sgro M, Shah V, Campbell D: *Canadian Paediatric Surveillance Program: challenge of early discharge: newborn assessment for jaundice,* 2005, available at www.cps.ca/English/Surveillance/CPSP/Resources/NHS.htm (accessed June 28, 2007).

Singh RH, Kable JA, Guerrero NV, et al: Impact of a camp experience on phenylalanine levels, knowledge, attitudes, and health beliefs relevant to nutrition management of phenylketonuria in adolescent girls, *J Am Diet Assoc* 100(7):797-803, 2000.

Sirkin A, Jalloh T, Lee L: Selecting an accurate point-of-care testing system: clinical and technical issues and implications in neonatal blood glucose monitoring, *J Spect Pediatr Nurs* 7(3):104-112, 2002.

Sperling MA: Hypoglycemia. In Kliegman RM, Behrman RE, Jenson HB, et al, editors, *Nelson textbook of pediatrics,* ed 18, Philadelphia, 2007, Saunders.

Sperling MA, Menon RK: Differential diagnosis and management of neonatal hypoglycemia, *Pediatr Clin North Am* 51(3):703-723, 2004.

Stier MF, Glick SA, Hirsch RJ: Laser treatment of pediatric vascular lesions: port wine stains and hemangiomas, *J Am Acad Dermatol* 58(2):261-285, 2008.

Stokowski LA: Fundamentals of phototherapy for neonatal jaundice, *Adv Neonat Care* 6(6):303-312, 2006.

Stoll BJ: Blood disorders. In Kliegman RM, Behrman RE, Jenson HB, et al, editors, *Nelson textbook of pediatrics,* ed 18, Philadelphia, 2007, Saunders.

Tappero E: Musculoskeletal system assessment. In Tappero E, Honeyfield MA, editors: *Physical assessment of the newborn: a comprehensive approach to the art of physical examination,* ed 4, Santa Rosa, Calif, 2009, NICU Ink.

Trefz FK, Burton BK, Longo N, et al: Efficacy of sapropterin dihydrochloride in increasing

phenylalanine tolerance in children with phenylketonuria: a phase III, randomized, double-blind, placebo-controlled study, *J Pediatr* 154(5):700-707, 2009.

Urbaniak SJ: Noninvasive approaches to the management of RhD hemolytic disease of the fetus and newborn, *Transfusion* 48(1):12-19, 2008.

Walter JH, White FJ: Blood phenylalanine control in adolescents with phenylketonuria,

Int J Adolesc Med Health 16(1):41-45, 2004.

Watchko JF: Identification of neonates at risk for hazardous hyperbilirubinemia: emerging clinical insights, *Pediatr Clin North Am* 56(3):671-687, 2009.

Zlatunich CO, Packman S: Galactosaemia: early treatment with an elemental formula, *J Inherit Metab Dis* 28:163-168, 2005.

The High-Risk Newborn and Family

Debbie Fraser Askin and David Wilson

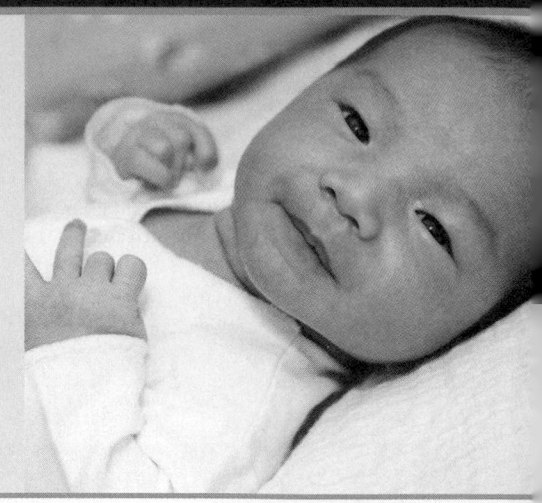

evolve WEBSITE

RELATED TOPICS

CHAPTER OUTLINE

GENERAL MANAGEMENT OF HIGH-RISK NEWBORNS

IDENTIFICATION OF HIGH-RISK NEWBORNS

The **high-risk neonate** is defined as a newborn, regardless of gestational age or birth weight, who has a greater-than-average chance of morbidity or mortality, usually because of conditions or circumstances superimposed on the normal course of events associated with birth and the adjustment to extrauterine existence. The high-risk period begins at the time of viability (the gestational age at which survival outside the uterus is believed to be possible, or as early as 23 weeks of gestation) up to 28 days after birth and includes threats to life and health that occur during the prenatal, perinatal, and postnatal periods.

There has been increased interest in late-preterm infants of 34 to 36⁶⁄₇ weeks of gestation who may receive the same treatment as term infants. Wang, Dorer, Fleming, and colleagues (2004) emphasize that late-preterm infants often experience similar morbidities to preterm infants: respiratory distress, hypoglycemia requiring treatment, temperature instability, poor feeding, jaundice, and discharge delays as a result of illness. Therefore assessment and prompt intervention in life-threatening perinatal emergencies often make the difference between a favorable outcome and a lifetime of disability. The nurse in the newborn nursery is familiar with the characteristics of neonates and recognizes the significance of serious deviations from expected observations. When providers can anticipate the need for specialized care and plan for it, the probability of successful outcome is increased.

Late-Preterm Infant

Within the past two decades, several significant changes have occurred in neonatal care. Early postpartum discharge for term and preterm infants gained popularity as health care institutions attempted to cut health care costs. Another change occurred in newborn care, as infants who appeared to be "near" term began to be treated much like term infants, thus avoiding the costs of neonatal intensive care for infants who appeared to be healthy. Experts have recommended that infants born between 34 and 36⁶⁄₇ weeks of gestation be referred to as **late-preterm infants** rather than *near-term infants* (Engle,

2006; Engle, Tomashek, Wallman, et al, 2007). Late-preterm infants may be able to make an effective transition to extrauterine life; however, such infants, by nature of their limited gestation, remain at risk for problems related to feeding, neurodevelopment, thermoregulation, hypoglycemia, hyperbilirubinemia, sepsis, and respiratory function (Bakewell-Sachs, 2007; Darcy, 2009). In one study children born at 34 to 36 weeks were more than three times as likely as children born at term to be diagnosed with cerebral palsy (CP) (Petrini, Dias, McCormick, et al, 2009). It is now estimated that late-preterm infants represent 70% of the total preterm infant population and that the mortality rate for this group is significantly higher than that of term infants (7.9 versus 2.4 per 1000 live births, respectively) (Tomashek, Shapiro-Mendoza, Davidoff, et al, 2007). Because late-preterm infants' birth weights often range from 2000 to 2500 g (4.4 to 5.5 lb) and they appear relatively mature in comparison to smaller preterm infants, they may be cared for in the same manner as healthy term infants, while risk factors for late-preterm infants are overlooked. Late-preterm infants are often discharged early from the birth institution and have a significantly higher rate of rehospitalization than term infants (Escobar, Clark, and Greene, 2006). Discussions regarding high-risk infants in this chapter also refer to late-preterm infants who are experiencing a delayed transition to extrauterine life.

The Association of Women's Health, Obstetric and Neonatal Nurses has published the *Late Preterm Infant Assessment Guide* (Askin, Bakewell-Sachs, Medoff-Cooper, et al, 2007) for the education of perinatal nurses regarding the late-preterm infant's risk factors and appropriate care and follow-up care (Table 10-1).

Classification of High-Risk Newborns

High-risk infants are most often classified according to birth weight, gestational age, and predominant pathophysiologic problems. The more common problems related to physiologic status are closely associated with the infant's state of maturity and usually involve chemical disturbances (e.g., hypoglycemia, hypocalcemia) and consequences of immature organs and systems (e.g., hyperbilirubinemia, respiratory distress, hypothermia). Box 10-1 outlines specific terminology describing the developmental status of the newborn.

Formerly, weight at birth reflected a reasonably accurate estimation of gestational age; that is, if an infant's birth weight

TABLE 10-1   LATE-PRETERM INFANT ASSESSMENT AND INTERVENTIONS

RISK FACTORS	ASSESSMENT	INTERVENTIONS*
Respiratory distress	Assess for cardinal signs of respiratory distress (nasal flaring, grunting, tachypnea, central cyanosis, retractions) and presence of apnea, especially during feedings. Assess for hypothermia, hypoglycemia.	Perform gestational age assessment. Observe for signs of respiratory distress; monitor oxygenation by pulse oximetry; provide supplemental oxygen judiciously.
Thermal instability	Monitor axillary temperature every 30 min immediately postpartum until stable; thereafter every 1-4 hr depending on gestational age and ability to maintain thermal stability.	Provide skin-to-skin care in immediate postpartum period for stable infant. Implement measures to avoid excess heat loss (adjust environmental temperature, avoid drafts). Bathe only after thermal stability has been maintained for 1 hr.
Hypoglycemia	Monitor for signs and symptoms of hypoglycemia. Assess feeding ability (latch-on, nipple-feeding). Assess thermal stability and signs and symptoms of respiratory distress. Monitor bedside glucose in infants with additional risk factors (IDM, prolonged labor, respiratory distress, poor feeding).	Initiate early feedings of human milk or formula. Avoid dextrose water or water feedings. Provide IV dextrose as necessary for hypoglycemia.
Jaundice	Observe for jaundice in first 24 hr. Evaluate maternal-fetal history for additional risk factors that may cause increased hemolysis and circulating levels of unconjugated bilirubin (Rh, ABO, spherocytosis, bruising). Assess feeding method, voiding and stooling patterns.	Monitor transcutaneous bilirubin and note risk zone on hour-specific nomogram (see Fig. 9-6).
Feeding problems	Assess suck-swallow and breathing. Assess for respiratory distress, hypoglycemia, thermal stability. Assess latch-on, maternal comfort with feeding method. Determine weight loss (should be ≤10% of birth weight).	Initiate early feedings (human milk or formula). Ensure maternal knowledge of feeding method and signs of inadequate feeding (sleepiness, lethargy, color changes during feeding, apnea during feeding, decreased or absent urine output).
Neurodevelopmental problems	Assess for respiratory distress, neonatal jaundice, hypoglycemia, and thermal instability. Assess neurodevelopmental status. Assess for seizure activity.	Perform newborn screening, including hearing test. Implement individualized developmental care. Encourage parents to keep follow-up appointments with primary care provider for evaluation of growth and development (including cognitive function and achievement of appropriate milestones).
Infection	Evaluate maternal-fetal history for risk factors that may contribute to neonatal septicemia. Assess for signs and symptoms of neonatal infection.	Use Standard Precautions, especially hand washing between infants and contact with surfaces that may harbor bacteria (e.g., keyboards, telephones). Maintain thermal stability. Administer hepatitis B vaccine. Encourage breast-feeding and assist mother-baby pair with breast-feeding. Encourage parents to decrease infant exposure to respiratory viruses postdischarge and obtain vaccines as appropriate to prevent development of respiratory viruses (e.g., influenza).

Portions adapted from Askin DF, Bakewell-Sachs S, Medoff-Cooper B, et al: *Late preterm infant assessment guide,* Washington, DC, 2007, Association of Women's Health, Obstetric and Neonatal Nurses.
IDM, Infant of diabetic mother; *IV,* intravenous.
*This is not an exhaustive list of nursing interventions; additional interventions include those discussed under the care of the high-risk infant in this chapter.

exceeded 2500 g (5.5 lb), the infant was considered to be mature. However, accumulated data have shown that intrauterine growth rates are not the same for all infants and that other factors (e.g., heredity, placental insufficiency, and maternal disease) influence intrauterine growth and the infant's birth weight. From these data a more definitive and meaningful classification system that encompasses birth weight, gestational age, and neonatal outcome has been developed. It has also been determined that the lowest perinatal mortality occurs in the infant who weighs between 3000 and 4000 g (6.4 and 8.8 lb) and whose gestational age is more than 36 weeks and less than 42 weeks (Walsh and Fanaroff, 2006). (See Fig. 8-2 for size comparison of newborn infants.)

Many perinatal problems can be anticipated before delivery. Prenatal testing and labor monitoring have reduced the incidence of perinatal mortality, and specialized care of the distressed newborn is improving the survival rate. If the infant is likely to require special therapy at or soon after birth, plans can be made for the delivery to take place at a hospital with the facilities to provide such care. This eliminates delay in initiating needed care and averts some of the hazards associated with transporting the sick newborn. Prenatal evaluation of fetal well-being and advanced surgical and anesthetic techniques have made intrauterine treatment of certain pathologic conditions possible, thus enhancing the neonate's chances for survival (Reed and Blumer, 2006).

BOX 10-1 CLASSIFICATION OF HIGH-RISK INFANTS

Classification According to Size

Low-birth-weight (LBW) infant—An infant whose birth weight is less than 2500 g (5.5 lb), regardless of gestational age

Very low–birth-weight (VLBW) infant—An infant whose birth weight is less than 1500 q (3.3 lb)

Extremely low–birth-weight (ELBW) infant—An infant whose birth weight is less than 1000 g (2.2 lb)

Appropriate-for-gestational-age (AGA) infant—An infant whose weight falls between the 10th and 90th percentiles on intrauterine growth curves

Small-for-date (SFD) or small-for-gestational-age (SGA) infant—An infant whose rate of intrauterine growth was slowed and whose birth weight falls below the 10th percentile on intrauterine growth curves

Intrauterine growth restriction (IUGR)—Found in infants whose intrauterine growth is retarded (sometimes used as a more descriptive term for the SGA infant)

Large-for-gestational-age (LGA) infant—An infant whose birth weight falls above the 90th percentile on intrauterine growth charts

Classification According to Gestational Age

Preterm (premature) infant—An infant born before completion of 37 weeks of gestation, regardless of birth weight

Full-term infant—An infant born between the beginning of 38 weeks and the completion of 42 weeks of gestation, regardless of birth weight

Postterm (postmature) infant—An infant born after 42 weeks of gestational age, regardless of birth weight

Late-preterm infant—An infant born between $34\frac{0}{7}$ and $36\frac{6}{7}$ weeks of gestation, regardless of birth weight

Classification According to Mortality

Live birth—Birth in which the neonate manifests any heartbeat, breathes, or displays voluntary movement, regardless of gestational age

Fetal death—Death of the fetus after 20 weeks of gestation and before delivery, with absence of any signs of life after birth

Neonatal death—Death that occurs in the first 27 days of life; early neonatal death occurs in the first week of life; late neonatal death occurs at 7 to 27 days

Perinatal mortality—Describes the total number of fetal and early neonatal deaths per 1000 live births

Postnatal death—Death that occurs at 28 days to 1 year after birth

INTENSIVE CARE FACILITIES

Rapid advances in our understanding of the pathophysiology of the neonate and increased capacity to apply this knowledge have emphasized the need for appropriate settings in which to care for the seriously ill infant. Advancements in electronics and biochemistry, new methods for monitoring cardiorespiratory function, microtechniques for biochemical determination from minute quantities of blood, noninvasive monitoring, and new methods for assisted ventilation and conservation of body heat have made it possible to effectively manage the newborn with serious illness.

Intensive care of the ill and immature newborn requires specialized knowledge and skill in a number of areas. Much of the equipment used in the care of the critically ill adult is unsuited to the singular needs of the very small infant; therefore equipment has been modified to meet these needs. Examples of modifications include ventilators that deliver small volumes of oxygen in the proper concentration and pressure, infusion pumps that accurately deliver very small amounts, and radiant heat warmers that provide a constant source of warmth and allow maximum access to the infant. Most important, advances in intensive care have created a need for highly skilled personnel trained in the art of neonatal intensive care.

The diversity of special care needs requires that the unit be arranged for graduated care of the infant population. There should be adequate facilities and skilled personnel to provide one-to-one nursing care for each seriously ill infant, as well as a means for graduation to one-to-three or one-to-four nursing care in a quieter area where infants require less intensive care until they are ready to be discharged to home. Family-centered care and a relatively quiet environment are often difficult to provide in a busy neonatal intensive care unit (NICU); therefore some units have developed step-down units and single-room units where high-risk infants may be observed by skilled staff. Such areas are designed for family-centered care along with appropriate neurodevelopmental care.

Organization of Services

The most efficient organization of services is a regionalized system of facilities within a designated geographic area. Neonatal intensive care facilities may provide three prescribed levels of care with special equipment, skilled personnel, and ancillary services concentrated in a centralized institution (American Academy of Pediatrics and American College of Obstetricians and Gynecologists, 2007):

Level I facility—Provides management of normal maternal and newborn care.

Level IIA facility—Provides a full range of maternity and newborn care and can provide care to infants born at more than 32 weeks of gestation and weighing more than 1500 g (3.3 lb) who are moderately ill with problems that are expected to resolve rapidly and who are not anticipated to need subspecialty care; or who are convalescing after intensive care.

Level IIB facility—In addition to the above, can provide mechanical ventilation for up to 24 hours and can provide continuous positive airway pressure (CPAP).

Level III facility—Neonatal intensive care
- Level IIIA units provide care for infants with birth weight of more than 1000 g (2.2 lb) and gestational age of more than 28 weeks. Life support is limited to conventional mechanical ventilation.
- Level IIIB units can provide care for extremely low–birth-weight (ELBW) infants with technology including high-frequency ventilation and inhaled nitric oxide, on-site access to pediatric medical subspecialists, and advanced diagnostic imaging and pediatric surgery available.
- Level IIIC units have the capabilities of a level IIIB NICU and, in addition, offer extracorporeal membrane oxygenation (ECMO) and surgical repair of serious congenital cardiac malformations.

Transporting High-Risk Newborns

When an at-risk infant is identified or anticipated, arrangements are made for care in the intensive care facility. The uterus is the ideal transport unit for the infant with anticipated difficulties; therefore, whenever possible, take the mother where special care is available for her delivery.

Some infants develop difficulties after a seemingly normal pregnancy and uncomplicated labor. Because it is impossible to always predict when infants will require intensive care, a coordinated system is needed to ensure them an optimum opportunity for survival. Each hospital that delivers infants should be able to provide for appropriate neonatal stabilization and arrange for transport to a tertiary care facility. The infant must be kept warm, be adequately oxygenated (including intubation if indicated), have vital signs and oxygen saturation monitored, and, when indicated, receive an intravenous (IV) infusion. The infant is transported in a specially designed incubator unit that contains a complete life-support system and other emergency equipment that can be carried by ambulance, van, plane, or helicopter.

The transport team may consist of one or more of the highly trained persons from the NICU: a neonatologist (or a fellow in neonatology), a neonatal nurse practitioner, a respiratory therapist, and one or more nurses. The professional assigned to accompany the infant must be constantly alert to every change in the infant's condition and able to intervene appropriately. The neonate who must be moved from one place to another within the hospital (e.g., to surgery, or from delivery room to nursery) is transported in an incubator or radiant warmer and accompanied by the necessary personnel and equipment.

NURSING CARE OF HIGH-RISK NEWBORNS

Because the majority of infants admitted to intensive care facilities are born before the estimated date of delivery, this chapter focuses primarily on the preterm infant. (See p. 344 for a description of the characteristics of preterm infants.) The incidence of neonatal complications (e.g., respiratory distress and hypoglycemia) is highest in this group, and often other high-risk factors (e.g., sepsis and congenital malformations) are found in association with prematurity. This chapter discusses nursing problems encountered in the intensive care nursery, then considers common complications. Nursing care of high-risk infants with more serious disorders is examined in relation to specific high-risk conditions.

ASSESSMENT

At birth the newborn is given a cursory yet thorough assessment to determine any apparent problems and identify those that demand immediate attention. This examination is primarily concerned with the evaluation of cardiopulmonary and neurologic functions. The assessment includes the assignment of an Apgar score (see Chapter 8) and an evaluation for any obvious congenital anomalies or evidence of neonatal distress. The infant is stabilized and evaluated before being transported to the NICU for therapy and more extensive assessment. (See Clinical Assessment of Gestational Age, Chapter 8.)

A thorough, systematic physical assessment is an essential component in the care of the high-risk infant (see Nursing Care Guidelines box). Subtle changes in feeding behavior, activity, color, oxygen saturation (SpO$_2$), or vital signs often indicate an underlying problem. The preterm infant, especially the ELBW infant, is not able to withstand prolonged physiologic stress and may die within minutes of exhibiting abnormal symptoms if the underlying pathologic process is not corrected. The alert nurse is aware of subtle changes and reacts promptly to implement interventions that promote optimum function in the high-risk neonate. The nurse notes changes in the infant's status through ongoing observations of the infant's adaptation to the extrauterine environment.

Observational assessments of the high-risk infant are made according to the infant's acuity (seriousness of condition); the critically ill infant requires close observation and assessment of respiratory function, including continuous pulse oximetry, electrolytes, and blood gases. Accurate documentation of the infant's status is an integral component of nursing care. With the aid of continuous, sophisticated cardiopulmonary monitoring, nursing assessments and daily care can be coordinated to allow for minimum handling of the infant (especially the very low–birth-weight [VLBW] or ELBW infant) to decrease the effects of environmental stress.

MONITORING PHYSIOLOGIC DATA

Most neonates under intensive observation are placed in a controlled thermal environment and monitored for heart rate, respiratory activity, and temperature. The monitoring devices are equipped with an alarm system that indicates when the vital signs are above or below preset limits. However, a "hands on" assessment, including auscultation of heart tones and breath sounds, is essential.

The placement of electrodes may be challenging because of the lack of flat areas on the neonate's chest, the limited space for alternating sites, the size of the electrodes, and irritation from the adhesive. Hydrogel electrodes are gentler on the skin and are easily removed by lifting an edge from the skin and moistening it with plain water to release the adhesive (Lund and Durand, 2006). If the same electrode is reapplied to the skin, rinse the hydrogel with plain water to remove accumulated sodium from perspiration, which can eventually irritate the skin. It is important to follow the manufacturer's directions for care and handling of electrodes to avoid malfunction or burns to sensitive skin.

Monitor blood pressure routinely in the sick neonate by either internal or external means. Direct recording with arterial catheters is often used but carries the risks inherent in any procedure in which a catheter is introduced into an artery. An umbilical venous catheter may also be used to monitor the neonate's central venous pressure. Oscillometry (Dinamap) or Doppler transcutaneous apparatus is a simple, effective means for detecting alterations in systemic blood pressure (hypotension or hypertension). Table 10-2 lists normal blood pressure ranges for healthy preterm infants. Infants who have birth asphyxia, have low Apgar scores, or are mechanically ventilated have lower systolic and diastolic pressures.

In the NICU frequent laboratory examinations and their interpretation are integral parts of the ongoing assessment of infants' progress. The nurse keeps accurate intake and output records on all acutely ill infants. An accurate output can be obtained by collecting urine in a plastic urine collection bag specifically made for preterm infants (see Urine Specimens, Chapter 27) or by weighing the diapers, which is the simplest and least traumatic means of measuring urinary output. The

NURSING CARE GUIDELINES

Physical Assessment

General Assessment

Using electronic scale, weigh daily or as the baby's condition dictates.

Measure length and head circumference periodically.

Describe general body shape and size, posture at rest, ease of breathing, presence and location of edema.

Describe any apparent deformities.

Describe any signs of distress (e.g., poor color, mottling, hypotonia).

Respiratory Assessment

Describe shape of chest (concave), symmetry, chest tubes, or other deviations.

Describe use of accessory muscles: nasal flaring or substernal, intercostal, or suprasternal retractions.

Determine respiratory rate and regularity.

Auscultate and describe breath sounds: stridor, crackles, wheezing, diminished sounds, areas of absence of sound, grunting, stridor, diminished air entry, equality of breath sounds.

Determine whether suctioning is needed.

Describe ambient oxygen and method of delivery; if intubated, describe size of tube, type of ventilator and settings, and method of securing tube.

Determine oxygen saturation by pulse oximetry and partial pressure of oxygen and carbon dioxide by transcutaneous oxygen (tcPO$_2$) and transcutaneous carbon dioxide (tcPCO$_2$).

Cardiovascular Assessment

Determine heart rate and rhythm.

Describe heart sounds, including any murmurs.

Determine the point of maximum intensity (PMI), the point at which the heartbeat sounds and palpates loudest (a change in the PMI may indicate a mediastinal shift).

Describe infant's color (abnormalities may be of cardiac, respiratory, or hematopoietic origin): cyanosis, pallor, plethora, jaundice, mottling.

Assess color of mucous membranes and lips.

Determine blood pressure. Indicate extremity used and cuff size.

Describe peripheral pulses, capillary refill (<2 to 3 seconds), peripheral perfusion (mottling).

Describe monitors, their parameters, and whether alarms are in "on" position.

Gastrointestinal Assessment

Determine presence of abdominal distention: increase in circumference, shiny skin, evidence of abdominal wall erythema, visible peristalsis, visible loops of bowel, status of umbilicus.

Determine any signs of regurgitation and time related to feeding; character and amount of residual if gavage fed; if nasogastric tube in place, describe type of suction, drainage (color, consistency, pH, guaiac).

Describe amount, color, and consistency of any emesis.

Palpate liver margin.

Describe amount, color, and consistency of stools; check for occult blood and/or reducing substances if ordered or indicated by appearance of stool.

Describe bowel sounds; presence or absence.

Genitourinary Assessment

Describe any abnormalities of genitalia.

Describe urine amount (as determined by weight), color, pH, labstick findings, and specific gravity (to screen for adequacy of hydration).

Check weight (the most accurate measure for assessment of hydration).

Neurologic-Musculoskeletal Assessment

Describe infant's movements (random, purposeful, jittery, twitching, spontaneous, elicited); level of activity with stimulation; evaluate based on gestational age.

Describe infant's position or attitude: flexed, extended.

Describe reflexes observed: Moro, sucking, Babinski, plantar, and other age-appropriate reflexes.

Determine level of response and consolability.

Determine changes in head circumference (if indicated); size and tension of fontanels, suture lines.

Determine pupillary responses in infant at or above 32 weeks of gestation.

Temperature

Determine axillary temperature.

Determine relationship to environmental temperature.

Skin Assessment

Describe any discoloration, reddened area, signs of irritation, blisters, abrasions, or denuded areas, especially where monitoring equipment, infusions, or other apparatus come in contact with skin; also check and note any skin preparation used (e.g., povidone-iodine).

Determine texture and turgor of skin: dry, smooth, flaky, peeling, etc.

Describe any rash, skin lesion, or birthmarks.

Determine whether intravenous infusion catheter or needle is in place, and observe for signs of infiltration.

Describe parenteral infusion lines: location, type (arterial, venous, peripheral, umbilical, central, peripherally inserted central catheter); type of infusion (medication, saline, dextrose, electrolytes, lipids, total parenteral nutrition); type of infusion pump and rate of flow; type of catheter or needle; and appearance of insertion site.

---

preweighed wet diaper is weighed on a gram scale, and the gram weight of the urine is converted directly to milliliters (e.g., 25 g = 25 ml).

Urine obtained from cloth diapers and disposable diapers containing absorbent gel material may yield inaccurate results for urine specific gravity, pH, and protein. Urine samples obtained from 100%-cotton cottonballs strategically placed in the diaper proved to be the most accurate.

> **NURSING TIP** When small volumes of urine are measured, superabsorbent disposable diapers, especially when kept closed, give more accurate volume measurements than cloth diapers because they are less affected by evaporative losses.

Blood examinations are a necessary part of the ongoing assessment and monitoring of the sick newborn's progress. The tests most often performed are blood glucose, bilirubin, electrolytes, calcium, hematocrit, and blood gases. Samples may be obtained by heel stick; venipuncture; arterial puncture; or an indwelling catheter in an umbilical vein, umbilical artery, or peripheral artery. (See Atraumatic Care box, Heel Punctures, in Chapter 8.) In one study, the use of an automated incision device for heel blood sampling resulted in the need for fewer heel pokes, less bruising of both the foot and the leg, and less inflammation than manual lancets (Vertanen, Fellman, Brommels, et al, 2001). When skilled phlebotomists are available, venipuncture for blood collections may be preferred. A Cochrane review comparing heel punctures to venipuncture

TABLE 10-2	BLOOD PRESSURE RANGES IN DIFFERENT WEIGHT GROUPS OF HEALTHY PRETERM INFANTS*	
BIRTH WEIGHT	**SYSTOLIC PRESSURE (mm Hg)**	**DIASTOLIC PRESSURE (mm Hg)**
501-750 g (1.1-1.6 lb)	50-62	26-36
751-1000 g (1.6-2.2 lb)	48-59	23-36
1001-1250 g (2.2-2.7 lb)	49-61	26-35
1251-1500 g (2.7-3.3 lb)	46-56	23-33
1501-1750 g (3.3-3.8 lb)	46-58	23-33
1751-2000 g (3.8-4.4 lb)	48-61	24-35

Modified from Hegyi T, Carbone MT, Anwar M, et al: Blood pressure ranges in premature infants, part I, The first hours of life, *J Pediatr* 124(4):630, 1994.
*Defined as infants without a history of maternal hypertension, Apgar scores of <3 at 1 min and <6 at 5 min, pneumothorax, hematocrit 0.32, serum pH 7.1, use of dopamine, infusion of erythrocytes or colloid, mechanical ventilation, or cardiopulmonary resuscitation.

found that infants receiving a venipuncture for blood collection demonstrated less pain response than those receiving a heel lance and that use of venipuncture reduced the need for repeated heel punctures (Shah and Ohlsson, 2007a).

When numerous blood samples must be drawn, it is important to maintain an accurate record of the amount of blood being removed, especially in ELBW and VLBW infants, who cannot afford to lose blood during the acute phase of their illness.

When infants require close monitoring of oxygenation, **pulse oximetry**, a noninvasive measurement of the saturation or percent of oxygen in the hemoglobin, is typically used. Although used less frequently than pulse oximetry, some situations warrant the monitoring of transcutaneous oxygen ($tcPo_2$) and carbon dioxide ($tcPco_2$). The nurse notes changes in oxygenation (or other aspects being monitored) associated with handling and adjusts the infant's care accordingly. The frequency of taking vital signs depends on the infant's acuity level and response to handling.

Safety Measures

The increased sophistication of supportive technology, including delivery systems, monitors, ventilator devices, and warmers, is both boon and bane. Although built-in safety systems and better engineering have made these devices more reliable and easier to use, our increasing reliance on them carries with it the additional risks of electrical biohazards and inaccurate function. Additionally, untrained or inexperienced operators confer an extra element of risk. Parents need instruction regarding safety precautions and observations. They are usually uncomfortable around the equipment and atmosphere of an intensive care unit and therefore appreciate an explanation of the purposes and functions of the devices and pertinent safety aspects. Although most NICUs are closed units, parents must also learn about specific safety measures designed to prevent neonatal abduction. Most institutions have their own protocols for preventing such an occurrence. (See Protect from Infection and Injury, Chapter 8.)

Respiratory Support

The primary objective in the care of high-risk infants is to establish and maintain respiration. Many infants require supplemental oxygen and assisted ventilation. All infants require appropriate positioning to ensure an open airway and to maximize oxygenation and ventilation. Oxygen therapy is provided on the basis of the infant's requirements and illness (see Respiratory Distress Syndrome, p. 347, and Oxygen Therapy, p. 352).

Thermoregulation

Concurrent with the establishment of respiration, the most crucial need of the low-birth-weight (LBW) infant is provision of external warmth. Prevention of heat loss in the distressed infant is absolutely essential for survival, and maintaining a neutral thermal environment is a challenging aspect of neonatal intensive nursing care. Heat production is a complicated process that involves the cardiovascular, neurologic, and metabolic systems, and the immature neonate has all the problems related to heat production that are faced by the full-term infant. (See Thermoregulation, Chapter 8.) However, LBW infants are placed at further disadvantage by a number of additional problems. They have an even smaller muscle mass and fewer deposits of brown fat for producing heat, lack insulating subcutaneous fat, and have poor reflex control of skin capillaries.

Pathophysiology

The immature neonate, unable to increase activity and lacking a shivering response, produces heat primarily through increased metabolic processes. Some heat continues to be generated by liver, heart, brain, and skeletal muscles, but the major source of increased heat production during cold stress is **nonshivering thermogenesis**. Norepinephrine, secreted by the sympathetic nerve endings in response to chilling, stimulates fat metabolism in the richly vascularized brown adipose tissue to produce internal heat, which is then conducted through the blood to surface tissues. A significant increase in metabolism requires increased oxygen consumption.

The consequences of cold stress that pose additional hazards to the neonate are (1) hypoxia, (2) metabolic acidosis, and (3) hypoglycemia. Increased metabolism in response to chilling creates a compensatory increase in oxygen and calorie consumption.

Norepinephrine, released in response to cold stress, causes pulmonary vasoconstriction, which further reduces the effectiveness of pulmonary ventilation. This decrease in oxygen intake diminishes the supply available for glucose metabolism. As a result, glucose is broken down by an alternate, hypoxic pathway (anaerobic glycolysis) that generates increased lactic acid. This, together with acid end-products of brown fat metabolism, contributes to the acidotic state. Anaerobic metabolism dissipates glycogen at a greatly increased rate over aerobic metabolism, thus precipitating hypoglycemia. This condition is especially marked when glycogen stores are diminished at birth and caloric intake is inadequate after birth.

Maintaining Thermoneutrality

To delay or prevent the effects of cold stress, at-risk newborns are placed in a heated environment immediately after birth, where they remain until they are able to independently maintain thermal stability—the capacity to balance heat production and conservation and heat dissipation. Because overheating produces an increase in oxygen and calorie consumption, the infant is also jeopardized in a hyperthermic environment. A neutral thermal environment is one that permits the infant to maintain a normal core temperature with minimum oxygen consumption and calorie expenditure. Studies indicate that optimum thermoneutrality cannot be predicted for every high-risk infant's needs (Blackburn, 2007; Blake and Murray, 2006).

VLBW and ELBW infants, with thin skin and almost no subcutaneous fat, can control body heat loss or gain only within a limited range of environmental temperatures. In these infants heat loss from radiation, evaporation, and transepidermal water loss is three to five times greater than in larger infants, and a decrease in body temperature is associated with an increase in mortality.

The three primary methods for maintaining a neutral thermal environment are the use of an incubator, a radiant warming panel, and an open bassinet with cotton blankets. The healthy, full-term infant dressed and under blankets can maintain a stable temperature within a wider range of environmental temperatures; however, the infant requiring close observation or treatments such as phototherapy may need to be cared for in an incubator or under radiant heat (Fig. 10-1). The incubator should always be prewarmed before placing an infant in it. The use of double-walled incubators significantly improves the infant's ability to maintain a desirable temperature and reduces energy expenditure related to heat regulation. The infant is clothed and warmly wrapped in blankets when removed from the warm environment of the incubator for feeding or cuddling. Inside or outside the incubator, head coverings are effective in preventing heat loss. A fabric-insulated cap is more effective than one fashioned from stockinette (Blackburn, 2007).

An effective means for maintaining the desired range of temperature in the infant is the use of an automatically controlled (servocontrolled) incubator. The mechanism, when set at the upper and lower limits of the desired circulating air temperature range, adjusts automatically in response to signals from a thermal sensor attached to the abdominal skin. If the infant's temperature drops, the warming device is triggered to increase heat output. The servocontrol is usually set to a desired skin temperature between 36° and 36.5° C (96.8° and 97.7° F) (Blake and Murray, 2006).

Convective heat loss occurs when infants are exposed to increased air flow velocity and turbulence (e.g., drafts from doors, ventilation system, opening and closing incubator portholes and side panels). The infant being cared for in a radiant warmer also experiences convective heat losses in response to ventilation drafts and traffic flow around the bed; these losses may be partially countered with plastic wrap placed directly on the infant's body or stretched over the side guards of the warmer unit (Fig. 10-2). Oxygen or any source of air, such as an oxygen mask or tube, should not blow directly on the infant's face. Oxygen concentrated around the head, such as that supplied to a hood, must be warmed and humidified.

Radiant heat loss is one of the greatest threats to temperature regulation in the incubator, since the temperature of circulating air within has no influence on heat loss to cooler surfaces without, such as windows, walls, or a lower nursery temperature. Such losses can be effectively reduced with the use of double-walled incubators; the infant radiates heat to the inner wall, which is surrounded by the warmed incubator air. The use of a cloth incubator cover further reduces radiant heat loss and provides some protection from exterior light sources.

A high-humidity atmosphere contributes to body temperature maintenance by reducing evaporative heat loss. Humidity is provided in some incubators by circulating air over a heated water reservoir, which has the additional advantage of decreasing heat loss by convection as the air flows over the infant. The water reservoir in older model incubators was often a source of water-borne bacteria, resulting in the need for frequent water changes. Newer technologies such as ultrasonic nebulizers may

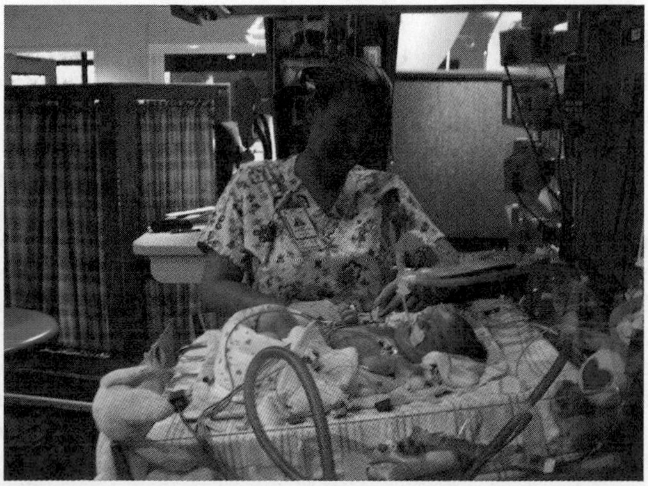

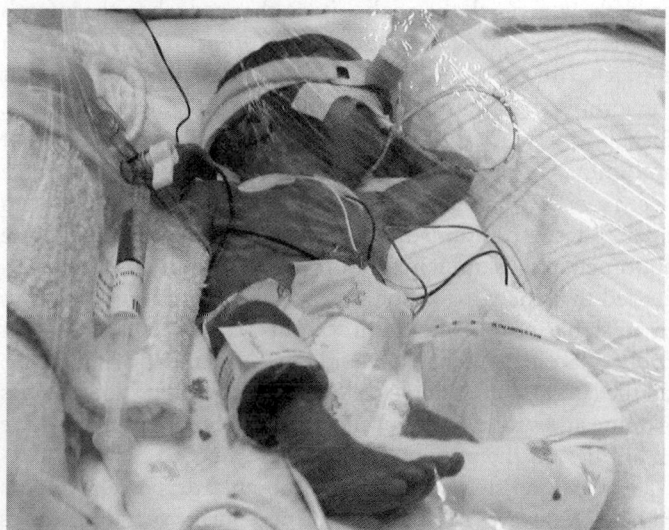

Fig. 10-1 Nurse caring for infant in radiant warmer. (Courtesy E. Jacobs, Texas Children's Hospital, Houston.)

Fig. 10-2 Infant under plastic wrap, which produces a draft-free environment. (Courtesy E. Jacobs, Texas Children's Hospital, Houston.)

reduce the risk of such infections. Follow manufacturer's recommendations in determining the frequency of water changes. The recommended humidity is 50% to 65%; higher humidity and a warmer environment are recommended for VLBW and ELBW infants.

A number of "microenvironments" may be used with the VLBW and ELBW infant to minimize evaporative and insensible water losses (IWLs). These include items such as bubble wrap blankets, humidified reservoirs for incubators, humidified tents, humidified Plexiglas boxes with plastic wrap coverings, polyethylene bags, and plastic wrap blankets. In cold-stressed infants, heat shields may be inappropriate because they may block heat from reaching the infant. The use of emollient cream to prevent transepidermal water loss has been used; however, this therapy has increased the risk of infection with coagulase-negative staphylococcus, and in preterm infants weighing 750 g or less, it should be used with caution (Association of Women's Health, Obstetric and Neonatal Nurses, 2007).

The nurse can reduce conductive heat loss by warming all items that come in direct contact with the infant, such as scales, radiographic film, blankets, and the hands of caregivers. For example, the nurse can store blankets in a warming unit ready for use and place a freestanding warming unit or a heat lamp over a scale before weighing an infant.

Although the open radiant warmer unit allows easier access to the infant, there is an inherent increase in evaporative water loss (and evaporative heat loss) from the skin, especially in ELBW and VLBW infants. Transepidermal water losses, a form of IWL, may be increased by as much as 50% to 200%, thus predisposing the infant to dehydration; daily fluid requirements are generally increased to compensate for such losses. The use of plastic wrap over the ELBW or VLBW infant in a radiant warmer will help reduce IWL and convective losses.

The infant being cared for in a radiant warmer is kept warm using the servocontrol method. Air temperature manual control should not be used because of the danger of overheating the infant. A reflective aluminum temperature probe cover is used to allow proper function of the servocontrol heating unit. Traditionally, the temperature probe is placed over a nonbony, well-perfused tissue area such as the abdomen, flank, or back. In general, the probe site is changed when the infant's position is changed to prevent the probe from coming in contact with the bed surface and potentially trapping heat at the probe site, causing an abnormal ambient temperature. Blackburn, De Paul, Loan, and colleagues (2001) found that abdominal and back skin temperatures varied considerably based on the infant's position and the probe position; when infants were positioned prone and the probe was on the abdomen, the skin temperature rose. The researchers concluded that changing probe sites with repositioning may result in unstable body temperatures, that a consistent method of probe placement is needed, and that placement of the probe on the lateral abdomen may allow for frequent position changes (supine and prone) without the difficulties that occur when the infant lies on the probe.

The use of sterile cloth or disposable drapes also blocks radiant heat waves in a radiant warmer; during such procedures the use of a warmed blanket under the infant is appropriate. Clothing an infant on servocontrol in an incubator or radiant warmer is not recommended; head covering and foot covering (socks or booties) may be used with discretion.

Prolonged exposure to cold stress in the sick or preterm infant, particularly the ELBW or VLBW infant, may have disastrous results from which recovery may not be possible. Thermoregulation measures in the labor and delivery area and during transport to the NICU are essential. The use of a plastic bag or plastic wrap; careful drying; prewarming of equipment such as scales, stethoscopes, and incubators; and prompt placement of the VLBW or ELBW newborn in a proper heat source are essential for the prevention of further morbidity.

Hyperthermia may cause equally untoward effects because high-risk infants typically have a limited ability to perspire, thus decreasing heat dissipation. In high-risk neonates hyperthermia is usually a result of overheating rather than hypermetabolism. Therefore knowledge of proper care and use of external heating devices, such as radiant warmers or incubators, is as important as knowing the conditions for which they are being used.

Protection from Infection

Protection from infection is an integral part of all newborn care, but preterm and sick neonates are particularly susceptible. Thorough, meticulous, and frequent hand washing is the foundation of a preventive program. This includes all persons who come in contact with infants and their equipment. After handling another infant or equipment, no one should ever touch an infant without first washing hands.

Personnel with infectious disorders are either barred from the unit until they are no longer infectious or are required to wear suitable shields, such as masks or gloves, to reduce the likelihood of contamination. Standard Precautions as a method of infection control are instituted in all nursery areas to protect the infants and staff. (See Chapter 27.)

Readmission of infants from home or admission of infants delivered in unsterile conditions or infants suspected of having communicable illnesses is handled per institutional protocol. Such infants should at least be initially physically isolated from other highly susceptible high-risk infants. (See American Academy of Pediatrics and American College of Obstetricians and Gynecologists [2007] for further infection control recommendations, including nursery care of infants with specific communicable diseases.)

Hydration

High-risk infants often receive supplemental parenteral fluids to supply additional calories, electrolytes, and/or water. Adequate hydration is particularly important in preterm infants because their extracellular water content is higher (70% in full-term infants and up to 90% in preterm infants), their body surface area is larger in comparison to their weight, and the capacity for osmotic diuresis is limited in their underdeveloped kidneys. Therefore these infants are highly vulnerable to fluid depletion.

Parenteral fluids may be given to the high-risk neonate via several routes depending on the nature of the illness, the duration and type of fluid therapy, and unit preference. Common routes of fluid infusion include peripheral, peripherally inserted central venous (or percutaneous central venous), surgically inserted central venous or arterial, and, at times, umbilical venous or umbilical arterial catheterization. The preferred sites for peripheral IV infusions in neonates are the peripheral veins on the dorsal surfaces of the hands or feet. Alternative sites are scalp veins and antecubital veins. Special precautions and frequent observations (at least once every hour) must accompany the use of peripheral lines with hypertonic solutions (dextrose 10% to 12%) and parenteral hyperalimentation solutions. In many neonatal centers the percutaneous central venous catheter, also commonly called the peripherally inserted central venous catheter, is used for IV hydration therapy and medication administration because of less expense and decreased neonatal trauma, and because of the ease of insertion (Bradshaw, Turner, and Pierce, 2006).

In most facilities NICU nurses insert peripheral IV catheters and maintain the infusions. IV fluids must always be delivered by continuous infusion pumps that deliver minute volumes at a preset flow rate. Secure the catheter to the skin with transparent tape or a specialized IV dressing, taking care not to cause undue pressure from the needle hub and tubing. Because ELBW and VLBW infants are highly vulnerable to any fluid shifts, infusion rates are carefully regulated and checked hourly to prevent tissue damage from extravasation, fluid overload, or dehydration (Kerr, Starbuck, and Block, 2006). Pulmonary edema, congestive heart failure, patent ductus arteriosus (PDA), and intraventricular hemorrhage (IVH) may occur with fluid overload. Dehydration may cause electrolyte disturbances (particularly sodium), with potentially serious central nervous system (CNS) effects.

> **! NURSING ALERT**
>
> Nurses should be constantly alert for signs of infiltration (e.g., redness, edema, or color change of tissue; blanching at site) and for signs of overhydration (weight gain of >30 g/24 hr [0.07 lb], periorbital edema, tachypnea, tachycardia, and crackles on lung auscultation).

Small, fragile peripheral blood vessels are subject to rupture and subsequent infiltration. This situation is compounded by the use of infusion pumps that continue to infuse fluid into surrounding tissues. Observations are especially important when using hypertonic solutions (calcium, sodium bicarbonate, parenteral hyperalimentation) and IV drugs (antibiotics and vasoactive drugs such as dopamine and dobutamine), which can cause serious tissue damage. With flexible catheters and small IV catheter shields, arm boards and limb restraints are usually unnecessary. If used, restraints should be checked frequently to ensure that no harm to the patient's extremity occurs and that peripheral circulation is adequate.

Infants who are ELBW, tachypneic, receiving phototherapy, or in a radiant warmer have increased IWL that require appropriate fluid adjustments. Nurses must monitor fluid status by taking daily (or more frequent) weights; accurately monitoring intake and output of all fluids, including medications and blood products; monitoring urine specific gravity as well as urine glucose and protein; and evaluating serum electrolyte levels. ELBW infants often require more frequent monitoring of these parameters because of their excessive transepidermal fluid loss, immature renal function, and propensity to dehydration or overhydration. Intolerance of even dextrose 5% is

not uncommon in the ELBW infant, with subsequent glycosuria and osmotic diuresis. Alterations in behavior, alertness, or activity level in these infants receiving IV fluids may signal an electrolyte imbalance, hypoglycemia, or hyperglycemia. The nurse is also observant for tremors or seizures in the VLBW or ELBW infant, since these may be a sign of hyponatremia or hypernatremia.

A common problem observed in infants who have an umbilical arterial catheter in place is vasoconstriction of peripheral vessels, which can seriously impair circulation. The response is triggered by arterial vasospasm caused by the presence of the catheter, the infusion of fluids, or injection of medication. Blanching of the buttocks, genitalia, or legs or feet is an indication of vasospasm. The problem is recognized promptly and reported to the practitioner. The nurse must also observe for signs of thrombi in infants with umbilical venous or arterial lines. The precipitation of microthrombi in the vascular bed with the use of such catheters is commonly manifested by a sudden bluish discoloration seen in the toes, called "cath toes." The problem is promptly reported to the practitioner because failure to alleviate the pathologic condition may result in permanent injury to the toes, foot, or leg.

Circulatory effects are observed first in the toes but may extend to include the legs and buttocks. The toes first flush and then turn a mulberry color; if the condition is not corrected, there may be serious complications involving the loss of a limb. The infant with an umbilical venous or arterial catheter should also be observed closely for catheter dislodgment and subsequent bleeding or hemorrhage; urinary output, renal function, and gastrointestinal function are also evaluated in these infants. Although the intent of such catheters is to effectively deliver IV fluids (and sometimes medications) and to obtain arterial blood gas samples, they are not without inherent complications.

Nutrition

Optimum nutrition is critical in the management of ELBW, VLBW, and LBW preterm infants, but difficulties arise in providing for their nutritional needs. The various mechanisms for ingestion and digestion of foods are not fully developed. The more immature the infant, the greater the problem.

Physiologic Characteristics

The preterm infant's need for rapid growth and daily maintenance must be met in the presence of several anatomic and physiologic disabilities. Although infants demonstrate some sucking and swallowing activities before birth, coordination of these mechanisms does not occur until approximately 32 to 34 weeks of gestation, and they are not fully synchronized until 36 to 37 weeks. Initial sucking is not accompanied by swallowing, and esophageal contractions are uncoordinated. As infants mature, the suck-swallow pattern develops but is slow and ineffectual, and these reflexes may easily become exhausted.

As with most full-term infants, preterm infants have poor muscle tone in the area of the lower esophageal (cardiac) sphincter. This causes milk in the stomach to be easily regurgitated into the esophagus, where it can trigger the chemoreceptors and cause apnea (vagal stimulation) and bradycardia and increase the risk of aspiration. The stomach has a limited capacity in preterm infants and is easily overdistended, further compromising respiration.

Physiologically, preterm infants (LBW, not ELBW or VLBW) have approximately the same capacity to digest and absorb protein as full-term infants. However, carbohydrates and fats are less well tolerated. The secretion of lactase, a late-developing enzyme, is low in infants born before 34 weeks of gestation; therefore formulas containing lactose may not be well tolerated. Although amylase is deficient in preterm infants, an alternative enzyme (glucoamylase) is able to compensate in most neonates so that they can tolerate moderate amounts of starch. Preterm infants are inefficient in digesting and absorbing lipids, especially the saturated triglycerides of cow's milk, because they have low levels of pancreatic lipase and low bile acid.

Nutritional Needs

The demand for nutrients in LBW infants is much higher than that in larger infants, and individual infants vary in activity level, ease of achieving basal energy expenditure, thermoneutrality, physical condition, and efficacy of nutrient absorption. The American Academy of Pediatrics, Committee on Nutrition (2009a), recommends an energy intake of 105 to 130 kcal/kg/day (taken enterally) for most preterm infants to achieve a satisfactory growth rate. It is estimated that for a daily weight gain of 15 g/kg, a caloric expenditure of 45 to 67 kcal/kg above the maintenance expenditure of 50 kcal/kg (Table 10-3) would be required (American Academy of Pediatrics, 2009a). Thus the amount of calories required for optimum growth in sick and VLBW infants is significantly higher than in their healthy full-term counterparts; the challenge of providing adequate calories for extrauterine growth in the preterm infant with limited capability to ingest and absorb nutrients is an important part of nursing care for this population.

Table 10-3 shows the caloric requirements of healthy, growing preterm infants at 3 to 4 weeks of age. The energy requirements for sick and VLBW infants remains unknown; estimates are an intake of up to 105 to 115 kcal/kg/day,

TABLE 10-3	ESTIMATED ENERGY REQUIREMENT IN LOW-BIRTH-WEIGHT INFANTS	
ENERGY EXPENDITURE	**AVERAGE ESTIMATION (kcal/kg/day)**
Total energy used	40-60
Resting metabolic rate	40-50*
Activity	0-5*
Thermoregulation	0-5*
Energy synthesis	15†
Stored energy	20-30†
Stool loss (energy)	15
Energy intake	90-120†

Adapted from American Academy of Pediatrics, Committee on Nutrition: *Pediatric nutrition handbook*, ed 6, Evanston, Ill, 2009, The Academy; and Committee on Nutrition of the Preterm Infant, European Society of Paediatric Gastroenterology and Nutrition: *Nutrition and feeding of preterm infants*, Oxford, 1987, Blackwell Scientific Publications.
*Energy required for maintenance.
†Energy expenditure for growth.

including a protein intake of 3 g/kg/day, for the ELBW infant (American Academy of Pediatrics, 2009a). Because most of the nutritional stores are accumulated in the final months of gestation, preterm infants also have low stores of calcium, iron, phosphorus, proteins, and vitamins A and C.

The infant's size and condition determine the amount and method of feeding. Nutrition can be provided by either the parenteral or enteral route or by a combination of the two.

Total parenteral nutritional support of acutely ill infants may be accomplished with commercially available IV solutions specifically designed to meet the infant's nutritional needs, including protein, amino acids, trace minerals, vitamins, carbohydrates (dextrose), and fat (lipid emulsion). Early protein intake (on day 1 of life) is also important in optimizing growth in LBW infants (Stephens, Walden, Gargus, et al, 2009). Daily monitoring of weight, electrolytes, renal function, calcium, and hydration status is carried out to ensure adequate therapy. As important as nutrition is the maintenance of adequate serum glucose homeostasis in sick preterm infants, who may depend on exogenous glucose sources for several days or weeks. Cornblath and Ichord (2000) recommend that in sick preterm infants an operational threshold blood glucose value of 45 to 50 mg/dl (2.6 to 2.8 mmol/L) be maintained.

Studies have revealed benefits to the early introduction of small amounts of enteral feedings in metabolically stable preterm infants (Hay, 2008). These minimum enteral feedings (MEFs; trophic feedings, gastrointestinal [GI] priming) have been shown to simulate the infant's GI tract, preventing mucosal atrophy and subsequent enteral feeding difficulties. They have also been shown to reduce the risk of sepsis. MEFs with as little as 0.1 to 4 ml/kg formula or breast milk may be given by gavage as early as day one of life or as soon as the infant is medically stable. In the past early introduction of milk feedings was thought to increase the risk of a devastating intestinal complication, necrotizing enterocolitis (NEC). NEC occurs more frequently in preterm infants, but the etiology of the disease remains unclear. No increased incidence of NEC in those VLBW infants given MEF has been found (Terrin, Passariello, Canani, et al, 2009; Berseth, Bisquera, and Paje, 2003).

A Cochrane review showed that infants receiving trophic feedings versus no feedings had an overall reduction in the number of days to full feedings and a shorter length of stay (Tyson and Kennedy, 2005). However, the researchers suggested that there was insufficient evidence to conclude that trophic feedings would indeed prevent NEC.

Controversy still exists regarding the type of enteral feeding that best meets the nutritional needs of LBW infants. The predominant view supports the use of milk from an infant's own mother. Alternatively, if breast milk is not available, commercial formulas designed specifically to meet the needs of small preterm infants that provide for adequate growth and metabolic stability can be used (Table 10-4). Prepared formulas have the advantage of allowing more concentrated feedings.

A number of studies regarding the effects of long-chain polyunsaturated fatty acids on cognitive development, visual acuity, and physical growth in full-term and preterm infants have prompted formula companies to add docosahexaenoic acid (DHA) and arachidonic acid (AA) to their infant formulas. AA and DHA are in human milk, and their presence has been

TABLE 10-4	PRETERM INFANT FORMULAS, HUMAN MILK FORTIFIERS, AND CALORIC ADDITIVES (DIET MODIFIERS)
FORMULA (MANUFACTURER)	**COMMENTS AND NUTRITIONAL CONSIDERATION**
EnfaCare (Mead Johnson)	22 kcal/fluid oz; iron fortified; contains nucleotides, AA and DHA; liquid
Similac NeoSure (Ross)	22 kcal/fluid oz; iron fortified; contains nucleotides; liquid; contains DHA and AA
Enfamil Premature with iron (Mead Johnson)	Available in 24 kcal/fluid oz; contains AA and DHA; liquid
Similac Special Care 24 (Ross); with Iron; High Protein; and Low Iron	24 kcal/fluid oz; iron fortified; liquid
Similac Special Care with Iron 20, 24, and 30 (Ross)	20, 24 and 30 kcal/fluid oz; liquid; contains DHA and AA; iron fortified; Low iron also available
Enfamil Human Milk Fortifier (Mead Johnson)	Powder; add to human milk—do not use as separate formula
Similac Human Milk Fortifier (Ross)	Powder; add to human milk—do not use as separate formula; fortification in excess of 1 package per 25 ml human milk not recommended
Polycose (Ross)	Powder used to augment caloric intake in formulas; 1 tsp powder = 8 kcal; glucose polymer; lactose- and gluten-free; infant formula additive only
Portagen (Mead Johnson)	Powder; 87% fat from MCT oil; *not* recommended as infant formula; indicated for use in children with defective mucosal fat absorption, decreased bile salts, and pancreatic lipase; long-term use not recommended; abdominal discomfort and diarrhea possible with initial use if not introduced gradually

AA, Arachidonic acid; *DHA,* docosahexaenoic acid.

assumed to lead to an increase in cognitive development in human milk–fed infants compared with infants fed a formula without these fatty acids (Gregory, 2004). One meta-analysis of four clinical trials demonstrated no clinically significant developmental benefits to supplementation of formula with AA and DHA in term and preterm infants at 18 months of age (Beyerlein, Hadders-Algra, Kennedy, et al, 2009).

Milk produced by mothers whose infants are born before term contains higher concentrations of protein, sodium, chloride, and immunoglobulin A (IgA). Thus mothers appear to be the preferred source of milk for their preterm infants. Growth factors, hormones, prolactin, calcitonin, thyroxine, steroids, and taurine (an essential amino acid) are also in human milk. The milk produced by mothers for their infants changes in content over the first 30 days postnatally, at which time it is similar to full-term human milk. Preterm infants who received human milk during their hospitalization demonstrated better intellectual performance scores at 7½ to 8 years of age compared with children who received formula (Schanler, 2001). Improved psychomotor development at 18 months has also been observed in preterm infants fed donor human milk compared with formula-fed preterm infants. Despite its benefits,

LBW infants (<1500 g [3.3 lb]) who are exclusively fed unfortified human milk demonstrate decreased growth rates and nutritional deficiencies even beyond the hospitalization period. These infants often have inadequacies of calcium, phosphorus, protein, sodium, vitamins, and energy (Schanler, 2001). Specially designed supplements for human milk have been developed to address these deficits. Preterm infants fed fortified human milk (FHM) have shorter hospital stays and less infection and NEC than infants given preterm formulas. Fortifiers are commercially available, usually as a liquid or powder containing protein; carbohydrate; calcium; phosphorus; magnesium; sodium; and varied amounts of zinc, copper, and vitamins. Because fortifiers do not contain sufficient iron, an exogenous source must be administered after enteral feeding. Fortifiers should be added to milk as close as possible to feeding time, and FHM should be refrigerated until it is used.

The antiinfectious attributes of human milk provide additional advantages for preterm infants. Secretory IgA concentration is higher in the milk from mothers of preterm infants than in the milk from mothers of full-term infants. IgA is important in the control of bacteria in the intestinal tract, where it inhibits adherence and proliferation of bacteria on epithelial surfaces. Additional protection from infection is provided by leukocytes, lactoferrin, and lysozyme, all of which are in human milk. Recent research suggests that administration of probiotics, live microbial supplements, decreases the incidence of NEC by normalizing intestinal flora, reducing intestinal permeability, and reducing gut inflammation (Alfaleh, Anabrees, and Bassler, 2009; Deshpande, Rao, and Patole, 2007).

NEC has been shown in several studies to be higher in formula-fed infants than in preterm infants fed human milk. Another report suggests that severity of NEC is lessened and the prevalence of intestinal perforation lowered when preterm infants are fed human milk (Schanler, 2001).

Preterm infants exclusively fed human milk have demonstrated significantly decreased NEC, fewer positive blood cultures, and decreased need for antibiotics. In one study infants fed human milk also received more skin-to-skin (STS) contact with their mothers and shorter hospital stays. Schanler (2001) suggests that STS contact might potentially stimulate the enteromammary immune system to produce specific antibodies against nosocomial pathogens in the nursery. Gastric emptying is improved with human milk feedings for preterm infants, primarily because of increased intestinal lactase and possibly decreased intestinal permeability. Finally, the psychologic advantages the mother gets from using her own milk cannot be overlooked.

For those infants who cannot be breast-fed but who also cannot survive except on human milk, banked donor milk is important. Because of the antiinfective and growth-promoting properties of human milk, as well as its superior nutrition, donor milk is used in many NICUs for preterm or sick infants when the mother's own milk is not available (American Academy of Pediatrics, 2005). Unprocessed human milk from unscreened donors is not recommended because of the risk of transmission of infectious agents (American Academy of Pediatrics, 2005).

The Human Milk Banking Association of North America (HMBANA; www.hmbana.org) has established guidelines for the operation of donor human milk banks (Human Milk Banking Association, 2008). Donor milk banks collect, screen, process (pasteurize), and distribute milk donated by breast-feeding mothers who are feeding their own infants and pumping a few extra ounces each day for the milk bank. All donors are screened both by interview and serologically for communicable diseases. Donor milk is stored frozen until it is heat processed to kill potential pathogens (bacteria and viruses), and then it is refrozen for storage until it is dispensed for use. The heat processing adds a level of protection for the recipient that is not possible with any other donor tissue or organ. Milk is dispensed only by prescription. A per-ounce fee is charged by the bank for processing, but the HMBANA guidelines prohibit payment to donors.

Although the timing of the first feeding has been controversial, most authorities now believe that early feeding (provided that the infant is medically stable) reduces the incidence of complicating factors such as hypoglycemia and dehydration and reduces the degree of hyperbilirubinemia. The feeding regimen used varies in different units. One strategy for the prevention of NEC that has been supported by research is the use of standardized feeding protocols. A meta-analysis of six studies found a significant reduction in NEC in infants fed by a standard protocol that included cautious advancement in feeding volumes (Patole and de Klerk, 2005).

Feeding tolerance and feeding success are not entirely the same concept. Feeding tolerance is evaluated by the following: (1) soft abdomen; (2) absence of abdominal distention or visible bowel loops on the skin surface; (3) minimum or no aspirated gastric residual; (4) presence of bowel sounds; (5) usual frequency, color, and consistency of stools; (6) minimum to no spitting up or vomiting; (7) infant's continued interest in feeding; and (8) consistent behavior pattern. Successful oral feeding should be safe, functional, and pleasurable. Feeding success can be measured by an infant's ability to (1) participate in feeding with energy, (2) coordinate sucking and swallowing with adequate pauses for breathing, (3) maintain vital signs and oxygenation within normal limits, (4) maintain normal muscle tone in face and body, (5) complete feeding in about 20 to 25 minutes, (6) manage a liquid bolus with minimum or no loss of liquid from mouth, (7) sustain alertness for feeding, (8) maintain strength and endurance for entire feeding, and (9) measure appropriate-for-age on standard growth curve. A preterm infant's success with feeding is first measured in terms of safety and functionality. Nurturing by holding close, but not socializing, during a feeding creates a warm and pleasurable experience. Later, after the infant is a competent feeder, socialization will enrich both parents' and infant's mealtime enjoyment.

Gavage Feeding

Gavage feeding is a safe means of meeting the nutritional requirements of infants who are not yet ready to feed orally. These infants are usually too weak to suck effectively, are unable to coordinate swallowing, or lack a gag reflex. A Cochrane review found that infants less than 1500 g (3.3 lb) fed by continuous tube-feeding took longer to reach full oral feeds than those fed intermittently; however, there was no difference in somatic growth or in the incidence of NEC (Premji and Chessell,

2003). Intermittent gavage feeding is used as an energy-conserving technique for infants learning to nipple-feed who become excessively tired, listless, or cyanotic.

A size 3.5, 5, 6, or 8 French feeding tube is usually used to instill the feeding, and the usual methods for determining correct placement are used. (See Chapter 27 for technique.) Although the more relaxed cardiac sphincter makes passage of the tube easier, the heart rate and blood pressure may change in response to vagal stimulation. The procedure is best accomplished when an infant is in a prone or a right side-lying position with the head slightly elevated. Small flexible nasogastric tubes (3.5 and 5 French) may be maintained as an indwelling feeding tube and used for prolonged periods without complications of intermittent removal and insertion.

The stomach is aspirated, the contents measured, and the aspirate returned as part of the feeding. However, this practice may vary, depending on circumstances and individual unit protocol.

> **! NURSING ALERT**
>
> An increase in gastric residuals, abdominal distention, bilious vomiting, temperature instability, apneic episodes, and bradycardia may indicate early NEC and should be called to the attention of the practitioner.

The feeding is allowed to flow by gravity, and the length of time varies. This procedure is not used as a timesaving method for the nurse. Complications of indwelling tubes include the obstructed nares, mucous plugs, purulent rhinitis, epistaxis, infection, and possible stomach perforation.

The infant may be held during gavage feedings by the caregiver or parent. Also, nonnutritive sucking (NNS) on a pacifier helps infants associate the sucking with the feeling of satiety. A Cochrane review of NNS demonstrated a significant reduction in length of stay in preterm infants receiving an NNS intervention. Other positive outcomes of NNS included enhanced transition from tube- to bottle-feeding and better bottle-feeding performance (Pinelli and Symington, 2005).

Oral Feeding

Vigorous infants can be fed orally with little difficulty, whereas compromised preterm infants require alternative methods. The amount to be fed is determined largely by the infant's weight gain and tolerance of previous feeding and is increased by small increments until a satisfactory caloric intake is ensured.

The rate of increase that is well tolerated varies from one infant to another, and determining this rate is often a nursing responsibility. Preterm infants require more time and patience to feed than full-term infants, and the oropharyngeal mechanism may be stressed by an attempt to feed too rapidly. It is important not to tire the infants or overtax their capacity to retain the feedings. When infants require a prolonged time (>30 minutes) to complete a feeding, gavage feeding may be considered for the next time.

The decision regarding when to start breast- or bottle-feeding is somewhat controversial. In many cases the decision is based on an evaluation of the infant's developmental maturity, weight, activity level, respiratory status (absence of apnea and adequate oxygen saturation levels), and sucking capabilities. Infant behavioral organizational skills, such as the ability to maintain a quiet alert state and display engagement cues, also influence the preterm infant's successful transition to oral feedings (Thoyre, Shaker, and Pridham, 2005). When infants are unable to tolerate breast- or bottle-feedings, intermittent feedings by gavage begin until they gain enough strength and coordination to use the nipple.

> ### ! NURSING ALERT
>
> Poor feeding behaviors such as apnea, bradycardia, cyanosis, pallor, and decreased oxygen saturation in any infant who has previously fed well may indicate an underlying illness in the preterm infant.

Although the nurse's role in relation to feeding depends on the institution, the following are suggested nursing responsibilities: (1) recognize feeding readiness cues; (2) identify feeding behaviors typical of preterm infants; (3) understand the infant's history and current medical condition; (4) consider environment, behavioral state, time of day, nipple type, and positioning; (5) understand rationale for different facilitation techniques and use appropriately; (6) evaluate feeding ability and tolerance; (7) identify infants with poor progress, structural defects, or abnormal feeding patterns who would benefit from specific therapy; and (8) play a supportive role for mothers who choose to breast-feed.

A developmental approach to feeding considers the individual infant's readiness rather than initiating feedings based on weight and age. Feeding readiness is determined by each infant's medical status, energy level, ability to sustain a brief quiet alert state, gag reflex (demonstrated with gavage tube insertion), spontaneous rooting and sucking behaviors, and functional sucking reflex (Hunter, 2001).

Oral feeding within a developmental framework involves three steps (Thoyre, Shaker, and Pridham, 2005):

1. Assessing individual physiologic, motor, and state behaviors during feeding
2. Individualizing the feeding plan based on specific infant cues
3. Fostering parental skill and confidence with feeding

The goal of feeding must be well understood. A key concept is recognizing the difference between a successful feeding (volume and time) and a successful feeder (infant ability and enjoyment). This is the difference between task and developmental feeding techniques. Planning the progression and nature of feedings requires close monitoring and careful documentation. Baseline assessment data are collected before each feeding and observed during and after the feeding to make a comparative evaluation of feeding success. Assessment is ongoing throughout the feeding, and facilitation techniques are chosen based on the individual infant's responses to improve the chance for feeding success and tolerance (Nye, 2008). Feeding stress and performance (Box 10-2) are evaluated and documented. Planning is done in collaboration with the health care team and family before the next feeding to determine appropriate strategies for the infant. Box 10-3 gives examples of ways to facilitate feeding.

BOX 10-2 FEEDING STRESS CUES

State Organization and Endurance
Decreased arousal
Awake but no energy
Irritable
Fatigues quickly within first 5 minutes

Physiologic
Tachypnea
Nasal flaring, retractions (increased work of breathing)
Decreased oxygen saturation
Apnea, bradycardia
Color change to dusky or pale

Oral-Motor
Unable to control fluid bolus (milk leaking out of mouth)
High-pitched sounds
Gulping
Coughing, choking
Multiple swallows without pausing for breath

Modified from Ancona J, Shaker CS, Puhek J, et al: Improving outcomes through a developmental approach to nipple feeding, *J Nurs Care Qual* 12(5):1-4, 1998.

BOX 10-3 FEEDING FACILITATION TECHNIQUES FOR PRETERM INFANTS

Environment
Prepare calm, quiet area with dim lighting and no distractions.
Ensure restful environment between feedings.

Direct Care
Avoid trial oral feedings after stressful procedures.
Choose slightly firm nipple with slower flow.
Gently arouse to alert state.
Swaddle in gentle flexion with infant's hands midline and toward face.
Support positioning with infant cradled close to body in semiupright or upright position, with neck in neutral to slightly flexed position.
Continuously observe physiologic, behavioral, and oral-motor functioning.
Provide adequate breathing and rest periods for infants who cannot pace themselves by gently removing nipple or, if that is too stressful, tipping bottle gently downward to drain milk from nipple.
Provide firm but gentle jaw and cheek support for problems with latching onto nipple (weak seal, loss of milk bolus).
Institute "developmental burping" on shoulder with postural support and gentle back rubbing in an upward motion to stimulate burp.
Recognize infant's limits and when to stop feeding.
Use gavage for the rest of the feeding as needed.
Schedule plenty of undisturbed rest between feedings.

Family Support and Education
Model appropriate feeding techniques.
Provide opportunity for feeding.
Educate on infant cues and how to measure feeding success.

Modified from Hunter J: The neonatal intensive care unit. In Case-Smith J, editor: *Occupational therapy for children,* ed 4, St Louis, 2001, Mosby.

Breast-Feeding

The American Academy of Pediatrics (2005) recommends human milk as the preferred food for all infants, including sick newborns and preterm infants (with rare exceptions). The academy recognizes that the choice of what to feed is the

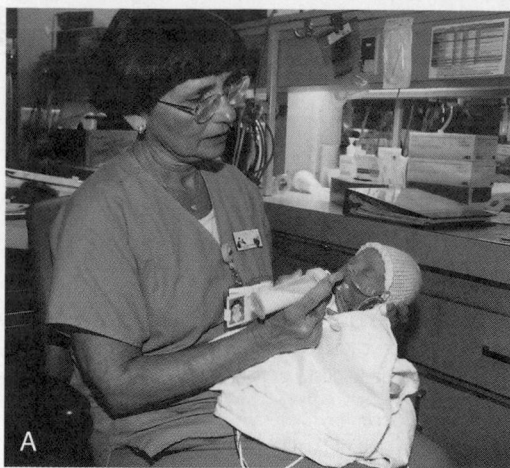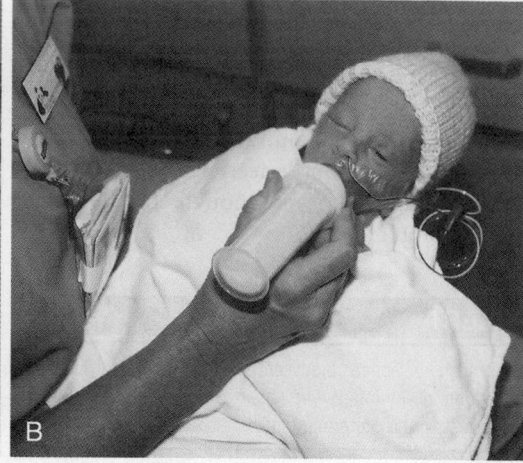

Fig. 10-3 Nipple-feeding the preterm infant. **A,** Infant is first brought to quiet alert state in preparation for feeding. **B,** After demonstrating readiness, infant is nipple-fed. (Courtesy Jeff Barnes, Education, and Eastern Oklahoma Perinatal Center, St. Francis Hospital, Tulsa.)

parents' prerogative but advises that providers give parents complete and accurate information on the benefits and methods of breast-feeding so they can make an informed decision. Barriers to initiation and continuation of breast-feeding include physician indifference, misinformation, lack of prenatal education about breast-feeding, distracting hospital policies, lack of follow-up, working mother, unsupportive work environment, lack of support from family or society, hospital discharge packs with formula or coupons for formula, and media portrayal of bottle-feeding.

Studies indicate that even small preterm infants are able to breast-feed if they have adequate sucking and swallowing reflexes and no other contraindications, such as respiratory complications or concurrent illness (Dougherty and Luther, 2008; Morton, 2002). Mothers who wish to breast-feed their preterm infants should pump their breasts until their infants are sufficiently stable to tolerate breast-feeding. Appropriate guidelines for the storage of expressed mother's milk should be followed to decrease the risk of milk contamination and destruction of its beneficial properties. (See Chapter 12.)

Preterm infants may be able to successfully breast-feed earlier than previously believed (28 to 36 weeks). In addition, preterm infants who are breast-fed rather than bottle-fed demonstrate fewer oxygen desaturation episodes; an absence of bradycardia; warmer skin temperature; and better coordination of breathing, sucking, and swallowing (Gardner, Snell, and Lawrence, 2006). The nurse should carefully evaluate the preterm infant for readiness to breast-feed, including assessment of behavioral state, ability to maintain body temperature outside an artificial heat source, respiratory status, and readiness to suckle at the mother's breast. The latter may be accomplished with NNS at the breast during STS (or kangaroo) contact so the mother and newborn can become accustomed to each other (Gardner, Snell, and Lawrence, 2006). Nasal cannula oxygen may also be provided during breast-feeding if the infant requires it.

Time, patience, and dedication on the part of the mother and the nursing staff are necessary to help infants breast-feed. The process starts slowly, beginning with one oral feeding daily and gradually increasing the feedings as the infant tolerates

them. Supplementary bottle-feeding is inefficient because the infant expends energy and calories to feed twice. Feeding more often and/or supplementing with gavage feeding is more energy and calorie efficient. Breast-feeding the preterm infant often requires additional guidance by a lactation consultant and continued support and encouragement by the nursing staff. In addition, postdischarge breast-feeding often requires further guidance, counseling, and support.

Social support for the mother is a major influence on the decision to breast-feed. To be effective advocates for mothers of all ethnicities, nurses must understand the cultural aspects that influence, whether positively or negatively, breast-feeding choices (McCarter-Spaulding, 2009; Gill, 2009). African-American women, for example, identify prenatal health care providers and friends as influential in decisions regarding breast-feeding. They tend to breast-feed less than women from other cultures and should be provided with appropriate information on breast-feeding by health care providers. Breast-feeding materials are available from organizations such as La Leche League International.*

Nipple-Feeding

The infant is positioned in the feeder's arms or placed semi-upright in the lap (Fig. 10-3) and is held with the back curved slightly to simulate the position assumed naturally by most full-term newborns. Stroking the infant's lips, cheeks, and tongue before feeding helps promote oral sensitivity.

Hill, Kurkowski, and Garcia (2000) used cheek and jaw support for preterm infants between 32 and 34 weeks of gestation to facilitate feeding. Supported infants had fewer and shorter pauses during feeding and had higher postfeeding oxygen saturations than infants not receiving oral support. The groups did not differ in terms of oxygen saturation, heart rate, and respiratory rate during feeding, indicating the technique is as safe as traditional feeding techniques. This technique uses the

---

*PO Box 4079, Schaumburg, IL 60618; 847-519-9585 (order department); www.llli.org. In Canada, La Leche League Canada, PO Box 700, Winchester, ON KOC 2KO; 613-774-4900; www.lalecheleaguecanada.ca.

thumb and index finger to provide gentle pressure (inward and forward) on the cheeks and the third finger to lift and stabilize the jaw under the mandible where the base of the tongue resides.

Bottle-feedings continue if infants are able to tolerate the feedings and take the required amount. The infant is best fed when fully alert. Drowsy infants feed more slowly, and liquid is more likely to fill the relaxed pharynx before the infant swallows, causing choking. It is believed that many digestive powers require signal stimulation to respond. Some preterm infants respond more slowly than full-term infants; therefore the feeding interval and amount are individualized. Preterm infants are often slow feeders and require patience, frequent rest periods, and burping (or bubbling).

A key ingredient for success is choosing an appropriate nipple. The nipple used should be relatively firm and stable. Although a high-flow, pliable nipple requires less energy to use, it may provide a flow rate that is too rapid for some preterm infants to manage without risk of aspiration. A firmer nipple facilitates a more "cupped" tongue configuration and allows for a more controlled, manageable flow rate.

Prodding techniques to encourage sucking can increase the risk of aspiration, especially if adequate breathing opportunities are not provided. The preterm infant has difficulty managing rapid or continuous milk flow with suck, swallow, and breathing coordination when the nipple is manipulated frequently by twisting or turning; the bottle is moved up and down or in and out of the mouth; or the infant's jaw is moved up and down (not the same as cheek and jaw support). The infant will try to continue to suck or swallow at the risk of physiologic and behavioral consequences.

Research by Law-Morstatt, Judd, Snyder, and colleagues (2003) has demonstrated that a paced bottle-feeding protocol that was structured to limit the length of sucking bursts and lengthen the duration of swallowing and breathing resulted in earlier emergence of organized sucking patterns than traditional approaches to feeding. Similar findings emerged from work by Fucile, Gisel, and Lau (2005), who found that a systematic protocol of oral motor stimulation resulted in enhanced tongue and jaw muscle strength and coordination.

Feeding Resistance

Any feeding technique that bypasses the mouth precludes the opportunity for the affected child to practice sucking and swallowing, or the opportunity to experience normal hunger and satiation cycles. Infants may demonstrate aversion to oral feedings by such behaviors as averting the head to the presentation of the nipple, extruding the nipple by tongue thrust, gagging, or even vomiting.

Developmental delays have occurred in perceptual-motor performance among infants with feeding refusal as measured by standard tests, although intellectual function remains within normal limits. Other observations include disinterest in or active resistance to oral play, diminished spontaneity and motivation, and shallow interpersonal relationships, probably related to the absence of some early incorporative patterns of normal oral experiences. The longer the period of nonoral feeding, the more severe the feeding problems, especially if this period occurs during a time when the infant progresses from

---

BOX 10-4	COMPONENTS OF A CARE PLAN TO PREVENT OR OVERCOME FEEDING RESISTANCE

- Simulate normal feeding interactions.
- Hold and cuddle infant in en face feeding position.
- Engage in eye contact with infant.
- Engage in verbal interaction with infant as tolerated.
- Help infant overcome oral hypersensitivity (sensitivity to intraoral stimulation).
- Provide oral stimulation.
- When external oral stimulation is tolerated, attempt gentle massage of gums and tongue (use finger or soft rubber item).
- Massage gums from center and move toward molar region, and move gradually from anterior to posterior.
- Withdraw stimulus and close child's mouth if child gags.
- Encourage oral exploration.
- Assist child in mouthing hands, fingers, toes, or soft rubber toys.
- Play oral games (e.g., blowing a kiss, kissing an object [toy animal]).
- Provide oral feedings.
- Introduce small volumes (even 3 to 5 ml) as early as possible.
- Offer feedings consistently (formula).
- Avoid force feeding.
- Provide feeding stimulation during tube-feedings.
- Hold child in feeding position.
- Provide nonnutritive sucking during bolus feedings.
- Give oral feedings before tube-feedings.
- Give bolus feedings in response to hunger when possible rather than on predetermined schedule.
- Provide nonnutritive sucking to encourage use of oral musculature.

Data from Orr MJ, Allen SS: Optimal oral experiences for infants on long-term total parenteral nutrition, *Nutr Clin Pract* 9:288-295, 1986.

---

reflexive to learned and voluntary feeding actions. During infancy the mouth is the primary instrument for reception of stimulation and pleasure.

Infants identified as being at risk for feeding resistance should receive regular oral stimulation based on the child's developmental level. Those who exhibit feeding aversion should begin a stimulation program to overcome resistance and acquire the ability to take nourishment by the oral route. Because management requires long-term commitment, successful implementation of a plan for oral stimulation depends on maximum parental involvement and promotion of primary nursing. Key components and interventions are in Box 10-4.

Skin Care

The skin of preterm infants is characteristically immature. Because of its increased sensitivity and fragility, no alkaline-based soap that might destroy the "acid mantle" of the skin is used. The increased permeability of the skin facilitates absorption of ingredients. All skin products (e.g., alcohol or povidone-iodine) are used with caution. The skin is rinsed with water afterward because these substances may cause severe irritation and chemical burns in LBW infants.

The skin is easily excoriated and denuded; therefore take care to avoid damage to the delicate structure. The total skin is thinner than that of full-term infants and lacks rete pegs, appendages that anchor the epidermis to the dermis. Therefore there is less cohesion between the thinner skin layers. Adhesives used after heel sticks or to secure monitoring equipment or IV infusions may excoriate the skin or adhere to the skin surface so well that the epidermis can be separated from the dermis and pulled away with the tape. The use of a zinc oxide–based tape such as Hy-Tape is encouraged to minimize epidermal stripping; the tape is flexible, waterproof, and, washable. The use of skin barriers protects healthy skin and helps excoriated skin heal.

Use scissors very carefully to remove dressings or tape from the extremities of very small and immature infants because it is easy to snip off tiny extremities or nick loosely attached skin. Avoid solvents to remove tape because they tend to dry and burn the delicate skin. Guidelines for skin care are given in the Nursing Care Guidelines box.

NURSING CARE GUIDELINES

Neonatal Skin Care

General Skin Care*
Assessment

Assess skin once each shift for redness, dryness, flaking, scaling, rashes, lesions, excoriation, or breakdown.

Consider using a validated skin assessment tool such as the Neonatal Skin Condition Score (Lund and Osborne, 2004).

Identify those infants at increased risk for skin breakdown.

Evaluate and report abnormal skin findings and analyze for possible causation.

Intervene according to interpretation of findings or physician order.

Bathing
Initial bath

Assess for stable temperature a minimum of 2 to 4 hours before first bath.

Use cleansing agents with neutral pH or minimum dyes or perfume, in water.

Do not completely remove vernix caeosa.

Bathe preterm infant (<32 weeks of gestation) in sterile water alone.

Routine

Decrease frequency of baths to every second or third day by daily cleansing of eye, oral and diaper areas, and pressure points.

Use cleanser or soaps no more than two or three times a week.

Avoid rubbing skin during bathing or drying.

Immerse stable infants fully (except head) in an appropriate-sized tub.

Use swaddled immersion bathing technique: slow unwrapping after gently lowering into water for sensitive, but stable, infants needing assistance with motor system reactivity.

Emollients

Follow hospital protocol or consider the following:
- Apply emollient as needed for dry, flaking skin.
- Use only emollients without perfumes, preservatives, or dyes.

Adhesives

Decrease use as much as possible.

Use transparent semipermeable adhesive dressings to secure intravenous lines, catheters, and central lines.

Use hydrogel electrodes.

Consider using pectin or hydrocolloid barriers beneath adhesives to protect skin.

Secure pulse oximeter probe or electrodes with elasticized dressing material (carefully avoid restricting blood flow).

Do not use adhesive remover, solvents, and bonding agents.

Avoid removing adhesives for at least 24 hours after application.

Adhesive removal can be facilitated using water, mineral oil, or petrolatum.

Remove adhesives or skin barriers slowly, supporting the skin underneath with one hand and gently peeling away the product from the skin with the other hand.†

Antiseptic Agents

Apply before invasive procedures.

Evaluate the risks and benefits of any antiseptic agent. Chlorhexidine gluconate and 10% povidone-iodine have both been shown to reduce skin bacterial counts in newborns. Povidone-iodine may be absorbed systemically.

Avoid use of alcohol.

Transepidermal Water Loss

Minimize transepidermal water loss and heat loss in small preterm infants (<30 weeks of gestation) by measuring ambient humidity during first weeks of life

and considering an increase in humidity to 70% for the first week of life by using one or more of the following options or hospital guidelines:
- Transparent dressings
- Servocontrolled humidifying incubator
- Supplemental conductive heat sources such as heated mattresses
- Polyethylene coverings (but avoid having plastic wraps in contact with skin surfaces for long periods)

Skin Breakdown*
Prevention

Decrease pressure from externally applied forces using water, air, or gel mattresses; sheepskin; or cotton bedding.

Provide adequate nutrition, including protein, fat, and zinc.

Apply transparent adhesive dressings to protect arms, elbows, and knees from friction injury.

Use tracheostomy and gastrostomy dressings for drainage and relief of pressure from tracheostomy or gastrostomy tube (Hydrasorb or Lyofoam).

Use emollient in the diaper area (groin and thighs) to reduce urine irritation.

Treating Skin Breakdown

Irrigate wound every 4 to 6 hours with warm half-strength normal saline using a 30 ml or larger syringe and 20-gauge Teflon catheter.

Culture wound and treat if signs of infection are present (excessive redness, swelling, pain on touch, heat, or resistance to healing).

Use petrolatum-based ointments for uninfected wounds.

Apply hydrogel with or without antibacterial or antifungal ointments (as ordered) for infected wounds (may need to moisten before removal).

Use hydrocolloid for deep, uninfected wounds (leave in place for 5 to 7 days) or as an ostomy barrier and to improve appliance adhesion; warm barrier in hand for several minutes to soften before applying to skin.

Avoid use of antiseptic solutions for wound cleansing (used for intact skin only).

Treating Diaper Dermatitis

Maintain clean, dry skin; use absorbent diapers and change often.

If mild irritation occurs, use petrolatum barrier.

For developing dermatitis, apply a generous quantity of zinc-oxide barrier.

For severe dermatitis, identify cause and treat (e.g., frequent stooling from spina bifida, severe opiate withdrawal, or malabsorption syndrome).

Treat *Candida albicans* with antifungal ointment or cream.

Avoid talcum powders and antibiotic ointments. (See Care of the Umbilicus and Circumcision, Chapter 8.)

Other Skin Care Concerns‡
Use of Substances on Skin

Evaluate all substances that come in contact with infant's skin.

Before using any topical agent, analyze components of preparation and:
- Use sparingly and only when necessary.
- Confine use to smallest possible area.
- Whenever possible and appropriate, wash off with water.
- Monitor infant carefully for signs of toxicity and systemic effects.

Use of Thermal Devices

Avoid heat lamps because of increased potential for burns. If needed, measure actual temperature of exposed skin every 15 minutes.

When using heating pads (Aqua-K pads):

NURSING CARE GUIDELINES—cont'd

Neonatal Skin Care

Other Skin Care Concerns—cont'd
Use of Thermal Devices—cont'd
- Change infant's position every 15 minutes initially and then every 1 to 2 hours.
- Preset temperature of heating pads to less than 40° C (104° F).

When using preheated transcutaneous electrodes:
- Avoid use on infants weighing less than 1000 g (2.2 lb).
- Set at lowest possible temperature (<44° C [111.2° F]) and secure with plastic wrap.
- Use pulse oximetry rather than transcutaneous monitoring whenever possible.

When prewarming heels before phlebotomy, avoid temperatures greater than 40° C.

Warm ambient humidity, and direct away from infant; use aerosolized sterile water and maintain ambient temperature so as not to exceed 40° C.
Document use of all heating devices.

Use of Fluid Therapy and Hemodynamic Monitoring
Be certain fingers or toes are visible whenever extremity is used for intravenous or arterial line.
Secure catheter or needle with transparent dressing or tape to promote easy visualization of site.
Assess site hourly for signs of ischemia, infiltration, and inadequate perfusion (check capillary refill).
Avoid use of restraints (e.g., arm boards); if used, check that they are secured safely and not restricting circulation or movement (check for pressure areas).
Use commercial intravenous protector (e.g., I.V. House) with minimum tape.

*From Association of Women's Health, Obstetric and Neonatal Nurses: *Evidence-based clinical practice guideline: neonatal skin care*, ed 2, Washington, DC, 2007, The Association.
†CAUTION: Scissors are not to be used for tape or dressing removal because of hazard of cutting skin or tiny digits.
‡Data from Taquino LT: Promoting wound healing in the neonatal setting: process versus protocol, *J Perinat Neonat Nurs* 14(1):108-118, 2000; and Malloy MB, Perez-Woods R: Neonatal skin care: prevention of skin breakdown, *Pediatr Nurs* 17(1):41-48, 1991.

During skin assessment of preterm infants, nurses are alert to the subtle signs that indicate zinc deficiency, a common problem in these infants. Breakdown usually occurs in the areas around the mouth, buttocks, fingers, and toes. In VLBW infants it may also occur in the creases of the neck, wrists, and ankles and around wounds. Zinc deficiency is most likely to appear in infants with sepsis, those experiencing nasogastric losses, or those who have had surgery. Report suspicious lesions to the practitioner so that zinc supplements can be prescribed. In most preterm infants the skin barrier properties resemble those of the term infant by 2 to 3 weeks postnatal age, regardless of gestational age at birth.

Although no studies comparing the effectiveness of different commercially available neonatal bedding have been done, a number of products are useful in minimizing skin problems. The Nursing Care Guidelines box gives general information about bedding. Particularly vulnerable areas of the skin, such as bony prominences, can be protected with transparent dressings. Gel pads or mattresses can also be used to prevent pressure ulcers (Association of Women's Health, Obstetric and Neonatal Nurses, 2007).

Skin injuries have been reported during use of phototherapy blankets. Caution is warranted in using these products with extremely preterm infants or infants with birth trauma, poorly perfused skin, or hypotension. Manufacturers of phototherapy blankets recommend the following during therapy: monitor skin color, observe for rashes or excoriation, keep skin clean with warm water, promptly clean perineum after stooling, reposition every 2 hours, carefully monitor cleanliness and skin integrity, and avoid direct contact of blanket with infant's skin.

Administration of Medications

Administration of therapeutic agents, such as drugs, ointments, IV infusions, and oxygen, requires judicious handling and meticulous attention to detail. The computation, preparation, and administration of drugs in minute amounts often require collaboration between nurses, physicians, and pharmacists to reduce the chance for error. In addition, the immaturity of an infant's detoxification mechanisms and inability to demonstrate symptoms of toxicity (e.g., signs of auditory nerve involvement from ototoxic drugs such as gentamycin) complicate drug therapy and require that nurses be particularly alert for signs of adverse reaction. (See Administration of Medication, Chapter 27.)

Nurses should be aware of the hazards of administering bacteriostatic and hyperosmolar solutions to infants. Benzyl alcohol, a common preservative in bacteriostatic water and saline, is toxic to newborns and should not be used to flush IV catheters or to dilute or reconstitute medications. It is recommended that medications with preservatives such as benzyl alcohol be avoided. Nurses must read labels carefully to detect the presence of preservatives in any medication administered to an infant.

Hyperosmolar solutions present a potential danger to preterm infants. Hyperosmolar solutions given orally to infants can produce clinical, physiologic, and morphologic alterations, the most serious of which is NEC. Oral or parenteral medications should be sufficiently diluted to prevent complications related to hyperosmolality.

Take caution to reduce adverse effects of medication administration in preterm infants. Strategies to heighten awareness and decrease unnecessary morbidity in such infants include having two registered nurses double check the dosages of potentially lethal medications (high-risk medications) and providing calculators in neonatal units to perform dosage calculations, double check unit dose medications, and check medications that are reconstituted by the nurse. Some other precautions are to have readily available quick-reference guides to weight-specific medication doses and appropriate dosages for preterm infants and to provide tables with medication cross-reactivity and incompatibility. One NICU developed a distinct neonatal formulary to reduce medication errors. Another strategy was to develop computerized guidelines for managing dose ranges based on the neonate's most recent weight so medications ordered outside the appropriate dose range could be reevaluated by the pharmacist and practitioner This concept was also applied to computer-generated emergency medication sheets, which are updated weekly (Lucas, 2004).

Information technology (e.g., computerized practitioner order entry and clinical participation by a clinical pharmacist) is available to reduce medication errors, yet this technology does not provide the entire solution (Taylor, Loan, Kamara, et al, 2008). The human factor involved in many root-cause analyses for medication errors involves systems and the humans involved in those systems. Nurses, physicians, and pharmacists are at times affected by internal and external environmental factors that lead to a medication error: excessive workload; distractions such as a monitor alarm or questions asked during medication administration; boredom; work hours (nighttime or daytime); lack of updated, consistent drug information; ambiguous drug labeling; and dosage calculation errors (Lefrak, 2002). The variables involved are numerous and multifaceted yet can be decreased by simple cautionary measures, extensive education, and verification of medication orders written.

Developmental Outcome

Neonatal intensive care and rapid improvements in technology are associated with improved survival of critically ill newborn and preterm infants. Survival rates have increased to 93% for VLBW infants (1001 to 1500 g [2.2 to 3.3 lb]), 85% for ELBW infants (751 to 1000 g [1.6 to 2.2 lb]), and about 50% for infants weighing 501 to 750 g [1.1 to 1.6 lb] (Msall and Tremont, 2000). With decreasing mortality, morbidity rates have remained stable. At highest risk for unfavorable outcomes are preterm infants compromised during the neonatal period by respiratory distress syndrome (RDS), bronchopulmonary dysplasia (BPD, or chronic lung disease), NEC, sepsis, anemia, IVH, hydrocephalus, meningitis, or seizures (McGrath, Sullivan, and Lester, 2000; Vohr, Widen, Cone-Wesson, et al, 2000). These serious sequelae of prematurity correlate with the degree of immaturity, demonstrating the relationship of increasing morbidity with decreasing gestational age. A greater incidence of CP, attention deficit hyperactivity disorder, visual-motor deficits, mild to severe cognitive disabilities, hearing loss, speech and language impairment, and neuromotor problems has been reported in outcome studies of preterm infants (van Baar, van Wassenaer, Briet, et al 2005; Wilson-Costello, 2007; Hack and Costello, 2008). Reduced language and visual-motor skills have been reported in former LBW infants at 7 years of age (Pietz, Peter, Graf, et al, 2004).

An increased need for special school services, especially in reading and math, has been reported in former LBW infants at 12 years of age (Luu, Ment, Schneider, et al, 2009). Another longitudinal study of 532 VLBW infants from four countries found that, when evaluated between 8 and 11 years of age, more than half of all cohorts required special educational assistance and/or repeated a grade (Saigal, den Ouden, Wolke, et al, 2003). Neurodevelopmental impairment also occurs in preterm infants who have been spared the complications of IVH, sepsis, and hypoxemia, moving through the NICU with seemingly few problems. Conversely, some preterm infants do well and function at age level without evidence of neurobehavioral limitations. Improved developmental outcomes are more likely for these survivors of early gestation and LBW when emphasis is placed on providing the finest medical and nursing care within a developmentally supportive framework. This philosophy requires caregivers to evaluate their own knowledge, skills, and attitudes and expand their thinking beyond the traditional medical and nursing models of care.

Developmental Assessment

One approach to NICU care is based on Als's (1982) synactive theory of infant development, which provides a framework for understanding the preterm infant's development. The model proposes a systematic method for observing NICU infants to collect information concerning each infant's competencies, vulnerabilities, and thresholds. This information forms the basis for planning individualized care appropriate for a particular infant (Table 10-5). The major assumption of this model is that infants, even ELBW infants, can communicate through physical and behavioral responses that provide us with the best information for planning their care. Communication by the infant is seen through three subsystems of function (autonomic, motor, and state) that can be readily observed in the clinical setting during rest, care, or procedures and during recovery from care or procedures. Responses by an infant's autonomic (physiologic), motor, and state systems to the environment, physical care, or procedures help the nurse make necessary adjustments in technique to optimize the infant's stability and function.

Individualized developmental care has had numerous positive effects on medical and neurobehavioral outcomes in high-risk newborn infants. Findings noted in a randomized controlled trial of developmental care for 92 preterm infants weighing less than 1250 g (2.7 lb) included shorter duration of parenteral feeding and time to full oral feeding; decreased time in intensive care and in hospital; lower incidence of NEC; improved weight, length, and head circumferences; enhanced autonomic, motor, state, attention, and self-regulatory function; and lowered family stress (Als, Gilkerson, Duffy, et al, 2003). In contrast, the Cochrane review done by Symington and Pinelli (2006) notes that, because of the inclusion of multiple interventions, it is difficult to ascribe specific benefits to the implementation of developmental care.

Because each infant is unique, supportive developmental care requires ongoing data collection of moment-by-moment responses and flexible care to address the infant's cues. For example, an infant who demonstrates altered vital signs and even apnea after being weighed might benefit from swaddled weighing to support the infant's competence and organization during a stressful procedure.

Knowledge of behavioral assessment and infant development assists the nurse in providing care that supports each infant's ongoing function in a manner consistent with current evidence. Nurses have the greatest impact on the daily routine experienced by their tiny patients. The CNS is undergoing rapid and significant change during the preterm infant's stay in the NICU. This vulnerable period of brain growth, differentiation, and organization is combined with the challenge of developing in environmental conditions that are not typical for the fetus and newborn (Blackburn, 2007). Brain organization peaks from about 20 weeks of gestation to several years after birth. The product of this complex process is establishment of an elaborate circuitry unique to the human brain.

Behavioral State Organization

Traditional nursing placed emphasis on interpreting physiologic data as the basis of caregiving. Developmentally support-

TABLE 10-5	SYNACTIVE THEORY OF DEVELOPMENT: NEUROBEHAVIORAL SUBSYSTEMS	
SUBSYSTEM	**SIGNS OF STRESS**	**SIGNS OF STABILITY**
Autonomic	Physiologic instability	Physiologic stability
Respiratory	Tachypnea, pauses, gasping, sighing	Smooth, stable respirations; regular rate and pattern
Color	Mottled, flushed, dusky, pale or gray	Pink, stable color
Visceral	Hiccups, gagging, choking, spitting up, grunting and straining as if having a bowel movement; coughing, sneezing, yawning	Absence of hiccups, gagging, spitting up, etc.
Autonomic	Tremors, startles, twitches	Absence of tremors, startles, twitches
Motor	Fluctuating tone; lack of control over movement, activity, and posture	Consistent tone; controlled or improved movement, activity, and posture
Flaccidity	Low tone in trunk; limp, floppy upper and lower extremities; limp, drooping jaw (gape face)	Tone consistent and appropriate for postmenstrual age
		Well-maintained posture
Hypertonicity	Arm or leg extensions, arm(s) outstretched with fingers splayed in salute gesture, fingers stiffly outstretched, trunk arching, neck hyperextended	Smooth, controlled movements
Hyperflexion activity	Trunk hyperflexion, hyperflexion of extremities, fisting; squirming; frantic diffuse activity or little or no activity or responsiveness	Successful motor strategies for self-regulation (see Self-Regulation below)
State	Disorganized quality to state behaviors, including range of available states, maintenance of state control, and transition from one state to another	Easy-to-read state behaviors that are maintained; calm, focused alertness, well-modulated sleep
Sleep	Whimpering sounds, facial twitching, irregular respirations, fussing, grimacing, restless appearance	Clear, well-defined sleep states; periods of quiet, restful sleep
Awake	Glazed unfocused look, staring, worried or pained expression, hyperalert or panicked appearance, eye roving, crying, "cry-face," actively averting gaze or closing eyes, irritability, prolonged awake periods, inconsolability, frenzy	Alert with bright, shiny eyes; focused attention on object or person; animated expression (e.g., cheek softening, frowning, "ooh-face," cooing, smiling)
	Abrupt or rapid state changes	Robust crying
		Good calming, consolability
		Smooth changes between states, full range of sleep-wake states
Other state-related behaviors and attention-interaction	Efforts to attend to and interact with environmental stimulation eliciting signs of stress and disorganized subsystem functioning	Responsive to auditory, visual, and social stimuli
Autonomic	Physiologic instability of varying degrees with autonomic, respiratory, color, and visceral responses	Responsiveness to stimuli well maintained and prolonged
Motor	Fluctuating tone, increased motor activity, progressively frantic diffuse activity if stimulation continues	Actively seeking auditory stimulus, minimum motor activity
State	Roving eyes, gaze averted, glazed-unfocused look or worried, panicked expression; weak cry; cry-face; irritability	Bright, shiny-eyed, alert, and attentive expression
	Closed eyes and sleeplike withdrawal	Sustained awake and alert state
	Abrupt state changes	Shifting attention smoothly to more than one type of stimulation
	Signs of stress when presented with more than one type of stimulus at a time	

Self-regulation—Infant's efforts to achieve, maintain, or regain a balanced, stable, and relaxed stated of subsystem functioning and integration. Success of these efforts will vary among infants depending on maturity, available self-regulatory skills, and overall subsystem organization. Examples of self-regulatory strategies include:

Motor—Foot bracing against a boundary or blanket nest, hand holding, clasping hands together, hand to mouth or face, grasping blanket, tubing, tucking trunk, sucking, position changes

State—Lowering state from high arousal to quiet alert or sleep state; releasing energy by rhythmic, robust crying; focused attention and orientation

Facilitation by caregivers—Environmental modifications or developmental care techniques to aid infant's own self-regulatory abilities when environmental challenges exceed infant's capabilities.

Modified from Als H: Toward a synactive theory of development: promise for the assessment and support of infant individuality, *Inf Mental Health J* 3(4):229-243, 1982; Als H: A synactive model of neonatal behavior organization: framework for the assessment of neurobehavioral development in the premature infant and for support of infants and parents in the neonatal intensive care environment, *Phys Occup Therap Pediatr* 6:3-55, 1986; and Hunter JG: The neonatal intensive care unit. In Case-Smith J, Allen AS, Pratt PN, editors: *Occupational therapy for children*, ed 4, St Louis, 2001, Mosby.

ive care uses both physiologic and behavioral information to better understand the needs of infants in the NICU setting. **Behavioral states** are highly individualized and formed by experience, maturation, circadian rhythms, and genetic inheritance. The emerging availability and regulation of arousal states mark a balancing of CNS inhibitory and excitatory processes

that affect attention states and also mark executive functions (prefrontal cortex) that influence information processing, learning, and socialization. **State organization** has been described as a gating mechanism that protects the cortex from overstimulation and promotes coordination between attentional, executive, and sensory cortical systems.

TABLE 10-6   AROUSAL STATES

STATE	DESCRIPTION
Deep sleep	Regular breathing; eyes closed with no movement of eyes under lid; relaxed face; little or no movement or activity except for possible startle response
Active sleep	Sometimes called light sleep; may see rapid eye movements under closed lids, low activity level, breathing regular or irregular, occasional sighing or smiling
Drowsy	Eyes open or closed, unfocused expression; activity level varied
Quiet awake	Different qualities of alerting
Robust	Bright, shiny appearance to eyes; focused attention; minimum motor activity
Low level	Dull or unfocused eyes; little energy; appears to look through object or caregiver
Hyperalert	Wide eyes, panicked expression; may fixate on object or caregiver intensely and have trouble breaking away
Active awake	Active; eyes open or closed; fussy but not crying robustly
Crying	Highest level of arousal; agitated, rhythmic, and robust crying

Modified from Als H: *Manual for the naturalistic observation of newborn behavior,* Newborn Individualized Developmental Care and Assessment Program (NIDCAP), Boston, 1995, Harvard Medical School.

Infant responsiveness to environmental stimuli depends on the quality, amount, and availability of particular states of arousal. States can be organized into five levels of arousal (Table 10-6). Transitional states such as drowsiness are not considered true states but are in-between levels of arousal in which the infant either moves toward wakefulness or back into sleep.

Distinct sleep and awake states are observable in infants between 25 and 27 weeks (Holditch-Davis and Blackburn, 2007). Young preterm infants spend 70% or more of their time in active sleep. Developmental maturation for the young preterm infant is seen by a decrease in the amount of active sleep with an increase in quiet sleep, awake periods, and crying. Around 30 to 32 weeks, quiet alert states with some focused attention can occur. Before 28 weeks, attempts to attend to stimuli may have physiologic consequences for the immature infant (Blackburn, 1998). Responsiveness to sound and touch is greater during active or light (rapid eye movement [REM]) sleep, resulting in longer periods of vulnerability to sleep disturbance (Holditch-Davis, 1998). Maturation continues throughout the first year of life. By 6 months, the amount of quiet sleep is greater than that of active sleep. By 1 year, infants usually sleep 10 to 12 hours at night and take one or two naps during the day. Preterm infants generally sleep for shorter periods at night and awaken more frequently than full-term infants. Other maturational changes include organization of the standard sleep cycle and electroencephalogram sleep patterns comparable to those of adults. Neurologic insults, severity of illness, hyperbilirubinemia, and prenatal exposure to drugs can alter behavioral state patterns.

Physiologic parameters vary depending on level of arousal. Heart rate is higher during waking periods but more variable during active sleep. Blood pressure is higher during wakefulness. Cerebral blood flow is greater during active sleep (greater during quiet sleep in full-term infants). Respiratory rates fluctuate more and are higher in active sleep. Arterial oxygen and carbon dioxide levels are lower in active sleep than in quiet sleep or awake states. Hypoventilation and poorly coordinated chest wall and abdominal movements are reported during active sleep. Apneic pauses of less than 20 seconds are more frequent in active than quiet sleep in preterm infants.

Nursing care should be timed to the responsiveness of the infant as much as possible to optimize the development of sleep organization and enhance alerting as it emerges. Sensory stimulation can influence behavioral state as seen by either increased or decreased infant arousal when presented with a stimulus and its removal; the type of stimulus (e.g., loud bell or soft lullaby) also is a factor. The quality of each state, its duration, and the movement between states provide information concerning how well organized the state is and how much state control the infant has. Protection of sleep is an important goal for both the preterm and full-term infant. Environmental modifications and timing of care to provide longer episodes of undisturbed sleep should be planned into care.

Nurses can also support transitions between states. Gentle arousal to wakefulness by soft speech or gentle touch before caregiving is preferable to the traditional model in which care is begun without warning and with abrupt disruption of sleep. Slow movements and gentle handling support quiet alerting or return to sleep without periods of arousal after care is over. Nurses should facilitate return to sleep or interact with a quietly alert infant after care events.

An infant's state of arousal allows for communication of responses that are valuable for individualized caregiving. Observing state patterns and individual responses of infants, nurses can better know their patients and support behavioral state organization. The nurse can also share this knowledge with parents to foster intimacy with the child.

Sensory System

Research with animal fetuses and infants has shown that atypical sensory experiences, whether overstimulating or depriving, can modify the developing brain (Glass, 2005; Lickliter, 2000a). In fact, much of the cerebral cortex is associated with the sensory system. Most sensory systems develop prenatally and are capable of functioning before birth. Onset of function of each sensory system proceeds in the same order for each individual (i.e., tactile, vestibular, gustatory-olfactory, auditory, and visual). The visual system becomes functional after birth. Sensory input provided before the stimulation would typically occur has been shown to interfere with perceptual and behavioral development (Lickliter, 2000b).

The normal experience for the preterm infant is within the womb and for the full-term infant is the home environment with a few primary caregivers. These environments are vastly different from the NICU. The NICU experience for the high-risk infant is made up of external conditions and interactions with caregivers. Often that experience is overstimulating to later-developing sensory systems (i.e., auditory and visual) and understimulating to earlier ones (i.e., tactile, vestibular, gustatory-olfactory). Alterations in the sensory environment may have developmental consequences. It is important for the nurse to consider the following while caring for high-risk infants: (1) timing of stimulation in relation to the infant's current developmental stage, (2) amount of stimulation provided or denied, (3) type of stimulation, and (4) the infant's response to the stimulation (Lickliter, 2000b).

By the age of viability, infants in the NICU have sophisticated perioral sensation and perceive pressure, pain, and temperature (Als, 1999). Touch in the NICU frequently involves routine, sometimes impersonal, caregiving and procedures that are either intrusive or painful. Even nonpainful care has been associated with adverse responses in preterm infants.

Preterm infants demonstrate cry expression, grimacing, and knee and leg flexion during major reposition changes. Hypoxemia, associated with nonpainful or routine caregiving activities such as suctioning, repositioning, taking vital signs, changing diapers, and removing electrodes, has been reported (Glass, 2005). Other physiologic changes involve blood pressure, heart rate, and respiratory rhythm and rate (Glass, 2005; Browne, 2000; Peters, 1999). Nursing activities that are painful or especially intrusive, such as needle puncture, suctioning, and chest physiotherapy, have resulted in acute decreases in SaO_2 and behavioral state changes in preterm infants ranging from 23 to 37 weeks of gestation (Zahr and Balian, 1995). Increased motor activity, agitation, crying, and startle reflex have also been described as negative behavioral responses to touch (Browne, 2000).

Touch is the first sensory system to develop and forms the basis for early communication between infants and caregivers. In particular, touch is a powerful means of emotional exchange for parents and infants. Positioning and handling techniques promote comfort and minimize stress, while creating a balance between nurturing care and necessary interventions.

Therapeutic Handling

Using the developmental model of supportive care, the nurse closely monitors physiologic and behavioral signs to promote organization and well-being of high-risk infants during handling (Box 10-5). The type, timing, and amount of handling are carefully considered in terms of the infant's current age, condition, vulnerabilities, thresholds for stress, and capabilities. Because touch can be disruptive to maturing sleep-wake states, avoid waking an infant for care or nurturing. Sleep deprivation may affect secretion of growth hormone and interfere with growth and development (Hunter, 2001).

Respectful approach before touching an infant allows more time for transition and adaptation from being alone to being handled. The nurse can use the infant's own cues to determine optimum times for caregiving rather than following a rigid schedule. The best time for care is when an infant is awake. If the care or procedure cannot be postponed, softly calling an infant by name and then gently placing a hand on the body signals care is beginning and avoids the abrupt interruption that frequently precedes caregiving. Abrupt transitions can disrupt even organized functioning of an infant's autonomic, motor, and state subsystems.

Infants who are unable to maintain a gently flexed position during repositioning or care procedures may benefit from containment. Gently holding the infant's arms and legs in a tucked, flexed position close to the body can be accomplished with

---

BOX 10-5 CONSIDERATIONS FOR TACTILE INTERVENTIONS IN THE NEONATAL INTENSIVE CARE UNIT

- Modify all handling and touch so that it is supportive and calming.
- Consider sleep-wake states and behavioral cues to determine optimum times for handling and touch.
- Adjust handling and touch based on continual observation of the infant's autonomic and behavioral responses.
- Ensure appropriate touch opportunities for parents aside from routine caregiving.
- Encourage parents to be primary providers of social touch.
- Avoid using massage with vulnerable high-risk infants (e.g., medically unstable, low-birth-weight infants less than 32 weeks of gestation; easily disorganized, low-threshold infants; chronically ill infants with chronic lung disease or cardiac disorders known to display physiologic and behavioral disorganization).
- Assist parents in identifying the most appropriate type of touch and handling for their infant.
- Teach infant cues to parents for monitoring responses to handling and touch.
- Weigh the risks and benefits for any tactile intervention.

---

hands or blanket swaddling. Facilitated tucking before ET suctioning was shown to decrease physiologic and behavioral distress in preterm infants as young as 23 weeks of gestational age (Ward-Larson, Horn, and Gosnell, 2004). Blanket swaddling and nesting or containment decreased physiologic and behavioral stress during routine care procedures such as bathing, weighing, and heel lance (Byers, 2003).

Because repositioning has been associated with significant physiologic distress in immature infants, avoid sudden postural changes. Slow turning while containing the infant's extremities in a gently tucked, midline position may reduce the impact of this procedure.

Stroking preterm infants who are not physiologically stable has been reported to result in behavioral signs of distress such as gasping, grunting, gaze aversion, and decreased $tcPO_2$ levels. Some infants experience apnea and bradycardia during massage or tactile-kinesthetic stimulation (Glass, 2005). Other researchers report positive benefits of gentle human touch, including heart rate and oxygen saturation stability (Modrcin-Talbott, Harrison, Groer, et al, 2003). Individual infants show varied responses to tactile intervention, further supporting the need for close monitoring of behavioral and physiologic parameters.

Investigators have reported positive benefits of massage on stable, growing, preterm infants. Beachy (2003) found that, when infant massage therapy is properly applied to stable preterm infants, they respond with increased weight gain, enhanced developmental scores, and shortened hospital stays. Parents of the preterm infant also benefit because infant massage enhances bonding with their child and increases confidence in their parenting skills. Dieter, Field, Hernandez-Reif, and colleagues (2003) studied 16 preterm infants (mean gestational age of 30 weeks) and found that after 5 days of receiving massage therapy, infants in the treatment group averaged a 53% greater weight gain and spent less time sleeping than control infants.

Vickers, Ohlsson, Lacy, and colleagues (2004) evaluated literature relevant to infant massage, gentle touch, and gentle human touch. The researchers concluded that available studies, although demonstrating advantages to massage for preterm infants, lack sound methodologic bases on which firm recommendations can be made to advocate wide-scale use of this intervention.

Kangaroo care, or STS holding, has been advocated for fostering neurobehavioral development and supporting parent-infant intimacy and attachment. STS contact is maintained with the diaper-clad infant resting prone and semiupright on the bare chest of either parent, who encloses the infant in his or her own clothing to maintain temperature stability. Kangaroo care is reported to reduce incidence of severe illness and nosocomial infection, support breast-feeding duration until discharge, improve maternal satisfaction (Conde-Agudelo, Diaz-Rossello, and Belizan, 2000) and parental interaction (Feldman, Eidelman, Sirota, et al, 2002), and accelerate neurologic maturation (Feldman and Eidelman, 2003). Hurst, Valentine, Renfro, and colleagues (1997) reported a significant increase in milk volume in mothers providing kangaroo care to stable, ventilated, LBW infants (mean 27.7 weeks of gestation) compared with a control group. Others have reported advantages that include maintenance of skin temperature, reduction of apnea and bradycardia, stable $tcPo_2$ level, increased frequency and duration of quiet sleep, less time crying, and lower activity levels during kangaroo care (Roberts, Paynter, and McEwan, 2000; Byers, 2003). Kangaroo care has been successfully initiated in stable preterm infants who weigh less than 1000 g (2.2 lb) (Neu, Browne, and Vojir, 2000).

However, in a study of preterm infants (mean gestational age of 29 weeks), kangaroo care was associated with a significant increase in bradycardia, less regular breathing, and hypoxemia. Temperatures increased (as measured rectally) every 2 hours (Bohnhorst, Heyne, Peter, et al, 2001). Although adverse effects are not usually associated with kangaroo care, monitoring to avoid potential harmful effects should include cardiorespiratory parameters, body temperature, and oxygenation.

Infants appear to be most vulnerable during the transfer from bed to parent and back to bed when kangaroo care is provided. Handling and repositioning necessary to prepare and move an infant into the STS position may result in similar disorganizing responses as previously described with routine nursing care.

Therapeutic Positioning

The American Academy of Pediatrics (2005) recommends the supine sleeping position for healthy infants in the first year of life as a preventive measure for sudden infant death syndrome (SIDS). Prone sleeping has decreased from more than 70% to about 13% in the United States since the guidelines were published in 1992. SIDS is the third highest cause of infant death after the neonatal period (28 days); the rate has decreased by more than 50% with the advent of supine sleeping. (See Sudden Infant Death Syndrome, Chapter 13.)

Parents of infants in the NICU should be educated on the safe sleeping position at home as part of discharge instructions. Supportive positioning in the NICU for acutely ill or recovering infants may look different from the academy's recommenda-

tions, depending on each infant's changing clinical condition, maturation, and readiness for the supine sleeping position and minimum bedding. It is important for staff to realize that routine care practices in the NICU may serve as a model for parents who, without proper instruction, may reproduce the environment and care techniques at home. Position and bedding choices in the unit, such as prone positioning, nests, and sheepskin, may be lethal for infants who have been discharged home.

Infants in the NICU are at increased risk for acquiring position-related deformities for a variety of reasons. Illness, weakness, low tone, immature motor control, the effects of gravity, and treatments such as ECMO or sedation are a few of the factors associated with prolonged immobility or decreased spontaneous movement (Hunter, 2001). Common position-related deformities include:

- Hyperabduction and flexion of the arms, causing upper extremity external rotation, resulting in a persistent W positioning of the arms; can interfere with later midline skills that form the foundation for feeding, crawling, reaching, and midline play with objects (Vaivre-Douret, Ennouri, Jrad, et al, 2004)
- Lower extremity external rotation deformities occurring when the trunk and pelvis are flat on the mattress, causing extreme hip abduction and outward rotation of the lower limbs, or the frog-leg appearance (Downs, Edwards, McCormick, et al, 1991)
- Neck extension and arching posture often observed in infants pulling away from ET tubes or nasal prongs during mechanical ventilation or nasal CPAP
- Motor asymmetries reported in preterm infants at 32 weeks of gestation or who are small for gestational age, occurring more often than in full-term infants even after 4 months corrected age (Samsom and de Groot, 2000, 2001)

Therapeutic positioning reduces the potential for acquired positional deformities that can affect motor development, play skills, attractiveness, and social attachment (Monterosso, Kristjanson, Cole, et al, 2003). Positioning can affect stability and comfort, and each infant must be observed for the effects of any position or repositioning. A position may also need to be adapted to accommodate necessary medical equipment or particular conditions, such as myelomeningocele, where the supine position is contraindicated before surgical repair of the defect. Deciding on which position and supportive aids to use requires the caregiver to consider the medical and developmental risks and benefits unique to a specific infant and situation (see Nursing Care Guidelines box).

The goal of therapeutic positioning for preterm and high-risk infants is to provide adequate support and containment as indicated to sustain flexed and midline postures, in an attempt to minimize positional deformities and assist infants in remaining calm and organized (Hunter, 2001).

The supine position requires support for the weak or immature infant. Because this position can create the most disorganization, make the position comfortable using positioning aids or blanket boundaries that support the head, trunk, and extremities according to the general positioning principles.

Although the prone position may appear to be the easiest to maintain, mistakes are often made with infants who are unable

General Considerations for Positioning

- Neutral or slightly flexed neck
- Gently rounded shoulders (no flattened posture against bed as in supine or prone positions)
- Elbows flexed
- Hands to face or midline as position allows
- Trunk slightly rounded with pelvic tilt
- Hips partially flexed and adducted to near midline (not medial or neutral alignment) and knee flexion (no frog leg or externally rotated hips flat against bed)
- Lower boundary secured for foot bracing

Modified from Biber P: When to seek consultation. In Creger PJ, Browne JV: *Developmental interventions for preterm and high-risk infants: self-study modules for professionals,* Tucson, 1995, Therapy Skill Builders.

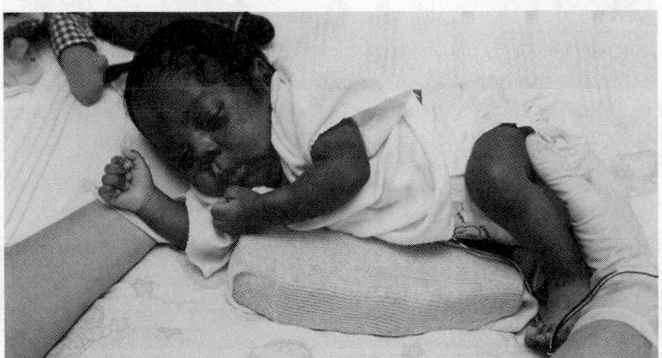

Fig. 10-4 Preterm infant slowly and gently transitioned to prone position on prone roll designed with stockinette-covered foam cut to individual specifications to prevent flattening of shoulders and pelvis against mattress and to support stable breathing base for the infant. (Courtesy Paul Vincent Kuntz, Halbouty Premature Nursery, Texas Children's Hospital, Houston.)

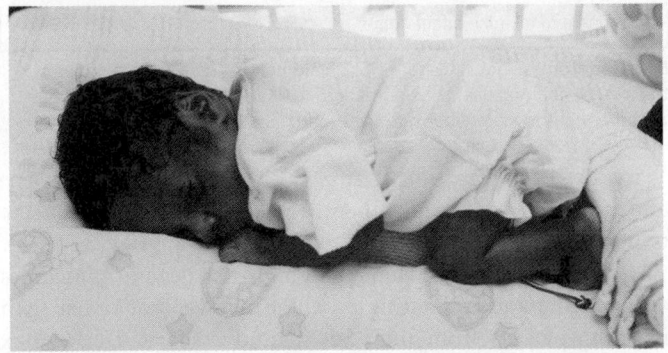

Fig. 10-5 Preterm infant positioned on prone roll. (Courtesy Paul Vincent Kuntz, Halbouty Premature Nursery, Texas Children's Hospital, Houston.)

to sustain rounded shoulders, trunk, and pelvis without assistance. Use of a postural support roll has been shown to prevent scapular-humeral tightness and shoulder retraction commonly seen as a result of this position (Figs. 10-4 and 10-5) (Monterosso, Kristjanson, Cole, et al, 2003).

Auditory Environment

The auditory system of the human fetus is mature enough for sound to produce physiologic effects as early as 23 weeks of gestation (Graven, 2000). Physical and behavioral responses to sudden, loud NICU noise have been observed in preterm and full-term infants (Philbin and Klaas, 2000; Bremmer, Byers, and Kiehl, 2003). Physiologic changes include apnea and bradycardia; fluctuations in heart and respiratory rates, blood pressure, and oxygen saturation; and changes in sleep-wake states (Philbin and Klaas, 2000, Bremmer, Byers, and Kiehl, 2003). These data demonstrate that infants in the NICU are capable of perceiving and responding to sounds around them.

The primary auditory environment in fetal life is made up of the maternal voice, respirations, heartbeat, and intestinal sounds. Soon after birth, newborn infants demonstrate preference for their own mother's voice and the language heard in utero (Gerhardt and Abrams, 2000). The acoustic environment of most NICUs is vastly different from the uterine and home milieu. Currently no data are available on the effects of long-term exposure to NICU noise levels. Of serious concern is the increased risk of sensorineural hearing loss (Cristobal and Oghalai, 2008) and language delays in infants born prematurely (Pietz, Peter, Graf, et al, 2004). NICU noise may interfere with developing auditory pathways and mask socially relevant sounds of the human voice necessary for language development.

Maintaining recommended sound levels (<45 dB) in the NICU may provide some or all of the following benefits: (1) increased physiologic stability, (2) improved growth, (3) more natural and consistent neurosensory maturation, (4) enhanced parent-infant interaction and subsequent attachment, and (5) fewer speech and language difficulties (Graven, 2000).

Visual Environment

Vision is the least mature of the newborn's senses. The preterm infant's eyes undergo significant maturation and differentiation of the retina and its connections to the visual cortex that typically occur in utero during the last trimester of pregnancy (Glass, 2005; Hunter, 2001). A current concern is that early, intense visual stimulation for preterm infants could adversely affect visual pathways and alter the developmental course for other sensory systems.

Visual function in preterm infants is more limited than that in full-term infants who, although limited in ability to focus (accommodation to near and far distances) and discriminate (acuity), will actively explore the environment. Preterm infants are less responsive to visual stimulation and have less acuity and accommodation than full-term infants. The ability to visually attend emerges around 30 to 32 weeks, and the infant may become stressed if the visual stimulus is intense and prolonged. Strong visual stimulation such as high-contrast black and white patterns can evoke an obligatory staring response by the immature infant who is unable to break away from it. This behavior is neither appropriate nor desired.

A variety of lighting conditions exist for NICUs from continuous 24-hour illumination, continuous dim lighting, day-night cycled lighting, or unpredictable periods of light-dark depending on staff or situations. Ambient lighting in some NICUs is reported to range from 40 to 150 foot-candles (ft-c) during the day with levels over 1500 ft-c if sunlight is added (Glass, 2005; Blackburn, 1998). These levels drop dramatically at night if light is cycled to reported levels of 5 to 9 ft-c (Fielder and Merrick, 2000).

BOX 10-6 VISUAL STIMULATION: CONSIDERATIONS FOR INFANTS

- Decrease ambient light levels by dimming lights or using incubator covers for lower-birth-weight and lower-gestational-age infants.
- Facilitate eye opening and visual attention in older preterm and term infants by dimming overhead lights.
- Direct procedure lights toward the necessary visual field and away from infants' eyes when performing tasks that require visual acuity such as intravenous catheter insertion.
- Shield infants' eyes from bright procedure lights or full ambient lighting as needed during examinations, treatments, or procedures.
- Avoid placing a cloth over the face or using eye patches that provide tactile irritation unless necessary for phototherapy or special circumstances.
- Ensure eye patches are securely in place during phototherapy.
- Introduce day-night cycling of lighting in the neonatal intensive care unit and intermediate nursery before discharge.
- Consider the human face the most appropriate visual stimulation in early infancy.
- Avoid leaving visual stimuli in the beds of infants who cannot escape from it.
- Provide appropriate visual stimuli or toys for recovering full-term or older infants.

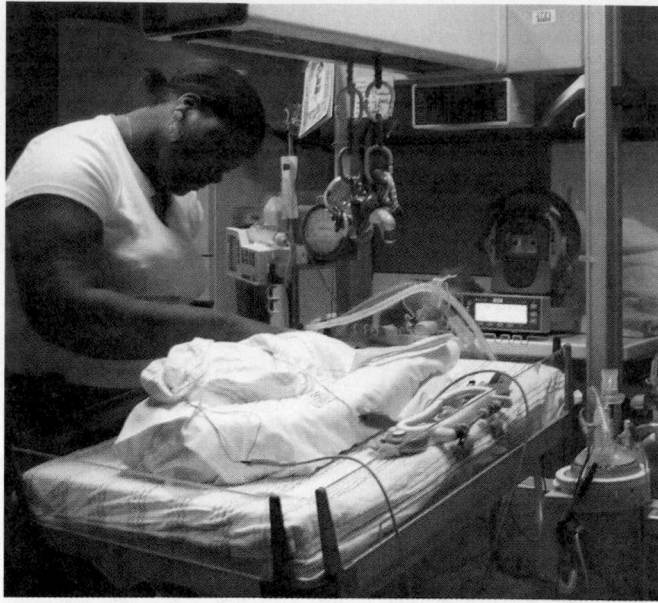

Fig. 10-6 Encouraging interaction of mother and her preterm infant in intensive care unit facilitates mother-infant attachment process. (Courtesy E. Jacobs, Texas Children's Hospital, Houston.)

Staff needs to carefully consider the impact of visual stimuli on the NICU infant. For preterm infants whose visual system is undergoing maturation, it is probably more prudent to provide stimulation to the earlier-developing senses first and minimize the impact of the NICU visual milieu. As attention and alerting emerge, the most appropriate visual stimulus is likely to be the human face, especially that of the parent. Box 10-6 provides some suggested approaches to visual stimulation in the NICU (Glass, 2005; Hunter, 2001; Mirmiran and Ariagno, 2000).

Facilitating Parent-Infant Relationships

Because of their physiologic instability, preterm infants are immediately separated from their mothers and surrounded by a complex, impenetrable barrier of glass windows, mechanical equipment, and special caregivers. Increasing evidence indicates that the emotional separation that accompanies the physical separation of mothers and infants interferes with the normal maternal-infant attachment process, discussed in Chapter 8. Maternal attachment is a cumulative process that begins before conception, strengthens by significant events during pregnancy, and matures through maternal-infant contact during the neonatal period.

When an infant is sick, the necessary physical separation appears to be accompanied by an emotional estrangement in the parents, which may seriously damage the capacity for parenting their infant. This detachment is further hampered by the tenuous nature of the infant's condition. When survival is in doubt, parents may be reluctant to establish a relationship with their infant. They prepare themselves for the infant's death while continuing to hope for recovery. This anticipatory grief (see Chapter 23) and hesitancy to embark on a relationship are evidenced by behaviors such as delay in giving the infant a name, reluctance to visit the nursery (or focusing on equipment and treatments rather than on their infant when they do visit),

BOX 10-7 PSYCHOLOGIC TASKS OF PARENTS OF A HIGH-RISK INFANT

- Work through the events surrounding labor and delivery.
- Acknowledge that the infant's life is endangered and begin the anticipatory grieving process.
- Recognize and confront feelings of inadequacy and guilt in not delivering a healthy child.
- Adapt to the neonatal intensive care environment.
- Resume parental relationships with the sick infant and initiate the caregiving role.
- Prepare to take the infant home.

Modified from Siegel R, Gardner SL, Merenstein GB: Families in crisis: theoretical and practical considerations. In Merenstein GB, Gardner SL: *Handbook of neonatal intensive care*, ed 6, St Louis, 2006, Mosby.

and hesitancy to touch or handle the infant when given the opportunity.

Comprehensive management of high-risk newborns includes encouraging and facilitating parental involvement rather than isolating parents from their infant and associated care (Box 10-7). This is particularly important in relation to mothers; to reduce the effects of physical separation, mothers are united with their newborns at the earliest opportunity (Fig. 10-6). Preparing the parents to see their infant for the first time is a nursing responsibility.

Before the first visit, the nurse prepares parents for their infant's appearance, the equipment attached to the child, and the general atmosphere of the unit. The initial encounter with the intensive care unit is stressful, and the frightening array of people, equipment, and activity is likely to be overwhelming. A book of photographs or pamphlets describing the NICU environment (infants in incubators or under radiant warmers, monitors, mechanical ventilators, and IV equipment) provides a useful and nonthreatening introduction to the NICU.

Encourage parents to visit their infant as soon as possible. Even if they saw the infant at the time of transport or shortly after birth, the infant may have changed considerably, especially if there are a number of medical and equipment requirements associated with the infant's hospitalization. At the bedside the nurse should explain the function of each piece of equipment and the role it plays in facilitating recovery. Explanations may often need to be patiently repeated because parents' anxiety over the infant's condition and the surroundings may prevent them from really "hearing" what is said. When possible, some items related to therapy can be removed; for example, photo-therapy can be temporarily discontinued and eye patches removed to permit eye-to-eye contact.

Parents appreciate the support of a nurse during the initial visit with their infant, but they may also want some time alone with the infant. It is important during the early visits to emphasize the positive aspects of their infant's behavior and development so that parents can focus on their infant as an individual rather than on the equipment that surrounds the child. For example, the nurse may describe the infant's spontaneous behaviors during care, such as grasp, sucking, and movement, or make comments about the infant's biologic functions. Most institutions promote family-centered care and have open visiting policies so that parents and siblings can visit as often as they wish.

Parents vary greatly in the degree to which they are able to interact with their infant. Some may wish to touch or hold their infant during the first visit, whereas others may not feel comfortable enough to even enter the nursery. Parents may not be receptive to early and extended infant contact because they need time to adjust to the impact of an infant with birth problems and must be helped to grieve before they can accept their infant.

The parents' inability to focus on their infant is a clue for the nurse to assist the parents in expressing feelings of guilt, anxiety, helplessness, inadequacy, anger, and ambivalence. Nurses can help parents deal with these distressing feelings and recognize that they are normal responses shared by other parents. It is important to point out and reinforce the positive aspects of parents' behavior and interactions with their infant.

Ward's (2001) research of parental needs in the NICU demonstrates the importance of nurses providing accurate information to the parent regarding treatment plan and procedures; answering parents' questions honestly; actively listening to parents' concerns, fears, and expectations; and helping parents understand infant responses to hospitalization.

Most parents feel shaky and insecure about initiating interaction with their infant. Nurses can sense parents' level of readiness and offer encouragement in these initial efforts. Parents of preterm infants follow the same acquaintance process as do parents of full-term infants. They may quickly proceed through the process or may require several days, or even weeks, to complete it. Parents begin by touching their infant's extremities with their fingertips and poking the infant tenderly, and then proceed to caresses and fondling (Fig. 10-7). Touching is the first act of communication between parents and child. Parents need to be prepared for their infant's exaggerated and generalized startle responses to touch so that they will not interpret these as negative reactions to their overtures. It may be neces-

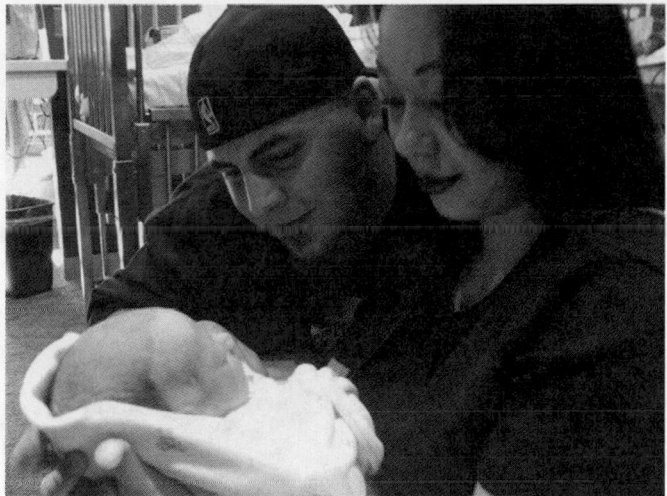

Fig. 10-7 Mother and father interact with their preterm infant. (Courtesy E. Jacobs, Texas Children's Hospital, Houston.)

sary to limit tactile stimuli when the infant is critically ill and labile, but the nurse can offer other options, such as speaking softly or sitting at the bedside.

Parents of acutely ill preterm infants may express feelings of helplessness and lack of control. Involving the parent in some type of caregiving activity, no matter how minor it may seem to the nurse, enables the parent to take on a more active role. Examples of such caregiving for the acutely ill infant who cannot be held and is seemingly not responding positively include moistening the infant's lips with a small amount of sterile water on a cotton-tipped swab or slipping the diaper from under the infant when it is wet or soiled.

The nurse encourages parents to bring in clothes, a toy, a stuffed animal, or a family snapshot for their infant, and the nurse can help parents set goals for themselves and for the infant. Parents may become involved by reading a children's storybook or nursery rhymes in a soft, soothing voice. The nurse encourages parents to visit at times when they can become involved in their infant's care (Figs. 10-8 and 10-9).

Throughout the parent-infant acquaintance process, the nurse listens carefully to what the parents say to assess their concerns and their progress toward incorporating their infant into their lives. The manner in which parents refer to their infant and the questions they ask reveal their worries and feelings and can serve as valuable clues to future relationships with the infant. The alert nurse is attuned to these subtle indications of parents' needs, which provide guidelines for nursing intervention. Often all that the parents need is reassurance that they will have the nurse's support during caregiving activities and that the behaviors about which they are concerned are normal reactions and will disappear as the infant matures (e.g., an exaggerated Moro reflex or inability to coordinate swallowing).

Parents need guidance in their relationships with their infant and assistance in their efforts to meet their infant's physical and developmental needs. The nursing staff must help parents understand that their preterm infant offers few behavioral rewards and show them how to accept small rewards from their infant. They need reassurance that avoidance behaviors are not a reflection on their parenting skills. Teach parents to recognize

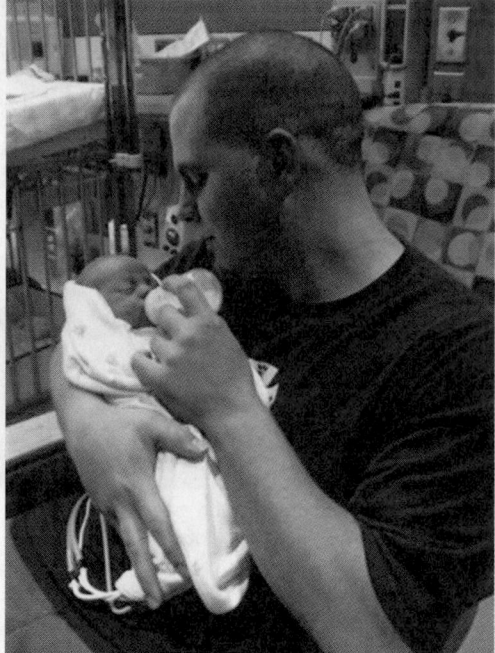

Fig. 10-8 Father feeding preterm infant. (Courtesy E. Jacobs, Texas Children's Hospital, Houston.)

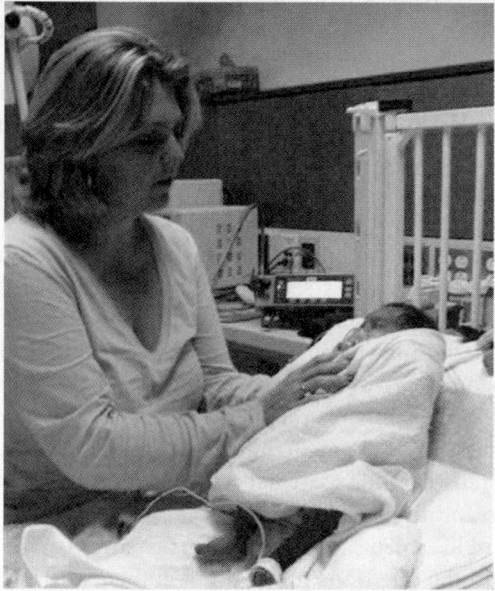

Fig. 10-9 Mother consoling preterm infant. (Courtesy E. Jacobs, Texas Children's Hospital, Houston.)

their infant's cues regarding stimulation, handling, and other interaction, especially aversive behaviors that indicate a need for rest. Nurses need to include parents in planning their infant's care.

Above all, nurses must encourage and reinforce parents during their caregiving activities and interactions with their infant to promote healthy parent-child relationships. It is also helpful for the parents to have contact and communication with the infant's primary nurse and associate primary nurse (according to unit model of nursing care). This decreases the

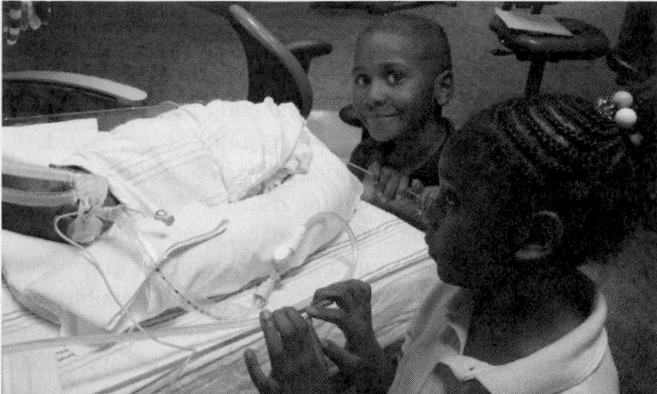

Fig. 10-10 Siblings visiting in the neonatal intensive care unit. (Courtesy E. Jacobs, Texas Children's Hospital, Houston.)

amount of different information given to parents and often instills confidence that, although the parents cannot be at their infant's bedside 24 hours a day, they can call competent and caring nurses to inquire about the infant's status. Periodic parent conferences involving the primary practitioner, primary nurse, and associate primary nurse serve to clarify misunderstandings or problems related to the infant's condition. Other members of the NICU team, such as the perinatal social worker, lactation consultant, discharge coordinator, or surgeon, may become involved as necessary.

Siblings
In the past, concerns about sibling visitation in the NICU focused on fears of infection and disruption of nursing routines. These fears have not been substantiated, and sibling visits should be a part of the normal operation of NICUs (Fig. 10-10).

The birth of a preterm infant is a difficult time for siblings, who rely on the support of understanding parents. When the happy anticipation changes to sadness, worry, and altered routines, siblings are bewildered and deprived of their parents' attention. They know something is wrong, but they do not completely understand what it is. Concern about the negative effects on visiting siblings of seeing the ill newborn has not been confirmed. Children have not hesitated to approach or touch the infant, and children less than 5 years of age have been less reluctant than older children. In addition, no measurable differences were found between previsit and postvisit behaviors.

The potential benefits of sibling visits must be weighed against the negatives of exposing the child to the NICU environment. Children must be prepared for the unfamiliar NICU atmosphere, but contact with the infant appears to have a positive effect on siblings by helping them deal with the reality rather than the bizarre fantasies that are characteristic of young children. Such visits also help bond the family as a unit.

Support Groups
Parents need to feel they are not alone. Parent support groups have been of immeasurable value to families of infants in the NICU. Some groups consist of parents who have infants in the hospital and share the same anxieties and concerns. Other

groups include parents who have had infants in the NICU and who have dealt with the crisis effectively. The groups are usually under the leadership of a staff person and may involve physicians, nurses, and social workers, but it is the parents who can offer other parents something that no one else can provide.

Family Support America* (formerly Family Resource Coalition) is a North American network of family support programs designed to help families of preterm infants. An excellent resource for parents of preterm infants is the book by J. Zaichkin, *Newborn Intensive Care: What Every Parent Needs to Know* (2009). This resource has technical and anecdotal information regarding different problems facing preterm infants, common treatments and therapies, preparation for home discharge, and home care for the preterm infant.

Discharge Planning and Home Care

Parents become apprehensive and excited as the time for discharge approaches. They have many concerns and insecurities regarding the care of their infant. They fear the child may still be in danger, that they will be unable to recognize signs of distress or illness, and that the infant may not be ready for discharge. Nurses need to begin early to assist parents in acquiring or increasing their skills in the care of their infant. Appropriate instruction must be provided and sufficient time allowed for the family to assimilate the information and learn the continuing special care requirements. Where rooming-in or other live-in arrangements are available, parents can stay for a few days and nights and assume the care of their infant under the supervision and support of the nursery staff.

There should be appropriate medical and nursing follow-up care, including developmental follow-up, and referrals to services that can benefit the family. Parents of preterm infants should also receive information about immunizations, including respiratory syncytial virus (RSV) prophylaxis, as well as other discharge planning information. Home health agencies provide nursing supervision, counseling, and referrals for nursing visits. With early discharge, many hospital-based home health care agencies become involved in the follow-up monitoring and care of the NICU "graduate" in the home. For an infant being discharged with equipment such as an oxygen tank, apnea monitor, or even a ventilator, discharge planning requires multidisciplinary, collaborative practice to ensure that the family has not only the appropriate resources but also the available assistance for dealing with the infant's needs. Many communities have organized support groups, including those discussed previously, those designed for parents of infants who require special care because of specific defects or disabilities, and those for parents of multiple births. (See Chapter 3.)

Car seat safety is an essential aspect of discharge planning. It is recommended that infants less than 37 weeks of gestation have a period of observation in an appropriate car seat to monitor for possible apnea, bradycardia, and decreased Sao_2 (Bull, Engle, and American Academy of Pediatrics, 2009). One study found that mean oxygen saturation levels decreased from 97% to 94% for both term and preterm infants who were observed in their car seats; 12% of the preterm infants in the study had significant apneic or bradycardic events in their car seats (Merchant, Worwa, Porter, et al, 2001). Despite this evidence, a Cochrane review of predischarge car seat testing failed to find evidence that such testing prevents morbidity or mortality (Pilley and McGuire, 2006) (see Family-Centered Care box).

🚼 FAMILY-CENTERED CARE
Preterm and Late-Preterm Infant Car Seat Evaluation

The American Academy of Pediatrics recommends that infants born before 37 weeks of gestation be evaluated for apnea, bradycardia, and oxygen desaturation episodes before hospital discharge. The academy suggests that facilities develop policies for implementing an evaluation program; however, few evidence-based practice recommendations have been published to date delineating specific requirements for such a program. Based on the available literature, suggestions for providing a car seat evaluation of infants born before 37 weeks of gestation include:

- Use the parents' car seat for the evaluation.
- Perform the evaluation 1 to 7 days before the infant's anticipated discharge.
- Secure infant in car seat per guidelines using blanket rolls on side.
- Set pulse oximeter low alarm at 88% (arbitrary).
- Set heart rate low alarm limit at 80 beats/min and apnea alarm at 20 seconds (cardiorespiratory monitor).
- Leave the infant undisturbed in car seat for 90 to 120 minutes *or* for the time parents state it takes to arrive at their home (if >90 minutes).
- Document infant's tolerance to car seat evaluation.
- An episode of desaturation, bradycardia, or apnea (≥20 seconds) constitutes a failure, and evaluation by the practitioner must occur before discharge.
- Repeat the test after 24 hours once modifications are made to the car seat, car bed, or infant's position in either restraint system.
- It is recommended that a certified car seat technician place the infant in the car seat (or bed) if a failure occurs (see National Highway Traffic Safety Administration website [www.nhtsa.dot.gov] for car seat inspection station). The technician will demonstrate appropriate positioning of the infant in the restraint device to the parents and have the parents do a return demonstration.
- Document the interventions, the infant's tolerance, and the parents' return demonstration.

Modified from Bull MJ, Engle WA, and American Academy of Pediatrics: Safe transportation of preterm and low birth weight infants at hospital discharge, *Pediatrics* 123(5):1424-1429, 2009; and American Academy of Pediatrics: Transporting children with special health care needs, *Pediatrics* 104(4):988-992, 1999.

Several car seat models can be adapted for small infants with the placement of blanket rolls on each side of the infant, but never behind, to support the head and trunk. For adequate support without slumping, the seat back-to-crotch strap distance must be 14 cm (5.5 inches) or less. A small rolled blanket may be placed between the crotch strap and the infant to reduce slouching. If the child's head drops forward because the position of the seat is upright, a roll cloth or blanket may be placed in the vehicle seat crease and under the safety base so the infant reclines at no more than a 45-degree angle. A car seat restraint without a shield is recommended; if the infant needs to be supine, a crash-tested car bed may be used (Bull, Engle, and American Academy of Pediatrics, 2009).

The rear-facing position provides support for the head, neck, and back, thereby reducing the stress to the neck and spinal cord in a vehicle crash. It is recommended that, before discharge from the hospital, the preterm infant have an evaluation in the designated car seat restraint by a staff member who is knowledgeable in car seat restraint positioning. Parents should learn how to properly restrain the child in the car seat for safe transportation (Bull, Engle, and American Academy of Pediatrics, 2009).

Additional guidelines are available from the American Academy of Pediatrics, including a videotape for the safe transportation of preterm and LBW infants. (See Chapter 12 for a discussion of infant car restraints and American Academy of Pediatrics website [www.aap.org] for a list of appropriate car seats for infants.)

An important part of discharge planning and care of the preterm infant is nutrition for continued growth; thus choice of feeding must be carefully addressed. Human milk should be fortified according to the infant's corrected age and physiologic needs. An enriched postdischarge formula (usually 22 kcal/oz) has been recommended for preterm infants born at less than 36 weeks to meet appropriate growth standards (see Table 10-4) (Lucas, Fewtrell, Morley, et al, 2001; Carver, Wu, Hall, et al, 2001). However, a Cochrane review of studies examining growth in preterm infants fed an enriched postdischarge formula did not find strong evidence of enhanced growth and development compared with infants fed standard formula (Henderson, Fahey, and McGuire, 2007).

The term vulnerable child syndrome is applied to physically healthy children who are perceived by their parents to be at high risk for medical or developmental problems. The syndrome has been observed in parents of children who had an illness or injury from which they had not been expected to recover. The family continues to perceive the child as fragile, vulnerable, and "different" and as having needs that warrant special status in the family, which adversely affects the child's and family's behavior. The parents may lack confidence in their parenting ability that persists beyond the illness. The parents may also become overly indulgent and have difficulty setting limits, resulting in interference with normal development. Consequently, the child becomes dependent, demanding, and out of control. Overprotection and frequent visits to the health care provider are characteristic.

Problems that may arise in the high-risk newborn include overfeeding, underfeeding, feeding resistance, aversion to human touch or interaction, and difficulty separating the child from the parent. To help parents deal with the stress of home care for the infant, nurses can help families discuss their fears and anxieties, which are exaggerated in parents of preterm infants, and encourage them to create a normal routine in caring for the infant. Parents need to learn the normal developmental delays expected of formerly preterm infants and the importance of setting disciplinary limits and schedules. Continued explanations and clarification of the infant's true health status and ongoing support of the parents' efforts are important aspects of follow-up care.

Neonatal Loss

The precarious nature of many high-risk infants makes death a real and ever-present possibility. Although infant mortality has been reduced sharply with improved technology, the mortality rate is still greatest during the neonatal period. Nurses in the NICU are the persons who must prepare the parents for an inevitable death and facilitate a family's grieving process after an expected or unexpected death.

The loss of an infant has special meaning for the grieving parents. It represents a loss of a part of themselves (especially for mothers), a loss of the potential for immortality that offspring represent, and the loss of the dream child that has been fantasized throughout the pregnancy. The parents have a sense of emptiness and failure. In addition, when an infant has lived for such a short time, they may have few, if any, pleasant memories to serve as a basis for the identification and idealization that are part of the resolution of a loss.

To help parents understand that the death is a reality, it is important that they be given the opportunity to hold their infant before death and, if possible, be present at the time of death so their infant can die in their arms if they choose.

Parents should have the opportunity to actually "parent" the infant in any manner they wish or are able to before and after the death. This may include seeing, touching, holding, caressing, and talking to their infant privately. The parents may also wish to bathe and dress the infant. If parents are hesitant to see their dead infant, it is advisable to keep the body in the unit for a few hours, since many parents change their minds after the initial shock of the death.

Parents may need to see and hold the infant more than once—the first time to say "hello" and the last time to say "good-bye." If parents wish to see the infant after the body has been taken to the morgue, the infant should be retrieved, wrapped in a blanket, rewarmed in a radiant warmer, and taken to the mother's room or other private place. The nurse should plan to stay with the parents but also provide them an opportunity for private time alone with their dead infant if they wish. Individual grief responses of the mother and father should be recognized and handled appropriately. Gender differences and cultural and religious beliefs will affect the parents' grief responses (Dyer, 2005).

Some units have implemented a hospice approach for families with infants for whom the decision has been made not to prolong life and who are receiving only palliative care. A special "family" room is set aside and contains all supportive equipment needed for the care of the infant. It also provides a homelike atmosphere for the family. All hospice services are available to the family, and the infant remains under the care and supervision of a primary nurse on the NICU staff. (See Chapter 23, End-of-Life Care, for further discussion of hospice care.)

A photograph of the infant taken before or after death is highly desirable. Parents may wish to have a special family portrait taken with the infant and other family members. This often helps personalize the experience and make it more tangible. The parents may not wish to see the photograph at the time of death, but the chance to refer to it later will help to make their infant seem more real, which is a part of the normal grieving process. A photograph of their infant being held by the hand or touched by an adult offers a more positive image than a morgue type of photograph. Many NICUs have a bereavement or memory packet made up for the grieving parents, which may include the infant's handprints and footprints, a lock of hair, the bedside name card, and, if appropriate to the family's religious beliefs, a certificate of baptism. The photographs and other personal effects of the deceased infant were perceived as critically important in the grieving process by one group of parents in a survey. Parents often indicated that the photographs were helpful in remembering the infant's actual appearance during this stressful period (Anderson, 2001; Gold, Dalton, and Schwenk, 2007). Naming the deceased infant is an important step in the grieving process. Some parents may hesitate to give the newborn a name that had been chosen during the pregnancy for their special "baby." However, it helps to have a tangible person for whom to grieve. In supporting parental responses to the loss of a child, care providers must understand and respect the cultural and religious practices.

A primary nurse who is familiar to the family should be present during the discussion about the dead or dying infant. A Resolve Through Sharing or bereavement counselor is often involved in helping the family through this difficult period. The nurse should talk with parents openly and honestly about funeral arrangements because few of them have had experience with this aspect of death. Many funeral homes now offer inexpensive arrangements for these special cases. Someone from the NICU should take the responsibility for acquiring this information. It is often helpful to parents for the NICU to have a list of local funeral homes, services offered, and prices. Families need to be informed of the options available, but a funeral is preferable because the ritual provides an opportunity for parents to feel the support of friends and relatives. A clergyman of the appropriate faith may be notified if the parents wish. Issues regarding an autopsy or organ donation (when appropriate) are approached in a multidisciplinary fashion (primary practitioner and primary nurse) with respect, tact, and consideration of the family's wishes. (See also "Grief and Perinatal Loss" in Merenstein and Gardner, 2006.)

Before the parents leave the hospital, the nurse should provide them with the telephone number of the unit (if they do not have it) and invite them to call any time they have any further questions. Many intensive care units make it a point to contact the parents after a neonatal death to assess the parents' coping mechanisms, evaluate the grieving process, and provide support as needed. Several organizations are available to offer support and understanding to families who have lost a newborn, including the Compassionate Friends* and Aiding Mothers and Fathers Experiencing Neonatal Death (AMEND).† (See Chapter 23 for further discussion of the family and the grieving process.)

Nurses who care for critically ill infants also experience grief. NICU nurses may feel helpless and sorrowful. It is important that such grief be allowed and that nurses attend the funeral or

memorial service as a part of working through the grieving process. Nurses may fear that showing emotion is unprofessional and that the expression of grief demonstrates "loss of control"; these fears are unfounded. Studies have demonstrated that to continue to be effective managers and providers of care, nurses must be allowed to grieve and support each other through the process (Jansen, 2003).

Education regarding bereavement, end-of-life care, and culturally sensitive care of families and their dying infants may help nurses comfort families during this stressful period (Engler, Cusson, Brockett, et al, 2004).

Baptism

Many Christian parents wish to have their child baptized if death is anticipated or is a decided possibility. Whenever possible, it is most desirable that a representative of the parents' faith (e.g., a Roman Catholic priest or a Protestant minister) perform such a ritual. When death is imminent, a nurse or a physician can perform the baptism by simply pouring water on the infant's forehead (a medicine dropper is a convenient means) while repeating the words, "I baptize you in the name of the Father and of the Son and of the Holy Spirit." This includes an infant of any gestational age, particularly when the parents are Roman Catholic.

When the faith of the parents is uncertain, a conditional baptism can be carried out by saying, "If you are capable of receiving baptism, I baptize you in the name of the Father and of the Son and of the Holy Spirit." The fact of the baptism is recorded in the infant's chart. Parents are informed at the first opportunity.

HIGH-RISK CONDITIONS RELATED TO DYSMATURITY

PRETERM INFANTS

Prematurity accounts for the largest number of admissions to an NICU. The immaturity not only places infants at risk for neonatal complications (e.g., hyperbilirubinemia and RDS, which has the highest incidence in preterm infants), but may also predispose the infant to problems that persist into adulthood (e.g., learning disabilities, growth deficiencies, asthma).

Etiology

A variety of maternal and pregnancy-related complications increase the risk of preterm delivery; however, the actual cause of prematurity is not known in most instances. The incidence of prematurity is lowest in the middle to high socioeconomic classes, in which pregnant women are generally in good health, are well nourished, and receive prompt and comprehensive prenatal care. The incidence is highest in the lower socioeconomic classes, in which a combination of deleterious circumstances is present. Other factors, such as multiple pregnancies, pregnancy-induced hypertension, and placental problems that interrupt the normal course of gestation before completion of fetal development, are responsible for a large number of preterm births.

The outlook for preterm infants is largely, but not entirely, related to the state of physiologic and anatomic immaturity of

*PO Box 3696, Oak Brook, IL 60522-3696; 630-990-0010, 877-969-0010; www.compassionatefriends.org.
†Contact Maureen Connelly, 4324 Berrywick Terr., St. Louis, MO 63128; 314-487-7582; e-mail: martha@amendgroup.com; www.amendgroup.com.

the various organs and systems at the time of birth. Infants at term have advanced to a state of maturity sufficient to allow a successful transition to the extrauterine environment. Infants born prematurely must make the same adjustments but with functional immaturity proportional to the stage of development reached at the time of birth. The degree to which infants are prepared for extrauterine life can be predicted to some extent by estimated gestational age. (See Clinical Assessment of Gestational Age, Chapter 8.) An understanding of prenatal development provides some concept of the status of the systems, at various stages of development, that must cope with functional changes that occur with birth.

Characteristics

Preterm infants have a number of distinct characteristics at various stages of development. Identification of these characteristics provides valuable clues to the gestational age and hence to the physiologic capabilities. The general, outward physical appearance changes as the fetus progresses to maturity. Characteristics of skin, general posture and tone, distribution of hair, and amount of subcutaneous fat provide clues to a newborn's physical development. Observation of spontaneous, active movements and response to stimulation and passive movement contributes to the assessment of neurologic status. The appraisal is made as soon as possible after admission to the nursery because much of the observation and management of infants depend on this information.

On inspection, preterm infants are very small and appear scrawny because they lack or have only minimum subcutaneous fat deposits and have a proportionately large head in relation to the body, which reflects the cephalocaudal direction of growth. The skin is bright pink (often translucent, depending on the degree of immaturity), smooth, and shiny (may be edematous), with small blood vessels clearly visible underneath the thin epidermis. The fine lanugo is abundant over the body (depending on gestational age) but is sparse, fine, and fuzzy on the head. The ear cartilage is soft and pliable, and the soles and palms have minimum creases, resulting in a smooth appearance. The bones of the skull and the ribs feel soft, and before 26 weeks the eyes may be fused. Male infants have few scrotal rugae, and the testes are undescended; the labia minora and clitoris are prominent in females. Fig. 10-11 compares the features of full-term and preterm infants.

In contrast to full-term infants' overall attitude of flexion and continuous activity, preterm infants are inactive and listless. The extremities maintain an attitude of extension and remain in any position in which they are placed. Physiologically immature, many preterm infants are unable to maintain body temperature, have limited ability to excrete solutes in the urine, and have increased susceptibility to infection. A pliable thorax, immature lung tissue, and an immature regulatory center lead to periodic breathing, hypoventilation, and frequent periods of apnea. These infants are more susceptible to biochemical alterations such as hyperbilirubinemia and hypoglycemia (see Chapter 9), and they have a higher extracellular water content that renders them more vulnerable to fluid and electrolyte imbalance. Preterm infants exchange fully half their extracellular fluid volume every 24 hours compared with one seventh of the volume turnover in adults.

The soft cranium is subject to characteristic unintentional deformation (dolichocephaly) caused by positioning from one side to the other on a mattress. The head looks disproportionately longer from front to back, is flattened on both sides, and lacks the usual convexity seen at the temporal and parietal areas. This positional molding is often a concern to parents and may influence their perception of the infant's attractiveness and their responsiveness to the infant. Frequent repositioning of the infant and positioning on a gel mattress can reduce or minimize cranial molding.

Late-preterm infants may not have the immature appearance so commonly observed in preterm infants born at a lower gestational age (<34 weeks' gestation). However, late-preterm infants are at risk for the development of some of the same physiologic adaptation problems as their preterm counterparts: respiratory distress syndrome, hyperbilirubinemia, thermoregulation difficulties, hypoglycemia, and feeding problems.

Therapeutic Management

When delivery of a preterm infant is anticipated, the intensive care nursery is alerted and a team approach implemented. Ideally, a neonatologist or a neonatal nurse practitioner, a staff nurse, and a respiratory therapist are present for the delivery. Infants who do not require resuscitation are immediately transferred in a heated incubator to the NICU, where they are weighed and where IV access, oxygen therapy, and other therapeutic interventions are initiated as needed. Resuscitation is conducted in the delivery area until infants can be safely transported to the NICU. Ongoing care is described elsewhere in the chapter.

Nursing Care Management

As with therapeutic management, individualize nursing care for each infant. See appropriate discussions under Nursing Care of High-Risk Newborns for details of care.

POSTTERM INFANTS

Infants born of a gestation that extends beyond 42 weeks as calculated from the mother's last menstrual period (or by gestational age assessment) are postterm, or postmature, regardless of birth weight. This constitutes 3.5% to 15% of all pregnancies. The cause of delayed birth is unknown. Some infants are appropriate for gestational age but show the characteristics of progressive placental dysfunction. These infants, often called postterm infants, display the characteristics of infants who are 1 to 3 weeks of age, such as absence of lanugo, little if any vernix caseosa, abundant scalp hair, and long fingernails. The skin is often cracked, parchmentlike, and desquamating. A common finding in postterm infants is a wasted physical appearance that reflects intrauterine nutritional deprivation. Depletion of subcutaneous fat gives them a thin, elongated appearance. The little vernix caseosa that remains in the skinfolds may be stained a deep yellow or green, which is usually an indication of meconium in the amniotic fluid.

Fetal and neonatal mortality increase significantly in postterm infants compared with those born at term. They are especially prone to fetal distress associated with the decreasing efficiency of the placenta, macrosomia, and meconium aspira-

CLINICAL EVALUATION

PRETERM	TERM

Posture—The preterm infant lies in a "relaxed attitude," limbs more extended; the body size is small, and the head may appear somewhat larger in proportion to the body size. The term infant has more subcutaneous fat tissue and rests in a more flexed attitude.

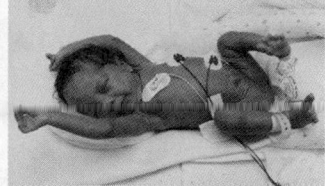 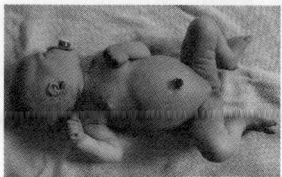

Ear—The preterm infant's ear cartilages are poorly developed, and the ear may fold easily; the hair is fine and feathery, and lanugo may cover the back and face. The mature infant's ear cartilages are well formed, and the hair is more likely to form firm, separate strands.

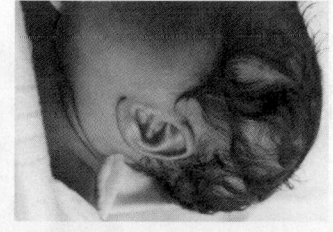 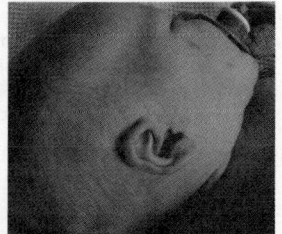

Sole—The sole of the foot of the preterm infant appears more turgid and may have only fine wrinkles. The mature infant's sole (foot) is well and deeply creased.

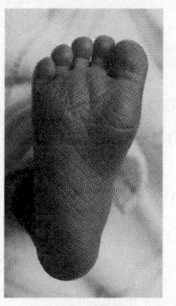 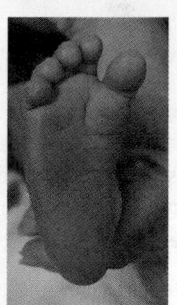

Female genitalia—The preterm female infant's clitoris is prominent, and labia majora are poorly developed and gaping. The mature female infant's labia majora are fully developed, and the clitoris is not as prominent.

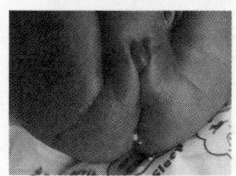 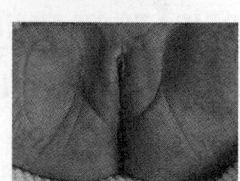

Male genitalia—The preterm male infant's scrotum is undeveloped and not pendulous; minimal rugae are present, and the testes may be in the inguinal canals or in the abdominal cavity. The term male infant's scrotum is well developed, pendulous, and rugated, and the testes are well down in the scrotal sac.

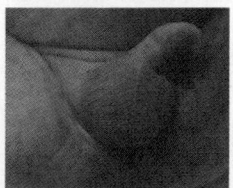 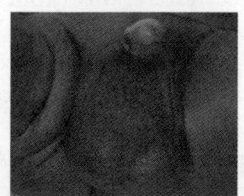

Scarf sign—The preterm infant's elbow may be easily brought across the chest with little or no resistance. The mature infant's elbow may be brought to the midline of the chest, resisting attempts to bring the elbow past the midline.

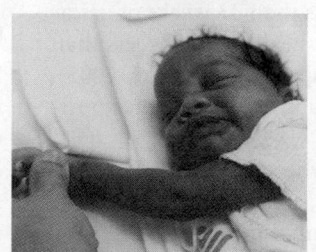 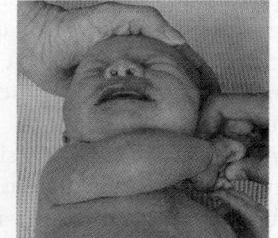

Fig. 10-11 Clinical and neurologic examinations comparing preterm and full-term infants. (Data from Pierog SH, Ferrara A: *Medical care of the sick newborn,* ed 2, St Louis, 1976, Mosby; photos courtesy Paul Vincent Kuntz, Texas Children's Hospital, Houston.)

Continued

NEUROLOGIC EVALUATION

PRETERM   TERM

Grasp reflex—The preterm infant's grasp is weak; the term infant's grasp is strong, allowing the infant to be lifted up from the mattress.

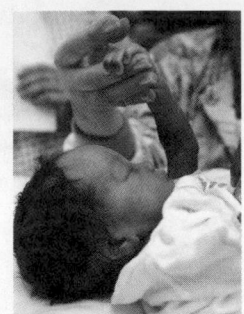
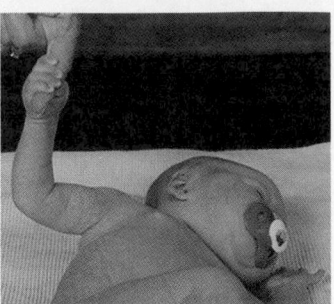

Heel-to-ear maneuver—The preterm infant's heel is easily brought to the ear, meeting with no resistance. This maneuver is not possible in the term infant, since there is considerable resistance at the knee.

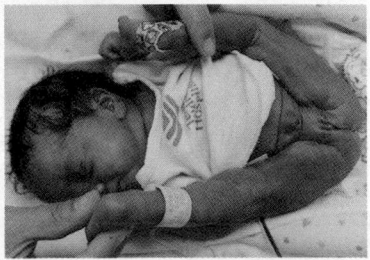

Fig. 10-11, cont'd.

tion syndrome (MAS). The greatest risk occurs during the stresses of labor and delivery, particularly in infants of primigravidas, or women delivering their first child. Induction of labor is usually recommended when infants are significantly overdue.

HIGH RISK RELATED TO DISTURBED RESPIRATORY FUNCTION

APNEA OF PREMATURITY

Characteristically, preterm infants are periodic breathers. They have periods of rapid respiration separated by periods of very slow breathing, and often short periods with no visible or audible respirations. Apnea is primarily an extension of this periodic breathing and can be defined as a lapse of spontaneous breathing for 20 or more seconds, or shorter pauses accompanied by hypotonia, bradycardia, or color change (Stokowski, 2005).

Apnea of prematurity (AOP) is a common phenomenon in the preterm infant. Rarely observed in full-term infants, apneic spells increase in prevalence the younger the gestational age. Approximately one third of infants less than 33 weeks of gestation and more than half of apparently healthy infants less than 30 weeks of gestation have apneic spells (Stokowski, 2005). Apnea usually resolves as the infant approaches 37 weeks postmenstrual age.

AOP may be further classified according to origin. The three recognized types are (1) central apnea, an absence of diaphragmatic and other respiratory muscle function that causes a lack of respiratory effort and occurs when the CNS does not transmit signals to the respiratory muscles; (2) obstructive apnea,

when air flow ceases because of upper airway obstruction, yet chest or abdominal wall movement is present; and (3) mixed apnea, a combination of central and obstructive apnea and the most common form of apnea seen in preterm infants (Poblano, Marquez, and Hernandez, 2006).

Pathophysiology

AOP reflects the immature and poorly refined neurologic and chemical respiratory control mechanisms in preterm infants. These infants are not as responsive to hypercarbia and hypoxemia, and their neurons have fewer dendritic associations than those of more mature infants. The respiratory reflexes of these infants are significantly less mature, which may be a contributing factor in the etiology. Overall weakness of the muscles of the thorax, diaphragm, and upper airway may also contribute to apneic episodes in the preterm infant. In addition, apnea is characteristically observed during periods of REM sleep. A variety of factors, including infection, intracranial hemorrhage (ICH), or PDA, can make apnea worse. Secondary causes of apnea should be investigated in infants with new-onset apnea or when there is a significant change in the frequency or severity of apneic episodes. Apnea in full-term infants should always be considered secondary and the cause investigated.

Clinical Manifestations

Factors that contribute to apnea in preterm neonates should be investigated and treated. Apnea can be anticipated in infants with a variety of conditions (Box 10-8); conversely, one of these disorders may be suspected in infants with persistent apneic spells. Although apnea is an expected event in preterm neonates, it should not be designated as being benign until all other causes have been ruled out. The observation of apnea is a reason to screen for any of the causes listed in Box 10-8.

BOX 10-8	POSSIBLE CAUSES OF APNEA OF PREMATURITY

- Prematurity
- Airway obstruction with mucus or milk, or poor positioning
- Anemia, polycythemia
- Dehydration
- Cooling or overheating
- Hypoxemia
- Hypercapnia or hypocapnia
- Hypoglycemia
- Hypocalcemia
- Hyponatremia
- Sepsis, meningitis
- Seizures
- Increased vagal tone (in response to suctioning nasopharynx, gavage tube insertion, reflux of gastric contents, endotracheal intubation)
- Central nervous system depression from pharmacologic agents
- Intraventricular hemorrhage
- Patent ductus arteriosus, congestive heart failure
- Depression following maternal obstetric sedation
- Respiratory distress as a result of pneumonia, inborn errors of metabolism such as hyperammonemia, congenital defects of the upper airways

Therapeutic Management

Administration of caffeine is often effective in reducing the frequency of primary apnea-bradycardia spells in newborns. Caffeine acts as a CNS stimulant to breathing. Neonates receiving caffeine must be closely observed for symptoms of toxicity. Caffeine has come to the forefront of pharmacologic therapy for AOP because it has fewer side effects than previously used aminophylline or theophylline, requires dosing once daily, has more predictable plasma concentrations, has slower elimination, and has a wider therapeutic range (trough, 5 to 20 mcg/ml). Caffeine citrate (Cafcit) has been approved for use in preterm infants with AOP. It is available in injectable and oral form. Weight and urinary output should be closely monitored because caffeine acts as a mild diuretic.

⚡ DRUG ALERT

Caffeine Toxicity

Signs of caffeine toxicity are tachycardia (>180 to 190 beats/min) at rest, vomiting, irritability, restlessness, diuresis, dysrhythmias, jitteriness, and gastritis (hemorrhagic).

Nasal CPAP and, more recently, nasal intermittent positive pressure ventilation have been used as an adjunct treatment for AOP. CPAP acts to maintain airway patency; hence it is most effective for obstructive or mixed apnea.

Nursing Care Management

Management of apnea consists of monitoring respiration and heart rate routinely in all preterm infants and preventing contributing conditions. Cardiorespiratory monitors alert the staff to cessation of respiration according to a preset delay time—usually 15 to 20 seconds. Effective monitoring devices do not eliminate the need for alert nursing observation. Nursing observation combined with monitoring is the most effective means of identifying neonatal apnea.

If begun early, gentle tactile stimulation (e.g., rubbing the back or chest gently, turning the infant to a supine position) will stop most apneic spells. If tactile stimulation fails to reinstitute respiration, flow-by oxygen and suctioning of the nose and mouth may be required. If breathing does not begin, the chin is raised gently to open the airway, and sufficient pressure is applied with a resuscitation mask and bag to lift the rib cage. The infant is never shaken. After breathing is restored, the infant is assessed for possible precipitating factors, such as unstable temperature, abdominal distention (if not observed earlier), and supplemental oxygen (if any) being delivered before the episode. The use of pulse oximetry has helped detect the onset of an apneic episode.

It is important that nurses maintain a careful record of episodes of apnea, including the number of apneic spells, the infant's appearance during and after the episode, and whether the infant self-recovers or whether tactile stimulation or other measures are needed to restore breathing. Subsequent investigation into the possible cause of the apneic episode is vital to the care of the preterm infant because it may signal an underlying condition such as sepsis or NEC.

❗ NURSING ALERT

When the alarm sounds, infants are first assessed for color and for presence of respiration. If they display the usual color and respirations, the nurse should investigate possible causes of a false alarm, such as faulty lead placement, detached or disconnected leads, improper alarm setting, or mechanical failure.

Persistent and repeated periods of apnea may be treated by mechanical ventilation or CPAP. Various methods devised to provide an intermittent stimulus for breathing, such as oscillating beds and water beds, have achieved variable success in the treatment of AOP.

RESPIRATORY DISTRESS SYNDROME

RDS refers to a condition of surfactant deficiency and physiologic immaturity of the thorax. The terms *respiratory distress syndrome* and *hyaline membrane disease* are most often applied to this severe lung disorder. It is seen almost exclusively in preterm infants but may also be associated with multifetal pregnancies, infants of diabetic mothers, cesarean section delivery, delivery before 37 weeks of gestation, precipitous delivery, cold stress, asphyxia, and a history of previous RDS (Dudell and Stoll, 2007). The disorder is rarely observed in drug-exposed infants or infants who have been subjected to chronic intrauterine stress (e.g., maternal preeclampsia or hypertension). Respiratory distress of a nonpulmonary origin in neonates may also be caused by sepsis, cardiac defects (structural or functional), exposure to cold, airway obstruction (atresia), IVH, hypoglycemia, metabolic acidosis, acute blood loss, and drugs. Pneumonia in the neonatal period is respiratory distress caused by bacterial or viral agents and may occur alone or as a complication of RDS.

Pathophysiology

Preterm infants are born before the lungs are fully prepared to serve as efficient organs for gas exchange. This appears to be a critical factor in the development of RDS. RDS results from a combination of structural and functional immaturity of the lungs.

Because the final unfolding of the alveolar septa, which increases the surface area of the lungs, occurs during the last trimester of pregnancy, preterm infants are born with numerous underdeveloped and many uninflatable alveoli. In addition, the fetal chest wall is highly compliant because of the predominance of cartilage rather than bone; and the diaphragm, the dominant respiratory muscle, is prone to fatigue.

Functionally, the fetal lungs are deficient in **surfactant**, a surface-active phospholipid secreted by type II cells in the alveolar epithelium. Surfactant is first produced at about 24 weeks of gestational age, but the type II cells in the lung do not fully mature until about 36 weeks of gestation (Fig. 10-12). Acting much like a detergent, this substance reduces the surface tension of fluids that line the alveoli and respiratory passages, resulting in uniform expansion and maintenance of lung expansion at low intraalveolar pressure. Immature development of these functions produces consequences that seriously compromise respiratory efficiency. Deficient surfactant production causes unequal inflation of alveoli on inspiration and the collapse of alveoli on end expiration. Without surfactant, infants are unable to keep their lungs inflated and therefore exert a great deal of effort to reexpand the alveoli with each breath. It has been estimated that each breath requires as much negative pressure (60 to 75 cm H_2O) as the initial lung expansion at birth. With increasing exhaustion they are able to open fewer and fewer alveoli. This inability to maintain lung expansion produces widespread atelectasis.

In the absence of alveolar stability (normal functional residual capacity) and with progressive atelectasis, pulmonary vascular resistance (PVR) increases, whereas with normal lung expansion it would decrease. Consequently, there is hypoperfusion to the lung tissue, with a decrease in effective pulmonary blood flow. The increase in PVR causes partial reversion to the

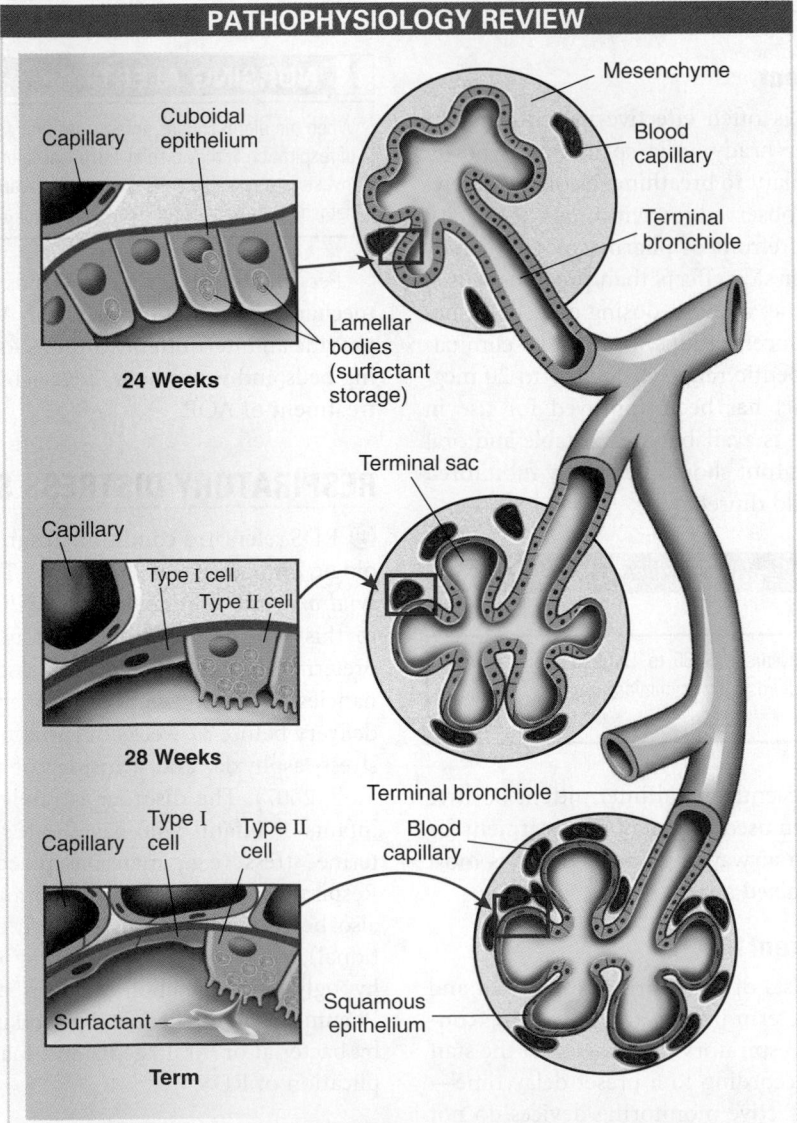

PATHOPHYSIOLOGY REVIEW

24 Weeks — Capillary, Cuboidal epithelium, Lamellar bodies (surfactant storage), Mesenchyme, Blood capillary, Terminal bronchiole

28 Weeks — Capillary, Type I cell, Type II cell, Terminal sac

Term — Capillary, Type I cell, Type II cell, Surfactant, Squamous epithelium, Terminal bronchiole, Blood capillary

Fig. 10-12 Prenatal development of the alveolar unit. (From McCance K, Huether S: *Pathophysiology: the biological basis for disease in adults and children*, ed 6, St Louis, 2010, Mosby.)

fetal circulation, with a right-to-left shunting of blood through the persisting fetal communications—the ductus arteriosus and foramen ovale.

Inadequate pulmonary perfusion and ventilation produce hypoxemia and hypercapnia. Pulmonary arterioles, with their thick muscular layer, are markedly reactive to diminished oxygen concentration. Thus a decrease in oxygen tension causes vasospasm in the pulmonary arterioles that is further enhanced by a decrease in blood pH. This vasoconstriction contributes to a marked increase in PVR. In normal ventilation with increased oxygen concentration, the ductus arteriosus constricts and the pulmonary vessels dilate to decrease PVR (Fig. 10-13).

Prolonged hypoxemia activates anaerobic glycolysis, which produces increased amounts of lactic acid. An increase in lactic acid causes metabolic acidosis; inability of the atelectatic lungs to blow off excess carbon dioxide produces respiratory acidosis. Lowered pH causes further vasoconstriction. With deficient pulmonary circulation and alveolar perfusion, Pao_2 continues to fall, pH falls, and the materials needed for surfactant production are not circulated to the alveoli.

Pulmonary edema observed in the early stages of RDS also contributes to impaired gas exchange. Factors believed to facilitate this fluid accumulation in the lungs include renal immaturity or insufficiency resulting from hypoxemia, high fluid intake and PDA, left ventricular dysfunction associated with papillary muscle necrosis, low serum protein concentration and low colloid osmotic pressure, increased alveolar surface tension that enhances the shift of interstitial fluid to alveolar spaces, oxygen toxicity, and high plasma vasopressin.

Pulmonary interstitial emphysema (PIE) may develop in preterm infants with RDS and immature lungs as a result of overdistention of distal airways. This condition further complicates adequate oxygenation in the immature airways (see Air Leak Syndromes, p. 358).

Deficiencies in other systems contribute to respiratory distress. For example, a high threshold of the respiratory center to afferent stimuli and weak or absent gag and cough reflexes reflect the immaturity of the nervous system. In addition, the persistence of fetal hemoglobin, so beneficial in prenatal existence, may place the infant at a disadvantage during respiratory distress. Although the binding power of fetal hemoglobin for oxygen is much greater than that of adult hemoglobin, this increased affinity also causes less oxygen to be released to the tissues at normal oxygen tension. In the newborn the arterial oxygen concentration must fall to a lower level for bound oxygen to be released from fetal hemoglobin.

A **hyaline membrane** is formed as hypoxemia and the increased pulmonary vascular pressure cause transudation of fluid into the alveoli. Necrotic cells from damaged alveoli plus the fibrin in the transudate form a membranous layer that lines the alveoli and inhibits gas exchange. The hyaline membrane contributes to respiratory difficulties by greatly diminishing **lung distensibility**, or compliance, the elastic quality of lung tissue that permits expansion in response to a given amount of applied pressure during inspiration. Affected lungs are stiffer and require far more pressure than do normal lungs to achieve an equal amount of expansion. Table 10-7 summarizes the major factors that produce RDS in immature infants.

Clinical Manifestations

Infants with RDS can develop respiratory distress either acutely or over a period of hours, depending on the acuity of pulmonary immaturity, associated illness factors, and gestational maturity. The observable signs produced by the pulmonary

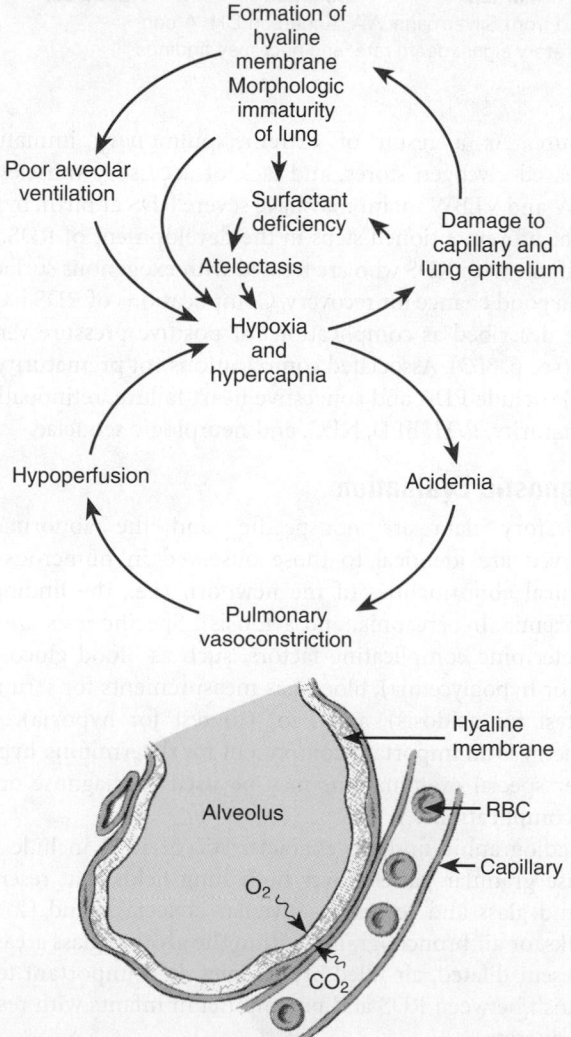

Fig. 10-13 Interdependent relationship of factors involved in pathology of respiratory distress syndrome. *CO₂,* Carbon dioxide; *O₂,* oxygen; *RBC,* red blood cell. (From Pierog SH, Ferrara A: *Medical care of the sick newborn,* ed 2, St Louis, 1976, Mosby.)

TABLE 10-7	MAJOR FACTORS IN RESPIRATORY DISTRESS SYNDROME
CAUSE	**EFFECT**
Increased pulmonary vascular resistance	Alveolar collapse; atelectasis; increased difficulty breathing
Impaired gas exchange	Hypoxemia and hypercapnia with respiratory acidosis
Increased transudation of fluid into lungs	Hypoperfusion of pulmonary circulation
Hypoperfusion (with hypoxemia)	Tissue hypoxia and metabolic acidosis
Hyaline membrane formation; impaired gas exchange	Increased surface tension of alveoli (surfactant deficiency)

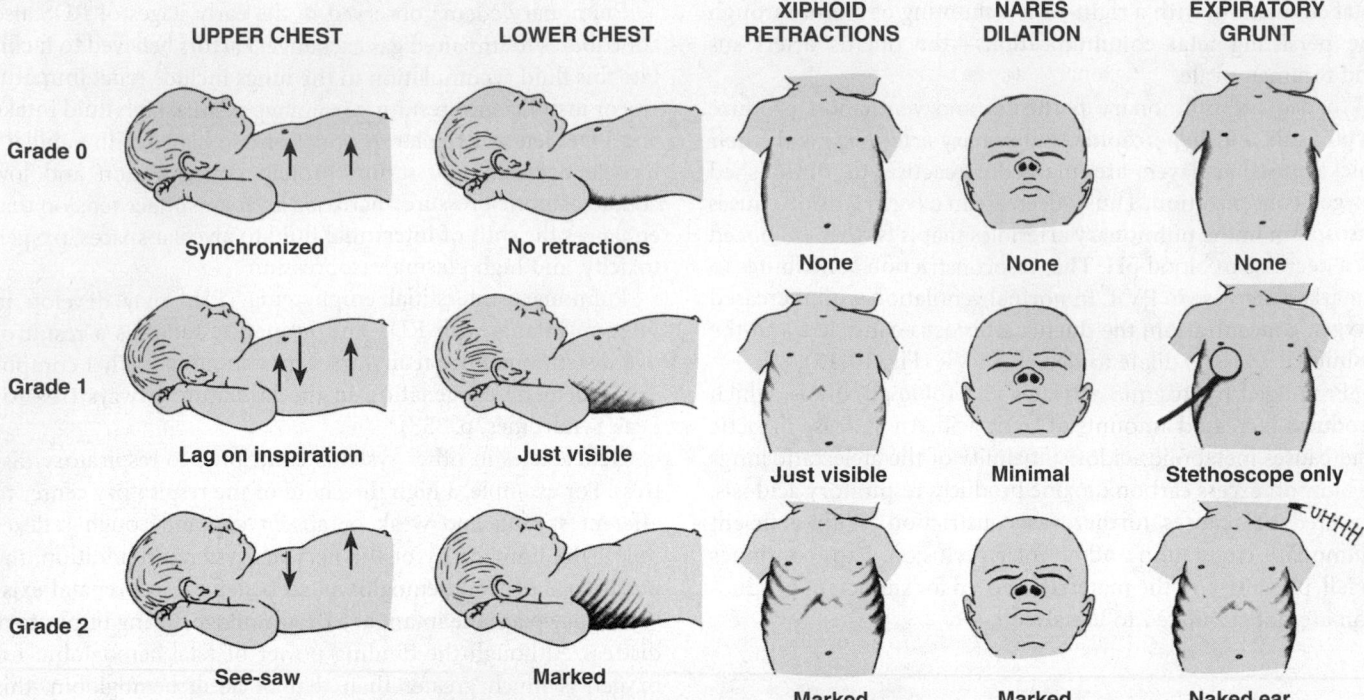

Fig. 10-14 Criteria for evaluating respiratory distress. (Modified from Silvermann WA, Anderson DH: A controlled clinical trial of effects of water mist on obstructive respiratory signs, death rate, and necropsy findings among premature infants, *Pediatrics* 17:1, 1956.)

changes usually begin to appear in infants who apparently achieve normal breathing and color soon after birth. In a matter of a few hours, breathing gradually becomes more rapid (>60 breaths/min). Infants may display retractions—suprasternal or substernal, and supracostal, subcostal, or intercostal—which result from a compliant chest wall. Weak chest wall muscles and the highly cartilaginous rib structure produce an abnormally elastic rib cage, resulting in indrawing, or retraction, of the skin between the ribs. During this early period the infant's color may remain satisfactory, and auscultation reveals air entry. Some of the criteria for evaluating respiratory distress in infants are illustrated in Fig. 10-14.

Within a few hours, respiratory distress becomes more obvious. The respiratory rate continues to increase (to 80 to 120 breaths/min), and breathing becomes more labored. It is significant to note that infants increase the rate rather than the depth of respiration when in distress. Substernal retractions become more pronounced as the diaphragm works hard in an attempt to fill collapsed air sacs. Fine inspiratory crackles can be heard over both lungs, and there is an audible expiratory grunt. This grunting, a useful mechanism observed in the earlier stages of RDS, serves to increase end-expiratory pressure in the lungs, thus maintaining alveolar expansion and allowing gas exchange for an additional brief period. Flaring of the nares is also a sign that accompanies tachypnea, grunting, and retractions in respiratory distress. Central cyanosis (a bluish discoloration of oral mucous membranes and generalized body cyanosis) is a late and serious sign of respiratory distress. Initially supplemental oxygen may eliminate cyanosis. The use of pulse oximetry and arterial blood gas sampling obviates the necessity for dependence on color to determine oxygen requirements.

Severe RDS is often associated with a shocklike state, as manifested by diminished cardiac inflow and low arterial blood pressure. As a result of extreme pulmonary immaturity, decreased glycogen stores, and lack of accessory muscles, the ELBW and VLBW infant may have severe RDS at birth, bypassing the aforementioned steps in the development of RDS.

Infants with RDS who are treated with exogenous surfactant have a good chance for recovery. Complications of RDS include those described as complications of positive pressure ventilation (see p. 353). Associated complications (of prematurity and RDS) include PDA and congestive heart failure, retinopathy of prematurity, IVH, BPD, NEC, and neurologic sequelae.

Diagnostic Evaluation

Laboratory data are nonspecific, and the abnormalities observed are identical to those observed in numerous biochemical abnormalities of the newborn (i.e., the findings of hypoxemia, hypercapnia, and acidosis). Specific tests are used to determine complicating factors, such as blood glucose (to test for hypoglycemia), blood gas measurements for serum pH (to test for acidosis), and Pao$_2$ (to test for hypoxia). Pulse oximetry is an important component for determining hypoxia. Other special examinations may be used to diagnose or rule out complications.

Radiographic findings characteristic of RDS include (1) a diffuse granular pattern over both lung fields that resembles ground glass and represents alveolar atelectasis and (2) dark streaks, or air bronchograms, within the ground glass areas that represent dilated, air-filled bronchioles. It is important to distinguish between RDS and pneumonia in infants with respiratory distress.

Prenatal Diagnosis

Fetal lung maturity depends on gestational age and maternal illnesses. Problems such as maternal diabetes delay fetal lung maturation, whereas fetuses exposed to chronic stress (intra-uterine growth restriction [IUGR], drug exposure) often have more mature lungs. Antenatal administration of glucocorticoids enhances fetal lung maturity, especially when combined with postnatal surfactant administration (Hintz, Poole, Wright, et al, 2005; Baud, 2004).

Functional maturity of the fetal lung can be determined by using surfactant phospholipids in amniotic fluid as indicators of maturity. The most commonly tested is the lecithin/sphingomyelin (L/S) ratio, which represents the relationship between these two lipids during gestation. Phospholipids are synthesized by fetal alveolar cells, and the concentrations in amniotic fluid change during gestation. Initially there is more sphingomyelin, but at approximately 32 to 33 weeks the concentrations become equal; sphingomyelin then diminishes and lecithin increases significantly until the fetus has developed sufficient surfactant to maintain alveolar stability at approximately 35 weeks. An **L/S ratio** of 2:1 in nondiabetic mothers indicates virtually no risk of RDS.

Other key surfactant compounds (also phospholipids) that are needed to stabilize surfactant are phosphatidylcholine (PC) and phosphatidylglycerol (PG). Without these compounds, lecithin is not functional as a surfactant. Concentrations of PC parallel those of lecithin, peaking at 35 weeks and then gradually decreasing. At 36 weeks PG appears in amniotic fluid and increases until term. By measuring these phospholipids—L/S ratio, PC, and PG—the clinician can estimate the maturity of the lungs with a high degree of accuracy. Other, less commonly used methods have been devised to provide rapid, inexpensive, and accurate measures of lung maturity. These include the "shake" or "bubble" test, in which stable foam or bubbles form when amniotic fluid is shaken in the presence of ethanol, and the tap test, in which abundant bubbles appear in a test tube of amniotic fluid with 6N-hydrochloric acid and diethyl ether.

Another test currently being used to evaluate fetal lung maturity is the TDx Fetal Lung Maturity (FLM) assay, which determines PG levels in amniotic fluid or neonatal tracheal aspirates. The FLM test is faster than L/S ratio determination (<1 hour versus 4 to 5 hours) and is reported to predict the absence of RDS with greater accuracy; a level of 50 or more is predictive of fetal lung maturity (Fantz, Powell, Karon, et al, 2002). TDx FLM may also be used in the postnatal period to determine the presence of RDS as a result of surfactant deficiency by collecting tracheal aspirate samples (Parvin, Kaplan, Chapman, et al, 2005).

Lamellar bodies, representing the storage form of surfactant, are found in amniotic fluid in increasing quantities with the advancement of gestational age and lung maturity. A quantitative count of lamellar bodies has been reported to be as accurate as the L/S ratio in determining fetal lung maturity. The count can be obtained faster than the L/S ratio, thus making it clinically appealing (Neerhof, Dohnal, Ashwood, et al, 2001; Wijnberger, Huisjes, Voorbij, et al, 2001).

Therapeutic Management

The treatment of RDS includes all the general measures required for any preterm infant, as well as those instituted to correct imbalances. The supportive measures most crucial to a favorable outcome are (1) maintain adequate ventilation and oxy-genation with an oxygen hood, continuous positive airway pressure (CPAP), or mechanical ventilation; (2) maintain acid-base balance; (3) maintain a neutral thermal environment; (4) maintain adequate tissue perfusion and oxygenation; (5) prevent hypotension; and (6) maintain adequate hydration and electrolyte status. Nipple and gavage feedings are avoided in any situation that creates a marked increase in respiratory rate because of the greater hazards of aspiration.

QUALITY PATIENT OUTCOMES: Neonatal RDS
- Room air or oxygen saturation ≥90%
- Respiratory rate <60 breaths/min
- Blood pH ≥7.35

Surfactant

The administration of exogenous surfactant to preterm neonates with RDS has become an accepted and common therapy in most neonatal centers worldwide. Numerous clinical trials involving the administration of exogenous surfactant to infants with or at high risk for RDS demonstrate improvements in blood gas values and ventilator settings, decreased incidence of pulmonary air leaks, decreased deaths from RDS, and an overall decreased infant mortality rate (Halliday, 2003; Soll, 2000, American Academy of Pediatrics, 2008). Exogenous surfactant comes from a natural source (e.g., porcine or bovine) or from the production of artificial surfactant. Commercially available surfactant products include beractant (Survanta), a bovine surfactant; and poractant alfa (Curosurf), a porcine surfactant.

Studies have shown mixed results in comparing one surfactant product with another. One study found fewer complications and earlier improvement with natural (versus synthetic) surfactant use (Soll and Blanco, 2001). Moya, Gadzinowski, Bancalari, and colleagues (2005) found that an investigational synthetic surfactant, lucinactant, mimics the action of human surfactant protein-B (SP-B), and it was more effective than beractant and colfosceril palmitate at reducing the RDS-related mortality rates by 14 days of life. BPD was significantly less common in infants at 36 weeks postmenstrual age who had received lucinactant.

Additional benefits of surfactant replacement therapy include decreased oxygen requirements and mean airway pressure (MAP) within hours of administration and an overall decrease in the incidence of pulmonary air leaks. To date, long-term improvement in the decrease of BPD and IVH has not been evidenced in all surfactant clinical trials.

Complications seen with surfactant administration include pulmonary hemorrhage and mucus plugging. Additional studies investigating the potential benefits of surfactant in infants with meconium aspiration found a reduction in the severity of respiratory illness and subsequent requirement of ECMO support (El Shahed, Dargaville, Ohlsson, et al, 2007). Other studies continue to investigate the potential benefits of exogenous surfactant for the treatment of infectious pneumonia and lung hypoplasia concomitant with congenital diaphragmatic hernia (Wiswell, 2001). Acute RDS/ALI may also respond favorably to surfactant administration (see Acute Respiratory Distress Syndrome/Acute Lung Injury, Chapter 32). Surfactant may be administered at birth as a prophylactic treatment of

RDS or later in the course of RDS as a rescue treatment. Studies found improved clinical outcomes and fewer adverse effects when surfactant is administered prophylactically to infants at risk for developing RDS (American Academy of Pediatrics, 2008). Surfactant is administered via the ET tube directly into the infant's trachea (Fig. 10-15); the exact number of doses

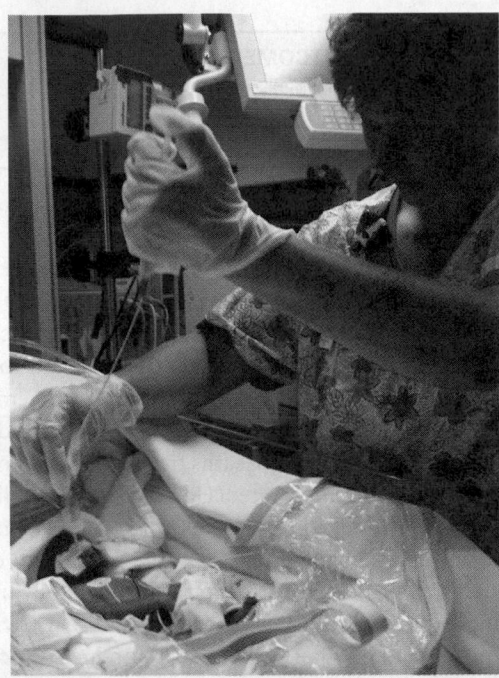

Fig. 10-15 Exogenous surfactant administration to infant on mechanical ventilation. (Courtesy E. Jacobs, Texas Children's Hospital, Houston.)

(single versus multiple) that is most effective has yet to be determined.

Nursing responsibilities with surfactant administration include assistance in the delivery of the product, collection and monitoring of arterial blood gases, scrupulous monitoring of oxygenation, and assessment of the infant's tolerance of the procedure. Once surfactant is absorbed, there is usually an increase in respiratory compliance that requires adjustment of ventilator settings to decrease MAP and prevent overinflation or hyperoxemia. Suctioning is usually delayed for an hour or so (depending on the type of surfactant, delivery system, and unit protocol) to allow maximum effects to occur. Current research is investigating the possibility of delivering an aerosolized surfactant. This method would decrease the problems associated with current delivery systems (contamination of the airway, interruption of mechanical ventilation, and loss of the drug in the ET tubing from reflux).

Oxygen Therapy

The goals of oxygen therapy are to provide adequate oxygen to the tissues, prevent lactic acid accumulation resulting from hypoxia, and, at the same time, avoid the potentially negative effects of oxygen toxicity. Numerous methods have been devised to improve oxygenation (Table 10-8). All require that the gas be warmed and humidified before entering the respiratory tract. If the infant does not require ventilatory assistance, oxygen can be given via a plastic hood placed over the head to supply variable concentrations of humidified oxygen. (See Oxygen Therapy, Chapter 31.) If oxygen saturation of blood cannot be maintained at a satisfactory level and the carbon dioxide level ($Paco_2$) rises, infants will require ventilatory assistance.

TABLE 10-8	COMMON METHODS FOR ASSISTED VENTILATION IN NEONATAL RESPIRATORY DISTRESS	
METHOD	**DESCRIPTION**	**HOW PROVIDED**
Conventional Methods		
Continuous positive airway pressure (CPAP)	Provides constant distending pressure to airway in spontaneously breathing infant	Nasal prongs Endotracheal tube Face mask
Positive end-expiratory pressure (PEEP)*	Provides increased end-expiratory pressure during expiration and between mandatory breaths, which prevents alveolar collapse; maintains residual airway pressure	Endotracheal intubation and either volume-limited or pressure-limited ventilator
Intermittent mandatory ventilation (IMV)*	Allows infant to breathe spontaneously at own rate but provides mechanical cycled respirations and pressure at regular preset intervals	Endotracheal intubation and ventilator
Synchronized intermittent mandatory ventilation (SIMV)	Mechanically delivers breaths synchronized to onset of spontaneous patient breaths; uses assist/control mode to facilitate full inspiratory synchrony; involves signal detection of onset of spontaneous respiration from abdominal movement, thoracic impedance, and airway pressure or flow changes	Patient-triggered infant ventilator with signal detector and assist/control mode; endotracheal tube
Volume guarantee ventilation	Delivers predetermined volume of gas using inspiratory pressure that varies according to infant's lung compliance (often used in conjunction with SIMV)	Volume guarantee ventilator with flow sensor; endotracheal tube
Alternative Methods		
High-frequency oscillatory ventilation (HFOV)	Application of high-frequency, low-volume, sine-wave flow oscillations to airway at rates between 480 and 1200 breaths/min	Variable-speed piston pump (or loudspeaker, fluidic oscillator); endotracheal tube
High-frequency jet ventilation (HFJV)	Uses separate, parallel, low-compliant circuit and injector port to deliver small pulses or jets of fresh gas deep into airway at rates between 250 and 900 breaths/min	May be used alone or with low-rate IMV; endotracheal tube

*Also referred to as conventional ventilation (versus HFOV).

Oxygen should be administered judiciously to preterm infants being stabilized in labor and delivery and for oxygenation maintenance in the NICU. Much attention has focused recently on high oxygen concentration and the effect of free oxygen radicals on the development of conditions such as NEC, BPD, and ROP. The current Neonatal Resuscitation Program guidelines recommend the use of oxygen concentrations between 21% and 100% in order to achieve an oxygen saturation of approximately 90% (American Academy of Pediatrics and American Heart Association, 2006). Finer and Leone (2009) recommend oxygen delivery to maintain an Spo$_2$ of 83% to 93% in preterm infants to decrease morbidity and mortality associated with liberal oxygen usage and high oxygen concentrations. Research indicates that optimal target ranges for maintaining adequate oxygenation while preventing ROP and BPD or other conditions is as yet unknown (Askie, Henderson-Smart, and Ko, 2009).

CPAP, the application of 3 to 8 cm H$_2$O (positive) pressure to the airway, uses the infant's spontaneous respiration to improve oxygenation by helping prevent alveolar collapse and increasing diffusion time. CPAP may be delivered via fitted face mask, nasal prongs, or an ET tube (Fig. 10-16). Ventilation with CPAP is done entirely by the infant. If oxygenation is not improved and the infant requires assisted ventilation, intermittent mandatory ventilation (IMV) is used with positive end-expiratory pressure (PEEP). This allows infants to breathe at their own rate but provides positive pressure with end-expiratory pressure to prevent alveolar collapse and overcome airway resistance. Additional components involved in IMV are peak inspiratory pressure (PIP) and rate (number of breaths per minute). The PIP is the maximum amount of positive pressure applied to the infant on inspiration. The total amount of pressure transmitted to the airway throughout an entire respiratory cycle is called the mean airway pressure (MAP). Increasing MAP in infants with severe RDS correlates positively with improved oxygenation by maintaining functional residual capacity and overcoming the resistive forces of the atelectatic lung. The MAP is affected by changes in the PEEP, PIP, and inspiratory/expiratory ratio. Although MAP is now recognized as the major determinant of oxygenation, this does not imply that simply increasing MAP alone will automatically improve oxygenation (Wood, 2003).

Improved technology has made available to preterm or sick neonates a form of mechanical ventilatory assistance previously used in adults: synchronized intermittent mandatory ventilation (SIMV). With this method breaths delivered by the ventilator are synchronized to the onset of spontaneous infant breaths. The net effect is to produce full respiratory synchrony rather than asynchronous respiratory efforts (commonly called "fighting the ventilator") that are believed to significantly impede the ability to adequately oxygenate infants without sedation or muscle paralysis. With SIMV, the operator sets the number of breaths per minute delivered by the ventilator, and the patient may breathe spontaneously between mechanical breaths. In the "assist-control" mode a mechanical breath is delivered each time a spontaneous respiration is detected; the "control" mode includes the delivery of a mechanical breath at a regular rate if the patient fails to initiate a spontaneous respiration. Additional benefits of SIMV are improved oxygenation, decreased incidence of pulmonary air leaks (pneumothorax), and decreased time on mechanical ventilation (Greenough, Dimitriou, Prendergast, et al, 2008).

If adequate oxygenation cannot be maintained and hypercarbia persists, infants may benefit from one of the two high-frequency ventilation (HFV) modalities. HFV delivers gas at very rapid rates to provide adequate minute volumes using lower proximal airway pressures by way of high-frequency oscillatory ventilation (HFOV) or high-frequency jet ventilation (HFJV). HFV was initially recommended for intractable respiratory failure, especially for infants with pulmonary air leaks and PIE. More recently, many clinicians are recommending earlier use of HFOV to prevent volutrauma to the lungs of very preterm infants (Ventre and Arnold, 2004).

Volutrauma is believed to be a key factor in the development of BPD. Courtney, Durand, Asselin, and colleagues (2002) reported that HFOV was associated with improved survival and a decreased need for supplemental oxygen at 36 weeks of postmenstrual age. HFJV is most often used in the treatment of full-term infants with meconium aspiration, persistent pulmonary hypertension, or air leak syndromes. The Cochrane review of HFJV use in preterm infants with RDS reports a similar benefit to that of HFOV in terms of pulmonary outcomes but cautions that sufficient studies have not been done to recommend the use of HFJV in preterm infants (Bhuta and Henderson-Smart, 2000).

Complications of Positive Pressure Ventilation

Although lifesaving, mechanical ventilation is not without hazards. Positive pressure introduced by mechanical apparatus has caused an increased incidence of air leaks that produce complications, such as PIE, pneumothorax, and pneumomediastinum (see p. 358). The avoidance of intubation and mechanical ventilation reduces the incidence of BPD (Verder, Bohlin, Kamper, et al, 2009). Other complications directly related to positive pressure include various problems associated with intubation, such as nasal, tracheal, or pharyngeal perforation; stenosis; inflammation; palatal grooves; subglottic stenosis; tube obstruction; and infection.

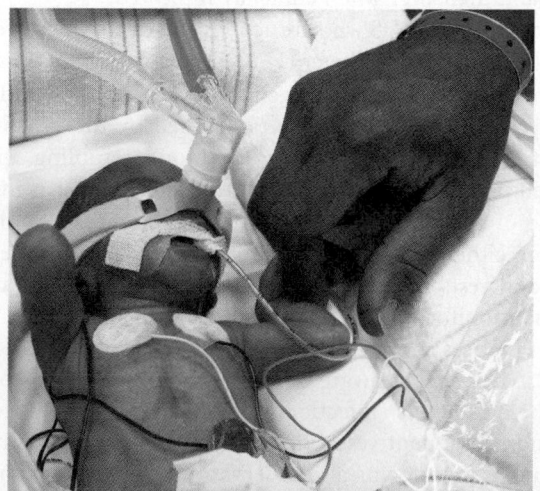

Fig. 10-16 Infant on nasal continuous positive airway pressure with father's finger in hand. (Courtesy E. Jacobs, Texas Children's Hospital, Houston.)

Nitric Oxide

Inhaled nitric oxide (NO) has emerged as a significant treatment modality for neonates with conditions that cause persistent pulmonary hypertension, pulmonary vasoconstriction, and subsequent acidosis and severe hypoxia. Infants with conditions such as MAS, pneumonia, sepsis, and congenital diaphragmatic hernia with pulmonary hypoplasia often require intervention in an attempt to reverse pulmonary hypertension. NO is a colorless, highly diffusible gas that causes smooth muscle relaxation and reduces pulmonary vasoconstriction and subsequent pulmonary hypertension when inhaled into the lungs. NO may be administered through the ventilator circuit and blended with oxygen. It attaches readily to hemoglobin and is thus deactivated so that systemic vasculature is not affected. NO is toxic in large quantities, but the amount required to induce pulmonary vasculature relaxation (6 to 20 ppm) is well below toxic levels.

Studies of term and near-term infants being treated with NO for respiratory failure have been positive (Finer and Barrington, 2006). In many cases reversal of persistent pulmonary hypertension of the newborn (PPHN) without ECMO has been achieved in infants with MAS, RDS, perioperative congenital heart disease, and sepsis (Konduri, 2004). One exception is the study of newborns with congenital diaphragmatic hernia who required ECMO after NO and whose morbidity and mortality were not significantly improved with inhaled NO (Field, 2005; Finer and Barrington, 2006). Surfactant replacement therapy may be performed in combination with inhaled NO therapy in infants with inadequate pulmonary maturity. Nursing care of the infant receiving inhaled NO is the same as for the newborn with PPHN; continuous assessment of respiratory status and response to treatment is essential.

The use of NO for preterm infants remains controversial. Some studies have proposed a role for NO in the treatment of RDS and respiratory failure in these infants, whereas others suggest no benefit (Barrington and Finer, 2006; Field, 2005; Hascoet, Fresson, Claris, et al, 2005; Mercier, Olivier, Loron, et al, 2009).

Medical Therapies

The treatment of the infant with RDS requires the establishment of one or more IV lines to maintain hydration and nutrition, monitor arterial blood gases, and administer medications. Systemic antibiotics may be administered during the acute phase if sepsis is suspected (see Sepsis, p. 362). The administration of morphine or fentanyl for pain and sedation is individualized according to the infant's response to illness. Caffeine may be administered to treat apnea and to prepare for weaning VLBW and ELBW infants from mechanical ventilation. Inotropes such as dopamine and dobutamine may be required to support the infant's systemic blood pressure and maintain effective cardiac output during the acute phase of illness.

Prevention

The most successful approach to prevention of RDS is prevention of preterm delivery, especially elective early delivery and cesarean section. Improved methods for assessing the maturity of the fetal lung by amniocentesis, although not a routine procedure, allow a reasonable prediction of adequate surfactant formation (see Diagnostic Evaluation, p. 350). Because estimation of a delivery date can be miscalculated by as much as 1 month, such tests are particularly valuable when scheduling an elective cesarean section. Studies indicate that the combination of maternal glucocorticoid administration before delivery and surfactant administration postnatally has a synergistic effect on neonatal lungs, with the net result being a decrease in infant mortality, incidence of IVH, pulmonary air leaks, and problems with PIE and RDS (Dudell and Stoll, 2007; Halliday, 2005).

Nursing Care Management

Care of infants with RDS involves all the observations and interventions previously described for high-risk infants. In addition, the nurse is concerned with the complex problems related to respiratory therapy and the constant threat of hypoxemia and acidosis that complicates the care of patients in respiratory difficulty.

The respiratory therapist, an important member of the neonatal intensive care team, is often responsible for maintenance and regulation of respiratory equipment. Nevertheless, nurses should understand the equipment and be able to recognize when it is not functioning correctly. The most essential nursing function is to observe and assess the infant's response to therapy. Continuous monitoring and close observation are mandatory because an infant's status can change rapidly and because oxygen concentration and ventilation parameters are prescribed according to the infant's blood gas measurements, $tcPo_2$, and pulse oximetry readings.

Changes in oxygen concentration are based on these observations. The nurse determines the amount of oxygen administered, expressed as the fraction of inspired air (Fio_2), on an individual basis according to pulse oximetry and/or direct or indirect measurement of arterial oxygen concentration. Capillary samples collected from the heel (see Chapter 27 for procedure) are useful for pH and $Paco_2$ determinations but not for oxygenation status. Continuous pulse oximetry readings are recorded at least hourly or more often as required. Blood sampling is performed after ventilator changes for the acutely ill infant and thereafter when clinically indicated.

In infants with RDS who are acutely ill or extremely preterm, an umbilical arterial catheter (UAC) may be used to draw arterial blood for monitoring oxygenation. This method, although initially invasive and therefore performed by the practitioner with sterile precautions, allows for blood sampling without repeated peripheral arterial punctures. The catheter is inserted via one of the umbilical arteries to the premeasured desired position (either at the level of the diaphragm, T6-10, or between L3-4) and rests in the descending aorta. Continuous arterial pressure monitoring may be carried out with an "in-line" transducer. Practices vary regarding medication administration via a UAC. The nurse is aware of the potential hazards associated with these catheters (infection, hemorrhage, thrombus formation and subsequent vessel occlusion, arterial vasospasm) and implements monitoring and observation strategies to promptly intervene should complications occur (see Hydration, p. 322). An umbilical venous catheter (UVC) may be used separately or in conjunction with the UAC, depending on the severity of the infant's illness, the fluid requirements, and preferred medical practice.

Mucus may collect in the respiratory tract as a result of the infant's pulmonary condition. Secretions interfere with gas flow and may obstruct the passages, including the ET tube. Suctioning should occur only when necessary and should be based on individual infant assessment, which includes auscultation of the chest, evidence of decreased oxygenation, excess moisture in the ET tube, or increased infant irritability. When nasopharyngeal passages, the trachea, or the ET tube is being suctioned, insert the catheter gently but quickly; intermittent suction is applied as the catheter is withdrawn. It is imperative that the catheter obstruct the airway for no more than 5 seconds, since continuous suction removes air from the lungs along with the mucus. It is recommended that, where possible, an in-line suction device be used on infants who are acutely ill and who do not tolerate any procedure without profound decreases in oxygen saturation, blood pressure, and heart rate. The purpose of suctioning an artificial airway is to maintain patency of that airway, not the bronchi. Suction applied beyond the ET tube can cause traumatic lesions of the trachea.

Research indicates that suctioning to a point where the catheter meets resistance and is then withdrawn causes trauma to the tracheobronchial wall. To remove secretions without damage to the tracheobronchial mucosa, the suction catheter is premeasured and inserted to a predetermined depth to avoid extension beyond the ET tube. The practice of suctioning patients on mechanical ventilation has undergone close scrutiny in recent years; further studies are needed to validate this practice and to determine the best methods for maintaining a patent airway without compromising the patient's well-being.

The most advantageous positions for facilitating an infant's open airway are with the infant on the side with the head supported in alignment by a small folded blanket or with the infant on the back, positioned to keep the neck slightly extended. With the head in the "sniffing" position, the trachea is opened to its maximum; hyperextension reduces the tracheal diameter in neonates (see Therapeutic Positioning, p. 336). The pulse oximeter is observed before, during, and after suctioning to provide an ongoing assessment of oxygenation status and to prevent hypoxemia.

> **! NURSING ALERT**
>
> Suctioning is not an innocuous procedure; it may cause bronchospasm, bradycardia because of vagal nerve stimulation, hypoxia, and increased intracranial pressure, predisposing the infant to IVH. It should never be carried out on a routine basis. Improper suctioning technique can also cause infection, airway damage, or even pneumothorax.

Inspection of the skin is part of routine infant assessment. Position changes and the use of gel mattresses are helpful in guarding against skin breakdown.

Mouth care is especially important when infants are receiving nothing by mouth, and the problem is often aggravated by the drying effect of oxygen therapy. The nurse can prevent drying and cracking by good oral hygiene using sterile water. Irritation to the nares or mouth that occurs from appliances used to administer oxygen may be reduced by the use of a water-soluble ointment (see Skin Care, p. 329; see Nursing Care Plan).

Nursing care of an infant with RDS is demanding. Pay meticulous attention to subtle changes in the infant's oxygenation status. The importance of attention to detail cannot be overemphasized, particularly in regard to medication administration.

MECONIUM ASPIRATION SYNDROME

Meconium aspiration occurs when a fetus has been subjected to asphyxia or other intrauterine stress that causes relaxation of the anal sphincter and passage of meconium into the amniotic fluid. The majority of meconium aspiration occurs with the first breath. However, a severely compromised fetus may aspirate in utero. At delivery of the chest and initiation of the first breath, infants inhale fluid and meconium into the nasooropharynx (Fig. 10-17).

Pathophysiology

MAS involves the passage of meconium in utero as a result of hypoxic stress. It occurs primarily in full-term and postterm infants but has been reported in infants at less than 37 weeks of gestation. Once the fetus ingests meconium, any gasping activity occurring as a result of intrauterine stress may cause the rather sticky and tenacious substance to become aspirated into the lower airways. The net results are partial airway obstruction, air trapping, hyperinflation distal to the obstruction, and atelectasis caused by surfactant deactivation. A "ball-valve" situation exists wherein gas flows into the lungs on inspiration but is trapped there on exhalation as a result of the small airway diameter. As the infant struggles to take in more air (air hunger), even more meconium may be aspirated. Hyperinflation, hypoxemia, and acidemia result in increased PVR.

In turn, shunting of blood through the ductus arteriosus (right to left) occurs because of increased resistance to blood flow through the pulmonary arteries (and to the lungs), leading

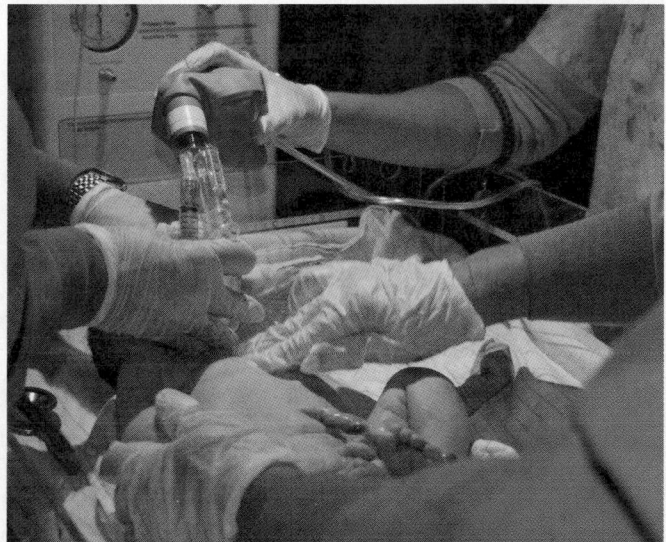

Fig. 10-17 Infant being resuscitated at birth. Note presence of meconium on abdomen, umbilical cord, and overbed warmer. (Courtesy Shannon Perry, Phoenix.)

to further hypoxemia and acidosis. Ductal shunting increases with hypoxia; some blood may enter the left atrium (LA) from the right atrium (RA) via the foramen ovale because there is a net decrease in blood returning to the LA via the pulmonary venous system, thus preventing closure of the foramen ovale. This pathologic process is essentially persistence of the fetal circulation, or PPHN, which is discussed later in this chapter. The air trapping of MAS causes overdistention of the alveoli and often air leaks. There is evidence that meconium contributes to the destruction of surfactant, thus increasing surface tension and further predisposing the alveoli to decreased functional capacity.

Clinical Manifestations

Infants who have released meconium in utero for some time before birth are stained from green meconium stools (those with more recent meconium passage may not be stained), tachypneic, hypoxic, and often depressed at birth. They develop expiratory grunting, nasal flaring, and retractions similar to those experienced by infants with RDS. They may initially be cyanotic or pale as well as tachypneic, and they may demon-strate the classic barrel chest from hyperinflation. The infants are often stressed, hypothermic, hypoglycemic, and hypocalcemic. Severe meconium aspiration progresses rapidly to respiratory failure. These infants exhibit profound respiratory distress with gasping, ineffective ventilations; marked cyanosis and pallor; and hypotonia.

Diagnostic Evaluation

At birth, meconium can often be visualized via laryngoscopy in the respiratory passages and vocal cords. Chest radiographs show uneven distribution of patchy infiltrates, air trapping, hyperexpansion, and atelectasis. Air leaks may be seen as the illness progresses. Oxygenation will be poor, as evidenced by pulse oximetry and arterial blood gases. These infants may quickly develop metabolic and respiratory acidosis. Echocardiography assists in the diagnosis of right-to-left shunting of blood away from the pulmonary system.

Therapeutic Management

Prevention of meconium aspiration begins with suctioning the mouth, nose, and posterior pharynx just after the head is

---

◎ NURSING CARE PLAN

The High-Risk Infant with Respiratory Distress

NURSING DIAGNOSIS	PATIENT OUTCOMES	NURSING INTERVENTIONS	RATIONALE
Ineffective Breathing Pattern related to pulmonary, neurologic, vascular, alveolar, and muscular immaturity	High-risk infant will maintain patent airway and ventilatory status adequate for oxygenation.	Position to facilitate airway expansion and prevent collection of secretions (prone position may be preferred initially in preterm infant to increase chest expansion and oxygenation).	To allow oxygen entry into bronchial tree and alveoli
Child's/Family's Defining Characteristics (Subjective and Objective Data)	**The Following NOC Concepts Apply to These Outcomes**	Closely monitor for deviations from desired breathing pattern—pulse oximetry, arterial blood gases, clinical signs of poor oxygenation, grunting, nasal flaring, apnea, tachypnea, retractions, cyanosis.	To facilitate proper oxygenation by implementing appropriate therapy such as supplemental oxygen, mechanical ventilation, or change of position
Decreased inspiratory and expiratory pressure	Respiratory Status: Ventilation	Monitor vital signs for change in condition or status such as decreased cardiac output (poor perfusion, mottling, deteriorating ventilation status).	To implement appropriate therapy such as suctioning, supplemental oxygen, or vasopressor drugs
Decreased minute ventilation	Respiratory Status: Gas Exchange	Assist with exogenous surfactant administration and monitor patient tolerance or change in status.	To increase alveolar expansion and enhance oxygen–carbon dioxide exchange
Use of accessory muscles to breathe	Tissue Perfusion: Pulmonary	Suction oropharynx, nasopharynx, trachea, or endotracheal tube only as necessary and based on respiratory assessment.	To remove secretions that may interfere with adequate ventilation and oxygenation
Nasal flaring		Perform gentle chest percussion, vibration, and postural drainage based on assessed need and infant tolerance.	To facilitate drainage and removal of secretions
Grunting			
Apnea		**The Following NIC Concepts Apply to These Interventions**	
Tachypnea		Vital Signs Monitoring	
Altered chest excursion		Newborn Monitoring	
Respiratory rate: <20 or >60 breaths/min		Acid-Base Management	
		Airway Management	
		Chest Physiotherapy	
		Oxygen Therapy	
		Airway Suctioning	
		Energy Management	
		Respiratory Monitoring	

NURSING CARE PLAN—cont'd

The High-Risk Infant with Respiratory Distress

NURSING DIAGNOSIS	PATIENT OUTCOMES	NURSING INTERVENTIONS	RATIONALE
Ineffective Thermoregulation related to immature neurologic and metabolic temperature control	Infant will maintain stable body temperature (specify range for age).	Place newborn in a thermally controlled incubator or radiant warmer.	To control environmental temperature and keep infant's temperature stable
Child's/Family's Defining Characteristics (Subjective and Objective Data)	**The Following NOC Concept Applies to These Outcomes** Thermoregulation: Newborn	Place knitted or cloth cap on head.	To prevent heat loss from exposed scalp
Reduction in body temperature below normal range		Use environmental controls for decreasing body heat loss—plastic heat shield, increased ambient temperature, servocontrol on warmer or incubator.	To regulate body temperature within acceptable range and minimize heat loss
Slow capillary refill Cool skin Increased respiratory rate Tachycardia		Monitor core temperature as often as necessary or per unit protocol.	To detect necessity for environmental temperature regulation and to determine infant's response to environmental thermoregulation
		Check temperature of newborn in relation to environmental temperature and temperature of heating element.	To detect change in thermoregulatory status, which may indicate a significant disease process such as sepsis
		Monitor vital signs and skin color, perfusion, pulses, and respiratory status.	To detect changes in status that require additional intervention for stabilization
		Monitor for signs of hyperthermia (flushing, tachycardia, altered level of consciousness) and hypothermia (decreased activity; respiratory distress [deterioration]; cool, mottled extremities).	To prevent untoward effects of hyperthermia (fluctuating cerebral perfusion, apnea, increased metabolism with decreased available glucose for vital functions) or hypothermia (increased glucose utilization, lactic acidosis, respiratory compromise)
		Monitor serum glucose levels as necessary or per unit protocol.	To ensure normoglycemia is maintained
		The Following NIC Concepts Apply to These Interventions Environmental Management Hypothermia Treatment	

NURSING DIAGNOSIS	PATIENT OUTCOMES	NURSING INTERVENTIONS	RATIONALE
Risk for Impaired Parent/Infant/Child Attachment	Parent(s) will form emotional bond or attachment with newborn.	Encourage parent(s) to hold and make eye contact with newborn as physical status allows.	To minimize effects of physical separation from newborn
Child's/Family's Defining Characteristics (Subjective and Objective Data)	**The Following NOC Concept Applies to These Outcomes** Parent/Infant/Child Attachment	Encourage parent-newborn skin-to-skin contact in delivery room as condition of newborn allows.	To facilitate parent-infant interaction that is meaningful and comforting
Risk Factors Separation Preterm infant Physical barriers		Explain to parents the newborn's illness in simple terms and expectations for recovery.	To enhance parental knowledge and decrease potential fear of unknown regarding infant's survival and recovery
		Encourage parents to name newborn.	To provide child individual identity
		Encourage parent participation in newborn care activities such as touching infant, expressing and storing maternal breast milk, and talking to infant.	To facilitate parental involvement in attaining the role of parents and decrease feelings of hopelessness
		The Following NIC Concepts Apply to These Interventions Infant Care Breastfeeding Assistance Anxiety Reduction Parent Education: Infant	

Additional nursing diagnoses that may be applicable to high-risk newborn with respiratory distress: Imbalanced Nutrition: Less Than Body Requirements; Risk for Imbalanced Body Temperature; Impaired Spontaneous Ventilation; Impaired Gas Exchange; and Ineffective Airway Clearance.

delivered while the chest is still compressed in the birth canal. After delivery, the need for tracheal suctioning is based on infant assessment. Infants who are vigorous with strong, stable respiratory effort, good muscle tone, and heart rate greater than 100 beats/min should not undergo tracheal suctioning but should be closely monitored (Kattwinkel, 2006). On the other hand, infants who demonstrate poor respiratory effort, low heart rate, and poor tone should be rapidly intubated, suctioned appropriately, and resuscitated according to clinical status after suctioning. These management protocols have been supported by ongoing research (Kabbur, Herson, Zaremba, et al, 2005).

Infants with respiratory distress are admitted to the NICU. Management of MAS consists of ventilatory support, exogenous surfactant administration, IV fluids, systemic antibiotics, and in some cases inotropes. Because these infants are prone to development of persistent pulmonary hypertension, they should be supported to maintain normal pH, carbon dioxide, and oxygen levels; they may be candidates for ECMO therapy, HFV, or NO (see Nitric Oxide, p. 354, and Persistent Pulmonary Hypertension of the Newborn, p. 359). Complications are managed symptomatically or as described under the specific disorder.

QUALITY PATIENT OUTCOMES: MAS
- Room air oxygen saturation ≥90%
- Maintains arterial/venous pH ≥7.35

Nursing Care Management

Nursing care management is the same as for any high-risk neonate (see nursing care in sections on oxygen therapy, persistent pulmonary hypertension, and other complications).

AIR LEAK SYNDROMES

Extraneous air syndromes, extraalveolar air accumulation, and air leaks are names applied to various clinically recognized disorders produced as a result of alveolar rupture and subsequent escape of air to tissues in which air is not normally present. Extraneous air collection (1) may occur spontaneously in normal neonates, (2) can result from congenital renal or pulmonary malformations, and (3) often complicates underlying respiratory disease and its therapy (e.g., positive pressure ventilation, especially when high distending pressures are required).

After alveolar rupture, air often vents directly into the pleural space to create a pneumothorax. Air may vent into the perivascular interstitium, a condition called pulmonary interstitial emphysema (PIE). PIE may be seen on radiographs as early as 2 to 3 hours after birth in ELBW and VLBW infants with severe RDS. Localized PIE may resolve by itself or may be a precursor to pneumothorax. HFV has been reported to improve the outcome in infants with PIE (Korones, 2003). Air can dissect along the perivascular sheaths to eventually enter the mediastinum and cause pneumomediastinum. More extensive leaks involve the pericardium (manifested as pneumopericardium) or emphysema in the cervical, subcutaneous, or retroperitoneal soft tissues.

Clinical Manifestations

Spontaneous pneumothorax usually occurs during the first few breaths after birth, primarily in full-term or postterm infants, and is evident by the gradual onset of symptoms of respiratory distress after arrival in the nursery. Use of positive pressure ventilation in resuscitation may cause air leaks. Mechanical positive pressure ventilation may contribute to an increase in the incidence of air leaks; however, in some cases, such as in extreme prematurity and meconium aspiration, air leaks may not be altogether preventable. The nurse suspects an air leak on the basis of respiratory manifestations and a shift in location of maximum intensity of heart sounds and absent or diminished breath sounds (although breath sounds may not be altered because of the small diameter of the chest and auscultation of referred breath sounds).

A tension pneumothorax occurs more frequently in infants requiring ventilatory assistance. In preterm infants being mechanically ventilated, an air leak may be demonstrated by hypotension, bradycardia, decreased or absent breath sounds unilaterally, decreased oxygenation (by pulse oximetry), and cyanosis, none of which responds to efforts for oxygenation (a resuscitation bag connected to the ET tube and provision of manual ventilations). There may also be chest asymmetry, altered cardiac sounds (diminished, shifted, or muffled), a palpable liver and spleen, and subcutaneous emphysema. Infants on HFV may demonstrate an air leak by a sudden decrease in systemic pressure or an absence of chest movement (because of difficulty in auscultation of the chest with such modalities). The otherwise healthy full-term infant may exhibit only mild to moderate signs of respiratory distress. The presence of an air leak has been identified as contributing to the risk of an adverse developmental outcome in preterm infants (Laptook, O'Shea, Shankaran, et al, 2005).

! NURSING ALERT

Early manifestations of pneumothorax include tachypnea, restlessness and irritability, lethargy, grunting, nasal flaring, and retractions. Pneumothorax during ventilatory assistance is evident from abrupt and profound duskiness or cyanosis; significant declines in heart rate, arterial blood pressure, and pulse pressure; and poor peripheral perfusion.

Therapeutic Management

Diagnosis is confirmed by transillumination of the chest with a fiberoptic light and/or radiographic examination. In symptomatic infants, treatment is urgent. Evacuation of trapped air is accomplished by chest tube insertion into the pleural space through a small chest incision. The chest tube is then attached to continuous water-seal drainage. A dry suction control drainage system not requiring water is also available. In situations requiring infant transport, a pocket-sized Heimlich valve may be used until an appropriate drainage system can be established; the valve is not effective when fluid drainage is required. Needle aspiration serves as an emergency measure until a chest tube can be inserted. Pneumomediastinum seldom requires treatment, but pneumopericardium is managed by needle aspiration or pericardial tube drainage. The full-term newborn with a small tension pneumothorax may require only oxygen therapy and IV nutrition for a brief period if respiratory distress is not severe.

Nursing Care Management

The most important nursing function, which is most effective for early detection, is close observation for the possibility of an air leak in susceptible infants. Nurses maintain a high level of suspicion in (1) infants with RDS with or without positive pressure ventilation, (2) infants with meconium-stained amniotic fluid or MAS, (3) infants with radiographic evidence of interstitial or lobar emphysema, (4) infants who required resuscitation at birth, or (5) infants receiving CPAP or positive pressure ventilation. For infants at risk, needle aspiration equipment (30-ml syringe, three-way stopcock, and 23- to 25-gauge needles) should be at the bedside for emergency use.

The general nursing care of the infant with an extraneous air syndrome is the same as that for all high-risk neonates. Respiratory management is similar to that for infants with RDS. Assessing breath sounds frequently, monitoring the efficacy of gas exchange, and regulating oxygen therapy according to the infant's needs are vital nursing functions. Attention to pain management with the procedure is vital in these preverbal and significantly stressed infants.

PERSISTENT PULMONARY HYPERTENSION OF THE NEWBORN

PPHN, formerly known as persistent fetal circulation, is a condition in which affected infants display severe pulmonary hypertension, with pulmonary artery pressure levels equal to or greater than systemic pressure, and large right-to-left shunts through both the foramen ovale and the ductus arteriosus. PPHN is a group of disorders having varied causes yet common presenting features and may be classified according to causative etiology (Konduri and Kim, 2009). Because full development of pulmonary arterial musculature occurs late in gestation, PPHN is primarily a condition of late-preterm, full-term, or postterm infants, many of whom were products of complicated pregnancies or deliveries. The condition is often associated with aspiration (especially meconium aspiration), congenital diaphragmatic hernia with severe respiratory distress, cold stress, respiratory distress (e.g., RDS or pneumonia), and septicemia (group B streptococci [GBS]). PPHN is believed to be precipitated by perinatal factors, such as perinatal asphyxia, that cause or contribute to constriction of the pulmonary vasculature.

PPHN can be either primary or secondary. Primary PPHN occurs when the pulmonary vascular system fails to open with the initial respiration at birth; secondary PPHN results from hypoxic stress that increases PVR and causes a return to fetal cardiopulmonary circulation. PPHN is most commonly observed in infants at 35 to 44 weeks of gestation who have a history of perinatal asphyxia, metabolic acidosis, or sepsis and respiratory distress within the first 24 hours. The infants become hypoxic and display marked cyanosis, tachypnea with grunting and retractions, and decreased peripheral perfusion. A loud pulmonary component of the second heart sound and, sometimes, a systolic ejection murmur are present. Diagnosis is established from clinical signs and diagnostic tests, including chest radiography, electrocardiogram, and echocardiography.

Therapeutic Management

Early recognition and management of conditions that contribute to or cause hypoxia and pulmonary vascular vasoconstriction are the primary goals in the prevention of PPHN. Additional treatment includes careful fluid regulation and evaluation of intravascular fluid volume. Supplemental oxygen reduces hypoxia and decreases pulmonary vasoconstriction. Assisted ventilation, often by HFV, is required if hypoxia is severe. Vasodilators, such as sildenafil (a phosphodiesterase [PDE5] inhibitor) or epoprostenol (prostacyclin), are sometimes prescribed to decrease PVR, thereby avoiding ECMO and NO. Sildenafil administered in intravenous or oral form has been shown to reduce PVR (hypertension) in neonates and improve oxygenation, but further controlled clinical trials are needed (Latini, Del Vecchio, De Felice, et al, 2008; Shah and Ohlsson, 2007b; Steinhorn, Kinsella, Pierce, et al, 2009).

Additional drug therapy used in the management of PPHN includes judicious use of sodium bicarbonate to maintain appropriate acid-base balance; volume expanders such as normal saline or lactated Ringer solution; and the vasopressors dopamine, dobutamine, and nitroprusside to increase systemic vascular resistance (Konduri, 2004). The use of inhaled NO has been successfully used to reverse pulmonary vascular vasoconstriction and is often attempted before other therapies such as ECMO (see Nitric Oxide, p. 354).

Another approach to management of infants with pulmonary complications is the use of ECMO with a modified heart-lung machine. Blood is shunted from a catheter in the right atrium or right internal jugular vein by gravity to a servoregulated roller pump; pumped through a membrane lung and a small heat exchanger; and returned to the systemic circulation via a major artery, such as the carotid artery, to the aortic arch. A venovenous approach (femoral vein) may be used, thus avoiding the need to ligate the carotid artery. ECMO provides oxygen to the circulation and allows the lungs to rest. The goal of ECMO is to "buy time" for the severely injured lung to heal while effectively oxygenating major organ systems, including the brain, heart, kidneys, and lungs (Fig. 10-18).

ECMO is labor intensive and thus expensive. Technical malfunctions may occur, requiring frequent monitoring of the equipment and the patient's response to treatment. Typically,

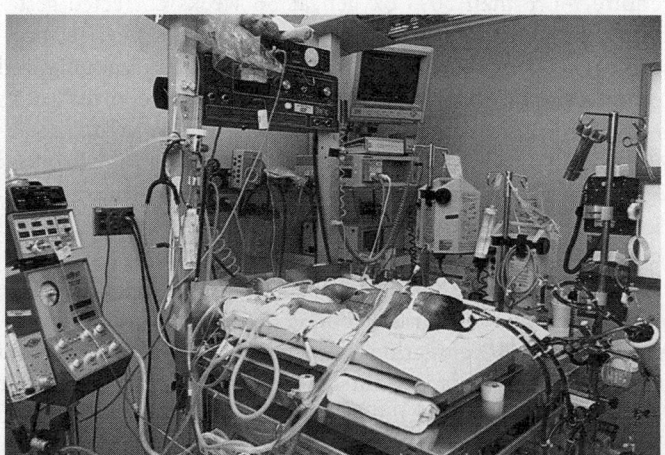

Fig. 10-18 Infant on extracorporeal membrane oxygenation (ECMO).

two nurses, or a nurse and a perfusionist, are required as minimum staffing for the ECMO patient; more staff, including a respiratory therapist, are required in the acute phase. ECMO requires heparinization of the blood and blood circuit; for this reason it is not used in infants at less than 35 weeks of gestation, who are prone to intraventricular hemorrhage. Bleeding is one of the major complications associated with ECMO. Overall the need for ECMO has decreased with increased use of exogenous surfactant, inhaled NO, and HFV for neonatal hypoxemic respiratory failure (Konduri and Kim, 2009).

Nursing Care Management

The nursing care for PPHN is the same as for infants with severe respiratory difficulties and infants supported by mechanical ventilation and cardiovascular support. The infant with PPHN is often the sickest on the unit, depending on the causative factors and reaction to treatment. Because handling for any reason causes a decrease in arterial oxygen concentration, the nurse must weigh the stresses imposed by routine care against the risk of iatrogenic hypoxia. It is important to decrease noxious stimuli that cause hypoxia and to use clustered nursing interventions that keep nonsedated infants calm. Continuous monitoring of oxygenation, temperature, central venous pressure, vital signs, blood pressure, and acid-base balance decreases the need for physical manipulation and disturbance. Infants are further assessed for response to treatments, including IV therapy, fluids, electrolytes, and exogenous glucose.

BRONCHOPULMONARY DYSPLASIA

BPD, sometimes referred to as chronic lung disease, is a pathologic process that develops primarily in ELBW and VLBW infants with RDS. BPD may also develop in infants with MAS, persistent pulmonary hypertension, pneumonia, and cyanotic heart disease. Infants who develop BPD are at risk for frequent hospitalization because of their borderline respiratory reserve, hyperactive airway, and increased susceptibility to respiratory infection.

Mild BPD is operationally defined the need for supplemental oxygen for 28 days or more but room air by 36 weeks corrected gestational age or at discharge. Moderate BPD is defined by the need for oxygen for 28 days or more and less than 30% oxygen at 36 weeks corrected gestational age. With severe BPD infants require more than 30% oxygen at 36 weeks corrected gestational age (Bhandari and Bhandari, 2009). An inverse relationship between incidence of BPD and birth weight is emphasized in the Vermont-Oxford Network report, which reported a 60% incidence for ELBW infants (501 to 750 g [1.1 to 1.6 lb]) versus 21% for infants weighing 1001 to 1250 g (2.2 to 2.7 lb). Risk factors for BPD include assisted ventilation, oxygen administration, prenatal and postnatal (nosocomial) infections, PDA, and fluid imbalance (Askin and Diehl-Jones, 2009a).

The more severe form of BPD usually begins with severe respiratory failure secondary to RDS or with pneumonia requiring mechanical ventilation with high airway pressure and oxygen supplementation during the first few days of life (Bancalari, 2001). Since the advent of antenatal glucocorticoid therapy, surfactant replacement, and new ventilator strategies, a "new" BPD is emerging (Greenough, 2008). These infants experience a milder initial respiratory course but continue to require ventilatory support or oxygen supplementation and show radiographic pulmonary changes characteristic of BPD.

Pathophysiology

The pathogenesis of BPD is complex and multifactorial. BPD begins with the immature lung that undergoes an initial injury leading to a chronic inflammatory process that results in recurrent injury and abnormal healing (Askin and Diehl-Jones, 2009a). A variety of mechanisms have been related to the initial injury: (1) prenatal infection (inflammatory process before birth), (2) mechanical ventilation (volutrauma, intubation), (3) supplemental oxygen (oxygen-derived free radicals), (4) increased pulmonary blood flow from PDA, or (5) postnatal infection.

The pulmonary changes are characterized by interstitial edema and epithelial swelling followed by thickening and fibrotic proliferation of the alveolar walls and squamous metaplasia of the bronchiolar epithelium. Areas of atelectasis and cystlike foci of hyperaeration are visible on radiographs between 10 and 20 days of life and persist for weeks; however, some infants may not demonstrate cystic foci. In addition, ciliary activity is paralyzed by high oxygen concentrations that interfere with the ability to clear the lung of mucus, thus aggravating airway obstruction and atelectasis. As the infant's lungs begin healing, the process is altered, possibly by continuous high oxygenation, inadequate nutrition, or vitamin E deficiency, resulting in decreased surface for oxygen and carbon dioxide exchange. The overall results of this process are hypercarbia, hypoxemia, and subsequent inability to wean successfully from oxygen.

As survival of immature preterm infants (<28 weeks of gestation) increases, the occurrence of BPD also increases.

In addition to BPD, other diseases associated with similar radiographic findings include congenital heart disease and viral pneumonia caused by cytomegalovirus. There are no laboratory alterations that confirm a diagnosis; diagnosis is made on the basis of radiographic findings, oxygen therapy or positive pressure ventilation after 28 days, signs of respiratory distress, and a history of requiring mechanical ventilation in the first week of life for more than 3 days.

Therapeutic Management

The first approach to management is prevention of the disorder in susceptible infants. Despite previous theorization that surfactant administration to preterm infants would eradicate BPD, studies so far have failed to show a significant decrease of BPD in infants less than 30 weeks receiving surfactant for prophylaxis or rescue (American Academy of Pediatrics, 2008). To reduce the risk of volutrauma when positive pressure ventilation is being used, maintain the lowest PIP necessary to obtain adequate ventilation, and use the lowest level of inspired oxygen to maintain adequate oxygenation. HFOV has been beneficial in reducing the risk of BPD, as has the administration of vitamin A (Shah, 2003). Fluid administration is carefully controlled and restricted. Drug or surgical intervention is indicated when there is significant shunting of blood through the PDA.

No specific treatment exists for BPD except to maintain adequate arterial blood gases with the administration of oxygen and to avoid progression of the disease. Corticosteroid (dexamethasone) therapy has been shown to benefit infants with BPD by decreasing the pulmonary inflammatory response and improving oxygenation and gas exchange, resulting in earlier weaning from mechanical assistance. However, with complications such as sepsis, hypertension, and hyperglycemia and an overall lack of decreased mortality in such infants, this therapy remains controversial. Other adverse effects of this long-acting, potent glucocorticoid have been reported: growth restriction, GI hemorrhage, and cardiomyopathy. In light of studies that show an increased incidence of periventricular leukomalacia, neuromotor abnormalities, CP, decreased cerebral cortical gray matter volume, and adverse long-term neurologic outcome, the benefits of this treatment may not outweigh the risks (American Academy of Pediatrics and Canadian Paediatric Society, 2002; Halliday, Ehrenkranz, and Doyle, 2009). Ongoing research is being done to determine whether an alternative dosing regimen of postnatal steroids can reduce the incidence of BPD without associated neurodevelopmental side effects (Onland, Offringa, De Jaegere, et al, 2009).

Weaning infants from oxygen is difficult and must be accomplished gradually. These infants do not tolerate excessive or even normal amounts of fluid well and have a tendency to accumulate interstitial fluid in the lungs, which aggravates the condition. Oral diuretics are used to control interstitial fluid. Nebulized or metered dose inhaler bronchodilators (albuterol) and inhaled steroids may be effective and promote improvement in infants with BPD. (See also Asthma, Chapter 32.) Oral electrolyte supplements are given to replace those lost with concurrent oral diuretics and renal water losses.

Growth and development are often delayed in infants with BPD, which is related in part to the difficulties in providing adequate nutrition and in part to the lack of normal sensory stimulation because of prolonged hospitalization. Children with BPD have metabolic needs far greater than those of the average infant. This can create a problem for the caregiver, who must meet the goals of adequate nutrition while avoiding overhydration, especially if the child is ill, eats poorly, or has cardiopulmonary instability. The infant may be further compromised by gastroesophageal reflux, a frequent complication in preterm infants. (See Chapter 33.) Adequate intake of protein is particularly important in preventing postnatal growth failure in LBW infants. Protein supplements may be necessary to ensure adequate intake.

Osteopenia may occur in infants with BPD and in preterm infants, with higher incidence among the infants with BPD, presumably because of low calcium and vitamin D intake secondary to the calciuric effects of diuretic therapy. Dietary supplementation with human milk fortifier, calcium and phosphorus, and vitamin D has reduced the incidence of osteopenia in preterm infants.

RSV prophylaxis with the monoclonal antibody palivizumab (Synagis) is effective in diminishing the complications of RSV. RSV is a common cause for hospitalization and death in growing preterm neonates, including those with BPD. Palivizumab is given intramuscularly to high-risk infants, does not interfere with immunizations, and has few side effects. Palivizumab is administered in a dose of 15 mg/kg once a month, usually beginning in October and ending in May. (See Respiratory Syncytial Virus, Chapter 32.)

Prognosis

Reports vary regarding the mortality rate for BPD. The hospital stay is often long because of the infant's need for supplemental oxygen, although home oxygen therapy provides selected infants the opportunity for discharge. A nasal cannula is an acceptable way to administer oxygen for the dependent infant to promote development of motor and social skills. Long-term problems seen in older children who had BPD as infants include growth failure, airway hyperreactivity, hyperexpansion, increased incidence of respiratory infections, and airway obstruction. A significant proportion of deaths occur after discharge from the hospital.

An 8-year follow-up study comparing the outcomes of preterm infants with BPD, preterm infants without BPD, and full-term infants without BPD found that BPD and duration on oxygen have long-term adverse effects on cognitive and academic achievement above and beyond the effects of VLBW alone. After controlling for birth weight and neurologic complications, BPD was associated with lower IQs; poorer perceptual organization, attention, and motor skills; reduced school achievement; and greater participation in special education such as physical and speech-language therapies (Short, Klein, Lewis, et al, 2003; Anderson and Doyle, 2008).

Nursing Care Management

Infants with BPD expend considerable energy in their efforts to breathe; therefore it is important that they receive plenty of opportunities for rest and additional calories. Growth records provide clues to the need for change in their diets, and some infants require nutritional supplements. Because these infants tire easily and because large quantities of formula might compromise respiration, small, frequent feedings are better tolerated. Reducing environmental stimuli and subsequent hypoxia is an important aspect in the care of these infants. Close attention to the infant's behavioral cues is important in the older infant with BPD because these cues may signal carbon dioxide retention.

Adequate hydration is extremely important because a large amount of fluid are lost through respiration, and secretions must be thinned sufficiently to facilitate removal by suctioning. However, because BPD increases lung permeability, many infants are subject to pulmonary edema and require fluid restriction. Nurses must be alert to signs of both overhydration and underhydration, such as changes in weight, electrolytes, output measurements, and urine specific gravity and signs of edema.

Because the growing infant with BPD has a restricted fluid intake, has higher than average caloric requirements, and often requires many oral medications, the nurse is challenged by the complexity of care involved. Infants with BPD may become difficult or maladaptive feeders if they are aware of hunger yet compromised by not being able to eat fast enough to satiate that hunger because of the increased labor of breathing. Individualized nursing care aimed at decreasing oxygenation requirements during feedings, decreasing environmental stimuli, fortifying feedings, and providing more contact with a primary caregiver may facilitate the infant's care. Feeding schedules should be individualized as much as possible. Oral medications that taste bad to the infant may be given at times separate from feedings to ensure that feeding time is pleasant. Adjustments to overall fluid administration requirements are made, taking into account that the oral medications are also fluids. Regurgitated medications and feedings need to be dealt with in regard to fluid and caloric needs and the amount of absorption of medication that occurs before emesis.

Parents are extremely anxious regarding the prognosis when their infant has BPD. In addition, the lengthy hospitalization interferes with parent-child relationships and deprives the infant of appropriate parental contact and stimulation. Nurses should encourage the parents to visit the infant and become involved in the routine care. The parents need to be informed regarding medical care, equipment, and procedures related to their infant and taught procedures such as suctioning and chest physiotherapy.

The older infant with BPD should have normal nurturing and developmental opportunities appropriate to the infant's condition and abilities. Careful monitoring of physiologic and behavioral systems during any activity is necessary so that activity can be stopped before the infant becomes irritable or tired. Opportunities out of bed in an infant seat or on a floor mat with a nurse or physical or play therapist provide one-on-one interaction that can enhance the infant's experience of the world and people.

Irritability has been associated with infants who have BPD, making their care often challenging and frustrating (see Developmental Outcome, p. 332). Some strategies to facilitate infant coping during prolonged hospitalization include (1) decreased number of unfamiliar caregivers, (2) increased access to parents, (3) predictability in schedule and caregivers, (4) consistency of care routines and practices, (5) pleasurable opportunities for play and socialization within physical tolerance, (6) adequate nutrition, and (7) uninterrupted rest cycles with diurnal variation to facilitate biologic rhythms. Parental involvement is critical because they are the one constant for the infant.

Home Care

Because the availability of home cardiac and apnea monitors and home oxygen therapy has increased, many infants with BPD can be discharged when they are gaining weight and their oxygen need is low. Home care is desirable to promote parent-infant bonding, minimize health care costs, and prevent nosocomial infections. Preparation for home care requires education and considerable reassurance. (See Chapter 25.) Management of home monitoring equipment and home oxygen therapy is stress provoking, but most families become comfortable with the machinery while their infant is still in the hospital. Families need reminders about their infant's increased risk of infection and about limiting contact with persons who have respiratory tract infections. Because of their minimum respiratory reserve, even a minor illness can threaten these infants.

Some infants are discharged with a tracheostomy on oxygen supplementation or home ventilators. Discharge teaching and home care nursing (minimum of 2 weeks to several months) is crucial to these infants' safe and successful transition into the community and home setting. Parents need to learn how to advocate for appropriate home care and supplies in anticipation of future needs.

Because of the high mortality rate in the first year, parents should learn cardiopulmonary resuscitation and how to manage any other emergency that might be anticipated for their infant. Helping families cope with their anxieties and reassuring them of their ability to manage the care of their infant are important nursing functions. Parents need follow-up visits in the home and the comfort of knowing that help is only a telephone call away.

HIGH RISK RELATED TO INFECTIOUS PROCESSES

SEPSIS

Sepsis, or septicemia, refers to a generalized bacterial infection in the bloodstream. Neonates are highly susceptible to infection as a result of diminished nonspecific (inflammatory) and specific (humoral) immunity, such as impaired phagocytosis, delayed chemotactic response, minimum or absent IgA and immunoglobulin M (IgM), and decreased complement levels. Because of the infant's poor response to pathogenic agents, there is usually no local inflammatory reaction at the portal of entry to signal an infection, and the resulting symptoms tend to be vague and nonspecific. Consequently, diagnosis and treatment may be delayed.

Although the mortality from sepsis has diminished, the incidence has not. Nursery epidemics are not infrequent, and the high-risk infant has a four times greater chance of developing septicemia than does the normal neonate. The frequency of infection is almost twice as great in male infants as in females and also carries a higher mortality for males. Other factors increasing the risk of infection are prematurity, congenital anomalies or acquired injuries that disrupt the skin or mucous membranes, invasive procedures such as placement of IV lines and ET tubes, administration of total parenteral nutrition, and nosocomial exposure to a number of pathogens in the NICU. Thorough hand washing is the single most important infection control measure in the NICU. Proper handling of formula and supplies such as syringes and gavage tubes is also vital to prevent infection.

Breast-feeding has a protective effect against infection and should be promoted for all newborns. It is of particular benefit to the high-risk neonate. Colostrum contains agglutinins that are effective against gram-negative bacteria. Human milk contains large quantities of IgA and iron-binding protein that exert a bacteriostatic effect on *Escherichia coli*. Human milk also contains macrophages and lymphocytes that promote a local inflammatory reaction.

Pathophysiology

The premature withdrawal of the placental barrier leaves infants vulnerable to most common viral, bacterial, fungal, and parasitic infections. Immune substances, primarily immunoglobulin G (IgG), are normally acquired from the maternal system and stored in fetal tissues during the final weeks of gestation to provide newborns with passive immunity to a variety of infectious agents. Early birth interrupts this transplacental transmission; thus preterm infants have a low level of circulating IgG;

the concentrations of immune substances directly relate to the length of gestation. IgA, which plays a role in defense against viral infections, and IgM, with properties that are most efficient in dealing with gram-negative organisms, are not transferred to the fetus, which leaves the infant highly vulnerable to invasion by these organisms.

Defense mechanisms of neonates are further hampered by a low level of complement, diminished opsonization ability, monocyte dysfunction, and a reduced number and inefficient function of circulating leukocytes. Furthermore, these leukocytes with diminished motility and phagocytic capacity are unable to concentrate their limited numbers selectively at the site of infection. In addition, a hypofunctioning adrenal gland contributes only a meager antiinflammatory response. Consequently, these deficiencies permit rapid invasion, spread, and multiplication of organisms. An immature gut mucosal barrier further predisposes the preterm infant to bacteria, which may easily cross the mucosa into the bloodstream.

Sources of Infection

Sepsis in the neonatal period can be acquired prenatally across the placenta from the maternal bloodstream or during labor from ingestion or aspiration of infected amniotic fluid. Prolonged rupture of the membranes always presents a risk for maternal-fetal transfer of pathogenic organisms. In utero transplacental transfer can occur with a variety of organisms and viruses such as cytomegalovirus, toxoplasmosis, and *Treponema pallidum* (syphilis), which cross the placental barrier during the latter half of pregnancy.

Early-onset sepsis (<3 days after birth) is acquired in the perinatal period. Infection can occur from direct contact with organisms from the maternal GI and genitourinary tracts. Organisms associated with early-onset infection include GBS, *E. coli,* and other gram-negative enteric organisms. Despite the development of maternal screening and prophylaxis, infection rates for early-onset GBS infection remain at approximately 0.3 per 1000 live births (Centers for Disease Control and Prevention, 2007). *E. coli,* which may be present in the vagina, accounts for approximately half of all cases of sepsis caused by gram-negative organisms. GBS is an extremely virulent organism in neonates, with a high (50%) death rate in affected infants. Other bacteria noted to cause early-onset infection include *Haemophilus influenzae, Citrobacter* and *Enterobacter* organisms, coagulase-negative staphylococci, and *Streptococcus viridans* (Stoll, Hansen, Higgins, et al, 2005). Other pathogens that are harbored in the vagina and may infect the infant include gonococci, *Candida albicans,* herpes simplex virus (type II), and chlamydia.

Late-onset sepsis (1 to 3 weeks after birth) is primarily nosocomial, and the offending organisms are usually staphylococci, *Klebsiella* organisms, enterococci, *E. coli,* and *Pseudomonas* or *Candida* species (Stoll, 2007). Coagulase-negative staphylococci, considered to be primarily a contaminant in older children and adults, is commonly found to be the cause of septicemia in ELBW and VLBW infants. Bacterial invasion can occur through sites such as the umbilical stump; the skin; mucous membranes of the eye, nose, pharynx, and ear; and internal systems such as the respiratory, nervous, urinary, and GI systems.

Postnatal infection is acquired by cross-contamination from other infants, personnel, or objects in the environment. Bacteria, such as *Klebsiella* and *Pseudomonas* organisms, that are commonly called "water bugs" (because they are able to grow in water) are found in water supplies; humidifying apparatus; sink drains; suction machines; most respiratory equipment; and indwelling venous and arterial catheters used for infusions, blood sampling, and monitoring vital signs. These organisms are often transmitted by personnel from person to person or object to person by poor hand washing and inadequate housecleaning.

Neonatal sepsis is most common in the infant at risk, particularly the preterm infant or the infant born after a difficult or traumatic labor and delivery, who is least capable of resisting such bacterial invasion.

Clinical Manifestations

A few neonatal infections (e.g., pyoderma, conjunctivitis, omphalitis, and mastitis) are easy to recognize. However, systemic infections are characterized by subtle, vague, nonspecific, and almost imperceptible physical signs. Often the only complaint concerns an infant's "failure to do well," not looking "right," or nonspecific respiratory distress. Rarely is there any indication of a local inflammatory response, which would suggest the portal of entry into the bloodstream. The presence of bacteria is indicated by a specific characteristic. For example, *Pseudomonas* organisms produce necrotic purplish skin lesions, and group B β-hemolytic streptococci usually result in severe respiratory distress, periods of apnea, and a chest radiograph similar to that of RDS.

All body systems tend to show some indication of sepsis, although often little correlation exists between the manifestations and the etiologic factors involved. For example, seizures and fever, a universal feature of infection in older children, may be absent in neonates. It is usually the nursing observation of subtle changes in appearance and behavior that leads to the detection of infection. The nonspecific, early signs are hypothermia and changes in color, tone, activity, and feeding behavior. In addition, sudden episodes of apnea and unexplained oxygen desaturation (hypoxia) may signal an infection. Significantly, similar signs may be manifestations of a number of clinical conditions unrelated to sepsis, such as hypoglycemia, hypocalcemia, heroin withdrawal, or a CNS disorder.

Preterm infants, particularly ELBW and VLBW infants, are highly susceptible to early sepsis and pneumonia occurring concurrently with RDS, since preterm delivery has been increasingly shown to be associated with a maternal bacterial pathogen. ELBW and VLBW infants are also highly susceptible to fungal and viral infections. Investigation for such agents should begin when sepsis is suspected in this population. Because meningitis is a common sequela of sepsis, the neonate is evaluated for bacterial growth in cerebrospinal fluid (CSF). Clinical signs of neonatal meningitis, particularly in VLBW infants, may not have typical features of older infants. Clinical signs that may indicate possible neonatal sepsis are listed in Box 10-9.

Diagnostic Evaluation

Because sepsis is easy to confuse with other neonatal disorders, the definitive diagnosis is established by laboratory and

BOX 10-9 MANIFESTATIONS OF NEONATAL SEPSIS

General Signs
Infant generally "not doing well"
Poor temperature control—hypothermia, hyperthermia (rare)

Circulatory System
Pallor, cyanosis, or mottling
Cold, clammy skin
Hypotension
Edema
Irregular heartbeat—bradycardia, tachycardia

Respiratory System
Irregular respirations, apnea, or tachypnea
Cyanosis
Grunting
Dyspnea
Retractions

Central Nervous System
Diminished activity—lethargy, hyporeflexia, coma
Increased activity—irritability, tremors, seizures
Full fontanel
Increased or decreased tone
Abnormal eye movements

Gastrointestinal System
Poor feeding
Vomiting
Diarrhea or decreased stooling
Abdominal distention
Hepatomegaly
Hemoccult-positive stools

Hematopoietic System
Jaundice
Pallor
Petechiae, ecchymosis
Splenomegaly

radiographic examination. Isolation of the specific organism is always attempted through cultures of blood, urine, and CSF. Blood studies may show signs of anemia, leukocytosis, or leukopenia. Leukopenia is usually an ominous sign because of its frequent association with high mortality. An elevated number of immature neutrophils (left-shift), decreased or increased total neutrophils, and changes in neutrophil morphologic characteristics also suggest an infectious process in the neonate. Other diagnostic data that are helpful in the determination of neonatal sepsis include C-reactive protein and interleukins, specifically interleukin-6 (Volante, Moretti, Pisani, et al, 2004; Laborada, Rego, Jain, et al, 2003).

Therapeutic Management

In addition to the institution of rigorous preventive measures such as good hand washing, early recognition and diagnosis are essential to increase the infant's chance for survival and reduce the likelihood of permanent neurologic damage. Diagnosis of sepsis is often based on suspicion of initial clinical signs and symptoms, and antibiotic therapy is initiated before laboratory results are available for confirmation and identification of the exact organism. Treatment consists of circulatory

support, respiratory support, and aggressive administration of antibiotics.

Supportive therapy usually involves administration of oxygen (if respiratory distress or hypoxia is evident), careful regulation of fluids, correction of electrolyte or acid-base imbalance, and temporary discontinuation of oral feedings. Blood transfusion may be needed to correct anemia; IV fluids for shock, electronic monitoring of vital signs, and regulation of the thermal environment are mandatory.

Antibiotic therapy is continued for 7 to 10 days if cultures are positive, discontinued in 36 to 72 hours if cultures are negative and the infant is asymptomatic, and most often administered via IV infusion. Antifungal and antiviral therapies are implemented as appropriate, depending on causative agents.

Prognosis

The prognosis for neonatal sepsis is variable. Severe neurologic and respiratory sequelae may occur in ELBW and VLBW infants with early-onset sepsis. Late-onset sepsis and meningitis may also result in poor outcomes for immunocompromised neonates.

The introduction of new markers for neonatal sepsis such as acute phase proteins, cytokines, cell surface antigens, and bacterial genomes may prove to be particularly helpful in early differentiation of true sepsis from RDS and in guidance for antibiotic therapy (Arnon and Litmanovitz, 2008). Future experimental methods being explored to combat infection in neonates include monoclonal antibody therapy, fibronectin infusion, and lymphokine enhancement.

Nursing Care Management

Nursing care of the infant with sepsis involves observation and assessment as outlined for any high-risk infant. Recognition of the existing problem is of paramount importance. It is usually the nurse who observes and assesses infants and identifies that "something is wrong" with them. Awareness of the potential modes of infection transmission also helps the nurse identify those at risk for developing sepsis. Much of the care of infants with sepsis involves the medical treatment of the illness. Knowledge of the side effects of the specific antibiotic and proper regulation and administration of the drug are vital. Antibiotics are usually administered via a special injection port near the infusion site. The appropriately diluted medication is administered slowly by mechanical pump.

Prolonged antibiotic therapy poses additional hazards for affected infants. Oral antibiotics, if administered, destroy intestinal flora responsible for the synthesis of vitamin K, which can reduce blood coagulability. In addition, antibiotics predispose the infant to growth of resistant organisms and superinfection from fungal or mycotic agents, such as *C. albicans.* Nurses must be alert for evidence of such complications. Nystatin oral suspension may be administered for prophylaxis against oral candidiasis.

Part of the total care of infants with sepsis is to decrease any additional physiologic or environmental stress. This includes providing an optimum thermoregulated environment and anticipating potential problems such as dehydration or hypoxia. Precautions are implemented to prevent the spread of infection to other newborns, but to be effective, activities must be carried out by all caregivers. Proper hand washing, the use of disposable equipment (e.g., linens, catheters, feeding supplies, and IV equipment), disposal of secretions (e.g., vomitus and stool), and adequate housekeeping of the environment and equipment are essential. Because nurses are the most consistent caregivers involved with sick infants, it is usually their responsibility to ensure that everyone maintains all phases of contact isolation or Standard Precautions.

Another aspect of caring for infants with sepsis involves observation for signs of complications, including meningitis and septic shock, a severe complication caused by toxins in the bloodstream.

A number of viral agents—namely, cytomegalovirus, herpes, hepatitis, and human immunodeficiency virus (HIV)—may also be transmitted to the fetus from the mother. When acquired prenatally (congenital), these viruses represent a serious threat to the infant's life. (See Table 10-11 for viral infections.)

NECROTIZING ENTEROCOLITIS

NEC is an acute inflammatory disease of the bowel with increased incidence in preterm and other high-risk infants; it is most common in preterm infants. Because the signs are similar to those observed in many other disorders of the newborn, nurses must constantly be aware of the possibility of this disease.

Pathophysiology

The precise cause of NEC is still uncertain, but it appears to occur in infants whose GI tract has suffered vascular compromise. Intestinal ischemia of unknown etiology, immature GI host defenses, bacterial proliferation, and feeding substrate are now believed to have a multifactorial role in the etiology of NEC. Prematurity remains the most prominent risk factor in this disease (Schurr and Perkins, 2008).

The damage to mucosal cells lining the bowel wall is great. Diminished blood supply to these cells causes their death in large numbers; they stop secreting protective, lubricating mucus; and the thin, unprotected bowel wall is attacked by proteolytic enzymes. Thus the bowel wall continues to swell and break down; it is unable to synthesize protective IgM, and the mucosa is permeable to macromolecules (e.g., exotoxins), which further hamper intestinal defenses. Gas-forming bacteria invade the damaged areas to produce intestinal pneumatosis, the presence of air in the submucosal or subserosal surfaces of the bowel.

Clinical Manifestations

The prominent clinical signs of NEC are a distended abdomen, gastric residuals, and blood in the stools. Because NEC closely resembles septicemia, the infant may "not look well." Nonspecific signs include lethargy, poor feeding, hypotension, apnea, vomiting (often bile stained), decreased urinary output, and hypothermia. The onset is usually between 4 and 10 days after the initiation of feedings, but signs may be evident as early as 4 hours of age and as late as 30 days. NEC in full-term infants almost always occurs in the first 10 days of life; late-onset NEC is confined primarily to preterm infants and coincides with the onset of feedings after they have passed through the acute phase of an illness such as RDS.

Diagnostic Evaluation

Radiographic studies show a sausage-shaped dilation of the intestine that progresses to marked distention and the characteristic intestinal pneumatosis—"soapsuds," or the bubbly appearance of thickened bowel wall and ultralumina. Air may be present in the portal circulation or free air observed in the abdomen, indicating perforation. Laboratory findings may include anemia, leukopenia, leukocytosis, metabolic acidosis, and electrolyte imbalance. In severe cases coagulopathy (disseminated intravascular coagulation) or thrombocytopenia may be evident. Organisms may be cultured from blood, although bacteremia or septicemia may not be prominent early in the course of the disease.

Therapeutic Management

Treatment of NEC begins with prevention. Oral feedings may be withheld for at least 24 to 48 hours from infants who are believed to have suffered birth asphyxia. Breast milk is the preferred enteral nutrient because it confers some passive immunity (IgA), macrophages, and lysozymes.

Minimum enteral feedings (trophic feeding, GI priming) in VLBW infants have gained acceptance. However, the question as to whether or not tropic feeding increases the incidence of NEC remains unanswered. Some studies have shown that such feedings may be protective against NEC in nonasphyxiated preterm infants (Schanler, Shulman, Lau, et al, 1999; Newell, 2000; Hay, 2008). Some researchers, however, suggest there is insufficient evidence to completely advocate for trophic feedings to prevent NEC (Tyson and Kennedy, 2005; Tyson, Kennedy, Lucke, et al, 2007). A study by Kamitsuka, Horton, and Williams (2000) demonstrated a reduction in NEC by 84% after implementation of a standardized feeding protocol in infants weighing 1250 to 2500 g (2.7 to 5.5 lb) who were less than 35 weeks of gestation.

The role of probiotics such as *Lactobacillus acidophilus* and *Bifidobacterium infantis* administered with enteral feedings for the prevention of NEC has yet to be explored fully enough to advocate widespread use in all VLBW infants. In some studies probiotics decreased the incidence of NEC (Alfaleh, Anabrees, and Bassler, 2009; Bin-Nun, Bromiker, Wilschanski, et al, 2005). There is evidence that human milk may have a protective effect against the development of NEC (Sisk, Lovelady, Gruber, et al, 2007). The administration of maternal antenatal steroids may prevent NEC in some infants by promoting early gut closure and maturation of the gut barrier mucosa (Thompson and Bizzarro, 2008).

Medical treatment of confirmed NEC consists of discontinuation of all oral feedings; institution of abdominal decompression via nasogastric suction; administration of IV antibiotics; and correction of extravascular volume depletion, electrolyte abnormalities, acid-base imbalances, and hypoxia. Replacing oral feedings with parenteral fluids decreases the need for oxygen and circulation to the bowel. Serial abdominal radiograph films (every 4 to 6 hours in the acute phase) are taken to monitor for possible progression of the disease to intestinal perforation.

With early recognition and treatment, medical management is increasingly successful. If there is progressive deterioration under medical management or evidence of perforation, surgical resection and anastomosis are performed. Extensive involvement may necessitate surgical intervention and establishment of an ileostomy, jejunostomy, or colostomy. Sequelae in surviving infants include short-bowel syndrome, colonic stricture with obstruction, fat malabsorption, and failure to thrive secondary to intestinal dysfunction. Various surgical interventions for NEC are available and depend on the extent of bowel necrosis, associated illness factors, and infant stability. Intestinal transplantation has been successful in some former preterm infants with NEC-associated short-bowel syndrome who had already developed life-threatening complications related to total parenteral nutrition. More than 50% of these patients survived with improved quality of life. Bowel lengthening procedures and intestinal transplantation may be lifesaving options for infants who previously faced high morbidity and mortality (Nucci, Burns, Armah, et al, 2008). Animal research is now under way using tissue-engineered small intestine as a possible lifesaving treatment for short-bowel syndrome (Guner, Chokshi, Petrosyan, et al, 2008).

Nursing Care Management

The nurse is a key factor in the prompt recognition of the early warning signs of NEC. When the disease is suspected, the nurse assists with diagnostic procedures and implements the therapeutic regimen. Vital signs, including blood pressure, are monitored for changes that might indicate bowel perforation, septicemia, or cardiovascular shock, and measures are instituted to prevent possible transmission to other infants. It is especially important to avoid rectal temperatures because of the increased danger of perforation. To avoid pressure on the distended abdomen and to facilitate continuous observation, infants are often left undiapered and positioned supine or on the side.

⚠ NURSING ALERT

Observe for indications of early development of NEC by checking the abdomen frequently for distention (measuring abdominal girth, measuring residual gastric contents before feedings, and listening for the presence of bowel sounds) and performing all routine assessments for high-risk neonates.

Conscientious attention to nutrition and hydration needs is essential, and antibiotics are administered as prescribed. The time at which oral feedings are reinstituted varies considerably but is usually at least 7 to 10 days after diagnosis and treatment. Sterile water or electrolyte solution may be given initially, followed by human milk (if available) or elemental formula such as Pregestimil.

Because NEC is an infectious disease, one of the most important nursing functions is control of infection. Strict hand washing is the primary barrier to spread, and confirmed multiple cases are isolated. Persons with symptoms of a GI infection should not care for these or any other infants.

The infant undergoing surgery requires the same careful attention and observation as any infant with abdominal surgery, including ostomy care (as applicable). This disorder is one of the most common reasons for performing ileostomies on newborns. Throughout the medical and surgical management of infants with NEC, the nurse is continually alert for signs of complications, such as septicemia, disseminated intravascular coagulation, hypoglycemia, and other metabolic derangements.

HIGH RISK RELATED TO CARDIOVASCULAR AND HEMATOLOGIC COMPLICATIONS

PATENT DUCTUS ARTERIOSUS

PDA is a common complication of severe respiratory disease in preterm infants. It occurs in the majority of preterm infants under 1200 g (2.6 lb), and the incidence diminishes in direct relationship to increasing birth weight. During fetal life the ductus remains patent through the vasodilatory action of prostaglandin, which is produced by the placenta and circulated to the fetus. Postnatally the increase in oxygen tension has a constricting effect on the ductus, but it may reopen in preterm infants in response to the lowered oxygen tension associated with respiratory impairment.

Lack of ductal smooth muscle in preterm infants also prolongs patency of the ductus arteriosus. Functional closure occurs usually within 3 to 4 days, but complete anatomic closure with fibrosis and permanent sealing of the lumen may take up to 2 to 3 weeks.

Clinical Manifestations

Signs of PDA may appear within the first week of life. Early signs are increased $Paco_2$, decreased Pao_2, increased Fio_2, increased work of breathing, and recurrent apnea. Other signs include bounding peripheral pulses; wide pulse pressure with decreased diastolic blood pressure; pericardial hyperactivity; cardiomegaly; and a systolic or continuous murmur usually referred to as a "machinery-type" murmur, heard loudest in systole. If the PDA is wide open, a murmur may not be heard. Spontaneous closure usually occurs within 12 weeks, but in infants with severe lung involvement, the left-to-right shunting of blood leads to pulmonary edema and may prevent timely weaning from mechanical ventilation. The diagnosis is confirmed by echocardiography.

Therapeutic Management

Therapy consists of careful fluid regulation; respiratory support; and administration of indomethacin or ibuprofen, which inhibit prostaglandin synthetase inhibitor. However, indomethacin inhibits platelet function and affects renal function in neonates, so close monitoring for bleeding and renal dysfunction is necessary if this drug is used. If a ductus reopens after cessation of therapy, readministration of the medication may produce a favorable response; as many as four doses may be used to accomplish ductal closure. Surgical ligation may be necessary if medical therapy is unsuccessful, since ductal shunting is perceived as an important contributor to respiratory distress and BPD.

Nursing Care Management

Nursing observations are important in the recognition and management of PDA. Assisting in early detection, carefully assessing cardiovascular status, and monitoring for complications after implementation of therapy are nursing responsibilities. Activities related to therapy include collection of specimens for laboratory examination, continued assessment of renal function (adequate urinary output, any abnormal laboratory findings such as blood urea nitrogen and creatinine levels), and observation for any bleeding tendencies (Hematest-positive stools or gastric aspirate, oozing from heel sticks or venipuncture sites, and laboratory evidence of clotting abnormalities).

Postoperative care includes monitoring for pneumothorax or atelectasis on the affected side, assessment for bleeding and signs or symptoms of infection, supportive respiratory care, and pain management. Other nursing observations and management are the same as for the high-risk infant and the infant with congenital heart disease. (See Chapter 34.)

ANEMIA

Preterm infants tend to develop anemia that is more severe and appears earlier than in more mature infants. It may be a result of hemorrhage during pregnancy or labor and delivery (loss of placental integrity, anomalies of the umbilical cord, fetomaternal hemorrhage), hemorrhage during the neonatal period (ICH, visceral trauma), or blood disorders (hemolytic disease, thrombocytopenia). Anemia may also be iatrogenic from blood withdrawn in the NICU for laboratory tests. Physiologic characteristics of prematurity tend to contribute to the development of anemia (i.e., a decreased red blood cell mass at birth, a drop in the production of hemoglobin, and shortened survival time of red blood cells). This lag in hematopoiesis during continued growth results in physiologic anemia, probably as a consequence of diminished erythropoietin values.

Fortunately, even VLBW infants are able to accommodate the GI absorption of iron required for their high needs. Iron is supplied in iron-fortified formulas or iron supplements as both a preventive and therapeutic measure. Transfusions with packed red blood cells are often required for severe anemia, usually for replacement of blood loss from iatrogenic measures. At 4 to 12 weeks of age, "physiologic anemia" reaches a peak, at which time infants sometimes display signs that suggest true anemia.

Nursing Care Management

One of the most common causes of anemia in acutely ill preterm infants is blood loss associated with frequent sampling for blood gas and metabolic analyses. Therefore an important nursing responsibility is careful monitoring and recording of all blood drawn for tests. It is surprising how easily and rapidly the small total blood volume of preterm infants is depleted by repeated withdrawals. In light of hepatitis and HIV transmission and the potential for other blood-borne pathogens, measures to reduce iatrogenic blood loss and to minimize the need for transfusions of blood products is an important consideration.

Observation for signs of anemia is a vital nursing function. The signs of anemia in the preterm infant are poor feeding, decreased oxygen saturation, systolic murmur, dyspnea, tachycardia, tachypnea, diminished activity, and pallor. However, some infants may not display all these signs. Poor weight gain may be an indication of a lowered hemoglobin level. (Chapter

35 discusses nursing precautions and observations during blood transfusion.)

POLYCYTHEMIA

The current definition of polycythemia is a venous hematocrit of 65% or more (Sarkar and Rosenkrantz, 2008). With a hematocrit above 65%, blood flow becomes increasingly sluggish and hyperviscous, resulting in hypoperfusion of organs. Polycythemia may result from in utero twin-to-twin transfusion and maternal-fetal transfusion, delayed cord clamping or stripping of the umbilical cord, maternal diabetes, or intrapartum asphyxia. The small-for-gestational-age infant is the most at risk for polycythemia; increased red blood cell consumption of glucose further predisposes the infant to hypoglycemia. Infants with polycythemia have a high incidence of cardiopulmonary distress symptoms (PPHN, cyanosis, and apnea), seizures, hyperbilirubinemia, and GI abnormalities.

Appropriate therapy for correcting metabolic disturbances (e.g., hypoxia, hypoglycemia, and hyperbilirubinemia) is implemented. Lowering blood viscosity by partial plasma exchange transfusion may be considered in symptomatic cases.

Nursing Care Management

Nursing care involves watching for signs of polycythemia (e.g., plethora, peripheral cyanosis, respiratory distress, lethargy, jitteriness or seizure activity, hypoglycemia, hyperbilirubinemia) and assisting with diagnostic tests and therapeutic procedures. (Care of the infant with hyperbilirubinemia is discussed in Chapter 9.)

RETINOPATHY OF PREMATURITY

Although often discussed in relation to respiratory dysfunction, retinopathy of prematurity (ROP) is a disorder involving immature retinal vasculature. Formerly known as retrolental fibroplasia, *ROP* is a term used to describe retinal changes observed in preterm infants. The incidence and severity of the disease correlates with the degree of the infant's maturity—the younger the gestational age, the greater the likelihood of the development of ROP, with extremely preterm infants being the group most at risk. However, cases have been documented of ROP in full-term infants who received no oxygen therapy (Korones, 2003).

In addition to immaturity, numerous factors have been implicated in the etiology of ROP, including hyperoxemia and hypoxemia, hypercarbia and hypocarbia, PDA, apnea, intralipid administration, IVH, infection, vitamin E and A deficiency, prenatal infection, exposure to light, and genetic factors (Askin and Diehl-Jones, 2009b). Previously considered an iatrogenic disease related to hyperoxia, ROP is now believed to be a complex disease of prematurity with multiple causes and therefore difficult to completely prevent.

Pathophysiology

Severe vascular constriction in the immature retinal vasculature, followed by hypoxia in those areas, is characteristic of ROP. This appears to stimulate vascular proliferation of retinal capillaries into the hypoxic areas, where veins become

BOX 10-10   STAGES OF RETINOPATHY OF PREMATURITY

1. A demarcation line (separates the avascular retina anteriorly from the vascularized retina posteriorly)
2. A ridge (formed from the demarcation line with the height and width, occupies volume, and extends beyond the plane of the retina)
3. A ridge with extraretinal fibrovascular proliferation
4. Partial retinal detachment
5. Total retinal detachment

"Plus" disease—increased dilation and tortuosity of peripheral retinal vessels (e.g., stage 2 plus retinopathy of prematurity)

Data from International Committee for the Classification of Retinopathy of Prematurity: The international classification of retinopathy of prematurity revisited, *Arch Ophthalmol* 123(7):991-999, 2005.

numerous and dilate. As new vessels multiply toward the lens, the aqueous humor and vitreous humor become turbid. The retina becomes edematous, and hemorrhages and scarring occurs, which separates the retina from its attachment. This extensive retinal detachment and scarring result in irreversible blindness.

Diagnostic Evaluation

A system of classification has been established to describe the location and extent of the developing vasculature involved (International Committee for the Classification of Retinopathy of Prematurity, 2005). Normal vascular growth proceeds in an orderly fashion from the optic disc toward the ora serrata, the irregular anterior margin of the retina. Box 10-10 outlines the stages of ROP. ROP is further classified by location of damage in the retina and by the extent of abnormally developing vascularization. U.S. guidelines recommend that all infants with a birth weight of less than 1500 g (3.3 lb) or a gestational age of less than 32 weeks, and selected infants who are believed to be at high risk, undergo ROP screening (American Academy of Pediatrics, American Association for Pediatric Ophthalmology and Strabismus, and American Academy of Ophthalmology, 2006). The frequency of follow-up examination is determined by the ophthalmologist and is outlined in the 2006 recommendations. With increased survival of extremely preterm infants, most authorities agree that the incidence of ROP is not likely to decrease until definitive causative factors are identified.

Therapeutic Management

Studies have demonstrated an association between the development of ROP and high arterial oxygen saturations in ELBW and VLBW infants. Fluctuations in arterial oxygen saturation in the first few weeks of life have also been implicated in the development of ROP. Although there is no consensus on the ideal arterial oxygen saturation in preterm infants—to prevent either hypoxemia or hyperoxemia—evidence is mounting that oxygen saturations of 100% are undesirable and may have a significant role in the development of ROP in preterm infants. Further studies are needed to clarify optimal arterial oxygen saturation (Pollan, 2009). Therefore the management and treatment of ROP are primarily aimed at preventing fluctuations in arterial concentrations of oxygen in preterm neonates. Studies also indicate that decreasing ambient light exposure in preterm

infants did not decrease the incidence of ROP (Phelps and Watts, 2001).

The early recognition of ROP, treatment, and follow-up care are essential components of disease management. Although prevention is the primary goal of therapeutic management, treatment of retinal pathologic conditions is directed toward arresting the proliferation process. Early treatment of high-risk prethreshold ROP significantly reduced unfavorable outcomes when evaluated at a corrected age of 9 months (Jones, MacKinnon, Good, et al, 2005). Cryotherapy ablation of the avascular retina and laser photocoagulation therapy are the most effective treatments for ROP. Laser photocoagulation is reported to be more effective than cryotherapy, and some studies indicate that early laser treatment produces better outcomes (Drenser and Capone, 2008).

Recently there has been increased interest in the administration of an antivascular endothelial growth factor (anti-VEGF) drug bevacizumab, which arrests the proliferation of vessels and prevents retinal detachment commonly seen in ROP. If successful this therapy may preclude the use of laser therapy (Mintz-Hittner and Best, 2009).

Nursing Care Management

The nursing care of extremely preterm infants and those at risk for development of ROP should focus on decreasing or avoiding events known to cause fluctuations in systemic blood pressure and oxygenation. The infant's oxygenation status should be carefully monitored and targeted Spo_2 ranges maintained for each infant. Individualized care of the preterm infant is essential to aid in further decreasing the incidence of ROP.

Intraoperative nursing care for the infant undergoing either cryotherapy or laser surgery involves proper infant identification, stabilization and monitoring of vital signs as required, monitoring of IV therapy, and administration of the necessary medications. Postoperative nursing care also includes monitoring the infant for signs of pain and appropriate pain management as needed. After surgery the infant's eyelids will be edematous and closed; the nurse informs the parents of this preoperatively. Eye medications are administered as needed, and the infant's tolerance of these medications is monitored closely. Most infants are able to bottle- or breast-feed once awake and alert in the postoperative period. When the infant suffers partial or complete visual impairment, the parents need a considerable amount of support and assistance in meeting his or her special developmental needs. (See Chapter 24.)

HIGH RISK RELATED TO NEUROLOGIC DISTURBANCE

Neurologic complications are observed with increased frequency in preterm infants and in infants born after a difficult labor and delivery. A disproportionately high incidence of perinatal encephalopathy and psychomotor delay occurs in the high-risk infant population, especially ELBW and VLBW infants. Preterm infants are also more vulnerable to cerebral insults (e.g., hypoxia) and chemical alterations (e.g., decreased blood glucose). In addition, fragility and increased permeability of capillaries and prolonged prothrombin time predispose the

Animation—Hypoxia

preterm infant's brain to trauma when delicate structures are subjected to increased pressure, such as the forces of labor, high ventilatory pressures, fluid and electrolyte imbalances, sepsis, acidosis, and seizure activity. All these factors contribute to intracranial insults, including traumatic bleeding in the newborn, which consists of four major types: intraventricular, subdural, primary subarachnoid, and intracerebellar.

PERINATAL HYPOXIC-ISCHEMIC BRAIN INJURY

Hypoxic-ischemic brain injury, or hypoxic-ischemic reperfusion injury, is the most common cause of neurologic impairment observed in term and preterm infants. The brain damage usually results from asphyxia before, during, or after delivery. Ischemia and hypoxemia may occur simultaneously, or one may precede the other. The fetal brain is somewhat protected against mild hypoxic events but may be damaged when there is a decrease in cerebral blood flow, systemic blood pressure, and oxygen and nutrients such as glucose. Subsequent reperfusion after the event may further result in bleeding of the fragile capillaries and tissue ischemia.

Hypoxic-ischemic encephalopathy (HIE) is the resultant cellular damage from hypoxic-ischemic injury that causes the clinical manifestations observed in each case. Such clinical manifestations are variable and may be mild, moderate, or severe. In some infants little or no residual damage may be observed. In general, hypoxia that is severe enough to cause HIE will also damage other organs such as the liver, kidneys, myocardium, and GI tract (Verklan, 2009; Hankins, Koen, Gei, et al, 2002). In the preterm infant HIE may occur in conjunction with IVH. As a consequence of prematurity and general organ and system immaturity, the preterm infant may also suffer hypoxic-ischemic brain damage in the neonatal period as a result of altered cerebral blood flow, systemic hypotension, and decreased cellular nutrients (blood glucose and oxygen).

The site of the hypoxic-ischemic injury varies according to the infant's gestational age. In the full-term infant the primary ischemic damage is parasagittal cerebral injury with cortical necrosis (deeper region of the brain). In the preterm infant the primary ischemic lesion is in the white matter near the ventricles, or periventricular, with resultant periventricular leukomalacia (Volpe, 2008).

Clinical Manifestations

The neurologic signs of encephalopathy appear within the first hours after the hypoxic episode, with manifestations of bilateral cerebral dysfunction. The infant may be stuporous or comatose. Seizures begin after 6 to 12 hours in approximately 50% of the infants, and they become more frequent and severe by 12 to 24 hours. Between 24 and 72 hours the level of consciousness may deteriorate, and after 72 hours persistent stupor, abnormal tone (usually hypotonia), and evidence of disturbances of sucking and swallowing may occur. Muscular weakness of the hips and shoulders occurs in full-term infants, and lower limb weakness occurs in preterm infants. Apneic episodes happen in approximately 50% of the affected infants.

Improvement in the neurologic deficiencies is highly variable and difficult to predict. Infants who demonstrate the most rapid initial improvement appear to have the best prognosis. Myocardial failure and acute tubular necrosis are frequent complications. The major long-term sequelae of hypoxic-ischemic injury are cognitive impairment, seizures, and CP.

Therapeutic Management

Treatment involves aggressive resuscitation at birth, supportive care to provide adequate ventilation and avoid aggravating the existing hypoxia, and measures to maintain cerebral perfusion and prevent cerebral edema. Recent research has shown that therapeutic hypothermia provided by either cooling the infant's head or the whole body reduces the severity of the neurologic damage when it is applied in the early stages of injury (first 6 hours after delivery) (Azzopardi, Strohm, Edwards, et al, 2009; Edwards and Azzopardi, 2006; Jacobs, Hunt, Tarnow-Mordi, et al, 2007; Laptook, 2009). Seizures are managed as described on p. 371. However, prevention is the most important therapy, and every effort should be made to recognize high-risk pregnancies, monitor the fetus, and initiate appropriate therapy early.

Nursing Care Management

Nursing care is primarily the same as for any high-risk infant: careful assessment and observation for signs that might indicate cerebral hypoxia or ischemia; monitoring of ventilatory and IV therapy; observation and management of seizures; and general supportive care to infants and parents, including guidelines for management in the event of cognitive impairment. During therapeutic hypothermia, the nurse directs care toward careful regulation of the infant's body temperature according to the parameters in the cooling protocol being used. The protocol also directs the frequency of blood work, vital signs, and other parameters to be monitored such as a continuous brain wave recording. (See Chapter 24.)

INTRAVENTRICULAR HEMORRHAGE

Germinal matrix–intraventricular hemorrhage is known by a variety of terms according to the locus of bleeding: intraventricular hemorrhage, periventricular hemorrhage, and subependymal-intraventricular hemorrhage. Most authorities use the term intraventricular hemorrhage (IVH) to describe this disorder, which is responsible for a significant percentage of seriously ill infants and neonatal mortality. The incidence of IVH ranges from 20% to 25% of VLBW infants (McCrea and Ment, 2008). IVH is extremely common in preterm infants, especially ELBW and VLBW infants less than 32 weeks of gestation; the degree of neonatal immaturity correlates with the incidence of hemorrhage, and subsequent neurologic handicap is not uncommon.

Pathophysiology

During the early months of prenatal development an extensive but fragile vascular network in the region of the ventricles receives a disproportionately large amount of cerebral blood flow. Blood is directed to the germinal matrix located in the periventricular region near the caudate nuclei of the cerebrum. Therefore preterm infants are subject to bleeding in this heavily vascularized region, especially during events that are likely to cause fluctuations in cerebral blood flow, such as hypoxic

TABLE 10-9	SEVERITY OF GERMINAL MATRIX—INTRAVENTRICULAR HEMORRHAGE
GRADE	**EXTENT OF HEMORRHAGE**
I	Germinal matrix hemorrhage with minimum to no IVH; <10% of the ventricle
II	IVH in roughly 10%-50% of ventricle
III	IVH with lateral ventricular distention; >50% of ventricle
III+*	IVH and periventricular hemorrhage

Data modified from Volpe JJ: *Neurology of the newborn*, ed 4, Philadelphia, 2008, Saunders.
IVH, Intraventricular hemorrhage.
*Another classification system considers this a grade IV involving parenchymal hemorrhage (Adams-Chapman and Stoll, 2007).

episodes and the associated increased venous pressure. In IVH the bleeding originates in these capillaries. The blood may rupture through the ependymal lining of the ventricles and fill all or part of the ventricular system. In severe cases the hemorrhage extends into the cerebral parenchyma. Bleeding in the cerebral parenchyma may lead to the development of cystic lesions referred to as periventricular leukomalacia, which is a significant risk factor for CP. Table 10-9 lists the classification of degrees of IVH.

Following bleeding in the ventricle, clots and other debris can obstruct the passages between the ventricles, causing the ventricles to dilate and resulting in the development of hydrocephalus.

Several clinical features are associated with IVH, such as birth asphyxia, early gestational age, LBW, respiratory distress, asynchronous breathing on ventilatory therapy, pneumothorax, low blood glucose, noxious stimulation, hypercarbia, coagulation and platelet disorders, and hypotension. Posthemorrhagic hydrocephalus and damage to the periventricular white matter of the brain (such as in grade III+) are major determinants of associated chronic problems and prognosis.

Clinical Manifestations

Volpe (2008) classifies clinical manifestations of IVH into three categories:

1. **Catastrophic deterioration**—Begins within minutes to hours of the insult with a coma or deep stupor, respiratory abnormalities such as apnea and hypoventilation, fixed pupils, decerebrate posturing, generalized tonic seizures, flaccid quadriparesis, and cardiac arrhythmias
2. **Saltatory deterioration**—More subtle; signs appear over several hours, may stop altogether, then reappear; signs consist of altered level of consciousness, hypotonia, subtle abnormal eye position and movements, decreased spontaneous or abnormal movements and an abnormally tight popliteal angle; respiratory abnormalities observed in some cases
3. **Clinically silent deterioration**—Often overlooked clinically, but a sudden unexplained decrease in hematocrit may be the only clinical sign of IVH

Approximately 50% of all IVHs occur on the first postnatal day of life, 25% on the second, 15% on the third, and 10% on or after the fourth day of life (Volpe, 2008).

Diagnostic Evaluation

When IVH is suspected or the infant is at risk, studies of intracranial structures are performed by ultrasonography, computed tomography (CT), or magnetic resonance imaging (MRI). In many NICUs screening with cranial ultrasonography is performed at the bedside (via the anterior fontanel) within hours of birth if there is suspicion of IVH or within 4 to 7 days for high-risk infants (<32 weeks of gestation). A positron emission tomography scan may also be helpful in identifying cerebral blood flow in and around the site of the hemorrhage.

Therapeutic Management

The treatment of IVH is aimed at prevention, particularly of prematurity and any events that may lead to IVH. The maintenance of adequate oxygenation by decreasing iatrogenic events is the key to keeping ELBW and VLBW infants neurologically intact. A number of factors associated with prematurity and RDS may predispose the preterm infant to IVH; these factors include acidosis, electrolyte imbalances and rapid fluid shifts (extracellular to intracellular), administration of hyperosmolar solutions (such as sodium bicarbonate), and hypotension followed by rapid volume expansion. Medical treatment aimed at preventing IVH with vitamin E, maternal vitamin K, pancuronium (to decrease blood pressure fluctuations), ibuprofen, phenobarbital, ethamsylate, magnesium sulfate, indomethacin, and surfactant (for RDS) has met with varying degrees of success. Antenatal betamethasone administration has played a significant role in the reduction of IVH in preterm infants (Volpe, 2008).

In the event of IVH, treatment is both preventive and supportive; prompt detection by clinical signs or periodic ultrasonography is a key element in implementing strategies to prevent further damage. Posthemorrhagic hydrocephalus is a common occurrence within 1 month of the event. Serial lumbar punctures may be used to decrease the amount of CSF and thus decrease ventricular size. A closed reservoir may be attached to an intraventricular shunt, with the reservoir tapped or drained intermittently to relieve pressure on the ventricles. Ventricular dilation (grade III to grade III+) may be managed with shunting (ventriculoperitoneal or subgaleal) or a temporary external ventricular drainage.

The long-term outcome of IVH is variable and unpredictable and is influenced by the size of the hemorrhage and the extent of parenchymal involvement. Infants with small lesions have an excellent prognosis for neurologic outcome (Hill, 2005).

Nursing Care Management

In addition to routine observations and management, the nurse also directs care toward prevention of fluctuations in cerebral blood flow. It has been observed that some nursing procedures increase intracranial pressure. For example, blood pressure increases significantly during ET suctioning in preterm infants, and head positioning produces measurable changes in intracranial pressure. Researchers have found that intracranial pressure is highest when infants are in the dependent position and decreases when the head is in a midline position and elevated 30 degrees.

Cerebral pressure is lower when infants are in a midline position as opposed to a right side-lying position. When the head is turned to the right without body alignment, the resulting venous congestion creates hydrostatic pressure fluctuations that increase intracranial pressure. Infants encumbered with tubes and monitoring equipment are more difficult to turn while maintaining head-body alignment.

Other interventions that may reduce the risk of increased intracranial pressure include avoiding interventions that cause crying (such as painful procedures). Crying (which essentially creates a Valsalva effect) can impede venous return, increase cerebral blood volume, and compromise cerebral oxygenation in LBW infants. Avoid rapid volume expansion following hypotension (primarily in preterms) and administration of hyperosmolar solutions such as sodium bicarbonate. Because air leaks such as pneumothorax produce variable cerebral blood flow, rapid detection and intervention are a key component of nursing care of the high-risk infant. Monitoring serum blood glucose levels and preventing hypoglycemia are also important factors in keeping the infant neurologically intact. Many units practice minimum handling of infants at high risk to avoid fluctuations in cerebral blood flow. In addition, research has implicated noxious external stimuli (e.g., pain and noise) as having a potential role in stimulation that may lead to IVH. Care includes evaluating manipulations and handling and administering analgesics to reduce discomfort.

INTRACRANIAL HEMORRHAGE

ICH in neonates, although manifested in the same ways as those described in older children, occurs with different frequencies and different degrees of severity.

Subdural Hemorrhage

A subdural hematoma is a life-threatening collection of blood in the subdural space. The stretching and tearing of the large veins in the tentorium cerebelli, the dural membrane that separates the cerebrum from the cerebellum, is the most common cause. With improved obstetric care this condition has become relatively uncommon; however, it is especially serious because of the inaccessibility of the hematoma to aspiration by subdural tap. Less commonly, hemorrhage occurs when veins in the subdural space over the surface of the brain are torn. (See Head Injury, Chapter 37.)

Subarachnoid Hemorrhage

Subarachnoid hemorrhage, the most common type of ICH, occurs in full-term infants as a result of trauma and in preterm infants as a result of the same types of events that cause IVH. Small hemorrhages are the most common. Bleeding is of venous origin, and underlying contusion may also occur.

Intracerebellar Hemorrhage

Intracerebellar hemorrhage is a common finding on postmortem examination of the preterm infant and can be a primary hemorrhage in the cerebellum associated with skull compression during abrupt, precipitous delivery, or it may occur secondary to extravasation of blood into the cerebellum from a

ventricular hemorrhage. In the full-term infant the bleeding may follow a difficult delivery.

Nursing Care Management

Nursing care is the same as care of the infant with IVH or with perinatal hypoxic-ischemic brain injury.

NEONATAL/PERINATAL STROKE

Neonatal stroke is reported to occur in 1 in 4000 live term births (Nelson and Lynch, 2004). Neonatal stroke has been defined to encompass all ischemic and hemorrhagic events that affect the venous and arterial distribution of blood supply from early gestation to the first 28 days of life (Golomb, Cvijanovich, and Ferriero, 2006). Perinatal stroke refers to strokes that occur between 28 weeks of gestation and the first 7 days of life, primarily as a result of altered arterial blood flow and ischemia (Nelson and Lynch, 2004). Fetal stroke may occur as early as 8 weeks' gestation (Kirton and deVeber, 2009).

Neonatal stroke is the second leading cause of seizures in term neonates and may be caused by arterial, thrombotic, or ischemic events that result in altered brain blood flow and infarction. Neonatal stroke is more predominant in males, and there is an increased tendency toward left-sided involvement. Known risk factors for neonatal and perinatal stroke include the presence of maternal and/or fetal factor V Leiden, antiphospholipid, and prothrombin factors (Curry, Bhullar, Holmes, et al, 2007; Simchen, Goldstein, Lubetsky, et al, 2009). Cerebral palsy, motor deficits, epilepsy, and language deficits, and visual deficits may occur as a result of neonatal stroke (Kirton and deVeber, 2009).

Diagnosis with MRI and venography is most accurate because head ultrasonography may be negative with an ischemic event; the electroencephalogram may be normal (Golomb, Cvijanovich, and Ferriero, 2006).

Because neonatal stroke can only be diagnosed retrospectively, it is important for the nurse to be vigilant for apnea or seizure activity in the first year of life, the time when clinical manifestations will appear.

NEONATAL SEIZURES

Seizures in the neonatal period are usually the clinical manifestation of a serious underlying disease. The most common cause of seizures in the neonatal period (for term and preterm infants) is HIE secondary to perinatal asphyxia (Volpe, 2008). Although not life threatening as an isolated entity, seizures constitute a medical emergency because they signal a disease process that may produce irreversible brain damage. Consequently, it is imperative to recognize a seizure and its significance so that the cause, as well as the seizure, can be treated (Box 10-11).

Pathophysiology

The features of neonatal seizures are different from those observed in the older infant or child. For example, the well-organized, generalized tonic-clonic seizures seen in older children are rare in infants, especially preterm infants. The newborn brain, with its immature anatomic and physiologic status and reduced cortical organization, is developmentally insufficient to

BOX 10-11   CAUSES OF NEONATAL SEIZURES

Metabolic
Hypoglycemia, hyperglycemia
Hypernatremia, hyponatremia
Hypocalcemia
Hypomagnesemia
Pyridoxine deficiency
Aminoacidurias (e.g., phenylketonuria, maple syrup urine disease)
Hyperammonemia

Toxic
Uremia
Bilirubin encephalopathy (kernicterus)

Prenatal Infections
Toxoplasmosis
Syphilis
Cytomegalovirus
Herpes simplex
Hepatitis

Postnatal Infections
Bacterial meningitis
Viral meningoencephalitis
Sepsis
Brain abscess

Trauma at Birth
Hypoxic brain injury
Intracranial hemorrhage
Subarachnoid, subdural hemorrhage
Intraventricular hemorrhage

Malformations
Central nervous system agenesis
Hydranencephaly
Panencephaly
Tuberous sclerosis

Miscellaneous
Degenerative disease
Benign familial neonatal seizures
Narcotic withdrawal
Stroke (fetal, perinatal, or neonatal)

TABLE 10-10   CLASSIFICATIONS OF NEONATAL SEIZURES

TYPE	CHARACTERISTICS
Clonic	Slow, rhythmic jerking movements
	Approximately 1-3/sec
Focal	Involves face, upper or lower extremities on one side of body
	May involve neck or trunk
	Infant is conscious during event
Multifocal	May migrate randomly from one part of the body to another
	Movements may start at different times
Tonic	Extension, stiffening movements
Generalized	Extension of all four limbs (similar to decerebrate rigidity)
	Upper limbs maintained in a stiffly flexed position (resembles decorticate rigidity)
Focal	Sustained posturing of a limb
	Asymmetric posturing of trunk or neck
Subtle	May develop in either full-term or preterm infants but more common in preterm
	Often overlooked by inexperienced observers
	Signs:
	• Horizontal eye deviation
	• Repetitive blinking or fluttering of the eyelids, staring
	• Sucking or other oral-buccal-lingual movements
	• Arm movements that resemble rowing or swimming
	• Leg movements described as pedaling or bicycling
	• Apnea (common)
	Signs may appear alone or in combination
Myoclonic	Rapid jerks that involve flexor muscle groups
Focal	Involves upper extremity flexor muscle group
	No electroencephalogram (EEG) discharges observed
Multifocal	Asynchronous twitching of several parts of the body
	No associated EEG discharges observed
Generalized	Bilateral jerks of upper and lower limbs
	Associated with EEG discharges

Adapted from Volpe J: Neonatal seizures. In Volpe J: *Neurology of the newborn*, ed 4, Philadelphia, 2008, Saunders.

allow ready development and maintenance of a generalized seizure. The advanced degree of development of limbic structures with connections to the diencephalon and brainstem probably accounts for the higher frequency of seizure manifestations (such as oral movements, oculomotor deviations, and apnea) that originate in these structures.

Clinical Manifestations

Seizures in newborns may be subtle and barely discernible or grossly apparent. Because most neonatal seizures are subcortical, they do not have the etiologic and prognostic significance of seizures in children. The type of seizure is seldom important because one may produce any of a variety of manifestations. Neonatal seizures can be divided into four major types: clonic, tonic, myoclonic, and subtle seizures. Table 10-10 lists these classifications in order of frequency (Volpe, 2008). Clonic, multifocal clonic, and migratory clonic seizures are more common in full-term infants.

Jitteriness or tremulousness in the newborn is a repetitive shaking of an extremity or extremities that may be observed with crying, may occur with changes in sleeping state, or may be elicited with stimulation. Jitteriness is relatively common in newborns, and in a mild degree may be considered normal during the first 4 days of life. Jitteriness can be distinguished from seizures by several characteristics: jitteriness is not accompanied by ocular movement as are seizures; the dominant movement in jitteriness is tremor, whereas seizure movement is clonic jerking that cannot be stopped by flexion of the affected limb; and jitteriness is highly sensitive to stimulation, whereas seizures are not. Further evaluation is indicated if jittery movements persist beyond the fourth day, if the movements are persistent and prolonged after a stimulus, or if they are easily elicited with minimum stimulus.

A **tremor** is repetitive movements of both hands (with or without movement of legs or jaws) at a frequency of two to five per second and lasting more than 10 minutes. It is common in newborn infants and has a variety of causes, including neurologic damage, hypoglycemia, and hypocalcemia. In most instances tremors are of no pathologic significance.

Diagnostic Evaluation

Early evaluation and diagnosis of seizures are urgent. In addition to a careful physical examination, the pregnancy and family histories are investigated for familial and prenatal causes. Blood is drawn for glucose and electrolyte examination, and CSF is obtained for examination for gross blood, cell count, protein, glucose, and culture. Electroencephalography may help identify subtle seizures but is less helpful in establishing a diagnosis. Other diagnostic procedures, such as CT, ultrasonography, and echoencephalography, may be indicated.

Therapeutic Management

Direct treatment toward the prevention of cerebral damage, correction of metabolic derangements, respiratory and cardiovascular support, and suppression of the seizure activity. The underlying cause is treated (e.g., glucose infusion for hypoglycemia, calcium for hypocalcemia, and antibiotics for infection). If needed, respiratory support is provided for hypoxia, and anticonvulsants may be administered, especially when the other measures fail to control the seizures. Phenobarbital is the drug of choice given intravenously or orally and is used if seizures are severe and persistent. Other drugs that may be used are fosphenytoin sodium, phenytoin (Dilantin), and lorazepam.

Nursing Care Management

The major nursing responsibilities in the care of infants with seizures are to recognize when the infant is having a seizure so that therapy can be instituted, to carry out the therapeutic regimen, and to observe the response to the therapy and any further evidence of seizures or other symptomatology. Assessment and other aspects of care are the same as for all high-risk infants. Parents need to be informed of their infant's status, and the nurse should reinforce and clarify the practitioner's explanations. The infant's behaviors need to be interpreted for the parents, and the infant's responses to the treatment must be anticipated and their significance explained. Encourage parents to visit their infant and perform the parenting activities consistent with the care plan. Seizures are frightening phenomena and generate a great deal of anxiety and fear, and the staff's concern, which is justifiable, can heighten that anxiety. Providing support and guidance is an important nursing function.

HIGH RISK RELATED TO MATERNAL CONDITIONS

INFANTS OF DIABETIC MOTHERS

Before insulin therapy, few women with diabetes were able to conceive; for those who did, the mortality rate for both mother and infant was high. The morbidity and mortality of infants of diabetic mothers (IDMs) have been significantly reduced as a result of effective control of maternal diabetes and an increased understanding of fetal disorders. However, the offspring of diabetic mothers are at risk for a large number of congenital anomalies. Central nervous system anomalies such as anencephaly, spina bifida, and holoprosencephaly occur at rates 10 times higher than any other population of mothers (Gabbe, Niebyl, and Simpson, 2007). Cardiac anomalies such as ventriculoseptal defects are increased fivefold in IDMs, and sacral agenesis and caudal regression occur almost exclusively in IDMs (Gabbe, Niebyl, and Simpson, 2007). Because infants born to women with gestational diabetes mellitus are at risk for many of the same complications as IDMs, the following discussion includes both types of infants.

The severity of the maternal diabetes affects infant survival. Several factors determine the severity: duration of the disease before pregnancy; age of onset; extent of vascular complications; and abnormalities of the current pregnancy such as pyelonephritis, diabetic ketoacidosis, pregnancy-induced hypertension, and noncompliance. *The single most important factor influencing fetal well-being is the mother's normoglycemic status.* Reasonable metabolic control that begins before conception and continues during the first weeks of pregnancy can prevent malformation in an IDM. Elevated levels of hemoglobin A_{1c} during the first trimester appear to be associated with a higher incidence of congenital malformations.

Effects of Diabetes on the Fetus

Hypoglycemia may appear a short time after birth and in IDMs is associated with increased insulin activity in the blood. A standardized definition for neonatal hypoglycemia remains elusive and controversial. At best, authorities agree that reliance on a single numeric value for every clinical situation is inadequate (see Therapeutic Management section). Hypoglycemia in the IDM is related to hypertrophy and hyperplasia of the pancreatic islet cells, causing a transient state of hyperinsulinism.

High maternal blood glucose levels during fetal life provide a continuous stimulus to the fetal islet cells for insulin production. This sustained hyperglycemia promotes fetal insulin secretion that ultimately leads to excessive growth and deposition of fat, which probably accounts for the infants who are large for gestational age, or macrosomic. When the neonate's glucose supply is removed abruptly at the time of birth, the continued production of insulin soon depletes the blood of circulating glucose, creating a state of hyperinsulinism and hypoglycemia within $1\frac{1}{2}$ to 4 hours, especially in infants of mothers with poorly controlled diabetes. Precipitous drops in blood glucose levels can cause serious neurologic damage or death. The birth defects observed in IDMs are thought to occur as a result of multifactorial teratogenic factors, rather than hyperglycemia alone (Leguizamon, Igarzabal and Reece, 2007).

Clinical Manifestations

IDMs have a characteristic appearance. They are usually macrosomic for their gestational age, very plump and full faced, liberally coated with vernix caseosa, and plethoric. The placenta and umbilical cord are also larger than average. However, infants of mothers with advanced diabetes may be small for gestational age, have IUGR, or be appropriate for gestational age because of the maternal vascular (placental) involvement. IDMs have an increased incidence of hypoglycemia, hypocalcemia, hyperbilirubinemia, hypomagnesemia, and RDS. Hyperglycemia in the diabetic mother and subsequent fetal hyperinsulinemia may be a factor in reducing fetal surfactant synthesis, thus contributing to the development of RDS.

Morbidities in IDMs are the result of exposure to elevated glucose and ketone levels, placental insufficiency, and prematurity. Although large, these infants may be delivered before term because of maternal complications or increased fetal size.

Therapeutic Management

The most effective management of IDMs is careful monitoring of serum glucose levels and observation for accompanying complications such as RDS. Examine these infants for any anomalies or birth injuries, and regularly obtain blood studies for determinations of glucose, calcium, hematocrit, and bilirubin. A common definition of hypoglycemia has not been established. Several authors have suggested the use of operational thresholds at which hypoglycemia should be closely monitored and treated. The researchers recommend close observation in infants with known risk factors such as maternal diabetes and close observation if plasma glucose values are below 45 mg/dl (2.5 mmol/L) (Cornblath, Hawdon, Williams, et al, 2000; Canadian Paediatric Society, 2004; Deshpande and Ward Platt, 2005). If a feeding fails to increase the glucose levels in such cases or if abnormal signs develop, IV glucose should be administered to maintain glucose levels above 45 mg/dl (2.5 mmol/L). A newborn with levels at or below 30 mg/dl should receive IV glucose. Cornblath, Hawdon, Williams, and colleagues (2000) further recommend that therapeutic glucose levels be kept at or above 60 mg/dl (3.3 mmol/L) in neonates with profound, recurrent, or persistent hyperinsulinemic hypoglycemia. Studies confirm the importance of maintaining serum glucose levels above 50 mg/dl (2.8 mmol/L) in hyperinsulinemic infants with hypoglycemia to prevent serious neurologic sequelae (Cowett and Loughead, 2002; Deshpande and Ward Platt, 2005).

Because the hypertrophied pancreas is so sensitive to blood glucose concentrations, the administration of oral glucose may trigger a massive insulin release, resulting in rebound hypoglycemia. Therefore feedings of breast milk or formula begin within the first hour after birth provided that the infant's cardiorespiratory condition is stable. Approximately half of IDMs do well and adjust without complications. Infants born to mothers with uncontrolled diabetes may require IV infusion of dextrose. Oral and IV intake may be titrated to maintain adequate blood glucose levels. Frequent blood glucose determinations are needed for the first 2 days of life to assess the degree of hypoglycemia present at any given time. Testing blood taken from the heel with point-of-care portable reflectance meters (glucometer) is a simple and effective screening evaluation that can then be confirmed by laboratory examination.

Nursing Care Management

The nursing care of IDMs involves early examination for congenital anomalies and signs of possible respiratory or cardiac problems, maintenance of adequate thermoregulation, early introduction of carbohydrate feedings as appropriate, and monitoring of serum blood glucose levels. The latter is of particular importance because many hypoglycemic infants may remain asymptomatic. IV glucose infusion requires careful monitoring of the site and the neonate's reaction to therapy; high glucose concentrations (>12.5%) should be infused via a central line instead of a peripheral one. Because macrosomic infants are at risk for problems associated with a difficult delivery, they are monitored for birth injuries such as brachial plexus injury and palsy, fractured clavicle, and phrenic nerve palsy. Additional monitoring of the infant for associated problems (RDS, polycythemia, hypocalcemia, poor feeding, and hyperbilirubinemia) is also a vital nursing function.

There is evidence that IDMs have an increased risk of acquiring metabolic syndrome (obesity, hypertension, dyslipidemia, and glucose intolerance) in childhood or early adulthood; therefore nursing care of IDMs should also focus on healthy lifestyle and prevention later in life (Boney, Verma, Tucker, et al, 2005).

DRUG-EXPOSED INFANTS*

Overview

In the 2002 to 2003 National Survey on Drug Use and Health, 4.3% of pregnant women ages 15 to 44 years reported illicit drug use within the past month (Substance Abuse and Mental Health Services Administration, 2005). Given the self-reporting nature of survey data, it is likely that this number is considerably lower than the actual number of substance-using pregnant women. Determining the effects of intrauterine drug and alcohol exposure is difficult for a variety of reasons. Many substance-using women ingest multiple drugs or a combination of drugs and alcohol, and some women who use drugs or alcohol may be undernourished or suffer from chronic medical conditions. Some may not seek prenatal care; for others, the drugs used may be cut with a variety of materials, and the strength, dose, and duration of exposure are likely to be unknown (Schempf, 2007).

Clinical Manifestations

Most infants of drug-dependent mothers appear normal at birth but may begin to exhibit signs of drug withdrawal within 12 to 24 hours, depending on the substance and the mother's pattern of use. If mothers have been taking methadone, the signs appear somewhat later—anywhere from 1 or 2 days to 2 to 3 weeks or more after birth. The clinical manifestations of withdrawal may fall into one or all of the following categories: CNS, GI, respiratory, and autonomic nervous system signs (Kuschel, 2007). The manifestations become most pronounced between 48 and 72 hours of age and may last from 6 days to 8 weeks (Box 10-12).

In a study of polydrug use during pregnancy the most prominent signs of withdrawal were increased tone, increased respiratory rate, disturbed sleep, fever, excessive sucking, and loose watery stools. Other signs observed included projectile vomiting, mottling, crying, nasal stuffiness, hyperactive Moro reflex,

---

*It is important to note that the term *addiction* is often associated with behaviors whereby the person seeks the drug to experience a high or euphoria, escape from reality, or satisfy a personal need. Newborns are not addicted in a behavioral sense, yet they may experience mild to strong physiologic signs as a result of the mother's drug use. Therefore to say that an infant born to a mother who uses substances is addicted is incorrect; *drug-exposed newborn* is a better term, which implies intrauterine drug exposure.

BOX 10-12 SIGNS OF WITHDRAWAL IN THE NEONATE

- Irritability
- Tachypnea (>60 beats/min)
- Tremors
- Excoriations (knees, face)
- Shrill cry
- Mottling (skin)
- Hypertonicity of muscles
- Sneezing
- Frantic sucking of hands
- Yawning
- Poor feeding
- Vomiting, often projectile
- Hyperactivity
- Temperature instability
- Perspiring
- Loose diarrheal stools
- Fever
- Seizures
- Nasal stuffiness
- Sleep disturbances

and tremors (D'Apolito and Hepworth, 2001). Although these infants suck avidly on fists and display an exaggerated rooting reflex, they are poor feeders with uncoordinated and ineffectual sucking and swallowing reflexes.

One observation in a large percentage of these infants is generalized perspiring, which is unusual in newborn infants. It is significant that, although drug-exposed infants may have some tachypnea, cyanosis, or apnea, they rarely develop RDS when born near term. Apparently, narcotics or stress factors in the intrauterine environment cause accelerated lung maturation even with a high incidence of prematurity.

Not all infants of narcotic-addicted mothers show signs of withdrawal. Because of irregular and varying degrees of drug use, quality of drug, and mixed drug usage by the mother, some infants display mild or variable manifestations. Most manifestations are the vague, nonspecific signs characteristic of infants in general; therefore it is important to differentiate between drug withdrawal and other disorders before instituting specific therapy. Other states (e.g., hypocalcemia, hypoglycemia, or sepsis) often coexist with the drug withdrawal.

A concern regarding substance abuse is that many of the mothers often use several drugs, such as tranquilizers, nicotine, sedatives, narcotics, amphetamines, phencyclidine (PCP), marijuana, and other psychotropic agents. Of increasing concern in the United States is the number of newborns who are exposed to methamphetamines and selective serotonin reuptake inhibitors in utero.

Therapeutic Management

The treatment of the drug-exposed infant initially consists of modulating the environment to decrease external stimuli. Drug therapies to decrease withdrawal side effects are implemented once **neonatal abstinence syndrome (NAS)** is identified.

Nursing Care Management

When possible, alert the nursery personnel to the likelihood of a drug-exposed infant requiring admittance. If the mother has had good prenatal care, the practitioner is aware of the problem and substance abuse treatment may have been instituted before delivery. However, a number of mothers deliver their infants without the benefit of adequate care, and the addiction is unknown to health care personnel at the time of delivery. The degree of narcosis or withdrawal is closely related to the amount of drug the mother has habitually taken, the length of time she has been taking the drug, and her drug level at the time of delivery. The most severe symptoms occur in the infants of mothers who have taken large amounts of drugs over a long period. In addition, the nearer to the time of delivery that the mother takes the drug, the longer it takes the child to develop withdrawal, and the more severe the manifestations. The infant may not exhibit withdrawal symptoms until 7 to 10 days after delivery.

Once the presence of NAS is identified in an infant, direct nursing care toward reducing external stimuli that might trigger hyperactivity and irritability (e.g., dimming the lights and decreasing noise levels), providing adequate nutrition and hydration, and promoting positive and nurturing maternal-infant relationships. Providing care on demand rather than on a fixed schedule may help reduce irritability for infants. Appropriate individualized developmental care is implemented, such as care with preterm infants to facilitate self-consoling and self-regulating behaviors (see Table 10-5). Some irritable and hyperactive infants respond to comforting, movement, containment, and close contact. Wrapping infants snugly and rocking and holding them tightly limit their ability to self-stimulate. The infant's arms should remain flexed with hands close to the mouth for sucking as appropriate; sucking on fingers or hands is a form of self-control and comfort. Arranging nursing activities to reduce disturbances helps decrease exogenous stimulation.

The Neonatal Abstinence Scoring System has been developed to monitor infants in an objective manner and evaluate the infant's response to clinical and pharmacologic interventions (Finnegan, 1985). This system also assists nurses and other health care workers in evaluating the severity of the infant's withdrawal symptoms.

Another scoring tool has been recently developed specifically aimed at measuring neurologic behavior and resultant effects on the neonate when substances are used during pregnancy. The NICU Network Neurobehavioral Scale, developed by the National Institutes of Health, provides an assessment of neurologic, behavioral, and stress-abstinence function in the neonate. The test combines items from other tests such as the Neonatal Behavioral Assessment Scale (NBAS); stress-abstinence items developed by Finnegan (1985); and a complete neurologic examination, which includes primitive reflexes and active and passive tone (Law, Stroud, LaGasse, et al, 2003).

Loose stools and poor intake and regurgitation after feeding predispose the infants to malnutrition, dehydration, and electrolyte imbalance. An oral opioid such as morphine may be administered to control loose watery stools (D'Apolito and Hepworth, 2001). It takes considerable time and patience to ensure that these infants receive a sufficient caloric and fluid intake.

Monitoring and recording the activity level and its relationship to other activities, such as feeding and preventing complications, are important nursing functions.

A valuable aid to anticipating problems in the newborn is recognizing drug abuse in the mother. Unless the mother is enrolled in a methadone rehabilitation program, she seldom risks calling attention to her habit by seeking prenatal care. Consequently, infants and mothers are exposed to the additional hazards of obstetric and medical complications resulting from the lack of adequate prenatal care. Moreover, the nature of heroin addiction makes the user susceptible to disorders such as infection (hepatitis B and HIV related to IV needle use), foreign body reaction, and the hazards of inadequate nutrition and preterm birth. Methadone treatment does not prevent withdrawal reaction in neonates, but the clinical course may be modified. Also, intensive psychologic support of mothers is a factor in the treatment and reduction of perinatal mortality. Experience has indicated that mothers are usually anxious and depressed, lack confidence, have poor self-image, and have difficulty with interpersonal relationships. They may have a psychologic need for the pregnancy and an infant.

Initial symptoms or the recurrence of withdrawal symptoms may develop after discharge from the hospital. Therefore it is important to establish rapport and maintain contact with the family so that they return for treatment if this occurs. The demands of the drug-exposed infant on the caregiver are enormous and unrewarding in terms of positive feedback. The infants are difficult to comfort, and they cry for long periods, which can be especially trying for the caregiver after the infant's discharge from the hospital. Long-term follow-up to evaluate the status of the infant and family is important.

An important aspect of nursing care is identification of an infant who was exposed to drugs in utero. Observation of signs mentioned previously may warrant further investigation so prompt treatment can be implemented. Newborn urine, rarely hair, or meconium sampling may be required to identify drug exposure and implement appropriate early interventional therapies aimed at minimizing the consequences of intrauterine drug exposure. Meconium sampling for fetal drug exposure provides more screening accuracy than urine, since drug metabolites accumulate in meconium (Kuschel, 2007). Urine toxicology screening has less accuracy because it only reflects recent substance intake by the mother (Huestis and Choo, 2002). Meconium testing for drug metabolites has the advantage of being easy to collect, noninvasive, and more accurate.

Pharmacologic treatment is usually based on the severity of withdrawal symptoms, as determined by an assessment tool. Drug therapies to decrease withdrawal side effects include administration of phenobarbital, morphine, diluted tincture of opium, methadone (Coyle, Ferguson, Lagasse, et al, 2002; Johnson, Gerada, and Greenough, 2003) buprenorphine (Kraft, Gibson, Dysart, et al, 2008), or clonidine (Agthe, Kim, Mathias, et al, 2009). A combination of these drugs may be necessary to treat infants exposed to multiple drugs in utero, and careful attention should be given to possible adverse effects of the treatment drugs (Johnson, Gerada, and Greenough, 2003).

Many problems relate to the disposition of infants of drug-dependent mothers. Those who advocate separation of mothers and children argue that the mothers are not capable of assuming responsibility for their infant's care, that child care is frustrating to them, and that their existence is too disorganized and chaotic. Others encourage the maternal-infant bond and recommend a protected environment such as a therapeutic community; a halfway house; or continuous ongoing, supportive services in the home after discharge. Careful evaluation and the cooperative efforts of a variety of health professionals are required, whether the choice is foster home placement or supportive follow-up care of mothers who keep their infants.

Opiate Exposure

Narcotics, which have a low molecular weight, readily cross the placental membrane and enter the fetal system. When the mother is a habitual user of narcotics, especially heroin or methadone, the unborn child may also become passively physiologically addicted to the drug, which places the infant at risk during the early neonatal period. NAS is the term used by many to describe the set of behaviors exhibited by the infant exposed to chemical substances in utero.

Prescription opioids such as oxycodone (Percodan) have been identified as increasingly popular drugs of abuse, which may cause withdrawal symptoms in neonates (Rao and Desai, 2002). Other chemical substances that may cause neonatal withdrawal include methadone, caffeine, and PCP.

Methadone Exposure

Methadone, a synthetic opiate, has been the therapy of choice for heroin addiction since 1965. Methadone crosses the placenta. An increasing number of infants have been born to methadone-maintained mothers, who seem to have better prenatal care and a somewhat better lifestyle than those taking heroin.

Some question exists concerning the benefits of methadone therapy during pregnancy because of its effect on the fetus. Methadone withdrawal resembles heroin withdrawal but tends to be more severe and prolonged. Signs of methadone withdrawal include tremors, irritability, state lability, hypertonicity, hypersensitivity, vomiting, mottling, and nasal stuffiness (Jansson, Velez, and Harrow, 2004). These infants exhibit a disturbed sleep pattern similar to that seen in heroin withdrawal. They have a higher birth weight than those infants in heroin withdrawal, usually appropriate for gestational age. No increased incidence of congenital anomalies is seen. The American Academy of Pediatrics, Committee on Drugs (2001), has revised its statement regarding breast-feeding for mothers who are in a methadone treatment program, suggesting such mothers be allowed to breast-feed regardless of the methadone dosage; follow-up counseling and monitoring of the mother and infant are recommended.

Late-onset withdrawal occurs at age 2 to 4 weeks and may continue for weeks or months. A higher incidence of SIDS also has been reported in these infants (Wagner, Katikaneni, Cox, et al, 1998). This factor is important for perinatal nurses who coordinate follow-up care for the infant and education for the mother or other caregiver. Community health nurses must know about the potential for withdrawal symptoms to occur.

Therapy for methadone withdrawal is similar to that for heroin withdrawal. The few available follow-up studies of these infants reveal a high incidence of hyperactivity, learning and behavior disorders, and poor social adjustment.

Cocaine Exposure

Cocaine, a commonly used illicit drug in the United States, has multiple modes of use. However, use of the relatively inexpensive and easily administered "crack" form increased significantly among pregnant women and women of childbearing age in the 1990s (Askin and Diehl-Jones, 2001; Eyler, Behnke, and Conlon, 1998). Because crack vaporizes at relatively low temperatures, it is smoked and absorbed in large quantities through pulmonary vasculature. The drug readily enters the placenta, placing the fetus at risk (Malanga and Kosofsky, 1999).

Cocaine is a CNS stimulant and peripheral sympathomimetic, and the effects on the fetus may be direct or indirect. Indirect effects include fetal hypoxemia secondary to impaired uterine blood flow. Cocaine also appears to affect fetal cardiac function and suppress the fetal immune system. The difficulties encountered by cocaine-exposed infants are compounded when the mother takes the drug in conjunction with other illicit drugs (Askin and Diehl-Jones, 2001). Studies have found that women who use cocaine in pregnancy are less likely to have adequate prenatal care, are more likely to smoke tobacco and consume alcohol, are more likely to be malnourished, and are more likely to have sexually transmitted infections than nonusers (Tronick and Beeghly, 1999). These variables compound the problem of drug exposure and effects on the fetus.

Clinical Manifestations

Infants who are exposed to cocaine in utero may demonstrate no immediate untoward effects. Previous reports of catastrophic neurologic effects have been published, yet the findings have considerable variability because of poor reliability of maternal history, maternal polydrug use, prematurity, poor social environment, and poor specificity in detecting cocaine exposure. A large meta-analysis of 15,208 pregnancies did not find an association between illicit drug use and congenital anomalies (van Gelder, Reefhuis, Caton, et al, 2009). It may be, however, that habitual cocaine use in pregnancy has negative effects that are too subtle to notice in the newborn and infancy period (Askin and Diehl-Jones, 2001).

Clinical manifestations of intrauterine cocaine exposure include IUGR, decreased head circumference, association with preterm delivery, NEC, cerebral infarcts, respiratory disturbances such as apnea, cardiac arrhythmias, transient electroencephalogram abnormalities, and IVH (Askin and Diehl-Jones, 2001; Chiriboga, Brust, Bateman, et al, 1999). Other findings related to neurobehavioral effects include sleep disturbances; increased tone; jitteriness; delayed language acquisition; behavior problems in school; poor impulse control; hypertonia; abnormal reflexes; poor NBAS scores; significant cognitive delays in the first 2 years; and poor responses to auditory, arousal, and visual stimuli (Chiriboga, Kuhn, and Wasserman, 2007; Chiriboga, Brust, Bateman, et al, 1999; Delaney-Black, Covington, Templin, et al, 1998; Eyler, Behnke, and Conlon, 1998; Schuler and Nair, 1999; Singer, Minnes, Short, et al, 2004; Levine, Liu, Das, et al, 2008). Environmental and sociodemo-

graphic factors likely play an important role in the outcome of children exposed to cocaine in utero.

Therapeutic Management

Infants exposed to cocaine alone are less likely than other drug-exposed infants to demonstrate signs of withdrawal. Regardless of the type of drug or substance to which the newborn was exposed, treatment begins with prompt identification of a potential problem by obtaining a comprehensive maternal history, identifying potential risks associated with exposure, and maintaining a safe environment. Newborn urine, hair (rarely), or meconium sampling may be required to identify intrauterine drug exposure and implement appropriate early interventional therapies aimed at minimizing the consequences.

Nursing Care Management

Nursing care of cocaine-exposed infants is similar to that of infants exposed to other drugs. Individualized assessment help determine appropriate intervention strategies. If the nurse identifies hypertonicity and sleep disturbance, the environment is modified accordingly to decrease noxious stimuli. The use of swaddling, containment, gentle rocking, NNS, and undisturbed periods of rest may help promote self-containment and state regulation. As previously noted, tissue samples may be required for identification of drug exposure. Because cocaine is easily passed in breast milk (Winecker, Goldberger, Tebbett, et al, 2001), mothers should be counseled regarding avoidance of breast-feeding. A fussy newborn may be interpreted by caretakers to be consistently hungry, and thus overfeeding and vomiting may be problematic. Provision of a safe environment in which the mother and newborn may interact is imperative. Opportunities for appropriate family bonding and attachment should be provided as with any other newborn. Because a large percentage of women who use cocaine during pregnancy have sexually transmitted infections, consider viral titers and hepatitis screening for the newborn (Askin and Diehl-Jones, 2001).

Referral to early intervention programs, including child health care, parental drug treatment, individualized developmental care, and parenting education, is essential in promoting optimum outcomes for these children. Children exposed to maternal cocaine use often live in impoverished conditions, putting them at high risk for cognitive delays, poor child health care, and inadequate nutrition; they would benefit from an early intervention program (Tronick and Beeghly, 1999, Singer, Minnes, Short, et al, 2004). Comprehensive health care services for both mother and child may be provided at one location in the "one-stop shopping" model (Tanney and Lowenstein, 1997). It is essential that nurses caring for these infants and their mothers understand the depth of the problem of prenatal drug exposure, have a positive attitude toward cocaine-using mothers and their children, be aware of community resources, and encourage positive parenting (Pokorni and Stanga, 1996).

Methamphetamine Exposure

The fetal and neonatal effects of maternal use of methamphetamines in pregnancy are not well known but appear to be dose related (Smith, Yonekura, Wallace, et al, 2003). LBW, preterm birth, and perinatal mortality may be consequences of higher doses used throughout pregnancy. In addition, a higher incidence of cleft lip and palate and cardiac defects has been reported in infants exposed to methamphetamines in utero (Plessinger, 1998). Behavioral changes in infants exposed prenatally to methamphetamines include decreased arousal, increased stress, and alterations in movement (Smith, Lagasse, Derauf, et al, 2008).

Methamphetamine use has increased significantly in the past 10 years in certain regions of the United States. In a 2003 study by Smith, Yonekura, Wallace, and colleagues, 63% of pregnant women using methamphetamines reported using the drug throughout the pregnancy. A higher incidence of preterm delivery and placental abruption was associated with methamphetamine use. In addition, fetal growth restriction (small for gestational age) was slightly higher in methamphetamine-exposed offspring; however, 80% of these neonates' mothers also had significant alcohol and tobacco use.

Study reports vary in the time of clinical manifestations of withdrawal from this drug; one study did not identify any signs of withdrawal in the first 3 days after birth, but long-term data were not collected (Smith, Yonekura, Wallace, et al, 2003). A study of infants exposed to methamphetamine in utero showed that such infants had significantly smaller head circumferences and birth weights than those not exposed. In addition, the exposed infants exhibited withdrawal signs of agitation, vomiting, and tachypnea, which were not observed in the unexposed infants (Chomchai, Na Manorom, Watanarungsan, et al, 2004). After birth, infants may experience bradycardia or tachycardia that resolves as the drug is cleared from the system. Lethargy may continue for several months, along with frequent infections and poor weight gain. Emotional disturbances and delays in gross and fine motor coordination may occur during early childhood.

The long-term effects of methamphetamine exposure on children living in households where the product is manufactured are not known, but there are early reports of burns in exposed children and concerns regarding the effects of the toxic by-products of methamphetamine production on small children. Skin rashes and respiratory tract illnesses are common problems seen in methamphetamine-exposed children; physical neglect and speech and language developmental delays are of significant concern as well (Crocker, 2005).

Marijuana Exposure

Marijuana has replaced cocaine as the most common illicit drug used by women ages 18 to 44 years (nonpregnant and pregnant) in the United States (Ebrahim and Gfroerer, 2003). Marijuana crosses the placenta. Some studies have shown that its use during pregnancy may result in a shortened gestation and a higher incidence of IUGR (Wagner, Katikaneni, Cox, et al, 1998). A review of studies examining the effects of marijuana during pregnancy found inconsistent results regarding the drug's effect on birth weight and gestational age (Schempf, 2007), but another study reported a strong association between the use of marijuana and a decrease in fetal growth and infant birth weight and length (Hurd, Wang, Anderson, et al, 2005). Other investigators have found a higher incidence of meconium staining (Bandstra and Accornero, 2006). Compounding the issue of the effects of marijuana, especially among women ages 18 to 30 years (Ebrahim and Gfroerer, 2003), is multidrug use,

which combines the harmful effects of marijuana, tobacco, alcohol, opiates, and cocaine. Long-term follow-up studies on exposed infants are needed.

Fetal Alcohol Spectrum Disorder

⊜ Infants and children exposed to alcohol in utero were previously reported to have characteristic facial features, prenatal and postnatal growth failure, and neurodevelopmental deficits. This triad of findings, termed fetal alcohol syndrome (FAS), was attributed to excessive ingestion of alcohol by the mother during pregnancy. It has since been shown that infants may not initially display the dysmorphic facial features. These are believed to be more well defined with increasing age during childhood. A number of terms (including *alcohol-related neurodevelopmental birth defects* and *fetal alcohol spectrum disorders*) have been proposed to describe the combination of findings. The umbrella term fetal alcohol spectrum disorder is now recommended to describe the continuum of defects seen in children affected by maternal alcohol intake, including classic FAS at the most severe end of the spectrum.

The three Centers for Disease Control and Prevention (2005) categories for diagnosis of FAS are (1) growth restriction, both prenatal and postnatal; (2) midfacial dysmorphic facial features; and (3) CNS involvement (structural, neurologic, or functional abnormality). Any single or multiple combination of these may be present in addition to confirmed or unknown history of maternal alcohol consumption. The Institute of Medicine has established diagnostic criteria (Welch-Carre, 2005), which include alcohol-related neurodevelopmental disorder (ARND) and alcohol-related birth defect (ARBD) criteria, but the Centers for Disease Control and Prevention criteria relate exclusively to FAS. The diagnosis of FAS is complicated by the absence of a specific single biologic marker and by manifestations that are often seen in other childhood conditions.

When possible, long-term disabilities are prevented by early evaluation and implementation of therapy. The family should learn any special handling techniques needed for the care of their infant and signs of complications or possible sequelae. When sequelae are inevitable, the family needs assistance in determining how to best cope with the problems, such as with home care assistance, referral to appropriate agencies, or placement in an institution for care.

The major goal of nursing care is prevention of these disorders through provision of adequate prenatal care for the expectant mother and precautions regarding exposure to potentially harmful infections.

FAS is recognized as the leading cause of cognitive impairment (American Academy of Pediatrics, 2000). The incidence of FAS is on the rise in the United States despite public warnings, including the U.S. surgeon general's warning that consumption of alcohol during pregnancy may cause cognitive impairment and other defects. The incidence of FAS (ARBD) in the United States is about 0.2 to 1.5 per 1000 live births (Centers for Disease Control and Prevention, 2005). The reported incidence of maternal alcohol consumption during pregnancy did not change substantially during the 1991 to 2005 period despite widespread education and information regarding periconceptional and gestational effects of drinking (Centers for Disease Control and Prevention, 2009). Among pregnant women ages 18 to 44 years, the average annual rates were 12.2% for alcohol use and 1.9% for binge drinking. In addition, among nonpregnant women any alcohol consumption was 53.7% while binge drinking was reported to be 12.1%. The Centers for Disease Control and Prevention (2009) found that pregnant women who were older, unmarried, more educated, and employed were more likely to use alcohol.

Alcohol (ethanol and ethyl alcohol) interferes with normal fetal development. The effects on the fetal brain are permanent, and even moderate use of alcohol during pregnancy may cause long-term postnatal difficulties, including impaired maternal-infant attachment. Because there is no known safe level of alcohol consumption in pregnancy, women should stop consuming alcohol at least 3 months before they plan to conceive.

Fetal abnormalities are not related to the amount of the mother's alcohol intake per se, but to the amount consumed in excess of the liver's ability to detoxify it. The liver's capacity to detoxify alcohol is limited and inflexible; when the liver receives more alcohol than it is able to handle, the excess is continually recirculated until the organ is able to reduce it to carbon dioxide and water. This circulating alcohol has a special affinity for brain tissue. There is no specific critical period at which alcohol toxicity may occur, although early gestation is considered the most vulnerable period; however, exposure at any period may cause subtle damage to the developing fetus (Brust, 2009). Other factors that contribute to the teratogenic effects include toxic acetyl aldehyde (a degradation byproduct of ethanol) and other substances that may be added to the alcohol. Poor nutritional state, smoking, polydrug intake, and infrequent or lack of prenatal care may compound the problem of alcohol abuse (Jones and Bass, 2003).

The effects on the fetal brain are reflected in CNS manifestations of FAS (Box 10-13). Cognitive and motor delays, hearing disorders, and a variety of defects in craniofacial development are prominent features (Fig. 10-19). MRI studies of children with diagnosed FAS revealed a high incidence of midbrain anomalies, including displacements in the corpus callosum, and changes in symmetry in the temporal lobes. Alcohol-exposed infants also demonstrate narrowing in the temporal region and reduced brain growth in portions of the frontal lobe (Riley, McGee, and Sowell, 2004). Some affected infants display physical features of the syndrome; behaviors, however, are nonspecific in newborns and may therefore pass undetected. These include difficulty in establishing respiration, irritability, lethargy, poor suck reflex, and abdominal distention.

Nursing Care Management

Nursing care of affected infants involves the same assessment and observations that are employed for any high-risk infant. Poor feeding is characteristic of infants with FAS and is a significant problem throughout infancy. Strategies to provide individualized developmental care are aimed at reducing noxious environmental stimuli and helping the infant achieve self-regulation (see Developmental Outcome, p. 332). Monitoring weight gain, analyzing feeding behaviors, and devising strategies to promote nutritional intake are especially important.

The effects of FAS have been identified in adolescents and young adults, primarily in relation to growth deficiencies,

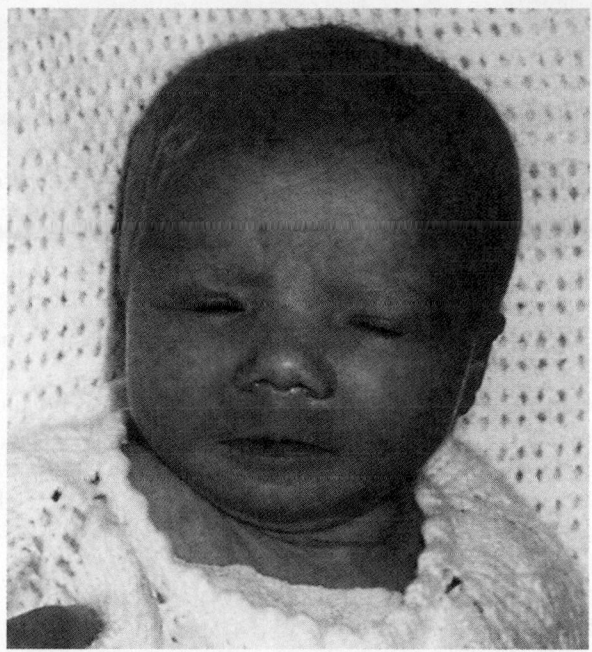

Fig. 10-19 Infant with fetal alcohol syndrome. (From Markiewicz M, Abrahamson E: *Diagnosis in color: neonatology*, St Louis, 1999, Mosby.)

BOX 10-13 MAJOR FEATURES OF FETAL ALCOHOL SYNDROME*

Facial Features
Short palpebral fissures
Hypoplastic or smooth philtrum (vertical ridge in upper lip)
Thinned upper lip (vermilion)
Short, upturned nose
Hypoplastic maxilla
Micrognathia or prognathia in adolescence
Retrognathia in infancy

Neurologic
Cognitive impairment
Motor delays
Microcephaly (head circumference below 10th percentile)
Poor coordination
Hypotonia
Hearing disorders

Behavior
Irritability (infancy)
Hyperactivity (child)

Growth
Disproportionately low weight to height
Prenatal growth restriction
Persistent postnatal growth lag

*For a comprehensive list of fetal alcohol related birth defects, see Fig. 1 in American Academy of Pediatrics, Committee on Substance Abuse and Committee on Children with Disabilities: Fetal alcohol syndrome and alcohol-related neurodevelopmental disorders, *Pediatrics* 106(2):358-361, 2000.

delayed motor development, and cognitive impairment. In one study children who were exposed to only small amounts of alcohol prenatally showed more aggressiveness, delinquent behavior, and attention problems at 6 to 7 years of age compared with unexposed controls (Sood, Delaney-Black, Covington, et al, 2001). Another study found that young adult offspring prenatally exposed to alcohol had significant alcohol-related problems by age 21 (Baer, Sampson, Barr, et al, 2003). Facial characteristics in adults tend to be more subtle than in infants and children.

Early diagnosis and intervention are reported to be beneficial for reducing the effects of alcohol exposure on the growing child (Stoler and Holmes, 2004); therefore nurses should be actively involved in identifying and referring children exposed to alcohol prenatally.

The dangers of heavy drinking are known, and *all* women should be counseled regarding the risks to the fetus. The nurse should emphasize to women of all ages that there is no known "safe" amount of alcohol intake during pregnancy that will preclude FASD. Furthermore, FASD is a totally preventable birth defect. A change in drinking habits even as late as the third trimester (when brain growth in the fetus is greatest) is associated with improved fetal outcome.*

Infants of Mothers Who Smoke

Cigarette smoking during pregnancy is clearly associated with significant birth weight deficits—up to 440 g (about 1 lb) in full-term newborns—and there is a definitive dose-response relationship between the number of cigarettes smoked by the mother and these deficits (Law, Stroud, LaGasse, et al, 2003). This dose-related response also affects the Apgar scores. The number of infants with low Apgar scores whose mothers smoked three packs per day is nearly four times higher than for infants whose mothers smoked none or only one pack per day. Large studies indicate that 21% to 39% of the incidence of LBW is attributable to maternal cigarette smoking.

The rate of preterm births is increased in mothers who smoke, but the infants are smaller at all stages of gestation. They show fetal growth restriction in length, weight, and chest and head circumference; these deficits are not related to maternal appetite or weight gain. The concentration of a pharmacologically active substance found in tobacco—nicotine—has been found to be higher in newborns of mothers who smoke than in the mothers themselves. Nicotine is metabolized to cotinine and secreted in breast milk and has a half-life of 70 to 80 minutes. In addition, it is now recognized that neonates may experience withdrawal symptoms after exposure to nicotine, whether in tobacco smoke or chewable form. It has also been shown that cigarette smoking has detrimental effects beyond the neonatal period, with deficits in growth, intellectual and emotional development, and behavior. Maternal smoking and passive smoking by household members has been correlated with an increased incidence of SIDS (Hunt and Hauck, 2006), respiratory tract illnesses (Jorgensen, 1999), spontaneous abortion, premature rupture of membranes, preterm delivery, and deficits in learning and behavior (Shea and Steiner, 2008). (See Environmental Tobacco Smoke Exposure, Chapter 32.)

---

*Further information is available from National Organization on Fetal Alcohol Syndrome, 900 17th St. NW, Washington, DC 20006; 202-785-4585; www.nofas.org; and Fetal Alcohol Syndrome Branch, National Center on Birth Defects and Developmental Disabilities, Centers for Disease Control and Prevention, Atlanta, www.cdc.gov/ncbddd/fas.

Nursing Care Management

Nurses are prime candidates for disseminating information to expectant mothers regarding smoking-related risks. Mothers who stop or substantially reduce smoking during pregnancy improve the quality of life for their unborn infants. In one study, infants of expectant mothers who were given information, support, encouragement, practical guidance, and behavior modification during pregnancy delivered infants with significantly higher birth weights than did controls. If mothers continue to smoke while breast-feeding, encourage them to do so immediately after breast-feeding to reduce the amount of nicotine and cotinine in the breast milk. Smoking decreases milk production in the breast-feeding mother (Lawrence and Lawrence, 2005). Parents should make all efforts to avoid second-hand smoke around all infants, but especially around those born with respiratory or cardiac problems and those born prematurely.

MATERNAL INFECTIONS

The range of pathologic conditions produced by infectious agents is large, and the difference between the maternal and fetal effects caused by any one agent is also great. Some maternal infections, especially during early gestation, can result in fetal loss or malformations because the fetus's ability to handle infectious organisms is limited and the fetal immunologic system is unable to prevent the dissemination of infectious organisms to the various tissues.

Not all prenatal infections produce teratogenic effects. Furthermore, the clinical picture of disorders caused by transplacental transfer of infectious agents is not always well defined. Some microbial agents can cause remarkably similar manifestations, and it is not uncommon to test for all when a prenatal infection is suspected. This is the so-called TORCHS complex, an acronym for:

T—Toxoplasmosis

O—Other (e.g., hepatitis B, parvovirus, HIV)

R—Rubella

C—Cytomegalovirus infection

H—Herpes simplex

S—Syphilis

To determine the causative agent in a symptomatic infant, perform tests to rule out each of these infections. The *O* category may involve testing for several viral infections (e.g., hepatitis B, varicella zoster, measles, mumps, HIV, human papillomavirus, and human parvovirus). Although this acronym has received substantial criticism because it does not cover the entire spectrum of congenital infections (Klein, Baker, Remington, et al, 2006), it is still used in clinical settings. Bacterial infections are not included in the TORCHS workup, since they are usually identified by clinical manifestations and readily available laboratory tests. Gonococcal conjunctivitis (ophthalmia neonatorum) and chlamydial conjunctivitis have been significantly reduced by prophylactic measures at birth. (See Chapter 8.) HIV infection is discussed in Chapter 35. The major maternal infections, their possible effects, and specific nursing considerations are outlined in Table 10-11.

TABLE 10-11 INFECTIONS ACQUIRED FROM MOTHER BEFORE, DURING, OR AFTER BIRTH*

FETAL OR NEWBORN EFFECT	TRANSMISSION	NURSING CONSIDERATIONS†
Human Immunodeficiency Virus (HIV) No significant difference between infected and uninfected infants at birth in some instances Embryopathy reported by some observers: • Depressed nasal bridge • Mild upward or downward obliquity of eyes • Long palpebral fissures with blue sclerae • Patulous lips • Ocular hypertelorism • Prominent upper vermilion border	Transplacental; during vaginal delivery; potentially in breast milk	Administer antiviral prophylaxis to the mother beginning at 14 wk of pregnancy. The choice of regimens is determined by examining a number of factors, including the mother's current treatment. Detailed recommendations can be obtained from Perinatal HIV Guidelines Working Group (2009). During labor *ZDV is recommended for all HIV-infected pregnant women, regardless of the antepartum treatment regimen.* HIV-exposed neonates should receive a 6-wk course of ZDV (consider addition of another antiretroviral drug based on maternal treatment and exposure). Cesarean section in HIV-positive mother is recommended to reduce transmission. For chemoprophylaxis against *Pneumocystis carinii* pneumonia in HIV-exposed infants, drug of choice is trimethoprim-sulfamethoxazole (Bactrim, Septra). Documented routine HIV education and routine testing with consent for all pregnant women in United States are recommended.
Chickenpox (Varicella-Zoster Virus [VZV]) Intrauterine exposure—congenital varicella syndrome: limb dysplasia, microcephaly, cortical atrophy, chorioretinitis, cataracts, cutaneous scars, other anomalies, auditory nerve palsy, motor and cognitive delays Severe symptoms (rash, fever) and higher mortality in infant whose mother develops varicella 5 days before to 2 days after delivery	1st trimester (fetal varicella syndrome); perinatal period (infection)	Use varicella zoster immunoglobulin (VariZIG) or IV immunoglobulin (IVIG) to treat infants born to mothers with onset of disease within 5 days before or 2 days after delivery. Institute Isolation Precautions in newborn born to mother with varicella up to 21-28 days (latter time if newborn received VariZIG or IVIG) after birth (if hospitalized). Prevention—universal immunization of children with varicella vaccine according to recommended schedule
Chlamydia Infection *(Chlamydia trachomatis)* Conjunctivitis, pneumonia	Last trimester or perinatal period	Standard ophthalmic prophylaxis for gonococcal ophthalmia neonatorum (topical antibiotics, silver nitrate, or povidone-iodine) is not effective in treatment or prevention of chlamydial ophthalmia. Treat with oral erythromycin for 14 days.
Coxsackievirus (Group B Enterovirus–Nonpolio) Poor feeding, vomiting, diarrhea, fever; cardiac enlargement, arrhythmias, congestive heart failure; lethargy, seizures, meningeal involvement Mimics bacterial sepsis	Peripartum	Treatment is supportive. Provide IVIG in neonatal infections.
Cytomegalovirus (CMV) Variable manifestation from asymptomatic to severe Microcephaly, cerebral calcifications, chorioretinitis Jaundice, hepatosplenomegaly Petechial or purpuric rash Neurologic sequelae—seizure disorders, sensorimotor deafness, cognitive impairment	Throughout pregnancy	Infection acquired at birth, shortly thereafter, or via human milk is not associated with clinical illness. Affected individuals excrete virus. Virus is detected in urine or tissue by electron microscopy. Avoid kissing affected child. Pregnant women should avoid close contact with known cases. To treat infection, administer IV antivirals such as ganciclovir to newborn.
Erythema Infectiosum (Parvovirus B19) Fetal hydrops and death from anemia and heart failure with early exposure Anemia with later exposure No teratogenic effects established Ordinarily, low risk of ill effect to fetus	Transplacental	First trimester infection has most serious effects. Pregnant health care workers should not care for patients who might be highly contagious (e.g., child with aplastic crisis). Routine exclusion of pregnant women from workplace where disease is occurring is not recommended.

CNS, Central nervous system; *HBsAg*, hepatitis B surface antigen; *IV*, intravenous.

*This table is not an exhaustive representation of all perinatally transmitted infections. For further information regarding specific diseases or treatment not listed here, refer to American Academy of Pediatrics, Committee on Infectious Diseases, Pickering L, editor: *2009 Red book: report of the Committee on Infectious Diseases*, ed 28, Elk Grove Village, Ill, 2009, The Academy.

†Isolation Precautions depend on institutional policy. (See Infection Control, Chapter 27.)

Continued

TABLE 10-11   INFECTIONS ACQUIRED FROM MOTHER BEFORE, DURING, OR AFTER BIRTH*—cont'd

FETAL OR NEWBORN EFFECT	TRANSMISSION	NURSING CONSIDERATIONS†
Gonococcal Disease (Neisseria gonorrhoeae) Ophthalmitis Neonatal gonococcal arthritis, septicemia, meningitis	Last trimester or perinatal period	Apply prophylactic medication to eyes at time of birth. Obtain smears for culture. To treat infection, administer penicillin.
Hepatitis B Virus (HBV) May be asymptomatic at birth Acute hepatitis, changes in liver function	Transplacental; contaminated maternal fluids or secretions during delivery	Administer hepatitis B immunoglobulin (HBIg) to all infants of HBsAg-positive mothers within 12 hr of birth; in addition, administer hepatitis B vaccine at separate site. Prevention—universal immunization of all infants with Hep B vaccine. (See Immunizations, Chapter 12.)
Herpes, Neonatal (Herpes Simplex Virus) Cutaneous lesions—vesicles at 6-10 days of age; may be no lesions Disseminated disease resembling sepsis—encephalitis in 60%-70% Visceral involvement—granulomas Early nonspecific signs—fever, lethargy, poor feeding, irritability, vomiting May include hyperbilirubinemia, seizures, flaccid or spastic paralysis, apneic episodes, respiratory distress, lethargy, or coma	History of genital infection in mother or partner in 50% of cases Transmitted intrapartum, either by ascending infection or direct contact, especially primary infection	Cesarean sections sometimes are preventive measure for mothers with active lesions. Vaginal delivery is recommended for infants of mothers with recurrent infection thought to be at lower risk. Infants should room-in with mother in private room. To treat infection, administer acyclovir (IV) to newborn.
Listeriosis (Listeria monocytogenes) Maternal infection associated with abortion, preterm delivery, and fetal death Preterm birth, sepsis, and pneumonia seen in early-onset disease; late-onset disease usually manifests as meningitis	Transplacental, by ascending infection or exposure at delivery	Hand washing is essential to prevent nosocomial spread. Treat infected newborn with antibiotics—ampicillin and gentamicin.
Rubella, Congenital (Rubella Virus) Eye defects—cataracts (unilateral or bilateral), microphthalmos, retinitis, glaucoma CNS signs—microcephaly, seizures, severe cognitive impairment Congenital heart defects—patent ductus arteriosus Auditory—high incidence of delayed hearing loss Intrauterine growth restriction Hyperbilirubinemia, meningitis, thrombocytopenia, hepatomegaly	1st trimester; early 2nd trimester	Pregnant women should avoid contact with all affected persons, including infants with rubella syndrome. Emphasize vaccination of all unimmunized prepubertal children, susceptible adolescents, and women of childbearing age (nonpregnant). Caution women against pregnancy for at least 3 mo after vaccination.
Syphilis, Congenital (Treponema pallidum) Stillbirth, prematurity, hydrops fetalis May be asymptomatic at birth and in 1st few weeks of life or may have multisystem manifestations: hepatosplenomegaly, lymphadenopathy, hemolytic anemia, and thrombocytopenia Copper-colored maculopapular cutaneous lesions (usually after 1st few weeks of life), mucous membrane patches, hair loss, nail exfoliation, snuffles (syphilitic rhinitis), profound anemia, poor feeding, pseudoparalysis of one or more limbs, dysmorphic teeth (older child)	Transplacental; can be anytime during pregnancy or at birth	This is most severe form of syphilis. Treatment consists of IV penicillin. Diagnostic evaluation depends on maternal serology testing and infant symptoms (American Academy of Pediatrics, 2009b).
Toxoplasmosis (Toxoplasma gondii) May be asymptomatic at birth (70%-90% of cases) or have maculopapular rash, lymphadenopathy, hepatosplenomegaly, jaundice, thrombocytopenia Hydrocephaly, cerebral calcifications, chorioretinitis (classic triad) Microcephaly, seizures, cognitive impairment, deafness Encephalitis, myocarditis, hepatosplenomegaly, anemia, jaundice, diarrhea, vomiting, purpura	Throughout pregnancy Predominant host for organism is cats May be transmitted through cat feces or poorly cooked or raw infected meats	Caution pregnant women to avoid contact with cat feces (e.g., emptying cat litter boxes). Administer sulfonamides (trimethoprim-sulfamethoxazole) or pyrimethamine (Daraprim).

CNS, Central nervous system; *HBsAg*, hepatitis B surface antigen; *IV*, intravenous.

*This table is not an exhaustive representation of all perinatally transmitted infections. For further information regarding specific diseases or treatment not listed here, refer to American Academy of Pediatrics, Committee on Infectious Diseases, Pickering L, editor: *2009 Red book: report of the Committee on Infectious Diseases,* ed 28, Elk Grove Village, Ill, 2009, The Academy.

†Isolation Precautions depend on institutional policy. (See Infection Control, Chapter 27.)

Nursing Care Management

One of the major goals in care of infants suspected of having an infectious disease is identification of the causative organism. Until the diagnosis is established, implement Standard Precautions according to institutional policy. In suspected cytomegalovirus and rubella infections, pregnant personnel are cautioned to avoid contact with the infant. Herpes simplex is easily transmitted from one infant to another; therefore risk of cross-contamination is reduced or eliminated by wearing gloves for patient contact. The American Academy of Pediatrics' *2009 Red Book: Report of the Committee on Infectious Diseases* (2009b) provides guidelines for the type and duration of precautions for most bacterial and viral exposures. Careful hand washing is the most important nursing intervention in reducing the spread of any infection.

Specimens need to be obtained for laboratory examinations, and the infant and parents need to be prepared for diagnostic procedures. When possible, long-term disabilities are prevented by early evaluation and implementation of therapy. Teach the family any special handling techniques needed for the care of their infant and signs of complications or possible sequelae. If sequelae are inevitable, the family will need assistance in determining how they can best cope with the problems, such as assistance with home care, referral to appropriate agencies, or placement in an institution for care. The major goal of nursing care is prevention of these disorders with provision of adequate prenatal care for the expectant mother and precautions regarding exposure to teratogenic infections.

KEY POINTS

- High-risk neonates may be defined as newborns, regardless of gestational age or birth weight, who have a greater than average chance of morbidity or mortality because of conditions or circumstances superimposed on the normal course of events associated with birth and adjustment to extrauterine existence.
- Identification of high-risk newborns may occur during any of the following stages: prenatal, natal, or postnatal.
- High-risk infants may be classified according to birth weight, gestational age, and morbidity factors.
- Late-preterm infants, by nature of their limited gestation, remain at risk for problems related to thermoregulation, hypoglycemia, hyperbilirubinemia, sepsis, and respiratory function.
- General management of the newborn entails immediate care, protection from infection, monitoring of physiologic data (including heart rate, respiratory activity, temperature, and blood pressure), laboratory data, and systematic assessment of the high-risk infant.
- Assessment of the high-risk newborn includes general, respiratory, cardiovascular, GI, genitourinary, neurologic-musculoskeletal, skin, and temperature assessments.
- Because many of their metabolic processes are immature, high-risk newborns are placed in a heated environment to help maintain thermal stability.
- Because of the immature, fragile skin of preterm infants, the nurse should use caution when applying topical preparations and, when possible, avoid adhesives.
- Meeting the high-risk infant's nutritional needs requires specific knowledge of physiologic characteristics, the infant's particular needs, and methods of feeding.

- Delayed development in high-risk neonates is a concern; developmental interventions are individualized to ameliorate the effects and increase infant well-being.
- Parental involvement in the care of high-risk infants is important, and nurses should encourage parent-infant relationships from birth to discharge.
- Prematurity accounts for the largest number of admissions to an NICU.
- Several severe respiratory conditions place the infant at high risk: AOP, RDS, MAS, air leak syndromes, and BPD.
- Therapeutic management of RDS includes oxygen therapy and assisted ventilation.
- Newborns are highly susceptible to infection, particularly septicemia.
- Cardiovascular complications in the high-risk infant may include PDA and PPHN.
- Neurologic disturbances in the high-risk newborn may include perinatal hypoxic-ischemic brain injury, IVH, ICH, neonatal seizures, and stroke.
- Nurses play an important role in end-of-life care of the family of the dying infant.
- Maternal conditions that pose a threat to the newborn include diabetes and substance abuse during pregnancy.
- Prenatal environmental conditions, especially selected maternal viral and bacterial infections and maternal alcohol ingestion, are responsible for high-risk problems in some newborns.

REFERENCES

Adams-Chapman I, Stoll BJ: Nervous system disorders. In Kliegman RM, Behrman RE, Jenson HB, Stanton BF, editors: *Nelson textbook of pediatrics*, ed 18, Philadelphia, 2007, Saunders.

Agthe AG, Kim GR, Mathias KB, et al: Clonidine as an adjunct therapy to opioids for neonatal abstinence syndrome: a randomized, controlled trial, *Pediatrics* 123(5):e849-e856. 2009.

Alfaleh K, Anabrees J, Bassler D: Probiotics reduce the risk of necrotizing enterocolitis in preterm infants: a meta-analysis, *Neonatology* 97(2):93-99, 2009.

Als H: Reading the premature infant. In Goldson E, editor: *Nurturing the premature infant: developmental interventions in the neonatal intensive care nursery,* New York, 1999, Oxford University Press.

Als H: Toward a synactive theory of development: promise for the assessment and support of infant individuality, *Inf Mental Health J* 3(4):229-243, 1982.

Als H, Gilkerson L, Duffy FH, et al: A three-center, randomized, controlled trial of individualized developmental care for very low birth weight preterm infants: medical, neurodevelopmental, parenting, and caregiving effects, *J Dev Behav Pediatr* 24(6):399-408, 2003.

American Academy of Pediatrics, Committee on Nutrition: *Pediatric nutrition handbook,* ed 6, Evanston, Ill, 2009a, The Academy.

American Academy of Pediatrics, Committee on Infectious Diseases, Pickering L, editor: *2009 Red book: report of the Committee on Infectious Diseases,* ed 28, Elk Grove Village, Ill, 2009b, The Academy.

American Academy of Pediatrics, Committee on Fetus and Newborn: Surfactant-replacement therapy for respiratory distress in preterm and term neonates, *Pediatrics* 121(2):419-432, 2008.

American Academy of Pediatrics: Breastfeeding and the use of human milk, *Pediatrics* 115(2):496-506, 2005.

American Academy of Pediatrics, Committee on Drugs: The transfer of drugs and other chemicals into human milk, *Pediatrics* 108(3):776-789, 2001.

American Academy of Pediatrics: Fetal alcohol syndrome and alcohol-related neurodevelopmental disorders, *Pediatrics* 106(2):358-361, 2000.

American Academy of Pediatrics, American Association for Pediatric Ophthalmology and Strabismus, American Academy of Ophthalmology: Screening examination of premature infants for retinopathy of prematurity, *Pediatrics* 117(2):572-576, 2006.

American Academy of Pediatrics, American College of Obstetricians and Gynecologists: *Guidelines for perinatal care,* ed 6, Elk Grove Village, Ill, 2007, The Academy and The College.

American Academy of Pediatrics and American Heart Association: *Textbook of neonatal resuscitation,* ed 5, Elk Grove Village, Ill, 2006, The Academy and The Association.

American Academy of Pediatrics, Canadian Paediatric Society: Postnatal corticosteroids to treat or prevent chronic lung disease in preterm infants, *Pediatrics* 109(2):330-338, 2002.

Anderson KV: The one thing you can never take away: perinatal bereavement photographs, *MCN* 26(1):123-128, 2001.

Anderson PJ, Doyle LW: Cognitive and educational deficits in children born extremely preterm, *Semin Perinatol* 32(1): 51-58, 2008.

Arnon S, Litmanovitz I: Diagnostic tests in neonatal sepsis, *Curr Opin Infect Dis* 21(3):223-227, 2008.

Askie LM, Henderson-Smart DJ, Ko H: Restricted versus liberal oxygen exposure for preventing morbidity and mortality in preterm or low birth weight infants, *Cochrane Database Syst Rev* 21(1):CD001077, 2009.

Askin DF, Bakewell-Sachs S, Medoff-Cooper B, et al: *Late preterm infant assessment guide,*

Washington, DC, 2007, Association of Women's Health, Obstetric and Neonatal Nurses.

Askin DF, Diehl-Jones W: Pathogenesis and prevention of chronic lung disease in the neonate. *Crit Care Nurs Clin North Am* 21(1):11-25, 2009a.

Askin DF, Diehl-Jones W: Retinopathy of prematurity. *Crit Care Nurs Clin North Am* 21(2):213-233, 2009b.

Askin DF, Diehl-Jones W: Cocaine: effects of in utero exposure on the fetus and neonate, *J Perinat Neonat Nurs* 14(4):83-102, 2001.

Association of Women's Health, Obstetric and Neonatal Nurses: *Evidence-based clinical practice guideline: neonatal skin care,* ed 2, Washington, DC, 2007, The Association.

Azzopardi DV, Strohm B, Edwards D, et al: Moderate hypothermia to treat perinatal asphyxial encephalopathy, *N Engl J Med* 361(14):1349-1358, 2009.

Baer JS, Sampson PD, Barr HM, et al: A 21-year longitudinal analysis of the effects of prenatal alcohol exposure on young adult drinking, *Arch Gen Psychiatry* 60(4):377-385, 2003.

Bakewell-Sachs S: Near-term/late preterm infants, *Newborn Infant Nurs Rev* 7(2): 67-71, 2007.

Bancalari E: Changes in the pathogenesis and prevention of chronic lung disease of prematurity, *Am J Perinatol* 18(1):1-5, 2001.

Bandstra ES, Accornero VH: Infants of substance abusing mothers. In Martin RJ, Fanaroff AA, Walsh MC, editors: *Neonatal-perinatal medicine: diseases of the fetus and infant,* ed 8, Philadelphia, 2006, Mosby.

Barrington K, Finer N: Inhaled nitric oxide for respiratory failure in preterm infants, *Cochrane Database Syst Rev* (1):CD000509, 2006.

Baud O: Antenatal corticosteroid therapy: benefits and risks, *Acta Paediatr Suppl* 93(444):6-10, 2004.

Beachy JM: Premature infant massage in the NICU, *Neonat Netw* 22(3):39-45, 2003.

Berseth CL, Bisquera JA, Paje VU: Prolonging small feeding volumes early in life decreases the incidence of necrotizing enterocolitis in very low birth weight infants, *Pediatrics* 111(3):529-534, 2003.

Beyerlein A, Hadders-Algra M, Kennedy K, et al: Infant formula supplementation with long-chain polyunsaturated fatty acids has no effect on Bayley developmental scores at 18 months of age—IPD meta-analysis of 4 large clinical trials, *J Pediatr Gastroenterol Nutr,* Oct 29, 2009 (Epub ahead of print).

Bhandari A, Bhandari V: Pitfalls, problems, and progress in bronchopulmonary dysplasia, *Pediatrics* 123(6):1562-1573, 2009.

Bhuta T, Henderson-Smart DJ: Elective high frequency jet ventilation versus conventional ventilation for respiratory distress syndrome in preterm infants, *Cochrane Database Syst Rev* (1):CD000328, 2000.

Bin-Nun A, Bromiker R, Wilschanski M, et al: Oral probiotics prevent necrotizing enterocolitis in very low birth weight neonates, *J Pediatr* 147(2):143-146, 2005.

Blackburn ST: *Maternal, fetal, and neonatal physiology: a clinical perspective,* ed 3, St Louis, 2007, Saunders.

Blackburn S: Environmental impact of the NICU on developmental outcomes, *J Pediatr Nurs* 13(5):279-289, 1998.

Blackburn S, De Paul D, Loan LA, et al: Neonatal thermal care, part 3, The effect of infant position and temperature probe placement, *Neonat Netw* 20(3):25-30, 2001.

Blackburn ST, Ditzenberger GR: Neurologic system. In Kenner C, Lott JW, editors: *Comprehensive neonatal care: a physiologic perspective,* ed 4, Philadelphia, 2007, Saunders.

Blake WW, Murray JA: Heat balance. In Merenstein GB, Gardner SL: *Handbook of neonatal intensive care,* ed 6, St Louis, 2006, Mosby.

Bohnhorst B, Heyne T, Peter CS, et al: Skin-to-skin (kangaroo) care, respiratory control, and thermoregulation, *J Pediatr* 138(2):193-197, 2001.

Boney CM, Verma A, Tucker R, et al: Metabolic syndrome in childhood: association with birth weight, maternal obesity, and gestational diabetes mellitus, *Pediatrics* 115(3):e290-e296, 2005.

Bradshaw WT, Turner BS, Pierce JR: Physiologic monitoring. In Merenstein GB, Gardner SL, editors: *Handbook of neonatal intensive care,* ed 6, St Louis, 2006, Mosby.

Bremmer P, Byers JF, Kiehl E: Noise and the premature infant: physiological effects and practice implications, *JOGNN* 32(4):447-454, 2003.

Browne JV: Considerations for touch and massage in the neonatal intensive care unit, *Neonat Netw* 19(1):61-64, 2000.

Brust JCM: The neurotoxicity of ethanol and related alcohols, In Dobbs MR, editor: *Clinical neurotoxicology: syndromes, substances, environments,* Philadelphia, 2009, Saunders.

Bull MJ, Engle WA, and American Academy of Pediatrics: Safe transportation of preterm and low birth weight infants at hospital discharge, *Pediatrics* 123(5):1424-1429, 2009.

Byers JF: Components of developmental care and the evidence for their use in the NICU, *MCN* 28(1):174-180, 2003.

Canadian Paediatric Society: Screening guidelines for newborns at risk for low blood glucose, *Paediatr Child Health* 9(10):723-729, 2004.

Carver JD, Wu PY, Hall RT, et al: Growth of preterm infants fed nutrient-enriched or term formula after hospital discharge, *Pediatrics* 107(4):683-689, 2001.

Centers for Disease Control and Prevention: Alcohol use among pregnant and nonpregnant women of childbearing age—United States, 1991-2005, *MMWR* 58(19):529-532, 2009.

Centers for Disease Control and Prevention: Perinatal group B streptococcal disease after universal screening recommendations—United States, 2003-2005, *MMWR* 56(28):701-705, 2007.

Centers for Disease Control and Prevention: Guidelines for identifying and referring persons with fetal alcohol syndrome, *MMWR* 54(RR11):1-10, 2005.

Chiriboga CA, Brust JC, Bateman D, et al: Drug-response effect on fetal cocaine exposure on newborn neurologic function, *Pediatrics* 103(1):79-85, 1999.

Chiriboga CA, Kuhn L, Wasserman GA. Prenatal cocaine exposures and dose-related cocaine effects on infant tone and behavior, *Neurotoxicol Teratol* 29(3):323-330, 2007.

Chomchai C, Na Manorom N, Watanarungsan P, et al: Methamphetamine abuse during pregnancy and its impact on neonates born at Siriraj Hospital, Bangkok, Thailand, *Southeast Asian J Trop Med Pub Health* 35(1):228-231, 2004.

Conde-Agudelo A, Diaz-Rossello JL, Belizan JM: Kangaroo mother care to reduce morbidity and mortality in low birthweight infants, *Cochrane Neonatal Rev* 2000, available at www.nichd.nih.gov/cochraneneonatal/Vickers/Vickers.htm (accessed August 2005).

Cornblath M, Hawdon JM, Williams AF, et al: Controversies regarding operational definition of neonatal hypoglycemia: suggested thresholds, *Pediatrics* 105(5):1141-1145, 2000.

Cornblath M, Ichord R: Hypoglycemia in the neonate, *Semin Perinatol* 24(2):136-149, 2000.

Courtney SE, Durand DJ, Asselin JM, et al: High-frequency oscillatory ventilation versus conventional mechanical ventilation for very-low-birth-weight infants, *N Engl J Med* 347(9):643-652, 2002.

Cowett RM, Loughead JL: Neonatal glucose metabolism: differential diagnoses, evaluation, and treatment of hypoglycemia, *Neonat Netw* 21(4):9-19, 2002.

Coyle MG, Ferguson A, Lagasse L, et al: Diluted tincture of opium (DTO) and phenobarbital versus DTO alone for neonatal opiate withdrawal in term infants, *J Pediatr* 140(5):561-564, 2002.

Cristobal R, Oghalai JS. Hearing loss in children with very low birth weight: current review of epidemiology and pathophysiology, *Arch Dis Child Fetal Neonatal Ed* 93(6):F462-F468, 2008.

Crocker E: Meth's burning issues, *Nurse Week, Heartland Ed* 6(8):22-23, 2005.

Curry CJ, Bhullar S, Holmes J, et al: Risk factors for perinatal arterial stroke: a study of 60 mother-child pairs, *Pediatr Neurol* 37(2):99-107, 2007.

D'Apolito K, Hepworth JT: Prominence of withdrawal symptoms in polydrug-exposed infants, *J Perinat Neonat Nurs* 14(4):46-60, 2001.

Darcy AE: Complications of the late preterm infant, *J Perinatal Neonatal Nurs* 23(1):78-86, 2009.

Delaney-Black V, Covington C, Templin T, et al: Prenatal cocaine exposure and child behavior, *Pediatrics* 102(4):945-950, 1998.

Deshpande G, Rao S, Patole S: Probiotics for prevention of necrotizing enterocolitis in preterm neonates with very low birthweight: a systematic review of randomized control trials, *Lancet* 369(9573):1614-1620, 2007.

Deshpande S, Ward Platt M: The investigation and management of neonatal hypoglycaemia, *Semin Fetal Neonatal Med* 10(4):351-361, 2005.

Dieter JN, Field T, Hernandez-Reif M, et al: Stable preterm infants gain more weight and sleep less after 5 days of massage therapy, *J Pediatr Psychol* 28(6):403-411, 2003.

Dougherty D, Luther M: Birth to breast—a feeding care map for the NICU: Helping the extremely low birth weight infant navigate the course. *Neonat Netw* 27(6):371-377, 2008.

Downs JA, Edwards AD, McCormick DC, et al: Effect of intervention on the development of hip posture in very preterm babies, *Arch Dis Child* 66(7):197-201, 1991.

Drenser KA, Capone A: Retinopathy of prematurity. In Yanoff M, Duker JS, editors: *Ophthalmology*, ed 3, St Louis, 2008, Mosby.

Dudell G, Stoll BJ: Respiratory tract disorders. In Kliegman RM, Behrman RE, Jenson HB, et al, editors: *Nelson textbook of pediatrics*, ed 18, Philadelphia, 2007, Saunders.

Dyer KA: Identifying, understanding, and working with grieving parents in the NICU, part I, Identifying and understanding loss and the grief response, *Neonat Netw* 24(3):35-46, 2005.

Ebrahim SH, Gfroerer J: Pregnancy-related substance use in the United States during 1996-1998, *Obstet Gynecol* 101(2):374-379, 2003.

Edwards AD, Azzopardi DV. Therapeutic hypothermia following perinatal asphyxia, *Arch Dis Child Fetal Neonatal Ed* 91(2):F127-F131, 2006.

El Shahed AI, Dargaville P, Ohlsson A, et al: Surfactant for meconium aspiration syndrome in full term infants, *Cochrane Database Syst Rev* (3):CD002054, 2007.

Engle WA: A recommendation for the definition of "late preterm" (near-term) and the birth weight–gestational age classification system, *Semin Perinatol* 30(1):2-7, 2006.

Engle WA, Tomashek KM, Wallman C, et al: Late-preterm infants: a population at risk, *Pediatrics* 120(6):1390-1401, 2007.

Engler AJ, Cusson RM, Brockett RT, et al: Neonatal staff and advanced practice nurses' perceptions of bereavement/end-of-life care of families of critically ill and/or dying infants, *Am J Crit Care* 13(6):489-498, 2004.

Escobar GJ, Clark RH, Greene JD: Short-term outcomes of infants born at 35 and 36 weeks gestation: we need to ask more questions, *Semin Perinatol* 30(1):28-33, 2006.

Eyler FD, Behnke M, Conlon M: Birth outcome from a prospective, matched study of prenatal crack/cocaine use, part 2, Interactive and dose effects on neurochemical assessment, *Pediatrics* 101(2):237-241, 1998.

Fantz CR, Powell C, Karon B, et al: Assessment of the diagnostic accuracy of the TDx-FLM II to predict fetal lung maturity, *Clin Chem* 48(5):761-765, 2002.

Feldman R, Eidelman AL: Skin-to-skin contact (kangaroo care) accelerates autonomic and neurobehavioral maturation in preterm infants, *Dev Med Child Neurol* 45:274-281, 2003.

Feldman R, Eidelman A, Sirota L, et al: Comparison of skin-to-skin (kangaroo) and

traditional care: parenting outcomes and preterm infant development, *Pediatrics* 110(1 pt 1):16-26, 2002.

Field DJ: Nitric oxide: still no consensus, *Early Hum Dev* 81(1):1-4, 2005.

Fielder AR, Merrick JM: Environmental light and the preterm infant, *Semin Perinatol* 24(4):291-298, 2000.

Finer NN, Barrington KJ: Nitric oxide for respiratory failure in infants born at or near term, *Cochrane Database Syst Rev* (4):CD000399, 2006.

Finer N, Leone T: Oxygen saturation monitoring for the preterm infant: the evidence basis for current practice, *Pediatr Res* 65(4):375-380, 2009.

Finnegan LP: Neonatal abstinence. In Nelson N, editor: *Current therapy in neonatal perinatal medicine 1985-1986*, Toronto, 1985, BC Decker.

Fucile S, Gisel EG, Lau C: Effect of an oral stimulation program on sucking skill maturation of preterm infants, *Dev Med Child Neurol* 47(3):158-162, 2005.

Gabbe SG, Niebyl JR, Simpson KL, editors: *Obstetrics: normal and problem pregnancies*, ed 5, London, 2007, Churchill Livingstone.

Gardner SL, Snell BJ, Lawrence RA: Breast-feeding the neonate with special needs. In Merenstein GB, Gardner SL, editors: *Handbook of neonatal intensive care*, ed 6, St Louis, 2006, Mosby.

Gerhardt KJ, Abrams RM: Fetal exposures to sound and vibroacoustic stimulation, *J Perinatol* 20(8 Pt 2):S21-S30, 2000.

Gill SL: Breastfeeding by Hispanic women, *J Obstet Gynecol Neonatal Nurs* 38(2):244-252, 2009.

Glass P: The vulnerable neonate and the neonatal intensive care environment. In MacDonald MG, Mullett MD, Seshia MK, editors: *Avery's neonatology: pathophysiology and management of the newborn*, ed 6, Philadelphia, 2005, Lippincott.

Gold KJ, Dalton VK, Schwenk TL. Hospital care for parents after perinatal death, *Obstet Gynecol* 109(5):1156-1166, 2007.

Golomb MR, Cvijanovich NZ, Ferriero DM: Neonatal brain injury. In Swaiman KF, Ashwal S, Ferriero DM, editors: *Pediatric neurology*, ed 4, Philadelphia, 2006, Mosby.

Graven SN: Sound and the developing infant in the NICU: conclusions and recommendations for care, *J Perinatol* 20(8 Pt 2):S88-S93, 2000.

Greenough A: Long-term pulmonary outcome in the preterm infant. *Neonatology* 93(4):324-327, 2008.

Greenough A, Dimitriou G, Prendergast M, et al: Synchronized mechanical ventilation for respiratory support in newborn infants, *Cochrane Database Syst Rev* (1):CD000456, 2008.

Gregory K: Update on nutrition for preterm and full-term infants, *JOGNN* 34(1):98-108, 2004.

Guner YS, Chokshi N, Petrosyan M, et al: Necrotizing enterocolitis—bench to bedside: novel and emerging strategies, *Semin Pediatr Surg* 17(4):255-265, 2008.

Hack M, Costello DW: Trends in the rates of cerebral palsy associated with neonatal intensive care of preterm children, *Clin Obstet Gynecol* 51(4):763-774, 2008.

Halliday HL: Evidence-based neonatal care, *Best Pract Res Clin Obstet Gynaecol* 19(1):155-166, 2005.

Halliday HL: Respiratory distress syndrome. In Greenough A, Milner AD, editors: *Neonatal respiratory disorders*, London, 2003, Arnold.

Halliday HL, Ehrenkranz RA, Doyle LW: Early postnatal (<96 hours) corticosteroids for preventing chronic lung disease in preterm infants, *Cochrane Database Syst Rev* (1):CD001146, 2009.

Hankins GD, Koen S, Gei AF, et al: Neonatal organ system injury in acute birth asphyxia sufficient to result in neonatal encephalopathy, *Obstet Gynecol* 99(5 Pt 1): 688-691, 2002.

Hascoet JM, Fresson J, Claris O, et al: The safety and efficacy of nitric oxide therapy in premature infants, *J Pediatr* 146(3):318-323, 2005.

Hay WW: Strategies for feeding the preterm infant, *Neonatology* 94(4):245-254, 2008.

Henderson G, Fahey T, McGuire W: Nutrient-enriched formula versus standard term formula for preterm infants following hospital discharge. *Cochrane Database Syst Rev* (4):CD004696, 2007.

Hill A: Neurological and neuromuscular disorders. In MacDonald MG, Mullett MD, Seshia MK, editors: *Avery's neonatology: pathophysiology and management of the newborn*, ed 6, Philadelphia, 2005, Lippincott.

Hill AS, Kurkowski TB, Garcia J: Oral support measures used in feeding the preterm infant, *Nurs Res* 49(1):2-10, 2000.

Hintz SR, Poole WK, Wright LL, et al (NICHD Neonatal Research Network): Changes in mortality and morbidities among infants born at less than 25 weeks during the post-surfactant era, *Arch Dis Child Fetal Neonatal Ed* 90(2):F128-F133, 2005.

Holditch-Davis D, Blackburn ST: Newborn and infant neurobehavioral development. In Kenner C, Lott J, editors: *Comprehensive neonatal nursing: a physiologic perspective*, ed 4, Philadelphia, 2007, Saunders.

Holditch-Davis D: Neonatal sleep-wake states. In Kenner C, Lott JW, Flandermeyer AA, editors: *Comprehensive neonatal care: a physiologic perspective*, ed 2, Philadelphia, 1998, Saunders.

Huestis MA, Choo RE: Drug abuse's smallest victims: in utero drug exposure, *Forensic Sci Int* 128(1-2):20-30, 2002.

Human Milk Banking Association: 2008 Guidelines for the Establishment and Operation of a donor human milk bank, 2008, available at www.hmbana.org (accessed July 5, 2009).

Hunt CE, Hauck FR: Sudden infant death syndrome, *CMAJ* 174(13):1861-1869, 2006.

Hunter J: The neonatal intensive care unit. In Case-Smith J, editor: *Occupational therapy for children*, ed 4, St Louis, 2001, Mosby.

Hurd YL, Wang X, Anderson V, et al: Marijuana impairs growth in mid-gestation fetuses, *Neurotoxicol Teratol* 27(2):221-229, 2005.

Hurst NM, Valentine CJ, Renfro L, et al: Skin-to-skin holding in the neonatal intensive care unit influences maternal milk volume, *J Perinatol* 17(3):213-217, 1997.

International Committee for the Classification of Retinopathy of Prematurity: The International Classification of Retinopathy of Prematurity revisited, *Arch Ophthalmol* 123(7):991-999, 2005.

Jacobs S, Hunt R, Tarnow-Mordi W, et al: Cooling for newborns with hypoxic ischaemic encephalopathy. *Cochrane Database Syst Rev* (4):CD003311, 2007.

Jansen JL: A bereavement model for the intensive care nursery, *Neonat Netw* 22(3):17-23, 2003.

Jansson LM, Velez M, Harrow C: Methadone maintenance and lactation: a review of the literature and current management guidelines, *J Hum Lact* 20(1):62-71, 2004.

Johnson K, Gerada C, Greenough A: Treatment of neonatal abstinence syndrome, *Arch Dis Child Fetal Neonatal Ed* 88(1):F2-F5, 2003.

Jones JG, MacKinnon B, Good WV, et al: The early treatment of ROP (ETROP) randomized trial: study results and nursing care adaptation, *Insight* 30(2):7-13, 2005.

Jones MW, Bass WT: Follow-up of the high-risk infant—fetal alcohol syndrome, *Neonat Netw* 22(3):63-70, 2003.

Jorgensen KM: The drug-exposed infant: physiology, signs and symptoms, *NANN Central Lines* 15(2):1-2, 8-9, 11, 1999.

Kabbur PM, Herson VC, Zaremba S, et al: Have the Year 2000 Neonatal Resuscitation Program Guidelines changed the delivery room management or outcome of meconium-stained infants? *J Perinatol* 25(11):694-697, 2005.

Kamitsuka MD, Horton MK, Williams MA: The incidence of necrotizing enterocolitis after introducing standardized feeding schedules for infants between 1250 and 2500 grams and less than 35 weeks gestation, *Pediatrics* 105(2):379-384, 2000.

Kattwinkel J, editor: *Textbook of neonatal resuscitation*, ed 5, Elk Grove Village, Ill, 2006, American Academy of Pediatrics and American Heart Association.

Kerr BA, Starbuck AL, Block SM: Fluid and electrolyte management. In Merenstein GB, Gardner SL, editors: *Handbook of neonatal intensive care*, ed 6, St Louis, 2006, Mosby.

Kirton A, deVeber G: Advances in perinatal ischemic stroke, *Pediatr Neurol* 40(3): 205-214, 2009.

Klein JO, Baker CJ, Remington JS, et al: Current concepts of infections of the fetus and newborn. In Remington JS, Klein JO, Wilson CJ, et al, editors: *Infectious diseases of the fetus and newborn infant*, Philadelphia, 2006, Saunders.

Konduri GG: New approaches for persistent pulmonary hypertension of newborn, *Clin Perinatol* 31(3):591-611, 2004.

Konduri GG, Kim UO. Advances in the diagnosis and management of persistent pulmonary hypertension of the newborn, *Pediatr Clin North Am* 56(3):579-600, 2009.

Korones SB: Complications: bronchopulmonary dysplasia, air leak syndromes, and retinopathy of prematurity. In Goldsmith JP, Karotkin EH, editors: *Assisted ventilation of the neonate*, ed 4, Philadelphia, 2003, Saunders.

Kraft WK, Gibson E, Dysart K, et al: Sublingual buprenorphine for treatment of neonatal abstinence syndrome: a randomized trial. *Pediatrics* 122(3):e601-e607, 2008.

Kuschel C: Managing drug withdrawal in the newborn infant. *Semin Fetal Neonatal Med* 212(2):127-133, 2007.

Laborada G, Rego M, Jain A, et al: Diagnostic value of cytokines and C-reactive protein in the first 24 hours of neonatal sepsis, *Am J Perinatol* 20(8):491-501, 2003.

Laptook AR: Use of therapeutic hypothermia for term infants with hypoxic-ischemic encephalopathy, *Pediatr Clin North Am* 56(3):601-616, 2009.

Laptook AR, O'Shea TM, Shankaran S, et al (NICHD Neonatal Network): Adverse neurodevelopmental outcomes among extremely low birth weight infants with a normal head ultrasound: prevalence and antecedents, *Pediatrics* 115(3):673-680, 2005.

Latini G, Del Vecchio A, De Felice C, et al: Persistent pulmonary hypertension of the newborn: therapeutic approach, *Mini Rev Med Chem* 8(14):1507-1513, 2008.

Law KL, Stroud LR, LaGasse L, et al: Smoking during pregnancy and newborn neurobehavior, *Pediatrics* 111(6):1318-1323, 2003.

Law-Morstatt L, Judd DM, Snyder P, et al: Pacing as a treatment technique for transitional sucking patterns, *J Perinatol* 23(6):483-488, 2003.

Lawrence RA, Lawrence RM: *Breastfeeding: a guide for the medical profession*, ed 6, St Louis, 2005, Mosby.

Lefrak L: Moving toward safer practice: reducing medication errors in neonatal care, *J Perinat Neonat Nurs* 16(2):73-84, 2002.

Leguizamon G, Igarzabal ML, Reece EA: Periconceptual care of women with diabetes mellitus, *Obstet Gynecol Clin North Am* 34(2):225-239, 2007.

Levine TP, Liu J, Das A, et al: Effects of prenatal cocaine exposure on special education in school-aged children. *Pediatrics* 122(1): e83-e91, 2008.

Lickliter R: Atypical perinatal sensory stimulation and early perceptual development: insights from developmental psychobiology, *J Perinatol* 20(8 Pt 2):S45-S54, 2000a.

Lickliter R: The role of sensory stimulation in perinatal development: insights from comparative research for care of the high-risk infant, *J Dev Behav Pediatr* 21(6):437-447, 2000b.

Lucas A: Improving medication safety in a neonatal intensive care unit, *Am J Health Syst Pharmacol* 61(1):33-37, 2004.

Lucas A, Fewtrell MS, Morley R, et al: Randomized trial of nutrient-enriched formula versus standard formula for postdischarge preterm infants, *Pediatrics* 108(3):703-711, 2001.

Lund CH, Durand DJ: Skin and skin care. In Merenstein GB, Gardner SL, editors: *Handbook of neonatal intensive care*, ed 6, St Louis, 2006, Mosby.

Lund CH, Osborne CW: Validity and reliability of the neonatal skin condition score, *J Obstet Gynecol Neonatal Nurs* 33(3):320-327, 2004.

Luu TM, Ment LR, Schneider KC, et al: Lasting effects of preterm birth and neonatal brain hemorrhage at 12 years of age, *Pediatrics* 123(3):1037-1044, 2009.

Malanga CJ, Kosofsky BE: Mechanism of action of drugs of abuse on the developing fetal brain, *Clin Perinatol* 26(1):17-37, 1999.

McCarter-Spaulding D: The influence of culture and health on the breastfeeding relationship, *J Obstet Gynecol Neonatal Nurs* 38(2):218, 2009.

McCrea HJ, Ment LR: The diagnosis, management, and postnatal prevention of intraventricular hemorrhage in the preterm neonate, *Clin Perinatol* 35(4):777-792, 2008.

McGrath MM, Sullivan MC, Lester MC: Longitudinal neurologic follow-up in neonatal intensive care unit survivors with various neonatal morbidities, *Pediatrics* 106(6):1397-1405, 2000.

Merchant JR, Worwa C, Porter S, et al: Respiratory instability of term and near-term healthy newborn infants in car safety seats, *Pediatrics* 108(3):647-652, 2001.

Mercier JC, Olivier P, Loron G, et al: Inhaled nitric oxide to prevent bronchopulmonary dysplasia in preterm neonates. *Semin Fetal Neonatal Med* 14(1):28-34, 2009.

Merenstein GB, Gardner SL, editors: *Handbook of neonatal intensive care*, ed 6, St Louis, 2006, Mosby.

Mintz-Hittner HA, Best LM: Antivascular endothelial growth factor for retinopathy of prematurity, *Curr Opin Pediatr* 21(2):182-187, 2009.

Mirmiran M, Ariagno RL: Influence of light in the NICU on the development of circadian rhythms in preterm infants, *Semin Perinatol* 24(4):247-257, 2000.

Modrcin-Talbott MA, Harrison LL, Groer MW, et al: The biobehavioral effects of gentle human touch on preterm infants, *Nurs Sci Q* 16(1):60-67, 2003.

Monterosso L, Kristjanson LJ, Cole J, et al: Effect of postural supports on neuromotor function in very preterm infants to term equivalent age, *J Paediatr Child Health* 39(3):197-205, 2003.

Morton JA: Strategies to support extended breastfeeding of the premature infant, *Adv Neonat Care* 2(5):267-282, 2002.

Moya FR, Gadzinowski J, Bancalari E, et al: A multicenter, randomized, masked, comparison trial of lucinactant, colfosceril palmitate, and beractant for the prevention of respiratory distress syndrome among very preterm infants, *Pediatrics* 115(4):1018-1029, 2005.

Msall ME, Tremont MR: Functional outcomes in self-care, mobility, communication, and learning in extremely low–birth weight infants, *Clin Perinatol* 27(2):381-401, 2000.

Neerhof MG, Dohnal JC, Ashwood ER, et al: Lamellar body counts: a consensus on protocol, *Obstet Gynecol* 97(2):318-320, 2001.

Nelson KB, Lynch JK: Stroke in newborn infants, *Lancet Neurol* 3(3):150-158, 2004.

Neu M, Browne JV, Vojir C: The impact of two transfer techniques used during skin-to-skin care on the physiologic and behavioral responses of preterm infants, *Nurs Res* 49(4):215-223, 2000.

Newell SJ: Enteral feeding the micropremie, *Clin Perinatol* 27(1):221-234, 2000.

Nucci A, Burns RC, Armah T, et al: Interdisciplinary management of pediatric intestinal failure: a 10-year review of rehabilitation and transplantation, *J Gastrointest Surg* 12(3):429-435, 2008.

Nye C: Transitioning infants from gavage to breast, *Neonat Netw* 27(1):7-13, 2008.

Onland W, Offringa M, De Jaegere AP, et al: Finding the optimal postnatal dexamethasone regimen for preterm infants at risk of bronchopulmonary dysplasia: a systematic review of placebo-controlled trials, *Pediatrics* 123(1):367-377, 2009.

Parvin CA, Kaplan LA, Chapman JF, et al: Predicting respiratory distress syndrome using gestational age and fetal lung maturity by fluorescent polarization, *Am J Obstet Gynecol* 192(1):199-207, 2005.

Patole SK, de Klerk N: Impact of standardized feeding regimes on incidence of neonatal necrotizing enterocolitis: a systematic review of meta-analysis of observational studies, *Arch Dis Child Fetal Neonatal Ed* 90:147-151, 2005.

Perinatal HIV Guidelines Working Group. Public Health Service Task Force recommendations for use of antiretroviral drugs in pregnant HIV-infected women for maternal health and interventions to reduce perinatal HIV transmission in the United States. April 29, 2009, available at http://aidsinfo.nih.gov/ContentFiles/PerinatalGL.pdf (accessed June 25, 2009).

Peters KL: Infant handling in the NICU: does developmental care make a difference? An evaluative review of the literature, *J Perinat Neonat Nurs* 13(3):83-109, 1999.

Petrini JR, Dias T, McCormick MC, et al: Increased risk of adverse neurological development for late preterm infants, *J Pediatr* 154(2):169-176, 2009.

Phelps DL, Watts JL: Early light reduction for preventing retinopathy of prematurity in very low birth weight infants, *Cochrane Neonatal Rev*, 2001, available at www.nichd.nih.gov/cochraneneonatal/Phelps/Phelps.htm (accessed December 4, 2009).

Philbin MK, Klaas P: Evaluating studies of the behavioral effects of sound on newborns, *J Perinatol* 20(8 part 2):61-67, 2000.

Pietz J, Peter J, Graf R, et al: Physical growth and neurodevelopmental outcome of nonhandicapped low-risk children born preterm, *Early Hum Dev* 79(2):131-143, 2004.

Pilley E, McGuire W: Pre-discharge "car seat challenge" for preventing morbidity and mortality in preterm infants. *Cochrane Database Syst Rev* (1):CD005386, 2006.

Pinelli J, Symington A: Non-nutritive sucking for promoting physiologic stability and nutrition in preterm infants, *Cochrane Database Syst Rev* (4):CD001071, 2005.

Plessinger M: Prenatal exposure to amphetamines, *Obstet Gynecol Clin North Am* 25(1):119-138, 1998.

Poblano A, Marquez A, Hernandez G: Apnea in infants, *Indian J Pediatr* 73(12):1085-1088. 2006.

Pokorni JL, Stanga J: Serving infants and families affected by maternal cocaine abuse, part I, *Pediatr Nurs* 22(5):439-442, 1996.

Pollan C: Retinopathy of prematurity: an eye toward better outcomes, *Neonat Netw* 28(2): 93-101, 2009.

Premji S, Chessell L: Continuous nasogastric milk feeding versus intermittent bolus milk feeding for premature infants less than 1500 grams, *Cochrane Database Syst Rev* (1):CD001819, 2003.

Rao R, Desai NS: OxyContin and neonatal abstinence syndrome, *J Perinatol* 22(4):324-325, 2002.

Reed MD, Blumer JL: Pharmacologic treatment of the fetus. In Martin RJ, Fanaroff AA, Walsh MC, editors: *Neonatal-perinatal medicine: diseases of the fetus and infant*, ed 8, Philadelphia, 2006, Saunders.

Riley EP, McGee CL, Sowell ER: Teratogenic effects of alcohol: a decade of brain imaging, *Am J Med Genet C Semin Med Genet* 127(1):35-41, 2004.

Roberts KL, Paynter C, McEwan B: A comparison of kangaroo mother care and conventional cuddling care, *Neonat Netw* 19(4):31-35, 2000.

Saigal S, den Ouden L, Wolke D, et al: School-age outcomes in children who were extremely low birth weight from four international population-based cohorts, *Pediatrics* 112(4): 943-950, 2003.

Samsom JF, de Groot L: Study of a group of extremely preterm infants (25-27 weeks): how do they function at 1 year of age? *J Child Neurol* 16(11):832-837, 2001.

Samsom JF, de Groot L: The influence of postural control on motility and hand function in a group of "high risk" preterm infants at 1 year of age, *Early Hum Dev* 60(2):101-113, 2000.

Sarkar S, Rosenkrantz TS: Neonatal polycythemia and hyperviscosity, *Semin Fetal Neonatal Med* 13(4):248-255, 2008.

Schanler RJ: The evidence for breastfeeding, *Pediatr Clin North Am* 48(1):207-219, 2001.

Schanler RJ, Shulman RJ, Lau C, et al: Feeding strategies for premature infants: randomized trial of gastrointestinal priming and tube-feeding method, *Pediatrics* 103(2):434-439, 1999.

Schempf AH: Illicit drug use and neonatal outcomes: a critical review. *Obstet Gynecol Surv* 62(11):749-757, 2007.

Schuler ME, Nair P: Brief report: frequency of maternal cocaine use during pregnancy and infant neurobehavioral outcome, *J Pediatr Psychol* 24(6):511-514, 1999.

Schurr P, Perkins EM. The relationship between feeding and necrotizing enterocolitis in very low birth weight infants, *Neonat Netw* 27(6):397-407, 2008.

Shah PS: Current perspectives on the prevention and management of chronic lung disease in preterm infants, *Pediatr Drugs* 5(7):463-468, 2003.

Shah V, Ohlsson A. Venepuncture versus heel lance for blood sampling in term neonates, *Cochrane Database Syst Rev* 17(4):CD001452, 2007a.

Shah PS, Ohlsson A: Sildenafil for pulmonary hypertension in neonates, *Cochrane Database Syst Rev* 18(3):CD005494, 2007b.

Shea AK, Steiner M: Cigarette smoking during pregnancy, *Nicotine Tob Res* 10(2):267-278, 2008.

Short EJ, Klein NK, Lewis BA, et al: Cognitive and academic consequences of bronchopulmonary dysplasia and very low birth weight: 8-year-old outcomes, *Pediatrics* 112(5):e359, 2003.

Simchen MJ, Goldstein G, Lubetsky A, et al: Factor V Leiden and antiphospholipid antibodies in either mothers or infants increase the risk for perinatal arterial ischemic stroke, *Stroke* 40(1):65-70, 2009.

Singer LT, Minnes S, Short E, et al: Cognitive outcomes of preschool children with prenatal cocaine exposure, *JAMA* 291(20):2448-2456, 2004.

Sisk PM, Lovelady CA, Gruber KJ, et al: Early human milk feeding is associated with a lower risk of necrotizing enterocolitis in very low birth weight infants, *J Perinatol* 27(7): 428-433, 2007.

Smith LM, Lagasse LL, Derauf C, et al: Prenatal methamphetamine use and neonatal neurobehavioral outcome, *Neurotoxicol Teratol* 30(1):20-28, 2008.

Smith L, Yonekura ML, Wallace T, et al: Effects of prenatal methamphetamine exposure on fetal growth and drug withdrawal symptoms in infants born at term, *J Dev Behav Pediatr* 24(1):17-23, 2003.

Soll RF: Synthetic surfactant for respiratory distress syndrome in preterm infants. *Cochrane Database Syst Rev* (2):CD001149, 2000.

Soll RF, Blanco F: Natural surfactant extract versus synthetic surfactant for neonatal respiratory distress syndrome. *Cochrane Database Syst Rev* (2):CD000144, 2001.

Sood B, Delaney-Black V, Covington C, et al: Prenatal alcohol exposure and childhood behavior at age 6 to 7 years, part I, Dose-response effect, *Pediatrics* 108(2):e34, 2001.

Steinhorn RH, Kinsella JP, Pierce C, et al: Intravenous sildenafil in the treatment of neonates with persistent pulmonary hypertension, *J Pediatr* 155(6): 841-847, 2009.

Stephens BE, Walden RV, Gargus RA, et al: First week protein and energy intakes are associated with 18-month developmental scores in extremely low-birth-weight infants. *Pediatrics* 123(5):1337-1343, 2009.

Stokowski L: A primer on apnea of prematurity, *Adv Neonatal Care* 5(3):155-170, 2005.

Stoler JM, Holmes LB: Recognition of facial features of fetal alcohol syndrome in the newborn, *Am J Med Genet C Semin Med Genet* 127(1):21-27, 2004.

Stoll BJ: Infections of the neonatal infant. In Kliegman RM, Behrman RE, Jenson HB, et al, editors: *Nelson textbook of pediatrics*, ed 18, Philadelphia, 2007, Saunders.

Stoll BJ, Hansen NI, Higgins RD, et al: Very low birth weight preterm infants with early onset neonatal sepsis: the predominance of gram-negative infections continues in the National Institute of Child Health and Human Development Neonatal Research Network, 2002-2003, *Pediatr Infect Dis J* 24(7):635-639, 2005.

Substance Abuse and Mental Health Services Administration: Substance use during pregnancy: 2002-2003 update. NSDUH Report. Rockville, Md, June 2, 2005, The Administration.

Symington A, Pinelli J: Developmental care for promoting development and preventing morbidity in preterm infants. *Cochrane Database Syst Rev* (2):CD001814, 2006.

Tanney MR, Lowenstein V: One-stop shopping: description of a model program to provide primary care to substance-abusing women and their children, *J Pediatr Health Care* 11(1):20-25, 1997.

Taylor JA, Loan LA, Kamara J, et al: Medication administration variances before and after implementation of computerized physician order entry in a neonatal intensive care unit, *Pediatrics* 121(1):123-128, 2008.

Terrin G, Passariello A, Canani RB, et al: Minimal enteral feeding reduces the risk of sepsis in feed-intolerant very low birth weight newborns, *Acta Paediatr* 98(2):31-35, 2009.

Thompson AM, Bizzarro MJ: Necrotizing enterocolitis in newborns: pathogenesis, prevention and management, *Drugs* 68(9): 1227-1238, 2008.

Thoyre SM, Shaker CS, Pridham KF: The early feeding skills assessment for preterm infants, *Neonat Netw* 24(3):7-16, 2005.

Tomashek KM, Shapiro-Mendoza CK, Davidoff MJ, et al: Differences in mortality between late-preterm and term singleton infants in the United States, 1995-2002, *J Pediatr* 151(5):450-456, 2007.

Tronick EZ, Beeghly M: Prenatal cocaine exposure, child development, and the compromising effects of cumulative risk, *Clin Perinatol* 26(1):151-171, 1999.

Tyson JE, Kennedy KA: Trophic feedings for parenterally fed infants. *Cochrane Database Syst Rev* (3):CD000504, 2005.

Tyson JE, Kennedy KA, Lucke JF, et al: Dilemmas initiating enteral feedings in high risk infants: how can they be resolved? *Semin Perinatol* 31(2):61-73, 2007.

Vaivre-Douret L, Ennouri K, Jrad I, et al: Effect of positioning on the incidence of abnormalities of muscle tone in low-risk, preterm infants, *Eur J Paediatr Neurol* 8(1):21-34, 2004.

van Baar AL, van Wassenaer AG, Briet JM, et al: Very preterm birth is associated with disabilities in multiple developmental domains, *Pediatr Psychol* 30(3):247-255, 2005.

van Gelder MM, Reefhuis J, Caton AR, et al: National Birth Defects Prevention Study: maternal periconceptional illicit drug use and the risk of congenital malformations, *Epidemiology* 20(1):60-66, 2009.

Ventre KM, Arnold JH: High frequency oscillatory ventilation in acute respiratory failure, *Paediatr Respir Rev* 5(4):323-332, 2004.

Verder H, Bohlin K, Kamper J, et al. Nasal CPAP and surfactant for treatment of respiratory distress syndrome and prevention of bronchopulmonary dysplasia, *Acta Paediatr* 98(9):1400-1408, 2009.

Verklan MT: The chilling details: hypoxic-ischemic encephalopathy, *J Perinat Neonatal Nurs* 23(1):59-68, 2009.

Vertanen H, Fellman V, Brommels M, et al: An automatic incision device for obtaining blood samples from the heels of preterm infants causes less damage than a conventional manual lancet, *Arch Dis Child Fetal Neonatal Ed* 84(1):F53-F55, 2001.

Vickers A, Ohlsson A, Lacy JB, et al: Massage for promoting growth and development of preterm and/or low birth-weight infants. *Cochrane Database Syst Rev* (2):CD000390, 2004.

Vohr BR, Widen JE, Cone-Wesson B, et al: Neurodevelopmental and functional outcomes of extremely low birth weight infants in the National Institute of Child Health and Human Development Neonatal Research Network, 1993-1994, *Pediatrics* 105(6):1216-1226, 2000.

Volante E, Moretti S, Pisani F, et al: Early diagnosis of bacterial infection in the neonate, *J Matern Fetal Med* 16(Suppl 2):13-16, 2004.

Volpe JJ: *Neurology of the newborn*, ed 5, Philadelphia, 2008, Saunders.

Wagner C, Katikaneni LD, Cox TH, et al: The impact of prenatal drug exposure on the neonate, *Obstet Gynecol Clin North Am* 25(1):169-194, 1998.

Walsh MC, Fanaroff AA: Epidemiology and perinatal services. In Martin RM, Fanaroff AA, Walsh MC, editors: *Neonatal-perinatal medicine: diseases of the fetus and infant*, ed 8, St Louis, 2006, Mosby.

Wang ML, Dorer DJ, Fleming MP, et al: Clinical outcomes of near-term infants, *Pediatrics* 114(2):372-376, 2004.

Ward K: Perceived needs of parents of critically ill infants in a neonatal intensive care unit (NICU), *Pediatr Nurs* 27(3):281-286, 2001.

Ward-Larson C, Horn RA, Gosnell F: The efficacy of facilitated tucking for relieving procedural pain of endotracheal suctioning in very low birthweight infants, *MCN Am J Matern Child Nurs* 29(3):151-156, 2004.

Welch-Carre E: The neurodevelopmental consequences of prenatal exposure, *Adv Neonat Care* 5(4):217-229, 2005.

Wijnberger LD, Huisjes AJ, Voorbij HA, et al: The accuracy of lamellar body count and lecithin/sphyngomyelin ratio in the prediction of neonatal respiratory distress syndrome: a meta-analysis, *Br J Obstet Gynecol* 108(6): 583-588, 2001.

Wilson-Costello D: Is there evidence that long-term outcomes have improved with intensive care? *Semin Fetal Neonatal Med* 12(5):344-354, 2007.

Winecker RE, Goldberger BA, Tebbett IR, et al: Detection of cocaine and its metabolites in breast milk, *J Forens Sci* 46(5):1221-1223, 2001.

Wiswell TE: Expanded uses of surfactant therapy, *Clin Perinatol* 28(3):695-711, 2001.

Wood BR: Physiologic principles. In Goldsmith JP, Karotkin EH, editors: *Assisted ventilation of the neonate*, ed 4, Philadelphia, 2003, Saunders.

Zahr LK, Balian S: Responses of premature infants to routine nursing interventions and noise in the NICU, *Nurs Res* 44(3):179-185, 1995.

Zaichkin J: *Newborn Intensive Care: What Every Parent Needs to Know*, ed 3, Elk Grove Village, Ill, 2009, American Academy of Pediatrics.

Conditions Caused by Defects in Physical Development

David Wilson, Barbara Montagnino, and Kristina Wilson

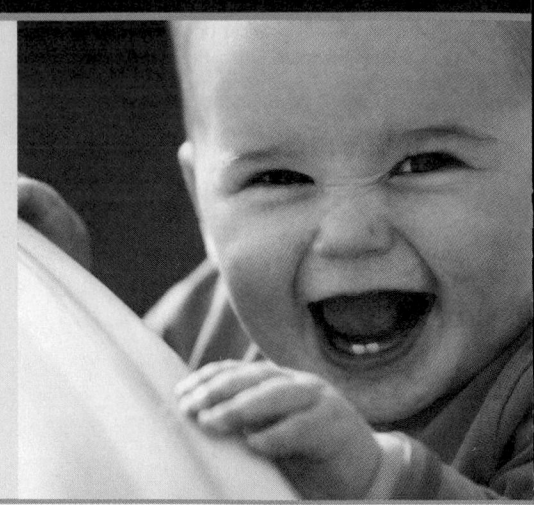

evolve WEBSITE

http://evolve.elsevier.com/wong/ncic

Animation
  Ventriculoperitoneal Shunt
Case Studies
  Cleft Lip and Palate
  Developmental Dysplasia of the Hip
  Hydrocephalus with Myelomeningocele
Critical Thinking Exercise
  Myelomeningocele
Key Points Audio Summaries
NCLEX Review Questions
Pediatric Assessment Video Clips
Spanish/English Translations
WebLinks

RELATED TOPICS

Alternative Feeding Techniques, **Ch. 27**
Anaphylaxis, **Ch. 29**
Assessment (Newborn), **Ch. 8**
Autosomal Inheritance Patterns, **Ch. 5**
Birth Injuries, **Ch. 9**
Birthmarks, **Ch. 9**
Cerebral Palsy, **Ch. 40**
Family-Centered Home Care, **Ch. 25**
Health Promotion of the Newborn and Family, **Ch. 8**
The High-Risk Newborn and Family, **Ch. 10**
Hypertrophic Pyloric Stenosis, **Ch. 33**
Multifactorial Disorders, **Ch. 5**
Neonatal Pain, **Ch. 7**
Osteogenesis Imperfecta, **Ch. 39**
Pain Assessment; Pain Management, **Ch. 7**
Preparation for Diagnostic and Therapeutic Procedures; Surgical Procedures, **Ch. 27**
Promotion of Parent-Infant Bonding (Attachment), **Ch. 8**

CHAPTER OUTLINE

DEFECTS IN PHYSICAL DEVELOPMENT

Congenital malformations, also called congenital anomalies or birth defects, may be caused by genetic or environmental factors, but not all congenital defects are malformations (e.g., inborn errors of metabolism that cause neurocognitive impairment). However, this chapter is primarily concerned with structural abnormalities and with the impact on the family of the birth of a child with a physical defect. The genetic basis of physical defects is discussed in Chapter 5, and other specific disorders are presented as appropriate throughout the book.

PRENATAL DEVELOPMENT

Fetal Growth and Differentiation

Development consists of two distinct but interrelated processes: growth and differentiation. Growth results when cells divide and synthesize new proteins and is reflected in increased size and weight. It is accomplished by two mechanisms: (1) hyperplasia (increase in cell number) and (2) hypertrophy (increase in cell size). Hyperplasia is the predominant form of growth during the embryonic period. Although the rate slows during later stages of gestation, cell division continues in variable degrees throughout childhood. Hypertrophy is more prominent during later periods of growth.

Each organ and tissue has a typical growth pattern, and all organs progress from a stage characterized by an increase in cell number to one of growth by increase in cell size. Any interference with this pattern of growth results in a reduction in the size and weight of that organ. However, the consequences of the inhibiting factor depend on whether the insult is inflicted during a period of hyperplasia or during a period of hypertrophy. Interference with growth during a period of cell proliferation is likely to cause irreversible growth restriction of that organ with a permanent deficit in overall cell numbers. Interruption of growth during cell enlargement is usually only temporary and can be overcome with proper intervention.

Differentiation is the process by which early cells are systematically modified and specialized to form all the tissues necessary to ensure an organized, coordinated individual. Each step in this process depends on successful completion of a previous step. Anything that interferes with one of these steps, such as a mutant gene or environmental agent, will cause an arrest in the development of that particular tissue or organ. Divergence from the normal course of development will result in maldevelopment of a part or, if it occurs at an early age, a sequence of distortions causing more severe or multiple malformations.

A relationship appears to exist between the incidence of one congenital anomaly and the presence of additional anomalies in an affected child. For example, malformed ears and kidney abnormalities have an association that reflects an event occurring at a common developmental stage. Knowledge of the stage of development for a variety of organs and systems provides a valuable clue for the examiner. When one defect is observed, closer scrutiny may reveal defects in another organ or system related to the same stage of development.

Extremely rapid development and change take place during the first 8 to 12 weeks of fetal life, and the beginnings of all major organ systems are formed (organogenesis). The embryo begins to acquire the specific functions needed to integrate these organs and organ systems into an organized, coordinated whole. It is also the period during which the organism is most vulnerable to structural disturbance from environmental hazards.

Sensitive Periods in Prenatal Development

Every organ, system, and body part goes through a period during which it experiences the most rapid cell division and differentiation. During this time the organism displays a marked susceptibility to injurious influences. These specific stages of crucial developmental advancement are termed sensitive or critical periods, and the major impact of environmental factors on development always coincides with these periods. The origin or method by which prenatal growth processes are disturbed to produce a structural or functional defect is termed teratogenesis (from the Greek *teratos*, "monster," and *genesis*, "production"). An agent capable of producing such an effect is a teratogen. (See Problems Caused by Perinatal Environmental Factors, Chapter 9.)

The sensitive periods for all organs or parts do not occur simultaneously. A part that is susceptible to adverse influences at one particular time may be resistant to the same influences at other periods of development, while another part may be highly sensitive at that moment. Susceptibility to environmental influences decreases as organ formation advances—the younger the organism and the fewer the cells, the greater is the extent of involvement when an adverse influence is applied.

During the period of intensive differentiation, most teratogenic agents are highly effective and may produce a variety of deformities. The type of defect produced depends on which organ is most susceptible at the time of application. The susceptibility of most tissues to teratogenic influences decreases rapidly in the later periods of development, which are characterized by growth and elaboration of established organs. However, some tissues, particularly those of the central nervous system (CNS), are sensitive to varying degrees throughout fetal life and even beyond. Fig. 11-1 illustrates the approximate times of critical differentiation for some of the major organs and systems.

BIRTH OF A CHILD WITH A PHYSICAL DEFECT

Parental Responses

Part of the preparation for childbirth involves fantasies and images of the expected infant. Normally, parents hope for a perfect child, but at the same time they fear that the infant will be abnormal. Parents often express this fear when they state that their concern is not whether the child is a girl or a boy, but just that the infant is healthy. One of the first things the mother wants confirmed at the time of birth is: "Is my baby all right?" In many instances some discrepancy exists between the parents' idealized child and the infant the mother delivers, as, for example, the birth of a boy when they had hoped for a girl. Resolution of this discrepancy is a developmental task of parenthood and is essential to the establishment of a healthy parent-child relationship. If this discrepancy is major, as when the infant has a birth defect or the wishes of the parents are unrealistic, the resulting emotional stress may be overwhelming.

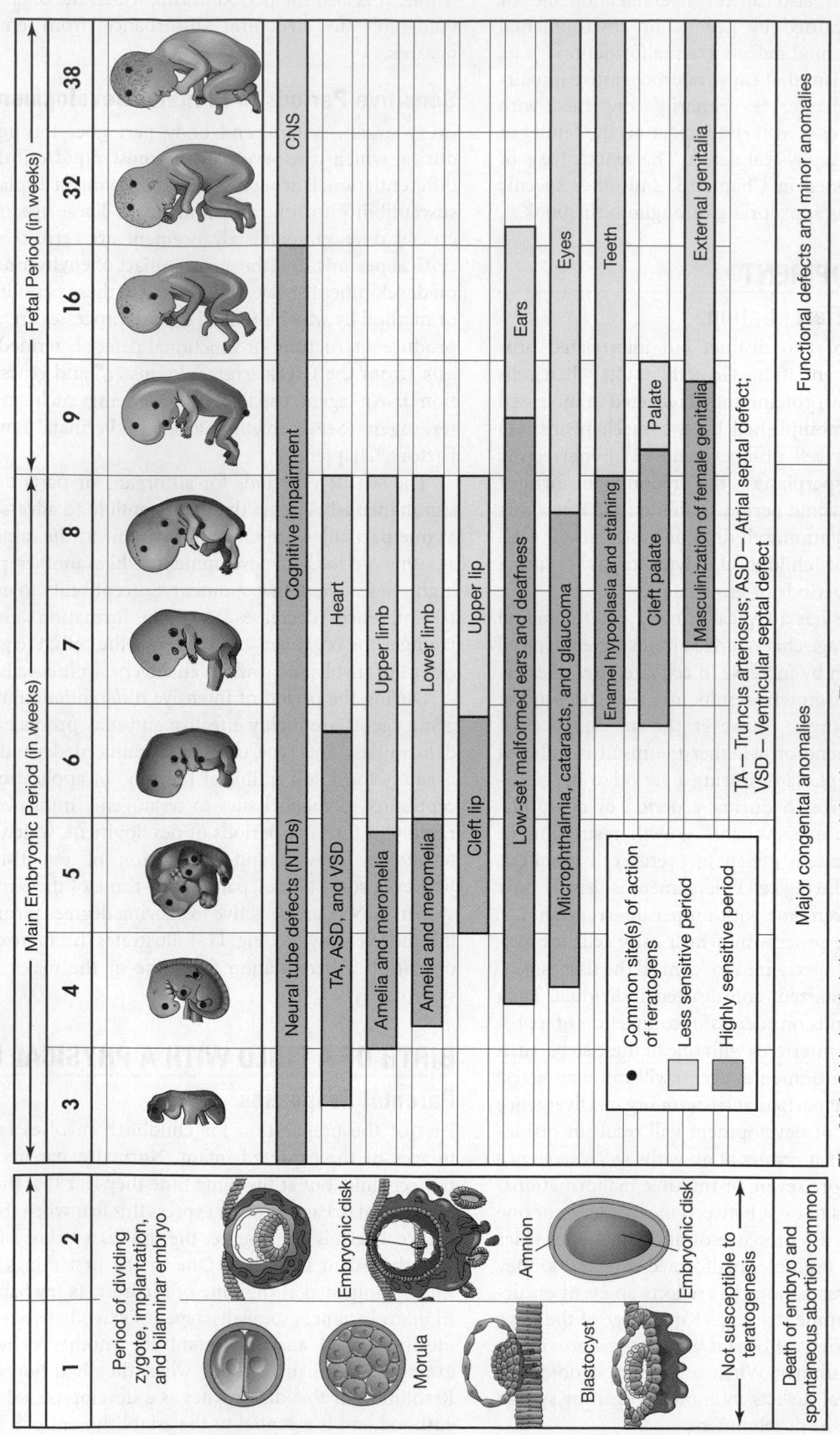

Fig. 11-1 Critical periods in human prenatal development. The mauve areas denote highly sensitive periods, when major defects may be produced. The green sections indicate stages that are less sensitive to teratogens, when minor defects may be induced. *CNS,* Central nervous system. (Modified from Moore KL, Persaud TVN: *Before we are born: essentials of embryology and birth defects,* ed 7, Philadelphia, 2008, Saunders.)

The more severe the defect, the greater the impact of the experience, especially for the mother. The birth of a child with a physical imperfection abruptly ends the psychologic attachment the mother has formed during pregnancy with the idealized child. She and the father must now deal with loss of the anticipated healthy child while they face meeting the demands of the affected child for care and affection. The birth of an infant with a defect evokes the same psychologic reaction as the death of a child. The parents' need to grieve for the loss of the expected child while adapting to the care of the child with a disability places overwhelming demands on them at a time when their own psychologic and physiologic resources have been depleted by the birth experience. The impact of this new and unexpected burden inhibits the accomplishment of the grief work that normally follows a loss.

The grief reaction experienced by parents at the birth of a child with a physical disability is the same as the response that follows the loss of any valued or significant object. The parents experience shock, frustration, and anger at what has happened to them, and they ask themselves, "Why? Why me?" Parents may feel shame and embarrassment, often with feelings of personal failure and guilt. Frequently the mother believes that she might have caused harm to the unborn child, and she may associate the condition with wrongdoing or evil thoughts, especially if the pregnancy was unwanted initially. She may believe the defect to be a result of passive or active attempts to terminate the pregnancy, such as deliberate attempts to induce abortion or failure to obtain prenatal care or comply with the practitioner's instructions. The father may react to the situation by becoming withdrawn from the newborn and the mother. Anger is common, and parents may direct it at health care workers involved in the child's care. Inwardly the father may blame himself for the child's "imperfection" yet project that blame to others. The mother may not understand the father's withdrawal, and this may compound her distress.

The phase of overwhelming shock is accompanied by weeping and feelings of helplessness. To deal with stress and anxiety, parents use defense mechanisms that have provided protection in the past. A common response is disbelief and denial, which may be short lived or may last for many months. They do not appear to "hear" what is told to them about their child, and they behave as though nothing is wrong with the child. Denial during the shock phase of the grief process can serve as a constructive means for parents to deal with the sudden and profound impact of the initial stress until they are better able to cope with the situation.

When parents are unable to face the reality of the infant's condition, they may withdraw from the situation either physically or emotionally. They frequently become incapacitated and unable to function in their usual manner. They may avoid interpersonal contacts. Unable to face relatives and friends for fear of the reactions they may encounter, parents choose the protection of isolation. They feel as though they are alone in a world all their own. Avoidance behaviors on the part of others, including health workers, contribute to this withdrawal and compound the loneliness that is so common in parents of an affected infant.

Parents may extend this avoidance behavior to include each other or the infant. They may seem unable to face the infant, and visits may become sporadic or nonexistent. It may take time for the parents to master their own feelings before they are able to deal constructively with the situation. A more subtle form of isolation occurs in parents who are objective in their behavior toward the infant and the defect. They are intellectually concerned with the infant's medical care but display no emotional involvement. Their attention is focused on the abnormality, not on the infant.

Parental reactions vary and include guilt, anger, anxiety, and sadness, which often last for years and depend to a large extent on the type and severity of the defect. A visible anomaly, especially one involving the face, usually elicits a more intense emotional response than one that is less apparent, such as a heart defect. The extent of the impairment does not determine the degree of parental reactions. Because of their limited contact with congenital defects, parents' perception of the abnormality and its implications may be distorted, and much depends on previous feelings they may have experienced with a similar abnormality. Therefore their reactions may seem out of proportion to the actual extent and severity of the impairment as viewed by health professionals.

Nursing Care Management

The attitudes and behaviors of nurses and other health care providers at the birth of a child with a birth defect significantly influence the effect of the situation on the parents. During this time parents are particularly sensitive and responsive to the behaviors of those with whom they are in contact. Therefore the reactions of health professionals toward the infant and the parents provide cues to the parents that can affect their feelings toward the infant and themselves. Parents exert the greatest influence on the child's growth and development, and their initial relationship with the child significantly affects the subsequent course of interaction.

Initial Contact

The first indication that all is not well often occurs at the time of delivery. The atmosphere of happy anticipation suddenly changes to one laden with anxiety. Even when the mother is unable to see the infant, she may be terrifyingly aware of the heightened tension in the room, which conveys to her that something is seriously wrong. Health professionals, unprepared for this disturbing experience, find it difficult to cope with their own feelings and react with frustration and resentment toward a situation that they are powerless to change. As a result, they may forget about or retreat from the parents, who at this moment are suffering the most.

Most practitioners believe it is their responsibility to inform the parents of a congenital anomaly. At the time of delivery, unless a pediatrician or nurse practitioner is in attendance, there is a delay while the practitioner is involved with the mother's care. During this period the mother, unable to see her child and feeling the tense atmosphere, will believe either that the child is normal but that others do not share her enthusiasm or that the child has a defect that is so terrible the professional people in the room are unable to talk about it. A nurse, the person who is most likely to be free to support the mother and who is familiar with most common congenital anomalies, can make truthful statements about the defect.

The manner in which nurses present the infant to the parents may well set the tone for the early parent-child relationship. It is probably best to explain briefly, in simple language, the nature of the defect and to reinforce and help clarify information given by the practitioner before the infant is shown to them. At this time they are more likely to "hear" what is said. Parents attach a great deal of meaning to the behavior of others during this critical period and will watch the facial expressions of others closely for signs of revulsion or rejection. Presenting the infant as something precious and emphasizing the well-formed aspects of the infant's body provide some reassurance to parents during this crisis period.

It is important to allow time and opportunity for the parents to express their initial response to the situation. Many issues may surface, such as the importance placed on this particular infant or the cultural significance of one sex over the other. Encourage parents to ask questions and to receive honest, straightforward answers without undue optimism or pessimism.

Family Support

Parents need time to grieve for the loss of the expected child before they are able to form an emotional attachment to the child they have. It is a nursing responsibility to help parents with their grief work and to facilitate the formation of a satisfactory adjustment to the child with a defect. They need help to see their infant as a person, support in coping with their situation, and guidance in physical care of the child.

Nurses who understand the grief response will be prepared to support the parents through this necessary process. This is particularly important with the birth of a child with a defect, since the parents may not begin to invest any feeling for the child until they are able to talk about and work through their feelings of disappointment, resentment, guilt, and helplessness. The supportive nurse creates and maintains an atmosphere that encourages expression of feelings. Open expression is difficult for many people, and the parent(s) may hesitate to display intense feelings. Containing those feelings expends considerable energy that would be better used later on to develop a relationship with the infant. Nurses therefore need to listen closely for cues that indicate areas of discomfort or readiness to talk.

Parents may not be ready to talk about their feelings during the first few days after the birth. Their dream has vanished, and when others avoid them, they often interpret it as another abandonment. Staying near and available tells them that they are not alone and that someone cares about them and their feelings. What is said to them is also important. Clichés such as "You will be able to have more children" or "It could be a lot worse" are not a comfort to the parents. Such behavior implies that this infant is not important, and this behavior may destroy the parents' trust. Parents may also attach inordinate significance to statements made by a health care worker about the prognosis of the infant; such statements may be recalled by the parent years later.

Initiating a discussion about matters that were of concern to others in a similar situation may help the parents to know that their feelings are natural. Parents need to be allowed silence and solitude if this is their wish. The parents are likely to be angry and often direct this anger at anyone nearby—physicians, nurses, friends, and families who have normal children. Directing their frustrations at a nonjudgmental target helps parents relieve some of their distress. Nurses must be prepared to accept any or all of the parental reactions and defenses—anger, hostility, rejection, dependency—without showing anger or withdrawing from the situation. If nurses make themselves available to the parents for support, they can often find nonthreatening ways to help and comfort. Most important, nurses need to promote communication and understanding within the family and help strengthen family interpersonal relationships.

Care of the Infant

Many parents are uneasy about handling their infant and require support and encouragement in their caregiving tasks. These parents need a longer period of dependency to muster their resources for coping. Although they should not feel forced to care for the infant until they are ready for the responsibility, they should be given opportunities to assume care as soon as possible to help them deal with the reality of the infant's condition. Parents' responses are highly individual and must be evaluated on this premise. However, all parents need sympathetic, patient, and understanding help to gain feelings of adequacy in the care of their child and to facilitate development of a positive relationship with the infant later on. As anxiety and the intensity of emotional responses decrease, parents begin to feel more comfortable with the infant and more confident in their ability to provide needed care.

Supplying Information

Parents need accurate, up-to-date information given to them early and in language they can understand. Because they do not hear everything the first time it is said, they need careful, repeated explanations about the child's defect, the treatments outlined, and what will be expected of them. Parents often misinterpret information, another reason for repeated explanations. Often the nurse's responsibility is to explain, interpret, and clarify and to answer questions about information that the practitioner has given. Following the basic concepts of informational needs assessment, the nurse determines what the parents know and proceeds from that point. One cannot assume that the parents' failure to ask questions means they understand. Most parents have little or no knowledge of basic anatomy or physiology; therefore use pictures and other tangible visual aids to explain both normal and deviant structures.

Teaching the parents to provide the special care that is frequently required for an infant with a physical defect is an important nursing responsibility. Nurses need to explain and demonstrate special feeding, holding, and positioning techniques. Anticipatory guidance regarding problems that are unique to each condition reduces apprehension and stimulates the parents to institute preventive measures and to make alert observations.

Numerous agencies and organizations offer services to families of children with congenital defects. Some provide services for a variety of conditions; others are devoted to specific disorders. They help families with ongoing problems and with anticipating problems, including financial burdens, they will encounter in raising a child with a defect. Many have local support groups. All have unique and specialized services to support the family and aid parents in problem solving. Among those that include most types of defects and conditions are the Easter Seals,* the March of Dimes,† and Birth Defect Research for Children, Inc.,‡ most of which have branches in all major cities and communities. The Centers for Disease Control and Prevention, National Center on Birth Defects and Developmental Disabilities has a website with information on birth defects.§

NURSING CARE OF THE SURGICAL NEONATE

Advances in early detection of defects (including prenatal diagnosis), surgical techniques, and anesthesia have made it possible for correction or amelioration of many physical defects in the newborn period. Fortunately, most malformations, even those with a dramatic presentation, are correctable with a high degree of success.

Preoperative Care

Most of the problems encountered with the infant undergoing surgery are discussed in relation to the high-risk infant (e.g., airway maintenance, cardiovascular support, thermoregulation, fluid and electrolyte balance, and nutritional needs). Electronic monitoring of cardiovascular and respiratory status is implemented and maintained, as are regular comprehensive assessments. (See Assessment, Chapter 10.) Monitoring and assessments are continued in the postoperative period. Some congenital defects are often associated with other anomalies; therefore assessment should include careful observation for evidence of complications related to these.

Before surgery the infant usually requires peripheral intravenous (IV) access for fluids and glucose. Any electrolyte problems, acid-base imbalance, and anemia are corrected. In some instances a blood product such as packed red blood cells or whole blood is placed on reserve in case blood loss is anticipated. Prophylactic antibiotic administration may begin before surgery, and the infant is observed and monitored for any evidence of infection. In addition to routine care, special attention is directed to specific defects, such as abdominal decompression, protection and management of open wounds, and specific measurements (e.g., abdominal girth, head dimensions). (See also discussion of specific defects.) A preoperative assessment of the infant's behavior is essential because postoperative deviations may be a manifestation of pain or unstable condition.

Compounding the initial shock of having an infant born with a physical defect, the parents are often further traumatized by the prospect of surgery, sometimes shortly after birth. Health care personnel provide parents with accurate information regarding the type of surgical procedure anticipated, method of anesthesia, and, most important, what to expect post-

operatively. (Parents are sometimes mentally unprepared for the infant's appearance postoperatively; some may have false hopes or expectations that the infant will be perfect in appearance after surgery.) The nurse also assures parents that the infant's pain management needs will be evaluated and met postoperatively.

When an infant is transported to a tertiary center for surgery shortly after birth, it is helpful for the nurse to stay in contact with the parents, especially the mother, regarding the infant's condition. Photographs and even videos, when possible, are helpful tools to relieve the mother's anxiety; without seeing her infant and without adequate communication, the mother's anxiety and fears about her infant's condition may be far worse than the reality. During this time the father may serve as the vital link of information between the mother, siblings, and the tertiary center where the infant is undergoing surgery.

Postoperative Care

Surgery imposes significant stresses on the neonate, especially the preterm or ill infant. The assessment and observations remain much the same as for preoperative care, with the additional problems related to surgery, such as anesthesia and pain. It is essential to maintain physiologic stability to avoid undesirable consequences. Because the neonate is subject to many adverse effects of stress in all physiologic parameters, continual vigilance is mandatory.

Many of the physiologic problems to which the neonate is vulnerable are discussed in relation to assessment and nursing care of the normal newborn (Chapter 8) and the high-risk infant (Chapter 10). Optimum ventilation, cardiac function, thermoregulation, fluid regulation, care of the operative site, and pain management are primary concerns (Table 11-1). Table 11-2 further outlines some of the possible reactions, their probable cause, and the nursing responsibilities.

Because of the respiratory characteristics of newborns, some compromising responses may occur. The newborn's poor chest wall stability, smaller and more reactive airways, fewer and smaller alveoli, and poorly developed accessory muscles contribute to respiratory dysfunction. Compression by intrapleural fluid, air, blood, or a distended abdomen can further compromise pulmonary efforts. Respiratory distress is a common problem in preterm infants. Many postoperative neonates require mechanical ventilation, which may be further influenced by the type, duration, and urgency of the surgery. Neonates are highly subject to acidosis and hypoxia and require continuous monitoring of oxygen and acid-base status. Preterm infants require close monitoring for respiratory complications from general anesthesia.

Cardiovascular support is of particular importance because the immature sympathetic innervation of the myocardium makes the neonate sensitive to vagal stimulation induced by many postoperative procedures, such as nasogastric (NG) tubes, endotracheal (ET) tubes, and tracheal suctioning. The nurse notes any evidence of early compensation for diminished cardiac output and implements interventions before decompensation occurs.

Careful management of fluid and electrolyte status is vital to neonatal surgical care. The natural tendency for rapid fluid shifts related to characteristics of the neonate (see Chapter 28)

*223 S. Wacker Drive, Suite 2400, Chicago, IL 60606-4802; 800-221-6827; **www.easterseals.com**. In Canada, **www.easterseals.org**.
†1275 Mamaroneck Ave., White Plains, NY 10605; 914-997-4488, 914-997-4488; **www.marchofdimes.com**. In Canada, **www.marchofdimes.ca**.
‡800 Celebration Ave., Suite 225, Celebration, FL 34747; 407-566-8304; e-mail: staff@birthdefects.org; **www.birthdefects.org**.
§1600 Clifton Road, Atlanta, GA 30333; 800-CDC-INFO; **www.cdc.gov/ncbddd/index.html**.

TABLE 11-1   CRITICAL GUIDELINES FOR NEONATAL POSTOPERATIVE CARE

NURSING RESPONSIBILITIES	RATIONALE
Airway Maintenance* Monitor respirations, especially if infant is extubated. Monitor oxygenation with pulse oximetry and arterial blood gases as necessary. Monitor and observe color.	Effects of anesthetics, surgery, and pain may decrease respiratory effort; alteration in acid-base balance may reflect early respiratory or metabolic response to surgical interventions.
Circulation* Monitor heart rate. Monitor peripheral perfusion; note color and temperature of extremities; capillary refill should be 2-3 sec. Monitor blood pressure.	Decrease in cardiac output may be seen peripherally before decrease in blood pressure because of compensatory mechanisms.
Fluids, Electrolytes, and Glucose Evaluate hydration status (overhydration versus dehydration) by weighing neonate postoperatively. Monitor electrolytes. Perform bedside glucose monitoring using glucometer.	Increase or decrease in fluids given intraoperatively is reflected in weight before external signs of hydration are evident. Change in electrolyte status often indicates hydration status. Stress response to surgery may be evidenced by elevated serum glucose; bedside monitoring is faster than laboratory analysis; physician's order may not be necessary.
Thermoregulation* Maintain neutral thermal environment. Monitor axillary temperature.	Effects of anesthetics, exposure to cold, and metabolic response to surgery may decrease body temperature.
Operative Site Observe surgical site and skin status. Observe dressings for drainage, bleeding, and amount of output from drainage tubes.	Loss of blood may require transfusion; chest tubes, catheters, gastrostomies not draining properly may impair operative site and status.
Pain Management Assess need for analgesics with neonatal pain scale (see Pain in Neonates, Chapter 7). Implement comfort measures. Administer analgesics as needed to prevent pain (see Pain Management, Chapter 7).	Neonate may not be capable of demonstrating pain response but is capable of perceiving pain. Major surgery without adequate anesthetics and analgesics can increase postoperative mortality and morbidity.

*Suggested interval for monitoring vital signs postoperatively in neonate: every 15 min for 4 hr; every 30 min for 2 hr; every 1 hr for 6 hr; then every 2 hr for 24 hr. More frequent monitoring may be needed based on nurse's judgment of infant's status.

TABLE 11-2   POSSIBLE EFFECTS OF SURGERY ON SELECTED SYSTEMS

PHYSIOLOGIC RESPONSE	NURSING RESPONSIBILITY
Cardiovascular System Hypotension related to: • Large doses of anesthetic • Vasodilation (narcotics) • Myocardial depression (anesthetic agents) • Impaired venous return Hypertension related to: • Hypervolemia, pain, hypercarbia • Increased intracranial pressure (ICP), vasoconstrictor drugs Tachycardia related to: • Compensation for hypovolemia • Pain • Certain drugs Bradycardia related to: • Hypoxemia (most common) • Vagal stimulation • Increased ICP (certain drugs) Vasoconstriction related to hypothermia	Observe for signs of low cardiac output: tachycardia, poor perfusion (prolonged capillary filling; normal is 2-3 sec in newborn), weak or absent peripheral pulses, decreased intensity of heart sounds, decreased urine specific gravity. Observe for signs of congestive heart failure: tachycardia, increased peripheral vasoconstriction (skin changes such as mottling), pulmonary venous engorgement (respiratory distress). Monitor laboratory data (glucose, electrolytes, acid-base balance, hemoglobin, hematocrit). Administer blood products, vasoactive drugs, cardiotonics as prescribed. Monitor and maintain fluid balance, including blood loss. Provide ventilatory support as needed.

TABLE 11-2	POSSIBLE EFFECTS OF SURGERY ON SELECTED SYSTEMS—cont'd
PHYSIOLOGIC RESPONSE	**NURSING RESPONSIBILITY**

Respiratory System

Increased respiratory rate related to physiologic characteristics

Airway obstruction related to:
- Bronchospasm
- Laryngeal edema
- Mucous plugs

Compressed lung tissue related to:
- Air, fluid, or blood in pleural cavities
- Anatomic defects of diaphragm
- Intrinsic pulmonary lesions

Ventilation/perfusion imbalance related to:
- Atelectasis
- Inadequate respiratory effort
- Pulmonary edema
- Pneumothorax

Hypoventilation related to:
- Termination of anesthesia
- Administration of narcotics, hypocarbia, cold stress, lack of surgical stimulus
- Extubation

Observe respiratory rate and symmetry, breath sounds (pitch, intensity, quality, duration, location), color, use of accessory muscles, signs of airway obstruction (decreased breath sounds, decreased P_{O_2}, respiratory distress, improper head alignment), signs of respiratory distress (marked retractions, nasal flaring, grunting, tachypnea, cyanosis), signs of impaired diaphragmatic movement (distended abdomen, constrictive dressings).

Monitor oxygenation/ventilation, laboratory data.

Administer oxygen in amount and manner prescribed.

Position for optimum ventilation.

Alleviate any impediment to diaphragmatic expansion.

Immune System

Subject to infection related to inability to generate rapid and effective immune defenses

Effects of anesthetics and surgery masking assessment data

Observe for evidence of sepsis (bradycardia, temperature instability, poor feeding, change in activity level, irregular respiration or apnea), gastrointestinal (GI) disturbances, evidence of abnormal clotting (bleeding from punctures, surgical sites).

Monitor for signs of pulmonary or cardiovascular compromise.

Monitor fluid administration to maintain vascular volume.

Administer antibiotics as ordered.

Endocrine System

Hypoglycemia related to:
- Surgical stress
- Rapid depletion of glycogen stores
- Decreased gluconeogenesis with stress

Hyperglycemia related to:
- Surgical stress
- Decreased insulin activity

Hypothermia

Hypocalcemia related to:
- Immaturity
- Stress
- Decreased parathyroid hormone secretion

Hypomagnesemia related to hypocalcemia

Observe for apnea, tachypnea, lethargy, pallor, tremors, or seizures.

Monitor serum glucose levels (bedside glucometer); verify abnormal values with laboratory sample.

Administer supplemental glucose as prescribed.

Monitor urinary output (1-2 ml/kg/hr).

Maintain neutral thermal environment.

Monitor serum calcium levels.

Observe for lethargy, vital sign instability, apnea, irritability, jitteriness, seizures.

Administer supplemental calcium if prescribed.

Observe for neuromuscular excitability (tetany, seizures).

Monitor serum magnesium levels in infants with above signs.

Renal System

Inability to concentrate urine and excrete waste related to:
- Immature renal function
- Decreased cardiac output
- Hypovolemia

Observe for amount and characteristics of urinary output.

Monitor renal function, drug levels, intravascular volume.

Gastrointestinal System

Abdominal distention related to:
- Hypoactive bowel
- Obstruction

Hypoactivity related to:
- Bowel surgery
- Peritonitis
- Perforation

Hyperactivity related to obstruction

Feeding modification related to GI surgery (see specific GI surgeries)

Monitor bowel sounds (hyperactivity or hypoactivity).

Observe for skin color and integrity (erythema of abdominal wall, prominent veins), abdominal distention (e.g., serial abdominal girth measurements).

Palpate abdomen for tenderness, organomegaly, evidence of masses.

Observe frequency, volume, and characteristics of vomiting and vomitus; frequency, volume, and characteristics of stools.

Delay enteral feedings if prescribed.

Monitor parenteral feedings and fluid therapy.

Provide alternative enteral feedings as prescribed (gavage, gastrostomy).

Begin and monitor oral feedings as prescribed.

Provide ostomy care if indicated.

Continued

TABLE 11-2   POSSIBLE EFFECTS OF SURGERY ON SELECTED SYSTEMS—cont'd

PHYSIOLOGIC RESPONSE	NURSING RESPONSIBILITY
Neurologic System Hypothermia (see Thermoregulation below) Seizures related to: • Hypoxemia • Hypoglycemia • Hypocalcemia Unresponsiveness Stress related to surgical procedure Pain (see Chapter 7)	See Thermoregulation below. Monitor serum calcium, glucose. Observe for any seizure activity, unresponsiveness, evidence of pain, signs of hypoglycemia or hypocalcemia (see Chapter 10). Administer sedatives, analgesics, antiepileptic drugs, glucose, calcium as prescribed.
Hematopoietic System Anemia related to blood loss Hyperviscosity related to: • Polycythemia • Decreased red blood cell deformability • Plasma protein abnormalities caused by third spacing Polycythemia related to chronic hypoxia Coagulation defects related to: • Inherited coagulation defects • Physiologic coagulation factor defects • Transitory coagulation disturbances • Platelet abnormalities	Monitor any blood loss. Monitor laboratory data. Administer blood or blood products as ordered. Observe for complications related to hematopoietic dysfunction and blood administration.
Fluid and Electrolyte Disturbances Abnormal fluid losses related to: • Blood loss • Fluid shifts (e.g., losses to interstitial tissues [third space]) • Transudated fluid • GI, renal, wounds, drains • Membrane injury from sepsis or injury • Insensible fluid losses from open wounds, exposed viscera, immature skin (prematurity)	Observe for evidence of dehydration or overhydration (see Chapter 28). Monitor laboratory data. Monitor blood pressure, central venous pressure. Weigh daily or more frequently as needed. Monitor vital signs. Monitor fluid and electrolyte administration. Administer albumin, electrolytes.
Acid-Base Balance Acid-base disturbance related to: • Cold stress • Respiratory embarrassment • GI disturbances • Infectious processes • Surgery • Immature buffering mechanisms Acidosis related to: • Ventilatory insufficiency (respiratory acidosis) • Ischemic tissue damage • Cold stress	Monitor acid-base status. Monitor respirations (see p. 396). Administer bicarbonate or other buffer as prescribed. Maintain neutral thermal environment (see Thermoregulation, below).
Thermoregulation Hypothermia related to: • Unstable regulatory mechanisms • Heat loss from large surface area, open wounds, defects • Depletion of glycogen stores and metabolism of brown fat • Immaturity of thermoregulation (see Thermoregulation, Chapter 10)	Monitor environmental and infant's core and skin temperatures. Maintain optimum thermal environment. Observe for evidence of hypothermia (peripheral vasoconstriction, apnea, cyanosis, decreased body temperature, respiratory distress, tachycardia). Minimize heat loss; conserve heat and provide external warmth as needed, including coverings for head and extremities. Warm any blood and irrigating solutions. Observe for seizure activity.

Data from Rushton CH: The surgical neonate: principles of nursing management, *Pediatr Nurs* 14:141-151, 1988.

may be aggravated by stress and any abnormal losses associated with some surgical procedures. (See Hydration, Chapter 10.)

Pain Management

During the postoperative period it is essential to assess and manage neonatal pain. This task is complicated by the vari-ability with which neonates respond to painful stimuli and the lack of physiologic responses that may occur as a result of anesthesia. The use of muscle-paralyzing agents may further mask physiologic manifestations of pain in the postoperative period. It is often noted that the more preterm or physiologically immature the infant, the more difficult it becomes to measure pain responses, particularly when major surgery is involved. Because infants of any gestational age are capable of experiencing pain and being adversely affected by it during and after operative procedures, it is important to advocate for appropriate pharmacologic therapy to improve neonatal pain. Both pharmacologic and nonpharmacologic pain management therapies may be used in the postoperative period to effectively reduce neonatal pain. (See Pain in Neonates, Chapter 7.)

MALFORMATIONS OF THE CENTRAL NERVOUS SYSTEM

DEFECTS OF NEURAL TUBE CLOSURE

Abnormalities that come from the embryonic neural tube (**neural tube defects [NTDs]**) constitute the largest group of congenital anomalies with multifactorial inheritance. Normally the spinal cord and cauda equina are encased in a protective sheath of bone and meninges (Fig. 11-2, *A*). Failure of neural tube closure produces defects of varying degrees (Box 11-1). They may involve the entire length of the neural tube or may be restricted to a small area.`

Etiology

Two of the defects, anencephaly and spina bifida (SB), occur in association with one another more often than would be expected by chance, suggesting a common origin. The CNS defects may alternate in siblings, which also tends to support the theory of a common origin. The incidence of SB is higher in girls than in boys, and it is three times more likely to occur in Caucasians than in African-Americans. In the United States, rates of NTDs declined by as much as 23% between 1995-1996 and 2000. NTD rates decreased an additional 6.9% between 2000 and 2005, primarily among African-American mothers. One concern is that NTD rates have not decreased among Hispanic and non-Hispanic Caucasian mothers since 1999 (Centers for Disease Control and Prevention, 2009). The decline in NTDs in the late 1990s has been attributed in large part to the addition of folic acid to cereal grain products (Honein, 2001). In 2005 the rates for SB were estimated by the Centers for Disease Control and Prevention to be 17.96 per 100,000 live births, thus making this one of the most common birth defects in the United States (Matthews, 2009; Wolff, Witkop, Miller, et al, 2009). Increased use of prenatal diagnostic techniques and termination of pregnancies have also affected the overall incidence of NTDs.

Most authorities believe that the primary defect in NTDs is a failure of neural tube closure during the embryo's early development (between the third and fourth week). However, evidence also implicates a multifactorial origin, including drugs, radiation, maternal malnutrition, chemicals, and possibly a genetic mutation in folate pathways in some cases, which may result in abnormal development (Kinsman and Johnston, 2007). Additional factors predisposing the infant to NTDs include prepregnancy maternal obesity, previous NTD pregnancy, and the use of antiepileptic drugs (e.g., valproic acid) in pregnancy (Frey and Hauser, 2003; Finnell, Gould, and Spiegelstein, 2003; Stothard, Tennant, Bell, et al, 2009). The degree of neurologic dysfunction depends on where the sac

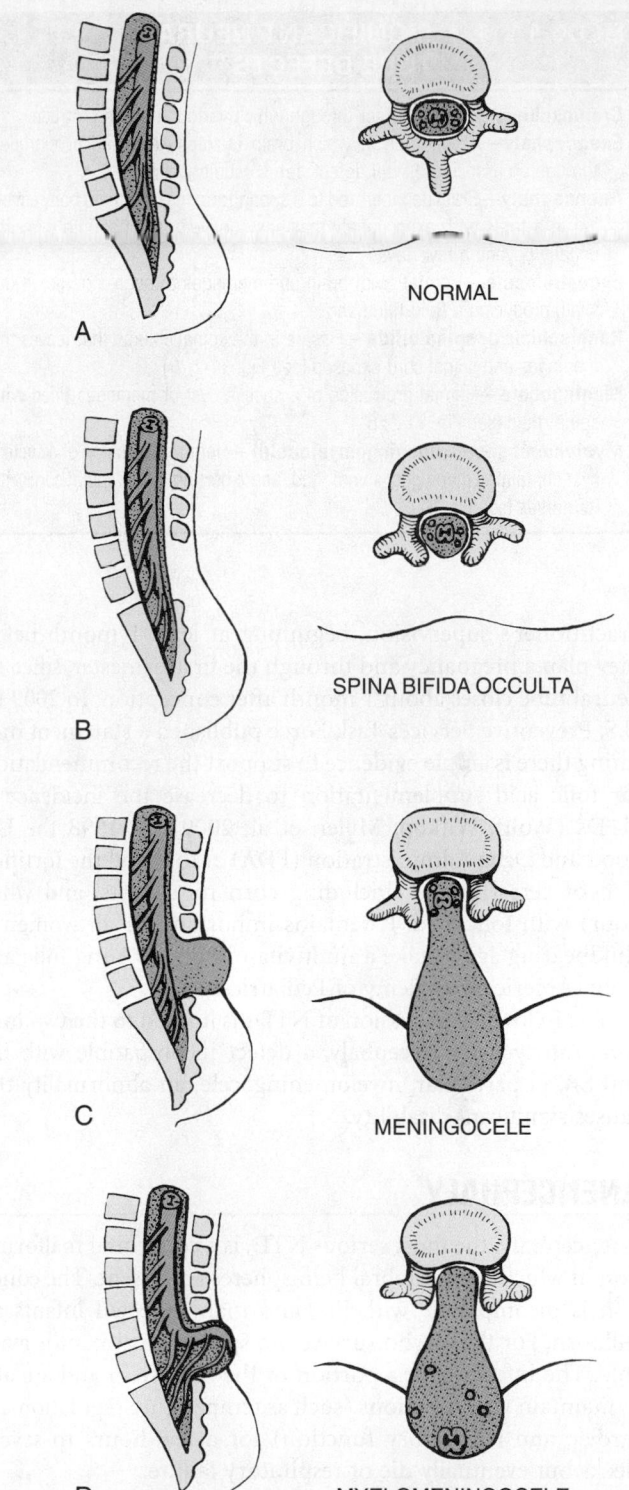

Fig. 11-2 A to D, Midline defects of osseous spine with varying degrees of neural herniations.

protrudes through the vertebrae, the anatomic level of the defect, and the amount of nerve tissue involved. Most myelomeningoceles involve the lumbar or lumbosacral area.

The American Academy of Pediatrics (2007) recommends daily intake of folic acid for all women of childbearing age. The recommended 0.4-mg daily dose is supplied safely in many multivitamin preparations. Because the greatest risk factor is a previous pregnancy affected by NTDs, women in this category should increase their daily folic acid dose to 4 mg, under a

---

BOX 11-1 **SIGNIFICANT NEURAL TUBE DEFECTS**

Cranioschisis—A skull defect through which various tissues protrude

Exencephaly—A condition in which brain is totally exposed or extruded through an associated skull defect; fetus usually aborted

Anencephaly—Brain degenerated to a spongiform mass with no bony covering in a fetus with exencephaly that has survived; incompatible with life usually beyond a few days

Encephalocele—Herniation of brain and meninges through a defect in the skull, producing a fluid-filled sac

Rachischisis or spina bifida—Fissure in the spinal column that leaves the meninges and spinal cord exposed (see Fig. 11-2, *B*)

Meningocele—Hernial protrusion of a saclike cyst of meninges filled with spinal fluid (see Fig. 11-2, *C*)

Myelomeningocele (meningomyelocele)—Hernial protrusion of a saclike cyst containing meninges, spinal fluid, and a portion of the spinal cord with its nerves (see Fig. 11-2, *D*)

---

practitioner's supervision, beginning at least 1 month before they plan a pregnancy and through the first trimester, since the neural tube closes about 1 month after conception. In 2009 the U.S. Preventive Services Task Force published a statement indicating there is ample evidence to support the recommendations for folic acid supplementation to decrease the incidence of NTDs (Wolff, Witkop, Miller, et al, 2009). In 1998 the U.S. Food and Drug Administration (FDA) authorized the fortification of cereal grains (including corn meal, grits, and wheat flour) with folic acid. It remains important for all women of childbearing age to take a multivitamin with 0.4 mg folic acid daily (American Academy of Pediatrics, 2007).

The following discussion of NTDs is limited to the two most common types: anencephaly, a defect incompatible with life; and SB, in particular, myelomeningocele, an abnormality that causes significant disability.

ANENCEPHALY

Anencephaly, the most serious NTD, is a congenital malformation in which both cerebral hemispheres are absent. The condition is incompatible with life, and many affected infants are stillborn. For those who survive, no specific treatment is available. The infants have a portion of the brainstem and are able to maintain vital functions (such as temperature regulation and cardiac and respiratory function) for a few hours to several weeks but eventually die of respiratory failure.

Traditionally these infants have been provided comfort measures, but with no effort at resuscitation. Ethical and moral questions are encountered regarding treatment and withdrawal of support systems (e.g., feedings) if the newborn survives the first few days of life, as well as use of the organs for donor transplants. During this time the family requires emotional support and counseling to cope with the birth of an infant with a fatal defect.

SPINA BIFIDA AND MYELODYSPLASIA

Myelodysplasia refers broadly to any malformation of the spinal canal and cord. Midline defects involving failure of the osseous (bony) spine to close are called spina bifida, the most common defect of the CNS. SB is categorized into two types: SB occulta and SB cystica.

SB occulta refers to a defect that is not visible externally. It occurs most commonly in the lumbosacral area (L5 and S1) (Fig. 11-2, *B*). Routine radiographic examinations indicate that the disorder may occur in as many as 10% to 30% of the general population. However, it may not be apparent unless there are associated cutaneous manifestations or neuromuscular disturbances. Superficial cutaneous indications include a skin depression or dimple (which may also mark the outlet of a dermal sinus tract that extends to the subarachnoid space); port-wine angiomatous nevi; dark tufts of hair; and soft, subcutaneous lipomas. These signs may be absent, appear singly, or be present in combination.

If associated neurologic involvement is present, the defect is known as occult spinal dysraphism. Fibrous bands and adhesions, an intraspinal lipoma (fatty tumor) or subcutaneous lipoma (lipomyelomeningocele), a dermoid or epidermoid cyst, diastematomyelia (spinal cord split in two), or a tethered cord can distort the spinal cord or roots. The usual cause is abnormal adhesion, or tethering, to a bony or fixed structure, resulting in traction on the spinal cord and cauda equina. (See Figs. 40-5 and 40-7 for areas innervated by specific spinal nerves.)

Neuromuscular disturbances usually consist of progressive or static changes in gait with foot weakness, foot deformity, or bowel and bladder sphincter disturbances. Some manifestations may not be evident until the child walks or is toilet trained.

Plain radiography is employed to disclose the precise bony defect in the symptomatic lesion and to establish the diagnosis in the suspected, nonsymptomatic occult variety. Magnetic resonance imaging (MRI) is the most sensitive tool for evaluating the defect. Computed tomography (CT), ultrasonography, and myelography are also used to differentiate between SB occulta and other spinal disorders.

SB cystica refers to a visible defect with an external saclike protrusion. The two major forms of SB cystica are meningocele, which encases meninges and spinal fluid, but no neural elements (Fig. 11-2, *C*), and myelomeningocele (or meningomyelocele), which contains meninges, spinal fluid, and nerves (Fig. 11-2, *D*). Neurologic deficit is not associated with meningocele but occurs in varying, often serious, degrees in myelomeningocele.

MYELOMENINGOCELE (MENINGOMYELOCELE)

Myelomeningocele develops during the first 28 days of pregnancy when the neural tube fails to close and fuse at some point along its length. It may be detected prenatally or at birth, accounts for 90% of spinal cord lesions, and may be located at any point along the spinal column. Usually the sac is encased in a fine membrane that is prone to tears through which cerebrospinal fluid (CSF) leaks. In other instances the sac may be covered by dura, meninges, or skin, in which case there is rapid and spontaneous epithelialization. The largest number (75%) of myelomeningoceles occur in the lumbar or lumbosacral area (Fig. 11-3). The location and magnitude of the defect determine the nature and extent of neurologic impairment. When the

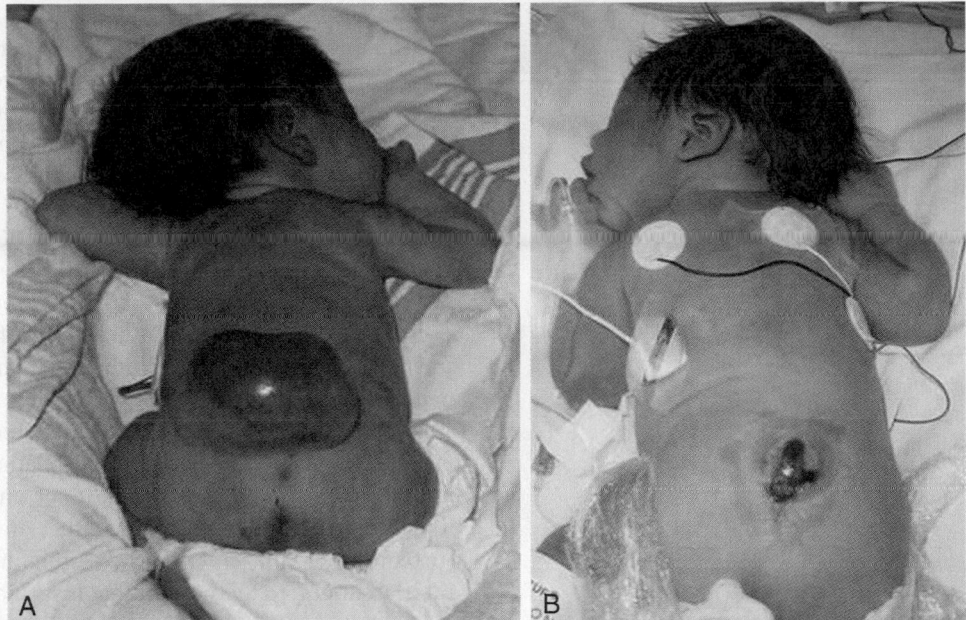

Fig. 11-3 A, Myelomeningocele with intact sac before surgery. **B,** Myelomeningocele with ruptured sac. (Courtesy Dr. Robert C. Dauser, Neurosurgery, Baylor College of Medicine, Houston.)

defect is below the second lumbar vertebra, the nerves of the cauda equina are involved, giving rise to symptoms such as flaccid, areflexic partial paralysis of the lower extremities and varying degrees of sensory deficit. Unlike a spinal cord injury, the degree of deficit is not necessarily uniform on both sides but may vary between extremities, depending on the compromise to specific nerves from malformation or tethering.

The anomaly most frequently associated with myelomeningocele is hydrocephalus; approximately 80% of children with SB develop hydrocephalus (Kinsman and Johnston, 2007). Although present at birth, hydrocephalus may not be apparent until shortly thereafter, or after the primary closure of the opening on the back. Careful monitoring of head circumference, fontanel tension, and ventricular size by head ultrasonography can indicate its presence. Hydrocephalus can occur because the NTD itself disrupts the flow of CSF. In many cases Chiari malformation (type II) is responsible (see p. 411). Type II Chiari malformation (a downward herniation of the brain into the brainstem) is present, though asymptomatic, in many children with SB. It can, however, adversely affect respiratory function, causing episodic apnea. Other clinical symptoms of problematic Chiari malformation include stridor, hoarse cry from vocal cord paralysis, feeding difficulties, aspiration pneumonia, and, in older children, upper extremity spasticity. The appearance of such symptoms should not be taken for granted; immediate referral is required to prevent further neurologic deterioration.

Pathophysiology

The pathophysiology of SB is best understood when related to the normal formative stages of the nervous system. At approximately 20 days of gestation a decided depression, the neural groove, appears in the dorsal ectoderm of the embryo. During the fourth week of gestation the groove deepens rapidly, and its elevated margins develop laterally and fuse dorsally to form the neural tube. Neural tube formation begins in the cervical region near the center of the embryo and advances in both directions—caudally and cephalically—until by the end of the fourth week of gestation the ends of the neural tube, the anterior and posterior neuropores, close.

Most authorities believe the primary defect in neural tube malformations is a failure of neural tube closure. However, some evidence indicates that the defects are a result of splitting of the already closed neural tube as a result of an abnormal increase in CSF pressure during the first trimester.

Clinical Manifestations

The manifestations of SB vary widely according to the degree of the spinal defect. The defect is readily apparent on inspection. The degree of neurologic dysfunction is directly related to the anatomic level of the defect and thus the nerves involved. Sensory disturbances usually parallel motor dysfunction. The upper level of sensory and motor impairment can be determined by observation of the infant's response to a pinprick over the legs and trunk. The infant responds to the sensory stimulus with limb movement, arousal, and crying. When withdrawal activity is used to determine the lowest level of spinal cord function, the response to pinprick should begin above the lesion.

Defective nerve supply to the bladder affects both sphincter and detrusor tone, which often causes constant dribbling of urine or produces overflow incontinence. This can often be mistaken for normal voiding patterns in the newborn. Some infants with SB, however, are able to void in a stream and achieve complete bladder emptying with each void.

Frequently the infant has poor anal sphincter tone and poor anal skin reflex, which result in lack of bowel control and sometimes rectal prolapse. Avoid taking rectal temperatures in affected infants. Because bowel sphincter function is frequently affected, the thermometer can cause irritation and rectal prolapse.

If the defect is below the third sacral vertebra, the infant has no motor impairment, but may have saddle anesthesia with bladder and anal sphincter paralysis.

Sometimes the denervation to the muscles of the lower extremities produces joint deformities in utero. These are primarily flexion or extension contractures, talipes valgus or varus contractures, kyphosis, lumbosacral scoliosis, and hip dislocations. The extent and severity of these associated orthopedic deformities again depend on the degree of nerve involvement. Most flexion deformities result from the pull of stronger, fully innervated muscles acting without the counterpull of their nonfunctioning paralyzed antagonists. See Box 11-2 for summary of clinical manifestations of SB cystica and occulta.

Diagnostic Evaluation

The diagnosis is made on the basis of clinical manifestations and examination of the meningeal sac. Diagnostic measures used to evaluate the brain and spinal cord include MRI, ultrasonography, CT, and myelography.

Laboratory examinations are used primarily to determine causative organisms in the major complications of myelomeningocele: meningitis and urinary tract infections. Infants with urinary incontinence require urinalysis, culture, and evaluation of blood urea nitrogen and creatinine clearance.

Prenatal Detection

It is possible to determine the presence of some major open NTDs prenatally. Ultrasonographic scanning of the uterus and elevated maternal concentrations of α-fetoprotein (AFP, or MS-AFP), a fetal-specific γ-1-globulin, in amniotic fluid may indicate the presence of anencephaly or myelomeningocele. (See Chapter 5.) The optimum time for performing these diagnostic tests is between 16 and 18 weeks of gestation, before AFP concentrations normally diminish and in sufficient time to permit a therapeutic abortion. It is recommended that such diagnostic procedures, as well as genetic counseling, be considered for all mothers who have borne an affected child, and testing is offered to all pregnant women (Kirkham, Harris, and Grzybowski, 2005). In addition, elective prelabor cesarean birth may result in less motor dysfunction. Chorionic villus sampling is also a method for prenatal diagnosis of NTDs; however, it carries certain risks (skeletal limb depletion) and is not recommended before 10 weeks of gestation.

Early surgical closure of the myelomeningocele sac through fetal surgery has been evaluated in relation to prevention of injury to the exposed spinal cord tissue and the improvement of neurologic and urologic outcomes in the affected child. Currently the Management of Myelomeningocele Study, a clinical trial supported by the National Institute of Health, is evaluating outcomes of fetal surgical correction of myelomeningocele at three sites in the United States; the results are expected to be published in 2011. The overall mortality rate from fetal surgery has been reported to be 4% to 6%, and complications include oligohydramnios, preterm delivery, and a smaller birth weight (Kaufman, 2004; Sutton, 2008).

Therapeutic Management

Management of the child who has a myelomeningocele requires a multidisciplinary team approach involving the specialties of neurology, neurosurgery, pediatrics, urology, orthopedics, rehabilitation, physical therapy, occupational therapy, and social services, as well as intensive nursing care in a variety of specialty areas. The collaborative efforts of these specialists focus on (1) the myelomeningocele and the problems associated with the defect—hydrocephalus, paralysis, orthopedic deformities, and genitourinary (GU) abnormalities; (2) possible acquired problems that may or may not be associated, such as Chiari II malformation, meningitis, seizures, hypoxia, and hemorrhage; and (3) other abnormalities, such as cardiac or gastrointestinal (GI) malformations. Many hospitals have routine outpatient care by multidisciplinary teams to provide the complex follow-up care needed for children with myelodysplasia.

Initial Care

Care of the newborn involves preventing infection; performing a neurologic assessment, including observation for associated anomalies; and dealing with the impact of the anomaly on the family. Although meningoceles are repaired early, especially if the sac is in danger of rupturing, the philosophy regarding skin closure of myelomeningocele varies. Most authorities believe that early closure, within the first 24 to 72 hours, offers the most favorable outcome. Surgical closure within the first 24 hours is recommended if the sac is leaking CSF (Kinsman and Johnston, 2007). Early closure, preferably in the first 12 to 18 hours, not only prevents local infection and trauma to the exposed tissues but also avoids stretching other nerve roots (which may occur as the meningeal sac expands during the first hours after birth), thus preventing further motor impairment. Broad-spectrum antibiotics are initiated, and neurotoxic substances such as povidone-iodine are avoided at the malformation.

A variety of neurosurgical and plastic surgical procedures are employed for skin closure without disturbing the neural elements or removing any portion of the sac. The objective is satisfactory skin coverage of the lesion and meticulous closure. Wide excision of the large membranous covering may damage functioning neural tissue.

Associated problems are assessed and managed by appropriate surgical and supportive measures. Shunt procedures provide relief from imminent or progressive hydrocephalus (see p. 409). When diagnosed, ventriculitis, meningitis, and urinary tract infection are treated with vigorous antibiotic therapy and supportive measures. Surgical intervention for Chiari II malformation is indicated only when the child is symptomatic (i.e., high-pitched crowing cry, stridor, respiratory difficulties, oral-motor difficulties, upper extremity spasticity).

Improved surgical techniques do not alter the major physical disability and deformity or chronic urinary tract infections that affect the quality of life for these children. Superimposed on these physical problems are the disorder's effects on family life and finances and on school and hospital services.

Musculoskeletal Considerations

According to most orthopedists, musculoskeletal problems that will affect later locomotion should be evaluated early and treatment, where indicated, instituted without delay. Neurologic assessment determines the neurosegmental level of the lesion, spasticity and progressive paralysis, potential for deformity, and functional expectations. Orthopedic and musculoskeletal management includes preventing joint contractures, correcting the existing deformity, preventing or minimizing effects of motor and sensory deficits, preventing skin breakdown, and obtaining the best possible function of affected lower extremities. Common musculoskeletal problems requiring attention in SB include deformities of the knees, hips, feet, and spine; fractures and insensate skin further complicate orthopedic care. Other problems that may occur later include kyphosis and scoliosis (Lazzaretti and Pearson, 2010). Because children with this condition often have decreased sensitivity in lower extremities, preventive skin care is important. A high percentage (60%) of children seen in a wound clinic for skin breakdown had myelomeningocele at birth (Samaniego, 2003).

The status of the neurologic deficit remains the most important factor in determining the child's ultimate functional abilities; however, many children with lumbar and sacral myelomeningocele are able to achieve functional ambulation (Kinsman and Johnston, 2007). With technologic advances, a variety of lightweight orthoses, including braces, special "walking" devices, and custom-built wheelchairs, are available to provide mobility to children with spinal cord lesions (see also Chapter 39). Early in infancy, intervention with passive range-of-motion exercises, positioning, and stretching exercises may help decrease the incidence of muscle contractures (Brown, 2001). Corrective surgical procedures, when indicated, are best initiated at an early age so that the child will not lag significantly behind age-mates in developmental progress. Where little hope exists for lower extremity function, surgery is seldom recommended unless it will improve sitting position in a wheelchair

and function for activities of daily living and mobility.

Physical therapy and musculoskeletal management of children with myelomeningocele is a continual process to achieve optimum function and ambulation when possible. Problems such as type II Chiari malformation, hydrocephalus, and a tethered spinal cord can complicate expectations.

Management of Genitourinary Function

Myelomeningocele is one of the most common causes of neuropathic (neurogenic) bladder dysfunction among children. Myelomeningocele affects approximately 1 in 1000 infants born in the United States, and as many as 90% experience subsequent voiding dysfunction. In infants the goal of treatment is to preserve renal function. In older children the goal is to preserve renal function and achieve optimum urinary continence. Urinary incontinence is a chronic, often debilitating problem for the child. In addition, the neuropathic bladder may produce urinary system distress, characterized by symptomatic urinary tract infections, ureterohydronephrosis, vesicoureteral reflux, or renal insufficiency. The characteristics of bladder dysfunction in children vary according to the level of the neurologic lesion and the influence of bony growth and development of the spine. In addition, the presence of type II Chiari malformation and subsequent hydrocephalus has the potential to affect bladder function, although spinal influences predominate.

During infancy, urinary incontinence is normally physiologic, but **urinary system distress** may occur. Ongoing urologic monitoring is essential. Evidence is growing that early intervention, based on evaluation during the neonatal period and before complications occur, has the following benefits: (1) improves bladder function, (2) reduces the subsequent risk of urinary system distress, and (3) reduces the need for reconstructive surgery of the lower urinary tract. Ultrasonography of the bladder and ureters and routine urinalysis (and urine cultures when indicated) are used to detect urinary system distress before renal function is compromised. In addition, urodynamic testing is used to identify bladder dysfunction that predisposes the child to urinary system distress (Gray and Moore, 2009). These conditions include high pressure detrusor hyperreflexia (reflex contractions of the detrusor muscle) with vesicosphincter dyssynergia (incoordination of detrusor and sphincter muscles), low bladder wall compliance (poor distensibility of the bladder wall causing increased intravesical pressures during urine filling and storage), or detrusor areflexia (absence of detrusor contractions caused by the spinal defect).

Infants may have one of several predominant neuropathic bladder disorders. Detrusor contractions associated with vesicosphincter dyssynergia are particularly common. Some infants are able to empty the bladder efficiently despite incoordination between the sphincter mechanism and detrusor, but the majority experience chronic residual urine, urinary tract infections, or more serious types of urinary system distress. A minority of infants have poor detrusor contraction strength or detrusor areflexia. This condition is particularly damaging to the urinary system when it coexists with low bladder wall compliance and an elevated detrusor leak point pressure. Low bladder wall compliance occurs when collagen or fibrosis causes stiffening of the bladder wall. This stiffened bladder wall raises intravesical pressures, obstructing the bladder, ureters, and, ultimately, the nephron. The impact of low bladder wall compliance is directly related to the influence of the bladder outlet. Among children with myelodysplasia, the urethral muscles are typically weakened, and collagen replaces much of the muscle tissue. As a result, the sphincter is fixed, so that it neither closes efficiently to prevent urinary leakage nor opens well to allow urinary flow with a detrusor contraction. When the magnitude of the pressure required to drive urine across the abnormal sphincter is greater than 40 cm H_2O (the detrusor leak point pressure) and the compliance of the bladder wall is low (<10 cm H_2O), the risk of urinary system distress is high.

In contrast, a small number of infants experience effective detrusor contractions without vesicosphincter dyssynergia. Effective bladder evacuation is likely among this group, and the incidence of urinary system distress during the first year of life is low.

As the child grows, detrusor hyperreflexia is often replaced by deficient detrusor contraction strength and stress urinary incontinence (SUI) (leakage produced by physical exertion). The bladder wall is often poorly compliant (producing chronically elevated intravesical pressures), and the bladder outlet, while incompetent, obstructs the outflow of urine. When the detrusor leak point pressure exceeds 40 cm H_2O, the child is predisposed to chronic urinary leakage and urinary distress symptoms, including recurrent urinary tract infections and reflux. When the detrusor leak point pressure is lower than 40 cm H_2O, urinary leakage is more severe, although the risk of urinary system distress is lessened. Thus the child with more severe urinary incontinence is less predisposed than the "drier" child to serious urinary tract infections.

Infants with myelomeningocele and a neurogenic bladder who are not at risk for urinary system distress are managed by diaper containment and watchful waiting. The infant empties the bladder into a diaper, the urine is routinely monitored for infection, and the upper urinary tracts are monitored for evidence of urinary system distress (dilation of the ureters, renal pelves, or collecting systems) via serial ultrasonography.

In contrast, children with evidence of urinary system distress, or those considered at risk based on early urodynamic testing, are placed on clean intermittent catheterization (CIC), typically in combination with an antispasmodic medication such as oxybutynin or propantheline (Gray and Moore, 2009; de Jong, Chrzan, Klijn, et al, 2008). Anticholinergic medications are prescribed because they reduce detrusor muscle tone and reduce bladder pressures during both urine filling and storage and during micturition. CIC is not intended to prevent spontaneous voiding. Instead, it ensures routine, regular bladder evacuation, further preventing deleterious elevation of intravesical pressures. Usually, the parents learn to catheterize the infant every 4 hours during the day and once each night. Follow-up evaluation, consisting of serial ultrasonography and urinalysis, is completed every 3 to 6 months as indicated.

Infants with significant urinary system distress and hostile neuropathic bladder dysfunction at birth sometimes require temporary urinary diversion to ensure adequate urine outflow and prevent further damage to the upper urinary tracts. A vesicostomy is a relatively simple procedure wherein the anterior bladder wall is brought to the abdominal wall, creating a small

stoma for urinary drainage. Urine is contained via a diaper, but double diapering or use of a larger diaper that can be placed higher on the abdomen is necessary for adequate urine containment. Meticulous skin care is necessary because the perineal skin is exposed to continuous urinary leakage.

Among older children the quest for continence typically begins with a CIC program. The parents learn the procedure, and teach the child to self-catheterize as soon as possible, usually by 6 years of age (Gray and Moore, 2009). The child with detrusor hyperreflexia and dyssynergia often responds well to antispasmodic medications and CIC. In contrast, the child with poor bladder wall compliance and SUI often requires a combination of antispasmodic medications to reduce intravesical filling pressures and an asympathetic agonist (such as imipramine, pseudoephedrine, or phenylpropanolamine) to enhance sphincter competence. Unfortunately, the combination of medications and CIC is typically only partially effective, and more aggressive interventions are often required to render the neuropathic bladder both continent and free from its predisposition toward producing urinary system distress.

When the child cannot attain continence by conservative measures, surgery is considered. Augmentation enterocystoplasty (or gastrocystoplasty) is a surgical procedure that increases bladder capacity, reverses or halts the negative effects of the poorly compliant bladder wall, and reduces harmfully high bladder pressures caused by detrusor hyperreflexia with vesicosphincter dyssynergia. A detubularized segment of large or small bowel or a wedge of the fundus of the stomach has been used to successfully augment bladder capacity. The choice of segment varies according to the surgeon's preference and the status of the patient's urinary and GI systems. Large and small bowel segments produce significant volumes of mucus that may clog catheters used for CIC. Augmentation with the stomach produces less mucus, and its acidic secretions may reduce the urinary system's predisposition to infection. The bladder must be irrigated to decrease mucus within the bladder; this also decreases the possible complications of infection, stones, and bladder perforation.

Even though augmentation of the bladder may improve or resolve urinary leakage related to detrusor hyperreflexia or urinary system distress caused by low bladder wall compliance, the SUI produced by the abnormal sphincter mechanism typically persists. Several surgical procedures help correct this intrinsic sphincter deficiency. The Mitrofanoff procedure uses the appendix to provide an alternative route for intermittent catheterization. The appendix is removed from the colon and used to create a continent conduit between the abdominal wall and the bladder. The resulting stoma is relatively small and produces minimum mucus. The ureter may be used as an alternative to the appendix for some children. If the appendix is insufficient, a segment of tapered intestine, ileum, or colon may be used to create a conduit (Monti tube) (Gray and Moore, 2009; Mitrofanoff and Liard, 2001). CIC through the easily accessible abdominal route fosters greater independence in children, especially in those unable to transfer from wheelchair to toilet to perform CIC.

When intrinsic sphincter deficiency produces only mild stress urinary leakage, the construction of a Mitrofanoff route alone may be sufficient to achieve continence between catheterization episodes. However, when SUI is more severe, a suburethral sling or suburethral collagen injection is used to alleviate intrinsic sphincter deficiency.

The suburethral sling is a slip of fascia or synthetic material that is placed below the proximal third of the urethra. The sling may be placed in a fashion that uses only slight tension to obstruct the urethra and prevent SUI. The sling may be used for both boys and girls, and the procedure can be completed at the same time the augmentation enterocystoplasty is constructed. After augmentation enterocystoplasty and placement of a suburethral sling, the patient can expect to evacuate the bladder by CIC of the appendiceal Mitrofanoff route or the urethra if a Mitrofanoff route has not been constructed.

Suburethral injection of glutaraldehyde cross-linked (GAX) collagen also may be used to alleviate or prevent SUI caused by intrinsic sphincter deficiency. Collagen is used to bulk or expand the urethral tissue, promoting coaptation (approximation) of the mucosa. The collagen implant complements the urethra's ability to form a watertight seal, rather than obstructing the urethral lumen. Collagen may be injected using different approaches. Transurethral collagen is injected through the working channel of a cystoscope. Transperineal collagen is directed underneath the urethra using a needle inserted through the perineal skin. In this case the location of the urethra is confirmed by simultaneous cystoscopic visualization of the urethra. The antegrade approach requires creation of a suprapubic cystostomy tract. A flexible cystoscope is then inserted through the cystostomy tract, and collagen is injected into the proximal urethra. Multiple injections may be required to achieve optimum continence. Subsequent injections may be required when the collagen is dissipated or resorbed by the body over a period of years.

The artificial urinary sphincter provides another alternative for the management of intrinsic sphincter deficiency in the child with myelomeningocele. The device consists of a urethral cuff, abdominal reservoir, and control pump. In the activated position, the cuff is filled, and the pressure of this cuff closes the urethral lumen. During micturition, the control pump is used to baffle fluid from the urethral cuff to the abdominal reservoir, opening the urethra for micturition or catheterization. However, because of the significant risk for infection, need for revision with growth, and mechanical failure, the popularity of the artificial urinary sphincter has declined.

Because of advances in neurogenic bladder management, adolescents and young adults with myelomeningocele and neurogenic bladders have been followed for up to 30 years without evidence of deterioration in renal function. Nevertheless, urinary and fecal incontinence are common, and these conditions lead to significant, and sometimes devastating, problems with growth and developmental tasks, including establishing independence and social and intimate relationships. This observation underscores the need to aggressively manage both continence and the threat of urinary system distress from an early age and to establish an expectation of social continence critical to providing these patients with the skills they need to thrive as adolescents and adults. Newborns with SB and normal urodynamics require close follow-up care during the first several years of life to prevent deterioration in urodynamic status as a result of neurologic deterioration.

Bowel Control

Some degree of fecal continence can be achieved in most children with myelomeningocele with diet modification, regular toilet habits, and prevention of constipation and impaction. It is frequently a lengthy process. Dietary fiber supplements (recommended 10 g/day), laxatives, suppositories, or enemas aid in producing regular evacuation. Older children and adolescents seeking more independence may attain bowel continence and higher quality of life after undergoing an antegrade continence enema procedure (Doolin, 2006). In a procedure similar to the Mitrofanoff, the appendix or ileum is used to create a catheterizable channel with attachment of the proximal end to the colon. The distal end of the channel exits through a small abdominal stoma. Every 1 or 2 days, a catheter is passed through the stoma, allowing enema solution to be instilled directly into the colon; this is called an antegrade colonic irrigation. After administration of the enema solution, the child sits on the toilet for 30 to 60 minutes as stool is flushed out through the rectum. Frequency of enemas and volume of solution used to completely evacuate the bowel vary among individuals.

Prognosis

The early prognosis for the child with myelomeningocele depends on the neurologic deficit present at birth, including motor ability, bladder innervation, and associated neurologic anomalies. Early surgical repair of the spinal defect, antibiotic therapy to reduce the incidence of meningitis and ventriculitis, prevention of urinary system dysfunction, and early detection and correction of hydrocephalus have significantly increased the survival rate and quality of life in such children. Many children with SB achieve partial independent living and gainful employment. Reports of survival rates vary, and many include adults who were born before medical advances and surgical techniques seen in the past 25 years. Coordinated care for adults with SB is essential; however, multidisciplinary adult care is often inadequate (Lazzaretti and Pearson, 2010). In children and adolescents with SB the achievement of urinary continence is associated with improved self-concept and esteem, especially among girls (Moore, Kogan, and Parekh, 2004). This chronic condition has an array of associated complications, including hydrocephalus and shunt malfunctions, scoliosis, bowel and bladder management issues, latex allergy, and epilepsy. However, based on current medical knowledge and ethical considerations, aggressive, early management is favored for the child with myelomeningocele.

Prevention

The Centers for Disease Control and Prevention (2009) continues to affirm that 50% to 70% of NTDs can be prevented by daily consumption of 0.4 mg of folic acid among women of childbearing age. The data indicate that serum folate concentrations among women of childbearing age decreased 16% from 2003 to 2004 in all ethnic groups studied. Lowest serum folate levels were seen in non-Hispanic Caucasians in 2003 to 2004; however, overall serum folate levels remained below recommended levels in non-Hispanic African-Americans during all three periods studied (Centers for Disease Control and Prevention, 2007). These results indicate that nurses and other health care workers have an important task in disseminating information that may decrease the incidence of birth defects in children by promoting maternal consumption of folic acid.*

To ensure adequate daily intake of the recommended amount of folic acid, women must take a folic acid supplement, eat a fortified breakfast cereal containing 100% of the recommended dietary allowance of folic acid (e.g., Kellogg's Product 19, General Mills Total, Multigrain Cheerios Plus), or increase their consumption of fortified foods (cereal, bread, rice, grits, pasta) and foods naturally rich in folate (green, leafy vegetables and citrus fruits). For women who have had a previous pregnancy affected by NTDs, folic acid intake is increased to 4 mg under supervision of a practitioner beginning 1 month before a planned pregnancy and continuing through the first trimester. Supplementation of 4 mg of folate should not be given solely in multivitamin preparations because of the risk of overdose of other vitamins. The only population in which folic acid has not been effective in decreasing the incidence of NTDs is in women taking antiepileptic medications during pregnancy (Finnell, Gould, and Spiegelstein, 2003).

Nursing Care Management

The basic needs of the infant with a myelomeningocele are essentially the same as for any newborn infant. (See Chapter 8.) Special needs related to the defect and potential complications are discussed in the following section. As the child matures, the problems increase and involve all aspects of daily living; therefore care is directly related to the child's habilitation at each stage of development.

Assessment

At the time of delivery an examination is performed to assess the intactness of the membranous cyst. During transport to the nursery, make every effort to prevent trauma to this protective covering. In addition to the routine assessment of the newborn (see Chapter 8), assess the infant for the level of neurologic involvement. Note movement of extremities or skin response, especially an anal reflex that might provide clues to the degree of motor or sensory impairment.

Care of the Myelomeningocele Sac

The infant is usually placed in an incubator or radiant warmer so that temperature can be maintained without clothing or covers that might irritate the CNS lesion. When an overhead warmer is used, the dressings over the defect require more frequent moistening because of the dehydrating effect of the radiant heat. Before surgical closure the myelomeningocele is kept from drying by the application of a sterile, moist, nonadherent dressing. The moistening solution is usually sterile normal saline. Dressings are changed frequently (every 2 to 4 hours), and the sac is closely inspected for leaks, abrasions, irritation, and signs of infection. The sac must be carefully cleansed if it becomes soiled or contaminated. Sometimes the

sac ruptures during delivery or transport, and any opening in the sac greatly increases the risk of infection to the CNS.

Positioning

One of the most important and challenging aspects of early care of the infant with myelomeningocele is positioning. Before surgery the infant remains in the prone position to minimize tension on the sac and the risk of trauma. The prone position allows for optimum positioning of the legs, especially in cases of associated hip dysplasia. A variety of aids, including diaper rolls, pads, or specially designed frames and appliances, are available to maintain the desired position.

The prone position affects other aspects of the infant's care. For example, in this position the infant is more difficult to keep clean, pressure areas are a constant threat, and feeding becomes a problem. The infant's head is turned to one side for feeding. Fortunately, most defects are repaired early, and the infant can be held for feeding soon after surgery. Physical therapy consultation may be necessary for difficult positioning problems. Speech-language pathologist consultation may be needed for difficulty with oral-motor skills that may indicate complications caused by a Chiari malformation.

General Care

Diapering the infant may be contraindicated until the defect has been repaired and healing is well advanced or epithelialization has taken place. The padding beneath the diaper area is changed as needed to keep the skin dry and free of irritation. When the nurse detects urinary retention (the bladder is still an abdominal organ in early infancy), CIC is employed. Because the bowel sphincter is frequently affected, there may be continual passage of stool, often misinterpreted as diarrhea, which is a constant irritant to the skin and a source of infection to the spinal lesion.

Areas of sensory and motor impairment are subject to skin breakdown and therefore require meticulous care. The infant may be placed on a pressure-reducing mattress or mattress to prevent pressure on the knees and ankles. (See Skin Care, Chapter 10, and Maintaining Healthy Skin, Chapter 27.)

Gentle range-of-motion exercises are carried out to prevent contractures, and stretching of contractures is performed when indicated. However, these exercises may be restricted to the foot, ankle, and knee joint. When the hip joints are unstable, stretching against tight hip flexors or adductor muscles, which act much like bowstrings, may aggravate a tendency toward subluxation. A physical therapy consultation is often necessary to develop a multidisciplinary plan to prevent long-term complications.

Some infants with unrepaired myelomeningocele are unable to be held in the arms and cuddled as unaffected infants are, so their need for tactile stimulation is met by caressing, stroking, and other comfort measures. To facilitate handling and reduce parental anxiety, the infant can recline on a pillow placed in the parent's lap. Black-and-white drawings or geometric shapes can be placed within the infant's view, and other stimulation usually provided for infants is appropriate. All infants respond to pleasant sounds. (See Developmental Outcome, Chapter 10.)

Ophthalmic complications may occur in children with SB and hydrocephalus. The appearance of a squint, other ocular motility, or papilledema usually denotes hydrocephalus and is

---

*Information is available from Centers for Disease Control and Prevention, National Center on Birth Defects and Developmental Disabilities, Division of Birth Defects and Developmental Disabilities, 1600 Clifton Road NE, MS E-86, Atlanta, GA 30333; 800-CDC-INFO; e-mail: cdcinfo@cdc.gov; www.cdc.gov/ncbddd/folicacid. And from March of Dimes Resource Center, 1275 Mamaroneck Ave., White Plains, NY 10605; www.marchofdimes.com.

reported. Ophthalmologic follow-up care, particularly in children with shunts, is generally included in the multidisciplinary care plan.

Postoperative Care

Postoperative care for the infant with myelomeningocele involves the same basic care as for any postsurgical infant: monitoring vital signs, weight, and intake and output; maintaining body temperature; assessing and relieving pain; providing nourishment; and observing for signs of infection. The wound is managed according to the surgeon's directions, and general care is continued as preoperatively.

The prone position is maintained after operative closure, although many neurosurgeons allow a side-lying or partial side-lying position unless it aggravates a coexisting hip dysplasia or permits undesirable hip flexion. This offers an opportunity for position changes, which reduces the risk of pressure sores and facilitates feeding. Once the effects of anesthesia have subsided and the infant is alert, feedings may resume unless there are other anomalies or associated complications.

Nursing assessments are carried out for implementation of comfort measures in the postoperative period. The infant can be held upright against the body, taking care to avoid pressure on the operative site. In the case of an unusually large defect, skin grafting may be required for wound closure; the infant must then be kept prone postoperatively with as little movement as possible to prevent tension on the skin graft.

The nurse can assist in determining the extent of neuromuscular involvement. Note movement of the extremities or skin response, especially an anal reflex, that might provide clues to the degree of motor or sensory status. Measure head circumference daily (see Chapter 6), and examine the fontanels for signs of tension or bulging. The nurse is also alert to early signs of infection, such as elevated or decreased temperature (axillary), irritability, and lethargy, and to signs of increased intracranial pressure (ICP). Urinary catheterization may be needed for urine retention. Although it may not have been a problem preoperatively, swelling around the operative site may cause transient urine retention, which resolves in 2 to 5 days.

Family Support and Home Care

As soon as the parents are able to cope with the infant's condition, encourage them to become involved in care. They need to learn how to continue at home the care that has been initiated in the hospital: positioning, feeding, skin care, and range-of-motion exercises when appropriate. Parents also need to learn CIC technique when prescribed. The family needs to know the signs of complications and how to reach assistance when needed.

As the child grows and develops, parents need guidance to encourage and stimulate the infant to accomplish age-appropriate developmental tasks within the limits imposed by the disabilities. Upper limb movement can be stimulated early by placing the infant on the floor in a prone position with toys within reach. Activities that encourage body consciousness, such as rolling over and pulling to a sitting position, are encouraged at the appropriate times. Creeping and crawling help the child explore the environment. The parents may need help to modify appliances and activities normally expected of a growing child. A standing table, frame, or parapodium is helpful for a variety of activities, and it is best for the child to begin supported weight bearing and standing as close as possible to the expected time for standing to occur.

It is important for the family to understand the nature of sensory deficit in a child with a spinal defect. The child will be insensitive to pressure or other sources of tissue injury. Therefore the family must be alert to hot or cold items that could cause thermal injury to tissues and remember to inspect the skin regularly for signs of pressure, especially over bony prominences. Because of sensory impairment, the child is unaware of bladder discomfort. Therefore signs of urinary tract infections may go unnoticed. Urinary tract infection is often considered when the child becomes ill.

The long-range planning with and support of the parents and newborn begin in the hospital and extend throughout childhood and even into young adulthood. The life expectancy of children with SB extends well into adulthood; therefore planning should involve long-term goals and plans for optimum function as an adult. Long-range planning goals should include a discussion of achievement of functional mobility, urinary continence, and as much bowel continence as much physically possible. Discussion about aspects of adulthood such as having a mate, sexual relationships, and bearing and rearing children is important and should not be overlooked (Barker, Saulino, and Caristo, 2002; Rowe and Jadhav, 2008). The unique service needs of adolescents with SB as they attempt to gain independence from family and establish a life of their own has not been adequately addressed in the literature yet is slowly emerging (Buran, McDaniel, and Brei, 2002; Rowe and Jadhav, 2008). Advances in neurology, orthopedics, and urology have enabled adolescents to progress into adulthood with fewer deficits than observed in previous decades; one key factor is the recognition of subtle signs of neurologic deterioration and rapid intervention (Rowe and Jadhav, 2008).

Nurses assume an important role as a central member of the health team. As a coordinator, the nurse reviews information with the family, takes responsibility for family teaching, and acts as a liaison between inpatient and outpatient services. The child may require numerous hospitalizations over the years, and each one will be a source of stress to which the younger child is especially vulnerable.

Changes in functional ability, particularly in the lower extremities, bowel, or bladder, may indicate the presence of a tethered cord, one that is bound down or restricted in an abnormal position by scar tissue. These symptoms usually occur after a growth spurt and can best be detected with MRI. Tethering can be repaired surgically but, unfortunately, may recur. **Hydromyelia**, a dilation of the central canal of the spinal cord and elevated fluid accumulation, may occur with SB; common symptoms include rapidly developing scoliosis, upper extremity weakness, spasticity, and lower extremity ascending motor strength changes (Barker, Saulino, and Caristo, 2002).

Habilitation involves solving not only problems of self-help and locomotion but also the most distressing problem of incontinence, which threatens the child's social acceptability. Assistance in preparing the child and the school regarding the special needs of children with disabilities helps the parents provide a better initial adjustment to broader social experiences. Numerous organizations and agencies offer assistance and support to children and families (see Family-Centered Care box). The Spina Bifida Association* provides services and support for families of children with spinal lesions.

FAMILY-CENTERED CARE

Additional References on Spina Bifida for Families and Professionals

Kriegsman KH, Zaslow EL, D'Zmura-Rechsteiner J: *Taking charge: teenagers talk about life and physical disabilities*, Bethesda, Md, 1992, Woodbine House.

Lutkenhoff M, editor: *Children with spina bifida: a parent's guide*, Bethesda, Md, 1999, Woodbine House.

Lutkenhoff M, Oppenheimer S, editors: *Spinabilities: a young person's guide to spina bifida*, Bethesda, Md, 1997, Woodbine House.

Rowley-Kelly F, Reigel D: *Teaching the student with spina bifida*, Baltimore, 1993, Paul H Brooks.

Sandler A: *Living with spina bifida: a guide for families and professionals*, Chapel Hill, NC, 1997, University of North Carolina Press.

The multiple aspects of care of the child with a disability are discussed in Chapter 22. Complex problems associated with partial or complete lower extremity paralysis are discussed in Chapters 39 and 40 and include bowel and bladder control; orthopedic appliances; and the observation and management of complications, especially urinary tract infections (see Chapter 30) and pressure necrosis (see Wounds, Chapter 18).

LATEX ALLERGY

Latex allergy, or latex hypersensitivity, was identified as being a serious health hazard when a report linked intraoperative anaphylaxis with latex in children with SB. Latex, a natural product derived from the rubber tree, is used in combination with other chemicals to give elasticity, strength, and durability to many products. Children with SB are at high risk for developing latex allergy because of repeated exposure to latex products during surgery and procedures. Children with chronic renal failure are also at an increased risk for latex allergy, and efforts should be made to decrease their exposure to latex products (Dehlink, Prandstetter, Eiwegger, et al, 2004). Allergic reactions range from urticaria, wheezing, watery eyes, and rashes to anaphylactic shock. More severe reactions tend to occur when latex comes in contact with mucous membranes, wet skin, the bloodstream, or an airway. There also can be cross-reactions to a number of foods (e.g., banana, avocado, kiwi, chestnut).

Latex hypersensitivity reactions have been diagnosed in infants. Symptoms included wheezing, facial swelling, facial rash, or anaphylaxis (Kimata, 2004). Allergic reactions to latex protein can also occur when the substance is transferred to food by food handlers wearing latex gloves, prompting several states to pass legislation that prohibits the use of latex gloves in food service. In addition to patients with SB, high-risk populations

BOX 11-3 MEDICAL CONDITIONS ASSOCIATED WITH RISK OF LATEX ALLERGY

- Spina bifida
- Urogenital anomalies
- Imperforate anus
- Esophageal atresia/tracheoesophageal fistula
- VATER association (*V*ertebral defects, imperforate *A*nus, *T*racheo*E*sophageal fistula, and *R*adial and *R*enal dysplasia); and VACTERL for *V*ertebral, *A*nal, *C*ardiac, *T*racheal, *E*sophageal, *R*enal, and *L*imb)
- Preterm infants
- Ventriculoperitoneal shunt
- Neurocognitive impairment
- Cerebral palsy
- Tetraplegia
- Multiple surgeries
- Atopy

Data from Slater JE: Latex allergy, *J Allergy Clin Immunol* 94:139-149, 1994; Alenius H, Palosuo T, Kelly K, et al: IgE reactivity to 14-kD and 27-kD natural rubber proteins in latex allergic children with spina bifida and other congenital anomalies, *Int Arch Allergy Immunol* 102:61-66, 1993; Centers for Disease Control and Prevention: Guidelines for prevention of transmission of human immunodeficiency virus and hepatitis B virus to health-care and public-safety workers, *MMWR* 38:9-10, 1989; and Landwehr LP, Lane G, Leung DYM: Latex allergy and intraoperative anaphylaxis in a child, *Am J Asthma Allergy Pediatr* 4:205-210, 1994.

include patients with urogenital anomalies or multiple surgeries and health care workers. See Box 11-3 for medical conditions associated with risk of latex allergy.

The most important goals are prevention of latex sensitivity and identification of children with a known hypersensitivity (see Nursing Care Guidelines box). High-risk and latex-allergic individuals must be managed in a latex-free environment. Take care that they do not come in direct or secondary contact with products or equipment containing latex at any time during medical treatment. Allergy testing can identify latex sensitivity with varying success. Skin prick testing and provocation testing carry the risk of allergic reaction or anaphylaxis. Several commercially available assays can be useful in confirming latex sensitivity. To date, none of these tests demonstrates complete

NURSING CARE GUIDELINES

Identifying Latex Allergy

- Does your child have any symptoms, such as sneezing, coughing, rashes, or wheezing, when handling rubber products (balloons, tennis or Koosh balls, adhesive bandage strips) or when in contact with rubber hospital products, such as gloves or catheters?
- Has your child ever had an allergic reaction during surgery?
- Does your child have a history of rashes, asthma, or allergic reactions to medication or foods, especially milk, kiwi, bananas, or chestnuts?
- How would you identify or recognize an allergic reaction in your child?
- What would you do if an allergic reaction occurred?
- Has anyone ever discussed latex or rubber allergy or sensitivity with you?
- Has the child had any allergy testing?
- When did the child last come in contact with any type of rubber product? Were you present?

Modified from Romanczuk A: Latex use with infants and children: it can cause problems, *MCN* 18(4):208-212, 1993.

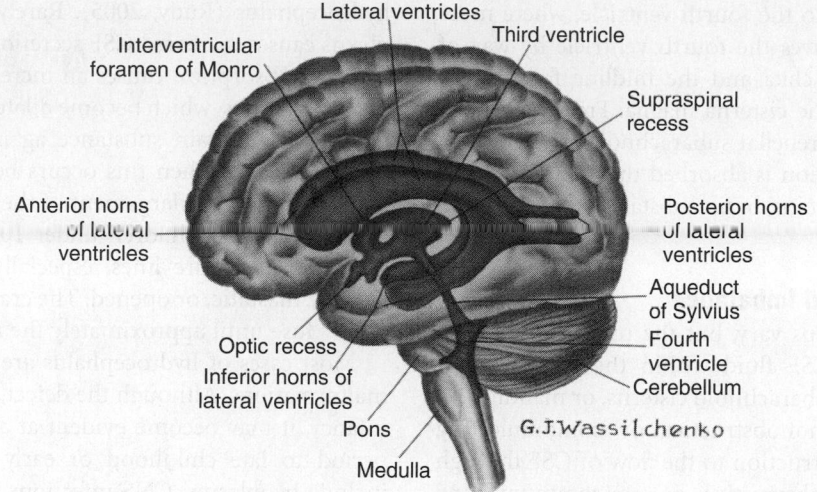

Fig. 11-4 Cerebral ventricular system. (From Thompson JM, McFarland G, Hirsch JE, et al: *Mosby's clinical nursing,* ed 5, St Louis, 2002, Mosby.)

diagnostic reliability, and they should not be the sole determinant of the presence or absence of an allergic response to latex.

The radioallergosorbent test (RAST) has been used to measure the serum level of latex-specific immunoglobulin E. The RAST has been shown to be 90% to 95% sensitive. Administration of antihistamines and steroids (dexamethasone) before and after surgery to reduce the possibility of a serious reaction remains controversial because it may interfere with healing.

Because children who have SB are prone to develop sensitivity to latex, reducing exposure, from birth on, may decrease the chance of allergy development. Nonlatex products lists are available to parents and health care workers; these products may be substituted for those containing latex. In the health care arena it is important to use products with the lowest potential risk of sensitizing patients and staff members. The FDA has proposed user labeling for latex-containing devices that come into contact directly or indirectly with live human tissue.*

The identification of those sensitive to latex is best accomplished through careful screening of all patients. During the health interview with the parent or child, ask *all* patients, not only those at risk, about sensitivity to latex. Be certain this is a routine part of all preoperative and preprocedural histories. Stress the importance of the allergy history to all personnel (e.g., phlebotomists). (See Nursing Care Guidelines box for questions related to latex allergy.) Children with latex hypersensitivity should carry some form of allergy identification, such as a Medic-Alert bracelet. Education programs regarding latex hypersensitivity are aimed at those who care for high-risk groups, such as children with SB, and may include relatives, school nurses, teachers, child care workers, and baby-sitters. In addition to educating caregivers about the child's exposure to medical products that contain latex, nurses need to inform them of common nonmedical latex objects such as water toys,

pacifiers, and plastic storage bags.† Items brought to the hospital, such as floral bouquets, are also screened for latex toys or balloons. Parents should also receive literature explaining signs and symptoms of latex hypersensitivity and appropriate emergency treatment. (See Anaphylaxis, Chapter 29.)

HYDROCEPHALUS

Hydrocephalus is not a single disease entity but rather a group of conditions, resulting from disturbances in the dynamics of cerebral circulation and CSF, which may be caused by various conditions. The advent of MRI and CT scanning has provided valuable information about the pathophysiology of hydrocephalus. The causes of hydrocephalus are diverse and include either congenital (myelomeningocele, intrauterine viral infection [cytomegalovirus, toxoplasmosis], aqueduct stenosis) or acquired conditions such as intraventricular hemorrhage, tumor, CSF infection, or head injury (Kestle, 2003; Kinsman and Johnston, 2007).

Pathophysiology

To appreciate the condition, an understanding of the dynamics of CSF and the relationship between the various structures that make up the ventricular and subarachnoid spaces is necessary (Fig. 11-4). The two mechanisms by which CSF is formed are secretion by the choroid plexuses and lymphatic-like drainage by the extracellular fluid of the brain. CSF circulates throughout the ventricular system and is then absorbed within the subarachnoid spaces by a mechanism that is not entirely clear.

Ventricular Circulation

The fluid flows from the lateral ventricles through the foramen of Monro to the third ventricle, where it combines with fluid secreted into the third ventricle. From there CSF flows through

---

*Additional information regarding latex allergy may be found at www. latex-allergy.org, and http://latexallergylinks.tripod.com. For a list of latex products and alternative products, see Latex List on the Spina Bifida Association home page, www.spinabifidaassociation.org.

†Latex-free product lists are available from the American Latex Allergy Association's online resource manual, available at www. latexallergyresources.org/ResourceManual/section1/index.cfm. American Latex Allergy Association, PO Box 198, Slinger, WI 53086; 888-972-5378; www.latexallergyresources.org.

the aqueduct of Sylvius into the fourth ventricle, where more fluid is formed; it then leaves the fourth ventricle by way of the lateral foramen of Luschka and the midline foramen of Magendie and flows into the cisterna magna. From there CSF flows to the cerebral and cerebellar subarachnoid spaces, where it is absorbed. A large portion is absorbed through the arachnoid villi, but the sinuses, veins, brain substance, and dura also participate in absorption.

Mechanisms of CSF Fluid Imbalance

The causes of hydrocephalus vary, but the result is either (1) impaired absorption of CSF fluid within the subarachnoid space, obliteration of the subarachnoid cisterns, or malfunction of the arachnoid villi (nonobstructive or communicating hydrocephalus); or (2) obstruction to the flow of CSF through the ventricular system (obstructive or noncommunicating hydrocephalus) (Kinsman and Johnston, 2007). The terms *communicating* and *noncommunicating hydrocephalus* traditionally referred to obstructive and nonobstructive types of hydrocephalus when pneumoencephalography was used to establish the diagnosis. Because other diagnostic methods are now used, the terms may be used only as a reference point in the diagnosis. Other authorities suggest that hydrocephalus be classified according to the cause as either congenital or acquired

hydrocephalus (Rudy, 2005). Rarely, a tumor of the choroid plexus causes increased CSF secretion. Any imbalance of secretion and absorption causes an increased accumulation of CSF in the ventricles, which become dilated (**ventriculomegaly**) and compress the brain substance against the surrounding rigid bony cranium. When this occurs before fusion of the cranial sutures, it causes enlargement of the skull, as well as dilation of the ventricles. In children under 10 to 12 years of age, previously closed suture lines, especially the sagittal suture, may become diastatic, or opened. The cranial sutures do not permanently fuse until approximately the age of 12 years or later.

Most cases of hydrocephalus are a result of developmental malformations. Although the defect usually is apparent in early infancy, it may become evident at any time from the prenatal period to late childhood or early adulthood. Other causes include neoplasms, CNS infections (e.g., meningitis, encephalitis), and trauma (e.g., shaken baby syndrome). An obstruction to the normal flow can occur at any point in the CSF pathway to produce increased pressure and dilation of the pathways proximal to the site of obstruction. Table 11-3 describes the most frequent sites of obstruction and the consequences.

Developmental defects (e.g., Chiari malformation [see following discussion], aqueduct stenosis, aqueduct gliosis, and atresia of the foramina of Luschka and Magendie [Dandy-

TABLE 11-3   SITES AND TYPES OF HYDROCEPHALUS

SITE	TYPE	CAUSES AND COMMENTS
Aqueduct of Sylvius—Accounts for 33% of hydrocephalus (Volpe, 2001)	Stenosis or atresia	Congenital (X-linked recessive in small number)
		Insidious onset of symptoms from birth to adulthood
	Gliosis	Postinflammatory, usually secondary to perinatal infection or hemorrhage
		Prenatal maternal infection (toxoplasmosis)
	Obstructive	Tumors of 3rd ventricle or midbrain
		Ependymitis from maternal toxoplasmosis
		Congenital aneurysm of Galen vein
	Posthemorrhagic	Blood from intraventricular hemorrhage in germinal matrix; most common type of hydrocephalus in preterm infants
4th ventricle or subarachnoid pathway—Intraventricular hemorrhage, postinflammatory conditions, or tumors	Posthemorrhagic	Blood from intraventricular hemorrhage in germinal matrix; most common type of hydrocephalus in preterm infants
4th ventricle and foramen magnum—Accounts for 50% of all hydrocephalus	Type I Chiari malformation	Accounts for 28%-40% of 4th ventricle obstructions
		Neural tube defect with herniation of medulla through foramen magnum; may be asymptomatic in childhood; similar to type II, but milder
	Type II Chiari malformation	More severe defect; downward displacement of brainstem, 4th ventricle, and lower parts of cerebellum through foramen magnum with fixed attachment of spinal cord at site of myelomeningocele
	Type III Chiari malformation (absence or occlusion of ventricles)	High cervical or occipitocervical myelomeningocele with cervical herniation through body defect
		Congenital (Dandy-Walker syndrome) caused by obstruction of foramina of Luschka and Magendie
		Tumors of posterior fossa (e.g., medulloblastoma) causing pressure on surrounding tissues to produce obstruction
		Less often—Subdural hematoma, bacterial or granulomatous meningitis
Arachnoid villi and cisterna magna—Obstruction by thick arachnoid membrane or meninges	Meningitis	Bacterial or granulomatous
		Acute phase—Clumping of purulent fluid in drainage channels
		Chronic phase—Organization of blood and exudate that results in fibrosis of subarachnoid spaces
	Prenatal maternal infections	Toxoplasmosis, cytomegalic inclusion disease, mumps
	• Meningeal malignancy	Secondary to leukemia or lymphoma
	• Arachnoid cyst	Located in basal cistern or (uncommon) over cerebral cortex
	• Tuberculosis, fungal or parasitic infection	More common in children ages 2-10 yr old

Walker malformation]) account for most cases of hydrocephalus from birth to 2 years of age. Dandy-Walker malformation involves a cystic expansion of the fourth ventricle and subsequent obstruction of CSF flow resulting in hydrocephalus (Kinsman and Johnston, 2007). Hydrocephalus is so often associated with myelomeningocele that all such infants should be observed for its development. In the remainder of cases there is a history of intrauterine infection (toxoplasmosis, cytomegalovirus), hemorrhage (posthemorrhagic hydrocephalus in preterm infant), and neonatal meningoencephalitis (bacterial or viral). In older children hydrocephalus is most often a result of intracranial masses (vascular anomalies, cysts, tumors), pre-existing developmental defects, intracranial infections, trauma, or hemorrhage.

Chiari Malformations

A Chiari malformation is a brain defect involving posterior fossa contents. Table 11-3 describes the major types. The type II Chiari malformation, seen almost exclusively with myelomeningocele, is characterized by herniation of a small cerebellum, medulla, pons, and fourth ventricle into the cervical spinal canal through an enlarged foramen magnum. The resulting obstruction of CSF flow causes the hydrocephalus.

Clinical Manifestations

The three factors that influence the clinical picture in hydrocephalus are the acuity of onset, timing of onset, and associated structural malformations. In infancy, before closure of the cranial sutures, head enlargement (increasing occipitofrontal circumference [OFC]) is the predominant sign, whereas in older infants and children the lesions responsible for hydrocephalus produce other neurologic signs through pressure on adjacent structures.

Infancy

In infants with hydrocephalus, the head grows at an abnormal rate, although the first signs may be bulging fontanels with or without head enlargement (Fig. 11-5). The anterior fontanel is tense, often bulging, and nonpulsatile. Scalp veins are dilated and markedly so when the infant cries. With the increase in intracranial volume, the bones of the skull become thin and the sutures become palpably separated to produce the cracked-pot sound (Macewen sign) on percussion of the skull. In severe cases there may be frontal protrusion, or frontal bossing, with depressed eyes, and the eyes may be rotated downward, producing a setting-sun sign, in which the sclera may be visible above the iris. Pupils are sluggish, with unequal response to light.

The infant is irritable and lethargic, feeds poorly, and may display changes in level of consciousness, opisthotonos (often extreme), and lower extremity spasticity. The infant cries when picked up or rocked and quiets when allowed to lie still. Early infantile reflexes may persist, and normally expected responses may not appear, indicating failure in the development of normal cortical inhibition.

Infants with Chiari malformation may exhibit behaviors that reflect cranial nerve dysfunction as a result of brainstem compression, including swallowing difficulties, stridor, apnea, aspiration, respiratory difficulties, and arm weakness.

The preterm infant with posthemorrhagic hydrocephalus may not exhibit any clinical signs and symptoms other than a gradual increase in head circumference. Alternatively, the nurse may note subtle seizure activity and alternating levels of consciousness. Assess ventricular size by ultrasonography or CT scanning in preterm infants at high risk for intraventricular hemorrhage.

If hydrocephalus is allowed to progress, development of lower brainstem functions is disrupted, as manifested by difficulty in sucking and feeding and a shrill, brief, high-pitched cry. Eventually the skull becomes enlarged, and the cortex is destroyed. If the hydrocephalus is rapidly progressive, the infant may display emesis, somnolence, seizures, and cardiopulmonary distress.

Childhood

The signs and symptoms in early to late childhood are caused by increased ICP, and specific manifestations are related to the focal lesion. Most commonly resulting from posterior fossa neoplasms and aqueduct stenosis, the clinical manifestations are primarily those associated with space-occupying lesions (i.e., headache on awakening with improvement following emesis or upright posture, papilledema, strabismus, and extrapyramidal tract signs such as ataxia [see Chapter 36]). As with

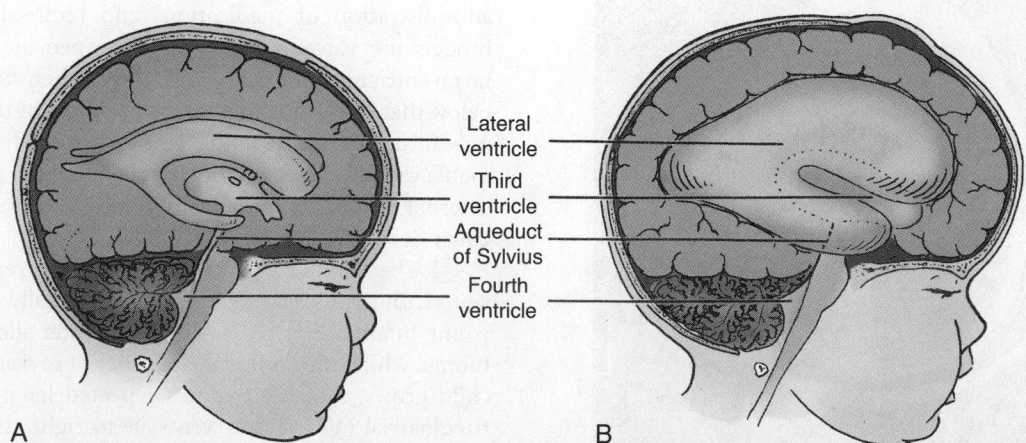

Lateral ventricle
Third ventricle
Aqueduct of Sylvius
Fourth ventricle

A   B

Fig. 11-5 Hydrocephalus: a block in flow of cerebrospinal fluid. **A,** Patent cerebrospinal fluid circulation. **B,** Enlarged lateral and third ventricles caused by obstruction of circulation—stenosis of aqueduct of Sylvius.

infants, the child is irritable, lethargic, apathetic, confused, and often incoherent. In one of the congenital defects with later onset (by age 3 months), the Dandy-Walker syndrome, characteristic manifestations are a bulging occiput, nystagmus, ataxia, and cranial nerve palsies.

Manifestations of Chiari malformation in children over 3 years of age are related to spinal cord dysfunction rather than brainstem compression as observed in infants. Scoliosis proximal to the level of the myelomeningocele (usually associated with Chiari malformation) and development of upper extremity spasticity, which may progress to weakness and atrophy, are common. Cranial nerve deficits are rare.

Diagnostic Evaluation

Antenatal diagnosis of hydrocephalus is possible with fetal ultrasonography as early as 14 to 15 weeks of gestation. Delivery is not currently recommended until fetal lung maturity has been achieved.

In infancy the diagnosis of hydrocephalus is based on head circumference that crosses one or more percentile lines on the head measurement chart within a period of 2 to 4 weeks and on associated neurologic signs that are progressive. However, other diagnostic studies are needed to localize the site of CSF obstruction. Routine daily head circumference measurements are carried out in infants with myelomeningocele, hemorrhage, or intrauterine viral or CNS infections. In evaluation of a preterm infant, specially adapted head circumference charts are consulted to distinguish abnormal head growth from rapid but normal head growth.

The primary diagnostic tools for detecting hydrocephalus in older infants and children are CT and MRI (Fig. 11-6). Mild sedation is usually required because the child must remain absolutely still for an accurate picture. Diagnostic evaluation of children who have symptoms of hydrocephalus after infancy is similar to that employed in those with a suspected intracranial tumor. In the neonate, echoencephalography is useful in comparing the ratio of lateral ventricle to cortex. Sometimes isotope ventriculograms are used to assess the flow and patency of existing shunts and to evaluate the size of the ventricles.

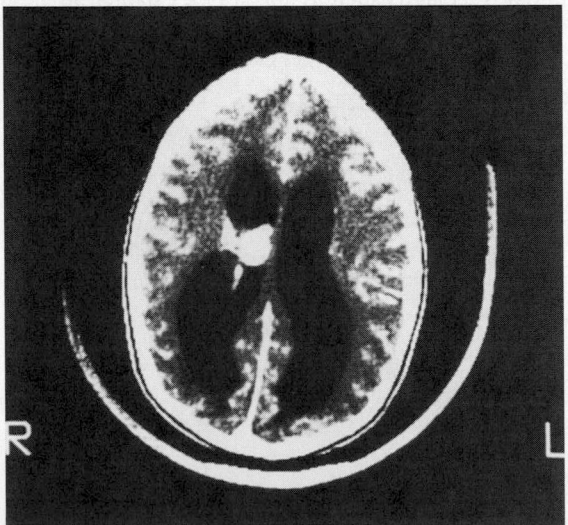

Fig. 11-6 Computed tomography scan reveals enlarged ventricles of child with hydrocephalus.

Problems in differential diagnosis are related to the child whose head circumference is greater than the 95th percentile but whose head growth parallels the normal growth curve. It is sometimes valuable to measure the parental OFC to detect a possible normal familial characteristic (benign familial megalencephaly). (See Table 37-2 for diagnostic tests for neurologic evaluation.)

Therapeutic Management

The treatment of hydrocephalus is directed toward (1) relief of ventricular pressure, (2) treatment of the cause of the ventriculomegaly, (3) treatment of associated complications, and (4) management of problems related to the effect of the disorder on psychomotor development. The treatment is, with few exceptions, surgical.

Medical therapy has been largely disappointing and inadequate. Many newborn infants with progressive cranial enlargement secondary to intracranial hemorrhage demonstrate spontaneous stabilization and resolution. Serial lumbar punctures and medications have been used with varying success but are recommended only until the preterm infant is stable enough to tolerate major surgery. The administration of acetazolamide and isosorbide or furosemide is somewhat beneficial in decreasing the production of CSF in selected cases of slowly progressive disease. The medication reduces the ICP until spontaneous arrest of hydrocephalus takes place or as a temporary measure when surgery is contraindicated.

Surgical Treatment

Improved neurosurgical techniques have established surgical treatment as the therapy of choice in almost all cases of hydrocephalus. This is accomplished by direct removal of an obstruction, such as resection of a neoplasm, cyst, or hematoma, or, in rare instances of fluid overproduction, by choroid plexus extirpation (plexectomy or electric coagulation). However, most children require a shunt procedure that provides primary drainage of the CSF from the ventricles to an extracranial compartment, usually the peritoneum.

Most shunt systems consist of a ventricular catheter, a flush pump, a unidirectional flow valve, and a distal catheter. All are radiopaque for easy visualization after placement, and all are tested for accuracy before insertion. A reservoir is frequently added to allow direct access to the ventricular system for administration of medications and removal of fluid. In all models the valves are designed to open at a predetermined intraventricular pressure and close when the pressure falls below that level, thus preventing backflow of fluid. Most shunts now in use have differential pressure and adjustable programmable valves with capability for changing the pressures with an external magnet, thus avoiding additional surgery (Chiafery, 2006; Kestle, 2003).

The standard procedure for many years has been the **ventriculoperitoneal (VP) shunt**, especially in neonates and young infants (Fig. 11-7). There is greater allowance for excess tubing, which minimizes the number of revisions needed as the child grows. Since it requires repeated lengthening, the ventriculoatrial (VA) shunt (ventricle to right atrium) is reserved for older children who have attained most of their somatic growth and children with abdominal pathologic conditions.

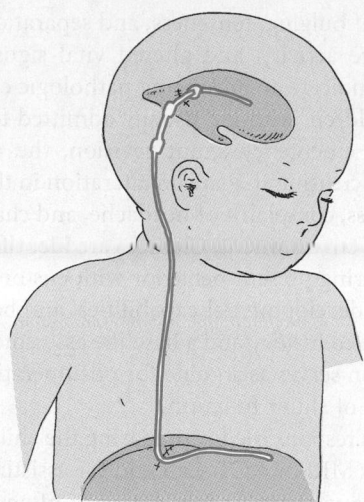

Fig. 11-7 Ventriculoperitoneal shunt. Catheter is threaded beneath skin.

The VA shunt is contraindicated in children with cardiopulmonary disease or elevated CSF protein.

Although placement of ventricular shunts (into the amniotic sac) in utero for ventricular enlargement is possible, results have not been as promising as shunting soon after birth (Golden and Bönnemann, 2007).

The initial shunt is placed when indicated on the basis of individual assessment. The timing of revisions varies widely. In most instances revisions are performed when physical signs indicate shunt malfunction (i.e., signs of elevated ICP). Sometimes revisions are planned for specific times during development. The initial success rate is relatively high. However, shunts are associated with complications that interfere with continued shunt function or that threaten the child's life.

Endoscopic third ventriculostomy (ETV) is a procedure that has potential for allowing greater independence from VA or VP shunting in children with hydrocephalus. In this procedure a small opening is made in the floor of the third ventricle, allowing CSF to flow freely through the previously blocked ventricle, thus bypassing the aqueduct of Sylvius. Children with SB, anatomic ventricular malformations, posthemorrhagic hydrocephalus (preterm infants), and postinfectious hydrocephalus are reportedly poor candidates for this procedure (Drake, 2008), as are children with bleeding disorders and those who have had previous radiotherapy. Reports of the success of ETV in children vary (see Research Focus box). Complications include CSF leak, hemorrhage from a perforated basilar artery, meningitis, cranial nerve injury, obstruction, and hypothalamic injury (Drake, 2008).

RESEARCH FOCUS

Endoscopic Ventriculostomy Success Based on Age

Several studies have reported that the younger the child, the lower the success rate of the endoscopic ventriculostomy; infants less than 6 months to 1 year of age reportedly have the lowest success rates (Drake, 2008; Kadrian, van Gelder, Florida, et al, 2008; Wagner and Koch, 2005), whereas others report success in infants as well as older children (Faggin, Bernardo, Stieg, et al, 2009; Fritsch, Kienke, Ankerman, et al, 2005).

Complications

The major complications of VP shunts are infection and malfunction. All shunts are subject to mechanical difficulties, such as kinking, plugging, or separation and migration of tubing. Malfunction is most often caused by mechanical obstruction either within the ventricles from particulate matter (tissue or exudate) or at the distal end from thrombosis or displacement as a result of growth. Functional obstruction of a shunt's anti-siphon device remains a common complication. Shunt malfunctions are reported to be 40% at 1 year and 50% at 2 years (Drake, 2008; Kestle, 2003). In a large study occurring over 13 years, at least one shunt revision was required in 58.5% of children; the median time to shunt failure or malfunction was 88 days (Mittler, 2005). The child with a shunt obstruction often is seen in an emergency visit with clinical manifestations of increased ICP, frequently accompanied by worsening neurologic status.

The most serious complication, shunt infection, can occur at any time, but the period of greatest risk is 1 to 2 months after placement. Shunt infection rates are reported to be approximately 10% (Drake, 2008). The infection may be a result of intercurrent infections at the time of shunt placement. Infections include sepsis, bacterial endocarditis, wound infection, shunt nephritis, meningitis, and ventriculitis. Brain abscess associated with colonic perforation and infection with a gram-negative enteric organism suggests an ascending shunt infection in a child who has a VP shunt. Meningitis and ventriculitis are of greatest concern because any complicating CNS infection is a significant predictor of subnormal intellectual outcome. Infection is treated with antibiotics administered intravenously or intrathecally for a minimum of 7 to 10 days. Antibiotic-impregnated shunts may decrease infection rates (Drake, 2008). A persistent infection may require removal of the shunt until the infection is controlled; however, this practice has been recently challenged (Drake, 2008). External ventricular drainage (EVD), or external ventriculostomy, is used until CSF is sterile. EVD allows removal of CSF from a tube placed in the child's ventricle that flows by gravity into a collection device.

The primary reasons for inserting an EVD include unstable status, increased ICP that is difficult to stabilize, or infection from an existing VP shunt. The EVD may drain CSF intermittently or continuously according to need. The EVD is a closed system made up of transparent pliable tubing, a collection bag, and, at times, a drip chamber between the tubing and the collection bag. The EVD is placed at the level of the child's external auditory meatus with the head at a 20- to 30-degree elevation, depending on physician preference. Elevating the EVD above this level decreases the flow of CSF, and placing the device below the level of the external meatus increases the flow. Ambulation or sitting up in bed or chair usually requires that the tubing be clamped to prevent imbalance in CSF drainage. In addition, the EVD is a closed sterile system and should be handled as such in relation to emptying the device or changing the scalp dressing. Accurate and frequent documentation of the incision site; amount, color, and consistency of drainage into the device; and the child's vital and neurologic signs are an important part of the nursing care.

Complications related to an EVD include infection, meningitis, hemorrhage, obstruction, malfunction (Ngo, Ranger,

Singh, et al, 2009), and, in some cases, tentorial herniation as a result of imbalance in CSF drainage (Pope, 1998). In preterm infants with intraventricular hemorrhage requiring CSF drainage, a ventricular access drain may be temporarily inserted. This system is similar to the EVD but has an access port for frequent taps and can be used to administer antibiotics and thrombolytic agents such as urokinase.

Another serious shunt-related complication is subdural hematoma caused by too rapid reduction of ICP and size. This usually can be averted by careful assessment of ICP before insertion of the shunt and use of correct valvular pressure. Other complications that may occur include peritonitis, abdominal abscesses, perforation of abdominal organs by catheter or trocar (at the time of insertion), fistulas, hernias, and ileus. Children often need shunt lengthening as body growth occurs. This procedure usually involves replacing the distal catheter below the valve during the toddler period and again before the growth acceleration of puberty.

Prognosis

The prognosis of children with treated hydrocephalus depends largely on the cause of the dilated ventricles before shunt placement and the amount of irreversible brain damage before shunting (Kinsman and Johnston, 2007). For example, malignant tumors have a high mortality rate regardless of other complicating factors.

Survivors have a high incidence of subnormal intellectual capacity, and a large majority have major physical and disabling neurologic handicaps such as ataxia, spastic diplegia, poor fine motor coordination, and perceptual deficits. Some children demonstrate aggressive or delinquent behavior, and those with myelomeningocele are likely to have accelerated pubertal development as a result of increased gonadotropin secretion with increased ICP (Kinsman and Johnston, 2007). Depression requiring treatment occurred in 45% of children in one survey; in the same survey 54% of the children with hydrocephalus required four or more shunt revisions (Gupta, Park, Solomon, et al, 2007).

Surgically treated hydrocephalus in patients with little or no evidence of irreversible brain damage has a survival rate of about 90%, with most deaths occurring within the first year of treatment. Those with poor outcomes included children shunted for posthemorrhagic hydrocephalus or meningitis, with 40% and 30%, respectively, showing cognitive impairment (Kestle, 2003). Of the surviving children, approximately two thirds are intellectually normal. The presence of additional medical problems in infancy, including ocular defects, is the most significant variable associated with a high likelihood of neurocognitive impairment. Most children who require shunting must depend on the shunt for the remainder of their life.

Nursing Care Management

The infant with suspected or confirmed hydrocephalus is observed carefully for signs of increasing ventricular size and increasing ICP. In infants the head is measured daily at the point of largest measurement—the OFC. (See Chapter 6 for technique.) To avoid the likelihood of wide discrepancies, the point at which the measurements are taken is indicated on the head with a marking pen. Fontanels and suture lines are palpated for size, signs of bulging, tenseness, and separation. Irritability, lethargy, seizure activity, and altered vital signs and feeding behavior may indicate an advancing pathologic condition.

In older children, who are usually admitted to the hospital for elective or emergency shunt revision, the most valuable indicators of increasing ICP are an alteration in the child's level of consciousness, complaint of headache, and changes in interaction with the environment. Changes are identified by observing and comparing present behavior with customary behavior, sleep patterns, developmental capabilities, and habits obtained through a detailed history and a baseline assessment. This baseline information serves as a guide for postoperative assessment and evaluation of shunt function.

The nurse is responsible for preparing the child for diagnostic tests such as MRI or a CT scan and for assisting with procedures such as a ventricular tap, which is often performed to relieve excessive pressure and to obtain CSF during the preoperative period. Sedation is required because the child must remain absolutely still during diagnostic testing. A variety of drugs are available for sedation. (See Chapter 27 for preparing children for procedures.) If surgery is anticipated, IV infusions should not be placed in a scalp vein.

Postoperative Care

In addition to routine postoperative care and observation, the infant or child is positioned carefully on the unoperated side to prevent pressure on the shunt valve. The child remains flat to help avert complications resulting from too rapid reduction of intracranial fluid. The surgeon indicates the position to be maintained and the extent of activity allowed.

The nurse continues observation for signs of increased ICP, which indicate obstruction of the shunt. Neurologic assessment includes pupil dilation (pressure causes compression or stretching of the oculomotor nerve, producing dilation on the same side as the pressure) and blood pressure (hypoxia to the brainstem causes variability in these vital signs). The nurse also observes for abdominal distention because CSF may cause peritonitis or a postoperative ileus as a complication of distal catheter placement.

Because infection is the greatest hazard of the postoperative period, nurses are continually on the alert for the usual manifestations of CSF infection, including elevated temperature, poor feeding, vomiting, decreased responsiveness, and seizure activity. There may be signs of local inflammation at the operative sites and along the shunt tract. Antibiotics are administered by the IV route as ordered, and the nurse may also need to assist with intraventricular instillation. Inspect the incision site for leakage, and test any suspected drainage for glucose, an indication of CSF.

Family Support

Specific needs and concerns of parents during periods of hospitalization are related to the reason for the child's hospitalization (shunt revision, infection, diagnosis) and the diagnostic and surgical procedures to which the child must be subjected. Parents may have little understanding of anatomy; therefore they need further explanation and reinforcement of information that was given to them by the physician and neurosurgeon, including information about what to expect. They are especially frightened of any procedure that involves the brain, and the fear of disability or brain damage is real and pervasive. Nurses can calm their anxiety with explanations of the rationale underlying the various nursing and medical activities such as positioning or testing and by simply being available and willing to listen to their concerns.

To prepare for the child's discharge and home care, instruct the parents on how to recognize signs that indicate shunt malfunction or infection. Active children may have injuries, such as a fall, that can damage the shunt, and the tubing may pull out of the distal insertion site or become disconnected during normal growth. Contact sports should be avoided, but swimming or tennis is appropriate. A helmet may be worn to protect the head in case of a fall or injury when outside play is vigorous (Chiafery, 2006). It is also important for the nurse to encourage families to enroll infants and toddlers with hydrocephalus into an early childhood development program. Depending on the degree of initial damage and the underlying cause, many children have normal intellectual development.

The management of hydrocephalus in a child is a demanding task for both the family and health professionals, and helping the family cope with the child's difficulties is an important nursing responsibility. Children with hydrocephalus have lifelong special health care needs. The nurse can provide optimum primary health care, including advice on immunizations, treatments for common infectious conditions, or child care and school precautions. The overall aim is to establish realistic goals and an appropriate educational program that will assist the child in achieving the maximum potential. Families can be referred to community agencies for support and guidance. The National Hydrocephalus Foundation (NHF)* and the Hydrocephalus Association† provide information on the condition for families, and the NHF assists interested groups in establishing local organizations.

Anticipatory guidance will prepare parents for possible problems and help them avoid being overprotective of the child. Few restrictions need be placed on the child's activities (mainly contact sports), and the child is encouraged to live as would any other youngster of the same age and abilities. Parents need support and encouragement in coping with the child and problems the child may encounter in relationships with peers and others. Reactions of other children when the child has a noticeably enlarged head or requires shaving at times of revision are stressful for both the child and the parents. (See Chapter 22 for problems and coping with a child with a disability.)

CRANIAL DEFORMITIES

In the normal newborn the cranial sutures are separated by membranous seams several millimeters wide. For the first few hours to 1 to 2 days after birth, the cranial bones are highly

---

*12413 Centralia Road, Lakewood, CA 90715-1653; 562-924-6666; www.nhfonline.org.
†870 Market St., Suite 705, San Francisco, CA 94102; 415-732-7040; www.hydroassoc.org. A booklet titled *About Hydrocephalus: A Book for Parents* is available in English or Spanish; also available is *Prenatal Hydrocephalus: A Book for Parents*. In Canada, contact the Spina Bifida and Hydrocephalus Association of Canada; 800-565-9488; www.sbhac.ca.

mobile, which allows the bones to mold and overlap one another, adjusting the circumference of the head to accommodate to the changing shape and character of the birth canal. The principal sutures in the infant's skull are the sagittal, coronal, and lambdoid sutures, and the major soft areas at the juncture of these sutures are the anterior and posterior fontanels. (See Fig. 8-7.)

After birth, growth of the skull bones occurs in a direction perpendicular (at right angles) to the line of the suture, and normal closure occurs in a regular and predictable order. Although the age at which closure takes place varies widely in individual children, solid union of all sutures is not completed until late childhood. Normally, sutures and fontanels are ossified by the following ages:

- Eight weeks—Posterior fontanel closed
- Six months—Fibrous union of suture lines and interlocking of serrated edges
- Eighteen months—Anterior fontanel closed
- Twelve years and older—Sutures not separable by ICP

Closure of a suture before the expected time inhibits the perpendicular growth. Since normal increase in brain volume requires expansion, the skull is forced to grow in a direction parallel to the fused suture. This alteration in skull growth always distorts the head shape when the underlying brain growth is normal. The small head with closed sutures and a normal shape is a result of deficient brain growth; the suture closure is secondary to this brain growth failure. Failure of brain growth is not secondary to suture closure.

Various types of cranial deformities are encountered in early infancy. These include the enlarged head with frontal protrusion, or **bossing** (characteristic of hydrocephalus); the parietal bossing that is seen in chronic subdural hematoma; the small head; and a variety of skull deformities (Fig. 11-8). Some occur during prenatal development. In others, head circumference is usually within normal limits at birth, and the deviation from normal development becomes apparent with advancing age.

MICROCEPHALY

Primary (genetic) microcephaly reflects a small brain and may be caused by an autosomal recessive disorder or a chromosomal abnormality (Kinsman and Johnston, 2007). **Secondary (nongenetic) microcephaly** can result from a variety of insults that occur during the third trimester of pregnancy, the perinatal period, or early infancy (Kinsman and Johnston, 2007). These stimuli may be irradiation (especially between 4 and 20 weeks of gestation), maternal infection (notably toxoplasmosis, rubella, or cytomegalovirus [see Maternal Infections, Chapter 10]), or chemical agents. Infection, trauma, metabolic disorders, and anoxia are all capable of causing decreased brain growth. Secondary microcephaly may also occur as a result of maternal diabetes and maternal hyperphenylalanemia. Fetal exposure to alcohol and tobacco use was shown to result in a 2.6-fold increase in the risk of isolated secondary microcephaly compared with other causes, including syndromes (Krauss, Morrissey, Winn, et al, 2003). Microcephaly is defined as an OFC greater than 3 standard deviations below the mean for age and sex (Kinsman and Johnston, 2007).

In both types the neurologic manifestations range from decerebration, complete unresponsiveness, and autistic

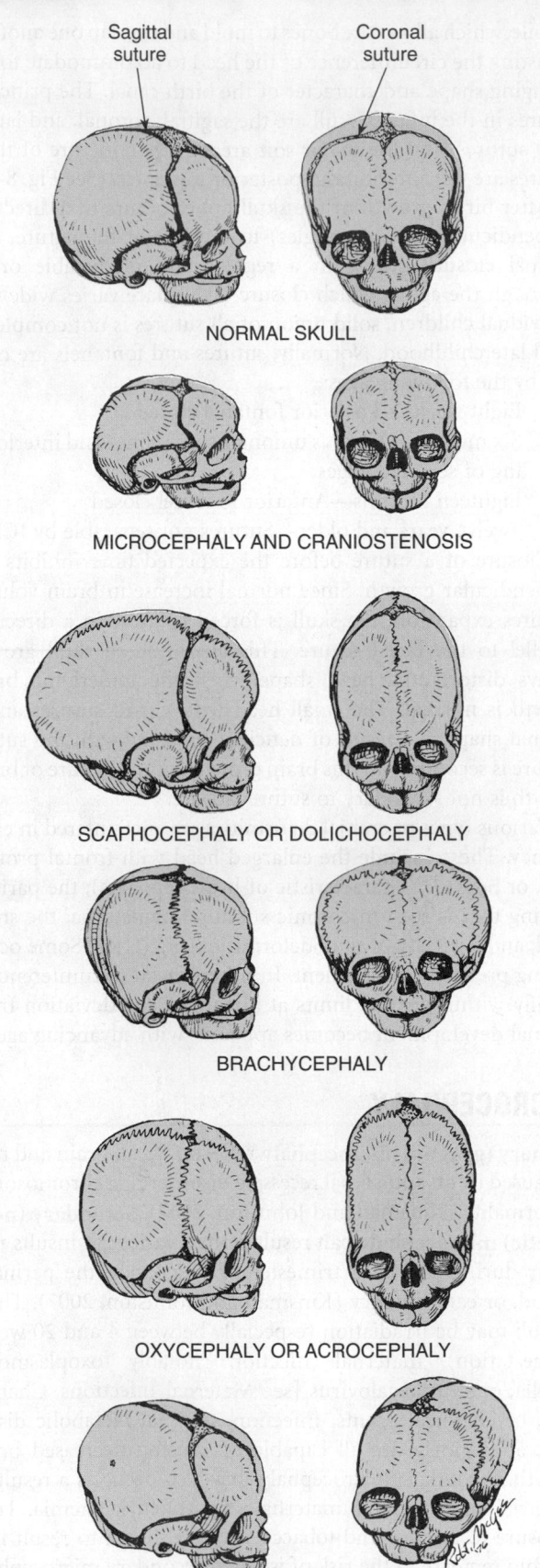

NORMAL SKULL

MICROCEPHALY AND CRANIOSTENOSIS

SCAPHOCEPHALY OR DOLICHOCEPHALY

BRACHYCEPHALY

OXYCEPHALY OR ACROCEPHALY

PLAGIOCEPHALY

Fig. 11-8 Craniostenosis. Abnormal head configuration resulting from premature closing of cranial sutures.

behavior to mild motor impairment, educable neurocognitive impairment, and mild hyperkinesis. There appears to be a decided relationship between microcephaly and cognitive delays of varying degrees; however, not all children with microcephaly have cognitive delays.

Nursing Care Management

There is no specific treatment. Nursing care is supportive and may be directed toward helping parents adjust to rearing a child with cognitive impairment when this condition is present. (See Chapter 24.)

CRANIOSTENOSIS

Craniostenosis is defined as the premature closure at birth of one or more cranial sutures (Kinsman and Johnston, 2007). The clinical picture depends on which sutures close, the duration of the closure process, and the success or failure of the other sutures to compensate by expansion (see Fig. 11-8). The condition may be divided according to the number of sutures involved; primary craniostenosis involves only one suture, whereas secondary craniostenosis involves two or more sutures (Kinsman and Johnston, 2007). Focal hydrodynamic mechanisms are involved in the compensatory skull changes seen in craniostenosis. Brain atrophy and an underlying motor delay account for the position-induced skull changes. Craniostenosis is also a common feature of children with Crouzon, Apert (Box 11-4), Pfeiffer, Carpenter, and Jackson-Weiss syndromes (Kinsman and Johnston, 2007). Potential risk factors for craniostenosis include maternal Caucasian race, advanced maternal age, male infant, use of nitrosatable drugs, fertility treatments, and certain paternal occupations (agriculture, repairmen, mechanics, forestry). Recently genetic mutations have been linked to the occurrence of craniostenosis, and in such cases genetic counseling is advised (Merritt, 2009). Diagnosis is established with CT scan, and MRI is useful in identifying accompanying brain abnormalities. Increased ICP is more frequent in children with more than one prematurely fused suture.

The most common form of craniostenosis is premature closure of the sagittal suture with resulting elongation of the

---

BOX 11-4 **CRANIAL ABNORMALITIES ASSOCIATED WITH ABNORMAL BONE GROWTH**

Crouzon syndrome—Craniofacial dysostosis (abnormal ossification of fetal cartilages) with shallow orbits and underdevelopment of the middle third of the face

Apert syndrome—Craniostenosis resulting in a prominent forehead; may be extracranial abnormalities, such as syndactyly (webbing) of fingers and toes and cardiac defects

Treacher Collins syndrome—Asymmetric facial deformity, including absent cheekbones, underslung jaw, and small chin; also downward slant of the eyes and other minor defects

Pierre Robin sequence—Displacement of the chin as a result of micrognathia (mandibular hypoplasia) or retrognathia (normal-sized mandible positioned posteriorly); also glossoptosis with obstruction of the airway and sometimes a cleft palate

skull in the anteroposterior direction. A similar head shape occurs as a result of postnatal position maintenance in some preterm infants; however, in this case there is no premature closure of sutures. Craniostenosis may cause an increase in ICP, which may or may not cause cognitive delays but can result in progressive papilledema, optic atrophy, and eventual blindness. Other complications include facial asymmetry and malocclusion.

Trigonocephaly, or metopic craniostenosis, represents a premature closure of the metopic suture in utero, a congenital problem that is familial and may not require surgical treatment. The metopic suture occurs where the right and left frontal bones meet on the forehead. Craniostenosis of the metopic suture may be an autosomal dominantly inherited disorder not associated with functional brain or other abnormalities.

Therapeutic Management

Treatment involves surgical excision of long bars of bone (strip craniectomy) along or parallel to the fused suture. Various surgical procedures are employed in an effort to release the fused suture and direct growth. Surgery is performed to achieve the best possible cosmetic effect and, in severe cases, to relieve cerebral pressure symptoms and complications. The advised timing of suture release is before 6 months of age for best cosmetic and neurodevelopmental results. An endoscopic strip craniectomy results in less blood loss than other types of craniectomy, and length of stay is decreased (Merritt, 2009).

Nursing Care Management

Nursing care primarily involves the early identification of persistent cranial molding weeks after regular birth molding would have resolved and referral for follow-up evaluation. In the postoperative period, nursing care includes observation for changes in neurologic status, hemorrhage, or infection.

Because of the type of bone surgery involved with craniostenosis, blood loss can be large. Therefore the nurse carefully monitors hematocrit and hemoglobin. Parents may also wish to provide a compatible blood donor for their infant. Nurses need to inform and guide parents through this blood bank procedure. With endoscopic surgery, blood loss is minimized, but the child must wear a cranial molding helmet for several months (Merritt, 2009). Instructions regarding compliance with the helmet and skin care are essential.

Most children have substantial swelling of the eyelids postoperatively; careful handling and talking to the child may help calm fears while the eyelids are swollen shut. Eye care should be limited to gentle cleansing with a moist cloth. Pain management measures should be instituted in infants experiencing postoperative pain as they would be for older children or adults. Fluids and adequate hydration are essential. Oral feedings resume as soon as possible for hydration and for the infant's nutritive sucking needs.

Early surgical management of craniostenosis allows proper expansion of the brain and the creation of an acceptable appearance. Parents require special support and education during this time, especially from other parents whose infants have undergone similar operations. The nurse can serve as a liaison for this type of parental support.

CRANIOFACIAL ABNORMALITIES

Craniofacial abnormalities are those deformities involving the skull and facial bones. They have a low incidence rate in the population, but their effects can be psychologically devastating to affected children and their families. Box 11-4 lists deformities caused by abnormal growth of cranial bone(s).

Most craniofacial anomalies are compatible with life, and all efforts are made to help the child and family live as normal a life as anyone else. Advances in microscopic, orthopedic, neurologic, and plastic reconstructive surgery techniques have made it possible for children with craniofacial anomalies not only to survive beyond childhood, but also to live a fulfilling life without the social stigmas of past decades. These children, however, may continue to face erroneous assumptions of cognitive impairment because of their appearance. Craniofacial multidisciplinary teams are dedicated to helping the child and family achieve optimum potential for intellectual growth, physical competence, and social acceptance.

Therapeutic Management

Craniofacial surgical correction involves peeling the patient's face away from the skull and remolding the understructures. Parts can be brought together, the skull reshaped and remodeled, and bone fragments removed or reshaped. Bone segments from the child's hip or ribs may be used to reshape the skull or facial features. The procedures are performed at various ages, depending on the anomaly, in craniofacial centers specializing in this pediatric problem. The timing of surgery is before school entry and is determined on an individual basis to ensure normal growth and development. Depending on the abnormality, other surgeries are performed, such as mandibular and digit correction. After surgery, continued growth conforming to the inborn abnormality is unlikely.

Nursing Care Management

Direct nursing efforts toward preparation for surgery (often several surgical procedures over time), postoperative care similar to care of any child with cranial surgery, and support of the child and family. Frequently this child and family must adjust to the unfamiliar body image, which may be as traumatic as the previous deformity. A helmet may be worn to protect the operative site and bone grafts for 6 months to 2 years. Follow-up care is important.

PIERRE ROBIN SEQUENCE

Pierre Robin sequence (PRS) is a defect characterized by retroposition of the tongue and mandible, which often results in neonatal respiratory and feeding problems. The condition has an incidence of 1 in 8500 to 14,000 live births, and about one half of those with PRS have other congenital anomalies (Buchenau, Urschitz, Sautermeister, et al, 2007). The tongue may be large (glossoptosis) and frequently falls over the neonate's airway, causing occlusion and respiratory distress. In severe upper airway obstruction a tracheostomy may be required. From a lateral view the infant's lower jaw can be seen to be positioned posterior (micrognathia) to the upper jaw. PRS may be diagnosed in the nursery when the infant has apnea and cyanosis, due primarily to the upper airway obstruction. The neonate is positioned to facilitate an open airway, and the practitioner is notified immediately. A tongue-lip adhesion is a common surgical procedure that repositions the tongue anteriorly (Bijnen, Don Griot, Mulder, et al, 2009). Surgical mandibular distraction is another technique used to correct the defect (Dauria and Marsh, 2008). There are usually no associated neurocognitive defects in isolated PRS.

POSITIONAL PLAGIOCEPHALY

Since the Back to Sleep campaign began in 1992 advocating nonprone sleeping for infants to prevent sudden infant death syndrome (SIDS), an increase in the incidence of positional plagiocephaly has been observed (American Academy of Pediatrics, 2005; Littlefield, Saba, and Kelly, 2004). Prevalence of positional plagiocephaly at 4 months is reported to range from slightly less than 20% to as much as 48% (Robinson and Proctor, 2009). The term plagiocephaly connotes an oblique or asymmetric head; *positional plagiocephaly, deformational plagiocephaly,* or *nonsynostotic plagiocephaly* implies an acquired condition that occurs as a result of cranial molding during infancy (Hummel and Fortado, 2005). Because the infant's sutures are not closed, the skull is pliable and, when the infant is placed on the back to sleep, the posterior occiput flattens over time (Fig. 11-9, *A*). A typical bald spot develops, which is usually transient. As a result of prolonged pressure on one side of the skull, that side becomes misshapen; mild facial asymmetry may develop. The sternocleidomastoid muscle may tighten on the preferential side, and torticollis may also develop. Congenital or acquired torticollis may cause plagiocephaly; other causes of deformational plagiocephaly include certain craniofacial syndromes. This discussion centers only on plagiocephaly caused by supine sleeping position.

Therapeutic Management

Treatment of torticollis and plagiocephaly initially involves exercises to loosen the tight muscle and switching head position sides during feeding, carrying, and sleep. If the plagiocephaly is not resolved within 4 to 8 weeks of physical therapy, a customized helmet may be worn to decrease the pressure on the affected side of the skull (Fig. 11-9, *B*). If no improvement occurs with physical therapy or a molded helmet over a given period, the infant may be referred to a pediatric neurosurgeon or craniofacial surgeon. In one study repositioning was not as helpful in reducing plagiocephaly as was the use of an orthotic helmet. Those treated with a helmet were older and had a longer treatment period, leading the authors to conclude that early detection and orthotic intervention were likely to be more successful (Graham, Gomez, Halberg, et al, 2005).

The helmet is worn 23 hours a day for a prescribed period (usually 3 months). Repositioning and physical therapy are said to be more effective when used before the infant can roll over or move his or her head alone (i.e., before approximately 3 to 4 months of age) (Robinson and Proctor, 2009). Reports of developmental delay in infants with positional plagiocephaly (nonsynostotic) vary in regard to outcomes, but current studies do not conclusively prove that such infants are at higher risk for developmental delays (Robinson and Proctor, 2009).

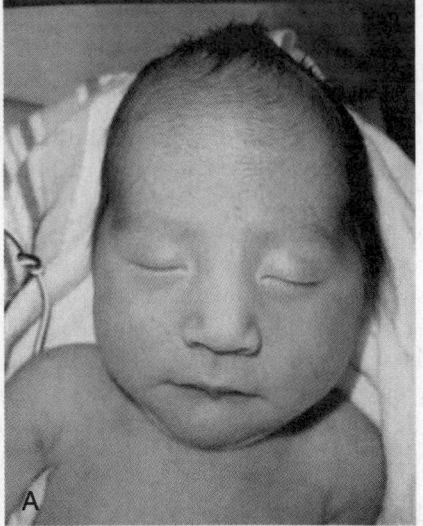

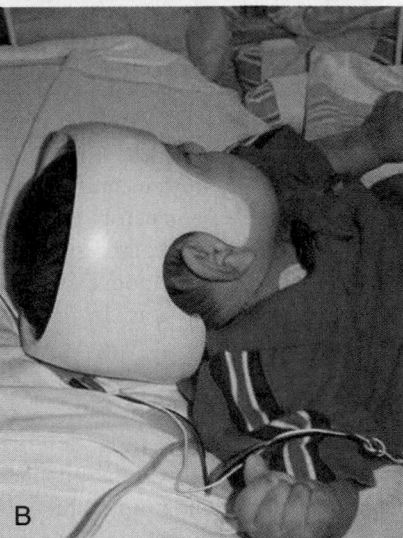

Fig 11-9 A, Plagiocephaly. **B,** Helmet used to correct plagiocephaly. (Courtesy Dr. Gerardo Cabrera-Meza, Department of Neonatology, Baylor College of Medicine, Houston.)

Nursing Care Management

Minor skull flattening is not considered significant, but parents should learn to prevent plagiocephaly by altering the infant's head position during sleep. Infants should be placed prone on a firm surface during awake time (tummy time), which prevents plagiocephaly and facilitates development of upper shoulder girdle strength; the latter helps in the progressive development of movements such as rolling over and starting to rise up on all fours, which are precursors to crawling and eventually walking. Thirty minutes of supervised tummy time per day in infants younger than 6 months of age is recommended (Robinson and Proctor, 2009).

Despite the perceived increase in the incidence of positional plagiocephaly, the supine sleeping position is still recommended because it has led to a significant decrease in loss of infant lives from SIDS (American Academy of Pediatrics, 2005). Additional measures to prevent plagiocephaly include avoiding excessive time spent in car restraint seats or infant seats and bouncers. Alternating the infant's head position for sleep times can also prevent unilateral molding. When a nurse or parent notices plagiocephaly, a consultation with the primary practitioner is recommended to evaluate the head shape and ascertain the need for early intervention.

Nurses are in a unique position in well-child care settings to encourage parents to follow guidelines for preventing plagiocephaly, to demonstrate alternating head placement for sleeping, to demonstrate sternocleidomastoid muscle exercises (as appropriate to the condition), and to encourage tummy time for infants during awake periods. Most important, nurses should continue to encourage parents to place the infant in a supine sleep position despite the development of plagiocephaly. Parents should not become so alarmed by plagiocephaly that they abandon supine sleeping position for the infant but should consult with the practitioner for further advice.

SKELETAL DEFECTS

This discussion is limited to those defects in development that are most common, that are amenable to therapy, and that involve nurses to a considerable extent. Less common defects and disorders are described in Table 11-4.

DEVELOPMENTAL DYSPLASIA OF THE HIP

The broad term **developmental dysplasia of the hip (DDH)** describes a spectrum of disorders related to abnormal development of the hip that may develop at any time during fetal life, infancy, or childhood. A change in terminology from *congenital hip dysplasia* and *congenital dislocation of the hip* to DDH more properly reflects the varying onset and types of hip abnormalities in which there is a shallow acetabulum, subluxation, or dislocation (Box 11-5).

The incidence of hip instability of some kind is approximately 1 to 1.5 per 1000 live births (Hosalkar, Horn, Friedman, et al, 2007). Approximately 30% to 50% of infants with DDH were born breech. The left hip is involved in 60% of cases, the right hip in 20%, and both hips in 20%. Eighty percent of those affected are female. Caucasian children have a higher incidence of DDH than other ethnic groups (Maher, Salmond, and Pellino, 2002).

Etiology and Pathophysiology

The cause of DDH is unknown, but certain factors such as gender, birth order, family history, intrauterine position,

TABLE 11-4	CONGENITAL DEFECTS INVOLVING THE SKELETON	
DISORDER	**DESCRIPTION AND ANATOMIC VARIATION**	**THERAPY**
Achondroplasia	Inherited (autosomal dominant)	None
	Defect in ossification at epiphyseal plate, resulting in short limbs, large head, and lordosis	
Osteogenesis imperfecta	Inherited (autosomal dominant, autosomal recessive)	Reduction of fractures
	Characterized by brittle, fragile, and easily fractured bones	Careful handling of extremities
	Intrauterine fractures may produce congenital deformities	See Chapter 39
Pes planus (flat foot)	Normal finding in infancy	Rarely indicated
	May be result of muscular weakness in older child	Wedge on inner side of heel and sole for persistent or severe cases
Pes valgus	Eversion of entire foot, but sole rests on ground	Exercises
Pes varus	Inversion of entire foot, but sole rests on ground	Exercises
Metatarsus valgus	Eversion of foot while heel remains straight	Passive exercises
	Also called toeing out or duck walk	
Talipes deformities	See p. 424	See p. 424
Supernumerary digits (polydactyly)	Excessive number of fingers, toes, or both; usually inherited (autosomal dominant)	No treatment, or amputation of extra digits to improve function or for cosmetic reasons
Genu varum (bowleg)	May be congenital, result of rickets, or caused by osteochondrosis of proximal tibial epiphysis	Corrective splinting
		Osteotomy in severe or neglected cases
Genu recurvatum (back knee)	Congenital, result of prenatal developmental defect or abnormal intrauterine position	Repeated corrective casting
	Developmental, result of postnatal trauma or infection	Exercises
Klippel-Feil syndrome	Absence of 1 or more cervical vertebrae and 2 or more fused together	Rarely indicated
	Neck short and limited in motion	Scapula brought down and fixed if marked deformity or loss of function
	Sometimes kyphosis and scoliosis	Bracing of spinal deformities
Arachnodactyly (Marfan syndrome)	Inherited (autosomal dominant)	Supportive measures
	Abnormal length of fingers, toes, and extremities; hypermobility of joints; defects of spine and chest (pigeon breast); other associated abnormalities	
Congenital spine deformities	Kyphosis, scoliosis, lordosis, hemivertebrae, or combination of these	Prevention of progression of defect with growth
		Casting, bracing
		Operative stabilization of affected vertebrae
		In some cases, exercise
Arthrogryposis multiplex congenita	Incomplete fibrous ankylosis of many or all joints (except spine and jaw) associated with hypoplasia of attached muscles	Bracing, splinting, corrective surgery, and rehabilitation efforts
	Contracture deformities—some extension, others flexion	

delivery method, joint laxity, and postnatal positioning affect the risk of DDH. Predisposing factors associated with DDH are divided into three broad categories: (1) physiologic factors, including maternal hormone secretion and intrauterine positioning; (2) mechanical factors; and (3) genetic factors. Mechanical factors involve breech presentation, multiple fetuses, oligohydramnios, and large infant size, as well as continued maintenance of the hips in adduction and extension, causing a dislocation (see Cultural Competence box). Genetic factors account for a higher incidence (6%) of DDH in siblings of affected infants, and an even greater incidence (36%) of recurrence if a sibling and one parent were affected.

BOX 11-5   DEGREES OF DEVELOPMENTAL DYSPLASIA OF THE HIP

Acetabular dysplasia (or preluxation)—The mildest form, in which there is neither subluxation nor dislocation. The dysplasia reflects an apparent delay in acetabular development evidenced by osseous hypoplasia of the acetabular roof, which is oblique and shallow, although the cartilaginous roof is comparatively intact. The femoral head remains in the acetabulum.

Subluxation—Accounts for the largest percentage of congenital hip dysplasias. Subluxation implies incomplete dislocation or disclosable hip and is sometimes regarded as an intermediate state in the progression from primary dysplasia to complete dislocation. The femoral head remains in contact with the acetabulum, but a stretched capsule and round ligament of femur cause the head of the femur to be partially displaced. Pressure on the cartilaginous roof inhibits ossification and produces a flattening of the socket.

Dislocation—The most severe form, in which the femoral head loses contact with the acetabulum and is displaced posteriorly and superiorly over the fibrocartilaginous rim. The round ligament of femur is elongated and taut.

DDH may be further categorized into two major groups: (1) typical, in which the infant is neurologically intact; and (2) teratologic, which involves a neuromuscular defect such as arthrogryposis or myelodysplasia. The teratologic forms usually occur in utero and are much less common.

Fig. 11-10 illustrates three degrees of DDH. They are also outlined in Box 11-5.

Clinical Manifestations

The diagnosis of DDH should be made in the newborn period if possible, since treatment initiated before 2 months of age achieves the highest rate of success. In the newborn period dysplasia usually appears as hip joint laxity rather than as outright dislocation. Subluxation and the tendency to dislocate can be demonstrated by the Ortolani or Barlow test. With the infant quiet and relaxed in the supine position on a firm surface and the legs facing the examiner, the hips are flexed (not forced) at right angles and the knees are flexed. The examiner places the middle finger of each hand over the greater trochanter and the thumbs on the inner side of the thigh at a point opposite the lesser trochanter. The knees are carried to midabduction, and each hip joint is submitted, one at a time, first to forward pressure exerted behind the trochanter and then to backward pressure exerted from the thumbs in front as the opposite joint is held steady. If the femoral head can be felt to slip forward into the acetabulum on pressure from behind, it is dislocated (Ortolani test) (Fig. 11-11, *D*).

Sometimes an audible "clunk" can be heard on exit or entry of the femur out of or into the acetabulum. If, on pressure from the front, the femoral head is felt to slip out over the posterior lip of the acetabulum and immediately slips back in place when pressure is released, the hip is said to be dislocatable or "unstable" (Barlow test). The audible clunk is not pathologic and occurs as a result of breaking surface tension across the hip joint, knee rotation, snapping of gluteal tendons, or patellofemoral motion.

❗ NURSING ALERT

The Barlow and Ortolani tests should be performed *only* by an experienced clinician to prevent damage to the hip. If these tests are performed too vigorously in the first 2 days of life, when the hip subluxates freely, persistent dislocation may occur.

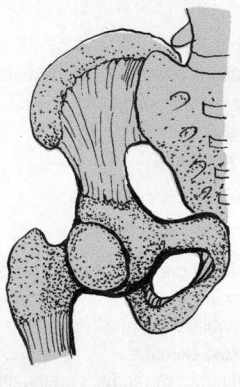
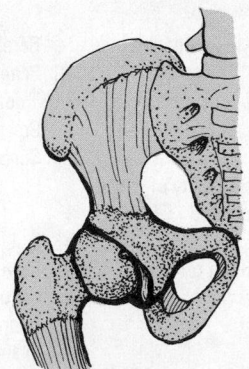
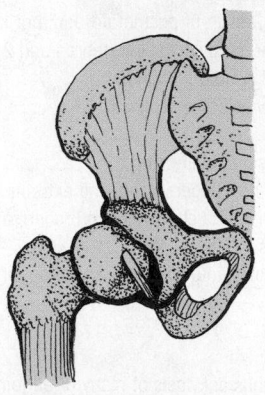
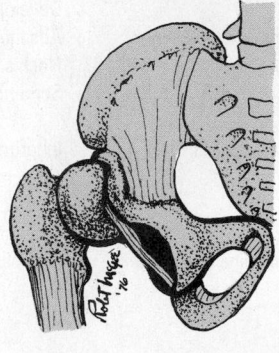

Normal   Dysplasia   Subluxation   Dislocation

Fig. 11-10 Configuration and relationship of structures in developmental dysplasia of hip.

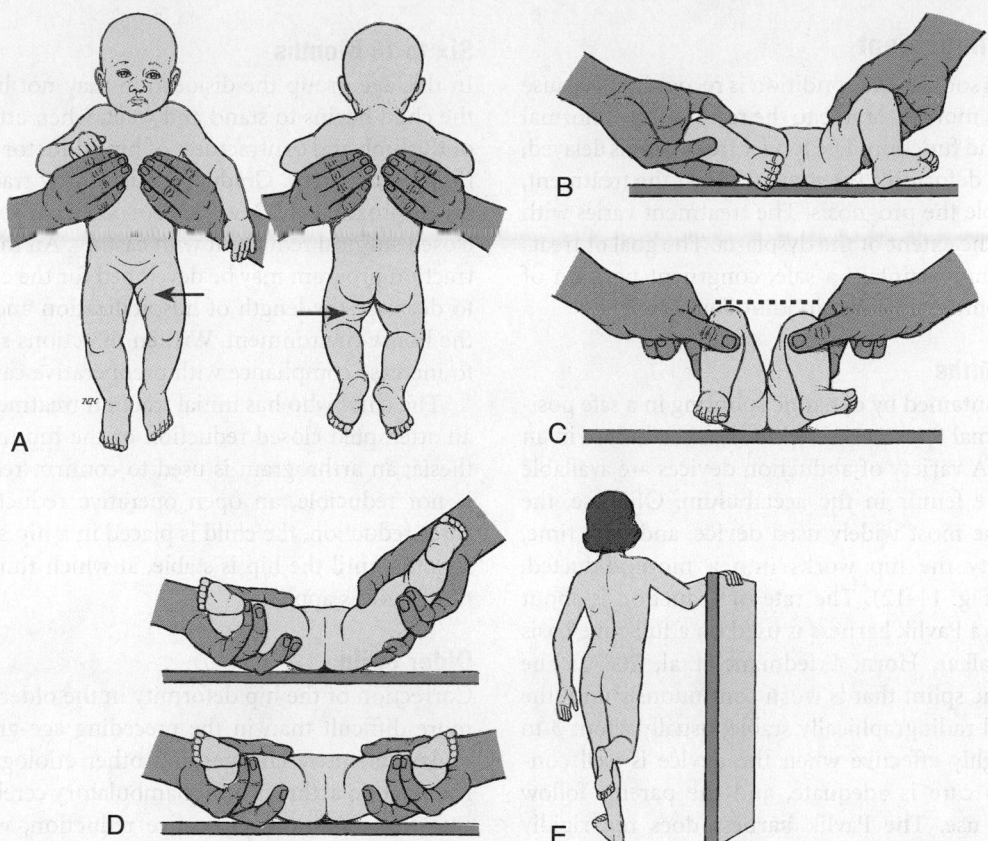

Fig. 11-11 Signs of developmental dysplasia of hip. **A,** Asymmetry of gluteal and thigh folds. **B,** Limited hip abduction, as seen in flexion. **C,** Apparent shortening of femur, as indicated by level of knees in flexion. **D,** Ortolani clunk (if infant is <4 weeks of age). **E,** Positive Trendelenburg sign (if child is weight bearing).

The Ortolani and Barlow tests are most reliable from birth to 2 or 3 months of age. Adduction contractures develop at about 6 to 10 weeks, and the Ortolani sign disappears. After this time the most sensitive test is limited hip abduction (Fig. 11-11, *B*). Other signs are shortening of the thigh on the affected side (Galleazzi sign) (Fig. 11-11, *C*), asymmetric thigh and gluteal folds (Fig. 11-11, *A*), and broadening of the perineum (in bilateral dislocation). Weight bearing may precipitate a transition from subluxation to dislocation in unrecognized cases.

A common cause of decreased hip abduction in the newborn is pelvic obliquity in which one side of the pelvis is higher than the other. This is caused by intrauterine positioning and will resolve on its own.

In the older infant and child the affected leg is shorter than the other, with telescoping or piston mobility; that is, the head of the femur can be felt to move up and down in the buttock when the extended thigh is first pushed toward the child's head and then pulled distally. Instability of the hip on weight bearing delays walking and produces a characteristic limp, waddling gait and toe walking. When the child stands first on one foot and then on the other (holding onto a chair, rail, or someone's hands), bearing weight on the affected hip, the pelvis tilts downward on the normal side instead of upward as it would with normal stability (positive Trendelenburg sign) (Fig. 11-11, *E*). The practitioner should test the child for at least 30 seconds. In both unilateral and bilateral dislocations the greater trochanter is prominent and appears above a line from the anterosuperior iliac spine to the tuberosity of the ischium. The child with bilateral dislocations has marked lordosis and a peculiar waddling gait.

Diagnostic Evaluation

DDH is often not detected at the initial examination after birth; thus all infants should be carefully monitored for hip dysplasia at follow-up visits throughout the first year of life. The primary diagnostic tools in the newborn period are the assessment techniques just described.

Radiographic examination in early infancy is not reliable because ossification of the femoral head does not normally take place until the third to sixth month of life. However, the cartilaginous head can be visualized directly with real-time high-resolution ultrasonography. There has been debate regarding the role of ultrasound technology in diagnosing DDH in early infancy, and widespread newborn screening has been suggested. However, numerous studies reveal this approach has a high rate of false positives and subsequent overtreatment. Once the proximal femoral epiphysis ossifies (usually 4 to 6 months), and in older children, radiographic examination is useful in confirming the diagnosis (Hosalkar, Horn, Friedman, et al, 2007). An upward slope in the roof of the acetabulum (the acetabular angle) greater than 40 degrees with upward and outward displacement of the femoral head is a frequent finding in older children. CT scan may be useful to assess the position of the femoral head relative to the acetabulum after closed reduction and casting.

Therapeutic Management

Treatment begins as soon as the condition is recognized because early intervention is more favorable to the restoration of normal bony architecture and function. The longer treatment is delayed, the more severe the deformity, the more difficult the treatment, and the less favorable the prognosis. The treatment varies with the child's age and the extent of the dysplasia. The goal of treatment is to obtain and maintain a safe, congruent position of the hip joint to promote normal hip joint development.

Newborn to 6 Months

The hip joint is maintained by dynamic splinting in a safe position with the proximal femur centered in the acetabulum in an attitude of flexion. A variety of abduction devices are available for maintaining the femur in the acetabulum. Of these, the Pavlik harness is the most widely used device, and with time, motion, and gravity the hip works into a more abducted, reduced position (Fig. 11-12). The rate of reduction is about 95% effective when a Pavlik harness is used on a full-time basis for 6 weeks (Hosalkar, Horn, Friedman, et al, 2007). The harness is a dynamic splint that is worn continuously until the hip is clinically and radiographically stable, usually about 3 to 5 months. It is highly effective when the device is well constructed, follow-up care is adequate, and the parents follow instructions in its use. The Pavlik harness does not rigidly immobilize the hip but acts to prevent hip extension or adduction. Because of the infant's rapid growth rate, the straps should be checked every 1 to 2 weeks for adjustments. Improper positioning may cause vascular or nerve damage.

When adduction contracture is present, other devices (such as skin traction) are employed to slowly and gently stretch the hip to full abduction, after which wide abduction is maintained until stability is attained. When maintaining stable reduction is difficult, a hip spica cast is applied and changed periodically to accommodate the child's growth. After 3 to 6 months, sufficient stability is acquired to allow transfer to a removable protective abduction brace. The duration of treatment depends on development of the acetabulum but usually lasts less than a year.

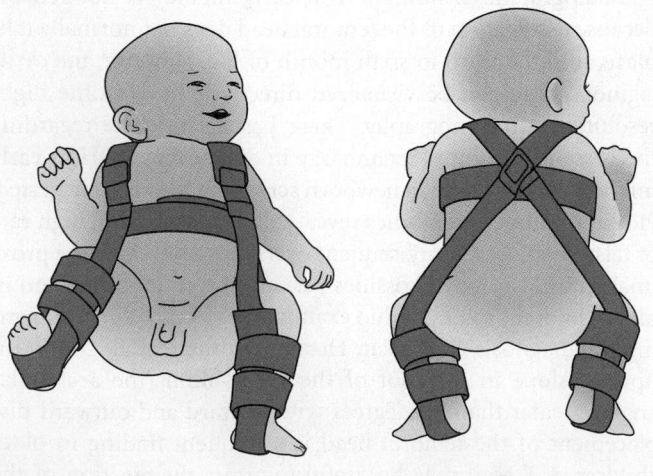

Front   Back

Fig. 11-12 Child in Pavlik harness. (From Ball JW: *Mosby's pediatric patient teaching guides*, St Louis, 1998, Mosby.)

Six to 18 Months

In this age-group the dislocation may not be recognized until the child begins to stand and walk, when attendant shortening of the limb and contractures of hip adductor and flexor muscles become apparent. Gradual reduction by traction may be used for approximately 3 weeks. An alternative to traction is the closed surgical reduction with casting. An individualized home traction program may be developed for the child preoperatively to decrease the length of hospitalization and keep the child in the home environment. Written directions should be provided to increase compliance with preoperative care.

The child who has initial traction treatment then undergoes an attempted closed reduction of the hip under general anesthesia; an arthrogram is used to confirm reduction. If the hip is not reducible, an open operative reduction is performed. After reduction, the child is placed in a hip spica cast for 2 to 4 months until the hip is stable, at which time a flexion-abduction brace is applied.

Older Child

Correction of the hip deformity in the older child is inherently more difficult than in the preceding age-groups because secondary adaptive changes and other etiologic factors (such as rheumatoid arthritis or nonambulatory cerebral palsy) complicate the condition. Operative reduction, which may involve preoperative traction, tenotomy of contracted muscles, and any one of several innominate osteotomy procedures designed to construct an acetabular roof, is usually required. After cast removal and before weight bearing is permitted, range-of-motion exercises help restore movement. Other rehabilitative measures may include muscle strengthening, a period of crutch walking, and gait training. Successful reduction and reconstruction become increasingly difficult after the age of 4 years and are usually impossible or inadvisable after age 6 because of severe shortening and contracture of muscles and deformity of the femoral and acetabular structures.

Hip dislocation is often observed in older children with SB and reportedly does not significantly interfere with ambulation. Reduction of the affected hip is not worthwhile in most of these children unless the dislocation is bilateral or there is significant flexion contracture (Rowe and Jadhav, 2008).

Nursing Care Management

Nurses are in a unique position to detect DDH in the newborn. During the infant assessment process and routine nurturing activities, the nurse inspects the hips and extremities for any deviations from normal. Observation for unequal gluteal and thigh folds is routine, and nurses who have been educated to perform the Ortolani and Barlow tests should refer the infant with a positive test result to the practitioner. The ambulatory child who displays a limp or waddling gait is referred for evaluation. This may indicate an orthopedic or neurologic problem. The nurse also assesses nonambulatory children with cerebral palsy for evidence of dislocation.

The former practice of double- or triple-diapering for DDH is controversial, but is generally not recommended because it promotes hip extension, thus exacerbating improper hip development.

Observations during routine care, such as diapering, provide an opportunity to observe the infant for limited movement and a wide perineum, which is an indication to assess for leg shortening, unequal gluteal and thigh folds, and limited abduction.

Care of the Child

The primary nursing goal is teaching parents to apply and maintain the reduction device. The Pavlik harness allows for easy handling of the infant and usually produces less apprehension in the parent than heavy braces and casts. It is important that parents understand the correct use of the appliance, which may or may not allow for its removal during bathing. If the infant has a harness that is not removed, a sponge bath is recommended.

The following instructions for preventing skin breakdown with the harness are stressed:

- Always put an undershirt (or a shirt with extensions that close at the crotch) under the chest straps and put knee socks under the foot and leg pieces to prevent the straps from rubbing the skin.
- Check frequently (at least two or three times a day) for red areas under the straps and the clothing.
- Gently massage healthy skin under the straps once a day to stimulate circulation. In general, avoid lotions and powders because they can cake and irritate the skin.
- Always place the diaper under the straps.

The parents are permitted to pad shoulder straps at pressure points if desired, but unbuckling or removal is determined on the basis of the family's level of understanding and the degree of hip deformity. In general, parents are not encouraged to adjust the harness without supervision. The practitioner should examine the child before any adjustment is attempted to ascertain that the hips are in correct position before the harness is resecured. Problems reported by parents included difficulty applying the harness after the bath, carrying the child, skin-crease dermatitis, feet slipping, and difficulty in clothing the child (Hassan, 2009). These findings highlight the importance of close follow up within the first few weeks of treatment and written take-home instructions for the parents to follow in managing the Pavlik harness.

The major challenges in the care of an infant or child in a cast or other device are related to maintaining the device and adapting nurturing activities to meet the patient's needs. Generally, treatment and follow-up care of these children are carried out in a clinic, practitioner's office, or outpatient unit. Hospitalization may be necessary for cast application or brace fitting but seldom exceeds 24 to 48 hours. Longer hospitalization is required for open reduction. (See also The Child in a Cast, Chapter 39.)

Casts offer more challenging nursing problems, since they cannot be removed for routine care. Care of an infant or small child with a cast requires nursing innovation to reduce irritation and to maintain cleanliness of both the child and the cast, particularly in the perineum and sacrum. The importance of spica cast care should be emphasized when providing instructions. The life of the cast should be prolonged to hold the legs and hips in proper position postoperatively and prevent an unnecessary cast change.

Chapter 39 discusses cast care and observation, so these are not elaborated on here. However, since DDH is almost the only reason for application of casts in early infancy, some of the problems specific to that age-group are mentioned.

Parents need to learn the proper care of the cast (or brace) and need help to devise means for maintaining cleanliness. A disposable newborn diaper is tucked beneath the entire perineal opening of the cast. A larger (toddler-size) diaper can be applied and fastened over the small diaper and cast. The goal is to absorb the urine while avoiding urine saturation or soiling of the cast.

For tightly fitting casts, transparent film dressing can be cut into strips as for petaling (see Chapter 39), and one edge can be applied to the cast edge and the other directly to the perineum; this forms a continuous waterproof bridge between the perineum and the cast to prevent leakage. An additional advantage to using this dressing material is that it keeps both the skin and the cast dry while allowing observation of the skin beneath the dressing.

Older infants and small children may stuff bits of food, small toys, or other items under the cast. Alert parents to this possibility so they can initiate suitable preventive measures, such as placing clothing over the cast.

Feeding the infant in a hip spica cast or brace offers problems of positioning. Very young infants can be fed in the supine position with the head elevated, and, with the infant's hips and legs supported on a pillow at the side, the parent can cuddle the infant during feeding. A somewhat similar position can be used for breast-feeding (i.e., with the infant supported on pillows or held in a "football" hold facing the mother with the legs behind her). An alternate position is to hold the infant upright on the mother's lap with the infant's legs astride the mother's legs.

Infants who are able to sit up can be fed in a feeding table or modified high chair. A padded tilt board with an adjustable chair may be adapted for the child in a hip spica cast. The table or chair provides an excellent place for the child to play in an upright position. The child's transportation in a safe car seat is also a vital consideration. Many hospitals have a child passenger safety program. A loan program for the appropriate automotive safety restraint or referral to an agency that provides this service may be offered by the discharge coordinator nurse or social worker.*

Family Support and Home Care

It is important for nurses, parents, and other caregivers to understand that children with DDH need to be involved in all the activities of any child in the same age-group. Toys are chosen that can be used in a prone position on the floor or in the seats devised for feeding and other activities. Confinement in a cast or appliance should not exclude children from family (or unit) activities. They can be held astride a lap for comfort and transported to areas of activity. The child may be allowed to walk in a cast or brace. An adapted wheelchair or stroller can

---

*For additional information contact the Automotive Safety Program, Riley Hospital for Children, Indiana University School of Medicine, 575 West Drive, Room 004, Indianapolis, IN 46202; 317-274-2977 (in Indianapolis), 800-543-6227; www.preventinjury.org.

offer mobility to the older infant or child. (See Chapter 39 for further discussion of care of a child in a spica cast.)

CONGENITAL CLUBFOOT

Congenital clubfoot is a complex deformity of the ankle and foot that includes forefoot adduction, midfoot supination, hindfoot varus, and ankle equinus. Also referred to as talipes equinovarus (TEV), congenital clubfoot involves bone deformity and malposition with soft tissue contracture (Fig. 11-13). This condition requires early evaluation and treatment for optimum correction. TEV is the most frequently occurring type of clubfoot (approximately 95%), although other variations may be seen and are generally described according to the position of the ankle and foot (Box 11-6). Unilateral clubfoot may occur as an isolated defect or in association with other disorders or syndromes, such as a chromosomal disorder, arthrogryposis (a generalized immobility of the joints), cerebral palsy, or SB.

The incidence of clubfoot in the general population is 1 to 2 per 1000 live births, with boys affected twice as often as girls. Bilateral clubfeet occur in 50% of the cases (Hosalkar, Spiegel, and Davidson, 2007). A positive family history is associated with increased incidence. Incidence varies with geographic location, with the lowest incidence in China and the highest in Polynesia.

Clubfoot may be further divided into three categories: (1) positional clubfoot (also called transitional, mild, or postural clubfoot), which is believed to occur primarily from intrauterine crowding and responds to simple stretching and casting; (2) syndromic (or teratologic) clubfoot, which is associated with other congenital abnormalities such as myelomeningocele (myelodysplasia) or arthrogryposis and is a more severe form of clubfoot that is often resistant to treatment; and (3) congenital clubfoot, also referred to as idiopathic or true clubfoot, which may occur in an otherwise normal child and has a wide

---

BOX 11-6	COMMON FOOT MALFORMATIONS

Talipes varus—An inversion or a bending inward
Talipes valgus—An eversion or a bending outward
Talipes equinus—Plantar flexion, in which the toes are lower than the heel
Talipes calcaneus—Dorsiflexion, in which the toes are higher than the heel

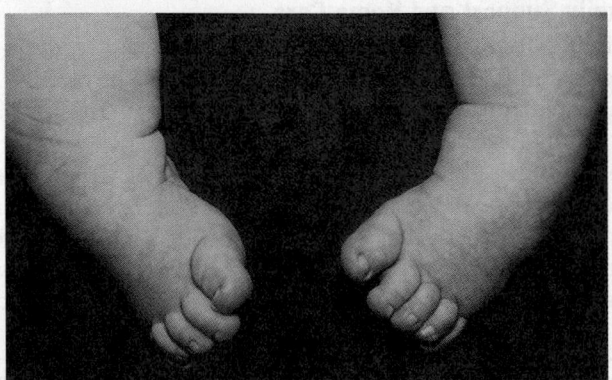

Fig. 11-13 Bilateral congenital talipes equinovarus (congenital clubfoot) in 2-month-old infant. (From Zitelli BJ, Davis HW: *Atlas of pediatric physical diagnosis,* ed 5, St Louis, 2007, Mosby.)

---

range of rigidity and prognosis. The third category may be detected in utero by ultrasonography and is the most common type of TEV seen.

The mild, or positional, clubfoot may correct spontaneously or may require passive exercise or serial casting. The infant has no bony abnormality, but may have tightness and shortening of the soft tissues medially and posteriorly. The teratologic clubfoot usually requires surgical correction and has a high incidence of recurrence. The congenital clubfoot almost always requires surgical intervention because of the bony abnormality.

Pathophysiology

The exact cause of clubfoot remains unknown. However, there is a strong familial tendency, with a 1 in 10 chance that a parent with clubfoot will have an affected offspring. Other possible theories as to the cause of clubfoot include arrested fetal developmental of skeletal and soft tissue during gestational weeks 9 to 10, when foot development occurs; abnormal neuromuscular dysfunction or muscle abnormalities; and possibly a defect in the primary germ plasma, resulting in ankle dysplasia. Cases of clubfoot have been observed as a possible result of distal limb amniotic banding, a condition in which the amnion forms constrictive bands around a limb in utero, cutting off the circulation to the limb and resulting in further abnormal or arrested development.

Diagnostic Evaluation

Clubfoot is readily apparent at birth if it has not been detected antenatally. Once it is detected, a careful yet comprehensive physical assessment of the affected foot (or feet) should be carried for appropriate decisions to be made regarding treatment and discussion of possible treatment plans and prognosis with the parents. The affected foot (or feet) is usually smaller and shorter, with an empty heel pad and a transverse plantar crease. When the defect is unilateral, the affected limb is usually shorter and some calf atrophy may be present. Anteroposterior and lateral (maximum dorsiflexion) radiographs are useful in determining the type and severity of clubfoot. Ultrasonography may also be used. The nurse should perform a thorough hip examination on all infants with a clubfoot. An increased risk of hip dysplasia is associated with clubfoot deformities.

Therapeutic Management

The goal of treatment for clubfoot is to achieve a painless, plantigrade, and stable foot. Once the diagnosis is established, treatment is ideally initiated in the newborn period and involves three stages: (1) correction of the deformity, (2) maintenance of the correction until normal muscle balance is regained, and (3) follow-up observation to avert possible recurrence of the deformity.

Serial casting begins immediately or shortly after birth. Successive casts allow for gradual stretching of skin and tight structures on the medial side of the foot (Fig. 11-14). Manipulation and casting are repeated frequently (every few days for 1 to 2 weeks, then at 1- to 2-week intervals) to accommodate the rapid growth of early infancy. The extremity or extremities are casted until maximum correction is achieved, usually within 8 to 12 weeks. A Denis Browne splint may be

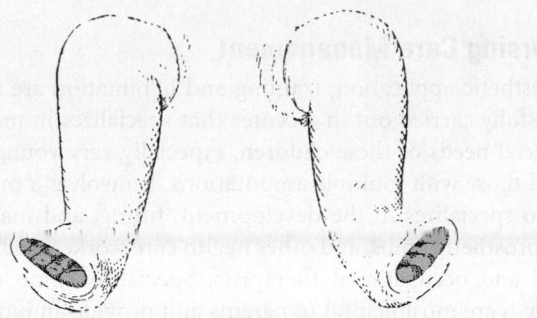

Fig. 11-14 Feet casted for correction of bilateral congenital talipes equinovarus. (From Brashear HR, Raney RB: *Handbook of orthopaedic surgery,* ed 10, St Louis, 1986, Mosby.)

used to manage feet that correct with casting and manipulation. A radiograph or ultrasound is then evaluated to see the relationship of the bones to each other. Failure to achieve normal alignment by 3 months indicates the need for surgical intervention, which may take place between 6 and 12 months of age. The foot (or feet) is immobilized postoperatively for approximately 6 to 12 weeks, and the child is allowed to walk after the cast is removed.

Surgical intervention for clubfoot involves pin fixation and the release of tight joints and tendons. Casting of the affected foot and leg is performed, and after 2 or 3 months a varus-prevention brace is used to maintain correction. With severe deformities, repeated surgical tendon or joint releases may be necessary.

In recent years several nonsurgical approaches to clubfoot have been reintroduced. These methods involve daily or weekly manipulation and stretching of tissues with either casting (Ponseti manipulation) or taping and splinting of the affected extremity (French physical therapy). A percutaneous Achilles tendon lengthening may be performed before the final casting at 6 to 7 weeks to correct the equinus deformity. With the French physical therapy treatment, a continuous passive motion machine may be used several hours daily to stretch and strengthen involved muscle groups (Faulks and Luther, 2005).

Prognosis

Some feet respond to treatment readily; some respond only to prolonged, vigorous, and sustained efforts; and the improvement in others remains disappointing even with maximum effort. Parents should realize that outcomes are not always predictable and depend on the severity of the deformity; age of the child at initial intervention; compliance with treatment protocols; and development of bones, muscles, and nerves. Surgical intervention may not restore the ankle to an entirely normal state, with the affected foot and leg remaining smaller and thinner than the unaffected side. Ankle range of motion after surgery may be even less than it was preoperatively. Many children with surgically corrected clubfoot, however, are able to walk without a limp and run and play.

Nursing Care Management

Nursing care of the child with nonsurgical correction of club-foot is the same as for any child who has a cast or corrective splint. (See Chapter 39.) The child spends considerable time in a corrective device, so nursing care plans include both long- and short-term goals. Careful observation of skin and circulation is particularly important in young infants because of their normally rapid growth rate.

Since treatment and follow-up care are handled in the orthopedist's office, clinic, or outpatient department, parent education and support are important in nursing care of these children. Parents need to understand the diagnosis, the overall treatment program, the importance of regular cast changes, and the role they play in the long-term effectiveness of the therapy. Nursing responsibilities include reinforcing and clarifying the orthopedic surgeon's explanations and instructions, providing emotional support, teaching parents about care of the cast or appliance (including vigilant observation for potential problems; see discussion of cast care on p. 423 and in Chapter 39), and encouraging parents to facilitate normal development within the limitations imposed by the deformity or therapy.

METATARSUS ADDUCTUS AND METATARSUS VARUS

Metatarsus adductus, sometimes also referred to as metatarsus varus when the forefoot is adducted and supinated (Hosalkar, Spiegel, and Davidson, 2007), is probably the most common congenital foot deformity. In most instances it is a result of abnormal intrauterine positioning and is usually detected at birth. It can occur bilaterally in 50% of newborns, and 10% of affected children will also have DDH. The deformity is characterized by medial adduction of the toes and forefoot, frequently associated with inversion, and convexity of the lateral border of the (kidney-shaped) foot. Metatarsus adductus can be divided into three categories: type I, in which the forefoot is flexible and corrects easily with manipulation; type II, in which the forefoot is only partially flexible and corrects passively past neutral position but only to neutral position with active manipulation; and type III, in which the forefoot is rigid and will not stretch to neutral position with manipulation. Unlike TEV, with which it is often confused, the angulation occurs at the tarsometatarsal joint, while the heel and ankle remain in a neutral position. Ankle range of motion is normal. This deformity often causes a pigeon-toed gait.

Management depends on the rigidity and type of the deformity. Correction can usually be accomplished by gentle manipulation and passive stretching of the foot with types I and II, which the parent is taught to perform. Repeated and consistent stretching is continued for the first 6 weeks, after which the treatment is based on the flexibility of the foot. With type III, the child usually requires serial manipulation and casting to correct the defect. Casting is performed every 1 to 2 weeks for 6 to 8 weeks after which a corrective shoe or orthosis may be used. Surgical correction is rarely required for the condition unless there is residual deformity at 4 years of age, at which time soft tissue release and serial casting are performed. Older children with deformity may require more extensive surgery (Hosalkar, Spiegel, and Davidson, 2007).

Nursing Care Management

The nursing role primarily involves identifying the defect so that early therapy and instruction of the parents can begin. The nurse teaches the parents how to hold the heel firmly and to stretch the forefoot. If casting is needed, the nurse instructs the parents in cast care and observation. (See Chapter 39.)

SKELETAL LIMB DEFICIENCY

Congenital limb deficiencies, or disruption defects, are manifested by destruction of a previously normal body part. Others may involve the loss of functional capacity of varying degrees. They are characterized by underdevelopment of skeletal elements of the extremities. The range of malformation can extend from minor defects of the digits to serious abnormalities such as amelia (absence of an entire extremity) or meromelia (partial absence of an extremity), which includes phocomelia (seal limbs), an interposed deficiency of long bones with relatively good development of hands and feet attached at or near the shoulder or the hips. Most disruption defects are primary defects of development of the limb, but prenatal destruction of the limb can occur, such as full or partial amputation of a limb in utero from constriction of an amniotic band (amniotic band syndrome).

Pathophysiology

Limb deficiencies are caused by both heredity and environment, and they can originate at any stage of limb development. Formation of limbs may be suppressed at the time of limb bud formation, or there may be interference in later stages of differentiation and growth. Heredity appears to play a prominent role, and prenatal environmental insults have been implicated in a number of cases, such as the well-publicized thalidomide tragedy in the late 1950s and early 1960s, which demonstrated a clear relationship between the time of exposure of the pregnant woman to the antiemetic drug and the presence and type of limb deformity in the newborn.

Therapeutic Management

An expert in dysmorphology, usually a genetic specialist, should evaluate children with congenital limb deficiencies. An extensive prenatal history and a pedigree are obtained. Extensive laboratory evaluation may be required.

The child with a limb deficiency is fitted with prosthetic devices whenever possible, and a functional replacement should be applied at the earliest possible stage of development in an attempt to match the infant's motor readiness. This favors natural progression of prosthetic use. For example, an infant with an upper extremity deficiency is fitted with a simple passive device such as a mitten prosthesis between 3 and 6 months of age, when limb exploration is active, sitting is beginning (with the extremities needed for support), and bilateral hand activities are encouraged. Lower limb prostheses are applied when the infant is ready to pull to a standing position.

In preparation for prosthetic devices, surgical modification is often necessary to ensure the most favorable use of the device, since severe deformity can interfere with its effective use. Phocomelic digits are preserved for controlling switches of externally powered appliances in the upper extremities. Digits (in both the upper and lower extremities) provide the child with surfaces for tactile exploration and stimulation. Prostheses are replaced to accommodate the child's growth and increasing capabilities.

Nursing Care Management

Prosthetic application, training and habilitation are most successfully carried out in a center that specializes in meeting the special needs of these children, especially very young children and those with multiple amputations. It involves a prosthetist, who specializes in the development, fitting, and maintenance of prosthetic limbs, and other health care workers such as physical and occupational therapists. Specialized limb deficiency clinics are most helpful to parents and provide an introduction to support groups for both parents and affected children. Parents must encourage the child in making age-commensurate adjustments to the environment. Although these children need assistance, overprotection may produce overdependency with later maladjustment to school and other situations.

Parents of children with limb deficiencies should always be referred for genetic counseling.

DISORDERS OF THE GASTROINTESTINAL TRACT

Congenital defects of the GI tract can involve any portion from the mouth to the anus. Most are apparent at birth or shortly thereafter and are anomalies in which normal growth ceased at a crucial stage of embryonic development, leaving the structure in an embryonic form or only partially completed. The result may be atresia, malposition, nonclosure, or any number of variations.

Atresia is absence of a normal opening or normally patent lumen. Atresia at any point along the length of the GI tract creates an obstruction to the normal progress of nutrients and secretions. The most common anomalies requiring surgical intervention are atresias of the esophagus, intestine, and anus. The congenital defects considered in this chapter include abnormalities of the lip and palate, esophagus, and anus. Some malformations of the GI tract are considered here rather than in Chapter 33 because they are identified at birth and are cause for considerable parental concern.

CLEFT LIP AND CLEFT PALATE

⊖ Cleft lip (CL) with or without cleft palate (CP) is the most common birth defect in the United States and occurs with a frequency of 1 in 600 live births (Cleft Palate Foundation, 2008). Isolated CP has an incidence of approximately 1 in 2500 live births (Tinanoff, 2007). CL with or without CP is more common in males, and CP alone is more common in females. CL appears more often in Native Americans and Asians and less frequently in African-Americans. Although the majority of clefts are nonsyndromic (have no associated identifiable syndrome), associated syndromes occur in varying frequencies according to the specific defect. It is estimated that 10% to 50% of children with CL/CP have an associated syndrome (Arosarena, 2007; Merritt, 2005). See Table 11-5 for a comparison of the two defects.

CL results from incomplete fusion of the embryonic structures surrounding the primitive oral cavity. The cleft may be unilateral or bilateral and is often associated with abnormal

TABLE 11-5 COMPARISON OF CLEFT LIP AND CLEFT PALATE

	CLEFT LIP	CLEFT PALATE
Incidence	1:600	1:2500
Inheritance	Multifactorial inheritance, environmental factors, familial occurrence Male predominance	Associated with syndromes (chromosomal), familial occurrence; environmental factors such as maternal alcohol ingestion, smoking, or teratogens Female predominance
Anatomy	Unilateral or bilateral May involve external nose, nasal cartilages, nasal septum, maxillary alveolar ridges, and dental anomalies	Soft palate and/or hard palate Midline of posterior palate May involve nostril and absence of nasal septal development (communication with oral and nasal cavity)
Management	Surgical repair at approximately 3 mo Early use of orthopedics	Surgical repair at 9-15 mo in many centers
Short-term problems (before repair)	Feeding and weight gain	Feeding (risk of aspiration); growth failure
Special postoperative care	Suture line protection and care Position on right side or upright in infant seat; avoid prone positioning to protect suture line Special feeding—breast-feeding, slow-flow nipple, plastic squeezable bottle, Haberman feeder, Pigeon bottle, syringe feeding—until suture line heals Care of scar in postoperative period with massage (after 2-3 wk) and tape	Feeding cup, syringe feeding, Haberman feeder, slow-flow nipple, Breck feeder; avoid spoon, fork (also tongue blade and other objects that could damage palatal suture line); possibly breast-feeding
Long-term problems	Social acceptance (depends on success of repair) Dental or orthodontic if associated with cleft palate	Speech, otitis media, middle ear effusion, possible hearing loss, upper respiratory tract infections Orthodontic or dental Feeding Social acceptance (voice changes, facial appearance if with cleft lip)

development of the external nose, nasal cartilages, nasal septum, and maxillary alveolar ridges. It may or may not be associated with CP. The extent of the cleft varies greatly from an indentation in the lip to a deep and wide fissure extending to the nostril. In CL, there is nasal slumping with collapse of the alar dome on the affected side. The columella is deviated to the *unaffected side*, pulling the nasal tip in that direction. In bilateral CL, the prolabium may be partially or completely separated from the lateral portion of the upper lip. This may extend into the gumline, separating the premaxilla from the remainder of the alveolar ridge. The premaxilla may deviate anteriorly outside of the oral cavity. Dental anomalies, such as missing, malpositioned, or deformed primary teeth, are common at the site of the cleft. Secondary teeth may or may not be affected, but will need bone in the alveolar cleft area in which to anchor during eruption.

CP occurs when the primary and secondary palatine plates fail to fuse during embryonic development. CPs vary greatly in degree and may involve only the soft palate or may extend into the hard palate. The cleft may occur on one side (unilateral) or both sides (bilateral). It can be incomplete or complete, or a combination of the two, independent of clefting of the lip. Wide central palatal clefts, often described as "horseshoe-shaped" clefts, may be associated with PRS. These children have associated micrognathia (retracted mandible) and airway issues related to the posterior positioning of the tongue. The cleft may occur only in the midline of the posterior palate or may extend to the nostril on one or both sides. When the lip is unattached and displaced forward, a portion of the alveolus is similarly detached. Occasionally, small clefts of the soft palate may be difficult to identify. A submucous CP may also

be difficult to identify initially because the palatal cleft is covered by the mucous membrane of the roof of the mouth. Classic stigmata of the submucous cleft include a bifid uvula, a bony notch in the hard palate, and a zona pellucida (a blue or whitish line that courses the midline of the soft palate). The submucous CP may be associated with speech problems and hypernasality in some cases. A bifid uvula, the smallest form of a velar cleft, is not in itself associated with speech or feeding problems.

Etiology

Many factors appear to be involved in the etiology of CL and CP, and evidence indicates that CL with or without CP is developmentally and genetically different from isolated CP. The majority of cases appear to be consistent with the concept of multifactorial inheritance as evidenced by an increased incidence in relatives and a higher concordance in monozygotic twins than in dizygotic twins. Siblings of children with CL with or without CP have an increased risk of the same anomaly but not of CP alone.

Many recognized syndromes include CL and CP as a feature. Some of these syndromes are a result of chromosomal abnormalities, and environmental factors or teratogens may be responsible for clefts at a critical point in embryonic development. Drugs such as phenytoin, valproic acid, thalidomide, and the pesticide dioxin can cause CL/CP. Maternal nutrition, especially folic acid deficiency, has been linked to clefting in humans, as have maternal alcohol ingestion and smoking during pregnancy. Alcohol consumption, specifically binge drinking (more than five drinks per sitting), increases the risk of having an infant with a cleft (DeRoo, Wilcox, Drevon, et al, 2008).

Evidence shows that maternal smoking early in pregnancy is associated with a 1.5- to 2-fold increase in the risk for orofacial clefts, especially isolated clefts, with the risk increasing proportionately with the number of cigarettes smoked (Little, Cardy, and Munger, 2004).

Pathophysiology

Development of the primary and secondary palates takes place at different times and involves different developmental processes. CL, or the primary palate, includes the upper lip and extends through the alveolar ridge. CP, or the secondary palate, starts posterior to the alveolar ridge and extends through the uvula. CL with or without CP results from failure of the maxillary processes to fuse with the nasal elevations on the frontal prominence, which normally occurs during the sixth week of gestation (Fig. 11-15, *A*). In some cases CP may occur as a result

of a rupture of unstable mesoderm layer resulting in a cleft. Merging of the upper lip at the midline is completed between the seventh and eighth weeks of gestation.

Fusion of the secondary palate (hard and soft palates) takes place later in development, between the seventh and twelfth weeks of gestation (Fig. 11-15, *B* to *D*). At the time the primary palate is completed, the two lateral palatine processes are situated in a vertical position at the side of the tongue. In the process of migrating to a horizontal position, they are, for a short time, separated by the tongue. With development of the neck and jaws, the tongue moves downward, allowing the palatine processes to fuse with one another and with the primary palate to form the roof of the mouth. If there is delay in this movement, or if the tongue fails to descend soon enough, the remainder of development proceeds but the palate never fuses.

Diagnostic Evaluation

A cleft that involves the lip with or without CP is readily apparent at birth and is a defect that may elicit significant distress in parents.

Palpation of the hard palate and soft palate, submucous palate, and uvula with a gloved finger and visual inspection of the oral cavity and its structures are important parts of the newborn physical examination. (See Chapter 8.) The degree of malformation of the CL or CP can then be evaluated (Figs. 11-16 and 11-17). Clefts of the lip may be unilateral or bilateral, and the extent of the cleft and degree of nasal deformity vary. As with CL, the degree of deformity with CP varies and may involve only the uvula or may extend through both the soft and hard palates. The severity of the CP has an impact on feeding problems; the infant is unable to generate negative pressure and create suction in the oral cavity. This impairs feeding even though in most cases the infant's ability to swallow is normal.

Therapeutic Management

Treatment of the child with isolated CL is surgical and involves the craniofacial multidisciplinary team. Depending on the severity of the CL, the team may include the surgeon, dentist or orthodontist, speech-language pathologist, nurse, and social worker. Management of CP also involves the cooperative efforts of a multidisciplinary health care team, including pediatrics, plastic surgery, orthodontics, otolaryngology, speech and language pathology, audiology, nursing, and social work. Treatment continues over a long time, but, even after completion of a program of health care, the child may retain defects of speech, facial appearance, and other problems related to the cleft. Management of both defects is directed toward surgical closure of the cleft, prevention of complications, and facilitation of normal growth and development of the child.

Surgical Correction: Cleft Lip

Closure of the lip defect precedes that of the palate, usually during the first few months of life. Many surgeons prefer the child to be 10 weeks of age and weigh 4.5 kg (10 lb); however, this varies. An important consideration in the timing of the surgery is the size of the cleft. Surgical correction is performed when the infant is free of any oral, respiratory, or systemic

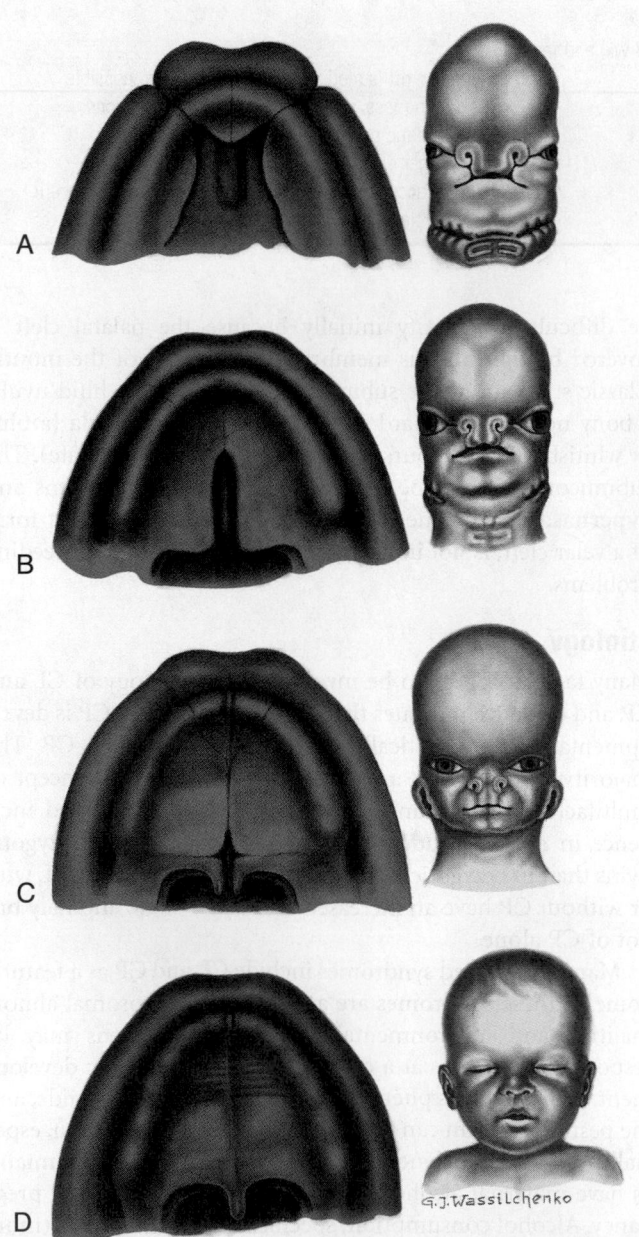

Fig. 11-15 A to D, Stages in palatine development. (See text for discussion.)

G.J.Wassilchenko

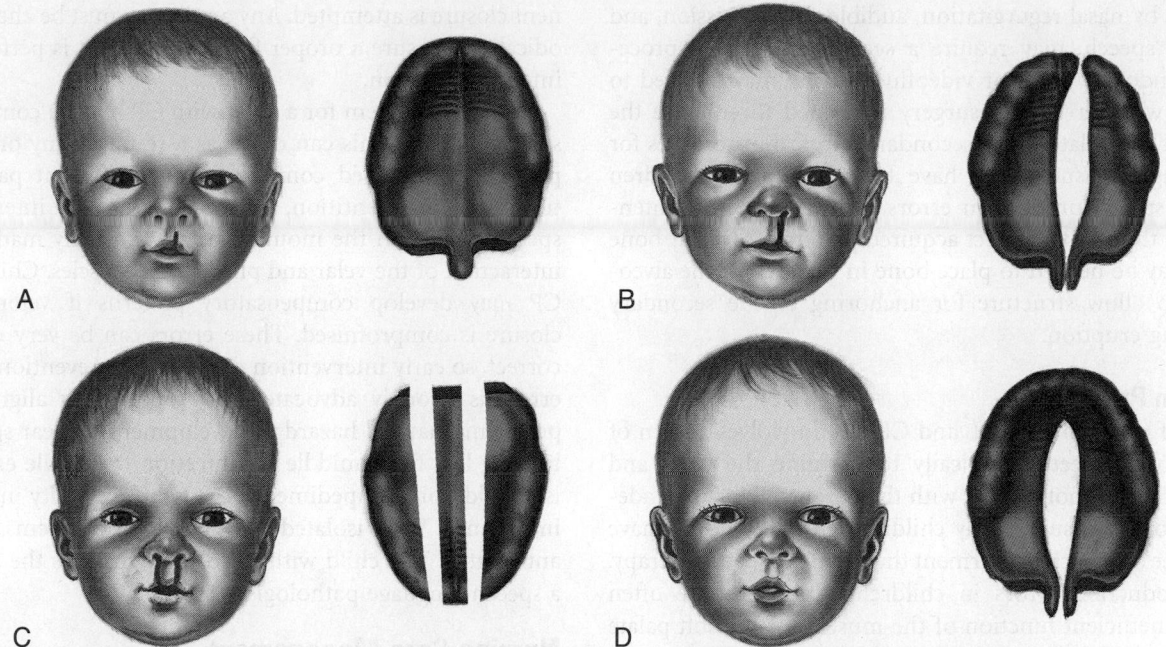

Fig. 11-16 Variations in clefts of lip and palate at birth. **A,** Notch in vermilion border. **B,** Unilateral cleft lip and cleft palate. **C,** Bilateral cleft lip and cleft palate. **D,** Cleft palate.

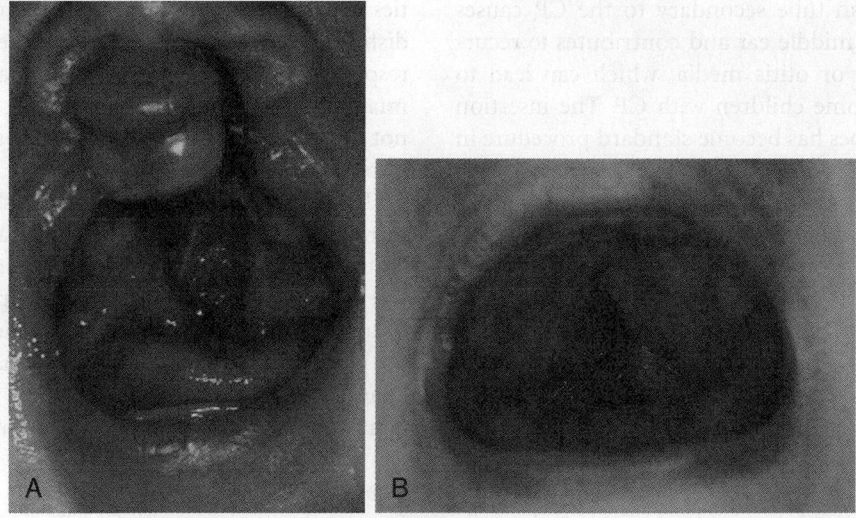

Fig. 11-17 A, Bilateral cleft lip with complete cleft palate. Cleft extends from soft to hard palate, exposing nasal cavity. **B,** Midline cleft of soft palate. (From Zitelli BJ, Davis HW: *Atlas of pediatric physical diagnosis,* ed 5, St Louis, 2007, Mosby; **B,** Courtesy Barbara Elster, Cleft Palate Center, Pittsburgh.)

infection. Repair of the CL involves a rotation advancement flap, resulting in a scar that mimics the philtrum column.

Improved surgical techniques have minimized deformity related to scar retraction, but optimum cosmetic results are difficult to obtain in severe defects. CL healing takes place with minimal scar formation. Optimal care in the postoperative period includes scar massage (approximately 2 weeks postoperatively) and the use of silicone tape and gels several weeks postoperatively. Remaining physical characteristics in the older child are residual nasal deformity, a mildly protruding lower lip secondary to midfacial hypoplasia, and a somewhat flattened lower third of the upper lip, usually with an abnormally shaped vermillion. Not infrequently, revisions may be required at a later age.

Surgical Correction: Cleft Palate

CP repair was previously postponed until a later age than repair of the CL to take advantage of palatal changes that occur with normal growth. However, the timing of repairs remains controversial and is typically performed at 9 to 15 months in most centers to maximize speech production and growth of the midface (Arosarena, 2007). Most CP teams prefer to close the cleft before the child develops compensatory speech patterns. Recent studies have shown that children who are younger and less advanced in terms of speech development exhibit better articulation and resonance than those who have their palates repaired when they are older and exhibit more speech and language development (Chapman, Hardin-Jones, Goldstein, et al, 2008). Persistent velopharyngeal insufficiency, manifested by nasal regurgitation, audible nasal emission, and hypernasal speech, may require a secondary surgical procedure. Nasendoscopy and/or videofluoroscopy may be used to determine whether further surgery is needed to enhance the function of the palate. Once secondary surgical procedures for velopharyngeal insufficiency have been completed, children exhibiting speech production errors will often require intensive speech therapy to correct acquired patterns. Alveolar bone grafting may be needed to place bone in the area of the alveolar cleft, to allow structure for anchoring of the secondary teeth during eruption.

Long-Term Problems

The care of children with CL and CP often involves a team of specialists who meet periodically to examine the child and consult with one another and with the parents. Even with adequate anatomic closure, many children with CL and CP have some degree of speech impairment that requires speech therapy. Speech production errors in children with clefts are often related to inefficient function of the muscles of the soft palate and nasopharynx (which lead to the development of compensatory speech patterns), improper tooth alignment, and varying degrees of hearing loss.

Improper drainage of the middle ear, as a result of inefficient function of the eustachian tube secondary to the CP, causes increased pressure in the middle ear and contributes to recurrent middle ear effusion or otitis media, which can lead to hearing impairment in some children with CP. The insertion of pressure-equalizing tubes has become standard procedure in the child with CL/CP and is often performed at the same time as other surgical procedures (such as CL repair) to facilitate fluid drainage from the middle ear and prevent middle ear effusion and recurrent otitis media.

Extensive orthodontics and prosthodontics are usually needed to correct malposition of the teeth and maxillary arches. Teeth may be missing, malformed, or malpositioned, which can interfere with speech and feeding. In addition, a significant number of these children have an inadequate nasal airway that forces them to breathe through the mouth, which also contributes to oral deformity. Children with both CL and CP often require several stages of orthodontic therapy. An orthopedic appliance is often worn 24/7 starting in the first week of life to align the maxillary segments into a near-normal relationship up until CL repair at 3 to 5 months. This is frequently done to facilitate a primary lip closure. The second stage (at 2 to 5 years) consists of palatal expansion and correction of a dental crossbite (a condition in which the upper teeth close inside the lower teeth) in an attempt to allow the primary teeth to develop in a normal relationship. The third stage of therapy (at 10 to 11 years) takes place during the mixed-dentition stage and involves correction of faulty occlusion. In the fourth stage (at 12 to 18 years) treatment of the permanent teeth is accomplished in much the same manner as for any adolescent except for alignment and spacing in the cleft area.

Often temporary or permanent dental prostheses are necessary to replace missing teeth. These assist in chewing and produce a more pleasing cosmetic effect. Special dental plates, called obturators, are sometimes used to mechanically close clefts in the palate to facilitate feeding and speech until permanent closure is attempted. Any appliance must be checked periodically to ensure a proper fit and see that it is performing its intended function.

A major problem for a child with CP may be compensatory speech pattern. This can occur as a result of any or all of the previously discussed complications: insufficient palate function, abnormal dentition, and hearing loss. CP interferes with speech sounds in the mouth that are normally made through interaction of the velar and pharyngeal muscles. Children with CP may develop compensatory patterns if velopharyngeal closure is compromised. These errors can be very difficult to correct, so early intervention focusing on prevention of speech errors is strongly advocated. Improper tooth alignment can pose a mechanical hazard to development of clear speech, and hearing loss from middle ear infection or middle ear effusion is an additional impediment because of difficulty in interpreting sounds. With isolated CL, no speech problems should be anticipated. The child with CP usually requires the services of a speech-language pathologist.

Nursing Care Management

The immediate nursing problems in the care of an infant with CL and CP deformities are related to feeding the infant and dealing with the parental reaction to the defect. Facial deformities are particularly disturbing to parents. CL, especially, is a disfiguring, visible defect that may generate a strong negative response in parents. During the initial phase after birth of an infant with CL or CP, it is important for the nurse to address not only the infant's physical needs but also the parents' emotional needs.

The nurse should encourage expression of parental grief and fears. Such expression may promote attachment in the preoperative period. It is especially important to emphasize the positive aspects of the infant's physical appearance and to express optimism regarding surgical correction while acknowledging the parents' concern. The manner of handling the infant should convey to the parents that the infant is indeed a precious human being. (See Birth of a Child with a Physical Defect, p. 391.)

Feeding

Feeding the newborn with CL/CP can be a challenge, and teaching the parent to successfully feed the child is perhaps one of the most significant and challenging nursing roles. Growth failure in these infants has been attributed to preoperative feeding difficulties; however, such difficulties can be overcome by increasing overall caloric intake with a higher-calorie formula, nutrition counseling, and evaluation. Weekly weight checks at the practitioner's office assist in monitoring the infant's weight preoperatively. After surgical repair most infants with isolated CL or CP and no associated syndrome gain weight successfully and achieve adequate weight and height for age.

Although some infants with isolated CL are typically able to breast-feed without difficulty, breast-feeding is a difficult process for most infants with an unrepaired CP. La Leche League International reports that "over time, lactation consultants have found that feeding exclusively at the breast is a difficult goal for all but a few infants with uncorrected cleft palates" (Cleft Palate Foundation, 2008). An infant with CP is unable to achieve adequate suction to extract breast milk directly from the breast. Clefts of the palate reduce the infant's ability to suck, which interferes with compression of the areola and renders breast-feeding and traditional bottle-feeding difficult. Standard bottle nipples may be unsuitable for these infants, who are unable to generate the suction required. Therefore special nipples or other feeding devices are needed. Liquid taken into the mouth tends to escape via the CP through the nose. Accepting that she may not be able to breast-feed can be difficult for a new mother. However, the Cleft Palate Foundation recommends that a mother of a child with a cleft should be encouraged to try the following strategies:

- She may try pumping her breast milk and providing the milk with an adapted bottle made for children with clefts.
- Skin-to-skin contact should be encouraged when possible.
- After bottle-feeding, the infant may be put to the mother's breast for nonnutritive sucking.

With appropriate adaptive bottles and positioning, infants with clefts can be efficient oral feeders. Feeding is best accomplished with the infant's head in an upright position, either held in the caregiver's hand or cradled in the arm.

A number of special feeding devices are available for feeding the infant with CL/CP, and some are more successful than others, depending on a number of factors (Fig. 11-18). One device is the Cleft Lip/Cleft Palate Nurser, which consists of a squeezable plastic bottle and a cross-cut nipple. The Haberman Special Needs Feeder may also be used successfully in infants with a poor or disorganized suck. The Haberman feeder has a specially designed valve and nipple to adjust the flow of milk to the infant and prevent choking or gagging. The nipple chamber of the Haberman bottle is large, which allows the feeder to provide extra assistance by squeezing the chamber if needed. The Pigeon bottle has a nipple with a Y-cut and is slightly larger and more bulbous to fit naturally into the oral cavity. A one-way back-flow valve prevents milk from flowing retrograde into the bottle to minimize the amount of air the infant swallows. The Pigeon bottle is not a squeezable feeding system.

Using these various types of nipples for feeding also has the advantage of helping to meet the infant's sucking needs. Muscle development is especially important for later development of speech. The Haberman and the Pigeon nipples work by compression, so the nipple is positioned in such a way that it is compressed by the infant's tongue and existing palate. If a single-slit nipple is used (such as the Haberman feeder), the slit is placed vertically so that the infant will be able to produce and stop the flow of milk by alternately opening and closing the opening. Regardless of the type of nipple used, the person doing the feeding should resist the temptation to remove the nipple because of the noise the infant makes or because of fear that the infant will choke. An indication that the infant needs to stop feeding momentarily is the facial signal, which involves elevated eyebrows and a wrinkled forehead; the nipple may be gently removed to allow the infant to swallow formula in the mouth without getting upset. These infants need frequent burping because they have a tendency to swallow excessive amounts of air.

Some CP specialists advocate for the use of feeding obturators to assist with feeding. However, these devices do not improve feeding efficiency or growth within the first year of life (Masarei, Wade, Mars, et al, 2007).

Regardless of the feeding method used, the mother should begin to feed the infant as soon as possible. In this way she is able to help determine the method best suited to her and the infant and to become adept in the technique before discharge.

Preoperative Care

In preparation for the surgical repair, instruct the parents to accustom the infant to some of the needs of the early postoperative period. Some craniofacial surgery teams encourage the transition to cup-feeding before CP surgery, and this feeding method is used postoperatively as well. Preoperative preparation, including medication, is determined by the surgeon and anesthesiologist.

Postoperative Care: Cleft Lip

The major efforts in the postoperative period are directed toward protecting the operative site. Avoid the prone position to prevent suture damage. After CL repair (**cheiloplasty**), some surgeons allow breast-feeding or syringe feeding once the child is awake and alert. Cheiloplasty is often performed on a day-of-surgery basis with discharge to home after ascertainment of adequate fluid intake.

Elbow restraints may be applied immediately after surgery to prevent the infant from rubbing the suture line, although many surgeons no longer support this practice.

Pain management should continue in the home setting, and parents are taught how to administer the appropriate dosage of analgesic. Clear liquids are offered when the infant has fully recovered from the anesthesia, and breast- or syringe-feeding is usually resumed as tolerated. A thin layer of antibiotic ointment may be prescribed for application to the suture line. Meticulous care of the suture line is a nursing responsibility. Inflammation or infection interferes with optimum healing and the ultimate cosmetic effect of the surgical repair.

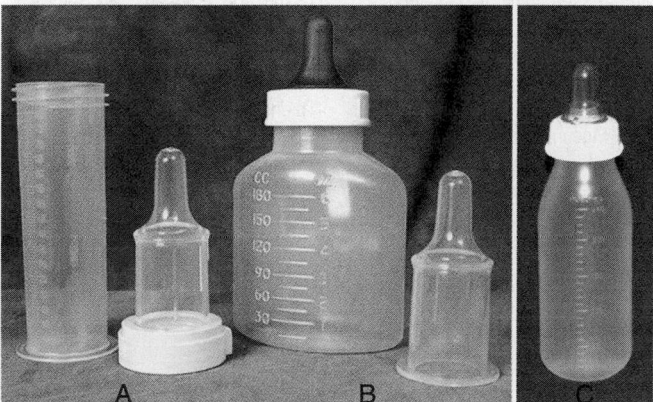

Fig. 11-18 A, Haberman feeder. **B,** Mead Johnson bottle used to feed an infant with cleft lip and palate. **C,** Pigeon bottle. (**A** and **B,** Courtesy Texas Children's Hospital, Houston. **C,** Courtesy Paul Vincent Kuntz, Texas Children's Hospital, Houston.)

> **! NURSING ALERT**
>
> Avoid the use of suction or objects in the mouth such as tongue depressors, thermometers, spoons, or straws.

The infant should be positioned to prevent airway obstruction by secretions, blood, or the tongue. Gentle aspiration of mouth and nasopharyngeal secretions may be necessary to prevent aspiration and respiratory complications. Because of vascularity of the lip and palate, postoperative care involves monitoring operative sites for bleeding. Excessive swallowing may be a sign of bleeding and swallowing blood.

Postoperative Care: Cleft Palate

The child with a CP repair (palatoplasty) can lie on the abdomen, especially immediately postoperatively. The child may resume feedings by special feeding device shortly after surgery. Acceptable feeding devices include soft-tip (like a nipple) sippy cups, an open cup, an oropharyngeal syringe, and specialized bottles with soft tubing.

The speech-language pathologist evaluates the child's individual needs and directs the parents in specific activities to facilitate speech development. The more children use speech, the sooner they will gain self-confidence and assurance in social situations.

Throughout the child's therapy, the ultimate goal should be the development of a healthy personality and self-esteem. Several agencies provide services and information for children with CL/CP and their families. These include the Cleft Palate Foundation,* Birth Defect Research for Children, Inc.,† and the March of Dimes.‡

---

*1504 E. Franklin St., Suite 102, Chapel Hill, NC 27514-2820; 919-933-9044; e-mail: info@cleftline.org; www.cleftline.org.

†800 Celebration Ave., Suite 225, Celebration, FL 34747; 407-566-8304, www.birthdefects.org.

‡1275 Mamaroneck Ave., White Plains, NY 10605; 914-997-4488, www.marchofdimes.com. In Canada, www.marchofdimes.ca.

Sometimes the infant has difficulty breathing after surgery because of swelling. Humidified air may be provided as blow-by to alleviate edema of the tissues, and the side-lying or semireclined positioning may be used to facilitate drainage of secretions.

Elbow restraints can keep the hands away from the mouth, and the parents should maintain this precaution at home until the palate is healed. When used the restraints may be removed with adequate supervision to allow the child to exercise the arms. Assess the infant for pain postoperatively. Opiates may be prescribed for the first 24 to 48 hours, or longer if needed, and acetaminophen may be given thereafter (see Nursing Care Plan).

The older infant is usually discharged on a blenderized or soft diet, and parents should continue the diet until the surgeon directs them to do otherwise. Caution them against allowing the child to eat hard items such as toast, hard cookies, or potato chips, which could damage the newly repaired palate.

Preparation for Discharge and Home Care

Parents should participate in the infant's care as soon as possible after surgery. They should learn the proper feeding method. Parents should also know how to cleanse the suture line to free any crust that might form and to replace elbow restraints (if used). Carefully evaluate and discuss car seat restraint appropriate to the infant's condition with the parents before discharge. Also discuss the infant sleep position based on the infant's condition and the American Academy of Pediatrics recommendation for supine sleeping in infants. (See Chapter 13.)

⊚ NURSING CARE PLAN

The Infant with Cleft Lip/Palate

NURSING DIAGNOSIS	EXPECTED PATIENT OUTCOMES	NURSING INTERVENTIONS	RATIONALE
Preoperative Care			
CL/CP—Impaired Swallowing related to impaired sucking and palatal cleft	Infant will breast-feed or bottle-feed successfully.	Suction nose and mouth with bulb syringe.	To maintain patent airway
		Position on right side with HOB elevated 30 degrees.	To facilitate drainage of secretions and/or feeding
Child's/Family's Defining Characteristics (Subjective and Objective Data)	**The Following NOC Concepts Apply to These Outcomes**	Assist mother with breast-feeding, if so desired.	To provide emotional and physical support
	Aspiration Control	Assess infant's ability to suckle at breast and maintain effective latch-on.	To promote optimum nutrition
Choking	Swallowing: Esophageal and Oral Phase		
Gagging		Use special CL/CP feeder such as CL/CP Nurser (Mead Johnson), Pigeon bottle, Ross Gravity Flow, or Haberman feeder as necessary; place device to back of oral cavity and adjust flow to infant's ability to swallow.	To ensure adequate intake of formula if not breast-feeding
Spitting breast milk or formula through nose and mouth			
		For feeding, position infant in semireclining position facing caregiver.	To prevent choking
			To minimize spitting up and assess tolerance of fluid intake
		The Following NIC Concepts Apply to These Interventions Parent Teaching Airway Suctioning Airway Management Positioning Risk Identification	

◎ **NURSING CARE PLAN—cont'd**

The Infant with Cleft Lip/Palate

NURSING DIAGNOSIS	EXPECTED PATIENT OUTCOMES	NURSING INTERVENTIONS	RATIONALE
Risk for Impaired Parent/Infant/ Child Attachment	Parents will demonstrate attachment behaviors and willingness to nurture infant.	Discuss with parents the infant's physical characteristics and positive attributes.	To promote acceptance of infant with birth defect
Child's/Family's Defining Characteristics (Subjective and Objective Data)	**The Following NOC Concept Applies to These Outcomes** Parenting	Provide nursing care as with any other infant.	To demonstrate acceptance of infant with birth defect
Infant with visible facial defect		Encourage parents to interact with infant through verbalizations and eye contact.	To promote normalization of the parent-infant relationship
		Involve parents in infant caregiving activities without restrictions or limitations.	To promote acceptance of infant as important family member
		Provide lactation consult and feeding assistance.	To promote closeness and bonding with infant
		Assist with feedings as necessary.	To promote nutrition and fluid intake
		Encourage parents to discuss feelings related to infant's appearance.	To allow feelings to be discussed in the open and assess areas for intervention
		Assess parents and other family members for signs of inadequate coping.	To provide early intervention as necessary
		Encourage siblings (as age appropriate) and other family members to visit and interact with infant.	To promote family integration
		The Following NIC Concepts Apply to These Interventions Infant Care Skin-to-Skin (Kangaroo) Care Normalization Promotion Anxiety Reduction Family Process Maintenance	

NURSING DIAGNOSIS	EXPECTED PATIENT OUTCOMES	NURSING INTERVENTIONS	RATIONALE
Imbalanced Nutrition, Less Than Body Requirements related to palatal defect	Infant will maintain adequate weight gain (stated goal per craniofacial team) until surgical repair of cleft occurs.	Weigh daily until discharge then every week or more often as necessary to monitor weight; use consistency in weighing process—same time of day, dry diaper only, and same scales.	To monitor weight as an indicator of nutritional status
Child's/Family's Defining Characteristics (Subjective and Objective Data)	**The Following NOC Concepts Apply to These Outcomes** Food and Fluid Intake	Assist parents with feeding; breast-feeding may require lactation consult; different positions may be required to achieve latch-on.	To promote parental involvement and adequate nutrient intake
Reported food intake less than RDA	Weight Management Nutritional Status: Adequate	Bottle-feed using specialized nipple such as Haberman, Ross Gravity Flow, Pigeon bottle, or Mead Johnson CL/CP Nurser.	To optimize feeding ability
Body weight 20% or more under ideal		Teach parents use of special feeding techniques or apparatus.	To promote parent and family involvement in care of infant
Weakness of muscles required for swallowing		Use patience and creativity during feeding.	To promote nutrient intake from mother and father
		Suction nose and mouth as necessary with bulb syringe or Yankauer suction set.	To maintain patent airway
		Encourage father's participation in feeding, whether breast or bottle, by helping position infant's cheeks and lip for optimum seal.	To promote family involvement
		Monitor for signs and symptoms of dehydration (dry buccal membranes and lips, loose dry skin, tenting, prolonged capillary refill [>3 sec], hypernatremia).	To detect early signs requiring intervention
		Teach parents signs and symptoms of inadequate caloric and fluid intake, dehydration.	To involve parents in care and prevent complications
		If medically indicated, use gavage to feed infant prescribed amount of breast milk or formula.	To ensure adequate caloric and fluid intake
		Allow parent(s) to hold infant during gavage feeding, and allow infant nonnutritive sucking.	To promote parent involvement in care
		The Following NIC Concepts Apply to These Interventions Vital Signs Monitoring Nutrition Management Lactation Counseling Fluid Management	

Continued

NURSING CARE PLAN—cont'd

The Infant with Cleft Lip/Palate

NURSING DIAGNOSIS	EXPECTED PATIENT OUTCOMES	NURSING INTERVENTIONS	RATIONALE
Postoperative Care CL/CP—Risk for Trauma to surgical site related to surgical procedure, developmental age of child, skin and mucous membrane fragility **Child's/Family's Defining Characteristics (Subjective and Objective Data)** Sutures exposed Skin delicate Developmental phase of oral exploration and gratification	Tissue integrity at surgical site will remain intact and undamaged. **The Following NOC Concept Applies to These Outcomes** Tissue Integrity: Skin and Mucous Membranes	Protect surgical site by doing the following: • Place infant supine. • Avoid straws, hard utensils or objects (hard pacifier, suction catheter, tongue depressor) in mouth (especially in infant with CP). • Use elbow restraints as indicated. • Cup or spoon feed as indicated. • Breast-feed as indicated (CL). • Gavage feed as indicated. • Cleanse surgical site with normal saline and use topical antibiotic ointment as indicated. Teach parents care of surgical incision. **The Following NIC Concepts Apply to These Interventions** Skin Care: Topical Infection Protection Oral Health Maintenance Nutrition Management	To promote healing of surgical repair site skin, mucosa To prevent injury to sutures and surrounding skin, mucosa To promote parental involvement in infant's care

NURSING DIAGNOSIS	EXPECTED PATIENT OUTCOMES	NURSING INTERVENTIONS	RATIONALE
Acute Pain related to surgical repair of CL/CP **Child's/Family's Defining Characteristics (Subjective and Objective Data)** Observed evidence Objective pain scale evaluation indicative of pain Sleep disturbance	Infant will be comfortable and rest quietly. **The Following NOC Concept Applies to These Outcomes** Pain Control	Administer oral or intravenous (as indicated) pain medication postoperatively on around the clock basis for 24 to 48 hr. Use objective pain scale to quantify pain. Encourage parents to use nonpharmacologic pain management measures such as rocking and cuddling, swaddling, singing, reading story. Teach parents to administer oral pain medication such as acetaminophen at home. **The Following NIC Concepts Apply to These Interventions** Medication Administration: Oral Analgesic Administration Positioning Presence Environmental Management: Comfort	To achieve optimum pain relief To ascertain requirement for additional dosage and strength of pain medication To involve parents in infant's care To decrease sense of helplessness To manage infant's pain and promote parental involvement in infant's care

CL, Cleft lip; *CP*, cleft palate; *HOB*, head of bed; *RDA*, recommended dietary allowance.

Long-Term Family Guidance

The problems of parents in the care of an infant with CP may extend well beyond the initial acceptance of and adjustment to the defect and surgical correction. These families need support and encouragement by health care professionals and guidance in activities that facilitate the most normal life for the child.

Parents often cite financial stressors as being the most difficult issue to deal with when the child has a craniofacial anomaly. However, with the combined efforts of the family and the health care team, the majority of these infants achieve a satisfactory long-term outcome.

Parents need to understand the therapy and the purpose of any appliance. They should learn proper care and placement of the device and that establishing good mouth care and proper brushing habits is especially important for these children.

Because of the increased risk of middle ear infection, the ears are examined regularly, and hearing tests are scheduled early and repeated periodically throughout childhood. It is important to emphasize the need for an ear examination when the child has symptoms of an upper respiratory tract infection. When treatment can be implemented early, the chances are greater that permanent damage to the ear can be avoided. Parents should be alert for signs of any hearing impairment in the child so they can obtain needed help and prevent progression of any deficit. (See Chapter 24.)

The parents also need guidance in helping the child develop normal speech. They should encourage the child's early attempts to make sounds. Some parents erroneously believe that the child may form poor speech habits if he or she tries to speak before the palate is repaired. Before palatal repair children

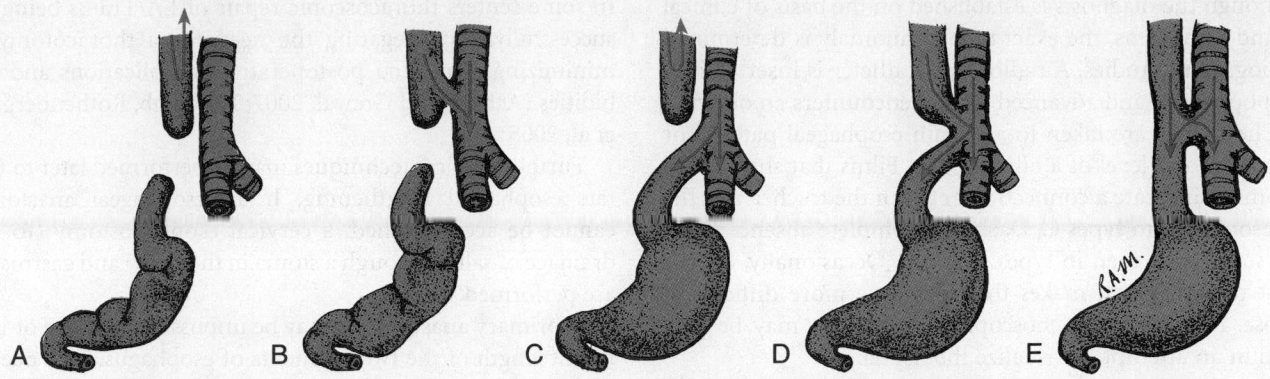

Fig. 11-19 A to E, Five most common types of esophageal atresia and tracheoesophageal fistula. (See text for discussion.)

should make the nasal consonants "m," "n," and "ng" (as "ing"), as well as "w" and "y" and most vowels. After palatal surgery children should attempt to produce most consonants, although speech therapy may be required to facilitate production of these sounds (see Nursing Care Plan).

ESOPHAGEAL ATRESIA AND TRACHEOESOPHAGEAL FISTULA

Congenital esophageal atresia (EA) and tracheoesophageal fistula (TEF) are rare malformations that represent a failure of the esophagus to develop as a continuous passage and a failure of the trachea and esophagus to separate into distinct structures. These defects may occur as separate entities or in combination, and without early diagnosis and treatment they pose a serious threat to the infant's well-being.

The incidence is estimated to be approximately 2 in 10,000 live births (Achildi and Grewal, 2007). There appears to be a slightly higher incidence in males, and the birth weight of most affected infants is significantly lower than average, with an unusually high incidence of preterm birth in infants with EA and a subsequent increase in mortality. A history of maternal polyhydramnios is common.

Approximately 50% of the cases of EA/TEF are a component of VATER or VACTERL association, acronyms used to describe associated anomalies (VATER for Vertebral defects, imperforate Anus, Tracheoesophageal fistula, and Radial and Renal dysplasia; and VACTERL for Vertebral, Anal, Cardiac, Tracheal, Esophageal, Renal, and Limb) (Orenstein, Peters, Khan, et al, 2007). Cardiac anomalies may also occur with EA/TEF; therefore all patients should undergo a workup for associated anomalies.

Pathophysiology

The esophagus develops from the first segment of the embryonic gut. During the fourth and fifth weeks of gestation, the foregut normally lengthens and separates longitudinally. Each longitudinal portion fuses to form two parallel channels (the esophagus and the trachea) that are joined only at the larynx. Anomalies involving the trachea and esophagus are caused by defective separation, incomplete fusion of the tracheal folds after this separation, or altered cellular growth during embryonic development.

The most commonly encountered form of EA and TEF (80% to 90% of cases) is one in which the proximal esophageal segment terminates in a blind pouch and the distal segment is connected to the trachea or primary bronchus by a short fistula at or near the tracheal bifurcation (Fig. 11-19, C). The second most common type (7% to 8%), or "pure EA," consists of a blind pouch at each end, widely separated and with no communication to the trachea (Fig. 11-19, A). An H-type EA refers to an otherwise normal trachea and esophagus connected by a fistula (4% to 5%) (Fig. 11-19, E). Extremely rare anomalies involve a fistula from the trachea to the upper esophageal segment (0.8%) (Fig. 11-19, B) or to both the upper and lower segments (0.7% to 6%) (Fig. 11-19, D).

Clinical Manifestations

The presence of EA is suspected in a newborn with frothy saliva in the mouth and nose, drooling, choking, and coughing. Respiratory distress may be mild or significant, depending on the type of defect and the infant's gestational age. If fed, the infant may swallow normally but suddenly cough and gag, with return of fluid through the nose and mouth. The infant may become cyanotic and apneic because of aspiration of formula or saliva.

In the infant who has EA with a distal TEF (type C), the stomach becomes distended with air, and thoracic and abdominal compression (especially during crying) cause the gastric contents to be regurgitated through the fistula and into the trachea, producing a chemical pneumonitis. When the upper segment of the esophagus opens directly into the trachea (types B and D), the infant is in danger of aspirating any swallowed material. Cyanosis or choking during feeding may be the only symptom of type E fistula (see Fig. 11-19). The child with this H type of EA may not manifest symptoms until later in life when he or she shows signs of chronic respiratory problems, recurrent pneumonia, and signs of gastroesophageal reflux (Orenstein, Peters, Khan, et al, 2007).

Diagnostic Evaluation

In a newborn who has symptoms suggestive of EA/TEF, an attempt is made to pass an NG-orogastric (OG) catheter into the esophagus. Inability to pass the catheter warrants further evaluation.

Although the diagnosis is established on the basis of clinical signs and symptoms, the exact type of anomaly is determined by radiographic studies. A radiopaque catheter is inserted into the hypopharynx and advanced until it encounters an obstruction. Chest films are taken to ascertain esophageal patency or the presence and level of a blind pouch. Films that show air in the stomach indicate a connection between the trachea and the distal esophagus in types C, D, and E. Complete absence of air in the stomach is seen in types A and B. Occasionally, fistulas are not patent, which makes their presence more difficult to diagnose. A careful bronchoscopic examination may be performed in an attempt to visualize the fistula.

The presence of polyhydramnios (accumulation of >2000 ml of amniotic fluid) prenatally is a clue to the possibility of EA in the unborn infant, especially with defect type A, B, or C. With these types of EA/TEF, amniotic fluid normally swallowed by the fetus is unable to reach the GI tract to be absorbed and excreted by the kidneys. The result is an abnormal accumulation of amniotic fluid, or polyhydramnios.

Therapeutic Management

The treatment of EA and TEF includes maintenance of a patent airway, prevention of pneumonia, gastric or blind pouch decompression, supportive therapy, and surgical repair of the anomaly.

When EA with a TEF is suspected, the infant is immediately deprived of oral intake, IV fluids are initiated, and the infant is positioned to facilitate drainage of secretions and decrease the likelihood of aspiration. Accumulated secretions are suctioned frequently from the mouth and pharynx. A double-lumen catheter should be placed into the upper esophageal pouch and attached to intermittent or continuous low suction. The infant's head is kept upright to facilitate removal of fluid collected in the pouch and to prevent aspiration of gastric contents. Broad-spectrum antibiotic therapy is often instituted if there is a concern about aspiration of gastric contents.

Surgical Correction

Most malformations can be corrected surgically in one operation or in two or more staged procedures. The success depends on early diagnosis before complications occur and on the presence and severity of associated anomalies and illness factors, including preterm birth. With measures instituted to prevent aspiration pneumonia and to ensure adequate hydration and nutrition, surgery may be postponed to allow for more effective treatment of pneumonia and physiologic stabilization so that the infant can better withstand the complex surgery. The delay also offers an opportunity for further evaluation and assessment to rule out any associated anomalies and to optimize respiratory support.

The surgery consists of a thoracotomy with division and ligation of the TEF and an end-to-end or end-to-side anastomosis of the esophagus. A chest tube may be inserted to drain intrapleural air and fluid. For infants who are not stable enough to undergo definitive repair or those with a lengthy gap between the proximal and distal esophagus, a staged operation is preferred that involves gastrostomy, ligation of the TEF, and constant drainage of the esophageal pouch. A delayed esophageal anastomosis is usually attempted after several weeks to months.

In some centers thoracoscopic repair of EA/TEF is being used successfully, thus negating the need for a thoracotomy and minimizing associated postoperative complications and morbidities (Achildi and Grewal, 2007; Holcomb, Rothenberg, Bax, et al, 2005).

Further surgical techniques may be performed later to facilitate esophageal lengthening. If an esophageal anastomosis cannot be accomplished, a cervical esophagostomy (to allow drainage of saliva through a stoma in the neck) and gastrostomy are performed.

A primary anastomosis may be impossible because of insufficient length of the two segments of esophagus. This occurs if the distance between the two segments is 3 to 4 cm (1.2 to 1.6 inches) or greater; this is often referred to as *long-gap EA* (Orenstein, Peters, Khan, et al, 2007). In these cases an esophageal replacement procedure using a part of the colon or gastric tube interposition may be necessary to bridge the missing esophageal segment.

Tracheomalacia may occur as a result of weakness in the tracheal wall that exists when a dilated proximal pouch compresses the trachea early in fetal life. It may also occur as a result of inadequate intratracheal pressure causing abnormal tracheal development. Clinical signs of tracheomalacia include barking cough, stridor, wheezing, recurrent respiratory tract infections, cyanosis, and, sometimes, apnea. Tracheomalacia may occur in up to as many as 75% of children with EA/TEF but may be clinically significant in only 10% to 20% of infants with EA/TEF; surgical intervention is required in severe cases (Achildi and Grewal, 2007).

Prognosis

The survival rate is nearly 100% in otherwise healthy children. Most deaths are the result of extreme prematurity or other lethal associated anomalies.

Potential complications after the surgical repair of EA and TEF depend on the type of defect and surgical correction. Complications of repair include an anastomotic leak, strictures caused by tension or ischemia, esophageal motility disorders causing dysphagia, respiratory compromise, and gastroesophageal reflux. Anastomotic esophageal strictures may cause dysphagia, choking, and respiratory distress. The strictures are often treated with routine esophageal dilation. Feeding difficulties are often present for months or years postoperatively, and the infant must be monitored closely to ensure adequate weight gain, growth, and development. In some cases laparoscopic fundoplication may be required. At times the infant must be fed via gastrostomy or jejunostomy to provide adequate caloric intake.

Nursing Care Management

The nursing process in the care of the infant with EA/TEF is described in the Nursing Care Plan on pp. 438-439.

Nursing responsibility for detection of this serious malformation begins immediately after birth. For the infant with the classic signs and symptoms of EA (see Clinical Manifestations, p. 435) the major concern is the establishment of a patent airway and prevention of further respiratory compromise. Cyanosis is usually a result of laryngeal spasm caused by overflow of saliva into the larynx from the proximal esophageal pouch or aspiration; it normally resolves after removal of the secretions from the oropharynx by suctioning. The passage of a small-gauge OG feeding tube via the mouth into the stomach during the initial nursing physical assessment is helpful to rule out EA or other obstructive defects. Additional stabilization and nursing care are discussed in the next section.

> **! NURSING ALERT**
>
> Any infant who has an excessive amount of frothy saliva in the mouth or difficulty with secretions and unexplained episodes of apnea, cyanosis, or oxygen desaturation should be suspected of having an EA/TEF and referred immediately for medical evaluation.

Preoperative Care

The nurse carefully suctions the mouth and nasopharynx and places the infant in an optimum position to facilitate drainage and avoid aspiration. The most desirable position for a newborn who is suspected of having the typical EA with a TEF (e.g., type C) is supine (or sometimes prone) with the head elevated on an inclined plane of at least 30 degrees. This positioning minimizes the reflux of gastric secretions at the distal esophagus into the trachea and bronchi, especially when intraabdominal pressure is elevated.

It is imperative to immediately remove any secretions that can be aspirated. Until surgery the blind pouch is kept empty by intermittent or continuous suction through an indwelling double-lumen or Replogle catheter passed orally or nasally to the end of the pouch. In some cases a percutaneous gastrostomy tube is inserted and left open so that any air entering the stomach through the fistula can escape, thus minimizing the danger of gastric contents being regurgitated into the trachea. The gastrostomy tube is emptied by gravity drainage. Feedings through the gastrostomy tube and irrigations with fluid are contraindicated before surgery in the infant with a distal TEF.

Nursing interventions include respiratory assessment, airway management, thermoregulation, fluid and electrolyte management, and parenteral nutritional support.

Often the infant must be transferred to a hospital with a specialized care unit and pediatric surgical team. The nurse advises the parents of the infant's condition and provides them with necessary support and information.

Postoperative Care

Postoperative care for these infants is the same as for any high-risk newborn. Adequate thermoregulation is provided, the double-lumen NG catheter is attached to low-suction or gravity drainage, parenteral nutrition is provided, and the gastrostomy tube (if applicable) is returned to gravity drainage until feedings are tolerated. If a thoracotomy is performed and a chest tube is inserted, attention to the appropriate function of the closed drainage system is imperative. Pain management in the postoperative period is important even if only a thoracoscopic approach is used. In the first 24 to 36 hours the nurse should provide pain management for the neonate just as for an adult undergoing a similar procedure. (See Neonatal Pain, Chapter 7.) Tracheal suction should only be done using a premeasured catheter and with extreme caution to avoid injury to the suture line.

If tolerated, gastrostomy feedings may be initiated and continued until the esophageal anastomosis is healed. Before oral feedings are initiated and the chest tube (if applicable) is removed, a contrast study or esophagram will verify the integrity of the esophageal anastomosis.

The nurse must carefully observe the initial attempt at oral feeding to make certain the infant is able to swallow without choking. Oral feedings are begun with sterile water, followed by frequent small feedings of breast milk or formula. Until the infant is able to take a sufficient amount by mouth, oral intake may need to be supplemented by bolus or continuous gastrostomy feedings. Ordinarily infants are not discharged until they can take oral fluids well. The gastrostomy tube may be removed before discharge or maintained for supplemental feedings at home.

Special Problems

Upper respiratory tract complications are a threat to life in both the preoperative and postoperative periods. In addition to pneumonia, the infants are in constant danger of respiratory distress resulting from atelectasis, pneumothorax, and laryngeal edema. Report any persistent respiratory difficulty after removal of secretions to the surgeon immediately. Monitor the infant for anastomotic leaks and signs of infection such as purulent chest tube drainage, an increased white blood cell count, and temperature instability.

In the infant awaiting esophageal replacement surgery, the upper esophageal segment may be drained by means of a cervical esophagostomy. An esophagostomy is difficult to care for because the skin may become irritated by moisture from the continuous discharge of saliva. Frequent removal of drainage followed by application of a layer of protective ointment, barrier dressing, and/or a collection device is usually sufficient treatment. An enterostomal nurse may provide helpful guidance in the prevention and treatment of skin breakdown.

For the infant who requires esophageal replacement, provide nonnutritive sucking with a pacifier. Sometimes food and fluid are given orally (sham feedings); the intake drains from the esophagostomy but allows the infant to develop mature sucking patterns and, with other appropriate oral stimulation, can prevent feeding resistance. (See Chapter 10.) Infants who take nothing by mouth (NPO) for an extended period and have not received oral stimulation frequently have difficulty eating by mouth after corrective surgery and may develop oral hypersensitivity and feeding aversion. They require patient, firm guidance in learning the techniques of taking food into the mouth and swallowing after repair. A referral to a multidisciplinary feeding behavior team may be necessary.

Family Support, Discharge Planning, and Home Care

One of the difficulties in TEF is the immediate transfer of the sick infant to the intensive care unit and sometimes lengthy hospitalization. Parent-infant bonding is facilitated by encouraging parents to visit the infant, participate in his or her care when appropriate, and express their feelings regarding the infant's condition. The nurse in the intensive care unit should assume responsibility for ensuring that the parents are fully informed of the infant's progress.

Preparing parents for discharge of their infant involves teaching the techniques that will be continued at home. The parents also learn signs of respiratory difficulty and of esophageal stricture (poor feeding, dysphagia, drooling, regurgitating undigested food) and gastroesophageal reflux.

Parents must be aware of dietary restrictions. Remind parents that it is particularly important to guard against the infant swallowing foreign objects. They should cut solid food into small pieces, teach the child to chew thoroughly, give frequent sips of liquid to help swallow food, and avoid foods such as whole hot dogs or large pieces of meat that may become lodged in the esophagus. (See Injury Prevention, Chapter 12.)

Many of these infants have some degree of tracheomalacia; therefore parents should be educated regarding the signs and symptoms. Discharge planning should include teaching parents and other caretakers infant cardiopulmonary resuscitation. Because many infants with EA and a TEF develop gastroesophageal reflux, precautions should be initiated. (See Gastroesophageal Reflux, Chapter 33.)

Discharge planning should include attainment of needed equipment and home nursing services to assist with ongoing assessment of the child and continuity of care (see Nursing Care Plan). (See Chapter 25.)

ANORECTAL MALFORMATIONS

Anorectal malformations are among the more common congenital malformations caused by abnormal development, with an incidence of approximately 1 in 5000 births (Levitt and Peña, 2007). These malformations may range from simple imperforate anus to include other associated complex anomalies of GU and pelvic organs, which may require extensive treatment for fecal, urinary, and sexual function. Anorectal malformations may occur in isolation or as a part of the VACTERL association (see p. 435). These anomalies are classified according to the newborn's gender and abnormal anatomic features, including GU defects (Box 11-7).

Rectal atresia and stenosis occur when the anal opening appears normal, there is a midline intergluteal groove, and usually no fistula exists between the rectum and urinary tract. **Rectal atresia** is a complete obstruction (inability to pass stool) and requires immediate surgical intervention. **Rectal stenosis** may not become apparent until later in infancy when the infant has a history of difficult stooling, abdominal distention, and ribbonlike stools.

A **persistent cloaca** is a complex anorectal malformation in which the rectum, vagina, and urethra drain into a common channel opening into the perineum (Fig. 11-20, A).

◎ NURSING CARE PLAN

The Infant with Esophageal Atresia/Tracheoesophageal Fistula

NURSING DIAGNOSIS	EXPECTED PATIENT OUTCOMES	NURSING INTERVENTIONS	RATIONALE
Preoperative Care			
Risk for Suffocation related to abnormal opening between esophagus and trachea	The child's airway will remain patent and respirations will be effective.	Suction mouth and nose as necessary to clear mucus.	To relieve and prevent airway obstruction
Child's/Family's Defining Characteristics (Subjective and Objective Data)	**The Following NOC Concepts Apply to These Outcomes**	Position supine or on right side with head elevated to at least 30 degrees.	To facilitate mucus drainage into stomach
	Aspiration Control	Monitor airway patency.	To detect signs of airway occlusion
Abundant mucus	Respiratory Status: Ventilation	Monitor vital signs, including pulse oximetry.	To determine oxygenation status
Choking	Family Coping	Place on cardiorespiratory monitor.	To monitor cardiac and respiratory status
Gagging and regurgitation	Parenting		
Episodes of cyanosis		Administer oxygen as needed per unit protocol.	To prevent hypoxia
Retractions		Keep NPO until cause of distress is determined.	To prevent airway obstruction and hypoxia
		Insert double-lumen NG tube and attach to gravity drainage or low suction.	To decompress stomach or remove mucus from blind pouch (diagnosis dependent)
		Establish peripheral intravenous access.	To maintain hydration and administer medications as necessary
		Keep parents informed of infant's status.	To decrease parents' anxiety and establish open lines of communication and trust
		Encourage parents to visit and touch (or hold) child as permissible.	To promote attachment
	The Following NIC Concepts Apply to These Interventions Airway Suctioning Airway Management Vital Signs Monitoring Environmental Management: Safety Fluid Monitoring		

◎ NURSING CARE PLAN—cont'd

The Infant with Esophageal Atresia/Tracheoesophageal Fistula

NURSING DIAGNOSIS	EXPECTED PATIENT OUTCOMES	NURSING INTERVENTIONS	RATIONALE
Risk for Impaired Parenting related to infant's physical defect and environmental factors causing parent-infant separation. **Child's/Family's Defining Characteristics (Subjective and Objective Data)** Infant is placed in an intensive care unit for care.	Parents will form an emotional bond with infant and demonstrate willingness to nurture infant. **The Following NOC Concepts Apply to These Outcomes** Parenting Parenting: Social Safety Parent-Infant Attachment	Encourage parents and siblings (per unit protocol) to visit infant. Encourage parents to hold and touch infant as condition permits. Involve parents in infant's care as much as possible in the preoperative and postoperative phases of care. Keep parents informed of infant's progress, complications, and care needs. Involve parents in decisions regarding infant's care. Educate parents on infant's home care needs, any special procedures required such as gastrostomy feedings, and potential complications or adverse effects to be alert for in care of infant at home. Teach parents infant CPR and choking relief. **The Following NIC Concepts Apply to These Interventions** Attachment Promotion Caregiver Support Anticipatory Guidance Infant Care Family Integrity Promotion	To promote bond with parents and siblings To promote sense of closeness To promote participation in nurturing child To maintain parental involvement in decision making To provide necessary information for home care of child To provide necessary skills for home care of child To promote child's well-being and possibly relieve parents' anxiety

NURSING DIAGNOSIS	EXPECTED PATIENT OUTCOMES	NURSING INTERVENTIONS	RATIONALE
Postoperative Care Risk for Disproportionate Growth related to inadequate nutritional intake secondary to surgical repair of TEF **Child's/Family's Defining Characteristics (Subjective and Objective Data)** Infant unable to take in adequate amounts of calories by mouth Swallowing impaired Lack of weight gain	Infant will achieve growth and developmental milestones for age. **The Following NOC Concept Applies to These Outcomes** Child Development: 6 and 12 months	Weigh daily. Provide nonnutritive sucking (NNS). If infant is fed via gastrostomy or NG tube, provide NNS during feeding. Ensure infant receives amount of calories prescribed at each feeding. Monitor for signs of feeding intolerance such as choking, spitting up, pneumonia (which may indicate TEF). Provide age-appropriate developmental care (specify). Involve parents in provision of developmental care interventions. **The Following NIC Concepts Apply to These Interventions** Risk Identification Bottle Feeding Parent Education: Infant Nutritional Monitoring Aspiration Precautions Breast Feeding Lactation Counseling	To monitor growth To promote and enhance oral and emotional satisfaction To provide oral satisfaction and prevent food refusal when able to take foods by oral route To promote growth To detect complications and implement therapy To promote development To promote attachment and parental involvement in decision making

NG, Nasogastric; *NPO*, nothing by mouth, *CPR*, cardiopulmonary resuscitation; *TEF*, tracheoesophageal fistula.

Imperforate anus includes several forms of malformation without an obvious opening (Fig. 11-21). Frequently a fistula (an abnormal communication) leads from the distal rectum to the perineum or GU system (Fig. 11-20, *B* and *C*). The fistula may be evidenced when meconium is evacuated through the vaginal opening, the perineum below the vagina, the male urethra, or the perineum under the scrotum. The presence of meconium on the perineum does not indicate anal patency. A fistula may not be apparent at birth, but as peristalsis increases, meconium is forced through the fistula into the urethra or onto the newborn's perineum.

Pathophysiology

During embryonic development the cloaca becomes the common channel for the developing urinary, genital, and rectal systems. The cloaca is divided at the sixth week of gestation into an anterior urogenital sinus and a posterior intestinal channel by the urorectal septum. After the lateral folds join the urorectal septum, separation of the urinary and rectal segments takes place. Further differentiation results in the anterior GU system and the posterior anorectal channel. An interruption of this development leads to incomplete migration of the rectum to its normal perineal position.

Diagnostic Evaluation

The diagnosis of an anorectal malformation is based on the physical finding of an absent anal opening. Other symptoms may include abdominal distention, vomiting, absence of meconium passage, or presence of meconium in the urine. Additional physical findings with an anorectal malformation are a flat perineum and the absence of a midline intergluteal groove. The appearance of the perineum alone does not accurately predict the extent of the defect and associated anomalies. GU and spinal-vertebral anomalies associated with anorectal malformations should be considered when an anomaly is noted. EA with or without TEF, cardiac defects, and spinal or vertebral anomalies may occur in association with anorectal malformations, and the infant should be carefully evaluated for the presence of these and other anomalies.

A perineal fistula (see Box 11-7) may be diagnosed by clinical observation. The presence of a prominent anal dimple and a band of skin tissue commonly known as a bucket handle is indicative of a perineal fistula (Levitt and Peña, 2007). Abdominal and pelvic ultrasonography is performed to further evaluate the infant's anatomic malformation. An IV pyelogram and a voiding cystourethrogram (VCUG) are performed to evaluate associated anomalies involving the urinary tract. Other diagnostic examinations that may be performed include a pelvic MRI, radiography, ultrasound, and fluoroscopic examination of pelvic anatomic contents and lower spinal anatomy.

Therapeutic Management

The primary management of anorectal malformations is surgical. Once the defect is identified, take steps to rule out associated life-threatening defects, which need immediate surgical intervention. Provided no immediate life-threatening problems exist, the newborn is stabilized and kept NPO for further evaluation. IV fluids are provided to maintain glucose and fluid and electrolyte balance. Current recommendation is that surgery be delayed at least 24 hours to properly evaluate for the presence of a fistula and possibly other anomalies (Levitt and Peña, 2007).

The surgical treatment of anorectal malformations varies according to the defect but usually involves one, or possibly a

---

BOX 11-7	CLASSIFICATION OF ANORECTAL MALFORMATIONS

Male Defects
Perineal fistula
Rectourethral bulbar fistula (see Fig. 11-20, *C*)
Rectourethral prostatic fistula
Rectovesicular (bladder neck) fistula
Imperforate anus without fistula
Rectal atresia and stenosis

Female Defects
Perineal fistula
Vestibular fistula
Imperforate anus without fistula
Rectal atresia and stenosis
Cloaca (see Fig. 11-20, *A*)

From Peña A, Hong A: Advances in the management of anorectal malformations, *Am J Surg* 180(5):370-376, 2000.

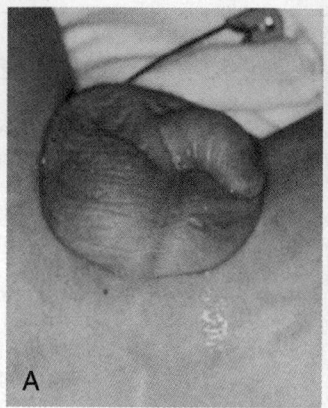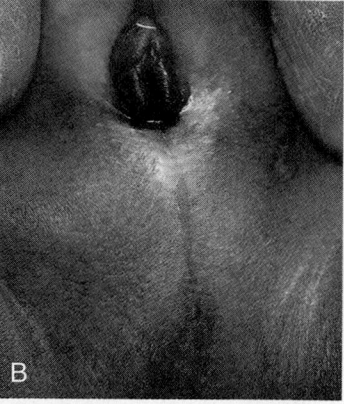

Fig. 11-21 A, No visible external opening is consistent with high imperforate anus defect; absence of intergluteal cleft is also common. **B,** Imperforate anus in female, commonly associated with cloacal anomaly, which manifests as a single perineal opening on perineum. (From Zitelli BJ, Davis HW: *Atlas of pediatric physical diagnosis*, ed 5, St Louis, 2007, Mosby.)

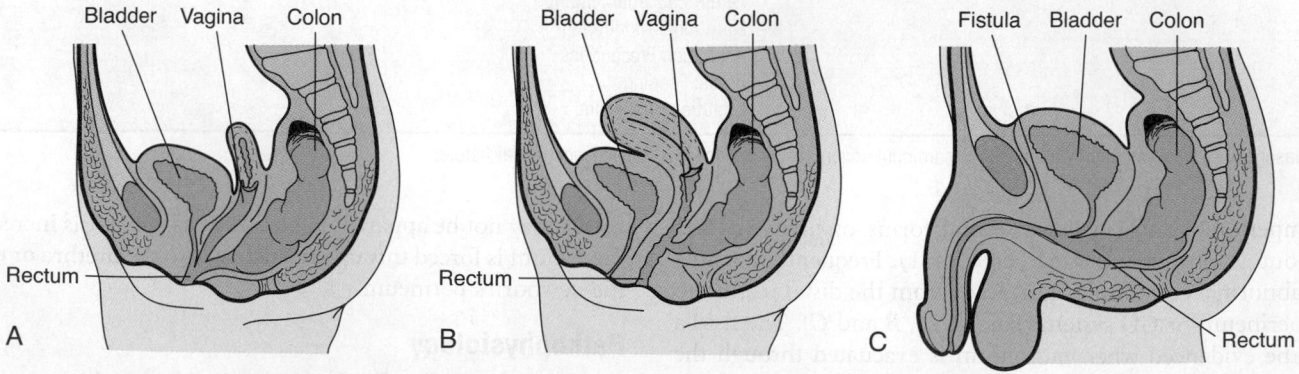

Fig. 11-20 Anorectal malformations. **A,** Typical cloaca (female). **B,** Low rectovaginal fistula (female). **C,** Rectourethral bulbar fistula (male).

combination of several, of the following procedures: anoplasty, colostomy, posterior sagittal anorectoplasty (PSARP) or other pull-through with colostomy, and colostomy (take-down) closure. The Nursing Care Management discussion below outlines some aspects of preoperative and postoperative care.

A primary laparoscopic repair (without colostomy) of some anorectal malformations is being performed successfully in some centers. This minimizes surgical risks, associated morbidity, and postoperative pain management.

Prognosis

The long-term prognosis depends on such factors as the type of defect, anatomy of the sacrum and vertebrae, quality of muscles, and the success of the surgery. Levitt and Peña (2005) emphasize that each defect has a different prognosis and that the prognosis varies according to individual presentation.

The presence of a flat or "rocker" bottom and no midline groove usually carries a poor prognosis for bowel continence because of associated neurologic, muscular, and anatomic problems. When the internal anal sphincter is absent, incontinence is a common long-term problem. These children may achieve socially acceptable continence over time with the aid of a bowel management program. Other potential complications after surgical treatment of anorectal anomalies include strictures, recurrent rectourinary fistula, mucosal prolapse, and constipation.

Nursing Care Management

The first nursing responsibility is assisting in identification of anorectal malformations. A newborn who does not pass stool within 24 hours after birth or has meconium that appears at a location other than the anal opening requires further assessment. Preoperative care includes diagnostic evaluation, GI decompression, bowel preparation, and IV fluids.

For the newborn with a perineal fistula, an anoplasty is performed, which involves moving the fistula opening to the center of the sphincter and enlarging the rectal opening. Postoperative nursing care after anoplasty is primarily directed toward healing the surgical site without other complications. A program of anal dilations is usually initiated when the child returns for the 2-week check-up. Feedings are started soon after surgical repair, and breast-feeding is encouraged because it causes less constipation.

In neonates with anomalies such as cloaca (female), rectourethral prostatic fistula (male), and vestibular fistula (female), a descending colostomy is performed to allow fecal elimination and avoid fecal contamination of the distal imperforate section and subsequent urinary tract infection in infants with urorectal fistulas. With a colostomy, postoperative nursing care is directed toward maintaining appropriate skin care at the stoma sites (both distal and proximal), managing postoperative pain, and administering IV fluids and antibiotics. Postoperative NG decompression may be required with laparotomy, and nursing care focuses on maintenance of appropriate drainage. (See Chapter 27 for colostomy care.)

The PSARP is a common surgical procedure for the repair of anorectal malformations in infants approximately 1 to 2 months after the initial colostomy. Preoperative PSARP care often involves irrigation of the distal stoma to prevent fecal contamination of the operative site. During this time parents must be given accurate yet simple information regarding the infant's appearance postoperatively and expectations as to their level of involvement in the child's care.

In the PSARP procedure the repair is made via a posterior midline sacral approach to dissect the different muscle groups involved without damaging strategic innervation of pelvic structures, so that optimum postoperative bowel continence is achieved. A laparotomy may be required if the rectum is unidentifiable by the posterior approach. Additional management after successful repair involves a program of anal dilations, colostomy closure, and a bowel management program.

Parents are instructed in perineal and wound care or care of the colostomy as needed. Anal dilations may be necessary for some infants. Parents should observe stooling patterns and observe for signs of anal stricture or complications. Information on dietary modifications and administration of medications is included in counseling. Nurses have a vital role in helping families of a child with anorectal malformations provide optimum care so that bowel management is successful and quality of life enhanced for the child and family.

Family Support, Discharge Planning, and Home Care

Long-term follow-up care is essential for children with complex malformations. Parents need reassurance when a colostomy is performed regarding the child's appearance and their ability to care for the child at home. With much patience and reassurance, parents learn how to provide optimum care of the skin and the appliance, while maintaining an appropriate bond with the child.

After the definitive pull-through procedure, toilet training may be delayed. Complete continence is seldom achieved at the usual age of 2 to 3 years. Bowel habit training, bowel management irrigation programs, diet modification, and administration of stool softeners or fiber help children improve bowel function and social continence. Some children never achieve bowel continence and must rely on daily bowel irrigations. Support and reassurance during the slow progression to normal, socially acceptable function are essential.

BILIARY ATRESIA

Biliary atresia, or extrahepatic biliary atresia (EHBA), is a progressive inflammatory process that causes both intrahepatic and extrahepatic bile duct fibrosis, resulting in eventual ductal obstruction. The incidence of biliary atresia is approximately 1 in 10,000 to 15,000 live births (A-Kader and Balistreri, 2007; Kelly and Davenport, 2007). Associated malformations include polysplenia, intestinal atresia, and malrotation of the intestine. Biliary atresia, if untreated, usually leads to cirrhosis, liver failure, and death in the first 2 years of life.

Pathophysiology

The exact cause of biliary atresia is unknown, although immune mechanisms or viral injury may be responsible for the progressive process that results in complete obliteration of the bile ducts. Biliary atresia is not seen in the fetus or stillborn or newborn infant. This suggests that biliary atresia is acquired late in gestation or in the perinatal period and is manifested a few weeks after birth. Congenital infections such as cytomegalovirus, rubella virus, Epstein-Barr virus, rotavirus, and reovirus type 3 have been implicated as a cause of hepatocellular damage leading to biliary atresia, yet no specific agent is identified in every case. Immune-mediated bile duct injury from viral exposure and immaturity of the neonatal immune system may play a role in the destruction of bile ducts and development of EHBA. Other potential causes include an early first trimester insult to the developing bile ducts or a postnatal viral insult; genetic factors may also play a role in the pathogenesis (Davenport, 2005). Early in the course of the disease, the intrahepatic ducts are patent from the interlobular ductules to the porta hepatis. The size of these structures is variable and is correlated with the infant's age and with bile excretion after surgical treatment. These structures are present in most affected infants under 2 months of age but gradually disappear over the next few months and by 4 months are completely replaced by fibrous tissue.

The degree of involvement of the extrahepatic biliary ducts is also variable. Most commonly the entire extrahepatic system is involved in the obliterative process, but some infants have a patent proximal portion of the extrahepatic duct or patency of the gallbladder, cystic duct, and common bile duct. Microscopic examination of the liver tissue reveals cholestasis with absent or diminished bile duct proliferation and fibrosis.

Clinical Manifestations

Many infants with biliary atresia are full term and appear healthy at birth. If jaundice persists beyond 2 weeks of age, especially if the direct (conjugated) serum bilirubin is elevated, the nurse should suspect biliary atresia. The urine may be dark, and the stools often become progressively acholic or gray, indicating absence of bile pigment. Hepatomegaly is present early in the course of the disease, and the liver is firm on palpation.

Diagnostic Evaluation

Early diagnosis is critical to the child with EHBA; the outcome in children surgically treated before 2 months of age is much better than in patients with delayed treatment. The diagnosis of biliary atresia is suspected on the basis of the history, physical findings, and laboratory studies. Laboratory tests include a complete blood count, serum bilirubin levels, and liver function studies. Additional laboratory analyses, including α_1-antitrypsin level, TORCH titers and other intrauterine infections (see p. 380), hepatitis serology, and urine cytomegalovirus, may be indicated to rule out other conditions that cause cholestasis and jaundice. An abdominal ultrasound is usually performed to identify potential causes of extrahepatic obstruction, such as a choledochal cyst. The patency of the extrahepatic biliary system will be demonstrated by a nuclear scintiscan using technetium 99m iminodiacetic acid (^{99m}Tc-IDA, or HIDA; HIDA scan). If there is no evidence of radioactive material excreted into the duodenum, biliary atresia is the most probable diagnosis. A percutaneous liver biopsy is probably the most useful method of diagnosing biliary atresia. The definitive diagnosis is further established during an exploratory laparotomy and an intraoperative cholangiogram that demonstrates complete obstruction at some level of the biliary tree.

Prognosis

Untreated biliary atresia results in progressive cirrhosis and death in most children by 2 years of age. The Kasai portoenterostomy improves the prognosis, but is not always a cure. Biliary drainage can often be achieved if the surgery is performed before the intrahepatic bile ducts are destroyed, usually by 8 weeks of age; otherwise the prognosis is poor. Long-term survival has been reported in children who underwent portoenterostomy before 8 weeks of age. However, even with successful bile drainage, many children ultimately develop liver failure and require liver transplantation. Davenport (2005) reports long-term symptom-free success rates of 10% to 15% in children after portoenterostomy. Reports vary for 10-year survival rates from centers in Japan, Europe, and the United States, with 27% to 68% success rates reported for children following portoenterostomy who survive with native liver (i.e., no transplant required) (Davenport, 2005).

The advances in surgical techniques for liver transplantation and the development of immunosuppressive and antifungal drugs have significantly improved the success of transplantation. Surgical techniques and immunosuppression have contributed to 1- and 5-year survival rates of 87% and 77%, respectively, in children who underwent transplant (Hurwitz and Cox, 2007). The major obstacle remains the shortage of suitable infant donors.

In infants with delayed diagnosis, or in children in whom surgery has failed to provide adequate bile drainage, liver disease progresses. Cirrhosis and splenomegaly occur with hypoalbuminemia, ascites, and coagulopathy. Malabsorption of fat and fat-soluble vitamins and malnutrition result in severe growth failure. Retained bile salts and cholesterol further contribute to pruritus (itching) and xanthomas, often requiring the administration of ursodeoxycholic acid. The severity of pruritus intensifies as the jaundice progresses as the result of disease advancement.

Therapeutic Management

Medical management of biliary atresia is primarily supportive. It includes nutritional support with infant formulas that contain medium-chain triglycerides and essential fatty acids. Supplementation with fat-soluble vitamins (A, D, E, K); a multivitamin; and minerals, including iron, zinc, and selenium, is usually required. Aggressive nutritional support in the form of continuous gastrostomy feedings or total parenteral nutrition may be indicated for moderate to severe growth failure; the enteral solution should be low in sodium. Phenobarbital may be prescribed after hepatic portoenterostomy to stimulate bile flow, and ursodeoxycholic acid may be used to decrease cholestasis and the intense pruritus from jaundice. In cases of advanced liver dysfunction, management is the same as in infants with cirrhosis. (See Chapter 33.)

The primary surgical treatment of biliary atresia is hepatic portoenterostomy (Kasai procedure). This surgical procedure involves dissection of the porta hepatis to expose an area through which bile may drain (Fig. 11-22). A Roux-en-Y jejunal limb is then anastomosed to the porta hepatis (a Y-shaped anastomosis performed to provide bile drainage without reflux). This procedure has several variations. In approximately 90% of infants with biliary atresia who are operated on when younger

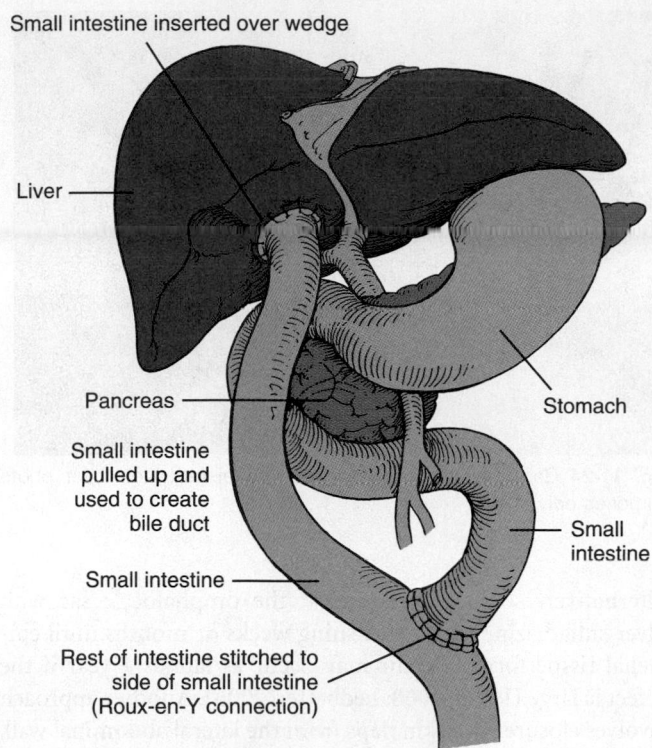

Fig. 11-22 Biliary atresia—Kasai procedure.

Small intestine inserted over wedge

Liver

Pancreas

Small intestine pulled up and used to create bile duct

Small intestine

Rest of intestine stitched to side of small intestine (Roux-en-Y connection)

Stomach

Small intestine

than 8 weeks of age, bile drainage is achieved. Complications after portoenterostomy include ascending cholangitis, cirrhosis, portal hypertension, and GI bleeding. Prophylactic antibiotics are given after the Kasai procedure to minimize the risk of ascending cholangitis.

After the Kasai procedure approximately one third of infants become jaundice free and regain normal liver function. Another one third of infants demonstrate liver damage; however, they may be supported by medical and nutritional interventions. A final third require liver transplantation. Liver transplantation is required for children who cannot regain bile flow and for those with end-stage liver disease or severe portal hypertension. Complications after liver transplantation include obstruction and bile leaks at the biliary anastomosis, portal hypertension, hemorrhage, infection, and rejection. Immunosuppressive drugs are required after transplantation.

Nursing Care Management

There are many important nursing interventions for the child with biliary atresia. The nurse should educate family members regarding all aspects of the treatment plan and the rationale for therapy. Immediately after a hepatic portoenterostomy, nursing care is similar to that following any major abdominal surgery. If an interrupted jejunal conduit has been performed, the family needs to learn how to care for the two stomas and how to refeed the bile after feedings. Teaching includes the proper administration of medications. Administration of nutritional therapy, including special formulas, vitamin and mineral supplements, gastrostomy feedings, or parenteral nutrition, is an essential nursing responsibility. Growth failure in such infants is common, and increased metabolic needs combined with ascites, pruritus, and nutritional anorexia constitute a challenge for care. The nurse teaches caregivers how to monitor and admin-

ister nutritional therapy in the home. Pruritus may be a significant problem that is addressed by drug therapy or comfort measures such as baths in colloidal oatmeal compounds and trimming of fingernails. The risk of complications of biliary atresia, such as cholangitis, portal hypertension, GI bleeding, and ascites, should be explained to the caregivers.

These children and their families require special psychosocial support. The uncertain prognosis, discomfort, and waiting for transplantation can produce considerable stress. (See Cirrhosis, Chapter 33.) In addition, extended hospitalizations, as well as pharmacologic and nutritional therapy, can impose significant financial burdens on the family, as with any chronic condition. The expertise of a multidisciplinary health care team, including surgeons, gastroenterologists, pediatricians, nurses, nutritionists, pharmacists, child life specialists, and social workers, is often necessary. Parent support groups can be beneficial as well. The Children's Liver Association for Support Services* and the American Liver Foundation† provide educational materials, programs, and support systems for parents of children with liver disease.

ABDOMINAL WALL DEFECTS

Gastroschisis and omphalocele are two of the more common forms of congenital abdominal wall defects. Gastroschisis occurs in varying incidences worldwide from about 0.4 to 3 in 10,000 births (Ledbetter, 2006), and omphalocele occurs in approximately 1 to 5 in 10,000 live births (Ledbetter, 2006; Stoll, 2007). Numerous reports cite an increase in the incidence of gastroschisis; the cause of this increased incidence is unknown (Islam, 2008). An omphalocele occurs when the abdominal contents herniate through the umbilical ring (hernia of the umbilical cord), usually with an intact peritoneal sac, whereas gastroschisis occurs when the herniation of intestine is lateral to the umbilical ring. This herniation is usually to the right of the umbilicus, and a peritoneal sac is not present.

Omphalocele

Omphalocele is related to a true failure of embryonic development. It occurs when there is failure of the caudal or lateral infolding of the abdominal wall at approximately the third week of gestation. With the deficiency in the abdominal wall, the bowel is unable to complete its return to the abdomen between the tenth and twelfth week of gestation.

The omphalocele is usually covered only by a translucent peritoneal sac (Fig. 11-23). The sac may contain only a small portion of the bowel or most of the bowel and other abdominal viscera, such as the liver. If the sac ruptures, the abdominal contents become exposed. Omphalocele often is associated with other anomalies (50% to 70% incidence of anomalies), including cardiac, neurologic, skeletal, and GU anomalies; imperforate anus; ileal atresia; and bladder exstrophy. Omphalocele is also associated with trisomies 13, 18, and 21 (Down syndrome) and with advanced maternal age (>30 years) (Ledbetter, 2006).

*25379 Wayne Mills Place, Suite 143, Valencia, CA 91355; 877-679-8256; www.classkids.org.
†75 Maiden Lane, Suite 603, New York, NY 10038; 212-668-1000; www.liverfoundation.org/education/info/biliaryatresia.

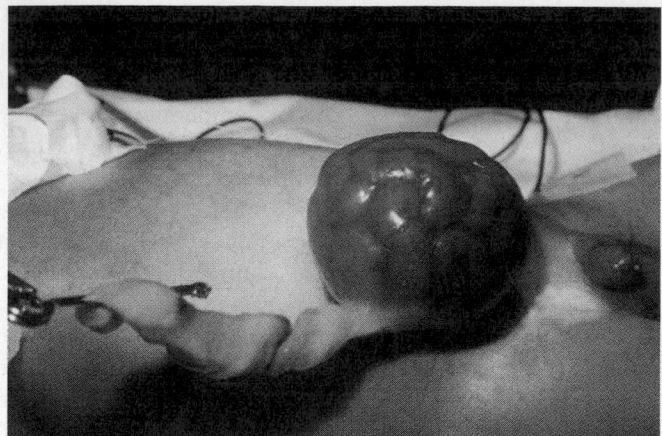

Fig. 11-23 Omphalocele in membranous sac.

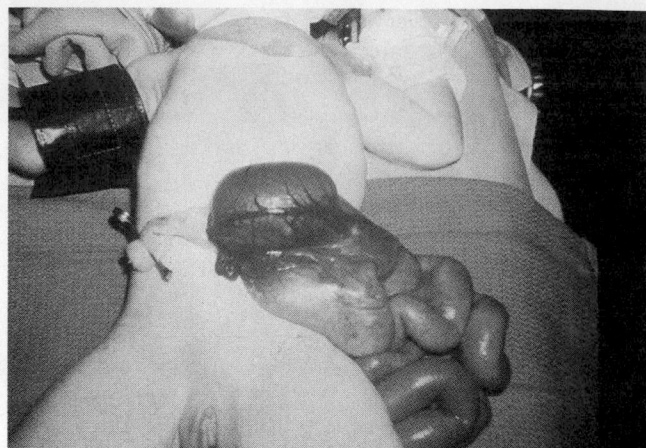

Fig. 11-24 Gastroschisis with exposed bowel (uncovered for photo purposes only).

A small omphalocele may go undetected at first glance and appear as a bulge in the umbilical cord. It is therefore imperative to inspect an unusually large umbilical cord for omphalocele before clamping to prevent possible damage to bowel tissue (Donlon, Furdon, and Clark, 2002). (See Care of the Umbilicus, Chapter 8.)

With the increasing frequency of and improvements in prenatal ultrasonography, some abdominal wall defects are being diagnosed prenatally. The benefits of prenatal ultrasonographic diagnosis include the ability to transfer the mother to a tertiary care center, where pediatric surgeons and a neonatal intensive care unit are available to assist with care after delivery.

Initial management after delivery includes inspection of the defect and any associated anomalies. If the bowel covering is intact, a nonadherent dressing is placed over the defect to prevent injury; if the bowel is exposed, the exposed abdominal contents and membranes are covered with a bowel bag or moist dressings and a plastic drape to prevent excessive fluid loss, drying, and temperature instability. IV fluids and antibiotics are administered, and a further evaluation for other associated anomalies is completed. Placement of a Silastic double-lumen catheter (NG-OG) is performed to accomplish gastric bowel decompression.

After initial medical management and stabilization, several surgical options may be carried out depending on the size of the defect, associated medical problems, and surgeon preference. Primary closure of the omphalocele is one option if the defect is small. The sac is resected, contents are reduced into the abdominal cavity, and an attempt is made to close the abdominal fascia with sutures. The abdominal wall may need to be stretched. If an intestinal atresia exists, a bowel resection may be performed, possibly involving a diverting stoma.

When primary closure of the defect is not possible because of the small size of the abdominal cavity or an extremely large omphalocele, staged reduction is accomplished. A silo mesh may be used to house the omphalocele. The silo may be suspended vertically using mild tension. An antibacterial ointment is applied to the silo and suture lines to prevent local infection. Usually the silo is compressed on a daily basis. Once the abdominal cavity is able to accommodate the viscera, the silo is removed and the defect is closed. Every effort is made to accomplish this within 7 to 10 days to minimize the risk of infection.

Alternatively some surgeons treat the omphalocele sac with silver sulfadiazine over the ensuing weeks or months until epithelial tissue forms. Repair may occur as late as 1 year if the defect is large (Islam, 2008; Ledbetter, 2006). Another approach involves closure with skin flaps from the lateral abdominal wall.

Postoperatively these infants may require mechanical ventilation and parenteral nutrition. Intraabdominal compression may prevent effective respiration and restrict blood flow to the lower extremities and abdominal organs. Feedings may resume once adequate bowel function is established. Postoperative complications involve many of those discussed below with omphalocele but also include infection, evisceration, intestinal volvulus, obstruction, and a ventral hernia.

Gastroschisis

Gastroschisis occurs when the bowel herniates through a defect in the abdominal wall to the right of the umbilical cord and through the rectus muscle (Fig. 11-24). There is no membrane covering the exposed bowel. Controversy exists regarding the etiology of gastroschisis. It has been suggested that at some point between the bowel's stay in the umbilical cord and the completion of fixation, a tear occurs at the base of the umbilical cord, allowing the intestine to herniate. The gap between the cord and the tear is filled in by skin, giving the appearance of a defect in the abdominal wall to the right of the umbilical cord. The base of the defect is narrow, and the lack of membranes results in thickening and foreshortening of the bowel. Gastroschisis is usually not associated with other major congenital anomalies (incidence of 10% to 20%); however, jejunoileal atresia, ischemic enteritis, and malrotation may occur as a result of the defect itself. Cryptorchidism in association with gastroschisis has also been reported to range from 24% to 55% (Williams, Butler, and Sundem, 2003). A teratogenic etiology (young maternal age, smoking, alcohol use, acetaminophen, aspirin, and pseudoephedrine) has been suggested as a possible contributor to this defect, as have environmental influences in certain cases (Ledbetter, 2006).

Initial management involves covering the exposed bowel with a transparent plastic bowel bag or loose, moist dressings. If the opening in the abdominal cavity through which bowel is protruding is small and strangulation of bowel is possible, the abdominal opening is enlarged at the bedside. IV fluids and antibiotics are administered, and a double-lumen NG tube is inserted for bowel decompression. Fluid replacement for gastroschisis is increased twofold to threefold because of large losses from the exposed viscera.

Adequate thermoregulation and fluid management are extremely important for both omphalocele and gastroschisis. During surgery the abdominal wall is stretched and the mass of bowel is replaced in the abdomen. If primary closure is not possible, a prefabricated, spring-loaded Silastic silo is placed over the unprotected bowel in labor and delivery or in the neonatal intensive care unit shortly after birth to protect the bowel and decrease fluid loss; primary surgical closure is attempted at a later date. The silo is reduced over several days, at which time it is removed surgically and the defect is closed.

Infants with gastroschisis have traditionally been operated on within 24 hours of birth because of temperature instability, risk of infection in the unprotected bowel, and fluid loss. Studies have shown that outcomes vary in regards to early surgical closure versus silo management and later surgical closure; some outcomes are heavily dependent on the amount of bowel to be replaced into the abdominal cavity and subsequent intraabdominal pressure with primary closure. However, the optimal time for closure has yet to be determined (Islam, 2008).

Postoperatively most infants require mechanical ventilation because of respiratory distress secondary to increased abdominal pressure. Pain management is imperative, especially in the first 72 hours. Morphine and fentanyl are effective opioid analgesics. Many infants also require prolonged nutritional support (parenteral and enteral) because of poor bowel function. Prolonged parenteral nutrition may cause liver failure. Exposure of the bowel to amniotic fluid in utero predisposes the infant to prolonged paralytic ileus and hypomotility. Other complications include infection, transient renal impairment, intestinal obstruction, vena cava compression, and a subsequent decrease in blood flow to the lower extremities.

Prognosis

Advanced surgical techniques, improved parenteral nutrition delivery systems, and better medical management have improved the prognosis for the newborn with an abdominal wall defect. Survival estimates for infants with gastroschisis range from 90% to 95% (Islam, 2008; Ledbetter, 2006). Survival rates for infants with an isolated omphalocele are reported to be 75% to 95% (Heider, Strauss, and Kuller, 2004; McNair, Hawes, and Urquhart, 2006). Because many newborns with omphalocele often have serious associated congenital anomalies, especially cardiac anomalies (40% to 50%), the prognosis for survival of such infants is often not as predictable or as positive as it is for those with gastroschisis (Ledbetter, 2006).

Nursing Care Management

Nursing care is similar to that for any high-risk infant. Infection is a constant threat before surgery, and careful positioning and handling are necessary to prevent rupture of the omphalocele sac or herniated bowel, or disturbance of the Silastic material used for gradual silo reduction. Viscera should be protected with moist dressings or a silo as described previously. Heat and fluid loss from the exposed viscera are major concerns in the preoperative period. Therefore thermoregulation and attention to adequate fluid volume are critical. Fluid replacement is vital and must compensate for losses. The GI tract is decompressed via an NG tube before surgery to aid in bowel reduction.

Postoperative care includes monitoring for signs of complications and assessment of bowel function; pain management with an opioid is also important in the recovery of the infant. Parenteral nutritional support may be necessary when ileus persists. It may require several days or weeks for normal bowel function to return and before full feedings can be achieved. Infants with a prolonged bowel recovery phase are prime candidates for the development of feeding resistance (see Feeding Resistance, Chapter 10); therefore consultation with a feeding specialist in the early postoperative period is recommended to enhance feeding success. Associated long-term problems with gastroschisis include bowel adhesions, bowel obstruction, necrotizing enterocolitis, and moderate to sometimes severe gastroesophageal reflux (Ledbetter, 2006).

Family Support, Discharge Planning, and Home Care

Because these abdominal defects are visible and may be shocking to parents, immediate emotional support at the time of birth is essential. The family needs a brief explanation of the defect and reassurance that their child is in no immediate danger (unless circumstances are different). After the parents have had time to interact with their newborn, inform them about the surgical treatment and postoperative care. At the time of discharge from the hospital, many of these infants are receiving oral feedings, but extended parenteral nutrition may be required if malabsorption and poor bowel function occur. The nurse can ensure continuity of care by referral to a home health care agency, especially if long-term nutritional support is required.

HERNIAS

A hernia is a protrusion of a portion of an organ or organs through an abnormal opening. The danger of herniation arises when the protrusion is constricted, impairing circulation, or when the protrusion interferes with the function or development of other structures. The herniations discussed in this section are those that protrude through the diaphragm, the abdominal wall, or the inguinal canal.

CONGENITAL DIAPHRAGMATIC HERNIA

Congenital diaphragmatic hernia (CDH) results when the diaphragm does not form completely, resulting in an opening between the thorax and the abdominal cavity. The most common type of CDH (90%) is a left posterolateral defect, also known as a Bochdalek hernia because the herniation occurs through the foramen of Bochdalek (Fig. 11-25). If the diaphragm does not form completely, the intestines and other abdominal structures, such as the liver, can enter the thoracic cavity, compressing the lung. Lung growth may be arrested on the affected side and to a lesser degree on the contralateral side. Ventilation is further compromised by hypoplasia and compression of the lung, including the airways and blood vessels. In addition to the anatomic defect, pulmonary hypoplasia and

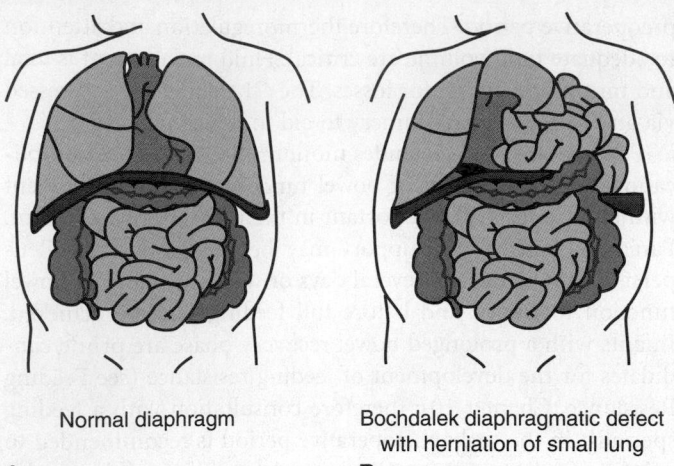

Normal diaphragm

Bochdalek diaphragmatic defect with herniation of small lung

A   **B**

Fig. 11-25 A, Normal diaphragm separating the abdominal and thoracic cavities. **B,** Diaphragmatic hernia with a small lung and abdominal contents in the thoracic cavity. (From Ehrlich PF, Coran AG: Diaphragmatic hernia. In Kliegman RM, Behrman RE, Jenson HB, et al, editors: *Nelson textbook of pediatrics*, ed 18, Philadelphia, 2007, Saunders.)

pulmonary hypertension have also been recently recognized as components in the pathology of CDH.

This serious defect requires prompt recognition and aggressive treatment to reduce its high mortality. The incidence of CDH is approximately 1 in 2000 to 5000 live births (Ehrlich and Coran, 2007). When stillbirths, intrauterine deaths, and elective abortions are included, the total incidence of CDH is higher than data observed in practice (Brownlee, Howatson, Davis, et al, 2009). Associated anomalies have occurred in as many as 30% of CDH, and CDH is observed in several chromosomal syndromes (Ehrlich and Coran, 2007).

Clinical Manifestations

The most common manifestation of CDH is acute respiratory distress in the newborn. Entrance of air into the intestines after birth further compromises respiration. Infants with a CDH may be dyspneic and cyanotic and have a scaphoid abdomen (because of abdominal contents in the chest). Cardiac output is impaired, and the infant exhibits signs and symptoms of shock. Some infants with small defects may not exhibit respiratory symptoms until later in infancy.

Diagnostic Evaluation

Prenatal diagnosis of CDH as early as the twenty-fifth week of gestation is possible. The three main features detected by ultrasonography that confirm the diagnosis are polyhydramnios, mediastinal shift, and loops of bowel in the chest cavity. In severe cases fetal hydrops is evident. Low MS-AFP levels are seen in cases of CDH; however, the finding is not specific for this anomaly.

Antenatal diagnosis of CDH is reported to have the following advantages: (1) counseling the family regarding pregnancy alternatives and potential problems of the neonatal period; (2) continuation of the pregnancy and further management, including possible antenatal treatment; and (3) transport of the fetus with a CDH in utero to a tertiary center for management. A multidisciplinary team of neonatologists, neonatal nurses,

and pediatric surgeons can intervene early in the acute phase to improve the infant's chances for survival and a positive outcome.

After birth, the diagnosis of CDH may depend on the type of hernia present. In the majority of cases the diagnosis is suspected on the basis of the clinical manifestations and is confirmed by a chest radiograph. The chest radiograph shows fluid- and air-filled loops of intestine in the affected side of the chest. The mediastinum may be shifted to the unaffected side, and auscultation may reveal decreased breath sounds on the affected side.

Therapeutic Management

Fetal Surgery

Advances in fetal diagnostic and surgical techniques led to intrauterine repair of CDH in the 1990s, but the outcomes were poor and prenatal surgery was discontinued for a period in the United States (Kays, 2006). Tracheal occlusion (TO) has been shown to expand the lungs and push the abdominal contents back into the abdomen, thus producing larger, functional lungs. Several surgical techniques, such as PLUG (plug the lung until it grows) and EXIT (ex utero intrapartum treatment), have been used in human fetuses to increase fetal lung growth and establish an effective airway for ventilation. Minimally invasive fetal surgical endoscopic tracheal occlusion techniques (FETENDO) in the United States have had moderate success (Jelin and Lee, 2009). Recently two outcome-prediction factors—intrathoracic liver position and lung (contralateral) area–to–head circumference ratio—have been used in combination with fetal endoscopic TO surgery in Europe with varying results (Deprest, Gratacos, Nicolaides, et al, 2009).

After Birth

Many infants with a CDH require immediate respiratory assistance, which includes endotracheal intubation and GI decompression with a double-lumen catheter to prevent further respiratory compromise. At birth, bag and mask ventilation is contraindicated to prevent air from entering the stomach and especially the intestines, further compromising pulmonary function. In infants with mild respiratory distress, oxygen may be given by hood. However, close attention to the infant's acid-base status is imperative in the management and prevention of pulmonary hypertension. Low ventilatory positive pressure and the lowest mean airway pressure possible, combined with rapid ventilatory rates (80 to 120 breaths/min), may reduce the incidence of pulmonary leaks from overinflation of the unaffected lung.

IV fluids are initiated during the stabilization period. A transcutaneous oxygen pressure monitor or pulse oximeter may be placed preductally (right hand) and postductally (left hand, arm, or either foot) to monitor the amount of ductal shunting through the patent ductus arteriosus. An umbilical arterial catheter will help monitor postductal arterial oxygen tension (Pao_2) and allow infusion of fluids, glucose, and electrolytes. Ductal shunting of deoxygenated blood occurs when pressure in the pulmonary artery is equal to or less than peripheral blood pressure. If pulmonary hypertension is severe with decreased pulmonary venous return, right atrial pressure will be greater than left atrial pressure, resulting in shunting of blood through the foramen ovale. The net results of these events cause further hypoxia, hypercarbia, and acidosis. (See Persistent Pulmonary Hypertension of the Newborn, Chapter 10.)

Because acidosis increases pulmonary hypertension and consequently shunting of unoxygenated blood away from the lungs, it is imperative to monitor acid-base status closely. Close attention to the infant's thermoregulatory status (maintaining a neutral thermal environment) and glucose requirements during the acute phase is another priority of care. Individualize ventilatory management on the basis of the infant's response and requirements. Surfactant replacement therapy may also be used to stabilize neonates with CDH, but outcomes have not demonstrated an overall advantage in relation to extracorporeal membrane oxygenation requirement and mortality (Kays, 2006). The use of inhaled nitric oxide to relieve pulmonary hypertension of CDH has also been used in some cases with mixed results (Kays, 2006). (See Nitric Oxide, Surfactant, and Persistent Pulmonary Hypertension of the Newborn, Chapter 10.)

Another strategy that has demonstrated considerable success in the management of CDH is the use of permissive hypercapnia wherein hyperventilation is not employed in order to reduce iatrogenic lung injury and barotrauma. Preductal Spo_2 is maintained at 90, Pco_2 is ignored, and metabolic acidosis is corrected with buffers instead of hyperventilation. Using lung protective ventilation (gentle ventilation) strategies aimed at decreasing mean inflation pressures (<25cm H_2O) and avoiding hyperventilation have demonstrated better overall outcomes and have significantly decreased pulmonary complications such as pneumothorax (Kays, 2006).

Operative treatment involves returning the abdominal organs to the abdomen and repairing the diaphragmatic defect. The timing of surgical repair may vary. Postoperative management involves continuation of ventilatory therapy, monitoring of acid-base balance, and allowing slight hypercapnea. In addition, gastric decompression, thermoregulation, sedation, and maintenance of adequate cardiac output and peripheral perfusion are continued. When muscle paralysis is required, pay careful attention to suctioning oropharyngeal secretions and maintaining intact skin is vital. If paralysis is continued in the postoperative period, appropriate pain management should not be overlooked.

Prognosis

CDH is a complex problem of pulmonary hypoplasia, immature lungs, and other associated problems. The overall mortality rates for CDH are decreasing as the pathophysiology is better understood in relation to current treatment modalities. Current data suggest overall survival rates of 80% to 90% in isolated CDH (Abdullah, Zhang, Sciortino, et al, 2009; Kays, 2006). Surgical repair of the defect alone does not resolve the infant's problems related to organ immaturity. Long-term complications of CDH include chronic lung disease, gastroesophageal reflux, feeding problems, recurrent diaphragmatic herniation, pneumonia, growth failure, sensorineural hearing loss, scoliosis, and impaired motor and cognitive function.

Nursing Care Management

Assessment of the infant at birth is an integral component of nursing care. This is accentuated in life-threatening cases such as CDH, where prompt recognition of neonatal respiratory distress, cyanosis, a scaphoid abdomen, and a possible mediastinal shift would alert the nurse to investigate further. Any one or a combination of these signs may signal the presence of CDH. A newborn in respiratory distress at birth who does not initially respond to resuscitation is further evaluated for CDH; endotracheal intubation is an option for providing adequate oxygenation until CDH is ruled out. If CDH is diagnosed prenatally and the infant is in distress, endotracheal intubation is required to prevent further accumulation of air in the stomach and intestines and subsequent respiratory compromise.

> **! NURSING ALERT**
>
> Any newborn infant with a scaphoid abdomen, moderate to severe respiratory distress, decreased breath sounds unilaterally, and a history of polyhydramnios should be suspected of having a CDH. Ventilation should not be given with bag and mask to prevent further intestinal air and subsequent respiratory compromise.

Preoperative care involves prompt recognition, resuscitation, and stabilization of the infant, including ventilatory support, blood gas monitoring, fluid volume maintenance, and administration of IV fluids and electrolytes. Gastric decompression is achieved with a double-lumen tube, and the infant is observed for signs of impaired cardiac output, acidosis, and hypoxemia.

Postoperative care includes the routine observations discussed in the care of the high-risk infant. Close observation to detect signs of respiratory distress or fluid and electrolyte imbalances is an important nursing function. Closely monitor the infant for signs of mediastinal shift, pulmonary air leak, and infection. Hypovolemia as a result of third spacing of intravascular fluids may occur. Also pay attention to skin care, since these infants often experience prolonged sedation, an increase in skin moisture, tubes and drains coming in contact with the skin, altered nutrition, and altered hemodynamics, all of which place the infant at risk for skin breakdown. Pain management and developmental needs must be met in addition to lifesaving therapy to ensure the infant has optimal development.

Nursing care of the infant with a CDH is also aimed at reducing stimulation either from care activities such as routine suctioning or from environmental factors such as noise and light. Measures that further reduce infant stress, such as management of pain, should be a routine aspect of care for the infant with a CDH.

Because of the serious nature of the condition and the urgency of treatment, the parents are in great need of ongoing support and education regarding postoperative care. The infant with a CDH may require long-term hospitalization and care. As soon as medically possible, the parents should be involved in the daily care of their child.

UMBILICAL HERNIA

The **umbilical hernia** is a common hernia observed in infants. It occurs when fusion of the umbilical ring is incomplete at the point where the umbilical vessels exit the abdominal wall. It affects African-Americans more often than Caucasians and

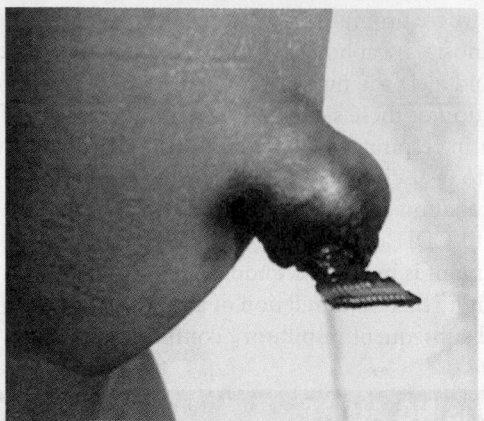

Fig. 11-26 Newborn with umbilical hernia. (From Zitelli BJ, Davis HW: *Atlas of pediatric physical diagnosis,* ed 5, St Louis, 2007, Mosby.)

low-birth-weight and preterm infants more often than full-term infants. An umbilical hernia usually is an isolated defect, but it may be associated with other congenital anomalies, such as Down syndrome (trisomy 21) and trisomies 13 and 18. The size of the defect is variable, and the protrusion is more prominent when the infant is crying (Fig. 11-26). Incarceration, in which the hernia is constricted and cannot be reduced manually, is rare; usually the defect resolves spontaneously by 3 to 5 years of age. If the hernia persists beyond this age, it is usually surgically corrected on an elective basis.

Nursing Care Management

The appearance of an umbilical hernia may be disconcerting to parents. Therefore they need reassurance that the defect usually is not harmful. Taping or strapping the abdomen to flatten the protrusion does not aid in resolution and can produce skin irritation.

Nursing care of the child with an umbilical hernia repair is essentially the same as that for other minor GI surgery. The procedure may be performed on an outpatient basis. Observe the child for complications related to a hematoma or infection. The child may resume a normal diet and activity postoperatively; however, strenuous activity or play is restricted for 2 to 3 weeks.

INGUINAL HERNIA

Inguinal hernias account for approximately 80% of all childhood hernias and occur more frequently in boys than in girls (roughly 6:1). An incidence of 3.5% to 5% is reported in term newborns; 9% to 11% in low-birth-weight and preterm infants, and 30% in very low–birth-weight infants (Aiken and Oldham, 2007).

Pathophysiology

Inguinal hernia comes from persistence of all or part of the processus vaginalis, the tube of peritoneum that precedes the testicle through the inguinal canal into the scrotum (in boys), or the round ligament into the labia (in girls), during the eighth month of gestation. After descent of the testicle, the proximal portion of the processus vaginalis normally atrophies and closes, whereas the distal portion forms the tunica vagina-

lis, which envelops the testicle in the scrotum. When the upper portion fails to atrophy, the abdominal fluid or an abdominal structure (bowel, ovary, Fallopian tubes) can be forced into it, creating a palpable bulge or mass. The persistent sac may end at any point along the inguinal canal; it may stop at the inguinal ring or extend all the way into the scrotum or labia (Fig. 11-27).

Clinical Manifestations

This common defect is asymptomatic unless the abdominal contents are forced into the patent sac. Most often it appears as a painless inguinal swelling that varies in size. It disappears during periods of rest or is reducible by gentle compression. It appears when the infant cries or strains or when the older child strains, coughs, or stands for a long time. The defect can be palpated as a thickening of the cord in the groin, and the silk glove sign can be elicited by rubbing together the sides of the empty hernial sac.

Sometimes the herniated loop of intestine becomes partially obstructed, producing variable symptoms that may include irritability, tenderness, anorexia, abdominal distention, and difficulty defecating. Occasionally the loop of bowel becomes incarcerated (irreducible), with symptoms of complete intestinal obstruction that, left untreated, will progress to strangulation and necrotic bowel. Incarceration occurs more often in infants under 10 months of age.

Therapeutic Management

The treatment for hernias is prompt, elective surgical repair in the healthy child as soon as the defect is diagnosed. However, an incarcerated hernia requires emergent surgical care. Because there was believed to be a significant incidence of bilateral involvement, many surgeons advocated exploration of both sides; however, this practice has gained disfavor due to complications occurring with open exploration and is seldom used (Brandt, 2008). Laparoscopic exploration of the contralateral side may be performed without risk of injury to the vas deferens (Brandt, 2008).

Nursing Care Management

Prompt recognition of an inguinal hernia is imperative. The hernia may first be noticed when the infant is crying or straining to stool (Valsalva maneuver). Nursing care of the infant or child with an inguinal hernia involves preoperative preparation of the infant and appropriate explanation to the parents of the child's expected postoperative status. Most hernia repairs can be managed on an outpatient basis. The preterm infant usually has hernia repair several days before discharge. The former preterm infant diagnosed after discharge is admitted the day of surgery and, after repair, is observed for 12 to 24 hours for apnea and bradycardia.

Postoperatively the incision is kept clean and dry, and the infant's pain is managed appropriately. In infants and small children who are not yet toilet trained, the wound may be covered with an occlusive dressing or left without a dressing. Changing diapers as soon as they become damp helps reduce the chance of irritation or infection of the incision.

No restrictions are placed on the infant's or toddler's activity, but older children are cautioned against lifting, pushing,

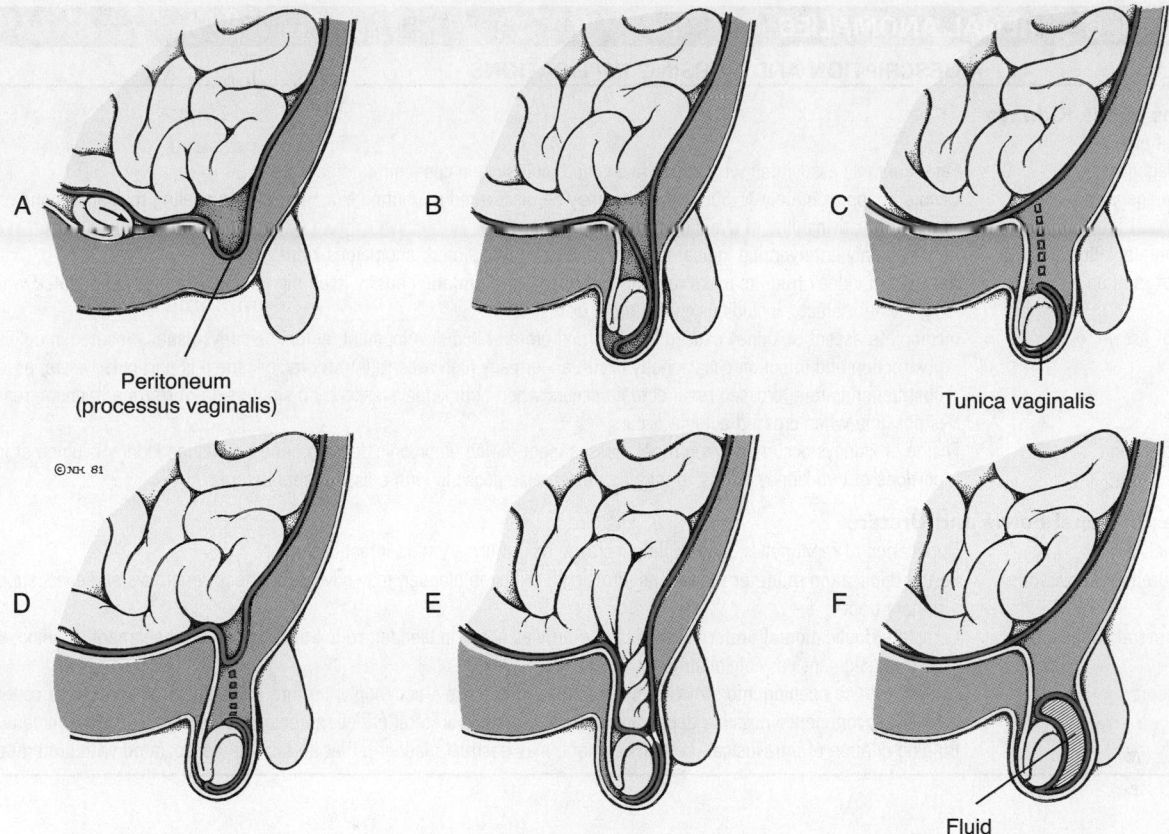

Peritoneum
(processus vaginalis)

Tunica vaginalis

© JXH 81

Fluid

Fig. 11-27 Development of inguinal hernias. **A** and **B,** Prenatal migration of processus vaginalis. **C,** Normal. **D,** Partially obliterated processus vaginalis. **E,** Hernia. **F,** Hydrocele.

wrestling or fighting, bicycle riding, and athletics for about 3 weeks.

If surgery is postponed, parents need to learn the signs of incarcerated hernia, simple measures to reduce it (a warm bath, avoidance of upright positioning, and comfort measures to reduce crying), and where to call for assistance if relief is not obtained in a reasonably short time.

FEMORAL HERNIA

Femoral hernias are rare in children, with a reported incidence of less than 1% (Brandt, 2008). The incidence is higher in girls than in boys. The hernia may manifest as a recurrent hernia following inguinal hernia repair (Brandt, 2008). Initial symptoms are swelling in the groin area associated with severe abdominal pain and cramping. Treatment and management are the same as for inguinal hernia. Incarceration and strangulation are frequent complications.

▌DEFECTS OF THE GENITOURINARY TRACT

External defects of the GU tract are usually obvious at birth. The anatomic location of these defects frequently causes more psychologic concern to parents than does the actual condition or treatment. The timing of medical and surgical procedures for correction of these defects has important implications for children. Surgery involving reproductive organs can be particularly disruptive to preschoolers, who fear punishment, retalia-

tion, body mutilation, or castration. Therefore the trend is toward early correction of visible genital defects, preferably without multiple-stage repairs. Table 11-6 describes renal anomalies, which are typically not obvious at birth.

PHIMOSIS

Phimosis is a narrowing or stenosis of the preputial opening of the foreskin that prevents retraction of the foreskin over the glans penis. It is a normal finding in infants and young boys and usually disappears as the child grows and the distal prepuce dilates. Occasionally the narrowing obstructs the flow of urine, resulting in a dribbling stream or even ballooning of the foreskin with accumulated urine during voiding.

Balanitis is an inflammation or infection of the phimotic foreskin, which occurs occasionally and is managed as any other inflammation or infection. Severe phimosis is treated surgically by circumcision.

Nursing Care Management

Proper hygiene of the phimotic foreskin in infants and young boys consists of external cleansing during routine bathing. The foreskin should not be forcibly retracted, since it may create scarring that can prevent future retraction. Furthermore, retraction of the tight foreskin can result in paraphimosis, a condition in which the retracted foreskin cannot be replaced in its normal position over the glans. This causes edema and venous congestion created by constriction by the tight band of

TABLE 11-6   RENAL ANOMALIES

ANOMALY	DESCRIPTION AND NURSING IMPLICATIONS
Anomalies of the Kidneys	
Anomalies of number	
Bilateral agenesis	Fatal anomaly associated with Potter facies and multisystem congenital defects
Unilateral agenesis	Occurs in approximately 1:1500 live births; may be discovered on routine examination; counseling for parents and child regarding advisability of avoiding contact sports
Supernumerary kidneys	Rare anomaly; intervention indicated if obstruction or infection of anomalous kidney occurs
Anomalies of rotation	Rotation of kidney from its usual relationship to spine; malrotation not by itself significant, but often associated with clinically significant defects, including renal ectopia or fusion
Anomalies of ascent	Incomplete ascent of kidney caused by abnormal ureteral bud development; ectopic kidneys usually located in pelvis; obstruction and infection occasionally occur; abnormally high ascent (intrathoracic kidney) is particularly rare; associated obstruction is rare; crossed renal ectopia occurs when both kidneys ascend on single side of retroperitoneum; renal fusion is possible when crossed ectopia occurs
Anomalies of fusion	Fusion of kidneys occurring when renal masses meet during embryonic development; horseshoe kidney is union of inferior portions of two kidneys crossing midline; fusion also possible with crossed renal ectopia
Anomalies of Renal Pelvis and Ureters	
Bifid renal pelvis	Duplication of renal pelvis; may slightly increase risk of urinary tract infections
Incomplete ureteral duplication	Partial duplication of ureter that opens into single orifice in bladder; may adversely affect peristalsis and evacuation of upper urinary tract
Complete ureteral duplication	Complete duplication of ureters with separate orifices noted in bladder; reflux of lower ureteral segment common; upper ureteral segment possibly obstructed
Ureteral ectopia	Ureteral orifice opening into structure other than bladder base—commonly, urethra and vagina; obstruction or continuous urinary incontinence possible depending on site of ectopic ureteral orifice; defects of associated kidney common
Ureterocele	Bulging dilation of intravesical ureteral segment; may obstruct bladder outlet and is often associated with ureteral duplication

foreskin—a urologic emergency that requires immediate evaluation.

HYDROCELE

Hydrocele is the presence of fluid in the processus vaginalis and is a result of the same developmental process as inguinal hernia (see Fig. 11-27, *F*). A hydrocele in which the upper segment of the processus vaginalis has been obliterated but the tunica vaginalis still contains peritoneal fluid is called a non-communicating hydrocele. This type of hydrocele is common in newborns and often subsides spontaneously as fluid is gradually absorbed.

A communicating hydrocele is one in which the processus vaginalis remains open and into which peritoneal fluid may be forced by intraabdominal pressure and gravity. The length of the hydrocele depends on the length of the processus vaginalis; it may extend into the tunica vaginalis within the scrotum. The hydrocele is asymptomatic except for a palpable bulge in the inguinal or scrotal area. Unlike a hernia, the hydrocele may not be reducible and may not be produced by a sudden increase in intraabdominal pressure (such as straining). The scrotum appears to be larger after an active day and smaller in the morning. Because a communicating hydrocele represents a patent processus vaginalis, it can predispose the child to herniation. Therefore surgical repair is indicated if spontaneous resolution does not take place by 1 year of age.

Nursing Care Management

The nursing care of the infant with a hydrocele is essentially the same as that for inguinal hernia. Advise parents that there is often temporary swelling and discoloration of the scrotum that resolves spontaneously.

CRYPTORCHIDISM (CRYPTORCHISM)

Cryptorchidism is failure of one or both testes to descend normally through the inguinal canal into the scrotum. Absence of testes within the scrotum can be a result of (1) undescended (cryptorchid) testes, (2) retractile testes, or (3) anorchism (absence of testes). Undescended testes can be categorized further according to location:

Abdominal—Proximal to the internal inguinal ring
Canalicular—Between the internal and external inguinal rings
Ectopic—Outside the normal pathways of descent between the abdominal cavity and the scrotum

The incidence of cryptorchidism is reported to be as high as 45% in preterm boys and less than 5% in full-term boys; by the age of 1 year the incidence decreases to less than 2% and does not change thereafter (Sijstermans, Hack, Meijer, et al, 2008).

Pathophysiology

Testicular development is influenced by a number of genes, but the dominant one is located on the Y chromosome. This gene stimulates the medullary sex cords of the embryonic gonad to differentiate into secretory Sertoli cells. Beginning around week 7, these cells secrete a glycoprotein, müllerian inhibiting substance, that leads to development of a male genital system. Testicular descent is a critical element of the development of the male genital system. This descent occurs in two phases; the first is dominated by müllerian inhibiting substance and the second phase by testosterone. Between weeks 8 and 15 a cord-like structure, the gubernaculum, extends from the developing testis (located in the lower abdomen) to the labioscrotal swelling. The fetus grows, but the length of this gubernaculum remains relatively fixed, anchoring the testis to the developing inguinal canal (transabdominal migration) in preparation for the second phase of descent. This second phase begins around weeks 25 to 30 and is characterized by shrinkage of the gubernaculum under the influence of testosterone, causing the testis to migrate down the inguinal canal and into a scrotal position (transinguinal migration). Descent is also characterized by protrusion of peritoneum, the processus vaginalis, that closes before birth.

Cryptorchidism occurs when one or both testes fail to descend through the inguinal canal and into the scrotum. Several processes may slow or arrest testicular descent, including endocrinologic abnormalities affecting the hypothalamic-pituitary-testicular axis, denervation of the genitofemoral nerve, traction of the gubernaculum, abnormal development of the epididymis, or preterm birth. Cryptorchid testes are often accompanied by congenital hernias and abnormal testes, and they are at risk for subsequent torsion.

An ectopic testis emerges outside the inguinal ring into the perineum or femoral area, or lies in a transverse scrotal or prepenile location. The most common site is the superficial inguinal pouch. Ectopia is postulated to occur because of obstruction of the scrotal inlet, scarring (fibrosis) of the gubernaculum, or other mechanical anomalies.

Anorchism is the complete absence of a testis. Anorchism is suspected whenever one or both testes cannot be palpated in the patient with apparent cryptorchidism. In some cases, bilateral anorchism is associated with genotypic and phenotypic abnormalities, but it is commonly associated with a normal karyotype (46,XY) and normal genital development. This observation supports the hypothesis that, in most cases, anorchism represents degeneration rather than agenesis of the testes (vanishing testes or testicular regression syndrome).

The cryptorchid or ectopic testis must be differentiated from anorchism because of the risk for malignant degeneration and subfertility when the testis is left in an extrascrotal location. This differentiation may be resolved by an imaging study, such as an ultrasound, or it may require laparoscopic or direct surgical exploration.

Retractile testes can be found at any level within the path of testicular descent, but they are most commonly identified in the groin. Fortunately, they are not truly cryptorchid. Instead, they are introverted to an inguinal or abdominal position because of an overactive cremasteric reflex. The cremasteric reflex, observed as withdrawal of the testis above the scrotum and into the inguinal canal in response to various stimuli, including exposure to cool temperatures, is active during infancy and peaks around age 4 to 5 years. Unlike the cryptorchid testis, the retractile testis can be gently moved into the scrotum without residual tension and does not require treatment.

Clinical Manifestations

A nonpalpable testis is typically observed by the parent or detected during routine physical examination by a nurse practitioner or physician. If one testis is not palpable, the affected hemiscrotum will appear smaller than the other. With bilateral nonpalpable testes, both hemiscrota appear small. In the case of retractile testes, the parents may report intermittently observing the testes in the scrotum, interspersed with periods when they cannot be visualized or palpated. Frequently, the retractile testis will be observed in the scrotum when child is being bathed in warm water.

Diagnostic Evaluation

It is important to differentiate the true undescended testis from the more common retractile testis. Retractile testes can be "milked" or pushed back into the scrotum, but truly undescended ones cannot. For examination, the nurse can obviate the cremasteric reflex by placing the child in a squatting position or by applying firm finger pressure on the external ring before palpating the abdomen or genitalia. (See Fig. 6-39.)

Undescended testes are palpable along the inguinal canal, but those in the abdominal cavity usually are not. Ultrasonography, CT, MRI, and abdominal laparoscopy are sometimes used to verify cryptorchidism in children undergoing orchiopexy. Laparoscopy is the most accurate means for locating nonpalpable testes (Gatti and Ostlie, 2007). Suggestions to employ in diagnostic examination include:

- An undescended testis is usually smaller and softer than its descended mate.
- A well-developed rugous scrotum usually indicates normal testicular descent (may be confused by the presence of a hydrocele or inguinal hernia).
- Retractile testes are usually bilateral (the cremasteric reflex is equally brisk on both sides).
- A testis can usually be distinguished from a lymph node by its elastic nature. A testis is mobile and can be massaged down into the scrotum, although it will spring back into the canal.
- Application of soap, cornstarch, or talcum powder to the tip of the examiner's fingers facilitates massaging the inguinal canal.

Acquired undescended testes in children who have had normally descended testes are relatively uncommon. Evaluation of the testes should continue to be a part of the routine physical assessment.

Therapeutic Management

Retractile testes that can be manipulated into the scrotum will eventually assume a satisfactory scrotal position without medical or surgical intervention. The diagnosis is not made at a single examination, and parents are asked if they have observed the testes in the scrotum at some time. If so, the anomaly probably represents the retractile variety and the parents can be reassured. By 1 year of age, retractile testes will descend spontaneously in approximately 75% of cases in both full-term and preterm infants. In contrast, true undescended testes rarely descend spontaneously after 1 year of age.

A trial of hormone therapy with luteinizing hormone–releasing hormone (nasal spray) and human chorionic gonadotropin (injection) may be attempted. This method is commonly used in Europe; however, a recent review of the evidence does not support the use of hormonal therapy to elicit testicular descent (Gapany, Frey, Cachat, et al, 2008). Surgical treatment is the preferred management in the United States. If the testes do not descend spontaneously, orchiopexy is performed before the child's second birthday, preferably between 1 and 2 years of age. Surgical repair is done to (1) prevent damage to the undescended testicle by exposure to the higher degree of body heat in the undescended location, thus maintaining future fertility; (2) decrease the incidence of malignancy formation, which is higher in undescended testicles; (3) avoid trauma and torsion; (4) close the processus vaginalis; and (5) prevent the cosmetic and psychologic handicap of an empty scrotum. Because of the increased propensity toward neoplastic changes (even after orchiopexy), cryptorchid testes are better observed in the scrotal position, where they can be routinely palpated.

The timing of the surgery is important, as it is in any genital surgery. Orchiopexy is usually performed between 6 and 24 months of age. Fewer psychologic effects and a higher rate of fertility may be achieved when repair takes place at an early age. Having both testes in the scrotum by school age prevents psychologic problems related to body image and peer-group embarrassment, since the empty scrotum is smaller in size and altered in shape.

In the routine surgical procedure for undescended testes, the testes are brought down into the scrotum and secured in that position without tension or torsion. A simple orchiopexy for a palpable testis can usually be performed in an outpatient surgical unit. Diagnostic laparoscopic surgery through the umbilicus is expected to improve outcomes in males with cryptorchid testes (Onal and Kogan, 2008). Intraabdominal testes require considerable surgical skill because of technical problems resulting from variations in the length of the spermatic cord, and overnight hospitalization may be necessary. In most cases the family can be reassured of normal testicular function in adulthood.

Nursing Care Management

Postoperative nursing care is directed toward preventing infection and instructing parents in home care of the child, including pain control. Infection is prevented by carefully cleansing the operative site of stool and urine. Observation of the wound for complications and activity restrictions are discussed. The child should avoid vigorous sports activities and use of toys that are straddled for 2 weeks postoperatively to prevent dislodgment of the testis from the scrotum. Parents are concerned about the child's future fertility, and the nurse counsels the family regarding the prognosis and the optimum time for discussing it with the child—ideally, as a part of sex education. Follow-up care for all boys with cryptorchidism is suggested, especially those in whom orchiopexy was delayed until after age 10 or 11 years or never performed, since these boys are nearly six times more likely than other boys to develop testicular cancer (Walsh, Dall'Era, Croughan, et al, 2007; Gapany, Frey, Cachat, et al, 2008). They should learn how to perform testicular self-examination.

HYPOSPADIAS

Hypospadias is a condition in which the urethral opening is located below the glans penis or anywhere along the ventral surface (underside) of the penile shaft (Fig. 11-28). The incidence of hypospadias is reported to be 1 out of 250 to 300 live births, with 10% to 15% of affected newborns having a first-degree male relative (sibling or father) with the same condition (Bukowski and Zeman, 2001; Gray and Moore, 2009). In mild cases the meatus is just below the tip of the penis. In the most

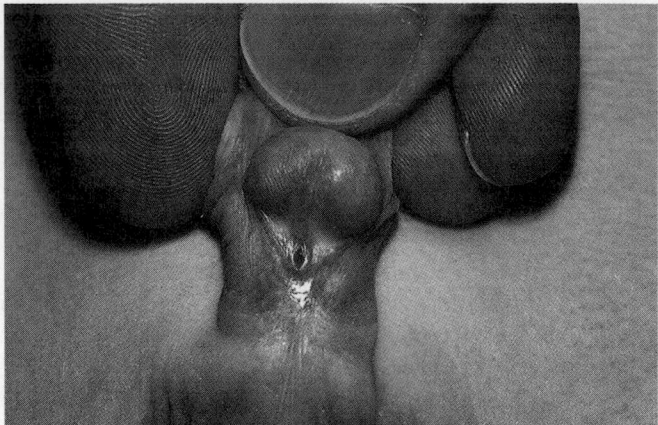

Fig. 11-28 Hypospadias. (Courtesy H. Gil Rushton, MD, Children's National Medical Center, Washington, DC.)

severe malformations the meatus is located on the perineum between the halves of the scrotum (bifid scrotum). Chordee, or ventral curvature of the penis, results from the replacement of normal skin with a fibrous band of tissue and usually accompanies more severe forms of hypospadias. In addition, the foreskin is usually absent ventrally and, when combined with chordee, gives the organ a hooded and crooked appearance. In severe cases the altered appearance may leave the infant's gender in doubt at birth because the perineal position of the meatus may be mistaken for a female urethra. Because undescended testes may also be present, the small penis may appear to be an enlarged clitoris. In any case of ambiguous genitalia, further study, such as chromosome analysis, is essential. (See Disorders of Sex Development, p. 457.)

Surgical Correction

The principal objectives of surgical correction are (1) to enhance the child's ability to void in the standing position with a straight stream, (2) to improve the physical appearance of the genitalia for psychologic reasons, and (3) to preserve a sexually adequate organ. Many procedures have been described that accomplish one or more of these goals. The choice of surgical procedure is affected primarily by the severity of the defect and the presence of associated anomalies.

Distal hypospadias (a defect noted on the glans penis) may be corrected by a meatal advancement and glanuloplasty (MAGPI) procedure or glans approximation procedure (GAP). The MAGPI requires a dorsal meatotomy with incision of the tissue between the urethral meatus and the glanular groove. The dorsal epithelium is then advanced distally, and care is taken to avoid disrupting the urethra. The ventral skin is then approximated, redundant tissue is carefully excised, and the defect is closed. The GAP requires approximation of the nonjoined urethral opening with lengthening of the urethra and deepithelialization of skin at the lateral edges of the defect. Although the procedure is relatively simple, the potential for urethrocutaneous fistula is significant.

More proximal hypospadias defects typically require alternative approaches. When sufficient ventral skin is present, a skin flap is mobilized that is large enough to reach the tip of the penis. The flap is freed with as much subcutaneous tissue attached as is feasible. Urethral reconstruction is accomplished by reversing the meatal-based flap distally to the glans penis. Specific strategies are used to provide adequate vascular supply to the mobilized skin grafts and to prevent fistula formation. When ventral skin volume is deficient, an island flap repair may be used. This procedure requires more extensive use of skin grafts to create the new urethra and close the defect.

The chordee that often coexists with a hypospadias defect is repaired by release of the ventral skin. When the chordee persists, additional procedures may be indicated. In many cases, a single operation will be all that is needed to correct hypospadias and chordee.

Increased surgical experience and improvements in technique have reduced the number of staged procedures needed for hypospadias defects. However, a staged procedure is indicated in particularly severe defects with marked deficits of available skin for mobilization of flaps and in rare cases when scrotal transposition occurs.

The preferred time for surgical repair is 6 to 12 months of age, before the child has developed body image. Occasionally a short course of testosterone is administered preoperatively to achieve additional penile size to facilitate the surgery.

Nursing Care Management

The nurse should examine every male newborn carefully for hypospadias. If the nurse suspects even mild hypospadias, this is reported to the practitioner. Traditionally the foreskin has been used to repair the hypospadias; however, newer surgical techniques do not require an intact foreskin for repair to be successful. In male infants who remain uncircumcised, the nurse should verify that the newborn's meatal opening is present on the glans penis, preferably without forcefully retracting the foreskin. Preparation of parents for the type of procedure to be done and the expected cosmetic result helps avert problems. Frequently parents are informed of what is to be surgically corrected but are not advised of what to expect as a reasonable consequence. More refined surgical techniques performed by surgeons specializing in pediatric urologic conditions have improved cosmetic and functional outcomes in these boys. If children are old enough to understand what is occurring, the nurse also prepares them for the operation and the expected outcome.

Hypospadias repair may require some type of urinary diversion with a silicone stent or feeding tube to promote optimum healing and to maintain the position and patency of the newly formed urethra. Sedation may be required for the excessively irritable or restless child, and pain is controlled with analgesics. Epidural anesthesia using a local anesthetic and/or analgesic may be used as an adjunct to general anesthesia for the repair and left in place for postoperative pain management.

The nurse teaches the parents to care for the indwelling catheter or stent and irrigation technique if indicated. They need to know how to empty the urine bag and how to avoid kinking, twisting, or blockage of the catheter or stent. Often the child is discharged with a catheter or stent emptying directly into the diaper. To prevent infection, a tub bath should be avoided until the stent has been removed. An antibacterial ointment may be applied to the penis daily for infection control. In older children a urine collection device can be used. Parents need to learn how to secure the drainage bag to the leg to allow

the child to be mobile, and they should be cautioned to never clamp off a catheter. A larger volume bedside urine bag should be used at night to prevent overfilling. Positioning the bag below the waist allows for proper drainage. An extra bag is sent home with the family in case of tears or leakage. The family should encourage the child to increase fluid intake. The child should avoid straddle toys, sandboxes, swimming, and rough activities until allowed by the surgeon.

EPISPADIAS AND EXSTROPHY COMPLEX

Epispadias is a defect of the urinary system characterized by failure of urethral canalization. Bladder exstrophy is a more severe defect characterized by externalization of the bladder, splaying of the urethra with failure of tubular formation, and diastasis (separation) of the pelvic bone (Figs. 11-29 and 11-30). Both these defects are part of a complex of congenital anomalies of GU development that range from relatively mild defects (such as glandular epispadias, or a defect on the dorsal surface [topside] of the penile shaft) to severe lower abdominal defects involving multiple organ systems (such as cloacal exstrophy). Fortunately, the incidence of exstrophy and epispadias complex anomalies is small. Bladder exstrophy, the most common of the defects, is estimated to occur in 1 of 50,000 live

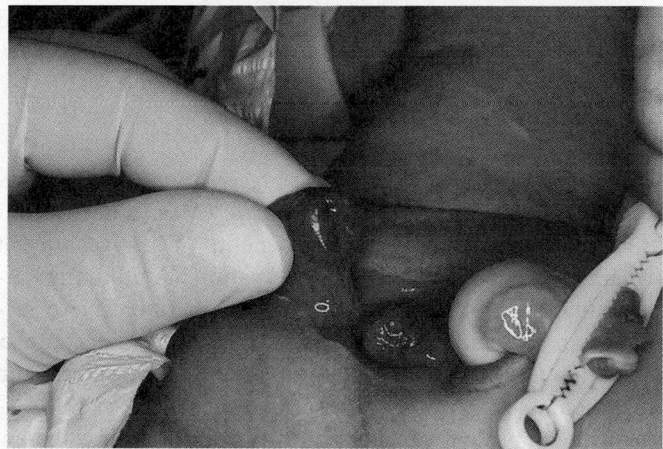

Fig. 11-29 Newborn with bladder exstrophy and epispadias. (Courtesy Tim Yankee, St. Francis Hospital, Tulsa.)

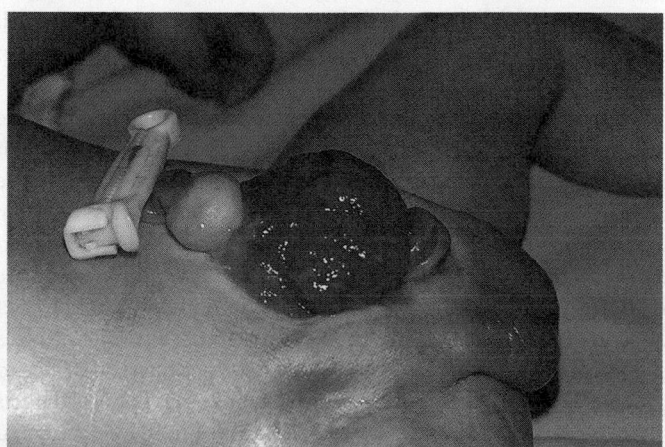

Fig. 11-30 Exstrophy of bladder. (Courtesy H. Gil Rushton, MD, Children's National Medical Center, Washington, DC.)

births; the defect is just as common in males and females (Nelson, Dunn, and Wei, 2005).

Pathophysiology

Exstrophy results from failure of the abdominal wall and underlying structures, including the ventral wall of the bladder, to fuse in utero. As a result, the lower urinary tract is exposed and the everted bladder appears bright red through the abdominal opening. This is accompanied by a constant seepage of urine from the exposed ureteral orifices, making the area malodorous and susceptible to infection. The constant accumulation of urine on the surrounding skin produces tissue ulceration and further infection. Progressive renal damage from infection and obstruction may cause renal failure if left untreated.

In males the defect is almost always associated with epispadias and may include other problems, such as undescended testes and inguinal hernias. Even after reconstruction the sexual handicap in males may be severe because the penis is shortened and does not hang dependently. In females the genitalia may be affected, with a cleft or bifid clitoris; a bifid uterus; completely separated labia; and a duplicate, exstrophic, or absent vagina. In either sex, separation of the pubic bones is generally corrected by pelvic osteotomy, resulting in a normal gait for these children (Nelson, King, Sponseller, et al, 2006). The upper urinary tract is usually normal, and fertility is possible in females but more complex in males, who may require assisted reproductive techniques such as percutaneous sperm aspiration and intracytoplasmatic sperm injection to achieve a pregnancy (D'Hauwers, Feitz, and Kremer, 2008).

Therapeutic Management

The objectives of treatment are (1) preservation of renal function, (2) attainment of urinary control, (3) adequate reconstructive repair for psychologic benefit, (4) prevention of urinary tract infections, and (5) preservation of optimum external genitalia with continence and sexual function. The correction of an epispadias or bladder exstrophy defect is complex and in the past has required multiple surgical procedures and ongoing management of the urinary system. Single-stage surgical closure of bladder exstrophy and epispadias repair with total mobilization is now being performed with varying degrees of success in infants who meet single-stage closure repair criteria (Gearhart, 2001; Husman, 2006; Mitchell, 2005). Widespread acceptance of this procedure began in 1998; therefore the full extent of its success or complications are not yet known (Husman, 2006).

For the child with exstrophy undergoing staged repair, the bladder is closed during the neonatal period, preferably within the first 1 to 2 days of life. Until closure is performed, the bladder is covered with clear plastic wrap or a thin film dressing without adhesive. Petroleum jelly is avoided because it tends to damage the bladder mucosa. After bladder closure, the neonate is monitored for urinary output and for signs of urinary tract or wound infection. At the time of closure, the pelvic diastasis is corrected with an osteotomy or an external fixation device to prevent the waddling gait that occurs when pelvic bone defects are not addressed. Inguinal herniorrhaphies may be completed with initial closure to reduce the risk of subsequent incarceration, particularly for boys.

During the next 3 to 5 years, urine drains freely from the urethra, which has no sphincter mechanism. This period should allow the bladder to gain capacity while the child grows and matures before subsequent surgical repair. The parents should learn to recognize the signs of urinary tract infection and monitor the urinary system regularly via urinalysis and ultrasonographic imaging.

The second stage of exstrophy management is repair of the epispadias and creation of a urethral sphincter mechanism. Epispadias repair attempts to lengthen and straighten the penis to a more dependent position and provide a distal urethra adequate for urination and ejaculation. Creation of a urethral sphincter mechanism requires reconstruction of the bladder neck and tubulization of the proximal urethra to accomplish these goals.

In some children, reconstruction (tightening) of the bladder neck may not provide sufficient resistance to achieve urinary continence. In these cases, suburethral collagen injections or implantation of an artificial urinary sphincter may be performed. Occasionally the bladder fails to achieve an adequate functional capacity, and augmentation enterocystoplasty is required. This procedure is typically combined with the creation of a Mitrofanoff appendiceal stoma because catheterization is particularly difficult after reconstruction of the proximal urethra (see p. 404).

Abnormalities of the genitalia are addressed to ensure optimal sexual function. In boys the testes are typically cryptorchid, and bilateral orchiopexy is combined with reconstruction of the bifid scrotum to preserve testicular function. In girls, surgical enlargement of the vaginal introitus may be needed to permit intercourse. In both genders, plastic surgery to reduce scarring of the genital area or to create an umbilicus may significantly improve the child's body image and emerging sexual identity.

Nursing Care Management

Physical care of the unrepaired defect includes meticulous hygiene of the bladder area to prevent infection and excoriation of the surrounding tissue. A sterile, nonadherent, moist dressing is placed over the exposed bladder area to prevent infection and to keep the diaper from adhering to the mucosa. Plastic wrap may be placed loosely over the dressing to protect the site and prevent drying of the dressing. A moisture barrier ointment may be prescribed for the surrounding skin to protect it from the constantly draining urine. After bladder closure, if external compression is used to immobilize the pelvis, the skin is inspected periodically for evidence of pressure necrosis.

Fluid management is critical because of the large insensitive water losses from the exposed viscera (Mercy and Brady-Fryer, 2004); therefore IV access is considered early. An umbilical arterial catheter may be inserted for blood specimen withdrawal and infusion of fluids (Mercy and Brady-Fryer, 2004).

Other aspects of preoperative care are similar to those for any major abdominal surgery. If a sterile specimen is needed for evaluation of existing infection, urine may be obtained by aspirating the specimen with a sterile syringe.

Nursing care after the complete primary repair is aimed at decreasing pain and agitation in the infant, preserving pelvic immobility, maintaining ureteric catheter patency, and maintaining the operative site intact. Abdominal distention from crying or other sources is avoided. NG tube decompression may be used to prevent abdominal distention. Dehiscence may occur postoperatively, and signs of suture separation or wound problems are promptly reported to the practitioner. The infant may require mummy wrapping or a spica cast, whereas the older child may have an external fixator in place to achieve pelvic stability and immobilization postoperatively (Nelson, King, Sponseller, et al, 2006). Skin care and care of the external fixation device to ensure appropriate function are essential components of nursing care of the child with exstrophy repair. Chapter 39 discusses nursing care of the child in a spica cast.

Postoperative nursing care after bladder neck reconstruction and antireflux surgery (ureteral reimplantation) includes routine wound care and careful monitoring of urinary output from the bladder and ureteral drainage tubes. Care after a penile lengthening, chordee release, and urethral reconstruction is similar to care after hypospadias repair.

Children who fail to attain urinary continence after bladder neck reconstruction are offered a continent diversion. Preoperatively, a bowel prep is required. In addition to routine postsurgical care, nursing after a continent diversion includes wound care, observation of NG suction (surgery requires bowel resection), and measurement and observation of urinary output. CIC is used to regularly empty the urinary reservoir. Most children are able to learn self-catheterization by age 6 or 7 years. Adult supervision is needed to ensure the child is compliant.

Family Support and Home Care

One of the most devastating aspects of exstrophy of the bladder is its appearance. Although the actual physical care is not difficult, it is not easy for parents to assume responsibility for what to them seems an enormous task because of the emotional impact of the defect.

The nurse should instruct parents regarding a realistic outcome of surgery because unrealistic expectations of the cosmetic and functional result may leave them disappointed and discouraged. Parents often worry about the child's sexual adjustment, even though they may not voice such concerns. Part of the nursing admission history is directed toward evaluating the parents' (and child's, if appropriate) expectation of the surgical repair, knowledge of the possibility of eventual urinary diversion, and feelings concerning this permanent change in body function.

When the infant is discharged with an unrepaired defect, plastic wrap is placed over the defect and diapers are changed frequently to prevent infection, ulceration, and odor. Parents learn to recognize the signs of urinary tract infection (see Chapter 30) and to report a suspected infection to the practitioner. General infant care remains unchanged except for sponge baths rather than immersion in water.

Even with improved reconstructive surgery for these patients, substantial psychologic support and guidance are needed to help them adjust to their fears of inadequate penile size; appearance of the genitalia; potential inability to procreate; and rejection by peers, especially the opposite sex. Ongoing discussion groups for parents and children are particularly useful in resolving these fears and promoting optimum psychologic adjustment, particularly during adolescence.

OBSTRUCTIVE UROPATHY

Structural or functional abnormalities of the urinary system can obstruct the normal flow of urine and compromise function. The area proximal to the site of obstruction is exposed to increased intraluminal pressure, dilation, and urinary stasis. For example, when the bladder outlet is obstructed, the renal pelves and both ureters may become distended, a condition called ureterohydronephrosis. However, if one ureterovesical junction is obstructed, the entire ureter and renal pelvis of that side will be affected and the contralateral system will remain normal in appearance and function. Similarly, if the ureteropelvic junction (UPJ) becomes obstructed, the renal pelvis and calyces will become dilated, a condition called **hydronephrosis**.

In children with end-stage renal disease, the most common types of obstructive uropathy reportedly include posterior urethral valves (PUVs); UPJ; obstructive megaureter, a type of urethral hypoplasia or atresia; ureterocele; and miscellaneous forms of obstruction (Hinds, 2004).

Obstruction may be congenital or acquired, unilateral or bilateral, complete or incomplete, and chronic or acute (Fig. 11-31). Boys are affected more commonly than girls, but obstructive uropathy is suspected whenever a child experiences a congenital urinary system defect. **Oligohydramnios** (decreased amount of amniotic fluid, usually defined as <500 ml) is often an indication of poor renal function in the fetus. Appropriate fetal pulmonary development is dependent on adequate renal function, and renal impairment may cause fetal pulmonary hypoplasia with resulting respiratory distress at birth (Hinds,

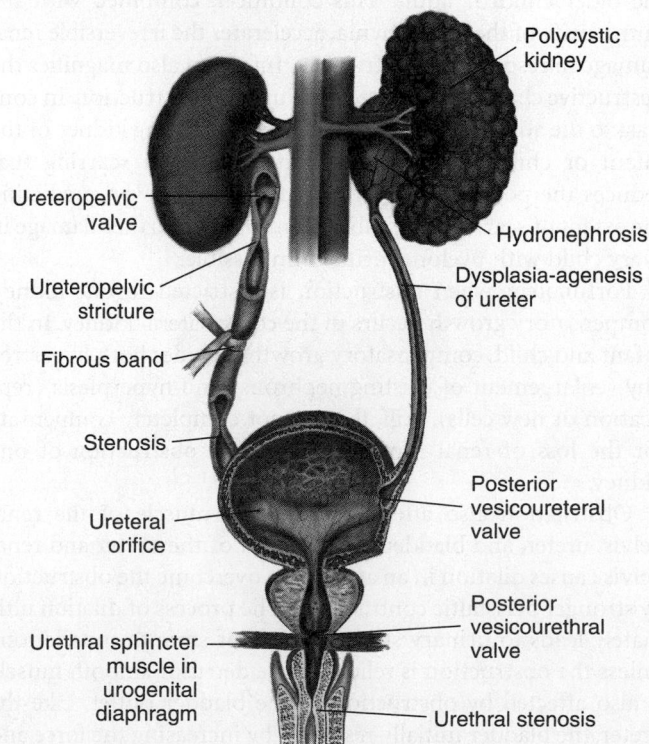

Fig. 11-31 Major sites of urinary tract obstruction.

TABLE 11-7	COMMON CAUSES OF OBSTRUCTIVE UROPATHY IN CHILDREN
OBSTRUCTIVE SITE	**DESCRIPTION AND NURSING IMPLICATIONS**
Calyx	Congenital infundibular stenosis, intrinsic blockage from a stone, inflammation, or tumor, causing calyceal dilation or diverticulum; obstructed calyx typically asymptomatic but clinically significant when it serves as a reservoir for infection
Ureteropelvic junction	Intrinsic stenosis or extrinsic blockage cause by anomalous blood vessel, kink, or fibrous band; often detected on prenatal ultrasonography or when diuresis causes acute-onset flank pain; radionuclide scan used to determine severity of obstruction and subsequent treatment
Ureterovesical junction	Congenital megaureter (congenital obstruction from unknown cause); acquired intrinsic blockage from stone, tumor, or inflammation; or extrinsic obstruction from tumor; megaureter may be asymptomatic or may cause urinary tract infection, hematuria, or abdominal mass
Bladder and urethra	Low bladder wall compliance or blockage of bladder outlet caused by bladder neck contracture or hypertrophy, urethral valves, urethral polyp; congenital urethral obstruction detected by observing infant's initial urination; straining or failure to urinate within first 12-24 hr of life indicative of potentially serious urinary system obstruction
Functional obstruction	Vesicosphincter dyssynergia caused by spinal anomalies (such as myelodysplasia or spinal injury) or functional causes (Hinman syndrome) often leading to ureterohydronephrosis, vesicoureteral reflux, and chronic voiding dysfunction

2004; Wu and Johnson, 2009). The leading causes of mortality in obstructive uropathy are pulmonary hypoplasia and preterm birth (Wu and Johnson, 2009). Table 11-7 summarizes common obstructive sites in children and their nursing implications.

Pathophysiology

The pathophysiologic changes produced by obstruction are influenced by the location and severity of the blockage and by the presence of complicating factors, such as infection. When the kidney is obstructed, the papilla is flattened; the distal nephron is dilated; and, if the obstruction persists, glomerular filtration is greatly diminished or arrested. Unless the obstruction is relieved, these changes become irreversible, leading to renal insufficiency and atrophy of the affected kidney.

Several factors may magnify the destructive changes associated with obstruction. During the neonatal period the immature kidneys have a higher vascular resistance than do the kidneys of the older child or adult. This condition, combined with the immaturity of the parenchyma, accelerates the irreversible renal damage in response to obstruction. Infection also magnifies the destructive changes associated with urinary obstruction. In contrast to the adult, pyelonephritis in the developing kidney of the infant or child increases the chances of renal scarring that reduces the potential for further growth. However, predicting the extent of scarring and subsequent risk for further damage in every child with pyelonephritis is impossible.

Fortunately, when obstruction is restricted to one kidney, compensatory growth occurs in the contralateral kidney. In the infant and child, compensatory growth includes both hypertrophy (enlargement of existing nephrons) and hyperplasia (replication of new cells). Still, this cannot completely compensate for the loss of renal function created by obstruction of one kidney.

Obstruction also affects the smooth muscle of the renal pelvis, ureter, and bladder. Obstruction of the ureter and renal pelvis causes dilation in an attempt to overcome the obstruction by stronger peristaltic contractions. The process of dilation ultimately leads to urinary stasis and loss of smooth muscle tone unless the obstruction is relieved. The detrusor smooth muscle is also affected by obstruction of the bladder outlet. Like the ureter, the bladder initially responds by increasing the force and duration of its contractions. However, when the obstruction

persists, the bladder wall becomes trabeculated and the effectiveness of the detrusor contractions is compromised. In addition to these changes, obstruction of the bladder causes neurologic changes that predispose the bladder to unstable (hyperactive) contractions and subsequent urge incontinence.

Clinical Manifestations

The clinical manifestations of obstructive uropathy depend on the location of the obstructing lesion, its severity, and the underlying cause. Maternal oligohydramnios may signal a renal problem in the developing fetus. Occasionally, UPJ obstruction is diagnosed when a child experiences flank pain, hematuria, and nausea after mild trauma or a urinary tract infection. However, these conditions are more frequently diagnosed on routine prenatal ultrasonographic examination or when a mass is observed during routine newborn examination. Congenital ureteral obstruction also may be asymptomatic, or the obstruction may cause urinary tract infections or an abdominal mass. In contrast, obstruction of the renal pelvis, ureter, or UPJ because of a urinary calculus produces a characteristic pain called renal colic. This pain is characterized by discomfort in the flank, lower back, or lower abdomen. The discomfort is typically intense and it is not relieved by changes in position. Renal colic typically occurs in the early morning hours and persists until the stone passes or is removed. Narcotic analgesia is frequently required to manage the pain produced by an obstructing stone.

Obstruction of the bladder produces lower urinary tract symptoms. These symptoms are closely related to those produced by other dysfunctional voiding conditions, including detrusor instability and urinary retention. Symptoms include poor force of urinary stream, intermittency of voided stream, feelings of incomplete bladder emptying, and postmicturition dribble. In addition, children with obstruction of the bladder or urethra may experience frequency of urination, nocturia, nocturnal enuresis, or urgency to urinate. Urge incontinence may occur, particularly when obstruction causes unstable contractions of the detrusor muscle.

Diagnostic Evaluation

Imaging studies are used to determine the level of the obstruction and the severity of the associated uropathy. Ultrasonography is used to define the anatomy of the obstruction, and radionuclide studies are frequently completed to determine the impact of the obstruction on renal function. Occasionally an IV pyelogram is used to provide a detailed evaluation of urinary tract function, but radionuclide scans or ultrasonography is generally preferred because it exposes the child to less radiation and carries no risk of adverse contrast reactions. The diethylenetriamine pentaacetic acid (DTPA) or mercaptoacetyltriglycine (MAG3) renal scan provides an estimate of renal function as well as renal and ureteral anatomy. The dimercaptosuccinic acid (DMSA) renal scan provides a superior method for determining individual kidney function, but this technique does not allow visualization of the renal pelves, ureters, or bladder. The VCUG is commonly performed to rule out reflux or to evaluate the posterior urethra in boys.

Prenatal detection of obstructive uropathy by sonogram and subsequent fetal surgery to relieve the obstruction in utero, thus preventing further damage as the kidneys develop, has met with varying success; in many cases renal function was not significantly improved (Chevalier, 2004; Salam, 2006). However, others report fewer fetal complications and morbidity with fetal surgical treatment of obstructive uropathy in large centers with more experience performing such procedures (Hofmann, Becker, Meyer-Wittkopf, et al, 2004; Wu and Johnson, 2009).

Therapeutic Management

The management of obstructive uropathy depends on the magnitude of the obstruction and the likelihood that renal function will be compromised unless aggressive intervention is undertaken. For example, UPJ obstruction causing hydronephrosis in the neonate may or may not require surgical intervention. In contrast, PUV obstruction requires aggressive intervention to prevent progressive, severe obstructive uropathy affecting the entire urinary system.

Whenever feasible, obstruction is treated by a surgical procedure that directly ablates the obstructive lesion. For example, UPJ obstruction is ideally treated by pyeloplasty or pyelotomy, urethral valves by endoscopic ablation, or obstructing calculi by extracorporeal or endoscopic shock-wave lithotripsy. Urinary flow is temporarily diverted during the postoperative period via a urethral catheter, ureteral stent, or pyelostomy tube (tube inserted directed into the renal pelvis) until postoperative edema subsides and adequate urinary outflow is achieved.

In contrast, transient or permanent urinary diversion may be required for the child with severe obstructive uropathy causing renal insufficiency who is not able to undergo surgery or who has irreversible damage to the lower urinary tract, posing an ongoing threat to renal function. Transient diversion can be created at the level of the renal pelvis (pyelostomy), the ureters (ureterostomy), or the bladder (vesicostomy), depending on the level of obstruction. The stomas created from these procedures are not typically pouched in the neonate. Instead, the infant's diaper may be placed higher on the abdomen or a two-diaper system may be used to ensure urinary containment. Permanent urinary diversion usually involves a continent urinary diversion that incorporates a segment of bowel, stomach, or ureter to increase bladder capacity. In contrast to transient diversions, this procedure is reserved for older children and requires ongoing intermittent catheterization.

Prognosis

The prognosis depends on the type of obstruction, the degree of irreversible renal damage, whether renal dysplasia is present, the age at diagnosis, and the severity of complications. Despite improvements in corrective surgery, some patients develop renal failure, which may evolve over a highly variable period that can extend into adulthood. Renal failure can result from hypoplasia-dysplasia, pyelonephritic scarring, and other proposed mechanisms that cause progressive nephron loss. Careful follow-up care should extend throughout childhood and adolescence, especially when any degree of renal insufficiency is present.

Nursing Care Management

Nursing goals in urinary tract obstruction include helping to identify cases, assisting with diagnostic procedures, and caring for children with complications. (See Chapter 30.) Preparing parents and children for procedures, especially urinary diversion procedures, is a major nursing responsibility. (See Preparation for Diagnostic and Therapeutic Procedures, Chapter 27.)

Parents and children need emotional support and counseling during the lengthy management of these disorders. Parents are the primary target during infancy and early childhood, when most reparative surgery is performed. They need assistance in managing the care of the child and in detecting subtle signs of urinary tract infection or renal failure. Parents may perform intermittent catheterizations in the home. Anticholinergics may also be used to decrease spasticity of smooth muscle of the bladder, and parents should be aware of the side effects of these medications (Hinds, 2004). Improved surgical techniques allow for the creation of urinary diversion systems that can be catheterized with greater ease, avoiding mechanical devices, which are often difficult to manage and impede normal everyday activities. (See also Management of Genitourinary Function, p. 403.)

Children with external diversional systems need psychologic support and guidance, especially as they reach adolescence and become more concerned with body image. Those with progressive renal deterioration may face the prospect of dialysis or transplantation and the emotional turmoil that accompanies these procedures.

DISORDERS OF SEX DEVELOPMENT (AMBIGUOUS GENITALIA)

Until recently, an infant born with ambiguous genitalia was referred to as having an intersex condition. Major advances in the identification of molecular genetic causes of abnormal sexual development, with heightened awareness of ethical issues and patient advocacy concerns, led to reexamination of the nomenclature. In 2006 the term disorders of sex development was proposed to indicate congenital conditions with atypical development of chromosomal, gonadal, or anatomic sex (Lee, Houk, Ahmed, et al, 2006).

The birth of a child with ambiguous genitalia constitutes a crisis quite different from that of other congenital anomalies. Uncertain gender is a potential lifetime social tragedy for the child and family. Furthermore, the electrolyte disturbances that accompany conditions such as congenital adrenal hyperplasia can be life threatening. The identification of appropriate gender must be done with precision and accuracy. The assignment of gender is a complex process; the newborn should be examined by a multidisciplinary team that includes a geneticist, a pediatric urologist, an endocrinologist, a pediatrician, a pediatric psychiatrist, and a pediatric surgeon. Although a rapid assignment of gender helps alleviate some of the parents' anxiety, an erroneous gender determination requiring a later change is even more stressful for the family. The parents may be advised to tell relatives and friends that the newborn has a congenital malformation of the external genitalia that will require some time for physicians to determine the child's sex.

Etiology

Genetic sex is determined at the time of conception and depends on whether the ovum is fertilized by a sperm bearing an X chromosome or one bearing a Y chromosome. The phenotypic evidence of gender depends on whether subsequent processes proceed normally: differentiation of primitive gonads, differentiation and development of internal duct systems, and differentiation and development of external genitalia. The normal order of events can be altered by abnormalities of the chromosomal complement, defects of embryogenesis, or biochemical (hormonal) abnormalities. Disturbances in any of these processes will lead to abnormal development evidenced by ambiguous genitalia at birth.

Normal Genitalia and Reproductive Organ Development

For the first 6 weeks of life the developing embryo is morphologically asexual, neither male nor female. The primitive, bipotential (able to form either a testicle or an ovary) gonad consists of an outer layer (the cortex) and an inner medulla. Differentiation into testes or ovaries takes place during the seventh and eighth weeks of gestation. At this time, in the male the medullary portion develops and the cortical zone regresses. In the female the cortex is preserved while the medulla regresses. Active factors from the male testes cause the müllerian duct system to regress. Without these factors the primitive gonad has an inherent tendency to feminize. The embryonic ovary develops in the absence of male hormone stimulation.

The final stage of genital and reproductive organ development is differentiation of the external genitalia, which in the early embryo consists of a urogenital sinus, two lateral labioscrotal swellings, and an anteriorly situated genital tubercle. Depending on the presence or absence of male hormones, the genital tubercle differentiates into a penis or a clitoris. In response to testicular androgens, the labiosacral folds fuse to form a scrotum and the ventral skin of the penis; the urethral folds form the perineal and penile urethra. Without the influence of masculinizing secretions, the urethral folds do not fuse and instead become the labia minora, the labiosacral folds remain unfused to separate into the labia majora, and the urogenital sinus differentiates into a lower vagina and the vaginal and urethral openings (Fig. 11-32).

Abnormal Genitalia and Reproductive Organ Development

Disturbances in the normal order of events in gender determination produce abnormal genitalia and reproductive organ development with the presence of ambiguous or indeterminate external genitalia at birth. Ambiguous genitalia can be variable and may often closely conform to one gender or the other. In some forms the external sexual structures represent those of a normal male or female, whereas the karyotype is the direct opposite. A situation in which the phenotypic gender differs from the chromosomal gender is a disorder of sex development.

A failure or abnormality in any of the four steps of genital and reproductive organ development can lead to abnormal development in subsequent stages. The mechanisms and sites of defective development include:

Abnormal gender determination—Chromosome abnormalities result in disturbance of secondary sexual characteristics and reproductive organ development. (See Chapter 5.)

Abnormal differentiation of gonads—When induction of the bipotential gonad fails, gender differentiation proceeds in the direction of the female phenotype, regardless of karyotype.

Abnormal differentiation of ductal systems—Biologic inactivity of androgenic male organizer substances or insensitivity of ductal tissue to the action of these substances results in a persistent female duct system, which leads to the presence of a uterus and uterine tubes.

Abnormal secretion of or tissue insensitivity to testicular androgen—Complete failure of male hormone secretion produces female external genitalia in a genetic male. Partial or incomplete failure results in incomplete masculinization with ambiguity of the external genitalia. The genetic female fetus exposed to large amounts of androgenic hormone may exhibit varying degrees of masculinization of the external genitalia (congenital adrenal hyperplasia).

Types of Abnormalities

Some disorders with abnormal genital development are not characterized by ambiguous genitalia in the newborn period. For example, the most common sex chromosome disorders do not become apparent until later childhood, adolescence, or even young adulthood, when the individual seeks medical attention because of problems of delayed development or infertility. The four conditions producing ambiguous genitalia in the newborn that require prompt and accurate evaluation are the masculinized female, the incompletely masculinized male, the presence of both male and female sexual organs, and mixed gonadal dysgenesis.

Ambiguous genitalia in the newborn is often a result of virilization in the female by adrenal androgens after the time of early gonadal differentiation. The most common type, **congenital adrenogenital hyperplasia (CAH)**, is an inherited deficiency of adrenal corticoid hormones. (See Chapter 38.) The resulting decrease in cortisol stimulates pituitary secretion of adrenocorticotropic hormone, which causes the adrenal cortex to increase production of adrenal hormones, including the androgens. Because the adrenal gland differentiates later than the gonadal duct system but before differentiation of the external genitalia, masculinization of the external genitalia is the predominant feature. The internal female anatomy is normal. Because even

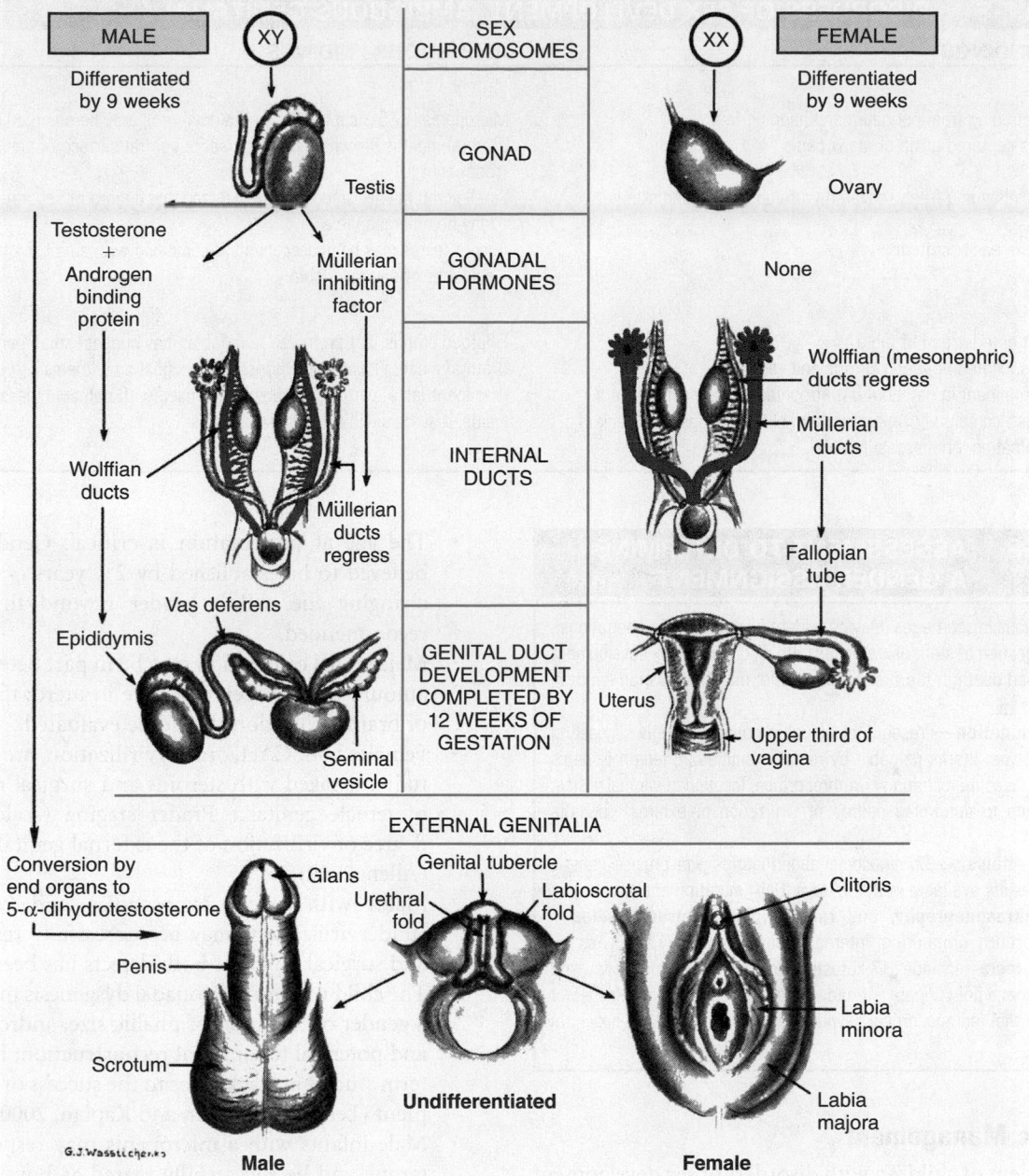

Fig. 11-32 Sex organ differentiation in male and female. (From Thompson JM, McFarland G, Tucker SM, et al: *Mosby's manual of clinical nursing,* ed 2, St Louis, 1989, Mosby.)

minor illnesses such as vomiting, diarrhea, and dehydration in the child with CAH can lead to life-threatening electrolyte disturbances, CAH should be considered in any situation where the child's gender is doubtful.

The external genitalia in the incompletely masculinized male may be incompletely male, ambiguous, or completely female. The complex nature of virilization offers numerous opportunities for disturbance in the process. Defects may be a result of deficient production of fetal androgen, deficiency in any of the enzymes needed for testosterone biosynthesis, or unresponsiveness or subresponsiveness of genital structures to testosterone. Individuals who may be either genetic males or females with both ovarian and testicular tissues, with an ovary on one side and a testis on the other or a combination of ovotestis, are rare.

The external genitalia may be male (possibly cryptorchid with a micropenis) or normal female, but are ambiguous in the majority of cases.

Mixed gonadal dysgenesis, in which affected infants are sex chromosome mosaics, is the second most common disorder. (See Sex Chromosome Aneuploidies, Chapter 5.) Genitalia vary greatly, but in those who appear predominantly female, the dysplastic testis may cause masculinization at puberty. Table 11-8 describes the external appearance of the genitalia.

Diagnostic Evaluation

Box 11-8 outline diagnostic tools and the significant findings that help determine sex and assist in making a gender assignment.

TABLE 11-8 DISORDERS OF SEX DEVELOPMENT (AMBIGUOUS GENITALIA)

NORMAL FINDINGS	AMBIGUOUS FINDINGS
Male	
Penile shaft protruding from perineum and hanging freely	Micropenis (<2.5-3 cm [1-1.2 inch] in newborn); may be enlarged clitoris
Urethral meatus centered at tip of glans penis	Urethral meatus anywhere along dorsal or ventral surface of penis, especially on perineum
Two scrotal sacs hanging freely, covered with loose, wrinkled skin	Small scrotum with smooth, tight skin and any degree of separation in midline; may be enlarged labia
Palpable testes in each scrotum	Absent testes may be undescended; if combined with small scrotum, may be evidence of enlarged labia
Female	
Small clitoris at anterior end of labia	Enlarged clitoris that protrudes from labia; may suggest small penis
Urethral meatus located between clitoris and vagina	Urethral meatus located in clitoris; may suggest small penis
Labia minora prominent in newborn but atrophied and almost absent in prepubertal girl; completely separated from clitoris to posterior vault of vagina; on palpation, no masses in labia	Prominent labia, partially or completely fused with palpable masses on each side; may be small scrotum with testes

---

BOX 11-8 ASSESSMENT TO DETERMINE A GENDER ASSIGNMENT

History—Previous miscarriages (may help identify chromosome aberrations); maternal ingestion of steroids; relatives with disorders of sex development or unexplained death in the first weeks of life; maternal ovarian tumor in pregnancy

Physical examination—Presence of palpable gonads strongly suggesting a male genotype; uterus palpable by rectal examination; length of penis stretched to measure location of urethral orifice; location of vaginal orifice; Prader staging to determine degree of virilization of external genitalia (Allen, 2009)

Chromosome analysis—Chromosome abnormalities and precise genetic karyotype; results available in 2 or 3 days; DNA mutation analysis

Endoscopy, ultrasonography, and radiographic contrast studies—Presence, absence, or nature of internal genital and urinary structures

Biochemical tests—Include 17-ketosteroids, 17-hydroxycorticoids, and urinary pregnanediol; urinary steroid excretion patterns to help detect several of the adrenocortical syndromes (congenital adrenogenital hyperplasia)

Therapeutic Management

The management of children with disorders of sex development has evolved in recent years as the traditional approach of assigning gender immediately followed by early surgical reconstruction has been challenged (Karkazis, 2006). Data describing long-term adjustment and quality-of-life issues for individuals with disorders of sex development are lacking. However, anecdotal reports from affected adults have influenced the standard of care. Decision making has become more complex now that endocrine, genetic, social, psychologic, and ethical elements of sex assignment have been integrated into the process. This multidisciplinary team approach, which includes parental participation, has led to the current practice of assigning gender while avoiding irreversible surgical interventions, realizing some children may change gender later in life.

The overall goal of management is to enable the affected child to grow into a well-adjusted, psychosocially stable person who is able to identify with the assigned gender and is content with same (Allen, 2009; Houk, Hughes, Ahmed, et al, 2006; Nabhan and Lee, 2007). Current recommendations for gender assignment involve a number of factors, including:

- The age at presentation is critical. Gender identity is believed to be established by 2½ years of age; therefore changing the child's gender beyond this age is not recommended.
- Male sexual orientation may be in part determined by the amount of androgen exposure in utero; therefore extent of brain virilization should be evaluated.
- Females with CAH, or overvirilization, are often successfully managed with steroids and surgical reconstruction of female genitalia. Prader staging (scale that reflects degree of virilization of the external genitalia) is essential (Allen, 2009).
- Males with severe hypospadias and cryptorchidism (undervirilization) may be successfully reared as males, and surgical repair of both defects has been successful.
- The child with mixed gonadal dysgenesis may be assigned a gender on the basis of phallic size, androgen exposure, and potential for surgical reconstruction; however, long-term studies are lacking as to the success of such management (Lerman, McAleer, and Kaplan, 2000).
- Male infants with a micropenis may respond to testosterone and be successfully reared as boys with the possible exception of those with cloacal exstrophy and penile agenesis (Lerman, McAleer, and Kaplan, 2000). However, a study suggests that even children with cloacal exstrophy may declare themselves as being male during puberty despite female gender assignment (surgically and socially) in the neonatal period (Reiner and Gearhart, 2004).

Clearly the decision for gender assignment in cases of ambiguous genitalia is a difficult one, and the "one size fits all" approach is not applicable. In some cases children may reach puberty and request gender reassignment (Phornphutkul, Fausto-Sterling, and Gruppuso, 2000; Migeon, Wisniewski, Brown, et al, 2002). Federman (2004) emphasizes that evidence in long-term studies suggests that a hormonal role in the sexualization of the brain is more significant than previously recognized. Each child must be considered individually with adequate input from family and extensive diagnostic evaluation. Families often require long-term counseling and follow-up to ensure the child's welfare and security in the assigned gender.

An evidence-based consensus statement on the management of disorders of sex development has been published and assists in providing a standard of care for these disorders, emphasizing quality of life and patient-centered decision making (Lee, Houk, Ahmed, et al, 2006).

Nursing Care Management

Families need a great deal of support and encouragement from nurses and other members of the health care team to cope with this emotionally charged situation.* Parents are confused, anxious, and overwhelmed by feelings of guilt and shame. They may pressure the health care team for immediate gender assignment because they are concerned about the child and the child's future and because they must face questioning relatives and friends. The best approach is honesty. The disorder should be treated as any other disorder, with no attempt to camouflage the problem. The sequence of embryologic events leading to the defect can be explained using correct terminology to describe abnormalities of genitalia and reproductive organs. An understanding of the anomaly assists parents in explaining the defect to others, just as with any other physical defect. It requires sympathy and understanding to deal with parental anxiety during this trying period and to guide them throughout the long-term management. (See Chapter 22.)

---

*Some parent and clinical resources may be found at the Accord Alliance website, www.accordalliance.org. *DSD Guidelines* and *Handbook for Parents* resources are available at www.dsdguidelines.org.

KEY POINTS

- Congenital malformations or anomalies, or "birth defects," are present at birth and are a result of genetic or nongenetic influences.
- Typical reactions of parents to an infant with a physical defect include grief over loss of a perfect child, shock, and withdrawal.
- The nurse's primary roles in care of an infant with a physical defect are caregiver, provider of family support, and supplier of information.
- Surgery initiates a number of physiologic responses, including cardiovascular, respiratory, endocrine, renal, GI, immune, neurologic, and fluid and electrolyte.
- One of the largest groups of congenital anomalies includes those associated with the embryonic neural tube, the most common of which are SB and myelomeningocele.
- When taken before and during pregnancy, folic acid supplementation may prevent as many as 50% to 70% of the cases of NTDs, anencephaly, and SB.
- Care of the infant and child with myelomeningocele requires both immediate and long-term professional supervision. Associated problems include infection, neurologic damage, impaired renal function, musculoskeletal impairment, and latex allergy.
- Hydrocephalus is a symptom of an underlying brain pathologic condition, demonstrated by impaired absorption of CSF or obstruction to the flow of CSF within the ventricles.
- Therapy for hydrocephalus involves relief of the ventricular dilation, treatment of the underlying brain pathologic condition, prevention and/or treatment of complications, and management of problems related to psychomotor development.
- Treatment of DDH involves maintaining the head of the femur correctly positioned in the acetabulum by means of an external device, usually the Pavlik harness.

- Treatment of clubfoot involves manual overcorrection of the deformity, maintenance of the correction until normal muscle balance is gained, and follow-up observation to detect possible recurrence of the deformity.
- CL deformities are repaired at the earliest opportunity; CP repair may be delayed to take advantage of growth changes.
- Management of CP involves a multidisciplinary approach involving professionals from surgery, medicine, nursing, social work, dentistry, speech-language pathology, and audiology.
- Major nursing challenges with infants born with either CL or CP involve feeding.
- TEF is an abnormal connection between the esophagus and the trachea, placing the untreated infant at risk for life-threatening pulmonary aspiration.
- Anorectal defects are often associated with other congenital anomalies, such as those involving the GI tract and kidneys.
- CDH may be diagnosed in the first trimester of pregnancy and usually causes moderate to severe respiratory distress at birth.
- Umbilical and inguinal hernias are common in children and require minor surgical intervention with excellent postoperative recovery.
- Abdominal wall defects, omphalocele and gastroschisis, require careful nursing care involving thermoregulation, fluid management, and prevention of infection preoperatively and postoperatively.
- GU defects are repaired early to promote normal function and psychosocial adjustment.
- In disorders of sex development, gender assignment is established after careful evaluation of prenatal and postnatal influences, karyotype, genitalia features, surgical possibilities, future fertility, and potential sexual function.

REFERENCES

Abdullah F, Zhang Y, Sciortino C, et al: Congenital diaphragmatic hernia: outcome review of 2,173 surgical repairs in US infants, *Pediatr Surg Int* Aug 30, 2009 (E-pub ahead of print).

Achildi A, Grewal H: Congenital anomalies of the esophagus, *Otolaryngol Clin North Am* 40(1):219-244, 2007.

Aiken JJ, Oldham KT: Inguinal hernias. In Kliegman RM, Behrman RE, Jenson HB, et al, editors: *Nelson textbook of pediatrics*, ed 18, Philadelphia, 2007, Saunders.

A-Kader HH, Balistreri WF: Cholestasis. In Kliegman RM, Behrman RE, Jenson HB, et al, editors: *Nelson textbook of pediatrics,* ed 18, Philadelphia, 2007, Saunders.

Allen L: Disorders of sexual development, *Obstet Gynecol Clin North Am* 36(2):25-45, 2009.

American Academy of Pediatrics, Committee on Genetics: Folic acid for the prevention of neural tube defects, *Pediatrics* 119(5):1031, 2007.

American Academy of Pediatrics, Task Force on Sudden Infant Death Syndrome: The changing concept of sudden infant death syndrome: diagnostic coding shifts, controversies regarding the sleeping environment, and new variables to consider in reducing risk, *Pediatrics* 116(5):1245-1255, 2005.

Arosarena OA: Cleft lip and palate, *Otolaryngol Clin North Am* 40(1):27-60, 2007.

Barker E, Saulino M, Caristo AM: Spina bifida, *RN* 66(12):33-38, 2002.

Bijnen CL, Don Griot PJW, Mulder W, et al: Tongue-lip adhesion in the treatment of Pierre Robin sequence, *J Craniofacial Surg* 20(2):315-320, 2009.

Brandt ML: Pediatric hernias, *Surg Clin North Am* 88(1):27-43, 2008.

Brown JP: Orthopaedic care of children with spina bifida: you've come a long way, baby! *Orthop Nurs* 20(4):51-58, 2001.

Brownlee EM, Howatson AG, Davis CRF, et al: The hidden mortality of congenital diaphragmatic hernia: a 20-year review, *J Pediatr Surg* 44(2):317-320, 2009.

Buchenau W, Urschitz MS, Sautermeister J, et al: A randomized clinical trial of a new orthodontic appliance to improve upper airway obstruction in infants with Pierre Robin sequence, *J Pediatr* 151(2):145-149, 2007.

Bukowski TP, Zeman PA: Hypospadias: of concern but correctable, *Contemp Pediatr* 18(2):89-109, 2001.

Buran CF, McDaniel AM, Brei TJ: Needs assessment in a spina bifida program: a comparison of the perceptions by adolescents with spina bifida and their parents, *Clin Nurs Spect* 16(5):256-262, 2002.

Centers for Disease Control and Prevention: Racial/ethnic differences in the birth prevalence of spina bifida—United States, 1995-2005, *MMWR* 57(53):1409-1413, 2009.

Centers for Disease Control and Prevention: Folate status in women of childbearing age, by race/ethnicity—United States, 1999-2000, 2001-2002, and 2003-2004, *MMWR* 55(51):1377-1380, 2007.

Chapman KL, Hardin-Jones MA, Goldstein JA, et al: Timing of palatal surgery and speech outcome, *Cleft Palate Craniofac J* 45(3):297-308, 2008.

Chevalier RL: Perinatal obstructive nephropathy, *Semin Perinatol* 28(2):124-131, 2004.

Chiafery M: Care and management of the child with shunted hydrocephalus, *Pediatr Nurs* 32(3):222-225, 2006.

Cleft Palate Foundation: *Factsheet: what about breastfeeding?* May 2008, The Foundation; available at www.cleftline.org (accessed June 2, 2009).

Dauria D, Marsh JL: Mandibular distraction osteogenesis for Pierre Robin sequence: what

percentage of neonates need it? *J Craniofac Surg* 19(9):1237-1243, 2008.

Davenport M: Biliary atresia, *Semin Pediatr Surg* 14(1):42-48, 2005.

Dehlink E, Prandstetter C, Eiwegger T, et al: Increased prevalence of latex-sensitization among children with chronic renal failure, *Allergy* 59(7):734-738, 2004.

de Jong TP, Chrzan R, Klijn AJ, et al: Treatment of the neurogenic bladder in spina bifida, *Pediatr Nephrol* 23(6):889-896, 2008.

Deprest JA, Gratacos E, Nicolaides K, et al: Changing perspectives on the perinatal management of isolated congenital diaphragmatic hernia in Europe, *Clin Perinatol* 36(2):329-347, 2009.

DeRoo LA, Wilcox AJ, Drevon CA, et al: First-trimester maternal alcohol consumption and the risk of infant oral clefts in Norway: a population-based case-control study, *Am J Epidemiol* 168(6):638-646, 2008.

D'Hauwers K, Feitz W, Kremer J: Bladder exstrophy and male fertility: pregnancies after ICSI with ejaculated or epididymal sperm, *Fertil Steril* 89(2):387-389, 2008.

Donlon CR, Furdon SA, Clark DA: Look before you clamp: delivery room examination of the umbilical cord, *Adv Neonat Care* 2(1):19-26, 2002.

Doolin E: Bowel management for patients with myelodysplasia, *Surg Clin North Am* 86(2): 505-514, 2006.

Drake JM: The surgical management of pediatric hydrocephalus, *Neurosurgery* 62(Suppl 2): 633-640, 2008.

Ehrlich PJ, Coran AG: Diaphragmatic hernia. In Kliegman RM, Behrman RE, Jenson HB, et al, editors: *Nelson textbook of pediatrics,* ed 18, Philadelphia, 2007, Saunders.

Faggin R, Bernardo A, Stieg P, et al: Hydrocephalus in infants less than six months of age: effectiveness of endoscopic third ventriculostomy, *Eur J Pediatr Surg* 19(4):216-219, 2009.

Faulks S, Luther B: Changing paradigm for the treatment of clubfeet, *Orthop Nurs* 24(1):25-30, 2005.

Federman DD: Three facets of sexual differentiation, *N Engl J Med* 350(4):323-324, 2004.

Finnell RH, Gould A, Spiegelstein O: Pathobiology and genetics of neural tube defects, *Epilepsia* 44(Suppl 3):14-23, 2003.

Frey L, Hauser WA: Epidemiology of neural tube defects, *Epilepsia* 44(Suppl 3):4-13, 2003.

Fritsch MJ, Kienke S, Ankerman T, et al: Endoscopic third ventriculostomy in infants, *J Neurosurg* 103(Pediatr 1):50-53, 2005.

Gapany C, Frey P, Cachat F, et al: Management of cryptorchidism in children: guidelines, *Swiss Med Weekly* 138(33-34):492-498, 2008.

Gatti J, Ostlie D: The use of laparoscopy in the management of nonpalpable undescended testes, *Curr Opin Pediatr* 19(3):349-353, 2007.

Gearhart JP: Complete repair of bladder exstrophy in the newborn: complications and management, *J Urol* 165(6 Pt 2):2431-2433, 2001.

Golden JA, Bönnemann CG: Developmental structural disorders. In Goetz CG, editor:

Textbook of clinical neurology, ed. 3, Philadelphia, 2007, Saunders.

Graham JM, Gomez M, Halberg A, et al: Management of deformational plagiocephaly: repositioning versus orthotic therapy, *J Pediatr* 146(2):258-262, 2005.

Gray M, Moore KN: *Urologic disorders: adult and pediatric care,* St Louis, 2009, Mosby.

Gupta N, Park J, Solomon C, et al: Long-term outcomes in patients with treated childhood hydrocephalus, *J Neurosurg* 106(Suppl 5): 334-339, 2007.

Hassan FA: Compliance of parents with regard to Pavlik harness treatment in developmental dysplasia of the hip, *J Pediatr Orthop B* 18(3):111-115, 2009.

Heider AL, Strauss RA, Kuller JA: Omphalocele: clinical outcomes in cases with normal karyotypes, *Am J Obstet Gynecol* 190(1): 135-141, 2004.

Hinds AC: Obstructive uropathy: considerations for the nephrology nurse, *Nephrol Nurs J* 31(2):166-180, 2004.

Hofmann R, Becker T, Meyer-Wittkopf M, et al: Fetoscopic placement of transurethral stent for intrauterine obstructive uropathy, *J Urol* 171(1):384-386, 2004.

Holcomb GW 3rd, Rothenberg SS, Bax KM, et al: Thoracoscopic repair of esophageal atresia and tracheoesophageal fistula: a multi-institutional analysis, *Ann Surg* 242(3):422-428, 2005.

Honein MA: Impact of folic acid fortification of the US food supply and occurrence of neural tube defects, *JAMA* 285(23):2981-2986, 2001.

Hosalkar HS, Horn D, Friedman JE, et al: The hip. In Kliegman RM, Behrman RE, Jenson HB, et al, editors: *Nelson textbook of pediatrics,* ed 18, Philadelphia, 2007, Saunders.

Hosalkar HS, Spiegel DA, Davidson RS: The foot and toes. In Kliegman RM, Behrman RE, Jenson HB, et al, editors: *Nelson textbook of pediatrics,* ed 18, Philadelphia, 2007, Saunders.

Houk C, Hughes I, Ahmed S, et al: Summary of consensus statement on intersex disorders and their management, *Pediatrics* 118(2):753-757, 2006.

Hummel P, Fortado D: Impacting infant head shapes, *Adv Neonat Care* 5(6):329-340, 2005.

Hurwitz M, Cox KL: Liver transplantation. In Kliegman RM, Behrman RE, Jenson HB, et al, editors: *Nelson textbook of pediatrics,* ed 18, Philadelphia, 2007, Saunders.

Husman D: Surgery insight: advantages and pitfalls of surgical techniques for the correction of bladder exstrophy, *Nat Clin Pract Urol* 3(2):95-100, 2006.

Islam S: Clinical care outcomes in abdominal wall defects, *Curr Opin Pediatr* 20(3):305-310, 2008.

Jelin E, Lee H: Tracheal occlusion for fetal congenital diaphragmatic hernia: the US experience, *Clin Perinatol* 36(2):349-361, 2009.

Kadrian D, van Gelder J, Florida D, et al: Long-term reliability of endoscopic third ventriculostomy, *Neurosurg* 62(Suppl 2): 614-621, 2008.

Karkazis K: Early genital surgery to remain controversial, *Pediatrics* 118(2):814-815, 2006.

Kaufman BA: Neural tube defects, *Pediatr Clin North Am* 51(2):389-419, 2004.

Kays DW: Congenital diaphragmatic hernia and neonatal lung lesions, *Surg Clin North Am* 86(2):329-352, 2006.

Kelly DA, Davenport M: Current management of biliary atresia, *Arch Dis Child* 92(12):1132-1135, 2007.

Kestle JP: Pediatric hydrocephalus: current management, *Neurol Clin North Am* 21(4):883-895, 2003.

Kimata H: Latex allergy in infants younger than 1 year, *Clin Exp Allergy* 34(12):1910-1915, 2004.

Kinsman SL, Johnston MV: Congenital anomalies of the central nervous system. In Kliegman RM, Behrman RE, Jenson HB, et al, editors: *Nelson textbook of pediatrics,* ed 18, Philadelphia, 2007, Saunders.

Kirkham C, Harris S, Grzybowski S: Evidence-based prenatal care, part I, General prenatal care and counseling issues, *Am Fam Physician* 71(7):1307-1316, 2005.

Krauss MJ, Morrissey AE, Winn HN, et al: Microcephaly: an epidemiologic analysis, *Am J Obstet Gynecol* 188(6):1484-1490, 2003.

Lazzaretti CC, Pearson C: Myelodysplasia. In Allen PJ, Vessey JA, Schapiro NA, editors: *Primary care of the child with a chronic condition,* ed 5, St Louis, 2010, Mosby.

Ledbetter DJ: Gastroschisis and omphalocele, *Surg Clin North Am* 86(2):249-260, 2006.

Lee P, Houk C, Ahmed S, et al: Consensus statement on management of intersex disorders, *Pediatrics* 118(2):e488-e500, 2006.

Lerman SE, McAleer IM, Kaplan GW: Sex assignment in cases of ambiguous genitalia and its outcome, *Urology* 55(1):8-11, 2000.

Levitt MA, Peña A: Anorectal malformations, *Orphanet J Rare Dis* 2:33, 2007.

Levitt MA, Peña A: Outcomes from the correction of anorectal malformations, *Curr Opin Pediatr* 17(3):394-401, 2005.

Little J, Cardy A, Munger RG: Tobacco smoking and oral clefts: a meta-analysis, *Bull World Health Org* 82(3):213-218, 2004.

Littlefield TR, Saba NM, Kelly KM: On the current incidence of deformational plagiocephaly: an estimation based on prospective registration at a single center, *Semin Pediatr Neurol* 11(4):301-304, 2004.

Maher AB, Salmond SW, Pellino TA: *Orthopaedic nursing,* ed 3, Philadelphia, 2002, Saunders.

Masarei AG, Wade A, Mars M, et al: A randomized control trial investigating the effect of presurgical orthopedics on feeding in infants with cleft lip and/or palate, *Cleft Palate Craniofac J* 44(2):182-193, 2007.

Matthews TJ: Trends in spina bifida and anencephalus in the United States, 1991-2006, Hyatsville, Md, 2009, National Center on Health Statistics, available at www.cdc.gov/nchs/products/pubs/pubd/hestats/spine_anen.pdf (accessed June 1, 2009).

McNair A, Hawes J, Urquhart H: Caring for the newborn with an omphalocele, *Neonat Netw* 25(5):319-327, 2006.

Mercy N, Brady-Fryer B: Bladder exstrophy: a challenge for nursing care, *J WOCN* 31(5):293-298, 2004.

Merritt L: Recognizing craniosynostosis, *Neonatal Network* 28(6):369-376, 2009.

Merritt L: Understanding the embryology and genetics of cleft lip and palate, part I, *Adv Neonat Care* 5(2):64-71, 2005.

Migeon CJ, Wisniewski AB, Brown TR, et al: Ambiguous genitalia with perineoscrotal hypospadias in 46,XY individuals: long-term medical, surgical, and psychosexual outcome, *Pediatrics* 110(3):e31, 2002.

Mitchell ME: Bladder exstrophy repair: complete primary repair of exstrophy, *Urology* 65(1):5-8, 2005.

Mitrofanoff P, Liard A: Bladder reconstruction and substitution. In Gearhart JP, Rink RC, Mouriquand PDE, editors: *Pediatric urology,* Philadelphia, 2001, Saunders.

Mittler MA: Time to failure of ventriculoperitoneal shunts (oral abstract), *J Neurosurg* 103(Suppl Pediatr 1):A103, 2005.

Moore C, Kogan BA, Parekh A: Impact of urinary incontinence on self-concept in children with spina bifida, *J Urol* 171(4):1659-1662, 2004.

Nabhan Z, Lee P: Disorders of sex development, *Curr Opin Obstet Gynecol* 19(5):440-445, 2007.

Nelson C, Dunn R, Wei J: Contemporary epidemiology of bladder exstrophy in the United States, *J Urol* 173(5):1728-1731, 2005.

Nelson C, King J, Sponseller P, et al: Repeat pelvic osteotomy in patients with failed closure of bladder exstrophy: applications and outcomes, *J Pediatr Surg* 41(6):1109-1112, 2006.

Ngo Q, Ranger A, Singh RN, et al: External ventricular drains in pediatric patients, *Pediatr Crit Care Med* 10(3):346-351, 2009.

Onal B, Kogan B: Additional benefit of laparoscopy for nonpalpable testes: finding a contralateral patent processus, *Urology* 71(6):1059-1063, 2008.

Orenstein S, Peters J, Khan S, et al: Congenital anomalies: esophageal atresia and tracheoesophageal fistula. In Kliegman RM, Behrman RE, Jenson HB, et al, editors: *Nelson textbook of pediatrics,* ed 18, Philadelphia, 2007, Saunders.

Phornphutkul C, Fausto-Sterling A, Gruppuso PA: Gender self-reassignment in an XY adolescent female born with ambiguous genitalia, *Pediatrics* 106(1):135-137, 2000.

Pope W: External ventriculostomy: a practical application for the acute care nurse, *J Neurosci Nurs* 30(3):185-190, 1998.

Reiner WG, Gearhart JP: Discordant sexual identity in some genetic males with cloacal exstrophy assigned to female sex at birth, *N Engl J Med* 350(4):333-341, 2004.

Robinson S, Proctor M: Diagnosis and management of deformational plagiocephaly: a review, *J Neurosurg Pediatrics* 3(4):284-295, 2009.

Rowe DE, Jadhav AL: Care of the adolescent with spina bifida, *Pediatr Clin North Am* 55(6):1359-1374, 2008.

Rudy C: Hydrocephalus, *J Pediatr Health Care* 19(2):111, 127-128, 2005.

Salam MA: Posterior urethral valve: outcome of antenatal intervention, *Int J Urol* 13(10):1317-1322, 2006.

Samaniego IA: A sore spot in pediatrics: risk factors for pressure ulcers, *Pediatr Nurs* 29(4):278-282, 2003.

Sijstermans K, Hack W, Meijer R, et al: The frequency of undescended testis from birth to adulthood: a review, *Int J Androl* 31(1):1-11, 2008.

Stoll B: The umbilicus. In Kliegman RM, Behrman RE, Jenson HB, et al, editors: *Nelson textbook of pediatrics,* ed 18, Philadelphia, 2007, Saunders.

Stothard KJ, Tennant PW, Bell R, et al: Maternal overweight and obesity and the risk of congenital anomalies: a systematic review and meta-analysis, *JAMA* 301(6):636-650, 2009.

Sutton LN: Fetal surgery for neural tube defects, *Best Pract Res Clin Obstet Gynaecol* 22(1):175-188, 2008.

Tinanoff N: Cleft lip and palate. In Kliegman RM, Behrman RE, Jenson HB, et al, editors: *Nelson textbook of pediatrics,* ed 18, Philadelphia, 2007, Saunders.

Volpe JJ: *Neurology of the newborn,* ed 4, Philadelphia, 2001, Saunders.

Wagner W, Koch D: Mechanisms of failure after endoscopic third ventriculostomy in young infants, *J Neurosurg* 103(Pediatr 1):43-49, 2005.

Walsh T, Dall'Era M, Croughan M, et al: Prepubertal orchiopexy for cryptorchidism may be associated with lower risk of testicular cancer, *J Urol* 178(4 Pt 1):1440-1446, 2007.

Williams T, Butler R, Sundem T: Management of the infant with gastroschisis: a comprehensive review of the literature, *NAINR* 3(2):55-63, 2003.

Wolff T, Witkop CT, Miller T, et al: Folic acid supplementation for the prevention of neural tube defects: an update of the evidence for the U.S. Preventive Services Task Force, *Ann Intern Med* 150(9):632-639, W112-W115, 2009.

Wu S, Johnson MP: Fetal lower urinary tract obstruction, *Clin Perinatol* 36(2):377-390, 2009.

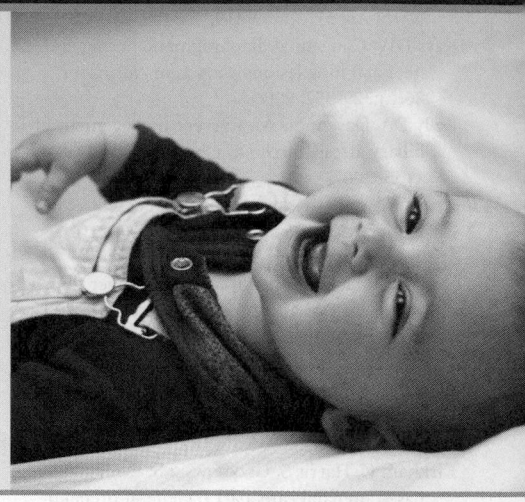

CHAPTER OUTLINE

PROMOTING OPTIMUM GROWTH AND DEVELOPMENT

BIOLOGIC DEVELOPMENT

At no other time in life are physical changes and developmental achievements so dramatic as during infancy. All body systems undergo progressive maturation. Concurrent development of skills allows infants to increasingly respond to the environment. Acquisition of these fine and gross motor skills occurs in an orderly head-to-toe and center-to-periphery (cephalocaudal-proximodistal) sequence.

Proportional Changes

Growth is rapid during the first year, especially during the initial 6 months. Infants gain 680 g (1.5 lb) per month until age 5 months, when the birth weight has at least doubled. An average weight for a 6-month-old child is 7.26 kg (16 lb). Weight gain decreases by half that amount during the second 6 months. By 1 year of age the infant's birth weight has tripled, to an average of 9.75 kg (21.5 lb). Infants who are breast-fed beyond 4 to 6 months of age typically gain less weight than those who are bottle-fed, yet head circumference is more than adequate (Lawrence and Lawrence, 2005). (See Family-Centered Care box, p. 263.)

Height increases by 2.5 cm (1 inch) per month during the first 6 months and by half that amount per month during the second 6 months. Increases in length occur in sudden spurts rather than in a slow, gradual pattern. Average height is 65 cm (25.5 inches) at 6 months and 74 cm (29 inches) at 12 months. By 1 year birth length has increased by almost 50%. This increase occurs mainly in the trunk rather than the legs and contributes to the characteristic physique of the older infant (see Fig. 12-8, A).

Head growth is also rapid and an important determinant of brain growth. Head circumference increases approximately 2 cm (0.75 inch) per month from birth to 3 months, 1 cm (0.4 inch) per month from 4 to 6 months, and 0.5 cm (0.2 inch) per month during the second 6 months. The average head size is 43 cm (17 inches) at 6 months and 46 cm (18 inches) at 12 months. By 1 year of age head size has increased by almost 33%. Closure of the cranial sutures occurs, with the posterior fontanel fusing by 6 to 8 weeks of age and the anterior fontanel closing by 12 to 18 months of age (the average age being 14 months).

It is important to note that genetic, metabolic, environmental, and nutritional factors strongly influence infant growth; thus the previous statements are general guidelines only. Use the appropriate growth charts reflecting weight for length and head circumference in each case to determine appropriate growth parameters.

Expanding head size reflects the growth and differentiation of the nervous system. By the end of the first year the brain has increased in weight approximately two and one half times. Maturation of the brain is exhibited in the dramatic developmental achievements of infancy (see Table 12-3). The primitive reflexes (see Table 8-4) are replaced by voluntary, purposeful movement, and new reflexes that influence motor development appear (Box 12-1 and Fig. 12-1).

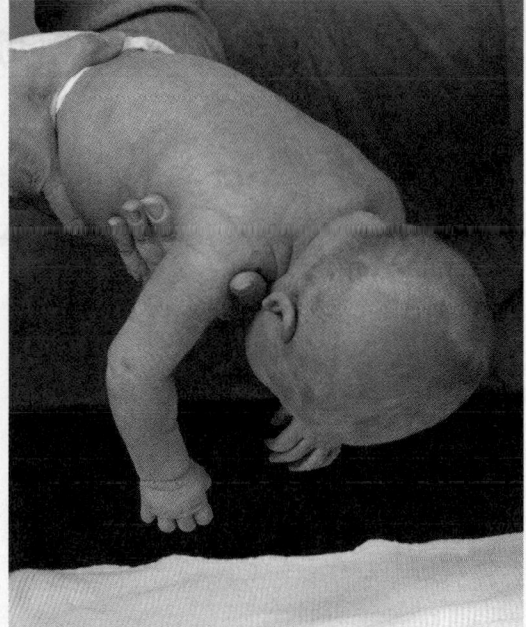

Fig. 12-1 Parachute reflex. (Courtesy Paul Vincent Kuntz, Texas Children's Hospital, Houston.)

BOX 12-1 NEUROLOGIC REFLEXES THAT APPEAR DURING INFANCY

Labyrinth righting—Infant in prone or supine position is able to raise head; appears at 2 months, strongest at 10 months

Neck righting—While infant is supine, head is turned to one side; shoulder, trunk, and finally pelvis will turn toward that side; appears at 3 months, until 24 to 36 months

Body righting—A modification of the neck-righting reflex in which turning hips and shoulders to one side causes all other body parts to follow; appears at 6 months, until 24 to 36 months

Otolith righting—When body of an erect infant is tilted, head is returned to upright, erect position; appears at 7 to 12 months, persists indefinitely

Landau—When infant is suspended in a horizontal prone position, the head is raised and legs and spine are extended; appears at 6 to 8 months, lasts until 12 to 24 months

Parachute—When infant is suspended in a horizontal prone position and suddenly thrust downward, hands and fingers extend forward as if to protect against falling (see Fig. 12-1); appears at 7 to 9 months, persists indefinitely

---

The chest assumes a more adult contour, with the lateral diameter becoming larger than the anteroposterior diameter. The chest circumference approximately equals head circumference by the end of the first year. The heart grows less rapidly than does the rest of the body. Its weight is usually doubled by 1 year of age, whereas body weight triples over the same period. The size of the heart is still large in relation to the chest cavity; its width is approximately 55% of the chest width.

Sensory Changes

During infancy, visual acuity gradually improves and binocular fixation is established. Box 12-2 lists the major developmental characteristics of vision during infancy. Binocularity, or the fixation of two ocular images into one cerebral picture (fusion), begins to develop by 6 weeks of age and should be well established by age 4 months (Fig. 12-2). Lack of binocular vision

BOX 12-2   MAJOR DEVELOPMENTAL CHARACTERISTICS OF VISION

Birth
Visual acuity: 20/100 to 20/400*
Pupillary and corneal (blink) reflexes present
Able to fixate on moving object in range of 45 degrees when held 20 to 25 cm (8 to 10 inches) away
Cannot integrate head and eye movements well (doll's eye reflex—eyes lag behind if head is rotated to one side; note that the presence of this reflex at any other time in childhood is abnormal and may indicate a neurologic problem)

4 Weeks
Can follow in range of 90 degrees
Can watch parent intently as he or she speaks to infant
Tear glands beginning to function
Visual acuity hyperoptic because of less spheric eyeball than in adult

6 to 12 Weeks
Has peripheral vision to 180 degrees
Has binocular vision beginning at age 6 weeks, well established by age 4 months
Convergence on near objects beginning by age 6 weeks, developed by age 3 months
Disappearance of doll's eye reflex

12 to 20 Weeks
Recognizes feeding bottle
Able to fixate on a 1.25-cm (0.5-inch) block
Looks at hand while sitting or lying on back
Able to accommodate to near objects

20 to 28 Weeks
Adjusts posture to see an object
Able to rescue a dropped toy
Develops color preference for yellow and red
Able to discriminate between simple geometric forms
Prefers more complex visual stimuli
Develops hand-eye coordination

28 to 44 Weeks
Can fixate on very small objects
Depth perception beginning to develop
Lack of binocular vision indicative of strabismus

44 to 52 Weeks
Visual acuity: 20/40 to 20/60
Visual loss developing if strabismus is present
Can follow rapidly moving objects

*Measurement of visual acuity differs according to testing procedures. (See Chapter 6.)

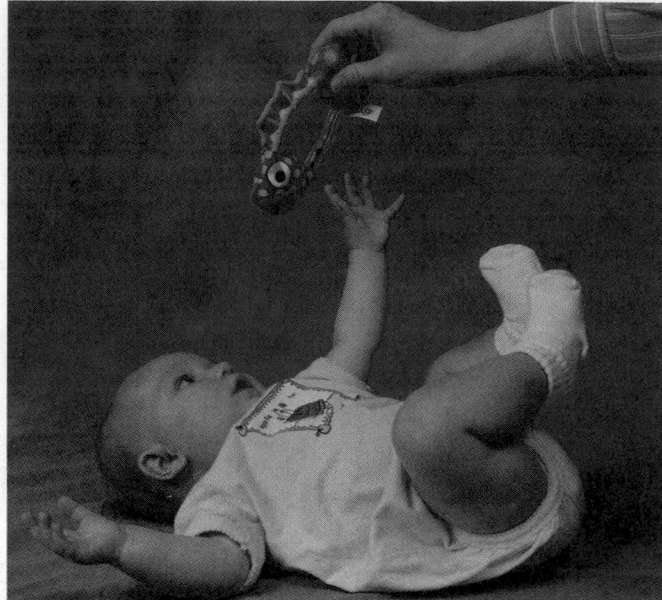

Fig. 12-2 Three-month-old infant focuses on visual object and reaches toward it. (Courtesy Paul Vincent Kuntz, Texas Children's Hospital, Houston.)

BOX 12-3   MAJOR DEVELOPMENTAL CHARACTERISTICS OF HEARING

Birth
Responds to loud noise by startle, or Moro, reflex
Responds to sound of human voice more readily than to any other sound
Quieting effect from low-pitched sounds, such as lullaby, metronome, or heartbeat

8 to 12 Weeks
Turns head to side when sound is made at level of ear

12 to 16 Weeks
Locates sound by turning head to side and looking in same direction

16 to 24 Weeks
Locates sound by turning head to side and then looking up or down

24 to 32 Weeks
Locates sounds by turning head in a curving arc
Responds to own name

32 to 40 Weeks
Localizes sounds by turning head diagonally and directly toward sound

40 to 52 Weeks
Knows several words and their meaning, such as "no," and names of family members
Learns to control and adjust own response to sound, such as listening for the sound to occur again

results in strabismus and must be detected early to prevent permanent blindness.

Depth perception (**stereopsis**) begins to develop by age 7 to 9 months but may exist earlier as an innate safety mechanism. At approximately 7 months the parachute reflex appears and may be a protective response during a fall (see Fig. 12-1 and Box 12-1).

Infants have a visual preference for looking at the human face; this preference also has a developmental sequence. At age 6 weeks infants show more interest in a picture of a face with eyes than in one without eyes. By 10 weeks of age a picture with both eyes and eyebrows elicits more response, and by 20 weeks of age the mouth is also necessary. By age 6 months infants respond to facial expressions and can distinguish between familiar and strange faces. This is about the time that separation anxiety begins to occur (see p. 480).

With progressive myelination of the auditory pathway, the specific responses of locating sound replace the generalized response of the neonate. Box 12-3 lists the major developmental characteristics of hearing. (For further discussion of hearing and the senses of smell, taste, and touch, see Chapter 8.)

Maturation of Systems

Other organ systems also change and grow during infancy. The respiratory rate slows somewhat (see inside back cover) and is relatively stable. Respiratory movements continue to be abdominal. Several factors predispose the infant to severe and acute respiratory problems. Given the proximity of the trachea to the bronchi and its branching structures, an infectious agent is rapidly transmitted from one anatomic location to another. The short, straight eustachian tube closely communicates with the ear, allowing infection to ascend from the pharynx to the middle ear. In addition, the immune system's inability to produce immunoglobulin (Ig) A in the mucosal lining provides less protection against infection in infancy than in later childhood. The entire respiratory tract's ability to produce mucus is diminished, decreasing the humidification of the large volume of inspired air.

Although the lumen of the trachea and bronchi enlarges during infancy, it remains small in comparison with the total size of the lung, maintaining high resistance to the volume of air inspired. The small airways are easily blocked by edema, mucus, or a foreign body. The pliant (flexible) rib cage has less elastic recoil, and during respiratory distress the work of breathing is increased. In addition, the volume of dead space (that amount of air needed to fill the respiratory passages with each breath) is large, requiring the infant to breathe approximately twice as fast as the adult to provide the body with the needed amount of oxygen.

As the infant grows, the heart rate slows (see inside back cover), and the rhythm is often sinus arrhythmia (rate increases with inspiration and decreases with expiration). Blood pressure also changes during infancy (see inside back cover). Systolic pressure rises during the first 2 months as a result of the left ventricle's increasing ability to pump blood into the systemic circulation. Diastolic pressure decreases during the first 3 months then gradually rises to values close to those at birth. Fluctuations in blood pressure occur during varying states of activity and emotion.

Significant hematopoietic changes occur during the first year (see Appendix D). Fetal hemoglobin (HgbF) is present up to the first 5 months, with adult hemoglobin steadily increasing through the first half of infancy. HgbF results in a shortened survival of red blood cells (RBCs) and thus a decreased number of RBCs. A common result at 2 to 3 months of age is physiologic anemia. High levels of HgbF depress the production of erythropoietin, a hormone released by the kidney that stimulates RBC production.

Maternally derived iron stores are present for the first 5 to 6 months and gradually diminish, which also accounts for lowered hemoglobin levels toward the end of the first 6 months. The occurrence of physiologic anemia is not affected by an adequate iron supply. However, when erythropoiesis is stimulated, iron stores are necessary for the formation of adequate amounts of hemoglobin.

The digestive processes are relatively immature at birth. Although full-term newborn infants have some limitations in digestive function, studies indicate that human milk has properties that partially compensate for decreased digestive enzymatic activity, thus enabling the infant to receive optimum nutrition during the first several months of life (Lawrence and Lawrence, 2005). The enzyme ptyalin (also called amylase) is present in small amounts but usually has little effect on the foodstuffs because of the small amount of time the food stays in the mouth. Gastric digestion in the stomach relies primarily on the action of hydrochloric acid and rennin, an enzyme that acts specifically on the casein in milk to cause the formation of curds (coagulated semisolid particles of milk). The curds cause the milk to be retained in the stomach long enough for digestion to occur.

Digestion also takes place in the duodenum, where pancreatic enzymes and bile begin to break down protein and fat. Secretion of the pancreatic enzyme amylase, which is needed for digestion of complex carbohydrates, is limited until about the fourth to sixth months of life. Lipase is also limited, and infants do not achieve adult levels of fat absorption until 4 to 5 months of age. Trypsin is secreted in sufficient quantities to catabolize protein into polypeptides and some amino acids.

The immaturity of the digestive processes is evident in the appearance of stools. During infancy, solid foods (e.g., peas, carrots, corn, and raisins) are passed incompletely broken down in the feces. An excessive quantity of fiber easily disposes the child to loose, bulky stools. During infancy the stomach enlarges to accommodate a greater volume of food. By the end of the first year the infant is able to tolerate three meals a day and an evening bottle and may have one or two bowel movements daily. However, with any type of gastric irritation the infant is vulnerable to diarrhea, vomiting, and dehydration. (See Chapters 28 and 29.)

The liver is the most immature of all the gastrointestinal organs throughout infancy. The ability to conjugate bilirubin and secrete bile is achieved after the first couple of weeks of life. However, the capacities for gluconeogenesis, formation of plasma protein and ketones, storage of vitamins, and deamination of amino acids remain relatively immature for the first year of life.

Maturation of the sucking, swallowing, and breathing reflexes and the later eruption of teeth parallel the changes in the gastrointestinal tract and prepare the infant for the introduction of solid foods.

Sucking activity can occur in utero as early as 15 to 18 weeks of gestation. Weak, disorganized mouthing movements may be noted at 27 to 28 weeks of gestation. Complete maturation of sucking, swallowing, and breathing patterns are usually synchronized by 36 to 38 weeks, although some sucking and swallowing synchrony is seen by 32 to 34 weeks (Blackburn, 2007). Sucking is further divided into nutritive and nonnutritive; the latter is observed in infants of all ages and is reported to be primarily for the purpose of satisfying the basic sucking urge. On the other hand, nutritive sucking has as its primary purpose the intake of food. *Suckling* is a term often used for breast-feeding (Lawrence and Lawrence, 2005), yet use of the term varies among different sources.

Swallowing (deglutition) is the ability to collect the food (bolus) and propel it into the esophagus. During the infantile (visceral) swallow reflex food lies in a shallow groove on the top (dorsum) of the tongue. As the tongue is pressed upward toward the palate, the milk flows by gravity down the sloping tongue and along the sides of the mouth in lateral furrows between the tongue, cheek, and gum pads. As the bolus moves downward, the posterior wall of the pharynx comes forward to displace the soft palate. This swallowing process is efficient for fluids but not for solids.

As the infant grows, the tongue becomes smaller in proportion to the oral cavity and attains greater motility, the orofacial muscles develop, and teeth erupt. Consequently, the mature (somatic) swallow reflex is significantly different. The tongue remains behind the central incisors, and the mandible no longer thrusts forward. The dorsum of the tongue is less concave and remains higher and parallel, not inclined, against the palate. The lateral furrows are absent because of tooth eruption. Tongue pressure and movement against the hard palate push the bolus back into the pharynx.

Infants also exhibit a special reflex called the Santmyer swallow. When a puff of air is directed at the face, the infant will exhibit a reflexive swallow. Because the infant cannot respond to a verbal command to swallow, this reflex is often useful in the administration of small amounts of fluids or medications.

The immunologic system undergoes numerous changes during the first year. The full-term newborn receives significant amounts of maternal IgG, which for approximately 3 months confers immunity against many antigens to which the mother was exposed. After birth IgG levels gradually fall as maternal IgG is catabolized and the newborn produces limited IgG. The lowest IgG levels occur at approximately 2 to 4 months, and levels remain low until approximately 6 months (Blackburn, 2007). Infants reach approximately 40% of adult levels by 1 year of age; therefore during the first 6 to 12 months of life the infant is at higher risk for infections. Significant amounts of IgM are produced at birth yet specificity is decreased, thus limiting recognition of certain pathogens. Adult levels of IgM are reached by 9 to 12 months of age. The production of IgA, IgD, and IgE is much more gradual, and maximum levels are not attained until early childhood.

Secretory IgA (sIgA) is not present at birth but is found in saliva and tears by 2 to 5 weeks. sIgA is present in large amounts in human colostrum. Researchers believe this has a protective role in the gastrointestinal tract against many bacteria such as *Escherichia coli* and viruses such as poliovirus. The development of the mucosa-associated lymphoid tissue (MALT) occurs during infancy. In part, this system prevents colonization and passage of bacteria across the infant's mucosal barrier (Lawrence and Lawrence, 2005). The function and quantity of T lymphocytes, lymphokines, interleukins, tumor necrosis factor alpha, interferon-γ, and complement are reduced in early infancy, thus preventing optimum response to certain bacteria and viruses. Prebiotic oligosaccharides found in breast milk produce probiotic bacteria such as bifidobacteria and lactobacilli, which in turn stimulate synthesis and secretion of sIgA. sIgA coats the gastrointestinal mucosa to further protect the infant from certain pathogens (Blackburn, 2007). Probiotics may have a significant role in helping the gastrointestinal tract establish a "good" bacterial colonization in the gut to prevent many illnesses, including possibly necrotizing enterocolitis in preterm infants (Caplan, 2009; Goldin and Gorbach, 2008).

There is evidence that vernix caseosa, a white oily substance that coats the term infant's body and is often found in abundance in the creases of the axillae and groin, has innate immunologic properties that serve to protect the newborn from infection (Narendran and Hoath, 2006).

During infancy thermoregulation becomes more efficient; the skin's ability to contract and of muscles to shiver in response to cold increases. The peripheral capillaries respond to changes in ambient temperature to regulate heat loss. The capillaries constrict in response to cold, conserving core body temperature and decreasing potential evaporative heat loss from the skin surface. The capillaries dilate in response to heat, decreasing internal body temperature through evaporation, conduction, and convection. Shivering (thermogenesis) causes the muscles and muscle fibers to contract, generating metabolic heat, which is distributed throughout the body. Increased adipose tissue during the first 6 months insulates the body against heat loss.

A shift in total body fluid occurs. At birth 78% of the infant's body weight is water, while a significant amount of that is extracellular fluid (ECF). As the percentage of body water decreases, so does the amount of ECF—from 44% at term to 20% in adulthood. The high proportion of ECF, which is composed of blood plasma, interstitial fluid, and lymph, predisposes the infant to more rapid loss of total body fluid and, consequently, dehydration. The loss of 5% to 10% of the term newborn's initial birth weight in the first 5 days of life is attributed to ECF compartment contraction, enhanced renal tubular function, and rapidly increasing glomerular filtration rate (Blackburn, 2007).

The immaturity of the renal structures also predisposes the infant to dehydration. Complete maturity of the kidney occurs during the latter half of the second year, when the cuboidal epithelium of the glomeruli becomes flattened. Before this time the filtration capacity of the glomeruli is reduced. Infants void urine frequently, and it has a low specific gravity (1.008 to 1.012). At term most infants produce and excrete approximately 15 to 60 ml/kg/24 hr, and an output of less than 0.5 ml/kg/hr after 48 hours of age is considered to be oliguria (Blackburn, 2007).

The endocrine system is adequately developed at birth, but its functions are immature. The interrelatedness of all the endocrine organs has a major effect on the function of any one gland. The lack of homeostatic control because of various functional deficiencies renders the infant especially vulnerable to imbalances in fluid and electrolytes, glucose concentration, and amino acid metabolism. For example, corticotropin (adrenocorticotropic hormone [ACTH]) is produced in limited quantities during infancy. ACTH acts on the adrenal cortices to produce their hormones, particularly the glucocorticoids and aldosterone. Because the feedback mechanism between ACTH and the adrenal cortex is immature during infancy, there is much less tolerance for stressful conditions, which affect fluid and electrolytes and the metabolism of fats, proteins, and carbohydrates. In addition, although the islets of Langerhans produce insulin and glucagon during fetal life and early infancy, blood glucose levels tend to remain labile, particularly under conditions of stress.

Fine Motor Development

Fine motor behavior includes the use of the hands and fingers in the prehension (grasp) of an object. Grasping occurs during the first 2 to 3 months as a reflex and gradually becomes voluntary. At 1 month of age the hands are predominantly closed, and by 3 months they are mostly open. By this time infants demonstrate a desire to grasp an object, but they "grasp" it more with the eyes than with the hands. If a rattle is placed in the hand, the infant will actively hold onto it. By 4 months of age the infant regards both a small pellet and the hands and then looks from the object to the hands and back again. By 5 months the infant is able to voluntarily grasp an object.

Gradually the palmar grasp (using the whole hand) is replaced with a pincer grasp (using the thumb and index finger). By 8 to 9 months of age the infant uses a crude pincer grasp (Fig. 12-3), and by 10 months of age the pincer grasp is sufficiently established to enable infants to pick up a raisin and other finger foods. By 11 months the infant has progressed to a neat pincer grasp (Fig. 12-4).

By 6 months of age infants have increased manipulative skill. They hold their bottle, grasp their feet and pull them to their mouth, and feed themselves a cracker. By 7 months they

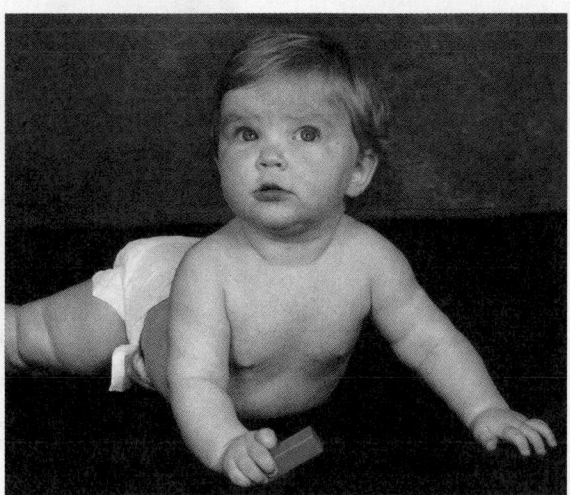

Fig. 12-3 Crude pincer grasp at 8 to 10 months of age. (Courtesy Paul Vincent Kuntz, Texas Children's Hospital, Houston.)

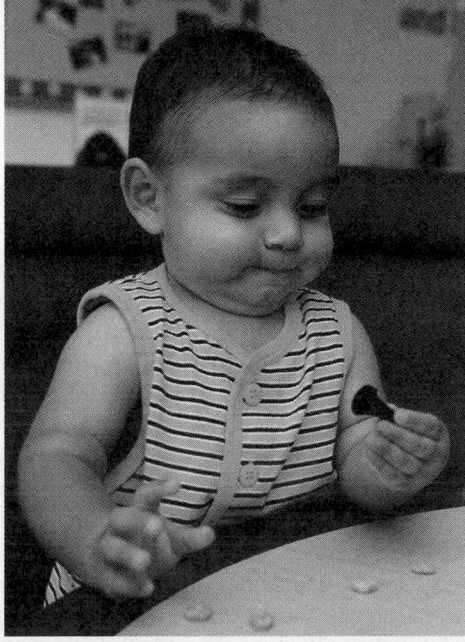

Fig. 12-4 Neat pincer grasp at 11 months of age. (Courtesy Paul Vincent Kuntz, Texas Children's Hospital, Houston.)

transfer objects from one hand to the other, use one hand for grasping, and hold a cube in each hand simultaneously. They enjoy banging objects and will explore the movable parts of a toy. By 10 months of age infants can deliberately let go of an object and will offer it to someone. By 11 months they put objects into a container and like to remove them. By age 1 year infants try to build a tower of two blocks but fail.

Gross Motor Development

Gross motor behavior includes developmental maturation in posture, head balance, sitting, creeping, standing, and walking. The full-term neonate is born with some ability to hold the head erect and reflexively assumes the postural tonic neck position when supine. Several of the primitive reflexes have significance in terms of development of later gross motor skills. The righting reflexes elicit certain postural responses, particularly of flexion or extension. They are responsible for certain motor activities, such as rolling over, assuming the crawl position, and maintaining normal head-trunk-limb alignment during all activities. The neck-righting reflex, which turns the body to the same side as the head, enables the child to roll over from supine to prone. Other reflexes, such as the otolith-righting and labyrinth-righting reflexes, enable the infant to raise the head (see Box 12-1).

The asymmetric tonic neck reflex, which persists from birth to 3 months, prevents the infant from rolling over. The symmetric tonic neck reflex, which is evoked by flexing or extending the neck, helps the infant assume the crawl position. When the head and neck are extended, the extensor tone of the upper extremities and the flexor tone of the lower extremities increase. The child extends the arms and bends the knees. Because of the strong flexor tone of the lower extremities, the infant may initially crawl backward before crawling forward. This reflex disappears when neurologic maturity allows actual crawling to occur because independent limb movement is required.

Head Control

The full-term newborn can momentarily hold the head in midline and parallel when the body is suspended ventrally and can lift and turn the head from side to side when prone (see Fig. 8-8). This is not the case when the infant is lying prone on a pillow or soft surface; infants do not have the head control to lift their head out of the depression of the object and therefore risk possible suffocation. (See Sudden Infant Death Syndrome, Chapter 13.) Marked head lag is evident when the infant is pulled from a lying to a sitting position. By 3 months of age infants can hold their head well beyond the plane of the body. By 4 months of age infants can lift the head and front portion of the chest approximately 90 degrees above the table, bearing their weight on the forearms. Only slight head lag is evident when the infant is pulled from a lying to a sitting position, and by 4 to 6 months head control is well established (Figs. 12-5 and 12-6).

Rolling Over

Newborns may roll over accidentally because of their rounded back. The ability to willfully turn from the abdomen to the back occurs at 5 months, and the ability to turn from the back to the abdomen occurs at 6 months. It is noteworthy that the

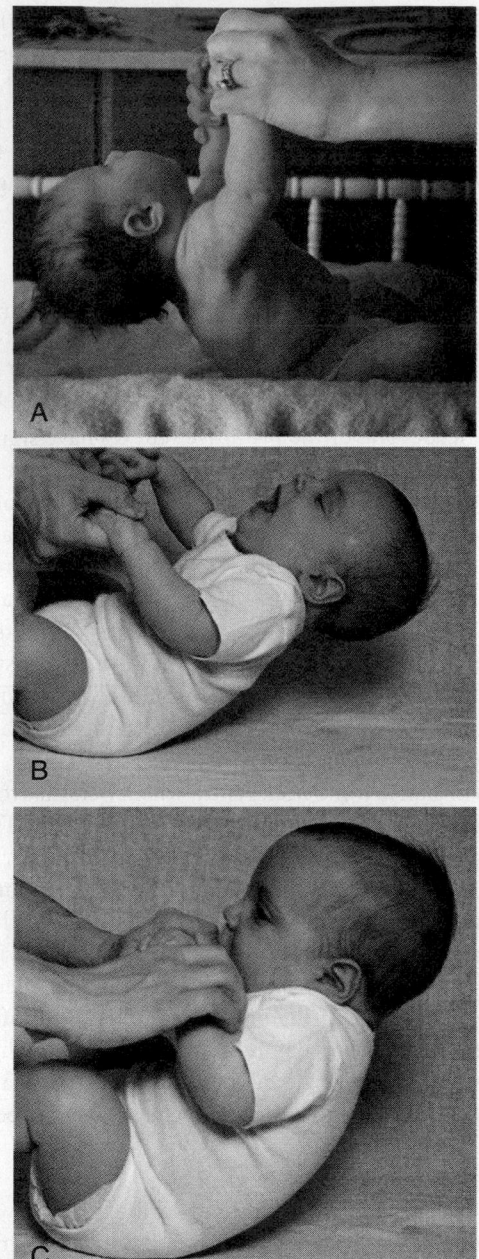

Fig. 12-5 Head control while pulled to sitting position. **A,** Complete head lag at 1 month. **B,** Partial head lag at 2 months. **C,** Almost no head lag at 4 months.

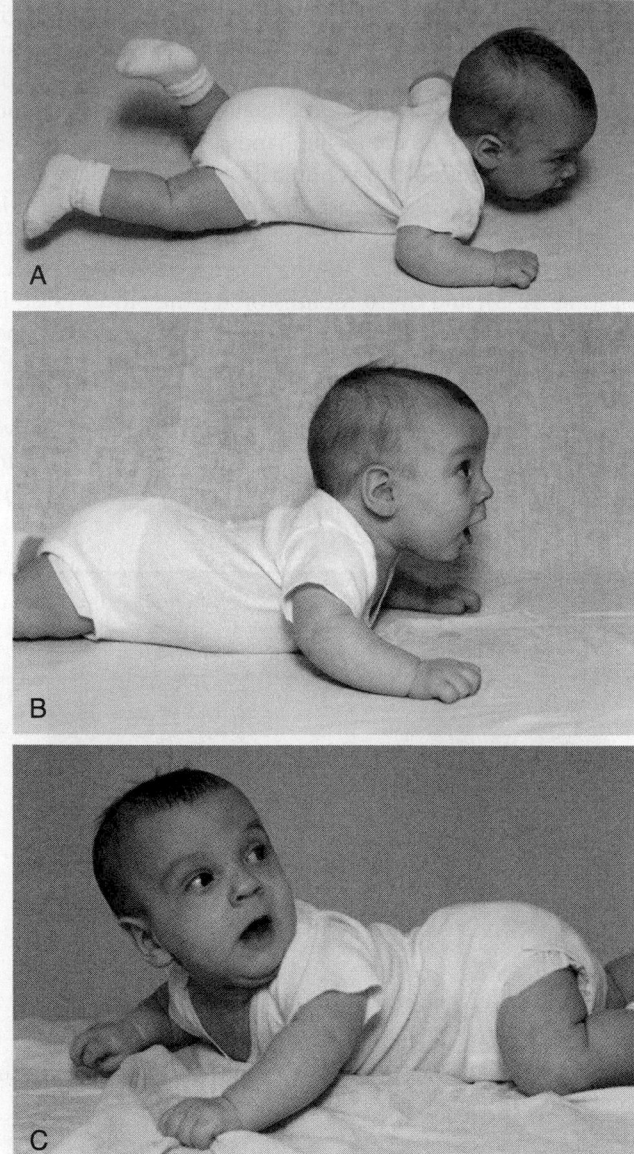

Fig. 12-6 Head control while prone. **A,** Infant momentarily lifts head at 1 month. **B,** Infant lifts head and chest 90 degrees and bears weight on forearms at 4 months. **C,** Infant lifts head, chest, and upper abdomen and can bear weight on hands at 6 months. Note how this position facilitates turning from abdomen to back.

parachute reflex (see Fig. 12-1), which elicits a protective response to falling, appears at 7 months.

Sitting

The ability to sit follows progressive head control and straightening of the back (Fig. 12-7). For the first 2 to 3 months the back is uniformly rounded. The convex cervical curve forms at approximately 3 to 4 months of age, when head control is established. The convex lumbar curve appears when the child begins to sit, at about age 4 months. As the spinal column straightens, the infant can be propped in a sitting position. By age 7 months infants can sit alone, leaning forward on their hands for support. By age 8 months they can sit well while

unsupported and begin to explore their surroundings in this position rather than in a lying position. By 10 months they can maneuver from a prone to a sitting position.

An infant who does not pull to a standing position by 11 to 12 months of age should be further evaluated for possible developmental dysplasia of the hip. (See Chapter 11.) Although infants vary considerably in regard to the achievement of these milestones, they provide guidelines for early intervention.

Locomotion

Locomotion involves acquiring the ability to bear weight, propel forward on all four extremities, stand upright with support, and, finally, walk alone (Fig. 12-8). Following a cepha-

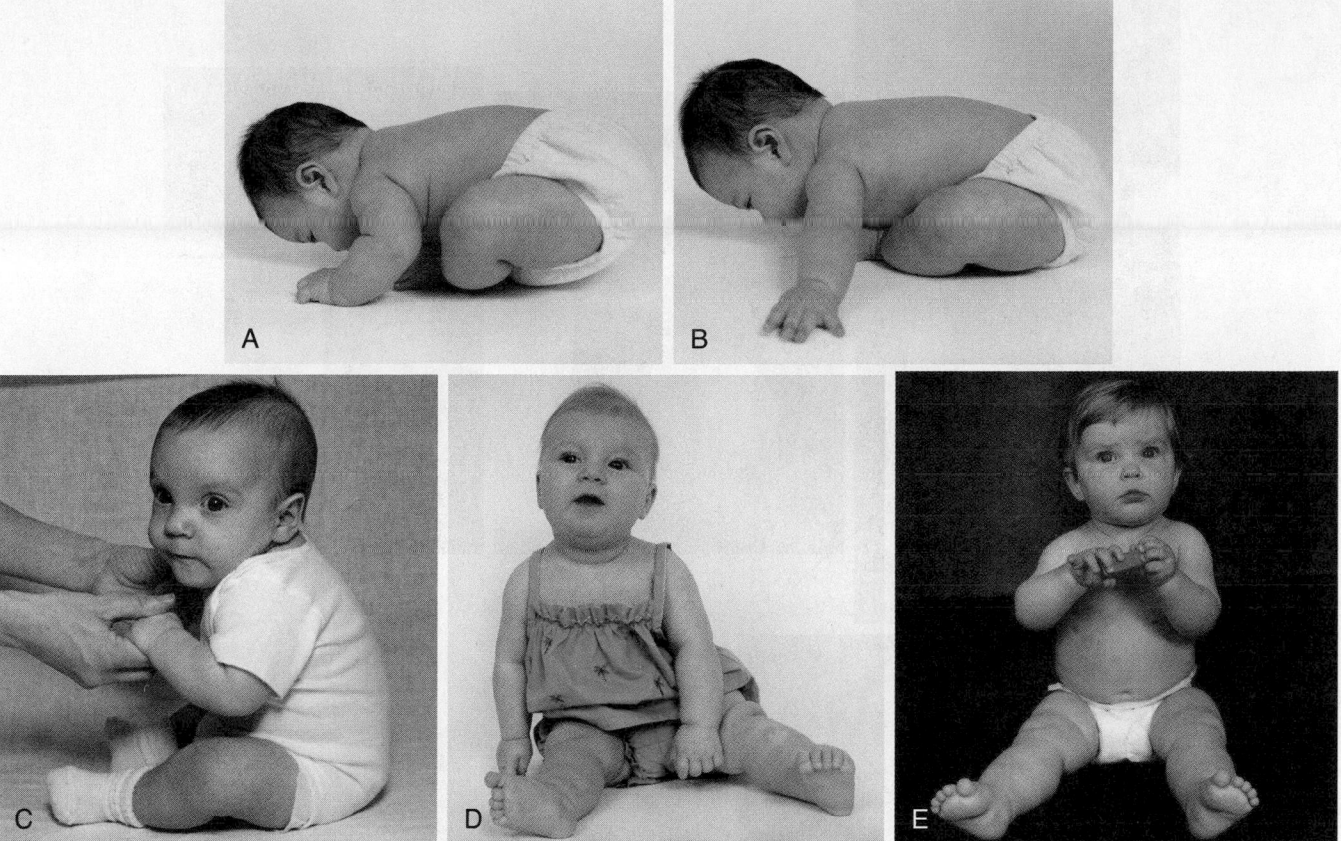

Fig. 12-7 Development of sitting. **A,** Back is completely rounded; infant has no ability to sit upright at 1 month. **B,** At 2 months, infant exhibits more control; back is still rounded, but infant can try to pull up with some head control. **C,** Back is rounded only in lumbar area; infant is able to sit erect with good head control at 4 months. **D,** Infant can sit alone, leaning on hands for support, at 7 months. **E,** Infant sits without support at 8 months. Note the transferring of objects that occurs at 7 months. (Courtesy Paul Vincent Kuntz, Texas Children's Hospital, Houston.)

locaudal pattern, infants 4 to 6 months old have increasing coordination in their arms. Initial locomotion results in infants propelling themselves backward by pushing with the arms. By 6 to 7 months of age they are able to bear all their weight on their legs with assistance. Crawling (propelling forward with belly on floor) progresses to creeping on hands and knees (with belly off floor) by 9 months. At this time they stand while holding onto furniture and can pull themselves to the standing position, but they are unable to maneuver back down except by falling. By 11 months they walk while holding onto furniture or with both hands held, and by age 1 year they may be able to walk with one hand held. A number of infants attempt their first independent steps by their first birthday.

Calculate an infant's motor age (development) by calculating a motor quotient (MQ) using the following formula:

$$MQ = \frac{Motor\ age\ (MA)}{Chronologic\ age} \times 100$$

For example, if a 12-month-old infant begins to creep, the motor quotient is 9 (MA for this skill) divided by 12 (chronologic age) times 100, which equals 75. Values above 85 are considered within normal limits, values below 70 are abnormal, and values between 70 and 85 are borderline (Johnson and Blasco, 1997).

PSYCHOSOCIAL DEVELOPMENT

⊜ Developing a Sense of Trust (Erikson)

Erik Erikson's (1963) phase I (birth to 1 year) is concerned with acquiring a sense of trust while overcoming a sense of mistrust. Erikson was a neo-Freudian who incorporated much of Freud's theory. (See Chapter 3.) The trust that develops is a trust of self, of others, and of the world. Infants "trust" that their feeding, comfort, stimulation, and caring needs will be met. The crucial element for the achievement of this task is the quality of both the relationship between the parent (or caregiver) and child and the care the infant receives. The provision of food, warmth, and shelter by itself is inadequate for the development of a strong sense of self. The infant and parent must jointly learn to satisfactorily meet their needs for mutual regulation of frustration to occur. When this synchrony fails to develop, mistrust is the eventual outcome. Frustration is heightened in situations in which the parent is emotionally immature and does not understand the infant's behavioral cues because of his or her own self-centered phase of development.

Failure to learn delayed gratification leads to mistrust. Mistrust can result from either too much or too little frustration. If parents always meet their children's needs before the children signal their readiness, infants will never learn to test

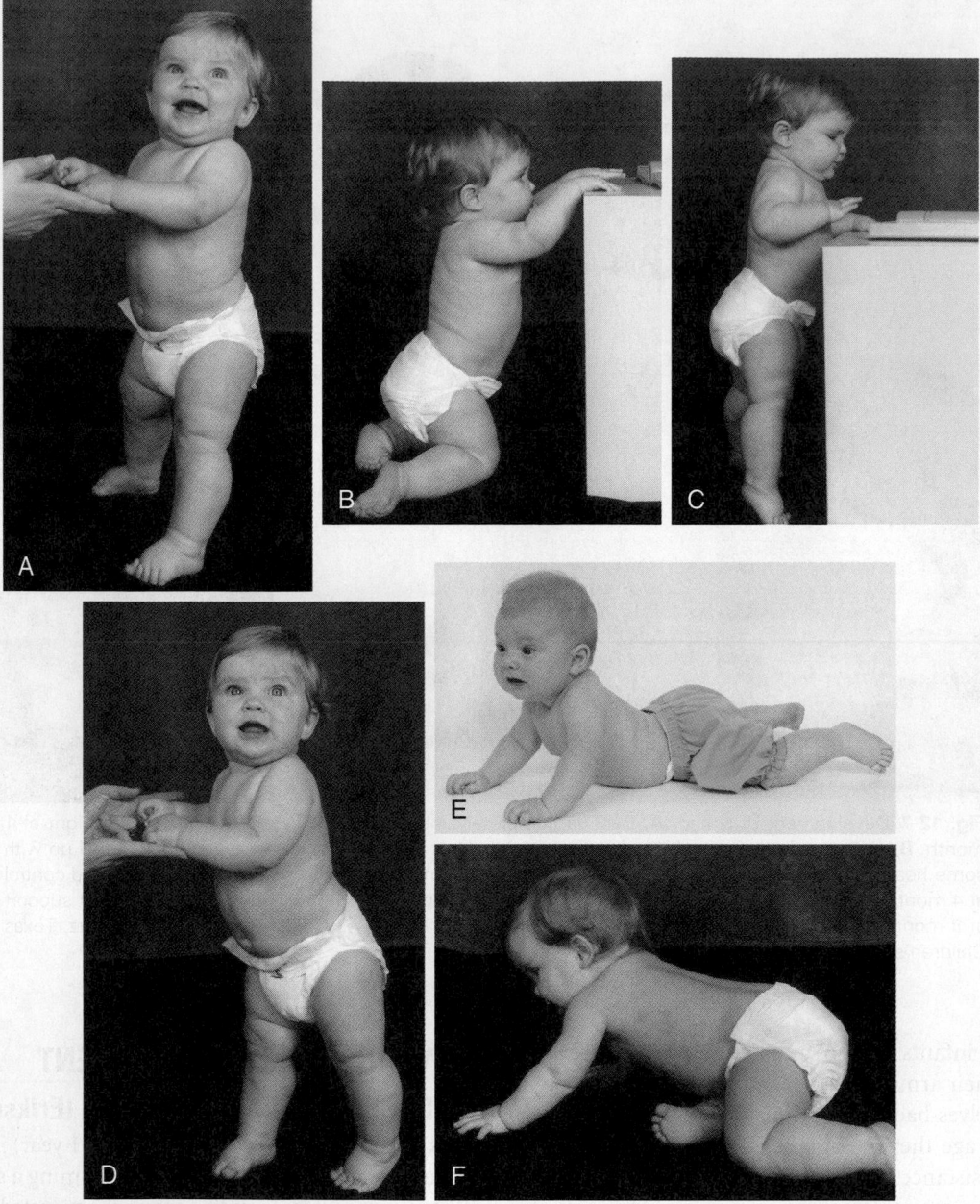

Fig. 12-8 Development of locomotion. **A,** Infant bears full weight on feet by 7 months. **B,** Infant can maneuver from sitting to kneeling position by 8 months. **C,** Infant can stand holding onto furniture at 8 to 9 months. **D,** While standing, infant takes deliberate step at 9 to 10 months. **E,** Infant crawls with abdomen on floor and pulls self forward and then, **F,** creeps on hands and knees at 9 months. (Courtesy Paul Vincent Kuntz, Texas Children's Hospital, Houston.)

their ability to control the environment. If the delay is prolonged, infants will experience constant frustration and eventually mistrust others in their efforts to satisfy them. Therefore consistency of care is essential.

The trust acquired in infancy provides the foundation for all succeeding phases. Trust allows infants a feeling of physical comfort and security, which assists them in experiencing unfamiliar, unknown situations with a minimum of fear. Erikson has divided the first year of life into two oral-social stages. During the first 3 to 4 months, food intake is the most important social activity in which the infant engages. The newborn can tolerate little frustration or delay of gratification. **Primary narcissism** (total concern for oneself) is at its height. However, as bodily processes such as vision, motor movements, and

vocalization become better controlled, infants use more advanced behaviors to interact with others. For example, rather than cry, infants may put their arms up to signify a desire to be held.

The next social modality involves a mode of reaching out to others through grasping. Grasping is initially reflexive, but even as a reflex it has a powerful social meaning for the parents. The reciprocal response to the infant's grasping is the parents' holding on and touching. There is pleasurable tactile stimulation for both the child and the parents.

Tactile stimulation is extremely important in the total process of acquiring trust. The degree of mothering skill, the quantity of food, or the length of sucking does not determine the quality of the experience. Rather, it is the total quality of the interpersonal relationship that influences the infant's formulation of trust.

During the second stage, the more active and aggressive modality of biting occurs. Infants learn that they can hold onto what is their own and can more fully control their environment. During this stage infants may be confronted with one of their first conflicts. If they are breast-feeding, they quickly learn that biting causes the mother to become upset and withdraw the breast. Yet biting also brings internal relief from teething discomfort and a sense of power or control.

This conflict has a variety of solutions. The mother may wean the infant from the breast and begin bottle-feeding, or the infant may learn to bite substitute "nipples," such as a pacifier, and retain pleasurable breast-feeding. The successful resolution of this conflict strengthens the mother-child relationship because it occurs at a time when infants are recognizing the mother as the most significant person in their life.

COGNITIVE DEVELOPMENT

Sensorimotor Phase (Piaget)

The theory most commonly used to explain cognition, or the ability to know, is that of Piaget (1952). The period from birth to 24 months is termed the sensorimotor phase and is composed of six stages. However, because this discussion centers on ages birth to 12 months, only the first four stages are discussed (Table 12-1; see Table 14-1 for the stages from 13 to 24 months).

During the sensorimotor phase, infants progress from reflexive behaviors to simple repetitive acts to imitative activity. Three crucial events take place during this phase. The first event involves separation, in which infants learn to separate themselves from other objects in the environment. They realize that others besides themselves control the environment and that certain adjustments must take place for mutual satisfaction to occur. This coincides with Erikson's concept of the formation of trust and mutual regulation of frustration.

The second major accomplishment is achieving the concept of object permanence, or the realization that objects that leave the visual field still exist. A typical example of the development of object permanence is when infants are able to pursue objects they observe being hidden under a pillow or behind a chair (Fig. 12-9). This skill develops at approximately 9 to 10 months of age, which corresponds to the time of increased locomotion skills.

The last major intellectual achievement of this period is the ability to use symbols, or mental representation. The use of symbols allows the infant to think of an object or situation

TABLE 12-1	SENSORIMOTOR PHASE DURING INFANCY*	
STAGE AND AGE	**COGNITIVE DEVELOPMENT**	**BEHAVIOR**
I. Use of reflexes (birth–1 mo)	Repetitious use of reflexes establishing pattern of experiences	Mostly reflective (sucking, swallowing, rooting, grasping, crying)
	Totally narcissistic (self-centered) being	Little or no tolerance for frustration of delayed gratification
II. Primary circular reactions (1-4 mo)	Use of reflexes gradually replaced by voluntary activity	Recognizes familiar faces and objects (e.g., bottle)
	Recognition of causality occurring when repetition of events causes one stimulus to produce consistent response	Shows anticipation before feeding
		Shows awareness of strange surroundings, indicating memory
	Beginning notion of temporal space of time as infant realizes progression of orderly sequence of events	Discovers parts of own body—plays with hands, fingers, feet
	Beginning separation of self from others	Becomes bored when left alone
	Learns from type of interaction between objects or individual rather than from object itself	Shows no separation anxiety unless caregiver's skill differs from usual routine
	Engages in activity for pleasure of the activity more than for its results	
III. Secondary circular reactions (4-8 mo)	Intentional activity replaces repetitive activity that did not produce desired result	Secures objects by pulling on string
		Searches for objects that have fallen
	Beginning of object permanence when object is beyond perceptual range	Shows separation anxiety
		Able to tolerate some frustration and delayed gratification
	Progressive idea of time; awareness of before and after in sequence of events	Imitates sounds and simple gestures
		Shows interest in mirror image (see Fig. 12-10)
	Able to imitate selective activity from several events	Beginning independence in self-feeding
	Further separation of self from environment	Shows displeasure if activity is inhibited
	Idea of quality and quantity	Language development; attracts attention by methods other than crying
	Beginning recognition of symbols as type of communication	Realizes that parents are present even if not in visual field
IV. Coordination of secondary schemas and their application to new situations (9-12 mo)	Concept of object permanence advancing; beginning of intellectual reasoning	Actively searches for hidden object (see Fig. 12-9)
		Comprehends meanings of words and simple commands
	Associates symbols with events, but classification is based on own experience	Know that gestures (bye-bye, kiss) have certain meanings
		Is able to put objects in container
	Distinguishes objects from related activity and perceives them as objects	Works to get toy that is out of reach
		Ventures away from parent to explore surroundings
	Distinguishes end products from their means; attempts to remove barriers to achieve the end	

*For phases during toddlerhood, see Table 14-1.

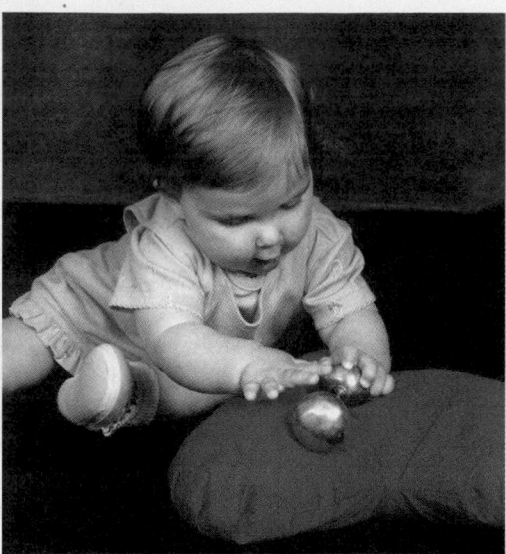

Fig. 12-9 Nine-month-old is able to find hidden object under pillow. (Courtesy Paul Vincent Kuntz, Texas Children's Hospital, Houston.)

without actually experiencing it. The recognition of symbols is the beginning of the understanding of time and space.

The first stage, from birth to 1 month, is identified by the infant's use of reflexes. At birth the infant expresses individuality and temperament through the physiologic reflexes of sucking, rooting, grasping, and crying. The repetitious nature of the reflexes is the beginning of associations between an act and a sequential response. When infants cry because they are hungry, a nipple is put in the mouth, and they suck, feel satisfaction, and sleep. They are assimilating this experience while perceiving auditory, tactile, and visual cues. This experience of perceiving certain patterns, or ordering, provides a foundation for the subsequent stages.

The second stage, primary circular reactions, marks the beginning of the replacement of reflexive behavior with voluntary acts. During the period from 1 to 4 months, activities such as sucking or grasping become deliberate acts that elicit certain responses. The beginning of accommodation is evident. Infants incorporate and adapt their reactions to the environment and recognize the stimulus that produced a response. Previously they would cry until the nipple was brought to the mouth. Now they associate the nipple with the sound of the parent's voice. They accommodate this new piece of information and adapt by ceasing to cry when they hear the voice—before receiving the nipple. What is taking place is a realization of causality and recognition of an orderly sequence of events. The infant takes in the environment with all the senses and with whatever motor ability is present.

The secondary circular reactions stage is a continuation of primary circular reactions and lasts until 8 months of age. In this stage the primary circular reactions are repeated and prolonged for the response that results. Grasping and holding now become shaking, banging, and pulling. Infants shake objects to hear a noise, not solely for the pleasure of shaking. Quality and quantity of an act become evident. "More" or "less" shaking produces different responses. Causality, time, deliberate intention, and separateness from the environment begin to develop.

Three new processes of human behavior occur. Imitation requires the differentiation of selected acts from several events. By the second half of the first year infants can imitate sounds and simple gestures. Play becomes evident as they take pleasure in performing an act after they have mastered it. Much of infants' waking hours are absorbed in sensorimotor play. Affect (outward manifestation of emotion and feeling) is evident as infants begin to develop a sense of permanency. During the first 6 months infants believe that an object exists only for as long as they can visually perceive it; in other words, out of sight, out of mind. A reaction to external objects is evident when the object continues to be remembered even though it is beyond the range of perception. Object permanence is a critical component of parent-child attachment and is seen in the development of separation anxiety at 6 to 8 months of age (p. 480).

During the fourth sensorimotor stage, coordination of secondary schemas and their application to new situations, infants use previous behavioral achievements primarily as the foundation for adding new intellectual skills to their expanding repertoire. This stage is largely transitional. Increasing motor skills allow for greater exploration of the environment. They begin to discover that hiding an object does not mean that it is gone but that removing an obstacle will reveal the object. This marks the beginning of intellectual reasoning. Furthermore, they can experience an event by observing it, and they begin to associate symbols with events (e.g., "bye-bye" with "Daddy goes to work"), but the classification is purely their own. In this stage they learn from the object itself. This is in contrast to the second stage, in which infants learn from the type of interaction between objects or individuals. Intentionality is further developed in that infants now actively attempt to remove a barrier to the desired (or undesired) action (see Fig. 12-9). If something is in their way, they attempt to climb over it or push it away, whereas previously they would have given up any attempt to achieve the desired goal.

DEVELOPMENT OF BODY IMAGE

The development of body image parallels sensorimotor development. Infants' kinesthetic and tactile experiences are the first perceptions of their body, and the mouth is the principal area of pleasurable sensations. Other parts of the body are primarily objects of pleasure—the hands and fingers to suck and the feet to play with. As physical needs are met, they feel comfort and satisfaction with their body. Messages conveyed by the caregivers reinforce these feelings. For example, when infants smile, they receive emotional satisfaction from others who smile back.

Achieving the concept of object permanence is basic to the development of self-image. By the end of the first year infants recognize that they are distinct from their parents. At the same time they have increasing interest in their image, especially in the mirror (Fig. 12-10). As motor skills develop, they learn that parts of the body are useful; for example, the hands bring objects to the mouth, and the legs help them move to different locations. All these achievements transmit messages to them about themselves. Therefore it is important to transmit positive messages to infants about their bodies.

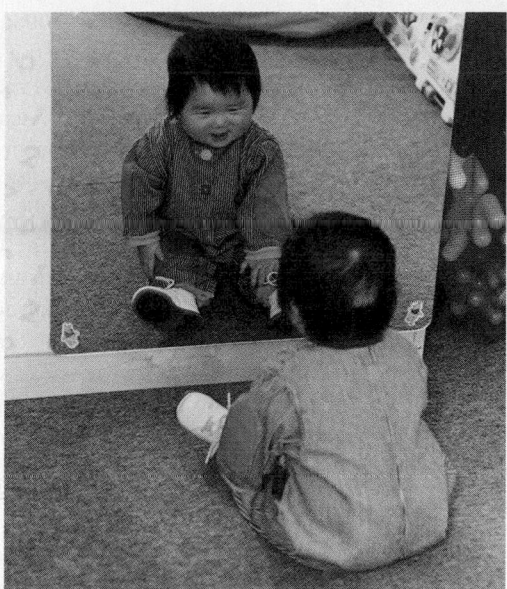

Fig. 12-10 Nine-month-old infant enjoying own image in mirror.

DEVELOPMENT OF GENDER IDENTITY

Gender identity is reported to begin in utero because of hormonal influences that are not entirely understood. At birth the child is named and significant others, especially the parents, act certain ways toward the infant because of its gender. Touch is crucial to infant development and plays a primary role in gender development. Infants have a great oral sensitivity, which is manifested through sucking and mouthing. They enjoy skin-to-skin contact and explore their own body for pleasure. Infants are capable of genital self-stimulation to orgasm; erections in male infants are common. Parents' responses to these early manifestations of sexuality influence children's evolving attitudes. Therefore a healthy, accepting response by parents is important.

SOCIAL DEVELOPMENT

Infants' social development is initially influenced by their reflexive behavior, such as the grasp, and eventually depends primarily on the interaction between them and the principal caregivers. Attachment to the parent is increasingly evident during the second half of the first year. In addition, infants make tremendous strides in communication and personal-social behavior. Play is a major socializing agent and provides the stimulation needed to learn from interactions with the environment.

Attachment

Human physical contact is extremely important. Parenting is not an instinctual ability but a learned, acquired process. The attachment of parent and child, which begins before birth and assumes even more importance at birth (see Chapter 8), continues during the first year. In the following discussion of attachment, the word *mother* is used in the broad context of the consistent caregiver with whom the child relates more than anyone else. However, in a society with a changing social climate and dissolving sex-role stereotypes, this person may well be the father, grandmother, or other family member.

Studies on father-child attachment demonstrate that stages similar to maternal attachment occur and that fathers are more involved in child care when mothers are employed (although mothers continue to do the majority of infant care) (Jones and Heermann, 1992). Additional research has shown that inexperienced, first-time fathers are as capable as experienced fathers of developing a close attachment with their infants (Ferketich and Mercer, 1995). Studies of fathers of high-risk infants demonstrate that fathers experience feelings of love and affection toward their offspring during the newborn period; fathers in one study verbalized more positive feelings of love and affection toward the newborn when they were able to have close physical contact such as holding the child (Sullivan, 1999). The father has also been reported to have a significant role in supporting the mother in the perinatal period; fathers of high-risk infants reported concern about their mates' well-being in addition to the status of the ill infant (Lundqvist and Jakobsson, 2003). Research demonstrates that fathers develop feelings of attachment with their offspring and that their relationship with the infant is an important factor in the mother's emotional well-being. Breast-feeding mothers reported in one study that the most important factor in establishing and maintaining breast-feeding in early infancy was the father's acceptance of breast-feeding and support for the mother (Arora, McJunkin, Wehrer, et al, 2000).

In one study children who had insecure attachment to their teenage mothers had a strong attachment to the grandmother who was also a primary caretaker (Patterson, 1997). With many single-parent families in existence, a grandmother (or other significant caretaker) may become the primary caretaker. It is important for nurses to recognize that infant-parent attachments may be present or absent in situations where caretaker roles are less well defined by those involved.

When the infant is not provided a safe haven and consistent and loving care, an insecure attachment develops; such infants do not feel they can trust the world in which they live. This insecure attachment may result in psychosocial difficulties as the child grows and may persist even into adulthood.

Attachment progresses during infancy, with the child assuming an increasingly significant role in the family. Two components of cognitive development are required for attachment: (1) the ability to discriminate the mother from other individuals and (2) the achievement of object permanence. Both these processes prepare the infant for an equally important aspect of attachment: separation from the parent. Separation-individuation should occur as a harmonious, parallel process with emotional attachment.

During the formation of attachment to the parent, the infant progresses through four distinct but overlapping stages. For the first few weeks infants respond indiscriminately to anyone. Beginning at approximately 8 to 12 weeks of age, they cry, smile, and vocalize more to the mother than to anyone else but continue to respond to others, whether familiar or not. At approximately 6 months of age, infants show a distinct preference for the mother. They follow her more, cry when she leaves, enjoy playing with her more, and feel most secure in her arms. About 1 month after showing attachment to the mother, many infants begin attaching to other members of the family, most often the father.

Infants acquire other developmental behaviors that influence the attachment process. These include (1) differential crying, smiling, and vocalization (more to mother than to anyone else); (2) visual-motor orientation (looking more at mother, even if she is not close); (3) crying when the mother leaves the room; (4) approaching through locomotion (crawling, creeping, or walking); (5) clinging (especially in presence of a stranger); and (6) exploring away from mother while using her as a secure base.

Effects of Prolonged Separation

Attachment is considered so critical to optimum child development that many researchers have documented the effects of prolonged and early separation on infants in the absence of high-quality parent substitutes. Some of the most famous research on emotional deprivation has been done by John Bowlby, John Robertson, and René Spitz. Bowlby (1969) studied the effects of the infant's separation from the mother and noted severe cognitive and physical impairment, particularly if emotional deprivation occurred during the first 3 years of life. He observed that progressive impairment could be arrested or reversed if no further emotional deprivation occurred after the first 2 years, whereas prolonged, severe deprivation beginning early in the first year and lasting for 3 years led to severe, permanent effects. Among these were the inability to form trusting, intimate interpersonal relationships; language impairment; and deficiency in abstract thinking. Robertson (1953) and Bowlby (1969) found typical behavioral reactions of infants who were hospitalized and separated from their mothers. (See Separation Anxiety, Chapter 26.)

Spitz (1945) studied the effects of emotional deprivation on children raised in foundling homes or institutions. The infants were cared for by one nurse who had responsibility for eight children. Although the caregiver might be a loving, motherly person, she lacked the time to devote individual attention and stimulation to each child. As a result, the children were delayed in physical growth, were more susceptible to disease, and demonstrated decreasing developmental quotients over a 2-year period. Spitz found that children developed normally if given one-to-one attention by a mother substitute.

Although these studies represent extreme examples of young children reared in environments essentially devoid of high-quality mothering, rather than temporary separation such as daycare, the question remains regarding the long-term effects of separation and other stresses on children.

Reactive attachment disorder (RAD) is a psychologic and developmental problem that stems from maladaptive or absent attachment between the infant and parent (or primary caregiver) and may persist into childhood and even adulthood (Wilson, 2001; Zeanah and Fox, 2004). Infants at risk for RAD include those who have been victims of physical or sexual abuse or neglect; infants exposed to parental alcoholism, mental illness, and substance abuse; and infants who have experienced the absence of a consistent primary caregiver as a result of foster care, institutionalization, parental abandonment, or parental incarceration. RAD is a form of extreme insecure attachment. Two different patterns of RAD have emerged: the emotionally withdrawn–inhibited pattern and an indiscriminate-disinhibited pattern (Hornor, 2008; Zeanah and Fox, 2004). Signs of RAD usually occur before the age of 5 years in infants who had insecure attachments to the mother or other primary caretaker (American Psychiatric Association, 2000). The child may manifest behaviors such as not being cuddly with parents, failing to make eye contact with significant others, having poor impulse control, and being destructive to self and others. Without early intervention, some of these children fail to develop a conscience and suffer from an antisocial personality disorder that may lead to criminal acts. The American Psychiatric Association (2002) Position Statement on RAD emphatically recommends against the use of coercive holding therapies or rebirthing techniques for the treatment of RAD. It is not within the scope of this text to discuss every attachment disorder and associated therapies.

Based on such findings, nurses need to assess each family with the understanding that stress may or may not be necessarily harmful and that children can adapt even under adverse conditions. The nurse evaluates individual risk factors that influence a child's coping ability, using tools such as the Revised Infant Temperament Questionnaire (see p. 478) to assess "goodness of fit." When parental separation occurs, make every effort to help the family provide suitable caregiver substitutes for the child. Individuals who are warm, responsive, and interactive with the infant during separation can significantly minimize the physiologic and behavioral effects. The nurse emphasizes the child's plasticity and resiliency in coping to minimize the family's feelings of responsibility and guilt.

Separation Anxiety

Between the ages of 4 and 8 months the infant progresses through the first stage of separation-individuation and begins to have some awareness of self and mother as separate beings. At the same time, object permanence is developing, and the infant is aware that the parent can be absent. Therefore **separation anxiety** develops and is manifested through a predictable sequence of behaviors.

During the early second half of the first year infants protest when placed in their crib, and a short time later they object when the mother leaves the room. Infants may not notice the mother's absence if they are absorbed in an activity. However, when they realize her absence, they protest. From this point on they become very alert to her activities and whereabouts. By 11 to 12 months they are able to anticipate her imminent departure by watching her behaviors, and they begin to protest before she leaves. At this point many parents learn to postpone alerting the child to their departure until just before leaving.

Stranger Fear

As infants demonstrate attachment to one person, they correspondingly exhibit less friendliness to others. Between ages 6 and 8 months fear of strangers and stranger anxiety become prominent and are related to infants' ability to discriminate between familiar and unfamiliar people. Behaviors such as clinging to the parent, crying, and turning away from strangers are common (Fig. 12-11). Suggestions for coping with stranger fear and separation anxiety are on p. 480.

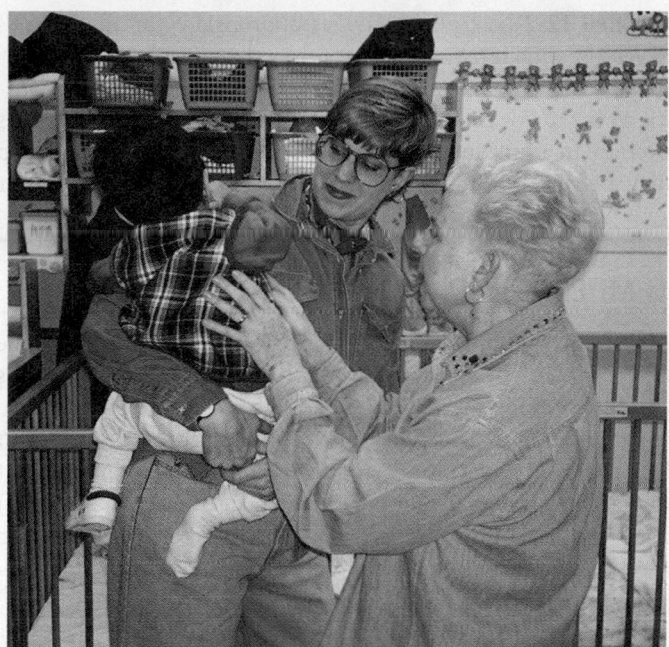

Fig. 12-11 Stranger fear behaviors include clinging to the parent and turning away from a stranger.

Language Development

The infant's first means of verbal communication is crying. Crying as a biologic sign conveys a message of urgency and signals displeasure, such as hunger. However, crying is also a social event that affects the development of the parent-infant relationship—either by its absence, which usually has a positive effect on parents, or its presence, which may evoke a negative response or persuade parents to minister to the child's physical or emotional needs.

In the first few weeks of life, crying has a reflexive quality and is mostly related to physiologic needs. Infants cry for 1 to 1½ hr/day up to 3 weeks of age and then build up to 2 hours and even 4 hours by 6 weeks. Crying tends to decrease by 12 weeks. It is thought that the increase in crying for no apparent reason during the first few months may be related to the discharge of energy and the maturational changes in the central nervous system. By the end of the first year infants cry for attention; from fear (especially stranger fear); and from frustration, usually in response to their developing but inadequate motor skills.

Many parents state that they can distinguish between different types of crying and from these messages are able to interpret the infant's needs. However, crying can be a source of acute distress for parents, especially the inconsolable crying of colic. (See Chapter 13.) Parents benefit from an explanation of the variability of crying among infants and an assurance that periods of "unexplained fussiness" are normal. Some parents may need guidance in consoling techniques, such as holding, swaddling, massaging, caressing, rocking, walking, or stimulating sucking.

Vocalizations heard during crying eventually become syllables and words (e.g., the "mama" heard during vigorous crying). Infants vocalize as early as 5 to 6 weeks of age by making small throaty sounds. By 2 months they make single vowel sounds such as *ah, eh,* and *uh.* By 3 to 4 months the consonants *n, k, g, p,* and *b* are added, and the infants coo, gurgle, and laugh aloud. By 6 months they imitate sounds; add the consonants *t, d,* and *w;* and combine syllables (e.g., "dada"), but they do not ascribe meaning to the word until 10 to 11 months of age (see Family-Centered Care box). By 9 to 10 months they comprehend the meaning of the word "no" and obey simple commands accompanied by gestures. By age 1 year they can say three to five words with meaning and may understand as many as 100 words. Because language development is based on expressive (ability to make thoughts, ideas, and desires known to others) and receptive skills (ability to understand the words being spoken), it is important that infants are exposed to expressive speech and that delays in achieving milestones are carefully evaluated for potential hearing loss. (See Universal Newborn Hearing Screening, Chapter 8.)

FAMILY-CENTERED CARE

Child's Developing Language Skills

During the acquisition of new language skills the child may temporarily stop using other recently learned sounds or words. This is often distressing for parents, who have waited in anticipation for the words "dada" or "mama." Because these sounds are commonly replaced by other vocalizations, they may not be repeated for several weeks. Nurses can reassure parents that the child will again say these special words and with increased meaning.

Personal-Social Behavior

Personal-social behavior includes the child's personal responses to the environment. It is the area most influenced by external stimuli but, as in the other fields of behavior, it follows certain developmental laws. Personal-social behavior implies communication with one's self and with others. It provides the foundation for the successful mastery of skills such as feeding, control of bodily functions, independence, and cooperativeness in play.

Infants have the ability to shape their environment and to elicit certain responses. Newborns show visual preference for the human face and, as early as 1 week of age, begin to watch the parent intently as he or she speaks to them. As they regard the parent's face, activity diminishes, their head bobs up and down, and their mouth moves, almost as if they were trying to say something.

By 6 to 8 weeks a social smile in response to pleasurable stimuli is present. This has a profound effect on family members and evokes continued responses from others. By 3 months infants show considerable interest in the environment—excitement when a toy is presented, refusal to be left alone, recognition of parent, and demonstration of pleasure by squealing. By 4 months they laugh aloud and enjoy strange, novel stimuli.

By 6 months infants are very personable. They play games such as peek-a-boo when their head is hidden in a towel, signal their desire to be picked up by extending their arms, and show displeasure when a toy is removed or their face is washed. They increasingly demonstrate their ability to control the environment. The acquisition of fine and gross motor skills allows much more independence in movement.

By the second half of the first year infants understand simple discipline, such as the meaning of the word "no" or a scolding remark. They comprehend different facial expressions and are sensitive to emotional changes in others. Imitation is developing during this time. They imitate actions and noises by 7 months, sounds by 8 months, and games such as pat-a-cake and peek-a-boo by 10 months.

From 11 months onward they are increasingly independent. They are learning to feed themselves; are using their fingers, spoon, and cup (with much spilling); and can help with dressing by putting the foot out for a shoe or pushing the arm through the sleeve. They not only comprehend the meaning of "no," but also shake their head to indicate "no." They can follow simple directions and gladly perform for others to attract and prolong attention.

Play

Play during infancy represents the various social modalities observed during cognitive development. Infants' activity is primarily narcissistic and revolves around their own body. As discussed under Development of Body Image, body parts are primarily objects of play and pleasure.

During the first year, play becomes more sophisticated and interdependent. From birth to 3 months, infants' responses to the environment are global and largely undifferentiated. Play is dependent; pleasure is demonstrated by a quieting attitude (1 month), a smile (2 months), and a squeal (3 months). From 3 to 6 months infants show more discriminate interest in stimuli and begin to play alone with a rattle or soft stuffed toy or with someone else. They interact much more during play. By 4 months of age they laugh aloud, show preference for certain toys, and become excited when food or a favorite object is brought to them. They recognize an image in a mirror, smile at it, and vocalize to it.

By 6 months to 1 year, play involves sensorimotor skills. Infants play actual games such as peek-a-boo and pat-a-cake. They demonstrate verbal repetition and imitation of simple gestures. Play is much more selective, not only in terms of specific toys but also in terms of "playmates." Although play is solitary or one sided, infants choose with whom they will interact. At 6 to 8 months they usually refuse to play with strangers. Parents are definite favorites, and infants know how to attract their attention. At 6 months they extend the arms to be picked up, at 7 months cough to make their presence known, at 10 months pull the parent's clothing, and at 12 months call them by name. This represents a tremendous advance from the newborn who signaled biologic needs by crying to express displeasure.

Stimulation is as important for psychosocial growth as food is for physical growth. Knowledge of developmental milestones allows nurses to guide parents regarding proper play for infants. It is not sufficient to place a mobile over a crib and toys in a playpen for a child's optimum social, emotional, and intellectual development. Play must provide interpersonal contact and recreational and educational stimulation. Infants need to be played with, not merely be allowed to play. Although the type of play infants engage in is called solitary, this is only a figurative, not literal, term to denote one-sided play. The types of toys given to the child are much less important than the quality of personal interaction that occurs.

Table 12-2 lists play activities appropriate for the infant's developmental level in terms of motor, language, and personal-social achievements. Although the activities are grouped according to the major mode of stimulation provided, many examples overlap. In addition, play activities suggested for one age-group may be appropriate for older infants but inappropriate for younger ones.

TEMPERAMENT

The infant's temperament or behavioral style influences the type of interaction that occurs between the child and parents and other family members. In assessing a child's temperament, it is the parents' perception of the child and the degree of fit between their expectations and the child's actual temperament that are important. The more dissonance (or lack of harmony) between the child's temperament and the parent's ability to accept and deal with the behavior, the greater the risk for subsequent parent-child conflicts.

Although many behavioral researchers agree that temperament has a strong biologic component, researchers also suggest that the environment, particularly the family, may modify temperament (Wilson, White, Cobb, et al, 2000). Family interaction with the infant is perceived as a circular process wherein each family member affects each other and the family as a unit. With these concepts in mind, the nurse has an important role in helping the family understand the infant's temperament as it relates to family dynamics and the eventual well-being of the child and family unit (Wilson, White, Cobb, et al, 2000).

Some researchers speculate that infant temperament may contribute to maternal depression. Indeed when there is a lack of reciprocity between the infant and the mother or when the infant's behavior does not meet maternal expectations, there is increased risk for discord. Beck's (2001) meta-analysis found that infant temperament was a mild risk factor for postpartum depression, whereas self-esteem, marital status, socioeconomic status, and unplanned or unwanted pregnancy were much more significant in predicting maternal depression. Recently, McGrath, Records, and Rice (2008) found that depressed mothers (versus nondepressed mothers) rated their infant's temperament at 2 and 6 months of age as more difficult. The researchers stress that depressed mothers need to be identified and assisted in making the transition to motherhood and in developing synchronicity with their newborn infants.

The Revised Infant Temperament Questionnaire (RITQ) (Carey and McDevitt, 1978) can be used as a screening tool with parents. The questionnaire focuses on nine temperament variables, with 95 questions related specifically to activities such as sleep, feeding, play, diapering, and dressing. The scores from the RITQ help identify the child's temperamental style. Use of the RITQ is well accepted by parents and should be accompanied by an adequate explanation of the results. In discussing the results, it is best to avoid descriptors such as "difficult" by describing such infants in terms of characteristics such as "intense" or "less predictable." The Early Infancy Temperament Questionnaire is a 76-item parent questionnaire that was adapted from the RITQ to evaluate temperament characteristics of infants 1 to 4 months old, whereas the RITQ is

TABLE 12-2   PLAY DURING INFANCY

AGE (mo)	VISUAL STIMULATION	AUDITORY STIMULATION	TACTILE STIMULATION	KINETIC STIMULATION
Suggested Activities				
Birth-1	Look at infant at close range. Hang bright, shiny object within 20-25 cm (8-10 inches) of infant's face and in midline. Hang mobiles with black-and-white designs.	Talk to infant; sing in soft voice. Play music box, tape, or compact disc. Have ticking clock or heartbeat doll nearby.	Hold, caress, cuddle. Keep infant warm. Swaddle infant with hands to face.	Rock infant; place in cradle. Use stroller for walks.
2-3	Provide bright objects. Make room bright with pictures or mirrors. Take infant to various rooms while doing chores. Place in infant seat for vertical view of environment (use a safe surface).	Talk to infant. Include infant in family gatherings. Expose to various environmental noises other than those of home. Use rattles, wind chimes.	Caress infant while bathing or changing diaper. Comb hair with a soft brush. Give massage.	Use infant swing. Take in car for rides. Exercise body by moving extremities in swimming motion. Use cradle gym.
4-6	Place infant in front of unbreakable mirror. Give brightly colored toys to hold (small enough to grasp).	Talk to infant; repeat sounds infant makes. Laugh when infant laughs. Call infant by name. Place rattle or bell in hand.	Give infant soft squeeze toys of various textures. Allow to splash in bath. Place nude on soft, furry rug and move extremities.	Use swing or stroller. Bounce infant in lap while holding in standing position. Support infant in sitting position; let infant lean forward to balance self. Place infant on floor to crawl, roll over, sit.
6-9	Give infant large toys with bright colors, movable parts, and noisemakers. Play peek-a-boo, especially hiding face in towel. Make funny faces to encourage imitation. Give ball of yarn or string to pull apart.	Call infant by name. Repeat simple words such as "dada," "mama," "bye-bye." Speak clearly. Name parts of body, people, and foods. Tell infant what you are doing. Use "no" only when necessary. Give simple commands. Show how to clap hands, bang a drum.	Let infant play with fabrics of various textures. Have bowl with foods of different sizes and textures to feel. Let infant "catch" running water. Encourage "swimming" in large bathtub or shallow pool. Give wad of sticky tape to manipulate.	Hold upright to bear weight and bounce. Pick up, say "up." Put down, say "down." Place toys out of reach; encourage infant to get them. Play pat-a-cake.
9-12	Show infant large pictures in books. Play ball by rolling it to child, demonstrate "throwing" it back. Demonstrate building a two-block tower.	Read infant simple nursery rhymes. Point to body parts and name each one. Imitate sounds of animals.	Give infant finger foods of different textures. Let infant mess and squash food. Let infant feel cold (ice cube) or warm objects; say what temperature each is. Let infant feel a breeze (fan blowing).	Give large push-pull toys. Turn in different positions.
Suggested Toys				
Birth-6	Nursery mobiles Unbreakable mirrors	Music boxes Musical mobiles Crib dangle bells Small-handled clear rattle	Stuffed animals Soft clothes* Soft or furry quilt* Soft mobiles	Rocking crib or cradle Weighted or suction toy Infant swing
6-12	Colored blocks Nested boxes or cups Books with rhymes and bright pictures Strings of big beads Simple take-apart toys Large ball Cup and spoon Large puzzles Jack-in-the-box	Rattles of different sizes, shapes, tones, and bright colors Squeaky animals and dolls Records with light, rhythmic music	Soft, different-texture animals and dolls Sponge toys, floating toys Squeeze toys Teething toys Books with textures and objects, such as fur and zipper	Activity box for crib Push-pull toys Wind-up swing

*Remove from crib when child is put to sleep to avoid possible suffocation (see p. 512).

best suited for infants 4 months old and older (Medoff-Cooper, Carey, and McDevitt, 1993).

With knowledge of the infant's temperament, nurses are better able to (1) provide parents with background information that will help them see their child in a better perspective, (2) offer a more organized picture of their child's behavior and possibly reveal distortions in their perceptions of the behavior, and (3) guide parents regarding appropriate childrearing techniques.

Childrearing Practices Related to Temperament

Most parents realize that their infant is born with unique characteristics, and few parents of difficult infants need to be told of the challenge of caring for them. However, most parents are unaware of the significance of the temperamental characteristics and of constructive approaches to dealing with them. The following are examples of interventions that promote more positive parenting of infants with different temperament styles.*

"Difficult" children may respond better to scheduled feedings and structured caregiving routines than demand feedings and frequent changes in daily routines. These children sleep less and may need more structured approaches to bedtime to prevent problems. Highly distractible children may require additional soothing measures such as swinging, rocking, or being carried in a pack that the parent wears across the chest or back. Children with high activity levels require vigilant watching, and parents need to take extra precautions in safeguarding the home. These children benefit from increased opportunities for gross motor activity to constructively channel their energy.

The child who is "slow to warm up" may demonstrate more stranger fear than other children and may require gradual and frequent preparation for new situations, such as substitute child care. Even the "easy child" can present problems in that the parents may need reminders to feed the child who sleeps for prolonged intervals and rarely cries. They may need to "retrain" the child because of the ease of developing habits such as keeping the child up late or sleeping with the young one, which may later become troublesome.

Appropriate counseling based on awareness of the child's temperament can greatly enhance the quality of interaction between parents and infant. Even just letting parents know that difficult traits are instinctive can relieve feelings of guilt and incompetence (see Temperament, Chapter 14).

Knowledge of the developmental sequence allows the nurse to assess normal growth and minor or abnormal deviations. It also helps parents gain realistic expectations of their child's ability, and provides guidelines for suitable play and stimulation. Parents who lack knowledge of child growth and development may set inappropriate behavioral expectations for their child. Emphasizing the child's developmental rather than chronologic age strengthens the parent-child relationship by fostering trust and lessening frustration. Therefore thorough

understanding and appreciation of children's growth and development are essential.

Because of the complexity of the developmental process during the first 12 months, Table 12-3 is presented to help organize and clarify the data already discussed. Although all milestones are important, some represent essential integrative aspects of development that lay the foundation for achievement of more advanced skills. These essential milestones are designated by a square (■) in the table. The table represents the average monthly age at which infants attain various skills. Remember that, although the sequence is the same, the rate will vary among children.

COPING WITH CONCERNS RELATED TO NORMAL GROWTH AND DEVELOPMENT

Separation Anxiety and Stranger Fear

A number of fears can appear during infancy. However, the fear that causes many parents concern is related to strangers and separation. Although some erroneously interpret this as a sign of undesirable, antisocial behavior, stranger fear and separation anxiety are important components of a strong, healthy parent-child attachment. Nevertheless, this period can present difficulties for the parent and child. Parents may be more confined to the home because the infant violently protests having a babysitter. To accustom the infant to new people, encourage parents to have close friends or relatives visit often. This provides other persons with whom the child is comfortable and who can give parents time for themselves.

Infants also need opportunities to safely experience strangers. Usually toward the end of the first year infants begin to venture away from the parent and demonstrate curiosity about strangers. If allowed to explore at their own rate, many infants eventually "warm up." If parents hold the child away from their face, the infant can observe while maintaining close physical contact.

A number of factors influence the intensity of a child's stranger fears:

Gender, age, and size of the stranger—Female, younger age, and smaller size (including kneeling or sitting rather than standing) is less stressful.

Approach—Loud, sudden, intrusive approach causes more distress.

Child's proximity to parent—Being closer to parent (on parent's lap rather than in infant seat) is less stressful.

Consequently, the best approach for the stranger (including the nurse) is to talk softly; meet the child at eye level (to appear smaller); maintain a safe distance from the infant; and avoid sudden, intrusive gestures, such as holding the arms out and smiling broadly.

Parents also may wonder whether they should encourage the child's clinging, dependent behavior, especially if there is pressure from others who view this as spoiling the child (see following discussion). Parents need reassurance that such behavior is healthy, desirable, and necessary for the child's optimum emotional development. If parents can reassure the infant of their presence, the infant will learn to realize that they are still there even if not physically present. Talking to infants

*Recommended resources for parents are Turecki SK, Tonner L: *The difficult child,* 2000, Bantam Books, New York, NY (www.randomhouse.com); and Chess S, Thomas A: *Know your child: an authoritative guide for today's parents,* Lanham, Md, 1996, Jason Aronson (www.aronson.com).

Text continued on p. 485.

TABLE 12-3 GROWTH AND DEVELOPMENT DURING INFANCY

AGE (mo)	PHYSICAL	GROSS MOTOR	FINE MOTOR	SENSORY	VOCALIZATION	SOCIALIZATION/COGNITION
1	Weight gain of 150-210 g (5-7 oz) weekly for first 6 mo Height gain of 2.5 cm (1 inch) monthly for first 6 mo Head circumference increases by 1.5 cm (0.6 inch) monthly for first 6 mo Primitive reflexes present and strong Doll's eye reflex and dance reflex fading Obligatory nose breathing (most infants)	■ Assumes flexed position with pelvis high but knees not under abdomen when prone (at birth, knees flexed under abdomen) ■ Can turn head from side to side when prone; lifts head momentarily from bed (see Fig. 12-6, A) Has marked head lag, especially when pulled from lying to sitting position (see Fig. 12-5, A) Holds head momentarily parallel and in midline when suspended in prone position Assumes asymmetric tonic neck reflex position when supine When held in standing position, is limp at knees and hips In sitting position, has uniformly rounded back, absence of head control	Hands predominantly closed Grasp reflex strong Clenches hand on contact with rattle	■ Able to fixate on moving object in range of 45 degrees when held at distance of 20-25 cm (8-10 inches) Visual acuity approaches 20/100* Follows light to midline Quiets when hears a voice	Cries to express displeasure Makes small, throaty sounds Makes comfort sounds during feeding	Is in sensorimotor phase, stage I, use of reflexes (birth— mo); and stage II, primary circular reactions (1-4 mo) Watches parent's face intently as she or he talks to infant
2	Posterior fontanel closed Crawling reflex disappears	■ Assumes less flexed position when prone—hips flat, legs extended, arms flexed, head to side Less head lag when pulled to sitting position (see Fig. 12-5, B) Can maintain head in same plane as rest of body when held in ventral suspension When prone, can lift head almost 45 degrees off table When held in sitting position, can hold head up, but bends forward (see Fig. 12-7, B) Assumes asymmetric tonic neck reflex position intermittently	Hands often open Grasp reflex fading	Binocular fixation and convergence to near objects beginning When supine, follows dangling toy from side to point beyond midline Visually searches to locate sounds Turns head to side when sound is made at level of ear	■ Vocalizes, distinct from crying Crying becomes differentiated Coos Vocalizes to familiar voice	■ Demonstrates social smile in response to various stimuli

■ Milestones that represent essential integrative aspects of development that lay the foundation for the achievement of more advanced skills.

*Degree of visual acuity varies according to vision measurement procedure used.

Continued

TABLE 12-3   GROWTH AND DEVELOPMENT DURING INFANCY—cont'd

AGE (mo)	PHYSICAL	GROSS MOTOR	FINE MOTOR	SENSORY	VOCALIZATION	SOCIALIZATION/COGNITION
3	Primitive reflexes fading	Able to hold head more erect when sitting, but still bobs forward Has only slight head lag when pulled to sitting position Assumes symmetric body positioning Able to raise head and shoulders from prone position to 45- to 90-degree angle from table; bears weight on forearms When held in standing position, able to bear slight fraction of weight on legs Regards own hand	Actively holds rattle but will not reach for it Grasp reflex absent Hands kept loosely open Clutches own hand; pulls at blankets and clothes	■ Follows objects to periphery (180 degrees) ■ Locates sound by turning head to side and looking in same direction Begins to have ability to coordinate stimuli from various sense organs	■ Squeals aloud to show pleasure Coos, babbles, chuckles Vocalizes when smiling "Talks" a great deal when spoken to Less crying during periods of wakefulness	Displays considerable interest in surroundings Ceases crying when parent enters room Can recognize familiar faces and objects, such as feeding bottle Shows awareness of strange situations
4	Drooling begins ■ Moro, tonic neck, and rooting reflexes disappeared	■ Has almost no head lag when pulled to sitting position (see Fig. 12-5, C) ■ Balances head well in sitting position (see Fig. 12-7, C) Back less rounded, curved only in lumbar area Able to sit erect if propped up Able to raise head and chest off surface to angle of 90 degrees (see Fig. 12-6, B) Assumes predominant symmetric position ■ Rolls from back to side	■ Inspects and plays with hands; pulls clothing or blanket over face in play Tries to reach objects with hand but overshoots Grasps object with both hands Plays with rattle placed in hand, shakes it, but cannot pick it up if dropped Can carry objects to mouth	Able to accommodate to near objects Binocular vision fairly well established Can focus on a 1.25-cm (0.5-inch) block Beginning eye-hand coordination	Makes consonant sounds n, k, g, p, b ■ Laughs aloud Vocalization changes according to mood	Is in stage III, secondary circular reactions Demands attention by fussing; becomes bored if left alone Enjoys social interaction Anticipates feeding when sees bottle or mother if breast-feeding Shows excitement with whole body, squeals, breathes heavily Shows interest in strange stimuli Begins to show memory
5	Beginning signs of tooth eruption Birth weight doubles	No head lag when pulled to sitting position When sitting, able to hold head erect and steady Able to sit for longer periods when back is well supported Back straight When prone, assumes symmetric positioning with arms extended ■ Can turn over from abdomen to back When supine, puts feet to mouth	■ Able to grasp objects voluntarily Uses palmar grasp, bidextrous approach Plays with toes Takes objects directly to mouth Holds one cube while regarding a second one	Visually pursues dropped object Is able to sustain visual inspection of object Can localize sounds made below ear	Squeals Makes cooing vowel sounds interspersed with consonant sounds (e.g., ah-goo)	Smiles at mirror image Pats bottle or breast with both hands More enthusiastically playful, but may have rapid mood swings Is able to discriminate strangers from family Vocalizes displeasure when object is taken away Discovers parts of body

Continued

Age (mo)	Physical	Gross Motor	Fine Motor	Sensory	Vocalization	Socialization
6	Growth rate may begin to decline Weight gain of 90-150 g (3-5 oz) weekly for next 6 mo Height gain of 1.25 cm (0.5 inch) monthly for next 6 mo ■ May begin teething with eruption of two lower central incisors ■ May chew and bite	When prone, can lift chest and upper abdomen off surface, bearing weight on hands (see Fig. 12-6, C) When about to be pulled to sitting position, lifts head Sits in high chair with back straight Rolls from back to abdomen When held in standing position, bears almost all of weight Hand regard absent	Resecures a dropped object Drops one cube when another is given Grasps and manipulates small objects Holds bottle Grasps feet and pulls to mouth	Adjusts posture to see object Prefers more complex visual stimuli Can localize sounds made above ear Will turn head to side, then look up or down	■ Begins to imitate sounds ■ Babbling resembles one-syllable utterances—*ma, mu, da, di, hi* Vocalizes to toys, mirror image Takes pleasure in hearing own sounds (self-reinforcement)	Recognizes parents; begins to fear strangers Holds arms out to be picked up Has definite likes and dislikes Begins to imitate (cough, protrusion of tongue) Excites on hearing footsteps Laughs when head is hidden in towel ■ Briefly searches for dropped object (object permanence beginning) Frequent mood swings from crying to laughing with little or no provocation
7	Eruption of upper central incisors Parachute reflex appears (see Fig. 12-1)	When supine, spontaneously lifts head off surface ■ Sits, leaning forward on both hands (see Fig. 12-7, D) When prone, bears weight on one hand Sits erect momentarily Bears full weight on feet (see Fig. 12-8, A) When held in standing position, bounces actively	■ Transfers objects from one hand to other (see Fig. 12-7, E) Has unidextrous approach and grasp Holds two cubes more than momentarily Bangs cubes on table Rakes at small object	■ Can fixate on very small objects Responds to own name Localizes sound by turning head in curving arch Beginning awareness of depth and space Has taste preferences	■ Produces vowel sounds and chained syllables—*baba, dada, kaka* Vocalizes four distinct vowel sounds "Talks" when others are talking	■ Increasing fear of strangers; shows signs of fretfulness when parent disappears Imitates simple acts and noises Tries to attract attention by coughing or snorting Plays peek-a-boo Demonstrates dislike of food by keeping lips closed Exhibits oral aggressiveness in biting and mouthing Demonstrates expectation in response to repetition of stimuli
8	Begins to show regular patterns in bladder and bowel elimination	■ Sits steadily unsupported (see Fig. 12-7, E) Readily bears weight on legs when supported; may stand holding onto furniture Adjusts posture to reach object	Has beginning pincer grasp using index, fourth, and fifth fingers against lower part of thumb Releases objects at will Rings bell purposely Retains two cubes while regarding third cube Secures object by pulling on string Reaches persistently for toys out of reach		Makes consonant sounds *t, d, w* Listens selectively to familiar words Utterances signal emphasis and emotion Combines syllables, such as *dada*, but does not ascribe meaning to them	Exhibits increasing anxiety over loss of parent, particularly mother, and fear of strangers Responds to word "no" Dislikes dressing, diaper change
9	Eruption of upper lateral incisor may begin	Creeps on hands and knees Sits steadily on floor for prolonged time (10 min) Recovers balance when leaning forward but cannot do so when leaning sideways ■ Pulls self to standing position and stands holding onto furniture (see Fig. 12-8, B and C)	■ Uses thumb and index finger in crude pincer grasp (see Fig. 12-3) Preference for use of dominant hand now evident Grasps third cube Compares two cubes by bringing them together	Localizes sounds by turning head diagonally and directly toward sound Depth perception increasing	Responds to simple verbal commands Comprehends "no-no"	Parent (mother) is increasingly important for own sake Shows increasing interest in pleasing parent Begins to show fears of going to bed and being left alone Puts arms in front of face to avoid having it washed

■ Milestones that represent essential integrative aspects of development that lay the foundation for the achievement of more advanced skills.

TABLE 12-3   GROWTH AND DEVELOPMENT DURING INFANCY—cont'd

AGE (mo)	PHYSICAL	GROSS MOTOR	FINE MOTOR	SENSORY	VOCALIZATION	SOCIALIZATION/COGNITION
10	Labyrinth-righting reflex strongest when infant in prone or supine position; is able to raise head	Can change from prone to sitting position Stands while holding onto furniture, sits by falling down Recovers balance easily while sitting While standing, lifts one foot to take step (see Fig. 12-8, *D*)	Crude release of an object beginning Grasps bell by handle		■ Says "dada," "mama" with meaning Comprehends "bye-bye" May say one word (e.g., "hi," "bye," "no")	Inhibits behavior to verbal command of "no-no" or own name Imitates facial expressions; waves bye-bye Extends toy to another person but will not release it ■ Develops object permanence Repeats actions that attract attention and cause laughter Pulls clothes of another to attract attention Plays interactive games such as pat-a-cake Reacts to adult anger; cries when scolded Demonstrates independence in dressing, feeding, locomotive skills, and testing of parents Looks at and follows picture in book
11	Eruption of lower lateral incisor may begin	When sitting, pivots to reach toward back to pick up an object ■ Cruises or walks holding onto furniture or with both hands held	Explores objects more thoroughly (e.g., clapper inside bell) Has neat pincer grasp Drops object deliberately for it to be picked up Puts one object after another into container (sequential play) Able to manipulate object to remove it from tight-fitting enclosure		Imitates definite speech sounds	Experiences joy and satisfaction when task is mastered Reacts to restrictions with frustration Rolls ball to another on request Anticipates body gestures when familiar nursery rhyme or story is being told (e.g., holds toes and feet in response to "This little piggy went to market") Plays games up-down, "so big," or peek-a-boo Shakes head for "no"
12	■ Birth weight tripled ■ Birth length increased by 50% Head and chest circumference equal (head circumference 46 cm [18 inches]) Has six to eight deciduous teeth Anterior fontanel almost closed Landau reflex fading Babinski reflex disappears Lumbar curve develops; lordosis evident during walking	■ Walks with one hand held Cruises well ■ May attempt to stand alone momentarily; may attempt first step alone Can sit down from standing position without help	Releases cube in cup Attempts to build two-block tower but fails Tries to insert pellet into narrow-necked bottle but fails Can turn pages in book, many at a time	Discriminates simple geometric forms (e.g., circle) Amblyopia may develop with lack of binocularity Can follow rapidly moving object Controls and adjusts response to sound; listens for sound to recur	■ Says three to five words besides "dada," "mama" Comprehends meaning of several words (comprehension always precedes verbalization) Recognizes objects by name Imitates animal sounds Understands simple verbal commands (e.g., "Give it to me," "Show me your eyes")	Shows emotions such as jealousy, affection (may give hug or kiss on request), anger, fear Enjoys familiar surroundings and explores away from parent Is fearful in strange situation; clings to parent May develop habit of "security blanket" or favorite toy Has increasing determination to practice locomotor skills ■ Searches for object even if it has not been hidden, but searches only where object was last seen

■ Milestones that represent essential integrative aspects of development that lay the foundation for the achievement of more advanced skills.

when leaving the room, allowing them to hear one's voice on the telephone, and using transitional objects (e.g., a favorite blanket or toy) reassures them of the parent's continued presence.

This is no less trying but a necessary time for infants, since parents cannot always be with them. An excellent example of necessary separation is bedtime. Fear of going to bed or being left alone in the dark commonly occurs during the second half of the first year. Fear at bedtime is only one of the many bedtime problems that can occur in young children (see p. 493 and Chapter 15).

Limit Setting and Discipline

As infants' motor skills advance and mobility increases, parents are faced with the need to set safe limits (see Nurse's Role in Injury Prevention, p. 516). Although numerous disciplinary techniques exist, some are more appropriate for this age than others. Parents can begin discipline using a negative voice and stern eye contact. When parents need to use more definitive measures, one of the most effective approaches is time-out. The basic principles are the same as those discussed in Chapter 3, except that the place for time-out needs to correspond with the child's abilities. For example, the playpen is better for most infants than a chair. Although parents may be concerned with instituting discipline during infancy, it is important to stress that the earlier effective disciplinary methods are employed, the easier it is to continue these approaches.

Parents must recognize the infant's cognitive and behavioral limitations and implement adequate protection from hazards because infants and toddlers do not understand a cause-and-effect relationship between dangerous objects and physical harm. Additionally, parents may need reassurance that their infant's behavior is exploratory, not oppositional (at this age) and primarily centered on needs for warmth, love, food, security, and comfort. Parents may verbalize that comforting the infant too much or meeting his or her needs will result in a spoiled child; there is no substantial evidence that meeting the infant's basic needs will result in such behaviors later in life. Children will innately test limits and explore during the exploratory phase of growth; instead of discouraging exploration, parents should provide safe alternatives, put away dangerous household items, and give children consistent discipline and nurturing. Effective teaching for injury prevention optimally begins in infancy by helping parents understand their child's normal development. It must be reiterated continually that infants cry because a need is not being met, not to intentionally irritate an adult. The fussy or irritable infant is a potential victim of shaken baby syndrome (or other bodily harm), since adults and caretakers may not understand the nature of the infant's crying.

A common concern of parents is that too much attention can spoil a child. Many of the recommendations for promoting attachment, such as attending to the infant's needs to establish trust, accepting fear of strangers and separation from parent, and holding and rocking the crying child, are described by parents as methods of spoiling. However, research on parents' response to crying during early infancy does not support the contention that picking up a crying baby leads to spoiling. Ainsworth (1982) found that the amount an infant cried during the first 3 months had no correlation with the frequency of

crying during the rest of the first year. However, the degree of maternal responsiveness to crying did. Parents who were less responsive, such as not picking up the infant immediately on crying, had infants who cried more than those of parents who responded promptly to crying. Parents of colicky infants less than 3 months old who responded to the crying with increased attention successfully decreased the overall crying time.

If too much attention does not cause spoiling in early infancy, parents need to understand what "spoiling" really is and how it differs from normal behavior that may mimic aspects of spoiling. The spoiled child syndrome has been defined as "excessive self-centered and immature behavior, resulting from the failure of parents to enforce consistent, age-appropriate limits" (McIntosh, 1989). Spoiled children demand to have their own way; are inconsiderate of others; and have intrusive, obstructive, and manipulative behavior. Indulging children, when combined with clear expectations and limits, does not cause spoiling. However, indulgence with failure to provide guidelines for acceptable behavior can result in a child who expects to get her or his way all the time. Such expectations are unrealistic and do not help the child in the transition to older childhood, adolescence, and adulthood.

Several age-related normal behaviors and child characteristics can be mistaken for evidence of spoiling:

- Crying during early infancy that may or may not be associated with colic
- Toddler behaviors such as negativism, persistent exploration, and temper tantrums
- Children with difficult temperaments or ADHD
- Children experiencing extreme stress from marital discord; physical, emotional, or sexual abuse; substance abuse; or mental illness in a parent

With anticipatory guidance regarding expected but challenging behaviors and situations that may produce extreme stress in children, parents should feel comfortable in loving their infant without fear of spoiling. However, as the infant gets older, parents may need assistance in providing limits that prevent normal, disruptive behaviors, such as temper tantrums, from becoming problems.

Alternative Child Care Arrangements

For many parents, especially working mothers, locating safe and competent child care facilities for the infant is a challenge—one that is compounded by the number of mothers working outside the home. Over the past 40 years a marked shift has occurred in child care arrangements, with fewer children cared for at home and more children cared for in group centers or other settings.

Types of Child Care

The basic types of care are in-home care, either in the parents' or caregivers' home (family daycare), and center-based care, usually in a daycare center. In-home care may consist of a full-time baby-sitter who lives in the home, a full-time baby-sitter who comes to the home, cooperative arrangements such as exchange baby-sitting, and family daycare. A licensed small family child daycare home typically provides care and protection for up to six children for part of a day and does not include informal arrangements such as exchange baby-sitting or caregivers in the child's own home. The six children include the family daycare provider's own children younger than 5 years of age living in the home. Large family child care homes may provide care for 8 to 12 children. Unfortunately, many family daycare homes operate without a license and may care for large numbers of infants without adequate staff and facilities.

Child center-based care usually refers to a licensed daycare facility that provides care for six or more children, for 6 or more hours a day. Work-based group care is another option that is becoming increasingly popular as employers recognize the benefit of providing high-quality and convenient child care to their employees. Sick-child care may also be available for times when the youngster is ill. Such programs are often located in community hospitals or in work settings.

Guiding Parents in Selecting Child Care

An important nursing responsibility is guiding parents in locating suitable facilities that have a well-qualified staff. State licensing agencies can help parents identify daycare centers that accept children of specific age-groups and are convenient to home and work. Their records are available to the public and provide reports from the health, safety, and fire departments; periodic evaluations from the licensing agency; complaints filed against the center; and qualification of the center's employees. State-licensed programs are supposed to follow established standards, which represent the minimum requirements and safeguards. However, enforcement of the standards is sometimes inadequate. Early childhood programs may also belong to a voluntary accreditation system, the National Academy of Early Childhood Programs/NAEYC,* which serves as a model for optimum care. References from other parents are also helpful, provided they have investigated the center carefully and have remained involved with the agency's activities.

Other areas for parents to evaluate are the center's daily program, teacher qualifications, nurturing qualities of caregivers, student-to-staff ratio, discipline policy, environmental safety precautions, provision of meals, sanitary conditions, adequate indoor and outdoor space per child, and fee schedule. Although fees vary considerably, a program that charges a minimum fee may also be providing minimum services. In terms of an overall evaluation, there is no substitute for personal observation of the facility. Parents should arrange to meet the director and some of the employees, especially those who would be caring for the child. Resources to familiarize parents with characteristics of quality child care and checklists to systematically evaluate the center and compare it with other facilities can help parents make successful choices. At all times

the parent should have the right to visit the child, and regular conferences should occur to review the child's progress.

Parents should apply the same conscientious attention to locating competent baby-sitters. References from other employers are essential, and there is no substitute for observing the interaction between the individual and the child. Although very young infants need little if any preparation for the introduction of a new caregiver, older infants may benefit from a gradual placement to reduce stranger fear. (See Preschool and Kindergarten Experience, Chapter 15.)

One of the areas that is increasingly important in selecting child care is the center's health practices; however, parents often do not check the center for health and safety features. Children in daycare centers, especially children under age 3 years, have more illnesses—including diarrhea, otitis media, respiratory tract infections (especially if the caregiver smokes), hepatitis A, meningitis, and cytomegalovirus—than children cared for in their home (National Institute of Child Health and Human Development Early Child Care Research Network, 2001). The strongest predictor of risk of illness is the number of unrelated children in the room. Proactive infection control measures and education of staff have been effective in reducing the incidence of upper respiratory tract infections, diarrhea, and rotavirus (Kotch, Isbell, Weber, et al, 2007). Families who have children in out-of-home child care lose an estimated 13 days of work per year as a result of infections (Brady, 2005). Parents should inquire about the center's policy regarding the attendance and care of sick children.

Nurses play an important role in infection control and injury prevention. Not only can they advise parents on evaluating a center's sanitary and safety practices, but they can also take an active part in educating staff in measures to minimize the transmission of infection and injury (Evers, 2002). For example, in centers caring for children who are not toilet trained, reducing environmental contamination with urine and feces is an important infection control issue. Guidelines for diapering and toileting recommended by the American Academy of Pediatrics, American Public Health Association, and Maternal and Child Health Bureau (2002) include (see Fig. 16-8):

- Washing hands by children and personnel after diaper changing and toileting
- Using disposable paper diapers, single-unit reusable cloth diapers with an inner cotton lining attached to an outer waterproof cover, or single-unit reusable systems with an inner cotton lining attached to an outer waterproof covering that are changed as a unit
- Changing diapers as soon as they are soiled
- Never rinsing reusable diapers, although fecal contents can be flushed down the toilet
- Sending soiled reusable diapers or clothing home in a sealed plastic bag
- Cleaning the diaper-changing surface properly after each use and using it only for this purpose
- Using child-sized toilets or access to steps and modified toilet seats that provide easier maintenance
- Sanitizing toilets, seats, potty chairs, and diaper-changing areas with a fresh solution of 1:64 dilution of household bleach (one quarter cup of bleach diluted in 1 gallon of water), applied for 2 minutes and rinsed

*Information about accreditation criteria and procedures of the National Academy for Early Childhood Program Accreditation/NAEYC is available from the National Association for the Education of Young Children, 1313 L St. NW, Suite 500, Washington, DC 20005; 800-424-2460 or 202-232-8777; www.naeyc.org. These criteria are excellent guidelines for evaluating child care facilities. Other resources are (1) *Child Care: What's Best for Your Family* and a number of other child care articles and pamphlets from American Academy of Pediatrics, 141 Northwest Point Blvd., Elk Grove Village, IL 60007; 847-434-4000; http://aap.org; and (2) Child Care Aware, 800-424-2246; www.childcareaware.org.

The American Academy of Pediatrics' *2009 Red Book: Report of the Committee of Infectious Diseases* (2009b) contains additional infection control guidelines regarding daycare hand washing; cleaning sleep equipment, toys, and food; care of pets; and conditions or illnesses for which children should be kept out of daycare to prevent the spread of illness.

The nurse should encourage parents to discuss their feelings regarding the child's separation from home. Practical ways of alleviating anxiety and improving the quality of time spent with the child include planning a household schedule that divides major chores into smaller ones and combining household duties with a childcare activity, such as cleaning the bathroom while the child is bathing. Providing time for relaxation and activity with the child is another way to reduce anxiety.

Thumb Sucking and Use of Pacifier

Sucking is the infant's chief pleasure and may not be satisfied by breast- or bottle-feeding. It is such a strong need that infants who are deprived of sucking, such as those with a cleft lip repair, will suck on their tongues. Some newborns are born with sucking blisters on their hands from in utero sucking activity.

Problems arise when parents are overly concerned about the sucking of the fingers, thumb, or pacifier and attempt to restrain this natural tendency. Before giving advice, nurses should investigate the parents' feelings and base guidance on this information.

Pacifier use, particularly in the early days after birth and in the birth hospital, has gained considerable attention in the scientific literature. Biancuzzo (2003) suggests that it cannot be stated with absolute certainty that pacifier use is bad in every situation but warns of a potential harm in the use of pacifiers based on available evidence. Furthermore, she cautions health care workers to be informed regarding potential harm in pacifier use and to inform parents of the potential. Lawrence and Lawrence (2005), as well as other experts in breast-feeding, recommend that health care workers not introduce pacifiers to breast-fed infants unless the parent requests it (see Research Focus box). Pacifier use is not recommended as part of the Baby-Friendly Hospital Initiative (see p. 261).

RESEARCH FOCUS

Pacifier Use and Breast-Feeding

O'Connor, Tanabe, Siadaty, and colleagues (2009) reviewed 29 studies and concluded that pacifier use did not adversely affect breast-feeding duration or exclusivity. They further concluded that pacifier use and shortened breast-feeding in many studies likely represented a number of other complex factors such as breast-feeding difficulties or intent to wean.

Pacifier use has been associated with an increased risk of otitis media in several studies (Niemela, Pihakari, Pokka, et al, 2000; Rovers, Numans, Langenbach, et al, 2008). The American Academy of Pediatrics and American Academy of Family Physicians recommend use of pacifier during the first 6 months because of the benefit in regard to pain management and prevention of sudden infant death syndrome (SIDS), but recommend the child be weaned from the pacifier during the second 6 months of life (Sexton and Natale, 2009). Pacifier use during

painful procedures in neonates has been shown to produce an analgesic effect. (See Chapter 7, Neonatal Pain.)

A review of studies by the Joanna Briggs Institute (2005) found an association between pacifier use in infancy and a reduction in breast-feeding and exclusive breast-feeding. However, the authors concluded that pacifier use did not cause a reduction in breast-feeding; rather it was a "marker for socioeconomic, demographic, psychosocial and cultural factors that determine pacifier use and breastfeeding." In addition, the researchers examined studies related to pacifier use and prevention of SIDS; infants put to sleep with a pacifier had a *reduced* risk of SIDS. Because of the limited number of studies correlating pacifier use and increased risk of infections or dental malocclusion, the authors were unable to make any recommendations for or against pacifier use in relation to these practices (Joanna Briggs Institute, 2005).

The American Academy of Pediatrics, Task Force on Sudden Infant Death Syndrome (2005), recommends limited pacifier use in infants, citing the strong evidence for pacifier use and its protective effect in SIDS reduction. The exact mechanism involved in the protection for SIDS is not known. Still, pacifier use should not replace actual feeding or suckling; prohibiting pacifier use will not ensure an increase in the length of breast-feeding; and there should be an emphasis on allowing the infant to control the pace, frequency, and termination of feeding rather than allowing the pacifier (or anything else) to become the focus of the interaction.

To decrease dependence on nonnutritive sucking in young infants, sucking pleasure can be increased by prolonging feeding time. Also, the parent's excessive use of the pacifier to calm the child should be explored. It is not unusual for parents to place a pacifier in the infant's mouth as soon as crying begins, thus reinforcing a pattern of distress-relief.

If the child uses a pacifier, stress safety considerations in purchasing one. Caution parents against altering a pacifier, thus making it more dangerous (see Aspiration of Foreign Objects, p. 510). During infancy and early childhood there is no need to restrain nonnutritive sucking of the fingers. Malocclusion may occur if thumb sucking persists past approximately 4 years of age, or when the permanent teeth erupt. Some parents may perceive pacifiers as less damaging because they are discarded by 2 to 3 years of age, whereas thumb sucking may persist well into school-age years. Both pacifier use and thumb sucking may also have significant cultural variations. Thumb sucking reaches its peak at age 18 to 20 months and is most prevalent when the child is hungry, tired, or feeling insecure. Persistent thumb sucking in a listless, apathetic child always warrants investigation. It may be a sign of an emotional problem between parent and child or of boredom, isolation, and lack of stimulation.

At the time of this writing, there is no evidence that pacifier use and nonnutritive sucking in *preterm infants* has any effect on the initiation and length of breast-feeding. Nonnutritive sucking should not be withheld from preterm infants, especially when used in conjunction with concentrated sucrose for pain management.

Teething

One of the more difficult periods in the infant's (and parents') life is the eruption of the deciduous (primary) teeth, often

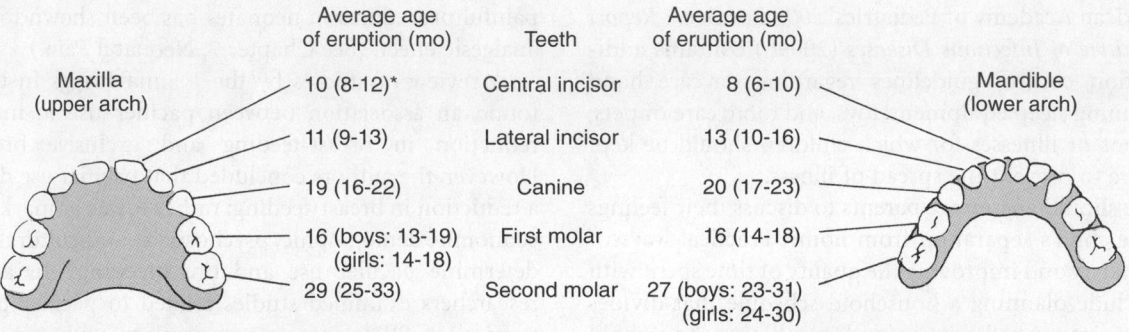

Fig. 12-12 Sequence of eruption of primary teeth. *Range represents ±1 standard deviation or 67% of subjects studied. (Data from McDonald RE, Avery DR: *Dentistry for the child and adolescent,* ed 6, St Louis, 1994, Mosby.)

referred to as teething. The age of tooth eruption shows considerable variation among children, but the order of their appearance is fairly regular and predictable (Fig. 12-12). The first primary teeth to erupt are the lower central incisors, which appear at approximately 6 to 8 months of age. These are followed closely by the upper central incisors. A quick guide to assessment of deciduous teeth during the first 2 years is: Age of the child in months − 6 = Number of teeth. For example: 8 months of age − 6 = 2 teeth at this time.

The exact mechanisms responsible for the eruption of teeth are not fully understood. The growth of the root, dentin, and pulp of the tooth; the pressure exerted against the periodontal tissue; and hormonal control of pituitary growth hormone and thyroid hormone are some of the theories under investigation.

Teething is a physiologic process. Some discomfort is common as the crown of the tooth breaks through the periodontal membrane. Some children show minimum evidence of teething, such as drooling, increased finger sucking, or biting on hard objects. Others are irritable and have difficulty sleeping, mild temperature elevation, ear rubbing, and decreased appetite for solid foods. Generally, signs of illness such as fever (>39° C [102° F]), vomiting, or diarrhea are not symptoms of teething but of illness and may warrant further investigation. Anderson (2004) suggests that frequent waking periods are related to environmental, behavioral, or developmental changes rather than teething.

Because teething pain is a result of inflammation, cold is soothing. Giving the child a frozen teething ring or an ice cube wrapped in a washcloth helps relieve the inflammation. Several nonprescription topical anesthetic ointments are available, such as Baby Orajel, although parents and health care workers should be aware of the risks of using topical anesthetic products (absorption rates vary in infants) (Anderson, 2004). The active ingredient in most of them is benzocaine. If such products are used, advise parents to apply them correctly. If persistent irritability affects sleeping and feeding, systemic analgesics such as acetaminophen or ibuprofen (if *age appropriate*) can be given for no more than 3 days (Anderson, 2004). However, parents should know that this is a temporary measure and should contact the practitioner if symptoms persist or if the child's condition changes. Discourage the use of teething powders or procedures such as cutting or rubbing the gums with aspirin because ingestion of the powder, infection or irritation of the

tissue, or aspiration of the aspirin can occur. Hard candy may cause accidental choking or aspiration and should be avoided at this age.

PROMOTING OPTIMUM HEALTH DURING INFANCY

NUTRITION

Ideally, discussion of optimum nutrition should begin prenatally with the decision to breast- or bottle-feed the newborn. The choice for either is highly individual and is discussed in Chapter 8. This section is primarily concerned with infant nutrition during the next 12 months, when growth needs and developmental milestones ready the child for the introduction of solid foods.

Despite adequate availability of optimum nutrient sources, experts are concerned that infants are not fed appropriately. Infants may be given solid foods when their digestive system is not ready to completely absorb such foods. In addition, drinks that are inappropriate for growing infants may be given in place of enriched infant milk and may only provide "empty" calories and contribute to childhood and adult obesity and place the infant at risk for iron deficiency anemia, vitamin D deficiency, and rickets. A recent survey of infant feeding practices found that about 40% of infants had consumed infant cereal, fruit, or vegetables by 4 months of age, despite recommendations that such foods not be introduced until 4 to 6 months (Grummer-Strawn, Scanlon, and Fein, 2008). In the same study 50% of infants were consuming cake, fried potatoes, candy, and cookies by age 12 months. There is some preliminary evidence that accelerated weight gain in the first 6 months of life may be correlated with obesity later in life (Taveras, Rifas-Shiman, Belfort, et al, 2009). Infant health practices, including nutrition, may have a far-reaching, long-term impact on the child's life. Growth and development could be negatively affected, as could the risk of acquiring certain chronic health conditions. Nurses must be proactive in teaching parents what constitutes appropriate infant nutrition and nutritional habits, which provide the child with an optimum opportunity to grow and develop into a healthy child and adult.

Health care professionals are concerned about the use of complementary and alternative medical therapies in children that may not be as beneficial as publicized in various media sources. One concern is children's intake of megavitamins and herbs. Parents may assume that the word *natural* in reference to ingredients means the product is safe, when this may not be the case. One report cited the home administration of star anise tea to treat colic as the cause of adverse neurologic reactions in seven infants (Ize-Ludlow, Ragone, Bruck, et al, 2004). It is important for nurses to be aware of the effects, availability, and practice of complementary therapies and to be able to cogently discuss their use with parents (Loman, 2003; Niggemann and Grüber, 2003).

The First 6 Months

Human milk is the most desirable complete diet for the infant during the first 6 months. The healthy term infant receiving breast milk from a well-nourished mother usually requires no specific vitamin and mineral supplements, with a few exceptions. Daily supplements of vitamin D and vitamin B_{12} may be indicated if the mother's intake of these vitamins is inadequate. The American Academy of Pediatrics (2008) issued a recommendation that all infants (including those exclusively breast-fed) receive a daily supplement of 400 international units of vitamin D beginning in the first few days of life to prevent rickets and vitamin D deficiency. Vitamin D supplementation should occur until the infant is consuming at least 1 L/day (or 1 quart/day) of vitamin D–fortified formula (American Academy of Pediatrics, 2008). Non-breast-fed infants who are taking less than 1 L/day of vitamin D–fortified formula should also receive a daily vitamin D supplement of 400 international units. If the infant is being exclusively breast-fed after 4 to 6 months (when fetal iron stores are depleted), iron supplementation, which may be accomplished with iron-fortified cereal, is recommended to offset the decrease in iron available in human milk at this time and to enhance erythropoiesis. Infants, whether breast- or bottle-fed, do not require additional fluids, especially water or juice, during the first 4 months of life. Excessive intake of water in infants may result in water intoxication and hyponatremia. Even in hot climates, additional water or fluids are not recommended for breast-fed infants.

Fluoride supplementation in exclusively breast-fed children is not required for the first 6 months because of the risk of dental fluorosis. However, fluoride supplementation may be necessary if the breast-feeding mother's water supply does not contain the required amount of fluoridation (see p. 495).

An acceptable alternative to breast-feeding is commercial iron-fortified formula. Like human milk, it supplies all nutrients needed by the infant for the first 6 months. Unmodified whole cow's milk, low-fat cow's milk, skim milk, other animal milks, and imitation milk drinks are not acceptable as a major source of nutrition for infants because of their limited digestibility, increased risk of contamination, and lack of components needed for appropriate growth. Whole milk can cause iron deficiency anemia in infants, possibly as a result of occult gastrointestinal blood loss. Pasteurized whole cow's milk is deficient in iron, zinc, and vitamin C and has a high renal solute load, which makes it undesirable for infants less than 12 months of age (American Academy of Pediatrics, 2009a). Dietary fat should not be restricted in infancy unless under medical supervision. Substituting skim or low-fat milk is unacceptable because the essential fatty acids are inadequate and the solute concentration of protein and electrolytes, such as sodium, is too high.

Honey should be avoided in the first 12 months because of the risk of botulism (see Chapter 40); pacifiers should not be coated with honey to encourage the infant to take it. Socializing the infant to food flavors of the family's culture is common in addition to continuing breast-feeding for 2 to 4 years (see Cultural Competence box). The amount of formula per feeding and the number of feedings per day vary among infants.

Employed mothers can continue breast-feeding with guidance and encouragement.* Encourage mothers to set realistic goals for employment and breast-feeding, with accurate information regarding the costs, risks, and benefits of available feeding options. Barriers encountered by working breast-feeding mothers include lack of employer or co-worker support, unavailable or inadequate facilities for pumping and storing milk, and insufficient time allowed during work time to pump (Rojjanasrirat, 2004). Important themes that emerged in the study by Rojjanasrirat (2004) of working breast-feeding mothers included support (emotional, informational, and instrumental), attitude, and psychologic distress. Many mothers may find that a program of breast-pumping when away from home and bottle-feeding the infant the expressed milk with or without formula supplementation is successful. Expressed breast milk may be stored in the refrigerator (4° C [39° F]) without danger of bacterial contamination for up to 5 days (Lawrence and Lawrence, 2005). Warming expressed milk in a microwave decreases the availability of antiinfective properties and vitamin C and causes a separation of milk layers, which affects fat content (Lawrence and Lawrence, 2005). To prevent oral burns from uneven warming of the milk, breast milk should never be thawed or rewarmed in a microwave oven. To thaw the frozen milk, either place container under a lukewarm water bath (40.5° C [105° F]), use a commercial breast milk warmer, or place in refrigerator overnight.

Although at home the infant may be fed on a demand basis, pumping milk away from home may be needed every 3 to 4 hours to maintain adequate supply. Breast milk may be expressed by hand or pump (manual or electric) and stored in an appropriate air-tight glass or plastic container. Expressed breast milk may be frozen (−18° C [0° F] or lower) for up to 12 months (depending on the type of freezer used), but take care to prevent freezer burn (see Appendix P, protocol no. 8, in

---

🌐 CULTURAL COMPETENCE

Multicultural Feeding Practices

Cultural beliefs and values often influence infant feeding practices. Health care professionals may benefit from understanding the multicultural feeding practices that parents choose for their infant. Traditional feeding practices include offering a variety of liquids or foods, such as sugared wine, water, or honey, during the first few days of life and thereafter.

---

*See also *The CDC Guide to Breastfeeding Interventions* (Shealy, Benton-Davis, and Grummer-Strawn, 2005), which includes information for working and breast-feeding.

Lawrence and Lawrence, 2005, for further guidelines on storing and freezing human milk).

In addition to efficient breast pumping, mothers also need child care by a trusted individual or agency and support and assistance from significant others. Like all breast-feeding mothers, these women must have proper nutrition and rest for adequate lactation. Maternal fatigue is considered the biggest threat to successful breast-feeding in employed mothers (Corbett-Dick and Bezek, 1997). With a schedule of work and child care, careful planning is required to successfully manage the demands of both responsibilities.

The addition of solid foods before 4 to 6 months of age is not recommended. During the early months solid foods are not yet compatible with the ability of the gastrointestinal tract and the infant's nutritional needs. Furthermore feeding solids exposes infants to food antigens that may produce food protein allergy. Despite these recommendations, and lacking scientific evidence to support such practices, many parents introduce solids as early as 2 weeks of age, often adding rice cereal to the formula so the infant will sleep better at night or to enhance weight gain (Morin, 2004).

Developmentally, infants are not ready for solid food. The extrusion (protrusion) reflex is strong and often causes food to be pushed out of the mouth. Infants instinctively suck when given food. Because of their limited motor abilities, infants are unable to deliberately push food away or avoid feeding. Therefore early introduction of solids is a type of forced feeding that may lead to excessive weight gain and increased predisposition to allergies and iron deficiency anemia. Caution parents concerning the excessive use of juices and nonnutritive drinks such as fruit-flavored drinks or carbonated beverages (soda or pop) during this period. Many juices and nonnutritive drinks, although readily available to consumers, do not provide sufficient and appropriate caloric intake for infants less than 12 months of age. Such drinks may replace the nutrients in milk (formula) and lead to growth or health problems. Fruit juices are not required in the first 6 months; there are no studies demonstrating benefits of giving fruit juice to infants.

Bottled water for mixing powdered or concentrated formula is a relatively safe alternative to tap water if available tap water has a high content of contaminants such as lead. Do not assume, however, that bottled water is sterile unless specifically stated on the container. Fluoridated bottled water is not necessary for mixing powdered formula unless the local water source is low in fluoride, in which case fluoride supplementation is recommended after age 6 months (see Dental Health, p. 495).

The Second 6 Months

During the second half of the first year human milk or formula continues to be the primary source of nutrition. Fluoride supplementation begins depending on the infant's intake of fluoridated tap water (see p. 495). If breast-feeding is discontinued, a commercial iron-fortified formula should be substituted. Formulas specially marketed for older infants, or follow-up formulas, offer no advantages over other infant formulas and provide excessive protein (American Academy of Pediatrics, 2009a).

Although microwaving formula bottles and baby food is not recommended (Akers and Groh-Wargo, 2005), it remains a

common practice. There is no scientific evidence that infants prefer warm milk (Akers and Groh-Wargo, 2005); however, most infants usually reject cold milk straight from the refrigerator. The nurse should give the family guidelines for microwave heating of refrigerated formula. These guidelines do not apply to human milk (see Family-Centered Care box).

FAMILY-CENTERED CARE
Microwave Heating of Refrigerated Infant Formula

Before Heating
Heat only 4 oz or more.
Heat only refrigerated formula.
Always stand the bottle up.
Always leave bottle top uncovered to allow heat to escape (steam may build up in a closed bottle or plastic bag).

Heating Instructions (Full Power)
For 4-oz bottles: Heat for no more than 30 seconds.
For 8-oz bottles: Heat for no more than 45 seconds.

Serving Instructions
Always replace nipple assembly; invert 10 times (vigorous shaking is unnecessary).
Formula should be cool to the touch; formula warm to the touch may be too hot to serve.
Always test formula; place several drops on your tongue or on top of the hand (not the inside wrist).

From Sigman-Grant M, Bush G, Anantheswaran R: Microwave heating of infant formula: a dilemma resolved, *Pediatrics* 90(3):414, 1992.

The major change in feeding habits is the addition of solid foods to the infant's diet. Physiologically and developmentally, the infant 4 to 6 months of age is in a transition period. By this time the gastrointestinal tract has matured sufficiently to handle more complex nutrients and is less sensitive to potentially allergenic foods. Tooth eruption is beginning and facilitates biting and chewing. The extrusion reflex has disappeared, and swallowing is more coordinated to allow the infant to accept solids easily. Head control is well developed, which permits infants to sit with support and purposely turn the head away to communicate a lack of interest in food. Voluntary grasping and improved eye-hand coordination gradually allow infants to pick up finger foods and feed themselves. Their increasing independence is evident in their desire to hold the bottle and try to "help" during feeding. The major developmental milestones associated with feeding are listed in Box 12-4.

Selection and Preparation of Solid Foods

The choice of solid foods to introduce first is variable but should meet the reasons for feeding solids, such as supplying nutrients not found in formula or breast milk. Iron-fortified infant cereal is generally introduced first because of its high iron content (7 mg/3 tbsp of prepared dry cereal). Commercially prepared ready-to-serve dry cereals for infants include rice, barley, oatmeal, and high-protein cereals. Rice is usually suggested as an initial food because of its easy digestibility and low allergenic potential. Some of the commercial baby cereals are combined with fruit. These preparations have little nutritional benefit and are more expensive. Parents should add new foods

BOX 12-4 DEVELOPMENTAL MILESTONES ASSOCIATED WITH FEEDING

Birth
Sucking, rooting, and swallowing reflexes
Feels hunger and indicates desire for food by crying; expresses satiety by falling asleep
Strong extrusion reflex

3 to 4 Months
Extrusion reflex fading
Beginning eye-hand coordination

4 to 5 Months
Can approximate lips to the rim of a cup but may spill contents

5 to 6 Months
Can use fingers to feed self a cracker

6 to 7 Months
Chews and bites
May hold own bottle, but may not drink from it (prefers for it to be held)

7 to 9 Months
Refuses food by keeping lips closed; has preferences
Holds a spoon and plays with it during feeding
May drink from a straw
Drinks from a cup with assistance

9 to 12 Months
Picks up small morsels of food (finger foods) and feeds self
Holds own bottle and drinks from it
Drinks from a cup but spills some of the contents
Uses a spoon with much spilling

one at a time; therefore parents should avoid cereal combinations when beginning a new grain.

Infant cereal may be mixed with formula in a bowl until whole milk is given. If the infant is breast-fed, the cereal is mixed with expressed breast milk or water. After 6 months of age, fruit juices can be mixed with the dry cereal. The vitamin C content of the juice enhances the absorption of iron in the cereal. Because of their benefit as a source of iron, continue infant cereals until the child is 18 months of age.

Parents can offer fruit juice from a cup as a rich source of vitamin C and as a substitute for milk for one feeding a day. Avoid certain juices (e.g., apple, pear, prune, sweet cherry, peach, and grape) because they contain high amounts of fructose and sorbitol and may cause abdominal pain, diarrhea, or bloating in some children. White grape juice (≤5 oz/day) is reported to be better absorbed and safe for infants this age without causing gastrointestinal distress (Calamaro, 2000). Some researchers have found fruit juice, particularly apple juice, to exacerbate colic and diarrhea, possibly because of carbohydrate malabsorption (Duro, Rising, Cedillo, et al, 2002; Moukarzel, Lesicka, and Ament, 2002). The American Academy of Pediatrics (2009a) recommends that fruit juice intake not exceed 4 to 6 oz/day in children 1 to 6 years of age and that juices not be given to infants less than 4 to 6 months old; only 100% fruit juice should be offered. Because heat destroys vitamin C, juice is not warmed. Juice containers are always kept covered and refrigerated to prevent further vitamin loss. In addition, fruit juice may be offered from a cup, rather than a bottle, to prevent the development of dental caries. (See Low-Cariogenic Diet, Chapter 14.)

The order of introduction of other foods is arbitrary. A common sequence is strained fruits followed by vegetables and, finally, meats. Some clinicians prefer to add vegetables before fruit. Only one solid is introduced every 5 to 7 days so that a reaction to a particular food can be distinguished. If foods are introduced early, citrus fruits, meats, and eggs are still delayed until after 6 months of age because of their potential to cause allergy. At 6 months foods such as a cracker or zwieback can be offered as finger and teething food. By 8 to 9 months junior foods and nutritious finger foods such as a firmly cooked vegetable, raw pieces of fruit (except grapes), or cheese can be given. By 1 year well-cooked table foods are served.

The introduction of solid foods into the infant's diet at this age is primarily for taste and chewing experience. The majority of the infant's caloric needs come from the primary milk source (human or formula); therefore solids should not be perceived as a substitute for milk until the child is older than 12 months. Portion sizes may vary according to the infant's taste. In general, 1 tbsp per year of age (i.e., ½ to ¾ tbsp for most infants under 12 months) is adequate for most infants. In most cases 2 tbsp may be served, but because of the infant's focus on the texture and feel of the food, smaller amounts than those served will be consumed. Another consideration for smaller portions is the concern over feeding habits in early childhood and obesity; early feeding of smaller portions may help prevent the "clean your plate" or "eat all your food or you can't get down from the table" concepts, which are known to contribute to overeating in later life. The addition of solids to the diet of exclusively breast-fed infants apparently does not significantly increase overall caloric intake or weight gain (Dewey, 2001).

In general, low-calorie milk and foods should be avoided in infants and toddlers unless a strict medically prescribed diet is required. The infant's growth during this phase is crucial to future development, and dietary fat should be curtailed with great caution. At the same time it is important to recognize that certain types of dietary fat are unacceptable for infants; fried potatoes, candy, ice cream, cake, soda pop and other sweetened drinks, and other such items do not constitute an appropriate amount of fat intake and may contribute to childhood obesity. One suggestion is to limit the *amount* (serving size) of dietary fat in foods provided rather than eliminate them altogether, especially during infancy.

Commercially prepared baby foods are the most common types of food served to infants in the United States. They are convenient and usually contain no added salt or sugar, but they are relatively expensive. An alternative is preparing baby foods at home, which is simple and inexpensive.

When solid foods are introduced, the safety and digestibility of the selections must be considered. Raw fruits with seeds, vegetables, and nuts are hazardous for infants and young children because of the danger of aspiration. Beans, grain cereals, and vegetables should be served well cooked and mashed during infancy (to prevent choking).

Preferably, home-prepared infant foods should be fresh or frozen, since canned foods, except for those prepared for infants, may contain excessive sodium or sugar. If sweetening is needed, refined sugar can be used, but avoid honey and corn syrup because of the risk of infant botulism.

Food Storage

Storage of commercial baby food requires a few simple rules. Unopened jars can remain on the shelf until the manufacturer's expiration date, which is on the container. Opened jars are refrigerated and can be used for a couple of days. If the infant does not finish a jar of food at one time, a portion of the food is removed from the jar using a clean spoon. Otherwise, if the infant is fed straight from the jar, the dirty spoon introduces bacteria and salivary enzymes that begin to digest unused portions of the food. Dried baby foods are prepared in individual portions, thus eliminating storage problems and waste of unused food.

Method of Introduction

When the spoon is first introduced, infants often push it away and appear dissatisfied. Some patience and skill are required to overcome this initial response. Food that is placed on the front of the tongue and pushed out is simply scooped up and refed. As infants become accustomed to the spoon, they will more eagerly accept the food and eventually open the mouth in anticipation (or keep it closed in dislike). Because the introduction of food is a new experience, spoon feeding should be attempted after ingestion of some breast milk or formula to associate this activity with a pleasurable and satisfying experience. Trying to introduce a food after the entire milk feeding is generally useless because the infant is satiated and has no inclination to try something new.

After several spoon feedings, food can be introduced at the beginning of a meal. Provided that atopy is not a concern, it is best to introduce many different foods during the first year, when the infant is more likely to eat them because of a hearty appetite resulting from a rapid growth rate. During the toddler years, eating becomes less of an adventure, and strong food preferences become evident.

Each new food item is introduced at an interval of 5 to 7 days to allow for identification of food allergies. New foods are fed in small amounts, from 1 tsp to a few tablespoons. As the amount of solid food increases, the quantity of milk decreases to less than 1 L/day to prevent overfeeding.

Because feeding is a learning process as well as a means of providing nutrition, new foods are given alone to allow the child to learn new tastes and textures. For healthy infants, food should not be mixed in the bottle and fed through a nipple with a large hole. This deprives the child of the pleasure of learning new tastes and developing a discriminating palate. It can also cause problems with poor chewing of food later in life because of lack of experience. The Family-Centered Care box gives guidelines for the introduction of new foods.

FAMILY-CENTERED CARE

Feeding During the First Year

Birth to 6 Months
Breast-Feeding
This is the most desirable complete diet for first half of the year.*
A recommended supplement is oral vitamin D (400 international units/day). (See Chapter 8, Human Milk.)

Formula
Iron-fortified commercial formula is a complete food for the first half of the year.*

6 to 12 Months
Breast- or Bottle-Feeding
After the child is 6 months of age, formula requires fluoride supplements (0.25 mg/day) when the concentration of fluoride in the drinking water is below 0.3 ppm.

Solid Foods
Solid foods may be started by 5 to 6 months of age.
First foods are strained, pureed, or finely mashed.
Finger foods such as teething crackers, raw fruit, or vegetables can be introduced by 6 to 7 months.
Chopped table food or commercially prepared junior foods can be started by 9 to 12 months.
With the exception of cereal, the order of introducing foods is variable; a recommended sequence is weekly introduction of a new food, beginning with fruit, then vegetables, and then meat. (Some clinicians prefer to introduce vegetables first.)
Avoid foods that have potential for choking: hot dogs, nuts, grapes, raw carrots, popcorn, and hard candies.

Method of Introduction
Introduce solids when infant is hungry.
Begin spoon feeding by pushing food to back of tongue because of infant's natural tendency to thrust tongue forward.

Use small spoon with straight handle; begin with 1 or 2 tsp of food; gradually increase to about 1 tbsp per year of age.
Introduce one food at a time, usually at intervals of 5 to 7 days, to identify food allergies.
Never introduce foods by mixing them with the formula in the bottle.

Cereal
Introduce commercially prepared iron-fortified infant cereals and administer daily until 18 months.
Rice cereal is usually introduced first because of its low allergenic potential.
Discontinue supplemental iron once cereal is given.

Fruits and Vegetables
Applesauce, bananas, and pears are usually well tolerated.
Avoid fruits and vegetables marketed in cans that are not specifically designed for infants because of variable and sometimes high lead content and addition of salt, sugar, and preservatives.
Offer diluted fruit juice only from a cup, not a bottle, to reduce the development of bottle caries (limit to ≤4 oz daily).

Meat, Fish, and Poultry
Avoid fatty meats (sausage, wieners).
Prepare by baking, broiling, steaming, or poaching.
Include organ meats such as liver, which has a high iron, vitamin A, and vitamin B complex content.
If soup is given, be sure all ingredients are familiar to child's diet.
Avoid commercial meat-vegetable combinations because protein is low.

Eggs and Cheese
Serve egg yolk hard boiled and mashed, soft cooked, or poached.
Introduce egg white in small quantities (1 tsp) toward end of first year to detect an allergy.
Use cheese as a substitute for meat and as finger food.

---

*Breast-feeding or commercial formula feeding for up to 12 months of age is recommended. After 1 year, whole cow's milk can be given if there is no history of atopy.

If older infants suddenly refuse to eat, the feeding process should be investigated. It is not unusual for an 11-month-old infant to become stubborn, push the spoon away, and refuse to open the mouth. The child may not be content with having a spoon to play with while someone else does the feeding. Helping parents understand the child's growing need for independence may prevent many temper tantrums and power struggles later on.

Weaning

Defined as the process of giving up one method of feeding for another, weaning usually refers to relinquishing the breast or bottle for a cup. In Western societies this is generally regarded as a major task for infants and is often seen as a potentially traumatic experience. It is psychologically significant because the infant is required to give up a major source of oral pleasure and gratification.

Other cultural groups define weaning in relation to significant life events (e.g., teething) or reaching a specific age. No one time for weaning is best for every child, but generally most infants show signs of readiness during the second half of the first year. It is recommended that weaning occur with the infant's needs as a guide (Lawrence and Lawrence, 2005). Infants have learned that good things come from a spoon. Their increasing desire for freedom of movement may lessen their desire to be held close for feedings. They are acquiring more control over their actions and can easily manipulate a cup to their lips (even if it is held upside down!). Imitation becomes a powerful motivator by age 8 or 9 months, and they enjoy using a cup or glass like others do.

Weaning should be gradual by replacing one bottle- or breast-feeding at a time. The nighttime feeding is usually the last feeding to be discontinued. It is advisable to never allow a child to take a bottle of milk to bed; this is a major cause of baby bottle caries in deciduous teeth. If breast-feeding ends before 5 or 6 months of age, weaning should be to a bottle to provide for the infant's continued sucking needs. If discontinued later, weaning can be directly to a cup, especially by age 12 to 14 months. Any liquid containing sucrose or other sugars, such as fruit juice, should be given in a cup.

SLEEP AND ACTIVITY

Sleep patterns vary among infants, with active infants typically sleeping less than milder children. Generally, by 3 to 4 months of age most infants have developed a nocturnal pattern of sleep that lasts from 9 to 11 hours. The total daily sleep is approximately 15 hours. In a study of Swiss children Iglowstein, Jenni, Molinari, and colleagues (2003) found that the average number of hours of sleep in 6 month olds was 14.2. Consolidation of nocturnal sleep hours occurred during the first 12 months with decreasing daytime sleep and increasing nighttime sleep (approximately 11.7 hours) by 1 year of age. The number of naps per day varies, but infants may take one or two naps by the end of the first year. Daytime naps usually decline during the toddler years to no daytime naps by preschool age. Breast-fed infants usually sleep for shorter periods, with more frequent waking, especially during the night, than do bottle-fed infants (Quillin and Glenn, 2004). Average total

sleep for 4-week-old infants in this study was 14 hours. (For a discussion of sleep position, see Sudden Infant Death Syndrome, Chapter 13.)

Most infants are naturally active and need no encouragement to be mobile. Problems can arise when devices such as playpens, strollers, commercial swings, and walkers are used excessively to limit the infant's naturally curious exploratory nature and activity or to be a "sitter" while the parent is otherwise occupied. These items restrict movement and prevent infants from exploring and developing necessary gross motor skills. Contrary to popular belief, walkers do not enhance coordination, and they are dangerous if tipped over or placed near the top of stairs, porches, decks, in-ground pools, floor furnaces, and other hazardous surfaces. The American Academy of Pediatrics, Committee on Injury and Poison Prevention (2001), recommended a ban on the sale of infant walkers with wheels because of the large number of injuries.

Sleep Problems

A number of sleep problems occur in small children. The two major categories are the dyssomnias: the child has trouble either falling or staying asleep at night, or has difficulty staying awake during the day. The second category, parasomnias, are characterized as confusional arousals, sleep-walking, sleep terrors, nightmares, and rhythmic movement disorders. These typically occur in children 3 to 8 years old (Ward, Rankin, and Lee, 2007) and decline in incidence as the child matures (Davis, Parker, and Montgomery, 2004). This discussion focuses on minor sleep issues in infants such as refusal to go to sleep or frequent waking during the night. Later the text will discuss other sleep disturbances such as obstructive sleep-disordered breathing and sleep terrors.

Concerns regarding sleep are common during infancy. Sometimes these concerns are as basic as parents' questioning whether the infant needs additional sleep. In this case it is best to investigate the reason for their concern, stressing the individual needs of each child. Infants who are active during wakeful periods and growing normally are sleeping a sufficient amount of time.

However, a number of more serious concerns require intervention. Sleep disturbances of physiologic origin are less common in infants with the exception of colic, which Chapter 13 discusses. The more common sleep disturbances are a learned pattern or developmental characteristic of some infants (Table 12-4). Although many families may report sleep problems typical of these patterns, interventions are offered only when the pattern is disruptive to the family.

Sleep problems in early infancy have also been positively correlated with higher maternal depression scores (Hiscock and Wake, 2001; Hawkins-Walsh, 2003). Therefore nurses must discuss infant sleep problems with the mother (and family) in addition to other developmental aspects of newborn care.

When a parent brings in a child with a sleeping problem, a careful assessment is essential. Charting sleep habits both before and after interventions is also an important strategy. Questions regarding the frequency and duration of waking, the usual bedtime routine, the number of nighttime feedings, the perceived problem (e.g., how much disruption the behavior generates), and the attempted interventions are important in

TABLE 12-4	SELECTED SLEEP DISTURBANCES DURING INFANCY AND EARLY CHILDHOOD
DISORDER AND DESCRIPTION	**MANAGEMENT**
Nighttime Feeding Child has a prolonged need for middle-of-night bottle- or breast-feeding. Child goes to sleep at breast or with bottle. Awakenings are frequent (may be hourly). Child returns to sleep after feeding; other comfort measures (e.g., rocking or holding) are usually ineffective.	Increase daytime feeding intervals to ≥4 hr (may need to be done gradually). Offer last feeding as late as possible at night; may need to gradually reduce amount of formula or length of breast-feeding. Offer no bottles in bed. Put to bed awake. When child is crying, check at progressively longer intervals each night; reassure child but do not hold, rock, take to parents' bed, or give bottle or pacifier.
Developmental Night Crying Child ages 6-12 mo with undisturbed nighttime sleep now awakens abruptly; may be accompanied by nightmares.	Reassure parents that this phase is temporary. Enter room immediately to check on child but keep reassurances brief. Avoid feeding, rocking, taking to parents' bed, or any other routine that may initiate trained night crying.
Refusal to Go to Sleep Child resists bedtime and comes out of room repeatedly. Nighttime sleep may be continuous, but frequent awakenings and refusal to return to sleep may occur and become a problem if parent allows child to deviate from usual sleep pattern.	Evaluate whether hour of sleep is too early (child may resist sleep if not tired). Assist parents in establishing consistent before-bedtime routine and enforcing consistent limits regarding child's bedtime behavior. If child persists in leaving bedroom, close door for progressively longer periods. Use reward system with child to provide motivation.
Trained Night Crying (Inappropriate Sleep Associations) Child typically falls asleep in place other than own bed (e.g., rocking chair or parents' bed) and is brought to own bed while asleep; on awakening, cries until usual routine is instituted (e.g., rocking).	Put child in own bed when awake. If possible, arrange sleeping area separate from other family members. When child is crying, check at progressively longer intervals each night; reassure child but do not resume usual routine.
Nighttime Fears Child resists going to bed or wakes during night because of fears. Child seeks parent's physical presence and falls asleep easily with parent nearby, unless fear is overwhelming.	Evaluate whether hour of sleep is too early (child may fantasize when nothing to do but think in dark room). Calmly reassure frightened child; keeping night-light on may be helpful. Use reward system with child to provide motivation to deal with fears. Avoid patterns that can lead to additional problems (e.g., sleeping with child or taking child to parents' room). If child's fear is overwhelming, consider desensitization (e.g., progressively spending longer time alone; consult professional help for protracted fears). Distinguish between nightmares and sleep terrors (confused partial arousals).

Modified from Ferber R: Behavioral "insomnia" in the child, *Psychiatr Clin North Am* 10(4):641-653, 1987.

planning effective approaches for the specific sleep problem. A common suggestion given for any type of sleep problem, "Let the child cry until falling asleep," is difficult to implement and inappropriate for certain conditions. Once the parents relent and console the child, they have only reinforced the crying.

In a study of children ages 5, 17, and 29 months old, the researchers found significant correlations between the child's lack of consolidated nighttime sleep, parental presence at bedtime, and feeding the child during the night if waking periods occurred (Touchette, Petit, Paquet, et al, 2005). Children who learn to fall asleep on their own at bedtime have longer sustained sleep periods than those who fall asleep with a parent present (Davis, Parker, and Montgomery, 2004). In addition, comforting children outside their own bed at night once they awaken was associated with poor sleep consolidation. Feeding the 5-month-old after awakening at night was associated with fewer consecutive sleep hours (Touchette, Petit, Paquet, et al, 2005). The authors of this study recommend parental presence at bedtime until the child is drowsy, then placing the child in his or her own bed for a night's sleep.

An equally effective approach to night crying, known as **graduated extinction**, is to let the child cry for progressively longer times between brief parental interventions that consist only of reassurance—not rocking, holding, or using the bottle or pacifier. For example, the parents may check on the child every 5 minutes during the first night and progressively extend this interval by 5 minutes on successive nights (Ferber and Kryger, 1995).

Families who cannot tolerate unexpected crying spells while everyone else is asleep can try the two-step approach. Graduated extinction is used during naps and at bedtime until the parents retire. If the child cries during the night, the parents use comforting measures. However, once the child is partially trained, step 2 is initiated—the use of graduated extinction at all times.

The best way to prevent sleep problems is to encourage parents to establish bedtime rituals that do not foster problematic patterns. One of the most constructive is placing infants awake in their own crib. When infants are accustomed to falling asleep somewhere else, such as in their parent's arms, and then being transferred to their crib, they awaken in unfamiliar surroundings and are unable to fall asleep until the routine is repeated. Also, the bed should be used for sleeping only, not as a playpen. It is advisable not to hang playthings over or on the bed; in this way the child associates the bed with sleep, not with activity. Although the interventions described previously and in Table 12-4 are usually successful, it is much easier to prevent the problem with appropriate counseling during the early months of the infant's life.*

DENTAL HEALTH

Good dental hygiene begins with appropriate maternal dental health and counseling during early infancy regarding dietary intake for the promotion of optimal oral hygiene (Douglass, Douglass, and Silk, 2004). Counsel parents early regarding feeding practices that increase the risk of poor dental health. Some of these, as previously mentioned, include avoiding propping the milk bottle or giving the milk bottle in the bed, and avoiding fruit juices in a bottle, especially before 6 months of age.

Once the primary teeth erupt, cleaning should begin. Parents should clean the teeth and gums initially by wiping with a damp cloth; toothbrushing is too harsh for the tender gingiva. The caregiver can stabilize the infant by cradling him or her with one arm and using the free hand to cleanse the teeth. Oral hygiene can be made pleasant by singing or talking to the infant. It is recommended that the infant have a brief oral health examination by 6 months of age from a qualified pediatric health practitioner; infants at high risk for caries are identified and oral health counseling is implemented. It is also recommended that the infant have an established dental home by 1 year of age (American Academy of Pediatric Dentistry, 2009). It is generally recommended that a small, soft-bristled toothbrush be used as more teeth erupt and the infant adjusts to the routine of cleaning. Water is preferred to toothpaste, which the infant will swallow (and if the toothpaste is fluoridated, the infant may ingest excessive amounts of fluoride).

Fluoride, an essential mineral for building caries-resistant teeth, is needed beginning at 6 months of age if the infant does not receive water with adequate fluoride content. The American Academy of Pediatrics, Committee on Nutrition (2009a), recommends that children 6 months to 3 years of age take 0.25 mg fluoride daily if water fluoride content is less than 0.3 ppm. The fluoride dosage has been decreased from earlier recommendations because of an increased occurrence of dental fluorosis from excessive fluoride ingestion. If bottled water is used to reconstitute powdered or concentrated formula, it should either be fluoride free or contain low levels of fluoride.

Dietary considerations are also important because habits begun during infancy tend to continue into later years. Avoid foods with concentrated sugar (sucrose) in the infant's diet. Parents need to be counseled regarding the detrimental effects of frequent and prolonged bottle- or breast-feeding during sleep, when the milk or other fluid, such as juice, bathes the

teeth, producing nursing caries. (See Chapter 14 for a more extensive discussion of dental care, including bottle caries.)

IMMUNIZATIONS

One of the most dramatic advances in pediatrics has been the decline of infectious diseases during the twentieth century because of the widespread use of immunization for preventable diseases. This trend has continued into the twenty-first century with the development of newer vaccines. Although many of the immunizations can be given to individuals of any age, the recommended primary schedule begins during infancy and, with the exception of boosters, is completed during early childhood. Therefore health promotion during infancy includes a discussion of childhood immunizations for diphtheria, tetanus, and pertussis (DTaP, using acellular pertussis); poliovirus; measles, mumps, and rubella (MMR); *Haemophilus influenzae* type b (Hib); hepatitis B virus (HBV); hepatitis A virus (HAV); meningococcal; pneumococcal conjugate vaccine (PCV); influenza (and H1N1); and chickenpox (Var). Selected vaccines generally reserved for children considered at high risk for the disease are discussed here and as appropriate throughout the text. (See Communicable Diseases, Chapter 16, for a discussion of several of the diseases for which vaccines are available.)

To facilitate an understanding of immunizations, key terms are listed in Box 12-5. Although in this discussion the terms *vaccination* and *immunization* are used interchangeably in reference to active immunization, they are not synonymous because the administration of an immunobiologic such as a vaccine cannot automatically be equated with the development of adequate immunity.

Schedule for Immunizations

In the United States two organizations, the Advisory Committee on Immunization Practices (ACIP) of the Centers for Disease Control and Prevention and the Committee on Infectious Diseases of the American Academy of Pediatrics, govern the recommendations for immunization policies and procedures. In Canada, recommendations are from the National Advisory Committee on Immunization under the authority of the Minister of Health and Public Health Agency of Canada. The policies of each committee are recommendations, not rules, and they change as a result of advances in the field of immunology. Nurses need to be knowledgeable about the purpose of each organization, view immunization practices in light of the needs of each individual child and the community, and keep informed of the latest advances and changes in policy.

The recommended age for beginning primary immunizations of infants is at birth or within 2 weeks of birth (Figs. 12-13 and 12-14). Children born preterm should receive the full dose of each vaccine at the appropriate chronologic age. A recommended catch-up schedule for children not immunized during infancy is available at the Centers for Disease Control and Prevention website (**www.cdc.gov/vaccines/recs/schedules/child-schedule.htm**). Table 12-5 describes immunization schedules for Canadian children.

Children who began primary immunization at the recommended age but fail to receive all the doses do not need to begin the series again but instead receive only the missed doses. For

---

*An excellent resource for parents is Ferber R: *Solve your child's sleep problems*, New York, 2006, Simon & Schuster (800-223-2336; **www.simonandschuster.com**). Also available in Spanish.

BOX 12-5   KEY IMMUNIZATION TERMS

Immunization—Inclusive term denoting the process of inducing or providing active or passive immunity artificially by administering an immunobiologic

Immunity—An inherited or acquired state in which an individual is resistant to the occurrence or the effects of a specific disease, particularly an infectious agent

Natural immunity—Innate immunity or resistance to infection or toxicity

Acquired immunity—Immunity from exposure to the invading agent, either bacteria, virus, or toxin

Active immunity—A state where immune bodies are actively formed against specific antigens, either naturally by having had the disease clinically or subclinically or artificially by introducing the antigen into the individual

Passive immunity—Temporary immunity obtained by transfusing immunoglobulins or antitoxins either artificially from another human or an animal that has been actively immunized against an antigen or naturally from the mother to the fetus via the placenta

Antibody—A protein, found mostly in serum, that is formed in response to exposure to a specific antigen

Antigen—A variety of foreign substances, including bacteria, viruses, toxins, and foreign proteins, that stimulate the formation of antibodies

Attenuate—Reduce the virulence (infectiousness) of a pathogenic microorganism by such measures as treating it with heat or chemicals or cultivating it on a certain medium

Immunobiologic—Antigenic substances (e.g., vaccines and toxoids) or antibody-containing preparations (e.g., globulins and antitoxins) from human or animal donors, used for active or passive immunization or therapy

  Vaccine—A suspension of live (usually attenuated) or inactivated microorganisms (e.g., bacteria, viruses, or rickettsiae) or fractions of the microorganism administered to induce immunity and prevent infectious disease or its sequelae

  Toxoid—A modified bacterial toxin that has been made nontoxic but retains the ability to stimulate the formation of antitoxin

  Antitoxin—A solution of antibodies (e.g., diphtheria antitoxin, botulinum antitoxin) derived from the serum of animals immunized with specific antigens and used to confer passive immunity and for treatment

  Immunoglobulin (Ig) or intravenous immunoglobulin (IVIG)—A sterile solution containing antibodies from large pools of human blood plasma; primarily indicated for routine maintenance of immunity of certain immunodeficient persons and for passive immunization against measles and hepatitis A

  Specific immunoglobulins—Special preparations obtained from blood plasma from donor pools preselected for a high antibody content against a specific antigen (e.g., hepatitis B immunoglobulin, varicella zoster immunoglobulin, rabies immunoglobulin, tetanus immunoglobulin, and cytomegalovirus immunoglobulin); as with Ig and IVIG, do not transmit hepatitis B virus, human immunodeficiency virus, or other infectious diseases

Vaccination—Originally referred to inoculation with vaccinia smallpox virus to make a person immune to smallpox; currently denotes physical act of administering any vaccine or toxoid

Herd immunity—A condition in which the majority of the population community is vaccinated and the spread of certain diseases is stopped, since the population that has been vaccinated protects those in the same population who are unvaccinated

Monovalent vaccine—Vaccine designed to vaccinate against a single antigen or organism

Conjugate vaccine—A carrier protein with proven immunologic potential combined with a less antigenic polysaccharide antigen to enhance the type and magnitude of the immune response (e.g., *Haemophilus influenza* type b [Hib])

Combination vaccine—Combination of multiple vaccines into one parenteral form

Polyvalent vaccine—Vaccine designed to vaccinate against multiple antigens or organisms (e.g., meningococcal polysaccharide vaccine [MPSV4])

---

situations in which there is doubt that the child will return for immunization according to the optimum schedule, HBV vaccine (HepB), DTaP, IPV (poliovirus vaccine), MMR, varicella, and Hib vaccines can be administered simultaneously. Parenteral vaccines are given in separate syringes in different injection sites (American Academy of Pediatrics, 2009b).

Recommendations for Routine Immunizations*
Hepatitis B Virus

HBV is a significant pediatric disease because HBV infections that occur during childhood and adolescence can lead to fatal consequences from cirrhosis or liver cancer during adulthood. Up to 90% of infants infected perinatally and 25% to 50% of children infected before age 5 years become HBV carriers. In addition, the incidence of HBV infection increases rapidly during adolescence (American Academy of Pediatrics, 2009b). It is recommended that newborns receive HepB before hospital discharge if the mother is hepatitis B surface antigen (HBsAg) negative. Monovalent HepB should be given as the birth dose, whereas combination vaccine containing HepB may be given for subsequent doses in the series (see also Fig. 12-13, footnote 1). Both full-term and preterm infants born to mothers whose HBsAg status is positive or unknown should receive HepB and hepatitis B immune globulin (HBIG), 0.5 ml, within 12 hours of birth at two different injection sites. Because the immune response to HepB is not optimum in newborns weighing less than 2000 g (4.4 lb), the first HepB dose should be given to such infants at 1 month, as long as the mother's HBsAg status is negative (American Academy of Pediatrics, 2009b). In the event that the preterm infant is given a dose at birth, the current recommendation is that the infant be given the full series (three additional doses) at 1, 2, and 6 months of age. The American Academy of Pediatrics (2009b) also encourages immunization of all children by age 11 years.

In the late 1990s HepB contained small amounts of mercury (thimerosal) as a preservative, which generated concern regarding possible mercury poisoning in infants and led to a subsequent decrease in HepB immunization rates in newborns. However, a preservative-free HepB (Recombivax HB, pediatric-adolescent formulation) is available, and the Centers for Disease Control and Prevention (2005a) strongly recommend that HepB immunization occur in newborns before discharge from the birth hospital. To date, studies have not found any association between thimerosal in vaccines and neurologic developmental disorders such as autism spectrum disorder (DeStefano, 2007; Heron, Golding, and ALSPAC Study Team, 2004).

The vaccine is given intramuscularly in the vastus lateralis in newborns or in the deltoid for older infants and children. Regardless of age, avoid the dorsogluteal site because it has been associated with low antibody seroconversion rates, indicating a

---

*Because of constant changes in the pharmaceutical industry, trade names of single and combination vaccines in this section may differ from those currently available. The reader is encouraged to access the vaccine page of the Center for Biologics Evaluation and Research (CBER) of the Food and Drug Administration for the latest licensed vaccine trade names: **www.fda.gov/BiologicsBloodVaccines/Vaccines/default.htm**.

Recommended Immunization Schedule for Persons Aged 0 Through 6 Years—United States • 2010
For those who fall behind or start late, see the catch-up schedule

Vaccine ▼ Age ►	Birth	1 month	2 months	4 months	6 months	12 months	15 months	18 months	19–23 months	2–3 years	4–6 years
Hepatitis B[1]	HepB	HepB				HepB					
Rotavirus[2]			RV	RV	RV[2]						
Diphtheria, Tetanus, Pertussis[3]			DTaP	DTaP	DTaP	see footnote[3]	DTaP				DTaP
Haemophilus influenzae type b[4]			Hib	Hib	Hib[4]	Hib					
Pneumococcal[5]			PCV	PCV	PCV	PCV				PPSV	
Inactivated Poliovirus[6]			IPV	IPV		IPV					IPV
Influenza[7]						Influenza (Yearly)					
Measles, Mumps, Rubella[8]						MMR		see footnote[8]			MMR
Varicella[9]						Varicella		see footnote[9]			Varicella
Hepatitis A[10]						HepA (2 doses)				HepA Series	
Meningococcal[11]										MCV	

Range of recommended ages for all children except certain high-risk groups

Range of recommended ages for certain high-risk groups

This schedule includes recommendations in effect as of December 15, 2009. Any dose not administered at the recommended age should be administered at a subsequent visit, when indicated and feasible. The use of a combination vaccine generally is preferred over separate injections of its equivalent component vaccines. Considerations should include provider assessment, patient preference, and the potential for adverse events. Providers should consult the relevant Advisory Committee on Immunization Practices statement for detailed recommendations: **http://www.cdc.gov/vaccines/pubs/acip-list.htm**. Clinically significant adverse events that follow immunization should be reported to the Vaccine Adverse Event Reporting System (VAERS) at **http://www.vaers.hhs.gov** or by telephone, **800-822-7967**.

1. **Hepatitis B vaccine (HepB).** (Minimum age: birth)
   At birth:
   - Administer monovalent HepB to all newborns before hospital discharge.
   - If mother is hepatitis B surface antigen (HBsAg)-positive, administer HepB and 0.5 mL of hepatitis B immune globulin (HBIG) within 12 hours of birth.
   - If mother's HBsAg status is unknown, administer HepB within 12 hours of birth. Determine mother's HBsAg status as soon as possible and, if HBsAg-positive, administer HBIG (no later than age 1 week).
   After the birth dose:
   - The HepB series should be completed with either monovalent HepB or a combination vaccine containing HepB. The second dose should be administered at age 1 or 2 months. Monovalent HepB vaccine should be used for doses administered before age 6 weeks. The final dose should be administered no earlier than age 24 weeks.
   - Infants born to HBsAg-positive mothers should be tested for HBsAg and antibody to HBsAg 1 to 2 months after completion of at least 3 doses of the HepB series, at age 9 through 18 months (generally at the next well-child visit).
   - Administration of 4 doses of HepB to infants is permissible when a combination vaccine containing HepB is administered after the birth dose. The fourth dose should be administered no earlier than age 24 weeks.
2. **Rotavirus vaccine (RV).** (Minimum age: 6 weeks)
   - Administer the first dose at age 6 through 14 weeks (maximum age: 14 weeks 6 days). Vaccination should not be initiated for infants aged 15 weeks 0 days or older.
   - The maximum age for the final dose in the series is 8 months 0 days
   - If Rotarix is administered at ages 2 and 4 months, a dose at 6 months is not indicated.
3. **Diphtheria and tetanus toxoids and acellular pertussis vaccine (DTaP).** (Minimum age: 6 weeks)
   - The fourth dose may be administered as early as age 12 months, provided at least 6 months have elapsed since the third dose.
   - Administer the final dose in the series at age 4 through 6 years.
4. ***Haemophilus influenzae* type b conjugate vaccine (Hib).** (Minimum age: 6 weeks)
   - If PRP-OMP (PedvaxHIB or Comvax [HepB-Hib]) is administered at ages 2 and 4 months, a dose at age 6 months is not indicated.
   - TriHiBit (DTaP/Hib) and Hiberix (PRP-T) should not be used for doses at ages 2, 4, or 6 months for the primary series but can be used as the final dose in children aged 12 months through 4 years.
*5. **Pneumococcal vaccine.** (Minimum age: 6 weeks for pneumococcal conjugate vaccine [PCV]; 2 years for pneumococcal polysaccharide vaccine [PPSV])
   - PCV is recommended for all children aged younger than 5 years. Administer 1 dose of PCV to all healthy children aged 24 through 59 months who are not completely vaccinated for their age.
   - Administer PPSV 2 or more months after last dose of PCV to children aged 2 years or older with certain underlying medical conditions, including a cochlear implant. See *MMWR* 1997;46(No. RR-8).

6. **Inactivated poliovirus vaccine (IPV)** (Minimum age: 6 weeks)
   - The final dose in the series should be administered on or after the fourth birthday and at least 6 months following the previous dose.
   - If 4 doses are administered prior to age 4 years a fifth dose should be administered at age 4 through 6 years. See *MMWR* 2009;58(30):829–30.
7. **Influenza vaccine (seasonal).** (Minimum age: 6 months for trivalent inactivated influenza vaccine [TIV]; 2 years for live, attenuated influenza vaccine [LAIV])
   - Administer annually to children aged 6 months through 18 years.
   - For healthy children aged 2 through 6 years (i.e., those who do not have underlying medical conditions that predispose them to influenza complications), either LAIV or TIV may be used, except LAIV should not be given to children aged 2 through 4 years who have had wheezing in the past 12 months.
   - Children receiving TIV should receive 0.25 mL if aged 6 through 35 months or 0.5 mL if aged 3 years or older.
   - Administer 2 doses (separated by at least 4 weeks) to children aged younger than 9 years who are receiving influenza vaccine for the first time or who were vaccinated for the first time during the previous influenza season but only received 1 dose.
   - For recommendations for use of influenza A (H1N1) 2009 monovalent vaccine see *MMWR* 2009;58(No. RR-10).
8. **Measles, mumps, and rubella vaccine (MMR).** (Minimum age: 12 months)
   - Administer the second dose routinely at age 4 through 6 years. However, the second dose may be administered before age 4, provided at least 28 days have elapsed since the first dose.
9. **Varicella vaccine.** (Minimum age: 12 months)
   - Administer the second dose routinely at age 4 through 6 years. However, the second dose may be administered before age 4, provided at least 3 months have elapsed since the first dose.
   - For children aged 12 months through 12 years the minimum interval between doses is 3 months. However, if the second dose was administered at least 28 days after the first dose, it can be accepted as valid.
10. **Hepatitis A vaccine (HepA).** (Minimum age: 12 months)
   - Administer to all children aged 1 year (i.e., aged 12 through 23 months). Administer 2 doses at least 6 months apart.
   - Children not fully vaccinated by age 2 years can be vaccinated at subsequent visits
   - HepA also is recommended for older children who live in areas where vaccination programs target older children, who are at increased risk for infection, or for whom immunity against hepatitis A is desired.
11. **Meningococcal vaccine.** (Minimum age: 2 years for meningococcal conjugate vaccine [MCV4] and for meningococcal polysaccharide vaccine [MPSV4])
   - Administer MCV4 to children aged 2 through 10 years with persistent complement component deficiency, anatomic or functional asplenia, and certain other conditions placing tham at high risk.
   - Administer MCV4 to children previously vaccinated with MCV4 or MPSV4 after 3 years if first dose administered at age 2 through 6 years. See *MMWR* 2009;58:1042–3.

The Recommended Immunization Schedules for Persons Aged 0 through 18 Years are approved by the Advisory Committee on Immunization Practices (**http://www.cdc.gov/vaccines/recs/acip**), the American Academy of Pediatrics (**http://www.aap.org**), and the American Academy of Family Physicians (**http://www.aafp.org**).

Department of Health and Human Services • Centers for Disease Control and Prevention

Fig. 12-13 Recommended immunization schedule for persons ages 0 through 6 years. *In March 2010 ACIP changed the recommendation for the pneumococcal vaccine; it is now recommended that PCV13 be administered to all children 2 to 59 months of age. PCV13 should replace PCV 7. (From Centers for Disease Control and Prevention: Recommended immunization schedules for persons aged 0 through 18 years—United States, 2010, *MMWR* 58[51-52]:1-4, 2010.)

Recommended Immunization Schedule for Persons Aged 7 Through 18 Years—United States • 2010
For those who fall behind or start late, see the schedule below and the catch-up schedule

Vaccine ▼ Age ►	7–10 years	11–12 years	13–18 years	
Tetanus, Diphtheria, Pertussis[1]		Tdap	Tdap	**Range of recommended ages for all children except certain high-risk groups**
Human Papillomavirus[2]	see footnote 2	HPV (3 doses)	HPV series	
Meningococcal[3]	MCV	MCV	MCV	
Influenza[4]	Influenza (Yearly)			**Range of recommended ages for catch-up immunization**
Pneumococcal[5]	PPSV			
Hepatitis A[6]	HepA Series			
Hepatitis B[7]	Hep B Series			
Inactivated Poliovirus[8]	IPV Series			**Range of recommended ages for certain high-risk groups**
Measles, Mumps, Rubella[9]	MMR Series			
Varicella[10]	Varicella Series			

This schedule includes recommendations in effect as of December 15, 2009. Any dose not administered at the recommended age should be administered at a subsequent visit, when indicated and feasible. The use of a combination vaccine generally is preferred over separate injections of its equivalent component vaccines. Considerations should include provider assessment, patient preference, and the potential for adverse events. Providers should consult the relevant Advisory Committee on Immunization Practices statement for detailed recommendations: http://www.cdc.gov/vaccines/pubs/acip-list.htm. Clinically significant adverse events that follow immunization should be reported to the Vaccine Adverse Event Reporting System (VAERS) at http://www.vaers.hhs.gov or by telephone, **800-822-7967.**

1. **Tetanus and diphtheria toxoids and acellular pertussis vaccine (Tdap).** (Minimum age: 10 years for Boostrix and 11 years for Adacel)
   - Administer at age 11 or 12 years for those who have completed the recommended childhood DTP/DTaP vaccination series and have not received a tetanus and diphtheria toxoid (Td) booster dose.
   - Persons aged 13 through 18 years who have not received Tdap should receive a dose.
   - A 5-year interval from the last Td dose is encouraged when Tdap is used as a booster dose; however, a shorter interval may be used if pertussis immunity is needed.
2. **Human papillomavirus vaccine (HPV).** (Minimum age: 9 years)
   - Two HPV vaccines are licensed: a quadrivalent vaccine (HPV4) for the prevention of cervical, vaginal and vulvar cancers (in females) and genital warts (in females and males), and a bivalent vaccine (HPV2) for the prevention of cervical cancers in females.
   - HPV vaccines are most effective for both males and females when given before exposure to HPV through sexual contact.
   - HPV4 or HPV2 is recommended for the prevention of cervical precancers and cancers in females.
   - HPV4 is recommended for the prevention of cervical, vaginal and vulvar precancers and cancers and genital warts in females.
   - Administer the first dose to females at age 11 or 12 years.
   - Administer the second dose 1 to 2 months after the first dose and the third dose 6 months after the first dose (at least 24 weeks after the first dose).
   - Administer the series to females at age 13 through 18 years if not previously vaccinated.
   - HPV4 may be administered in a 3-dose series to males aged 9 through 18 years to reduce their likelihood of acquiring genital warts.
3. **Meningococcal conjugate vaccine (MCV4).**
   - Administer at age 11 or 12 years, or at age 13 through 18 years if not previously vaccinated.
   - Administer to previously unvaccinated college freshmen living in a dormitory.
   - Administer MCV4 to children aged 2 through 10 years with persistent complement component deficiency, anatomic or functional asplenia, or certain other conditions placing them at high risk.
   - Administer to children previously vaccinated with MCV4 or MPSV4 who remain at increased risk after 3 years (if first dose administered at age 2 through 6 years) or after 5 years (if first dose administered at age 7 years or older). Persons whose only risk factor is living in on-campus housing are not recommended to receive an additional dose. See *MMWR* 2009;58:1042–3.

4. **Influenza vaccine (seasonal).**
   - Administer annually to children aged 6 months through 18 years.
   - For healthy nonpregnant persons aged 7 through 18 years (i.e., those who do not have underlying medical conditions that predispose them to influenza complications), either LAIV or TIV may be used.
   - Administer 2 doses (separated by at least 4 weeks) to children aged younger than 9 years who are receiving influenza vaccine for the first time or who were vaccinated for the first time during the previous influenza season but only received 1 dose.
   - For recommendations for use of influenza A (H1N1) 2009 monovalent vaccine. See *MMWR* 2009;58(No. RR-10).
5. **Pneumococcal polysaccharide vaccine (PPSV).**
   - Administer to children with certain underlying medical conditions, including a cochlear implant. A single revaccination should be administered after 5 years to children with functional or anatomic asplenia or an immunocompromising condition. See *MMWR* 1997;46(No. RR-8).
6. **Hepatitis A vaccine (HepA).**
   - Administer 2 doses at least 6 months apart.
   - HepA is recommended for children aged older than 23 months who live in areas where vaccination programs target older children, who are at increased risk for infection, or for whom immunity against hepatitis A is desired.
7. **Hepatitis B vaccine (HepB).**
   - Administer the 3-dose series to those not previously vaccinated.
   - A 2-dose series (separated by at least 4 months) of adult formulation Recombivax HB is licensed for children aged 11 through 15 years.
8. **Inactivated poliovirus vaccine (IPV).**
   - The final dose in the series should be administered on or after the fourth birthday and at least 6 months following the previous dose.
   - If both OPV and IPV were administered as part of a series, a total of 4 doses should be administered, regardless of the child's current age.
9. **Measles, mumps, and rubella vaccine (MMR).**
   - If not previously vaccinated, administer 2 doses or the second dose for those who have received only 1 dose, with at least 28 days between doses.
10. **Varicella vaccine.**
   - For persons aged 7 through 18 years without evidence of immunity (see *MMWR* 2007;56[No. RR-4]), administer 2 doses if not previously vaccinated or the second dose if only 1 dose has been administered.
   - For persons aged 7 through 12 years, the minimum interval between doses is 3 months. However, if the second dose was administered at least 28 days after the first dose, it can be accepted as valid.
   - For persons aged 13 years and older, the minimum interval between doses is 28 days.

The Recommended Immunization Schedules for Persons Aged 0 through 18 Years are approved by the Advisory Committee on Immunization Practices (http://www.cdc.gov/vaccines/recs/acip), the American Academy of Pediatrics (http://www.aap.org), and the American Academy of Family Physicians (http://www.aafp.org).

Department of Health and Human Services • Centers for Disease Control and Prevention

Fig. 12-14 Recommended immunization schedule for persons ages 7 through 18 years. (From Centers for Disease Control and Prevention: Recommended immunization schedules for persons aged 0 through 18 years—United States, 2010, *MMWR* 58[51-52]:1-4, 2010.)

TABLE 12-5 ROUTINE IMMUNIZATION SCHEDULE FOR INFANTS AND CHILDREN: CANADA, 2006

A. INFANTS AND CHILDREN

AGE AT VACCINATION	DTaP-IPV[a]	Hib[b]	MMR[c]	Var[d]	HB[e]	Pneu–C-7[f]	Men-C[g]	Tdap[h]	Inf[i]
Birth					X				
2 mo	X	X				X	X		
4 mo	X	X				X	(X)		
6 mo	X	X			Infancy	X	X or		X 6-23 mo
12 mo			X	X	3 doses	X 12-15 mo	X if not yet given		1-2 doses
18 mo	X	X	X						
4-6 yr	X		or X		or				
14-16 yr					X Preteen/teen 2-3 doses		X if not yet given	X	

B. CHILDREN <7 YEARS OF AGE NOT IMMUNIZED IN EARLY INFANCY

TIMING	DTaP-IPV	Hib	MMR	Var	HB	Pneu–C-7	Men-C	Tdap
First visit	X	X	X	X	X	X	X	
2 mo later	X	(X)	X		X	(X)	(X)	
2 mo later	X					(X)		
6-12 mo later	X	(X)			X			
4-6 yr of age	(X)							
14-16 yr of age								X

C. CHILDREN ≥7 YEARS OF AGE UP TO 17 YEARS OF AGE NOT IMMUNIZED IN EARLY INFANCY

TIMING	Tdap	IPV[j]	MMR	Var	HB	Men-C
First visit	X	X	X	X	X	X
2 mo later	X	X	X	(X)	(X)	
6-12 mo later	X	X			X	
10 yr later	X					

Modified from Public Health Agency of Canada: *Canadian immunization guide*, ed 7, Ottawa, Ontario, Canada, 2006, The Agency. Parentheses imply that these doses may not be required, depending on the age of the child or adult.

[a]**Diphtheria, tetanus, acellular pertussis, and inactivated polio virus vaccine (DTaP-IPV):** DTaP-IPV (±Hib) vaccine is the preferred vaccine for all doses in the vaccination series, including completion of the series in children who have received one or more doses of DPT (whole cell) vaccine (e.g., recent immigrants). In schedules *A* and *B*, the 4- to 6-yr dose can be omitted if the fourth dose was given after the fourth birthday.

[b]*Haemophilus influenzae* **type b conjugate vaccine (Hib):** The Hib schedule shown is for the *Haemophilus* b capsular polysaccharide–polyribosylribitol phosphate (PRP) conjugated to tetanus toxoid (PRP-T). For catch up, the number of doses depends on the age at which the schedule is begun. Not usually required past age 5 yr.

[c]**Measles, mumps, and rubella vaccine (MMR):** A second dose of MMR is recommended for children at least 1 mo after the first dose for the purpose of better measles protection. For convenience, options include giving it with the next scheduled vaccination at 18 mo of age or at school entry (4-6 yr) (depending on the provincial/territorial policy) or at any intervening age that is practical. In the catch-up schedule *(B)*, the first dose should not be given until the child is ≥12 mo old. MMR should be given to all susceptible adolescents and adults.

[d]**Varicella vaccine (Var):** Children ages 12 mo to 12 yr should receive one dose of varicella vaccine. Susceptible individuals ≥13 yr of age should receive two doses at least 28 days apart.

[e]**Hepatitis B vaccine (HB):** Hepatitis B vaccine can be routinely given to infants or preadolescents, depending on the provincial/territorial policy. For infants born to chronic carrier mothers, the first dose should be given at birth (with hepatitis B immunoglobulin); otherwise, the first dose can be given at 2 mo of age to fit more conveniently with other routine infant immunization visits. The second dose should be administered at least 1 mo after the first dose, and the third at least 2 mo after the second dose, but these may fit more conveniently into the 4- and 6-mo immunization visits. A two-dose schedule for adolescents is an option.

[f]**Pneumococcal conjugate vaccine–7-valent (Pneu–C-7):** Recommended for all children <2 yr of age. The recommended schedule depends on the age of the child when vaccination is begun.

[g]**Meningococcal C conjugate vaccine (Men-C):** Recommended for children <5 yr of age, adolescents, and young adults. The recommended schedule depends on the age of the individual and the conjugate vaccine used. At least one dose in the primary infant series should be given after 5 mo of age. If the provincial/territorial policy is to give Men-C to persons ≥12 mo of age, one dose is sufficient.

[h]**Diphtheria, tetanus, acellular pertussis vaccine—adult/adolescent formulation (Tdap):** A combined adsorbed "adult type" preparation for use in people ≥7 yr of age; contains less diphtheria toxoid and pertussis antigens than preparations given to younger children and is less likely to cause reactions in older people.

[i]**Influenza vaccine (Inf):** Recommended for all children 6-23 mo of age and all persons ≥65 yr of age. Previously unvaccinated children <9 yr of age require two doses of the current season's vaccine with an interval of ≥4 wk. The second dose within the same season is not required if the child received one or more doses of influenza vaccine during the previous influenza season.

[j]**Inactivated polio virus (IPV)**

reduced immune response. No data exist regarding the sero-conversion when the ventrogluteal site is used. The vaccine can be safely administered simultaneously at a separate site with DTaP, MMR, and Hib vaccines.

Hepatitis A Virus

Hepatitis A has been recognized as a significant child health problem, particularly in communities with unusually high infection rates. HAV is spread by the fecal-oral route and from person-to-person contact, by ingestion of contaminated food or water, and rarely by blood transfusion. The illness has an abrupt onset, with fever, malaise, anorexia, nausea, abdominal discomfort, dark urine, and jaundice being the most common clinical signs of infection. In children under 6 years of age, who represent approximately one third of all cases of hepatitis A, the disease may be asymptomatic, and jaundice is rarely evident.

HepA vaccine is now recommended for all children beginning at age 1 year (i.e., 12 months to 23 months). The second dose in the two-dose series may be administered no sooner than 6 months after the first dose. Since the implementation of widespread childhood HepA vaccination, infection rates among children ages 5 to 14 years have declined significantly (Centers for Disease Control and Prevention, 2006a). For further information, see Fig. 12-13, footnote 10.

Diphtheria

Although cases of diphtheria are rare in the United States, the disease can result in significant morbidity. Respiratory manifestations include respiratory nasopharyngitis or obstructive laryngotracheitis with upper airway obstruction. The cutaneous manifestations of the disease include vaginal, otic, conjunctival, or cutaneous lesions, which are primarily seen in urban homeless persons and in the tropics (American Academy of Pediatrics, 2009b). Administer a single dose of equine antitoxin intravenously to the child with clinical symptoms because of the often fulminant progression of the disease (American Academy of Pediatrics, 2009b). Diphtheria vaccine is commonly administered (1) in combination with tetanus and pertussis vaccines (DTaP) or DTaP and Hib vaccines for children younger than 7 years of age, (2) in combination with a conjugate *H. influenzae* type B vaccine (see Fig. 12-13), (3) in a combined vaccine with tetanus (DT) for children younger than 7 years of age who have some contraindication to receiving pertussis vaccine, (4) in combination with tetanus and acellular pertussis (Tdap) for children 11 years and older, or (5) as a single antigen when combined antigen preparations are not indicated. Although the diphtheria vaccine does not produce absolute immunity, protective antitoxin persists for 10 years or more when given according to the recommended schedule, and boosters are given every 10 years for life (see discussion below for adolescent diphtheria and acellular pertussis and tetanus toxoid recommendation). Several vaccines contain diphtheria toxoid (Hib, meningococcal, pneumococcal), but this does not confer immunity to the disease.

Tetanus

Three forms of tetanus vaccine—tetanus toxoid, tetanus immunoglobulin (TIG) (human), and tetanus antitoxin (equine antitoxin)—are available; however, tetanus antitoxin is no longer available in the United States. Tetanus toxoid is used for routine primary immunization, usually in one of the combinations listed for diphtheria, and provides protective antitoxin levels for approximately 10 years.

Tetanus and diphtheria toxoids along with acellular pertussis vaccine (Tdap, adolescent formulation) are now recommended for children ages 11 to 12 years who have completed the recommended DTaP/DTP vaccine series but have not received the tetanus (Td) booster dose. Adolescents 13 to 18 years of age who have not received the Td/Tdap booster should receive a single Tdap booster, provided the routine DTaP/DTP childhood immunization series has been previously received. It is recommended that children receive subsequent Td boosters every 10 years (American Academy of Pediatrics, 2009b) (see Fig. 12-13, footnote 3). Boostrix (Tdap) is currently licensed for children 10 to 18 years of age, whereas Adacel (Tdap) is licensed for individuals 11 to 64 years of age.

For wound management, passive immunity is available with TIG. Persons with a history of two previous doses of tetanus toxoid can receive a booster dose of the toxoid. Separate syringes and different sites are used when tetanus toxoid and TIG are given concurrently. Table 12-6 summarizes the recommended procedure for tetanus prophylaxis in wound management.

For children over 7 years who require wound prophylaxis, tetanus immunization may be accomplished by administering Td (adult-type diphtheria and tetanus toxoids). If TIG is not

TABLE 12-6	GUIDE TO TETANUS PROPHYLAXIS IN ROUTINE WOUND MANAGEMENT			
HISTORY OF ABSORBED TETANUS TOXOID (DOSES)	**CLEAN, MINOR WOUNDS**		**ALL OTHER WOUNDS[a]**	
	Td[b] OR Tdap[c]	**TIG[d]**	**TD[e] OR Tdap[c]**	**TIG[d]**
Unknown or <3	Yes	No	Yes	Yes
≥3[e]	No[f]	No	No[g]	No

Data from American Academy of Pediatrics, Committee on Infectious Diseases, Pickering L, editor: *2009 Red book: report of the Committee on Infectious Diseases*, ed 28, Elk Grove Village, Ill, 2009, The Academy.

Td, Adult-type diphtheria and tetanus toxoids; *TD*, pediatric diphtheria and tetanus toxoids; Tdap, tetanus toxoid, reduced diphtheria toxoid, acellular pertussis; *TIG*, tetanus immunoglobulin.

[a]Such as, but not limited to, wounds contaminated with dirt, feces, soil, and saliva; puncture wounds; avulsions; and wounds resulting from missiles, crushing, burns, and frostbite.

[b]For children <7 yr old: DTaP (diphtheria-tetanus–acellular pertussis) (or DT [diphtheria-tetanus], if pertussis vaccine is contraindicated) is preferred to tetanus toxoid alone. For persons >7 yr of age, Td is preferred to tetanus toxoid alone.

[c]Tdap is preferred to Td vaccine for adolescents who never have received Tdap vaccine. Td is preferred to tetanus toxoid (TT) vaccine in adolescents who formerly received Tdap vaccine or when Tdap is not available.

[d]Immune globulin intravenous should be used when TIG is not available

[e]If only three doses of fluid toxoid have been received, then a fourth dose of toxoid, preferably an adsorbed toxoid, should be given. Although licensed, fluid tetanus toxoid is rarely used.

[f]Yes, if ≥10 yr since last tetanus-containing dose.

[g]Yes, if >5 yr since last tetanus-containing dose. (More frequent boosters are not needed and can accentuate side effects.)

available, the equine antitoxin (not available in the United States) may be administered after appropriate testing for sensitivity. The antitoxin is administered in a separate syringe and at a separate intramuscular site if given concurrently with tetanus toxoid.

Pertussis

Pertussis vaccine is recommended for all children 6 weeks through 6 years of age (up to the seventh birthday) who have no neurologic contraindications to its use. Concerns over outbreaks of the disease in the past decade have prompted discussion about vaccinating infants and adults. Many cases of pertussis have occurred in children less than 6 months or persons over 7 years, both groups falling in the category for which pertussis immunization previously was not recommended (Centers for Disease Control and Prevention, 2005c). The tetanus and diphtheria toxoids and acellular pertussis vaccine (Tdap) is now recommended at ages 11 to 12 years for children who have completed the DTaP/DTP childhood series. The Tdap is also recommended for adolescents 13 to 18 years old who have not received a tetanus booster (Td) or Tdap dose and have completed the childhood DTaP/DTP series. When the Tdap is used as a booster dose, it may be administered 5 years from the last Td dose or earlier if pertussis immunity is necessary (Centers for Disease Control and Prevention, 2009).

Currently, two forms of pertussis vaccine are available in the United States. The whole-cell pertussis vaccine is prepared from inactivated cells of *Bordetella pertussis* and contains multiple antigens. In contrast, the acellular pertussis vaccine contains one or more immunogens derived from the *B. pertussis* organism. The highly purified acellular vaccine is associated with fewer local and systemic reactions than those occurring with the whole-cell vaccine in children of similar age. The acellular pertussis vaccine is recommended by the American Academy of Pediatrics (2009b) for the first three immunizations and is usually given at 2, 4, and 6 months of age with diphtheria and tetanus (DTaP). Several forms of acellular pertussis vaccine are currently licensed for use in infants: Daptacel, Pediarix, Kinrix (DTaP and IPV), and Infanrix (diphtheria, tetanus toxoid, and acellular pertussis conjugate). Pentacel is licensed for use in infants 4 weeks old and older; in addition to acellular pertussis, diphtheria, and tetanus, this vaccine also contains inactivated poliovirus (IPV) and Hib conjugate. Either the acellular or whole-cell vaccine may be given for the fourth and fifth doses, but the acellular is preferred. It is also recommended that the first three DTaP vaccinations be from the same manufacturer. The fourth dose may be from a different manufacturer. The child who has received one or more whole-cell vaccines may complete the series of five with the acellular vaccine.

Health care workers who may be susceptible to pertussis as a result of waning immunity and who have potential exposure to children or adults with pertussis should take the necessary protective precautions against droplet contamination (wear procedural or surgical masks and practice hand washing). The diagnosis of pertussis may be missed or delayed in unvaccinated infants, who often are seen with respiratory distress and apnea without the typical cough (Centers for Disease Control and

Prevention, 2005c). Additional guidelines for prevention and treatment of pertussis among health care workers and close contacts are given in the *2009 Red Book: Report of the Committee on Infectious Diseases* (American Academy of Pediatrics, 2009b).

Polio

An all-IPV (inactivated poliovirus vaccine) schedule for routine childhood polio vaccination is now recommended for children in the United States. All children should receive four doses of IPV at 2 months, 4 months, 6 to 18 months, and 4 to 6 years of age (American Academy of Pediatrics, 2009b).

The change from the exclusive use of oral polio vaccine (OPV) to the exclusive use of IPV is related to the rare risk of vaccine-associated polio paralysis (VAPP) from OPV. The exclusive use of IPV eliminates the risk of VAPP but is associated with an increased number of injections and increased cost. Since IPV usage was instituted in the United States in 2000, no new indigenously acquired cases of VAPP have occurred. Pediarix is a **combination vaccine** containing DTaP, hepatitis B, and IPV. This may be used as the primary immunization beginning at 2 months of age. Kinrix may be used for the fourth booster dose of IPV and fifth booster dose of DTaP at 4 to 6 years of age (American Academy of Pediatrics, 2009b).

Measles

The measles (rubeola) vaccine is given at 12 to 15 months of age. During the course of measles outbreaks, the vaccine can be given any time after 6 months of age, followed by a second inoculation after age 12 months. The second measles immunization is recommended at 4 to 6 years of age (at school entry) but may be given earlier provided that 4 weeks have elapsed since the administration of the previous dose. Revaccination should occur by 11 to 12 years of age if the measles vaccine was not administered at school entry (4 to 6 years). Any child who is vaccinated before 12 months of age should receive two additional doses beginning at 12 to 15 months and separated by at least 4 weeks (American Academy of Pediatrics, 2009b). Revaccination should include all individuals born after 1956 who have not received two doses of measles vaccine after 12 months of age. Individuals born before this date are thought to be immune from exposure to natural measles virus. Because of the continuing occurrence of measles in older children and young adults, identify potentially susceptible adolescents and young adults and immunize them if two doses of measles vaccine have not been administered previously or the person had a confirmed case of the illness.

The MMRV vaccine (measles, mumps, rubella, and varicella) is an attenuated live virus vaccine and may be given to children 12 months to 12 years of age concurrent with other vaccines. Recent concerns for increased risk of febrile seizures in children 12 months to 23 months of age after administration of MMRV has prompted the ACIP (Centers for Disease Control and Prevention, 2008b) to remove its recommendation for MMRV being the preferred vaccine (versus separate injections of MMR and varicella vaccines) (American Academy of Pediatrics, 2009b).

Vitamin A supplementation has been effective in decreasing the morbidity and mortality associated with measles in developing countries. A Cochrane review of studies wherein a single dose of vitamin A was administered to children with measles found no decrease in mortality. However, children with measles under the age of 2 years who received two doses of vitamin A (200,000 international units) on consecutive days did have decreased mortality rates and a reduced rate of pneumonia-specific mortality (Huiming, Chaomin, and Meng, 2005).

Mumps

Mumps virus vaccine is recommended for children at 12 to 15 months of age and is typically given in combination with measles and rubella. It should not be administered to infants younger than 12 months because persisting maternal antibodies can interfere with the immune response. Because of continued occurrence of the disease, especially in children 10 to 19 years of age, mumps immunization is recommended for all individuals born after 1957 who may be susceptible to mumps (i.e., those who have no history of having had the disease or vaccine and who have no laboratory evidence of immunity).

Rubella

Rubella is a relatively mild infection in children, but in a pregnant woman the actual infection presents serious risks to the developing fetus. Therefore the aim of rubella immunization is actually protection of the unborn child rather than the recipient of the immunization.

Rubella immunization is recommended for all children at 12 to 15 months of age and is administered in a combined form with measles and mumps vaccine. Increased emphasis should also be placed on vaccinating all unimmunized prepubertal children and susceptible adolescents and adult women in the childbearing age-group. Because the live attenuated virus may cross the placenta and theoretically present a risk to the developing fetus, rubella vaccine is currently not given to any pregnant woman. Although this is standard practice, current evidence from women who received the vaccine while pregnant and delivered unaffected offspring indicates that the risk to the fetus is negligible. In addition, there is no reported danger of administering rubella vaccine to a child if the mother is pregnant.

Haemophilus influenzae Type b

Hib conjugate vaccines protect against a number of serious infections caused by Hib, especially bacterial meningitis, epiglottitis, bacterial pneumonia, septic arthritis, and sepsis (Hib is not associated with the viruses that cause influenza, or "flu"). Hib vaccines that are currently available include PedvaxHIB, Pentacel, and Comvax, which are combination vaccines; HibTITER; and ActHIB. Pentacel is described in the previous section on Pertussis. These conjugate vaccines connect Hib to a nontoxic form of another organism, such as meningococcal protein or diphtheria protein. There is no antibody response to these nontoxic proteins, but they significantly improve the antibody response to Hib, especially in infants. The use of combination vaccines provides equivalent immunogenicity and decreases the number of injections an infant receives. However, it is important that they be given to the appropriate-age child.

The 2009 Centers for Disease Control and Prevention immunization guidelines indicate there is limited data for administering the HiB vaccine to persons 5 years and older; however, the guidelines suggest that children with sickle cell disease, leukemia, or human immunodeficiency virus (HIV) infection, or children who have had a splenectomy, may benefit from one dose of the Hib vaccine (Centers for Disease Control and Prevention, 2009).

When possible, the Hib conjugate vaccine used at the first vaccination should be used for all subsequent vaccinations in the primary series. All Hib vaccines are administered by intramuscular injection using a separate syringe and at a site separate from any concurrent vaccinations.

The use of meningococcal and diphtheria proteins in combination vaccines does not mean the child has received adequate immunization for meningococcal or diphtheria illnesses. The child must be given the appropriate vaccine for that specific disease.

Varicella

Administration of the cell-free live-attenuated varicella vaccine is recommended for any susceptible child (one who lacks proof of varicella vaccination or has a reliable history of varicella infection). A single dose of 0.5 ml should be given by subcutaneous injection. The first dose of varicella vaccine is recommended for children ages 12 to 15 months, and to ensure adequate protection a second varicella vaccine is recommended for children at 4 to 6 years of age. The second varicella vaccine may be administered before 4 years of age as long as a period of 3 months occurs between the first and second doses. Children 13 years of age or older who are susceptible should receive two doses administered at least 4 weeks apart. Children in the same age-group who have received only one previous varicella vaccine should receive a second varicella vaccine. MMRV is not licensed for use in children ages 13 years or older (American Academy of Pediatrics, 2009b). The American Academy of Pediatrics (2009b) reports that the two-dose regimen was adopted to protect children who did not have adequate protection with one dose, not because of waning immunity to the vaccine.

According to the American Academy of Pediatrics (2009b), children who have received two doses of the varicella vaccine are one third less likely to have breakthrough illness in the first 10 years of immunization in comparison with those who have received one dose. Children who do contract varicella after immunization reportedly have milder cases with fewer vesicles, lower degree of fever, and faster recovery. Antibodies persist for at least 8 years (American Academy of Pediatrics, 2009b).

Keep the vaccine frozen in the lyophilic form (stable particles that readily go into solution) and use it within 30 minutes of being reconstituted to ensure viral potency.

Varicella vaccine may be administered simultaneously with MMR. However, separate syringes and injection sites should be used. If they are not administered simultaneously, the interval between administration of varicella vaccine and MMR should be at least 1 month. Varicella vaccine may also be given simultaneously with DTaP, IPV, HepB, or Hib (American Academy of Pediatrics, 2009b).

Pneumococcal

A seven-valent *Streptococcus pneumoniae* conjugate vaccine (PCV7, or Prevnar) has been used for children under 2 years of age since 2000. In February 2010 the Food and Drug Administration approved a new 13-valent pneumococcal vaccine, Prevnar 13, which replaces PCV7 (Prevnar). PCV13 was approved for children 6 weeks to 71 months of age (Centers for Disease Control and Prevention, 2010). Streptococcal pneumococci are responsible for a number of bacterial infections in children under 2 years, which may cause serious morbidity and mortality. Among these are generalized infections such as septicemia and bacterial meningitis or localized infections such as otitis media, sinusitis, and pneumonia. These illnesses are particularly problematic in children who attend daycare facilities (the incidence in daycare children is two to three times higher than in children not attending out-of-home daycare) and in those who are immunocompromised.

The vaccine is administered at 2, 4, and 6 months, with a fourth dose at 12 to 15 months of age. Children 7 to 11 months old may receive three doses as long as they are 6 to 8 weeks apart and a fourth dose at 12 to 15 months. Children 12 to 23 months who have not been immunized with the pneumococcal vaccine may be given two doses, 6 to 8 weeks apart. PCV13 is also recommended for all children under 24 months and in older children (24 to 71 months) with sickle cell disease; functional or anatomic asplenia; nephrotic syndrome or chronic renal failure; conditions associated with immunosuppression, such as solid organ transplantation, drug therapy, or cytoreduction therapy (including long-term systemic corticosteroid therapy); diabetes mellitus; cochlear implants; congenital immunodeficiency; HIV infection; cerebrospinal fluid leaks; chronic cardiovascular disease (e.g., congestive heart failure or cardiomyopathy); chronic pulmonary disease (e.g., emphysema or cystic fibrosis, but not asthma); chronic liver disease (e.g., cirrhosis); or exposure to living environments or social settings in which the risk of invasive pneumococcal disease or its complications is very high (e.g., Alaskan Native, African-American, and certain Native American populations) (American Academy of Pediatrics, 2009b). Low-birth-weight infants (≤1500 g [3.3 lb]) should receive the vaccine when they reach a chronologic age of 6 to 8 weeks regardless of calculated gestational age. The PCV7 vaccine may be administered in conjunction with all other immunizations in a separate syringe and at a separate intramuscular site.

The PPV (pneumococcal polysaccharide [23-valent] vaccine) is not recommended for children younger than 24 months who do not have one of the high-risk conditions described previously.

Influenza

The influenza vaccine is now recommended annually for children 6 months to 18 years. Influenza vaccine (trivalent inactivated influenza vaccine [TIV]) may be given to any healthy children 6 months old and older. Children who have a reported anaphylactic hypersensitivity to eggs should not receive the vaccine. The vaccine is administered in early fall before the flu season begins and is repeated yearly for ongoing protection. The intramuscular vaccine is administered as two separate doses 4 weeks apart in first-time recipients under the age of 9 years. The dose is 0.25 ml for children ages 6 to 35 months and 0.5 ml for children 3 years and above. The vaccine may be given simultaneously with other vaccines but at a separate site. The vaccine is administered yearly because different strains of influenza are used each year in the manufacture of the vaccine.

The live attenuated influenza vaccine (LAIV) is an acceptable alternative to the intramuscular trivalent vaccine in specific age-groups. The vaccine is given nasally as two doses at least 28 days apart in healthy persons ages 2 to 49 years. Although it is an alternative to the injection, it costs more and may not be covered by insurance companies. Either TIV or LAIV may be given to healthy, nonpregnant persons ages 2 to 49 years (American Academy of Pediatrics, 2009c). Yearly influenza vaccine should be administered to health care workers and to children ages 6 to 59 months with medical conditions (including asthma, cardiac disease, HIV, diabetes, and sickle cell disease) that place them at risk for influenza-related complications.

The H1N1 virus (swine flu) is a subtype of influenza type A. Previous outbreaks of H1N1 influenza occurred in 1918, and the mortality rates were significant both in the United States and worldwide (American Academy of Pediatrics, 2009b). The pandemic of H1N1 caused significant morbidity and mortality worldwide, but particularly in Mexico and the United States. **Antigenic shift** occurs when influenza A viruses undergo significant changes that result in new infection subtypes; such is the case in the current pandemic. The signs and symptoms of H1N1 flu are the same as those mentioned below for influenza. Oseltamivir (Tamiflu) has been approved for infants 3 months of age and older who are symptomatic and in infants 0 to 3 months if the practitioner feels it is absolutely critical to the child's well being. In the United States the 2011-2012 winter influenza vaccines (LAIV and TIV) contain protection against the H1N1 influenza strain as well as other influenza strains. The most updated information on the status of this disease may be found at the websites for the Centers for Disease Control and Prevention (**www.cdc.gov**) and the World Health Organization (**www.who.int/csr/disease/swineflu/en/index.html**).

Meningococcal

Invasive meningococcal disease continues to be the cause of high morbidity in children in the United States. Infants younger than 1 year of age are particularly susceptible, yet the highest fatalities occur in adolescents (approximately 20%). There is also evidence that the risk of meningococcal infections is high in college freshmen living in dormitories. Meningococcal infections are also responsible for significant morbidities, including limb or digit amputation, skin scarring, hearing loss, and neurologic disabilities (American Academy of Pediatrics, 2009b).

Neisseria meningitidis is the leading cause of bacterial meningitis in the United States. It is now recommended that children 2 to 10 years old at increased risk for meningococcal disease receive either the quadrivalent conjugate vaccine MCV4 (Menactra) or MenACY-CRM (Menveo). Adolescents who received a single meningococcal vaccine prior to the age of 16 years should receive a single booster of meningococcal quadrivalent vaccine (Centers for Disease Control and Prevention, 2011). Children in certain high-risk groups such as those with terminal complement component deficiency, anatomic or functional asplenia, or HIV and children who travel to or reside in countries where *N. meningitidis* is hyperendemic or epidemic should also receive one of the quadrivalent meningococcal vaccines (American Academy of Pediatrics, 2009b). Children and adolescents 11 to 18 years of age should receive a single immunization of MCV4. Others at high risk who should receive MCV4 include college freshmen living in dormitories and military recruits (American Academy of Pediatrics, 2009b).

Persons who are at high risk for the disease and previously received MPSV4 3 or more years previously should be vaccinated with MCV4. The vaccine protects against meningococcal disease caused by serogroups A, C, Y, and W-135. MCV4 is administered as an intramuscular injection (0.5 ml) and may be administered in conjunction with other vaccines in a separate syringe and at a separate site. Immunization with MCV4 is contraindicated in persons with hypersensitivity to any components of the vaccine, including diphtheria toxoid, and to rubber latex (part of vial stopper).

Reports of an association between MCV4 (Menactra) and cases of Guillain-Barré syndrome in vaccinated persons ages 11 to 19 years of age have been addressed. Onset of symptoms occurred within 2 to 23 days of vaccination. A preliminary survey by the Centers for Disease Control and Prevention (2006b) indicates there are insufficient data to change the 2005 recommendation for adolescents, college freshmen residing in dormitories, and other high-risk populations.

Recommendations for Selected Immunizations

Two additional vaccines are recommended for children and adolescents at high risk for particular diseases. Two rotavirus vaccines, RotaTeq and Rotarix, have been licensed by the U.S. Food and Drug Administration for distribution in the United States. Rotavirus is one of the leading causes of severe diarrhea in infants and young children. RotaTeq is licensed for administration to infants at 6 to 12 weeks of age, with two additional doses administered at 4- to 10-week intervals but not after 32 weeks of age. The dose is 2 ml, and the product must be protected from light until administration (American Academy of Pediatrics, 2009b). Rotarix (1 ml) may be administered beginning at 6 weeks of age with a second dose at least 4 weeks after the first dose, but before 24 weeks of age. Both vaccines are administered orally.

A quadrivalent human papillomavirus (HPV) vaccine, Gardasil, has been approved and is recommended for female children and adolescents to prevent HPV-related cervical cancer. The vaccine is administered intramuscularly in three separate doses; the first dose in the series may be given at 11 to 12 years of age (minimum age 9 years), the second dose is administered 2 months after the first, and the third dose is given 6 months after the first dose (Centers for Disease Control and Prevention, 2007b). (See Fig. 12-14, footnote 2.)

Immunizations that may be used in older children and adolescents in the future and that are being evaluated include vaccines for preventing diseases such as herpes simplex virus, human cytomegalovirus, and Epstein-Barr virus. Others, such as the rabies vaccine, are discussed elsewhere in this text.

Reactions

Vaccines for routine immunizations are among the safest and most reliable drugs available. However, minor side effects do occur after many of the immunizations, and, rarely, a serious reaction may result from the vaccine. A number of inactive components are incorporated in vaccines to enhance their effectiveness and safety. Some of these components include preservatives, stabilizers, adjuvants, antibiotics (e.g., neomycin), and purified culture medium proteins (e.g., egg) to enhance effectiveness. A child may react to the preservative in the vaccine rather than the vaccine component; an example of this is the hepatitis B vaccine, which is prepared from yeast cultures. Yeast hypersensitivity therefore would preclude one from receiving that particular vaccine without consulting an allergist. Trace amounts of neomycin are used to decrease bacterial growth within certain vaccine preparations, and persons with documented anaphylactic reactions to neomycin should avoid those vaccines. Most vaccine preparations now contain vial stoppers with a synthetic rubber to prevent latex allergy reactions. In the event that an individual has a severe reaction to a vaccine and subsequent immunizations are required, an allergist may be consulted to determine the best course of action.

Some vaccines contain a preservative, thimerosal, which contains ethylmercury. Concerns regarding possible mercury poisoning in the 1990s prompted many to put off vaccination of infants and small children for fear of childhood developmental problems such as autism. A number of manufacturers have since stopped producing vaccines containing thimerosal. No local hypersensitivity reactions to thimerosal have been recorded, and studies on thimerosal and the potential link to autism or any other pervasive developmental disorder failed to establish a causal relationship between the two (DeStefano, 2007; Hviid, Stellfeld, Wohlfahrt, et al, 2003; Parker, Schwartz, Todd, et al, 2004). The Institute of Medicine (2004), following an in-depth 3-year study, issued a report concluding that there is no link between autism and the MMR vaccine or vaccines containing the preservative thimerosal. The H1N1 vaccines do not contain any additives such as thimerosal.

With inactivated antigens, such as DTaP, side effects are most likely to occur within a few hours or days of administration and are usually limited to local tenderness, erythema, and swelling at the injection site; low-grade fever; and behavioral changes (drowsiness, fretfulness, eating less, prolonged or unusual cry). Local reactions tend to be less severe when a needle of sufficient length to deposit the vaccine in the muscle is used (see Atraumatic Care box). Rarely, more severe reactions may occur, especially with pertussis and varicella. Reactions to DTaP tend to be more severe if they occurred with a previous immunization.

Hib vaccine is one of the safest vaccines available but may be associated with low-grade fever and mild local reactions at the site of injection, which resolve rapidly.

Unlike the inactivated antigens, live attenuated virus vaccines such as MMR multiply for days or weeks, and unfavorable

ATRAUMATIC CARE

Immunizations

Needle length is an important factor and must be considered for each individual child; fewer reactions to immunizations are observed when the vaccine is given deep into the muscle rather than into subcutaneous tissue. Contrary to previous belief, deep intramuscular tissue has a better blood supply and fewer pain receptors than adipose tissue, thus providing an optimum site for immunizations with fewer side effects (Zuckerman, 2000).

To minimize local reactions from vaccines:
- Recommended needle length for newborn to 2 months is 16 mm (⅝ inch).
- Select a needle of adequate length (25 mm [1 inch] in infants) to deposit the antigen deep in the muscle mass.
- Toddlers and older children require a needle length of 16 to 25 mm (⅝ to 1 inch) for deltoid, or 25 to 32 mm (1 to 1¼ inches) for vastus lateralis (Schechter, Zempsky, Cohen, et al, 2007).
- Adolescents require a needle length of 25 to 51 mm (1 to 2 inches) in deltoid or vastus lateralis (Schechter, Zempsky, Cohen, et al, 2007).
- Inject into the vastus lateralis or ventrogluteal muscle; the deltoid may be used in children 18 months of age or older.
- Use an air bubble to clear the needle after injecting the vaccine (theoretically beneficial but unproved).

Use one or more of the following techniques to minimize pain:
- Apply the topical anesthetic EMLA (lidocaine-prilocaine) to the injection site and cover with an occlusive dressing for at least 1 hour.*
- Apply the topical anesthetic LMX4 (4% lidocaine) to the injection site 30 minutes before the injection; there is no evidence that an occlusive dressing is required except to prevent ingestion or accidental application to the eyes in infants (Wong, 2003). To date, the studies for LMX4 have only discussed pain from procedures such as venipuncture, not injections.
- Apply a vapocoolant spray (e.g., ethyl chloride or FluoriMethane) directly to the skin or to a cotton ball, which is placed on the skin for 15 seconds immediately before the injection (Reis and Holubkov, 1997).
- There is evidence that a concentrated oral sucrose solution (24%) and nonnutritive sucking (NNS) (pacifier) decrease the pain related to minor

invasive procedures in neonates (Stevens, Johnston, Franck, et al, 1999; Stevens, Yamada, and Ohlsson, 2001). Most studies have focused on heel lance, venipuncture, and circumcision (neonatal period), but one institution has incorporated a neonatal oral sucrose pain protocol for painful procedures, including injections (Thompson, 2005). Hatfield (2008) found that 2- and 4-month-old infants who received a 0.6 ml/kg dose of 24% sucrose and NNS 2 minutes before immunization administration had decreased pain behavioral responses in comparison to a control group of infants who only received sterile water and NNS 2 minutes before the injection. Therefore it is recommended that a concentrated oral sucrose solution (1 to 2 ml) be administered orally 2 minutes before the injection, during the injection, and up to 3 minutes after the procedure to decrease neonatal pain with immunizations.
- In preschool children, use distraction, such as telling the child to "take a deep breath and blow and blow and blow until I tell you to stop."
- Two studies in adult patients receiving intramuscular injections documented a decrease in pain sensation at the time of the injection when manual pressure was applied to the site before the injection; pressure was applied for 10 seconds in both studies (Barnhill, Holbert, Jackson, et al, 1996; Chung, Ng, and Wong, 2002). To date, there are no published studies involving the use of this technique in children.
- A needleless system that delivers lidocaine to the skin has been used in older children for venipuncture; the J-tip delivers 1% buffered lidocaine, which numbs the skin within 1 to 3 minutes (Jimenez, Bradford, Seidel, et al, 2006; Spanos, Booth, Koenig, et al, 2008; Zempsky, 2008). To date, there is no literature supporting the use of the J-tip with immunizations.
- NOTE: Changing the needle on the syringe after drawing up the vaccine and before injecting it has not been shown to decrease local reactions. In children 4 to 6 years of age, the administration of sequential injections or simultaneous injections of vaccines did not alter their perceptions of distress, but parents preferred the simultaneous method (Horn and McCarthy, 1999).

*The use of the EMLA patch before administration of diphtheria-tetanus–acellular pertussis–inactivated poliovirus–*Haemophilus influenzae* type b (DTaP-IPV-Hib) and hepatitis B vaccines did not decrease antibody titers in immunized infants and was effective in reducing pain in 6-month-old children (Halperin, Halperin, McGrath, et al, 2002). The EMLA patch is no longer commercially available in the United States.

---

reactions and vaccine-associated disorders can occur up to 30 to 60 days later. These reactions are usually mild, although reactions to rubella tend to be more troublesome in older children and adults.

Contraindications and Precautions

Nurses need to be aware of the reasons for withholding immunizations—both for the child's safety in terms of avoiding reactions and for the child's maximum benefit from receiving the vaccine. Unfounded fears and lack of knowledge regarding contraindications can needlessly prevent a child from gaining protection from life-threatening diseases. Issues that have surfaced regarding vaccines include the misconception that administering combination vaccines may overload the child's immune system. The combined vaccines have undergone rigorous study in relation to side effects and immunogenicity rates following administration. Give parents appropriate information regarding vaccine safety, benefits, and risks so they can make informed decisions regarding vaccinations for their children. The advantage of widespread information on television and the Internet is that it is readily available at any given moment. The disadvantage is that some of this information may be incorrect, incomplete, or misleading and may influence parents to make

decisions that could harm their children's health. Parents may also receive information regarding vaccines from antivaccine groups, which advocate changes in the mass vaccination system in the United States. At times such groups may publicize information related to extremely rare events occurring after a child is immunized.

The general contraindication for all immunizations is a severe febrile illness. This precaution avoids adding the risk of adverse side effects from the vaccine to an already ill child or mistakenly identifying a symptom of the disease as having been caused by the vaccine. The presence of minor illnesses such as the common cold is not a contraindication. Live virus vaccines are generally not administered to anyone with an altered immune system, since multiplication of the virus may be enhanced, causing a severe vaccine-induced illness.

Another contraindication to live virus vaccines (MMR and varicella) is the presence of recently acquired passive immunity through blood transfusions, immunoglobulin, or maternal antibodies. Administration of MMR and varicella should be postponed for a minimum of 3 months after passive immunization with immunoglobulins and blood transfusions (except washed RBCs, which do not interfere with the immune response). Suggested intervals between administration of immunoglobulin preparations and MMR and varicella depend on the type of immune product and dosage. If the vaccine and immunoglobulin are given simultaneously because of imminent exposure to disease, the two preparations are injected at sites far from each other. Vaccination should be repeated after the suggested intervals unless there is serologic evidence of antibody production.

Pregnancy is a contraindication to MMR vaccines, although the risk of fetal damage is primarily theoretic. Breast-feeding is not a contraindication for any vaccine.

A final contraindication is a known allergic response to a previously administered vaccine or a substance in the vaccine. MMR vaccines contain minute amounts of neomycin; measles and mumps vaccines, which are grown on chick embryo tissue cultures, are not believed to contain significant amounts of egg cross-reacting proteins. Therefore only a history of anaphylactic reaction to neomycin, gelatin, or the vaccine itself is considered a contraindication to their use. To identify the rare child who may not be able to receive the vaccines, take a careful allergy history. (See Nursing Care Guidelines box, "Taking an Allergy History," Chapter 6.) If the child has a history of anaphylaxis, report this to the practitioner before administering the vaccine. Contact dermatitis in reaction to neomycin is not considered a contraindication to immunization. Evidence indicates that children who are egg-sensitive are not at increased risk for untoward reactions to MMR vaccine. Furthermore, skin testing of egg-allergic children with vaccine has failed to predict immediate hypersensitivity reactions (American Academy of Pediatrics, 2009b).

A family history of seizures, allergies to duck meat or duck feathers, and a family history of SIDS are not considered contraindications to receiving childhood vaccines (American Academy of Pediatrics, 2009b).

Nurses are at the forefront in providing parents with appropriate information regarding childhood immunization benefits, contraindications, and side effects and the effects of nonvaccination on the child's health. Some suggestions for communicating with parents about the benefits of immunizations in childhood include (portions adapted from Coyer, 2002; Fredrickson, Davis, and Bocchini, 2001; Rosenthal, 2004):

- Provide accurate and user-friendly information on vaccines (the necessity for each one, the disease each prevents, potential adverse effects).
- Realize that the parent is expressing concern for the child's health.
- Acknowledge the parent's concerns in a genuine, empathetic manner.
- Be knowledgeable about the benefits of individual vaccines, the common adverse effects, and how to minimize those effects.
- Give the parent the **vaccine information statement (VIS)** beforehand and be prepared to answer any questions that may arise.
- Help the parent make an informed decision regarding the administration of each vaccine.
- Be flexible and provide parents options regarding the administration of multiple vaccines, especially in infants, who must receive multiple injections at 2, 4, and 6 months (i.e., allow parents to space the vaccinations at different

visits to decrease the total number of injections at each visit; make provisions for office visits for immunization purposes only [does not incur a practitioner fee except for administration of vaccine], provided the child is healthy).
- Involve the parent in minimizing the potential adverse effects of the vaccine (e.g., administering an appropriate dose of acetaminophen 45 minutes before administering the vaccine [as warranted]; applying a topical analgesic such as lidocaine-prilocaine [EMLA] or 4% lidocaine [LMX4] to the injection sites before going to the administration site [see Atraumatic Care box, p. 505]; following up to check on the child if untoward reactions have occurred in the past or parent is especially anxious about the child's well-being).
- Respect the parent's ultimate wishes.

Administration

The principal precautions in administering immunizations include proper storage of the vaccine to protect its potency and institution of recommended procedures for injection. The nurse must be familiar with the manufacturer's directions for storage and reconstitution of the vaccine. For example, if the vaccine is to be refrigerated, it should be stored on a center shelf, not in the door, where frequent temperature increases from opening the refrigerator can alter the vaccine's potency. For protection against light the vial can be wrapped in aluminum foil. Periodic checks are established to ensure that no vaccine is used after its expiration date.

The DTP (or DTaP) vaccines contain an adjuvant to retain the antigen at the injection site and prolong the stimulatory effect. Because subcutaneous or intracutaneous injection of the adjuvant can cause local irritation, inflammation, or abscess formation, excellent intramuscular injection technique must be used (see Atraumatic Care box, p. 505).

The total series requires several injections, and every attempt is made to rotate the sites and administer the injections as painlessly as possible. (See discussion on intramuscular injections, Chapter 27.) When two or more injections are given at separate sites, the order of injections is arbitrary. Some practitioners suggest injecting the less painful one first. Some believe this is DTP (or DTaP), whereas others suggest the MMR or Hib vaccine. Still others advocate injecting at two sites simultaneously (requires two operators) (see Research Focus box).

RESEARCH FOCUS

Order of Injections

Ipp, Parkin, Lear, and colleagues (2009) evaluated the administration order of the vaccines diphtheria-tetanus–acellular pertussis–*Haemophilus influenzae* type b (DTaP-Hib) and pneumococcal conjugate vaccine (PCV) and pain perception in 120 infants 2 to 6 months of age. The infants who were given the primary DTaP-Hib vaccine before the PCV vaccine had significantly lower pain scores as measured by the Modified Behavioral Pain Scale than those who received the PCV vaccine first. Both groups of infants were given both vaccines. Additional pain measures included crying as measured by video recording and parent perception of child pain using the visual analog scale. The researchers recommend giving the primary DTaP-Hib vaccine before the PCV to reduce pain in infants receiving routine immunizations.

Because allergic reactions can occur after injection of vaccines, take the appropriate precautions. (See Nursing Alert on anaphylactic reaction, Chapter 36.)

One of the most important features of injecting vaccines is adequate penetration of the muscle for deposition of the drug intramuscularly, not subcutaneously. In two studies, the use of longer needles in administering vaccines to a group of infants significantly decreased the incidence of localized edema and tenderness (Diggle and Deeks, 2000; Diggle, Deeks, and Pollard, 2006) (see Evidence-Based Practice box).

EVIDENCE-BASED PRACTICE

Appropriate Site, Technique, Needle Size, and Dose for Intramuscular Injections in Infants, Toddlers, and Small Children*

ASK THE QUESTION

In infants, toddlers, and small children what is the best site, technique, needle size and gauge, and dosage for intramuscular (IM) injections?

SEARCH FOR THE EVIDENCE

Search strategies

Literature from 1990 to 2009 was reviewed to obtain clinical research studies related to this issue.

Databases used

CINAHL, PubMed

CRITICALLY ANALYZE THE EVIDENCE

GRADE criteria: Evidence quality low; recommendation strong (Guyatt, Oxman, Vist, et al, 2008)

The searches reviewed were mostly small studies. There were no randomized trials, double-blinded trials, or large clinical studies addressing the subject of IM injections in children.

- Studies in adults indicate that injection pain can be minimized by deep IM administration, since muscle tissue has fewer nerve endings and medications are absorbed faster than those administered subcutaneously (Zuckerman, 2000). Immunizations such as diphtheria-tetanus–acellular pertussis (DTaP) and hepatitis A and B contain an aluminum adjuvant that, if injected into subcutaneous tissue, increases the incidence of local reactions. Inadvertent injection into subcutaneous tissue may be caused by use of a needle too short to reach IM tissue (Zuckerman, 2000).
- One study found that 4-month-old infants experienced fewer local side effects (redness, tenderness, and swelling) when immunizations were administered into the anterior aspect of the thigh with a 25-mm (1-inch) needle as opposed to the shorter 16-mm (⅝-inch) needle (Diggle and Deeks, 2000).
- Another study comparing needle length and injection method found that a longer needle (25 mm) was preferred for injection when bunching the skin and injecting, whereas a shorter needle (16 mm) was perceived as causing fewer localized reactions when the injection was administered with the skin being held taut (Groswasser, Kahn, Bouche, et al, 1997). However, the study's conclusions fail to address whether needle lengths were applicable to both the deltoid and vastus lateralis muscles.
- Cook and Murtagh (2002) made ultrasound measurements of the subcutaneous and muscle layer thickness in 57 children ages 2, 4, 6, and 18 months. These researchers concluded that a 16-mm needle was sufficient to penetrate the anterolateral thigh muscle if the needle is inserted at a 90-degree angle without pinching the muscle, whereas thigh measurements demonstrated that a 25-mm needle was necessary to penetrate the muscle when a 45-degree injection technique was employed. This study supports the concept of longer needle length to fully deposit the medication into the muscle.
- In a study by Davenport (2004), needle length proved to be the most significant variable for local reactions in children after injection with 16-mm and 25-mm needles; the 25-mm needle was associated with fewer localized reactions.
- Diggle, Deeks, and Pollard (2006) likewise found that when long needles (25 mm) were used for infant immunizations, localized vaccine reactions were significantly reduced in comparison to the shorter needles (16 mm).
- Beecroft and Redick (1990) cited numerous differences of opinion regarding IM injection technique among pediatric nurses, highlighting how little agreement there is among nursing texts evaluated in regards to injection site and technique.
- In a nursing journal column a nurse noted discrepancies in IM administration technique when injections were given to her child, further highlighting the differences in opinion regarding IM injection technique among pediatric nurses (Winslow and Jacobson, 1997).
- In a study of diphtheria-tetanus-pertussis (DTP) immunizations administered to infants 7 months and younger, only 84.6% of injections were administered at the correct site (anterior thigh); an alarming number were given in the dorsogluteal (5.1%) and deltoid (2.6%) muscles (Daly, Johnston, and Chung, 1992).
- Beecroft and Kongelbeck (1994) evaluated pediatric IM injections and concluded that the ventrogluteal site is the site of choice in children of all ages; they found no reports of complications at this site in the literature. The ventrogluteal site is relatively free of important nerves and vascular structures, the site is easily identified by landmarks, and the subcutaneous tissue is thinner in that area. To date, no reports can be found in the literature to refute the claims made by these researchers.
- The American Academy of Pediatrics (2009) and the Centers for Disease Control and Prevention (2002) recommend that vaccines containing adjuvants such as aluminum (DTaP, hepatitis A and B, diphtheria-tetanus [DT or Td]) be given deep into the muscle to prevent local reactions. In addition, a 16-mm needle may be adequate for injections in small infants, and a 22- to 25-mm (⅞ to 1 inch) needle can be used in infants 4 months and older. The Centers for Disease Control and Prevention (2002) recommends that toddlers receive injections with a 22- to 38-mm (⅞- to 1¼-inch) needle in the deltoid if muscle size is adequate; a minimum of a 25-mm long needle is recommended for anterolateral thigh injection in toddlers. Both the American Academy of Pediatrics (2009) and the Centers for Disease Control and Prevention (2002) recommend a 22- to 25-mm needle for all IM childhood immunizations. The deltoid muscle may be used for immunizations in toddlers, older children, and adolescents.
- Diggle (2003) recommends the deltoid muscle for IM injections in children over 1 year of age. When multiple vaccines are given, two may be given in the thigh (anterior and lateral) because of its larger size. The American Academy of Pediatrics (2009) recommends that injections in the anterolateral thigh be given at least 2.5 cm (1 inch) apart so local reactions are less likely to overlap. The dorsogluteal muscle should be avoided in infants and toddlers, and perhaps even in smaller preschoolers with smaller muscle mass, because of the possibility of damaging the sciatic nerve.

---

*See also Intramuscular Administration, Chapter 27.

Continued

EVIDENCE-BASED PRACTICE—cont'd

Appropriate Site, Technique, Needle Size, and Dose for Intramuscular Injections in Infants, Toddlers, and Small Children*

No research or supportive data were found regarding the amount of medication to be given at the different sites in infants and toddlers. In general, 1 ml of medication is recommended for infants less than 12 months; however, no data can be found to refute or support such a recommendation. Furthermore, small and preterm infants may only tolerate up to 0.5 ml in each muscle to prevent local complications.

In summary, some discrepancy remains in actual clinical practice regarding IM injection sites, amount of drug injected, and needle size in infants and toddlers. Further research is needed to address the following issues:

- What is the appropriate muscle in which an IM injection can be administered with fewest adverse effects in infants and toddlers?
- What is the appropriate needle size based on the infant or toddler's age and weight?
- What is the largest safe amount of medication that can be given to infants and toddlers based on weight and muscle size?

APPLY THE EVIDENCE: NURSING IMPLICATIONS

Based on the evidence in the literature, the recommendation is to continue administering IM injections to children in the anterolateral thigh (<12 months old), deltoid (≥12 months old), and ventrogluteal site.

Needle length is an important factor in decreasing local reactions; the length should be adequate to deposit the medication into the muscle for IM injections. Recommendations are for a 25-mm (1-inch) needle in infants, 25- to 32-mm (1- to 1¼-inch) needle for toddlers, and 38- to 51-mm (1½- to 2-inch) needle for older children; preterm and small emaciated infants may require a shorter needle (16 to 25 mm [⅝ to 1 inch]) based on weight and muscle mass size.

References

American Academy of Pediatrics, Committee on Infectious Diseases, Pickering L, editor: *2009 Red book: report of the Committee on Infectious Diseases,* ed 28, Elk Grove Village, Ill, 2009, The Academy.

Beecroft PC, Kongelbeck SR: How safe are intramuscular injections? *AACN Clin Issues* 5(2):207-215, 1994.

Beecroft PC, Redick SA: Intramuscular injection practices of pediatric nurses: site selection, *Nurs Educ* 15(4):23-28, 1990.

Centers for Disease Control and Prevention: General recommendations on immunization, *MMWR* 51(RR-2):12-14, 2002.

Cook IF, Murtagh J: Needle length required for intramuscular vaccination of infants and toddlers: an ultrasonographic study, *Austral Fam Phys* 31(3):295-297, 2002.

Daly JM, Johnston W, Chung Y: Injection sites utilized for DPT immunizations in infants, *J Comm Health Nurs* 9(2):87-94, 1992.

Davenport JM: A systematic review to ascertain whether the standard needle is more effective than a longer or wider needle in reducing the incidence of local reaction in children receiving primary immunization, *J Adv Nurs* 46(1):66-77, 2004.

Diggle L: The administration of child vaccines, part 11, Childhood vaccinations, *Practice Nurse* 25(12):63-69, 2003.

Diggle L, Deeks J: Effect of needle length on incidence of local reactions to routine immunisation in infants aged 4 months: randomised controlled trial, *BMJ* 321(7266):931-933, 2000.

Diggle L, Deeks JJ, Pollard AJ: Effect of needle size on immunogenicity and reactogenecity of vaccines in infants: randomized controlled trial, *BMJ* 333(7568):571, 2006.

Groswasser J, Kahn A, Bouche B, et al: Needle length and injection technique for efficient intramuscular vaccine delivery in infants and children evaluated through an ultrasonographic determination of subcutaneous and muscle layer thickness, *Pediatrics* 100(3 Pt 1):400-403, 1997.

Guyatt GH, Oxman AD, Vist GE, et al: GRADE: an emerging consensus on rating quality of evidence and strength of recommendations, *BMJ* 336: 924-926, 2008.

Winslow EH, Jacobson AF: Research for practice: pediatric IM injections: one size does not fit all, *Am J Nurs* 97(11):20, 1997.

Zuckerman J: The importance of injecting vaccines into muscle, *BMJ* 321(7271):1237-1238, 2000.

*See also Intramuscular Administration, Chapter 27.

Because nurses often administer vaccines, they may have the responsibility for adequately informing parents of the nature, prevalence, and risks of the disease; the type of immunization product to be used; the expected benefits and risk of side effects of the vaccine; and the need for accurate immunization records. Referring to immunizations as "baby shots" and limiting the discussion to vague statements about the vaccines are unacceptable practices.

Another important nursing responsibility is accurate documentation. Each child should have an immunization record for parents to keep, especially for families who move frequently. Although immunization rates have increased significantly, health professionals should use every opportunity to encourage complete immunization of all children (see Community Focus box). Blank immunization records may be downloaded from a number of websites, including the Immunization Action Coalition (www.immunize.org), which has vaccine information and records in a number of languages.

Document the following information on the medical record: day, month, and year of administration; manufacturer and lot number of vaccine; and name, address, and title of the person administering the vaccine. Additional data to record are the site and route of administration and evidence that the parent or legal guardian gave informed consent before the immunization was administered. Report any adverse reactions after the administration of a vaccine to the Vaccine Adverse Event Reporting System (www.vaers.hhs.gov; 800-822-7967).

An additional source of vaccine information that must be given to parents (as required by the National Childhood Vaccine Injury Act, 1986) before the administration of vaccines is the VIS for the particular vaccine being administered. Practitioners are required by law to fully inform families of the risks and benefits of the vaccines. VISs are designed to provide updated information to the adult vaccinee or parents or legal guardians of children being vaccinated regarding the risks and benefits of each vaccine. The practitioner should answer questions regarding the information in the VISs. VISs are available for the following vaccines: anthrax, tetanus, diphtheria, pertussis, MMR, IPV, HPV, varicella, Hib, H1N1 influenza, influenza, meningococcal, pneumococcal, rabies, rotavirus, shingles, smallpox, yellow fever, Japanese encephalitis, typhoid, and hepatitis A and B. An updated VIS should be provided to the primary caregiver, and documentation in the patient's chart should include the VIS title and the VIS publication date. VISs are available from state or local health departments, the Immunization Action Coalition (www.immunize.org/vis), and the

Centers for Disease Control and Prevention (http://www.cdc.gov/vaccines/pubs/vis/default.htm; 800-232-4636).

In response to the concerns of manufacturers, practitioners, and parents of children with serious vaccine-associated injuries, the National Childhood Vaccine Injury Act of 1986 and the Vaccine Compensation Amendments of 1987 were passed. These laws are designed to provide fair compensation for children who are inadvertently injured and provide greater protection from liability for vaccine manufacturers and providers. (See American Academy of Pediatrics, 2009b, for further details of this program.)

Bioterrorism and Vaccines

A number of events, including those of September 11, 2001, have precipitated changes in family's lives across the United States. The threats of anthrax and smallpox germ warfare have prompted public safety and health care officials to reevaluate disasters and threats to the general population's health. Children are aware of media stories discussing potential threats and may have concerns and fears regarding their personal, family's, and friends' safety and health. A common theme expressed among adolescents after the September 11 attack and various wide-scale shootings in high schools was concern and fear for personal safety and the general fear of the unknown outcome in the event of another attack in their community or school.

Nurses are in a position to help families deal effectively with children's fears and concerns related to events that may affect their mental and physical health. It is not within the scope of this text to discuss the many strategies for counseling children about natural and man-made disasters, but it is important to be knowledgeable about health issues related to vaccines should

an event occur that requires wide-scale inoculation of children and adults.

The American Academy of Pediatrics offers a number of resources regarding disasters (**www.aap.org/disasters/resources.cfm**), including a free *Family Readiness Kit* that may help parents discuss disaster issues with children (**www.aap.org/family/frk/frkit.htm**). Starr (2002) provides a number of strategies for helping children of different ages cope with disaster and numerous excellent resources for parents and nurses helping children.

Nurses working with children may use these resources and others to help families and children become knowledgeable about disasters and vaccines developed for the protection of children and adults in the event of exposure to toxic agents.

INJURY PREVENTION

Injuries are a major cause of death during infancy, especially for children 6 to 12 months old. According to some surveys (Agran, Anderson, Winn, et al, 2003; Pickett, Streight, Simpson, et al, 2003), the leading causes of injury to infants are falls, ingestion injuries (poison and medications), and burns. In a Canadian survey (Pickett, Streight, Simpson, et al, 2003), the top leading causes of injury to infants were falls, ingestion injuries, and burns. The three leading causes of accidental death injury in infants in the United States were suffocation, motor vehicle–related accidents, and drowning (Centers for Disease Control and Prevention, 2007a). Mack, Gilchrist, and Ballesteros (2007) report that fall-related injuries in the home were the most common reason for emergency department visits in infants ages 0 to 12 months; according to these authors one infant is injured every $1\frac{1}{2}$ minutes. In a similar study of infants

treated for accidents, the bed was commonly listed as being involved, whereas car seat at 2 months of age and stairs at 12 months were reported to be the cause of the accidental injury (Mack, Gilchrist, and Ballesteros, 2008). Constant vigilance, awareness, and supervision are essential as the child gains increased locomotor and manipulative skills that are coupled with an insatiable curiosity about the environment. Box 12-6 lists the major developmental achievements of each period during infancy and the appropriate injury prevention plan.

Aspiration of Foreign Objects

Asphyxiation by foreign material in the respiratory tract, combined with mechanical suffocation, is one of the leading causes of fatal injury in children younger than 1 year. Both food and nonfood items are among the most common foreign bodies ingested and found in the gastrointestinal tract (Agran, Anderson, Winn, et al, 2003). The size, shape, and consistency of foods or objects are important determinants of fatal obstruction. For example, small spheric or cylindric and pliable objects (<3.2 cm [1.2 inches]) are more likely to completely obstruct the airway.

Toys are the most common cause of aspiration; therefore all toys must be carefully inspected for potential danger. Many toys that make noise or rattle, for example, have small beads inside. A broken or cracked toy can be dangerous because the beads can easily be aspirated while the infant has the toy in the mouth. Stuffed animals are potentially dangerous if any of the parts, such as the eyes or nose, are removable buttons or plastic pieces. Front buttons on infant clothes can easily be pulled off and swallowed. An active infant can grab a low-hanging mobile and quickly chew off a small piece. As soon as the infant crawls or plays on the floor, the floor must be kept free of any small articles that can be picked up and swallowed, such as coins and buttons.

Food items are the second most common cause of aspiration, and the most common offenders are hot dogs, candy, nuts, and grapes. When new foods are given to the child, nuts, hard candies, marshmallows, large amounts of peanut butter, or fruits with pits or seeds are avoided. If given to young children, hot dogs must be cut into small, irregular pieces rather than served whole or sliced into sections because their size (diameter), round shape, and consistency allow for complete occlusion of the airway. Perhaps the most dangerous foods are dried beans, which, if aspirated, enlarge when they come in contact with the wet mucosa and block the airway.

Pacifiers can also be dangerous because the entire object may be aspirated if it is small, or the nipple and shield may become detached from the handle and become lodged in the pharynx. Improvised pacifiers, such as those made from a padded nipple, also present dangers. The nipple may separate from the plastic collar and be aspirated. Thus only safe commercial pacifiers should be used, if at all. Candy pacifiers pose dangers because the candy portion can dislodge from the circular base and be aspirated. To be safe, pacifiers should have:

- Sturdy, one-piece construction with material that is non-toxic, flexible, and firm but not brittle
- An easily grasped handle
- A mouthguard that cannot be separated from the nipple, has two ventilating holes, and is too large to be aspirated
- No detachable ribbon or string
- A label warning against tying the pacifier around the infant's neck

---

BOX 12-6 INJURY PREVENTION DURING INFANCY

Birth to 4 Months
Major Developmental Accomplishments
Involuntary reflexes, such as the crawling reflex, may propel infant forward or backward; the startle reflex may cause the body to jerk
May roll over
Has increased eye-hand coordination and voluntary grasp reflex

Injury Prevention
Aspiration
This is not as great a danger to this age-group, but parents should begin practicing safeguarding early (see under 4 to 7 Months).
Never shake baby powder directly on infant; place powder in hand and then on infant's skin; store container closed and out of infant's reach.
Hold infant for feeding; do not prop bottle.
Know emergency procedures for choking.
Use pacifier with one-piece construction and loop handle.

Suffocation and Drowning
Keep all plastic bags stored out of infant's reach; discard large plastic garment bags after tying in a knot.
Do not cover mattress with plastic.
Use firm mattress and loose blankets; no pillows.
Make certain crib design follows federal regulations and mattress fits snugly— crib slats 6 cm (2.375 inches) apart.*
Position crib away from other furniture and away from radiators.
Do not tie pacifier on a string around infant's neck.
Remove bibs at bedtime.
Never leave infant alone in bath.

Do not leave infant under 12 months alone on adult or youth mattress or "beanbag" type pillows.
Do not leave infant in a car on warm day.

Falls
Always raise crib rails.
Never leave infant on a raised, unguarded surface.
When in doubt as to where to place child, use floor.
Restrain child in infant seat and never leave child unattended while the seat is resting on a raised surface.
Avoid using a high chair until child can sit well with support.

Poisoning
This is not as great a danger to this age-group, but begin practicing safeguards early (see under 4 to 7 Months).

Burns
Install smoke detectors in home.
Use caution when warming formula in microwave oven; always check temperature of liquid before feeding.
Check bath water.
Do not pour hot liquids when infant is close by, such as sitting on lap.
Beware of cigarette ashes that may fall on infant.
Do not leave infant in sun for more than a few minutes; keep exposed areas covered.
Wash flame-retardant clothes according to label directions.
Use cool-mist vaporizers.
Do not leave child in parked car.
Check surface heat of car restraint before placing child in seat.

BOX 12-6 INJURY PREVENTION DURING INFANCY—cont'd

Motor Vehicles

Transport infant in federally approved, rear-facing car seat, preferably in back seat.

Do not place infant on seat of car or in lap.

Do not place child in a carriage or stroller behind a parked car.

Do not place infant or child (in car seat) in front passenger seat with an air bag unless air bag is deactivated.

Bodily Damage

Keep sharp, jagged objects out of child's reach.

Keep diaper pins closed and away from infant.

4 to 7 Months
Major Developmental Accomplishments

Rolls over

Sits momentarily

Grasps and manipulates small objects

Resecures a dropped object

Has well-developed eye-hand coordination

Can focus on and locate small objects

Can push up on hands and knees

Crawls backward

Places objects in mouth (hand-to-mouth)

Injury Prevention
Aspiration

Keep buttons, beads, syringe caps, and other small objects out of infant's reach.

Keep floor free of any small objects.

Do not feed infant hard candy, nuts, food with pits or seeds, or whole or circular pieces of hot dog.

Exercise caution when giving teething biscuits, since large chunks may be broken off and aspirated.

Do not feed infant while he or she is lying down.

Inspect toys for removable parts.

Keep baby powder, if used, out of reach.

Suffocation

Keep all latex balloons out of reach.

Remove all crib toys that are strung across crib or playpen when child begins to push up on hands or knees or is 5 months old.

Falls

Restrain in a high chair.

Keep crib rails raised to full height.

Poisoning

Make sure that paint for furniture or toys does not contain lead.

Place toxic substances on a high shelf or in locked cabinet.

Keep medication vials and bottles locked in a secure place.

Hang plants or place on high surface rather than on floor.

Avoid storing large quantities of cleaning fluid, paints, pesticides, and other toxic substances.

Discard used containers of poisonous substances.

Do not store toxic substances in food containers.

Keep cosmetic and personal products out of child's reach.

Discard used button-size batteries; store new batteries in safe area.

Know telephone number of local poison control center (usually listed in front of telephone directory).

Burns

Keep faucets out of reach.

Place hot objects (cigarettes, candles, incense) on high surface.

Limit exposure to sun; apply sunscreen.

Motor Vehicles

See under Birth to 4 Months

Bodily Damage

Give toys that are smooth and rounded, preferably made of wood or plastic.

Avoid long, pointed objects as toys.

Avoid toys that are excessively loud.

Keep sharp objects out of infant's reach.

8 to 12 Months
Major Developmental Accomplishments

Crawls, creeps

Stands holding onto furniture

Stands alone

Cruises around furniture

Walks

Climbs

Pulls on objects

Throws objects

Picks up small objects; has pincer grasp

Explores by putting objects in mouth

Dislikes being restrained

Explores away from parent

Has increasing understanding of simple commands and phrases

Injury Prevention
Aspiration

Keep lint and small objects off floor, off furniture, and out of reach of children.

Take care in feeding solid table food to give very small pieces.

Do not use beanbag toys or allow child to play with dried beans.

See also under 4 to 7 Months.

Suffocation and Drowning

Keep doors of ovens, dishwashers, refrigerators, coolers, and front-loading clothes washers and dryers closed at all times.

If storing an unused appliance, such as a refrigerator, remove the door.

Supervise contact with inflated balloons, immediately discard popped balloons, and keep uninflated balloons out of reach.

Fence swimming pools.

Always supervise when near any source of water, such as cleaning buckets, drainage areas, or toilets.

Keep bathroom doors closed.

Eliminate unnecessary pools of water.

Keep one hand on child at all times when in tub.

Falls

Avoid walkers, especially near stairs.

Ensure that furniture is sturdy enough for child to pull self to standing position and cruise.

Fence stairways at top and bottom if child has access to either end.

Dress infant in safe shoes and clothing (soles that do not "catch" on floor, tied shoelaces, pant legs that do not touch floor).

Poisoning

Administer medications as a drug, not as a candy.

Do not administer medications unless prescribed by a practitioner.

Replace medications and poisons immediately after use; replace caps properly if a child-protector cap is used.

Keep phone number for poison control center readily available.

Burns

Place guards in front of or around any heating appliance, fireplace, or furnace.

Keep electrical wires hidden or out of reach.

Place plastic guards over electrical outlets; place furniture in front of outlets.

Keep hanging tablecloths out of reach (child may pull down hot liquids or heavy or sharp objects).

*Information on many items such as cribs or walkers available from U.S. Consumer Product Safety Commission, 800-638-2772; **www.cpsc.gov.**

Using a syringe to accurately measure and dispense oral liquid medications to young children has become common practice. However, a syringe with a cap becomes a potential aspiration hazard. The newer medication administration syringes for children do not have a removable cap. Other items that can easily be aspirated include soda and fruit juice bottle tops or caps, aluminum soda can pop-top rings that tear off easily, and small key rings (<1.5 inches in diameter).

Suffocation

According to one survey, accidental suffocation and strangulation rates among infants quadrupled between 1984 and 2004 in the United States; African-American boys under the age of 4 months were most affected (Shapiro-Mendoza, Kimball, Tomashek, et al, 2009). Schnitzer (2006) indicates that almost 67% of injury deaths in infants are due to suffocation. Mechanical suffocation includes suffocation by covering of the airway (i.e., mouth and nose); by pressure on the throat and chest; and by exclusion of air, such as by refrigerator entrapment. Nonfood items cause the majority of deaths in young children. Latex balloons, whether partially inflated, uninflated, or popped, are the leading cause of pediatric choking deaths from children's products. They should be kept away from infants and young children.

The bed or crib poses a number of hazards. An infant who is placed in a bed under tucked-in blankets and sheets can be caught under them and unable to wriggle free. (See Sudden Infant Death Syndrome, Chapter 13.) Bumper crib pads are a common cause of death in infants either as a result of suffocation or strangulation on the bumper ties (Thach, Rutherford, and Harris, 2007). Baby pillows filled with plastic foam beads that make them resemble small bean bags are dangerous; very young infants are suffocated when the pillow contours to the face and blocks the airway. There are potential dangers in adults sleeping with an infant because of the possibility of their rolling over and smothering the child (overlaying), especially when alcohol, tobacco, or recreational drugs are involved. According to U.S. federal regulations, the distance between crib slats should not be more than 6 cm (2.375 inches), roughly the width of three adult fingers. Mattresses should fit snugly against the slats; bumper pads are no longer recommended. A general rule is that the mattress is too small if two adult fingers can be placed between the mattress and crib or bed side. A temporary solution is to place large, rolled towels in the space to create a snug fit.

Corner post extensions on cribs are another source of strangulation. Children have died when their clothing caught on raised corner posts as they climbed out of the crib. Voluntary manufacturing standards state that corner post extensions not exceed $\frac{1}{16}$ inch. However, the safety of any extension is questionable. Decorative extensions need to be removed from cribs. Ideally, information regarding correct crib design should be given prenatally, before parents have purchased or borrowed a crib.*

---

*A number of parent education pamphlets—such as *Crib Safety Tips* and *Is Your Used Crib Safe?*—are available in English and Spanish from the U.S. Consumer Product Safety Commission, Publication Request, Washington, DC 20207; 800-638-2772; www.cpsc.gov.

Mesh-sided playpens and cribs can result in death if the sides are left in the lowered position. Infants have suffocated when they fell off the edge of the mattress and the head or chest was compressed between the floorboard and mesh side. Cribs should be located away from windows, where drape or blind cords can become wrapped around the infant's neck.

Another cause of suffocation is plastic bags. Large plastic bags used over garments are lightweight and can easily and quickly be wrapped around the head of an active infant or pressed against the face. For this reason, pillows and mattresses should not be covered with plastic. Older infants may play with a plastic bag and accidentally pull it over their heads. Because plastic is nonporous, suffocation occurs in a matter of minutes.

Cords located near the infant or tied around the infant's neck can potentially cause strangulation. Bibs are removed after meals, and objects such as pacifiers are never hung on a string around the infant's neck. This is a common practice in some cultures that can be remedied by tying a short string to a pacifier and pinning the string to the child's shirt.

Toys that have strings attached, such as a telephone, or toys that are tied to cribs or playpens can be hazards because the string can become wrapped around the child's neck or the child can become entrapped in the toy. As a precaution, all cords should be less than 30 cm (12 inches) long. Crib toys should be hung high enough that the infant cannot become entangled in them and should no longer be used once the child is able to reach them.

Motor Vehicle Injuries

Automobile injuries are the leading cause of accidental death in children between the ages of 1 and 9 years (Centers for Disease Control and Prevention, 2007a). A significant number of nonfatal vehicle-related injuries in children between 1 and 4 years of age occur as a result of back-over while children are playing in a driveway (Centers for Disease Control and Prevention, 2005b). In addition, a significant number of infants are injured or die from improper restraint within the vehicle, most often from riding on the lap of another occupant. Desapriya, Joshi, Subwarzi, and colleagues (2008) found that falls accounted for a significant proportion of injuries (98%) in infants from birth to 4 months of age as a result of inappropriate use of a car restraint system. Reports indicate that child restraint use decreases with increasing age of children and increasing number of occupants. Lack of proper child restraint continues to be a major factor in fatal accidents involving children. All infants must be secured in a federally approved restraint rather than held or placed on the seat of the car. There is no safe alternative.

Infant restraints are designed either as an infant-only model or as a convertible infant-toddler model. Either restraint is a semireclined seat that faces the rear of the car. A rear-facing car seat provides the best protection for the disproportionately heavy head and weak neck of an infant (Fig. 12-15). This position minimizes the stress on the neck by spreading the forces of a frontal crash over the entire back, neck, and head; the spine is supported by the back of the car seat. If the seat were faced forward, the head would whip forward because of the force of the crash, creating enormous stress on the neck. A recent study indicated that children 0 to 3 years of age riding properly restrained in the middle of the back seat had a 43%

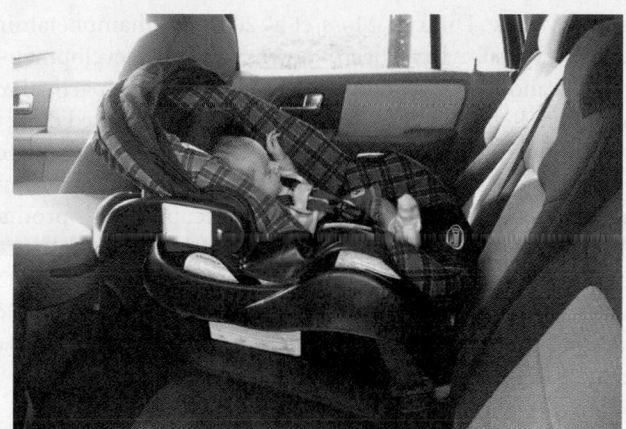

Fig. 12-15 Rear-facing infant seat in rear seat of car. (Courtesy Brian and Mayannyn Sallee, Las Vegas.)

lower risk of injury than children riding in the outboard (window) seat during a crash (Kallan, Durbin, Arbogast, et al, 2008). Another study showed that children 0 to 23 months riding in a rear-facing restraint were less likely to be injured than those riding in a forward-facing restraint (Henary, Sherwood, Crandall, et al, 2007).

The restraint is anchored to the vehicle with the vehicle's seat belt, and the restraint has a harness system for securing the infant. Some harness systems require a clip to keep the shoulder straps correctly positioned. Newer vehicles (manufactured after 1999) have tether straps that attach to anchors in the car seat to better secure the seat and minimize forward movement of the forward-facing convertible seats in the event of an accident. The LATCH (lower anchor and tether for children) system provides car seat anchors between the front cushion and backrest so that the seat belt does not have to be used. Some automobiles have tether straps for rear-facing infant-only seats as well. (See Chapter 14.) Although many infant restraints can be recliners, they are used in the car only in the position specified by the manufacturer.

It is now recommended that all infants and toddlers ride in a rear-facing car safety seat until they have reached the age of 2 years or they reach the highest weight or height recommended by the car seat manufacturer (American Academy of Pediatrics, 2011).

Rear-facing infant safety seats must not be placed in the front seats of cars equipped with an air bag on the passenger side. If an infant safety seat is placed in the passenger seat with an air bag, the child could be seriously injured if the air bag is released, since rear-facing infant seats extend closer to the dashboard. Severe injuries and deaths in children have occurred from air bags deploying on impact in the front passenger seat. The back seat is the safest area of the car. If the back seat is not an option, an infant restraint may be positioned in the front seat provided that the seat belt can be locked into position and there is no passenger-side air bag. If there is a passenger-side air bag and the child has special health care needs or constant observation is recommended by the practitioner and no other adult is available to ride in the back seat with the child, an on/off switch may be installed to prevent the air bag from deploying and injuring the child riding in the front seat. In vehicles without a back seat, it is best to place the front passenger seat as far back as possible and use appropriate child safety restraint. The new, "smart" air bags include features that make it possible to deactivate the air bag temporarily if an infant must ride in the front seat. Remind parents to reactivate the airbag once the infant is no longer riding in the front seat.* (See discussion of air bag safety in Chapter 14.)

For restraints to be effective, they must be used properly. Dressing the infant in an outfit with sleeves and legs allows the harness to hold the child securely in the seat. A small blanket or towel rolled tightly can be placed on either side of the head to minimize movement and keep the infant's hips against the back of the seat. Padding between the infant's legs and crotch can prevent slouching. Thick, soft padding is not placed under the infant or behind the back because during the impact the padding will compress, leaving the harness straps loose. Preterm infants being discharged home should be secured in an appropriate car seat restraint as it would be placed in the car and the infant's oxygen saturations monitored for a determined period to detect any potential problems with airway occlusion. (For further discussion of car seat restraints, see Chapter 14; for preterm infant car restraint test guidelines, see Family-Centered Care box, p. 341.)

Another automobile-related hazard for infants is overheating (hyperthermia) and subsequent death when left in a vehicle in hot weather (>26.4° C [80° F]). Infants dissipate heat poorly, and an increase in body temperature may cause death in a few hours. Caution parents against leaving infants in a vehicle alone for *any reason*. A small sign or placard has been designed to hang in the rear-view mirror to remind the parent that there is a child in the back seat. Busy parents may forget the child in the back when preoccupied with errands, children's school and extracurricular activities, and busy work schedules.

Falls

Residential injuries, especially falls, accounted for the highest incidence of unintentional injuries to children seen in emergency departments in the United States (Phelan, Khoury, Kalkwarf, et al, 2005). A study of childhood injuries found that beginning at the age of 3 to 5 months, the incidence of falls increased dramatically with increasing age, peaking at 15 to 17 months of age. Most falls were from heights such as furniture, stairs, and buildings (Agran, Anderson, Winn, et al, 2003). A large percentage of infants have fallen as a result of being dropped or falling out of car seats, down stairs, or from child walkers (Pickett, Streight, Simpson, et al, 2003; Dedoukou, Spyridopoulos, Kedikoglou, et al, 2004). Falls from shopping carts and bunk beds also contribute to a significant number of injuries in small children (Wright, Griffin, MacLennan, et al, 2008; D'Souza, Smith, and McKenzie, 2008).

Infant walkers are responsible for a number of different types of injuries that occur when the walker tips over or falls down stairs. Warn parents of these dangers and encourage them to keep constant watch on their child's activities; discourage the use of walkers. The American Academy of Pediatrics

*An air bag safety fact sheet is available from the American Academy of Pediatrics, 141 Northwest Point Blvd., Elk Grove Village, IL 60007; www.aap.org. Car seat information is available at www.aap.org/family/carseatguide.htm; and from the Insurance Institute for Highway Safety, 1005 N. Glebe Road, Suite 800, Arlington, VA 22201; 703-247-1500; fax: 703-247-1588; www.iihs.org. The National Highway Traffic Safety Administration, www.nhtsa.gov, also provides child passenger safety and air bag safety information for parents.

(2001) does not recommend the use of walkers with wheels. One alternative is to use a stationary play station with a seat similar to that of a walker. There is no evidence that infant walkers help infants walk sooner.

Once infants are mobile, they should not be allowed to crawl unsupervised on any raised surface, near stairs, or near any water reservoir. Gates should be used at the bottom and top of stairs, since both present dangers to the crawling and climbing infant. As children begin to pull themselves to a standing position, heavy objects, such as unsturdy furniture, televisions, compact disc players, or any freestanding item (e.g., wrought iron fish tank stands or concrete birdbath), can be extremely dangerous if pulled down on top of the child. To prevent injury from furniture tipping over, place televisions on lower furniture and as far back as possible. Angle braces or anchors can secure furniture to walls.

Poisoning

Poisoning is one of the major causes of death in children younger than 5 years of age. The highest incidence occurs in the 2-year-old group, with the second highest incidence occurring in 1-year-old children. Infants who do not crawl are relatively free from the danger of poisonous agents because they are immobile. However, once they become mobile, danger from poisoning is almost everywhere. The average home contains more than 500 toxic substances, and approximately one third of all poisonings occur in the kitchen.

The major reason for ingestion of poisons is improper storage. To protect the infant, toxic agents should not be placed on a low shelf, table, or floor. Plants are another source of poisoning for infants. Plants are commonly placed on the floor, and the leaves or flowers are attractive and easy to pull off. More than 700 species of plants are known to cause illness or death. Common household over-the-counter medications such as acetaminophen and cold and cough preparations, cosmetics and personal care products, and cleaning products are also sources of childhood poisoning (Wilkerson, Northington, and Fisher, 2005).

Another danger is ingestion of the button-sized batteries used in devices such as hearing aids, calculators, watches, and cameras. Because they are bright and shiny, they are attractive to children. However, they can cause severe morbidity, even death, if lodged in the esophagus. The strong alkali in a battery can leak and cause a severe caustic burn. As a precaution, small batteries must be safely stored and discarded where young children cannot easily retrieve them.

Not all poisonings result from ingestion; another possible route is inhalation, such as inhaling chlorine vapors from household cleaning or pool supplies. Passive cocaine toxicity has occurred in young children exposed to freebase cocaine ("crack") smoking by adults. The production of methamphetamines, a common central nervous system stimulant also known as ice, speed, or crystal, involves a number of chemicals that may be toxic alone (contact or ingestion) or during the production (cooking) of the drug itself. Methamphetamine laboratories are commonly in household areas where children may be exposed to harmful inhalants and to open fires where meth is "cooked." Methamphetamine laboratories are also often mobile, and children may be similarly exposed to dangerous chemicals (Farst, Duncan, Moss, et al, 2007). Methamphetamine use and exposure have been shown to cause developmental problems and short- and long-term brain damage, particularly in children. Reports of the number of children exposed daily to methamphetamine laboratories in the United States and Canada are alarming. Such children are also at high risk for abuse and neglect because their caretakers are preoccupied with production, sale, and use of the drug (Bellemare, 2008; Matteucci, Auten, Crowley, et al, 2007; Mecham and Melini, 2002). Children should be protected from environments in which inhaled toxins exist. (See Chapter 32 for discussion of effects of chemical substances on the fetus and neonate.)

! **NURSING ALERT**

Parents should know the telephone number of the local poison control center—**800-222-1222**—and call this number in the event of a suspected poisoning. Ipecac, used to induce vomiting, is no longer a standard recommendation. If the child is not breathing, the parent should call 911 immediately.

The only certain way to prevent poisoning is to remove toxic agents, which means placing containers out of the infant's reach or contact. Because crawling infants soon become climbing toddlers, it is best to keep all toxic agents, especially drugs, in a locked cabinet. Special plastic hooks can be attached to the inside of cabinet doors to keep them securely closed. Firm thumb pressure is required to unlatch the hook, and small children are usually unable to manipulate them. Locks are best, but for frequently used cleaning agents, such as those often kept under a kitchen sink, hooks are a practical alternative.

With several hundred toxic substances in each house, locking them all up can present a problem. Potentially hazardous substances should not be stored in any type of food container. A popular container used to store toxic liquids is a soda or pop bottle. A child who is unaware of the dangerous contents is vulnerable to poisoning. Parents should know the telephone number of local poison control centers and call in the event of a suspected poisoning. Chapter 16 discusses emergency measures for poisoning.

Burns

Scalding from water that is too hot; excessive sunburn; and burns from house fires, electrical wires, sockets, and heating elements such as radiators, registers, and floor furnaces cause a significant number of deaths and many more injuries in infants. The infant's skin is particularly sensitive to irritation, and the mechanisms for temperature perception are not completely developed. As a general precaution, all homes should have smoke alarms installed near the bedroom areas and on each level of the building.

Scald burns from hot tap water can be prevented by lowering the hot water heater to a safe temperature of 49° C (120° F). In addition, parents should check the bath water before placing the infant in it. The two most common types of scald injury are from the child pulling a hot pan of water off a stove or elevated surface or overturning a container of hot water on herself or himself (Drago, 2005). The handles of cooking utensils should be turned toward the back of the stove. When the infant is underfoot, caretakers should avoid pouring hot liquids and cooking with hot oil. Hanging tablecloths should also be out of the infant's reach to prevent pulling hot items off the table.

Scalds can also occur from bathing infants in the kitchen sink when the garbage disposal, occluded with debris, causes the draining dishwasher effluent to back up into the sink. The temperature of the effluent from a dishwasher is typically that of the maximum water temperature of the household water heater, but many dishwashers are equipped with heating elements that heat water to an even higher temperature. As a precaution, instruct caregivers to avoid bathing small children in the kitchen sink while the dishwasher is running.

If formula or food is warmed in a microwave oven, parents must check it before feeding because the container may remain cool while the contents are hot. Oropharyngeal burns from the contents of baby bottles heated in a microwave have been reported. Another danger is explosion of the bottle from the buildup of steam. Because of these dangers, parents should avoid microwaving infant formula or food or do it using the guidelines in the Family-Centered Care box on p. 490.

Sunburn can be a source of a first- or second-degree burn. Exposure to direct sunlight should be avoided for the first 6 months. When infants are in the sun, the body, especially the face and head, should be covered. Sunscreen can be used on older infants but should be used on small areas of the body and sparingly in infants under 6 months. (See Sunburn, Chapter 18.) Although dark-skinned infants burn less readily, their thin skin can become sunburned and needs protection.

Electrical outlets should be covered with protective plastic caps that prevent the child from sucking on the outlet or putting metal objects into it. Live wires are placed out of reach so that curious infants cannot chew on them and break the rubber coating. Infants should not be allowed to play near television sets, stereo units, or other appliances, whether these units are turned on or off, because infants cannot determine when the appliance is safe.

Any heat-producing element should have a guard in front of it. Fireplaces should be well screened because they are appealing and within easy access. Small portable heaters should be placed on a high surface. Floor furnaces should have barrier gates to prevent children from crawling or walking over them. Burning cigarettes, candles, and incense should be kept out of reach, and infants should not be held by a smoking adult because falling ashes are a hazard, especially to the eyes. Heated-mist vaporizers are a source of burns and should not be used. If humidity is needed, only cool mist vaporizers are safe.

By law, all infant sleepwear must be flame retardant. Unfortunately, this does not apply to all infant clothing. Flame-retardant fabric is not the ultimate protection against burns. Repeated washing reduces the flame-retardant properties, and the use of soap or bleach destroys the protection. If sleepwear is home sewn, advise parents to look for specially treated, flame-retardant fabric.

Another type of thermal injury occurs when children are exposed to excessive heat during confinement in poorly ventilated vehicles. The practice of leaving the windows open a couple of inches is not protective. The nurse should caution parents never to leave children in parked cars, especially when the automobile is in direct sunlight.

Children can also be burned by overheated metal hardware and vinyl seats in cars parked in the sun. As a precaution, the surface heat of car restraints should be determined before placing children in them. Covering the restraints and hardware (such as metal latches on seat belts) may be necessary to prevent skin burns. An additional safeguard is buying a light-colored restraint, which absorbs less heat.

Drowning

Drowning in this age-group can occur in just an inch or 2 of water. Consequently, infants should always be supervised in a bathtub and near a source of water such as a swimming pool, lake, toilet, or bucket. A survey found that most drownings among infants younger than age 1 year took place in a toilet, bathtub, or bucket (Lassman, 2002). Five-gallon buckets are particularly dangerous because the child may inadvertently fall in head first and, because of the weight of the upper body at this age, may be unable to withdraw from the bucket. Somers, Chiasson, and Smith (2006) noted that 72% of pediatric bathtub drownings occurred in infants under 12 months of age, and inadequate adult supervision was the leading associated factor (89% of cases). Organized swimming instruction is not recommended for children younger than 4 years of age, since it may lead to a false sense of security (American Academy of Pediatrics, 2003). Infants cannot learn the elements of water safety or react appropriately in an emergency. Therefore all young children need to be considered at risk when near water. Infants and toddlers are also at increased risk of infection and seizures from swallowing large amounts of water.

Bodily Damage

Injuries can occur in numerous ways. Sharp, jagged-edged objects can cause wounds in the skin. Long-pointed items, such as a toothpick or fork, can be poked into the eye or ear, causing serious damage. Such articles should be safely stored away from the infant's reach. Forks are best avoided for self-feeding until the child has mastered the spoon, usually by age 18 months.

In addition to hazards such as aspiration, infants can place small articles in the ear or nose, and excessive noise from toys can result in sensorineural hearing loss. Although toys with the highest noise levels are model airplanes, air guns, and toy cap guns, even common squeaking toys used by young children may be harmful if placed close to the ear.

A Centers for Disease Control and Prevention report (2008a) highlights the fact that in 2005 to 2006, 19% of child maltreatment fatalities in the United States occurred in infants less than 1 year of age. Homicide statistics suggest the fatality risk is highest in the infant's first week of life. Nonfatal maltreatment data for the same period indicate that 38.8% of infants maltreated were less than 1 month of age; 84% of those were less than 1 week old. Neglect and physical abuse were the most frequently reported forms of maltreatment. A high rate of battering injury has been reported in infants 0 to 5 months (Agran, Anderson, Winn, et al, 2003).

Another commonly unrecognized danger to infants is animal attacks. As newcomers to the home, helpless infants can provoke jealousy in animals, especially dogs and cats. Parents must be aware and protect the child from household pets and farm animals. (See Mammal Bites, Chapter 18.)

Nurse's Role in Injury Prevention

The task of injury prevention begins to be appreciated only when the potential environmental dangers to which infants are vulnerable are considered. Injury prevention and parent education should be handled on a growth and developmental basis. It is simply impossible to completely protect infants and small children from all potential dangers without placing them in a sterile, impractical environment. However, a large percentage of childhood deaths continue to occur as a result of preventable injuries (Martin, Kochanek, Strobino, et al, 2005). Nurses must be aware of the possible causes of injury in each age-group to provide anticipatory, preventive teaching. For example, the nurse should discuss guidelines for injury pre-

---

🏠 FAMILY-CENTERED CARE

Child Safety Home Checklist

Safety: Fire, Electrical, Burns

☐ Guards in front of or around any heating appliance, fireplace, or furnace (including floor furnace)*
☐ Electrical wires hidden or out of reach*
☐ No frayed or broken wires; no overloaded sockets
☐ Plastic guards or caps over electrical outlets; furniture in front of outlets*
☐ Hanging tablecloths out of reach, away from open fires*
☐ Smoke detectors tested and operating properly
☐ Kitchen matches stored out of child's reach*
☐ Large, deep ashtrays throughout house (if used)
☐ Small stoves, heaters, and other hot objects (cigarettes, candles, coffee pots, slow cookers) placed where they cannot be tipped over or reached by children
☐ Hot water heater set at 49° C (120° F) or lower
☐ Pot handles turned toward back of stove, center of table
☐ No loose clothing worn near stove
☐ No cooking or eating hot foods or liquids with child standing nearby or sitting in lap
☐ All small appliances, such as iron, turned off, disconnected, and placed out of reach when not in use
☐ Cool, not hot, mist vaporizer used
☐ Fire extinguisher available on each floor and checked periodically
☐ Electrical fuse box and gas shutoff accessible
☐ Family escape plan in case of a fire practiced periodically; fire escape ladder available on upper-level floors
☐ Telephone number of fire or rescue squad and address of home with nearest cross street posted near phone

Safety: Suffocation and Aspiration

☐ Small objects stored out of reach*
☐ Toys inspected for small removable parts or long strings*
☐ Hanging crib toys and mobiles placed out of reach
☐ Plastic bags stored away from young child's reach; large plastic garment bags discarded after tying in knots*
☐ Mattress or pillow not covered with plastic or in manner accessible to child*
☐ Crib design according to federal regulations (crib slats <6 cm [2.375 inches] apart) with snug-fitting mattress*
☐ Crib positioned away from other furniture or windows*
☐ Portable playpen gates up at all times while in use*
☐ Accordion-style gates not used*
☐ Bathroom doors kept closed and toilet seats down*
☐ Faucets turned off firmly*
☐ Pool fenced with locked gate
☐ Proper safety equipment at poolside
☐ Electric garage door openers stored safely and garage door adjusted to rise when door strikes object
☐ Doors of ovens, trunks, dishwashers, refrigerators, and front-loading clothes washers and dryers kept closed*
☐ Unused appliance, such as a refrigerator, securely closed with lock or doors removed*

☐ Food served in small, noncylindric pieces*
☐ Toy chests without lids or with lids that securely lock in open position*
☐ Buckets and wading pools kept empty when not in use*
☐ Clothesline above head level
☐ At least one member of household trained in basic life support (cardiopulmonary resuscitation), including first aid for choking (See Chapter 31.)

Safety: Poisoning

☐ Toxic substances, including batteries, placed on a high shelf, preferably in locked cabinet
☐ Toxic plants hung or placed out of reach*
☐ Excess quantities of cleaning fluid, paints, pesticides, drugs, and other toxic substances not stored in home
☐ Used containers of poisonous substances discarded where child cannot obtain access
☐ Telephone number of local poison control center and address of home with nearest cross street posted near each phone
☐ Medicines clearly labeled in childproof containers and stored out of reach
☐ Household cleaners, disinfectants, and insecticides kept in their original containers, separate from food and out of reach
☐ Smoking in areas away from children

Safety: Falls

☐ Nonskid mats, strips, or surfaces in tubs and showers
☐ Exits, halls, and passageways in rooms kept clear of toys, furniture, boxes, or other items that could be obstructive
☐ Stairs and halls well lighted, with switches at both top and bottom of stairs
☐ Sturdy handrails for all steps and stairways
☐ Nothing stored on stairways
☐ Treads, risers, and carpeting in good repair
☐ Glass doors and walls marked with decals
☐ Safety glass used in doors, windows, and walls
☐ Gates on top and bottom of staircases and elevated areas, such as porch, fire escape*
☐ Guardrails on upstairs windows with locks that limit height of window opening and access to areas such as fire escape*
☐ Crib side rails raised to full height; mattress lowered as child grows*
☐ Restraints used in high chairs, walkers, or other baby furniture; preferably walkers not used*
☐ Scatter rugs secured in place or used with nonskid backing
☐ Walks, patios, and driveways in good repair

Safety: Bodily Injury

☐ Knives, power tools, and unloaded firearms stored safely or placed in locked cabinet
☐ Garden tools returned to storage racks after use
☐ Pets properly restrained and immunized for rabies
☐ Swings, slides, and other outdoor play equipment kept in safe condition
☐ Yard free of broken glass, nail-studded boards, other litter
☐ Cement birdbaths placed where young child cannot tip them over*

Federal regulations are available from U.S. Consumer Product Safety Commission, 800-638-2722; www.cpsc.gov.
*Safety measures are specific for homes with young children. All safety measures should be implemented in homes where children reside and visit frequently, such as those of grandparents or baby-sitters.

vention during infancy (see Box 12-6) before the child reaches the susceptible age-group. Preventive teaching ideally begins during pregnancy.

Two thirds of all injuries to children occur in the home, and therefore safety is essential to emphasize with parents. The nurse can give parents a home safety checklist to increase their awareness of danger areas in the home and assist them in implementing safety devices and practices before an injury occurs (see Family-Centered Care box). Hands-on displays such as cabinet latches or toilet seat locks can familiarize parents with inexpensive, commercial devices that can be used in the home to prevent injuries.

To help parents appreciate the dangers present in their home to young children, suggest that they get eye level with the floor to survey the environment from a curious child's view.

Injury prevention requires protection of the child and education of the caregiver. Nurses in ambulatory care settings; health maintenance centers; and home health, public health, or visiting nurse agencies are in a most favorable position for injury education. This does not exclude nurses in inpatient facilities, who could use visiting times for discussing this topic. Although early postpartum discharge may be restrictive, this is an excellent opportunity to introduce the family to infant safety and safety for other children in the household as well. Pamphlets, safety checklists, and brief information sessions describing potential dangers and remedies aimed at preventing injury can help the new family get off to a good beginning with the new infant.

One approach to teaching injury prevention is to relate why children in various age-groups are prone to specific types of injuries. Stressing prevention is just as important as emphasizing why the injury occurs. However, injury prevention must also be practical. Asking parents for their ideas leads to realistic suggestions they can follow.

Parents need to remember that infants and young children cannot anticipate danger or understand when it is or is not present. Although parents can always explain to the child why something is dangerous, they also must remember that small children need to be physically removed from the situation. It is not easy to teach safety, supervise closely, and refrain from saying "no" a hundred times a day. Parents become acutely aware of this dilemma as soon as the infant learns to crawl and pull up to furniture. Preventing injuries is usually the first reason for limit setting and discipline, but limits are also set to prevent damage to valuable household objects. When small children are in the home, parents must remove or guard dangerous objects and place valuable articles out of reach.

When children learn the meaning of "no," they should also learn what "yes" means. Parents should praise children for playing with suitable toys, reinforce their efforts at behaving or listening, and provide innovative and creative recreational toys for them. Infants love to tear paper and avidly pursue books, magazines, or newspapers left on the floor. Instead of always scolding them for destroying a valued book, keep child-safe books (such as those constructed of fabric) available for them to play with. If they enjoy pots and pans, a cabinet can be arranged with safe utensils for them to explore.

One additional factor must be stressed concerning injury prevention and education. Children are imitators; they copy what they see and hear. Thus practicing safety teaches safety, a rule that applies to parents and their children and to nurses and their clients. Saying one thing but doing another confuses children and can lead to difficulties as the child grows older.

ANTICIPATORY GUIDANCE— CARE OF FAMILIES

Childrearing is no easy task; it presents challenges to both new and seasoned parents. With society's changing roles and mores, combined with a highly mobile population, traditional role models and time-honored methods of raising children are declining. As a result, parents look to professionals for guidance. Nurses are in an advantageous position to render assistance and offer suggestions. Every phase of a child's life has its particular traumas—toilet training for toddlers, unexplained fears for preschoolers, and identity crises for adolescents. For parents of an infant some challenges center around dependency, discipline, increased mobility, and safety. Major areas for parental guidance during the first year are listed in the Family-Centered Care box.

👪 FAMILY-CENTERED CARE

Guidance During Infant's First Year

Birth to 6 Months

Teach parents about car safety with use of federally approved restraint, facing rearward, in the middle of the back seat—not in a seat with an air bag.

Understand each parent's adjustment to newborn, especially mother's postpartum emotional needs.

Teach care of infant and help parents to understand the infant's individual needs and temperament and that the infant expresses wants through crying.

Reassure parents that infant cannot be spoiled by too much attention during the first 4 to 6 months.

Encourage parents to establish a schedule that meets needs of child and themselves.

Help parents understand infant's need for stimulation in environment.

Support parents' pleasure in seeing child's growing friendliness and social response, especially smiling.

Plan anticipatory guidance for safety.

Stress need for immunization.

Prepare for introduction of solid foods.

6 to 12 Months

Prepare parents for child's "stranger anxiety."

Encourage parents to allow child to cling to them and avoid long separation from either parent.

Guide parents concerning discipline because of infant's increasing mobility.

Encourage use of negative voice and eye contact rather than physical punishment as a means of discipline.

Encourage showing most attention when infant is behaving well, rather than when infant is crying.

Teach injury prevention because of child's advancing motor skills and curiosity.

Encourage parents to leave child with suitable caregiver to allow some free time.

Discuss readiness for weaning.

Explore parents' feelings regarding infant's sleep patterns.

KEY POINTS

- The child's biologic development encompasses proportional changes; sensory changes, including binocularity, depth perception, and visual preference; maturation of biologic systems; fine motor development; and gross motor development.

- Erikson's theory of psychosocial development states that, from birth to 1 year, the infant is concerned with acquiring a sense of trust while overcoming a sense of mistrust.

- Piaget's theory of cognitive development, as it applies to the infant, focuses on the sensorimotor phase, which includes the use of reflexes, primary circular reactions, secondary circular reactions, and coordination of secondary schemas and their application to new situations.

- Development of body image begins in infancy; by 1 year of age infants recognize that they are distinct from their parents.

- Social development of the infant is guided by attachment, language development, personal-social behavior, and participation in play.

- Temperament influences the type of interaction that occurs between the child, parents, and siblings.

- Parents face many concerns, including infant fears, daycare, limit setting and discipline, thumb sucking and pacifier use, teething, and choice of infant shoes.

- Breast milk is the most desirable food for the infant for the first 6 to 12 months. Commercial iron-fortified formula is an acceptable choice for infant nutrition when breastfeeding is not an option, followed by gradual introduction of solid food during the second 6 months. Whole milk is not recommended until after 12 months.

- Common sleep problems that develop during infancy—and that are easily prevented—are associated with night crying and feeding. Nurses should instruct the parents, after careful assessment, in strategies to deal with the specific problem.

- Cleaning the gums and teeth regularly and appropriate dietary intake promote good dental health.

- Recommended routine immunizations include those for hepatitis B, hepatitis A, diphtheria, tetanus, pertussis, polio, measles, mumps, rubella, pneumococcal, chickenpox, meningococcal, influenza, and *H. influenzae* type b.

- Combination vaccines are effective and decrease the total amount of injections a child must receive.

- Because injuries are a major cause of death during infancy, parents should be alerted to dangers of aspiration of foreign objects, suffocation, falls, poisoning, burns, motor vehicle injuries, and bodily damage, as well as preventive actions needed to make the environment safe for infants.

REFERENCES

Agran PF, Anderson C, Winn D, et al: Rates of pediatric injuries by 3-month intervals for children 0 to 3 years of age, *Pediatrics* 111(6):e683-e692, 2003.

Ainsworth M: Early caregiving and later patterns of attachment. In Klaus M, Robertson M, editors: *Birth, interaction, and attachment*, Skillman, NJ, 1982, Johnson & Johnson Baby Products.

Akers SM, Groh-Wargo SL: Normal nutrition during infancy. In Samour PQ, Helm KK, Lang CE, editors: *Handbook of pediatric nutrition*, ed 2, Sudbury, Mass, 2005, Jones & Bartlett.

American Academy of Pediatric Dentistry: Guideline on infant oral health care, *Clin Guidelines Ref Man 2008-2009* 30(7):90-92, 2009; available at www.aapd.org/media/Policies_Guidelines/G_InfantOralHealthCare.pdf (accessed June 17, 2009).

American Academy of Pediatrics, Committee on injury, violence, and poison prevention: Policy statement—Child passenger safety, *Pediatrics* 127(4):788, 2011.

American Academy of Pediatrics, Committee on Nutrition: *Pediatric nutrition handbook*, ed 6, Elk Grove Village, Ill, 2009a, The Academy.

American Academy of Pediatrics, Committee on Infectious Diseases, Pickering L, editor: *2009 Red book: report of the Committee on Infectious Diseases*, ed 28, Elk Grove Village, Ill, 2009b, The Academy.

American Academy of Pediatrics: Policy statement—recommendations for the prevention and treatment of influenza in children, 2009-2010, *Pediatrics* 124(4):1216-1226, 2009c.

American Academy of Pediatrics: Prevention of rickets and vitamin D deficiency in infants, children, and adolescents, *Pediatrics* 122(5): 1142-1148, 2008.

American Academy of Pediatrics, Task Force on Sudden Infant Death Syndrome: The changing concept of sudden infant death syndrome: diagnostic coding shifts, controversies regarding the sleeping environment, and new variables to consider in reducing risk, *Pediatrics* 116(5):1245-1255, 2005.

American Academy of Pediatrics, Committee on Injury, Violence, and Poison Prevention: Prevention of drowning in infants, children and adolescents, *Pediatrics* 92(2):292-294, 2003.

American Academy of Pediatrics, American Public Health Association, Maternal and Child Health Bureau: *Caring for our children: national health and safety performance standards: guidelines for out-of-home child care programs*, ed 2, Elk Grove Village, Ill, 2002, The Academy.

American Academy of Pediatrics, Committee on Injury and Poison Prevention: Injuries associated with infant walkers, *Pediatrics* 108(3):790-792, 2001.

American Psychiatric Association: Position statement: reactive attachment disorder, 2002, available at www.psych.org/public_info/libr_publ/position.cfm (accessed June 2005).

American Psychiatric Association: *Diagnostic and statistical manual of mental disorders*, ed 4, Washington, DC, 2000, The Association.

Anderson JE: "Nothing but the tooth": dispelling myths about teething, *Contemp Pediatr* 21(7):75-83, 2004.

Arora S, McJunkin C, Wehrer J, et al: Major factors influencing breastfeeding rates: mother's perception of father's attitude and milk supply, *Pediatrics* 106(5):e67, 2000.

Barnhill BJ, Holbert MD, Jackson NM, et al: Using pressure to decrease the pain of intramuscular injections, *J Pain Symptom Manage* 12(1):52-58, 1996.

Beck CT: Predictors of postpartum depression: an update, *Nurs Res* 50(5):275-285, 2001.

Bellemare S: Dangers for children in the care of drug users, *CMAJ* 179(2):164, 2008.

Biancuzzo M: *Breastfeeding the newborn: clinical strategies for nurses*, ed 2, St Louis, 2003, Mosby.

Blackburn ST: *Maternal, fetal, and neonatal physiology: a clinical perspective*, ed 3, Philadelphia, 2007, Saunders.

Bowlby J: *Attachment and loss*, vol 1, New York, 1969, Basic Books.

Brady MT: Infectious disease in pediatric out-of-home child care, *Am J Infect Control* 33(5):276-285, 2005.

Calamaro CJ: Infant nutrition in the first year of life: tradition or science? *Pediatr Nurs* 26(2):211-215, 2000.

Caplan MS: Probiotic and prebiotic supplementation for the prevention of neonatal necrotizing enterocolitis, *J Perinatol* 29(Suppl 2):S2-S6, 2009.

Carey WB, McDevitt SC: Revision of the infant temperament questionnaire, *Pediatrics* 61(5):735-739, 1978.

Centers for Disease Control and Prevention: Licensure of a meningococcal conjugate vaccine for children aged 2 through 10 years and updated booster dose guidance for adolescents and other persons at increased risk for meningococcal disease—Advisory Committee on Immunization Practices (ACIP), 2011, *MMWR Weekly* 60(30):1018-1019, 2011.

Centers for Disease Control and Prevention: Licensure of a 13-valent pneumococcal conjugate vaccine (PCV13) and recommendations for use among children—Advisory Committee on Immunization Practices (ACIP, 2010), *MMWR Weekly Rep* 59(9):258-261, 2010.

Centers for Disease Control and Prevention: Recommended immunization schedules for persons aged 0 through 18 years—United States, 2009, *MMWR* 57(51):Q-1-Q-4, 2009.

Centers for Disease Control and Prevention: Nonfatal maltreatment of infants—United States, October 2005–September 2006, *MMWR* 57(13):336-339, 2008a.

Centers for Disease Control and Prevention: Update: recommendations from the Advisory Committee on Immunization Practices (ACIP) regarding administration of combination MMRV vaccine, *MMWR* 57(10):258-260, 2008b.

Centers for Disease Control and Prevention: Fatal injuries among children by race and ethnicity—United States, 1999-2002, *MMWR* 56(SS05):1-16, 2007a.

Centers for Disease Control and Prevention: Quadrivalent human papillomavirus vaccine, *MMWR* 56(RR-2):1-24, 2007b.

Centers for Disease Control and Prevention: Prevention of hepatitis A through active or passive immunization, *MMWR* 55(RR07):1-23, 2006a.

Centers for Disease Control and Prevention: Update: Guillain-Barré syndrome among recipients of Menactra meningococcal conjugate vaccine—United States, June 2005–September 2006, *MMWR* 55(41):1120-1124, 2006b.

Centers for Disease Control and Prevention: A comprehensive immunization strategy to eliminate transmission of hepatitis B virus infection in the United States, *MMWR* 54(RR16):1-23, 2005a.

Centers for Disease Control and Prevention: Nonfatal motor-vehicle-related backover injuries among children—United States, 2001-2003, *MMWR* 54(06):144-146, 2005b.

Centers for Disease Control and Prevention: Outbreaks of pertussis associated with hospitals—Kentucky, Pennsylvania, and Oregon, 2003, *MMWR* 54(03):67-71, 2005c.

Chung JWY, Ng WMY, Wong TKS: An experimental study on the use of manual pressure to reduce pain in intramuscular injections, *J Clin Nurs* 11:457-461, 2002.

Corbett-Dick P, Bezek SK: Breastfeeding promotion for the employed mother, *J Pediatr Health Care* 11(1):12-19, 1997.

Coyer SM: Understanding parental concerns about immunizations, *J Pediatr Health Care* 16(4):193-196, 2002.

Davis KF, Parker K, Montgomery GL: Sleep in infants and young children, part 2, Common sleep problems, *J Pediatr Health Care* 18(3):130-137, 2004.

Dedoukou X, Spyridopoulos T, Kedikoglou S, et al: Incidence and risk factors for fall injuries among infants: a study in Greece, *Arch Pediatr Adolesc Med* 158(10):1002-1006, 2004.

Desapriya EB, Joshi P, Subwarzi S, et al: Infant injuries from child restraint safety seat misuse at British Columbia Children's Hospital, *Pediatr Int* 50(5):674-678, 2008.

DeStefano F: Vaccines and autism: evidence does not support a causal association, *Clin Pharmacol Ther* 82(6):756-759, 2007.

Dewey KG: Nutrition, growth, and complementary feeding of the breastfed infant, *Pediatr Clin North Am* 48(1):87-105, 2001.

Diggle L, Deeks J: Effect of needle length on incidence of local reactions to routine immunizations in infants aged 4 months: randomized controlled trial, *BMJ* 321(7266):931-993, 2000.

Diggle L, Deeks JJ, Pollard AJ: Effect of needle size and immunogenicity and reactogenecity of vaccines in infants: a randomized controlled trial, *BMJ* 333(7568):571, 2006.

Douglass JM, Douglass AB, Silk HJ: A practical guide to infant oral health, *Am Fam Physician* 70(11):2113-2120, 2004.

Drago DA: Kitchen scalds and thermal burns in children 5 years and younger, *Pediatrics* 115(1):10-16, 2005.

D'Souza AL, Smith GA, McKenzie LB: Bunk bed–related injuries among children and adolescents treated in emergency departments in the United States, 1990-2005, *Pediatrics* 121(6):e1696-e1702, 2008.

Duro D, Rising R, Cedillo M, et al: Association between infantile colic and carbohydrate malabsorption from fruit juices in infancy, *Pediatrics* 109(5):797-805, 2002.

Erikson E: *Childhood and society,* New York, 1963, WW Norton.

Evers DB: The pediatric nurse's role as health consultant to a child care center, *Pediatr Nurs* 28(3):231-235, 2002.

Farst K, Duncan JM, Moss M, et al: Methamphetamine exposure presenting as caustic ingestions in children, *Ann Emerg Med* 49(3):341-343, 2007.

Ferber R, Kryger M: *Principles and practice of sleep medicine in the child,* Philadelphia, 1995, Saunders.

Ferketich SL, Mercer RT: Paternal-infant attachment of experienced and inexperienced fathers during pregnancy, *Nurs Res* 44(1):31-37, 1995.

Fredrickson DD, Davis TC, Bocchini JA: Explaining the risks and benefits of vaccines to parents, *Pediatr Ann* 30(7):400-406, 2001.

Goldin BR, Gorbach SL: Clinical indications for probiotics: an overview, *Clin Infect Dis* 46(Suppl 2):S96-S100, 2008.

Grummer-Strawn LM, Scanlon KS, Fein SB: Infant feeding and feeding transitions during the first year of life, *Pediatrics* 122(Suppl 2):S36-S42, 2008.

Halperin BA, Halperin SA, McGrath P, et al: Use of lidocaine-prilocaine patch to decrease intramuscular injection pain does not adversely affect the antibody response to diphtheria-tetanus–acellular pertussis–inactivated poliovirus–*Haemophilus influenzae* type b conjugate and hepatitis B vaccines in infants from birth to 6 months of age, *Pediatr Infect Dis* 21(5):399-405, 2002.

Hatfield LA: Sucrose decreases infant neurobehavioral pain response to immunizations: a randomized controlled trial, *J Nurs Scholarship* 40(3):219-225, 2008.

Hawkins-Walsh E: A behavioural infant sleep intervention resolved sleep problems, *Evid Based Nurs* 6(1):10-12, 2003.

Henary B, Sherwood CP, Crandall JR, et al: Car safety seats for children: rear facing for best protection, *Inj Prev* 13(6):398-402, 2007.

Heron J, Golding J, ALSPAC Study Team: Thimerosal exposure in infants and developmental disorders: a prospective cohort study in the United Kingdom does not support a causal association, *Pediatrics* 114(3):577-583, 2004.

Hiscock H, Wake M: Infant sleep problems and postnatal depression: a community-based study, *Pediatrics* 107(6):1317-1322, 2001.

Horn MI, McCarthy AM: Children's responses to sequential versus simultaneous immunization injections, *J Pediatr Health Care* 13(1):18-23, 1999.

Hornor G: Reactive attachment disorder, *J Pediatr Health Care* 22(4):234-239, 2008.

Huiming Y, Chaomin W, Meng M: Vitamin A for treating measles in children, *Cochrane Database Syst Rev* (4):CD001479, 2005.

Hviid A, Stellfeld M, Wohlfahrt J, et al: Association between thimerosal-containing vaccine and autism, *JAMA* 290(13):1763-1766, 2003.

Iglowstein I, Jenni OG, Molinari L, et al: Sleep duration from infancy to adolescence: reference values and generational trends, *Pediatrics* 111(2):302-307, 2003.

Institute of Medicine: *Immunization safety review: vaccines and autism,* Washington, DC, 2004, National Academies Press.

Ipp M, Parkin PC, Lear N, et al: Order of vaccine injection and infant pain response, *Arch Pediatr Adolesc Med* 163(5):469-472, 2009.

Ize-Ludlow D, Ragone S, Bruck IS, et al: Neurotoxicities in infants seen with the consumption of star anise tea, *Pediatrics* 114(5):e653, 2004.

Jimenez N, Bradford H, Seidel KD, et al: A comparison of a needle-free injection system for local anesthesia versus EMLA for intravenous catheter insertion in the pediatric patient, *Anesth Analag* 102(2):411-414, 2006.

Joanna Briggs Institute: Early childhood pacifier use in relation to breastfeeding, SIDS, infection, and dental occlusion, *Best Practice* 9(3):1-6, 2005.

Johnson CP, Blasco PA: Infant growth and development, *Pediatr Rev* 18(7):224-242, 1997.

Jones L, Heermann J: Parental division of infant care: contextual influences and infant characteristics, *Nurs Res* 41(4):228-234, 1992.

Kallan MJ, Durbin DR, Arbogast KB et al: Seating patterns and corresponding risk of injury among 0- to 3-year-old children in child safety seats, *Pediatrics* 121(5):e1342-e1347, 2008.

Kotch JB, Isbell P, Weber DJ, et al: Hand-washing and diapering equipment reduces disease among children in out-of-home child care centers, *Pediatrics* 120(1):e29-e36, 2007.

Lassman J: Water safety, *J Emerg Nurs* 28(3): 241-243, 2002.

Lawrence RA, Lawrence RM: *Breastfeeding: a guide for the medical profession*, ed 6, St Louis, 2005, Mosby.

Loman DG: The use of complementary and alternative health care practices among children, *J Pediatr Health Care* 17(2):58-63, 2003.

Lundqvist P, Jakobsson L: Swedish men's experiences of becoming fathers to their preterm infants, *Neonat Netw* 22(6):25-31, 2003.

Mack KA, Gilchrist J, Ballesteros MF: Injuries among infants treated in the emergency departments in the United States, 2001-2004, *Pediatrics* 121(5):930-937, 2008.

Mack KA, Gilchrist J, Ballesteros MF: Unintentional injuries among infants age 0-12 months, *J Safety Res* 38(5):609-612, 2007.

Martin JA, Kochanek KD, Strobino DM, et al: Annual summary of vital statistics—2003, *Pediatrics* 115(3):619-634, 2005.

Matteucci MJ, Auten JD, Crowley B, et al: Methamphetamine exposures in young children, *Pediatr Emerg Care* 23(9):638-640, 2007.

McGrath JM, Records K, Rice M: Maternal depression and infant temperament characteristics, *Infant Behav Dev* 31(1):71-80, 2008.

McIntosh B: Spoiled child syndrome, *Pediatrics* 83(1):108-114, 1989.

Mecham N, Melini J: Unintentional victims: development of a protocol for the care of children exposed to chemicals at methamphetamine laboratories, *Pediatr Emerg Care* 18(4):327-332, 2002.

Medoff-Cooper B, Carey WB, McDevitt SC: The Early Infancy Temperament Questionnaire, *J Dev Behav Pediatr* 14(4):230-231, 1993.

Morin K: Infant nutrition: solids—when and why, *MCN* 29(4):259, 2004.

Moukarzel AA, Lesicka H, Ament ME: Irritable bowel syndrome and nonspecific diarrhea in infancy and childhood: relationship with juice carbohydrate malabsorption, *Clin Pediatr* 41(3):145-150, 2002.

Narendran V, Hoath SB: The skin. In Martin RJ, Fanaroff AA, Walsh MC, editors: *Fanaroff and Martin's neonatal-perinatal medicine*, ed 8, St Louis, 2006, Mosby.

National Institute of Child Health and Human Development Early Child Care Research Network: Child care and common communicable illnesses: results from the National Institute of Child Health and Human Development Study of Early Child Care, *Arch Pediatr Adolesc Med* 155(4):481-488, 2001.

Niemela M, Pihakari O, Pokka, et al: Pacifier as a risk factor for acute otitis media: a randomized, controlled trial of parental counseling, *Pediatrics* 106(3):483-488, 2000.

Niggemann B, Grüber C: Side-effects of complementary and alternative medicine, *Allergy* 58(8):707-716, 2003.

O'Connor NR, Tanabe KO, Siadaty MS et al: Pacifiers and breastfeeding: a systematic review, *Arch Pediatr Adolesc Med* 163(4):378-382, 2009.

Parker SK, Schwartz B, Todd J, et al: Thimerosal-containing vaccines and autistic spectrum disorder: a critical review of published original data, *Pediatrics* 114(3):793-804, 2004.

Patterson DL: Adolescent-mothering: child-grandmother attachment, *J Pediatr Nurs* 12(4):228-237, 1997.

Phelan KJ, Khoury J, Kalkwarf H, et al: Residential injuries in U.S. children and adolescents, *Pub Health Rep* 120(1):63-70, 2005.

Piaget J: *The origins of intelligence in children*, New York, 1952, International University Press.

Pickett W, Streight S, Simpson K, et al: Injuries experienced by infant children: a population-based epidemiological analysis, *Pediatrics* 111(4 Pt 1):e365-e370, 2003.

Quillin SI, Glenn LL: Interaction between feeding method and co-sleeping on maternal-newborn sleep, *JOGNN* 33(5):580-588, 2004.

Reis EC, Holubkov R: Vapocoolant spray is equally effective as EMLA cream in reducing immunization pain in school-aged children, *Pediatrics* 100(6):1025, 1997.

Robertson J: Some responses of young children to the loss of maternal care, *Nurs Times* 49:382-386, 1953.

Rojjanasrirat W: Working women's breastfeeding experiences, *MCN* 29(4):222-227, 2004.

Rosenthal P: Overcoming skepticism toward vaccines: a look at the real benefits and risks, *Consult Pediatr* Nov-Dec (Suppl):S3-S7, 2004.

Rovers MM, Numans ME, Langenbach E, et al: Is pacifier use a risk factor for otitis media? A dynamic cohort study, *Fam Pract* 25(4):233-236, 2008.

Schechter NL, Zempsky WT, Cohen LL, et al: Pain reduction during pediatric immunizations: evidence-based review and recommendations, *Pediatrics* 119(5):e1184-e1198, 2007.

Schnitzer PG: Prevention of unintentional childhood injuries, *Am Fam Physician* 74(11):1864-1869, 2006.

Sexton S, Natale R: Risks and benefits of pacifiers, *Am Fam Physician* 79(8):681-685, 2009.

Shapiro-Mendoza CK, Kimball M, Tomashek KM, et al: US infant mortality trends attributable to accidental suffocation and strangulation in bed from 1984 through 2004: are rates increasing? *Pediatrics* 123(2):533-539, 2009.

Shealy KR, Benton-Davis S, Grummer-Strawn LM: The CDC guide to breastfeeding interventions, Atlanta, 2005, Centers for Disease Control and Prevention, available at www.cdc.gov/breastfeeding/pdf/breastfeeding_interventions.pdf (accessed July 30, 2009).

Somers GR, Chiasson DA, Smith CR: Pediatric drowning: a 20-year review of autopsied cases, part III, Bathtub drownings, *Am J Forensic Med Pathol* 27(2):113-116, 2006.

Spanos S, Booth R, Koenig H, et al: Jet injection of 1% buffered lidocaine versus topical ELA-Max for anesthesia before peripheral intravenous catheterization in children: a randomized controlled trial, *Pediatr Emerg Care* 24(8):511-515, 2008.

Spitz RA: Hospitalism: an inquiry into the genesis of psychiatric conditioning in early childhood. In Fenichel O, Greenacre P, Hartmann H, editors: *Psychoanalytic studies of the child*, vol 1, New York, 1945, International University Press.

Starr NB: Helping children and families deal with the psychological aspects of disaster, *J Pediatr Health Care* 16(1):36-39, 2002.

Stevens B, Johnston C, Franck L, et al: The efficacy of developmentally sensitive interventions and sucrose for relieving procedural pain in very low birth weight neonates, *Nurs Res* 48(1):35-43, 1999.

Stevens B, Yamada J, Ohlsson A: Sucrose for analgesia in newborn infants undergoing painful procedures, *Cochrane Database Syst Rev* (4):CD001069, 2001.

Sullivan JR: Development of father-infant attachment in fathers of preterm infants, *Neonat Netw* 18(7):33-39, 1999.

Taveras EM, Rifas-Shiman SL, Belfort MB, et al: Weight status in the first 6 months of life and obesity at 3 years of age, *Pediatrics* 123(4):1177-1183, 2009.

Thach BT, Rutherford GW Jr, Harris K: Deaths and injuries attributed to infant crib bumper pads, *J Pediatr* 151(3):271-274, 2007.

Thompson DG: Utilizing an oral sucrose solution to minimize neonatal pain, *JSPN* 10(1):3-10, 2005.

Touchette E, Petit D, Paquet J, et al: Factors associated with fragmented sleep at night across early childhood, *Arch Pediatr Adolesc Med* 159(3):242-249, 2005.

Ward TM, Rankin S, Lee KA: Caring for children with sleep problems, *J Pediatr Nurs* 22(4): 283-296, 2007.

Wilkerson R, Northington LD, Fisher W: Ingestion of toxic substances by infants and children: what we don't know can hurt, *Crit Care Nurs* 25(4):35-44, 2005.

Wilson ME, White MA, Cobb B, et al: Family dynamics, parental-fetal attachment and infant temperament, *J Adv Nurs* 31(1): 204-210, 2000.

Wilson S: Attachment disorders: review and current status, *J Psychol* 135(1):37-51, 2001.

Wong DL: Topical local anesthetics: two products for pain relief during minor procedures, *Am J Nurs* 103(6):42-45, 2003.

Wright JW, Griffin R, MacLennan PA, et al: The incidence of shopping cart–related injuries in the United States, 2002-2006, *Accid Annal Prev* 40(3):1253-1256, 2008.

Zeanah CH, Fox NA: Temperament and attachment disorders, *J Clin Child Adolesc Psychol* 33(1):82-87, 2004.

Zempsky WT: Pharmacologic approaches for reducing venous access pain in children, *Pediatrics* 122(Suppl 3):S140-S153, 2008.

Zuckerman J: The importance of injecting vaccines into muscle, *BMJ* 321(7271):1237-1238, 2000.

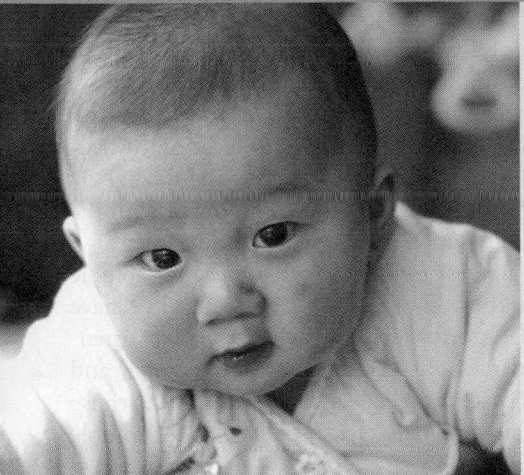

Health Problems During Infancy

David Wilson

CHAPTER OUTLINE

NUTRITIONAL DISTURBANCES

VITAMIN DISTURBANCES

Although true vitamin deficiencies are rare in the United States, subclinical deficiencies are commonly seen in population subgroups in which either maternal or child dietary intake is imbalanced and contains inadequate amounts of vitamins. **Vitamin D–deficiency rickets**, once rarely seen because of the widespread commercial availability of vitamin D–fortified milk, increased before the turn of the century. Populations at risk include:

- Children who are exclusively breast-fed by mothers with an inadequate intake of vitamin D or are exclusively breast-fed longer than 6 months without adequate maternal vitamin D intake or supplementation
- Children with dark skin pigmentation who are exposed to minimal sunlight because of socioeconomic, religious,

or cultural beliefs or housing in urban areas with high levels of pollution

• Children with diets that are low in sources of vitamin D and calcium

• Individuals who use milk products not supplemented with vitamin D (e.g., yogurt,* raw cow's milk) as the primary source of milk

The American Academy of Pediatrics (2008) now recommends that infants who are exclusively breast-fed should receive 400 international units of vitamin D beginning shortly after birth to prevent rickets and vitamin D deficiency. Vitamin D supplementation should continue until the infant is consuming at least 1 L/day (or 1 quart/day) of vitamin D–fortified formula (American Academy of Pediatrics, 2008). Non-breast-fed infants who are taking less than 1 L/day of vitamin D–fortified formula should also receive a daily vitamin D supplement of 400 international units. Inadequate maternal ingestion of cobalamin (vitamin B_{12}) may contribute to infant neurologic impairment when exclusive breast-feeding (past 6 months) is the only source of the infant's nutrition (Centers for Disease Control and Prevention, 2003).

Children may also be at risk secondary to disorders or their treatment. For example, vitamin deficiencies of the fat-soluble vitamins A and D may occur in malabsorptive disorders. Preterm infants may develop rickets in the second month of life as a result of inadequate intake of vitamin D, calcium, and phosphorus. Children receiving high doses of salicylates may have impaired vitamin C storage. Environmental tobacco smoke exposure has been implicated in decreased concentrations of ascorbate in children; therefore increased intake of sources of vitamin C should be encouraged even in children minimally exposed to environmental tobacco smoke (Preston, Rodriguez, and Rivera, 2006; Preston, Rodriguez, Rivera, et al, 2003). Children with chronic illnesses resulting in anorexia, decreased food intake, or possible nutrient malabsorption as a result of multiple medications should be carefully evaluated for adequate vitamin and mineral intake in some form (parenteral or enteral).

Children with sickle cell disease are reported to have suboptimal intakes (according to dietary reference intake [DRI] recommendations) of vitamins E and D, folate, calcium, and fiber, which decrease significantly with increasing age. Poor dietary intake was a significant factor in the study's findings (Kawchak, Schall, Zemel, et al, 2007).

Vitamin A deficiency has been reported with increased morbidity and mortality in children with measles. However, a Cochrane review of studies wherein a single dose of vitamin A was administered to children with measles found no decrease in mortality. Children with measles under the age of 2 years who received two doses of vitamin A (200,000 international units) on consecutive days did have decreased mortality rates and a reduced rate of pneumonia-specific mortality (Huiming, Chaomin, and Meng, 2005). Complications from diarrhea and infections are often increased in infants and children with vitamin A deficiency. Although scurvy (caused by a deficiency of vitamin C) is rare in developed countries, cases have been

reported in children who were fed an organic diet deficient in vegetables and fruits (Burk and Molodow, 2007).

An excessive dose of a vitamin is generally defined as 10 or more times the recommended dietary allowance (RDA), although the fat-soluble vitamins, especially A and D, tend to cause toxic reactions at lower doses. With the addition of vitamins to commercially prepared foods, the potential for hypervitaminosis has increased, especially when combined with the excessive use of vitamin supplements. Hypervitaminosis of A and D presents the greatest problems, since these fat-soluble vitamins are stored in the body. High intakes of vitamin A have been linked to physeal growth arrest, which can lead to osteoporosis, fracture, and metaphyseal irregularity (Saltzman and King, 2007). Vitamin D is the most likely of all vitamins to cause toxic reactions in relatively small overdoses. The water-soluble vitamins, primarily niacin, B_6, and C, can also cause toxicity. Poor outcomes in infants (e.g., fatal hypermagnesemia) have been associated with megavitamin therapy with high doses of magnesium oxide (McGuire, Kulkarni, and Baden, 2000), and severe anemia and thrombocytopenia have resulted from megadoses of vitamin A (Perrotta, Nobili, Rossi, et al, 2002).

One vitamin supplement that is recommended for all women of childbearing age is a daily dose of 0.4 mg of folic acid, the usual RDA. Folic acid taken before conception and during early pregnancy can reduce the risk of neural tube defects such as spina bifida by as much as 70%. Drugs such as oral contraceptives and antidepressants may decrease folic acid absorption; thus adolescent females taking such medications should consider supplementation. (See Spina Bifida and Myelodysplasia, Chapter 11.) General nursing care management is discussed on p. 524.

COMPLEMENTARY AND ALTERNATIVE MEDICINE

The misuse or overuse of vitamins as a part of complementary and alternative medicine (CAM) places some children at risk for health problems. One survey found that a relatively small group of parents routinely gave their children megavitamin therapy; however, the researcher recommends further research to ascertain a realistic number of children using multivitamin preparations (Loman, 2003). Sawni, Ragothaman, Thomas, and colleagues (2007) noted that of persons reportedly using CAM, the most common CAM remedies reportedly used in children seen in the emergency department for other health problems were home or folk remedies (59%), herbs (41%), prayer for healing (14%), and massage therapy (10%). A survey in a Women, Infants, and Children (WIC) clinic found that child herbal use was common, especially among Hispanic children attending the clinic. Some of the herbs used by the children in the survey (St. John's wort, dong quai, and kava) have questionable safety (Lohse, Stotts, and Priebe, 2006).

There is concern among health care workers that terms often used to market supplements such as megavitamins may mislead parents regarding the actual benefits (or harm) of such therapies. The intention herein is not to discredit the use of CAM such as vitamin supplements; rather, it is to ensure safety and efficacy in children and to avoid inadvertent harm. The use of various herbal therapies, or intake of herbs, is also becoming

---

*Yogurt does not contain adequate amounts of vitamins A and D yet is an acceptable source of calcium and phosphorus.

more popular; many of these supplements have been a part of medicine since early days and are beneficial in some cases.

The use of herbs by lactating mothers to increase breast milk supply is reportedly increasing. The galactogogues fenugreek, blessed thistle, fennel, and chaste tree have been purported to increase maternal milk supply; however, few studies support the efficacy or safety of these herbs in breast-feeding infants. Fenugreek has been the most widely studied, yet it may have adverse effects such as colic and diarrhea in breast-feeding infants (Conover and Buehler, 2004; Lawrence and Lawrence, 2005). For a discussion of galactogogues, including those mentioned previously, see Appendix P in Lawrence and Lawrence (2005).

Herbs known to have adverse effects in children include ephedra, comfrey, and pennyroyal; some herbs may not be harmful taken alone but may counteract or potentiate prescription medications when taken concurrently (Loman, 2003). Parents should be fully informed of the use of herbs to ensure they confer more benefit than potential harm. Health care workers also need to be knowledgeable about the benefits or potential harm in herbs so that they can appropriately counsel parents and address their concerns. Little research has been performed in children on many over-the-counter herbal medicines, yet some herbs are known to cause harm in children (Kemper and Gardiner, 2007; Lanski, Greenwald, Perkins, et al, 2003; Loman, 2003). Parents should be cautioned not to exceed the upper limits of vitamin intake according to the new DRI (see p. 524).*

MINERAL DISTURBANCES

A number of minerals are essential nutrients. The macrominerals are those with daily requirements greater than 100 mg, including calcium, phosphorus, magnesium, sodium, potassium, chloride, and sulfur. Microminerals, or trace elements, have daily requirements of less than 100 mg and include several essential minerals and those whose exact role in nutrition is still unclear. The greatest concern with minerals is deficiency, especially iron deficiency anemia. (See Chapter 35.) However, other minerals that may be inadequate in children's diets, even with supplementation, include calcium, phosphorus, magnesium, and zinc. Low levels of zinc can cause nutritional growth failure (failure to thrive).

The regulation of mineral balance in the body is a complex process. Dietary extremes of mineral intake can cause a number of mineral-mineral interactions that could result in unexpected deficiencies or excesses. For example, excessive amounts of one mineral, such as zinc, can result in a deficiency of another mineral, such as copper, even if sufficient amounts of copper are ingested. This is thought to be a result of competition in the process of absorption because of (1) displacement of one mineral by another on the molecule necessary for their uptake from the lumen in the intestinal cell or (2) competition for pathways through the intestinal wall or into the bloodstream.

Therefore megadose therapy with one mineral may not cause adverse effects from an excess but rather from a deficiency in a competing mineral.

Deficiencies can also occur when various substances in the diet interact with minerals. For example, iron, zinc, and calcium can form insoluble complexes with phytates or oxalates (substances found in plant proteins), which impairs the bioavailability of the mineral. This type of interaction is important in vegetarian diets because plant foods, such as soy, are high in phytates. Contrary to popular opinion, spinach is not a rich source of iron or calcium because of its high oxalate content.

Children with certain illnesses are at greater risk for growth failure, especially in relation to bone mineral deficiency as a result of the treatment of the disease, decreased nutrient intake, or decreased absorption of necessary minerals. Those at risk for such deficiencies include children who are receiving or have received radiation and chemotherapy for cancer; children with human immunodeficiency virus (HIV), sickle cell disease, cystic fibrosis, gastrointestinal (GI) malabsorption, or nephrosis; and very low–birth-weight (VLBW) preterm infants.

Box 13-1 lists factors that affect iron absorption. General nursing care management is discussed below, and specific interventions are discussed in the table.

VEGETARIAN DIETS

Vegetarian diets have become increasingly popular in the United States because people are concerned about hypertension; cholesterol; obesity; cardiovascular disease; the animal rights movement; and cancer of the stomach, intestine, and colon. In one survey, adolescent vegetarians were more likely than nonvegetarians to meet the Healthy People 2010 objectives for overall nutrient consumption (Perry, McGuire, Neumark-Sztainer, et al, 2002). According to the Vegetarian Resource Group (Stahler, 2005), approximately 3% of children ages 8 to 18 years in the United States are vegetarians. The American

---

*Helpful websites for health care and consumer information concerning herbs are National Center for Complementary and Alternative Medicine, www.nccam.nih.gov; American Botanical Council, www.herbalgram.org; and Herb Research Foundation, www.herbs.org.

BOX 13-1   FACTORS THAT AFFECT IRON ABSORPTION

Increased Absorption
Acidity (low pH)—Administer iron between meals (gastric hydrochloric acid)
Ascorbic acid (vitamin C)—Administer iron with juice, fruit, or multivitamin preparation
Vitamin A
Calcium
Tissue need
Meat, fish, poultry
Cooking in cast iron pots

Decreased Absorption
Alkalinity (high pH)—Avoid any antacid preparation
Phosphates—Milk unfavorable vehicle for iron administration
Phytates—Found in cereals
Oxalates—Found in many fruits and vegetables (plums, currants, green beans, spinach, sweet potatoes, tomatoes)
Tannins—Found in tea, coffee
Tissue saturation
Malabsorptive disorders
Disturbances that cause diarrhea or steatorrhea
Infection

Dietetic Association and Dietitians of Canada (2003) issued a statement endorsing vegetarian diets for adults and children; the statement further notes that well-planned vegetarian diets are adequate for all stages of the life cycle and promote normal growth. Children and adolescents on vegetarian diets have the potential for lifelong healthy diets and have been shown to have lower intakes of cholesterol, saturated fat, and total fat and higher intakes of fruits, fiber, and vegetables than nonvegetarians (American Dietetic Association and Dietitians of Canada, 2003).

The major types of vegetarianism are:

Lacto-ovo vegetarians, who exclude meat from their diet but consume dairy products and rarely fish

Lactovegetarians, who exclude meat and eggs but drink milk

Pure vegetarians (vegans), who eliminate any food of animal origin, including milk and eggs

Macrobiotics, who are even more restrictive than pure vegetarians, allowing only a few types of fruits, vegetables, and legumes

Semivegetarians, who consume a lacto-ovo vegetarian diet with some fish and poultry (an increasingly popular form of vegetarianism that poses little or no nutritional risk to infants unless dietary fat and cholesterol intake are severely restricted)

Many individuals who are concerned about healthy diets subscribe to vegetarian diets that may not be typified by these categories. Therefore during nutritional assessment it is necessary to clearly list exactly what the diet includes and excludes.*

The major deficiencies that may occur in the stricter vegan diets are inadequate protein for growth; inadequate calories for energy and growth; poor digestibility of many of the bulky natural, unprocessed foods, especially for infants; and deficiencies of vitamin B_6, niacin, riboflavin, vitamin D, iron, calcium, and zinc. Strict vegan diets also require supplements of vitamin B_{12} and vitamin D. Vitamin D is essential if exposure to sunlight is inadequate (<5 to 15 min/day on the hands, arms, and face of light-skinned persons; slightly more in darker pigmented individuals) or in persons who are dark-skinned or who live in northern latitudes or cloudy or smoky areas. A multivitamin-mineral supplement can be given to avoid many of these deficiencies in children who are not consuming 100% of the RDA of vitamins and minerals (Dunham and Kollar, 2006) (see Cultural Competence box).

Children on strict vegetarian and macrobiotic diets should be evaluated for iron deficiency anemia, zinc deficiency, and rickets; this may occur as a result of consuming plant foods such as unrefined cereals, which impair the absorption of iron, calcium, and zinc. Other factors that affect iron absorption are listed in Box 13-1.

NURSING CARE MANAGEMENT

Evaluation of adequacy of nutrient intake is the initial nursing goal and requires assessment based on a dietary history and

⊕ CULTURAL COMPETENCE
Vegetarian Diets

In the United States strict vegetarian diets are common among members of Black Muslim or Seventh-Day Adventist faiths and among immigrant population groups such as Asians and East Indians. Achieving a nutritionally adequate vegetarian diet is not difficult, but it requires careful planning and knowledge of nutrient sources. For children the lacto-ovo vegetarian diet is nutritionally adequate; however, the vegan diet requires supplementation with vitamins D and B_{12}, particularly for children ages 2 to 12 years. Infants on a vegan diet should be breast-fed for the first 6 months and preferably for 1 year, fed solid foods after about 4 months, and receive iron-fortified cereal for at least 18 months. The use of juices containing vitamin C with foods high in iron will further improve iron absorption. If cow's or human milk is not given, fortified soy milk is recommended. Other approaches to increase vitamin D and calcium intake are inclusion of fatty fish (herring, salmon, sardines, trout, tuna) and less fiber, since high fiber intake limits mineral absorption by decreasing intestinal transit time and binding calcium, iron, and other minerals.

physical examination for signs of deficiency or excess. Once assessment data are collected, this information is evaluated against standard intakes to identify areas of concern. (See Nutritional Assessment, Chapter 6.)

The DRIs† (see also Chapter 6) are quantitative estimates of nutrient requirements for planning and evaluating diets for healthy infants and are made of four categories, including estimated average (EA) requirements for age and gender categories, tolerable upper-limit (TUL) nutrient intakes that are associated with a low risk of adverse effects, adequate intakes (AIs) of nutrients, and new standard RDAs. The guidelines present information about lifestyle factors that may affect nutrient function, such as caffeine intake and exercise, and about how the nutrient may be related to chronic disease. DRIs currently published include calcium, magnesium, phosphorus, vitamin D, and fluoride. Additional groups of nutrients include folate and other B vitamins, dietary antioxidants, micronutrients, macronutrients, trace elements, electrolytes, and food components such as dietary fiber. The comprehensive set of guidelines covers nutrient needs across the life span, including infancy. An important factor in the development of the DRIs that affects children, particularly infants 0 to 6 months, is that the AIs are based on the nutrient intake of term, healthy, breast-fed infants (by well-nourished mothers), which now represents the gold standard for infant nutrition in this age-group. This represents a major change in infant nutrition recommendations; specific needs to meet the nutrient requirements for formula-fed infants were not included in DRI reports (Devaney and Barr, 2002; Institute of Medicine, 2000).

The American Heart Association Dietary Guidelines, patterned after the 2005 Dietary Guidelines for Americans, may also be used to encourage healthy dietary intakes designed to decrease obesity and cardiovascular risk factors and subsequent cardiovascular disease, which is now known to occur in both young children and adults (Gidding, Dennison, Birch, et al,

---

*Further information regarding vegetarian diets may be found at the Vegetarian Resource Group, PO Box 1463, Baltimore, MD 21203; 410-366-8343; www.vrg.org.

†For information on the DRIs go to the Institute of Medicine website, **www.iom.edu,** and click on the link for Food and Nutrition; or call 202-334-2352.

2005; Gidding, Lichtenstein, Faith, et al, 2009). The American Heart Association guidelines have been endorsed by the American Academy of Pediatrics (2006), but it is important to note that these guidelines are for children ages 2 years and older. The guidelines encourage a variety of fruits, vegetables, whole grains, and low-fat dairy and nonfat dairy products, in addition to fish, beans, and lean meat.

In 2011 the United States Department of Agriculture replaced the Food Guide Pyramid (MyPyramid) with MyPlate (http://www.choosemyplate.gov/) (Figure 6-4). This colorful plate shows the 5 main food groups—fruits, grains, vegetables, protein, and dairy—with the intended purpose to involve children and their families in making appropriate food choices for meals and decrease the incidence of overweight and obesity in the United States. MyPlate provides an online interactive feature that allows the individual to select (click on) an individual food group and see choices for foods in that group. Approximate serving sizes are suggested and vegetarian substitutions are also provided.

A vegetarian food pyramid (rainbow for Canadian vegetarians) developed by the American Dietetic Association and Dietitians of Canada includes guidelines for meeting the minimum recommendations for nutrients, including protein, iron, zinc, calcium, vitamin D, riboflavin, and iodine. The new food guide can be adapted to different types of vegetarian diets according to specific needs (American Dietetic Association and Dietitians of Canada, 2003; Messina, Melina, and Mangels, 2003).

Achieving a nutritionally adequate vegetarian diet is not difficult (except with the strictest diets), but it requires careful planning and knowledge of nutrient sources. For children the lacto-ovo vegetarian diet is nutritionally adequate; however, the vegan diet requires supplementation with vitamins D and B_{12} for children ages 2 to 12 years. Infants should be breast-fed for the first 6 months and preferably for 1 year, be introduced to some solid foods after about 4 to 6 months, and receive iron-fortified cereal for at least 18 months. Vitamin B_{12} supplementation of breast-feeding infants is recommended if the mother's intake of the vitamin is inadequate and she is not taking vitamin supplements (Dunham and Kollar, 2006). Solids may be introduced to vegetarian infants using the same guidelines as for other children (see p. 492). The American Dietetic Association and Dietitians of Canada (2003) and American Academy of Pediatrics (2009) recommend iron supplementation in infants exclusively breast-fed after 4 to 6 months by vegetarian mothers and no dietary fat restrictions in vegetarian children younger than 2 years. The use of vitamin C juices (in moderate amounts, not as a milk substitute) with foods high in iron further improves iron absorption. If cow's or human milk or commercial infant formula is not given, fortified soy formula is recommended. A variety of foods should be introduced during the early years to ensure a well-balanced intake. A registered dietitian is a good resource for assisting with meal planning for vegetarian infants and children.

To ensure sufficient protein in the diet, foods with incomplete proteins (those that do not have all the essential amino acids) must be eaten at the same meal with other foods that supply the missing amino acids. The three basic combinations of foods consumed by vegetarians that generally provide the appropriate amounts of essential amino acids are:

1. Grains (cereal, rice, pasta) and legumes (beans, peas, lentils, peanuts)
2. Grains and milk products (milk, cheese, yogurt)
3. Seeds (sesame, sunflower) and legumes

Additional dietary considerations for young children are found in Chapters 12 and 14.

The nurse has an important role in evaluating the food intake of infants, children, and adolescents and may serve as a resource for parents; *the overall nutritional goal should be to provide the best sources of vitamin and mineral intake through food intake rather than rely on supplemental vitamins,* which may not always be as well absorbed as food products.

Based on current recommendations, the infant who is exclusively breast-feeding for the first 4 to 6 months (the latter is preferred) should receive a vitamin D supplement of 400 international units; at approximately 6 months the breast-fed infant should begin receiving an iron supplement (elemental iron, 1 mg/kg/day), or iron requirements may be met with iron-fortified cereal (average of 2 servings of ½ oz of dry cereal per serving) (American Academy of Pediatrics, 2009). Fruit juice is not necessary for adequate growth in infants but may be given after 6 months in amounts not to exceed 4 oz/day. Low iron formula is not recommended for infants.

PROTEIN-ENERGY MALNUTRITION (SEVERE CHILDHOOD UNDERNUTRITION)

Malnutrition continues to be a major health problem in the world today, particularly in children under 5 years of age. However, lack of food is not always the primary cause for malnutrition. In many developing and underdeveloped nations, diarrhea (gastroenteritis) is a major factor. Additional factors are bottle-feeding (in poor sanitary conditions), inadequate knowledge of proper child care practices, parental illiteracy, economic and political factors, climate conditions, cultural and religious food preferences, and simply the lack of adequate food. Müller and Krawinkel (2005) point out that poverty is the underlying cause of malnutrition. The most extreme forms of malnutrition, or **protein-energy malnutrition** (PEM), are kwashiorkor and marasmus. Some authorities suggest that severe malnutrition encompasses more than protein energy deficits and thus prefer the term *severe childhood undernutrition (SCU)* (Heird, 2007). Entities such as the World Health Organization continue to use the term *protein energy malnutrition.* SCU may also be subdivided into edematous (kwashiorkor) and nonedematous (marasmus) types (Heird, 2007).

In the United States milder forms of PEM are seen as a result of primary malnutrition, although the classic cases of marasmus and kwashiorkor may also occur. Unlike in developing countries, where the main reason for PEM is inadequate food, in the United States PEM occurs despite ample dietary supplies (see Growth Failure [Failure to Thrive], p. 534). PEM may also be seen in persons with chronic health problems such as cystic fibrosis, renal dialysis, cancer, and GI malabsorption; in the elderly who have chronic malnutrition; or in persons with acute illnesses such as prolonged, untreated anorexia nervosa. Kwashiorkor has been reported in the United States in children fed only a rice beverage diet (Rice Dream) and few solid foods (Katz, Mahlberg, Honig, et al, 2005). The rice drink contains 0.13 g of protein per ounce (compared with the 0.5 g found in human milk and infant formulas) and is an inadequate source of nutrition for children. Other reported cases of kwashiorkor in developed countries involved infants who were fed nonstandard infant diets such as flour water, corn porridge, molasses, and nondairy creamer (Katz, Mahlberg, Honig, et al, 2005). Kwashiorkor has also been reported in the United States when infants have been fed inappropriate food as a result of parental (caretaker) nutritional ignorance, a perceived cow's milk–based formula intolerance, family social chaos, or cow's milk intolerance (Liu, Howard, Mancini, et al, 2001). Therefore it is important that health care workers not assume that PEM cannot occur in developed countries; a comprehensive dietary history should be obtained in any child with clinical features resembling PEM.

Kwashiorkor

Kwashiorkor has been defined as primarily a deficiency of protein with an adequate supply of calories. A diet consisting mainly of starch grains or tubers provides adequate calories in the form of carbohydrates but an inadequate amount of high-quality proteins. Some evidence, however, supports a multifactorial etiology, including cultural, psychologic, and infective factors that may interact to place the child at risk for kwashiorkor. Penny (2003) suggests that kwashiorkor may result from the interplay of nutrient deprivation and infectious or environmental stresses, which produces an imbalanced response to such insults. Kwashiorkor often occurs subsequent to an infectious outbreak of measles and dysentery. There is further evidence that oxidative stress occurs in children with kwashiorkor, resulting in free radical damage, which may precipitate cellular changes, resulting in edema and muscle wasting (Penny, 2003). The role of the essential fatty acid arachidonic acid in lipid metabolism, altered leukotriene production, and oxidative stress in kwashiorkor has yet to be fully understood, but arachidonic acid seems to have an interactive role in its development (Penny, 2003).

Taken from the Ga language (Ghana), the word *kwashiorkor* means "the sickness the older child gets when the next baby is born" and aptly describes the syndrome that develops in the first child, usually between 1 and 4 years of age, when weaned from the breast after the second child is born.

The child with kwashiorkor has thin, wasted extremities and a prominent abdomen from edema (ascites). The edema often masks severe muscular atrophy, making the child appear less debilitated than he or she actually is (Fig. 13-1). The skin is scaly and dry and has areas of depigmentation. Several dermatoses may be evident, partly resulting from the vitamin deficiencies. Permanent blindness often results from the severe lack of vitamin A. Mineral deficiencies are common, especially iron, calcium, and zinc. Acute zinc deficiency is a common complication of severe PEM and results in skin rashes, loss of hair, impaired immune response and susceptibility to infections, digestive problems, night blindness, changes in affective behavior, defective wound healing, and impaired growth. Its depressant effect on appetite further limits food intake. The hair is thin, dry, coarse, and dull. Depigmentation is common, and patchy alopecia may occur.

Diarrhea (persistent diarrhea malnutrition syndrome) commonly occurs from a lowered resistance to infection and further

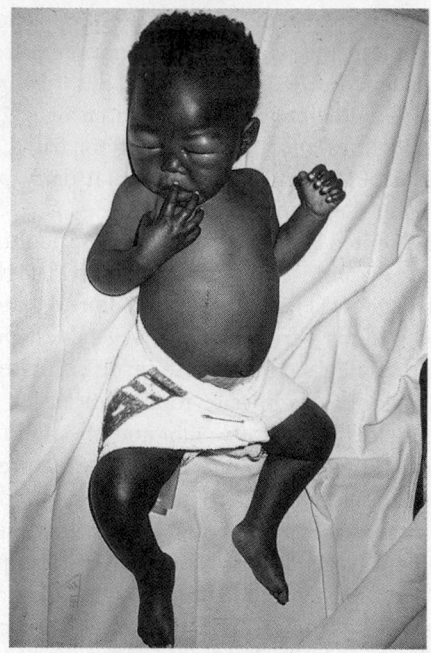

Fig. 13-1 Kwashiorkor. The infant shows generalized edema, seen in the puffiness of the face, arms, and legs. (From Kumar V, Abbas A, Fausto N, et al: *Robbins basic pathology*, ed 8, Philadelphia, 2007, Saunders.)

complicates the electrolyte imbalance. Low levels of cytokines (protein cells involved in the primary response to infection) have been reported in children with kwashiorkor, suggesting that such children have a blunted immune response to infection. A large number of deaths in children with kwashiorkor occur in those who develop HIV infection. GI disturbances such as fatty infiltration of the liver and atrophy of the acini cells of the pancreas occur. Anemia is also a common finding in malnourished children. Protein deficiency increases the child's susceptibility to infection, which eventually results in death. Fatal deterioration may be caused by diarrhea and infection or by circulatory failure.

Marasmus

Marasmus results from general malnutrition of both calories and protein. It is common in underdeveloped countries during times of drought, especially in cultures where adults eat first; the remaining food is often insufficient in quality and quantity for the children.

Marasmus is usually a syndrome of physical and emotional deprivation and is not confined to geographic areas where food supplies are inadequate. It may be seen in children with growth failure in whom the cause is not solely nutritional but primarily emotional. Marasmus may be seen in infants as young as 3 months of age if breast-feeding is not successful and there are no suitable alternatives. Marasmic kwashiorkor is a form of PEM in which clinical findings of both kwashiorkor and marasmus are evident; the child has edema, severe wasting, and stunted growth. In marasmic kwashiorkor the child suffers from inadequate nutrient intake and superimposed infection. Fluid and electrolyte disturbances, hypothermia, and hypoglycemia are associated with a poor prognosis.

Marasmus is characterized by gradual wasting and atrophy of body tissues, especially of subcutaneous fat. The child appears to be very old, with loose and wrinkled skin, unlike the child with kwashiorkor, who appears more rounded from the edema. Fat metabolism is less impaired than in kwashiorkor; thus deficiency of fat-soluble vitamins is usually minimal or absent. In general, the clinical manifestations of marasmus are similar to those seen in kwashiorkor with the following exceptions: with marasmus there is no edema from hypoalbuminemia or sodium retention, which contributes to a severely emaciated appearance; no dermatoses caused by vitamin deficiencies; little or no depigmentation of hair or skin; moderately normal fat metabolism and lipid absorption; and smaller head size and slower recovery after treatment.

The child is fretful, apathetic, withdrawn, and so lethargic that prostration frequently occurs. Intercurrent infection with debilitating diseases such as tuberculosis, parasitosis, HIV, and dysentery is common.

Therapeutic Management

The treatment of PEM includes providing a diet with high-quality proteins, carbohydrates, vitamins, and minerals. When PEM occurs as a result of persistent diarrhea, three management goals are identified:

1. Rehydration with an oral rehydration solution that also replaces electrolytes
2. Administration of medications such as antibiotics and antidiarrheals
3. Provision of adequate nutrition by either breast-feeding or a proper weaning diet

Local protocols are used in developing countries to deal with PEM. Penny (2003) proposes a three-phase treatment protocol: (1) acute or initial phase in the first 2 to 10 days, involving initiation of treatment for oral rehydration, diarrhea, and intestinal parasites; prevention of hypoglycemia and hypothermia; and subsequent dietary management; (2) recovery or rehabilitation (2 to 6 weeks), focusing on increasing dietary intake and weight gain; and (3) follow-up phase, focusing on care after discharge in an outpatient setting to prevent relapse and promote weight gain, provide developmental stimulation, and evaluate cognitive and motor deficits. In the acute phase care is taken to prevent fluid overload; the child is observed closely for signs of food or fluid intolerance. The refeeding syndrome may occur if intake progresses too rapidly; cardiac failure may cause sudden death in the child who has been malnourished and refed too rapidly.

Vitamin and mineral supplementation are required in most cases of PEM; vitamin A, zinc, and copper are recommended; iron supplementation is not recommended until the child is able to tolerate a steady food source. In addition, the child is observed for signs of skin breakdown, which should be treated to prevent infection. Breast-feeding is encouraged if the mother and child are able to do so effectively; in some cases partial supplementation with a modified cow's milk–based formula may be necessary (Penny, 2003).

The World Health Organization (2006) issued a statement recognizing the importance of breast-feeding for the first 6 months in developing countries where HIV is prevalent among childbearing women and children. The World Health Organization recognizes that appropriate sources of food and water for infants may not be available once the 6 months are concluded and that the risk for malnutrition is greater among such children than the theoretical risk of HIV. However, the organization does recommend that breast-feeding continue after 6 months with the introduction of complementary foods, provided these are safe for child consumption. In severely malnourished children a modest energy food source is given initially, followed by a high-protein and energy food source; severely malnourished children will not tolerate a high-energy and high-protein source initially. A number of food sources may be provided to treat PEM. They include oral rehydration solutions (ReSoMal), amino acid–based elemental food, and ready-to-feed foods that do not require the addition of water (to minimize contaminated water consumption); parenteral and oral antibiotics are often part of the standard treatment for PEM (Ciliberto, Sandige, Ndehka, et al, 2005; Amadi, Mwiya, Chomba, et al, 2005) (see Cultural Competence box).

⊕ CULTURAL COMPETENCE

World Health Organization Child Growth Standards

The World Health Organization (2006) has published new growth standards for children that are based on the growth of healthy breast-fed infants throughout the first year of life. The World Health Organization growth standards are designed to evaluate the growth of children aged birth to 5 years. The growth charts were compiled from a multicenter project conducted in Brazil, Ghana, India, Norway, Oman, and the United States, which included 8440 children raised in environments that promoted healthy growth habits, such as having been breastfed and being born to nonsmoking mothers. The growth standards are representative of an international standard of growth designed to promote healthy eating and living habits in all countries. The growth charts and additional information may be accessed at **www.who.int/ childgrowth/standards/en**.

World Health Organization: *WHO child growth standards,* The Organization, 2006, Geneva, Switzerland, available at www.who.int/childgrowth/en (accessed July 2, 2009).

Nursing Care Management

Because PEM appears early in childhood, primarily in children 6 months to 2 years of age, and is associated with early weaning, low-protein diet, delayed introduction of complementary foods, and frequent infections (Müller and Krawinkel, 2005), it is essential that nursing care focus on prevention of PEM through parent education about feeding practices during this crucial period. Breast-feeding is the optimal method of feeding for the first 6 months. The immune properties naturally found in breast milk not only nourish the infant but also help prevent opportunistic infections, which may contribute to PEM. Providing for essential physiologic needs, such as appropriate nutrient intake, protection from infection, adequate hydration, skin care, and restoration of physiologic integrity, is paramount. Additional nursing care focuses on education about and administration of childhood vaccinations to prevent illness, promotion of nutrition and well-being for the lactating mother, encouragement and participation in well-child visits for infants and toddlers, appropriate food sources for children being weaned from the breast, and education regarding sanitation practices to prevent childhood GI diseases.

Poor skin integrity further increases the chance of infections, hypothermia, water loss, and skin breakdown. Tube feedings may be required in infants too weak to breast- or bottle-feed. Oral rehydration with an approved oral rehydration solution is commonly used in cases of PEM in which diarrhea and infection are not immediately life threatening.

One approach that has gained acceptance for treating childhood malnutrition in developing countries is the home-based use of ready-to-use therapeutic food (RUTF). The RUTF is a paste based on peanut butter and dried skim milk with vitamins and minerals; it requires no mixing with water or milk. The packaged RUTF can be stored without refrigeration. Studies have demonstrated improved survival rates in malnourished children (Amthor, Cole, and Manary, 2009; Ciliberto, Sandige, Ndehka, et al, 2005). Some of the reported advantages of home-based treatment include that children are not exposed to hospital-acquired infections and may receive the RUTF from village health aides (Kapil, 2009).

It is imperative that nurses be at the forefront in educating and reinforcing healthy nutrition habits in parents of small children to prevent malnutrition. Because children with marasmus may suffer from emotional starvation as well, care should be consistent with care of the child with growth failure (p. 534).

The World Health Organization has published guidelines for the treatment and management of children with severe malnutrition (Ashworth, Khanum, Jackson, et al, 2003). These guidelines include a two-phase program with a 10-step guide to treating the child with malnutrition.

FOOD SENSITIVITY

Food sensitivity is a general term that includes any type of adverse reaction to food or food additives. The terms *food sensitivity, hypersensitivity, allergy,* and *intolerance* are often used interchangeably. The American Academy of Allergy, Asthma and Immunology further suggests defining food-induced reactions according to the following: adverse food reactions, food hypersensitivity (allergy), food anaphylaxis, food intolerance, food idiosyncrasy, food toxicity or poisoning, anaphylactoid reaction to food, pharmacologic food reaction, and metabolic food reaction (American Academy of Pediatrics, 2009). Approximately 6% of children may experience food allergic reactions in the first 3 years of life; 1.5% will have an allergy to eggs and 0.6% to peanuts (Sampson and Leung, 2007a).

The clinical manifestations of food hypersensitivity may be divided as follows (American Academy of Pediatrics, 2009):

Systemic—Anaphylactic, growth failure
GI—Abdominal pain, vomiting, cramping, diarrhea
Respiratory—Cough, wheezing, rhinitis, infiltrates
Cutaneous—Urticaria, rash, atopic dermatitis

Food hypersensitivities usually occur either as an immunoglobulin E (IgE)–mediated or non–IgE-mediated immune response; some toxic reactions may occur as a result of a toxin found within the food (Sampson, 2004). Food allergy is caused by exposure to allergens, usually proteins (but not the smaller amino acids) that are capable of inducing IgE antibody formation (sensitization) when ingested. Sensitization refers to the initial exposure of an individual to an allergen, resulting in an immune response; subsequent exposure induces a much stronger response that is clinically apparent. Consequently, food

hypersensitivity typically occurs after the food has been ingested one or more times.

Oral allergy syndrome occurs when a food allergen (commonly fruits and vegetables) is ingested and there is subsequent edema and pruritus involving the lips, tongue, palate, and throat. Recovery from symptoms is usually rapid. Immediate GI hypersensitivity is an IgE-mediated reaction to a food allergen; reactions include nausea, abdominal pain, cramping, diarrhea, vomiting, anaphylaxis, or all of these. Additional food hypersensitivities seen in young children include allergic eosinophilic esophagitis, allergic eosinophilic gastroenteritis, food protein–induced proctocolitis, and food protein–induced enteropathy (milk [cow or soy] protein intolerance, celiac disease).

Food hypersensitivity may also be classified according to the interval between ingestion and the manifestation of symptoms: immediate (within minutes to hours) or delayed (2 to 48 hours) (American Academy of Pediatrics, 2009).

Allergens can produce an allergic response when inhaled or injected, but these routes rarely apply to food allergens. (See also Asthma, Chapter 32.) The most common food allergens in children are eggs, cow's milk, and peanuts (Sampson and Leung, 2007a); soy, wheat, corn, tree nuts, shellfish, and fish allergies are more common in adults (Sicherer, 2003; Sampson, 2004) (Box 13-2).

Food allergies can occur at any time but are common during infancy, since the immature intestinal tract is more permeable to proteins than the mature intestinal tract, thus increasing the likelihood of an immune response. Allergies in general demonstrate a genetic component: children who have one parent with allergy have a 50% or greater risk of developing allergy; children

---

BOX 13-2   HYPERALLERGENIC FOODS AND SOURCES

Milk*—Ice cream, butter, margarine (if it contains dairy products), yogurt, cheese, pudding, baked goods, wieners, bologna, canned creamed soups, instant breakfast drinks, powdered milk drinks, milk chocolate

Eggs*—Mayonnaise, creamy salad dressing, baked goods, egg noodles, some cake icing, meringue, custard, pancakes, French toast, root beer

Wheat*—Almost all baked goods, wieners, bologna, pressed or chopped cold cuts, gravy, pasta, some canned soups

Legumes—Peanuts,* peanut butter or oil, beans, peas, lentils

Nuts*—Some chocolates, candy, baked goods, cherry soda (may be flavored with a nut extract), walnut oil

Fish or shellfish*—Cod liver oil, pizza with anchovies, Caesar salad dressing, any food fried in same oil as fish

Soy*—Soy sauce, teriyaki or Worcestershire sauce, tofu, baked goods using soy flour or oil, soy nuts, soy infant formulas or milk, soybean paste, tuna packed in vegetable oil, many margarines

Chocolate—Cola beverages, cocoa, chocolate-flavored drinks

Buckwheat—Some cereals, pancakes

Pork, chicken—Bacon, wieners, sausage, pork fat, chicken broth

Strawberries, melon, pineapple—Gelatin, syrups

Corn—Popcorn, cereal, muffins, cornstarch, corn meal, corn bread, corn tortilla; many processed foods also contain corn syrup

Citrus fruits—Orange, lemon, lime, grapefruit; any of these in drinks, gelatin, juice, or medicines

Tomatoes—Juice, some vegetable soups, spaghetti, pizza sauce, catsup

Spices—Chili, pepper, vinegar, cinnamon

*Most common allergens.

who have both parents with allergy have up to a 100% risk of developing allergy. Allergy with a hereditary tendency is referred to as atopy. Some infants with atopy can be identified at birth from elevated levels of IgE in cord blood.

Deaths have been reported in children who suffered an anaphylactic reaction to food. Onset of the reactions occurred shortly after ingestion (5 to 30 minutes). In most of the children the reactions did not begin with skin signs, such as hives, red rash, and flushing, but rather mimicked an acute asthma attack (wheezing, decreased air movement in airways, dyspnea). Watch children with food anaphylaxis closely because a biphasic response has been recorded in a number of cases in which there is an immediate response, apparent recovery, then acute recurrence of symptoms (Simons, 2009). Children with extremely sensitive food allergies should wear a medical identification bracelet and have an injectable epinephrine cartridge (EpiPen) readily available. (See Anaphylaxis, Chapter 29.) Any child with a history of food allergy or previous severe reaction to food should have a written emergency treatment plan, as well as an EpiPen and liquid diphenhydramine (Benadryl) or cetirizine (Zyrtec) (Sampson and Leung, 2007b).

! NURSING ALERT

Indications for the administration of intramuscular epinephrine in a child with a life-threatening anaphylactic reaction, or one who is experiencing severe symptoms, include any one of the following (Wang and Sampson, 2007):

- Itching sensation or tightness in throat; hoarseness
- "Barky" cough
- Difficulty swallowing; dyspnea
- Wheezing
- Cyanosis
- Respiratory arrest; mild dysrhythmia or mild hypotension
- Severe bradycardia, hypotension, or cardiac arrest; or loss of consciousness

---

⚡ DRUG ALERT

Emergency Management of Anaphylaxis*

Drug: Epinephrine 0.001 mg/kg up to 0.3 mg
Dose: EpiPen Jr (0.15 mg) IM for child 8 to 25 kg (17.5 to 55 lb)
EpiPen (0.3 mg) IM for child over 25 kg (55 lb)
Observe for adverse reactions: tachycardia, hypertension, irritability, headaches, nausea, and tremors.

*Sampson and Leung, 2007b.

Educate parents, teachers, and daycare workers regarding signs and symptoms of food hypersensitivity reactions. People with food sensitivity should avoid unfamiliar foods and restaurants that do not disclose food ingredients. New labeling guidelines require that food additives such as spices and flavoring be clearly labeled on commercially sold, store-bought foods. Hidden ingredients in prepared foods are also a potential source of food hypersensitivity.

Children with a history of food allergy may spend a considerable amount of time in daycare; therefore persons working in daycare centers and other children's settings need to be properly educated regarding recognition and management of severe anaphylactic reactions (Bansal, Marsh, Patel, et al, 2005).

Although the reason is unknown, many children "outgrow" their food allergies. About 80% of all infants who are intolerant to cow's milk usually develop tolerance by the fourth birthday (Sampson, 2004). More than half (60%) of infants have an IgE-mediated reaction to cow's milk, and 25% will retain sensitivity until the second decade of their life. About 35% develop other food allergies (Sampson, 2004). Children who are allergic to more than one food may develop tolerance to each food at a different time. The most common allergens, such as peanuts, are outgrown less readily than other food allergens. Because of the tendency to lose the hypersensitivity, reintroduce allergenic foods into the diet after a period of abstinence (usually ≥1 year) to evaluate whether the food can be safely added to the diet. Foods that are associated with severe anaphylactic reactions, however, continue to present a lifelong risk and must be avoided.

The only way to positively establish the diagnosis of food allergy is by eliminating the suspected food from the diet for approximately 10 to 14 days (for IgE-mediated allergy; longer for cell-mediated disorder), then following with a food challenge. Food challenges should only be performed by an allergist who has the appropriate equipment and training to manage anaphylaxis (Sampson and Leung, 2007a).

Because children with food allergies (usually two or more) are at risk for inadequate nutrient intake and growth failure, it is recommended that they have an annual nutritional assessment to prevent such problems (Christie, Hine, Parker, et al, 2002).

Breast-feeding is now considered a primary strategy for avoiding atopy in families with known food sensitivities; however, there is no evidence that maternal avoidance (during pregnancy or lactation) of cow's milk protein or other dietary products known to cause food hypersensitivity will prevent atopy in children (American Academy of Pediatrics, 2009). Researchers indicate that delaying the introduction of highly allergenic foods past 4 to 6 months may not be as protective for atopy as previously believed (Greer, Sicherer, Burks, et al, 2008). Likewise studies have shown that soy formula does not prevent allergic disease in infants and children (American Academy of Pediatrics, 2009). The strategies listed in the Nursing Care Guidelines box are those recommended by most authorities for infants with a family history of atopy.*

Cow's Milk Allergy

Cow's milk allergy (CMA) is a multifaceted disorder representing adverse systemic and local GI reactions to cow's milk protein. Approximately 2.5% of infants develop cow's milk hypersensitivity; 80% of those children may outgrow the hypersensitivity by 4 years of age (Sampson, 2004). Recent studies reveal that milk allergy may persist and some children may not

---

*Further information for parents of infants with food allergies is available from the American Academy of Allergy, Asthma and Immunology, 555 E. Wells St., Suite 1100, Milwaukee, WI 53202; 414-272-6071; www.aaaai.org. Additional helpful websites for information on food allergy include MedlinePlus (sponsored by U.S. National Library of Medicine and National Institutes of Health), http://medlineplus.gov; Food Allergy and Anaphylaxis Network, 800-929-4040, www.foodallergy.org; National Institute of Allergy and Infectious Diseases, www3.niaid.nih.gov; and www.allergicchild.com.

NURSING CARE GUIDELINES*

Preventing Atopy in Children

Identify Children at Risk
Family history of allergy
Increased immunoglobulin E in cord blood and postnatal serum
Dry, flaky skin

Prenatal Precautions (Last Trimester)
Avoid any known food allergens.
Avoid milk and other dairy products, peanuts, and eggs.
Minimize ingestion of other hyperallergenic foods (see Box 13-2).

Postnatal Precautions
Provide breast milk or casein–whey hydrolysate formula (e.g., Nutramigen, Pregestimil, Alimentum) or amino acid–based formula (Neocate, EleCare) exclusively for at least 6 months, possibly up to 12 months if family history indicates a high risk for atopy.
In infants at high risk for atopy, breast-feeding mothers eliminate peanuts and tree nuts from diet and consider eliminating eggs, cow's milk, and fish.
Offer no solid food for first 6 months.
Offer no cow's milk or soy formula for 12 months.
In infants at high risk for atopy, delay introducing eggs until 24 months, and peanuts, tree nuts, and fish until 3 years of age.
Add one new food at 5- to 7-day intervals to identify possible reaction.

Environmental Control
Limit exposure to dust mites, molds, furry animals, and cigarette smoke.

Data from Johnstone D: Strategy for intervention of food allergy in infants, *Int Pediatr* 4(4):319-325, 1989; Zeiger R, Heller S, Mellon M, et al: Effectiveness of dietary manipulation in the prevention of food allergy in infants, part 2, *J Allergy Clin Immunol* 78(1 Pt 2):224-238, 1986; Wood RA: Prospects for the prevention of allergy in children, *Curr Opin Pediatr* 8(6):601-605, 1995; and American Academy of Pediatrics, Committee on Nutrition: *Pediatric nutrition handbook*, ed 5, Elk Grove Village, Ill, 2004, The Academy.
*Recently Greer, Sicherer, Burks, et al (2008) noted that some of these interventions may not prevent atopy in children; however, they admitted there is no harm in implementing some of these preventive measures.

BOX 13-3 **COMMON CLINICAL MANIFESTATIONS OF COW'S MILK SENSITIVITY**

Gastrointestinal
Diarrhea
Vomiting
Colic
Wheezing
Gastroesophageal reflux
Bloody stools
Rectal bleeding

Respiratory
Rhinitis
Bronchitis
Asthma
Sneezing
Coughing
Chronic nasal discharge

Other Signs and Symptoms
Eczema
Excessive crying
Pallor (from anemia secondary to chronic blood loss in gastrointestinal tract)
Fussiness, irritability

---

be able to tolerate milk until they are 16 years of age (American Academy of Pediatrics, 2009). (This discussion centers on cow's milk protein contained in commercial infant formulas; whole milk is not recommended for infants <12 months of age.) The hypersensitivity may be manifested within the first 4 months of life through a variety of signs and symptoms that may appear within 45 minutes of milk ingestion or after several days (Box 13-3). The diagnosis may initially be made from the history, although the history alone is not diagnostic. The timing and diversity of clinical manifestations vary greatly. For example, CMA may be manifested as colic (see p. 532), diarrhea, vomiting, GI bleeding, gastroesophageal reflux, chronic constipation, or sleeplessness in an otherwise healthy infant.

Diagnostic Evaluation

A number of diagnostic tests may be performed, including stool analysis for blood, eosinophils, and leukocytes (both frank and occult bleeding can occur from the colitis); serum IgE levels; skin-prick or scratch testing; and radioallergosorbent test (RAST) (measures IgE antibodies to specific allergens in serum by radioimmunoassay). Both skin testing and RAST may help identify the offending food, but the results are not always conclusive. No single diagnostic test is considered definitive for the diagnosis (American Academy of Pediatrics, 2009).

The most definitive diagnostic strategy is elimination of milk in the diet, followed by challenge testing after improvement of symptoms. A clinical diagnosis is made when symptoms improve after removal of milk from the diet and two or more challenge tests produce symptoms (Ewing and Allen, 2005). Challenge testing involves reintroducing small quantities of milk in the diet to detect resurgence of symptoms; at times it involves the use of a placebo so that the parent is unaware of (or "blind" to) the timing of allergen ingestion. A **double-blind placebo-controlled food challenge** is the gold standard for diagnosing food allergies such as CMA, yet it may not be used often for diagnosing CMA because of the expense, time involved, and risk for further exposure and anaphylactic reaction (Ewing and Allen, 2005). Careful observation of the child is required during a challenge test because of the possibility of anaphylactic reaction.

Therapeutic Management

Treatment of CMA is elimination of cow's milk–based formula and all other dairy products. For infants fed cow's milk formula, this primarily involves changing the formula to a casein hydrolysate milk formula (Pregestimil, Nutramigen, or Alimentum), in which the protein has been broken down into its amino acids through enzymatic hydrolysis. Although the American Academy of Pediatrics (2009) recommends the use of extensively hydrolyzed formulas for CMA, many practitioners may start a soy formula instead because of the expense of the hydrolyzed formulas. Approximately 50% of infants who are sensitive to cow's milk protein also demonstrate sensitivity to soy, yet soy is less expensive than protein hydrolysate formula. Other choices for children who are intolerant to cow's milk–based formula are the amino acid–based formulas Neocate or EleCare, yet their cost is a major consideration. Goat's milk is not an acceptable substitute because it cross-reacts with cow's milk protein, is deficient in folic acid, and is unsuitable as the only source of calories. Anaphylactic reaction to goat's milk has been noted in an infant who was also allergic to cow's milk (Pessler and Nejat, 2004). Infants usually remain on the milk-free diet for 12 months, after which time small quantities of milk are reintroduced.

Children who have CMA may tolerate extensively heated cow's milk (Nowak-Wegrzyn, Bloom, Sicherer, et al, 2008).

Nursing Care Management

The principal nursing objectives are identification of potential CMA and appropriate counseling of parents regarding substitute formulas. Parents often interpret GI symptoms such as spitting up and a loose stool or fussiness as an indication that the infant is allergic to cow's milk and switch the infant to a variety of formulas in an attempt to resolve the problem.

Parents need much reassurance regarding the needs of nonverbal infants with such an array of symptoms. Endless nights of lost sleep and a crying infant may promote feelings of parenting inadequacy and role conflict, thus aggravating the situation. Nurses can reassure parents that many of these symptoms are common and the reasons are often never found, yet the child does achieve appropriate growth and development. Report acute symptoms to the practitioner for further evaluation. Parents need reassurance that the infant will receive complete nutrition from the new formula and will suffer no ill effects from the absence of cow's milk.

Once solid foods are started, parents need guidance in avoiding milk product (see Box 13-3). Carefully reading all food labels helps avoid exposure to prepared foods containing milk products.

Lactose Intolerance

Lactose intolerance refers to at least four different entities that involve a deficiency of the enzyme lactase, which is needed for the hydrolysis or digestion of lactose in the small intestine; lactose is hydrolyzed into glucose and galactose. Congenital lactase deficiency occurs soon after birth after the newborn has consumed lactose-containing milk (human milk or commercial formula). This inborn error of metabolism involves the complete absence or severely reduced presence of lactase. It is rare and requires lifelong lactose-free or extremely reduced lactose diet.

Primary lactase deficiency, sometimes referred to as *late-onset lactase deficiency*, is the most common type of lactose intolerance and is manifested usually after 4 or 5 years of age, although the time of onset varies. Ethnic groups with a high incidence of lactase deficiency include Asians, southern Europeans, Arabs, Israelis, and African-Americans, whereas Scandinavians tend to have the lowest. Lactose malabsorption manifests as lactose intolerance and is characterized by an imbalance between the ability of lactase to hydrolyze the ingested lactose and the amount of lactose ingested (Heyman and American Academy of Pediatrics, 2006).

Secondary lactase deficiency may occur secondary to damage of the intestinal lumen, which decreases or destroys the enzyme lactase. Cystic fibrosis; sprue; celiac disease; kwashiorkor; or infections such as giardiasis, HIV, or rotavirus may cause temporary or permanent lactose intolerance.

Developmental lactase deficiency refers to the relative lactase deficiency observed in preterm infants of less than 34 weeks of gestation (Heyman and American Academy of Pediatrics, 2006).

The primary symptoms of lactose intolerance include abdominal pain, bloating, flatulence, and diarrhea after the ingestion of lactose. The onset of symptoms occurs within 30 minutes to several hours of lactose consumption. Lactose intolerance is often perceived as an allergy; and in several studies with reports of acute GI symptoms ascribed to lactose intolerance, measurement of lactase activity is normal (Goldberg, Folta, and Must, 2002).

Lactose intolerance may be diagnosed on the basis of the history and improvement with a lactose-reduced diet. The breath hydrogen test is used to positively diagnose the condition. Breath samples in lactose-deficient individuals yield a higher percentage of hydrogen (≥ 20 ppm above baseline). In infants lactose malabsorption may be diagnosed by evaluating fecal pH and reducing substances; fecal pH in infants is usually lower than in older children, but an acidic pH may indicate malabsorption (Heyman and American Academy of Pediatrics, 2006).

Treatment of lactose intolerance involves elimination of offending dairy products; however, some advocate decreasing amounts of dairy products rather than total elimination, especially in small children (Heyman and American Academy of Pediatrics, 2006; Goldberg, Folta, and Must, 2002). In infants lactose-free or low-lactose formula offers no special advantages over lactose-containing formula, except in the severely malnourished (Heyman and American Academy of Pediatrics, 2006).

One concern is that dairy avoidance in children and adolescents with lactose intolerance contributes to reduced bone mineral density and osteoporosis (Sibley, 2004). There is evidence that dietary lactose enhances calcium absorption and that lactose-free diets may negatively affect bone mineralization (Heyman and American Academy of Pediatrics, 2006). Individuals with lactose maldigestion who do not experience lactose intolerance symptoms should continue to consume small amounts of dairy products with meals to prevent reduced bone mass density and subsequent osteoporosis (Sibley, 2004). In one study a decreased intake of calcium-containing dairy foods in early adolescent girls with perceived lactose intolerance resulted in lower spinal bone mineral content than in girls without perceived milk intolerance; the researchers cautioned that decreased dairy intake in persons with lactose intolerance may increase the risk of osteoporosis in later life (Matlik, Savaiano, McCabe, et al, 2007). One option to meet calcium intake needs of adolescents with dairy restriction due to lactose intolerance is to consume one half to one and a half servings of calcium-fortified citrus juice per day; vitamin D supplementation and increased physical activity are also recommended to increase bone health (Gao, Wilde, Lichtenstein, et al, 2006). There is evidence that probiotics (food preparations containing microorganisms such as *Lactobacillus*, which alter the GI microflora and thus are beneficial to the host) improve lactose intolerance when live cultures are fermented in dairy products (de Vrese and Schrezenmeir, 2008; Zeisel and Erickson, 2003). The positive attributes of probiotics for those with lactose maldigestion include delayed GI transit (slower than milk), positive effects on intestinal and colonic microflora, and a reduction of maldigestion symptoms.

Most people are able to tolerate small amounts of lactose even in the presence of deficient lactase activity (Heyman and American Academy of Pediatrics, 2006) and should be encouraged to continue their intake of dairy products in small amounts to obtain much-needed nutrients. Milk taken at meals may be better tolerated than when taken alone (see Family-Centered Care box). Pretreated milk (with microbial-derived lactase) is reported to be effective in improving lactose absorption. Because dairy products are a major source of calcium and vitamin D, supplementation of these nutrients is needed to prevent deficiency. Yogurt contains inactive lactase enzyme, which is activated by the temperature and pH of the duodenum; this lactase activity substitutes for the lack of endogenous lactase. Fresh, plain yogurt may be tolerated better than frozen or flavored yogurt; hard cheeses, lactase-treated dairy products, and lactase tablets taken with dairy products are also viable options. An important distinction between lactose intolerance and food hypersensitivity is that lactose intolerance does not manifest as an anaphylactic-type reaction.

FAMILY-CENTERED CARE

Controlling Symptoms of Lactose Intolerance

- In infants substitute soy-based formula for cow's milk–based formula or human milk.
- Limit milk consumption to one glass at a time.
- Drink milk with other foods rather than alone.
- Eat hard cheese, cottage cheese, or yogurt instead of drinking milk.
- Use enzyme tablets (Lactaid, Lactrase, Dairy Ease) to predigest the lactose in milk or supplement the body's own lactase (add tablets to milk or sprinkle on dairy products such as ice cream).
- Eat small amounts of dairy foods daily to help colonic bacteria adapt to ingested lactose.

Nursing Care Management

Nursing care is similar to the interventions discussed for CMA: explaining the dietary restrictions to the family; identifying alternate sources of calcium such as yogurt and calcium supplementation; explaining the importance of supplementation; and discussing sources of lactose, especially hidden sources such as its use as a bulk agent in certain medications, and ways of controlling the symptoms (see Family-Centered Care box). Parents are advised to check with the pharmacist regarding this possibility when obtaining medication.*

CONDITIONS RELATED TO FEEDING

IMPROPER FEEDING TECHNIQUE

A common cause of feeding problems is improper feeding technique. A satisfactory feeding requires a number of mechanical skills, such as placing the infant to the breast properly (see Breast-Feeding, Chapter 8); holding the bottle at an angle that allows fluid, not air, to flow into the nipple; understanding and responding to the infant's cues for burping or satiation; and holding the infant during feeding, rather than propping the

*Parents may find updated resources on lactose intolerance at www. allallergy.net.

bottle. A number of other problems can also occur singly or in combination, such as:

- Feeding too much or too little food
- Feeding too often, especially during the night, or too infrequently
- Selecting inappropriate foods for the infant's physiologic and motor development
- Incorrectly preparing formula

Although such feeding problems are more common for first-time inexperienced parents, they can also occur with seasoned parents who are unprepared for an infant who has different needs or exhibits less clear cues of hunger or satiation. Improper feeding may also occur in caretakers (parents) who are too immature to understand the infant's need for human contact during feeding and thus misinterpret hunger and satiation cues. It also occurs in parents who have an infant with a difficult temperament (see Temperament, Chapter 12) and in parents who may be impaired as a result of recreational drugs such as methamphetamines (see Drug-Exposed Infants, Chapter 10). Improper feeding is also a potential concern in family situations where an older child is left to care for a younger sibling when there is social disruption, dysfunction, and no responsible adult to intervene.

Most of these feeding problems are easily corrected with reassurance, guidance, and demonstration. Early assessment is essential to prevent complex problems from developing between parent and child at mealtime.

REGURGITATION AND "SPITTING UP"

The return of small amounts of food after a feeding is common during infancy. Do not confuse this with actual vomiting, which can be associated with a number of disturbances that may be insignificant or serious. It is usually benign, although persistent regurgitation necessitates medical evaluation to rule out gastroesophageal reflux. For clarification, the following terms are defined:

Regurgitation—Return of undigested food from the stomach, usually accompanied by burping

Spitting up—Dribbling of unswallowed formula from the infant's mouth immediately after a feeding

The nurse should explain the normal occurrence of regurgitation or spitting up to parents, especially those who are unduly concerned about it. Regurgitation can be reduced by some simple measures, such as frequent burping during and after feeding, minimum handling during and after feeding, and positioning the child on the right side with the head slightly elevated after feeding. The inconvenience of spitting up can be managed with absorbent bibs on the infant and protective cloths on the parent.

Sometimes frequent dribbling of formula causes excoriation of the corners of the mouth, chin, and neck. Keeping the area dry promotes healing but can be difficult to maintain.

COLIC (PAROXYSMAL ABDOMINAL PAIN)

Colic is reported to occur in 15% to 40% of all infants (Morin, 2009), yet has no particular affinity in regard to the gender, race, or socioeconomic status (Ellett, 2003). An organic cause may be identified in less than 5% of infants seen by physicians because of excessive crying (Roberts, Ostapchuk, and O'Brien, 2004). The condition is generally described as abdominal pain or cramping that is manifested by loud crying and drawing the legs up to the abdomen. Other definitions include variables such as duration of cry greater than 3 hours a day, occurring more than 3 days per week, and for more than 3 weeks and parental dissatisfaction with the child's behavior. Some studies report an increase in symptoms (fussiness and crying) in the late afternoon or evening (Morin, 2009); however, in some infants the onset of symptoms occurs at another time. Colic is more common in young infants under the age of 3 months than in older infants, and infants with difficult temperaments are more likely to be colicky.

Despite the obvious behavioral indications of pain, the infant with colic gains weight and usually thrives. There is no evidence of a residual effect of colic on older children, except perhaps a strained parent-child relationship in some cases. In other words, infants who are colicky grow up to be normal children and adults. Colic is self-limiting and in most cases resolves as the infant matures, generally around 12 to 16 weeks of age (Lobo, Kotzer, Keefe, et al, 2004; O'Connor, 2009).

Etiology

Among the theories investigated as potential causes are too rapid feeding, overeating, swallowing excessive air, improper feeding technique (especially in positioning and burping), and emotional stress or tension between parent and child. Although all these may occur, there is no evidence that one factor is consistently present. Infants with CMA symptoms have a high rate of colic (44%), and eliminating cow's milk products from the infant's diet can reduce the symptoms. However, there is considerable controversy about the role of allergy and colic because there does not appear to be an increased incidence of atopy in infants with colic (Sicherer, 2003).

Parental smoking, strained parent-infant interaction, lactase deficiency, difficult infant temperament, difficulty regulating emotions, overstimulation, central nervous system immaturity, and neurochemical dysregulation in the brain have also been proposed as potential causes of colic (Ellett, 2003; Neu and Robinson, 2003). A positive association between consumption of fruit juices (carbohydrate malabsorption) and colic has been demonstrated in some cases (Duro, Rising, Cedillo, et al, 2002). Some experts have suggested that gastroesophageal reflux is a cause of colic, but studies have not supported this theory (St. James-Roberts, 2008). The consensus of many experts who study colic is that it is multifactorial and that no single treatment for every colicky infant will be effective in alleviating the symptoms.

Therapeutic Management

Management of colic should begin with an investigation of possible organic causes, such as CMA, intussusception, or other GI problem. If a sensitivity to cow's milk is strongly suspected, a trial substitution of another formula such as an extensively hydrolyzed (Nutramigen, Alimentum, Pregestimil), whey hydrolysate, or amino acid (Neocate, EleCare) formula is warranted. Soy formulas are usually avoided because of the possibility of sensitivity to soy protein as well (American Academy of Pediatrics, 2009). Oral administration of *Lactobacillus reuteri* to colicky breast-fed infants decreased symptoms within 1 week of initiation in one small study (Savino, Pelle, Palumeri, et al, 2007).

When no specific inciting agent can be found, the supportive measures discussed under Nursing Care Management are employed.

The use of drugs, including sedatives, antispasmodics, antihistamines, and antiflatulents, is sometimes recommended. The most commonly used sedatives are phenobarbital, hydroxyzine hydrochloride (Atarax), and chloral hydrate. Simethicone (Mylicon) may also help allay the symptoms of colic. However, in most controlled studies none of these drugs completely reduced the symptoms of colic. Herbal (chamomile) tea offered at the onset of crying and up to three times daily has proved effective in relieving the symptoms of colic in some infants (Weizman, Alkrinawi, Goldfarb, et al, 1993); however, parents are to be cautioned regarding the unknown safety of this treatment (Crotteau, Wright, and Eglash, 2006). Behavioral interventions have not proved effective at reducing symptoms of colic but have helped parents deal with the crying infant in a more positive manner. The addition of lactase to infant formula has produced mixed results as far as abatement of overall symptoms.

One study found that a combination of interventions—massage, herbal tea, sucrose solution, and hydrolyzed formula—decreased crying in reported colicky infants; the administration of the hydrolyzed formula achieved best results, whereas massage was least effective at reducing crying (Arikan, Alp, Gozum, et al, 2008).

An extensive review of a wide variety of interventions for colic indicates there are no specific safe remedies to alleviate symptoms of colic in every infant. Dietary changes, such as eliminating cow's milk protein from the lactating mother's diet, and behavioral interventions were shown to be effective in helping parents reduce stimulation and respond to the infant's crying, yet these interventions are perceived only as moderately effective (Joanna Briggs Institute, 2008). Administering sucrose was effective at reducing crying in colicky infants for a short period (3 to 30 minutes) (Joanna Briggs Institute, 2008).

The literature on colic contains many behavioral remedies for treatment; however, none has proved entirely effective at reducing the symptoms of colic in all infants treated. Studies on infant massage for relieving the symptoms of colic demonstrated no advantage, and the practice is not recommended (Roberts, Ostapchuk, and O'Brien, 2004). The Internet offers a variety of remedies for colic. Parents should be aware of the sources of information and use home remedies such as herbal teas or natural remedies touted for colic relief cautiously.

A survey of pediatric nurse practitioners (PNPs) and pediatricians managing infants with colic found that the PNPs were more likely to suggest behavioral or environmental modification strategies, whereas the pediatricians predominantly suggested pharmacologic interventions or formula changes (Lobo, Kotzer, Keefe, et al, 2004). The study emphasized the lack of understanding and consensus regarding the etiology and management of infant colic.

Nursing Care Management

The initial step in managing colic is to take a thorough, detailed history of the usual daily events. Areas that should be stressed include (1) the infant's diet; (2) the diet of the breast-feeding mother; (3) the time of day when crying occurs; (4) the relationship of crying to feeding time; (5) the presence of specific family members during crying and habits of family members, such as smoking; (6) activity of the mother or usual caregiver before, during, and after crying; (7) characteristics of the cry (duration, intensity); (8) measures used to relieve crying and their effectiveness; and (9) the infant's stooling, voiding, and sleeping patterns. Of special emphasis is a careful assessment of the feeding process via demonstration by the parent.

If cow's milk sensitivity is suspected, breast-feeding mothers should follow a milk-free diet (see Box 13-3) for a minimum of 3 to 5 days in an attempt to reduce the infant's symptoms. Caution mothers that some nondairy creamers may contain calcium caseinate, a cow's milk protein. If a milk-free diet is helpful, lactating mothers may need calcium supplements to meet the body's requirement. Bottle-fed infants may improve with the same dietary modifications as for the child with CMA (see p. 530).

One important nursing intervention (before or after organic cause has been eliminated) is reassuring both parents they are not doing anything wrong and that the infant is not experiencing any physical or emotional harm. Parents, especially mothers, become easily frustrated with the infant's crying and perceive this as a sign that something is horribly wrong. Additionally, colicky infants may be at increased risk for being shaken by the caregiver and experiencing traumatic brain injury. A survey of fathers of colicky infants revealed that professional assistance was limited. The fathers described the experience of having a colicky infant as like falling into an abyss from which they had to climb with the assistance of family and friends, thus reinforcing the importance of empathetic nurses (Ellett, Appleton, and Sloan, 2009). An empathetic, gentle, and reassuring attitude, in addition to suggestions for treatment, will help allay parents' anxieties, which are usually exacerbated by loss of sleep and preoccupation over the infant's welfare. Colic disappears spontaneously, usually by 3 to 4 months of age, although guarantees should never be given, since it may continue for much longer. Other support persons and extended family members may be enlisted to support the parents during this difficult time.*

When no specific organic or behavioral cause can be identified, it is preferable to determine the time of the onset of crying and attempt to manipulate the circumstances associated with it. For example, some infants have episodes of colic around the family's dinner time, when all household members are home and often tired and busy. The overstimulating, tense atmosphere may upset the infant. Changing the evening routine, such as encouraging someone other than the mother or primary

*Parents may find helpful resources at www.colicnet.com. Additional resources for parents include the following: Jones S, Ziedrich L, Thompson M: *Crying Baby, Sleepless Nights: Why Your Baby Is Crying and What You Can Do About It*, Cambridge, Mass, 1992, Harvard Common Press; and Sears W, Sears M: *The Fussy Baby Book: Parenting Your High-Need Child from Birth to Five*, New York, 1996, Little Brown.

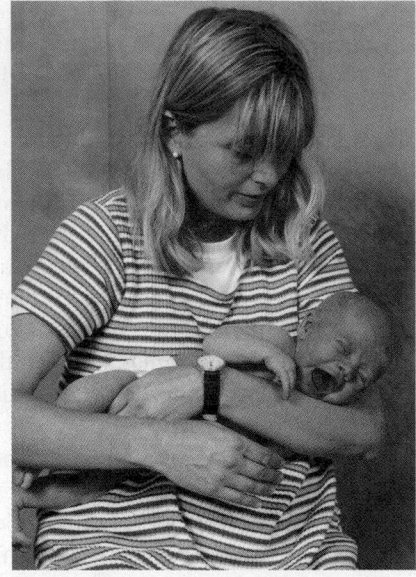

Fig. 13-2 The "colic carry" may be comforting to an infant with colic. (Courtesy Paul Vincent Kuntz, Texas Children's Hospital, Houston.)

caregiver to prepare dinner, preparing dinner earlier in the day, and feeding the infant in a quieter area of the house, may help. Other approaches for relieving colic are listed in the Family-Centered Care box and shown in Fig. 13-2. Encourage parents to try as many of these approaches as possible, since not all are effective for every infant.

One author suggests that a problem-solving discussion with the parents, in addition to acknowledgment that the infant has colic, is an optimal strategy for helping parents manage the infant with colic until a cure is found (Ellett, 2003). Nurses must also be aware that once colic symptoms are resolved, family function may be negatively impacted by residual feelings and emotions experienced during the acute phase of the colic (Ellett, Schuff, and Davis, 2005). Practical parental support interventions include the provision of a colic hotline (mother-to–nurse practitioner or nurse) and nurse-managed colic support groups (Ellett, Schuff, and Davis, 2005).

GROWTH FAILURE (FAILURE TO THRIVE)

Growth failure, or failure to thrive (FTT), is a sign of inadequate growth resulting from inability to obtain or use calories required for growth. FTT has no universal definition, although one of the more common criteria is a weight (and sometimes height) that falls below the 5th percentile for the child's age. Another definition of FTT includes a weight for age (and height) z value of less than −2.0 (a z value is a standard deviation value that represents anthropometric data normalizing for sex and age with greater precision than growth percentile curves [Markowitz, Watkins, and Duggan, 2008]). A third way to define FTT is a weight curve that crosses more than 2 percentile lines on the National Center for Health Statistics growth charts after previous achievement of a stable growth pattern. Growth measurements alone are not used to diagnose children with FTT. Rather, the finding of a pattern of persistent deviation from established growth parameters is cause for concern. In addition to lack of consensus on the precise definition of FTT,

FAMILY-CENTERED CARE

Relieving Colic

- Place infant prone over a covered hot-water bottle, heated towel, or covered heating pad.
- Gently massage infant's abdomen.
- Respond immediately to the crying.
- Change infant's position frequently; walk with child's face down and with body across parent's arm, with parent's hand under infant's abdomen, applying gentle pressure (see Fig. 13-2).
- Use a front carrier for transporting infant.
- Swaddle infant tightly with a soft, stretchy blanket.
- Place infant in a wind-up swing.
- Take infant for car rides or outside for a change in environment.
- Use bottles that minimize air swallowing (curved bottle or inner collapsible bag).
- Use a commercial device* in the crib that simulates the vibration and sound of a car ride or plays soothing "noise," in utero sounds, or music.†
- Provide smaller, frequent feedings; burp infant during and after feedings with the infant in the shoulder position or sitting upright, and place infant in an upright seat after feedings.
- Introduce a pacifier for added sucking.
- In breast-fed infants, mother should avoid all milk and other dairy products for a trial period.
- If household members smoke, avoid smoking near infant; preferably confine smoking activity to outside of home.
- Give appropriate dose of acetaminophen elixir or suppository if suggested by health professional; not recommended for daily use.
- If nothing reduces the crying, place infant in crib and allow to cry; periodically hold and comfort child and put down again.‡

*Sweet Dreems, Inc., Sleep Tight Order Department, 800-662-6542; www.colic.com.
†Suggested infant relaxation music: "Heartbeat Lullabies" by Terry Woodford. Available from Baby-Go-To-Sleep Center, Audio-Therapy Innovations, Inc., PO Box 550, Colorado Springs, CO 80901; 800-537-7748; www.babygotosleep.com.
‡Helpful information may also be found at www.colichelp.com.

there are those who advocate for a change in terminology; thus terms such as *growth failure* and *pediatric undernutrition* are used in the literature for FTT (Locklin, 2005).

Some experts suggest that the previously used classifications of *organic FTT* and *nonorganic FTT* are too simplistic because most cases of growth failure have mixed causes; they suggest that FTT be classified according to pathophysiology in the following categories (Krugman and Dubowitz, 2003):

Inadequate caloric intake—Incorrect formula preparation, neglect, food fads, excessive juice consumption, poverty, behavioral problems affecting eating, or central nervous system problems affecting intake

Inadequate absorption—Cystic fibrosis, celiac disease, vitamin or mineral deficiencies, biliary atresia, or hepatic disease

Increased metabolism—Hyperthyroidism, congenital heart defects, or chronic immunodeficiency

Defective utilization—Genetic anomaly such as trisomy 21 or 18, congenital infection, or metabolic storage diseases

The cause of growth failure is often multifactorial and involves a combination of infant organic disease, dysfunctional parenting behaviors, subtle neurologic or behavioral problems, and disturbed parent-child interactions (Block, Krebs, and

Committee on Child Abuse and Neglect and Committee on Nutrition [American Academy of Pediatrics], 2005).

Infants who are born preterm and with VLBW or extremely low birth weight (ELBW), as well as those with intrauterine growth restriction, are often referred for growth failure within the first 2 years of life because they typically do not grow physically at the same rate as term cohorts, even after discharge from the acute care facility. Catch-up growth has been shown to be much more difficult to achieve in ELBW and VLBW infants. As children, former VLBW and ELBW infants are more likely to have small stature and demonstrate lower cognitive and academic achievement scores than term cohorts (Casey, Whiteside-Mansell, Barrett, et al, 2006).

Other factors that can lead to inadequate caloric intake in infancy include poverty, health or childrearing beliefs such as fad diets, inadequate nutritional knowledge, family stress, feeding resistance, and insufficient breast milk intake.

Diagnostic Evaluation

Diagnosis is initially made from evidence of growth failure. If FTT is recent, the weight, but not the height, is below accepted standards (usually the 5th percentile); if FTT is longstanding, both weight and height are low, indicating chronic malnutrition. Perhaps as important as anthropometric measurements are a complete health and dietary history (including perinatal history), physical examination for evidence of organic causes, developmental assessment, and family assessment. A dietary intake history, either a 24-hour food intake or a history of food consumed over a 3- to 5-day period, is also essential. In addition, explore the child's activity level, parental height, perceived food allergies, and dietary restrictions. An assessment of household organization and mealtime behaviors and rituals is important in the collection of pertinent data. It is often helpful to obtain the growth patterns of the affected child's parents and siblings; these can be compared with norm-referenced standards to evaluate the child's growth (Markowitz, Watkins, and Duggan, 2008). An assessment of the home environment and child-parent interaction may be helpful as well. Other tests (lead toxicity, anemia, stool-reducing substances, occult blood, ova and parasites, alkaline phosphatase, and zinc levels) are selected only as indicated to rule out organic problems. In most cases laboratory studies are of little diagnostic value (American Academy of Pediatrics, 2009). To prevent the overuse of diagnostic procedures, consider FTT early in the differential diagnosis. To avoid the social stigma of FTT during the early investigative phase, some health care workers use the term *growth delay* (or *failure*) until the actual cause is established.

Therapeutic Management

The primary management of FTT is aimed at reversing the cause of the growth failure. If malnutrition is severe, the initial treatment is directed at reversing the malnutrition. The goal is to provide sufficient calories to support "catch-up" growth—a rate of growth greater than the expected rate for age. The following formula may be used to calculate required caloric intake:

$$\text{kcal/kg required} = \frac{\text{RDA for age (kcal/kg)} \times \text{Ideal weight for height}}{\text{Actual weight}}$$

In this formula ideal weight for height is the median weight for the child's height based on the current National Center for Health Statistics weight-for-height growth charts.

In addition to adding caloric density to feedings, the child may require multivitamin supplements and dietary supplementation with high-calorie foods and drinks. Any coexisting medical problems are treated.

In most cases of FTT an interdisciplinary team of physician, nurse, dietitian, child life specialist, occupational therapist, pediatric feeding specialist, and social worker or mental health professional is needed to deal with the multiple problems. Make efforts to relieve any additional stresses on the family by offering referrals to welfare agencies or supplemental food programs. In some cases family therapy may be required. Temporary placement in a foster home may relieve the family's stress, protect the child, and allow the child some stability if insurmountable obstacles are preventing appropriate family function. Behavior modification aimed at mealtime rituals (or lack thereof) and family social time may be required. Hospitalization admission is indicated for (1) evidence (anthropometric) of severe acute malnutrition, (2) child abuse or neglect, (3) significant dehydration, (4) caretaker substance abuse or psychosis, (5) outpatient management that does not result in weight gain, and (6) serious intercurrent infection (American Academy of Pediatrics, 2009; Block, Krebs, and Committee on Child Abuse and Neglect and Committee on Nutrition [American Academy of Pediatrics], 2005).

Prognosis

The prognosis for FTT is related to the cause. If the parents have simply not understood the infant's needs, teaching may remedy the child's limited caloric intake and permanently reverse the growth failure. Inadequate or infrequent feeding periods by the infant's primary caretaker, in conjunction with family disorganization, are often observed to be the cause of FTT.

Few long-term studies provide data on the prognosis for children with FTT; however, some studies indicate that children who had FTT as infants had shorter heights, lower weights, and lower scores on measures of psychomotor development than peers (Black, Dubowitz, Krishnakumar, et al, 2007; Rudolf and Logan, 2005). Factors related to poor prognosis are severe feeding resistance, lack of awareness in and cooperation from the parent(s), low family income, low maternal educational level, adolescent mother, preterm birth, intrauterine growth restriction, and early age of onset of FTT. Because later cognitive and motor function is affected by malnourishment in infancy, many of these children are below normal in intellectual development, have poorer language development and less well-developed reading skills, attain lower social maturity, and have a higher incidence of behavioral disturbances (Markowitz, Watkins, and Duggan, 2008). Such findings indicate that a long-term plan and follow-up care are needed for the optimum development of these children.

Nursing Care Management

Caring for the child with FTT presents many nursing challenges, whether treatment takes place in the hospital, clinic, or home. Providing a positive feeding environment, teaching the parent successful feeding strategies, and supporting the child and family are essential components of care.

Nurses play a critical role in the diagnosis of FTT through their assessment of the child, parents, and family interactions. Knowledge of the characteristics of children with FTT and their families is essential in helping identify these children and hastening the confirmation of a diagnosis. Accurate assessment of initial weight and height and daily weight, as well as recording of all food intake, is mandatory. The nurse documents the child's feeding behavior and the parent-child interaction during feeding, other caregiving activities, and play. One available feeding observation instrument is the Nursing Child Assessment Satellite Training (NCAST) Feeding Scale, which is designed to assess the feeding interaction of infants up to 12 months of age (Barnard, Hammond, Booth, et al, 1993).* (See Nutritional Assessment, Chapter 6.)

The nurse should assess the approximate developmental age on admission by administering an appropriate developmental test. Only after objective measurements are available is a care plan for stimulation outlined. The nursing admission history and ongoing assessment should also focus on the following characteristics that have been identified in many of these children and their parents.

The Child

Besides showing signs of malnutrition and delayed social development, children with FTT may exhibit altered behavioral interactions. They may display intense interest in inanimate objects, such as a toy, but much less interest in social interactions. They are often watchful of people at a distance but become increasingly distressed as others come closer. They may dislike being touched or held and avoid face-to-face contact. However, when held, they protest briefly on being put down and are apathetic when left alone.

Children with growth failure may have a history of difficult feeding, vomiting, sleep disturbance, and excessive irritability. Patterns such as crying during feedings; vomiting; hoarding food in the mouth; ruminating after feeding; refusing to switch from liquids to solids; and displaying aversion behavior, such as turning from food or spitting food, become attention-seeking mechanisms to prolong the attention received at mealtime. In some cases the child may use feeding as a control mechanism in a poorly organized or chaotic family situation; parents may allow the child to dictate the norms for behavior and feeding because of inexperience with parenting or poor parenting role models. Thus refusing to eat or only eating high sugar foods may be the child's norm. In such cases family therapy is essential to reverse the trend and assist the parents and child in understanding each others' roles.

The Parents

Some parents are at increased risk for attachment problems because of (1) isolation and social crisis; (2) inadequate support systems, such as for teenage and single mothers; and (3) poor

---

*Training is required to use the feeding scale. For information, contact NCAST Programs, University of Washington, PO Box 357920, Seattle, WA 98195; 206-543-8528; e-mail: ncast@u.washington.edu; www.ncast.org.

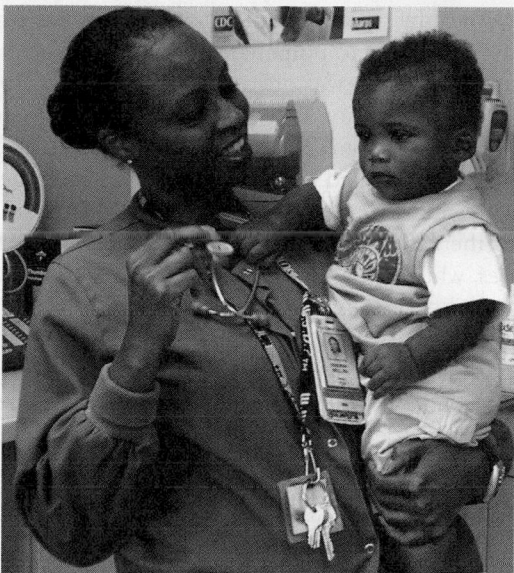

Fig. 13-3 A consistent nurse is important in developing trust with infants who have growth failure.

parenting role models as a child. Other factors that should be considered are lack of education; physical and mental health problems such as physical and sexual abuse, depression, or drug dependence; immaturity, especially in adolescent parents; and lack of commitment to parenting, such as giving priority to entertainment or employment. Often these parents and their families are under stress and in multiple chronic emotional, social, and financial crises.

Because part of the difficulty between parent and child is dissatisfaction and frustration, the child should have a primary core of nurses (Fig. 13-3). The nurses caring for the child can learn to perceive the child's cues and reverse the cycle of dissatisfaction, especially in the area of feeding. Depending on the cause of FTT, children may be treated on an outpatient basis.

Because many of these children are responding to stimuli that have led to the negative feeding patterns, the first goal is to structure the feeding environment to encourage eating. Initially staff members and a feeding specialist may need to feed these children to thoroughly assess the difficulties encountered during the feeding process and to devise strategies that eliminate or minimize such problems. General guidelines for the feeding process are outlined in the Nursing Care Guidelines box.

Nutritional Management

Four primary goals in the nutritional management of FTT are to (1) correct nutritional deficiencies and achieve ideal weight for height, (2) allow for catch-up growth, (3) restore optimum body composition, and (4) educate the parents or primary caregivers regarding the child's nutritional requirements and appropriate feeding methods (Corrales and Utter, 2005; Maggioni and Lifshitz, 1995). For infants, 24 kcal/oz formulas may be provided to increase caloric intake; older children (1 to 6 years) may benefit from a 30 kcal/oz formula (American Academy of Pediatrics, 2009). Other carbohydrate additives include fortified rice cereal and vegetable oil. Because vitamin and mineral deficiencies may occur, multivitamin supplemen-

tation, including zinc and iron, is recommended. For toddlers, a high-calorie milk drink such as PediaSure may be used to increase caloric intake. Carefully monitor for signs of intolerance to the formula. Usually only in extreme cases of malnourishment are tube feedings or intravenous therapy required.

Because maladaptive feeding practices often contribute to growth failure, give parents specific step-by-step directions for formula preparation, as well as a written schedule of feeding times. Avoid juices in children with growth failure until adequate weight gain has been achieved with appropriate milk sources; thereafter give no more than 4 oz/day of juice.

Behavior-modification techniques may be used with older infants and toddlers to interrupt poor feeding patterns. Feeding times may actually involve "struggles of will" in cases of maladaptive feedings that result in FTT. These behaviors are different from the occasional toddler behavior of food refusal, which is primarily developmental, not pathologic. The association of appropriate food with good or bad behaviors and consequent rewards may be part of the complex problem. In severe cases of malnourishment, tube feedings or intravenous therapy may be required.

In addition to attending to the child's physical needs, the interdisciplinary team must plan care for appropriate developmental stimulation. After an approximate developmental age is established, a planned program of play is begun. Ideally a child life specialist is involved to implement and supervise the stimulation program. Every effort is made to teach the parent how to play and interact with the child.

Nursing care of these children involves a "family systems" approach. In other words, for the entire family to become healthy, each member must be helped to change. Care of the parents is aimed at helping them improve their self-esteem by acquiring positive, successful parenting skills. Initially this necessitates providing an environment in which they feel welcomed and accepted. Depending on the cause of FTT, many children are treated on an outpatient basis.

SKIN DISORDERS

DIAPER DERMATITIS

Diaper dermatitis is common in infants and one of several acute inflammatory skin disorders caused either directly or indirectly by wearing diapers. Diaper dermatitis is a form of irritant contact dermatitis, which may also involve secondary bacterial or yeast infection. The peak age for diaper dermatitis is 9 to 12 months, and the incidence is greater in bottle-fed infants than in breast-fed infants. Prevalence rates vary among sources; Noonan, Quigley, and Curley (2006) reported a prevalence rate of 17% in one hospital. Others report prevalence rates as high as 42% (McLane, Bookout, McCord, et al, 2004).

Pathophysiology and Clinical Manifestations

Diaper dermatitis is caused by prolonged and repetitive contact with an irritant, principally urine, feces, soaps, detergents, ointments, and friction. Although the obvious irritant in the majority of incidences is urine and feces, the specific components that contribute to irritation include a combination of factors (Fig. 13-4).

Prolonged contact of the skin with diaper wetness affects several skin properties. Continuous moisture exposure enhances permeability to exogenous materials, produces maceration, increases susceptibility to friction damage, increases transepidermal permeability, and increases microbial counts. Irritant exposure also affects the epidermal barrier structure and function, further increasing permeability and inflammation.

Therefore healthy skin, specifically the stratum corneum, becomes less resistant to potential irritants.

Although ammonia was once thought to cause diaper rash because of the association between the strong odor on diapers and dermatitis, ammonia alone is not sufficient. The irritant quality of urine is related to an increase in pH from the breakdown of urea in the presence of fecal urease. The increased pH promotes the activity of fecal enzymes, principally proteases and lipases, which act as irritants. Fecal enzymes also increase the permeability of skin to bile salts, another potential irritant in feces. Researchers believe the decreased incidence of diaper dermatitis in breast-fed infants is related to this interaction between pH and fecal enzymes, since feces from breast-fed infants have lower fecal enzyme activity and lower pH.

The eruption of diaper dermatitis occurs primarily on convex surfaces or in the folds (intertriginous areas), and the lesions can represent a variety of types and configurations. Eruptions commonly involve the skin in most intimate contact with the diaper (e.g., the convex surfaces of buttocks, inner thighs, mons pubis, and scrotum). However, lesions not involving the folds are likely to be caused by chemical irritants, especially from urine and feces (Fig. 13-5). Other causes are detergents or soaps from inadequately rinsed cloth diapers or the chemicals (alcohol) in disposable wipes. Dyes in disposable diapers have also been cited as causing diaper dermatitis.

Perianal involvement is usually the result of chemical irritation from feces, especially diarrheal stools. *Candida albicans* infection produces bright red, confluent lesions with raised borders and often with satellite lesions (Fig. 13-6). The infected area usually includes the folds and is painful. Risk factors for development of *Candida* infection are an altered immune status and antibiotic therapy.

Therapeutic Management

Treatment is primarily aimed at prevention of diaper dermatitis. A number of interventions are discussed under Nursing Care Management. For inflammations that do not respond to these interventions, topical glucocorticoid preparations are sometimes required. If steroids are prescribed, their use is limited to low-potency preparations, such as a 0.5% or 1% hydrocortisone cream. Potential side effects include striae, epidermal atrophy, suppression of the pituitary-adrenal axis, cessation of longitudinal growth, and Cushing syndrome from chronic use. Topical antifungals are used to treat candidal infections and include

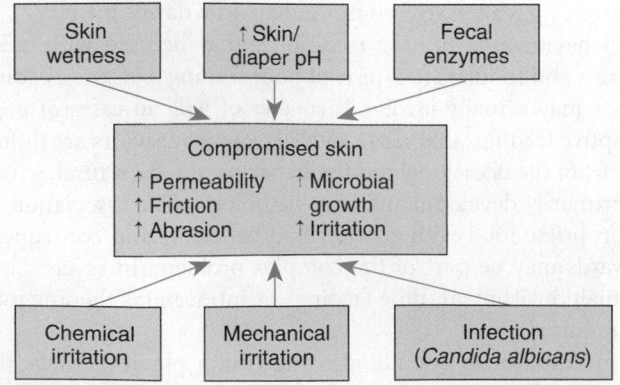

Fig. 13-4 Principal factors involved in development of diaper dermatitis.

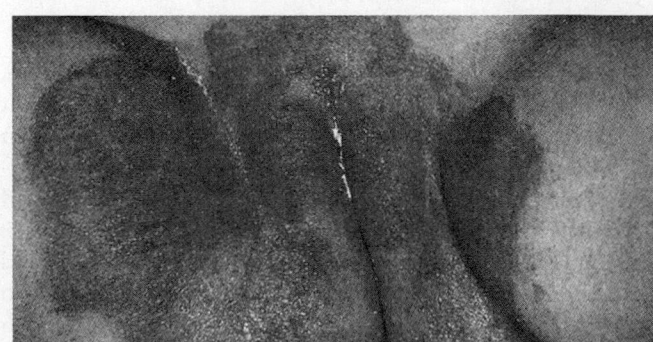

Fig. 13-5 Irritant diaper dermatitis. Note sharply demarcated edges. (From Habif TP: *Clinical dermatology: a color guide to diagnosis and therapy,* ed 3, St Louis, 1996, Mosby.)

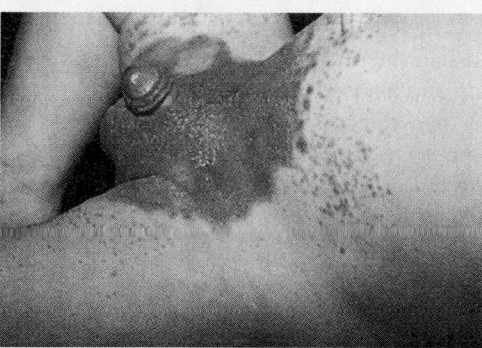

Fig. 13-6 Candidiasis of diaper area. Note beefy red central erythema with satellite pustules. (From Weston WL, Lane AT, Morelli JG: *Color textbook of pediatric dermatology*, ed 4, St Louis, 2007, Mosby.)

clotrimazole, miconazole, ketoconazole, and nystatin ointment. When *C. albicans* is present elsewhere, oral administration of a fungicide is advised because the GI tract is usually the source of infection. (See Candidiasis, Chapter 9.)

⚡ DRUG ALERT

Combination Antifungals/Topical Steroids

Avoid combined antifungals with potent halogenated topical steroids, such as clotrimazole–betamethasone disproprionate (Lotrisone) and nystatin-triamcinolone (Mycolog), because their use on compromised thin skin increases systemic absorption (Visscher, 2009).

Nursing Care Management

Nursing interventions are aimed at altering the three factors considered to produce dermatitis: wetness (hydration), pH, and fecal irritants. The most significant factor amenable to intervention is the moist environment created in the diaper area. Changing the diaper as soon as it becomes wet eliminates a large part of the problem, and removing the diaper to expose intact skin to air facilitates drying as long as fecal contamination of the skin does not occur, in which case the skin is again exposed to possible injury. However, avoid rubbing or washing the skin frequently (unless fecal matter is present), since frequent washing or rubbing may also disrupt the barrier function of the skin. Many commercial diaper wipes contain alcohol and other products that are detrimental to the natural skin barrier and should be avoided.

The use of a hair dryer or heat lamp is not recommended because they can cause burns. Also, on denuded skin, dry heat delays healing. Instead, occlusive (barrier) ointments or dressings are applied to provide a moist healing environment for open wounds and to protect the skin from further irritation. (See Ostomies, Chapter 27.) Recommended barrier ointments include white petrolatum ointment, Aquaphor (contains lanolin), and zinc oxide. A protective barrier such as zinc oxide prevents skin injury and allows the skin to heal. In the event of diaper dermatitis caused by fungal and contact irritants, a layer of antifungal powder (nystatin [Mycostatin] powder) or cream *under* a zinc oxide–based skin barrier ointment may be used, but providers must take care to avoid mixing the two preparations together. A combination of products may provide better results for some children; combining a protective powder such as Stomahesive Protective Powder with karaya or cornstarch

powder may be helpful (Borkowski, 2004). Some diaper pastes called butt balm or cream may be helpful with some cases of diaper dermatitis, but parents should check to ensure that the ingredients are safe for use in this age-group. Also, such pastes are often expensive (Borkowski, 2004). A Cavilon No-Sting Barrier Film may be used on infants older than 30 days (Baharestani, 2007). Other products include iLEX Skin Protectant Paste and Sureprep No-Sting Protective Barrier Wipe. Once a barrier paste has been applied, it is recommended that the paste not be removed when soiling occurs because this further disrupts the integrity of the skin; instead wipe off the stool or contaminated portion only, leaving as much barrier paste intact as possible.

A 1:1 mixture of iLEX paste and petroleum jelly applied liberally to the affected area is reported to be very effective in healing diaper dermatitis within 24 to 48 hours; as noted above, wipe off only excess stool, leaving as much paste in place as possible, and then reapply more as necessary (Hodge, 2009).

Diaper construction has a significant impact on the incidence and severity of diaper dermatitis. Superabsorbent disposable diapers reduce diaper dermatitis because they contain an absorbent gelling material that binds water tightly to decrease skin wetness, maintains pH control by providing a buffering capacity, and decreases skin irritation by preventing mixing of urine and feces in the diaper (Visscher, 2009). The improved containment of urine and feces is also an important factor in decreasing contamination of the environment, such as in daycare centers, and spread of disease.

Another advance in diapers is the addition of an inner layer or top sheet that is impregnated with petrolatum or zinc oxide. The liner transfers the petrolatum to the skin, where it acts as a barrier to moisture and irritants. Guidelines for controlling diaper rash are presented in the Family-Centered Care box.

Some caregivers may choose to apply a powder that may contain either talc or cornstarch. A common misconception about using cornstarch on skin is that it promotes the growth of *C. albicans*. Both cornstarch and talc do not support growth of the fungi under conditions normally found in the diaper area; however, the use of powders in the hospital nursery is not recommended (Association of Women's Health, Obstetric and Neonatal Nurses, 2007).

An objective assessment of diaper dermatitis may be performed using the scale in Box 13-4.

SEBORRHEIC DERMATITIS

Seborrheic dermatitis is a chronic, recurrent, inflammatory reaction of the skin that occurs most commonly on the scalp (cradle cap) but may involve the eyelids (blepharitis), external ear canal (otitis externa), nasolabial folds, and inguinal region. The cause is unknown, although it is more common in early infancy when sebum production is increased and is thought to be linked to the overgrowth of *Malassezia* yeast (O'Connor, McLaughlin, and Ham, 2008).

Seborrheic dermatitis in infants has historically been identified as occurring as a result of poor personal care and hygiene; however, such is not the case. The condition may also occur in adolescence but is localized to the scalp and intertriginous areas; pruritus is more common when the condition occurs in

---

BOX 13-4 **TYPES OF DIAPER DERMATITIS**

Type 1—Epidermis intact and no candidal infection present
Type 2—Epidermis intact and candidal infection present
Type 3—Epidermis not intact and no candidal infection present
Type 4—Epidermis not intact and candidal infection present

From Noonan C, Quigley S, Curley MAQ: Skin integrity in hospitalized infants and children: a prevalence survey, *J Pediatr Nurs* 21(6):445-453, 2006.

FAMILY-CENTERED CARE

Controlling Diaper Rash

- Avoid prolonged exposure to urine and feces.
- Use superabsorbent disposable diapers to reduce skin wetness.
- If using cloth diapers, only use overwraps that allow air to circulate; avoid rubber pants.
- Change diapers as soon as soiled, especially with stool, whenever possible and preferably once during the night.
- Expose healthy or only slightly irritated skin to air, not heat, to dry completely.
- Apply a barrier ointment, such as zinc oxide or white petrolatum, in a thick layer to protect skin, especially if skin is very red or has moist, open areas.
- Avoid removing skin barrier cream with each diaper change; remove waste material and reapply skin barrier cream.
- To completely remove ointment, especially zinc oxide, use mineral oil; do not wash vigorously.
- Avoid overwashing the skin, especially with perfumed soaps or commercial wipes that may be irritating.
- Use a moisturizer or nonsoap cleanser, such as cold cream or Cetaphil, to wipe urine from skin.
- Avoid the use of baby talc powder.*
- Gently wipe stool from skin using water and a mild, fragrance-free cleanser.
- When possible allow perineal (diaper-free time) exposure to open air.

*Powder helps keep the skin dry, but talc is dangerous if breathed into the lungs. Plain cornstarch or cornstarch-based powder is safer. When using any powder product, shake it first into your hand, then apply it to the diaper area. Store the container away from the infant's reach; keep container closed when not in use.

adolescents (Morelli, 2007). The lesions are characteristically thick, adherent, yellowish, scaly, oily patches that may or may not be mildly pruritic. If pruritus is present, the infant may be irritable. Unlike AD, seborrheic dermatitis is not associated with a positive family history for allergy, is common in infants shortly after birth, and is also common after puberty. Diagnosis is made primarily by the appearance and location of the crusts or scales.

Nursing Care Management

When seborrheic lesions are present, direct the treatment mainly at removing the crusts. White petrolatum may be applied to the scalp to assist with the removal of the scaly patches; another remedy involves soaking the scalp several hours in vegetable oil then removing the scales (O'Connor, McLaughlin, and Ham, 2008). Tar-containing shampoos are more expensive but may be effective. Teach parents the appropriate procedure to clean the scalp, which may necessitate a demonstration. Shampooing should be done daily with a mild soap or commercial baby shampoo. Medicated shampoos are

usually not needed, but an antiseborrheic shampoo containing sulfur and salicylic acid may be used. The shampoo is applied to the scalp and allowed to remain on until the crusts are softened, and then the scalp is thoroughly rinsed. Using a fine-tooth comb or a soft facial brush after shampooing helps remove the loosened crusts from the strands of hair. If shampoos are not effective, an antifungal cream (ketoconazole) or shampoo may be helpful.

ATOPIC DERMATITIS (ECZEMA)

Atopic dermatitis (AD), or eczema, is a chronic inflammatory skin condition that usually begins during infancy and is associated with allergy with a hereditary tendency (atopy). AD occurs as a result of complex interactions between genetic host factors, infectious and environmental agents, defects in skin barrier function, and immunologic inflammatory responses, which result in chronic skin inflammation (Leung, 2007; Wasserbauer and Ballow, 2009). AD affects approximately 10% to 20% of children worldwide (Leung, 2007). AD is commonly referred to as the "rash that itches" because of the intense pruritus. Because the disease often begins within the first 6 months of life, this discussion is restricted to the infantile form of AD.

The diagnosis of AD is based on a combination of history and morphologic findings (Box 13-5 and Fig. 13-7). Children with the disease have a lower threshold for cutaneous itching, and some authorities believe the dermatologic manifestations appear subsequent to scratching from the intense pruritus. Lesions often disappear if the scratching is stopped.

The majority of children with AD have a family history of eczema, asthma, food allergies, or allergic rhinitis, which strongly supports a genetic predisposition. In addition, approximately 50% of children with AD subsequently develop asthma (Boguniewicz, 2005). The cause is unknown but may be related to an immune reaction with abnormal function of the skin, including alterations in perspiration, peripheral vascular function, and heat tolerance. Patients with AD have dry skin and evidence of increased transepidermal water loss; a defect in the ceramide cells, which help retain water and provide a barrier function; and increased colonization of the skin with *Staphylococcus aureus* (Boguniewicz, 2005). The chronic disease is better in humid climates and worse in fall and winter, when homes are heated and environmental humidity is lower. The disorder can be controlled but not cured. House dust mites, certain foods, mold, and animal hair may play a role in the etiology of AD. Many children with AD have elevated toxic-specific IgE levels, and a T-cell dysfunction is currently believed to be a major factor in the development of AD (Boguniewicz, 2005). In addition, some evidence suggests that abnormally low levels of the protein filaggrin may have a role in altering the protective barrier function of the skin, thus increasing transepidermal water loss and increasing inflammation (Ong and Boguniewicz, 2008). Leung (2007) describes two types of AD: atopic, which is IgE mediated and affects the majority of children with AD (70% to 80%), and nonatopic eczema, which is not associated with IgE-mediated sensitization. Approximately 30% to 40% of children with moderate AD have IgE-mediated food reactions (Ong and Boguniewicz, 2008). Therefore it is

BOX 13-5 CLINICAL MANIFESTATIONS OF ATOPIC DERMATITIS

Distribution of Lesions
Infants—Generalized, especially cheeks, scalp, trunk, and extensor surfaces of extremities (see Fig. 13-7)
Older child—Flexural areas (antecubital and popliteal fossae, neck), wrists, ankles, and feet
Adolescents—Face, sides of neck, hands, feet, and antecubital and popliteal fossae (to a lesser extent)

Appearance of Lesions
Infants
Erythema
Vesicles
Papules
Weeping
Oozing
Crusting
Scaling
Often symmetric

Children
Symmetric involvement
Clusters of small erythematous or flesh-colored papules or minimally scaling patches
Dry; may be hyperpigmented
Lichenification (thickened skin with accentuation of creases)
Keratosis pilaris (follicular hyperkeratosis) common

Adolescents and Adults
Same as childhood manifestations
Dry, thick lesions (lichenified plaques) common
Confluent papules

Other Manifestations
Intense itching
Unaffected skin dry and rough
African-American children likely to exhibit more papular or follicular lesions than Caucasian children
May exhibit one or more of the following:
- Lymphadenopathy, especially near affected sites
- Increased palmar creases (many cases)
- Atopic pleats (extra line or groove of lower eyelid)
- Tendency toward cold hands
- Pityriasis alba (small, poorly defined areas of hypopigmentation)
- Facial pallor (especially around nose, mouth, and ears)
- Bluish discoloration beneath eyes ("allergic shiners")
- Increased susceptibility to unusual cutaneous infections (especially viral)

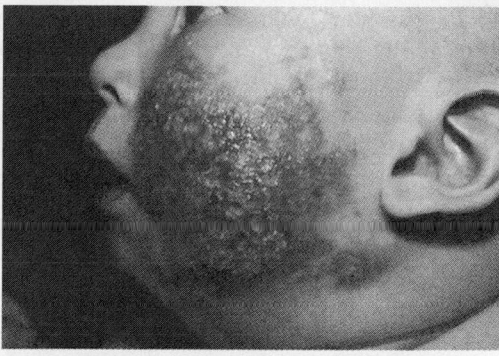

Fig. 13-7 Atopic dermatitis with oozing and crusting of lesions. (From Weston WL, Lane AT, Morelli JG: *Color textbook of pediatric dermatology,* ed 4, St Louis, 2007, Mosby.)

- Avoiding skin moisture loss
- Improving skin hydration
- Administering medications such as topical steroids

There are a number of ways to enhance skin hydration and prevent dry, flaky skin, depending on the child's skin characteristics and individual needs. A tepid bath with a mild soap (Dove or Neutrogena), no soap, or an emulsifying oil, followed immediately by application of an emollient (within 3 minutes), assists in preventing moisture loss. Avoid bubble baths and harsh soaps. The bath may need to be repeated once or twice daily, depending on the child's status. Excessive bathing without emollient application only dries out the skin. Some lotions are not effective, and emollients should be chosen carefully to prevent excessive skin drying. Aquaphor, Cetaphil, and Eucerin are acceptable for skin hydration. A nighttime bath, followed by emollient application and dressing in soft cotton pajamas, may alleviate much of the nighttime pruritus.

Moderate or severe pruritus is usually relieved by administration of oral antihistamine drugs (hydroxyzine or diphenhydramine), with the amount tailored to the individual child. Nonsedating antihistamines such as loratadine (Claritin) or fexofenadine (Allegra) may be preferred for daytime pruritus relief. Because pruritus increases at night, a mildly sedating antihistamine may be needed.

Topical corticosteroids are now considered first-line treatment for AD (Leung, 2007; Williams, 2005). Occasional flare-ups require the use of topical steroids to diminish inflammation. Low-, moderate-, or high-potency topical corticosteroids are prescribed, depending on the degree of involvement, the body area to be treated, the child's age, potential for local side effects (striae, skin atrophy, and pigment changes), and the type of vehicle to be used (e.g., cream, lotion, ointment). Medical management of secondary skin infections with systemic antibiotics is an important part of the treatment of AD. Coal tar preparations may also be used to hydrate the skin yet are considered cumbersome because they stain clothing.

Two calcineurin inhibitors (immunomodulators) used in children with AD are tacrolimus and pimecrolimus (Elidel). Tacrolimus is available in two ointment strengths (0.03% and 0.1%); these have been approved for use in children 2 years of age and older. Pimecrolimus is available in a 1% cream that has no systemic accumulation or effects; this drug has been approved for children ages 2 years and older.

suggested that those with a family history of atopy follow feeding guidelines in early infancy discussed earlier in this chapter.

Therapeutic Management

The major goals of management are to (1) hydrate the skin, (2) relieve pruritus, (3) reduce flare-ups or inflammation by avoiding triggers, (4) prevent and control infection, and (5) live as near as normal a childhood as possible. Most of the general measures for managing AD serve to reduce pruritus and other aspects of the disease. General management includes:

- Avoiding exposure to skin irritants or allergens
- Avoiding overheating

Acute flare-ups may require the use of wet wraps. One method is to apply a light coat of topical corticosteroid, then wrap the child in cool wet towels for 10 minutes (warm towels slightly in the winter to prevent heat loss). Once the towels are removed, the steroid ointment is reapplied, followed by a moisturizer. Be careful, however, not to use excessive wet wraps, since these may cause skin maceration and secondary infections.

Controversy exists regarding prevention of AD by limiting the exposure of infants at risk to allergens both prenatally and postnatally. Studies have shown a decrease in atopic eczema in infants at risk for atopy whose mothers breast-fed at least 4 months; avoiding highly allergenic foods during lactation may or may not help reduce the incidence of atopy. Infants who are not breast-fed and who are at risk for AD may benefit from extensively hydrolyzed formula (Greer, Sicherer, Burks, et al, 2008). Although conclusive evidence for preventive strategies is lacking, the precautions in the Nursing Care Guidelines box on p. 530 may be recommended.

Nursing Care Management

The child with AD presents a nursing challenge. Controlling the intense pruritus is imperative if the disorder is to be successfully managed, since scratching leads to the formation of new lesions and may cause secondary infection. In addition to the medical regimen, other measures can prevent or minimize the scratching. Keep fingernails and toenails short and clean, and file them frequently to prevent sharp edges. Gloves or cotton socks can be placed over the hands and pinned to shirtsleeves.

Also, eliminate conditions that increase itching when possible. Remove woolen clothes or blankets, rough fabrics, and furry stuffed animals. Because heat and humidity cause perspiration, which intensifies the itching, proper dress for climatic conditions is essential. Pruritus is often precipitated by exposure to the irritant effects of certain components of common products such as soaps, detergents, fabric softeners, perfumes, diaper wipes, and powders. Most children experience less itching when soft cotton fabrics are worn next to the skin. Avoid exposure to latex products, such as gloves and balloons. Launder clothes and sheets in a mild liquid detergent and rinse them thoroughly in clear water (without fabric softeners or antistatic chemicals); use a second rinse cycle to further reduce residual detergent. The use of skin cleansers with minimal defatting activity and a neutral pH is preferred over the usual soaps.

Preventing infection is usually accomplished by preventing scratching. Maintain personal hygiene as described previously. Give baths as prescribed, keeping the water tepid, and avoid soaps (except as indicated), bubble baths, oils, and powders. Skinfolds and diaper areas need frequent cleansing with plain water. A room humidifier or vaporizer may benefit children with extremely dry skin. The lesions are examined for signs of infection—usually honey-colored crusts with surrounding erythema. Report any signs of infection to the practitioner.

Wet soaks or compresses are applied as needed, and medications for pruritus or infection are administered as directed. The nurse gives the family explicit written instructions on the preparation and use of soaks, special baths, and topical medications, including the order of application if more than one is pre-scribed. If children have difficulty remaining still for a 10- or 15-minute soak, bath, or dressing application, perform these at nap time or when the child is watching television, listening to a story, or playing with tub toys.

No particular diet is recommended for children with AD. When a hypoallergenic diet is prescribed, parents need help in understanding the reason for the diet and guidelines for avoiding hyperallergenic foods (see Box 13-2). Because hypoallergenic diets take time before visible effects are apparent, parents need reassurance that results may not be seen immediately. If airborne allergens also worsen the eczema, the family is counseled regarding measures to "allergy proof" the home. (See Asthma, Chapter 32.)

Family Support*

The nurse can assure parents that the lesions will not produce scarring (unless secondarily infected) and that the disease is not contagious. However, the child will be subject to repeated exacerbations and remissions. Spontaneous and permanent remission takes place at approximately 5 years of age in most children, though they may have an occasional relapse in adolescence or adulthood (Leung, 2007).

During periods of acute exacerbation, when the physical problems may seem insurmountable, the emotional stress becomes intense for family members. They need time to discuss negative feelings and to be reassured that these feelings are expected, normal, acceptable, and healthy, provided they have an emotional outlet to dissipate pent-up energy. During acute phases, efforts aimed at relieving anxiety in both parents and child have a beneficial emotional and physical effect because stress tends to aggravate the severity of the condition.

DISORDERS OF UNKNOWN ETIOLOGY

SUDDEN INFANT DEATH SYNDROME

Sudden infant death syndrome (SIDS) is defined as the sudden death of an infant younger than 1 year of age that remains unexplained after a complete postmortem examination, including an investigation of the death scene and a review of the case history. Since 1992, the incidence of SIDS in the United States has decreased by 53% to an all-time low of 0.57 per 1000 live births in 2002 (American Academy of Pediatrics, 2005). The dramatic decrease is attributed to the Back to Sleep campaign.† SIDS is the third leading cause of infant deaths (birth to 12 months) and the first leading cause of postneonatal deaths (between 1 and 12 months). SIDS claimed the lives of 2162 infants in the United States in 2003 (Heron and Smith, 2007).

The SIDS rate remained fairly static between 1999 and 2001. This has been attributed to improved death scene investigation

---

*Parents may also find helpful information at the American Academy of Dermatology, 866-503-7546; www.aad.org; and for pamphlets www.aad.org/public/publications/pamphlets/skin_eczema.html; and the National Eczema Association, 800-818-7546; www.nationaleczema.org.
†Back to Sleep materials may be ordered by contacting NICHD Information Resource Center, Back to Sleep, PO Box 3006, Rockville, MD 20847; 800-370-2943; fax: 866-760-5947; www.nichd.nih.gov/sids.

TABLE 13-1	EPIDEMIOLOGY OF SUDDEN INFANT DEATH SYNDROME
FACTORS	**OCCURRENCE**
Incidence	54.5 per 100,000 live births (2006) (Heron M, Hoyert DL, Murphy SL, et al, 2009)
Peak age	2-3 mo; 95% occur by 6 mo; preterm infants die from sudden infant death syndrome (SIDS) at mean age of 6 wk later than mean age of death from SIDS for term infants
Sex	Higher percentage of males affected
Time of death	During sleep
Time of year	Increased incidence in winter
Racial	Greater incidence in African-Americans, Native Americans, and Hispanics. In 2001 rate of SIDS in African-Americans was 2.5 times higher than in Caucasians; prone positioning rates were also higher in African-Americans in 2001 (21% in African-Americans versus 11% in Caucasians).
Socioeconomic	Increased occurrence in lower socioeconomic class
Birth	Higher incidence in: • Preterm infants, especially infants of extremely and very low birth weight • Multiple births* • Neonates with low Apgar scores • Infants with central nervous system disturbances and respiratory disorders such as bronchopulmonary dysplasia • Increasing birth order (subsequent siblings as opposed to firstborn child)
Health status	Higher incidence in infants with a recent history of illness
Sleep habits	Highest risk associated with prone position; use of soft bedding; overheating (thermal stress); cosleeping with adult, especially on sofa, or noninfant bed Infants cosleeping with adult at higher risk if <11 wk old
Feeding habits	Lower incidence in breast-fed infants
Pacifier	Lower incidence in infants put to sleep with pacifier
Siblings	May have greater incidence in siblings of SIDS victims
Maternal	Young age; cigarette smoking, especially during pregnancy; poor prenatal care; substance abuse (heroin, methadone, cocaine). A few studies have shown an increased risk in infants exposed to second-hand environmental tobacco smoke.

Data from American Academy of Pediatrics, Task Force on Sudden Infant Death Syndrome: The changing concept of sudden infant death syndrome: diagnostic coding shifts, controversies regarding the sleeping environment, and new variables to consider in reducing risk, *Pediatrics* 116(5):1245-1255, 2005; American Academy of Pediatrics, Task Force on Infant Sleep Position and Sudden Infant Death Syndrome: Changing concepts of sudden infant death syndrome: implications for infant sleeping environment and sleep position, *Pediatrics* 105(3):650-656, 2000.
*Although a rare event, simultaneous death of twins from SIDS can occur.

and determination of non-SIDS causes of postneonatal mortality. In addition, there is speculation that deaths attributed to SIDS during the period of 1992 to 2001 may have been a result of other causes (American Academy of Pediatrics, 2005). Table 13-1 summarizes the major epidemiologic characteristics of SIDS.

There has been much debate over the term *SIDS*, yet the definition noted above remains for the time being. Other terms have been developed to explain sudden deaths in infants. Sudden unexpected early neonatal death (SUEND) and sudden unexpected death in infancy (SUDI) share similar features but differ in regards to the timing of death: SUDI is considered a death in the postneonatal period, whereas SUEND occurs in the first week of life.

Etiology

Numerous theories have been proposed regarding the etiology of SIDS; however, the cause remains unknown. One compelling hypothesis is that SIDS is related to a brainstem abnormality in the neurologic regulation of cardiorespiratory control. This maldevelopment affects arousal and physiologic responses to a life-threatening challenge during sleep (American Academy of Pediatrics, 2005). Abnormalities include prolonged sleep apnea, increased frequency of brief inspiratory pauses, excessive periodic breathing, and impaired arousal responsiveness to increased carbon dioxide or decreased oxygen. However, *sleep apnea is not the cause of SIDS*. The vast majority of infants with apnea do not die, and only a minority of SIDS victims have

documented apparent life-threatening events (ALTEs) (see Apnea and Apparent Life-Threatening Events, p. 546). Numerous studies indicate that there is no association between SIDS and any childhood vaccine.

A genetic predisposition to SIDS has been postulated as a cause. In one study a genetic mutation on chromosome 6q 22.1-22.31 was positively linked to a syndrome of SIDS and dysgenesis of the testis (Puffenberger, Hu-Lince, Parod, et al, 2004).

Recently there has been increased interest in infection and inflammation as a possible cause of SIDS (Blood-Siegfried, 2009; Highet, 2008; Mitchell, 2009).

Maternal smoking during pregnancy has emerged in numerous epidemiologic studies as a major factor in SIDS, and tobacco smoke in the infant's environment after birth has also been shown to have a possible relationship to the incidence of SIDS (American Academy of Pediatrics, 2005). Data show that exposure to tobacco smoke increased an infant's risk for SIDS 1.9 times over infants not exposed; 59% of SIDS deaths in smoke-exposed infants were attributed to maternal smoking (Anderson, Johnson, and Batal, 2005). It has been postulated that 12% of all SIDS deaths could be prevented with prenatal maternal smoking cessation (Pollack, 2001). One mechanism that has been proposed as a link between maternal smoking and SIDS is a decrease in the ability to arouse to auditory stimuli in infants of mothers who smoked prenatally (Franco, Groswasser, Hassid, et al, 1999). Exposure to maternal smoking has recently been positively correlated with decreased arousal potential in infants (Richardson, Walker, and Horne, 2009). Increased nicotine concentrations in lung tissue were found in children who died from SIDS compared with a group of control children (McMartin, Platt, Hackman, et al, 2002).

Cosleeping, or an infant sharing a bed with an adult or older child on a noninfant bed, has been reported to have a positive association with SIDS. One survey found a high association between infant deaths, nonstandard beds (sofa, day bed), and bed sharing; a large percentage of infants were found dead on their backs when bed sharing, suggesting suffocation (Unger, Kemp, Wilkins, et al, 2003). A study from Scotland indicates that the risk for SIDS when bed sharing is significantly increased for infants less than 11 weeks of age (Tappin, Ecob, and Brooke, 2005). Vennemann, Bajanowski, Brinkmann, and colleagues (2009) identified infant sleeping in the house of a friend or relative and sleeping in the family living room as significant risk factors for SIDS. Other studies correlated higher incidences of SIDS and infant cosleeping with maternal smoking, cosleeping with multiple family members, sleeping on a couch, use of a pillow in the infant's bed, maternal overweight, soft bedding, and unintentional asphyxiation resulting from adult intoxication (overlaying) (American Academy of Pediatrics, 2000, 2005; Blair, Sidebotham, Evason-Coombe, et al, 2009; Hauck, Herman, Donovan, et al, 2003; Carroll-Pankhurst and Mortimer, 2001; Li, Zhang, Zielke, et al, 2009; Person, Lavezzi, and Wolf, 2002; McGarvey, McDonnell, Chong, et al, 2003).

A study by Hauck, Herman, Donovan, and colleagues (2003) found that bed sharing and SIDS correlated positively only in cases where the infant was sleeping with someone other than the parent; a high number of SIDS cases involved sleeping on a sofa. There are reports of a greater incidence of SIDS among African-American and non-Caucasian infants. In a population-based study Hauck, Herman, Donovan, and colleagues (2003) found that SIDS occurred more frequently among African-American infants. The prone sleep position was associated with twice (2.4% odds ratio) the rate of SIDS compared with infants placed nonprone to sleep. It has been suggested that the higher SIDS deaths among non-Caucasian infants is related to a higher incidence of prone sleep positioning (American Academy of Pediatrics, 2005; Hauck, Herman, Donovan, et al, 2003).

Cosleeping with infants in the age range when most SIDS deaths occur has not been shown to be preventive. The latest recommendation for cosleeping from the American Academy of Pediatrics (2005) is that the infant's crib or bassinette be placed in close proximity to the mother's bed and that the infant be placed in the adult bed only for breast-feeding, then placed to sleep in his or her own crib once the feeding session is completed.

Mesich (2005) notes that the current scientific literature fails to provide definitive guidance regarding mother-infant sleeping together in relation to safety or nonsafety; certain sleep environments (prone sleeping, tobacco smoke exposure, soft bedding, noninfant bed surface, use of certain drugs by cosleeper, and thermal stress), however, are known to increase the risk for SIDS.

Studies from countries other than the United States link sleep habits with an increased risk of SIDS. Prone sleeping may cause oropharyngeal obstruction or affect thermal balance or arousal state. One study found that healthy full-term infants had significantly impaired arousal from active and quiet sleep states when sleeping prone (Horne, Ferens, Watts, et al, 2001). Rebreathing of carbon dioxide by infants in the prone position is also a possible cause for SIDS. Infants sleeping prone and on soft bedding may not be able to move their heads to the side, thus increasing the risk of suffocation and lethal rebreathing. Evidence from other countries and the United States shows an increased incidence of SIDS in infants placed in a side-lying position; thus the side-lying position is no longer recommended for infants sleeping at home, daycare, or hospitals (unless medically indicated). Most preterm infants being discharged from the hospital should be placed in a supine sleeping position unless special factors predispose them to airway obstruction.

One postulated cause of SIDS has been a prolonged Q-T interval; however, there has been no strong evidence to support this as a cause of SIDS or universal testing of newborns for prolonged Q-T interval (American Academy of Pediatrics, 2005).

Soft bedding such as waterbeds, sheepskins, beanbags, pillows, or quilts should be avoided for infant sleeping surfaces. Bedding items such as stuffed animals or toys should be removed from the crib while the infant is asleep. Head covering by a blanket has also been found to be a risk factor for SIDS, thus supporting the recommendation to avoid extra bed linens or other items (Mitchell, Thompson, Becroft, et al, 2008).

One study indicated that breast-feeding during the first 16 weeks of life decreased the likelihood of SIDS (Alm, Wennergren, Norvenius, et al, 2002). Some studies have found pacifier use in infants to be a protective factor against the occurrence of SIDS; the data for pacifier use in infants in the first year of life are said to be more compelling than data linking pacifier use to the development of dental complications and the inhibition of breast-feeding (American Academy of Pediatrics, 2005). Therefore the American Academy of Pediatrics recommends using a pacifier at naptime and bedtime, using a pacifier only if the infant is breast-feeding successfully, not using a sweetened coating on the pacifier, and avoiding forcing the infant to use the pacifier.

The American Academy of Pediatrics (2005) recommends that healthy infants be placed to sleep in the supine (on the back) position. Since the Back to Sleep campaign in 1992 advocating nonprone sleeping for infants, an increased incidence of positional plagiocephaly has been observed. (See Chapter 11 and Fig. 11-9.) It is recommended that an infant's head position be alternated during sleep time to prevent plagiocephaly. Infants may be placed prone during awake periods to prevent positional plagiocephaly and to encourage development of upper shoulder girdle strength (American Academy of Pediatrics, 2005).

Although the cause of SIDS is unknown, autopsies reveal consistent pathologic findings, such as pulmonary edema and intrathoracic hemorrhages that confirm the diagnosis. Consequently, autopsies should be performed on all infants suspected of dying of SIDS, and findings should be shared with the parents as soon as possible after the death. Postmortem findings in SIDS and accidental suffocation or intentional suffocation such as in Munchausen syndrome by proxy (see Child Maltreatment, Chapter 16) are practically the same. Individuals with less experience and training in performing autopsies, such as coroners instead of medical examiners, may not correctly identify some deaths as SIDS. Therefore mortality statistics can vary in different regions.

Infants at Risk for SIDS

Certain groups of children are at increased risk for SIDS:

- Low birth weight
- Low Apgar scores
- Recent viral illness
- Siblings of two or more SIDS victims
- Male sex
- Infants of Native American or African-American ethnicity

Factors that are often listed as being protective against SIDS include:

- Immunizations up to date
- Pacifier use at nap and bedtime
- Breast-feeding
- Placed to sleep in supine position

No diagnostic tests exist to predict which infants, including those in the above groups, will survive, and home monitoring is no guarantee of survival. Whether subsequent siblings of one SIDS infant are at increased risk for SIDS is unclear. Even if the risk is increased, families have a 99% chance that their subsequent child will *not* die of SIDS. A review of sibling deaths attributed to SIDS in England failed to ascertain a precise risk of recurrence; previous studies suggested a recurrence risk range of 1.7 to 10.1, yet the researchers concluded the studies had too many methodologic flaws to draw any firm conclusions (Bacon, Hall, Stephenson, et al, 2008). Others report that recurrence risks for a SIDS death in a family with a previous infant SIDS death range from 2% to 6% (American Academy of Pediatrics, 2005). Home monitoring is not recommended for this group of children, but it is often used by practitioners and may even be requested by parents (American Academy of Pediatrics, 2005). Monitoring is best initiated on an individual basis.

Nursing Care Management

Nurses have a vital role in preventing SIDS by educating families about the risk of prone sleeping position in infants from birth to 6 months of age, the use of appropriate bedding surfaces, the association with maternal smoking, and the dangers of cosleeping on noninfant surfaces with adults or other children. Additionally nurses have an important role in modeling behaviors for parents to foster practices that decrease the risk of SIDS: placing infants in a supine sleeping position in the hospital and using a pacifier at nap and bedtime. Data indicate that a small percentage of nurses still place healthy infants in a side-lying position in the hospital (Bullock, Mickey, Green, et al, 2004; Thompson, 2005). Statistics for infants being placed in a prone sleeping position in the United States decreased from 70% in 1992 to 13% in 2004 (American Academy of Pediatrics, 2005). One study of neonatal intensive care nurses indicated that 52% routinely provided discharge instructions that promote supine sleep positions at home; common nonsupine positions recommended by the nurses included either supine or side or exclusive side-lying sleep position (Aris, Stevens, Lemura, et al, 2006). Nurses must be proactive in further

decreasing the incidence of SIDS; postpartum discharge planning, newborn discharges, follow-up home visits, well-baby clinic visits, and immunization visits provide excellent opportunities to educate parents in these matters.

Many health care workers are concerned that infants placed on the back to sleep will aspirate emesis or mucus, yet studies fail to show an increase in infant deaths, spitting up during sleep, aspiration, asphyxia, or respiratory failure as a result of supine sleep positioning (Malloy, 2002; Tablizo, Jacinto, Parsley, et al, 2007).

Loss of a child from SIDS presents several crises with which the parents must cope. In addition to grief and mourning the death of their child, the parents must face a tragedy that was sudden, unexpected, and unexplained. The psychologic intervention for the family must deal with these additional variables. This discussion focuses primarily on the objectives of care for families experiencing SIDS, rather than on the process of grief and mourning, which is explored in Chapter 23.

Research findings have important implications for practices that may reduce the risk of SIDS, such as avoiding smoking during pregnancy and near the infant; using the supine sleeping position; avoiding soft, moldable mattresses, blankets, and pillows; avoiding bed sharing; breast-feeding; and avoiding overheating during sleep. The infant's head position should be varied to prevent flattening of the skull (positional plagiocephaly).

The first persons to arrive at the scene may be the police and emergency medical service personnel. They should handle the situation by asking few questions; giving no indication of wrongdoing, abuse, or neglect; making sensitive judgments concerning any resuscitation efforts for the child; and comforting the family members as much as possible. A compassionate, sensitive approach to the family during the first few minutes can help spare them some of the overwhelming guilt and anguish that commonly follow this type of death.

The medical examiner or coroner may go to the home or place of death and make the death pronouncement; until then the sleep environment should remain as it was when the infant was initially found (Koehler, 2008). If the infant is not pronounced at the scene, he or she may be transported to the emergency department to be pronounced dead by a physician. Usually there is no attempt at resuscitation in the emergency department. While they are in the emergency department, parents are asked only factual questions, such as when they found the infant, how he or she looked, and whom they called for help. The nurse avoids any remarks that may suggest responsibility, such as "Why didn't you go in earlier?" "Didn't you hear the infant cry out?" "Was the head buried in a blanket?" or "Were the siblings jealous of this child?" It is the coroner's responsibility to document these findings at the scene rather than have parents recount the experience in the emergency department (Koehler, 2008). Parents may also express feelings of guilt about administering cardiopulmonary resuscitation (CPR) correctly or the timing of CPR in relation to finding the infant.

At this time the physician should initiate the discussion of an autopsy, often with the nurse being present to support the family. The physician or medical examiner, depending on the circumstances, emphasizes that a diagnosis cannot be confirmed until the postmortem examination is completed. Nurses may balk at the idea of requesting an autopsy because of the parents' emotional state; however, an autopsy may clear up possible misconceptions regarding the death. Instructions about the autopsy and funeral arrangements may need to be repeated or put in writing. If the mother was breast-feeding, she needs information about abrupt discontinuation of lactation. The nurse or physician should contact the primary care practitioner for the infant and the mother to avoid any miscommunications or telephone calls at a later date inquiring about the child's health status.

A review of 60 studies shows that parents experiencing perinatal death perceive health care workers' responses as having a significant impact on the parents' grieving process; parents perceived the behavior of many health care workers as thoughtless or insensitive. The findings suggest that nurses and physicians would benefit from more bereavement training (Gold, 2007).

An important aspect of compassionate care for these parents is allowing them to say good-bye to their child. These are the parents' last moments with their child, and they should be as quiet, meaningful, peaceful, and undisturbed as possible. Encourage parents to hold their infant before leaving the emergency department. Because the parents leave the hospital without their infant, it is helpful to accompany them to the car or arrange for someone else to take them home. A debriefing session may help health care workers who dealt with the family and deceased infant to cope with emotions that are often engendered when a SIDS victim is brought into the acute care facility. Comprehensive guidelines have been published for health professionals involved in SIDS investigations to assist the family and at the same time to determine that the infant's death was not the result of other factors such as child maltreatment (American Academy of Pediatrics, 2001).

When the parents return home, a competent, qualified professional should visit them as soon after the death as possible. They should receive printed material that contains excellent information about SIDS (available from the national organizations*).

During the initial visit help the parents gain an intellectual understanding of the condition. The nursing objectives are to assess what the parents have been told about SIDS; what they think happened; and how they explained this to the other siblings, family members, and friends. One question that the nurse will never be able to answer and therefore should not attempt to is, "Why did this happen to our baby?" or "Who is responsible for this tragedy?" These and other questions may linger in the parents' minds for months or even years.

When the unexpected death of a child occurs, it is not uncommon for one parent to blame the other for the child's death. Parents may also experience guilt over the child's death; if they had checked earlier, the child might still be alive. It is important that the nurse assist parents in working through these feelings to prevent marital disruption in addition to the loss of the loved child.

Some parents are able to discuss their feelings openly, and the nurse supports this coping skill. However, others may be reluctant to express their grief, and the nurse can encourage the expression of emotions by asking about crying and feeling sad, angry, or guilty. This is an attempt to provoke a display of emotion, not just an admission of a feeling. During this session, help the parents explore their usual coping mechanisms and, if these are ineffectual, to investigate new approaches. For example, one parent may refrain from discussing the death for fear of upsetting the other parent, but each may need to hear how the other feels.

Ideally, the number of visits and plans for subsequent intervention need to be flexible. Parents facing the question of a subsequent child will need support. Both the birth of a subsequent child and the survival of that child, especially past the age of death of the previous child, are important transitional stages for parents.

APNEA AND APPARENT LIFE-THREATENING EVENTS

Apnea is defined as a cessation of breathing for 20 seconds. **Apnea of infancy** is defined as an unexplained respiratory pause of 20 seconds or more, or pauses of less than 20 seconds that are accompanied by pallor, cyanosis, bradycardia, or hypotension in the term infant. The latter is distinct from **apnea of prematurity**, which is the cessation of breathing longer than 20 seconds, or any period if accompanied by bradycardia and cyanosis; it is not associated with any predisposing conditions (Dudell and Stoll, 2007). An **ALTE**, formerly referred to as *aborted SIDS death* or *near-miss SIDS*, generally refers to an event that is sudden and frightening to the observer, in which the infant exhibits a combination of apnea, change in color (pallor, cyanosis, redness), change in muscle tone (usually hypotonia), choking, gagging, or coughing, and which usually involves a significant intervention and even CPR by the caregiver who witnesses the event (National Institutes of Health Consensus Development Conference, 1987). The definition of ALTE may include apnea, but ALTE may occur without apnea (Silvestri and Weese-Mayer, 2003). It is erroneous to characterize ALTE as a near-miss SIDS incident (Adams, Good, and Defranco, 2009).

Apnea during infancy can be a symptom of any one of many disorders—including sepsis, seizures or other neurologic disorder, upper or lower airway infection or abnormality, gastroesophageal reflux, hypoglycemia or other metabolic problems, and impaired regulation of breathing during sleep or feeding—or a result of intentional harm by an adult caregiver. Delayed ventilatory responses to hypercapnia and hypoxia were observed in one study of 69 infants with apnea of infancy (Katz-Salamon, 2004). Abusive head injury has been reported in a small percentage (2.5%) of children with ALTE (Altman, Brand, Forman, et al, 2003). Intentional suffocation and Munchausen syndrome by proxy cases have also been reported with ALTE (Hall and Zalman, 2005). However, in about half the cases of ALTE no cause is identified.

*American SIDS Institute, 509 Augusta Drive, Marietta, GA 30067; 800-232-SIDS, 770-426-8746; www.sids.org; First Candle, 1314 Bedford Ave., Suite 210, Baltimore, MD 21208; 800-221-7437; www.sidsalliance.org; National Sudden and Unexpected Infant/Child Death and Pregnancy Loss Resource Center, Georgetown University, Box 571272, Washington, DC 20057-1272; 866-866-7437, 202-687-7466; www.sidscenter.org.

Infants with a history of ALTEs may be at increased risk for SIDS, but these children constitute only approximately 7% to 12% of all SIDS victims. Most infants with ALTE are less than 6 months of age, and although there has been a significant decrease in SIDS since 1992, the incidence of ALTE has not changed (Hall and Zalman, 2005). A diagnosis of apnea of infancy or idiopathic ALTE is often made when no cause is found.

One European study found that infants with ALTE demonstrated behavioral abnormalities in the first weeks of life that included episodes of cyanosis, repeated episodes of apnea, pallor, and difficulty feeding (Kiechl-Kohlendorfer, Hof, Peglow, et al, 2005). Others have noted that a significant number of ALTEs in their emergency department were associated with accidental poisoning; over-the-counter medications were identified in toxicology screens (Pitetti, Whitman, and Zaylor, 2008).

Results from the Collaborative Home Infant Monitoring Evaluation study found that apnea and bradycardia occurred at conventional and extreme alarm thresholds in *all* groups of infants studied: siblings of SIDS infants, infants with ALTEs, symptomatic (of apnea and bradycardia) and asymptomatic preterm infants weighing less than 1750 g (3.8 lb) at birth, and healthy term infants. The researchers concluded that many infants in each of these groups experience apnea and bradycardia yet do not die (Jobe, 2001; Ramanathan, Corwin, Hunt, et al, 2001). Furthermore, it was reported that apnea does not appear to be an immediate precursor to SIDS *and that cardiorespiratory monitoring is not an effective tool for identifying infants at greater risk for SIDS* (American Academy of Pediatrics, 2003). CHIME data indicate that infants with ALTE did not have some of the typical characteristics associated with SIDS infants; these include fewer infants with low birth weight and who are small for gestational age at birth, fewer teenage pregnancies, and a younger infant age at the time of ALTE. The researchers concluded that despite some similar characteristics between ALTE and SIDS, the differences warrant a separate focus on ALTE events (Esani, Hodgman, Ehsani, et al, 2008).

Diagnostic Evaluation

An essential component of the diagnostic process includes a detailed description of the event—who witnessed the event, where the infant was during the event, and what, if any, activities were involved (such as during or after a feeding, riding in a car seat restraint, presence of siblings or any minor children, what clothing the infant was wearing). In addition, a prenatal and postnatal history must be obtained. A short period of observation in the emergency department may be appropriate to observe the infant's respiratory pattern and response to feeding. A careful evaluation of the preterm infant in the car restraint currently in use is essential; upper airway occlusion and subsequent apnea and cyanosis may occur if the infant is not positioned properly. Reported diagnoses in infants with ALTE include a neurologic event such as a seizure (30% of cases seen); GI problem, including gastroesophageal reflux (50%); respiratory conditions (20%); and metabolic conditions, cardiac anomaly, or child abuse (each <5%). In some cases, multiple diagnoses may be made (Hall and Zalman, 2005).

In the event that an underlying diagnosis such as those mentioned previously is not established, home monitoring may be recommended. The most commonly used monitoring is continuous recording of cardiorespiratory patterns (cardiopneumogram, or pneumocardiogram). Four-channel pneumocardiograms (or multichannel pneumogram) monitor heart rate, respirations (chest impedance), nasal airflow, and oxygen saturation. A more sophisticated test, polysomnography (sleep study), also records brain waves, eye and body movements, esophageal manometry, and end-tidal carbon dioxide measurements. However, none of these tests can predict risk. Some children with normal results may still have subsequent apneic episodes.

Therapeutic Management

The treatment of the infant with an ALTE depends on the underlying condition (see above). Treatment of recurrent apnea (without an underlying organic problem) usually involves continuous home monitoring of cardiorespiratory rhythms and in some cases the use of methylxanthines (respiratory stimulant drugs, such as theophylline or caffeine). The decision to discontinue the monitoring is based on the infant's clinical condition. A general guideline for discontinuation is when infants with ALTEs have gone 2 or 3 months without significant numbers of episodes requiring intervention.

Newer home apnea monitors allow download of information that assists the practitioner in deciding when to discontinue home monitoring. It is imperative to remember, however, that the home apnea monitor will not predict or prevent SIDS deaths. Furthermore, impedance-based monitors detect chest wall movement and will not detect obstructive apnea unless the episode involves significant bradycardia (see Family-Centered Care box).

Nursing Care Management

The diagnosis of an ALTE engenders great anxiety and concern in parents, and the institution of home monitoring presents additional physical and emotional burdens. Parents of infants on home apnea monitors report experiencing emotional distress, especially depression and hostility, during the first few weeks after hospital discharge (Abendroth, Moser, Dracup, et al, 1999). For parents of a SIDS victim who have a new infant on home apnea monitoring, the anxiety is compounded by the uncertainty of the future of the living child and grief for the lost child. Home apnea monitoring may offer some predictability and control over the current child's survival through the period of uncertainty.

If home monitoring is required, the nurse can be a major source of support to the family in terms of education about the equipment; education regarding observation of the infant's status; and instructions regarding immediate intervention during apneic episodes, including CPR. Several reports indicate that the first week to month after discharge is the most stressful for parents, particularly when the rate of false alarms is high (Bennett, 2002). To help the family cope with the numerous procedures they must learn, adequate preparation before discharge and written instructions are essential. In the first few weeks after discharge, parents may benefit by having a practitioner readily available to answer questions regarding false

FAMILY-CENTERED CARE

Using Apnea Monitors

Use the monitor as instructed by the practitioner and the manufacturer.

Do not adjust the monitor to eliminate false alarms. Adjustments could compromise the monitor's effectiveness.

Place the monitor on a firm surface away from the crib and drapes; plug power cord directly into a wall socket with a three-pronged outlet.

Do not sleep in the same bed as a monitored infant.

Keep pets and children away from the monitor and infant.

Keep the monitor away from possible electrical interferences such as appliances (e.g., electric blankets, televisions, air conditioners, remote telephones).

Check the monitor several times a day to ensure the alarm is working and that it can be heard from room to room. Be certain the caregiver can reach the monitor quickly (in <30 seconds).

Periodically check the monitor's breath detection indicator and battery or charger connections.

Be aware that strong signals from nearby radio and television stations, airports, ham radios, cellular phones, or police stations could interfere with the monitor. Check for proper monitor functioning if any of these are in use.

Read the monitor's user manual carefully; report problems promptly.

Inform community utility and rescue squads of home monitoring as appropriate.

Keep emergency numbers near phones in the home.

Practice safety precautions:

- Remove leads when infant is not attached to the monitor.
- Unplug the power cord from the electrical outlet when the cord is not plugged into the monitor.
- Use safety covers on electrical outlets to prevent children from inserting objects into a socket.

Data primarily from FDA Safety Alert: *Important tips for apnea monitor users,* Rockville, Md, 1990, US Department of Health and Human Services.

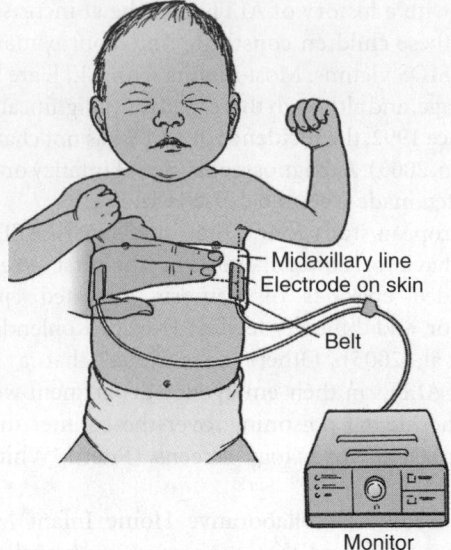

Fig. 13-8 Electrode placement for apnea monitoring. In small infants, one fingerbreadth may be used.

alarms and for other technical assistance (Abendroth, Moser, Dracup, et al, 1999).

Several types of home monitors are available and are set up by either a home monitor equipment company or home health staff. Nurses, especially those involved in the care at home, must become familiar with the equipment, including its advantages and disadvantages. Safety is a major concern because monitors can cause electrical burns and electrocution. The following precautions are recommended:

- Remove leads from infant when not attached to monitor.
- Unplug power cord from electrical outlet when cord is not plugged into monitor.
- Use safety covers on electrical outlets to discourage children from inserting objects into a socket.

Siblings should also be supervised when near the infant and taught that the monitor is not a toy. Other safety practices include informing local utility and rescue squads of the home monitoring in case of an emergency. Telephone numbers for these services should be posted near all telephones in the home.

! NURSING ALERT

If the infant is apneic, gently stimulate the trunk by patting or rubbing it. If the infant is prone, turn to the back and flick the feet. If there is still no response, begin CPR and activate the emergency medical service—"Call 911!" Never vigorously shake the child. No more than 10 to 15 seconds are spent on stimulation before implementing CPR.

Caregivers need detailed information regarding proper attachment of the electrodes to the infant's chest with impedance monitors that detect chest movement. The electrodes are placed in the midaxillary line, at a space one or two fingerbreadths below the nipple. For home use, electrodes attached to a belt that is placed around the child's trunk are preferred (Fig. 13-8). The belt is positioned so that the electrodes contact the skin in the same area. Monitors may have memory chips that allow for event recording, which can be an effective tool in evaluating the use of the monitor, events immediately before and after the ALTE, and reported frequency of alarms.

Monitors are effective only if they are used. They do not prevent death but alert the caregiver to the ALTE in time to intervene. The need to use the monitor and to respond appropriately to alarms must be stressed. Noncompliance can result in the infant's death.

Family Support

Many of the stresses observed during the monitoring period are characteristic of those of families with chronically ill children. The child with an apnea or cardiorespiratory monitor may have additional health care needs such as a gastrostomy, tracheostomy, ostomy, and myriad medications or treatments that exacerbate the parents' stress. Parents report increased stress, including concern for the child's survival, fear of incompetence in assuming home responsibility, inadequate respite care, lack of time for other children and spouse, social isolation from friends and extended family, constant work, and fatigue. The monitored child is at risk for vulnerable child syndrome, which may lead to lack of parental separation and preferential treatment, causing further family disruption (Bennett, 2002). To deal with these potential effects, nurses need to employ the same interventions as those discussed for children with chronic illness and be aware of the need for referral when difficulties are suspected.

To lessen the continuous responsibility of monitoring, other family members, such as grandparents, should be taught how to manipulate the equipment, read and interpret the signals, and administer CPR. They are encouraged to stay with the infant for regular periods to allow parents respite. Support groups of other families who have successfully completed monitoring can also be of benefit. Because reliable baby-sitters are difficult to locate, support group members or nursing students may be potential sources of qualified caregivers.

KEY POINTS

- Common nutritional disturbances of infancy include vitamin and mineral disturbances, some types of vegetarian diets, childhood malnutrition, and food hypersensitivity or intolerance.
- Mineral disturbances may be caused by mineral-mineral interactions and mineral-diet interactions.
- Nurses should counsel parents to provide the RDA of vitamins and minerals through appropriate foods instead of depending on supplements.
- Nutrient consumption varies among vegetarians; therefore a detailed dietary assessment is essential for planning AIs, particularly in children and pregnant and lactating women.
- PEM (SCU) may occur as a complication of social unrest when the child lacks food as a result of an underlying disease, a fad diet, lack of parental education about infant nutrition, inappropriate management of food allergy, incorrect preparation of formula, or poor food storage and handling.
- Food intolerance encompasses food allergies and food sensitivities during infancy, the most serious of which is CMA.
- Food hypersensitivity may cause a severe anaphylactic reaction in some children; a ready-to-administer dose of intramuscular epinephrine should be carried at all times by such children.
- Common feeding difficulties in the infant include regurgitation, spitting up, and colic.
- Treatment of colic may involve change in feeding practices, correction of a stressful environment, and support of the parent. Medications may or may not relieve some of the symptoms of colic.
- Behavioral interventions aimed at helping parents deal with the colicky infant may be more helpful than changing feeding practices or medications.
- Common skin disorders of infancy are diaper dermatitis, seborrheic dermatitis, and AD.
- Growth failure, or FTT, may occur in children who have a chronic illness, or it may occur in a family environment wherein healthy infant feeding practices are poorly managed or understood. FTT is not always associated with a pattern of disturbed maternal-infant relationship.
- SIDS is the third leading cause of infant death in the United States.
- Factors that place the infant at high risk for SIDS include prone sleeping position, soft bedding, sleeping in a noninfant bed with an adult or older child, and maternal prenatal smoking.
- The primary nursing responsibility in care associated with sudden infant death is educating the family of newborns about the risks for SIDS, modeling appropriate behaviors in the hospital such as placing the infant in a supine sleep position, and providing emotional support of the family that has experienced a SIDS loss.
- Infants with ALTEs are carefully evaluated for clues to the underlying cause.
- Home apnea or cardiorespiratory monitors do not prevent SIDS.

REFERENCES

Abendroth D, Moser DK, Dracup K, et al: Do apnea monitors decrease emotional distress in parents of infants at high risk for cardiopulmonary arrest? *J Pediatr Health Care* 13(2):50-57, 1999.

Adams SM, Good MW, Defranco GM: Sudden infant death syndrome, *Am Fam Physician* 79(10):870-874, 2009.

Alm B, Wennergren G, Norvenius SG, et al: Breast-feeding and the sudden infant death syndrome in Scandinavia, 1992-1995, *Arch Dis Child* 86(6):400-402, 2002.

Altman RL, Brand DA, Forman S, et al: Abusive head injury as a cause of apparent life-threatening events in infancy, *Arch Pediatr Adolesc Med* 157(10):1011-1015, 2003.

Amadi B, Mwiya M, Chomba E, et al: Improved nutritional recovery on an elemental diet in Zambian children with persistent diarrhoea and malnutrition, *J Trop Pediatr* 51(1):5-10, 2005.

American Academy of Pediatrics: *Pediatric nutrition handbook*, ed 6, Elk Grove Village, Ill, 2009, The Academy.

American Academy of Pediatrics: Prevention of rickets and vitamin D deficiency in infants, children, and adolescents, *Pediatrics* 122(5):1142-1148, 2008.

American Academy of Pediatrics: Dietary recommendations for children and adolescents: a guide for practitioners, *Pediatrics* 117(2):544-559, 2006.

American Academy of Pediatrics: The changing concept of sudden infant death syndrome: diagnostic coding shifts, controversies regarding the sleeping environment, and new variables to consider in reducing risk, *Pediatrics* 116(5):1245-1255, 2005.

American Academy of Pediatrics, Committee on Fetus and Newborn: Apnea, sudden infant death syndrome, and home monitoring, *Pediatrics* 111(4):914-917, 2003.

American Academy of Pediatrics, Committee on Child Abuse and Neglect: Distinguishing sudden infant death syndrome from child abuse fatalities, *Pediatrics* 107(2):437-441, 2001.

American Academy of Pediatrics, Task Force on Infant Sleep Position and Sudden Infant Death Syndrome: Changing concepts of sudden infant death syndrome: implications for infant sleeping environment and sleep position, *Pediatrics* 105(3):650-656, 2000.

American Dietetic Association, Dietitians of Canada: Position of the American Dietetic Association and Dietitians of Canada: vegetarian diets, *J Am Diet Assoc* 103(6):748-765, 2003.

Amthor RE, Cole SM, Manary MJ: The use of home-based therapy with ready-to-use therapeutic food to treat malnutrition in a rural area during a food crisis, *J Am Diet Assoc* 109(3):464-467, 2009.

Anderson ME, Johnson DC, Batal HA: Sudden infant death syndrome and prenatal maternal smoking: rising attributed risk in the Back to Sleep era, *BMC Med* 3(1):4, 2005.

Arikan D, Alp H, Gozum S, et al: Effectiveness of massage, sucrose solution, herbal tea or hydrolyzed formula in the treatment of infantile colic, *J Clin Nurs* 17(13):1754-1761, 2008.

Aris C, Stevens TP, Lemura C, et al: NICU nurses' knowledge and discharge teaching related to infant sleep position and risk of SIDS, *Adv Neonatal Care* 6(5):281-294, 2006.

Ashworth A, Khanum S, Jackson A, et al: Guidelines for the inpatient treatment of severely malnourished children, Geneva, 2003, World Health Organization, available at www.who.int/nutrition/publications/severemalnutrition/9241546093_eng.pdf (accessed July 2009).

Association of Women's Health, Obstetric and Neonatal Nurses: *Neonatal skin care: evidence-based clinical practice guideline*, ed 2, Washington, DC, 2007, The Association.

Bacon CJ, Hall DB, Stephenson TJ, et al: How common is repeat sudden infant death syndrome? *Arch Dis Child* 93(4):323-326, 2008.

Baharestani MM: An overview of neonatal and pediatric wound care knowledge and considerations, *Ostomy Wound Manage* 53(6):34-55, 2007.

Bansal PJ, Marsh R, Patel B, et al: Recognition, evaluation, and treatment of anaphylaxis in the child care setting, *Ann Allergy Asthma Immunol* 94(1):55-59, 2005.

Barnard K, Hammond MA, Booth CL, et al: Measurement and meaning of parent-child interaction. In Morrison F, Lord C, Keating D, editors: *Applied developmental psychology*, vol 3, New York, 1993, Academic Press.

Bennett AD: Home apnea monitoring for infants: a discussion of primary care issues, *Adv Nurs Pract* 10(3):48-53, 2002.

Black MM, Dubowitz H, Krishnakumar A, et al: Early intervention and recovery among children with failure to thrive: follow-up at age 8, *Pediatrics* 120(1):59-69, 2007.

Blair PS, Sidebotham P, Evason-Coombe C, et al: Hazardous cosleeping environments and risk factors amenable to change: case-control study of SIDS in south west England, *BMJ* 339:b3446, 2009.

Block RW, Krebs NF, Committee on Child Abuse and Neglect and Committee on Nutrition (American Academy of Pediatrics): Failure to thrive as a manifestation of child neglect, *Pediatrics* 116(5):1234-1237, 2005.

Blood-Siegfried J: The role of infection with inflammation in sudden infant death syndrome, *Immunopharmacol Immunotoxicol* 31(4):516-523, 2009.

Boguniewicz M: Atopic dermatitis: beyond the itch that rashes, *Immunol Allergy Clin North Am* 25(2):333-351, 2005.

Borkowski S: Diaper rash care and management, *Pediatr Nurs* 30(6):467-470, 2004.

Bullock LF, Mickey K, Green J, et al: Are nurses acting as role models for the prevention of SIDS? *MCN* 29(3):172-177, 2004.

Burk CJ, Molodow R: Infantile scurvy: an old diagnosis revisited with a modern dietary twist, *Am J Clin Dermatol* 8(2):103-106, 2007.

Carroll-Pankhurst C, Mortimer EA: Sudden infant death syndrome, bedsharing, parental weight, and age of death, *Pediatrics* 107(3):530-536, 2001.

Casey PH, Whiteside-Mansell L, Barrett K, et al: Impact of prenatal and/or postnatal growth problems in low birth weight preterm infants on school-age outcomes: an 8-year longitudinal evaluation, *Pediatrics* 118(3):1078-1086, 2006.

Centers for Disease Control and Prevention: Neurologic impairment in children associated with maternal dietary deficiency of cobalamin—Georgia, 2001, *MMWR* 52(4):61-64, 2003.

Christie L, Hine RJ, Parker JG, et al: Food allergies in children affect nutrient intake and growth, *J Am Diet Assoc* 102(11):1648-1651, 2002.

Ciliberto MA, Sandige H, Ndekha MJ, et al: Comparison of a home-based therapy with ready-to-use therapeutic food with standard therapy in the treatment of malnourished Malawin children: a controlled, clinical effectiveness trial, *Am J Clin Nutr* 81(4):864-870, 2005.

Conover E, Buehler BA: Use of herbal agents by breastfeeding women may affect infants, *Pediatr Ann* 33(4):235-240, 2004.

Corrales KM, Utter SL: Growth failure. In Samour PQ, King K, editors: *Handbook of pediatric nutrition*, ed 3, Sudbury, Mass, 2005, Jones & Bartlett.

Crotteau CA, Wright ST, Eglash A: What is the best treatment for infants with colic? *J Fam Pract* 55(7):634-636, 2006.

Devaney BL, Barr SI: DRI, EAR, RDA, AI, UL: making sense of this alphabet soup, *Pediatr Basics* 97(Winter):2-9, 2002.

de Vrese M, Schrezenmeir J: Probiotics, prebiotics, and synbiotics, *Adv Biochem Eng Biotechnol* 111:1-66, 2008.

Dudell GG, Stoll BJ: Respiratory tract disorders. In Kliegman RM, Behrman RE, Jenson HB, et al, editors: *Nelson textbook of pediatrics*, ed 18, Philadelphia, 2007, Saunders.

Dunham L, Kollar L: Vegetarian eating for children and adolescents, *J Pediatr Health Care* 20(1):27-34, 2006.

Duro D, Rising R, Cedillo M, et al: Association between infantile colic and carbohydrate malabsorption from fruit juices in infancy, *Pediatrics* 109(5):797-805, 2002.

Ellett MLC: What is known about colic? *Gastroenterol Nurs* 26(2):60-65, 2003.

Ellett ML, Appleton MM, Sloan RS: Out of the abyss of colic: a view through the father's eyes, *MCN* 34(3):164-171, 2009.

Ellett M, Schuff A, Davis JB: Parental perceptions of the lasting effects of infant colic, *MCN* 30(1):127-132, 2005.

Esani N, Hodgman JE, Ehsani N, et al: Apparent life-threatening events and sudden infant death syndrome: comparison of risk factors, *J Pediatr* 152(3):A2, 2008.

Ewing WM, Allen PJ: The diagnosis and management of cow's milk protein intolerance in the primary care setting, *Pediatr Nurs* 31(6):486-492, 2005.

Franco P, Groswasser J, Hassid S, et al: Prenatal exposure to cigarette smoking is associated with a decrease in arousal in infants, *J Pediatr* 135(1):34-38, 1999.

Gao X, Wilde PE, Lichtenstein AH, et al: Meeting adequate intake for dietary calcium without dairy foods in adolescents aged 9 to 18 years (National Health and Nutrition Examination Survey 2001-2002), *J Am Diet Assoc* 106(11):1759-1765, 2006.

Gidding SS, Dennison BA, Birch LL, et al: Dietary recommendations for children and adolescents: a guide for practitioners: consensus statement from the American Heart Association, *Circulation* 112(13):2061-2075, 2005.

Gidding SS, Lichtenstein AH, Faith MS, et al: Implementing American Heart Association pediatric and adult nutrition guidelines, *Circulation* 119(8):1161-1175, 2009.

Gold KJ: Navigating care after a baby dies: a systematic review of parent experiences with health providers, *J Perinatol* 27(4):230-237, 2007.

Goldberg JP, Folta SC, Must A: Milk: can a "good" food be so bad? *Pediatrics* 110(4):826-831, 2002.

Greer FR, Sicherer SH, Burks AW, et al: Effects of early nutritional interventions on the development of atopic disease in infants and children: the role of maternal dietary restriction, breastfeeding, timing of introduction of complementary foods, and hydrolyzed formulas, *Pediatrics* 121(1):183-191, 2008.

Hall KL, Zalman B: Evaluation and management of apparent life threatening events in children, *Am Fam Physician* 71(12):2301-2308, 2005.

Hauck FR, Herman SM, Donovan M, et al: Sleep environment and the risk of sudden infant death syndrome in an urban population: the Chicago Infant Mortality Study, *Pediatrics* 111(5):1207-1214, 2003.

Heird WC: Food insecurity, hunger, and undernutrition. In Kliegman RM, Behrman RE, Jenson HB, et al, editors: *Nelson textbook of pediatrics*, ed 18, Philadelphia, 2007, Saunders.

Heron M, Hoyert DL, Murphy SL, et al: Deaths: final data for 2006, *Natl Vital Stat Rep* 57(14):1-134, 2009.

Heron MP, Smith BL: Deaths: leading causes for 2003, *Natl Vital Stat Rep* 55(10):1-92, 2007.

Heyman MB, American Academy of Pediatrics, Committee on Nutrition: Lactose intolerance in infants, children, and adolescents, *Pediatrics* 118(3):1279-1286, 2006.

Highet AR: An infectious aetiology of sudden infant death syndrome, *J Appl Microbiol* 105(3):625-635, 2008.

Hodge D: *Diaper dermatitis: iLEX and Vaseline*, Personal Communication, Nashville, Tenn, December 29, 2009, Vanderbilt Children's Hospital.

Horne RS, Ferens D, Watts AM, et al: The prone sleeping position impairs arousability in term infants, *J Pediatr* 138(6):793-795, 2001.

Huiming Y, Chaomin W, Meng M: Vitamin A for treating measles in children, *Cochrane Database Syst Rev* (4):CD001479, 2005.

Institute of Medicine, Food and Nutrition Board: *Dietary reference intakes: applications in dietary assessment*, Washington, DC, 2000, National Academy Press.

Joanna Briggs Institute: Best practice: the effectiveness of interventions for infant colic, *Best Practice Information Sheet* 12(6):1-4, 2008, available at www.joannabriggs.edu.au/pdf/BPIScolic.pdf (accessed July 20, 2009).

Jobe AH: What do home monitors contribute to the SIDS problem? (editorial), *JAMA* 285(17):2244-2245, 2001.

Kapil U: Ready to use therapeutic food (RUTF) in the management of severe acute malnutrition in India, *Indian Pediatr* 46(5): 381-382, 2009.

Katz KA, Mahlberg MA, Honig PJ, et al: Rice nightmare: kwashiorkor in two Philadelphia-area infants fed Rice Dream beverage, *J Am Acad Dermatol* 52(5 Suppl 1):S69-S72, 2005.

Katz-Salamon M: Delayed chemoreceptor responses in infants with apnoea, *Arch Dis Child* 89(3):261 266, 2004.

Kawchak DA, Schall JI, Zemel BS, et al: Adequacy of dietary intake declines with age in children with sickle cell disease, *J Am Diet Assoc* 107(5):843-848, 2007.

Kemper KJ, Gardiner P: Herbal medicines. In Kliegman RM, Behrman RE, Jenson HB, et al, editors: *Nelson textbook of pediatrics*, ed 18, Philadelphia, 2007, Saunders.

Kiechl-Kohlendorfer U, Hof D, Peglow UP, et al: Epidemiology of apparent life threatening events, *Arch Dis Child* 90(3):297-300, 2005.

Koehler SA: Sudden infant death syndrome deaths: the role of forensic nurses, *J Forensic Nurs* 4(3):141-142, 2008.

Krugman SD, Dubowitz H: Failure to thrive, *Am Fam Physician* 68(5):879-886, 2003.

Lanski SL, Greenwald M, Perkins A, et al: Herbal therapy in a pediatric emergency department population: expect the unexpected, *Pediatrics* 111(5 Pt 1):981-985, 2003.

Lawrence RA, Lawrence RM: *Breastfeeding: a guide for the medical profession*, ed 6, Philadelphia, 2005, Saunders.

Leung DYM: Atopic dermatitis (atopic eczema). In Kliegman RM, Behrman RE, Jenson HB, et al, editors: *Nelson textbook of pediatrics*, ed 18, Philadelphia, 2007, Saunders.

Li L, Zhang Y, Zielke RH, et al: Observations on increased accidental asphyxia deaths in infancy while cosleeping in the state of Maryland, *Am J Forensic Med Pathol* 30(4):318-321, 2009.

Liu T, Howard RM, Mancini AJ, et al: Kwashiorkor in the United States: fad diets, perceived and true milk allergy, and nutritional ignorance, *Arch Dermatol* 137(5):630-636, 2001.

Lobo ML, Kotzer AM, Keefe MR, et al: Current beliefs and management strategies for treating infant colic, *J Pediatr Health Care* 18(3):115-122, 2004.

Locklin M: The redefinition of failure to thrive from a case study perspective, *Pediatr Nurs* 31(6):474-479, 495, 2005.

Lohse B, Stotts JL, Priebe JR: Survey of herbal use by Kansas and Wisconsin WIC participants reveals moderate, appropriate use and identifies herbal education needs, *J Am Diet Assoc* 106(2):227-237, 2006.

Loman DG: The use of complementary and alternative health care practices among children, *J Pediatr Health Care* 17(2):58-63, 2003.

Maggioni A, Lifshitz F: Nutritional management of failure to thrive, *Pediatr Clin North Am* 42(4):791-810, 1995.

Malloy MH: Trends in postneonatal aspiration deaths and reclassification of sudden infant death syndrome: impact of the "Back to Sleep" program, *Pediatrics* 109(4):661-665, 2002.

Markowitz R, Watkins JB, Duggan C: Failure to thrive: malnutrition in the pediatric outpatient setting. In Markowitz R, Watkins JB, Duggan C, editors: *Nutrition in pediatrics*, ed 4, Hamilton, Ontario, 2008, BC Decker.

Matlik L, Savaiano D, McCabe G, et al: Perceived milk intolerance is related to bone mineral content in 10- to 13-year- old female adolescents, *Pediatrics* 120(3):e669 e677, 2007.

McGarvey C, McDonnell M, Chong A, et al: Factors relating to the infant's last sleep environment in sudden infant death syndrome in the Republic of Ireland, *Arch Dis Child* 88(12):1058-1064, 2003.

McGuire JK, Kulkarni MS, Baden HP: Fatal hypermagnesemia in a child treated with megavitamin/megamineral therapy, *Pediatrics* 105(2):414, 2000.

McLane KM, Bookout K, McCord S, et al: The 2003 national pediatric pressure ulcer and skin breakdown prevalence survey: a multisite study, *J Wound Ostomy Continence Nurs* 31(4):168-178, 2004.

McMartin KI, Platt MS, Hackman R, et al: Lung tissue concentrations of nicotine in sudden infant death syndrome, *J Pediatr* 140(2):205-209, 2002.

Mesich HM: Mother-infant co-sleeping: understanding the debate and maximizing infant safety, *MCN* 30(1):30-37, 2005.

Messina V, Melina V, Mangels AR: A new food guide for North American vegetarians, *J Am Diet Assoc* 103(6):771-775, 2003.

Mitchell EA: What is the mechanism of SIDS? Clues from epidemiology, *Dev Psychobiol* 51(3):215-222, 2009.

Mitchell EA, Thompson JM, Becroft DM, et al: Head covering and the risk for SIDS: findings from the New Zealand and German SIDS case-control studies, *Pediatrics* 121(6):e1478-e1483, 2008.

Morelli J: Eczematous disorders. In Kliegman RM, Behrman RE, Jenson HB, et al, editors: *Nelson textbook of pediatrics*, ed 18, Philadelphia, 2007, Saunders.

Morin K: The challenge of colic in infants, *MCN* 34(3):192, 2009.

Müller O, Krawinkel M: Malnutrition and health in developing countries, *CMAJ* 173(3):279-286, 2005.

National Institutes of Health Consensus Development Conference on Infantile Apnea and Home Monitoring, Sept 29 to Oct 1, 1986, *Pediatrics* 79(2):292-299, 1987.

Neu M, Robinson JA: Infants with colic: their childhood characteristics, *J Pediatr Nurs* 18(1):12-20, 2003.

Noonan C, Quigley S, Curley MAQ: Skin integrity in hospitalized infants and children: a prevalence survey, *J Pediatr Nurs* 21(6):445-453, 2006.

Nowak-Wegrzyn A, Bloom KA, Sicherer SH, et al: Tolerance to extensively heated milk in children with cow's milk allergy, *J Allergy Clin Immunol* 122(2):342-347, 2008.

O'Connor NR: Infant formula, *Am Family Physician* 79(7):565-570, 2009.

O'Connor NR, McLaughlin MR, Ham P: Newborn skin, part I, Common problems, *Am Fam Physician* 77(1):47-52, 2008.

Ong PY, Boguniewicz M: Atopic dermatitis, *Primary Care* 35(1):105-117, 2008.

Penny ME: Protein-energy malnutrition: pathophysiology, clinical consequences, and treatment. In Walker WA, Watkins JB, Duggan C, editors: *Nutrition in pediatrics*, ed 3, Hamilton, Ontario, 2003, BC Decker.

Perrotta S, Nobili B, Rossi F, et al: Infant hypervitaminosis A causes severe anemia and thrombocytopenia: evidence of a retinol-dependent bone marrow cell growth inhibition, *Blood* 99(6):2017-2022, 2002.

Perry CL, McGuire MT, Neumark-Sztainer D, et al: Adolescent vegetarians: how well do their dietary patterns meet the healthy people 2010 objectives? *Arch Pediatr Adolesc Med* 156(5):426-427, 2002.

Person TL, Lavezzi WA, Wolf BC: Cosleeping and sudden unexpected death in infancy, *Arch Pathol Lab Med* 126(3):343-345, 2002.

Pessler F, Nejat M: Anaphylactic reaction to goat's milk in a cow's milk–allergic infant, *Pediatr Allergy Immunol* 15(2):183-185, 2004.

Pitetti RD, Whitman E, Zaylor A: Accidental and nonaccidental poisonings as a cause of apparent life-threatening events in infants, *Pediatrics* 122(2):e359-e362, 2008.

Pollack HA: Sudden infant death syndrome, maternal smoking during pregnancy and effectiveness of smoking cessation intervention, *Am J Pub Health* 91(3):432-436, 2001.

Preston AM, Rodriguez C, Rivera CE: Plasma ascorbate in a population of children: influence of age, gender, vitamin C intake, and smoke exposure, *P R Health Sci J* 25(2):137-142, 2006.

Preston AM, Rodriguez C, Rivera CE, et al: Influence of environmental tobacco smoke on vitamin C status in children, *Am J Clin Nutr* 77(1):167-172, 2003.

Puffenberger EG, Hu-Lince D, Parod JM, et al: Mapping of sudden infant death with dysgenesis of the testis syndrome (SIDDT) by a SNP genome scan and identification of TSPYL loss of function, *Proc Natl Acad Sci USA* 101(32):11,689-11,694, 2004.

Ramanathan R, Corwin MJ, Hunt DE, et al: Cardiorespiratory events recorded on home monitors: comparison of healthy infants with those at increased risk for SIDS, *JAMA* 285(17):2199-2243, 2001.

Richardson HL, Walker AM, Horne RS: Maternal smoking impairs arousal patterns in sleeping infants, *Sleep* 32(4):515-521, 2009.

Roberts DM, Ostapchuk M, O'Brien J: Infantile colic, *Am Fam Physician* 70(4):735-740, 741-742, 2004.

Rudolf MCJ, Logan S: What is the long term outcome for children who fail to thrive? A systematic review, *Arch Dis Child* 90(9):925-931, 2005.

Saltzman MD, King EC: Central physeal arrests as a manifestation of hypervitaminosis A, *J Pediatr Orthop* 27(3):351-353, 2007.

Sampson HA: Update on food allergy, *J Allergy Clin Immunol* 113(5):805-819, 2004.

Sampson HA, Leung DYM: Adverse reactions to foods. In Kliegman RM, Behrman RE, Jenson

HB, et al, editors: *Nelson textbook of pediatrics*, ed 18, Philadelphia, 2007a, Saunders.

Sampson HA, Leung DYM: Anaphylaxis. In Kliegman RM, Behrman RE, Jenson HB, et al, editors: *Nelson textbook of pediatrics*, ed 18, Philadelphia, 2007b, Saunders.

Savino F, Pelle E, Palumeri E, et al: *Lactobacillus reuteri* (American type culture collection strain 55730) versus simethicone in the treatment of infantile colic: a prospective randomized study, *Pediatrics* 119(1):e124-e130, 2007.

Sawni A, Ragothaman R, Thomas RL, et al: The use of complementary/alternative therapies among children attending an urban pediatric emergency department, *Clin Pediatr* 46(1): 36-41, 2007.

Sibley E: Carbohydrate intolerance, *Curr Opin Gastroenterol* 20(2):162-167, 2004.

Sicherer SH: Clinical aspects of gastrointestinal food allergy in children, *Pediatrics* 111(6 Pt 3):1609-1616, 2003.

Silvestri JM, Weese-Mayer DE: Disorders of respiratory control: apnea and SIDS. In Rudolph CD, Rudolph AM, Hostetter MK, editors: *Rudolph's pediatrics*, ed 21, New York, 2003, McGraw-Hill.

Simons FE: Anaphylaxis: recent advances in assessment and treatment, *J Allergy Clin Immunol* 124(4):625-636, 2009.

Stahler C: How many youth are vegetarian? *Vegetarian J* (4):1-2, 2005; available at www.vrg.org/journal/vj2005issue4/vj2005issue4youth.htm (accessed July 3, 2009).

St. James-Roberts I: Infant crying and sleeping: helping parents to prevent and manage problems, *Primary Care* 35(3):547-567, 2008.

Tablizo MA, Jacinto P, Parsley D, et al: Supine sleeping position does not cause clinical aspiration in neonates in hospital newborn nurseries, *Arch Pediatr Adolesc Med* 161(5): 507-510, 2007.

Tappin D, Ecob R, Brooke H: Bedsharing, roomsharing, and sudden infant death syndrome in Scotland: a case-control study, *J Pediatr* 147(1):32-37, 2005.

Thompson DG: Safe sleep practices for hospitalized infants, *Pediatr Nurs* 31(5):400-403, 409, 2005.

Unger B, Kemp JS, Wilkins D, et al: Racial disparity and modifiable risk factors among infants dying suddenly and unexpectedly, *Pediatrics* 111(2):e127-e131, 2003.

Vennemann MM, Bajanowski T, Brinkmann B, et al: Sleep environment risk factors for sudden infant death syndrome: the German Sudden Infant Death Syndrome Study, *Pediatrics* 123(4):1162-1170, 2009.

Visscher MO: Recent advances in diaper dermatitis: etiology and treatment, *Pediatr Health* 3(1):81-98, 2009, available at www.medscape.com/viewarticle/589066_print (accessed April 14, 2009).

Wang J, Sampson HA: Food anaphylaxis, *Clin Exp Allergy* 37(5):651-660, 2007.

Wasserbauer N, Ballow M: Atopic dermatitis, *Am J Med* 122(2):121-125, 2009.

Weizman Z, Alkrinawi S, Goldfarb D, et al: Efficacy of herbal tea preparation in infantile colic, *J Pediatr* 122(4):650-652, 1993.

Williams HC: Atopic dermatitis, *N Engl J Med* 352(22):2314-2324, 2005.

World Health Organization: *HIV and infant feeding update*, Geneva, 2006, The Organization.

Zeisel SH, Erickson KE: Dietary supplements (nutraceuticals). In Walker WA, Watkins JB, Duggan C, editors: *Nutrition in pediatrics*, ed 3, Hamilton, Ontario, 2003, BC Decker.

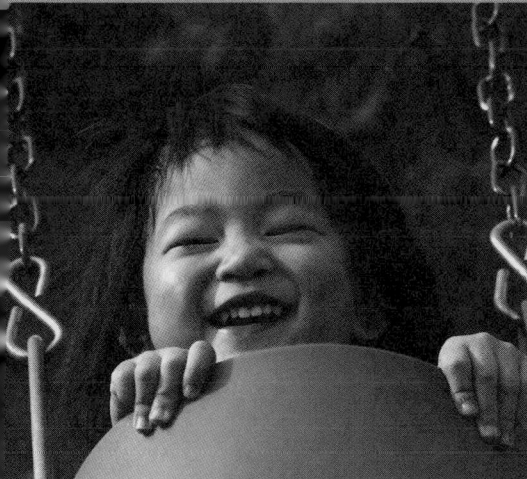

Health Promotion of the Toddler and Family

David Wilson

PROMOTING OPTIMUM GROWTH AND DEVELOPMENT

The term *terrible twos* has often been used to describe the toddler years, the period from 12 to 36 months of age. It is a time of intense exploration of the environment as children attempt to find out how things work; what the word "no" means; and the power of temper tantrums, negativism, and obstinacy. "Getting into things" is their way of learning about their world, especially relationships. Successful mastery of the tasks of this age requires a strong foundation of trust during infancy and frequently necessitates guidance from others when parent and toddler face the struggles of toilet training, limit setting, and sibling rivalry. Nurses who understand the dynamics of growth and development of the toddler can help families deal effectively with the tasks of this age.

BIOLOGIC DEVELOPMENT

Proportional Changes

Growth slows considerably during toddlerhood. The average weight at 2 years is 12 kg (26.5 lb). The average weight gain is 1.8 to 2.7 kg (4 to 6 lb) per year. By 2½ years of age, toddlers have quadrupled their birth weight. The rate of increase in height also slows. The usual increment is an addition of 7.5 cm (3 inches) per year and occurs mainly in elongation of the legs rather than the trunk. The average height of a 2-year-old is 86.6 cm (34 inches). In general, adult height is about twice the child's height at 2 years of age. Accurate measurement of height and weight during the toddler years should reveal a steady growth curve that is steplike rather than linear (straight), which is characteristic of the growth spurts during the early childhood years.

The rate of increase in head circumference slows somewhat by the end of infancy, and head circumference is usually equal to chest circumference by 1 to 2 years of age. The usual total increase in head circumference during the second year is 2.5 cm (1 inch). Then the rate of increase slows until age 5 years, when the increase is less than 1.25 cm (0.5 inch) per year. The anterior fontanel closes between 12 and 18 months of age.

Chest circumference continues to increase and exceeds head circumference during the toddler years. Its shape also changes as the transverse (or lateral) diameter exceeds the anteroposterior diameter. After the second year the chest circumference exceeds the abdominal measurement, which, in addition to the growth of the lower extremities, gives the child a taller, leaner appearance. However, the toddler retains a squat, "pot-bellied" appearance because of the less well-developed abdominal musculature and short legs (Fig. 14-1). The legs retain a slightly bowed or curved appearance during the second year from the weight of the relatively large trunk.

Sensory Changes

Visual acuity of 20/40 is considered acceptable during the toddler years. Full binocular vision is well developed, and any evidence of persistent strabismus should receive professional attention as early as possible to prevent amblyopia. Depth perception continues to develop, but because of the child's lack

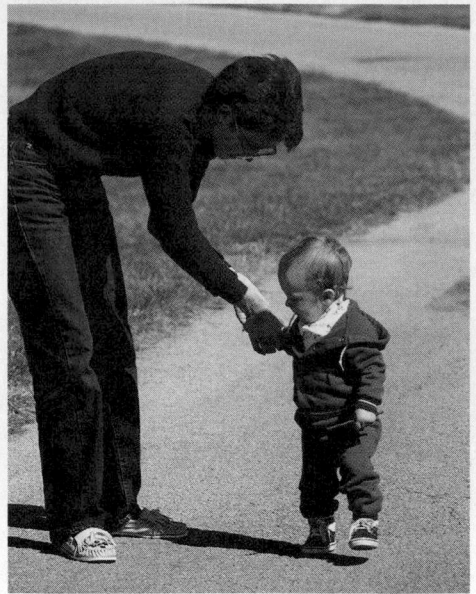

Fig. 14-1 Typical toddling gait.

of motor coordination, falls from heights remain a persistent danger.

The senses of hearing, smell, taste, and touch become increasingly well developed, coordinated with each other, and associated with other experiences. Toddlers use all the senses to explore the environment. Toddlers visually inspect an object by turning it over; they may taste it, smell it, and touch it several times before they are satisfied with their investigation. They will shake it to see if it makes noise and vigorously test its durability.

Another example of the integrated function of the senses is the toddler's development of specific taste and texture preferences. The child is much less likely than infants to try a new food because of its appearance or smell, not just its taste. Likewise a toddler is likely to reject a new food because of its texture. Nonsensory associations with objects also take on significance. For example, if parents refuse a particular food because of their dislike, they will transfer this negative connotation to the child before the child has had an opportunity to taste it. Awareness of these factors is important in several areas of childrearing, such as feeding, teaching socially acceptable habits, and reinforcing appropriate behavioral responses to various situations.

Touch continues to be important to the toddler. Descending development of the spinal tract is evidenced by increased sensation in the lower extremities, such as ticklish feet. Pleasant tactile sensations soothe and comfort the toddler, especially in times of stress or fatigue.

Maturation of Systems

Most of the physiologic systems are relatively mature by the end of toddlerhood. By the end of the first year, all the brain cells are present but continue to increase in size. Myelination of the spinal cord is almost complete by 2 years of age, which parallels the completion of most of the gross motor skills associated with locomotion. Brain growth is 75% completed by the end of 2 years.

Development of various areas of the brain seems to correspond with the child's progressive intellectual capacity. As development progresses, specific changes take place in various areas of the cerebral cortex, such as the Broca area for speech and cortical areas for control of the legs, hands, feet, and sphincters. Because this neuromotor organization is so inclusive, complex, and intricate, the child is limited in the ability to attend to any one aspect of behavior for more than a few minutes.

Between 2 and 3 years of age, coordination and consolidation of these voluntary functions allow the toddler to listen better, look longer, and have an extended attention span. Although postural control is increasingly developed as myelination of the spinal cord advances, the immaturity of this control, combined with the child's limited experiences and lack of visual perception, makes it difficult to do simple acts such as seating oneself in a chair or climbing down stairs.

Volume of the respiratory tract and growth of associated structures continue to increase during early childhood, lessening some of the factors that predisposed the child to frequent and serious infections during infancy. However, the internal structures of the ear and throat continue to be short and straight, and the lymphoid tissue of the tonsils and adenoids continues to be large. As a result, otitis media, tonsillitis, and upper respiratory tract infections are common. The respiratory and heart rates slow, and the blood pressure increases (see inside back cover). Respirations continue to be abdominal.

The digestive processes are fairly complete by the beginning of toddlerhood. The acidity of the gastric contents continues to increase and has a protective function because it destroys many types of bacteria. Stomach capacity increases to allow for the usual schedule of three small meals a day.

One of the more prominent changes of the gastrointestinal system is the voluntary control of elimination. With complete myelination of the spinal cord, the toddler gradually achieves control of anal and urethral sphincters. The physiologic ability to control the sphincters occurs somewhere between ages 18 and 24 months. Bladder capacity also increases considerably. By 14 to 18 months of age the child is able to retain urine for up to 2 hours or longer.

The skin functionally matures during early childhood. The epidermis and dermis are more tightly bound together, increasing their resistance to infection and irritation and creating a more effective barrier against fluid loss. Production of sebum is minimal, which contributes to the development of dry skin. The eccrine glands are functional during early childhood and react to changes in temperature, but they produce minimum amounts of sweat. Hair grows thicker and coarser and usually darkens and loses some curliness. Fine hair is evident on the lower arms and legs. Production of adipose tissue declines as hyperplasia of muscle cells increases. With the concurrent growth of the lower extremities, the child assumes more adult-like proportions.

Under conditions of moderate variation in temperature, the toddler rarely has the difficulties of the young infant in maintaining body temperature. The capillaries are able to conserve core body temperature by constricting in response to cold and dilating in response to heat. Shivering, an involuntary act that results in rhythmic muscle contraction, which increases cellular metabolism and produces heat, is much more effective as a source of thermogenesis. The child also learns mechanisms to control body temperature—putting on clothing when cold or removing it when warm.

The defense mechanisms of the tissues and blood, particularly phagocytosis, are much more efficient in the toddler than in the infant. The production of antibodies is well established. Immunoglobulin G, which neutralizes microbial toxins, reaches adult levels by the end of the second year of life. Passive immunity from maternal transfer during fetal life disappears by the beginning of toddlerhood. Immunoglobulin M, which responds to artificial immunizing techniques and combats serious infection, attains adult levels during late infancy. Immunoglobulins A, D, and E increase gradually, not reaching eventual adult levels until later childhood. Many young children demonstrate a sudden increase in colds and minor infections when entering daycare or preschool because of exposure to new antigens.

Gross and Fine Motor Development

The major gross motor skill during the toddler years is the development of locomotion. By 12 to 13 months of age toddlers walk alone, using a wide stance for extra balance; by age 18 months they try to run but fall easily. Between 2 and 3 years of age, refinement of the upright, biped position is evident in improved coordination and equilibrium. By age 2 years toddlers can walk up and down stairs, and by age 2½ years they jump using both feet, stand on one foot for a second or two, and manage a few steps on tiptoe. By the end of the second year they stand on one foot, walk on tiptoe, and climb stairs with alternate footing.

Fine motor development is demonstrated in increasingly skillful manual dexterity. Once toddlers achieve pincer grasp, usually at 9 to 10 months of age, they combine this skill with other developing sensory and cognitive abilities. For example, by age 12 months they are able to grasp a very small object. By age 15 months they can drop a pellet into a narrow-necked bottle. Casting or throwing objects and retrieving them become an almost obsessive activity at about 15 months. By 18 months of age they can throw a ball overhand without losing their balance.

Visual perception of geometric shapes is also evident at this time. At age 12 months children selectively look at a round hole in a special form board but are unable to insert a round object. By age 15 months they promptly place the round object in the hole, even if the board is revised or turned upside down. Spatial relations also are evident in their ability to build a tower with blocks: by age 18 months, a tower of three or four blocks; by age 24 months, a tower of six or seven blocks; and by age 30 months, a tower of eight blocks or more.

Fine motor skill and visual ability are demonstrated in toddlers' progressive adeptness in manipulating a pencil or crayon. By age 15 months they scribble spontaneously, and by age 24 months they imitate a circular stroke and a vertical line. By the end of the toddler period, the child can copy a circle and imitate a cross.

Mastery of gross and fine motor skills is evident in all phases of the child's activity, such as play, dressing, language comprehension, response to discipline, social interaction, and propensity for injuries. Activities occur less in isolation and more in conjunction with other physical and mental abilities to produce a purposeful result. For example, the toddler walks to reach a new location, releases a toy and picks it up again or chooses a new one, and scribbles to look at the image produced. The possibilities of the exploration, investigation, and manipulation mastery of the environment—and its hazards—are endless.

PSYCHOSOCIAL DEVELOPMENT

Toddlers are faced with the mastery of several important tasks. If the need for basic trust has been satisfied, they are ready to give up dependence for control, independence, and autonomy. Some of the specific tasks include:

- Differentiation of self from others, particularly the mother or primary caregiver
- Toleration of separation from parents
- Ability to withstand delayed gratification
- Control over bodily functions
- Acquisition of socially acceptable behavior
- Verbal means of communication
- Ability to interact with others in a less egocentric manner

Mastery of these goals is only begun during late infancy and the toddler years, and such tasks as developing interpersonal relationships with others may not be completed until adolescence. However, crucial foundations for successful completion of such developmental tasks are laid during these early formative years.

Developing a Sense of Autonomy (Erikson)

According to Erikson (1963), the developmental task of toddlerhood is acquiring a sense of autonomy while overcoming a sense of doubt and shame. As infants gain trust in the predictability and reliability of their parents, environment, and interaction with others, they begin to discover that their behavior is their own and that it has a predictable, reliable effect on others. However, although they are aware of their will and control over others, they are confronted with the conflict of exerting autonomy and relinquishing the much enjoyed dependence on others. Exerting their will has definite negative consequences, whereas retaining dependent, submissive behavior is generally rewarded with affection and approval. On the other hand, continued dependency creates a sense of doubt regarding their potential capacity to control their actions. This doubt is compounded by a sense of *shame* for feeling this urge to revolt against others' will and a fear that they will exceed their own capacity for manipulating the environment. The latter fear is a basis for instituting limit setting and consistent discipline at this age. Without appropriate limits on what is acceptable versus unacceptable behavior, children have no guidelines for establishing the end points of their ability to control.

Just as the infant has the social modalities of grasping and biting, the toddler has the newly gained modality of holding on and letting go. Holding on and letting go are evident in how the toddler uses the hands, mouth, eyes, and, eventually, sphincters when toilet training is begun. Children constantly express these social modalities in play activities such as casting or throwing objects; taking objects out of boxes, drawers, or cabinets; holding

on tighter when someone says, "No, don't touch"; and spitting out food as taste preferences become strong.

Several characteristics, especially negativism and ritualism, are typical of toddlers in their quest for autonomy. As toddlers attempt to express their will, they often act with negativism, giving a negative response to requests. The words "no" or "me do" can be the sole vocabulary. Toddlers express emotions strongly, usually in rapid mood swings. One minute toddlers can be engrossed in an activity, and the next minute they might be violently angry because they were unable to manipulate a toy or open a door. If scolded for doing something wrong, they can have a temper tantrum and almost instantaneously pull at the parent's legs to be picked up and comforted. Understanding and coping with these swift changes is often difficult for parents. Many parents find the negativism exasperating and, instead of dealing constructively with it, give in to it, which further threatens the child's search for acceptable methods of interacting with others (see p. 568).

In contrast to negativism, which frequently disrupts the environment, ritualism, the need to maintain sameness and reliability, provides a sense of comfort. Toddlers can venture out with security when they know that familiar people, places, and routines still exist. One can easily understand why change, such as hospitalization, represents such a threat to these children. Without the comfortable rituals, they have little opportunity to exert autonomy. Consequently, dependency and regression occur (see p. 569).

Erikson focuses on the development of the ego, which may be thought of as reason or common sense, during this phase of psychosocial development. The child struggles to deal with the impulses of the id, tolerate frustration, and learn socially acceptable ways of interacting with the environment. The ego becomes evident as the child is able to delay gratification.

This stage also sees a rudimentary beginning of the superego, or conscience, which is the incorporation of the morals of society and the process of acculturation. With the development of the ego, children further differentiate themselves from others and expand their sense of trust in self. But as they begin to develop awareness of their own will and capacity to achieve, they also become aware of their ability to fail. This ever-present awareness of potential failure creates doubt and shame. Successful mastery of the task of autonomy necessitates opportunities for self-mastery while withstanding the frustration of necessary limit setting and delayed gratification. Opportunities for self-mastery are present in appropriate play activities, toilet training, the crisis of sibling rivalry, and successful interactions with significant others.

COGNITIVE DEVELOPMENT

Sensorimotor Phase (Piaget)

The period from 12 to 24 months of age is a continuation of the final two stages of the sensorimotor phase (Table 14-1). During this time the cognitive processes develop rapidly and at times seem similar to mature thinking. However, reasoning skills are still primitive and need to be understood to effectively deal with the typical behaviors of this age child. The main cognitive achievement of early childhood is the acquisition of language, which represents mental symbolism.

TABLE 14-1	SENSORIMOTOR AND PREOPERATIONAL PHASES DURING TODDLERHOOD*	
STAGE AND AGE	**COGNITIVE DEVELOPMENT**	**BEHAVIOR**
Sensorimotor		
V. Tertiary circular reactions (13-18 mo)	Active experimentation to achieve previously unattainable goals	Insatiable curiosity about environment
	Increased concept of object permanence	Uses all sensory cues for exploration
	Differentiation of oneself from objects	Ventures away from parent for longer periods
	Early traces of memory	Uses physical skills to achieve particular goal
	Beginning awareness of spatial, causal, and temporal relationships	Can find hidden objects, but only in first location
	Able to enter into an action at any point without reproducing entire sequence	Able to insert round object into hole
		Fits smaller objects into each other (nesting)
		Gestures "up" and "down"
		Puts objects into container and takes them out
		Realizes that "out of sight" is not out of reach; opens doors and drawers to find objects
		Gains comfort from parent's voice even if parent is not visible
VI. Invention of new means through mental combinations (19-24 mo)	Awareness of object permanence regardless of number of invisible displacements	Searches for object through several hiding places
	Can infer a cause only while experiencing the effect	Will infer cause by associating two or more experiences (such as candy missing, sister smiling)
	Imitation increasingly symbolic	Imitates words and sounds of animals
	Beginning sense of time in terms of anticipation, memory, and ability to wait	Imitates adult behavior (domestic mimicry)
	Egocentrism in thought and behavior	Follows directions and understands requests
	Global organization of thought	Uses words "up," "down," "come," and "go" with meaning
		May sit and wait for meals at table for short period
		Has some sense of time; waits in response to "just a minute"; may use word "now"
		Refers to self by name
		Engages in parallel play; demonstrates awareness of ownership
		Concerned with ritualistic, routinized schedule
Preoperational		
2-4 yr	Increased use of language as mental symbolization	Uses two- or three-word phrases
	Egocentrism still present in thought, play, and behavior	Increased vocabulary
	Increased sense of time, space, causality	Refers to self by pronoun
	See Box 14-1	Possessive of own toys; uses word "mine"
		Begins to use past tense of verbs
		Uses phrases "going to," "in a minute," "today," "all done"
		Uses many future-oriented words, such as "tomorrow," "next day," "afternoon," but has poor concept of passage of time
		Follows directions using prepositions, such as "up," "behind," "under," "in back of"

*For the previous four stages during early infancy, see Table 12-1.

In the fifth stage, tertiary circular reactions (from 13 to 18 months of age), the child uses active experimentation to achieve previously unattainable goals. Newly acquired physical skills are increasingly important for the function they serve rather than for the acts themselves. The child incorporates the old learning of secondary circular reactions and applies the combined knowledge to new situations, with emphasis on the results of the experimentation. In this way there is the beginning of rational judgment and intellectual reasoning. During this stage the child further differentiates self from objects. This is evident in the child's increasing ability to venture away from the parent and to tolerate longer periods of separation.

Awareness of a causal relationship between two events is apparent. After flipping a light switch, toddlers are aware that a response occurs. However, they are not able to transfer that knowledge to new situations. Therefore every time they see what appears to be a light switch, they must reinvestigate its function. Such behavior demonstrates the beginning of categorizing data into distinct classes, subclasses, and so on. Innumerable examples of this type of behavior occur as toddlers repeatedly explore the same object each time it appears in a new place. A classic example is their curiosity about electrical outlets. Even if they receive a shock from one of them, they will adamantly poke and inspect every other outlet. This inability to transfer information leaves toddlers particularly vulnerable to injuries. However, traces of memory are evident because they usually avoid the outlet where the shock occurred.

Because classification of objects is still basic, the appearance of an object indicates its function. For example, if the child's toys are stored in a paper bag or large container, the toddler does not perceive a difference between that toy receptacle and the garbage pail or laundry basket. If allowed to turn over the toy receptacle, the child will just as quickly do the same to other similar objects because, in the child's mind, there is no difference. Expecting toddlers to judge which receptacles are permissible to explore and which are not is inappropriate for this age-group. Instead, the forbidden object, such as the garbage pail, should be placed out of reach. This has significant implications for prevention of accidents and accidental ingestion of injurious agents.

The discovery of objects as objects leads to an awareness of their spatial relationships. Children are able to recognize different shapes and their relationship to each other. For example, they can fit slightly smaller boxes into each other (nesting) and can place a round object into a hole, even if the board is turned around, upside down, or reversed. However, they cannot do the same thing with a square until 2 years of age. Children are also aware of space and the relationship of their body to dimensions such as height. They will stretch, stand on a low stair or stool, and pull a string to reach an object.

Object permanence has also advanced. Although they still cannot find an object that has been displaced and is no longer visible or has been moved from under one pillow to another without their seeing the change, toddlers are increasingly aware of the existence of objects behind closed doors, in drawers, and under tables. Parents are usually acutely aware of this developmental achievement because they find high places and locked cabinets to be the only areas inaccessible to toddlers. Parents also experience toddlers' protest behaviors when the parents leave because toddlers are aware that their parents are absent when they cannot see them.

During ages 19 to 24 months the child is in the final sensorimotor stage, invention of new means through mental combinations. This stage completes the more primitive, autistic thought processes of infancy and prepares the way for more complex mental operations during the phase of preoperational thought. One of the most dramatic achievements of this stage is in the area of object permanence. Children will now actively search for an object in several potential hiding places. In addition, they can infer a cause when only experiencing the effect. They can infer that an object was hidden in any number of places even if they only saw the original hiding place.

Imitation displays deeper meaning and understanding. Earlier, imitation was concrete and action oriented. For example, "bye-bye" was a behavioral response more than a conceptual gesture of departure. Now it has a broader meaning, such as Daddy is going to work, it is time for a walk, or something is no longer present. There is greater symbolization to imitation.

One type of symbolic imitation is domestic mimicry, the imitation of household activity. Toddlers are acutely aware of others' actions and attempt to copy them in gestures and in words. They can imitate the parents' performance of a household task both physically and verbally (Fig. 14-2). Parents often remark how accurately they see themselves when the child engages in domestic mimicry. Such activity is part of the child's learning sex-role behavior. Identification with the parent of the same sex becomes apparent by the second year and represents the child's intellectual ability to differentiate models of behavior and to imitate them appropriately.

The concept of time is still embryonic, but children have some sense of timing in terms of anticipation, memory, and the limited ability to wait. They may listen to the command, "Just a minute," and behave appropriately. However, their sense of timing is exaggerated—1 minute can last an hour. Toddlers' limited attention spans also indicate their sense of immediacy and concern for the present.

Egocentrism, or the inability to envision situations from perspectives other than one's own, is evident in all aspects of

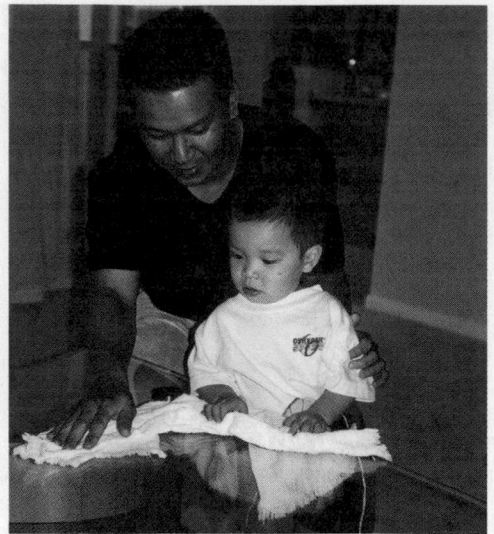

Fig. 14-2 Domestic mimicry is common during toddlerhood.

toddlers' behavior. They see, experience, and live every event in reference to themselves. A common example of egocentric behavior is the toddler who takes a toy away from another child. The toddler is concerned only with playing with the toy and is unable to conceptualize that taking the toy away will make the other child unhappy.

Preoperational Phase (Piaget)

At approximately 2 years of age the child enters the preconceptual phase of cognitive development, which lasts until about age 4 years. The preconceptual phase is a subdivision of the preoperational phase, which spans ages 2 to 7 years. The preconceptual phase is primarily one of transition that bridges the purely self-satisfying behavior of infancy and the undeveloped socialized behavior of latency. The principal characteristics of this stage are egocentric use of language and dependence on perception in problem solving.

From ages 2 to 4 years children learn a variety of words and increasingly use language. In fact, toddlers talk a lot. Speech is primarily of two types: egocentric or socialized. Egocentric speech consists of repeating words and sounds for the pleasure of hearing oneself and is not intended to communicate. This collective monologue reflects the child's lingering self-centeredness.

Socialized speech is for communication; however, it is still egocentric in that children communicate about themselves to others. Before age 3 most speech is directed at self-fulfillment or self-reference, such as, "Want drink," or "I do," and is directed mostly toward adults. Because children think that everyone else's world is the same as theirs, they expect others to understand their verbal messages even when limited information is conveyed.

Preoperational thinking implies that children cannot think in terms of operations—the ability to manipulate objects in relation to each other in a logical fashion. Rather, toddlers think primarily based on their perception of an event. Problem solving is based on what they see or hear directly rather than on what they recall about objects and events (Box 14-1).

BOX 14-1   CHARACTERISTICS OF PREOPERATIONAL THOUGHT

Egocentrism—Inability to envision situations from perspectives other than one's own
- Example—If a person is positioned between the toddler and another child, the toddler, who is facing the person, will explain that both children can see the middle person's face. The toddler is unable to realize that the other child views the middle person from a different perspective, the back.

Transductive—Reasoning from the particular to the particular
- Example—Child refuses to eat a food because something previously eaten did not taste good.

Global organization—Belief that changes in any one part of the whole changes the entire whole
- Example—Child refuses to sleep in room because location of bed is changed.

Centration—Focusing on one aspect rather than considering all possible alternatives
- Example—Child refuses to eat a food because of its color, even though its taste and smell are acceptable.

Animism—Attributing lifelike qualities to inanimate objects
- Example—Child scolds stairs for making child fall down.

Irreversibility—Inability to undo or reverse the actions initiated physically
- Example—When told to stop doing something, such as talking, child is unable to think of opposite activity.

Magical—Believing that thoughts are all-powerful and can cause events
- Example—Child wishes someone dead; then if the person dies, child feels at fault because of the "bad" thought that made the death happen.
- Example—Calling children "bad" because they did something wrong makes children feel as though they are bad.

Inability to conserve—Inability to understand the idea that a mass can be changed in size, shape, volume, or length without losing or adding to the original mass (instead, children judge what they see by the immediate perceptual clues given to them)
- Example—If two lines of equal length are presented in such a way that one appears longer than the other, the child will state that one line is longer even if he or she measures both lines with a ruler and finds that they are the same length.

Within the second year the child increasingly uses language symbolically and is concerned with the "why" and "how" of things. For example, a pencil is "something to write with" and food is "something to eat." However, such mental symbolization is closely associated with prelogical reasoning. For instance, a needle is "something that hurts." Such painful experiences take on new significance because memory is associated with the specific event and fears are likely to develop, such as resistance to people who wear uniform scrubs or rooms that look like the practitioner's office. Sometimes parents and health care personnel underestimate the child's ability to recall events and give little thought to preparation for visits to a practitioner's office or other health facility, resulting in fears that can last a lifetime. Because of the vulnerability of these early years, it is essential to prepare children for new experiences, whether it is a new baby-sitter, a primary practitioner, or a visit to the dentist.

MORAL DEVELOPMENT: PRECONVENTIONAL OR PREMORAL LEVEL

Toddlers' development of moral judgment is at the most basic level. They have little, if any, concern for why something is wrong. Kohlberg's theory of moral development is influenced by Piaget's theory of moral thought; the first phase of Kohlberg's theory is called the preconventional phase, and it involves punishment and obedience. Young children behave in accordance with the freedom or restriction that is placed on actions. In the punishment and obedience orientation, whether an action is good or bad depends on whether it results in reward or punishment. If children are punished for it, the action is bad. If they are not punished, the action is good, regardless of the meaning of the act. For example, if parents allow hitting, the child will perceive that hitting is good because it is not associated with punishment. By the age of 36 months, developmental aspects of conscience may be present.

The type of discipline also affects children's moral development. When parents use power to control behavior, such as physical punishment or withholding privileges, children receive a negative view of morals, especially toward authority figures, such as law enforcement officials. When parents withdraw love or attention, children behave primarily because of guilt, rather than from an internalization of morals. However, when parents give explanations for the misbehavior and try to help children change through positive approaches, such as consequences or rewards, children feel less hostility and are more likely to base their actions on an analysis of why an act may be wrong. Of course, the effect of discipline is not limited to the toddler years, and the sole use of explanation is inappropriate during this period. Because parents usually establish disciplinary techniques at this time, the use of constructive approaches should begin early. (See Limit Setting and Discipline, Chapter 3.)

SPIRITUAL DEVELOPMENT

Spiritual development in children is often discussed in terms of the child's developmental level because the evolution of spirituality often parallels cognitive development (Elkins and Cavendish, 2004). The child's family and environment strongly influence the child's perception of the world around him or her, and this often includes spirituality. Furthermore, family values, beliefs, customs, and expressions of these will influence the child's perception of his or her spiritual self (Elkins and Cavendish, 2004). The relationship between spirituality, illness in childhood, and nursing has been studied in the context of suffering, terminal illness such as cancer, and end-of-life care (McSherry, Kehoe, Carroll, et al, 2007; Bull and Gillies, 2007). In the past two decades there has been an increased interest in and focus on spiritual care in adults and children as further understanding of the influence of one's spirituality on health, illness, and well-being has progressed.

Toddlers learn about God through the words and the actions of those closest to them. They have only a vague idea of God and religious teachings because of their immature cognitive processes; however, if God is spoken about with reverence, young children associate God with something special. During this period the designation of powerful religious symbols and images is strongly influenced by the manner in which they are presented; therein lies the potential for the development of guilt and fear or, conversely, love and companionship with religious symbols (Roehlkepartain, Benson, King, et al, 2006).

Developmentally toddlers are unable to clearly distinguish between fantasy, make-believe, and factual representations; therefore the manner in which spiritual symbols and images are represented to them by the primary caretakers is extremely important in the ultimate development of the child's sense of self and a higher power (Roehlkepartain, Benson, King, et al, 2006).

Toddlers begin to assimilate behaviors associated with the divine (e.g., folding hands in prayer). Routines such as saying prayers before meals or at bedtime can be important and comforting. Near the end of toddlerhood, when children use preoperational thought, there is some advancement of their understanding of God. Religious teachings, such as reward or fear of punishment (heaven or hell) and moral development (see Chapter 15), may influence their behavior (Fosarelli, 2003).

DEVELOPMENT OF BODY IMAGE

As in infancy, the development of body image closely parallels cognitive development. With increasing motor ability, toddlers recognize the usefulness of body parts and gradually learn their respective names. They also learn that certain body parts have various meanings; for example, during toilet training, the genitalia become significant and cleanliness is emphasized. By 2 years of age toddlers recognize gender differences and refer to self by name and then by pronoun. By age 3 years, toddlers have developed gender identity. Also by this time the child begins to remember events with reference to their personal significance, forming an autobiographic memory that helps establish a continuous identity throughout life's events.

Once they begin preoperational thought, toddlers can use symbols to represent objects, but their thinking may lead to inaccuracies. For example, if someone who is pregnant is called "fat," they will describe all "fat" ladies (sometimes even men!) as having babies. They have a beginning recognition of words used to describe physical appearance, such as "pretty," "handsome," or "big boy." Such expressions eventually influence how children view their own bodies, and such labeling (negative or positive) becomes part of their body image.

Although little research has been done on body image development in young children, it is evident that body integrity is poorly understood and that intrusive experiences are threatening (Dahlquist, Busby, Slifer, et al, 2002). For example, toddlers forcefully resist procedures such as examining the ear or mouth and taking an axillary temperature. The procedure itself (e.g., taking vital signs) does not hurt the child, but it represents an intrusion into the child's personal space, which elicits a strong protest. Toddlers also have unclear body boundaries and may associate nonviable parts, such as feces, with essential body parts. This can be seen in a toddler who is upset by flushing the toilet and watching the stool disappear.

Nurses can help parents foster a positive body image in their child by encouraging them to avoid negative labels, such as "skinny arms" or "chubby legs"; such self-perceptions are internalized and can last a lifetime. Body parts, especially those related to elimination and reproduction, should be called by their correct names. Respect for the body should be practiced.

DEVELOPMENT OF GENDER IDENTITY

Just as toddlers explore their environment, they also explore their bodies and find that touching certain body parts is pleasurable. Genital fondling (masturbation) can occur and involves manual stimulation, as well as posturing movements (especially in young girls) such as tightening of the thighs or mechanical pressure applied to the pubic or suprapubic area. Other demonstrations of pleasurable activities include rocking, swinging, and hugging people and toys. Parental reactions to toddlers' sexual behavior influence the children's own attitudes and should be accepting rather than critical. If such acts are performed in public, parents should not condone or bring attention to the behavior, but should teach the child that it is more acceptable to perform the behavior in private (Meyer, 2002).

Children in this age-group are learning vocabulary associated with anatomy, elimination, and reproduction. Certain associations between words and functions become significant and can influence future sexual attitudes. For example, if parents refer to the genitalia as dirty, especially in the context of elimination, this association between "genitalia" and "dirty" may be transferred to sexual functions. Sex-role differences become obvious to children and are evident in much of their imitative play. A sense of maleness or femaleness, or gender identity, is formed by age 3 years, and the child's feelings about being male or female begin to form (Fonseca and Greydanus, 2007). Early attitudes are formed about affectionate behaviors between adults from observing parental and other adult sexual or sensual activities. (See also Sex Education, Chapter 15.) The quality of relationships with parents is important to the child's capacity for sexual and emotional relationships later in life (DeLamater and Friedrich, 2002).

SOCIAL DEVELOPMENT

Separation and Individuation

A major task of the toddler period is differentiation of self from significant others, usually the mother. The differentiation process consists of two phases: separation, the children's emergence from a symbiotic fusion with the mother; and individuation, those achievements that mark children's assumption of their individual characteristics in the environment. Although the process begins during the latter half of infancy, the major achievements occur during the toddler years.

Toddlers have an increased understanding and awareness of object permanence and some ability to withstand delayed gratification and tolerate moderate frustration. They begin to lose some of their resistance to separation yet appear even more concerned about the parent's whereabouts. They have learned from experience that parents exist when physically absent. Repetition of events such as going to bed without the parents but waking to find them again reinforces the reliability of such brief separations. Consequently, toddlers are able to venture away from their parents for brief periods because of the security of knowing that the parents will be there when they return. Verbal and visual reassurance from the parent gradually replaces some of the previous need to be physically close for comfort.

Toddlers also show less fear of strangers, but only when their parents are present. When left alone with a stranger, they are fearful and acutely anxious; manifest depressive behavior, such as crying and withdrawal; and may become restless, hyperactive, or passive, reverting to regressive behaviors. Such reactions may be evident when a child is left with a baby-sitter; is beginning kindergarten, preschool, or daycare; or is hospitalized. (See Chapter 26.)

These behaviors are not pathologic or harmful if parents realize how desperately their children need them. Indiscriminate friendliness toward strangers and lack of anxiety during separation from parents may be reasons for concern. Sensitive, perceptive parents will be aware of the child's need for increased love, affection, and attention when they are together. An attitude such as "They will get used to the baby-sitter" will not help young children positively tolerate separation.

According to Harpaz-Rotem and Bergman (2006), the separation-individuation phase encompasses the phenomenon of rapprochement; as the toddler separates from the mother and begins to make sense of experiences in the environment, the child is drawn back to the mother for assistance in verbally articulating the meaning of the experiences. Developmentally the term *rapprochement* means the child moves away and returns for reassurance. If the mother's response to the toddler is inappropriate, the toddler may experience insecurity and confusion.

Parents often need help in realizing the necessity of preparing children for an inevitable separation. Particularly with the firstborn, parents tend to overprotect children, shield them from any anxiety-producing experience, and insulate them from less than immediate gratification. Although this is not necessarily harmful, especially if opportunities for independence are allowed later, it does not prepare children for unexpected events. A typical example is the birth of a sibling. The child is faced with the crisis of sibling rivalry and separation from the parent. Allowing children to experience brief periods of separation during early infancy prepares them for such experiences later. Indeed, they may still manifest the typical behaviors of protest, but they will also have learned that their mother or father always returns. Therefore it is easy to appreciate the tremendous loss that the death of a parent represents for young children; unlike their other experiences with separation, this time the parent will not return.

Transitional objects, such as a favorite blanket or toy, provide security for young children, especially when they are separated from parents, are dealing with a new stress, or are just fatigued (Fig. 14-3). Security objects often become so important to toddlers that they refuse to let them be taken away. Such behavior is normal; there is no need to discourage this tendency. During separations, such as daycare, hospitalization, or even overnight stays with a relative, transitional objects should be provided to minimize any feelings of fear or loneliness.

Learning to tolerate and master brief periods of separation are important developmental tasks of children in this age-group. In addition, it is a necessary component of parenting because brief periods of separation from their children allow parents to recoup their energy and patience and to avoid directing their irritations and frustrations at the children.

Language Development

The most striking characteristic of language development during early childhood is the increasing level of comprehen-

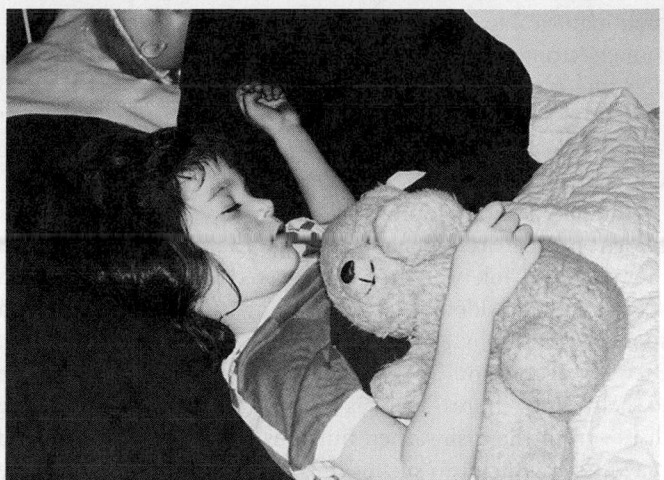

Fig. 14-3 Transitional objects, such as a warm and fuzzy stuffed animal, are sources of security to a toddler.

sion. Although the number of words acquired—from about 4 at 1 year of age to approximately 300 at age 2 years—is notable, the ability to understand speech is much greater than the number of words the child can say. Bilingual children can also achieve their early linguistic milestones in each language at the same time and produce a substantial number of semantically corresponding words in each of their two languages from the first words or signs (Petitto, Katerlos, Levy, et al, 2001).

At age 1 year the child uses one-word sentences, or holophrases. The word "up" can mean "pick me up" or "look up there." For the child the one word conveys the meaning of a sentence, but to others it may mean many things or nothing. At this age about 25% of the vocalizations are intelligible. By the age of 2 years the child uses multiword sentences by stringing together two or three words, such as the phrases, "mama go bye-bye" or "all gone," and approximately 65% of the speech is understandable. At 30 months the toddler knows her or his full name. By 3 years the child puts words together into simple sentences, begins to master grammatical rules, acquires five or six new words daily, knows his or her age and gender, and can count three objects correctly (Feigelman, 2007). Looking at books during this period provides an ideal setting for further language development (Feigelman, 2007). Authorities have evaluated the impact of television viewing on toddler language development and found that those who started watching television at less than 12 months and who watched longer than 2 hours per day had significant language delays (Chonchaiva and Pruksananonda, 2008). Adult-child conversations with infants and toddlers have been shown to positively affect language development; the researchers recommend reading, storytelling, and interactive adult-child communication (Zimmerman, Gilkerson, Richards, et al, 2009).

Gestures (such as putting phone to ear or pointing) precede or accompany each of the language milestones up to 30 months of age. Once language is sufficiently mastered, gestures phase out and the pace of word learning increases (Bates and Dick, 2002).

Personal-Social Behavior

One of the most dramatic aspects of development in the toddler is personal-social interaction. Parents frequently wonder why their manageable, docile, lovable infant has turned into a determined, strong-willed, volatile-tempered little "tyrant." In addition, the tyrant can swiftly and unpredictably revert back to the adorable infant. All this is part of growing up and is evident in such areas as dressing, feeding, playing, and establishing self-control.

Toddlers are developing skills of independence, which are evident in all areas of behavior. By age 15 months children feed themselves, drink well from a covered cup, and manage a spoon, with considerable spilling. By age 24 months they use a spoon well, and by age 36 months they may be using a fork. Between ages 2 and 3 years they eat with the family and like to help with chores such as setting the table or removing dishes from the dishwasher, but they lack table manners and may find it difficult to sit through the family's entire meal (see Table 14-3).

In dressing, toddlers also demonstrate strides in independence. The 15-month-old child helps by putting the arm or foot out for dressing and pulls shoes and socks off. The 18-month-old child removes gloves, helps with pullover shirts, and may be able to unzip. By age 2 years the toddler removes most articles of clothing and puts on socks, shoes, and pants without regard for right or left and back or front. Toddlers still need help to fasten clothes.

Toddlers also begin to develop concern for the feelings of others and develop an understanding of how adult expectations for behavior apply to specific situations (e.g., causing a sibling to cry while playing rough). As their understanding increases, they develop control. Age-appropriate discipline contributes to healthy social and emotional development. Positive reinforcement, redirection, and time-out are appropriate for most toddlers. It is recognized that social and emotional problems can develop in the youngest children. Early screening and intervention promote more positive outcomes as the young child grows and develops.

Play

Play magnifies toddlers' physical and psychosocial development. Interaction with people becomes increasingly important. The solitary play of infancy progresses to parallel play—the toddler plays alongside, not with, other children. Although sensorimotor play is still prominent, there is much less emphasis on the exclusive use of one sensory modality. The toddler inspects the toy, talks to the toy, tests its strength and durability, and invents several uses for it.

Play assumes many forms and serves several functions. Toddlers benefit from a wide variety of play interactions (alone, with other children, with adults), environments (own home, other children's homes, park), and activities (active, quiet, organized, unstructured).

Imitation is one of the most distinguishing characteristics of play and enriches children's opportunity to engage in fantasy. With less emphasis on sex-stereotyped toys, play objects such as dolls, carriages, dollhouses, dishes, cooking utensils, child-sized furniture, trucks, and dress-up clothes are used by both sexes; however, boys may be more interested than girls in activities related to trucks, trailers, cars, miniature plastic soldiers or superheroes, and building blocks, whereas girls may prefer doll-related activities (Fig. 14-4).

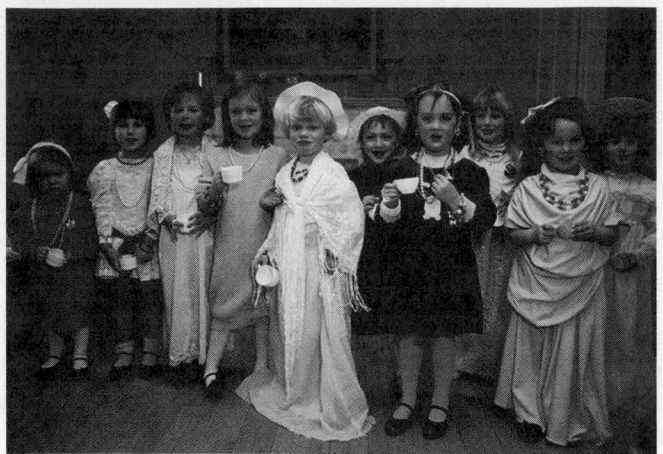
Fig. 14-4 Young children enjoy dressing up.

Increased locomotive skills make push-pull toys; stick horses; straddle trucks or cycles; a small, low gym and slide; variously sized balls; and rocking horses appropriate for the energetic toddler. Finger paints, thick crayons, chalk, chalkboard, paper, and puzzles with large, simple pieces use the child's developing fine motor skills. Interlocking blocks in varied sizes (but large enough to avoid aspiration) and shapes provide hours of fun and, during later years, are useful objects for creative and imaginative play. The most educational toy is the one that fosters the interaction of an adult with a child in supportive, unconditional play. Parents and other providers are encouraged to allow children to play with a variety of simple toys that foster creative thinking (such as blocks, dolls, and clay), rather than passive toys that the child observes (battery-operated or mechanical). Active play time should also be encouraged over the use of computer or video games, which are more passive (Ginsburg and American Academy of Pediatrics, 2007). Toys are never substitutes for the attention of devoted caregivers, but toys can enhance these interactions (Glassy, Romano, and Committee on Early Childhood, Adoption, and Dependent Care, 2003).

Certain aspects of play are related to emerging linguistic abilities. Talking is a form of play for toddlers who enjoy musical toys such as age-appropriate cassette players, talking dolls and animals, and toy telephones. Appropriate children's television programs are excellent for children in this age-group, who learn to associate words with visual images. However, parents should limit total media time to 1 to 2 hours of high-quality programming per day (American Academy of Pediatrics, 2001). Toddlers also enjoy "reading" stories from a picture book and imitating the sounds of animals.

Tactile play is also important for the exploring toddler. Water toys, a sandbox with pail and shovel, finger paints, soap bubbles, and clay provide excellent opportunities for creative and manipulative recreation. Adults sometimes forget the fascination of feeling slippery textures such as mud, catching airy bubbles, squeezing and reshaping clay, or smearing paints. These types of unstructured activities are as important as educational play to allow children freedom of expression.

TOYS

Toys are the inanimate objects with which children interact, and cognitive development appears to be related to the variety and accessibility of objects for children to explore, experiment with, and come to know. Access to playthings, particularly during the earlier years, correlates with the accessibility of caregivers who make objects available, react to children's responses to the objects, encourage further exploration, and talk about what is happening. Consequently, although they can be significant in themselves, playthings assume an especially important aspect as a medium of social interchange.

Selecting Toys

The type of toys chosen by and provided for children can facilitate learning and development in the areas just described. Toys that are small replicas of the culture and its tools help children assimilate their culture and learn gender and occupational roles. Toys that require pushing, pulling, rolling, and manipulating teach children about the physical properties of the items and help develop muscles and coordination. Such toys also allow toddlers to use newly developed fine and gross motor skills; children can push, pull and bang away on such objects and release frustration rather than acting out with inappropriate behavior. Toddlers can learn rules and the basic elements of cooperation and organization through board games.

Because they can be employed in a variety of ways, raw materials or multidimensional toys are best for enhancing skills and stimulating the imagination. Through manipulation, playthings such as boxes, clay, and blocks can assume a multitude of symbolic forms and inspire creative impulses. For example, building blocks can be used to construct a variety of structures, to count, and to learn shapes and sizes. "Educational" toys such as puzzles are less flexible. Families can encourage children's toy play in a number of ways.

Play materials do not need to be expensive or elaborate. Infants and small children get enjoyment from simple kitchen utensils such as wooden spoons and small plastic plates to bang, pot lids to clang together, and a nest of measuring spoons to rattle. Empty cartons, especially oversized ones used to ship furniture, can assume the function of clubrooms, hideaways, and other private places. For older toddlers, a mound of dirt can become a place for rolling toy cars and balls and digging holes during summer and a place for sliding in winter. Paper is a fascinating and versatile raw material for children of any age, and most books on toy materials include recipes for play dough and finger paint.

Toy Safety

The selection of toys and play equipment is a joint effort between parents and children, but evaluating their safety is the adult's responsibility. Government agencies do not inspect and police all toys on the market. Therefore adults who purchase play equipment, supervise purchases, or allow children to use play equipment need to evaluate its safety, including toys that are gifts or those that are purchased by the children themselves. Adults should also be alert to notices of defective toys and manufacturer recalls. Parents and health care workers can obtain information on a variety of recalled products and can report potentially dangerous toys and child products to the U.S. Consumer Product Safety Commission* or, in Canada, the Canadian Toy Testing Council.† Printable tips on toy safety are also available from Safe Kids Worldwide (www.safekids.org).

TEMPERAMENT

Temperamental characteristics of children during infancy tend to predominate during toddlerhood. Most difficult infants remain difficult during early childhood, but the easy infants also become less easy. Parents often perceive toddlers as more challenging, especially considering the typical negativistic traits of this age-group. Parents of easy infants may be particularly distressed by the behavior change, whereas parents of difficult children may be more prepared, because of a previously troublesome year, or be overwhelmed by the additional behaviors. The use of the Toddler Temperament Scale can assist in identifying temperamental characteristics that benefit from individualized approaches to childrearing (Stein, Carey, and Snyder, 2004). The Toddler Behavior Assessment Questionnaire has also proved to be a reliable assessment of toddler temperament and behaviors. For practitioners in a busy setting, asking parents about their impression of the child's temperament can help professionals understand the parent-child interactional process.

Stein, Carey, and Snyder (2004) emphasize that an important step in the clinical management of a child with a difficult or adverse temperament is to help the parents understand and cope with the child's behavior. The authors suggest that the recognition and discussion of temperament often elicits a positive response in the parent. Parents are often concerned that their child with an adverse temperament will develop a behavioral dysfunction that persists for a lifetime. The lack of fit between the child's temperament and the parents' expectations is often a source of conflict that may escalate if providers do not intervene (Stein, Carey, and Snyder, 2004). These authors point out that behavioral problems in children can be managed appropriately, but the child's temperament cannot be changed.

Although temper tantrums are common in toddlers, certain temperament characteristics make some children more prone to such outbursts. Active, intensely responding children are apt to yell, scream, and fling items during tantrums. Discipline is also influenced by temperament. Easy children generally respond well to mild forms of discipline, including a stern voice and sustained eye contact. However, difficult children often need more structured types of discipline, such as time-out, physical containment, or rewards, and the effectiveness of one approach may be short lived. Efforts at preventing misbehavior are especially important with children who have persistent natures. (See Limit Setting and Discipline, Chapter 3.) Without "friendly warnings" such children often have difficulty terminating an activity. These children may be punished for behavior that is merely typical of their temperament, and if the unwarranted punishment continues, the pattern can develop into a behavior problem. Slow-to-warm-up children may also present

---

*800-638-2772; www.cpsc.gov (assistance is also available in Spanish).
†1973 Baseline Road, Ottawa, Ontario K2C 0C7 Canada; 613-228-3155; fax: 613-228-3242; www.toy-testing.org.

challenges, especially when this characteristic is combined with the toddler's usual fear of strangers. These children require gradual introduction to new situations, such as daycare and baby-sitters.

COPING WITH CONCERNS RELATED TO NORMAL GROWTH AND DEVELOPMENT

Table 14-2 summarizes the major features of growth and development for the age-groups of 15, 18, 24, and 30 months. The key developmental ages are 18 and 24 months, although the chronologic ages of 15 and 30 months are also significant. Fifteen months of age is a particularly integrative period of developmental achievement because it represents the completion or fruition of many skills that were unperfected at 1 year of age.

TOILET TRAINING

One of the major tasks of toddlerhood is **toilet training.** Voluntary control of the anal and urethral sphincters is achieved sometime after the child is walking, probably between ages 18 and 24 months. However, complex psychophysiologic factors are required for readiness. The child must be able to recognize the urge to let go and hold on and be able to communicate this sensation to the parent. In addition, the child may require some motivation in the desire to please the parent by holding on, rather than pleasing oneself by letting go.

Schmitt (2004) notes that comparative studies over the past five decades indicate that children in the 1990s in the United States were toilet trained at a later age (18 months in the 1960s versus 36 months in the 1990s). One possible contributing factor is the availability and convenience of disposable diapers. Another study showed that the child's average age at initiation of toilet training was 20.6 months (Horn, Brenner, Rao, et al, 2006).

Five markers signal a child's readiness to toilet train: bladder readiness, bowel readiness, cognitive readiness, motor readiness, and psychologic readiness (Schmitt, 2004). According to some experts, physiologic and psychologic readiness is not complete until ages 22 to 30 months (Schum, Kolb, McAuliffe, et al, 2002). Choby and George (2008) suggest that the mastery of skills required for training are not present before 24 months

TABLE 14-2 GROWTH AND DEVELOPMENT DURING THE TODDLER YEARS

PHYSICAL	GROSS MOTOR	FINE MOTOR	SENSORY	LANGUAGE	SOCIALIZATION/ COGNITION
Age 15 Mo					
Steady growth in height and weight Head circumference 48 cm (19 inches) Weight 11 kg (24 lb) Height 78.7 cm (31 inches)	Walks without help (usually since age 13 mo) Creeps up stairs Kneels without support Cannot walk around corners or stop suddenly without losing balance Assumes standing position without support Cannot throw ball without falling	Constantly casting objects to floor Builds tower of two cubes Holds two cubes in one hand Releases pellet into narrow-necked bottle Scribbles spontaneously Uses cup well but often rotates spoon	Able to identify geometric forms; places round object into appropriate hole Binocular vision well developed Displays intense and prolonged interest in pictures	Uses expressive jargon Says four to six words, including names Asks for objects by pointing Understands simple commands May shake head to denote "no" Uses "no" even while agreeing to the request Uses common gestures such as putting cup to mouth when empty	Tolerates some separation from parent Less likely to fear strangers Beginning to imitate parents, such as cleaning house (sweeping, dusting), folding clothes May discard bottle Manages spoon but rotates it near mouth Kisses and hugs parents; may kiss pictures in book Expresses emotions; has temper tantrums
Age 18 Mo					
Physiologic anorexia from decreased growth needs Anterior fontanel closed Physiologically able to control sphincters	Runs clumsily; falls often Walks up stairs with one hand held Pulls and pushes toys Jumps in place with both feet Seats self on chair Throws ball overhand without falling	Builds tower of three or four cubes Release, prehension, and reach well developed Turns two or three pages in book at a time In drawing, makes stroke imitatively Manages spoon without rotation		Says 10 or more words Points to common object, such as shoe or ball, and to two or three body parts Forms word combinations Forms gesture-word combinations (points while naming) Forms gesture-gesture combinations	Great imitator (domestic mimicry) Takes off gloves, socks, and shoes, and unzips zippers Temper tantrums may be more evident Beginning awareness of ownership ("my toy") May develop dependency on transitional objects, such as security blanket

TABLE 14-2   GROWTH AND DEVELOPMENT DURING THE TODDLER YEARS—cont'd

PHYSICAL	GROSS MOTOR	FINE MOTOR	SENSORY	LANGUAGE	SOCIALIZATION/ COGNITION
Age 24 Mo					
Head circumference 49-50 cm (19.5-20 inches)	Goes up and down stairs alone with two feet on each step	Builds tower of six to seven cubes	Accommodation well developed in geometric discrimination; able to insert square block into oblong space	Has vocabulary of approximately 300 words	Stage of parallel play
Chest circumference exceeds head circumference	Runs fairly well, with wide stance	Aligns two or more cubes like a train		Uses two- or three-word phrases	Has sustained attention span
Lateral diameter of chest exceeds anteroposterior diameter	Picks up object without falling	Turns pages of book one at a time		Uses pronouns "I," "me," "you"	Temper tantrums decreasing
Usual weight gain of 1.8-2.7 kg (4-6 lb)	Kicks ball forward without overbalancing	In drawing, imitates vertical and circular strokes		Understands directional commands	Pulls people to show them something
Usual gain in height of 10-12.5 cm (4-5 inches)		Turns doorknob, unscrews lid		Gives first name; refers to self by name	Increased independence from parent
Adult height approximately double height at 2 yr				Verbalizes need for toileting, food, or drink	Dresses self in simple clothing
May be ready to begin daytime control of bowel and bladder				Talks incessantly	Develops visual recognition and verbal self-reference ("me big")
Primary dentition of 16 teeth				Able to remember and imitate arbitrary sequences of manual actions and gestures	Develops awareness that feelings and desires of others may be different and begins to explore implications and consequences
Age 30 Mo					
Birth weight quadrupled	Jumps with both feet	Builds tower of eight cubes		Gives first and last name	Separates more easily from parent
Primary dentition (20 teeth) completed	Jumps from chair or step	Adds chimney to train of cubes		Refers to self by appropriate pronoun	In play, helps put things away; can carry breakable objects; pushes with good steering
May have daytime bowel and bladder control	Stands on one foot momentarily	Good hand-finger coordination; holds crayon with fingers rather than fist		Uses plurals	Begins to notice gender differences; knows own gender
	Takes a few steps on tiptoe	In drawing, imitates vertical and horizontal strokes; makes two or more strokes for cross; draws circles		Names one color	May attend to toilet needs without help except for wiping
					Emotions expand to include pride, shame, guilt, embarrassment

of age and that there is no benefit to intensive training before 27 months of age. However, Schmitt (2004) emphasizes that parents should begin preparing the child for toilet training earlier than 30 months. By this time the child has mastered the majority of essential gross motor skills, can communicate intelligibly, is in less conflict with parents in terms of self-assertion and negativism, and is aware of the ability to control the body and please the parent. There is no universal right age to begin toilet training or an absolute deadline to complete training. One of the nurse's most important responsibilities is to help parents identify the readiness signs in their child (see Nursing Care Guidelines box).* On average, girls are developmentally ready to begin toilet training 2 to 2½ months before boys (Schum, Kolb, McAuliffe, et al, 2002).

Nighttime bladder control normally takes several months to years after daytime training. This is because the sleep cycle needs to mature so the child can awaken in time to urinate. Few children have night wetting episodes after achieving daytime dryness. However, those children who do not have nighttime dryness by the age of 6 years are likely to require intervention (Mercer, 2003).

Bowel training is usually accomplished before bladder training because of its greater regularity and predictability. The sensation for defecation is stronger than that for urination and easier for the child to recognize. A well-balanced diet that includes dietary fiber helps keep stool soft and supports the development and maintenance of regular bowel movements.

*A helpful book is *Guide to Toilet Training*, available from the American Academy of Pediatrics, 847-434-4000; www.aap.org/bookstore. Additional resources are listed in the Schmitt (2004) reference.

NURSING CARE GUIDELINES
Assessing Toilet Training Readiness

Physical Readiness
Voluntary control of anal and urethral sphincters, usually by ages 22 to 30 months
Ability to stay dry for 2 hours; decreased number of wet diapers; waking dry from nap
Regular bowel movements
Gross motor skills of sitting, walking, and squatting
Fine motor skills to remove clothing

Mental Readiness
Recognition of urge to defecate or urinate
Verbal or nonverbal communication skills to indicate when wet or has urge to defecate or urinate
Cognitive skills to imitate appropriate behavior and follow directions

Psychologic Readiness
Expressing willingness to please parent
Ability to sit on toilet for 5 to 8 minutes without fussing or getting off
Curiosity about adults' or older sibling's toilet habits
Impatience with soiled or wet diapers; desire to be changed immediately

Parental Readiness
Recognition of child's level of readiness
Willingness to invest the time required for toilet training
Absence of family stress or change, such as a divorce, moving, new sibling, or imminent vacation

 CULTURAL COMPETENCE
Toilet Training

Cultural practices influence the timing, method, and significance of toilet training. For many families in China, the timing is liberal, the method is distinct, and the significance is low. Children are diapered during infancy. Once they are walking, they wear loose pants with a long slit between the legs, and they eliminate on the ground. This practice may continue until the child is 5 years of age. In cold weather, a piece of cloth, like a "curtain," may be inserted. However, the Chinese have a concept that the buttocks are not susceptible to cold, so this is not a common practice.

A number of techniques are helpful when initiating training, and cultural differences should be considered (see Cultural Competence box). In the United States some of the options recommended by practitioners include the Brazelton child-oriented approach, the American Academy of Pediatrics guidelines (which are similar to Brazelton method), Dr. Spock's training method, and the intensive "toilet-training-in-a-day" (operant conditioning) approach by Azrin and Foxx (Choby and George, 2008). An extensive study and review by the Agency for Healthcare Research and Quality in 2006 (Klassen, Kiddoo, Lang, et al, 2006) concluded that the child-oriented method and the Azrin and Foxx methods were effective at toilet training healthy children (Choby and George, 2008). The following discussion of toilet training methods includes suggestions from the child-oriented approach.

Parents should begin the readiness phase of toilet training by teaching the child about how the body functions in relation to voiding and having a stool. Schmitt (2004) suggests that parents talk about how adults and animals perform such functions on a routine basis. Another suggestion is to make toilet training as easy and simple as possible. Important considerations are the selection of the child's clothing and the potty chair or use of the toilet. A freestanding potty chair allows children a feeling of security (Fig. 14-5, *A*). Planting the feet firmly on the floor also facilitates defecation. Another option is a portable seat attached to the regular toilet, which may ease the transition from potty chair to regular toilet. Placing a small bench under the feet helps stabilize the child's position. It is probably best to keep the potty in the bathroom and to let the child observe the excreta being flushed down the toilet to associate these activities with usual practices. If a potty chair is not available, having the child sit facing the toilet tank provides added support (Fig. 14-5, *B*). Practice sessions should be limited to 5 to 8 minutes, and a parent should stay with the child, practicing sanitary habits after every session. Parents should

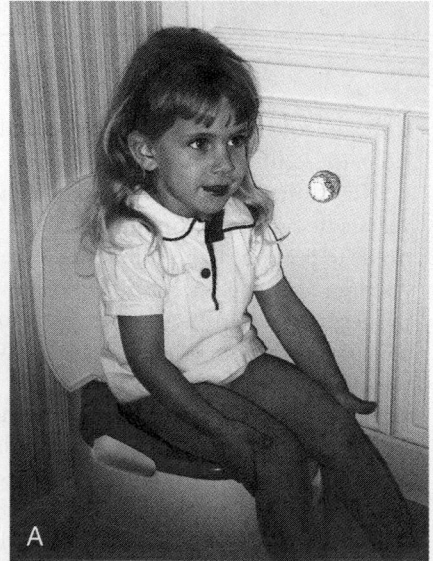
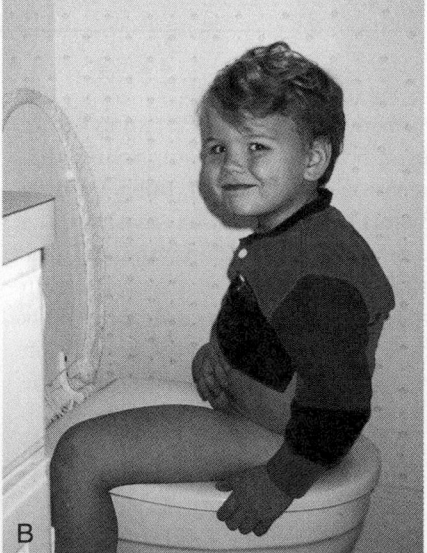

Fig. 14-5 A, Children may begin toilet training sitting on a small toilet. **B,** Sitting in reverse fashion on a regular toilet provides additional security to a young child.

praise children for cooperative behavior and successful evacuation. Dressing children in easily removed clothing; using training pants, "pull-on" diapers, or panties; and encouraging imitation by watching others are other helpful suggestions.

When the child begins to show regular daytime dryness, parents may experiment with underwear during the day. Daytime accidents are common, particularly during periods of intense activity. Recognizing the child's facial expressions when the need to urinate or defecate and suggesting a practice run to the potty is helpful. Young children become so engrossed in play activity that if they are not reminded, they will wait until it is too late to reach the bathroom. Therefore frequent reminders and trips to the toilet are necessary.

As the child develops each step of toileting (discussion, undressing, going, wiping, dressing, flushing, and hand washing), he or she gains a sense of accomplishment that parents should reinforce. If the parent-child relationship becomes strained, both may need a break to focus on enjoyable activities together. Regression may coincide with a stressful family situation or occur if the child is being pushed too hard and too fast. Regression is a normal part of toilet training and does not mean failure but should be viewed as a temporary setback to a more comfortable place for the child.

Daycare providers also play a role in the support and education of parents regarding toilet training practices. It is important for parents to inform all caregivers of their individual family values and the child's specific needs when planning for training away from home. Ensuring consistency in care of the toddler and ensuring healthy practices in a sanitary environment allow for safe and effective toilet practices in all settings.

SIBLING RIVALRY

The term **sibling rivalry** refers to the natural jealousy and resentment of children to a new child in the family. It typically involves the arrival of a new infant but may be associated with anyone who joins the family. A common example is the merging of stepfamilies (**blended families**). However, the following discussion focuses on the sibling's response to the birth of a newborn.

Toddlers do not hate or resent the infant but do resent the changes that this additional sibling brings, especially the separation from the mother during the birth. The parents now share their love and attention with someone else, the usual routine is disrupted, and toddlers may lose their crib or room—all at a time when they thought they were in control of their world. Sibling rivalry tends to be most pronounced in the firstborn, who experiences "dethronement" (loss of sole parental attention). It also seems to be most difficult for young children, particularly in terms of mother-child interaction.

Preparation of children for the birth of a sibling is individual, but age dictates some important considerations. Time is a vague concept for toddlers. A good time to start talking about the new baby is when toddlers become aware of the pregnancy and the changes occurring in the home in anticipation of the new member. Jealousy can develop from feeling left out; because fantasy dictates reality, fear of the unknown can lead to fear of abandonment, separation anxiety, and insecu-

rity. To avoid additional stresses when the newborn arrives, parents should perform anticipated changes, such as moving the toddler to a different room or bed, well in advance of the birth.

Toddlers need to have a realistic idea of what the newborn will be like. Telling them that a new playmate will come home soon sets up unrealistic expectations. Rather, parents should stress the activities that will take place when the baby arrives home, such as diapering, bottle- or breast-feeding, bathing, and dressing. At the same time, parents should emphasize which routines will stay the same, such as reading stories or going to the park. If toddlers have had no contact with an infant, it is a good idea to introduce them to one, if feasible. Providing a doll on which toddlers can imitate parental behaviors is another excellent strategy. They can tend to the doll's needs (diapering, feeding) at the same time the parent is performing similar activities for the infant, then progress to helping with the sibling (Fig. 14-6).

When the newborn arrives, toddlers keenly feel the changed focus of attention. Visitors may initiate problems when they inadvertently shower the infant with attention and presents while neglecting the older child. Parents can minimize this by alerting visitors to the toddler's needs, having small presents on hand for the toddler, and including the child in the visit as much as possible. The toddler can also help with the care of the newborn by getting diapers and doing other small tasks. It is important to involve toddlers in their new sibling's care, since even young infants learn to respond to the sounds of their siblings' voices.

How children exhibit jealousy is complex. Some openly hit the infant, push the child off the mother's lap, or pull the bottle or breast from the infant's mouth. More often the expressions of hostility and resentment are more subtle and covert. Toddlers

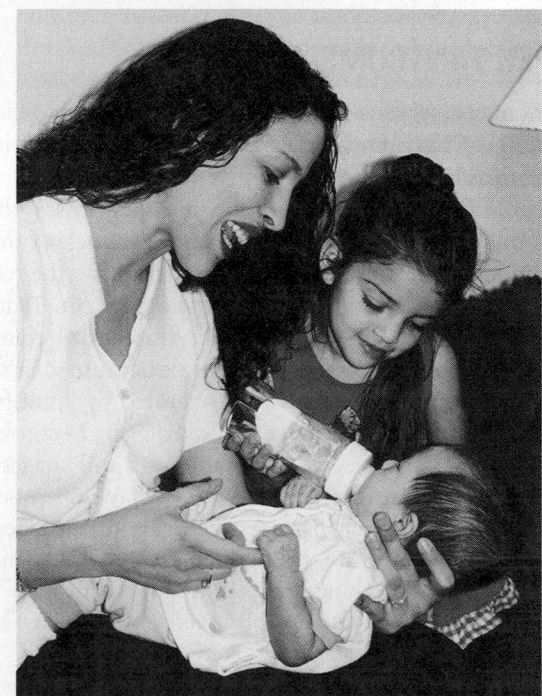

Fig. 14-6 To minimize sibling rivalry, parents should include the toddler during caregiving activities.

may verbally express a wish that the infant "go back inside Mommy," or they will revert to more infantile forms of behavior, such as demanding a bottle, soiling their diaper, clinging for attention, using baby talk, or aggressively acting out toward others. The latter is particularly common in preschoolers, who may seem to accept the new sibling at home but behave poorly in daycare or preschool. This is a form of displacement that says, "I can't let my parents know how I feel, so I will tell you." Encouraging parents to explore how their older child is acting with other caregivers is an important aspect of intervention.

Regardless of how well adjusted and accepting toddlers or preschoolers appear, infants must be protected by supervising the interaction between siblings. Other safety considerations are "baby proofing" the house and instructing children regarding the dangers to infants of small, sharp, or pointed objects. Parents should keep crib rails fully raised and the mattress lowered to discourage toddlers from picking up the infant. Infant seats or bassinets should be on the floor so that young children cannot pull them off a raised surface to see or play with the baby.

The first few weeks at home with a newborn and toddler can be challenging for parents. Assuring them that this period will pass, that the toddler will learn to accept the changes in lifestyle, and that the newborn will sleep through the night is part of the intervention. Allowing parents to talk about their feelings of ambivalence and frustration and suggesting ways of dealing with the sibling jealousy help all members of the family with this experience. Indeed, sibling rivalry is so common, regardless of the children's ages, that it is a part of family life. Suggestions such as spending time with each child, letting children settle their arguments, and accepting angry feelings while teaching children appropriate ways to express hostility are general guidelines for dealing with the eventual conflicts between brothers and sisters.

TEMPER TANTRUMS

Toddlers may assert their independence by violently objecting to discipline. They may lie down on the floor, kick their feet, and scream as loud as possible. Some have learned the effectiveness of holding their breath until the parent relents. Although holding one's breath may cause fainting from lack of oxygen, the accumulation of carbon dioxide will stimulate the respiratory control center, resulting in no physical harm. Tantrums are an indication of the child's inability to control emotions; toddlers are particularly prone to tantrums because their strong drive for mastery and autonomy is frustrated by adult figures or lack of motor and cognitive skills. Potegal, Kosorok, and Davidson (2003) analyzed temper tantrums and suggest that they are a result of two emotional and behavioral processes: anger and distress. Anger increases rapidly and peaks near the beginning of the tantrum; components of distress, such as crying and comfort seeking, increase as anger subsides. Three fourths of the temper tantrums observed in the study lasted 5 minutes or less.

The best approach toward tapering temper tantrums requires consistency and developmentally appropriate expectations and rewards. Ensuring consistency among all caregivers in expecta-

tions, prioritizing what rules are important, and developing consequences that are reasonable for the child's level of development help manage the behavior. For example, a popular time for a tantrum is before bed. Active toddlers often have trouble slowing down and, when placed in bed, resist staying there. Parents can reinforce consistency and expectations by stating, "After this story it is bedtime." Starting at 18 months, *time-outs* work well for managing temper tantrums.

During tantrums ignore the behavior, provided the behavior is not injurious to the child, such as violently banging the head on the floor. Continue to be present to provide a feeling of control and security to the child once the tantrum has subsided. At this time a toy or a favorite activity can be substituted for the request. (See also Limit Setting and Discipline, Chapter 3.) During periods of no tantrums, practice developmentally appropriate positive reinforcement.

Other suggestions for handling tantrums include (Needlman, Howard, and Zuckerman, 1995):

- Offering the child options instead of an "all or none" position
- Picking one's battles carefully and ignoring small skirmishes over unimportant issues
- Giving comfort once the child is able to control emotions but not giving in to the original request
- Praising the child for positive behavior when he or she is not having a tantrum

Temper tantrums are common during the toddler years and essentially represent normal developmental behaviors. However, temper tantrums can be signs of serious problems. Nurses should be alert to situations that require further evaluation (see Nursing Care Guidelines box).*

NURSING CARE GUIDELINES
Identifying Problem Tantrums in Children

- Parents express concern; feel angry, sad, and helpless; or report nothing positive about the child.
- Child is younger than 1 year or older than 4 years.
- Tantrums occur regularly in school.
- Tantrums are associated with aggressive, violent behavior (e.g., injuries to self or others).
- There is a history of other concerns, such as sleep disorders, food refusal, or extreme difficulty with separation from parent.
- Child holds breath and faints during tantrums.
- Child displays unusual flirtatiousness or extreme modesty (suggests possible sexual abuse).

Modified from Needlman R, Howard B, Zuckerman B: Helping parents get beyond the terrible 2's, *Patient Care* 29(1):52-61, 1995.

NEGATIVISM

One of the more difficult aspects of rearing toddlers is related to their persistent negative response to every request. The negativism is not an expression of being stubborn or disrespectful, but a necessary assertion of control. One method of dealing with negativism is by reducing the opportunities for a "no"

---

*The American Academy of Pediatrics offers a helpful brochure: *Temper Tantrums: A Normal Part of Growing Up*; 847-434-4000; www.aap.org/bookstore.

answer. Asking the child, "Do you want to go to sleep now?" is almost certain to be met with an emphatic "no." A more appropriate approach is to tell the child when it will be time to go to sleep (preferably within a specific time frame, such as "after reading a story") and proceed accordingly.

In their attempt to exert control, children like to make choices. When confronted with appropriate choices, such as "You can have a peanut butter–and-jelly sandwich or chicken noodle soup for lunch," they are more likely to choose one than to automatically say no. However, if their response is negative, parents should make the choice for the child. This behavior is frustrating for both the child and the parent. Parents need to respond in a calm, reassuring manner. Many of the suggestions for preventing misbehavior in Chapter 3 also help minimize negativism.

STRESS

Adults rarely think of young children as being exposed to stress or suffering its consequences. However, the normal demands of growing up coupled with the usual pressures most families experience mean that few, if any, young children grow up stress free. Small amounts of stress are beneficial during the early years to help children develop effective coping skills. However, excessive stress is destructive, and young children are especially vulnerable because of their limited ability to cope.

To deal with stress in their children's lives, parents must be aware of the signs of stress and be able to identify the source. The normal stresses of toddlerhood are listed in Box 14-2. Any number of other stresses may be imposed on children, such as

alternative caregiving arrangements, birth of a sibling, separation and divorce, relocation, or illness. Watching children at play can help identify stressors. For example, one child was seen pounding on a doll, yelling "Go away! Go away!" The parent was quick to observe that the child's recent irritability was probably caused by the stress of a new sibling. Other signs of increased stress in a toddler's life may include increased thumb sucking, aggressive behavior, and biting.

The best approach to dealing with stress is prevention—monitoring the amount of stress in children's lives so that levels do not exceed their coping ability. In many instances this is as simple as increasing the child's rest periods to allow for quiet recovery time. Often it involves adequately preparing the child for change, such as daycare or a new sibling. It also requires helping the child cope with stress. Unsupervised play is an excellent vehicle for releasing anger or frustration, and toys such as drums, play nails and hammer, clay, and play dough provide alternative methods of dissipating anxiety. They also begin to teach socially acceptable ways of dealing with such feelings. Another approach is the use of relaxation and imagery. Even young children can learn to "let their bodies go limp like a rag doll" or "imagine floating on a cloud."

Regression is a retreat from a present pattern of functioning to past levels of behavior. It usually occurs in instances of stress, when one attempts to cope by reverting to patterns of behavior that were successful in earlier stages of development. Regression is common in toddlers because almost any additional stress lessens their ability to master present developmental tasks. Any threat to their autonomy, such as illness, hospitalization, separation, or adjustment to a sibling, represents a need to revert to earlier forms of behavior, such as increased dependency. This can include refusal to use the potty chair; temper tantrums; demand for the bottle or crib; and loss of newly learned motor, language, social, and cognitive skills.

At first, such regression appears acceptable and comfortable for children, but on closer inspection it becomes evident that the loss of newly acquired achievements is frightening and threatening, since children are aware of their total helplessness in the recent past. Parents, too, become concerned about regressive behavior and may force the child to cope with an additional source of stress: the pressure of living up to expected standards. Brazelton (1999) suggests that these predictable times of regression, or *touchpoints*, are an opportunity to prepare parents for the next step in their child's development.

When regression does occur, the best approach is to ignore it while praising existing patterns of appropriate behavior. The child is saying, "I can't cope with this present stress and accomplish this new skill as well, but I will eventually if given patience and understanding." For this reason, it is advisable not to introduce new areas of learning when an additional crisis is present or expected, such as beginning toilet training shortly before a sibling is born or during a brief hospitalization.

Fears are common during this age and include fear of annihilation, going to sleep, animals, and engines, with the greatest fear continuing to be fear of strangers and separation from parents or other caregivers. Because fear of strangers and separation begins in infancy, it is discussed in Chapter 12. The other fears often escalate in the preschool period and consequently are discussed in Chapter 15.

BOX 14-2   SOURCES OF STRESS IN TODDLERS

Negativism—Does not like to take orders; may be contrary

Regression—Fears losing newly learned skills; may feel helpless

Rigidity—Wants own way; is upset when rituals are disrupted; dislikes interference; has difficulty coping with disrupted family routines (e.g., divorce, daycare, maternal employment)

Lack of sociability—Engages in solitary or parallel play but is generally uninterested in socializing

Self-centeredness—Believes the world revolves around her or him; does not want to share; seen with arrival of sibling

Separation anxiety—Fears being separated from parent

Stranger anxiety—Fears strangers; is shy

Toilet training—Especially if begun before the child is ready

Bedtime—Dislikes being ordered to bed; may fear bedwetting or separation from parents; may have terrifying dreams

Tantrums—May revert to temper tantrums or destructive behavior; may hit or bite

Security object—May have a security object that, if lost or misplaced, leads to great emotional upset

Overdoing—May become overstimulated or overtired

Fears—In particular, may include animals or anything that makes a loud noise

Illness and hospitalization—Source of many stressors: separation, pain, regression, rigidity, fears, and so on

Violence—Exposure to family or community violence or excessive exposure to media violence

Modified from Kuczen B: *Childhood stress: don't let your child be a victim,* New York, 1987, Dell.

PROMOTING OPTIMUM HEALTH DURING TODDLERHOOD

NUTRITION

The Feeding Infants and Toddlers Study (FITS) conducted in 2002 found that almost 70% of the energy in diets of infants and toddlers was provided by milk or formula, juices, and fruit-flavored drinks (Devaney, Kalb, Briefel, et al, 2004). Approximately one fourth of the toddlers consumed no vegetables, and about the same number consumed no fruit during the day. The food items most consumed by toddlers were cheese, breads, cookies, bananas, white potatoes, and processed meats such as hot dogs. Stang (2006) emphasizes that the FITS data indicate the diets of children in the United States place them at risk for inadequate intake of some vitamins and minerals and excessive consumption of added fats and sugars, which are poor in nutritional value. Nurses have an important role in assisting parents in making appropriate choices in foods and drinks for toddlers to promote optimal growth and prevent childhood obesity and subsequent cardiovascular disease and disability.

During the period from 12 to 18 months of age, the growth rate slows, decreasing the child's need for calories, protein, and fluid. However, the protein (13 g/day) and energy requirements are still relatively high to meet the demands for muscle tissue growth and high activity level. Estimated energy requirements (EER) for toddlers vary by age, gender, and feeding method; for example, an 18-month-old boy weighing 11.7 kg (25.8 lb) would have an EER of 961 kcal/day, whereas an 18-month-old girl with a weight of 10.9 kg (24 lb) would have an EER of 899 kcal/day (Institute of Medicine, 2005). The need for minerals such as iron, calcium, and phosphorus may be difficult to meet, considering the characteristic food habits of children in this age-group. For the toddler, fluid needs drop to approximately 115 ml/kg, representing a decrease in the relative total body water and an increase in fluid within the cells (intracellular fluid).

At approximately 18 months of age, most toddlers manifest this decreased nutritional need with a decrease in appetite, a phenomenon known as **physiologic anorexia**. They become picky, fussy eaters with strong taste preferences. Toddlers are increasingly aware of the nonnutritive function of food: the pleasure of eating, the social aspect of mealtime, and the control of refusing food. They are influenced by factors other than taste when choosing food. If a family member refuses to eat something, toddlers are likely to imitate that response. If the plate is overfilled, they are likely to push it away, overwhelmed by its size. In essence, mealtime is more closely associated with psychologic components than with nutritional ones.

Many authorities consider this period of picky eating to be a developmental phase and stress that most toddlers will consume the necessary amount of food required for growth (Cathey and Gaylord, 2004).

Developmentally, by 12 months of age most children are eating the same food prepared for the rest of the family. Some may have mastered using a cup with occasional spilling, although most cannot adeptly use a spoon until 18 months of age or later and generally prefer using their fingers. Because toddlers have unpredictable table manners, it is best to use plastic dishes and cups, for both economic and safety reasons.

The emphasis on preventing childhood obesity and cardiovascular disease in the United States has prompted a number of changes in dietary recommendations for children and adults alike. It is now recognized that lifetime eating habits may be established in early childhood, and health care workers are increasingly emphasizing the role of food selection choices, exercise, stress reduction, and other lifestyle choices (tobacco and alcohol use) on the quality of adult life and survival. The 2005 American Heart Association Dietary Guidelines for Americans encourage eating a variety of foods; maintaining ideal body weight; consuming adequate starch and fiber; and limiting intake of fat, cholesterol, sugar, salt, and alcohol. The American Heart Association recently published a scientific statement with guidelines for implementing the 2005 guidelines in children, adolescents, and adults with greater emphasis on cardiovascular disease and stroke prevention (Gidding, Lichtenstein, Faith, et al, 2009). The Dietary Guidelines for Children are appropriate for children ages 1 to 18 years, and examples of recommended choices and food serving sizes are available at the American Heart Association website (see Fig. 6-4; www.americanheart.org). In addition to these guidelines the United States Department of Agriculture recently introduced MyPlate (http://www.choosemyplate.gov/) to replace MyPyramid for Kids (see also p. 134). This colorful plate shows the 5 main food groups—fruits, grains, vegetable, protein, and dairy—with the intended purpose to involve children and their families in making appropriate food choices for meals and decrease the incidence of overweight and obesity in the United States. MyPlate provides an online interactive feature which allows the individual to select (click on) an individual food group and see choices for foods in that group. Approximate serving sizes are suggested and vegetarian substitutions are also provided (see also Dietary Intake, Chapter 6).

The requirements for most vitamins and minerals increase slightly during toddlerhood. The need for minerals such as iron, calcium, and phosphorus may be difficult to meet, considering the characteristic food habits of children in this age-group. Nutrition during toddlerhood involves a transition as a young toddler is weaned off milk- or formula-based diets. Milk intake, the chief source of calcium and phosphorus, should average two or three servings (24 to 30 oz) a day. More than a quart of milk consumption daily considerably limits the intake of solid foods, resulting in a deficiency of dietary iron and other nutrients. After 2 years of age children can be given low-fat milk to reduce daily total fat to less than 30% of calories, saturated fatty acids to less than 10% of calories, and cholesterol to less than 300 mg. Fat restriction, other than trans fatty acids and saturated fats, is not appropriate for toddlers (Allen and Myers, 2006). Other measures to reduce dietary fat include using lean meats, fat-modified products (such as low-fat cheese), and low-fat cooking. Because less fat in children's diet can also mean fewer calories and nutrients, caregivers must know what kinds of food to choose.

Iron-fortified cereals and iron-rich foods are recommended for all children beyond 6 months of age. Parents are encouraged to provide an iron-rich diet that includes heme and nonheme iron sources (red meats, poultry, fish, green leafy vegetables, dried fruit, beans) and limit whole-milk consumption. Iron supplementation may be necessary in some cases.

Calcium and vitamin D are essential for healthy bone development. Adequate intake of calcium for the child 1 to 3 years of age is 500 mg. Whole milk, cheese, yogurt, legumes (beans), and vegetables (broccoli, collard greens, kale) are good sources for calcium. Popular calcium-fortified foods include waffles, cereals and cereal bars, orange juice, and some white breads. Adequate vitamin D intake is essential to prevent rickets; it is now recommended that children and adolescents have an intake of at least 400 international units of vitamin D daily (American Academy of Pediatrics, 2009). Multivitamin preparations containing 400 international units of vitamin D are adequate if food intake is poor or exposure to sunlight is minimal; vitamin D–only preparations containing 400 international units are also available commercially (Wagner, Greer, and American Academy of Pediatrics, 2008). Sources of vitamin D include fish, fish oils, and egg yolks; additionally, the consumption of 1 quart of vitamin D–fortified milk provides 400 international units of vitamin D. Fortified cereals, dairy products, and meat are also good sources of zinc and vitamin E.

The American Heart Association (Gidding, Dennison, Birch, et al, 2005) recommends that toddlers have 1 cup of fruit each day. Vitamin C enhances iron absorption. Toddlers should consume approximately 4 to 6 oz of 100% fruit juice per day. It tastes good to toddlers and is readily available. A 6-oz glass of fruit juice equals one fruit serving; however, juices lack the fiber of whole fruit and should not be used as a substitute. High intake of juice can contribute to diarrhea, overnutrition or undernutrition, and the development of caries; thus only 4 to 6 oz of 100% fruit juice per day are recommended (American Academy of Pediatrics, 2009). Fruit-flavored drinks advertised as juices may not actually contain 100% juice and should be avoided.

Nutritional Counseling

Eating habits established in the first 2 to 3 years of life tend to have lasting effects on subsequent years. If food is used as a sign of approval, a child may overeat for nonnutritive reasons. If parents force food and mealtime is consistently unpleasant, the usual pleasure associated with eating may not develop. Mealtimes should be enjoyable rather than times for discipline or family arguments. The social aspect of mealtime may be distracting for young children; therefore an earlier feeding hour may be appropriate. Young children are unable to sit through a long meal and become restless and disruptive. This is particularly common when children are brought to the table just after active play. Calling them in 15 minutes before mealtime allows them to get ready for eating while settling down their active minds and bodies.

Frequent, nutritious, *planned* snacks can replace a meal; however, these should not replace a regular sit-down meal. "Grazing"—nibbling and snacking—is a good way to ensure proper nutrition, provided that appropriate foods are offered and this does not fill up the child just prior to a regular meal.

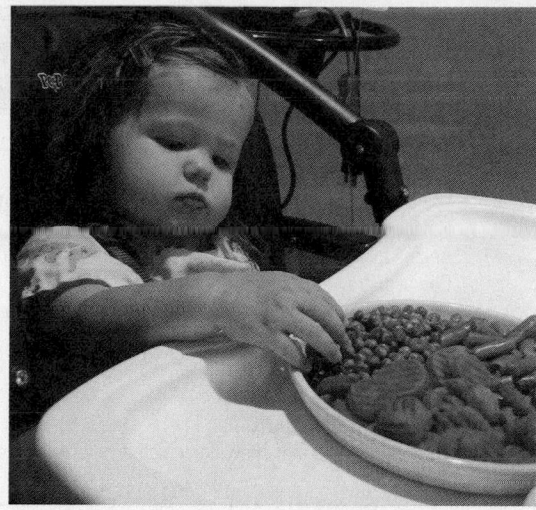

Fig. 14-7 Toddlers enjoy finger foods such as green peas. (Courtesy E. Jacobs, Texas Children's Hospital, Houston.)

Between-meal snacks can provide significant nutrition, especially calories, protein, carbohydrate, calcium, and vitamin C. For snacks, parents can place several small pieces of food (carrot sticks, cheese blocks, raisins, crackers, sliced cold meat, apple slices) in an ice cube tray for a pick-and-choose menu. Toddlers like to eat with their fingers and enjoy foods of different colors and shapes (Fig. 14-7).

The method of serving food also takes on more importance during this period. Toddlers need to feel in control and to have a sense of achievement. Giving them large, adult-size portions contributes to their feeling overwhelmed. In general, what is eaten is much more significant than how much is consumed. Small amounts of meat and vegetables supply greater food value than a large consumption of bread or potato. Parents can provide substitutions for foods children do not enjoy, although this practice should not cater to all their desires.

Serving sizes need to be appropriate for age. It is often a good idea to offer less than toddlers may eat and let the child ask for more. A general guide to the serving size of food is 1 tbsp of solid food per year of age or one fourth to one third the adult portion size. Use the tablespoon guide for easily measured foods such as vegetables or rice. Use the fraction guide for milk, bread, or fruit.

The ritualism of this age also dictates certain principles in feeding practices. Toddlers like to have the same dish, cup, or spoon every time they eat. They may reject a favorite food simply because it is served in a different dish. If one food touches another, they often refuse to eat it. Mixed foods, such as stews or casseroles, are rarely favorites. Because toddlers have unpredictable table manners, it is best to use plastic dishes and cups, for both economic and safety reasons. For some children a regular mealtime schedule also contributes to their desire and need for predictability and ritualism.

Appetite and food preferences are sporadic during these years. A child may enjoy one food for 3 days in a row and then suddenly refuse to eat it again for days. Such food fads (or "jags") do not ensure a well-balanced diet, but attempts to alter them are met with resentment and obstinacy. It is preferable to accept such extremes and offer other foods in small portions.

TABLE 14-3	DEVELOPMENTAL MILESTONES ASSOCIATED WITH FEEDING
AGE (mo)	**DEVELOPMENT**
12-18	Drools less
	Drinks well from cup with lid but may drop it when finished
	Holds cup with both hands
	Begins to use spoon but turns it before reaching mouth
24	Can use straw and cup
	Chews food with mouth closed, and shifts food in mouth
	Distinguishes between finger and spoon foods
	Uses spoon correctly but with some spilling
36	Spills small amount from spoon
	Begins to use fork; holds it in fist
	Uses adult pattern of chewing, which involves rotary action of jaw

Generally, the child will choose another "favorite food" that may compensate for the nutritional inadequacy.

Developmentally, by 12 months of age most children are eating the same food prepared for the rest of the family. Some may have mastered using a cup with occasional spilling, although most cannot adeptly use a spoon until 18 months of age or later (Table 14-3) and generally prefer using their fingers. Some children find weaning easy and voluntarily relinquish the breast or bottle by the first birthday. Others are unable to give up that pleasure and require a bottle before bedtime or occasionally during the day. Allowing children to give up the bottle when they are ready is preferable to forcing the issue.

This period can be trying for parents and child alike. Because eating habits established in early life affect not only the child's future eating habits but also the child's health as an adolescent and adult, it is recommended that toddlers not be forced to eat foods they are reluctant to eat. Evidence indicates that toddlers are able to regulate their hunger and satiety needs internally and that forcing foods during this period may lead to future eating problems (Cathey and Gaylord, 2004).

SLEEP AND ACTIVITY

Total sleep time decreases only slightly during the second year and averages about 11 to 12 hours. Most toddlers take one nap a day, and by the end of the second or third year many relinquish this habit. The activity level is high, and rarely is there a problem with too little physical exercise, provided that inappropriate restrictions are not instituted. Recently, however, there has been concern that decreased time spent in actual physical play and more time involved with computers and television watching has increased the tendency toward being overweight. This is especially true in large urban centers during the winter months where there may not be adequate "safe" play and physical exercise space. With increasing numbers of young children being cared for outside the home, attention to the kinds of activity provided is important. For example, children with high activity levels may benefit from an environment that encourages vigorous play whether outside or in a large indoor play area.

Toddlers are more prone to having bedtime resistance (refusal to go to bed) and frequent night waking; during later toddlerhood this group of children may become more resistant about going to bed and express fears about monsters (Meltzer and Mindell, 2006). Sleep problems, especially going to bed and falling asleep, are common and are probably related to fears of separation. Bedtime rituals (same hour of sleep, snack, quiet activity) are helpful, and transitional objects, such as a favorite stuffed animal or blanket, can ease the insecurity at bedtime. For problems that persist, parents should employ the interventions outlined in Table 12-4.

DENTAL HEALTH

Regular Dental Examinations

The American Academy of Pediatric Dentistry (2009) now recommends that every child have an oral health examination by a practitioner by the age of 12 months. Initial visits to the dentist should be nontraumatizing. Because toddlers react negatively to new and potentially frightening experiences, the initial visit can center around meeting the dentist, seeing the equipment, and sitting in the chair. If the child is cooperative, the dentist may just look at the teeth but reserve a more thorough examination for another visit. Modeling, in which the child observes procedures performed on the parent or a cooperative sibling, can also be effective but may not work with all toddlers.

Removal of Plaque

Oral hygiene measures should be implemented as noted above to remove plaque, soft bacterial deposits that adhere to the teeth and cause **dental caries** (decay or cavities) and **periodontal** (gum) **disease**. Poor oral hygiene and poor dietary habits are associated with the development of caries in children. The most effective methods for plaque removal are brushing and flossing. Several brushing techniques exist, although there is no universal agreement regarding the best method. One that is suitable for cleaning the primary teeth is the scrub method. The tips of the bristles are placed firmly at a 45-degree angle against the teeth and gums and moved back and forth in a vibratory motion. The ends of the bristles should be wiggling but not moving forcefully back and forth, which can damage the gums and enamel. All the surfaces of the teeth are cleaned in this manner except the lingual (inner) surfaces of the anterior teeth. To clean these surfaces, the toothbrush is placed vertical to the teeth and moved up and down. Only a few teeth are brushed at one time, using six to eight strokes for each section. A systematic approach is used so that all surfaces are thoroughly cleaned (Fig. 14-8).

For young children, the most effective cleaning is done by parents (Fig. 14-9). Several positions can be used that facilitate access to the mouth and help stabilize the head for comfort:

- Stand with child's back toward adult. (When done in front of a bathroom mirror, both child and adult can see what is being done in the mirror.)
- Sit on a couch or bed with child's head resting in adult's lap.
- Sit on the floor or a stool with child's head resting between adult's thighs.

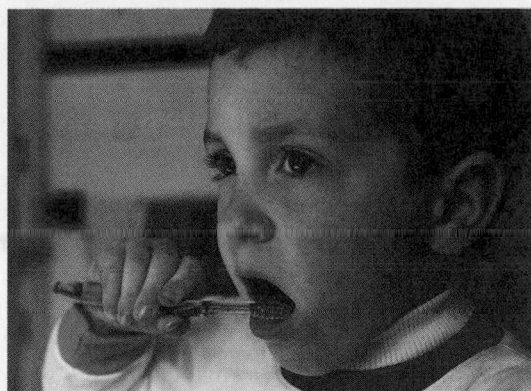

Fig. 14-8 Young children can participate in toothbrushing.

TABLE 14-4	DIETARY FLUORIDE SUPPLEMENTATION		
	WATER FLUORIDE CONTENT (ppm)		
AGE	**<0.3**	**0.3-0.6**	**>0.6**
Birth-6 mo	0	0	0
6 mo-3 yr	0.25	0	0
3-6 yr	0.50	0.25	0
6-16 yr	1.00	0.50	0

From American Academy of Pediatric Dentistry: *Reference manual, 2009-2010: guideline on fluoride therapy,* 31(6):128-129, 2009, available at www.aapd.org/media/Policies_Guidelines/G_FluorideTherapy.pdf (accessed January 6, 2010).

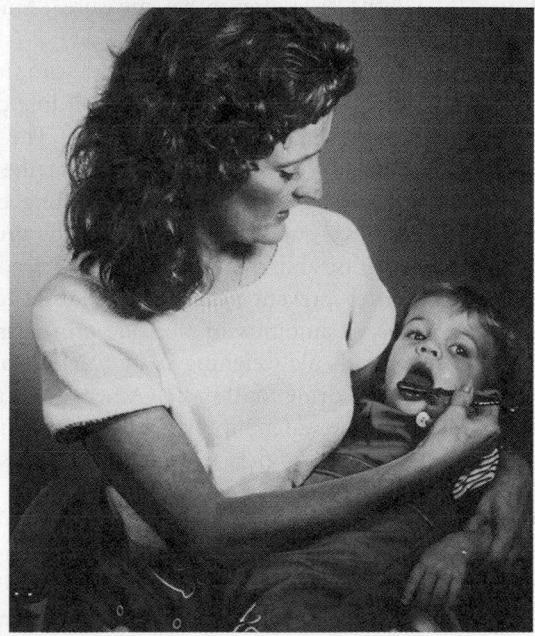

Fig. 14-9 The most effective cleaning of the teeth is done by parents.

Use one hand to cup the chin and the other to brush the teeth. For easier access to back teeth, hold the mouth partially open.

For effective cleaning, a small toothbrush with soft, rounded, multitufted nylon bristles that are short and uniform in length is recommended. Nylon bristles dry more rapidly after use and retain their shape better than natural bristles. Toothbrushes are replaced as soon as the bristles are frayed or bent. With young children, brushing may be more easily accomplished using only water, since many children dislike the foam from toothpaste and the foam interferes with visibility. There is also the danger of swallowing fluoridated toothpaste (see following discussion under Fluoride). When using toothpaste, children should select the flavor they like to encourage the brushing habit.

After the teeth have been cleaned, the teeth are flossed with dental floss to remove plaque and debris from between the teeth and below the gum margin, where brushing is ineffective. Since young children do not have the dexterity to manipulate the floss, parents are taught the procedure.

A disclosing agent is helpful in identifying those areas of the teeth where plaque accumulates. It also helps motivate children to clean their teeth because plaque is difficult to see. After cleaning, the mouth is inspected to ensure that all traces of plaque have been removed. Where plaque remains, the teeth are rebrushed.

Ideally, the teeth should be cleaned after each meal and especially before bedtime, and the child should be given nothing to eat or drink after the night brushing except water. When brushing is impractical, the "swish-and-swallow" method of cleaning the mouth is taught: with a mouthful of water the child rinses the mouth and swallows, repeating the procedure three or four times.*

Fluoride

Consider fluoride supplementation for any child over the age of 6 months whose drinking water is deficient in fluoride. Supplementation based on fluoride concentration of water supply at less than 0.3 ppm is 0.25 mg for a child age 6 months to 3 years of age (American Academy of Pediatric Dentistry, 2009).

Fluoride, a mineral, is found in water, foods, or drinks in which fluoridated water is used as part of the processing system. Because the water fluoridation process and manufacturing of fluoride toothpaste are almost impossible to standardize in the United States, the dosage of fluoride supplements has been lowered to reduce the incidence of fluorosis, a condition characterized by an increase in the degree and extent of the enamel's porosity (Table 14-4). Increased fluoride ingestion leads to enamel protein retention, hypomineralization of the enamel and dentin, and disturbance of crystal formation. Fluorosis can cause staining of the teeth (chalky white to yellow or brown), barely discernible white fiberlike lines, or, in more severe forms, spots to gray-brown stains or pitted areas (see Community Focus box).

Fluoride toothpaste reduces caries even further when the water supply is fluoridated, since it imparts a topical benefit to the teeth. However, a concern with fluoride toothpaste used in conjunction with other sources of fluoride is excessive fluoride ingestion by young children and the possibility of fluorosis. To prevent excessive intake, only a smear of toothpaste should be used for children under 2 years and for children aged 2 to 5 years a pea-sized amount (0.25 g) of toothpaste (American

*More detailed information can be obtained from the American Academy of Pediatric Dentistry, **www.aapd.org**.

COMMUNITY FOCUS

An Optimum Fluoride Regimen in Young Children

Base recommendations on the fluoride concentration in child's drinking water, including bottled water, filtered water, and well water.

If the water is fluoridated, encourage use of tap water for drinking and for preparation of formula (except soy formula, which has twice the fluoride of regular formula), frozen-concentrated juices, powdered mixes, soups, ice, and gelatin.

If the water is nonfluoridated or contains less than 0.3 ppm (ages 6 months to 3 years) or less than 0.6 ppm (ages 3 to 6 years) fluoride, or if child refuses to drink tap water or refuses drinks or foods made with tap water, consider fluoride supplements.

If the water, such as water from some wells or springs, has a concentration of fluoride above the recommended level, encourage use of bottled nonfluoridated water for drinking.

Encourage supervision of toddler when brushing teeth or using a fluoridated mouth rinse to prevent overingestion of fluoridated topical supplement.

Use fluoridated toothpaste only in children 2 years old and older.

Consider other sources of fluoride from diet, such as tea.

If fluoride supplements are needed, give special instructions to family, including:

- Give supplements on an empty stomach without calcium-rich products, such as milk or cheese.
- Do not give food or drink for at least 30 minutes after taking the supplement.
- Place drops on tongue; it should be mixed with saliva and swished around in the mouth so that fluoride comes in contact with the teeth.
- Chewable tablets should be chewed and then mixed with saliva and swished in mouth for 30 seconds so that fluoride comes in contact with the teeth.
- Store fluoride products away from toddlers to avoid overingestion.
- Keep only a 4-month supply.
- Administer supplement at same time daily; post reminders if necessary.

Stress that dental appointments should be scheduled every 6 months for professional topical fluoride treatment.

Fluoride rinses are usually only suggested for children at high cariogenic risk or over the age of 6 years.

Modified from American Academy of Pediatric Dentistry: *Reference manual 2009-2010: guideline on fluoride therapy,* 31(6):128-129, 2009, available at www.aapd.org/media/Policies_Guidelines/G_FluorideTherapy.pdf (accessed January 6, 2010).

Academy of Pediatric Dentistry, 2009). Fluoride may also be recommended by the dentist as a mouth rinse for children old enough to swish the rinse in the mouth and spit it out instead of swallowing the rinse. Although the prevalence of dental enamel fluorosis in children has increased over the past 30 years (American Academy of Pediatrics, 2009), a specific cause in each case has yet to be identified (Erdal and Buchanan, 2005). There are concerns that the increased amount of fluoride found in community drinking water, in addition to fluoride in water-based beverages such as reconstituted formula, may be a contributing factor (American Academy of Pediatrics, 2009; Marshall, Levy, Warren, et al, 2004). Ismail and Hasson (2008) examined a number of studies and found only weak and inconsistent evidence that fluoride supplements prevent dental caries in primary teeth, but the effect on permanent teeth was significant; the researchers also noted that the children under 3 years of age who used fluoride supplements had a mild to moderate increase in dental fluorosis.

The American Academy of Pediatrics (2009) does not recommend the use of fluoridated toothpaste in children 2 years of age and younger.

Caution parents against regular use of fluoridated water or infant beverages containing fluoride if the community water supply already has an adequate amount of fluoride (see Table 14-4). Fluorosis is not a health concern but may be a cosmetic concern for affected children. Ingesting excessive fluoride after age 5 or 6 years does not result in fluorosis, since the permanent teeth, except for the third-year molars, are completely calcified.

If children primarily consume water from another source other than the public water supply (e.g., bottled water), a fluoride supplement or rinse may be required. Professional fluoride treatments may be administered to children at risk for caries at routine dental visits as a preventive measure (American Academy of Pediatric Dentistry, 2009).

Nurses have a responsibility to ensure an optimum fluoride regimen for children and to counsel families regarding correct use of fluoride mouth rinses and supplements. The nurse should have knowledge of the fluoride content of the community water supply and instruct parents regarding correct administration of fluoride supplements. All fluoride products (toothpaste, supplements, and rinse) need to be stored away from young children to prevent poisoning. Fluoride toxicity may occur if significant amounts of fluoride are ingested; a toxic dose for a 12-month-old weighing 10 kg (22 lb) would be 50 ml of a 1000 ppm fluoride toothpaste (American Academy of Pediatrics, 2009). If the water supply is fluoridated, encourage parents to use tap water to prepare drinks and foods.

Dietary Factors

Nutrition is critical to developing good teeth because the carious process depends primarily on fermentable sugars, especially sucrose. Refined table sugar is not the only concentrated sweet food that is cariogenic. Natural foods, including honey, molasses, corn syrup, and dried fruits such as raisins, are highly cariogenic. Complex carbohydrates, such as breads, potatoes, and pasta, also contribute to caries because they lower the plaque pH. (See Dental Disorders, Chapter 18.)

The more cariogenic foods are those that are sticky or hard because they remain in the mouth longer. Thus sucking on lollipops is more cariogenic than eating a chocolate bar. The consumption of sweetened carbonated beverages has increased among children and these drinks have significant potential for causing caries. Sometimes the source of the sugar is "hidden," as in numerous prescription and nonprescription drugs and in many popular cereals, including the "all-natural" variety. Reading food labels is essential in identifying and eliminating sources of sucrose. Ideally, parents should eliminate foods containing high amounts of sucrose. However, since this is impractical, some suggestions can be helpful. First, the frequency with which sugar is consumed is more important than the total amount eaten. Sweets are less damaging if consumed immediately after a meal rather than as a snack between meals. When sweets are served as the dessert, the teeth can be cleaned afterward, decreasing the amount of time the sugar is in the mouth.

These suggestions can help parents plan "treats" in a way that is less damaging to the teeth. In addition, parents should be aware of foods that are good snacks and that contribute less to tooth decay. Some snacks do not contribute to tooth decay and may actually protect against it. Aged cheeses, such as cheddar, may alter the pH and retard bacterial growth. Sugarless gum chewed for about 20 minutes after eating may also protect against cavities by stimulating saliva that neutralizes acid, and saliva itself may have caries-protective factors. The artificial sweeteners saccharin and aspartame are noncariogenic, and sorbitol has low cariogenic potential.

! NURSING ALERT

The response to an accidental dislodgment (avulsion, when a tooth is knocked out of the socket) of a primary tooth in a toddler is to place the tooth in milk, saline, or saliva and notify the child's dentist. The dentist may be able to replace the tooth in the socket; however, current guidelines suggest that replantation of a completely avulsed primary tooth may cause more harm than benefit to the child (Flores, Malmgren, Andersson, et al, 2007) (see Emergency Treatment box). If necessary, a temporary removable appliance may be indicated.

✚ EMERGENCY TREATMENT

Dental Trauma

- Keep the child calm.
- Clean the bleeding wound with a saline solution (0.9%) or tap water.
- Stop bleeding by applying pressure with a cotton ball or gauze sponge for 5 minutes.
- Some skin injuries to the mouth, lips, or gum may require suturing (see primary care physician).
- For minor dental injuries such as a chipped tooth or a tooth knocked out of the socket, see a pediatric dentist.

Modified from Flores MT: Traumatic injuries in the primary dentition, *Dental Traumatol* 18(6):287-298, 2002.

A special form of tooth decay in children between 18 months and 3 years of age is **early childhood caries (ECC)** (historically called *nursing caries* or *baby bottle tooth decay*). This often occurs when the child is routinely given a bottle of milk or juice at naptime or bedtime or uses the bottle as a pacifier while awake. Frequent nocturnal breast-feeding for prolonged periods also leads to extensive destruction of the teeth. The practice of coating pacifiers in honey can also contribute to caries and may be a potential source of botulism poisoning. As the sweet liquid pools in the mouth, the teeth are bathed for several hours in this cariogenic environment. Prolonged bottle-feeding well into toddler years in the Mexican-American culture may contribute to significant ECC (Brotanek, Schroer, Valentyn, et al, 2009). In one group prolonging bottle-feeding into toddlerhood was perceived as "buying time" to decrease the child's crying (Freeman and Stevens, 2008). The maxillary (upper) incisors and sometimes molars are affected most because the mandibular (lower) teeth are protected by the lower lip, tongue, and saliva (Fig. 14-10). Severely decayed teeth may require the application of stainless steel crowns, with or without white fronts, to preserve the spacing until the permanent teeth erupt.

ECC is now considered to be an infectious disease of childhood. There is evidence that *Streptococcus mutans* is a highly cariogenic bacteria (American Academy of Pediatrics, 2009).

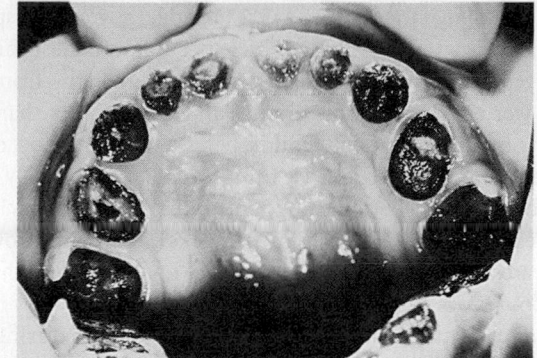

Fig. 14-10 Nursing caries. Note extensive carious involvement of maxillary primary incisors. (Courtesy Bruce Carter, DDS, Texas Children's Hospital, Houston.)

One of the early origins of *S. mutans* is the mother's saliva; infants of mothers with high counts of the bacteria have a greater incidence of ECC. Therefore it is important to discuss oral hygiene with pregnant women because of its impact on the child's tooth development. Exposure to tobacco smoke has also been linked to an increased incidence of caries in children (Shenkin, Broffitt, Levy, et al, 2004).

Prevention involves eliminating the bedtime bottle completely, feeding the last bottle before bedtime, substituting a bottle of water for sweet liquids, not using the bottle as a pacifier, and never coating pacifiers in sweet substances. Discourage juice in bottles, especially commercially available ready-to-use bottles, since the beverage is especially damaging because the sugar is more readily converted to acid. Juice should always be in a cup to avoid prolonging the bottle-feeding habit.

Nurses are in an excellent position to counsel parents regarding this habit, especially if it occurs during hospitalization. Although the child may need the comfort of the bottle at this stressful time, nurses can show parents photographs depicting the typical tooth destruction and give them literature about the condition.* Over an extended hospital stay, children can be gradually weaned from the bedtime bottle or given a bottle of water.

INJURY PREVENTION

🌐 According to recent data from the Centers for Disease Control and Prevention (Borse, Gilchrist, Delinger, et al, 2008), children ages 1 to 4 years had the second highest rate of deaths from accidental injuries in the United States during the period from 2000 to 2006; the group with the highest number of deaths (56%) from accidental injuries were children ages 15 to 19 years. Males were involved almost twice as often as females in deaths attributed to unintentional injury. Among children ages

---

*Sources of information about nursing caries and other aspects of child dental health include the National Institute of Dental and Craniofacial Research, National Institutes of Health, Bethesda, MD 20892-2190; 301-496-4261; www.nidcr.nih.gov; American Academy of Pediatric Dentistry, 211 E. Chicago Ave., Suite 1700, Chicago, IL 60611; 312-337-2169; www.aapd.org; American Dental Association, 211 E. Chicago Ave., Chicago, IL 60611; 312-440-2500; www.ada.org; and Canadian Dental Association, 1815 Alta Vista Drive, Ottawa, Ontario K1G 3Y6; 613-523-1770; www.cda-adc.ca.

Skill—Instructing Families in Child Safety

1 to 4 years of age the leading causes for death were transportation related (including motor vehicle occupant, pedestrian, and pedal cyclist), drowning, and fires or burns. Deaths from poisoning were higher among infants and adolescents than toddlers. Nonfatal injuries in children ages 1 to 4 years of age occurred as a result of falls (leading cause), followed by being struck by or against something, and bites or stings (including dog bites and bee or other insect attacks). Nonfatal drowning injury rates and nonfatal poisoning were higher among children ages 1 to 4 years than any other age-group.

A major factor in the critical increase of injuries during early childhood compared with the number in preschoolers and school-aged children is the unrestricted freedom achieved through locomotion combined with an unawareness of danger within the environment. Specific categories of injuries and appropriate prevention are best understood by associating them with the major developmental achievements of young children. The discussions of injuries in Chapters 1, 12, and 15 are also relevant to safety concerns at this age.

Motor Vehicle Injuries

Motor vehicle injuries cause more accidental deaths in all pediatric age-groups after age 1 year than any other type of injury or disease and are responsible for a significant number of all accidental deaths among children ages 1 to 4 years. Many of the deaths are caused by injuries within the car when restraints have not been used or age-related guidelines have not been properly followed. Unrestrained children riding in the vehicle's front seat are at the highest risk for injury (Durbin, Chen, Smith, et al, 2005). Approved restraints properly installed and applied can reduce the majority of fatalities and injuries (American Academy of Pediatrics, 2010; Schnitzer, 2006).

Nurses are responsible for educating parents regarding the importance of car restraints and their proper use. Five types of restraints are available: (1) infant-only devices, (2) convertible models for both infants and toddlers, (3) boosters, (4) safety belts, and (5) devices for children with special needs (see Chapter 22). Chapter 12 discusses the infant-type restraints; convertible restraints and boosters are included here. The convertible restraint is suitable for infants in the rearward-facing position (Fig. 14-11). It has been recently recommended that children ride in a convertible seat in a rear-facing position to the highest weight or height allowed by the manufacturer of the seat; this recommendation includes children aged 12 to 23 months of age (Bull and Durbin, 2008).

One study showed that children from birth to 23 months experienced fewer injuries when riding in rear-facing car restraints (Henary, Sherwood, Crandall, et al, 2007). Another study indicated that children 0 to 3 years of age riding properly restrained in the middle of the back seat had a 43% lower risk of injury than children riding in the outboard (window) seat during a crash (Kallan, Durbin, and Arbogast, 2008).

A convertible safety seat is positioned semireclined and facing the rear of the car for a child younger than 1 year weighing less than 9 kg (20 lb). The seat is positioned upright and facing forward for an older and heavier child (up to 18 kg [40 lb]). Convertible safety seats should be used until the child weighs at least 13.6 kg (30 lb) or more regardless of age and as long as the child fits properly into the seat (American Academy of Pediatrics, 2010). Convertible restraints use different types of harness systems: a five-point harness that consists of a strap over each shoulder, one on each side of the pelvis, and one between the legs (all five come together at a common buckle); and a padded shield that uses shoulder straps attached to a shield that is held in place by a crotch strap. With both the infant and toddler restraints, it is important not to add extra blankets, head cushions, or padding between the child and the restraint straps that did not come as original equipment because these "add-ons" create spaces of air between the child and the restraint and decrease support for the back, head, and neck.

Cars with free-sliding latch plates on the lap or shoulder belt require the use of a metal locking clip to keep the belt in a tight-holding position. The locking clip is threaded onto the belt above the latch plate (Fig. 14-12, *A*). If parents have newer cars with automatic lap and shoulder belts, they need to have additional lap belts installed to properly secure the restraint.

Booster seats are not restraint systems like the convertible devices because they depend on the vehicle belts to hold the child and booster seat in place. Three booster models have been approved by the National Highway Traffic Safety Administration: the high-back belt-positioning seat (Fig. 14-12, *B*), which provides head and neck support for the child riding in a vehicle seat without a head rest; the no-back belt-positioning seat, which should be used only if the vehicle seat has a head rest; and a combination seat, which converts from a forward-facing toddler seat to a booster seat. This last model is equipped with a harness for use by toddlers; the harness may be removed and a shoulder-lap belt used when the child outgrows the harness. Booster seats are used for children who are less than 145 cm (4 feet, 9 inches) tall and who weigh 15.9 kg to 36.3 kg (35 to 80 lb, depending on the type of booster seat), typically those between 4 and 8 years of age (National Highway Traffic Safety Administration, 2009). A booster seat should be used until the child is able to sit against the back of the seat with feet hanging down and legs bent at the knees. The belt-positioning booster model raises a child higher in the seat, moving the shoulder part of the belt off the neck and the lap portion of the belt off the abdomen onto the pelvis. Children who outgrow the convertible restraint may still be able to ride safely in a booster seat until the midpoint of the head is higher than the vehicle seat back.

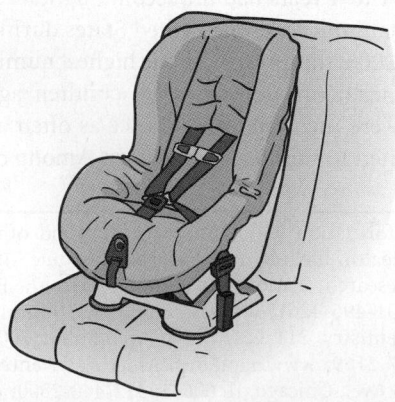

Fig. 14-11 Convertible seat in forward-facing position for older infants and children.

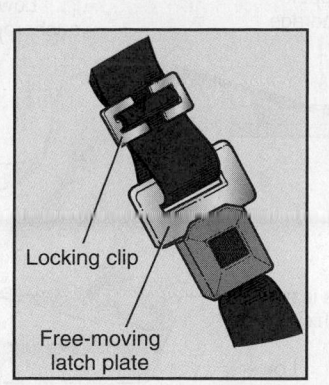

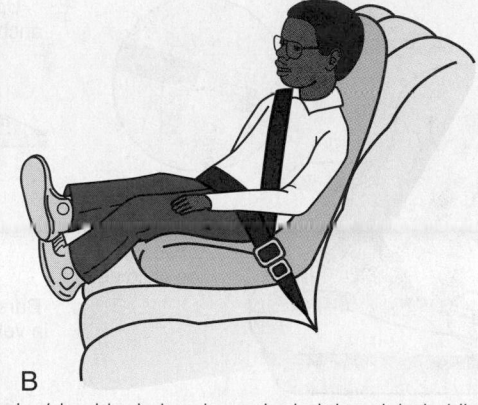

Locking clip

Free-moving
latch plate

A   B

Fig. 14-12 A, Locking clip used with free-sliding lap/shoulder belt to keep the belt in a tight-holding position. **B,** Automobile booster seat. Note placement of shoulder strap (away from neck and face).

Children should use specially designed car restraints until they are 145 cm (4 feet, 9 inches) in height or are 8 to 12 years old (American Academy of Pediatrics, 2010). Shoulder-lap safety belts should be worn low on the hips, snug, and not on the abdominal area. Children should be taught to sit up straight to allow for proper fit. The shoulder belt is used only if it does not cross the child's neck or face (see Family-Centered Care box).

FAMILY-CENTERED CARE

Summary of Car Seat Safety Guidelines for Infants and Toddlers

Infants
Infant-Only Seat
Ride facing rear of car until 1 year old, weight 9 to 10 kg (20 to 22 lb, depending on the model)
Safest in back seat
No activated front air bag if in front passenger seat; rear-facing infant seat if in front
Three- and five-point harness: adjust so clips are not at neck or throat level; should be at midchest level

Convertible Seat
Ride facing rear until 1 year old, weight 9 to 10 kg (20 to 22 lb, depending on the model)
Safest in back seat
No activated front air bag if in front passenger seat (consult manufacturer recommendation for side air bag)
Five-point harness or overhead shield

Toddlers
Convertible Seat
Must be at least 1 year old and weigh at least 9 kg (20 lb)
Convertible seat (usually up to 18 kg [40 lb]) or booster seat
Ride facing forward
No activated front air bag if in front passenger seat (consult manufacturer recommendation for side air bag)
Harness straps at or above child's shoulders

Booster Seat
Ride facing forward
No activated air bag if in front passenger seat
Lap belt low and snug across the thighs, not the stomach
Shoulder belt lying across the middle of the chest and shoulder, not neck or throat

Shoulder-only automatic belts are designed to protect adults. Children should use the manual shoulder belts in the rear seat. Air bags do not take the place of child safety seats or seat belts and can be lethal to young children. The safest area of the car for children is the back seat. Children who must ride in the passenger side of the front seat with an air bag should be positioned as far back as possible.

Built-in seats are available in some cars and vans. They may be used for children who are at least 1 year of age and weigh at least 9 kg (20 lb). Built-in seats eliminate installation problems. However, weight and height limits vary. Reinforce that owners must verify with vehicle manufacturers details about built-in seats.

For any restraint to be effective, it must be used consistently and properly. Examples of misuse include misrouting the vehicle seat belt through the restraint; failing to use the vehicle seat belt to secure the restraint; failing to use a tether strap; failing to use the restraint's harness system; and incorrectly positioning the child, especially by facing infants forward instead of rearward. To address these issues, nurses must stress correct use of car restraints and rules that ensure compliance (see Family-Centered Care box). Children riding in car safety seats are generally much better behaved than children left unrestrained, which can be a major benefit to parents and should be emphasized as an additional advantage of restraints. Additional information about child safety restraints is available from various sources.*

The LATCH (Lower Anchors and Tethers for Children) universal child safety seat system was implemented as a requirement starting in 2002 for all new automobiles and child safety seats. This system provides uniform anchorage consisting of two lower anchorages and one upper anchorage in the rear seat of the vehicle (Fig. 14-13). When used appropriately, the top anchor (tether) strap prevents the child from pitching forward in a crash. If the tether strap is not used, up to 90% of the restraint's protection is lost. Instructions for proper installation

---

*American Academy of Pediatrics, 141 Northwest Point Blvd., Elk Grove Village, IL 60007; 847-434-4000; www.aap.org; and local division of traffic safety or National Highway Traffic Safety Administration, 1200 New Jersey Ave. SE, West Building, Washington, DC 20590; 888-327-4236; www.nhtsa.dot.gov.

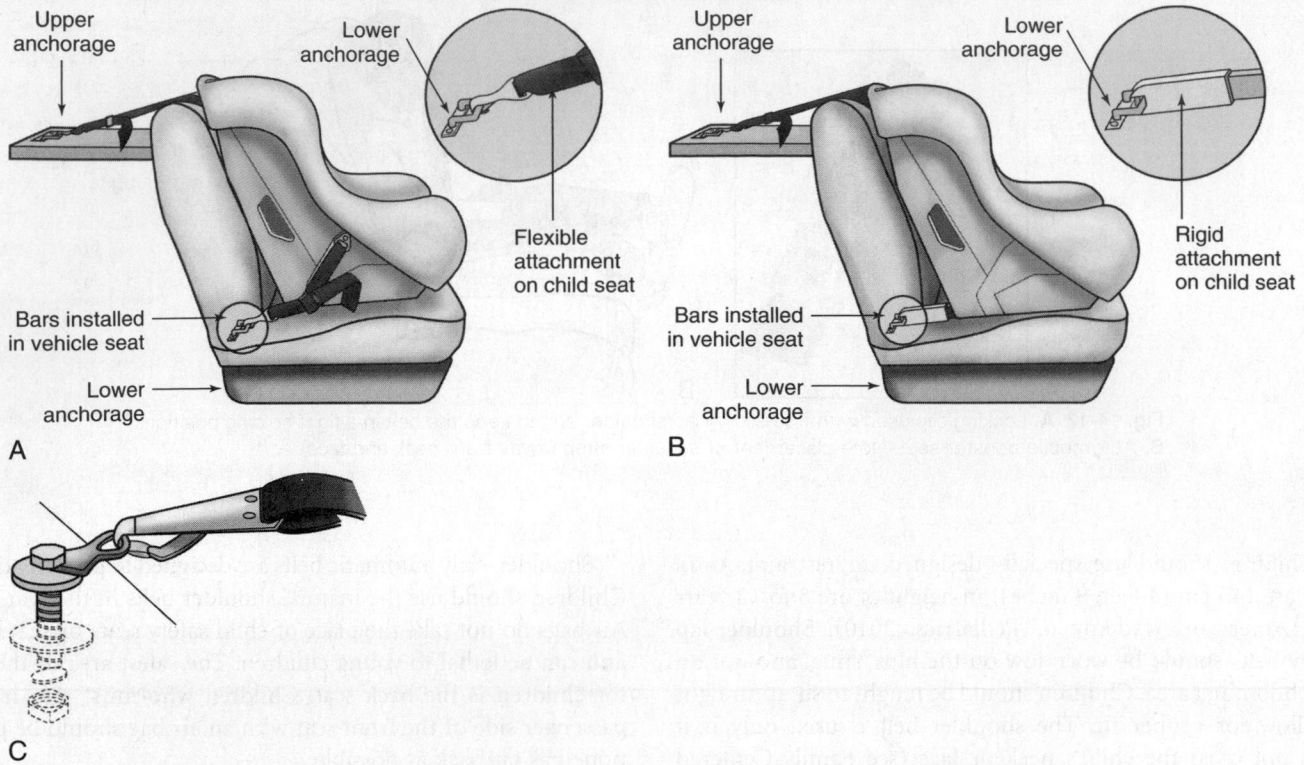

Fig. 14-13 Lower anchors and tethers for children (LATCH). **A,** Flexible two-point attachment with top tether. **B,** Rigid two-point attachment with top tether. **C,** Top tether. (Courtesy US Department of Transportation, National Highway Traffic Safety Administration.)

FAMILY-CENTERED CARE

Using Car Safety Seats

- Read manufacturer's directions and follow them exactly.
- Anchor safety seat securely to car's seat and apply harness (depending on model) snugly to child.
- Do not start car until everyone is properly restrained.
- Always use the restraint, even for short trips.
- If child begins to climb out or undo harness, firmly say, "no." It may be necessary to stop the car to reinforce the expected behavior. Use rewards, such as stars or stickers, to encourage cooperative behavior.
- Allow child to hold favorite toy, blanket, or stuffed animal in car seat.
- Encourage child to help attach buckles, straps, and shields.
- Decrease boredom on long trips. Keep special toys in car for quiet play; talk to child; point out objects and teach child about them. Stop periodically. If child wishes to sleep, make certain child stays in restraint.
- Insist that others who transport children also follow these safety rules.

---

of the tether strap and permanent bracket are included with the car restraint. New child safety seats have a hook, buckle, strap, or other connector that attaches to the anchorage. Seat belts are no longer used to anchor child safety seats to newer vehicles. The first phase required all new cars to have an upper anchorage. After fall 2002, all new cars were required to have the entire LATCH system.

Children with special needs may require a restraint system that secures them appropriately in the event of a crash. Examples of such devices include car bed restraints for infants who cannot tolerate a semireclining position and specially adapted molded-plastic chairs for children who have spica casts. The E-Z-On vest is a special safety harness for larger children with poor

trunk control. Additional safety restraints and a list of distributors are available at the SafetyBeltSafe U.S.A. website (www.carseat.org). See also Chapter 27 for discussion of preterm infants being discharged home and car seat evaluation.

Children should never ride in the open back of a truck. The danger of falls can be compounded by another vehicle striking the child or by the truck rolling over. In addition, leaving children unsupervised in a parked vehicle, especially in a private driveway, provides an opportunity for a child to release the brake or put the car in gear. The child also can be injured from a collision to or a fall from a bicycle-towed trailer or bicycle-mounted child seat.

Toddlers are often involved in pedestrian traffic injuries. Because of their gross motor skills of walking, running, and climbing and their fine motor skills of opening doors and fence gates, they are likely to be in hazardous areas unsupervised. Unaware of danger and unable to estimate the speed of a car, children are hit by moving vehicles. Running after a ball, playing in a pile of leaves or snow or inside a cardboard box, riding a tricycle, and playing behind a parked car or near the curb are common activities that may result in a vehicular tragedy.

A precaution when children are playing in driveways is to attach to the tricycle a pole with a bright flag that is high enough to be visible through an automobile's back window. Other safeguards include a device that beeps when the vehicle is driven in reverse to alert children to the oncoming car, van, or truck. Some vehicles now include a rearview video camera. Physical barriers (fences or barricades) limiting children from playing near vehicles help prevent these injuries.

Another type of injury that has become more common occurs when children crawl into an open trunk and pull it closed. Asphyxia may occur in such cases; therefore car trunks should not be left open when children are unsupervised. Some cars are equipped with a safety switch that can be activated from inside the trunk to open a closed trunk door.

Another automobile-related hazard for toddlers is overheating (hyperthermia) and subsequent death when left in a vehicle in hot weather (>27° C [80° F]). Small children dissipate heat poorly, and an increase in body temperature can cause death in a few hours. From 1998 to 2009 (July), a total of 431 children died from hyperthermia when left alone in a parked car; in 2008 the total number of child deaths was 43, and it is estimated that an average of 37 children die each year from overheating in a car (McLaren, Null, and Quinn, 2005; Null, 2009). It is estimated that with the ambient temperature at 22° to 35.5° C (72° to 96° F), the vehicle interior temperature rises by 10.5° to 11° C (19° to 20° F) for each 10 minutes, even with a window cracked (Null, 2009). In a study of 171 child fatalities from overheating in a car, 50% of adults who left a child in a car either forgot or were unaware that the child was still in the car. A significant number of those children (32) were left by family members who intended to take the child to daycare but forgot the child in the car at the workplace; 22 children were left in the car by a daycare worker or driver (Guard and Gallagher, 2005). Parents are cautioned against leaving infants alone in a vehicle for *any reason.*

Preventing vehicular injuries involves protecting and educating children about the danger of moving or parked vehicles. Although preschool children are too young to be trusted to always obey, the parent should emphasize looking for moving vehicles before crossing the street, recognizing the stop and go colors of traffic lights, and following traffic officers' signals. Physical barriers limiting children from playing near vehicles help prevent these injuries. Most important, what is preached must be practiced. Children learn through imitation, and consistency reinforces learning.

Drowning

Drowning ranks second among boys and third among girls ages 1 to 4 years as a cause of accidental death. Drowning rates in toddlers have changed little despite prevention strategies. With well-developed skills of locomotion, toddlers are able to reach potentially dangerous areas, such as bathtubs, swimming pools, wading pools, irrigation ditches, post holes, hot tubs, ponds, and lakes. Even unlikely sources of water, such as toilets and 5-gallon buckets, are dangerous (Brenner and American Academy of Pediatrics, 2003). As inquisitive toddlers lean over the rim of the receptacle, their large, heavy head, limited strength, and poor coordination make it difficult for them to extricate themselves. Therefore water in containers should be removed immediately after use. Toddlers' intense drive for exploration and investigation, combined with an unawareness of the danger of water and their helplessness in water, makes drowning always a threat. Also, death occurs within minutes, diminishing the chance for rescue and survival. Near-drowning is one of the leading causes of a vegetative state in young children. Half of all children who receive cardiopulmonary resuscitation (CPR) and survive have permanent neurologic impairment (Brenner and American Academy of Pediatrics, 2003).

Supervising children when near any source of water is essential. Participation in formal swimming lessons was associated with an 88% reduction in the risk of drowning in one study of 1- to 4-year-old children (Brenner, Taneja, Haynie, et al, 2009). In contrast, previously it was suggested that teaching children under age 4 years to swim does not provide "drown proofing" and may lead to a false sense of security (Brenner and American Academy of Pediatrics, 2003). Four-sided fencing should surround the pool and have a child-proof latch. Parents should know CPR and have a telephone and U.S. Coast Guard–approved emergency equipment at the poolside.

Burns

Toddlers' ability to climb, stretch, and reach objects above their heads makes any hot surface a potential source of danger. Children pulling pots with hot liquids, especially oil and grease, on top of themselves are a major source of burns. As a precaution, turn pot handles toward the back of the stove, and electric pots (e.g., coffee maker, frying pan, slow cooker, popcorn maker), including cords, should be placed out of reach. Ideally, the knobs for controlling the range burners should be out of reach, not on the front panel where nimble fingers can turn them on and accidentally touch the hot burner.

Other sources of heat, such as radiators, fireplaces, accessible furnaces, kerosene heaters, or wood-burning stoves, should have guards placed in front of them. The tops of some of these heaters are designed to become hot enough to boil water to provide humidity. They are hazardous if touched or if the pan of water is spilled. Portable electric heaters must be placed in a high area, well out of reach of climbing young children.

Hot objects such as candles, incense, hot embers and ashes, cigarettes, pots of tea or coffee, or irons must be placed away from children. Ashtrays with a center well are preferred to prevent the cigarette from falling off the rim, and adults should try not to smoke, cook, or drink hot liquids when children are nearby. If tablecloths are used, place the edges out of reach to prevent injuries from both burns and falling objects. When children are near smoldering fires (campfires, brush fires, fires buried on the beach), wearing shoes can help protect the feet from burns.

Flame burns represent one of the most fatal types of burns and commonly occur when children play with matches and accidentally set themselves (and the home) on fire (Fig. 14-14). All matches must be stored safely away from children, and parents need to teach children the dangers of playing with matches. In addition, all homes should have smoke detectors installed to alert the occupants of a fire. A safety plan for immediate escape is also essential.

Electrical burns represent an immediate danger to children. With the ability to manipulate small, thin objects, they are able to insert hairpins or other conductive articles into electrical sockets. Young toddlers may explore outlets and wires by mouthing them. Because saliva is an excellent conductor, the chance for a severe circumoral electrical burn is great. Electrical outlets should have protective guards plugged into them when not in use or be made inaccessible by placing furniture in front of them when feasible (Fig. 14-15). Children should not be allowed to play with electrical cords, appliances, or batteries, which should be kept out of reach as much as possible.

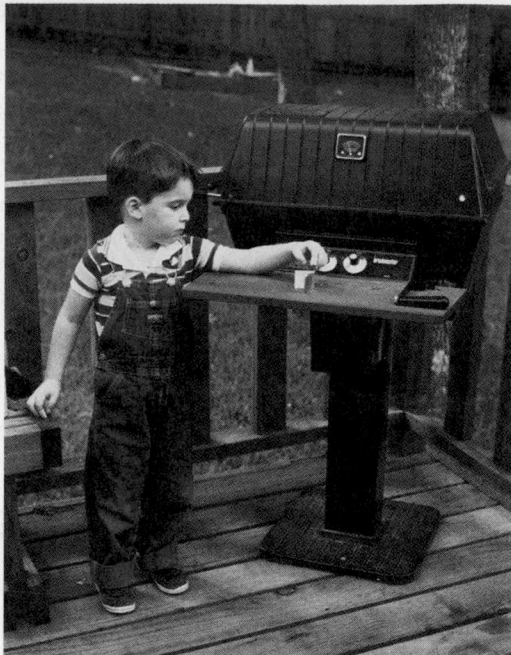

Fig. 14-14 Matches are a potentially deadly hazard for young children.

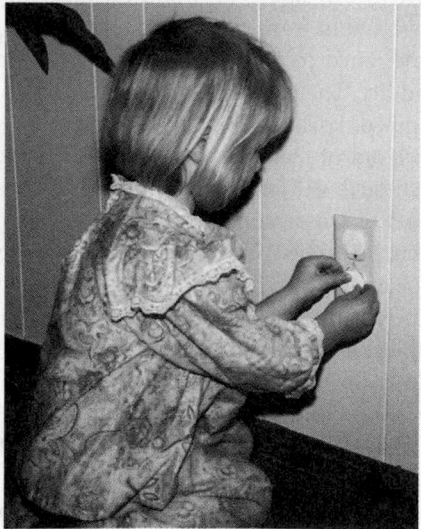

Fig. 14-15 Special plastic caps in electrical sockets prevent young fingers from exploring dangerous areas.

Scald burns are the most common type of thermal injury in children, especially 1- and 2-year-olds (Drago, 2005). Scalding often occurs because the child is reaching to a stove or other surface and pulling hot water onto herself or himself, or because the child has spilled a hot liquid container (such as a parent's coffee or tea) onto herself or himself (Drago, 2005). Scalding can also occur from children coming into contact with high-temperature tap water by turning on the hot-water faucet, falling into a bathtub of hot water, or suffering deliberate abuse. Besides the obvious prevention of always supervising children when they are near tap water and checking bathwater temperatures, a recommended passive prevention is to set the water heater to limit household water temperatures to less than 49° C (120° F). At this temperature it takes 10 minutes for

exposure to the water to cause a full-thickness burn. Conversely, water temperatures of 54° C (130° F), the usual setting of most water heaters, expose household members to the risk of full-thickness burns within 30 seconds. Nurses can help prevent such burns by advising parents of this common household danger and recommending that they adjust the water heater to a safe temperature. An easy-to-read hot-water gauge that changes color to show water temperatures between 49° and 65.5° C (120° and 150° F) is available; it shows "hot," "cool," or "OK" water temperature. A special device can also be added to the faucet that reduces the water flow if the set temperature is reached.

Sunburns are a special concern for this age group. Children spend a large amount of time outdoors, and their increased mobility makes it difficult to prevent sun exposure. Sunburn can be prevented by applying a sunscreen with a sun protection factor (SPF) of 15 or greater, dressing in protective clothing (wide-brimmed hat, protective cotton clothing with a tight weave), and avoiding sun exposure between 10 AM and 2 PM.

Poisoning

Although in many instances poisoning does not result in death, it may cause significant morbidity, such as esophageal stricture from lye ingestion. Mouthing activity increases toddlers' risk of poisoning; exploring objects by tasting them is part of children's curious investigation. Because of their curious nature, children under 6 years of age are more likely to eat unusual, distasteful substances. Recent attention has focused on the use of over-the-counter (OTC) medications used for cough and colds as a common cause of accidental poisonous ingestion in toddlers. Ingestion of acetaminophen is also a common cause of morbidity because it is found in many combination OTC products; caregivers may unknowingly administer a dose of acetaminophen in addition to an OTC drug containing the product without knowing the danger.

Although young children may be able to identify some items as poisonous, they do not understand the toxic effects of ingesting excessive amounts of a familiar drug, such as vitamins or iron. Many household products, medications, and plants can be poisonous if swallowed, if in contact with the skin or eyes, or if inhaled. Almost every nonfood substance is potentially harmful, and by 2 years of age toddlers are able to climb most heights, open most drawers or closets, and unscrew most lids. By trial and error, they also manage to undo tops of bottles, plastic containers, aerosol cans, and jars.

However, they are most likely to ingest substances that are on their level, such as plants, cleaning agents stored under sinks, rat poison, or diaper pail deodorants, especially when stored in the kitchen, bathroom, laundry, or garage. Child-resistant tops are required on some substances, such as prescription drugs, but many young children have opened such "safe" caps. In addition, pharmacists often transfer drugs to regular containers for the elderly, who may have difficulty with child-resistant closures. Cosmetics and drugs found in a purse are common agents ingested by toddlers.

The major reason for poisoning is improper storage (Fig. 14-16). The guidelines suggested in Chapter 12 apply to children in this age-group as well. However, unlike infants, who are unable to reach certain heights or unlatch inventive locks,

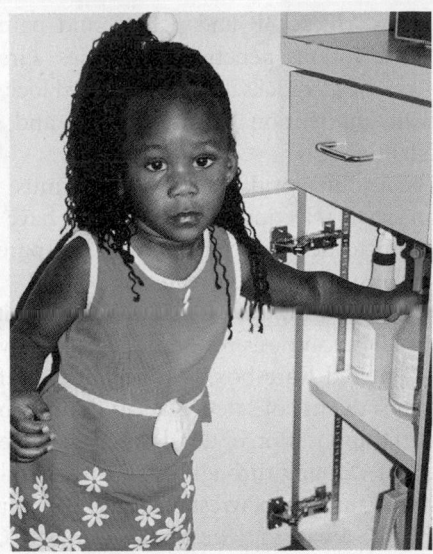

Fig. 14-16 Children are most likely to ingest substances that are on their level, such as cleaning agents stored under sinks, rat poison, plants, or diaper pail deodorants.

young children manage to find access to many high-level, tight-security places. For this age-group, only a locked cabinet is safe.

Ipecac syrup is no longer recommended as an antidote for poisoning in children (American Academy of Pediatrics, 2003) because it has not been shown to improve the eventual outcome in affected children and may prolong the incidence of vomiting when other ingestion therapies are necessary. (See Evidence-Based Practice box: Gastric Lavage in Children, Chapter 16.)

Parents should have ready access to the telephone number for the poison control center and be prepared to act on the center's advice.* Emergency and preventive measures for accidental poisoning are in Chapter 16.

Falls

Falls are still a hazard to children in this age-group, although by the later part of early childhood, gross and fine motor skills are well developed, decreasing the incidence of falls down stairs or from chairs. However, playground injuries are common. Children need to learn safety at play areas, such as no horseplay on high slides or jungle gyms, sitting on swings, and staying away from moving swings.

The climbing and running activity of the typical toddler is complicated by total neglect for and lack of appreciation of danger, immature coordination, and a high center of gravity. Falling from furniture is a major cause of injury, with more children in this age-group sustaining head injuries than older children. Gates must be placed at both ends of stairs. Accessible windows that are left open during warm weather must be guarded with a rail. Falling from open windows is a major cause

of accidental death in urban lower socioeconomic groups; screens are not designed to prevent falls. Doors leading to stairwells or porches must be locked. A convenient type of lock is a sliding bar or hook that can be attached to the door and frame at a level higher than the child can reach, provided that inventive youngsters do not pull a chair over to unlatch the device.

Another site of falls is from cribs and vehicles. In addition to crib rails being fully raised, the mattress should remain at the lowest position, and toys or bumper pads that may be used as steps to climb out should be removed. Ideally, the floor should be carpeted. Once children reach a height of 89 cm (35 inches), they should sleep in a bed rather than a crib. If a bunk bed is selected, parents should be aware of possible dangers: falls and head entrapment between the mattress and guardrail or between the supporting mattress slats. If the beds are constructed of tubular metal or if the brackets holding the mattress are metal, parents should check for breaks or cracks in the metal and welds, which may lead to collapse and injury. Children who sleep on the top bunk should be 6 years or older.

Children can fall from high chairs, shopping carts, carriages, and car seats if not properly restrained or if balance changes when the place where they are sitting is weighed down with heavy objects. Therefore proper restraint and adequate supervision are essential.

Clothing can also increase the chance of falling. Slippery shoes or socks, rubber-soled shoes that "catch" on the floor and rug, and loose or cuffed pants can easily make a child fall. Simple safety measures, such as checking clothing and shoes, keeping shoelaces tied with double knots, or using self-adhering closures, can prevent such needless injuries.

Falls in hospitalized children have received little attention in the scientific literature but are known to occur. Research is currently in progress to identify fall risk factors specific to hospitalized children.

Aspiration and Suffocation

Usually by 1 year of age children chew well, but they may have difficulty with large pieces of food, such as meat or whole hot dogs, and with hard foods, such as nuts or dried beans. Small items such as colored beads, green peas, pellets, or beans are often placed into the nose by toddlers and may present a danger if aspirated into the airway. Young children cannot discard pits from fruit or bones from fish like older children. Therefore implement the same precautions as discussed for infants regarding food selection. (See Chapter 12.)

Play objects for toddlers must still be chosen with an awareness of the danger of small parts. Large, sturdy toys without sharp edges or removable parts are safest. Coins, paper clips, pull tabs on cans, thumbtacks, nails, screws, jewelry (especially pierced earrings), and all types of pins are common household objects that can cause significant harm if swallowed or aspirated. Because of the danger of aspiration, parents should know emergency procedures for choking. (See Airway Obstruction, Chapter 31.)

Suffocation is less frequent from causes seen during infancy but is an ever-present threat from old refrigerators, car trunks, ovens, and other large appliances. Toddlers can climb inside these appliances and, if they close the door behind them, can become trapped inside. Discarding old appliances and removing all doors during storage prevents such tragic injuries. Toddlers may also suffocate when toy boxes with heavy, hinged lids accidentally close on their head or neck. Advise parents of this danger and encourage them to buy storage chests with lightweight, removable covers.

Bodily Harm

Toddlers are still clumsy in many of their skills and can seriously harm themselves when walking while holding a sharp or pointed object or having food or objects such as spoons in their mouths. Preventing such occurrences is the best approach with toddlers. Teach the child that, when walking with a pointed object, such as a fork, knife, or scissors, he or she needs to hold the pointed end away from the face. Dangerous garden or workshop equipment and all firearms should be stored in a locked cabinet. Power lawn mowers are especially dangerous, and young children should not be allowed in an area where a mower is being used, nor should they be taken for a ride on a mower or allowed to operate the device.

Toddlers are often unable to understand that all pets are not as safe as their own; because of the toddlers' height, they are often at the eye level of some dogs and may be bitten on the face. It is imperative to teach pet safety to toddlers and keep animals at a safe distance because even the most loving pet may perceive a threat and react accordingly.

Safety education should include respect for firearms and their proper and appropriate use, including nonpowder guns, such as air guns, rifles (BB and pellet), and paintball guns, which can cause serious penetrating injuries. Firearm safety devices such as a trigger locks and personalized locks are necessary to prevent unintentional firing of guns and subsequent injuries or fatalities.

Toys can be a source of danger, and safety must be a prime consideration when selecting toys. Most toys have age ranges written on them to designate their safety, but parents should also consider the specific child's readiness.

Strategies for ensuring safety in households with toddlers include the usual precautions recommended for any age-group (see Family-Centered Care box). An additional safeguard for young children is the use of safety glass in doors, windows, and tabletops and the application of decals on glassed areas to lessen the likelihood of running through glass. Also, children should not be allowed to run, jump, wrestle, or play ball in areas where glass litter may be a hazard. (See Bodily Damage, Chapter 12; Mammal Bites, Chapter 18.)

ANTICIPATORY GUIDANCE— CARE OF FAMILIES

Understanding toddlers is fundamental to successful child-rearing. Nurses, particularly those in ambulatory or child health centers, are in a most favorable position to assist parents in meeting the tasks and needs of children in this age-

---

FAMILY-CENTERED CARE

Guidance During Toddler Years

12 to 18 Months

Prepare parents for expected behavioral changes of toddler, especially negativism and ritualism.

Assess present feeding habits and encourage gradual weaning from bottle and increased intake of solid foods.

Stress expected feeding changes of physiologic anorexia, presence of food fads and strong taste preferences, need for scheduled routine at mealtimes, inability to sit through an entire meal, and lack of table manners.

Assess sleep patterns at night, particularly habit of a bedtime bottle, which is a major cause of dental caries, and procrastination behaviors that delay hour of sleep.

Prepare parents for potential dangers, particularly motor vehicle, poisoning, and falling injuries; give appropriate suggestions for childproofing the home.

Discuss need for firm but gentle discipline and ways to deal with negativism and temper tantrums; stress positive benefits of appropriate discipline.

Emphasize importance for both child and parents of brief, periodic separations.

Discuss toys that use developing gross and fine motor, language, cognitive, and social skills.

Emphasize need for dental supervision, types of basic dental hygiene at home, and food habits that predispose the child to caries; stress importance of supplemental fluoride.

18 to 24 Months

Stress importance of peer companionship in play.

Explore need for preparation for additional sibling; stress importance of preparing child for new experiences.

Discuss present discipline methods, their effectiveness, and parents' feelings about child's negativism; stress that negativism is important aspect of developing self-assertion and independence and is not a sign of spoiling.

Discuss signs of readiness for toilet training; emphasize importance of waiting for physical and psychologic readiness.

Discuss development of fears, such as fear of darkness or loud noises, and of habits, such as security blanket or thumb sucking; stress normalcy of these transient behaviors.

Prepare parents for signs of regression in time of stress.

Assess child's ability to separate easily from parents for brief periods under familiar circumstances.

Allow parents opportunity to express their feelings of weariness, frustration, and exasperation; be aware that it is often difficult to love toddlers at times when they are not asleep!

Point out some of the expected changes of the next year, such as longer attention span, somewhat less negativism, and increased concern for pleasing others.

24 to 36 Months

Discuss importance of imitation and domestic mimicry and need to include child in activities.

Discuss approaches toward toilet training, particularly realistic expectations and attitude toward accidents.

Stress uniqueness of toddlers' thought processes, especially through their use of language, poor understanding of time, causal relationships in terms of proximity of events, and inability to see events from another's perspective.

Stress that discipline still must be structured and concrete and that relying solely on verbal reasoning and explanation leads to confusion, misunderstanding, and even injuries.

Discuss investigation of preschool or daycare center toward completion of second year.

group. Anticipatory guidance in each of the areas presented in the Family-Centered Care box can prevent future problems. Advice is sometimes not the sole answer. Actual assistance, such as being available for home visiting or telephone consulting, should be a part of the nurse's flexible repertoire of interventions. Whether parents are experiencing the challenges of rearing a first or a subsequent child, they benefit from sharing their feelings, frustrations, and satisfactions. They need adult companionship, shared childrearing responsibilities, and periodic separation from their children. For single parents such goals can be especially difficult to achieve. Part of a nurse's responsibility is to provide opportunities for parents to express their feelings and to meet their emotional and physical needs.

KEY POINTS

- The toddler stage, extending over ages 12 to 36 months, is a period of intense exploration of the environment.
- Biologic development during the toddler years is characterized by the acquisition of fine and gross motor skills that allow children to master a wide variety of activities.
- Although most of the physiologic systems are mature by the end of toddlerhood, development of certain areas of the brain is still occurring, allowing for greater intellectual capacity.
- Locomotion is the major gross motor skill acquired during toddlerhood, followed by increased eye-hand coordination.
- Specific tasks in the psychosocial development of a toddler include differentiating self from others, tolerating separation from parent, coping with delayed gratification, controlling bodily functions, acquiring socially acceptable behavior, communicating verbally, and interacting with others in a less egocentric manner.
- According to Erikson, the major developmental task of toddlerhood is acquiring a sense of autonomy while overcoming a sense of doubt and shame.
- In Piaget's sensorimotor and preconceptual phases of development, the toddler experiments by incorporating the old learning of secondary circular reactions with new skills and applies this knowledge to new situations. The toddler experiences the beginning of rational judgment, an understanding of causal relationships, and discovery of objects as objects.
- Preconceptual thought is characterized by centration, global organization of thought processes, animism, and irreversibility.
- Language is the major cognitive achievement in toddlerhood.
- The most striking characteristic of language development during early childhood is the increasing level of comprehension.
- Discipline, or a punishment-obedience orientation, aids in children's moral development.
- Development of body image occurs with increasing motor ability, at which point toddlers recognize the importance and capacity of body parts.
- The two phases of differentiation of self from significant others are separation and individuation.
- Parental concerns during the toddler years include toilet training, sibling rivalry, temper tantrums and negativism, and stress.
- Nutrition is important at this stage because eating habits established in toddlerhood tend to have lasting effects in subsequent years.
- Regular dental examinations, fluoride supplementation, removal of plaque, and provision of foods and beverages that have low cariogenic potential promote optimum dental health.
- Because of increased locomotion, toddlers are at high risk for sustaining injuries. Fatal injuries are primarily the result of motor vehicle accidents, drownings, and burns.
- Drowning was the second leading cause of accidental death in children ages 1 to 4 between 2000 and 2006.
- Children should never be left alone in a car when the environmental temperature is above 27° C (80° F).

REFERENCES

Allen RE, Myers AL: Nutrition in toddlers, *Am Fam Physician* 74(9):1527-1532, 2006.

American Academy of Pediatric Dentistry: *Reference manual 2009-2010: guideline on fluoride therapy*, 31(6):128-129, 2009, available at www.aapd.org/media/Policies_Guidelines/G_FluorideTherapy.pdf (accessed January 6, 2010).

American Academy of Pediatrics: *Car safety seats: information for families for 2010*, 2010, available at www.healthychildren.org/English/safety-prevention/on-the-go/pages/Car-Safety-Seats-Information-for-Families-2010.aspx (accessed January 5, 2010).

American Academy of Pediatrics, Committee on Nutrition: *Pediatric nutrition handbook*, ed 6, Elk Grove Village, Ill, 2009, The Academy.

American Academy of Pediatrics: Poison treatment in the home, *Pediatrics* 112(5):1182-1185, 2003.

American Academy of Pediatrics, Committee on Public Health: Children, adolescents, and television, *Pediatrics* 107(2):423-426, 2001.

Bates E, Dick F: Language, gesture, and the developing brain, *Dev Psychobiol* 40(3):293-310, 2002.

Borse NN, Gilchrist J, Delinger AM, et al: *CDC Childhood Injury Report: patterns of unintentional injuries among 0-19 year olds in the United States, 2000-2006*, Atlanta, 2008, Centers for Disease Control and Prevention.

Brazelton TB: How to help parents of young children: the touchpoints model, *J Perinatol* 19(6 Pt 2):S6-S7, 1999.

Brenner RA, American Academy of Pediatrics, Committee on Injury, Violence, and Poison Prevention: Prevention of drowning in infants, children, and adolescents, *Pediatrics* 112(2):437-439, 2003.

Brenner RA, Taneja GS, Haynie DL, et al: Association between swimming lessons and drowning in childhood: a case-control study, *Arch Pediatr Adolesc Med* 163(3):203-210, 2009.

Brotanek JM, Schroer D, Valentyn L, et al: Reasons for prolonged bottle-feeding and iron deficiency among Mexican-American toddlers: an ethnographic study, *Acad Pediatr* 9(1):17-25, 2009.

Bull A, Gillies M: Spiritual needs of children with complex healthcare needs in hospital, *Paediatr Nurs* 19(9):34-38, 2007.

Bull MJ, Durbin DR: Rear-facing car safety seats: getting the message right, *Pediatrics* 121(3):619-620, 2008.

Cathey M, Gaylord N: Picky eating: a toddler's continuing approach to mealtime, *Pediatr Nurs* 30(2):101-107, 2004.

Choby BA, George SA: Toilet training, *Am Family Physician* 78(9):1059-1064, 2008.

Chonchaiva W, Pruksananonda C: Television viewing associates with delayed language development, *Acta Paediatr* 97(7):977-982, 2008.

Dahlquist LM, Busby SM, Slifer KJ, et al: Distraction for children of different ages who undergo repeated needle sticks, *J Pediatr Oncol Nurs* 19(1):22-34, 2002.

DeLamater J, Friedrich WN: Human sexual development, *J Sex Res* 39(1):10-14, 2002.

Devaney B, Kalb L, Briefel R, et al: Feeding Infants and Toddlers Study: overview of the study design, *J Am Diet Assoc* 104(1 Suppl 1):S8-S13, 2004.

Drago DA: Kitchen scalds and thermal burns in children 5 years and younger, *Pediatrics* 115(1):10-16, 2005.

Durbin DR, Chen I, Smith R, et al: Effects of seating position and appropriate restraint use on the risk of injury to children in motor vehicle crashes, *Pediatrics* 115(3):e305-e309, 2005.

Elkins M, Cavendish R: Developing a plan for pediatric spiritual care, *Holistic Nurs Pract* 18(4):179-184, 2004.

Erdal S, Buchanan SN: A quantitative look at fluorosis, fluoride exposure, and intake in children using a health risk assessment approach, *Environ Health Perspect* 113(1): 111-117, 2005.

Erikson EH: *Childhood and society*, ed 2, New York, 1963, Norton.

Feigelman S: The second year. In Kliegman RM, Behrman RE, Jenson HB, et al, editors: *Nelson textbook of pediatrics*, ed 18, Philadelphia, 2007, Saunders.

Flores MT, Malmgren B, Andersson L, et al: Guidelines for the management of traumatic dental injuries, part III, Primary teeth, *Dent Traumatol* 23(4):196-202, 2007.

Fonseca H, Greydanus DE: Sexuality in the child, teen, and young adult: concepts for the clinician, *Prim Care Clin Office Pract* 34(2):275-292, 2007.

Fosarelli P: Children and the development of faith: implications for pediatric practice, *Contemp Pediatr* 20(1):85-98, 2003.

Freeman R, Stevens A: Nursing caries and buying time: an emerging theory of prolonged bottle-feeding, *Community Dent Oral Epidemiol* 36(5):425-433, 2008.

Gidding SS, Dennison BA, Birch LL, et al: Dietary recommendations for children and adolescents: a guide for practitioners: consensus statement from the American Heart Association, *Circulation* 112(13):2061-2075, 2005.

Gidding SS, Lichtenstein AH, Faith MS, et al: Implementing American Heart Association pediatric and adult nutrition guidelines, *Circulation* 119(8):1161-1175, 2009.

Ginsburg KR, American Academy of Pediatrics, Committee on Communications: The importance of play in promoting healthy child development and maintaining strong parent-child bonds, *Pediatrics* 119(1):182-191, 2007.

Glassy D, Romano J, and Committee on Early Childhood, Adoption, and Dependent Care: Selecting appropriate toys for young children: the pediatrician's role, *Pediatrics* 111(4):911-913, 2003.

Guard A, Gallagher SS: Heat related deaths in young children in parked cars: an analysis of 171 fatalities in the United States, 1995-2002, *Inj Prev* 11(1):33-37, 2005.

Harpaz-Rotem I, Bergman A: On an evolving theory of attachment: rapprochement—theory of a developing mind, *Psychoanal Study Child* 61:170-189, 2006.

Henary B, Sherwood CP, Crandall JR, et al: Car safety for children: rear facing for best protection, *Inj Prev* 13(6):398-402, 2007.

Horn IB, Brenner R, Rao M, et al: Beliefs about the appropriate age for initiating toilet training: are there racial and socioeconomic differences? *J Pediatr* 149(2):165-168, 2006.

Institute of Medicine: *Dietary reference intakes for energy, carbohydrate, fiber, fat, fatty acids, cholesterol, protein, and amino acids*, Washington, DC, 2005, The Institute, National Academies Press.

Ismail AI, Hasson H: Fluoride supplements, dental caries and fluoride: a systematic review, *J Am Dent Assoc* 139(11):1457-1468, 2008.

Kallan MJ, Durbin DR, Arbogast KB: Seating patterns and corresponding risk of injury among 0- to 3-year-old children in child safety seats, *Pediatrics* 121(5):e1342-e1347, 2008.

Klassen TP, Kiddoo D, Lang ME, et al: The effectiveness of different methods of toilet training for bowel and bladder control, *Evid Rep Technol Assess (Full Rep)*, 147:1-57, 2006.

Marshall TA, Levy SM, Warren JJ, et al: Association between intakes of fluoride from beverages during infancy and dental fluorosis of primary teeth, *J Am Coll Nutr* 23(2):108-116, 2004.

McLaren C, Null J, Quinn J: Heat stress from enclosed vehicles: moderate ambient temperatures cause significant temperature rise in enclosed vehicles, *Pediatrics* 116(1): e109-e112, 2005.

McSherry M, Kehoe K, Carroll JM, et al: Psychosocial and spiritual needs of children living with a life-limiting illness, *Pediatr Clin North Am* 54(5):609-629, 2007.

Meltzer LJ, Mindell JA: Sleep and sleep disorders in children and adolescents, *Psych Clin North Am* 29(4):1059-1076, 2006.

Mercer R: Treating nocturnal enuresis, *Adv Nurs Pract* 11(2):26-31, 2003.

Meyer TL: Unveiling the secrecy behind masturbation, *Pediatr Rev* 23(4):148-149, 2002.

National Highway Traffic Safety Administration: *A parent's guide to booster seats* (pamphlet), Washington, DC, 2009, The Administration, available at www.nhtsa.gov.org (accessed July 10, 2009).

Needlman R, Howard B, Zuckerman B: Helping parents get beyond the terrible 2's, *Patient Care* 29(1):52-61, 1995.

Null J: *Hyperthermia deaths of children in vehicles*, 2009, San Francisco State University, Department of Geosciences, available at www.ggweather.com/heat (accessed July 2009).

Petitto LA, Katerlos M, Levy BG, et al: Bilingual signed and spoken language acquisition from birth: implications for the mechanisms underlying early bilingual language acquisition, *J Child Lang* 28(2):453-496, 2001.

Potegal M, Kosorok MR, Davidson RJ: Temper tantrums in young children, part 2, Tantrum duration and temporal organization, *J Dev Behav Pediatr* 24(3):148-154, 2003.

Roehlkepartain EC, Benson PL, King PE, et al, editors: *The handbook of spiritual development in childhood and adolescence*, Thousand Oaks, Calif, 2006, Sage.

Schmitt BD: Toilet training: getting it right the first time, *Contemp Pediatr* 21(3):105-108, 111-112, 115-116, 2004.

Schnitzer PG: Prevention of unintentional childhood injuries, *Am Fam Physician* 74(11):1864-1869, 2006.

Schum TR, Kolb TM, McAuliffe TL, et al: Sequential acquisition of toilet-training skills: a descriptive study of gender and age differences in normal children, *Pediatrics* 109(3):e48, 2002.

Shenkin JD, Broffitt B, Levy SM, et al: The association between environmental tobacco smoke and primary tooth caries, *J Pub Health Dent* 64(3):184-186, 2004.

Stang J: Improving the eating patterns of infants and toddlers, *J Am Diet Assoc* 106(1 Suppl):S7-S9, 2006.

Stein MT, Carey WB, Snyder DM: Is this a behavior problem or normal temperament? *J Dev Behav Pediatr* 25(5 Suppl):S1-S7, 2004.

Wagner CL, Greer FR, and American Academy of Pediatrics, Section on Breastfeeding and Committee on Nutrition: Prevention of rickets and vitamin D deficiency in infants, children, and adolescents, *Pediatrics* 122(5):1142-1150, 2008.

Zimmerman FJ, Gilkerson J, Richards JA, et al: Teaching by listening: the importance of adult-child conversations to language development, *Pediatrics* 124(1):342-349, 2009.

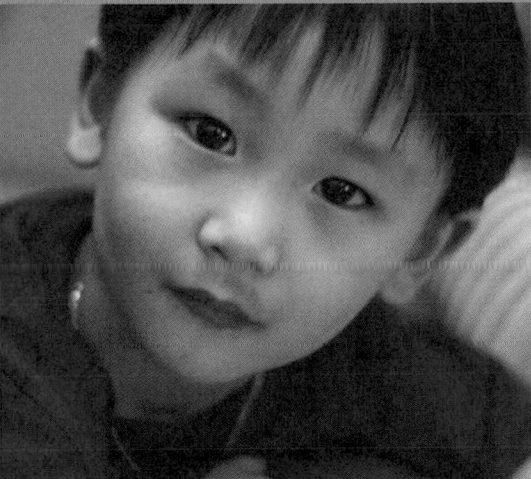

Health Promotion of the Preschooler and Family

Rebecca A. Monroe

evolve WEBSITE

http://evolve.elsevier.com/wong/ncic

Case Study
  Sleep Problems
Critical Thinking Exercise
  Imitative Play
Key Points Audio Summaries
NCLEX Review Questions
Pediatric Assessment Video Clips
Spanish/English Translations
WebLinks

RELATED TOPICS

CHAPTER OUTLINE

PROMOTING OPTIMUM GROWTH AND DEVELOPMENT

The combined biologic, psychosocial, cognitive, spiritual, and social achievements during the preschool period (3 to 5 years of age) prepare preschoolers for their most significant change in lifestyle: entrance into school. Their control of bodily systems, experience of brief and prolonged periods of separation, ability to interact cooperatively with other children and adults, use of language for mental symbolization, and increased attention span and memory prepare them for the next major period: the school years. Successful achievement of previous levels of growth and development is essential for preschoolers to refine many of the tasks that were mastered during the toddler years.

BIOLOGIC DEVELOPMENT

The rate of physical growth slows and stabilizes during the preschool years. The average weight is 14.5 kg (32 lb) at 3 years, 16.5 kg (36.5 lb) at 4 years, and 18.5 kg (41 lb) at 5 years. The average weight gain remains approximately 2 to 3 kg (4.5 to 6.5 lb) per year.

Growth in height also remains steady at a yearly increase of 6.5 to 9 cm (2.5 to 3.5 inches). The legs of a preschooler, rather than the trunk, increase in length. The average height is 95 cm (37.5 inches) at 3 years, 103 cm (40.5 inches) at 4 years, and 110 cm (43.5 inches) at 5 years.

Physical proportions no longer resemble those of the squat, pot-bellied toddler. The preschooler is slender but sturdy, graceful, agile, and posturally erect. There is little difference in physical characteristics according to sex, except in factors such as dress and hairstyle.

Most organ systems can adjust to moderate stress and change. During this period, most children are toilet trained. For the most part, motor development consists of increases in strength and refinement of previously learned skills, such as walking, running, and jumping. However, muscle development and bone growth are still far from mature. Excessive activity and overexertion can injure delicate tissues. Good posture, appropriate exercise, and adequate nutrition and rest are essential for optimum development of the musculoskeletal system.

Gross and Fine Motor Behavior

By 36 months, preschoolers are walking, running, climbing, and jumping well. Refinement in eye-hand and muscle coordination is evident in several areas. At age 3, the preschooler rides a tricycle, walks on tiptoe, balances on one foot for a few seconds, and broad jumps. By age 4, the child skips and hops proficiently on one foot (Fig. 15-1) and catches a ball reliably. By age 5, the child skips on alternate feet, jumps rope, and begins to skate and swim.

Achievement in fine motor development is evident in the child's increasingly skillful manipulation. Drawing shows several advancements in the perception of shape and the development of fine muscle coordination. The 3-year-old child copies a circle and imitates a cross and vertical and horizontal lines. He or she holds the writing instrument with the fingers rather than the fist. The child scribbles or scrawls drawings but can name what has been drawn. The 3-year-old is not able to draw a complete stick figure but draws a circle, later adds facial features, and by age 5 or 6 years can draw several parts (head, arms, legs, body, and facial features). Between 4 and 5 years of age, the child can trace a cross and copy a square. The triangle and diamond are usually the last geometric figures to be mastered, sometime between ages 5 and 6.

As children progress from scribbling to picture making, they advance through four distinguishable stages (Kellogg, 1969). In the placement stage, 15-month-old children place their earliest spontaneous scribblings on the paper in a specific placement pattern, such as in the center, all over, across the lower half, or across the page in a diagonal direction (Fig. 15-2). Approximately 17 different placement patterns appear by age 2 years and, once developed, are never lost.

By 3 years of age, children are in the shape stage. They draw single-line outline forms such as rectangles, circles, ovals, crosses, and other odd shapes. As soon as they draw diagrams, they almost immediately progress to the design stage, in which simple forms are drawn together to make structured designs. When two diagrams are united, the resulting design is called a *combine*. Three or more united diagrams produce an aggregate. Between the ages of 4 and 5, most children enter the pictorial stage, in which their designs are recognizable as familiar objects. Early pictorial drawings are suggestive of human figures, houses, animals, and trees. Later pictorial drawings are more clearly defined and recognizable; they are not representations of the actual object but aesthetically satisfying structures that resemble

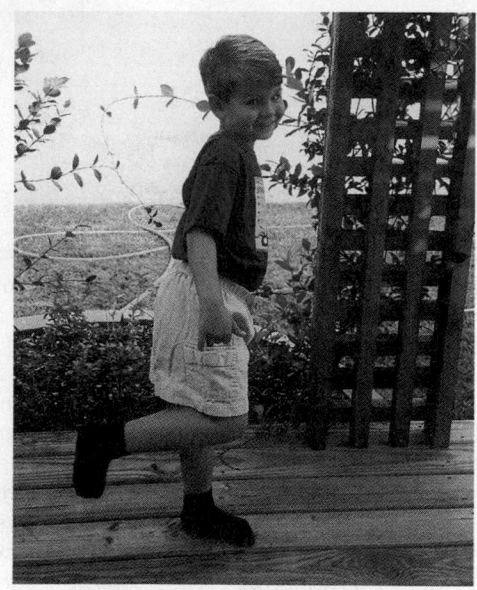

Fig. 15-1 A 4-year-old child has sufficient balance to hop on one foot.

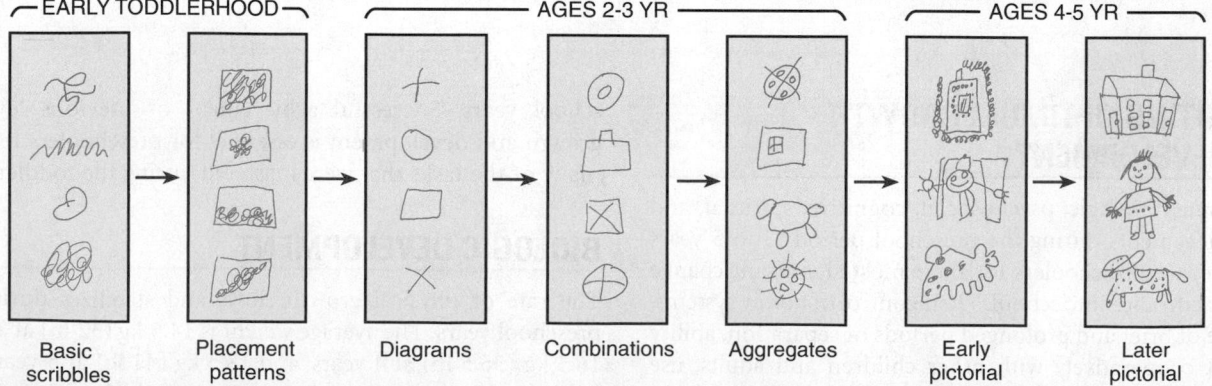

Fig. 15-2 Sequential development in self-taught art. (From Kellogg R: Understanding children's art. In *Readings in psychology today*, Del Mar, Calif, 1969, Communications/Research/Machines.)

familiar objects. For example, the initial human figure drawing is a circle with arms attached to the head. It is more an aggregate drawing than any attempt to copy a human figure. Drawings of animals follow the human figure drawing but are only a slight modification, such as attaching ears to the top of the head.

Kellogg (1969) suggests that uninhibited scribbling and drawing are necessary for children to learn to read and that children who have been free to experiment and produce abstract forms have developed the mental set required for learning symbolic language. Scribbling and drawing also help develop the fine muscle skills and eye-hand coordination eventually required for making precise letters and numbers.

Drawing is also a tool used for assessing intelligence, personality development, and psychosocial adjustment. The precise value of using drawing to measure such concepts is still a nebulous science. However, children (especially school-age children) do reveal thoughts about themselves in their drawings. It is generally not necessary to have in-depth knowledge of children's drawings to make assumptions about their significance. Being receptive to all the clues, both verbal and nonverbal, is essential to understanding how and what children are communicating to others (see Cultural Competence box).

 CULTURAL COMPETENCE

Drawings

Children's drawings before age 6 years are strikingly similar universally, suggesting that some inherent neurologic mechanisms influence the type of self-taught art forms. After age 6, cultural and environmental influences, particularly from parents and teachers, shape much of what children draw. For example, drawings of physical characteristics (skin color, hair type, and facial features), style of dress, type of housing, and scenery may reflect ethnic or geographic variations. Therefore nurses need to consider children's backgrounds when interpreting drawings.

PSYCHOSOCIAL DEVELOPMENT

Developing a Sense of Initiative (Erikson)

If preschoolers have mastered the tasks of the toddler period, they are ready to face the developmental challenges of the preschool period. Erikson maintained that the chief psychosocial task of this period is acquiring a sense of initiative. Children are in a stage of energetic learning. They play, work, and live to the fullest and feel a real sense of accomplishment and satisfaction in their activities. Conflict arises when children overstep the limits of their ability and inquiry and experience guilt for not having behaved appropriately. Feelings of guilt, anxiety, and fear may also result from thoughts that differ from expected behavior.

A particularly stressful thought is wishing one's parent dead. As a sense of rivalry or competition develops between the child and the same-sex parent, the child may think of ways to get rid of the interfering parent. In most situations, this contest is resolved when the child strongly identifies with the same-sex parent and peers during the school years. However, if that parent dies before the identification process is completed, the preschooler can be overwhelmed with guilt for having wished and therefore "caused" the death. Clarifying for children that

wishes cannot make events occur is essential in helping them overcome their guilt and anxiety.

Development of the superego, or conscience, starts toward the end of the toddler years and is a major task for preschoolers. Learning right from wrong and good from bad is the beginning of morality (see Cultural Competence box). Children in this age-group are generally unable to understand why something is acceptable or unacceptable. They are aware of appropriate behavior primarily through punishment or reward and rely almost completely on parental principles for developing their own moral judgment. Verbal enforcement of limits is much more effective in this age-group than with toddlers. For example, to prevent injuries, parents need to supervise toddlers, keep them contained within protected areas, and tell them not to run into the street. The preschooler still needs close supervision but is much more aware of danger and can listen and obey in most instances. If allowed to disagree and question, they will develop socially acceptable behavior and independence in thought and action.

 CULTURAL COMPETENCE

Learning Sociocultural Mores

Developing a conscience implies learning the sociocultural mores of the family's heritage. Depending on the type of attitudes conveyed, children will learn not only appropriate behaviors but also tolerant, biased, or prejudicial values concerning their ethnic, religious, and social background and those of other groups. Much of this influence may remain dormant until they associate with children or adults of a different heritage. Then, depending on the particular group, they may be accepted or excluded for their attitudes.

Oedipal Stage (Freud)

As soon as children comprehend their separateness as persons, they begin to realize that there are categories of objects, such as things, people, males, females, children, and adults. One of the principal goals in further differentiation of oneself from others is learning sex differences and sexually appropriate behavior.

Freud described this goal in psychosexual terms and labeled the period the *oedipal*, or *phallic*, stage. He believed that conflict arises when a boy realizes that his father is much stronger and more powerful than he. Subconsciously, he wishes that his father were dead so he could marry his mother (Oedipus complex). Concurrently, he notices physical sexual differences, specifically that boys have a penis and girls do not. In his mind, he supposes that girls have lost their penis for some wrongdoing. His guilt regarding his feelings toward his father makes him fear the same punishment of mutilation, resulting in the castration complex. Girls have similar wishes to marry their father and kill their mother (the Electra complex). However, girls do not fear castration; rather they experience penis envy (desire to have a penis). The resolution of the Oedipus or Electra complex is identification with the same-sex parent.

COGNITIVE DEVELOPMENT

One of the tasks related to the preschool period is readiness for school and scholastic learning. Many of the thought processes of this period are crucial for achieving such readiness, and it is intentional that the child begins school between ages 5 and 6 rather than earlier.

Preoperational Phase (Piaget)

Piaget's cognitive theory does not include a period specifically for children 3 to 5 years old. The preoperational phase covers the age span from 2 to 7 years and is divided into two stages: the preconceptual phase, ages 2 to 4, and the phase of intuitive thought, ages 4 to 7. One of the main transitions during these two phases is the shift from totally egocentric thought to social awareness and the ability to consider other viewpoints (Fig. 15-3). Egocentricity, however, is still evident. Children are able to think and verbalize their mental processes without having to act out their thinking. They can think of only one idea at a time and are unable to think of all parts in terms of the whole.

Language continues to develop during the preschool period. Speech remains primarily a vehicle of egocentric communication. Preschoolers assume that everyone thinks as they do and that a brief explanation of their thinking makes them understood by others. Because of this self-referenced, egocentric verbal communication, it is often necessary to explore and understand young children's thinking through other, nonverbal approaches. For children in this age-group, the most enlightening and effective method is play, which becomes the child's way of understanding, adjusting to, and working out life's experiences. Because of a child's rich imagination and unlimited ability to invent and imitate, all types of play hold therapeutic and communicative value.

Preschoolers increasingly use language without comprehending the meaning of words, particularly concepts of right and left, causality, and time. Children may use the concepts correctly but only in the circumstances in which they have learned them. For example, they may know how to put on shoes by remembering that the buckle is always on the outside of the foot. However, if different shoes have no buckles, they cannot reason which shoe fits which foot. They do not understand the concept of right and left.

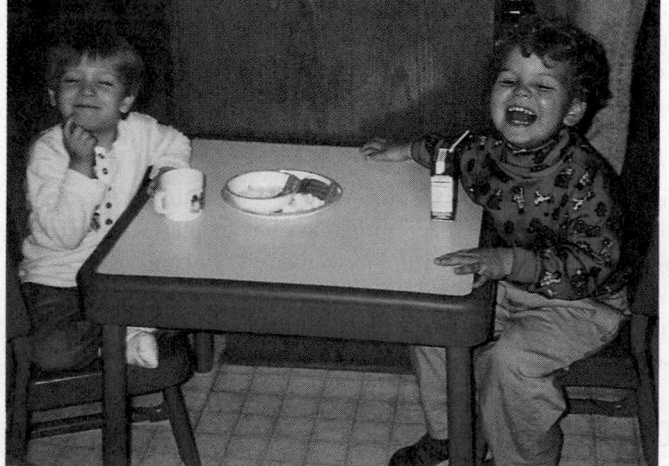

Fig. 15-3 Preschool children enjoy friends and often use nonverbal messages to communicate.

Superficially, causality resembles logical thought. Preschoolers explain a concept as they have heard it described by others, but their understanding is limited. For example, since preschoolers do not completely understand time, they interpret it according to their own frame of reference, such as "A long time means until Christmas." Consequently, time is best explained in relation to an event, such as "Your mother will visit you after you finish your lunch." Avoiding words such as "yesterday," "tomorrow," "next week," or "Tuesday" to express when an event is expected to occur and associating time with usual expected daily occurrences help children learn about temporal relationships while increasing their trust in others' predictions.

Preschoolers' thinking is often described as magical thinking. Because of their egocentrism and transductive reasoning, they believe that thoughts are all powerful. Such thinking places them in the vulnerable position of feeling guilty and responsible for bad thoughts that may coincide with the occurrence of a wished event. A typical example is wishing a new sibling dead. If that sibling does die, young children think their wish caused the death. Their inability to reason the cause and effect of illness or injury makes it especially difficult for them to understand such events.

Preschoolers believe in the power of words and accept their meaning literally. A significant example of this type of thinking is calling children "bad" because they did something wrong. In their minds, telling children that they are bad means that they are bad. For this reason, it is better to relate such words to the act by saying, for example, "That was a bad thing to do."

MORAL DEVELOPMENT (KOHLBERG)

Moral development theory is based on cognitive development theory and consists of three major levels: preconventional, conventional, and postconventional (Kohlberg, 1968). Young children's development of moral judgment is at the most basic level. They have little, if any, concern for why something is wrong. They behave because of the freedoms or restrictions placed on actions. In the punishment and obedience orientation, children (approximately ages 2 to 4 years) judge whether an action is good or bad according to whether it results in reward or punishment. If children are punished for it, the action is bad. If they are not punished, the action is good, regardless of its meaning. For example, if parents allow hitting, the child will perceive that hitting is good because it is not associated with punishment.

From approximately 4 to 7 years of age, children are in the stage of naive instrumental orientation, in which actions are directed toward satisfying their needs and, less commonly, the needs of others. They have a concrete sense of justice and fairness during this period of development.

SPIRITUAL DEVELOPMENT

Children learn about faith and religion from significant others in their environment, usually from parents and their religious beliefs and practices. However, cognitive level influences young children's understanding of spirituality. Preschoolers have a concrete conception of a God with physical characteristics, often like an imaginary friend. They understand simple stories and memorize short prayers, but have limited understanding of the meaning of these rituals. They benefit from concrete representations of religious practices, such as picture books and small statues.

Development of the conscience is strongly linked to spiritual development. At this age, children are learning right from wrong and behave correctly to avoid punishment. Wrongdoing provokes guilt, and preschoolers often misinterpret illness as punishment for real or imagined transgressions. It is important that children view God as one who bestows unconditional love, rather than as a judge of good or bad behavior. Observing religious traditions and participating in a religious community often help children and their families cope during stressful periods, such as illness and hospitalization (Speraw, 2006).

DEVELOPMENT OF BODY IMAGE

The preschool years play a significant role in the development of body image. With increasing comprehension of language, preschoolers recognize that individuals have undesirable and desirable appearances. They recognize differences in skin color and racial identity and are vulnerable to learning prejudices and biases. They are aware of the meaning of words such as "pretty" or "ugly," and they reflect the opinions of others regarding their own appearance. By 5 years of age, children compare their size with that of their peers and can become conscious of being large or short, especially if others refer to them as "so big" or "so little" for their age. Research indicates that negative associations between weight status and self-concept are present in girls as young as 5 years of age, and weight status can affect the psychologic well-being of both males and females (Wardle and Cooke, 2005).

Despite the advances in body image development, preschoolers have poorly defined body boundaries and little knowledge of their internal anatomy. Intrusive experiences are frightening, especially those that disrupt the integrity of the skin (e.g., injections and surgery). They fear that all their blood and "insides" can leak out if the skin is "broken." Therefore preschoolers may believe it is critical to use bandages after an injury.

DEVELOPMENT OF SEXUALITY

Sexual development during the preschool years is important to a person's overall sexual identity and beliefs. Preschoolers form strong attachments to the opposite-sex parent while identifying with the same-sex parent. Sex typing, or the process by which an individual develops the behavior, personality, attitudes, and beliefs appropriate for his or her culture and sex, occurs through several mechanisms during this period. Probably the most powerful mechanisms are childrearing practices and imitation. The ways in which parents dress, hold, cuddle, caress, discipline, and talk to their child express some aspect of sexually oriented behavior. Gender identification is a result of complex prenatal and postnatal psychologic factors, as well as biologic, social, and genetic influences. It is believed that most children are aware of their sex and the expected set of related behaviors by $1\frac{1}{2}$ to $2\frac{1}{2}$ years of age. Although toddlers might be aware of their particu-

lar sex, they do not possess the language and cognitive skills to investigate sexual identity as fully as preschoolers.

As sexual identity develops beyond gender recognition, modesty and fears of mutilation may become a concern. Sex-role imitation and "dressing up" like Mommy or Daddy are important activities. Attitudes and responses of others to role-playing can condition the child to adopt particular views of self or others. For example, comments such as "Boys shouldn't play with dolls" can influence a boy's masculine self-concept.

Sexual exploration may be more pronounced now, particularly in terms of exploring and manipulating the genitalia. Preschoolers' may have questions about sexual reproduction as they search for understanding. (See Sex Education, p. 596, and also Chapters 17 and 19.)

SOCIAL DEVELOPMENT

During the preschool period, the separation-individuation process is completed. Preschoolers have overcome much of their anxiety associated with strangers and the fear of separation of earlier years. They relate to unfamiliar people easily and tolerate brief separations from parents with little or no protest. However, they still need parental security, reassurance, guidance, and approval, especially when entering preschool or elementary school. Prolonged separation, such as that imposed by illness and hospitalization, is difficult; however, preschoolers respond well to anticipatory preparation and concrete explanation. They can cope with changes in daily routine much better than toddlers but may develop more imaginary fears. They gain security and comfort from familiar objects such as toys, dolls, or photographs of family members. They are able to work through many of their unresolved fears, fantasies, and anxieties through play, especially if guided with appropriate play objects (e.g., dolls or puppets) that represent family members, health professionals, and other children.

Language

Language becomes more sophisticated and complex during the preschool years. Both cognitive ability and environment, particularly consistent role models, influence vocabulary, speech, and comprehension. Language becomes a major mode of communication and social interaction. Vocabulary increases dramatically, from 300 words at age 2 to more than 2100 words at the end of 5 years. Sentence structure, grammatical usage, and intelligibility also advance to a more adult level. Preschool children may even become bilingual (see Cultural Competence box).

CULTURAL COMPETENCE

Bilingual Children

Many children in the United States are bilingual. Children who learn two languages simultaneously or develop bilingualism in early childhood reach language milestones at similar stages to monolinguals (Werker and Byers-Heinlein, 2008). If a child has a language disability, it will manifest in both languages, although a language disability is not a result of becoming bilingual (American Speech-Language-Hearing Association, 2009). Nurses should inquire about each child's language repertoire and identify the child's primary language, especially when assessing a child's development.

Children between the ages of 3 and 4 years form sentences of approximately three or four words and include only the words most essential to convey meaning. Such speech is often termed telegraphic because of its brevity. Three-year-old children ask many questions and use plurals, correct pronouns, and the past tense of verbs. They name familiar objects (such as animals and parts of the body), relatives, and friends. They can give and follow simple commands. They talk incessantly, regardless of whether anyone is listening to or answering them. They enjoy musical or talking toys or dolls and imitate new words proficiently.

From ages 4 to 5 years, preschoolers use longer sentences of four or five words and use more words to convey a message, such as prepositions, adjectives, and a variety of verbs. They follow simple directional commands, such as "Put the ball on the chair," but can carry out only one request at a time. They answer questions such as "What do you do when you are hungry?" by describing the appropriate action. The pattern of asking questions is at its peak, and children usually repeat the question until they receive an answer.

By age 6, children can use all parts of speech correctly, except for deviations from the rule. They can define simple objects and actions by describing their use, shape, or general category of classification, rather than simply describing their outward appearance. For example, they can define a ball as "round, something you bounce, or a toy," rather than only describing its color. They can give some opposites, such as "If Mommy is a woman, Daddy is a man." They can also describe an object according to its composition, such as "A spoon is made of metal."

Personal-Social Behavior

The pervasive ritualism and negativism of toddlerhood gradually diminish during the preschool years. Although self-assertion is still a major theme, preschoolers demonstrate their sense of autonomy differently. They are able to verbalize their request for independence and perform independently because of their much-refined physical and cognitive development. By 4 or 5 years of age, they need little if any assistance with dressing, eating, or toileting (Fig. 15-4). They can also be trusted to obey warnings of danger, although 3- or 4-year-old children may exceed their boundaries at times.

Preschoolers are much more sociable and willing to please than toddlers. They have internalized many of the standards and values of the family and culture. However, by the end of early childhood they begin to question parental values and compare them with those of their peer group and other authority figures. As a result, they may be less willing to abide by the family's code of conduct. Preschoolers become increasingly aware of their position and role within the family. Although this is a more secure age for experiencing the addition of another sibling, relinquishing the position of first or youngest is still difficult and requires appropriate preparation. (See Sibling Rivalry, Chapter 14.)

Play

Various types of play are typical of this period, but preschoolers especially enjoy associative play, group play in similar or identical activities but without rigid organization or rules. Play

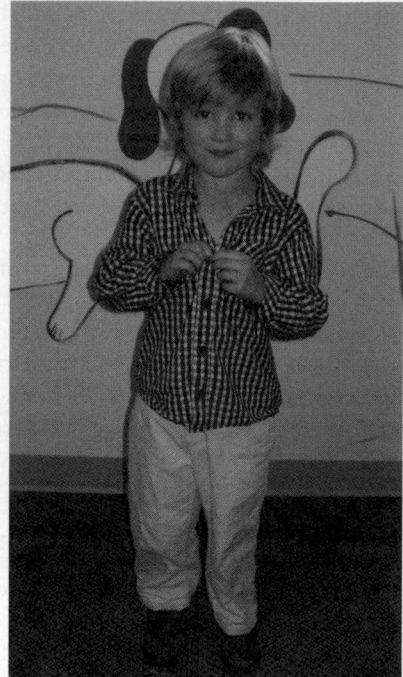

Fig. 15-4 Most preschoolers are able to dress themselves but need help with more difficult items of clothing.

should provide for physical, social, and mental development (see Table 15-1).

Play activities for physical growth and the refinement of motor skills include jumping, running, and climbing. Tricycles, wagons, gym and sports equipment, sandboxes, wading pools, and winter sleds can help develop muscles and coordination. Activities such as swimming, skating, and skiing teach safety and can also help develop muscles and coordination.

Manipulative, constructive, creative, and educational toys provide for quiet activities, fine motor development, and self-expression. Easy construction sets, large blocks of various sizes and shapes, a counting frame, alphabet or number flash cards, paints, crayons, simple carpentry tools, musical toys, illustrated books, simple sewing or handicraft sets, large puzzles, and clay are suitable toys (Fig. 15-5). Electronic games and computer programs are especially valuable in helping children learn basic skills, such as letters and simple words. Although their attention span is still short, preschoolers are beginning to enjoy crafts, especially with the guidance and assistance of adults. A helpful rule in planning creative activities is one simple project per year of age. For example, a 3-year-old child usually has the patience to decorate three eggs but will become bored and restless with more.

Probably the most characteristic and pervasive preschooler activity is imitative, imaginative, and dramatic play. Dress-up clothes, dolls, housekeeping toys, dollhouses, telephones, farm animals and equipment, village sets, trains, trucks, cars, planes, hand puppets, and medical kits provide hours of self-expression (Fig. 15-6). Probably more than any other age-group, 4- and 5-year-old children are absorbed in the reproduction of the behavior of significant adults. Toward the end of the preschool period, children are less satisfied with make-believe or pretend objects and enjoy actually doing the activity, such as cooking and carpentry.

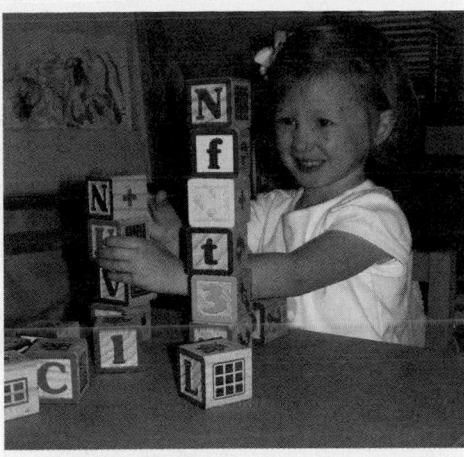

Fig. 15-5 Preschoolers enjoy a sense of accomplishment from activities such as stacking blocks.

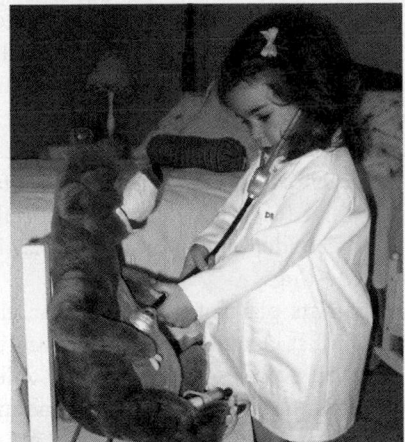

Fig. 15-6 Imaginative and imitative play is typical of preschoolers.

Television and DVDs also have their place in children's play, although each should be only one part of their total repertoire of social and recreational activities. Parents and other caregivers should supervise the selection of programs, watch and discuss programs with their children, schedule limited hours for television viewing, and set a good example of television viewing (American Academy of Pediatrics, 2007). Children enjoy and learn from educational programs; however, television viewing may limit time spent in other meaningful activities such as reading, physical activity, and socialization (American Academy of Pediatrics, 2007). Television can become an interactive activity when adults view programs with children and discuss program content.

Play is so much a part of the young child's life that reality and fantasy become blurred. The make-believe is reality during play and becomes fantasy only when toys are put away or dress-up clothes are removed. It is no wonder that imaginary playmates are so much a part of this age period. Imaginary companions usually appear between the ages of 2½ and 3 years and, for the most part, last until the child enters school. Preschool girls have a higher incidence of creating imaginary companions, whereas preschool boys tend to impersonate characters (Carlson and Taylor, 2005). Imaginary companions serve many purposes; they become friends in times of loneliness, they

accomplish what the child is still attempting, and they experience what the child wants to forget or remember. It is not unusual for the "friend" to have myriad vices and be blamed for wrongdoing. Sometimes the child hopes to escape punishment by saying, "My friend Brian broke the glass." At other times the preschooler may fantasize that the "companion" misbehaved and play the role of parent. This becomes a way of assuming control and authority in a safe situation.

Parents often worry about their child having imaginary playmates, not realizing how normal and useful they are. Parents should be reassured that the child's fantasy is a sign of health that helps differentiate between make-believe and reality. Parents can acknowledge the presence of the imaginary companion by calling him or her by name and even agreeing to simple requests such as setting an extra place at the table, but they should not allow the child to use the playmate to avoid punishment or responsibility. For example, if the child blames the companion for messing up a room, the parents need to state clearly that the child is the only person they see, and therefore the child is responsible for cleaning up (see Critical Thinking Exercise).

? CRITICAL THINKING EXERCISE

Imaginary Playmates

Mrs. Petner tells you, the nurse, that her 2½-year-old daughter, Kimberly, has an imaginary playmate named Allison. She was not concerned about this until Kimberly started asking her to put a plate on the table for Allison at mealtimes. What is your response?

1. Evidence—Is there sufficient evidence to draw any conclusions about Kimberly's mental state at this time?
2. Assumptions—Describe the underlying assumptions about each of the following:
   a. Kimberly's developmental level
   b. The possibility of needing a referral to a mental health professional
   c. Mrs. Petner's hesitancy to comply with Kimberly's request to include her imaginary playmate at mealtimes
3. What implications for nursing care can be drawn at this time?
4. Does the evidence support your nursing interventions?

Children also benefit from play that occurs between them and a parent. Mutual play fosters development from birth through the school years and provides enriched opportunities for learning. Through mutual play, parents can provide tactile and kinesthetic experiences, can maximize verbal and language abilities, and can offer praise and encouragement for exploration of the world. Additionally, mutual play encourages positive interactions between the parent and child, strengthening their relationship. Recommendations for mutual play should reflect the child's developmental level and can incorporate readily available items found in the home or community (musical CDs, puppets, games, and puzzles).

TEMPERAMENT

Temperament influences children's social development and interactions. Chapters 12 and 14 discuss the importance of temperament during early childhood. Because temperamental characteristics tend to remain stable, the same considerations in terms of childrearing apply during the preschool years.

One major concern in the preschool age-group is the effect of temperament on adjustment in group situations, especially school, and the long-term consequences of temperamental characteristics. In particular, the degree of adaptability to new situations, intensity of response, distractibility, amount of persistence, mood, and activity level may influence a child's chances for success in school. Consequently, parents can benefit from suggestions that can promote preschoolers' adjustment. For example, children who are slow to warm up need gradual introduction to new situations and may benefit from the parent's presence until they have settled in. Children with high activity levels tend to adjust better to environments that allow freedom of movement, rather than a structured or regimented classroom. The more aware parents are of their children's unique behaviors, the better they are able to inform teachers or other caregivers of the children's needs and successful approaches to handling the youngsters.

The Behavioral Style Questionnaire helps identify temperamental characteristics in children from 3 to 7 years old (McDevitt and Carey, 1978). Simply asking parents to rate their child as being much easier than, easier than, as easy as, more difficult than, or much more difficult than the average child may also be a valuable screening method.

Table 15-1 summarizes the major developmental achievements for children 3, 4, and 5 years old.

COPING WITH CONCERNS RELATED TO NORMAL GROWTH AND DEVELOPMENT

Preschool and Kindergarten Experience

Some children are home-schooled, but many children attend some type of early childhood program, usually preschool or a daycare center. Group care has become commonplace with the large number of parents currently employed outside the home. The effects of early education and stimulation on children have increasingly gained recognition. Because social development widens to include age-mates and other significant adults, preschool provides an excellent vehicle for expanding children's experiences with others. It is also excellent preparation for entrance into elementary school.

In preschool or daycare centers, children have opportunities to learn about group cooperation; adjustment to sociocultural differences; and coping with frustration, dissatisfaction, and anger. In preschool centers, activities often provide for mastery and achievement, which makes children increasingly feel success, self-confidence, and personal competence. Whether structured learning is imposed is less important than the social climate, type of guidance, and attitude toward the children that is fostered by the teacher or leader. With a teacher who is aware of preschoolers' developmental abilities and needs, children will learn from the activity provided. Most programs incorporate a daily schedule of quiet play, outdoor activity, group activities such as games and projects, creative or free play, and snack and rest periods.

Preschool is particularly beneficial for children who lack a peer-group experience, such as an only child, and for children from impoverished homes. It provides extensive stimulation for language, physical, and social development. It is also excellent preparation for kindergarten. For a child from an underprivileged home, elementary school can be so overwhelming that the sensory overload impedes all learning. Regular school places many more demands on children for prolonged attention, self-disciplined behavior, and demonstrated progress in performance and achievement than does the less-structured atmosphere of preschool.

One of the issues that parents face is the child's readiness for preschool or kindergarten. School readiness is influenced by myriad elements, including a child's social, emotional, and physical development; health status; ability and desire to learn; life experiences; family environment; and parental support. There are no absolute indicators for school readiness. The child's social maturation, especially attention span, is as important as academic readiness.

The use of developmental screening tools and readiness testing varies by state and local district. Developmental screening differs from readiness testing, and there is controversy over the most beneficial form of evaluation in determining a child's readiness to enter school. Readiness testing focuses on evaluation of skill acquisition, whereas developmental screening focuses on the potential to learn. Developmental screening tools address cognitive (especially language), social, and physical milestones and can identify children who may benefit from further diagnostic testing.

Schools and parents play integral roles in a child's school readiness. Schools must be able to assist children with varying learning and physical abilities and should be able to provide diverse learning situations that serve as a foundation for continued growth and maturation. Parents should promote a positive attitude toward learning, read to their children, encourage their children to participate in a variety of activities to explore their talents and interests, and choose appropriate child care or preschool programs (Hagan, Shaw, and Duncan, 2008).

Nurses can help parents assess children's readiness in terms of age, physical ability, and cognitive and social development (see Table 15-1). For example, a group experience may be difficult for young children with short attention spans. These children may require a different type of experience with more individualized attention.

Health care providers can also be helpful in guiding parents in selecting enriched social and educational early intervention programs, schools, and childcare centers. Careful selection of early childhood education is fundamental to future learning and development. Licensed and regulated programs must follow established standards, which represent minimum requirements and safeguards. Regulation is important to protect children from harm and to promote the conditions essential for a child's healthy development and learning. The National Association for the Education of Young Children supports early childhood regulation on all levels.*

---

*Information about the accreditation criteria and procedures of the NAEYC Academy for Early Childhood Program Accreditation is available from the National Association for the Education of Young Children, 1313 L St. NW, Suite 500, Washington, DC 20005; 800-424-2460 or 202-232-8777; www.naeyc.org.

TABLE 15-1	GROWTH AND DEVELOPMENT DURING PRESCHOOL YEARS				
PHYSICAL	**GROSS MOTOR**	**FINE MOTOR**	**LANGUAGE**	**SOCIALIZATION**	**FAMILY RELATIONSHIPS**
Age 3 Yr					
Usual weight gain of 1.8-2.7 kg (4-6 lb)	Rides tricycle	Builds tower of 9-10 cubes	Has vocabulary of about 900 words	Dresses self almost completely if helped with back buttons and told which shoe is right or left	Is in preconceptual phase
Average weight of 14.5 kg (32 lb)	Jumps off bottom step	Builds bridge with three cubes	Uses primarily "telegraphic" speech		Is egocentric in thought and behavior
Usual gain in height of 7.5 cm (3 inches) per year	Stands on one foot for few seconds	Adeptly places small pellets in narrow-necked bottle	Uses complete sentences of three or four words	Pulls on shoes	Has beginning understanding of time; uses many time-oriented expressions, talks about past and future as much as about present, pretends to tell time
Average height of 95 cm (3 feet, 1½ inches)	Goes up stairs using alternate feet; may still come down using both feet on step	In drawing, copies circle, imitates cross, names what has been drawn; cannot draw stick figure but may make circle with facial features	Talks incessantly regardless of whether anyone is paying attention	Has increased attention span	Is less jealous of younger sibling; may be opportune time for birth of additional sibling
May have achieved nighttime control of bowel and bladder	Broad jumps		Repeats sentence of six syllables	Feeds self completely	Is aware of family relationships and sex-role functions
	May try to dance, but balance may not be adequate		Asks many questions	Can prepare simple meals, such as cold cereal and milk	Boys tend to identify more with father or other male figure
				Can help set table; can dry dishes without breaking any	Has increased ability to separate easily and comfortably from parents for short periods
				May have fears, especially of dark and going to bed	
				Knows own gender and gender of others	
				Play is parallel and associative; begins to learn simple games, but often follows own rules; begins to share	

Continued

TABLE 15-1 GROWTH AND DEVELOPMENT DURING PRESCHOOL YEARS—cont'd

PHYSICAL	GROSS MOTOR	FINE MOTOR	LANGUAGE	SOCIALIZATION	COGNITION	FAMILY RELATIONSHIPS
Age 4 Yr						
Pulse and respiration rates decrease slightly	Skips and hops on one foot	Uses scissors successfully to cut out picture following outline	Has vocabulary of 1500 words or more	Very independent	Is in phase of intuitive thought	Rebels if parents expect too much, such as impeccable table manners
Growth rate is similar to that of previous year	Catches ball reliably	Can lace shoes but may not be able to tie bow	Uses sentences of four or five words	Tends to be selfish and impatient	Causality is still related to proximity of events	Takes aggression and frustration out on parents or siblings
Average weight of 16.5 kg (36.5 lb)	Throws ball overhead	In drawing, copies square, traces cross and diamond, adds three parts to stick figure	Questioning is at peak	Aggressive physically as well as verbally	Understands time better, especially in terms of sequence of daily events	Do's and don'ts become important
Average height of 103 cm (3 feet, 4½ inches)	Walks downstairs using alternate footing		Tells exaggerated stories	Takes pride in accomplishments	Unable to conserve matter	May have rivalry with older or younger siblings; may resent older sibling's privileges and younger sibling's invasion of privacy and possessions
Length at birth is doubled			Knows simple songs	Has mood swings	Judges everything according to one dimension, such as height, width, or order	May "run away" from home
Maximum potential for development of amblyopia			May be mildly profane if associates with older children	Shows off dramatically, enjoys entertaining others	Immediate perceptual clues dominate judgment	Identifies strongly with parent of opposite sex
			Obeys prepositional phrases, such as "under," "on top of," "beside," "in back of," or "in front of"	Tells family tales to others with no restraint	Is beginning to develop less egocentrism and more social awareness	Is able to run simple errands outside the home
			Names one or more colors	Still has many fears	May count correctly but has poor mathematic concept of numbers	
			Comprehends analogies, such as, "If ice is cold, fire is ___"	Play is associative	Obeys because parents have set limits, not because of understanding of right or wrong	
				Imaginary playmates common		
				Uses dramatic, imaginative, and imitative devices		
				Sexual exploration and curiosity demonstrated through play, such as being "doctor" or "nurse"		

Age 5 Yr

Physical	Gross Motor	Fine Motor	Language	Socialization/Cognition		
Pulse and respiration rates decrease slightly	Skips and hops on alternate feet	Ties shoelaces	Has vocabulary of about 2100 words	Less rebellious and quarrelsome than at age 4 yr	Begins to question what parents think by comparing them with age-mates and other adults	Gets along well with parents
Average weight of 18.5 kg (41 lb)	Throws and catches ball well	Uses scissors, simple tools, or pencil well	Uses sentences of six to eight words, with all parts of speech	More settled and eager to get down to business	May notice prejudice and bias in outside world	May seek out parent more often than at age 4 yr for reassurance and security, especially when entering school
Average height of 110 cm (3 feet, 7½ inches)	Jumps rope	In drawing, copies diamond and triangle; adds seven to nine parts to stick figure; prints a few letters, numbers, or words, such as first name	Names coins (e.g., nickel, dime)	Not as open and accessible in thoughts and behavior as in earlier years	Is more able to view other's perspective, but tolerates differences rather than understanding them	Begins to question parents' thinking and principles
Eruption of permanent dentition may begin	Skates with good balance		Names four or more colors	Independent but trustworthy, not foolhardy; more responsible	May begin to show understanding of conservation of numbers through counting objects regardless of arrangement	Strongly identifies with parent of same sex, especially boys with their fathers
Handedness is established (about 90% are right-handed)	Walks backward with heel to toe		Describes drawing or pictures with much comment and enumeration	Has fewer fears; relies on outer authority to control world	Uses time-oriented words with increased understanding	Enjoys activities such as sports, cooking, and shopping with parent of same sex
	Jumps from height of 12 inches and lands on toes		Knows names of days of week, months, and other time-associated words	Eager to do things right and to please; tries to "live by the rules"	Cautious about factual information regarding world	
	Balances on alternate feet with eyes closed		Knows composition of articles, such as "A shoe is made of _____."	Has better manners		
			Can follow three commands in succession	Cares for self totally, occasionally needing supervision in dress or hygiene		
				Not ready for concentrated close work or small print because of slight farsightedness and still unrefined eye-hand coordination		
				Play is associative; tries to follow rules but may cheat to avoid losing		

Other areas to evaluate are the facility's daily program, teacher qualifications, staff/student ratio, discipline policy, environmental safety precautions, provision of meals, sanitary conditions, amount of indoor and outdoor space per child, and fee schedule. References from other parents help to evaluate a facility, but personal observation of the facility is recommended. Encourage parents to meet the director and some of the employees at a few facilities to make an informed choice.

Evaluation of the facility's health practices is extremely important. Children in daycare centers have more illnesses than children not in daycare centers, especially gastrointestinal tract infections; respiratory tract infections; and hepatitis A, varicella-zoster virus, and cytomegalovirus infections (Nesti and Goldbaum, 2007). Health care providers can advise parents regarding the evaluation of a facility's sanitary practices and can actively participate in educating staff in measures to minimize infection.

Preparing the Child

Children need preparation for the preschool or kindergarten experience.* For young children, these programs represent a change from their usual home environment and prolonged separation from their parents. Even if children have been cared for by a baby-sitter or in a group setting, preschool and kindergarten differ because there is less individualized attention, programs are more structured, and learning is usually expected.

Before children begin school, parents should present the idea as exciting and pleasurable. Talking to them about activities such as painting, building with blocks, or enjoying swings and other outdoor equipment allows children to fantasize about the forthcoming event in a positive manner. When the first day of school arrives, parents should behave confidently. Such behavior requires parents to have resolved their own feelings regarding the experience.

Parents should introduce their child to the teacher and the facility. In some instances, it is helpful for parents to remain for at least part of the first day until the child is comfortable. If parents stay, they should be available to the child but inconspicuous. A full-day routine is often too overwhelming for a child and could be shortened to a morning or afternoon session if possible. To decrease separation anxiety, parents can provide the school with detailed information about the child's home environment, such as familiar routines, favorite activities, food preferences, names of siblings or pets, and personal habits. Such information helps the child feel at ease in the strange surroundings. A school that automatically requests this information demonstrates the staff's awareness of each child's needs, and the parent has a valuable clue to evaluating the quality of the program. Transitional objects, such as a favorite toy, may also help the child bridge the gap from home to school.

Sex Education

Preschoolers have assimilated a tremendous amount of information during their short lifetimes. Although their thinking may not be mature, they search constantly for explanations and reasons that are logical and reasonable to them. The word "why" seems to supplant the word "no," which was common in toddlerhood. It is only natural that as they learn about "me," they will also want to know "why me," and "how me." Questions such as "Where do babies come from?" are as casual as "Why is the sky blue?" "What makes it rain?" or "Who is that?" It is the *way* in which adults answer questions about procreation that conditions children, even the youngest, to separate these questions from others about their world. If adults answer these questions honestly and as matter-of-factly as any other inquiry, children will continue to search for answers. If they are answered with a "tall tale" or an anxious "You are too young to know about that," children will learn to keep such questions to themselves. Unfortunately, as they harbor these silent mysteries, they formulate their own theories to explain birth. Because magical thinking need not be based on logic or fact, any fantastic and often terrifying explanation can substitute for the truth.

Two rules govern answering sensitive questions about topics such as sex. The first is to *find out what children know and think*. By investigating the theories children have produced as a reasonable explanation, parents can not only give correct information but also help children understand why their explanation is inaccurate. Another reason for ascertaining what the child thinks before offering any information is to avoid giving an "unasked for" answer. For example, 4-year-old Lauren asked her father, "Where did I come from?" Both parents quickly took this inquiry as a clue for offering sex education. After the explanation, Lauren exclaimed, "I don't know about all that! All I know is Mary came from New York, and I want to know where I was born."

The second rule for giving information is to *be honest*. True, the preschooler will forget or misunderstand much of the correct information, but the correct information can be restated until the child absorbs and comprehends the facts. Even though the correct anatomic words may be hard to pronounce or difficult to remember, they become important for explaining other concepts later on. Nurses have the opportunity to contribute to early sex education by conveying accurate information regarding genital terms during physical examinations.

Honesty does not imply imparting every fact of life or allowing excessive permissiveness in sexual curiosity. A child who asks one question is looking for one answer. When they are ready, children will ask about the other "unfinished" parts of the story. Sooner or later they will wonder how the "sperm meets the egg" and "how the baby gets out," but it is best to wait until they ask.

If parents offer too much information, the child will simply become bored or end the conversation with an irrelevant question. Parents worry a great deal about whether they can "harm" their children with "too much" information or tell them things they will not understand. In general, knowledge is not harmful when delivered in a developmentally appropriate manner. It is likely that children may not comprehend everything parents explain initially; they will process information at their own pace. What matters is that parents are approachable and do not dismiss their child's inquiries. It is also important for parents to recognize that children's sex education is affected not only

---

*Resources for developmental and learning activities can be found at Teacher Created Resources, 6421 Industry Way, Westminster, CA 92683; 800-662-4321; www.teachercreated.com.

by the information they receive verbally but also by the relationship and sexual behavior they see their parents modeling and by the sexual content they are exposed to in their everyday environment (e.g., television, magazines, movies).

When a child does not ask questions, parents and health professionals should take advantage of natural opportunities to discuss reproduction, such as talking about someone who is pregnant or discussing a television program or movie about biologic aspects. Many excellent books on sex education are available for preschool children at public libraries, and the Sexuality Information and Education Council of the United States,* local chapters of Planned Parenthood Federation of America,† and the American Academy of Pediatrics‡ have bibliographies of suggested reading material. Parents should read the book before giving or reading it to a child.

Regardless of whether children are given sex education, they will engage in games of sexual curiosity and exploration. At approximately 3 years of age, children are aware of the anatomic differences between the sexes and are concerned with how the other "works." This is not really "sexual" curiosity because many children are still unaware of the reproductive function of the genitalia. They are curious about the eliminative function of the anatomy. Little boys wonder how girls can urinate without a penis, so they watch girls go to the bathroom. Because they cannot see anything but the stream of urine coming out, they want to observe further. "Doctor play" is often a game invented for just such investigation. Little girls are no less curious about boys' anatomy. They find it intriguing to inspect this "thing" that girls do not have.

Parents often wonder how to handle such sexual curiosity. A positive approach is to neither condone nor condemn the behavior but to tell the children that, if they have questions, they should ask the parents; the parents should then encourage the children to engage in some other activity. In this way, children understand that they can satisfy their sexual curiosity in ways other than playing investigative games. This in no way condemns the act but stresses alternative methods by which to seek solutions and answers. Allowing children unrestricted permissiveness only intensifies their anxiety and concern, since exploring and searching usually yield little evidence to satisfy their curiosity.

Occasionally, parents are faced with special dilemmas (e.g., when a child accidentally witnesses sexual intercourse). When such an event occurs, parents must remember that sex education is much more than textbook facts. It is part of a broader concept called *sexuality;* two people unite intimately because of the special relationship they have together. Intercourse is not a physical act apart from feeling or emotion but a private act that two people share to express caring and for pleasure. Offering such an explanation teaches appropriate social behavior and, in particular, stresses the meaningful, intimate relationship

between two adults. When children witness sexual acts, parents should use the opportunity immediately to communicate that sex is part of a healthy and natural adult relationship. However, to prevent subsequent interruptions, children are cautioned to always knock first; if they are too young to understand or comply, a lock on the door is appropriate.

Another concern for some parents is masturbation, or self-stimulation of the genitalia. This occurs at any age for a variety of reasons and, if not excessive, is normal and healthy. For preschoolers, it is part of sexual curiosity and exploration. An important feature of normal childhood masturbation is that the child stops masturbating when distracted (Mallants and Casteels, 2008). If parents are concerned about their child masturbating, it is essential for nurses to investigate the circumstances associated with the activity. Masturbation can be associated with a genitourinary condition, or it may be an expression of anxiety, anger, or boredom; however, in the case of excessive sexual behavior, it may be associated with sexual abuse and emotional or behavioral problems (Mallants and Casteels, 2008). Management of normal childhood masturbation includes parent education and reassurance; redirection of the child to other activities, if masturbation is taking place openly and publicly; and avoidance of punishment, which may reinforce the behavior (Yang, Fullwood, Goldstein, et al, 2005). In addition, parents should emphasize that masturbation is a private act, thus teaching children socially acceptable behavior.

Gifted Children

The importance of identifying gifted children and their needs is increasingly being recognized. Although the definition of *gifted* varies, **giftedness** is traditionally defined as a minimum intelligence quotient (IQ) of 130 (Lovett and Lewandowski, 2006). A broader view, reflected in the term *gifted-talented,* considers signs of giftedness to include specific academic aptitudes, advanced memory skills, creative thinking, ability in the visual or performing arts, and psychomotor ability, either individually or in combination. Children may be identified as gifted when they enter school or are referred by parents or teachers and receive IQ tests. However, parents and caregivers should be aware that giftedness may be present in both academic and nonacademic areas. Therefore not all gifted children are identified when IQ tests alone are used to determine giftedness, which may result in the tragic loss of the opportunity to develop a child's full potential (Lovett and Lewandowski, 2006). It is also important to recognize that giftedness can exist in children who have learning disabilities (Lovett and Lewandowski, 2006) or attention deficit hyperactivity disorder (Antshel, Faraone, Stallone, et al, 2007). Nurses who are aware of the behavioral and developmental characteristics of giftedness can assess children's mental and physical capabilities and assist in early identification (Box 15-1).

Gifted children can present unique challenges to parents. They often demand increased stimulation as infants and continue to seek a great deal of attention from their parents. Their high energy level and persistence can lead to discipline problems similar to those seen in children with difficult temperaments. Parents may be intimidated by having a child smarter than themselves and be hesitant to set limits. However, gifted

---

*90 John St., Suite 704, New York, NY 10038; 212-819-9770; fax: 212-819-9776; www.siecus.org.

†National office: 434 W. 33rd St., New York, NY 10001; 212-541-7800 or 800-230-7526; fax: 212-245-1845; www.plannedparenthood.org.

‡American Academy of Pediatrics Publications, 141 Northwest Point Blvd., Elk Grove Village, IL 60007; 847-434-4000 or 866-843-2271 fax: 847-434-8000; www.aap.org.

- Asynchrony across developmental domains
- Advanced language and reasoning skills
- Conversation and interests similar to those of older children and adults
- Insatiable curiosity; perceptive questions
- Rapid and intuitive understanding of concepts
- Impressive long-term memory
- Ability to hold problems in mind that are not yet figured out
- Ability to make connections between one concept and another
- Interest in patterns and relationships
- Advanced sense of humor (for age)
- Courage in trying new pathways of thinking
- Pleasure in solving and posing new problems
- Capacity for independent, self-directed activities
- Talent in a specific area: drawing, music, games, math, reading
- Sensitivity and perfectionism
- Intensity of feeling and emotion

From Robinson NM, Olszewski-Kubilius PM: Gifted and talented children: issues for pediatricians, *Pediatr Rev* 17(12):428, 1996. Used with permission. American Academy of Pediatrics.

children are children first and have the same needs for love, security, and consistent boundaries as other youngsters.

Sometimes children's advanced skills in one area cause adults to exaggerate their abilities in all areas and thus expect excessively mature behavior. Parents may mislabel slower achievement in a particular skill as lack of trying, when really it represents children's natural progression of abilities. These children benefit from academic settings that provide enrichment and accelerated learning commensurate with their capabilities. Consequently, early identification of gifted-talented children and appropriate parental guidance are critical to their optimum development and emotional adjustment (Liu, Lien, Kafka, et al, 2005).

Informational materials on parenting gifted and talented children is available from the National Association for Gifted Children,* the Council for Exceptional Children,† and local associations.

Aggression

The term *aggression* refers to behavior that attempts to hurt a person or destroy property. Aggression differs from anger, which is a temporary emotional state, but anger may be expressed through aggression. Hyperaggressive behavior in preschoolers is characterized by unprovoked physical attacks on other children and adults, destruction of others' property, frequent intense temper tantrums, extreme impulsivity, disrespect, and noncompliance.

A complex set of biologic, sociocultural, and familial variables influence aggression. Evidence indicates that gender differences exist and that boys exhibit more physical aggression than girls during preschool years (Bendersky, Bennett, and

*1707 L St. NW, Suite 550, Washington, DC 20036; 202-785-4268, fax: 202-785-4248; www.nagc.org.
†1110 N. Glebe Road, Suite 300, Arlington, VA 22201; 888-232-7733 or 703-620-3660; fax: 703-264-9494; www.cec.sped.org.

Lewis, 2006; Benzies, Keown, and Magill-Evans, 2009); however, preschool girls exhibit more relational aggression than preschool boys (Ostrov and Bishop, 2008). Sociocultural factors that are associated with childhood aggression include exposure to community violence and violence in the media (Reebye, 2005). Familial variables such as maternal depression, low level of maternal education, and low socioeconomic status contribute to childhood aggression (Miner and Clarke-Stewart, 2008). Negative parenting practices, including coercive parent-child interactions (McKee, Colletti, Rakow, et al, 2008), low levels of positive interactions and warmth (McKee, Colletti, Rakow, et al, 2008), physical abuse (Sheehan and Watson, 2008), and punitive interactions such as yelling and threatening (Sheehan and Watson, 2008), also contribute to childhood aggression. Other factors that tend to increase aggressive behavior are frustration, modeling, and reinforcement.

Frustration, or the continual thwarting of self-satisfaction by parental disapproval, humiliation, punishment, and insults, can lead children to act out against others as a means of release. These children displace their anger on others, particularly peers and other authority figures, especially if they fear their parents. This type of aggression often applies to the child who is well behaved at home but a discipline problem at school or a bully among playmates.

Modeling, or imitating the behavior of significant others, is a powerful influencing force in preschoolers. Children who see their parents as physically abusive are observing behavior that they come to know as acceptable and therefore may exhibit this behavior with others (Benzies, Keown, and Magill-Evans, 2009). Also, early harsh discipline may lead to aggressive behavior (Miner and Clarke-Stewart, 2008). Another aspect of modeling is establishing a double-standard for acceptable conduct. For example, in some families aggression is synonymous with masculinity, and boys are encouraged to defend themselves. Although defending one's rights is to be encouraged for both sexes, at times the principle of "being tough" or "standing up for yourself" is not tempered with judgment, fairness, or equality but becomes an excuse for ruling and dominating others. Such permissive aggression can produce extreme anxiety in children because it makes them feel out of control, even though outwardly they may appear to be the "boss" or "bully."

Another significant source for modeling is television. Numerous studies have found a positive correlation between viewing violent programs and developing aggression; therefore parents need encouragement to supervise programming, especially for children with aggressive tendencies (Brown and Hamilton-Giachritsis, 2005). The American Academy of Pediatrics (2007) offers a list of recommendations for healthy television viewing.

Reinforcement can also shape aggressive behavior and is closely associated with modeling "masculine" behavior. Sometimes the reward for aggressive behavior is negative (e.g., punishment or disapproval) yet reinforcing because it brings attention. For example, children who are ignored by their parents until they hit a sibling learn that this act attracts attention. Additionally, parents who permit aggressive behavior by not interfering communicate silent, implicit approval of such acts.

One of the tasks of preschoolers is learning socially acceptable behavior and the ability to control aggression and redirect their anger. Parents can help children by modeling the appropriate behavior and encouraging children to express themselves verbally. For example, rather than condoning the hitting of another child for taking a toy, parents can suggest that the child state how he or she feels, such as "I am angry when you take my ball. Please give it back."

Children should not be made to feel guilty or ashamed for being angry or frustrated. When children recognize these feelings, they are better able to channel them into constructive, not destructive, outlets. One of the earliest demonstrations of aggression is temper tantrums. (See Chapter 14.) Parents can handle them constructively by not attending to or reinforcing them and by helping children find control through appropriate play situations. In this way, young children learn to acknowledge such feelings and express them in alternate ways, such as pounding on clay or hitting a punching bag. When children are out of control, they may need to be physically restrained or removed from the scene to prevent them from hurting themselves or others.

Sometimes the type of discipline used to extinguish other forms of unacceptable behavior actually promotes aggressive behavior. For example, if a child is spanked for an aggressive act, aggression is being used to "teach" a lesson against aggression. In addition to physically aggressive discipline, inconsistency in disciplinary practices may also foster aggressiveness in children (Ostrov and Bishop, 2008). The use of time-out and solitary play is an effective intervention for aggression. Additionally, minimizing anger and frustration can lead to fewer opportunities for acting-out behavior.

When a child exhibits extreme behaviors, such as aggression, parents are often concerned about the need for professional help. Generally, the difference between normal and problematic behavior is not the behavior itself but its quantity (number of occurrences), severity (interference with social or cognitive functioning), distribution (different manifestations), onset (when the behavior started), and duration (at least 4 weeks). When aggressive tendencies are evaluated, these factors are assessed to distinguish between behaviors typically seen at various ages and those that may represent an underlying problem. Extreme aggression requires professional treatment and is often difficult to change.*

Speech Problems

The most critical period for speech development occurs between 2 and 4 years of age. During this period, children are using their rapidly growing vocabulary faster than they can produce the words. A failure to master sensorimotor integration results in stuttering or stammering as children try to say the word they are already thinking about. This dysfluency in speech pattern is called developmental stuttering and is common during language development in children ages 2 to 5 years (Nelson, 2008). Stuttering affects boys more frequently than girls, has been shown to have a genetic link, and usually resolves during childhood (Prasse and Kikano, 2008). The National Institute on Deafness and Other Communication Disorders (2008) encourages parents and caregivers of children who stutter to speak slowly and clearly, refrain from correcting or criticizing the child's speech, resist completing the child's sentences, and take time to listen attentively. When parents or other significant caregivers place undue emphasis on a child's stuttering, they may exacerbate the problem. A speech evaluation is indicated if stuttering persists for longer than 6 months with no improvement (Hagan, Shaw, and Duncan, 2008).

The best therapy for speech problems is prevention and early detection. Common causes of speech problems are hearing loss, developmental delay, autism, and lack of verbal or psychosocial stimulation (Feldman, 2005). Referral for further evaluation and treatment may be necessary to prevent a problem from interfering with learning. Anticipatory preparation of parents for expected developmental norms may calm caregiver anxiety.

Children pressured into producing sounds ahead of their developmental level may develop dyslalia (articulation problems) or revert to using infantile speech. Prevention involves educating parents regarding the usual achievement of speech production during childhood. The Denver Articulation Screening Examination is an excellent tool for assessing articulation skills in the child and for explaining to parents the expected progression of sounds. (See Appendix A.)

Stress

Although for parents the preschool years generally are less troublesome than toddlerhood, this period presents children with many unique stresses. Some are innate and stem from preschoolers' unique understanding of the world, such as fears. Others are imposed, such as beginning school. Although minimum amounts of stress are beneficial during the early years to help children develop effective coping skills, excessive stress is harmful. Young children are especially vulnerable because of their limited capacity to cope.

To help parents deal with stress in their child's life, they must be aware of signs of stress and be helped to identify the source (Box 15-2). Any number of stresses may be present, such as the birth of a sibling, marital discord, relocation, or illness. The best approach to dealing with stress is prevention. It is important to monitor the amount of stress in the child's life so that levels do not exceed ability to cope. In many instances, structuring the child's schedule to allow rest and preparing the child for change, such as entering school, are sufficient measures.

Because stress is a constant aspect of daily living, it is not too early to help preschool children learn to cope with it. They can learn the meaning of the word *stress* and recognize physical signs of a stress reaction, such as a rapid pulse, a pounding heart, or fatigue. Teaching children relaxation and imagery is effective. Young children can learn to "let their bodies go limp like a rag doll." Parents can use stories to help their child imagine pleasurable events. As language skills improve, encourage preschoolers to talk about their feelings and explore other ways of expressing emotions. Play is an excellent vehicle for venting anger or frustration, and toys such as drums, clay, and

---

*Information on child development and behavior can be obtained through Developmental Behavioral Pediatrics Online, www.dbpeds.org.

BOX 15-2   SOURCES OF STRESS IN PRESCHOOLERS

Age 3 Years

Stubbornness—Despite developing interest in social relationships and a concept of "we," may lapse into uncooperative behavior

Belongings—Guards possessions

Jealousy—Particularly when it comes to parents' love

Separation anxiety—Difficulty leaving the parent

Stranger anxiety—Expresses fear being around someone unknown

Confusion—Cannot always discriminate between fantasy and reality

Fears—May be precipitated by imagination; may also fear dogs or other animals

Speech—May stutter or stumble over words

Activity level—Seems to be in perpetual motion; may exhaust himself or herself

Mealtime—May forget to eat or lose interest in food

Nap or bedtime—May fear bad dreams, the dark, or missing out on some fun while asleep

Destructiveness—May damage or destroy objects

Questions—Continually asks "why," and is upset if trusted adults do not respond or do not know the answer

Age 4 Years

Insecurity—May develop nervous habits such as nail biting, facial tics, thumb sucking, genital manipulation, eye blinking, or nose picking; may insist on bringing a familiar item from home to preschool

Companionship—Enjoys interacting with friends, although they may quarrel

Belongings—Protects possessions

Sex—Interested in the human body; may engage in exhibitionism

Activity level—Enjoys running, jumping, and slamming doors; may be punished for disruptive behavior

Fears—Picks up fears from adults; may fear dark room or anything perceived as "creepy"

Attention—Likes to talk and is frustrated if ignored or put off

Age 5 Years

Approval—Parents' love and acceptance are vital; seeks praise

School—May have difficulty adjusting to kindergarten

Separation anxiety—Particularly fears loss of mother

Worrying—May develop irrational fears; take information out of context; or fret over a misinterpreted, overheard conversation

Belongings—Protects possessions

Procrastination—Delays completing chores or activities

Name calling—Insults others to boost self-image but is upset when he or she is the victim of mockery

Modified from Kuczen B: *Childhood stress: don't let your child be a victim,* New York, 1982, Delacorte.

---

punching bags provide alternative methods of dissipating anxiety and teach socially acceptable ways of dealing with such feelings.

Fears

The greatest number and variety of real and imagined fears are present during the preschool years. Preschoolers may fear the dark, being left alone (especially at bedtime), animals (particularly large dogs and snakes), ghosts, sexual matters (castration), and objects or persons associated with pain. The exact cause of children's fears is unknown. Freudians believe that the upsurge of fears during the preschool years results from the anxiety of being injured and mutilated (castration complex). Piaget views fears as a product of the type of thinking in this age-group;

preschoolers are caught between the egocentric thinking of infants, which protects them from imagined fears, and the more logical thought processes of school-age children, which help explain and dispel potential fears. Children in the preconceptual stage still engage in egocentric thought but are now able to imagine an event without actually experiencing it. For example, seeing someone hurt is sufficient for realizing what the hurt must be like and for consequently fearing that hurt. This is commonly observed in medical practice. When watching another child get an injection, the preschooler may become upset, almost as if he or she received the injection.

The concept of animism (ascribing life-like qualities to inanimate objects) helps explain why children fear objects. For example, a child may refuse to use the toilet after watching a television commercial in which the toilet bowl is portrayed as turning into a monster.

One fear peculiar to this age is fear of annihilation. Because of poorly defined body boundaries and improved cognitive abilities, young children develop concerns related to loss of body parts, such as their body going down the drain. Because preschool children cannot understand concepts of size, they cannot understand that their body is too large to disappear down the drain.

Preschoolers are also likely to develop parent-induced fears. When parents demonstrate their fears, these concerns are communicated to the children. Such fears tend to be long lasting and difficult to dispel.

The best way to help children overcome their fears is by actively involving them in finding practical methods to deal with frightening experiences. This may be as simple as keeping a dim night-light in the child's bedroom for reassurance or letting the child bathe a doll so that the child can observe that large objects cannot go down the drain. In this way, the experience that created the fear in the child can be reconstructed without involving the child directly as the victim. The child is allowed alternative methods by which to feel in control while overcoming fear.

Exposing children to the feared object in a safe situation provides a type of conditioning, or desensitization. For instance, children who are afraid of dogs should never be forced to approach or touch one, but they may be gradually introduced to the experience by watching other children play with the animal. This type of modeling, having others demonstrate fearlessness, can be effective if children are allowed to progress at their own rate.

Usually by 5 or 6 years of age, children relinquish many of their fears. Explaining the developmental sequence of fears and their gradual disappearance may help parents feel more secure in handling preschoolers' fears. However, sometimes fears do not subside with simple measures or developmental maturation. When children experience severe fears that disrupt family life, professional help is required. Successful training programs may include (1) muscle relaxation; (2) guided imagery; (3) positive self-talk or recitation of brave statements; or (4) thought stopping, or repetition of reassuring statements that block fearful thoughts. Rewards or "tokens" may be given for "bravery" and not being afraid. Nurses can apply such interventions in clinical settings to reduce fears (e.g., of being alone or of painful procedures).

PROMOTING OPTIMUM HEALTH DURING THE PRESCHOOL YEARS

NUTRITION

Healthy nutrition during childhood should include eating a variety of foods and consuming sufficient energy to promote growth and development, while avoiding the development of obesity (Kleinman, 2009). For preschoolers, the requirement for calories per unit of body weight decreases slightly to 90 kcal/kg, for an average daily intake of 1800 calories. Fluid requirements may also decrease slightly (to approximately 100 ml/kg/day) but depend on activity level, climatic conditions, and state of health. Protein requirements increase with age; the recommended intake for preschoolers is 13 to 19 g/day (0.45 to 0.67 oz/day) (Otten, Hellwig, and Meyers, 2006). In children over 2 years of age, intake of dietary fiber should equal the child's age plus 5 in grams per day (Kleinman, 2009).

The American Academy of Pediatrics Committee on Nutrition recommends the following guidelines for children over the age of 2 years: saturated fatty acid consumption should be less than 10% of total caloric intake, total fat over several days should be 20% to 30% of total caloric intake, and cholesterol consumption should be less than 300 mg/day (Kleinman, 2009). Evidence supports the efficacy of following these recommendations, and negative health effects have not been reported (American Heart Association, Gidding, Dennison, et al, 2006). These efforts are important in the prevention of childhood obesity, cardiovascular disease, diabetes, and metabolic syndrome. While limiting fat consumption, it is also important to ensure the diet contains adequate nutrients. This can be done simultaneously as in the following example regarding calcium. The recommendation for daily calcium intake for children 1 to 3 years old is 500 mg, and the recommendation for children 4 to 8 years old is 800 mg (Otten, Hellwig, and Meyers, 2006). Milk and dairy products provide a major source of calcium. Eating less fat does not necessarily require drinking less milk or eating fewer dairy products but instead replacing higher fat milk, cheese, and yogurt with lower fat or nonfat choices.

Excessive consumption of fruit juices and other sweetened beverages has been associated with adverse health effects such as dental caries, gastrointestinal conditions such as chronic diarrhea, and diets poor in nutritive value (Allen and Myers, 2006). The American Academy of Pediatrics recommends limiting the intake of 100% fruit juice to 4 to 6 oz/day for children ages 1 to 6 years (American Heart Association, Gidding, Dennison, et al, 2006). Nurses should counsel moderation in fruit juice consumption and at the same time provide suggestions for more appropriate sources of nutrients such as ascorbic acid, folate, magnesium, and potassium.

In 2008 the US Department of Agriculture released a new food guide system called MyPyramid for Preschoolers, created specifically for children age 2 to 5 years (US Department of Agriculture, 2009). This new system is comprehensive and provides information for developing a healthy lifestyle at an early age. MyPyramid for Preschoolers includes customizable eating plans and offers information on growth during the preschool years, healthy eating habits, physical activity, and food safety.

Parents can use this information to assist their children in making healthy lifestyle choices and to help prevent adverse health conditions secondary to poor nutrition.

> ### ! NURSING ALERT
>
> Obesity in young children has increased over the past two decades. Efforts to provide a healthy diet and to encourage physical activity should begin early to help children achieve optimum health (American Heart Association, Gidding, Dennison, et al, 2006). The 5-2-0-1 framework described by Joy (2008), and inspired by American Academy of Pediatrics recommendations, provides a foundation for patient education regarding healthy lifestyle choices. This framework refers to five servings of fruits and vegetables per day, 2 hours or less of screen time, 0 servings of sugar-sweetened beverages, and 1 hour of physical activity per day.

Some preschoolers still have food habits typical of toddlers, such as food fads and strong taste preferences. When children reach 4 years of age, they seem to enter another period of finicky eating, which is generally characteristic of the more rebellious behavior of children in this age-group. By age 5 years, children are more agreeable to trying new foods, especially if encouraged by an adult who allows the child to help with food preparation or experiments with a new taste or different dish (Fig. 15-7). Mealtime can become a battle if parents expect excellent table manners. A 5-year-old child is usually ready for the "social" side of eating, but the younger child still has difficulty sitting quietly through a long family meal.

The amount and variety of foods young children eat vary greatly from day to day. Consequently, parents sometimes worry about the quantity and quality of food consumed by preschoolers. In general, the quality is much more important than the quantity, which nurses should stress during nutritional counseling. There is some evidence that children self-regulate their caloric intake. If they eat less at one meal, they compensate at another meal or snack.

One approach toward lessening parental concern is advising parents to keep a weekly record of everything the child eats. In particular, stress the need to measure the amount of food, such as setting aside ½ cup of vegetables and serving the child from

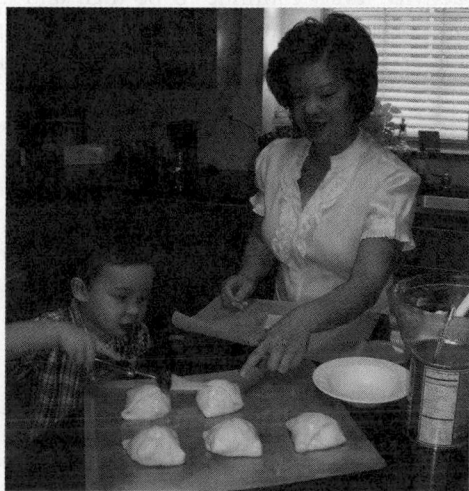

Fig. 15-7 Preschool children enjoy helping adults and are more likely to try new foods if they are included in the preparation.

this premeasured amount, to provide a more accurate estimate of food intake at each meal. When parents look at the food chart at the end of the week, they are usually amazed at how much the child consumed. In general, preschoolers eat only slightly more than toddlers, or approximately half of an adult's portion. Resources are available for the health care provider and the caregiver to help build healthy eating habits for children* (see Critical Thinking Exercise).

? CRITICAL THINKING EXERCISE
Nutrition

Mrs. Pierce reports that she thinks her 3-year-old daughter, Hannah, is not eating enough and she is concerned about her overall nutrition. Mealtimes are difficult, and sometimes it takes an hour to get Hannah to eat what is on her plate. She seems to only want to eat chicken nuggets. Mrs. Pierce feels discouraged that mealtimes are such a battle but knows it is important for Hannah to get the nutrients she needs for growth. Many times she uses activities to entice Hannah to eat such as allowing her to watch her favorite video while eating or allowing her to bring her doll to the table. Today, Hannah weighed 14.2 kg (31.3 lb), and her height was 94.1 cm (3 feet, 1 inch). She has been growing along the 50th percentile on growth curves for both height and weight for the past 1½ years. Her assessment reveals a healthy, well-nourished, well-developed preschooler.

1. Evidence—Is there sufficient evidence to draw any conclusions about Hannah's nutritional status at this time?
2. Assumptions—Describe the underlying assumptions about each of the following:
   a. Hannah's eating habits
   b. The family's mealtime routine
   c. Hannah's growth
3. What implications for nursing care can be drawn at this time?
4. Does the evidence support your nursing interventions?

SLEEP AND ACTIVITY

Sleep patterns vary widely, but the average preschooler sleeps approximately 12 hours a night and infrequently takes daytime naps. Waking during the night is common throughout early childhood and may be related to social rather than developmental factors (Moore, Meltzer, and Mindell, 2008).

Motor activity levels continue to be high and allow preschoolers to explore their environment, begin learning physical games and sports, and interact with others. Motor activity is therefore encouraged. Quiet activities, such as television and video games, are increasingly appealing and can become an unhealthy substitute for active play.

Preschoolers' increased gross motor abilities and coordination allow them to engage in many physical activities, if only at a novice level. Whether young children should begin formalized training in an activity at this early age is controversial. Training programs must consider the child's physical and psychologic

immaturity, and readiness must be determined individually. The American Academy of Pediatrics (2006) encourages free play and a variety of physical activities. However, the Academy also supports organized play when it is developmentally appropriate and occurs in a nonthreatening, fun, and safe environment.

Sleep Problems

The preschool years are a prime time for sleep disturbances. As toddlers and preschoolers cope with separation anxiety and increasing autonomy, they may begin to have more sleep problems (Jenni, Fuhrer, Iglowstein, et al, 2005; Moore, Meltzer, and Mindell, 2008). Some have trouble going to sleep, especially after so much activity and stimulation during the day. Others may develop bedtime fears, wake during the night, or have nightmares or sleep terrors. Still others may prolong the inevitable bedtime through elaborate rituals.

Recommendations for handling a sleep disturbance are offered only after a thorough assessment. Cultural traditions may dictate sleep practices contrary to certain well-accepted professional recommendations. Therefore parents may not perceive particular sleep habits as problematic (see Cultural Competence box).

🌐 CULTURAL COMPETENCE
Cosleeping

Many experts recommend that infants and children be trained to always sleep in their own crib or bed. However, cosleeping, or the "family bed" (in which parents allow the children to sleep with them), is an accepted cultural practice among many African-American, Hispanic, and Asian families (Owens, 2008). Others who have adopted cosleeping include parents who think that cosleeping promotes parent-child bonding, parents who think that cosleeping diminishes their child's nighttime fears or other sleep disturbances, and mothers who are breast-feeding. Cosleeping may be a practical solution to limited numbers of bedrooms or beds in lower socioeconomic families. Controversy exists regarding the medical, developmental, and social advantages and disadvantages of cosleeping. Parents who are considering cosleeping should fully investigate the potential risks and benefits, and health care providers should be proactive in discussing sleeping arrangements with families at each visit to ensure children's safety.

Interventions differ greatly; for example, nightmares and sleep terrors require different approaches (Table 15-2). For children who delay going to bed, a recommended approach involves counseling parents about the importance of a consistent bedtime ritual and emphasizing the normalcy of this type of behavior in young children. Parents should ignore attention-seeking behavior, and the child should not be taken into the parents' bed or allowed to stay up past a reasonable hour. Other measures that may be helpful include keeping a light on in the room, providing transitional objects such as a favorite toy, or leaving a drink of water by the bed.

Helping children slow down before bedtime also reduces resistance to going to bed. One approach is to establish limited rituals that signal readiness for bed, such as a bath or story. Parents can reinforce the pattern by stating, "After this story, it is bedtime," and consistently carrying through the routine. If

---

*A nutritional resource for the health care provider is American Academy of Pediatrics, Committee on Nutrition: *Pediatric nutrition handbook*, Elk Grove, IL, 2009, The Academy. A nutritional resource for parents and caregivers is *Food Fights*. To order, contact the American Academy of Pediatrics, 866-843-2271; www.aap.org.

TABLE 15-2   COMPARISON OF NIGHTMARES TO SLEEP TERRORS

CHARACTERISTIC	NIGHTMARES	SLEEP TERRORS
Description	A scary dream; takes place during rapid-eye-movement (REM) sleep and is followed by full waking	A partial arousal from very deep (state IV, non-REM) sleep
Time of distress	After dream is over, child wakes and cries or calls; not during nightmare itself	During terror itself, as child screams and thrashes; afterward is calm
Time of occurrence	In second half of night, when dreams are most intense	Usually 1-4 hr after falling asleep, when non-REM sleep is deepest
Child's behavior	Crying in younger children, fright in all; behaviors persistent even though child is awake	Initially may sit up, thrash, or run in bizarre manner, with eyes bulging, heart racing, and profuse perspiring; may cry, scream, talk, or moan; shows apparent fright, anger, or obvious confusion, which disappears when child is fully awake
Responsiveness to others	Is aware of and reassured by another's presence	Is not very aware of another's presence, is not comforted, and may push person away and scream and thrash more if held or restrained
Return to sleep	May be considerably delayed because of persistent fear	Usually rapid; often difficult to keep child awake
Description of dream	Yes (if old enough)	No memory of a dream or of yelling or thrashing
Interventions	Accept dream as real fear. Sit with child; offer comfort, assurance, and sense of protection. Avoid forcing child back to his or her own bed. Consider professional counseling for recurrent nightmares unresponsive to above approaches.	Observe child for a few minutes, *without interfering*, until child becomes calm or wakes fully. Intervene only if necessary to protect child from injury. Guide child back to bed if needed. Stress to parents that sleep terrors are a normal, common phenomenon in preschoolers that requires relatively little intervention.

Modified from Ferber R: *Solve your child's sleep problems,* New York, 1985, Simon & Schuster.

anticipated extra stimulation (e.g., having visitors arrive at the children's bedtime) disrupts this routine, it is advisable to settle children in bed beforehand.

Television viewing just before bedtime can also contribute to bedtime resistance and delay sleep onset. Research has revealed a direct correlation between extensive television viewing and sleep problems in children (Johnson, Cohen, Kasen, et al, 2004). Specific sleep problems related to television exposure include decreased sleep length, night wakings, impaired sleep quality, sleep onset problems, and sleep-wake transition disorders (Paavonen, Pennonen, Roine, et al, 2006). In addition to limiting the duration of television viewing, parents should ensure that television shows and other types of media are age appropriate and are not too frightening or over-stimulating. Nurses should incorporate assessment of sleep patterns and education about the development of healthy sleep behaviors into every well-child visit.

DENTAL HEALTH

By the beginning of the preschool period, the eruption of the deciduous (primary) teeth is complete. Dental care is essential to preserve these temporary teeth and to teach good dental habits. (See Chapter 14.) Although preschoolers' fine motor control is improved, they still require assistance and supervision with brushing, and parents should perform flossing. Professional care and routine prophylaxis, especially fluoride supplements, should continue. The frequency of professional dental care should be based on a child's individual risk assessment, including family history, socioeconomic status, dental development, presence or absence of dental disease, special health care needs, and dietary habits (Kagihara, Niederhauser, and Stark, 2009). Primary care providers are in an ideal situation to perform dental screenings and risk assessments and refer children to a dental home (Section on Pediatric Dentistry and Oral Health, 2008). The American Academy of Pediatric Dentistry offers a Caries-Risk Assessment Tool for health care providers (www.aapd.org/media/Policies_ Guidelines/P_CariesRiskAssess.pdf), and the American Academy of Pediatrics provides a training program for pediatric health care professionals that presents information on dental screenings, risk assessments, and triage (www.aap.org/ oralhealth/cme).

Trauma to teeth during this period is not uncommon, and prompt evaluation by a dentist is necessary if oral trauma occurs. Preservation of the space previously occupied by an avulsed tooth is necessary for proper eruption of the secondary tooth.

INJURY PREVENTION

Because of improved gross and fine motor skills, coordination, and balance, preschoolers are less prone to falls than toddlers. They tend to be less reckless; listen more to parental rules; and are aware of potential dangers, such as hot objects, sharp instruments, and dangerous heights. Putting objects in the mouth as part of exploration has all but ceased, but poisoning is still a danger. Cognitive ability may play a role in injury avoidance, especially in girls, who are less daring and risk taking. Inform parents that children as young as $4\frac{1}{2}$ years old have been shown to engage in risk-taking behaviors. Intervention strategies targeted at high-risk populations need to be part of safety education. Pedestrian motor vehicle injuries increase because of activities such as playing in the street, riding tricycles, running after balls, or forgetting safety regulations when crossing streets.

In general, the guidelines suggested for injury prevention in Box 12-6 may apply to children in this age-group as well. However, emphasis is now on protection and education for safety and potential hazards. Because preschoolers are great imitators, it is essential that parents set a good example by "practicing what they preach." Children quickly observe discrepancies between what they are told to do and what they observe. Establishing habits at this time, such as wearing bicycle helmets, can create long-term safety behaviors.

ANTICIPATORY GUIDANCE—CARE OF FAMILIES

The preschool years present fewer childrearing difficulties than the earlier years, and this stage of development is facilitated by appropriate anticipatory guidance in the areas already discussed

(see Family-Centered Care box). Injury prevention also shifts from protection to education. For example, at this age the use of electrical outlet caps may be discontinued, with verbal explanations given of why danger exists and how to avoid it.

During this period, an emotional transition between parent and child occurs. Although children are still attached to their parents and accept all their values and beliefs, they are nearing the period of life when they will question previous teachings and prefer the companionship of peers. Entry into school marks a separation for both parents and children. Parents may need help in adjusting to this change, particularly if one parent has focused his or her daily activities on home responsibilities. As a child begins preschool or elementary school, parents may need to seek activities outside the home, such as community involvement or a career. In this way, all family members are adjusting to change, which is part of the process of growth and development.

FAMILY-CENTERED CARE

Guidance During Preschool Years

Age 3 Years

Prepare parents for the child's increasing interest in widening personal relationships.

Encourage enrollment in preschool or other socialization activities.

Emphasize importance of setting limits.

Prepare parents to expect exaggerated tension-reduction behaviors, such as need for "security blanket."

Encourage parents to offer the child choices.

Prepare parents to expect marked changes at 3½ years, when the child becomes insecure and exhibits emotional extremes.

Prepare parents for normal dysfluency in speech and advise them to avoid focusing on the pattern.

Prepare parents to expect extra demands on their attention as a reflection of the child's emotional insecurity and fear of loss of love.

Warn parents that the equilibrium of a 3-year-old will change to the aggressive, out-of-bounds behavior of a 4-year-old.

Prepare parents to handle anger appropriately and constructively.

Inform parents to anticipate a more stable appetite with more food selections.

Stress the need for protection and education of the child to prevent injury. (See Injury Prevention, Chapter 14.)

Age 4 Years

Prepare parents for more aggressive behavior, including motor activity and offensive language.

Prepare parents to expect resistance to parental authority.

Explore parental feelings regarding the child's behavior.

Suggest some type of respite for primary caregivers, such as placing the child in preschool for part of the day.

Prepare parents for the child's increasing sexual curiosity.

Emphasize the importance of realistic limit setting on behavior and appropriate disciplinary techniques.

Prepare parents for the highly imaginative 4-year-old who indulges in "tall tales" (to be differentiated from lies) and develops imaginary playmates.

Prepare parents to expect nightmares or an increase in them.

Provide reassurance that a period of calm begins at 5 years of age.

Age 5 Years

Inform parents to expect a tranquil period at 5 years.

Help parents prepare the child for entrance into the school environment.

Make certain immunizations are up to date before entering school.

Encourage parents to establish safety rules regarding interaction with strangers.

Suggest that unemployed mothers or fathers consider own activities when child begins school.

Suggest swimming lessons for child.

Encourage parents to limit television viewing and to preview shows and movies for inappropriate content.

KEY POINTS

- The preschool years encompass the period from 3 to 5 years of age—a time considered critical for emotional and psychologic development.
- Biologic development in the preschool period is characterized by mature organ systems and refinement in gross and fine motor behavior, as evidenced by participation in activities such as running, riding a tricycle, and drawing.
- According to Erikson, acquiring a sense of initiative is the chief psychosocial task of the preschooler. Development of the superego occurs during this period, and the conscience begins to emerge.
- According to Freudian theory, preschoolers are in the oedipal stage. Resolution of this stage occurs when children strongly identify with the parent of the same sex.

- According to Piaget, the preschool age is characterized by intuitive or prelogical thinking and a move toward logical thought processes through advanced and complex learning, language, and understanding of causality.
- The seeds of moral development are planted during the preschool period. According to Kohlberg, these children are in the stage of naive instrumental orientation, in which they are concerned with satisfying their own needs and, less frequently, the needs of others.
- Social development includes further separation-individuation; more sophisticated language; greater independence; and more complex, imaginative forms of play.
- Areas of special concern to parents during the preschool period are the preschool and kindergarten experience, sex education, speech problems, stress, and fears.

- In selecting a school, parents should inquire about daily programs, teacher qualifications, accreditation, staff/student ratio, safety, meals, fees, and health practices. Licensing, regulation, and accreditation are intrinsic factors to look for when selecting early education programs.
- Two rules that govern answering questions about sex and other sensitive issues are finding out what the child thinks and being honest.

- Preschool aggression may result from frustration, modeling behavior, and reinforcement.
- Fears are a great part of the preschool period; fear of objects or potential annihilation and parent-induced fears are common.
- Health promotion includes proper nutrition, adequate sleep, proper dental care, and injury prevention.

ANSWERS TO CRITICAL THINKING EXERCISES

Imaginary Playmates

1. **Yes.** The situation that Mrs. Petner reported describes appropriate preschool behavior. Imaginative play and imaginary playmates are often part of preschoolers' play activities and do not indicate a mental illness.

2. **a.** Imaginary playmates are typical for children this age. They may serve as companions in times of loneliness, such as for only children or those with a vast age discrepancy between siblings; they may comfort children in times of distress; and they allow children an avenue to process unresolved conflicts or interactions.
   b. Since there is no mention of abnormal activity or behavior, it is reasonable to conclude that a referral to a mental health professional is not necessary.
   c. Mrs. Petner may believe that if she complies with Kimberly's request, she will be affirming the presence of an imaginary person, and she may worry that this is not healthy.

3. The nurse can take this opportunity to educate Mrs. Petner regarding imaginary play and imaginary playmates during the preschool years. The nurse should reassure Mrs. Petner that she can acknowledge the presence of an imaginary companion as long as Kimberly does not use the playmate to avoid responsibility or discipline. Kimberly will likely abandon this type of play as she enters the school-age years.

4. **Yes.** The evidence supports implementing this care plan. You should not dismiss the parent's concern but use this occasion to educate the parent about normal preschool development and play. Also explore whether other factors contribute to the parent's concern regarding the child's development.

Nutrition

1. **Yes.** Hannah's growth measurements indicate that she is obtaining adequate nutrition to sustain her growth. However, other items that could offer more insight into Hannah's nutritional status include a diet history and blood work, such as electrolytes and a protein panel. Although Hannah is displaying some normal preschool behavior in regard to nutrition, it is concerning that mealtimes have become such a point of contention between Hannah and her mother.

2. **a.** Hannah is exhibiting selective food choices, often called food jags, which are typical of this age-group. New or distasteful foods and large servings could potentially contribute to Hannah's refusal to eat all the items on her plate.
   b. Mealtimes could be more pleasant and less distracting by eliminating activities that draw attention away from eating. Making changes to improve the mealtime environment could affect Hannah's willingness to eat.
   c. Hannah's growth is not concerning. She has maintained her growth in height and weight.

3. Mrs. Pierce's concern regarding proper nutrition is a healthy parental concern. However, this is a good opportunity to educate Mrs. Pierce about normal preschool appetite, food jags, neophobia, and appropriate serving sizes. Mrs. Pierce should be encouraged to supplement meals with healthy snacks between mealtimes instead of trying to meet all Hannah's nutritional requirements in three large meals. She should offer a variety of foods but be aware that preschool children do not usually like trying new foods, and it may take several attempts before Hannah will eat them. Hannah may be more interested in trying new foods if she is included in the meal preparation. Mrs. Pierce should also be encouraged to make mealtimes more pleasant. She can reduce distractions by turning off the television and not allowing toys at the table. The family should sit down and eat together. This time serves as an occasion for preschoolers to observe others eating and socializing. Hannah should be encouraged to feed herself and not be pressured to eat more than she wants. Mrs. Pierce can be reassured regarding Hannah's growth and development with a review of her growth chart. Sometimes a visual display of a child's growth will ease parents' concern. Also, Mrs. Pierce can be advised to maintain a diet history of Hannah's food intake over 1 week, including accurate measurements of food and fluid volume intake. The record should also include the number and type of snacks that Hannah consumes. High-calorie snacks and drinks could contribute to Hannah's lack of interest in eating at mealtimes. Review of the diet record may provide reassurance once Mrs. Pierce is able to see how much Hannah has eaten cumulatively over the entire week.

4. **Yes.** Information obtained from Hannah's growth and physical assessments support these interventions. Additionally, knowledge about preschool nutrition supports these interventions.

REFERENCES

Allen RE, Myers AL: Nutrition in toddlers, *Am Fam Physician* 74(9):1527-1532, 2006.

American Academy of Pediatrics: *TV and your family*, 2007, The Academy, available at www.aap.org/publiced/BR_TV.htm (accessed March 9, 2009).

American Academy of Pediatrics, Committee on Sports Medicine and Fitness and Committee on School Health: Active healthy living: prevention of childhood obesity through increased physical activity, *Pediatrics* 117(5):1832-1842, 2006.

American Heart Association, Gidding SS, Dennison BA, et al: Dietary recommendations for children and adolescents: a guide for practitioners, *Pediatrics* 117(2):544-559, 2006.

American Speech-Language-Hearing Association: *The advantages of being bilingual*, 2009, The Association, available at www.asha.org/about/news/tipsheets/bilingual.htm (accessed March 7, 2009).

Antshel KM, Faraone SV, Stallone K, et al: Is attention deficit hyperactivity disorder a valid diagnosis in the presence of high IQ? Results from the MGH Longitudinal Family Studies of ADHD, *J Child Psychol Psychiatry* 48(7):687-694, 2007.

Bendersky M, Bennett D, Lewis M: Aggression at age 5 as a function of prenatal exposure to cocaine, gender, and environmental risk, *J Pediatr Psychol* 31(1):71-84, 2006.

Benzies K, Keown L, Magill-Evans J: Immediate and sustained effects of parenting on physical aggression in Canadian children aged 6 years and younger, *Can J Psychiatry* 54(1):55-64, 2009.

Brown KD, Hamilton-Giachritsis C: The influence of violent media on children and adolescents: a public-health approach, *Lancet* 365(9460):702-710, 2005.

Carlson SM, Taylor M: Imaginary companions and impersonated characters: sex differences in children's fantasy play, *Merrill-Palmer Q* 51(1):93-118, 2005.

Feldman HM: Evaluation and management of language and speech disorders in preschool children, *Pediatr Rev* 26(4):131-142, 2005.

Hagan JF, Shaw JS, Duncan PM, editors: *Bright futures: guidelines for health supervision of infants, children, and adolescents*, ed 3, Elk Grove Village, Ill, 2008, American Academy of Pediatrics.

Jenni OG, Fuhrer HZ, Iglowstein I, et al: A longitudinal study of bed sharing and sleep problems among Swiss children in the first 10 years of life, *Pediatrics* 115(1):233-240, 2005.

Johnson JG, Cohen P, Kasen S, et al: Association between television viewing and sleep problems during adolescence and early adulthood, *Arch Pediatr Adolesc Med* 158(6):562-568, 2004.

Joy EA: Practical approaches to office-based physical activity promotion for children and adolescents, *Curr Sports Med Rep* 7(6):367-372, 2008.

Kagihara LE, Niederhauser VP, Stark M: Assessment, management, and prevention of early childhood caries, *J Am Acad Nurse Pract* 21(1):1-10, 2009.

Kellogg R: Understanding children's art. In *Readings in psychology today*, Del Mar, Calif, 1969, Communications/Research/Machines.

Kleinman RE, editor: *Pediatric nutrition handbook*, ed 6. Elk Grove Village, Ill, 2009, American Academy of Pediatrics.

Kohlberg L: Moral development. In Sills DL, editor: *International encyclopedia of the social sciences*, New York, 1968, MacMillan.

Liu YH, Lien J, Kafka T, et al: Discovering gifted children in pediatric practice, *Devel Behav Pediatr* 26(5):366-369, 2005.

Lovett BJ, Lewandowski LJ: Gifted students with learning disabilities: who are they? *J Learning Disabil* 39(6):515-527, 2006.

Mallants C, Casteels K: Practical approach to childhood masturbation: a review, *Eur J Pediatr* 167(10):1111-1117, 2008.

McDevitt S, Carey W: The measurement of temperament in 3-7 year old children, *J Child Psychol Psychiatry* 19(3):245-253, 1978.

McKee L, Colletti C, Rakow A, et al: Parenting and child externalizing behaviors: are the associations specific or diffuse? *Aggress Violent Behav* 13(3):201-215, 2008.

Miner JL, Clarke-Stewart KA: Trajectories of externalizing behavior from age 2 to age 9: relations with gender, temperament, ethnicity, parenting, and rater, *Devel Psychol* 44(3):771-786, 2008.

Moore M, Meltzer LJ, Mindell JA: Bedtime problems and night wakings in children, *Primary Care Clin Office Pract* 35(3):569-581, 2008.

National Institute on Deafness and Other Communication Disorders, National Institutes of Health: Stuttering, 2008, available at www.nidcd.nih.gov/health/voice/stutter.htm (accessed March 22, 2009).

Nelson A: *Stuttering*, 2008, KidsHealth, available at http://kidshealth.org/parent/medical/ears/stutter.html (accessed March 22, 2009).

Nesti MMM, Goldbaum M: Infectious diseases and daycare and preschool education, *J Pediatria* 83(4):299-312, 2007.

Ostrov JM, Bishop CM: Preschoolers' aggression and parent-child conflict: a multiinformant and multimethod study, *J Experiment Child Psychol* 99(4):309-322, 2008.

Otten JJ, Hellwig JP, Meyers LD, editors: *Dietary reference intakes: the essential guide to nutrient requirements*. Washington, DC, 2006, National Academies Press.

Owens J: Classification and epidemiology of childhood sleep disorders, *Primary Care Clin Office Pract* 35(3):533-546, 2008.

Paavonen EJ, Pennonen M, Roine M, et al: TV exposure associated with sleep disturbances in 5- to 6-year-old children, *J Sleep Res* 15(2):154-161, 2006.

Prasse JE, Kikano GE: Stuttering: an overview, *Am Fam Physician* 77(9):1271-1276, 2008.

Reebye P: Aggression during early years—infancy and preschool, *Can Child Adolesc Psychiatry Rev* 14(1):16-20, 2005.

Section on Pediatric Dentistry and Oral Health: Preventive oral health intervention for pediatricians, *Pediatrics* 122(6):1387-1394, 2008.

Sheehan MJ, Watson MW: Reciprocal influences between maternal discipline techniques and aggression in children and adolescents, *Aggress Behav* 34(3):245-255, 2008.

Speraw S: Spiritual experiences of parents and caregivers who have children with disabilities or special needs, *Issues Mental Health Nurs* 27(2):213-230, 2006.

US Department of Agriculture, Center for Nutrition Policy and Promotion: *MyPyramid for preschoolers*, 2009, available at www.mypyramid.gov/preschoolers (accessed March 20, 2009).

Wardle J, Cooke L: The impact of obesity on psychological well-being, *Best Pract Res Clin Endocrinol Metab* 19(3):421-440, 2005.

Werker JF, Byers-Heinlein K: Bilingualism in infancy: first steps in perception and comprehension, *Trends Cogn Sci* 12(4):144-151, 2008.

Yang ML, Fullwood E, Goldstein J, et al: Masturbation in infancy and early childhood presenting as a movement disorder: 12 cases and a review of the literature, *Pediatrics* 116(6):1427-1432, 2005.

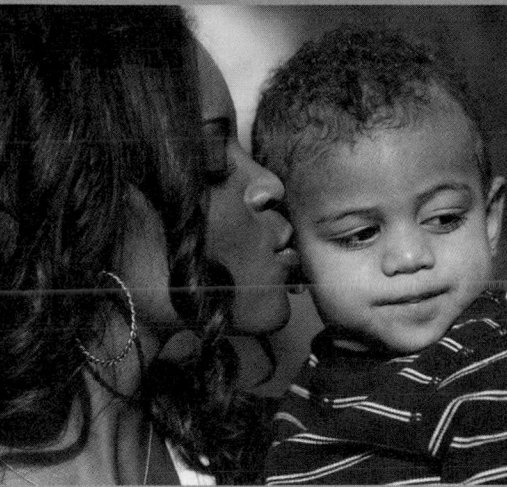

Health Problems of Early Childhood

Marilyn J. Hockenberry and Lisa Creamer

INFECTIOUS DISORDERS

COMMUNICABLE DISEASES

The incidence of childhood communicable diseases has declined significantly since the advent of immunizations. The use of antibiotics and antitoxins has further reduced serious complications resulting from such infections. However, infectious diseases do occur, and nurses must be familiar with the infectious agent to recognize the disease and to institute appropriate preventive and supportive interventions (Table 16-1).

Text continued on p. 614.

Case Study—Chickenpox (Varicella)

TABLE 16-1 COMMUNICABLE DISEASES OF CHILDHOOD

DISEASE	CLINICAL MANIFESTATIONS	THERAPEUTIC MANAGEMENT AND COMPLICATIONS	NURSING CARE MANAGEMENT
Chickenpox (Varicella) (Fig. 16-1) **Agents**—Varicella-zoster virus (VZV) **Source**—Primary secretions of respiratory tract of infected persons; to a lesser degree, skin lesions (scabs not infectious) **Transmissions**—Direct contact, droplet (airborne) spread, and contaminated objects **Incubation period**—2-3 wk, usually 14-16 days **Period of communicability**—Probably 1 day before eruption of lesions (prodromal period) to 6 days after first crop of vesicles when crusts have formed	**Prodromal stage**—Slight fever, malaise, and anorexia for first 24 hr; rash highly pruritic; begins as macule, rapidly progresses to papule and then vesicle (surrounded by erythematous base; becomes umbilicated and cloudy; breaks easily and forms crusts); all three stages (papule, vesicle, crust) present in varying degrees at one time **Distribution**—Centripetal, spreading to face and proximal extremities but sparse on distal limbs and less on areas not exposed to heat (i.e., from clothing or sun) **Constitutional signs and symptoms**—Elevated temperature from lymphadenopathy, irritability from pruritus	**Specific**—Antiviral agent acyclovir (Zovirax); varicella-zoster immune globulin (VariZIG) or immune globulin intravenous (IGIV) after exposure in high-risk children **Supportive**—Diphenhydramine hydrochloride or antihistamines to relieve itching; skin care to prevent secondary bacterial infection **Complications**—Secondary bacterial infections (abscesses, cellulitis, necrotizing fasciitis, pneumonia, sepsis) Encephalitis Varicella pneumonia (rare in normal children) Hemorrhagic varicella (tiny hemorrhages in vesicles and numerous petechiae in skin) Chronic or transient thrombocytopenia **Preventive**—Childhood immunization	Maintain Standard, Airborne, and Contact Precautions if hospitalized until all lesions are crusted; for immunized child with mild breakthrough varicella, isolate until no new lesions are seen. Keep child in home away from susceptible individuals until vesicles have dried (usually 1 wk after onset of disease), and isolate high-risk children from infected children. Administer skin care: give bath and change clothes and linens daily; administer topical calamine lotion; keep child's fingernails short and clean; apply mittens if child scratches. Keep child cool (may decrease number of lesions). Lessen pruritus; keep child occupied. Remove loose crusts that rub and irritate skin. Teach child to apply pressure to pruritic area rather than scratching it. Avoid use of aspirin (possible association with Reye syndrome).

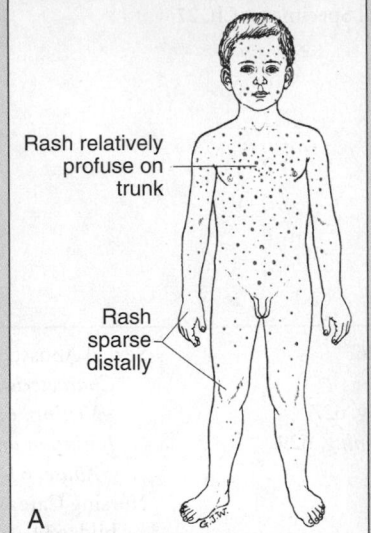

Rash relatively profuse on trunk

Rash sparse distally

A

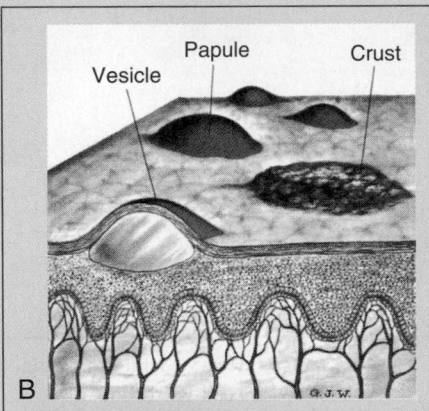

Vesicle   Papule   Crust

B

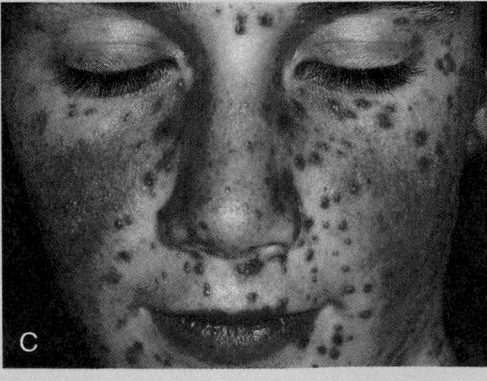

C

Fig. 16-1 Chickenpox (varicella). **A,** Progression of disease. **B,** Simultaneous stages of lesions. **C,** Clinical view. (**C,** From Habif TP: *Clinical dermatology: a color guide to diagnosis and therapy,* ed 4, St Louis, 2004, Mosby.)

TABLE 16-1	COMMUNICABLE DISEASES OF CHILDHOOD—cont'd		
DISEASE	**CLINICAL MANIFESTATIONS**	**THERAPEUTIC MANAGEMENT AND COMPLICATIONS**	**NURSING CARE MANAGEMENT**
Diphtheria **Agent**—*Corynebacterium diphtheriae* **Source**—Discharges from mucous membranes of nose and nasopharynx, skin, and other lesions of infected person **Transmission**—Direct contact with infected person, a carrier, or contaminated articles **Incubation period**—Usually 2-5 days, possibly longer **Period of communicability**—Variable; until virulent bacilli are no longer present (identified by three negative cultures); usually 2 wk but as long as 4 wk	Vary according to anatomic location of pseudomembrane **Nasal**—Resembles common cold, serosanguineous mucopurulent nasal discharge without constitutional symptoms; may have frank epistaxis **Tonsillar-pharyngeal**—Malaise; anorexia; sore throat; low-grade fever; pulse increased above expected for temperature within 24 hr; smooth, adherent, white or gray membrane; lymphadenitis possibly pronounced ("bull's neck"); in severe cases, toxemia, septic shock, and death within 6-10 days **Laryngeal**—Fever, hoarseness, cough, with or without previous signs listed; potential airway obstruction; apprehensive; dyspneic retractions; cyanosis	Equine antitoxin (usually intravenously); preceded by skin or conjunctival test to rule out sensitivity to horse serum Antibiotics (penicillin G procaine or erythromycin) in addition to equine antitoxin Complete bed rest (prevention of myocarditis) Tracheostomy for airway obstruction Treatment of infected contacts and carriers **Complications**—Toxic cardiomyopathy (2nd-3rd week) Toxic neuropathy **Preventive**—Childhood immunization	Follow Standard and Droplet Precautions until two cultures are negative for *C. diphtheriae*; use Contact Precautions with cutaneous manifestations. Administer antibiotics in timely manner. Participate in sensitivity testing; have epinephrine available. Administer complete care to maintain bed rest. Use suctioning as needed. Observe respiration for signs of obstruction. Administer humidified oxygen as prescribed.
Erythema Infectiosum (Fifth Disease) (Fig. 16-2) **Agent**—Human parvovirus (HPV) B19 **Source**—Infected persons, mainly school-age children **Transmission**—Respiratory secretions and blood, blood products **Incubation period**—4-14 days; may be as long as 21 days **Period of communicability**—Uncertain but before onset of symptoms in children with aplastic crisis	Rash appears in three stages: **I**—Erythema on face, chiefly on cheeks ("slapped face" appearance); disappears by 1-4 days **II**—About 1 day after rash appears on face, maculopapular red spots appear, symmetrically distributed on upper and lower extremities; rash progresses from proximal to distal surfaces and may last ≥1 wk **III**—Rash subsides but reappears if skin is irritated or traumatized (sun, heat, cold, friction) In children with aplastic crisis, rash usually absent and prodromal illness includes fever, myalgia, lethargy, nausea, vomiting, and abdominal pain Child with sickle cell disease may have concurrent vaso-occlusive crisis	**Symptomatic and supportive**—Antipyretics, analgesics, antiinflammatory drugs Possible blood transfusion for transient aplastic anemia **Complications**—Self-limited arthritis and arthralgia (arthritis may become chronic); more common in adult women May result in serious complications (anemia, hydrops) or fetal death if mother infected during pregnancy (primarily second trimester) Aplastic crisis in children with hemolytic disease or immunodeficiency Myocarditis (rare)	Isolation of child is not necessary, except hospitalized child (immunosuppressed or with aplastic crises) suspected of HPV infection is placed on Droplet Precautions and Standard Precautions. Pregnant women need not be excluded from workplace where HPV infection is present; they should not care for patients with aplastic crises. Explain low risk of fetal death to those in contact with affected children; assist with routine fetal ultrasound for detection of fetal hydrops.

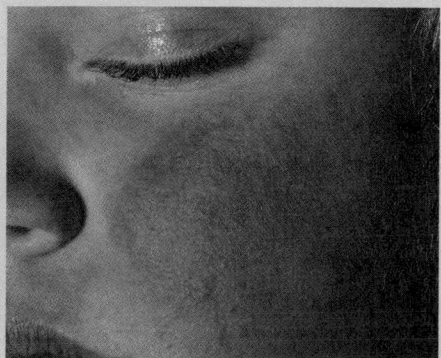

Fig. 16-2 Erythema infectiosum (fifth disease). (From Habif TP: *Clinical dermatology: a color guide to diagnosis and therapy*, ed 4, St Louis, 2004, Mosby.)

Continued

TABLE 16-1   COMMUNICABLE DISEASES OF CHILDHOOD—cont'd

DISEASE	CLINICAL MANIFESTATIONS	THERAPEUTIC MANAGEMENT AND COMPLICATIONS	NURSING CARE MANAGEMENT
Exanthem Subitum (Roseola Infantum) (Fig. 16-3) **Agent**—Human herpesvirus type 6 (HHV-6; rarely HHV-7) **Source**—Possibly acquired from saliva of healthy adult person; entry via nasal, buccal, or conjunctival mucosa **Transmission**—Year round; no reported contact with infected individual in most cases (virtually limited to children <3 yr but peak age is 6-15 mo) **Incubation period**—Usually 5-15 days **Period of communicability**—Unknown	Persistent high fever for 3-4 days in child who appears well Precipitous drop in fever to normal with appearance of rash **Rash**—Discrete rose-pink macules or maculopapules appearing first on trunk, then spreading to neck, face, and extremities; nonpruritic; fades on pressure; lasts 1-2 days **Associated signs and symptoms**—Cervical and postauricular lymphadenopathy, inflamed pharynx, cough, coryza	Nonspecific Antipyretics to control fever **Complications**—Recurrent febrile seizures (possibly from latent infection of central nervous system that is reactivated by fever) Encephalitis (rare)	Teach parents measures for lowering temperature (antipyretic drugs); ensure adequate parental understanding of specific antipyretic dosage to prevent accidental overdose. If child is prone to seizures, discuss appropriate precautions and possibility of recurrent febrile seizures.

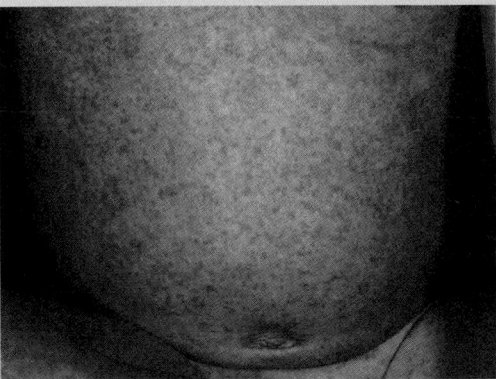

Fig. 16-3 Exanthem subitum (roseola infantum). (From Habif TP: *Clinical dermatology: a color guide to diagnosis and therapy*, ed 4, St Louis, 2004, Mosby.)

ⓔ Animation—Mumps

ⓔ Mumps

Agent—Paramyxovirus **Source**—Saliva of infected persons **Transmission**—Direct contact with or droplet spread from an infected person **Incubation period**—14-21 days **Period of communicability**—Most communicable immediately before and after swelling begins	**Prodromal stage**—Fever, headache, malaise, and anorexia for 24 hr, followed by "earache" that is aggravated by chewing **Parotitis**—By third day, parotid gland(s) (either unilateral or bilateral) enlarges and reaches maximum size in 1-3 days; accompanied by pain and tenderness; other exocrine glands (submandibular) may also be swollen	**Preventive**—Childhood immunization **Symptomatic and supportive**—Analgesics for pain and antipyretics for fever Intravenous fluid if needed for child who refuses to drink or vomits because of meningoencephalitis **Complications**—Sensorineural deafness Postinfectious encephalitis Myocarditis Arthritis Hepatitis Epididymoorchitis Oophoritis Pancreatitis Sterility (extremely rare in adult men) Meningitis	Maintain isolation during period of communicability; institute Droplet and Contact Precautions during hospitalization. Encourage rest and decreased activity during prodromal phase until swelling subsides. Give analgesics for pain; if child is unwilling to swallow pills or tablets medication, use elixir form. Encourage fluids and soft, bland foods; avoid foods requiring chewing. Apply hot or cold compresses to neck, whichever is more comforting. To relieve orchitis, provide warmth and local support with tight-fitting underpants.

TABLE 16-1   COMMUNICABLE DISEASES OF CHILDHOOD—cont'd

DISEASE	CLINICAL MANIFESTATIONS	THERAPEUTIC MANAGEMENT AND COMPLICATIONS	NURSING CARE MANAGEMENT
Measles (Rubeola) (Fig. 16-4) **Agent**—Virus **Source**—Respiratory tract secretions, blood, and urine of infected person **Transmission**—Usually by direct contact with droplets of infected person; primarily in the winter **Incubation period**—10-20 days **Period of communicability**—From 4 days before to 5 days after rash appears, but mainly during prodromal (catarrhal) stage	**Prodromal (catarrhal) stage**—Fever and malaise, followed in 24 hr by coryza, cough, conjunctivitis, Koplik spots (small, irregular red spots with a minute, bluish white center first seen on buccal mucosa opposite molars 2 days before rash); symptoms gradually increasing in severity until second day after rash appears, when they begin to subside **Rash**—Appears 3-4 days after onset of prodromal stage; begins as erythematous maculopapular eruption on face and gradually spreads downward; more severe in earlier sites (appears confluent) and less intense in later sites (appears discrete); after 3-4 days assumes brownish appearance, and fine desquamation occurs over area of extensive involvement **Constitutional signs and symptoms**—Anorexia, abdominal pain, malaise, generalized lymphadenopathy	**Preventive**—Childhood immunization. Vitamin A supplementation (see p. 616) **Supportive**—Bed rest during febrile period; antipyretics Antibiotics to prevent secondary bacterial infection in high-risk children **Complications**—Otitis media Pneumonia (bacterial) Obstructive laryngitis and laryngotracheitis Encephalitis (rare but has high mortality)	Maintain isolation until fifth day of rash; if child is hospitalized, institute Airborne Precautions. Encourage rest during prodromal stage; provide quiet activity. **Fever**—Instruct parents to administer antipyretics; avoid chilling; if child is prone to seizures, institute appropriate precautions. **Eye care**—Dim lights if photophobia present; clean eyelids with warm saline solution to remove secretions or crusts; keep child from rubbing eyes. **Coryza, cough**—Use cool-mist vaporizer; protect skin around nares with layer of petrolatum; encourage fluids and soft, bland foods. **Skin care**—Keep skin clean; use tepid baths as necessary.

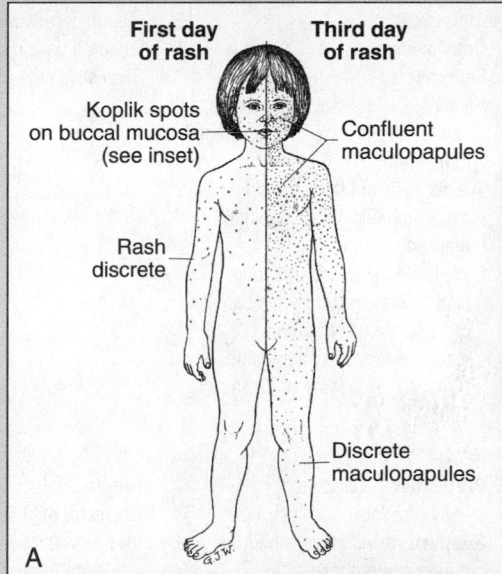

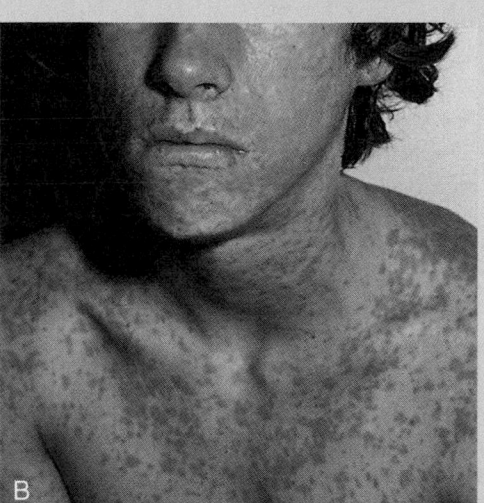

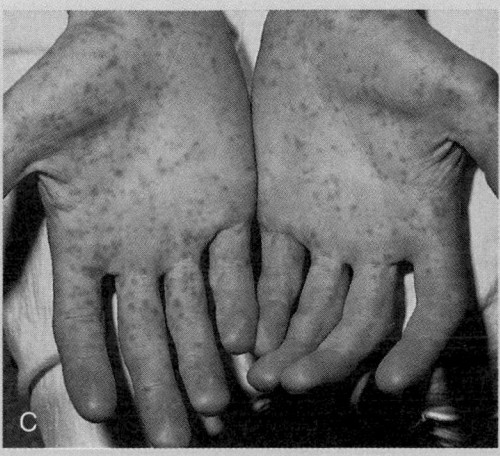

Fig. 16-4 Measles (rubeola). **A,** Progression of disease. **B,** Exanthem first appears at the hairline and spreads from head to toe over 3 days. **C,** Measles ultimately involves the palms and soles. (**B** and **C,** From Zitelli BJ, Davis HW: *Atlas of pediatric physical diagnosis,* ed 5, St Louis, 2007, Mosby; courtesy Dr. Michael Sherlock, Lutherville, Md.)

Continued

TABLE 16-1 COMMUNICABLE DISEASES OF CHILDHOOD—cont'd

DISEASE	CLINICAL MANIFESTATIONS	THERAPEUTIC MANAGEMENT AND COMPLICATIONS	NURSING CARE MANAGEMENT
Pertussis (Whooping Cough) **Agent**—*Bordetella pertussis* **Source**—Discharge from respiratory tract of infected persons **Transmission**—Direct contact or droplet spread from infected person; indirect contact with freshly contaminated articles **Incubation period**—6-20 days; usually 7-10 days **Period of communicability**—Greatest during catarrhal stage before onset of paroxysms	**Catarrhal stage**—Begins with symptoms of upper respiratory tract infection, such as coryza, sneezing, lacrimation, cough, and low-grade fever; symptoms continue for 1-2 wk, when dry, hacking cough becomes more severe **Paroxysmal stage**—Cough most common at night, consists of short, rapid coughs followed by sudden inspiration associated with a high-pitched crowing sound or "whoop"; during paroxysms, cheeks become flushed or cyanotic, eyes bulge, and tongue protrudes; paroxysm may continue until thick mucous plug is dislodged; vomiting frequently follows attack; stage generally lasts 4-6 wk, followed by convalescent stage Infants <6 mo may not have characteristic whoop cough, but have difficulty maintaining adequate oxygenation with amount of secretions, frequent vomiting of mucus and formula or breast milk Pertussis may occur in adolescents and adults with varying manifestations; cough and whoop may be absent, however, as many as 50% of adolescents may have a cough for up to 10 wk (American Academy of Pediatrics, 2009) Additional symptoms in adolescents include difficulty breathing, and posttussive vomiting (See also Immunization, Chapter 10, for discussion of pertussis immunization schedule.)	**Preventive**—Immunization; current belief is that childhood immunizations for pertussis do not confer lifelong immunity to adolescents and adults, so a pertussis booster is recommended for adolescents (see Chapter 10, Immunization Schedule) Antimicrobial therapy (e.g., erythromycin, clarithromycin, azithromycin) **Supportive**—Hospitalization sometimes required for infants, children who are dehydrated, or those who have complications Increased oxygen intake and humidity Adequate fluids Intensive care and mechanical ventilation if needed for infants <6 mo **Complications**—Pneumonia (usual cause of death in younger children) Atelectasis Otitis media Seizures Hemorrhage (scleral, conjunctival, epistaxis; pulmonary hemorrhage in neonate) Weight loss and dehydration Hernias (umbilical and inguinal) Prolapsed rectum Complications reported among adolescents include syncope, sleep disturbance, rib fractures, incontinence, and pneumonia (American Academy of Pediatrics, 2009)	Maintain isolation during catarrhal stage; if child is hospitalized, institute Droplet Precautions. Obtain nasopharyngeal culture for diagnosis. Encourage oral fluids; offer small amount of fluids frequently. Ensure adequate oxygenation during paroxysms; position infant on side to decrease chance of aspiration with vomiting. Provide humidified oxygen; suction as needed to prevent choking on secretions. Observe for signs of airway obstruction (increased restlessness, apprehension, retractions, cyanosis). Encourage compliance with antibiotic therapy for household contacts. Encourage adolescents to obtain pertussis booster (Tdap) (see also Immunizations, Chapter 10). Use Standard Precautions and mask in health care workers exposed to children with persistent cough and high suspicion of pertussis.
Poliomyelitis **Agent**—Enteroviruses, three types: type 1, most frequent cause of paralysis, both epidemic and endemic; type 2, least frequently associated with paralysis; type 3, second most frequently associated with paralysis **Source**—Feces and oropharyngeal secretions of infected persons, especially young children **Transmission**—Direct contact with persons with apparent or inapparent active infection; spread via fecal-oral and pharyngeal-oropharyngeal routes	May be manifested in three different forms: **Abortive or inapparent**—Fever, uneasiness, sore throat, headache, anorexia, vomiting, abdominal pain; lasts a few hours to a few days **Nonparalytic**—Same manifestations as abortive but more severe, with pain and stiffness in neck, back, and legs **Paralytic**—Initial course similar to nonparalytic type, followed by recovery and then signs of central nervous system paralysis	**Preventive**—Childhood immunization **Supportive**—Complete bed rest during acute phase Mechanical or assisted ventilation in case of respiratory paralysis Physical therapy for muscles after acute stage **Complications**—Permanent paralysis Respiratory arrest Hypertension Kidney stones from demineralization of bone during prolonged immobility	Institute Contact Precautions. Administer mild sedatives as necessary to relieve anxiety and promote rest. Participate in physical therapy procedures (use of moist hot packs and range-of-motion exercises). Position child to maintain body alignment and prevent contractures or skin breakdown; use footboard or appropriate orthoses to prevent footdrop; use pressure mattress for prolonged immobility. Encourage child to perform activities of daily living to capability; promote early ambulation with assistive devices; administer analgesics for maximum comfort during physical activity; give high-protein diet and bowel management for prolonged immobility.

TABLE 16-1	COMMUNICABLE DISEASES OF CHILDHOOD—cont'd		
DISEASE	**CLINICAL MANIFESTATIONS**	**THERAPEUTIC MANAGEMENT AND COMPLICATIONS**	**NURSING CARE MANAGEMENT**
Poliomyelitis—cont'd Vaccine-acquired paralytic polio may occur as a result of the live oral polio vaccination (no longer available in the United States) **Incubation period**—Usually 7-14 days, with range of 5-35 days **Period of communicability**—Not exactly known; virus present in throat and feces shortly after infection and persists for about 1 wk in throat and 4-6 wk in feces			Observe for respiratory paralysis (difficulty talking, ineffective cough, inability to hold breath, shallow and rapid respirations); report such signs and symptoms to practitioner.
Rubella (German Measles) (Fig. 16-5) **Agent**—Rubella virus **Source**—Primarily nasopharyngeal secretions of person with apparent or inapparent infection; virus also present in blood, stool, and urine **Incubation period**—14-21 days **Period of communicability**—7 days before to about 5 days after appearance of rash **Constitutional signs and symptoms**—Occasionally low-grade fever, headache, malaise, and lymphadenopathy	**Prodromal stage**—Absent in children, present in adults and adolescents; consists of low-grade fever, headache, malaise, anorexia, mild conjunctivitis, coryza, sore throat, cough, and lymphadenopathy; lasts 1-5 days, subsides 1 day after appearance of rash **Rash**—First appears on face and rapidly spreads downward to neck, arms, trunk, and legs; by end of first day, body is covered with discrete, pinkish red maculopapular exanthema; disappears in same order as it began and is usually gone by third day	**Preventive**—Childhood immunization No treatment necessary other than antipyretics for low-grade fever and analgesics for discomfort **Complications**—Rare (arthritis, encephalitis, or purpura); most benign of all childhood communicable diseases; greatest danger is teratogenic effect on fetus	Institute Droplet Precautions. Reassure parents of benign nature of illness in affected child. Use comfort measures as necessary. Avoid contact with pregnant woman. Monitor rubella titer in pregnant adolescent.

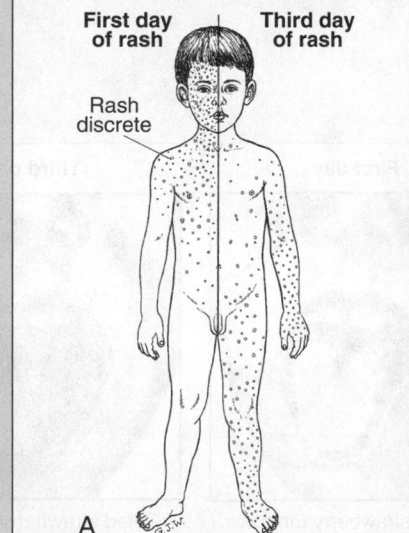
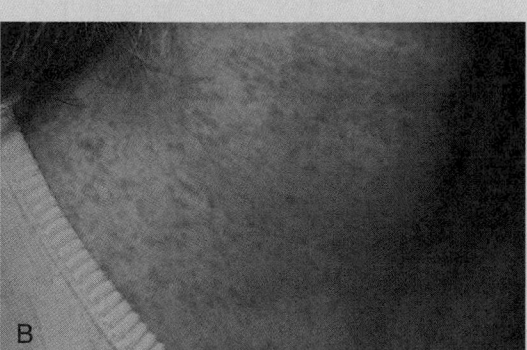

Fig. 16-5 Rubella (German measles). **A,** Progression of rash. **B,** Clinical view. (**B,** From Zitelli BJ, Davis HW: *Atlas of pediatric physical diagnosis*, ed 5, St Louis, 2007, Mosby; courtesy Dr. Michael Sherlock, Lutherville, Md.)

Continued

TABLE 16-1 **COMMUNICABLE DISEASES OF CHILDHOOD—cont'd**

DISEASE	CLINICAL MANIFESTATIONS	THERAPEUTIC MANAGEMENT AND COMPLICATIONS	NURSING CARE MANAGEMENT
Scarlet Fever (Fig. 16-6) **Agent**—Group A β-hemolytic streptococci **Source**—Usually from nasopharyngeal secretions of infected persons and carriers **Transmission**—Direct contact with infected person or droplet spread; indirectly by contact with contaminated articles or ingestion of contaminated milk or other food **Incubation period**—2-5 days, with range of 1-7 days **Period of communicability**—During incubation period and clinical illness, approximately 10 days; during first 2 wk of carrier phase, although may persist for months	**Prodromal stage**—Abrupt high fever, pulse increased out of proportion to fever, vomiting, headache, chills, malaise, abdominal pain, halitosis **Enanthema**—Tonsils enlarged, edematous, reddened, and covered with patches of exudates; in severe cases appearance resembles membrane seen in diphtheria; pharynx is edematous and beefy red; during first 1-2 days tongue is coated and papillae become red and swollen (white strawberry tongue); by fourth or fifth day white coat sloughs off, leaving prominent papillae (red strawberry tongue); palate is covered with erythematous punctate lesions **Exanthema**—Rash appears within 12 hr after prodromal signs; red pinhead-sized punctate lesions rapidly become generalized but are absent on face, which becomes flushed with striking circumoral pallor; rash more intense in folds of joints; by end of first wk desquamation begins (fine, sandpaper-like on torso; sheetlike sloughing on palms and soles), which may be complete by 3 wk or longer	Full course of penicillin (or erythromycin in penicillin-sensitive children) or oral cephalosporin Antibiotic therapy for newly diagnosed carriers (nose or throat cultures positive for streptococci) **Supportive**—Rest during febrile phase, analgesics for sore throat; antipruritics for rash if bothersome **Complications**—Peritonsillar and retropharyngeal abscess Sinusitis Otitis media Acute glomerulonephritis Acute rheumatic fever Polyarthritis (uncommon)	Institute Standard and Droplet Precautions until 24 hr after initiation of treatment. Ensure compliance with oral antibiotic therapy; intramuscular benzathine penicillin G [Bicillin] may be given. Encourage rest during febrile phase; provide quiet activity during convalescent period. Relieve discomfort of sore throat with analgesics, gargles, lozenges, antiseptic throat sprays, and inhalation of cool mist. Encourage fluids during febrile phase; avoid irritating liquids (certain citrus juices) or rough foods (chips); when child is able to eat, begin with soft diet. Advise parents to consult practitioner if fever persists after beginning therapy. Discuss procedures for preventing spread of infection—discard toothbrush; avoid sharing drinking and eating utensils.

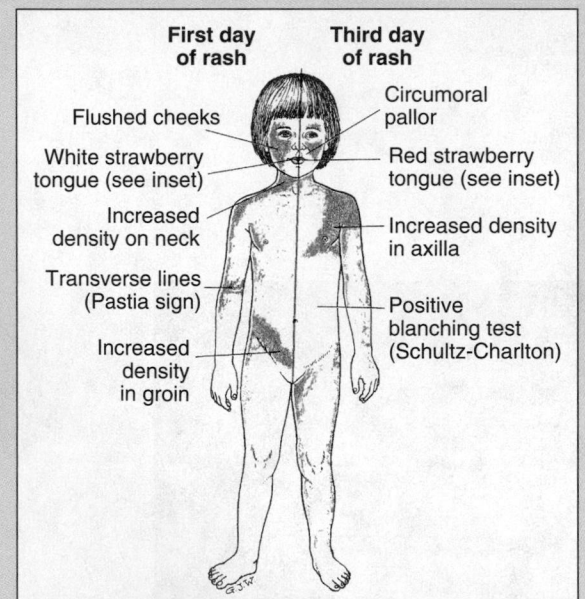

First day of rash — Flushed cheeks, White strawberry tongue (see inset), Increased density on neck, Transverse lines (Pastia sign), Increased density in groin

Third day of rash — Circumoral pallor, Red strawberry tongue (see inset), Increased density in axilla, Positive blanching test (Schultz-Charlton)

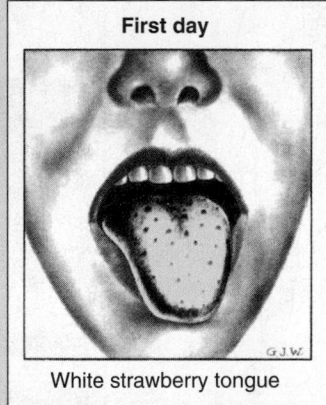

First day — White strawberry tongue

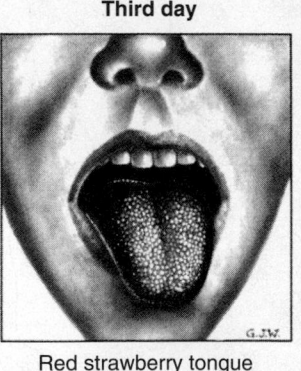

Third day — Red strawberry tongue

Fig. 16-6 Scarlet fever.

(See also Chapter 18 for a discussion of nursing care for dermatologic conditions.)

Nursing Care Management

Table 16-1 describes the more common communicable diseases of childhood, their therapeutic management, and specific nursing care. The following is a general discussion of nursing care management for communicable diseases.

Identification of the infectious agent is of primary importance to prevent exposure to susceptible individuals. Nurses in ambulatory care settings, child care centers, and schools are often the first persons to see signs of a communicable disease, such as a rash or sore throat. The nurse must operate under a high index of suspicion for common childhood diseases to identify potentially infectious cases and to recognize diseases that require medical intervention. An example is the common complaint of sore throat. Although most often a symptom of a minor viral infection, it can signal diphtheria or a streptococcal infection, such as scarlet fever. Each of these bacterial conditions requires appropriate medical treatment to prevent serious complications.

When the nurse suspects a communicable disease, it is important to assess:

- Recent exposure to a known case
- Prodromal symptoms (symptoms that occur between early manifestations of the disease and its overt clinical syndrome) or evidence of constitutional symptoms, such as a fever or rash (see Table 16-1)
- Immunization history
- History of having the disease

Immunizations are available for many diseases, and infection usually confers lifelong immunity; therefore the possibility of many infectious agents can be eliminated based on these two criteria.

Prevent Spread

Prevention consists of two components: prevention of the disease and control of its spread to others. Primary prevention rests almost exclusively on immunization. (Chapter 12 discusses the nurse's role in immunization of children.)

Control measures to prevent spread of disease should include techniques to reduce risk of cross-transmission of infectious organisms between patients and to protect health care workers from organisms harbored by patients. If the child is hospitalized, follow the facility's policies for infection control. (See Chapter 27.) The most important procedure is hand washing. Persons directly caring for the child or handling contaminated articles must wash their hands and practice effective Standard Precautions in care of their patients.

Instruct the child to practice good hand-washing technique after toileting and before eating. For those diseases spread by droplets, the nurse instructs parents in measures to reduce airborne transmission. The child who is old enough should use a tissue to cover the face during coughing or sneezing; otherwise, the parent should cover the child's mouth with a tissue and then discard it. Stress the usual hygiene measures of not sharing eating and drinking utensils to the family.

> **! NURSING ALERT**
>
> If a child is admitted to the hospital with an undiagnosed exanthema, institute strict Transmission-Based Precautions (contact, airborne, and droplet) and Standard Precautions until a diagnosis is confirmed. Childhood communicable diseases requiring these precautions include diphtheria, chickenpox, measles, tuberculosis, adenovirus, *Haemophilus influenzae* type b, influenza, mumps, *Mycoplasma pneumoniae* infection, pertussis, plague, streptococcal pharyngitis, pneumonia, or scarlet fever (American Academy of Pediatrics, 2009).

Prevent Complications

Although most children recover without difficulty, certain groups are at risk for serious, even fatal, complications from communicable diseases, especially the viral diseases chickenpox and erythema infectiosum (EI) (fifth disease) caused by human parvovirus (HPV) B19.

Children with immunodeficiency—those receiving steroid or other immunosuppressive therapy, those with a generalized malignancy such as leukemia or lymphoma, or those with an immunologic disorder—are at risk for viremia from replication of the varicella-zoster virus (VZV)* in the blood. VZV is so named because it causes two distinct diseases: varicella (chickenpox) and zoster (herpes zoster or shingles). Varicella occurs primarily in children younger than 15 years of age. However, it leaves the threat of herpes zoster, an intensely painful varicella that is localized to a single dermatome (body area innervated by a particular segment of the spinal cord). In children the dermatomes most likely affected by herpes zoster are the cervical and sacral dermatomes (Leung, Robson, and Leong, 2006). Immunocompromised patients and healthy infants younger than 1 year of age (who also have reduced immunity) are at a higher risk for reactivation of VZV causing herpes zoster, probably as a result of a deficiency in cellular immunity (American Academy of Pediatrics, 2009; Galea, Sweet, Beninger, et al, 2008). Complications of herpes zoster virus in children include secondary bacterial infection, depigmentation, and scarring. Postherpetic neuralgia in children is uncommon (Leung, Robson, and Leong, 2006).

The use of varicella-zoster immune globulin (VariZIG) or immune globulin intravenous (IGIV) is recommended for children who are immunocompromised, who have no previous history of varicella, and who are likely to contract the disease and have complications as a result (American Academy of Pediatrics, 2009). The antiviral agent acyclovir (Zovirax) may be used to treat varicella infections in susceptible immunocompromised persons. It is effective in decreasing the number of lesions; shortening the duration of fever; and decreasing itching, lethargy, and anorexia. Consider oral acyclovir for immunocompromised children without a history of varicella disease, newborns whose mother had varicella within 5 days before delivery or within 48 hours after delivery, and hospitalized preterm infants with significant varicella exposure (American Academy of Pediatrics, 2009).

Children with hemolytic disease, such as sickle cell disease, are at risk for aplastic anemia from EI. HPV B19 infects and lyses red blood cell precursors, thus interrupting the production of red blood cells. Therefore the virus may precipitate a severe aplastic crisis in patients who need increased red blood cell production to maintain normal red blood cell volumes. Thrombocytopenia and neutropenia may also occur as a result of HPV B19 infection. The fetus has a relatively high rate of red blood cell production and an immature immune system; it may develop severe anemia and hydrops as a result of maternal HPV infection. Fetal death rates as a result of HPV B19 have been estimated to be between 2% and 6% (American Academy of Pediatrics, 2009).

> **! NURSING ALERT**
>
> Refer children at risk for contracting these communicable diseases to the practitioner immediately in case of known exposure or outbreaks.

---

*Educational materials may be obtained from the National Shingles Foundation, 590 Madison Ave., 21st Floor, New York, NY 10022; 212-222-3390; www.vzvfoundation.org.

Case Study—Varicella in Spite of Vaccine

In the past decade incidence of pertussis has increased, particularly in infants less than 6 months old and in children 10 to 14 years of age. Early clinical manifestations of pertussis in infants may include gagging, coughing, emesis, and apnea; the typical "whoop" associated with the disease is absent (Wood and McIntyre, 2008). In older children the disease may manifest as a common cold (see Table 16-1). There is now a recommendation that children ages 11 to 18 receive a booster pertussis vaccine (Tdap) to prevent the disease. (See Immunizations, Chapter 12.) Because pertussis is contagious, especially among close household members, identify pertussis early and initiate treatment for the child and those who have been exposed. Azithromycin (for infants <1 month) and erythromycin, clarithromycin, or azithromycin are administered to infants and children with pertussis (Wood and McIntyre, 2008).

Prevention of complications from diseases such as diphtheria, pertussis, and scarlet fever requires compliance with antibiotic therapy. With oral preparations, stress the need to complete the entire course of therapy. (See Compliance, Chapter 27.)

Evidence suggests that vitamin A supplementation reduces both morbidity and mortality in measles and that all children with severe measles should receive vitamin A supplements. A single oral dose of 200,000 international units for children at least 1 year old is recommended (use half that dose for children 6 to 12 months of age). The higher dose may be associated with vomiting and headache for a few hours. The dose should be repeated the next day and at 4 weeks for children with ophthalmologic evidence of vitamin A deficiency (American Academy of Pediatrics, 2009).

> **! NURSING ALERT**
>
> Although the risk of vitamin A toxicity from these doses (they are 100 to 200 times the recommended dietary allowance) is relatively low, nurses should instruct parents on safe storage of the drug. Ideally, vitamin A should be dispensed in the age-appropriate unit dose to prevent excessive administration and possible toxicity.

Provide Comfort

Many communicable diseases cause skin manifestations that are bothersome to the child. The chief discomfort from most rashes is itching, and measures such as cool baths (usually without soap) and lotions (e.g., calamine) are helpful.

> **! NURSING ALERT**
>
> When lotions with active ingredients such as diphenhydramine in Caladryl are used, they are applied sparingly, especially over open lesions, where excessive absorption can lead to drug toxicity. Use these lotions with caution in children who are simultaneously receiving an oral antihistamine. Cooling the lotion in the refrigerator beforehand often makes it more soothing on the skin than at room temperature.

To avoid overheating, which increases itching, children should wear lightweight, loose, nonirritating clothing and keep out of the sun. If the child persists in scratching, keep the nails short and smooth or use mittens and clothes with long sleeves or legs. For severe itching, antipruritic medication, such as diphenhydramine (Benadryl) or hydroxyzine (Atarax), may be required, especially when the child has trouble sleeping because of itching. Loratadine, cetirizine, and fexofenadine do not cause drowsiness and may be preferred for urticaria during the day.

An elevated temperature is common, and both antipyretic medicine (acetaminophen or ibuprofen) and environmental manipulation are implemented. (See Controlling Elevated Temperatures, Chapter 27.) The acetaminophen is effective in lowering the fever but does not significantly reduce the symptoms of itching, anorexia, abdominal pain, fussiness, or vomiting.

A sore throat, another frequent symptom, is managed with lozenges, saline rinses (if the child is old enough to cooperate), and analgesics. Because most children are anorectic during an illness, bland foods and increased liquids are usually preferred. During the early stages of the disease, children voluntarily curtail their activity, and although bed rest is beneficial, it should not be imposed unless specifically indicated. During periods of irritability, quiet activity (e.g., reading, music, television, video games, puzzles, coloring) helps distract children from the discomfort.

Support Child and Family

Most communicable diseases are benign, but may produce considerable concern and anxiety for parents. Often the occurrence of a disease such as chickenpox is the first time the child is acutely uncomfortable. Parents need assistance to cope with manifestations of the illness, such as intense itching. The family and child need reassurance that recovery is generally rapid. However, visible signs of the dermatosis may be present for some time after the child is well enough to resume usual activities.

> **! NURSING ALERT**
>
> The occurrence of a communicable disease provides the opportunity to ask parents about the child's immunization status and reinforce the benefits of vaccines for children.

CONJUNCTIVITIS

Acute **conjunctivitis** (inflammation of the conjunctiva) occurs from a variety of causes that are typically age related. In newborns conjunctivitis can occur from infection during birth, most often from *Chlamydia trachomatis* (inclusion conjunctivitis) or *Neisseria gonorrhoeae*. These organisms, as well as herpes simplex virus (HSV), cause serious ocular damage. In infants recurrent conjunctivitis may be a sign of nasolacrimal (tear) duct obstruction. A chemical conjunctivitis may occur within 24 hours of instillation of neonatal ophthalmic prophylaxis; the clinical features include mild lid edema and a sterile, nonpurulent eye discharge (Fuloria and Kreiter, 2002). In children the usual causes of conjunctivitis are viral, bacterial, allergic, or related to a foreign body. Bacterial infection accounts for most instances of acute conjunctivitis in children. Diagnosis is made primarily from the clinical manifestations (Box 16-1), although cultures of purulent drainage may be needed to identify the specific cause.

BOX 16-1 CLINICAL MANIFESTATIONS OF CONJUNCTIVITIS

Bacterial Conjunctivitis ("Pink Eye")
Purulent drainage
Crusting of eyelids, especially on awakening
Inflamed conjunctiva
Swollen lids

Viral Conjunctivitis
Usually occurs with upper respiratory tract infection
Serous (watery) drainage
Inflamed conjunctiva
Swollen lids

Allergic Conjunctivitis
Itching
Watery to thick, stringy discharge
Inflamed conjunctiva
Swollen lids

Conjunctivitis Caused by Foreign Body
Tearing
Pain
Inflamed conjunctiva
Usually only one eye affected

Therapeutic Management

Treatment of conjunctivitis depends on the cause. Viral conjunctivitis is self-limiting, and treatment is limited to removal of the accumulated secretions. Bacterial conjunctivitis has traditionally been treated with topical antibacterial agents such as polymyxin and bacitracin (Polysporin), sodium sulfacetamide (Sulamyd), or trimethoprim and polymyxin (Polytrim). However, in one study of children with acute infective conjunctivitis treated by placebo versus topical chloramphenicol, there was little difference in cure rates; the authors concluded that most children will get better without antibiotic treatment (Rose, Harnden, Brueggemann, et al, 2005). Fluoroquinolones, approved for children ages 1 year and older, are viewed by ophthalmologists as the best ophthalmic antimicrobial agents available (Lichtenstein, Rinehart, and Levofloxacin Bacterial Conjunctivitis Study Group, 2003). Drops may be used during the day and an ointment at bedtime because the ointment preparation remains in the eye longer but blur the vision. Corticosteroids are avoided because they reduce ocular resistance to bacteria.

Nursing Care Management

Nursing care includes keeping the eye clean and properly administering ophthalmic medication. Remove accumulated secretions by wiping from the inner canthus downward and outward, away from the opposite eye. Warm, moist compresses, such as a clean washcloth wrung out with hot tap water, are helpful in removing the crusts. Compresses are *not* kept on the eye because an occlusive covering promotes bacterial growth. Instill medication immediately after the eyes have been cleaned and according to correct procedure. (See Chapter 27.)

Prevention of infection in other family members is an important consideration with bacterial conjunctivitis. Keep the child's washcloth and towel separate from those used by others. Discard tissues used to clean the eye. Instruct the child to refrain from rubbing the eye and to use good hand-washing technique.

! NURSING ALERT

Signs of serious conjunctivitis include reduction or loss of vision, ocular pain, photophobia, exophthalmos (bulging eyeball), decreased ocular mobility, corneal ulceration, and unusual patterns of inflammation (e.g., the perilimbal flush associated with iritis or localized inflammation associated with scleritis). If a patient has any of these signs, refer him or her immediately to an ophthalmologist (Lederman and Lederman, 2003).

STOMATITIS

Stomatitis is inflammation of the oral mucosa, which may include the buccal (cheek) and labial (lip) mucosa, tongue, gingiva, palate, and floor of the mouth. It may be infectious or noninfectious and may be caused by local or systemic factors. In children aphthous stomatitis and herpetic stomatitis are typically seen. Children with immunosuppression and those receiving chemotherapy or head and neck radiotherapy are at high risk for developing mucosal ulceration and herpetic stomatitis.

Aphthous stomatitis (aphthous ulcer, canker sore) is a benign but painful condition whose cause is unknown. Its onset is usually associated with mild traumatic injury (biting the cheek, hitting the mucosa with a toothbrush, or a mouth appliance rubbing on the mucosa), allergy, or emotional stress. The lesions are painful, small, whitish ulcerations surrounded by a red border. They are distinguished from other types of stomatitis by healthy adjacent tissues, absence of vesicles, and no systemic illness. The ulcers persist for 4 to 12 days and heal uneventfully.

Herpetic gingivostomatitis (HGS) is caused by HSV, most often type 1, and may occur as a primary infection or recur in a less severe form known as **recurrent herpes labialis** (commonly called *cold sores* or *fever blisters*). The primary infection usually begins with a fever; the pharynx becomes edematous and erythematous; and vesicles erupt on the mucosa, causing severe pain (Fig. 16-7). Cervical lymphadenitis often occurs, and the breath has a distinctly foul odor. In the recurrent form the vesicles appear on the lips, usually singly or in groups. The precipitating factors for the cold sores include emotional stress, trauma (often related to dental procedures), immunosuppression, or exposure to excessive sunlight. The disease can last 5 to 14 days, with varying degrees of severity.

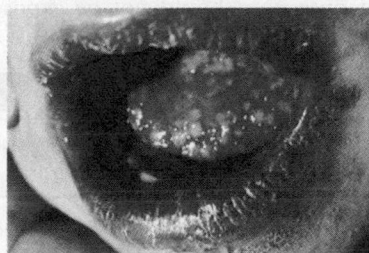

Fig. 16-7 Primary gingivostomatitis. (From Thompson JM, McFarland GM, Hirsch JE, et al: *Mosby's clinical nursing*, ed 5, St Louis, 2002, Mosby.)

Stomatitis may occur as a manifestation of hand-foot-and-mouth disease and herpangina; both manifest with scattered vesicles on the buccal mucosa and are commonly caused by the nonpolio enteroviruses (primarily coxsackieviruses). Children with either hand-foot-and-mouth or herpangina often have poor intake as a result of the mouth sores.

Therapeutic Management

Treatment for all types of stomatitis is aimed at relief of symptoms, primarily pain. Acetaminophen and ibuprofen are usually sufficient for mild cases, but with more severe HGS, stronger analgesics such as codeine may be needed. Topical anesthetics are helpful and include over-the-counter preparations such as Orabase, Anbesol, and Kank-A. Lidocaine (Xylocaine Viscous) can be prescribed for the child who can keep 1 tsp of the solution in the mouth for 2 to 3 minutes and then expectorate the drug. A mixture of equal parts of diphenhydramine elixir and Maalox (aluminum and magnesium hydroxide) provides mild analgesia, antiinflammatory properties, and a protective coating for the lesions. Sucralfate can also be used as a coating agent for oral mucous membranes. Specific treatment for children with severe cases of HGS is the use of antiviral agents such as acyclovir (Phillips, 2008). A recent systematic review found weak evidence that acyclovir is effective in reducing the number of oral lesions, preventing development of new lesions, and decreasing difficulty with eating and drinking (Nasser, Fedorowicz, Khoshnevisan, et al, 2008).

Nursing Care Management

The chief nursing goals for children with stomatitis are relief of pain and prevention of spread of the herpes virus. Analgesics and topical anesthetics are used as needed to provide relief, especially before meals to encourage food and fluid intake. For younger infants and toddlers who cannot swish and swallow, apply the diphenhydramine and Maalox solution with a cotton-tipped applicator before feedings to minimize pain. Educating parents regarding the use of these medications is important to maintain adequate hydration in the child whose mouth is too sore to take liquids. Drinking bland fluids through a straw is helpful in avoiding the painful lesions. Encourage mouth care; the use of a very soft bristle toothbrush or disposable foam-tipped toothbrush provides gentle cleaning near ulcerated areas.

Careful hand washing is essential when caring for children with HGS. Because the infection is autoinoculable, children should keep their fingers out of the mouth; contaminated hands can infect other body parts. Very young children may require elbow restraints to ensure compliance. Articles placed in the mouth are cleaned thoroughly. Newborns and individuals with immunosuppression should not be exposed to infected children.

> **! NURSING ALERT**
>
> When examining herpetic lesions, wear gloves. The virus easily enters breaks in the skin and can cause herpetic whitlow of the fingers.

Because herpes infection is often associated with sexual transmission, explain to parents and older children that HGS is usually caused by type 1 HSV, the type not associated with sexual activity.

INTESTINAL PARASITIC DISEASES

Intestinal parasitic diseases, including helminths (worms) and protozoa, constitute the most frequent infections in the world. In the United States the incidence of intestinal parasitic disease, especially giardiasis, has increased among young children who attend daycare centers. Young children are especially at risk because of typical hand-mouth activity and uncontrolled fecal activity.

Various infecting organisms cause intestinal parasitic diseases in humans. This discussion is limited to the two most common parasitic infections among children in the United States: giardiasis and pinworms. Table 16-2 describes the outstanding features of selected helminths that belong to the family of nematodes.

GENERAL NURSING CARE MANAGEMENT

Nursing responsibilities related to intestinal parasitic infections involve assistance with identification of the parasite, treatment of the infection, and prevention of initial infection or reinfection. Laboratory examination of substances containing the worm, its larvae, or ova can identify the organism. Most are identified by examining fecal smears from the stools of persons suspected of harboring the parasite. Fresh specimens are best for revealing parasites or larvae; therefore take collected specimens directly to the laboratory for examination. If this is not possible, place the specimen in a container with a preservative. Parents need clear instructions on obtaining an adequate sample and the number of samples required. (See Stool Specimens, Chapter 27.) In most parasitic infections, other family members, especially children, may be examined to identify those who are similarly affected.

After the diagnosis is confirmed and appropriate treatment is planned, parents need further explanation and reinforcement. Compliance in terms of drug therapy and other measures, such as thorough hand washing, is essential for eradication of the parasite. The family needs to understand the nature of transmission and that in some cases the medication must be repeated in 2 weeks to 1 month to kill organisms hatched since initial treatment.

The nurse's most important function is preventive education of children and families regarding hygiene and health habits. Thorough hand washing before eating or handling food and after using the toilet is the most important precautionary method. The Family-Centered Care box lists other preventive practices.

GIARDIASIS

Giardiasis is caused by the protozoan *Giardia lamblia* (also called *Giardia intestinalis, Giardia duodenalis,* and *Lamblia intestinalis*). It is the most common intestinal parasitic pathogen in the United States. Child care centers and institutions providing care for persons with developmental disabilities are common sites for urban giardiasis, and the children may pass cysts for months. Also consider giardiasis in those with a history of recent travel to an endemic area (Yoder and Beach, 2007; Shields, Gleim, and Beach, 2008).

TABLE 16-2   SELECTED INTESTINAL PARASITES

CLINICAL MANIFESTATIONS	COMMENTS
Ascariasis—*Ascaris lumbricoides* (Common Roundworm) Light infections—Asymptomatic Heavy infections—Anorexia, irritability, nervousness, enlarged abdomen, weight loss, fever, intestinal colic Severe infections—Intestinal obstruction, appendicitis, perforation of intestine with peritonitis, obstructive jaundice, lung involvement (pneumonitis)	Transferred to mouth by way of contaminated food, fingers, or toys Largest of the intestinal helminths Affects principally young children 1-4 yr of age Prevalent in warm climates
Hookworm Disease—*Necator americanus* Light infections in well-nourished individuals—No problems Heavier infections—Mild to severe anemia, malnutrition May be itching and burning followed by erythema and a papular eruption in areas to which the organism migrates	Transmitted by discharging eggs on the soil, which are picked up, causing infection from direct skin contact with contaminated soil Recommend wearing shoes, although children playing in contaminated soil expose many skin surfaces
Strongyloidiasis—*Strongyloides stercoralis* (Threadworm) Light infection—Asymptomatic Heavy infection—Respiratory signs and symptoms; abdominal pain, distention; nausea and vomiting; diarrhea (large, pale stools, often with mucus) Life threatening in children with weakened immunologic defenses	Transmission is same as for hookworm except autoinfection common Older children and adults affected more often than young children Severe infections may lead to severe nutritional deficiency
Visceral Larva Migrans—*Toxocara canis* (Dogs) **Intestinal Toxocariasis—*Toxocara cati* (Cats)** Depends on reactivity of infected individual May be asymptomatic except for eosinophilia Specific diagnosis difficult	Transmitted by direct contamination of hands from contact with dog, cat, or objects or by ingestion of soil Keep dogs and cats away from areas where children play; sandboxes especially important transmission areas Periodic deworming of diagnosed dogs and cats Control of dog and cat population
Trichuriasis—*Trichuris trichiura* (Whipworm) Light infections—Asymptomatic Heavy infections—Abdominal pain and distention, diarrhea	Transmitted from contaminated soil, vegetables, toys, and other objects Most frequent in warm, moist climates Occurs most often in undernourished children living in unsanitary conditions

FAMILY-CENTERED CARE
Preventing Intestinal Parasitic Disease

- Always wash hands and fingernails with soap and water before eating and handling food and after toileting.
- Avoid placing fingers in mouth and biting nails.
- Discourage children from scratching bare anal area.
- Use superabsorbent disposable diapers to prevent leakage.
- Change diapers as soon as soiled and dispose of diapers in closed receptacle out of children's reach.
- Do not rinse cloth or disposable diapers in toilet.
- Disinfect toilet seats and diaper-changing areas; use dilute household bleach (10% solution) or ammonia (Lysol) and wipe clean with paper towels.
- Drink only treated water or bottled water, especially if camping.
- Wash all raw fruits and vegetables and food that have fallen on the floor.
- Avoid growing foods in soil fertilized with human or untreated animal excreta.
- Teach children to defecate only in a toilet, not on the ground.
- Keep dogs and cats away from playgrounds or sandboxes.
- Avoid swimming in pools frequented by diapered children.
- Wear shoes outside.

BOX 16-2   CLINICAL MANIFESTATIONS OF GIARDIASIS

Infants and young children:
- Diarrhea
- Vomiting
- Anorexia
- Growth failure (failure to thrive)—if chronic exposure

Children older than 5 years of age:
- Abdominal cramps
- Intermittent loose stools
- Constipation

Stools that are malodorous, watery, pale, and greasy
Spontaneous resolution of most infections in 4 to 6 weeks

Rare, chronic form:
- Intermittent loose, foul-smelling stools
- Possibility of abdominal bloating, flatulence, sulfur-tasting belches, epigastric pain, vomiting, headache, and weight loss

The potential for transmission is great, because the cysts—the nonmotile stage of the protozoa—can survive in the environment for months. Chief modes of transmission are person to person; food; and animals, especially puppies. Contaminated water, especially in mountain lakes and streams and swimming or wading pools frequented by diapered infants, are common sources of transmission. In children, person-to-person transmission is the most likely cause. Recent studies indicate swimming pool filters and interactive water fountains to be sites of contamination (Eisenstein, Bodager, and Ginzl, 2008; Shields, Gleim, and Beach, 2008). Although individuals infected with giardiasis may be asymptomatic, common symptoms include abdominal cramps and diarrhea (Box 16-2).

Diagnosis of giardiasis may be made by microscopic examination of stool specimens or duodenal fluid, or by identification of *G. lamblia* antigens in these specimens by techniques such as enzyme immunoassay (EIA). Because the *Giardia* organisms live in the upper intestine and are excreted in a highly variable pattern, repeated microscopic examination of stool specimens may be required to identify trophozoites (active parasites) or cysts. Duodenal specimens are obtained by direct aspiration, biopsy, or the string test. In the string test, the child swallows a gelatin capsule with a nylon string attached. Several hours later, the string is withdrawn and the contents are sent for laboratory analysis. With the availability of EIA techniques to identify *Giardia* antigens in stool specimens, other tests are being used less often.

Therapeutic Management

The drugs of choice for treatment of giardiasis are metronidazole (Flagyl), tinidazole (Tindamax), and nitazoxanide (Alinia). Tinidazole is said to have an 80% to 100% cure rate after a single dose (American Academy of Pediatrics, 2009). Metronidazole and tinidazole have a metallic taste and gastrointestinal side effects, including nausea and vomiting; nitazoxanide has no bitter taste and should be taken with food to avoid gastrointestinal symptoms. Albendazole is also used to treat the disease and reportedly has fewer side effects than metronidazole (American Academy of Pediatrics, 2009).

Nursing Care Management

The most important nursing consideration is prevention of giardiasis and education of parents, child care center staff, and those who assume the daily care of small children. Attention to meticulous sanitary practices, especially during diaper changes, is essential (see Family-Centered Care box and Fig. 16-8). Nurses can play an important role in educating parents of small

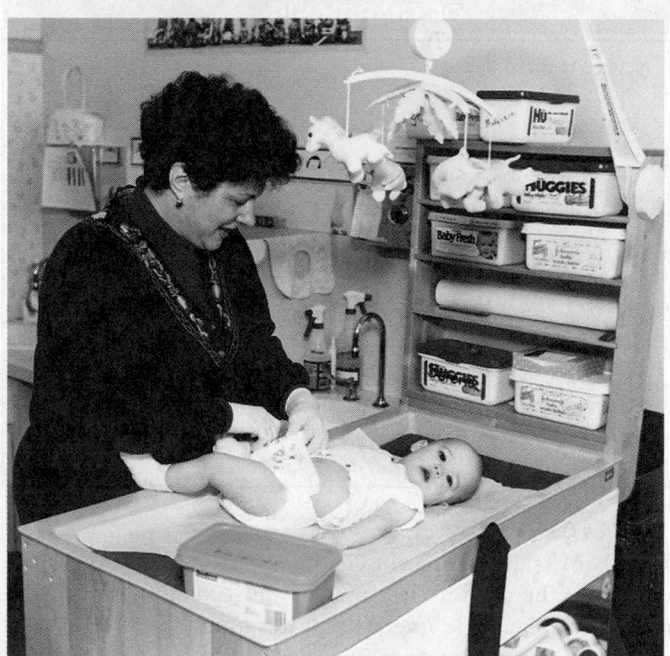

Fig. 16-8 Prevention of giardiasis, especially in daycare centers, requires sanitary practices during diaper changes, such as discarding paper diapers in a covered receptacle, changing paper covers on the diaper-changing surface, and having facilities for hand washing nearby. NOTE: Soiled cloth diapers and clothing should be stored in a plastic bag for transport home.

children and daycare staff regarding appropriate sanitation practices. (See Alternative Child Care Arrangements, Chapter 12.) In addition, discourage young children who are infected or who have diarrhea from swimming in community or private pools until they are infection-free. Lakes and streams may contain high numbers of *Giardia* spore cysts, which can be swallowed in the water. Discourage children from swimming in stagnant bodies of water, and in water where there are known infected children swimming when there is a high chance of swallowing water. *Giardia* organisms are said to be resistant to chlorine (Eisenstein, Bodager, and Ginzl, 2008). Encourage parents to take small children to the restroom frequently when swimming, to avoid letting children in diapers in swimming areas, and to change diapers away from the water source. (See also Centers for Disease Control information on recreational water illnesses [www.cdc.gov/healthyswimming].) After children are infected, family education regarding drug administration is essential.

ENTEROBIASIS (PINWORMS)

Enterobiasis, or pinworms, caused by the nematode *Enterobius vermicularis,* is the most common helminthic infection in the United States. It is universally present in temperate climatic zones and may infect more than 30% of all children at any one time. Crowded conditions, such as in classrooms and daycare centers, favor transmission.

Infection begins when the eggs are ingested or inhaled (the eggs float in the air). The eggs hatch in the upper intestine, then mature and migrate through the intestine. After mating, adult females migrate out the anus and lay eggs (American Academy of Pediatrics, 2009). The movement of the worms on skin and mucous membrane surfaces causes intense itching. As the child scratches, eggs are deposited on the hands and underneath the fingernails. The typical hand-to-mouth activity of youngsters makes them especially prone to reinfection. Pinworm eggs persist in the indoor environment for 2 to 3 weeks, contaminating anything they contact, such as toilet seats, doorknobs, bed linen, underwear, and food. Except for the intense rectal itching associated with pinworms, the clinical manifestations are nonspecific (Box 16-3).

Diagnostic Evaluation

Diagnosis is most commonly made from the tape test (see Nursing Care Management). Repeated tests to collect eggs may

---

BOX 16-3   CLINICAL MANIFESTATIONS OF PINWORMS

Intense perianal itching is the principal symptom. Evidence of itching in young children includes:
- General irritability
- Restlessness
- Poor sleep
- Bed-wetting
- Distractibility
- Short attention span
- Perianal dermatitis and excoriation secondary to itching
- If worms migrate, possible vaginal (vulvovaginitis) and urethral infection

be necessary, and if there is a possibility that other family members may be infected, perform a tape test on them.

Therapeutic Management

The drugs available for treatment of pinworms include mebendazole (Vermox), pyrantel pamoate (Pin-Rid, Antiminth), and albendazole. The drug of choice is mebendazole, which is safe, effective, and convenient, with few side effects. However, it is not recommended for children younger than 2 years of age. If pyrvinium pamoate is prescribed, advise parents that the drug stains stool and vomitus bright red, as well as clothing or skin that comes in contact with the drug; it is available without prescription and should not be used in children under 2 years without consulting the primary practitioner. Because pinworms are easily transmitted, all household members are treated. The dose of antiparasitic medication should be repeated in 2 weeks to completely eradicate the parasite and prevent reinfection.

Nursing Care Management

Direct nursing care at identifying the parasite, eradicating the organism, and preventing reinfection. Parents need clear, detailed instructions for the **tape test**. A loop of transparent (not "frosted" or "magic") tape, sticky side out, is placed around the end of a tongue depressor, which is then firmly pressed against the child's perianal area. A convenient, commercially prepared tape is also available for this purpose. Pinworm specimens are collected in the morning as soon as the child awakens and *before* the child has a bowel movement or bathes. The procedure may need to be performed on 3 or more consecutive days before eggs are collected. Parents are instructed to place the tongue blade in a glass jar or loosely in a plastic bag so that it can be brought in for microscopic examination. For specimens collected in the hospital, practitioner's office, or clinic, place the tape smoothly on a glass slide, sticky side down, for examination.

Adherence to the drug regimen is usually excellent since only one or two doses are needed. The family should be reminded of the need to take a second dose in 2 weeks to ensure eradication of the eggs.

To prevent reinfection, washing all clothes and bed linens in hot water and vacuuming the house may be recommended. However, there is little documentation on the effectiveness of these measures, since pinworms survive on many surfaces. Helpful suggestions include hand washing after toileting and before eating, keeping the child's fingernails short to minimize the chance of ova collecting under the nails, dressing children in one-piece sleeping outfits, and daily showering rather than tub bathing. Inform families that recurrence is common. Treat repeated infections in the same manner as the first one.

INGESTION OF INJURIOUS AGENTS

Since the passage of the Poison Prevention Packaging Act of 1970, which requires that certain potentially hazardous drugs and household products be sold in child-resistant containers, the incidence of poisonings in children has decreased dramatically. However, despite these advances, poisoning remains a significant health concern, with most cases (51% in 2007) occurring in children younger than 6 years of age (Bronstein,

Spyker, Cantilena, et al, 2008). The home environment lends itself to injury in this vulnerable age-group of children (Dessypris, Dikalioti, Skalkidis, et al, 2009). Although pharmaceuticals such as analgesics, cough and cold preparations, topical preparations, antibiotics, vitamins, gastrointestinal preparations, hormones, and antihistamines are frequently the agents of poisonings, a variety of other substances can still poison children. The most frequently ingested poisons include (Bronstein, Spyker, Cantilena, et al, 2008; Franklin and Rodgers, 2008)*[1]

- Cosmetics and personal care products (perfume, cologne, aftershave)
- Cleaning products (hypochlorite [household] bleach, pine oil disinfectants)
- Plants (nontoxic gastrointestinal irritants, oxalates) (Box 16-4)
- Foreign bodies, toys, and miscellaneous substances (desiccants, thermometers, bubble-blowing solutions)

Children are exposed to toxic substances more frequently than any other age-group (Eldridge, Van Eyk, and Kornegay, 2007). Many poisonings reflect the ready accessibility of the product in the home, where more than 90% of poisonings occur. A significant number of poisonings take place elsewhere, such as in a grandparent's or friend's home, in a school, or in a health care facility.

The developmental characteristics of young children predispose them to poisoning by ingestion. Infants and toddlers explore their environment through oral experimentation. Because their sense of taste is not discriminating at this age, they ingest many unpalatable substances. In addition, toddlers and preschoolers are developing autonomy and initiative, which increase their curiosity and noncompliant behavior. Imitation is also a powerful motivator, especially when combined with lack of awareness of danger.

This section is primarily concerned with the immediate emergency treatment of ingestion of injurious agents. Box 16-5 summarizes specific management of corrosive, hydrocarbon, acetaminophen, salicylate, iron, and plant poisoning. Because of the importance of lead poisoning among young children, ingestion of lead is discussed separately. Appropriate suggestions for poison prevention are discussed on p. 625 and in Chapter 14.

PRINCIPLES OF EMERGENCY TREATMENT

A poisoning may or may not require emergency intervention, but in every instance medical evaluation is necessary to initiate appropriate action. Advise parents to call the **poison control center** (PCC) *before* initiating any intervention. Parents should post the local PCC telephone number (usually listed in the front of the telephone directory) near each phone in the house† (see Critical Thinking Exercise and Emergency Treatment box).

---

*The most common substances in each category are in parentheses. Substances ingested are not necessarily the most toxic but often are readily available.
†Also available by calling 800-222-1222 or online at American Association of Poison Control Centers, **www.aapcc.org**.

BOX 16-4 POISONOUS AND NONPOISONOUS PLANTS

Poisonous Plants (Toxic Parts)
Apple (leaves, seeds)
Apricot (leaves, stem, seed pits)
Azalea (all parts)
Buttercup (all parts)
Castor (bean or seeds—extremely toxic)
Cherry (wild or cultivated) (twigs, seeds, foliage)
Daffodil (bulbs)
Dumbcane (dieffenbachia) (all parts)
Elephant ear (all parts)
English ivy (all parts)
Foxglove (leaves, seeds, flowers)
Holly (berries and leaves)
Hyacinth (bulbs)
Ivy (leaves)
Mistletoe* (berries, leaves)
Oak tree (acorn, foliage)
Philodendron (all parts)
Plum (pit)
Poinsettia† (leaves)
Poison ivy, poison oak (leaves, stems, sap, fruit, smoke from burning plants)
Pokeweed, pokeberry (roots, berries, leaves [when eaten raw])
Pothos (all parts)
Rhubarb (leaves)
Tulip (bulbs)

Water hemlock (all parts)
Wisteria (seeds, pods)
Yew (all parts)

Nonpoisonous Plants
African violet
Aluminum plant
Asparagus fern
Begonia
Boston fern
Christmas cactus
Coleus
Gardenia
Grape ivy
Jade plant
Piggyback begonia
Piggyback plant
Prayer plant
Rubber tree
Snake plant
Spider plant
Swedish ivy
Wax plant
Weeping fig
Zebra plant

*Eating one or two berries or leaves is probably nontoxic.
†Mildly toxic if ingested in massive quantities.

❓ CRITICAL THINKING EXERCISE

Poisoning

Mrs. Berry, a neighbor, calls you. She is upset because her 2-year-old son has eaten several chewable multivitamins with iron. She asks you if she should give her son ipecac. What should you advise her to do?
1. Evidence—Is there sufficient evidence to formulate an answer for Mrs. Berry?
2. Assumptions—Describe some underlying assumptions about the following:
   a. What is the best initial response when a child ingests a potentially poisonous substance?
   b. What is ipecac?
   c. What are the dangers involved in the use of ipecac?
3. What is the priority for nursing care at this time?
4. Does the evidence support your conclusion?

➕ EMERGENCY TREATMENT

Poisoning

1. Assess the victim:
   • Initiate cardiorespiratory support if needed (airway, breathing, circulation).
   • Take vital signs; reevaluate routinely.
   • Treat associated complications.
2. Terminate exposure:
   • Empty mouth of pills, plant parts, or other material.
   • Flush eyes continuously with normal saline (or room-temperature tap water at home) for 15 to 20 minutes.
   • Flush skin and wash with soap and a soft cloth; remove contaminated clothes, especially if a pesticide, acid, alkali, or hydrocarbon is involved.
   • Bring victim of an inhalation poisoning into fresh air.
3. Identify the poison:
   • Question the victim and witnesses.
   • Look for environmental clues (empty container, nearby spill, odor on breath) and save all evidence of poison (container, vomitus, urine).
   • In absence of other evidence, be alert to signs and symptoms of potential poisoning, including symptoms of ocular or dermal exposure.
   • Call poison control center or other competent emergency facility for immediate advice regarding treatment.
4. Prevent poison absorption:
   • Place child in side-lying, sitting, or kneeling position with head below chest to prevent aspiration.
   • Administer activated charcoal if ordered (unless used repeatedly, usual dose is 1 g/kg unless amount of toxin is known), administer drug antidote, or perform gastric lavage.

Based on the initial telephone assessment, the PCC counsels the parents to begin treatment at home or to take the child to an emergency facility. When a call is taken, the name and telephone number of the caller is recorded to reestablish contact if the connection is interrupted. Because most poisonings are managed in the home, expert advice is essential in minimizing adverse effects. When the exact quantity or type of ingested toxin is not known, admission to a health care facility with pediatric emergency treatment services for laboratory evaluation and surveillance during the time after ingestion is critical.

Assessment

The first and most important principle in dealing with a poisoning is to treat the child first, not the poison. This requires

BOX 16-5 SELECTED POISONINGS IN CHILDREN

Corrosives (Strong Acids or Alkalis)
Drain, toilet, or oven cleaners
Electric dishwasher detergent (liquid, because of higher pH, is more hazardous than granular)
Mildew remover
Batteries
Clinitest tablets
Denture cleaners
Bleach

Clinical Manifestations
Severe burning pain in mouth, throat, and stomach
White, swollen mucous membranes; edema of lips, tongue, and pharynx (respiratory obstruction)
Violent vomiting (hemoptysis)
Drooling and inability to clear secretions
Signs of shock
Anxiety and agitation

Comments
Household bleach is a frequently ingested corrosive but rarely causes serious damage.
Liquid corrosives cause more damage than granular preparations.

Treatment
Inducing emesis is contraindicated (vomiting redamages the mucosa).
Contact poison control center (PCC) immediately. If PCC or medical advice and treatment are not immediately available, it may be appropriate to dilute corrosive with water or milk (usually ≤120 ml [4 oz]).
Do not neutralize. Neutralization can cause an exothermic reaction (which produces heat and causes increased symptoms or produces a thermal burn in addition to a chemical burn).
Maintain patent airway as needed.
Administer analgesics.
Do not allow oral intake.
Esophageal stricture may require repeated dilations or surgery.

Hydrocarbons
Gasoline
Kerosene
Lamp oil
Mineral seal oil (found in furniture polish)
Lighter fluid
Turpentine
Paint thinner and remover (some types)

Clinical Manifestations
Gagging, choking, and coughing
Nausea
Vomiting
Alterations in sensorium, such as lethargy
Weakness
Respiratory symptoms of pulmonary involvement
- Tachypnea
- Cyanosis
- Retractions
- Grunting

Comments
Immediate danger is aspiration (even small amounts can cause bronchitis and chemical pneumonia).
Gasoline, kerosene, lighter fluid, mineral seal oil, and turpentine cause severe pneumonia.

Treatment
Inducing emesis is generally contraindicated
Gastric decontamination and emptying are questionable, even when the hydrocarbon contains a heavy metal or pesticide; if gastric lavage must be performed, a cuffed endotracheal tube should be in place before lavage because of a high risk of aspiration.
Symptomatic treatment of chemical pneumonia includes high humidity, oxygen, hydration, and antibiotics for secondary infection.

Acetaminophen
Clinical Manifestations
Occurs in four stages:
1. Initial period (2 to 4 hours after ingestion)
   - Nausea
   - Vomiting
   - Sweating
   - Pallor
2. Latent period (24 to 36 hours)
   - Patient improves
3. Hepatic involvement (may last up to 7 days and be permanent)
   - Pain in right upper quadrant
   - Jaundice
   - Confusion
   - Stupor
   - Coagulation abnormalities
4. Patients who do not die in hepatic stage gradually recover.

Comments
This is the most common accidental drug poisoning in children.
It occurs from acute ingestion.
Toxic dose is 150 mg/kg or greater in children.
Because of multiple formulations and concentrations, chronic acetaminophen toxicity is a significant problem.
Parents should be counseled to read product packaging carefully and to consult a health care professional to avoid inappropriate dosing.

Treatment
Antidote N-acetylcysteine (Mucomyst) can usually be given orally but is first diluted in fruit juice or soda because of the antidote's offensive odor.
Given as 1 loading dose and usually 17 maintenance doses in different dosages.
May be given intravenously, but use is investigational.

Aspirin (Acetylsalicylic Acid [ASA])
Clinical Manifestations
Acute poisoning
- Nausea
- Disorientation
- Vomiting
- Dehydration
- Diaphoresis
- Hyperpnea
- Hyperpyrexia
- Oliguria
- Tinnitus
- Coma
- Convulsions

Chronic poisoning
- Same as above but subtle onset (often mistaken for viral illness)
- Dehydration, coma, and seizures may be more severe
- Bleeding tendencies

Comments
May be caused by acute ingestion (severe toxicity occurs with 300 to 500 mg/kg).
May be caused by chronic ingestion (i.e., >100 mg/kg/day for 2 or more days); can be more serious than acute ingestion.
Time to peak serum salicylate level can vary with enteric aspirin or the presence of concretions (bezoars).

Continued

BOX 16-5	SELECTED POISONINGS IN CHILDREN—cont'd

Aspirin (Acetylsalicylic Acid [ASA])—cont'd

Treatment

Hospitalization is necessary for severe toxicity.

Emesis, lavage, activated charcoal, or cathartic may be used.

Lavage will not remove concretions of ASA.

Activated charcoal is important early in ASA toxicity.

Sodium bicarbonate transfusions are used to correct metabolic acidosis, and urinary alkalinization may be effective in enhancing elimination; urinary alkalinization is difficult to achieve.

Be aware of the risk for fluid overload and pulmonary edema.

Use external cooling for hyperpyrexia.

Administer anticonvulsants.

Provide oxygen and ventilation for respiratory depression.

Administer vitamin K for bleeding.

In severe cases, hemodialysis (not peritoneal dialysis) is used.

Iron

Mineral supplement or vitamin containing iron

Clinical Manifestations

Occurs in five stages:

1. Initial period ($\frac{1}{2}$ to 6 hours after ingestion; if child does not develop gastrointestinal symptoms in 6 hours, toxicity is unlikely)
   - Vomiting
   - Hematemesis
   - Diarrhea
   - Hematochezia (bloody stools)
   - Gastric pain
2. Latency (2 to 12 hours): patient improves
3. Systemic toxicity (4 to 24 hours)
   - Metabolic acidosis
   - Fever
   - Hyperglycemia
   - Bleeding
   - Shock
   - Death (may occur)
4. Hepatic injury (48 to 96 hours)
   - Seizures
   - Coma
5. Rarely, pyloric stenosis develops at 2 to 5 weeks

Comments

Factors related to frequency of iron poisoning include:
- Widespread availability
- Packaging of large quantities in individual containers
- Lack of parental awareness of iron toxicity
- Resemblance of iron tablets to candy (e.g., M&Ms)

Toxic dose is based on the amount of elemental iron in various salts (sulfate, gluconate, fumarate), which ranges from 20% to 33%; ingestions of 60 mg/kg are considered dangerous.

Treatment

Use emesis or lavage.

For toxic doses lavage may be necessary for all chewable tablets or liquids if spontaneous vomiting has not occurred.

Chelation therapy with deferoxamine is used in severe intoxication (may turn urine red to orange).

If intravenous deferoxamine is given too rapidly, hypotension, facial flushing, rash, urticaria, tachycardia, and shock may occur; stop the infusion, maintain the intravenous line with normal saline, and notify the practitioner immediately.

Plants

Plants listed in Box 16-4

Clinical Manifestations

Depends on type of plant ingested

May cause local irritation of oropharynx and entire gastrointestinal tract

May cause respiratory, renal, and central nervous system symptoms

Topical contact with plants can cause dermatitis

Comments

Plants are some of most frequently ingested substances.

They rarely cause serious problems, although some plant ingestions can be fatal.

Plants can also cause choking and allergic reactions.

Treatment

Induce emesis.

Wash from skin or eyes.

Provide supportive care as needed.

---

an immediate concern for life support. Vital signs are taken, and respiratory or circulatory support is instituted as needed. The child's condition is routinely reevaluated. Because shock is a complication of several types of household poisons, particularly corrosives, measures to reduce the effects of shock are important, beginning with the ABCs (airway, breathing, circulation) of resuscitation. Establishing and maintaining vascular access for rapid intravascular volume expansion is vital in the treatment of pediatric shock.

The emergency department nurse's responsibility is to be prepared for immediate intervention with all of the necessary equipment. Because time and speed are critical factors in recovery from serious poisonings, anticipation of potential problems and complications may mean the difference between life and death.

Gastric Decontamination

Although pediatric poison ingestions are common, they rarely result in significant morbidity or mortality (Greene, Harris, and Singer, 2008). Consider using gastrointestinal decontamination (GID) only after careful evaluation of the potential toxicity of the poison and the risks versus benefits. When GID is needed, the immediate treatment is to remove the ingested poison by adsorbing the toxin with activated charcoal, performing gastric lavage, or increasing bowel motility (catharsis). Because of continuing controversy regarding the use of these methods, treat each toxic ingestion individually (Madden, 2008; Eldridge, Van Eyk, and Kornegay, 2007). Specific antidotes may be administered for certain poisonings.

Syrup of ipecac, an emetic that exerts its action through irritation of the gastric mucosa and by stimulation of the vomiting center, is no longer recommended for routine treatment of poison ingestion (American Academy of Pediatrics, 2009; Greene, Harris, and Singer, 2008; Sheffield and Serwint, 2008; Criddle, 2007). Box 16-6 lists the certain situations when ipecac may be of benefit.

> **! NURSING ALERT**
>
> Ipecac is not recommended for routine poison treatment intervention in the home (American Academy of Pediatrics, 2009; Greene, Harris, and Singer, 2008; Sheffield and Serwint, 2008; Criddle, 2007).

BOX 16-6   INDICATIONS FOR IPECAC USE IN THE HOME

Ipecac may be helpful in the home environment after consultation with a health care professional or poison control center in the following circumstances:

- There is no contraindication to ipecac use.
- There is substantial risk of serious toxicity (e.g., colchicines, calcium-channel antagonists, digoxin).
- There is no alternative therapy available or effective means to decrease gastrointestinal absorption.
- There will be a delay of more than 60 minutes before the patient arrives at an emergency department.
- Ipecac can be administered within 30 minutes of the poison ingestion.
- Ipecac will not adversely affect more definitive treatment.

From Greene S, Harris C, Singer J: Gastrointestinal decontamination of the poisoned patient, *Pediatr Emerg Care* 24(3):176-189, 2008.

Medications such as calcium channel blockers and benzodiazepines either produce a rapid onset of adverse symptoms (e.g., sedation, seizures, coma) or exaggerate the vagal response induced by gagging, which can lead to significant bradycardia. Under either circumstance, uncontrolled vomiting becomes an undesirable and unsafe event.

A more commonly used method of gastrointestinal decontamination is the use of activated charcoal (AC), an odorless, tasteless, fine black powder that adsorbs many compounds, creating a stable complex (Sheffield and Serwint, 2008). AC should be used in the following situations:

- Poison is potentially toxic.
- No contraindications exist to using AC.
- Poison ingested is bound by charcoal.
- Poison is likely to be in the gastrointestinal tract at the time of AC administration.
- Gastrointestinal tract is intact.
- No safer or more effective alternative therapy is available.

AC is mixed with water or a saline cathartic to form a slurry. Slurries are neither gritty nor distasteful but resemble black mud. To increase the child's acceptance of AC, the nurse should mix it with diet soda and serve it through a straw in an opaque container with a cover (such as a disposable coffee cup and lid) or an ordinary cup covered with aluminum foil or placed inside a small paper bag. In one small study, healthy adolescents preferred the taste of AC mixed with cola or chocolate milk mixture instead of water (Cheng and Ratnapalan, 2007). For small children a nasogastric tube may be required to administer AC (Greene, Harris, and Singer, 2008).

There is discussion of the use of AC in the home for pediatric poison ingestion. The evidence is not clear regarding the risk versus benefit of home AC administration (Eldridge, Van Eyk, and Kornegay, 2007). Potential complications from the use of AC include aspiration (usually in patients with impaired gag reflexes), constipation, and intestinal obstruction (in multiple doses) (Sheffield and Serwint, 2008). Superactivated charcoal products for gastric decontamination are often more palatable and just as effective (Criddle, 2007).

If the child is admitted to an emergency facility, gastric lavage may be performed to empty the stomach of the toxic agent; however, this procedure can be associated with serious complications (gastrointestinal perforation, hypoxia, aspiration) and it is no longer recommended in all cases of ingestion. There is no conclusive evidence that gastric lavage decreases morbidity (Greene, Harris, and Singer, 2008; Sheffield and Serwint, 2008; Criddle, 2007). In addition, gastric lavage may be of little benefit if used later than 1 hour after ingestion (Greene, Harris, and Singer, 2008). Conditions that may be appropriate for the use of gastric lavage include presentation within 1 hour of ingestion of a toxin, ingestion in patient who has decreased gastrointestinal motility, the ingestion of a toxic amount of sustained-release medication, and a massive or life-threatening amount of poison (Madden, 2008; Criddle, 2007). When gastric lavage is used, the patient requires a protected airway, possible sedation, and the largest-diameter tube that can be inserted to facilitate passage of gastric contents. The Evidence-Based Practice box reviews recent literature on the use of gastric lavage in comparison to AC when a child has ingested poison.

In a minority of poisonings, specific antidotes are available to counteract the poison. They are highly effective and should be available in all emergency facilities. The supply of antidotes should be checked routinely and replaced as used or according to expiration dates. Antidotes available to treat toxin ingestion include *N*-acetylcysteine for acetaminophen poisoning, oxygen for carbon monoxide inhalation, naloxone for opioid overdose, flumazenil (Romazicon) for benzodiazepines (diazepam [Valium], midazolam [Versed]) overdose, digoxin immune Fab (Digibind) for digoxin toxicity, amyl nitrate for cyanide, and antivenin for certain poisonous bites.

Prevention of Recurrence

The ultimate objective is to prevent poisonings from occurring or recurring. Home safety education improves poison-prevention practices (Kendrick, Smith, Sutton, et al, 2008). Research supports the effectiveness of parent education on preventing unintentional injuries (Kendrick, Barlow, Hampshire, et al, 2007; Kendrick, Coupland, Mulvaney, et al, 2007). One effective counseling method is first to discuss the difficulties of constantly watching and safeguarding young children (see Family-Centered Care box). In this way the challenging task of raising children can lead to a discussion of injury prevention as part of the parental role. This approach also incorporates contributory causes for the incident, such as inadequate support systems; marital discord; discipline techniques (especially use of physical punishment); and any disruption in the family or family activities, such as vacations, moves, visitors, illnesses, or births. A visit to the home, especially after repeat poisonings, is recommended as part of the follow-up care to assess hazards, including family factors, and to evaluate appropriate injury-proofing measures. One method of identifying risk areas is to ask specific questions or to have the parent complete a questionnaire designed to isolate factors that predispose children to poisoning. Another approach is to encourage parents to bend down to the child's eye level and survey the home environment for potential hazards. Have the parents try to open cabinets and reach shelves to access poisons.

Passive measures (those that do not require active participation) have been the most successful in preventing poisoning and include using child-resistant closures and limiting the

EVIDENCE-BASED PRACTICE   *Curt Roberts, RN, and Danna Salinas, RN, BSN*

Gastric Lavage in Children

ASK THE QUESTION

What is the effect of gastric lavage in reducing systemic absorption of toxic substances compared with the administration of activated charcoal or forced emesis?

SEARCH FOR THE EVIDENCE

Search strategies

Keywords included gastric lavage, gastric decontamination, activated charcoal, and toxic ingestion. Searches were limited to English articles with human subjects.

Databases used

PubMed, STAT!Ref, UpToDateOnline, CINAHL, EMBASE, D.A.R.E, Cochrane Library, National Guideline Clearinghouse (AHRQ)

CRITICALLY ANALYZE THE EVIDENCE

GRADE criteria: Evidence quality moderate; recommendation strong (Guyatt, Oxman, Vist, et al, 2008)

Eddleston, Juszczak, and Buckley (2003) reviewed the literature to determine whether gastric lavage pushes poisons beyond the pylorus to assist with faster elimination of toxins from the body. The review examined two studies designed to measure movement of substances through the stomach and into the small intestine after gastric lavage. One study randomized 40 patients to gastric emptying by forced emesis or gastric lavage and maintained a control group of 20 patients in whom gastric emptying was not necessary. Either radiopaque pellets or radiolabeled water was used as a marker. There were no significant differences in the number of pellets in the small bowel between the emesis group and the control group or between the gastric lavage group and the control group. The second study consisted of five volunteers who were subjected to gastric lavage on three occasions. Less poison was found in the small bowel after gastric lavage than after no intervention. The researchers concluded there was no evidence that gastric lavage drives toxins into the small intestine.

Other studies have demonstrated that gastric lavage is equivalent to forced emesis as a method of gastric emptying (American Academy of Clinical Toxicology and European Association of Poisons Centres and Clinical Toxicologists, 2005; Smilkstein, 2002). A randomized crossover study with 12 volunteers who ingested paracetamol 50 mg/kg 1 hour after a standard meal demonstrated that activated charcoal administered within 1 hour of ingestion was more effective than gastric lavage followed by charcoal because of the delay in administration of the activated charcoal (Christophersen, Levin, Hoegberg, et al, 2002). Forced emesis was superior to gastric lavage when the goal was to remove large particles and fragments. However, the literature supports that gastric emptying has limited benefit in gastrointestinal decontamination because administration of activated charcoal appears to be more effective (Greene, Harris, and Singer, 2008; Sheffield and Serwint, 2008; American Academy of Clinical Toxicology and European Association of Poisons Centres and Clinical Toxicologists, 2005; Smilkstein, 2002).

Numerous complications are reported with both gastrointestinal lavage and activated charcoal. Complications of orogastric or nasogastric intubation include esophageal tears or perforation, nasal injury, oropharyngeal injury, gastric perforation, and inadvertent tracheal intubation (Eldridge, Van Eyk, and Kornegay, 2007; American Academy of Clinical Toxicology and European Association of Poisons Centres and Clinical Toxicologists, 2005; Smilkstein, 2002; Caravati, Knight, Linscott, et al, 2001). The American Academy of Clinical Toxicology and the European Association of Poisons Centers and Clinical Toxicologists (2005) have not recommended the routine use of gastric lavage in the management of toxic ingestions since 1997. Contraindications to the administration of charcoal also exist, including in patients who have ingested corrosive materials and in those at risk for hemorrhage or perforation due to structural abnormalities or recent surgery.

APPLY THE EVIDENCE: NURSING IMPLICATIONS

Gastric lavage has little or no effect in reducing absorption, especially when used as an intervention more than 1 hour after ingestion. Single-dose or multidose activated charcoal is most effective when administered within 1 hour of ingestion but may have an effect up to 4 hours after ingestion, depending on the substance. Administration of activated charcoal should not be delayed by the use of forced emesis or gastric lavage.

References

American Academy of Clinical Toxicology, European Association of Poisons Centres and Clinical Toxicologists: Position paper: single-dose activated charcoal, *J Toxicol Clin Toxicol* 43:61-87, 2005.

Caravati EM, Knight HH, Linscott MS, et al: Esophageal laceration and charcoal mediastinum complicating gastric lavage, *J Emerg Med* 20(3):273-276, 2001.

Christophersen AB, Levin D, Hoegberg LCG, et al: Activated charcoal alone or after gastric lavage: a simulated large paracetamol intoxication, *Br J Clin Pharmacol* 53(3):312-317, 2002.

Eddleston M, Juszczak E, Buckley N: Does gastric lavage really push poisons beyond the pylorus? A systematic review of the evidence, *Ann Emerg Med* 42(3):359-364, 2003.

Eldridge DL, Van Eyk J, Kornegay C: Pediatric toxicology, *Emerg Med Clin North Am* 25(2):283-308, 2007.

Greene S, Harris C, Singer J: Gastrointestinal decontamination of the poisoned patient, *Pediatr Emerg Care* 24(3):176-189, 2008.

Guyatt GH, Oxman AD, Vist GE, et al: GRADE: an emerging consensus on rating quality of evidence and strength of recommendations, *BMJ* 336:924-926, 2008.

Sheffield P, Serwint JR: Emetics, cathartics and gastric lavage, *Pediatr Rev* 29:214-215, 2008.

Smilkstein MJ: Techniques used to prevent gastrointestinal absorption of toxic compounds. In Goldfrank LR, Flomenbaum NE, Lewin NA, et al, editors: *Goldfrank's toxicologic emergencies*, ed 7, New York, 2002, McGraw-Hill.

number of tablets in one container. However, these measures alone are not sufficient to prevent poisoning, since most toxic agents in the home do not have safety closures. Therefore active measures (those that require participation) are essential. The Nursing Care Guidelines box lists the guidelines for preventing the occurrence or recurrence of a poisoning.

HEAVY METAL POISONING

Heavy metal poisoning can occur from the ingestion of a variety of substances, the most common being lead. Other sources that are important in terms of children are iron and mercury. Mercury toxicity, a rare form of heavy metal poisoning, has occurred in children from a variety of sources, such as broken thermometers or thermostats, broken fluorescent light bulbs, disk batteries, topical medications, gas regulators, cathartics, and interior latex house paint (Clifton, 2007). Elemental mercury (also called metallic mercury or quicksilver) is nontoxic if ingested and if the gastrointestinal tract is healthy (e.g., has no fistulas). However, mercury is volatile at room temperature and enters the bloodstream after it is inhaled, causing toxicity (tremors, memory loss, insomnia, gingivitis, diarrhea,

FAMILY-CENTERED CARE

Poisoning

A poisoning is more than a physical emergency for the child—it usually represents an emotional crisis for the parents, particularly in terms of guilt, self-reproach, and insecurity in the parenting role. The emergency department is no place to admonish the family for negligence, lack of appropriate supervision, or failure to injury-proof the home. Rather, it is a time to calm and support the child and parents, while unaccusingly exploring the circumstances of the injury. If the nurse prematurely attempts to discuss ways of preventing such an incident from recurring, the parents' anxiety will block out any suggestions or offered guidance. Therefore it is preferable for the nurse to delay the discussion until the child's condition is stabilized or, if the child is discharged immediately after emergency treatment, to make a public health referral or send a packet of information.

NURSING CARE GUIDELINES

Poison Prevention

- Assess possible contributing factors in occurrence of injury, such as discipline, parent-child relationship, developmental ability, environmental factors, and behavior problems.
- Institute anticipatory guidance for possible future injuries based on child's age and developmental level.
- Initiate referral to appropriate agency to evaluate home environment and need for injury-proofing measures.
- Provide assistance with environmental manipulation, such as lead removal, when necessary.
- Educate parents regarding safe storage of toxic substances.
- Advise parents to take drugs out of sight of children.
- Teach children the hazards of ingesting nonfood items.
- Advise parents against using plants for teas or medicine.
- Discuss problems of discipline and children's noncompliance and offer strategies for effective discipline.
- Instruct parents regarding correct administration of drugs for therapeutic purposes and to discontinue drug if there is evidence of mild toxicity.
- Advise parents to contact the poison control center, 800-222-1222, or practitioner immediately when a poisoning occurs.
- Tell them to post number of regional poison control center with emergency phone list by telephone.
- They should include by the telephone the home address with nearest cross street in case an ambulance is needed. (In an emergency, family members may not remember the house address, and baby-sitters may not be aware of the information.)

NURSING ALERT

Mercury thermometers are no longer recommended because, if they are broken, the inhaled vapors can cause toxicity. To prevent inhalation, clean up spilled mercury quickly, using disposable towels and rubber gloves and washing the hands well afterward.

anorexia, weight loss). The classic form of mercury poisoning is called acrodynia (or "painful extremities").

Heavy metals have an affinity for certain essential tissue chemicals, which must remain free for adequate cell functioning. When metals are bound to these substances, cellular enzyme systems are inactivated. Treatment involves chelation, use of a chemical compound that combines with the metal for rapid and safe excretion.

BOX 16-7 SOURCES OF LEAD

- Lead-based paint in deteriorating condition
- Lead solder
- Lead crystal
- Battery casings
- Lead fishing sinkers
- Lead curtain weights
- Lead bullets
- Some of these may contain lead:
  - Ceramic ware
  - Water
  - Pottery
  - Pewter
  - Dyes
  - Industrial factories
  - Vinyl mini-blinds
  - Playground equipment
  - Collectible toys
- Some imported toys or children's metal jewelry
- Artists' paints
- Pool cue chalk
- Occupations and hobbies involving lead:
  - Battery and aircraft manufacturing
  - Lead smelting
  - Brass foundry work
  - Radiator repair
  - Construction work
  - Bridge repair work
  - Painting contracting
  - Mining
  - Ceramics work
  - Stained-glass making
  - Jewelry making

LEAD POISONING

Poisoning from lead has been a problem throughout history and throughout the world. In the United States the problem became apparent in the early 1900s when white lead was added to paints and when tetraethyl lead was added to gasoline as an antiknock compound. Lead content in paint was decreased in 1950, and in 1978 the use of lead in household paint was banned. The use of lead in paint and leaded gasoline has been banned in the United States. After this change in policy, the average blood lead level (BLL) in the United States for people ages 1 to 74 years dropped from 12.8 mcg/dl in 1980 to 1.9 mcg/dl in 1999 (American Academy of Pediatrics, 2005). However, children continue to be exposed to lead; an estimated 1.6% of U.S. children had BLLs of more than 10 mcg/dl in 2002, and almost 14% had BLLs of 5 to 9 mcg/dl (Levin, Brown, Kashtock, et al, 2008).

Causes of Lead Poisoning

Although there are numerous sources of lead (Box 16-7), in most instances of acute childhood lead poisoning, the source is nonintact lead-based paint in an older home or lead-contaminated bare soil in the yard. Microparticles of lead gain entrance into a child's body through ingestion or inhalation and, in the case of an exposed pregnant woman, by placental transfer. When measured, a mother's lead level is nearly the same as that of her unborn child. However, though the level of lead may not be harmful to an adult woman, it can be harmful to the fetus.

Inhalation exposure usually occurs during renovation and remodeling activities in the home, whereas ingestion happens during normal day-to-day play and mouthing activities. Sometimes a child will actually swallow loose chips of lead-based paint because it has a sweet taste. Water and food may also be contaminated with lead. A child does not need to eat loose paint chips to be exposed to the toxin; normal hand-to-mouth behavior, coupled with the presence of lead dust in the environment that has settled over the decades, is the usual method of poisoning (Frazer, 2008; American Academy of Pediatrics, 2005; Erickson and Thompson, 2005).

Because of family, cultural, or ethnic traditions, a source of lead may be a routine part of life for a child. Nurses must educate themselves about the practices of their patients and identify when such products may be a source of lead. The use of pottery or dishes containing lead may be an issue, as may the use of folk remedies for stomachaches or the use of some cosmetics (see Cultural Competence box). Children of immigrants and internationally adopted children may have been exposed to sources of lead before arrival in the United States and should also be carefully evaluated for lead exposure (Woolf, Goldman, and Bellinger, 2007). Other risk factors for having an elevated BLL include living in poverty, being less than 6 years of age, dwelling in urban areas, and living in older rental homes where lead decontamination may not be a priority. Nurses are often in a position to observe or elicit information about these practices and educate families about their potential harm.

 CULTURAL COMPETENCE

Sources of Lead

In some cultures the use of traditional ethnic remedies that contain lead may increase children's risk of lead poisoning. These remedies include:

Azarcon (Mexico)—For digestive problems; a bright orange powder; usual dose is 0.25 to 1 tsp, often mixed with oil, milk, or sugar or sometimes given as a tea; sometimes a pinch is added to a baby bottle or tortilla dough for preventive purposes

Greta (Mexico)—A yellow-orange powder, used in the same way as azarcon

Paylooah (Southeast Asia)—Used for rash or fever; an orange-red powder given as 0.5 tsp straight or in a tea

Surma (India)—Black powder applied to the inner lower eyelid that is used as a cosmetic to improve eyesight

Unknown ayurvedic (Tibet)—Small, gray-brown balls used to improve slow development; two balls given orally three times a day

Tamarindo jellied, fruit candy (Mexico)—Fruit candy packaged in paper wrappers that contain high lead levels

Lozeena (Iraq)—A bright orange powder used to color meat and rice

Modified from Centers for Disease Control and Prevention: Lead poisoning associated with use of traditional ethnic remedies—California, 1991-1992, *MMWR* 42(27):521-524, 1993; Centers for Disease Control and Prevention: Lead poisoning associated with imported candy and powdered food coloring—California and Michigan, *MMWR* 47(48):1041-1043, 1998; Centers for Disease Control and Prevention: Childhood lead poisoning associated with tamarind candy and folk remedies—California, 1992-2000, *MMWR* 51(31):684-686, 2002.

Pathophysiology and Clinical Manifestations

Lead can affect any part of the body, including the renal, hematologic, and neurologic systems (Fig. 16-9). Of most concern for young children is the developing brain and nervous system, which are more vulnerable than those of an older child or adult. Lead in the body moves via an equilibration process between the blood, the soft tissues and organs, and the bones and teeth. Lead ultimately settles in the bones and teeth, where it remains inert and in storage. This makes up the largest portion of the body burden, approximately 75% to 90%. At the cellular level it competes with molecules of calcium, interfering with the regulating action of calcium. In the brain, lead disrupts the biochemical processes and may have a direct effect on the release of neurotransmitters, may cause alterations in the

blood-brain barrier, and may interfere with the regulation of synaptic activity (Lidsky and Schneider, 2006).

There is a relationship between anemia and lead poisoning. Children who are iron deficient absorb lead more readily than those with sufficient iron stores. Lead can interfere with the binding of iron onto the heme molecule. This sometimes creates a picture of anemia, even though the child is not iron deficient. Lead toxicity to the erythrocytes leads to the release of the enzyme erythrocyte protoporphyrin (EP). Because EP is not sensitive to BLLs of less than about 16 to 25 mcg/dl, it is no longer used as a screening test. Therefore the BLL test is currently used for screening and diagnosis. However, elevation of the EP level (>35 mcg/dl of whole blood) is a good indicator of toxicity from lead and reflects the length of exposure and body burden of lead in the individual child.

Although adults have been shown to suffer adverse renal effects from occupational lead exposure, few studies document renal effects in children except at extremely high lead levels. One can hypothesize that lead can affect the renal integrity of children as well as adults. Therefore the renal system of a child is still considered a potential target for the harmful effects of lead.

The lead levels identified in children have declined since the initiation of screening for children at risk for lead poisoning. With earlier intervention, the most prevalent effects have changed. Since the late 1960s, children have rarely died of lead poisoning, and seizures or cognitive impairment have become less likely. However, even mild and moderate lead poisoning can cause a number of cognitive and behavioral problems in young children, including aggression, hyperactivity, impulsivity, delinquency, disinterest, and withdrawal. Long-term neurocognitive signs of lead poisoning include developmental delays, lowered intelligence quotient (IQ), reading skill deficits, visual-spatial problems, visual-motor problems, learning disabilities, and lower academic success. Chronic lead toxicity may also affect physical growth and reproductive efficiency (Woolf, Goldman, and Bellinger, 2007).

! **NURSING ALERT**

Acute signs of lead poisoning include nausea, vomiting, constipation, anorexia, and abdominal pain. Additional clinical manifestations are hypophosphatemia, glycosuria, and aminoaciduria (Erickson and Thompson, 2005).

Diagnostic Evaluation

Children with lead poisoning rarely have symptoms, even at levels requiring chelation therapy. A diagnosis of lead poisoning is based only on the lead testing of a venous blood specimen from a venipuncture. The collection process is important. Blood must be collected carefully to avoid contamination by lead on the skin. The level of concern for an elevated BLL has dropped from 80 mcg/dl in 1950 to 10 mcg/dl today (Heavey, 2008).

Anticipatory Guidance

Anticipatory guidance lends support to primary prevention efforts. The Centers for Disease Control and Prevention (2005)

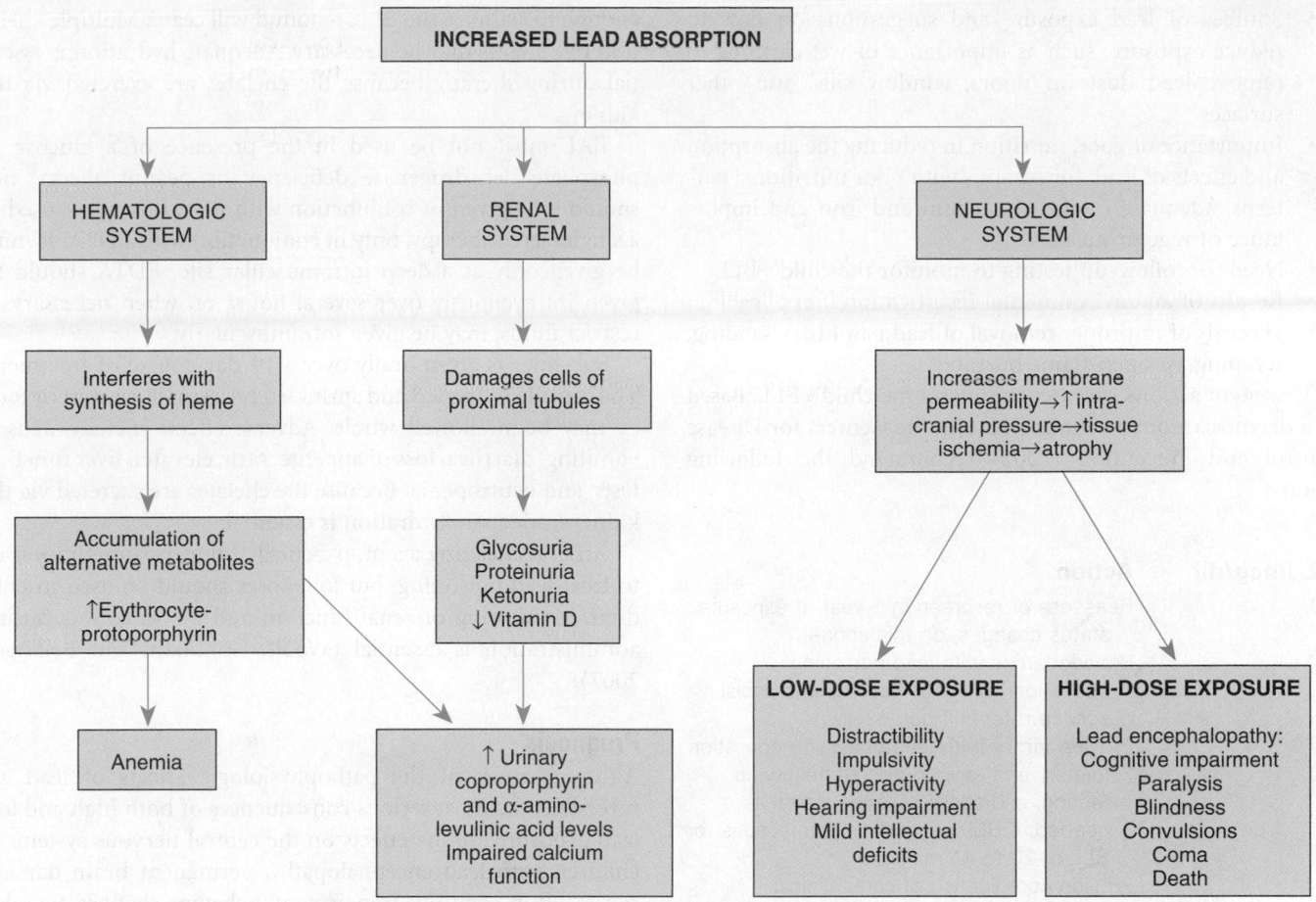

Fig. 16-9 Main effects of lead on body systems.

recommend that the following information be made available to families beginning during prenatal care, at 3 to 6 months, and at 1 year of age:

- Hazards of lead-based paint in older housing
- Ways to control lead hazards safely
- How to choose safe toys
- Hazards accompanying repainting and renovation of homes built before 1978
- Other exposure sources, such as traditional remedies, that might be relevant for a family

There has been recent concern regarding toys and other imported items children play with which were found to contain lead. Parents should carefully evaluate the source of the toy (manufacturer) or item the child may play with and not assume it is safe because it is sold in a U.S. market. The U.S. Consumer Product Safety Commission (www.cpsc.gov) is an excellent resource for parents and caregivers concerned about the safety of a given toy or product that may be harmful.

Screening for Lead Poisoning

When primary prevention fails, secondary prevention screening efforts for elevated BLLs can identify children much earlier than in the past. Guidelines recommend universal or targeted screening (Levin, Brown, Kashtock, et al, 2008). This need is established using blood lead surveillance and other risk factor data collected over time to establish the status and risk of children throughout the state. In areas without available data, universal screening is recommended.

Universal screening should be done at ages 1 and 2 years. Any child between the ages of 3 and 6 years who has not been previously screened should also be tested. Screen any child with risk factors more often.

Targeted screening is acceptable when an area has been determined by existing data to have less risk. Children should be screened when they live in a high-risk geographic area or are members of a group determined to be at risk (e.g., Medicaid recipients), or if their family cannot answer "no" to the following personal risk questions:

- Does your child live in or regularly visit a house that was built before 1950?
- Does your child live in or regularly visit a house built before 1978 with recent or ongoing renovations or remodeling within the past 6 months?
- Does your child have a sibling or playmate who has or did have lead poisoning?

Therapeutic Management

The degree of concern, urgency, and need for medical intervention changes as the lead level increases. Education is one of the most important elements of the treatment process. Several areas that the nurse needs to discuss with the family of every child who has an elevated BLL (≥10 mcg/dl) include (Heavey, 2008; Levin, Brown, Kashtock, et al, 2008):

- The child's BLL and what it means
- Potential adverse health effects of an elevated BLL

- Sources of lead exposure and suggestions on how to reduce exposure, such as importance of wet cleaning to remove lead dust on floors, window sills, and other surfaces
- Importance of good nutrition in reducing the absorption and effects of lead; for persons with poor nutritional patterns, adequate intake of calcium and iron and importance of regular meals
- Need for follow-up testing to monitor the child's BLL
- Results of an environmental investigation if applicable
- Hazards of improper removal of lead paint (dry sanding, scraping, or open-flame burning)

Treatment actions vary depending on the child's BLL. Based on a diagnosis from a venous BLL test, the Centers for Disease Control and Prevention (2002) recommend the following actions:

BLL (mcg/dl)	Action
<10	Reassess or rescreen in 1 year. If exposure status changes, do this sooner.
10-14	Provide family with lead poisoning education, follow-up testing, and social service referral if necessary.
15-19	Provide family with lead poisoning education (dietary and environmental), follow-up testing, and social service referral as needed; if BLL persists, initiate actions for BLL of 20 to 44 mcg/dl.
20-44	Provide coordination of care, clinical management, environmental investigation, and lead hazard control.
45-69	Within 48 hours, provide coordination of care and clinical management, including treatment, environmental investigation, and lead hazard control. The child must not remain in a lead-hazardous environment if resolution is to occur.
≥70	*Immediately* provide medical treatment and begin coordination of care, clinical management, environmental investigation, and lead hazard control.

Chelation Therapy

Chelation is the term used for removing lead from circulating blood and, theoretically, some lead from organs and tissues. It is unclear whether chelation affects lead stores in bones. Although not an antidote in the truest sense, it does serve a similar purpose in that the toxic substance or poison is removed from the body. However, chelation does not counteract any effects of the lead.

Historically two chelating agents have been used consistently: calcium disodium edetate ($CaNa_2EDTA$, or calcium EDTA) and succimer (Chemet, *meso*-2,3-dimercaptosuccinic acid [DMSA]). British antilewisite (BAL, dimercaprol, dimercaptopropanol) is used in conjunction with EDTA. All the agents have potential toxic side effects and contraindications. Monitor renal, hepatic, and hematologic parameters.

Because of the equilibration process between blood, soft tissues, and other sites in the body, there is often a rebound of the BLL after chelation. After the body burden of lead is reduced

enough to stabilize the BLL, rebound will cease. Multiple chelation treatments may be necessary. Adequate hydration is essential during therapy because the chelates are excreted via the kidneys.

BAL must not be used in the presence of a glucose 6-phosphate dehydrogenase deficiency or peanut allergy, nor should it be given in conjunction with iron. It is never used as a single-agent therapy, only in conjunction with EDTA. It must be given only at a deep intramuscular site. EDTA should be given intravenously over several hours or, when necessary to restrict fluids, may be given intramuscularly.

Succimer is given orally over a 19-day course of treatment. The capsule is opened and sprinkled on a small amount of food or may be swallowed whole. Adverse effects include nausea, vomiting, diarrhea, loss of appetite, rash, elevated liver function tests, and neutropenia. Because the chelates are excreted via the kidneys, adequate hydration is essential.

An oral chelating agent, D-penicillamine, is sometimes used to treat lead poisoning, but low doses should be used in children. Monitoring of renal function and blood counts during administration is essential (Woolf, Goldman, and Bellinger, 2007).

Prognosis

Although most of the pathophysiologic effects of lead are reversible, the most serious consequences of both high and low lead exposure are the effects on the central nervous system. In children with lead encephalopathy, permanent brain damage can result in cognitive impairment, behavior changes, possible paralysis, and seizures. However, moderate- to low-dose exposure may also cause permanent neurologic deficits. Increased distractibility, short attention span, impulsivity, reading disabilities, and school failure have been associated with lead exposure. There is some evidence that treatment of moderate levels of lead poisoning can result in cognitive improvement (American Academy of Pediatrics, 2005).

Nursing Care Management

The primary nursing goal in lead poisoning is to prevent the child's initial or further exposure to lead. For children with low-level exposure, this requires identifying the sources of lead in the environment. Careful history taking is the most useful and most valuable tool and should concentrate on the personal risk questions (see p. 629). Suggestions for reducing lead in the child's environment are listed in the Community Focus box.

For children who undergo chelation therapy, the nurse prepares them for the injections and makes all efforts to reduce injection pain. Chelating agents are administered deeply into a large muscle mass (see Atraumatic Care box). To lessen the pain from EDTA, the local anesthetic procaine is injected with the drug. Rotation of sites is essential to prevent the formation of painful areas of fibrotic tissue. Because EDTA and lead are toxic to the kidneys, keep records of intake and output, and assess the results of urinalysis to monitor renal functioning.

Discharge planning for children with lead poisoning must include thorough education of families regarding safety from lead hazards, clear instructions regarding medication administration and follow-up, and confirmation that the child will be discharged to a home without lead hazards. Although the nurse

🏠 COMMUNITY FOCUS

Reducing Blood Lead Levels

- Make certain child does not have access to peeling paint or chewable surfaces painted with lead-based paint, especially window sills and wells.
- If a house was built before 1960 (possibly before 1980) and has hard-surface floors, wet mop them at least once per week. Wipe other hard surfaces (e.g., window sills, baseboards). If there are loose paint chips in an area, such as a window well, use a wet disposable cloth to pick up and discard them. Do not vacuum hard-surfaced floors or window sills or wells, since this spreads dust. Use vacuum cleaners with agitators to remove dust from rugs rather than vacuum cleaners with suction only. If a rug is known to contain lead dust and cannot be washed, it should be discarded.
- Wash and dry child's hands and face frequently, especially before eating.
- Wash toys and pacifiers frequently.
- If soil around home is or is likely to be contaminated with lead (e.g., if home was built before 1960 or is near a major highway), plant grass or other ground cover; plant bushes around outside of house so that child cannot play there.
- During remodeling of older homes, follow correct procedures. Be certain children and pregnant women are not in the home, day or night, until process is completed. After deleading, thoroughly clean house, using cleaning solution to damp mop and dust before inhabitants return.
- In areas where lead content of water exceeds the drinking water standard and a particular faucet has not been used for 6 hours or more, "flush" the cold-water pipes by running the water until it becomes as cold as it will get (30 seconds to >2 minutes). The more time water has been sitting in pipes, the more lead it may contain.
- *Use only cold water* for consumption (drinking, cooking, and especially for reconstituting powder infant formula). Hot water dissolves lead more quickly than cold water and thus contains higher levels of lead. It is all right to use first-flush water for nonconsumption uses.
- Have water tested by a competent laboratory. This action is especially important for apartment dwellers; flushing may not be effective in high-rise buildings or in other buildings with lead-soldered central piping.
- Do not store food in open cans, particularly if cans are imported.
- Do not use pottery or ceramic ware that was inadequately fired or is meant for decorative use for food storage or service. Do not store drinks or food in lead crystal.
- Avoid folk remedies or cosmetics that contain lead.
- Make certain that home exposure is not occurring from parental occupations or hobbies. Household members employed in occupations such as lead smelting should shower and change into clean clothing before leaving work. Construction and lead abatement workers may also bring home lead contaminants.
- Ensure child eats regular meals, since more lead is absorbed on an empty stomach.
- Ensure child's diet contains sufficient iron and calcium and not excessive fat.

Modified from Centers for Disease Control and Prevention: *Preventing lead poisoning in young children*, Atlanta, 2005, The Centers.

ATRAUMATIC CARE

Lead Chelation Therapy

To lessen the pain from intramuscular injection of calcium disodium edetate (CaNa$_2$EDTA, or calcium EDTA), the local anesthetic procaine is injected with the drug. Apply topical anesthetic cream such as eutectic mixture of local anesthetic (e.g., lidocaine-prilocaine [EMLA]) or LMX4 (4% lidocaine) over the puncture site before the injection of EDTA and British antilewisite (BAL) (time per manufacturer's guidelines). Administer intravenous EDTA whenever possible.

❗ NURSING ALERT

Use extreme caution with chelating agents. Incidences of child death from hypocalcemia have been recorded when Na$_2$EDTA was substituted for CaNa$_2$EDTA and used as a chelating agent (Centers for Diseases Control and Prevention, 2006).

❗ NURSING ALERT

Calcium EDTA is always administered when there is adequate urinary output. Children receiving the drug intramuscularly must be able to maintain adequate oral intake of fluids.

must use caution to avoid alarming parents unnecessarily, it is important that they know the risk implications for their child's behavior and cognitive functions. Nurses should observe the development and behavior of children who are hospitalized. Thoroughly evaluate any concerns that are identified. Referral to a child development or speech and language specialist may be necessary.

As in any situational crisis, parents need support and understanding if their child is treated for lead poisoning. Many families at the highest risk for lead poisoning have the fewest resources to comply with measures such as relocation or removal of lead from the environment where the child experiences exposure.

CHILD MALTREATMENT

The broad term **child maltreatment** includes intentional physical abuse or neglect, emotional abuse or neglect, and sexual abuse of children, usually by adults. It is one of the most significant social problems affecting children. In 2007 Child Protective Service (CPS) agencies in the United States confirmed that an estimated 794,000 children were victims of child maltreatment. Of the confirmed cases, about 11% suffered physical abuse, 8% sexual abuse, 60% neglect, and 4% psychologic maltreatment or emotional abuse. In 2007 there were an estimated 1760 child fatalities as a result of child abuse and neglect (US Department of Health and Human Services, 2009). Reported statistics only partially represent the actual incidence of child maltreatment, since many cases are believed to go unreported.*

CHILD NEGLECT

Child neglect is the most common form of maltreatment. More than half of all reported cases are associated with deprivation of necessities, and 34% of deaths from maltreatment are in this group (US Department of Health and Human Services, 2009). Neglect is generally defined as the failure of a parent or other person legally responsible for the child's welfare to provide for the child's basic needs and an adequate level of care.

---

*Additional information is available from the Children's Bureau, Administration for Children and Families, 370 L'Enfant Promenade SW, Washington, DC 20447; 800-422-4453; **www.acf.hhs.gov/ programs/cb**.

Nursing Care Plan—The Child Who Is Maltreated

Important contributing factors for child neglect are lack of knowledge of child's needs, lack of resources, and caregiver substance abuse. For example, neglectful parents often demonstrate poor parenting skills. They may be unaware that an infant needs to be fed every 3 to 4 hours, may not know what to feed the child, and may have insufficient funds to buy food. The most serious lack of knowledge is failure to recognize emotional nurturing as an essential need of children. (See also Growth Failure [Failure to Thrive], Chapter 13.)

Types of Neglect

Neglect takes many forms and can be classified broadly as physical or emotional maltreatment. **Physical neglect** involves the deprivation of necessities, such as food, clothing, shelter, supervision, medical care, and education. **Emotional neglect** generally refers to failure to meet the child's needs for affection, attention, and emotional nurturance.

Neglect may also include lack of intervention for or fostering of maladaptive behavior, such as delinquency or substance abuse. **Emotional abuse** or **psychologic maltreatment**, an even more difficult aspect of maltreatment to define, refers to the deliberate attempt to destroy or significantly impair a child's self-esteem or competence. Emotional abuse may take the form of rejecting, isolating, terrorizing, ignoring, corrupting, verbally assaulting, or overpressuring the child (Nelms, 2001).

PHYSICAL ABUSE

The deliberate infliction of physical injury on a child, usually by the child's caregiver, is termed *physical abuse*. Legal definitions of physical abuse are found in state and federal statutes. The Child Abuse Prevention and Treatment Act of 1996 defines abuse as "any recent act or failure to act that results in imminent risk of serious harm, death, serious physical or emotional harm of a child (<18 years) by a parent or caregiver who is responsible for the child's welfare." Each state defines abuse according to its reporting laws. Minor physical injury is responsible for more reported cases of maltreatment than major physical injury, but major physical abuse causes more deaths. Despite the importance of the problem, a universally accepted definition of what constitutes minor and major physical abuse does not exist. Rather, each state in the United States defines abuse according to its individual reporting laws.

Shaken Baby Syndrome

Shaken baby syndrome (SBS) is a serious form of child abuse caused by violent shaking of infants and young children and is one form of abusive head trauma. Physicians commonly use more general terms, including *abusive head trauma, inflicted head injury,* or *neuroinflicted brain injury;* these terms do not assume the mechanism of injury, but rather describe the injury itself (Chiesa and Duhaime, 2009). This violent shaking would be easily recognized by others as dangerous (American Academy of Pediatrics, 2001) and is most often a result of the caregiver's frustration with crying (Castiglia, 2001). Every year in America an estimated 1200 to 1400 children are shaken, and of these victims 25% to 30% die as a result of their injuries. The rest have life-long complications (National Center on Shaken Baby Syndrome, n.d.).

It is important to understand what happens in SBS. Infants have a large head-to-body ratio, weak neck muscles, and a large amount of water in the brain. Violent shaking causes the brain to rotate within the skull, resulting in shearing forces that tear blood vessels and neurons. The characteristic injuries that occur are intracranial bleeding (subdural and subarachnoid hematomas) and, in approximately 85% of cases, retinal hemorrhages, which are classic results of repetitive acceleration-deceleration head trauma (Levin, 2009). Injuries may also include fractures of the ribs and long bones. Most often there are no signs of external injury. SBS is often not an isolated event, and in one study 45% of the children with inflicted traumatic brain injury caused by shaking showed some evidence of prior injury (Ewing-Cobb, Kramer, Prasad, et al, 1998). Victims of SBS can be seen with a variety of symptoms, from generalized flulike symptoms to unresponsiveness with impending death (Miehl, 2005). Many of the presenting symptoms, such as vomiting, irritability, poor feeding, and listlessness, are often mistaken for common infant and childhood ailments. In more severe forms presenting symptoms may include seizures, posturing, alterations in level of consciousness, apnea, bradycardia, or death. The long-term outcomes of SBS include seizure disorders; visual impairments, including blindness; developmental delays; hearing loss; cerebral palsy; and mild to profound mental, cognitive, or motor impairments (Walls, 2006). Nurses can take an active role in prevention of SBS by teaching all caregivers about crying and techniques to cope with inconsolable crying (Carbaugh, 2004).

> **! NURSING ALERT**
>
> Stress to parents the danger of shaking infants (shaking can cause SBS). Education must include coping mechanisms on caring for children with inconsolable crying.

Munchausen Syndrome by Proxy

Munchausen syndrome by proxy (MSBP), also known as medical child abuse or factitious disorder by proxy, is a rare but serious form of child abuse in which caregivers deliberately exaggerate or fabricate histories and symptoms or induce symptoms. It is a form of child maltreatment that may include physical, emotional, and psychologic abuse for the gratification of the caregiver. In most cases the perpetrator is the biologic mother, with some degree of health care knowledge and training. Health care providers can become easily misled and unknowingly enable the perpetrator (Leider, Irving, Mauricio, et al, 2005). Because of the history of symptoms provided by the caregiver, the child endures painful and unnecessary medical testing and procedures. Common symptoms presented are seizures, nausea and vomiting, diarrhea, and altered mental status; they are usually witnessed only by the perpetrator.

Considerations when determining whether a child is a victims of MSBP include:

- Is the child's condition consistent with the reported history?
- Does diagnostic evidence support the reported history?
- Has anyone other than the caregiver witnessed the symptoms?

- Is treatment being provided primarily because of the caregiver's demands?

The resolution of symptoms after separation from the perpetrator confirms the diagnosis.

Factors Predisposing to Physical Abuse

The causes of child abuse are multifaceted. Child maltreatment occurs across all socioeconomic, religious, cultural, racial, and ethnic groups (Goldman, Salus, Wolcott, et al, 2003). Three risk factors are commonly identified in child abuse: parental characteristics, characteristics of the child, and environmental characteristics. However, no single factor or group of factors is predictive of abuse. Rather, the interaction of these factors is thought to increase the risk of abuse occurring in a particular family.

Parental Characteristics

Some identified characteristics occur more frequently in parents who abuse their children and are therefore considered risk factors. Younger parents more often are abusers of their children. Single-parent families are at higher risk for abuse, and in single-parent families that include an unrelated partner, the partner is sometimes the abuser, although a biologic parent is most commonly the perpetrator (US Department of Health and Human Services, 2009).

Abusive families are often socially isolated and have few supportive relationships. They often have additional stressors such as low-income circumstances, with little education. Parents with substance abuse problems pose a greater risk for abuse and neglect due to a variety of factors. The additional stressors of substance abuse with the demands of normal care of children create situations where abuse and neglect can occur, since these parents have impaired judgment and may react with violence while under the influence of drugs or alcohol (Wells, 2009). With little or no available support system and concurrent stressors imposed by the child or environment, these parents are vulnerable to additional crises of any nature and may strike out at the child as a method of releasing their frustration and anxiety.

Other factors identified in abusive parents include low self-esteem and little knowledge of appropriate parenting skills. Parenting skills are learned behaviors, and parents who grew up with poor parental role models may have difficulty parenting their own children. Approximately one third of parents who were maltreated as children will subject their children to similar maltreatment (Gara, Allen, Herzog, and other, 2000).

Characteristics of the Child

The onus for child abuse is always on the abuser. However, children who are abused do have some common characteristics. Children from birth to 1 year of age are at highest risk for being abused (US Department of Health and Human Services, 2009). Infants and small children require constant attention and must have all their needs met by others. This can result in parental or caregiver fatigue that results in striking out at the child with physical force, shaking the child, or ignoring the child's needs.

The physical and emotional demands placed on the parents or caregiver of an unwanted, brain-damaged, hyperactive, or physically disabled child may overwhelm them, resulting in

abuse. Disabled children may not understand that abusive behaviors are not appropriate, so do not tell others or defend themselves. Premature infants may be at risk for maltreatment due to failure of parent-child bonding during early infancy, increased physical needs, or irritability. One child may be singled out in an abusive family. Removing that child from the home often places the other siblings at risk for abuse. Therefore no child is safe if left in the abusive environment unless the parents can be helped to learn new parenting skills, to meet the children's needs, and to release their frustration through alternatives other than attacking their children.

Environmental Characteristics

The environment is a significant part of the potentially abusive situation. A typical environment is one of chronic stress, including problems of divorce, poverty, unemployment, poor housing, frequent relocation, alcoholism, and drug addiction. Increased exposure between children and parents, such as that which occurs in crowded living conditions, also increases the likelihood of abuse.

Although most reporting of abuse has been from lower socioeconomic populations, as stated before, child abuse is not a problem of any one societal group. Stresses imposed by poverty predispose lower socioeconomic families to abusive situations, and abuse in these groups is more likely to be reported. However, concealed crises may also be present in upper-class families. Families who have substitute caregivers such as daycare providers and baby-sitters may also be at risk for child abuse, especially if the family has not fully evaluated the caregiver. Nurses need to be aware of all these factors to identify the less obvious examples of child abuse and neglect.

SEXUAL ABUSE

Sexual abuse is one of the most devastating types of child maltreatment, and estimates indicate that it has increased significantly during the past decade (US Department of Health and Human Services, 2009). Some of the apparent increase is due to increased awareness (Putnam, 2003).

As with all forms of child maltreatment, no universal definition for sexual abuse exists. Definitions of sexual abuse cover a range of acts including involvement of children in sexual acts they do not understand, to which they cannot give consent, or that violate social taboos (Finkel and DeJong, 2001). The Child Abuse and Prevention Act defines **sexual abuse** as "the use, persuasion, or coercion of any child to engage in sexually explicit conduct (or any simulation of such conduct) or producing any visual depiction of such conduct, or rape, molestation, prostitution, or incest with children."

Sexual abuse includes the following types of sexual maltreatment (see also Rape, Chapter 20):

Incest—Any physical sexual activity between family members; blood relationship is not required (abusers can include stepparents, unrelated siblings, grandparents, uncles, and aunts); does not include sexual relations between legally sanctioned partners, such as spouses

Molestation—A vague term that includes "indecent liberties," such as touching, fondling, kissing, single or mutual masturbation, or oral-genital contact

Exhibitionism—Indecent exposure, usually exposure of the genitalia by an adult man to children or women

Child pornography—Arranging and photographing, in any media, sexual acts involving children, alone or with adults or animals, regardless of consent by the child's legal guardian; also may denote distribution of such material in any form with or without profit

Child prostitution—Involving children in sex acts for profit and usually with changing partners

Pedophilia—Literally means "love of child" and does not denote a type of sexual activity but the preference of an adult for prepubertal children as the means of achieving sexual excitement

Characteristics of Abusers and Victims

Anyone, including siblings and mothers, can be sexual abusers, but a typical abuser is a male whom the victim knows. Offenders come from all levels of society. Adults comprise 80% of sexual abuse offenders, with the remaining 20% being made of adolescents and preadolescents (Johnson, 2004). Many offenders hold full-time jobs, are active in community affairs, and may not have prior criminal records (Finkel and DeJong, 2001). Offenders often are employed (or volunteers) in positions such as teaching or coaching that will bring them into contact with young girls and boys. Child sexual abuse may be generational unless discovered and stopped (Johnson, 2004). Offenders may commit many assaults before being caught.

Incestuous relationships between father or stepfather and daughter are generally prolonged, and the victims are usually reluctant to report the situation because of fear of retaliation and fear that they will not be believed. Typically, incestuous relationships begin later than other forms of child abuse. The eldest daughter is usually abused, but in her absence another sister may be substituted. Sibling incest may also occur. Sexual abuse by relatives with a strong emotional bond with the victim, like a parent, is often the most devastating to the child.

Boys are also victims of both intrafamilial and extrafamilial abuse. Compared with female victims, male victims are much less likely to report abuse, and they may suffer much greater emotional harm from incestuous relationships. Boys are likely to be subjected to anal penetration and oral-genital contact. They often have subtle physical findings and are abused by a father, stepfather, or mother's boyfriend.

Significant risk factors for child sexual abuse include parental unavailability, lack of emotional closeness and flexibility, social isolation, emotional deprivation, and communication difficulties. Most sexual abuse is committed by men and by persons known to the child, with family members constituting up to two thirds of the perpetrators (Christian, Lavelle, DeJong, et al, 2000). Around 20% to 25% of child sexual abuse cases involve penetration or oral-genital contact. In 2007, over 35% of sexual abuse victim were between 12 to 15 years of age (US Department of Health and Human Services, 2009).

Initiation and Perpetuation of Sexual Abuse

The cycle of sexual abuse often starts insidiously unless it involves an isolated attack, such as rape. Often offenders spend time with the victims to gain their trust before initiating any sexual contact. Most victims are then pressured into being an accessory to the sexual activity through various means and may be unaware that sexual activity is part of the offer. Children may not reveal the truth for fear that their parents would not believe them if they told, especially if the offender is a trusted member of the family. Some fear that they will be blamed for the situation, and many young children with limited vocabulary have difficulty describing the activity when they do have the courage or opportunity to reveal the abuse.

Methods used to pressure children into sexual activity include:

- The child is offered gifts or privileges, or has privileges withheld.
- The adult misrepresents moral standards by telling the child that it is "okay to do."
- Isolated or emotionally and socially impoverished children are enticed by adults who meet their needs for warmth or human contact.
- The successful sex offender pressures the victim into secrecy by describing it as a "secret between us" that other people would take away if they found out.
- The offender plays on the child's fears, including the fear of punishment by the offender, fear of repercussions if the child tells, and fear of abandonment or rejection by the family.

Incest most frequently occurs between fathers and daughters, but may be between grandfather and granddaughter, or brother and sister. Brother-sister incest has been found to be just as damaging as father-daughter abuse (Cyr, Wright, McDuff, et al, 2002). Victims may take years to disclose this abuse. However, not all incestuous relationships follow this pattern of silence. Reports of father-daughter incest during child custody conflicts have become more common and have raised serious concerns regarding the possibility of false accusation. Rather than tolerating or denying the child's sexual abuse, the other parent (usually the mother) is typically the chief accuser.

NURSING CARE OF THE MALTREATED CHILD

A critical responsibility of health professionals is identifying abusive situations as early as possible. Nurses who increase their knowledge of the different types of abuse and neglect and underlying causes will enhance their ability to identify, intervene, and prevent children from maltreatment and neglect (Giardino and Giardino, 2003). The characteristics that may predispose members of some families to commit abuse can serve as a framework for assessing vulnerability, but are never predictive of actual abuse. A careful, detailed history and interview combined with a thorough physical examination are the diagnostic tools needed to identify abuse. Nurses have a special role because they may be the first person to see the child and parent and are the consistent caregivers if the child is hospitalized (see Nursing Care Guidelines box).

In interviewing the child and family, the nurse must be careful to avoid biasing the child's retelling of the events. Some experts suggest that health professionals limit the interview to

📋 **NURSING CARE GUIDELINES**

Talking with Children Who Reveal Abuse

- Provide a private time and place to talk.
- Do not promise not to tell; tell them that you are required by law to report the abuse.
- Do not express shock or criticize their family.
- Use their vocabulary to discuss body parts.
- Avoid using any leading statements that can distort their report.
- Reassure them that they have done the right thing by telling.
- Tell them that the abuse is not their fault, that they are not bad or to blame.
- Determine their immediate need for safety.
- Let the child know what will happen when you report.

BOX 16-8   WARNING SIGNS OF ABUSE

- Child has physical evidence of abuse or neglect, including previous injuries.
- History is incompatible with the pattern and/or degree of injury, such as bilateral skull fractures after being dropped.
- Explanation of how injury occurred is vague, or parent or guardian is reluctant to provide information.
- Patient is brought in with minor, unrelated complaint and significant trauma is found.
- Histories are contradictory among caregivers.
- Mechanism of injury provided is not possible given age or developmental level of patient, such as 6-month old turning on hot water.
- Bruising or other injury is present in a nonmobile patient.
- Patient's affect is inappropriate in relation to extent of injury.
- Evidence of abusive or neglectful parent-child interaction is present.
- Parent, guardian, or custodian disappears after bringing patient in for trauma or patient with suspicious injury is brought in by an unrelated adult.
- Patient has multiple fractures of differing ages.
- There was a delay in seeking care.
- Parent or caregiver discloses that abuse has or may have occurred.
- Patient makes an outcry of abuse or neglect.

---

the child's physical and mental health concerns and leave topics of the family's social, legal, or other problems to the police or the CPS (McClain, Giardet, Lahoti, et al, 2000). If this is not possible, make an effort to coordinate the interview process so that all pertinent health care professionals can be present for the interview.

Recognition of abuse or neglect necessitates a familiarity with both physical and behavioral signs that suggest maltreatment (Box 16-8). No one indicator can be used to diagnose maltreatment. It is a pattern or combination of indicators that should arouse suspicion and lead to further investigation. It is important to note that some situations, such as bleeding disorders, osteogenesis imperfecta, or sudden infant death syndrome, may be misinterpreted as abuse. Also, some cultural practices, such as cupping or coin rubbing (see Health Practices, Chapter 2), may mimic physical abuse. Unintentional injuries, such as burns from metal buckles on car seats, bruising from seat belts, or spiral fractures from a twist and fall injury, may also be wrongly diagnosed as abuse. Normal variants, such as mongolian spots and congenital anomalies of genitalia, can be mistaken for abuse.

Caregiver-Child Interaction

The nurse can use the initial contact with the family to assess the interaction between the caregiver and the child. Observations of the caregivers should include emotional support for the child, attentiveness to the child's needs, and concern for the child's injury. Although caregivers and children may vary in responses to a stressful event, note an unusual caregiver-child relationship and factor this into the overall evaluation of the child.

Certain behavioral responses of the parents to their child and to the interviewer should alert the nurse to the possibility of maltreatment. Abusive parents may have difficulty showing concern toward their child. They may be unable or unwilling to comfort the child. Abusers may blame the child for the injuries or belittle him or her for being clumsy or stupid. When interacting with the health care workers, the parent may become hostile or uncooperative. During the child's hospitalization they may not participate in the child's care and may show little concern for his or her progress, eventual discharge, or need for follow-up care.

Abused children's responses to their parents or the injury may also support the suspicion of abuse. Although no one pattern is typical, extremes of behavior may be observed. Children may be unresponsive to the parent or excessively clinging and intolerant of separation. They may be overly attached to the abusive parent, possibly in the hope of preventing any upset that may precipitate anger and another attack. During care of the injury, children may be passive and accepting of the discomfort or uncooperative and fearful of any physical contact. They may avoid eye contact. Some children maintain a wary watchfulness of all strangers; some shy away from strangers as if frightened; others are unusually affectionate and outgoing.

History and Interview
Child Physical Abuse

It is often difficult to distinguish child maltreatment from accidental injuries. Caregivers whose history of events may be deceptive or incomplete and children who are nonverbal may make the assessment more complex. A purposeful, skilled history and appropriate interview questions will help the nurse ensure the right course of action. Knowledge of mechanism of injury and child development is essential. Cases of abuse are often detected when the child or caregiver history of events do not match with physical findings. Children who are verbal can often give a history of the injury. Separating the child from the caregiver may provide a more reliable history. It is important to ask nonleading, open-ended questions. The history should include a narrative of the injury from both caregiver and child (if verbal). Date, time, and location where injury took place along with who was present at the time of the injury are essential questions. Family history for bleeding or bone disorders is important. Box 16-8 outlines areas of history that are concerning for abuse.

Neglect and Emotional Abuse

Each child may manifest different responses to neglect, depending on the situation and developmental age of the child. The

BOX 16-9   CLINICAL MANIFESTATIONS OF POTENTIAL CHILD MALTREATMENT

Physical Neglect

Suggestive Physical Findings

Growth failure

Signs of malnutrition, such as thin extremities, abdominal distention, lack of subcutaneous fat

Poor personal hygiene

Unclean or inappropriate dress

Evidence of poor health care, such as delayed immunization, untreated infections, frequent colds

Frequent injuries from lack of supervision

Suggestive Behaviors

Dull and inactive affect; excessively passive or sleepy

Self-stimulatory behaviors, such as finger sucking or rocking

Begging or stealing food

Absenteeism from school

Substance abuse

Vandalism or shoplifting

Emotional Abuse and Neglect

Suggestive Physical Findings

Growth failure

Eating or feeding disorder

Enuresis

Sleep disorder

Suggestive Behaviors

Self-stimulatory behaviors, such as biting, rocking, sucking

During infancy, lack of social smile and stranger anxiety

Withdrawal from environment and people

Unusual fearfulness

Antisocial behavior, such as destructiveness, stealing, cruelty to animals or people

Extremes of behavior, such as overcompliant and passive, or aggressive and demanding

Lags in emotional and intellectual development, especially language

Suicide attempts

Physical Abuse

Suggestive Physical Findings

Bruises and welts (may be in various stages of healing)

- On face, lips, mouth, back, buttocks, thighs, or areas of torso
- Regular patterns descriptive of object used, such as belt buckle, hand, wire hanger, chain, wooden spoon, squeeze or pinch marks
- May be present in various stages of healing

Burns

- On soles, palms, back, or buttocks
- Patterns descriptive of object used, such as round cigar or cigarette burns; sharply demarcated areas from immersion in scalding water; rope burns on wrists or ankles from being bound; burns in the shape of an iron, radiator, or electric stove burner
- Absence of "splash" marks and presence of symmetric burns
- Stun gun injury: lesions circular, fairly uniform ($\leq$0.5 cm), and paired about 5 cm apart

Fractures and dislocations

- Skull, nose, or facial structures
- Injury denoting type of abuse, such as spiral fracture or dislocation from twisting of an extremity or whiplash from shaking the child
- Multiple new or old fractures in various stages of healing

Lacerations and abrasions

- On backs of arms, legs, torso, face, or external genitalia
- Unusual symptoms, such as abdominal swelling, pain, and vomiting from punching
- Descriptive marks such as from human bites or pulling out of hair

Chemical

- Unexplained repeated poisoning, especially drug overdose
- Unexplained sudden illness, such as hypoglycemia from insulin administration

Suggestive Behaviors

Wary of physical contact with adults

Apparent fear of parents or going home

Lying very still while surveying environment

Inappropriate reaction to injury, such as failure to cry from pain

Lack of reaction to frightening events

Apprehension when hearing other children cry

Indiscriminate friendliness and displays of affection

Superficial relationships

Acting-out behavior, such as aggression, to seek attention

Withdrawal behavior

Sexual Abuse

Suggestive Physical Findings

Bruises, bleeding, lacerations, or irritation of external genitalia, anus, mouth, or throat

Torn, stained, or bloody underclothing

Pain on urination or pain, swelling, and itching of genital area

Penile discharge

Sexually transmitted infection, nonspecific vaginitis

Difficulty in walking or sitting

Unusual odor in the genital area

Recurrent urinary tract infections

Presence of sperm

Pregnancy in young adolescent

Suggestive Behaviors

Sudden emergence of sexually related problems, including excessive or public masturbation, age-inappropriate sexual play, promiscuity, or overtly seductive behavior

Withdrawn behavior, excessive daydreaming

Preoccupation with fantasies, especially in play

Poor relationships with peers

Sudden changes, such as anxiety, loss or gain of weight, clinging behavior

In incestuous relationships, excessive anger at mother for not protecting daughter

Regressive behavior, such as bed-wetting or thumb sucking

Sudden onset of phobias or fears, particularly fears of the dark, men, strangers, or particular settings or situations (e.g., fear of leaving the house or staying at the daycare center or the baby-sitter's house)

Running away from home

Substance abuse, particularly of alcohol or mood-elevating drugs

Profound and rapid personality changes, especially extreme depression, hostility, and aggression (often accompanied by social withdrawal)

Rapidly declining school performance

Suicidal attempts or ideation

goal of the interview is to determine whether the child is in a safe environment and whether the caregiver has the skills and resources to care for the child. It is often difficult to determine whether the circumstances constitute poor parenting skills or true neglect. Box 16-9 lists flags for behaviors to look for in neglected and abused children.

Sexual Abuse

An essential component to identifying sexual abuse is the interview. Several dynamics may impede the child's revelation of sexual abuse. Child sexual abuse is often perpetrated by someone known to the child, including family members. In some cases, the child may have been sworn to secrecy. The child may have been told that no one will believe the story or that his or her family would be harmed if he or she told someone about the abuse. Small children may imitate behaviors they have had perpetrated on themselves or have seen others do. The nurse must be able to recognize normal, age-related sexual curiosity and self-stimulating behaviors. Typically, children do not act out specific details of the sexual act or perform intrusive acts on others unless they have sexual knowledge beyond their normal age-related development. (Johnson, 2004).

Children's reports of sexual abuse may vary from contradictory stories to unwavering versions of the experience. Stories that sound contradictory may reflect the child's experiences in several instances of abuse. Also, children who repeatedly tell identical facts may have been prompted to do so.

Increasing evidence suggests that the types of interrogation children are exposed to after reports of sexual abuse shape their thinking. To avoid biasing the interaction, nurses must be skillful interviewers when questioning children who may be victims of abuse. Medical records should include verbatim statements made by the child and interviewer that reflect appropriate non-leading questions and statements (Hornor, 2001; McClain, Girardet, Lahoti, et al, 2000). The child may not be emotionally ready to discuss the abuse. Establishing rapport with the child is essential to gaining his or her trust. Interviews should not be rushed. Engaging the child in play activities while encouraging conversation may help the child discuss the abuse. It may take several interviews or psychologic counseling for the child to be forthcoming about the abuse. Information regarding the last sexual contact is important because it determines the need for a forensic evaluation. Children who have been sexually abused within the past 72 to 96 hours should be considered for forensic testing.

Unfortunately, there is no typical profile of the victim, and the nurse must have a high index of suspicion to identify these children. Physical signs vary and may include any of those listed for sexual abuse. The victim may exhibit various behavioral manifestations, but none of these behaviors is diagnostic. When abused children exhibit these behaviors, the signs may be incorrectly attributed to the normal stresses of childhood, especially in older school-age children or adolescents. Even signs considered most predictive of sexual abuse, such as certain genital findings, sexually inappropriate behavior for age, enactment of adult sexual activity, and intense focus on sexual activity (e.g., masturbation), do not always indicate that sexual abuse has occurred. Conversely, abused children may not demonstrate more knowledge of sexual activity than nonabused children. However, one difference in the abused children's explanation of sexual activity may be unusual affective responses. For example, abused children may have an increased incidence of sleep disorders, temper tantrums, and depression (Calam, Horne, Glasgow, et al, 1998).

> **! NURSING ALERT**
>
> When children report potentially sexually abusive experiences, take their reports seriously, but also cautiously to avoid alarming the child or falsely accusing someone.

Physical Assessment
Child Physical Abuse

The goal of the physical assessment for child physical abuse is identification of all injuries. A system approach ensures the whole body is evaluated. In instances of severe abuse and injuries, the assessment should begin with a rapid assessment of airway, breathing, circulation, and neurologic systems. A systematic head-to-toe examination follows. Attention to areas often overlooked, such as the scalp, behind the ears, and the frenulum, is essential. The child's exterior genital area and posterior surface should be completely examined.

Record the location and a detailed description of all injuries. Note color, size, and location of all bruising. Burn documentation should include location, pattern, demarcation lines, and presence of eschar or blisters. Diagrams of the injuries using a body diagram form are helpful. If possible, obtain photographs of the injuries using a measurement tool.

Not all forms of physical abuse have obvious signs. Intraabdominal organ injury from blunt trauma to the abdomen can occur without signs of external abdominal bruising. Nurses should consider intraabdominal injury in infants and children who have any other signs of abuse.

> **! NURSING ALERT**
>
> Incompatibility between the history and the injury is probably the most important criterion on which to base the decision to report suspected abuse.

All evidence collected must adhere to strict guidelines for legal purposes; chain of custody must be appropriately maintained with local law enforcement personnel. Documentation on the chain of custody form should include the names of persons collecting and receiving evidence (such as photographs and DNA samples), types of evidence collected and received, and date of receipt (Kaczor, Pierce, Makoroff, et al, 2006).

Neglect and Emotional Abuse

Neglect from deprivation of necessities is easier to identify than emotional neglect or psychologic maltreatment because physical signs are usually evident. Assessment of the child's height, weight, nutritional status, hygiene, and age-appropriate interactions is important for the overall picture of potential neglect. Emotional maltreatment may be readily suspected, but it is difficult to substantiate. Physical signs are often nonspecific, and nurses must rely on behavioral indicators, which range from depression to acting-out behavior, to help identify a possibly abusive situation. Any persistent and unexplained change in the child's behavior is an important clue to possible emotional abuse.

Sexual Abuse

Identifying instances of sexual abuse is particularly difficult because, often, few if any obvious physical indications of the activity exist. Physical signs vary and may include any of those listed in Box 16-9 for sexual abuse. The goal of the physical examination is to document genital findings. In most cases, the genital examination is normal, which does not mean that sexual abuse did not occur. Fondling or genital-to-genital contact without penetration may leave no physical findings. Forensic evidence obtained directly from a prepubertal victim's body diminishes greatly after 24 hours, with the best chance for evidence collection coming from bed linens or the child's underwear (Christian, Lavelle, DeJong, et al, 2000). The female genital examination should include a description of the vulva, hymen, and surrounding tissue. Abnormal findings of concern are injuries to the posterior vulva or the lower half of the hymeneal ring, or abrasions, bruising, or bleeding of the genital or anal tissue. It is often helpful to use a magnifying instrument (colposcope) to detect subtle injuries. There are many variants of normal findings for female genital anatomy, so it is recommended that the examination be done by a practitioner experienced with these type of cases. Contrary to popular myth, the size of the hymeneal opening is not predictive of the likelihood of sexual abuse (Christian and Rubin, 2002). For male victims, swelling, abrasions, or bruising of the genital tissue raises concerns for abuse. Examine the anal area for symmetry, tone, fissures, or scars. Genital tissue heals very quickly and most often without scars. Therefore, unless the child is seen within a few days of injury, the genital tissue may appear normal. In addition, the vaginal and anal mucosa is elastic; therefore penetration without disruption of tissue is possible. This defies another myth that there is always evidence of female virginity. Consider the collection of specimens for determining the presence of sexually transmitted infections, which may have been contracted during the sexual contact.

A number of nursing diagnoses are prominent in the nursing care of the maltreated child and family, and others specific to individual cases become evident. The Nursing Care Plan on p. 640 describes the expected outcomes.

Nursing Care Management
Protect Child from Further Abuse
Initially, identification of instances of suspected abuse or neglect is essential. The nurse may come in contact with abused children in an emergency department, practitioner's office, home, daycare center, or school.

> ### ! NURSING ALERT
>
> The priority is to remove the child from the abusive situation to prevent further injury.

All states and provinces in North America have laws for mandatory reporting of child maltreatment. Suspected child abuse is reported to the local authorities.* Referrals usually come to the state child welfare department and are assigned to a caseworker in an agency such as CPS. After a referral has been made, a caseworker is assigned to investigate the report. Based on the findings, the child is left in the home or temporarily removed.

A court proceeding may be necessary before the child can be placed outside the home or when parental rights are to be terminated. When the courts are involved, they usually require

---

*Telephone numbers are usually listed under "Child Abuse" in the business white pages of the local directory, or call the emergency child abuse hotline: 800-422-4453 (800-4-A-CHILD).

firsthand testimony by the referring parties. Nurses may be subpoenaed to appear in court, or their notes may be introduced as evidence in court hearings. Accurate and factual documentation is essential. Behaviors are described, not interpreted, and are recorded daily to establish a progress record (see Nursing Care Guidelines box). Conversations among the nurse, child, and parent are recorded verbatim as much as possible.

NURSING CARE GUIDELINES
Recording Assessment Data in Suspected Abuse

History of Injury
Date, time, and place of occurrence
Sequence of events with recorded times
Presence of witnesses, especially person caring for child at time of incident
Time lapse between occurrence of injury and initiation of treatment
Interview with child when appropriate, including verbal quotations and information from drawing or other play activities
Interview with parent, witnesses, or other significant persons, including verbal quotations
Description of parent-child interactions (verbal interactions, eye contact, touching, parental concern)
Name, age, and condition of other children in home (if possible)

Physical Examination
Location, size, shape, and color of bruises; approximate location, size, and shape on drawing of body outline
Distinguishing characteristics, such as a bruise in the shape of a hand or a round burn (possibly caused by cigarette)
Symmetry or asymmetry of injury; presence of other injuries
Degree of pain; any bone tenderness
Evidence of past injuries; general state of health and hygiene
Developmental level of child; screening test (see Developmental Assessment, Chapter 6)

Support Child
Children suspected of being abused are often hospitalized for medical management of their injuries and to allow further assessment of their safety needs. The needs of these children are the same as those of any hospitalized child. The child should be treated as a child with the usual physical needs, developmental tasks, and play interests—not as a victim of abuse. The goal of the nurse-child relationship is to provide a role model for the parents in helping them to relate positively and constructively to their child and to foster a therapeutic environment for the child in his or her reprieve from the abusing situation.

Support Family
The nurse also encourages the child's relationship with nonoffending parents. The nurse does not become a substitute parent, but rather acts as a role model for parents in helping them to relate positively and constructively to their child. When parental ignorance of childrearing practices has played a part in the abuse, the nurse can educate the parent regarding children's physical and emotional needs. Because of the parents' own childrearing, they may not be aware of nonviolent methods of discipline, such as time-out. They may also need help in dealing with their frustration so that they do not vent anger on the child. Because these parents may be sensitive to criticism or resistant to authority figures, teaching is implemented through demonstration and example rather than through lecturing.

Praise any competent parenting abilities they demonstrate to promote their sense of parental adequacy.

Advise family members to encourage the child to resume normal activities and observe the child for signs of distress. (See Posttraumatic Stress Disorder, Chapter 18.) Children express their feelings primarily through behavior. Parents should be alert for changes in behavior that indicate distress resulting from the incident, such as remaining in the house, refusal to go to school, changes in sleeping patterns, and frequency of dreams and nightmares.

Referral to appropriate social service agencies is also essential. Many abusive parents live in poverty, and the daily stresses imposed by their circumstances are overwhelming. Seek resources for financial aid, improved housing, and child care. Self-help groups also provide important services. Groups such as Parents Anonymous* (a group for parents who have abused or fear that they may abuse their child, but only in terms of physical abuse, not sexual abuse).

Plan for Discharge

Discharge planning should begin as soon as the legal disposition for placement has been decided, which may be temporary foster home placement, return to the parents, or permanent termination of parental rights. The latter is the most drastic solution, but it is necessary in situations of life-threatening abuse. Whenever children are sent to a foster home or juvenile institution, they must be allowed an opportunity to express their feelings. No matter how severe the abuse, they usually mourn the loss of their parents. They need help to understand why they must not return home and that this new home is in no way a punishment. Whenever possible, foster parents are encouraged to visit in the hospital, and the nurse should take an active role in helping these new parents understand the child, as well as the child's health care needs, since studies have shown that the health care needs of children in foster care often go unmet (Mekonnen, Noonan, and Rubin, 2009).

Prevent Abuse

Prevention of child maltreatment has been an extremely difficult goal. However, nurses have played an important role in such programs. For example, home visits to primiparas who were either teenagers, unmarried, or of low socioeconomic status was noted to be an effective preventive measure (Eckenrode, Ganzel, Henderson, et al, 2000; McMillian, 2000). The nurses provided information on normal child growth and development and routine health care needs, served as informal support persons, and referred families to appropriate services when a need for assistance was identified. The Nurse-Family Partnership is one such program that has demonstrated evidence-based interventions resulting in the prevention of child maltreatment (Donelan-McCall, Eckenrode, and Olds, 2009).

Nurses in a variety of settings can implement similar activities. For example, nurses in prenatal clinics can prepare expectant families for adjustment to parenthood. Nursery and postpartum nurses can foster the attachment process by encouraging parents to hold and look at their infant, as well as teaching

coping mechanisms for prolonged crying. Nurses in neonatal intensive care units can minimize the effects of separation by encouraging parents to visit and can help parents become comfortable caring for their child. Nurses in ambulatory settings can teach parents appropriate methods of bathing, feeding, toileting, disciplining, and preventing injuries, while stressing the normal needs and developmental characteristics of children. Nurses must be sensitive to parental needs for attention, reassurance, and reinforcement, and refer parents to community services and self-help groups.

Unlike preventive efforts for neglect and physical abuse, which have been aimed at the potential offender, prevention of child sexual abuse has centered on education of children to protect themselves. Materials are available for parents that describe sexual abuse and its prevention.† Helpful games such as "What

---

👪 FAMILY-CENTERED CARE
Preventing or Dealing with Sexual Abuse of Children

Sexual assault of children is much more common than most people realize. It may be preventable if children have good preparation. To provide protection and preparation:

- Pay careful attention to who is around children. (Unwanted touch may come from someone liked and trusted.)
- Back up a child's right to say no.
- Encourage communication by taking seriously what children say.
- Take a second look at signals of potential danger.
- Refuse to leave children in the company of those not trusted.
- Include information about sexual assault when teaching about safety.
- Provide specific definitions and examples of sexual assault.
- Remind children that even "nice" people sometimes do mean things.
- Urge children to tell about *anybody* who causes them to be uncomfortable.
- Prepare children to deal with bribes, threats, and possible physical force.
- Virtually eliminate secrets between children and parents.
- Teach children how to say no, ask for help, and control who touches them and how.
- Model self-protective and limit-setting behavior for children.

Should it ever become necessary to help a child recover from a sexual assault:

- Listen carefully to understand the child.
- Support the child for telling through praise, belief, sympathy, and lack of blame.
- Know local resources and choose help carefully.
- Provide opportunities to talk about the assault.
- Provide opportunities for the entire family to go through a recovery process.

Sexual assault affects everyone. To help deal with this social problem:

- Provide care and support to those who have been victimized.
- Recognize that offenders may not change behavior even with intervention.
- Organize neighborhood programs to support each other's efforts to protect children.
- Encourage schools to provide information about sexual assault as a problem of health and safety.
- Organize community groups to support educational treatment and law enforcement programs.

Modified from Adams C, Fay J: *No more secrets: protecting your child from sexual assault,* San Luis Obispo, Calif, 1981, Impact.

---

*675 W. Foothill Blvd., Suite 220, Claremont, CA 91711; 909-621-6184; www.parentsanonymous.org.

†Sources of information are Prevent Child Abuse America, 228 S. Wabash Ave., 10th Floor, Chicago, IL 60604; 312-663-3520 or 800-Children; www.preventchildabuse.org; and American Humane, 63 Inverness Drive East, Englewood, CO 80112; 800-227-4645 (outside Colorado) or 303-792-9900; www.americanhumane.org.

NURSING CARE PLAN

The Child Who Is Maltreated

NURSING DIAGNOSIS	EXPECTED PATIENT OUTCOMES	NURSING INTERVENTIONS	RATIONALE
Risk for Trauma related to the child, care giver(s) environment	Child will not experience any maltreatment.	Observe child for physical and behavioral evidence of abuse.	To detect abuse and protect the child
Child's/Family's Defining Characteristics (Subjective and Objective Data)	Child will be protected from further abuse.	Report suspicions to appropriate authorities.	To comply with laws requiring health care providers to report suspicions of maltreatment to child protective services
Physical Neglect	Child and family will receive adequate support.		
Failure to thrive	Child will be able to express feelings about returning to the home or foster home.	Assist in removing child from unsafe environment.	To prevent further injury or neglect
Malnutrition		Refer family to social agencies.	To provide assistance for physical needs that may help prevent neglect and abuse
Poor hygiene	Child and family, including foster parents if appropriate, will be prepared for discharge.		
Poor health care			
Frequent injuries			To provide counseling and education so that parents learn appropriate parenting skills
Emotional Neglect	**The Following NOC Concepts Apply to These Outcomes**		
Failure to thrive	Abuse Protection Support	Collaborate with multidisciplinary team.	To allow several disciplines to provide expertise in prevention of future neglect or abuse
Enuresis	Abuse Recovery: Physical, Sexual		
Sleep disorders	Anxiety Control	Keep factual, objective records of child and parental behaviors.	To facilitate documentation and action planning by authorities
Physical Abuse	Fear Control		
Bruises	Coping	Be aware of signs for continued abuse or neglect.	To prevent further injury or neglect
Burns	Safety Behavior:		
Fractures or dislocation	Personal	Help families identify circumstances that precipitate an abusive act.	To promote more effective parenting skills
Lacerations	Home Physical Environment		
Intracranial hemorrhage		Assist families in realizing abuse has occurred.	To promote awareness with what has happened
Sexual Abuse			
Torn or bloody underclothing		**The Following NIC Concepts Apply to These Interventions**	
Bruises, bleeding, lacerations of external genitalia, anus, mouth or throat		Abuse Protection Support: Child	
Genital discharge or odor		Coping Enhancement	
Recurrent urinary tract infection		Environment Management: Violence Prevention	

NURSING DIAGNOSIS	EXPECTED PATIENT OUTCOMES	NURSING INTERVENTIONS	RATIONALE
Fear/Anxiety related to negative interpersonal interaction, repeated maltreatment, powerlessness, potential loss of parents	Child will exhibit minimal fear and anxiety.	Provide consistent caregiver during hospitalization.	To promote trust
	Child will engage in positive relationships with caregivers.	Demonstrate acceptance of the child.	To minimize feelings of shame and guilt
Child's/Family's Defining Characteristics (Subjective and Objective Data)	Child will grieve loss of parent.	Praise child's abilities.	To promote self-esteem
		Treat child as one with a specific physical problem, not as "abused" victim.	To promote self-esteem and minimizes feelings of guilt
Withdrawn and depressed	**The Following NOC Concepts Apply to These Outcomes**	Avoid asking too many questions.	To avoid upsetting child by probing investigation; to avoid interfering with interrogation
Change in behavior	Anxiety Control		
Inappropriate responses	Fear Control		
Fear of strangers	Coping	Use play to communicate.	To allow child to communicate thoughts and feelings
Lack of engagement with others			
No response to painful interventions		Encourage child to talk about feelings.	To facilitate coping
May not cry or ask for food when hungry		Provide a private time and place to talk.	To foster trust
		Help child grieve for loss of parents if parental rights are terminated.	To support child who will likely be attached to parents despite the abuse
		Encourage introduction of foster parents before placement if possible.	To give child time to adjust
		Offer and encourage food intake at usual times.	To promote adequate nutrition
		The Following NIC Concepts Apply to These Interventions	
		Active Listening	
		Calming Technique	
		Counseling	
		Presence	
		Therapeutic Play	
		Distraction	

if the baby-sitter wants to wrestle and hug but tells you to keep it a secret?" can be used to explore dangerous situations in advance and help children learn the importance of saying "no." They need reassurance that no matter what the other person says or does, the parents want to know about it and will not punish them. Even if children participate in the activity before telling the parents, they must be reassured that it was not their fault. It is equally important to teach children safety in terms of potential risk situations. Several suggestions for parents regarding protecting and educating children against possible molestation are presented in the Family-Centered Care box. The nurse is frequently in a position to discuss the topic of abuse with parents and to provide guidelines. In addition, parents need to be made aware that "nice" people, including

friends and relatives, can be offenders; parents should carefully observe how others act toward the child. A sudden change in the child's behavior and a response such as "I don't like Uncle anymore" are clues to investigate the relationship. In the event of any doubt, prevent further solitary encounters with this person and the child. It is sometimes to the child's great misfortune that parents do not take certain comments seriously, such as "He hugs me too tight" or "I don't want to go with him." Casual parental statements such as "He just loves you" or "You do whatever adults tell you to do" can place children in jeopardy. Health professionals must alert parents to such dangers and guide them toward an appreciation of the problem, providing concrete guidelines toward child education and protection (see Nursing Care Plan).

KEY POINTS

- Common infectious disorders during early childhood include communicable diseases, intestinal parasitic infections, conjunctivitis, and stomatitis.
- Nursing goals in the treatment of a communicable disease are identification, prevention of transmission, provision of comfort, and prevention of complications.
- Intestinal parasitic diseases constitute the most common infections in the world; giardiasis and enterobiasis are the most widespread parasitic infections among children in the United States.
- Although the incidence of poisoning has decreased in the past 30 years as a result of more stringent packaging regulations, childhood poisoning remains a serious health concern.
- The major principles of treatment for poisoning include assessment and the ABCs of resuscitation (airway, breathing, and circulation), minimization of poison absorption, prevention of complications, family support, and prevention of recurrence.
- Communication with the area PCC is essential in the treatment of any poisoning.

- Acetaminophen poisoning is the most common accidental drug poisoning among children and occurs primarily from acute overdose.
- The most important factor contributing to lead poisoning is its availability in the child's environment. Lead-based paint is the most toxic source of lead.
- Because of increasing awareness of the detrimental effects of low levels of lead on the developing nervous system, acceptable BLLs have been decreasing and now are at less than 10 mcg/dl.
- Child maltreatment may take the form of physical abuse or neglect, emotional abuse or neglect, or sexual abuse.
- Parental, child, and environmental characteristics are criteria that may predispose children to maltreatment.
- Identification of abuse entails securing evidence of maltreatment, taking a history pertaining to the incident, and assessing parental and child behaviors.
- The reported incidence of sexual abuse has increased in the past decade; common forms are incest, molestation, rape, exhibitionism, child pornography, child prostitution, and pedophilia.

ANSWERS TO CRITICAL THINKING EXERCISE

Poisoning

1. Yes, there is sufficient evidence to formulate an answer for Mrs. Berry.
2. **a.** When a child ingests a poisonous substance, the initial goal is to limit the absorption of the poison in the gastrointestinal system and enhance elimination. Specific actions that are taken to limit absorption and enhance elimination of poisons are to administer an agent that neutralizes the poison such as activated charcoal. Multiple administrations of activated charcoal may also enhance excretion of the poison through the gastrointestinal tract, thus limiting absorption.
   b. Ipecac is an emetic that induces vomiting by producing an irritant effect on the gastric mucosa. In the past, ipecac was recommended for home treatment of some cases of ingestion. However, ipecac is no longer recommended for routine home treatment of poisoning.

   c. Ipecac induces emesis, which may predispose the child to aspiration if level of consciousness is affected. In addition, emesis may be prolonged beyond the desired time when oral hydration is desirable. In the event that hydrocarbons or corrosive substances are ingested, inducing vomiting with ipecac may cause esophageal damage and aspiration into the lungs.
3. The first priority for nursing care is to advise Mrs. Berry to call the poison control center immediately to obtain guidance. Each ingestion is treated individually, and information from the poison control center is essential to determine the most appropriate action. The most toxic ingredient in a chewable multivitamin is iron, which produces symptoms after several hours. Therefore treatment, if needed, should begin long before symptoms appear.
4. Yes, there is sufficient information to formulate an answer for Mrs. Berry.

REFERENCES

American Academy of Pediatrics, Committee on Infectious Diseases, Pickering L, editor: *Red book: 2009 report of the Committee on Infectious Diseases,* ed 28, Elk Grove Village, Ill, 2009, The Academy.

American Academy of Pediatrics, Committee on Environmental Health: Lead exposure in children: prevention, detection, and management, *Pediatrics* 116(4):1036-1046, 2005.

American Academy of Pediatrics, Committee on Child Abuse and Neglect: Shaken baby syndrome: rotational cranial injuries (technical report), *Pediatrics* 108(1):206-210, 2001.

Bronstein AC, Spyker DA, Cantilena LR Jr, et al: 2007 Annual report of the American Association of Poison Control Centers' National Poison Data System (NPDS): 25th annual report, *Clin Toxicol (Phila)* 46(10):927-1057, 2008.

Calam R, Horne L, Glasgow D, et al: Psychological disturbances and child sexual abuse: a follow-up study, *Child Abuse Negl* 22(9):901-913, 1998.

Carbaugh SF: The long road home: understanding shaken baby syndrome, *Adv Neonatal Care* 4:105-117, 2004.

Castiglia R: Shaken baby syndrome, *J Pediatr Health Care* 15(2):78-80, 2001.

Centers for Disease Control and Prevention: Deaths associated with hypocalcemia from chelation therapy—Texas, Pennsylvania, and Oregon, 2003-2005, *MMWR* 55(08):204-207, 2006.

Centers for Disease Control and Prevention: *Statewide plan for childhood blood lead screening,* Atlanta, 2005, The Centers.

Centers for Disease Control and Prevention: *Managing elevated blood lead levels among young children: recommendations from the Advisory Committee on Childhood Lead Poisoning Prevention,* Atlanta, 2002, The Centers.

Cheng A, Ratnapalan S: Improving the palatability of activated charcoal in pediatric patients, *Pediatr Emerg Care* 23(6):384-386, 2007.

Chiesa A, Duhaime A: Abusive head trauma, *Pediatr Clin North Am* 56(2):317-331, 2009.

Christian CW, Lavelle JM, DeJong AR, et al: Forensic evidence findings in prepubertal victims of sexual assault, *Pediatrics* 106:100-104, 2000.

Christian CW, Rubin DM: Sexual abuse. In Giardino AP, Giardino ER, editors: *Recognition of child abuse for the mandated reporter,* St Louis, 2002, GW Medical Publishing.

Clifton JC: Mercury exposure and public health, *Pediatr Clin North Am* 54(2):237-269, 2007.

Criddle LM: An overview of pediatric poisonings, *AACN Adv Crit Care* 18(2):109-118, 2007.

Cyr M, Wright J, McDuff P, et al: Intrafamilial sexual abuse: brother-sister incest does not differ from father-daughter incest and stepfather-stepdaughter incest, *Child Abuse Negl* 26(9):957-973, 2002.

Dessypris N, Dikalioti SK, Skalkidis I, et al: Combating unintentional injury in the United States: lessons learned from the ICD-10 classification period, *J Trauma* 66(2):519-525, 2009.

Donelan-McCall N, Eckenrode J, Olds D: Home visiting for the prevention of child maltreatment: lessons learned during the past 20 years, *Pediatr Clin North Am* 56(2):389-403, 2009.

Eckenrode J, Ganzel B, Henderson C, et al: Preventing child abuse and neglect with a program of nurse home visitation: the limiting effects of domestic violence, *JAMA* 284(11):1385-1391, 2000.

Eisenstein L, Bodager D, Ginzl D: Outbreak of giardiasis and cryptosporidiosis associated with a neighborhood interactive water fountain—Florida, 2006, *J Environ Health* 71(3):18-22, 2008.

Eldridge DL, Van Eyk J, Kornegay C: Pediatric toxicology, *Emerg Med Clin North Am* 25(2):283-308, 2007.

Erickson L, Thompson T: A review of a preventable poison: pediatric lead poisoning, *J Soc Pediatr Nurs* 10(4):171-182, 2005.

Ewing-Cobb L, Kramer L, Prasad M, et al: Neuroimaging, physical, and developmental findings after inflicted and noninflicted traumatic brain injury in young children, *Pediatrics* 102:300-307, 1998.

Finkel MA, DeJong AR: Medical findings in child sexual abuse. In Reece RM, Ludwig S, editors: *Child abuse medical diagnosis and management,* Philadelphia, 2001, Lippincott Williams & Wilkins.

Franklin RL, Rodgers GB: Unintentional child poisonings treated in United States hospital emergency departments: national estimates of incident cases, population-based poisoning rates, and product involvement, *Pediatrics* 122(6):1244-1251, 2008.

Frazer L: Soil in the city: a prime source of lead. *Environ Health Perspect* 116(12):A522, 2008.

Fuloria M, Kreiter S: The newborn examination, part I, Emergencies and common abnormalities involving the skin, head, neck, chest, and respiratory and cardiovascular systems, *Am Fam Physician* 65(1):61-68, 2002.

Galea SA, Sweet A, Beninger P, et al: The safety profile of varicella vaccine: a 10-year review, *J Infect Dis* 197(Suppl 2):S165-S169, 2008.

Gara MA, Allen LA, Herzog EP, et al: The abused child as parent: the structure and content of physically abused mothers' perceptions of their babies, *Child Abuse Negl* 24(5):627-639, 2000.

Giardino ER, Giardino AP, editors: *Nursing approach to the evaluation of child maltreatment,* St Louis, 2003, GW Medical Publishing.

Goldman J, Salus MK, Wolcott D, et al: What factors contribute to child abuse and neglect? In *A coordinated response to child abuse and neglect: the foundation for practice,* 2003, Child Welfare Information Gateway, available at www.childwelfare.gov/pubs/usermanuals/

foundation/foundatione.cfm (accessed June 4, 2007).

Greene S, Harris C, Singer J: Gastrointestinal decontamination of the poisoned patient, *Pediatr Emerg Care* 24(3):176-189, 2008.

Heavey E: Lead poisoning in children: still a threat, *Nursing* 38(12):17-18, 2008.

Hornor G: Repeated sexual abuse allegations: a problem for primary care providers, *J Pediatr Health Care* 15(2):71-76, 2001.

Johnson CF: Child sexual abuse, *Lancet* 364(9432):462-470, 2004.

Kaczor K, Pierce MC, Makoroff K, et al: Bruising and physical child abuse, *Clin Pediatr Emerg Med* 7(3):153-160, 2006.

Kendrick D, Barlow J, Hampshire A, et al: Parenting interventions for the prevention of unintentional injuries in childhood, *Cochrane Database Syst Rev* Oct 17(4):CD006020, 2007.

Kendrick D, Coupland C, Mulvaney C, et al: Home safety education and provision of safety equipment for injury prevention, *Cochrane Database Syst Rev* Jan 24(1): CD005014, 2007.

Kendrick D, Smith S, Sutton A, et al: Effect of education and safety equipment on poisoning-prevention practices and poisoning: systematic review, meta-analysis and meta-regression, *Arch Dis Child* 93(7):599-608, 2008.

Lederman C, Lederman M: Ophthalmologic emergencies. In Crain EF, Gershel JC, editors: *Clinical manual of emergency pediatrics,* ed 4, New York, 2003, McGraw-Hill.

Leider HS, Irving SY, Mauricio R, et al: Munchausen syndrome by proxy: a case report, *AACN Clin Issues* 16(2):178-184, 2005.

Leung AK, Robson WL, Leong AG: Herpes zoster in childhood, *J Pediatr Health Care* 20(5):1783-1785, 2006.

Levin A: Retinal hemorrhages: advances in understanding, *Pediatr Clin North Am* 56(2):333-344, 2009.

Levin R, Brown MJ, Kashtock ME, et al: Lead exposures in U.S. children, 2008: implications for prevention, *Environ Health Perspect* 116(10):1285-1293, 2008, available at www.ncbi.nlm.nih.gov/pmc/articles/PMC2569084/?tool=pubmed (accessed February 1, 2010).

Lichtenstein SJ, Rinehart M: Levofloxacin Bacterial Conjunctivitis Study Group: Efficacy and safety of 0.5% levofloxacin ophthalmic solution for the treatment of bacterial conjunctivitis in pediatric patients, *J AAPOS* 7(5):317-324, 2003.

Lidsky TI, Schneider JS: Adverse effects of childhood lead poisoning: the clinical neuropsychological perspective, *Environ Res* 100(1):284-293, 2006.

Madden MA: Responding to pediatric poisoning, *Nursing* 38(8):52-55, 2008.

McClain N, Giardet R, Lahoti S, et al: Evaluation of sexual abuse in the pediatric patient, *J Pediatr Health Care* 14(3):93-102, 2000.

McMillian H: Child maltreatment: what we know in the year 2000, *Can J Psychiatry* 45(8):702-709, 2000.

Mekonnen R, Noonan K, Rubin D: Achieving better healthcare outcomes for children in foster care, *Pediatr Clin North Am* 56(2):405-415, 2009.

Miehl NJ: Shaken baby syndrome, *J Forensic Nurs* 1(3):111-117, 2005.

Nasser M, Fedorowicz Z, Khoshnevisan MH, et al: Acyclovir for treating primary herpetic gingivostomatitis, *Cochrane Database Syst Rev* Oct 8(4): CD006700, 2008.

National Center on Shaken Baby Syndrome: *All about SBS/AHT*, n.d., available at www.dontshake.org/sbs.php?topNavID=2&subNavID=10 (accessed May 29, 2009).

Nelms BC: Emotional abuse: helping prevent the problem, *J Pediatr Health Care* 15(3):103-104, 2001.

Phillips B: Towards evidence-based medicine for paediatricians, *Arch Dis Child Educ Pract Ed* 93(4):129, 2008.

Putnam FW: Ten year update review: child sexual abuse, *J Am Acad Child Adolesc Psychiatry* 42(3):269-278, 2003.

Rose PW, Harnden A, Brueggemann AB, et al: Chloramphenicol treatment for acute infective conjunctivitis in children in primary care: a randomized double-blind placebo-controlled trial, *Lancet* 366(9479):37-43, 2005.

Sheffield P, Serwint JR: Emetics, cathartics, and gastric lavage, *Pediatr Rev* 29(6):214-215, 2008.

Shields JM, Gleim ER, Beach MJ: Prevalence of *Cryptosporidium* spp. and *Giardia intestinalis* in swimming pools, Atlanta, Georgia, *Emerg Infect Dis* 14(6):948-950, 2008.

US Department of Health and Human Services, Administration on Children, Youth and Families: *Child maltreatment 2007,* Washington, DC, 2009, US Government Printing Office.

Walls C: Shaken baby syndrome education: a role for nurse practitioners working with families of small children, *J Pediatr Health Care* 20(5):304-310, 2006.

Wells K: Substance abuse and child maltreatment, *Pediatr Clin North Am* 56(2):354-362, 2009.

Wood N, McIntyre P: Pertussis: review of epidemiology, diagnosis, management and prevention, *Paediatr Respir Rev* 9(3):201-212, 2008.

Woolf AD, Goldman R, Bellinger DC: Update on clinical management of childhood lead poisoning, *Pediatr Clin North Am* 54(2):271-294, 2007.

Yoder JS, Beach MJ: Centers for Disease Control and Prevention (CDC): Giardiasis surveillance—United States, 2003-2005, *MMWR Surveill Summ* 56(7):11-18, 2007.

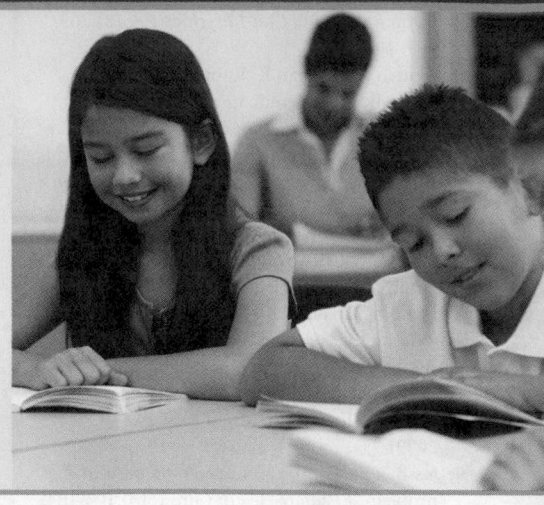

PROMOTING OPTIMUM GROWTH AND DEVELOPMENT

The segment of the life span that extends from age 6 years to approximately age 12 years has a variety of labels, each of which describes an important characteristic of the period. The middle years are most often referred to as school age or the school years. This period begins with entrance into the wider sphere of influence represented by the school environment, which has a significant impact on development and relationships.

Physiologically the middle years begin with the shedding of the first deciduous tooth and end at puberty with the acquisition of the final permanent teeth (with the exception of the wisdom teeth). In the 5 to 6 years before the school-age period, children progressed from helpless infants to sturdy, complicated individuals with the capacity to communicate, conceptualize in a limited way, and become involved in complex social and motor behavior. Physical growth was been equally rapid. In contrast, the period of middle childhood—between the rapid growth of early childhood and the prepubescent growth spurt—is a time of gradual growth and development, with more even progress in both physical and emotional aspects.

BIOLOGIC DEVELOPMENT

During middle childhood, growth in height and weight assumes a slower but steady pace compared with the earlier years. Between the ages of 6 and 12 years, children grow an average of 5 cm (2 inches) per year to gain 30 to 60 cm (1 to 2 feet) in height and will almost double in weight, increasing 2 to 3 kg (4.4 to 6.6 lb) per year. The average 6-year-old child is about 116 cm (46 inches) tall and weighs about 21 kg (46.3 lb); the average 12-year-old child stands about 150 cm (59 inches) tall and weighs approximately 40 kg (88.2 lb). During this age period girls and boys differ little in size, although boys tend to be slightly taller and somewhat heavier than girls. Toward the end of the school-age years both boys and girls begin to increase in size, although most girls begin to surpass boys in both height and weight, to the acute discomfort of both sexes.

Physical Changes

School-age children are more graceful than they were as preschoolers, and they are steadier on their feet. Their bodies take on a slimmer look with longer legs, varying body proportions, and a lower center of gravity. Posture improves over that of the preschool period to facilitate locomotion and efficiency in using the arms and trunk. These proportions make climbing, bicycle riding, and other activities much easier. Fat gradually diminishes, and its distribution patterns change, which contributes to the thinner appearance of children during the middle years.

Accompanying the skeletal lengthening and fat diminution is an increase in the percentage of body weight represented by muscle tissue. By the end of this age period, both boys and girls have doubled their strength and physical capabilities, and their steady and relatively consistent acquisition of refined coordination increases their poise and skill. However, this increased strength is often misleading. Although strength increases, muscles are still functionally immature when compared with

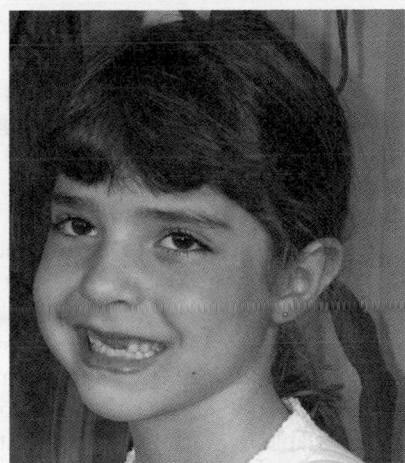

Fig. 17-1 Middle childhood is the stage of development when deciduous teeth are shed.

those of the adolescent, and they are more readily injured by overuse.

The most pronounced changes that seem best to indicate increasing maturity in children are a decrease in head circumference in relation to standing height, a decrease in waist circumference in relation to height, and an increase in leg length related to height. These indicators often provide a clue to a child's degree of maturity and have proved useful in predicting readiness for meeting the demands of school. There appears to be a correlation between physical indicators of maturity and success in school.

Certain physiologic and anatomic characteristics are typical of school-age children. Facial proportions change as the face grows faster in relation to the remainder of the cranium. The skull and brain grow very slowly during this period and increase little in size thereafter. Because all of the primary (deciduous) teeth are lost during this age span, middle childhood is sometimes known as the age of the loose tooth (Fig. 17-1) and the early years of middle childhood as the ugly duckling stage, when the new secondary (permanent) teeth appear to be much too large for the smaller face.

Maturation of Systems

As the gastrointestinal system matures, the child has fewer stomach upsets; better maintenance of blood sugar levels; and an increased stomach capacity, which permits retention of food for longer periods. The school-age child does not need to be fed as carefully, as promptly, or as frequently as before. Caloric needs are lower than they were in the preschool years and lower than they will be during the coming adolescent growth spurt.

Physical maturation occurs in other body tissues and organs. Bladder capacity, although differing widely among individual children, is generally greater in girls than in boys. There are individual variations in frequency of urination and differences in the same child according to circumstances such as temperature, humidity, time of day, amount of fluids ingested, and emotional state.

The heart grows more slowly during the middle years and is smaller in relation to the rest of the body than at any other period of life. Heart and respiratory rates steadily decrease, and blood pressure increases between ages 6 to 12 (see inside back cover).

The immune system becomes more competent in its ability to localize infections and produce an antibody-antigen response. Because of increased exposure to others in school classes, children can have several infections in the first 1 to 2 years of school while immunity develops.

Bones continue to ossify throughout childhood, but because mineralization is not completed until maturity, children's bones resist pressure, and muscles pull less than with mature bones. Consequently, parents must be careful to prevent alterations in bone structure and provide children with well-fitted shoes and with chairs and desks that allow correct sitting posture with the feet able to reach the floor and the hips able to fit well back in the seat. Children should have ample opportunity to move around and be cautious about carrying heavy loads. For example, they should shift books and/or tote bags from one arm to the other. Back packs, when worn correctly, distribute weight more evenly.

Wider differences between children are seen at the end of middle childhood than at the beginning; such differences are sometimes striking. These differences become increasingly apparent and, if extreme or unique, may create emotional problems. The nurse should explain the associated characteristics of height and weight relationships, rapid or slow growth, and other important features of development to children and their families. Physical maturity is not necessarily correlated with emotional and social maturity. Seven-year-old children who look like 10-year-old children will think and act like 7-year-olds. To expect behavior appropriate for 10-year-old children from them is unrealistic and can be detrimental to their development of competence and self-esteem. Conversely, to treat 10-year-old children as though they were 7 years old is an equal disservice to them.

Prepubescence

Preadolescence is the period that begins toward the end of middle childhood and ends with the thirteenth birthday. Puberty signals the beginning of the development of secondary sex characteristics, and prepubescence, the 2-year period that precedes puberty, typically occurs during preadolescence.

Toward the end of middle childhood the discrepancies in growth and maturation between boys and girls become apparent. On the average, there is a difference of approximately 2 years between girls and boys in the age of onset of pubescence. For many, especially for girls, preadolescence is a period of rapid growth. For others, mostly boys, it is generally a period of continued steady growth in height and weight.

There is no universal age at which children assume the characteristics of preadolescence. The first physiologic signs appear at about 9 years (particularly in girls) and are usually clearly evident in 11- to 12-year-old children. Although preadolescent children do not want to be different, variability in physical growth and physiologic changes among children of the same sex, and between the two sexes, is often striking at this time. This variability, especially in relation to the onset of secondary sex characteristics, is of utmost concern to the preadolescent. Either early or late appearance of these characteristics is a source of embarrassment and uneasiness to both sexes.

Early appearance of secondary sex characteristics in girls is often associated with dissatisfaction with physical appearance, greater general unhappiness, and lower self-esteem. Late-developing boys often have a negative self-concept. Both early appearance of physical characteristics in girls and late appearance in boys have been linked to participation in risk-taking behaviors (early sexual activity, substance use, and reckless vehicle use).

Preadolescence is a time when considerable overlapping of developmental characteristics occurs, with elements of both middle childhood and early adolescence apparent. However, there are sufficient unique characteristics to set this period apart as an age category. Generally, puberty begins no earlier than 10 years in girls and 12 years in boys, but its onset in either sex after the age of 8 years is considered normal. The average age of puberty is 12 years in girls and 14 years in boys. Boys experience little sexual maturation during preadolescence.

PSYCHOSOCIAL DEVELOPMENT

Middle childhood is the period of psychosexual development that Freud described as the latency period, a time of tranquility between the oedipal phase of early childhood and the eroticism of adolescence. During this time children experience relationships with same-sex peers following the indifference of earlier years and preceding the heterosexual fascination that occurs for most boys and girls in puberty.

Developing a Sense of Industry (Erikson)

Successful mastery of Erikson's first three stages of psychosocial development is probably the most important accomplishment in terms of development of a healthy personality (Erikson, 1963). Successful completion of these stages requires a loving environment within a stable family unit that has prepared the child to engage in experiences and relationships beyond this intimate group. During childhood, children affiliate with age-mates, receive the systematic instruction prescribed by their individual cultures, and develop the skills needed to become useful, contributing members of their social communities.

A sense of industry, or a stage of accomplishment, occurs somewhere between age 6 years and adolescence. The goal of this stage of development is to achieve a sense of personal and interpersonal competence through the acquisition of technologic and social skills. School-age children are eager to build skills and participate in meaningful and socially useful work. Interests expand, and, with a growing sense of independence, children want to engage in tasks that they can complete (Fig. 17-2). Failure to develop a sense of accomplishment may result in a sense of inferiority.

Many aspects of industry contribute to the child's sense of competence and mastery. Intrinsic motivation is associated with increased competence in mastering new skills and assuming new responsibilities. Children gain a great deal of satisfaction from independent behavior in exploring and manipulating their environment and from interaction with peers. Extrinsic sources of reinforcement in the form of grades, material rewards, additional privileges, and recognition provide encouragement and stimulation. Often the acquisition of skills is a

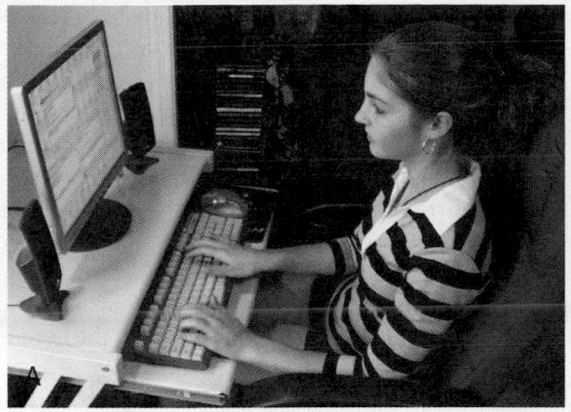 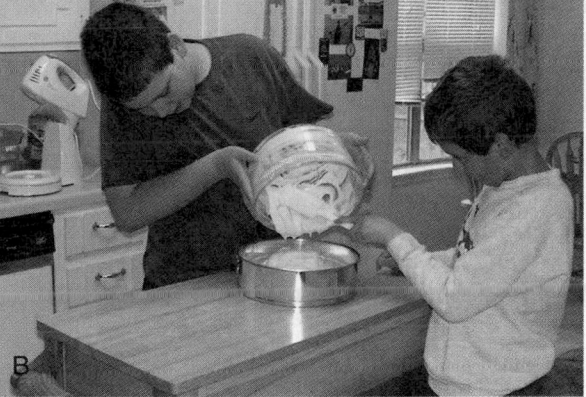

Fig. 17-2 School-age children are motivated to complete tasks. **A,** Working alone. **B,** Working with others.

means for achieving success in special activities such as athletics or social organizations. Peer approval is a strong motivating factor.

The danger inherent in this period of personality development is the occurrence of situations that might result in a sense of inadequacy or inferiority. This may happen if the previous stages have not been successfully mastered or if a child is incapable of or unprepared to assume the responsibilities associated with developing a sense of accomplishment. Feelings of inferiority or lack of worth come from children themselves or from the social environment. Children with physical or mental limitations are sometimes at a disadvantage for acquisition of certain skills. When the reward structure is based on evidence of mastery, children who are incapable of developing these skills are at risk for feeling inadequate and inferior.

Even children without chronic disabilities show such a wide range of individual differences in capabilities and preferences that they experience feelings of inadequacy in some areas. No child is able to do well in everything, and children must learn that they will not be able to master each skill that they attempt. All children, even children who in most instances have positive attitudes toward work and their own capabilities, feel some degree of inferiority in regard to a specific skill that they cannot master.

For some children, success or aptitude in one area may compensate for failure or ineptitude in another. However, the differences in reinforcement provided for success in various areas have significant effects on feelings of adequacy. For example, in the United States, reading proficiency is more highly rewarded than the mechanical aptitude needed for tinkering with broken automobile engines. Society places a higher value on success in team sports than on success in repairing a bicycle. Compensating for the inability to excel in more socially valued skills through mastery of other, less valued skills is difficult for children. If the social environment places a negative value on any failure, feelings of inferiority may be increased in the less capable child. Repeated failures can generate such strong feelings that eventually the child is reluctant to attempt any new task or is fearful of not being able to perform as well as his or her peers. Thus intrinsic motivation toward engaging in a task for the pleasure of the challenge conflicts with the external forces that cause feelings of doubt and inferiority. Consequently, the child may no longer try.

A child's concept of success or failure is important. Children who aspire to more than they are capable of usually experience failure. In contrast, children who set their aspirations lower than their level of achievement are likely to experience success. Most accomplishments during the school years are very public. Family, teachers, and peers are all aware of success or failure in school. In school and sometimes at home, feelings of inferiority may be produced through comparisons with others that suggest the child is not as good as a peer, sibling, or member of another group. This inadequacy becomes a source of embarrassment. The child may even be shamed for the failure. Earlier conflicts of doubt and guilt are closely associated with feelings of inferiority.

A sense of accomplishment also involves the ability to cooperate, to compete with others, and to cope effectively with people. Middle childhood is the time when children learn the value of doing things with others and the benefits derived from division of labor in the accomplishment of goals. Children need and want real achievement. When they can accomplish tasks that need to be done and perform well despite individual differences in capacities and emotional development, and when they are suitably rewarded, children develop a sense of industry and accomplishment that prepares them for establishing a stable identity later in life.

TEMPERAMENT

The reactivity patterns or temperamental traits identified in infancy may continue to influence behavior in middle childhood. Analyzing behavioral patterns observed in past situations can provide clues to the way that a child may react to new situations, although long-range projections are not always successful. Through interaction with the environment, experiences, motives, and abilities, many children change. In some children major temperamental characteristics persist into adolescence; in others they do not.

Many children tend to be identified with one of three broad temperament categories: easy, slow to warm up, and difficult. Parents and teachers are in an excellent position to assess a child's behavioral style and to try to make their demands and expectations consonant with the individual child's temperamental characteristics. With easy children this rarely poses a problem. They adapt readily to many childrearing programs and new situations. School entry and other changes usually go smoothly and are accomplished with minimal stress. Difficulties arise with children who are slow to warm up or are difficult or easily distracted.

Slow-to-warm-up children usually exhibit discomfort when introduced to new situations and need time to become accustomed to a new environment, authority figures, and expectations. These children may respond with tears, somatic complaints, or other maneuvers to avoid the event. The nurse should encourage them to try new experiences but allow them to adapt to their surroundings at their own speed. Pressure to move quickly into new situations only strengthens the tendency to withdraw. After-school activities can be a cause for reaction, but attending with a friend or contracting for permission to withdraw after a trial of a specified number of times may provide them with sufficient incentive to try (see Critical Thinking Exercise).

> ### ❓ CRITICAL THINKING EXERCISE
> #### *Temperament in the School-Age Child*
>
> Mary's teacher asks the school nurse for guidance. Mary is 8 years old and has just entered the third grade. In the classroom Mary is quiet and passive, and she frequently cries when the teacher talks with her. Mary's mother describes her daughter as a healthy child who has always required more time and effort to adapt to changes in her routine. In counseling Mary's teacher, what should the nurse encourage the teacher to do?
>
> 1. Evidence—Is there sufficient evidence to draw any conclusions about Mary's behavior?
> 2. Assumptions—Describe the underlying assumptions about each of the following:
>   a. Factors and timing related to establishment of a child's temperament
>   b. Ease or difficulty of adapting to new situations in relation to temperament
>   c. Helping the slow-to-warm-up child adjust to new situations
> 3. What priorities for nursing care can be drawn from this situation?
> 4. Does the evidence support your conclusion?

Difficult or easily distracted children may benefit from "practice" sessions in which they are prepared for a given event by role playing, visiting the site, or reading or listening to stories, or use of other methods to acquaint them with what to expect. Children who are persistent need to know when to stop what they are doing so that the signal to stop will not come as a surprise or trigger a reaction. Nurses need to handle children with difficult temperaments with exceptional patience, firmness, and understanding so that they can learn appropriate behavior in their interactions with others. If possible, teachers' styles and characteristics should match the temperament of children to ensure a good fit.

COGNITIVE DEVELOPMENT (PIAGET)

When they enter the school years, children begin to acquire the ability to relate a series of events and actions to mental representations that they can express both verbally and symbolically. This is the stage that Piaget describes as **concrete operations**,

when children are able to use their thought processes to experience events and actions. The term *operation* implies an action that is performed on an object or set of objects; thus a mental operation is an alteration or transformation that an individual carries out in thought rather than in action. Toddlers or preschool children can perform acts that involve ordering, such as correctly arranging a graduated set of circles from largest to smallest on a stick, and can find their way to a friend's house, but they are unable to verbalize the actions involved in the process. School-age children are able to articulate the process and perform the actions mentally without the need to carry out the behaviors.

As children move from the preschool years into the school years, their conceptual abilities become increasingly flexible. During the concrete operational period, they acquire the ability to perform cognitive operations and apply these new skills when thinking about objects, situations, and events. Their rigid, egocentric outlook is replaced by thought processes that allow them to see things from another's point of view. They become aware of a variety of perspectives and become more sensitive to the fact that others do not always perceive events exactly as they do. They are able to delay an action until they have evaluated alternative responses to situations. Their steady reduction in egocentricity helps form the basis for logical thought and the development and maturation of morality.

The concrete operational stage occurs between the ages of 7 and 11 years. During this stage children develop an understanding of relationships between things and ideas. They progress from making judgments based on what they see (perceptual thinking) to making judgments based on what they reason (conceptual thinking). They are increasingly able to master symbols and to use their memory store of past experiences to evaluate and interpret the present.

One of the major cognitive tasks of school-age children is mastering the concept of **conservation**—that physical matter does not appear and disappear by magic. They learn that certain properties of the environment are not changed simply by altering their disposition in space. They are able to resist perceptual cues that suggest alterations in the physical state of an object.

The nurse can use commonplace items to demonstrate the conservation of liquid, mass, number, length, area, and volume (Fig. 17-3). To explain the observation that the mass of the clay in the figure has not been altered, children use one of three concepts:

1. Identity—Because nothing has been added and nothing has been taken away, the pancake is still the same clay. Nothing has changed but the shape.
2. Reversibility—The clay can be reshaped into its original form (a ball).
3. Reciprocity—Although the pancake appears larger in circumference, the ball is much thicker. In this instance the child demonstrates the ability to deal with two dimensions at the same time and to comprehend that a change in one dimension compensates for a change in another.

When children are able to use the concepts of identity, reversibility, and reciprocity, they can conserve along any physical dimension. They perceive the concept of volume in relation to container size and shape, recognize that size is not necessarily

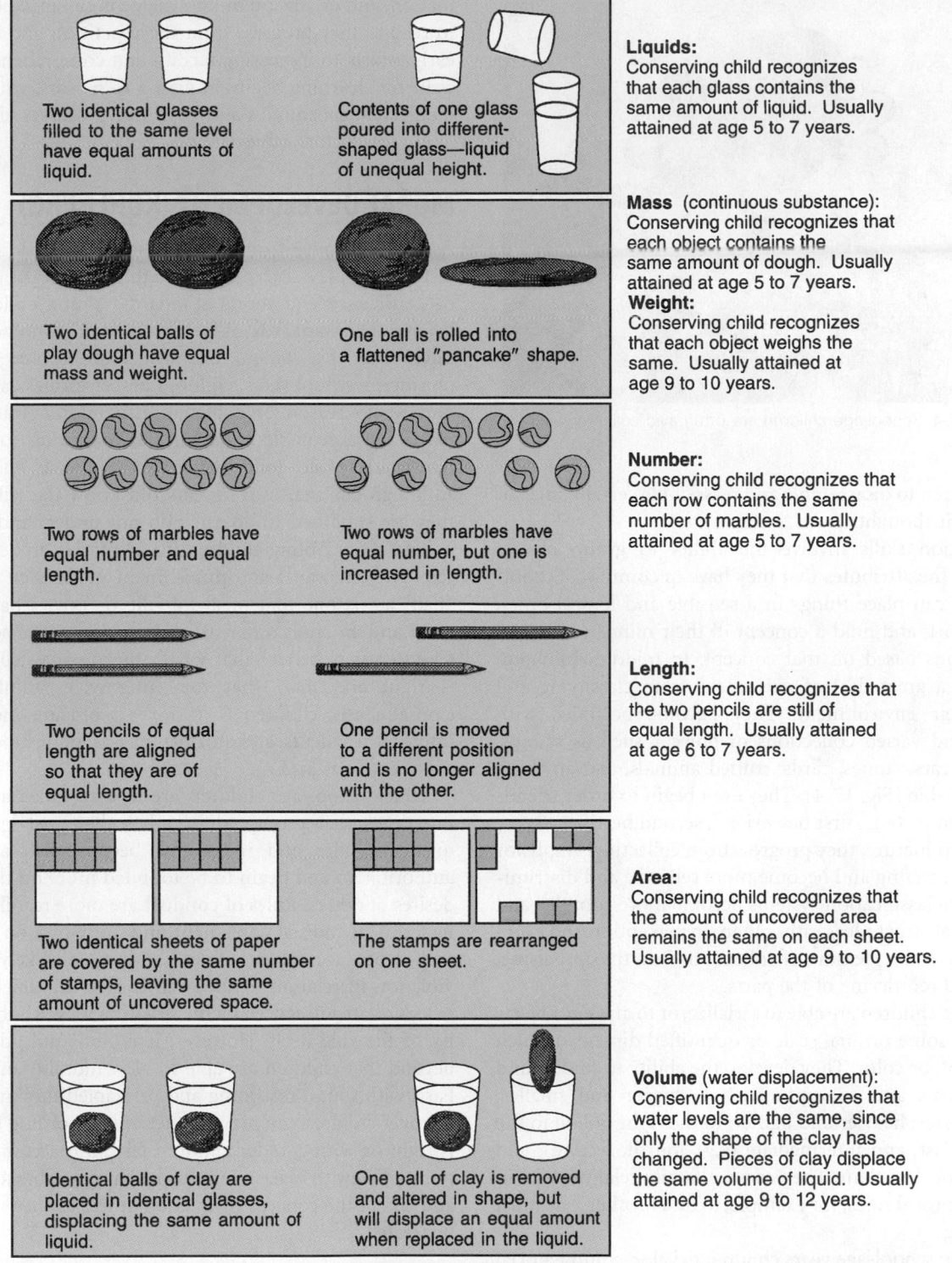

Liquids:
Conserving child recognizes that each glass contains the same amount of liquid. Usually attained at age 5 to 7 years.

Two identical glasses filled to the same level have equal amounts of liquid.

Contents of one glass poured into different-shaped glass—liquid of unequal height.

Mass (continuous substance):
Conserving child recognizes that each object contains the same amount of dough. Usually attained at age 5 to 7 years.

Weight:
Conserving child recognizes that each object weighs the same. Usually attained at age 9 to 10 years.

Two identical balls of play dough have equal mass and weight.

One ball is rolled into a flattened "pancake" shape.

Number:
Conserving child recognizes that each row contains the same number of marbles. Usually attained at age 5 to 7 years.

Two rows of marbles have equal number and equal length.

Two rows of marbles have equal number, but one is increased in length.

Length:
Conserving child recognizes that the two pencils are still of equal length. Usually attained at age 6 to 7 years.

Two pencils of equal length are aligned so that they are of equal length.

One pencil is moved to a different position and is no longer aligned with the other.

Area:
Conserving child recognizes that the amount of uncovered area remains the same on each sheet. Usually attained at age 9 to 10 years.

Two identical sheets of paper are covered by the same number of stamps, leaving the same amount of uncovered space.

The stamps are rearranged on one sheet.

Volume (water displacement):
Conserving child recognizes that water levels are the same, since only the shape of the clay has changed. Pieces of clay displace the same volume of liquid. Usually attained at age 9 to 12 years.

Identical balls of clay are placed in identical glasses, displacing the same amount of liquid.

One ball of clay is removed and altered in shape, but will displace an equal amount when replaced in the liquid.

Fig. 17-3 Common examples that demonstrate the child's ability to conserve (ages are approximate).

related to weight or volume, and are able to manipulate or "see" in a concrete manner. They recognize that logical operations move in two directions (such as addition and subtraction or multiplication and division) and that certain properties are invariant (e.g., 7 remains 7 whether it is represented by 3 + 4, 2 + 5, seven buttons, seven stars, or seven boys).

There appears to be a developmental sequence in children's capacity to conserve matter. Children usually grasp conservation of numbers (ages 5 to 6) before conservation of substance. Conservation of liquids, mass, and length usually is accom-

plished at about ages 6 to 7, conservation of weight sometime later (ages 9 to 10), and conservation of volume or displacement last (ages 9 to 12).

Children use reversibility in selecting a course of action, which thus provides greater control over themselves and their environment. They have the ability to think through an action sequence, anticipate the consequences, and, if needed, return to the beginning and rethink the action in a different direction. They no longer need to experience an action before they can anticipate the results. Reversibility allows mental action and

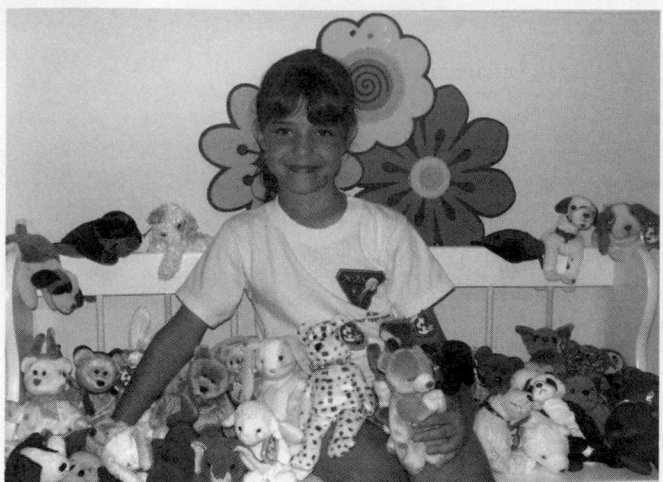

Fig. 17-4 School-age children are often avid collectors.

enables children to disassemble and reassemble certain kinds of things in their thoughts.

Classification skills involve the ability to group objects according to the attributes that they have in common. School-age children can place things in a sensible and logical order, group and sort, and hold a concept in their minds while they make decisions based on that concept. In middle childhood children get a great deal of enjoyment from classifying and ordering their environment. They become occupied with numerous and varied collections of objects, such as stamps, shells, dolls, cars, stones, cards, stuffed animals, and anything that is classifiable (Fig. 17-4). They even begin to order friends and relationships (e.g., first best friend, second best friend).

As children mature, they progress from collecting simply for the sake of collecting and become more selective and discriminating. Their classification systems become more complex and are based on abstract ideas rather than on perception and experience. Much of the pleasure of collections is in the appraising, ordering, and reordering of the parts.

School-age children are able to serialize, or to arrange objects according to some ordinal scale or quantified dimension such as size, weight, or color. They develop the ability to understand relational terms and concepts, such as bigger and smaller; darker and paler; heavier and lighter; to the right of and to the left of; first, last, and intermediate (e.g., fourth, second); and more than and less than. They can see family relationships in terms of reciprocal roles; for example, to be a brother, one must have a sibling.

During the school-age years children develop combinatorial skills—the ability to manipulate numbers and to learn the skills of addition, subtraction, multiplication, and division. They learn to apply the basic operations to any object or quantity. They learn the alphabet and the ever-widening world of symbols called words that can be arranged in terms of structure and their relationship to the alphabet. They learn to tell time, to see the relationship of events in time (history) and places in space (geography), and to combine time and space relationships (geology and astronomy).

The most significant skill, the ability to read, is acquired during the school years and becomes the most valuable tool for independent inquiry. Children's capacity for exploration, imag-ination, and expansion of knowledge is enhanced by the ability to read as they progress from the repetition and confusion of early efforts to increasing facility and comprehension. Formal academic learning begins at ages 5 to 6 years, when children's intellectual capabilities and cognitive processes allow them to attain intellectual achievements.

MORAL DEVELOPMENT (KOHLBERG)

As children move from egocentrism to more logical patterns of thought, they also move through stages in the development of conscience and moral standards. Young children do not believe that standards of behavior come from within themselves but that others establish and enforce these rules. During preschool years, children perceive rules as definite and require no reason or explanation. Children learn the standards for acceptable behavior, act according to these standards, and feel guilty when they violate the standards. Although children 6 or 7 years old know the rules and what they are supposed to do, they do not understand the reasons behind them. Young children usually judge an act by its consequences. Rewards and punishment guide their judgment; a "bad" act is one that breaks a rule or causes harm. When a child and an adult differ in judging an act, the adult is right. Children may believe that what other people tell them to do is right and that what they themselves think is wrong. Consequently, children 6 or 7 years old are more likely to interpret accidents and misfortunes as punishment for misdeeds or "bad" acts.

Older school-age children are able to judge an act by the intentions that prompted it rather than just by the consequences. Rules and judgments become less absolute and authoritarian and begin to be founded more on the needs and desires of others. Rules of conduct are more readily considered in terms of mutual agreement and are based on cooperation and respect for others. Older children will likely view a rule violation in relation to the total context in which it appears; reactions are influenced by the situation as well as by the morality of the rule itself. However, it is not until adolescence or beyond that children are able to view morality on an abstract basis with sound reasoning and principled thinking. Although younger children can judge an act only according to whether it is right or wrong, older children take into account a different point of view to make a judgment. They are able to understand and accept the concept of treating others as they would like to be treated.

SPIRITUAL DEVELOPMENT

Children at this age think in very concrete terms but are avid learners and have a great desire to learn about their God or deity. They picture God as human and use adjectives such as "loving" and "helping" to describe their deity. They are fascinated by heaven and hell and, with a developing conscience and concern about rules, they fear going to hell for misbehavior. School-age children want and expect to be punished for misbehavior and, if given the option, tend to choose a punishment that "fits the crime." Often they view illness or injury as a punishment for a real or imagined misdeed. The beliefs and ideals

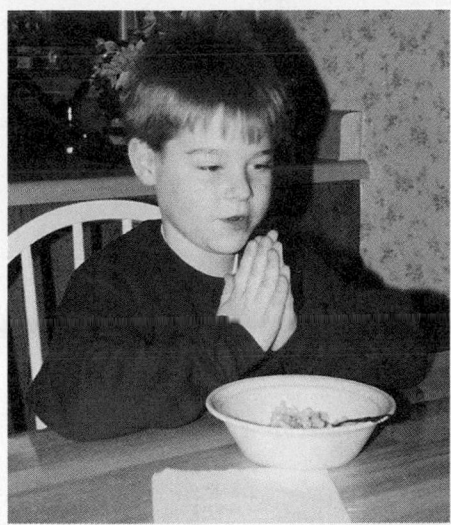
Fig. 17-5 Children are comforted by prayer or other religious rituals.

of family and religious personages are more influential than those of their peers in matters of faith.

School-age children begin to learn the difference between the natural and the supernatural but have difficulty understanding symbols. Consequently, religious concepts must be presented to them in concrete terms. They try to relate phenomena in the world in a logical, systematic manner, which is both satisfying and occasionally disheartening. Religion is a means whereby children can relate to their deity in a direct and personal way.

Prayer and other religious rituals are often a comfort to children, and if these activities are a part of children's daily lives, they can help children cope with threatening situations (Fig. 17-5). Their petitions to their God in prayers tend to be for tangible rewards. Although younger children expect their prayers to be answered, as children get older they begin to recognize that this does not always occur and become less concerned when prayers are not answered. They are able to discuss their feelings about their faith and how it relates to their lives (see Cultural Competence box).

🌐 **CULTURAL COMPETENCE**

Religious Orientation

Many schools and communities have a Judeo-Christian orientation toward prayer, holidays, and values. This may result in conflict and discomfort for children of other religious and ethnic groups. Schools should exercise sensitivity so as not to offend and confuse children from other religious backgrounds, such as the Buddhist, Hindu, and Muslim faiths.

LANGUAGE DEVELOPMENT

Children enter middle childhood with remarkably efficient language skills, but they make many important linguistic achievements during the school-age years. During the elementary school years they learn to correct previous syntactic errors and begin to use more complex grammatical forms, such as correct past tenses for irregular verbs, correct plurals for irregular nouns, and correct personal pronouns.

Word usage and the ability to find and retrieve words quickly when called on to produce what they know in a relatively short time grow considerably during the school years. Children learn to apply the minimum-distance principle—the rule that the subject of a verb in an active sentence is the noun or pronoun that immediately precedes it. For example, a 6-year-old child will understand the sentence "Ask Mary her last name" but until age 9 or 10 years will be confused by the sentence "Ask Mary what to bring to the party."

Narrative skills improve markedly. School-age children are increasingly able to provide directives that others can correctly interpret without visual data (e.g., explain directions over the telephone). By age 10 to 12 years the child should be able to use factitive words (such as *know, think,* and *believe*), as well as complex pronouns and conjunctions, and be able to form grammatically correct sentences. School-age children gradually become more proficient at making inferences about meanings and learn the subtle exceptions to grammatical rules. This makes them less likely to engage in literal interpretation of messages.

They rapidly develop metalinguistic awareness—an ability to think about language and to comment on its properties. This enables them to appreciate jokes, riddles, and puns that involve play on words, sounds, or double meanings. They are beginning to understand metaphors and figurative statements, such as "A stitch in time saves nine." The acquisition of cognitive skills enables them to think about the quality of their own and others' speech and to evaluate and clarify messages.

SOCIAL DEVELOPMENT

At the beginning of middle childhood, children enter a period of less intense emotions, secure in their dependency on their parents and family and with self-confidence tempered by a more realistic perspective. They have the energy to explore the environment beyond the family, to gradually increase the scope of interpersonal interactions, and to invest their curiosity in understanding the world.

Identification with peers is a strong influence in children's gaining independence from parents. The aid and support of peers provides children with enough security to risk the moderate parental rejection brought about by each small victory in their development of independence.

Questions of masculinity and femininity take on importance as sex-role learning assumes more prominence. Boys associate with boys, and girls with girls, each group pursuing its own interests, with communication between the sexes confined to that which is necessary. Much of the child's concept of the appropriate sex role is acquired through relationships with peers. During the early school years there is little difference relative to sex in the play experiences of children. Both girls and boys share games and other activities. However, in the later school years the differences become marked.

Social Relationships and Cooperation

Daily relationships with age-mates provide the most important social interactions for school-age children. For the first time, children are able to join in group activities with unrestrained enthusiasm and steady participation. Previously, interactions were limited to short periods under considerable adult supervision. With increased skills and wider opportunities, children become involved with one or several peer groups in which they can gain status as respected members.

Valuable lessons are learned from daily interaction with age-mates. First, children learn to appreciate the numerous and varied points of view that are represented in the peer group. As they play together, children discover that there are many occupations for fathers and mothers, more than one version of the same song, different rules for the same game, and different customs for celebrating the same holiday. As children interact with peers who see the world in ways that are somewhat different from their own, they become aware of the limits of their own point of view. Because age-mates are peers and are not forced to accept one another's ideas as they are expected to accept those of adults, other children have a significant influence on decreasing the egocentric outlook of the individual child. Consequently, children learn to argue, persuade, bargain, cooperate, and compromise to maintain friendships.

Second, children become increasingly sensitive to the social norms and pressures of the peer group. The peer group establishes standards for acceptance and rejection, and children may be willing to modify their behavior to be accepted by the group. They are judged by the physical impression they convey, the skills they possess, and other abilities they can demonstrate. The need for peer approval becomes a powerful influence toward conformity. Children learn to dress, talk, and otherwise behave in a manner acceptable to the group. A variety of roles, such as class joker or class hero, may be assumed by the individual child to gain approval from the group. However, no child can adapt perfectly to all the requirements of the peer group. If some children find differences between the values of the peer group and the values of their families to be too great, they may relinquish the pleasure of interaction with the group to abide by the regulations established in the home. Thus, to diminish conflict within the family, some children may be forced into a position outside the peer group.

Third, the interaction among peers leads to the formation of intimate friendships between same-sex peers (Fig. 17-6). School age is the time when children have "best friends" with whom they share secrets, private jokes, and adventures; they come to one another's aid in times of trouble. In the course of these friendships, children also fight, threaten, break up, and reunite. These dyadic relationships, in which children experience love for and closeness with a peer, seem to be important as a foundation for heterosexual relationships in adulthood. The conflicts encountered in the relationship are usually resolved in terms that children are able to control. Because neither child has authority over the other, as in an adult-child relationship, children must work through their differences within the framework of their commitment to each other.

Clubs and Peer Groups

One of the outstanding characteristics of middle childhood is the formation of formalized groups or clubs. Initially, children in the early middle years merely hang around the periphery of the formalized group, watching, learning, practicing various

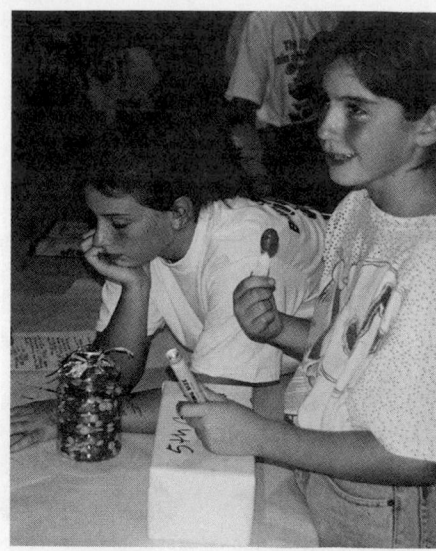

Fig. 17-6 School-age children enjoy engaging in activities with a "best friend."

skills, and participating in group activities whenever the members of the group allow them to do so. As they age, children eventually take their places as full-fledged participating group members.

A prominent feature of middle childhood groups is the code of rigid rules imposed on the members. Exclusiveness is evident in the selection of persons given the privilege of joining. Acceptance in the group often depends on a pass-fail basis according to social or behavioral criteria. Conformity is the core of the group structure. There are often secret codes, shared interests, special modes of dress, and special words that signify membership in the group. Each child must follow a standard of behavior established by the group. Conforming to the rules provides children with feelings of security and relieves them of the responsibility of making decisions.

Membership in the group provides children with a comfortable place in society. Many of the qualities valued by the group, such as physical strength, daring, ingenuity, and comradeship, have not been stressed in the family. However, these are values that contribute to an individual child's total personality. By merging their identity with the identities of their peers, children move from the family group to an outside group as a step toward further independence. They substitute conformity to a peer-group pattern for conformity to a family pattern while they are still too insecure to function independently.

During the early school years, groups are small and loosely organized, with changing membership and little formal structure. They do not demonstrate the elements of give and take, cooperation, and order that are seen in groups of older children. As a rule, girls' groups are less formalized than boys' groups, and although there may be a mixture of both sexes in groups in the earlier school years, those of later school years are composed predominantly of children of the same sex. Common interests are frequently the central element around which a group is structured.

Children's strong desire not to be different creates problems for those who are, for various reasons, unable to meet the accepted standards of the peer group. Children with disabilities or those who are in some way unable to compete have a difficult time. Children become self-consciousness when they are unable to dress like other children, do not have spending money like other children, or appear different from other children.

Children who have physical characteristics that are obviously different (such as birthmarks, ears that "stick out," or physical defects) may be set apart from the peer group and become a target for the criticism and ridicule. Peer-group identification and association are essential to socialization.

Poor relationships with peers and a lack of group identification can also contribute to bullying behavior. Bullying is the infliction of repetitive physical, verbal, or emotional abuse by one or more individuals intended to harm or bother another who is perceived as being less physically or psychologically powerful than the aggressor(s). Bullying can occur in varying degrees of severity in a physical, social, or emotional context. Boys usually participate in more direct or physical acts of bullying, whereas girls are commonly more involved with indirect acts such as spreading rumors or social exclusion. Although bullying can occur in any setting, it usually takes place in a classroom or on the playground when supervision is minimal (Vreeman and Carroll, 2007). Approximately 25% of students engage in bullying or are victims of bullying during elementary school, with bullying peaking on transition from elementary to secondary school (Jenson and Dieterich, 2007). Children who are bullies are often defiant, antisocial, impulsive, easily frustrated, and likely to break school rules.

Bullies and victims of bullying are at risk for long-term psychologic disturbances and psychiatric symptoms. Future problems of bullies include a higher risk for conduct problems, hyperactivity, school drop-out, and participation in criminal behavior (Gini, 2007; Jenson and Dieterich, 2007). Victims of bullying are at increased risk for low self-esteem; anxiety; feelings of insecurity; poor academic performance; and psychosomatic complaints such as feeling tense, tired, or dizzy (Gini, 2007; Jenson and Dieterich, 2007). Bullying can be reduced or prevented through supportive relationships with family, intervention of school personnel, and involvement with positive peer groups.* Many school districts have developed bullying prevention programs in response to local circumstances; however, these programs have yet to be critically evaluated for their effectiveness.

Although peer-group identification and association are essential to a child's emergence into the world, dangers are inherent in strong peer-group attachment. Peer pressure may force children into taking risks, even against their better judgment. Peer-group activities that result in unacceptable, unlawful, or criminal gang violence are increasing in the United States and represent a significant challenge for health professionals and teachers who work with children (see Community Focus box).

---

*For information on bullying and how to prevent it in the school setting, contact Educators for Social Responsibility, 23 Garden St., Cambridge, MA 02138; 617-492-1764 or 800-370-2515; www. esrnational.org.

🏠 COMMUNITY FOCUS

Providing Guidance About Gangs

Parents of school-age children often worry about the informal and unstructured social groups that their children are attracted to and wish to join. Parents of boys seem particularly concerned about "boys only" groups and the possibility that such groups could become gangs and participate in violent activities.

To help parents cope with these fears, nurses can encourage parents to become aware of any gang-related activities in their community. Typically, activities of organized gangs are illegal, and children involved in gang activities may experience frequent accidents or trips to the emergency department or police station. In addition, gang members frequently have characteristics that parents can identify, such as graffiti, a particular clothing style, unique tattoos, hand signals, or violent illegal initiation rituals. Nurses can also encourage parents to become acquainted with their child's friends and to become involved in providing positive recreational activities for their children.

The community's awareness of gangs that promote violence is essential to stop the spread of gang membership among youth. The media can inform the community of gang influx, identification, and activities to raise parents' awareness of the potential dangers to their children. Community services that promote a sense of belonging among children and offer structured recreational and social events can help youth find alternatives to being a gang member.

Relationships with Families

Although the peer group is highly influential and necessary to normal child development, parents are the primary influence in shaping children's personalities, setting standards for behavior, and establishing value systems. Family values usually predominate when parental and peer value systems come into conflict. Although children may appear to reject parental values while testing the new values of the peer group, ultimately they retain and incorporate many parental values into their own value systems. Peer associations seem to remain within the social class system.

As children move into a wider world of peer-group relationships, parents are faced with the task of letting go of control. Parents may find it difficult to face the rejection that children demonstrate as they become more involved with their peer groups. Children may want to spend more time in the company of their peers, may seem eager to leave the house, and often prefer activities of the peer group to family activities. During this time, children discover that parents can be wrong, and they begin to question the knowledge and authority of the parents who previously were considered to be all-knowing and all-powerful. Parents can best serve the interests of their children through tolerant understanding and support.

Although increased independence is the goal of middle childhood, children are not yet prepared to abandon parental control. Children need and want restrictions placed on their behavior; they are not yet prepared to cope with all of the problems of their expanding environment. They feel more secure knowing that there is an authority greater than themselves to implement controls and restrictions. Children may complain loudly about the restrictions and try to break down parental barriers, but they are uneasy if they succeed in doing so. Children feel secure with reasonable, consistent controls. They respect the adults on whom they can rely to prevent them from acting on each and every urge. Children see this behavior as an expression of love and concern for their welfare.

Children also need their parents as adults, not as "pals." Sometimes parents, hurt by their children's rejection, attempt to maintain their children's love and gratitude by assuming the role of pal. Children need the stable, secure strength provided by mature adults to whom they can turn during troubled relationships with peers or stressful changes in their world. During a disruption in their lives, such as times of failure, periods of illness, or a move that separates them from the security of friends, children need the firm, secure anchor of parental interest and concern. With a secure base in a loving family, children are able to develop the self-confidence and maturity needed to stand independently.

Children's relationships with siblings change during the middle years. Children view siblings as equal in power and status. In earlier years, older siblings were influential in the younger siblings' learning. In the middle years the relationship becomes one of companionship. Positive emotional tone increases, but sibling conflict also increases as the siblings get older. Middle childhood is a period of transition for sibling relationships, a juncture between the open bickering of early childhood and the supportive relationships observed in adult siblings.

DEVELOPMENT OF SELF-CONCEPT

Closely associated with developing a sense of industry is developing a concept of one's value and worth. With the emphasis on skill building and broadened social relationships, children are continually occupied in the process of self-evaluation. Children's self-concepts are composed of their own critical self-assessments plus their interpretations of the opinions of others. Self-concept refers to a conscious awareness of a variety of self-perceptions, such as one's physical characteristics, abilities, values, and self-ideals, and one's idea of self in relation to others.

Body Image

Body image is what children think about their bodies. School-age children are knowledgeable about the human body, and social development during this period focuses to a large extent on the body and its capabilities. School-age children can draw a recognizable human figure, although individually their portrayal of body parts may vary considerably. They are acutely aware of their own bodies as well as those of their peers and those of adults. It is important that children know body functions and that adults correct any misinformation children have about the body (e.g., what is fat).

During the school years, children focus on peer relationships and conform to group norms. They evaluate how their physical appearance, body configuration, and coordination compare with those of their peers. The head is the most noticeable and, to them, important part of the body. They also model themselves after their parents and compare themselves to favored peers and images observed in the media.

Children are aware of physical disabilities in others, and it is not unusual for them to believe that their own bodies are not the right size or the right shape or are in some way defective.

They respond to such concerns in a variety of ways. For example, they will conceal perceived shortcomings of body or performance, as in the obese child who refrains from going swimming, the child who conveniently forgets a gym suit, the child who conceals an imagined defect, or the child with enuresis who declines invitations to slumber parties. Children seldom express these concerns to families. However, they need reassurance about both the uniqueness and the sameness of their bodies while their privacy is respected and they are allowed appropriate protective strategies. Children who are different become aware of the differences and may find themselves excluded from the group. When children are teased or criticized about being different, the effect can last even into adulthood.

Self-Esteem

Self-esteem is children's pictures of their individual worth and consists of both positive and negative qualities. Children actively strive to achieve internalized goals. At the same time, they continually receive feedback on the quality of their performance from individuals they consider to be authorities. By the time they reach school age, children have received messages regarding the extent to which they are able to accomplish tasks that have been delegated to them. For example, one child may have been given prestigious responsibilities at home or at school or received special commendation for an achievement. On the other hand, another child may have been sent to a special class for slow learners or may have been the last person selected when children chose sides for a game. These and other signs serve as clues to social worth that children incorporate as part of their self-evaluation.

Children approach the process of self-evaluation from a framework of either self-confidence or self-doubt. Children who have mastered the maturational crises of autonomy and initiative are able to face the world with feelings of pride rather than shame. At first, children's self-concepts are formed exclusively from their perceptions of their parents' evaluation of them. During middle childhood the opinions of peers and teachers are important. Criticisms and peer approval are additional sources of data for evaluation. Parents and other adults are no longer the only persons who respond to their skills, talents, and abilities; peers also identify skills and capabilities. Each child soon begins to internalize these outside opinions. If children regard themselves as worthwhile or satisfactory persons, they have high self-esteem, self-confidence, and a positive self-concept. If they view themselves as worthless, they have low self-esteem.

Pets also influence a child's self-esteem. Pets can have a positive effect on physical and emotional health and can teach children the importance of nurturing and nonverbal communication (Podberscek, 2006).

Children encounter difficulties assessing their own abilities because they rely on their own expectations or on the expectations expressed by others regarding their performance. They depend almost entirely on external evidence of worth, such as school grades, teachers' comments, and parental and peer approval. Children do not yet have the capacity to develop their own independent criteria to evaluate their own accomplishments. It is especially difficult for them to assess their achievement in abstract skills.

Nothing succeeds like success. Significant adults in children's lives can often manage to manipulate the environment so that children meet with success. Each small success can improve a child's self-image. The more positive children feel about themselves, the more confident they feel in trying again for success. All children profit from feeling that they are special to significant adults. A positive self-image makes them feel likable, worthwhile, and capable of valuable contributions. Such feelings lead to self-respect, self-confidence, and a general feeling of happiness. Parents can help their school-age children develop self-esteem by being honest, by providing opportunities for creativity, by helping them succeed in activities, and by providing positive reinforcement. Nurses can enhance self-esteem by fostering supportive relationships between children and members of their families and by emphasizing children's strengths and positive aspects of their behavior (see Community Focus box).

🏠 COMMUNITY FOCUS

Socialization of Boys and Girls

Health professionals have long been aware that boys and girls are socialized differently by parents and teachers. Girls are encouraged to express their emotions and to be sensitive and responsive to others. Boys, on the other hand, are often told to hide their feelings and are criticized if they are "too sensitive." In school, boys are encouraged to take the most challenging courses, to do well in math and science, and to participate in athletic endeavors. Girls may be discouraged from taking math and science, ostracized socially if they take typically "male" courses, and penalized for joining athletic teams. These differences in socialization may contribute to stereotypic behavior and the way that boys and girls relate to each other. Boys may feel entitled to life's opportunities and benefits, and girls may think that they need to be submissive and deferential to succeed. Such beliefs may ultimately influence participation in risk-taking behaviors in adolescence.

To prevent the development of a sense of entitlement in boys and to foster self-reliance in girls, parents can encourage boys to be socially and interpersonally sensitive and responsive to others, and teach boys that interrupting girls is rude and inappropriate behavior. Teachers can encourage girls, as well as boys, to take the challenging courses in math and science, foster cooperation between boys and girls on school projects, and facilitate the development of athletic endeavors for not only boys but also girls. Some schools are providing same-sex courses to provide a more neutral and nurturing environment for students.

DEVELOPMENT OF SEXUALITY

Evidence indicates that many children experience some form of sex play during or before preadolescence as a response to normal curiosity, not as a result of love or sexual urge. Children are experimentalists by nature, and this play is incidental and transitory. Adverse emotional consequences or guilt feelings depend on how the parents manage the behavior and whether children view their actions as wrong in the eyes of significant persons, particularly their parents.

Children's attitudes toward sex are acquired indirectly at an early age and affect the way they respond to sexual information presented later. Many parents discourage sexual exploration, either through subtle substitution of activities that divert their children's attention from the genitalia or by expressions of anger or disgust at their children's behavior. These tactics clearly communicate to children that they should not engage in such activities, discourage questions about sex, and limit the sources of information.

Sex Education

Parents may not teach young children the correct terminology for sexual organs or sexual feelings. Often the only vocabulary available to children is one that identifies sexual organs with excretory functions. If children learn that excretory organs and functions are dirty, they may associate "dirtiness" with the reproductive organs and functions. If children learn the correct terminology for the organs and their functions, this will eliminate or reduce this association.

Because parents often either repress or avoid their children's sexual curiosity, sexual information received in childhood may be acquired almost entirely from peers. Such information is often transmitted in secret conversations and contains considerable misinformation. These communications can also create anxiety in children and inhibit spontaneous expressions or questioning of their parents.

Although middle childhood is an ideal time for formal sex education, this subject has created considerable controversy. Many parents and groups are unconditionally opposed to the inclusion of sex education in the schools. Others believe that information relating to sexual maturation and the process of reproduction should be presented as naturally as information about other natural phenomena, such as the growth of plants, the changing seasons, and the migratory habits of birds. When sex education is presented from a life span perspective and treated as a normal part of growth and development, the information is less likely to contain overtones of uncertainty, guilt, or embarrassment that could in turn produce anxiety in children.

Sex education programs have been successfully incorporated into a number of elementary school curricula. In many of these programs, sexuality is presented in the context of its central role as a biologic mechanism for the survival of the culture. Children learn that sexual maturation and reproduction represent each individual's contribution to the natural order of things. This approach provides a natural entry into discussion of sexuality as a basis for family units, marriage, and attitudes toward children, as well as an entry into a presentation of the biologic facts of sexuality. Many sex education programs also emphasize that sexual intimacy is part of a close, personal relationship and a means of conveying love, as well as a means for ensuring the survival of the species.

Nurse's Role in Sex Education

No matter where nurses practice, they can provide information on human sexuality to both parents and children. To discuss the topic adequately, nurses must understand the physiologic aspects of sexuality; know the common myths and misconceptions associated with sex and the reproductive process; understand cultural and societal values; and be aware of their own attitudes, feelings, and biases.

When nurses present sexual information to children, they should treat sex as a normal part of growth and development. Nurses should answer questions honestly, matter-of-factly, and at the child's level of understanding. School-age children may be more comfortable when boys and girls are segregated for discussions; however, each group needs information about both sexes.

Children need help to differentiate sex and sexuality. Exercises focused on clarifying values, identifying role models, solving problems, and accepting responsibility are important to prepare school-age children for early adolescence and puberty. In addition, care providers need to explain sexual information that is discussed via the media or jokes. A comprehensive sex education program including information about abstinence, contraception, and birth control methods should be presented during the middle school years (Eisenberg, Bernat, Bearinger, et al, 2008). Teaching a child to be sexually responsible is an important component of sex education. Health care providers should supply specific information concerning sexually transmitted infections, human immunodeficiency virus (HIV), and acquired immunodeficiency syndrome (AIDS). Anticipatory guidance should include information about prevention, transmission, and implications of sexually transmitted infections.

Preadolescents need precise and concrete information that will allow them to answer questions such as "What if I start my period in the middle of class?" or "How can I keep people from telling I have an erection?" It is important to tell them what they want to know and what they can expect to happen as they mature sexually.

During encounters with parents, nurses can be open and available for questions and discussion. They can set an example by the language they use in discussing body parts and their function and by the way in which they deal with problems that have emotional overtones, such as exploratory sex play and masturbation. Parents need help to understand normal behaviors and to view sexual curiosity in their children as a part of the developmental process. Assessing the parents' level of knowledge and understanding of sexuality provides cues to their need for supplemental information that will prepare them for increasingly complex explanations as their children grow older.

Children with developmental disabilities need emotional and sexual relationships. Parents of children with developmental disabilities may need special assistance and help with sex education. In 1996 the American Academy of Pediatrics developed specific guidelines that discuss ways to teach these children about human anatomy, pubertal changes, expression of physical affection, protection from sexual abuse or exploitation, and independence in personal hygiene and self-care. Sex education for children with disabilities requires individualized techniques, depending on the type and degree of disability (Murphy and Young, 2005). Nurses must bring the issue of sexuality out in the open and promote the idea that sexuality is a part of every individual's identity in order to address educational needs (Murphy and Young, 2005).

Sometimes participation in short classes or group discussions can help parents address disturbing behaviors and anticipate their children's questions and learning needs. It is wise to include both parents in such activities when possible. Both parents should assume responsibility for sex education in the home so that the children will not acquire a distorted view of either the male or the female role that may alter relationships with the opposite sex in later life.

PLAY

As children enter the school years, their play takes on new dimensions that reflect a new stage of development. Not only does play involve increased physical skill, intellectual ability, and fantasy, but as children form groups and cliques, they begin to evolve a sense of belonging to a team or club. To belong to a group is of vital importance. Clubs, societies, and organizations are important parts of the culture of childhood.

Rules and Rituals

The need for conformity in middle childhood is strongly manifested in the activities and games so important in the life of school-age children. Up to this point, they have either played games they have invented themselves or have played in the company of a friend or an adult, and rules more or less evolved with the game. Now they begin to see the need for rules, and the games they play have fixed and unvarying rules that may be bizarre and extraordinarily rigid (especially those made up by the group). But part of the enjoyment of the game is knowing the rules, because knowing means belonging. Once the rules are established and agreed on, the demand for conformity is strong (Fig. 17-7).

Conformity and ritual characterize the play of school-age children, not only in games, but also in behavior and language. Childhood is full of chants and taunts, such as "Eeny, meeny, miney, mo," "Last one is a rotten egg," and "Step on a crack,

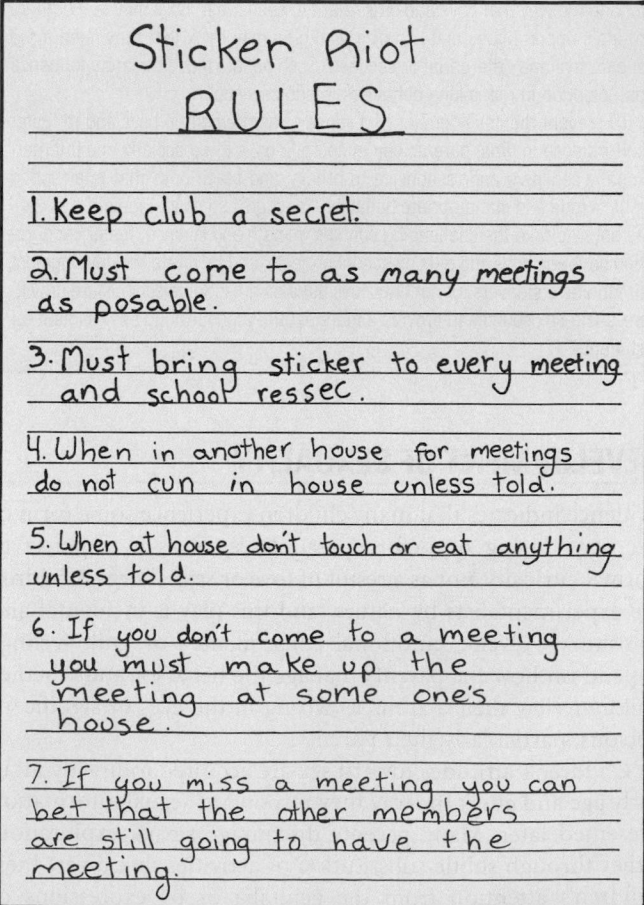

Sticker Riot
RULES

1. Keep club a secret.

2. Must come to as many meetings as posable.

3. Must bring sticker to every meeting and school ressec.

4. When in another house for meetings do not cun in house unless told.

5. When at house don't touch or eat anything unless told.

6. If you don't come to a meeting you must make up the meeting at some one's house.

7. If you miss a meeting you can bet that the other members are still going to have the meeting.

Fig. 17-7 A list of club rules compiled by a group of 9-year-old children.

break your mother's back." Children receive a great deal of pleasure and power from such sayings, which have been handed down with few changes through generations.

Team Play

A more complex form of group play that develops from the need for peer interaction involves the team games and sports that are part of the school years. Such games may require a referee, umpire, or person of authority so the rules can be followed more accurately. Team membership has several characteristics that promote child development during the middle years.

Children learn to subordinate personal goals to group goals. Team membership means that each child is accountable to the other team members and that each member's acts may affect the success or failure of the entire group. Each member's behavior is open to public evaluation, and children risk ostracism, ridicule, or scapegoating if they contribute to a team loss. Although individual skills are recognized, team successes and failures are shared by all members. Children learn the concept of interdependence and the reliance of all players on one another.

Children learn that division of labor is an effective strategy for the attainment of a goal. Each person on a team has a specific function, which increases the team's chances of winning. Once children learn that certain goals are best accomplished by dividing tasks among several individuals, they can transfer this knowledge to other social situations. Children also learn that some children are best equipped to perform one part of the task and other children are best suited to another aspect of the task.

Team play helps children learn about the nature of competition. In all team play there is a winning side and a losing side. Because losing is often interpreted as failure, children go to great lengths to avoid the public embarrassment and personal shame that accompany failure. The more a child identifies with the team and values membership in the group, the more distasteful losing becomes. Fear of losing and the failure it implies are strong incentives for group commitment; however, winning is not universally given high value. Some cultures and subcultures emphasize the game and consideration for one's companions rather than the outcome.

Team play also contributes to children's social, intellectual, and skill growth. Children work hard to develop the skills needed to become members of a team, to improve their contribution to the group effort, and to anticipate the consequences of their behavior for the group. Team play helps stimulate cognitive growth as children are called on to learn many complex rules, make judgments about those rules, plan strategies, and assess the strengths and weaknesses of members of their own and the opposing teams (Fig. 17-8).

Quiet Games and Activities

Although the play of school-age children can be highly active, they also enjoy many quiet and solitary activities. The middle childhood years are the time for collections, and young school-age children's collections are an odd assortment of unrelated objects in messy, disorganized piles. Collections of later years are more orderly and selective and often are organized neatly in scrapbooks, on shelves, or in boxes.

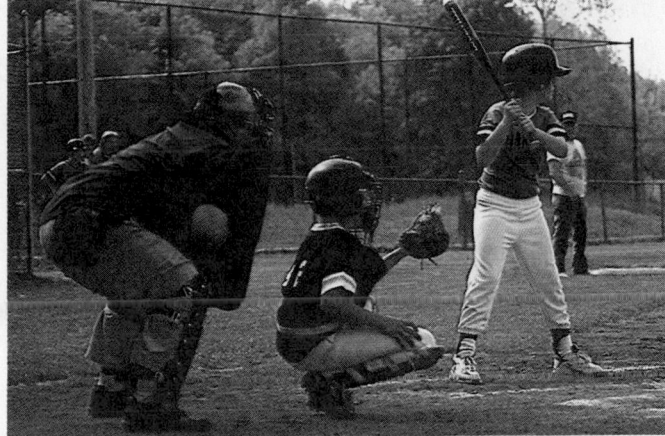

Fig. 17-8 Activities engaged in by school-age children, such as Little League baseball, vary according to each child's interest and opportunity.

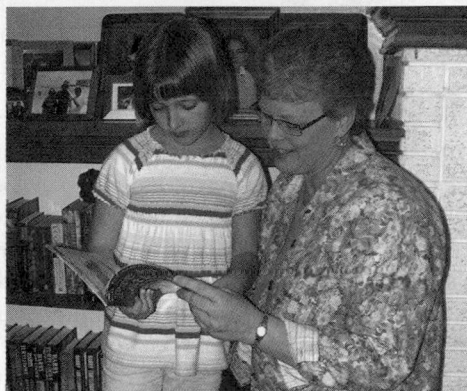

Fig. 17-9 Selecting a book with the assistance of an adult.

School-age children become fascinated with increasingly complex board, card, and computer games. Children play these games alone or in groups. As in all games, the adherence to rules is fanatic. There is usually much discussion and argument, but children easily resolve disagreement by learning the appropriate rules of the game.

The newly acquired skill of reading becomes increasingly satisfying as school-age children begin to expand their knowledge of the world through books (Fig. 17-9). School-age children never tire of stories, and, like preschool children, they love to have stories read aloud. They also enjoy sewing, cooking, carpentry, gardening, and creative endeavors such as painting. Many creative skills, such as those involving music and art, and athletic skills, such as swimming, riding, hiking, dancing, and karate, are acquired during childhood and continue to be enjoyed into adolescence and adulthood (Fig. 17-10).

Hero worship is another characteristic of children and adolescents. The object of the adoration can be a friend, relative, teacher, or national sports or entertainment figure. However, problems can arise when the idol proves to be an inappropriate role model.

Ego Mastery

Play also affords children the means to acquire representational mastery over themselves, their environment, and other persons. Through play, children can feel as big, as powerful, and as

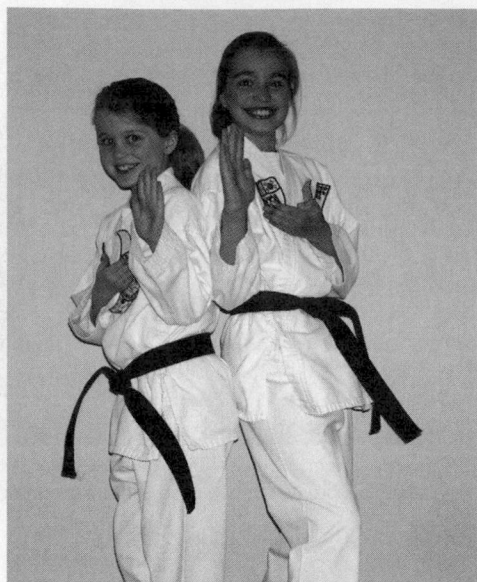

Fig. 17-10 School-age children take pride in learning new skills.

skillful as their imaginations will allow, and they can attain vicarious mastery and power over whomever and whatever they choose. They need to feel in control in their play. School-age children still need the opportunity to use large muscles in exuberant outdoor play and the freedom to exert their newfound autonomy and initiative. They need space in which to exercise large muscles and to work off tensions, frustrations, and hostility. Physical skills practiced and mastered in play help to develop a feeling of personal competence, which contributes to a sense of accomplishment and helps provide a place of status in the peer group.

Table 17-1 presents a summary of growth and development in middle childhood. Because each child has a unique developmental pattern, any descriptions of the typical child of any age-group can represent only an average and should not be considered as absolute criteria for any given child.

COPING WITH CONCERNS RELATED TO NORMAL GROWTH AND DEVELOPMENT

SCHOOL EXPERIENCE

School serves as an agent for transmitting societal values to each succeeding generation of children and as a setting for many peer relationships. As a socializing agent second only to the family, school exerts a profound influence on the social development of children.

School entrance causes a sharp break in the structure of a child's world. For some children it is their first experience in conforming to a group pattern imposed by an adult who is not a parent and who has responsibility for too many children to be constantly aware of each child as an individual. Children want to go to school and usually adapt to the new environment with little difficulty. Successful adjustment is directly related to the child's physical and emotional maturity and the parents' readiness to accept the separation associated with school entrance. Cooperation among parents and support for the

child are successful ways of coping with school entry stress. Unfortunately, some parents express their unconscious attempts to delay their child's maturity by clinging behavior, particularly with their youngest child.

Anticipatory Socialization

By the time they enter school, most children have a fairly realistic concept of what school involves. They receive information regarding the role of pupil from parents, playmates, and the media. In addition, most children have had experience with daycare or preschool and kindergarten.

Children's attitudes toward school and the extent of their adjustment are strongly influenced by their parents' attitudes. Middle-class children have fewer adjustments to make and less to learn about expected behavior because the school tends to reflect dominant middle-class customs and values, although this may be tempered by the school's location and predominant teachers and student body. Parents who view school as a place that they have helped to create and support and that is directed toward the same objectives for socialization as their own usually prepare their children with useful anticipatory socialization and furnish them with confidence to meet the challenge. Parents who view the school as an alien culture and one that they have little, if any, power to affect may unknowingly teach their children to be fearful and resentful toward school, even though the parents agree with its purposes and objectives.

The television, which influences the acquisition of information and attitudes, also provides anticipatory socialization. Television viewing has the potential to increase a child's vocabulary, extend the child's horizons, and enrich the school experience. However, television relies heavily on images to convey information. Consequently, it is difficult to explore complex issues by this medium. Extensive television viewing may also encourage children to seek simple answers to tough problems and to believe that violence is the most effective and quick solution to conflict.

Although most children have had some experience with schooling before they enter the first grade, the extent to which early childhood education prepares children for primary school varies. Some preschool programs provide custodial care; others also emphasize emotional, social, and intellectual development. Early childhood programming that stresses cognitive more than social aspects appears to be more effective in facilitating later academic achievement.

Role of the Teacher

To facilitate the transition from home to school, teachers should have personality characteristics that allow them to deal with the needs of young children. Because they react to the teacher on the basis of past experience, children respond best to teachers with attributes that they would find in a warm, loving parent. As a parental surrogate, teachers in the early grades perform many of the activities formerly assumed by the parents, such as recognizing the children's personal needs (e.g., a need to go to the bathroom or for assistance with clothing) and helping to develop their social behavior (e.g., manners).

Teachers, like parents, are concerned about the psychologic and emotional welfare of children. Although the functions of teachers and parents differ, both place constraints on behavior,

TABLE 17-1 GROWTH AND DEVELOPMENT DURING SCHOOL-AGE YEARS

PHYSICAL AND MOTOR	MENTAL	ADAPTIVE	PERSONAL-SOCIAL
Age 6 Yr Height and weight gain continues slowly Weight—16-26.3 kg (35.5-58 lb); height—106.7-123.5 cm (42-49 inches) Central mandibular incisors erupt Loses first tooth Demonstrates gradual increase in dexterity Active age; constant activity Often returns to finger feeding More aware of hand as a tool Likes to draw, print, color Vision reaches maturity	Develops concept of numbers Can count 13 pennies Knows whether it is morning or afternoon Defines common objects such as fork and chair in terms of their use Obeys triple commando in succession Knows right and left hands Says which is pretty and which is ugly of a series of drawings of faces Describes the objects in a picture rather than simply enumerating them Attends first grade	At table, uses knife to spread butter or jam on bread At play, cuts, folds, pastes paper toys; sews crudely if needle is threaded Takes bath without supervision; performs bedtime activities alone Reads from memory; enjoys oral spelling game Likes table games, checkers, simple card games Giggles a lot Sometimes steals money or attractive items Has difficulty owning up to misdeeds Tries out own abilities	Can share and cooperate better Has great need for children of own age Will cheat to win Often engages in rough play Often jealous of younger brother or sister Does what adults are seen doing May have occasional temper tantrums Is a boaster Is more independent, probably influence of school Has own way of doing things Increases socialization
Age 7 Yr Begins to grow at least 5 cm (2 inches) in height per year Weight—17.7-30 kg (39-66 lb); height—111.8-129.5 cm (44-51 inches) Maxillary central incisors and lateral mandibular incisors erupt More cautious in approaches to new performances Repeats performances to master them Jaw begins to expand to accommodate permanent teeth	Notices that certain items are missing from pictures Can copy a diamond Repeats three numbers backward Develops concept of time; reads ordinary clock or watch correctly to nearest quarter hour; uses clock for practical purposes Attends second grade More mechanical in reading; often does not stop at the end of a sentence, skips words such as *it, the,* and *he*	Uses table knife for cutting meat; may need help with tough or difficult pieces Brushes and combs hair acceptably without help May steal Likes to help and have a choice Is less resistant and stubborn	Is becoming a real member of the family group Takes part in group play Boys prefer playing with boys; girls prefer playing with girls Spends a lot of time alone; does not require a lot of companionship
Ages 8-9 Yr Continues to gain 5 cm (2 inches) in height per year Weight—19.6-39.6 kg (43-87 lb); height—116.8-141.8 cm (46-56 inches) Lateral incisors (maxillary) and mandibular cuspids erupt Movement fluid; often graceful and poised Always on the go; jumps, chases, skips Increased smoothness and speed in fine motor control; uses cursive writing Dresses self completely Likely to overdo; hard to quiet down after recess More limber; bones grow faster than ligaments	Gives similarities and differences between two things from memory Counts backward from 20 to 1; understands concept of reversibility Repeats days of the week and months in order; knows the date Describes common objects in detail, not merely their use Makes change out of a quarter Attends third and fourth grades Reads more; may plan to wake up early just to read Reads classic books, but also enjoys comics More aware of time; can be relied on to get to school on time Can grasp concepts of parts and whole (fractions) Understands concepts of space, cause and effect, nesting (puzzles), conservation (permanence of mass and volume) Classifies objects by more than one quality; has collections Produces simple paintings or drawings	Makes use of common tools such as hammer, saw, screwdriver Uses household and sewing utensils Helps with routine household tasks such as dusting, sweeping Assumes responsibility for share of household chores Looks after all of own needs at table Buys useful articles; exercises some choice in making purchases Runs useful errands Likes pictorial magazines Likes school; wants to answer all the questions Is afraid of failing a grade; is ashamed of bad grades Is more critical of self Takes music and sports lessons	Is easy to get along with at home Likes the reward system Dramatizes Is more sociable Is better behaved Is interested in boy-girl relationships but will not admit it Goes about home and community freely, alone or with friends Likes to compete and play games Shows preference in friends and groups Plays mostly with groups of own sex but is beginning to mix Develops modesty Compares self with others Enjoys organizations, clubs, and group sports

Continued

TABLE 17-1	GROWTH AND DEVELOPMENT DURING SCHOOL-AGE YEARS—cont'd		
PHYSICAL AND MOTOR	**MENTAL**	**ADAPTIVE**	**PERSONAL-SOCIAL**
Ages 10-12 Yr			
Boys—Slow growth in height and rapid weight gain; may become obese in this period	Writes brief stories	Makes useful articles or does easy repair work	Loves friends; talks about them constantly
Weight—24.3-58 kg (54-128 lb); height—127-162.6 cm (50-64 inches)	Attends fifth to seventh grades	Cooks or sews in small way	Chooses friends more selectively; may have a "best friend"
	Writes occasional short letters to friends or relatives on own initiative	Raises pets	Enjoys conversation
Girls—Pubescent changes may begin to appear; body lines soften and round out	Uses telephone for practical purposes	Washes and dries own hair	Develops beginning interest in opposite sex
Remainder of teeth erupt and tend toward full development (except wisdom teeth)	Responds to magazine, radio, or other advertising	Is responsible for a thorough job of cleaning hair, but may need reminding to do so	Is more diplomatic
	Reads for practical information or own enjoyment—stories or library books of adventure or romance, animal stories	Is sometimes left alone at home for an hour or so	Likes family; family really has meaning
		Is successful in looking after own needs or those of other children left in his or her care	Likes mother and wants to please her in many ways
			Demonstrates affection
			Likes father, who is admired and may be idolized
			Respects parents

and both are in a position to enforce standards of conduct. However, the teacher's primary responsibility is stimulating and guiding children's intellectual development as opposed to providing for their physical welfare beyond the school setting.

Teachers share the parental influence in shaping a child's attitudes and values. They serve as models with whom children can identify and whom they try to emulate. Children seek a teacher's approval and avoid a teacher's disapproval. The teacher is a significant person in the life of the early school-age child, and hero worship of a teacher may extend into late childhood and preadolescence. It is not uncommon for the first or second grader to be heartbroken and tearful at leaving a familiar teacher at the end of the school term or to be upset when faced with a substitute teacher for even a short period.

Children's interest in school and learning and much of their social interaction and self-concept are related to interactions with the teacher (Fig. 17-11). The differential systems of reward and punishment administered by teachers affect the emotional adjustment and self-concept of children and how they respond to school in general.

The interaction between the teacher and an individual pupil affects the pupil's acceptance by other children, which in turn affects the child's self-concept. Behaviors praised by the teacher usually acquire a positive value, whereas those viewed negatively by the teacher are devalued by the children. In this way the teacher exerts considerable influence in a number of areas, such as attitudes toward minority groups, the disabled, or less favorably endowed children. Teacher approval of children and their self-acceptance are closely related.

The teacher sets the emotional tone of the classroom. Those who are able to establish a positive social climate are usually concerned about the mental health and social dynamics of children. Feeling a responsibility for personality development in their pupils, they are alert and sensitive to a child's anxieties, peer-group relationships, self-concepts, and general attitudes toward school. Learner-centered behaviors, such as supportive statements that reassure or commend children,

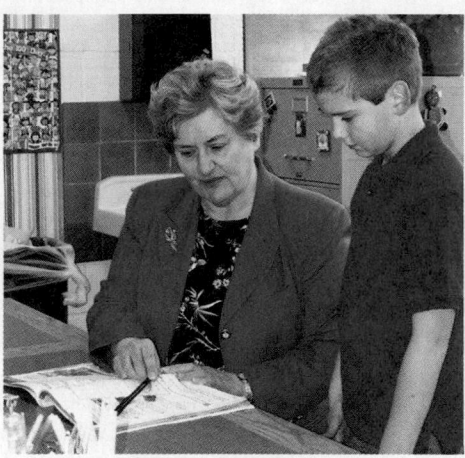

Fig. 17-11 School represents an important change in a child's life, and teachers exert a significant influence on the child.

accepting and clarifying statements that help them refine ideas and feelings to provide a sense of being understood, and constructive assistance that aids them with their own problem solving, contribute to the expansion and development of a positive self-concept.

Role of the Parents

Parents share responsibility with the schools for helping children achieve their maximum potential. Parents can supplement the school program in numerous ways (see Family-Centered Care box). Cultivating responsibility is the goal of parental assistance. Being responsible for schoolwork helps children learn to keep promises, meet deadlines, and succeed at their jobs as adults. Responsible children may occasionally ask for help (e.g., with a spelling list), but usually they like to think through their work by themselves. Excessive pressure or lack of encouragement from parents may inhibit the development of these desirable traits.

👪 FAMILY-CENTERED CARE
Helping Children in School

General Guidelines

Be supportive; through companionship, share ideas and thoughts.

Be positive; every child should experience some success each day.

Share an interest in reading; use the library, discuss books they are reading.

Support and encourage activity rather than passivity.

Encourage originality; help children make their own projects from discarded articles or other available materials.

Foster the development of hobbies and collections.

Encourage children to wonder and reflect during free time.

Encourage family experiences and trips to places of interest.

Encourage questions; help children discover sources for information or places to explore and investigate.

Stimulate creative thinking and problem solving; help children try out new solutions to problems without fear of making mistakes.

Use rewards rather than punishment.

Specific Guidelines

Meet the teacher at the beginning of school and plan to visit the school to see what is taught and expected.

Send the child to school every day. Teachers are concerned when parents make other plans for their children; it conveys the impression that school is unimportant.

Demonstrate an interest in what the child is learning.

Demonstrate an interest in content and growth more than in grades.

Make it clear to the child that schoolwork is between the child and the teacher; teacher and child should set goals for better school performance to allow the child to feel responsible for school successes and failures.

Take advantage of situations that support and reinforce school learning.

Share information with teachers that will help them understand the child better.

Communicate with the teacher if there appears to be a problem; avoid waiting for a scheduled conference.

Provide a quiet, well-lit area for study that is safe from interruption; do not allow television or radio.

Avoid dictating a study time, but do enforce rules, such as no television until homework is done; accept the child's word that work is complete.

Help with homework should focus on explaining the question, not giving the answer.

Teach the child to break large tasks (such as a report) into smaller, manageable tasks spread over the allotted time rather than to attempt the entire project the night before it is due.

Request special help for children with learning problems.

Support the school staff by showing respect for both the school system and the teacher, at least in the child's presence.

DISCIPLINE

Numerous factors influence the amount and manner of discipline imposed on school-age children: the parents' psychosocial maturity, their own childrearing experiences during childhood, the children's temperament, the context of the children's misconduct, and the children's response to rewards and punishments. Discipline serves many purposes: (1) to help the child interrupt or inhibit a forbidden action; (2) to point out a more acceptable form of behavior so that the child knows what is right in a future situation; (3) to provide some reason, understandable to the child, that explains why one action is inappropriate and another action is more desirable; and (4) to stimulate the child's ability to empathize with the victim of a misdeed.

As children are increasingly able to see a situation from the point of view of another, they are able to understand the effects of their reactions on others and themselves. Disciplinary techniques should help children control their own behavior.

To be effective, discipline should take place in an environment characterized by positive, supportive parent-child relationships and should involve strategies that instruct and guide desired behaviors and eliminate undesired or ineffective behaviors (Towe-Goodman and Teti, 2008). Parents should not use punitive actions or corporal punishment, since these methods are of limited value and are associated with increasingly disruptive behavior in children. Negative outcomes associated with corporal punishment are discussed in Chapter 3. In particular, physically aggressive parenting practices that involve spanking are linked to children with poor psychologic adjustment, including depression, anxiety, hopelessness, and destructive behavior such as aggression and violence (Durrant, 2008). Reasoning, on the other hand, is an effective disciplinary technique for school-age children; however, use of a time-out may be necessary to stop the behavior acutely (Towe-Goodman and Teti, 2008).

As their cognitive skills advance, school-age children are able to benefit from more complex disciplinary strategies. For example, withholding privileges, requiring recompense, imposing penalties, and contracting can be used with great success. Problem solving is the best approach to limit setting, and children themselves can be included in the process of determining appropriate disciplinary measures.

Dishonest Behavior

During middle childhood, children may engage in what is considered to be antisocial behavior. Lying, stealing, and cheating may become manifest in previously well-behaved children. This is especially disturbing to parents, who may have difficulty coping with such behavior.

Lying can occur for a number of reasons. Preschool children often have difficulty distinguishing between fact and fantasy. They do not have the cognitive capacity to deliberately mislead. Sometimes they misperceive or fail to remember an event. By the time they reach school age, they still tell stories but can distinguish between what is real and what is make-believe. If not, they need to learn to distinguish between fantasy and reality. Often children will exaggerate a story or situation as a means to impress their family or friends.

Young children lie to escape punishment or get out of some difficulty, even when the evidence of their misbehavior is before their eyes. Lying is more common in families in which punishment is severe. When parents model honesty and veracity, the children will often behave in the same way. If parents lie, the children will emulate their behavior. Older children may lie to meet expectations set by others to which they have been unable to measure up. They may also lie because of low self-esteem or as a means of getting ahead or acquiring something with little effort. However, most children are concerned with the wrongfulness of lying and cheating—especially in their friends. They are quick to tell on others when they detect cheating.

Parents need to be reassured that all children lie sometimes and that they often have difficulty separating fantasy from reality. Providers should help parents to understand the importance of their own behavior as role models and of being truthful in their relationships with children. Parents can discuss the issue with the children directly to impress on them how much of their own security and respect is lost when they are not believed.

Cheating is most common in young children, ages 5 to 6 years. They find it difficult to lose at a game or contest, and they cheat to win. They have not yet acquired the full realization of the wrongfulness of this behavior and do it almost automatically. It usually disappears as they mature. However, when children observe parental behaviors such as boasting about cheating on income taxes, they assume this to be appropriate behavior. Parents need to be aware of the types of behaviors they model for their children. When they set examples of honesty, children are more likely to conform to these standards.

As with other ethically related behavior, stealing is not an unexpected event in the younger child. Between ages 5 and 8 years, children's sense of property rights is limited; they tend to take something simply because they are attracted to it, or they take money for what it will buy. They are equally likely to give away something valuable that belongs to them. When young children are caught and punished, they are penitent—they "didn't mean to" and promise "never to do it again," but they may well repeat the performance the following day. Often they not only steal but lie about it as well or attempt to justify the act with excuses. It is seldom helpful to trap children into admission by asking directly if they did the offensive thing. Children do not take on such responsibility until nearer the end of middle childhood.

Children steal for several reasons: lack of a sense of property rights, an attempt to acquire the means with which to bribe other children for favors, a strong desire to own the coveted item, or a wish for revenge to "get back at someone" (usually a parent) for what they consider to be unfair treatment. Older children may steal to supplement an inadequate income from other sources. Sometimes stealing is an indication that something is seriously wrong or lacking in the child's life. Children may steal to make up for a perceived lack of love or another satisfaction.

In some settings in which living arrangements are crowded, children have little privacy, and much of the family property is communal, children may fail to develop a sense of property rights. Sometimes parents unintentionally confuse children with seemingly conflicting values. In an attempt to teach unselfishness, they may force children to share belongings with others, with the result that the children fail to understand property rights.

If children are told not to take money from their mother's purse or their father's pocket but observe the parents doing the same thing, they receive conflicting messages. Parents may go through a child's pockets or other private areas at night and even discard, without explanation, items of which they do not approve. Children should have a place that is private to them alone that other family members respect. If children's personal rights are respected, they are more likely to respect the rights of others.

It is difficult for many parents to cope with stealing by their children. In most situations it is best not to attempt to find a hidden or deep meaning to the stealing. A reprimand, together with an appropriate and reasonable punishment, such as having the older child pay back the money or return the stolen items, will ordinarily take care of most cases. Most children can learn to respect the property rights of others with little difficulty despite temptations and opportunities. Some children simply need more time to learn the importance of the culture's rules regarding private property.

COPING WITH STRESS

Children today experience more stress than children in previous generations. This stress comes from a variety of sources. Other sections in this book discuss dealing with specific types of stresses, especially those in which nurses assume a major role, such as hospitalization, illness, abuse, disabling injuries, and death or the threat of death.

In the normal course of growing up, children are pressured by their peers to identify with their friends; to eat, dress, and look like their friends; to talk about the same things that their friends talk about; to engage in the same activities as their friends; and yet to compete with them. They are pressured by parents to excel in school, in athletics, and in social situations at ever-younger ages. Children in the middle school years are often over-programmed with activities such as ballet lessons, music lessons, athletics, and other activities until the cumulative effect is overwhelming.

Although children receive better treatment than in earlier times, when beatings and child labor were common, their physical and emotional well-being is threatened by different stresses, especially violence. Children are stressed by conflict within the home. The high divorce rate and the number of single-parent families result in altered relationships and increasing responsibilities for children.

Children's exposure to domestic violence is a significant problem in the United States. Approximately 3.3 million children in the United States witness domestic violence every year (Murrell, Christoff, and Henning, 2007). Children who are exposed to domestic violence are 15 times more likely to be physically abused or neglected than children without exposure (Holt, Buckley, and Whelan, 2008). Parents of violent households may be unable to meet their children's needs and may have ineffective relationships with their children (Holt, Buckley, and Whelan, 2008). These children are often more aggressive, participate in delinquent behaviors, experience developmental and academic deficits, and have difficulties maintaining peer relationships (Murrell, Christoff, and Henning, 2007). In addition, longitudinal studies have shown that children exposed to domestic violence are more likely to display antisocial behavior and become involved in violent crimes and substance abuse as adults (Holt, Buckley, and Whelan, 2008).

Exposure to violence in the family, school, or community affects children's ability to concentrate and function. Children may be traumatized by witnessing violence and develop fear, insecurity, and a sense of helplessness (Fredland, 2008). Children exposed to repeated violence can display hyperarousal symptoms leading to posttraumatic stress disorder and symptoms such as nightmares, flashbacks, a fatalistic orientation to the future, depression, and anxiety (Fowler, Tompsett, Braciszewski, et al, 2009).

School itself is stressful for many children, and school has become a more violent environment. A recent national survey found that 6.5% of students brought a weapon such as a gun, knife, or club to school in the last 30 days, and 8% of students reported being threatened or injured with a weapon (Fredland, 2008). Nearly 30% of students reported that their property was stolen or damaged one or more times while at school (Fredland, 2008).

The school environment may also pose a threat to the middle schooler's self-image. School-age children have a high fear of failure and criticism (Weems and Costa, 2005). Competing with classmates for grades and teacher recognition, failing an examination, being teased or made fun of in school, or being labeled as "stupid" or "learning disabled" all result in emotional distress. Teachers or parents may not always recognize or appreciate the worries or sources of stress for school-age children.

Students' interactions with their teachers are an important component of the school day and can affect student behavior (Eisenbraun, 2007). Children become distressed when teachers raise their voices, yell or scream, or use fear of physical punishment in the classroom. Students exposed to such behavior may show symptoms of stress, express excessive worry about school, demonstrate negative self-perceptions, and verbalize fear of

physical harm by the teacher. Although parents and nurses should be cautious in interpreting such behaviors (they are in many ways similar to school phobia; see Chapter 18), a high degree of suspicion might be justified if the symptoms are not explained by other factors or if they represent a marked change from previous patterns.

Some children are encouraged to feel, think, and behave at a level of maturity far beyond what could reasonably be expected of individuals their age. They are expected to take on many adult-type responsibilities, to make decisions they are not really able to make, and to achieve more. A school's emphasis on high test score achievement can increase stress. Children have little time for being young and enjoying the spontaneous activities of childhood.

When asked to describe sources of worry, school-age children identified concerns such as social threats (e.g., being teased), personal harm, medical procedures, punishment, death, and school performance (Weems and Costa, 2005). Girls are often more sensitive to critical comments at school or other social settings than boys (Li and Prevatt, 2007). Other potential sources of stress are listed in Box 17-1.

BOX 17-1 POTENTIAL SOURCES OF STRESS IN MIDDLE CHILDHOOD*

Sources of Stress for the 6-Year-Old

Expectations—Parents, teachers, and other adults beginning to demand more

School—First grade introduces the child to the more formal, academic setting; may be the child's first experience away from home all day

Activity level—May find it difficult to sit still for long periods; may have frequent accidents, such as spilling milk

Competition—Wants to be "first" or best

Shyness—May initially be shy in a new situation but usually recovers quickly

Aggression—May become hostile or aggressive; temper tantrums peak

Sensitivity—Begins to read body language or facial expressions and becomes upset when sensing disapproval

Teasing—Engages in teasing but becomes upset when on the receiving end

Decisions—Has difficulty coping with increasing independence

Jealousy—Sibling rivalry is common

Fears—Usually center around newly found independence and might include fear of getting lost or fear of making an embarrassing social blunder

Sources of Stress for the 7-Year-Old

Moodiness—Is often moody, unhappy, or pensive

Approval—Continues to need praise and approval from peer group and parents

Modesty—Demands privacy when in the bathroom or dressing

Organization—Is comfortable with rules, regulations, routines, and order; becomes upset when they are disrupted

Interruptions—Hates to be disturbed when intensely involved in an activity

Idols—Has a desire to be more like an admired idol

Friendship—Becomes more selective about playmates

Sources of Stress for the 8-Year-Old

Self-criticism—Is very critical of personal ability and performance

Parental authority—Is beginning to resent parental authority

Loneliness—Likes frequent interaction with friends; may hate to miss school

Praise—Continues to seek approval but can identify when praise is not genuine

Independence—May begin to stay alone for brief periods while parents run errands, with resulting feelings of uneasiness

Sources of Stress for the 9-Year-Old

Rebelliousness—Occasionally tests independence by rebelling

Opposite sex—Engages in sex-segregated play; expresses an aversion to the opposite sex

Fair play—Has a keen sense of what is fair and is vehement in demanding personal rights when a situation is perceived as unfair

Interruptions—Continues to dislike interruptions but will usually resume an activity after an interruption

Propriety—Has a sense of propriety and will often be upset if siblings or parents offend the child's notion of decorum or dignity

Sources of Stress for the 10- to 12-Year-Old

Sexual maturation—Girls, in particular, may become self-conscious regarding obvious signs of development

Social issues—A new level of awareness can generate concern regarding pressing societal problems

Stature—Both boys and girls may be upset by the fact that the girls are taller; the extremely small or extremely large child may be concerned about his or her size

Shyness—If the child already has a problem in this area, it is likely to become more pronounced at this stage

Opposite sex—May become interested, yet shy, around members of the opposite sex

Confusion—Too much freedom can cause the child to flounder

Health—May become a hypochondriac during this period of development

Money—Is anxious to earn and handle money but often uses poor judgment

Competition—Continues to be highly competitive and looks to peer group for prestige

Burnout—May become vigorously involved in so many activities that he or she finally becomes exhausted

Self-concept—May engage in teasing, scapegoating, or vicious attacks to temporarily boost his or her self-image; guilt often ensues; may be self-conscious about attempting a new skill

Parents—Often becomes highly critical or intolerant of parents

Idols—Continues hero worshipping

Fair play—Continues to have a highly developed sense of fair play

Drugs and sex—May be tempted to experiment with drugs or sex because "everyone" is doing it

Peer pressure—Becomes a powerful motivating force

Self-criticism—May be highly critical of personal performance

From Kuczen B: *Childhood stress: don't let your child be a victim*, New York, 1982, Delacorte Press.
*Violence is a universal stress at all ages (see text).

Children respond to stress by using coping mechanisms that include internalizing symptoms such as withdrawal, delaying tactics, and daydreaming, along with externalizing symptoms such as aggression and delinquency (Fowler, Tompsett, Braciszewski, et al, 2009). Variables that contribute to children's ability to cope with stress include socioeconomic status, family relationships, social support, gender, and previous life experiences.

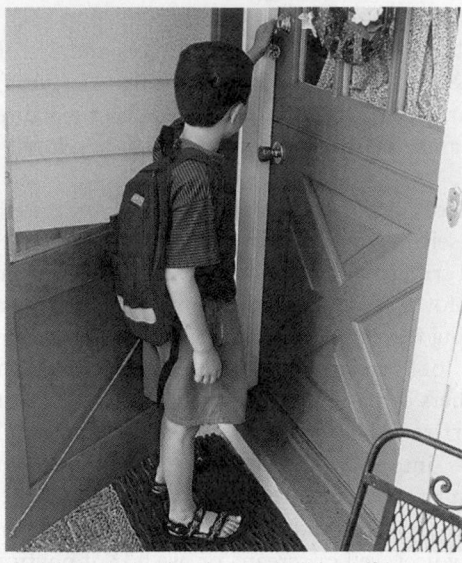

Fig. 17-12 A child unlocks the door to let himself into his home after school.

> **! NURSING ALERT**
>
> The nurse who observes the following signs of stress in a child should explore the situation further:
> - Stomach pains or headache
> - Sleep problems
> - Bed-wetting
> - Changes in eating habits
> - Aggressive or stubborn behavior
> - Reluctance to participate
> - Regression to earlier behaviors (e.g., thumb sucking)

To help children cope with the stresses in their lives, the parent, teacher, or health care worker must recognize signs that indicate that a child is undergoing stress (see Box 17-1) and identify the source promptly. Children need to learn how to recognize signs of stress in themselves, such as a pounding heart, rapid breathing, or "butterflies" in the stomach. Once they are able to recognize that they are stressed, they can employ techniques for managing their stress. Probably the most useful technique is to help them plan a process for dealing with any stress through problem solving.

Children can learn relaxation techniques such as deep-breathing exercises, progressive relaxation of muscle groups, and positive imagery. Encouraging them to "blow off steam" through physical activity reduces tension and anxiety. Children need to learn to identify their stress reactions. Those involving situations or actions of others are easy to identify. Feelings within themselves are sometimes more difficult. Alternative actions must be explored. Children should list all possibilities, including those that they know will not work. They need to examine what might happen as a consequence of each alternative. The final step is to select what they perceive to be the best option. It is sometimes helpful to have children model their behavior after that of someone they know who has successfully coped with a similar problem. When children work through this process a few times, they are able to apply problem solving automatically.

Fears

Several anxiety symptoms, including fear of the dark, excessive worry about past behavior, self-consciousness, social withdrawal, and an excessive need for reassurance, are considered normal developmental events for children. School-age children are less fearful of body safety than they were as preschoolers, although they still fear being hurt, kidnapped, or having to undergo surgery. They also fear death and are fascinated by all aspects of death and dying. They have less fear of noises, darkness, storms, and dogs. Most new fears that trouble school-age

children are related to school and family (e.g., fear of failing, fear of teachers and bullies, or fear of something bad happening to their parents).

Parents and other persons involved with children should discuss children's fears with them individually or through group activities. Their viewpoints must be respected, and their need to communicate their concerns should be recognized. Sometimes school-age children are inclined to hide their fears to avoid being ridiculed or labeled as a "baby" or "chicken." Hiding fears does not end them, and children who are afraid to communicate their fears may develop displaced fears or phobias. Children need to know that their concerns are heard and understood. Parents who convey this to their children without becoming overprotective help their children to feel less lonely and less frightened.

Latchkey Children

The term latchkey children is used to describe children in elementary school who are left to care for themselves before or after school without supervision of an adult (Fig. 17-12). The increasing numbers of single-parent families and working mothers, together with a lack of available child care, have created a stress-provoking situation for many school-age children. Some latchkey children may have a chronic illness as well.

Inadequate adult supervision after school leaves children at greater risk for injury and delinquent behavior. Latchkey children feel more lonely, isolated, and fearful than children who have someone to care for them. To cope with their fears and anxieties while alone, these children may devise strategies such as hiding (in a bathroom, closet, or shower or under a bed), playing the television loudly to drown out noises, and using pets as a comfort.

Many communities and persons concerned about such children's welfare are trying to help children and their parents deal with this potentially serious problem. School-age child care programs have been implemented by some communities and

FAMILY CENTERED-CARE

Latchkey Children

Safety

Teach the child not to display keys and to always lock doors.

Tell the child not to enter the house after school if the door is ajar, a window is open, or anything appears unusual.

Talk through the after-school routine with the child.

Consult with public safety officials about burglar-proofing and fireproofing the home.

Teach the child first-aid procedures.

Teach safety rules to the child who is expected to cook (microwave ovens are safest).

Emphasize fire safety rules and conduct practice fire drills.

Teach and reinforce traffic and bicycle safety.

Teach the child weather-related safety (e.g., stay inside but do not take a bath during an electrical storm; go to and stay in a storm cellar during a tornado warning).

Teach and reinforce water safety practices (e.g., warn the child not to go swimming alone; caution about safe bathing methods and keeping the toilet lid down when infants or toddlers are in their care).

Keep firearms securely locked away and teach the child that they are for adult use only.

Teach the child not to open the door to anyone.

Telephone Use

Teach the child his or her home telephone number, address, and parents' names.

Teach the child to tell callers that parents are "busy"; instruct the child not to tell a caller that parents are not at home.

Teach the child not to tell casual callers the home address; instruct the child to tell the caller that the parents cannot come to the phone right now and will call back later.

Keep a list of emergency numbers by the telephone. Make certain that the child knows how to report emergencies.

Have a list of telephone numbers of friends or neighbors who are available for help with emergencies.

Ask public safety officials to offer classes about when and how to call them.

If a telephone hotline for latchkey children exists, teach the child how to use it.

After-School Activities

Arrange for the child to spend some afternoons with friends.

Provide structured activities for the child.

Have the child attend a public library–sponsored activity rather than watch television at home.

Discuss with the child things to do after school.

Emphasize positive aspects of independence and resourcefulness, but do not demand too much from the child.

Help the child feel successful in self-care.

Consider the potential problems of letting an older child assume care of younger ones before the child is developmentally ready.

Loneliness

Help the child talk about experiences and feelings about being alone after school.

Consider getting a pet to help provide company for the child.

Be punctual in arriving home. A child's anxiety level accelerates when parents are not home when expected.

Call the child if there is a delay in arriving home.

Leave a tape-recorded message for the child to play on arrival home from school.

Form a group of parents with flex-time so that children can be cared for by one of the group after school.

---

employers. Some guidelines appropriate for presentation to parents and/or children to help alleviate their stress and increase the children's safety are listed in the Family-Centered Care box. Other types of programs include those designed to teach self-help skills to children, hotlines that provide telephone check-in and reassurance programs for children, and programs that link latchkey children with reassuring older persons in their community.

Nurses should be aware of services in their communities designed to meet the needs of latchkey children and include this information in anticipatory guidance of school-age children and their families. It is vital that children have adequate supervision and companionship.

PROMOTING OPTIMUM HEALTH DURING THE SCHOOL YEARS

HEALTH BEHAVIORS

During the middle childhood years, children acquire increased cognitive skills that allow them to make decisions about health behaviors they will select and pursue. By the end of middle childhood, children should be able to assume personal responsibility for self-care in the areas of hygiene, nutrition, exercise, recreation, sleep, and safety.

Little is known about how school-age children acquire positive health behaviors. However, both boys and girls view themselves as healthy and can manage their own care in the areas of seat belt use, exercise, emergency situations, and dental health.

Health education is a primary component of comprehensive health care, and health education programs should promote desired health behavior through guided learning and modeling. An optimum program helps children learn about their bodies and about the effect of their behavior on their health.

Health promotion projects teach school-age children that social decision making to promote health is important. Children who attain skills in self-control, social awareness, and problem solving through classroom discussions and practice may engage in fewer risk-taking behaviors.

Children can also learn to take a more active role in relationships with health care providers. If asked what they would like to ask the health practitioner, most children are able to formulate several questions related to the reason for their visit. Providers can also teach children how to ask these questions so they can learn about their health during well-child visits to the pediatrician, nurse practitioner, or school nurse.

NUTRITION

Although caloric needs are diminished in relation to body size during middle childhood, resources are being laid down for the

BOX 17-2 SCHOOL-BASED INTERVENTIONS TO PROMOTE NUTRITION EDUCATION

- Have young children collect pictures of healthy foods and make a poster for display in the school cafeteria.
- Make healthy foods (fruits, vegetables, whole grains, low-fat snacks) available in school vending machines and at school sporting events.
- Discourage the use of high-fat foods (candy bars) as part of school fund-raising projects.
- Avoid the use of food as rewards for behavior; use verbal praise and token gifts to reinforce healthy eating and physical activity.
- Have teachers and school personnel model healthy eating habits.
- Ask children to select foods from a fast-food restaurant menu and to identify those foods high in fat, cholesterol, and sodium.
- Ask each child to keep a diary of foods eaten in 1 day; using MyPlate, evaluate these foods.
- Incorporate nutrition education into other classes (such as using a computer to analyze the nutritional content of foods).
- Have students keep a diary to identify cues for their eating behavior (e.g., hunger, stress, other people, social situations).
- Teach students how to read and discuss the nutrition labels on foods.
- Ask students to examine television commercials, magazine advertisements, and billboards to identify social influences on eating and physical activities.
- Use role playing to help students learn to cope with social and peer pressures to eat specific foods.
- Have students identify environmental barriers to healthy eating.
- Have students prepare nutritious foods, plan menus, and develop a recipe book of healthy foods.
- Involve parents in nutrition education through homework assignments or by inviting parents to attend student-led nutrition fairs.

Modified from Center for Communicable Diseases: Guidelines for school programs to promote lifelong healthy eating, *J Sch Health* 67:9-26, 1996.

increased growth needs of the adolescent period. It is important to impress on children and their parents the value of a balanced diet to promote growth (Box 17-2). When children enter school, they develop an eating style that is increasingly independent from parental influence and scrutiny. Parents do not know what their children eat when they are away from home. A parent may pack a lunch to be eaten at school but be unaware of how much is eaten, traded, sold, or thrown away.

Mealtime continues to be a central issue in many families. Although it should be a pleasant part of a child's day, parents' concern and emphasis on manners often make it a battleground. Likes and dislikes established at an early age continue in middle childhood, although the inclination for single-food preferences begins to end and children acquire a taste for an increasing variety of foods. Because children usually eat as the family does, the quality of their diet depends to a large extent on their family's pattern of eating. Other interests and participation in outside activities often compete with mealtime.

Outside Influences

With the influence of the mass media and the temptation of an immense variety of "junk food," it is all too easy for children to fill up on empty calories—foods that do not promote growth, such as sugars, starches, and excess fats. They have more freedom to move without parental supervision and often have small amounts of money to spend on candy, soft drinks, and other easily accessible treats. Midafternoon snacks are common, and it is wise to encourage consumption of fruit, nuts, and other wholesome finger foods to meet this need. Nutrition is a joint responsibility of both the child and the family.

The popularity of fast-food restaurants has aroused the interest of nutritionists and other health care professionals concerned with children's nutrition. The restaurants provide fast service, they are relatively inexpensive and appealing to children, and their convenience makes them attractive to busy parents as an alternative to eating at home. Because the nutritional content of fast foods is usually available, it is easier for nutrition-conscious parents to help children select appropriate items from the available menu. Nurses can support consumer advocate groups to encourage restaurants to offer items higher in nutritional value (such as skimmed milk, broiled meats, and fresh fruits and vegetables) and to list ingredients on the menu as required for packaged foods.

Childhood obesity is an increasingly prevalent health problem in school-age children. It is estimated that approximately 17% of American children ages 6 to 11 years are overweight (Centers for Disease Control and Prevention, 2009b). The easy availability of high-calorie foods, the tendency toward more sedentary activities (such as watching television and playing or working at a computer), and the trend away from walking or cycling and toward transportation by automobile and bus have reduced caloric expenditure. The consumption of a high-fat diet also contributes to obesity. The problem of childhood obesity is discussed further in Chapter 21. Given the threat of obesity and a diet-conscious society, many school-age children start to diet in an effort to prevent obesity or lose weight or to conform to peer behaviors and pressures. Children need education about food selection and the importance of body-building nutrients as opposed to empty caloric intake.

School Programs

Working parents assume that their children are sufficiently mature and frequently leave the responsibility of meal preparation to them. Although most older school-age children are capable of preparing simple meals, all too often breakfast and lunch may be inadequate, makeshift, or nonexistent. In recognition of this problem, the federal government has established the National School Lunch Program and the School Breakfast Program in many areas. These meals must meet specified nutritional requirements and furnish one third of the daily recommended dietary allowance for children in the United States. Most schools subscribe to the programs, and although the results are difficult to measure directly, it is believed that these school meal programs positively influence the behavior and learning capacity of children. However, the average school lunch may also exceed the recommended dietary guidelines for saturated and total fat. In addition, children who purchase school lunches often select only the items they want. In general, food choices of American children do not meet recommended intakes outlined in the U.S. Department of Agriculture MyPyramid. Many Americans consume too many foods and drinks high in fat and carbohydrates and too little nutrient-dense foods and drinks such as fruits, vegetables, and low-fat milk (Wells and Buzby, 2008).

BOX 17-3 SAMPLE MENU FOR SCHOOL-AGE CHILDREN BASED ON MYPLATE

Breakfast
Cold cereal (1 cup bran flakes, 1 cup fat-free milk, 1 small banana)
1 slice whole wheat toast with 1 tsp soft margarine
1 cup prune juice

Lunch
Tuna fish sandwich (2 slices rye bread, 3 oz tuna [packed in water, drained], 2 tsp mayonnaise, 1 tbsp diced celery, ¼ cup shredded romaine lettuce, 2 slices tomato)
1 medium pear
1 cup fat-free milk

Dinner
3 oz boneless skinless chicken breast, roasted
1 large baked sweet potato
½ cup peas and onions with 1 tsp soft margarine
1 oz whole wheat dinner roll with 1 tsp soft margarine
1 cup leafy salad greens with 3 tsp sunflower oil and vinegar dressing

Snack
¼ cup dried apricots
1 cup low-fat fruited yogurt

Average Servings
Bread, cereal, rice, pasta: 6
Vegetable: 2.5
Fruit: 2
Milk, yogurt, cheese: 3
Meat, poultry, fish, dried beans, nuts: 5.5

http://www.choosemyplate.gov/foodgroups/downloads/Sample_Menus-2000Cals-DG2010.pdf

Nutrition Education

Nutrition education should be integrated throughout the school years into classroom learning. In school, children can learn daily food choices, serving sizes, portion control, and the elements of a wholesome diet using MyPlate (Box 17-3). (See Chapter 6.) Guidelines from the U.S. Department of Agriculture (2009) include the following:

- Balance food and physical activity: choose a lifestyle that combines sensible eating with regular physical activity.
- Choose a diet with plenty of nutrient-dense foods such as grain products, vegetables, and fruits.
- Choose a diet low in fat, saturated fat, and cholesterol.
- Choose protein foods that are lean.
- Eat a variety of foods.
- Choose a diet moderate in salt and sugar.
- Choose calcium-rich foods.

The school nurse should take an active role in nutrition education and work with teachers to implement nutrition instruction that is relevant and interesting to children (see Box 17-2 and Critical Thinking Exercise). The U.S. Department of Agriculture also maintains a website called Team Nutrition that provides nutrition education information and resources for schools, students, parents, and communities.*

*U.S. Department of Agriculture, Food and Nutrition Service, 3101 Park Center Drive, Alexandria, VA 22302; 703-305-1624; www.fns. usda.gov/tn.

? CRITICAL THINKING EXERCISE
Physical Growth in the School-Age Child

Janie, an 8-year-old girl, has just received her annual school physical examination. Janie weighs 30 kg (66 lb) and is 127 cm (50 inches) tall. Janie has gained 4.5 kg (10 lb) since last year and is otherwise reported as in good health with no acute illnesses.

1. Evidence—Is there sufficient evidence to draw conclusions about this situation?
2. Assumptions—Describe the underlying assumption about each of the following:
   a. Changing eating patterns among children
   b. Genetic, environmental, and societal risk factors associated with becoming overweight and obese
   c. Comorbidities associated with overweight and obesity in children
   d. Healthy food choice education for the school-age child
3. What implications for nursing care can be drawn from this situation?
4. Does the evidence support your conclusion?

SLEEP AND REST

The amount of sleep and rest required during middle childhood is highly individualized. The specific amount of needed sleep depends on the child's age, activity level, and other factors such as health status. The growth rate has slowed; therefore less energy is expended in growth than during the preceding periods.

Sleep requirements decrease during school-age years; 5-year-olds generally require 11 hours of sleep, whereas 13-year-olds require approximately 9 hours of sleep (Smaldone, Honig, and Byrne, 2007). School-age children usually do not require a nap. Fewer bedtime problems occur during these years, but occasional difficulties are still associated with the necessary bedtime ritual.

Usually children 6 and 7 years old have few problems, and encouraging quiet activity before bedtime, such as coloring and reading, can facilitate the task of going to bed. Although most children in middle childhood must be reminded to go to bed, 8- to 9-year-old children and 11-year-old children are particularly resistant, with approximately 25% of all school-age children showing reluctance to go to bed (Spruyt, O'Brien, Cluydts, et al, 2005). Often children are unaware that they are tired; if they are allowed to remain up later than usual, they are fatigued the following day. Sometimes parents can resolve bedtime resistance by allowing a later bedtime in deference to their advancing age. Twelve-year-old children usually offer no difficulty in relation to bedtime. Some even retire early to enjoy slow preparations for bed, to read, or to listen to music.

A firm approach to bedtime is usually the most successful. Parents can help children by giving them a little advance warning, but children should realize that when the final bedtime is announced, the parents mean it.

Sleep Problems

During middle childhood, nighttime sleep is usually continuous, and the child has developed a repertoire of tactics (such as reading or playing quietly without involving the parents) to deal with occasional difficulties in falling asleep. If a child has a sleep problem, a thorough assessment may be necessary to plan appropriate interventions.

The cause of bedtime resistance is not always clear. For some children it is related to normal fears of their age, such as fear of the dark, strange noises, intruders, or other imagined phenomena. Children who are subject to frightening dreams are hesitant to retire, and their sleep is more likely to be disturbed after emotional stimulation before bedtime. Sometimes children are unwilling to give up an exciting or interesting activity, or they are reluctant to leave the protective social circle of the family. Another factor associated with reluctance to go to bed is related to status. For example, older children are given the privilege of a later bedtime than younger children. Promotion to a later bedtime is highly prestigious, and age-mates compare their bedtimes. This may explain why children who believe that playmates enjoy a more privileged position strongly oppose parental decisions. In some situations going to bed is used as a method of control. When going to bed early is imposed as a punishment or when staying up late is a reward, children may view bedtime as punitive or status degrading.

Some children resort to multiple "curtain calls," such as wanting a drink of water, asking for one more story, needing to go to the bathroom, or wanting to watch television. Some children persist in coming out of their rooms repeatedly after being put back to bed. Some voice fears, such as "there is someone outside the window." Parents may have difficulty determining whether the fear is legitimate or whether the behavior is a bid for attention. Consistent reassurance and limit setting usually resolve the problem. Children feel tense and insecure when limits are applied inconsistently, such as when parents grant permission one night and punish the next for the same behavior.

The night terrors of preschool children may be replaced by sleepwalking and sleep talking. Like night terrors, sleepwalking is associated with the transition from stage 4 to stage 1 of non–rapid eye movement sleep. When children arouse from stage 4 sleep, it is often difficult for them to reach a fully alert, wakeful state rapidly. Sleepwalking occurs in the first 3 to 4 hours of sleep. Children often have no memory of sleepwalking in the morning. The episode begins when the child sits up abruptly and walks. During sleepwalking, movements are clumsy and repetitive; parents often observe finger and hand movements. Most commonly, children move about restlessly, then lie down and return to sleep. However, they may get out of bed and engage in nonpurposeful walking. They rarely perform purposeful acts during sleepwalking. Any attempts to communicate with the child elicit only mumbled and slurred responses. Sleep talking, like sleepwalking, is not purposeful, and speech is usually incomprehensible and monosyllabic.

The best approach is to leave sleepwalking children alone unless they are in danger or may endanger others. However, clumsiness and stereotyped movements can make sleepwalking very dangerous. If the environment is not safe, children can get hurt. Instruct parents to gently redirect children back to bed without waking them, if possible. If children must be wakened, it is best to call them by name slowly and softly, orient them to where they are, explain that they were walking in their sleep, and assure them that it will not happen when they are more relaxed. Preventive measures include avoiding over-fatigue in children, making certain they get adequate rest, employing relaxation techniques, and relieving any stress the children may be experiencing.

Sleepwalking is usually self-limiting and requires no treatment. Persistent sleepwalking occurs in some older children and adolescents who are well behaved and tend to repress strong emotions, such as anger. They may benefit from learning to express their feelings and from doing self-relaxation before bedtime.

Nightmares are a part of the normal developmental process; 70% to 90% of young adults reported experiencing nightmares at some time during childhood (Schredl, Biemelt, Roos, et al, 2008). However, repetitive nightmares or increased nightmare frequency may indicate a specific underlying conflict or stressor that is strongly influencing the child's behavior and thought. Resolving worries or stress will often reduce nightmares. If nightmares become chronic, parents should consider professional counseling (Schredl, Biemelt, Roos, et al, 2008).

A traumatic event often produces posttraumatic nightmares, which are anxiety provoking and literal in their depiction of the trauma. As time goes on, the dreams of affected children may consist of "modified repetitions" that may add more current material to the recurrent dreams (e.g., involving others who were not a part of the traumatic event). Current external stresses, movies, or stories may also precipitate a nightmare by reactivating old traumas. (For a comparison of nightmares and night [or sleep] terrors, see Table 15-2.)

PHYSICAL ACTIVITY

Exercise is essential for muscle development and tone, refinement of balance and coordination, gaining of strength and endurance, and stimulation of body functions and metabolic processes. Throughout middle childhood, children's increasing capabilities and adaptability permit greater speed and effort in motor activities. Larger, stronger muscles with greater efficiency and skill permit longer and increasingly strenuous play without exhaustion. During this period children acquire the coordination, timing, and concentration that are required to participate in adult-type activities, even though they may lack the strength, stamina, and control of the adolescent and adult. Consequently, parents should expect and encourage a larger amount of physical activity during the school years.

Children should have opportunities that provide satisfying experiences to meet individual likes and dislikes. Children need space to run, jump, skip, and climb as well as safe facilities and equipment to use both inside and outside. Appropriate activities that promote coordination and development include running, rope skipping, swimming, roller skating, ice skating, and bicycle riding. Positive reinforcement achieved by experiencing increasingly smooth, rhythmic, and efficient use of the body conditions the child toward regular physical activity. However, one must keep in mind that although school-age children are large and appear to be strong, they may not be prepared for strenuous competitive athletics.

Most children need little encouragement to engage in physical activity. They have so much energy that they seldom know when to stop. However, children with disabilities or those who hesitate to become involved in active play, such as obese children, require special assessment and help in determining activities that appeal to them, are compatible with their limitations, and meet their developmental needs. Parents also need to limit television viewing to encourage outside activities.

Physical Fitness

The development of physical fitness is a goal for all children. This goal was easy to accomplish in the past when school-age children spent a considerable amount of time each day playing on playgrounds, walking to school, and participating in games or sports at school or in their communities. With the advent of technology and the information age, many children are less active physically and spend large portions of their day in front of a computer or television (see Research Focus box).

RESEARCH FOCUS

Strategies to Increase Physical Activity in Children

Strategies focusing on increasing physical activity and reducing sedentary behavior have become a priority; however, only 8% of elementary schools and 6% of middle schools in America provide daily physical education classes (Bagby and Adams, 2007). Recent studies show less than 25 minutes of school time is spent in moderate to vigorous physical activity each week (Bagby and Adams, 2007). Furthermore, some students offset any increased activity during school with little to no exercise outside of school (Cawley, Meyerhoefer, and Newhouse, 2007).

Counseling should include developing goals, identifying fun and safe physical activities, addressing potential barriers, and encouraging support from family and friends. Nurses can further promote efforts to include physical fitness in school programs and encourage children to engage in aerobic physical activities during their free time. Such activities provide cardiopulmonary benefits, maintain normal weight, and have the potential to contribute to lifelong fitness.

Sports

Much controversy has surrounded the trend toward earlier participation in competitive athletics and the amount and type of competitive sports that are appropriate for children in the elementary grades. The current view is that virtually every child is suited for some type of sport, and authorities do not discourage participation if children are matched to the type of sport appropriate to their abilities and to their physical and emotional constitutions. School-age children enjoy competition, and when teachers, parents, and coaches understand children's physical limitations and teach them the proper techniques and safety measures to avoid injury to developing bones and muscles, a safe and appropriate sport can be found for even the most unskilled and uncompetitive child.

During middle childhood, girls have the same basic structure as boys and thus have a similar response to systematic exercise training. At puberty, when boys become larger and have more muscle mass, it is usually recommended that girls compete only against other girls. Before puberty there is no essential difference in strength and size between girls and boys, which makes these precautions unnecessary.

BOX 17-4 GOALS OF ORGANIZED ATHLETICS FOR PREADOLESCENT CHILDREN

Organized extracurricular athletic programs for preadolescent children should focus on helping children to develop:
- Enjoyment of sports and fitness that will be sustained through adulthood
- Physical fitness
- Basic motor skills
- A positive self-image
- A balanced perspective on sports in relation to the child's school and community life
- A commitment to the values of teamwork, fair play, and sportsmanship

Modified from American Academy of Pediatrics, Committee on Sports Medicine and Committee on School Health: Organized athletics for preadolescent children, *Pediatrics* 107(6):1459-1462, 2001.

BOX 17-5 SAFEGUARDS FOR ATHLETIC PROGRAMS

Every athletic program should require the following:
- Participation physical examinations at least every 2 years
- Warm-up procedures
- The availability of a medically trained person who is competent in recognizing significant injuries during practices and games of contact sports
- The establishment of policies for first aid, referral of injured participants, treatment, rehabilitation, and certification for return to participation
- Suitable and well-maintained sports facilities
- Appropriate protective equipment
- Strict enforcement of rules concerning safety
- A formal surveillance method to ensure that goals are met

Modified from American Academy of Pediatrics, Committee on Sports Medicine and Committee on School Health: Organized athletics for preadolescent children, *Pediatrics* 107(6):1459-1462, 2001.

Well-organized extracurricular sports programs based in the community or school encourage enjoyment of sports and fitness in childhood (Box 17-4). Preadolescence is a time to teach fundamental motor skills; develop fitness in a practical, safe, and gradual manner; and promote desired attitudes and values. Activities should include practice sessions and unstructured play. The actual game or event should be managed in a manner that stresses mastery of the sport and enhancement of self-image rather than winning or pleasing others. All children should have an opportunity to participate, and special ceremonies should recognize all participants rather than individuals.

In addition to ensuring the interest, suitability, and safety (Box 17-5) of the sport, parents must make certain that coaches (if involved in the sport) are skillful in managing children and do not engage in abusive behavior. Coaches, parents, and others involved in children's sports play critical roles in shaping children's self-esteem. Any sport for children should emphasize the pleasure of the activity. It is wise to expose children to a variety of individual sports. The overall emphasis of both team and individual sports should be on playing and learning. Parents who pressure their children to perform beyond their capabilities run the risk of the child's being injured, developing a dislike for the activity, and developing a lowered self-image (see Family-Centered Care box).

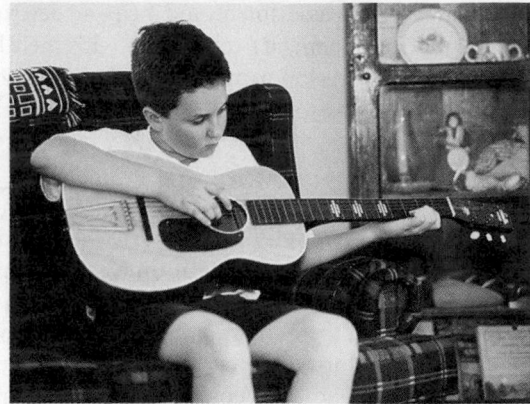

Fig. 17-13 Music is a favorite form of expression for school-age children.

The same principles described in the preceding paragraphs apply to children with chronic illnesses, such as diabetes, epilepsy, asthma, or allergies, if the disorder is mild and can be controlled with medication. Children with cognitive impairment do not need to be excluded from sports competition if they are matched evenly against other children of equal abilities and provided with skilled supervision and coaching. Some activities need to be modified to accommodate the skills of these children.

Acquisition of Skills

School-age children demonstrate increasing capacity in fine muscle facility and complex artistic skills. Handedness is well established by the beginning of the school years, and children make great strides in writing and drawing during this age period. It is a time of energetic and vibrant creative productivity. With the tools of language and reading, children can create poems, stories, and plays. With more advanced fine motor skills, they are able to master an unlimited variety of handicrafts, such as ceramics, needlework, wood carving, and beadwork. They avidly pursue these skills in solitude, with a friend, or in programs offered through organizations such as boys' or girls' clubs or special interest groups that use crafts as a means to occupy, entertain, and educate children.

Music is a favorite form of expression in middle childhood (Fig. 17-13). Music stimulates and invigorates school-age children. They can sing in harmony, play instruments in orchestras and bands, and manage music at a more complex level. They can compose original songs, learn lyrics almost effortlessly, and turn any empty moment into an occasion for singing.

School-age children are capable of assuming responsibility for their own needs, although their distaste for soap and water and "dress" clothes is legendary. School-age children can and want to assume their share of household tasks, which usually are related to the male and female roles that have been defined by their culture (Fig. 17-14). Many also assume responsibility for tasks outside the home, such as baby-sitting, yard work, or paper routes.

Television, Videogames, and the Internet

For some time, child development specialists and parents have been concerned about the effect of media on child development

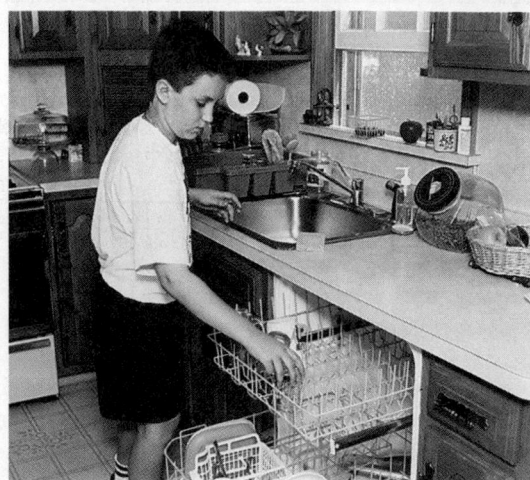

Fig. 17-14 Children can assume responsibility for a variety of household tasks.

and behavior. Children spend a significant amount of time each day involved in media-related activities, including the use of television, computers, videogames, and CD players. Children ages 8 to 18 years spend close to 4 hours every day watching television or videos, with 20% of these children watching more than 5 hours a day (Rideout, Roberts, and Foehr, 2005). Because of the long periods of exposure, the media have more time to develop children's attitudes than do parents and teachers.

There is no doubt that children learn from television, but the values and attitudes depicted on television are not always realistic and may conflict with values that children were previously taught. School-age children can distinguish fantasy from reality, and some have had sufficient life experience to view television programs with skepticism. However, television rarely depicts the reality of day-to-day situations that confront children. When children view characters they admire using violence, such as Superheroes, it can teach them to become more violent (Christakis and Zimmerman, 2007). In addition, repeated exposure to violence can desensitize children to violence, can convey a message that violence is acceptable, and can teach children that initiating violent behavior is a way to protect themselves (Christakis and Zimmerman, 2007).

Violence in the media can also increase fear and anxiety in children. Events such as the 9/11 terrorist attacks and the war in Iraq have infiltrated television, frequently exposing children to real-life violence. Viewing violence in the news causes more fear and worry in children than viewing the same content in a fictional setting (Van Der Molen and Bushman, 2008).

Parents should make the ultimate decisions about which programs their child will watch. To reduce exposure to violence and maximize the beneficial effects of television, parents are advised to monitor program selection, view programs with their children, and discuss program content when the programs are finished (Christakis and Zimmerman, 2007). (See Chapter 2 for a more in-depth discussion of children and television.)

Videogames have been both criticized and supported in relation to their effect on children and adolescents. Critics maintain that videogames keep children from schoolwork and can cause tension, sleeplessness, and violence. Others support the activity as a means for improving eye-hand coordination and as a substitute for the inactivity of passive television viewing. Benefits may also include development of inductive reasoning (drawing generalizations from specific observations), improving spatial perception, and learning to handle multiple variables that interact simultaneously.

Research suggests that videogames may affect physical and psychologic functioning. Physical effects may include triggering of epileptic seizures. (See seizure discussion, Chapter 37.) However, research has noted some positive applications of videogames with dyslexic children (American Psychological Association, 2005).

Computers and the Internet are becoming a popular means for obtaining educational and recreational information. Children with home computers increased from 73% in 2000 to 86% in 2005, and an estimated 45 million U.S. children ages 10 to 17 years use the Internet every day (Rideout, Roberts, and Foehr, 2005; Williams and Guerra, 2007). Although the Internet provides valuable educational opportunities for children, there are also many risks that parents must acknowledge before children access the Internet. Major risks include exposure to inappropriate, dangerous, or illegal material; exposure to harassment through e-mail or chat rooms; revelation of financial information that leads to negative consequences; and safety issues relating to sharing personal information or meeting strangers (McColgan and Giardino, 2005). The best way to eliminate potential risks is to educate parents and children about the Internet and to provide adult supervision when children use the Internet.

Parent and teacher education relating to television, videogames, and the Internet should include recommendations to limit playing time, monitor game selection and content, and increase access to games and information that are educational.

DENTAL HEALTH

The first permanent (secondary) teeth erupt at about 6 years of age. Before their appearance they have been developing in the jaw beneath the deciduous (primary) teeth. The roots of the latter are gradually absorbed, so that when a deciduous tooth is shed, only the crown remains. At 6 years of age, all of the

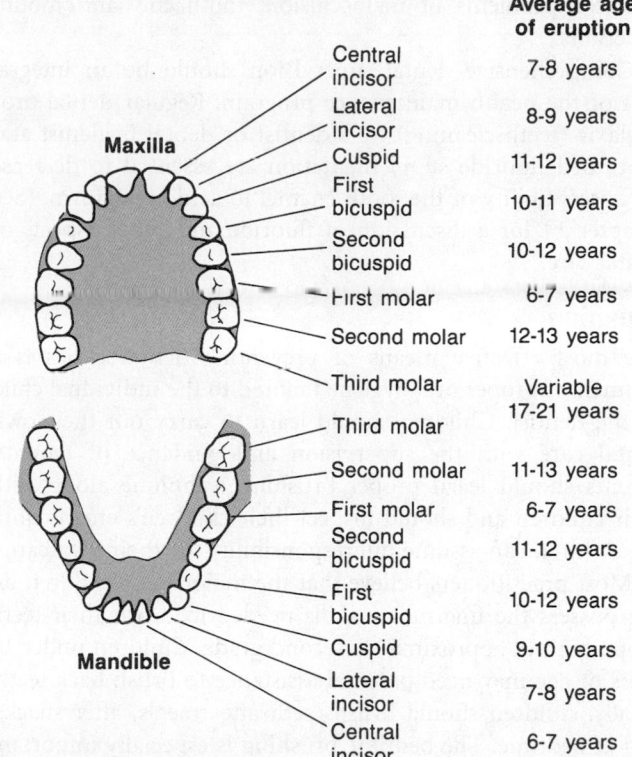

	Average age of eruption
Maxilla	
Central incisor	7-8 years
Lateral incisor	8-9 years
Cuspid	11-12 years
First bicuspid	10-11 years
Second bicuspid	10-12 years
First molar	6-7 years
Second molar	12-13 years
Third molar	Variable 17-21 years
Mandible	
Third molar	
Second molar	11-13 years
First molar	6-7 years
Second bicuspid	11-12 years
First bicuspid	10-12 years
Cuspid	9-10 years
Lateral incisor	7-8 years
Central incisor	6-7 years

Fig. 17-15 Sequence of eruption of secondary teeth. (Data from Dean JA, McDonald RE, Avery DR: *McDonald and Avery dentistry for the child and adolescent,* ed 9, St Louis, 2011, Mosby.)

primary teeth are present, and those of the secondary dentition are relatively well formed. Eruption of the permanent teeth begins with the 6-year molar, which erupts posterior to the deciduous molars. The others appear in approximately the same order as in eruption of the primary teeth and follow shedding of the deciduous teeth (Fig. 17-15).

The pattern of shedding of primary teeth and eruption of secondary teeth is subject to wide variation among children. To allow the larger permanent teeth to occupy the limited space left by shed primary teeth, a series of complicated changes must take place in the jaws. At this time many of the difficulties created by crowding of teeth become apparent. With the appearance of the second permanent (12-year) molars, most of the permanent teeth are present. The third permanent molars, or wisdom teeth, may erupt from 18 to 25 years of age or later. Permanent dentition is somewhat more advanced in girls than in boys.

Because permanent teeth erupt during the school-age years, good dental hygiene and regular attention to dental caries are vital parts of health supervision during this period. Caries is a common problem, affecting as many as 57% of American school-age children (Wagner and Oskouian, 2008). Children of this age tend to become careless about oral hygiene unless they are carefully supervised. Although children are assuming more responsibility for their own care, they are not as motivated by improved appearance and odor as they will be during adolescence. School nurses should be alert for opportunities to teach correct brushing and flossing techniques; to reinforce avoidance of fermentable carbohydrates and sticky sweets; and to be alert for problems of malocclusion, toothache, and mouth infections.

Comprehensive dental supervision should be an integral part of the health maintenance program. Regular dental prophylaxis (teeth cleaning) by a dentist or dental hygienist and continued fluoride supplementation are essential to decrease the susceptibility of the tooth enamel to acid breakdown. (See Chapter 14 for a discussion of fluoride and other aspects of dental care.)

Brushing

The most effective means of preventing dental caries is a regimen of proper oral hygiene tailored to the individual child by the dentist. Children should learn to carry out their own dental care with the supervision and guidance of parents. Parents should learn proper brushing technique along with their children and should inspect their children's efforts until the children can assume full responsibility for their own care.

Most practitioners believe that the majority of children do not possess the fine motor skills needed to brush their teeth properly until approximately second grade. Children under 10 years of age may need parental assistance to brush back teeth. Ideally, children should brush teeth after meals, after snacks, and at bedtime. The bedtime brushing is especially important because there is more time overnight for interaction between oral bacteria and unremoved substrate on the tooth substance. Children who brush their teeth frequently and become accustomed to the feel of a clean mouth at an early age usually maintain the habit throughout life.

The thoroughness of plaque removal (cleaning) can be checked using a plaque-disclosing agent that stains any remaining plaque red. The child should inspect the teeth closely with the aid of a mirror and under adequate light. The teeth then are again cleansed with a fluoridated dentifrice to remove the remaining plaque and provide further protection. This procedure may be carried out regularly or occasionally, according to instructions from the child's dentist. Toothpastes recommended by the American Dental Association Council on Dental Therapeutics carry a seal of approval, which is easily identified on the package. They have been submitted to testing and demonstrate the ability to reduce the incidence of dental caries when used correctly.

For school-age children with mixed and permanent dentition, the best toothbrush is one with soft nylon bristles and an overall length of about 21 cm (8 inches). There are numerous methods of brushing the teeth for children, but no conclusive evidence indicates that one method is superior to another. The thoroughness of the cleaning is more important than the specific technique used. The dentist will assess all factors, such as the child's manipulative skills and special needs, and suggest the most appropriate brushing technique and regimen. Flossing follows brushing. Parents usually floss until children acquire the manual dexterity needed. Most children are not able to floss properly until about 8 or 9 years of age.

SCHOOL HEALTH

Child health maintenance is ultimately the responsibility of parents; however, public schools and health departments in the United States have contributed to the improvement of child health by providing a healthful school environment, health services, and health education functions that emphasize sound health practices. These functions constitute major components of community health services and involve large amounts of public funds and many health professionals, including nurses.

A safe and healthful school environment is an essential element of any school health program. Conditions within the school must contribute to the physical, mental, and social development and well-being of the children. One model that has been used to provide information about the essential components of school health is the Coordinated School Health Program (Centers for Disease Control and Prevention, 2008). The eight basic components of this program are a healthy school environment; health services; health education; nutrition services; counseling, psychologic, and social services; health promotion for staff; physical education; and family and community involvement in school health (Centers for Disease Control and Prevention, 2008). See Boxes 17-6 and 17-7 for factors that contribute to a healthful school setting and for characteristics of school health programs.

Health Education

Health education of school-age children focuses on providing knowledge of health and influencing habits, attitudes, and conduct in relation to health (Box 17-8). A viable health education program is based on sound health concepts but should be adjusted to meet specific local needs, objectives, and legal

---

BOX 17-6 COMPONENTS OF A COORDINATED SCHOOL HEALTH PROGRAM

Healthy school environment—A clean, safe environment that meets Occupational Safety and Health Administration regulations, addresses sanitation measures, identifies environmental irritants, enforces disciplinary measures, and monitors safety risks

Health services—Services provided to students to protect and promote health through health appraisals, prevention and control of communicable diseases, emergency care, and educational counseling

Health education—A planned, sequential, kindergarten to grade 12 curriculum that addresses physical, mental, emotional, and social dimensions of health

Nutrition services—Food service that conforms to U.S. Department of Agriculture guidelines and ensures balanced diets and, when needed, special diets

Counseling, psychologic, and social services—Services provided to students to improve mental, emotional, and social health through on-site counseling services or referral to such services

Health promotion for staff—Services to promote health and wellness (e.g., blood pressure screening, stress reduction programs, fitness activities) among school staff

Physical education—Physical education for students in kindergarten to grade 12 that provides cognitive learning and physical fitness experiences with a variety of activities

Family and community involvement—Dynamic partnerships with school, parents, and community groups to enhance the health and well-being of students

From Centers for Disease Control and Prevention: *Healthy youth! Coordinated school health programs,* 2008, available at www.cdc.gov/healthyyouth/CSHP/index.htm (accessed February 26, 2009).

BOX 17-7   **CONTENT OF SCHOOL HEALTH SERVICES**

Health appraisal—Screening tests (vision, hearing); measurements (height, weight); and medical, dental, and psychologic examinations

Health promotion—Teaching healthy lifestyles and encouraging avoidance of health risks through promotion and awareness programs

Emergency care and safety—Emergency treatment (first aid), notification of parents, and transportation of the ill or injured child to home or hospital

Communicable disease control—Detection and exclusion of affected children and policies for readmission and attendance at school (immunizations required in most states before school entry)

Counseling and guidance—Health guidance, referral, and follow-up for parents and children with special health needs

Adjustment to individual student needs

BOX 17-8   **RECOMMENDATIONS FOR SCHOOL HEALTH PROGRAMS**

- Health and safety education should be taught as part of basic education and deserves the same priority in the curriculum as traditional subjects.
- Planned integrated programs of comprehensive health and safety education should be a requirement for students from kindergarten through grade 12 and should be taught by specially qualified teachers or those certified to teach health education.
- Health and safety education should include the active participation of students for the most effective learning of sound health concepts.
- Financial support for health and safety education programs must be ensured. Proper funding is critical to the development of effective programs, and the agencies responsible must be convinced to continue or increase funding.
- Comprehensive health and safety education programs should be directed by qualified health educators who function in consultation and cooperation with school personnel and administrators.
- The programs should be monitored by a well-organized school health committee composed of representative parents, students, pediatricians, and health agency personnel (e.g., public health nurses) in the community.
- Health and safety education should be a part of every elementary school and secondary school teacher's training program.
- School districts, other public agencies, the medical community, and private agencies should intensify their health and safety education program for adults as part of a coordinated community health and safety education effort, and pediatricians should make health and safety education a regular component of child health supervision and routine illness visits.
- Research studies to evaluate the impact of such programs on students must be carried out at local and national levels.

Data from American Academy of Pediatrics: *Health, mental health and safety guidelines for schools,* 2009, available at www.nationalguidelines.org (accessed March 15, 2009).

---

requirements. Parents must understand and approve the health education curriculum so that its teaching will be reinforced at home. A comprehensive approach to health education is more successful in developing positive health practices than one in which the subjects are taught in isolation. Many topics presented in health education classes are associated with differing social and cultural attitudes and should be presented accurately and with sensitivity to these attitudes.

Health education concerning AIDS is a specific example. Most authorities agree that AIDS education should begin in the elementary grades to prevent high-risk behaviors. However, educational programs concerning AIDS must be developmentally appropriate and, to be effective, must be implemented with parental and community support. Young children need information on how HIV is transmitted, in simple, accurate terms without elaborate, unnecessary discussions of sex. Misconceptions that increase children's anxiety about contracting the virus should be corrected. Although many children have heard that sex and drugs cause AIDS, some children also have misconceptions about AIDS. Children need information that HIV is transmitted through infected blood on shared drug needles and that the virus is not spread through common forms of expressing affection such as hugging and holding hands.

School Nursing Services

School nurses assume a major role in the school health program and can affect the lives of school-age children significantly. Working in collaboration with others in the school and community, school nurses provide health supervision, health counseling, and health education. The responsibilities of the school nurse can include providing education and interventions for acute and chronic illness, injuries, communicable diseases, obesity and nutrition, mental health, dental disease, and sexually transmitted infections (American Academy of Pediatrics, 2008b). These functions are not necessarily limited to the confines of the school environment but extend into the community in which the students live. As a health practitioner, the school nurse is in a position to promote and evaluate health services throughout the community as they affect children and to collaborate with agencies in planning for health and safety. For some children, especially those in poverty, the school nurse may be the only contact with illness prevention and health promotion. For children with chronic health conditions, the school nurse provides leadership within the school health team and assesses the student's health status, identifies potential barriers of the educational process, and develops an individualized health care plan (American Academy of Pediatrics, 2008b).

Traditionally, school nurses have been viewed from a limited perspective that placed them in the role of disease detector, applier of bandages, and official caregiver in cases of illness and injury. Although these are still important functions, this traditional role has acquired much broader dimensions. School nurses develop, implement, and evaluate health care plans and programs. In some settings a school-based health center is near or within a school to provide additional health services. In these centers, school nurse practitioners provide primary health care, including assessment of physical, psychomedical, psychoeducational, behavioral, and learning disorder problems, as well as comprehensive well-child care (American Academy of Pediatrics, 2008b).

The minimum qualifications for a school nurse should include a baccalaureate degree from an accredited college or university and licensure as a registered nurse (American Academy of Pediatrics, 2008b). Unlicensed assistive personnel (UAP) may be a part of the school health care team. These paraprofessionals have a state certification and are trained to assist a professional but must be supervised by the school nurse (American Academy of Pediatrics, 2008b). The school nurse must use good assessment and professional judgment in deciding which procedures may be delegated to UAP.

> ### ! NURSING ALERT
>
> In the delegation or transfer of responsibility for the performance of an activity to an assistant, the nurse remains accountable for the outcome.

The passage of Public Laws 94-142 and 99-457 required the integration of children with chronic illness or disability into regular classrooms. School nurses are responsible for the medical and nursing needs of these children in the school setting. School nurses assess and monitor all health problems in children who come into the school and compile a health care list of all of these problems and their associated therapies. The nurse may call the parents of the child and arrange a visit to the home, made by either the school nurse or a public health nurse. After gathering information, the nurse can develop a nursing care plan for use in the school. The nurse collaborates with the family and includes their suggestions in the care plan. The nurse then discusses the plan with the child's teachers and provides any needed education. School nurses are the only ones in the school system qualified to deal with medical problems. However, in many instances school nurses can collaborate with teachers to provide atraumatic care (see Community Focus box).

> ### 🏠 COMMUNITY FOCUS
> #### *Collaboration Between School Nurse and Teachers*
>
> - All students should have health cards completed by their parents.
> - All teachers should receive a list of students who have health problems.
> - Teachers should have a code to highlight students with health needs in their grade books so that substitute teachers can recognize these students and intervene immediately if problems occur in the classroom.
> - Teachers should schedule students who miss physical education into an adaptive physical education class if possible.
> - All students with asthma should have their metered-dose inhalers available to them for emergency use in physical education and all other classes.
> - Adult volunteers should serve as team captains for games; selections of team members should be supervised so that one team is not stacked with all the good players.
> - In physical education, evaluation of a skill or activity should be repeated several times if some students score extremely high and others extremely low, since every child has good and bad days.
> - Teachers should never question a child's ability in front of other students.
> - Nurses should maintain privacy for height and weight checks and for vision and hearing tests (students should be taken into the nurse's office individually so other students do not hear the test results).

Suggestions submitted by Linda L. Smith, Health/Physical Education Teacher.

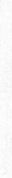

Sometimes all that is required is conducting an assessment and making the teacher aware that the child has a health problem. In other cases more complex teaching is needed, such as how to observe for certain signs (e.g., insulin reaction), how to perform certain techniques (e.g., tracheostomy suctioning, gastrostomy or nasogastric tube feedings), and how to manage emergencies (e.g., care of a child during a seizure). School nurses instruct teachers in the necessary procedures and review their performance.

The American Academy of Pediatrics (2008a) has established guidelines for emergency medical care of children in schools. These guidelines include developing emergency policies and procedures, clarifying school staff roles, collecting emergency data on all school children, making emergency equipment and medication easily accessible, and adequately training staff. It is recommended that at least one staff member, in addition to the school nurse, have cardiopulmonary resuscitation, first aid, and automated external defibrillator training (American Academy of Pediatrics, 2008a).

A child who must take medication at school needs written authorization from his or her attending physician and/or written permission from the parents allowing the nurse to administer or supervise the administration of the medication. The medication must be brought to the school in a container appropriately labeled by the pharmacist or physician. Medications are kept locked up in the nurse's office; usually the child is not allowed to carry medications at school. The policy may vary in some school districts or situations. For example, some children may be allowed to carry metered-dose inhalers that contain their asthma medication, provided that their physician and a parent provide the required authorization. Guidelines for administration of medications in schools are also available from the National Association of School Nurses.*

INJURY PREVENTION

⊖ Because school-age children have developed more refined muscular coordination and control and can apply their cognitive capacities to select a more judicious course of action, the incidence of unintentional injury is diminished in children in this age-group compared with the incidence in early childhood. School-age children have exposure to more environments in which they need protection, they acquire skills and interests that expose them to new perils, they have less supervision, and they take more responsibility as they begin to participate in the adult world.

Injuries most prevalent in school-age children reflect their developmental stage. Table 17-2 outlines the developmental characteristics and accomplishments of middle childhood that predispose children to physical injury and offers guidelines for injury prevention.

The incidence of injury during middle childhood is significantly higher in school-age boys than in school-age girls, and their death rate is twice that of girls. (See Chapter 1.) Most injuries occur in or near the home or school. The prevalence of injury depends on the dangers present in the environment, the protection offered by adults, and the behavior patterns of the children. Although school-age children are conscious of rules and frequently impose them in relationships with peers, they also tend to challenge established rules. It is often difficult to maintain a balance between the level of supervision and restriction needed by children and their need for freedom and independence.

*8484 Georgia Ave., Suite 420, Silver Springs, MD 20910; 866-627-6767; e-mail: nasn@nasn.org; www.nasn.org.

Vertical text in left margin: Critical Thinking Exercise—Injury Prevention | Case Study—Injury Prevention

TABLE 17-2	INJURY PREVENTION DURING SCHOOL-AGE YEARS
DEVELOPMENTAL ABILITIES RELATED TO RISK OF INJURY	**INJURY PREVENTION**
	Motor Vehicle Accidents
Is increasingly involved in activities away from home Is excited by speed and motion Is easily distracted by environment Can be reasoned with	Educate child regarding proper use of seat belts while a passenger in a vehicle. Maintain discipline while the child is a passenger in a vehicle (e.g., ensure that child keeps arms inside, does not lean against doors or interfere with driver). Remind parents and children that no one should ride in the bed of a pickup truck. Emphasize safe pedestrian behavior. Insist that child wear safety apparel (e.g., helmet) when applicable, such as riding bicycle (see Family-Centered Care box, p. 678), motorcycle, moped, or all-terrain vehicle (see Family-Centered Care box, p. 677).
	Drowning
Is apt to overdo May work hard to perfect a skill Has cautious, but not fearful, gross motor actions Likes swimming	Teach child to swim. Teach basic rules of water safety. Select safe and supervised places to swim. Check sufficient water depth for diving. Caution child to swim with a companion. Ensure that child uses an approved flotation device in water or boat. Advocate for legislation requiring fencing around pools. Learn cardiopulmonary resuscitation.
	Burns
Has increasing independence Is adventurous Enjoys trying new things	Make sure smoke detectors are in homes. Set water heaters to 48.9° C (120° F) to avoid scald burns. Instruct child regarding behavior in areas involving contact with potential burn hazards (e.g., gasoline, matches, bonfires or barbecues, lighter fluid, firecrackers, cigarette lighters, cooking utensils, chemistry sets). Instruct child to avoid climbing or flying kite around high-tension wires. Instruct child in proper behavior in the event of fire (e.g., fire drills at home and school). Teach child safe cooking (use low heat; avoid any frying; be careful of steam burns, scalds, or exploding foods, especially from microwaving).
	Poisoning
Adheres to group rules May be easily influenced by peers Has strong allegiance to friends	Educate child regarding hazards of taking nonprescription drugs and chemicals, including aspirin and alcohol. Teach child to say no if offered illegal or dangerous drugs or alcohol. Keep potentially dangerous products in properly labeled receptacles, preferably out of reach.
	Bodily Damage
Has increased physical skills Needs strenuous physical activity Is interested in acquiring new skills and perfecting attained skills Is daring and adventurous, especially with peers Frequently plays in hazardous places Confidence often exceeds physical capacity Desires group loyalty and has strong need for friends' approval Attempts hazardous feats Accompanies friends to potentially hazardous facilities Delights in physical activity Is likely to overdo Growth in height exceeds muscular growth and coordination	Help provide facilities for supervised activities. Encourage playing in safe places. Keep firearms safely locked up except with adult supervision. Teach proper care of, use of, and respect for potentially dangerous devices (e.g., power tools, firecrackers). Teach children not to tease or surprise dogs, invade their territory, take dogs' toys, or interfere with dogs' feeding. Stress use of eye, ear, or mouth protection when using potentially hazardous objects or devices or when engaged in potentially hazardous sports. Do not permit use of trampolines except as part of supervised training. Teach safety regarding use of corrective devices (glasses); if child wears contact lenses, monitor duration of wear to prevent corneal damage. Stress careful selection, use, and maintenance of sports and recreation equipment, such as skateboards and in-line skates (see Family-Centered Care box, p. 678). Emphasize proper conditioning, safe practices, and use of safety equipment for sports or recreational activities. Caution against engaging in hazardous sports, such as those involving trampolines. Use safety glass and decals on large glassed areas, such as sliding glass doors. Use window guards to prevent falls. Teach name, address, and phone number and emphasize that child should ask for help from appropriate people (e.g., cashier, security guard, police) if lost; have identification on child (e.g., sewn in clothes, inside shoe). Teach safety and stranger awareness: • Avoid personalized clothing in public places. • Never go with a stranger. • Tell parents if anyone makes child feel uncomfortable in any way. • Say no when confronted with uncomfortable situations. Always listen to child's concerns regarding others' behavior.

The incidence of transportation-related injuries is higher in school-age children than in younger children, and the incidence of bicycle injury not involving a motor vehicle is higher than that in teenagers and preschool children. Injuries from burns and poisonings are lowest in school-age children. However, physically active school-age children are highly susceptible to cuts and abrasions, and the incidence of childhood fractures, strains, and sprains is impressive.

Risk-Taking Behavior

Achieving social acceptance is a primary objective for school-age children. They often attempt dangerous acts (sometimes extreme behaviors) to prove themselves worthy of acceptance and improve their status in the peer group. Peer pressure is a normal part of psychologic development, but it is also a major contributor to risk-taking behaviors. Peer challenges often encourage problem behaviors that place children at risk for injury or hazardous habits. School-age children are in the process of moving from preoperational to concrete operational thinking and are only beginning to understand causal relationships. Therefore they may attempt certain activities without planning or evaluating the consequences.

Children who are risk takers may have inadequate self-regulatory behavior. These children need to learn the motivation or the incentives for such behavior and to visualize the possible consequences if the risk-taking behavior ends in a tragic outcome.

Motor Vehicle Injury

As in all other age-groups, the most common cause of severe accidental injury and death in school-age children is involvement in motor vehicle accidents—either as a pedestrian or as a passenger. In 2007 approximately 18% of traffic-related fatalities involved pedestrians (National Highway Traffic Safety Administration, 2007). Most of the injuries occur when children misinterpret traffic signs or disobey common traffic safety regulations, cross the street against a red light, cross at places other than designated crosswalks, dart into the street, or walk in the same direction as the traffic. Parents consistently overestimate the street-crossing skills of young children ages 5 to 6 years and need education about their children's developmental abilities and competence as pedestrians. Nurses can help parents to develop more realistic expectations of their children's behavior and teach them to model safe street-crossing behaviors through pedestrian skills training programs.

Use of restraint systems, door-lock mechanisms, and appropriate passenger seating and behavior are simple but effective measures for eliminating noncrash injuries and reducing the severity of crash injuries. The importance of the correct use of seat restraints is essential. School-age children do not usually require special car seats. However, despite evidence that safety belt use saves lives and prevents injury, estimates of seat belt use in school-age children are still discouragingly low.

In 2006, 1335 children ages 0 to 14 years died in motor vehicle accidents and 184,000 received injuries requiring emergency department treatment (Centers for Disease Control and Prevention, 2009a). Investigations of motor vehicle accidents showed deployment of passenger-side air bags critically or fatally injured children seated in the right front seat (Newgard and Lewis, 2005). Therefore the National Highway Traffic Safety Administration recommends that children under age 13 years not ride in the front passenger seat of vehicles with air bags.* The American Academy of Pediatrics reiterates this view and strongly emphasizes that the rear seat of any vehicle is the safest place for children to ride. When in the car, school-age children should always be buckled properly in a weight-, height-, and age-appropriate seat. If the child weighs more than 18 kg (40 lb), a convertible safety seat that is positioned in the semiupright and forward-facing position may be used if the child fits in it well. If the child has outgrown the convertible safety seat but is still too small for a regular lap-shoulder belt, a booster seat restraint device equipped with a combination lap-shoulder belt should be used.

Injuries to children ages 5 to 9 years restrained in adult-type seat belts are related to anatomic differences between adults and children. The child's sitting height is less than the adult's, and the child's center of gravity is located above the level of the lap belt. Consequently, the greater proportion of body mass above the belt may cause more forward motion and jackknifing over the belt, which increases the risk of head injury from impact with interior vehicle parts. The child's smaller and less developed iliac crests are not suited to serve as an anchor for belts designed to restrain adults, and their intra-abdominal organs are less protected by the bony pelvis. The natural behavior of children, such as readjusting the seating position, moving about, and otherwise altering the fit of the restraint, also influences its effectiveness.

When children use adult-type seat belts, parents should make certain that the restraints are fitted to their children and fastened correctly. To reduce their risk of sliding beneath the standard seat belt during a collision, children should sit up straight and well back in the seat, and the seat should be moved forward until the feet fit firmly against the toe board. Caution children against assuming alternate seating positions, such as tailor fashion, while riding in the car. (See Chapter 14 for a comprehensive discussion of safety restraints.)

Each year 23.5 million children are transported to and from school on school buses. The majority of school travel–related injuries and deaths occur from passenger vehicles, while only 4% of school travel injuries and 2% of school travel deaths occur in school buses (American Academy of Pediatrics, 2007). However, the National Highway Traffic Safety Administration and the American Academy of Pediatrics have developed minimum standards to enhance school bus safety. These standards state that all children should travel to and from school in an age-appropriate, properly secured child-restraint system; all school buses should be equipped with lap-shoulder restraint systems that can accommodate safety seats, booster seats, and harness systems; and school districts should encourage appropriate education on safety devices (American Academy of Pediatrics, 2007).

---

*Guidelines for car seat safety are also available in Wilson D and Hockenberry MJ: *Wong's clinical manual of pediatric nursing,* ed 7, St Louis, 2008, Mosby.

All-terrain vehicles (ATVs), designed for off-road use by children and adolescents, are popular with children under 16 years of age but are responsible for a significant number of childhood injuries. These vehicles have a short wheelbase and low profile, which makes them relatively unstable and unable to be seen easily. The vehicles can also achieve substantial speed. Most injuries occur when the driver loses control of the vehicle, is thrown from the vehicle, or collides with fixed objects or other vehicles. Immature judgment and poorly developed motor skills also contribute to injury. The American Academy of Pediatrics views ATVs as a major hazard to the health of children, opposes their use by children younger than 16 years of age, and has created a safety bill outlining requirements to enhance ATV safety (Killingsworth, Tilford, Parker, et al, 2005). However, for parents who allow their use, the committee provides safety guidelines (see Family-Centered Care box).

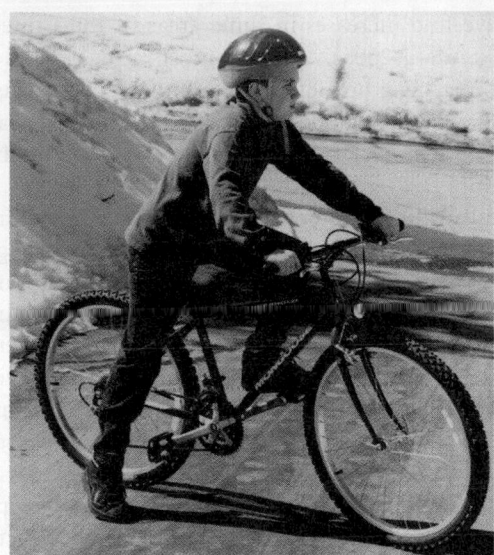

Fig. 17-16 The right-size bike is important; the child should be able to sit on the bike and place the balls of both feet on the ground. The foot should comfortably reach and manipulate the pedal in the down position. Wearing a protective helmet is mandatory for safe cycling. The helmet should sit on top of the head in a level position and should not rock back and forth or from side to side. The strap should always be fastened securely under the chin.

 FAMILY-CENTERED CARE

Safe Use of All-Terrain Vehicles

- Children under the age of 16 years should not operate an off-road vehicle.
- Vehicles should be sturdy and stable; quality construction is essential.
- Riders should receive instruction from a mature, experienced cyclist or a certified instructor.
- Riding should be supervised and allowed only after the rider has demonstrated competence in handling the machine on familiar terrain (preferably require licensing).
- Riders should wear approved helmets, eye protection, and protective reflective clothing (e.g., trousers, boots, gloves).
- Parents should prohibit street use of off-road vehicles.
- Riding should be restricted to familiar terrain.
- Nighttime riding should not be allowed.
- Vehicle should not carry more than one person.
- Vehicles should include seat belts, roll bars, and automatic headlights.

Modified from Killingsworth J, Tilford J, Parker J, et al: National hospitalization impact of pediatric all-terrain vehicle injuries, *Pediatrics* 115(3):e316-e321, 2005.

Bicycle Injury

The majority of school-age children have bicycles and love riding them, but this increases their risk of injury on streets and byways. In 2008 bicycle injuries in children ages 5 to 15 years accounted for approximately 13,000 nonfatal injuries and 89 fatal injuries (National Highway Traffic Safety Administration, 2008).

Many injuries are related to violations of traffic laws by the bicyclist, including wrong-way riding (facing traffic), failure to yield the right of way, and turning violations. Others are related to road conditions described as hazardous: bumps, potholes, and gravel. Bicycle-related injuries occur in young children playing in their own neighborhoods and in older children using their bicycles for transportation on streets with heavy traffic.

In addition to major injuries, cuts and bruises from falls and collisions account for a large number of injuries. Other injuries include trauma to internal organs. These injuries initially seem trivial, but injured children can develop serious symptoms (e.g., pain, vomiting, or collapse) hours later.

Many of the injuries to school-age children on bicycles occur because of the child's developmentally limited range of vision and their inability to process perceptions of road situations sufficiently well and quickly enough to ride safely in traffic. Other important factors are lack of instruction in use of the equipment, lack of safety equipment, and unfamiliarity with the bicycle (e.g., having ridden the bicycle for less than a month).

To prevent bicycle injuries, both parents and children should learn and periodically review bicycle safety. Children need bicycles that are suited to their size and age; they should be able to stand with the balls of both feet on the ground when seated on the bicycle, be able to place both feet flat on the ground when straddling the center bar, and be able to grasp the brake lever comfortably and easily enough to apply sufficient pressure to brake the bicycle. Discourage parents from buying their child a bicycle that the child can "grow into."

Because head injury is the major cause of bicycle-related fatalities, the single most important aspect of bicycle safety is to encourage the rider to wear a protective helmet (Fig. 17-16). Helmet use has caused an 88% reduction in head and brain injury and 65% reduction in face-related injuries (Okun and Adam, 2008). Hard-shelled helmets lined with expanded polystyrene (Styrofoam) provide the best head protection. The helmet should be one that can be adjusted to the individual child's head, fits securely, and does not limit the child's vision or hearing. A brightly colored helmet improves visibility. The helmet should carry a seal indicating that it is approved by the U.S. Consumer Product Safety Commission. All helmets should be replaced after any damage or crash.

Legislative interventions and educational campaigns have significantly increased children's usage of bicycle helmets, with two- to five-fold increases in some areas of the United States (Okun and Adam, 2008). Although most young riders acknowledge that wearing a helmet is important for safety, reasons for not wearing them include discomfort (especially heat), presumed lack of importance for casual riding, lack of style, and peer pressure.

Parental attitudes and behaviors also influence children's use of bicycle helmets. Parental nonuse of a helmet is strongly associated with lack of intention to require the children to use helmets. Parents, as well as children, need to be educated on safety. The American Academy of Pediatrics recommends that (1) parents be informed of the dangers of riding without a helmet, (2) retail outlets carry inexpensive helmets available at the time of bicycle purchase, (3) state and local governments continue to enact legislation requiring helmet use by all bicyclists, (4) parents and community-based programs promote bicycle safety and helmet use, and (5) the media depict helmet use in all programs and promotional materials.

Schools, hospital emergency departments, and communities have developed numerous bicycle helmet promotion programs. Programs that are most successful are those that address the cost of helmets and peer pressure and combine multimedia public education announcements with the support of community organizations. The Family-Centered Care box lists guidelines for bicycle safety, and the Critical Thinking Exercise discusses bicycle helmets.

❓ CRITICAL THINKING EXERCISE

Bicycle Helmets

During the past month in your school district, one child died and another sustained a serious head injury from bicycle-vehicle collisions. Neither child wore a bicycle helmet. As a school nurse, you are considering effective approaches to increase the students' use of bicycle helmets.

1. Evidence—Is there sufficient evidence to draw any conclusions?
2. Assumptions—Describe the underlying assumption about each of the following:
   a. Potential hazards to children associated with bicycling
   b. Intrinsic and extrinsic risk factors for bicycle injuries
   c. Factors associated with deciding whether to wear a bicycle helmet
   d. Strategies for pediatricians and nurses to help decrease bicycle-related injuries
3. What implications for nursing care can be drawn from this situation?
4. Does the evidence support your conclusion?

Other Vehicle-Related Injuries

After a short period of decline, skateboards are again becoming popular, with an accompanying resurgence of related injuries. Although the majority of injuries involve the extremities, severe injuries of the head and neck can occur. School-age children often use their skateboards on streets and highways, which increases the likelihood of high-speed collisions with objects or vehicles. Recommendations for safe skateboard use are in the Family-Centered Care box.

👪 FAMILY-CENTERED CARE

Bicycle Safety

- Always wear a properly fitted helmet that is approved by the U.S. Consumer Product Safety Commission; replace a damaged helmet.
- Ride bicycles with traffic and away from parked cars.
- Ride single file.
- Walk bicycles through busy intersections and at crosswalks.
- Give hand signals well in advance of turning or stopping.
- Keep as close to the curb as practical.
- Watch for drain grates, potholes, soft shoulders, and loose dirt or gravel.
- Keep both hands on handlebars except when signaling.
- Never ride double on a bicycle.
- Do not carry packages that interfere with vision or control; do not drag objects behind bike.
- Watch for and yield to pedestrians.
- Watch for cars backing up or pulling out of driveways; be especially careful at intersections.
- Look left, right, then left before turning into traffic or roadway.
- Never hitch a ride on a truck or other vehicle.
- Learn rules of the road and respect for traffic officers.
- Obey all local ordinances.
- Wear shoes that fit securely while riding.
- Wear light colors at night, and attach fluorescent material to clothing and bicycle.
- Be certain the bicycle is the correct size.
- Equip the bicycle with proper lights and reflectors.
- Have the bicycle inspected to ensure good mechanical condition.
- When riding as a passenger, wear appropriate-size helmet and sit in a specially designed protective seat.

Modified from American Academy of Pediatrics, Committee on Injury and Poison Prevention: Bicycle helmets, *Pediatrics* 108(4):1030-1032, 2001.

👪 FAMILY-CENTERED CARE

Skateboard and In-Line Skate Safety

- Children younger than 10 years of age should not use skateboards without close supervision by an adult. They are not developmentally prepared to protect themselves from injury.
- The age when children are ready to use in-line skates safely is not known because of differences in the ability to acquire the skills needed to participate in the sport. Novice skaters should learn indoors on a flat, smooth surface.
- Children who use skateboards and in-line skates should wear helmets and protective padding, especially on wrists, knees, and elbows, to prevent injury.
- Skateboards and in-line skates should never be ridden near traffic. Their use should be prohibited on streets and highways. Activities that bring skateboards or in-line skates and cars together (e.g., "catching a ride") are especially dangerous.
- Some types of use, such as riding homemade ramps on hard surfaces, may be particularly hazardous.

Modified from McGeehan J, Shields BJ, and Smith GA: Children should wear helmets while ice-skating: a comparison of skating-related injuries, *Pediatrics* 114(1):124-128, 2004.

Like skateboard injuries, roller skate or in-line skate injuries involve predominantly the upper extremities (especially the wrist and forearm) as children attempt to break a fall with outstretched arms. Safety measures are basically the same as for skateboards. Parents should carefully evaluate the skill level of the child before allowing the child to use skates. Younger children sustain injuries more frequently than older children. Some authorities believe that parents should not encourage children to engage in these activities until their bone strength and skills are sufficiently mature to decrease the risk of fracture.

Ride-on mower and other power mower injuries also occur among school-age children. Approximately 9400 children under the age of 18 years require emergency care for lawn mower–related injuries in the United States each year (Vollman and Smith, 2006). These injuries occur when children are allowed to operate a mower, when they are run over or backed over by another driver, or when they fall from a mower or from a trailer pulled by a mower. Although there are no age-specific criteria for the use of lawn mowers, children should not operate lawn mowers until they have appropriate levels of judgment, strength, coordination, and maturity, which is usually over the age of 12 years for walk-behind mowers and over the age of 16 years for riding mowers (Samson, 2006).

Similar injuries occur with snowmobiles. Most deaths and injuries involving snowmobiles occur when the vehicle collides with a stationary object or when riders fall or are ejected from the vehicle. The American Academy of Pediatrics recommends that persons under 16 years of age be prohibited from operating or riding snowmobiles (Nayci, Stavlo, Zarroug, et al, 2006).

Injuries at School

The risk of injury at school is relatively low, despite the amount of time children spend in that environment. Some injuries occur in gyms, shops, and laboratories, as well as on playgrounds and playing fields. Most injuries occur on the way to and from school. Many are related to sports activities. (See Chapter 39.) Persons concerned with child safety should be alert to hazards in the school environment and should become involved in efforts to make the environment safe in every aspect—physical facilities, equipment, training practices, and supervision.

Trampolines are popular with young children, and continue to cause significant injuries. In 2005 approximately 88,500 children suffered a trampoline related injury, with 66% of these patients ranging from 5 to 12 years old (Linakis, Mello, Machan, et al, 2007). Fractures, sprains, and head injuries have all been attributed to trampolines.

Farm Injuries

Many school-age children are involved in farm activities and play in the farm environment. They may be children of migrant workers, and as such, they constitute a significant proportion of agricultural workers. Most injuries take place during the summer when children are home from school and in the autumn when farming activity is brisk. Health facilities are also more scattered and less accessible for emergency treatment in farming areas than they are in urban communities.

Health workers need to be aware of the problems and to emphasize to the farm family the hazards related to their environment and ways to prevent injuries, especially when children are present. Rural schools should provide safety education regarding machinery operation, safety procedures, and injury prevention. Nurses in rural areas can be advocates for farm safety programs and for revision of the current farm safety legislation.

Other Injuries

Falls are still a source of injury in school-age children but less so than in preschool children and toddlers. "Flipping," a popular activity in which children jump from an elevated surface and perform an aerial flip with the idea of landing upright, has resulted in serious injuries to the face and head and places children at risk for back and spinal cord injury. Seasonal injuries such as sledding accidents are common and more likely to occur when children ride sleds without adult supervision and in streets, as opposed to parks. Horseback riding injuries are another source of concern for parents of school-age children. The most common cause of death from horseback riding activities is head injury, followed by injuries to the chest and abdomen. Before enrolling children for riding lessons, parents should determine the instructor's safety record with students, verify that safety helmets will be used, and confirm that the instructor is certified by a recognized organization. Injuries at public playgrounds and amusement parks (especially water slides) and around the home (power tools, ladders, fireworks) are ongoing concerns of parents and health care providers.

Injuries to eyes and teeth are a constant threat to school-age children involved in rough play. (See Chapter 24 [eyes] and Chapter 18 [teeth].) The normally shallow bony orbit of children in this age-group makes them particularly vulnerable to eye trauma, especially during contact sports or activities such as baseball or softball. Wearing protective eye and mouth gear is essential (Merriman, 2009).

Injuries have been reported from a variety of toys (slingshots, water balloons, lawn darts, chemistry sets) and household equipment (mowers, lawn trimmers). Gunshot wounds have become a significant problem during past years. The overall rate of firearm-related homicides for U.S. children younger than 15 years of age is nearly 12 times greater than that found in 25 other industrialized countries (Guralnick and Serwint, 2007). So-called toy firearms (air guns and air rifles) also cause frequent firearm injuries to children. Most of these injuries involve the face or eyes.

Nurse's Role in Injury Prevention

Nurses are primary advocates for preventive care and guidance. Safety education and anticipatory guidance for both parents and school-age children can be incorporated in all nursing interventions. The most effective means of prevention is education of the child and family regarding the hazards of risk-taking behavior and improper use of equipment. No piece of equipment is safe unless a child is physically and mentally equipped to use it. A careful history and knowledge of normal growth and development serve as guidelines for both planned and impromptu education.

Parents are often unaware of hazards to their children at various ages, especially those related to normal developmental progress. Susceptibility to injuries and understanding of safety issues are influenced by children's developmental level. Nurses who understand the growth and development of school-age children can provide effective safety education to parents and children and can correct misconceptions before injuries occur.

School nurses should be alert to hazards in the school and instrumental in evaluating safety risks and implementing safety programs. Characteristics of the school-age child and preventive measures are outlined in Table 17-2.

ANTICIPATORY GUIDANCE—CARE OF FAMILIES

The parents of the school-age child find themselves in the position of sharing their child's time and interests with the increasingly important peer group. As a child feels the need to fit into a peer group and gain a sense of industry through individual and cooperative production and performance, he or she moves away from the close, familiar relationships of the family group. It is through these early peer relationships that children prepare for moving from narrow, sheltered family relationships to a broader world of relationships and increased independence. Parents must learn to provide support as unobtrusively as possible without feeling rejected, hurt, or angry. The nurse can help parents of the school-age child by providing anticipatory guidance and reassurance throughout this period of child development and maturation (see Family-Centered Care box).

FAMILY-CENTERED CARE

Guidance During School Years

Age 6 Years
Prepare parents to expect strong food preferences and frequent refusal of specific food items.
Prepare parents to expect increasingly ravenous appetite.
Prepare parents for emotional reactions as child experiences erratic mood changes.
Help parents anticipate continued susceptibility to illness.
Teach injury prevention and safety, especially bicycle safety.
Encourage parents to respect child's need for privacy and to provide a separate bedroom for child, if possible.
Prepare parents for child's increasing interests outside the home.
Help parents understand the need to encourage child's interactions with peers.

Ages 7 to 10 Years
Prepare parents to expect improvement in health with fewer illnesses, but warn them that allergies may increase or become apparent.
Prepare parents to expect an increase in minor injuries.
Emphasize caution in selecting and maintaining sports equipment and reemphasize safety.
Prepare parents to expect increased involvement with peers and interest in activities outside the home.
Emphasize the need to encourage independence while maintaining limit setting and discipline.
Prepare mothers to expect more demands at 8 years.

Prepare fathers to expect increasing admiration at 10 years; encourage father-child activities.
Prepare parents for prepubescent changes in girls.

Ages 11 to 12 Years
Help parents prepare child for body changes of pubescence.
Prepare parents to expect a growth spurt in girls.
Make certain child's sex education is adequate with accurate information.
Prepare parents to expect energetic but stormy behavior at 11 years, with child becoming more even tempered at 12 years.
Encourage parents to support child's desire to "grow up" but to allow regressive behavior when needed.
Prepare parents to expect an increase in masturbation.
Instruct parents that the child may need more rest.
Help parents educate child regarding experimentation with potentially harmful activities.

Health Guidance
Help parents understand the importance of regular health and dental care for child.
Encourage parents to teach and model sound health practices, including diet, rest, activity, and exercise.
Stress the need to encourage children to engage in appropriate physical activities.
Emphasize providing a safe physical and emotional environment.
Encourage parents to teach and model safety practices.

KEY POINTS

- Middle childhood, also known as the school years, is a comfortable period of life that extends from 6 to 12 years of age.
- Although growth is slower than in previous years, there is a steady gain in height and weight with maturation of body systems; primary teeth are lost and replaced by permanent teeth.
- Skeletal lengthening, an increase in the ratio of muscle mass to fat, and maturation of the gastrointestinal system are major components of biologic development during middle childhood.
- Developing a sense of industry or accomplishment is a major task during the middle years (Erikson).
- Piaget's theoretical stage of concrete operations refers to the school-age period, when children are able to use their thought processes to experience events and actions and make judgments based on what they reason.
- Through identity, reversibility, and reciprocity, children master the cognitive task of conservation.

- Children develop a conscience and are able to understand and adhere to rules and standards set by others.
- Spiritual development entails curiosity about deities, knowledge of the difference between the natural and the supernatural, and reliance on prayers or other religious rituals.
- Entertaining different points of view, becoming sensitive to social norms of peers, and forming peer friendships are the most important features of social development in the middle years.
- Children develop a self-concept from their own self-assessment and feedback from others.
- Increased socialization, earlier pubertal development, and constant media exposure make the school years an ideal time for sex education.
- Cooperative play, team activities, and acquisition of skills are prime elements of play during the school years; rules and rituals assume greater importance.

- Optimum nutrition is often hampered by an affinity for and availability of junk foods, irregular family meals, and schedules of working parents.
- Typical parental concerns during middle childhood include dishonest behavior, lying, cheating, stealing, and school-related stress.
- The school years are an ideal time for children to begin to take responsibility for their own health.
- School health centers ideally offer programs that include health appraisal, emergency care, safety education, communicable disease control, counseling, guidance, and health education, with adjustment to individual student needs.
- The major sources of accidental injury during middle childhood include a variety of conveyances, including motor vehicles, bicycles, skateboards, and in-line skates.
- Direct injury prevention toward safety education, provision of safe play areas and equipment, and good supervision of sports activities.

ANSWERS TO CRITICAL THINKING EXERCISES

Temperament in the School-Age Child

1. Although many of Mary's symptoms may be associated with her slow-to-warm-up temperament, it is difficult to rule out other health-related problems. Mary's mother reports that she is in good health, but Mary could have an emotional or chronic illness that has not been identified. The nurse should encourage Mary's mother to visit with her pediatrician if she has not done so already. The nurse should also instruct the teacher and parents about Mary's temperament and offer suggestions to encourage Mary.

2. **a.** By the time a child reaches school-age years, his or her temperament has been defined. Most characteristics of a child's temperament are innate; however, some characteristics can be modified by experiences and interactions with other people and with their environment, by their motives and abilities, and by the child's health.
   b. A child's behavioral adjustment can depend greatly on his or her temperament. Easy children adapt to new environments and people quickly; children who are slow to warm up may initially withdraw when encountering new situations; and difficult children usually adapt to new situations poorly, with explosive or stubborn behavior.
   c. Possible interventions include preparing the child for the specific activity in advance, allowing a friend to assist with the activity, offering praise and encouragement when the activity is completed, providing opportunities to do things the child is good at, and allowing the child extra time to get ready for the activity.

3. The first priority for the school nurse should be to discuss the situation with Mary's mother to ensure that all potential causes of Mary's behavior have been evaluated. If there is no evidence of other causes, Mary's temperament characteristics should be discussed. The school nurse should educate Mary's teachers and parents about her slow-to-warm-up temperament so that Mary's needs can be accommodated to allow her to excel in all situations. The school nurse should evaluate what events are difficult for Mary and provide appropriate interventions for the teacher and parents to use when encountering these situations.

4. **Yes.** The information about Mary's behavior provides a conclusion that Mary is either a slow-to-warm-up child or has an emotional or chronic illness. If emotional and chronic illnesses are ruled out, Mary's behavior can be attributed to her temperament. Mary's behavior fits into the slow-to-warm-up category and can be managed by assisting her in dealing with new situations.

Physical Growth in the School-Age Child

1. **Yes.** There is sufficient evidence to conclude that Janie is overweight. School-age children do not grow as quickly as they did in the preschool years; therefore caloric needs are diminished. Growth during school-age years is more even and steady with an average weight gain per year of 2.5 kg (5.5 lb). The 50th percentile for weight and height in an 8-year-old girl is 25.3 kg (55.8 lb) and 127 cm (50 inches), respectively.

2. **a.** Children's eating patterns include increased restaurant food consumption, larger portion sizes, shifts in beverage consumption, and changes in meal patterns and meal frequency. Children are not eating the recommended servings of fruits, vegetables, and grains but are eating a diet high in fat, sweetened beverages, and salty foods.
   b. Risk factors include genetic factors such as high birth weight, maternal diabetes, and obesity in family members; environmental factors such as low economic status, lack of access to healthy food choices, and parental food choices; and societal factors such as increasingly sedentary leisure activities and decreased physical activity required in schools.
   c. Comorbidities include high blood pressure, insulin resistance and type 2 diabetes, hypercholesterolemia, dyslipidemia, and mental health issues such as depression and low self-esteem.
   d. Although parents exert a big influence on children's attitudes and food choices, school-age children are starting to make decisions on their own. Parents do not know what or how much their children eat when they are away from home, such as during school lunch or at a friend's house. Therefore educating the child about healthy food choices is essential so that the child can make appropriate food choices for his or her growing body.

3. Nursing care should include extensive education about nutrition and physical activity. This information should be shared with Janie and her family. Appropriate food consumption should include healthy eating patterns with nutritious snacks and suitable food portion sizes. Information about the importance and benefits of physical exercise should also be discussed, along with ideas for potential activities.

4. **Yes.** The data support the conclusion that Janie is overweight. Information about Janie's food consumption and physical activity should be evaluated so that appropriate interventions can be identified.

Bicycle Helmets

1. **Yes.** There is a lack of bicycle helmet usage among children in your school district that is causing an increased risk for injury and deaths. Bicycling is one of the most popular recreational sports among children; however, it is also the leading cause of sports-related injuries when preventive gear is not used.

2. **a.** Hazards to children include serious brain injury, head injury, facial injury, broken bones, and abrasions.

   b. Intrinsic factors include children exceeding their ability level when riding or attempting to perform stunts; extrinsic factors include swerving to avoid a motor vehicle, striking a fixed object, and not wearing protective gear.

   c. The most influential factors associated with bicycle helmet use include helmet use by an accompanying parent and a state mandatory helmet law. Other factors include discomfort (especially heat), perceived lack of importance for casual riding, lack of style, and peer pressure.

   d. Pediatricians and nurses should serve as community and legislative advocates to encourage legislation requiring helmet use; encourage school districts to mandate helmet use when riding bicycles to and from school; assist in developing and implementing community- and school-based education programs to promote bicycle safety; urge retail stores to include helmets in the purchase of every new bicycle sold; and urge the media to consistently show helmets whenever bicycle riding is portrayed.

3. The major implication for nursing is the need to educate children and families on the importance of wearing helmets and other bicycle safety information.

4. **Yes.** Educating children and families about bicycle safety can reduce the number of bicycle-related injuries. Use of bicycle helmets can lessen the severity of brain injury and head trauma when used correctly. Other safety educational strategies add to the prevention of further injury.

REFERENCES

American Academy of Pediatrics, Council on School Health: Medical emergencies occurring at school, *Pediatrics* 122(4):887-894, 2008a.

American Academy of Pediatrics, Council on School Health: Role of the school nurse in providing school health services, *Pediatrics* 121(5):1052-1056, 2008b.

American Academy of Pediatrics, Committee on Injury, Violence, and Poison Prevention and Council on School Health: School transportation safety, *Pediatrics* 120(1):213-220, 2007.

American Psychological Association: *Undoing dyslexia via video games*, 2005, available at www.psychologymatters.org/dyslexia.html (accessed February 26, 2009).

Bagby K, Adams S: Evidence-based practice guideline: increasing physical activity in schools—kindergarten through 8th grade, *J Sch Nurs* 23(3):137-143, 2007.

Cawley J, Meyerhoefer C, Newhouse D: The impact of state physical education requirements on youth physical activity and overweight, *Health Economics* 16:1287-1301, 2007.

Centers for Disease Control and Prevention: *Motor vehicle safety*, 2009a, available at www.cdc.gov/MotorVehicleSafety/Child_Passenger_Safety/childseat-spot.html (accessed March 1, 2009).

Centers for Disease Control and Prevention: *Overweight and obesity*, 2009b, available at www.cdc.gov/nccdphp/dnpa/obesity/childhood/prevalence.htm (accessed February 22, 2009).

Centers for Disease Control and Prevention: *Healthy youth! Coordinated school health programs*, 2008, available at www.cdc.gov/HealthyYouth/CSHP (accessed February 26, 2009).

Christakis D, Zimmerman F: Children and television: a primer for pediatricians, *Contemp Pediatr* 24(3):31-42, 2007.

Durrant J: Physical punishment, culture, and rights: current issues for professionals, *J Dev Behav Pediatr* 29(1):55-66, 2008.

Eisenberg M, Bernat D, Bearinger L, et al: Support for comprehensive sexuality education: perspectives from parents of school-age youth, *J Adolesc Health* 42:352-359, 2008.

Eisenbraun K: Violence in schools: prevalence, prediction, and prevention, *Aggression Violent Behav* 12:459-469, 2007.

Erikson EH: *Childhood and society*, ed 2, New York, 1963, Norton.

Fowler P, Tompsett C, Braciszewski J, et al: Community violence: a meta-analysis on the effect of exposure and mental health outcomes of children and adolescents, *Dev Psychopathol* 21:227-259, 2009.

Fredland N: Nurturing hostile environments: the problem of school violence, *Fam Commun Health* 31(Suppl 1):S32-S41, 2008.

Gini G: Association between bullying behaviour, psychosomatic complaints, emotional and behavioural problems, *J Paediatr Child Health* 44(9):492-497, 2007.

Guralnick S, Serwint J: Firearms, *Pediatr Rev* 28(10):396-397, 2007.

Holt S, Buckley H, Whelan S: The impact of exposure to domestic violence on children and young people: a review of the literature, *Child Abuse Negl* 32(8):797-810, 2008.

Jenson J, Dieterich W: Effects of a skills-based prevention program on bullying and bully victimization among elementary school children, *Prev Sci* 8(4):285-296, 2007.

Killingsworth J, Tilford J, Parker J, et al: National hospitalization impact of pediatric all-terrain vehicle injuries, *Pediatrics* 115(3):e316-e321, 2005.

Li H, Prevatt F: Fears and related anxieties across three age groups of Mexican American and white children with disabilities, *J Genetic Psychol* 168(4):381-400, 2007.

Linakis J, Mello M, Machan J, et al: Emergency department visits for pediatric trampoline-related injuries: an update, *Acad Emerg Med* 14:539-544, 2007.

McColgan MD, Giardino AP: Internet poses multiple risks to children and adolescents, *Pediatr Ann* 34(5):405-414, 2005.

Merriman J: Wearing protective sports gear, *Contemp Pediatr* 26(2):34, 2009.

Murphy N, Young P: Sexuality in children and adolescents with disabilities, *Dev Med Child Neurol* 47:640-644, 2005.

Murrell A, Christoff K, Henning K: Characteristics of domestic violence offenders: associations with childhood exposure to violence, *J Fam Violence* 22:523-532, 2007.

National Highway Traffic Safety Administration: *Traffic safety facts, bicyclists and other cyclists*, 2008, available at www.nrd.nhtsa.dot.gov/Pubs/811156.PDF (accessed February 1, 2010).

National Highway Traffic Safety Administration: *Traffic safety facts, children*, 2007, available at www.nhtsa.gov (accessed March 1, 2009).

Nayci A, Stavlo P, Zarroug A, et al: Snowmobile injuries in children and adolescents, *Mayo Clin Proc* 81(1):39-44, 2006.

Newgard CD, Lewis RJ: Effects of child age and body size on serious injury from passenger air-bag presence in motor vehicle crashes, *Pediatrics* 115(6):1579-1585, 2005.

Okun A, Adam H: Safety on bicycles, skateboards, scooters, and skates, *Pediatr Rev* 29(10):366-367, 2008.

Podberscek AL: Positive and negative aspects of our relationship with companion animals, *Vet Res Commun* 30(S1):21-27, 2006.

Rideout V, Roberts D, Foehr U: *Generation M: media in the lives of 8-18 year olds*, 2005, Kaiser Family Foundation, available at www.kff.org/entmedia/7251.cfm (accessed February 26, 2009).

Samson Z: Lawn-mowing fraught with danger, *Am Acad Pediatr News* 27(8):29-30, 2006.

Schredl M, Biemelt J, Roos K, et al: Nightmares and stress in children, *Sleep Hypnosis* 10(1):19-25, 2008.

Smaldone A, Honig J, Byrne M: Sleepless in America: inadequate sleep and relationships to health and well-being of our nation's children, *Pediatrics* 119(S1):S29-S37, 2007.

Spruyt K, O'Brien L, Cluydts R, et al: Odds, prevalence and predictors of sleep problems in school-age normal children, *J Sleep Res* 14:163-176, 2005.

Towe-Goodman N, Teti D: Power assertive discipline, maternal emotional involvement, and child adjustment, *J Fam Psychol* 22(3):648-651, 2008.

US Department of Agriculture: *MyPlate*, 2011, available at www.choosemyplate.gov (accessed September 8, 2011).

Van Der Molen JH, Bushman BJ: Children's direct fright and worry reactions to violence in fiction and news television programs, *J Pediatr* 153:420-424, 2008.

Vollman D, Smith GA: Epidemiology of lawn mower–related injuries to children in the United States, *Pediatrics* 118(2):e273-e278, 2006.

Vreeman RC, Carroll AE: A systematic review of school-based interventions to prevent bullying, *Arch Pediatr Adolesc Med* 161:78-88, 2007.

Wagner R, Oskouian R: The ECG epidemic, *Contemp Pediatr* 25(9):60-79, 2008.

Weems CF, Costa NM: Developmental differences in the expression of childhood anxiety symptoms and fears, *J Am Acad Child Adolesc Psychiatry* 44(7):656-663, 2005.

Wells HF, Buzby JC: *Dietary assessment of major trends in U.S. food consumption*, 2008, US Department of Agriculture, available at www.ers.usda.gov (accessed March 8, 2009).

Williams KR, Guerra NG: Prevalence and predictors of Internet bullying, *J Adolesc Health* 41(6):S14-S21, 2007.

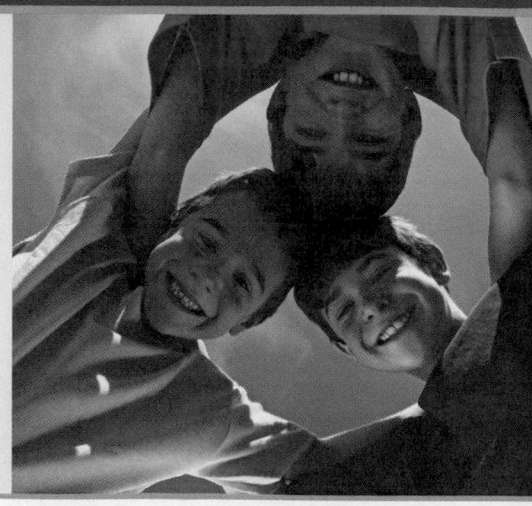

evolve WEBSITE

RELATED TOPICS

CHAPTER OUTLINE

DISORDERS AFFECTING THE SKIN

Skin of Younger Children

The major skin layers arise from different embryologic origins. Early in the embryonic period, a single layer of epithelium forms from the ectoderm, while simultaneously the corium develops from the mesenchyme. In the infant and small child the epidermis is still loosely bound to the dermis, partly because the rete pegs are flat. This poor adherence causes the layers to separate readily and form blisters during an inflammatory process. This is especially true in preterm infants, who have an even greater propensity to blister formation and separation during careless handling (such as removal of adhesive tape). The skin is thinner than in older children, and the cells of all strata are more compressed.

Several characteristics influence skin responses in infants and young children. Their skin is far more susceptible to superficial bacterial infection compared with older children and adults. They are more likely to have associated systemic symptoms with some infections and are more apt to react to a primary irritant than to a sensitizing allergen. Infants and young children are more frequently affected by chronic atopic dermatitis (eczema). The infant's skin is much more prone to develop a toxic erythema as a result of skin eruptions or drug reactions and is subject to maceration, infection, and the moisture retention associated with diaper rash.

SKIN LESIONS

Lesions of the skin can result from a variety of etiologic factors. In general, skin lesions originate from (1) contact with injurious agents such as infectious organisms, toxic chemicals, and physical trauma; (2) hereditary factors; (3) an external factor that produces a reaction in the skin (e.g., allergens); or (4) a systemic disease in which the lesions are a cutaneous manifestation (e.g., measles, lupus erythematosus, nutritional deficiency diseases). Responses are highly individual. An agent that may be harmless to one individual may be damaging to another, and a single agent may produce various types of responses in different individuals.

Another factor involved in the etiology of skin manifestations is the child's age. For example, infants are subject to "birthmark" malformations and atopic dermatitis that appear early in life, the school-age child is susceptible to ringworm of the scalp, and acne is a characteristic skin disorder of puberty. Contact dermatitis, such as that caused by poison ivy, occurs only where the noxious agent is touched. Similarly, insect bites are associated with life-cycle and seasonal activities. Tension and anxiety may produce, modify, or prolong many skin conditions, although this is less common in children.

Pathophysiology of Dermatitis

More than half of dermatologic problems are various forms of dermatitis. This implies a sequence of inflammatory changes in the skin that are grossly and microscopically similar but diverse in course and causation. Acute responses produce intercellular and intracellular edema, the formation of intradermal vesicles, and an initial minimum infiltration of inflammatory cells into the epidermis. In the dermis there is edema, vascular dilation, and early perivascular cellular infiltration. The location and manner of these reactions produce the lesions characteristic of each disorder. The changes are reversible, and the skin ordinarily recovers without blemish and completely intact unless complicating factors such as ulceration from the primary irritant, scratching, and infection are introduced or underlying vascular disease develops. In chronic conditions permanent effects are seen that vary according to the disorder, the general condition of the affected individual, and available therapy.

Clinical Manifestations and Diagnostic Evaluation

The following discussion first explores the history and symptoms, but also notes some objective findings simultaneously. One of the more advantageous aspects of skin lesions is that often the diagnosis is readily established after simple, careful inspection.

History and Symptoms

Many cutaneous lesions are associated with local symptoms, the most common of which is itching (**pruritus**) that varies in kind and intensity. Pain or tenderness often accompanies some skin lesions, and other sensations may be described as burning, prickling, stinging, or crawling. Alterations in local feeling or sensation include absence of sensation (**anesthesia**); excessive sensitivity (**hyperesthesia**); diminished sensation (**hypesthesia**); and abnormal sensation, such as burning or prickling (**paresthesia**). These symptoms may remain localized or may migrate. They may also be constant or intermittent and may be aggravated by a specific activity or circumstance, such as exposure to sunlight.

Determining whether the child has had an allergic condition such as asthma or hay fever or has had previous skin disease is also important. Atopic dermatitis, often associated with allergies, frequently begins in infancy. It should be determined when the lesion or symptom first became apparent and whether it is related to ingestion of a food or other substance, including any medication the child might be taking. Keep in mind that the condition may be related to an activity such as contact with plants, insects, or chemicals.

Objective Findings

The skin lesion's distribution, size, and morphologic characteristics provide significant information. The usual extrinsic causes are physical, chemical, or allergic irritants or infectious agents such as bacteria, fungi, viruses, or animal parasites. Intrinsic causes such as a specific infection (e.g., measles or chickenpox), drug sensitization, or other allergic phenomena can produce skin manifestations. Other diagnostic tools include medical and laboratory studies.

Laboratory Studies

When it is suspected that a skin problem might be related to a systemic disease, such as one of the collagen diseases or an immunodeficiency disease, studies are needed to rule out these possibilities. Diagnostic modalities include microscopic examination, cultures, skin scrapings or biopsy, cytodiagnosis, patch testing, and Wood light examination. Allergic skin testing and various other laboratory tests (blood count, sedimentation rate) are used when indicated.

WOUNDS

Wounds are structural or physiologic disruptions of the integument that call for normal or abnormal tissue repair responses. All wounds can be classified as acute or chronic. Acute wounds are those that heal uneventfully within the usual time frame. Chronic wounds are those that do not heal in the expected time frame or are associated with many complications. In children most wounds are acute and can be prevented from becoming chronic through appropriate nursing care. Wounds are classified in the same manner as burns: partial-thickness, full-thickness, and complex wounds that include muscle and/or bone. Wounds that often become chronic are burns and pressure ulcers, localized areas of cellular necrosis that develop when soft tissue is compressed between a bony prominence and a firm surface. (See Burns, Chapter 29, and Maintaining Healthy Skin, Chapter 27.)

Some types of acute wounds are the following:

Abrasion—Removal of the superficial layers of skin by rubbing or scraping

Avulsion—Forcible pulling out or extraction of tissue

Laceration—Torn or jagged wound; accidental cut wound

Incision—Division of the skin made with a sharp object; cut

Penetrating wound—Disruption of the skin surface that extends into underlying tissue or into a body cavity

Puncture—Wound with a relatively small opening compared with the depth

Process of Wound Healing
Epidermal Injuries

Abrasions are the most common epidermal wounds of childhood, usually in the form of a skinned knee or elbow. In most injuries the margins of the abraded area are superficial, involving only the outer layers of epidermis, although the central portion may extend into the dermis. Initially the defect is

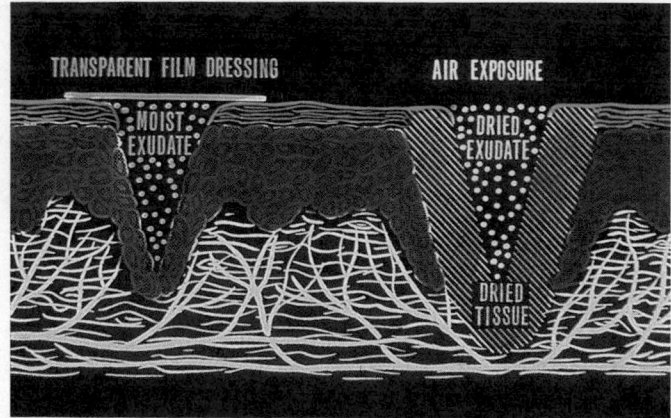

Fig. 18-1 Process of epithelialization is facilitated by maintaining a moist environment as opposed to a dry, open environment. In a moist environment, epithelial cells freely migrate across the wound surface. (Courtesy ConvaTec, Princeton, NJ.)

filled by a blood clot and necrotic debris, which subsequently dehydrate to form a scab. Epithelial tissue is composed of labile cells, which are constantly destroyed and replaced throughout life. Injury to these tissues results in **regeneration** (i.e., rapid replacement by similar cells).

The epithelial wound heals by migration and proliferation of epithelial cells from the wound margin and from cells surviving in transected skin appendages. This response begins within 24 to 48 hours after the wound is incurred. Cell migration ceases when migrating cells make contact with epithelial cells migrating from all other sites. Fixed basal cells adjacent to the wound edge and in skin appendages begin to divide rapidly to replace the migrated cells. As resurfacing is accomplished, the migrated cells begin to divide and thicken the new epithelial layer.

Epithelial cells advance over the wound surface by "flowing." The first cell advances, anchors, and then moves no more. Instead, a cell from behind advances over it, anchors, and subsequently is overridden by other cells that advance over both of the primary cells—similar to a leapfrog movement. Epithelial cells move most rapidly in moist environments, such as when the wound is covered with a transparent or other occlusive-type dressing, and the rate of epithelialization depends on a variety of factors, particularly the amount of oxygen supplied to the wound. Allowing the skin to dry and form an **eschar** or crust (scab) impedes the migration of epithelial cells (Fig. 18-1). In addition, fluid may collect and infection may occur under the eschar.

Injury to Deeper Tissues

Tissues composed of permanent cells, such as muscle and some nerve cells, are unable to regenerate. Therefore these tissues repair themselves by substituting fibrous connective tissue for the injured tissue. This fibrous tissue, or scar, serves as a patch to preserve or restore the continuity of the tissue. Wounds involving permanent cells include surgical incisions, lacerations, ulcers, evulsions, and full-thickness burns. Injured cells of glandular organs and bones, composed of stable cells, multiply less vigorously and heal more slowly. (See Bone Healing and Remodeling, Chapter 39.) With some wounds an overgrowth of nerve endings may occur, resulting in allodynia, or the sensation of pain from normally nonpainful stimuli, such as light touch.

Mechanism of Wound Healing

The nonspecific repair mechanism of wound healing with scar formation involves the processes of inflammation, fibroplasia, scar contraction, and scar maturation. The initial response at the site of injury is inflammation, a vascular and cellular response that prepares the tissues for the subsequent repair process. There is a transient constriction of transected blood vessels, lasting 5 to 10 minutes, followed by active vasodilation of all local small vessels and increased blood flow to the area. This is accompanied by increased permeability of small venules, which allows plasma to leak into surrounding tissues (edema). A blood clot is formed along wound edges, providing a framework for future growth of capillaries (angiogenesis) and epithelial cells.

At the same time, vessel walls become lined with leukocytes, primarily neutrophils, which pass through the walls and concentrate at the injured site, where they ingest bacteria and debris (phagocytosis). Neutrophils are superseded by macrophages, which continue phagocytosis, and also by growth factors needed for skin repair and angiogenesis. Fibroblasts attracted to the area from blood vessels deposit fibrin throughout the clot. Adjacent capillaries begin to form buds that stretch across the supporting fibrin threads, and epithelial cells secrete a fibrolytic enzyme that allows their advancement across the wound. This initial phase of wound healing takes place during the first 3 to 5 days after injury. The wound is weakest at this time.

Fibroplasia (granulation or proliferation), the second phase of healing, lasts from 5 days to 4 weeks. Fibroblasts, immature connective tissue cells, migrate to the healing site and begin to secrete collagen into the meshwork spaces. Granulation tissue is highly vascular, "beefy" red, shiny connective tissue that organizes and restructures, forming thicker, stronger fibers arranged in orderly layers. A thin layer of epithelial tissue is regenerated over the surface of the wound, and leukocytes gradually disappear from the area. The wound is fragile at this time, and granulation tissue bleeds profusely if disturbed.

During contraction and maturation, the third and fourth phases of wound healing, collagen continues to be deposited and organized into layers, compressing the new blood vessels and gradually stopping blood flow across the wound. Fibroblasts disappear as the wound becomes stronger. Fibroblast movement causes contraction of the healing area, which helps to bring wound edges closer together. A mature scar is then formed. Initially the scar is pink and raised. With maturation, the scar becomes pale, does not tan when exposed to sunlight, will not sweat or produce hair, and may cause itching. The maturation process may continue for years, and the extent to which the scar remodels and matures varies among individuals.

Children heal aggressively with abundant scar tissue, especially during growth spurts. Because of its highly elastic quality, children's skin pulls on wounds, which defend against the pull by aggressive scarring. Consequently, the child's skin heals with more scar tissue than the less elastic skin of the adult.

First intention (clean incision)

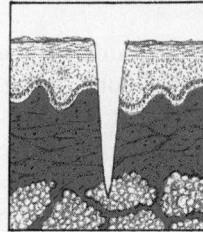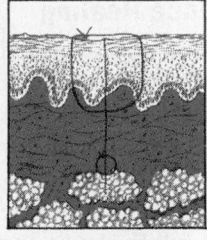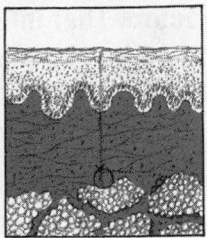

Second intention (wide, irregular wound)

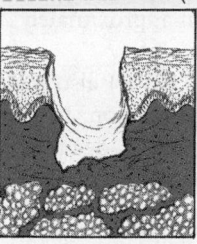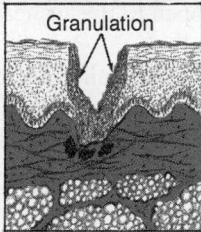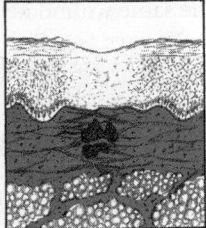

Granulation

Third intention (puncture wound)

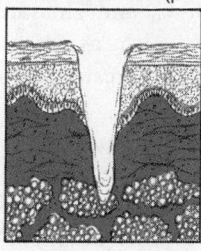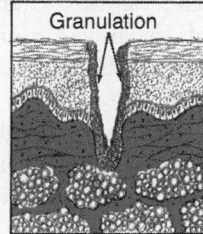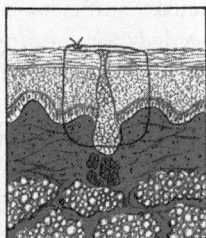

Granulation

Fig. 18-2 Types of wound healing.

Types of Wound Healing

Repair healing takes place in one of three ways: by primary, secondary, or tertiary intention (Fig. 18-2). Primary intention healing takes place when all layers of the wound margins (skin, subcutaneous tissue, and muscle) are neatly approximated, as with a surgical incision. Unless infection interferes or the wound edges separate, these wounds heal with a minimum of scarring.

Repair by secondary intention takes place in wounds that occur from ulceration and lacerations in which the edges cannot be approximated, such as an avulsion or a third-degree burn. The inflammatory reaction may be greater, and the chance of infection is increased. Often debris, cells, and exudate must be cleaned away (débrided) before healing can take place. Healing takes place from the edges inward and from the bottom of the wound upward until the defect is filled. More granulation tissue and a larger scar are formed than in healing by primary intention.

Repair by tertiary intention takes place when suturing is delayed after injury or the wound later breaks down and is sutured or resutured when granulation is present. More granulation tissue is formed than in healing by primary intention, and there is a greater chance that microorganisms will invade the wound. Frequently, suturing of a contaminated wound is deliberately delayed to afford better removal of infection before closing. Healing of wounds by tertiary intention results in a larger and deeper scar than healing by primary intention.

Factors That Influence Healing

During the past two decades, understanding of wound healing has revolutionized the interventions used to promote healing. Emphasis has shifted from interventions directed at maintaining a dry environment that promotes eschar formation to those that promote a moist, crust-free environment that enhances the migration of epithelial cells across the wound and facilitates resurfacing. An acute full-thickness wound kept in a moist environment usually reepithelializes in 12 to 15 days, whereas the same wound kept open to the air heals in approximately 25 to 30 days (see Fig. 18-1).

Eschar (thick, fibrin-containing necrotic tissue) also interferes with healing by preventing wound contraction. In most situations it is best to remove eschar and other dead tissue from the wound. Repeated application of occlusive dressings mobilizes the body's own enzymes to lyse the eschar, a process known as autolysis.

Adequate nutrition is essential for wound healing. In particular, sufficient protein, calories, vitamin C, and zinc are needed for healing of extensive wounds, such as burns. Supplemental nutrition is an integral aspect of treatment of severe wounds.

Numerous factors delay healing (Table 18-1). Some traditional practices are ineffective or even harmful; for example, antiseptics that were once used to help prevent infections (hydrogen peroxide and povidone-iodine [Betadine] solutions) are now known to have cytotoxic effects on healthy cells and minimal effect on controlling infections. Povidone-iodine may be absorbed through the skin in neonates and young children and must be used with caution in patients with thyroid or renal disease.

GENERAL THERAPEUTIC MANAGEMENT

The human body tends to heal; therefore direct treatment is directed toward eliminating or ameliorating factors that interfere with normal healing processes. Some disorders may demand aggressive therapy, but by and large the major aim of any treatment is to prevent further damage, eliminate the cause, prevent complications, and provide relief from discomfort while tissues undergo healing. When possible, eliminate factors that contribute to the dermatitis and prolong the course of the disease. The most common offenders in pediatrics are environmental factors (such as soaps, bubble baths, shampoos, rough or tight clothing, wet diapers, blankets, and toys) and natural elements (such as dirt, sand, heat, cold, moisture, and wind). Dermatitis can also be aggravated by home remedies and medications.

Dressings

No one dressing meets the needs of all wounds. The traditional *dry* gauze dressing should not be used on open wounds, since it allows the wound surface to dry, does little to prevent bacterial invasion, and adheres to the dried scab so that removal disturbs the newly regenerating epithelial cells. In most instances, traditional gauze dressings have been replaced by moist wound healing dressings. Moist wound healing increases the rate of collagen synthesis and reepithelialization and

TABLE 18-1	FACTORS THAT DELAY WOUND HEALING
FACTOR	**EFFECT ON HEALING**
Dry wound environment	Allows epithelial cells to dry out and die; impairs migration of epithelial cells across wound surface
Nutritional deficiencies	
Vitamin A	Results in inadequate inflammatory response
Vitamin B_1	Results in decreased collagen formation
Vitamin C	Inhibits formation of collagen fibers and capillary development
Protein	Reduces supply of amino acids for tissue repair
Zinc	Impairs epithelialization
Immunocompromise	Results in inadequate or delayed inflammatory response
Impaired circulation	Inhibits inflammatory response and removal of debris from wound area
	Reduces supply of nutrients to wound area
Stress (pain, poor sleep)	Releases catecholamines that cause vasoconstriction
Antiseptics	
Hydrogen peroxide	Toxic to fibroblasts; can cause subcutaneous gas formation (mimics gas-forming infection)
Povidone-iodine	Toxic to white and red blood cells and fibroblasts
Chlorhexidine	Toxic to white blood cells
Medications	
Corticosteroids	Impair phagocytosis
	Inhibit fibroblast proliferation
	Depress formation of granulation tissue
	Inhibit wound contraction
Chemotherapy	Interrupts the cell cycle
	Damages DNA or prevents DNA repair
Antiinflammatory drugs	Decrease the inflammatory phase
Foreign bodies	Increase inflammatory response
	Inhibit wound closure
Infection	Increases inflammatory response
	Increases tissue destruction
Mechanical friction	Damages or destroys granulation tissue
Fluid accumulation in area	Inhibits tissues from approximating
Radiation	Inhibits fibroblastic activity and capillary formation
	May cause tissue necrosis
Diseases	
Diabetes mellitus	Inhibits collagen synthesis
	Impairs circulation and capillary growth
	Hyperglycemia impairs phagocytosis
Anemia	Reduces oxygen supply to tissues
Peripheral vascular disease	Reduces oxygen supply to wounds
Uremia	Decreases collagen and granulation tissue

DNA, Deoxyribonucleic acid.

decreases pain and inflammation. It also creates an environment for autolytic débridement of necrotic tissue, which creates a clean wound bed and enhances granulation. However, a balance must be achieved between creating a moist wound bed and maintaining a dry periwound area that protects the skin and wound from maceration. The dressing type and frequency of dressing changes help to achieve this balance. The frequency of dressing changes depends on the presence or absence of infection, the type of dressing, the location of the wound, and the amount of drainage. Dressings should always be changed

TABLE 18-2   DRESSING CATEGORY DEFINITIONS AND EXAMPLES OF PRODUCTS

CATEGORY	DESCRIPTION	EXAMPLES
Gauze or sponge for external use	Nonresorbable Sterile or nonsterile Strip, piece, or pad Woven or nonwoven mesh cotton cellulose Simple chemical derivatives of cellulose Intended for medical purposes	Pads Island dressings
Hydrophilic wound dressing	Sterile or nonsterile Nonresorbable Material with hydrophilic properties No added drugs or biologics Intended to cover wound and absorb exudate	Alginate dressings Foam dressings Hydropolymer dressings Sheet gel dressings Hydrocolloid dressings Composite dressings Hydrogel dressings
Occlusive wound dressing	Sterile or nonsterile Nonresorbable Synthetic polymeric material with or without adhesive backing Intended to cover wound, provide or support moist wound environment, and allow exchange of gases	Transparent adhesive dressings Thin film dressings Foam dressings Hydrocolloid dressings Composite dressings Hydropolymer dressings
Hydrogel wound dressing	Sterile or nonsterile Nonresorbable Matrix of hydrophilic polymers or other material combined with at least 50% water Intended to cover wound; absorb wound exudates; control bleeding or fluid loss; and protect against abrasion, friction, desiccation, and contamination	Alginate dressings Hydropolymer dressings Hydrogel dressings Gauze dressings impregnated with hydrogel (without active ingredients)
Porcine wound dressing	Made from pigskin Temporary burn dressing	

From van Rijswijk L: Recommendations to change the FDA classification of various wound dressings, *Ostomy Wound Manage* 45(3):31, 1999. Used with permission.

when they are loose or soiled. They should be changed more frequently in areas where contamination is likely (e.g., the sacral area, the buttocks, the tracheal area) or when wound infection is suspected or confirmed.

Dressings serve the following functions: (1) provide a moist healing environment, (2) protect the wound from infection and trauma, (3) provide compression in the event of anticipated bleeding or swelling, (4) apply medication, (5) absorb drainage, (6) débride necrotic tissue, (7) reduce pain, and (8) control odor. To ensure a moist environment, cover wounds with an occlusive ointment or dressing (Table 18-2).

Occlusive dressings can be classified according to their degree of permeability. The term *occlusive* is synonymous with impermeable, *semiocclusive* is synonymous with semipermeable, and *nonocclusive* is synonymous with permeable. No one dressing meets the needs of all types of wounds. The traditional gauze dressing is a permeable dressing that reduces the moisture content in a wound by absorbing exudate and allowing it to evaporate. Traditional gauze dressings should not be used on open wounds because they allow wounds to dehydrate, are permeable to bacteria, increase the probability of wound sepsis, and adhere to the wound when removed, which causes additional trauma to newly regenerating epithelial cells. In many situations traditional gauze dressings have been replaced by new "active occlusive" dressings, which allow for moist wound healing. The use of silver in wound care has reemerged.

Silver is impregnated in various dressing vehicles such as foam, hydrocolloid dressings, and wound gels. Several studies suggest that silver decreases the bacteria and bioburden in the wound, which allows optimal wound conditions for granulation and healing (Ovington, 2004). Since the absorption of these products in infants and children is unknown, use caution when applying these dressings in the pediatric population.

Topical Therapy

A variety of agents and methods are available for treatment of dermatologic problems. In selecting a therapeutic program, the practitioner considers (1) the active ingredient of the agent, (2) the vehicle or base, (3) the cosmetic effect, (4) the cost, and (5) instructions for the agent's use. In addition, keep several basic concepts in mind. Avoid overtreatment. For example, when the dermatitis is acute, topical applications should be mild and bland to avoid further irritation. Broken or inflamed skin, especially in children, is more absorbent than intact skin, and chemicals that are nonirritating to intact skin may be quite irritating to inflamed skin.

Topical applications may be used to treat the disorder, reduce the itching associated with many diseases, decrease external stimuli, or provide external heat or cold. The emollient action of soaks, baths, and lotions provides a soothing film over the skin surface that reduces external stimuli. Ordinarily, tepid or cool applications offer the greatest relief.

Topical Corticosteroid Therapy

The glucocorticoids are the therapeutic agents used most widely for skin disorders. Their local antiinflammatory effects are merely palliative, so the medication must be applied until the disease state undergoes a remission or the causative agent is eliminated. Corticosteroids are applied directly to the affected area. Because they are essentially nonsensitizing and have only minor side effects, they can be applied over prolonged periods with continuing effectiveness. As with any steroids, their use in large amounts may mask signs of infection, and symptoms may be exacerbated after termination of the drug. Caution families that the medication cannot be used for all skin disorders. At the concentrations available without prescription, they are not adequate for some stubborn conditions (e.g., psoriasis) and may lead to worsening of inflammation caused by fungus or bacteria. Most parents and children apply too much topical hydrocortisone; therefore counsel them that it is both effective and economical to apply only a thin film and to massage it into the skin. Also advise parents and children to use the medication for no more than 5 to 7 days because these agents may cause depigmentation and other changes in the skin.

Other Topical Therapies

Other topical treatments include chemical cautery (especially useful for warts), cryosurgery, electrodesiccation (chiefly used for warts, granulomas, and nevi), ultraviolet therapy (primarily used in psoriasis and acne), laser therapy (especially for birthmarks), and special acne therapies such as dermabrasion and chemical peels. New drugs called topical immunomodulators are effective in reducing the itching of atopic dermatitis (eczema) and preventing flare-ups. Recently, chronic use of immunomodulators in transplant patients has been linked to possible skin cancer and lymphoma. The U.S. Food and Drug Administration (FDA) has issued a black box warning cautioning against the use of these topicals as first-line treatments in children younger than 2 years of age (Dohil and Eichenfield, 2005). A recent study by Papp, Breuer, Meurer, and colleagues (2005) on the use of pimecrolimus cream (Elidel) in infants and children concluded that there was no apparent effect on the antibody responses in these patients.

Systemic Therapy

Systemic therapeutic agents are often used as an adjunct to topical therapy in dermatologic disorders, and those most frequently used therapeutically are the corticosteroids and the antibiotics. The corticosteroid hormones, with their capacity to inhibit inflammatory and allergic reactions, are valuable in the treatment of severe skin disorders. Dosage is carefully adjusted and gradually tapered to the minimum that is effective and tolerated. In infants and children, the dosage is larger than is usually calculated from body weight ratios. However, prolonged use may temporarily suppress growth.

Antibiotics, which interfere with the growth of microorganisms, are used in cases of severe or widespread skin infection. However, because they tend to produce a hypersensitivity in the patient, they are used with caution. Antifungal agents are the only means for treating systemic fungal infections.

NURSING CARE OF THE CHILD WITH A SKIN DISORDER

To help establish a diagnosis, it is important for nurses to accurately describe any deviation in the character of the skin, using both inspection and palpation. Note the color, shape, and distribution of the lesions or wounds. Describe the individual lesions using the accepted terminology and may consist of more than one type, such as a maculopapular rash. Assess wounds for depth of tissue damage, evidence of healing, and signs of infection.

To confirm or amplify the findings made by inspection, gently palpate the skin to detect characteristics such as temperature, moisture, texture, elasticity, and the presence of edema. Indicate whether the findings are restricted to the area of the lesion(s) or are generalized.

QUALITY PATIENT OUTCOMES: Skin Disorder
- Early, accurate diagnosis of the skin lesion or disorder
- Effective treatment and symptom relief
- Prevention of spread if contagious

The child's symptoms provide additional information. Older children are able to describe the condition as painful, itching, or tingling or in other descriptive terms. However, the nurse can determine much by noting the younger child's behavior and the parents' account of these reactions. Does the child scratch? Is the child restless or irritable? Does the child favor or avoid using a body part? A careful history may provide clues. Has the child had access to chemicals or been in the woods or around a woodpile? Has the child eaten a new food? Is the child taking medication? Does the child have any known allergy? Do any playmates have a similar lesion? An uncertain diagnosis is frequently confirmed on the basis of the history.

Therapeutic programs are usually designed to provide general measures, such as rest, protection, and relief of discomfort; and specific treatments, such as a definitive medication or physical technique. Because only a few skin diseases are contagious, it is usually not necessary to isolate the affected child unless there is a danger of the child's acquiring a secondary infection (e.g., the child who is receiving large doses of corticosteroids or other immunosuppressant drugs or the child with an immunologic deficiency disorder). If the skin manifestation is a viral exanthem, such as measles or chickenpox, the child is prevented from exposing other susceptible children.

Wound Care

Parents can generally manage small wounds to the skin at home. Instruct parents to wash their hands and then wash the wound gently with mild soap and water, or normal saline. Caution them to avoid povidone-iodine, alcohol, and hydrogen peroxide because these products are toxic to wounds. To prevent possible tattooing, an abrasion from which the dirt cannot be removed requires wound cleaning with the patient receiving topical anesthesia. Wounds covering a very large area (>15% of the body) need medical attention with the child undergoing conscious sedation and analgesia. (See Chapter 7.) Open wounds are covered with a dressing, such as a commercial adhesive bandage, although larger wounds may benefit from the use of occlusive dressings (see Table 18-2). If occlusive dressings are applied, instruct the parents on their correct application and removal. For example, hydrocolloid dressings adhere best if a wide margin is left around the wound and the dressing is pressed against intact skin until it adheres. The edges of the dressing can be secured to the skin with waterproof tape. The dressings are removed if leakage occurs or after a specific time interval, usually 7 days.

Dressings are removed carefully to protect intact skin and the epithelial surface of the wound from damage. To remove transparent or hydrocolloid dressings, raise one edge of the dressing and pull parallel to the skin to loosen the adhesive. The longer the dressings are left on, the easier they are to remove. Use of a nonalcohol skin barrier protects the skin from epidermal stripping on tape removal. Or the wound may be "picture-framed" with strips of a skin barrier dressing (DuoDERM, Coloplast) on the skin and the adhesive tape secured to the skin barrier. This technique protects the underlying skin with dressing changes. If a dressing sticks to the wound base when it is being removed, saturate the dressing with normal saline, water, or wound cleanser to loosen it.

> ! **NURSING ALERT**
>
> Don't put anything in a wound that you wouldn't put in your eye. The safest solution is normal saline.

> ! **NURSING ALERT**
>
> Advise parents that the yellow gel forming under hydrocolloid dressings may look like pus and has a distinct odor (somewhat fruity) but is normal leakage.

Lacerations present a special challenge. The injured child and family are usually distressed by the bleeding and are in variable degrees of shock. Parental guilt usually accompanies the injury. Because scalp lacerations bleed so profusely, they are especially frightening. The initial nursing intervention is to apply pressure to the area and attempt to calm the child before further examination. Unless there is bleeding from a severed artery, the wound can be cleansed with a forced jet of sterile tepid water or saline (via syringe) and examined for extent; depth; and foreign material such as dirt, glass, or fabric fragments.

> ! **NURSING ALERT**
>
> Hydrogen peroxide and povidone-iodine are contraindicated for cleaning fresh, open wounds. Hydrogen peroxide can cause formation of subcutaneous gas when applied under pressure.

The location of the wound also dictates assessment. For example, wounds over bony areas may contain bone chips, and clear fluid seeping from severe head wounds may indicate cerebrospinal fluid leakage. Apply a pressure dressing for transfer to medical care; prepare the child in a medical facility for suturing. Soak puncture wounds that do not require a tetanus booster in warm water and soap for several minutes. Causing the wound to rebleed may be helpful. Apply an adhesive bandage if desired. Puncture wounds of the head, chest, or abdomen or those that could still contain a portion of the puncturing object must be evaluated.

Caution parents against opening blisters or kissing a wound "to make it better." The wound can easily become contaminated from germs in the human mouth. If scabs form, they are allowed to slough off without assistance; picking or early removal may cause scarring. Advise parents to seek medical help if there is evidence of infection.

Relief of Symptoms

Most of the therapeutic regimens are directed toward relief of pruritus, the most common subjective complaint. Itching is believed to often result from stimulation of C fibers at the dermoepidermal junction. These fibers are similar to but distinct from pain fibers. Substances released within the skin, histamine and endopeptidases, also elicit itching, although their release triggers are unknown (Barnett, 2001).

Cooling the affected area and increasing the skin pH with measures such as cool baths or compresses to reduce external stimuli to the area, as well as alkaline applications such as baking soda baths to increase skin pH, help to prevent scratching. Clothing and bed linen should be soft and lightweight to decrease the irritation from friction and stimulation.

During any type of treatment, both affected and unaffected skin is protected from damage and secondary infection. Preventing scratching is of primary importance. Older children usually cooperate, although they may need to be reminded to stop scratching or rubbing. In smaller and uncooperative children, techniques and devices such as mittens (especially during sleep) or special coverings are required. Keeping fingernails short, well trimmed, and clean helps reduce the chance of secondary infection.

Antipruritic medications, such as diphenhydramine (Benadryl) or hydroxyzine (Atarax), may be prescribed for severe itching, especially if it disturbs the child's rest. Pain and discomfort are usually managed with nonpharmacologic measures and mild analgesia. Severe pain requires more potent medication. Occlusive dressings over wounds reduce pain. For

Evidence-Based Practice—Wound Care

suturing wounds a topical anesthetic, tissue adhesive, or intradermal buffered lidocaine can be used. Pain medications should be given before dressing changes and cleansing, with adequate time allowed for the medicine to take effect. (See Pain Management, Chapter 7.)

Topical therapy usually involves application of some type of topical agent, and the mode of application depends on the nature and location of the lesion being treated. For example, soothing lotions, creams, and intermittent wet dressings or soaks help cool and moisten; ointments, lotions, and creams soften and lubricate dry, scaling areas. Nurses and parents are responsible for the application of topical therapeutic agents.

It is especially important to wash the hands before and after application of topical therapies. Assess the skin before the treatment or application of medication and reassess after the treatment is completed. Note any changes and describe them.

Wet compresses or dressings cool the skin by evaporation, relieve itching and inflammation, and cleanse the area by loosening and removing crusts and debris. Any of a variety of ingredients, such as plain water or Burow solution (available without a prescription), can be applied on Kerlix gauze, plain gauze, or (preferably) soft cotton cloths such as freshly laundered handkerchiefs or strips from cloth diaper, sheeting, or pillowcase material.

Dressings immersed in the desired solution are wrung out slightly and applied to the affected area wet but not dripping. They are applied flat and smooth and in such a way that motion is not totally restricted; fingers are wrapped separately, and arms and legs are wrapped so that elbows and knees can bend. Dressings are kept in place by Kerlix or other cotton wrap, tubular stockinette, mittens, or socks (two pairs—one to hold the dressings in place, the other to take up movement) but are left uncovered. When evaporation begins to dry them, the dressings are removed, rewet in the solution, and reapplied to the area using aseptic technique. The solution is not poured or syringed directly over the dressings. As fluid evaporates, the solution becomes increasingly concentrated and thus stronger, which may damage sensitive lesions.

Fresh solution at room temperature is applied at 2-, 3-, or 4-hour intervals and is allowed to remain on the lesion from 30 to 90 minutes. Wet dressings are seldom continued after about 48 hours. The child must be guarded against chilling during treatment, and no more than 20% of the body should be covered at one time to avoid the risk of hypothermia. After treatment, the skin is dried thoroughly by patting with a towel. Application of lotion or other medication may be ordered at this time.

When children are uncooperative in the use of wet dressings, soaks are often used for removal of crusts and for their mild astringent action. The same solution as for wet compresses is used. Gaining young children's cooperation for hand or foot soaks is difficult unless the procedure is made attractive to them through play. Older infants and toddlers delight in playing with brightly colored objects or poker chips scattered over the bottom of the receptacle, and preschoolers can be challenged to hold a floating item beneath the water's surface. These activities require supervision; infants and small children often place items in their mouths, and children can easily lose control with

water play. Washing dishes, cars, dolls, or doll clothes will occupy many children for some time.

Although older children are able to cooperate, they need something to do during the procedure, such as listening to music or a story, or watching television or a video. A single extremity (a foot or a hand) can be easily soaked by placing the solution and the extremity in a sealable plastic bag. The closure is then zipped snugly around the limb.

Baths are especially useful in the treatment of widespread dermatitis because they evenly distribute the soothing antipruritic and antiinflammatory solution, usually an oatmeal or mineral oil preparation. The solution is added to a tub of water. The temperature of the bath is tepid, and the treatment usually lasts 15 to 30 minutes. Therapeutic baths are always more interesting when the child has toy boats or other items for water play.

Topical agents are applied to skin lesions to ease discomfort, prevent further injury, and facilitate healing. Most preparations are placed directly on the skin and left uncovered; some may be applied under an occlusive dressing. A thin application of the ointment or cream is covered with plastic film and anchored with adhesive or covered with a commercial transparent dressing. Occlusive dressings promote moisture retention and decrease evaporation of the preparation, which increases the penetration of the medication. Apply topical applications systematically with the contour of the body surface (not simply up and down). Children love to be "painted," so lotion applications can be fun when an ordinary paintbrush is employed.

Regardless of the type of preparation used, parents need detailed information on how to apply it and how long the preparation should remain on the skin or under an occlusive dressing.

> **! NURSING ALERT**
>
> Provide written instructions and demonstrate to parents the correct amount of topical medication to apply (e.g., size of a pea; thin film to cover). If more than one preparation is to be applied, mark the containers 1 and 2 to help parents remember the correct order. Stress that more is not necessarily better with some medications, such as steroids.

Recombinant growth factors are human platelet–derived growth factors that are engineered outside the body. They foster the formation of new granulation tissue by stimulating the migration of fibroblasts, macrophages, smooth muscle cells, and capillary endothelial cells to the wound site (Beaumont and Anderson-Dam, 1998). Becaplermin (Regranex) is the only recombinant growth factor currently approved by the FDA; however, the safety of this product has not been established for children under 16 years of age.

The vacuum-assisted closure (VAC) device uses a subatmospheric technique that involves placing an open-cell foam dressing into the wound, covering with an occlusive dressing, and applying suction. The negative force of the suction is applied from the foam dressing to the wound surfaces. The mechanical force removes excess fluids from the wound, stimulates formation of granulation tissue, restores capillary flow, and fosters closure of the wound (Patel, Kinsey, Koperski-

Moen, et al, 2000). VAC has been used to prepare wounds for a skin graft and to treat surgical wounds, burns, and pressure ulcers (Kinetic Concepts, 2003). Recently, VAC therapy has been used in pediatrics. Despite case reports indicating this therapy is beneficial in infants and children, prospective, randomized trials are needed to determine the safety and efficacy of the VAC technique for these age-groups (McCord, Naik-Mathuria, Murphy, et al, 2007; Bookout, McCord, and McLane, 2004).

Home Care and Family Support

Dermatologic conditions always involve the family. Because few situations require hospitalization and children who are hospitalized will complete a therapy program at home, the family must carry out the treatment plan; therefore their cooperation is essential. Regimens that are simple to accomplish in the hospital or office may be frustrating and baffling at home. The family often needs assistance in adapting equipment available in the home to the therapy.

It is important to give the child and family as detailed explanations as possible about both the expected and the unexpected results of treatment, including any ill effects that might occur. Direct the family to discontinue treatment and report the reactions to the appropriate person(s) if unexplained reactions do develop. Discourage the use of over-the-counter medicines unless these have first been approved by the attending practitioner.

Because the skin is the most visible portion of the body, defects in its surface that alter its appearance are sometimes a source of distress to the child and a source of revulsion and rejection by others. Parents of other children may fear that their children will "catch" the disorder. Occasionally the affected child's own family members reduce their interaction with the child, especially close physical contact, or otherwise demonstrate a distaste for the condition, which the child may interpret as rejection. This is seldom a difficulty with dermatitis of short duration, but chronic conditions can create problems and affect the child's self-concept (see Family-Centered Care box).

FAMILY CENTERED CARE

Skin Lesions and Self-Esteem in the School-Aged Child

When I was 8 years old, a lot of small, oval, tannish brown spots developed, especially around my neck and waist. The dermatologist said it was a rare condition and that it should disappear by the time I was 11 or 12. They actually disappeared when I was 10. Because the spots were kind of unusual, the dermatologist invited me to attend a dermatology meeting where people with strange skin problems were placed in private clinic rooms and doctors came in and looked at each person's skin. They were all nice, but I felt a little like an animal in the zoo. The thing I mostly remember about the spots was that I always tried to keep them covered. People stared, and kids made fun of me. The spots didn't hurt or itch, but I always knew they were there. I would not wear a two-piece swimsuit, even though my friends wore them. My mom and I tried to think of anything that might have caused the spots, but I never knew why they developed on me. I remember thinking it wasn't fair that it happened to me. I learned that many times, people cannot prevent the bad things that happen to them.

Marissa, age 16
Tulsa, Oklahoma

INFECTIONS OF THE SKIN

BACTERIAL INFECTIONS

Normally, the skin harbors a variety of bacterial flora, including the major pathogenic varieties of staphylococci and streptococci. The degree of their pathogenicity depends on the invasiveness and toxigenicity of the specific organism, the integrity of the skin (the host's barrier), and the host's immune and cellular defenses. Children with congenital or acquired immune disorders such as acquired immunodeficiency syndrome (AIDS), children in a debilitated condition, those receiving immunosuppressive therapy, and those with a generalized malignancy such as leukemia or lymphoma are at risk for developing bacterial infections.

The characteristic "walling-off" process of the inflammatory reaction (abscess formation) makes staphylococci more difficult to attack, and the local infected area is associated with an increase in the numbers of bacteria all over the skin surface, which serves as a source of continuing infection. Staphylococcal infections occur most often in children in the younger age-groups; the incidence decreases with advancing age. All these factors point up the importance of careful hand washing and cleanliness when caring for infected children and their lesions to prevent spread of the infection and as an essential prophylactic measure when caring for infants and small children. Table 18-3 outlines common bacterial skin disorders.

Nursing Care Management

The major nursing functions related to bacterial skin infections are to prevent the spread of infection and to prevent complications. Impetigo contagiosa and methicillin-resistant *Staphylococcus aureus* (MRSA) infection can easily spread by self-inoculation; therefore caution the child against touching the involved area. Hand washing is mandatory before and after contact with an affected child. Also emphasize hand washing to both the child and the family. Many children with atopic dermatitis are colonized with MRSA in the nares and under the fingernails (Rosenthal, 2004). For many bacterial infections and for MRSA infection in particular, the child should be provided with washcloths and towels separate from those of other family members. The child's pajamas, underwear, and other clothes should be changed daily and washed in hot water. Razors used for shaving should be discarded after each use and not shared. To prevent recurrence, some infectious disease specialists recommend bathing in a chlorine bath once or twice weekly. A 5-minute soak of 2.5 ml of bleach diluted in 13 gallons of water, or 1/2 cup of bleach diluted in a standard 50-gallon tub one fourth filled with water, could decrease community-acquired MRSA colonies by more than 99.9% (Fisher, Chan, Hair, et al, 2008; Kaplan, 2008). In addition, mupirocin can be applied to the nares of patients and families twice daily for 2 to 4 weeks to prevent reinfection (Lee, Rios, Aten, et al, 2004; Dohil and Eichenfield, 2005).

Children and parents are often tempted to squeeze follicular lesions. They must be warned that squeezing will not hasten the resolution of the infection and that there is a risk of making the lesion worse or spreading the infection. Children should not

Case Study—Impetigo

TABLE 18-3 BACTERIAL INFECTIONS

DISORDER AND ORGANISM	MANIFESTATIONS	MANAGEMENT	COMMENTS
Impetigo contagiosa— Staphylococci (Fig. 18-3)	Begins as a reddish macule Becomes vesicular Ruptures easily, leaving superficial, moist erosion Tends to spread peripherally in sharply marginated irregular outlines Exudate dries to form heavy, honey-colored crusts Pruritus common Systemic effects—Minimal or asymptomatic	Careful removal of undermined skin, crusts, and debris by softening with 1:20 Burow solution compresses Topical bactericidal ointment Oral or parenteral antibiotics (penicillin) in cases of severe or extensive lesions	Tends to heal without scarring unless secondary infection occurs Autoinoculable and contagious Very common in toddlers, preschoolers May be superimposed on eczema
Pyoderma—Staphylococci, streptococci	Deeper extension of infection into dermis Tissue reaction more severe Systemic effects—Fever, lymphangitis	Soap and water cleansing Wet compresses Bathing with antibacterial soap as prescribed	Autoinoculable and contagious May heal with or without scarring
Folliculitis (pimple), furuncle (boil), carbuncle (multiple boils)—Staphylococcus aureus, methicillin-resistant S. aureus (MRSA)	Folliculitis—Infection of hair follicle Furuncle—Larger lesion with more redness and swelling at a single follicle Carbuncle—More extensive lesion with widespread inflammation and "pointing" at several follicular orifices Systemic effects—Malaise, if severe	Skin cleanliness Local warm, moist compresses Topical antibiotic agents Systemic antibiotics in severe cases Incision and drainage of severe lesions, followed by wound irrigations with antibiotics or suitable drain implantation MRSA infections: • 5-inch soak of ½ cup bleach diluted in a standard 50-gallon tub one fourth filled with water once or twice weekly • No sharing of towels or washcloths, changing of clothes and underwear daily, and laundering in hot water • Disposal of razors after one use • Application of mupirocin to nares bid for 2-4 wk	Autoinoculable and contagious Furuncle and carbuncle tend to heal with scar formation Lesion should never be squeezed
Cellulitis—Streptococci, staphylococci, Haemophilus influenzae (Fig. 18-4)	Inflammation of skin and subcutaneous tissues with intense redness, swelling, and firm infiltration Lymphangitis "streaking" frequently seen Involvement of regional lymph nodes common May progress to abscess formation Systemic effects—Fever, malaise	Oral or parenteral antibiotics Rest and immobilization of both affected area and child Hot moist compresses	Hospitalization may be necessary for child with systemic symptoms Otitis media may be associated with facial cellulitis
Staphylococcal scalded skin syndrome—S. aureus	Macular erythema with "sandpaper" texture of involved skin Epidermis becomes wrinkled (in 2 days or less), and large bullae appear	Systemic administration of antibiotics Gentle cleansing with saline, Burow solution, or 0.25% silver nitrate compresses	Infants subject to fluid loss, impaired body temperature regulation, and secondary infection, such as pneumonia, cellulitis, and septicemia Heals without scarring

puncture the surface of the pustule with a needle or sharp instrument. A child with a stye may waken with the eyelids of the affected eye sealed shut with exudate. Instruct the child or the parents to gently wipe the lid from the inner to the outer edge with warm water and a clean washcloth until the exudate has been removed.

The child with limited cellulitis of an extremity is usually managed at home on a regimen of oral antibiotics and warm compresses. Teach the parents the procedures and instruct them in administration of the medication. Children with more extensive cellulitis, especially around a joint with lymphadenitis or on the face, or with lesions larger than 5 cm (2 inches), may be admitted to the hospital for parenteral antibiotics, incision, and drainage (Fisher, Chan, Hair, et al, 2008; Kaplan, 2008). Nurses are responsible for teaching the family to administer the medication and to apply compresses.

VIRAL INFECTIONS

Viruses are intracellular parasites that produce their effect by using the intracellular substances of the host cells. Composed of only a deoxyribonucleic acid or ribonucleic acid core enclosed

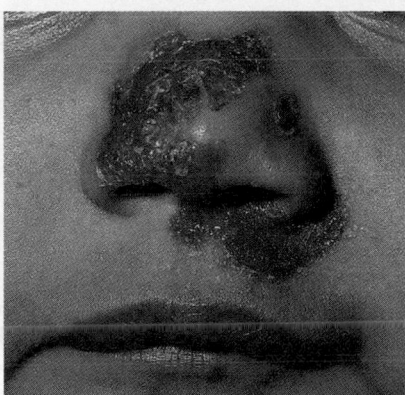

Fig. 18-3 Impetigo contagiosa. (From Weston WL, Lane AT: *Color textbook of pediatric dermatology,* ed 4, St Louis, 2007, Mosby.)

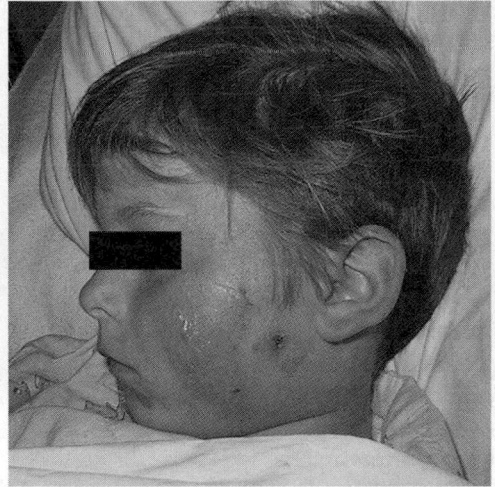

Fig. 18-4 Cellulitis of the cheek from a puncture wound. (From Weston WL, Lane AT: *Color textbook of pediatric dermatology,* ed 4, St Louis, 2007, Mosby.)

in an antigenic protein shell, viruses are unable to provide for their own metabolic needs or to reproduce themselves. After a virus penetrates a cell of the host organism, it sheds the outer shell and disappears within the cell, where the nucleic acid core stimulates the host cell to form more virus material from its intracellular substance. In a viral infection the epidermal cells react with inflammation and vesiculation (as in herpes simplex) or by proliferating to form growths (warts).

Most of the communicable diseases of childhood are associated with rashes, and each rash is characteristic. The type of lesion and the configuration of the viral exanthems of rubeola, rubella, and chickenpox are described in Table 16-1. Other common viral disorders of the skin are in Table 18-4.

DERMATOPHYTOSES (FUNGAL INFECTIONS)

The **dermatophytoses** (ringworm) are infections caused by a group of closely related filamentous fungi that invade primarily the stratum corneum, hair, and nails. These are superficial infections by organisms that live on, not in, the skin. These microbes are confined to the dead keratin layers and are unable to survive in the deeper layers. Because keratin is being shed constantly, the fungus must multiply at a rate that equals the

rate of keratin production to maintain itself; otherwise the organism would be shed with the discarded skin cells. Table 18-5 outlines common dermatophytoses.

Three principal types of fungi are responsible for dermatophyte infections: Trichophyton, Microsporum, and Epidermophyton. They are designated by the Latin word *tinea,* with further designation relating to the area of the body where they are found (e.g., tinea capitis [ringworm of the scalp]) (Fig. 18-5, *A*). Dermatophyte infections are most often transmitted from one person to another or from infected animals to humans. Atopic individuals (those with a tendency to develop allergy) are more susceptible to dermatophyte infections. Fungi exert their effect by means of an enzyme that digests and hydrolyzes the keratin of hair, nails, and the stratum corneum. Dissolved hair breaks off to produce the bald spots characteristic of tinea capitis. In the annular lesions the fungi principally appear in the edge of the inflamed border as they move outward from the inflammation. Diagnosis is made from microscopic examination of scrapings taken from the advancing periphery of the lesion, which almost always produces scale.

Nursing Care Management

When teaching families about the care of children with ringworm, the nurse should emphasize good health and hygiene. Both 2% ketoconazole and 1% selenium sulfide shampoos may reduce colony counts of dermatophytes. These shampoos can be used in combination with oral therapy to reduce the transmission of the disease to others. The shampoo should be applied to the scalp for 5 to 10 minutes at least three times per week (Roberts and Friedlander, 2005). The child may return to school once therapy is initiated. Because of the infectious nature of the disease, affected children should not exchange with other children any grooming items, headgear, scarves, or other articles of apparel that have been in proximity to the infected area. Infected children should use their own towels and wear a protective cap at night to avoid transmitting the fungus to bedding, especially if they sleep with another person. Because the infection can be acquired by animal-to-human transmission, all household pets should be examined for the disorder. Other sources of infection are seats with headrests (e.g., airplane seats), seats in public transportation, helmets, and gymnasium mats.

Treatment with the drug griseofulvin frequently continues for weeks or months, and because symptoms subside, children or parents may be tempted to decrease or discontinue the drug. The nurse should emphasize to family members the importance of maintaining the prescribed dose and schedule and of taking the medication with high-fat foods for best absorption. Also inform them about possible side effects of the drug, such as headache, gastrointestinal upset, fatigue, insomnia, and photosensitivity. For children who take the drug over many months, periodic testing is required to monitor for leukopenia and assess liver and renal function. Newer antifungal drugs such as terbinafine, itraconazole, and fluconazole may be used when there are adverse reactions to griseofulvin. Currently, these drugs are being studied to determine their efficacy and safety in treating tinea capitis in children but are not approved by the FDA for this indication at this time.

TABLE 18-4   VIRAL INFECTIONS

DISORDER AND ORGANISM	MANIFESTATIONS	MANAGEMENT	COMMENTS
Verruca (warts)—Human papillomavirus (various types)	Usually well-circumscribed, gray or brown, elevated, firm papules with a roughened, finely papillomatous texture Occur anywhere, but usually appear on exposed areas such as fingers, hands, face, and soles May be single or multiple Asymptomatic	Not uniformly successful Local destructive therapy, individualized according to location, type, and number—surgical removal, electrocautery, curettage, cryotherapy (liquid nitrogen), caustic solutions (lactic acid and salicylic acid in flexible collodion, retinoic acid, salicylic acid plasters), x-ray treatment, laser	Common in children Tend to disappear spontaneously Course unpredictable Most destructive techniques tend to leave scars Autoinoculable Repeated irritation will cause to enlarge Topical anesthetic EMLA can be applied
Verruca plantaris (plantar wart)	Located on plantar surface of feet and, because of pressure, are practically flat; may be surrounded by a collar of hyperkeratosis	Caustic solution applied to wart, foam insole worn with hole cut to relieve pressure on wart; soaked 20 min after 2-3 days; procedure repeated until wart comes out	Destructive techniques tend to leave scars, which may cause problems with walking Topical anesthetic EMLA can be applied
Cold sore, fever blister—Herpes simplex virus type 1 **Genital herpes**—Herpes simplex virus type 2	Grouped burning and itching vesicles on inflammatory base, usually on or near mucocutaneous junctions (lips, nose, genitalia, buttocks) Vesicles dry, forming a crust, followed by exfoliation and spontaneous healing in 8-10 days May be accompanied by regional lymphadenopathy	Avoidance of secondary infection Burow solution compresses during weeping stages Topical therapy (penciclovir [Denavir]) can shorten duration of cold sores Oral antiviral (acyclovir [Zovirax]) for initial infection or to reduce severity in recurrence Valacyclovir (Valtrex), an oral antiviral used for episodic treatment of recurrent genital herpes, reduces pain, stops viral shedding, and has a more convenient administration schedule than acyclovir	Heal without scarring unless secondary infection Type 1 cold sores can be prevented by using sunscreens protecting against ultraviolet A and ultraviolet B light to prevent lip blisters Aggravated by corticosteroids Positive psychologic effect from treatment May be fatal in children with depressed immunity
Herpes zoster, shingles—Varicella zoster virus	Caused by same virus that causes varicella (chickenpox) Virus has affinity for posterior root ganglia, posterior horn of spinal cord, and skin; crops of vesicles usually confined to dermatome following along course of affected nerve Usually preceded by neuralgic pain, hyperesthesias, or itching May be accompanied by constitutional symptoms	Symptomatic Analgesics for pain Mild sedation sometimes helpful Local moist compresses Drying lotions may be helpful Ophthalmic variety—Systemic corticotropin (adrenocorticotropic hormone) or corticosteroids Acyclovir Lidocaine (Lidoderm) topical anesthetic	Pain in children usually minimal Postherpetic pain does not occur in children Chickenpox may follow exposure; isolate affected child from other children in a hospital or school May occur in children with depressed immunity; can be fatal
Molluscum contagiosum (small, benign tumors)—Poxvirus	Flesh-colored papules with a central caseous plug (umbilicated) Usually asymptomatic	Cases in well children resolve spontaneously in about 18 mo Treatment reserved for troublesome cases Application of topical anesthetic EMLA and removal with curette Tretinoin gel 0.01% or cantharidin (Cantharone) liquid Curettage or cryotherapy	Common in school-age children Spread by skin-to-skin contact, including autoinoculation and fomite-to-skin contact

EMLA, Eutectic mixture of local anesthetics.

SCABIES

Scabies is an endemic infestation caused by the scabies mite, *Sarcoptes scabiei.* Lesions are created as the impregnated female scabies mite burrows into the stratum corneum of the epidermis (never into living tissue), where she deposits her eggs and feces.

Clinical Manifestations

The inflammatory response causes intense pruritus that leads to punctate discrete excoriations secondary to the itching.

Maculopapular lesions are characteristically distributed in intertriginous areas: interdigital surfaces, the axillary-cubital area, popliteal folds, and the inguinal region. There is variability in the lesions. Infants often develop an eczematous eruption; therefore the observer must look for discrete papules, burrows, or vesicles (Fig. 18-6). A mite is identified as a black dot at the end of a minute, linear, grayish brown, threadlike burrow. In children older than 2 years of age, most eruptions are on the hands and wrists. In children younger than 2 years, they are often on the feet and ankles. Children with Down syndrome

TABLE 18-5   DERMATOPHYTOSES (FUNGAL INFECTIONS)

DISORDER AND ORGANISM	MANIFESTATIONS	MANAGEMENT	COMMENTS
Tinea capitis—*Trichophyton tonsurans, Microsporum audouinii, Microsporum canis* (see Fig. 18-5, *A*)	Lesions in scalp but may extend to hairline or neck Characteristic configuration of scaly, circumscribed patches or patchy, scaling areas of alopecia Generally asymptomatic, but severe, deep inflammatory reaction may occur that manifests as boggy, encrusted lesions (kerions) Pruritic Diagnosis—Microscopic examination of scales	Oral griseofulvin Oral ketoconazole for difficult cases Selenium sulfide shampoos Topical application of antifungal agents (e.g., clotrimazole, haloprogin, miconazole)	Person-to-person transmission Animal-to-person transmission Rarely, permanent loss of hair *M. audouinii* transmitted from one human to another directly or from personal items; *M. canis* usually contracted from household pets, especially cats Atopic individuals more susceptible
Tinea corporis—*Trichophyton rubrum, Trichophyton mentagrophytes, M. canis, Epidermophyton* organisms (see Fig. 18-5, *B*)	Generally round or oval, erythematous scaling patch that spreads peripherally and clears centrally; may involve nails (tinea unguium) Diagnosis—Direct microscopic examination of scales Usually unilateral	Oral griseofulvin Local application of antifungal preparation such as tolnaftate, haloprogin, miconazole, clotrimazole; applied 2.5 cm (1 inch) beyond periphery of lesion; application continued 1-2 wk after no sign of lesion	Usually of animal origin from infected pets Majority of infections in children caused by *M. canis* and *M. audouinii*
Tinea cruris ("jock itch")—*Epidermophyton floccosum, T. rubrum, T. mentagrophytes*	Skin response similar to that in tinea corporis Localized to medial proximal aspect of thigh and crural fold; may involve scrotum in males Pruritic Diagnosis—Same as for tinea corporis	Local application of tolnaftate liquid Wet compresses or sitz baths may be soothing	Rare in preadolescent children Health education regarding personal hygiene

Tinea pedis ("athlete's foot")—*T. rubrum, Trichophyton interdigitale, E. floccosum*	On intertriginous areas between toes or on plantar surface of feet
	Lesions vary:
	  • Maceration and fissuring between toes
	  • Patches with pinhead-sized vesicles on plantar surface
	Pruritic
	Diagnosis—Direct microscopic examination of scrapings
		Oral griseofulvin
		Local application of tolnaftate liquid and antifungal powder containing tolnaftate
		Acute infections—Compresses or soaks followed by application of glucocorticoid cream
		Elimination of conditions of heat and perspiration by use of clean, light socks and well-ventilated shoes; avoidance of occlusive shoes
			Most frequent in adolescents and adults; rare in children, but occurrence increases with wearing of plastic shoes
			Transmission to other individuals rare despite general opinion to contrary
			Ointments not successful

Candidiasis (moniliasis)—*Candida albicans*	Grows in chronically moist areas Inflamed areas with white exudate, peeling, and easy bleeding Pruritic Diagnosis—Characteristic appearance	Application of amphotericin B, nystatin ointment, or other antifungal preparations	Common form of diaper dermatitis Oral form common in infants (see Chapter 9) Vaginal form in older females May be disseminated in immunosuppressed children

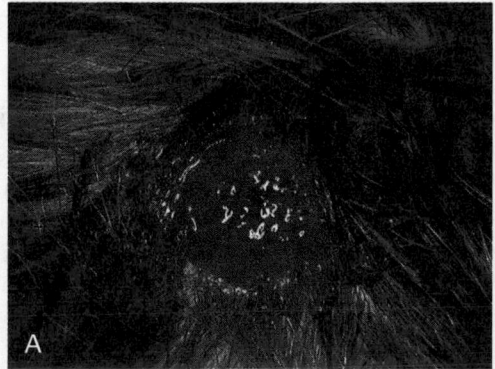 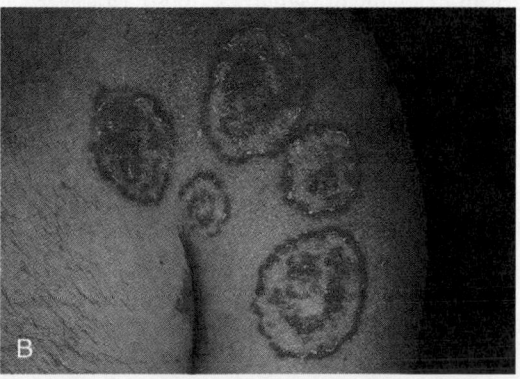

Fig. 18-5 A, Tinea capitis. **B,** Tinea corporis. Both infections are caused by *Microsporum canis,* the "kitten" or "puppy" fungus. (From Habif TP: *Clinical dermatology: a color guide to diagnosis and therapy,* ed 4, St Louis, 2004, Mosby.)

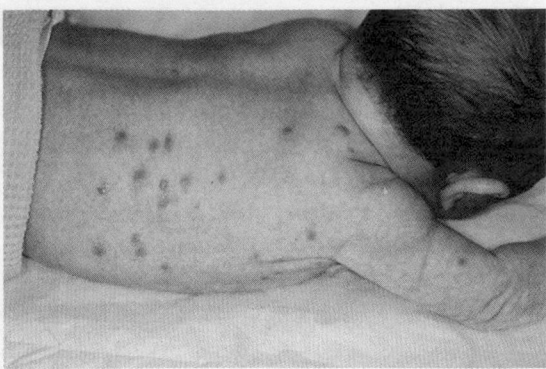

Fig. 18-6 Scabies. (From McCance K, Huether S: *Pathophysiology: the biological basis for disease in adults and children*, ed 6, St Louis, 2010, Mosby.)

may not complain of itching; therefore they can get a severe infestation before it is recognized.

The inflammatory response and itching occur after the host becomes sensitized to the mite, approximately 30 to 60 days after initial contact. (In persons previously sensitized to the mite, the inflammatory response occurs within 48 hours after exposure.) After this time, anywhere the mite has traveled will begin to itch and develop the characteristic eruption. Consequently, mites will not necessarily be located at all sites of eruption. A person needs prolonged contact with the mite to become infested. It takes about 45 minutes for the mite to burrow under the skin; consequently, transient body contact is less likely to cause transfer of the mite. The diagnosis is made by microscopic identification from scrapings of the burrow.

Therapeutic Management

The treatment of scabies is the application of a scabicide. The drug of choice in children and infants older than 2 months is permethrin 5% cream (Elimite). Alternative drugs are 10% crotamiton, ivermectin, or 1% lindane cream or lotion. Lindane can be neurotoxic and is contraindicated in several age-groups. Lindane should be reserved for treatment of patients who fail to respond to other preparations (American Academy of Pediatrics, 2009).

Ivermectin, an oral medication, may be used to treat scabies in patients with secondary excoriations for whom topical scabicides are irritating and not well tolerated or whose infestation is refractory (American Academy of Pediatrics, 2009). However, the safety and efficacy of ivermectin for children younger than 5 years of age or children weighing less than 15 kg (33 lb) has not been established.

Because of the length of time between infestation and physical symptoms (30 to 60 days), all persons who were in close contact with the affected child need treatment. This may include boyfriends or girlfriends, baby-sitters, grandparents, and immediate family members. The objective is to treat as thoroughly as possible the first time. Enough medication for the entire family should be prescribed, with 2 oz allowed for each adult and 1 oz for each child.

Nursing Care Management

Nurses instructing families in the use of the scabicide should emphasize the importance of following the directions carefully.

If lindane lotion is prescribed, it is applied to cool, dry skin—not following a hot bath. It is applied over the entire cutaneous surface from the neck down and is left on for the recommended time, usually 4 hours for infants and 6 hours for older children and adults. Because scabies is a superficial skin disorder, penetration need not be promoted. One liberal application is sufficient.

When permethrin 5% is used, the cream should be thoroughly and gently massaged into all skin surfaces (not just the areas that have a rash) from the head to the soles of the feet. Skin surfaces between the fingers and toes, the folds of the wrist and waist, the umbilicus, and the cleft of the buttocks should not be missed. A toothpick can be used to apply permethrin cream beneath the fingernails and toenails. Take care to avoid contact with the eyes. If permethrin cream accidentally gets into the eyes, they should be flushed immediately with water. Permethrin cream should remain on the skin for 8 to 14 hours, after which time it can be removed by bathing and shampooing.

Touching and holding the child should be minimized until treatment is completed, and the hands should be washed carefully after contact is made. Nurses should wear gloves when caring for the child. Following treatment, freshly laundered bed linen and clothing should be used, and bedclothes and previously worn clothing should be washed in very hot water and dried at the high setting in the dryer. Aggressive housecleaning is not necessary. Families need to know that although the mite will be killed, the rash and the itch will not be eliminated until the stratum corneum is replaced, which takes approximately 2 to 3 weeks. Soothing ointments or lotions, antihistamines, and topical corticosteroids can be used for itching. Antibiotics may be given for secondary infection.

PEDICULOSIS CAPITIS

Pediculosis capitis (head lice) is an infestation of the scalp by *Pediculus humanus capitis,* a common parasite in school-age children. These lice infestations create embarrassment and concern in the family and community. They can also cause a child to be ridiculed by other children.

The louse is a blood-sucking organism that requires approximately five meals a day. The adult louse lives only about 48 hours when away from a human host, and the life span of the average female is 1 month. The female lays her eggs at night at the junction of a hair shaft and close to the skin because the eggs need a warm environment. The nits, or eggs, hatch in approximately 7 to 10 days.

Clinical Manifestations and Diagnostic Evaluation

Itching, caused by the crawling insect and insect saliva on the skin, is usually the only symptom. Common sites of involvement are the occipital area, behind the ears, and at the nape of the neck. Observation of the white eggs (nits) firmly attached to the hair shafts confirms the diagnosis. Because of their brief life span and mobility, adult lice are difficult to locate. Nits must be differentiated from dandruff, lint, hair spray, and other items of similar size and shape. On inspection, nits are seen attached to the hair shaft. Scratch marks and/or inflammatory papules caused by secondary infection may be found on the scalp in the vulnerable areas (Fig. 18-7).

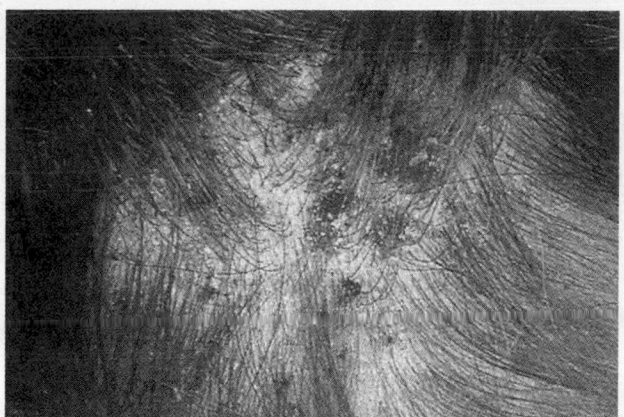

Fig. 18-7 Pediculosis capitis. (From Habif TP, Campbell JL, Chapman MS, et al: *Skin disease: diagnosis and treatment,* ed 2, St Louis, 2005, Mosby.)

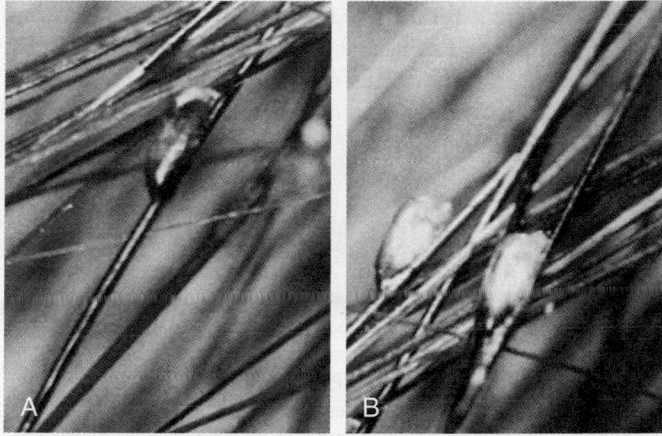

Fig. 18-8 A, Empty nit case. **B,** Viable nits. (From *The contemporary approach to the control of head lice in schools and communities,* Pittsburgh, 1991, SmithKline Beecham.)

Therapeutic Management

Treatment consists of the application of pediculicides and manual removal of nit cases. Because of its efficacy and lack of toxicity, the drug of choice for infants and children is permethrin 1% cream rinse (Nix), which kills adult lice and nits (American Academy of Pediatrics, 2009). This product and preparations of pyrethrin with piperonyl butoxide (RID or A-200 pyrinate) can be obtained without a prescription and are more effective and safer than lindane. Most experts advise a second treatment at 7 to 10 days to ensure a cure (America Academy of Pediatrics, 2009; Leung, Fong, and Pinto-Rojas, 2005). However, pyrethrin products are contraindicated for individuals with contact allergy to ragweed or turpentine. If neither permethrin nor pyrethrin products are effective, the prescription drug 0.5% malathion, which has been approved for treatment of head lice, can be used. However, malathion contains flammable alcohol, must remain in contact with the scalp for 8 to 12 hours, and is not recommended for children younger than 2 years of age.

Because of concerns that head lice may be developing resistance to chemical shampoos and that repeated exposure of children to strong chemicals on the scalp may be unwise, effective nonchemical control measures are essential. Daily removal of nits from a child's hair with a metal nit or flea comb is an essential control measure following treatment with the pediculicide. The child's entire head should be completely combed every day until no more nits are found. In most instances, a nit comb removes most of the nits. However, in some instances, nits need to be removed by scraping them off strands of hair with the fingernail or using tweezers. Several nit combs are currently available at community pharmacies.

Lice are small and grayish tan, have no wings, and are visible to the naked eye. The nits, or eggs, appear as tiny whitish oval specks adhering to the hair shaft about 6 mm (0.25 inch) from the scalp. The adherent nature of the nits distinguishes them from dandruff, which falls off readily. Empty nit cases, which indicate hatched lice, are translucent rather than white and are located more than 0.25 inch from the scalp (Fig. 18-8).

If evidence of infestation is found, it is important to perform the treatment according to the directions on the label of the pediculicide. Advise parents to read the directions carefully before beginning treatment. Instructions indicate that dead lice and remaining nits are to be removed with an extra-fine-tooth comb (included with many preparations).

Make the child as comfortable as possible during the pediculicide application process, since the agent must remain on the scalp and hair for several minutes. Playing "beauty parlor" during the shampoo is a useful strategy. The child lies supine, with the head over a sink or basin, and covers the eyes with a dry towel or washcloth. This prevents medication, which can cause chemical conjunctivitis, from splashing into the eyes. If eye irritation occurs, flush the eyes well with tepid water.

Live lice survive for up to 48 hours away from the host, but nits are shed into the environment and are capable of hatching in 7 to 10 days. Therefore parents must take measures to prevent further infestation (see Community Focus box). Spraying with

---

🏠 COMMUNITY FOCUS

Preventing the Spread and Recurrence of Pediculosis

- Machine wash all washable clothing, towels, and bed linens in hot water and dry in a hot dryer for at least 20 minutes. Dry-clean nonwashable items.
- Thoroughly vacuum carpets, car seats, pillows, stuffed animals, rugs, mattresses, and upholstered furniture.
- Seal nonwashable items in plastic bags for 14 days if unable to dry-clean or vacuum.
- Soak combs, brushes, and hair accessories in lice-killing products for 1 hour or in boiling water for 10 minutes.
- In daycare centers, store children's clothing items such as hats and scarves and other headgear in separate cubicles.
- Discourage the sharing of items such as hats, scarves, hair accessories, combs, and brushes among children in group settings such as daycare centers.
- Avoid physical contact with infested individuals and their belongings, especially clothing and bedding.
- Inspect children in a group setting regularly for head lice.
- Provide educational programs on the transmission, detection, and treatment of pediculosis.

From Benenson AS, editor: *Control of communicable diseases manual,* Washington, DC, 1995, American Public Health Association.

insecticide is not recommended because of the danger to children and animals. Families should also be advised that the pediculicide is relatively costly, especially when several members of the household require treatment. Families may be inclined to try home remedies to treat the lice (see Research Focus box).

The psychologic effects of lice infestations are stressful to children. They are influenced by the reactions of others, including their parents, school nurses, and officials. Some children feel ashamed or guilty. Parents are strongly cautioned against cutting a child's hair or, worse, shaving a child's head. Lice infest short hair as readily as long hair, and these actions only compound the child's distress and serve as a continual reminder to their peers, who are prone to taunt children who have a different appearance.

Nursing Care Management

Nurses should emphasize that anyone can get pediculosis; it has no respect for age, socioeconomic level, or cleanliness. The louse does not jump or fly, but it can be transmitted from one person to another on personal items. Children are cautioned against sharing combs, hair ornaments, hats, caps, scarves, coats, and other items used on or near the hair. Children who share lockers are more likely to contract an infestation, and slumber parties place children at risk. Lice are not carried or transmitted by pets.

Nurses or parents should carefully inspect a child who scratches the head more than usual for bite marks, redness, and nits. The hair is systematically spread with two flat-sided sticks or tongue depressors, and the scalp is observed for any movement that indicates a louse. Nurses should wear gloves when examining the hair and use new tongue depressors or examining sticks for each child.

Prevention

The increasing incidence of pediculosis in schoolchildren has become a serious concern for school nurses, parents, and community health agencies. School nurses usually coordinate school-community prevention and control programs for pediculosis (see Research Focus box). The National Pediculosis Association* offers education and advocates a "no-nit" policy for the reentry of treated children into school (see Evidence-Based Practice box).

*PO Box 610189, Newton, MA 02461; 800-323-1305, ext 7971; fax: 800-235-1305; e-mail: npa@headlice.org; www.headlice.org.

SYSTEMIC DISORDERS RELATED TO SKIN LESIONS

SYSTEMIC MYCOTIC (FUNGAL) INFECTIONS

Systemic mycotic (or deep fungal) infections have the capacity to invade the viscera as well as the skin. The best known of these are primarily lung diseases, which are usually acquired by inhalation of fungal spores. The fungi produce a variable spectrum of disease, and some are common in certain geographic areas. They are not transmitted from person to person but appear to reside in the soil, from which their spores are airborne. The cutaneous lesions are granulomatous and appear as ulcers, plaques, nodules, fungating masses, and abscesses. The course of deep fungal diseases is chronic, with slow progression that favors sensitization (Table 18-6).

RICKETTSIAL INFECTIONS

Rickettsiae are intracellular parasites, similar in size to bacteria that inhabit the alimentary tract of a wide range of natural hosts. Except in Q fever, mammals become infected only through the bites of infected insects (lice and fleas) or arachnids (ticks and mites), which serve as both infectors and reservoirs. Rickettsial diseases are more common in temperate and tropical climates and in areas where humans live in association with arthropods. Infection in humans is incidental (except in epidemic typhus) and is not necessary for the survival of the rickettsial species. However, once the organism invades a human, it causes a disease that varies in intensity from a benign self-limiting illness to a fulminating and frequently fatal one. Table 18-7 outlines some rickettsial infections.

LYME DISEASE

Lyme disease is the most common tick-borne disorder in the United States. It is caused by the spirochete *Borrelia burgdorferi*, which enters the skin and bloodstream through the saliva and feces of ticks, especially the deer tick *Ixodes dammini* (also known as *Ixodes scapularis*) in the Midwest and Northeast and *Ixodes pacificus* in the Pacific Northwest regions of the United States. The ticks are clear to light brown and are very small, 2 to 4 mm (0.08 to 0.16 inch) in length (the size of a sesame seed), which makes detection difficult.

Clinical Manifestations

The disease may be initially seen in any of three stages. Stage 1, early localized disease, consists of the tick bite at the time of

EVIDENCE-BASED PRACTICE

No-Nit School Policies

ASK THE QUESTION

In schoolchildren, are pediculosis policies ("no-nit" policies) effective methods to decrease lice infestation?

SEARCH FOR THE EVIDENCE

Search strategies

Search terms used were head lice in children, pediculosis, head lice and school-age children, and policies for head lice.

Databases used

MEDLINE, PubMed, Ovid, CINAHL.

CRITICALLY ANALYZE THE EVIDENCE

GRADE criteria: Evidence quality moderate; recommendation strong (Guyatt, Oxman, Vist, et al, 2008)

To determine how often children were excluded from school inappropriately because of head lice, health care providers and nonspecialists were invited to submit to the Harvard School of Public Health specimens that they found in children's hair when they suspected head lice (Pollack, Kiszewski, and Spielman, 2000). Analysis of 614 specimens revealed that lice and eggs were present in less than two thirds of these specimens, and only 53% of the specimens contained a live louse or viable eggs. Health professionals as well as nonspecialists overdiagnosed pediculosis capitis and failed to distinguish active from extinct infestations. Eighty-two percent of the schools involved in this study had a no-nits policy, and noninfested children were excluded as often as children with active infestations.

In a study evaluating the presence of head lice in 1729 school-age children, a total of 28 children (1.6%) were found to have lice and 63 (3.6%) had nits with no lice (Williams, Reichert, MacKenzie, et al, 2001). Repeat assessment 2 weeks later revealed that only 18% of the children with nits alone developed lice. These researchers stated that having five or more nits within 6 mm (0.25 inch) of the head increased the risk of nit conversion, but most children with nits had no lice. The researchers concluded that school policies that excluded children with nits alone from school were not warranted.

The American Academy of Pediatrics established guidelines for diagnosis and treatment of pediculosis in 2002. These guidelines state that no-nit policies in schools are detrimental, causing lost time in the classroom and inappropriate allocation of the school nurse's time, and that such a response is not warranted because pediculosis is not a serious medical condition (Frankowski, 2004).

No-nit policies state that when a school nurse finds head lice in a child's hair, that child is promptly sent home from school with directions for the parents to shampoo the child's hair and remove the lice. Parents comply with these directions and send the child back to school after shampooing and meticulously combing the child's hair. If the school nurse finds a single egg or nit remaining in the child's hair, the school's no-nit policy demands that the nurse exclude the child from school until the eggs or nits are completely removed. The problem is that the treatment does not eliminate all nits, but the nits left after treatment are inactive or dead, and harmless. Remnants of dead nits may remain attached to the hair for months or years. If the eggs are dead, there is no reason for a child to miss school. In addition, no-nit policies have not been proven to be effective in reducing transmission and are not recommended (American Academy of Pediatrics, 2009).

APPLY THE EVIDENCE: NURSING IMPLICATIONS

A no-nit policy inflates the risks associated with lice infestations, increases the probability of overusing pediculicides, and may hinder academic performance by excluding children from school. Several practice implications can be derived from the studies:

1. School nurses should receive training and a microscope or magnifying glass to help them identify head lice correctly.
2. A diagnosis of head lice should be based on observation of live lice rather than dead eggs, dandruff, or other suspicious material in a child's hair.
3. A no-nit policy should be invoked only as a last resort.
4. Repeated failure of parents to rid a child's hair of nits is not a sound basis for suspecting neglect or abuse or instituting legal action against the parents.

References

American Academy of Pediatrics, Committee on Infectious Diseases, Pickering LK, editor: *2009 Red book: report of the Committee on Infectious Diseases*, ed 28, Elk Grove Village, Ill, 2009, The Academy.

Frankowski BL: American Academy of Pediatrics guidelines for the prevention and treatment of head lice infestation, *Am J Managed Care* 10(9):S269-S272, 2004.

Guyatt GH, Oxman AD, Vist GE, et al: GRADE: an emerging consensus on rating quality of evidence and strength of recommendations, *BMJ* 336:924-926, 2008.

Pollack RJ, Kiszewski AE, Spielman A: Overdiagnosis and consequent management of head louse infestations in North America, *Pediatr Infect Dis J* 19(8):689-693, 2000.

Williams LK, Reichert A, MacKenzie WR, et al: Lice, nits, and school policy, *Pediatrics* 107:1011-1015, 2001.

inoculation, followed in 3 to 30 days by the development of erythema migrans at the site of the bite. The lesion begins as a small erythematous papule that enlarges radially up to 30 cm (12 inches) over a period of days to weeks. It results in a large circumferential ring with a raised, edematous doughnut like border resulting in a bull's eye appearance (Fig. 18-10). The thigh, groin, and axilla are common sites. The lesion is described as "burning," feels warm to the touch, and occasionally is pruritic. The single annular rash may be associated with fever, myalgia, headache, or malaise.

Stage 2, early disseminated disease, occurs 3 to 10 weeks after inoculation. Many patients develop multiple smaller, secondary annular lesions without the indurated center. They may occur anywhere except on the palms and soles, and in untreated patients they disappear in 3 to 4 weeks. Constitutional symp-

toms, including fever, headache, malaise, fatigue, anorexia, stiff neck, generalized lymphadenopathy, splenomegaly, conjunctivitis, sore throat, abdominal pain, and cough, are often observed. A focal neurologic finding of cranial nerve palsy (seventh nerve palsy) occurs in 3% to 5% of cases.

Stage 3, the most serious stage of the disease, is characterized by systemic involvement of neurologic, cardiac, and musculoskeletal systems that appears 2 to 12 months after inoculation. Lyme arthritis is the most common manifestation with pain, swelling, and effusion. In children the arthritis is characterized by intermittently painful swollen joints (primarily the knees), with spontaneous remissions and exacerbations. Rare neurologic features of pediatric Lyme disease may include chronic demyelinating encephalitis, polyneuritis, and memory problems (Kest and Pineda, 2008).

TABLE 18-6 SYSTEMIC MYCOSES

DISORDER AND ORGANISM	SKIN MANIFESTATIONS	SYSTEMIC MANIFESTATIONS	TREATMENT	COMMENTS
North American blastomycosis—*Blastomyces dermatitidis*	Chronic granulomatous lesions and microabscesses on any part of body Initial lesion is a papule; undergoes ulceration and peripheral spread	Pulmonary symptoms, such as cough, chest pain, weakness, and weight loss Possible skeletal involvement, with bone destruction and formation of cutaneous abscesses	Intravenous (IV) administration of amphotericin B	Usual portal of entry is lungs Source of infection unknown Noninfectious Pulmonary infections may be mild and self-limiting and require no treatment Progressive disease often fatal
Cryptococcosis—*Cryptococcus neoformans (Torula histolytica)*	Usually on face; acneiform, firm, nodular, painless eruption	Central nervous system (CNS) manifestations—Headache, dizziness, stiff neck, and signs of increased intracranial pressure Low-grade fever, mild cough, lung infiltration	IV amphotericin B; may be administered intrathecally for CNS involvement 5-Fluorocytosine for meningitis Excision and drainage of local lesions	Acquired by inhalation of dust but may enter through skin Prognosis serious Noninfectious Increased incidence in persons receiving corticosteroids with lymphoreticular malignancies, or type 2 diabetes
Histoplasmosis—*Histoplasma capsulatum*	Not distinctive or uniform but most appear as punched-out or granulomatous ulcers	General systemic symptoms may include pallor, diarrhea, vomiting, irregular spiking temperature, hepatosplenomegaly, and pulmonary symptoms Any tissue of body may be involved with related symptoms	IV amphotericin B for severe cases Oral ketoconazole	Organism cultured from soil, especially where contaminated with fowl droppings Fungus enters through skin or mucous membranes of mouth and respiratory tract Endemic in Mississippi and Ohio River valleys Disseminated diseases most common in infants and children
Coccidioidomycosis (valley fever)—*Coccidioides immitis*	Erythema nodosum Erythema multiforme Erythematous maculopapular rash	Primary lung disease usually asymptomatic May be sign of acute febrile illness Disseminated disease is very serious	IV amphotericin B IV miconazole (synthetic imidazole) Intraventricular miconazole plus oral ketoconazole for CNS involvement Surgical resection of persistent pulmonary cavities	Inhalation of aerospores from soil Endemic in southwestern United States Usually resolves spontaneously Increased incidence in dark-skinned races (African-American, Hispanic, Asian)

TABLE 18-7 ERUPTIONS CAUSED BY RICKETTSIAE

DISORDER, ORGANISM, AND HOST	MANIFESTATIONS	MANAGEMENT	COMMENTS
Rocky Mountain spotted fever—*Rickettsia rickettsii* Arthropod—Tick Transmission—Tick Mammal source—Wild rodents; dogs	Gradual onset—Fever, malaise, anorexia, myalgia Abrupt onset—Rapid temperature elevation, chills, vomiting, myalgia, severe headache Maculopapular or petechial rash primarily on extremities (ankles and wrists) but may spread to other areas, characteristically on palms and soles (Fig. 18-9)	Control—Protection from tick bite by wearing proper apparel, tick repellent Tetracycline or chloramphenicol Vigorous supportive therapy	Usually self-limiting in children Onset in children may resemble that of any infectious disease Severe disease rare in children Children and dogs should be inspected regularly if they play in wooded areas See Table 18-10 for management of ticks
Epidemic typhus—*Rickettsia prowazekii* Arthropod—Body louse Transmission—Infected feces into broken skin Mammal source—Humans	Abrupt onset of chills, fever, diffuse myalgia, headache, malaise Maculopapular rash becomes petechial 4-7 days later, spreading from trunk outward	Control—Immediate destruction of vectors Tetracycline or chloramphenicol Supportive treatment	Isolate patient until deloused See discussion on p. 699 for management of pediculosis Excreta from infected lice also in dust—patient's clothing, bedding, and possessions should be disinfected and washed in hot water
Endemic typhus—*Rickettsia typhi* Arthropod—Rat fleas or lice Transmission—Flea bite; inhalation or ingestion of flea excreta Mammal source—Rats	Headache, arthralgia, backache followed by fever; may last 9-14 days Maculopapular rash after 1-8 days of fever; begins in trunk and spreads to periphery; rarely involves face, palms, soles	Control—Eliminate rat reservoir, insect vectors, or both Tetracycline or chloramphenicol Supportive treatment	Fairly common in United States Shorter duration than epidemic typhus Mild, seldom fatal illness Difficult to distinguish from epidemic typhus
Rickettsialpox—*Rickettsia akari* Arthropod—Mouse mite Transmission—Mite Mammal source—House mouse	Maculopapular rash following primary lesion; eschar at site of bite; fever, chills, headache	Control—Eradication of rodent reservoir and mite vector Tetracycline or chloramphenicol Supportive treatment	Self-limiting, nonfatal disease Endemic in New York City Found in many cities in United States

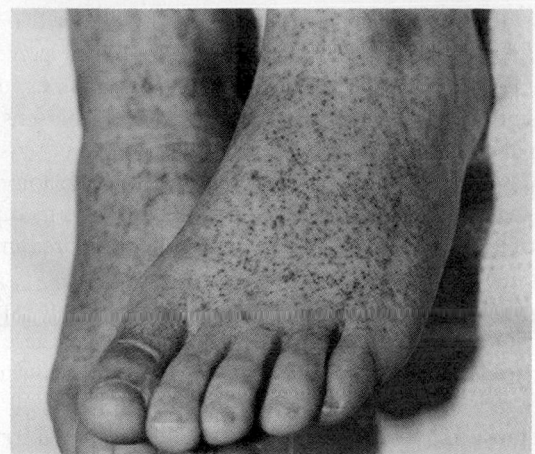

Fig. 18-9 Petechial rash of Rocky Mountain spotted fever.

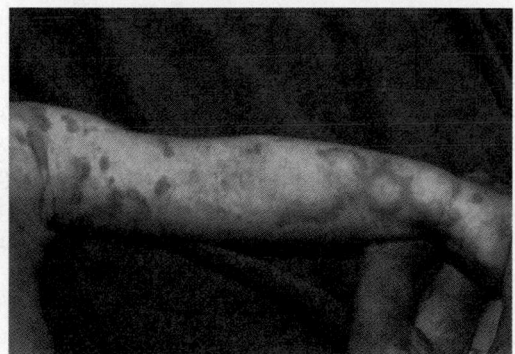

Fig. 18-10 Lyme disease. Note annular red rings in erythema chronicum migrans. (From Weston WL, Lane AT: *Color textbook of pediatric dermatology*, St Louis, 1991, Mosby.)

Cardiac complications, which may appear in a small percentage of persons 4 to 5 weeks after erythema chronicum migrans, are commonly acute atrioventricular conduction abnormalities and may result in severe heart block (Wormser, Dattwyler, Shapiro, et al, 2006). Patients may be asymptomatic but can develop syncope, palpitations, dyspnea, chest pain, and severe bradycardia.

Diagnostic Evaluation

The diagnosis is based primarily on the history, observation of the lesion, and clinical manifestations. Serologic testing for Lyme disease at the time of a recognized tick bite is not recommended (Fix, Strickland, and Grant, 1998). Serologic testing is not standardized, and there is a high frequency of false-negative and false-positive results (Seltzer and Shapiro, 1996), which may lead to unnecessary treatments. Laboratory diagnosis can be established in later stages with a two-step approach that includes the enzyme-linked immunosorbent assay (ELISA) screening test and, if it is positive, Western Blot testing, as outlined by the Centers for Disease Control and Prevention (2009a) and adopted by the American Academy of Pediatrics.

Therapeutic Management

At the time the rash appears or shortly thereafter, children over 8 years of age are treated with oral doxycycline or amoxicillin, and children under 8 years of age are given amoxicillin. For patients who are allergic to penicillin, alternative drugs include cefuroxime and erythromycin (Wade, 2000; Centers for Disease Control and Prevention, 2009a).

The length of treatment depends on the clinical response and other disease manifestations, but it usually lasts from 14 to 21 days (American Academy of Pediatrics, 2009). The treatment is effective in preventing second-stage manifestations in most cases. Neurologic, cardiac, and arthritic manifestations are managed with intravenous or intramuscular antibiotics, such as ceftriaxone or penicillin G. For patients in whom tetracycline is contraindicated or who have allergies to penicillin, parenterally administered ceftriaxone is as effective as doxycycline in the treatment of acute disseminated Lyme disease (Dattwyler, Luft, Kunkel, et al, 1997). Follow-up care is important in ensuring that treatment is initiated or terminated as needed.

Nursing Care Management

The major thrust of nursing care should be educating parents to protect their children from exposure to ticks. In endemic areas tick habitats can include yards and parks, in addition to wooded areas.

Children should avoid tick-infested areas or wear light-colored clothing so that ticks can be spotted easily, tuck pant legs into socks, and wear a long-sleeved shirt tucked into pants when in wooded areas. Children should avoid grass and shrubbery where ticks may be lurking, and children and adults should walk in the center of trails. Parents and children need to perform regular tick checks when they are in infested areas. After a hike, a bare skin check (with special attention to the scalp, neck, armpits, and groin areas) is important to spot any ticks and remove them (see Table 18-10).

Parents should also be alert for signs of the skin lesion, especially if their children are known to have been exposed to the tick vector.

The use of insect repellents such as those containing diethyltoluamide (DEET) or permethrin can protect against insects. Advise parents to use them cautiously. DEET is absorbed through the skin and can cause toxicity in infants and children. These preparations can be used as directed by product insert in children as young as 2 months of age (American Academy of Pediatrics, 2009). The preparation should be sprayed on the child's clothing, not directly on the skin. Information about Lyme disease is available from the Centers for Disease Control and Prevention.*

CAT SCRATCH DISEASE

Cat scratch disease is the most common cause of regional lymphadenitis in children and adolescents. It usually follows the scratch or bite of an animal (a cat or kitten in 90% of cases) and is caused by *Bartonella henselae*, a gram-negative bacterium (Margileth, 2000; Rombaux, M'Bilo, Badr-el-Din, et al, 2000). The disease is usually a benign, self-limiting illness that resolves spontaneously in 2 to 4 months.

The usual manifestations are a painless, nonpruritic erythematous papule at the site of inoculation, followed by regional

---

*800-CDC-INFO; CDCinfo@cdc.gov; **www.cdc.gov**.

lymphadenitis. The lymph nodes most commonly involved are axillary epitrochlear, cervical, submandibular, inguinal, and preauricular. The disease may persist for several months before gradual resolution. In some children, especially those who are immunocompromised, the adenitis may progress to suppuration. Some children may develop serious complications that include encephalitis, hepatitis, and Parinaud oculoglandular syndrome. This syndrome is characterized by granulomatous lesions on the palpebral conjunctiva associated with swelling of the ipsilateral preauricular nodes.

Diagnosis is made on the basis of (1) a history of contact with a cat or kitten, (2) the presence of regional lymphadenopathy for several days, and (3) serologic identification of the causative organism by indirect fluorescent antibody assay or polymerase chain reaction test (St. Geme, Haslam, and Ditmar, 1997).

Treatment is primarily supportive. Antibiotics do not shorten the duration or prevent progression to suppuration, but may be helpful in severe forms of the disease. Trimethoprim-sulfamethoxazole, ciprofloxacin, gentamicin, and rifampin have shown some benefit in uncontrolled clinical studies (St. Geme, Haslam, and Ditmar, 1997).

Activity is limited to prevent trauma to the large lymph nodes, and bed rest is indicated for children with fever. Analgesics are given for discomfort. Most children can continue normal activities during the disease. The animals are not ill during the time they transmit the disease, and most authorities do not recommend disposal of a cherished pet.

SKIN DISORDERS RELATED TO CHEMICAL OR PHYSICAL CONTACTS

CONTACT DERMATITIS

Contact dermatitis is an inflammatory reaction of the skin to chemical substances, natural or synthetic, that evoke a hypersensitivity response or to those agents that cause direct irritation. The initial reaction occurs in an exposed region, most commonly the face and neck, backs of the hands, forearms, male genitalia, and lower legs. There is characteristically a sharp delineation between inflamed and normal skin early in the reaction that ranges from a faint, transient erythema to massive bullae on an erythematous swollen base. Itching is a constant symptom.

The cause may be a primary irritant or a sensitizing agent. A primary irritant is one that irritates any skin. A sensitizing agent produces an irritation on those who have encountered the irritant or something chemically related to it, have undergone an immunologic change, and have become sensitized. A sensitizer irritates in relatively low concentrations only persons who are allergic to it.

The clinical course is relatively short (1 to 4 weeks) if the causative agent is eliminated. Whether or not there are complications from secondary invasion or reactions to topical therapy depends on the severity of the original reaction.

Sensitizing reactions are acquired by repeated or prolonged exposure, and the sensitizing capacity of different substances varies widely. Strong sensitizers require only one or two exposures and provoke sensitivity reactions in a higher percentage of individuals; weak sensitizers require numerous exposures, and a smaller percentage of those exposed will be sensitized. The length of time from exposure to development of sensitivity varies and may be as short as a week or much longer. Sometimes with repeated exposure and reactions the skin loses its capacity to return to normal, or secondary factors become predominant and produce a chronic inflammatory process.

The major goal in treatment is to prevent further exposure of the skin to the offending substance. Provided there is no further irritation, the skin's normal recuperative powers will produce satisfactory results without treatment.

The most frequent offenders are plant and animal irritants, the prototype of which is poison ivy (see discussion later). In infants the most common contact dermatitis occurs on the convex surfaces of the diaper area as a result of chemical irritation from putrefactive fecal enzymes acting on urine or laundry products. (See Diaper Dermatitis, Chapter 13.) Other agents that frequently produce dermatologic responses from contact are animal irritants such as wool, feathers, lanolin, and furs and vegetable irritants such as oleoresins, oils, and turpentine. Chemicals of all kinds, including synthetic fabrics (e.g., shoe components), dyes, metals, cosmetics, perfumes, soaps (including bubble baths), baby wipes, and moist towelettes, are also irritants (Nijhawan, Matiz, and Jacob, 2009).

Several cosmetic products advertised as safe for children may be responsible for skin irritation. These include a cream hair relaxer marketed especially for children that contains lye and must be used with extreme care. Because children's hair is more resistant to artificial curling or straightening, pediatric preparations contain chemicals as strong as or stronger than those intended for use on adults.

Nursing Care Management

A thorough history is necessary to determine the causative agent or allergen associated with the patient's dermatitis. Nurses frequently detect evidence of contact dermatitis during routine physical assessments. Skin manifestations in specific areas suggest limited contact, such as around the eyes (mascara), areas of the body covered by clothing but not protected by undergarments (wool), or areas of the body not covered by clothing (ultraviolet injury). Generalized involvement is more likely to be caused by bubble bath or soap. Often nurses are able to identify the offending agent and counsel families regarding management. If the lesions persist, are extensive, or show evidence of infection, medical evaluation is indicated.

POISON IVY, OAK, AND SUMAC

Contact with the dry or succulent portions of any of three poisonous plants (ivy, oak, or sumac) produces localized, streaked or spotty, oozing, and painful impetiginous lesions. Poison ivy grows almost everywhere east of the Rockies, poison oak is found primarily west of the Rockies, and poison sumac is usually restricted to swamp areas of the Southeast. Only Nevada, Hawaii, and Alaska (and regions above 4000 feet) appear to be free of the plants.

The offending substance in these plants is an oil, urushiol, that is extremely potent. Sensitivity to urushiol is not inborn but is developed after one or two exposures and may change over a lifetime. Repeated exposures appear to lower the reaction; exposure after long periods away from it may elicit a heightened response. Some highly sensitive persons may suddenly become resistant, whereas resistant persons may become sensitive. All parts of the plants, including dried leaves and stems, contain urushiol. Even smoke from burning brush piles can produce a reaction. There is widespread contact with the skin from the smoke of burning plants, and lung reactions from smoke inhalation can be life threatening.

Animals do not seem to be affected by the oil; dogs or other animals that have run or played in the plants may carry the sap on their fur, and animals that eat the plants can transfer the oil in saliva. Shoes, tools, and toys can transfer the oil. Golf balls that have been in the rough can be sources of contact.

Clinical Manifestations

Urushiol has an effect as soon as it touches the skin. It penetrates through the epidermis as a mixture of compound molecules called catechols. These catechols bond skin proteins, where it initiates an immune response (Fig. 18-11, *A*). The full-blown reaction is evident after about 2 days, with redness, swelling, and itching at the site of contact. Several days later, streaked or spotty blisters oozing serum from damaged cells produce the characteristic impetiginous lesions (Fig. 18-11, *B*). The lesions dry and heal spontaneously, and itching stops by 10 to 14 days.

Therapeutic Management

Treatment of the lesions includes application of calamine lotion, soothing Burow solution compresses, and/or Aveeno baths to relieve discomfort. Topical corticosteroid gel is

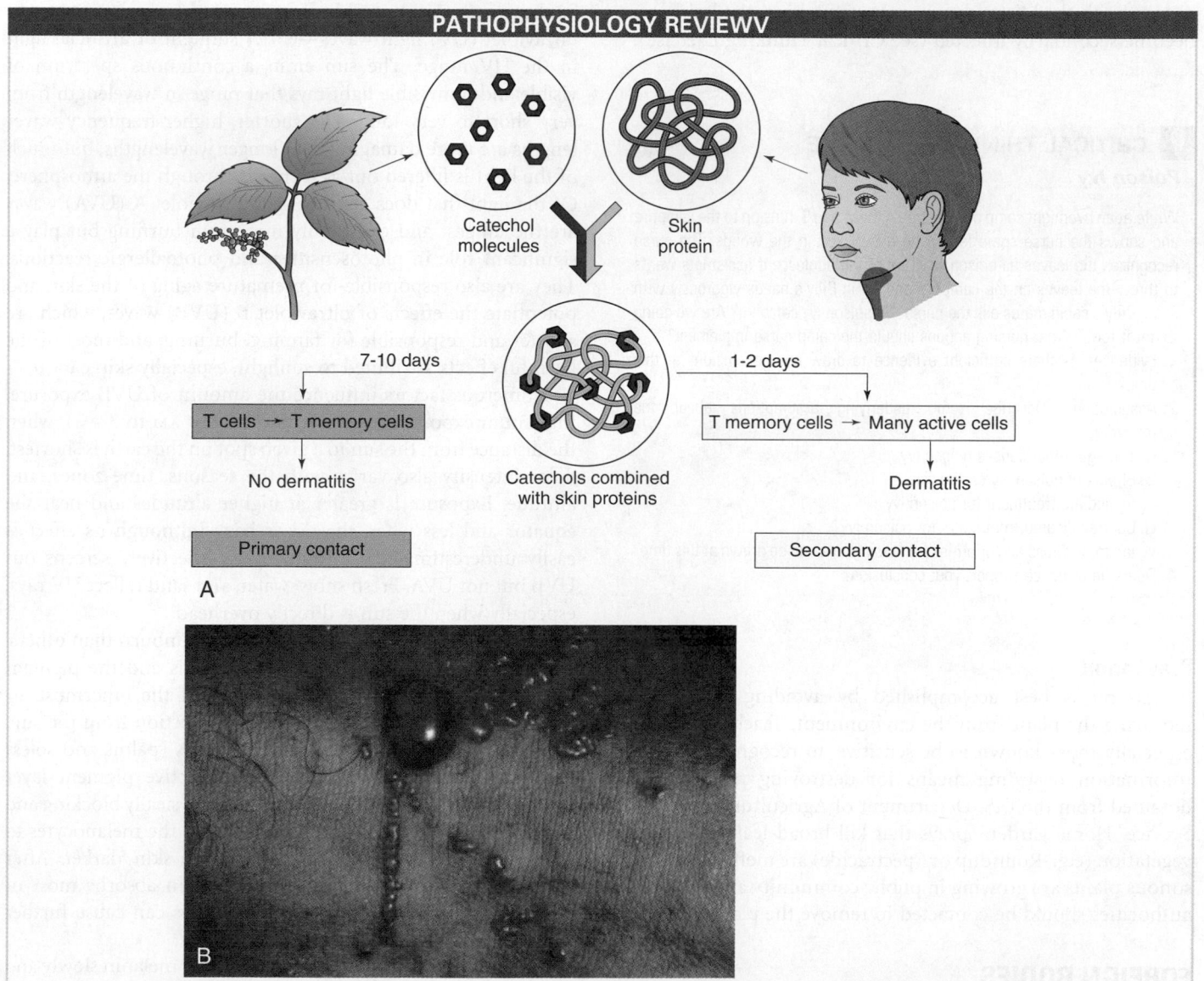

PATHOPHYSIOLOGY REVIEW

Catechol molecules

Skin protein

7-10 days

T cells → T memory cells

No dermatitis

Primary contact

A

Catechols combined with skin proteins

1-2 days

T memory cells → Many active cells

Dermatitis

Secondary contact

B

Fig. 18-11 A, Development of allergic contact dermatitis. **B,** Poison ivy lesions; note "streaked" blisters surrounding one large blister. (**A,** From McCance K, Huether S: *Pathophysiology: the biological basis for disease in adults and children,* ed 6, St Louis, 2010, Mosby. **B,** From Habif TP: *Clinical dermatology: a color guide to diagnosis and therapy,* ed 4, St Louis, 2004, Mosby.)

effective for prevention or relief of inflammation, especially when applied before blisters form. Oral corticosteroids may be needed for severe reactions, and a sedative such as diphenhydramine may be ordered.

Nursing Care Management

When the child has made contact with the plant, flush the area immediately (preferably within 15 minutes) with cold running water to neutralize the urushiol not yet bonded to the skin. If there is a stream nearby, an effective method is to have the child enter the water (clothes and all) and allow the water to rinse the oil from both skin and clothing. Use of harsh soap is contraindicated because it removes protective skin oils and dilutes the urushiol, allowing it to spread. Hard scrubbing irritates the skin. All clothing that has come in contact with the plant is removed with care and thoroughly laundered in hot water and detergent. Every effort is made to prevent the child from scratching the lesions. Although the lesions do not spread by contact with the blister serum or by scratching, the lesions can become secondarily infected (see Critical Thinking Exercise).

 CRITICAL THINKING EXERCISE

Poison Ivy

While at an overnight camp near a stream, Billy, age 9, runs up to the campfire and shows the nurse some leaves he has picked in the woods. The nurse recognizes the leaves as poison ivy. One of the adolescent assistants wants to throw the leaves on the campfire and scrub Billy's hands vigorously with soap. Billy's cabin mates ask the nurse: "Is poison ivy catching? Are we going to get it too?" What nursing actions should the camp nurse implement?

1. Evidence—Is there sufficient evidence to draw any conclusions at this time?
2. Assumptions—Describe some underlying assumptions about the following:
   a. The agent that causes poison ivy
   b. Effects of poison ivy on the skin
   c. Immediate treatment for poison ivy
   d. Contraindicated treatments for poison ivy
3. What implications and priorities for nursing care can be drawn at this time?
4. Does the evidence support your conclusion?

Prevention

Prevention is best accomplished by avoiding contact and removing the plant from the environment. Teach all children, especially those known to be sensitive, to recognize the plant. Information regarding means for destroying plants can be obtained from the U.S. Department of Agriculture or Forestry Service. Home garden sprays that kill broad-leaf plants or all vegetation (e.g., Roundup or Spectracide) are ineffective. If poisonous plants are growing in public community areas, the local authorities should be contacted to remove the plants.

FOREIGN BODIES

Small wooden splinters can be removed with a needle and tweezers that have been sterilized with alcohol or a flame. The area around the sliver is washed with soap and water before removal is attempted. The sliver is exposed with the needle and then grasped firmly by the tweezers and pulled out. Some foreign bodies, such as fishhooks, pieces of glass, difficult-to-see objects, or deeply embedded objects (such as a needle in a foot or near a joint), require medical evaluation.

Cactus Spines

Small cactus prickles or spines are troublesome to remove, and attempts are distressing to the child and family. Large spines or clumps can be removed with tweezers. Smaller prickles or spines may be removed by the following methods:

- Apply a thin layer of water-soluble household glue and cover with gauze; when the glue dries, peel off the gauze.
- Apply hair removal wax, let dry, and remove.
- Place cellophane tape, sticky side down, over the spines and lift off.

SUNBURN

Sunburn is a common skin injury caused by overexposure to ultraviolet (UV) light waves—either sunlight or artificial light in the UV range. The sun emits a continuous spectrum of visible and nonvisible light rays that range in wavelength from very short to very long. The shorter, higher-frequency wavelengths are more damaging than longer wavelengths, but much of the light is filtered out as it travels through the atmosphere. Of the light that does get through, ultraviolet A (UVA) waves are the longest and cause only minimum burning but play a significant role in photosensitive and photoallergic reactions. They are also responsible for premature aging of the skin and potentiate the effects of ultraviolet B (UVB) waves, which are shorter and responsible for tanning; burning; and most of the harmful effects attributed to sunlight, especially skin cancer.

Numerous factors influence the amount of UVB exposure. Maximum exposure occurs at midday (10 AM to 3 PM), when the distance from the sun to a given spot on the earth is shortest. Solar intensity also varies with the seasons, time zones, and altitude. Exposure is greater at higher altitudes and near the equator and less when the sky is hazy (although its effect is easily underestimated). Window glass effectively screens out UVB but not UVA. Fresh snow, water, and sand reflect UV rays, especially when the sun is directly overhead.

Some persons are more susceptible to sunburn than others. The fibrous keratin of the outer epidermis and the pigment melanin, produced by the melanocytes of the innermost, or basal, layer of the epidermis, provide protection from the sun. Areas of the body with thick keratin layers (palms and soles) enjoy the greatest protection. The protective pigment layer decreases the intensity of all UV light by physically blocking and scattering the radiation. UV rays stimulate the melanocytes to produce more melanin, which turns the skin darker. After several days of exposure, the dark melanin absorbs most of the incoming UV radiation before the rays can cause further damage.

Persons with light skin and eyes produce melanin slowly and are more prone to burning, whereas those with very dark skin are able to tolerate more rays without damage. People with certain diseases (e.g., porphyria, lupus erythematosus) are more sensitive to the sun's rays. Some substances increase the skin's sensitivity; these include numerous medications (e.g., barbiturates, oral contraceptives, sulfonamides, antiepileptics), topical products (e.g., retinoic acid [Retin-A], antiseptic soap, after-shave lotions, perfumes, colognes), and certain foods containing photosensitizing chemicals (e.g., carrots, parsley, limes).

UV rays penetrate the skin surface, precipitate a chemical change in the cell molecules, and produce toxic by-products that irritate surrounding tissues. The result is redness, tissue swelling, increased capillary permeability, and the tenderness characteristic of superficial (first-degree) burns and the coagulation, necrosis, and blistering of partial thickness (second degree) burns. (See Burns, Chapter 29.) Sunburned skin is exquisitely sensitive, and severe sunburn may be accompanied by nausea, chills, fever, abdominal cramping, and headache. Dehydration may occur.

Excessive or long-term exposure to the sun permanently damages the skin. Ninety percent of skin cancers occur in areas of the skin that are exposed to sunlight, and rates of skin cancers are higher in parts of the world where sunlight is more intense. Studies have also shown that childhood is a crucial time for sun exposure. Children who immigrate to sunny climates after 10 years of age develop cancer at lower rates than native-born children. In general, children receive three times as much sun exposure as adults. Teenagers spend even more time in the sun than school-age children, and their desire for the "perfect tan" places their skin at high risk for sun damage.

Nursing Care Management

Treatment involves stopping the burning process, decreasing the inflammatory response, and rehydrating the skin. Local application of cool tap water soaks or immersion in a tepid water bath (temperature slightly below 36.7° C [98° F]) for 20 minutes or until the skin is cool limits tissue destruction and relieves the discomfort. After the cool applications, a bland oil-in-water moisturizing lotion can be applied, but petrolatum-based products that trap radiant heat in the tissues should be avoided. Acetaminophen is recommended for relief of discomfort. Partial-thickness burns are treated the same as those from any heat source.

Prevention

Protection from sunburn is the major goal of management, and the harmful effects of the sun on the delicate skin of infants and children have been receiving increased attention. Protection can be achieved by physical means (e.g., protective clothing and a hat) or by chemical means. Two types of products are available for sun protection: topical sunscreens, which partially absorb UV light, and sun blockers, which block out UV rays by reflecting sunlight. The most frequently recommended sun blockers are zinc oxide and titanium dioxide ointments.

Sunscreens are products with a sun protective factor (SPF) based on evaluation of effectiveness against UV rays. The SPF is indicated by a number such as 15. If individuals normally burn in 10 minutes without a sunscreen, use of a sunscreen with an SPF of 15 allows them to remain in the sun for 15 times 10, or 150 minutes (2½ hours), before acquiring the same degree of burn. Most sunscreens have an SPF ranging from 2 to more than 30; the higher the number, the greater the protection. Waterproof sunscreens with a minimum SPF of 15 are recommended. The SPF provides information primarily in relation to

the effects of UVB, not UVA. Claims such as "broad spectrum" or "UVA-UVB sun block" are usually unsubstantiated. One agent that affords protection against UVA is Parsol 1789, found in Photoplex and Shade UVA Guard.

The most effective sunscreens against UVB contain p-aminobenzoic acid (PABA) and PABA esters. PABA is more effective than PABA esters. It penetrates the outer layer of skin and may accumulate with repeated use; thus it provides protection even when the child is swimming or sweating. PABA may stain clothing; PABA esters are less likely to do so. However, PABA can cause an allergic response in sensitive persons, manifested as redness and itching 24 hours after application. Benzophenones also offer protection against UVA but are less effective than the PABA preparations and wash off easily. For best results, the sunscreen should be effective against both UVA and UVB.

> ### ! NURSING ALERT
>
> Sunscreens are not recommended for infants under 6 months of age. However, infants under 6 months of age may have sunscreen applied over small areas of skin such as the backs of the hands that may not be adequately covered by clothing when they are in the sun. Encourage parents to use many types of sun protection, not just sunscreen (Hall, Jorgensen, McDavid, et al, 2001). Infants should be kept out of the sun or physically shaded from it. Fabric with a tight weave, such as cotton, offers good protection.

The range of sunscreens available offers the consumer access to a type and combination to meet any need. Sunscreens are applied evenly to all exposed areas, with special attention to skinfolds and areas that might become exposed as clothing shifts. The FDA recommends a layer of sunscreen that is 2 mg/cm². Direct parents to read labels of sunscreen products carefully for the SPF and follow the manufacturer's directions for application.

Individuals who work in the community, such as teachers, daycare workers, coaches, youth group leaders, and children's relatives, should all be made aware of sun safety for children. Sunscreens must be applied liberally.

It is wise to avoid direct sun exposure when solar radiation is at maximum intensity. The strongest radiation occurs when the sun is at its highest (directly overhead). Earlier or later in the day, when the sun is at a 45-degree angle, the earth's atmosphere provides protection equivalent to an SPF of 2.4.

Sun damage is cumulative. Although most long-term effects (cancer, wrinkling) are not evident until adulthood, skin care must begin in childhood. Nurses should teach skin care as a basic practice that becomes a part of the child's life, much the same as tooth brushing (see Community Focus box). Sun-protection behaviors should also be included in existing school health curricula and result in knowledge and a potential change in behavior (Geller, Rutsch, Kenausis, et al, 2003).

COLD INJURY

Cold injuries are most commonly seen in very cold regions. The nature of the heat-regulating mechanisms of the body are such that the inner portion of the body, or core, produces heat and the periphery, or outer area, conserves or dissipates the heat.

When the body attempts to conserve heat, the outer tissues are subjected to low temperatures, and local trauma may result.

Chilblain, redness and swelling of the skin, occurs when extremities, usually the hands, are exposed intermittently to temperatures of 1.1° to 15.5° C (30° to 60° F). The response may vary but is characterized by intense vasodilation that increases the temperature of involved tissues above that of unaffected tissue and produces edematous, reddish blue patches that itch and burn. As warming takes place, the sensations become more intense but ordinarily subside in a few days.

Frostbite is the term used to describe tissue damage caused when excessive heat loss to local tissues allows ice crystals to form in tissues. The mechanisms of slow and rapid freezing differ. Slow freezing causes ice crystals to form in the extracellular fluid, which leads to increased osmolality and movement of water from the cells. This causes cellular dehydration and destruction. Rapid freezing produces both extracellular and intracellular freezing and immediate cellular destruction. Rapid freezing takes place at high altitudes or with high conductivity from cold water immersion.

When frozen tissues thaw, the tissue damage is like that from a high-temperature burn—red blood cell aggregation, stasis, venous thrombosis, tissue edema and ischemic damage, increased tissue pressure, and death and necrosis of surrounding tissues. The frostbitten part appears white or blanched, feels solid, and is without sensation.

Rapid rewarming is associated with less tissue necrosis than slow thawing. It restores blood flow and shortens the period of cellular damage. Rewarming produces a flush (sometimes deep purple) and a return of sensation, which is extremely painful. Large blisters may appear 24 to 48 hours after rewarming and begin to resorb within 5 to 10 days, followed by the formation of a hard black eschar. Superficial injury often heals satisfactorily.

Therapeutic Management

Rewarming is accomplished by immersing the part in well-agitated water at 37.8° to 42.2° C (100° to 108° F). Discomfort is managed with analgesics and sedatives. Care of blistered skin is similar to that described for burns. It is seldom possible to estimate the extent of tissue loss until new skin layers are revealed after the eschar layer separates. Therefore amputation of extremities is usually delayed for 60 to 90 days unless there is evidence of gangrene.

Nursing Care Management

Transfer the frostbite victim to the nearest emergency treatment center. Protect injured parts from trauma and handle gently. Prevent the patient from ambulating on injured feet. Rubbing injured tissues is contraindicated and can cause damage by rupture of crystallized cells. After rewarming, apply a loose dressing. Dry heat is not applied. (See Burns, Chapter 29, and Pain Management, Chapter 7.)

HYPOTHERMIA

Hypothermia is defined as the cooling of the body's core temperature (pulmonary artery or esophageal temperature) to injurious levels, usually identified as below 35° C (95° F). Hypothermia occurs in environmental settings when heat production by exercise and metabolism is less than heat lost by convection, conduction, or radiation. There is a 6% drop in blood flow for each 1° C (1.8° F) decrease in core temperature. Very young children with a large surface area relative to body mass and thin persons are at the greatest risk for hypothermia.

The body in positive heat balance conserves heat by alternating vasoconstriction and vasodilation in extremities. Threat of prolonged or severe cold exposure causes the body to conserve core temperature at the expense of the extremities by shunting warm blood to the core after it passes through the muscles of the extremities. Shivering contributes to warming by raising the metabolic rate to increase the heat of blood before it returns to the core. Clinical manifestations related to degree of hypothermia are listed in Table 18-8.

Therapeutic Management

Rewarming is the major objective of therapy. For mild hypothermia (30° to 35° C [86° to 95° F]), only external application of heat lamps or immersion in water (38° to 42° C [100.4° to 107.6° F]) is necessary to restore core temperature with little risk of complications. Lower temperatures require core rewarming by any of several modalities: delivery of warm humidified oxygen, intravenous infusion of fluids, rectal lavage or peritoneal lavage (dialysis) with warm fluids, hemodialysis,

TABLE 18-8	PHYSICAL EFFECTS OF HYPOTHERMIA
TEMPERATURE	**CHARACTERISTICS**
35° C (95° F)	Increased respiratory rate, decreased intestinal motility; vigorous shivering; may be conscious and alert; task performance often impaired
32° C (90° F)	May continue uncontrollable shivering or may begin to show muscular rigidity; decreased respiratory rate; atrial fibrillation; may still be conscious but sensorium changes evident; impaired cognition, reasoning, and speech; loss of manual skills and dexterity; brief vasodilation that causes flushes and warm sensation and possible confusion
30° C (86° F)	Decreased cerebral blood flow; may show increased blood pressure (may be difficult to measure), tachycardia, and tachypnea; may have supraventricular arrhythmia, premature ventricular contractions, and T-wave inversion; usually conscious, but a loss of consciousness is preceded by irritability
27° C (80.6° F)	Bradycardia and slowed respiratory rate; metabolic rate decreased by 50%; decreased oxygen uptake, CO_2 production; ventricular fibrillation; rigid extremities
25° C (77° F)	Hypotension; glomerular filtration and blood flow to kidneys reduced by 30%
20° C (68° F)	Unconscious; nonfunctioning reflexes; unresponsive pupils; respirations barely detectable or undetectable; extremities and trunk cold to touch; abnormal electrocardiogram; pulse may decrease to 4 per min, progressing to cardiac standstill; flat electroencephalogram; dead appearance
18° C (64.4° F)	Injury to peripheral tissue

application of external warmth to core circulation areas (groin, axilla, posterior neck region), and/or extracorporeal blood rewarming.

Supportive therapy includes maintenance of ventilation, cardiac monitoring, monitoring of renal function, and correction of fluid and acid-base imbalances. The prognosis is directly correlated with the degree of hypothermia, method of rewarming, and presence of underlying medical conditions.

Nursing Care Management

Nursing care consists of monitoring vital functions and assisting with therapies. Obtaining a history from the family or other observers, including outside environmental temperature, length of exposure to elements, location of exposure site (e.g., outside or inside a vehicle or structure), and any care that may have been given, is essential. If trauma is associated with the hypothermia, ascertain the mechanism and circumstances of injury.

Prevention

Anticipation of cold conditions and knowledge of cold survival techniques are the basis of prevention. Children living in cold climates should have adequate protection when outdoors. Multiple layers of warm clothing are more effective than a single heavy layer for reducing the rate of heat loss, although they do not prevent it. Families living in cold climates should take precautions against unexpected prolonged exposure to cold (e.g., store extra blankets, food rations, and other equipment in

their vehicles in the event of an unexpected mechanical breakdown).

Loss of central core heat can be reduced by 50% when an individual assumes the fetal position or when a person in water remains still. A person suspected of having hypothermia should be moved to a sheltered area, and wet clothing should be removed and replaced with dry, warm garments. Administration of warm, high-calorie liquids is important if the person is conscious.

SKIN DISORDERS RELATED TO DRUG SENSITIVITY

DRUG REACTIONS

Adverse reactions to drugs are seen more often in the skin than in any other organ, although drugs can affect any organ of the body. The reaction may be a result of toxicity related to drug concentration, individual intolerance to the average dosage of the drug, or an allergic or idiosyncratic response. The manifestations may be associated with side effects or secondary effects of a drug, either of which are unrelated to its primary pharmacologic actions.

> **! NURSING ALERT**
>
> Intravenous drugs are more likely to cause a reaction than oral drugs. Stop the drug but maintain the infusion with normal saline.

Although any drug is capable of producing almost any form of reaction in the susceptible individual, some have a tendency to produce a particular reaction consistently, and some are more likely than others to produce an untoward effect. Many such effects are allergenic responses following a prior administration of the drug, even a topical application. Other factors influence response to a drug in a particular individual. For example, the incidence of reaction increases with the amount and the number of drugs given.

Manifestations of drug reactions may be delayed or immediate. A period of 7 days is usually required for a child to develop sensitivity to a drug that has never been administered previously. With prior sensitivity the manifestations appear almost immediately. Rashes—exanthematous, urticarial, or eczematoid—are the most common manifestation of adverse drug reactions in children. However, individual drug reactions may vary from a single lesion to extensive, generalized epidermal necrosis. Cutaneous manifestations can resemble almost any skin disease and can be seen in almost any degree of severity. With few exceptions, the distribution of a drug eruption is widespread (because it results from a circulating agent); appears as an inflammatory response with itching; is sudden in onset; and may be associated with constitutional symptoms such as fever, malaise, gastrointestinal upset, anemia, and liver and kidney damage.

Another common response is a fixed eruption (i.e., a recurrent eruption at the same site with each readministration of the drug). The lesion, a purplish red round or oval plaque with a sharp border seen most frequently on the extremities, disappears slowly, and the pigmentation deepens with each episode.

In most cases treatment for simple cutaneous reactions consists of discontinuation of the drug. Sometimes a decision is made to continue the drug (such as an antibiotic in an infant or small child) until the cause of the rash is clearly indicated. In urticarial-type eruptions, antihistamines may be ordered, and for widespread and severe lesions corticosteroids are beneficial. Severe anaphylactic reactions are a medical emergency. (See Anaphylaxis, Chapter 29.)

Nursing Care Management

The most effective means of management is prevention. Parents always remember a severe response. A careful history taking will elicit evidence of a previous drug reaction. The history should include the name of the drug, nature of the reaction, drug dose, and how soon after administration the reaction occurred. (See History Taking, Chapter 6.)

Nurses who suspect that medication is the cause of the rash should withhold any further dose and report the eruption to the practitioner. Frequent offenders in drug reactions are penicillin and sulfonamides, and nurses must be alert to this possibility. However, even commonplace drugs such as aspirin and barbiturates, chemical agents in some foods, flavoring agents, and preservatives are capable of producing an undesired response. Persons who have severe reactions should wear a medical identification bracelet or necklace in case of emergency or inadvertent administration of the offending agent.

ERYTHEMA MULTIFORME

Erythema multiforme is an acute cutaneous disorder that may be associated with infections (usually viral) or ingestions of drugs. The characteristic lesion consists of an urticarial plaque with a dusky or vesicular center, which appears primarily on the palms, soles, and extensor surfaces.

Treatment involves discontinuing the drug, applying wet compresses for erosive lesions, and administering analgesics for discomfort. Antihistamines may be prescribed for pruritus.

ERYTHEMA MULTIFORME EXUDATIVUM (STEVENS-JOHNSON SYNDROME)

Stevens-Johnson syndrome is the severe form of erythema multiforme characterized by lesions of the skin and mucous membranes, fever, and multiple systemic symptoms. The disease is presumed to be a hypersensitivity reaction to certain drugs, although the reaction may follow an upper respiratory tract infection. The disorder is relatively rare, occurs at any age, and is more common in males than in females.

The syndrome begins with flulike symptoms: malaise, sore throat, fever, and severe headache. Inflammation of the glans penis (balanitis), eyes (conjunctivitis), or mouth and pharynx (stomatitis) appears next, followed in a few days by an erythematous papular rash. The lesions can involve any cutaneous surface, including the palms and soles, but usually spare the scalp. They can be scattered or confluent. The initial lesions enlarge by peripheral expansion with a vesicular center that

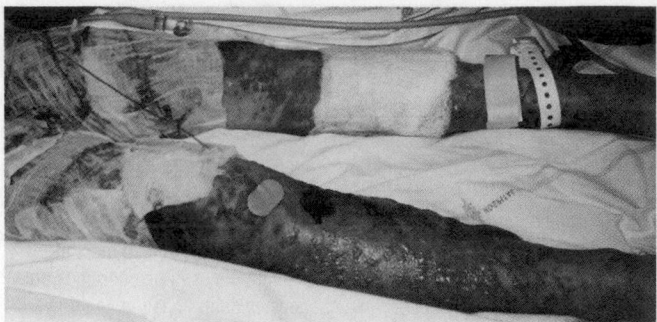

Fig. 18-12 Stevens-Johnson syndrome.

often becomes bullous (Fig. 18-12). Mucous membrane ulceration often becomes severe enough to interfere with eating, and many patients have pulmonary involvement.

Mild disease requires only symptomatic treatment. However, severe disease necessitates hospitalization. Fluid and nutritional requirements are high, and patients often respond to topical lidocaine to relieve oral pain and a liquid diet. Intravenous opioids, such as morphine, and parenteral feedings may be needed for extensive oral involvement. Meticulous mouth care is important, and skin care frequently requires management in a burn unit. (See Stomatitis, Chapter 16, and Burns, Chapter 29.) Daily ophthalmologic examination is advised. Dry eyes are a problem, as is risk of chronic mild symblepharon (adhesion of lids to the eyeball). Eye lubricants promote moisture and comfort. Antibiotics are administered to patients with positive culture results, but the use of corticosteroids is controversial.

The mortality is estimated at 10% to 15% during the acute phase, especially in patients with pulmonary involvement. The disease is self-limiting, and the skin lesions gradually disappear without scarring in 2 to 3 weeks but may recur on reexposure to an offending drug. Wound care usually consists of cleansing with normal saline and providing a moist environment to promote wound healing. Hydrogel dressings (gauze impregnated with gel) are usually soothing and do not stick to the wound with removal (see Wound Care section, p. 691). The family needs emotional support to cope with the life-threatening nature of the disease.

TOXIC EPIDERMAL NECROLYSIS (LYELL DISEASE)

Toxic epidermal necrolysis is a drug-induced injury to the skin characterized by a generalized erythematous rash that rapidly evolves into bullae and peeling. It appears to be a hypersensitivity reaction with precipitating factors similar to those responsible for erythema multiforme. The more common offending drugs are phenobarbital, phenytoin, allopurinol, sulfonamides, and penicillin. In children the clinical appearance is the same as that seen in staphylococcal scalded skin syndrome.

The disease begins with a prodromal period of fever and malaise. Symptoms include a generalized erythematous rash that rapidly evolves into bullae and extensive epidermal peeling, and oral lesions similar to those observed in Stevens-Johnson syndrome. Treatment consists of withdrawal of the offending drug, fluid and electrolyte replacement, and skin management as for severe burns. The disease can be protracted, and mortality can range from 25% to 50%. It is essential that families of children receiving antiepileptics or sulfonamides be informed of the significance of a rash and the importance of promptly reporting it to their health professional.

MISCELLANEOUS AND CONGENITAL SKIN PROBLEMS

A number of other skin disorders also occur in children (Table 18-9). Psoriasis can occur in children younger than 16 years of age, and photosensitivity eruptions associated with inherited diseases appear early in childhood. Ichthyoses are a heterogeneous group of disorders characterized by scaling that creates challenging treatment problems.

NEUROFIBROMATOSIS 1

Neurofibromatosis 1 (NF1), or von Recklinghausen disease, is a relatively common disorder with an autosomal dominant inheritance pattern. It occurs in 1 in 3000 persons and has a high mutation rate. The manifestations are highly variable and appear to result from a defect that alters peripheral nerve differentiation and growth.

Initial clinical presentation involves small, discrete, flat, pigmented skin lesions with smooth edges (café-au-lait spots, pigmented nevi) (Fig. 18-13) and/or axillary or inguinal freckling that develops in early infancy or childhood. Slow-growing cutaneous and subcutaneous neurofibromas that grow along the course of a peripheral nerve appear in later childhood or adolescence and increase in number with age. Lisch nodules, dome-shaped clear to yellow or brown elevations on the iris surface, develop before puberty in most affected individuals. Elephantiasis (thickening and enfolding of the skin) may also occur.

Other characteristics include developmental delay, cognitive impairment, seizures, scoliosis or kyphosis, short stature, macrocephaly, speech defects, learning disabilities, and problems with fine and gross motor skills (Johnson, Saal, Lovell, et al, 1999). Severity varies within the same family: one family member may have only café-au-lait spots or axillary freckling, whereas another may have more severe manifestations.

Diagnosis is established by physical findings based on National Institutes of Neurofibromatosis Fact Sheet (Box 18-1). A family history is elicited to determine whether the specific case is inherited or represents a new mutation. Risk for transmitting the disorder to offspring is 50%. Therapy is limited to excision of tumors that produce pain or impair function and symptomatic management of manifestations.

Nursing Care Management

Nursing care involves recognition of signs that indicate a possibility of the disease, referral for diagnosis, and family counseling and support. It is important that a diagnosis be made, even when the only manifestations are a few café-au-lait spots. The family needs to know the genetic implications and be alert for signs that indicate the child is developing more serious characteristics of the disease. Cancer occurs in patients with the dis-

order, although the rates vary widely. Other members of the family should be assessed for evidence of the disorder.

In addition, families need to know that children with NF1 have a significantly increased risk for learning, social, and emotional problems. Parents need to receive written materials about these problems that they can share with teachers and other adults who interact with the child. Children with NF1 should be screened using systematic standardized tests, and more aggressive and intensive treatment should be provided for speech, motor, and cognitive deficits that may contribute to social and emotional problems (Johnson, Saal, Lovell, et al, 1999).

The Children's Tumor Foundation* is an organization dedicated to increasing public awareness of NF1, providing help and support to families affected by the disorder, and stimulating research.

BITES AND STINGS

ARTHROPOD BITES AND STINGS

Arthropods include insects and arachnids (mites, ticks, spiders, and scorpions). Manifestations and management of skin lesions caused by arthropods are given in Table 18-10.

Some proteins in insect venom are species specific; others are common to a number of species, and crossover reactivity is common. The usual local response to a sting is sharp pain; a local wheal (<5 cm [2 inches] in diameter); and erythema accompanied by intense itching at the site, lasting less than 24 hours. The reaction is produced by enzymes; cytotoxic proteins; and vasoactive compounds, primarily histamine and kinins.

Systemic reactions can occur and, in some instances, can be life threatening. More benign systemic reactions begin several minutes to several hours after the sting and consist of simple urticaria, erythema, pruritus, and angioedema. Serious, life-threatening reactions usually begin within 5 to 10 minutes after the sting and include airway obstruction secondary to laryngeal edema, bronchospasm, hypotension, and cardiovascular collapse.

To prevent contact with stinging and biting insects, teach children behaviors that reduce the likelihood of injury. In addition, topical insect repellents generally provide safe and effective protection for several hours. The best all-purpose repellents contain the active ingredient DEET, which is effective for a variety of insects and arachnids, including mosquitoes, chiggers, ticks, fleas, deerflies, and sand flies. Protection may last from 1 to several hours, but effectiveness is influenced by the concentration of active ingredients. The product must be reapplied after sweating, swimming, wiping, or exposure to rain. Because adverse effects have been reported in young children and because long-term effects of DEET are unknown, parents are advised against excessive application or prolonged use, especially of products with high concentrations of DEET. The insect repellent should not be applied to children's hands because it may be rubbed into the eyes. It should be removed with soap and water when the child is brought inside.

---

*95 Pine St., 16th Floor, New York, NY 10005; 800-323-7938 or 212-344-6633; fax: 212-747-0004; e-mail: info@ctf.org; www.ctf.org.

TABLE 18-9 MISCELLANEOUS SKIN DISORDERS

DISEASE AND CAUSATIVE AGENT	LOCAL MANIFESTATIONS	MANAGEMENT	COMMENTS
Urticaria—Usually allergic response to drugs or infection	Development of wheals Vary in size and configuration and tend to appear quickly, spread irregularly, and fade within a few hours May be constant or intermittent, sparse or profuse, small or large, discrete or confluent May be acute, chronic, or recurrent in acute attacks	Topical soothing and antipruritic agents Antihistamines Epinephrine or ephedrine Cortisone in severe cases Severe upper respiratory tract involvement may require tracheostomy	Known etiologic agents should be avoided May be accompanied by malaise, fever, lymphadenopathy Severe cases may involve mucous membranes, internal organs, and joints Obstruction to air passages constitutes medical emergency (see Chapter 32)
Intertrigo—Mechanical trauma and aggravating factors of excessive heat, moisture, and sweat retention	Red, inflamed, moist, partially denuded, marginated areas, the shape of which is determined by location Appears where opposing skin surfaces rub together, such as intergluteal folds, groin, neck, and axilla Excessive moisture and obesity are often factors	Maintenance of cleanliness and dryness of affected areas Application of a generous supply of nonmedicated powder to keep skinfolds separated Exposure to air and light Removal of excess clothing	A form of diaper irritation Prevent recurrence by keeping susceptible areas clean and dry Frequently associated with overheating from too much clothing Common in tracheostomy patients with short necks and copious secretions
Psoriasis—Cause unknown; hereditary predisposition; may be triggered by stress	Round, thick, dry, reddish patches covered with coarse, silvery scales over trunk and extremities; first lesions commonly appear in scalp; facial lesions more common in children than in adults Affected cells proliferate at a much more rapid rate than normal cells	Tar preparations in combination with ultraviolet B light or natural sunlight Topical corticosteroids Topical vitamin D analog calcipotriene Phenol and saline solutions followed by a tar shampoo to remove scales Keratolytic agents (salicylic acid) Acitretin Emollients may provide relief	Uncommon in children younger than 6 yr Affected patients are otherwise healthy Coal tar acts synergistically with ultraviolet light Keratolytic agents enhance absorption of corticosteroids Humidifiers may help in winter
Alopecia			
Alopecia areata	Sudden onset of asymptomatic, noninflammatory, round, bald patches in hairy parts of body	Psychologic support Inducement of allergic contact dermatitis to stimulate growth of hair Minoxidil (peripheral vasodilator)	Family history in 10%-26% of cases Some concern regarding drug therapy safety Refer to support groups*
Traumatic alopecia	Traction alopecia around scalp margins from tight hair styles (e.g., braids, ponytails, corn rows)	Counseling regarding hair styling, use of hair cosmetics, hot combs, rollers	More prevalent in African-American children and adolescents Prolonged traction can produce fibrosis of hair root and permanent loss
Trichotillomania	Compulsive hair pulling	Determination and treatment of cause	Chronic hair pulling may require psychologic therapy
Tinea capitis	See Table 18-5	See Table 18-5	See Table 18-5
Erythema multiforme (Stevens-Johnson syndrome)—Cause unknown; associated with ingestion of some drugs; often follows upper respiratory tract infection	Erythematous papular rash Lesions enlarge by peripheral expansion, develop central vesicle Involves most skin surfaces except scalp May extend to mucous membranes, especially oral, ocular, and urethral	Symptomatic and supportive Maintenance of adequate intake of fluids (oral or intravenous), calories, and protein Moist wound care, hydrogels such as CarraGauze, Vaseline, or Aquaphor Appropriate treatment of complications Diligent monitoring of urine volume and specific gravity, hemoglobin and hematocrit, serum electrolyte levels, total body weight	Rash often preceded by fever and malaise Complications include renal failure and severe eye disease Respiratory involvement in a number of cases Self-limiting, but recovery may extend for weeks; skin lesions may subside without scarring; mucous membrane lesions may persist for months Recurrence rate 20%; mortality as high as 10% High mutation rate
Neurofibromatosis—Inherited disorder; autosomal dominant inheritance pattern	Café-au-lait spots, pigmented nevi, axillary freckling Slow-growing cutaneous and subcutaneous neurofibromas	Symptomatic treatment of associated manifestations (e.g., speech defects, seizures, skeletal defects [scoliosis, kyphosis], learning disabilities) Surgical removal of troublesome tumors	Refer to support groups† Family needs to know about genetic implications

*National Alopecia Areata Foundation, 14 Mitchell Blvd., San Rafael, CA 94903; 415-472-3780; fax: 415-472-5343; e-mail: info@naaf.org; **www.naaf.org**.
†Children's Tumor Foundation (see p. 711 for contact information).

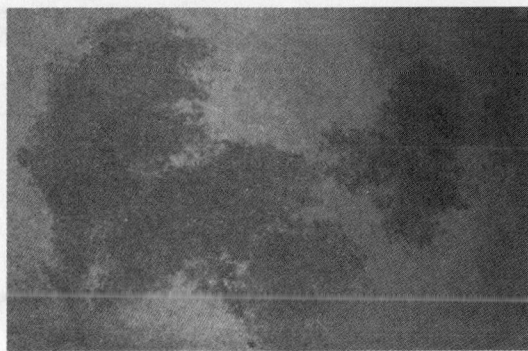

Fig. 18-13 Café-au-lait patches. (From Seidel HM, Ball JW, Daines JE, et al: *Mosby's guide to physical examination,* ed 6, St Louis, 2006, Mosby.)

BOX 18-1 **CRITERIA FOR DIAGNOSIS OF NEUROFIBROMATOSIS 1**

An individual with two or more of the following clinical signs meets the criteria for neurofibromatosis 1 (NF1):

- Six or more café-au-lait spots larger than 5 mm (0.2 inches) in diameter in prepubertal children and larger than 15 mm (0.6 inch) in postpubertal individuals
- Two or more neurofibromas of any type or one plexiform neurofibroma
- Freckling in the axillary or inguinal region
- Optic glioma
- Two or more Lisch nodules
- A distinctive osseous lesion (e.g., sphenoid dysplasia or thinning of long bone cortex with or without pseudoarthrosis)
- A first-degree relative with NF1 according to the criteria listed above

TABLE 18-10 SKIN LESIONS CAUSED BY ARTHROPODS

MECHANISM AND CHARACTERISTICS	MANIFESTATIONS	MANAGEMENT
Insect Bites—Flies, Gnats, Mosquitoes, Fleas		
Mechanism—Foreign protein in insects' saliva introduced when skin is penetrated for a blood meal Distribution: 　Almost everywhere—Fleas, mosquitoes, ants 　Suburbs and rural areas—Bees 　Urban areas—Hornets, wasps, yellow jackets	Hypersensitivity reaction Papular urticaria Firm papules; may be capped by vesicles or excoriated Little or no reaction in nonsensitized person	Treatment: 　Use antipruritic agents and baths 　Administer antihistamines 　Prevent secondary infection Prevention: 　Avoid contact 　Remove focus, as by treating furniture, mattresses, carpets, and pets where insects may live 　Apply insect repellent when exposure is anticipated
Chiggers—Harvest Mites		
Mechanism—Attach with claws and secrete a digestive substance that liquefies the host's epidermis	Erythematous papules Intense itching Favor warm areas of body, especially intertriginous areas and areas covered with clothing	Treatment—May require systemic steroids for extensive bites Prevention: 　Avoid contact, especially in areas of tall grass and underbrush 　Apply insect repellent when exposure is anticipated 　Spray insecticides such as diazinon in yards
Hymenopterans—Bees, Wasps, Hornets, Yellow Jackets, Fire Ants		
Mechanism: 　Injection of venom through stinging apparatus 　Venom contains histamine; allergenic proteins; and often a spreading factor, hyaluronidase 　Severe reactions caused by hypersensitivity or multiple stings	Local reaction—Small red area, wheal, itching, and heat Systemic reactions—May be mild to severe, including generalized edema, pain, nausea and vomiting, confusion, respiratory embarrassment, and shock	Treatment: 　Carefully scrape off stinger or pull out stinger as quickly as possible 　Cleanse with soap and water 　Apply cool compresses 　Apply common household product (e.g., lemon juice, paste made with aspirin or baking soda) 　Administer antihistamines 　Severe reactions—Administer epinephrine, corticosteroids; treat for shock Prevention: 　Teach child to wear shoes; to avoid wearing bright clothing, flowery prints, shiny jewelry, or perfumed grooming products (cologne, scented hairspray), which might attract the insect; and to avoid places where the insect may be contacted 　Hypersensitive children should wear medical identification to indicate allergy and therapy needed; family should keep emergency medication and be taught its administration

Continued

TABLE 18-10	SKIN LESIONS CAUSED BY ARTHROPODS—cont'd	
MECHANISM AND CHARACTERISTICS	**MANIFESTATIONS**	**MANAGEMENT**
Black Widow Spiders Mechanism—Venom injected through a clawlike appendage; has neurotoxic action Characteristics: Spider is shiny black, with a body about 1.25 cm (0.5 inch) long and a red or orange hourglass-shaped marking on underside Avoids light and bites in self-defense	Mild sting at time of bite Swelling, pain, and erythema developing in area of bite Dizziness, weakness, and abdominal pain Possible delirium, paralysis, seizures, and (if large amount of venom absorbed) death	Treatment: Cleanse wound with antiseptic Apply cool compresses Administer antivenin Administer muscle relaxant, such as calcium gluconate; analgesics or sedatives; hydrocortisone or diazepam intravenously Prevention—Teach children to avoid places that harbor the spider (e.g., woodpiles)
Brown Recluse Spiders Mechanism: Venom injected via fangs Venom contains powerful necrotoxin Characteristics: Spider is slender, with long legs and body length of 1-2 cm (0.4-0.8 inch); color is fawn to dark brown; recognized by fiddle-shaped mark on head Shy; bites only when annoyed or surprised Prefers dark areas where seldom disturbed	Mild sting at time of bite Transient erythema followed by bleb or blister; mild to severe pain in 2-8 hr; purple, star-shaped area in 3-4 days; necrotic ulceration in 7-14 days (Fig. 18-14) Systemic reactions—May include fever, malaise, restlessness, nausea, vomiting, and joint pain Generalized petechial eruption Wounds heal with scar formation	Treatment: Apply cool compresses locally Administer antibiotics, corticosteroids Relieve pain Wound may require skin graft Prevention—Teach children to avoid possible nesting sites
Scorpions Mechanism: Venom injected via a hooked caudal stinger Venom of more poisonous species contains hemolysins, endotheliolysins, and neurotoxins Characteristics—Usual habitat is southwestern United States	Intense local pain, erythema, numbness, burning, restlessness, vomiting Ascending motor paralysis with seizures, weakness, rapid pulse, excessive salivation, thirst, dysuria, pulmonary edema, coma, and death Some species produce only local tissue reaction with swelling at puncture site (distinctive) Symptoms subside in a few hours Deaths occur among children <4 yr old, usually in first 24 hr	Treatment: Delay absorption of venom by keeping child quiet; place involved area in dependent position Administer antivenin Relieve pain Admit to pediatric intensive care unit for surveillance Prevention—Teach children to avoid possible nesting sites
Ticks ⊖ Mechanism—In process of sucking blood, head and mouth parts are buried in skin Characteristics: Feed on blood of mammals Significant in humans because of pathologic organisms carried May be vectors of various infectious diseases, such as Rocky Mountain spotted fever, Q fever, tularemia, relapsing fever, Lyme disease, tick paralysis Must attach and feed for 1-2 hr to transmit disease Usual habitat is very wooded area	Tick usually attached to skin, head embedded Firm, discrete, intensely pruritic nodules at site of attachment Possible urticaria or persistent localized edema	Treatment: Grasp tick with tweezers (forceps) as close as possible to point of attachment Pull straight up with steady, even pressure; if bare hands, use a tissue to touch tick during removal; wash hands thoroughly with soap and water Remove any remaining part (e.g., head) with sterile needle Cleanse wound with soap and disinfectant Prevention: Teach children to avoid areas where prevalent Inspect skin (especially scalp) after being in wooded areas

Animation—Tick Paralysis

Most bites are managed by simple symptomatic measures such as use of cool compresses, application of calamine lotion, and prevention of secondary infection. Often treatment consists of application of a substance that relieves the swelling and discomfort and can be made from common household products.

Hymenoptera Stings

When a hymenopteran (a bee, in particular) stings, its barbed stinger penetrates into the skin. The stinger also contains a nerve ganglion, muscles, and a venom sac. As long as the stinger remains in the skin, the muscles push the stinger deeper, and venom is pumped into the wound. A study of different methods of extracting the stinger revealed that the method of removal did not influence the amount of venom injected into the wound. There was no difference in the amount of venom injected when the stinger was removed by external compression with forceps and when the stinger was flicked or scraped off the skin. The influencing factor was the amount of time from the bee sting

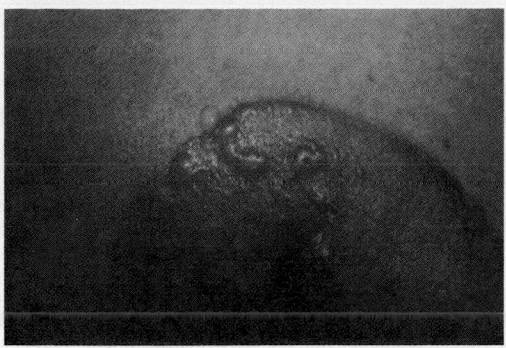

Fig. 18-14 Brown recluse spider bite; note central necrosis surrounded by purplish area and blisters. (From Weston WL, Lane AT: *Color textbook of pediatric dermatology,* St Louis, 1991, Mosby.)

to removal of the stinger; the longer the time interval, the greater the amount of venom injected (Visscher, Vetter, and Camazine, 1996). The best approach is to remove the bee stinger as quickly as possible and to get away from the vicinity of other bees to prevent further injury.

Children need to know how to avoid contact with bees and to recognize the insect (e.g., it is not part of the flower). For those who have become sensitized to hymenoptera stings and demonstrate a severe life-threatening systemic response, intramuscular administration of epinephrine provides immediate relief, and the drug must be available for emergency use. For hypersensitive children, a kit must be available that contains epinephrine, a hypodermic syringe, and perhaps ephedrine and an antihistamine preparation. Hypersensitive children should wear medical identification, such as a bracelet. Nurses should remind parents to frequently check the expiration date on the kit and replace an outdated one. Families should find out whether a nurse is available at the school; if not, someone at the school should be designated to inject the epinephrine in case of an emergency.

Children with a history of generalized reactivity to an insect sting should undergo skin testing with the radioallergosorbent test and possibly immunotherapy with venous extract (desensitization) to prevent serious or fatal reactions. In the United States venous extracts are available for the honeybee, yellow jacket, yellow hornet, and wasp.

Arachnid Bites

Most arachnids in the United States, including tarantulas, are relatively harmless. All spiders produce venom that is injected via fangs. Some are unable to pierce the skin; others produce a venom that is insufficiently toxic to be harmful. A local tissue reaction is relieved by cool compresses or the methods described for hymenoptera stings.

Only scorpions and two spiders—the brown recluse and the black widow—inject venom deadly enough to require immediate attention. Children bitten by these arachnids must receive medical attention as soon as possible.

Ticks are troublesome because they become partially imbedded in the skin as they feed. The recommended method for removal is to grasp the tick with curved forceps as close as possible to the point of attachment and pull straight up with a steady, even pressure. If a portion of the body (e.g., the head)

remains, it can be removed with a sterile needle in the same manner as a sliver. The bite is cleansed with soap and a disinfectant after removal.

To avoid ticks, children should wear long pants tucked into the socks and a long-sleeved shirt when walking in infested areas, especially in the spring and summer. Ticks can also be picked up by dogs and other household pets. Parents are advised to check their children carefully for the organisms when their children have been in areas where ticks might be acquired.

MAMMAL BITES

Nonhuman

Nonhuman mammal bites are common injuries and are inflicted by both wild and domestic animals. Wild animal bites are discussed in relation to rabies in Chapter 37, and these wounds are treated in the same way as the bites of domestic animals such as dogs, cats, hamsters, and mice. The present discussion is directed primarily toward dog bites.

Approximately half the victims of dog bites are younger than 5 years of age; boys are bitten more frequently than girls (Bernardo, Gardner, O'Connor, et al, 2000). Stray dogs are seldom involved in attacks; most dogs involved are owned by the family of the victim or by a neighbor. Most dog attacks occur in or adjacent to the owners' yards, and the attack is usually preceded by verbal or physical contact with the animal (Bernardo, Gardner, O'Connor, et al, 2000). This problem is increasing because of a growing trend of acquiring large, aggressive guard dogs. Most animal bites are caused by dogs. Cat bites are less frequent, although cat scratches are extremely common (see Cat Scratch Disease, p. 703). Most injuries caused by dogs and cats are to the upper extremities. Small children are more likely to receive bites or scratches to the head, face, and neck because they tend to put their heads near the animal's head and flail their arms rather than protecting their heads.

Animal bites are potentially serious because of the likelihood of significant infection. Injuries vary in intensity from small puncture wounds to complete avulsion of tissue that is associated with significant crush injury. Dog bites are seen as lacerations or evulsions; cats exert less biting force, but their sharp teeth penetrate more deeply, inoculating organisms deep into tissues.

The location of a bite influences the incidence of infection. Injuries to the arm and hand tend to become infected more often than those on the legs, scalp, and face. Redness, swelling, and tenderness develop around the site of injury, often accompanied by purulent or serosanguineous drainage. It may be difficult to assess hand infection because most lymphatic drainage is contained in the dorsal subcutaneous space, and swelling occurs in this area when the injury may be elsewhere.

Therapeutic Management

General wound care consists of rinsing the wound with copious amounts of saline or Ringer's lactate delivered under pressure via a large syringe and washing the surrounding skin with mild soap. A clean pressure dressing is applied, and the extremity is elevated if the wound is bleeding. Medical evaluation is advised because of the danger of tetanus and rabies, although dogs in most urban areas are required to be immunized against rabies. Bites from wild animals, such as raccoons, skunks, foxes, and bats, are potentially dangerous. (See Rabies, Chapter 37.)

Prophylactic antibiotics are indicated for puncture wounds and wounds in areas where infection could result in cosmetic or functional impairment. Extensive lacerations are débrided and loosely sutured to allow for drainage in the event of infection. Primary closure of jagged, irregular wounds with associated crush injury and devitalized tissue is contraindicated, except for facial wounds because of cosmetic reasons. Tetanus toxoid is administered according to standard guidelines (see Chapter 12), and rabies protocol is followed. Injuries to poorly vascularized areas such as the hands are more likely to become infected than those in more vascularized areas such as the face. Puncture wounds are more likely to become infected than are lacerations.

Nursing Care Management

The most important aspect related to animal bites is prevention. Children should understand animal behavior and develop respect for animals. It is vital that they learn how to treat animals and how to react to them. Parents should monitor their children's behavior with dogs and instruct them not to tease or surprise a dog, invade its territory, interfere with its feeding or sleeping, take its toy, or interact with a sick or injured dog or a dog with pups (Humane Society of the United States, 1998).

Parents who are considering getting a pet, especially a dog, for themselves or their children should select a dog that is least likely to be a danger to their children. The level of sociability with children is the key to a selection, and dogs range from dangerous and unsuitable to tolerant of children and well behaved.

Parents should obtain dogs from a reputable source that breeds dogs for good temperament. After the dog is purchased, obedience training and socialization should begin to prevent the dog from developing behaviors that are undesirable to the family and neighborhood. Such training is often provided through veterinary services or animal shelters (Bernardo, Gardner, O'Connor, et al, 2000). Prevention programs should educate families about preventing bites and responsible ownership (i.e. training, socializing, neutering).

Human

Children often acquire lacerations from the teeth of other humans in rough play, during fights, or as victims of child abuse. Many preschool children bite others out of frustration or anger. Because human dental plaque and gingiva harbor pathogenic bacteria, all human bite wounds should receive attention. Delaying treatment increases the risk of infection.

If the laceration is less than 6 mm (0.25 inch) long, the wound can be treated at home. The wound is washed vigorously with soap and water, and a pressure dressing is applied to stop bleeding. Ice applications minimize discomfort and swelling. Increased pain or redness at the wound site is an indication that the child should receive medical attention for antibiotic therapy. Tetanus toxoid is needed if the child is insufficiently immunized. Wounds larger than 6 mm should receive medical attention.

SNAKEBITES

In spring snakes emerge from winter hibernation hungry for food and water. The best prevention for snake bites is to avoid snakes, since most people are bitten when trying to handle them. Approximately 1600 venomous bites from domestic snakes were reported to the American Association of Poison Control Centers in 1998 (Litovitz, Klein-Schwartz, Caravati, et al, 1999). Asian and African snakes are far more dangerous than those in the United States and Europe. The major families in the United States are the Crotalidae (pit vipers), which include rattlesnakes, copperheads, and cottonmouths, and the Elapidae, which include coral snakes and cobras. Most bites are attributed to the Crotalidae species.

The manifestations and morbidity are highly variable and depend on the species and size of the snake, the amount of venom injected, the time of year, the child's age and size, and the location of the bite. Not every bite from a poisonous snake injects venom (Schexnayder and Schexnayder, 2000).

The initial action after snakebite is to move the victim away from the area, attempt to calm the child, and place the child at rest. A loose tourniquet applied proximal to the bite delays the flow of lymph, which can carry the venom to the systemic circulation. It should not be tight enough to occlude circulation; a pulse should be palpable distal to the bite. Remove any constricting items of clothing or jewelry from the affected limb. Apply a splint to immobilize the limb, and transport the victim to the nearest medical facility.

If the child has been bitten by a large snake, if less than 30 minutes (some authorities say 5 minutes) has elapsed since the child was bitten, and if medical help is more than 30 minutes away, suction may be beneficial. Suction should be applied by a suction device such as the Sawyer extractor, which is very effective if used within 3 minutes.

> **! NURSING ALERT**
>
> Do not apply ice to the snakebite, since doing so decreases the blood supply to the envenomated site, which allows the venom to work more destruction and decreases the effect of antivenom on the natural immune mechanisms.

If possible, the dead snake should be transported with the patient for identification. If there is any possibility that a child has been bitten by a coral snake, aggressive use of antivenom is indicated; once symptoms occur, it is difficult to stop the respiratory paralysis and death.

DENTAL DISORDERS

DENTAL CARIES

Dental caries (cavities) is one of the most common chronic diseases that affect individuals at all ages; it is the principal oral problem in children and adolescents. Although the overall incidence of dental caries in children has decreased since the introduction of fluoridation, reducing the incidence and consequences of the disorder remains important. Dental caries, if untreated, results in total destruction of the involved teeth. The ages of greatest vulnerability are 4 to 8 years for the primary dentition and 12 to 18 years for the secondary or permanent dentition. (See Figs. 12-13 and 17-15 for sequence of tooth eruption.)

Pathophysiology

Dental caries is a multifactorial disease. It involves a number of elements: (1) the host, (2) microorganisms, (3) substrate, and (4) time.

Host

The prevalence of caries is directly related to the tooth size and morphologic characteristics and to the consistency, composition, and amount of saliva. The incidence of caries is increased in teeth that are improperly developed, crowded, or deeply fissured. The areas most subject to attack by bacteria are grooves and fissures, interdermal areas, gum margins, and other smooth surfaces. Newly erupted teeth that have not yet acquired sufficient surface minerals are more susceptible to decay than those that have been erupted for 2 years or longer. Hereditary factors influence resistance and susceptibility, and similar patterns and anatomic characteristics often appear in successive generations. Salivary flow can mechanically clean away bacteria and food debris. It also contains buffering systems, lysozymes, peroxidases, and immunoglobulins that influence the development of caries.

Microorganisms

Certain types of microflora that produce different effects contribute to the formation of dental caries. Acidogenic bacteria act on fermentable carbohydrates in dental plaque to produce organic acids that decalcify hard surface tooth enamel. With the inner organic matrix exposed, proteolytic organisms and acids digest and destroy the inner tooth structure. These destructive organisms are harbored and protected in a gelatinous plaque formed on the tooth surface by another group of bacteria that are thought to play no primary role in production of decay.

Substrate

Caries formation is strongly influenced by the two concurrent processes that continually operate on enamel surfaces: acid production and acid neutralization by saliva. The material on which the acid-forming bacteria act consists essentially of carbohydrates. Among the fermentable carbohydrates, sucrose has been consistently implicated as the most cariogenic. Sucrose-containing substances, especially in forms that cling (such as chewy candy) or that promote prolonged contact with the teeth (such as hard candy and lollipops), when ingested between meals, contribute markedly to the development of dental caries. Saliva, some foods, and chewing gum after a meal tend to help neutralize much of the acid formed from sucrose.

Time and Other Factors

Bacterial enzymes act on salivary glycoproteins to produce a tenacious protein matrix on the tooth surface. This substance, along with the microorganisms, forms dental plaque. If plaque removal is inadequate or nonexistent for a significant length of time (a few days), the plaque is metabolized by the bacteria to form acid, which initiates the demineralization of enamel.

Other factors that contribute to caries formation are heredity, the amount of fluoride in drinking water, and the child's general state of health. Hereditary factors influence both resistance and susceptibility to dental caries. For example, structural defects, such as deep fissures on occlusal surfaces, predispose the teeth to decay, and individuals in whom acid formation exceeds neutralization are prone to caries. The effectiveness of the buffering action of saliva is highly variable among individuals.

Poor oral hygiene that permits the accumulation of food debris on tooth surfaces allows acid-forming bacteria to thrive and proliferate. Removal of food particles and bacteria-laden plaque inhibits destructive acid formation.

The susceptibility to dental decay is also influenced by the child's general health. Children who suffer from chronic debilitating disease show increased caries activity, as do children with systemic conditions that alter the quality and quantity of saliva produced.

Diagnostic Evaluation

Because the permanent teeth erupt during middle childhood, children are more susceptible to the development of dental caries during this time than at any other age. Caries penetrates the vulnerable teeth rapidly at this age, whereas carious activity is slower and more irregular at later ages.

Caries on visible surfaces are easily detected by oral inspection. Large, extensive caries are apparent to the untrained eye, but small, beginning lesions are best identified by trained professionals. Caries between the teeth may not be located without x-ray examination. A common site of decay is the fissures of the molars.

Therapeutic Management

Well-informed health care professionals can provide dental information and make periodic dental assessments. However, dentists are prepared to provide both of these services and are the only ones qualified to treat most dental problems. Prophylaxis, including hygiene and fluoride treatment, is the major thrust of dental therapy. (See Chapter 14.) Plasticized sealant, applied to the deep fissures and grooves of healthy teeth, is effective in blocking cavity formation. Treatment of dental caries involves removal of all carious portions of the tooth as soon as decay is detected, preparation of a retentive cavity, and replacement of the lost portion of the tooth with a material that is durable in the mouth environment. This restoration of involved teeth not only prevents progression of established caries but also reduces the number of bacteria in the oral cavity to decrease the danger to uninvolved teeth.

Nursing Care Management

Oral inspection is an integral part of the nursing assessment of the child. If there is evidence of dental caries or another unhealthy state, the child is referred for dental services. Many families have a family dentist or a pedodontist who can provide needed care. However, an alarming number of children do not receive regular dental supervision, and a significant number reach adulthood without being examined or treated by a dentist. Nurses can be active members of preventive educational programs and serve as counselors to families regarding the importance of regular dental care, oral hygiene, and dietary management.

Nurses should encourage good oral hygiene and teach correct tooth cleaning to both children and their parents. The random brushing allowed during the early childhood years should be replaced by more careful and methodic cleaning techniques. Children should brush their teeth and use dental floss according to the method recommended by their dentists. (See Chapter 14.) Regular administration of fluoride is also important. (See Chapter 14.) Families should be aware of the fluoride content of their drinking water, including bottled water if it is used. School-age children can usually manage the chewable tablets, which have both a topical and a systemic effect.

Restriction of cariogenic foods is important to prevent dental caries, but this should be viewed as an activity in which all family members are involved and not simply a directive for the child to obey. It should not be communicated in such a way that the child interprets the withholding of sweets as a punishment.

Concern has been generated about the sugar content of children's pharmaceutical products, especially because children with chronic conditions such as seizure disorders, asthma, and recurrent urinary tract or ear infections must take medications over a period of years. Children with chronic illness who regularly take medications containing sugar are cautioned to brush their teeth after taking the medication, just as they would after eating any carbohydrate substance. Children taking tricyclic antidepressants are also prone to develop dental caries.

The greatest task for nurses is counseling children and families to develop sound dental hygiene and nutritional practices. School nurses have an excellent opportunity to participate in community detection of dental needs, to educate children in dental hygiene, to make referrals, and to motivate children to comply with prophylaxis and treatment.

Children should be prepared for dental services in such a way that visits to the dentist are a positive experience. Keeping appointments and following through on recommended treatments and practices are habits that extend beyond childhood.

PERIODONTAL DISEASE

Periodontal disease, an inflammatory and degenerative condition involving the gums and tissues supporting the teeth, often begins in childhood and accounts for a significant amount of tooth loss in adulthood. The more common periodontal problems are gingivitis (simple inflammation of the gums) and periodontitis (inflammation of the gums and loss of connective tissue and bone in the supporting structures of the teeth). An uncommon condition is acute necrotizing ulcerative gingivitis ("trench mouth").

The most prevalent periodontal disease, gingivitis, is a reversible inflammatory disease that begins very early in many children and is most often associated with the buildup of plaque on the teeth. Changes take place in the plaque bacteria, in both the type and number of organisms, that cause them to release a variety of destructive exotoxins, enzymes, and other noxious agents. These agents produce an inflammatory reaction in the gingival tissues, which causes the gums to become red, edematous, tender, and subject to bleeding at slight irritation.

Management is directed toward prevention by conscientious brushing and flossing and by depriving the bacteria of the substrates required to produce the disease. The implementation and maintenance of preventive dental practice, including the use of fluoride, and conscientious brushing and flossing are effective in preventing both caries and periodontal disease.

Nursing Care Management

Nursing care of the child with periodontal disease is primarily supportive; it includes education regarding dental hygiene and regular inspection of the gingival tissues for signs of early inflammation. Advise the child to see the dentist at any sign of inflammation or irritation.

Nurses caring for teenagers should observe for the use of chewing tobacco. The easily detectable clinical lesions appear as tooth erosion, periodontal destruction, and red or white mucosal alterations. The primary site of lesions is the anterior mandibular mucobuccal fold region.

MALOCCLUSION

When teeth of the upper and lower dental arches do not approximate in the proper relationships, the physiologic function of mastication is less effective, and the cosmetic effect is less pleasing. Teeth that are uneven, crowded, or overlapping or are otherwise unable to meet their opponents in the opposite jaw in the appropriate relationships may be predisposed to dental disease. More than half of children 12 to 17 years of age suffer from malocclusions that could be corrected.

The most common cause of malocclusion is hereditary factors, but abnormal growth and habits such as thumb sucking and tongue thrusting also contribute to the disordered alignment and occlusion of the teeth. Treatment of malocclusion includes eliminating habits that aggravate the deformity and initiating corrective therapy at the optimum time. Orthodontic treatment is usually most successful when it is started in the later school-age years or the early adolescent years, after the last primary teeth have been shed and before growth ceases. However, because some deformities can be corrected at an earlier age, referral should be made as soon as malocclusion is evident. For example, removal of extra teeth or impacted teeth or prosthetic replacement of missing teeth can prevent problems from developing.

Nursing Care Management

The nurse who detects malocclusion is obligated to recommend that the teeth be examined by a dentist. The sooner the child is evaluated, the sooner treatment can begin.

Although orofacial appearance is a subjective phenomenon, it can have an adverse effect on a child's self-esteem and body image. Poorly aligned teeth can be a source of both psychologic and physical stress to affected children. Many children with severe malocclusion are teased by their peers or siblings.

If fixed appliances or braces are applied, the child is advised that there will be some discomfort for a few days. During the period of orthodontic treatments, which averages 18 to 30 months, proper oral hygiene is vital. Although the bands or brackets protect the teeth they cover, plaque can collect on the unprotected surfaces or under loose-fitting bands. The teeth should be brushed with a fluoride toothpaste after every meal and snack and at bedtime, using the method recommended by the dentist. Some orthodontists recommend using an oral irrigating device to remove food from between the teeth and around the braces. However, the device does not remove plaque and is not a substitute for thorough brushing. Some foods can damage the braces; others may be difficult to remove from the teeth during cleaning. Forbidden foods include chewing gum, ice, nuts, toffee and hard candy, corn on the cob, uncut apples, hard taco shells, nachos, and popcorn.

Occasionally, tooth movement or poking at the braces with a pencil or other object may cause an arch wire to break or protrude. If this happens, instruct the child to cover the broken portion with a special wax provided by the dentist and schedule an appointment as soon as possible. Regular visits are usually scheduled every 3 to 6 weeks. After the braces are taken off, a removable or permanent retainer must be used to maintain the desired position of the teeth. Placement of a permanent wire behind the front teeth requires no compliance from the youngster.

Sometimes children need considerable reinforcement for compliance with orthodontic treatment. It may be difficult for some to relate the present barriers of discomfort, inconvenience, and embarrassment to the future reinforcers of improved appearance and dental health. Teenagers with a heightened awareness of body image and physical attractiveness are especially at risk for noncompliance. (See Chapter 27 for a discussion of compliance.)

TRAUMA

Dental injury is not uncommon in childhood. Most injuries occur after bicycle and playground mishaps and include fractures of varying degrees of severity, chipping, dislocation, or avulsion. All tooth injuries require prompt treatment by a competent dentist to prevent permanent displacement or loss. Delayed examination and diagnosis of tooth damage can result in infection or pulp involvement. Because it can affect the remaining teeth, loss of a permanent tooth requires professional attention to maintain normal alignment and position of teeth.

Trauma usually involves the maxillary incisors, and children with protruding teeth, craniofacial abnormalities, or neuromuscular disorders are more likely to sustain dental injuries.

Nursing Care Management: Tooth Avulsion

A permanent tooth that is avulsed (evulsed, exarticulated, or "knocked out") should be reimplanted by the child, parent, or nurse and stabilized as soon as possible so that the blood supply to the tooth can be reestablished and the tooth kept alive (American Academy of Pediatric Dentistry, 2009) (see Emergency Treatment box). If the tooth is replaced within 15 minutes, there is a better chance that it will become reattached and the roots will not resorb or the crown exfoliate. Avulsed primary teeth are usually not reimplanted.

✚ EMERGENCY TREATMENT

Avulsed Tooth

1. Recover tooth.
2. Hold tooth by crown; avoid touching root area.
3. If tooth is dirty, rinse it gently under running water or saline; be sure to insert stopper in sink or basin (to avoid losing the tooth).
4. Insert tooth into socket.
5. Have child hold tooth in place.
6. Transport child to dentist immediately.
7. Avoid sudden stops or sharp turns to prevent dislodging tooth

If Reluctant to Reimplant Tooth

1. Place avulsed tooth in suitable medium for transport:
   - Cold milk
   - Saliva—under child's or parent's tongue
2. If child is holding tooth in mouth, avoid sudden stops to prevent swallowing of tooth.
3. *Don't forget to take tooth!*

Before reimplantation it is important to carefully rinse a dirty tooth in milk or saline solution or under running water to avoid disturbing the adhering periodontal membrane, which is essential to the success of the reimplantation. The tooth is held by the crown, not the root, while rinsing, with the drain plugged. The tooth is then fit back into its socket as atraumatically as possible (Troupe, 1995). If the tooth is reimplanted almost immediately, excessive pressure is not needed; however, it becomes extremely difficult after clot formation (in approximately 10 minutes). The tooth is held in place by the child during transportation to a dentist. If the child or parents are reluctant to reimplant the tooth, the next best alternative is to place the tooth in Viaspan, Hank's Balanced Salt Solution, cold milk, saliva, contact lens solution, saline, or water for transport to the dentist (American Academy of Pediatric Dentistry, 2009). Cold milk has precisely the osmolality needed to maintain fluid balance within the tissues surrounding the tooth. Water is the least desirable storage medium because the hypotonic environment causes rapid cell lysis.

After reimplantation, the tooth usually becomes firmly attached, although endodontic therapy is often required. If reimplantation is not permanent, the tooth may be retained anywhere from 6 months to 12 years and facilitates normal development and occlusion, since loss of teeth during the period of permanent tooth eruption may adversely affect such development.

As with all mouth trauma, tooth avulsion causes a large amount of bleeding, which is frightening to children and their families. The nurse or anyone faced with dental trauma should be prepared to cope with the emotionality that accompanies tooth avulsion. Using a calm approach and providing gentle reassurance to the child are often successful in reducing anxiety.

DISORDERS OF CONTINENCE

ENURESIS

Enuresis (bed-wetting) is a common and troublesome disorder that is defined as intentional or involuntary passage of urine into the bed (usually at night) or into clothes during the day in children who are beyond the age when voluntary bladder control should normally have been acquired. The inappropriate voiding of urine must occur at least twice a week for a minimum of 3 months, and the chronologic or developmental age of the child must be at least 5 years (see Cultural Competence box). In addition, the urinary incontinence must not be related to the direct physiologic effects of a substance (e.g., diuretics) or a general medical condition (e.g., diabetes mellitus or diabetes insipidus, spina bifida, seizure disorder, or sickle cell disease).

🌐 CULTURAL COMPETENCE

Enuresis

The age at which children attain urinary continence varies widely. For example, white children in the United States tend to achieve continence earlier than African-American children. In addition, children in Great Britain and Sweden appear to attain continence slightly earlier than children in the United States. Therefore practitioners should be sensitive to the differences among cultural groups before assessing a child as enuretic.

Enuresis can also be defined as primary (bed-wetting in children who have never been dry for extended periods) or secondary (the onset of wetting after a period of established urinary continence). The passage of urine may occur only during night-time sleep (nocturnal), only during the waking hours (diurnal), or during both times of the day. The nocturnal type is most common.

Enuresis is more common in boys, and nocturnal bed-wetting usually ceases between 6 and 8 years of age (American Academy of Pediatrics, 2003). Although most children with enuresis do not have coexisting psychopathology, some children do have other developmental disorders, learning problems, or behavior difficulties, such as increased motor activity and aggression.

Enuresis can cause serious psychologic problems. The degree of impairment is related to the effect on the child's social life, such as not being able to attend overnight camps, and the effect on others, who may ostracize or ridicule the youngster. Adolescents with enuresis have described themselves as being tense, having difficulty sleeping, and having bad dreams. Children state that they are embarrassed about the disorder and are often hesitant to sleep at other children's homes. Avoiding overnight excursions can impede normal socialization or self-esteem. Enuresis can influence self-esteem if parental response to the disorder is harsh or punitive. In some instances, enuresis may serve as a trigger for child abuse. Although behavior problems can be associated with these psychologic effects, research suggests that adults treated for enuresis as children have normal psychologic profiles.

Etiology and Pathophysiology

No clear cause for enuresis has been determined. However, predictive factors have been noted, including longer duration of sleep in infancy, a positive family history, and a slower rate of physical development in children up to 3 years of age. There is a high concordance rate of enuresis in monozygotic (identical) twins and an even higher one in dizygotic (nonidentical) twins, which suggests more than a pure genetic link in the dis-

order. Approximately 75% of all children with functional enuresis have a first-degree relative who has, or has had, the disorder.

Enuresis is primarily an alteration of neuromuscular bladder functioning and as such is benign and self-limiting. Emotional factors may influence the symptom. Some children exhibit temporary regressive behavior resulting in enuresis after the birth of a sibling or other trauma. Other children, such as those with attention deficit hyperactivity disorder (ADHD), may have occasional "accidents" when they become so involved in play that they are unaware of a full bladder or "forget" to empty the bladder. In other children enuresis may be related to problems with toilet training, such as the age at which training began; the emotional atmosphere surrounding the training situation; or an excessive amount of emotional dependence on the parent, usually the mother. Occasionally enuresis can be a behavioral manifestation of a personality disorder.

Although several theories have been proposed, no one theory thoroughly explains enuresis. The sleep theory stems from parental reports that these children sleep more soundly and are difficult to arouse from sleep.

Another theory relates to functional bladder capacity, the volume of urine voided after maximum delay of micturition. Although there is evidence that some children with enuresis have a smaller bladder capacity than unaffected children, other evidence suggests that this is not the cause. For example, children without enuresis but with a smaller bladder capacity awaken during the night to void, whereas children with enuresis do not awaken.

The nocturnal polyuria theory suggests that the kidneys of these children fail to concentrate urine during sleep because of insufficient secretion of antidiuretic hormone (ADH). The ADH circadian rhythm may thus be a significant biologic marker in enuresis, but additional research must be conducted to clarify its role.

The dysfunctional detrusor activity theory suggests that an unstable bladder detrusor muscle spontaneously contracts to produce bed-wetting, either because of abnormal innervation or as a result of other, unknown reasons. Studies to explore this theory have yielded contradictory and inconclusive results; more research is needed to clarify these contradictions and to determine whether there is a relationship between ADH production and detrusor activity.

Clinical Manifestations

The predominant symptom of enuresis is urgency that is immediate and accompanied by acute discomfort, restlessness, and sometimes urinary frequency. With nocturnal enuresis, the child may or may not feel urgency. If awareness of the urgency is present, the child often reports difficulty awakening to urinate. Spontaneous voiding during sleep occurs, which usually results in multiple nightly incidents. Spontaneous remission of nocturnal enuresis occurs in approximately 15% of cases. However, in some cases nocturnal enuresis continues into adolescence and adulthood.

Diagnostic Evaluation

During the initial phases of evaluation, a routine physical examination is performed to rule out physical causes, such as urinary tract infection, structural disorders, major neurologic deficits, nocturnal epilepsy, disorders that increase the normal output of urine (e.g., diabetes mellitus and diabetes insipidus), and disorders that impair the concentrating ability of the kidneys (e.g., chronic renal failure or sickle cell disease). The examination may include diagnostic evaluation of functional bladder capacity. Normal bladder capacity (in ounces) is the child's age plus 2; therefore normal bladder capacity for 6-year-old is 8 oz (237 ml). Functional bladder capacity is determined by having the child hold off voiding until the strongest urgency is felt, at which time the child voids into a measurement container. A bladder volume of 300 to 350 ml (10 to 12 oz) is sufficient for retention of a night's urine.

If psychologic difficulties are evident or a personality disorder is suspected, seek a routine psychiatric evaluation.

A history of wetting behavior is obtained, including information about the toilet-training process. Assess parental attitudes by listening and asking parents how they have attempted to cope with the wetting. An important feature of assessment is a baseline count of enuretic incidents and the time of day when each occurs. This is necessary not only to establish diagnostic reliability but also to confirm outcome success after treatment. The baseline information is gathered for 1 to 2 weeks by the child and family. It usually consists of a chart or calendar given to the family on which they indicate the date of the incident, the time of the incident, and the approximate volume of the urinary output.

Therapeutic Management

Enuresis not resulting from known organic causes has been treated in several ways. No single method has achieved universal endorsement. Frequently, more than one technique is employed. In some cases, a spontaneous decrease in bed-wetting occurs with age and irrespective of the treatments used (American Academy of Pediatrics, 2003). Successful treatment is defined as a specified period of dry nights, varying from 7 to 28 consecutive dry nights.

Conditioning therapy involves training the child to awaken to urinate after a stimulus is given, especially with a urine alarm. The device consists of a moisture-sensitive wire pad that is placed inside the underpants and is attached to a bell or buzzer. When the system detects moisture, the bell or buzzer sounds, which fully awakens the child. The child is thus conditioned to awaken at the initiation of micturition or to the stimulus of the bell or buzzer and eventually learns to continue voiding in the toilet. The urine alarm can be very effective, but children may relapse once they stop using it. Relapse is addressed by reinstituting the alarm during sleep. This method is inexpensive compared with drug therapy and has no side effects.

Retention control training was developed after the observation of reduced functional bladder capacity in children who were bed wetters. The child drinks fluids and delays urination as long as can be tolerated to stretch the bladder to accommodate increasingly larger volumes of urine. The use of Kegel, or pelvic muscle, exercises may be helpful in children with daytime enuresis.

In the waking schedule treatment, the child is awakened during the night at intervals to void. This method has been successful in reducing, but not eliminating, wetting incidents.

Drug therapy is increasingly being prescribed to treat enuresis. Three types of drugs are used: tricyclic antidepressants, antidiuretics, and antispasmodics. The selection depends on the interpretation of the cause. The drug used most frequently is the tricyclic antidepressant imipramine (Tofranil), which exerts an anticholinergic action in the bladder to inhibit urination. The dosage and time of administration are individualized, and the drug is given in amounts sufficient to lighten sleep but not to cause wakefulness. Some practitioners prescribe low doses, which reduces bed-wetting in two thirds of children. However, it is important to note that almost all children relapse when the medication is stopped. The suggested length of treatment is 6 to 8 weeks, followed by gradual withdrawal over 4 weeks. Because this drug is dangerous in overdosage, caution parents about safe use and the need to keep supplies of the drug from the reach of younger siblings.

Anticholinergic drugs, especially oxybutynin, reduce uninhibited bladder contractions and may be helpful for children with daytime urinary frequency. Success has also been achieved with desmopressin acetate (DDAVP) nasal spray, an analog of vasopressin, which reduces nighttime urinary output to a volume less than functional bladder capacity. Typically, the child receives two sprays before bedtime. The medication is generally well tolerated but may cause nasal irritation or, rarely, headache or nausea. A preparation of desmopressin acetate is also available in tablet form. This preparation is as effective and safe as the nasal spray but avoids the problem of nasal irritation.

One of the challenges of using the drug therapeutically is the difficulty in simulating the normal circadian rhythm of ADH secretion. Another concern is the expense of the treatment. Although DDAVP is effective in reducing the number of wet nights, only about 25% of children become completely dry, and the relapse rate is about 80% to 90% (Bosson and Lynn, 2001).

Other therapies and treatment options include stream interruption, paired associations, overlearning, reinforcement systems, and self-monitoring (motivation therapy). Frequently these therapies are coupled with other treatment modalities. In conclusion, alarms are the most effective treatment for enuresis, but desmopressin may provide temporary relief (Glazener, Evans, and Petro, 2004a, 2004b). Counseling may be beneficial in helping the child, and sometimes the family, adjust to the bed-wetting.

It is imperative that punishment not be used to correct enuresis. Supportive therapy such as teaching the child to change pajamas and bed linens, as well as restriction of fluids before bedtime, should be used in place of punishment. Behavior modification techniques, such as placing stars or stickers on a chart for each dry night and providing rewards for achieving a certain goal, are also helpful. Token or social reinforcement can also be used to enhance the rewards for success.

Nursing Care Management

No matter what techniques are used, the nurse can help both children and parents understand the problem of enuresis, the treatment plan, and the difficulties they may encounter in the process. Essential to the success of any method is the supportive management of parents and their children. Both need encouragement and patience. The problem is discussed with both the parent and the child, since any treatment involves and requires the child's active participation. In some treatment interventions the child is in charge of the intervention; therefore parents must learn to support the child rather than intervene themselves. For example, children can strip their wet covers, limit fluids, and use the toilet before bedtime (American Academy of Pediatrics, 2006).

Parents should also be taught to observe for side effects of any medications used. All children with primary enuresis should be encouraged to void before bedtime. Diapering should be avoided. Positive reinforcement in the form of keeping diaries to record dry nights has been effective in fostering motivation in children.

The most important predictor for the outcome of treatment is family difficulties. Family disturbances influence the initial arrest of the enuresis, the relapse rate, and the long-term success rate.

Many parents believe that enuresis is caused by an emotional disturbance and fear that they have somehow produced the situation by improper childrearing practices. They need reassurance that the bed-wetting is not a manifestation of emotional disturbance and does not represent willful misbehavior. Parents need to understand that punishment such as scolding, shaming, and threatening is contraindicated because of their negative emotional impact and limited success in reducing the behavior. Encourage parents to be patient, to be understanding, and to communicate love and support to the child.

Communication with children is directed toward eliminating the emotional impact of the problem; relieving feelings of shame, guilt, and the burden of parental disapproval; building self-confidence; and motivating them toward independent control. More important, the nurse can provide consistent support and encouragement to help children through the inconsistent and unpredictable treatment process. Children need to believe that they are helping themselves and to maintain feelings of confidence and hope.

ENCOPRESIS

Encopresis is repeated voluntary or involuntary passage of feces of normal or near-normal consistency in places not appropriate for that purpose according to the individual's own sociocultural setting. The event must occur at least once a month for a minimum of 3 months, and the child's chronologic or developmental age must be at least 4 years. The fecal incontinence must not be caused by physiologic effects of a substance (e.g., laxatives) or a general medical condition except through a mechanism involving constipation. The consistency of the stool may vary from normal or near-normal to liquid, with a more liquid stool seen especially in individuals who have overflow incontinence secondary to fecal retention.

A child 4 years of age or older who has never achieved fecal continence is said to have primary encopresis. This type is more frequently observed as a result of neglect, lax training methods, mental subnormalities, and familial causes. Secondary encopresis is fecal incontinence occurring in a child over 4 years of age after a period of established fecal continence. The disorder is more common in males than in females.

Etiology

One of the most common causes of encopresis is constipation, which may be precipitated by environmental change, such as having a new sibling, moving to a new house, changing schools, or even having to use new or unfamiliar toilet facilities. Chronic, severe constipation has a tendency to impair the usual movement and contractions of the colon, which can lead to fecal obstruction. Abnormalities in the digestive tract (e.g., Hirschsprung disease, anorectal lesions, malformations, and rectal prolapse) and medical conditions such as hypothyroidism, hypokalemia, hypercalcemia, lead intoxication, myelomeningocele, cerebral palsy, muscular dystrophy, and irritable bowel syndrome are also associated with constipation, which can lead to encopresis (Coughlin, 2003). Voluntary retention of stool may also follow an incident of painful defecation (e.g., in a child with anal fissures). Involuntary retention may be produced by emotional problems caused by the encopresis, which sets up a fear-pain cycle and results in learned abnormal defecation patterns. Psychogenic encopresis, in which the soiling is caused by emotional problems, is often related to a disturbed mother-child relationship.

Normally, children and adolescents have one or two soft-formed stools per day. Children with soiling problems tend to form large-bore stools, which are painful to excrete. Therefore they tend to avoid defecation and withhold stooling. Stool held in the rectum and sigmoid colon loses water and progressively hardens, which causes successively more painful bowel movements and a stretched rectal vault. Over time the child will lose the urge to defecate on his or her own (Montgomery, 2008). A pain-retention-pain cycle is established. Many children have diarrhea or loose leakage in their clothing and pass small amounts of hard stool, which suggests leakage around an impaction.

Children may experience exacerbations with transitions in the school setting. Some reasons for developing retentive tendencies at this time are fear of using school bathrooms, a busy schedule, and the interruption of an established time schedule for bowel evacuation. Children may also react to stress with bowel dysfunction.

Clinical Manifestations

The manifestation of simple constipation is painful expulsion of hard, pelletlike stools. Voluntary retention is usually temporary, with a history of a painful precipitating episode and blood-streaked stools. Involuntary retention is associated with a history of abdominal pain, distention, moodiness, poor appetite, and accumulation of stools with periodic passage of voluminous stools. Children display a characteristic posturing during suppression of colonic signals to defecate—stiffening, standing in a corner with straight legs and a bright red face, "doing a little dance," "crawling," or hiding behind furniture or behind a tree when playing outdoors. They typically hide soiled underwear. It is not unusual for soiling to take place after bathing because of reflex stimulation.

The child with encores often feels ashamed and may wish to avoid situations (e.g., camp or school) that might lead to embarrassment. School performance and attendance are affected as the child's offensive odor becomes a target for scorn and derision by classmates. The child is not well liked by peers and may be severely rejected by the parents as a result of the symptom. Rejection by peers and parents causes further withdrawal and other behavioral manifestations.

Therapeutic Management

Direct treatment toward the cause of the soiling. To determine the cause, perform a complete physical examination, including a rectal examination. An abdominal x-ray film may be obtained to determine the severity of impaction. Diet, lubricants, and a toilet ritual that encourages the child to establish normal defecation are used. Fecal impaction is relieved by lubricants such as mineral oil; osmotic laxatives such as lactulose, sorbitol, or polyethylene glycol (PEG or MiraLax); and magnesium hydroxide. Customary dosages are usually insufficient. Mineral oil should be avoided in children who have dysphagia or vomiting to prevent risk of aspiration. Dietary changes may be helpful, including elimination of milk and dairy products and consumption of increased amounts of high-fiber foods, such as fruits, vegetables, and cereals, as well as increased fluids. Behavior therapy may be indicated to eliminate any fear that has developed as a result of painful defecation. Psychotherapeutic intervention with the child and the family may become necessary.

Nursing Care Management

A thorough history of the soiling is essential—when soiling began, how often it occurs and under what circumstances, and whether the child uses the toilet successfully at all. Because the parents and child are reluctant to volunteer information, direct questioning about the soiling is more successful.

Education regarding the physiology of normal defecation, toilet training as a developmental process, and the treatment outlined for the particular family is a prerequisite to a successful outcome. The regimen prescribed for stimulating elimination is explained to parents. Bowel retraining with mineral oil, a high-fiber diet, and a regular toileting routine is essential in treating encopresis or chronic constipation.

Encourage the child to sit on the toilet 10 to 15 minutes after meals for intervals of 10 minutes. Placing a footstool below the feet may relax the abdomen and make the child more comfortable. Enemas may be needed for impactions, but long-term use prevents the child from assuming responsibility for defecation. Initially lubricants are given liberally, but stimulant cathartics often cause abdominal cramps that can frighten the child. Positive reinforcement such as giving stickers, praising the child, and awarding special activities may encourage the child to participate in the bowel regimen.

Family counseling is directed toward reassurance that most problems resolve successfully, although the child may have relapses during periods of stress, such as vacations or illness (see Family-Centered Care box). If encopresis persists beyond occasional relapses, the condition needs to be reevaluated. Behavior modification techniques are explained, and the family is assisted with a plan suited to the particular situation.

👪 FAMILY-CENTERED CARE
Helping Families Understand Encopresis

The prevailing attitude of nurses toward the family of a child with encopresis should be one of no fault, to relieve the guilt of both parents and child. Because parents and children are often reluctant to volunteer information, direct questioning about the soiling is more successful. Family education about the condition can be very helpful. Parents are usually relieved to know that other families share this problem and are surprised to learn that functional changes that take place as the condition develops make control of seepage impossible. Many parents complain that their children soil because they do not take time from play for a bowel movement. Actually, the children may be unaware of a prior sensation and unable to control the urge once it begins. They may be so accustomed to bowel accidents that they are unable to smell or feel anything and even deny soiling when it occurs.

DISORDERS WITH BEHAVIORAL COMPONENTS

ATTENTION DEFICIT HYPERACTIVITY DISORDER

ⓔ ADHD refers to developmentally inappropriate degrees of inattention, impulsiveness, and hyperactivity. Some hyperactive-impulsive or inattentive symptoms must have been present before age 7 years and must be present in at least two settings. Prevalence rates for ADHD vary but range from approximately 4% to 12%, depending on whether they are based on school samples or community samples (American Academy of Pediatrics, 2000). ADHD is seen more frequently in boys than in girls. The symptoms of ADHD were first recognized in the early 1900s. Several different names have been applied to the disorder. ADHD was originally called *minimal brain damage,* then *minimal brain dysfunction,* and in the mid-1900s the term *hyperkinetic reaction of childhood* was given to the symptoms. Currently the term *attention deficit hyperactivity disorder* has been adopted by the American Psychiatric Association (2000).

Difficulties associated with ADHD are most often school related or academic. Family and social relationships can also be affected if aggressive behavior and mood lability interfere with peer relationships, cause difficulties in social interactions, or make discipline difficult. Children with ADHD are at greater risk for conduct disorders, oppositional defiant disorders, depression, anxiety disorders, and developmental disorders such as speech and language delays and learning disabilities than are children without ADHD (American Academy of Pediatrics, 2000).

Early identification of affected children is important because the characteristics of ADHD significantly interfere with the normal course of emotional and psychologic development. Many children develop maladaptive behavior patterns that hinder psychosocial adjustment. Their behavior evokes negative responses from others, and repeated exposure to negative feedback adversely affects the child's self-concept (see Research Focus box).

Etiology

The exact cause of ADHD is unknown. A combination of organic, genetic, and environmental factors is probably

Case Study—Attention Deficit Hyperactivity Disorder

involved. A variety of factors put a child at risk for symptoms of ADHD. ADHD is seen more often in children who have family members with ADHD, especially the father, a brother, or an uncle. There is also an increased incidence of substance abuse, conduct disorders, learning disabilities, depression, and antisocial personality disorder in families of children with ADHD. Chromosomal or genetic abnormalities such as fragile X syndrome have been implicated in ADHD. Girls with Turner syndrome have a high incidence of impaired spatial abilities and right-left directional sense, and a large number of boys with Klinefelter syndrome have learning, behavior, or peer problems. A sex-linked factor may be operating because the disorder is much more common in boys than in girls.

Other risk factors include exposure to toxins or medications, perinatal complications, chronic otitis media, head trauma, meningitis, neurologic infections, and mental disorders such as the affective disorders.

Another popular theory is the concept of a developmental lag. Distractibility, short attention span, and impulsiveness are normal characteristics of children at a much younger developmental level. However, research indicates that symptoms of ADHD do not diminish with age. Symptoms such as inattentiveness and impulsivity last into adolescence and young adulthood in many affected individuals (King, 2000). In addition, hyperactivity may be a normal variant of innate temperament in some children who represent the extreme end of the normal distribution curve for activity.

Support for a neurochemical etiology is suggested by the fact that many children with ADHD respond to medications that affect the central nervous system. Some children may have an absence or insufficiency of norepinephrine, dopamine, and serotonin. These neurotransmitters normally occur in high concentrations in the brain and affect activity level, mood, and awareness. It is hypothesized that children who lack these neurotransmitters experience learning difficulties in reading, math, and language and are prone to impulsivity. Many of these children respond to treatment with psychostimulants such as methylphenidate hydrochloride, which increases dopamine and norepinephrine levels (American Academy of Pediatrics, 2001). The fact that some children with ADHD manifest decreased symptoms in stressful situations (such as in the physician's or principal's office) provides additional support for this theory, since stress increases the level of norepinephrine.

Another neurochemical theory suggests that symptoms result from an excess of norepinephrine and/or an alteration in the reticular activating system of the midbrain, an area that controls consciousness and attention. This excess or abnormality interferes with the function of filtering out extraneous stimuli. Consequently, children are unable to focus on one stimulus and are compelled to respond to every stimulus in the environment. They demonstrate hyperactive behaviors that result from cognitive "flooding" and exaggerated arousal that overwhelms the attention filters and overrides inhibitory processes. Other theories maintain that symptoms of ADHD result from dysfunction in the brain circuits of the behavioral inhibition system; structural abnormalities in the prefrontal cortex, caudate, and thalamus; and a gene variant known to code for a receptor for dopamine.

Interest in diet as a factor in hyperactivity continues to generate controversy. Some believe that the observed behavior patterns are related to an innate sensitivity to food items such as sucrose or food additives such as aspartame (NutraSweet). This theory does not have widespread support and has not been validated by empirical studies. Nevertheless, some children do show improvement when certain foods are eliminated from the diet, particularly those that cause hyperallergic reactions, such as chocolate, cow's milk, and eggs. A recent study by Konofal, Lecendreux, Arnulf, and colleagues (2004) suggests that low iron stores may contribute to ADHD because iron is a coenzyme of dopamine synthesis and that these children may benefit from iron supplementation.

Clinical Manifestations

The behaviors exhibited by the child with ADHD are not unusual aspects of child behavior. The difference lies in the quality of motor activity and the developmentally inappropriate inattention, impulsivity, and hyperactivity that the child displays. The manifestations may be numerous or few, mild or severe, and vary with the child's developmental level. Any given child will not have every manifestation that is characteristic of the syndrome, and the degree of severity is highly variable. Mild manifestations of the symptoms may not be apparent in some educational and family environments, whereas severe symptomatology will be recognizable in most environments. Every child with ADHD is different from all other children with ADHD (Box 18-2).

Most behavioral manifestations are apparent at an early age, but the learning disabilities may not become evident until the child enters school. The disorder is unpredictable; it may remit spontaneously at any age, and the number of years that a child will require treatment is unknown.

A major clinical manifestation is distractibility. The stimuli may come from external sources or internal sources. Children frequently demonstrate immaturity relative to chronologic age. Selective attention is often seen, in which the child has difficulty attending to "nonpreferred" tasks, such as completing chores or finishing homework. The child may not consider the consequences of behavior, may take excessive physical risks (often beginning early in life), and may demonstrate inappropriate social skills.

Children with ADHD demonstrate one of three subtypes (American Psychiatric Association, 2000).

1. Combined type—Six (or more) symptoms of inattention and six (or more) symptoms of hyperactivity-impulsivity have persisted for at least 6 months. Most children and adolescents with the disorder have the combined type.

2. Predominantly inattentive type—Six (or more) symptoms of inattention (but fewer than six symptoms of

BOX 18-2 DIAGNOSTIC CRITERIA FOR ATTENTION DEFICIT HYPERACTIVITY DISORDER

A. Either (1) or (2):

(1) Six (or more) of the following symptoms of inattention have persisted for at least 6 months to a degree that is maladaptive and inconsistent with developmental level:

Inattention

(a) Often fails to give close attention to details or makes careless mistakes in schoolwork, work, or other activities

(b) Often has difficulty sustaining attention in tasks or play activities

(c) Often does not seem to listen when spoken to directly

(d) Often does not follow through on instructions and fails to finish schoolwork, chores, or duties in the workplace (not because of oppositional behavior or failure to understand instructions)

(e) Often has difficulty organizing tasks and activities

(f) Often avoids, dislikes, or is reluctant to engage in tasks that require sustained mental effort (such as schoolwork or homework)

(g) Often loses things necessary for tasks or activities (e.g., toys, school assignments, pencils, books, or tools)

(h) Is often easily distracted by extraneous stimuli

(i) Is often forgetful in daily activities

(2) Six (or more) of the following symptoms of hyperactivity-impulsivity have persisted for at least 6 months to a degree that is maladaptive and inconsistent with developmental level:

Hyperactivity

(a) Often fidgets with hands or feet or squirms in seat

(b) Often leaves seat in classroom or in other situations in which remaining seated is expected

(c) Often runs about or climbs excessively in situations in which it is inappropriate (in adolescents or adults, may be limited to subjective feelings of restlessness)

(d) Often has difficulty playing or engaging in leisure activities quietly

(e) Is often "on the go" or often acts as if "driven by a motor"

(f) Often talks excessively

Impulsivity

(g) Often blurts out answers before questions have been completed

(h) Often has difficulty awaiting turn

(i) Often interrupts or intrudes on others (e.g., butts into conversations or games)

B. Some hyperactive-impulsive or inattentive symptoms that caused impairment were present before age 7 years.

C. Some impairment from the symptoms is present in two or more settings (e.g., at school [or work] and at home).

D. There must be clear evidence of clinically significant impairment in social, academic, or occupational functioning.

E. The symptoms do not occur exclusively during the course of a pervasive developmental disorder, schizophrenia, or other psychotic disorder and are not better accounted for by another mental disorder (e.g., mood disorder, anxiety disorder, dissociative disorder, or personality disorder).

Code based on type:

314.01 Attention-Deficit/Hyperactivity Disorder, Combined Type: if both Criteria A1 and A2 are met for the past 6 months

314.00 Attention-Deficit/Hyperactivity Disorder, Predominantly Inattentive Type: if Criterion A1 is met but Criterion A2 is not met for the past 6 months

314.01 Attention-Deficit/Hyperactivity Disorder, Predominantly Hyperactive-Impulsive Type: if Criterion A2 is met but Criterion A1 is not met for the past 6 months

Coding note: For individuals (especially adolescents and adults) who currently have symptoms that no longer meet full criteria, "in partial remission" should be specified.

From American Psychiatric Association: *Diagnostic and statistical manual of mental disorders (DSM-IV-TR)*, ed 4, text revision, Washington, DC, 2000, The Association.

hyperactivity-impulsivity) have persisted for at least 6 months.

3. Predominantly hyperactive-impulsive type—Six (or more) symptoms of hyperactivity-impulsivity (but fewer than six symptoms of inattention) have persisted for at least 6 months. Inattention may often still be a significant clinical feature in such cases.

Course of ADHD

ADHD is relatively stable throughout early adolescence for most children. Some children experience decreased symptoms during adolescence and adulthood, but a significant number of these children carry symptoms into adulthood. The goal for children with learning disabilities is to help them identify areas of weakness and learn to compensate for them.

Diagnostic Evaluation

The basic characteristics outlined in Box 18-2 are used to establish a clinical diagnosis of ADHD. It is important to emphasize the need for a complete and thorough multidisciplinary evaluation of the child, incorporating the efforts of the pediatrician (often a developmental pediatrician or pediatric neurologist), psychologist, pediatric nurse, classroom teacher, reading and math specialist, special education teacher, possibly a speech therapist, and the child's parents. The clinicians and profession-

als must first determine whether the child's behavior is age appropriate or truly problematic.

A history, both medical and developmental, and a description of the child's behavior should be obtained from as many observers of the child as possible, especially the parents and teachers, along with the health professionals involved. Descriptions of the child's behavior in home and school situations should be included. In obtaining descriptive material, the interviewer must question the observers carefully, because some persons, especially parents, may be so concerned with gross behaviors that they overlook less distressing but equally important symptoms. For example, parents may report a "colicky" infant, a child who began to run soon after walking, a toddler who was compelled to touch everything in sight, and a child who resisted sleep until exhausted. A pregnancy and birth history may provide clues to a situation that might have produced an episode of hypoxia.

A physical examination, including vision and hearing screening and a detailed neurologic evaluation, will help rule out any severe neurologic disorders. Psychologic testing, especially projective tests, is valuable in identifying visual-perceptual difficulties, problems with spatial organization, and other phenomena that suggest cortical or diencephalic involvement, and it helps to identify the child's intelligence and achievement levels.

Behavioral checklists and adaptive scales are also helpful in measuring social adaptive functioning in children with ADHD. Psychiatric disorders, medical problems, and traumatic experiences are ruled out, including lead poisoning, seizures, partial hearing loss, psychosis, and witnessing of sexual activity and/or violence.

Therapeutic Management

Management of the child with ADHD involves many approaches, including family education and counseling, medication, proper classroom placement, environmental manipulation, and behavior therapy and/or psychotherapy for the child (see Research Focus box).

RESEARCH FOCUS

Treatment for Attention Deficit Hyperactivity Disorder

The National Institute of Mental Health conducted a large multicenter randomized study of several of these approaches to the treatment of attention deficit hyperactivity disorder (ADHD). This investigation, called the MTA study, examined the long-term effectiveness of (1) medication, (2) intensive behavioral treatment with a therapist, (3) a combination of medication plus behavior therapy, and (4) routine community care for the treatment of ADHD in children (Jensen, 1999). More than 579 children with ADHD, ages 7 to 9 years, were randomly assigned to one of these four types of therapy and received the therapy for 14 months. Although all four approaches produced some improvement, the medication-only group and the combined treatment group had superior outcomes with regard to the core symptoms of ADHD. However, the medication-only approach was superior to the behavior therapy–only approach and the community approach (Jensen, 1999; MTA Cooperative Group, 1999).

Behavior Therapy and Psychotherapy

Behavior therapy focuses on the prevention of undesired behavior. Families are helped to identify new appropriate contingencies and reward systems to meet the child's developing needs. They may also receive instruction in effective parenting skills, such as delivering positive reinforcement, rewarding small increments of desired behaviors, and providing age-appropriate consequences (e.g., time-out, response cost). Through collaborative teamwork, parents learn techniques to help the child become more successful at home and in school.

Use of organizational charts for completing self-care activities and use of a word processor instead of manually writing out assignments are emphasized.

Pharmacologic Therapy

The most frequently used medications are the psychostimulants: methylphenidate hydrochloride (Ritalin) and dextroamphetamine sulfate (Dexedrine) (American Academy of Pediatrics, 2001). The majority of ADHD cases are treated with the psychostimulant methylphenidate. Psychostimulants cause an increase in dopamine and norepinephrine levels that leads to stimulation of the inhibitory system of the central nervous system. Children are given a small dosage initially, and the dosage is gradually increased until the desired response is achieved. Children who receive stimulants should be monitored carefully for the development of tics during initial treatment, and stimulants should be avoided in children who have a history of ticlike behaviors, a family history of Tourette syndrome (TS), or ADHD combined with TS.

Other medications used in the treatment of ADHD include the tricyclic antidepressants, primarily imipramine, desipramine (Norpramin), and nortriptyline (Pamelor). The tricyclic antidepressants block norepinephrine and serotonin at the nerve endings and increase the action of these substances in nerve cells. Clonidine, used occasionally in the treatment of ADHD, has been recommended primarily for children with ADHD and coexisting conditions such as sleep disturbances (American Academy of Pediatrics, 2001).

Regularly scheduled reevaluation of the child is essential with all of these medications to determine medication effectiveness, detect and evaluate any side effects, monitor development and health status (especially growth and blood pressure), and assess family interaction.

Nursing Care Management

Nurses, especially school nurses, are active participants in all aspects of management of the child with ADHD. Nurses in the community setting work with families in the home on a long-term basis to help plan and implement therapeutic regimens and to evaluate the effectiveness of therapy. They coordinate services and serve as a liaison between health and education professionals directly involved in the child's therapy program. School nurses understand the child's special needs and work with teachers. Nurses in any setting (community, school, hospital, practitioner's office) provide support and guidance to children and families during the difficult period of the child's growing up with a disabling condition.

Management begins with an explanation to the parents and the child about the diagnosis, including the nature of the problem and the practitioner's concept of the underlying central nervous system basis for the disorder. Most parents are confused and feel some measure of guilt. To some parents, a diagnosis of ADHD is confirmation of the fear that their child has some irreversible, serious disease; to others it is a relief. All need the opportunity to vent their feelings and suspicions. A common complaint of parents is that health professionals do not listen to what they have to say about their child. The health professional should focus on building self-esteem by encouraging the family to focus on developing their child's strengths (e.g., sport, hobbies, and talents) rather than just weaknesses (Jellinek, 2008).

Parents need information about the prognosis and an understanding of the treatment plan. The greater their understanding of the disorder and its effects, the more likely they will be to carry out the recommended program of therapy. It is important that they understand that the therapy is not necessarily a panacea and that it will extend over a long period. This has particular significance for changes they need to make in environmental management. Reading material to help the child and family is available from a variety of sources.

Medication

Psychostimulants are prescribed for administration on a variety of schedules, but the most common schedule is twice daily, usually in the morning at breakfast and at noon. Many school-age children take their medication at home in the morning before going to school and at lunchtime in the school health suite. Both parents and school nurses should be sensitive to the issue of peer stigma and the feelings that children have in rela-

FAMILY-CENTERED CARE
A Child's Perception of Taking Ritalin at School

I feel embarrassed by having to leave class early to go take my medication. The other kids always ask where I'm going and why. It would be better if we could leave class at the same time as everyone else, go take the medication, and then just be a little late to the next class. Students don't ask why people are late for class, only why they leave early. It also bothers me when kids tell other kids, "Go take a pill," and other mean things just because someone is acting up.

What could nurses and teachers do to help? Most kids do not understand why other kids have to take medication. I think it would help if a nurse or teacher talked with the other kids and explained why some children take the medication and how attention deficit hyperactivity disorder affects people. That way there would be more understanding among all kids.

Marissa, age 16
Tulsa, Oklahoma

CRITICAL THINKING EXERCISE
Attention Deficit Hyperactivity Disorder

Johnnie, age 8 years, is a third-grader who was recently diagnosed with attention deficit hyperactivity disorder (ADHD). He has been taking the drug methylphenidate (Ritalin) for about a month. In the short time that Johnnie has been on this medication, his math teacher has noticed an improvement in his performance in math class. He is receiving a grade of B instead of his previous grades of D on most math quizzes. The math teacher has also noted that Johnnie is socializing more with his classmates and that he now has a "best friend" in math class. Johnnie usually receives his methylphenidate from the school nurse before lunch. Yesterday Johnnie's mother told the school nurse that he has not eaten his lunch for the past week and that he is not hungry.

What important issues regarding Johnnie's medication should the nurse consider in her discussions with Johnnie's mother?

1. Evidence—Is there sufficient evidence to draw conclusions about Johnnie's medication from his behavior?
2. Assumptions—Describe some underlying assumptions about the following:
   a. Pharmacologic action of methylphenidate in ADHD
   b. Side effects of methylphenidate
   c. Management of side effects
3. What implications for nursing care can be drawn at this time?
4. Does the evidence objectively support your conclusion?

tion to taking these medications at school (see Family-Centered Care box).

Some medications are begun at low dosage and increased until the desired effect is attained. When the child's response to the medication is evaluated, it is helpful to obtain reports from the teacher, as well as from the parents, because the parents may see the child when the effects of the drug are wearing off. Observing the child's behavior through visits to the home and school is useful for assessing attention span, interactional patterns with others at school, and performance on academic tasks. The nurse can consult with the teacher and analyze data needed to regulate dosage based on recorded, systematic observations of the child's behaviors.

Parents need to be informed of the possible side effects of medications. The psychostimulants have similar side effects that include weight loss, abdominal pain, headaches, decreased appetite, sleeplessness, increased crying and irritability, nervous stimulation, and cardiovascular stimulation (see Critical Thinking Exercise). The use of caffeine decreases the efficacy of these drugs, and insulin requirements may also be altered. If decreased appetite is a concern, giving the psychostimulants with or after meals rather than before, encouraging consumption of nutritious snacks in the evening when the effects of the medication are decreasing, and serving frequent small meals with healthy "on the go" snacks are helpful interventions. Sleeplessness is reduced by administering medication early in the day.

Children taking tricyclic antidepressants display a dramatic increase in the incidence of dental caries. The marked anticholinergic action of the drugs increases saliva viscosity and produces a dry mouth. Emphasis on rigorous dental hygiene, conscientious home fluoride treatments, regular visits to the dentist, limited intake of refined carbohydrates, and use of artificial saliva is an important nursing function. The child should drink plenty of fluids and be well hydrated.

The issue of continuous administration of psychostimulants and their relationship to growth suppression is another area of concern for parents. Long-term use of dextroamphetamine may result in suppression of growth. Although some practitioners have suggested "drug holidays" on the weekends and during summer vacations, children who respond well to medi-

cation often benefit from continuous therapy. For many children, the symptoms of ADHD do not disappear on the weekends or during vacations. For these children, continuous medication may provide an enhancement that allows them not only to succeed in school but also to function successfully in other social situations and to develop a positive self-image.

Parents often express concern that their child will become addicted to the psychostimulants or the antidepressant drugs. Both types of drugs have the potential for abuse, and all children taking these drugs should be monitored closely for psychologic dependence, tolerance, depression, and other adverse behavior changes or idiosyncratic effects. Most children with ADHD are not interested in abusing their drugs because the effect of the drugs in these children is opposite that produced in normal individuals. However, caution parents to keep these drugs safely stored away from young children who may inadvertently ingest them and adolescents who may abuse these drugs.

Environmental Manipulation

Encourage families to learn how to modify the environment to allow the child to be more successful. Consistency is especially important for children with ADHD. Consistency between families and teachers in terms of reinforcing the same goals is essential. Fostering improved organizational skills requires a more highly structured environment than most children need. The child should be encouraged to make more appropriate choices and to take responsibility for his or her actions.

Other helpful interventions include teaching parents how to make organizational charts (e.g., listing all activities that must be performed before leaving for school) and decrease distractions in the environment while the child is completing homework (e.g., turning the television off, having a consistent study area equipped with needed supplies) and helping parents to understand ways to model positive behaviors and problem solving. The focus is on strategies to help the child succeed and cope with deficits while emphasizing strengths.

Appropriate Classroom Placement

Children with ADHD need an orderly, predictable, and consistent classroom environment with clear and consistent rules. Homework and classroom assignments may need to be reduced, and more time may need to be allotted to allow the child to complete tests. Verbal instructions should be accompanied by visual references such as written instructions on the blackboard. Schedules may need to be arranged so that academic subjects are taught in the morning when the child is experiencing the effects of the morning dose of medication. Low-interest and high-interest classroom activities should be intermingled to maintain the child's attention and interest. Regular and frequent breaks in activity are helpful because sitting in one place for an extended time may be difficult. Computers are helpful for children who have difficulty with written assignments and fine motor skills.

If learning disabilities exist, special training activities may be accomplished in self-contained classes limited to six to eight children, in special resource rooms with equipment and teaching teams, by mobile consultants who move from room to room to provide assistance to teachers and children, and in special first-grade programs in which high-risk children receive special attention to prevent or reduce the need for services as they progress. The purpose of programs for children with special learning disabilities is to assist them toward more successful achievement, personal adjustment, and retention in the regular classroom.

Psychiatric, Psychologic, and Social Therapies

Counseling or therapy can be helpful for children who demonstrate signs of anxiety or depression. Therapy can help the child develop a healthier self-esteem and practice problem-solving strategies. The adolescent may benefit from group work focusing on social skill development. Parents of children with ADHD can face a lot of stress, and therapy may be indicated for parents and other family members.

LEARNING DISABILITY

Learning disorders exist when the individual's achievement on individually administered, standardized tests in reading, mathematics, or written expression is substantially below that expected for age, schooling, and level of intelligence. The learning problems significantly interfere with academic achievement or activities of daily living that require reading, mathematics, or writing skills (Kelly, 2005). Not included are learning problems that result primarily from visual, hearing, or motor disabilities; cognitive impairment; emotional disturbances; or environmental disadvantage. The types of disabilities include dyslexia (difficulty with reading, letter reversal), dysgraphia (difficulty with writing), dyscalculia (difficulty with calculation), right-left confusion, and short attention span.

A comprehensive battery of tests is needed to confirm a learning disability. These include intelligence tests (these children tend to have normal or above-average intelligence); hand-eye coordination tests; and measurements of auditory and visual perception, comprehension, and memory. Often a wide gap exists between verbal and performance scores on intelligence tests.

Therapeutic Management

Special training activities in the schools can assist in areas of deficit such as visual and auditory perception and other areas involving integration and coordination. Programs for children with special learning disabilities assist them in successful achievement, personal adjustment, and eventual retention in the regular classroom (Lambros and Leslie, 2005). According to Public Law 94-142, the Education for All Handicapped Children Act, children with learning disorders must receive free public education in the least restrictive environment possible. (See Chapters 1 and 22.)

Nurses must understand which type of learning disability a child has to best provide direction for the child, parents, and teachers. Children with an auditory perceptual deficit appear unable to follow directions or to comprehend large amounts of verbal teaching. These children need to learn with diagrams, pictures, demonstration, and written lists. Children with a visual perceptual deficit may have difficulty reading, lining up numbers for mathematical operations, or judging distance. These children may have dyslexia and may do better with demonstration and a verbal approach. Children with an integrative deficit may have difficulty sequencing data or storing and retrieving sensory data. Multisensory techniques should be used, and comprehension should be checked frequently throughout instruction. Children with motor deficits may need to use computers or typewriters in the classroom because their handwriting will not improve. They may need to find alternatives to physical competition that requires coordination of movement (Selekman and Snyder, 2000). The Learning Disabilities Association of America* provides information and support to families who have a child with a learning disability. An online interactive website (www.ldonline.org) is also available for parents, teachers, and children with learning disabilities.

Children with learning disorders grow up to be adults with learning disorders. The goal is to help them identify their area of weakness and to compensate for it.

TIC DISORDERS

A **tic** is an involuntary, recurrent, random, rapid, highly stereotyped movement or vocalization. Tics occur in 10% to 35% of all children (Table 18-11). Tics can be simple or complex and can involve eye movements, other motor movements, or vocalizations (Box 18-3). Tics decrease during concentration, are markedly diminished during sleep, and become more exaggerated when the affected children are experiencing stress or excitement. Obsessive-compulsive behaviors, in the form of ritualistic activities, may also be present and can occur in individuals free of tics. A number of medications can precipitate or exacerbate tics.

*4156 Library Road, Pittsburgh, PA 15234; 412-341-1515; fax: 412-344-0224; e-mail: info@LDAAmerica.org; www.ldaamerica.org.

TABLE 18-11 SPECTRUM OF TIC DISORDERS

	MILD	↔	CHRONIC
Duration	Acute	Subacute	Chronic
Motor tics	Simple	Complex	Obscene gestures
	Few		Multiple
Vocal tics	None	Noises	Coprolalia
Suppressible	Yes		No

BOX 18-3 TYPES OF TICS

Simple motor—Eye blinking, grimacing, neck jerking, shoulder jerking

Complex motor—Jumping, squatting, stamping the foot, thrusting out the arm, hitting or biting self, ritualistic movements (smelling an object, touching own or another's body, obsessive or compulsive patterns of behavior), grooming behaviors

Simple vocal—Throat clearing, sniffing, grunting, coughing, snorting, lip noises

Complex vocal—Echolalia (repeating last-heard sound, word, or phrase of another), palilalia (repeating own sounds or words), coprolalia (use of socially unacceptable words, often obscene), shouting of words out of context

Almost all mild, transient tic disorders of childhood are self-limiting and disappear within a few months, usually less than a year. The most common tics involve the eyes, head, and face, and treatment does not affect recovery. Tic disorders can begin at any time during childhood. Boys are affected at least three times more often than girls, and transient tic disorders are observed in other family members (see Research Focus box).

RESEARCH FOCUS

Streptococcal Infections and Tics

A study of Italian children points to a possible connection between group A streptococcal infections and the development of tics (Cardona and Orefici, 2001). Results of this study indicated a relationship between the severity of a tic disorder and the magnitude of serologic response to group A streptococcal antigens. The authors postulate that group A streptococcal infections may trigger a specific neurobehavioral disorder such as a tic.

Motor or vocal tics are considered chronic if they persist for longer than 1 year (Shapiro, 2002). The most severe of the chronic tic disorders is Gilles de la Tourette syndrome, more commonly referred to as just Tourette syndrome. Diagnosis of a tic disorder is based on clinical observations.

Most tic disorders resolve by late childhood or adolescence without treatment and cause no physical harm to the child. Therapeutic management consists primarily of support to the child and family, reassurance about the prognosis, and education regarding expectations (of the child) for control. Although the child is able to suppress the manifestations to some degree, persistent pressure for control constitutes an additional stress to an affected child. Medications may provide some relief of symptoms of chronic tics. Genetic counseling is advisable for families of children with chronic tics.

TOURETTE SYNDROME

TS is the most complex and severe of the tic disorders. It begins between ages 2 and 16 years, persists throughout life, and is characterized by rapidly repetitive multiple motor and vocal movements. The cause is uncertain; most theories implicate abnormalities of various neurotransmitters or a dysregulation in brain circuits that connect the basal ganglia to the motor cortex. TS is an inheritable disorder that is three times more likely to occur in boys than in girls (Centers for Disease Control and Prevention, 2009b).

The manifestations of TS wax and wane in intensity and exhibit a continuing pattern of change in which old tics disappear and new tics develop (Box 18-4). The onset is usually mild, and the initial tic is of brief duration. The minor tics then come and go, becoming more intense and lasting longer. Some tics may be severe from the onset, often with no symptom-free periods. A high percentage of children with TS have associated obsessive-compulsive symptoms (e.g., recurring thoughts or the need to arrange and rearrange objects, repeatedly turn the light switch off and on, tie and retie their shoes, and so on). Other problems associated with TS include ADHD, disruptive behavior, and learning disabilities (Shapiro, 2002). For some children, these associated symptoms may be more disturbing than the tics. Diagnosis is based on clinical observations, especially if other family members are affected. The tics do not lead to physical deterioration or affect the child's life expectancy.

Therapeutic Management

Treatment of TS is primarily symptomatic and consists of child and family education and support. Children with more severe tics sometimes obtain symptomatic relief from medications. Various α-adrenergic agonists, neuroleptics, SSRIs, tricyclic antidepressants, and stimulants may be prescribed depending on the most significant symptoms to be alleviated. Psychostimulants and tricyclic antidepressants have been used to treat the coexisting symptoms of ADHD. Antidepressant medications such as clomipramine (Anafranil), fluoxetine (Prozac), and sertraline (Zoloft), which block the reuptake of serotonin in the brain, have also been used to treat

BOX 18-4 DIAGNOSTIC CRITERIA FOR TOURETTE SYNDROME

A. Both multiple motor and one or more vocal tics have been present at some time during the illness, although not necessarily concurrently. (A tic is a sudden, rapid, recurrent, nonrhythmic, stereotyped motor movement or vocalization.)

B. The tics occur many times a day (usually in bouts) nearly every day or intermittently throughout a period of more than 1 year, and during this period there was never a tic-free period of more than 3 consecutive months.

C. The disturbance causes marked distress or significant impairment in social, occupational, or other important areas of functioning.

D. The onset is before age 18 years.

E. The disturbance is not due to the direct physiologic effects of a substance (e.g., stimulants) or a general medical condition (e.g., Huntington disease or postviral encephalitis).

From American Psychiatric Association: *Diagnostic and statistical manual of mental disorders (DSM-IV-TR)*, ed 4, text revision, Washington, DC, 2000, The Association.

obsessive-compulsive symptoms associated with TS. The goal is to use the lowest dose of medication that reduces symptoms to an acceptable level while enhancing the child's development (Shapiro, 2002; Zinner 2004). Genetic counseling is also advised.

Nursing Care Management

Education of children, families, teachers, and others involved in children's everyday life is a major aspect of therapy. Punishment for the behaviors is inappropriate because they are involuntary. Affected children are often quick to anger, have a low tolerance of frustration, and may engage in temper tantrums. These children need to be guided toward acceptable substitute behaviors to develop normally, both socially and emotionally. For example, suggesting that a child retire to a quiet area to gain control of emotions or providing a pillow, stuffed toy, or punching bag on which to vent feelings is often helpful.

Influential persons in the children's lives must help foster feelings of self-esteem. Children with TS are in a constant, ongoing battle to control their impulses and need positive relationships with their parents to become well adjusted. A child's self-concept can be damaged if parents react to the disability with controlling behaviors, guilt, anger, or hostility.

School nurses can help children with TS cope with teasing by their classmates, can advocate to ensure they are not barred from extracurricular activities, and can educate teachers and classmates about the effects of TS and which behaviors the child can and cannot control in the classroom. Many children with TS experience difficulty writing and benefit from using a tape recorder or computer in the classroom. They may also need extra time when taking standardized tests.

Nurses can assist families in long-term monitoring of symptoms, which includes establishing the waxing and waning pattern and determining whether symptoms interfere with development and adaptation or require more intensive therapy. Families of children taking medication need to be alert to possible side effects, including lethargy, personality change, increased appetite and overweight, depression, parkinsonian symptoms (tremor; muscle rigidity; shuffling gait; hypokinesia; and difficulty chewing, swallowing, and speaking), and anticholinergic symptoms (confusion, excitement, dilated pupils, blurred vision, dry mouth, and dysphagia).

The family may benefit from referral to health agencies such as the local health departments, social services, and parent groups. The Tourette Syndrome Association* is active in research and education and provides services to affected children and their families.

POSTTRAUMATIC STRESS DISORDER

Posttraumatic stress disorder (PTSD) refers to the development of characteristic symptoms after exposure to an extremely traumatic experience or catastrophic event. The traumatic experience or catastrophic event is typically life threatening to self or a significant other and may involve grotesque mutilation or death, serious injury, or physical coercion. An accident; an

assault or victimization; a natural disaster (earthquake, flooding, train wreck, plane crash); sexual abuse; or witnessing of a suicide, homicide, beating, shooting, or other act of violence can lead to PTSD. It is important to note that PTSD is not limited to children who have lived in war-torn countries. Events such as automobile, school, and recreational accidents and bullying have been identified as causes of PTSD (Sundelin-Wahlsten, Ahmad, and von Knorring, 2001).

The response to the event must involve intense fear, helplessness, or horror. In children the response must involve disorganized or agitated behavior. The characteristic symptoms include persistent reexperiencing of the traumatic event, persistent avoidance of stimuli associated with the trauma, numbing of general responsiveness, and persistent symptoms of increased arousal. The response to the event occurs in three stages. The initial response to the stressor is intense arousal, which usually lasts from a few minutes to 1 or 2 hours, depending on the stressor and the individual. The stress hormones are at the maximum as the individual prepares for "fight or flight." A prolonged arousal phase may indicate psychosis.

The second phase, which lasts approximately 2 weeks, is one in which defense mechanisms are mobilized. It is a period of calm in which the event appears to have produced no impression. The victim feels numb, and stress hormone secretion is absent. The reaction is outside the individual's awareness, is not well controlled, and involves some type of behavior pattern. Defense mechanisms are less adaptive to specific situations and may not be what the situation demands. Denial that anything is wrong is a frequently observed defense mechanism.

The third phase is one of coping, which normally extends over 2 to 3 months. This is a phase of consciously directed inquiry. The victim wants to know what happened and appears to be getting worse, when actually he or she is getting better. Numerous psychologic symptoms such as depression, repetitive phenomena, phobic symptoms, anxiety symptoms, and conversion reactions may be apparent. Children frequently display repetitive actions. They play out the situation over and over again in an attempt to come to terms with their fear. Flashbacks are common. This phase can be self-perpetuating, and a prolonged reaction can develop into an obsession with the traumatic event. Some traumatic effects remain indefinitely.

Nursing Care Management

Children need to deal with any traumatic event; much hinges on the intensity of the event and their reactions to it. Children's reactions depend heavily on their social environment and the way in which their caretaking adults react to the event. Children usually react in the same manner as their caregivers (contagious pathology); therefore it is important to be aware of these reactions. In the second, or defense, phase of the PTSD the appropriateness of the defense mechanism must be assessed, and children must be assisted in the application of their defense. If children do not engage in some catharsis or if their defense phase is prolonged, they may need referral for special psychologic help.

Coping is a learned response, and children in the third phase can be helped to use their coping strategies to deal with their fears. Children usually are willing to accept reasoning. Those

---

*42-40 Bell Blvd., Suite 205, Bayside, NY 11361; 718-224-2999; e-mail: ts@tsa-usa.org; www.tsa-usa.org.

who are assisted in their catharsis and allowed expression will survive without serious lasting effects. Encourage them to play out the stress and/or discuss their feelings about the event. If they are unable to do this, they may become obsessed with the traumatic event and need professional help. Conversion reactions are common obsessive behaviors in children suffering from PTSD.

Children need professional help if any of the phases of PTSD are prolonged. Boys tend to have a prolonged defense phase more often than do girls. Occasionally the precipitating event will go unrecognized, and the affected child will engage in what is considered to be unusual behavior. Children exhibiting any sudden change in behavior need to be assessed for exposure to a traumatic event. When the change in behavior is determined to be caused by a traumatic event, treatment can be implemented.

SCHOOL PHOBIA

Children other than beginning students who resist going to school or who demonstrate extreme reluctance to attend school for a sustained period as a result of severe anxiety or a fear of school-related experiences are said to have school phobia. The terms *school refusal* and *school avoidance* are also used to describe this behavior. School phobia occurs in children of all ages, but it is more common in children 10 years of age and older. School avoidance behaviors occur in both boys and girls and in children from all socioeconomic levels.

Anxiety that frequently verges on panic is a constant manifestation, and children can develop symptoms as a protective mechanism to keep them from facing the situation that distresses them. Physical symptoms are prominent and may affect any part of the body—anorexia, nausea, vomiting, diarrhea, dizziness, headache, leg pains, or abdominal pains. The children may even develop a low-grade fever. A striking feature of school phobia is the prompt subsiding of symptoms when it is evident that the child can remain at home. Another significant observation is absence of symptoms on weekends and holidays, unless they are related to other places such as Sunday school or parties. Occasional mild reluctance to attend school is not uncommon among schoolchildren, but if the fear continues for longer than a few days, it must be considered a serious problem.

The onset is usually sudden and precipitated by a school-related incident. By taking a careful history, nurses find out whether a poor attendance record is due to trivial reasons.

Etiology

A number of factors can cause school phobia. Sometimes the complaints are related to a transient, specific cause, such as fear of a mismatched or overcritical teacher; fear of failing an examination or giving an oral recitation for a painfully shy child; or discrimination based on race, dress, or physical defect. Sometimes it may be related to a school bully or threatening gang. An insecure home situation in which children fear that they may be deserted by a parent may be the basis of anxiety, especially if the parent has previously threatened to leave.

A frequent source of fear is separation anxiety growing out of a strong, dependent relationship between the mother and child in which the child is reluctant to leave the mother and she is equally reluctant to have the child leave her (although this feeling may be unconscious on the mother's part). The intense need for closeness between mother and child is normal in infancy, but the persistence of this type of relationship into childhood is inappropriate.

Characteristically, these children are not afraid to go to school; rather, they are afraid to leave home. They fear that something dreadful might happen while they are separated from their families. No event is required to trigger the associated behaviors. However, symptoms may be precipitated by a situation that intensifies the mutual dependency between the mother and the child, such as illness, arrival of a new baby, a move to a strange neighborhood or a new school, or parental discord.

In some instances children have an unrealistic, exaggerated view of their abilities and achievements. When they feel threatened by incidents that challenge their estimates of themselves, such as a minor episode that leads to embarrassment, return to school after an absence, transfer to another class, or even imagined social or academic failure, they become anxious and withdraw, frequently seeking proximity to the mother. Sometimes the step-up in expectations at school or change of important personnel at school (e.g., teacher or principal) is a contributing factor. Occasionally the child may be suffering from an undiagnosed learning disability.

Therapeutic Management

The treatment for school phobia depends on the cause. If the reason for the problem is an examination, a relationship with a bully, or a mismatch between teacher and child, it can be dealt with accordingly. When the child is helped to understand and cope with the fear, the symptoms usually disappear. In severe cases when returning to school is unsuccessful, professional psychiatric consultation is usually desirable to help identify possible distorted family relationships or a personality disturbance in the child and to help both the child and the family understand the sources of the problem.

Some children with a moderately severe separation anxiety disorder and school refusal may be treated with a tricyclic antidepressant. However, psychiatric evaluation is almost always required before anxiolytic agents are prescribed.

Nursing Care Management

Treatment of school phobia depends on the cause. The primary goal is to return the child to school. The longer the child is permitted to stay out of school, the more difficult it is to reenter. Parents must be convinced gently but firmly that immediate return is essential and that it is their responsibility to insist on school attendance.

A school reentry protocol may be necessary for a child with severe symptoms. In reentry programs, the child role-plays routines that are involved in getting ready for school and that occur at school. Relaxation techniques are also useful. The child usually goes to school for a half-day initially and then progresses to a full day. Children may be rewarded with points for each period during the day that they are able to remain in school. These points are then redeemed for rewards (e.g., playing with favorite toys or social rewards). Often the school nurse can provide both the teacher and the parents with support in carrying out this plan.

Prevention

School phobia and other dependency problems can be avoided by encouraging independence at appropriate times during infancy and early childhood. For example, by 6 months of age children can be left with a baby-sitter during a parents' night out. Two-year-olds can be left at home (while awake) with a sitter. By 3 years of age children should experience being left somewhere other than their home (e.g., grandparents' home). As soon as they are able, they should be able to feed, dress, and wash themselves. By 3 to 4 years of age children can be allowed to play in the yard by themselves, and later they should be allowed to play in the neighborhood by themselves.

Specific clues indicate that a child may be experiencing first-time fear of school and may need help to cope. Extra preparation may be needed for children who are fearful, have trouble adjusting to new situations, or are clinging. Many individuals continue to manifest some form of fear throughout the school years. When the problem is identified early and treated effectively, negative emotions surrounding school are minimized, and the child is less likely to carry residual fears throughout life.

For most first-time school fears, simple reassurances and a little advance preparation are all that is necessary. Direct contact with the school and teachers is an excellent way to allay anticipatory anxiety. Parents can take the child to visit the school about a month before school starts, introduce the child to the teacher, and let the child experience the classroom firsthand.

Bedtime is also an excellent time to help children resolve first-day jitters. Bedtime stories and books suited to the occasion are available from bookstores and libraries. Several videotapes and tape recordings are also available to help children cope with a variety of common fears (dark, nightmares, baby-sitters, doctors, dentists, monsters).

Parents who suspect that their child may be especially frightened may want to accompany the child to school and wait outside the classroom the first day. A gradual breakaway over succeeding days should relieve their child's and their own anxiety. If the distress extends over a long period, professional help may be necessary.

RECURRENT AND FUNCTIONAL ABDOMINAL PAIN

Recurrent abdominal pain (RAP) is a complaint of childhood that is often attributed to psychogenic causes, although it can be a symptom of either psychosomatic or organic disease. RAP is traditionally defined as three or more separate episodes of abdominal pain at least 3 months before diagnosis that interferes with functioning. This condition has subclassified functional abdominal pain (FAP), and a list of criteria has been developed to assist in the diagnosis of FAP (Yacob and Di Lorenzo, 2009). The disorder affects school-age children 4 to 18 years of age but is more common in children over the age of 8 and occurs in girls more often than in boys (Scholl and Allen, 2007).

Etiology and Pathophysiology

Only a minority of youngsters with RAP have an organic basis for their pain. Organic causes include inflammatory bowel disease, peptic ulcer disease, lactose intolerance, pelvic inflammatory disease, urinary bladder infection, and pancreatitis. Psychogenic causes of abdominal pain, such as school phobia, depression, acute reactive anxiety, and conversion reaction, account for a small number of cases. Most children with RAP suffer from FAP.

In cases in which no organic disorder is identifiable, the abdominal pain of RAP has been attributed to dysfunction (Smith, 2001). Dysfunctional conditions causing RAP include constipation, chronic stool retention, overeating, irritable colon, and intestinal gas with heightened awareness of intestinal motility or dysmotility. Normally, intestinal contents arrive at the distal portion of the intestine with a relatively high fluid content, and fluid is extracted in the distal colon and rectum. If the normally relaxed distal intestine fails to relax and prevents the flow of its contents toward the rectum, the resulting excessive distention and spasms of the distal intestinal musculature produce pressure on nerve endings, causing pain.

The symptoms of RAP may result from multiple causes, and it is important to assess a number of factors that could place a child at risk for this condition. These include (1) somatic predisposition, dysfunction, or disorder; (2) lifestyle and habit, including routines, diet, and life tempo; (3) temperament and learned response patterns, such as the child's behavior style, personality, and learned coping skills; and (4) milieu and critical events (i.e., the child's intimate surroundings [familial, social, and cultural norms] and unexpected sources of stress or gratification).

Children at risk for RAP tend to be high achievers who have extensive personal goals or whose parents have unusually high expectations. They are described as being more mature and sensitive than others or as worriers. At risk are children who are overly concerned about what others think about them but have difficulty meeting the expectations of parents, teachers, and others. They are uncomfortable with expressions of anger or argument, especially directed at those persons who are significant in their lives. School attendance is adversely affected, and these children generally exhibit poor learning performance. It is not uncommon for symptoms to be aggravated during school days.

Clinical Manifestations

Children with RAP have real pain that is usually located in the periumbilical and/or epigastric area. On palpation the pain is more likely to be experienced in the epigastric area or in the lower right or left quadrant and is accompanied by vague tenderness without muscle guarding. The pain is irregular in time, duration, and intensity and is associated with either loose or pellet-formed stools. Other symptoms that may accompany the abdominal pain are headache, flushing, pallor, dizziness, and fatigue. Nausea, vomiting, diarrhea, and dysuria are sometimes part of the syndrome. The symptoms reflect the heightened intensity of response to stimulation of the autonomic bowel sites. Loose stools are a result of the exaggerated propulsive motility, and the pain is caused by the sharply increased mechanical tension in the gut.

Diagnostic Evaluation

Diagnosis is based on a complete family history, the child's health history, physical examination, and laboratory tests. The family history may provide evidence of a hereditary disorder or mimicry of adult symptoms. The child is evaluated for evidence of an organic basis for symptoms, such as pain that radiates to the back, pain that awakens the child from sleep, persistent right upper or right lower quadrant pain, unexplained or recurrent fever, weight loss, gastrointestinal blood loss, significant vomiting, chronic severe diarrhea, or family history of inflammatory bowel disease (American Academy of Pediatrics, 2005). Pain is assessed for location, quality, frequency, duration, any associated symptoms, alleviating factors, and exacerbating factors (Smith, 2001).

Therapeutic Management

Treatment involves providing reassurance and reducing or eliminating symptoms. Hospitalization may be necessary, and the child frequently shows improvement in the hospital environment. Initial efforts are directed toward ruling out organic causes of the pain, relieving discomfort, and attempting to determine the situations that precipitate attacks.

Emphasize a high-fiber diet, psyllium bulk agents, lubricants such as mineral oil, and bowel training for pain associated with bowel patterns. Treatment may also include acid-reduction therapy for pain associated with dyspepsia; antispasmodic agents, smooth muscle relaxants, or low doses of psychotropic agents for pain. Dietary modifications may include removal of dairy products, fructose, and gluten for 2 to 3 weeks to rule out lactose intolerance, sensitivity to high sugar content, and celiac disease. Other treatments include cognitive-behavior therapy and biofeedback.

Nursing Care Management

The nurse can be instrumental in assessment and management of RAP in children. Many techniques used in a routine assessment elicit information that might help identify factors that contribute to the child's symptoms. Evaluate the child's social and psychologic adjustment, and obtain the details of the pain directly from the child. Questions that provide clues to parent-child relationships and the way the family deals with angry feelings provide information for diagnosis and management. Relationships with peers, school problems, and other concerns of the child need to be explored. Note any evidence of depression.

Once the diagnosis has been established, the parents and the child need an explanation of the pain, which can be compared to a skeletal muscle cramp, "charley horse," or headache for easier comprehension. Reassurance that the symptoms are not unique to their child and that the pain is rarely associated with a severe disease can help relieve parental fears and anxieties.

Discuss a high-fiber diet with the child and family (see Chapter 33), and emphasize bowel training. The child is encouraged to establish a pattern of sitting on the toilet for 10 to 15 minutes immediately after breakfast to take advantage of the increased colonic activity following meals. If necessary, have the child use stimulatory suppositories to induce early morning defecation.

Once parents are reassured that there is no organic cause for the pain, they need guidance on what to do during a pain episode. Often they feel helpless and anxious, which tends to compound the child's distress. The simple measure of having the child rest in a peaceful, quiet environment and providing comfort will often relieve the symptoms in a short time. Application of a heating pad may also ease the discomfort. (See Nonpharmacologic [Pain] Management, Chapter 7.) If pain is not relieved by these simple measures, teach parents how to administer antispasmodics, if prescribed. For example, if pain is precipitated by meals, having the child take the medication 20 to 30 minutes before mealtime may prevent an episode.

The most valuable assistance that the nurse can provide is support and reassurance to the family. When open communication is established and families are able to see a relationship between stress-provoking situations and the child's symptoms, the chance for remedial action is enhanced. Follow-up care and continued support are essential because the symptoms tend to remit and exacerbate; therefore the availability of a supportive health professional can be a source of comfort to the child and family.

CONVERSION REACTION

Conversion reaction, also known as hysteria, hysterical conversion reaction, and childhood hysteria, is a psychophysiologic disorder with a sudden onset that can usually be traced to a precipitating environmental event. The disorder is observed with equal frequency in both sexes in childhood, but affected girls outnumber affected boys during adolescence. The manifestations involve primarily the voluntary musculature and special senses and include abdominal pain, fainting, pseudoseizures, paralysis, headaches, and visual field restriction. Once considered rare in childhood, the disorder occurs more frequently than has generally been acknowledged. The most commonly observed symptom is seizure activity, which can be differentiated from symptoms of neurogenic origin by formal tests, the most useful of which is the finding of a normal electroencephalogram.

Many children with conversion reaction have experienced a major family crisis before the onset of symptoms, such as loss of a parent or other significant person through death, divorce, or moving. The families of children with conversion reaction characteristically display problems in communication and depression or hypochondriasis in a parent.

Educating the child and family regarding the cause of emotional stresses or feelings and alternative approaches to coping with stress may alleviate the child's symptoms. If deep personality problems are evident, psychiatric consultation is indicated. Nursing care is similar to that for the child with RAP.

CHILDHOOD DEPRESSION

Depression in childhood is often difficult to detect because children may be unable to express their feelings and tend to act out their problems and concerns. Authorities agree that childhood depression exists, but the manifestations may differ from those in depressed adults. The characteristics of depression are largely determined by parallel developments in symbolism, language, and cognitive development. Younger children demonstrate a more cause-and-effect relationship between the stressors and the depressive manifestations. In older children the relationships between stressful events and depression are

BOX 18-5	CHARACTERISTICS OF CHILDREN WITH DEPRESSION

Behavior

Predominantly sad facial expression with absent or diminished range of affective response

Solitary play or work; tendency to be alone; disinterest in play

Withdrawal from previously enjoyed activities and relationships

Lowered grades in school; lack of interest in doing homework or achieving in school

Diminished motor activity; tiredness

Tearfulness or crying

Dependent and clinging or aggressive and disruptive behavior

Internal States

Utterance of statements reflecting lowered self-esteem, sense of hopelessness, or guilt

Suicidal ideations

Physiologic Manifestations

Constipation

Nonspecific complaints of not feeling well

Change in appetite resulting in weight loss or gain

Alterations in sleeping pattern, sleeplessness, or hypersomnia

---

less clear. Their reactions are less physiologic and more cognitively complex, and the observed behaviors tend to be age specific. Depressed children exhibit a distinctive style of thinking characterized by low self-esteem, hopelessness, and a tendency to explain negative events in terms of personal shortcomings.

Some states of depression are temporary (e.g., acute depression precipitated by a traumatic event). The causative event might be a period of hospitalization, loss of a parent through death or separation, or loss of a significant relationship with something (a pet), someone (a friend or family member), or a place (move from a familiar home, neighborhood, or city). The easily identified manifestations include a sad, downcast face; tearfulness; irritability; and withdrawal from previously enjoyed activities and relationships. The child tends to spend more time in solitary activities, especially television viewing. Schoolwork is impaired. Some children become more dependent and clinging; others become more aggressive and disruptive. Sleeplessness or hypersomnia, changes in appetite or weight (either increased or decreased), constipation, tiredness, and nonspecific complaints of not feeling well are common reactions. Responses are not sustained and can be modified with social and family support.

More serious and less common are depressive responses to more chronic stress and loss. These are frequently observed in children with chronic illness or disability. There is no apparent precipitating event, but a history of frequent disruptions in important relationships often occurs. A history of depressive illness in one or both parents during the child's lifetime is also common. The manifestations are similar to those seen in acute reactions. Box 18-5 outlines some of the primary and associated symptoms that are observed in depressed children and that are included in the criteria of the *Diagnostic and Statistical Manual of Mental Disorders* (American Psychiatric Association, 2000) currently used for establishing a diagnosis of major depression. Major depressive disorders in childhood have a number of similarities with several other psychologic disorders.

Therapeutic Management

Depressed children are managed by a health team specially trained in the care of children with mental disorders. Treatment is highly individualized and should be undertaken in the least constrictive environment, usually an outpatient setting. Suicidal children are admitted to the hospital for protection if the family is unable to provide constant monitoring. Hospitalization may also be advised for children with associated disruptive behavior, such as fighting with peers or family. Most therapeutic regimens focus on various combinations of counseling, psychotherapy, family therapy, cognitive therapy, education (teaching social and life skills that facilitate coping), environmental improvement, and pharmacotherapy.

Pharmacotherapy may involve tricyclic antidepressants or SSRIs such as fluoxetine, trazodone (Desyrel), sertraline, and paroxetine (Paxil), as well as bupropion (Wellbutrin) and venlafaxine (Effexor). There have been reports that antidepressant medications may cause increased suicidal thinking and behaviors in pediatric patients. This prompted the FDA to require black box drug labeling detailing potential suicide-related risks for pediatric patients.

Nursing Care Management

Nurses should be aware that depression is a problem that can easily be overlooked in the school-age child and one that can interrupt normal growth and development. Recognizing depression and making appropriate referrals is an important nursing function. Identification of the depressed child requires a careful history taking (health, growth and development, social, and family health); interviews with the child; and observations by the nurse, parents, and teachers. If antidepressants are prescribed, the child and family need to know that antidepressants must be at a therapeutic level for 2 to 4 weeks to achieve a beneficial effect. The child and family also need to monitor the child for side effects of the specific drug prescribed and any interactions with other drugs. (See Chapter 21 for a discussion of suicide, since suicidal ideation is common during depression.)

CHILDHOOD SCHIZOPHRENIA

Childhood schizophrenia refers to severe deviations in ego functioning and is generally reserved for psychotic disorders that appear in children younger than 15 years of age. Childhood schizophrenia is a very rare illness among children in the general population; only about 2 in every 1000 children with mental illness have childhood schizophrenia.

The cause of schizophrenia is unknown, but three risk factors have been identified: genetic characteristics, gestational and birth complications, and winter birth. Biologic relatives of affected individuals have an increased chance of developing the disorder. For example, the risk for the children if both parents have schizophrenia is 40%. The rate of concordance is 10% for dizygotic (nonidentical) twins and 40% to 50% for monozygotic (identical) twins. Current thinking is that altered development of the central nervous system is an etiologic factor. Psychosocial theories, especially those focusing on the parent-child relationship, have not been supported, but certain social and environmental factors may play a role in a child's vulnerability to developing schizophrenia.

Childhood schizophrenia is characterized by symptoms that last at least 6 months and that seriously interfere with the child's functioning at school, at home, or in other social situations. However, the basic core disturbance is a lack of contact with reality and the subsequent development by the child of a world of his or her own.

The most common manifestations are language disturbances, impaired interpersonal relationships, and inappropriate affect (outward expression of emotion) (Box 18-6). Treatment involves management of symptoms, prevention of relapse, and social and occupational rehabilitation of the young person. In some individuals drug therapy produces dramatic improvement in symptoms and social adjustment. Antipsychotic drugs that may be used include haloperidol, clozapine, chlorpromazine, and risperidone. Family interventions and family therapy often result in improvements in psychotic symptoms, thought disorders, and social functioning among children with schizophrenia.

Nursing Care Management

Nursing of psychotic children is a highly specialized area, but because such problems are occurring with increasing frequency, nurses should recognize children who consistently demonstrate abnormal behavior and refer them for evaluation.

Nurses should also instruct family members of children taking antipsychotic drugs to observe for possible side effects. Common side effects of these drugs include dizziness, drowsi-

> **BOX 18-6 SOME CHARACTERISTICS OF CHILDHOOD SCHIZOPHRENIA**
>
> - Bizarre behavior patterns and stereotyped movements such as robotlike walking, whirling, or graceful gyrations
> - Periods of hypoactivity alternating with periods of hyperactivity
> - Inappropriate affect that ranges from flatness to explosiveness
> - Common occurrence of temper tantrums
> - Language disturbances such as speaking in fragmented sentences, parrot-like repetition of words, development of a private language, and altered tone of voice; for some schizophrenic children, muteness or uttering only a single word on rare occasions
> - Distorted time orientation with a blending of past, present, and future
> - Distorted sense of and use of the body
> - Apparent denial of the human quality in people, such as attempting to use a person as a step stool to reach an object
> - Conveying of a nonhuman identity by action, sounds, or posture, such as barking or calling self a vacuum cleaner
> - Frequent occurrence of compulsive behavior and phobias

ness, tachycardia, hypotension, and extrapyramidal effects such as abnormal movements and seizures. Agranulocytosis occurs in 1% of patients who take clozapine in the first few months of treatment. Therefore a mandatory monitoring program requires that patients taking clozapine have a white blood cell (WBC) count performed every week during the first 6 months of therapy and every other week for the second 6 months of therapy. Pharmacies and clinicians report the weekly WBC count and cannot dispense clozapine to the patient without evidence of a safe WBC count.

KEY POINTS

- Middle childhood is a relatively healthy period, and most problems encountered are not considered serious.
- The skin serves several important functions: protection, prevention of loss of body fluids, heat regulation, and sensation.
- It is important for nurses to be able to describe skin lesions accurately.
- The process of wound healing consists of inflammation, fibroplasia, scar contraction, and scar maturation.
- Wound healing occurs by primary, secondary, or tertiary intention.
- Bacterial, viral, and fungal infections are common in childhood.
- Prevention of infection or reinfection is the primary goal in management of pediculosis.

- Contact dermatitis may involve a reaction to a primary irritant or sensitization.
- Teaching prevention of thermal injury, especially sunburn, is an important nursing function.
- Adverse reactions to drugs occur more often in the skin than in any other organ.
- Dental care is essential in middle childhood; the most frequent problems that arise are dental caries and malocclusion.
- The behavior disorders of childhood are primarily ADHD and tic disorders.
- Other major behavior or mental disorders involving school-age children include school phobia, RAP, conversion reaction, depression, and schizophrenia.

ANSWERS TO CRITICAL THINKING EXERCISES

Poison Ivy

1. **Yes.** There is sufficient evidence to determine an effective intervention.
2. **a.** The leaves and stems of the poison ivy plant contain urushiol, an oil that produces an immune reaction in the skin.
   b. When urushiol comes in contact with the skin, it penetrates the epidermis and bonds with the dermal layer. After

about 2 days, localized, oozing, and painful impetiginous lesions are produced in the skin.
c. When a child has contact with any part of the poison ivy plant, the skin areas should be immediately flushed with cold running water to neutralize the urushiol, and calamine lotion should be applied. Clothing that has come in contact with the plant should be removed and thoroughly laundered in hot water and detergent.

d. Use of harsh soap is contraindicated because it removes the protective skin oils and dilutes the urushiol, which allows it to spread; hard scrubbing irritates the skin.

3. The most important immediate intervention is to rinse Billy's hands in cool water and apply calamine lotion. Because Billy's camp is near a stream, he can enter the water where it is shallow and allow the water to rinse the oil of the poison ivy from his hands and clothes. The leaves should not be burned because contact with the smoke can cause a skin reaction and is also dangerous to the lungs if it is inhaled. Billy's clothes should be washed in hot water with detergent. Poison ivy lesions are not contagious, so the camp nurse should tell Billy's cabin mates that they will not "catch" his poison ivy.

4. **Yes.** The evidence supports these interventions.

Attention Deficit Hyperactivity Disorder

1. **Yes.** There is sufficient evidence to arrive at a possible conclusion.

2. a. Methylphenidate is a stimulant that increases dopamine and norepinephrine levels, which leads to stimulation of the inhibitory system of the central nervous system.

   b. Common side effects of methylphenidate include nausea, anorexia, decreased appetite, and insomnia.

c. Although the absorption rate of methylphenidate is increased when the drug is taken with meals, side effects such as decreased appetite may become more pronounced with this schedule of administration. Side effects can be alleviated by changing the times that the drug is administered or by switching to a sustained-release form of the drug that is taken once per day in the morning.

3. Although Johnnie seems to have responded favorably to his medication and has demonstrated several positive effects of methylphenidate (improvement in math class and increasing self-confidence in social skills), the nurse should be concerned about the fact that Johnnie has not eaten his lunch for the past week and that he is not hungry. Decreased appetite is a negative side effect of methylphenidate.

4. **Yes.** The data indicate that Johnnie is currently experiencing a decrease in his appetite. Because decreased appetite is a common side effect of methylphenidate, there is a high probability that this symptom is related to Johnnie's medication. However, adjusting or changing the times the medication is administered can often alleviate this side effect. Another option is to ask Johnnie's doctor to switch his medication to a sustained-release form of methylphenidate that can be given once per day in the morning.

REFERENCES

American Academy of Pediatric Dentistry: Decision tree for an avulsed tooth: resource section, 2009, available at www.aapd.org (accessed May 13, 2009).

American Academy of Pediatrics, Committee on Infectious Diseases, Pickering LK, editor: *2009 Red book: report of the Committee on Infectious Diseases,* ed 28, Elk Grove Village, Ill, 2009, The Academy.

American Academy of Pediatrics: *Bedwetting.* Elk Grove Village, Ill, 2006, The Academy.

American Academy of Pediatrics: Chronic abdominal pain in children, *Pediatrics* 115(3):812-815, 2005.

American Academy of Pediatrics: *Caring for your school age child (5-12):* encopresis and enuresis. Elk Grove Village, Ill, 2003, The Academy.

American Academy of Pediatrics: Clinical practice guideline: treatment of the school-aged child with attention-deficit/hyperactivity disorder, *Pediatrics* 108(4):1033-1044, 2001.

American Academy of Pediatrics: Clinical practice guideline: diagnosis and evaluation of the child with attention-deficit/hyperactivity disorder, *Pediatrics* 105(5):1158-1170, 2000.

American Psychiatric Association: *Diagnostic and statistical manual of mental disorders (DSM-IV-TR),* ed 4, text revision, Washington, DC, 2000, The Association.

Barnett NK: Pruritus. In Hoekelman RA, Adam HM, Nelson NM, et al, editors: *Primary pediatric care,* ed 4, St Louis, 2001, Mosby.

Beaumont E, Anderson-Dam M: Technology scorecard. Wound care science at the crossroads, *Am J Nurs* 98(12):16-21, 1998.

Bernardo LM, Gardner MJ, O'Connor J, et al: Dog bites in children treated in a pediatric emergency department, *J Soc Pediatr Nurs* 5(2):87-95, 2000.

Bookout K, McCord S, McLane K: Case studies of an infant, a toddler, and an adolescent treated with a negative pressure wound treatment system, *J Wound Ostomy Continence Nurs* 31(4):184-192, 2004.

Bosson S, Lynn N: Nocturnal enuresis. In Barton S, editor: *Clinical evidence issues.* London, 2001, BMJ Publishing.

Cardona F, Orefici G: Group streptococcal infections and tic disorders in an Italian pediatric population, *J Pediatr* 138:71-75, 2001.

Centers for Disease Control and Prevention: *Lyme disease,* 2009a, available at www.cdc.gov/ncidod/dvbid/lyme/index.htm (accessed February 11, 2010).

Centers for Disease Control and Prevention: Prevalence of diagnosed Tourette syndrome in persons aged 6-17 years—United States, 2007, *MMWR* 58(21):581-585, 2009b.

Coughlin EC: Assessment and management of pediatric constipation in primary care, *Pediatr Nurs* 29(4):296-301, 2003.

Dattwyler RJ, Luft BJ, Kunkel MJ, et al: Ceftriaxone compared with doxycycline for the treatment of acute disseminated Lyme disease, *N Engl J Med* 337(5):289-294, 1997.

Dohil MA, Eichenfield LF: A treatment approach for atopic dermatitis, *Pediatr Ann* 34(3):201-210, 2005.

Dumas D, Pelletier L: Perception in hyperactive children, *MCN Am J Matern Child Nurs* 24(1):12-19, 1999.

Fisher RG, Chan RL, Hair PS, et al: Hypochlorite killing of community-acquired methicillin-resistant *Staphylococcus aureus. Pediatr Infect Dis J* 27(10):934-935, 2008.

Fix AD, Strickland GT, Grant J: Tick bites and Lyme disease in an endemic setting:

problematic use of serologic testing and prophylactic antibiotic therapy, *JAMA* 279:206-210, 1998.

Geller AC, Rutsch L, Kenausis K, et al: Can an hour or two of sun protection education keep the sunburn away? Evaluation of the environmental protection and Sunwise School Program. *Environ Health* 2(1):13, 2003.

Glazener CMA, Evans JA, Petro RE: Complex behavioral and educational interventions for nocturnal enuresis in children, *Cochrane Database Syst Rev* (2):CD004558, 2004a.

Glazener CMA, Evans J, Petro RE: Treating nocturnal enuresis in children: review of the evidence, *J Wound Ostomy Continence Nurs* 31(4):223-233, 2004b.

Hall HI, Jorgensen CM, McDavid K, et al: Protection from sun exposure in US white children ages 6 months to 11 years, *Public Health Rep* 116(4):353-361, 2001.

Humane Society of the United States: *Preventing and avoiding dog bites,* Washington, DC, 1998, The Society.

Jellinek M: ADHD Treatments. Going beyond the meds. *Contemp Pediatr* 25(5):39-48, 2008.

Jensen PS: Fact versus fancy concerning the multimodal treatment study for attention deficit hyperactivity disorder, *Can J Psychiatry* 44(10):975-980, 1999.

Johnson NS, Saal HM, Lovell AM, et al: Social and emotional problems in children with neurofibromatosis type 1: evidence and proposed interventions, *J Pediatr* 134:767-772, 1999.

Kaplan SL: Commentary: prevention of recurrent staphylococcal infections, *Pediatr Infect Dis J* 27(10):935-937, 2008.

Kelly DP: Learning disorders, *Pediatr Ann* 34(4):259-262, 2005.

Kest HE, Pineda C: Lyme disease: prevention, diagnosis, and management, *Contemp Pediatr* 25(6):56-64, 2008.

Kinetic Concepts: *The V.A.C. therapy guidelines: a reference source for clinicians,* San Antonio, 2003, Author.

King DE: Attention deficit disorder isn't just for kids, *Nurs Spect* 10(25DC):24-25, 2000.

Konofal E, Lecendreux M, Arnulf I, et al: Iron deficiency in children with attention-deficit/hyperactivity disorder, *Arch Pediatr Adolesc Med* 158:1113-1115, 2004.

Lambros KM, Leslie LK: Management of the child with a learning disorder, *Pediatr Ann* 34(4):275-287, 2005.

Lee MC, Rios AM, Aten MF, et al: Management and outcome of children with skin and soft tissue abscesses caused by community-acquired methicillin-resistant *Staphylococcus aureus, Pediatr Infect Dis J* 23(2):123-127, 2004.

Leung A, Fong J, Pinto-Rojas A: Pediculosis capitis, *J Pediatr Health Care,* 19(6):369-373, 2005.

Litovitz TL, Klein-Schwartz W, Caravati EM, et al: 1998 Annual report of the American Association of Poison Control Centers Toxic Exposure Surveillance System, *Am J Emerg Med* 17:435-487, 1999.

Margileth AM: Recent advances in diagnosis and treatment of cat scratch disease, *Curr Infect Dis Rep* 2(2):141-146, 2000.

McCord SS, Naik-Mathuria BJ, Murphy KM, et al: Negative pressure wound therapy is effective to manage a variety of wounds in the pediatric population, *J Wound Healing Regen* 15(3), 296-301, 2007.

Montgomery DF: Management of constipation and encopresis in children. *J Pediatr Health Care* 22(3):199-204, 2008.

MTA Cooperative Group, Multimodal Treatment Study of Children with ADHD: A 14-month randomized clinical trial of treatment strategies for attention-deficit/hyperactivity

disorder. *Arch Gen Psychiatry* 56(12):1073-1086, 1999.

Nijhawan RI, Matiz CM, Jacob SE: Contact dermatitis: from basics to allergodromes. *Pediatr Ann* 38(2):99-108, 2009.

Ovington L: Silver, fact or fiction: utilizing the antibacterial mechanisms of silver in wound care, *Ostomy Wound Manage* 50(9a):1S-16S, 2004.

Papp KA, Breuer K, Meurer M, et al: Long-term control of atopic dermatitis with pimecrolimus cream 1% in infants and young children: a 2-year study, *J Am Acad Dermatol* 52(3):247-253, 2005.

Patel CTC, Kinsey GC, Koperski-Moen KJ, et al: Vacuum-assisted wound closure: changing atmospheric pressure assists wound healing, *Am J Nurs* 100(12):45-48, 2000.

Pearlman DL: A simple treatment for head lice: dry on, suffocation-based pediculicide, *Pediatrics* 114(3):e275-e279, 2004.

Price JH, Burkhart CN, Burkhart CG, et al: School nurses' perceptions of and experiences with head lice, *J Sch Health* 69(4):153-158, 1999.

Roberts BJ, Friedlander S: Tinea capitis: a treatment update, *Pediatr Ann* 34(3):191-200, 2005.

Rombaux P, M'Bilo T, Badr-el-Din A, et al: Cervical lymphadenitis and cat scratch disease (CSD): an overlooked disease? *Acta Otorhinolaryngol Belg* 54(4):491-496, 2000.

Rosenthal M: Bacterial colonization, hyperresponsive immune systems conspire in eczema: diagnosing dermatological disorders, *Infect Dis Child* 17(3):47-48, 2004.

Schexnayder SM, Schexnayder RE: Bites, stings, and other painful things, *Pediatr Ann* 29(6):354-358, 2000.

Scholl J, Allen PJ: A primary care approach to functional abdominal pain, *Pediatr Nurs* 33(3):247-259, 2007.

Selekman J, Snyder M: Learning disabilities and/or attention deficit disorder. In Jackson PL,

Vessey JA, editors: *Primary care of the child with a chronic condition,* ed 3, St Louis, 2000, Mosby.

Seltzer EG, Shapiro ED: Misdiagnosis of Lyme disease: when not to order serologic tests, *Pediatr Infect Dis J* 15:762-763, 1996.

Shapiro NA: "Dude, you don't have Tourette's": Tourette's syndrome, beyond the tics, *Pediatr Nurs* 22(3):1-15, 2002.

Smith JC: Abdominal pain. In Hoekelman RA, Adam HM, Nelson NM, et al, editors: *Primary pediatric care,* ed 4, St Louis, 2001, Mosby.

St. Geme JW, Haslam DB, Ditmar MF: Infectious diseases. In Polin RA, Ditmar MF, editors: *Pediatric secrets,* ed 2, Philadelphia, 1997, Mosby.

Sundelin-Wahlsten V, Ahmad A, von Knorring AL: Traumatic experiences and post-traumatic stress reactions in children from Kurdistan and Sweden, *Acta Paediatr* 90:563-568, 2001.

Troupe M: Clinical management of the avulsed tooth, *Dent Clin North Am* 39(1):93-112, 1995.

Visscher PK, Vetter RS, Camazine S: Removing bee stings, *Lancet* 348(9023):301-302, 1996.

Wade CF: Keeping Lyme disease at bay: an integrated approach to prevention, *Am J Nurs* 100(7):26-31, 2000.

Wormser GP, Dattwyler RJ, Shapiro ED, et al: The clinical assessment, treatment, and prevention of Lyme disease, human granulocytic anaplasmosis, and babesiosis: clinical practice guidelines by the infections diseases society of America, *Clin Infect Dis* 43(9):1089-1143, 2006.

Yacob D, Di Lorenzo C: Functional abdominal pain: all roads lead to Rome (criteria), *Pediatr Ann* 38(5):253-258, 2009.

Zinner SH: Tourette syndrome—much more than tics: Moving beyond misconceptions to diagnosis, *Contemp Pediatr* 21(8):22-49, 2004.

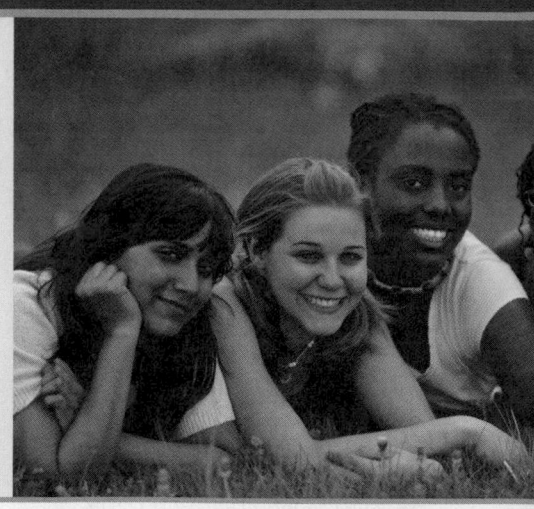

CHAPTER OUTLINE

PROMOTING OPTIMUM GROWTH AND DEVELOPMENT

Adolescence is a period of transition between childhood and adulthood, a time of profound biologic, intellectual, psychosocial, and economic change. During this period individuals reach physical and sexual maturity, develop more sophisticated reasoning abilities, and make educational and occupational decisions that will shape their adult careers. The changes of adolescence have important implications for understanding the kinds of health risks to which young people are exposed, the health-enhancing and risk-taking behaviors in which they engage, and the major opportunities for health promotion among this population.

In the process of examining widely accepted theories of adolescent development, researchers have challenged many popular notions. For example, a common belief is that teenagers' behaviors are overwhelmingly determined by "raging hormones," and that adolescence is a period when rebellious and risky behavior is the norm. Both notions are misguided, but these mistaken beliefs are not benign. They may have detrimental effects on attitudes and interactions with individual adolescents and on policy and program development. Although current research supports a more positive view of this life period, it also confirms that adolescence involves a complex interplay of biologic, cognitive, psychologic, and social change, perhaps more so than at any other time of life. Unfortunately, some perceive that the United States as a society often has provided little help to individuals as they try to cope with the normal changes of adolescence.

Change during adolescence occurs on multiple levels. On the individual level, changes include biologic maturation, cognitive development, and psychologic development. Change also occurs in the social contexts of adolescents' families, peer groups, schools, and workplaces. Adolescence involves three distinct subphases: early adolescence (ages 11 to 14), middle adolescence (ages 15 to 17), and late adolescence (ages 18 to 20). The changes, opportunities, pressures, skills, and resources available to young people differ during these subphases. For example, early adolescence is characterized primarily by the changes of puberty and responses to those changes. Middle adolescence is characterized by transition to a dominant peer orientation, with all the stereotypic adolescent preoccupations of music, technology, dress and appearance, language, and behavior. Late adolescence involves transition into adulthood, including taking on adult work roles and developing adult relationships (Table 19-1).

BIOLOGIC DEVELOPMENT

⊜ Neuroendocrine Events of Puberty

The fundamental biologic changes of adolescence are collectively referred to as puberty. Puberty involves a predictable sequence of hormonal and physical changes that occur universally over a defined period of time. It encompasses both sexual maturation and physical growth. It is generally accepted that the events of puberty are triggered by hormonal influences and are controlled by the anterior pituitary gland in response to a stimulus from the hypothalamus.

Puberty begins as some not completely understood cluster of events triggers the production of gonadotropin-releasing hormone (GnRH) by the hypothalamus (Fig. 19-1). GnRH travels through a network of capillaries to the anterior pituitary gland, where it stimulates the production and secretion of follicle-stimulating hormone (FSH) and luteinizing hormone (LH). Increasing levels of FSH and LH in the blood stimulate gonadal response. For females, FSH stimulates growth of ovarian follicles and production of estrogen. LH initiates ovulation, the formation of the corpus luteum, and progesterone production. For males, LH acts on testicular Leydig cells, prompting maturation of the testicles and testosterone production. FSH, acting with LH, stimulates sperm production. The sex steroids—estrogen, progesterone, and testosterone and other androgens—are released from the gonads and effect biologic changes in various organs, including muscles, bones, skin, and hair follicles. Increasing serum levels of sex steroids also provide feedback to the hypothalamus, causing decreases in GnRH secretion. When serum sex hormone levels decrease, the hypothalamus is stimulated to increase GnRH secretion, again initiating the sequence that produces the appropriate gonadal responses.

Initiation of Puberty

The precise mechanism that institutes the changes at puberty is not completely understood. Although the pituitary gland and gonads are capable of mature function and can respond to stimuli at any age, the hypothalamic-pituitary-gonadal system is kept in a dormant state throughout childhood by some central nervous system inhibitory mechanism in the region of the hypothalamus. It is believed that the receptor sites in the hypothalamus are so highly sensitive that the most minute quantities of circulating sex hormones are sufficient to inhibit the secretion of GnRH during childhood. The hypothalamus loses this negative sensitivity at puberty, which allows the hypothalamic-pituitary-gonadal mechanism to attain full secretory function. As puberty progresses, the pituitary and gonads become increasingly sensitive to positive hormonal stimulation.

Changes in Reproductive Hormones
Females

The primary sexual characteristic in girls is the development and release of an egg, or ovum, from the ovaries approximately every 28 days. Beginning in early puberty, FSH stimulates estrogen production by the ovaries. However, concentrations of estrogen do not reach levels high enough to cause ovulation. By the time girls reach midpuberty, the body produces estrogen in larger amounts. This quantity of estrogen production results in the building of an endometrial lining of the uterus and first menstruation, or menarche. At menarche, ova still do not generally mature enough to be released. However, as puberty progresses, usually one ovarian follicle becomes dominant during each menstrual cycle and produces increasing amounts of estrogen during the early-cycle, follicular phase. This follicle then releases an ovum, a process termed *ovulation,* around day 14 of the menstrual cycle. After ovulation the follicle involutes and its estrogen production decreases. This leads to a drop in

TABLE 19-1   GROWTH AND DEVELOPMENT DURING ADOLESCENCE

EARLY ADOLESCENCE (11-14 yr)	MIDDLE ADOLESCENCE (15-17 yr)	LATE ADOLESCENCE (18-20 yr)
Growth		
Rapidly accelerating growth	Growth decelerating in girls	Physically mature
Reaches peak velocity	Stature reaches 95% of adult height	Structure and reproductive growth almost complete
Secondary sexual characteristics appear	Secondary sexual characteristics well advanced	
Cognition		
Explores newfound ability for limited abstract thought	Developing capacity for abstract thinking	Established abstract thought
Clumsy groping for new values and energies	Enjoys intellectual powers, often in idealistic terms	Can perceive and act on long-range options
Comparison of "normality" with peers of same sex	Concern with philosophic, political, and social problems	Able to view problems comprehensively
		Intellectual and functional identity established
Identity		
Preoccupied with rapid body changes	Modifies body image	Body image and gender-role definition nearly secured
Trying out of various roles	Self-centered; increased narcissism	Mature sexual identity
Measurement of attractiveness by acceptance or rejection by peers	Tendency toward inner experience and self-discovery	Phase of consolidation of identity
Conformity to group norms	Has rich fantasy life	Increase in self-esteem
Decline in self-esteem	Idealistic	Comfortable with physical growth
	Able to perceive future implications of current behavior and decisions; variable application	Social roles defined and articulated
Relationships with Parents		
Defining independence-dependence boundaries	Major conflicts over independence and control	Emotional and physical separation from parents completed
Strong desire to remain dependent on parents while trying to detach	Low point in parent-child relationship	Independence from family with less conflict
No major conflicts over parental control	Greatest push for emancipation; disengagement	Emancipation nearly secured
	Final and irreversible emotional detachment from parents; mourning	
Relationships with Peers		
Seeks peer affiliations to counter instability generated by rapid change	Strong need for identity to affirm self-image	Peer group recedes in importance in favor of individual friendship
Upsurge of close, idealized friendships with members of same sex	Behavioral standards set by peer group	Testing of romantic relationships against possibility of permanent alliance
Struggle for mastery within peer group	Acceptance by peers extremely important—fear of rejection	Relationships characterized by giving and sharing
	Exploration of ability to attract opposite sex	
Sexuality		
Self-exploration and evaluation	Multiple plural relationships	Forms stable relationships and attachment to another
Limited dating, usually group	Internal identification of heterosexual, homosexual, or bisexual attractions	Growing capacity for mutuality and reciprocity
Limited intimacy	Exploration of "self-appeal"	Dating as a romantic pair
	Feeling of "being in love"	May publicly identify as gay, lesbian, or bisexual
	Tentative establishment of relationships	Intimacy involves commitment rather than exploration and romanticism
Psychologic Health		
Wide mood swings	Tendency toward inner experiences; more introspective	More constancy of emotion
Intense daydreaming	Tendency to withdraw when upset or feelings are hurt	Anger more likely to be concealed
Anger outwardly expressed with moodiness, temper outbursts, and verbal insults and name calling	Vacillation of emotions in time and range	
	Feelings of inadequacy common; difficulty asking for help	

serum estrogen and progesterone. The pituitary gland responds to the drop in these hormone levels with increased production of FSH, initiating the start of a new menstrual cycle.

By direct action, estrogens cause growth and development of the vagina, uterus, and fallopian tubes. The skin of the labia majora, as well as that of the breast areola and nipples, grows and darkens under the influence of estrogen. Estrogen is responsible for breast enlargement. Estrogen also promotes the growth of pubic and axillary hair, and widening of the hips. At low levels estrogen tends to stimulate skeletal growth in both boys and girls, but at higher levels it inhibits growth.

Males

The primary male sexual characteristic is the development of viable sperm. During puberty, FSH acts on testicular cells, stimulating the production of viable sperm. FSH and LH also act on a different group of testicular cells, resulting in increased production and secretion of testosterone. In this process of sexual development, boys do not experience a discrete event analogous to menstruation or ovulation in girls. However, just as the production of a mature ovum tends to occur 1 year or more after menarche in girls, the production of viable sperm tends to follow boys' first ejaculations. The capacity to ejaculate appears relatively early in boys' sexual development, approximately 1 year after initial testicular enlargement and the appearance of pubic hair. From a clinical perspective, however, an adolescent should be considered potentially fertile with a first menstrual period or a first ejaculation.

Testosterone and other androgens have a direct impact on growth of the penis, scrotum, prostate, and seminal vesicles of the testicles. The tremendous growth-promoting properties of these hormones also result in rapid increases in muscle mass, skeletal growth, bone age, and bone density. In both sexes androgens are responsible for the development of pubic, axillary, facial, and body hair. Clinically, increased activity of androgens is associated with pubertal conditions such as acne, body odor, deepening of the voice, a spurt in height, and an increase in red blood cell levels.

Pubertal Sexual Maturation

Increases in reproductive hormones are responsible for dramatic changes in secondary sexual characteristics that occur during puberty. As with general growth, development of secondary sexual characteristics occurs in a predictable sequence. This sequence has been divided into a series of five phases termed the Tanner stages (Box 19-1 and Figs. 19-2 to 19-6). Although the sequence of sexual development is predictable, the ages at which these changes occur and the rate of developmental progression vary considerably among individuals. Over the course of pubescence, many young people have questions about the timing, rate, and normalcy of their body changes. These concerns provide nurses with a prime opportunity to discuss health-related topics such as puberty, sexuality, birth control, prevention of sexually transmitted infections (STIs), nutrition, exercise, and safe methods of weight control.

Sexual Maturation in Girls

In four out of five girls, changes in the nipple and areola and development of a small bud of breast tissue (thelarche) are the

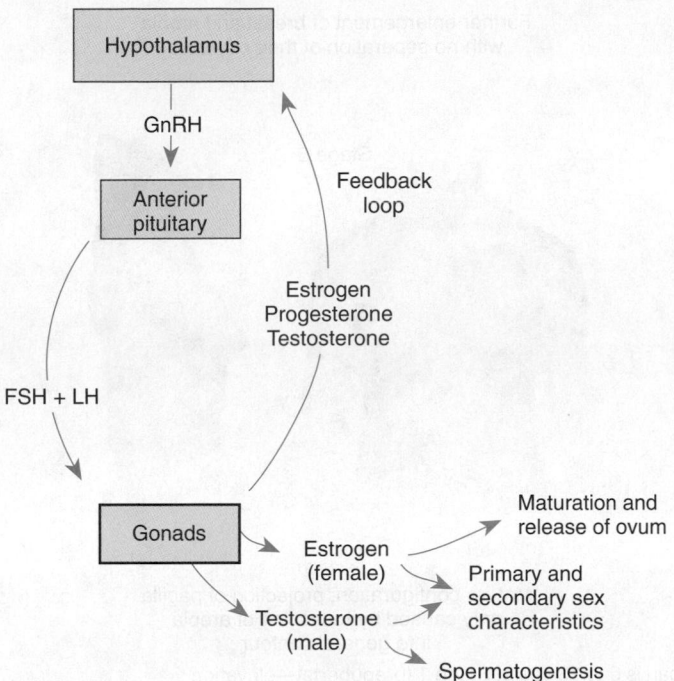

Fig. 19-1 Hormonal interaction between hypothalamus, pituitary, and gonads. *GnRH*, Gonadotropin-releasing hormone; *FSH*, follicle-stimulating hormone; *LH*, luteinizing hormone.

BOX 19-1   TANNER STAGES

The Tanner stages were developed by Dr. J.M. Tanner and colleagues. Tanner stages describe the stages of pubertal growth and are numbered from stage 1 (immature) to stage 5 (mature) for both males and females. In females the Tanner stages describe pubertal development based on breast size and the shape and distribution of pubic hair. In males the Tanner stages describe pubertal development based on the size and shape of the penis and scrotum and the shape and distribution of pubic hair.

Tanner JM: *Growth of adolescents*, Oxford, 1962, Blackwell Scientific Publications.

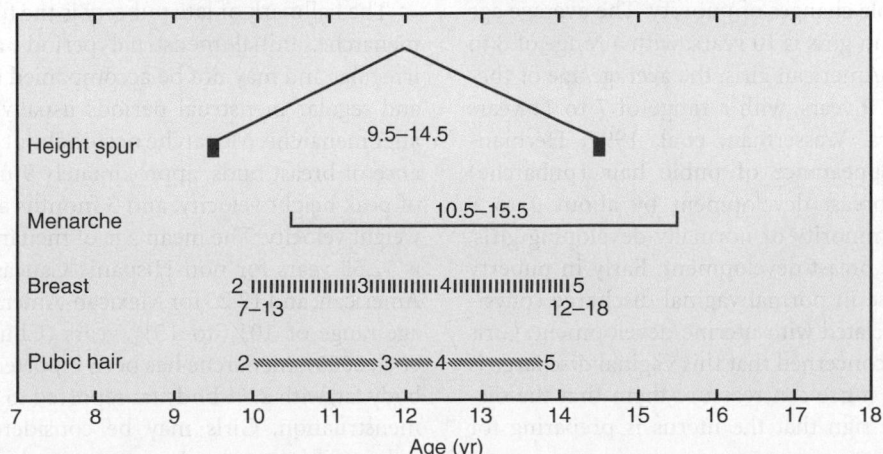

Fig. 19-2 Approximate timing of developmental changes in girls. Numbers indicate stages of development. Range of ages during which some of the changes occur is indicated by inclusive numbers below them. See Figs. 19-3 and 19-4 for explanation. (Based on revised data from Herman-Giddens M, Slora EJ, Wasserman RC, et al: Secondary sexual characteristics and menses in young girls seen in office practice: a study from the Pediatric Research in Office Settings Network, *Pediatrics* 99(4):505-512, 1997.)

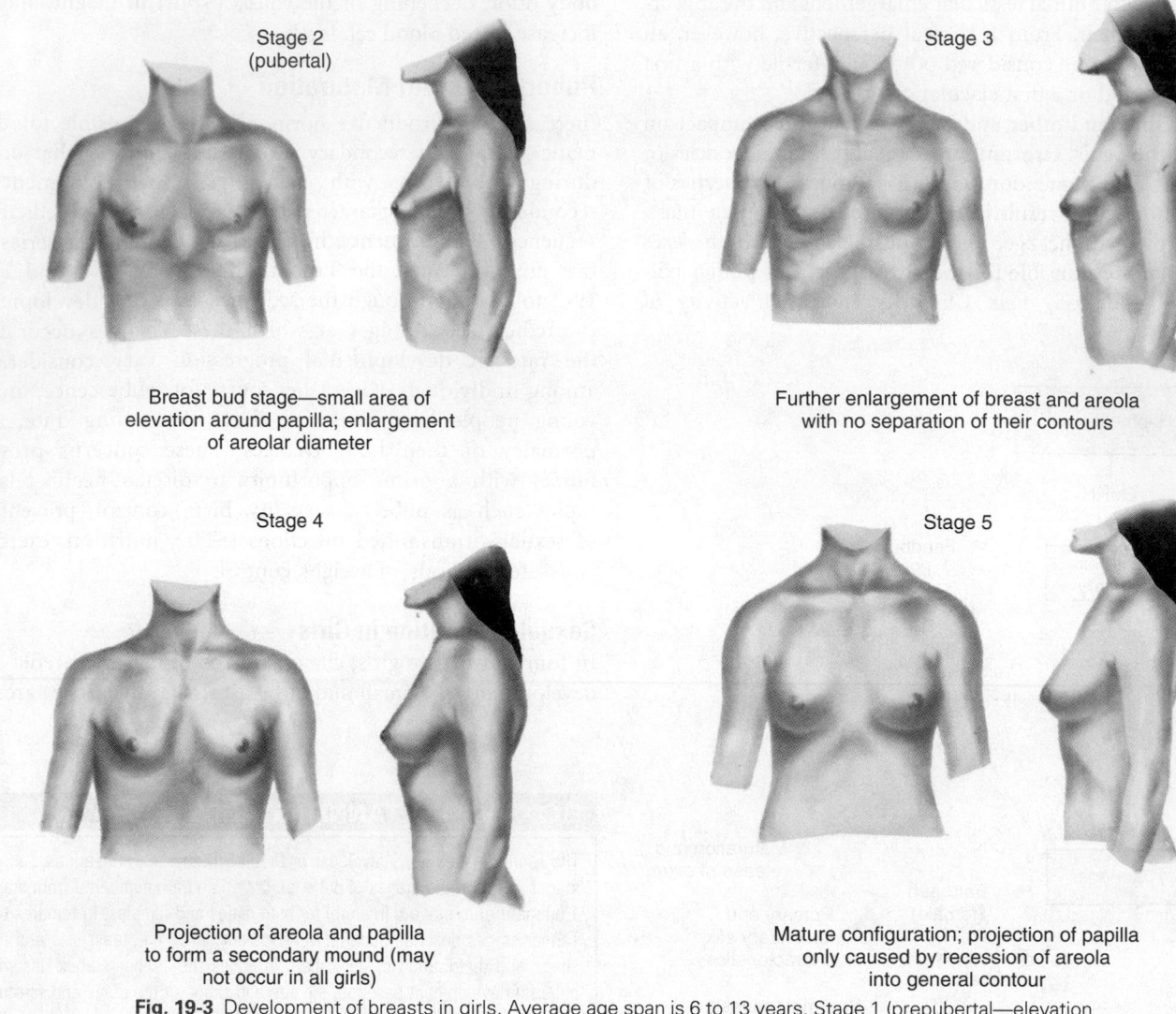

Stage 2
(pubertal)

Breast bud stage—small area of
elevation around papilla; enlargement
of areolar diameter

Stage 3

Further enlargement of breast and areola
with no separation of their contours

Stage 4

Projection of areola and papilla
to form a secondary mound (may
not occur in all girls)

Stage 5

Mature configuration; projection of papilla
only caused by recession of areola
into general contour

Fig. 19-3 Development of breasts in girls. Average age span is 6 to 13 years. Stage 1 (prepubertal—elevation of papilla only) is not shown. (Modified from Marshall WA, Tanner JM: Variations in pattern of pubertal changes in girls, *Arch Dis Child* 44(235):291-303, 1969; and Daniel WA, Paulshock BZ: A physician's guide to sexual maturity, *Patient Care* 13:122-124, 1979.)

earliest, most easily visible changes of puberty. The average age of thelarche for Caucasian girls is 10 years, with a range of 8 to 12.75 years; for African-American girls, the average age of thelarche is earlier, around 9 years, with a range of 7 to 11 years (Herman-Giddens, Slora, Wasserman, et al, 1997; Herman-Giddens, 2006). The appearance of pubic hair (pubarche) usually follows initial breast development by about 2 to 6 months; however, in a minority of normally developing girls, pubic hair may precede breast development. Early in puberty there is often an increase in normal vaginal discharge (physiologic leukorrhea), associated with uterine development. Girls or their parents may be concerned that this vaginal discharge is a sign of infection. The nurse can reassure them that the discharge is normal and a sign that the uterus is preparing for menstruation.

During midpuberty, breast enlargement occurs, and pubic hair progresses to adult-type sexual hair covering the mons pubis and labia majora. Most girls reach their peak height velocity and peak weight velocity in midpubescence.

The hallmark of late puberty is the first menstrual period, or menarche. Initial menstrual periods are usually scanty and irregular and may not be accompanied by ovulation. Ovulation and regular menstrual periods usually begin 6 to 14 months after menarche. Menarche occurs about 2 years after the appearance of breast buds, approximately 9 months after attainment of peak height velocity, and 3 months after attainment of peak weight velocity. The mean age of menarche in the United States is 12.55 years for non-Hispanic Caucasian, 12.06 for African-American, and 12.25 for Mexican-American girls, with a normal age range of $10\frac{1}{2}$ to $15\frac{1}{2}$ years (Chumlea, Schubert, Roche, et al, 2003). Menarche has been reported to occur at about 17% body fat, with 22% body fat reported to be required to maintain menstruation. Girls may be considered to have precocious puberty if breast development or pubic hair occurs before age 7 years for Caucasian girls or age 6 years for African-American girls, or if menarche occurs before age 10 years (Kaplowitz and Oberfield, 1999). Girls may be considered to have pubertal delay if breast development has not occurred by age 13 or if

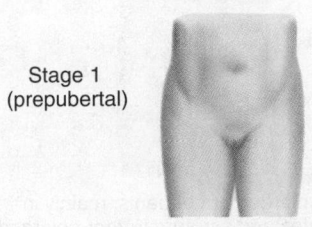

Stage 1
(prepubertal)

No pubic hair; essentially the same as
during childhood; no distinction between
hair on pubis and over the abdomen

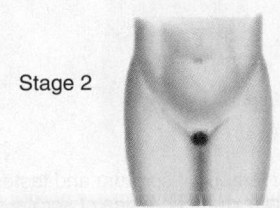

Stage 2

Sparse growth of long, straight, downy, and
slightly pigmented hair extending along labia;
between stages 2 and 3 begins to appear on pubis

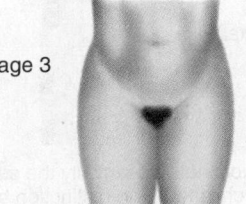

Stage 3

Hair darker, coarser, and curly and
spread sparsely over entire pubis in
the typical female triangle

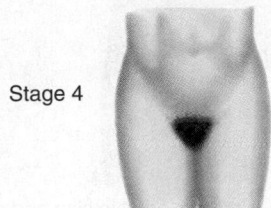

Stage 4

Pubic hair denser, curled, and adult in distribution
but less abundant and restricted to the pubic area

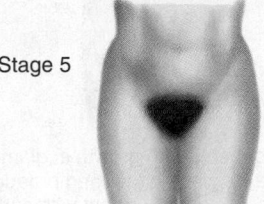

Stage 5

Hair adult in quantity, type, and pattern
with spread to inner aspect of thighs

Fig. 19-4 Growth in pubic hair in girls. Average age span for stages 2 through 5 is 11 to 14 years. (Modified from Marshall WA, Tanner JM: Variations in pattern of pubertal changes in girls, *Arch Dis Child* 44(235):291-303, 1969; and Daniel WA, Paulshock BZ: A physician's guide to sexual maturity, *Patient Care* 13:122-124, 1979.)

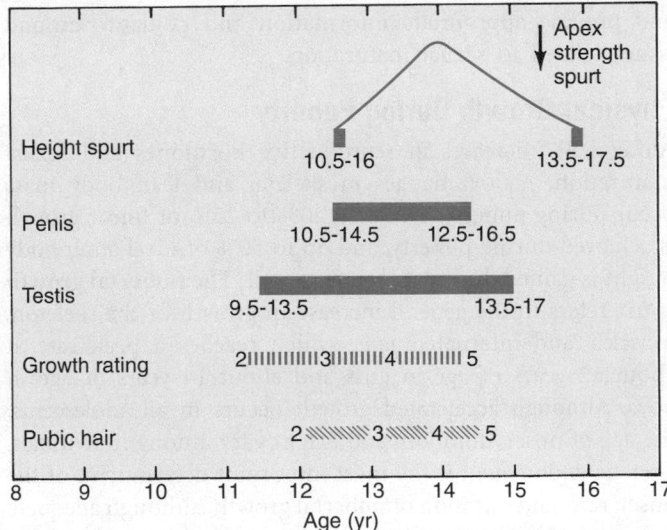

Fig. 19-5 Approximate timing of developmental changes in boys. Numbers indicate stages of development. Range of ages during which some of the changes occur is indicated by inclusive numbers below them. See Fig. 19-6 for explanation. (From Marshall WA, Tanner JM: Variations in the pattern of pubertal changes in boys, *Arch Dis Child* 45(239):13-23, 1970.)

menarche has not occurred within 2 to 2½ years of the onset of breast development.

In the United States and most developed countries, the mean age of menarche has gradually decreased over the past century, corresponding to population improvements in nutrition, sanitation, and control of infectious diseases. This decline in the average age of menarche appears to have leveled off in recent years (Patton and Viner, 2007). Internationally, a decline in the average age at first menses has not been seen in countries where children are more likely to be malnourished and suffer from chronic illness.

Sexual maturation influences young peoples' satisfaction with their appearance, but the effects appear to differ for girls and boys. For girls, physical maturation can lead to greater dissatisfaction with their appearance. For example, recent studies indicate that adolescent girls are more dissatisfied with their appearance and significantly more likely to identify themselves as being overweight than adolescent boys, even when they are at a normal weight for height (Smith, Stewart, Peled, et al, 2009). Normal increases in weight and fat deposition that accompany puberty among girls conflict with cultural norms that emphasize a slender look. Early-maturing girls suffer most because they begin to develop at a time when their age-mates still exemplify prepubertal slimness. Unfortunately, an all-too-common response to changes in body shape among teenage girls is to engage in extensive dieting at a time when nutritional requirements are at a peak. For some, the focus on slimness and dieting may trigger the development of eating disorders. (See Chapter 21.) Consequently, health promotion efforts related to pubertal growth, eating behaviors, and body image are important for adolescent girls, especially early-maturing girls.

Sexual Maturation in Boys

The first pubescent changes in boys are testicular enlargement accompanied by thinning, reddening, and increasing looseness of the scrotum. These events usually occur between 9½ and 14 years of age. Early puberty is also characterized by the initial appearance of pubic hair. Penile enlargement begins,

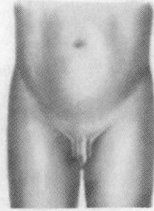

Stage 1
(prepubertal)

No pubic hair; essentially the same as
during childhood; no distinction between
hair on pubis and over the abdomen

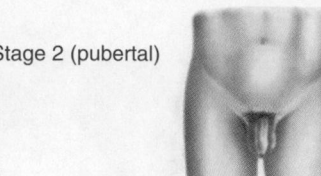

Stage 2 (pubertal)

Initial enlargement of scrotum and testes;
reddening and textural changes of scrotal skin;
sparse growth of long, straight, downy, and
slightly pigmented hair at base of penis

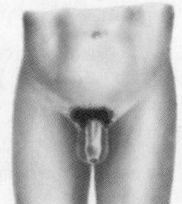

Stage 3

Initial enlargement of penis, mainly in
length; testes and scrotum further enlarged;
hair darker, coarser, and curly and spread
sparsely over entire pubis

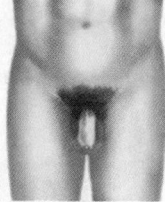

Stage 4

Increased size of penis with growth in diameter and
development of glans; glans larger and broader; scrotum
darker; pubic hair more abundant with curling but
restricted to pubic area

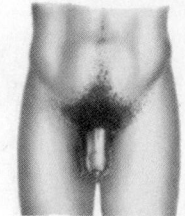

Stage 5

Testes, scrotum, and penis adult in size and shape;
hair adult in quantity and type with spread to inner
surface of thighs

Fig. 19-6 Developmental stages of secondary sexual characteristics and genital development in boys. Average age span is 12 to 16 years. (Modified from Marshall WA, Tanner JM: Variations in the pattern of pubertal changes in boys, *Arch Dis Child* 45(239):13-23, 1970; and Daniel WA, Paulshock BZ: A physician's guide to sexual maturity, *Patient Care* 13:122-124, 1979.)

and testicular enlargement and pubic hair growth continue throughout midpuberty. During this period boys also undergo increasing muscularity, early voice changes, and development of early facial hair. Gynecomastia (breast enlargement and tenderness) is common during midpuberty. It occurs in up to one third of boys and is usually temporary. The spurts in height and weight occur concurrently toward the end of midpuberty. For most boys, breast enlargement disappears within 2 years. By midpuberty, there is a definite increase in the length and width of the penis, testicular enlargement continues, and first ejaculation occurs. Axillary hair develops, and facial hair extends to cover the anterior neck. Final voice changes occur secondary to the growth of the larynx.

Precocious puberty in boys may be a concern if secondary sexual characteristics occur before age 9. Concerns about pubertal delay should be considered for boys who exhibit no enlargement of the testes or scrotal changes by ages 13½ to 14, or if genital growth is not complete 4 years after the testicles begin to enlarge.

Changes in the size and shape of the penis and testicles and changes in genital functioning can be areas of great concern for adolescent boys. Although the ability for penile erection is present at birth, only with pubertal maturation do boys have seminal emissions. Ejaculation may occur spontaneously as a nocturnal emission, or "wet dream"; as a result of self-stimulation (masturbation); or during sexual activity with others. Unless they are prepared, boys may find spontaneous ejaculations puzzling, troublesome, and embarrassing. Pubertal changes and related concerns create important opportunities for health promotion among young teenage boys. Health care professionals can be a resource for boys

and provide appropriate information and guidance around issues related to sexual maturation.

Physical Growth During Puberty

Along with increases in reproductive hormones and sexual maturation, major changes in skeletal and lean body mass occur during puberty. The final 20% to 25% of linear growth is achieved during puberty, and up to 50% of ideal adult body weight is gained during this time as well. The **pubertal growth spurt** refers to the general increase in growth of the skeleton, muscles, and internal organs, which reaches a peak rate at about 12 years of age in girls and about 14 years of age in boys. Although accelerated growth occurs in all adolescents, the age of onset, duration, and extent vary among individuals. Genetic endowment is the most important determinant of the onset, rate, and duration of pubertal growth, although adequate nutrition also plays a role.

Normal Patterns of Growth

Once the process of growth begins, the sequence of changes is progressive and usually predictable. Awareness of this sequence is not only important for reassuring concerned adolescents and parents but also useful in diagnosing conditions associated with abnormal growth. In general, girls begin puberty and reach maturity about 1½ to 2 years earlier than boys. The pubertal growth spurt begins as early as 9½ years or as late as 14½ years in girls, and as early as 10½ years and as late as 16 years in boys.

General growth includes accumulation of body mass, along with increases in height and weight. Lean body mass, primarily muscle mass, increases in both girls and boys during early puberty. For girls, the rate of muscle mass growth peaks at menarche and then slows. For boys, muscle mass continues to increase throughout puberty, resulting in the attainment of significantly higher lean body mass in boys than in girls. In girls, gain in fat mass increases markedly early in puberty and continues to increase after menarche. In boys there is a peak deceleration in the rate of fat mass accumulation at the time of their growth spurt, and thereafter a slower and much less dramatic increase than in girls.

The rate of linear growth (height) (Fig. 19-7) begins to increase in girls during early puberty, whereas in boys the rate does not increase until midpuberty. Peak height velocity (PHV) occurs at about 12 years of age in girls, around 6 to 12 months before menarche. PHV is used as a predictor of menarche; height at menarche is a predictor of ultimate adult height. Few girls grow more than 5 cm (2 inches) in height after menarche. Growth in girls' height usually ceases 2 to 2½ years after menarche. Boys typically reach PHV at about 14 years of age, after growth of the testicles and penis and the appearance of axillary and mature pubic hair. Among most boys, growth in height ceases at 18 or 20 years of age. Increases in leg length tend to precede growth of the trunk by about 6 to 9 months and that of the shoulders and chest by about 1 year. In short, teenagers tend to follow a linear growth pattern in which they outgrow their shoes first, then their pants, and finally their shirts. Peak weight velocity occurs about 6 months after PHV in girls. In contrast, weight and height spurts occur simultaneously for boys. On average, girls gain 5 to 20 cm (2 to 8 inches) in height and 7 to 25 kg (15.5 to 55 lb) in weight during adolescence, and boys gain 10 to 30 cm (4 to 12 inches) in height and 7 to 30 kg (15.5 to 66 lb) in weight during adolescence.

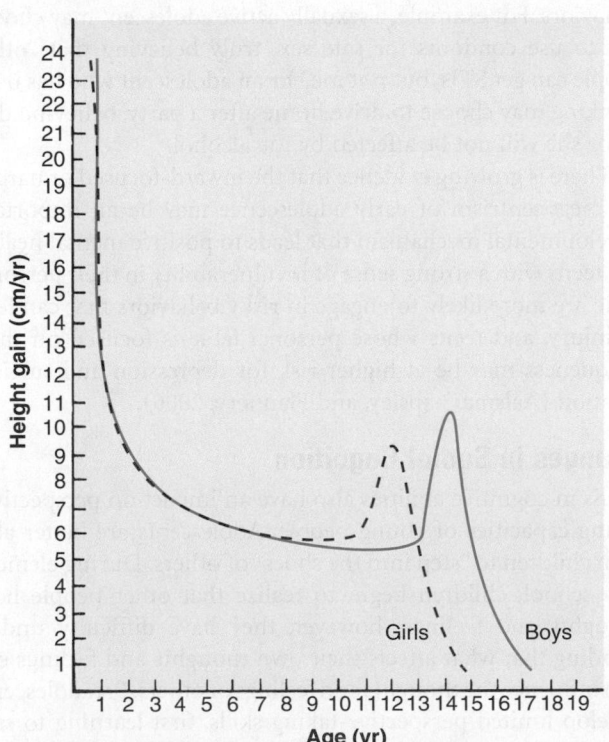

Fig. 19-7 Linear growth in centimeters per year. (From Tanner JM, Whitehouse RH, Takaishi M: Standards from birth to maturity for height, weight, height velocity and weight velocity: British children, 1965, *Arch Dis Child* 41:454-471, 1966.)

Other Physiologic Changes

In addition to the characteristic changes of puberty already discussed, numerous others occur. The size and strength of the heart, blood volume, and systolic blood pressure increase, whereas the heart rate decreases. Consistent with the general developmental timetable, these changes appear earlier in girls, who establish a slightly higher pulse rate and a slightly lower systolic blood pressure than boys. Blood volume, which has increased steadily during childhood, reaches higher levels in boys than in girls, a fact that may be related to the increased muscle mass in pubertal boys. Adult values are reached for all formed elements of the blood. For instance, there is a marked increase in serum iron, the number of red blood cells, hemoglobin, and hematocrit in boys, but not in girls.

The lungs increase in both diameter and length during puberty. The respiratory rate, decreasing steadily throughout childhood, reaches the adult rate in adolescence. Respiratory volume, vital capacity, and other physiologic properties related to respiratory function are increased, and to a greater extent in boys than in girls. The differences between the sexes are a result of the greater lung growth associated with boys' increased shoulder and chest size.

The rate of steady decline in basal metabolic rate from birth to adulthood slows during puberty, coinciding with the growth spurt in both sexes, reflecting the increase in physiologic activities. A slightly higher metabolic rate in boys than in girls is probably a function of differences in androgenic hormones. Basal body temperature gradually decreases with age in both sexes, reaching adult values by 12 years of age in girls and somewhat later in boys.

Adolescence is also a time of continued brain growth. Although the number of neurons does not increase, there is a proliferation of the support cells that brace and nourish the neurons, and an increase in the number of neural connections. Development of these connections within the cortex of the brain continues during adolescence and may not reach adult levels until after age 20. In addition, the growth of the myelin sheath around the nerve cells continues through and beyond puberty, enabling faster neural processing. This "fine tuning" of the neural system coincides with development of the more advanced cognitive capacities of youth, but continues into early adulthood. Recent studies have shown, for example, that the frontal cortex areas of the brain, associated with executive functions, continue myelinization into the twenties, and may not be complete until as late as age 25.

COGNITIVE DEVELOPMENT

Emergence of Formal Operational Thought (Piaget)

Jean Piaget (1972) described the shift from childhood to adolescence as a movement from concrete to formal operational thought. Children's thinking is oriented to things and events that they can observe directly. Unable to think in terms of abstract possibilities, they process information based on what is directly observable. For most young people, emergence of formal operational thinking occurs between the ages of 11 and 14. **Formal operational thought** includes being able to think in abstract terms, think about possibilities, and think through hypotheses. Young people become able to think about abstractions; thus they can symbolically associate behaviors with abstract concepts such as attractiveness, adult status, or happiness. Adolescents also become capable of using a future time perspective rather than being tied to the here-and-now thinking of childhood. They are able to imagine possibilities, such as a sequence of future events that might occur, including college or occupational opportunities, or how current situations, such as relationships with parents or friends, could change to meet an imagined ideal.

Hypothetical reasoning is aligned with thinking about possibilities. To think through hypotheses, one needs to see beyond what is directly observable and reason in terms of what might be possible. Hypothetical thinking allows adolescents to systematically generate alternative possibilities and explanations and to compare what they actually observe with what they believe is possible. In practical terms, being able to plan ahead and identify future consequences of possible actions are skills dependent on being able to think hypothetically.

The health care provider's ability to assess an adolescent's level of cognitive development has important implications for health promotion. Older adolescents may be able to consider some of the symbolic and long-term implications of their behaviors. Thus they may respond to health promotion efforts that require a future time perspective or attention to symbolic rewards. For young people who primarily use concrete thinking (i.e., younger teenagers), health promotion efforts should emphasize immediate risks or benefits of the behavior.

Along with cognitive development, decision-making abilities increase over the adolescent period. Young people develop the ability to consider hypothetical risks and benefits of possible behaviors, along with potential consequences of such behaviors. In addition, the likelihood of teenagers consulting with adult experts, mentors, and role models increases over the junior and senior high school years. By middle adolescence, most teenagers are able to reason as well as adults. Health promotion efforts, especially those aimed at younger adolescents, should offer learning strategies that enhance decision-making skills. Such efforts might include discussions emphasizing health-promoting norms for behavior among young people and alternatives to unhealthy behaviors, along with opportunities to practice skills necessary to resist unhealthy behaviors.

Even with the best framework for health promotion, persons who are capable of formal operational thought and reasoned decision making do not use these processes all the time. When faced with time pressures, personal stress, or overwhelming peer pressure, young people are more likely to abandon rational thought processes. Thoughts about unfamiliar or emotionally arousing topics also tend to be less sophisticated and more vulnerable to the effects of stress and pressure. Unfortunately, many of the health-related decisions adolescents confront, such as those related to substance use or sexual behavior, involve issues that are personally stressful, emotion laden, or new. Under such conditions, people tend not to use their capacities for abstract formal reasoning, even if they typically use advanced decision-making skills.

Adolescent Conceptions of Self

With development of formal operational thought, adolescents become able to describe the self more abstractly. Compared with children, they are more psychologic in their self-descriptions, focusing on personal and interpersonal characteristics, beliefs, and emotional states. They also develop a more differentiated self-concept, recognizing that their behavior and performance vary from setting to setting. With time, they become able to integrate these disparate observations of self into abstract personal characterizations (e.g., "I am a sensitive person").

Psychologic theories help explain how teens use these powerful new cognitive tools to make the transition to adult roles and relationships (Elkind, 1978; Lapsley, 1993). Being able to think about one's own thoughts and emotions can lead to periods of extreme self-absorption, what Elkind called *adolescent egocentrism*. This self-absorption has also been described by Lapsley as a way of imagining and "trying on" various personas and practicing hypothetical interactions in an attempt to develop a separate sense of self.

Two common patterns of thinking help explain some of the health-related beliefs and behaviors of youth. The first, the imaginary audience, involves having such a heightened sense of self-consciousness that an adolescent imagines that everyone notices and is focused on his or her behavior. For example, a teen who has diabetes may worry about injecting insulin at school because "everybody will notice." The second pattern of thinking, called the personal fable, is the belief that one's feelings and experiences are completely unique, or that one is all-knowing or invulnerable. This helps explain the common accusation from younger teens towards adults, "You just don't understand!" as well as some of their decisions around risk behaviors. For example, a sexually active adolescent may choose not to use condoms for safe sex, truly believing that "other people can get STIs, but not me," or an adolescent who has been drinking may choose to drive home after a party, believing that he or she will not be affected by the alcohol.

There is growing evidence that the inward-focused or narcissistic egocentrism of early adolescence may be an important developmental mechanism that leads to positive mental health, but teens with a strong sense of invulnerability in their personal fable are more likely to engage in risky behaviors that can lead to injury, and teens whose personal fable is focused on their uniqueness may be at higher risk for depression and suicidal ideation (Aalsma, Lapsley, and Flannery, 2006).

Changes in Social Cognition

Gains in cognitive abilities also have an impact on perspective-taking capacities of young people. Adolescents are better able than children to "step into the shoes" of others. During elementary school, children begin to realize that other people have thoughts and feelings; however, they have difficulty understanding that what affects their own thoughts and feelings can also influence the thoughts and feelings of others. Preadolescents develop limited perspective-taking skills, first learning to step into the shoes of best friends, then peers and family members, and finally people of other ages and backgrounds.

Perspective-taking capacities develop further as adolescents become able to engage in mutual role taking. In other words, teenagers can both understand the perspectives of others and see how the thoughts or actions of one person can influence those of others. Role-taking capabilities continue to expand throughout adolescence. They are able to discuss various issues highlighting points of importance to people in various social roles (e.g., "From a parent's perspective, having a curfew is important because ..."). Older adolescents also realize that the perspectives people hold are complicated in that they are influenced by a range of intrapersonal, interpersonal, and sociocultural factors.

Ultimately, gains in perspective-taking skills that take place during adolescence lead to an increased capacity to learn from the experiences of others. Older adolescents are able to consider the choices, behaviors, and outcomes experienced by others in making their own health-related choices. This newfound capacity significantly expands the opportunities to learn health-promoting behaviors.

DEVELOPMENT OF VALUE AUTONOMY

With advances in cognitive development, adolescents' beliefs become more abstract and increasingly rooted in general ideologic principles. At the same time, young people are gaining increasing emotional independence from parents, relying less on their parents' beliefs and values than they did as children. Adolescents also progress toward greater behavioral independence, encountering situations and decisions they have not previously experienced. With these new capacities and experiences, young people face a variety of cognitive conflicts as they compare the advice of parents and friends and deal with competing pressures to behave in given ways. These conflicts may prompt young people to consider, in serious and thoughtful terms, what they themselves really believe. Whereas earlier in life they may have merely accepted the decisions or points of view of adults, adolescents begin to substitute a set of values distinct from those of significant adults in their lives. This struggle to clarify values, created in part by an expanded behavioral independence, is a large part of the process of developing what has been termed value autonomy (Steinberg, 1990). The development of a personal value system is a gradual process, with evidence that value autonomy occurs relatively late in adolescence, between the ages of 18 and 20 (Steinberg, 1990).

Moral Development

Moral development parallels advances in reasoning and social cognition. With the attainment of abstract thought and the realization that people's perspectives and opinions may differ, the ways adolescents approach moral issues change. According to one theory of moral development (Kohlberg and Gilligan, 1972), older children and young adolescents function at a conventional level of moral reasoning in which absolute moral guidelines are seen to emanate from authorities such as parents or teachers. Thus judgments of right and wrong are made according to a set of concrete rules. A major concern is to act or behave in ways that will gain or maintain the approval of others. The correctness of society's rules is not questioned—one "does one's duty" by upholding and respecting the social order.

Elements of principled moral reasoning emerge during adolescence. With this level of reasoning, adolescents question absolutes and rules and view moral standards as subjective and based on points of view that are subject to disagreement. One may have a moral duty to abide by social standards for behavior, but only insofar as those standards support and serve human ends. Thus occasions arise in which social conventions ought to be questioned and when principles such as justice, caring, or quality of life take precedence over established social norms. Empirical research on Kohlberg's theory has demonstrated that aspects of both conventional and principled reasoning are present during adolescence, and different levels of reasoning are used at different times and in different situations.

Kohlberg's scheme of moral development focuses on an orientation to justice. This orientation holds as its ideal a morality based on reciprocity and equal respect. From this orientation the most important consideration in making moral decisions would be whether the individuals involved were treated "fairly" by the ultimate decision. Gilligan (1982) proposes that an equally valid alternative to the justice orientation is one that emphasizes caring. From this perspective, the ideal is a morality of attention to others and responses to human need. As opposed to the justice orientation, which assumes that moral decisions are best made from a detached position of objectivity, the caring orientation is rooted in the belief that moral decisions should be shaped by attachments and responsiveness to others. Studies have found that although both men and women are capable of approaching moral problems from the perspectives of justice and caring, women may be more likely to give caring-oriented responses before justice-oriented ones, whereas men are more likely to follow the opposite pattern (Gilligan, 1986; Walker, de Vries, and Trevethan, 1987).

Spiritual Development

Religious beliefs also become more abstract and principled during the adolescent years. Specifically, adolescents' beliefs become more oriented toward spiritual and ideologic matters and less oriented toward rituals, practice, and the strict observance of religious customs. Compared with children, adolescents place more emphasis on the internal aspects of religious commitment, such as what a person believes, and less on the external manifestations, such as whether an individual attends religious worship (Elkind, 1978).

Generally, the stated importance of participation in organized religion declines somewhat during the adolescent years. More high school students than postsecondary school young people attend religious services regularly, and, not surprisingly, the younger the adolescents, the more likely they are to view religion as being important to them. Among older adolescents, the importance of organized religion declines more among college students than among those not in college. Late adolescence appears to be a time when individuals reexamine and reevaluate many of the beliefs and values of their childhood. Consistent with developmental changes in value autonomy, the religious beliefs of young people are likely to become more personalized and less bound to the traditional religious practices they may have been exposed to when they were younger.

Although religious cults and dramatic religious conversion have attracted a great deal of attention in the media, they remain rare phenomena among American adolescents and often reflect nonreligious concerns. Membership in a religious cult is often associated with a preceding period of psychologic stress, identity diffusion, rootlessness, and dissatisfaction with mainstream societal values.

PSYCHOSOCIAL DEVELOPMENT

Identity Development

The task of identity formation is to develop a stable, coherent picture of oneself that includes integrating one's past and present experiences with a sense of where one is headed in the future. Before adolescence the child's identity is like pieces of a puzzle scattered on a table. Both cognitive development and social situations encountered during adolescence push individuals to combine puzzle pieces—to reflect on their place in society, the way others view them, their own sense of self-worth, and their options for the future. For most individuals, puzzle pieces first form a coherent whole sometime during late adolescence and early adulthood. Erik Erikson, one of the most influential theorists in the area of psychosocial development, describes identity achievement as one of the main psychosocial tasks of the adolescent years. According to Erikson (1968), "From among all possible and imaginable relations [the adolescent] must make a series of ever-narrowing selections of personal, occupational, sexual, and ideological commitments."

Social forces play a large role in shaping an adolescent's sense of self. Erikson (1968) argues that the key to identity achievement lies in adolescents' interactions with others. The people with whom a young person interacts serve as mirrors that reflect information back to the adolescent about whom she or he is and who she or he ought to be. During the period of identity formation, adolescents also learn from others what they ought to keep doing and what they ought not to do. Society also plays an important role in determining the range of available alternatives open to young people involved in identity formation. Optimally, adolescents have the opportunity to explore a range of possible options related to ideologic, occupational, and interpersonal roles before making an identity commitment.

The status of personal commitments in occupational, social, and ideologic domains can measure progress towards identity achievement. The status of personal commitments has four proposed levels: achievement, moratorium, foreclosure, and diffusion (Marcia, 1966). Individuals who demonstrate identity achievement have established a coherent identity after actively exploring possible alternatives; individuals currently engaged in this exploration are in moratorium. Foreclosure refers to making identity commitments without a period of exploration or experimentation, and identity diffusion refers to a lack of firm identity commitments, along with a lack of effort to make those commitments. During adolescence, many individuals progress from diffusion to moratorium to identity achievement, or, alternatively, from diffusion to foreclosure.

Experiences and opportunities within one's social environment influence both the content of identity and progression toward identity achievement. Among ethnic minority adolescents, identity foreclosure may be more common than among teenagers from the majority culture because of restricted opportunities to explore alternative roles. Identity diffusion also appears to be more common among minority boys and men than among other groups. Possible barriers to identity formation among minority youth may include conflicting values between their minority ethnic group and the broader society, a lack of adult role models who exemplify positive ethnic identity, and inadequate preparation for stereotyping and prejudice that are frequently experienced. However, many ethnic minority adolescents develop effective bicultural identities and abilities to navigate the cultural expectations of home and society, and positive connections to cultural identities can foster healthy adolescent development.

Development of Autonomy

Becoming an autonomous, self-governing person is another of the fundamental psychosocial tasks of adolescence. Autonomy includes emotional, cognitive, and behavioral components. Emotional autonomy is that aspect of independence related to changes in an individual's close relationships, and behavioral autonomy is the capacity to make independent decisions and follow through with them. Generally, emotional and behavioral autonomy are likely to surface as psychosocial concerns somewhat earlier during adolescence than value autonomy, which usually does not become a prominent concern until middle or late adolescence.

Individuals generally begin the process of emotional autonomy during early adolescence by becoming more emotionally independent from their parents but less separate from their friends. In the process of separating from their parents, younger adolescents often shift a portion of their emotional ties to other adults, often developing "crushes" on teachers, coaches, celebrities, or the parent of a best friend. By the end of adolescence, individuals are less emotionally dependent on their parents than they were as children. This emotional autonomy can be seen in several ways. First, older adolescents do not generally rush to their parents when they are worried or upset. Second, they no longer see their parents as all-knowing or all-powerful. Third, teenagers often have more emotional energy invested in relationships outside their families. Finally, older adolescents are able to see and interact with their parents as people, not just as their parents.

As adolescents increasingly find themselves in situations where adults are not present and where they must make decisions and take responsibility for their own actions, the extent to which they are capable of independent decision making and autonomous behavior takes on added importance. An individual who is behaviorally autonomous is able to turn to others for advice when it is appropriate, weigh alternative courses of action based on his or her own judgment and the suggestions of others, and reach an independent conclusion about how to behave. Behavioral autonomy includes the ability to make independent decisions based on one's own choices rather than conforming to the opinions of others. Decision-making abilities improve over the adolescent years, with older adolescents being more likely than younger adolescents to be aware of risks and benefits involved with a particular decision, to consider future consequences, to turn to "experts" for advice, and to realize when vested interests may influence the advice of others. Conformity to parents' opinions declines during early adolescence. However, conformity to peer influence increases during this time. During middle and late adolescence, conformity to both parent and peer opinions declines, allowing for genuine behavioral autonomy. Subjective feelings of self-reliance increase steadily over the adolescent years.

In contrast to popular stereotypes, the development of autonomy during adolescence does not typically involve rebellion, nor is it usually accompanied by strained or tense family relationships. In households where guidelines for adolescent behavior are clear and consistently enforced; where changes in guidelines are open to discussion; and where an atmosphere of interpersonal warmth, concern, and fairness exists, family relationships nurture a gradual and smooth maturational process over the course of the adolescent years. Problems in the development of autonomy are often understandable reactions to excessively controlling circumstances or to growing up in the absence of clear standards. In addition to dispelling the myths that major parent-child conflicts and adolescent rebellion are essential to the development of autonomy, research has shown that parent and peer influences are not necessarily opposing forces but can play complementary roles in the development of a healthy degree of individual independence.

Achievement

Another set of psychosocial tasks encountered during adolescence centers around achievement. Broadly speaking, achievement concerns the development of motives, capabilities, interests, and behaviors related to performance in evaluative situations. The study of achievement during adolescence has focused almost exclusively on young people's performance in educational settings and on the development and implementation of plans for future scholastic and occupational careers. Various theories have attempted to explain why some young people achieve at higher levels in school. Some have focused on differences in individuals' motivations to succeed. Others have examined young people's beliefs about success and failure. Still others have pointed to differences in adolescents' opportunities for success and to the roles of important adults and peers in their lives. Various indicators of achievement are highly interrelated. For example, success in school during the early elementary years leads to later success in school; doing well in school generally leads to higher levels of educational attainment, which in turn lead to more challenging forms of employment with greater earning power.

Although there are distinct differences among different occupations, the actual process leading toward occupational achievement can be a lengthy one in contemporary society. Because career options have expanded and changed so dramatically, and because increasing numbers of individuals enter college after completing high school, many people do not decide on a career until well into adulthood.

A definite relationship exists between social class and both educational and occupational achievement. A significant problem facing those interested in promoting achievement during adolescence is socioeconomic disparities in educational

and occupational achievement. Beginning in early childhood, through no action of their own, many individuals find themselves on an educational course that directs them toward low levels of academic achievement, curtailed schooling, and limited occupational mobility. They reach adulthood with little hope and few dreams for their future. Understanding how this course is set in motion and identifying factors that help individuals from economically disadvantaged backgrounds succeed despite tremendous barriers are necessary steps in building interventions that promote the development and health of these young people.

Sexuality

Adolescence represents a critical time in the development of sexuality. Hormonal, physical, cognitive, and social changes that occur during adolescence all have an impact on sexual development. Of all the developmental changes that affect adolescent sexuality, none is more obvious than the impact of puberty. Adolescents must come to terms with hormonal influences, physiologic manifestations such as menstruation and ejaculation, and physical changes such as breast and genital development. All these changes have a profound impact on the way teenagers perceive their bodies (i.e., body image). In addition to transitions in body image, increasing levels of pubertal hormones contribute to increased levels of sexual motivation among both boys and girls. Evidence also suggests that early development of secondary sexual characteristics is associated with early sexual activity. For example, some early-maturing girls begin dating earlier and may have sexual intercourse at younger ages than their peers (Doswell, Millor, Thompson, et al, 1998). Even when physical development occurs at an average onset and pace, the degree to which adolescents feel comfortable with their bodies may affect sexual behaviors.

Changes in sexual motivations and feelings, happening at the same time as shifts in cognitive skills, contribute to painful conjectures ("Is what I'm feeling normal?"), self-conscious concern ("Am I good looking enough?"), and hypothetical thinking ("What if she wants to have sex?"). The emergence of formal operational thinking also increases adolescents' decision-making capabilities concerning sexual issues. As they mature, teenagers become better able to think through potential risks and benefits of sexual behaviors before they engage in them. Older adolescents may also be able to conceptualize more long-term consequences of present behaviors. One of the important tasks of adolescence is to incorporate sexuality successfully into intimate relationships (Sullivan, 1953). This task is made possible by the advanced cognitive abilities that emerge over the course of adolescence.

Part of adolescent identity formation involves the development of sexual identity. As they begin to integrate changes involved with puberty, young adolescents also develop emotional and social identities separate from their families. For young adolescents, the process of sexual identity development usually involves forming close friendships with same-sex peers, with whom they may experiment sexually, often to satisfy curiosity. Sexual activity among young teenagers varies by gender. Masturbation provides an opportunity for sexual self-exploration; participation in this behavior is influenced by learned cultural attitudes and sex-role expectations. Boys typically begin masturbating during early adolescence; the age of first masturbation varies greatly for girls. Although some girls begin masturbating during early adolescence, many do not masturbate until after they have had intercourse. Similarly, a small number of teens may engage in oral sex during early adolescence, but the percentage of teens who report oral sex at each age is similar to the percentage of teens who report sexual intercourse, suggesting that oral sex does not necessarily precede intercourse (Brewster and Tillman, 2008; Smith, Stewart, Peled, et al, 2009). Although the age of initiating sexual intercourse has been getting older among teens in the past decade in the United States, about one third of teens have had sexual intercourse by age 15. These young people are at high risk for STIs and pregnancy.

Many teenagers begin to make a shift from relationships with same-gender peers to intimate relationships with opposite-gender partners during middle adolescence (Fig. 19-8). Opposite-gender relationships typically begin with peer activities involving both boys and girls. Pairing off as couples becomes more common as middle adolescence progresses. The type and degree of seriousness of partner relationships vary. Initial relationships are usually noncommittal, extremely mobile, and seldom characterized by any deep romantic attachments. Sexual activity (whether with same- or opposite-gender partners) becomes more common during middle to late adolescence. Nationally, approximately 38% of ninth-grade boys and 27% of girls report having had sexual intercourse. By twelfth grade, 62% of boys and 68% of girls report having had intercourse (Eaton, Kann, Kinchen, et al, 2008). Around 11% of girls and 5% of boys report same-gender sexual partners (Mulye, Park, Nelson, et al, 2009).

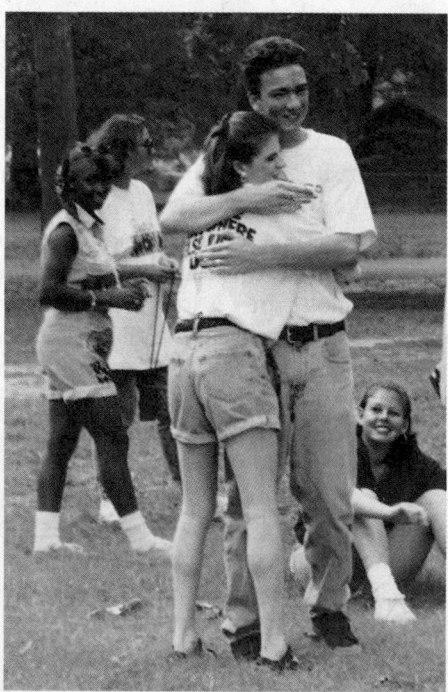

Fig. 19-8 Romantic relationships are an important part of adolescence.

The relationship between love and sexual expression is brought into focus during middle adolescence. Most young people oppose exploitation, pressure, or force in sex as well as sex solely for the sake of physical enjoyment without a personal relationship. Many adolescents find it hard to believe that sex can exist without love; therefore they view each relationship as real love. However, some teen social groups have embraced norms that include sexual relationships with friends who are not considered exclusive romantic partners, but rather "friends with benefits."

The meaning and implication of sexual activity as it affects psychosocial development may be quite different for adolescent boys and girls; that is, sexual socialization differs for males and females in our society. Typically, adolescent boys' first sexual experiences are in early adolescence through masturbation. Before adolescent boys begin dating, they have generally already experienced orgasm and know how to arouse themselves sexually. For boys, the development of sexuality during adolescence revolves around efforts to integrate the formation of close relationships into an already existing sense of sexual capability. Girls' first sexual experiences are likely to be different and to carry different meanings. Masturbation is a less prevalent activity among girls, and it is less regularly practiced. The adolescent girl, in contrast to the adolescent boy, is more likely to experience sexual intercourse for the first time in a perceived close relationship. For girls, the development of sexuality involves the integration of sexual activity into an existing capacity for emotional involvement.

An integrated sexual identity often emerges during late adolescence as individuals incorporate sexual experiences, feelings, and knowledge. For most, this identity is consistent with their own physical and mental capacities and with societal limits and expectations. Most older adolescents identify themselves as being predominantly heterosexual or mostly heterosexual, with a smaller number self-identifying as bisexual, or gay or lesbian; an even smaller group is still unsure of their sexual orientation, although this varies somewhat by ethnicity (Russell, Seif, and Truong, 2001; Saewyc, Poon, Wang, et al, 2007). Whatever their sexual orientation, most older teenagers possess the capacity to have intimate relationships that satisfy the emotional and sexual needs of both partners.

Sexual orientation is an important aspect of sexual identity. **Sexual orientation** is defined as a pattern of sexual arousal or romantic attraction toward persons of the opposite gender (heterosexual), of the same gender (homosexual, often called gay or lesbian), or of both genders (bisexual). Sexual orientation encompasses several dimensions, including attraction, fantasy, actual sexual behavior, and self-labeling or group affiliation. In individuals the direction and intensity of each dimension are not necessarily consistent with any of the others. For example, individuals may be attracted most strongly to their same gender, fantasize about both genders, have sexual activity only with the opposite gender, and identify as gay or lesbian. Other individuals may engage in same-gender sexual behavior, fantasize about both genders, but identify as heterosexual. As with all aspects of sexual identity, cultural meaning and expectation, gender, peer groups, opportunities for intimacy, and other environmental contexts all influence sexual orientation. Research has suggested that the trajectory of developing sexual orientation may be different for boys and girls, and that girls' sexual behaviors and attractions may be more fluid (Diamond, 2000).

Adolescence is the period during which individuals commonly begin to identify their sexual orientation as part of their developing sexual identity. However, cultural beliefs and values, societal and family pressures, or a lack of similar peers can influence this identification process. The majority of adolescents eventually report an orientation toward exclusively heterosexual relationships. For adolescents whose orientation encompasses any same-gender dimensions, the identity process during adolescence can be complicated, especially when community norms disapprove of orientations other than heterosexual. Adolescents who have witnessed harassment or violence directed at gay, lesbian, and bisexual people, for example, may be reluctant to self-identify, even when their attractions and behaviors are exclusively same-gender or bisexual. In several population-based studies throughout the 1990s, researchers found approximately 1% to 5% of adolescents identify as gay, lesbian, or bisexual, whereas 3% to 12% report same-gender or bisexual orientation in one or more of the other dimensions of sexual orientation (Reis and Saewyc, 1999).

The development of sexual orientation as part of sexual identity includes several developmental milestones during late childhood and throughout adolescence. These milestones do not necessarily occur in the same order for everyone, nor are they completed in the same amount of time (Rosario, Meyey-Bahlburg, Hunter, et al, 1996). They include (1) the realization of romantic or erotic attraction to people of one (or both) genders; (2) erotic daydreaming about one or both genders; (3) romantic partners or dates without sexual activity; (4) sexual activity with people of the preferred gender or genders (also, for some teens, sexual activity with a nonpreferred gender, due to curiosity or social pressure); (5) self-identification of the orientation that best fits one's current circumstances and understanding; (6) publicly self-identifying that orientation, usually to intimate friends and family first, then the wider social group; and (7) an intimate, committed sexual relationship with a person of the gender appropriate to one's orientation.

The order of these milestones varies greatly among adolescents, but adolescents who identify as gay, lesbian, or bisexual tend to publicly self-identify later than their heterosexual peers. Without positive gay, lesbian, or bisexual role models or a supportive peer group, sexual minority teens can feel isolated, and they may not share their orientation with anyone for fear of rejection or violence (see Critical Thinking Exercise). When adolescents who would otherwise identify as bisexual can only find a peer group of gay and lesbian teens, they may focus on their same-gender dimensions of orientation and adopt the label of lesbian or gay; later, they may self-label as bisexual. Likewise, some gay and lesbian adolescents may first identify as heterosexual, then bisexual, before identifying as gay or lesbian. In studies among self-identified gay, lesbian, bisexual, and heterosexual adolescents, many of the adolescents report changing their self-labels one or more times during their adolescence and beyond (Rosario, Meyey-Bahlburg, Hunter, et al, 1996; Diamond, 2000).

> ### ❓ CRITICAL THINKING EXERCISE
> #### *Discussing Sexual Orientation with Adolescents*
>
> John, a 17-year-old adolescent, comes into the school-based clinic and tells the nurse practitioner that he thinks he is gay. What is the most appropriate response for the nurse practitioner?
> 1. Evidence—Is there sufficient evidence to draw any conclusions about John's sexual orientation at this time?
> 2. Assumptions—Describe an underlying assumption about each of the following issues:
>   a. Sexual orientation in adolescents
>   b. Society's reaction to homosexuality
>   c. Health care professionals and sexuality
> 3. What implications and priorities for nursing care can be drawn at this time?
> 4. Does the evidence support your argument (conclusion)?

Although only a few states in the United States, some European countries, and Canada legally recognize same-gender marriages at present, some religious faiths and social groups do celebrate committed same-gender couples' relationships. There is no evidence that gay, lesbian, or bisexual adults are more or less likely to create long-term, stable relationships than are heterosexual couples. It should be noted that bisexual adolescents and adults do not generally engage in sexual relationships with both genders concurrently; self-identification as bisexual usually refers to the ability to be attracted to either gender but does not imply that such a person requires partners of both genders, or that one must be equally attracted to and have sexual experience with both genders in order to be bisexual.

Intimacy

Intimate relationships are emotional attachments between two people characterized by concern for each other's well-being; a willingness to disclose private, possibly sensitive topics; and a sharing of common interests and activities. Intimate relationships are distinct from sexual relationships. It is possible for individuals to have close relationships without becoming sexually involved. At the same time, people can be involved in sexual relationships that are not particularly intimate.

It is not until adolescence—a time characterized by pubertal changes, advances in social cognitive abilities, and broadening of social worlds—that truly intimate relationships first emerge. Adolescents' close friendships are more likely to include a strong emotional foundation in which individuals understand and care about each other. The development of intimacy during adolescence involves changes in the adolescent's needs for intimacy and in the capacity and opportunities to have intimate friendships. Puberty and its resultant changes in sexual impulses often raise new issues and concerns requiring serious, intimate discussions. Over the course of the adolescent years, individuals become more capable of and interested in emotional closeness with other people. The greater degree of behavioral independence often accompanying the transition into adolescence provides more opportunities for teenagers to be alone with friends and to come into meaningful contact with adults outside their families. Although research on intimacy during adolescence has focused on peer friendships, intimate relationships are by no means limited to peers. Teenagers may also develop intimate relationships with parents, siblings, and adults who are not part of their immediate families.

Harry Stack Sullivan (1953) was among the first to describe the developmental course of intimacy. Usually adolescents develop the capacity for intimacy through preadolescent and early adolescent relationships with same-gender peers. Intimate relationships with opposite-sex peers develop relatively late during adolescence. Opposite-gender friendships may play a more important role in the development of intimacy among boys than among girls, who may develop and experience intimacy with other girls earlier in adolescence.

Individuals move through a series of stages in their close relationships with others. Many adolescents move into role-focused friendships, behaving in ways that are dominated by conventional norms. In their close relationships, individuals at this level attempt to avoid controversy and control their emotions. Role-focused persons are generally more concerned with conforming to the appropriate roles and norms in a relationship (e.g., what the "good" girlfriend does) than with a friend as an individual. It is not until later in adolescence that people develop the capacity for having individuated-connected friendships. With this level of friendship, individuals form intimate relationships with others that acknowledge the complexity and contradictions in close relationships. Differences in outlook between individuals are not only tolerated but encouraged as part of what makes the relationship vital.

Although teenagers may begin dating during early adolescence, these early dating relationships are not usually psychosocially intimate. Early dating relationships typically follow highly ritualized "scripts," in which adolescents are more likely to play stereotypic roles than to really be themselves. Participating in mixed-gender group activities, such as going to parties or other events, may have a positive impact on young teenagers' well-being. One-on-one dating during early adolescence, however, with a lot of time spent alone, may lead to sexual intimacy before a teen is ready. A moderate degree of dating, with serious relationships delayed until late adolescence, may be the ideal pattern of interpersonal involvement.

SOCIAL ENVIRONMENTS

Although all adolescents experience similar biologic and cognitive changes and face similar psychosocial tasks, the health-related effects of these changes are not the same for all people. Why aren't individuals affected in the same ways by puberty, by changes in thinking patterns, and by changes in social and legal status? The answer lies in the fact that biologic, cognitive, and social changes of adolescence are shaped by the social environment in which the changes take place (Bronfenbrenner, 1979). The social environment provides the opportunities, barriers, role models, and support for individuals' development and health. Systems within the social environment, including family, peers, schools, community (including Internet-based community), and the larger society, all contribute uniquely to an adolescent's development and health.

The nurse can use an ecologic model as a way of understanding adolescents' social environments (Bronfenbrenner, 1979). In this model the social environment is divided into proximal and more distal systems. The social environment includes microsystems, mesosystems, exosystems, and macrosystems.

Microsystems are the most proximal social contexts in which adolescents participate directly, such as family, peer groups, school, and the workplace. All these contexts have substantial influences on the development and health-related behaviors of adolescents (Perry, Kelder, and Komro, 1993).

The next layer of social environment, mesosystems, is formed by linkages between microsystems. The extent to which individuals in one microsystem are involved in other systems determines the strength or "richness" of the mesosystem. For example, regular interactions between family members and school personnel, which have positive effects on student achievement and school performance, reflect a rich mesosystem.

The third layer of social environment, exosystems, consists of settings that influence adolescent behavior and development but in which they do not directly participate. Many community-level influences fall within this layer. These include opportunities within a community for health-enhancing or health-compromising behaviors, such as the availability of age-appropriate activities for young people that do not include alcohol, tobacco, or drugs.

The most distal social environment, macrosystems, consists of culturally based belief systems and economic and political systems. These systems can have profound effects on young people's health-related behaviors and development, mostly through their influences on more proximal systems. Social systems are embedded within each other, and what happens within one system can influence what happens in others. To have the most impact on adolescent health promotion, interventions must address multiple environmental systems.

Families

Over the past several decades, changes have taken place within the family microsystem that have important implications for adolescent health. Higher rates of divorce and remarriage, increasing numbers of single-parent or blended families, and greater percentages of working mothers have become characteristic of contemporary U.S. society. The "ideal" family consisting of an employed father, an at-home mother, and two or more school-age children is no longer the norm for American society. Higher rates of divorce and the decisions of single women to have children have increased the number of U.S. children spending at least part of their childhood in a single-parent family. Correspondingly, many young people find themselves in blended families, thus developing relationships with stepparents during their adolescent years. A growing number of same-gender couples are raising their own or adopted children as well; in the 2000 census, an estimated 250,000 households were headed by same-gender partners (Bennett and Gates, 2004). Changes in family structure have been accompanied by changes in parent work patterns and a dramatic increase in the percentage of mothers who work outside the home (Gottfried and Gottfried, 1994). (See Family Structure, Chapter 3.)

These changes in family structure and parent employment have resulted in young people having more time unsupervised by adults with increased time alone or with peers. Although for mature adolescents little risk may be involved with minimum supervision, for less competent teenagers, decreased adult supervision may result in more risk-taking behaviors, such as substance use and sexual intercourse. Poorly monitored teenagers may also socialize with peers who engage in risky behaviors. Lack of adult supervision also decreases adolescents' opportunities for communication and intimacy with a parent or other supportive adults. Although quantity of time does not guarantee quality, sufficient quantity is necessary for communication and the development of intimate relationships.

Consistently, adolescents who feel close to their parents show more positive psychosocial development and behavioral competence, less susceptibility to negative peer pressure, and lower tendencies to be involved in risk-taking behaviors (Resnick, Bearman, Blum, et al, 1997; Smith, Stewart, Peled, et al, 2009). In many situations lack of direct adult supervision may be counterbalanced by parent monitoring and communication about adolescents' activities during parental absence.

On the other hand, in dysfunctional or abusive families, spending greater amounts of time with parents may compromise the health of teenagers. In these situations the type and content of communication may be the most important factors to address.

In addition to adult supervision, the overall parenting style affects adolescent development. Both effective conflict resolution within families and family cohesion create environments conducive to healthy adolescent development. These two characteristics, along with parent expectations for mature behavior on the part of the adolescent and the practice of setting and enforcing reasonable limits for behavior, form the basis of effective parenting. This parenting style, termed **authoritative parenting**, is related to greater psychosocial maturity and school performance and less substance abuse among young people.

Adolescents from low-income households are more likely than other adolescents to spend less supervised time with adults, to have parents working at more than one job, to drop out of high school, and to experience violence in their homes and communities. Although disorder within their larger social environments often creates a need for a buffer, which could include spending quality time with adults, poor adolescents often experience fewer of these health-enhancing activities.

Nurses should be cautious, however, in attributing differences in adolescent risk behaviors to racial or ethnic group membership, socioeconomic status, or family structure.

Peer Groups

One hallmark of adolescence is the increasing value young people place on friendships and relationships with peers (Fig. 19-9). Adolescents spend more time with their peers than do children. Compared with children, their peer groups are more autonomous and are more likely to include members of the opposite sex. Because of the changes that have taken place within family systems in contemporary society, peer groups play a significant role in the socialization of adolescents.

Peers serve as credible sources of information, role models of new social behaviors, sources of social reinforcement, and bridges to alternative lifestyles. Close and supportive peer friendships have beneficial effects for young people (Fig. 19-10). However, adolescents with greater peer identification than parental identification, especially when peers model and support

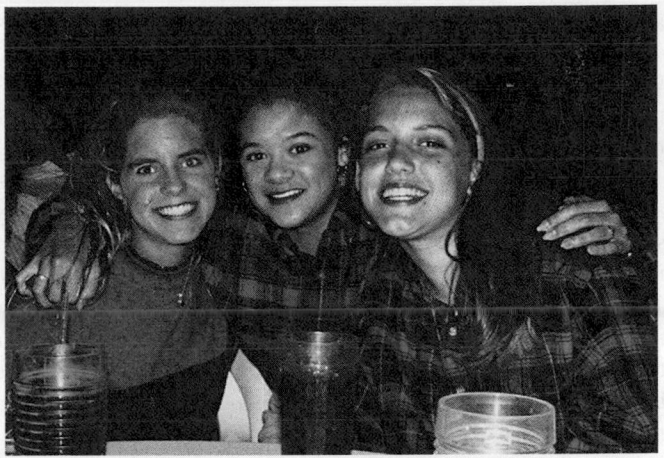

Fig. 19-9 The peer group is a major influence in adolescent development.

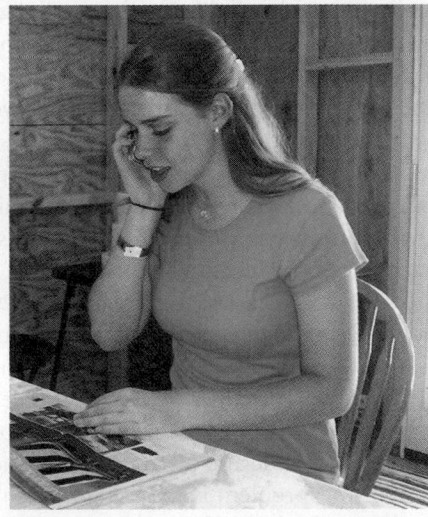

Fig. 19-10 The cell phone allows adolescents to talk or text message for hours with peers.

problem behaviors, are more prone to negative and health-compromising behaviors. Thus the transition to greater peer involvement, like other developmental transitions of adolescence, is a process requiring guidance; skills; and, optimally, a prolonged time to complete the transition. At a time when they are developing interpersonal skills to deal with peer pressure, young adolescents who lack adult supervision and opportunities for communication with adults may be more susceptible to peer influences and at a higher risk for poor peer-group selection than teenagers who have close relationships with caring adults.

The heightened value placed on adolescent peer relationships leads to questions about the quality and nature of peer influence. Rather than thinking of all peer influence as either good or bad, it is important to recognize that the influence of peers varies from one adolescent to another, from one peer group to another, and across different societies and cultures. Adolescents' selection of peer groups seems to be most strongly influenced by sociodemographic factors and by common patterns of behavior, including, for example, substance use, school achievement, and religious participation. Peers can have either positive or negative effects on adolescent behavior. Negative effects include increased substance use, gang membership, and violent behaviors. Positive effects include an orientation supporting academic achievement, an environmental commitment, or a commitment to religious or social youth groups.

Peers can also be a positive force in health promotion. Same-age and older adolescents can encourage healthy behavior by serving as positive role models and promoting positive health norms in the peer group (Rosenfeld, Keenan, Fox, et al, 2000; Tuttle, Bidwell-Cerone, Campbell-Heider, et al, 2000). For most adolescents, prosocial pressures from peers are greater than antisocial ones, and adolescents are influenced more by prosocial or neutral pressures than by pressures toward misconduct.

Schools

In contemporary society, schools play an increasingly important role in preparing young people for adulthood. Schooling is essential for a successful future for both boys and girls. Failure to complete high school reduces employment opportunities and the probability of earning an adequate income. Yet many schools in the United States do not meet the developmental needs of all young people.

Many minority-group members are not at appropriate grade levels for their age, and the dropout rate among minority students is higher than among nonminority students. However, gains have been made in educational attainment in the past 30 years; in 2004, 93% of Caucasian adults ages 25 to 29 years had graduated from high school, as had 88% of African-American young adults, and the number of African-Americans attending college and completing bachelor's degrees doubled over the same time period (US Census Bureau, 2004). Dropout rates are still highest among Hispanic and Native American adolescents.

Another important problem is the lack of parental involvement in schools. Parental involvement increases the effectiveness of schools at all levels. However, with the larger number of single-parent and two–working parent families, parents have less time for involvement in schools.

The timing of school transition may be important, especially if the school environment is not appropriate to the adolescent's developmental needs. In particular, the transition into a middle or junior high school at age 12 or 13 typically occurs at the same time as the rapid physical changes of puberty.

Another characteristic of school that may have negative effects is a system of grading that acknowledges few young people for their academic successes. Teenagers whose grades fall below average may spend much of their time in environments in which they perceive negative evaluations by adult authorities. As a result, they may feel alienated from school. Subgroups of adolescents may unite and develop countercultures or exhibit antisocial behavior. This process may be most intense for young people from poorer families who attend schools that include students from a broad range of socioeconomic classes.

In addition, students who repeat one or more grades exhibit greater emotional distress than those who do not repeat grades (Resnick, Bearman, Blum, et al, 1997). Students with below-average grades are more likely to be engaged in health-compromising behaviors such as tobacco and alcohol use, unprotected sexual intercourse, and suicide attempts.

The social environment of schools has an impact on student outcomes. Small classroom size and small school size are both related to higher-quality social environments within schools. Safety and respect for all students are critical issues, since students have difficulty learning in unsafe environments, where bullying occurs and is not addressed. In many schools, violence and harassment of students on the basis of race, gender, or sexual orientation is common, affecting more than half of all students (Saewyc, Singh, Reis, et al, 2000). Students targeted for repeated teasing and harassment are more likely to skip school, to report symptoms of depression, and to attempt suicide (Eisenberg and Aalsma, 2005). Equally troubling, teens who are regularly harassed or bullied are also more likely to bring weapons to school to feel safe. In 2007, 20% of adolescents nationwide reported carrying a weapon one or more days in the past month, which is a decline since 1991, when 27% of youth reported carrying a weapon (Mulye, Park, Nelson, et al, 2009). School practices and conditions that lead to better student outcomes stress the importance of supportive environments that foster positive peer group relationships, promote health and fitness, encourage family involvement in school, and strengthen connections between schools and communities.

Work

For the majority of young people in the United States, the workplace becomes a fourth microsystem. Most teenagers are employed in a relatively restricted array of jobs as restaurant workers, cashiers, sales clerks, clerical assistants, and unskilled laborers. The jobs tend to be monotonous, require little initiative or decision making, and rarely use skills learned in school. Furthermore, some are highly stressful, requiring work under extreme time pressure.

Adolescent work as it exists today may negatively affect development. The typical teenager's job fails to provide continuity to adult employment or links to adults who could serve as vocational mentors. In addition, the monotonous nature of many adolescent jobs is neither intellectually stimulating nor related to role experimentation involved in identity development. Rather, involvement in work may take time away from other activities that could contribute to identity development. Greater involvement in work can also lead to fatigue, decreased interest in school, reduced extracurricular involvement, and poorer grades. Detrimental effects are especially likely for adolescents who work more than 20 hours a week.

Although much work done by teenagers may not contribute to healthy development, jobs that allow young people to develop intellectual and social skills, to have some autonomy, or to feel that their contributions matter can be positive experiences. Jobs that provide adolescents with experiences relevant to future employment or that link them to adults who can serve as vocational mentors may be especially valuable.

Technology as a Social Environment

In the past decade a number of emerging technologies have influenced adolescent social relationships and development. The widespread availability of the Internet and access to social networking websites such as FaceBook, chatrooms, free e-mail, blogs, and Twitter have created "virtual" communities and ways for young people to interact with others; web cameras even allow those interactions to include real-time video communication. Cellular telephones offer more mobile opportunities to talk on the phone, send text messages, send photos, or use video phone capabilities. Young people are no longer limited in their friendships or communities to those who live geographically close. But how do adolescents use these technologies, and how do they influence health and risk behaviors?

Recent studies show increasingly universal access to the Internet and computers. A study in 2004 found that nearly two thirds of urban youth in New York had computer access at home (Bleakley, Merzel, VanDevanter, et al, 2004), whereas a population study in 2008 found that 99% of students in a western Canadian province had access to a computer at home (Smith, Stewart, Peled, et al, 2009).

The Internet chatrooms and social networking sites have created a more public arena for trying out identities and developing interpersonal skills with a wider network of people, occasionally with anonymity. This can create opportunities for young people who have a limited access to friends (because of rural location, shyness, or rare chronic conditions) to interact with people like themselves. However, most adolescents appear to be using the online social environment to interact with the same peers they spend their day with at school.

Text messaging via cell phones has become a common activity and can sometimes be disruptive during school. In addition, both the online and text environment can create opportunities for cyberbullying, where teens engage in insults, harassment, and publicly humiliating statements online or on cell phones. These can evoke responses as distressing as those to bullying in the school setting; there are reports of youth committing suicide after being the target of cyberbullying, and estimates of the prevalence of cyberbullying are similar to reports of in-person bullying and harassment.

Another problematic form of technology use is "sexting," or the electronic transmission of sexual comments, suggestive pictures, or even sexually explicit photos, primarily via cell phones. Although teens may intend to send the picture or comment only to a boyfriend or girlfriend, they cannot control what happens to the photo after that, whether it is shared with others or even posted online. Some states and countries have laws that consider the transmission of such photos of teens as distributing child pornography and have responded with criminal charges. It is important to help teens think about the possible consequences of posting images on websites or sending them to friends.

Studies have noted that teens are not only enthusiastic technology users, but frequently use multiple types of media at the same time. They may be listening to music on their digital music player while the television is on, and they are surfing the Internet to do their homework and texting friends on their cell phone or on their computer. It is unclear at present how this multitasking and multiple media exposure will affect development of the brain and attention, but frequent media use has been associated with late nights and sleep deprivation. In addition, there are some demonstrated affective and behavioral effects among adolescents who are exposed to high levels of violence or sexual content in the media they use, which can become a cause of concern for health promotion (Brown, L'Engle, Pardun, et al, 2006).

There is increased concern focusing on adolescent vehicle driving and concurrent handheld cellular phone usage. Studies have shown that drivers using handheld devices are considerably more distracted and spend less time looking at the road or paying attention to driving conditions (Hosking, Young, and Regan, 2009). Many states have outlawed the use of handheld mobile devices while actively operating a vehicle (McCartt, Hellinga, and Bratiman, 2006).

Community and Society

Society influences adolescent health and development indirectly through the structures of social institutions, division of economic wealth, and construction and implementation of public policies. Society also provides a dominant set of values and expectations for behavior to which adolescents are exposed. These values and expectations are transmitted through the mass media, local institutions, and social networks.

In the United States, adolescence is a time during which individuals are expected to make the transition from childhood to adulthood. Adolescents are given more autonomy than children and are also expected to show more responsible behavior. Young people are given more personal control over health-related behaviors but often fail to receive necessary guidance, support, or access to positive adult role models. At the same time, society seeks to limit adolescents' involvement in some risk-taking behaviors that may convey adult status, such as alcohol and tobacco use or sexual behaviors. Many of these same behaviors are glamorized through media programming and advertising campaigns directed at teenagers. For some teenagers faced with societal expectations to "grow up," risk-taking behaviors take on specific functional meanings. Behaviors such as substance use or unsafe sex may offer adolescents opportunities to challenge social authority, demonstrate autonomy, or gain social approval.

Local communities, as part of the broader societal context, also influence adolescents' capacity for healthy development. The local community has a more proximal influence on adolescents' motivations and opportunities to engage in health-enhancing or risk-taking behaviors. For example, adults within the community serve as direct role models, affecting adolescents' expectations concerning their likely roles and activities as adults. Communities with a high proportion of employed, well-educated, financially successful adults provide a different array of models than impoverished neighborhoods predominated by poor households, chronic illness, and drug abuse, where the financially successful adults are those involved in illicit activities. Such environmental characteristics affect young people's expectations for the future, their perceptions of how current behavior could jeopardize future chances, and, consequently, their motivation to avoid high-risk behavior.

A community's economic resources play a significant role in the health and well-being of young people. Resources affect opportunities for health promotion (e.g., by influencing the quality of local schools and health-related services). Schools in wealthy areas can provide high-quality education that will enhance students' interest in school and their chances of future success. Wealthy communities also provide opportunities for alternative, health-enhancing activities through community clubs and organizations. Thus community resources influence the type and number of health risks young people face and the local capacity for health promotion.

PROMOTING OPTIMUM HEALTH DURING ADOLESCENCE

Health promotion involves empowering individuals, families, and communities to take developmentally and contextually appropriate actions toward realizing their potential. It includes physical, cognitive, emotional, and social dimensions. For adolescents, health promotion involves helping youth acquire the power (including knowledge, attitudes, and skills), authority (permission to use their power), and opportunities to make choices that increase the likelihood of their creating positive expressions of health for themselves in their contexts.

A comprehensive approach to health promotion combines activities aimed at individuals with interventions focused on changing norms, attitudes, and behaviors of peer groups, families, communities, and society at large. For example, prevention of tobacco use involves more than a teacher's lecture on the consequences of cigarette and smokeless tobacco use, a ban on tobacco use in schools, a parent's admonition not to smoke, or a nurse's question to an adolescent about smoking history. In reality, it requires all these components and more. Effective health promotion requires the support of many individuals and institutions that affect the lives of adolescents.

The rationale for focusing on these health issues becomes obvious when one examines the major sources of mortality and morbidity during adolescence. The primary causes of mortality during adolescence are injuries, homicide, and suicide; together these three causes are responsible for 75% of all adolescent deaths. Major causes of adolescent morbidity include the use of motor and recreational vehicles, sexual and physical abuse, sexual activity such as unwanted pregnancy and STIs, and substance use. Mental disorders, chronic illness, eating disorders, and oral health problems are other important sources of morbidity (Eaton, Kann, Kinchen, et al, 2008). Chapters 20 and 21 provide further information about threats to adolescent health and well-being.

A number of inequities exist in relation to health status among subsets of the U.S. population. Adolescents are one subgroup that experiences health inequities. For example, a substantial gap in life expectancy exists between African-American and Caucasian adolescents. African-American and Native American males have a higher risk of premature death than any other racial or ethnic group. Adolescent males die at a rate more than twice that of girls. Mortality rates increase by more than 200% between early and late adolescence. There are also age differences in the causes of death, with a shift toward more violent deaths occurring in late adolescence. Among Caucasian adolescents a dramatic increase in suicide occurs during later adolescence, making it the second leading cause of death in this group. For older African-American adolescents, homicide ranks as the most likely cause of death. Similar to mortality, patterns of morbidity vary within the adolescent population. For example, rates of vehicular injury are high among males, whereas for females morbidities associated with "quietly disturbed" behaviors such as eating disorders and emotional distress are common (Eaton, Kann, Kinchen, et al, 2008).

ADOLESCENTS' PERSPECTIVES ON HEALTH

To be most effective, adolescent health promotion efforts must incorporate adolescents' perspectives on what health means. Such efforts also must focus on adolescents' concerns and priorities related to health and health care services. From a positive perspective, adolescents' developmentally based sense of curiosity and movement toward autonomy provide opportunities for health promotion that should not be wasted.

Adolescents define health in much the same way as adults: health means being able to live up to one's potential; being able to function physically, mentally, and socially; and experiencing positive emotional states. The content of their definitions often goes beyond an "absence of illness" and includes what can be done to maintain and enhance health.

Adolescents' health-related interests and concerns include stress and anxiety, relationships with adults and peers, weight, acne, and feelings of sadness or depression. Health concerns are often consistent with the immediate developmental tasks that teenagers face. For example, younger adolescents—in the midst of the physical changes of puberty—have a particular interest in issues related to growth and development. In the process of making transitions from middle or junior high school to senior high school, middle adolescents have questions and concerns related to peer-group acceptance, relationships with friends, and physical appearance. Older adolescents focus increasingly on school performance, future career and employment plans, and emotional health issues.

Among the behaviors that adolescents view as risky are substance use, sexual activity, and the use of recreational and motor vehicles. Adolescents also identify health threats that primarily involve psychologic issues, such as clinical depression and eating or weight problems. Other perceived health threats include violence and pollution and threats within the more immediate social environment, including school problems and conflicts with parents, teachers, and friends. When adolescents are asked about general threats to youth, they respond differently than if asked about how their own personal behaviors produce certain risks. Like adults, adolescents tend to underestimate the potentially negative consequences of their own behaviors.

Although young people identify health risks and concerns that are primarily social and psychologic, many are reluctant to seek health services for problems they do not consider to be organic, despite the fact that they indicate they would like help with these problems. A variety of factors influence an adolescent's reluctance to seek health care, including perceived availability of confidential services, characteristics of health care providers, geographic access, and financial limitations (Smith, Stewart, Peled, et al, 2009).

The availability of confidential services is particularly important to adolescents, especially when they have concerns related to sensitive issues such as sexual or substance use behaviors. Many teenagers are unwilling to seek health care related to sensitive topics if their parents will know about the visit (Reddy, Fleming, and Swain, 2002). Although most states have provisions for confidential care for problems related to substance abuse and sexual health, adolescents often do not know whether and where they can receive confidential health care. Laws also vary by state, and since 2001, a number of states have either enacted or are considering laws requiring parental notification for a variety of health care services for teens, including reproductive health care. Adolescents may be more likely to participate in health care services when such services are delivered by caring, respectful providers.

FACTORS THAT PROMOTE ADOLESCENT HEALTH AND WELL-BEING

Even when they are exposed to risk factors such as poverty, neighborhood violence, parental abuse or neglect, or divorce of parents, most adolescents become competent, healthy adults. It is important to understand how this group of young people succeeds despite odds against them. Health promotion efforts with adolescents should focus on nurturing such protective factors in addition to reducing risk factors. Indeed, a large body of research has shown that fostering protective factors can reduce a wide range of health risk behaviors, so it may be more effective than health promotion efforts solely focused on reducing the problem behavior.

A variety of protective factors characterize children and youth who cope successfully when faced with adverse life situations such as poverty, parental alcoholism or psychopathology, or poor relationships between parents. The protective factors include individual personal attributes, attributes of families, and attributes of the larger social environment (Resnick, 2000). One protective personal factor is the ability to adapt to new persons and situations.

Adolescents who cope successfully in the midst of adverse circumstances are often supported by caring, cohesive families in which the parents are concerned with the well-being of their children. This family support can also be provided by some other caring adult, such as a grandparent, in the absence of a supportive parent. Protective factors within the community include connections with adults outside the family, with the school, or with a church group (Resnick, 2000). For example, health care providers who are able to connect with adolescents help support successful coping. Schools that are comfortable, safe, and intellectually engaging can make a difference in the health and well-being of young people. Involvement with healthy peer groups, guided by caring adults who are good role models, also prevents poor outcomes. Community engagement where young people think their involvement is meaningful, and they are listened to, is associated with better adjustment during adolescence.

The potential positive impact of social interactions suggests guidelines for making changes in adolescent environments that support overall health and well-being. Nurses involved with adolescents can develop interventions that shift the balance for young people from vulnerability to resilience by decreasing exposures to health risks or stressful life events (i.e., the impact of parental alcoholism or threats of violence) and by increasing the number of protective factors (i.e., communication and problem-solving skills or sources of emotional support).

Contexts for Adolescent Health Promotion

A consensus is growing that the most effective adolescent health promotion efforts involve multiple systems and address multiple issues. Interventions integrating programs and expertise from health care, school, and community-based settings can effectively increase adolescents' prevention skills, improve their access to health care services, build adult motivation and support for adolescent prevention practices, and change physical environments and social norms to support healthy behavior. Such a comprehensive approach to health promotion requires a great deal of cooperation and coordination on the part of complex institutions. On the other hand, by not limiting the responsibility for adolescent health to one person or one setting, multiple opportunities for health promotion arise. Individual efforts reinforce important themes and become an integral part of an overall health promotion strategy. For example, a plan for smoking cessation devised by a teenager with the help of a nurse is most likely to be successful if the teenager is encouraged by peers and family members to abstain, and if use and access to tobacco products are discouraged through policy interventions such as smoke-free schools and bans on cigarette vending machines.

Schools

Schools are a primary site for adolescent health promotion and disease prevention. Large numbers of young people can be affected by school-based health promotion efforts, since virtually all teenagers attend school at least through the early adolescent years. Group interventions offer adolescents a sense of anonymity, which they prefer when obtaining information about sensitive topics. School personnel often have special expertise and experience with health education. Through daily contact, school staff can develop supportive relationships with a limited number of students. Parent-teacher associations and school boards also link schools with the larger community in ways that can be used to expand the scope of adolescent health promotion efforts.

School-based health promotion interventions include classroom health education, school-level policies, and environmental changes. Classroom programs often include components that focus on building students' knowledge and skills and establishing peer support for health-enhancing behaviors. Some programs effectively use classroom peer leaders as positive role models and social support for healthy behaviors. Out-of-class assignments often involve parents or other admired adults, emphasizing the roles that adults play as resources regarding health issues. Classroom programs have been designed to address health-related issues, including healthy eating and exercise habits (Fig. 19-11), nonviolent conflict resolution, substance use and abuse prevention, and responsible sexual behavior.

Other school-level interventions involve changing the school environment itself, including improving physical education and food service programs or adopting tobacco-free school policies. School-wide environmental changes reinforce classroom programs aimed at promoting health-enhancing behavior.

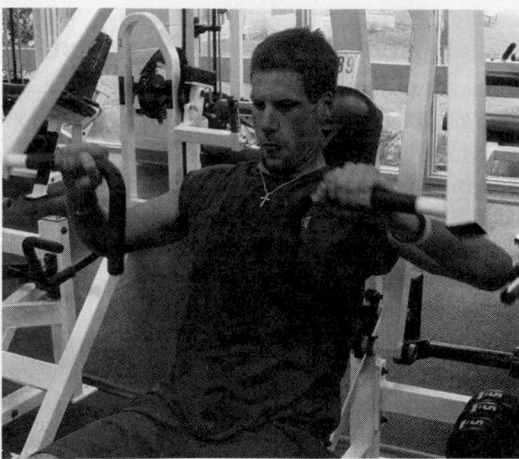

Fig. 19-11 Adolescents should be encouraged to participate in activities that contribute to lifelong physical fitness.

School-Based and School-Linked Health Services

Another avenue for health promotion is school-based and school-linked clinics. School-based clinics (SBCs) are located on school grounds and serve adolescents within a specific school. School-linked clinics (SLCs) may be located off school grounds or on school campuses but serve more than one school. Originally designed to address issues related to adolescent pregnancy, SBCs and SLCs have expanded to address a broad range of health problems and psychosocial issues. In combination, school-linked health services and traditional school-based health promotion efforts provide a comprehensive approach to health promotion that integrates health care, education, and environmental support.

Several private foundations, as well as state and local governments, have provided considerable resources to initiate school-linked health services that offer adolescents confidential services at minimum cost. Parental consent for services is usually obtained on a blanket basis before adolescents seek services. These services increase adolescents' access to preventive and primary care services through highly visible locations, convenient hours, affordability, and confidential care. SLCs have made a concerted effort to provide the services of a multidisciplinary team of health professionals—which may include nurses, nurse practitioners, health educators, medical assistants, physicians, psychologists, nutritionists, and social workers—skilled in meeting both the mental and physical health needs of adolescents. Adolescents are receptive to services offered by SLCs, especially when they address emotionally charged issues such as depression.

Communities

Community-level approaches to adolescent health promotion, involving both media campaigns and initiatives on the part of community groups, offer the advantage of reaching a broad audience. Specifically, community-based approaches can reach adolescents who do not attend school or have no source of preventive health care. This type of approach directly addresses changing social environments where high-risk behaviors occur. For example, violence prevention may be more effectively addressed by changing community-wide standards related to issues such as conflict resolution than by focusing on the individual. Community-based approaches have the potential to be most effective when they involve various sectors of the community (including adolescents) and include persons representing a variety of youth-serving agencies. With the involvement of multiple sectors, adolescents have the opportunity to hear consistent health messages across a variety of social contexts.

Media campaigns can be an effective but somewhat costly way to reach adolescents in community-level health promotion efforts. Adolescents receive considerable information from sources such as television, the Internet, radio, and magazines. Messages can also be targeted to appeal to parents and other adults who have an impact on the health-related behavior of youth. Media campaigns use brief images and provide short, superficial coverage of specific issues. Podcasts and youth-created videos uploaded to public websites such as YouTube are other ways of using media for health promotion efforts (see The Internet and Other Technologies, below).

Coalitions and task forces are another setting in which nurses can raise awareness about health issues or influence the larger environments for health promotion. This is an opportunity to partner with parents, community agencies, and concerned community groups. The goal of initiatives launched by parent and community groups is often to build climates within communities that support health-enhancing behaviors. Such initiatives create social contexts in which teenagers encounter more health-promoting messages and norms.

Health Care Settings

Consistent, supportive, one-on-one interactions over time between adolescents and members of the health care team provide significant opportunities for health promotion. These relationships can create "safe environments" in which adolescents can disclose sensitive information related to health risk. In turn, this information should be incorporated into preventive interventions specific to individual adolescent needs.

Health care settings offer the advantage of being able to provide confidential services, which are especially important in sensitive situations such as those involving substance use and sexual behavior. Interventions provided through health care settings can include parents and help to create social environments that support adolescents' health-enhancing behaviors. Another advantage is that health care settings have resources available to address various components of health, including physical, emotional, and social needs.

However, health promotion interventions provided in health care settings have limitations. Individual care is time-consuming, limiting the number of adolescents who can be reached in one-on-one encounters. Although one-on-one interventions can foster health-enhancing attitudes and behaviors of individual adolescents, they do not address changes in social environments, such as peer groups and communities, that may be necessary to support these attitudes and behaviors.

To be effective, health care services for adolescents must be accessible and appropriate. To be accessible, services must be available, affordable, and approachable. Services must include outreach to adolescents and their parents, informing them of the availability of services. Mechanisms for low- or no-cost services must be developed, since cost is a major barrier to adolescents receiving appropriate care. Locating health care services in places such as schools, youth services centers, shopping malls, and detention facilities and offering convenient clinical hours are two strategies that increase accessibility for teenagers who may not use traditional services.

Research has shown that adolescent-focused care can be cost-effective and improve health outcomes (Bensussen-Walls and Saewyc, 2001). To be appropriate, services must take into consideration the cultural contexts and adolescents' needs for confidential, developmentally appropriate care that addresses their specific health concerns.

The Internet and Other Technologies

A growing number of health promotion activities use the communication technologies that adolescents surround themselves with. Health-related websites designed to appeal to youth (often designed with youth) offer extensive information on nearly every topic that can affect adolescent health, although the accuracy and quality of such websites varies greatly. Programs for helping youth manage their chronic conditions can include a web-based or electronic "health passport," with information about their condition, their medications, and their health regimen. Social networking sites have been created to help youth with specific health issues. For example, Beyond Blue is a website in Australia about depression that includes therapist-monitored online support groups (see www.beyondblue.org). Some youth clinics offer text message reminders of appointments and cell phone calls to return for STI testing results. Other programs even offer text message or e-mail encouragements for youth who are trying to quit smoking; reminders about safer sex practices; or tips to improve nutrition, exercise, and weight management. Although clinicians need to consider carefully the levels of privacy and confidentiality in the use of different forms of technology, there is growing evidence of effectiveness in engaging youth through the technology they use to communicate.

Adolescent Health Screening

One vehicle for health promotion used by nurses and other professionals in health care settings is one-on-one health screening. Through information gained during a health screening interview, the health professional can identify both assets and threats to an adolescent's health and well-being. The health screening interview also offers an opportunity for health professionals to build trusting relationships with adolescents. This sense of trust may be critical for adolescents to act on information, attitudes, and skills that are shared to help them successfully negotiate particular stressors.

In addition, the health screening interview provides an opportunity for teaching adolescents self-advocacy skills. Nurses in schools and clinic settings can use several specific strategies to promote self-advocacy skills. These strategies include (1) maintaining an up-to-date file of handouts, pamphlets, and websites to show adolescents during "teachable moments"; (2) directing adolescents to resources in their community and to appropriate, accurate sources of health information on the Internet; and (3) teaching adolescents how the health care system works, how to schedule their health care appointments, and how to keep their own personal health records of immunizations, allergies, and health care encounters.

Interview Process

The development of trust between the adolescent and the health professional is vital to a health screening interview. Within the context of trusting relationships, adolescents are able to disclose sensitive and personal information, and nurses are able to transmit information, attitudes, and skills necessary for adolescents to take health-promoting actions. Three critical elements in establishing trusting relationships are active listening, responding to the adolescent's emotions, and ensuring confidentiality and privacy.

Active listening involves seeking to understand what is being said without imposing judgment. It includes paying attention to teenagers' nonverbal cues and noting inconsistencies between verbal and nonverbal communication. Finally, active listening requires listening for understanding rather than truth. For example, when an adolescent states, "My mother hates me," a nurse who is listening for understanding may reply, "That must be very hard for you," rather than "What does your mother do to make you think that?" Listening to understand the psychoemotional context of situations can be a difficult skill to master because the cultural milieu in which health care services are provided often encourages getting "just the facts." However, in noncrisis situations this approach is a critical element in encouraging communication and establishing trusting relationships.

Responding to an adolescent's emotions includes verbalizing concern about nonverbal cues that are observed. It also involves expressing empathy and support. Furthermore, it includes respecting adolescents' rights and abilities to make decisions and acknowledging potential issues related to developmental stage, cultural and religious values, beliefs and practices, gender, and sexual orientation.

A third critical element in establishing trusting relationships is ensuring confidentiality and privacy. In general, adolescents have the right to confidential communication with providers unless they are being abused or a life-threatening situation arises. Health care providers need to become familiar with the legal rights of adolescent patients in their state and their obligations to adolescent patients and families.

The nurse should establish the boundaries around confidentiality and privacy at the beginning of the interview so that adolescents feel they can discuss sensitive topics. A brief, clear explanation of confidentiality can clarify that the nurse will not share most things discussed during the interview with others and that life-threatening issues that need to be shared (e.g., report of ongoing abuse, suicidal or homicidal plans) will not be shared without the adolescent's prior knowledge. To allow for private conversation, complete most of the health screening interview with parents out of the room (Fig. 19-12).

The Nursing Care Guidelines box lists several other considerations related to the interview process. To convey an interest in adolescents' perspectives, nurses can begin interviews by asking teenagers to explain their reasons for the visit. At the beginning of the interview, give adolescents a nonthreatening explanation of why questions are asked, such as "I'll be asking you questions, including some that some people find personal

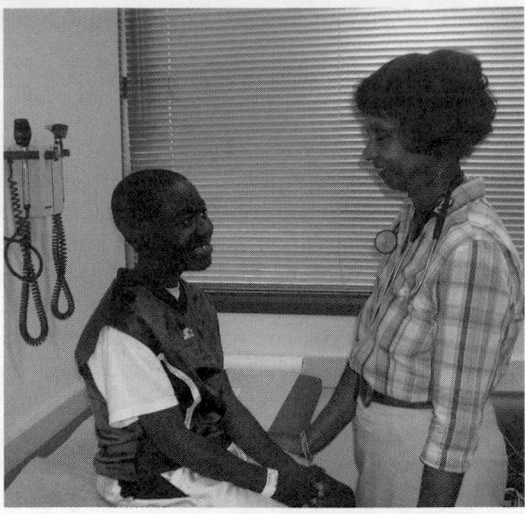

Fig. 19-12 Most of the health screening interview with the adolescent can be completed with parents out of the room.

or even embarrassing, so that I can better understand your health." To increase adolescents' comfort in disclosing sensitive information, nurses should avoid lectures and questions that convey judgmental attitudes. Asking open-ended questions and avoiding assumptions (e.g., all teenagers have supportive families, all teenagers are heterosexual) give adolescents opportunities to share more of their psychosocial contexts. Any medical language used during the interview should be clarified, and adolescents should be asked to explain any terms they use that are unfamiliar. Restating issues that adolescents may verbalize during an interview allows for a mutual understanding of their concerns.

NURSING CARE GUIDELINES

Interviewing Adolescents

- Ensure confidentiality and privacy; interview adolescent without parents.
- Explain the limits of confidentiality (e.g., legal duty to report physical or sexual abuse, or to get others involved if patient is suicidal).
- Show concern for the adolescent's perspective: "First, I'd like to talk about your main concerns" and "I'd like to know what you think is happening."
- Offer a nonthreatening explanation for the questions you ask: "I'm going to ask a number of questions to help me better understand your health."
- Maintain objectivity; avoid assumptions, judgments, and lectures.
- Ask open-ended questions when possible; move to more directive questions if necessary.
- Begin with less sensitive issues and proceed to more sensitive ones.
- Use language that both the adolescent and you understand.
- Restate: reflect back to the adolescent what he or she has said, along with feelings that may be associated with the descriptions.

Interview Content

Reviewing the major morbidities and mortalities of youth reveals that many threats to adolescent health are psychosocial and behavioral. Therefore, given the limited time available during routine clinical encounters, place emphasis on assessment of social, personal, and behavioral factors that underlie the major threats to the health and well-being of adolescents. This approach to assessment will help to identify the majority of adolescents who are coping well, those who require simple health information or counseling, and those who have significant psychosocial problems requiring referral to appropriate resources.

The mnemonic device SAFE TIMES can be used to guide interview questions. As shown in Box 19-2, each letter represents an important issue in preventive care. The less sensitive issues are toward the bottom (i.e., safety, education). It is best to begin the interview with less sensitive topics, ending with more sensitive areas such as sexuality.

HEALTH CONCERNS OF ADOLESCENCE

Several professional organizations have published guidelines aimed at improving and maintaining health care for adolescents and young adults. The American Academy of Pediatrics, American Academy of Family Physicians, American Medical Association, Bright Futures, and U.S. Preventive Services Task Force have similar guidelines for health supervision of adolescents. These guidelines emphasize the need to provide health services to adolescents that meet their physical and emotional needs. They place great import on provision of health care by health care providers who are trained in meeting the adolescents' needs (Jenkins, 2007). The American Medical Association issued a comprehensive set of recommendations, the *Guidelines for Adolescent Preventive Services* (GAPS), intended to provide a framework for providers who have one-on-one contact with adolescents in clinical settings (American Medical Association, 1997). The following discussion is an overview of the GAPS topics and provides specific recommendations related to screening, guidance, and immunizations.

Parenting and Family Adjustment

Having family members who are emotionally available and appropriately involved in their lives has proved to be a key factor in adolescents' well-being. On the other hand, family dysfunction can be a strong contributor to many adolescent problems, including depression, alcohol and other drug abuse, eating disorders, and school failure. A wide variety of family disorders, including parental discord, alcohol or drug abuse, mental illness, and sexual and physical abuse, can lead to additional stresses in teenagers coping with the tasks of adolescence.

Screening questions such as "Who is in your family?" "How are things going at home?" and "Who in your family could you talk with about problems you are having?" help to give a general sense of family relationships. More directed questions that give insight into family functioning include "How does your family generally solve disagreements?" "What are some of the rules in your family related to (issues such as underage drinking, curfew, friends)?" "Who sets these rules?" and "Are you currently having conflicts with your family?"

Many parents are interested in, concerned about, and involved in the lives of their adolescent. Parents who are appropriately involved serve as an important protective influence, and efforts to exclude parents from adolescent health services are both unrealistic and unwise. In providing health care, a

BOX 19-2 SAFE TIMES: A METHOD FOR HEALTH-SCREENING INTERVIEWS WITH ADOLESCENTS

NOTE: In clinical interviewing, SAFE TIMES is best used in reverse order.

S—Sexuality
Pubertal development, menstrual history (girls)
Extent of sexual activity, type of relationships, symptoms of sexually transmitted infections (STIs)
Pregnancy and STI prevention methods
Sexual orientation issues (attractions, behaviors)
History of sexual abuse

A—Affect
Symptoms of depression ("feeling down or blue") or hopelessness ("discouraged about the future")

Abuse
Use of tobacco, alcohol, marijuana, cocaine, other drugs

F—Family
Who the patient lives with and whether there are any family conflicts or problems
Family history (medical, psychiatric)

E—Examination
Breast or testicular self-examination (middle to late adolescence)
Explain pelvic examination (if indicated)

T—Timing of Development
For younger adolescents, "Is your development going too fast, too slow, or at about the right speed?" and "Do you feel too tall, too short, or about the right height?"
For all, "Do you feel too thin, too heavy, or about the right weight?"

I—Immunization
Diphtheria-tetanus-pertussis (Tdap) booster needed at 11 to 12 years of age or on entry to high school (15 years) if not given at 11 to 12 years
Measles-mumps-rubella unless two vaccines given during childhood or unless girl is pregnant
Hepatitis B vaccine, if not current
Hepatitis A vaccine, if not current
Tuberculin skin test yearly for high-risk groups
Pneumococcal vaccine if chronic disease (See Chapter 12, Immunizations.)
Yearly influenza; H1N1 as appropriate
Meningococcal vaccine, if not current
HPV vaccine to prevent cervical cancer and genital warts (optional)

M—Minerals
Iron—Supplementation required if less than two servings of meats daily or low hemoglobin
Calcium—Supplementation required (e.g., Tums, three or four tablets daily) for those who drink less than two or three glasses of milk daily (especially for girls)
Cholesterol—intake of fats, lipid levels

E—Education, Employment
If in school, what grades attained, any problems
Work history and future plans

S—Safety
Especially car safety, use of seat belts, drinking and driving, or accepting rides from drivers using alcohol or drugs
Motorcycles, mopeds, all-terrain vehicles
Handguns in the home, handgun availability

Modified from Schubiner H: Preventive health screening in adolescent patients, *Prim Care* 16:211-230, 1989.

balance must be sought between the individual adolescent's growing autonomy and the parents' diminishing control over, and responsibility for, the adolescent.

Offer parents health guidance at least once during their child's early adolescence, once during middle adolescence, and once during late adolescence. Such guidance can include information about normative adolescent development, along with signs and symptoms of troubled adolescents. Engage parents in discussion of parenting behaviors that promote healthy adolescent adjustment, including maintaining open communication, setting age-appropriate limits, monitoring their child's social and recreational activities, and acting as role models for health-enhancing behaviors. Encourage parents to discuss health-related behaviors with their adolescents (see Family-Centered Care and Community Focus boxes and the Family-Centered Care box, p. 772).

👪 FAMILY-CENTERED CARE

Communication with Teens: The Art of Listening

Conflicts between parents and their adolescents are often a result of a natural characteristic of parenthood: the desire to protect one's offspring—from harm or from simply doing something "stupid," something embarrassing, or something they may later regret. Teens sometimes bounce their thoughts and ideas off adults. At times they really want feedback; at other times they simply want to elicit a reaction.

I found it easy to listen openly, thoughtfully, and without interrupting when my teenager's friends discussed troublesome topics. However, one day, when one of my own teenagers had a similar conversation with me, the parent part kicked in. I felt responsible and spoke my piece on the spot. This brought communication to a halt and resulted in defensiveness. It was a long time before my child tried to talk to me about anything controversial again.

The next time one of my teenagers started a similar conversation, I decided to try to trick myself. Throughout the entire conversation, I told myself over and over again to act as though this were not my teenager, but rather someone else's child. I found this worked well, and I was able to listen without interrupting. I continue to use the system, sometimes with more success than at other times.

—Mother of four

🏠 COMMUNITY FOCUS

Rules for Adolescents

U.S. society does little to help adolescents mature and separate. Americans have remarkably few rites of passage that mark the stages of life. Few ceremonies and tests are practiced to determine eligibility for specific adult privileges. Obtaining a driver's license, graduating from high school, and reaching legal age for drinking are among the few that exist. U.S. society also does not have many generally agreed-on social dictums. When is the right age to begin dating? What is a reasonable curfew? Should an 18-year-old be allowed to stay out all night? There are few areas of general agreement. Every family makes up its own rules, influenced, but uninstructed, by the society at large. Many families have great difficulty with this process.

Modified from Prothrow-Stith D: *Deadly consequences: how violence is destroying our teenage population and a plan to begin solving the problem,* New York, 1993, HarperCollins.

Generally, if an adolescent is doing well in school, relates well to peers, and is able to resolve areas of conflict with family members, family intervention is not necessary. Nurses can support positive conflict resolution around minor issues between adolescents and their families, such as curfew hours and appropriate limit setting. Families dealing with major conflicts or dysfunctional relationships should be referred to a family therapist or other mental health professional.

Psychosocial Adjustment

As adolescents experience the many changes of adolescence, they redefine who they are and what they want out of life. Most individuals progress through the changes of their adolescent years with minimum emotional upheaval, countering the belief that this period in life is one of "storm and stress." Some adolescents, however, do have difficulty coping and exhibit emotional distress, especially when multiple normative events happen simultaneously and are combined with nonnormative life events.

Adolescence is characterized by change within multiple domains. Changes associated with pubertal development typically take place during the early adolescent years. Early- and late-maturing adolescents, who feel they are "out of synch" with their age-mates' growth patterns, may have a more difficult time emotionally than those who develop "on time" with their peers. Another normative change, typically occurring during middle adolescence, is the transition from middle or junior high school to high school. With this transition, adolescents often are increasingly concerned about same- and opposite-sex peer relationships. School transitions may also expose teenagers to social environments that are larger, less individualized, and less capable of providing adult support and supervision. During older adolescence, psychosocial concerns focus on school achievement and future career plans.

Questions such as "Do you think that your development is going too fast, too slow, or at about the right speed?" may allow young adolescents to discuss issues related to physical development. Questions about feeling cared for and connected to teachers, counselors, students, and others at school, along with questions about their involvement in school-related activities, give teenagers an opportunity to talk about strengths and deficits they experience within their school environments. Questions about the quality of peer relationships may help identify teenagers who feel socially isolated. Finally, questions about future plans related to education and employment or career choices may give older youths the chance to talk through significant sources of stress.

As sources of credible information, support, and encouragement, nurses can help adolescents cope with the changes and challenges they face. To promote both emotional health and psychosocial adjustment, nurses and other health care professionals can encourage adolescents to develop (1) skills to cope with stress and change and (2) skills to become involved in personally meaningful activities.

Intentional and Unintentional Injury

Injuries kill more U.S. adolescents than any other single cause, with unintentional injury, homicide, and suicide accounting for 70% of deaths among teens 10 to 24 years old in 2005 (Mulye, Park, Nelson, et al, 2009). (See Childhood Mortality, Chapter 1.) Motor vehicle crashes are the single greatest source of unintentional injury and death in young people. Many factors contribute to the higher rate of crashes among teen drivers, including lacking driving experience and maturity, following

too closely, driving too fast, having other teen passengers in the car, and using alcohol. Homicide, a form of intentional injury, is the second leading cause of death among all U.S. adolescents; for African-American teenagers it is the most likely cause of death. In the United States, homicides among teenagers are most likely to involve firearms and to occur among friends or gangs. In 2007, 82% of all homicides for persons 13 through 19 years of age were firearm related (Mulye, Park, Nelson, et al, 2009).

In addition to being the leading cause of death, injuries also account for substantial morbidity among youth. The leading causes of injury-related morbidity include vehicular crashes, firearms, drownings, poisonings, burns, and falls. Certain behaviors increase the risk of unintentional injury. For example, 11% of high school students nationwide report rarely or never using seat belts. When asked about their practices over the past 30 days, nearly one third (30%) of U.S. high school students reported riding with a driver who had been drinking, and 3.5% of students had driven a vehicle after drinking alcohol (Mulye, Park, Nelson, et al, 2009). The majority of adolescents who use in-line skates or ride bicycles, skateboards, and snowboards do not wear helmets, despite the risk of traumatic brain injury that accidents can cause with these forms of recreation or transportation.

Behaviors that contribute to intentional injury are also prevalent among young people. For example, in 2007, 18% of U.S. high school students reported carrying a weapon (e.g., a gun, knife, or club) at some point during the previous month, with 6% noting that they carried a weapon on school property during that same time period. Nationwide, 36% of students reported being in a physical fight during the year (Mulye, Park, Nelson, et al, 2009). Many adolescents have easy access to a gun in their home, and such accessibility is significantly associated with involvement in violent behavior and with fatal suicide attempts among adolescents.

During an interview, the segment addressing injury prevention should include screening and counseling related to motor vehicle crashes, firearm use, and suicide. In relation to prevention of motor vehicle injury, one might initially ask how the adolescent "gets around town." Further questions and health education might focus on seat belt or helmet use and the practice of drinking and driving or riding with drivers who have been drinking. Ask adolescents whether they have access, at home or elsewhere, to firearms; whether they carry a gun; and whether they ever use alcohol or other substances in combination with handling guns.

Health education related to firearm injury prevention should include advising parents to limit their children's household access to firearms, counseling on nonviolent ways to resolve conflicts, and discouraging use of weapons. Family members and acquaintances are a common source of guns for young people. Having a gun in the home increases the risk of adolescent suicide and homicide. Assess all families for the presence of a gun in the home and inform them of the increased risk for suicide and homicide. Gun availability in the general population is linked to increased gun death among children (Glatt, 2005; Miller, Azrael, and Hemenway, 2002). When guns are present in the home, families must take preventive action to be certain that the guns are never loaded, that they are locked up in a safe place, and that ammunition is locked up in a separate location accessible only to appropriate adults.

Dietary Habits, Eating Disorders, and Obesity

Puberty marks the beginning of accelerated physical growth, which can as much as double adolescents' nutritional requirements for iron, calcium, zinc, and protein. At the same time, growing independence, the need for peer acceptance, concern with physical appearance, and an active lifestyle may affect eating habits, food choices, nutrient intake, and thus nutritional status. Although problems related to overt nutritional deficiencies (excluding iron deficiencies) have decreased since the 1940s, they have been replaced by problems of dietary imbalances and excess. Excess intake of calories, sugar, fat, cholesterol, and sodium is common among adolescents and is found in all income and racial or ethnic groups and both genders (Fig. 19-13). Inadequate intake of certain vitamins (folic acid, vitamin B₆, vitamin A) and minerals (iron, calcium, zinc) is also evident, particularly among girls and teenagers of low socioeconomic status. In combination with other factors, these dietary patterns could result in increased risk for obesity and chronic diseases such as heart disease, osteoporosis, and some types of cancer later in life. Girls, in particular, may be susceptible to iron deficiency at menarche. Maximum bone mass is also acquired during adolescence; therefore the calcium deposited during these years determines the risk of osteoporosis.

In terms of weight concerns and weight control behaviors, the number of adolescents who are overweight has increased significantly over the past decade, with 18% of 12- to 19-year-olds qualifying as overweight (Mulye, Park, Nelson, et al, 2009). Female adolescents who are normal weight are also more likely to be currently attempting to lose weight, whereas male adolescents are more often trying to gain weight (Smith, Stewart, Peled, et al, 2009). Although most teens trying to lose weight exercise or diet, a small percent of students (around 5%) engage in risky weight-loss practices such as vomiting after meals or taking laxatives (Smith, Stewart, Peled, et al, 2009).

Currently in the United States, obesity and overweight among adolescents are increasing. Adolescent obesity poses both immediate and long-term problems for adolescents.

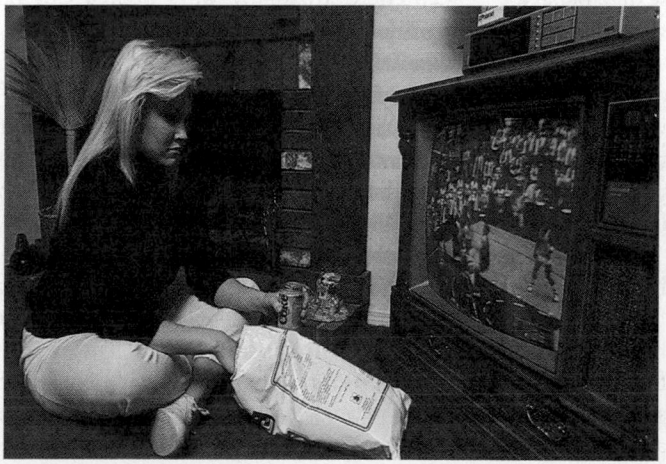

Fig. 19-13 Snacking on empty calories is common among adolescents, especially during inactivity.

Anorexia nervosa and bulimia nervosa also commonly occur during the adolescent and young adult years. If left untreated, these disorders, like obesity, can lead to considerable morbidity and mortality. (See Obesity and Eating Disorders, Chapter 21.)

Routine nutrition screening for all adolescents should include questions about meal patterns, dieting behaviors, consumption of high-fat and high-salt foods, and recent changes in weight. In 2007, one third of adolescents reported drinking sweetened soda daily, and only 22% ate the recommended five or more servings of fruits and vegetables (Mulye, Park, Nelson, et al, 2009). Discuss healthy dietary habits with all adolescents, including the benefits of a healthy diet; ways to consume foods rich in calcium, iron, and other vitamins and minerals; and safe weight management.

A screening hemoglobin or hematocrit is recommended at the first encounter with an adolescent, at the end of puberty, or at both screening visits and at the end of pubertal development. The American Academy of Pediatrics (2007) recommends annual measures of weight and height, along with calculation and plotting of body mass index (BMI [weight in kilograms divided by height in meters squared]). Reference BMI values for adolescent males and females are given in Table 19-2. Along with height and weight measurements, an appropriate screening or interview question related to obesity and eating disorders might be, "Do you feel that you are too heavy, too thin, or about the right weight?"

The American Medical Association Expert Committee on the Assessment, Prevention, and Treatment of Child and Adolescent Overweight and Obesity recently published recommendations for the assessment and management of children and adolescents who are either at risk for or are overweight or obese (Rao, 2008). These recommendations include a comprehensive assessment and review of the child or adolescent's lifestyle habits, family history, physical examination, and laboratory evaluation. Adolescents with a family history of obesity, type 2 diabetes, hypertension, or cardiovascular disease should be carefully screened for risk or presence of health habits that place them at further risk for overweight and obesity (Rao, 2008). Adolescents with a BMI between the 85th and 94th percentiles are considered overweight, whereas adolescents with a BMI equal to or greater than the 95th percentile for age and gender are considered obese. Adolescents who are overweight should have an in-depth dietary and health assessment to determine psychosocial effects and risk for future cardiovascular and metabolic disease. (See Chapter 21 for a comprehensive discussion of the management of obesity.)

Physical Fitness

Nationwide, in 2007 nearly two thirds (64%) of all high school students reported that they had participated in activities that made them "sweat and breathe hard for at least 20 minutes" (i.e., vigorous physical activity) three or more times in the past week. Male students were more likely than female students to engage in vigorous physical activity (Mulye, Park, Nelson, et al, 2009). Participation in school physical education classes declines with age, since schools often do not have mandatory requirements past grade 9 or 10.

High levels of physical activity and fitness may reduce cardiovascular disease risk factors during adolescence, including

TABLE 19-2	ADOLESCENT BODY MASS INDEX PERCENTILE RANKINGS									
	MALES					FEMALES				
AGE (yr)	5th	25th	50th	85th	95th	5th	25th	50th	85th	95th
11	15	16	17	20	23	15	16	18	21	25
12	15	16	18	21	24	15	17	18	22	26
13	16	17	19	22	25	15	17	19	22	26
14	16	17	19	22	26	16	17	19	23	27
15	16	18	20	23	27	16	18	20	24	28
16	17	19	22	24	27	17	18	20	25	29
17	18	20	22	25	28	17	19	21	25	30

Data from Centers for Disease Control and Prevention: *Body mass index–for-age percentiles growth charts*, Atlanta, 2000, The Centers, available at www.cdc.gov/growthcharts/clinical_charts.htm (accessed January 29, 2010).

obesity, high blood pressure, and hyperlipidemia. In addition, routine exercise may reduce adolescents' risk for depression and emotional distress. Although only some evidence supports a positive relationship between a person's level of physical activity and fitness during adolescence and this level as an adult, the association between exercise and physical fitness and reduced risk for cardiovascular disease during adulthood is well documented.

Routine screening related to exercise should include questions about frequency, intensity, and type of physical activity. Health care organizations such as the American Academy of Pediatrics (2006) recommend discussing the emotional, social, and physical benefits of exercise with all adolescents. Furthermore, encourage all adolescents to engage in safe exercise on a regular basis. Nurses should encourage all adolescents to be physically active daily, or nearly every day, as part of play, games, sports, work, transportation, recreation, physical education, or other planned exercise.

Sedentary activities, such as watching television, playing video games, and using a computer to surf the Internet or engage with friends, can also contribute to obesity and cardiovascular health problems in later life. Youth should limit their "screen time" in order to get enough exercise. Some new forms of video games include equipment for more active involvement, such as dance or musical performance video games or "virtual" sports. It is unclear if these will offer levels of aerobic activity equivalent to those of more traditional forms of sports and exercise, or if they are temporary fads among youth.

Sexual Behavior, Sexually Transmitted Infections, and Unintended Pregnancy

Sexual activity significantly decreased among U.S. youth in the 1990s through 2005, and among those who are sexually active, responsible sexual behavior had increased until recently. As a result, unintended pregnancy and birth among teens reached the lowest rates ever measured in the United States in 2005, although birth rates increased between 2005 and 2006 and increased again between 2006 and 2007 (Santelli, Orr, Lindberg, et al, 2009). Nationwide, in 2007 less than half (45.9%) of ninth through twelfth graders reported having had sexual intercourse ever during their lifetime, and 35.6% of students reported having had sexual intercourse in the previous 3 months. Rates of STIs and human immunodeficiency virus (HIV) infection

among teens have increased, although this may be partly due to increased testing and better sensitivity of STI testing.

Many sexually active young people engage in behaviors that put them at risk for STIs or pregnancy, such as having sex with multiple partners and having sex without using condoms or other forms of contraception. Approximately 14% of U.S. high school students reported having had four or more sexual partners during their lifetime. Among the sexually active students, nearly two thirds reported using a condom during their most recent experience of intercourse, and 16% reported using birth control pills at the time of their most recent experience of intercourse. Since 2003, however, rates of oral contraceptive use have been declining, especially among Hispanic and African-American adolescents, and condom use appears to be decreasing as well, which helps explain the reversing trend in teen pregnancy (Santelli, Orr, Lindberg, et al, 2009).

Obtaining a sexual history can be an important step in promoting sexual health and preventing STIs and unintended pregnancies among young people. Given their sensitive nature, questions about sexuality should be prefaced by an explanation of their purpose and the limits of confidentiality. Initial questions can cover less sensitive topics, such as milestones in pubertal development and, for girls, the menstrual history (including the age at menarche, timing of menstrual cycles, duration of menstrual flow, and symptoms of dysmenorrhea). Questions should also address dating behavior, same- and opposite-gender attractions, and same- and opposite-gender sexual behavior (e.g., "There are many ways people can be sexual with others, such as kissing; touching; and having oral, vaginal, and anal sex. In what ways have you been sexual with others?"). Adolescents should be asked about a history of uninvited or nonconsensual sexual contact (e.g., "Has anyone ever touched you in a sexual way that felt uncomfortable or when you did not want them to? Has anyone ever forced you to have sex?").

Sexually active youth should be asked about their consistency and motivation to use condoms or other barrier methods for preventing STIs; use of birth control pills or other forms of hormonal contraception; the number of sexual partners they have had over the past 6 months; and the use of alcohol or other substances in connection with sexual activity. Sexually active adolescents should also be asked about any history of pregnancies or STIs. Adolescents who reveal a history of physical or sexual abuse, who admit to heavy use of alcohol or other drugs, or who have unstable social or economic support systems should also be asked whether they have ever exchanged sex for money, shelter, or drugs.

Sexually active adolescents should be screened for STIs with laboratory tests for gonorrhea, chlamydia, and, for females, a Papanicolaou (Pap) test to detect human papillomavirus (HPV) infection or other cervical dysplasia. Both males and females should be evaluated for HPV by visual inspection and should also be asked about whether they have received the HPV vaccine series. Sexually active teenagers should have a serologic test for syphilis if they have lived in an area endemic for syphilis, have had other STIs, have had more than one sexual partner within the past 6 months, have exchanged sex for drugs or money, or are males who have had sex with other males.

One of the newly proposed goals for *Healthy People 2020* is to increase the number of adolescents who have been tested for HIV (US Department of Health and Human Services, 2009). Adolescents at risk for HIV infection should be offered confidential HIV screening tests. HIV risk status includes having a history of injecting drug use (including anabolic steroid injections), having sexual intercourse in an area with a high prevalence of HIV infection, having other STIs, having more than one sexual partner in the past 6 months, exchanging sex for drugs or money, being a male and engaging in sex with other males, or having a sexual partner who is at risk for HIV infection. The frequency of laboratory screening for STIs and HIV depends on the sexual practices and STI history of individual adolescents.

All adolescents should receive medically accurate health guidance regarding responsible sexual behaviors, including abstinence. Adolescents should receive information on how STIs, including HIV, are transmitted and on possible consequences of infection. Counsel sexually active adolescents about ways to reduce their risk of STIs and unwanted pregnancy, including limiting the number of sexual partners, using condoms and barrier methods consistently, using appropriate methods of birth control, and avoiding substance use in connection with sexual activity. Counseling should include instruction on how to use condoms and other methods of birth control effectively. Despite extensive government funding available to provide "abstinence-only" sexual health education over the past decade, research evidence shows most such programs are not effective in delaying sexual behavior and may actually increase unprotected sex among adolescents once they become sexually active (Kirby, 2008). Adolescents should receive positive reinforcement for responsible sexual behaviors, including abstinence, consistent condom use, and appropriate use of birth control. Adolescents should also be counseled on ways to reduce their risk of sexual exploitation. Techniques for counseling adolescents to reduce risky sexual behaviors are discussed in detail in Chapter 20.

Gay, lesbian, and bisexual teens are as likely to be sexually active as their heterosexual peers, although the age of sexual debut is more likely to be during early adolescence, in part because of a higher risk for sexual abuse (Saewyc, Skay, Reis, et al, 2006). These youths may engage in heterosexual intercourse as a way to blend in with their peers. This strategy can even include pregnancy and teen parenting in an attempt to avoid detection as gay, lesbian, or bisexual. Recent studies have found sexual minority teens are more likely to be involved in a pregnancy during their adolescent years than their heterosexual peers (Saewyc, Poon, Homma, et al, 2008) and may be more likely to be a teen parent (Forrest and Saewyc, 2004).

Nurses need to acknowledge the possibility of same-gender and bisexual attractions and relationships in their work with adolescents. Screening questions regarding sexual attractions and experiences should be phrased in ways that allow adolescents to discuss same- and opposite-gender attractions, such as using the term *partner* rather than *boyfriend* or *girlfriend*. Gay, lesbian, and bisexual adolescents need the same sexuality education and information on pregnancy prevention and STI transmission and prevention that is appropriate for all other adolescents.

Use of Tobacco, Alcohol, and Other Substances

Statistically, experimentation with substances is common among U.S. adolescents. By the twelfth grade, the majority of students have used alcohol, just under half have smoked, a similar percentage have tried cannabis, and much smaller proportions have tried other illicit drugs. Substance use increases with age, with older teens more likely to use alcohol and cannabis than younger teens, but the rates have generally declined over the past 15 years. Among twelfth graders, for example, 43% used alcohol in the past month, but this is a decline since the early 1990s. One in five smoked cigarettes in the past month, 10% report smoking daily (Mulye, Park, Nelson, et al, 2009), and 5% use cannabis daily. Heavy use of alcohol and tobacco is not uncommon, although the prevalence of binge drinking and tobacco use among high school students is declining. Only about 10% of high school students ages 12 to 17 report binge drinking (having had five or more drinks in a row) at least once in the past month, while among twelfth graders, 25% have done so. However, rates among late adolescents and young adults (ages 18 to 24) increase dramatically compared to teens.

In contemporary U.S. society, adolescents may use tobacco, alcohol, and marijuana because these substances provide an opportunity to challenge authority, demonstrate autonomy, gain entry into a peer group, or simply relieve the stress of growing up. Although use may be accepted among many U.S. teenagers, there are substantive, documented consequences of early experimentation with alcohol, tobacco, and other drugs. Drinking and driving is the leading cause of death among teenagers. Persons who begin smoking at younger ages are more likely to become heavier smokers and are at increased risk for illness and death attributable to smoking (Rojas, Killen, Haydel, et al, 1998). Substance use has also been associated other health-challenging behaviors, such as delinquency, absenteeism, dropping out of school, lower academic achievement, and early sexual behavior.

In terms of health screening, the nurse can ask adolescents whether they or their friends have ever used tobacco, alcohol, marijuana, or other substances. They should also be asked about their current use and current use patterns among peers. The nurse should assess practices of drinking and driving or riding with someone who has been drinking. If answers to these initial questions indicate some problem use, the nurse should ask about the amount and frequency of use; frequency of getting "high" or "wasted"; use in relation to sexual activity; and difficulties with peers, school, parents, or the law in relation to use.

Adolescents who have begun experimenting or who engage in low-level use need to be made aware of other options that can help them achieve the same goals, and of the risks of higher-level use. Furthermore, they need to know the short-term effects of alcohol, tobacco, or other drugs, particularly in relation to driving and school or work performance. Offer cessation plans to adolescents who use tobacco products. Adolescents whose substance use patterns endanger their health should be referred to an appropriate mental health provider. Chapter 21 includes an in-depth discussion of etiology, prevention strategies, and nursing considerations related to adolescent substance use.

Depression and Suicide

A national survey of ninth through twelfth grade students found that 34% of the boys and 22% of girls reported feeling sad or hopeless almost every day for greater than or equal to 2 weeks in a row (Fig. 19-14). Nearly 15% of high school students reported seriously considering suicide during the past year, with female students (19%) being more likely than male students (10%) to have considered a suicide attempt. Around 7% of U.S. high school students reported actually having attempted suicide during the previous 12 months, with girls (9%) being more likely than boys (5%) to have attempted suicide (Mulye, Park, Nelson, et al, 2009).

A brief psychologic screening is necessary during the course of a routine health visit. Screening for depression or suicidal risk should be done with adolescents who note declining school grades; chronic melancholy; family dysfunction; alcohol or other drug use; gay, lesbian, or bisexual orientation; a history of abuse; or previous suicide attempts. Most adolescents who are depressed respond affirmatively to the question, "Have you been feeling down or blue lately?" although they may not necessarily "look" depressed. Refer nonsuicidal adolescents who report commonly feeling "blue," "down," or "depressed" to a psychologist, psychiatrist, or other mental health professional who works with young people (Shain and Committee on Adolescence, 2007).

It is crucial to explore thoughts about and possible plans for suicidal acts with all troubled adolescents. Once an assessment of the immediate risk of suicide is completed, the nurse can construct a management scheme. If the adolescent has a specific plan, immediate referral for acute intervention with a psychiatrist or other mental health professional is indicated. (See Chapter 21 for further discussion of suicide.)

Physical, Sexual, and Emotional Abuse

Adolescents who have been physically, sexually, or emotionally abused during childhood or adolescence face challenges to healthy development. Over the past 2 decades, reported cases of physical and sexual abuse first increased dramatically, then declined in the late 1990s, and have remained fairly stable between 2001 and 2003 (US Department of Health and Human Services, 2005). In anonymous school-based surveys of adolescents, the proportion of teens reporting abuse appears to have been declining from the 1990s, although in some recent surveys, rates have plateaued or begun to increase again (Smith, Stewart, Peled, et al, 2009). Around one in four adolescents reports having been physically abused by family members. Approximately 3% to 5% of boys and 10% to 15% of girls report experiencing sexual abuse, most often by someone outside the family, less commonly by incest (sexual abuse by a family member), or both types of abuse (Saewyc, Pettingell, and Magee, 2003). Certain groups of adolescents, such as gay, lesbian, or bisexual youth (Saewyc, Skay, Hynds, et al, 2007) or those who are developmentally delayed, may be especially vulnerable to abuse.

A common constellation of symptoms among adolescents who have been victims of sexual abuse includes substance abuse, depression, withdrawn mood, suicidal ideation, and somatic complaints (Frederickson, 1999). Adolescents who have been abused are more likely than nonabused adolescents to engage in health-compromising behaviors such as self-mutilation, suicide attempts, injection drug use, and early sexual activity (Saewyc, Pettingell, and Magee, 2003) and are at higher risk of being sexually exploited (Widom and Kuhns, 1996). Adolescents with a history of sexual abuse are also more likely to become pregnant or father a child during their teen years (Saewyc, Pettingell, Skay, et al, 2004).

Early identification of abuse can protect adolescents who have been victims of physical, sexual, and emotional trauma. For this reason, questions about abuse should be part of routine adolescent health visits. Ensure privacy before inquiring about abuse. If an adolescent reports a history of sexual or physical abuse, further questions should be directed toward any ongoing abuse; the circumstances surrounding the abuse incident; and the presence of physical, emotional, or behavioral sequelae, including involvement in risk-taking behaviors. Once a history of maltreatment is suspected or disclosed, health care providers have a legal responsibility to report the case to the appropriate child protection agency. The more acute the problem, the more quickly the report must be made. Adolescents reporting abuse should always be informed about steps in the reporting process before information is disclosed to local authorities.

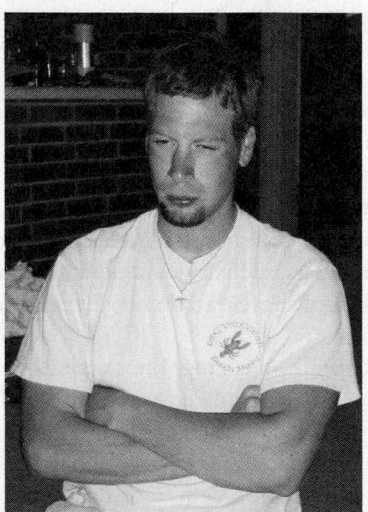

Fig. 19-14 Adolescents use being alone as a method of coping with stress. Health care professionals need to assess whether this also indicates an attempt to cope with depression.

Adolescents who live in homes where there is constant conflict may run away, sometimes to a friend's home. The conflict may be real (interpersonal) or perceived (intrapersonal), and escalation to abuse or the fear of abuse may prompt the adolescent to leave home. In addition, an adolescent who encounters difficulty with authority figures in the home may leave home believing this will solve the problem. The adolescent may stay in school and maintain close ties with less threatening family members and friends; the term *couch surfing* is used in some circles to refer to the adolescent who spends time at different friends' houses sleeping on the couch or in an available spare room to "crash" temporarily. Such adolescents are often at higher risk for further abuse and neglect.

School and Learning Problems

In 2007, 16% of U.S. youth between the ages of 16 and 24 years of age (almost 6.2 million persons) dropped out before completing high school (Center for Labor Market Studies, 2009). Dropout rates vary by ethnicity. In 2007, 30% of dropouts were Hispanic, 18.8% were African-Americans, and 12% were Caucasians (Center for Labor Market Studies, 2009). Among in-school adolescents, a low grade point average has been associated with higher levels of emotional distress; cigarette, alcohol, and marijuana use; and earlier onset of sexual activity. School problems and dropping out of school can also be markers for difficulties such as learning disabilities, language barriers, family problems, lack of supportive relationships at school, and employment needs. In contemporary U.S. society, education is critical to economic self-sufficiency. Teenagers who drop out of school can expect to earn approximately $400,000 less over a lifetime (ages 18 to 64 years) than those who graduate. Males who drop out of school may earn $500,000 less over the same time period (Center for Labor Market Studies, 2009).

Questions about recent grades, school absences, suspensions, and any history of repeating a grade in school can be used to screen for school-related problems. Specific management plans for youth who note school problems should be coordinated with school personnel and with the adolescent's parents or caregivers if possible.

Hypertension

As adolescents experience sexual maturation, along with increases in height and weight, blood pressure increases from the onset of adolescence and continues to rise until the end of pubertal growth. This trend is especially apparent among males. Approximately 1% of adolescents have sustained hypertension, defined as a blood pressure greater than the 95th percentile of standards. (See inside back cover for blood pressure tables and Chapter 34 for an in-depth discussion of hypertension in children and adolescents.) The detection of hypertension during adolescence is important because hypertension is one of the major preventable risk factors for adult cardiovascular disease. With increasing levels of obesity, there have been reports of increasing incidence of hypertension among adolescents (Hansen, Gunn, and Kaelber, 2007). To detect early hypertension, all adolescents should have blood pressure taken annually (American Academy of Pediatrics, 2007).

Hyperlipidemia

Along with hypertension, smoking, and obesity, elevated serum cholesterol and triglyceride levels are major risk factors for the development of adult cardiovascular disease. Results of several studies suggest that 23% to 35% of young adolescents have at least one cardiovascular disease risk factor; approximately 5% to 10% have two or more risk factors.

The American Academy of Pediatrics (Daniels, Greer, and Committee on Nutrition, 2008) recommends that children and adolescents with a family history of dyslipidemia or premature cardiovascular disease be screened for total blood cholesterol level (nonfasting) at least once after 2 years of age but no later than 10 years of age. The American Heart Association (McCrindle, Urbina, Dennison, et al, 2007) recommends that adolescents with borderline elevated total cholesterol (170 to 200 mg/dl) have a fasting cholesterol level repeated to monitor low-density lipoprotein (LDL) and high-density lipoprotein (HDL). Diet therapy is recommended for adolescents with elevated LDL levels (borderline high, 110 to 129 mg/dl; high, ≥130 mg/dl). LDL cholesterol–lowering drug therapy is recommended for children and adolescents whose LDL remains elevated after 6 months to 1 year on a restricted fat diet (Daniels, Greer, and Committee on Nutrition, 2008; McCrindle, Urbina, Dennison, et al, 2007; Zapalla and Gidding, 2009).

Infectious Diseases and Immunizations

Immunization updates are a significant part of adolescent preventive care. Adolescents 11 to 18 years of age should receive a single tetanus-diphtheria–acellular pertussis (Tdap) vaccine if they have received the recommended childhood series of DTaP immunizations. This vaccine is now required because of the increased incidence of pertussis seen in adolescents and adults who were previously immunized with the DTaP series yet developed the condition as adolescents. The adolescent who has received Td but not Tdap vaccine should also receive a single dose of the Tdap vaccine, provided 5 years have elapsed between the Td and Tdap vaccination (American Academy of Pediatrics, 2009). Meningococcal vaccine (MCV4) should be given to adolescents 11 to 12 years of age or at 15 years of age if previous immunization with MPSV4 occurred in childhood and at least 3 to 5 years have passed since primary immunization. The MCV4 vaccine is now preferred over the MPSV4 vaccine. College students living in dormitories are at increased risk for meningococcal disease and should therefore be immunized with MCV4 (American Academy of Pediatrics, 2009).

Two HPV vaccines are currently licensed for use in the United States. HPV4 (Gardasil) is recommended in females starting at ages 11 to 12 years for the prevention of cervical, vaginal, and vulvar cancers, and in males ages 9 to 18 for the prevention of genital warts. HPV2 (Cervacil) is recommended for females starting at age 11 or 12 years to prevent cervical cancers. Both are given in a series of three vaccines.

With the exception of pregnant teenagers, all adolescents should receive a second measles-mumps-rubella (MMR) vaccine unless they have documentation of two MMR vaccinations during childhood.

All adolescents who have not previously received three doses of hepatitis B vaccine should be vaccinated against hepatitis B virus. The hepatitis A vaccine should be given to all adolescents as part of the routine immunization schedule; the two-dose series may be completed in childhood, and a catch-up schedule for those who have not been previously immunized is recommended. Annual influenza vaccination with either the live attenuated influenza vaccine or trivalent influenza vaccine is now encouraged for all children and adolescents. All adolescents should also be assessed for previous history of varicella infection or vaccination. Vaccination with the varicella vaccine is recommended for those with no previous history; for adolescents 13 years or older with no previous infection or history, the varicella vaccine may be given in two doses 4 or more weeks apart (American Academy of Pediatrics, 2009). Any adolescent who has not completed the immunization series for hepatitis A, hepatitis B, poliovirus, and influenza should receive these immunizations according to the latest catch-up schedule. (See also Immunizations, Chapter 12.)

Adolescents should receive a tuberculin skin test if they have been exposed to active tuberculosis (TB), have lived in a homeless shelter, have been incarcerated, have lived in or come from an area with a high prevalence of TB, or currently work in a health care setting. Among adolescents who are at high risk for infection, an induration of 10 mm or more at the skin test site is considered positive. Adolescents with a positive skin test should be referred for evaluation for active TB. The frequency of TB testing depends on the risk factors for the individual adolescent. (See Tuberculosis, Chapter 32.)

H1N1 influenza (also called swine flu) became widespread throughout the world and the United States, reaching pandemic status by late summer of 2009, with adolescents and young adults appearing to have no previously acquired immunity to the new strain. The H1N1 vaccine was distributed in the United States beginning in late fall of 2009; the live-attenuated H1N1 influenza vaccine (LAIV) is available as nasal spray given once, whereas the inactivated influenza (H1N1) monovalent vaccine is administered by intramuscular route. Targeted candidates to receive the first supplies of vaccine available included pregnant women and persons aged 6 months to 24 years, health care and emergency workers, persons living with or providing care for infants less than 6 months of age, and persons aged 25 to 64 years who have medical conditions that place them at higher risk for influenza-related complications (Centers for Disease Control and Prevention, 2009). Nurses should provide general health teaching about preventing the spread of influenza through regular hand washing; staying out of public places when one has flulike symptoms; and sneezing or coughing into one's sleeve, rather than the hand.

Body Art

Body art (piercing and tattooing) has become a major factor in some adolescents' identity formation. The skin has become one of the latest sources of parent-adolescent conflict. The adolescent often seeks body art as an expression of his or her personal identity and style. Tattoos are often obtained to mark significant life events such as new relationships, births, and deaths. Piercing the ear, nose, nipple, navel, genitalia, or tongue may sometimes create a health problem in the uninformed teenager. It is a nursing responsibility to caution girls and boys against having piercing performed by friends, parents, or themselves. In addition, health education regarding the health risks of tattoos must be provided to youth and their families during routine health care visits (Betz, 2009). Although most cases of piercing are accompanied by few if any serious side effects, there is always a danger of complications such as infection, abscess formation, cyst or keloid formation, bleeding, dermatitis, or metal allergy. Using the same unsterilized needle to pierce body parts of multiple teenagers presents the same risk of HIV, hepatitis C, and hepatitis B virus transmission as with other needle-sharing activities.

A qualified operator using proper sterile technique should perform the procedure. This is especially important if the individual has a history of diabetes, allergies, or skin disorders. Adolescents should be informed about the approximate time for healing after body piercing and the care of the pierced area during and after healing. Some body sites need extra precautions. For example, cartilage (ear, nose) has a poor blood supply and heals slowly and scars easily; nipple piercing puts the adolescent at risk for breast abscess. Finally, migration of the piercing is common with naval and other flat skin surface piercing. Piercing guns should not be used for piercing anything other than the earlobe because guns place the piercing too deeply.

Studies of distinct populations of young adults and adolescents report body art rates as high as 23% (Braverman, 2006). Professional and amateur artists administer tattoos. The risk to the adolescent receiving a tattoo is low. The greatest risk is for the tattoo artist who comes in contact with the client's blood. Adolescents who are amateur tattoo artists benefit from discussions about Standard Precautions and the hepatitis B vaccination. Many states either have no regulations or do not enforce existing regulations of piercing and tattooing facilities. The local health department is a source of information about local regulatory requirements. The Centers for Disease Control and Prevention has an excellent website that outlines safety concerns for persons performing and receiving body art (www.cdc.gov/Features/BodyArt).

Sleep Deprivation and Insomnia

The changing social environment of adolescents can often change their sleep patterns, at a time when their growth and development requires additional sleep for health. Although adolescents should generally get around 9 hours of sleep each night, early morning school scheduling, extracurricular activities, homework, employment, and desired social time with peers or on the Internet can make it difficult for them to get sufficient sleep. Recent studies into sleep among adolescents have shown that nearly half may not get the recommended amounts of sleep, and as many as 1 in 4 is regularly sleep-deprived, that is, reports 6 hours or less of sleep per night (Roberts, Roberts, and Duong, 2009). Sleep deprivation can affect physical and mental health and has been associated with higher rates of depression, somatic complaints such as headaches and stomachaches, fatigue, and difficulties with concentration. These physical and psychologic effects of inadequate sleep can also affect school performance and thus contribute to school problems.

Homeless and street-involved youth, youth who go to bed hungry because of insufficient access to food, and those with anxiety disorders are all more likely to experience sleep disturbances. However, the high rate of young people who do not get enough sleep, and the health consequences of inadequate sleep, suggest that nurses should regularly assess all adolescents for the amount and quality of sleep they are getting. Health teaching and health promotion should include information to promote sufficient sleep.

Tanning

The desire to be attractive leads many teenagers to excessive sunbathing and artificial means for tanning. However, this practice has serious long-term risks, and the adolescent should be educated regarding the detrimental effects of sunlight on the skin. (See Sunburn, Chapter 18.) Long-term effects include premature aging of the skin, increased risk of skin cancer, and, in susceptible individuals, phototoxic reactions.

The increasing popularity of artificial tanning has prompted concern among health professionals regarding the use of sunlamps and tanning machines. The long-term effects of tanning machines are similar to those of the sun; dermatologists do not recommend tanning by these means. Those who insist on using tanning equipment should be warned that goggles must be worn in tanning booths to prevent serious corneal burning. Education on the use of sunscreens, including hypoallergenic products, with a sun protective factor (SPF) of at least 15 and a nonalcohol base without lanolin, parobens, or fragrance is important. Broad-spectrum sunscreens that protect against both ultraviolet A and B are the most effective. Self-tanning creams safely simulate the appearance of a tan; however, teens using these products should be cautioned that sun protection is still required. Targeting health education messages to adolescents and incorporating information on sun protection behaviors in school health curricula and in health care visits will increase adolescent knowledge and awareness.

A large cross-sectional study of 12- to 18-year-olds in the United States found that teens are not following these recommendations; only 34% used sunscreen routinely in the past summer and 14% used a tanning bed at least once (Geller, Colditz, Oliveira, et al, 2002). Cutaneous melanoma, the most common fatal form of skin cancer, is associated with ultraviolet light exposure and continues to affect a significant amount of individuals yearly (Geller and Annas, 2003; Leiter and Garbe, 2008; Rigel, 2008).

HEALTH PROMOTION AMONG SPECIAL GROUPS OF ADOLESCENTS

Certain groups of adolescents—including adolescents of color; gay, lesbian, and bisexual youth; and adolescents living in rural areas—experience health problems at disproportionate rates and face barriers to health care because of a lack of financial resources, limited availability of appropriate resources, or other factors.

Minority Adolescents

Minority children (i.e., children of African-American, Latino-Hispanic, Asian, Native American, and Alaskan Native descent) are the fastest-growing population within the United States. It is estimated that by 2020 roughly 40% of the U.S. child population will be made up of minorities. In 2003, 34% of African-American children and 30% of Hispanic children lived in families with incomes below the poverty level (ChildTrends Data Bank, 2003). Large numbers of Native American children also live in poverty; unemployment on some reservations is estimated at 80%. The disproportionate levels of health problems experienced by adolescents from these racial, ethnic, and tribal groups can be attributed, at least in part, to the effects of poverty and the lack of access to health care that is associated with being poor.

Most of these children grow and develop normally and successfully meet the challenges of adolescence and young adulthood. Research has begun to identify factors that promote resiliency among minority adolescents from disadvantaged backgrounds, including those who grow up in poverty. Often these young people have come from families and communities that provide nurturing, supportive, and culturally rich environments (Isaacs, 1993). To be most effective, future health promotion interventions must include strategies that increase these protective factors in the lives of other adolescents growing up in high-risk environments.

However, too many minority adolescents experience predictable outcomes associated with living in environments where risk factors outweigh protective factors. Compared with nonminority children, higher percentages of minority children and adolescents have learning, emotional, or physical disabilities. They are more likely to drop out of school and have limited opportunities for higher education, become parents at an early age, are incarcerated in youth detention facilities, or die as a result of homicide or unintentional injuries before reaching adulthood. The increase in health risk behaviors during adolescence, in combination with limited access to health care and effective preventive services, places these adolescents at significantly higher risk for adolescent pregnancy, STIs, HIV infection and acquired immunodeficiency syndrome, chronic or other infectious diseases (i.e., hypertension, TB, and hepatitis), substance abuse, emotional problems, and violence. All these health problems, which often lead to premature death or chronic disorders, are preventable.

Effective health promotion programs can make important contributions to the prevention of health problems among minority adolescents. A consensus is growing that health promotion programs will be most effective if they are culturally competent. A culturally competent approach is one that both recognizes the importance of culture and incorporates—at all levels—the assessment of relations across cultures, with attention to dynamics that result from cultural differences, the expansion of cultural knowledge, and the adaptation of programs to meet culture-specific needs (Schorr, 1997). Nurses, working with other health care professionals and community leaders, can develop or adapt culture-specific health promotion interventions (see Cultural Competence box).

⊕ **CULTURAL COMPETENCE**

The Adolescent Years

Other societies in which adolescence is seen as part of the life cycle may have ideas very different from those of American culture about how the adolescent years are to be spent. For example, some societies discourage contact between adolescent boys and girls. Sexual experimentation is out-lawed, and all grown children, males and females, remain in the homes of their parents until they wed. In America we tend to believe that the way our culture is organized is the way all cultures are or should be organized, but of course this is not so. Each society is unique. The way we describe adoles-cence, the way we experience it, and the predisposition of our adolescents toward violence are peculiar to our American culture.

Modified from Prothrow-Stith D: *Deadly consequences: how violence is destroying our teenage population and a plan to begin solving the problem,* New York, 1993, HarperCollins.

Several basic principles can guide the development of culturally appropriate health promotion efforts (Isaacs, 1993):

- Health promotion messages are most effective when they are conveyed through multiple community institutions. The content of these messages should be consistent across agencies, culturally appropriate, and couched in terms that deal with health-destructive behaviors in a pragmatic rather than a judgmental manner.
- Health promotion efforts should involve peer groups, schools, communities, and families. In particular, fami-lies must be recognized as a positive source of cultural strength and a primary source of information, education, and support for young people. Because "family" is defined differently by different cultures, a culture-specific defini-tion of family must be the basis of developing inter-ventions involving families. For example, prevention strategies that involve concerned relatives and friends have proved highly successful in reaching Hispanic youth involved in high-risk behavior. The willingness of family and friends to be involved is rooted in Hispanic values of familialism and community.
- Those who develop strategies for minority adolescents and communities must draw on community-based values, traditions, and customs and work with knowl-edgeable persons from the community in developing focused interventions and communication channels. The challenge for professionals, whose culture may be differ-ent from that of the target audience, is to develop col-laborative relationships with community members that enable communities to identify health problems and their underlying causes and to design and evaluate programs that address identified needs.
- Health promotion interventions focused on minority adolescents may be most effective if they provide a generic framework and skills for developing relation-ships and problem solving that can be applied to any health-related decision. There is an emerging belief that this type of generic approach can be more effective than interventions focused on specific problems (i.e., STIs, pregnancy, or substance use), since the behaviors that lead to many adolescent health problems are highly interrelated.

- Health promotion and prevention strategies must be developed and implemented in places where these ado-lescents are found. Adolescents who have left the school system are often at greater risk for health problems than those who remain in school. Health promotion messages must be incorporated into shelters for homeless and runaway youth, detention centers, residential programs, and community recreation centers to reach young people at highest risk.

To date, there has been little systematic evaluation of the effectiveness of health promotion interventions among minor-ity adolescents. Interventions that work must be documented so that these efforts can be disseminated and adapted for other communities of color.

Gay, Lesbian, and Bisexual Adolescents

The population of gay, lesbian, and bisexual adolescents has unique developmental issues and health challenges. Although adolescents may participate in same-gender sexual activity or have same-gender attractions, they do not necessarily become gay, lesbian, or bisexual adults. Assigning sexual orientation labels to adolescents is complex and should be approached cau-tiously, but most studies conclude that between 3% and 10% of adolescents are lesbian or gay and a larger percentage are bisexual in orientation (Saewyc, Skay, Hynds, et al, 2007).

Most of the health challenges of sexual minority teens are responses to negative societal attitudes and messages about homosexual or bisexual orientation. The stigma associated with gay, lesbian, or bisexual identity makes adolescents reluctant to acknowledge or identify their orientation to themselves and others. For those who try to manage this stigma by keeping their same-gender attractions hidden, the isolation and fear of disclosure can create emotional distress. They may use alcohol and other substances to escape their anxieties, and they are at much greater risk for suicidal behaviors than their heterosexual peers. In several population-based studies, nearly one third of gay, lesbian, and bisexual adolescents report attempting suicide one or more times (Saewyc, Skay, Hynds, et al, 2007). Although nurses should screen all youth about suicidal thoughts and history of suicide attempts, it is especially critical for an adoles-cent who identifies as gay, lesbian, or bisexual or one who is questioning his or her orientation.

Publicly disclosing a gay, lesbian, or bisexual orientation during adolescence ("coming out") brings additional chal-lenges. Many adolescents face hostility and even violence from their families when they first come out. Some families physically or sexually assault the adolescent, whereas others seek psychologic counseling or treatment to "change" their teen's orientation (D'Augelli, Hershberger, and Pilkington, 1998). The American Psychological Association (2006) and the American Academy of Pediatrics have both issued state-ments that "reparative therapy," or treatment designed to alter sexual orientation, shows no evidence of effectiveness but does show evidence of psychologic harm and is therefore unethical.

Some families are so distressed and angry after their teen's disclosure of a homosexual or bisexual identity that they throw the adolescent out of the house. A disproportionate number of homeless and street youth are gay, lesbian, or bisexual (Smith,

Saewyc, Albert, et al, 2007). Others are rejecting in more subtle ways, but even these nonsupportive responses can have an effect on adolescents' healthy development; those who are rejected by their families are at increased risk for suicide attempts and substance abuse (Ryan, Huebner, Diaz, et al, 2008).

Nurses should not encourage teens to disclose their sexual orientation to their families without first forming a safety plan in case the reaction is not supportive. For teenagers who question their sexual orientation, the nurse should not reassure them that these feelings are only a passing phase. For the majority of young people, referral to an agency providing support services or social opportunities for gay, lesbian, and bisexual adolescents is appropriate. In many high schools, Gay Straight Alliances (GSAs), after-school advocacy and social groups, can be a source of peer and social support as well. Parents who seek assistance in adjusting to their son or daughter's disclosure can be referred to a local chapter of Parents, Families and Friends of Lesbians and Gays (www.pflag.org), which provides information and support for parents and family members.

Teens who acknowledge same-gender attractions or relationships are also at risk for violence and harassment from schoolmates, neighbors, and even strangers. Gay, lesbian, and bisexual adolescents who are homeless face additional risks of physical and sexual violence. They may be forced to exchange sex for shelter or food or to avoid assault and may not be able to negotiate safer sex practices. As a result, they may be at increased risk for sexual abuse, STIs, and pregnancy.

Given their pervasive experiences of negative attitudes and potential violence, sexual minority adolescents may fear similar uncaring attitudes among health care providers and might avoid disclosing their orientation during health assessments. Many gay, lesbian, and bisexual adolescents have experienced insensitive behaviors from health care providers, and they may avoid needed health care as a result (Ryan and Futterman, 1997). To provide sensitive, professional care for gay, lesbian, and bisexual adolescents, nurses should be sensitive in their choice of language and be nonjudgmental and caring in their communication. Placing a poster or brochure about local services for gay, lesbian, and bisexual youth in a prominent position in the clinic setting sends the message it is safe to talk about such issues at the clinic. Health professionals who work with teenagers regarding sexual orientation issues are encouraged to seek out additional information and resources that address health needs and services for gay, lesbian, and bisexual adolescents (Ryan and Futterman, 1997).

Rural Adolescents

Except for higher rates of accidental injuries (related in part to farm accidents) and lower rates of delinquency among rural adolescents compared with urban ones, few known differences in health problems exist. Research on the health status of rural adolescents is limited, but rural adolescents experience many of the same health problems as adolescents in metropolitan areas. However, rural adolescents face barriers to health promotion, since they have more limited access to appropriate health care services.

Rural adolescents' access to health care is limited by shortages of professionally staffed mental and physical health services, inadequately trained providers, transportation problems, and less access to Medicaid in rural states. Rural communities often lack adequately trained nurses, physicians, dentists, psychologists, social workers, and allied health professionals, in addition to modern equipment. Rural health professionals often feel inadequately prepared to address adolescents' physical and psychosocial health issues. In metropolitan areas providers who are unwilling or unable to address adolescents' concerns can refer to colleagues with expertise in adolescent health issues. The absence of adolescent health specialists, combined with a limited network of agencies focused on adolescent health promotion, exacerbates rural youths' problems in obtaining appropriate services. Finally, rural adolescents who live in poverty are less likely than their low-income urban counterparts to be covered by Medicaid and to have financial coverage for health care services.

In addition to health promotion topics addressed with other populations of adolescents, prevention efforts focused on rural adolescents must include efforts to improve the safety of farm machinery and farming practices. Innovative efforts are needed to increase rural adolescents' access to health care services, including development and funding for school-linked health services, improvements in transportation, use of nonprofessionals and adult community members, better dissemination of information about availability of local health services, and access to further education in adolescent health for health care providers.

NURSING CARE MANAGEMENT

With continued increases in the numbers of adolescents in the United States and rising rates of health-related problems of youth, there is an unprecedented need for adolescent health promotion. Nursing professionals can make significant contributions to health promotion among adolescents and their families. Because nurses understand the biologic, cognitive, psychosocial, and social transitions of adolescence and their impact on health behavior, they can address adolescents' developmental and health needs. Working with colleagues from other disciplines, community members, parents, and adolescents themselves, nurses must become part of a comprehensive approach that delivers consistent messages across clinical, school, and community-based settings. Nurses should be at the forefront of developing and disseminating culturally appropriate health promotion interventions among special populations, including adolescents of color; gay, lesbian, and bisexual youths; and rural teenagers.

Parents are often confused and perplexed about the changes and behaviors of adolescence. They need support and guidance to help them through this time. They need to understand the changes taking place and to accept the expected behaviors that accompany the process of detachment, to be prepared to "let go," and to promote the changed relationship from one of dependency to one of mutuality. Suggestions for anticipatory guidance of parents of adolescents are listed in the Family-Centered Care box.

FAMILY-CENTERED CARE

Guidance During Adolescence

Encourage parents to:
- Accept adolescent as a unique individual.
- Respect adolescent's ideas, likes and dislikes, and wishes.
- Be involved with school functions and attend adolescent's performances, whether it is a sporting event or a school play.
- Listen and try to be open to adolescent's views, even when they disagree with parental views.
- Avoid criticism about no-win topics.
- Provide opportunity for choosing options and accepting natural consequences of these choices.
- Allow young person to learn by doing, even when choices and methods differ from those of adults.
- Provide adolescent with clear, reasonable limits.
- Clarify house rules and consequences for breaking them.
- Let society's rules and consequences teach responsibility outside the home.
- Allow increasing independence within limitations of safety and well-being.
- Be available for conversation but avoid pressing adolescent too far.
- Respect adolescent's privacy.

- Try to share adolescent's feelings of joy or sorrow.
- Respond to feelings as well as words.
- Be available to answer questions, give information, and provide companionship.
- Try to make communication clear.
- Avoid comparisons with siblings.
- Assist adolescent in selecting appropriate career goals and preparing for adult role.
- Welcome adolescent's friends into the home and treat them with respect.
- Provide unconditional love.
- Be willing to apologize when mistaken.

Be aware that adolescents:
- Are sometimes subject to turbulent, unpredictable behavior
- Are struggling for independence
- Are extremely sensitive to feelings and behaviors that affect them
- May receive a different message from what was sent
- Consider friends extremely important
- Have a strong need to belong

KEY POINTS

- Adolescence is characterized by important biologic, cognitive, psychologic, and social change.
- The biologic events of puberty result in hormonal changes; changes in height, weight, strength, and endurance; and development of secondary sexual characteristics.
- During adolescence most individuals move from patterns of concrete thinking to abstract, hypothetical thinking.
- Major psychologic tasks of adolescence involve establishing a sense of identity along with behavioral, emotional, and value autonomy.
- According to Kohlberg's theory of moral development, adolescents begin to question existing moral values and learn to make choices. Gilligan observed differences in the way males and females make moral decisions.
- Spiritual development is characterized by the questioning of family values and ideals, a move to more philosophic thinking, and emphasis on personal religion.
- As adolescents establish identities separate from those of parents and families, relationships with peers often become more important.

- Biologic, cognitive, and psychosocial changes all affect sexual activity and sexual identity development of adolescents.
- Gay, lesbian, and bisexual youth have unique issues to cope with in identity formation.
- The three primary causes of death during adolescence are injuries, homicide, and suicide.
- Motor vehicle injuries are the greatest causes of mortality from unintentional injuries in this age-group.
- Major causes of adolescent morbidity include injury; STIs; unintended pregnancy; and mental health problems, including depression, chronic illness, and eating disorders.
- To be most effective, adolescent health promotion efforts must actively involve teenagers at all stages.
- The availability of confidential health services is particularly important to adolescents.
- Certain groups of adolescents—including youth of color; rural youth; and gay, lesbian, and bisexual youth—experience health problems at disproportionate rates and face barriers to health care because of limited access to appropriate, affordable resources.

ANSWERS TO CRITICAL THINKING EXERCISE

Discussing Sexual Orientation with Adolescents

1. **Yes.** There is sufficient information to arrive at a conclusion about John's sexual orientation.
2. **a.** Studies of gay, lesbian, and bisexual people indicate that adolescence is the time when individuals become aware of same-gender attraction. Gay and bisexual youths are at risk for health-damaging behaviors such as early initiation of sexual behavior, substance abuse, suicide, and running away from home.
   b. Gay, lesbian, and bisexual youths are often confronted with anti-gay attitudes and values in society. This reaction

makes it difficult for these youths to grow up and become healthy physically and mentally.
   c. Health care professionals who work with adolescents should consider the adolescent's increasing independence and responsibility while ensuring confidentiality.
3. The nurse's first priority in this situation is to give John permission to discuss his feelings about this topic. He has come to the nurse practitioner to discuss this matter, and he probably feels comfortable sharing this information with her. The nurse practitioner needs to be open and nonjudgmental in her interactions with John. He needs

to know that the nurse practitioner will maintain confidentiality, appreciate his feelings, and remain sensitive to his need to talk about this topic. An example of an appropriate response for the nurse practitioner might be, "John, tell me more about how you came to this conclusion."

4. Yes. The information about sexual orientation in adolescence and the role of the health care professional support this conclusion.

REFERENCES

Aalsma MC, Lapsley DK, Flannery DJ: Personal fables, narcissism, and adolescent adjustment, *Psychol Schools* 43:481-491, 2006.

American Academy of Pediatrics, Committee on Infectious Diseases, Pickering L, editor: *2009 Red book: report of the Committee on Infectious Diseases,* ed 28, Elk Grove Village, Ill, 2009, The Academy.

American Academy of Pediatrics: Recommendations for preventive health care, *Pediatrics* 120(6):1376-1377, 2007.

American Academy of Pediatrics: Active healthy living: prevention of childhood obesity through increased physical activity, *Pediatrics* 117(5):1834-1842, 2006.

American Medical Association: *Guidelines for adolescent preventive services,* ed 4, Chicago, 1997, The Association, available at www. ama-assn.org/ama/upload/mm/39/gapsmono. pdf (accessed January 29, 2010).

American Psychological Association: Just the facts about sexual orientation and youth: a primer for principals, educators and school personnel, *APA Online,* 2006, available at www.apa.org/pi/lgbc/publications/justthefacts. html (accessed February 18, 2006).

Bennett L, Gates GJ: *The cost of marriage inequality to children and their same-sex parents,* 2004, Human Rights Campaign Foundation, available at www.hrc.org (accessed March 2005).

Bensussen-Walls W, Saewyc EM: Teen-focused vs adult-focused prenatal care models for high-risk pregnant adolescents, *Pub Health Nurs* 18(6):424-435, 2001.

Betz C: To tattoo or not: that is the question, *J Pediatr Nurs* 24(4):241-243, 2009.

Bleakley A, Merzel CR, VanDevanter NL, et al: Computer access and Internet use among urban youths, *Am J Pub Health* 94:744-746. 2004.

Braverman PK: Body art: piercing, tattooing, and scarification, *Adolesc Med* 17:505-519, 2006.

Brewster KL, Tillman KH: Who's doing it? Patterns and predictors of youths' oral sexual experiences, *J Adolesc Health* 42(1):73-80, 2008.

Bronfenbrenner U: *The ecology of human development,* Cambridge, Mass, 1979, Harvard University Press.

Brown JD, L'Engle KL, Pardun CJ, et al: Sexy media matter: exposure to sexual content in music, movies, television and magazines predicts black and white adolescents' sexual behavior, *Pediatrics* 117:1018-1027, 2006.

Center for Labor Market Studies: *Left behind in America: the nation's dropout crisis,* 2009, Northeastern University, available at www. clms.neu.edu/publication/documents/ CLMS_2009_Dropout_Report.pdf (accessed September 11, 2009).

Centers for Disease Control and Prevention: 2009 H1N1 monovalent influenza vaccine dosage, administration, and storage, Atlanta, 2009, The Centers, available at www.cdc.gov/ h1n1flu/vaccination/dosage.htm (accessed December 2009).

ChildTrends Data Bank: *Children in poverty, 2003,* 2003, available at www.childtrensdatabank.org (accessed January 5, 2010).

Chumlea WC, Schubert CM, Roche AF, et al: Age at menarche and racial comparisons in US girls, *Pediatrics* 111(1):110-115, 2003.

Daniels SR, Greer FR, Committee on Nutrition: Lipid screening and cardiovascular health in childhood, *Pediatrics* 122(1):198-208, 2008.

D'Augelli AR, Hershberger SL, Pilkington NW: Lesbian, gay, and bisexual youth and their families: disclosure of sexual orientation and its consequences, *Am J Orthopsychiatry* 68(3):361-371, 1998.

Diamond LM: Sexual identity, attractions, and behavior among young sexual minority women over a 2 year period, *Dev Psychol* 36(2):241-250, 2000.

Doswell WM, Millor GK, Thompson H, et al: Self-image and self-esteem in African-American preteen girls: implications for mental health, *Issues Mental Health Nurs* 19(1):71-94, 1998.

Eaton DK, Kann L, Kinchen S, et al: Youth risk behavior surveillance—United States, 2007, *MMWR Surv Summ* 57(SS04):1-131, 2008.

Eisenberg M, Aalsma M: Bullying and peer victimization: position paper of the Society for Adolescent Medicine, *J Adolesc Health* 36(1):88-91, 2005.

Elkind D: Understanding the young adolescent, *Adolescence* 13(49):128-134, 1978.

Erikson E: *Identity: youth in crisis,* New York, 1968, Norton.

Forrest R, Saewyc E: Sexual minority teen parents: demographics of an unexpected population, *J Adolesc Health* 34(2):122, 2004.

Frederickson D: Maltreatment of children, *Child Family Nurs* 2(6):393-401, 1999.

Geller AC, Annas GD: Epidemiology of melanoma and nonmelanoma skin cancer, *Semin Oncol Nurs* 19(1):2-11, 2003.

Geller AC, Colditz G, Oliveira S, et al: Use of sunscreen, sunburning rates and tanning bed use among more than 10,000 U.S. children and adolescents, *Pediatrics* 109(6):1009-1014, 2002.

Gilligan C: *Adolescent development reconsidered,* paper presented at Invitational Conference on Health Futures of Adolescents, Daytona Beach, Fla, 1986.

Gilligan C: *In a different voice,* 1982, Cambridge, Mass, 1982, Harvard University Press.

Glatt K: Child-to-child unintentional injury and death from firearms in the United States:

what can be done? *J Pediatr Nurse* 20(6):448-452, 2005.

Gottfried AE, Gottfried AW: *Redefining families: implications for children's development,* New York, 1994, Plenum Press.

Hansen ML, Gunn PW, Kaelber DC: Underdiagnosis of hypertension in children and adolescents, *JAMA* 298(8):874-879, 2007.

Herman-Giddens ME: Recent data on pubertal milestones in United States children: the secular trend toward earlier development, *Int J Androl* 29(1):241-246, 2006.

Herman-Giddens M, Slora EJ, Wasserman RC, et al: Secondary sexual characteristics and menses in young girls seen in office practice: a study from the Pediatric Research in Office Settings Network, *Pediatrics* 99(4):505-512, 1997.

Hosking SG, Young KL, Regan MA: The effects of text messaging on young drivers, *Hum Factors* 51(4):582-592, 2009.

Isaacs M: Developing culturally competent strategies for adolescents of color. In Elster A, Panzarine S, Holt K, editors: *American Medical Association State of the Art Conference on Adolescent Health Promotion: proceedings,* Arlington, Va, 1993, National Center for Education in Maternal and Child Health.

Jenkins RR: Adolescent medicine. In Kliegman RM, Behrman RE, Jenson HB, et al, editors, *Nelson textbook of pediatrics,* ed 18, Philadelphia, 2007, Saunders.

Kaplowitz P, Oberfield SE: Reexamination of the age limit for defining when puberty is precocious in girls in the United States: implications for evaluation and treatment: Drug and Therapeutics and Executive Committees of the Lawson Wilkins Pediatric Endocrine Society, *Pediatrics* 104(4 Pt 1): 936-941, 1999.

Kirby D: The impact of abstinence and comprehensive sex and STI/HIV education programs on adolescent sexual behavior, *Sexual Res Soc Policy* 5(3):18-27, 2008.

Kohlberg L, Gilligan C: The adolescent as philosopher: the discovery of the self in a post-conventional world. In Kagan J, Coles R, editors: *Twelve to sixteen: early adolescence,* New York, 1972, Norton.

Lapsley DK: Toward an integrated theory of adolescent ego development: the "new look" at adolescent egocentrism, *Am J Orthopsychiatry* 63(4):562-571, 1993.

Leiter U, Garbe C: Epidemiology of melanoma and nonmelanoma skin cancer—the role of sunlight, *Adv Exp Med Biol* 624(1):89-103, 2008.

Marcia J: Development and validation of ego identity status, *J Perspec Soc Psychol* 3(5):551-558, 1966.

McCartt AT, Hellinga LA, Bratiman KA: Cell phones and driving: a review of research, *Traffic Inj Prev* 6(2):89-106, 2006.

McCrindle BW, Urbina EM, Dennison BA, et al: AHA scientific statement: drug therapy of high-risk lipid abnormalities in children and adolescents: a scientific statement from the American Heart Association Atherosclerosis, Hypertension, and Obesity in Youth Committee, Council of Cardiovascular Disease in the Young, with the Council on Cardiovascular Nursing, *Circulation* 115(14):1948-1967, 2007.

Miller M, Azrael D, Hemenway D: Firearm availability and unintentional firearm deaths, suicide and homicide among 5-14 year olds, *J Trauma* 52:267-275, 2002.

Mulye TP, Park MJ, Nelson CD, et al: Trends in adolescent and young adult health in the United States, *J Adolesc Health* 45:8-24, 2009.

Patton GC, Viner R: Adolescent health, part 1, Pubertal transitions in health, *Lancet* 369:1130-1139, 2007.

Perry C, Kelder S, Komro K: The social world of adolescents: family, peers, schools, and the community. In Millstein S, Petersen A, Nightingale E, editors: *Promoting the health of adolescents: new directions for the twenty-first century*, New York, 1993, Oxford University Press.

Piaget J: Intellectual evolution from adolescence to adulthood, *Hum Dev* 15:1-12, 1972.

Rao G: Childhood obesity: highlights of AMA Expert Committee recommendations, *Am Acad Fam Physician* 78(1):56-63, 65-66, 2008.

Reddy DM, Fleming R, Swain C: Effect of mandatory parental notification on adolescent girls' use of sexual health care services, *JAMA* 288(6):710-714, 2002.

Reis E, Saewyc EM: *83,000 youth: selected findings of eight population-based studies as they pertain to anti-gay harassment and the safety and well-being of sexual minority students*, Seattle, 1999, Safe Schools Coalition of Washington.

Resnick MD: Protective factors, resiliency and healthy youth development, *Adolesc Med* 11(1):157-165, 2000.

Resnick MD, Bearman PS, Blum RW, et al: Protecting adolescents from harm: findings from the National Longitudinal Study of Adolescent Health, *JAMA* 278(10):823-831, 1997.

Rigel DS: Cutaneous ultraviolet exposure and its relationship to the development of skin cancer, *J Am Acad Dermatol* 58(5 Suppl 2): S129-S132, 2008.

Roberts RE, Roberts CR, Duong HT: Sleepless in adolescence: prospective data on sleep deprivation, health and functioning, *Adolescence* 23:1045-1057, 2009.

Rojas NL, Killen JD, Haydel KF, et al: Nicotine dependence among adolescent smokers, *Arch Pediatr Adolesc Med* 152(2):151-156, 1998.

Rosario M, Meyey-Bahlburg H, Hunter J, et al: The psychosexual development of urban lesbian, gay, and bisexual youth, *J Sex Res* 33(2):113-126, 1996.

Rosenfeld SL, Keenan PM, Fox DJ, et al: Youth perceptions of comprehensive adolescent health services through the Boston HAPPENS program, *J Pediatr Health Care* 14(2):60-67, 2000.

Russell ST, Seif H, Truong N: School outcomes of sexual minority youth in the United States: evidence from a national study, *J Adolesc Health* 24(1):111-127, 2001.

Ryan C, Futterman D: *Lesbian and gay youth: care and counseling*, New York, 1997, Columbia University Press.

Ryan C, Huebner D, Diaz R, et al: Family rejection as a predictor of negative health outcomes in white and Latino lesbian, gay, and bisexual young adults. *Pediatrics* 123:346-352, 2008.

Saewyc EM, Pettingell S, Magee LL: The prevalence of sexual abuse among adolescents in school, *J School Nurs* 19(5):266-272, 2003.

Saewyc EM, Pettingell S, Skay C, et al: Teen pregnancy among sexual minority youth in population-based surveys of the 1990s: countertrends in a population at risk, *J Adolesc Health* 34(2):125-126, 2004.

Saewyc EM, Poon C, Homma Y, et al: Stigma management? The links between enacted stigma and teen pregnancy trends among gay, lesbian and bisexual students in British Columbia. *Can J Hum Sex* 17(3):123-131, 2008.

Saewyc E, Poon C, Wang N, et al: *Not yet equal: the health of lesbian, gay, and bisexual youth in BC*. Vancouver, 2007, McCreary Centre Society.

Saewyc EM, Singh N, Reis E, et al: The intersection of racial, gender and orientation harassment in school and health risk behaviors among adolescents (abstract), *J Adolesc Health* 26(2):148, 2000.

Saewyc EM, Skay CL, Hynds P, et al. Suicidal ideation and attempts among adolescents in North American school-based surveys: are bisexual youth at increasing risk? *J LGBT Health Res* 3:25-36, 2007.

Saewyc EM, Skay CL, Reis E, et al: Hazards of stigma: the sexual and physical abuse of gay, lesbian, and bisexual adolescents in the U.S. and Canada, *Child Welfare* 58(2):196-213, 2006.

Santelli JS, Orr M, Lindberg LD, et al: Changing behavioral risk for pregnancy among high school students in the United States, 1991-2007, *J Adolesc Health* 45(1):25-32, 2009.

Schorr LB: *Common purpose: strengthening families and neighborhoods to rebuild America*, New York, 1997, Anchor Books.

Shain B, Committee on Adolescence: Suicide and suicide attempts in adolescents, *Pediatrics* 120(3):669-676, 2007.

Smith A, Saewyc E, Albert M, et al: *Against the odds: a profile of marginalized and street-involved youth in BC*, Vancouver, 2007, McCreary Centre Society.

Smith A, Stewart D, Peled M, et al: *A picture of health: highlights of the 2008 British Columbia Adolescent Health Survey*, Vancouver, 2009, McCreary Centre Society.

Steinberg L: Autonomy, conflict and harmony in the family relationship. In Feldman S, Elliot G, editors: *At the threshold: the developing adolescent*, Cambridge, Mass, 1990, Harvard University Press.

Sullivan H: *The interpersonal theory of psychiatry*, New York, 1953, Norton.

Tuttle J, Bidwell-Cerone S, Campbell-Heider N, et al: Teen club: a nursing intervention for reducing risk-taking behavior and improving well-being in female African-American adolescents, *J Pediatr Health Care* 14(3):103-108, 2000.

US Census Bureau: *Educational attainment in the United States*, 2004, detailed tables: Table 1a, 2004, available at www.census.gov/population/www/socdemo/education/cps2004.html (accessed January 5, 2010).

US Department of Health and Human Services, Administration on Children, Youth, and Families: *Child maltreatment 2003*, Washington, DC, 2005, US Government Printing Office.

US Department of Health and Human Services: *Healthy people 2020: the road ahead*, Washington, DC, 2009, The Department, available at www.healthypeople.gov/HP2020/default.asp (accessed December 2009).

Walker L, de Vries B, Trevethan S: Moral stages and moral orientations in real-life and hypothetical dilemmas, *Child Dev* 58:842-858, 1987.

Widom C, Kuhns J: Childhood victimization and subsequent risk for promiscuity, prostitution and teen pregnancy: a prospective study, *Am J Pub Health* 86(11):1607-1611, 1996.

Zapalla FR, Gidding SS: Lipid management in children, *Endocrinol Metab Clin North Am* 38(1):171-183, 2009.

Physical Health Problems of Adolescence

Linda M. Kollar

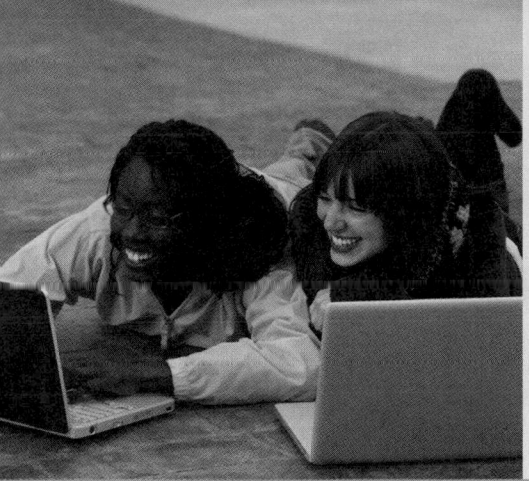

⊝volve WEBSITE

RELATED TOPICS

CHAPTER OUTLINE

COMMON HEALTH CONCERNS OF ADOLESCENCE

ACNE

⊝ Adolescents are subject to the same skin conditions that affect the school-age child, such as bacterial, viral, and fungal infections; contact dermatitis; and drug reactions. However, one skin disorder, although not limited to the adolescent age-group, appears predominantly at this time: acne vulgaris (common acne). Acne is the most common skin problem treated by physicians. Acne involves important anatomic, physiologic, biochemical, genetic, immunologic, and psychologic factors.

More than half the adolescent population will have had acne by the end of the teenage years, and many children have evidence of the disorder before age 10. Acne usually occurs in middle to late adolescence, at age 16 to 17 years in girls and 17 to 18 years in boys. The disorder is more common in boys than in girls. After this age period the disease usually decreases in severity, but it may persist well into adulthood. Early acne occurs in the midface region (midforehead, nose, and chin) and later spreads to the lateral cheeks, lower jaw, back, and chest. The degree to which acne affects an individual may range from nothing more than a few isolated comedones to a severe inflammatory reaction. Although the disease is self-limiting and is not life threatening, its significance to the affected adolescent is great, and it is a mistake to underestimate its impact on teens.

Etiology

Numerous factors affect the development and course of acne. Research has shown a familial aspect to acne vulgaris, with a high occurrence of severe acne and increased sebum secretion among monozygotic twins. Forty-five percent of adolescent boys with acne have a positive family history, whereas only 8% of adolescent boys without acne have a positive family history. Premenstrual flares of acne occur in nearly 70% of girls, suggesting a hormonal cause. Scientific studies do not demonstrate a clear association between stress and acne; however, adolescents commonly cite stress as a cause for acne outbreaks. Cosmetics containing lanolin, petrolatum, vegetable oils, lauryl alcohol, butylstearate, and oleic acid can increase comedone production. Exposure to oils in cooking grease can be a precursor to acne in adolescents working in fast-food restaurants. There is no known link between dietary intake and the development or worsening of acne lesions.

Pathophysiology

Acne is a disease that involves the pilosebaceous unit, which consists of the sebaceous glands and hair follicles. Acne is most commonly found on the face, chest, upper back, and neck because of the large quantity of sebaceous glands on these skin areas. There are nearly 900 glands per square centimeter on the skin surfaces of the face, chest, neck, and upper back, compared with 100 glands per square centimeter on the rest of the body.

Three pathophysiologic factors have the greatest influence on acne development: excessive sebum production, comedogenesis, and the overgrowth of *Propionibacterium acnes* (Olutunmbi, Paley, and English, 2008). Increased sebum production begins at the time of adrenocortical maturation and subtly continues to increase until the late teens. Acne severity is proportional to the sebum secretion rate, which is genetically determined.

Comedogenesis (formation of comedones) results in a noninflammatory lesion that may be either an open comedone (blackhead) or a closed comedone (whitehead). Inflammation occurs with the proliferation of *P. acnes,* which draws in neutrophils, causing inflammatory papules, pustules, nodules, and cysts (Fig. 20-1). The traditional ice pick scarring results from macrophages that digest the inflamed skin along with the normal dermis in the process.

Psychosocial Ramifications

Adolescents are acutely aware of their physical appearance, and their cognitive development results in the feeling that they are constantly on stage. In one survey one third of teenagers reported that pimples were the first thing people noticed about them (Gupta and Gupta, 2003). A population-based study found that older adolescents with acne had lower self esteem,

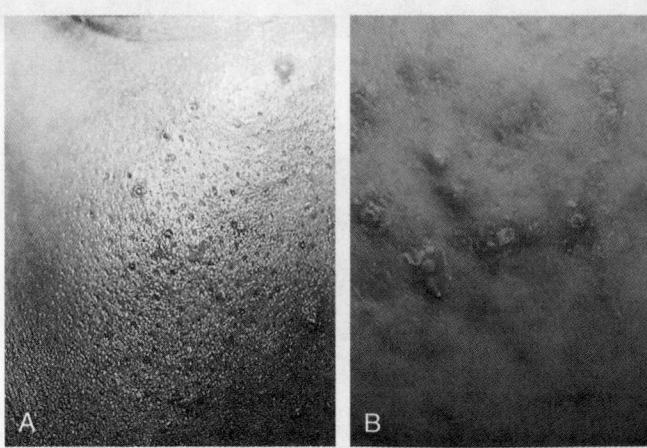

Fig. 20-1 Acne vulgaris. **A,** Comedonal acne with open comedones. **B,** Papulopustular acne. (From Zitelli BJ, Davis HW: *Atlas of pediatric physical diagnosis,* ed 5, St Louis, 2007, Mosby.)

lower self-worth, and less body satisfaction than those without acne (Dalgard, Gieler, Holm, et al, 2008). The amount of psychologic stress does not directly correlate to the clinical severity of the acne. The importance of timely treatment has been underscored by research demonstrating the long-term psychologic impact of living with acne over critical developmental periods of life (Gupta and Gupta, 2003).

Therapeutic Management

Successful management of acne depends on a cooperative effort between the care provider, adolescent, and parents. The care provider must determine the adolescent's goals and increase understanding of the cause and treatment of acne. Unlike many dermatologic conditions, the acne lesions resolve slowly, and improvement may not be apparent for at least 6 weeks. Individual comedones may take several weeks to months to resolve, and papules and pustules usually resolve in about 1 week.

The multifactorial causes of acne require a combined approach for successful treatment. Treatment consists of general measures of care and specific treatments determined by the type of lesions involved.

General Measures

The practitioner provides the adolescent with an overall explanation of the disease process, emphasizing the patient's individual requirements. Parents should be present at the initial discussion to ensure their cooperation, understanding, and support. Remind adolescents that acne occurs, to some degree, in almost all teenagers.

Improvement of the adolescent's overall health status is part of the general management. Adequate rest, moderate exercise, a well-balanced diet, reduction of emotional stress, and elimination of any foci of infection are all part of general health promotion. Review general skin care considerations, including limiting sun exposure and the use of noncomedogenic moisturizers and sunscreens.

Cleansing

Acne is not caused by dirt or oil on the surface of the skin. Gentle cleansing with a mild cleanser once or twice daily is usually sufficient. Antibacterial soaps are ineffective and may be drying when used in combination with topical acne medications. For some adolescents, hygiene of the hair and scalp appears to be related to the clinical activity of acne. Acne on the forehead may improve with brushing the hair away from the forehead and more frequent shampooing.

Medications

Treatment success depends on commitment from the adolescent. Before prescribing treatment, the clinician should determine the adolescent's level of comfort and readiness to begin treatment. The teen should be reminded that clinical improvement may take weeks to months. Those who are impatient with speed of recovery may discontinue the medication or apply too much. Discussion about acne treatment should begin in early puberty. In young girls the early development of acne is the best predictor of future severe acne. Early intervention, most often with topical medications, may prevent the development of more severe acne.

Topical retinoids are the only drugs that effectively interrupt the abnormal follicular keratinization that produces microcomedones, the invisible precursors of the visible comedones. Retinoids are recommended as the first line of treatment for most forms of acne. Tretinoin has been the gold standard for topical retinoids and is available as a cream, gel, or liquid. The cream is less irritating than the gel, which is less irritating than the liquid. Newer formulations contain tretinoin trapped within porous copolymer microspheres that localize the medication to the follicle. These are less irritating to the skin because the medication is released over time, reducing the concentration on the skin (Guttman, 2009). The next-generation topical retinoids adapalene and tazarotene became available in the late 1990s. A comparison trial of the two medications found them to have similar efficacy, but adapalene gel 0.3% was better tolerated. After 12 weeks of treatment more than 50% of subjects in both treatment arms reported marked improvement or near clearing of acne (Thiboutot, Arsonnaud, and Pascale, 2008).

A gel combining 0.25% tretinoin and 1.2% clindamycin phosphate (Ziana gel) has been recently approved by the U.S. Food and Drug Administration (FDA). This gel has been shown to be more effective in treating acne than tretinoin or clindamycin monotherapy (Eichenfield and Wortzman, 2009).

Instruct the patient to begin with a pea-sized dot of medication, which is divided into the three main areas of the face and then gently rubbed into each area. The patient should not apply the medication until at least 20 to 30 minutes after washing to decrease the burning sensation. A daily moisturizer should be used along with retinoid treatment. Since sun exposure may easily result in severe sunburn, advise adolescents to avoid sun, apply the medication at night, and use a sunscreen with a sun protective factor (SPF) of at least 15 in the daytime.

Topical benzoyl peroxide is an antibacterial agent that inhibits the growth of *P. acnes*. Benzoyl peroxide is effective against both inflammatory and noninflammatory acne and is an effective first-line agent. The medication is available as a cream, lotion, gel, or wash. Using benzoyl peroxide is less likely to result in the development of antibiotic-resistant strains of *P. acnes*, which makes it an ideal adjunct when topical or oral antibiotic treatment is employed (Bowe and Shalita, 2008).

Benzoyl peroxide soaps are convenient because they can be applied in the shower and assist in the treatment of acne on the chest and back. Benzoyl peroxide and salicylic acid are the most common ingredients in popular and effective acne treatment kits available over the counter. Patient education should include information regarding the bleaching effect of the peroxide on sheets, bedclothes, and towels. The adolescent can be reassured that skin bleaching will not occur. The drying effects of the medication can be accommodated with gradual increases in strength and frequency of application.

When inflammatory lesions accompany the comedones, a topical antibacterial agent may be prescribed. These agents are used to prevent new lesions and to treat preexisting acne. Clindamycin, erythromycin-metronidazole, and azelaic acid are currently available topical antibiotics. Side effects of these medications include erythema, dryness, and burning; using the medications every other day will decrease the adverse effects. Topical antimicrobials combined with benzoyl peroxide are more effective than either product alone. Retinoids in combination with antimicrobials also improve the penetration of these topical agents and are the only means to address three of the pathogenic causes of acne: keratinization, *P. acnes*, and inflammation. Combination therapy is usually more effective than either component alone (Krakowski, Stendardo, and Eichenfield, 2008).

Systemic antibiotic therapy is initiated when moderate to severe acne does not respond to topical treatments. The foundation for using systemic antibiotics in acne treatment has been the elimination of the inflammatory effects of *P. acnes* by suppressing the bacteria. Tetracycline, erythromycin, minocycline, doxycycline, and amoxicillin are systemic antibiotics used to treat acne (Olutunmbi, Paley, and English, 2008; Yan, 2006). They are relatively free of side effects with the exception of occasional gastrointestinal upset, photosensitivity, or vaginal candidiasis. Minocycline is more expensive but is less likely to cause gastrointestinal side effects and is very effective against severe inflammatory acne. Resistance to antibiotics may develop, especially with tetracycline and erythromycin. Judicious use of oral antibiotics and avoidance of topical antibiotics in combination with oral treatment can prevent resistance. Providers should avoid use of multiple antibiotic classes and shorten the course by using the full dose of systemic antibiotics for 1 month and then begin to taper the dosage. The adolescent can then be maintained on topical treatment (Krakowski, Stendardo, and Eichenfield, 2008).

Girls with mild to moderate acne may respond to topical treatment and the addition of an oral contraceptive pill (OCP). OCPs reduce the endogenous androgen production and decrease the bioavailability of the woman's circulating androgens. Combination OCPs containing levonorgestrel, gestodene, and desogestrel as the progestin decrease acne in women. The FDA has approved multiple combination OCPs for the treatment of acne in girls. Visible improvement may take up to 4 months.

Isotretinoin 12-*cis*-retinoic acid (Accutane), a potent and effective oral agent, is reserved for severe, cystic acne that has not responded to other treatments. Isotretinoin is the only agent available that affects all factors in the development of acne. Only physicians who have taken a comprehensive educational program about the medication, necessary monitoring of patients, and parameters for pregnancy prevention may manage treatment with isotretinoin. Adolescents with multiple, active, deep dermal or subcutaneous cystic and nodular acne lesions are treated for 20 weeks. Long-term remissions occur with this highly effective drug. However, multiple cutaneous side effects can occur, which vary from mild to moderate in severity. Dry skin, dry eyes, dry mucous membranes, nasal irritation, decreased night vision, photosensitivity, arthralgia, headaches, mood changes, depression, and suicidal ideation may occur. There is some concern that isotretinoin may be associated with increased incidence of depression and suicide despite several findings to the contrary (Webster, 2009). Careful monitoring for signs of depression among all adolescents taking isotretinoin is recommended as part of all health visits for acne treatment (Hull and D'Arcy, 2003; Jacobs, Deutsch, and Brewer, 2001). The most significant side effects are the teratogenic effects, causing limb and skull abnormalities. Isotretinoin is absolutely contraindicated in pregnant women. Sexually active young women must use an effective contraceptive method during treatment and for 1 month after treatment. Providers should also monitor patients receiving isotretinoin for elevated cholesterol and triglyceride levels. Significant elevation may require discontinuation of the medication.

Scarring begins early in all types of acne, from papulopustular to nodulocystic. Most of the scarring is a result of loss of tissue rather than thickening. Chemical peels have been traditionally used for the treatment of scarring in acne. Only the mildest acne scarring will actually resolve with chemical peels. Fractional photothermolysis using laser technology is considered to be as effective as carbon dioxide lasers for treating acne scarring; some side effects are associated with carbon dioxide laser therapy (Chapas, Brightman, Sukai, et al, 2008; Walgrave, Ortiz, MacFalls, et al, 2009).

Nursing Care Management

The health screening interview should contain questions regarding the adolescent's concern about acne. Because acne is so common and its appearance may seem so mild, the health care provider may underestimate the relative importance of the disease to the adolescent. The nurse should assess the individual adolescent's level of distress, current management, and perceived success of any regimen before initiating a referral. If the adolescent does not perceive the acne to be a problem, he or she may lack motivation to follow the treatment plan. The primary care provider can manage most cases of acne without referral to a dermatologist.

The nurse can provide ongoing support for the adolescent when a treatment plan has been initiated. Encourage the family to support the adolescent in his or her efforts. Discuss the use of the medications and basic skin care information in detail with the adolescent. Written information to accompany the discussion is helpful. Inform patients that it will take 6 to 8 weeks to appreciate improvement in their skin. Information to dispel myths regarding the use of abrasive cleansing products as a means of removing blackheads can prevent unnecessary costs and trauma to the skin. Teenagers also need to be educated about factors that may aggravate acne and damage skin, such as too vigorous scrubbing. Picking, squeezing, and manual expression with fingernails breaks down ductal walls and causes acne to worsen. Mechanical irritation, such as vinyl helmet straps that rub areas predisposed to acne, can cause the development of lesions.

VISION CHANGES

Vision changes are common during the teenage years. The onset of refractory errors or worsening of previous errors peaks in adolescence as a result of the growth spurt. Other than myopia, new eye problems in this age-group are rare. Vision screening is usually performed in the school by nurses, and referrals are made as required to correct vision problems. The main goal is to detect new refractive errors. Adolescents with vision changes are referred for contacts or glasses as appropriate.

HEALTH PROBLEMS OF THE MALE REPRODUCTIVE SYSTEM

PENILE PROBLEMS

Common congenital anomalies of the penis are almost always detected and corrected in infancy or early childhood. In some cases boys who need an operative procedure to repair hypospadias (the most common congenital deformity of the penis) may reach adolescence with a penis that looks different from those of their friends. A few who have received no medical care have uncorrected deformities that can cause serious psychologic problems during this sensitive period of development. These young boys need to be identified for surgical repair of the defect.

Uncircumcised males may encounter some problems during adolescence related to a tight foreskin that cannot be retracted over the enlarging glans; some males may not cleanse the area properly. These boys are at risk for more frequent infections. Penile carcinoma is associated with human papillomavirus types 16 and 18 (HPV 16, 18). Although HPV is a common sexually transmitted infection (STI) among American males, penile carcinomas are rare in the United States and most Western countries.

Trauma to the penis, including burns and accidental injuries, can occur in various ways. The frenulum (the fold on the lower surface of the glans that connects it with the prepuce) can be torn after retraction of the foreskin, unusually rough masturbation, or coitus. It can be frightening to the young boy but usually heals spontaneously with minimum care. However, any extensive bleeding may require suturing of the tissues. Penile fracture is a rupture of the corpus cavernosum as a result of blunt trauma to the erect penis, usually during vigorous sexual intercourse or manipulation. The condition is considered a urological emergency, and surgical repair is recommended to prevent further complications (Al-Shaiji, Amann, and Brock, 2009; Maruschke, Lehr, and Hakenberg, 2008).

Drugs such as trazodone (Desyrel), taken alone or in combination with cocaine or Ecstasy (MDMA [3-4 methylene-dioxymethamphetamine]), may cause a prolonged erection (priapism), which can be extremely uncomfortable and in some cases may require surgical intervention to release blood trapped in the corpus cavernosum. Drugs available to adults for erectile dysfunction or other drugs not intended for recreational uses may have unintentional and undesirable side effects (James and Mendelson, 2004).

TESTICULAR TUMORS

Tumors of the testes are not a common condition but are usually malignant when found in adolescence. Testicular carcinomas account for 7% of the malignancies that occur in 15- to 19-year-olds in the United States (Reaman and Bleyer, 2006). Testicular cancer is the most common solid tumor in males 15 to 34 years of age. The usual presenting symptom is a heavy, hard, painless mass that is palpable on the anterior or lateral aspect of a testis. The tumor may be smooth or nodular and does not transilluminate unless accompanied by a hydrocele. The involved testicle hangs lower and is therefore more susceptible to trauma. Although not all scrotal masses are malignant, any firm swelling of the testes demands immediate evaluation. If a firm swelling is noted, the adolescent should be evaluated by ultrasonography and immediately referred for direct biopsy if the mass is found to be solid.

Treatment for testicular cancer consists of surgical removal of the affected testicle (orchiectomy) and the adjacent lymph nodes if they are affected. If metastases are evident in more distant nodes or organs, chemotherapy and radiotherapy are implemented. (See Chapter 36.)

Nursing Care Management

To supplement routine health assessment, every adolescent boy should learn to perform monthly testicular self-examination (TSE). This provides an opportunity for the adolescent to familiarize himself with his own anatomy and to ensure early detection of any abnormality. In the TSE each testicle is examined individually, preferably after a warm bath or shower, when scrotal skin is more relaxed, using the thumbs and fingers of both hands and applying a small amount of firm, gentle pressure. The normal testicle is a firm organ with a smooth, egg-shaped contour. The epididymis can be palpated as a raised swelling on the superior aspect of the testicle and should not be confused with an abnormality. The nurse can play an important role in providing anticipatory guidance to all adolescent boys. This guidance includes an explanation of the rationale for TSE and how to perform this procedure (see Critical Thinking Exercise).

VARICOCELE

A varicocele is characterized by elongation, dilation, and tortuosity of the veins of the spermatic cord superior to the testicle. The finding is rare in prepubertal children, but the incidence increases dramatically at the onset of puberty. Idiopathic varicocele is the most common treatable cause of male-related impaired fertility, especially if caught and treated early (Zampieri, Mantovani, Ottolenghi, et al, 2009). Varicoceles occur most often on the left side because of the greater length of the left spermatic vein and its entry into the left renal artery; the right spermatic vein enters the vena cava directly and at a

lesser angle, which may be a source of future difficulty. A varicocele can be palpated as a wormlike mass situated above the testicle that decreases in size when the male is recumbent and becomes distended and tense when he is upright. Some males may experience discomfort during sexual stimulation.

In pubertal boys the left testicle is usually larger than the right. However, when there is an associated varicocele, the left testicle is usually smaller than the right. Testicular size and levels of dihydrotestosterone in seminal plasma decrease with increasing duration of the varicocele. Varicocelectomy is indicated in adolescents when there is growth arrest of the affected testicle or when there is pain associated with the varicocele. Currently, improvement in testicular volume is the main outcome measure following varicocelectomy in children and adolescents. Several recent studies have shown significant catch-up growth after surgical treatment (Sakamoto, Ogawa, and Yoshida, 2008; Sakamoto, Saito, Ogawa, et al, 2008). Surgical repair of varicoceles in adult men is less successful than in children and adolescents. There is no statistical difference in catch-up growth postoperatively for males between 10 and 24 years of age (DeCastro, Shabsigh, Poon, et al, 2009). Whether there is a correlation between testicular catch-up growth and testicular function is still to be determined.

EPIDIDYMITIS

Epididymitis is an inflammatory reaction of the epididymis of the testicle as a result of an infection (bacterial or viral), a chemical irritant (urine), or a nonspecific cause (local trauma). The clinical presentation is an insidious (slow) onset of unilateral scrotal pain, redness, and swelling. Associated symptoms include urethral discharge, dysuria, fever, and pyuria. Epididymitis is not associated with gastrointestinal symptoms as found in testicular torsion. The causative factor in males less than 35 years of age is thought to be predominantly *Chlamydia trachomatis*, although nearly 90% do not have laboratory evidence of the bacteria from urethral swab (Tracy, Steers, and

---

? CRITICAL THINKING EXERCISE

Testicular Self-Examination

At a recent faculty meeting, Paul, the pediatric nurse practitioner who runs the school-based health clinic, presented his plan for a class on testicular self-examination (TSE) to be delivered to the sophomore boys. Several teachers questioned the value of providing such a class when there is limited time to deliver content relating to "routine academic subjects." What important issues regarding testicular cancer and TSE should Paul use to justify providing this class to the sophomore boys?

1. Evidence—Is there sufficient evidence to justify teaching sophomore boys about TSE?
2. Assumptions—Describe the underlying assumption about each of the following:
   a. Detection of testicular cancers in adolescence
   b. Usual presenting symptom of testicular cancer
   c. Knowledge of genital anatomy among adolescent boys
   d. Ways to teach adolescent boys about their anatomy
3. What priorities for nursing care can be drawn at this time?
4. Does the evidence support your nursing intervention?

Costabile, 2008). Mild presentation of symptoms may mimic testicular torsion, which requires immediate surgical intervention. Therefore immediate evaluation by a practitioner is indicated. Treatment consists of analgesics, scrotal support, bed rest, and appropriate antibiotic therapy. Conduct an assessment for other STIs, including human immunodeficiency virus (HIV), for adolescent males who test positive for chlamydia.

TESTICULAR TORSION

Intravaginal torsion of the testicle is a condition in which the tunica vaginalis, which normally encases the testicle, fails to do so and the testis hangs free from its vascular structures. This condition can result in partial or complete venous occlusion with rotation around this vascular axis. In severe torsion the organ can become swollen and painful; the scrotum becomes red, warm, and edematous and appears to be immobile or fixed as a result of spasm of the cremasteric fibers.

Testicular torsion occurs in 1 in every 4000 males, with a peak onset at 13 years of age. Rapid growth and increasing vascularity of the testicle are thought to be precursors to torsion, accounting for the occurrence at puberty (Gatti and Murphy, 2008). Testicular torsion is the most common cause of testicular loss in young males (Adelman and Joffe, 2000; Mansbach, Forbes, and Peters, 2005). Typically, the adolescent complains of pain that was either acute or insidious in onset and that has radiated to the groin. Nausea, vomiting, and abdominal pain may accompany the pain; the cremasteric reflex is often absent. Fever and urinary symptoms are generally not present. The history often reveals that similar painful episodes have occurred previously, resolving spontaneously. Emergency surgery is often necessary to preserve the testicle.

Nursing Care Management

Nurses should be alert to the possibility of testicular torsion in adolescents who complain of scrotal pain. Because torsion often results from trauma to the scrotum, school nurses are likely to encounter such injuries and should refer the adolescent for medical evaluation immediately.

❗ NURSING ALERT

Refer any male patient with signs of testicular torsion (red, painful, swollen scrotum) for immediate medical evaluation.

GYNECOMASTIA

Some degree of bilateral or unilateral breast enlargement occurs frequently in young boys during puberty. Approximately half of adolescent boys have transient gynecomastia, which usually lasts less than 1 year. When gynecomastia has a prepubertal onset, the adolescent should be evaluated for rare adrenal or gonadal tumors, liver disease, or Klinefelter syndrome. Gynecomastia may also be drug induced; calcium channel blockers, cancer chemotherapeutic agents, histamine$_2$-receptor blockers, and oral ketoconazoles have all been shown to cause the disorder. Some report that marijuana causes gynecomastia.

If gynecomastia persists or is extensive enough to cause embarrassment, plastic surgery is indicated for cosmetic and psychologic reasons. Administration of testosterone has no effect on breast development or regression and may even aggravate the condition.

Nursing Care Management

Management usually consists of assuring the adolescent and his parents that this situation is benign and temporary. The adolescent may benefit from the knowledge that it occurs in more than 50% of his peers.

HEALTH PROBLEMS OF THE FEMALE REPRODUCTIVE SYSTEM

GYNECOLOGIC EXAMINATION

Whether it is her first experience or one of many, adolescent girls are often apprehensive before a pelvic examination. Adolescents are self-conscious about their bodies and the changes taking place. The adolescent needs anticipatory guidance regarding what to expect and what she can do to help herself relax during the procedure. Many fears and apprehensions are a result of information she has obtained from family members and friends. The discussion should begin by addressing these anxieties.

The ideal time to begin preparing a girl for examination of the genitalia is as she is entering puberty. External genitalia examination should always be included as part of a routine physical assessment; excluding the genitalia reinforces the attitude that sexuality is something to be avoided.

The timing of the initial pelvic examination is controversial; the ultimate decision depends on the adolescent and the health care provider. Indications for a pelvic examination during adolescence are listed in Box 20-1. The advent of effective urine based STI tests has added to the controversy, since assessment for many STIs can be done without the use of the speculum.

The pelvic examination provides an excellent opportunity for teaching about hygiene, body functions, and sexuality. Encourage the girl to ask questions about changes in her body and the implications. The pelvic examination also allows an opportunity to discuss practicing safer sex, preventing STIs, and postponing sexual involvement. Lack of knowledge is a factor in risky sexual experimentation in adolescence.

BOX 20-1 INDICATIONS FOR PELVIC EXAMINATION OF ADOLESCENT FEMALES

Menstrual disorders:
- Amenorrhea
- Irregular uterine or vaginal bleeding
- Dysmenorrhea unresponsive to therapy

Undiagnosed abdominal pain
Suspected pelvic mass
Rape
Request by patient
Virginal 21-year-old woman

The pelvic examination should be as nonstressful as possible. Nurses should attempt to make the initial pelvic examination a positive experience for the adolescent, since this can increase the likelihood of compliance with annual visits. The teenager should have the option of choosing a supportive person to be present during the examination. Suggested individuals might include a parent, best friend, boyfriend, or other health professional. The use of models and drawings and a display of equipment to be used facilitate understanding. Allowing the adolescent to handle the speculum may help decrease some of the fear. The adolescent is given the choice of wearing a gown or her own clothing during the examination. A description of the examination, including information about the procedure and words that describe anticipated feelings and sensations experienced during the examination, may reduce anxiety. Of major concern to the adolescent is fear of discovery of a pathologic pelvic condition. Reassurance regarding normal physical findings is extremely important.

Most girls favor a semisitting position, which has the additional advantage of allowing eye contact during the procedure. Sometimes a pillow helps the patient feel more comfortable and less vulnerable. The provision of a mirror for the girl to see what is taking place if she so desires helps the examiner explain various aspects of anatomy. When possible, it is important to respect the adolescent's request for a female provider.

Numerous techniques have been described to teach women to relax during a pelvic examination, including breathing exercises, imagery, and other strategies for reducing stress. (See Pain Management, Chapter 7.) However, these techniques are not effective with all individuals. When the examination is finished, the provider discusses the findings with the adolescent and makes referrals if indicated. Written materials are useful educational materials.

MENSTRUAL DISORDERS

The mean age of menarche in the United States is 12.55 years for non-Hispanic Caucasian, 12.06 for African-American, and 12.25 for Mexican-American girls, with 80% of girls beginning between 11 and 13.75 years of age (Chumlea, Schubert, Roche, et al, 2003). Pubertal development proceeds in a predictable sequence and tempo. When evaluating an adolescent with amenorrhea, the nurse requires an accurate history of the timing of development of secondary sexual characteristics. Primary amenorrhea is defined as no menses by age 15. An evaluation is necessary at age 13 if the girl has no secondary sexual characteristics or if menarche does not follow within 3 years of the onset of secondary sexual characteristics. Secondary amenorrhea is no menses for 6 months in a previously menstruating female when pregnancy has been excluded. Secondary amenorrhea is much more common than primary amenorrhea.

It is not unusual for an adolescent to have irregular menses when establishing ovulatory cycles. This is a result of an immature hypothalamic-pituitary-ovarian axis. In general, the later menarche occurs, the longer the period of anovulation. Two thirds of adolescent girls establish regular menstrual cycles by 2 years after menarche. Oligomenorrhea (abnormally light or infrequent menstruation) early after menarche is not uncommon. After a careful examination to rule out any physical abnormalities, including signs of androgen excess and congenital defects of the genital tract, the young girl and parent can be given reassurance with no additional evaluation.

Amenorrhea

The causes of amenorrhea can be divided into organ system and estrogen status. The most common cause of amenorrhea is pregnancy. A pregnancy test is an essential part of the evaluation for all females with amenorrhea, regardless of the sexual history. The next most prevalent causes of amenorrhea in adolescents are polycystic ovary syndrome and hypothalamic amenorrhea. For girls who are more than 2 or 3 years past menarche, the most common hypothalamic causes of amenorrhea are eating disorders, excessive exercise, medication, and stress (Wiksten-Almstromer, Hirschberg, and Hagenfeldt, 2007).

Polycystic ovary syndrome (PCOS) is a common endocrine disorder. There are no formal diagnostic criteria for teens with PCOS, and the cause is unclear. The characteristic findings are hyperandrogenism, chronic anovulation, and polycystic ovaries. Other ovarian causes of amenorrhea include gonadal dysgenesis; the most common form is Turner syndrome. Girls with Turner syndrome have delayed puberty, short stature, webbed neck, widely spaced nipples, and cardiac and kidney abnormalities. Premature ovarian failure, galactosemia, and ovarian tumor are other ovarian causes of amenorrhea.

Thyroid disease is not uncommon in adolescents and is more common in females than males. Both hypothyroidism and hyperthyroidism may result in menstrual irregularities, with the latter more likely to cause amenorrhea.

Adrenal causes of amenorrhea include congenital adrenal hyperplasia, which is an autosomal recessive disorder of steroidogenesis. Nonclassic adrenal hyperplasia is characterized in adolescents by hirsutism or amenorrhea. Pituitary causes of amenorrhea include prolactinoma, Cushing syndrome, and sarcoidosis.

Primary amenorrhea in an adolescent complaining of periodic (usually monthly) lower abdominal pain with evidence of estrogen production and sexual maturation may be related to an imperforate hymen, closed hymen from female circumcision, or transverse vaginal septum. The treatment is simple surgical perforation and drainage. Other anatomic causes of the amenorrhea include intrauterine adhesions and congenital absence of a uterus.

Menstrual Irregularities in the Female Athlete

The most common clinical indications of potentially adverse effects of exercise on an adolescent's reproductive cycle include (1) delayed menarche, (2) anovulation associated with dysfunctional uterine bleeding, and (3) oligomenorrhea or amenorrhea with hypoestrogenic states. Researchers have not been able to identify the exact mechanism of these menstrual changes. The most probable cause is at the hypothalamic level as a result of an imbalance of the amount of energy in (food) compared to the energy out (exercise). Amenorrhea is so common among female athletes that it is misinterpreted as normal by athletes, coaches, and some health care providers. Prevalence of amenorrhea has been found to be as high as 69% among ballet dancers and 65% among distance runners. Eating disorders are often part of the syndrome with exercise-induced amenorrhea (Warren and Chua, 2008). Adolescents who exercise intensely and have menstrual bleeding more frequently than every 21 days or at intervals of 35 to 120 days are likely to have chronic anovulation. They usually produce estrogen but have inadequate levels of progesterone. Unopposed estrogen can lead to endometrial hyperplasia and theoretic risk of endometrial adenocarcinoma.

In addition to menstrual dysfunction, female athletes also may be at risk for eating disorders and decreased bone mineral density (Joy, Van Hala, and Cooper, 2009). Any adolescent athlete who becomes amenorrheic requires medical evaluation to rule out other causes of amenorrhea and to assess for disordered eating (Sherman and Thompson, 2004). Sometimes a trial of decreasing the intensity or duration of exercise and improving nutrition will relieve irregularities. Careful evaluation by a health care provider who specializes in the treatment of eating disorders and athletes is essential. (See Chapter 39.)

Dysmenorrhea

Dysmenorrhea is defined as painful menstrual flow. Primary dysmenorrhea is painful menses without any identifiable pathologic disorder. Primary dysmenorrhea is the most common cause of painful menses in adolescents. Secondary dysmenorrhea is defined as painful menses with a pathologic condition such as endometriosis, salpingitis, or congenital anomalies of the müllerian system. The incidence of dysmenorrhea increases as adolescents mature; at age 12 years the prevalence is reported at 38%, and it increases to 66% to 77% by age 17 (Slap, 2003). It is a leading cause of recurrent absence from work and school.

Etiology

The factor present in all instances of primary dysmenorrhea is the onset of ovulatory cycles. Although it is not invariable, the symptoms do not occur during the first few postmenarchal months or during months of irregular anovulatory menses. After the progesterone withdrawal before menstruation, prostaglandins and leukotrienes are released in the uterus, causing an inflammatory response. This response is the cause of cramping and the systemic symptoms of nausea, vomiting, bloating, and headaches. Levels of prostaglandins are higher in the menstrual fluid of women with dysmenorrhea (Harel, 2008).

Clinical Manifestations

Typical complaints of the adolescent with dysmenorrhea are lower abdominal cramping and pain or discomfort. About 50% of girls also have systemic symptoms, including nausea and vomiting, fatigue, nervousness, diarrhea, and headache. The pain usually begins several hours before the appearance of visible vaginal bleeding, is most severe on the first day of menstruation, and may last from a few hours to a day or more but seldom exceeds 2 or 3 days. The symptoms and degree of discomfort vary considerably from one individual to another and from one period to another in the same female. The pain may be only a mild, fleeting discomfort or so severe as to be incapacitating, requiring absence from school. After adolescence the menstrual discomfort decreases with age, and it may resolve completely after childbirth.

Therapeutic Management

A careful history, including a menstrual and sexual history, is necessary. In addition, a careful review of gastrointestinal and genitourinary systems is necessary to rule out problems. A thorough gynecologic examination is carried out to exclude any pelvic abnormalities. The pelvic examination may not be indicated in an adolescent who is not sexually active and who responds to medical therapy.

The treatment of choice for adolescents is the administration of nonsteroidal antiinflammatory drugs (NSAIDs). These drugs block the formation of prostaglandins, leading to a reduction in uterine activity and prevention of pain. Antiprostaglandins are taken for only 2 or 3 days of the menstrual cycle. Prophylactic use of NSAIDs has proved effective when begun a few days before the onset of the menses, approximately 11 days after ovulation. The relief appears to be a result of prostaglandin inhibition rather than analgesic effect.

A variety of drugs that are taken at the onset of symptoms are available without prescription, such as ibuprofen and naproxen. The fenamates have the additional benefit of antagonizing the action of already-formed prostaglandins. If NSAIDs are unsuccessful in relieving the pain or if the adolescent desires contraception, cyclic estrogen therapy to prevent ovulation can provide dramatic and predictable relief from pain. Oral contraceptives are effective in approximately 90% of cases.

Transcutaneous electrical nerve stimulation, which reduces the perception of pain, has been an effective nonpharmacologic source of relief of pain associated with dysmenorrhea but less effective than NSAIDs. Insufficient evidence is available to prove whether acupuncture is effective. Small clinical studies have demonstrated positive effects, but randomized, placebo-controlled trials are needed (Yang, Liu, Chen, et al, 2008). Exercise is widely believed to alleviate dysmenorrhea by improving pelvic blood flow and stimulating the release of β-endorphins, which have an analgesic effect.

Nursing Considerations

The nurse may be the person to whom a young woman turns for advice regarding menstrual problems. The nurse should provide anticipatory guidance concerning menstrual physiology and hygiene and the importance of a well-balanced diet, exercise, and general health maintenance. Adolescents need information regarding availability of effective treatment for dysmenorrhea. Only about 50% of females with dysmenorrhea take medication to relieve the symptoms, even though effective treatment is available. The nurse should review correct dosing, since many adolescents use subtherapeutic doses of medication. Timing of the onset of the treatment requires the use of a menstrual calendar.

Most of the prostaglandin inhibitors are available without prescription. Whatever drug the adolescent chooses, she needs to be told how the drug produces its effect, how to take the drug for maximum effect, and the side effects. The drug should be taken with food and a full glass of water. If no satisfactory relief is achieved, refer the adolescent for further evaluation.

ENDOMETRIOSIS

Dysmenorrhea that is not substantially relieved within 6 months of taking OCPs and NSAIDs requires an evaluation with laparoscopy to rule out endometriosis. The disease is much more common in adolescents than was previously thought, with incidence rates ranging from 47% to 67% (Templeman, 2009).

Endometriosis is defined as the presence of endometrial glands and stroma outside the normal intrauterine endometrial cavity. The etiology is still unclear; risk factors include early menarche and late menopause. Research now suggests there is a genetic component to the etiology. The use of OCPs is protective and decreases the risk of endometriosis for up to 1 year after the method is discontinued. The presentation of endometriosis is variable, but women with surgical diagnosis of endometriosis are more likely to have dysmenorrhea, dyspareunia, pelvic pain, and menorrhagia. In addition, women with endometriosis are likely to have subfertility or infertility (Ballard, Seaman, de Vries, et al, 2008).

Treatment is medical, surgical, or a combination. The goal of treatment is pain control and suppression of the disease. The patient and family need to understand that the recurrence rate is high and that currently no cure is available for the disease.

Nursing Care Management

Adolescents require careful counseling about the use of the medications prescribed. The hormonal treatments have common side effects that are not well tolerated by adolescents, requiring education and support throughout the course of treatment.

PREMENSTRUAL SYNDROME

Although **premenstrual syndrome (PMS)** was first described in 1931, after several decades of research it remains poorly defined. The natural history of PMS is not known. It has more than 200 reported symptoms, and, with no confirmatory laboratory test, providers are hesitant to initiate treatment (Braverman, 2007). Research about PMS in adolescents is sparse; pharmacologic treatment trials have not included adolescent subjects. The symptoms are stable across cycles, occur regularly in the late luteal phase, and resolve within days of onset of menstrual bleeding. The manifestations most frequently cited are irritability, mood swings, headache, anxiety, and depression with the physical complaints of bloating, fatigue, and breast tenderness.

PMS is very common, occurring at some point in most women's reproductive lives. When specific diagnostic criteria are used, about 30% of women are significantly affected by moderate to severe symptoms. Only 5% to 8% of women meet the criteria for premenstrual dysphoric disorder (PMDD) (Rapkin and Mikacich, 2008). PMDD is characterized by symptoms of marked and persistent anger, irritability, mood swings, anxiety, and affective lability sufficient to cause significant impairment in one's ability to function occupationally or socially during the week preceding menses (Vigod, Ross, and Steiner, 2009).

Accurate diagnosis of PMS requires a thorough history and careful physical examination to exclude other medical or psychiatric conditions. A daily report form enables the young woman to pinpoint symptoms, which allows for monitoring during treatment. The diagnosis is made when at least one disabling physical or psychologic symptom is present up to 2 weeks before menses with remission when the menstrual flow begins (Rapkin and Mikacich, 2008). Currently, few well-controlled studies demonstrate effective treatment. Treatment options vary depending on the type and severity of symptoms.

Nutritional supplements have long been recommended as a treatment for PMS. Supplementation with 1200 mg/day of calcium and vitamin D has been demonstrated to reduce water retention, food craving, and pain (Bertone-Johnson, Hankinson, Bendich, et al, 2005). There is no clear evidence that dietary supplements such as vitamin B_6, primrose oil, or multivitamins are effective in the treatment of PMS. High-intensity aerobic exercise improves symptoms of PMS in adult studies.

An OCP containing a new progestin called drospirenone in a regimen of 24 active and four inactive pills has been demonstrated to be effective in the treatment of PMDD (Rapkin and Mikacich, 2008). Case reports have shown that adolescents with PMDD respond well to fluoxetine given in the luteal phase (Hetrick, Merry, McKenzie, et al, 2007).

> ### ⚡ DRUG ALERT
> #### *Selective Serotonin Reuptake Inhibitors*
>
> Since 2004, the FDA has issued a "black box warning" for the use of selective serotonin reuptake inhibitors in adolescents. These medications should be managed with a psychiatrist or adolescent medicine specialist.

The nurse can provide information regarding direct-care measures, adequate rest, good nutrition, and regular exercise. Families often have questions about the myriad treatment options available. The nurse can provide information about current recommended therapies. The nurse can teach patients to cope with the psychosocial aspect of the syndrome through stress reduction techniques, counseling, and support groups.

DYSFUNCTIONAL UTERINE BLEEDING

Dysfunctional uterine bleeding (DUB) is abnormal vaginal bleeding that occurs in the absence of pregnancy, infection, neoplasms, or any other demonstrable pathologic condition or disease. DUB is usually associated with anovulation and is the most frequent urgent gynecologic problem for adolescents. During adolescence, abnormalities in the menstrual flow's timing (intervals of <20 or >40 days), length (>8 days' duration), and amount (>80 ml) can occur frequently. This irregularity is usually attributed to immaturity of the positive feedback mechanism between the hypothalamic-pituitary-gonadal axis and absence of the luteinizing hormone surge late in the menstrual cycle. The result is anovulatory cycles in which the production of estrogen is unopposed because of a lack of progesterone. The effect of the estrogen is an increase in the thickness of the endometrial lining without structural integrity. Without progesterone, menstrual flow is not limited. Not all anovulatory females have DUB. One contributing factor is the amount of endogenous estrogen.

A comprehensive health history and physical examination, including a pelvic examination, are indicated to ascertain the cause of bleeding. The initial assessment should include the amount of blood loss and the possible need for hospitalization. Common causes of vaginal bleeding need to be ruled out before the diagnosis of DUB can be established. The most common reason for vaginal bleeding in adolescence is pregnancy. Other causes of vaginal bleeding can be related to anatomic anomalies, foreign bodies, endocrine disease, STIs, chronic illness, or previously undetected familial bleeding disorders (e.g., von Willebrand disease).

Treatment of vaginal bleeding depends on determination of the underlying mechanism. The initial management depends on the amount of blood lost and the patient's symptoms. If the bleeding is infrequent and not associated with anemia, reassurance and a menstrual calendar for follow-up monitoring are often sufficient.

When moderate anemia occurs, hormonal therapy, in the form of OCPs or cyclic medroxyprogesterone, has been beneficial. The adolescent needs to know that, at completion of the recommended regimen, a heavy flow with cramping will probably occur for 3 or 4 days. Without this information, she may believe that her condition is worse and assume that the treatment was ineffective. Untreated patients are at increased risk for endometrial hyperplasia and adenocarcinoma from the persistent, unopposed estrogen stimulation of the endometrium. The OCPs are continued for several months, after which bleeding irregularities seldom recur. DUB may persist for up to 2 years in more than half the cases.

Dilation and curettage may be necessary to control hemorrhage in severe cases or in those that do not respond to more conservative management. Supplemental iron is sometimes needed to correct anemia. Normally menstruating females average a loss of 1 mg of iron daily; thus blood loss of more than 80 ml/month is a significant risk factor for the development of iron deficiency anemia and signifies the need for oral iron therapy (Ferrara, Coppola, Coppola, et al, 2006).

Nursing Care Management

Ordinarily, only reassurance and attention to general health status are needed, with emphasis on a well-balanced diet, adequate rest, and moderate exercise. The nurse should instruct the adolescent to use a menstrual calendar to track improvement and guide future interventions. When OCPs are prescribed, the adolescent and her parents need careful explanation of the use of these medications. The high-dose estrogen OCPs can result in nausea and vomiting. Anticipatory supportive care includes preparation for procedures if these are a possibility.

VAGINITIS AND VULVITIS (VULVOVAGINITIS)

A small quantity of vaginal mucus is normal and in adolescent girls usually increases at the time of ovulation and before the onset of menstruation. It is characteristically clear and, except in rare instances when it appears in large amounts, causes no discomfort. However, some teenagers mistakenly believe that the discharge is a sign of vaginal infection. After an examination the girl can generally be reassured and given anticipatory guidance about hygiene and the increased secretions associated with sexual excitement.

Leukorrhea is the term used to describe a glutinous, gray-white discharge, which can be caused by physical, chemical, or infectious agents. Physical causes include foreign bodies such as a forgotten tampon. Irritation from pinworms, bubble bath, douching, deodorant pads or tampons, or improper wiping after defecation can also cause leukorrhea. The resulting discharge may be purulent, blood tinged, or brown with an offensive odor. Removal of the offending material is usually all that is necessary.

The normal vaginal flora is predominantly composed of *Lactobacillus acidophilus,* which produces lactic acid and hydrogen peroxide to maintain an acidic environment. Vaginitis occurs when pathogens or changes in the environment disrupt this balance. Oral antibiotics, oral and vaginal contraceptive agents, sexual intercourse, douching, and stress may allow pathogen proliferation and the development of vaginitis.

Vulvovaginal candidiasis results when *Candida* organisms begin to proliferate, resulting in overgrowth and infection. The most common organism is *Candida albicans,* accounting for 80% to 90% of infections; *Candida glabrata* occurs in 10% to 20% of cases. Susceptibility to candidiasis can be increased by a number of factors, including estrogen status, presence of glycogen, and the loss of protective bacterial flora from broad-spectrum antibiotics. A small percentage of women have recurrent yeast infections, four or more episodes in a year, and would benefit from culture identification of the *Candida* species. The nurse should be alert to risk factors for HIV, since recurrent or persistent vulvovaginal candidiasis may be the first symptom of the infection.

The adolescent with vulvovaginal candidiasis generally has vaginal pruritus and sometimes dysuria. The presence of the classic thick "cottage cheese–like" discharge is seen in a minority of patients. Most females have a minimum amount of an uncharacteristic discharge. The diagnosis is easy to confirm with microscopic evaluation.

First-line treatment of candidiasis remains the administration of over-the-counter topical antifungal drugs. The medications are available in cream, lotion, suppository, and tablet formulations. Shorter treatment regimens are associated with increased compliance; those with recurrence may benefit from a longer course (7 to 14 days). Oral 1-day treatment regimens are safe and as effective as topical treatments but may result in more systemic side effects. Treatment of the male partner in sexually active adolescents is not necessary unless the glans penis is inflamed. The adolescent should be advised to expect decreased symptoms in 24 to 72 hours and complete resolution in 6 to 8 days, regardless of treatment type.

Trichomonas vaginalis is an anaerobic parasitic protozoan involved in 20% to 30% of all cases of vaginitis. It is the most prevalent nonviral STI in adolescents. The infection was once considered a nuisance infection but is now recognized to play a role in several poor health outcomes. Females with *T. vaginalis* are more likely to acquire HIV, herpes, and pelvic inflammatory disease (PID). Infection with *T. vaginalis* doubles the risk of persistent HPV infection in women and increases the shedding of HIV among both men and women with HIV infection (Pattullo, Griffeth, Ding, et al, 2009).

The infection is often asymptomatic and self-limiting in men. Women may be asymptomatic, but many have a vaginal discharge and vulvovaginal soreness. Dysuria and an odor may accompany the symptoms. *T. vaginalis* diagnosis has traditionally been made by microscopic visualization of the motile trichomonads from a vaginal wet mount specimen. This has low sensitivity depending on the clinician's skills with microscopy and the length of time from specimen collection to observation. Culture is the gold standard but is expensive, is not widely available, and requires 4 days for a final reading. More commercially available tests for *T. vaginalis* are now offered; these are more sensitive than wet prep and less costly than culture.

Metronidazole or tinidazole is used for the treatment of *T. vaginalis*, in either a 2-g single dose or 500 mg twice daily for 7 days. Single-dose treatment is ideal in the adolescent population. Tinidazole has fewer gastrointestinal side effects than metronidazole. Sexual partners should also be treated and should abstain from sexual intercourse until 7 days after treatment is completed.

Bacterial vaginosis (BV) is a common vaginal infection in young women. The infection is noninflammatory and caused by an overgrowth of a variety of organisms. The symptoms include a thin, homogeneous, malodorous vaginal discharge. Providers commonly use the Amsel criteria for the diagnosis of bacterial vaginosis. It requires three out of four positive findings: homogeneous thin, gray vaginal discharge; pH more than 4.5; more than 20% clue cells on wet mount; and a positive Whiff test (fishy odor after application of potassium hydroxide). BV is associated with abnormal Papanicolaou (Pap) smears, PID, premature rupture of membranes, preterm labor, and postoperative infections. BV is not an STI; however, sexual transmission occurs as a result of disruption of normal vaginal flora. Other associated factors are smoking, oral receptive sex, and douching.

Treatment is recommended only for symptomatic women or those undergoing gynecologic surgery or abortion. The most effective treatment is metronidazole, 500 mg twice daily for 7 days, or as an intravaginal preparation for 5 days. Single-dose therapy is not recommended. Treatment of the male sexual partner is not necessary. Instruct the adolescent to abstain from sexual intercourse while taking the medication. Recurrence of BV is not uncommon.

Nursing Care Management

The adolescent who comes in for treatment of a vaginal discharge provides an opportunity for health teaching. Teach the young woman how to differentiate normal vaginal discharge from a potential infection. The discussion may elicit questions and concerns the adolescent has regarding other aspects of her developing body and sexuality. The nurse should stress the importance of an evaluation whenever the adolescent notices a change in her normal vaginal discharge.

When an infection is identified, the nurse can explain how the etiologic agents produced the irritation and the principles behind management. The prescription of a vaginal cream requires a careful explanation and demonstration of use. Girls who have never used a tampon will be less familiar with insertion of the vaginal applicator. Instruct the adolescent to apply the cream before bedtime to avoid leakage of the medication while in an upright position. The use of oil-based vaginal creams may break down the latex condom.

Health teaching should include the prevention of future infections. Teach girls at an early age to wipe front to back after toileting. Avoiding tight fitting clothes and nylon panties can assist in prevention. Douching is a common practice among adolescents and should be discouraged because it leads to changes in the normal vaginal microflora. Also, stress the use of condoms for prevention of *T. vaginalis* and other STIs.

HEALTH PROBLEMS RELATED TO SEXUALITY

The biologic maturation that forms the foundation of adolescent development and the transition to adulthood is accompanied by conflicting feelings, attitudes, and social practices related to developing sexuality. During adolescence the sexual drive emerges, and adolescents begin to explore their ability to attract a partner. The physical urges often precede emotional maturity.

The Youth Risk Behavior Surveillance System from the Centers for Disease Control and Prevention conducts a national school-based survey to monitor key health-risk behaviors among youth. The 2007 survey results found that 47.8% of students had had sexual intercourse, with 7.1% having their first sexual encounter before the age of 13. Not all young people who have ever had sexual intercourse are currently sexually active; in this survey 35% of the students had sexual intercourse with at least one person during the 3 months before the survey. Among those students, 61.5% used a condom during the last sexual intercourse (Centers for Disease Control and Prevention, 2008).

The causes of adolescent sexual risk taking are multifactorial. There is great social pressure to experiment with sex, and enticements by the media to enhance physical attractiveness conflict with traditional religious and societal expectations for chastity. Easy access to cars, unsupervised time at home, and changing family composition also contribute to the incidence of sexual experimentation among the adolescent population. Egocentrism and the concept of the personal fable (feelings of omnipotence, invulnerability, and immortality) lead to risk taking and experimentation. Past research has found that low self-esteem in females was associated with intercourse at an early age; more recent studies have reported similar findings for adolescent males (Spencer, Zimet, Aalsma, et al, 2002; Laflin, Wang, and Barry, 2008).

Family influences can delay the initiation of sexual activity. Adolescents who have at least one warm, supportive parent engage in less risky behavior. Effective parent-child communication about sexual topics can delay the onset of sexual intercourse. In addition, supervision of the adolescent's social activities and peer group, frequently referred to as *parental monitoring*, has consistently been shown to postpone sexual involvement. However, parents often underestimate the level of risk for their child and may not provide the appropriate monitoring and communication to assist in postponing sexual involvement (O'Donnell, Stueve, Duran, et al, 2008).

The social environment also has an effect on sexual risk-taking behavior. Adolescents who attend schools where they feel connected and involved in the programming are more likely to postpone sexual involvement. Youth with high academic achievement are more likely to postpone sexual involvement as well (Laflin, Wang, and Barry, 2008). Community support, resources, and supervision will also decrease risk taking among adolescents. Current data suggest that personal and perceived peer norms about sexual intercourse, condom use, and oral sex along with the use of alcohol and other drugs are strong predictors of initiation of sexual intercourse among adolescents (Santelli, Kaiser, Hirsch, et al, 2004; Potard, Courtois, and Rusch, 2008).

Prevention strategies must be comprehensive to decrease high-risk sexual behaviors. Delaying sexual intercourse, using condoms, choosing partners carefully, limiting sexual partners, and using reliable contraception help to reduce the impact of sexual activity on the adolescent. Nurses working with individual adolescents benefit from taking a sexual history so that prevention strategies are appropriate for the level of risk. Questioning adolescents who have not initiated sexual intercourse about their intention to initiate it is helpful, since their intentions are positively associated with actual sexual initiation in boys and girls (Gray, Austin, Huang, et al, 2008). Instruction in the skills needed to resist sexual intercourse has a stronger influence on reducing sexual activity than simply providing information on acquired immunodeficiency syndrome (AIDS) or birth control methods.

ADOLESCENT PREGNANCY

In recent years the teenage pregnancy rate has shown a continual downward trend. Between 1990 and 2004, birth rates for teenagers 15 to 19 years of age declined nationally for all races and Hispanic-origin populations. The rates for younger teens have declined more than the rate for older teens (Ventura, Abma, Mosher, et al, 2008). However, adolescent birth rates still remain high in the United States compared with those in other developed countries (American Academy of Pediatrics, 2005).

Contraception use among adolescents is variable, with decisions made within the context of the relationship. The less familiar an adolescent is with his or her partner, the less likely it is that they will use contraception during intercourse. Contraception use increases among girls as the duration of the relationship increases. A hormonal method (OCPs, contraceptive patch, injectable progesterone) is more likely to be used in later relationships than in first sexual relationships. Discontinuation of contraception is common; 46% of women have discontinued at least one method because of dissatisfaction (Moreau, Cleland, and Trussell, 2007).

In most cases, with early prenatal care, teenage pregnancy is no longer considered to be biologically disadvantageous to the child. However, teenage parenting is still regarded as socially, educationally, psychologically, and economically disadvantageous to both mother and child. Poverty is often the result of teenage childbearing (Aquilino and Bragadottir, 2000). African-American and Hispanic adolescents were more likely to become pregnant than their Caucasian counterparts. Eighty-two percent of all teenage pregnancies are unplanned (Alan Guttmacher Institute, 2006). Many of these social risk factors can be improved if a second pregnancy is prevented during the adolescent years or if the second pregnancy does not occur until 26 months postpartum. Other predictors of maternal success include participation in a program for pregnant teens, a social support system, and a sense of control over one's life (American Academy of Pediatrics, 2001).

Medical Aspects

Adolescents often receive delayed or inadequate prenatal care. Prenatal care may be delayed because the adolescent does not realize she is pregnant or denies the pregnancy until the second or third trimester. Health care providers working with adolescents should have a high index of suspicion for pregnancy. She may or may not have considered the possibility of pregnancy no matter how at risk for pregnancy she is. A pregnant adolescent may give vague reports of irregular periods or missed periods; the bleeding that occurs with implantation may be mistaken for a period, further delaying the diagnosis. Lacking adequate care, adolescent mothers and their unborn infants are at greater risk for low-birth-weight infants and infant deaths. It remains unclear whether this is a result of biologic immaturity or sociodemographic factors.

The obstetric risk and risk to the infant during a second pregnancy for the teenager is much higher. An adolescent with a poor outcome in the first pregnancy has a threefold risk of repeating the poor outcome in the second pregnancy. In teenagers the risk for a preterm delivery recurring is double the rate found in mature women. However, the mean birth weight for second deliveries is higher, related to an increase in the maternal prepregnancy body mass index (BMI).

Diagnosis of Pregnancy

A detailed menstrual and sexual history should be a routine part of health care for adolescents. Review specific symptoms of pregnancy, including amenorrhea, breast tenderness, urinary frequency, fatigue, and nausea. Absence of these symptoms does not exclude pregnancy. It is best not to perform a pregnancy test without the adolescent's knowledge. Before the pregnancy test, discuss with the adolescent what she will do if the test is positive and determine who else is aware she is sexually active and possibly pregnant.

After confirming that a pregnancy test is positive, inform the adolescent privately. Common reactions are ambivalence, shock, fear, or apparent apathy. The nurse should be supportive at this time and assure her the feelings are normal. Review the facts about the pregnancy, including the duration of pregnancy and anticipated due date. The next step is to determine who she plans to inform and, if she is under 18, how she would like to tell her parents. Some girls may want to take some time before notifying their parent. The nurse should schedule a follow-up appointment in 24 to 48 hours to assist with parental notification. Usually, the adolescent informs her parent on her own terms during this period. The nurse can assist with notification by offering to tell the parent for the teen or to be present when she tells her parent. Nonjudgmental support is critical at this time for the safety of the teen and her pregnancy.

Complications of Pregnancy

Bleeding is common in early pregnancy (occurring in 20% to 25% of cases), and about half of these pregnancies end in spontaneous abortion. Most spontaneous abortions occur in the first trimester as a result of abnormal chromosomal complement, uterine or cervical abnormalities, maternal systemic illness, or infection. Ultrasound evaluation can assist in determining the prognosis for the pregnancy. Bed rest is usually recommended when bleeding occurs; however, there is little evidence to demonstrate its effectiveness in preventing spontaneous abortions (Sotiriadis, Papatheodorou, and Makrydimas, 2004).

When a young woman is seen with bleeding and abdominal pain, an ectopic pregnancy must be ruled out. Ectopic pregnancy occurs when the fertilized egg implants outside of the uterus, usually in the fallopian tube. Damage to the fallopian tube is the most frequent cause of ectopic pregnancy. This damage occurs as a result of tubal surgery, PID, and previous ectopic pregnancy. Smoking is another risk factor for ectopic pregnancy; however, the mechanism is not known (Vichnin, 2008). When ectopic pregnancy is suspected, prompt evaluation and treatment are necessary. If the adolescent is seen with hypotension and abdominal pain, the ectopic pregnancy may have ruptured and emergency surgery is indicated.

Structural Factors

Labor may be prolonged in younger teenagers, particularly those 12 to 16 years of age; this is directly related to fetopelvic incompatibility and is a reflection of the teenager's smaller stature and incomplete growth process. The incidence of prolonged labor is highest in girls younger than age 14. Girls who are 12 to 13 years old have the highest rate of cesarean births, primarily because of cephalopelvic disproportion. However, older adolescents, 15 to 21 years of age, and especially those who have previously delivered a baby, often have labors that are shorter than average. The transition between pelvic disproportion and pelvic adequacy appears to occur around 15 years of age in the average adolescent.

Nutritional Needs

Caloric requirements during adolescence closely parallel the growth curve, and the need for protein, calcium, and iron is increased. Young adolescents tolerate caloric restriction poorly, and the anabolic need for calories during pregnancy places an added burden on their bodies. The preconception weight is a major determinant of birth weight for infants born to adolescents. Weight gain recommendations for pregnant girls should be based on their weight-for-height percentile or BMI, not on their age. Primiparous adolescents are more likely than first time adult pregnant women to gain more than 18 kg (40 lb). Excessive weight gain during pregnancy is associated with labor and delivery complications, preterm labor, maternal anemia, and infant mortality. Excessive weight gain during pregnancy is also linked with postpartum obesity and the associated health risks (American Academy of Pediatrics, 2009). Recommended weight gain in pregnancy varies according to the woman's prepregnancy BMI; a higher weight gain is recommended for thin women and a lower weight gain for women who are overweight or obese (American Academy of Pediatrics, 2009).

> **! NURSING ALERT**
>
> All pregnant women should take a vitamin and mineral supplement to ensure the recommended dietary allowance for folic acid (0.4 mg [400 mcg] daily) to help prevent neural tube defects. (See Myelomeningocele [Meningomyelocele], Prevention, Chapter 11.) Initiation before pregnancy has shown to have the most benefit. Consider a multivitamin for all sexually active women.

Because of the marked variation in the dietary needs of individual teenagers, there are no hard-and-fast rules to describe an adequate diet for all pregnant girls. The diet must provide sufficient nutrients to meet growth needs of both the prospective mother and the unborn child without the threat of excessive weight gain or fetal malnutrition. An additional 340 kcal/day (second trimester) to 452/day kcal (third trimester) are recommended for nutritional intake (American Academy of Pediatrics, 2009). The best guides for determining nutritional needs for the adolescent and pregnant adolescent are the Recommended Dietary Allowances and the Dietary Guidelines for Americans; the dietary reference intakes (DRIs) from the Institute of Medicine include recommended intakes of vitamins, minerals, and macronutrients for women of all ages and for those who are pregnant.* (See also Nutritional Assessment, Chapter 6.) Pregnant teenagers exhibit food preferences, eating behaviors, and lifestyle habits that are similar to those of their nonpregnant peers. Frequent snacking on foods high in fat and sugar and low in essential nutrients results in less than the recommended intake of calcium; iron; zinc; folic acid; and vitamins B_6, A, and C—nutrients of special concern during pregnancy.

Social and Economic Aspects

Poor school performance usually precedes adolescent pregnancy. Unable to achieve academically, the girl views motherhood as a rite of passage into adult status. Adolescents with high educational expectations are less likely than others to become pregnant. Another significant aspect of school dropout and accelerated maturity is the girl's alienation and isolation from her peers during a stage of development when identity formation is closely allied with peer identification. She is deprived of the interrelationship with the adolescent social system that is so essential to the development of a sense of identity. The girl may believe that she no longer "belongs" to the peer group and does not qualify for membership in the older peer group of mothers. On the other hand, the pregnancy may give the adolescent an entrance into a peer group. One study found that absenteeism and dropout rates were lower when adolescents received prenatal care in a school-based health center in an alternative school. Programs such as this can help reduce the long-term negative outcomes of adolescent parenting (Barnet, Arroyo, Devoe, et al, 2004).

Mother-Infant Relationship

Adolescents often have unrealistic expectations for the child. The young mother may view the infant as a plaything or a love object for herself. Children of adolescent mothers experience

---

*See DRIs at www.nal.usda.gov/fnic/etext/000105.html, or access the Institute of Medicine home page, www.iom.edu.

more developmental problems than children of adult mothers. The amount of cognitive stimulation in the child's early home environment is associated with the child's level of cognitive attainment. Many children of adolescents are raised by a grandparent. Although living with a grandparent may have positive effects on child outcomes, coresidence with the grandmother may have negative effects if the mother and grandmother are in conflict. Nurses need to stress the importance of the adolescent caring for the child even when other adults (e.g., mother or grandmother) are involved. The other adults present need education and support to allow optimum development of the infant and adolescent mother.

Several factors influence the mother-infant relationship. Maternal stresses, including changes in circumstances, influence coping ability and sensitivity to the infant's needs. Teenage mothers may consider an argument with a parent, boyfriend, or husband stressful, whereas adult mothers focus on problems directly involving the infant. Vocational and educational disadvantages of both teenage mothers and fathers further affect their coping abilities. It is important to recognize that not all adolescent mothers are alike. Some teenagers adjust well to the stresses and responsibilities of parenting, whereas others may lack the maturity or confidence to nurture optimally.

When socioeconomic status is controlled for, it has been found that younger adolescent mothers have lower acceptance of their children compared with older adolescent mothers. Studies in the literature indicate that specific family variables, including the mother's age (<19 years), are risk indicators for child abuse and neglect (Lounds, Borkowski, and Whitman, 2006; Murray, Baker, and Lewin, 2000).

A positive correlation exists between the total amount of social support and the frequency of appropriate maternal behavior. An assessment of whom the adolescent thinks she receives the most support from (her family, her partner, his family, or a close friend) allows the nurse to help the young mother benefit from this support (see Family-Centered Care box).

FAMILY-CENTERED CARE

Adolescent Pregnancy

The vast majority of adolescent girls who make the decision to continue a pregnancy will choose to parent the infant rather than release the newborn for adoption. Research has demonstrated that many of these young mothers have successful childrearing skills. One key factor is the amount of assistance the mother receives from her family of origin. This assistance may be in the form of financial support or child care assistance. Family support allows the young mother to complete her education and acquire vocational skills while still meeting her child's needs.

Nurses can increase the young mother's sense of competence by providing feedback about positive parenting skills and referring the teenager to community resources, such as parenting classes and infant stimulation programs. Nurses can also initiate and lead support groups for adolescent parents to foster self-confidence and parenting skills.

The cognitive development of the adolescent influences the development of attitudes and realistic expectations regarding childbearing. To cope effectively and solve situational dilemmas, pregnant teenagers must be able to use the problem-solving approach to assess and evaluate consequences. The concrete thought and egocentrism of early adolescence can influence the mother's ability to evaluate the infant's needs. Adolescent mothers lack knowledge of normal infant growth and development. This deficit may directly affect their perception, interpretation, and responsiveness to infant cues.

Infant characteristics also influence parental behavior. Teenage parents view their children as more temperamentally difficult than do adult parents. Temperamentally difficult infants have an adverse effect on the parents' sensitivity and responsiveness. Parent-infant interaction that is not mutually satisfying can also alter the parents' feelings of effectiveness and self-worth.

Adolescent Fathers

Little information is available about adolescent fathers. Most studies have small sample sizes and rely on reporting from the mother rather than the young man himself. Most teen fathers are involved with and interested in their children (Savio Beers, and Hollo, 2009). This involvement has positive effects on the mother's self-esteem and decreases her level of distress and depression. The teen mother and her mother largely influence the level of participation a teen father has with his children. Social supports and parenting classes are often lacking for adolescent fathers. The nurse should take advantage of opportunities to involve young fathers in educational programs.

Nursing Care Management

It is evident from the preceding discussion that nurses play a central role in meeting the needs of pregnant teenagers. The nurse may be the one to whom the young girl turns for help and guidance in her dilemma and on whom she relies for support and reassurance.

The first goal in nursing care of the pregnant teenager is to help her obtain health care whether she elects to continue or terminate the pregnancy. Typically, adolescents are reluctant to seek medical help, in part because of anxiety but more often because of a tendency to deny the pregnancy. Early prenatal care is essential for the welfare of both mother and infant. For guidelines, teaching, and general support measures during pregnancy, the reader is directed to the excellent textbooks available on nursing care throughout the maternity cycle.

Basic to the implementation of any care program is communication and the establishment of a trusting relationship. Initially the adolescent may appear apathetic and display little interest in discussing her pregnancy. The nurse must make every effort to put the adolescent at ease and avoid undue pressure. The young girl may have encountered rejection and open criticism from authority figures and peers. Conveying a nonjudgmental and genuine caring acceptance of the adolescent and her goals will assist the nurse in gaining the adolescent's confidence and trust.

Communication takes time and patience. Asking open-ended questions and listening for cues will help identify physical, emotional, social, and cultural influences that might affect the adolescent's progress through the maternity cycle. Factors that might affect her physical status, such as smoking, drug use, and nutritional state and habits, need to be explored and confronted. Each teenager represents a unique situation in terms of background, lifestyle, support structure, and coping mechanisms. Listening to the teenager and understanding the situation from her perspective are essential for a trusting relationship and effective communication.

Nutrition assessment should focus on the dietary adequacy of iron and calcium; multivitamins with folic acid are prescribed. Refer the adolescent for food supplement programs and other financial assistance, such as Women, Infants, and Children; Medicaid; Temporary Assistance for Needy Families (formerly Aid to Families with Dependent Children); and housing. Social work referral for thorough psychosocial assessment and planning may be initiated. Programs that have been most successful are comprehensive and use an interdisciplinary team concept.

The adolescent needs to know what is happening to her, what is expected of her, and how she can help in developing a care plan. Adolescents have their own ideas about the type of help and support they need. Nurses should consult with them and provide them an opportunity to share their ideas. It is important to jointly choose goals that the adolescent believes are beneficial, attainable, and able to be maintained over time. When developing a plan with a teen parent, the nurse should include the family, school, and community; involve the young father early in the relationship; and respect and understand the grandmothers' role.

The adolescent needs help to improve her altered self-image, a crucial factor in adolescence. Giving her as much individual attention as possible; being a sympathetic listener; providing the opportunity for her to know, support, and be supported by other girls in the same situation; and helping her experience success will facilitate progress toward achieving this goal.

The nurse should involve the family whenever possible. The parents of the adolescent mother and the father of the child need to express feelings and attitudes about the situation. The nurse should not make assumptions about whether the girl wishes to have these persons involved in her decisions and care.

Direct postpartum care of adolescents to prevent subsequent pregnancies and enhance life outcomes for the teen parents and child. Health care programs that provide contraceptive services for the young mother at the time of her child's appointment are helpful. Merely dispensing contraception is not enough. Comprehensive programs to promote positive parenting, self-esteem, vocational or academic assessment, career goals, and family cohesiveness are necessary.

ADOLESCENT ABORTION

In 1973 the landmark U.S. Supreme Court case *Roe v. Wade* concluded that individuals had the right to a first-trimester abortion. This right was not absolute but subject to certain state restrictions. Abortion is one of the most controversial moral issues in the United States. For example, many Americans believe that a pregnant woman should be able to obtain an abortion if her own life is endangered, if there is a strong chance that the fetus has a serious defect, or if the pregnancy is a result of a rape. However, some Americans do not believe that a woman should be able to have an abortion for any reason. The right to an abortion is also legally determined by the stage of pregnancy.

Many pregnant adolescents choose to continue their pregnancies and parent the child. The abortion rate has fallen more quickly than the drop in the pregnancy rate for adolescents. There are many possible explanations for this trend, including the possibility that access to abortion services for teens has decreased, that those who truly do not want to parent are abstaining from intercourse or using more effective methods of contraception, and that there is more social support for parenting among adolescents (Henshaw and Feivelson, 2000).

Under current federal constitutional law, minors have the right to obtain first-trimester abortions without parental consent unless otherwise specified by state law. (See the concept of "mature minor" and informed consent in Chapter 27. See also the Alan Guttmacher Institute website [**www.guttmacher. org**] for an update on state policies regarding adolescent abortion and state notification.) Legislation that mandates parental involvement as a requirement for adolescents who seek an abortion has generated considerable controversy. U.S. Supreme Court rulings have held that it is not unconstitutional for states to impose parental notification requirements as long as pregnant adolescents who believe that this involvement would not be in their best interests are allowed to go to court without involving their parents and are legally permitted to make their own decisions. The American Academy of Pediatrics (1996) and several other health care organizations have reached a consensus that minors should not be compelled or required to involve their parents in this decision but should be encouraged to discuss their pregnancies with their parents and other responsible adults.

Abortion is a controversial and emotional issue and one that frequently confronts health care professionals involved in delivery of services to pregnant adolescents. Because the law in this area is unsettled and varies by state, nurses must stay informed of legal changes as they relate to reproductive rights of minors in the state in which they practice (Tillett, 2005).

Other barriers to receiving an abortion include distance to the clinic, cost, and antiabortion harassment. Abortion services in the United States are offered primarily at freestanding abortion clinics, usually in major population centers. Abortions are not covered by many insurers, and the cost may be prohibitive to many women, especially adolescents.

The medical safety of a legal abortion has been well established. The mortality rate associated with teenage full-term pregnancy is much higher than the rate with abortion. A discussion of surgical procedures available is beyond the scope of this text. First-trimester abortions are performed as outpatient procedures and require local anesthesia or mild sedation only. Complication rates have been reported to be 1% or less. Problems that arise after abortion are endometritis, hemorrhage, Rh sensitization, genital tract injury, retained fetal elements, and (in rare cases) pulmonary embolism or death. Second-trimester abortions are more complicated and are associated with greater risk from hemorrhage. Women who have an induced abortion are no more likely than other women to experience problems in bearing a healthy baby in subsequent pregnancies.

In 2000 the FDA approved mifepristone for medical abortion. This oral medication provides women the option of a nonsurgical abortion procedure at 49 days or less of pregnancy.

The drug prevents receptor binding of endogenous or exogenous progesterone, which causes an abortion. The cervix is softened and the myometrium is sensitized to the contraction-inducing activity of prostaglandins. The medication can be used from the time of detection of pregnancy up to 49 days since the last menstrual period (Meier, 2000). The abortion completion rate is 92% to 95% in pregnancies less than 49 days (Grimes, 2000).

Numerous studies have examined the mental health risks associated with obtaining an abortion. There is no empirical evidence that women of any age who choose to have a legal first-trimester abortion experience psychologic problems or regret. Most of the studies have examined the effects up to 2 years after the abortion (Major, Cozzarelli, Cooper, et al, 2000).

Nursing Care Management

Early identification of pregnancy is essential, and nurses are in an optimum position to provide counseling on pregnancy options. Whatever option the adolescent chooses, initiate referral as quickly as possible to eliminate risk. Pelvic ultrasound may be indicated to assess gestational age correctly for those adolescents who cannot recall the date of their last menstrual period and when a bimanual examination is inconclusive.

Patient education regarding the medical aspects of the abortion should be conducted verbally, and the patient should be provided with written instructions before the procedure. Reviewing relaxation strategies that can be used during the procedure is helpful. Encourage the parents or other significant adults to be present during the medical procedure.

Conduct discussions about future contraceptive needs before the abortion. The adolescent may be started on a hormonal method of contraception immediately after the abortion. The young woman should be seen 3 weeks after an abortion to receive medical, contraceptive, and psychologic follow-up care.

CONTRACEPTION

Family planning services have developed and expanded during recent years. Contraceptive use among adolescents continues to increase. Contraceptive options have expanded over the past decade as well. Although all teenagers need sexuality education, not all of them are candidates for contraception. Among the large adolescent population, some have made the decision to postpone sexual involvement, some are in exclusively same-sex relationships, and some also may wish to have a child.

Confidentiality is a critical issue when discussing contraception with adolescents. Privacy is important to adolescents as they struggle to forge a personal identity and establish social relationships. Adolescents are particularly concerned about the judgments of others. The American Medical Association, Society for Adolescent Medicine, American Academy of Pediatrics, and American College of Obstetricians and Gynecologists have written policy statements in support of a minor's right to confidential health care. All agree that, although parental involvement is desirable, confidentiality may be central to encouraging teens to access needed health advice and treatment. Health delivery systems must be structured to allow confidentiality, including methods for appointment scheduling, billing, record keeping, and follow-up, that ensures privacy rights for adolescents. Family-centered care and parental involvement in contraceptive choice are ideal for patient compliance. However, there are adolescents who need confidential care. The predominant belief among many health professionals is that parental notification is important but that the "parents' rights" view is not necessarily sensitive to the health needs and basic rights of youth. No evidence substantiates the belief that providing contraceptive guidance contributes to sexual irresponsibility and promiscuity. In fact, a request for contraceptive information indicates a responsible effort on the part of the teenager to avoid an unplanned pregnancy.

Contraceptive Methods

To be safe and effective, a contraceptive method must be suited to the individual. The choice is based on the adolescent's preference after being informed of all the benefits and disadvantages of the methods available. The adolescent must be motivated to use whatever method is chosen. Factors associated with successful use of contraception include education, expectations, availability, cost, parent education level, perception of high likelihood of pregnancy, perception of disadvantages of having a pregnancy, and low rate of disadvantages of birth control methods.

Providing a birth control device is only part of a comprehensive sex education program. Partner involvement, when possible, is important to enhance user compliance. To make truly informed choices about contraception, adolescents need to know not only the efficacy of methods as they are actually used but also their efficacy when used consistently. Contraceptive efficacy is a representation of the number of unintended pregnancies that occur per year while using a particular method. Sexual intercourse with no protection is estimated to result in 85% of the women becoming pregnant. Table 20-1 outlines the advantages and disadvantages of various contraceptive methods recommended for use in adolescents.

Nonprescription Methods

Sometimes, despite the effectiveness of prescription methods, teenagers use less effective methods to avoid side effects and the necessity for medical screening and supervision inherent in the use of prescription methods. Adolescents may report the use of withdrawal and reliance on "safe" periods in the menstrual cycle as their current method of contraception. Using the method of periodic abstinence, or the rhythm method, is very risky. When the couple breaks the rules in this method, they are having unprotected sexual intercourse at times during the menstrual cycle when pregnancy is most likely to occur. Providing factual information about condoms and clarifying myths and misinformation about pregnancy prevention helps reduce the incidence of unwanted pregnancy.

Because of the high incidence of STIs in the adolescent population, discuss condom use with all adolescents seeking contraceptive advice. The adolescent can then be assisted in choosing an additional method to prevent pregnancy.

The lack of female-controlled barrier methods known to protect against infection with STIs has led to the development of the female condom. The contraceptive efficacy of the female

TABLE 20-1	ADVANTAGES AND DISADVANTAGES OF CONTRACEPTIVE METHODS IN ADOLESCENTS	
METHOD	**ADVANTAGES**	**DISADVANTAGES**
Behavioral Methods		
Abstinence	100% effective in preventing sexually transmitted infections (STIs) and pregnancy	Peer pressure to conform
		Relatively high failure rate from noncompliance
Withdrawal (coitus interruptus)	No medical visit necessary	High failure rate
Withdrawal of penis before ejaculation		Some seminal fluid often released before ejaculation
		Ejaculate at vaginal orifice may enter vagina
		No STI protection
Calendar method	Teaches adolescent girls about their menstrual cycle	High failure rate
Refrain from intercourse during fertile period (time of ovulation)	Encourages couple participation	Requires a regular, predictable menstrual cycle (irregular menses are common for first 2 yr after menarche)
		No STI protection
Barrier Methods		
Condom	Minimal side effects	Requires consistent use
	Easy to use	Requires premeditated intent for sexual union
	Available without prescription	May decrease sensation
	Portable	Misuse results in failure
	Provides protection against STIs	Decreased spontaneity
Male—Penile covering to trap sperm	Spermicidal condoms increase effectiveness for pregnancy and STI prevention	Latex sensitivity or allergies in small percentage of people
	Inexpensive in comparison to female condom	Improper use may lead to pregnancy or development of STI
Female—Inserted into vagina with base covering part of perineum; may be inserted 8 hr before intercourse	Female participation	May be difficult to insert
	Made of polyurethane; no latex sensitivities and can be used with oil-based lubricants	Noisy
	Provides protection from STIs	Requires premeditated intent for sexual union
Diaphragm	Can be fitted in virgins	High failure rate in adolescents because of inconvenience of use
Cervical covering to prevent sperm from reaching egg	Low failure rate when used correctly	Requires consistent use
Must be used in conjunction with spermicidal jelly	Few contraindications	Requires fitting and instruction by medical personnel
May be inserted 4-6 hr before intercourse	May be reused	Requires premeditated intent for sexual union
If inserted early, should be checked for placement before coitus		Requires body awareness and comfort with touching oneself for insertion
		Little STI protection
		May increase incidence of UTIs
Lea's shield	No latex allergies	May increase incidence of UTIs
Reusable vaginal contraceptive made of silicone	Reusable	Less effective in women who have delivered a baby
Elliptical bowl placed in vagina up to 48 hr before sexual intercourse and removed 8 hr after intercourse	Very effective in nulliparous women	Requires prescription
	Simple fitting—no sizing required	No STI protection
		More effective if spermicidal cream is used
		Must be replaced annually
Cervical cap	May be inserted hours before intercourse	Available in only four sizes
Soft rubber dome with a firm but pliable rim; fits over base of the cervix close to the junction of the cervix and vaginal fornices	Insertion and removal similar to those of a diaphragm	Must remain in place at least 6 hr after intercourse, but no more than 48 hr
		Not recommended for women with abnormal Papanicolaou test, history of toxic shock syndrome, or difficulty with proper fitting
		No STI protection
Chemicals		
Spermicidal foam, jelly, cream, and suppositories	Available without prescription	High failure rate unless combined with condom
Substance inserted into vagina to kill sperm	Inexpensive	Possible for sperm to be ejaculated directly into uterine os, bypassing spermicide in vagina
	Easy to use	Must be used shortly before coitus; therefore requires interruption of sexual experience
	No major health concerns	Repeated sexual union requires repeated application
		Requires premeditated intent for sexual union
		Messy
		Nonoxynol-9 associated with increased transmission of HIV to females; should not be used with anal sex in male partner sex for same reason

HIV, Human immunodeficiency virus; *UTIs*, urinary tract infections.

Continued

TABLE 20-1	ADVANTAGES AND DISADVANTAGES OF CONTRACEPTIVE METHODS IN ADOLESCENTS—cont'd	
METHOD	**ADVANTAGES**	**DISADVANTAGES**
Hormonal Methods		
Oral contraceptives Estrogen and progesterone-like compounds Inhibit ovulation by blocking release of gonadotropins from anterior pituitary gland	99% effective if used correctly Safe for adolescents Method of choice for most adolescents Administered by mouth Becomes a ritual not associated with sexual activity Regulates menses, decreases dysmenorrhea and acne, decreases menstrual flow Prevents ovarian and endometrial cancers Prevents functional ovarian cysts	Higher failure rate in adolescents than in older women Need to follow precise instructions; requires continued motivation, consistent use Requires prescription Price substantial for teenager No STI protection Possible side effects include headaches, missed or scanty periods, breakthrough bleeding, blood clot Increased rates of chlamydia
Medroxyprogesterone acetate (Depo-Provera) Progestin that suppresses hormonal cycle and prevents ovulation Injection given every 3 months	No interruption of sex Invisible method	No STI protection Possible side effects include significant weight gain, decreased bone density, decreased high-density lipoproteins (HDLs), irregular menses or amenorrhea, decreased libido, depression Fertility perhaps delayed after discontinuation Must return to care provider every 3 months for injection U.S. Food and Drug Administration recommends discontinuation after 2 yr because of decreased bone density
Ethinyl estradiol and norelgestromin transdermal system (Ortho Evra) Hormonal patch 4.5 cm (1.8 inches) square applied to skin weekly for 3 wk per month Suppresses ovulation, thickens cervical mucus, and thins endometrium	88.2% effective in perfect users Simple to use Regular menstrual cycles Not associated with sexual activity Avoids first-pass metabolism, resulting in more constant levels	Not recommended for women >90 kg (198 lb) Possible side effects include skin reaction at site, nausea, headache, dysmenorrhea, and breast tenderness Slight increased risk of blood clot formation compared with combination oral contraceptive pill Patch may be visible No STI protection
Etonogestrel plus ethinyl estradiol (NuvaRing) Soft, flexible, transparent ring placed in vagina for 3 wk Suppresses ovulation	99.3% effective Immediate return to ovulation at discontinuation May leave in place during sexual intercourse Avoids first-pass metabolism, resulting in more constant levels No spermicide needed No vaginal erosion No weight gain	Device may be felt by female or partner during sexual intercourse Device may fall out Possible side effects include headache, vaginitis, leukorrhea, nausea, and breakthrough bleeding May have late withdrawal bleeding requiring placement of ring during menses No STI protection
Levonorgestrel intrauterine system (Mirena) T-shape intrauterine device that releases 20 mcg/day of levonorgestrel Inserted within 7 days of menses and remains in place for 5 yr Thickens cervical mucus; inhibits sperm mobility and function	>99% effective Effectively prevents fertilization, resulting in low rates of ectopic pregnancy Reduced length and quantity of menstrual bleeding Reduced dysmenorrhea No weight gain	Risk of perforation at time of insertion 2%-12% expulsion rate Not recommended in nulliparous women or women not in monogamous relationships Possible side effects include abdominal pain, headache, vaginal discharge, and breast pain No STI protection
Etonogestrel implant (Implanon) 40 × 2 mm implanted rod Progestin-only method Suppresses ovulation	>99% effective Efficacy not user dependent Provides 3 yr of protection Single rod insertion and removal Palpable but not visible after insertion	Irregular menstrual bleeding Other less common side effects include headache, vaginitis, weight gain (1.7 kg [3.7 lb] at 2 yr) No STI protection
Emergency or Postcoital Contraception		
Progestin-only pill given within 72 hr of intercourse Emergency contraception works in one of three ways: by suppressing or delaying ovulation, by preventing the meeting of sperm and egg, or by preventing implantation *or* **Insertion of a copper-releasing intrauterine device** up to 7 days after unprotected intercourse	Useful in unplanned sexual intercourse or contraceptive failure May be given in advance for emergency use Available without prescription for adults	No STI protection May cause nausea if combination method used May change timing of next menstrual cycle

HIV, Human immunodeficiency virus; *UTIs*, urinary tract infections.

condom during typical use is similar to that of the diaphragm or cervical cap. The female condom is nearly as effective in preventing pregnancy as the male condom without spermicidal lubricant. The female condom appears to have great potential for giving a woman control in reducing her risk of HIV infection; however, there is no scientific evidence to prove this because efficacy studies of HIV transmission are unethical. Currently only one female condom is approved by the FDA for use in the United States. The female condom has been poorly used because of expense, problems with insertion, and slippage during sexual intercourse. A new female condom has been developed and is in the final stages of testing before potential acceptance by the FDA. Research has found that the PATH (Program for Appropriate Technology in Health) Woman's condom is preferred over the current female condom in a comparative crossover study with both methods (Schwartz, Barnhart, Creinin, et al, 2008).

The spermicide nonoxynol-9 does not protect against STIs, including HIV, and may actually increase the risk of HIV transmission because of the irritation it causes to the vagina and rectum. The Centers for Disease Control and Prevention (2006a) recommends not using spermicides and condoms with nonoxynol-9.

Prescription Methods

The recommendation of a prescription method of contraception requires a careful medical history and assurance that the adolescent understands the method. A discussion of the pros and cons of each method helps dispel myths and helps the adolescent find the right method for her current situation. The clinician should provide accurate, unbiased information about the benefits and risks, effectiveness, and return to fertility for each contraceptive method.

Use of Contraception

The birth control pill and condoms remain the most popular methods for adolescents. Adolescents commonly delay seeking contraceptive information. The typical interval from onset of sexual intercourse until the first visit for contraception is 1 year. A pregnancy scare is usually the precipitating event for the contraception appointment. Fear of the pelvic examination is a common reason that girls postpone seeking contraception. The World Health Organization, American College of Obstetricians and Gynecologists, and Planned Parenthood Federation of America have all recommended unbundling these services. Box 20-2 lists additional reasons adolescents give for not making better use of contraception.

Emergency contraception (ECP) is the administration of an effective contraceptive method after sexual intercourse. It is appropriate to use after any unprotected sexual intercourse, after condom breakage, when it is too late for injectable contraception, after missed pills, or after rape. The FDA has approved a progestin-only method for ECP (levonorgestrel [Plan B]) with high effectiveness and low rates of side effects. ECP must be given within 3 days (72 hours) of unprotected sexual intercourse, with highest efficacy closest to the time of sexual intercourse. There are no contraindications to use of the progestin-only method. Plan B is available to adult women over the counter without a prescription.

BOX 20-2   REASONS FOR NOT SEEKING OR USING BIRTH CONTROL

Responses of teenagers at initial interview for contraception in order of frequency:

- Dangerous to use
- Waiting for closer relationship with partner
- Afraid family would find out
- Not having sex
- Afraid of examination
- Did not think had sex often enough for pregnancy
- Did not expect to have sex
- Thought wanted pregnancy
- Thought too young to get pregnant
- Partner objected
- Thought it cost too much
- Thought had to be older to get birth control

Modified from Zabin LS, Stark HA, Emerson MR: Reasons for delay in contraceptive clinic visit: adolescent clinic and nonclinic populations compared, *J Adolesc Health* 12:225-232, 1991.

Compliance in contraceptive use is related to many factors, including those discussed in the following sections.

Lack of Information

Sometimes health professionals have a tendency to confuse a teenager's sophistication with knowledge. Although adolescents are acutely aware of their sexuality, their understanding of reproductive anatomy and physiology is often incomplete. If they are using contraception, they often do so with little or no instruction and with only vague understanding. Misinformation is commonplace. Lacking a fundamental understanding of fertility, they often believe they are too young or have sex too infrequently to become pregnant.

Anxiety Regarding Contraception

Some adolescents are concerned that their parents will be notified. Many have exaggerated ideas about the hazards of prescription methods, which correlate with misguided fears in the adult population. Myths about undesirable side effects prevail even after educational courses about contraception.

Conflict About Sexual Activity

Many teenagers feel ambivalent regarding their sexual activity and avoid many contraceptives because their use seems too premeditated and implies that sex is planned rather than a spontaneous activity. Most of these girls believe that sex is all right if it is not planned. This may also play a role in those adolescents who delay contraception, waiting for a relationship that is "close enough." A close relationship would allow the adolescents to accept and acknowledge their sexual activity.

Desire for Pregnancy

Some teens are seeking pregnancy and fail to use an effective method of contraception or use a prescribed method improperly. Some adolescents seek pregnancy as a rite of passage into adulthood or as a misdirected attempt to have someone to love them. Careful counseling and assistance with decision-making skills are essential when counseling the adolescent desiring pregnancy.

Nursing Care Management

Much of contraceptive education and service are delivered by nurses as part of sex education programs, family planning services, or postpartum health services. The introduction of contraceptive methods should ideally be associated with ongoing sex education. When they are included in this education process, sexually active adolescents will consider contraceptives as a natural and logical part of intercourse. Education about sexuality, conception, and contraception should be accurate, straightforward, and nonjudgmental.

Although sexual abstinence is highly desirable as a form of contraception, it is difficult for many adolescents to "just say no." Postponing sexual involvement requires effective communication and decision-making skills. Adolescents benefit from role-playing refusal skills in a safe environment. The nurse should also discuss with the adolescent how to introduce condoms into an existing or new relationship. Young women who have asked a partner to use a condom are more likely to use a condom consistently than women who have never made the request. The nurse plays an important role in offering appropriate education, helping build confidence in adolescents' ability to make requests of their partners, and providing social support to the sexually active adolescent.

To make an informed decision, the adolescent needs a careful review of all methods available, including their advantages and disadvantages. Discontinuation rates of prescription methods are high among all women, particularly adolescents. A critical aspect of counseling about a contraceptive method is education about use, noncontraceptive benefits, and expected side effects. Clear verbal explanations and demonstrations with the actual methods assist the concrete thinker in understanding the complicated instructions. Whenever possible, the parent or partner should be included in the teaching. Provide written instructions and a phone number for questions. When adolescents choose hormonal methods, they should also use condoms for the prevention of STIs (see Community Focus box). The nurse should demonstrate the correct use of condoms to all sexually active adolescents. Frequent follow-up with a review of side effects, usage patterns, and an opportunity to voice concerns increases the likelihood that the adolescent will continue to use contraception effectively.

An organization that provides education and services for adolescents, including both individual and group counseling, is the Planned Parenthood Federation of America.* It has branches in most cities in the United States.

RAPE

Adolescents and young adults have the highest rates of rape and other sexual assaults of any age-group. The majority of sexual assaults in the adolescent age-group are perpetrated by an acquaintance or relative of the teen (Kaufman and American Academy of Pediatrics, 2008). Females are more likely to report these experiences than males. In each instance the victim is potentially subjected to serious physical or emotional harm. There is no typical victim. Sexual assault victims are of all ages,

*434 W. 33rd St., New York, NY 10001; 212-541-7800 or 800-230-7526; **www.plannedparenthood.org**.

---

ethnic groups, and economic groups and are of either gender, although adolescents and children with a physical or developmental disability are more vulnerable to sexual abuse than their peers.

Legal definitions of rape vary from state to state but include the following categories: completed rape, attempted rape, and statutory rape. Many current definitions of rape have been expanded to include all forms of sexual victimization, including anal, oral, and genital penetration. Sexual assault is not restricted to vaginal or anal penetration but includes every form of sexual activity, including voyeurism.

Statutory rape may be charged when the victim is unable to give consent legally by virtue of age (age varies from state to state but is usually <16 years); mental deficiency; psychosis; or an altered state of consciousness caused by sleep, drugs, or illness.

Assailants

Three relationships are identified for assault: stranger, non-stranger, and incest. Although all can have serious and long-lasting effects, they are presumed to be different in a number of important ways: in the nature of the dominant psychologic and cognitive behaviors they provoke, in the issues they raise for service providers and other potential helpers, and in the techniques that may be helpful for treating existing and new cases.

Nonstranger Rapist

The majority of rapes are committed by a nonstranger. This is often referred to as acquaintance rape. The acquaintance may be a date, someone who lives near the adolescent, someone who has contact with the victim through recreational activities, or someone in an official association with the teenager. Some assailants wait for an opportunity when the victim is defenseless, such as the teenager at home alone with an uncle or cousin or the baby-sitter being driven home.

The assailant may be another teenager known through social activity. The nature of sex-role learning in most cultures associates females with softness, nonassertiveness, and dependence on men. Young women are socialized to be alluring yet sexually unavailable and to assume the role of pacesetter in sexual situations. Males are conditioned to be strong, powerful, and aggressive (measures of masculinity) and to be aggressors in sexual situations.

Stranger Rapist

It is believed that stranger rapes probably account for nearly 50% of all rapes reported to the police. Victims are frequently selected at random because they are apparently helpless.

Incest

The most commonly reported incestuous relationships are between a daughter and a father or stepfather (or other man in a caretaking role). The victim's participation is gained through the application of authority, subtle pressure, persuasion, or misrepresentation of moral standards. (For a further discussion of sexual abuse, see Child Maltreatment, Chapter 16.)

Clinical Manifestations

Adolescents who have been raped arrive at the emergency department or practitioner's office under a variety of circumstances. They are usually brought in by parents, friends, or the police, but some girls may seek medical help on their own. They may display a variety of manifestations, such as hysterical crying or giggling; agitation; feelings of degradation, rage, or helplessness; nervousness; and rapid mood swings. Adolescents may alternately appear calm and controlled, masking inner turmoil; they may be angry, confused, and filled with self-blame.

The rape victim may manifest evidence of physical force, including roughness, nonbrutal beating (slapping), brutal beating (slugging, kicking), and choking or gagging. The predominant reaction of the victim is fear of the rape and of injury. Thus the victim is faced with the dilemma of submission or resistance. Resistance increases the victim's chance of escape but also increases the likelihood of violence against the victim.

Therapeutic Management

It is advisable to obtain parental consent for examination, but the examination may be performed without consent if the adolescent is legally mature or the parents are unavailable. A female observer should be present during the history taking and examination of female victims who are examined by a male practitioner. Whether a parent should be present during the examination is determined on an individual basis. The parent's presence is usually encouraged, but only if the parent is supportive. Often the presence of a parent or a police officer inhibits the person's ability to describe the incident.

The medical assessment of the sexual assault victim includes the assessment and treatment of physical injury with focus on the genitalia. Pregnancy assessment and prevention, as well as evaluation and treatment for STIs, are performed. Obtaining forensic evidence requires training and should be conducted as soon after the incident as possible. Psychologic assessment and ongoing support are essential.

Initial Contact

The interrogation and associated activities, including the initial medical evaluation, have the potential to add to the trauma of the sexual assault. The initial contact with the rape victim must be supportive, and the fundamental goal is to do no further harm. Establishing a trusting relationship is an important step to decrease the victim's anxiety. The victim needs to know that she is (1) all right and (2) not being blamed for the situation. The first approach is not one of repeated interrogation but an attempt to reduce the victim's stress.

History

Although it is important to obtain a clear account of the circumstances of an alleged rape, it is also essential to minimize any further psychologic trauma that might occur if the adolescent is forced to relive a painful experience. The adolescent has probably been questioned by family and the police. If the person is too upset, the detailed history may be delayed. The adolescent should not be further victimized by insensitive care and unnecessary trauma.

The history should be as complete as possible and must be taken and presented in the patient's own words, including any account of force or threats. Information includes the date, time, location, and an accurate description of all types of sexual contact. All related activities are included. For example, evidence can be altered if the victim has bathed, urinated, defecated, douched, or changed clothing; therefore these activities are recorded. Use of a condom by the assailant can alter evidence. For adequate care, other important data include the date of the last menstrual period, the date of last intercourse, use of contraception, and any possibility of a preexisting pregnancy or STI. Also record the victim's behavior and emotional state.

Examination

The physical examination and collection of evidence are carried out as soon as possible because physical evidence deteriorates rapidly. Practitioners specially trained for rape examination should be used when possible. Nurses are often members of this group and are known as sexual assault nurse examiners (SANEs) (Stermac, Dunlap, and Bainbridge, 2005). The adolescent is always told in advance in understandable terms exactly what to expect in the way of tests and procedures, and the explanation is accompanied by emotional support. The victim is examined thoroughly, including nongenital areas, for evidence of injury that might substantiate the use of force. Photographs are taken of bruises, lacerations, or scratches for evidence, and rips or tears in clothing and the presence of dirt or grass stains are noted and recorded. Perineal, vaginal, or rectal lacerations suggest rape.

It is not uncommon for adolescent rape victims to delay seeking help, especially in cases of acquaintance or date rape. Nurses can be most supportive by acknowledging the painful and sometimes confusing feelings that surround such experiences and by focusing on the fact that the victim is seeking assistance now.

Treatment

Assessment of injury and management of pain are the first steps. Any injuries sustained by the victim that require surgical treatment are repaired. Most care providers prescribe prophylactic antibiotics at the initial examination. Pregnancy prophylaxis with ECPs is offered to the victim who was not previously pregnant or using a contraceptive method.

Nursing Care Management

Many of the approaches described for the sexually abused child apply to the adolescent. (See Chapter 16.) Sexual assault is a devastating experience with long-lasting effects. The primary goal of nursing care is to not inflict further stress on the victim, who is often angry, confused, frightened, embarrassed, and filled with self-blame. Young rape victims fear pregnancy, bodily injury, and the reactions of their parents and peers. Some believe that their bodies are permanently damaged and may even fear death as a consequence of the experience.

The nurse must do everything possible to reduce the stress of the interrogation and examination. Application of stress reduction techniques during the process can help the adolescent manage the immediate experience. Although most health professionals and law enforcement officers are sensitive to the needs of the victim and attempt to make the process as nonstressful as possible, the nurse acts as the advocate for the adolescent and is alert for cues that the victim is being overstressed.

Follow-up care of the rape victim extends over a long time. Rape victims typically show high levels of distress within the first week, which peak in severity by 3 weeks after the assault, continue at high levels for the next month, and then begin to decrease by 2 to 3 months after the assault. Make a referral to a public health agency or mental health agency as soon as possible. Victims who live in areas with established rape crisis centers are referred to these facilities.*

Aside from the universal need for emotional support, no firm guidelines exist for meeting the needs of rape victims. Trauma-focused cognitive behavioral therapy has been shown to be helpful for adolescents who have been abused or assaulted (Kaufman and American Academy of Pediatrics, 2008). In general, their needs vary widely and depend on the nature of the incident, when it took place, the physical and emotional injuries sustained, actions being considered as a result, resources available for informal support, and anticipated reactions of persons in the informal support network (see Family-Centered Care box). Posttraumatic stress disorder occurs in many victims of rape. (See Chapter 18.) Acquaintance rape is as devastating to the victim as stranger rape. There are few reliable predictors of positive readjustment among rape survivors. In general, a young age at the time of assault is associated with increased distress. Women victimized in childhood are more likely than nonvictims to be assaulted as adults.

Prevention

With the increasing incidence of rape in some communities in the United States, many professionals are looking for additional means for preventing rape at all ages. Many schools and orga-

---

*For information about local organizations, contact National Organization for Victim Assistance, 510 King St., Suite 424, Alexandria, VA 22314; 800-879-6682 or 703-535-6682; e-mail: NOVA@trynova.org; www.trynova.org.

 FAMILY-CENTERED CARE
Supporting the Rape Victim's Parents

In addition to the needs of the adolescent rape victim, the nurse should also be sensitive to the needs and reactions of the youngster's parents. Some will be angry and blame the adolescent; others will feel guilty and embarrassed. Many reactions can be expected at the time of the incident, ranging from despair to extreme agitation. Frequently the parents require as much support and reassurance as the victim. Agitated, angry, or incapacitated parents are unable to provide support for their youngster. Meeting parental needs can facilitate their ability to support the teenager during the crisis.

---

nizations arrange for classes on how to avoid an attack and how to behave in the event of an attempted rape. Rape trauma centers and most law enforcement agencies provide this service to groups. Every effort should be made to protect children and adolescents from injury and to teach them how to avoid situations that may promote an attack and how to behave in a threatening situation.

Nurses can be advocates for improving the community environment and street lighting, providing safe housing and transportation, and improving the effectiveness of the criminal justice system. They can work to educate adolescents about the relationship of risk-taking behaviors and sexual attack. These behaviors include drinking, taking drugs, and hitchhiking.

Nurses can also play a role in identifying intimate partner violence. Only a small percentage of victims initiate a discussion about partner violence with their health care provider. One step toward increasing safety is to begin to ask adolescents about safety in their current relationship. Offer adolescents antiviolence information as routinely as other messages about pregnancy prevention, driving safety, and prevention of STIs.

Display information about dating violence in the waiting room, examining room, and bathroom. Awareness of local resources for adolescents who experience violence allows the nurse to assist in referring those teens in need of help. At a broader level, nurses can also provide community education about intimate partner violence, including antiviolence presentations that target young men.

SEXUALLY TRANSMITTED INFECTIONS

STIs represent one of the major causes of morbidity during adolescence and young adulthood and annually afflict approximately 10 million persons under the age of 25 years. Teenagers represent one of the groups at highest risk. The actual prevalence rates among adolescents is underestimated, since the most prevalent STIs in adolescents, chlamydial infection and HPV infection, are not required to be reported to the Centers for Disease Control and Prevention.

Several unique characteristics—biologic, developmental, and environmental—place adolescents at risk for acquisition of STIs. Biologically, the immature adolescent female cervix is composed of columnar epithelium on the exocervix (cervical ectopia). The thin layer of columnar cells appears to favor attachment of infectious agents (especially *C. trachomatis* and HPV), which accounts in part for the increased prevalence of these infections in adolescents. The unchallenged immune system does not provide localized antibody response at the cervical level when exposed repeatedly to infectious agents. During anovulatory cycles, estrogen predominates, as demonstrated by the clear and watery cervical discharge. This may facilitate the transport of pathogens to the upper genital tract.

Developmentally, teenagers experience biologic discontinuities when pubertal maturation precedes psychologic and cognitive maturity. As the average age of menarche has declined, the age of sexual debut has also declined. An earlier age at sexual initiation results in increased numbers of sexual partners. The absence of planning is often evident in the failure to see the implications of current behavior on future outcome, such as condom use to prevent an STI or pregnancy or the need to return for follow-up visits for contraceptive refill or STI treatment.

Adolescents lack the knowledge that many STIs can be asymptomatic, or they fail to recognize the symptoms when they occur. Adolescents also fail to recognize that oral or rectal sex may be a source of STIs. A substantial number of adolescents engage in sexual intercourse other than penile-vaginal intercourse.

Adolescents perceive themselves as at low risk for acquiring STIs, even when infected with the disease. Young people who do not perceive a risk are not likely to use condoms to protect themselves or seek testing for diseases (Ford, Jaccard, Millstein, et al, 2004). Studies have shown that as young women have more sexual partners, their use of hormonal contraception increases; at the same time, the use of condoms declines. Adolescents diagnosed with an STI have a 40% risk of acquiring another STI in the same year (Orr, Johnston, Brizendine, et al, 2001; Peterman, Tian, Metcalf, et al, 2006). Without behavioral changes, these adolescents are at significant risk for additional STIs.

Designing health care systems and providing in-service education for all health care personnel are essential to providing services that meet the needs of adolescents. Environmental barriers to health care use by teenagers include high cost, lack of insurance, inconvenient timing of appointments, and inconvenient location of health facilities. Services need to be easily accessible and sensitive to the adolescent's developmental needs and desire for confidentiality.

Gonorrhea
Epidemiology

Several demographic factors place teenagers at risk for acquiring gonorrhea. Adolescents 15 to 19 years of age have the highest overall incidence of gonococcal infection compared with any other age-group when rates are adjusted for sexual activity. Gonorrhea among non-Caucasians is 10 times more frequent than among Caucasians. Part of this discrepancy is due to the fact that non-Caucasians are more likely to attend public health clinics, where reporting of the disease is better than in the private sector. Other known risk factors are low socioeconomic status, urban residence, early onset of sexual activity, single marital status, previous history of gonorrhea, and multiple sexual partners.

Epidemiologic evidence suggests the existence of a core group, or cluster of individuals, who are never treated or are inadequately treated and thus serve as a reservoir for reinfec-

tion. This emphasizes the need for partner identification and appropriate treatment to interrupt this cycle of reinfection. Prior infection is an important marker and should alert the clinician that the individual is at risk for reinfection.

Gonorrhea is almost always sexually transmitted, except when it appears in the conjunctiva, in which case vertical transmission from the maternal cervix to the newborn's conjunctiva is the usual mode of infection. The incidence of gonococcal ophthalmia has decreased in developed countries as a result of the routine application of prophylactic antibiotics to the eyes of newborn infants. (See Chapter 8.) Gonococcal infections do not confer lifelong immunity; therefore individuals are subject to reinfection.

Pathophysiology

The causative organism is *Neisseria gonorrhoeae*, a gram-negative diplococcus. The organisms have specific survival requirements, preferring a moist, alkaline environment (pH 7.2 to 7.6) and a temperature of 35° to 36° C (95° to 96.8° F). The gonococci survive only on the columnar and transitional epithelium; stratified epithelium is resistant to the onslaught. The organism spreads along the mucosa from the point of entry. It penetrates between the epithelial cells and, when dead, liberates an irritant that produces the inflammatory response, characterized by localized capillary dilation, edema, and leukocytosis. This process accounts for the purulent discharge and erosive balanitis and cervicitis sometimes observed in affected persons.

Clinical Manifestations

Symptoms can appear as early as 1 day or as late as 2 weeks after sexual contact. Gonococcal infection can manifest in many diverse ways, with four basic presentations: asymptomatic, uncomplicated symptomatic, complicated symptomatic, and disseminated disease. The infection can involve a number of organs and a wide range of manifestations (Table 20-2). PID in females simulates the inflammatory process caused by other bacterial infections, and differential diagnosis is made for more definitive medical treatment. Because a large percentage of affected persons are asymptomatic, consider gonorrhea in the evaluation of all sexually active adolescents. Lack of clinical symptoms is especially characteristic of rectal and pharyngeal infections.

Diagnostic Evaluation

Diagnosis has traditionally been made by culture taken from the urethra in males or the cervix in females. The development of nucleic acid amplification tests (NAATs) has given clinicians the ability to provide sensitive testing from a variety of collection methods with rapid return of results, although these are more expensive than the traditional Gram stain or culture (Swygard, Seña, and Cohen, 2005). A pelvic examination is no longer the only option for testing females. Urine testing is highly sensitive although slightly less sensitive than cervical testing for women. Another valid alternative is a self-collected vaginal swab. For males a urine sample is adequate for diagnosis; the male should obtain a freshly voided urine sample *without* prepping the urethra before obtaining the specimen. A large array of tests are available for gonorrhea and chlamydia; they differ in requirements for storage and specimen source (urine,

TABLE 20-2	COMPARISON BETWEEN GONORRHEA AND CHLAMYDIAL INFECTION	
CHARACTERISTICS	**GONORRHEA**	**CHLAMYDIA**
Incubation period	2-6 days; rare cases 10-16 days	8-21 days
Major site of infection	Urethritis (male)	Urethritis (male)
	Cervicitis (female)	Cervicitis (female)
Local complications	Epididymitis, bartholinitis, salpingitis, prostatitis, pelvic inflammatory disease, conjunctivitis, pharyngitis proctitis	Epididymitis, bartholinitis, salpingitis, postpartum endometriosis, pelvic inflammatory disease, conjunctivitis (trachoma), proctitis
Systemic complications	Septicemia with resulting arthritis, dermatitis, endocarditis, meningitis, perihepatitis, peritonitis	Arthritis, perihepatitis, chronic conjunctivitis
Carrier state	Recognized, especially in women; can last for months; primary reservoir is cervix; male urethra is minor site	Recognized, especially in women; can last for months; primary reservoir is cervix; male urethra is minor site
Effects of maternal infection	Less well established; ophthalmia neonatorum	Well known; inclusion conjunctivitis and pneumonia in newborn
Treatment	Ceftriaxone or cefixime	Azithromycin single-dose treatment
	Single-dose treatment	Treat sexual contacts
	Treat for possible chlamydial infection if reliable tests not available	
	Treat sexual contacts	

urethra, throat, vagina, cervix), and the nurse should follow labeling instructions.

Therapeutic Management

Uncomplicated gonorrhea is treated with a single dose of cefixime, 400 mg orally, or ceftriaxone may be administered as a one-time intramuscular dose of 125 mg (Centers for Disease Control and Prevention, 2006a). Azithromycin is added to cover chlamydial infection if a reliable test for chlamydia has not ruled out a coexisting chlamydial infection. Treatment failure is rare, and a test of cure after completion of antibiotics is not necessary. Sexual partners must be treated, and instruct the teen to abstain from sexual intercourse for 7 days after treatment (Centers for Disease Control and Prevention, 2006a).

Prevention

Until a genuine prophylaxis against gonorrheal infections is available, direct preventive efforts toward finding and treating affected persons, locating and examining contacts of affected persons, and educating young people regarding the facts of the disease and its spread. Latex condoms prevent transmission of the infection.

Chlamydial Infection

Chlamydial infection is the most common bacterial STI in the United States. Rates are highest among adolescents and young adults. The sequelae of untreated chlamydial infections include PID, ectopic pregnancy, epididymitis, and infertility. Infants born to infected mothers may be born prematurely and develop conjunctivitis and pneumonia. Annual screening of all sexually active adolescent females for chlamydia is recommended (American College of Obstetricians and Gynecologists, 2006; US Preventive Services Task Force, 2007).

Pathophysiology

The disease is caused by the bacterium *C. trachomatis*. Like viruses, chlamydiae are intracellular parasites during part of their life cycle. The organisms consist of alternating forms: the extracellular, or elementary, body and the intracellular, or

initial, body. The elementary body attaches to the host cell, where it induces active phagocytosis and is ingested in a vesicle that serves as a setting for the next stage of the cycle.

Unlike other phagocytosed organisms, *C. trachomatis* is able to circumvent host cell defenses and become a part of the cell. Within the host cell the elementary body reorganizes into the larger initial body, which uses the cell's synthetic functions and energy sources for its own metabolic needs. It divides to produce microcolonies of chlamydiae. After 18 to 24 hours the initial bodies again reorganize into elementary bodies and exit from the disrupted host cell to infect new cells. The entire process takes about 40 hours, and the result is a slow, steady accumulation of intracellular inclusions that are diagnostic of the infection.

Clinical Manifestations

The most common symptoms for females are vaginal discharge or dysuria. As the infection ascends to the endometrium and fallopian tubes, menstrual irregularities and lower abdominal pain may develop. Symptomatic males have a urethral discharge or dysuria. Rectal infections are generally asymptomatic; however, symptoms of proctitis may occur.

Diagnostic Evaluation

The diagnosis has traditionally been confirmed by culture media; the emergence of NAATs has improved the testing options and sensitivity for chlamydia as well as for gonorrhea.

Therapeutic Management

The recommended treatment for uncomplicated chlamydial infections is azithromycin, 1 g by mouth as a single dose. The alternate therapy is doxycycline, 100 mg by mouth twice daily for 7 days. The single-dose treatment is preferred for compliance. A test of cure is not necessary. All sexual partners must be treated, and the adolescent should abstain from sexual intercourse for 7 days after treatment. Females should be rescreened in 3 months because recurrent chlamydial infections are more likely to result in PID (Centers for Disease Control and Prevention, 2006a).

Pelvic Inflammatory Disease

PID is an infection of the upper genital tract (endometrium, fallopian tubes, and ovaries), most commonly caused by sexually transmitted bacteria, such as *N. gonorrhoeae, C. trachomatis,* and a variety of other anaerobic bacteria.

The long-term effects of PID include infertility because of tubal scarring, ectopic pregnancy, and chronic abdominal pain. It is estimated that each year 1 million females of reproductive age experience an episode of PID, with approximately 20% of cases occurring in teenagers. Women under the age of 25 years have a one in eight chance of experiencing PID, compared with a 1 in 8 risk in those over age 25 years. Menstruation at the time of initial infection can increase the risk for the development of PID. The loss of the mucous plug allows the infecting organism to ascend to the upper tract more readily. The blood itself acts as a culture medium for growth of the infecting organisms. Other mechanical factors such as douching may increase the risk of PID; sperm and motile *Trichomonas* organisms may also carry other infections up the genital tract. Another risk factor for adolescents is lack of access to health care that is affordable, convenient, and confidential. Lack of access results in delays of diagnosis and treatment of abdominal pain, which increases the risk for severe PID (Banikarim and Chacko, 2004).

PID can have acute complications, such as tubo-ovarian abscess and the Fitz-Hugh–Curtis syndrome. This syndrome occurs in about 5% to 20% of women who have acute salpingitis (infection of the fallopian tubes). The same organisms that cause the salpingitis produce an acute inflammation of the covering surrounding the liver (the hepatic capsule) and the peritoneum in contact with the hepatic capsule. The Fitz-Hugh–Curtis syndrome causes acute or chronic right upper quadrant abdominal pain and can lead to chronic adhesions between the hepatic capsule and the peritoneum. In some individuals the pain and tenderness associated with this syndrome may be more pronounced than the pelvic signs and symptoms.

Symptoms in the adolescent may be generalized, with lower abdominal pain; urinary tract symptoms; and vague influenza-like manifestations, such as malaise, nausea, diarrhea, or constipation. A pelvic examination to evaluate the possibility of PID is indicated for every sexually active female who complains of lower abdominal pain.

The diagnosis of PID is based on clinical findings. The 2006 STI guidelines (Centers for Disease Control and Prevention, 2006a) list the minimum criteria for diagnosis as uterine or adnexal tenderness and cervical motion tenderness. Additional criteria to support the diagnosis include oral temperature of 38° C (100.4° F), abnormal cervical discharge, presence of white blood cells on wet mount, elevated erythrocyte sedimentation rate or elevated C-reactive protein, and laboratory documentation of chlamydia or gonorrhea.

The potential for sequelae even after one episode of PID is as high as 25%. The adolescent with PID is at increased risk for infertility, ectopic pregnancy, and recurrent PID. Chronic pelvic pain and dyspareunia are not uncommon after an episode of PID.

The risk of sequelae requires aggressive management of PID in the adolescent. The two outpatient treatment recommendations are ofloxacin, 400 mg twice daily for 14 days, or levofloxacin, 500 mg once daily for 14 days, with or without metronidazole, 500 mg twice daily for 14 days; an alternative is ceftriaxone, 250 mg given intramuscularly, or cefoxitin, 2 g given intramuscularly, plus doxycycline, 100 mg orally twice daily for 14 days, with or without metronidazole. Inpatient therapy includes intravenous antibiotics such as cefoxitin, cefotetan, doxycycline, clindamycin, or gentamicin. On discharge, the adolescent receives a 14-day course of oral doxycycline or metronidazole.

Adolescents with PID need counseling to prevent future infections. Partner notification and treatment are necessary to avert recurrent infection. The adolescent should be instructed to abstain from sexual intercourse while taking the medication and until after her partner is treated. A discussion of negotiating condom usage is beneficial for the prevention of future infections.

Human Papillomavirus

Anogenital warts, caused by HPV infection, are the most common STI in the United States. The highest prevalence of HPV is among women 18 to 24 years of age. Persistent HPV infection is associated with cervical dysplasia and cervical cancer. HPV deoxyribonucleic acid (DNA) has been found in 99.7% of cervical cancer tissues (Kahn and Hillard, 2004). HPV types are classified by genomes with almost 120 genotypes described, 40 of which infect the genital tract. The HPV types are classified as low risk or high risk based on their potential for causing cancer. Either of the risk types may regress spontaneously. Risk factors for HPV infection include sexual behavior (multiple partners), lack of condom use, young age at first sexual intercourse, and history of prior infection (Kahn, Rosenthal, Succop, et al, 2002).

The most visible type of wart is condyloma acuminatum, a raised, polypoid mass with an irregular fingerlike surface and fissures, commonly described as having a "cauliflower" appearance. In females these warts are most commonly seen on the external genitalia or the vagina, cervix, or rectum. The shaft of the penis is the most common site in males, but warts may also appear on the meatus, anus, and scrotum. The presence of warts on the rectum or anus of males is frequently associated with anal intercourse; anal warts in females can be associated with autoinoculation.

Subclinical genital HPV infection is much more common than the warts that are exophytic (growing outward from surface). The previously common practice of treating areas that give a white appearance after application of acetic acid is no longer recommended. Acetowhitening is not a specific test for HPV. Subclinical infections often regress spontaneously without treatment.

Cytologic screening techniques provide high sensitivity in the diagnosis of cervical dysplasia, especially high-grade dysplasia. These liquid-based screening tests filter out the noncellular debris, thus allowing a single layer of cells on the slide. The liquid supernatant may be used to test for HPV DNA. Screening guidelines from the American Cancer Society recommend initiating Pap screening in adolescents 3 years after initiation of sexual intercourse or by age 21; thereafter it is recommended women have annual screening with traditional Pap smears or every 2 years with liquid-based cervical cytologic screening (Saslow, Runowicz, Solomon, et al, 2002). Recent American

College of Obstetricians and Gynecologists guidelines recommend that women receive their first cervical cancer screening at age 21 instead of 3 years after initiation of sexual intercourse. In addition, women aged 21 to 30 years should be screened once every 2 years, and women aged 30 years and older who have had three negative cervical cancer tests may be screened once every 3 years (American College of Obstetricians and Gynecologists, 2009).

Therapeutic Management

The treatment of external warts on females and males consists of both patient-applied and provider-administered options. The patient-applied option includes (1) podofilox, 0.5% solution applied with a cotton swab twice daily for 3 days followed by 4 days without therapy; this cycle is repeated as needed for a total of four cycles; or (2) imiquimod, 5% cream applied every day for 3 days a week for 16 weeks. The provider-administered option includes (1) cryotherapy with liquid nitrogen every 1 to 2 weeks; (2) podophyllin resin, 10% to 25% in benzoin, repeated weekly; or (3) 80% to 90% trichloroacetic acid applied weekly (Centers for Disease Control and Prevention, 2006a).

Patient education regarding the use of medication and the importance of follow-up care is essential and should be ongoing. When parents are aware of the infection, their participation in the education may be beneficial to the adolescent. The concrete aspects of HPV and cervical dysplasia may be more easily understood by the adolescent; however, the abstract concepts of asymptomatic infections and the relationship of cigarette smoking to cervical cancer are more difficult to comprehend. The nurse plays an important role in educating the adolescent about the disease process, assisting with smoking cessation, and providing information regarding procedures and treatments. Vaccination against HPV is an important addition to the prevention education for females and males. Current immunization guidelines recommend initiating HPV vaccine at the 11- or 12-year-old well-child visit (see Immunizations, Chapter 12).

Human Immunodeficiency Virus Infection and Acquired Immunodeficiency Syndrome

Preliminary surveillance data from the Centers for Disease Control and Prevention (2006b) indicate that the number of deaths from AIDS in U.S. children younger than 13 years declined from 945 in 1992 to 55 in 2004; preliminary data show a further decrease to an estimated 28 cases in 2007 (Centers for Disease Control and Prevention, 2009). In 2006 a study of 50 states estimated that 56,300 new cases of HIV were diagnosed in adolescents and adults, for an overall rate of 22.8 per 100,000. The most significant increase in new HIV cases was reported among African-Americans males (Centers for Disease Control and Prevention, 2009). In 2006 estimates indicated that the rate of new HIV infections in African-Americans was seven times the rate in Caucasians. Seventy-three percent of all newly diagnosed cases were in men, and 27% were in women; 53% of the new cases were transmitted via males having sex with males, and 31% were transmitted through high-risk heterosexual contact (Hall, Song, Rhodes, et al, 2008). (See Human Immunodeficiency Virus Infection and Acquired Immunodeficiency Syndrome, Chapter 35.)

HIV Diagnostic Testing

Since 2006, the Centers for Disease Control and Prevention has recommended universal testing for everyone 13 to 64 years of age regardless of risk factors in all health care settings, unless the patient opts out. Retesting should be done when the patient has a new partner and with any STI assessment (Centers for Disease Control and Prevention, 2006c). Traditional enzyme immunoassay venipuncture testing, rapid testing from fingerstick, and oral swab home testing kits are available. Nurses in traditional health care office settings can assist in implementing universal testing in primary care.

Hepatitis B Virus

Hepatitis B virus (HBV) is an infection of the liver that affects 300,000 persons annually, 10,000 of whom require hospitalization. (See Chapter 33.) Major concerns have been voiced because of the increased rate of infection, particularly among high-risk populations: intravenous drug users, sexual partners of HBV-infected individuals, homosexual males, and infants of HBV-infected pregnant women. It is estimated that infants whose mothers are positive for HBV have a 70% to 90% chance of becoming infected, and nearly all these infants develop chronic HBV carrier status. Another area of concern is transmission of HBV through contaminated body fluids to health care workers.

Many potential negative outcomes can be avoided through immunization. Current immunization guidelines recommend beginning the hepatitis B vaccine series at birth or, in unimmunized children, at 11 to 12 years of age. (See Immunizations, Chapter 12.) The immunization consists of a series of three intramuscular injections. The goal of universal immunization is to target uninfected infants and adolescents before the onset of high-risk behaviors.

Other Sexually Transmitted Genital Infections

Many sores or lesions that appear on the genitalia are the result of STIs. Experienced clinicians can correctly diagnose these lesions by visual examination only about half of the time. A complete health history, physical examination, and appropriate diagnostic cultures are needed to determine the causative factors. Nurses who interact with adolescents are in a primary position to obtain a health history and refer any sexually active adolescent for appropriate evaluation. Follow-up health education regarding any treatment regimen and prevention strategies is a major nursing role. Because many of the lesions are viral, nurses can assist the adolescent with communication techniques to inform future sexual partners about the potential for infection with an STI. Table 20-3 summarizes the most common genital lesions seen in adolescents.

Nursing Care Management

Nursing responsibilities encompass all aspects of STI education, prevention, and treatment. Primary prevention by avoiding exposure is the least expensive and most effective approach. The nurse can play a role in offering this education to young people before they initiate sexual intercourse. Sexuality education should include information about these diseases, such as their symptoms or lack of symptoms and treatment, and information

TABLE 20-3   GENITAL LESIONS IN ADOLESCENTS

DISEASE	MANIFESTATIONS	THERAPY	NURSING CONSIDERATIONS
Herpes simplex (viral)	Prodrome—Intense burning or itching at site of outbreak; often flulike symptoms Painful, enlarged inguinal lymph nodes First lesions—Clear, raised vesicles, very painful Recurrent lesions resolve more quickly and are less painful	Acyclovir (oral) or famciclovir Shortens clinical course in first episode Prophylaxis decreases recurrence rate	Immunocompromised patient at risk for overwhelming infection Sexual partner treated only if lesion present Can be transmitted to infant during birth Education and support needed for adolescents Increased risk for human immunodeficiency virus (HIV) with open lesion
Primary syphilis	Chancre—Hard, nontender, red, sharply defined lesion with indurated base, raised border, eroded surface, and scanty yellow discharge Nonpainful, enlarged lymph nodes	Penicillin	Affected person more infectious during first yr of disease May be transmitted to fetus Partner treatment necessary Increased risk for HIV with open lesion
Molluscum (viral)	Solitary clusters of raised, pearly white, firm, nontender papules Umbilicated dimpled lesions	Excision and expression of core material Imiquimod Cryotherapy Laser surgery	No known complications Sex partner treated only if lesions persist

dispelling the myths associated with their mode of transmission. These diseases are not contracted from toilet seats, drinking glasses, or bath towels. Most teens are uninformed or misinformed about STIs.

Promoting the inclusion of STI information, access to care, and interpersonal and social skill building in school sexuality education programs is an important function of the nurse. No matter what their area of practice, nurses are in a position to disseminate information, identify probable cases of STIs, and refer these cases for treatment.

The increasing incidence of STIs in young people is influenced to a great extent by the number of adolescents who engage in sexual activity. Improvements in testing methods and availability of testing for diseases will result in increased reporting of STIs. The hormonal contraceptive methods provide no protection against STIs. Unfortunately, many girls using these methods mistakenly believe they are also protected against STIs. To decrease the likelihood of infection, encourage sexually active adolescents to always use a condom.

Essential measures for control of the disease include treating the disease, reporting it promptly, and tracking and treating contacts. When working with adolescents, nurses need highly developed interviewing skills and a nonjudgmental approach to elicit an accurate sexual history. Several characteristics of teenagers influence the way health professionals address specific issues related to STIs. Teenagers are often concrete thinkers, which affects the way they process information. Teenagers also have limited coping mechanisms to draw on to assist in dealing with such information. To gain the adolescent's cooperation and trust, the nurse must convey acceptance and assure the adolescent of confidentiality. The nurse should always consider the early involvement of parents with permission from the adolescent. Family support may make access to health services easier and decrease the emotional stressors associated with acquiring an STI.

For additional information on STIs and abortion, refer to a women's health or maternity text such as Perry, Hockenberry, Lowdermilk, and colleagues (2010).

KEY POINTS

- Adolescent health-seeking behaviors center on skin problems, abdominal discomfort, menstrual symptoms, and anxieties about physical development and sexual changes.
- Acne is prevalent in the adolescent years; medication and gentle facial cleansing are the treatments of choice.
- The most frequent problems related to the male reproductive system are infections, scrotal conditions, and gynecomastia.
- The most frequent problems of the female reproductive system involve menstruation delays, irregularities, discomfort, and infections.
- Adolescent pregnancy has profound social, educational, psychologic, and economic ramifications. The pregnancy necessitates special attention to nutrition and psychologic and emotional support for the mother and father.
- Abortion as an alternative to birth is a highly controversial issue; there is evidence that it has no long-term psychologic sequelae for most women.
- Adolescents often do not use contraception because of lack of information, anxiety regarding use, conflict over sexual activity, or desire for pregnancy.
- Rape is a serious problem among adolescents; common forms are rape by a nonstranger, rape by a stranger, and incest.
- STIs are the most frequently occurring infectious diseases and a major cause of adolescent morbidity. HIV infection is an increasingly important adolescent health problem.

ANSWERS TO CRITICAL THINKING EXERCISES

Testicular Self-Examination

1. **Yes.** Although testicular cancer is not common in adolescence, when it does occur, it is generally malignant. Testicular cancer is very curable if detected early.

2. **a.** The best way to detect testicular tumors is by performing TSE every month.

   b. The usual presenting symptom for testicular cancer is a heavy, hard painless mass (either smooth or nodular) that is palpated on the testis.

   c. Adolescent boys are often self-conscious about their genital anatomy. Adolescent boys may joke about their genital anatomy because of peer influence, but many adolescent males will not admit that they have limited knowledge of their actual genital anatomy and its relation to health.

   d. As a pediatric nurse practitioner at the school-based clinic, Paul is in an excellent position to teach young men how to perform this examination. It is highly probable that he has already won their trust and confidence through his routine daily nursing activities, such as providing sports physicals and treating their episodic illnesses. Paul will be able to present the class in a manner that is respectful of the boys, while also allaying their anxieties and providing them with an important health skill. The class should be presented in a matter-of-fact way, with an explanation of both the characteristics of the normal testicle and a description of abnormal findings.

3. The first priority is to make certain that all adolescent boys with health problems feel comfortable visiting the health suite and sharing their concerns with the nurse practitioner. The ultimate goal is to ensure that no adolescent boy with a potential testicular tumor fails to get an immediate assessment and referral for treatment.

4. **Yes.** The information about testicular cancer and the importance of detecting it early provide a definite rationale for the class.

REFERENCES

Adelman WP, Joffe A: The adolescent with a painful scrotum, *Contemp Pediatr* 17(3):111-127, 2000.

Alan Guttmacher Institute: *In brief: facts on American teens' sexual and reproductive health,* New York, 2006, The Institute.

Al-Shaiji TF, Amann J, Brock GB: Fractured penis: diagnosis and management, *J Sex Med* 6(12):3231-3234, 2009.

American Academy of Pediatrics: *Pediatric nutrition handbook,* ed 6, Elk Grove Village, Ill, 2009, The Academy.

American Academy of Pediatrics, Committee on Adolescence: Adolescent pregnancy: current trends and issues, *Pediatrics* 116(1):281-286, 2005.

American Academy of Pediatrics: Care of adolescent parents and their children, *Pediatrics* 107(2):429-434, 2001.

American Academy of Pediatrics, Committee on Adolescence: The adolescent's right to confidential care when considering abortion, *Pediatrics* 97(5):746-751, 1996.

American College of Obstetricians and Gynecologists: Practice Bulletin No. 109: Cervical cytology screening, *Obstet Gynecol* 114(6):1409-1420, 2009.

American College of Obstetricians and Gynecologists, Committee on Gynecologic Practice: Primary and preventive care: periodic assessments. *Obstet Gynecol* 108:1615-1622, 2006.

Aquilino ML, Bragadottir H: Adolescent pregnancy, *MCN* 25(4):192-197, 2000.

Ballard KD, Seaman HE, de Vries CS, et al: Can symptomatology help in the diagnosis of endometriosis? Findings from a national case-control study, *BJOG* 115:1382-1391, 2008.

Banikarim C, Chacko MR: Pelvic inflammatory disease in adolescents, *Adolesc Med* 15(2): 273-285, 2004.

Barnet B, Arroyo C, Devoe M, et al: Reduced school dropout rates among adolescent mothers receiving school-based prenatal care, *Arch Pediatr Adolesc Med* 138:262-268, 2004.

Bertone-Johnson ER, Hankinson SE, Bendich A, et al: Calcium and vitamin D intake and risk of incident premenstrual syndrome, *Arch Intern Med* 165:1246-1252, 2005.

Bowe WP, Shalita AR: Effective over the counter acne treatments, *Semin Cutan Med Surg* 27(3):170-176, 2008.

Braverman PK: Premenstrual syndrome and premenstrual dysphoric disorder, *J Pediatr Adolesc Gynecol* 20(1):3-12, 2007.

Centers for Disease Control and Prevention: *HIV/AIDS surveillance report, 2007,* Atlanta, 2009, The Centers, available at www.cdc.gov/hiv/topics/surveillance/resources/reports/2007report/cover.htm (accessed January 31, 2010).

Centers for Disease Control and Prevention: Youth risk behavior surveillance—United States, *MMWR* 7(SS-4):1-131, 2008.

Centers for Disease Control and Prevention: 2006 STD treatment guidelines, *MMWR* 55(RR11):1-94, 2006a.

Centers for Disease Control and Prevention: Cases of HIV infection and AIDS in the United States, 2004, *HIV/AIDS Surv Rep* 16:2006b, available at www.cdc.gov/hiv/topics/surveillance/resources/reports/2004report/default.htm (accessed March 8, 2006).

Centers for Disease Control and Prevention: Updated guidelines for HIV testing, *MMWR* 55(RR44):1-17, 2006c.

Chapas AM, Brightman L, Sukai S, et al: Successful treatment of acneiform scarring with CO_2 ablative fractional resurfacing, *Lasers Surg Med* 40(6):381-386, 2008.

Chumlea WC, Schubert CM, Roche AF, et al: Age at menarche and racial comparisons in US girls, *Pediatrics* 111(1):110-115, 2003.

Dalgard F, Gieler U, Holm JO, et al: Self-esteem and body satisfaction among late adolescents with acne: results from a population survey, *J Am Acad Dermatol* 59(5):746-751, 2008.

DeCastro GJ, Shabsigh A, Poon SA, et al: Adolescent varicocelectomy: is the potential for catch-up growth related to age and/or Tanner stage? *J Urology* 181(1):322-327, 2009.

Eichenfield LF, Wortzman M: A novel gel formulation of 0.25% tretinoin and 1.2% clindamycin phosphate: efficacy in acne vulgaris patients aged 12 to 18 years, *Pediatr Dermatol* 26(3):257-261, 2009.

Ferrara M, Coppola L, Coppola A, et al: Iron deficiency in childhood and adolescence: retrospective review, *Hematology* 11(3):183-186, 2006.

Ford CA, Jaccard J, Millstein SG, et al: Perceived risk of chlamydial and gonococcal infection among sexually experienced young adults in the United States, *Perspect Sexual Reprod Health* 36(6):258-264, 2004.

Gatti JM, Murphy JP: Acute testicular disorders, *Pediatr Rev* 29(7):235-240, 2008.

Gray SH, Austin SB, Huang B, et al: Predicting sexual initiation in a prospective cohort study of adolescents, *J Arch Pediatr Adolesc Med* 162(1):55-59, 2008.

Grimes DA: FDA approval of mifepristone: an overview, *Contracep Rep* 11(4):4-11, 2000.

Gupta MA, Gupta AK: Psychiatric and psychological co-morbidity in patients with dermatologic disorders, *Am J Clin Dermatol* 4(12):833-842, 2003.

Guttman C: The future is now: nanotechnology creates promising new tretinoin formulation, *Dermatol Times* 30(11):39, 2009.

Hall HI, Song R, Rhodes P, et al: Estimation of HIV incidence in the United States, *JAMA* 300(5):520-529, 2008.

Harel Z: Dysmenorrhea in adolescents, *Ann NY Acad Sci* 1135:185-195, 2008.

Henshaw SK, Feivelson DJ: Teenage abortion and pregnancy statistics by state, 1996, *Fam Plan Perspect* 32(6):272-280, 2000.

Hetrick S, Merry S, McKenzie J, et al: Selective serotonin reuptake inhibitors for depressive disorders in children and adolescents, *Cochrane Database Syst Rev* 3:CD004851, 2007.

Hull PR, D'Arcy C: Isotretinoin use and subsequent depression and suicide, *Am J Clin Dermatol* 4:493-505, 2003.

Jacobs DG, Deutsch NL, Brewer M: Suicide, depression, and isotretinoin: is there a causal link? *J Am Acad Dermatol* 45(5):S168-S175, 2001.

James SP, Mendelson WB: The use of trazodone as a hypnotic: a critical review, *J Clin Psychiatry* 65(6):752-755, 2004.

Joy EA, Van Hala S, Cooper L: Health-related concerns of the female athlete: a lifespan approach, *Am Fam Physician* 79(6):489-495, 2009.

Kahn JA, Hillard PA: Human papillomavirus and cervical cytology in adolescents, *Adolesc Med Clin* 15(2):301-321, 2004.

Kahn JA, Rosenthal SL, Succop PA, et al: Mediators of the association between age of first sexual intercourse and subsequent human papillomavirus infection, *Pediatrics* 109(1):e5, 2002.

Kaufman M, American Academy of Pediatrics: Care of the adolescent sexual assault victim, *Pediatrics* 122(2):462-470, 2008.

Krakowski AC, Stendardo S, Eichenfield LF: Practical considerations in acne treatment and the clinical impact of topical combination therapy, *Pediatr Dermatol* 25(Suppl 1):1-14, 2008.

Laflin MT, Wang J, Barry M: A longitudinal study of adolescent transition from virgin to nonvirgin status, *J Adolesc Health* 42(3):228-236, 2008.

Lounds JJ, Borkowski JG, Whitman TL: The potential for child neglect: the case of adolescent mothers and their children, *Child Maltreat* 11(3):281-294, 2006.

Major B, Cozzarelli C, Cooper ML, et al: Psychological responses of women after first-trimester abortion, *Arch Gen Psychiatry* 57(8):777-784, 2000.

Mansbach JM, Forbes P, Peters C: Testicular torsion and risk factors for orchiectomy, *Arch Pediatr Adolesc Med* 159(12):1167-1171, 2005.

Maruschke M, Lehr C, Hakenberg OW: Traumatic penile injuries—mechanisms and treatment, *Urol Int* 81(3):367-369, 2008.

Meier E: RU-486 and implications for use among adolescents seeking an abortion, *Pediatr Nurs* 26(1):93-94, 2000.

Moreau C, Cleland K, Trussell J: Contraception discontinuation attributed to method dissatisfaction in the United States, *Contraception* 76(4):267-272, 2007.

Murray SK, Baker AW, Lewin L: Screening families with young children for child maltreatment potential, *Pediatr Nurs* 26(1):47-54, 65, 2000.

O'Donnell L, Stueve A, Duran R, et al: Parenting practices: parents' underestimation of daughters' risks and alcohol and sexual behaviors of urban girls, *J Adolesc Health* 42(5):496-502, 2008.

Olutunmbi BA, Paley K, English JC: Adolescent female acne: etiology and management, *J Pediatr Adolesc Gynecol* 21(4):171-176, 2008.

Orr DP, Johnston K, Brizendine E, et al: Subsequent sexually transmitted infection in urban adolescents and young adults, *Arch Pediatr Adolesc Med* 155(8):947-953, 2001.

Pattullo L, Griffeth S, Ding L, et al: Stepwise diagnosis of *Trichomonas vaginalis* infection in adolescent women, *J Clin Microbiol* 47(1):59-63, 2009.

Perry SE, Hockenberry MJ, Lowdermilk D, et al: *Maternal child nursing care*, ed 4, St Louis, 2010, Mosby.

Peterman TA, Tian LH, Metcalf CA, et al: High incidence of new sexually transmitted infections in the year following a sexually transmitted infection: a case for rescreening, *Ann Intern Med* 145(8):564-572, 2006.

Potard C, Courtois R, Rusch E: The influence of peers on risky sexual behaviour during adolescence, *Eur J Contracept Reprod Health Care* 13(3):264-270, 2008.

Rapkin AJ, Mikacich JA: Premenstrual syndrome and premenstrual dysphoric disorder in adolescents, *Curr Opin Obstet Gynecol* 20:455-463, 2008.

Reaman GH, Bleyer WA: Infants and adolescents with cancer: special considerations. In Pizzo PA, Poplack DG, editors: *Principles and practice of pediatric oncology*, ed 5, Philadelphia, 2006, Lippincott Williams & Wilkins.

Sakamoto H, Ogawa Y, Yoshida H: Relationship between testicular volume and varicocele in patients with infertility, *Urology* 71:104-109, 2008.

Sakamoto H, Saito K, Ogawa Y, et al: Effects of varicocele repair in adults on ultrasonographically determined testicular volume and on semen profile, *Urology* 71:485-489, 2008.

Santelli JS, Kaiser J, Hirsch L, et al: Initiation of sexual intercourse among middle school adolescents: the influence of psychosocial factors, *J Adolesc Health* 34(3):200-208, 2004.

Saslow D, Runowicz CD, Solomon D, et al: American Cancer Society guideline for the early detection of cervical neoplasia and cancer, *Cancer J Clin* 52:342-362, 2002.

Savio Beers LA, Hollo RE: Approaching the adolescent-headed family: a review of teen parenting, *Curr Probl Pediatr Adolesc Health Care* 39(9):216-233, 2009.

Schwartz JL, Barnhart K, Creinin MD, et al: Comparative crossover study of the PATH woman's condom and the FC female condom, *Contraception* 78(6):465-473, 2008.

Sherman RT, Thompson RA: The female athlete triad, *J Sch Nurs* 20(4):197-202, 2004.

Slap GS: Menstrual disorders in adolescence, *Best Pract Res Clin Obstet Gynecol* 17(1):75-92, 2003.

Sotiriadis A, Papatheodorou S, Makrydimas G: Threatened miscarriage: evaluation and management, *BMJ* 329(7458):152-155, 2004.

Spencer JM, Zimet GD, Aalsma MC, et al: Self-esteem as a predictor of initiation of coitus in early adolescents, *Pediatrics* 109(4):581-584, 2002.

Stermac L, Dunlap H, Bainbridge D: Sexual assault services delivered by SANEs, *J Forensic Nurs* 1(3):124-128, 2005.

Swygard H, Seña AC, Cohen MC: *Neisseria gonorrhoeae* infections in men, *UpToDate*, 2005, available at www.uptodate.com (accessed July 1, 2005).

Templeman C: Adolescent endometriosis, *Obstet Gynecol Clin North Am* 36(1):177-185, 2009.

Thiboutot D, Arsonnaud S, Pascale S: Efficacy and tolerability of adapalene 0.3% gel compared to tazarotene 0.1% gel in the treatment of acne vulgaris, *J Drugs Dermatol* 4(5):S3-S10, 2008.

Tillett J: Adolescents and informed consent: ethical and legal issues, *J Perinat Neonatal Nurs* 19(2):112-121, 2005.

Tracy CR, Steers WD, Costabile R: Diagnosis and management of epididymitis, *Urol Clin North Am* 35:101-108, 2008.

US Preventive Services Task Force: Screening for chlamydia infection: US Preventive Services Task Force recommendation statement, *Ann Intern Med* 147:128-134, 2007.

Ventura SJ, Abma JC, Mosher WD, et al: Estimated pregnancy rates by outcome for the United States, 1990-2004. *Natl Vital Stat Rep* 56(15):1-25, 2008.

Vichnin M: Ectopic pregnancy in adolescents, *Curr Opin Obstet Gynecol* 20(5):475-478, 2008.

Vigod SN, Ross LE, Steiner M: Understanding and treating premenstrual dysphoric disorder: an update for the women's health practitioner, *Obstet Gynecol Clin North Am* 36(4):907-924, 2009.

Walgrave SE, Ortiz AE, MacFalls HT, et al: Evaluation of a novel fractional resurfacing device for treatment of acne scarring, *Lasers Surg Med* 41(2):122-127, 2009.

Warren MP, Chua AT: Exercise-induced amenorrhea and bone health in the adolescent athlete, *Ann NY Acad Sci* 1135:244-252, 2008.

Webster GF: Acne: tips and tricks for the pediatrician, *Pediatr Ann* 38(2):80-83, 2009.

Wiksten-Almstromer M, Hirschberg AL, Hagenfeldt K: Menstrual disorders and associated factors among adolescent girls visiting a youth clinic. *Acta Obstet Gynecol Scand* 86:65-72, 2007.

Yan AC: Current concepts in acne management, *Adolesc Med Clin* 17(3):613-637, 2006.

Yang H, Liu CZ, Chen X, et al: Systematic review of clinical trials of acupuncture related therapies for primary dysmenorrhea, *Acta Obstet Gynecol Scand* 87(11):1114-1122, 2008.

Zampieri N, Mantovani A, Ottolenghi A, et al: Testicular catch up growth after varicocelectomy: does surgical technique make a difference? *Urology* 73:289-292, 2009.

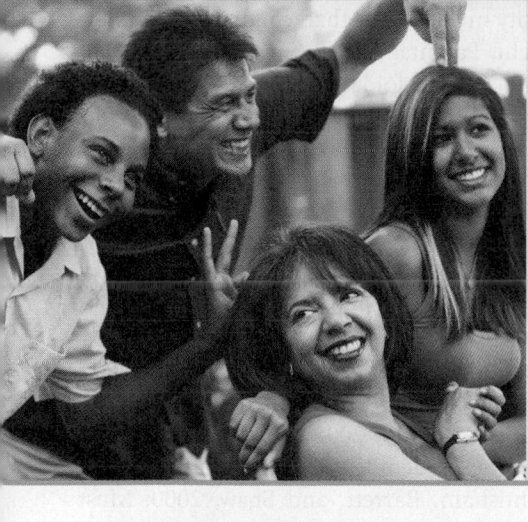

CHAPTER OUTLINE

Adolescence is a significant period of transition from childhood to young adulthood. This is the period when the precepts that govern the person's life in adulthood are established. Adolescents may find it difficult to cope with the inward conflict of becoming independent from parental support and rules yet at the same time meeting expectations imposed by peers and society. This chapter focuses on conditions that adolescents may be facing that have a profound effect on their lives as adults. As health care providers, nurses can have a significant impact in helping adolescents make an effective transition to adulthood.

OBESITY

The growth and development that occurs during adolescence can affect youth's interaction with food, nutrition, and physical activity.

Few health problems in adolescence are so obvious to others, are so difficult to treat, and have such long-term effects as obesity. It is the most common nutritional disturbance of children and one of the most challenging contemporary health problems at all ages.

In a 2001 report the U.S. surgeon general stated that in the year 2000 the total annual cost of obesity in the United States was $117 billion (US Surgeon General, 2001). The direct health costs of childhood overweight can only be estimated, since the major impact is likely to be felt in the next generation (Lobstein, Baur, and Uauy, 2004). However, reports indicate that for the first time in U.S. history, the current generation of children will have a shorter life expectancy than their parents (Olshansky, 2005).

Approximately 12.5 million children are overweight or obese (Ogden, Carroll, and Flegal, 2008). Numerous studies dating back to the early 1960s have documented childhood overweight through comprehensive evaluations of dietary intake, physical activity, and anthropometric measures (Centers for Disease Control and Prevention using the various National Health Examination Surveys [NHANES], I, II, III, and IV) (Ogden, Carroll, and Flegal, 2008; Ogden, Kuczmarski, Flegal, et al, 2002; Ogden, Troiano, Briefel, et al, 1997). In children ages 6 to 11 years the prevalence of childhood overweight remained fairly constant in between 1963 and 1974 at approximately 4% and 5.5%, respectively. However, recent NHANES surveys have seen those numbers steadily climb to reach 17% in both 6- to 11-year-olds and 12- to 19-year-olds (Ogden, Carroll, and Flegal, 2008) (Fig. 21-1). African-American and Hispanic children youth are disproportionately represented by a higher prevalence of overweight and obesity (23.1% and 21.0%, respectively) when compared with non-Hispanic Caucasian children (15.9%) (Ogden, Carroll, and Flegal, 2008). A study of 9464 Native American schoolchildren ages 5 to 18 years found that 39% were overweight, and a further review of tribes across the United States found that 30% to 46% of Native Americans were at risk for overweight (Hardy, Harrell, and Bell, 2004).

Because adult obesity is associated with increased mortality and morbidity from a variety of complications, both physical and psychologic, adolescent obesity is a serious condition. Overweight children and adolescents are at risk of continuing to be obese as adults, thereby experiencing the health and social consequences of obesity much earlier than children and adolescents of normal weight. Parental obesity increases the risk of overweight by twofold to threefold (Baker, Barlow, Cochran, et al, 2005). The probability that overweight school-age children will become obese adults is estimated at 50%, whereas the likelihood that overweight adolescents will become obese adults is estimated at 70% to 80% (National Institute for Health Care Management Foundation, 2003).

Obesity in childhood and adolescence has been related to elevated blood cholesterol, high blood pressure, asthma and other respiratory tract disorders, orthopedic conditions, cholelithiasis, some types of adult-onset cancer (MacKenzie, 2000), nonalcoholic fatty liver disease (Baker, Barlow, Cochran, et al, 2005; Lavine, 2000; Angulo, 2002), and an increase in type 2 diabetes mellitus (Fagot-Campagna, Narayan, and Imperatore, 2001; Ehtisham, Barrett, and Shaw, 2000; Must and Anderson, 2003).

Overweight refers to the state of weighing more than average for height and body build. Overweight status is defined as an age- and gender-specific body mass index (BMI) between the 85th percentile and the 94th percentile based on the 2000 Centers for Disease Control and Prevention Growth Charts for the United States. Obesity is defined as an age- and gender-specific BMI at or above the 95th percentile for children of the same age and sex (US Preventive Services Task Force, 2010). Obesity is an increase in body weight resulting from an excessive accumulation of body fat relative to lean body mass (Barlow and Expert Committee, 2007).

Currently, the BMI measurement is recommended as the most accurate method for screening children and adolescents for obesity by the Expert Committee on Pediatric Obesity (Barlow and Expert Committee, 2007), the US Preventive Services Task Force (2010), and the National Institute for Health Care Management Foundation (2003). (See Appendix B.) The BMI measurement is strongly associated with subcutaneous and total body fat and also with skinfold thickness measurements. It is also highly specific for children with the greatest amount of body fat (MacKenzie, 2000). A subset of children may have a high BMI because of increased muscle mass rather than fat mass (Swallen, Reither, Haas, et al, 2005).

Etiology and Pathophysiology

Obesity results from an energy imbalance (i.e., caloric intake that consistently exceeds caloric requirements and expenditure) and may involve a variety of interrelated influences, including metabolic, hypothalamic, hereditary, social, cultural, and psychologic factors. Because the etiology of obesity is multifactorial, the treatment requires multilevel interventions. Fig. 21-2 illustrates an ecological approach to understanding the multitude of risk factors associated with childhood and adolescent obesity. This framework suggests that the dominant factors, such as the availability of fast-food restaurants, may influence food choices of the children and adolescents who live there. An ecological approach helps promote a better understanding of the role that institutional, community, and societal factors play in the development of children's eating practices and activity levels, thereby taking some of the blame off children for their overweight (Neumark-Sztainer, 2003).

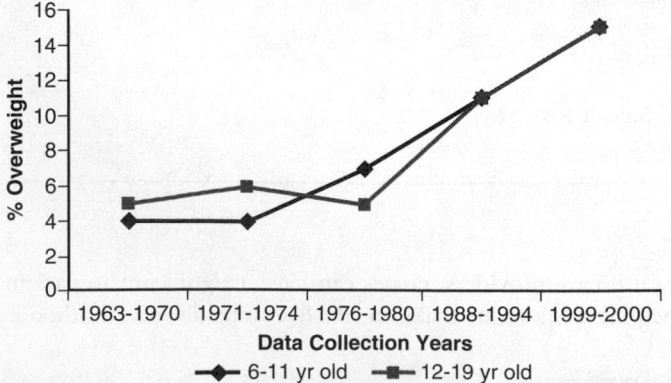

Fig. 21-1 Increasing incidence of overweight in children (National Health Examination Survey [NHANES] 1963-2000). Data collected using measured height and weight. The y-axis signifies the percent of obese children, overweight being defined as ≥95th percentile of age- and sex-specific body mass index.

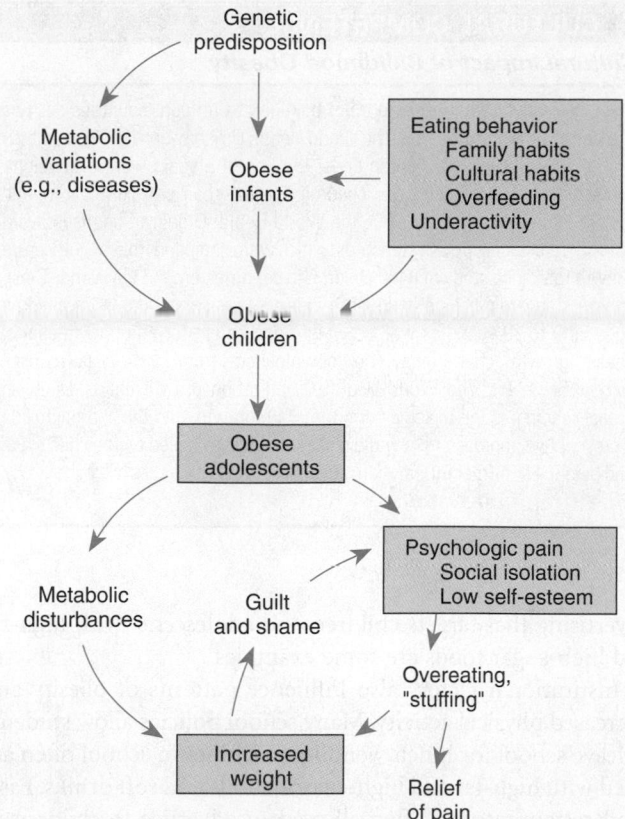

Genetic
predisposition

Metabolic
variations
(e.g., diseases)

Obese
infants

Eating behavior
Family habits
Cultural habits
Overfeeding
Underactivity

Obese
children

Obese
adolescents

Metabolic
disturbances

Guilt
and shame

Psychologic pain
Social isolation
Low self-esteem

Overeating,
"stuffing"

Increased
weight

Relief
of pain

Fig. 21-2 Complex relationships in adolescent obesity.

Birth weight does not seem to be a long-term contributing factor in detection and prediction of childhood obesity (Kain, Corvalán, Lera, et al, 2009). There is, however, a high correlation between childhood adiposity and parental adiposity (Li, Kaur, Choi, et al, 2005; Boney, Verma, Tucker, et al, 2005; Bouchard, 2009).

Energy Balance

A balance between energy intake and energy expenditure is a critical factor in regulating body weight. Factors that raise energy intake or decrease energy expenditure by even small amounts can have a long-term impact on the development of overweight and obesity. For example, a positive balance of one serving of a sweetened juice or soft drink (about 120 kcal) per day would produce a 50 kg (110 lb) increase in body mass over a 10-year period (Hill, Wyatt, Reed, et al, 2003).

Genetic Factors

Familial influence is an epidemiologic consideration in regard to a child weight. Twin studies suggest that approximately 35% to 50% of the tendency toward obesity is inherited (Beaty, 2007). Twin studies have also suggested that this tendency is a combination of genetic and environmental factors. Mothers seem to play a greater role in the gestational weight of a child (Jaquet, Swaminathan, Alexander, et al, 2005). When both parents are obese, there is a 60% to 80% increase in the likelihood of the child becoming obese (Koeppen-Schomerus, Wardle, and Plomin, 2001). The specific influences of genes and environment within the developing child is not well defined.

The increasing rates of obesity within genetically stable populations suggest that environmental and some perinatal factors (e.g., bottle-feeding) are contributors to the current increases in childhood obesity (National Institute for Health Care Management Foundation, 2003). More research is needed to better understand the influences of family behavior and adolescent overweight.

Diseases

Fewer than 5% of the cases of childhood obesity can be attributed to an underlying disease. Such diseases include hypothyroidism; adrenal hypercorticoidism; hyperinsulinism; and dysfunction or damage to the central nervous system as a result of tumor, injury, infection, or vascular accident. Obesity is a frequent complication of muscular dystrophy, paraplegia, Down syndrome, spina bifida, and other chronic illnesses that limit mobility.

Several congenital syndromes have obesity as a feature, including Laurence-Moon-Biedl, Prader-Willi, and Alström syndromes and pseudohypoparathyroidism. The most common of these is Prader-Willi syndrome, a disorder characterized by hypogonadism; slow intellectual development; short stature; and dysmorphic facial features, including a narrowed bifrontal diameter, almond-shaped eyes, and triangular mouth. These children are hypotonic and hyperphagic. They lack the internal mechanism that regulates satiety and as a result go to great lengths to obtain food.

Molecular, Metabolic, and Endocrine Factors: Regulators of Appetite

A major focus of obesity research has been appetite and its regulation. The expression of appetite is chemically coded in the hypothalamus by distinctive circuitry. Orexigenic substances produce signals that promote eating behaviors, and anorexigenic substances promote the cessation of eating behaviors. Feedback loops between signals have been identified where one signal peptide is able to alter the secretion of another signal peptide. No one signal has been identified as the gatekeeper of appetite. It is apparent that an entire network of signals, including their frequency and amplitude, is responsible for triggering eating behaviors.

This network of appetite signals explains the behavioral observations that appetite and food consumption patterns are dynamic and influenced by biologic, environmental, and psychologic events. Internal cues such as habitual intake, memories of food-related activities, and anticipation of consumption easily modify human eating behaviors. External cues that modify the perception of appetite include food aroma, appearance, anticipation, and the number food choices (Feldman, Friedman, and Sleisenger, 2002).

Researchers have identified a number of hormones and proteins that regulate appetite and weight in animal models. It is likely that these same mechanisms apply to humans. However, the role of hormones and neurotransmitters in determining overweight in humans remains unknown. Only a small number of enzyme abnormalities and metabolic defects have been identified, and these cannot account for the rapid increase in childhood obesity over the past three decades (Baker, Barlow, Cochran, et al, 2005).

There is little evidence to support a relationship between obesity and "low metabolism." There may be small differences in regulation of dietary intake or metabolic rate between obese and nonobese children that could lead to an energy imbalance and inappropriate weight gain, but these small differences are difficult to accurately quantify. However, research by Leahy, Birch, Fisher, and colleagues (2008) indicated that children can self-regulate intake when presented with high- and low-calorie food choices. Obese children tend to be less active than lean children, but it is uncertain whether inactivity creates the obesity or obesity is responsible for the inactivity. Obesity in adolescents and children can be caused by overeating, low activity levels, or both. Obese adolescents have actually been found to have higher total daily energy expenditure and resting energy expenditure than nonobese adolescents. This would seem to suggest that obese children need to eat more to maintain their higher weight. No differences in basal metabolic rate, sleeping metabolic rate, respiratory quotient, heart rate, or total energy expenditure have been found in normal weight children with or without a familial predisposition to overweight (Baker, Barlow, Cochran, et al, 2005).

Caloric Equilibrium: Sociocultural Factors

The tendency toward obesity occurs whenever environmental conditions are favorable toward excessive caloric intake, such as an abundance of food, limited access to nutrient-dense foods, reduced or minimum physical activity, and snacking combined with excessive screen (computer, television, video games) time. Family and cultural eating patterns, as well as psychologic factors, play an important role. Some families and cultures consider fat to be an indication of good health, a status symbol, or an indication of affluence. It is not uncommon for obese children to have families that emphasize large portion sizes, admonish children for leaving food on their plates, or use food as a reward or punishment. Parents may not have a concept of the amount of food children require and expect them to eat more than they need.

In countries such as the United States and Western Europe, the prevalence of obesity shows a marked difference between upper- and lower-class children, with differences often becoming apparent before 6 years of age. Lower socioeconomic groups have a greater prevalence of obesity, especially in girls. Sociocultural factors also influence physical activity. Results of a recent study indicate that activity and inactivity patterns differ by ethnicity, and minority adolescents (non-Hispanic African-Americans, Hispanics, and Filipinos) engage in less physical activity and more inactivity than their non-Hispanic Caucasian counterparts (Iannotti, Kogan, Janssen, et al, 2009) (see Cultural Competence box).

Community and Institutional Contributors

Some community factors that influence activity patterns include a lack of a built environment (sidewalks, parks, bike paths) or affordable and accessible facilities for low-income youth to be active, thus limiting their opportunities to participate in physical activities. Social policies also contribute to obesity. The increased availability of energy-dense foods, pricing strategies that promote unhealthy food choices, and overzealous food

CULTURAL COMPETENCE
Cultural Impact of Childhood Obesity

Child overweight and obesity are not confined to affluent countries such as the United States and Europe. The World Health Organization (2009) estimates that in 2007, 22 million children under the age of 5 years were overweight. More than two thirds of these children live in urban settings in low- and middle-income countries. In 2006 the World Health Organization made available new childhood growth standards, which were compiled from a Multicentre Growth reference study of 8440 children in countries around the world. These growth standards include body mass index reference standards for children ages birth to 19 years, as well as weight and height for age growth charts. These growth charts may be downloaded from **www.who.int/ growthref/en**. The World Health Organization growth charts establish breast-feeding as the biologic norm for infant growth, and the charts provide a prescriptive approach to how the child should grow based on the child's age and height. For further information, go to **www.who.int/childgrowth/ launch/en/index.html**.

advertising that targets children and adolescents with high-fat and high-sugar foods are some examples.

Institutional factors also influence patterns of obesity and decreased physical activity. Many school policies allow students to leave school for lunch. Vending machines in school often are filled with high-fat and high-calorie foods and soft drinks. Fast-food restaurants are often allowed to advertise to children in schools. Although well-balanced, nutritious school lunches may be available to students, they will often opt for no lunch or one that is of less nutritious choices such as high-fat and high-sugar snacks.

Physical inactivity has also been identified as an important contributing factor in the development and maintenance of childhood overweight. There is little doubt that physical activity has decreased in elementary and secondary schools in the United States. The percentage of high school students who attended physical education classes daily decreased from 42% in 1991 to 25% in 1995 and remained stable at that level until 2007 (30%). In 2007, 40% of ninth grade students but only 24% of twelfth grade students attended physical education class daily (Centers for Disease Control and Prevention, 2008). Consequently, most of a child's physical activity must occur within the family or outside of school. Decreased physical activity within the family and community is a powerful influence on children, since children model their parents and other adults.

The growing attraction and availability of many sedentary activities, including television, video games, computers, and the Internet, have greatly influenced the amount of exercise that children get. Children ages 8 and over were found in 2005 to consume an average of an additional hour of media content per day compared with 1999. On average one fourth (26%) of their media use time was spent "media multitasking," or using more than one medium at a time (Roberts, Foehr, and Rideout, 2006). Cross-sectional studies have shown the association between TV use and obesity among children (Robinson, 2006; Neumark-Sztainer, 2003; Gable, Chang, and Krull, 2007).

Other Influences

Psychologic factors also affect eating patterns. Infants experience relief from discomfort through feeding and learn to associate eating with a sense of well-being, security, and the comforting presence of a nurturing person. Eating is soon associated with the feeling of being loved. In addition, the pleasurable oral sensation of sucking provides a connection between emotions and early eating behavior. Many parents use food as a positive reinforcer for desired behaviors. This practice may become a habit, and the child may continue to use food as a reward, a comfort, and a means of dealing with feelings of depression or hostility. Many individuals eat when they are not hungry or in response to stress, boredom, loneliness, sadness, depression, or tiredness. Difficulty in determining feelings of satiety can lead to weight problems and may compound the factor of eating in response to emotional rather than physical hunger cues.

Meta-analyses of observational studies have found that obesity risk at school age was reduced by 15% to 25% with early breast-feeding compared with formula-feeding (Arenz, Ruckerl, Koletzko, et al 2004; Owen, Martin, Whincup, et al, 2005; Harder, Bergmann, Kallischnigg, et al, 2005). In one of these, one month of breast-feeding was associated with a 4% decrease in risk for obesity (Harder, Bergmann, Kallischnigg, et al, 2005). This effect lasted for up to 9 months of breast-feeding and was independent of the definition of overweight and age at follow-up. Researchers have suggested several possible explanations, including a lower insulinemic response compared with bottle-fed infants, lower energy and protein intake, and ability of breast-fed infants to self-regulate their energy intake from both breast milk and solid foods (Heinig, Nommsen, Peerson, et al, 1993).

Frequency of family meals has consistently been shown to be a protective factor for obesity (Utter, Scragg, Schaaf, et al, 2008; Fulkerson, Neumark-Sztainer, Hannan, et al, 2008). Family meals tend to provide access to a variety of nutrient-rich foods, particularly fruits and vegetables. Family meals also create a forum for increased family communication and connectedness, both of which promote healthy weight behaviors.

Leptin is a hormone synthesized by adipocytes. As adipocytes enlarge, leptin secretion increases; it decreases when the person is fasting. Leptin receptors are located in the hypothalamus. However, the true role of the leptin receptor in human obesity remains obscure (Baker, Barlow, Cochran, et al, 2005). The leptin signal may serve as an anorexin by its ability to alter secretion of orexins and anorexins. Obese individuals have appropriately elevated leptin levels, but it is not clear if this is the result of obesity or if this could relate to a pathologic cause of obesity (Feldman, Friedman, and Sleisenger, 2002). Researchers continue to explore the network of appetite signals and their effects on food consumption and weight.

Complications of Obesity

Adults with longstanding obesity are at risk for medical complications that include hypertension, diabetes, coronary heart disease, stroke, fatty liver disease, and colorectal cancer. Although obesity-related complications occur frequently in adults, children and adolescents are experiencing significant health consequences as well. Health care providers, researchers, and government agencies are beginning to discover that children and adolescents are developing these complications sooner rather than later in adult life. Childhood obesity has become an increasingly important medical problem, resulting in hyperten-

sion, type 2 diabetes, pulmonary complications (e.g., asthma, sleep apnea), growth acceleration, dyslipidemia, musculoskeletal problems, fatty liver disease, and a potential for psychosocial problems. Diagnostic evaluations of children and adolescents who are at risk for being overweight and children and adolescents who are overweight have expanded to screen for these complications.

Physical Complications of Obesity

Insulin Resistance and Type 2 Diabetes. Along with obesity, type 2 diabetes mellitus is reaching epidemic proportions in children and adolescents. One out of three newly diagnosed type 2 diabetics are adolescents. Inactivity and obesity influence insulin resistance. Insulin resistance syndrome, also known as syndrome X, is characterized by hyperinsulinemia, obesity, hypertension, and dyslipidemia and develops before any of these conditions develops.

Insulin is necessary for the metabolism of fats, proteins, and carbohydrates and must be present for glucose to enter the fat and muscle cells. Insulin facilitates the storage of glucose in the form of glycogen in the liver and muscle cells and further prevents the mobilization of fat from fat cells. The cell membrane has special receptor sites for insulin. Once the receptor site has been established, a chemical reaction results and glucose enters the cell. If the amount of insulin is inadequate, glucose cannot enter the cell. In response to elevated levels of glucose in the body, the pancreas increases the production of insulin, resulting in hyperinsulinemia. Type 2 diabetes develops when the pancreas is no longer able to lower the blood glucose level by hypersecretion of insulin.

Persons with insulin resistance sometimes have decreased high-density lipoprotein cholesterol levels, increased serum very low–density lipoprotein cholesterol, increased triglyceride levels, and increased or sometimes decreased low-density lipoprotein cholesterol levels (Rao, 2001; Yensel, Preud'Homme, and Curry, 2004; Bremer, Auinger, and Byrd, 2009).

Fatty Liver Disease. Recently, a growing number of children and adolescents have been diagnosed with nonalcoholic fatty liver disease (NAFLD), which has been recognized as one of the leading causes of chronic liver disease in the general population. Children account for approximately 2.5% of the population diagnosed with NAFLD, and between 20% and 77% of these children are considered obese (Imhof, Kratzer, Boehm, et al, 2007). NAFLD is liver damage that ranges from steatosis, steatohepatitis, and advanced fibrosis to cirrhosis. Nonalcoholic steatohepatitis (NASH) is a stage within the spectrum of NAFLD. The pathology of NASH is consistent with that seen in alcohol-induced liver injury, but occurs in persons who have not abused alcohol. NAFLD is the most common reason for elevated aminotransferase levels. It has been estimated that about 25% of obese children have elevated serum aminotransferases. The increased prevalence of NAFLD in the pediatric population appears to coincide with the increasing prevalence of obesity.

Although the disease process is not completely understood, some factors contribute to the development of NASH. These include insulin resistance; free-radical damage to fatty acids in the body, leading to inflammation and eventual tissue death and liver fibrosis; and dietary habits that cause blood fats to accumulate in the liver. People with NASH may feel healthy and show no outward signs of liver disease. However, NASH is progressive and can lead to cirrhosis and end-stage liver disease, which may require liver transplantation. Not everyone with elevated liver enzymes has liver damage. It also appears that serum aminotransferase levels are poor predictors of the severity of NAFLD. The only way to distinguish NASH from other forms of fatty liver disease, at this time, is with a liver biopsy (Patton, Sirlin, Behling, et al, 2006).

Pulmonary Complications. Childhood obesity is related to pulmonary complication, including sleep apnea, exercise intolerance, and asthma. Asthma and exercise intolerance can in turn worsen obesity by limiting physical activity and causing further weight gain. Chu, Chen, Wang, and colleagues (2009) examined the relationship between obesity and asthma in a study of more than 170,000 children in middle school. They found that significantly higher weight children had a 1.5 to 2.0 fold increase in the risk of asthma. This difference in obesity between asthmatics and nonasthmatics was significant for both sexes.

Sleep-disordered breathing is another significant problem with severely obese adults and children. Airway obstructions such as enlarged tonsils and adenoids may require assessment and intervention by an ear, nose, and throat specialist. Continuous positive airway pressure (CPAP) and bilevel positive airway pressure (BiPAP) are used for obese children requiring additional nighttime respiratory support.

Musculoskeletal and Abnormal Growth Acceleration. Obesity has been associated with musculoskeletal problems resulting from increased body weight on the supporting structures of the hips, knees, and feet. Slipped capital femoral epiphysis is the most common hip disorder among young teenagers and occurs when the cartilage plate (epiphysis) at the top of the femur slips out of place. Blount disease, another orthopedic problem, is the overgrowth of the medial aspect of the proximal tibial metaphysis that causes the lower leg to angle inward (tibia vara). The inner part of the tibia, just below the knee, fails to develop normally, resulting in angulation of the bone. The incidence of Blount disease is low. The cause is unknown, but it is thought to be due to the effects of weight on the growth plate. Approximately two thirds of patients with Blount disease are obese (Dietz, 1998), and one study has shown a dose-response relationship between BMI and Blount disease (Pirpiris, Jackson, Farng, et al, 2006).

Obesity is the most common cause of abnormal growth acceleration in childhood. Overweight children tend to be taller with advanced bone age and mature earlier than children who are not overweight. Longitudinal studies of children who became overweight have shown that height accelerates either with or shortly after excessive weight gain (Garn and Clark, 1976). Some data indicate that females with an elevated BMI achieve earlier pubertal milestones than their counterparts with a normal BMI (Rosenfield, Lipton, and Drum, 2009).

Psychologic and Social Complications of Obesity

Studies of the psychologic and social components of obesity have revealed a mixture of findings. Childhood obesity has been associated not only with metabolic health risk, but also with problems in social interactions and relationships. Obese children become targets of early and systematic discrimination.

Early studies reported that children at a young age are sensitized to obesity and have begun to incorporate the culture's preference for thinness.

Dietz (1998) found that in spite of the negative impressions of obesity, overweight young children do not appear to have negative self-image or low self-esteem. However, this differs for adolescents. Obesity status is inversely related to several self-perception factors (Strauss, 2000). Many appear to develop a negative self-image that persists into adulthood. Several researchers have found body dissatisfaction to be associated with lowered self-esteem in some populations (Mirza, Davis, and Yanovski, 2005; Muris, Meesters, van de Blom, et al, 2005).

Janssen, Craig, Boyce, and colleagues (2004) did a study that examined the association between overweight and obesity and bullying in school-aged children. They found that overweight children are more frequently the victims of bullying compared with children of normal weight. Bullying behaviors included name calling, teasing, threats, physical harm, rejection, rumors, and sexual harassment. Because adolescents are extremely reliant on their peers for social support, identity, and self-esteem, they are particularly at risk for the negative consequences of bullying and victimization.

Some studies have found that social problems among obese adolescents are quite prevalent and predictive of both short- and long-term psychologic outcomes. Studies have found that being overweight during adolescence has an effect on high school performance. Overweight adolescents have also been found to have lower household incomes as adults than their normal weight peers (Janssen, Craig, Boyce, et al, 2004).

More studies are needed to better understand the effects of overweight and obesity on the psychologic and social functioning of children and adolescents.

Diagnostic Evaluation

For some time, assessment and treatment of obesity in children consisted of little more than weighing and dietary counseling. With increasing knowledge of the potential health risks of obesity, a more thorough evaluation may be indicated. A careful history is obtained regarding the development of obesity, and a physical examination is performed to differentiate simple obesity from increased fat that results from organic causes. A family history of obesity, diabetes, coronary heart disease, and dyslipidemia should be obtained for all children who are overweight or at risk for overweight. Specific information from the patient and family about the effects of obesity on daily functioning—for example, problems with nighttime breathing and sleep, daytime sleepiness, pain in the joints, ability to keep up with family activities and peers at school—is helpful. The physical examination should focus on identifying comorbid conditions and identifiable causes of obesity. For some, psychologic assessment, by interviews and standardized personality tests, may provide insight into the personality and emotional problems that contribute to obesity and that might interfere with therapy.

It is useful to estimate the degree of obesity to determine the component of body weight that can be modified. All the following methods have been used to assess obesity: BMI, body weight, weight-height ratios, weight-age ratios, hydrostatic weight, dual energy x-ray absorptiometry (DXA), skinfold measurements, bioelectrical analysis, computed tomography (CT), magnetic resonance imaging (MRI), and neutron activation. Each of these methods has advantages and disadvantages. Hydrostatic, or underwater, weighing provides the most accurate measurement of lean body weight. In hydrostatic weighing, total body density is determined by total submersion in a water-filled tank. However, this method is not practical in clinical settings. Skinfold thickness with special calipers defines obesity as skinfold thickness greater than or equal to the 85th percentile. Human error is a problem with this method; results can vary greatly for health care professionals who do not perform these measurements frequently.

The bioelectrical impedance method determines body fat from measures of impedance of electrical current by way of electrodes attached to the arm and leg. CT is used to estimate subcutaneous and intraabdominal fat deposition. MRI provides clear images of fat deposits compared with tissues containing water and other components. Total-body neutron activation provides an estimation of water and fat, as well as calcium, protein, and other components. These techniques are expensive and are typically used in specialized clinical setting (Gibson, 2005).

BMI is currently considered the best method to assess weight in children and adolescents (Barlow and Expert Committee, 2007). The calculation is based on the individual's height and weight. In adults, BMI definitions are fixed measures without regard for sex and age. The BMI in children and adolescents varies to accommodate age- and gender-specific changes in growth. The formula for BMI calculation can be found in the footnote on p. 142. BMI measures in children and adolescents are plotted on growth charts that enable heath care professionals to determine BMI-for-age for the patient. (See Appendix B.)

The initial assessment of obese children and adolescents should include screening to evaluate for comorbidities. The history is an important guide to determine the workup. A complete physical examination is important. Some areas to focus on include (1) skin for stretch markings and discolorations (e.g., acanthosis nigricans), (2) joints for swelling and evidence of pain, and (3) airway for evidence of obstruction and enlarged tonsils. Basic laboratory studies include a fasting lipid panel; fasting insulin level; fasting glucose hepatic enzymes, including a γ-glutamyltransferase (GGT); and, in some institutions, hemoglobin A_{1c}. Other studies, such as a polysomnogram (sleep study), metabolic studies, and radiographic evaluations, may be added based on the history and physical examination. These assessments may determine whether the patient needs a referral to specialty services for more focused evaluation and treatment, such as endocrinology (insulin resistance, diabetes), hepatology (elevated liver enzymes, NAFLD), orthopedics (Blount disease), or pulmonary medicine (sleep-disordered breathing, CPAP).

Therapeutic Management

The best approach to the management of obesity is a preventive one. Early recognition and control measures are essential before the child or adolescent reaches an obese state. Health care providers need to educate families about the medical complications of obesity.

Currently, the only treatments recommended for children are diet, exercise, behavior modification, and in some situations

pharmacologic agents such as sibutramine and orlistat. The treatment of obesity is difficult. Many approaches do not achieve long-term success. The average individual only loses about 5% to 10% of his or her weight with the current available therapies. Losing weight can have a significant positive effect on many comorbidities, but unfortunately the lost weight is frequently regained in a year or two (Yanovski and Yanovski, 2002). A number of multidisciplinary programs offer interventions combining medical, dietary, exercise, and psychologic support. This therapy is labor intensive and fairly costly.

Researchers continue searching for medications that will successfully treat obesity. The U.S. Food and Drug Administration has approved sibutramine, an appetite suppressant, for use in adolescents 16 years old and older for the treatment of obesity (US Preventive Services Task Force, 2010). There are currently no drugs approved for use in overweight or obese children under the age of 12 years. Many medical centers are studying surgical approaches to the management of obesity. Surgical techniques have seen growing use in adults, but their application in children is being cautiously evaluated.

Diet

Diet modification is an essential part of weight-reduction programs. Dietary counseling focuses on improving the nutritional quality of the diet rather than on dietary restriction. Children should avoid fad diets. Most dietitians and nutrition experts recommend a diet with no trans fats, low-saturated fat, moderate total fat (<30%), and nine servings of fruits and vegetables, consistent with MyPlate. Also, promoting high-fiber foods and avoiding highly refined starches and sugars will decrease caloric intake. Many programs recommend using a food diary as a helpful tool to increase awareness of food choices and eating behaviors. The goal is to encourage the individual to make healthier choices in foods selection and discourage using food by habit or to appease boredom. Box 21-1 contains helpful suggestions.

Many dietitians recommend encouraging parents to take charge of family meals to improve their nutritional quality. Getting families to sit down together at the table, away from distractions such as television, makes dinner time more than just eating. Dinner time becomes a time to share the events of

---

BOX 21-1   RECOMMENDED BEHAVIORS FOR PREVENTING OBESITY

In counseling adolescents whose body mass index is between the 5th and 84th percentiles, physicians and health care providers should recommend the following steps to prevent obesity:

- Limit consumption of sugar-sweetened beverages.
- Consume recommended quantities of fruits and vegetables.
- Limit television and other screen time to no more than 2 hours per day.
- Remove television and computer screens from primary sleeping areas.
- Eat breakfast daily.
- Limit eating at restaurants.
- Have frequent family meals in which parents and youth eat together.
- Limit portion sizes.

Adapted from Davis DM, Gance-Cleveland B, Hassink S, et al: Recommendations for prevention of childhood obesity, *Pediatrics* 120:S229-S253, 2007.

the day and build relationships (Baker, Barlow, Cochran, et al, 2005).

Special Diets

In patients with severe obesity, strict diets have been used, such as the protein-sparing modified fast, hypocaloric, ketogenic diet, that are designed to provide enough protein to minimize loss of lean body mass during weight loss. These diets need to be closely monitored and should be used only with multidisciplinary teams that include a physician, nutritionist, and behavior therapist. Generally, the diet consists of 1.5 to 2.5 g of protein per kilogram. The intake of carbohydrates is low enough to induce ketosis. The benefits of the diet are relatively rapid weight loss and anorexia induced by ketosis. Potential complications include protein losses, hypokalemia, hypoglycemia, inadequate calcium intake, and orthostatic hypotension. Potassium and calcium supplements and adequate calorie-free beverages can minimize these complications (Baker, Barlow, Cochran, et al, 2005). It is difficult to sustain these diets over the long term, and the long-term outcomes of using these diets have not been established.

Physical Activity

Regular physical activity is incorporated into all weight-reduction programs. Any form of increased physical activity is beneficial, provided that the activities are age appropriate and enjoyable. Recommendations for physical activity need to consider the patient's current health status and developmental level. Current recommendations encourage children to be physically active for 60 minutes or more a day. The best choice for exercise is any form that is enjoyable and likely to be sustainable. Aerobic and endurance exercises help oxidize body fats. Light exercises like walking may provide an opportunity for the family to increase time together and increase caloric expenditure. Weight training can increase basal metabolic rate and replace fat mass with muscle mass. However, weight training is not generally recommended for prepubertal children until they have reached physical and skeletal maturity. In prepubertal children increasing outdoor playtime is likely to be beneficial. Many children find exercise videos and treadmills boring and may not continue these activities. Behavioral research supports that individuals are more likely to exercise when they have a choice (Thompson and Wankel, 1980; Martin, Dubbert, Katell, et al, 1984). Individuals can choose from a large variety of physical activities, including team sports and individual sports such as yoga, dance, bike riding, swimming, and karate.

Limiting sedentary behaviors such as television viewing is the most effective way to encourage physical activity (Robinson, 1999, 2001). The American Academy of Pediatrics (2006) recommends limiting television viewing to less than 2 hours a day. Box 21-2 shows more strategies to increase physical activities.

Behavior Modification

Behavior modification approaches to weight loss are based on the observation that obese individuals have abnormal eating practices that can be altered. Attention is focused not on food but on the social and behavioral aspects surrounding food consumption. Successful behavior modification weight programs help adolescents identify and eliminate inappropriate eating habits and include a problem-solving component that enables adolescents to identify problems and determine solutions. Combining behavioral modifications with pharmacologic therapy in children 12 years and older has produced mixed results with regard to total weight loss maintained over a significant period of time (US Preventive Services Task Force, 2010). Reports suggest modest benefits with moderate-to-high behavioral interventions (measured in number of contact hours) in decreasing mean BMI of children and adolescents involved in such programs over a period of 6 to 12 months (Whitlock, O'Connor, Williams, et al, 2010). Programs including family-based behavioral modification, dietary modification, and exercise have been shown to be successful in reducing obesity in some children (American Academy of Pediatrics, 2006). Behavior modification is an important part of multidisciplinary intervention programs.

Drugs

A number of medications have been used in adults with varying results. Currently, multicenter clinical trials are being conducted to evaluate the effects of medications on weight loss in children. To date the only drug approved for use in adolescents is the appetite suppressant sibutramine. Orlistat, a lipase inhibitor, has been approved for use in children 12 years and older. Currently no long-term data are available regarding the benefits of such drugs for obesity management in children and adolescents (US Preventive Services Task Force, 2010). Some drugs have been used to promote weight loss in children with certain conditions such as metformin in obese adolescents with insulin resistance and hyperinsulinemia, octreotide for hypothalamic obesity caused by intracranial tumors, growth hormone in children with Prader-Willi syndrome, and leptin for congenital leptin deficiency (Baker, Barlow, Cochran, et al, 2005; Freemark and Bursey, 2001; Myers, Carrel, Whitman, et al, 2000; Farooqi, Jebb, Langmark, et al, 1999).

BOX 21-2 **STRATEGIES TO INCREASE PHYSICAL ACTIVITIES**

1. Start by identifying how much time is spent in sedentary activities (e.g., television, computer, video games).
2. Decrease television and sedentary activities to 1 to 2 hours per day or less.
3. Put more physical activities into your daily routine.
   - Walk the dog.
   - Walk with friend instead of talking on the phone.
   - Walk to school.
   - Consider purchasing a pedometer ($10 to $15) and aim for 10,000 to 22,000 steps daily.
   - Take classes—dance, karate, swimming, tennis.
   - Take aerobic classes or use tapes.
   - Participate in team sports.
   - Jump rope.
   - Ride bicycles or scooters.
4. Consider an hour of activity after school before sitting down for homework.
5. Younger children should play outdoors daily or play indoors with Nerf ball, scooter toys, etc.
6. Buy active toys rather than computer games and videotapes.

Surgical Techniques

Surgical techniques (bariatric surgery) that bypass portions of the intestine or occlude a segment of the stomach to produce a marked diet restriction and weight loss are hazardous and cause many metabolic complications. These complications include severe water and electrolyte depletion, persistent diarrhea, vitamin deficiency, internal herniation, and fatty infiltration and degeneration of the liver. In the recent past, these procedures were considered contraindicated for pediatric patients. Surgical intervention for children and adolescents is being reevaluated in the context of the significant increase in the prevalence of obesity and concomitant comorbidities within this population.

Bariatric surgery may be the only practical alternative for increasing numbers of severely overweight adolescents who have failed organized attempts to lose or maintain weight loss through conventional nonoperative approaches and who have serious life-threatening conditions. There are few studies in adults and no information for adolescents that suggest surgical weight loss improves the early mortality of patients with severe obesity. Therefore, in general, bariatric surgery should be reserved for severely obese adolescents with comorbidities after careful consideration. Physicians must define clear, realistic, and restrictive guidelines to apply with younger patients when surgery is considered. Candidates for surgery should be referred to centers that offer a multidisciplinary team experienced in the management of childhood and adolescent obesity. The surgery should be performed by surgeons who have participated in subspecialty training in bariatric medical and surgical care as detailed by the American College of Surgeons and the American Society for Metabolic and Bariatric Surgery.

It is recommended that a pediatric review process be in place to carefully screen patients. Candidates should undergo complete medical assessments and psychologic evaluations that include the patient and parents. The most important ethical considerations for bariatric surgery in an adolescent are whether (1) the patient's health is severely compromised by severe obesity, (2) the patient has failed more conservative treatment options, and (3) the patient (adolescent) has the ability to make this decision. Current criteria for bariatric surgery include (1) failed attempt at weight loss for at least 6 months as determined by the primary care physician; (2) attainment of physical maturity (Tanner stage IV); (3) BMI of at least 40 with serious obesity-related comorbidities, or BMI of at least 50 with less severe comorbidities (Box 21-3); (4) demonstrated commitment to comprehensive medical and psychologic evaluations both before and after surgery; (5) agreement to avoid pregnancy for at least 1 year postoperatively; (6) ability and willingness to adhere to nutritional guidelines; (7) ability to give informed consent to surgical treatment; and (8) a supportive family environment (Inge, Krebs, Garcia, et al, 2004).

In addition, recent recommendations state that bariatric surgery should be limited to youth (12 to 18 years old) with a BMI of 40 or more. Surgery is appropriate only for those with severe to moderate degrees of comorbidities, such as diabetes with hemoglobin A_{1c} greater than 9, regardless of therapy. Only the most severe degree of hypertension is an appropriate criterion for this group. Elevated lipids and sleep apnea, regardless of level of treatment, are also appropriate criteria for surgery in

adolescents. Chronic joint pain in its most severe state, venous stasis disease, and impaired quality of life are also considered appropriate criteria for this young age-group (Yermilov, McGory, Shekelle, et al, 2009). Laparoscopic adjustable gastric banding surgery was effective in reducing weight by as much as 55% at 1- and 2-year follow-up in 73 obese pediatric patients aged 13 to 17 years (Nadler, Youn, Ren, et al, 2008).

Surgical treatment options for adolescents should be chosen carefully and with the support of the multidisciplinary team, the patient, and the family. More will be learned about outcomes of this approach with time and careful study and evaluations. It is strongly recommended that all patients who have bariatric surgery be monitored throughout their lives. Knowledge about appropriate timing and better surgical and postoperative management of adolescent surgical patients depends on the rigorous collection of high-quality outcome data (Inge, Krebs, Garcia, et al, 2004).

BOX 21-3   COMORBIDITIES THAT MAY BE IMPROVED WITH BARIATRIC SURGERY

Serious Comorbidities
Type 2 diabetes mellitus
Obstructive sleep apnea
Pseudotumor cerebri

Less Serious Comorbidities
Hypertension
Dyslipidemias
Nonalcoholic steatohepatitis
Venous stasis disease
Significant impairment in activities of daily living
Intertriginous soft-tissue infections
Stress urinary incontinence
Gastroesophageal reflux disease
Weight-related arthropathies that impair physical activity
Obesity-related psychosocial distress

From Inge TH, Krebs NF, Garcia VF, et al: Bariatric surgery for severely overweight adolescents: concerns and recommendations, *Pediatrics* 114(1):217-223, 2004.

QUALITY PATIENT OUTCOMES: Childhood and Adolescent Overweight
BMI for age is maintained between 5th and 84th percentiles.

Nursing Care Management

Nurses play a key role in the adherence and maintenance phases of many weight-reduction programs. Nurse practitioners assess, manage, and evaluate the progress of many overweight adolescents. They also play an important role in recognizing potential weight problems and assisting parents and adolescents in preventing obesity.

The presence of obesity may not be obvious from appearance alone. Regular assessment of height and weight and computation of the BMI facilitate early recognition. There are published guidelines for childhood obesity prevention and treatment (Barlow and Expert Committee, 2007). Evaluation

BOX 21-4 PEDIATRIC OBESITY PREVENTION PROTOCOL FOR PRIMARY CARE

Step 1: Assess
Explain and conduct assessments of:
- Weight, height, and body mass index percentile
- Dietary intake (fruit, vegetables, sweetened beverages, and fast food)
- Activity (screen time, moderate-to-vigorous activity)
- Eating behaviors (breakfast, portion sizes, family meals)

Provide and elicit feedback on body mass index and behaviors found to be inside and outside the optimal range.

Step 2: Set Agenda
Explore interest in changing behaviors not in the optimal range.
Agree on target behaviors with the patient and caregiver.

Step 3: Assess Motivation and Confidence
With regard to interest in changing weight status or behaviors, assess:
- Willingness
- Perceived importance
- Confidence in having success

Probe the patient regarding ratings of willingness, perceived importance, and confidence to explore the advantages and disadvantages of changing.

Step 4: Summarize and Probe Possible Changes
Summarize the advantages and disadvantages of change.
Query possible next steps.
Offer ideas for getting started in making a change as needed.
Summarize the change plan.
Provide positive feedback.

Step 5: Schedule Follow-Up Visit
If a change plan is made, agree on a follow-up appointment within a specified number of weeks or months.
If no change plan is made, agree to revisit the topic within a specific number of weeks or months.

Adapted from Davis DM, Gance-Cleveland B, Hassink S, et al: Recommendations for prevention of childhood obesity, *Pediatrics* 120:S229-S253, 2007.

BOX 21-5 STAGES OF CHANGE MODEL

Precontemplation—Not yet acknowledging that there is a problem behavior that needs to be changed
Contemplation—Acknowledging there is a problem but not yet ready or sure of wanting change
Preparation/determination—Getting ready to change
Action/willpower—Changing behavior
Maintenance—Maintaining the behavior change
Relapse—Returning to older behaviors and abandoning the new changes

From Prochaska JO, DiClemente CC: *The transtheoretical approach: crossing traditional boundaries of change,* Homewood, Ill, 1984, Dorsey Press.

includes a height and weight history of the adolescent and family members, eating habits, appetite and hunger patterns, and physical activities. A psychosocial history is also helpful in understanding the impact of obesity on the child's life. Davis, Gance-Cleveland, Hassink, and colleagues (2007) describe steps to approaching behavior change with youth (Box 21-4).

Before initiating a treatment plan, it is important to be certain that the family is ready for change. Lack of readiness may result in failure, frustration, and reluctance to address the problem in the future. It may be wiser to defer treatment until the family is ready (Box 21-5). The nurse should explore with adolescents the reasons behind the desire to lose weight because motivation to lose weight is the key to success. Adolescents need to take a personal responsibility for dietary habits and physical activity. Teens who are forced by their parents to seek help are seldom motivated, become rebellious, and are unwilling to control their dietary intake.

Nutritional Counseling

Preventing an increase in body fat during growth is a realistic approach. This is often accomplished by adjusting four aspects of eating: (1) reducing the quantity eaten by purchasing, preparing, and serving smaller portions; (2) altering the quality consumed by substituting low-calorie, low-fat foods for high-calorie foods (especially for snacks); (3) eating regular meals and snacks, particularly breakfast; and (4) altering situations by severing associations between eating and other stimuli, such as eating while watching television. Nutrition counseling incorporates health behavior theories to help motivate and maintain behavior change. The most successful changes are those that are attainable, reasonable, and sustainable.

The nurse teaches adolescents and parents how to incorporate favorite foods into their diet and to select satisfying substitutes. To maintain a healthy diet, it is necessary to encourage the consumption of nutrient-dense foods such as fruits, vegetables, whole grains, and low-fat dairy protein products. Calories and fat should be kept to a healthy level without being significantly restricted. To be successful, a dietary program should be nutritionally sound with sufficient satiety value, produce the desired weight loss, and be accompanied by nutrition education and continued support.

Behavior Therapy

Altering eating behavior and eliminating inappropriate eating habits are essential to weight reduction, especially in maintaining long-term weight control. Most behavior modification programs include the following concepts:

- A description of the behavior to be controlled, such as eating habits
- Attempts to modify and control the stimuli that govern eating
- Development of eating techniques designed to control speed of eating
- Positive reinforcement for these modifications through a suitable reward system that does not include food

Box 21-1 includes specific strategies to modify eating habits.

Group Involvement

Commercial groups (e.g., Weight Watchers) or diet workshops are usually directed to adults; a group of other adolescents is often more effective. Teenage groups include summer camps designed for obese young people and conducted by health professionals, school groups organized and led by a school nurse or health professional, and groups associated with special clinics.

These groups are concerned not only with weight loss but also with the development of a positive self-image, social support, and the encouragement of physical activity. Nutrition education, diet planning, and the improvement of social skills are essential components of these groups. Improvement is determined by positive changes in all aspects of behavior.

Family Involvement

There is a definite connection between family environment, interaction, and obesity. The nurse needs to educate parents in the purposes of the therapeutic measures and their role in management. The family needs nutrition education and counseling regarding the reinforcement plan, alterations in the food environment, and ways to maintain proper attitudes. They can support their child in efforts to change eating behaviors, food intake, and physical activity.

Prognosis

Lifelong eating habits and psychologic problems make weight reduction difficult. Weight reduction is more successful in older adolescents who have lean parents, a good academic performance, no affective disorder, and no recent stressful life event (such as parents' divorce or a death).

Prevention

Reducing adolescent obesity has been identified as a national public health priority by the Institute of Medicine and numerous other expert groups. In 2005 the Institute of Medicine Committee on Prevention of Obesity in Children and Youth (Koplan, Liverman, and Kraak, 2005) developed guidelines for the prevention of childhood obesity. These guidelines suggest federal, state, local community, industry, and media changes that can positively affect childhood obesity in the United States. Weight loss programs do not enjoy the success of therapeutic interventions for other disorders. Gradual accumulation of adipose tissue during childhood establishes a pattern of eating that is difficult to reverse in adolescence. Prevention of obesity should begin in early childhood with the development of healthy eating habits, regular exercise patterns, and a positive relationship between parents and children. Prevention of adolescent obesity is best accomplished by early identification of obesity in the preschool, school-age, and preadolescent periods. Health care professionals should encourage frequent health care visits for children who are overweight or obese and incorporate a dietary history and counseling into each well-infant, well-child, and well-adolescent visit.

EATING DISORDERS

Eating disorders affect an estimated 5 million Americans every year. These psychologic illnesses include anorexia nervosa (AN), bulimia nervosa (BN), binge eating, and variations of these. Eating disorders are characterized by serious disturbances in eating and distortion of the body image that is manifested by restriction of intake or bingeing and an obsessive concern about body shape or body weight. These behaviors have the potential to cause serious health problems resulting from the physiologic sequelae brought on by altered nutritional status and purging. Often there is a significant delay in the diagnosis and treatment that relates to the nature of the illness; however, those with AN have one of the highest mortality rate of all psychiatric illnesses (Marcus, 2007; Neumarker, 1997). Persons with eating disorders frequently hide their symptoms because of a lack of awareness of the effects on their health, the shame of discussing their symptoms with others, and an unwillingness to give up these harmful behaviors (Becker, Grinspoon, Klibanski, et al, 1999).

ANOREXIA NERVOSA AND BULIMIA NERVOSA

AN is a complex illness that results in significant morbidity and mortality. It is a disorder with social, psychologic, behavioral, cultural, and physiologic components. AN is characterized by a strong fear of becoming fat, a distorted body image, and progressive weight loss. The disorder is a clinical diagnosis listed in the *Diagnostic and Statistical Manual of Mental Disorders* (DSM-IV-TR) (American Psychiatric Association, 2000) (Box 21-6).

Bulimia refers to an eating disorder somewhat similar to AN. BN is characterized by repeated episodes of binge eating followed by inappropriate compensatory behaviors, such as self-induced vomiting; misuse of laxatives, diuretics, or other medications; fasting; or excessive exercise (American Psychiatric Association, 2000). The binge behavior consists of secretive, frenzied consumption of large amounts of high-calorie (or "forbidden") foods during a brief time (usually <2 hours). The binge is counteracted by a variety of weight control methods (purging), including self-induced vomiting, diuretic and laxative abuse, and rigorous exercise. These binge-purge cycles are followed by self-deprecating thoughts, a depressed mood, and an awareness that the eating pattern is abnormal (Box 21-7).

Binge eating disorder (BED) is currently recognized as a diagnostic category in need of further study and as a type of *eating disorder not otherwise specified* (EDNOS). It is characterized by recurrent binge eating (overeating accompanied by loss of control occurring on average at least twice weekly for 6 months)

BOX 21-6　DIAGNOSTIC CRITERIA FOR ANOREXIA NERVOSA

1. Refusal to maintain body weight at or above a minimally normal weight for age and height (e.g., weight loss leading to maintenance of body weight less than 85% of that expected; or failure to make expected weight gain during period of growth, leading to body weight less than 85% of that expected)
2. Intense fear of gaining weight or becoming fat, even though underweight
3. Disturbance in the way in which one's body weight or shape is experienced, undue influence of body weight or shape on self-evaluation, or denial of the seriousness of the current low body weight
4. In postmenarcheal females, amenorrhea (i.e., the absence of at least three consecutive menstrual cycles). A woman is considered to have amenorrhea if her periods occur only following hormone (e.g., estrogen) administration.

Specify type:
- Restricting type: During the current episode of anorexia nervosa, the person has not regularly engaged in binge-eating or purging behavior (i.e., self-induced vomiting or the misuse of laxatives, diuretics, or enemas).
- Binge-eating/purging type: During the current episode of anorexia nervosa, the person has regularly engaged in binge-eating or purging behavior (i.e., self-induced vomiting or the misuse of laxatives, diuretics, or enemas).

From American Psychiatric Association: *Diagnostic and statistical manual of mental disorders*, ed 4 (text revision) (DSM-IV-TR), Washington, DC, 2000, The Association.

and marked distress in the absence of regular compensatory behaviors (American Psychiatric Association, 2000). Binge episodes may be associated with a cluster of symptoms, including eating rapidly; eating until uncomfortably full; eating large amounts in the absence of hunger; eating in secret due to embarrassment; and feeling disgusted, depressed, or guilty after eating.

Epidemiology

The incidence of AN in adolescent females in the United States has been estimated at 0.5%, and between 1% and 5% of these girls meet the criteria for bulimia (American Academy of Pediatrics, 2003). However, estimates of the prevalence of disordered eating reaches up to 65% of females and 35% of males (Croll, Neumark-Sztainer, Story, et al, 2002). The incidence is approximately 5 to 10 in 100,000 population per year. The incidence in males is one tenth of that of females.

The epidemiology of these eating disorders is difficult to accurately assess because of changes in diagnostic criteria over time and because the methods of detection, primarily self-report, may not be reliable in an illness characterized by denial and secrecy. Most resources report an increase in the incidence of AN and BN over the past 50 years, but the prevalence in the past 20 years is debated. The highest incidence occurs in 15- to 19-year-olds. The onset of the disorder appears to have two peaks: at age 14 and age 18 (Foreman, 2009). BED is reported among 20% to 35% of youth seeking weight loss treatment (Eddy, Celio Doyle, Hoste, et al, 2008). The incidence of AN, in particular, is increasing in emerging economies or non-Western societies (Latzer, Azaiza, and Tzischinsky, 2009; Preti, Girolamo, Vilagut, et al, 2009). Although most people with AN

recover completely or partially, about 5% die of the condition and 20% develop a chronic eating disorder (Lock and Fitzpatrick, 2009).

Pathophysiology

No consensus exists on the pathophysiology of AN and BN. It has been shown that AN, BN, and BED patients do not differ from each other in their level of shape and weight concern, but do differ from those without eating disorders (Devlin, Goldfein, and Dobrow, 2003). A combination of genetic, neurochemical, psychodevelopmental, and sociocultural factors appear to cause the disorder (Becker, Grinspoon, Klibanski, et al, 1999; Hudson, Hiripi, Pope, et al, 2007). Dieting appears to be common to the initiation of both AN and BN. Also characteristic is a childhood preoccupation with being thin reinforced by sociocultural and environmental factors supporting the concepts of ideal body shape. Many sports and artistic endeavors that emphasize leanness (e.g., ballet and running) and sports in which the scoring is partly subjective (e.g., skating and gymnastics) have been associated with a higher incidence of eating disorders. The term *female athlete triad,* characterized by eating disorder, amenorrhea, and osteoporosis, has been applied to young women with restrictive eating disorders and amenorrhea (Rome, Ammerman, Rosen, et al, 2003).

The prominent physiologic changes that occur as a result of weight loss have raised suspicion for a prominent physiologic disturbance as causative factor. Since most of these physiologic disturbances resolve with the normalization of body weight, this argues against their role as a primary cause. The neurotransmitter serotonin affects appetite control, sexual and social behavior, stress responses, and mood and possibly accounts for some of the changes seen in patients with AN. BED is also associated with dopamine in the nucleus accumbens portion of the brain that is programmed for reward and motivation. Neuroimaging studies using MRI and, more recently, positron emission tomography scans have demonstrated subtle changes, but the significance of these changes and their connection to eating disorders are not well understood (Rome, Ammerman, Rosen, et al, 2003; Foreman, 2009; Chial, McAlpine, and Camilleri, 2002; Van den Eynde and Treasure, 2009; Avena, 2009).

Familial transmission is an area that has attracted research attention, but there are no strong empirical data to indicate that one particular family prototype is responsible for the development of an eating disorder. However, many experts have associated the development of an eating disorder with family characteristics such as an adolescent perception of high parental expectations for achievement and appearance, difficulty managing conflict, poor communication styles, enmeshment and occasionally estrangement between family members, devaluation of the mother or the maternal role, marital tension, and mood and anxiety disorders. Families struggling with an eating disorder have been characterized as often having difficulties responding positively to the changing physical and emotional needs of the adolescent. Family stress of any kind may become a significant factor in the development of an eating disorder (Foreman, 2009; Lilenfeld, Kaye, Greeno, et al, 1998; Hudson, Laird, Betensky, et al, 2001; Strober, Freeman, Lampert, et al, 2007).

Results of twin studies suggest that both genetic and environmental factors contribute to the development of AN. A concordance rate for AN appears higher in monozygotic twins compared with dizygotic twins (Chial, McAlpine, and Camilleri, 2002). There also appears to be a higher prevalence of affective disorders and alcoholism in first-degree relatives of patients with eating disorders (Hudson, Laird, Betensky, et al, 2001; Foreman, 2009).

Individuals with eating disorders commonly have psychiatric problems, including affective disorder, anxiety disorder, obsessive-compulsive disorder, and personality disorder. Adult women with eating disorders were found to have higher rates of obsessive-compulsive behavior traits in their childhood. Persons with eating disorders have also been found to have higher reported rates of substance abuse, with alcohol problems being more common in those with BN than AN (Foreman, 2009). It is important to note that many of the clinical findings are directly related to the state of starvation and improve with weight gain.

Research continues in an effort to better understand the etiology and pathogenesis of eating disorders.

Clinical Manifestations

The most obvious manifestation of AN is the severe and profound weight loss induced by self-imposed starvation (see Box 21-6). The adolescents identify with this skeleton-like appearance and do not regard it as abnormal or ugly. Adolescents with AN often eat small amounts of food or play with food on their plates to give the impression that they are eating adequately and not experiencing disturbances in their eating habits. This can lead friends and family to disregard the possibility of AN. The adolescents can display a marked preoccupation with food—preparing meals for others, talking about food, hoarding food. Some become obsessed with fasting and engage in frequent strenuous exercise, self-induced vomiting, or laxative usage to speed up the weight-loss process (Lock and Fitzpatrick, 2009).

These young people tend to withdraw from peer relationships and engage in self-imposed social isolation. They continually strive for perfection, which may be demonstrated in other compulsive behaviors. They are usually overachievers, and their school work is very important to them.

In the wake of the severe weight loss, these girls and young women exhibit physical signs of altered metabolic activity. They develop secondary amenorrhea, bradycardia, lowered body temperature, decreased blood pressure, and cold intolerance. They have dry skin and brittle nails and develop lanugo. The changes are usually reversible with adequate weight gain and improved nutritional status.

Bulimia is more common in older adolescent girls and young women; males with bulimia are less common. BN patients may be of average or slightly above average weight. The diagnosis is confirmed, according to American Psychiatric Association's DSM-IV-TR (2000) (see Box 21-7), by at least two binge-eating episodes per week for the preceding 3 months. Although persons with bulimia have many issues in common with those who have other eating disorders, impulse control and satiety regulation are important problems in bulimia. Many individuals with bulimia begin with only occasional binges and purges "just for fun," enjoying the control over their weight while eating amounts of food that would normally produce obesity. As the disease progresses, the frequency of binges increases, the amount of food consumed increases, and they gradually lose control over the binge-purge cycle. The purging provides relief from feelings of guilt resulting from the enormous amounts of food consumed. The family becomes angry, and the individual with bulimia becomes frightened, frustrated, and increasingly guilt ridden, which only increases the symptoms in the self-destructive cycle.

The frequency of bingeing can be anywhere from once per week to seven or eight times per day. Because persons with bulimia usually binge on high-calorie foods, especially sweets, ice cream, and pastries, insulin production is stimulated to cope with the added carbohydrates. When the food is vomited, the unused insulin stimulates hunger and the desire to eat.

Diagnostic Evaluation

Diagnosis is made on the basis of clinical manifestations and conformity to the criteria established by the American Psychiatric Association (2000) (see Boxes 21-6 and 21-7). The DSM-V will be published in 2012, and these diagnoses criterion will likely change slightly. Table 21-1 lists the differences between AN and BN. A diagnosis of bulimia may first be suspected from the presence of complications.

Screening Tools

All patients in high-risk categories for eating disorders should be screened during routine office visits. The medical history is most important for diagnosing eating disorders, since the physical examination may be normal, especially early in the illness. A number of screening questionnaires are available to assist with the interview. For example, with the Scoff Questionnaire, 1 point is scored for every "yes." A score of 2 or more indicates a likely case of AN or BN. The questions related to the mnemonic SCOFF are (1) Do you make yourself *sick* because you feel uncomfortably full? (2) Do you worry that you have lost *control* over how much you eat? (3) Have you recently lost more than 6.4 kg (14 lb, or *one* stone) in a 3-month period? (4) Do you believe yourself to be *fat* when others say that you are too thin? (5) Would you say that *food* dominates your life? (Morgan, Reid, and Lacey, 1999).

History and Physical Examination

A complete history and physical examination are important to rule out other causes for weight loss. The medical assessment of an eating disorder focuses on the complications of altered nutritional status and purging. A careful history assesses weight changes, dietary patterns, and the frequency and severity of purging and excessive exercise. Purging behaviors include vomiting or other methods such as abuse of laxatives, enemas, diuretics, anorexic drugs, caffeine, or other stimulants. Measure the patient's weight and height and evaluate it for appropriateness according to standard weight for height, age, and sex determined according to the percentile of his or her expected body weight or BMI.

Particularly important parts of the physical examination are vital sign measurement (heart rate and blood pressure both supine and standing, and body temperature). Hypotension, bradycardia, and hypothermia are often seen in association

TABLE 21-1   CHARACTERISTICS OF INDIVIDUALS WITH EATING DISORDERS

FACTORS	ANOREXIA NERVOSA	BULIMIA
Food	Turns away from food to cope	Turns to food to cope
Personality	Introverted	Extroverted
	Avoids intimacy	Seeks intimacy
	Negates feminine role	Aspires to feminine role
Behavior	"Model" child	Often acts out
	Obsessive-compulsive	Impulsive
School	High achiever	Variable school performance
Control	Maintains rigid control	Loses control
Body image	Body image distortion	Less frequent body image distortion
Health	Denies illness	Recognizes illness
		Health fluctuates
Weight	Body weight <85% of expected norm	Within 2.3-7 kg (5-15 lb) of normal body weight or may be overweight
Sexuality	Usually not sexually active	Often sexually active

with extremely low weight. Dry skin, lanugo, acrocyanosis, and breast atrophy are findings that have been associated with AN. Distinctive hand lesions (Russell sign) have also been observed; the backs of the hands are often scarred and cut from repeated abrasion of the skin against the maxillary incisors during self-induced vomiting (Lock and Fitzpatrick, 2009). Other findings include swelling of the parotid and submandibular glands and erosion of the enamel of the anterior teeth because of chronic acid exposure from vomiting.

Prolongation of the QT interval may be detected in some patients. Mitral valve prolapse (MVP) may also develop. An abdominal examination is important to detect intestinal dilation from chronic severe constipation as a result of decreased intestinal motility. Finally, a neurologic examination assesses for other causes of weight loss or vomiting such as evidence of brain tumor.

Laboratory Assessments

The initial laboratory assessment for a patient with an eating disorder should include a complete blood count to evaluate for anemia and other hematologic abnormalities. An erythrocyte sedimentation rate or C-reactive protein may be ordered to detect evidence of inflammation. These levels should be low in an eating disorder. Electrolytes should be measured, along with calcium, magnesium, phosphorus, blood urea nitrogen, and creatinine, if the patient appears to be dehydrated or if purging is suspected. A human chorionic gonadotropin measurement is done to rule out pregnancy in patients with prolonged amenorrhea. A urinalysis to assess the specific gravity helps to detect water loading, since many patients attempt to increase their weight this way. In females with amenorrhea, thyroid function tests and measurement of serum prolactin and follicle-stimulating hormone can help rule out prolactinoma (hormone-secreting pituitary tumor), hyperthyroidism, hypothyroidism, or ovarian failure. A bone density study may be ordered to detect bone loss, which is a complication of AN. Other tests are included based on findings of the physical examination.

Complications of Eating Disorders

Many potential complications can occur as a result of starvation and persistent purging. Some of these are osteoporosis, cardiac

impairments, cognitive changes, difficulties in psychologic functioning, gastrointestinal dysfunction (e.g., slowed motility, symptoms of nausea and bloating), endocrinologic changes, electrolyte abnormalities (especially hypokalemia and metabolic alkalosis), dental erosions, enlarged salivary glands, and infertility.

The pathogenesis of osteoporosis is not completely understood but is believed to be associated with estrogen deficiency, inadequate vitamin D and calcium intake, and the nutritional effects on bone loss.

AN has been associated with MVP, possible QT interval prolongation, and heart failure. MVP is a common finding in patients with AN, affecting 32% to 60% of patients compared with 6% to 22% in the general population. This may be because of an increased ability to detect the disorder in patients with intravascular volume depletion consistent with the state of starvation.

The risk of heart failure is greatest in the first 2 weeks of refeeding in patients with an eating disorder. Patients with moderate to severe AN (e.g., >10% below ideal body weight) are at risk for the refeeding syndrome during the first 2 to 3 weeks of treatment. Refeeding syndrome consists of cardiovascular, neurologic, and hematologic complications that occur because of shifts in phosphate from extracellular to intracellular spaces in individuals who have total body phosphorus depletion as a result of malnutrition. Refeeding syndrome can cause cardiac arrest and delirium. The risk is reduced by slower refeeding, replacing phosphorus, and carefully avoiding a high sodium intake. Carefully monitoring serum electrolytes and observing for signs of edema or congestive heart failure are important during refeeding.

Amenorrhea occurs in 90% of women with AN as a result of low levels of follicle-stimulating hormone and luteinizing hormone. Menses is usually restored within 6 months of achieving 90% of the ideal body weight.

Therapeutic Management

The treatment and management of AN involve three major thrusts: (1) reinstitution of normal nutrition or reversal of the severe state of malnutrition, (2) resolution of disturbed patterns of family interaction, and (3) individual psychotherapy to correct deficits and distortions in psychologic functioning.

BOX 21-8 CRITERIA FOR HOSPITAL ADMISSION

Anorexia Nervosa

At or below 75% ideal body weight or ongoing weight loss despite intensive management

Refusal to eat

Body fat less than 10%

Heart rate less than 50 beats/min in daytime and less than 45 beats/min at night

Systolic pressure less than 90 mm Hg

Orthostatic changes in pulse (>20 beats/min) or blood pressure (>10 mm Hg)

Temperature less than 35.5° C (96° F)

Arrhythmia

Bulimia Nervosa

Syncope

Serum potassium concentration less than 3.2 mmol/L

Serum chloride concentration less than 88 mmol/L

Esophageal tears

Cardiac arrhythmias, including prolonged QT interval

Hypothermia

Suicide risk

Intractable vomiting

Hematemesis

Failure to respond to outpatient treatment

From American Academy of Pediatrics, Committee on Adolescence: Identifying and treating eating disorders, *Pediatrics* 111(1):204-211, 2003.

Because of the psychogenic nature of the disorder, the treatment may be long.

Most adolescents with AN are treated on an outpatient basis. However, adolescents who have severe malnutrition, electrolyte disturbances, vital sign abnormalities, or psychiatric disturbances (e.g., severe depression or suicidal ideation) may require hospitalization (Box 21-8). Therapy for the adolescent with AN requires interventions delivered by a multidisciplinary team that includes dietitians, physicians, nurses, counselors, and psychologists or psychiatrists.

Nutrition

The initial goal is to treat the life-threatening malnutrition with strict adherence to dietary requirements, which may necessitate intravenous or tube feeding in severe situations. Dietary interventions are combined with family psychotherapy to improve the underlying psychologic misconception about the weight loss. Weight gain alone cannot be considered a cure for the disease and is an unreliable sign of progress. Relapses are frequent as the person reverts to previous eating patterns when removed from the therapeutic environment.

The dietitian should be experienced in working with children and adolescents and understand how to implement a dietary plan with sufficient calories needed for weight restoration. The plan needs to be firm but flexible. Letting the patient participate in setting up a food plan and teaching food exchanges to patients and parents is important so they can make food choices that will promote weight restoration. The goals of weight restoration are to avoid serious medical complications and restore cognitive functioning to derive the maximum benefit from psychotherapy. Methods that have been used include oral, nasogastric, and intravenous feedings. The least intrusive method for weight restoration should be used, only resorting to nasogastric or intravenous feeds when other strategies have failed. A reasonable goal for weight gain is approximately 1 kg (2 lb) per week. Pushing for more rapid weight gain can result in increasing anxiety or depression and result in bulimia.

Psychotherapy

Psychotherapy is central to the treatment of eating disorders. Patients need to be active participants in the treatment process to better understand the impulses, feelings, and needs that have resulted in their eating disorder. Weight restoration is a primary goal in recovery, since patients obtain only minimum benefit from psychotherapy when their weight is low. They do not process information well and have a decreased ability to concentrate. Weight restoration as an outpatient is accomplished with behavioral contracts negotiated between the therapists and patient. The goal is to increase the patient's feelings of control and responsibility toward achieving recovery. The contract can stipulate at what weight tube feedings will be implemented. Realistic goals are set with the patient, including rewards for achievement that include special privileges or outings and consequences such as restrictions on exercise or increased consumption of a feared food. For inpatients, the contract for foods might be negotiated as food exchanges or number of calories. One suggested approach begins with 1200 calories and increases by 100-calorie increments each day. Inpatients need to be closely supervised by the nursing staff during the meal and for 1 to 1½ hours after the meal. If the agreed on number of calories is not consumed, there might be a provision for the intake of a nutritional supplement (Mikhail, 2001; Schmidt, 2009).

Eating disorders are complex and multifaceted. Because patients often deny their illness, they may refuse the treatment efforts of health providers. The treatment plan needs to be developed carefully. Power struggles with patients may escalate the eating disorder symptomatology in that control issues are often central to the development of eating disorders. Implementing less intrusive interventions first and allowing them time to develop is important before applying more restrictive interventions. A contract is helpful to clarify for patients at what point tube feeding may be implemented so they make informed decisions about their actions. The team needs to agree about the treatment philosophy and protocol to avoid sending mixed messages to the patient. It is important to treat eating disorder patients with respect and support preservation of their self-esteem to promote a successful recovery (Mikhail, 2001; Schmidt, 2009).

It is essential that adolescents rely on their own thinking, become more realistic in self-appraisal, and become capable of living as self-directed, competent individuals who enjoy life without manipulating the body and its functions. Psychotherapy focuses on helping the young person resolve the adolescent identity crisis, particularly when it results in a distorted body image.

The family therapist's goal is to address dysfunctional roles, conflicts, alliances, and patterns that the eating disorder is precipitating or maintaining while helping family members deal with the eating disorder. Some targets for intervention include control, individuation, communication, expression of feelings, realistic expectations, perfectionism, performance, achievement, marital relationship, and parental attitudes toward dieting and exercise (Mikhail, 2001; Schmidt, 2009).

Pharmacotherapy

Pharmacotherapy in the treatment of AN has been disappointing so far. The few studies that have been done have primarily evaluated medications' efficacy in the treatment of comorbid disorders such as obsessive-compulsive disorders and depression. Anxiolytic medications may be helpful before meals to relieve some patients' anxiety. American Psychiatric Association guidelines have discouraged using medication as the only therapy. Appetite stimulants have not been particularly helpful (Foreman, 2009; Mikhail, 2001; Powers and Bruty, 2009).

Tricyclic antidepressants and fluoxetine belong to a group of medications known as selective serotonin reuptake inhibitors (SSRIs), which have been more successful when used with BN. There is also some evidence that tricyclic antidepressants such as desipramine, imipramine, and amitriptyline; monoamine oxidase inhibitors; and buspirone are more effective compared with a placebo in decreasing bingeing and vomiting in patients with BN. Topiramate, an antiepileptic agent, and the selective serotonin antagonist ondansetron may have some benefit in treating BN. As with AN, pharmacotherapy should be an adjunct to psychotherapy. Clearly more research is needed to clarify whether medications have a role in the treatment of eating disorders (Foreman, 2009; Mikhail, 2001; Powers and Bruty, 2009).

Prognosis

Most of the outcome studies on eating disorders have looked at AN. Some studies have found that 50% of AN patients have good outcomes when evaluated by the criteria of return of menses and weight gain. Another 25% have some weight regain and some relapse, and 25% were characterized as having a poor outcome. Predictors of more favorable outcome are (1) having BN, rather than AN; (2) having a purging type of AN, rather than a restricting type; (3) having a short duration of illness; and (4) having a higher discharge weight after hospitalization. Poor outcomes have been associated with (1) long duration of illness, (2) low body weight at time of initial treatment, (3) high creatinine levels (>1.5 mg/dl), (4) premorbid obesity (for BN), (5) premorbid problems with sociability, (6) compulsion to exercise, and (7) disturbed family relationships (Rome, Ammerman, Rosen, et al, 2003).

AN is associated with significant mortality. One study found a 6.6% mortality rate overall. The reasons given for death in one study were complications of the eating disorder in 54%, suicide in 27%, and unknown causes in 19% (Foreman, 2009).

Although the changes associated with AN are often reversible, the physical complications can involve every organ system in the body, and the effects of severe malnutrition are often obvious for many years. For example, adolescents with eating disorders are at risk of developing osteopenia or osteoporosis associated with a twofold to sevenfold higher fracture risk in later life. Most of the bone mass is built up during adolescence. Most studies of AN are retrospective. Further investigation is necessary to determine the functional significance of these abnormalities and the extent to which they return to normal after nutritional rehabilitation (Herpertz-Dahlmann, 2009).

Nursing Care Management

The nursing process for care of the adolescent with an eating disorder is outlined in the Nursing Care Plan. A number of nursing interventions are included in the following discussion.

Nurses need to adopt and maintain a kind and supportive yet firm manner in managing the care of the adolescent with AN without creating a passive-dependent attitude. The individual requires sustained support and reassurance to cope with ambivalent feelings related to body concept and the desire to be seen as cooperative, reliable, and worthy of receiving kindness. Encouraging the adolescent with education and activities that strengthen self-esteem facilitates the resocialization process and promotes social acceptance among peers.

It is important that nurses be aware of the physical side effects of AN. Patients with AN often limit their fluid intake. Urinary tract problems are frequent, and ketones and proteins are commonly detected in the urine as a result of fat and protein breakdown. Vital sign instability can be severe and can include orthostatic hypotension; the pulse becomes irregular and may decrease markedly. Bradycardia and hypothermia can result in cardiac arrest.

Diet

The patient should avoid rapid weight gain because it has been associated with severe metabolic abnormalities in some patients, such as refeeding syndrome as previously described. Deaths associated with AN have also occurred during rehabilitation as a result of cardiovascular overload. Restoration of body weight to a target weight or end point within 10% of the patient's ideal body weight should be one of the main goals of nutritional rehabilitation (Schneider and Fisher, 2001).

Establishing a "maintenance weight range" of about 1 kg (2 lb) over or under the target weight helps the adolescent feel in control, encourages maintenance of weight through healthy dietary habits, and teaches the adolescent that uncontrollable weight gain is not inevitable when a normal diet is consumed.

Behavior Therapy

The use of behavior modification in the treatment of AN has met with varying degrees of success. Providing privileges or activities for weight gain or positive eating behaviors may be successful, but treatment should also address the conflict precipitating the disorder. Communicate a clearly defined behavior modification plan to the young person and maintain it through a unified team approach by all persons involved in care.

The team responsible for the management of young people with AN arranges a carefully structured environment. First, there must be consistency. The team decides on an approach and adheres to it. The plan is structured with reality testing regarding caloric intake and body-image perception as an essential component. The team members provide a unified front to avoid any possibility of manipulation or inconsistency. Second, all team members are involved; responsibility for the program cannot be left to one person. The role and boundaries

NURSING CARE PLAN

The Adolescent with an Eating Disorder

NURSING DIAGNOSIS	EXPECTED PATIENT OUTCOMES	INTERVENTIONS	RATIONALE
Imbalanced Nutrition: Less Than Body Requirements related to altered self-image, inadequate nutrient intake, and chronic vomiting	Nutrient intake will be sufficient to maintain optimum cellular and metabolic function.	If adolescent's life is in immediate danger as a result of malnutrition, implement plan for restoring physiologic homeostasis: electrolyte and fluid replacement, enteral feedings as required, and monitoring of vital signs and fluid and electrolyte balance.	To prevent death or multiorgan failure To restore fluid and electrolyte balance
Adolescent's/Family's Defining Characteristics (Subjective and Objective Data)	**The Following NOC Concepts Apply to These Outcomes** Weight Gain Behavior Nutritional Status: Food and Fluid Intake		
Body weight 20% or more under ideal Reported food intake less than recommended dietary allowance Perceived inability to ingest food Aversion to eating Poor muscle tone Excessive hair loss Misconceptions		Work collaboratively with multidisciplinary health care team (dietitian, mental health counselor, physician, nurse) to establish consistent care plan for the adolescent with identified disordered eating.	To provide optimal care in all aspects—physical, mental, emotional—of adolescent's life
		Develop a mutually agreeable targeted daily caloric intake goal.	To give adolescent sense of control over nutrient intake and establish realistic plan for weight gain
		Observe eating behaviors and monitor nutritional intake and behavior thereafter for 1 to 1½ hours.	To detect detrimental habits such as purging or bingeing
		Monitor vital signs as warranted by patient status.	To detect physiologic changes that may be life threatening
		Monitor fluid and electrolyte status.	To detect life-threatening conditions such as dehydration or hyponatremia
		Set mutually agreeable target intake of fluids per day.	To prevent dehydration
		Establish mutually agreeable targeted goal for daily exercise that is congruent with nutrient intake and weight gain.	To prevent further weight loss
		Monitor activities for detrimental behaviors such as administering enemas, purging, bingeing (bulimic), and exercising excessively.	To prevent self-harm
		Set limits and clearly define expectations in relation to therapeutic plan to increase nutrient intake.	To clarify expectations and provide limits for control of behaviors that are not acceptable
		Develop a behavioral contract for nutrient intake and cessation of behaviors related to eating that are detrimental.	To establish a mutually agreed on plan for nutrient intake and weight gain
		Monitor for signs of relapse: weight loss, muscle wasting, alopecia, signs of fluid and electrolyte imbalance.	To implement lifesaving strategies
		The Following NIC Concepts Apply to These Interventions Vital Signs Monitoring Weight Management Nutrition Therapy Behavior Modification Nutritional Counseling Nutritional Monitoring	

Continued

⊚ **NURSING CARE PLAN—cont'd**

The Adolescent with an Eating Disorder

NURSING DIAGNOSIS	EXPECTED PATIENT OUTCOMES	INTERVENTIONS	RATIONALE
Disturbed Body Image related to altered self-perception	Adolescent will display evidence of developing and maintaining a positive self-image.	Encourage adolescent to verbalize feelings and concerns regarding view of self in relation to peers and family members.	To promote verbalization of concerns and fears
Adolescent's/Family's Defining Characteristics (Subjective and Objective Data)	**The Following NOC Concepts Apply to These Outcomes**		To promote expression of perceptions about self within family and identify any distorted patterns of interaction that require clarification or modification
Negative feelings about body	Child Development: Adolescence		
Verbalization of feelings that reflect an altered perception of body appearance	Self-Esteem	Provide opportunity for adolescent to engage in activities that have potential to build self-esteem.	To enhance self-esteem and alter misconception of self in relation to others
		Encourage self-care in relation to dietary management and weight control.	To promote self-esteem
		Encourage discussion of maladaptive behaviors surrounding food and fluid intake: bingeing, purging, laxative use, excessive exercise.	To set limits for behavior To provide consistency in therapy and allow mutual discussion
		Provide a therapeutic discussion (over time) of personal attributes perceived as positive.	To enhance reality-based self-perception
		Involve adolescent in activities designed to promote positive image of self-worth and accomplishment.	To promote sense of accomplishment and enhance self-image
	The Following NIC Concepts Apply to These Interventions Emotional Support Socialization Enhancement Body Image Enhancement Self-Esteem Enhancement Mutual Goal Setting Values Clarification		

of each member are clearly spelled out. Third, continuity of team members is important; it is helpful to have the same team members all the time.

Fourth, communication among team members is essential. Communication with the patient regarding what is expected is also important. Sometimes the limit setting may seem unreasonable. If the adolescent does not understand the rationale for the limits, he or she may sabotage the entire program. It is also important to communicate with the family. Fifth, the plan must provide for support of the adolescent, the family, and team members. Support the adolescent's efforts, and provide positive feedback for accomplishments made in normalizing eating habits. Meetings are held to discuss the feelings and concerns of the patient, immediate caregivers, and team members.

All individuals involved in therapy must remember that the adolescent's distorted sense of body image and self-awareness, feelings of self-doubt, ineffectiveness, helplessness, and lack of control prompt the self-damaging behavior. The underlying principle in many behavior modification programs for hospitalized adolescents is to grant privileges only as a reward for weight gain. Adolescents who view these programs as coercive and become depressed by this approach seldom maintain

weight gain outside the hospital environment (Varchol and Cooper, 2009).

Family therapy is often used in the treatment of adolescent eating disorders, specifically in the treatment of AN. In particular, the Maudsley approach aims to help parents rediscover their own resources and take an active role in their children's recovery. Encourage families to explore how it has become problematic to follow the normal developmental course of their family life cycle by looking at how the eating disorder and the interactional patterns in the family have become entangled. Sharing experiences among families and the intensity of this treatment program set it apart from the experience that is more typical of outpatient family therapy (Dare and Eisler, 1997; Eisler, Le Grange, and Asen, 2003; Le Grange, 2005).

A behavioral contract, an agreement that the adolescent makes with another to change a maladaptive behavior, has proved effective in some cases. The written contract is constructed by the therapeutic team and approved and signed by the adolescent. Unless the adolescent agrees to its terms, the contract can become the source of a power struggle. However, it can be an effective tool that places the responsibility for weight gain or other behavior change on the adolescent.

Nursing care of the adolescent with BN is similar to care of the patient with AN. Acute care involves careful monitoring of fluid and electrolyte alterations and observation for signs of cardiac complications. Nutritional consultation and follow-up care are essential. The nurse should encourage the adolescent and family members to structure the environment to reduce the bingeing behavior. Getting rid of binge foods; restricting eating to one room of the house; not engaging in other activities while eating; and substituting exercise, crafts, visualization, and relaxation techniques for bingeing are helpful interventions.

Nurses, patients, and families can find assistance and information from several organizations. The American Anorexia/Bulimia Association, Inc.,* provides information, referrals, counseling, and activities aimed at combating eating disorders. The National Association of Anorexia Nervosa and Associated Eating Disorders† provides counseling, referral, and self-help programs for young people with AN. The National Eating Disorders Association‡ provides information and support services for both patients and families.

Cost of Care (Insurance)

Treatment programs are characterized by multidisciplinary teams and involve stages and phases over time, which can become expensive. More difficult cases require long-term care and can involve multiple hospitalizations. Families find that insurance companies begin to deny coverage or, in the interest of managing costs, begin to insist on alternative treatment programs that may be inferior. For many families, the costs of care result in serious financial problems. Insufficient treatment may result in chronicity, invalidism, and even death. Nurses must understand the barriers to care and become advocates for their patients. They need to be educated about the unique characteristics of eating disorders to be better patient advocates (Rome, Ammerman, Rosen, et al, 2003).

Prevention

There are no easy ways to prevent AN. However, public and professional awareness of signs and symptoms can facilitate early identification and treatment to prevent or reduce the long-term adverse consequences. Additionally, media literacy on the societal drive for thinness and overall nutrition education may help. Box 21-9 outlines the early signs of AN.

SUBSTANCE ABUSE

OVERVIEW

Although experimentation with alcohol and other drugs during adolescence is fairly common, the majority of teens do not become high-risk users. National and statewide surveys indicate that although more than half of adolescents will have tried tobacco, alcohol, and marijuana before they are out of their

*800-522-2230; http://americananorexiabulimiaassociationinc.visualnet.com.
†Hotline 630-577-1330; e-mail: anadhelp@anad.org; www.anad.org.
‡603 Stewart St., Suite 803, Seattle, WA 98101; 800-931-2237; www.nationaleatingdisorders.org.

BOX 21-9 EARLY SIGNS OF ANOREXIA NERVOSA

The adolescent:

- Consumes an inappropriate diet (excessively strict) or may refuse to eat altogether
- Develops peculiar eating habits such as toying with food, performing food "rituals," preparing and forcing food on family members without eating any herself
- Engages in excessive exercise, such as compulsive jogging, running up and down stairs, rigorous calisthenics to burn off calories—often to the point of exhaustion
- Withdraws from social interaction; starts to spend all her time in her room studying, exercising, or otherwise occupied
- Ceases to have menstrual periods after sudden or excessive weight loss, sometimes almost as soon as dieting begins
- Takes laxatives, diuretics, or enemas to speed intestinal transit time, to lose added weight, and to empty intestines to flatten abdomen
- Vomits deliberately; may go to bathroom after a meal and turn on faucets to avoid being heard
- Denies hunger even after eating practically nothing for days or even weeks
- Develops a distorted body image; states she "feels fat" as she becomes increasingly thin
- Loses weight; fails to achieve the 25th percentile on normal growth curves

---

teens, fewer than one adolescent in eight has tried illicit stimulants and inhalants; fewer than 1 in 10 has ever tried "hard" drugs such as hallucinogens, sedatives, or crack cocaine; and a tiny percentage use injection drugs such as heroin. Adolescents at greatest risk are not the majority of high school students who have tried alcohol or marijuana, but rather the estimated 2% to 4% who report daily use of alcohol or marijuana during the past 30 days; the 5% to 10% who used narcotics like oxycodone (OxyContin) in the past year; and the 1% or so who report using illicit drugs such as crystal methamphetamine, heroin, crack cocaine, or 3-4-methylenedioxymethamphetamine (MDMA, or Ecstasy) at least once in the past month (Johnston, O'Malley, Bachman, et al, 2008).

The etiology of substance abuse is not completely understood. Current research focuses on biopsychosocial risk and protective factors, but some emerging research has begun to explore genetics and physiologic mechanisms. For the majority of adolescents, experimentation with drugs occurs during a period in which they are trying out a variety of behaviors and then discarding them when the fit is not right. There are a number of theories about pathways leading to the abuse of substances. Research has identified risk factors such as the presence of an enzyme (aldehyde dehydrogenase [ALDH]) that makes decomposition of ethanol in the body possible (Patton, 1995), family history of drug abuse and dependence (Baer, Barr, Brookstein, et al, 1998; Kosterman, Hawkins, Guo, et al, 2000), a history of child maltreatment or other traumas affecting the biologic stress response systems (De Bellis, 2002), and genetic inheritance and individual psychopathology (Carlson, Iacono, and McGue, 2002; Angold, Costello, and Erkanli, 1999). However, no single factor explains the cause of adolescent substance abuse. The enormous impact of poverty and ready availability of substances, combined with biogenetic predispositions for abuse, are likely factors to consider in understanding the cause. Although there is much to learn about what leads an adolescent to abuse substances, most experts agree with a diathesis-stress model, which presumes a biologic predisposition accompanied by psychosocial risk factors.

An adolescent abusing alcohol or other drugs often does so as a means of coping with depression, anxiety, restlessness, or chronic feelings of boredom or emptiness (Harrison, Fulkerson, and Beebe, 1997). Because denial is often associated with substance abuse, nurses, other health care professionals, and parents may not be aware of the abuse problem.

Definitions

Considerable misinformation and confusion are related to the terms applied to substance use and substance abuse. The most important differences among these terms are the distinctions between *voluntary* and *involuntary* behavior and between *culturally defined* and *physiologically identified* events. Drug abuse, misuse, and addiction are all culturally defined terms and are voluntary behaviors. Drug tolerance and physical dependence are involuntary physiologic responses to the pharmacologic characteristics of drugs, such as opioids and alcohol. Consequently, an individual can be "addicted" to a narcotic with or without being physically dependent, and a person may be physically dependent on a narcotic without being addicted (e.g., patients who use opioids to control pain).

The broad term *drug abuse,* which is often applied to all forms of drug misuse, is confusing and does not necessarily define the problem related to drug use. Many substances are controlled by law and involve severe penalties for any illegal use. Others are sanctioned from a legal, social, and medical standpoint, but their excessive use may cause physical or social problems for the adolescent. Problems concerning drug use are defined as follows:

Legal—The drug being taken is strictly controlled by law and is accompanied by severe penalties for its use or possession.

Social—Use of a substance leads to disruptive or bizarre behavior that alienates the user from the rest of society; this results in a social problem.

Medical—Current or continued use of a substance may adversely affect the adolescent's physical or mental health.

Individual—This focuses on the role that drug use plays in the individual's life and factors that contribute to the individual's need for the drug.

Patterns of Drug Use

Many factors influence the extent to which teenagers use drugs. The type of drug used, mode of administration, duration of use, frequency of use, and single- or multiple-drug use must be considered in determining the severity of the individual drug problem. Most drug use begins with experimentation. The drug may be tried only once, may be used occasionally, or may become an integral part of a drug-centered lifestyle. Identification of the pattern of drug use in an individual facilitates the formulation of an approach to the problem. Patterns have been observed based on dose and frequency of use.

Adolescents who use drugs fall into two broad categories: experimenters and compulsive users. Between these groups on opposite ends of a continuum is a broad range of recreational users, principally of drugs such as marijuana, cocaine, alcohol, and prescription drugs. For many the goal is typically peer acceptance. These users fit more closely with the experimenting, intermittent users. For others the goal is intoxication or the sustained intense effects from using the particular drugs; these users resemble the compulsive users. They may engage in periodic heavy use, or binges. The groups of greatest concern to health care workers are those whose patterns of use involve high doses or mixed drugs with the danger of overdose or other harms that can occur when bingeing, and those compulsive users with the threat of dependence, withdrawal syndromes, and altered lifestyle.

Types of Drugs Abused

Any drug can be abused, and most are potentially harmful to adolescents still going through formative life experiences. Although rarely considered drugs by society, the chemically active substances most commonly used are the xanthines and theobromines contained in chocolate, tea, coffee, colas and energy drinks (of which caffeine is the most common). Ethyl alcohol and nicotine are others that, although recognized as drugs, are sanctioned by society for use by adults. Any of these substances can produce mild to moderate euphoric or stimulant effects and can lead to physical or psychologic dependence.

Many factors determine personal preferences for gratification. Many drugs are not harmful for all teenagers, and some, used intermittently, will probably not produce ill effects or result in dependence. Reactions vary according to the drug used, its purity, the user's expectations, the route of administration, and the context in which the drug is used. These factors determine to a great extent whether the experience is pleasant or unpleasant. The type of drugs used also varies according to geographic location, socioeconomic status, urban versus suburban areas, and various historical periods.

A drug that is popular with one "generation" of adolescents may not be attractive to another. Changing trends are influenced by the adolescent's search for new and different experiences, as well as availability, costs, and perceived risks. Since 2000, declines have occurred in teenagers' use of most drugs, including alcohol, tobacco, marijuana, and drugs that had seen sharp increases between 1998 and 2001, such as MDMA (Johnston, O'Malley, Bachman, et al, 2008). The level of drug use among teens in the United States still creates a number of potential health risks; ongoing concerns include the use of alcohol, marijuana, tobacco, MDMA, inhalants, prescription drugs, and cocaine.

Drugs with mind-altering capacity that are available on the black market and are of medical and legal concern are the hallucinogenic, narcotic, hypnotic, and stimulant drugs. In addition, health care professionals are concerned about the use of various volatile substances such as gasoline, model airplane cement, and organic solvents such as butane. These substances are inhaled by the user to achieve an altered sensation, and the most recent surveillance has indicated only a slight decline in use, after a modest increase in use starting in 2003 (Johnston, O'Malley, Bachman, et al, 2008). More recently, abuse of prescription drugs such as oxycodone and methylphenidate has received added attention. Drugs available on the street are often mixed with other compounds and fillers so that the purity of the drug, its strength, and the nature of the additives are highly variable. Table 21-2 outlines some of the more commonly abused substances and their general manifestations.

TOBACCO

Cigarette smoking has continued to decline since the late 1990s, dropping by more than half in the decade between 1996 and 2007 (Johnston, O'Malley, Bachman, et al, 2008). These declines are due in part to increased costs for cigarettes because of added taxes, changes in community attitudes about smoking and laws restricting smoking in public places, and increased antismoking advertising as a result of the government lawsuits against tobacco companies. In 2007, 7.1% of eighth grade teens reported smoking once or more in the past 30 days, whereas 21.6% of twelfth graders did so. Daily smoking is less common, with 4.4% of eighth graders and 15.6% of twelfth graders reporting smoking at least one cigarette daily in the past month. African-American youth are less likely to smoke than Hispanic or Caucasian adolescents.

Although the number of adult and adolescent smokers has declined in recent years, cigarette smoking is still considered the chief avoidable cause of death. The hazards of smoking at any age are undisputed. However, a preventive approach to teenage

Case Study—Teen Smoking

TABLE 21-2	MAJOR SUBSTANCES ABUSED BY ADOLESCENTS			
CHEMICAL AGENT	**ROUTE**	**PHYSICAL SIGNS**	**BEHAVIOR**	**COMPLICATIONS**
Opiates				
Heroin, morphine, meperidine, hydromorphone, fentanyl, methadone, oxycodone	Injected subcutaneously or intravenously (IV), intranasal (sniffing), oral	Constricted pupils, respiratory depression, cyanosis Needle marks	Initial euphoria, tranquilization, lethargy, coma	Overdose—Coma, respiratory arrest, death Injection site infection, hepatitis, abscesses, septicemia, tetanus, pulmonary complications, acquired immunodeficiency syndrome (AIDS) Withdrawal—Muscle and stomach cramps, diarrhea, runny nose and eyes, restlessness, seizures, death Dental caries
Depressants				
Barbiturates—Secobarbital, amobarbital, pentobarbital, amobarbital-secobarbital	Oral, IV	Slurred speech, ataxia, slowed reflexes, dilated pupils (glutethimide)	Short attention span, impaired judgment, combativeness, violence	Overdose—Respiratory depression, coma, death Injection site infection, hepatitis, septicemia, AIDS Withdrawal—Hyperreflexia, irritability, seizures, death
Nonbarbiturates—Methaqualone (Quaalude), ethchlorvynol (Placidyl)	Oral	Poor coordination, tremors, ataxia, confusion, slurred speech, hyperreflexia, diplopia, general muscle weakness	Hyperexcitability; euphoria of methaqualone similar to opiate experience	Overdose—Delirium and coma, convulsions, hepatic damage, respiratory arrest, death Withdrawal—Similar to barbiturates and alcohol
Alcohol (ethanol)	Oral	Poor coordination	Impaired judgment and perception, loss of inhibitions, emotional lability, quarrelsomeness, aggressiveness, hostility, lethargy	Hazards related to impaired judgment (e.g., automobile accidents, fights) Nutritional deficiencies Gastritis Overdose—Coma, death, especially when used in combination with barbiturates Withdrawal—Anxiety, tremors, hallucinations, hyperreflexia, seizures, death
Minor Tranquilizers				
Chlordiazepoxide (Librium), diazepam (Valium), meprobamate	Oral	Nonspecific	Decreased anxiety and tension Occasional disinhibition	Similar to barbiturates but with reduced intensity

Continued

TABLE 21-2	MAJOR SUBSTANCES ABUSED BY ADOLESCENTS—cont'd			
CHEMICAL AGENT	**ROUTE**	**PHYSICAL SIGNS**	**BEHAVIOR**	**COMPLICATIONS**
Organic Solvents				
Hydrocarbons and fluorocarbons (inhalants)—Glue, cleaning fluid, lighter fluid, aerosol sprays, nail polish, gasoline, paint thinner, butane, varnish	Sniffed or inhaled	Nonspecific (may include sore throat, cough, runny nose)	Euphoria, dysphoria, confusion, impaired perception and coordination, restlessness, loss of consciousness	Asphyxia from plastic bags used to inhale fumes Lead poisoning Possible irreversible damage to central nervous system, kidneys, liver, and bone marrow
Stimulants				
Amphetamines—Amphetamine sulfate, dextroamphetamine, methamphetamine	Oral, subcutaneous, IV, smoke, sniffed	Hypertension, weight loss, dilated pupils Sweating (when injected)	Psychologic and motor stimulation Hyperactivity, false bravado, euphoria, increased alertness, insomnia, anorexia, irritability, personality change	Injection site infection Paranoia, severe depression with suicidal tendency when drug stopped
Hallucinogens				
Cocaine	Intranasal, IV, smoke	Hypertension, tachycardia, hyperreflexia	Restlessness, hyperactivity, intense euphoria	Nausea, vomiting Inflammation or perforation of nasal septum
Cannabis—Marijuana, hashish	Smoke, oral	Occasional tachycardia, delayed response time, poor coordination	Simple euphoria, mild intoxication, heightened sensory awareness, drowsiness	Occasionally depressive or anxiety reactions
Lysergic acid diethylamide (LSD), phencyclidine (PCP), dimethyltryptamine (DMT), 3,5-dimethoxy-4-methylamphetamine (STP), tetrahydrocannabinol (THC), mescaline	Oral	Dilated pupils, reddened eyes, occasionally hypertension, hyperthermia, piloerection	Euphoria, heightened sensory awareness, increased appetite, hallucinations, confusion, paranoia	Primary psychiatric; may intensify latent psychotic tendencies; panic, suicide possible, flashbacks

smoking is especially important. Because of its addictive nature, smoking begun in childhood and adolescence can result in a lifetime habit, with increased morbidity and early mortality. Smoking in adolescence has also been related to other risk behaviors for weight management, including vomiting after meals and use of amphetamines (Parkes, Saewyc, Cox, et al, 2008). Smoking has also been associated with marijuana use, multiple sexual partners, and binge drinking (Escobedo, Reddy, and DuRant, 1997).

Etiology

Teenagers begin smoking for a variety of reasons. Factors related to the onset of smoking can be categorized as social, sociodemographic, psychosocial, and biologic. Once smoking behavior is established, smoking itself produces enough reinforcement to sustain the practice without the initial pressure.

Social Factors

Social pressures to smoke include imitation of the smoking behavior and attitudes of parents and other adults. The association of smoking with maturity or mature behavior; pressures from peers who view smoking as the popular thing to do; and the use of smoking as an outlet for school, social, or home pres-

sures are also factors. Other pressures come from advertisements aimed directly at teens, although the United States has limited such advertisements in recent years.

Previous research has indicated some parental influence on tobacco use in children; that is, adolescents who smoke are more likely to have parents who smoke (Institute of Medicine, 1994). Parental disapproval of smoking may influence adolescents not to smoke (Sargent and Dalton, 2001), but only if the parents themselves do not smoke (Chassin, Presson, and Sherman, 2005). Parenting style may also play a role. In the study by Chassin, Presson, and Sherman, teens with parents who were warm and accepting but also regularly monitored their teens' behavior, with consistent rules and discipline—the authoritarian style of parenting—were significantly less likely to start smoking than teens whose parents were disengaged (low monitoring, but also low levels of acceptance and attention). In their study, general parenting style had more overall influence than parental attitudes and antismoking messages, especially if the parents smoked. This makes sense, since teens will notice the "do as I say, not as I do" discrepancy between parents' behaviors and their words.

The influence of peers or friends on smoking initiation has been documented in several studies (Bertrand and Abernathy, 1993; Flay, Hu, Siddiqui, et al, 1994). In particular, the effects of friends' smoking have been found to be greater for females than for males, leading to greater peer pressure for young girls to start smoking (Hu, Flak, Hedeker, et al, 1995).

The mass media have contributed to the initiation of smoking in adolescents. In advertisements smokers are engaged in activities and dressed in clothes suitable for adolescents, and smoking is associated with fun, risk taking, sexual adventure, maturity, and autonomy. The ads also imply an association between smoking and youthful vigor; a slim figure; good looks; and personal, social, and professional acceptance and success. The number of major actors who smoke cigarettes in movies and television shows also appears to influence smoking behavior in teens.

Some uses of the media have been helpful in increasing adolescent exposure to antismoking messages. Mass media antismoking campaigns in general have been effective. However, tobacco companies have funded and developed smoking prevention advertising that has had opposite effects on smoking-related beliefs and intentions of adolescents (Wakefield, Terry-McElrath, Emery, et al, 2006).

Sociodemographic Factors

Sociodemographic factors that relate to levels of smoking include socioeconomic status, gender, sexual orientation, history of trauma, and performance in school. A consistent, negative association has been observed between socioeconomic status and smoking (especially among boys), and there is a positive correlation between low academic goals and performance and smoking. Gay, lesbian, and bisexual adolescents are more likely to smoke than their heterosexual peers (Austin, Ziyadeh, Fisher, et al, 2004), possibly as a way of coping with unique stressors of stigmatization, rejection, and violence from family, school, and community (D'Augelli, 2004). Similarly, youth who report a history of physical or sexual abuse are more likely to smoke (Al Mamun, Alati, O'Callaghan, et al, 2007). Rates of smoking are highest among homeless and street-involved youth, as well as adolescents who did not complete high school. Students who focus on schoolwork and who have high educational goals for themselves are significantly less likely than their peers to develop a long-term smoking habit.

Psychosocial Factors

Although theories explaining the relationship between personality and smoking behavior have been suggested, research has not documented any significant differences between adolescents who smoke and those who do not smoke. Rather than enabling us to discriminate between likely smokers and non-smokers, personality traits such as anxiety have been shown to predict how much adolescents will smoke once they begin the habit. Although depression does not seem to be related to heavy cigarette smoking in adolescents, current use is a determinant in the development of depressive symptoms (Goodman and Capitman, 2000).

Research has examined the development of different personality characteristics of adolescents at the time of the onset of tobacco use and with continued use. Youthful smokers (seventh grade) have been found to be extroverted and involved with their peers, whereas older smokers are often depressed and withdrawn (Stein, Newcomb, and Bentler, 1996). This research supports the hypothesis that smoking takes on different psychosocial meanings with continued use.

Biologic Factors

Studies have begun to identify the genetic predispositions for tobacco use and to try to explain the complex interplay of genetics, environment, and behavior that can lead to smoking. For example, youth with attention deficit hyperactivity disorder (ADHD) are twice as likely to smoke cigarettes as their peers, to start at younger ages, and to smoke more regularly and in greater amounts (Laucht, Hohm, Esser, et al, 2007). However, the main component of this increased risk is from the influence of substance-using peers, with some small contribution of genetics.

Biologic factors serve both to encourage and to deter further experimentation by would-be smokers. The initial harshness, nausea, and irritation may influence many youngsters not to try smoking again. For others, however, such symptoms are a challenge to overcome.

Smoking has been found to lower endurance by decreasing breathing capacity or ventilatory muscle endurance. Cigarette smoking is also associated with mild airway obstruction and slowed growth of lung function in adolescents. The detrimental effects of smoking on growth of lung function may be more pronounced in adolescent girls. Cigarette smoking showed a dose-response relationship with the development of sleep problems in a group of more than 3000 adolescents (Patten, Choi, Gillin, et al, 2000).

Dependence is a result of nicotine, the primary alkaloid in tobacco. Nicotine exerts both stimulating and sedating effects on the central and peripheral nervous systems and on several organ systems. Attempts to stop smoking are accompanied by severe craving and withdrawal symptoms.

Process of Becoming a Smoker

The process of becoming a smoker involves three stages: initiation (trying the first cigarette), experimental smoking (less than weekly), and regular smoking (at least weekly). Some researchers also recognize a preparation stage in which psychosocial, environmental, and possibly biologic factors prepare some youngsters to be smokers. Regardless of reason, the fact remains that 75% of teenage smokers will smoke regularly as adults (Moolchan, Ernst, and Henningfield, 2000), in part because of the addictive nature of nicotine in the tobacco (Chassin, Presson, and Sherman, 2005).

Smokeless Tobacco

The term *smokeless tobacco* refers to tobacco products that are placed in the mouth or inhaled through the nose but not ignited (e.g., snuff and chewing tobacco). This substitute for cigarettes continues to pose a hazard to adolescents, although use has declined by about 50% since the peak prevalence in 1995, with only 15.1% of teens in 2007 having tried smokeless tobacco by the twelfth grade (Johnston, O'Malley, Bachman, et al, 2008). Although a much smaller percent reported using smokeless tobacco in the past month (6.6%), nearly half of them reported using it daily (2.8%). More boys (13.4%) than girls (2.3%) in 2007 used smokeless tobacco within the past 30 days, and Caucasian males were far more likely to use smokeless tobacco

(18.0%) than African-American males (2.0%) or Hispanic males (6.7%) (Centers for Disease Control and Prevention, 2008). Many children and adolescents believe that smokeless tobacco is a safe alternative to cigarette smoking and is not addictive, and they believe they can stop using it at any time. However, the number of adolescents who identify it as a health risk has increased since the mid-1990s, with nearly half now agreeing it has health risks (Johnston, O'Malley, Bachman, et al, 2008). These products have also been proved to be carcinogenic, and regular use can cause dental problems, foul-smelling breath, and tooth erosion or loss.

Nursing Care Management

Prevention of regular smoking in teenagers is the most effective way to reduce the overall incidence of smoking. A variety of methods have been employed. Posters, charts, displays, statistics, and the use of examples of actual damaged lungs to communicate the hazards of smoking all have their supporters and doubters. Some schools also use films and demonstrations in science classes.

For the most part, smoking-prevention programs that focus on the negative, long-term effects of smoking on health, such as lung cancer and heart disease, have been ineffective. Youth-to-youth programs and those emphasizing the immediate effects are more effective, but primarily in improving the teenagers' attitudes toward not smoking. Because smoking and smoking-related behaviors are social symbols, antismoking campaigns must address the norms of potential smokers. Anything that ridicules or threatens the social norms of the peer group can be unproductive or counterproductive. Investigators have found that teaching resistance to peer pressure to smoke is effective in early adolescence. Although the effects of these programs may decrease with time, the effects can be enhanced in older adolescents by using a curriculum instead of simply handing out written material to the students (Adelman, Duggan, Hauptman, et al, 2001).

Two areas of focus for antismoking programs are peer-led programs and use of media in smoking prevention (e.g., videotapes and films). Peer-led programs emphasizing the social consequences of smoking have proved most successful. If a significant number of influential peers can "sell" their classmates on the idea that the habit is not popular, the followers will imitate their behavior. Such programs emphasize short-term rather than long-term consequences (e.g., the effects of smoking on personal appearance, such as unattractive stains on teeth and hands and unpleasant odor of breath and clothing, as well as lower sperm counts in young males).

The impact of school-based antismoking programs can be strengthened by expanding these programs to include parents, mass media, youth groups, and community organizations. For example, mass media efforts that involve antismoking radio campaigns have been identified as the most cost-effective mass media intervention. Many public schools have used the American Lung Association's smoking cessation program Not-on-Tobacco (NOT; www.notontobacco.com) with modest results (Horn, Dino, Kaselkar, et al, 2004).

Smoking bans in schools also accomplish several goals: (1) they discourage students from starting to smoke, (2) they reinforce knowledge of the health hazards of cigarette smoking and exposure to environmental tobacco smoke, and (3) they promote a smoke-free environment as the norm.

ALCOHOL

Acute or chronic misuse of alcohol (ethanol), a socially accepted depressant, is responsible for many acts of violence, suicide, accidental injury, and death. Ethanol reduces inhibitions against risky behaviors, aggression, and sexual behavior; it slows reflexes and impairs judgment in driving and other activities that require skill to avoid injury. Abrupt withdrawal is accompanied by severe physical and psychologic symptoms, and long-term use leads to slow tissue destruction, especially of the brain and liver cells.

Teenage drinking is not a new phenomenon. Because of its social acceptance, peer pressure, and easy accessibility, alcohol is the drug of choice for many adolescents. It is the most widely accepted drug, can be purchased legally by adults, and is relatively inexpensive. It is often part of a meal (wine, beer), approved by adults throughout the world when used in moderation, and is even promoted as a health benefit under certain circumstances. Young people may not even consider it a drug. Many have been exposed to alcohol all their lives.

Although there are racial, ethnic, and gender differences, the pattern of frequent, heavy drinking among those who will develop this pattern is likely to begin in high school. Drinking increases with age. By age 18 years, 85% of all adolescents have used alcohol. In 2007 the monthly prevalence of alcohol use was 54.9% among high school seniors, with 36.5% of these youths reporting episodic heavy drinking (Centers for Disease Control and Prevention, 2008). The rates of ever using alcohol, as well as daily use, have declined over the past several years, and so has binge drinking (Johnston, O'Malley, Bachman, et al, 2008).

Although the majority of adolescents who experiment with alcohol do not become heavy users, social drinking remains a great concern, primarily because of the troubling rates of morbidity and mortality related to drinking. Alcohol-related motor vehicle accidents are the leading cause of unintentional injury and death among adolescents (Mulye, Park, Nelson, et al, 2009). About one in three adolescents reports being a passenger in a vehicle with a driver who had been drinking, and just over 10% acknowledge drinking and driving.

The most noticeable effects of alcohol occur within the central nervous system and include changes in cognitive and autonomic functions such as judgment, memory, and learning ability. Marked mood changes are characteristic of adolescent drinkers, who are described as hard to live with and unable to make up their minds. They can be identified by the way in which they use alcohol. Adolescent alcoholics often drink alone; cannot predictably control their use of alcohol; and protect their supply, afraid that they will be caught without anything to drink.

Adolescents who misuse alcohol often rely on it as a defense against depression, anxiety, fear, and anger. They become increasingly tolerant and need to drink more to experience the same effects. Some abusers have difficulty remembering things done while intoxicated and often intend to swear off the drug or cut down on its use. Not all these characteristics are observed in the alcoholic, but if several of the signs are evident, individuals should be considered at risk and detoxification therapy should be initiated.

Answers to questions and information about alcohol can be obtained by calling the Alcohol Hotline (800-ALCOHOL). Several support groups such as Al-Anon, Ala-Teen, and Ala-Tot also help children and families who have an alcoholic family member. Information about these groups can be obtained from Alcoholics Anonymous listings in local telephone directories.

Etiology
Social Factors

Parents, siblings, and peers have a significant impact on adolescent alcohol use. Adolescents who develop drinking problems tend to come from families with negative communication patterns, inconsistent parental discipline, marital discord, and an absence of parent-child closeness. Although family genetic influences have been identified for alcoholism and other substance abuse (Krueger, Hicks, Patrick, et al, 2002), parental and older sibling drinking practices and parental attitudes about alcohol also influence adolescent alcohol use, especially during early adolescence (Hoffmann and Su, 1998). Several studies assessing family structure have found a relationship between adolescent substance abuse and the over-involvement of one parent, accompanied by distancing from the other (see Family-Centered Care box).

FAMILY-CENTERED CARE
Adolescent Alcohol Abuse

The two primary tasks of parenting an adolescent are nurturing the child and setting appropriate limits (Hagan, Shaw, and Duncan, 2008). Research on families with alcohol-abusing adolescents reveals serious deficiencies in one or both of these areas. There is nothing to be gained by explicitly or implicitly blaming the parents. Alcohol abuse also has a strong genetic factor (Krueger, Hicks, Patrick, et al, 2002), and family assessment often reveals the parents' own history of neglect and substance abuse problems. One of the most difficult yet important challenges for health care professionals is to establish a trusting relationship with families while attempting to help the adolescent who is struggling with a substance abuse problem. The services and referrals provided must be determined by the unique needs and circumstances of the individuals whom nurses are serving.

Although the family environment may provide the kindling for adolescent alcohol abuse, peers provide the spark. An association with substance-using peers is the strongest predictor of an adolescent's continued use (Hoffmann and Su, 1998). Peer association does not cause adolescent substance abuse, but in most cases adolescents who drink have friends who also drink, and young people whose friends would be upset if they got drunk are significantly less likely to drink or to binge drink (Smith, Stewart, Peled, et al, 2009). The impact of peers on drug use has been demonstrated among African-Americans, Asian Americans, and Hispanics.

Sociodemographic Factors

Frequency of alcohol use is influenced by several sociodemographic factors. Adolescents in different regions of the United States and across the world drink at different levels, often dependent on the general community acceptance of alcohol use. Girls and boys report a similar onset and course of experimentation with alcohol, although boys more often become heavy users. Homeless and street-involved youth report high levels of alcohol use, often starting at a very young age (Smith, Saewyc, Albert, et al, 2007). Gay, lesbian, and bisexual teens are at increased risk for alcohol use and problems associated with drinking (Marshall, Friedman, Stall, et al, 2008). A commitment to education reduces risk; in contrast, school failure is associated with alcohol abuse. School dropouts are at particularly high risk and have been shown to drink more than high school graduates. However, binge drinking is highest among college students.

Psychosocial Factors

Research on personality and alcohol abuse in adolescence has investigated the interplay of complex factors that determine risk for alcohol abuse. Although aggressiveness early in life predicts subsequent alcohol use, only one third of boys with aggressive behavior continue to be aggressive into adulthood (White, Brick, and Hansell, 1993). Children with hyperactivity, particularly when combined with conduct problems, are at risk for abuse of drugs, including alcohol. Personality traits associated with alcohol abuse include excessive and consistent rebelliousness and rejection of social norms.

In his research, Jessor (1991) examined several psychosocial factors and developed the Problem Behavior Theory for understanding adolescent drug and alcohol use. This theory identified several domains of psychosocial variation: the personality system, the perceived environmental system, the social system, and the behavior system. These systems are interrelated and constitute the risk of occurrence of problem behaviors. A common dimension within these systems that distinguishes drug users from nonusers is conventionality versus unconventionality. In reference to the personality system, for example, an adolescent who is disconnected from conventional institutions such as school or religious faith community is at greater risk for involvement with drugs and alcohol. Conversely, adolescents who embrace conventional values such as academic achievement and community involvement are less likely to engage in drug use.

Jessor (1991) also identified protective factors that enable at-risk adolescents to resist pressures to use drugs and alcohol. Protective factors can be defined as those personal attributes and environmental influences that buffer, neutralize, and interact with risk factors to prevent, limit, or reduce drug use. Protective factors do not imply the absence of risk but are viewed as distinctly different from risk factors (Scheier, Newcomb, and Skager, 1994). Protective factors include a caring and supportive family, peer models for conventional behavior, connectedness to school and community organizations, social support in the form of perceptions that adults outside the family care about the youth, and the availability of people to talk to about problems (Resnick, Bearman, Blum, et al, 1997; Smith, Stewart, Peled, et al, 2009). A host of studies since Jessor's original model have modified and nuanced the list of assets and protective factors that reduce initiation of substance use, identifying protective factors specific to a diverse groups of adolescents (Oman, Vesley, Aspy, et al, 2004).

Biologic Factors

The interplay of personality, environment, and genetic factors influencing alcohol abuse has also come under scrutiny (Krueger, Hicks, Patrick, et al, 2002). Twin studies comparing the concordance of alcoholism in monozygotic and dizygotic twins indicate a significantly higher rate of concordance for alcoholism in monozygotic twins than in dizygotic twins (Morrison, Rogers, and Thomas, 1995). This finding holds true even if the twins were reared separately early in life. Other longitudinal population-based twin studies have explored the link between substance abuse and other externalizing behaviors such as conduct disorder or ADHD and have concluded that genetic inheritance determines about 80% of the likelihood of developing substance abuse in late adolescence and young adulthood, with the remainder of the risk in environmental influences of the family or community (Krueger, Hicks, Patrick, et al, 2002).

ALDH is an enzyme that assists with the breakdown of ethanol in the body. The absence of ALDH significantly reduces the likelihood that alcoholism will develop (Patton, 1995). Other genetic studies have indicated an association between the dopamine D2 receptor gene *(DRD2)* and alcoholism. This gene may confer susceptibility to at least one form of alcoholism (Blum, Noble, Sheridan, et al, 1990; Patton, 1995). Other studies of brainwave patterns and alcoholism or other substance abuse disorders among adolescents further support the genetic susceptibility findings (Carlson, Iacono, and McGue, 2002).

Research has also documented a relationship between early sexual maturation and alcohol use, smoking, and cannabis use, especially among adolescent girls (Patton and Viner, 2007). This association may be an external manifestation of the emotional reaction that occurs in girls who feel physically different because of early biologic maturation, or it may be due to altered patterns of sensation seeking or affiliations with older peers. However, research shows the link between early puberty and alcohol use may not continue into adulthood, as studies have found no association between early development and higher levels of adult substance use (Patton and Viner, 2007).

ADDITIONAL DRUGS

The majority of adolescents limit their experimentation with drugs to alcohol, tobacco, and marijuana (also called cannabis). A smaller proportion try other drugs that have serious consequences, including cocaine and other amphetamines, inhalants, barbiturates, narcotics, and hallucinogens. Approximately 15% of adolescents report using any illicit substance other than marijuana in the past year (Johnston, O'Malley, Bachman, et al, 2008), and the rates of use for most substances have been declining since the 1980s. Adolescent abuse of inhalants declined through the last half of the 1990s and the first few years of the new century, but in 2003 and 2004 lifetime prevalence of inhalant use increased slightly, one of the few drugs to increase, and then began to decline among eighth and twelfth graders (Johnston, O'Malley, Bachman, et al, 2008). Inhalant abuse is generally a "younger teen" drug, possibly because of its readier accessibility; up to 15.6% of eighth graders reported ever using inhalants in 2007, whereas only 10.5% of twelfth graders did

(Johnston, O'Malley, Bachman, et al, 2008). Prescription drugs are another growing concern; in 2007, 2% of eighth graders and nearly 10% of twelfth graders reported using narcotics such as oxycodone and hydrocodone at least once in the past year; 2% to 4% reported using methylphenidate without a prescription. Although crystal methamphetamine ("crystal meth," "ice") has received a lot of media attention in the past several years, fewer than 2% of teens in any grade reported using it in the past year, and only 3% had used it by grade 12.

Drug users have developed a specialized terminology or slang for the substances they use. This vocabulary varies in different localities at different times, and new descriptive terms arise spontaneously wherever drugs are part of the environment. This can create challenges for nurses in assessing drug use.

Cocaine

Cocaine is the most potent antifatigue agent known. Although pharmacologically not a narcotic, it is legally categorized as such. Cocaine is available in two forms: (1) water-soluble cocaine hydrochloride administered by insufflation (snorting) and intravenous injection, and (2) a nonsoluble alkaloid (freebase) used primarily for smoking. Crack, or rock, is a purer and more problematic form of the drug; it can be produced cheaply and smoked in either water pipes, mentholated cigarettes, or specialized "crack pipes." Cocaine taken by injection is associated with the highest levels of dependence, crack smoking has intermediate levels, and intranasal forms of cocaine have the lowest levels of dependence (Gossop, Griffiths, Powis, et al, 1994). Signs of serious use include an imbalance in sensory neurons causing a feeling of insects crawling under the skin; calluses and superficial burns on hands caused by repetitive use of a crack pipe to melt and smoke crack cocaine; and brown-black sputum, shortness of breath, and even pneumonia from the residues of the crack smoke.

Cocaine creates a sense of euphoria, or an indefinable high. It is intense but short acting, with the high lasting 15 to 30 minutes for cocaine and 5 to 10 minutes for crack. Withdrawal does not produce the dramatic symptoms observed during withdrawal from other substances. The effects are those more commonly seen in depression, including a lack of energy and motivation, irritability, appetite changes, psychomotor retardation, and irregular sleep patterns. More serious symptoms include cardiovascular manifestations and seizures. Physical withdrawal is not to be confused with the so-called crash after a cocaine high, which consists of a long period of sleep.

In 2007, 7.2% of high school students reported ever having tried cocaine (Centers for Disease Control and Prevention, 2008). Hispanic students (10.9%) were more likely to report ever using cocaine than Caucasian students (7.4%) or African-American students (1.8%). Around 3% reported using cocaine in the past month. Answers to questions about the health risks of cocaine can be obtained by calling the National Cocaine Hotline (800-COCAINE). It also provides referrals to support groups and treatment centers.

Narcotics

Narcotics include opiates, such as heroin, morphine, oxycodone and hydrocodone, as well as opioids (opiate-like drugs), such as hydromorphone (Dilaudid), fentanyl, meperidine (Demerol), and codeine. The narcotics produce a state of euphoria by removing painful feelings and creating a pleasurable experience of a specific quality and a sense of success accompanied by clouding of consciousness and a dreamlike state. Narcotics can be ingested or injected intravenously.

Physical signs of narcotic abuse include constricted pupils, respiratory depression, and often cyanosis. Needle marks may be visible on the arms or legs of chronic users. Physical withdrawal from opiates is extremely unpleasant unless controlled with supervised tapering doses of the opiate or substitution of methadone.

Perhaps more important are the indirect consequences related to the illegal status of narcotic use and the problems associated with securing the drug—health-compromising and often illegal methods used to meet the high cost of the doses, such as prostitution and drug dealing. Health problems result from self-neglect of physical needs (nutrition, cleanliness, dental care); overdose; contamination; and infection from risky sexual transactions and from shared needles, including human immunodeficiency virus and hepatitis B and C. Although different countries have different philosophic approaches to addressing injection drug use, evidence from Canada and Europe suggests needle-exchange programs and nurse-staffed safe injection sites can reduce the risks of overdose and infectious disease transmission, and may also increase the chance an injection drug user will seek drug treatment (Wood, Tyndall, Montaner, et al, 2006). This approach is called *harm reduction*, and there are increasing examples of its effectiveness in reducing the consequences of serious drug use.

Central Nervous System Depressants and Stimulants

Central nervous system depressants include a variety of hypnotic drugs that produce physical dependence and withdrawal symptoms on abrupt discontinuation. They create a feeling of relaxation and sleepiness but impair general functioning. Drugs in this category include barbiturates, nonbarbiturates (e.g., methaqualone [Quaalude]), and alcohol. Barbiturates combined with alcohol produce a profound depressant effect.

Barbiturates and other sedatives have also been associated with attempted and successful suicides. Flunitrazepam (Rohypnol), known as the "date rape drug," is a recent hypnotic drug abused by adolescents. Many women report being raped after unknowingly being given flunitrazepam in a drink. Flunitrazepam is 10 times more powerful than diazepam (Valium). It produces prolonged sedation, a feeling of well-being, and short-term memory loss. The drug is illegally imported into the United States. Recent alterations to the tablets include a dye that makes the drug visible if slipped into a drink. Flunitrazepam use is fairly rare among adolescents, with only about 1% reporting past year use (Johnston, O'Malley, Bachman, et al, 2008). A newer date rape drug, with similar effects, is γ-hydroxybutyric acid, or GHB. It dissolves instantly in water and other drinks and is colorless. Combined with alcohol, it has potent risk for coma, respiratory depression, and amnesia. In 2007 fewer than 1% of twelfth graders reported using GHB in the past year, a rate that has decreased since 2004 (Johnston, O'Malley, Bachman, et al, 2008).

The central nervous system stimulants, amphetamines and cocaine, do not produce strong physical dependence and can be withdrawn without much danger. However, psychologic dependence is strong, and acute intoxication can lead to violent, aggressive behavior or psychotic episodes manifested by paranoia, uncontrollable agitation, and restlessness. When combined with barbiturates, these stimulants have euphoric effects that are particularly addictive.

Methamphetamine can be snorted, injected, swallowed, or smoked and produces a burst of energy along with intense, alternating attacks of boldness and paranoia. It provokes an excitement far more intense than that caused by crack and cocaine. The drug, with the street names *crank, meth, ice,* and *crystal meth,* is inexpensive and has a longer period of action than that of cocaine. The drug is readily made from ephedrine and pseudoephedrine found in cold medications and diet pills, and the number of homemade "meth labs" in rural areas has increased significantly over the past several years. Some pharmacies have begun to limit access to over-the-counter medications containing pseudoephedrine, and some pharmaceutical companies have substituted other decongestants for pseudoephedrine in their cold medications. The effects of methamphetamine are more intense than those of cocaine. Instead of the short (few minutes) high achieved with crack, a user can remain "up" for hours on a similar dose of crystal meth. After persistent use, dependence makes the effects much more difficult to achieve, and higher doses are generally needed, which leads to bingeing; overdose can cause seizures, cardiovascular collapse, stroke, myocardial infarction, hyperthermia, and amphetamine psychosis. Because methamphetamine also suppresses appetite, thirst, and sleep, this can lead to malnutrition and dehydration. Like cocaine, the crash that occurs as the drug clears the system can be intense. In 2007, just over 3% of twelfth grade students reported trying methamphetamine or crystal meth, and 1.6% used it in the past year (Johnston, O'Malley, Bachman, et al, 2008).

A specific variant of the methamphetamine that is becoming common in certain groups is MDMA. It can be found as tablets imprinted with logos like butterflies or other pictures, as powder sprinkled on pacifiers or suckers, or as a powder that is snorted or smoked. The euphoria, psychedelic effects, and increased tactile sensitivity associated with MDMA use contribute to its popularity at dance club settings, but it can lead to exhaustion and dehydration after long hours of nonstop dancing. In addition, police laboratory testing of drugs seized in Canada and the United States has found that pills sold as Ecstasy often contain crystal methamphetamine in addition to MDMA. In 2007, 5.8% of high school students reported using Ecstasy at least once in their lifetimes (Centers for Disease Control and Prevention, 2008).

Inhalants

Inhalants include glue "sniffing" and the inhalation of plastic cement, spray paint, and other volatile substances (e.g., gasoline, nitrous oxide, and air "dusters" used to remove dust from computers and camera lenses). These dusters contain chemical solvents, usually a form of Freon, that can cause fatal cardiac arrhythmias. Inhalant abuse is most common in the early teenage years. A recent survey noted that 15.6% of adolescents in eighth grade in the United States had abused inhalants at least once in their lives (Johnston, O'Malley, Bachman, et al, 2008). Young teens are often completely unaware of the inherent dangers of "sniffing" or "huffing." They breathe the inhalants directly or place them in paper or plastic bags or soda cans from which they rebreathe the fumes, which produces an immediate euphoria and altered consciousness. Although these substances give the teen an inexpensive euphoric or "high" feeling, they are extremely dangerous and can cause rapid loss of consciousness and respiratory arrest. In addition, visual-spatial difficulties, visual scanning problems, language deficiencies, motor instability, memory deficits, and attention and concentration problems may occur.

Hallucinogens

Mind-altering drugs or hallucinogens (psychedelic, psychotomimetic, psychotropic, or illusionogenic) are drugs that produce vivid hallucinations and euphoria. These drugs do not produce physical dependence and therefore can be abruptly withdrawn without ill effect. However, the acute and long-term effects are variable, and in some individuals the dissociative behavior may be unduly protracted. This category includes cannabis (marijuana, hashish), psilocybin mushrooms, and lysergic acid diethylamide (LSD).

In some parts of the United States and Canada, marijuana has replaced tobacco as the second most widely used drug by teens, after alcohol (Centers for Disease Control and Prevention, 2008; Smith, Stewart, Peled, et al, 2009). Nationwide, they appear nearly equal: in 2007, 19.7% of high school students nationwide reported using marijuana once or more in the past 30 days, while 20.0% reported similar use of cigarettes (Centers for Disease Control and Prevention, 2008).

THERAPEUTIC MANAGEMENT

Adolescents experiencing toxic drug effects or withdrawal symptoms are commonly seen in emergency departments. Experienced emergency department personnel are familiar with the management of acute drug toxicosis; the signs, symptoms, and behavior characteristics of a variety of substances; and the differences and similarities among them. When the drug is questionable or unknown, knowledge of these factors facilitates handling of the youngster and implementation of a treatment regimen.

The treatment for drug toxicity or withdrawal varies according to the drug and the method used. Make every effort to determine the type and amount of drug taken, the time it was taken, the mode of administration, and factors related to the onset of presenting symptoms.

It is helpful to know the patient's pattern of use. For example, if two types of drugs are involved, they may require different treatments. Gastric lavage may be employed when the drug has been ingested recently and the cough reflex is intact but would be of little value when the drug has been administered by the intravenous ("mainlined") or intranasal ("sniffed") route. Because the actual content of most street drugs is highly questionable, other pharmaceutical agents are administered with caution, except perhaps the narcotic antagonists in cases of suspected opiate overdose. It is necessary to assess for possible trauma sustained while the patient was under the influence of the drug.

Rehabilitation from illicit drug use may require withdrawing the adolescent from both the environment and the chemical agent. Programs must be suited to the individual and may involve foster home placement or a residential treatment setting, although many adolescents are handled in an ambulatory setting. Programs often include group sessions with other adolescents. Adolescents can also obtain information regarding help from the Center for Substance Abuse Treatment hotline (800-662-HELP).

NURSING CARE MANAGEMENT

Nurses in almost every setting are increasingly likely to have contact with adolescents who misuse alcohol and other drugs; nurses are in a position to serve as educators and patient advocates. Nurses can be listeners, confidants, and counselors to troubled teens. They are essential members of health care teams whose efforts are directed toward short- and long-term therapy for adolescents with substance abuse disorders, and in some limited situations, they may provide harm reduction services as part of a needle-exchange program or safer injection facility for injection drug users. Most often, however, nurses encounter adolescents who are under the influence of alcohol or other drugs in acute care settings, such as emergency departments and urgent care clinics.

Observation or a description of the behavior often is more valuable than a report by patients or friends as to the chemical agent taken. For example, aggressive behavior and disorientation are often seen in barbiturate, alcohol, stimulant, or hallucinogen intoxication but not in opiate intoxication. Overdose from barbiturates, inhalants, or opiates can result in respiratory failure and coma. Pinpoint pupils are seen only in opiate toxicity. Nurses must be alert for life-threatening consequences of drug toxicity. Equipment and personnel should be available, or the patient should be transferred to facilities that are prepared to provide supportive measures for physiologic depression and psychogenic phenomena.

Keep stimulation to a minimum for agitated, frightened teens. Treatments or tests not immediately required should be postponed. These teens primarily need psychologic support in a nonthreatening environment and close contact with a caring, understanding person who can stay with them and help them maintain social contact. Intoxicated adolescents may be aggressive, and nurses need to be aware of possible risk for injury. Calm, soothing environments can reduce this response.

School nurses play an essential role because they may be the only health care professionals with an opportunity to identify many adolescents with substance abuse problems who appear anxious, depressed, or angry. Assessment of potential substance abuse problems is an important part of evaluation. By ensuring confidentiality within appropriate limits and in a straightforward manner, nurses enable many adolescents to discuss problems involving substance abuse openly.

Obstetric and nursery personnel encounter drug dependence and withdrawal in newborn infants or in a mother with substance abuse disorders. Affected infants are at risk and require special surveillance for complications of withdrawal.

Therefore nurses should be aware of the possibility of drug dependence in mothers who come to the hospital for delivery. (See Chapter 10.)

Long-Term Management

A major factor in the treatment and rehabilitation of young teens with substance abuse disorders is careful assessment in the nonacute stage to determine the function that the drug plays in these teens' lives. Several standardized instruments can be used to identify and screen for substance abuse. These instruments include the HEADSS interview questions, which assess the topics of home, education, activities, drugs, sex, and suicide; and the CAGE AID questionnaire, which assesses alcohol use and abuse (Ewing, 2008; Norris, 2007). Before they can embark on a rehabilitation program, adolescents need help in identifying the issues that motivated them to use drugs and in recognizing their own role in self-destructive, inappropriate drug-abuse behavior.

The motivation phase of treatment is directed toward exploring the factors that influence drug use. It also involves establishing in the teen a feeling of self-worth and a commitment to self-help. It requires a trusting relationship between the adolescent and the health care team and involves a thorough physical examination and assessment of psychologic, educational, and vocational status. A realistic appraisal of the adolescent's potential and efforts aimed at short-term goals, along with building self-esteem, lays the groundwork for a successful rehabilitation program.

Rehabilitation begins when teens decide that they can and are willing to change. Rehabilitation involves fostering healthy interdependent relationships with caring and supportive adults and exploring alternate mechanisms for problem solving while simultaneously reducing or eliminating drug use. Persons working with troubled young people must be prepared for recidivism, or the tendency to relapse, and maintain a plan for reentry into the treatment process.

The majority of treatment programs for adolescent substance abusers are based on adult 12-step models such as Alcoholics Anonymous. Research is needed to determine whether applying adult models to adolescents is effective. ToughLove (www.toughlove.com) is one such program. The ToughLove philosophy, first employed by Alcoholics Anonymous and Al-Anon, is based on the conviction that parents have the right and the responsibility to be the policy-makers in the family, set limits on their children's behavior, and take control of the household from out-of-control teenagers. The premise is that allowing teenagers to experience the negative consequences of their behavior will bring them closer to accepting help and changing their behavior. Adolescents are offered the choice of (1) getting treatment for their mental health or drug problem or (2) finding another place to live.

Pieper and Pieper (1992) criticize the ToughLove approach, contending that the uncompromising position adopted by parents is harmful to both parents and child. In contrast, they believe treatment emphasizing self-caretaking is more useful as a long-term approach. Depending on the substance, treatment approaches may include tapered withdrawal or medications to assist with the dependence and cravings. For adolescents with ADHD, who are at higher risk of substance abuse, encour-

aging appropriate medication adherence may prevent self-medication with illicit substances (Wilens, Faraone, Biederman, et al, 2003). Similarly, youth with a history of sexual abuse and similar traumas are at higher risk for substance abuse disorders. Addressing abuse trauma may be necessary as part of or before effective substance abuse treatment (Saewyc, 2007).

The fact remains that effective approaches to the treatment of adolescent substance abuse have limited evidence at present. Treatments sensitive to the developmental transitions of adolescence and the variety of biopsychosocial factors affecting substance use need to be further developed and rigorously evaluated.

Prevention

Given the difficulty of treating substance abusers, prevention is the most effective policy. In recent years a variety of programs have been applied with promising results. Successful programs for reducing substance abuse risk have promoted parenting skills, social skills among children with ADHD, academic achievement, and skills to resist peer influence. Prevention programs are often provided in the school setting, as a way of reaching most youth; however, not all prevention programs are equally effective. The Drug Abuse Resistance Education (DARE) program, for example, which trains police officers to provide the curriculum in schools, is popular and has been rigorously evaluated, but unfortunately has not been shown to be effective in preventing alcohol and drug use (West and O'Neal, 2004).

Peer pressure has been used effectively in prevention efforts. For example, Students Against Destructive Decisions (SADD) (www.sadd.org; formerly known as Students Against Drunk Driving) is an organization of young people who work to eliminate teenage drunk driving and other destructive behaviors. Techniques used by this group include peer counseling, the development of parental guidelines for teenage parties, and community awareness efforts. Nurses should encourage the formation of a SADD chapter in high schools in their communities.

Nurses can also play an important role in other preventive efforts. Young people need to be educated regarding the appropriate use of substances. Health care professionals associated with adolescents should listen to what they are saying, determine what is bothering them, and try to help meet their needs before they resort to drugs.

Prevention programs carry the implicit assumption that poor outcomes facing children at risk can be forestalled or at least reduced. In the past, prevention research has focused on the identification of risk factors and their relationship to drug use. More recently, research has begun to investigate the protective forces that contribute to resisting drug use, such as family, school, and cultural connectedness. Other studies are testing interventions that foster protective factors and assets as a strategy for preventing or reducing alcohol and other drug use. It is important for nurses to consider the multiple risk and protective factors and their interactions in influencing drug use and abuse. Preventive and clinical interventions should attempt to increase the protective factors as well as reduce the risk factors. Nurses in a variety of settings are in a position to identify emerging risk factors, to refer problems for assessment and management, and to foster those parenting skills and interpersonal skills that may be protective against substance abuse.

SUICIDE

Suicide is defined as the deliberate act of self-injury with the intent that the injury results in death. Most experts distinguish between suicidal ideation, suicide attempt, and suicide. Suicidal ideation involves a preoccupation with thoughts about committing suicide and may be a precursor to suicide. Although it is not uncommon for adolescents to experience occasional suicidal thoughts, nurses should take expressions of suicidal preoccupation seriously and conduct an assessment for appropriate referral. A suicide attempt is intended to cause injury or death but is unsuccessful. Some acts of self-injury or self-harm may not be direct suicide attempts, although self-harm behaviors may occur along with suicidal thoughts or intent. Some researchers and clinicians prefer to use the term *self-harm* to refer to these behaviors because it makes no reference to intent and a person's motive may be too difficult or complex to ascertain. Take all self-harm activity seriously.

> **! NURSING ALERT**
>
> A history of a previous suicide attempt is a serious indicator for possible suicide completion in the future. Studies of adolescent suicides have found that as many as half had made previous attempts.

A survey of U.S. high school students in 2007 indicated that 9.3% of females and 4.6% of males had attempted suicide in the previous 12 months. However, 19% of females and 10% of males had serious suicidal ideation during the 12 months preceding the survey (Centers for Disease Control and Prevention, 2008). In the United States, the suicide rate for adolescents increased dramatically in the 1970s and 1980s, declined from 1990 to 2002, and increased again from 2003 to 2005, in part due to changes in treatment patterns for depression among adolescents. In 2006 the suicide rate was 7.1 per 100,000 young people ages 10 to 24. Suicide is currently the third leading cause of death for adolescents 10 to 24 years of age (Mulye, Park, Nelson, et al, 2009).

The major tasks of adolescence are (1) developing a coherent sense of personal identity, (2) establishing a clear gender and sexual identity, (3) establishing autonomy from parents, (4) beginning to master the ability to be in intimate relationships, (5) acquiring coping skills, (6) consolidating values, and (7) developing educational or vocational goals. It is likely that the onset of depression and suicide during adolescence is due to cognitive development and the newly developed capacity for self-observation and future orientation. Some young people experience a pervasive sense of despair when they look into the future and are faced with a discrepancy between what they have been led to anticipate and what they are truly able to obtain. Self-hate and hopelessness may result. In part, the despair is a consequence of adolescents' newly developed cognitive ability to consider the abstract and hypothetical, which may paint a bleak picture of their lives in the future. As adolescents struggle to establish their sense of self, they constantly seek external

validation and confirmation of who they are. Introspection becomes a prominent part of this process. Social experiences and peer relationships become more important during the adolescent years, and the increased need to belong and conform leads to an increased vulnerability to depression and suicidal thought. In the context of this intrapersonal and interpersonal searching, self-esteem becomes pivotal, moderating hopelessness and developing a strong sense of self.

Young people also focus on mastering empathy during the teen years. The ability to truly empathize with others creates a new awareness of the suffering of others. The capacity to passionately feel both joy and sorrow is exciting, yet frightening. For some, the pain seems overwhelming. Because they most likely have not lived through intensely painful experiences, they have not developed the means to cope with deep emotions. They may feel alone in experiencing pain and sorrow and unable to recognize or express their need for support. For adolescents who have not had guidance and experience in problem solving and coping with sorrow, suicide may represent a means of escape and seem the only option.

Many of today's young people have been desensitized to death by constantly viewing it on television, in the movies, and in video games. Suicide may be romanticized and inaccurately portrayed. The frequency of contagion suicides, or copycat suicides, among young people (i.e., an increase in youth suicides after the suicide of one teenager is publicized) may indicate an adolescent perception of suicide as glamorous. Simultaneously, changes in families have insulated teens from other kinds of death experiences. Improvements in health care and geographic mobility in the United States isolate family members from one another, and young people are not as likely to participate in the painful emotional realities of sickness and death among older family members.

Over several decades the increasing youth suicide rate paralleled increasing rates of child poverty, violence, and parental divorce and decreasing parental involvement and support. As adolescents strive for healthy autonomy from their parents and master the skills required for interdependence with others, they begin to question and criticize their parents. They attempt to discover their own identity and discern which qualities of their parents they want to incorporate into their lives. This questioning and criticizing process can generate a sense of guilt, insecurity, fear, and conflict. Even though they may rebel against their parents, young people need to feel needed, wanted, and loved by their families. Studies indicate that young people who believe that their families care about them are less likely to show suicidal behaviors (Resnick, Bearman, Blum, et al, 1997).

The changing roles of young people in society have also had an impact on adolescent suicidality. The period of adolescence is prolonged in the United States, and roles for young people are unclear and difficult to formulate. The earlier onset of puberty and the growing need for higher educational attainment has increased the period of adolescence from 6 years to potentially 14 years or longer. This extended time between childhood and adulthood has created greater role confusion. Today the majority of parents are employed at jobs away from home. Consequently, young people do not have the opportunity to see their parents as vocational role models. The higher percentage of adolescents within the total population and the increased difficulties adolescents have in obtaining jobs and being admitted to college also contribute to a higher youth suicide rate.

Although most people emerge from adolescence with a healthy sense of who they are and where they are headed, the widespread belief that adolescence is a time of turmoil—of storm and stress—has created a sense that hopelessness and despair are a normal part of the second decade of life. This is not so. Most young people do not experience adolescence as a time of despair. Depressive symptoms, acting-out behaviors, and talk of suicide need to be taken seriously. They are not a common phase of adolescence—they are a call for help that requires the response of nurses and other professionals.

INCIDENCE

The incidence of youth suicide varies greatly by gender and racial or ethnic background. In 2006, for every 100,000 young people ages 10 to 24 in the United States, the suicide rates were 11.4 for males and 2.4 for females (Centers for Disease Control and Prevention, 2006). The rates were lower for African-American and Asian-American male adolescents compared with Caucasian adolescents: 7.6 for African-American males, 8.35 for Asian-American males, compared to 12.1 for Caucasian males. However, suicide rates were higher for Asian-American females (2.9) than either African-American females (1.3) or Caucasian females (2.5). Native American–Alaskan Native–Native Hawaiian adolescents have the highest rates of suicide attempts, at 25.4 per 100,000 among males, and 7.9 among females.

Although Native Americans have a high rate of suicide compared with other racial and ethnic groups in the United States, there is great variation among tribes. Tribes with less social integration, less adherence to tribal traditions, and a high degree of individuality generally have higher suicide rates than tribes that are tightly integrated and adhere to traditional values and practices. Family, school, and tribal connectedness has been shown to be a protective factor associated with lower rates of hopelessness and suicidality among high-risk Native American adolescents (Dexheimer-Pharris, Resnick, and Blum, 1997).

Incarcerated youths in public correctional facilities have a higher suicide rate than adolescents in the general population. Minors detained in adult jails are at especially high risk for suicide.

Even though the statistics reveal hopelessness and despair among young people, the true incidence of completed suicides in children and adolescents is not known because of general underreporting. Deaths by suicide often are reported as accidental because of pressures exerted by the family and society to avoid the cultural and religious stigma associated with self-destruction. The high accident rate in this age-group may reflect suicides masked by accidental death or homicide. In the United States the mortality patterns for suicide and homicide among youths follow similar trends. It is possible that these forms of violent death in youths share common antecedents.

The incidence of suicide attempts, as opposed to suicide completions, is even more difficult to measure. There is no national reporting system for suicide attempts, although national surveys of youth in school such as the Centers for Disease Control and Prevention's Youth Risk Behavior Survey do ask for self-report of suicide attempts. Although more males than females complete suicide, suicide attempts are far more common in females than in males. In 2007, 9.3% of females compared to 4.6% of males reported they had attempted suicide once or more in the past year (Centers for Disease Control and Prevention, 2008). The major difference between suicide attempts and suicide completions is often whether a lethal weapon is available. Successful suicide is more likely when alcohol and firearms are involved. Thus a higher incidence of youth suicide occurs in societies in which alcohol and lethal weapons are readily available to youths. Firearms were more likely to be present in the homes of suicide completers than in those of youths who attempted suicide or had suicidal ideation (Shain and Committee on Adolescence, 2007).

FACTORS ASSOCIATED WITH SUICIDE RISK

An effective research methodology that studies the risk factors associated with suicide is psychologic autopsy, which involves data collection from the deceased person's family, friends, teachers, counselors, spiritual advisers, and educational and health care records. Psychologic autopsies reveal several factors associated with adolescent suicide: depression or other affective disorders, drug and alcohol abuse, family conflict, prior suicide attempt, antisocial or aggressive behavior, a family history of suicidal behavior, and the availability of a firearm (Box 21-10). Another approach is to examine the factors associated with self-reported suicide attempts among youth in population-based school surveys. Although this will not capture the experiences of teens who are homeless or have dropped out of school, the large representative nature of the sample can be useful for understanding risks reported by the teens themselves, which may not have been revealed to friends, family, or others.

Individual Factors

The single most important individual factor associated with an increased risk of suicide is the presence of an active psychiatric disorder (e.g., affective disorders such as depression and bipolar disorder, substance abuse, and conduct disorder). Several studies have documented the relationship between psychiatric illness and suicide. Shaffer, Gould, Fisher, and colleagues (1996) found that more than 90% of the children and adolescents who committed suicide were retrospectively found to meet the criteria for at least one major psychiatric diagnosis. Depression is the predominant affective disorder that represents a major risk for suicide.

Psychiatric illness is also associated with an increased potential for suicidal ideation or suicide attempts. In a random sample of 1285 children and adolescents, Gould, King, Greenwald, and colleagues (1998) noted that the rate of suicide attempts was 22% among children with one psychiatric illness (major depression). For children with two or more psychiatric disorders, the rate of suicide attempts was 18 times higher, and the rate of suicidal ideation was eight times higher than the rate in healthy children.

Comorbidity of an affective disorder and substance abuse also increases the risk for suicide (Jellinek and Snyder, 1998). Alcohol use in particular has been associated with more than

BOX 21-10 FACTORS ASSOCIATED WITH SUICIDE RISK

History
Previous suicide attempt
Suicide attempt by a family member or friend
History of physical or sexual abuse or of neglect
Past psychiatric hospitalization
Death of a parent when child was young

Individual Factors
Hopelessness
Marked, persistent depression
Alcohol or drug abuse
Impulsiveness
Difficulty tolerating frustration
Feelings of self-hatred, excessive guilt, or humiliation
Thinking disorder (wishing to join a deceased person, hearing voices telling to kill self)
Physical or body image problems and behavior and developmental problems (delayed puberty, chronic illness, disability, attention deficit hyperactivity disorder, learning disorders)
Gender identity or sexual orientation concerns; gay, lesbian, bisexual, or transgender in an unsupportive environment
Seeing self as totally helpless, a victim of fate
A need to do things perfectly

Family Factors
Difficult home situation; long, bitter parent-child conflict
Hostile parents
Overt rejection by one or both parents
Divorce or separation of parents
Recent or impending move
Family breakup or parental loss
Exposure to unrealistically high parental expectations
Parental indifference with low expectations

Social and Environmental Factors
Firearms in the home
Incarceration
Lack of effective social support system
Isolation
Exposure to suicide of another
Few social, vocational, or educational opportunities

tity, and who experience high levels of harassment or violence. Parent and family responses when adolescents disclose their orientation ("coming out") are also important: a recent study found that teens who thought their parents were rejecting (even if the parent did not intend his or her response to be rejecting) were eight times more likely to attempt suicide in later adolescence (Ryan, Huebner, Diaz, et al, 2009). In assessing for level of risk, the youths' knowledge, feelings, and experience in the area of sexual orientation and identity are important. The amount of accurate knowledge and the level of support youths feel directly affect their risk for depression, substance abuse, and suicidality. By providing care that enhances support systems and nurtures opportunities for the healthy development of self-esteem in gay, lesbian, and bisexual adolescents and their families, nurses can play a significant role in reducing youth suicide rates in the United States.

Additional individual risk factors for suicidal behavior include poor academic progress, a history of being a victim of sexual abuse, learning disabilities, attention deficit disorder, chronic illness, disability, and antisocial behavior (especially assaultive behavior, which when experienced with suicidal feelings, provides a strong risk indicator for suicide potential).

In the context of these major risk factors, adolescents' maturity, particularly their cognitive development, may determine the likelihood of suicidal behavior. Adolescents who have developed and mastered problem-solving and social skills, have an internal locus of control, and have a positive sense of their future will be less likely to turn to suicide, even when faced with extreme stressors. In contrast, youths who see themselves as totally helpless, as victims of fate, or who are impulsive, unable to tolerate frustration, filled with self-hatred, experiencing excessive guilt, suffering from humiliation, withdrawn and aloof, or aggressive and impulsive will be more likely to take their own life.

Family Factors

Families hold the greatest potential for protecting young people from suicidal behavior. Families who respect individuality, are cohesive and caring, balance discipline with a supportive and understanding relationship, have good systems of communication, and have at least one attentive and caring parent available to the child protect adolescents from suicidal outcomes. In contrast, family risk factors for suicide include:

- Parental loss
- Family disruption
- A family history of suicidality, substance abuse, or emotional disturbance
- Child abuse or neglect
- Unavailable parents
- Poor communication
- Isolation within an inflexible family system
- Family conflict
- Unrealistically high parental expectations
- Parental indifference with low expectations

Nursing interventions should be designed to enhance family cohesiveness (Box 21-11). However, in working with families who have experienced the loss of a child through suicide, nurses should remember that although the risk of suicide is higher in families that are under stress and less cohesive, youth suicide

50% of suicides (Shain and Committee on Adolescence, 2007). For some teens, suicide becomes the final pathway for release from their psychiatric and social problems (Jellinek and Snyder, 1998). Childhood and adolescent suicide victims are reported to have higher rates not only of depression but also conduct disorders; bipolar disorders; substance abuse; interpersonal problems with parents; and a family history of depression, substance abuse, and suicidal behavior.

Gay, lesbian, and bisexual adolescents are at particularly high risk for suicide attempts, especially if raised in an environment where they are denied support systems (Russell and Joyner, 2001; Saewyc, Skay, Hynds, et al, 2007). When gay, lesbian, or bisexual young persons grow up in a community and family that do not accept their orientation, they are likely to internalize the homophobia and feel self-hate, which often turns into suicidal feelings. This alienating social context challenges self-esteem. Youths most at risk are those who struggle with sexual orientation, who have not yet disclosed their iden-

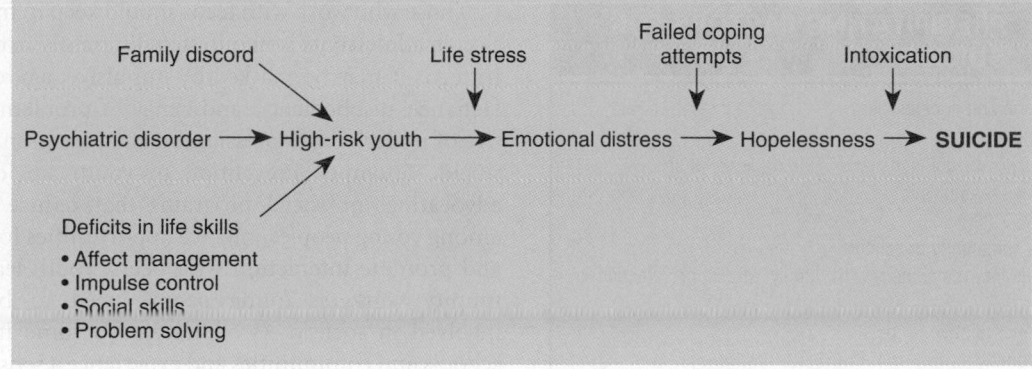

Fig. 21-3 Pathway from risk factors to completed suicide. (From Hoberman H: Completed suicide in children and adolescents: a review, *Resid Treat Child Youth* 7:61-88, 1989.)

BOX 21-11 PROTECTIVE FACTORS FOR YOUTH SUICIDE

- Warm and caring family environment
- Self-esteem, internal locus of control, self-confidence
- Social skills
- Problem-solving skills
- Regular attendance at religious or spiritual services or ceremonies (except for gay, lesbian, or bisexual youth whose religious community holds negative values about nonheterosexual orientations)
- An adult who listens to the adolescent
- Perception of school personnel as caring
- Parental support
- Parents with realistic, high expectations
- A family that pays a lot of attention to the adolescent
- Cohesive family environment
- Supportive friendships
- Ability to manage a negative affect, tolerate frustration and unfavorable events, think things through, actively problem solve, easily form close relationships, celebrate good things, and feel pleasure
- Family respect for individuality

---

can and does happen in the context of a caring and cohesive family environment.

Social and Environmental Factors

Important social and environmental influences that protect adolescents from suicidal behavior include good peer relationships, regular participation in religious services (unless the religious beliefs or community is rigid and unsupportive, especially for gay, lesbian, or bisexual youth), strong social support within the community or school system, and available options for vocational and educational development. In contrast, factors associated with increased suicide risk include incarceration, social isolation, acute loss of a boyfriend or girlfriend, lack of future options, and the availability of firearms in the home.

METHODS

Completed Suicide

Firearms are the most commonly used instruments in completed suicides among male and female adolescents (Shain and

Committee on Adolescence, 2007). For adolescent males the second and third most common means of suicide are hanging and overdose; for adolescent females the second and third most common means are overdose and strangulation (Centers for Disease Control and Prevention, 2006).

Suicide Attempt

The most common method of suicide attempt is overdose or ingestion of a potentially toxic substance, such as drugs. The second most common method of suicide attempt is self-inflicted laceration. It has been suggested that some automobile crashes may actually be suicide attempts rather than accidents; however, unless the teen discloses this intent, there is no clear evidence of intending self-harm, and such crashes are identified and counted as unintentional rather than intentional injuries.

PRECIPITATING FACTORS

Although suicide is often an impulsive act, it takes place against a backdrop of individual, family, and social risk factors and is often carried out in response to an exacerbation of longstanding stressors or in reaction to an acute precipitating factor. The most common factors precipitating adolescent suicide are a fight with a close friend; the breakup of an important relationship; failure in an important area (e.g., school activities); changing schools or moving; involvement in the legal system; discovery of pregnancy plus family crisis or rejection by boyfriend; and the death of a close friend, relative, or pet.

Fig. 21-3 presents a model for understanding the dynamics of the pathway from risk factors to completed suicide. This model incorporates multiple factors related to individual differences, as well as family and social contexts (Box 21-12).

NURSING CARE MANAGEMENT

Prevention

Nurses play a pivotal role in reducing youth suicide. Nurses have the opportunity to provide anticipatory guidance to parents and adolescents. They can teach parents to be supportive and to develop positive communication patterns that help teens feel connected with and loved by their families. To foster healthy development, encourage parents to provide teens with

---

BOX 21-12 PRECIPITATING FACTORS FOR SUICIDE

- Increased depression and hopelessness
- Fight with close friend
- Failure to achieve specific goals in school, job, or personal life
- Breakup of important relationship
- Friend moving away
- Relocation to new community or school
- Discovery of pregnancy combined with family stress or rejection by boyfriend
- Death of close friend, relative, or pet
- Argument within family
- Shameful or humiliating experience
- Trouble with police

BOX 21-13 WARNING SIGNS OF SUICIDE

- Preoccupation with themes of death; focusing on morbid thoughts
- Wanting to give away cherished possessions
- Talking of own death, desire to die
- Loss of energy, loss of interest, listlessness
- Exhaustion without obvious cause
- Changes in sleep patterns (too much or too little)
- Increased irritability, argumentativeness, or stubbornness
- Physical complaints (e.g., recurrent stomachaches, headaches)
- Repeated visits to physician, nurse practitioner, or emergency department for treatment of injuries
- Reckless behavior
- Antisocial behavior (drinking, using drugs, fighting, committing acts of vandalism, running away from home, becoming sexually promiscuous)
- Sudden change in school performance (lowered grades, cutting classes, dropping out of activities)
- Resisting or refusing to go to school
- Remaining distant, sad, remote; flat affect, frozen facial expression
- Describing self as worthless
- Sudden cheerfulness following deep depression
- Social withdrawal from friends, activities, interests that were previously enjoyed
- Impaired concentration
- Dramatic change in appetite

---

creative outlets and to assist young people in accepting strong emotions—pain, anger, and frustration—as a normal part of the human experience.

Given what is known about youth suicide, nurses should ask parents, especially those of at-risk teenagers, if firearms are available in the house and, if so, recommend their removal. Parents must ensure that their children—especially children who are depressed, have poor problem-solving skills, or use drugs or alcohol—do not have access to firearms. Parents must be educated on the warning signs of suicide (Box 21-13).

Nurses working in the community are in a strategic position to conduct educational programs in schools, places of worship, and community centers to help young people develop healthy, effective coping mechanisms and problem-solving skills. Nurses can teach teens and their parents, teachers, and youth workers about youth depression and stress. Informed parents are more likely to seek help in the form of psychologic evaluation and treatment for young people who report persistent, deep feelings of sadness, hopelessness, and suicidal feelings.

Those who work with teens should keep in mind that depression in adolescents is manifested differently from that in adults. In teens it may be masked by impulsive, aggressive behaviors. Defiance, disobedience, and behavior problems can be indicative of underlying depression, suicidal ideation, and impending suicide attempts. Prevention of youth suicide also involves advocating for social programs that reduce social isolation among young people; enhance opportunities for social support; and promote interaction with peers, youth leaders, and community workers. Young people need to be meaningfully involved in society. As adolescents become involved in their schools and communities and experience a sense of competence and confidence in these roles, they become capable of coping with sadness, despair, and stressful life events.

Universal school-based screening for suicidal ideation and attempts has recently been recommended as a strategy to prevent suicides, since most youth attend school. Such screening has been effective in identifying at-risk youth. Although some school staff and parents may express concern that asking about suicidal thoughts and prior attempts might precipitate suicidal behavior from someone who is depressed, studies have tested this possibility and have shown that, in fact, screening appears to lower emotional distress and suicidality among depressed students (Gould, Marrocco, Kleinman, et al, 2005).

The clustering of suicides ("copycat" suicides) requires a specific response from television and newspaper reporters. Suicide needs to be portrayed as a poor means of coping with life's stressors and, at times, a response to underlying psychiatric disorders (see Community Focus box). In addition, to reduce copycat suicides, schools and communities must provide counseling programs when a suicide has occurred. The nurse can obtain information from the American Association of Suicidology.*

Health care professionals must be alert to the warning signs of adolescent suicide. No threat of suicide should be ignored. Too often, suicidal threats or minor attempts are confused with bids for attention. It is a mistake to be lulled into a false sense of security when an adolescent's depression is apparently relieved. The improvement in attitude may mean that the adolescent has made the decision and found the method to carry out the threat.

In educating youth, nurses should include the following in their teaching plan: the importance of seeking help when feeling sad or depressed, sources of available help for depression, warning signs of suicide (see Box 21-13), the importance of informing a responsible adult if a friend is talking about suicide, and how to access local suicide prevention services. Peers are valuable observers and excellent sources of information. They are able to sense when a friend has undergone a marked personality change. It is important to emphasize that the peer who detects any change in a friend is a "potential rescuer" and should not remain quiet about the observations. Teach all youths that, when a peer talks of suicide, they must alert someone who is in a position to help, such as a parent, teacher, or guidance counselor. Suicide prevention education should be incorporated into a comprehensive adolescent health curriculum.

---

*5221 Wisconsin Ave., NW, Washington, DC 20015; 202-237-2280; www.suicidology.org.

Working with the Media to Prevent Youth Suicide Clustering

A small percentage of adolescent suicides occur in clusters after the suicide of another adolescent has been highly publicized. Excessive media coverage after the suicide of an adolescent is believed to contribute to copycat, or contagion, suicides, particularly if the suicide is romanticized and the good points of the person's life are overemphasized while the struggles are not mentioned.

In the face of this tendency to sensationalize youth suicide, nurses, public health professionals, teachers, and community officials can work with the media to ensure responsible reporting. Responsible reporting of suicides should include the following elements (American Foundation for Suicide Prevention, 2009):

- Minimizing sensationalism by limiting the details of the suicide; instead call it a death
- Avoiding use of the word *suicide* in the headlines
- Refraining from describing the technical details regarding the method of suicide and from displaying dramatic photos related to the suicide
- Minimizing the reporting of public expressions of grief (e.g., memorial services, public eulogies, creation of memorials at the site)
- Not overemphasizing the positive aspects of the person's life while deleting mention of his or her problems
- Emphasizing that the precipitating event was not the only cause of the suicide
- Including information on identifying persons at risk for suicide and resources for adolescents who are feeling depressed or suicidal
- Including information that effective treatments for these mental illness conditions are available

⚠ NURSING ALERT

The National Suicide Prevention Lifeline (800-273-TALK) offers someone to talk to 24/7.

Screening for Suicidality

Routine assessment of adolescents should include questions that assess the presence of suicidal thought or intent. The nurse can ask the following questions (Greydanus and Pratt, 1995):

1. Do you consider yourself more a happy person, an unhappy person, or somewhere in the middle?
2. Have you ever been so unhappy or upset that you felt like being dead?
3. Have you ever thought about hurting yourself?
4. Have you ever developed a plan to hurt yourself or kill yourself?
5. Have you ever attempted to kill yourself?

If adolescents answer "yes" to questions 2, 3, or 4, they should be asked if they feel that way now to assess for current suicidality. If teens say they have attempted suicide in the past, assess the number of times and ask them to describe what they were feeling, which method they used, what happened, if they would make a similar attempt, and how they would handle their despair now. Any previous suicide attempt indicates an increased risk for a future attempt. The risk of a suicide attempt in the near future increases as the frequency of suicidal ideation increases.

Adolescents who do not currently have a plan for suicide but who struggle with frequent thoughts of suicide should be asked what they would do if they felt suicidal. They should have a plan

to access immediate help. Many nurses contract with such youths, asking them to sign an agreement that they will not attempt suicide during an agreed-on period and that they will call the 24-hour crisis line immediately if they feel they cannot keep the contract. The amount of time for which a youth feels comfortable contracting may be an indication of his or her level of risk and stability.

For youths who have suicidal thoughts, are depressed, and abuse substances, the nurse should discuss safety issues with the parent or guardian. Give clear instructions to remove any firearms from the home (not just locking them up, since adolescents are adept at opening locked gun cabinets) and to remove all prescription medications and over-the-counter medications such as acetaminophen and aspirin. Encourage parents to contract with their children, asking them to inform the parents if they are feeling suicidal. Youths will usually honor such contracts and welcome the support and monitoring by parents.

Youths who are actively suicidal need inpatient care, monitoring, and treatment. Medications for depression and bipolar disorder often take several weeks to reach therapeutic dosages. The time until medications and therapy begin to take effect can be trying for the adolescent and the family. It is important to encourage families to support their teen in adherence to the regimen prescribed.

In 2004 the U.S. Food and Drug Administration ordered "black box" warnings placed on the labels of SSRIs used to treat depression in young people, indicating a potential risk of suicide attempts among children and youth. Although subsequent reanalyses of the data suggest there is no added risk from the medications, families were reluctant to accept SSRI treatment, and prescriptions dropped 19%. Unfortunately, the same years that SSRI prescriptions decreased in the United States and Europe saw an unexpected rise in suicides among youth (Gibbons, Brown, Hur, et al, 2007). Teens who are taking such medications need careful, frequent monitoring. Youths who are suffering from psychiatric disorders (major depression, bipolar disorder, and psychoses) and substance abuse need a comprehensive treatment referral that incorporates mental health and chemical dependency treatment.

Care of the Suicidal Adolescent

In caring for young persons who express suicidal feelings, the nurse's first responsibility is to ensure their safety. The nurse must take any suicidal remarks seriously and not leave the young persons alone until the degree of suicidality is assessed. A mnemonic for the assessment process is SLAP: specificity, lethality, accessibility, and proximity. The first step (specificity) is to ask adolescents whether they feel suicidal or as though they would like to take their own life. If so, have they chosen a means of suicide, and do they have a specific plan? The second stage of assessment (lethality) involves determining the lethality of the methods available to them. Do they plan to use a gun or knife? Have they chosen highly lethal medications, hanging, or carbon monoxide poisoning? The third stage (accessibility) involves determining the availability of the means of suicide, and the fourth stage (proximity) involves assessing whether they have determined a time to commit suicide and when.

Confidentiality cannot be honored in the case of self-destructive behaviors. The nurse must report suicidal behaviors to the family and other professionals and should inform the adolescent that this will be done. Such action conveys an important message to the adolescent—that the nurse understands and cares about his or her safety.

The nurse's demonstration of understanding and caring is extremely therapeutic. Adolescents have a deep need to be normal and will only feel more depressed and suicidal if they are stigmatized. Expressing a commitment to keep them safe until they no longer feel so terribly sad and assuring them that they will indeed feel better with time are helpful nursing actions. A person who feels extremely suicidal will welcome the security of being restrained if it is presented as an act of care, not punishment. Feeling actively suicidal is a frightening experience, and the adolescent should not be left alone. By demonstrating care, open communication, and understanding, the nurse is modeling appropriate behavior for the young person's family. Time spent listening to family members and helping them understand will reduce the incidence of future suicidal actions.

The attempted and, especially, the completed suicide of an adolescent is a major family crisis. In an attempted suicide the family and teenager have an opportunity to obtain help. Because these families are often already in conflict and at risk, nurses play an important role in referring them to appropriate mental health services. They should stress to parents the seriousness of the attempt and that this crisis offers the opportunity to avoid the tragedy of completed suicide. (See Care of the Family Experiencing Unexpected Childhood Death, Chapter 23.)

KEY POINTS

- Obesity in adolescence is a significant risk factor for adult obesity.
- Diet, exercise, and behavior modification are the hallmarks of treatment for obesity.
- The nurse's involvement in obesity control includes nutritional counseling, behavior therapy, group programs, and family counseling.
- AN, a disorder characterized by severe weight loss in the absence of obvious physical cause, consists of three areas of disordered psychologic functioning: disturbed body image and body concept of delusional proportions, inaccurate and confused perception and interpretation of inner stimuli, and a paralyzing sense of ineffectiveness that pervades all aspects of daily life.
- Therapeutic management of AN involves reinstitution of normal nutrition or reversal of malnutrition, resolution of the disturbed patterns of family interaction, and individual psychotherapy to correct distortions in psychologic functioning.
- Individuals with BN can be classified into two categories: (1) those who consume vast quantities of food followed by purging but who, if unable to purge, still consume large amounts; and (2) those who restrict their caloric intake, especially when unable to purge.
- Smoking tobacco is a declining problem among teenagers, but tobacco, binge drinking, marijuana, and other drug use are ongoing concerns. Reasons for substance use include social pressures, mass media influence, and attempts to cope with stress.
- Substance abuse can be a severe problem in adolescence; abusers include experimenters and compulsive users.
- Common types of drugs abused include alcohol, inhalants, hallucinogens, narcotics, central nervous system depressants, and central nervous system stimulants.
- Suicide, the deliberate act of self-injury with the intent to kill, may occur in adolescents because of psychiatric disorders, primarily depression; family discord; and difficulties in coping with stress.
- Suicide is much more likely to occur if the adolescent has access to a firearm or has been drinking alcohol or using drugs.

REFERENCES

Adelman WP, Duggan AK, Hauptman P, et al: Effectiveness of a high school smoking cessation program, *Pediatrics* 107(4):e50, 2001.

Al Mamun A, Alati R, O'Callaghan M, et al: Does childhood sexual abuse have an effect on young adults' nicotine disorder (dependence or withdrawal)? Evidence from a birth cohort study, *Addiction* 102(4):647-654, 2007.

American Academy of Pediatrics: Active healthy living: prevention of childhood obesity through increased physical activity, *Pediatrics* 117(5):1834-1842, 2006.

American Academy of Pediatrics, Committee on Adolescence: Identifying and treating eating disorders, *Pediatrics* 111(1):204-211, 2003.

American Foundation for Suicide Prevention: Report on suicide: recommendations for the media, New York. 2009, The Foundation, available at www.afsp.org/index.cfm?page_id= 0523D365_A314-431E-A925C03E13E762B1 (accessed September 14, 2009).

American Psychiatric Association: *Diagnostic and statistical manual of mental disorders,* ed 4 (text revision) (DSM-IV-TR), Washington, DC, 2000, The Association.

Angold A, Costello EJ, Erkanli A: Cormorbidity, *J Child Psychol Psychiatr* 40(1):57-87, 1999.

Angulo P: Nonalcoholic fatty liver disease, *N Engl J Med* 346(16):1221-1231, 2002.

Arenz S, Ruckerl R, Koletzko B, et al: Breastfeeding and childhood obesity: a systematic review, *Int J Obes Relat Metab Disord* 28:1247-1256, 2004.

Austin SB, Ziyadeh N, Fisher LB, et al: Sexual orientation and tobacco use in a cohort study of US adolescent girls and boys, *Arch Pediatr Adolesc Med* 158(4):317-322, 2004.

Avena NM: Binge eating: neurochemical insights from animal models. *Eat Disord* 17(1):89-92, 2009.

Baer JS, Barr HM, Brookstein FL, et al: Prenatal alcohol exposure and family history of alcoholism in the etiology of adolescent alcohol problems, *J Stud Alcohol* 59(5):533-543, 1998.

Baker S, Barlow S, Cochran W, et al: Overweight children and adolescents: a clinical report of the North American Society for Pediatric Gastroenterology, Hepatology and Nutrition, *J Pediatr Gastroenterol Nutr* 40:533-543, 2005.

Barlow SE, Expert Committee: Expert Committee recommendations regarding the prevention, assessment, and treatment of child and adolescent overweight and obesity: summary report, *Pediatrics* 120(Suppl 4):S164-S192, 2007.

Beaty TH: Invited commentary: two studies of genetic control of birth weight where large data sets were available, *Am J Epidemiol* 165: 753-755, 2007.

Becker AE, Grinspoon SK, Klibanski A, et al: Eating disorders, *N Engl J Med* 340(14):1092-1098, 1999.

Bertrand LD, Abernathy TJ: Predicting cigarette smoking among adolescents using cross-sectional and longitudinal approaches, *J Sch Health* 63(2):98-103, 1993.

Blum K, Noble EP, Sheridan PJ, et al: Allelic association of human dopamine D2 receptor gene in alcoholism, *JAMA* 263(15):2055-2060, 1990.

Boney C, Verma A, Tucker R, et al: Metabolic syndrome in childhood: association with birth weight, maternal obesity, and gestational diabetes mellitus, *Pediatrics* 115:290-296, 2005.

Bouchard C: Childhood obesity: are genetic differences involved? *Am J Clin Nutr* 89(5):1494S-1501S, 2009.

Bremer AA, Auinger P, Byrd RS: Relationship between insulin resistance–associated metabolic parameters and anthropometric measurements with sugar-sweetened beverage intake and physical activity levels in US adolescents: findings from the 1999-2004 National Health and Nutrition Examination Survey, *Arch Pediatr Adolesc Med* 163(4): 328-335, 2009.

Carlson S, Iacono W, McGue M: P300 amplitude in adolescent twins concordant and discordant for alcohol use disorders, *Biol Psychol* 61:203-227, 2002.

Centers for Disease Control and Prevention, National Center for Injury Prevention and Control: Web-based Injury Statistics Query and Reporting System (WISQARS), injury mortality data, 2006, available at www.cdc.gov/ncipc/wisqars.2009 (accessed June 12, 2009).

Centers for Disease Control and Prevention: Youth Risk Behavior Surveillance—United States, 2007, *MMWR* 57(SS-4):1-31, 2008.

Chassin L, Presson CC, Sherman SJ: Adolescent cigarette smoking: a commentary and issues for pediatric psychology, *J Pediatr Psychol* 30(4):299-303, 2005.

Chial HJ, McAlpine DE, Camilleri M: Anorexia nervosa: manifestations and management for the gastroenterologist, *Am J Gastroenterol* 97(2):257-269, 2002.

Chu YT, Chen WY, Wang TN, et al: Extreme BMI predicts higher asthma prevalence and is associated with lung function impairment in

school-aged children, *Pediatr Pulmonol* 44(5):472-479, 2009.

Croll J, Neumark-Sztainer D, Story M, et al: Prevalence and risk and protective factors related to disordered eating behaviors among adolescents: relationship to gender and ethnicity, *J Adolesc Health* 31(2):166-175, 2002.

Dare C, Eisler I: Family therapy for anorexia nervosa. In Garner DM, Garfinkel PE, editors: *Handbook of psychotherapy for anorexia nervosa and bulimia*, ed 2, New York, 1997, Guilford Press.

D'Augelli AR: High tobacco use among lesbian, gay, and bisexual youth: mounting evidence about a hidden population's health risk behavior, *Arch Pediatr Adolesc Med* 158(4):310-311, 2004.

Davis DM, Gance-Cleveland B, Hassink S, et al: Recommendations for prevention of childhood obesity, *Pediatrics* 120:S229-S253, 2007.

De Bellis MD: Developmental traumatology: a contributory mechanism for alcohol and substance abuse disorders, *Psychoneuroendocrinology* 27:155-170, 2002.

Devlin MJ, Goldfein JA, Dobrow I: What is this thing called BED? Current status of binge eating disorder nosology, *Int J Eat Disord* 34:S2-S18, 2003.

Dexheimer-Pharris M, Resnick MD, Blum RW: Protecting against hopelessness and suicidality in sexually abused American Indian adolescents, *J Adolesc Health* 21(6):400-406, 1997.

Dietz WH: Health consequences of obesity in youth: childhood predictors of adult disease, *Pediatrics* 101(3 Suppl):518-525, 1998.

Eddy KT, Celio Doyle A, Hoste RR, et al: Eating disorder not otherwise specified in adolescents. *J Am Acad Child Adolesc Psychiatry* 47(2):156-164, 2008.

Ehtisham S, Barrett TG, Shaw NJ: Type 2 diabetes mellitus in UK children: an emerging problem, *Diabetes Med* 17(12):867-871, 2000.

Eisler I, Le Grange D, Asen E: Family interventions. In Treasure J, Schmidt U, Van Furth E, editors. *Handbook of eating disorders*, Chichester, United Kingdom, 2003, John Wiley & Sons.

Escobedo LG, Reddy M, DuRant RH: Relationship between cigarette smoking and health risk and problem behaviors among US adolescents, *Arch Pediatr Adolesc Med* 151(1):66-71, 1997.

Ewing JA: The CAGE questionnaire for detection of alcoholism: a remarkably simple but useful tool, *JAMA* 300(17):2054-2056, 2008.

Fagot-Campagna A, Narayan KMV, Imperatore G: Type 2 diabetes in children: exemplifies the growing problem of chronic diseases. *BMJ* 322:377-378, 2001.

Farooqi IS, Jebb SA, Langmark G, et al: Effects of recombinant leptin therapy in a child with congenital leptin deficiency, *N Engl J Med* 341(12):879-884, 1999.

Feldman M, Friedman LS, Sleisenger MH: Obesity: a historical perspective and disease prevalence estimates. In Feldman M, Friedman LS, Sleisenger MH, editors,

Sleisenger and Fordtran's gastrointestinal and liver disease, ed 7, Philadelphia, 2002, Saunders.

Flay BR, Hu FB, Siddiqui O, et al: Differential influence of parental smoking and friends' smoking on adolescent initiation and escalation of smoking, *J Health Soc Behav* 35(3):248-265, 1994.

Foreman SF: Eating disorders: epidemiology, pathogenesis, and clinical features, *UpToDate*, 2009, available at www.uptodate.com (accessed December 2009).

Freemark M, Bursey D: The effects of metformin on body mass index and glucose tolerance in obese adolescents with fasting hyperinsulinemia and a family history of type 2 diabetes, *Pediatrics* 107(4):e55, 2001.

Fulkerson JA, Neumark-Sztainer D, Hannan PJ, et al: Family meal frequency and weight status among adolescents: cross-sectional and 5-year longitudinal associations, *Obesity* 16(11): 2529-2534, 2008.

Gable S, Chang Y, Krull JL: Television watching and frequency of family meals are predictive of overweight onset and persistence in a national sample of school-aged children, *J Am Diet Assoc* 107(1):53-61, 2007.

Garn SM, Clark DC: Trends in fatness and the origins of obesity, *Pediatrics* 57(4):443-456, 1976.

Gibbons RD, Brown CH, Hur K, et al: Early evidence on the effects of regulators' suicidality warnings on SSRI prescriptions and suicide in children and adolescents, *Am J Psychiatry* 164(9):1356-1363, 2007.

Gibson RS: Anthropometric assessment of body composition. In Gibson RS, editor: *Principles of nutritional assessment*, ed 2, New York, 2005, Oxford University Press.

Goodman E, Capitman J: Depressive symptoms and cigarette smoking among teens, *Pediatrics* 106(4):748-755, 2000.

Gossop M, Griffiths P, Powis B, et al: Cocaine: patterns of use, route of administration, and severity of dependence, *Br J Psychiatry* 164(5):660-664, 1994.

Gould MS, King R, Greenwald S, et al: Psychopathology associated with suicidal ideation and attempts among children and adolescents, *J Am Acad Child Adolesc Psychiatr* 37(9):915-923, 1998.

Gould MS, Marrocco FA, Kleinman M, et al: Evaluating iatrogenic risk of youth suicide screening programs, *JAMA* 295(13):1635-1643, 2005.

Greydanus DE, Pratt HD: Emotional and behavioral disorders of adolescence, part II, *Adolesc Health Update* 8(1):1-8, 1995.

Hagan JF, Shaw JS, Duncan PM, editors: *Bright futures: guidelines for health supervision of infants, children and adolescents*, ed 3, Elk Grove Village, Ill, 2008, American Academy of Pediatrics.

Harder T, Bergmann R, Kallischnigg G, et al: Duration of breastfeeding and risk of overweight: a meta-analysis, *Am J Epidemiol* 162:397-403, 2005.

Hardy LR, Harrell JS, Bell RA: Overweight in children: definitions, measurements, confounding factors, and health consequences, *J Pediatr Nurs* 19(6):376-383, 2004.

Harrison PA, Fulkerson JA, Beebe TJ: Multiple substance use among adolescent physical and sexual abuse victims, *Child Abuse Negl* 21:529-539, 1997.

Heinig MJ, Nommsen LA, Peerson JM, et al: Intake and growth of breast-fed and formula-fed infants in relation to the timing of introduction of complementary foods: the DARLING study, *Acta Paediatr* 82:999-1006, 1993.

Herpertz-Dahlmann, B: Adolescent eating disorders: definitions, symptomatology, epidemiology and comorbidity. *Child Adolesc Psychiatr Clin North Am* 18(1):31-47, 2009.

Hill JO, Wyatt HR, Reed GW, et al: Obesity and the environment: where do we go from here? *Science* 299(5608):853-855, 2003.

Hoffmann JP, Su SS: Parental substance use disorder, mediating variables and adolescent drug use: a non-recursive model, *Addiction* 93(9):1351-1364, 1998.

Horn KA, Dino GA, Kaselkar ID, et al: Appalachian teen smokers: not on tobacco 15 months later, *Am J Pub Health* 94(2):181-184, 2004.

Hu FB, Flak BR, Hedeker D, et al: The influences of friends' and parental smoking on adolescent smoking behavior: the effects of time and prior smoking, *J Appl Soc Psychol* 25(22):2018-2047, 1995.

Hudson JI, Hiripi E, Pope HG Jr, et al: The prevalence and correlates of eating disorders in the National Comorbidity Survey Replication, *Biol Psychiatry* 61(3):348-358, 2007.

Hudson JI, Laird NM, Betensky RA, et al: Multivariate logistic regression for familial aggregation of two disorders, part II, Analysis of studies of eating and mood disorders, *Am J Epidemiol* 153(5):506-514, 2001.

Iannotti RJ, Kogan MD, Janssen I, et al: Patterns of adolescent physical activity, screen-based media use, and positive and negative health indicators in the U.S. and Canada, *J Adolesc Health* 44(5):493-499, 2009.

Imhof A, Kratzer W, Boehm B, et al: Prevalence of non-alcoholic fatty liver and characteristics in overweight adolescents in the general population, *Eur J Epidemiol* 22:889-897, 2007.

Inge TH, Krebs NF, Garcia VF, et al: Bariatric surgery for severely overweight adolescents: concerns and recommendations, *Pediatrics* 114(1):217-223, 2004.

Institute of Medicine, Committee on Preventing Nicotine Addiction in Children and Youths, Lynch BS, Bonnie RJ, editors: *Growing up tobacco free*, Washington, DC, 1994, National Academy Press.

Janssen I, Craig WM, Boyce WF, et al: Association between overweight and obesity with bullying behaviors in school-aged children, *Pediatrics* 113(5):1187-1194, 2004.

Jaquet D, Swaminathan S, Alexander GR, et al: Significant paternal contribution to the risk of small for gestational age, *BJOG* 112:1539, 2005.

Jellinek MS, Snyder JB: Depression and suicide in children and adolescents, *Pediatr Rev* 19(8):255-264, 1998.

Jessor R: Risk behavior in adolescence: a psychosocial framework for understanding and action, *J Adolesc Health* 12:597-605, 1991.

Johnston LD, O'Malley PM, Bachman JG, et al: *Monitoring the Future national results on adolescent drug use: Overview of key findings, 2007*, NIH Pub No 08-6418, Bethesda, Md, 2008, National Institute on Drug Abuse.

Kain J, Corvalán C, Lera L, et al: Accelerated growth in early life and obesity in preschool Chilean children, *Obesity* 17(8):1603-1608, 2009.

Koeppen-Schomerus G, Wardle J, Plomin R: A genetic analysis of weight and overweight in 4 year old twin pairs, *Int J Obesity Related Metab Dis* 25(6):838-844, 2001.

Koplan JP, Liverman CT, Kraak VA: *Preventing childhood obesity: health in the balance*, Washington, DC, 2005, National Academy of Science.

Kosterman R, Hawkins JD, Guo J, et al: The dynamics of alcohol and marijuana initiation: patterns and predictors of first use in adolescence, *Am J Pub Health* 90(3):360-366, 2000.

Krueger RF, Hicks BM, Patrick CJ, et al: Etiologic connections among substance dependence, antisocial behavior, and personality: modeling the externalizing spectrum, *J Abnorm Psych* 111(3):411-424, 2002.

Latzer Y, Azaiza F, Tzischinsky O: Eating attitudes and dieting behavior among religious subgroups of Israeli-Arab adolescent females, *J Relig Health* 48(2):189-199, 2009.

Laucht M, Hohm E, Esser G, et al: Association between ADHD and smoking in adolescence: shared genetic, environmental, and psychopathological factors, *J Neural Transm* 114:1097-1104, 2007.

Lavine JE: Vitamin E treatment of nonalcoholic steatohepatitis in children: a pilot study, *J Pediatr* 136(6):734-738, 2000.

Le Grange D: The Maudsley family-based treatment for adolescent anorexia nervosa, *World Psychiatry* 4(3):142-146, 2005.

Leahy KE, Birch LL, Fisher JO, et al: Reductions in entrée energy density increase children's vegetable intake and reduce energy intake, *Obesity* 16(7):1559-1565, 2008.

Li C, Kaur H, Choi WS, et al: Additive interactions of maternal prepregnancy BMI and breast-feeding on childhood overweight, *Obesity Res* 13:362-371, 2005.

Lilenfeld LR, Kaye WH, Greeno CG, et al: A controlled family study of anorexia nervosa and bulimia nervosa: psychiatric disorders in first-degree relatives and effects of proband comorbidity, *Arch Gen Psychiatry* 55(7): 603-610, 1998.

Lobstein T, Baur L, Uauy R: Obesity in children and young people: a crisis in public health, *Obesity Rev* 5(Suppl 2):4-104, 2004.

Lock J, Fitzpatrick KK: Anorexia nervosa, *Clin Evid (Online)* March 10, 2009, pii:1011.

MacKenzie NR: Childhood obesity: strategies for prevention, *Pediatr Nurs* 26(5):527-530, 2000.

Marcus MD: Eating disorders. In Goldman L, Ausiello D, editors: *Cecil medicine*, ed 23, Philadelphia, 2007, Saunders/Elsevier.

Marshall M, Friedman M, Stall R, et al: Sexual orientation and adolescent substance use: a meta-analysis and methodological review, *Addiction* 103:546-556, 2008.

Martin JE, Dubbert PM, Katell AD, et al: Behavioral control of exercise in sedentary adults: studies 1 through 6, *J Consult Clin Psychol* 52:795-811, 1984.

Mikhail C: Anorexia nervosa and bulimia nervosa. In Lifschitz CH, editor: *Pediatric gastroenterology and nutrition in clinical practice*, New York, 2001, Marcel Dekker.

Mirza NM, Davis MS, Yanovski J: Body dissatisfaction, self-esteem, and overweight among inner-city Hispanic children and adolescents. *J Adolesc Health* 36(3):267, 2005 (e16-e20).

Moolchan ET, Ernst M, Henningfield JE: A review of tobacco smoking in adolescents: treatment implications, *J Am Acad Child Adolesc Psychiatr* 39(6):682-693, 2000.

Morgan JF, Reid F, Lacey JH: The SCOFF questionnaire: assessment of a new screening tool for eating disorders, *BMJ* 319(7223): 1467-1468, 1999.

Morrison SF, Rogers PD, Thomas MH: Alcohol and adolescents, *Pediatr Clin North Am* 42(2):371-387, 1995.

Mulye TP, Park MJ, Nelson CD, et al: Trends in adolescent and young adult health in the United States, *J Adolesc Health*, 45:8-24, 2009.

Muris P, Meesters C, van de Blom W, et al: Biological, psychological, and sociocultural correlates of body change strategies and eating problems in adolescent boys and girls, *Eating Behaviors* 6:11-22, 2005.

Must A, Anderson SE: Effects of obesity on morbidity in children and adolescents, *Nutr Clin* 6(1):4-11, 2003.

Myers SE, Carrel AL, Whitman BY, et al: Sustained benefit after 2 years of growth hormone on body composition, fat utilization, physical strength and agility and growth in Prader-Willi syndrome, *J Pediatr* 137:42-49, 2000.

Nadler EP, Youn HA, Ren CJ, et al: An update on 73 US obese pediatric patients treated with laparoscopic adjustable gastric banding: comorbidity resolution and compliance data, *J Pediatr Surg* 43(1):141-146, 2008.

National Institute for Health Care Management Foundation: *Childhood obesity: advancing effective prevention and treatment: an overview for health professionals, prepared for National Institute for Health Care Management Foundation Forum*, Washington, DC, April 9, 2003.

Neumark-Sztainer DN: Childhood and adolescent obesity: an ecological perspective, *Pediatr Basics* 101(1):12-20, 2003.

Neumarker KJ: Mortality and sudden death in anorexia nervosa, *Int J Eat Disord* 21:205-212, 1997.

Norris ML: HEADSS up: adolescents and the internet, *Paediatr Child Health* 12(3):211-216, 2007.

Ogden CL, Carroll MD, Flegal KM: High body mass index for age among US children and adolescents, 2003-2006, *JAMA* 299(20):2401-2405, 2008.

Ogden CL, Kuczmarski RJ, Flegal KM, et al: Centers for Disease Control and Prevention 2000 growth charts for the United States: improvements to the 1977 National Center for Health Statistics version, *Pediatrics* 109(1):141-142, 2002.

Ogden CL, Troiano RP, Briefel RR, et al: Prevalence of overweight among preschool children in the United States, 1971 through 1994, *Pediatrics* 99(4):e1, 1997.

Olshansky SJ: Projecting the future of U.S. health and longevity, *Health Aff* 24(Suppl 2W5R): 86-89, 2005.

Oman RF, Vesley S, Aspy CB, et al: The potential protective effect of youth assets on adolescent alcohol and drug use, *Am J Pub Health* 94(8):1425-1430, 2004.

Owen CG, Martin RM, Whincup PH, et al: Effect of infant feeding on the risk of obesity across the life course: a quantitative review of published evidence, *Pediatrics* 115:1367-1377, 2005.

Parkes S, Saewyc EM, Cox DN, et al: The relationship between body image and stimulant use among Canadian adolescents, *J Adolesc Health* 43(6):616-618, 2008.

Patten CA, Choi WS, Gillin JC, et al: Depressive symptoms and cigarette smoking predict development and persistence of sleep problems in US adolescents, *Pediatrics* 106(2):e23, 2000.

Patton GC, Viner R: Pubertal transitions in health, *Lancet* 369(9567)1130-1139, 2007.

Patton HM, Sirlin C, Behling C, et al: Pediatric nonalcoholic fatty liver disease: a critical appraisal of current data and implications for future research, *J Pediatr Gastroenterol Nutr* 43(4):413-427, 2006.

Patton LH: Adolescent substance abuse, *Pediatr Clin North Am* 42(2):283-293, 1995.

Pieper MH, Pieper WJ: It's not tough, it's tender love: problem teens need compassion that the "tough love" approach to childrearing doesn't offer them, *Child Welfare* 71:369-377, 1992.

Pirpiris M, Jackson KR, Farng E, et al: Body mass index and Blount disease, *J Pediatr Orthop* 26:659-663, 2006.

Powers PS, Bruty H: Pharmacotherapy for eating disorders and obesity. *Child Adolesc Psychiatr Clin North Am* 18(1):175-187, 2009.

Preti A, Girolamo GD, Vilagut G, et al: The epidemiology of eating disorders in six European countries: results of the ESEMeD-WMH project, *J Psychiatr Res* 43(14):1125-1132, 2009.

Rao G: Insulin resistance syndrome, *Am Fam Physician* 63(6):1159-1166, 2001.

Resnick MD, Bearman PS, Blum RW, et al: Protecting adolescents from harm: findings from the National Study on Adolescent Health, *JAMA* 278(10):823-832, 1997.

Roberts DF, Foehr UG, Rideout V: *Generation M: media in the lives of 8-18 year olds*, Menlo Park, Calif, 2006, Kaiser Family Foundation.

Robinson TN: Obesity prevention in primary care, *Arch Pediatr Adolesc Med* 160(2):217-218, 2006.

Robinson TN: Television viewing and childhood obesity, *Pediatr Clin North Am* 48:1017-1025, 2001.

Robinson TN: Reducing children's television viewing to prevent obesity: a randomized controlled trial, *JAMA* 282:1561-1567, 1999.

Rome ES, Ammerman S, Rosen DS, et al: Children and adolescents with eating disorders: the state of the art, *Pediatrics* 111(1):e98-e108, 2003.

Rosenfield RL, Lipton RB, Drum ML: Thelarche, pubarche, and menarche attainment in children with normal and elevated body mass index, *Pediatrics* 123(1):84-88, 2009.

Russell ST, Joyner K: Adolescent sexual orientation and suicide risk: evidence from a national study, *Am J Pub Health* 91:1276-1281, 2001.

Ryan C, Huebner D, Diaz RM, et al: Family rejection as a predictor of negative health outcomes in white and Latino lesbian, gay, and bisexual young adults, *Pediatrics* 123: 346-352, 2009.

Saewyc E: Substance abuse among non-mainstream youth. *In Substance abuse in Canada: focus on youth,* Ottawa, 2007, Canadian Centre on Substance Abuse.

Saewyc EM, Skay CL, Hynds P, et al. Suicidal ideation and attempts among adolescents in North American school-based surveys: are bisexual youth at increasing risk? *J LGBT Health Res* 3:25-36, 2007.

Sargent JD, Dalton M: Does parental disapproval of smoking prevent adolescents from becoming established smokers? *Pediatrics* 108(6):1256-1262, 2001.

Scheier LM, Newcomb MD, Skager R: Risk protection, and vulnerability to adolescent drug use: latent-variable models of three age groups, *J Drug Educ* 24(1):49-82, 1994.

Schmidt, U: Cognitive behavioral approaches in adolescent anorexia and bulimia nervosa. *Child Adolesc Psychiatr Clin North Am* 18(1):145-157, 2009.

Schneider MB, Fisher MM: Anorexia and bulimia nervosa. In Hoekelman RA, editor: *Primary pediatric care,* ed 4, St Louis, 2001, Mosby.

Shaffer D, Gould MS, Fisher P, et al: Psychiatric diagnosis in child and adolescent suicide, *Arch Gen Psychiatr* 53:339-348, 1996.

Shain BN, Committee on Adolescence: Suicide and suicide attempts in adolescents, *Pediatrics* 120(3):669-676, 2007.

Smith A, Saewyc E, Albert M, et al: *Against the Odds: A Profile of Marginalized and Street-Involved Youth in BC,* Vancouver, 2007, McCreary Centre Society.

Smith A, Stewart D, Peled M, et al: *A picture of health: highlights of the 2008 British Columbia Adolescent Health Survey,* Vancouver, 2009, McCreary Centre Society.

Stein JA, Newcomb MD, Bentler PM: Initiation and maintenance of tobacco smoking: changing personality correlates in adolescence and young adulthood, *J Appl Soc Psychol* 26(2):160-187, 1996.

Strauss RS: Childhood obesity and self-esteem, *Pediatrics* 105(1):e15, 2000.

Strober M, Freeman R, Lampert C, et al: The association of anxiety disorders and obsessive-compulsive personality disorder with anorexia nervosa: evidence from a family study with discussion of nosological and neurodevelopmental implications. *Int J Eating Disorders* 40:S46-S51, 2007.

Swallen KC, Reither EN, Haas SA, et al: Overweight, obesity and health-related quality of life among adolescents: the national longitudinal study of adolescent health, *Pediatrics* 115(2):340-347, 2005.

Thompson CE, Wankel LM: The effects of perceived activity choice upon frequency of exercise behavior, *J Appl Soc Psychol* 10:436-443, 1980.

US Preventive Services Task Force: Screening for obesity in children and adolescents: US Preventive Services Task Force recommendation statement, *Pediatrics* 125(2):361-367, 2010.

US Surgeon General: *Overweight and Obesity: Health Consequences,* Rockville: Md, 2001, available at www.surgeongeneral.gov/topics/obesity/calltoaction/fact_consequences.htm (accessed April 25, 2009).

Utter J, Scragg R, Schaaf D, et al: Relationships between frequency of family meals, BMI and nutritional aspects of the home food environment among New Zealand adolescents, *Int J Behav Nutr Phys Act* 5:50, 2008.

Van den Eynde F, Treasure J: Neuroimaging in eating disorders and obesity: implications for research, *Child Adolesc Psychiatr Clin North Am* 18(1):95-115, 2009.

Varchol L, Cooper H: Psychotherapy approaches for adolescents with eating disorders, *Curr Opin Pediatr* 21(7):457-464, 2009.

Wakefield M, Terry-McElrath Y, Emery S, et al: Effect of televised, tobacco company–funded smoking prevention advertising on youth smoking-related beliefs, intentions, and behavior, *Am J Pub Health* 96(12):2154-2160, 2006.

West SL, O'Neal KK: Project D.A.R.E. outcome effectiveness revisited, *Am J Pub Health* 94(6):275-336, 2004.

White HR, Brick J, Hansell S: Longitudinal investigation of alcohol use and aggression in adolescence, *J Stud Alcohol* 11:62-77, 1993.

Whitlock EP, O'Connor EA, Williams SB, et al: Effectiveness of weight management interventions in children: a targeted systematic review for the USPSTF, *Pediatrics* 125(2):e396-e418, 2010.

Wilens TE, Faraone SV, Biederman J, et al: Does stimulant therapy of attention-deficit/hyperactivity disorder beget later substance abuse? A meta-analytic review of the literature, *Pediatrics* 111(1):179-185, 2003.

Wood E, Tyndall MW, Montaner JS, et al: Summary of findings from the evaluation of a pilot medically supervised safer injecting facility, *CMAJ* 175(11):1399-1404, 2006.

World Health Organization: Childhood obesity and overweight. Geneva, 2009, The Organization, available at www.who.int/dietphysicalactivity/childhood/en/index.html (accessed September 14, 2009).

Yanovski SZ, Yanovski JA: Obesity, *N Engl J Med* 346(8):591-602, 2002.

Yensel CS, Preud'Homme D, Curry DM: Childhood obesity and insulin-resistant syndrome, *J Pediatr Nurs* 19(4):238-246, 2004.

Yermilov I, McGory ML, Shekelle PW, et al: Appropriateness Criteria for Bariatric Surgery: Beyond the NIH Guidelines, *Obesity* 17(8):1521-1527, 2009.

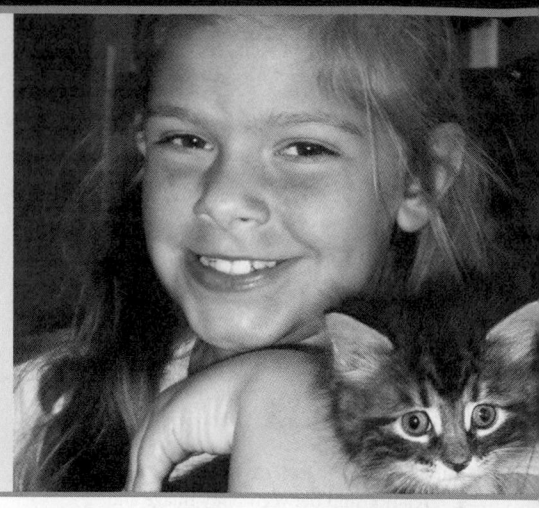

evolve WEBSITE

http://evolve.elsevier.com/wong/ncic
Key Points Audio Summaries
NCLEX Review Questions
Spanish/English Translations
WebLinks

RELATED TOPICS

Birth of a Child with a Physical Defect, **Ch. 11**
The Child with Cognitive, Sensory, or Communication
    Impairment, **Ch. 24**
Childhood Morbidity, **Ch. 1**
Communicating with Families, **Ch. 6**
Developmental Assessment, **Ch. 6**
Discharge Planning and Home Care (High-Risk Newborn), **Ch. 10**
Facilitating Parent-Infant Relationships (High-Risk
    Newborn), **Ch. 10**
Family-Centered Care, **Ch. 1**
Family-Centered Care of the Child During Illness and
    Hospitalization, **Ch. 26**
Family-Centered End-of-Life Care, **Ch. 23**
Family-Centered Home Care, **Ch. 25**
Family Structure, **Ch. 6**
Health Promotion: Infant, **Ch. 12;** Toddler, **Ch. 14;** Preschooler,
    Ch. 15; School-Age Child, **Ch. 17;** Adolescent, **Ch. 19**
School Phobia, **Ch. 18**
Social, Cultural, and Religious Influences on Child Health
    Promotion, **Ch. 2**

CHAPTER OUTLINE

PERSPECTIVES IN THE CARE OF CHILDREN WITH SPECIAL NEEDS

SCOPE OF THE PROBLEM

Significant changes in the health care system have increased the need for services and benefits to children with chronic illness or disability (Stein, Shenkman, Wegener, et al, 2003). A major obstacle in the effort to provide these services has been the issue of how best to define populations of children with chronic conditions. For many years a number of terms have been used to classify and describe children with special health care needs (Box 22-1).

More recently there has been a drive to develop a definition of children with special health care needs that could be used by federal and state programs to facilitate planning of comprehensive, family-centered, community-based services for this population (Jackson, 2009; Beers, Kemeny, Sherritt, et al, 2003; Miller, Recsky, and Armstrong, 2004). To date, children with special health care needs, as defined by the federal Maternal and Child Health Bureau (Msall, Avery, Tremont, et al, 2003), are "children who have or are at increased risk for a chronic physical, behavioral, developmental, or emotional condition and who also require health and related services of a type or amount beyond that required by children in general."

Each year in the United States, 6 million children ranging from newborns to 17-year-olds are hospitalized for a variety of conditions, and the average length of stay for those patients is approximately $3\frac{1}{2}$ days (Weiner, 2008). Advances in biomedical science and technology have resulted in dramatic improvement in the health care of pediatric chronic conditions (Varni, Limbers, and Burwinkle, 2007). There is now improved management of infectious diseases, identification of children with previously unrecognized illnesses, and implementation of preventive and public health measures (Jackson, 2009). With these medical advances and decreasing patient lengths of stay, many more patients are requiring care in the home setting. The burden of care is then carried by the family and outpatient care facilities to provide services required.

For example, the median life expectancy of children with cystic fibrosis today is more than 30 years, in contrast to 5 years in 1955. In 1955, 90% of children born with spina bifida died in infancy. Today 90% survive infancy and have a normal life expectancy if they have appropriate and timely medical intervention such as improved surgical advances and management of urinary tract infections (Jackson, 2009). In addition, advances in combination antiretroviral therapy have resulted in a decreased mortality rate for children infected with human immunodeficiency virus (HIV) (Fahrner and Mario, 2009; Yogev and Chadwick, 2007). Infants with very low birth weight and extreme prematurity are living longer (Jackson, 2009), and more than 80% of children diagnosed with cancer today will be cured of their disease (Gurney and Bondy, 2010; Horner, Ries, Krapcho, et al, 2008).

The dramatic decline in mortality rates has led to an increase in the number of children with special health care needs and has implications for the provision of comprehensive, long-term health care services for these patients (Jackson, 2009; Palfrey and Richmond, 2005). Chronic illness has surpassed acute illness as the major health concern for children (Perrin, Bloom, and Gortmaker, 2007). In the United States an estimated 18% of children (12.6 million) have a chronic illness or disability that requires health care services beyond those usually required by children (Perrin, Bloom, and Gortmaker, 2007; Arango, 2005; Newacheck, McManus, Fox, et al, 2000).

The most common chronic childhood conditions causing disability are respiratory diseases (primarily asthma), impairments of speech and sensory functions, and mental and nervous system disorders (Arango, 2005). Asthma is the single most prevalent cause of disability in children and has been largely responsible for much of the recent increase in childhood disability. Mental and nervous system disorders account for about one sixth of all childhood disability. The prevalence of disability is higher in boys, in children older than 5 years of age, and in children from single-parent and low-income families (Newacheck and Halfon, 2000; Schiller, Adams, and Nelson, 2005).

The impact of chronic illness and disability on children's health and functional status is profound. Children with disabilities spend three times as many days ill in bed and days absent from school as other children. They make 26 million more visits per year to the physician than typical children and spend 5 million more days in the hospital annually (Arango, 2005). They are limited in their daily activities for slightly more than 2 weeks each year, and one tenth of all children with disabilities are unable to play or attend school (Arango, 2005). In addition, children with disabilities are more likely to be a victim of emotional or sexual abuse, have behavioral problems, drop out of school, and be involved in the juvenile justice system than are their peers without disabilities (Perrin, Bloom, and Gortmaker, 2007).

BOX 22-1	KEY TERMS RELATING TO CHILDREN WITH SPECIAL HEALTH CARE NEEDS

Chronic illness—A condition that interferes with daily functioning for more than 3 months in a year, causes hospitalization of more than 1 month in a year, or (at the time of diagnosis) is likely to do either of these

Congenital disability—A disability that has existed since birth but is not necessarily hereditary

Developmental delay—A maturational lag; an abnormal, slower rate of development in which a child demonstrates a functioning level below that observed in normal children of the same age

Developmental disability—Any mental and/or physical disability that is manifested before age 22 years and is likely to continue indefinitely

Disability—A long-term reduction in the child's ability to engage in day-to-day activities (e.g., playing, attending school) because of a chronic condition

Handicap—A condition or barrier imposed by society, the environment, or one's own self; not a synonym for disability

Impairment—A loss or abnormality of structure or function

Technology-dependent child—A child between the ages of birth and 21 years with a chronic disability that requires the routine use of a medical device to compensate for the loss of a life-sustaining bodily function; requires daily ongoing care and/or monitoring by trained personnel

Modified from Westbrook LE, Silver EJ, Stein RE: Implications for estimates of disability in children: a comparison of definitional components, *Pediatrics* 101(6):1025-1030, 1998; and Newacheck PW, Halfon N: Prevalence and impact of disabling chronic conditions in childhood, *Am J Public Health* 88(4):610-617, 1998.

Chronic illness and disability have substantial effects on family functioning. Chronic conditions present most families with additional tasks, responsibilities, and concerns such as the additional caretaking needs of the child, identification of and access to educational and medical services, payment for services, uncertainty about the future, emotional grieving, stigmatizing reactions from the community, social isolation, and lost social opportunities. These demands can be grouped according to their personal impact on a parent, the financial impact on the family, and the impact on social and family relationships.

Parents are caught in a juggling act of meeting their child's normal growth and development needs and dealing with the consequences of the chronic illness (Sullivan-Bolyai, Knafl, Sadler, et al, 2004). Parents of children with disabilities are more likely to report depression than parents of children without disabilities (Sullivan-Bolyai, Sadler, Knafl, et al, 2003). Family members of children with disabilities are more likely to experience behavioral and psychologic symptoms. Parents may miss days from work, experience financial strain, and be challenged both physically and emotionally while they deal with caring for a child with a chronic illness or disability. Siblings may experience a wide range of feeling and concerns and often have to identify and deal with these concerns in the absence of the parent, who is either physically separated or emotionally unavailable to the well sibling (Pearson, 2005). Frequently, siblings' lives reflect the routines imposed by the affected child's chronic condition.

The increased prevalence of chronic illness and disability in children and the far-reaching effects on the child and family members have many implications for nursing. Nurses need to take an active role in early screening, case finding, and assessment and provide supportive and educational interventions that decrease the disruptive effects of the chronic condition on the child and family members. In addition, nurses should attempt to prevent disabling conditions by removing their known causes; this entails encouraging adherence with immunization programs, identifying infants and mothers at risk, recognizing the disability early, fostering injury prevention programs and policies, and providing innovative health education programs. Skilled case management is necessary to ensure that the family of a child with special needs has the support to successfully adapt to the consequences of the child's chronic condition. This includes providing community-based, comprehensive, and culturally appropriate care to the child with special needs (McPherson, Weissman, Strickland, et al, 2004).

TRENDS IN CARE

Because of advances in technology, economic effects, and the demand for more meaningful models of care, care has changed not only in the types of services and care children receive, but also in where services are provided and by whom.

Developmental Focus

Using a developmental approach rather than one based on chronologic age when caring for children with special health care needs helps the nurse to determine where children are at present and to understand their response to the chronic illness or disability. Developmental changes in the child continue despite the added stress of coping with a chronic illness. The chronic condition imposes a dimension of behavioral and developmental risk (Rittey, 2003). Because children with chronic conditions are more alike than different, a noncategorical approach emphasizing the commonalities of these children, rather than solely the illness, is beneficial. Referring to children by the names of their disabilities or illnesses affects professional and parental attitudes, as well as the assessment of the child's present abilities and future expectations (Green, 2003). Therefore parents and the health care team should work jointly for the benefit of the child who has an illness rather than allowing the illness to define the child. Knowledge of the developmental theory perspective is paramount in providing the support necessary for children to successfully adjust to a stressful life experience such as a chronic illness or disability.

Family Development

A developmental approach also includes an assessment of family development. The family life cycle focuses on the changing ages and developmental tasks of both children and adults and on the changing external demands as the family grows older. Families are expected to accomplish certain tasks at various stages (e.g., finding, furnishing, and maintaining their first home during the married couple stage). A diagnosis of chronic illness in a family member has a profound effect on every member of the family unit (Sullivan-Bolyai, Sadler, Knafl, et al, 2003). As with individual development, family development may be interrupted or even regress to a previous level of functioning. For example, having a child with a chronic illness may impose an added stress on the newly married couple who are in the midst of establishing a family identity. Nurses can apply family developmental theory when planning interventions for families of children with special health care needs. (See Developmental Theory, Chapter 3.)

Family-Centered Care

Family-centered care is paramount in the care of children with special health needs. Over the past 40 years significant changes have occurred in parents' responsibilities for providing and coordinating the care of their ill child. Today families of chronically ill children have comprehensive and complex caretaking responsibilities in the hospital and at home (Sullivan-Bolyai, Knafl, Sadler, et al, 2004).

The increasing numbers of chronically ill children and the families who are assuming the major burden of coordinating their children's care have reinforced the demand for new approaches in the health care system. The outcome has been the emergence of family-centered care to reflect, recognize, and facilitate the changing roles of families in care delivery. Because a cure is not likely for a number of chronic conditions, health care professionals must focus their efforts on care.

The federal legislation Public Law (PL) 99-457, which affords states the opportunity to extend the benefits of PL 94-142 (Education for All Handicapped Children Act of 1975) to children from birth to age 5 years, targets family-centered care. This legislation establishes a process whereby families become active participants in decision making about the care of their children.

The goal of care is to minimize the manifestations of the illness and maximize the child's cognitive, physical, and psychosocial potential. Advocating a family-centered approach to care facilitates attainment of this goal (Vessey and Mebane, 2009). (See Family-Centered Care, Chapter 1.) Integrating family-centered care in practice requires health professionals to (1) acknowledge and respect the family's individuality and strengths, (2) foster the family's competence and confidence in caring for the child, and (3) empower the family to advocate for the child when dealing with the health care system (Vessey and Mebane, 2009). In the family-centered framework, consistent attention is given to the effects of the child's chronic illness on all family members, not only on the affected child. This is paramount, because the best predictors of the well-being of children with special health needs include factors associated with family functioning.

As parents become knowledgeable about their child's special health needs, they frequently become experts in providing care. As part of the health care team, nurses are adjuncts in the child's care and need to build alliances with parents, respecting and drawing on their expertise. One of the key principles in family-centered care is the involvement of family members in decision making about their child's physical care. Collaboration—consistent sharing of information about the illness, responsibility, and decision making—is necessary to establish effective and trusting partnerships with parents.

Care conferences with the child's family and members of the health care team, including nurses, offer opportunities for mutual sharing of thoughts and concerns about the child's care. Being attentive the parent's observations helps assure them that their role is valued and their opinions important.

In fostering effective family-centered care, the nurse not only acknowledges that the family is a key component of the child's care and illness experience but also recognizes and respects the family's expertise in caring for the child within and outside of the hospital milieu. In the absence of the child's family during hospitalization, the nurse should try to maintain routines established by the family. In the family's presence, the nurse, child, and parent form a relationship in which the process of care negotiation occurs. This relationship is pivotal to the needs of the child and family and is where roles are defined and guidelines are developed. Through open communication, the nurse values the parents' roles by viewing them as the ultimate experts in caring for their child. Simultaneously the family looks to the nurse for empowerment, support, education, and expertise in caring for their child (Fazil, Wallace, Singh, et al, 2004; Sullivan-Bolyai, Knafl, Sadler, et al, 2004).

Normalization

Normalization refers to establishing a normal pattern of living (see Nursing Care Guidelines box, p. 855). Normalization occurs on several levels. It implies child and family access to services in as usual a fashion and environment as possible, with a focus placed on the home and community. Application of the principles of normalization means that daily routines for the child with illness or disability should be fitted to the family's schedule, rather than vice versa. Age-appropriate expectations for the child's behavior should be applied. As necessary, the environment should be structured to encourage the child's engagement in age-appropriate activities. Thus consequences of the illness are minimized, and the child and family live as normal a life as possible given the disability.

Nurses can facilitate the normalization process for families of children with special needs by acknowledging their normalcy, strengths, and weaknesses. Being supportive of the child's illness and treatment and actively including the family in all aspects of the care will improve their self-esteem and promote further development (Shepard and Mahon, 2009).

Home Care

Along with the trend toward normalization, there has also been a trend of earlier discharge of children from acute or chronic care facilities to the family and community. Home care refers to the return to a system and set of priorities whereby family values are as significant in the care of a child with a chronic illness as they are in the care of healthy children. The primary incentive for home care of children with special health needs was a parental need to keep these children at home and professionals' willingness to work with families to attain this goal. The goal of home care is to:

- Normalize the life of the child with special needs, including the child with technologically complex care, in a community and family setting
- Lessen the disruptive impact of the child's condition on the family
- Promote the child's maximum growth and development

With appropriate support and training, families today can accomplish complex treatments and procedures in the home. Parents are challenged to maintain a homelike setting in the midst of ventilators, monitors, and other sophisticated equipment. Throughout this text home care is discussed as appropriate for specific conditions. Chapter 25 focuses on family-centered home care; the process of transition from the hospital to the home setting is described in Chapter 26.

Mainstreaming

Mainstreaming refers to a process of integrating children with special needs into regular classrooms and child care centers. Attending school allows these children to acquire a sense of self and understanding of their place with respect to their peers. It also provides important opportunities for socialization with nondisabled children, which enables the latter group to develop respect for and acceptance of their peers with special needs. A crucial developmental task for children 5 years of age and older is to move beyond the family environment into the school community, where social competence, academic achievement, and regular attendance are important goals (Vessey and Jackson, 2009). A variety of supplemental programs exist in the school system to accommodate children with special needs and thereby afford them equal educational opportunity.

For the most part this change facilitating normalization for these children has resulted from the passage of PL 94-142, the Education for All Handicapped Children Act of 1975, which provides children with "free and appropriate public education," including special education and related services, rendered at public expense, under public supervision, and without charge, that meet the standards of the state educational agency (Vessey and Jackson, 2009). The 1990 amendment to this law, PL 101-

476, changed the name of the act to the Individuals with Disabilities Education Act (IDEA). Passage of PL 101-476, along with current federal child care mandates and increasing public concern about child care, demonstrates a national commitment to the concept that early services are crucial if children with disabilities are to achieve their full potential. In December 2004 PL 108-446 was passed, resulting in a major reauthorization and revision of IDEA. This reauthorized state and local aid for special education and related services for children with disabilities, specifically in development and maintaining early intervention programs for infants and toddlers with disabilities.

PL 94-142 requires states to identify, diagnose, teach, and provide related services to children with disabilities from 5 to 18 years of age. In 1977 the age range was extended to include children 3 to 21 years of age, with services for children ages 3 to 5 years optional. In accordance with this law, a multidisciplinary team writes an individualized education program (IEP), which includes specific therapeutic and educational goals and strategies for each eligible child referred for special education. Parents may intervene in educational decisions and have the right to a hearing when they believe the team's decision is harmful or inappropriate. Because many parents are unaware of this or other laws providing rights for disabled children, it is imperative that nurses inform them of what the laws are and where to obtain information. Nurses may also be involved in formulating IEPs.

Early Intervention

Early intervention includes any systematic and sustained effort to assist young, disabled, and developmentally vulnerable children from birth to 3 years of age. PL 99-457, the Education of the Handicapped Act Amendments of 1986, directs states to develop and enact statewide coordinated, comprehensive, multidisciplinary interagency programs of early intervention services for infants and toddlers with disabilities, in addition to support services for their families.

An important component of the law's implementation is the individualized family service plan (IFSP). As a product of collaboration between professionals and families, the IFSP consists of information relating to the infant's or toddler's current level of development, family needs and strengths for improving development, main outcomes anticipated, services required, designation of a case manager, and transition steps to preschool services. All outcomes and services concern the needs of the child and family. The IFSP represents a commitment to families and children that their strengths will be acknowledged and built on, that their needs will be satisfied in a manner that respects their values and beliefs, and that their aspirations will be fostered and empowered.

Nurses can provide many services for children covered by PL 99-457. Implementation of family-centered care and clinical expertise in practice provide nurses with a role in early identification and assessment of children at risk for disability, in multidisciplinary assessment, and in case management. Nurses can assess children in preschool settings, implement ongoing staff and patient education, coordinate care with the heath care team, become actively involved in community nursing networks, and develop health promotion programs for school personnel and family members.

Managed Care

Managed care health plans have become the primary form of health care coverage in the United States (Jackson, 2009; Smucker, 2001). An evaluation of out-of-pocket expenditures for insured versus uninsured children with special health care needs revealed higher out-of-pocket burden and financial problems among the uninsured (Jeffrey and Newacheck, 2006). Not only has managed care expanded rapidly, particularly for Medicaid-eligible patients, but the roles and responsibilities of state Title V programs for children with special health needs have changed as well (McPherson, Weissman, Strickland, et al, 2004; Inkelas, 2005). Provision of direct services by specialty clinics funded through Title V were reduced while managed care systems attempted to provide services to children within the managed care organization.

Implementing managed care for children with disabilities differs from providing care for adults with disabilities in three ways (McPherson, Weissman, Strickland, et al, 2004): (1) the changing dynamics of child development affect the needs of these children at various developmental stages and change their anticipated outcomes; (2) the prevalence and epidemiology of childhood disabilities, with few common conditions and many low-incidence or rare ones, vary considerably from those of adults, for whom there are many common conditions and few rare ones; and (3) because of children's need for adult guidance and protection, their development and health rely heavily on their families' socioeconomic status and health. These differences have implications for monitoring care provided to children with chronic conditions in managed care settings. The diverse effects of managed care on these children are seen in seven major domains: access to care, use of services, quality of care, satisfaction with care, cost of care, health outcomes, and family impact (Newacheck, Hung, and Wright, 2002; van Dyck, Kogan, Heppel, et al, 2004).

Families offer four basic suggestions for improving services for their children with chronic conditions: (1) reduce barriers to programs and services; (2) improve the quality of services; (3) improve the training given to families, health care professionals, and the community relating to chronic conditions and their management; and (4) increase the availability and quality of community-based services (van Dyck, Kogan, Heppel, et al, 2004). All of these suggestions require two factors: universality of care and adequate funding (Vessey and Jackson, 2009). Health care providers play an important role in working jointly with the leaders of managed care programs to ensure high-quality care for children with chronic conditions.

CULTURAL ISSUES

Increasing migration around the world in the past 10 years has led to heterogeneity in many nations, including the United States. For this reason, cultural competence is an important goal of nursing practice.

For many minority and ethnic populations, cultural understanding of disability and illness, social roles for disabled individuals, the structure of family life, and other factors associated with the perception of children vary from those of "mainstream" American culture. These factors may affect family choices regarding the care of the child with special needs.

Although culture cannot fully define how an individual will act and think, knowledge of cultural perspectives can assist nurses in anticipating and understanding why families make certain decisions. Cultural attributes, including beliefs and values concerning disability or illness and its causes, family structure, social roles for the disabled, the role of children, childrearing practices, spirituality, and time orientation, also influence a family's reaction to a chronic condition. Although eliciting health beliefs and negotiating interventions can be challenging, it is necessary for compliance, collaboration, patient/family satisfaction, and optimal care (see Nursing Care Guidelines box).

NURSING CARE GUIDELINES

Identifying Cultural Influences on Health Beliefs

Asking parents about the following perceptions can help identify cultural health beliefs:
- Perception of the cause of the illness
- Understanding of what the illness does to the child
- Perception of the seriousness or severity of the illness or disability
- Length of time the illness is expected to last
- Type(s) of treatment that the family would prefer to have used
- Results to be expected from the type(s) of treatment preferred
- Concerns or worries about the condition

Modified from Carrillo JE, Green AR, Betancourt JR: Cross-cultural primary care: a patient-based approach, *Ann Intern Med* 130(10):829-834, 1999.

Recognizing the growing cultural diversity in our society, nurses must incorporate cultural competence in their clinical practice to promote delivery of effective and sensitive care to children with chronic illness and their families. Care should be consistent with the cultural practices and beliefs of the child's family whenever possible; increasing cultural competence will improve communication and promote respect for human diversity (Rehm, 2009) (see Cultural Competence box).

 CULTURAL COMPETENCE

Using Interpreters

When parents who do not speak English are informed of their child's chronic illness, interpreters familiar with both their culture and language should be used. Children, family members, and friends of the family should not be used as translators because their presence may prevent parents from openly discussing the issues. In addition, accurate information translated by family members is at risk of being misinterpreted as a protective coping mechanism.

IMPACT OF CHRONIC ILLNESS OR DISABILITY ON THE CHILD

A child's reaction to chronic illness or disability depends largely on his or her developmental level. Knowledge of developmental stages is essential for nurses to understand how children interpret events. Because children's cognitive abilities change as they grow, they require varied explanations of their chronic illness as they mature. Normal development should occur in the context of the child's temperament, intelligence, motor skills, and relationships with family and friends. Identifying the child's coping strategies and promoting successful adaptation to the illness are essential. Factors influencing coping include the developmental stage, age, gender, type and duration of illness, and family cohesion (Schmidt, Petersen, and Bullinger, 2003). Caring for the child involves health education efforts, normalization principles, and assistance to the growing child in planning realistic future goals.

PROMOTING NORMAL DEVELOPMENT

Normative developmental tasks throughout childhood center on developing a sense of self and acquiring autonomy in all areas of life (Turkel and Pao, 2007). The impact of a chronic illness or disability on a child is affected by the child's age at the onset of the illness or disability (Vessey and Mebane, 2009). Chronic illness can affect children of all age-groups, although each age-group faces its own specific challenges. Children redefine their illness and its implications as they develop and grow. Accordingly, nurses must plan and implement care that promotes the child's successful progression from one stage of development to the next.

In addition to learning about the illness and its effects on the child's abilities, the family needs to acquire strategies to promote appropriate development in their child. Even with delays in achievement of developmental milestones, nurses need to be instrumental in teaching parents how best to help their child reach his or her developmental potential (Vessey and Mebane, 2009). Table 22-1 describes developmental aspects of chronic illness or disability in children and accompanying supportive interventions.

Infant

During infancy the child is establishing trust and learning about the environment through sensorimotor exploration (Vessey and Mebane, 2009). However, the diagnosis of a chronic illness, accompanied by a disruption in routines and physical discomfort, may compromise the dependability and consistency of an infant's environment and hinder the development of basic trust. Disability or chronic illness frequently impairs the child's motor abilities, restricting the child to a crib and decreasing contact with the environment. Illness may influence the infant's growth and developmental parameters by its effects on mobility, sleeping, feeding, and sensory functions. Separation of infant and parent as a result of frequent hospitalizations may prevent attachment and the emergence of a trusting relationship for the infant.

For the infant with a painful illness, exploration of his or her environment is restricted, which further curtails development (Vessey and Mebane, 2009). Messages transmitted to infants about their bodies are affected by the amount of pain and discomfort they experience. Associating pain with touch can lessen the infant's ability to give and receive affection. Lack of pleasant sensations can result in an irritable and unhappy child. Parents may interpret this behavior as indicative of their inadequacy in satisfying the child's emotional and physical needs, which further affects the parent-child relationship and the

TABLE 22-1	DEVELOPMENTAL ASPECTS OF CHRONIC ILLNESS OR DISABILITY IN CHILDREN	
DEVELOPMENTAL TASKS	**POTENTIAL EFFECTS OF CHRONIC ILLNESS OR DISABILITY**	**SUPPORTIVE INTERVENTIONS**
Infancy		
Develop a sense of trust	Multiple caregivers and frequent separations, especially if hospitalized	Encourage consistent caregivers in hospital or other care settings.
	Deprivation of consistent nurturing	Encourage parental presence, "rooming in" during hospitalization, and participation in care.
Bond or attach to parent	Delay in attachment because of separation; parental grief for loss of "dream" child; parental inability to accept the condition, especially a visible defect	Emphasize healthy, perfect qualities of infant. Help parents learn special care needs of infant so they will feel competent.
Learn through sensorimotor experiences	Increased exposure to painful experiences over pleasurable ones	Expose infant to pleasurable experiences through all senses (touch, hearing, sight, taste, movement).
	Limited contact with environment from restricted movement or confinement	Encourage age-appropriate developmental skills (e.g., bottle holding, finger feeding, crawling)
Begin to develop a sense of separateness from parent	Increased dependency on parent for care	Encourage all family members to participate in care to prevent overinvolvement of one member
	Overinvolvement of parent in care	Encourage periodic respite from demands of care responsibilities
Toddlerhood		
Develop autonomy	Increased dependency on parent	Encourage independence in as many areas as possible (e.g., toileting, dressing, feeding).
Master locomotor and language skills	Limited opportunity to test own abilities and limits	Provide gross motor skill activity and modification of toys or equipment, such as modified swing or rocking horse.
Learn through sensorimotor experience; begin to develop preoperational thought	Increased exposure to painful experiences	Give choices to allow simple feeling of control (e.g., choice of what book to look at, what kind of sandwich to eat).
		Institute age-appropriate discipline and limit setting.
		Recognize that negative and ritualistic behaviors are normal.
		Provide sensory experiences (e.g., water play, sandbox play, finger painting).
Preschool Age		
Develop initiative and purpose	Limited opportunities for success in accomplishing simple tasks or mastering self-care skills	Encourage mastery of self-help skills.
Master self-care skills		Provide devices that make task easier (e.g., self-dressing).
Begin to develop peer relationships	Limited opportunities for socialization with peers; may appear "like a baby" to age-mates	Encourage socialization (e.g., play dates with friends, daycare experience, trips to park). Provide age-appropriate play, especially associative play opportunities.
	Protection within tolerant and secure family, which may cause child to fear criticism and withdraw	Emphasize child's abilities; dress appropriately to enhance desirable appearance. Encourage relationships with same-sex and opposite-sex peers and adults.
Develop sense of body image and sexual identification	Awareness of body that may center on pain, anxiety, and failure	Help child deal with criticisms; realize that too much protection prevents child from facing realities of world.
	Sex-role identification focused primarily on mothering skills	Clarify that cause of child's illness or disability is not his or her fault or a punishment.
Learn through preoperational thought (magical thinking)	Guilt (thinking he or she caused the illness or disability or is being punished for wrongdoing)	
School Age		
Develop a sense of accomplishment	Limited opportunities to achieve and compete (e.g., many school absences, inability to join regular athletic activities)	Encourage school attendance; schedule medical visits at times other than school; encourage child to make up missed work. Educate teachers and classmates about child's condition, abilities, and special needs.
Form peer relationships	Limited opportunities for socialization	Encourage sports activities (e.g., Special Olympics).
Learn through concrete operations	Incomplete comprehension of the imposed physical limitations or treatment of the disorder	Encourage socialization (e.g., Girl Scouts, Campfire Girls, Boy Scouts, 4-H Club; club membership or association with peers). Provide child with knowledge about his or her condition. Encourage creative activities (e.g., VSA arts).

TABLE 22-1	DEVELOPMENTAL ASPECTS OF CHRONIC ILLNESS OR DISABILITY IN CHILDREN—cont'd	
DEVELOPMENTAL TASKS	**POTENTIAL EFFECTS OF CHRONIC ILLNESS OR DISABILITY**	**SUPPORTIVE INTERVENTIONS**
Adolescence		
Develop personal and sexual identity	Increased sense of feeling different from peers and less capability to compete with peers in appearance, abilities, special skills	Realize that many of the difficulties the teenager is experiencing are part of normal adolescence (rebelliousness, risk taking, lack of cooperation, hostility toward authority).
Achieve independence from family	Increased dependency on family; limited job and career opportunities	Provide instruction on interpersonal and coping skills.
Form heterosexual relationships	Limited opportunities for heterosexual friendships; less opportunity to discuss sexual concerns with peers	Encourage socialization with peers, including peers with special needs and those without special needs.
	Increased concern with issues such as why he or she got the disorder, whether he or she can marry and have a family	Provide instruction on decision making, assertiveness, and other skills necessary to manage personal plans. Encourage increased responsibility for care and management of the disease or condition (e.g., assuming responsibility for making and keeping appointments, ideally alone; sharing assessment and planning stages of health care delivery; contacting resources).
Learn through abstract thinking	Hindrance in achieving level of abstract thinking because of decreased opportunity for attaining earlier stages of cognition	Encourage activities appropriate for age (e.g., attending mixed-sex parties and sports activities, driving a car). Be alert to cues that signal readiness for information regarding implications of condition on sexuality and reproduction. Emphasize good appearance and wearing stylish clothes, use of makeup. Understand that adolescent has same sexual needs and concerns as any other teenager. Discuss planning for future and how condition can affect choices.

development of trust. Illness may threaten the parents' feelings of confidence and competence in their newly acquired parenting roles.

The presence of a visible or serious defect can hinder parental attachment while the parents mourn the loss of the perfect child. They may gain little comfort from trying to satisfy their child's basic needs despite their best efforts. Physical deformity or fatigue may influence a child's responsiveness to his or her parents, who may in turn react differently to their child. A poor prognosis for the child may cause some parents to emotionally detach themselves from their infant to protect themselves from future emotional pain (Vessey and Mebane, 2009).

Nurses can be pivotal in helping parents care for their infant with special needs. They may need assistance in learning how best to meet their infant's needs, for example, how to hold a flaccid or rigid infant, how to comfort an irritable infant, how to feed a child with dyspnea or tongue thrust, or how to stimulate a child unable to develop common skills.

Nurses should advocate for practices and policies that support the developmental needs of the infant and the family. Twenty-four-hour visitation in the neonatal intensive care unit and other infant units is paramount and lessens the infant's experience of separation. In addition, nurses need to limit the number of caregivers for the infant to enhance consistency and continuity of care. Showing parents how to hold and touch their infant will foster their competence and confidence. Kangaroo care (with skin-to-skin contact) has been demonstrated to be both beneficial and safe for the infant. (See Chapter 10.) Give support to mothers who want to breast-feed, and provide a private room with refrigerated storage for the woman who pumps or nurses. Promote sibling visitation as well.

Toddler

The toddler is acquiring a sense of autonomy, developing self-control, and forming symbolic representation through language acquisition. The need for parental involvement in managing the child's illness may interfere with the toddler's need for increasing independence and impede his or her sense of autonomy and self-control. Mobility is possibly the primary tool used by the toddler to experiment with attaining control. For the toddler who is incapacitated, a sense of helplessness results that is difficult to overcome at a later time.

If a child's chronic illness prevents daily activities, this may impede autonomy in tasks such as feeding, toileting, and building larger social networks. Developmental tasks that have just been mastered are often easily lost in the toddler suffering from an acute exacerbation of the illness. Behavioral regression, commonly seen in toddlers, is worsened by stress related to pain and separation.

Because of the toddler's desire for autonomy, the mastery of language and locomotor skills is very important. The child learning to talk and walk progresses toward being a separate individual, both psychologically and physically. A toddler's limited ability to verbally communicate thoughts and feelings makes it especially difficult for the child to cope with the stresses imposed by a chronic illness. In the presence of disability or illness, mobility to explore and master the environment is impeded, and the child is prevented from acquiring these skills. Within the constraints of the illness or disability, the nurse should help parents provide safe opportunities that foster independence in these and other areas for their toddler, both at home and in the hospital (Fig. 22-1).

Illness can impose separations that cause anxiety in the toddler. A disability or chronic illness can entail frequent painful procedures and hospitalizations. The latter may hinder the normal development of trusting relationships within the family. If the hospital does not help maintain the parent-child relationship, the child may become depressed and eventually detach from parents. Children appear to have a great ability to withstand stress as long as they retain their attachment to the parent.

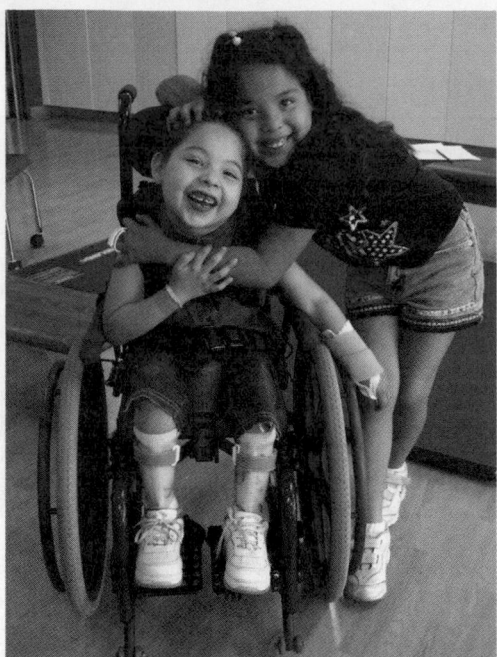

Fig. 22-1 Wheelchairs designed for children can help a child with disabilities gain mobility and promote growth and development.

Toddlers are especially sensitive to changes in familiar routines, in addition to hospitalizations. They may perceive disruption of normal daily activities and hospitalization as punishment. If invasive and painful medical procedures are required in the treatment of the child's illness, this perception is further validated. Therefore encourage parents to bring in familiar toys for the toddler during hospitalization, and establish routines so the child can become acclimated.

Parents of toddlers may seek out daycare or respite care, which can be difficult to find for the child with special needs.* Caregivers need time away from caring for their child to allow for their own growth and development. The Americans with Disabilities Act (ADA) requires that daycare providers make "reasonable modifications" for equal access to program participation (Mahoney, Wheeden, and Perales, 2004). Special medical daycare facilities are emerging in some areas (Mahoney, Wheeden, and Perales, 2004).

Preschooler

The preschooler is focused on acquiring a sense of initiative to successfully meet the challenges of his or her growing world. Preschoolers with a chronic illness may lack the resources or energy to plan and engage in such activities; thus opportunities for building social relationships, learning about the environment, and developing a sense of purpose and self-confidence are often limited. Illness may restrict the preschooler to the home and cause the child to fall behind in social skills beneficial in school or group settings.

It may be difficult for preschoolers to build a healthy sexual identity and body image, especially if most of their body awareness is linked with pain and disability. Children's understanding of their body is confined to what they see, feel, and use. In the presence of a chronic illness, their body awareness may be focused on the anxiety and pain elicited. The chronically ill child may lose control over newly acquired bowel and bladder function, which results in feelings of embarrassment and inferiority. The child with a disability may find it difficult to form a mental image of impaired body parts, for example, paralyzed extremities. This poorly developed sense of body integrity causes children to be particularly fearful of mutilating or intrusive experiences, which can occur frequently during a lengthy illness. Thus before any medical procedure children should be given a brief, honest explanation of what the procedure is, how it will be performed, and the duration and intensity of any accompanying pain.

When the young child has a disability that affects motor development, there is the risk of shifting to development of compensatory intellectual pursuits before the child is ready. This could compromise attainment of initiative and autonomy and place the child at risk for emotional problems. Thus intervention must focus on providing activities that allow maximum motor development. For example, if a child has paraplegia, it is not enough to strengthen the upper extremities to compensate for the lower ones. Rather, the activity must consider the child's need for a sense of control over the body, social interaction, feeling of achievement and competence, and outlet for aggression. Appropriate activities may include ball throwing; play with building blocks; water and swimming activities such as bubble blowing, splashing, and racing; or pounding with a hammer.† Children with disabilities may be able to ride a tricycle with minor changes such as self-adhering straps to protect the hands or feet.

One of the more crucial effects of chronic illness or disability on preschoolers is the feeling of guilt that they "caused" the illness through an imagined or real misdeed. This is less of an issue if the child is born with the condition than if it occurs during the preschool period. Such guilt can significantly affect the child's developing but fragile self-esteem, especially if the child experiences frequent insults. In contrast, the child with a temporary physical disability has added opportunities for attaining mastery and overcoming feelings of inferiority and guilt. Structuring situations to foster success can assist a child in developing a sense of confidence and competence.

Another critical component for normal child development is discipline. Discipline is essential to the child's sense of security because boundaries are necessary for the child to test behavior. It also teaches the child socially acceptable behavior. Applying appropriate discipline to the child who is chronically ill or disabled can also limit the resentment and hostility that can develop among siblings if parents apply different standards to each child. The nurse's responsibility is to help parents learn successful methods of guiding the child.

When a chronic illness imposes restrictions that cause difficulty with mastery, it can inflict a lasting sense of failure. Preschoolers are egocentric and have naive reasoning, which

---

*Access to Respite Care and Help (ARCH) is available at www.archrespite.org.

†Information on individual toy selection and toy lending libraries for children with sensory deficits, motor disabilities, and developmental delay are available from the National Lekotek Center at 800-366-PLAY; www.lekotek.org.

may affect their interpretation and understanding of their illness.

Because preschoolers need to explore and acquire experience with pretend situations and objects before they really experience them, nurses need to facilitate opportunities for imaginative play (e.g., using dolls and syringes) and to give simple answers to children's questions about their illness and treatment.

School-Age Child

School-age children focus on increasing mastery over their environment and independence. A lack of physical stamina may prevent the child with a chronic illness from engaging in school and extracurricular activities and result in feelings of inferiority or inadequacy. These activities help the child acquire social skills, develop a sense of achievement, gain the skills to achieve self-sufficiency, and learn to effectively deal with stress. School-age children should be involved as much as possible in their own care and in decision making about their treatment to facilitate their sense of control and mastery.

School-age children are mostly concerned with learning to take initiative. School initiates the processes of working toward independence from parents, gaining academic skills, and building peer relationships. Along with the family, school is the major context in which children develop their sense of self and understanding of their place relative to their peers.

During the school-age period, the child is increasingly able to distinguish fantasy from reality, self from others, and he or she advances to inductive reasoning and beginning logic. Coupled with this limited sense of causality comes a deeper understanding of differences. Children with an illness that is not obvious may try to hide its existence once they realize that it differentiates them from their peers (Vessey and Mebane, 2009).

School-age children also begin active inquiry. They are usually verbal regarding their condition and ask for information about all phases of the illness and treatment. In addition, they experience pride after they learn the correct label for the illness, treatment, and medication. From the beginning, nurses should respond to the child's questions in a simple, direct manner.

The school-age child separates from parents more easily and becomes more active in peer relationships. Peers strongly influence school-age children's opinions of themselves and their self-esteem (Murray, 2000). If not provided with the required skills to disseminate information about their illness to peers, school-age children may withdraw with a diminished self-concept (Vessey and Mebane, 2009).

The number of children with chronic illnesses who return to school continues to increase (Kliebenstein and Broome, 2000). Children need preparation before entering or resuming school. Having a tutor in the hospital or home as soon as children are physically able helps them realize that school will continue and gives them time to consider this prospect. They need to investigate possible answers to the many questions others will ask. One method of anticipatory preparation is to role-play, with the child as the "returned pupil" and the nurse as "other schoolmates." The nurse asks questions about the reason for the child's absence, the name of the disease, and so on. The child is provided with a safe opportunity to explore possible answers and to experience some of the possible reactions of others. If the child returns to school with some obvious physical change, such as hair loss, an amputation, or a visible scar, the nurse might also ask questions about these alterations to prompt preparatory responses from the child.

Initially the child may find it easier to attend half-day school sessions or to participate in a limited number of activities. It is preferable to plan the school program with as much participation and leadership from the child as possible. Once the child returns, regular assessments of the child's progress in various areas (academic, social, physical) are essential to ensure a satisfactory adjustment.

Classroom peers also need preparation, and a joint plan involving the schoolteacher, nurse, parents, and child is best. At a minimum the classmates should be given a description of the child's condition, prepared for any visible changes in the child, and allowed an opportunity to ask questions. The child should have the option to attend this session. As the child's condition changes, particularly if the illness is potentially fatal, school personnel, including the students, need periodic apprisal of the child's status and preparation for what to expect. (See Chapter 23.)

Children with special needs should maintain or reestablish relationships with peers and to participate according to their capabilities in any age-appropriate activities. Alternative activities may be substituted for those that are impossible or that place a strain on their health. It is important for these children to have the opportunity to interact with healthy peers, as well as to engage in activities with groups or clubs composed of similarly affected age-mates. Such organizations as ostomy clubs, diabetic clubs, and cerebral palsy groups share information and provide support related to the special problems the members face.

Programs such as the Special Olympics (www.specialolympics.org) offer children with physical disabilities an opportunity to compete with their peers and to achieve athletic skill. Summer camps* also provide children unique opportunities to associate with similarly affected peers and to develop a wide variety of skills, including increased independence in activities of daily living and self-care associated with their condition. With creativity, parents can make many adaptations in children's environments to increase their mobility and independence.† Technology is rapidly advancing, especially in the application of computers, and parents should be directed to the latest developments that may help their child.

Children with special needs obtain enormous benefits from expressive activities, such as art, music, poetry, dance, and drama. With adaptive equipment and imagination, children can participate in a variety of activities. Organizations such as

---

*A directory of camps for children with a variety of chronic illnesses and general physical disabilities is available at American Camp Association, www.ACAcamps.org; Candlelighters Childhood Cancer Foundation, www.candlelighters.org; and Easter Seals, www.easterseals.com.
†Excellent publications on adapting the environment for children with disabilities are available from National Rehabilitation Information Center, www.naric.com.

VSA (vision, strength, and artistic expression) arts* encourage children to celebrate and share their accomplishments.

Adolescent

Adolescence marks the transitional period from childhood to adulthood and is characterized by important changes in intellectual, physical, social, and psychologic growth and development. Adolescence is the time for achieving independence. This may be difficult for adolescents with chronic illness, especially those who are dependent on others for daily care or therapy.

Chronic illness may impose the additional burden of hospitalization, pain, surgery, extensive diagnostic testing, medications, school absences, and activity restrictions on the adolescent. Such stressors may provoke many anxieties, fears, and grief reactions. Illness-related fears include loss of physical integrity, inability to separate successfully from one's parents, loss of control, being different from peers, and death. They must cope not only with complex normative developmental tasks but also with the stress related to the diagnosis and treatment of life-threatening or long-term illness (see Research Focus box).

RESEARCH FOCUS

Hospitalized Children's Fears

In a recent study asking children about their fears when hospitalized, children listed their greatest fears regarding hospitalization as being separated from family and friends, being in an unfamiliar environment, receiving investigations or treatments, and losing self-determination or choices (Coyne, 2006).

Adolescents are striving for autonomy, which is threatened by the forced dependence, need for compliance, and loss of control associated with an illness and treatment. Consequently, dealing with the illness may be more difficult and adolescents may be at greater risk for depression, anxiety, and adjustment problems. Many adolescents wish to assume total responsibility for their care despite their inexperience; however, their extensive care needs may prevent this from occurring (Newacheck, Wong, Galbraith, et al, 2003). If the chronic illness is associated with mobility limitations forcing dependence on caregivers for basic needs, it may compromise the emergence of a secure sexual and physical identity and peer relationships.

Adolescence is a time for achieving independence from the family and planning for future goals and responsibilities. Adolescents with long-term chronic illness may be less future directed and less independent than well peers. Enforced dependency from physical impairment can exacerbate the parent-child conflicts surrounding independence. Lack of understanding by both parties can result in bitter feelings and intrafamilial turmoil. The tendency toward rebellion may be directed at the disorder and reflected in decreased compliance with treatment; denial of the disorder to preserve a sense of normalcy with peers; and risk-taking behavior that can place the teenager in jeopardy, such as driving a car despite a disorder that increases the chance of an accident. Such behaviors can further strain an already tense parent-child relationship.

On the other hand, parents can promote independence by giving the adolescent a greater role in his or her own treatment regimen, encouraging the adolescent to develop a relationship with the physicians and nurses that is not mediated by parents, and promoting normalization principles.

During adolescence hormonal changes accompany the onset of puberty and a simultaneous preoccupation with body image. The major task of the adolescent is to develop his or her own identity. Hormone-related changes must be integrated into the self-image while the adolescent is gaining mastery and control over sexuality and increased physical abilities. During early adolescence this process occurs mostly within the peer group. The beginning of puberty, a period of uncertainty and rapid change, is even more confusing for teenagers with chronic illnesses.

Most adolescents are embarrassed by their appearance and emerging sexuality. For chronically ill adolescents the illness or its treatment may be most embarrassing and may influence their body image and hinder their sense of mastery and control over a changing body. It is difficult for the adolescent with a disability to incorporate the disability into a changing self-concept and body image. The young person who has a disability or is diagnosed with an illness during the critical adolescent years has more difficulty accomplishing these tasks than does the adolescent who has been affected since childhood. The earlier the onset of a limiting illness, the better the individual is able to adjust to it. The youngster with a newly acquired condition has the added task of grieving the loss while adapting to the changes occurring as a natural course of events. The adolescent often feels rejected because of personal appearance or inability to participate in activities expected of a healthy teenager.

Adolescence is a most difficult period to be seen as different by one's peers, and some adolescents may withdraw from social relationships and activities that foster healthy psychosexual development. Appearance, abilities, and skills are highly regarded by peers; an adolescent who is limited in any of these qualities is subject to rejection by this influential group. A sense of feeling different from peers can cause isolation, loneliness, and depression. To be accepted by peers, some adolescents may decide to participate in risky behaviors such as unprotected sex and smoking, despite the possible harmful effects. Participation in groups of teenagers with chronic illnesses or disabilities can alleviate feelings of isolation and ease the transition to a meaningful relationship with one person in adulthood.

The topic of sexuality related to the effects of the illness is an important concern of adolescents, although they seldom initiate a discussion of this sensitive subject. Discuss any likely interference in sexual function due to the disability candidly and openly with the adolescent. Unfortunately, many nurses are reluctant to discuss sexual issues with teenagers. Adults often underestimate the degree to which adolescents participate in unrealistic fantasies about sexual activities and related matters, or even in sexual activity itself.

Nurses can facilitate the adolescent's striving for autonomy by allowing and encouraging the adolescent's participation in medical decisions by signing an assent as part of the informed consent document. Within the confines of the specific treatment center, the adolescent can be given control over the scheduling of procedures and treatments, allowed to view test results

---

*VSA arts is an international organization that creates learning opportunities through the arts for individuals with disabilities; **www.vsarts. org**.

or radiographs, and included in discussions of alternative therapies. Adolescents should assume increasing responsibility for management of their illness consistent with their developmental stage, level of maturity, and understanding of their illness. Areas of responsibility may include monitoring their condition, assessing indicators of exacerbation and change, self-medicating, asking for assistance, and maintaining insurance coverage (Newacheck, Wong, Galbraith, et al, 2003).

HELPING THE CHILD COPE

Through ongoing contact with the child, the nurse (1) observes the child's reactions to chronic illness or disability, ability to function, and adaptive behaviors within the environment and with significant others; (2) explores the child's own understanding of his or her illness; and (3) provides support while the child learns to cope with his or her feelings. Encourage children to verbalize their concerns rather than allowing others to verbalize for them, since open discussions may lessen anxiety.

Parents often express concern because their child cannot communicate the anxieties he or she is feeling. If the child will not or cannot speak, the child may need to play out his or her feelings. Toys can be provided to facilitate expression of the meaning of stressful or threatening emotions. The nurse may realize that the child responds best to telling stories or drawing pictures. (See Chapter 6.)

Coping Mechanisms

Children's innate and learned coping mechanisms are crucial in their ability to cope with their condition. Children with special needs are likely to use distinct coping patterns (Box 22-2). Children with more accepting and positive attitudes about their chronic illness use a more adaptive coping style, characterized by competence, optimism, and compliance. They display fewer behavior problems at school and at home.

BOX 22-2 COPING PATTERNS USED BY CHILDREN WITH SPECIAL NEEDS

Develops competence and optimism—Accentuates the positive aspects of the situation and concentrates more on what he or she has or can do than on what is missing or on what he or she cannot do; is as independent as possible

Feels different and withdraws—Sees self as being different from other children because of the chronic health condition; views being different as negative; sees self as less worthy than others; focuses on things he or she cannot do and sometimes overrestricts activities needlessly

Is irritable and moody and acts out—Uses proactive and self-initiated coping behaviors, although these are usually counterproductive in that the behaviors are not ego enhancing or socially responsible and do not result in desired outcomes; acts out irritability, which may or may not be associated with condition's symptoms

Complies with treatment—Takes necessary medications and treatments; adheres to activity restrictions; also uses behaviors that indicate developing independence (e.g., assumes responsibility for taking medication)

Seeks support—Talks with adults, children, physicians, and nurses; develops plans to handle problems as they occur; uses downward comparison (i.e., realizes that others have it worse)

Modified from Austin J, Patterson J, Huberty T: Development of the Coping Heath Inventory for children, *J Pediatr Nurs* 6(3):166-174, 1991.

Because it is often easier to recognize children who cope poorly with illness or disability, it is helpful to describe those behaviors typical of well-adjusted children. Well-adapted children gradually learn to accept their physical limitations.

Normalization

One of the most important interventions to promote coping is alleviating the child's feeling of being different and normalizing his or her life as much as possible. The principles in the Nursing Care Guidelines box are fundamental in implementing the normalization process. The nurse can help parents assess the child's daily routine for indications of normalizing practices. For example, the child who remains in a bedroom all day needs a restructured daily routine to provide activities in different parts of the house, such as eating in the kitchen with the family, and the inclusion of social, recreational, and academic activities in the care plan.

 NURSING CARE GUIDELINES

Promoting Normalization

Preparation—Prepare the child in advance for changes that may occur from the illness or disability; for example, tell the child in advance of the possible side effects of drug therapy.

Participation—Include the child in as many decisions as possible, especially those relating to his or her care plan; for example, the child is responsible for taking medications or scheduling home treatments.

Sharing—Allow both family members and the child's peers to be a part of the care regimen whenever possible; for example, give the child his or her medication when the other siblings receive their vitamins; the parent cooks the same menu for the whole family; if the child is invited to another's home, the parent advises the family of the child's dietary restrictions.

Control—Identify areas in which the child can be in control to decrease feelings of uncertainty, passivity, and helplessness; for example, the child identifies activities that are appropriate for his or her energy level and chooses to rest when fatigued.

Expectations—Apply the same family rules to the child with a chronic illness or disability as to the well siblings or peers; for example, the child is disciplined, expected to fulfill household responsibilities, and attends school in accordance with abilities.

Positive attitude—Focus, and help the child to focus, on areas of ability and competence to build self-esteem.

Children who are concerned that their condition detracts from their physical attractiveness need attention focused on the normal aspects of appearance and capabilities. Health professionals can help parents strengthen the child's self-image by emphasizing the normal, while at the same time allowing children to express anger, isolation, fear of rejection, sadness, and loneliness. Parents should encourage anything that might improve attractiveness and contribute to a positive self-image, such as makeup for a teenager with a scar, clothing that disguises a prosthesis, or a hairstyle or wig to cover a deformity or lost hair.

The parent's behavior, particularly in relation to childrearing, is one of the most critical influences on the child's adaptation to chronic illness. For example, children who are raised by parents who establish reasonable limits are likely to develop independence that is appropriate for their age and achievement equal to their limitations. They frequently exhibit confidence and pride in their ability to cope successfully with the challenges resulting from their condition. On the other hand, children whose parents are overprotective are likely to show fearfulness, marked dependency, and inactivity and to have few outside interests. Using anticipatory guidance and encouragement of normalizing practices, the nurse may assist parents in facilitating positive adaptation in their children. Normalization is important because it focuses on the child, not the condition.

Nurses can demonstrate the process of normalization to the child's family by acknowledging the strengths and weaknesses of the family unit, by being supportive and open about the child's condition and treatment, and by actively including the family in all aspects of care (Shepard and Mahon, 2009). If the child's family adopts a normalized view of management of the chronic illness, the child may be more confident in the home as well as in social and community situations. Thus the family's perception of the impact and the integration of the chronic illness may directly or indirectly improve the child's adaptation (Sullivan-Bolyai, Knafl, Sadler, et al, 2004).

Nurses also can assist parents by identifying and building on family strengths, promoting family and child competence, and fostering the development of a nurturing environment that addresses the needs of siblings and parents, as well as of the child with special needs.

Hopefulness

Children, especially adolescents, are sensitive to the presence or absence of hope. From a psychologic perspective, Erikson's theory of psychosocial growth and development proposes that hope is a basic ego quality that is initially experienced in infancy and is the positive outcome of successful resolution of the developmental stage of trust versus mistrust (Ritchie, 2001).

Hopefulness helps protect the adolescent from incapacitating despair and assists the adolescent in coping with unmet personal needs. A sense of hopefulness can result in increased participation in health-seeking behaviors and an improved sense of well-being. Nurses can be instrumental in fostering hopefulness through environmental and interpersonal means (see Nursing Care Guidelines box).

📋 NURSING CARE GUIDELINES

Fostering Hopefulness

- Give honest reports of conditions or events.
- Encourage and participate with the child in physical activities (e.g., arrange activities, play games, or go for walks together).
- Convey a fond, personal interest in the child (give hugs, ask follow-up questions from previous discussions).
- Introduce conversations on neutral, non-disease-related, or less sensitive topics (discuss child's favorite sports, tell stories).
- Convey competence and gentleness when delivering care.
- Provide information about other children in similar situations who are doing well.
- Encourage the child to think ahead to more comfortable and preferred natural times.
- Be lighthearted and initiate or respond to teasing or other playful interactions with the child.

Modified from Hinds P, Martin J, Vogel RJ: Nursing strategies to influence adolescent hopefulness during oncologic illness, *J Assoc Pediatr Oncol Nurs* 4(1/2):14-22, 1987.

Health Education and Self-Care

Health education teaches children self-care behaviors and self-advocacy skills for dealing with the health care community. These are important skills for children and adolescents with chronic conditions to master because they are likely to use the health care system frequently throughout their lives (Vessey and Mebane, 2009). Active participation in care requires comprehensive family and patient education. Empowerment of individuals with disabilities is the philosophy that is currently advocated for provision of services. Gaining access to information helps the individual make informed decisions and acquire some control over the environment.

Children need information about how the body works, the characteristics of their condition, the treatment plan, the impact of illness or therapy, and, when age-appropriate, the intricacies of the health care system. Education is a primary component of self-care, and teaching methods must be modified to meet the child's developmental age. In addition, children near puberty need to understand the maturation process and how their disability may change this event. For example, the child with Crohn disease should know that this illness is linked with delayed puberty and growth failure. The child with diabetes needs to understand that increased growth needs and hormonal changes will change insulin and food requirements at this time. The sexually active girl with systemic lupus erythematosus or sickle cell anemia needs to be aware of the risks of pregnancy. The information should not be provided during a single teaching session but rather timed appropriately to meet the child's changing needs, and it should be described and repeated as frequently as the situation warrants.

For young children the information presented needs to be concise, simple, and honest, even if the news is not positive. Answer questions openly, since children need answers to the questions they are able to ask. If they have no confidence in the answer provided or are ignored, the only alternative left to them is to relate their experience to something fantasized or seen on television. If young children state that they do not want to learn more, then respect their wishes.

Developing the judgment and expertise for participating in self-care of chronic illness or disability is a process that occurs gradually. Self-care necessitates negotiation between child and parents. Nurses are instrumental in providing information on strategies for teaching children of various ages in self-care.

Realistic Future Goals

Because medical advances have led to prolonged survival for children with many chronic illnesses, these individuals are confronted with new decisions and problems such as employment,* marriage, medical and dental care access, and insurance coverage. Adolescents usually look forward to what their lives will be like in the future.

For some chronic illnesses or severe disabilities, one of the most difficult adjustments is establishing realistic goals for the

---

*Information about employment is available from the Office of Disability Employment Policy (www.dol.gov/odep). The Job Accommodation Network (www.jan.wvu.edu) provides information about job accommodations and the employability of individuals with disabilities.

child and for those involved in the child's continual care. Occasionally the impact of these decisions does not surface until the child graduates from school or the parents move toward retirement, when a crisis can arise because of disruptions in the family roles and relationships that maintained stability.

For children with severe disabilities, preparing for the future should be a gradual process. All along the child and parents should consider realistic vocational options. For example, children with physical disabilities can be directed to artistic, intellectual, or musical pursuits. Children with developmental disabilities can be instructed in manual skills. Thus the child's development progresses to self-support through gainful employment.

Unfortunately, vocational pursuits and independence are not realistic goals for all individuals. Persons with multiple or severe disabilities may require lifelong care and assistance. In these situations parents must look to the time when they will no longer be able to care for their child. Advance financial planning should be considered. Residential placement may be difficult unless the family mutually participates in the decision-making and planning processes. Parents should not view care outside the home as abandonment. Often it is the only way to preserve the family unit. The nurse should help the family investigate suitable placements, discuss their feelings regarding this decision, and explore measures to maintain meaningful communication with the member who has a disability. The nurse can take a larger advocacy role in educating the public regarding persons with special needs and helping normalize the experience for the child, the family, and the community.

Determining readiness for transfer to adult providers is a primary consideration. Arbitrary transfer to adult services based solely on an age criterion can compromise both psychosocial and physical care for some young adults. Many adolescents have received care in the same medical setting since birth and have established a trusting relationship with practitioners and staff. Moreover, age is not an indicator of adolescent readiness for transfer to an adult care provider. Important factors include (Reiss, Gibson, and Walker, 2005):

- Knowledge of the condition and its management
- Readiness to assume responsibility for treatment management
- Prior involvement in and compliance with the treatment regimen
- Demonstration of responsible and independent judgment
- Prior response to emergency situations
- Coping ability
- Attitude of pediatric provider to transition

Nurses can take steps to help the adolescent prepare for the transition. These include presenting the idea of transfer; assessing the readiness of the adolescent and parent; coordinating a meeting with the adolescent, the family, and both pediatric and adult care providers; and formally acknowledging the transfer (Reiss, Gibson, and Walker, 2005).

Nurses are instrumental in assisting and supporting adolescents in assuming responsibility for managing their own care as much as possible. Adolescents should actively participate in the planning and decision-making processes for transi-

tion to adult care. In addition, nurses can foster continuity of care by providing information to adult health care providers about the adolescent's needs relating to disease management and his or her compliance with the treatment regimen. The ultimate goal of transition care to adulthood for the adolescent with a chronic illness is to promote the achievement of responsible self-care and linkages to adult health care services and thus to provide the best prospects for educational options, social networks and relationships, community living, and employment.

THE FAMILY OF THE CHILD WITH SPECIAL NEEDS

A major goal in working with the family of a child with special needs is to support the family's coping and help them function as best as they can throughout the child's life. Long-term, comprehensive, family-centered approaches extend beyond supporting the child and family during the crucial periods of diagnosis and hospitalization. Comprehensive care involves building parent-professional partnerships that can support a family's adaptation to the many changes that may be necessary in everyday life, defining expectations of and for the child, and providing a long-term perspective (Box 22-3).

ASSESSING FAMILY STRENGTHS AND ADJUSTMENT

The purpose of a family assessment is to determine what assistance a family may need or want in managing their child's care. Ideally the nurse should initiate an assessment as soon as the family learns the diagnosis. Integral to the family-centered care philosophy is the conception that the family should be an active participant in the process. Sample questions designed to elicit information for assessing the family's adjustment are listed in Table 22-2. Family members should always be informed of the purpose of the assessment, including the rationale for asking personal questions. They should be afforded the opportunity to participate or not as they choose.

A number of instruments can be used to assess the family's overall functioning and support system. In addition, specific tools have been developed for families of children with chronic illness or disability. For example, the Coping Health Inventory for Parents (CHIPTS) is an 80-item checklist that provides self-report information about how parents perceive their overall

BOX 22-3	ADAPTIVE TASKS OF PARENTS OF CHILDREN WITH CHRONIC CONDITIONS

- Accept the child's condition.
- Manage the child's condition on a day-to-day basis.
- Meet the child's normal developmental needs.
- Meet the developmental needs of other family members.
- Cope with ongoing stress and periodic crises.
- Assist family members in managing their feelings.
- Educate others about the child's condition.
- Establish a support system.

From Canam C: Common adaptive tasks facing parents of children with chronic conditions, *J Adv Nurs* 18:46-53, 1993.

TABLE 22-2 ASSESSMENT OF FACTORS AFFECTING FAMILY ADJUSTMENT	
FACTORS AFFECTING ADJUSTMENT	**ASSESSMENT QUESTIONS**
Available support system • Status of marital relationship • Availability of alternate support systems • Ability to communicate	Whom do you talk to when you have something on your mind? (If answer is not the spouse, ask for the reason.) When something is worrying you, what do you do? What helps you most when you are upset? Does talking seem to help when you feel upset?
Perception of the illness or disability • Previous knowledge of disorder • Influence of religion and culture • Beliefs about cause of disorder • Effects of illness or disability on family	Have you ever heard the word (name of diagnosis) before? Tell me about it (if answer is yes). Has your religion, faith, or cultural practice been of help to you? Tell me how (if answer is yes). What are your thoughts about the causes of the disorder? How has your child's illness or disability affected you and your family?
Coping mechanisms • Reactions to previous crises • Reactions to the child • Childrearing practices • Attitudes	How has your lifestyle changed? Tell me about a time you've had another crisis (problem, bad time) in your family. How did you solve that problem? Do you find yourself being a little more cautious with this child than with your other children? Do you feel as comfortable disciplining this child as disciplining your other children? How is this child different from the siblings or other children of similar age? Describe your child's personality. Is it easy, difficult, or in between? When you think of your child's future, what thoughts come to mind?
Available resources	What parts of your child's care are causing the most difficulty for you and/or your family? What services are available to help? What services do you need that presently are not available?
Concurrent stresses	What other problems are you facing now? (Be specific; ask about financial, marital, sibling, and extended family or friend concerns.)

response to the management of family life with a child with a chronic illness. Coping behaviors (e.g., "believing that my child[ren] will get better" or "talking with the hospital staff [nurses, social workers] when we visited the medical center") are listed, and parents are asked to rate how helpful the coping items are to them in managing the home situation. Chapter 25 describes tools that a family can use to assess the home environment and resources.

Regardless of the approach, assessment is a continual process. Because support systems and the perception of events may change at any time during an illness, nurses must assist families on an ongoing basis in evaluating the effectiveness of changes and interventions in support needs.

ACCEPTING THE CHILD'S CONDITION AND RECEIVING SUPPORT AT THE TIME OF DIAGNOSIS

The impact of a child's developmental or medical condition is often experienced as a crisis at the time of diagnosis, which may be during birth, after a long period of psychologic and/or physical testing, or soon after a tragic injury. It may also begin before the diagnosis, when parents know that something is wrong with their child but there has been no medical confirmation.

Interventions facilitating the parents' adjustment to the diagnosis of their child's chronic illness or disability and their ability to care for their child include planning the setting for informing parents, assessing the family's prior knowledge of and experience with chronic conditions (see Family-Centered Care box), selecting strategies that best meet the family's needs and situation, evaluating the family's understanding of the information presented, and providing ongoing follow-up. Effectively discussing the diagnosis provides a vital foundation

FAMILY-CENTERED CARE
Meaning of the Chronic Illness or Disability

The meaning and significance that a family places on the child's condition are influenced by individual perceptions of the diagnosis. Nurses can help families evaluate how their previous knowledge about and imagined causes of the disorder, religious beliefs, and culture influence their perceptions and coping strategies.

Although parents may be shocked to learn that their child has a serious illness or disability, they usually have some prior knowledge of the disorder from previous reading or associations. Nurses can help families explore the accuracy and completeness of their previous knowledge. Some people, for example, think that cancer is always terminal.

Although the causes of many disorders are unknown, people commonly feel a need to supply a reason for an illness or disability. Sometimes reasons are associated with cultural or religious beliefs, but they may also be influenced by previous events. Children, for example, may interpret the illness as a punishment for disobedience. Parents may be convinced that the condition was inherited or due to behaviors during pregnancy. Once the imagined cause is revealed, family members can be helped to consider the implications of that thinking and to move beyond feelings of guilt, blame, or anger.

Religious beliefs and spirituality are a source of meaning and support for many people. For some, healing and faith are synonymous, and any criticism of the family's spirituality can weaken their trust in medical care. For others, religious beliefs may intensify feelings of guilt, shame, or punishment. Some may ask, "What have I done to deserve this?" or "God, why are you punishing me in this way?" Always take such statements seriously and help the person to explore the reason why he or she believes the condition is a punishment.

Culture influences the understanding of illness or disability and appropriate treatment strategies. The nurse can help families express their culturally related beliefs about the causes and severity of the condition and treatments that may be culturally specific or that may conflict with cultural beliefs. A respectful approach has the goal of both explaining the beliefs and approaches of health care providers and supporting the family's culturally determined needs.

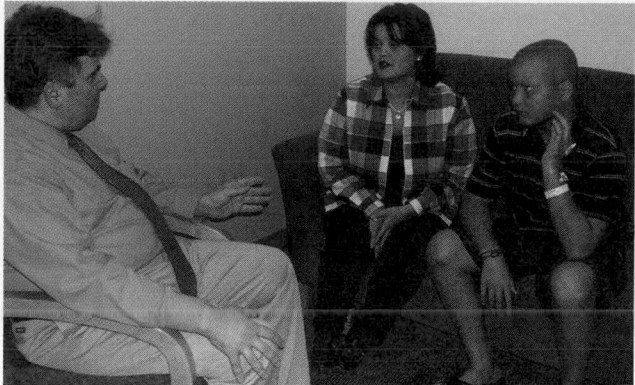

Fig. 22-2 Informing sessions should take place in a private, comfortable setting free of distractions and interruptions.

for a strong collaborative relationship between parents and health care providers that will be needed in the future.

The physician or advanced practice nurse usually informs the family of the child's diagnosis. Nurses are also responsible for providing follow-up information and coordinating services with other agencies. Whatever role nurses assume, they can follow the guidelines in the Nursing Care Guidelines box during disclosure of the diagnosis to offer the family support at this crucial time.

The informing conference should take place in a private, comfortable setting free of interruptions and distractions (Fig. 22-2). The environment should be one in which parents feel free to show their emotions. If parents can express their emotions openly, the nurse will be able to determine their need for additional counseling. Parents often sense a certain attitude of rejection, acceptance, hope, or despair that may affect their ability to assimilate the shock and begin adapting to the implications of the illness for their future.

The parents' emotional needs at the time of diagnosis are acknowledged by exhibiting acceptance of such expressions as sadness, crying, disappointment, and anger. Emotional support is provided by having tissues available if a family member cries and by showing through body and facial language that indeed this is a painful and difficult time. Even though touching is a strong expression of empathy, it must be used cautiously. For example, it can prematurely terminate free expression of feelings, particularly when combined with statements such as, "Everything will be all right." Nurses should also be cognizant of cultural sensitivity regarding touching. (See Chapter 2.)

Nurses should observe the responses of family members on hearing the diagnosis. Their facial expressions, their ability to maintain eye contact with the nurse, the times they look down, behaviors that indicate they are avoiding what the nurse is saying (such as turning their heads, looking away, or looking around), and any other activities that demonstrate they are dealing with a difficult matter are observed.

One of the most supportive interventions is to accept the family's emotional reactions to the diagnosis in a nonjudgmental manner. Although all families react differently and with varying degrees of intensity, three reactions are common and are frequently poorly managed: guilt, denial, and anger.

Parents should receive the kind of information they want. Most parents prefer a simple, clear explanation of the diagnosis, including what is and is not known about the diagnosis, a

NURSING CARE GUIDELINES
Informing the Family of a Serious Condition

Initial Discussion

Discuss suspicions of a problem with parents when waiting for a definite diagnosis to help prepare them for a potentially serious diagnosis.

Have both parents present or have a friend or family member accompany a single parent.

Let the practitioner who knows the family best present the diagnosis with the primary nurse present.

Share information about the child's diagnosis:
- Use the correct terminology for the diagnosis.
- Avoid using names of symptoms that immediately have negative connotations to define the disorder. For example, instead of saying, "Down syndrome involves retardation," say, "Down syndrome is a chromosome abnormality." Once the dialogue has begun, tell parents other characteristics of the condition (e.g., "A characteristic of Down syndrome is cognitive impairment").
- Mention alternative names for the condition.
- Discuss the possible range of functioning.
- Explain other medical problems and how these are or are not related to the child's diagnosis.

Be willing to repeat information if necessary.

Convey kindness and understanding by sitting down near the parents, touching a parent's hand or shoulder, having tissues available, calling the child by name, and saying the parents' names during the conversation.

Stress the personhood of the child by showing love, concern, and respect for the child as an individual.

Allow parents to express emotion and to work through feelings naturally.

Encourage the parents to ask questions and provide a telephone number for them to call if they have questions later or if they just want to talk more.

Be patient if the parents continue to ask the same questions.

Help the parents feel competent and in control:
- Assure the parents that they will be kept informed to enable them to participate effectively in decision making regarding their child's treatment and care.
- Provide the parents with information about parent support groups, family resource centers, services, resources, and financial assistance programs.
- Ask for permission to call and give their names and phone number to a parent self-help organization, so that the organization can reach out to them.
- Discuss the siblings and assure the parents that siblings tend to do well, especially if kept informed and included in the child's care.

Ongoing Information

Share complete information with the parents on an ongoing basis.

Share information in manageable doses. Ask the parents what information they want to receive at a given time to determine readiness and to avoid overload.

Be sensitive to the parents' reactions.

Listen carefully when the parents identify their needs, remembering that they may not always know the level of service they require (e.g., that respite service is having someone else take over for a while so they can get some rest).

Provide technical information in understandable terms, yet link these explanations with medical terminology.

Explain why certain questions are being asked.

Offer to share information with the child or with others involved in the child's care (e.g., brothers, sisters, grandparents, other extended family members, teachers, caregivers).

Provide information on family support programs, referrals for specialty consultations and intervention programs, and opportunities to meet other parents with a child with a similar condition.

prediction of possible prospects for the child, advice on what to do next, an opportunity to ask questions, a sympathetic and warm listener, and, most important, time. Determine the family's level of understanding and expectations. Assess comprehension of explanations with questions such as, "Is this clear to you?" or "Do you see what I mean?" Take notes for the family to refer to in the future. Provide parents with supplemental written information or a written summary of the diagnosis in keeping with their emotional readiness.

A crucial task for parents is to decide when, what, and how to tell their child about the diagnosis. Like parents, children later remember vividly what happened when the diagnosis was disclosed. Ideally the parents should be responsible for sharing this information with their child. However, they need much guidance in communicating information about the nature of the illness and the changes imposed on physical appearance and energy using a calm and honest approach. This is because parents frequently use euphemisms and try to protect their child from the harsh realities of the diagnosis and illness. Nurses can promote open communication between parents and ill child by providing them with information about how young children think and respond to illness and to changes in their parents (crying or increased concern).

The informing conference should not only include the presentation of devastating news, but emphasize the child's strengths and potential for development. Also assure the parents that the nurse will be available to answer questions and to provide further assistance as needed. Because of the need for long-term follow-up of chronic conditions, the initial informing conference is only one in a series of ongoing discussions. In all interactions the family's input is requested and included in the care plan (see Nursing Care Guidelines box, p. 872).

MANAGING THE CONDITION ON AN ONGOING BASIS

Promoting the family's adaptation to the day-to-day management of the child's condition involves education about the child's condition, general health care, and developmental needs and about realistic goal setting. Emotional support and assessment of the family also play a pivotal role in adaptation. Encourage families to articulate their goals and approaches to managing their children's condition, which provides vital information on how to intervene more thoughtfully with families based on their treatment approach.

Because the majority of mothers and fathers of children with special needs have little or no experience with children who have chronic or disabling conditions, the nurse can remind them of their child's many strengths and normal traits. Mothers and fathers need to experience happiness, success, and pride with regard to their child. The nurse can model appropriate interventions with the child. Most important, the nurse should ensure that the siblings and parents learn to perceive the child as a child first, with unique and individual needs and characteristics. The nurse needs to convey an accepting, humanistic attitude toward the child so that the parents can observe this acceptance. This attitude of having concern for, liking, and demonstrating acceptance of the child should begin in early infancy and continue throughout the child's life.

Special Information Needs

Educating the family about the child's condition is actually a continuation of the diagnostic talk (see Nursing Care Guidelines box, p. 859). Education involves providing technical information regarding management of the condition, such as how to administer insulin injections, and assessing both parental skills and understanding. In childhood cancer, educational components may include understanding and following a chemotherapy protocol, administering chemotherapy medications at home, anticipating and treating side effects, managing the child's adjustment to the illness, and arranging support and care from home health agencies and community resources (Hockenberry and Kline, 2010). Discussions with parents must also address the impact of the condition on the child. For example, children who have lost a limb require more than an explanation about the prosthetic leg. They need to know what restrictions it imposes on their activity level and how to function with it.

Parents also need guidance on how the child's condition may interfere with activities of daily living, such as dressing, eating, toileting, and sleeping* (see Family-Centered Care box). Common nutritional problems include overnutrition, which results from a caloric intake in excess of energy expenditure and may be related to boredom and lack of stimulation in other areas, and undernutrition, usually caused by inappropriate restriction of food, vomiting, loss of appetite, increased metabolic needs, or motor deficits that interfere with feeding. Although the child has the same basic needs as other children, the daily requirements may vary. Special nutritional considerations are discussed throughout the text.

🏃 FAMILY-CENTERED CARE
Identifying Family Needs

> To ensure an effective care plan, attention to basic family-identified needs and priorities is essential before understanding the nuances of the child's chronic condition.

Another major area in which modifications are necessary is car transportation. Children with conditions such as orthopedic, respiratory, or neuromuscular problems or low birth weight often cannot safely use conventional car restraints. For example, children with hip spica casts are unable to sit properly in child safety seats. (See Developmental Dysplasia of the Hip, Chapter 11.) Alterations can be made to some commercial models,† and for older children a special vest‡ is available that secures the child in a lying-down position to the back seat. Children in wheelchairs present special challenges because the wheelchair should be anchored with four points of attachment to the vehicle (two in front and two behind) and should always face forward. The family should contact the wheelchair manufacturer for specific instructions to ensure safe car transportation.

---

*Home care instruction sheets, which may be copied and given to families, are available in Hockenberry MJ: *Wong's clinical manual of pediatric nursing,* St Louis, ed 6, 2004, Mosby.
†Information on restraints for children with special needs is available from Automotive Safety Program, Riley Hospital for Children, www.preventinjury.org.
‡E-Z-On vest is available from E-Z-On Products, Inc., www.ezonpro.com.

Children with special needs require the usual primary health care recommended for any child. Anticipatory guidance, including attention to immunizations, injury prevention, dental health, and regular physical examinations, is important. Nurses play a pivotal role in reminding parents regarding these issues that are so frequently neglected when the concern is focused on the child's specific illness or disability. (See General Approaches Toward Examining the Child, Chapter 6, for information on assessing the general aspects of health maintenance. Specific discussions of sleep and activity, nutrition, dental health, and injury prevention are presented in the chapters on health promotion for particular age-groups. See Chapter 12 for a discussion of immunizations.)

Parents also need to be aware of the importance of communicating the child's condition in the event of an emergency. Young children are unable to give information regarding their condition, and older children may be unable or unwilling to speak after an accident. Thus all children with any type of chronic condition that may affect medical care should carry some type of identification, such as a medical alert bracelet (www.medicalert.org), which lists the medical condition and a collect telephone number for access to emergency medical records and other vital information.

Family Management Styles

Families who have a child with a chronic illness often face multiple challenges. This includes making sense of the illness in regard to its meaning for their life, mastering demanding treatment regimens, accommodating the family budget and routine to the demands of the illness, creating a normal life for the child despite the illness, and negotiating with school and health care professionals.

Family management style is the configuration formed by individual family members, the management behaviors they engage in with regard to the chronic condition, and the sociocultural context in which these behaviors occur (Shepard and Mahon, 2009). Five distinct family management styles have been identified: thriving, accommodating, enduring, struggling, and floundering.

Thriving and accommodating families perceive the condition and the child as "normal." Parents are confident in their ability to manage the illness; children see themselves as "healthy." Accommodating families differ from thriving families in that they perceive their situation as essentially normal but view it somewhat more negatively. They also take a more compliant approach to illness management. Enduring families view having a child with a chronic illness as difficult and as having major consequences for family life, and describe illness management as a burden. In contrast to families with thriving and accommodating management styles, these families perceive their child as a tragic figure, someone whose life chances have been irreparably compromised because of the illness, and are more protective of the child. Struggling families are characterized by conflict over how best to manage their child's condition. Struggling parents perceive less support and mutuality from one another; this is especially true of mothers, who feel that they receive inadequate support from their spouses in illness management. In floundering families the overriding theme is confusion. Parents view the illness negatively and perceive the child

as a tragic figure. They are uncertain about the best management approaches, and they view illness management as burdensome and difficult (Shepard and Mahon, 2009).

Understanding the various ways in which families may respond to a chronic illness—specifically, how they define the situation, manage daily life, handle conflict, and work jointly—can help nurses develop interventions tailored to the unique problems individual families encounter in managing the illness and the strengths on which they can draw. Tailored interventions may best foster optimal adaptation (see the discussion of coping strategies, p. 867).

MEETING THE CHILD'S NORMAL DEVELOPMENTAL NEEDS

General strategies for meeting a child's normal developmental needs in both the home and school settings include normalizing practices such as emphasizing abilities, deemphasizing limitations, structuring the environment to promote age-appropriate development, and providing appropriate discipline (see earlier discussion of these issues under Impact of Chronic Illness or Disability on the Child, p. 849).

For parents the task of meeting the child's normal developmental needs is integrally related to accepting the child's condition. Thus helping a family become aware of their reactions to the diagnosis and their reactions to managing the condition can help them evaluate their readiness to support the child's needs (see Table 22-2 for assessment questions).

While questioning parents about their reactions and understanding, the nurse can help them focus on the child's and sibling's knowledge of the condition. It is not uncommon for parents who appear knowledgeable and well adjusted to acknowledge that they have never told the children the truth about the illness. Conflict arises when the siblings or child learns of the diagnosis from nonparental sources. Parents may need assistance in deciding how best to explain a condition to children of various ages. (See Awareness of Dying in Children with Life-Threatening Illness, Chapter 23.)

Special challenges are present when assessing children's feelings about having a disability. The discussion on communication techniques in Chapter 6 focuses on a number of approaches to encourage children to discuss feelings regarding their diagnosis and future. For example, using play and drawing as a method of communication is appropriate for any child dealing with difficult feelings or a child who lacks verbal skills.

School is the second most important setting for a child. Teachers have a profound influence on the child's developmental progress, learning ability, feelings of self-esteem, and formation of social relationships. Whenever possible, nurses should ask parents for permission to visit the school to observe the child's interaction and behavior with classmates and teachers. A summary of objectives for home and school visits is given in the Nursing Care Guidelines box.

MEETING DEVELOPMENTAL NEEDS OF OTHER FAMILY MEMBERS

Each family that has a child with special needs is affected by the experience. The effects on the parents and their responses are

NURSING CARE GUIDELINES

Assessing the Child's Home and School Environment

- Observe the child's home and classroom behaviors, such as the ability to sit, follow directions, and comply with requests; observe the child's responses to questions; and determine the child's independence in functioning.
- Gather data on reported behavioral problems such as "hyperactivity," "non-compliance," or "stubbornness."
- Observe the child's interactions with siblings and peers.
- Observe the child's behaviors in structured and nonstructured activities.
- Observe the parents' and teacher's appropriate and inappropriate interactions with the child.
- Observe the parents' and teacher's teaching strategies with the child. (Are school strategies consistent with home teaching?)
- Observe the child's relationships with adults.
- Determine the parents' and teacher's concerns and expectations of the child.
- Administer standardized screening tools with the parent or teacher.
- Observe the child's energy level and any illness-related symptoms in relation to the daily schedule.
- Observe the child's behavior before, during, and after a medication regimen.
- Observe the child's eating patterns at home and at school.
- Collaborate with the parents and teacher in future planning for the child.
- Determine the effectiveness of programs of care for the child.
- Coordinate parents', teacher's, and others' plans for the child.
- Assess the teacher's and school nurse's understanding of the child's disorder.

BOX 22-4   STRESSES OF FAMILIES WITH A CHILD WITH SPECIAL NEEDS

Day-to-Day Stresses
Constant attention required by the child
Reactions of other children and the larger community
Social relations
Effect on siblings
Marital relations

Life Maintenance Stresses
Financial stress, insurance
Housing
Transportation
Clothing and appliances
Worries about the future
Future children
Schooling and vocational training
Residential care

Anticipated Parental Stress
Diagnosis of the condition—Requires considerable education, as well as dealing with emotional response
Developmental milestones—May be delayed or not attained
Entry into school—Appropriate learning may not take place in a regular classroom
Adolescence—Must address issues such as sexuality and independence
Future placement—Must decide about placement when the child becomes an adult or when the parents can no longer care for the child
Death of the child

Anticipated Sibling Stress
Birth of another child—May react to the birth of the affected sibling or the subsequent birth of an unaffected child
Diagnosis of the condition—Times of remission or exacerbations
Entry into school—May experience particular stress if friends reject the child with special needs
Adolescence—May be embarrassed to bring peers home
Future placement—May worry about responsibility for the affected sibling, especially if the parents are ill or die
Death of the child

so critical that they directly influence the other members' reactions and the child's own coping.

Parents

Grieving for the loss of a perfect child and managing the demands of caregiving can place many strains on parents (Box 22-4). In addition, parents may or may not receive positive feedback from interactions with their child. Many parents of children with special needs feel satisfaction and fulfillment from the parenting role. Adequate information, parent-to-parent support, collaboration with health care providers, and other resources can support and empower many parents. However, for others, parenting a child with a disability or chronic illness may be a series of unrewarding experiences that continually undermine the parents' feelings of adequacy and competence. These responses may be most evident in parents who are responsible for the child's care. For example, they may become preoccupied with their ability to carry out certain procedures, perhaps overlooking the child's personal comfort and satisfaction or failing to offer praise for anything less than perfect cooperation or performance. For these parents several strategies may be helpful: education regarding what can reasonably be expected of their child, assistance in identifying the child's strengths, praise for a parental job well done, and help in finding respite care so that the parent can renew his or her own energies.

Parental Roles

Caring for a child with chronic illness or disability may place tremendous demands on the parents' energy, time, and financial resources. In many cases the mother performs the bulk of the traditional child care and household responsibilities, and

the father shoulders the financial responsibilities. However, with changing gender roles these responsibilities may be shared, and parents may divide the tasks according to their level of comfort or skills. For example, the parent with patience for waiting may be the logical person to bring the child for tests, procedures, and examinations. In contrast, the parent who deals best with the illness and side effects of therapy can prepare the home for the child's return. On the other hand, involving both parents in decision making and in education regarding the care of the child with special needs can decrease some of the burden of care often placed inadvertently on mothers.

In some families, changing gender roles signify additional responsibilities for one parent. For example, the working mother may feel the need to remain employed to help pay expenses, but this adds to the burden of increased home and child care responsibilities. This may result in conflict, because one parent may perceive an unequal sharing of tasks with the partner.

In addition, the parent who is not involved in the caregiving activities may feel neglected because much attention is directed toward the child and resentful that he or she is not adequately informed to be competent in the care. Without active participation in the care of the child, the parent may have little understanding of the time and energy needed to perform those activities. When the less competent parent makes an effort to become involved, the other parent often criticizes the less skillful efforts. As a result, communication may break down, and neither is able to support the other.

Nurses can help parents avoid role conflict by providing anticipatory guidance early in the child's diagnosis. Teaching should address the stressors often identified as having an impact on the marriage: (1) home care with the burden assumed primarily by one parent, (2) the financial burden, (3) fear of the child's dying, (4) pressure from relatives, (5) the hereditary nature of the illness (if applicable), and (6) fear of pregnancy. Other causes of marital stress may concern the inconveniences related to care, for example, long waiting times for appointments, lack of overnight accommodations, and lack of parking near health care facilities. These stressors are certainly within the realm of health care professionals to minimize, if not eliminate, for parents.

Mother-Father Differences

Clarke, McCathy, Downie, and colleagues (2009) recently published a systematic review of 30 articles on gender differences in role perceptions; illness beliefs; psychologic distress; coping strategies; and perceptions of marital, family, and child functioning. Findings in relation to parent psychologic distress and preferred coping strategies were mixed, with trends toward increased distress, more emotion-focused coping, and greater need for social support in mothers.

To foster communication between parents who are adjusting to their child's chronic illness, the nurse can encourage them to recognize and accept differences in coping behaviors. This may increase mutual support and effect positive outcomes for their child's care.

Fathers

Fathers of children with chronic illness or disability face formidable challenges that are distinct from those of mothers (see Research Focus box). Fathers must reexamine priorities, come to terms with losses, and develop and strengthen caretaking abilities. Many fathers experience feelings of guilt and failure and may suffer from isolation because fewer social supports are available for men than for women. Feelings of isolation can be intensified by a health care system that frequently excludes, disenfranchises, and disregards men. Nurses can be instrumental in helping fathers of children with special needs overcome these challenges by addressing their concerns and engaging them in becoming supportive and important figures in the lives of their children (see Nursing Care Guidelines box).

Because the traditional paternal role, particularly with sons, emphasizes joint recreation over caregiving, fathers appear to have more difficulty adjusting to a son with special needs than to a daughter with special needs. With today's increasing emphasis on fathers' involvement in the lives of their children, this loss is felt more profoundly than in the past. However, fearful of losing control or being perceived as ineffectual or weak, a father may hide his feelings and exhibit an outward confidence that can lead others to believe that everything is fine (Goble, 2004).

RESEARCH FOCUS
Paternal Response to a Child with Chronic Illness

A study by Goble (2004) found that fathers were profoundly affected by their child's chronic illness in every aspect of their lives. Financial strain, limited social life, lack of intimacy, being primary caregiver for the healthy child, and concerns about the future were identified as the most common themes during their child's illness. These fathers coped with stress by working more and not complaining (Goble, 2004). Some fathers escape into their work as a way of dulling the pain. Others perceive having a child with special needs as a challenge to overcome, with the biggest worry being the ability to care for the child as a chronically ill adult (Goble, 2004).

NURSING CARE GUIDELINES
Encouraging the Involvement of Fathers in Caring for Children

- Be willing to include men in the care of the child, even when it appears they are not interested.
- Include fathers in education regarding the illness.
- Provide flexible clinic schedules.
- Foster fathers' strengths.
- Provide opportunities for men to embrace their children.
- Encourage men to talk with their own fathers, if possible.
- Provide a private place for men to grieve their loss.
- Encourage men to speak with other men.

Traditionally the mother and child have actively participated in and received professional care, whereas the father and siblings have been excluded. However, for the family unit to achieve optimum functioning, each member must be included. This means scheduling home and office visits at times when other family members can be present, which may dictate early morning, early evening, or late afternoon hours. Fathers often adjust their work schedule to meet with a health care professional once an invitation is offered.

Approach the task of including other members of a family in a visit positively. If they have not been included in the past, they may view such an invitation as a sign of more bad news or an indication of their own problems. One approach for welcoming others to participate is to remark that, after hearing so often about the father and the other siblings, the nurse wishes to meet them. This carries a friendly connotation and is nonthreatening.

Single-Parent Families

The field of pediatric chronic illness has not kept pace with the demographic changes that now characterize our society, changes that have the potential to profoundly affect child and family functioning (Brown, Wiener, Kupst, et al, 2008). Single-parent families of children with special needs are of particular concern. The proportion of children in two-parent families has decreased from 85% to 69% in the last 30 years; thus nearly 3 in 10 children live in single-parent homes (Shudy, de Almeida, Ly, et al, 2006). A parent may be absent due to death, divorce, or the parents never having married. Make special efforts to assist the single parent in obtaining support and financial services that can lessen the burden of care. Nurses can also be advocates for the single parent by suggesting helping roles for which friends and relatives can be enlisted. Some single parents are reluctant to join support groups because they feel out of place if the group is largely composed of married couples. Nurses need to assist single parents in mobilizing a positive social support network and must be empathetic to the concerns of single parents by locating appropriate resources to meet their needs.

Foster or Adoptive Families

Foster or adoptive families may benefit from information and support to encourage effective early adaptation to a chronic illness or developmental disability in the child. Information on the child's condition, unique needs, available services, warning signs of problems, and sources of both respite and support care can assist families in coping. Supporting foster families may promote longer-term placements or adoption of children with special needs.

Siblings

Many parents express concern regarding when and how to inform the other children in the family about the disability of a newborn sibling. The answer depends on each child's level of understanding and sophistication. Adolescents and even younger siblings routinely use the Internet to obtain information. What siblings piece together or overhear is often much worse than the truth. Often they imagine gruesome things regarding the experiences related to a sibling's illness, treatment, and hospitalization (Shepard and Mahon, 2009). Health care professionals need to anticipate questions and provide answers to children about the medical condition of their siblings in an age-appropriate manner that respects their constant need for information. Children need to be informed throughout the course of their sibling's illness. Parents are usually in the best position to impart this information, although they are often overwhelmed with the medical crisis at hand (Fleitas, 2000). Nurses can encourage parents to talk with the siblings about how they perceive their sick brother or sister and to be accepting of the siblings' feelings. Provisions should be made to allow siblings to visit the child in the hospital.

Nurses also can provide information to parents about teaching children of various ages and developmental stages. If the parents are unable to talk to the siblings, it is essential to find someone else who can do so in an appropriate manner. Nurses are ideal individuals to educate and counsel siblings during the course of their brother's or sister's illness (Shepard and Mahon, 2009).

Siblings must be prepared for the physical changes that their brother or sister will experience and for the possible role changes occurring in the family. Siblings must realize that their concerns, thoughts, and questions are important and acceptable. This includes jealousy toward the sick child and feelings of anger toward their parents. Siblings need reassurance that they will be kept abreast of their brother's or sister's treatment progress and, when possible, be involved in the care. When treatment necessitates parental absence from home or hospitalization of the sick child, a regularly scheduled time should be arranged for the siblings and parents to speak by telephone. This helps decrease separation anxiety and allows the siblings a sense of consistency, belonging, and involvement in the sick child's care (see Critical Thinking Exercise).

? CRITICAL THINKING EXERCISE

Impact of the Child with Special Needs on the Sibling

After the mother spends 2 weeks in the hospital with a severely disabled 9-year-old son, the previously quite cooperative 5-year-old brother suddenly becomes irritable, disruptive, defiant, and aggressive toward the mother.

1. Evidence—Is there sufficient evidence to draw conclusions about the 5-year-old sibling's behavioral change after the hospitalization stay of the disabled brother and mother?
2. Assumptions—Describe an underlying assumption about each of the following:
   a. Sibling's reaction to the 2-week absence of the mother and disabled brother
   b. Five-year-old's limited understanding of the 2-week absence of the mother and disabled brother
3. What priorities for nursing care should be established regarding the sibling's reaction?
4. Does the evidence support your nursing intervention?

Some siblings, particularly younger male or older female children, develop behavior or adjustment difficulties. Younger children tend to become irritable and withdrawn, whereas older siblings tend to act out. Some common difficulties include bed-wetting, headaches and other physical complaints, school phobia, changes in school performance, proneness to injury, sleep problems, depression, and severe separation anxiety.

Some problems for siblings arise from demands imposed by the child's condition. For example, at diagnosis the child with special needs by necessity becomes the focus of parental concern and attention. Frequent visits to a health care facility or hospitalizations disrupt the family routine. Siblings are pushed to the background, often staying at the homes of friends and relatives. The affected child's condition may interfere with vacations, holiday celebrations, and other special events. Siblings may resent these intrusions, which often require self-sacrifice. For a while parents may miss the siblings' ball games, school functions, or other activities and at times may be emotionally and physically unavailable to them. The family's emotional and financial resources may be directed toward the child with special needs. When this happens, there is often not only a decrease in normal family activities but a decrease in personal items and attention for the other children as well. Feelings of jealousy, anger, and resentment are not uncommon (see Research Focus Box). Siblings may worry about "catching" the condition or worry that playing rough with their brother or sister or even thinking bad thoughts about the sibling caused the condition. Nurses need to reassure siblings that their emotions are acceptable, but correct any misconceptions.

RESEARCH FOCUS

Sibling Response to Chronic Illness

Fleitas (2000) compiled data from interviews with siblings of hospitalized children and comments from other siblings who responded on a website titled "Band-Aids and Blackboards: When Chronic Illness . . . or Some Other Medical Problem . . . Goes to School." Feelings reported by siblings in response to having a brother or sister with medical problems were loneliness, responsibility, fear, jealousy, guilt, and resentment.

Feelings of resentment are also reported by siblings when their brother or sister with special needs becomes the focus of parental attention or is overprotected, indulged, or permitted to exhibit unacceptable behaviors. Parents may not realize that they are applying different standards to their children or they may feel that the child's condition calls for leniency.

Discipline provides structure and limits and should be consistent between siblings and within families (see Family-Centered Care box). When a child becomes seriously ill or disabled, the entire family is affected and role changes occur. Siblings, particularly older sisters, are often asked to assume increased responsibilities.

When children have complex disabilities or medical needs, particularly those that involve some degree of physical difference (e.g., hair loss), siblings must cope with the responses of others to these differences in appearance or behavior. This causes embarrassment for the siblings; however, at the same time they want to protect their brother or sister from the sarcastic remarks or stares of others (Fleitas, 2000). Having a child in the family who is disfigured, ill, or disabled labels the family as "different" (see Family-Centered Care box). When siblings perceive an illness to be life threatening, the power of the unspoken sibling bond is manifested. The child may demonstrate feelings of sadness when their future together as siblings is threatened. Finally, siblings report confusion arising from lack of information and poor communication with them about their brother's or sister's condition (Fleitas, 2000).

FAMILY-CENTERED CARE

Helping Parents Establish Expectations

Parents whose children have had prolonged or chronic illnesses sometimes have difficulty setting the boundaries of acceptable behavior with the child. The nurse has an opportunity to model behavior for the parent as care is delivered. For example, the nurse can establish a level of expectation that the child will perform age-appropriate self-care activities. It is important that expectations be established within an environment of respect for the child and the parent. When a child has been acutely ill, it is often a signal to the family that the nurse thinks the child is getting better if the child is expected to wash his or her face, brush his or her teeth, or pick up the toys in the room.

Chronically ill children can and should have age-appropriate assigned chores for which they are held responsible. Further, children should be knowledgeable about and participate in the management of their own health care regimen. Parents can learn what parts of the regimen can be delegated to the child and what parts must remain under the parents' control. The nurse can be a model for this type of parental behavior and a mentor as the parent learns where to set boundaries.

Often overlooked is the positive caring that exists between children with special needs and their brothers and sisters. Siblings feel pride and satisfaction in their own contributions to the family, happiness and excitement in their brother's or sister's achievements, and genuine love. Some siblings express that they sense more closeness in their families.

Research has shown positive aspects of sibling resilience when a child is ill. Children in families in which a sibling has a disability exhibit greater independence and maturity than do their peers. These children acknowledge feeling good about themselves and are proud of their patience and sense of responsibility. They also have a great appreciation of family closeness and health (Fleitas, 2000). Parental attitudes about the child and efforts promoting normalization are crucial in the development of positive reactions in siblings.

Nurses must be aware of and responsive to the reactions of siblings to their brother's or sister's illness or disability. Screening for sibling social support, mood, and self-esteem, both at the time of diagnosis and periodically, may help prevent mental health problems in siblings.

Focusing on strengths rather than problems requires nurses to impart an appreciation of how family members proceed with their lives despite the presence of a child with a chronic illness. Whenever possible, nurses need to intervene to foster positive adaptation. Siblings often state that they are expected to assume additional responsibilities to help parents care for the child. It is not unusual for them to display a positive reaction to taking on the extra duties but a negative reaction to feeling unappreciated for doing so. The nurse can help minimize such feelings by encouraging the siblings to discuss this with the parents and by advocating ways of showing gratitude, such as an increase in allowance, special privileges, and, most important, verbal praise (see Family-Centered Care box).

Extended Family Members and Friends

In addition to parents and siblings, a child's chronic illness or disability can have an impact on significant family members or friends. Although extended family relationships are often helpful to parents in rearing a child with special needs, they may also be sources of stress. For example, grandparents or other well-meaning relatives may attempt to reassure the parents that the child "will grow out of" his or her slowness at a time when parents are struggling to accept reality.

The nurse must be aware of the family's cues concerning sources of stress from extended family members such as grandparents. Encourage parents, when appropriate, to provide literature or to invite the grandparents to be present during one of the child's visits to the outpatient health care facility during the diagnostic period or during a conference with the health care team. Including grandparents in a discussion in which they can share their concerns may assist them in coping with their feelings and thereby lessen stress on the entire family. Grandparents may adapt even less well than parents because they lack adequate information, have limited involvement in decision making, and have less responsibility for the child's care. Often they feel helpless to provide assistance. Grandparents' feelings of anger and blame should be openly discussed. Grandparents can be helped to understand the impact of their behavior on the family with an appropriate statement such as, "Your son is presently experiencing a lot of pain and anguish. We realize that this is difficult for you, as well as your son; however, you can be of great help by being supportive of him."

Most grandparents experience some ambivalence because they love their grandchild yet feel personal disappointment when a diagnosis is made. They often experience two types of grief: for their grandchild who is ill and for their child, the parent, who is suffering. The future is now unpredictable, not only for the grandchild but for the child's parents as well. Behavioral disturbances such as poor decision making, disorganization, and disorientation, already seen in some older adults, may be intensified during grief. Grandparents do not

FAMILY-CENTERED CARE
Supporting Siblings of Children with Special Needs

Promote Healthy Sibling Relationships

Value each child individually and avoid comparisons. Remind each child of his or her positive qualities and contribution to other family members.

Help siblings see the differences and similarities between themselves and a child with special needs. Create a climate in which children can achieve successes without feeling guilty.

Teach siblings ways to interact with the child.

Seek to be fair in terms of discipline, attention, and resources; require the affected child to do as much for himself or herself as possible.

Let siblings settle their own differences; intervene only to prevent siblings from hurting one another.

Legitimize reasonable anger. Even children with special needs behave badly sometimes.

Respect a sibling's reluctance to be with or to include the child with special needs in activities.

Help Siblings Cope

Listen to siblings to let them know that their thoughts and suggestions are valued.

Praise siblings when they have been patient, have sacrificed, or have been particularly helpful. Do not expect siblings always to act in this manner.

Acknowledge the personal strengths siblings have and their ability to cope with stress successfully.

Provide age-appropriate information about the condition of the ill or disabled child and update when appropriate.

Let teachers know what is happening so they can be understanding and helpful.

Recognize special stress times for siblings and plan to minimize negative effects.

Schedule special time with siblings; have a friend or family member substitute when a parent is unavailable.

Encourage siblings to join or help establish a sibling support group.

Use the services of professionals when needed. If a parent feels that such a service is necessary, it should be provided in a vigorous a manner as a service for the child with special needs.

Involve Siblings

Seek out ways to realistically include siblings in the care and treatment of the child with special needs.

Limit caregiving responsibilities and give recognition when siblings fulfill them.

Develop a library of children's books on special needs.

Invite siblings to attend meetings to develop plans for the child with special needs (e.g., individualized education program, individualized family service plan).

Discuss future plans with them.

Solicit their ideas on treatment and service needs.

Have them visit professionals who work with the child.

Help them develop competencies to teach the child new skills.

Provide opportunities for siblings to advocate for the child.

Allow siblings to set their own pace for learning and involvement.

Modified from Powell T, Ogle P: *Brothers and sisters: a special part of exceptional families*, Baltimore, 1985, Paul H Brooks; Spokane Washington Deaconess Medical Center, Pediatric Oncology Unit: Tips for dealing with siblings, *Candlelighters Childhood Center Found Q Newsl* 11(3,4):7, 1987; and Carlson J, Leviton A, Mueller M: Services to siblings: an important component of family-centered practice, *ACCH Advocate* 1(1):53-56, 1993.

often admit these emotions, and they are left to adjust on their own. Although support groups for grandparents are uncommon, they can be helpful. Special support may be needed for the grandparent assuming the role of a primary caregiver for the child.

Significant stress can also arise from nonfamilial sources, such as neighbors, friends, or strangers. Neighbors display various reactions to the child's diagnosis. Some turn away, some pry, and some ask inappropriate questions or make insensitive remarks. Inability to deal with comments about the condition or curious stares by others may promote the tendency to protect and isolate the child in the home. The family needs guidance in preparing for these inevitable encounters. One approach is encouraging parents to dress the child as much as possible like his or her peers. Good grooming is extremely important in minimizing differences in appearance. Through role playing, parents can rehearse responses to comments such as, "Is your child retarded?" or "Has he always been crippled?" Parent groups can allow family members to share experiences and learn from each other about dealing with unkind remarks or probing questions. They also provide a type of support parents cannot obtain from relatives, friends, and neighbors.

Some neighbors and friends will not allow their children to play with the child or siblings for fear of contagion or formation of a close friendship with a child who might die. For some parents friendships may be difficult to maintain because they have little time and energy for social gatherings. Friends may withdraw for a number of reasons, such as being uncomfortable with the situation and feeling unable to help.

Parents have to decide how much and what to tell relatives, friends, baby-sitters, and teachers. Concerns regarding discrimination are very real for parents and must be balanced with the need to share information so that the child receives proper care.

Nurses can address the issue of discrimination by asking parents if they have worries about how to inform others of the child's condition. Intervention strategies not only must focus on problems confronting children and families but also must discreetly consider the many sources from which discrimination may develop. Nurses may also be able to provide suggestions regarding essential education for others who will care for the child.

COPING WITH ONGOING STRESS AND PERIODIC CRISES

Families of children with chronic conditions face ongoing stress associated with factors such as the child's condition and financial concerns (see Box 22-4). They also may undergo periodic crises, including uncertainty regarding the diagnosis and the need to cope with recurrent hospitalizations. Some families are strengthened by being able to deal with these stresses. Others become overwhelmed when stresses exceed resources. The increasing stress can overwhelm family resources and result in a financial crisis (Goble, 2004). Concurrent stresses such as out-of-pocket expenditures related to the chronic condition pose additional challenges (Newacheck and Kim, 2005).

Health care professionals can assist families in coping with stress by providing anticipatory guidance, offering emotional support, helping the family to assess and recognize specific stressors, assisting the family in developing problem-solving strategies and coping mechanisms, continuing efforts to meet developmental needs, encouraging spiritual beliefs to find hope and meaning, and working collaboratively with parents so they become empowered in the process.

Concurrent Stresses Within the Family

The ability to cope with the overwhelming stresses of a lifelong illness or disability is challenged further when additional stresses are present. Ongoing stresses and strains in the family accumulate, increasing the family's vulnerability and lessening its ability to adapt to a child with special needs. For some family members, non-illness-related stressors are perceived as more stressful than those related to a child's chronic condition.

Stressors may be developmental or situational. They may be associated with sibling needs, marital discord, homelessness, or social isolation. Even the more minor stresses, such as managing the home, arranging care for siblings, and commuting to distant treatment centers, can challenge a family's ability to cope successfully (see Box 22-4).

Family or child developmental stressors exacerbate situational stresses. For example, a common developmental stressor in the family life cycle is the birth of a child, an event that necessitates adjustment by the parents. The birth of a child with a congenital health problem adds situational stress to the equation.

The majority of families, regardless of their insurance coverage or income, have financial concerns. The costs of caring for a child with special needs can be overwhelming. Children with functional limitations account for one third of child hospital days, and their hospital stays are twice as long; they also visit physicians twice as often as children without limitations. Direct medical expenses, transportation costs, nonprescription medication, wigs or cosmetics to conceal the effects of the illness or treatment, parking, meals, housing, and child care can consume a high percentage of a family's income.

Additional loss of family income occurs when parents take time off work or quit a job to care for a child.* The family breadwinner may also have to sacrifice career opportunities to remain close to the child's treatment center.

Nurses can make appropriate referrals to case managers and social workers to assist a family in reviewing various options for financial assistance, including insurance, health maintenance organization or managed care policies, Medicaid, the Supplemental Security Income (SSI) program, Women, Infants, and Children (WIC) program, the state program for children with special health needs, disease-related associations, and local philanthropic organizations.

Coping Mechanisms

Coping mechanisms are those behaviors directed at reducing the tension elicited by a crisis. Approach behaviors are coping mechanisms resulting in movement toward adjustment and resolution of the crisis. Avoidance behaviors result in movement away from adjustment or maladaptation to the crisis. Several approach and avoidance behaviors used in coping with a chronic illness or disability are listed in the Nursing Care Guidelines box. None of the indicators can be used alone to assess possible success or failure in resolving the crisis. Each behavior must be seen in the context of all of the variables

influencing the family. For example, the observation of many avoidance behaviors in an emotionally healthy family may indicate significantly less risk to the successful resolution of the crisis than an equal number of avoidance behaviors in an individual who has few available supports.

NURSING CARE GUIDELINES

Assessing Coping Behaviors

Approach Behaviors

Asks for information regarding diagnosis and present condition

Seeks help and support from others

Anticipates future problems; actively seeks guidance and answers

Shares burden of disorder with others

Plans realistically for the future

Acknowledges and accepts child's awareness of diagnosis and prognosis

Expresses feelings, such as sorrow, depression, and anger, and realizes reason for the emotional reaction

Realistically perceives child's condition; adjusts to changes

Recognizes own growth through passage of time, such as earlier denial and nonacceptance of diagnosis

Verbalizes possible loss of child

Avoidance Behaviors

Fails to recognize seriousness of child's condition despite physical evidence

Refuses to agree to treatment

Intellectualizes about the illness, but in areas unrelated to child's condition

Is angry and hostile to members of the staff, regardless of their attitude or behavior

Avoids staff, family members, or child

Entertains unrealistic future plans for child, with little emphasis on the present

Is unable to adjust to or accept a change in progression of disease

Continually looks for new cures with no perspective toward possible benefit

Refuses to acknowledge child's understanding of disease and prognosis

Uses magical thinking and fantasy; may seek "occult" help

Places complete faith in religion to point of relinquishing own responsibility

Withdraws from outside world; refuses help

Punishes self because of guilt and blame

Makes no change in lifestyle to meet needs of other family members

Resorts to excessive use of alcohol or drugs to avoid problems

Verbalizes suicidal intention

Is unable to discuss possible loss of child or previous experiences with death

Two long-term coping strategies of familial adaptation to severe and chronic childhood illness have been found to be significantly related to a high level of family functioning. The first is the parents' ability to assign the illness meaning within an existing medical-scientific or spiritual philosophy of life. They have an optimistic belief that things work out for the best and an emphasis on the positive qualities of the situation. Statements such as "God has chosen our family to care for this special child" reflect the religious philosophy.

The second long-term coping strategy of family adaptation is an ability to share the burdens imposed by the illness with individuals both inside and outside the family network. Intrafamilial relationships promote togetherness of the family members and support a mutual recognition that all members are vital contributors to the family unit. Extrafamilial supports help preserve meaningful external contacts and provide needed assistance to the family.

The chronic illness trajectory model recognizes that chronic conditions have a course that changes over time (Corbin and Strauss, 1995). The course of the illness is influenced by several

---

*Information regarding financial issues is available from Family Voices, Inc., a grassroots advocacy network of parents and professionals; www.familyvoices.org.

psychologic and medical factors, including resources (interpersonal, intrapersonal, and instrumental), technology, motivation, experience, the type and severity of the illness, lifestyle, and the social climate. Most chronic illness management occurs in the home, not in the hospital. This model advocates that the goal of nursing care in chronic illness is to assist the family in shaping the course of the illness medically while maintaining quality of life for the child and family. This is achieved through assessment, teaching, monitoring, and initiation of referrals.

Fostering normalization, teaching coping skills, and assisting the family in using or further defining their social support networks are other nursing interventions that can encourage and empower the parents and promote positive adaptation in the family and optimum mental health for the child.

Parental Empowerment

Empowerment can be viewed as a personal process through which individuals develop and use the necessary knowledge, confidence, and competence to make their voices heard. Nurses can provide resources and support to parents of chronically ill children based on their individual level of empowerment. Nurses can also encourage parent membership on staff, boards, and committees and include parents in presentations at conferences and meetings. Nurses can help keep parents abreast of pending legislation on child health issues and take action when appropriate.*

ASSISTING FAMILY MEMBERS IN MANAGING THEIR FEELINGS

Considerable individual variation is seen in reactions to the diagnosis, use of defense mechanisms, and time frames for coming to terms with a diagnosis. It is imperative that professionals recognize and respect the vast range of reactions and coping mechanisms. In fact, members of a family of a child with chronic illness or disability may experience many difficult emotions, such as guilt, fear, anger, resentment, and anxiety (see Nursing Care Guidelines box). Support from health professionals, extended family members, and friends can help family members deal with their feelings. When parents are able to cope successfully with the stress of caring for their disabled child, all family members experience positive outcomes such as a sense of increased love and warmth within the family, discovery of meaning for one's life, a strong sense of having done a good job

NURSING CARE GUIDELINES

Encouraging Expression of Emotion

- Describe the behavior: "You seem angry at everyone."
- Give evidence of understanding: "Being angry is only natural."
- Give evidence of caring: "It must be difficult to endure so many painful procedures."
- Help focus on feelings: "Maybe you wonder why this happened to your child."

*An excellent resource for becoming involved in political action is the *Public Affairs Public Issues Handbook,* available from the American Cancer Society, www.cancer.org; and Family Voices, Inc., see footnote on p. 867.

parenting, a sense of pride in the disabled child's achievements no matter how small, and discovery of meaning in the presence of a disabled child in the family.

Shock and Denial

The initial diagnosis of a chronic illness or disability is often met with intense emotion characterized by shock, disbelief, and sometimes denial, especially if the disorder is not obvious, such as in chronic illness. Denial as a defense mechanism is a necessary cushion to prevent disintegration and is a normal response to grieving for any type of loss. Probably all family members experience various degrees of adaptive denial as they learn of the impact that the diagnosis has on their lives.

Shock and denial can last from days to months, sometimes even longer. Manifestations of denial that may occur at the time of diagnosis include (1) physician shopping; (2) attributing the symptoms of the actual illness to a minor condition; (3) refusing to believe the diagnostic test results; (4) delaying in agreeing to treatment; (5) acting happy and optimistic despite the revealed diagnosis; (6) refusing to tell or talk to anyone about the condition; (7) insisting that no one is telling the truth, regardless of others' attempts to do so; (8) denying the reason for hospital admission; and (9) asking no questions about the diagnosis, treatment, or prognosis. Generally, these behaviors should be respected as short-term responses that allow individuals to protect themselves from a tremendous emotional impact and to collect and mobilize their energies toward goal-directed, problem-solving behaviors.

In some instances, various indicators of denial can actually be adaptive behaviors. Searching for another professional opinion may mean that parents cannot obtain answers to their questions or that they are looking for a different approach to treatment that better meets the needs of their child and family. When parents discuss their strengths and the benefits they derive from caring for their child with special needs, it does not necessarily reflect refusal to accept their difficult circumstances. Sometimes a delay in making decisions or a failure to ask questions simply reflects a lack of information.

Families with children who have life-threatening conditions commonly exhibit partial denial, such as seeking additional professional consultations or occasionally acting as if nothing were wrong. Without such a temporary protective mechanism, few people could survive the constant emotional drain of anticipating their own death or the death of a family member. Partial denial allows the child and family to absorb stressful information or "dose" themselves in amounts they can personally manage at the time.

In children denial has repeatedly been demonstrated as an important factor in their positive coping with the diagnosis. Denial allows the child to maintain hope in the face of overwhelming odds and to function adaptively and productively. Like hope, denial may be an adaptive mechanism for dealing with loss that persists until the family or patient is ready or needs other responses.

Denial is probably the reaction that is least understood and most poorly handled. Health care professionals commonly label denial as maladaptive and act inappropriately by attempting to strip it away through repeated and often blunt explanations of the prognosis. Because denial is based on fear, nurses need to address parental feelings of inadequacy. It is imperative that health professionals understand that denial is a necessary coping mechanism.

Denial becomes maladaptive only when it impedes recognition of treatment or rehabilitative goals essential for the child's optimum development or survival. For example, protracted denial may be evident in the response of a family to cognitive impairment. As long as the family can maintain a function of normality and manage the difference within the existing familial values and roles, they may not recognize the diagnosis. Rather, the problem is explained as an easily treated condition or as slow maturation. The child's social development may strengthen the denial, which disguises the degree of speech and motor impairment. Not uncommonly, this ability to rationalize delayed development is successful until the child begins school and is compared with other children, which makes his or her differences apparent. At this point the family may start to perceive the illness as a crisis and respond with shock and disbelief. Denial is no longer beneficial to the family, and other coping mechanisms must be used.

Adjustment

For most families, adjustment gradually follows shock and is usually characterized by an open admission that the condition exists. Adjustment may be accompanied by a number of responses that are normal components of the adaptation process. Perhaps the most universal of these feelings are guilt and self-accusation. Guilt is often greatest when the cause of the condition is linked directly to the parent, such as in genetic disorders or accidental injuries. However, it can arise even without any realistic or scientific basis for parental responsibility. Often the guilt develops from a false assumption that the disability is a result of personal wrongdoing or failing, such as not doing something correctly during the pregnancy or the birth. Guilt may be associated with religious or cultural beliefs as well. Some parents are convinced that they are being punished for some earlier misdeed. Others may perceive the condition as a sacrifice required by God to test their religious faith and strength. With appropriate information, support, and time, most parents deal with self-accusation and guilt. The ability to cope with resentful and self-accusatory feelings of having "caused" the child's condition is a critical factor in determining the parents' acceptance of their child.

Children also may perceive their serious illness as retribution for past misbehavior. The nurse should be particularly aware of the child who passively accepts all painful procedures. This child may believe that such acts are inflicted because of deserved punishment. It is always best to assure children that the goal during diagnosis or treatment is to make them feel better.

Other common reactions to a diagnosis of chronic illness or disability are anger and bitterness. Anger is a normal and expected reaction to chronic illness that arises when an individual realizes that certain needs, wishes, and plans for the future can no longer be satisfied due to limitations imposed by an illness. An intense feeling of unfairness consequently leads to feelings of frustration and anger. Anger directed inward may be manifested as punitive or self-reproaching behavior, such as verbally degrading oneself and neglecting one's health. In contrast, anger directed outward may be revealed in either open arguments or withdrawal from communication with several individuals, such as the child, siblings, and spouse. Passive anger toward the child may be manifested in refusal to believe how sick the child is, inability to provide comfort, or decreased visiting. Among the most common targets for parental anger are members of the health care team. Parents may complain about the lack of time physicians spend with them, the nursing care, or the lack of qualified individuals to draw blood or start intravenous infusions (see Critical Thinking Exercise).

❓ CRITICAL THINKING EXERCISE

Parental Anger

The mother of an obese adolescent who was recently diagnosed with type 2 diabetes begins to argue with you about the insulin injection. The mother angrily shouts, "Why does my child have to take painful insulin injections anyway?"

1. Evidence—Is there sufficient evidence to draw conclusions about the mother's reactions regarding her child's recent diagnosis of type 2 diabetes?
2. Assumptions—Describe an underlying assumption about each of the following:
   a. Parent's reaction to her adolescent's recent diagnosis of type 2 diabetes
   b. Parent's reaction to the cause of type 2 diabetes in an obese adolescent
   c. Parent's feelings toward the medical provider and insulin treatment
3. What priorities for nursing care should be established with regard to the mother's reactions?
4. Does the evidence support your nursing intervention?

Children are likely to respond with anger, and this includes the ill child and the healthy siblings. Children are aware of the loss caused by their illness or disability and may react angrily to the feelings of being different from their peers or to the limitations instituted. Siblings may also feel resentment and anger toward the ill child and parents for the loss of parental attention and daily routines in the home. It is difficult for older children and almost impossible for younger children to understand the plight of the ill child. Their perception is of a sister or brother who has the undivided attention of their parents, is showered with toys and other gifts, and is the focus of everyone's concern.

Children of various ages exhibit anger differently. Young children may display their uncooperativeness by screaming, yelling, and physically fighting off the adversary. In contrast, older children use abusive language. Passive anger, expressed in such statements as "I don't know" or "I don't care," usually elicits anger in others and may be misconstrued as an obnoxious, sullen, or hostile response. As a result, these statements are effective in keeping people at a distance, when the hidden message really is "I need to talk. Please help me understand what is happening."

During the period of adjustment, four types of parental reactions to the child affect the child's eventual response to the condition: (1) overprotection, in which the parents fear allowing the child to achieve any new skill, avoid all discipline, and cater to every desire to impede frustration; (2) rejection, in

BOX 22-5	CHARACTERISTICS OF PARENTAL OVERPROTECTION

- Sacrifices self and rest of family for the child
- Continually helps the child, even when the child is capable
- Is inconsistent with regard to discipline or employs no discipline; frequently applies different rules to the other siblings
- Is dictatorial and arbitrary, making decisions without considering the child's wishes, such as keeping the child from attending school
- Hovers and offers suggestions; calls attention to every activity, overdoing praise
- Protects the child from every possible discomfort
- Restricts play, often because of fear that the child will be injured
- Denies the child opportunities for growing up and assuming responsibility, such as learning to give own medications or perform treatments
- Does not understand the child's capabilities and sets goals too high or too low
- Monopolizes the child's time, such as sleeping with the child, permitting few friends, or refusing participation in social or educational activities

BOX 22-6	CONCEPT OF FUNCTIONAL BURDEN

Impact of Child with Special Needs
Child's need for medical and nursing care
Child's fixed deficits
Child's age-appropriate dependency in activities of daily living
Disruptions in the family routine caused by the care
Competing demands for family members' time and energy
Psychologic burden of the prognosis on the family

Family Resources and Ability to Cope
Family's physical resources
Family's emotional resources
Family's educational resources
Family's social supports and available help

which the parents detach themselves emotionally from the child but usually constantly nag and scold the child and provide adequate physical care; (3) denial, in which the parents act as if the condition does not exist or attempt to have the child overcompensate for it; and (4) gradual acceptance, in which the parents place realistic and necessary limitations on the child, foster reasonable social and physical activities, and promote self-care. Overprotection (Box 22-5) is such a common parental reaction that it behooves the nurse to assess for its presence and to begin anticipatory guidance with the family when appropriate. Many of these characteristics are also seen in the vulnerable child syndrome and could occur or persist should the child recover from injury or illness. (See Chapter 10.)

Reintegration and Acknowledgment

For many families the adjustment process concludes in the development of realistic expectations for the child and reintegration of family life with the disability or illness in a manageable perspective. Because a significant portion of this phase is one of grief for a loss, total resolution is not possible until the child dies or leaves home as an independent adult. Thus one can regard adjustment as "increased comfort" with day-to-day living rather than as a complete resolution.

This adjustment phase also involves social reintegration in which the family broadens its activities to include relationships outside the home, with the child as a participating and acceptable member of the group. This latter criterion often distinguishes the reaction of gradual acceptance during the adjustment period from total acceptance or possibly is more descriptive of the acknowledgment process.

During the acknowledgment phase of adjustment, individuals take stock of what remains rather than focusing on what is lost and begin to establish new goals for their lives. It is a time when the family is particularly motivated to learn about the restrictions imposed by the child's illness and to decide how they want to function within those confines. Nursing interventions that emphasize self-control are particularly beneficial because they promote the highest level of function possible and increase a sense of self-worth.

Many parents of children with special needs experience chronic sorrow, an emotional reaction exhibited throughout the span of the parent-child interaction. Chronic sorrow occurs while parents redefine parental expectations and the parameters for appraising the child's achievements. External events, such as the passage of a child's expected date of graduation, trigger resurgences of chronic sorrow when the parent is again reminded of what could have been.

ESTABLISHING A SUPPORT SYSTEM

The diagnosis of a serious health problem or disability in a child is a major situational crisis affecting the entire family. However, families can experience positive outcomes while they successfully cope with the many challenges that accompany a child with chronic illness or disability. One nursing goal is to assess which families are at lesser or greater risk for succumbing to the effects of the crisis. A number of variables, including available support systems, reactions to the child, perception of the illness or disability, coping mechanisms, available financial resources, and concurrent stresses within the family, may affect the resolution of a crisis. Although most families do cope, the needs of families at risk are considerable. If they receive guidance and emotional support early in the crisis, there is an increased possibility that they will cope successfully.

Although it is easy to assume that families of children with the most severe illnesses or disabilities will have the poorest adjustment, the severity of the condition is only one part of the overall picture. The level of adjustment is greatly influenced by the functional burden on the family. The issues associated with caring for and living with the child must be considered in relation to the family's resources and coping ability (Box 22-6). The family of a child with multiple disabilities warranting complex care that has many coping strategies and resources may adjust more successfully to the child's situation than the family of a child with a less serious condition and few resources to counterbalance it.

Intrafamilial resources, social support from friends, parent-to-parent support, parent-professional partnerships, and community resources intertwine to provide a flexible web of support for the family of a child with a chronic condition.

Intrafamilial Resources

Family members' experience or maturity, education, intelligence, ability and willingness to learn how to provide the child's care, sense of humor, and sense of optimism are resources they can bring to a situation. Resources within the family, such as adaptability, cohesion, a sense of coherence, and hardiness, can greatly facilitate the family's adjustment.

The marital relationship is a primary source of potential support and overall is the best predictor of coping behavior and adjustment. Conflicts in parental role definition and differences in paternal and maternal coping patterns can place a strain on the marital relationship. Most health care professionals assume that the rate of family dissolution is greater due to increased familial stress from the presence of a chronic condition in a family member. These families may experience more conflict and strain over the roles of their members, as well as fewer exchanges of affection. Parents of chronically ill children, however, are not more likely to experience higher levels of marital dissatisfaction, economic problems, or depression than families of healthy children (Emerson, 2003). When partners can openly discuss their feelings, there appears to be much less guilt, blame, anger, and indecision. Each crisis during the lengthy period of chronic illness is successfully resolved, which reduces the overlapping and accumulation of multiple stresses.

Social Support Systems

The significant others who are available to individuals for emotional strength during periods of crisis constitute their support system. Support systems may be available through various relationships and may include one significant other, such as a spouse, or a group of significant others, such as the health care team or the extended family. The amount and type of social support received by families is a crucial factor in their adjustment to the child's chronic condition.

The source of support is a determining factor in the effectiveness of certain forms of support. For example, emotional or expressive support is best provided by individuals with whom one has strong ties and who are like oneself. The ability to verbalize feelings such as guilt, anger, fear, or anxiety helps individuals deal with the particular emotion. Verbalization allows for the validation of thoughts and feelings. When professionals develop a strong therapeutic relationship with the family, they also can be appropriate sources of emotional support (see Parent-Professional Partnerships later in the chapter).

On the other hand, instrumental support can often be provided by those to whom the family has weaker ties and can link the family to a more diverse and broader social network. For example, the most appropriate sources of informational support are both professionals who have practical and theoretic knowledge, and nonprofessionals or parents whose experience makes them experts.

Coping with illness or disability may be a new experience for a family and their support system, and the family may benefit from recommendations on effective ways to use their support system to meet their needs. Providing parents with written information they can share with extended family can often help them reach out to others during a stressful time. In addition, helping family members identify members of their support system and consider practical tasks for which to request assistance (e.g., laundry, care of siblings, and transportation) can mobilize resources.

Health care providers should assess the type of support needed before planning interventions. They may assist families early in the diagnostic and treatment processes by encouraging them to plan for and use helpful resources. Parents may also benefit from the suggestion that it is okay to refuse certain types of well-intended support from friends and family (Shepard and Mahon, 2009). Families often state that they need help finding recreational activities and community resources for their children with chronic conditions. Health care providers can help by identifying the types of support that may be most helpful to the family and by being culturally sensitive and informed about parents' groups and community resources.

Because of withdrawal and social isolation, some individuals may not be able to reach out to others for practical or emotional support. These individuals are more likely to feel overwhelmed and may benefit from consultation with a social worker or therapist.

Parent-to-Parent Support

The support a parent receives from another parent is unique and cannot be obtained from any other source. Veteran parents provide something that other support systems cannot in shared experiences. They have intimately known the stress related to diagnosis; weathered the many transitional times, such as moving from one program to another; and have sifted through services so that they have a practical knowledge of resources. A growing number of clinics and hospitals now have on staff a parent with a child who is chronically ill or disabled. The services these parents provide are invaluable for parents of children with special needs who are likely to experience lengthy and repeated hospitalizations and many routine outpatient visits.

Just being with another parent who has shared similar experiences can be beneficial. It is not always necessary for this parent to have a child with the same diagnosis. Parents walk a common path in the process of adjusting to a child with special needs or finding respite services, rehabilitative or educational services, special equipment vendors, or financial counseling.

If the child's treatment center does not have a parent staff position, the nurse can contact parent groups, who will usually send a representative. Another intervention is to ask another parent with a chronically ill or disabled child to talk with the parents. The nurse should seek out a parent who has a nonjudgmental approach to differences in families, is a good listener, and has good problem-solving and advocacy skills.

The parent self-help group is another approach to fostering parent-to-parent support.* Group members feel less alone and have the opportunity to observe both mastery role modeling and coping in other members. Parents' groups are rich resources for information. Even if parents cannot attend meetings, they can still benefit from the group newsletters and other literature

---

*Information about self-help groups, as well as books and pamphlets, is available from the National Self-Help Clearinghouse, 365 5th Ave., Suite 3300, New York, NY 10016; 212-817-1822; fax: 212-817-2990; e-mail: info@selfhelpweb.org; www.selfhelpweb.org.

that often accompany membership. The nurse can promote parent participation in self-help groups by serving as a group advisory board member, a referral agent, a resource person, or an assistant in finding a group. Often all that is necessary to start a group is identifying one or two parents as leaders; sharing with them the names, addresses, and telephone numbers of other families; and guiding them in how to organize the first meeting.

Parent-Professional Partnerships

One important component of family-centered care is parent-professional collaboration. By their nature, collaborative relationships show respect and therefore support for families. Collaboration reflects a change from the traditional models of care. For this reason nurses must examine their attitudes to determine their ability to participate in parent-professional partnerships. A basic characteristic is the belief that parents are experts concerning their child. The partnership is based on trust and communication. The Nursing Care Guidelines box offers strategies for developing successful partnerships with parents.

 NURSING CARE GUIDELINES

Developing Successful Parent-Professional Partnerships

- Promote primary nursing; in nonhospital settings designate a case manager.
- Acknowledge parents' overall competence and their unique expertise with their child.
- Respect parents' time as having value equal to that of other members of the child's health care team.
- Explain or define any medical, technical, or discipline-specific terms.
- Tell families, "I am not sure" or "I don't know," when appropriate.
- Facilitate family's effectiveness in team meetings (e.g., provide parents with same information as other participants).

Throughout the lengthy process of caring for a child with special needs, family members become experts in managing their child's care. Unfortunately, this expertise is not always acknowledged by health care providers, who tend to be directive rather than collaborative in their approach to the family. This is particularly common during periods of hospitalization, when role confusion occurs. At home parents are expected to care for their child, yet in the hospital they may be disregarded as participants in care. Provision of a supportive atmosphere must include respect for parents' knowledge, coordination of care with family members, and willingness to include their suggestions in the treatment plan.

Partnership depends on good communication. A nurse's classification or perception of the "difficult" family can influence nurse-family communication. A family whose child is ill responds along what health care providers may perceive as a continuum from the "good" to the "difficult" family stereotype. Nurses readily establish relationships with the "good" family, who perceive staff as having control or power and accept this hierarchy. However, often this is not the case with a family that is considered "difficult" and is characterized as being overinvolved or underinvolved in the child's care.

Nurses also display patterns of behavior with regard to parents of ill children. First, facilitative nurses acknowledge the parents' crucial roles and attempt to remove barriers to their involvement in care. Second, nurses who desire a high degree of control over their work may become "rule enforcers" with parents. Third, nurses may establish collegial relationships with parents over time, with respect for the parents as experts regarding their child. Finally, nurses may avoid a parent whose values differ from their own or a parent who is overly demanding from the nurses' perspective.

The nurse and family come to have explicit and implicit expectations of one another, form views of one another, and negotiate roles in the child's care. Levels of trust and control are central to their interactions.

Parents who mistrust professionals act differently from those who have trust in the health care team. Nurses trust parents differently as well, based on their judgments of the parenting they observe.

Community Resources

In the past, if coping strategies could not be used to reduce the disruption and stress of maintaining the child in the home, the seriously affected child may have been permanently placed outside the home in a residential facility. Such placements are increasingly difficult to secure. Options vary from one location to another; however, many possibilities can be considered: in-home care by nursing personnel, medical daycare, respite care, transitional and long-term care, and medical or specialized foster care.

A family's acknowledgment that caring for their child is burdensome is not necessarily maladjustment. Alternative placements may be the only option that will maintain the family's integrity. Aging parents may be forced to accept such alternatives because of progressive inability to meet the demands of a child's severe disability. When most of the child's care is given over to others, abandoning the role of primary caregiver may be followed by an initial sense of loss, guilt, relief, and ambivalence, patterns of reactions not unlike those seen after the death of a terminally ill child. (See Chapter 23.) Besides out-of-home placement options, other community resources, such as parent support groups, health care resources, financial assistance, rehabilitation services, respite care, alternatives for schooling, equipment, and educational facilities and recreational programs,* are major elements in family adjustment.

Local and national disease-oriented organizations may provide needed support and assistance to families that qualify. Many of these organizations are identified elsewhere in the text under discussion of the specific diagnosis. Federal and state departments of health, social services, mental health, and labor may be able to help locate appropriate regional resources. For example, state programs for children with special health needs (formerly crippled children's services) offer financial assistance for children with various disabling conditions. Nurses should become familiar with those in their communities and with vocational programs for special groups.

---

*A general source of information is the National Dissemination Center for Children with Disabilities, www.nichcy.org. A comprehensive list of books and pamphlets for parents and teachers is available from Easter Seals, www.easterseals.com.

Although community resources may exist, it is often difficult for parents to find appropriate services, and coordination among many agencies may be lacking. Fragmented care is a key complaint of families, and specific problems of delayed referral and negative experiences with agency personnel are identified as other concerns. Therefore community networking for improved services is essential.

> **! NURSING ALERT**
>
> Be aware that many families may not have a telephone. Some families may have a telephone but may be reluctant to reveal the telephone number. To overcome these difficulties, use the following strategies:
> 1. Help the family identify telephone access close to home (e.g., neighbor's home, nearby store).
> 2. Explore methods of obtaining telephone service for the family (e.g., social service agencies, charitable organizations).
> 3. Be sensitive to the family's concern for privacy when asking for a telephone number; explain the reason for needing the number and to whom it will be given.
>
> Case management is a crucial service for families of children with special needs. Effective case management can result in both the use of more community services and improved financial assistance for families.

KEY POINTS

- Trends in the care of children with chronic illness or disability include increased focus on developmental stages, family development, family-centered care, normalization, mainstreaming, early intervention, and managed care.
- Promoting normal development in the child with a chronic condition or disability involves a variety of individualized strategies of support, normalization, and problem solving at each developmental stage.
- Providers and parents can play an active role in helping the child with a chronic condition or disability to cope. Acknowledging positive and negative coping strategies, applying principles of normalization, fostering hope, providing age-appropriate health education, and assisting the older child in setting realistic future goals are some key strategies.
- The family should play an active role in assessing needs and strengths.
- Supporting the family at the time of diagnosis includes planning the setting, becoming aware of the family's experiences and background, individualizing support strategies, and ensuring that family members receive the information they want and need.
- Family tasks in adjusting to the child's condition include managing the child's condition on a daily basis, meeting the developmental needs of all family members, coping with stress, managing a wide range of feelings stemming from the diagnosis and other stresses, and developing personal and professional supports.
- As families confront the challenges of caring for a child with a chronic condition, nurses can help families realize their abilities and strengths, identify problems, develop problem-solving strategies, and identify new coping strategies. The goal is optimal family functioning, as defined by the family.
- A family-centered approach to care that strengthens parent-professional collaboration empowers parents and provides the best opportunity for appropriate intervention strategies that meet the unique needs of all family members.

ANSWERS TO CRITICAL THINKING EXERCISES

Impact of the Child with Special Needs on the Sibling

1. **Yes.** The 5-year-old boy's behavioral change occurs after a 2-week period without his mother and disabled sibling, which is a disruption in his usual family routine.
2. **a.** The 5-year-old resents the 2-week loss of the mother and brother and develops separation anxiety.
   b. The 5-year-old understands that the mother went away with the disabled child and left him behind.
3. The first priority is to encourage communication between the mother and the 5-year-old son by considering when and how to inform him of the purpose of the disabled sibling's hospitalization in an age-appropriate manner. Encourage the mother to accept the child's feelings, and allow the child to express his feelings of sadness, anger, fear, guilt, and loneliness in an acceptable manner. If feasible, encourage the mother to have the child brought to the hospital to visit with the mother and disabled sibling. Encourage the mother to spend time with the 5-year-old while a relative, friend, or hospital volunteer remains with the disabled child.

4. **Yes.** The 5-year-old boy's acting out is a way of pleading with the mother for an understanding of the loss of her and the sibling's presence from his daily routine.

Parental Anger

1. **Yes.** The mother of an obese adolescent newly diagnosed with type 2 diabetes expressed anger and bitterness as she questions the need for insulin injections.
2. **a.** The mother's anger and bitterness represent universal feelings expressed by parents of a child newly diagnosed with a chronic illness.
   b. Parental guilt develops regarding the cause of the type 2 diabetes.
   c. The parent may target his or her feelings of frustration, anger, and unfairness of the treatment toward the nurse.
3. The first priority is to encourage the expression of the mother's anger and bitterness through open-ended questions (e.g., "You sound angry about this"). Also encourage expression of the adolescent's concerns. Encourage the family to discuss the impact of the adolescent's chronic

illness on the marriage, family structure, finances, and plans. Reiterate and repeat the pathophysiology and treatment plan as needed. Interview the parent, adolescent, and family to determine whether their needs and concerns have been adequately addressed.

4. **Yes.** The first priority is to allow the parent to express his or her thoughts and feelings. The next essential nursing education opportunity is to make sure the parent understands the importance of insulin for the child.

REFERENCES

Arango P: Special health care needs. In Cosby AG, Greenberg RE, Southward LH, et al, editors: *About children: an authoritative resource on the state of childhood today,* Elk Grove Village, Ill, 2005, American Academy of Pediatrics.

Beers NS, Kemeny A, Sherritt L, et al: Variations in state-level definitions: children with special health care needs, *Public Health Rep* 118(5): 434-447, 2003.

Brown RT, Wiener L, Kupst MJ et al: Single parenting and children with chronic illnesses: understudied phenomenon, *J Pediatr Psychol* 33(4):404-421, 2008.

Clarke NE, McCathy MC, Downie P, et al: Gender differences in the psychosocial experience of parents of children with cancer: A review of the literature, *Psychooncology* 18(9):907-915, 2009.

Corbin JS, Strauss A: A nursing model for chronic illness management based upon the trajectory framework, *Sch Inq Nurs Pract* 3(3):155-174, 1995.

Coyne I: Children's experiences of hospitalization, *J Child Health Care* 10(4):326-336, 2006.

Emerson E: Mothers of children and adolescents with intellectual disability: social and economic situation, mental health status, and the self-assessed social and psychological impact of the child's difficulties, *J Intellect Disabil Res* 47(Pt 4/5):385-399, 2003.

Fahrner R, Mario EB: HIV infection and AIDS. In Jackson-Allen PL, Vessey JA, Schapiro M, editors: *Primary care of the child with a chronic condition,* ed 5, St Louis, 2009, Mosby.

Fazil Q, Wallace LM, Singh G, et al: Empowerment and advocacy: reflections on action research with Bangladeshi and Pakistani families who have children with severe disabilities, *Health Soc Care Commun* 12(5):389-397, 2004.

Fleitas J: When Jack fell down . . . Jill came tumbling after: siblings in the web of illness and disability, *MCN Am J Matern Child Nurs* 25(5):267-273, 2000.

Goble LA: The impact of a child's chronic illness on fathers, *Issues Compr Pediatr Nurs* 27(3): 153-162, 2004.

Green SE: "What do you mean 'what's wrong with her?'": stigma and the lives of families of children with disabilities, *Soc Sci Med* 57(8): 1361-1374, 2003.

Gurney JG, Bondy ML: Epidemiologic research methods and childhood cancer. In Pizzo PA, Poplack DG, editors: *Principles and practice of pediatric oncology,* ed 6, Philadelphia, 2010, Lippincott Williams & Wilkins.

Hockenberry MJ, Kline NE: Nursing support of the child with cancer. In Pizzo PA, Poplack DG, editors: *Principles and practice of pediatric oncology,* ed 6, Philadelphia, 2010, Lippincott Williams & Wilkins.

Horner MJ, Ries LAG, Krapcho M, et al: SEER Cancer Statistics Review, 1975-2006, Bethesda, Md, 2008, National Cancer Institute, available at http://seer.cancer. gov/csr/1975_2006/, based on November 2008 SEER data submission (accessed July 8, 2009).

Inkelas M: Incentives in a Medicaid carve-out: impact on children with special health care needs, *Health Serv Res* 40(1):79-102, 2005.

Jackson PL: The primary care provider and children with chronic conditions. In Jackson-Allen PL, Vessey JA, Schapiro M, editors: *Primary care of the child with a chronic condition,* ed 5, St Louis, 2009, Mosby.

Jeffrey, AE, Newacheck, PW: Role of insurance for children with special health care needs: a synthesis of the evidence, *Pediatrics* 118(4): e1027-e1038, 2006.

Kliebenstein MA, Broome ME: School re-entry for the child with chronic illness: parent and school personnel perceptions, *Pediatr Nurs* 26(6):579-583, 2000.

Mahoney G, Wheeden CA, Perales F: Relationship of preschool special education outcomes to instructional practices and parent-child interaction, *Res Dev Disabil* 25(6):539-558, 2004.

McPherson M, Weissman G, Strickland BB, et al: Implementing community-based systems of services for children and youths with special health care needs: how well are we doing? *Pediatrics* 113(5):1538-1544, 2004.

Miller AR, Recsky MA, Armstrong RW: Responding to the needs of children with chronic health conditions in an era of health services reform, *CMAJ* 171(11):1366-1367, 2004.

Msall ME, Avery RC, Tremont MR, et al: Functional disability and school activity limitations in 41,300 school-age children: relationships to medical impairments, *Pediatrics* 111(3):548-553, 2003.

Murray JS: Understanding sibling adaptation to childhood cancer, *Issues Compr Pediatr Nurs* 23:39-47, 2000.

Newacheck PW, Halfon N: Prevalence, impact, and trends in childhood disability due to asthma, *Arch Pediatr Adolesc Med* 154:287-293, 2000.

Newacheck PW, Hung Y, Wright KK: Racial and ethnic disparities in access to care for children with special health care needs, *Ambul Pediatr* 2(4):247-254, 2002.

Newacheck PW, Kim SE: A national profile of health care utilization and expenditures for children with special health care needs, *Arch Pediatr Adolesc Med* 159(4):10-17, 2005.

Erratum in *Arch Pediatr Adolesc Med* 159(4):318, 2005.

Newacheck PW, McManus M, Fox HB, et al: Access to health care for children with special health care needs, *Pediatrics* 105(4):760-766, 2000.

Newacheck PW, Wong ST, Galbraith AA, et al: Adolescent health care expenditures: a descriptive profile, *J Adolesc Health* 32(6 Suppl):3-11, 2003.

Palfrey JS, Richmond JB: Health services: past, present, and future. In Cosby AG, Greenberg RE, Southward LH, et al, editors: *About children: an authoritative resource on the state of childhood today,* Elk Grove Village, Ill, 2005, American Academy of Pediatrics.

Pearson LJ: Children's hospitalization and other health-care encounters. In Rollins JA, Bolig R, Mahan CC, editors: *Meeting psychosocial needs across the health-care continuum,* ed 1, Austin, 2005, Pro-Ed.

Perrin JM, Bloom SR, Gortmaker SL: The increase of childhood chronic conditions in the United States. *JAMA* 297(24):2755-2759, 2007.

Rehm RS: Family culture and chronic conditions. In Jackson-Allen PL, Vessey JA, Schapiro M, editors: *Primary care of the child with a chronic condition,* ed 5, St Louis, 2009, Mosby.

Reiss JG, Gibson RW, Walker LR: Health care transition: youth, family, and provider perspectives, *Pediatrics* 115(1):112-120, 2005.

Ritchie MA: Self-esteem and hopefulness in adolescents with cancer, *J Pediatr Nurs* 16(1):35-42, 2001.

Rittey CD: Learning difficulties: what the neurologist needs to know, *J Neurol Neurosurg Psychiatry* 74:30-36, 2003.

Schiller JS, Adams PF, Nelson ZC: *Summary health statistics for the U.S. population: National Health Interview Survey, 2003,* Vital and Health Statistics Series 10, No 224, Washington, DC, 2005, US Government Printing Office.

Schmidt S, Petersen C, Bullinger M: Coping with chronic disease from the perspective of children and adolescents: a conceptual framework and its implications for participation, *Child Care Health Dev* 29(1): 63-75, 2003.

Shepard MP, Mahon MM: Chronic conditions and the family. In Jackson-Allen PL, Vessey JA, Schapiro M, editors: *Primary care of the child with a chronic condition,* ed 5, St Louis, 2009, Mosby.

Shudy M, de Almeida ML, Ly S, et al: Impact of pediatric critical illness and injury on families: A systematic literature review. *Pediatrics* 118(Suppl 3):S203-S218, 2006.

Smucker JMRL: Managed care and children with special health care needs, *J Pediatr Health Care* 15(1):3-9, 2001.

Stein REK, Shenkman E, Wegener DH, et al: Health of children in Title XXI: should we worry? *Pediatrics* 112(2):e112-e118, 2003.

Sullivan-Bolyai S, Knafl KA, Sadler L, et al: Great expectations: a position description for parents as caregivers: part II, *Pediatr Nurs* 30(1):52-56, 2004.

Sullivan-Bolyai S, Sadler L, Knafl KA, et al: Great expectations: a position description for parents as caregivers: part I, *Pediatr Nurs* 29(6):457-461, 2003.

Turkel S, Pao M: Late consequences of pediatric chronic illness, *Psychiatr Clin North Am* 30(4):819-835, 2007.

van Dyck P, Kogan MD, Heppel D, et al: The National Survey of Children's Health: a new data resource, *Matern Child Health J* 8(3):183-188, 2004.

Varni JW, Limbers CA, Burwinkle TM: Impaired health-related quality of life in children and adolescents with chronic conditions: a comparative analysis of 10 disease clusters and 33 disease categories/severities utilizing the PedsQL(tm) 4.0 generic core scales, *Health Qual Life Outcomes* 5:43, 2007.

Vessey JA, Jackson PL: School and the child with a chronic condition. In Jackson-Allen PL, Vessey JA, Schapiro M, editors: *Primary care of the child with a chronic condition*, ed 5, St Louis, 2009, Mosby.

Vessey JA, Mebane DJ: Chronic conditions and child development. In Jackson-Allen PL, Vessey JA, Schapiro M, editors: *Primary care of the child with a chronic condition*, ed 5, St Louis, 2009, Mosby.

Weiner, P: Educational consultant for children with a chronic illness. In Hicks M, editor: *Child life beyond the hospital*, ed 1, Rockville, Md, 2008, Child Life Council.

Yogev R, Chadwick EG: Acquired immunodeficiency syndrome. In Kliegman RM, Behrman RE, Jenson HB, et al, editors: *Nelson textbook of pediatrics*, ed 18, Philadelphia, 2007, Saunders.

CHAPTER

23

Family-Centered End-of-Life Care

Angela M. Ethier

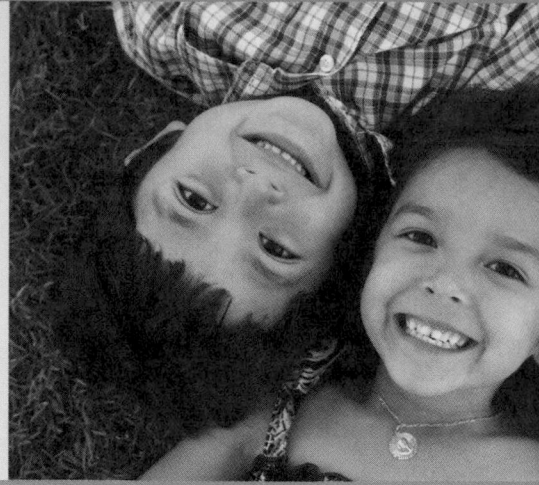

PALLIATIVE CARE IN CHILDHOOD TERMINAL ILLNESS

SCOPE OF THE PROBLEM

In 2007 more than 53,000 children from birth to 19 years of age died in the United States (Heron, Sutton, Xu, et al, 2010). Nearly 70% of 29,241 infant deaths resulted from congenital malformations, low birth weight, sudden infant death syndrome (SIDS), maternal complications, accidents, cord and placental complications, newborn respiratory distress and bacterial sepsis, neonatal hemorrhage, and circulatory system diseases (Heron, Sutton, Xu, et al, 2010). Accidents (unintentional injuries), followed by assault (homicide), cancer, and intentional self-harm (suicide), are the leading causes of death for all children 1 to 19 years of age (Heron, Sutton, Xu, et al, 2010). (See Chapter 1.)

In addition to the children who die each year, approximately another 400,000 children in the United States are living with a life-threatening illness (Calabrese, 2007). The number of children living with chronic, life-limiting illnesses has increased exponentially as advances in technology and pharmacology have led to improved treatments (Palfrey, Tonniges, Green, et al, 2005). These chronic conditions often result in substantial health care needs and increase the possibility of death during childhood (Box 23-1) (Himelstein, Hilden, Boldt, et al, 2004). Although the number of children who die of any one illness is small, those children who will not survive their illness need a significant amount of care. The majority of these children die in a hospital setting, most frequently in an intensive care unit (Feudtner, Silveira, and Christakis, 2002), having been mechanically ventilated (Feudtner, Christakis, Zimmerman, et al, 2002), and often experiencing acute and chronic pain and other distressing symptoms (McCulloch and Collins, 2006; Pritchard, Burghen, Srivastava, et al, 2008; Zhukovsky, Herzog, Kaur, et al, 2009) (see Evidence-Based Practice box).

Fortunately, increasing attention has been given in recent years to the needs of children who have experienced irreversible trauma or who have incurable diseases or disorders. The American Academy of Pediatrics (2000) released a statement on the need to incorporate principles of palliative care in pediatric practice. In addition, a number of national and international specialty groups have published suggested guidelines for the care of children with life-threatening and terminal illnesses (Bowden, Conway-Orgel, Dulzack, et al, 2003; Hazinski, Markenson, Neish, et al, 2004; Masera, Spinetta, Jankovic, et al, 1999; World Health Organization, 1998a; National Hospice and

Palliative Care Organization, 2000). Unfortunately, currently health care professionals lack clinical education in the principles of making the transition with children from curative to palliative care or methods of adequately managing the pain and suffering experienced by children and their families during the dying process (Hilden, Emanuel, Fairclough, et al, 2001; Zhukovsky, Herzog, Kaur, et al, 2009). It is clear, however, that as our ability to treat disease, disability, and trauma advances, we must also improve our care of those children who live with the specter of chronic, life-threatening illness and premature death.

PRINCIPLES OF PALLIATIVE CARE

Palliative care involves an interdisciplinary approach to the management of a child's life-threatening or life-limiting illness from diagnosis through death when cure may not be possible, and focuses on preventing or relieving the child's symptoms

---

> **BOX 23-1   CONDITIONS CONTRIBUTING TO CHILDHOOD DEATH**
>
> Cancer
> Complications of prematurity
> Congenital anomalies
> - Trisomy 13, 18
> - Anencephaly
> - Holoprosencephaly
> - Lissencephaly
> - Inborn errors of metabolism
> Cystic fibrosis
> Human immunodeficiency virus infection/acquired immunodeficiency syndrome
> Major organ dysfunction or failure
> - Congenital or acquired heart disease or defects
> - Liver defects
> - Renal failure
> Neurodegenerative diseases
> - Muscular dystrophy
> - Spinal muscular atrophy
> - Adrenoleukodystrophy
> - Ataxia-telangiectasia
> Severe neurologic and/or physical disability
> Severe gastrointestinal disorder or malformation
> Epidermolysis bullosa
> Severe immunodeficiencies
> Severe forms of osteogenesis imperfecta
> Trauma
> - Accidents

EVIDENCE-BASED PRACTICE

Pediatric Pain and Symptom Management at the End of Life

ASK THE QUESTION

In children, what is the pain and symptom experience at the end of life?

SEARCH FOR THE EVIDENCE

Search strategies

Published studies from 2005 to 2009 using the subject terms infant or child, palliative care or end of life, pain, and symptoms were identified and examined. Retrospective descriptive studies characterizing infants' and children's end-of-life experiences through the use of medical record reviews and provider and parental surveys dominated the findings. Most studies examined the symptom experience of the infant or child with cancer.

Database used

PubMed

CRITICALLY ANALYZE THE EVIDENCE

GRADE criteria: Evidence quality moderate; recommendation strong (Guyatt, Oxman, Vist, et al, 2008)

Children experienced an average of nine symptoms near the end of life (Theunissen, Hoogerbrugge, van Achterberg, et al, 2007; Zhukovsky, Herzog, Kaur, et al, 2009) Pain, dyspnea, fatigue, loss of motor function, changes in behavior, changes in appearance, not eating, vomiting, cough, diarrhea, mouth sores, sadness, difficulty talking with others about their feelings, fear, and anxiety were the most frequently acknowledged symptoms experienced by most children at the end of life (Bradshaw, Hinds, Lensing, et al, 2005; Hechler, Blankenburg, Friedrichsdorf, et al, 2008; Hendricks-Ferguson, 2008; Jalmsell, Kreicbergs, Onelov, et al, 2006; Lavy, 2007; Pritchard, Burghen, Srivastava, et al, 2008; Theunissen, Hoogerbrugge, van Achterberg, et al, 2007; Zhukovsky, Herzog, Kaur, et al, 2009). Children and their parents reported high distress over pain and symptoms at the end of life. Parents reported the child's pain and suffering as one of the most important factors in deciding to withhold or withdraw their child from life support in the pediatric intensive care unit (Sharman, Meert, and Sarnaik, 2005).

Helpful interventions to manage symptoms included physical comfort, time spent with child and family, and pharmacologic agents (Hechler, Blankenburg, Friedrichsdorf, et al, 2008; Hendricks-Ferguson, 2008; Pritchard, Burghen, Srivastava, et al, 2008). Morphine, diamorphine, and fentanyl were the most common pain medication; the most common routes of pain medication administration were oral, intravenous, subcutaneous, rectal, and transdermal (Hewitt, Goldman, Collins, et al, 2008). Most studies reported a lack of documented symptom assessment and intervention, as well as inadequate symptom management (Hechler, Blankenburg, Friedrichsdorf, et al, 2008; Lavy, 2007; Zhukovsky, 2009; Zhukovsky, Herzog, Kaur, et al, 2009), particularly the psychological symptoms of the dying child (Hechler, Blankenburg, Friedrichsdorf, et al, 2008; Theunissen, Hoogerbrugge, van Achterberg, et al, 2007).

APPLY THE EVIDENCE: NURSING IMPLICATIONS

Although the philosophy of palliative care encompasses pain and symptom management for infants and children who may not outlive their disease, the provision of that care to ease physical and psychologic suffering and provide comfort to those who will die continues to lag. Studies show that children experience significant pain and other distressing symptoms at the end of life that are not well managed. Discrepancies in the assessment of infant and child pain and suffering continue to exist between providers and parents. Improvements are needed in the management of pain and symptoms at the end of life for infants and children.

References

Bradshaw G, Hinds PS, Lensing S, et al: Cancer-related deaths in children and adolescents, *J Palliat Med* 8(1):86-95, 2005.

Guyatt GH, Oxman AD, Vist GE, et al: GRADE: an emerging consensus on rating quality of evidence and strength of recommendations, *BMJ* 336:924-926, 2008.

Hechler T, Blankenburg M, Friedrichsdorf SJ, et al: Parents' perspective on symptoms, quality of life, characteristics of death and end-of-life decisions for children dying from cancer, *Klin Padiatr* 220(3):166-174, 2008.

Hendricks-Ferguson V: Physical symptoms of children receiving pediatric hospice care at home during the last week of life, *Oncol Nurs Forum* 35(6):E108-E115, 2008.

Hewitt M, Goldman A, Collins GS, et al: Opioid use in palliative care of children and young people with cancer, *J Pediatr* 152(1):39-44, 2008.

Jalmsell L, Kreicbergs U, Onelov E, et al: Symptoms affecting children with malignancies during the last month of life: a nationwide follow-up, *Pediatrics* 117(40):1314-1320, 2006.

Lavy V: Presenting symptoms and signs in children referred for palliative care in Malawi, *Palliat Med* 21:333-339, 2007.

Pritchard M, Burghen E, Srivastava DK, et al: Cancer-related symptoms most concerning to parents during the last week and last day of their child's life, *Pediatrics* 212(5):e1301-e1309, 2008.

Sharman M, Meert KL, Sarnaik AP: What influences parents' decisions to limit or withdraw life support? *Pediatr Crit Care Med* 6(5):513-518, 2005.

Theunissen JMJ, Hoogerbrugge PM, van Achterberg T, et al: Symptoms in the palliative phase of children with cancer, *Pediatr Blood Cancer* 49(1):160-165, 2007.

Zhukovsky DS: The impact of palliative care consultation on symptom assessment, communication needs, and palliative interventions in pediatric patients with cancer, *J Palliat Med* 12(4):343-349, 2009.

Zhukovsky DS, Herzog CE, Kaur G, et al: Impact of palliative care consultation on symptom assessment, communication needs, and palliative interventions in pediatric patients with cancer, *J Palliat Med* 12(4):333-339, 2009.

and support of the child and family (Hubble, Ward-Smith, Christenson, et al, 2008; Johnston, Nagel, Friedman, et al, 2008). The World Health Organization (1998c) defines pediatric palliative care as being the "active total care of the child's body, mind, and spirit, and also involv[ing] giving support to the family. It begins when illness is diagnosed, and continues regardless of whether or not a child receives treatment directed at the disease." Palliative care interventions do not serve to hasten death; rather, they provide pain and symptom management, attention to issues faced by the child and family with regard to death and dying, and promotion of optimal functioning and quality of life during the time the child has remaining. The implementation of neonatal and pediatric palliative care consulting services within hospitals has led to enhanced quality of life and end-of-life care for children and their families and support for their care providers (Hubble, Ward-Smith, Christenson, et al, 2008; Jennings, 2005; Pierucci, Kirby, and Leuthner, 2001).

Several principles are the hallmarks of palliative care. The child and family are the unit of care. The death of a child is an extremely stressful event for a family because it is out of the natural order of things. Children represent health and hope, and their death calls into question the understanding of life. An interdisciplinary team of health care professionals consisting of social workers, chaplains, nurses, personal care aides, and physicians skilled in caring for children with life threatening or life-limiting conditions assists the family by focusing care on the complex interactions between physical, emotional, social, and spiritual issues.

Palliative care seeks to create a therapeutic environment, as homelike as possible, if not in the child's own home. Through education and support of family members, an atmosphere of open communication is provided regarding the child's dying process and its impact on all members of the family.

DECISION MAKING AT THE END OF LIFE

Discussions concerning the possibility that a child's illness or condition is not curable and that death is an inevitable outcome causes everyone involved a great deal of stress. Physicians, other members of the health care team, and families consider all information regarding the child's situation and make decisions to which all parties agree and which will have a profound impact on the child and family.

Ethical Considerations in End-of-Life Decision Making

A number of ethical concerns arise when parents and health care professionals are deciding on the best course of care for the dying child (Table 23-1). Many parents and health care providers are concerned that not offering treatment that would cause potential pain and suffering, but might extend life, would be considered euthanasia or assisted suicide. To eliminate such concerns, one must understand the various terms. **Euthanasia** involves an action carried out by a person other than the patient to end the life of the patient suffering from a terminal condition. This action is based on the belief that the act is "putting the person out of his or her misery." This action has also been called *mercy killing*. **Assisted suicide** occurs when someone provides the patient with the means to end his or her life and the patient uses that means to do so. The important distinction between these two actions is who is actually acting to end the person's life.

TABLE 23-1	COMMON ETHICAL DILEMMAS IN CARING FOR TERMINALLY ILL CHILDREN
RATIONALE IN PROVIDING TO PATIENT	**RATIONALE IN WITHHOLDING FROM PATIENT**
Pain Control	
Comfort (the primary goal)	Side effects of opioids
Improved quality of life	Decreased level of cognition
Easier dying process if child is pain free	Fear of addiction (unfounded for terminally ill patients)
Chemotherapy or Experimental Therapy	
Prolonged life span	Decreased blood counts, increased risk of infection, bleeding
Possible increase in quality of life	Side effects of treatment that may be painful, uncomfortable
Provision of sense that family has done everything they can to save the child	
Supplemental Nutrition and Hydration (Intravenous, Nasogastric, Gastrostomy Tube)	
Belief that the child is hungry or thirsty	Supplemental feedings beyond what child can ingest may actually cause nausea or vomiting
Inability or unwillingness of child to eat	Increase in tumor growth (feeding of the tumor)
Fear that child will "starve" to death	Increase in fluid volume may result in congestive heart failure, increased respiratory secretions, and/or
Primary role of parent to feed and nourish child	pulmonary congestion, which leads to questions of whether to implement diuresis
Parental guilt	Increased risk of skin breakdown if child is incontinent, due to increased urinary output
	Risk of third spacing
	More comfortable and natural death
	Complaint of thirst is associated with dying process, not level of hydration (Zerwekh, 1997)
Resuscitation	
Unwillingness of family to give up	Allows nature to take its course
Conflicts with cultural or religious beliefs	Family believes child has suffered enough, does not want aggressive intervention
Denial that child is actually going to die	Relieves family of responsibility to stop interventions that might prolong life
Autopsy	
Research to help other children	Religious, cultural belief
Ability to check genetic link	Family emotions
	Belief that body will be desecrated for funeral viewing (an unfounded fear)

Modified from Hockenberry-Eaton M, Bottomley S, Dahl KL, et al: *Essentials of pediatric oncology nursing: a core curriculum*, Glenview, Ill, 1998, Association of Pediatric Oncology Nurses.

The American Nurses Association Code for Ethics (2005) does not support the active intent on the part of a nurse to end a person's life. However, it does permit the nurse to provide interventions to relieve symptoms in the dying patient even when the interventions involve substantial risks of hastening death. When the prognosis for a patient is poor and death is the expected outcome, it is ethically acceptable to withhold or withdraw treatments that may cause pain and suffering and to provide interventions that promote comfort and quality of life. Therefore providing palliative care for patients is the ethically correct choice in such a circumstance.

Physician and Health Care Team Decision Making

Physicians often make decisions about care on the basis of the progression of the disease or amount of trauma, the availability of treatment options that would provide cure from disease or restoration of health, the impact of such treatments on the child, and the child's overall prognosis (Davis and Eng, 1998). Often the main determinants prompting physicians to discuss end-of-life issues and options for children with critical illnesses are the child's age, premorbid cognitive condition and functional status, pain or discomfort, probability of survival, and quality of life (Masri, Farrell, Lacroix, et al, 2000). When the physician discusses this information openly with families, a shared decision-making process can occur and decisions can be made regarding do-not-resuscitate (DNR) orders and care that is focused on the comfort of the child and family during the dying process (see Table 23-1). However, uncertainty of the child's prognosis among health care providers is frequently a barrier to the provision of optimal palliative care (Davies, Sehring, Partridge, et al, 2008; Thompson, Knapp, Madden, et al, 2009). As a result, many families do not always receive the option of shifting the focus of treatment to the child's comfort and quality of life when cure is unlikely (see Research Focus box).

RESEARCH FOCUS

Palliative Care

Results of studies of physician decision making regarding when to change the focus of care to palliation and comfort continue to show high variability across physicians and settings (Randolph, Zollo, Egger, et al, 1999; Thompson, Knapp, Madden, et al, 2009). This reluctance to change to a focus on palliative care by physicians occurs for a number of reasons, including the belief that not being able to "save" a child is a "failure." Also, the physician and other members of the health care team may lack knowledge of and experience with the principles of palliative care (Davies, Sehring, Partridge, et al, 2008; Hubble, Ward-Smith, Christenson, et al, 2008; Thompson, Knapp, Madden, et al, 2009).

The current approach by palliative care experts promotes the inclusion of palliative care along the continuum of care from diagnosis through treatment, not merely at the end of life (Field and Behrman, 2004; Himelstein, Hilden, Boldt, et al, 2004; Hubble, Ward-Smith, Christenson, et al, 2008), and sometimes after the child's birth in the neonatal intensive care unit (Carter, 2004; De Lisle-Porter and Podruchny, 2009).

Family Decision Making

Rarely are families prepared to cope with the numerous decisions that must be made when a child is dying. When the death is unexpected, as in the case of an accident or trauma, the confusion of emergency services and possibly an intensive care setting presents challenges to parents as they are asked to make difficult choices. Determination of parental decision-making preferences, which may be active or independent, collaborative or shared between parents and provider, or passive or authoritarian, can help providers support parents (Higgins and Kayser-Jones, 1996; Hinds, Oakes, Furman, et al, 2001; Pyke-Grimm, Degner, Small, et al, 1999). If the child has experienced a life-threatening illness such as cancer or lived with a chronic illness that has now reached its terminal phase, parents are often unprepared for the reality of their child's impending death (see Family-Centered Care box).

FAMILY-CENTERED CARE

Family of the Dying Child

No matter whether you have a PhD or many children, when your child dies, it is a new experience and nothing can prepare you for it. Like so many things in life, experience is the best teacher.

Three of our children have died, and by the time the third was dying, we handled many things differently. We learned a lot about dignity and the rights of the child and family. For example, at first, we didn't know that we had a right to have our child die at home. We also didn't understand pain medications and that if children are taking these medicines and are still in agony, they have not overdosed on the medication.

We learned a lot about case management. With our first two children, lots of different people were making decisions and disagreeing about what was best and what should be done. No one had primary authority. With our third child, one doctor took a primary role. Any questions and problems were handled by one person. I could call him 24 hours a day. It made a lot of difference, and I felt our concerns and needs were better heard and respected.

The nurses caring for our third child at home enabled me to step back and just be his mommy. When I could do this, I realized that we were fighting so hard for his life that we weren't really letting him die. His nurses had worked with him for a long time and really loved him. It was hard for them when we decided to let him die. In his last several days we wanted a lot of family time with our son, and I think the nurses felt left out. Something about their reaction to our increased time with him in the last few days made us feel guilty. If we had all been able to communicate a little more openly, I would have understood that they needed more time with him at the end, too. Everyone's needs could have been met.

Jeni Stepanek
Mother
Upper Marlboro, Maryland

Earlier acknowledgment by both physicians and parents that children have no realistic chance for cure is associated with earlier implementation of DNR orders, less use of aggressive therapies, and greater provision of palliative care measures (Wolfe, Klar, Grier, et al, 2000). Additional factors found to influence parents' decisions to limit or withdraw life-sustaining measures include parents' prior end-of-life decision making for loved ones; observations of pain and suffering of their child and other hospitalized children; various emotions, including guilt and sorrow; and awareness of their child's desire to forego life-sustaining measures (Sharman, Meert, and Sarnaik, 2005). The use of a pediatric advance directive for older minors may raise awareness of children's wishes as part of the family decision-making process (Knapp, Huang, Madden, et al, 2009; Zinner, 2009) (see Research Focus box).

RESEARCH FOCUS

Importance of Honest Communication

Numerous studies have found that families facing the impending death of a child depend on information provided to them by the health care team, particularly an honest appraisal of the child's prognosis, to make difficult decisions regarding care options for their child (Hinds, Oakes, Furman, et al, 1997; James and Johnson, 1997; Sharman, Meert, and Sarnaik, 2005) and care measures after life-sustaining measures were eliminated (Sharman, Meert, and Sarnaik, 2005).

As the group of health professionals who are most involved with families, nurses are in an excellent position to ensure that families know the options available to them (Box 23-2). The nurse's first responsibility is to explore the family's wishes. This is best done with the physician, but at times nurses need to initiate the process. When discussing difficult issues, nurses are open to the child's or family's indirect comments that communicate uncertainty or concerns about the course of care. Nurses answer questions honestly, and if they do not know the answer, reassure the family that they will arrange for a discussion with the physician. It is important to address any fantasies or misunderstandings by seeking to clarify what the family has heard. Finally, it is important for the nurse to remain neutral and avoid giving personal opinions or experiences. The goal of communication is to facilitate the identification of the family's wishes, based on their unique values and beliefs (Table 23-2).

BOX 23-2	COMMUNICATING WITH FAMILIES

Listen for an "invitation" to talk about the situation.
"Sometimes I wonder if I am doing the right thing."
"What have other parents done in this situation?"
"Do you know of other children who have survived this?"
"I think the doctor is not telling me everything."
Use open-ended, nonjudgmental questions to explore families' wishes.
"Can you tell me more about how you are feeling?"
"What questions do you (or your child) have that I can answer for you?"
"What are your concerns (or worries, fears) right now?"
"What is important to you (or your child, family) at this time?"

AWARENESS OF DYING IN CHILDREN WITH LIFE-THREATENING ILLNESS

One of the initial reactions of parents (and some health care professionals) to the discovery of a life-threatening illness is to protect the child from the impact of the diagnosis. Often they do not have the knowledge or energy to help the child (Bluebond-Langner, 1978; Dyregrov, 2004; Kirwin and Hamrin, 2005; Zhukovsky, Herzog, Kaur, et al, 2009). However, it is now

TABLE 23-2	COMMUNICATING BAD NEWS TO FAMILIES
APPROACH	**EFFECTIVE TECHNIQUES**
Provide a setting conducive to communication.	Ensure privacy; use appropriate body language; make eye contact. Have parents choose who will attend.
Determine what the parent knows.	Ask questions ("What have you made of all this?" or "What were you told?"). Listen to the vocabulary and comprehension of the parents. Recognize denial but do not acknowledge it at this stage.
Determine what the parent wants to know.	Obtain a clear invitation to share information (if this is what the parent wants). Use questions such as, "Are you the sort of person who likes to know every detail, or just the basic facts?"
Give information (aligning and educating).	Start at level of parents' comprehension and use the same vocabulary. Give information slowly, concisely, and in simple language. Avoid medical jargon. Check regularly to be certain that content is understood.
Respond to parents' reactions.	Acknowledge all reactions and feelings, particularly using the emphatic response technique (identifying emotion, identifying cause of emotion, and responding appropriately). Expect tears, anger, and other strong emotions.
Close.	Briefly summarize major areas discussed. Ask parents if they have other important issues to discuss at this time. Make an appointment for the next meeting.

Modified from Buchman R, Baile W: *How to break bad news to patients with cancer: a practical protocol for clinicians*, Spring Education Book, Alexandria, Va, 1998, American Society of Clinical Oncology.

widely understood that terminally ill children develop an awareness of the seriousness of their diagnosis, even when protected from the truth (Bluebond-Langner, 1978; Spinetta, 1974). The avoidance of talking openly and honestly with children with life-threatening illnesses and their siblings can lead to fear, guilt, misconceptions, and the pain of grieving alone. Surviving siblings may experience psychiatric sequelae as children and into adulthood (Kirwin and Hamrin, 2005; Schoen, Burgoyne, and Schoen, 2004).

Discussing Death with Children

Children need honest and accurate information about their illness, treatments, and prognosis. This information needs to be given in clear, simple language. In most situations this best occurs as a gradual process, characterized by increasingly open dialogue among parents, professionals, and the child (Hockley, 2000; Lee and Johann-Liang, 1999). Providing an atmosphere of open communication early in the course of an illness facilitates answering difficult questions as the child's condition worsens. Providing appropriate literature about the disease, as well as about the experience of illness and possible death, is also helpful. Exactly how and when to involve children in decisions regarding care during their dying process and death is an individual matter. In general, the nurse should ask parents how they would like their child to be told of the prognosis and how they want to be included in their child's care. Some parents may request that their child not be told that he or she is dying, even if the child asks. This often places health care providers in a difficult situation. Children, even at a young age, are perceptive. Despite not being told outright that they are dying, they realize that something is seriously wrong and that it involves them. Children deserve to be provided with the truth.

Often, helping parents understand that honesty and shared decision making between them and their child at this time are important for the emotional health of the child and family will encourage parents to allow discussion of dying with their child. The truth provides answers for future questions and fosters trust. It is difficult to encourage children to be honest, confide in others, and openly discuss their fears if parents refuse to do the same.

Honesty is certainly not the easiest solution; the truth may prompt children to ask other distressing questions. The question many parents and health professionals dread the most is, "Am I going to die?" When children have the answer to this question, the next question is, "When?" Children need answers that are straightforward, yet caring. In telling children that a cure is no longer possible, one must also leave room for hope. The hope is redirected from cure to quality of life and comfort.

Adults need to be prepared to assist children in understanding and coping with the emotions of dealing with their own death and to reassure children that it is all right to express their feelings as they choose. If given the opportunity to ask questions, children will tell others how much they want to know. Asking questions such as, "If the disease came back, would you want to know?" or "Do you want others to tell you everything, even if the news is not good?" helps children set the limits of how much truth they can accept and handle. Children need time to process feelings and information so that they can assimilate and ideally accept the inevitable fact of mortality. As the child and family move through the dying process, it is important for the family to share their beliefs regarding noncorporeal continuation and to reassure the child that he or she will not be alone at the time of death, and that the child will always be loved and remembered (Stevens, 1998).

Parents may require professional support and guidance in this process from a nurse, social worker, or child life specialist who has a good relationship with the child and family. Certain principles and guidelines can assist nurses and families in determining how to present facts about possible death and hope to a child in a way that fosters trust, enhances meaningful communication, and offers emotional support (Table 23-3 and Box 23-3). Professionals may also provide information to parents about their child(ren)'s general developmental understanding of and reactions to death and how to explain death in a developmentally appropriate manner and offer to assist parents when speaking with their terminally ill child and siblings.

- Encourage parents to approach the discussion of death with a child gently. *What* is said is important, but *how* it is said is critical to how a child is able to accept, within their abilities, the reality of death.

TABLE 23-3 COMMUNICATING WITH DYING CHILDREN

APPROACH	EFFECTIVE TECHNIQUE
Discuss at the child's level.	Gear information to the child's developmental age, remembering that younger children tend to be concrete thinkers, whereas older children are capable of abstract thought.
	Begin with the child's experiences ("You've told us how tired you've been lately").
Let the child's questions guide.	Begin the conversation with basic information, and let the child's questions direct the conversation.
Provide opportunities for the child to express feelings.	Look for clues that the child is open to communication.
	Be accepting of whatever emotion is expressed.
Encourage feedback.	Ask the child to summarize what has been heard. This provides the opportunity to clarify misunderstandings.
Use other resources.	Use books and movies to encourage dialogue.
	Ask the child to name the people with whom he or she can discuss problems.
Use the child's natural expressive means to stimulate dialogue.	Use books, games, art, play, and music to provide a means of expression.

Modified from Doka KJ: *Living with life-threatening illness: a guide for patients, their families, and caregivers,* Lexington, Mass, 1993, Lexington Books.

BOX 23-3 THE DYING CHILD'S RIGHT TO REFUSE TREATMENT

Traditionally, minor children (the age of minority varies with state law) have not had the legal right to give informed consent for treatment or to refuse treatment. However, support is growing for ensuring that children in the end stage of a fatal disease have a voice in their care. One of the major issues is the age at which children have the cognitive ability to understand the medical information, consider and comprehend the consequences of a decision (death), and choose freely among the options (Leikin, 1989). Depending on children's development level, a mature understanding of death does not occur until approximately 9 years of age, but experience with death and an awareness of one's own impending death may affect the ability to understand (Martinson, 1995). Centers that have developed protocols for allowing informed choice by children document that youngsters as young as 6 years of age understand the implications of their disease as incurable and death as irreversible (Nitschke, Humphrey, Sexauer, et al, 1982). These findings are consistent with those of Bluebond-Langner (1978, 1989), who found that fatally ill children progress through a series of stages that shape their understanding of their disease and death.

Other issues raised by opponents include concerns about dispelling hope in the child once death is pronounced as imminent, parents' guilt if they later question the decision, and possible conflict between the child's and parents' wishes (Shumway, Grossman, and Sarles, 1983; Stanfill and Strong, 1985). Although there is insufficient research to answer these concerns, it seems unlikely that these situations will occur if the family is allowed to choose therapeutic alternatives in an atmosphere of professional support and with sufficient information. In addition, staff members need to assess each child's capacity to understand the implications of refusing treatment, with documentation of the words and actions of the child that support their conclusions (Foley, 1985).

- Advise parents to begin the discussion with a child by using a nonthreatening example such as trees and leaves and how long they live.
- Allow the child's questions to guide the discussion and avoid unnecessary information; speak on the child's developmental level; provide basic information slowly, directly, and honestly using simple, concrete, age-appropriate words, including "die"; avoid the use of euphemisms (e.g., pass away, lost).
- Clarify misconceptions and let the child know he or she did not cause the illness or death; allow the child to express his or her feelings and accept whatever emotions are expressed by the child; provide warmth and support during the discussion and speak with a calm and reassuring voice.
- Ask the child to repeat what has been discussed to clarify any misunderstandings.
- Encourage family members to discuss the child's impending death openly and honestly with the child, siblings, and other family members (Ethier, 2008).

The nurse can facilitate ongoing and open communication about death and dying through the use of various resources, including books (e.g., *The Fall of Freddie the Leaf* by Leo Buscaglia) and movies (e.g., *The Velveteen Rabbit* by Margery Williams) (Auvrignon, Leverger, and Lasfargues, 2008; Ethier, 2005). Play and art activities (e.g., music, drawing, painting, writing) offer a vehicle for expression of emotions that are often difficult for children to put into words (Rollins and Riccio, 2002).

CHILDREN'S UNDERSTANDING OF AND REACTIONS TO DYING

Studies, although limited, have found a child's concept of death to be influenced by their age and cognitive development, nationality, religion, life-limiting illness, personal experiences with death, and family members' explanations and attitudes surrounding death (Silverman, 2000; Slaughter, 2005; Speece and Brent, 1996; Spinetta, 1974). By approximately 7 years of age most children understand the key bioscientific components of death (Box 23-4). Studies have found children ranging in age from 4 to 12 years to have an adultlike understanding of death. However, anyone working with children must be aware of significant developmental variations related to their understanding and fears of death. These variations are discussed in detail on pp. 883-885 (Speece and Brent, 1996). Cultural, national, and religious differences in beliefs about an afterlife have also been found to influence a child's understanding of death (Speece and Brent, 1996). Sensitive assessment of the child's developmental understanding of death and the family's cultural and spiritual beliefs related to dying and death is an important but often overlooked aspect of care (Bull and Gillies, 2007; Feudtner, Haney, and Dimmers, 2003; Heilferty, 2004; Kagawa-Singer, 1998).

Infants and Toddlers

Exactly how preverbal children view death is a mystery, since there is no way of reliably assessing their views of death. On the

---

BOX 23-4   CHILDREN'S DEVELOPMENT OF THE SUBCONCEPTS OF DEATH

Universality
- All living things eventually die.
- Death is all inclusive; everyone dies.
- Death is inevitable, unavoidable.
- Death is unpredictable; exact timing is unknown.

Before universality
- They themselves, children in general, and/or their family or friends may be viewed as excluded
- Understanding that *they* will die precedes understanding that *everyone* will die.
- Death is avoidable if you are clever.
- Death occurs in the remote future only.

Irreversibility
- Once the physical body dies, it cannot be made alive again.

Before irreversibility
- Death is temporary (e.g., falling asleep and waking up, leaving for and returning from a trip) and reversible.

Nonfunctionality
- Once a living thing dies, all life-defining capabilities (e.g., eating, sleeping, seeing, hearing) of the body cease.

Before nonfunctionality
- The dead continue external functions (e.g., eating, speaking).

Causality
- External and internal events can cause one's death.

Before causality
- Death results from unrealistic causes (e.g., misbehaving), concrete causes (e.g., poison, guns), or external causes (e.g., accidents, murder).

Noncorporeal continuation
- Some form of personal continuation exists after death of the physical body (e.g., reincarnation, ascension of the soul to heaven).

Before noncorporeal continuation
- Unknown.

Adapted from Speece MW, Brent SB: The development of children's understanding of death. In Corr CA, Corr DM, editors: *Handbook of childhood death and bereavement*, New York, 1996, Springer.

---

basis of their cognitive abilities, it is likely that they have no concept of death. The egocentricity of toddlers and their vague separation of fact and fantasy make it impossible for them to comprehend absence of life. Although they may repeat what initially sounds like a correct definition of death, such as, "Grandpa is dead; he went to heaven," they may expect Grandpa's return for several months before accommodating themselves to the absence. They can perceive events only in terms of their own frame of reference: living.

Reactions to Dying

Separation from parents and alterations in their routine represent threats to the toddler who is seriously ill and to the well toddler sibling. Behavioral responses may include regression to less independent levels of behavior related to speech, toileting, eating, drinking, crying, clinging, biting, hitting, withdrawal, and physical illness. Toddlers may perceive the seriousness of their condition from the parents' reactions of anxiety, sadness, depression, or anger. Although young children are unaware of the reason for such emotions, they often find their parents' behavior disturbing and upsetting. Helping parents deal with their feelings allows them more emotional reserve to meet the needs of their children. Encouraging parents to stay in the hospital as much as possible and to participate in the child's care promotes the parents' and child's adjustment to a serious, potentially fatal illness or injury. Helpful interventions for infants and toddlers include providing the child with physical comfort (e.g., being held or rocked), consistent providers, consistent routines, and familiar objects (e.g., favorite blanket or toy) (Ethier, 2008; Himelstein, Hilden, Boldt, et al, 2004).

Preschool Children

Several characteristics of preschoolers' cognitive and psychologic development affect their concept of death. Because they are egocentric at this age, they often have a tremendous sense of self-power and omnipotence. Therefore they believe that their thoughts are sufficient to cause events. The consequence of such magical thinking is feelings of guilt, shame, and punishment (Speece and Brent, 1996).

Concept of Death

Children between 3 and 5 years of age have usually heard the word *death* and have some sense of its meaning. They see death as a departure, possibly as a type of sleep. They may recognize the fact of physical death, but do not separate it from living abilities. The dead person in the coffin still breathes, eats, and sleeps. Death is temporary and reversible; life and death can change places with one another. Because of the immature concept of time, they have no real understanding of the universality and inevitability of death. Words such as *forever* and *everyone* have meaning only in the child's egocentric thinking. Waiting until Christmas may be "forever," and anybody the child denotes is "everyone." Children of this age take the literal meaning of words, and euphemisms are avoided. Preschoolers who are told that Grandma has "gone to sleep" may fear going to sleep themselves.

Reactions to Dying

If preschoolers become seriously ill, they may conceive of the illness as punishment for their thoughts or actions. The usual diagnostic and treatment procedures, in combination with enforced hospitalization, can confirm their belief that they are being punished. If their parents do not stay with them during hospitalization or prevent the traumatic procedures, they may believe that the parents are retaliating for previous misdeeds or bad thoughts (Fig. 23-1).

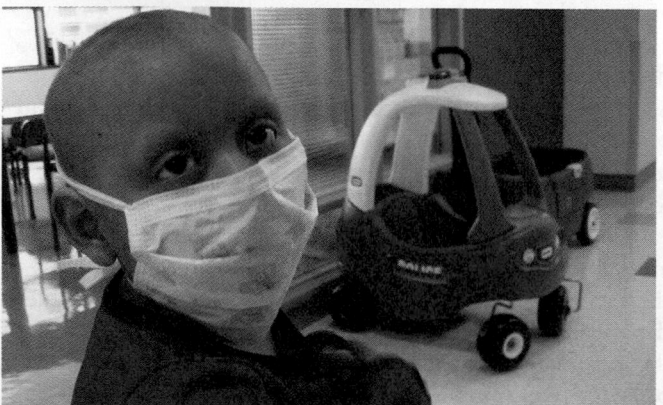

Fig. 23-1 Young children's greatest fear concerning death is separation from parents.

The same principles of magical thinking and omnipotence affect preschoolers when a sibling becomes critically ill or dies. One of the most significant types of death is SIDS. Because it occurs unexpectedly to a healthy infant (who may have been rejected and unwanted by a jealous sibling), preschoolers find no evidence to support a physical cause of death. Indeed, the parents often are unaware of the reason for the fatality and may question any possible cause. If preschoolers are in any way accused or suspected of having harmed the infant, they may feel extremely guilty and responsible for the tragedy. On observing their parents' acute grief, they may interpret the anger or depression as a rejection of them.

When a child becomes ill, the healthy siblings experience the loss of routine and parental attention. It is natural for them to resent such disruptions and blame the changes on the ill child. However, preschoolers have less ability than older children to understand the reasons for the parents' prolonged absence from home. Although parents may explain how ill the sibling is, what the hospital is like, and why they must be there, preschoolers see only the special attention and material rewards that the ill sister or brother is receiving. Because they are also unable to differentiate causes for separation of the parents and ill child, they may fear that the parents will never return. If they should learn that the ill child may not get well or come home, they may interpret this to mean that the parents will also never return. Their greatest fear concerning death is separation from parents (Silverman, 2000). Asking repeated questions; complaining about stomachaches, headaches, and other physical symptoms; displaying intensified fears and emotional outbursts; and showing signs of regression are common behavioral responses to death among preschoolers. They may appear indifferent about the death of a sibling, but this is a normal response related to their limited coping abilities. Play provides the preschooler with relief from the feelings of grief, but unknowing caregivers may misunderstand this. Helpful interventions for preschoolers include minimizing separation from parents; clarifying misconceptions of illness and death as punishment; using accurate, simple language repeated as often as the child needs; and providing the opportunity to play (Ethier, 2008; Speece and Brent, 1996).

School-Age Children

Although school-age children have a better understanding of causality, less egocentricity, and an advanced perception of time, they may still associate misdeeds or bad thoughts with causing death and feel intense guilt and responsibility for the event. However, because of their higher cognitive abilities, they respond well to logical explanations and comprehend the figurative meaning of words better than children in younger age-groups. Although they are less likely to interpret explanations in a purely literal sense, they are still prone to self-referenced definitions. For this reason, it is important for adults to clarify the meanings of statements and to repeatedly ask the children what they think.

Concept of Death

Much of the discussion on the preschool child's understanding of death also relates to the younger school-age child. However, these children have a deeper understanding of death in the concrete sense. According to Nagy (1948), children of this age attempt to ascribe a more comprehensible meaning to the event by personifying death as a devil, God, ghost, or bogeyman. Naturalistic-physiologic explanations of why death occurs and what happens to the dead body may also be a preoccupation in this age-group. Factual explanations, such as, "When you die, your body decays in the ground," are consistent with their concrete thinking.

By age 7 years, most children have an increasingly adult concept of death. They realize that it is universal, irreversible, and nonfunctional. Some studies suggest that children with cancer gain a more mature, biologic understanding of death at an earlier age than their well peers (Silverman, 2000). Their attitudes toward death are greatly influenced by the reactions and attitudes of others, particularly their parents.

Reactions to Dying

The increased ability of school-age children to comprehend and reason poses additional risks for them. They may fear the reason for the illness, communicability of the disease to themselves or others, consequences of the disease on their functioning and relationships with others, and the process of dying and death itself. They tend to fear the expectation of the event more than its realization. Their fear of the unknown is greater than that of the known. Like preschoolers, their fantasy explanations for the unexpected or the unknown are usually much more frightening and extreme than the actual situation. For this reason, anticipatory preparation is both necessary and effective. These children respond well to explanations of the disease, names of drugs, and so on. The developmental task of this age is industry; thus helping children who may be facing their own death to maintain control over their body—by understanding what is happening to them and participating in what is done to them—allows them to achieve independence, self-worth, and self-esteem and to avoid a sense of inferiority.

The realization of impending death or failure to recover is a tremendous threat to school-age children's sense of security and ego strength. These children are likely to exhibit their fear more through verbal uncooperativeness. Health care professionals may erroneously interpret this behavior as rude, impolite, insolent, or stubborn. In reality the words are conveying the same meaning as physical attempts to run away or fight off others. This verbal "flight or fight" reaction to stress is a plea for some control and power. Additional behavioral responses for the well sibling may include worrying about the health and safety of other family members and having problems in school. Encouraging children to talk about their feelings, allowing control where possible and appropriate, and providing outlets for aggression through play are means of dealing with this expression of anger and fear.

Adolescents

By the time most children reach adolescence, they have a mature understanding of death. As abstract thinking develops, there is more questioning of death and related topics, such as the religious meaning of afterlife. However, other developmental needs, especially formation of the child's own identity, make this an exceptionally difficult time for young people to cope with the loss of a loved one or with their own impending death.

Concept of Death

Although adolescents have a mature understanding of death, they tend to think they will not die as a young person. The search for the spiritual meaning of what follows death is typical at this age.

Reactions to Dying

Adolescents may have a great deal of difficulty in coping with death. Although they have reached the level of adult comprehension of the concept of death, they are least likely of all age-groups to accept cessation of life, particularly their own. Developmentally, the rejection of death is understandable because adolescents' tasks are to establish an identity by finding out who they are, what their purpose is, and where they belong. Any suggestion of being different or of not being is a tremendous threat to this task.

Adolescents strive for group acceptance and independence from parental constraints. As a result, they rely on peer rules and beliefs for personal direction and reject opposing parental demands. However, when faced with the crisis of serious illness, they may consider themselves alienated from peer associations and unable to communicate with their parents for emotional support. Therefore they may feel virtually alone in their struggle. Support groups or other means of networking with adolescents facing death may be useful.

Healthy adolescents must deal with several maturational crises, such as the acceptance of bodily changes and socialization of intensifying sexual impulses. Any threat to either task increases their vulnerability to the stress of coping with such crises. The devastation of a terminal illness and the effects of chemotherapy may be greater concerns than the prospect of dying. Adolescents' orientation to the present compels them to worry about physical changes even more than the prognosis for future recovery.

Nurses are in a key position in working with terminally ill adolescents. In the hospital setting they spend the greatest amount of time with them. They can structure the hospital admission to allow for maximum self-control and independence while allowing the adolescent the opportunity to get to know the nurse. Answering adolescents' questions honestly; treating them as mature individuals; and respecting their needs for privacy, solitude, and personal expressions of emotions such as anger, sadness, or fear convey to adolescents the adult's true concern for their physical and emotional welfare. Nurses can help parents to communicate with adolescents by providing information on typical adolescent responses and coping patterns; acting as role models; avoiding alliances with either parent or child; and allowing parents the opportunity to vent their feelings of frustration, incompetence, or failure in an atmosphere of acceptance and without judgment (see Box 23-3).

DELIVERY OF PALLIATIVE CARE SERVICES

Once the health care team and family have discussed the likelihood of death as the outcome of a child's medical condition or illness, it is necessary to determine the child and family's preference for the location of palliative care. The circumstances of the child's illness may influence the location in which palliative care is provided. For instance, traumatic injury or acute illness often leads to death in the emergency department or intensive care unit setting. Children with progressive chronic illnesses or disabilities may initially receive palliative care services through a coordination of services between outpatient visits to their primary physician and care provided by a community agency (home health or hospice) in the home. As the illness progresses, the family may cease to come to the clinic or hospital and depend solely on care provided at home by the community agency as directed by the primary physician. Regardless of the circumstances of the illness or the location of care, it is important to focus on interventions that address all aspects of the child's and family's comfort. This requires attention to the child's physical comfort and the social, emotional, and spiritual needs of the child and family. Based on the decision by the child and family regarding their wishes for care, the family has several options from which to choose.

Hospital

Families may choose to remain in the hospital to receive care if the child's illness or condition is unstable and home care is not an option, or the family is uncomfortable with providing care at home. If a family chooses to remain at the hospital for terminal care, make the setting as homelike as possible. Families can bring familiar items from the child's room at home. In addition, develop a consistent and coordinated care plan for the child's and family's comfort.

Home Care

Some families may prefer to take their child home and receive services from a home care agency. Generally, these services entail periodic nursing visits, medications, equipment, and supplies. The primary physician continues to direct the child's care (Ferrell and Coyle, 2002). Physicians and families often choose home care because of the traditional view that a child must be considered to have a life expectancy of fewer than 6 months to be referred to hospice care. Fortunately, a number of hospice organizations are expanding their services to children, basing admission on the presence of a life-limiting disease process for which cure is not possible, rather than on the sole criterion of a limited 6-month prognosis. Dussell, Kreicbergs, Hilden, and colleagues (2008) found parents whose children received home care had honest, open, end-of-life communication from the physician. Parents, were more likely to plan the location of their child's death as the home and to report favorable outcomes. Unfortunately, only a limited number of hospitals and hospices in the United States provide palliative end-of-life care for children (Johnston, Nagel, Friedman, et al, 2008).

Hospice Care

Hospice care is another option for families who wish to take their child home during the final phases of an illness. Hospice is a community health care program that specializes in the care of dying patients by combining the hospice philosophy with the principles of palliative care. Hospice philosophy regards dying as a natural process and views the care of dying patients as including management of the physical, psychologic, social, and spiritual needs of the patient and family. A multidisciplinary group of professionals provide care in the patient's home or an inpatient facility that follows the hospice philosophy. Hospice care for children was introduced in the 1970s (Martinson, 1993), and a number of community hospice organizations now accept children into their care (Faulkner and Armstrong-Dailey, 1997).* Collaboration between the child's primary treatment team and the hospice care team is essential to the success of hospice care. Families may continue to see their primary care physicians as they choose.

The goal of hospice care is for children to live life to the fullest without pain, with choices and dignity, in the familiar environment of their homes, and with the support of their families. Hospice care is covered under state Medicaid programs and by most insurance plans. The service provides home nursing visits and visits from social workers, chaplains, and, in some cases, physicians. For children, the hospice concept has most commonly been implemented in the home, which benefits the family in a variety of ways. Children who are dying are allowed the opportunity to remain with those they love and with whom they feel secure. Many children who were thought to be in imminent danger of death have gone home and lived longer than expected. Siblings can feel more involved in the care and often have more positive perceptions of the death. In addition to the care and support provided through the dying process to the child and family, hospice is concerned with the family's postdeath adjustment, and bereavement care may continue for a year or more.

Parental adaptation may be more favorable, as is shown by their perceptions of how the experience at home affected their marriage, social reorientation, religious beliefs, and views on the meaning of life and death.

If the home is chosen for hospice care, the child may or may not die in the home. One study revealed that 55% of children enrolled in hospice died in the home (Knapp, Shenkman, Marcu, et al, 2009). Reasons for final admission to a hospital vary but may be related to the parents' or siblings' wish to have the child die outside the home; exhaustion on the part of the caregivers; and physical problems such as sudden acute pain or respiratory distress.

Location and Participation in Child's Care

The location of the child's terminal care and death and the participation of parents in their child's terminal care influences parental bereavement. Parents whose child died in the home rather than the hospital setting and who participated in caring for their child have consistently reported better bereavement outcomes (e.g., adaptive coping; family cohesion; less anxiety, stress, and depression) than parents whose children died in the hospital setting and/or who were not actively involved in their child's care (Goodenough, Drew, Higgins, et al, 2004; Lauer, Mulhern, Schell, et al, 1989; Rando, 1983). The grief work of fathers in particular seems to be facilitated when their children die in the home setting. This finding may be related to the

---

*National Hospice and Palliative Care Organization, 1731 King St., Suite 100, Alexandria, VA 22314; 703-837-1500; fax: 703-837-1233; www.nhpco.org; and Children's Hospice International, 1101 King St., Suite 360, Alexandria, VA 22314; 703-684-0330, 800-2-4-CHILD; fax: 703-684-0226; www.chionline.org.

greater opportunity for working fathers to provide care to and spend time with their children at home than in the hospital setting. In contrast, a recent study suggests that parental opportunity to plan the location of their child's death, whether death occurred in the home or in the hospital, may be a more relevant outcome variable than the child's actual location of death (Dussell, Kreicbergs, Hilden, et al, 2008).

NURSING CARE OF THE CHILD AND FAMILY AT THE END OF LIFE

MANAGEMENT OF PAIN AND SUFFERING

The presence of unrelieved pain and other distressing symptoms in a terminally ill child, unfortunately, are commonly reported (Hendricks-Ferguson, 2008; Pritchard, Burghen, Srivastava, et al, 2008; Zhukovsky, Herzog, Kaur, et al, 2009). Distressing symptoms can have detrimental effects on the child's quality of life and long-lasting negative effects on the family after the child's death. Parents have reported that having their child in pain was unendurable and resulted in feelings of helplessness and a sense that they must be present and vigilant to get the necessary pain medications (Ferrell, 1995). Persistent pain also has an impact on the family as a whole. Nurses can alleviate the fear of pain and suffering by providing interventions aimed at treating the pain and symptoms associated with the terminal process in children.

Pain and Symptom Management

When the pain and symptoms experienced by dying children are being managed, it is important to clearly communicate the intent of any interventions proposed. For example, many children with progressive cancer may be given "palliative chemotherapy" or "palliative radiotherapy." The health care team and family must understand that the goal of these treatments is either to increase comfort by slowing the progression of an incurable tumor (palliative chemotherapy) or to reduce swelling or pressure from a tumor that is causing pain (palliative radiation). The family should understand that these treatments will not ultimately change the outcome of death for the child. This understanding reduces the chance of confusion among family members and health care providers regarding the focus of care and its aim toward palliation. In addition, providers consider the benefit versus risk of any suggested interventions in relation to the child's current quality of life.

The child's and family's views of quality of life, religious and cultural values, and level of acceptance of the terminal prognosis will shape the types of interventions considered as symptoms occur. One family may choose to continue blood-product support if the child is otherwise comfortable and active but has fatigue and shortness of breath related to anemia. Another child and family may forgo transfusions to avoid having to return to the hospital or clinic. The child and family should be aware of potential side effects of any proposed treatments and consequences of choosing not to intervene and are provided with options that are consistent with their values and goals for the child's comfort. Health care practitioners must respect each individual family's choice regarding their child's care.

Nurses should use a holistic approach to symptom management that includes pharmacologic and nonpharmacologic interventions when possible to optimize treatment. For instance, in addition to giving lorazepam for anxiety, instruct the child and family in nonpharmacologic techniques such as distraction or relaxation breathing and encourage them to explore and communicate fears to further alleviate feelings of anxiety.

Carefully consider the route of medication administration used for pain and symptom management. Generally the nurse should use the least traumatic method of administration. Children may present a special challenge for administration of medication depending on their age, level of cooperation, and temperament. If taking medicine becomes a struggle, children and parents may underreport the severity of pain and symptoms to avoid the trauma of administering the medication. Most medications can be administered orally, sublingually, transdermally, or by intravenous or subcutaneous infusion. Compounding pharmacists can be helpful in making medications in a form that is palatable or can be delivered with less distress.

Give pain control for children in the terminal stages of illness or injury the highest priority. Despite ongoing efforts to educate physicians and nurses on pain management strategies in children, studies have reported that children continue to be undermedicated for their pain (Wolfe, Grier, Klar, et al, 2000; Wolfe, Hammel, Edwards, et al, 2008). Nearly all children experience some amount of pain in the terminal phase of their illness. The current standard for treating children's pain is according to the World Health Organization's analgesic and side effect stepladder (World Health Organization, 1998b), which takes into account the intolerable side effects of opioids (Riley, Ross, Gretton, et al, 2007) (Fig. 23-2). This approach promotes individualizing the pain interventions to children's level of reported pain. Children's pain is assessed frequently, and medications adjusted as necessary. Pain medications are given on a regular schedule, and extra doses for breakthrough pain are available to maintain comfort. Opioid drugs such as morphine are given for severe pain, and the dosage is increased as necessary to maintain optimum pain relief. Techniques such as distraction, relaxation techniques, and guided imagery (Lambert, 1999) are combined with drug therapy to provide the child and family with strategies to control pain (Russell and Smart, 2007). (See Chapter 7 for further discussion of pain assessment and management strategies.)

Occasionally children require very high doses of opioids to control pain. This may occur for several reasons. The child on long-term opioid pain management can become tolerant of the drug, so more drug must be given to maintain the same level of pain relief. This is not to be confused with addiction, which is a psychologic dependence on the side effects of opioids. Addiction is not a factor in managing terminal pain in children. Other reasons for increasing dosages of opioids include progression of disease and other physiologic causes of pain. It is important to understand that there is no maximum dosage that can be given to control pain. However, nurses often express concern that administering dosages of opioids that exceed those with which they are familiar will hasten the child's death. The **principle of double effect** addresses such concerns (Box 23-5). It provides an ethical standard that supports the use of interventions that

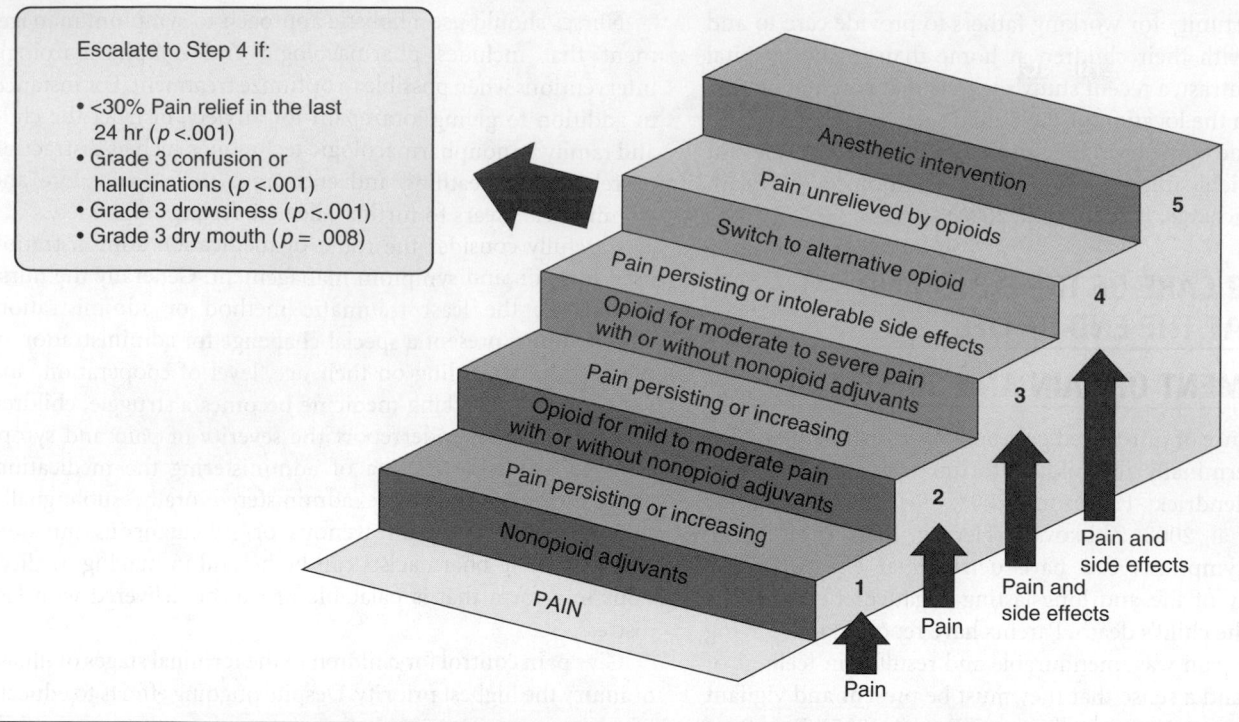

Escalate to Step 4 if:

• <30% Pain relief in the last 24 hr (p <.001)
• Grade 3 confusion or hallucinations (p <.001)
• Grade 3 drowsiness (p <.001)
• Grade 3 dry mouth (p = .008)

Anesthetic intervention
Pain unrelieved by opioids
Switch to alternative opioid
Pain persisting or intolerable side effects
Opioid for moderate to severe pain with or without nonopioid adjuvants
Pain persisting or increasing
Opioid for mild to moderate pain with or without nonopioid adjuvants
Pain persisting or increasing
Nonopioid adjuvants
PAIN

5
4
3
2
1

Pain and side effects
Pain and side effects
Pain
Pain

Grade 0: Not at all	Grade 1: A little	Grade 2: Quite a bit	Grade 3: Very much

Fig. 23-2 Overview of proposed five-step World Health Organization analgesic and side effect ladder. (From Riley J, Ross JR, Gretton SK, et al: Proposed five-step World Health Organization analgesic and side effect ladder, *Eur J Pain* [Suppl S]:23-30, 2007.)

BOX 23-5   ETHICAL PRINCIPLE OF DOUBLE EFFECT

An action that has one good (intended) and one bad (unintended but foreseeable) effect is permissible if the following conditions are met:

• The action itself must be good or indifferent. Only the good consequences of the action must be sincerely intended.
• The good effect must not be produced by the bad effect.
• There must be a compelling or proportionate reason for permitting the foreseeable bad effect to occur.

---

have the intention of relieving pain and suffering even though there is a foreseeable possibility that death may be hastened (Siever, 1994). In cases in which the child is terminally ill and in severe pain, using large doses of opioids and sedatives to manage pain is justified when no other treatment options are available that would relieve the pain but make the possibility of death less likely (Fleischman, 1998). (See Chapter 7 for an extensive discussion of pain assessment and management.)

In addition to pain, children experience a variety of other symptoms during their terminal course, either as a result of their disease process or as a side effect of medicines used to maintain their comfort (Box 23-6). The underlying disease and previous treatment history will contribute to the types and severity of symptoms the individual child experiences during the dying process. Nurses caring for children who are receiving palliative care for a terminal condition or illness assess frequently for any symptoms that are causing the child physical distress. Assessment includes information regarding

the symptom's onset, severity, duration, and effect on the child's quality of life.

These symptoms are consistently managed with appropriate medications or treatments and interventions such as repositioning, relaxation, massage, and other measures to maintain the child's comfort and quality of life. (For further information on pain and symptom management for children, see the Cancer Pain Management in Children [www.childcancerpain.org] and End-of-Life Care for Children [www.childendoflifecare.org] websites.)

PARENTS' AND SIBLINGS' NEED FOR EDUCATION AND SUPPORT THROUGH THE CAREGIVING PROCESS

Often, as the child's illness worsens, parents and other family members are the primary caregivers while the child is at home. This role can create physical, emotional, and financial strain on the larger family system. Therefore parents and other family members caring for dying children have a number of educational and support needs.

Educational Needs

Family caregivers need comprehensive education about various aspects of the care that they are providing to their child. This preparation can ease feelings of helplessness and anxiety and provide a sense of competence as they move from caring for an ill child to caring for a dying child. This education begins early in the transition from curative to palliative care. Table 23-4

BOX 23-6 COMMON SYMPTOMS EXPERIENCED BY DYING CHILDREN

Pain
Visceral pain
Bone pain
Neuropathic pain

Gastrointestinal
Anorexia
Nausea and vomiting
Constipation
Diarrhea

Genitourinary
Urinary tract infections
Urinary retention

Hematologic
Anemia
Bleeding

Respiratory
Cough
Congestion
Shortness of breath
Wheezing

Central Nervous System
Fevers, chills
Sleep disturbance
Restlessness, agitation
Seizures

Integumentary
Dry skin
Rash, itching
Pressure sores
Edema

Emotional
Fear
Anxiety
Depression

⊕ CULTURAL COMPETENCE
Cultural Considerations in Dying and Death

Culture influences perceptions, coping styles, and family dynamics in every arena of life. A death in the family is no exception. When language and cultural barriers exist, families may seek less support during the process of dying, death, and bereavement. This can result in unfortunate outcomes. When health care providers have a poor understanding of cultural influences on family dynamics and the family's perception of an illness, death, and grief, they cannot give optimum support when help is sought. To provide comprehensive care, health care professionals must take both language differences and cultural influences seriously.

Data from Prong LL: Childhood bereavement among Cambodians: cultural considerations, *Hospice* 10(2):51-64, 1995; and Saiki SC, Martinson IM, Inano M: Japanese families who have lost children to cancer: a primary study, *J Pediatr Nurs* 9(4):239-250, 1994.

Spiritual and Religious Support

Meeting the spiritual or religious needs of the child and family is as important as teaching caregiving techniques, and the degree to which these needs are met successfully may determine how well the child and family cope with the dying process. It is important for nurses working with dying children and their families to assess the family's spiritual or religious needs (Heilferty, 2004; National Cancer Institute, 2009), model comfort when discussing the family's spiritual issues, facilitate the family's spiritual or religious rituals (e.g., prayer), refrain from disclosing their own beliefs, inform family members of a hospital's multifaith chapel or quiet area for prayer, note signs of spiritual distress (e.g., "Why my child?"; "Why aren't my prayers being answered?"), inform family members of the chaplain role, and offer chaplaincy referral (Robinson, Thiel, Backus, et al, 2006). Referral to a hospital chaplain are indicated when a family member requests prayer, sacraments, ritual, devotional materials, or a faith perspective during their process of decision-making; when a family member expresses spiritual or religious objections to the child's treatment; when a provider notes signs of spiritual distress by a family member; and when a provider observes spiritual or religious solicitation (Robinson, Thiel, Backus, et al, 2006).

Sibling Support

It is important to consider the needs of siblings experiencing the death of a brother or sister (Fig. 23-3). As mentioned earlier, the developmental stage and level of maturity of the siblings will have a strong influence on the feelings and behaviors exhibited as their brother's or sister's illness progresses and their care intensifies. Siblings may feel isolated and displaced during the time that a brother or sister is dying (Nolbris and Hellstrom, 2005). Parents devote the majority of their time to the care and comfort of the dying child, which causes siblings to feel left out (Nolbris and Hellstrom, 2005). Siblings may become resentful of their sick brother or sister and begin to feel guilty or ashamed about such feelings (Murray, 1999; Nolbris and Hellstrom, 2005). Nurses can assist the family by helping the parents identify ways to involve the siblings in the caring process and provide honest, developmentally appropriate information to siblings (Giovanola, 2005; Nolbris and Hellstrom, 2005). Encourage

provides some common areas of educational needs of family caregivers and suggestions on how nurses can assist families in meeting these needs. Education about physical care is best provided as the need arises. Instructing parents too early in the signs and symptoms of respiratory distress or the method of stopping a nosebleed can increase the parents' anxiety.

Emotional Support

Members of the family can be overwhelmed by powerful emotions that can threaten their ability to cope. Anger, guilt, anxiety, and helplessness are normal feelings that many parents experience and often project onto other members of the family or health care team. Nurses assisting these families cannot prevent parents from feeling this way; however, they can assist the family in recognizing the normalcy of these emotions and in identifying ways in which to cope. Encourage families to seek assistance outside of the family circle and to arrange for periods of respite care when available (see Cultural Competence box).

TABLE 23-4 PREPARATION AND EDUCATION OF FAMILY CAREGIVERS

NEEDS OF FAMILY CAREGIVERS	PROFESSIONAL INTERVENTIONS
Practical Needs	
Is home care, hospice care, or care in the hospital appropriate for my child?	Explore the family's preferences for home care or hospice as appropriate.
How will we pay for end-of-life care at home, in the hospital, or in hospice?	Evaluate the family's funding source and provide resources and assistance as necessary.
Where do I get equipment and supplies?	Provide the family with appropriate telephone numbers and contact people for questions about equipment and medical care.
How does the equipment work?	
Who do I call if equipment malfunctions?	
How should we arrange our house to best meet the needs of our child?	Plan for availability of caregivers (i.e., parents, family, friends, professionals) and help coordinate a schedule for provision of care.
Will there be help available to us at home?	
Whom do I call for medical questions?	Provide a contact person for the family to call with concerns or questions.
Personal Care	
How do I give my child a bed bath?	Instruct all caregivers about providing daily care to the child.
How do I wash my child's hair in bed?	Provide written instruction and reference material for caregivers to review.
How do I change linen with my child in bed?	
How do I perform skin care?	
How do I perform mouth care?	
How do I administer medications?	
What do I do if my child does not want to eat?	Assess the child's nutritional status and parents' view on supplemental nutrition.
Is there something I can do to get my child to eat?	Educate the family on decreased nutritional needs and potential complications from overfeeding or overhydration.
Does my child need supplements or a special diet?	
Physical Care	
How do I assess my child's pain?	Assess the child's current comfort status and educate the family on current interventions.
When should I give pain medications?	
What do I do when pain management is ineffective?	Educate the family about assessing the child's comfort level.
	Instruct the family that the child may be uncomfortable for a variety of reasons (e.g., constipation, anxiety, fever, headache, muscle cramp, disease) and educate the family about the appropriate interventions for particular circumstances.
What should I do when our child is constipated or has diarrhea?	Provide an accessible supply of medications that can help alleviate discomfort (i.e., laxatives, sedatives, antipyretics).
How do I control nausea and vomiting?	
What do I do if my child has a fever?	Encourage the caregiver to telephone a contact person about questions or ineffective interventions.
What do I do if my child has seizures?	
What do I do if my child has trouble breathing?	
Activity and Social Interactions	
Can we safely travel and enjoy family gatherings with our child?	Encourage the family to engage in fun and memorable activities with the child.
In which activities can we engage our child?	
Should friends and family be encouraged to visit?	Encourage visitors when appropriate.
What interventions can I do to help my child relax and rest comfortably?	Encourage the family to use relaxation techniques that have previously been beneficial to the child.

From Brown-Hellsten M, Hockenberry-Eaton M, Lamb D, et al: *End of life care for children,* Austin, 1999, Texas Cancer Council. Reprinted with permission.

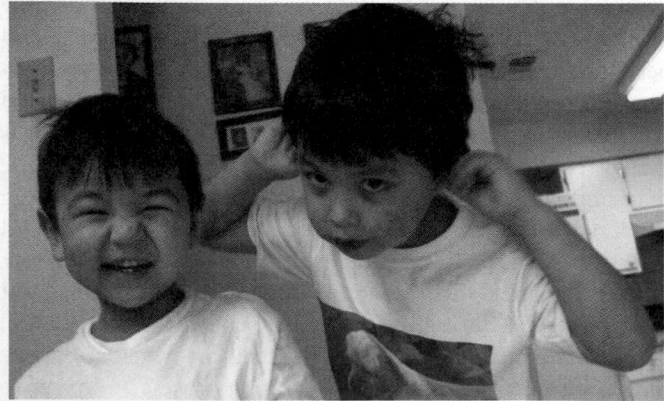

Fig. 23-3 It is important to consider the needs of siblings experiencing the death of a brother or sister.

parents to spend time with the other children during which the focus is on them. Nurses can assist the parents by helping them identify a trusted friend or family member who can sit with the ill child for a short time.

Caregiver Support

As the care of the dying child becomes the primary focus of the parent, personal and household needs often take on secondary significance. These tasks, however, can become burdensome and increase the family's stress if not attended to. Nurses can help the family identify ways for friends, community service organizations, and extended family members to assist with tasks such as household chores, shopping, meal preparation, and laundry.

CARE AT THE TIME OF DEATH

Few parents have cared for a dying child, and thus parents are not prepared to lead their child through the dying process (Fig. 23-4). Awareness that the child's death is near allows the parents and family to determine the location and circumstance of the child's death. This allows the family to create a meaningful death for their child, which improves their ability to cope in the difficult days, weeks, and years after the child has died. Nurses have an important role in helping parents recognize the changes in their child that signal that death may be near (see Nursing Care Guidelines box).

 NURSING CARE GUIDELINES

Supporting Grieving Families*

General
Stay with the family; sit quietly if they prefer not to talk; cry with them if desired.
Accept the family's grief reactions; avoid judgmental statements (e.g., "You should be feeling better by now").
Avoid offering rationalizations for the child's death (e.g., "You should be glad your child isn't suffering anymore").
Avoid artificial consolation (e.g., "I know how you feel," or "You are still young enough to have another baby").
Deal openly with feelings such as guilt, anger, and loss of self-esteem.
Focus on feelings by using a feeling word in the statement (e.g., "You're still feeling all the pain of losing a child").
Refer the family to an appropriate self-help group or to professional help if needed.

At the Time of Death
Reassure the family that everything possible is being done for the child, if they wish lifesaving interventions.
Do everything possible to ensure the child's comfort, especially relief of pain.
Provide the child and family the opportunity to review special experiences or memories in their lives.
Express personal feelings of loss or frustration (e.g., "We will miss him so much," or "We tried everything; we feel so sorry that we couldn't save him").
Provide information that the family requests and be honest.
Respect the emotional needs of family members such as siblings, who may need brief respites from being with the dying child.
Make every effort to arrange for family members, especially parents, to be with the child at the moment of death, if they wish to be present.
Allow the family to stay with the dead child for as long as they wish and to rock, hold, or bathe the child.
Provide practical help when possible, such as collecting the child's belongings.
Arrange for spiritual support, such as clergy; pray with the family if they wish it and if no one else can stay with them.

After the Death
Attend the funeral or visitation if there was a special closeness with the family.
Initiate and maintain contact (e.g., send cards, telephone, invite the family back to the unit, or make a home visit).
Refer to the dead child by name; discuss shared memories with the family.
Discourage the use of drugs or alcohol as a method of escaping grief.
Encourage all family members to communicate their feelings rather than remaining silent to avoid upsetting another member.
Emphasize that grieving is a painful process that often takes years to resolve.

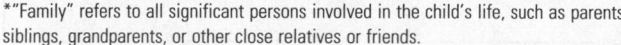
*"Family" refers to all significant persons involved in the child's life, such as parents, siblings, grandparents, or other close relatives or friends.

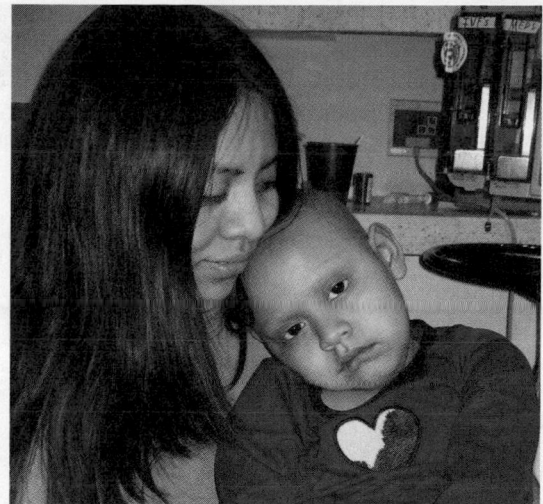
Fig. 23-4 For the dying child there is no greater comfort than the security and closeness of a parent.

Physical Changes

Physical changes occur more often in children dying of prolonged illness or disability and can vary widely among children. Generally, as the child progresses through the dying process, there is an overall decline in the child's physical condition. This decline may be interspersed with brief spurts of energy or periods of alertness and can cause parents to become exhausted and overwhelmed in "waiting for the inevitable." Often parents ask "how long" their child has to live. Initially this question may represent the parents' attempt to determine what special activities or events the family should try to accomplish. As the dying process progresses, this question may reveal a wish to know how long they and their child will have to endure the dying process.

As the child moves closer to his or her actual death, some general physical changes occur (Box 23-7). Initially the child may begin to sleep more. Appetite decreases, and the child begins to take only small bites of favorite foods or sips of fluids. As the child begins to eat and drink less, urinary frequency declines and the urine becomes more concentrated. In the final few days before death, the child most likely becomes less responsive. Breathing may become slow and shallow, with periodic deep sighs. Urinary output may decrease or stop. As the child nears the final hours before death, breathing becomes more irregular, deep, and gasping, with long periods of apnea (Cheyne-Stokes respirations). The skin may have a pale, grayish blue color and may be cool to the touch. The child's eyes may be slightly open, with a fixed gaze. It is important to prepare the family for these changes and to provide them with caregiving activities that promote a loving presence in the child's care (Box 23-8). Reassure parents that this is a normal process and that the child is not suffering.

Emotional Changes

As children approach death, they may begin to recall events that were important with their families. They may want to draw pictures or leave messages for important friends and family. Often children begin to reassure their parents and other significant people that they are not afraid and are ready to die.

During the final few days to hours of death, children may experience visions of "angels" or people and talk with them

BOX 23-7 PHYSICAL SIGNS OF APPROACHING DEATH

Increased sleeping

Loss of sensation and movement in the lower extremities, progressing toward the upper body

Sensation of heat although body feels cool

Mottling of skin

Loss of senses:
- Tactile sensation decreases
- Sensitivity to light develops
- Hearing is last sense to fail

Confusion, loss of consciousness, slurred speech

Muscle weakness

Decreased urination, more concentrated urine

Loss of bowel and bladder control

Decreased appetite and thirst

Difficulty swallowing

Change in respiratory pattern:
- Cheyne-Stokes respirations (waxing and waning of depth of breathing with regular periods of apnea)
- "Death rattle" (noisy chest sounds from accumulation of pulmonary and pharyngeal secretions)

BOX 23-8 CARE DURING THE TERMINAL PHASE

Physical Support

Provide frequent mouth care to prevent drying, cracking, and bleeding of lips and mucous membranes.

Maintain good hygiene by giving bed baths and using skin lotion as tolerated.

Continue necessary medications to manage symptoms and maintain comfort using intravenous infusion (if access is easily established) or subcutaneous infusion.

Discontinue unnecessary medications and procedures (e.g., measuring vital signs).

Emotional Support

Encourage the family to discuss the impending death openly with the child and other family members.

Encourage the family to continue to speak to the child in a calm, reassuring voice.

Provide familiar surroundings or objects.

Encourage caregivers to provide each other with periods of respite.

Allow the performance of spiritual and cultural rituals as desired.

Allow the family time with the child after the death and participation in the preparation of the body if they choose.

(Ethier, 2005). They may mention that they are not afraid and that someone is waiting for them. Often these visions are of family members or friends who have preceded them in death. In most instances these visions provide a comforting presence and reassurance for the child and family. Not all children will express these types of experiences.

As the child's death approaches, the family may begin the "death vigil," which is a natural phenomenon in which family and friends gather at the bedside. Rarely is the child left alone for any length of time. During this time families may read favorite books, recite prayers, light candles, or play music that is special to the child. Spiritual, religious, or family rituals surrounding the time of death are important, and nurses involved in the care of the family at this time are sensitive to such needs (Heilferty, 2004; National Cancer Institute, 2009) (see Nursing Care Plan).

NURSING CARE PLAN

End-of-Life Care in Children

NURSING DIAGNOSIS	EXPECTED PATIENT OUTCOMES	NURSING INTERVENTIONS	RATIONALE
Death Anxiety: Anxiety related to fear or worry about dying	Child and family will receive appropriate emotional support and information during the terminal phase of child's illness.	Encourage family to remain near child as much as possible.	To provide support through the presence of a loved one
Child's/Family's Defining Characteristics (Subjective and Objective Data)	**The Following NOC Concepts Apply to These Outcomes**	Encourage child to talk about feelings; help family as they encourage child to express feelings.	To provide a sense of closeness and understanding among family members
Unstable emotions Aggressive behavior Withdrawn behavior Depression	Anxiety Self-Control Coping Fear Level: Child	Provide safe, acceptable outlets for aggression or for grieving.	To establish that anger and sadness are normal reactions
		Answer questions as honestly as possible while maintaining a positive, hopeful approach.	To promote trust as a major strength for therapeutic relationships
		Explain progression of physical symptoms as child nears the end of life.	To decrease anxiety
		Explain all procedures and therapies, especially physical effects child will experience.	To decrease fear of the unknown, which may be more of a concern than the actual procedure or therapy
		Help child distinguish between consequences of treatment and manifestations of the disease.	To focus on interventions that can minimize discomfort
		Structure hospital or home environment to allow for maximum self-control and independence within limitations imposed by child's developmental level and physical condition.	To minimize fear and loss of control
		The Following NIC Concepts Apply to These Interventions Active Listening Coping Enhancement Simple Relaxation Therapy Touch	

NURSING CARE PLAN—cont'd

End-of-Life Care in Children

NURSING DIAGNOSIS	EXPECTED PATIENT OUTCOMES	NURSING INTERVENTIONS	RATIONALE
Pain related to disease process **Child's/Family's Defining Characteristics (Subjective and Objective Data)** Crying Withdrawal Aggression Fear of touch Fear of movement	Child will exhibit minimal or no evidence of physical discomfort. **The Following NOC Concepts Apply to These Outcomes** Comfort Level Pain Control	Assess child's level of comfort. Provide pain management around the clock. Assess child for symptoms associated with pain or its treatment. Provide stool softener, laxative, or diphenhydramine as needed. Provide nonpharmacologic interventions child prefers. Administer anticholinergic drugs as needed. Encourage family to provide comfort measures child prefers. Provide soothing surroundings for child. Avoid excessive noise or light. Provide pleasant smell, touch, temperature. Place all commodities within easy reach of child. Use gentle touch when required to perform physical procedures. Avoid pressure on painful areas or bony prominences. Use pillows or other supports to prop child in comfortable position. Place absorbent pads under hips if child is incontinent. Limit care to essential needs. **The Following NIC Concepts Apply to These Interventions** Analgesic Administration Patient-Controlled Analgesia Assistance Positioning Simple Massage Sleep Enhancement Simple Relaxation Therapy	To ensure child is treated for changes in pain To prevent recurrence or escalation of pain To ensure child is treated for symptoms accompanying pain or its management To prevent untoward side effects related to pain treatment To aid pharmacologic management of pain, helping to prevent recurrence or escalation of pain and accompanying symptoms To reduce secretions and lessen "death rattle," which can be distressing to family To provide comfort To minimize irritation and maximize comfort To minimize discomfort from movement To minimize pain when possible To make it easier for child to breathe To prevent skin breakdown by keeping child clean and dry To minimize fatigue
NURSING DIAGNOSIS	**EXPECTED PATIENT OUTCOMES**	**NURSING INTERVENTIONS**	**RATIONALE**
Grieving related to anticipated loss **Child's/Family's Defining Characteristics (Subjective and Objective Data)** Parents' feelings and physical responses of loss and depression Parents' feelings of loss of control and uncertainty Child's and siblings' feelings and physical responses of loss and depression Child's and siblings' feelings of loss of control and uncertainty	Family will express fears, concerns, and any special desires for terminal care and will seek resources to assist them during the grieving process. Family will demonstrate an understanding of their child's needs and be actively involved in the care. **The Following NOC Concepts Apply to These Outcomes** Family Coping Grief	Discuss with family and child the grieving process and differences in grieving among men, women, and children. Provide opportunities for family members to express emotions independently or together as desired. Facilitate child's and siblings' expression of emotions through art or play activities. Help parents and siblings deal with their feelings about child's death. Encourage parents to remain as near child as possible. Provide family with information regarding child's status. Help parents to understand behavioral reactions of their children. Encourage family's assistance with child's care. Encourage family to maintain own health care needs. Provide as much privacy as possible without isolating family from nurse's care. Assist family in assessing their needs for referral services.	To facilitate understanding of what family members are feeling and experiencing To provide an outlet for their emotions To provide opportunities to express their emotions To provide support To allow parents to feel they are doing something for their child To promote understanding and communication To provide understanding of their children's behaviors To assist with coping and minimize loss of control To prevent families from becoming ill To provide dignity for grieving process To facilitate support for families

Continued

◎ NURSING CARE PLAN—cont'd

End-of-Life Care in Children

NURSING DIAGNOSIS	EXPECTED PATIENT OUTCOMES	NURSING INTERVENTIONS	RATIONALE
Grieving related to anticipated loss—cont'd		Encourage parents to honestly answer children's questions about dying.	To decrease children's fear and anxiety
		Provide resources for family to facilitate discussions with children about dying.	To provide support and facilitate parents' discussion
		Encourage parents to share their moments of sorrow with their children.	To promote grief expression of children
		Assist family and child with memory-making opportunities.	To facilitate emotions and sharing between family and child.
		Assist child as needed to complete any unfinished business.	To facilitate support of child
		Discuss with parents appropriate involvement of siblings.	To prevent siblings from feeling excluded
		Identify family's religious and cultural beliefs related to death.	To provide support and spiritual care
		Provide preparation for postdeath services.	To provide support and guidance
		Discuss with parents the frequent need of children to be given permission to die.	To provide support and guidance
		Discuss with family their preferences for care if death is imminent.	To allow families to be in control
		Facilitate appropriate spiritual care in accordance with family's beliefs or affiliations.	To provide support
		Provide support for families who choose home care for their child.	To allow families to choose where the child is to die and provide guidance for this to occur
		The Following NIC Concepts Apply to These Interventions Anticipatory Guidance Anxiety Reduction Caregiver Support Counseling Family Support Family Therapy	

POSTMORTEM CARE

The final moments of a child's life are often extremely stressful as the family waits for the child to die. Families often depend on trusted health care professionals, particularly nurses, to help them recognize the exact moment of the child's death. Once the nurse has observed that the child is no longer showing signs of life, the child is pronounced dead (registered nurse pronouncement is allowed by the state practice act). Initially the family may show joy and relief that the child is no longer struggling. They may have many varied emotions in the immediate moments after the child's death, and the nurse must be prepared for a range of reactions. Generally all that is necessary is a supportive presence at this time. In rare instances, particularly in more conflicted families, there may be strong outbursts of anger. It is important for the nurse to be aware of families in which this situation may occur and respond by assuring them that appropriate resources (social worker, chaplain, security personnel) are readily available to ensure that the situation does not escalate.

Once the initial reaction to the moment of death has occurred, the family may move away from the bedside and enter a phase of relaxation. One or both of the parents may stay with the child while others in attendance make brief visits to view the child. Nursing care at this time is to facilitate the parents' ability to spend time with their child as they wish. Allow the family the time needed to say good-bye.

When the parents are ready, the nurse offers to bathe and dress the body for removal from the home or hospital room. The parents may wish to undertake this task, may participate with the nurse, or may ask the nurse to do the bathing for them. If the death was at home and the body is prepared for removal and the parents are ready, contact the funeral home. Often hospice organizations have arrangements with the medical examiners in their area that allow the body to be directly removed by a funeral director. In some instances it may be necessary for the police to make a report before the release of the child's body. It is important for the nurse to explain to the parents the requirements of their local area for removal of a body. This allows the parents to be prepared for questions or information that may be required. Hospital deaths require the parents to leave the child, and the body is taken to the morgue. Some parents may ask to go with the body to the morgue, and nurses work within their institutions' regulations to try to honor such requests if possible.

The final separation of the child's body from the parents and family is often the most emotional and traumatic time. The nurse should offer support to the parents and ensure that other family members or friends are available in the coming hours to continue to provide support and assistance to the parents and siblings.

CARE OF THE FAMILY EXPERIENCING UNEXPECTED CHILDHOOD DEATH

In cases of long-term, potentially fatal illnesses, families may experience anticipatory grief. Parents mourn the loss of their child long before the death. They are reminded of their child's uncertain future each time they see the pain the child must endure or experience the sudden loss of hope during a relapse. This prolonged period of anticipatory grief provides families with the opportunity to complete "unfinished business," such as helping the child and siblings understand and cope with a fatal prognosis. Many families reflect on their changed perspective of time after learning of the diagnosis, particularly their heightened awareness of the value of each day.

In contrast, after sudden, unexpected death, the family is deprived of any of the advantages of anticipatory grief. They have no opportunity to prepare themselves or others for the death, and the initial denial may be very strong. Many families feel great guilt and remorse for not having done something additional or different with the child. For example, they may berate themselves for depriving the child of some desired material object or privilege or, more painfully, for not having prevented the sudden death in some way. "If only I'd been a better parent" is a common feeling at this time. Without proper support, the risk of complicated grief responses may be high (Oliver and Fallat, 1995; Rando, 1993). Mothers experiencing the sudden, unexpected death of their child have reported a more prolonged grief response compared with mothers who anticipated their child's death (Seecharan, Andresen, Norris, et al, 2004).

Death resulting from accident or trauma or from acute illness in settings such as the emergency department or intensive care unit often requires the active withdrawal of some form of life-supporting intervention, such as a ventilator or bypass machine. These situations often raise difficult ethical issues (Savage, 1997), and parents are often less prepared for the actual moment of death (Box 23-9). Nurses can assist parents by providing detailed information about what will happen as supportive equipment is withdrawn, ensuring that appropriate pain medications are administered to prevent pain during the dying process, and allowing the parents time before the start of the withdrawal to be with and speak to their child. It is important that the nurse attempt to control the environment around the family at this time by providing privacy; asking if they would like to play music; softening lights and monitoring noises; and arranging for any spiritual, religious, or cultural rituals that the family may want performed. After the child's death, the family is allowed to remain with the body and hold or rock the child if they desire. Once the nurse has removed all tubes and equipment from the body, give parents the option of assisting with the preparation of the body, such as bathing and dressing.

BOX 23-9   STRATEGIES FOR INTERVENTION WITH SURVIVORS AFTER SUDDEN CHILDHOOD DEATH

Arrival of the Family

Meet the family immediately and escort to a private area.

A health care worker with bereavement training should remain with the family.

Provide information about the extent of illness or injury and treatment efforts.

If the health care worker must leave the family or if the family requests privacy, return in 15 minutes so the family does not feel forgotten.

Provide tissues, telephone, coffee, and a Bible.

Pronouncement of Death

When available, the family's own physician should inform them of the child's death.

Alternatively, the physician or nurse should introduce himself or herself and establish calm, reassuring eye contact with the parents.

Honest, clear communication that avoids misinterpretation is essential.

Nonverbal communication such as hugging, touching, or remaining with the family in silence may be most empathetic.

Acknowledge the family's guilt, attempt to alleviate it, and deal openly and nonjudgmentally with anger.

Provide information, answer questions, and offer reassurance that everything possible was done for the child.

Viewing of the Body

Offer the parents the opportunity to see the body; repeat the offer later if they decline.

Before viewing, inform the parents of bodily changes they should expect (tubes, injuries, cold skin).

A single staff member should accompany the family but remain inconspicuous.

Offer the opportunity to hold the child.

Allow the family as much time as they need.

Offer parents the opportunity for siblings to view the body.

Formal Concluding Process

Discuss and answer questions concerning autopsy and funeral arrangements; obtain signatures on the body release and autopsy forms.

Provide anticipatory guidance regarding symptoms of grief response and their normalcy.

Provide written materials about grief symptoms.

Escort the family to the exit or to their car if necessary.

Provide a follow-up phone call in 24 to 48 hours to answer questions and provide support.

Provide referral for community health nursing visit.

Provide referrals to local support and resource groups (e.g., bereavement groups, bereavement counselors, sudden infant death syndrome groups, Parents of Murdered Children, Mothers Against Drunk Driving).

Modified from Back K: Sudden, unexpected pediatric death: caring for the parents, *Pediatr Nurs* 17(6):571-574, 1991.

Community-Based Follow-Up

A community health or visiting nurse referral may be helpful after a sudden, unexpected pediatric death. Some families have reported that this was a missing piece in their care (Dent, Condon, Blair, et al, 1996). During several home visits the nurse can answer the families' questions, provide information about the grief process, assess and support coping mechanisms, and give appropriate referrals to support groups (Box 23-10) (Buckalow and Esposito, 1995).

Families who experience a child's sudden death may have recurrent memories of both the child and the death experience

BOX 23-10 ASPECTS OF HOME HEALTH NURSING VISITS FOR SUDDEN INFANT DEATH SYNDROME

- Express condolences.
- Involve as many family members as possible in the visit.
- Clarify any misconceptions about the circumstances of death.
- Provide and interpret information about sudden infant death syndrome (SIDS).
- Provide information about the grief process.
- Offer suggestions on future coping: holidays, birthdays, anniversaries.
- Evaluate and support coping strategies.
- Assist the family in identifying their support network.
- Reinforce parental ability to care for the other children.
- Offer information about children's grief process.
- Provide information on siblings, risk factors, and monitoring.
- Obtain signatures, if necessary, for autopsy consent form.
- Provide referrals, as desired by family, to crisis intervention, SIDS organizations, and mental health resources.

Modified from Buckalow PG, Esposito CM: The role of the home health nurse in sudden infant death syndrome, *Home Health Care Pract* 7(3):36-45, 1995.

and may long grieve over missed opportunities. Support and resource groups that may be useful to families include the First Candle (previously SIDS Alliance),* National Sudden and Unexpected Infant/Child Death and Pregnancy Loss Resource Center,† American SIDS Institute,‡ Mothers Against Drunk Driving,§ and National Organization of Parents of Murdered Children, Inc.||

SPECIAL DECISIONS AT THE TIME OF DYING AND DEATH

Rarely are people prepared to cope with the numerous decisions that must be made when a loved one is dying or dies. When the death is expected, there is the opportunity to make plans in advance, such as where the child should spend the last days or what type of funeral arrangements are desired. When death is unexpected, the shock is sufficient to render the survivors incapable of making even simple decisions. Those in attendance at the death and those caring for the dying child can be instrumental in initiating decisions that may facilitate the grief process. The following is a brief review of selected instances in which nurses can guide parents in making decisions related to the expected or unexpected death.

*1314 Bedford Ave., Suite 210, Baltimore, MD 21208; 800-221-7437, 410-653-8226; fax: 410-653-8709; www.firstcandle.org.
†2115 Wisconsin Ave., NW, Suite 601, Washington, DC 20007; 866-866-7437, 202-687-7466; fax: 202-784-9777; e-mail: info@sidscenter.org; www.sidscenter.org.
‡509 Augusta Drive, Marietta, GA 30067; 770-426-8746, 800-232-SIDS; fax: 770-426-1369; www.sids.org.
§511 E. John Carpenter Freeway, Suite 700, Irving, TX 75062; 214-744-6233, 800-438-6233; www.madd.org.
||100 E. Eighth St., Suite 202, Cincinnati, OH 45202; 513-721-5683, 888-818-POMC; fax: 513-345-4489; www.pomc.com.

RIGHT TO DIE AND DO-NOT-RESUSCITATE ORDERS

One of the benefits of hospice has been the recognition of patients' right to die as they wish, with emphasis on the quality of life. Unfortunately, this is not always the focus of care, especially in the traditional hospital setting. Many families are not given the option of terminating treatment when cure is unlikely, and staff may be reluctant to raise the question of "no code" or DNR orders (withholding cardiopulmonary resuscitation in response to cardiac arrest).

Guidelines have been established for discontinuing mechanical ventilation and life-support measures for infants whose parents and providers consider care futile (De Lisle-Porter and Podruchny, 2009; Sine, Sumner, Gracy, et al, 2001). Such plans must carefully encompass preplanning, educational, discharge, and postextubation procedures and the needs of the family and health care staff and unit. If parents choose DNR, they must be aware of exactly what will and will not be done for the child and be assured that this does not mean "no care." For example, the family may wish that oxygen be given to the child for difficult breathing but does not want active resuscitation. Once a decision is made, it must be communicated to all members of the health team, and a written medical order for the use or withholding of lifesaving measures must be included. An order to "slow" or "delay" code is not legal. Because the child's condition or the family's wishes may change, review DNR orders regularly. Respect orders even if it is difficult to follow them at the moment of death (Martinson, 1995).

VIEWING OF THE BODY

Although most institutions recognize the need for parents to hold and spend time with the dead child, a dilemma may arise when the body is mutilated. Although the memory of the child's disfigurement can be extremely upsetting and can generate concern regarding how much the child suffered, not seeing the body can leave the parents with imagined ideas of how their child looked that can be worse than the reality and can delay the acceptance of the death. When family members choose to view the body, they need preparation for this upsetting experience. The nurse should inform them about what to expect and why certain parts of the body are covered or bandaged. It is desirable to place the body in a private room, without medical apparatus, and make it as presentable as the situation allows. Some people appreciate the presence of a nurse in the room with them; others desire privacy. Regardless of how badly the body is harmed, parents may want to hold the child. Offer and respect such options. Give family members as much time as they need to say good-bye; for many, viewing the body is a sign of closure—an opportunity to finish their good-byes and leave the hospital.

ORGAN OR TISSUE DONATION AND AUTOPSY

Many states have legislated a mandatory request for organ or tissue donation when a child dies. For some families this may be a meaningful act—one that benefits another human being despite the loss of their child. Unfortunately, initiating a discussion about tissue donation is often stressful for staff, and there may be confusion regarding whose responsibility this is. In centers in which transplants are performed, a full-time transplant coordinator is usually available to inform the family about organ donation and to take care of details. If such services are not available, the staff determines which members should discuss this topic with the family. Ideally the person who knows the family best, knows when the death is expected, or has the opportunity to spend time with the family when the death is unexpected takes the role. Often nurses are in an optimum position to suggest tissue donation after consultation with the attending physician. When possible, the topic is raised before death occurs. Make the request in a private and quiet area of the hospital. Be simple and direct, with questions such as, "Are you a donor family?" or "Have you ever considered organ donation?"

Written consent from the family is required before donation can proceed. When requests for organ donation are made, health care practitioners must address common misunderstandings families have about brain death and organ donation (Bellali and Papadatou, 2007; Franz, DeJong, Wolfe, et al, 1997). Training of health care professionals regarding sensitive approaches to request organ donation has shown to increase families' willingness to consent to organ donation (Bellali and Papadatou, 2007; Evanisko, Beasley, Brigham, et al, 1998). Discussion of the option to donate organs is always separate from communication of impending or actual death.

Nurses need to be aware of common questions about organ donation so they can help families make an informed decision. Healthy children who die unexpectedly are excellent candidates for organ donation. Children who have cancer, chronic disease, or infection or who have suffered prolonged cardiac arrest may not be suitable candidates, although this is individually determined. The nurse inquires whether organ donation was discussed with the child or whether the child ever expressed such a wish. Any number of body tissues or organs can be donated (skin, corneas, bone, kidney, heart, liver, pancreas), and their removal does not mutilate or desecrate the body or cause any suffering. The family may have an open casket, and there is no delay in the funeral. There is no cost to the donor family, but organ donation does not eliminate funeral or cremation responsibilities. Most religions permit organ donation as long as the recipient benefits from the transplant, although Orthodox Judaism forbids it.

In cases of unexplained death, violent death, or suspected suicide, autopsy is required by law. In other instances it may be optional, and the nurse should inform parents of this choice. Explain the procedure, as well as forms that require signing. Inform the family that the child can be in an open casket following an autopsy.

SIBLINGS' ATTENDANCE AT FUNERAL SERVICES

One of the most frequent concerns of parents is whether young or school-age children should attend funeral or burial services (see Research Focus box). Sharing moments of deep signifi-

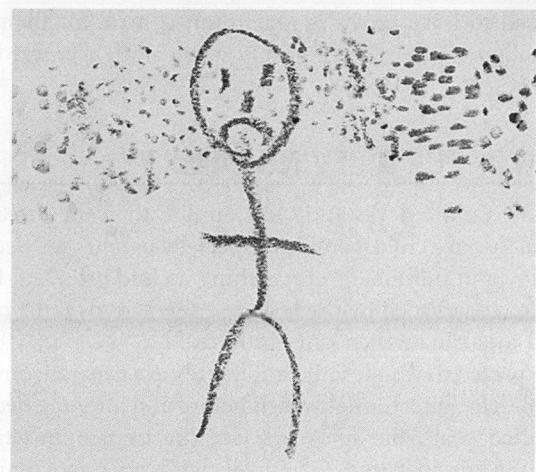

Fig. 23-5 Drawing made by a 7-year-old child whose sister died in a car crash. The drawing shows the boy sad and crying (dots are tears) because he was not allowed to see his dead sibling.

cance with parents helps children understand the experience and deal with their own feelings, and depriving them of this opportunity may leave children with lifelong regrets (Fig. 23-5). However, a child is never to be forced to attend a postdeath service. Children need preparation for postdeath services (Pearson, 2005). They should be told what to expect, particularly how the deceased person will look if the coffin is open. Ideally a parent explains the details to the child; if the parent's grief prevents this communication, a significant family member or friend should substitute.

RESEARCH FOCUS

Children's Involvement in the Death Process

Unfortunately, little research has focused on the difference in adjustment between children who do and those who do not attend postdeath services. However, one study provided substantial evidence of the benefit of involving children in the experience of their dying sibling. Lauer, Mulhern, Bohne, and colleagues (1985) compared children's perceptions of their sibling's death at home versus death in the hospital. The home care group (ages 5 to 23 years) reported that they were prepared for the impending death, received consistent information and support from their parents, were involved in most activities, found the funeral experience comforting, and viewed their own involvement as the most important aspect of the experience. The non–home care group (ages 2 to 26 years) had opposite perceptions. Another study found that greater participation in the child's care and death, including funeral attendance, was associated with higher self-esteem in the siblings (Michael and Lansdown, 1986). Among adolescents, Kuntz (1991) found that seeing a parent who had died and being involved with the rituals surrounding the death promoted adaptive grieving. Thus it appears that children benefit from increased involvement with the death, rather than isolation and "protection."

It is often helpful to bring children to the funeral service before many visitors arrive. They are allowed private time to say good-bye but are spared some of the unpredictable emotional reactions of others, which can be distressing to them. Children are allowed to stay as long as they wish, but respecting their need to leave provides maximum control for them over their ability to grieve comfortably (see Family-Centered Care box).

CARE OF THE GRIEVING FAMILY

No event is more devastating for families than the threatened or actual loss of a child. Families, especially parents, are deprived of the joy and fulfillment of watching a child grow. All family members are affected by the loss, and their needs must be recognized to facilitate their grief process.

In expected death the child and family are generally involved in the plan for interventions both before and after the death. In unexpected death the survivors face the tremendous task of integrating the loss into their lives, with no opportunity for anticipatory grief. In either situation nurses can facilitate the grief process by having a basic understanding of the process; being aware of expected reactions; talking with family members; ascertaining their needs; and supporting their efforts to cope, adapt, and grieve (see Nursing Care Guidelines box). Applying the principles of family-centered care is as important at this time as at any other.

 FAMILY-CENTERED CARE

Children Need to Say Good-Bye

As a nurse–grief counselor, I conduct grief workshops with children who have experienced the death of someone special. Children often communicate their feelings of being excluded through drawings. They may draw a picture of the dying person in a hospital bed that is raised too high for them to see the person's face clearly. Sometimes children reveal that they did not get to say good-bye because a family member told them, for example, "You don't want to see your grandma this way. She is too sick for you to visit." If the special person died at home, the children had to stay in their room when the funeral home staff took away the body.

I have learned never to underestimate the importance of allowing children to be involved with the dying person and the significance of a child's loss. Once, when I asked a 6-year-old girl to draw a picture with the theme "This is what I was doing when my _____ died," she drew a picture and completed the sentence with "when my *home* died." Her grandmother had been like her mother; to the child, her home was gone. We need to give children the choice of being included in the family's activities of saying good-bye.

Barbara Bilderback, MS, MA, RN
Bereavement Supervisor
Saint Francis Hospice
Tulsa

 NURSING CARE GUIDELINES

Communicating with the Bereaved Family

Examples of Nontherapeutic Statements

Advice
You should get out more.
Stop feeling sorry for yourself.
You need to be strong for your family.

Cheerfulness
Now, now, don't cry; cheer up.
Cheer up, you can always have another baby.

Interpretation
It was God's will.
It's better now because she is at peace.

Reassurance
I know how you feel.
God never gives us more than we can handle.
Don't worry, everything will work out.
At least you still have the rest of your family.

Argument
How can you say that?
It's wrong to blame anyone.
You should be glad his suffering is over.

Ignoring the Loss
Remember, you're young and can still have another baby.
It could be worse; he could have lived with severe brain damage.

Examples of Therapeutic Statements

Focus on Feelings
You seem confused and angry.

You are still feeling the pain.
Tell me more about how you are feeling.

Nonjudgmental Questions
Can I be of any help?
Have you decided who the pallbearers will be?

Clarification
Correct me if I'm wrong, but you intend to make all the arrangements.
You believe the accident was your husband's fault?
I'm not sure I understand. Tell me more about _____.

Explanations
You can touch her and hold her if you wish.

Concern, Support, Empathy
Your daughter's birthday is near. That must be painful to deal with.
It's OK to cry.
It sounds like you have been doing some painful thinking.

Support, Silence
I'm here if you want to talk. (Silence)
Hello. (Touch, silence)

Assessment of Coping and Support
Do you have friends and family who can help you now?
You have been through a lot. How are you doing now?
Is there someone who can drive you home?

Validation of Loss
You have been through a very tough time.
He was a special boy to all the staff. I will miss him.

Data from Davidowitz M, Myrick R: Responding to the bereaved: an analysis of "helping statements," *Death Educ* 8:1-10, 1984; Johnson L, Mattson S: Communication: the key to crisis prevention in pediatric death, *Crit Care Nurs* 12(8):23-27, 1992; and Segal S, Fletcher M, Meekison W: Survey of bereaved parents, *CMAJ* 134(1):38-42, 1986.

GRIEF

Grief is a process, not an event, of experiencing physiologic, psychologic, behavioral, social, and spiritual reactions to the loss of a child (Rando, 1993). Grief is highly individualized, encompassing a broad range of manifestations from person to person. It is a natural and expected reaction to loss. It is neither orderly nor predictable. Grieving in any form is necessary for healing to occur. When death is the expected or a possible outcome of a disorder, the child and family members may experience anticipatory grief. Anticipatory grief may be manifested in varying behaviors and intensities and may be characterized by denial, anger, depression, and other psychologic and physical symptoms (Rando, 1986). Anticipatory guidance may assist grieving family members. Health care professionals emphasize that grief reactions such as hearing the dead person's voice, feeling distant from others, or seeking reassurance that they did everything possible for the lost person are normal, necessary, and expected. These reactions in no way signify poor coping, insanity, or an approaching mental breakdown. On the contrary, such behaviors signify that the survivor is working through the acute grief. They are a necessary part of grief work. Anticipatory guidance regarding the mourning process may be helpful to families so that they can recognize the normalcy of their experiences.

It is important to recognize that some family members may experience "complicated" grief. Complicated grief reactions (those that continue more than a year after the loss) include such symptoms as intense intrusive thoughts, pangs of severe emotion, distressing yearnings, feelings of being excessively alone and empty, unusual sleep disturbance, and maladaptive levels of loss of interest in personal activities (Horowitz, Siegel, Holen, et al, 1997). An unexpected, sudden death is a risk factor for complicated grief (Keesee, Currier, and Neimeyer, 2008). Bereaved persons experiencing such prolonged and complicated grief are referred to an expert in grief and bereavement counseling.

Parental Grief

The grief of parents after the death of a child has been found to be a more intense, complex, long-lasting, and fluctuating grief experience than that of other bereaved individuals (Rando, 1986). Although parents experience the primary loss of their child, many secondary losses are felt, such as the loss of part of one's self, hopes and dreams for the child's future, the family unit, prior social and emotional community supports, and often spousal support. It is common for parents of the same child to experience different grief reactions.

Studies involving bereaved parents have shown that grieving does not end by the severing of the bond with the deceased child, but rather involves a continuing bond between the parent and the dead child (Klass, 2001). Parental resolution of grief is a process of integrating the deceased child into daily life in which the pain of losing a child is never completely gone but lessens. There are occasions of brief relapse, but not to the degree experienced when the loss initially occurred. Thus parental grief work is never completed and is a timeless process

of accepting the new reality of being without a child, as it changes over time (Davies, 2004). Although parents are expected to grieve the loss of their child, parental grief is often minimized, which leaves parents to work through their grief in isolation and silence (Rando, 1993).

Parental grief can be stressful on a marriage. As parents become lost in their grief, they are unable to perform many of their roles within the family. For instance, a mother who is generally the nurturing parent now finds herself immobilized by grief and unable to nurture and support her husband and surviving children. Her husband functions in the family as the provider and protector; however, he could not "fix" his dying child. He may now feel the need to "fix" the other members of his family. In addition, he may not have the resources to express his grief, which leads him to postpone his grief by keeping busy at work or around the house. This "tabling" of emotion can lead to outbursts of anger and emotional distancing. Parents often need guidance in understanding each other's needs during their grief process. Not only may the parents be unavailable to each other, they may also be so lost in their own grief that they cannot easily respond to their children's grief.

Sibling Grief

Each child grieves in his or her own way and on his or her own timeline. Children, even adolescents, grieve differently from adults. Adults and children differ more widely in their reactions to death than in their reactions to any other phenomenon. Children of all ages grieve the loss of a loved one, and their understanding and reactions to death depends on their age and developmental level (Table 23-5). Children often grieve for a longer duration than adults, revisiting their grief as they grow and develop new understandings of death. However, they do not grieve 100% of the time. They grieve in spurts and can be emotional and sad one moment and then, just as quickly, off and playing.

Children express their grief through play and behavior. Children can be exquisitely attuned to their parents' grief and try to protect them by not asking questions and avoiding upsetting them. This can set the stage for the sibling to try to become the "perfect child." Children exhibit many of the grief reactions of adults, including physical sensations and illnesses, anger, guilt, sadness, loneliness, withdrawal, acting out, regression, sleep disturbances, isolation, and search for meaning. Again, nurses are attentive for signs that siblings are struggling with their grief and provide guidance to parents when possible (see Critical Thinking Exercise).

MOURNING
Shock and Disbelief

Shock, numbness, and disbelief are seen during the immediate phase of grief. As one parent described, "We were as prepared for our son's death as anyone could be, but it was a shock when in a moment his life was finished. I just can't get over the rapidity with which life ends." This temporary numbness protects the survivors from the overwhelming pain associated with grief.

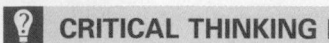

CRITICAL THINKING EXERCISE

Preschool Siblings and Death

Parents consult you about the preschool-age sibling of an infant who recently died. Which of the following behaviors, which are of concern to the parents, represent normal responses?
1. "Our daughter cut her knee and said it was because the baby died."
2. "Our daughter used to enjoy preschool but now clings to us every morning and doesn't want to go."
3. "Our daughter sometimes asks where the baby is and when she'll come home."
4. "Our daughter lost a stuffed rabbit at the park and was distraught."

Questions
1. Evidence—Are there sufficient data to support your decision?
2. Assumptions—Describe some underlying assumptions about the following:
   a. Young children and death
   b. Common behaviors seen in young children experiencing a loss
3. What are the priorities of care for the preschool-age sibling at this time?
4. Does the evidence support your conclusion?

Decisions are often made automatically, and only certain details are remembered.

Expression of Grief

When the numbness fades, a period of intense grief begins, characterized by loneliness and yearning for the deceased. During this stage many of the signs of acute grief are evident, and physical complaints such as appetite changes and an inability to sleep are common. There is a tendency to review the events of the deceased's life and to evaluate the relationship with the loved one. Feelings of guilt and anger are common at this time.

Disorganization and Despair

During the stage of disorganization and despair the pain of the loss is replaced primarily by emptiness, apathy, and deep depression. There is a feeling that life has no meaning and that the pain will never end. This is particularly relevant for parents. For example, mothers often comment that they feel

TABLE 23-5	CHILDREN'S UNDERSTANDING OF AND REACTIONS TO DEATH	
CONCEPTS OF DEATH	**REACTIONS TO DEATH**	**INTERVENTIONS**
Infants and Toddlers		
Death has least significance to children younger than 6 mo of age.	With the death of someone else, they may continue to act as though the person is alive.	Help parents deal with their feelings, allowing them more emotional reserve to meet the needs of their children.
After parent-child attachment and the development of trust is established, the loss, even if temporary, of the significant person is profound.	As children grow older, they will be increasingly able and willing to let go of the dead person.	Encourage parents to remain as near to the child as possible, yet be sensitive to the parents' needs.
Prolonged separation during the first several years is thought to be more significant in terms of future physical, social, and emotional growth than at any subsequent age.	Ritualism is important; a change in lifestyle could be anxiety producing.	Maintain as normal an environment as possible to retain ritualism.
Toddlers are egocentric and can only think about events in terms of their own frame of reference—living.	This age-group reacts more to the pain and discomfort of a serious illness than to the probable fatal prognosis. This age-group also reacts to parental anxiety and sadness.	If a parent has died, encourage the establishment of a consistent caregiver for the child. Promote primary nursing.
Their egocentricity and vague separation of fact and fantasy make it impossible for them to comprehend absence of life.		
Instead of understanding death, this age-group is affected more by any change in lifestyle.		
Preschool Children		
Children of this age believe their thoughts are sufficient to cause death; the consequence is a feeling of guilt, shame, and punishment.	If they become seriously ill, they conceive of the illness as a punishment for their thoughts or actions.	Help parents deal with their feelings, allowing them more emotional reserve to meet the needs of their children.
Their egocentricity implies a tremendous sense of self-power and omnipotence.	They may feel guilty and responsible for the death of a sibling.	Help parents to understand behavioral reactions of their children.
They usually have some sense of the meaning of death.	Their greatest fear concerning death is separation from their parents.	Encourage parents to remain near the child as much as possible, to minimize the child's great fear of separation from parents.
Death is seen as a departure, a kind of sleep.	They may engage in activities that seem strange or abnormal to adults.	If a parent has died, encourage establishment of a consistent caregiver for the child.
They may recognize the fact of physical death but do not separate it from living abilities.	With fewer defense mechanisms to deal with loss, young children may react to a less significant loss with more outward grief than to the loss of a significant person.	Promote primary nursing.
Death is seen as temporary and gradual; life and death can change places with one another.	The loss is so deep, painful, and threatening that the child must deny it for the time being to survive its overwhelming impact.	
There is no understanding of the universality and inevitability of death.	Behavioral reactions such as giggling, joking, attracting attention, or regressing to earlier developmental skills indicate children's need to distance themselves from tremendous loss.	

TABLE 23-5	CHILDREN'S UNDERSTANDING OF AND REACTIONS TO DEATH—cont'd	
CONCEPTS OF DEATH	**REACTIONS TO DEATH**	**INTERVENTIONS**
School-Age Children These children still associate misdeeds or bad thoughts with causing death and feel intense guilt and responsibility for the event. Because of their higher cognitive abilities, they respond well to logical explanations and comprehend the figurative meaning of words. They have a deeper understanding of death in a concrete sense. They particularly fear the mutilation and punishment they associate with death. They personify death as the devil, a monster, or the bogeyman. They may have naturalistic-physiologic explanations of death. By age 9 or 10, children have an adult concept of death, realizing that it is inevitable, universal, and irreversible.	Because of their increased ability to comprehend, they may have more fears, for example: • The reason for the illness • Communicability of the disease to themselves or others • Consequences of the disease • The process of dying and death itself • Fear of the unknown, which is greater than their fear of the known The realization of impending death is a tremendous threat to their sense of security and ego strength. They are likely to exhibit fear through verbal uncooperativeness rather than actual physical aggression. They are interested in postdeath services. They may be inquisitive about what happens to the body.	Help parents deal with their feelings, allowing them more emotional reserve to meet the needs of their children. Encourage parents to remain near the child as much as possible, yet be sensitive to the parents' needs. Because of children's fear of the unknown, anticipatory preparation is very important. Because the developmental task of this age is industry, interventions of helping children maintain control over their bodies and increasing their understanding allow them to achieve independence, self-worth, and self-esteem and avoid a sense of inferiority. Encourage children to talk about their feelings and provide aggressive outlets. Encourage parents to honestly answer questions about dying rather than avoiding questions or fabricating euphemisms. Encourage parents to share their moments of sorrow with their children. Provide preparation for postdeath services.
Adolescents Adolescents have a mature understanding of death. They are still very much influenced by remnants of magical thinking and are subject to feelings of guilt and shame. They are likely to see deviations from accepted behavior as the reason for their illness.	Adolescents straddle transition from childhood to adulthood. They have the most difficulty in coping with death. They are least likely to accept the cessation of life, particularly if it is their own. Concern for the present is much greater than for the past or the future. They may consider themselves alienated from their peers and unable to communicate with their parents for emotional support, feeling alone in their struggle. Adolescents' orientation to the present compels them to worry about physical changes even more than the prognosis. Because of their idealistic view of the world, they may criticize funeral rites as barbaric, money making, and unnecessary.	Help parents deal with their feelings, allowing them more emotional reserve to meet the needs of their children. Avoid alliances with either parent or child. Structure hospital admission to allow for maximum self-control and independence. Answer adolescents' questions honestly, treating them as mature individuals and respecting their needs for privacy, solitude, and personal expressions of emotions. Help the parents understand their child's reactions to death and dying, especially that concern for present crises, such as loss of hair, may be much greater than concern for future ones, including possible death.

they have suffered a double loss—loss of their child and loss of the mothering role. Feelings of estrangement from other loved ones are common, and social isolation may foster the depression.

Reorganization

Reorganization refers to recovery from the loss. During this gradual process the survivors again find meaning in living, readjust to life without the deceased, develop new or renewed relationships, and learn to live with the memory of the deceased with much less pain. This never means that the loved one is forgotten and the pain is gone. There always remains a deep ache that is never totally replaced with happiness and one that returns more intensely, for example, on holidays or anniversaries.

BEREAVEMENT PROGRAMS

Part of the difficulty in helping the bereaved family is lack of opportunity for follow-up in the traditional health care system. Consequently, many families never receive the support and guidance that could help them in their grief work. At a minimum, one follow-up phone call or meeting with the family is arranged, possibly 1 month after the child's death, to give the family time to overcome the phase of shock and disbelief. Families can also be referred to self-help groups, such as the Compassionate Friends,* an international

---

*PO Box 3696, Oak Brook, IL 60522-3696; 630-990-0010, 877-969-0010; fax: 630-990-0246; www.compassionatefriends.org.

organization for bereaved families, parents, and siblings. When such groups are not available, nurses can be instrumental in helping families network or facilitating parent and sibling groups.

A formal bereavement program or bereavement counseling may help family members to work through their grief. Comprehensive bereavement programs begin at the time of the child's death and continue for as long as the family desires. The purpose of a bereavement program is to assist and support families in the process of coping with the devastating impact of the loss of a child and hopefully with grief resolution. The components of such a program include initial contact and support by knowledgeable staff, information and reading materials relevant to the grief process, follow-up contacts by phone or mail, parent and sibling support groups, and referrals for counseling if indicated (Stewart, 1995). Give parents the option of participating in such a program, when available, but do not judge negatively the desire not to participate, since grief work is an individual process.

THE NURSE AND THE CHILD WITH LIFE-THREATENING ILLNESS

NURSES' REACTIONS TO CARING FOR CHILDREN WITH LIFE-THREATENING ILLNESSES

Nurses experience grief and moral distress as they become aware that a child's death is inevitable (Davies, Clarke, Connaughty, et al, 1996). Furthermore, nurses experience compassion fatigue as a result of cumulative losses over time as children they care for die. Reflection on these experiences and feelings, knowledge of the grief process, and care of oneself are essential for the nurse to provide effective care to dying children and their families (Maytum, Heiman, and Garwick, 2004).

Denial

When children are admitted to a pediatric unit with a suspected diagnosis of a serious illness, the initial response from some nurses is shock and denial. However, their behavioral reaction may be withdrawal from the child and family. They choose the "cure" philosophy over the "care" philosophy as a method of distancing themselves from the implications of emotional involvement. Because of their own dependency on denial, some nurses may inappropriately support denial in parents. There are several methods of conveying this message, such as emphasizing only optimistic "survival statistics," negating the seriousness of the illness, focusing on "cheering up" the family, and engaging in casual conversation to avoid meaningful dialogue. Although this increases nurses' comfort in caring for the dying child, it does little to help family members progress beyond denial and begin anticipatory grieving.

Some denial is as important for nurses as it is for the child or parents. It protects nurses from the overwhelming reality of death. It would be extremely difficult to participate in the treatment plan without some expectation of a cure. Denial is also necessary to prevent feelings of failure. In general, nursing and medical goals emphasize curing illness and saving lives, not allowing patients to die. However, denial loses its beneficial functions when nurses refuse to admit the failure of treatment efforts and insist on adhering to the "curing" regimen, regardless of its effectiveness or value. Failure of treatment is not to be equated with personal failure or failure to provide optimum nursing care.

Anger and Depression

Some nurses may be angry for having been assigned to the "leukemia case," for example, because the very exposure to potential failure in a fatal illness is extremely threatening. Others may feel angry for having to subject the child to painful procedures or for being unable to relieve the child's physical and emotional suffering. Instead of anger, some nurses may feel depression for any of these reasons.

Without understanding the reason for the emotion, however, nurses may project the anger onto others, particularly family members. They may be unable to tolerate the child's uncooperative behavior or the parents' continual requests for information. Anger fuels more anger, and parents react with hostility and think the members of the nursing staff are rejecting them. A vicious circle of resentment, mistrust, and frustration may result.

Depression also has adverse effects on the therapeutic relationship, since nurses may withdraw from the child and parents as a method of controlling their sadness. Unaware of the reason for the avoidance, family members interpret it as evidence of inadequate care. This reaction also fosters a nonsupportive cycle of avoidance, withdrawal, resentment, and frustration. However, the messages are usually more covert than when the nurses' reaction is anger and may prevent a climax that could result in a solution to the problem.

Guilt

Nurses who feel unable to deal with fatal illness in a child often experience guilt. Nurses who become angry or depressed when caring for a dying child often reveal that they are uncomfortable with this response but are unable to choose a more direct and constructive approach. They express guilt for having been intolerant of the child's or parents' behaviors and, even more important, realize the missed opportunity to provide these individuals with professional support and guidance.

The one important difference between a dying child and an ill child is that there may be no second chance to meet the needs of the dying child. This finality is difficult to comprehend but can lead to a better understanding of one's own responses to dying. For example, when guilt makes an individual uncomfortable enough to seek alternate behavior patterns, there is an opportunity for change, provided the individual is given some assistance and support.

Ambivalence

One of the most universal reactions of nurses is ambivalence in their feelings toward a dying child. There is the fluctuating adherence to hope for a cure and fear of a relapse.

Sometimes the motivations for both are more for personal needs. For example, the nurse may hope that the child recovers to avoid readmissions. Or the nurse may wish for a remission so that discharge is ensured. Such thoughts are certainly understandable in light of the emotional toll of nursing a dying child.

Ambivalence may be demonstrated in a particular type of bargaining. Rather than bargaining for extra time, nurses may hope that their colleagues are assigned to the patient or that a death may occur on a shift other than their own. Bargaining for a temporary absence from the dying child is a healthy response, because it demonstrates nurses' awareness of their own emotional limits. Nurses who are unable to recognize their personal emotional limits are in danger of seeking to have the professional relationship meet their needs for gratification, achievement, and fulfillment. This results in the loss of an objective evaluation of therapeutic interventions and the increased potential for subjective overinvolvement with the family.

COPING WITH STRESS

Pediatric critical care and oncology nurses surveyed about work stresses rank patient death as their most stressful yet one of their most rewarding experiences (Bond, 1994; Kushnir, Rabin, and Azulai, 1997; Olson, Hinds, Euell, et al, 1998). The less experienced the nurse, the more likely that death is rated as a stressor. Furthermore, nurses overestimated the percentage of deaths on their units, which suggests that the experience overwhelms them.

One stress-related outcome of caring for dying children is **burnout**—a state of physical, emotional, and mental exhaustion. It occurs as a result of prolonged involvement with individuals in situations that are emotionally demanding. Nurses working in intensive care units are particularly prone to this occupational hazard, but staff nurses also can experience it when dealing with certain groups of children, such as those who may die. Avoiding burnout and coping constructively, effectively, and therapeutically with children who are dying and their families requires a deliberate and concerted effort on the part of the nurse.

Self-Awareness

The initial step in effectively caring for a dying child is making a deliberate choice to become involved. Many nurses react negatively to the word *involvement* because they believe that professionals must remain uninvolved to maintain objectivity. Involvement does not displace objectivity. On the contrary, allowing oneself to feel with the other person expands one's ability to comprehend the meaning and depth of their emotion (see Family-Centered Care box). Ideally the nurse achieves detached concern, which allows sensitive, understanding care because the nurse is sufficiently detached to make objective, rational decisions.

Knowledge and Practice

Intervening therapeutically with terminally ill children and their families demands more than self-awareness. It also requires

---

FAMILY-CENTERED CARE

A Dying Child: A Nurse's Perspective

Claire was unresponsive with slow, gasping breathing. Her mother asked me what I thought was happening. I replied honestly, "Your baby is dying because of her brain tumor." The mother put her arms around me and cried. We arranged for Claire to be baptized.

Honesty. Painful as the loss of a child is, my job is to assist the family through this experience. Although I usually wait until a private moment, such as driving home, I found tears streaming down my face as family and friends gathered for Claire's baptism. I went into the kitchen to compose myself, only to find several of my colleagues crying as well. Saying good-bye to a dying child will always be a difficult but shared experience.

Jeanne O'Connor Egan, RN, MSN
Pediatric Clinical Specialist
Children's Hospital
Washington, DC

---

that nursing practice be based on sound theoretic formulations and empirical observations that provide a general, concise analysis of the typical reactions of families.

Involvement does carry the potential risk of clouding objectivity, but awareness of one's reactions and investments in the care of a dying child minimizes this hazard. Developing awareness requires the willingness to investigate one's motivations for choosing to work in such an area, to understand the stresses inherent in the role, to review one's resolution of past losses, and to contemplate one's own fears of death. Often nurses who have a cold, impersonal reaction to dying patients come to realize that their reaction stems from previous unresolved conflicts or losses. Once they are able to talk about such experiences, they are usually able to gain insight into their behavior and begin to develop alternative methods of reacting.

Nurses also must explore ethical issues surrounding the definition of death, the use of extraordinary and lifesaving measures versus allowing the child to die, and patients' rights to know and choose their own destinies. Once nurses have soundly formulated the principles by which to practice, they need opportunities for decision making. When a team approach is used, nurses can be valuable members of the group if their own values have been clarified and they have critically assessed the family's responses. (See Ethical Decision Making, Chapter 1.)

Support Systems

Support systems are essential to continued functioning in a high-stress environment. They allow nurses to regenerate energies by sharing feelings and concerns with others. Dealing with feelings about death in isolation can lead to repressed feelings such as denial, anger, and depression. These feelings may be manifested in poor interactions among staff, inappropriate or nonsupportive interactions with families, an inability to evaluate care plans or advocate for families, and a need to control (Hammer, Nichols, and Armstrong, 1992). Support is an important catalyst for processing feelings about death.

Social supports may be personal family members such as parents or spouses, extended relatives, and friends. Professional supports include colleagues, consultants, teachers, and supervisors. Peers may be sources of technical and practical advice. Because the death of a patient is more stressful for a less-experienced nurse, a mentoring relationship between a senior nurse and the less-experienced nurse may provide support and role modeling and assist in the development of effective coping strategies (Gardner, 1999). Forums for staff support and opportunities for debriefing after deaths have been shown to facilitate adaptive coping responses and enhance provider-patient relationship (Contro, Larson, Scofield, et al, 2004).

Other Strategies

Any number of other strategies may be used to reduce stress. These include maintaining good general health practices, especially regular exercise, and participating in diversionary activities that are of personal interest beyond the workplace. Distancing techniques are also effective, such as leaving work at work, informing other staff not to contact one on one's days off, periodically assuming less demanding assignments, and taking time off when needed. Mindfulness-based meditation may be another effective strategy to decrease stress and regain a sense of control among nurses experiencing compassion fatigue and burnout (Davies, 2008).

A final technique is to focus on the positive aspects of the caregiving role. Despite the difficult times in caring for these children and families, many rewarding experiences must be remembered. Dedicated efforts reap numerous rewards, and these must not be forgotten or minimized. Reflection on positive feedback from appreciative families can revitalize self-esteem and job satisfaction.

Some nurses find shared remembrance rituals useful in resolving grief. Similarly, attending the funeral services can be a supportive act for both the family and the nurse and in no way detracts from the professionalism of care. For the family it conveys a sense of worth and caring by the nurse. For the nurse it can provide a sense of closure with the family and facilitate the grief process (Box 23-11).

BOX 23-11 NURSES EXPERIENCING THE STRESS OF CAREGIVING: STRATEGIES THAT HELP

Recognize the inevitability of the child's death—One's own unrealistic expectations can cause the greatest grief due to the belief that something more should or could have been done to prevent the child's death. Shift the focus of care to providing guidance and comfort for the child and family to increase a sense of accomplishment. Avoid self-blame for situations over which you have no control.

Develop knowledge and apply it—Increase personal knowledge about caring for dying children and their families. Apply this knowledge to provide the best possible care to the patient and family.

Identify ways the work setting can provide support—Ask for relief from highly emotional or conflicted situations, take time off and vacation, seek mentorship, make use of institutional support services such as multidisciplinary team meetings or employee assistance personnel.

Provide briefings—Inform others involved in the child's care about the child's condition and changes as they occur. After the death, notify caregivers who were closely involved to allow them the opportunity to grieve for the child.

Provide debriefings—Organize staff remembrance services to share experiences and feelings, "bereavement" rounds, multidisciplinary team review of care.

Find meaning—Accept that even the death of a child is a part of life and find meaning in the caregiving experience with the child and family. Reflect on the experience, what it meant, how it influenced your view on nursing care.

Separate work and personal life—Develop strategies to leave work behind when at home with family. Avoid trips to the hospital on off days.

Take care of yourself—Recognize the stress of caring for dying children and find healthy activities to help manage that stress. Exercise, good nutrition, and rest are important when work stress is high.

Say good-bye—Identify comfortable ways to say good-bye to the dead child. Attending memorial or funeral services, keeping a memento, journaling, making plantings, and so on are all individual ways to acknowledge the importance of the child to the caregiver.

Modified from Brown-Hellsten M, Hockenberry-Eaton M, Lamb D, et al: *End of life care for children*, Austin, 1999, Texas Cancer Council.

KEY POINTS

- A family-centered approach to care of the child and family facing life-threatening illness or death respects the central role of the family and emphasizes communication, collaboration, and cultural sensitivity.

- There are common phases of family reactions to a life-threatening illness such as cancer. These phases correspond to the progression of the disease and the status of treatment.

- Special decisions at the time of dying and death may involve hospital or hospice care, the child's right to die and DNR orders, viewing of the body, organ and tissue donation, autopsy, and siblings' attendance at the funeral.

- Special needs of the family facing the unexpected death of a child include support while awaiting news of the child's status; a sensitive pronouncement of death; acknowledgment of feelings of denial, guilt, and anger; an opportunity to view the body; closure; and referrals for support.

- To counsel families and children regarding death, nurses need to understand children's perceptions of death, the fears in each age-group, and personal meanings of death and bereavement during developmental stages.

- Toddlers' egocentricity and vague separation of fact from fantasy make death incomprehensible; they may still refer to a dead person as though the person exists.

- Because of their sense of precausality and self-power, preschoolers may believe that their thoughts actually cause another person's death.

- With their reasoning power and fear of the unknown, school-age children may feel intense guilt and responsibility for someone's death.

- Adolescents have difficulty accepting death because of their preoccupation with developing a sense of identity.

- Nurses may offer the following assistance in education about death: counseling parents about children's age-specific understanding of death, encouraging parents to help children become familiar and comfortable with loss, taking part in organized death education in schools, and serving as a resource to answer families' and children's questions.

- What children are told about their serious illness is the family's decision and can be based on several general principles regarding developmental age, previous knowledge, and honesty.
- Siblings have special needs, including the need for information, reassurance about their own health status, assurance that they are not responsible for the illness or death, and support for their own grieving process.
- Acute grief is a syndrome with psychologic and somatic symptomatology that may appear after the crisis or may be

delayed, exaggerated, or apparently absent. "Distorted" reactions may represent one aspect of the syndrome and can be transformed into normal grief work.

- Mourning, or grief work, consists of four phases that do not necessarily proceed in sequence and may recur at any time: shock and disbelief, expression of grief, disorganization and despair, and reorganization.
- Formal bereavement programs may assist families in coping with the loss of a child and in the process of grief resolution.
- In dealing with stress related to the dying patient, the nurse can cope successfully through self-awareness, knowledge and practice, available support systems, maintenance of general good health, and focus on the positive rewards of involvement with dying children and their families.

ANSWERS TO CRITICAL THINKING EXERCISE

Preschool Siblings and Death

1. Any of the described reactions of a preschool child may be normal responses to the death of a sibling and reflect correct assumptions related to the concept of death in children of different ages.
2. **a.** Young children may feel guilty and responsible for a sibling's death or may interpret illness or injury as a punishment for their thoughts about the sibling (response 1).
   b. Regression to earlier behaviors is common, and separation from parents is a particular concern (response 2). Preschoolers are not as likely as toddlers to think that a person who has died is still alive, but they may deny the

loss for a time (response 3). After a significant loss, a young child may express more outward grief at small losses because of their weaker defense mechanisms (response 4).

3. Siblings may feel isolated and displaced after a brother or sister has died. Priorities include ensuring that parents do not forget the siblings during their grieving process. Support that allows the parents to grieve and at the same time provide comfort to their other children is essential.
4. **Yes.** The developmental stage and level of maturity of the siblings has a strong influence on the feelings and behaviors exhibited after the death of a sibling.

REFERENCES

American Academy of Pediatrics, Committee on Bioethics and Committee on Hospital Care: Palliative care of children, *Pediatrics* 106(2):351-357, 2000.

American Nurses Association: *Code of ethics for nurses with interpretive statements*, 2005, American Nurses Publishing, available at http://nursingword.org/ethics/code/protected_nwcoe813.htm#1.1 (accessed April 18, 2009).

Auvrignon A, Leverger G, Lasfargues G: How to discuss death with a dying child: can a story help? (abstract), *Bull Acad Natl Med* 192(2):393-400, 2008.

Bellali T, Papadatou D: The decision-making process of parents regarding organ donation of their brain dead child: a Greek study, *Soc Sci Med* 64(2):439-450, 2007.

Bluebond-Langner M: Worlds of dying children and their well siblings, *Death Stud* 13:1-16, 1989.

Bluebond-Langner M: *The private words of dying children*, Princeton, NJ, 1978, Princeton University Press.

Bond DC: The measured intensity of work-related stressors in pediatric oncology nursing, *J Pediatr Oncol Nurs* 11(2):44-52, 1994.

Bowden VR, Conway-Orgel M, Dulzack S, et al: Precepts of palliative care for children, adolescents and their families, *Last Acts*, October 2003, available at www.apon.org/

files/public/last_acts_precepts.pdf (accessed March 9, 2006).

Buckalow PG, Esposito CM: The role of the home health nurse in sudden infant death syndrome, *Home Health Care Pract* 7(3):36-45, 1995.

Bull A, Gillies M: Spiritual needs of children with complex healthcare needs in hospital, *Pediatr Nurs* 19(9):34-38, 2007.

Calabrese CL: ACT: for pediatric palliative care, *Pediatr Nurs* 33(6):532-534, 2007.

Carter BS: Providing palliative care for newborns, *Pediatr Ann* 33(11):770-777, 2004.

Contro NA, Larson J, Scofield S, et al: Hospital staff and family perspectives regarding quality of pediatric palliative care, *Pediatrics* 114(5):1248-1252, 2004.

Davies B, Clarke D, Connaughty S, et al: Caring for dying children: nurses' experiences, *Pediatr Nurs* 22(6):500-507, 1996.

Davies B, Sehring SA, Partridge JC, et al: Barriers to palliative care for children: perceptions of pediatric health care providers, *Pediatrics* 121(2):282-288, 2008

Davies R: New understandings of parental grief: literature review, *J Adv Nurs* 46(5):506-513, 2004.

Davies WR: Mindful meditation: healing burnout in critical care nursing, *Holist Nurs Pract* 22(1):32-36, 2008.

Davis B, Eng B: Special issues in bereavement and staff support. In Doyle D, Hanks GWC, MacDonald N, editors: *Oxford textbook of palliative medicine*, ed 2, New York, 1998, Oxford University Press.

De Lisle-Porter M, Podruchny AM: The dying neonate: family-centered end-of-life care, *Neonatal Netw* 28(2):75-83, 2009.

Dent A, Condon L, Blair P, et al: A study of bereavement care after a sudden and unexpected death, *Arch Dis Child* 74(6):522-526, 1996.

Dussell V, Kreicbergs U, Hilden JM, et al: Looking beyond where children die: determinants and effects of planning a child's location of death, *J Pain Symptom Manage* 37(1):33-43, 2008.

Dyregrov K: Bereaved parents' experience of research participation, *Soc Sci Med* 58(2):391-400, 2004.

Ethier AM: Care of the dying child and the family. In Tomlinson D, Kline N, editors: *Pediatric oncology nursing: advanced clinical handbook*, ed 2, New York, 2008, Springer-Verlag.

Ethier AM: Death-related sensory experiences, *J Pediatr Oncol Nurs* 22(2):104-111, 2005.

Evanisko MJ, Beasley CL, Brigham LE, et al: Readiness of critical care physicians and nurses to handle requests for organ donation, *Am J Crit Care* 7(1):4-12, 1998.

Faulkner KW, Armstrong-Dailey A: Care of the dying child. In Pizzo PA, Poplack DG, editors: *Principles and practice of pediatric oncology,* ed 3, Philadelphia/New York, 1997, Lippincott-Raven.

Ferrell BR: The impact of pain on quality of life: a decade of research, *Nurs Clin North Am* 30(4):609-624, 1995.

Ferrell BR, Coyle N: An overview of palliative nursing care, *Lippincotts Case Manag* 7(4):163-168, 2002.

Feudtner C, Christakis DA, Zimmerman FJ, et al: Characteristics of deaths occurring in children's hospitals: implications for supportive care services, *Pediatrics* 109(5):887-893, 2002.

Feudtner C, Haney J, Dimmers MA: Spiritual care needs of hospitalized children and their families: a national survey of pastoral care providers' perceptions, *Pediatrics* 111:e67-e72, 2003, available at http://pediatrics. aappublications.org/cgi/reprint/111/1/e67?ma xtoshow=&HITS=10&hits=10&RESULTFOR MAT=&fulltext=spiritual+care&searchid=1&F IRSTINDEX=0&sortspec=relevance&resourcet ype=HWCIT (accessed April 18, 2009).

Feudtner C, Silveira MJ, Christakis DA: Where do children with complex chronic conditions die? Patterns in Washington State, 1980-1998, *Pediatrics* 109(4):656-660, 2002.

Field MJ, Behrman RE, editors: *When children die: improving palliative and end-of-life care for children and their families,* Washington, DC, 2004, National Academies Press.

Fleischman AR: Commentary: ethical issues in pediatric pain management and terminal sedation, *J Pain Symptom Manage* 15(4):260-261, 1998.

Foley GV: Conflicts in practice: the argument, *J Assoc Pediatr Oncol Nurses* 2(3):22-24, 1985.

Franz HG, DeJong W, Wolfe SM, et al: Explaining brain death: a critical feature of the donation process, *J Transpl Coord* 7(1):14-21, 1997.

Gardner JM: Perinatal death: uncovering the needs of midwives and nurses and exploring helpful interventions in the United States, England, and Japan, *J Transcult Nurs* 10(2):120-130, 1999.

Giovanola J: Sibling involvement at the end of life, *J Pediatr Oncol Nurs* 22(4):222-226, 2005.

Goodenough B, Drew D, Higgins S, et al: Bereavement outcomes for parents who lose a child to cancer: are place of death and sex of parent associated with differences in psychological functioning? *Psychooncology* 13(11):779-791, 2004.

Hammer M, Nichols DJ, Armstrong L: A ritual of remembrance, *MCN Am J Matern Child Nurs* 17(6):310-313, 1992.

Hazinski MF, Markenson D, Neish S, et al: Response to cardiac arrest and selected life-threatening medical emergencies: the medical emergency response plan for schools: a statement for healthcare providers, policymakers, school administrators, and community leaders, *Pediatrics* 113(1):155-168, 2004.

Heilferty CM: Spiritual development and the dying child: the pediatric nurse practitioner's role, *J Pediatr Health Care* 18:271-275, 2004.

Hendricks-Ferguson V: Physical symptoms of children receiving pediatric hospice care at home during the last week of life. *Oncol Nurs Forum* 35(6):E108-E115, 2008.

Heron M, Sutton PD, Xu J, et al: Annual summary of vital statistics, *Pediatrics* 125(1):4-15, 2010.

Higgins SS, Kayser-Jones J: Factors influencing parent decision making about pediatric cardiac transplantation, *J Pediatr Nurs* 11(3):152-160, 1996.

Hilden JM, Emanuel EJ, Fairclough DL, et al: Attitudes and practices among pediatric oncologists regarding end-of-life care: results of the 1998 American Society of Clinical Oncology Survey, *J Clin Oncol* 19(1):205-212, 2001.

Himelstein BP, Hilden JM, Boldt AM, et al: Pediatric palliative care, *N Engl J Med* 350:1752-1762, 2004.

Hinds PS, Oakes L, Furman W, et al: End-of-life decision making by adolescents, parents, and healthcare providers in pediatric oncology: research to evidence-based practice guidelines, *Cancer Nurs* 24(2):122-134, 2001.

Hinds PS, Oakes L, Furman W, et al: Decision making by parents and healthcare professionals when considering continued care for pediatric patients with cancer, *Oncol Nurs Forum* 24(9):1523-1528, 1997.

Hockley J: Psychosocial aspects in palliative care: communicating with the patient and family, *Acta Oncol* 39(8):905-910, 2000.

Horowitz MJ, Siegel B, Holen A, et al: Diagnostic criteria for complicated grief disorder, *Am J Psychiatry* 154(7):904-910, 1997.

Hubble RA, Ward-Smith P, Christenson K, et al: Implementation of a palliative care team in a pediatric hospital, *J Pediatr Health Care* 23(2):126-131, 2008.

James L, Johnson B: The needs of parents of pediatric oncology patients during palliative care phase, *J Pediatr Oncol Nurs* 14(2):83-95, 1997.

Jennings PD: Providing pediatric palliative care through a pediatric supportive care team, *Pediatr Nurs* 31(3):195-200, 2005.

Johnston DL, Nagel K, Friedman DL, et al: Availability and use of palliative care and end-of-life services for pediatric oncology patients, *J Clin Oncol* 26(28):4646-4650, 2008.

Kagawa-Singer M: The cultural context of death rituals and mourning practices, *Oncol Nurs Forum* 25(20):1752-1756, 1998.

Keesee NJ, Currier JM, Neimeyer RA: Predictors of grief following the death of one's child: the contribution of finding meaning, *J Clin Psychol* 64(10):1145-1163, 2008.

Kirwin KM, Hamrin V: Decreasing the risk of complicated bereavement and future psychiatric disorders in children, *J Child Adolesc Psychiatr Nurs* 18(2):62-78, 2005.

Klass D: The inner representation of the dead child in the psychic and social narratives of bereaved parents. In Neimeyer RA, editor: *Meaning reconstruction and the experience of loss,* Washington, DC, 2001, American Psychological Association.

Knapp C, Huang I, Madden V, et al: An evaluation of two decision-making scales for children with life-limiting illnesses (abstract), *Palliat Med* 23(6): 518-525, 2009.

Knapp CA, Shenkman EA, Marcu MI, et al: Pediatric palliative care: describing hospice users and identifying factors that affect hospice expenditures (abstract), *J Palliat Med* 12(3):223-229, 2009.

Kuntz B: Exploring the grief of adolescents after death of a parent, *J Child Adolesc Psychiatr Ment Health Nurs* 4(3):105-109, 1991.

Kushnir T, Rabin S, Azulai S: A descriptive study of stress management in a group of pediatric oncology nurses, *Cancer Nurs* 20(6):414-421, 1997.

Lambert S: Distraction, imagery, and hypnosis techniques for management of children's pain, *J Child Fam Nurs* 2(1):5-15, 1999.

Lauer ME, Mulhern RK, Bohne JB, et al: Children's perceptions of their sibling's death at home or hospital: the precursors of differential adjustment, *Cancer Nurs* 8(1):21-27, 1985.

Lauer ME, Mulhern RK, Schell MJ, et al: Long-term follow-up of parental adjustment following a child's death at home or hospital, *Cancer* 63(5):988-994, 1989.

Lee CL, Johann-Liang R: Disclosure of the diagnosis of HIV/AIDS to children born of HIV-infected mothers, *AIDS Patient Care* 13(1):41-45, 1999.

Leikin S: A proposal concerning decisions to forego life-sustaining treatment for young people, *J Pediatr* 115(1):17-22, 1989.

Martinson IM: Improving care of dying children, *West J Med* 163:258-262, 1995.

Martinson IM: Hospice care for children: past, present, and future, *J Pediatr Oncol Nurs* 10(3):93-98, 1993.

Masera G, Spinetta JJ, Jankovic M, et al: Guidelines for assistance to terminally ill children with cancer: a report of the SIOP working committee on psychosocial issues in pediatric oncology, *Med Pediatr Oncol* 32:44-48, 1999.

Masri C, Farrell CA, Lacroix J, et al: Decision making and end-of-life care in critically ill children, *J Palliat Care* 16(Suppl):S45-S52, 2000.

Maytum JC, Heiman MB, Garwick AW: Compassion fatigue and burnout in nurses who work with children with chronic conditions and their families, *J Pediatr Health Care* 18(4):171-179, 2004.

McCulloch R, Collins JJ: Pain in children who have life-limiting conditions, *Child Adolesc Psychiatr Clin North Am* 15(3):657-682, 2006.

Michael S, Lansdown R: Adjustment to the death of a sibling, *Arch Dis Child* 61:278-283, 1986.

Murray JS: Siblings of children with cancer: a review of the literature, *J Pediatr Oncol Nurs* 16(1):25-34, 1999.

Nagy M: The child's view of death, *J Genet Psychol* 73:3-27, 1948.

National Cancer Institute: Spirituality in cancer care, 2009, National Cancer Institute, available at www.cancer.gov/cancertopics/ pdq/supportivecare/spirituality/ HealthProfessional (accessed May 2, 2009).

National Hospice and Palliative Care Organization, Children's International Project on Palliative/Hospice Services: *Compendium of pediatric palliative care,* Alexandria, Va, 2000, The Organization.

Nitschke R, Humphrey GB, Sexauer CL, et al: Therapeutic choices made by patients with end-stage cancer, *J Pediatr* 101(3):471-476, 1982.

Nolbris M, Hellstrom AL: Siblings' needs and issues when a brother or sister dies of cancer, *J Pediatr Oncol Nurs* 22(4):227-233, 2005.

Oliver RC, Fallat ME: Traumatic childhood death: how well do parents cope? *J Trauma* 39(2):303-307, 1995.

Olson MS, Hinds PS, Euell K, et al: Peak and nadir experiences and their consequences described by pediatric oncology nurses, *J Pediatr Oncol Nurs* 15(1):13-24, 1998.

Palfrey JS, Tonniges TF, Green M, et al: Introduction: addressing the millennial morbidity—the context of community pediatrics, *Pediatrics* 115(4):1121-1123, 2005.

Pearson LJ: The child who is dying. In Rollins JA, Bolig R, Mahan CC, editors: *Meeting children's psychosocial needs across the heath-care continuum,* Austin, 2005, Pro-Ed.

Pierucci RL, Kirby RS, Leuthner SR: End-of-life for neonates and infants: the experience and effects of a palliative care consultation service, *Pediatrics* 108(3):653-660, 2001.

Pritchard M, Burghen E, Srivastava DK, et al: Cancer-related symptoms most concerning to parents during the last week and day of their child's life, *Pediatrics* 121(5):e1301-e1309, 2008.

Pyke-Grimm KA, Degner L, Small A, et al: Preferences for participation in treatment decision making and information needs of parents of children with cancer: a pilot study, *J Pediatr Oncol Nurs* 16:13-24, 1999.

Rando TA: *Treatment of complicated mourning,* Champaign, Ill, 1993, Research Press.

Rando TA, editor: *Parental loss of a child,* Champaign, Ill, 1986, Research Press.

Rando TA: An investigation of grief and adaptation in parents whose children have died from cancer, *J Pediatr Psychol* 8(1):3-20, 1983.

Randolph AG, Zollo MB, Egger MJ, et al: Variability in physician opinion on limiting pediatric life support, *Pediatrics* 103:e46, 1999.

Riley J, Ross JR, Gretton SK, et al: Proposed five-step World Health Organization analgesic

and side effect ladder, *Eur J Pain* (Suppl S): 23-30, 2007.

Robinson MR, Thiel MM, Backus MM, et al: Matters of spirituality at the end of life in the pediatric intensive care unit, *Pediatrics* 118:e719-e729, 2006.

Rollins JA, Riccio LL: ART is the heART: a palette of possibilities for hospice care, *Pediatr Nurs* 28(4):355-362, 2002.

Russell C, Smart S: Guided imagery and distraction therapy in paediatric hospice care, *Paediatr Nurs* 19(2):24-25, 2007.

Savage TA: Ethical decision making for children, *Crit Care Nurs Clin North Am* 9(1):97-105, 1997.

Schoen AA, Burgoyne M, Schoen SF: Are the developmental needs of children in America adequately addressed during the grief process? *J Instructional Psych* 31(2):143-148, 2004.

Seecharan GA, Andresen EM, Norris K, et al: Parents' assessment of quality of care and grief following a child's death, *Arch Pediatr Adolesc Med* 158(6):515-520, 2004.

Sharman M, Meert KL, Sarnaik AP: What influences parents' decisions to limit or withdraw life support? *Pediatr Crit Care Med* 6(5):513-518, 2005.

Shumway CN, Grossman LS, Sarles RM: Therapeutic choices by children with cancer (letter), *J Pediatr* 103(1):168, 1983.

Siever BA: Pain management and potentially life-shortening analgesia in the terminally ill child: the ethical implications for pediatric nurses, *J Pediatr Nurs* 9(5):307-312, 1994.

Silverman PR: Research, clinical practice, and the human experience: putting the pieces together, *Death Stud* 24(6):469-478, 2000.

Sine D, Sumner L, Gracy D, et al: Pediatric extubation: "pulling the tube," *J Palliat Med* 4(4):519-524, 2001.

Slaughter V: Young children's understanding of death, *Austral Psychol* 40(3):1-8, 2005.

Speece MW, Brent SB: The development of children's understanding of death. In Corr CA, Corr DM, editors: *Handbook of childhood death and bereavement,* New York, 1996, Springer.

Spinetta JJ: The dying child's awareness of death: a review, *Pscyhol Bull* 81(4):256-260, 1974.

Stanfill P, Strong C: Conflicts in practice: the argument against, *J Assoc Pediatr Oncol Nurs* 2(3):25-26, 1985.

Stevens MM: Care of the dying child and adolescent: family adjustment and support. In Doyle D, Hanks GWC, MacDonald N, editors: *Oxford textbook of palliative medicine,* ed 2, New York, 1998, Oxford University Press.

Stewart ES: Family-centered care for the bereaved, *Pediatr Nurs* 21(2):181-184, 1995.

Thompson LA, Knapp C, Madden V, et al: Pediatricians' perceptions of preferred timing for pediatric palliative care, *Pediatrics* 123:e777-e782, 2009.

Wolfe J, Grier HE, Klar N, et al: Symptoms and suffering at the end of life in children with cancer, *N Engl J Med* 342(5):326-333, 2000.

Wolfe J, Hammel JF, Edwards KE, et al: Easing suffering in children with cancer at the end of life: is care changing? *J Clin Oncol* 26(10):1717-1723, 2008.

Wolfe J, Klar N, Grier HE, et al: Understanding of prognosis among parents of children who died of cancer: impact on treatment goals and integration of palliative care, *JAMA* 284(19):2469-2475, 2000.

World Health Organization: *Cancer pain relief and palliative care,* Geneva, 1998a, The Organization.

World Health Organization, with International Association for the Study of Pain: Cancer pain relief and palliative care in children, Order No. 11500459, Geneva, 1998b, The Organization.

World Health Organization: *WHO definition of palliative care,* 1998c, available at www.who. int/cancer/palliative/definition/en (accessed August 24, 2008).

Zerwekh JV: Do dying patients really need IV fluids? *Am J Nurs* 3:26-30, 1997.

Zhukovsky DS, Herzog CE, Kaur G, et al: The impact of palliative care consultation on symptom assessment, communication needs, and palliative interventions in pediatric patients with cancer, *J Palliat Med* 12(4):343-349, 2009.

Zinner SE: The use of pediatric advance directives: a tool for palliative care physicians, *Am J Hosp Palliat Med* 25(6):427-430, 2009.

The Child with Cognitive, Sensory, or Communication Impairment

Rosalind Bryant

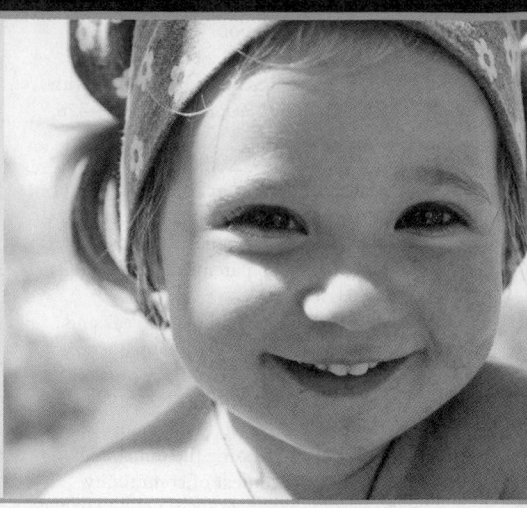

evolve WEBSITE

RELATED TOPICS

CHAPTER OUTLINE

COGNITIVE IMPAIRMENT

GENERAL CONCEPTS

Cognitive impairment (CI) is a general term that encompasses any type of intellectual disability. The term *intellectual disability* is increasingly being used instead of mental retardation (Schalock, Luckasson, Shogren, et al, 2007). In this chapter CI is used synonymously with *intellectual disability* and the out-

dated term *mental retardation*. Although the family's needs and concerns are a primary focus throughout the chapter, the reader should review Chapter 22, which details the family's adjustment to disabilities in general.

The definition of intellectual disability developed by the American Association on Intellectual and Developmental Disabilities (AAIDD), formally known as American Association on Mental Retardation, includes diagnostic criteria that place increased emphasis on the child's functional strengths and weaknesses and the environmental supports the child needs (Schalock, Luckasson, Shogren, et al, 2007; Wehmeyer, Buntinx, Lachapelle, et al, 2008). Classification using the AAIDD definition requires a description of intellectual functioning and functional strengths and weaknesses in a number of real-world adaptive skills; onset of the condition must be before 18 years of age. The child must manifest subaverage intellectual functioning, which in practical terms means an intelligence quotient (IQ) of 70 to 75 or below. In addition, the American Psychiatric Association's *Diagnostic and Statistical Manual of Mental Disorders*, fourth edition, text revision (DMS-IV-TR), which is the diagnostic standard, states that the child with CI (intellectual disability) must demonstrate functional impairment in at least two of the following adaptive skill domains: communication, self-care, home living, social skills, use of community resources, self-direction, health and safety, functional academics, leisure, and work (American Psychiatric Association, 2000).

The AAIDD definition of CI (intellectual disability) emphasizes abilities, environments, supports, and empowerment. The intensity of support required is classified as intermittent, limited, extensive, or pervasive. The underlying assumption is that when appropriate supports are given over a prolonged period, the ability of the person with CI to function each day will generally improve. For educational purposes, the mildly impaired group encompasses about 85% of all people with CI, and the children with moderate levels of CI account for about 10% of the intellectual disabled population (American Psychiatric Association, 2000; Johnson and Walker, 2006) (Table 24-1).

The central role of the family in caring for the child with CI cannot be overlooked. Principles of family-centered care are key. (See Chapters 6, 22, and 25.) Nurses are instrumental in helping to socialize families of children with CI toward a collaborative model of care, which is critical in efforts to teach these children functional skills.

Diagnosis

The diagnosis of CI is usually made after a period of suspicion by professionals or the family that the child's developmental progress is delayed. In some cases it is made at birth when distinct syndromes such as Down syndrome are recognized, or when severe to profound delays in development are apparent. At the other extreme, it may be made after the child begins school and does poorly. In all cases a high index of suspicion for developmental disability is necessary for early diagnosis, and routine developmental screening can assist in early identification. (See Chapter 6.) Delays occur most commonly in language and cognitive skills, although delays in fine and gross motor skills are also typical. **Developmental disability** can be described as any significant lag or delay in a child's physical, cognitive, behavioral, emotional, or social development, when compared against developmental norms. CI is an impairment encompassing intellectual ability and adaptive behavior that are functioning significantly below average.

Results of standardized tests are helpful in making the diagnosis of CI. The most commonly used test for infants is the Bayley Scales of Infant Development, although the Mullen Scales of Early Learning is also used for this population. (See also Chapter 6.) The Harris Infant Neuromotor Test (HINT) is another valid and reliable screening tool for identification of potential motor and cognitive developmental disorders in infants. A recent study suggested that the HINT norms developed from the data collected from Canadian infants may be applicable to U.S. infants (McCoy, Bowman, Smith-Blockley, et al, 2009). During the school years the Wechsler Intelligence

TABLE 24-1	CLASSIFICATION OF COGNITIVE IMPAIRMENT		
LEVEL—IQ	**PRESCHOOL (BIRTH–5 yr)— MATURATION AND DEVELOPMENT**	**SCHOOL AGE (6-21 yr)—TRAINING AND EDUCATION**	**ADULT (≥21 yr)—SOCIAL AND VOCATIONAL ADEQUACY**
Mild—50 to approximately 70-75	Often not noticed as delayed by casual observer but is slower to walk, feed self, and talk than most children; follows same developmental sequence as normal children	Can acquire practical skills and useful reading and arithmetic to a third to sixth grade level with special education; can be guided toward social conformity; achieves mental age of 8-12 yr	Can usually achieve social and vocational skills adequate for self-maintenance; may need occasional guidance and support when under unusual social or economic stress; can adjust to marriage but not childrearing
Moderate—36-49	Noticeable delays in motor development, especially in speech; responds to training in various self-help activities	Can learn simple communication, elementary health and safety habits, and simple manual skills; does not progress in functional reading or arithmetic; achieves mental age of 3-7 yr	Can perform simple tasks under sheltered conditions; participates in simple recreation; travels alone in familiar places; usually incapable of self-maintenance
Severe—20-35	Marked delay in motor development; little or no communication skills; may respond to training in elementary self-care (e.g., self-feeding)	Usually walks, barring specific disability; has some understanding of speech and some response; can profit from systematic habit training; achieves mental age of toddler	Can conform to daily routines and repetitive activities; needs continuing direction and supervision in protective environment
Profound—<20	Gross delay; minimum capacity for functioning in sensorimotor areas; needs total care	Obvious delays in all areas of development; shows basic emotional responses; may respond to skillful training in use of legs, hands, and jaws; needs close supervision; achieves mental age of young infant	May walk; needs complete custodial care; has primitive speech; usually benefits from regular physical activity

Data modified from American Psychiatric Association: *Diagnostic and statistical manual of mental disorders (DSM-IV-TR)*, ed 4, text rev, Washington, DC, 2000, The Association; and Rittey CD: Learning difficulties: what the neurologist needs to know, *J Neurol Neurosurg Psychiatry* 74(Suppl 1):30-36, 2005.
IQ, Intelligence quotient.

Scale for Children, fourth edition, is most often used. The Differential Ability Scales, Stanford-Binet Intelligence Scale, and Kaufman Assessment Battery for Children are additional tests that can be used from toddlerhood through school age. Specialized tests such as the Leiter International Performance Scale, revised edition, can be useful for assessing children who speak a different language, nonverbal children, or those with significant language or motor impairment. All of these tests are individually administered (never given as a group test) in a standardized manner under favorable conditions by specially trained clinicians, such as psychologists, psychometrists, or child development specialists. Tests for assessing adaptive behavior functioning include the Vineland Adaptive Behavior Scales and the AAMR Adaptive Behavior Scale. Informal appraisal of adaptive behavior may be made by those fully acquainted with the child (e.g., teachers, parents, or other care providers). Frequently these observations lead parents to seek a developmental evaluation.

When a family suspects a diagnosis of CI, it can be devastating. Nurses should take care to provide support from sensitive professionals at the time of diagnosis. (See Chapter 22.) Provide information to address any misconceptions and answer parental questions and concerns. Make referrals for counseling or additional information if appropriate or desired. Nurses can be an important resource as parents sort through an often confusing array of educational, health, and therapeutic services to determine how best to meet the needs of their child.

Etiology

The etiology of CI includes familial, social, environmental, organic, and unknown causes. Among individuals with severe CI, chromosomal disorders and prenatal toxin exposure are common, with Down syndrome, fragile X syndrome, and fetal alcohol syndrome accounting for a sizable proportion of cases. Other identifiable disorders or syndromes, such as severe cerebral palsy, microcephaly, or infantile spasms, are also associated with CI. Box 24-1 lists the prenatal, perinatal, and postnatal causes of CI.

Prevention

Currently there is much concern about prevention of CI. Primary prevention strategies—those designed to avoid conditions that cause CI—include avoidance of prenatal rubella infection; maintenance of current immunizations; genetic counseling, especially regarding risk of Down or fragile X syndrome; use of folic acid supplements during pregnancy to prevent neural tube defects; education regarding the dangers of smoking or ingesting alcohol during pregnancy and ingesting lead during childhood; adequate prenatal care and childhood nutrition; and reduction of head injuries. In the future, gene therapy for selected conditions will probably be a significant advance in preventing genetic disorders, such as phenylketonuria.

Secondary prevention activities—those designed to identify the condition early and initiate treatment to avert cerebral damage—include prenatal diagnosis or carrier detection of disorders such as Down syndrome and newborn screening for treatable inborn errors of metabolism, such as congenital hypothyroidism, phenylketonuria, and galactosemia.

BOX 24-1 CAUSES OF COGNITIVE IMPAIRMENT

Infections and intoxications—Any conditions associated with abnormalities or malformations, such as rubella, syphilis, toxoplasmosis, maternal drug consumption (including alcohol), exposure to smoking prenatally or to industrial chemicals, increased blood levels of lead, Rh incompatibility resulting in kernicterus, and maternal disorders such as eclampsia

Trauma or physical agents—Injury to brain suffered during prenatal, perinatal, or postnatal period, including physical injury, lack of oxygen, or exposure to radiation

Metabolic or nutritional abnormalities—Imbalances in fat, carbohydrates, and amino acids; inadequate nutrition; and metabolic or endocrine disorders, such as phenylketonuria or congenital hypothyroidism

Gross postnatal brain diseases—Diseases characterized by skin eruptions, lesions, and tumors, such as neurofibromatosis and tuberous sclerosis

Unknown prenatal conditions—Cerebral, spinal, and craniofacial malformations, such as microcephaly, hydrocephalus, meningomyelocele, and craniostenosis

Chromosomal abnormalities—Chromosomal aberrations resulting from radiation, virus infection, chemical exposure, parental age, and genetic mutations, such as Down syndrome and fragile X syndrome

Gestational disorders—Associated with prematurity, low birth weight, and postmaturity

Psychiatric disorders with onset during child's developmental period—For example, autism

Environmental influences—Deprived environment associated with a history of cognitive impairment among parents and siblings

---

Tertiary prevention strategies—those concerned with treatment to minimize long-term consequences—include early identification of conditions and provision of appropriate therapies and rehabilitation services. These include medical treatment of coexisting problems, such as hearing and visual impairment in Down syndrome, and programs for infant stimulation, parent training, preschool education, and counseling services to preserve the integration of the family unit.

NURSING CARE OF CHILDREN WITH COGNITIVE IMPAIRMENT

The goal of caring for children with CI is to promote their optimum social, physical, cognitive, and adaptive development as individuals within a family and community. General guidelines for coping with and adjusting to the child with special needs are in Chapter 22.

Nurses play a major role in identifying children with CI. In the newborn and early infancy period, few signs are present, except in various syndromes that have distinctive features, such as Down syndrome. Delayed developmental milestones are the major clues to CI. In addition, nurses must have a high index of suspicion for early signs suggestive of CI (Box 24-2). Take parental concerns, such as delayed development compared with siblings, seriously. All children should receive regular developmental assessment, and the nurse is often the person responsible for performing such assessments. (See Chapter 6.) When delays are found, the nurse must use sensitivity and discretion in revealing this finding to parents.

Nurses play a role in developing and implementing the individualized education plan for each child with special needs in the school system and the individualized family service plan

<table>
<tr><td>

BOX 24-2 EARLY SIGNS SUGGESTIVE OF COGNITIVE IMPAIRMENT

- Dysmorphic features (e.g., Down syndrome, microcephaly)
- Irritability or nonresponsiveness to contact
- Abnormal eye contact during feeding
- Gross motor delay
- Decreased alertness to voice or movement
- Language difficulties or delay
- Feeding difficulties

Modified from Shapiro B, Batshaw M: Mental retardation (intellectual disability). In Kliegman RM, Behrman RE, Jenson HB, editors: *Nelson textbook of pediatrics*, ed 18, Philadelphia, 2007, Saunders.

</td></tr>
</table>

designed for the family and child with special needs in an early intervention program (American Academy of Pediatrics, 2000) (see Community Focus box).

 COMMUNITY FOCUS

Key Terms to Know in Special Education and Early Intervention

ADA—Americans with Disabilities Act (Public Law [PL] 101-336) prohibits discrimination against individuals with disabilities. The act applies to adults and children and affects many businesses and services, including stores, hotels, public transportation terminals, parks, museums, employers, schools, and daycare centers.

IDEA—Individuals with Disabilities Education Act (PL 101-476) is based on the Education for All Handicapped Children Act (PL 94-142). Children enrolled in special education (criteria vary by state) may be eligible to receive special education and related services mandated by IDEA. Covered disabilities range widely and include severe visual and hearing impairments, speech impairment, cognitive impairment, emotional problems, learning disabilities, physical disabilities, and other health impairments.

IEP—Individualized education plan is required under IDEA. Based on a multidisciplinary evaluation and shared with parents, the IEP outlines special education and other related services to be received by the child with special needs. Related services can include transportation, developmental services (speech, audiology, physical therapy, occupational therapy), supportive services (psychologic services, social work), and medical services as required to assist the child in benefiting from special education. Provision of the educational services is initiated by a formal letter submitted by the medical provider.

IFSP—Individualized family service plan, called for in PL 99-457, is based on the IEP concept but has other components, including a developmental assessment, identification of family strengths, a plan for supporting the child's development, early intervention services to be provided for the child and the family, expected outcomes, a designated case manager, and a plan for transition to school services.

Education of the Handicapped Act Amendments of 1986 (PL 99-457) were passed to address the needs of young children with disabilities. Title I (Part H) asks states to coordinate early intervention services for children from birth through age 2 years 11 months. Title II extends the provisions of PL 94-142, a special education law, to children 3 to 5 years of age and notes that the services can be provided in the home or in other settings.

Copyright Elizabeth Ahmann, ScD, RN, and modified from Lambros KM, Leslie LK: Management of the child with a learning disorder, *Pediatr Ann* 34(4):278-279, 2005.

Standards of care have been developed for physicians and nurses working with persons with developmental disabilities or CI (Lambros and Leslie, 2005; Ranweiler, 2009) and also for nurses working in early intervention programs. Nursing organizations concerned with developmental disabilities are listed in Box 24-3.

<table>
<tr><td>

BOX 24-3 NURSING ORGANIZATIONS FOR DEVELOPMENTAL DISABILITIES

American Association on Intellectual and Developmental Disabilities (Nursing Division)
501 3rd St., NW, Suite 200
Washington, DC 20001
202-387-1968, 800-424-3688
Fax: 202-387-2193
www.aamr.org

Developmental Disabilities Nurses Association
PO Box 536489
Orlando, FL 32853-6489
407-835-0642, 800-888-6733
Fax: 407-426-7440
www.ddna.org

</td></tr>
</table>

Educate the Child and Family

To teach children with CI, one must investigate their learning abilities and deficits. This is important for the nurse who may be involved in a home care type of program or who may be caring for the child in a school or health care setting. The nurse who understands how these children learn can effectively teach them basic skills or prepare them for various health-related procedures.

Children with CI have a marked deficit in their ability to discriminate between two or more stimuli because of difficulty in recognizing the relevance of specific cues. However, these children can learn to discriminate if the cues are presented in an exaggerated, concrete form and if all extraneous stimuli are eliminated. For example, the use of colors to emphasize visual cues or the use of singing or rhymes to stress auditory cues can help them learn. Their deficit in discrimination also implies that concrete ideas are much easier to learn effectively than abstract ideas. Therefore demonstration is preferable to verbal explanation, and the nurse should direct learning toward mastering a skill rather than understanding the scientific principles underlying a procedure.

Another cognitive deficit is in short-term memory. Whereas children of average intelligence can remember several words, numbers, or directions at one time, children with CI are less able to do so. Therefore they need simple one-step directions. Learning through a step-by-step process requires a task analysis, in which each task is separated into its necessary components and each step is taught completely before proceeding to the next activity (Box 24-4). Considerable repetition and review of new instructional information is important for long-term retention.

One critical area of learning that has had a tremendous impact on the education of cognitively impaired individuals is motivation, or the use of positive reinforcement to encourage the accomplishment of specific tasks or the development of specific behaviors. Two techniques are especially important with this group of learners: fading and shaping. Fading is physically taking the child through each sequence of the desired activity and gradually fading out physical assistance so that the child becomes more independent. Shaping is waiting for the child to give a response that approximates the desired behavior, then reinforcing successive approximations of the end goal

BOX 24-4   SAMPLE TASK ANALYSIS: SPOON FEEDING

1. Orients to the food by looking at it
2. Delivers the spoon to the bowl
3. Lowers the spoon into the food
4. Scoops food onto the spoon
5. Lifts the spoon
6. Delivers the spoon to the mouth
7. Opens the mouth
8. Inserts the spoon into the mouth
9. Moves the tongue and mouth to receive the food
10. Closes the lips and chews food
11. Swallows the food
12. Returns the spoon to the bowl

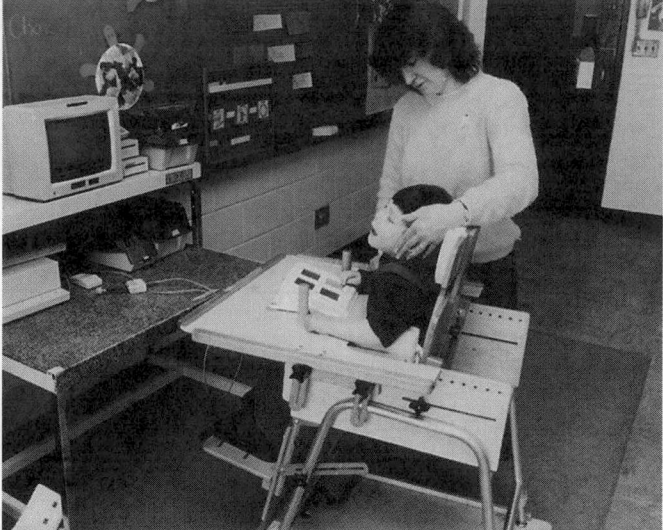

Fig. 24-1 A push panel allows a child with cognitive impairment to turn a computer on and off.

through the use of praise or tangible reinforcers. Repetition plays an important part in learning. As the child gains mastery, reinforcement gradually decreases. Such principles are easy to implement in the home in teaching self-help skills. Maintaining feelings of success in accomplishing specified goals also promotes self-esteem in the child. If a learning program does not move forward successfully, both parent and nurse can reevaluate the last sequence the child mastered to see if they are expecting too much too soon.

When behavior modification is employed, it is crucial to reinforce desirable behavior, because it has a considerable impact on the education of the cognitively impaired child. Employing positive reinforcement for specific tasks or behaviors tends to enhance the child's ability to learn.

Advances in technology have greatly assisted in providing reinforcement, especially for children who have severe CI and physical disabilities that limit their range of capabilities. For example, specially designed switches give children control of some event in the environment, such as turning on the computer (Fig. 24-1). Activation of the computer becomes reinforcement for pushing the switch. Repetitive use of these switches provides an early, simplistic association with a technical device that may progress to the use of increasingly complex aids.

Early intervention programs have been widely promoted for children with developmental disabilities, and there is considerable evidence that these programs are valuable for children with CI. **Early intervention program** is a systematic program of therapy, exercises, and activities designed to address developmental delays in disabled children to help achieve their full potentials (American Academy of Pediatrics, 2001a; Hartway, 2009a; National Down Syndrome Society, 2009d). Nurses working with families of disabled children need to be aware of the types of programs available in their community. Early intervention programs are provided by a number of organizations. Under Public Law 101-476, the Individuals with Disabilities Education Act of 1990, states are encouraged to provide full early intervention services* and are required to

provide educational opportunities for all children with disabilities from birth to 21 years of age. Early intervention services may be provided by each state, such as through programs for children with special health needs (formerly crippled children's programs) or Head Start, or by private organizations such as Easter Seals† and the ARC of the United States (formerly the Association for Retarded Citizens of the United States).‡ Local school districts provide educational services that begin when the child reaches age 3 years. Parents should inquire about these programs by contacting the appropriate agencies. To promote optimum outcomes, education should begin as soon as possible, not at 5 or 6 years of age. As children grow older, their education can focus on vocational training that prepares them for as independent a lifestyle as possible within their scope of abilities (American Academy of Pediatrics, 2001a; Johnson, Kastner, and American Academy of Pediatrics, 2005; Shapiro and Batshaw, 2007).

Promote the Child's Optimum Development

Optimum development requires appropriate guidance for establishing acceptable social behavior and personal feelings of self-esteem, worth, and security. These attributes are not simply learned through a stimulating program but must arise from the genuine love and caring that exists among family members. However, families may need guidance in providing an environment that fosters optimum development. Often it is the nurse who can provide assistance in these areas of childrearing.

Another important area for promoting optimum development and self-esteem is ensuring the child's physical well-being. Any congenital defects, such as cardiac, gastrointestinal, or orthopedic anomalies, should be repaired. Plastic surgery may be considered when the child's appearance can be substan-

---

*Information on early intervention programs in each state is available from the National Down Syndrome Society, 666 Broadway, New York, NY 10012; 800-221-4602; fax: 212-979-2873; e-mail: info@ndss.org; www.ndss.org.

†233 S. Wacker Drive, Suite 2400, Chicago, IL 60606; 312-726-6200, 800-221-6827; fax: 312-726-1494; TTY: 312-726-4258; www.easterseals.com.

‡1660 L St., NW, Suite 301, Washington, DC 20036; 202-534-3700, 800-433-5555; fax: 202-534-3731; www.thearc.org.

tially improved. Dental health is significant, and orthodontic and restorative procedures can immensely improve facial appearance.

Communication

Development of verbal skills is often delayed more than development of other physical skills. Speech requires adequate hearing and interpretation of sounds (receptive skills) and facial muscle coordination (expressive skills). Both receptive and expressive skills may be significantly impaired, so frequent audiometric testing should be conducted, and hearing aids should be provided to children with hearing difficulties. Other children may require training in controlling their facial muscles. For example, some children may need tongue exercises to correct tongue thrust or gentle reminders to keep the lips closed.

For some of these children, nonverbal methods of communication should be employed. The choice of an assistive device often depends on the child's cognitive level and physical abilities. For the child without associated physical disabilities, a talking picture board is helpful. For children with physical limitations, several adaptations to and types of communication devices are available to facilitate selection of the appropriate picture or word. Some children may learn sign language or Blissymbolics, a system of graphic symbols representing words, ideas, and concepts. The symbols are typically arranged on a board, and the individual points or uses a selector to communicate a message.

Discipline

Discipline must begin early. Limit-setting measures must be simple, consistent, and appropriate for the child's mental age. Control measures are based primarily on teaching a specific behavior, rather than on developing an understanding of the reasons behind it. Stressing moral lessons is of little value to a child who lacks the cognitive skills to learn from self-criticism and evaluation of previous mistakes. Behavior modification, especially reinforcement of desired actions and the use of time-out procedures, is an appropriate form of behavior control. (See Chapter 3.) Avoid aversive strategies.

Socialization

Acquisition of social skills is complex. Active rehearsal (with role playing and practice sessions) and positive reinforcement for desired behavior are successful approaches. Encourage parents early to teach their child socially acceptable behavior: waving good-bye, saying hello and thank you, responding to his or her name, and greeting visitors. The teaching of socially acceptable sexual behavior is especially important to minimize sexual exploitation. Parents also need to expose the child to strangers so that manners can be practiced, since transfer of learning from one situation to another is not automatic.

Social acceptance and self-esteem are enhanced when a child is appropriately dressed and well-groomed. Clean, stylish, well-fitting clothing that has self-adhering fasteners and elastic openings facilitates self-dressing and social acceptance.

Opportunities for social interaction and training should begin at an early age. Encourage parents to enroll their child in infant stimulation programs and other appropriate preschool programs as soon as possible. These programs provide education, training, and opportunities for social interaction with other children and adults.

As children grow older, they should have peer experiences similar to those of other children, including participation in group outings, sports, and organized activities such as scouts and Special Olympics. These children often enjoy participating in developmentally appropriate peer activities such as dance and karate classes (American Academy of Pediatrics, 2004; Rehm and Bradley, 2006; Shapiro and Batshaw, 2007). A close relationship with a best friend can be encouraged. Vacations, family outings, dances, and dating are important social opportunities.

Sexuality

Adolescence may be a particularly difficult time for parents, especially in terms of the child's sexual behavior, possibility of pregnancy, future plans to marry, and ability to be independent. Often, minimal anticipatory guidance is available to parents to prepare the child for physical and sexual maturation, and the degree of the adolescent's interest in and experience with sex has been underestimated.

The question of contraceptive protection for female adolescents is often a parental concern. Permanent contraception through sterilization is a special dilemma because of moral and ethical questions, as well as psychologic effects on the adolescent. State laws vary; some allow no sterilization, whereas others permit review of requests. Intramuscular injection of medroxyprogesterone acetate (Depo-Provera) is a contraceptive choice that provides long-term protection, requires little compliance, and often produces amenorrhea.

Parents of these adolescents are often concerned about the advisability of marriage between two individuals with significant CI. There is no conclusive answer; each situation must be judged individually. In many instances marriage would help the couple achieve a mutually satisfying and supportive relationship, meaningful companionship, and a more normal social and sexual adjustment. Under the Fourteenth Amendment to the Constitution, every individual has the right to marry and have a family, regardless of his or her mental capacity (Silber and Batshaw, 2004). The nurse should discuss this topic with parents and with the prospective couple, stressing the need for suitable living accommodations and use of appropriate contraceptive methods to prevent pregnancy. If children are conceived, these parents require specialized assistance and guidance in learning to meet the needs of their offspring (Johnson and Walker, 2006; Silber and Batshaw, 2004).

Nurses can help in this area by providing parents with information about sex education that is geared to the child's developmental level. For example, the adolescent female needs a simple explanation of menstruation and instructions on personal hygiene during the menstrual cycle.*

---

*Sources of information on sexuality and conception include Planned Parenthood Federation of America, 434 W. 33rd St., New York, NY 10001; 212-541-7800, 800-230-7526; fax: 212-245-1845; www.plannedparenthood.org; and the ARC of the United States (see footnote on p. 912).

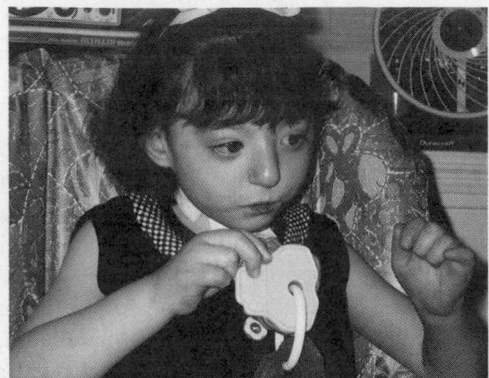

Fig. 24-2 A favorite toy provides stimulation for a young child.

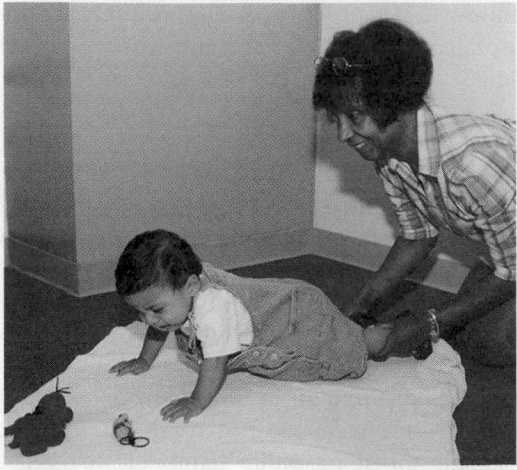

Fig. 24-3 Placing an attractive object outside of the child's reach encourages crawling movements. (Courtesy James DeLeon, Texas Children's Hospital, Houston.)

These adolescents also need practical sexual information regarding anatomy, physical development, and conception. Because they are easy to persuade and lack judgment, they need a well-defined, concrete code of conduct with specific instructions for handling certain situations. Girls should know never to go alone anywhere with any person they do not know well. Boys should be warned of intimate advances from other males. Sexual assault of a cognitively impaired adolescent should be treated and investigated by law enforcement personnel (Eastgate, 2005).

Play and Exercise

Children who are cognitively impaired have the same need for play as any other children. Exercise is beneficial for development of coordination, cardiovascular fitness, and weight management. Because of the child's slower development, however, parents may be less aware of the need to provide for such activities. They may also feel inadequate in playing with the child because the usual reciprocal interaction and resulting satisfaction between child and parent may be slower in developing.

In addition, children who are cognitively impaired may not be able to initiate appropriate play activities on their own. They may resort to self-stimulatory behavior, such as rocking, twirling, masturbating, or finger sucking, and self-injurious behaviors, such as head banging or biting, hitting, or scratching themselves (Murray, 2003; Shapiro and Batshaw, 2007). The nurse should inquire as to what precipitates the behaviors and review the parent's techniques used to manage the behaviors (Johnson and Walker, 2006). The nurse may also guide parents toward selection of suitable toys and interactive activities (Fig. 24-2).

The type of play is based on the child's developmental age, although the need for sensorimotor play may be prolonged. Parents should use every opportunity to expose the child to as many different sounds, sights, and sensations as possible. Appropriate toys include musical mobiles, stuffed toys, floating toys, a rocking chair or horse, a swing, bells, and rattles. The child should be taken on outings, such as trips to the grocery store or shopping center. Other people should visit in the home, and individuals should relate directly to the child, through such means as cuddling, holding, and talking to the child in the face-to-face position.

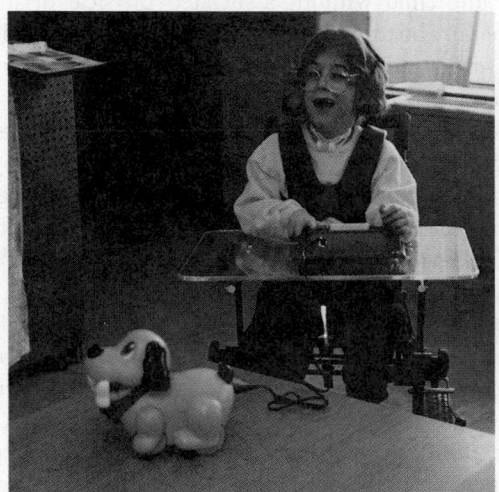

Fig. 24-4 An electric switch allows a child with physical impairment to play with a battery-operated toy.

Parents should select toys for their recreational and educational value. For example, a large inflatable beach ball is a good water toy; encourages interactive play; and can be used to learn motor skills such as balance, rocking, kicking, and throwing. Attractive toys encourage a child to reach, thus assisting in the development of motor skills (Fig. 24-3). Musical toys that mimic animal sounds or respond with social phrases are excellent ways of encouraging speech. A doll with removable clothes and different types of closures can help the child learn dressing skills. Toys should be simple in design so that the child can learn to manipulate them without help. For children with severe cognitive or physical impairment, electronic switches can be used to allow them to operate toys (Fig. 24-4).

Suitable physical activity is based on the child's size, coordination, physical fitness and maturity, motivation, and health. Some children may have physical problems that prevent participation in certain sports, such as atlantoaxial instability in children with Down syndrome. Children with CI often have greater success in individual and dual sports than in team sports and enjoy themselves most with children of the same develop-

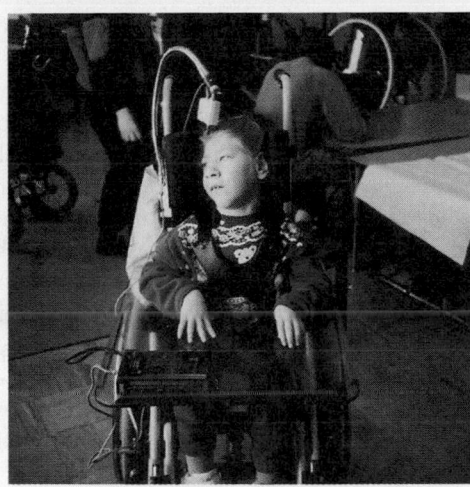

Fig. 24-5 A child with cognitive and physical impairments can play a tape recorder by moving a device near her head.

mental level. The Special Olympics* provides a unique competitive opportunity.

Safety is a major consideration in selecting recreational and exercise activities. Some toys that may be appropriate developmentally may present dangers to a child who is strong enough to break them or use them incorrectly.

Promote Independent Self-Help Skills

When a child with CI is born, parents often need assistance in promoting normal developmental skills that other children learn easily. There is no way to predict when a child should be able to master self-help skills; wide variability exists in the ages at which these children accomplish such functions (see Table 24-3). Parents need support, both as the primary caretakers and teachers of the child, and they need detailed written descriptions of a jointly developed training program. Parents should also receive information about commercially available devices that can aid in achievement of independence (Fig. 24-5).

Feeding

Self-feeding is the first major self-help skill that children learn. It involves the integration of fine and gross motor skills and visual perception. Most parents take for granted that they will be successful in teaching their children to feed themselves. Therefore the nurse and other team members must be especially sensitive to the needs of the parent, as well as the child, if assistance is offered.

Before beginning a self-feeding program, the nurse and parent should do a task analysis, breaking the process of feeding into its smallest components (see Box 24-4). It is important to observe the child in an eating situation to determine whether he or she has mastered any self-feeding skills.

Along with a task analysis, the nurse assesses a number of other factors, such as the shape of the child's mouth and the

*1133 19th St., NW, Washington, DC 20036-3604; 202-628-3630, 800-700-8585; fax: 202-824-0200; www.specialolympics.org (website includes listing of state offices). In Canada: Special Olympics Canada, 60 St. Clair Ave. E, Suite 700, Toronto, Ontario M4T 1N5, Canada; 416-927-9050; fax: 416-927-8475; www.specialolympics.ca.

child's control of mouth, lip, and tongue movements (whether the tongue moves forward and backward or from side to side, whether there are rotary movements). The presence of teeth determines the textures and consistencies of foods that the child can eat. The child's developmental readiness for self-feeding, such as the ability to maintain head and trunk support and to sit without support, the level of eye-hand coordination, the firmness of the grasp, and the ability to reach for an object, hold it, and release it, is examined. If the child has any physical impairments that interfere with holding or grasping the utensil, specially designed utensils can be substituted or homemade modifications can be used. For example, the handle can be built up with a sponge or piece of wood or bent to accommodate arm movement.

The nurse obtains further data from the parent by asking specifically about the family's approach to feeding. For example, who feeds the child regularly? Is the child fed when hungry or according to a prescribed schedule? What are the child's appetite patterns? Does the parent know when the child is full? What foods does the child like? How long does feeding take? A short feeding time, such as 10 minutes, might indicate that the child is being deprived of sensory experiences or appropriate interactions; a long time might indicate frustration and fatigue on the parent's part. Is the feeding environment described as quiet and nondistracting? The nurse also helps determine the best time to begin teaching this new task. If the family is going on vacation, if someone is visiting, or if there has been a major stress in the family, this may not be the ideal time to begin a teaching program.

Also consider preparation for the feeding activity, such as proper placement of the child at the table and protection of the area against spills. Feeding should fit in with family life. (See Chapter 22.) For example, the child is fed in the kitchen, at the table, or in a high chair in a sitting position, and with other family members whenever possible. Food should be offered in separate servings, not pureed or mixed together; should be served at the appropriate temperature; and should be of sufficient variety and texture from each of the basic food groups.

Once the feeding program begins, the nurse is in an important position to give parents supportive feedback. The nurse acknowledges the parents' observational skills and their ability to share observations, keep records of the child's progress, and establish goals that are appropriate and realistic for both the child and the parents.

Toileting

Independent toileting is another major self-help skill that parents can teach using behavior modification principles. It usually begins after self-feeding because this is the normal sequence of development. Plans for a toileting program begin by assessing the child's physical and psychologic readiness. (See Chapter 14.) Because of physical or developmental limitations, certain signals may not be possible. For example, children who cannot walk can be trained once they are able to sit with good balance, and children with poor speech may need to rely on hand gestures to signal their toileting needs.

Interview parents regarding their readiness to pursue a toilet-training program. Readiness is characterized by a positive, consistent, individualized, nonpunitive, nonpressured style of teaching. It is important to explore with parents the time they have to invest in the program, the advantages they see, the inconveniences that toilet training may cause them, the reason they wish to start, and whether this is the best time for both the parents and the child to begin.

Review any past attempts at toilet training the child: When and why did the parents start training? What methods did they use? Did they experience frustration, indifference, or discomfort? How long did they attempt training, and what were their reasons for discontinuing training efforts? Were their efforts consistent? Looking back, how did they view the experience for themselves and the child? If the parents acknowledge using punishment in any form, including spanking, scolding, withholding privileges, using suppositories, withholding fluid, or getting the child up in the middle of the night, the nurse offers positive alternatives.

As part of the procedure for determining the readiness of both parents and child to become involved in a successful toilet-training program, ask parents to keep detailed records for 7 days. They should discontinue record keeping if the child becomes ill or if fluid intake is changed. Record keeping includes documentation of:

- Oral intake
- Behavioral indicators (e.g., the child was noticeably quieter or louder, started fussing or tugging at clothes, pointed toward the bathroom, cried, or squirmed)
- Positive parenteral feedback related to toileting behaviors only, in the form of praise, concrete rewards, affection, or approval
- Parental criticism in the form of scolding, threatening, or spanking if the child had wet or soiled the underclothes or did not tell them before eliminating
- Indication by the child of the need to go to the toilet by either gestures or words
- Observation that the child had dry underclothes
- Observation that the child had wet underclothes

If possible, a toilet-training program should begin after such records are completed because they show how parents are responding to the child's behaviors and at what times the child is most likely to eliminate.

The objective of any toilet-training program is to help the child achieve small goals and experience comfort and success and to help the parents simultaneously experience feelings of adequacy, minimum tension, and success. Parents should understand that they will be capitalizing on the times the child is most likely to eliminate and that they should respond immediately to any cues indicating this need.

A task analysis for toileting includes the same type of discrete steps as outlined for feeding (see Box 24-4). A positive and relaxed attitude toward toilet training is important and differs little from the approach used with other children. (See Chapter 14.)

Dressing

Although dressing skills develop without special instruction in most children, special training is necessary to promote this skill in children with CI. Factors that interfere with spontaneous learning include immature motor skills, lack of motivation, physical impairments, and lack of opportunity.

The level of independence in dressing varies according to the degree of CI. Children with mild to moderate CI and no accompanying physical limitations can become independent in all dressing skills, except for more complex tasks such as color coordination. Those who have moderate CI can master most dressing skills, except fastening complicated closures such as buttons or ties. Those who have profound CI are usually able to assist in undressing and dressing but achieve no independent skills.

Children are considered developmentally ready for dressing training if they can sit quietly for 3 to 5 minutes while working on a task; can watch what they are doing while working on a task; can follow physical gestures or cues; can follow verbal commands; and can relate clothing to the appropriate body part, such as socks to feet. As with other self-help skills, the child may not be able to master every task but should be evaluated for evidence of willingness to participate at his or her level of readiness. The use of teaching devices, such as dolls with clothing with mock closures, and reinforcement for success in managing the fasteners can increase the child's manipulative skills, which may be transferred to ready-to-wear clothing.

Grooming

The child usually learns self-grooming along with other independence-promoting skills, such as washing hands during toilet training. As with self-dressing, a major factor in learning independent grooming is the opportunity to practice the skills.

Dental hygiene is especially important. An odor-free mouth and clean teeth are essential in promoting a positive image. In addition, healthy teeth are necessary for proper chewing and speech. Missing teeth interfere with proper tongue positioning for clear speech. Most dental problems are preventable with the dental hygiene practices discussed in Chapter 14.

If the child has physical impairments that limit the ability to brush, special devices may be necessary, such as a larger-handled or curved toothbrush, to reach all surfaces of the teeth. Any strategies that help motivate the child to brush are used. For example, the parent can place a special calendar on the wall and mark each date with stars to represent the number of brushings per day. After earning a specified number of stars, the child can receive a special reward.

The child should routinely see a dentist. It is important to prepare the child for such visits, because it is much more difficult to change an unsatisfactory experience than to prevent one. The nurse can assist families by locating dentists who are familiar with treating children with CI and by discussing with parents procedures for preparing the child for the visit.

Help Families Adjust to Future Care

Not all families are able to cope with home care of children who are cognitively impaired, especially those who have severe or profound CI or multiple disabilities. Older parents may not be able to continue with care responsibilities once they reach retirement or old age. The decision regarding residential placement is difficult for families, and the availability of such facilities varies widely. The nurse's role includes assisting parents in investigating and evaluating programs and helping parents adjust to the decision for placement. Guidelines for assessing out-of-home care facilities are given in the Nursing Care Guidelines box (also see Community Focus box).

Care for the Child During Hospitalization

Caring for the child during hospitalization can be a special challenge. Frequently nurses are unfamiliar with children who

NURSING CARE GUIDELINES

Assessing Out-of-Home Care Facilities

- Assess the environment for adequacy of stimuli for the residents.
- Determine the appropriateness of the amount of stimulation in the environment.
- Observe care provider–to–resident ratios.
- Observe care personnel interacting with residents in a variety of teaching and learning situations.
- Determine the appropriateness of the setting for the person being considered for placement.
- Observe the quality of physical care administered.
- See whether the residents are attended to regularly and consistently, instead of when inappropriate behaviors occur.
- Determine whether activities are age-appropriate for the residents.
- Determine whether structured and unstructured activities are provided.
- Determine whether individual care plans are available and implemented.
- Determine the functional levels of those who reside in the settings (e.g., Are they ambulatory and is speech encouraged?).
- Determine whether speech, physical, and occupational therapies are available.
- Determine whether each person is perceived as unique and distinct and whether care is given to residents according to their needs.
- Determine whether and to what degree official standards of care are met.
- Meet with parents of those who reside in special settings to hear their comments, both positive and negative.

COMMUNITY FOCUS

Long-Term Care

Long-term care for a dependent with cognitive impairment is a concern for many parents, particularly those who are aging. Some parents have concerns about quality of care in institutions and group homes. Changes in the health care system, human service systems, and the disability field may leave parents wondering what the future holds. Many organizations recommend that parents write a detailed plan outlining their preferences in each area of their child's life to be followed after the parents die. Parents may also be interested in building a network of relationships to provide ongoing support to the child with cognitive impairment.

are cognitively impaired, and they may cope with their insecurity and fear by ignoring or isolating the child. Not only is this approach nonsupportive, it may also be destructive to the child's sense of self-esteem and optimum development and may impair the parents' ability to cope with the stress of the experience. To prevent engaging in this nontherapeutic approach, nurses can use the mutual participation model in planning the child's care. Parents should stay with their child and assist with care, but they should not be made to feel as if the responsibility is totally theirs. Ideally the family should visit the hospital before admission. A visit minimizes the unfamiliarity of the hospital setting and is an opportunity for staff members to allay any fears the parents or child may have. When the child is admitted, a detailed history is taken, with special focus on all self-care abilities. (See Chapter 26.) During the interview the child's developmental age is assessed.

Questions about the child's abilities are approached positively. For example, rather than asking, "Is your child toilet trained yet?" the nurse may say, "Tell me about your child's toileting habits." The assessment should also focus on any special devices the child uses, effective measures of limit setting,

unusual or favorite routines, and any behaviors that may require intervention. For example, if the parent states that the child engages in self-stimulatory or self-injurious activities, the nurse inquires about events that precipitate them and techniques the parents use to manage them. Once the child's functional level is known, encourage him or her to be as independent as possible in the hospital setting.

The nurse can help the child feel less lonely during the hospital stay by making certain that the child has toys, is engaged in other activities, and has a roommate of approximately the same developmental age. The nurse should treat the child with dignity and respect in a manner that promotes acceptance and understanding of the child by children, parents, or others with whom the child comes into contact in the hospital.

Explain procedures to the child using methods of communication that are at the appropriate cognitive level. Generally explanations should be simple, short, and concrete, emphasizing what the child will physically experience. Demonstration either through actual practice or with visual aids is preferable to verbal explanation. Include parents in preprocedural teaching to aid in the child's learning and to help the nurse learn effective methods of communicating with the child.

During hospitalization the nurse should also focus on growth-promoting experiences for the child. For example, hospitalization may be an excellent opportunity to emphasize to parents abilities the child does have but has not had the opportunity to practice, such as self-dressing. It may also be an opportunity for social experiences with peers, group play, or new educational or recreational activities. For example, one child who had the habit of screaming and kicking demonstrated a definite decrease in these behaviors after learning to pound pegs and use a punching bag. Through social services the parents may become aware of specialized programs for the child. Nutritional counseling is available if the child is overweight or has evidence of specific deficiencies, such as iron deficiency. Hospitalization may also offer parents a respite from everyday care responsibilities and an opportunity to discuss their feelings with a concerned professional.

DOWN SYNDROME

Down syndrome is the most common chromosomal abnormality of a generalized syndrome, occurring in 1 in 733 live births (Hall, 2007; Descartes and Carroll, 2007; National Down Syndrome Society, 2009d). It occurs slightly more often in Caucasians than in African-Americans, although the incidence does not vary with socioeconomic class.

Etiology

The cause of Down syndrome is not known. A number of theories have been proposed, including genetic predisposition to nondisjunction, exposure to radiation before conception, immunologic problems, and infection, but none of the hypotheses has been substantiated. Recent reports of cytogenetic and epidemiologic studies support the concept of multiple causality.

Although the etiology is unclear, the cytogenetics of the disorder is well established. Approximately 97% of all cases of Down syndrome are attributable to an extra chromosome 21 (group G), hence the name *nonfamilial trisomy 21*. Although

TABLE 24-2	RELATION BETWEEN MATERNAL AGE AND ESTIMATED RISK OF DOWN SYNDROME
AGE (yr)	**RISK OF DOWN SYNDROME**
20	1 : 2000
25	1 : 1200
30	1 : 900
35	1 : 350
40	1 : 100
45	1 : 30
49	1 : 10

National Down Syndrome Society: *About Down syndrome: incidences and maternal age,* New York, 2009, The Society, available at www.ndss.org/index.php?option=com_content&view=article&id=61&Item id=78 (accessed March 16, 2009).

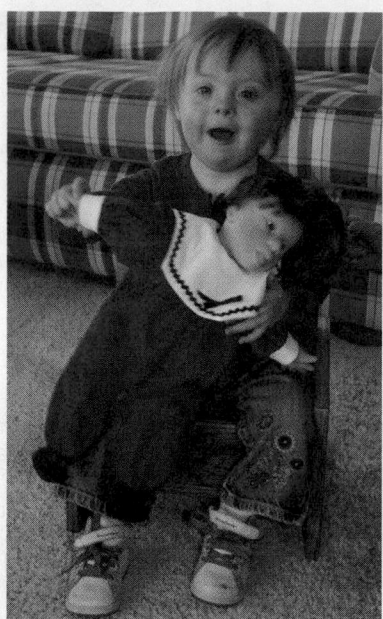

Fig. 24-6 A young child with Down syndrome holding a doll with Down syndrome.

children with trisomy 21 are born to parents of all ages, there is a statistically greater risk for older women, particularly those over 35 years of age (Table 24-2). For example, the incidence of Down syndrome is about 1 in 350 live births to women 35 years of age, but about 1 in 100 live births to women 40 years old. However, 80% of infants with Down syndrome are born to women under age 35 years because younger women have higher fertility rates (National Down Syndrome Society, 2009c). In less than 5% of cases, paternal age is a factor, especially if the father is 55 years of age or older (Grech, 2001; National Down Syndrome Society, 2009d).

Some 3% to 4% of cases may be caused by translocation of chromosome 21, which means chromosome 21 is attached to another chromosome. The majority of translocations in Down syndrome are fusions at the centromere between chromosomes 13, 14, 15, or 21; this is known as Robertsonian translocation (Descartes and Carroll, 2007; Hartway, 2009b; Ranweiler, 2009). About one-third of the translocation cases in Down syndrome are hereditary and are not associated with advanced parental age (Hartway, 2009b; National Down Syndrome Society, 2009c; Ranweiler, 2009). From 1% to 3% of affected persons demonstrate mosaicism, in which cell populations with both normal and abnormal chromosomes are present. The degree of physical and cognitive impairment is related to the percentage of cells with the abnormal chromosomal makeup. (For a discussion of the genetics involved in Down syndrome, see Chapter 5.)

Except for mosaicism, the mechanism by which the syndrome occurs has little effect on the characteristics displayed by the affected child and the management of the disorder. However, it is significant for purposes of genetic counseling. Whereas nondisjunction is usually a sporadic event associated with a low risk of recurrence (0.5% to 1%), a hereditary translocation is associated with a higher risk of recurrence (5% to 15%) (Hartway, 2009b; National Down Syndrome Society, 2009a). In Down syndrome caused by translocation, testing of the parents is necessary to identify the carrier and offer genetic counseling.

Clinical Manifestations

Down syndrome can usually be diagnosed by the clinical manifestations alone, although no one physical feature is diagnostic (Box 24-5 and Fig. 24-6), and there is considerable variation in phenotypic expression. In addition, some infants may have characteristics of Down syndrome, such as epicanthal folds, a narrow palate, short broad hands, and a transpalmar crease, but may be cytogenetically normal. A chromosomal analysis is therefore performed to confirm the genetic abnormality. The following are other outstanding features of the syndrome:

Intelligence—Mental capacity varies from severe CI to low-average intelligence but is generally within the mild to moderate range of CI and may be related to parental intelligence (National Down Syndrome Society, 2009a). Initial development may appear near normal. Although abilities can vary considerably, relative strengths often occur in visual over auditory processing, with relative weaknesses in grammar and expressive language and delays in motor development (National Down Syndrome Society, 2009a; Shapiro and Batshaw, 2007).

Social development—Development may be 2 to 3 years beyond the mental age, especially during early childhood. Temperamental characteristics show the same range as those found in unaffected peers. However, there is a relative strength in sociability (American Academy of Pediatrics, 2001a; Johnson and Walker, 2006) and a trend toward the easy-child pattern that may facilitate parent-child attachment and assist in integration with peers at school and in the community.

Congenital anomalies—About 40% to 45% have congenital heart disease (CHD), especially septal defects. Other structural defects include renal agenesis, duodenal atresia, Hirschsprung disease, and tracheoesophageal fistula. Skeletal defects include patella dislocation, hip subluxation, and atlantoaxial instability (instability of the first and second cervical vertebrae) in some children.

Sensory problems—Ocular problems include strabismus, nystagmus, astigmatism, myopia, hyperopia, head tilt, excessive tearing, and cataracts. Hearing loss occurs in a

BOX 24-5 CLINICAL MANIFESTATIONS OF DOWN SYNDROME

Head
Separated sagittal suture*
Brachycephaly
Rounded and small skull
Flat occiput
Enlarged anterior fontanel
Sparse hair (variable)

Face
Flat profile

Eyes
Oblique palpebral fissures (upward, outward slant)*
Inner epicanthal folds
Speckling of iris (Brushfield spots)
Short, sparse eyelashes
Blepharitis

Nose
Small nose*
Depressed nasal bridge (saddle nose)*

Ears
Small ears
Short pinna (vertical ear length)
Overlapping upper helixes
Narrow canals
Conductive hearing loss

Mouth
High, arched, narrow palate*
Small osseous orbit
Protruding tongue, may be fissured at lip and furrowed on surface
Hypoplastic mandible
Downward curve (especially noted when crying)
Mouth kept open

Teeth
Delayed eruption
Alignment abnormalities (common)
Microdontia
Periodontal disease

Chest
Shortened rib cage
Twelfth rib anomalies
Pectus excavatum, pectus carinatum

Neck
Excess and lax skin*
Short, broad neck

Abdomen
Protrusion
Lax and flabby muscles
Diastasis recti abdominis
Umbilical hernia

Genitalia
Small penis
Cryptorchidism
Bulbous vulva

Hands
Broad, short hands
Stubby fingers
Incurved fifth finger (clinodactyly)
Transverse palmar crease

Feet
Wide space between big and second toes*
Plantar crease between big and second toes*
Broad, stubby, short feet

Musculoskeletal
Short stature
Hyperflexibility*
Muscle weakness*
Hypotonia
Atlantoaxial instability

Skin
Dry, cracked skin and frequent fissuring
Cutis marmorata (mottling)

Other
Reduced birth weight
Learning difficulty (average intelligence quotient of 50)
Early-onset dementia (in one third)
Impaired immune function
Increased risk of leukemia

*Most common findings (Pueschel, 1999).

large percentage of children with Down syndrome. Conductive, sensorineural, and mixed losses each account for approximately one third of the diagnoses. Frequent otitis media, narrow canals, and impacted cerumen may contribute to the hearing problems.

Other physical disorders—These children have altered immune function, which contributes to numerous other conditions (Rittey, 2003). Respiratory tract infections are prevalent; when combined with cardiac anomalies, they are the chief cause of death, particularly during the first year. Because a high incidence of CHD is associated with trisomy 21, echocardiography is recommended at the time of initial diagnosis (American Academy of Pediatrics, 2001a; Bernstein, 2007). The incidence of leukemia is several times more frequent than expected in the general population, and in about half of the cases the type is acute megakaryoblastic leukemia. Thyroid dysfunction, including Graves disease, goiter, chronic lymphocytic thyroiditis, and hypothyroidism, is common. Acquired thyroid dysfunction also occurs frequently.

Growth—Growth in both height and weight is reduced, but weight gain is more rapid than growth in stature, which often results in overweight by 36 months of age. Deficient growth is most marked during infancy and adolescence. Growth of children with moderate or severe CHD is more affected than growth of those with mild or no CHD.

Sexual development—Development may be delayed, incomplete, or both. Male genitalia and secondary sexual characteristics such as facial hair may be underdeveloped. Breast development in females is mild to moderate. Menstruation usually occurs at the average age, and postpubertal women can be fertile; a small number have had offspring, the majority of whom were born with some type of abnormality. Men with Down syndrome have significantly lower overall fertility rate than other men of comparable ages (Descartes and Carroll, 2007; National Down Syndrome Society, 2009b).

Therapeutic Management

Although Down syndrome has no cure, these children may require surgery to correct serious congenital anomalies, and they benefit from regular health care. Evaluation of sight and hearing is essential, and treatment of otitis media is required to prevent hearing problems, which can influence cognitive function. Neonatal and subsequent periodic testing of thyroid function is recommended, especially if growth is delayed. Special growth charts are available to monitor nutrition, height, weight, and general aspects of well-child care. Growth hormone therapy may be considered to increase height. Plastic surgery to alter phenotypic stigma is performed in some cases.

Fifteen percent to twenty percent of children with Down syndrome have occipitoatlantal and atlantoaxial instability. Symptoms of the disorder include neck pain, weakness, and torticollis; however, most affected children are asymptomatic. The American Academy of Pediatrics (2004) recommends screening children with Down syndrome for atlantoaxial instability with a neurologic examination and radiography after their second birthday and before they engage in physically energetic exercise or sports or undergo surgery or rehabilitative procedures; however, this recommendation is controversial (Thompson, 2007). If children are diagnosed with atlantoaxial instability, surgery may be required, and they should refrain from participating in activities that may involve stress on the head and neck. If children become symptomatic, they should receive prompt attention because they are at risk for spinal cord compression.

! NURSING ALERT

Report immediately any of the following signs of spinal cord compression in a child:
- Persistent neck pain
- Loss of established motor skills and bladder or bowel control
- Changes in sensation

Prognosis

Life expectancy for those with Down syndrome has significantly increased in recent years but remains lower than for the general population (Wiseman, Alford, Tybulewicz, et al, 2009). More than 80% of individuals with Down syndrome survive to age 55 years and beyond. As the prognosis continues to improve for these individuals, it will be important to provide for their long-term health care, social, and leisure needs.

Nursing Care Management
Support the Family at the Time of Diagnosis

Because of the distinctive physical characteristics, the infant with Down syndrome is usually diagnosed at birth. Generally parents wish to know the diagnosis as soon as possible. Most parents prefer that both of them be present during the informing interview so they can support each other emotionally.

TABLE 24-3	DEVELOPMENTAL MILESTONES AND SKILLS IN CHILDREN WITH DOWN SYNDROME	
	AVERAGE (mo)	RANGE (mo)
Milestone		
Smiling	2	1½-4
Rolling over	8	4-22
Sitting alone	10	6-28
Crawling	12	7-21
Creeping	15	9-27
Standing	20	11-42
Walking	24	12-65
Talking, words	16	9-31
Talking, phrases	28	18-96
Skill		
Eating		
Finger feeding	12	8-28
Using spoon or fork	20	12-40
Toilet Training		
Bladder	48	20-95
Bowel	42	28-90
Dressing		
Undressing	40	29-72
Putting on clothes	58	38-98

Modified from Pueschel SM: The child with Down syndrome. In Carey WB, Crocker AC, Elias ER, et al, editors: *Developmental-behavioral pediatrics*, ed 4, Philadelphia, 2009, Saunders.

Parental responses to the child may greatly influence decisions regarding future care (see Cultural Competence box). Whereas some families willingly plan to take the child home, others consider foster care or adoption. Institutionalization is no longer an option. The nurse must answer questions regarding developmental potential carefully, since the responses may influence the parents' decision. It is obvious from ranges such as those given in Table 24-3 that the potential for developmental achievement varies greatly. Therefore it would be inaccurate and unfair to predict the child's intellectual capacity at birth. It is important to stress that a decision regarding placement will affect all of the family members' lives and need not be made at the time of diagnosis (see Critical Thinking Exercise). The nurse should emphasize every available source of assistance, such as parent groups, professional counseling, and literature, to help the family learn about Down syndrome and deal with childrearing problems.*

Assist the Family in Preventing Physical Problems

Many of the physical characteristics of Down syndrome present challenges. The hypotonicity of muscles and hyperex-

*For the ARC and National Down Syndrome Society contact information, see footnotes, p. 912. It may also be helpful for parents to know that studies of families who choose to rear their child at home report many favorable responses. Parental feelings toward the child usually are very positive; parents believe the experience of having this special child makes them stronger and more accepting of others. Behavioral problems among the siblings are similar to those found among families without children with Down syndrome.

Importance of Cultural Factors in Coping

The importance of cultural factors in parental coping with a child's disability cannot be overstated. Perceptions of illness or disability and its meaning are culturally influenced. Styles of interacting with health care professionals may have cultural determinants. Cultural values and practices may influence approaches to treatment and intervention, including the use of alternative or adjunctive therapies.

Finally, cultural background often influences coping styles. Becoming aware of these variables, appreciating and respecting cultural diversity, and learning about the values and practices of different cultural groups can augment nursing practice in any setting.

❓ **CRITICAL THINKING EXERCISE**

Diagnosis of Down Syndrome

The parents of Melissa, a newborn diagnosed as having Down syndrome, ask the nurse, "What are we supposed to do with her?" They further state that they already have three other children at home.

1. Evidence—Is there sufficient evidence to draw conclusions about the parents' concerns regarding their newborn daughter?
2. Assumptions—Describe an underlying assumption about each of the following:
   a. Newborn diagnosed with Down syndrome
   b. Parental care of a newborn with Down syndrome
   c. Newborn with Down syndrome and older siblings
3. What priorities for the nursing response should be established?
4. Does the evidence support your nursing intervention?

tensibility of joints complicate positioning. The limp, flaccid extremities resemble the posture of a rag doll; as a result, holding the infant is difficult and cumbersome. Sometimes parents perceive this lack of molding to their bodies as evidence of inadequate parenting. The extended body position promotes heat loss because more surface area is exposed to the environment. Encourage parents to swaddle the infant (wrap him or her tightly in a blanket) before picking up the infant to provide security and warmth. The nurse also discusses with parents their feelings concerning attachment to the child, emphasizing that the child's lack of clinging or molding is a physical characteristic, not a sign of detachment or rejection.

Decreased muscle tone compromises respiratory expansion. In addition, the underdeveloped nasal bone causes a chronic problem of inadequate drainage of mucus. The constant stuffy nose forces the child to breathe by mouth, which dries the oropharyngeal membranes and thus increases the susceptibility to upper respiratory tract and ear infections. Measures to lessen infection include clearing the nose with a bulb-type syringe, rinsing the mouth with water after feedings, increasing fluid intake and using a cool-mist vaporizer to keep the mucous membranes moist and the nasal secretions liquefied, changing the child's position frequently, and practicing good hand-washing technique. If antibiotics are ordered, the importance of completing the full course of therapy for successful eradication of the infection and prevention of growth of resistant organisms is stressed. Because hearing impairment is common

and can interfere with development, the nurse should emphasize the importance of auditory testing.

Feeding difficulties may occur. The large, protruding tongue and hypotonia interfere with breast-feeding, bottle-feeding, and introduction of solid foods. Parents need to know that the tongue thrust does not indicate refusal to feed but is a physiologic response. Advise parents to use a small but long, straight-handled spoon to push the food toward the back and side of the mouth. If food is thrust out, it should be refed. At times the family may require the assistance of a specially trained individual, such as a lactation expert or occupational therapist, to guide them in dealing with feeding problems.

Dietary intake, especially of solid foods, needs supervision. Decreased muscle tone affects gastric motility, predisposing the child to constipation. Dietary measures such as increased fiber and fluid intake promote evacuation. The child's eating habits need careful monitoring to prevent obesity. Obtain height and weight measurements on a serial basis and plot them on specialized growth charts, especially during infancy, because excessive weight gain can impede motor development. The child should receive calories in accordance with height and weight, not chronologic age.

During infancy the child's skin is pliable and soft. However, it gradually becomes rough and dry and is prone to cracking and infection. Skin care involves minimum use of soap and application of lubricants. Apply lip balm to the lips, especially when the child is outdoors, to prevent excessive chapping.

Promote the Child's Developmental Progress

Hypotonicity affects muscular development. Supporting skills, such as rolling over, sitting up, standing, or pulling oneself to a sitting or standing position, may be delayed. These children should be involved in an early stimulation program that provides physical therapy to help them learn motor skills.

Assess the child's developmental progress at regular intervals, and encourage therapeutic adherence to a stimulation program. Developmental screening tests are inadequate to evaluate indications of progress such as increased strength, balance, coordination, or muscle tone. Therefore keep detailed written records of the child's motor abilities to distinguish subtle changes in functioning. Periodic formal testing should also occur.

Parents can investigate appropriate daycare programs for the child as soon as possible. They should also investigate the public school system for special education classes, including early intervention programs and preschools. The nurse should give attention to preventing the problem of overprotection and including family members, especially the father and siblings, in the caring role.

Assist in Prenatal Diagnosis and Genetic Counseling

Prenatal diagnosis of Down syndrome is possible through chorionic villus sampling and amniocentesis, since chromosomal analysis of fetal cells can detect the presence of trisomy or translocation. Sporadic cases occur in young mothers that are not identified because there is no indication for prenatal testing. However, maternal testing for low serum α-fetoprotein levels, high chorionic gonadotropin levels, and low unconjugated estriol levels may identify potential cases, and these women can then undergo amniocentesis (Descartes and Carroll, 2007; Hall, 2007).

Offer prenatal testing and genetic counseling to women of advanced maternal age or those with a family history of Down syndrome. Although many women elect to have testing, some do not. If testing is conducted and the fetus is affected, the nurse must allow the parents to express their feelings concerning elective abortion and support their decision to terminate or proceed with the pregnancy. It is important for nurses to be aware of their own attitudes regarding testing and related decisions.

FRAGILE X SYNDROME

Fragile X syndrome is the most common inherited cause of CI and the second most common genetic cause of CI or intellectual disability after Down syndrome. It has been described in all ethnic groups and races. Fragile X syndrome occurs in 1 in 2000 to 5000 live births and affects males more severely than females (Menon, Leroux, White, et al, 2004; Rapaport, 2007). Fragile X syndrome occurs approximately 1 in 4000 males and 1 in 8000 females (National Fragile X Foundation, 2009). Because its identification as a disorder is relatively rare, many health care professionals and educators lack the necessary familiarity with the manifestations for appropriate referral and management once it is diagnosed.

The syndrome is caused by an abnormal mutation in the fragile X mental retardation 1 protein gene *(FMR1)* on the lower end of the long arm of the X chromosome (National Fragile X Foundation, 2009). Chromosomal analysis may demonstrate a fragile site (a region that fails to condense during mitosis and is characterized by a nonstaining gap or narrowing) in the cells of affected males and females and in carrier females. Since 1991, direct deoxyribonucleic acid (DNA) analysis for the *FMR1* gene mutation causing fragile X syndrome has greatly increased the accuracy of diagnostic testing of both affected and carrier individuals; this testing also permits prenatal diagnosis. However, when cognitively impaired individuals without an established family history of fragile X syndrome are being evaluated, cytogenetic and DNA studies should be performed to determine whether another chromosomal abnormality may be the cause of the CI.

This fragile site is caused by a gene mutation that results in excessive repeats of nucleotide base pairs in a specific DNA segment of the X chromosome. The number of repeats in a normal individual is between 5 and about 40 times. An individual with 55 to 200 base pair repeats is said to have an *FMR1* premutation and is therefore a carrier. When passed from a parent to a child, these base pair repeats can expand from 200 to 2000 or more, which is termed a *full mutation*. This expansion occurs only when a carrier mother passes the mutation to her offspring; it does not occur when a carrier father passes the mutation to his daughters. Most males (80%) with a full mutation are affected (e.g., have the physical and behavioral features and intellectual disability); however, only 30% of females with a full mutation are affected. Interestingly, even females with a full mutation who do not appear to be affected, as well as carrier males and females with normal intelligence, may exhibit some learning disabilities and psychosocial disorders. This inheri-

tance pattern has been termed *X-linked dominant with reduced penetrance*. It is in distinct contrast to the classic X-linked recessive pattern, in which all carrier females are normal, all affected males have symptoms of the disorder, and no males are carriers. Consequently, genetic counseling of affected families is more complex than that for families with a classic X-linked disorder such as hemophilia. Prenatal diagnosis of the fragile X gene mutation is possible through direct DNA testing in a family with an established history of the disorder, using amniocentesis or chorionic villus sampling (Hall, 2007; National Fragile X Foundation, 2009). Affected members of both sexes are capable of transmitting the fragile X disorder.

Clinical Manifestations

The classic pattern of physical findings in adult males with fragile X syndrome consists of a long face with a prominent jaw (prognathism); large, protruding ears; and large testes (macroorchidism). However, these features may be less obvious in prepubertal children, and behavioral manifestations may initially suggest the diagnosis (Box 24-6). Developmental delay and language delay are common. Autism-like behavior (e.g., rocking, talking to self, spinning, hand flapping, hand biting, poor eye contact, echolalia) occurs in some individuals with fragile X syndrome (Chiu, Wegelin, Blank, et al, 2007; Hatton, Sideris, Skinner, et al, 2006; Wiesner, Cassidy, Grimes, et al, 2004). Some individuals also show social anxiety, whereas others have appropriate social skills and adaptive behavior, which means they may function or appear to function at a higher level than their IQ scores would predict.

In carrier females the clinical manifestations are extremely varied. Carrier and affected females may exhibit psychosocial

---

BOX 24-6   CLINICAL MANIFESTATIONS OF FRAGILE X SYNDROME

Physical Features

Long, wide, or protruding ears
Long, narrow face with prominent jaw
In postpubertal males, enlarged testicles
Long palpebral fissures
High, arched palate
Strabismus
Increased head circumference
Mitral valve prolapse, aortic root dilation
Hypotonia
Hyperextensible finger joints
Transpalmar crease
Pes planus (flat feet)

Behavioral Features

Mild to severe cognitive impairment (occasional normal intelligence quotient with learning disabilities)
Possible greater delay in expressive language than in receptive language; this pattern may increase with age
Speech delay; speech may be rapid, with stuttering and repetition of words
Short attention span, hyperactivity
Mouthing beyond expected age for this behavior
Hypersensitivity to taste, sounds, touch
Intolerance to change in routine
Autism-like behaviors: social anxiety, gaze aversion, sensitivity to sensory stimulation
Possible aggressive behavior

deficits such as anxiety, withdrawal, and depression (Roberts, Mirrett, and Burchinal, 2001). In fact, some evidence suggests that low-expressing fragile X may be associated with personality changes in the absence of cognitive deficits (Goodlin-Jones, Tassone, Gane, et al, 2004).

Therapeutic Management

Fragile X syndrome has no cure. Medical treatment may include the use of serotonin agents such as carbamazepine (Tegretol) or fluoxetine (Prozac) to control violent temper outbursts, and central nervous system (CNS) stimulants to improve attention span and decrease hyperactivity. The use of folic acid, which affects the metabolism of CNS transmitters, is controversial. Medical treatment also addresses physical problems associated with the syndrome, which may include musculoskeletal concerns, mitral valve prolapse, recurrent otitis media, and seizures.

All affected children require early speech and language therapy, occupational therapy, and special educational assistance. Without appropriate intervention, a progressive decline in IQ can occur. Children with fragile X syndrome mimic the behavior of other children. Therefore mainstreaming them with children of similar age may improve their behavior.

Prognosis

Individuals with fragile X syndrome are expected to live a normal life span. Their CI may improve with behavioral and educational interventions, which should begin in preschool. Newborn inexpensive screening methods for fragile X syndrome is being researched in the United States, in line with the broadening of newborn screening criteria to include neurodevelopmental disorders that would benefit from early intervention (Bailey, Beskow, Davis, et al, 2006; Tassone, Pan, Amiri, et al, 2008). The availability of this test will likely facilitate expansion of the newborn screening in other high-risk populations (Hagerman, Berry-Kravis, Kaufmann, et al, 2009).

Nursing Care Management

Because CI is a fairly consistent finding in individuals with fragile X syndrome, the care for these families is the same as that for any child with intellectual disability. Because the disorder is hereditary, genetic counseling is important to inform parents and siblings of the risks of transmission. In addition, any male or female with unexplained or nonspecific mental impairment should be referred for chromosomal analysis and DNA testing, as well as appropriate genetic counseling. Families with a member affected by the disorder should be referred to the National Fragile X Foundation.*

▌SENSORY IMPAIRMENT

HEARING IMPAIRMENT

Hearing impairment is one of the most common disabilities in the United States. An estimated 3 in 1000 infants have hearing

*925-938-9300, 800-688-8765; fax: 925-938-9315; www.fragilex.org.

loss of varying degrees (Gregg, Wiorek, and Arvedson, 2004; Tierney and Brown, 2008). For those patients admitted to the neonatal intensive care unit, the incidence rises to approximately 2 to 4 per 100 neonates (Cunningham, Cox, Committee on Practice and Ambulatory Medicine, et al, 2003). There are about 1 million children with hearing impairment ranging in age from birth to 21 years in the United States. Almost a third of these children have other disabilities, such as visual or cognitive impairments.

Definition and Classification

Hearing impaired is a general term indicating the presence of disability that may range in severity from slight to profound hearing loss. *Severe to profound hearing loss* describes a person whose hearing disability precludes successful processing of linguistic information through audition, with or without use of a hearing aid. *Slight to moderately severe hearing loss* describes a person who has residual hearing sufficient to enable successful processing of linguistic information through audition, generally with the use of a hearing aid. Hearing-impaired persons who are speech impaired tend not to have a physical speech defect other than that caused by the inability to hear.

Hearing defects may be classified according to etiology, pathology, or symptom severity. Each is important in terms of treatment, possible prevention, and rehabilitation.

Etiology

A number of prenatal and postnatal conditions can cause hearing loss. It is often associated with a family history of childhood hearing impairment, anatomic malformations of the head or neck, low birth weight, severe perinatal asphyxia, perinatal infection (cytomegalovirus, rubella, herpes, syphilis, toxoplasmosis, and bacterial meningitis), maternal prenatal substance abuse, chronic ear infection, cerebral palsy, Down syndrome, or administration of ototoxic drugs (Haddad, 2007; Smith, Bale, and White, 2005). In addition, high-risk neonates who survive once-fatal prenatal or perinatal conditions may be susceptible to hearing loss from the disorder or its treatment. For example, sensorineural hearing loss may result from exposure to the continuous humming noises or high noise levels associated with incubators, oxygen hoods, or intensive care units, especially when combined with the use of potentially ototoxic antibiotics.

Environmental noise is a special concern. Sounds loud enough to damage sensitive hair cells of the inner ear can produce irreversible hearing loss. Very loud, brief noise, such as gunfire, can cause immediate, severe, and permanent loss of hearing. Longer exposure to less intense but still hazardous sounds, such as loud persistent music via headphones, sound systems, concerts, or industrial noises, can also produce hearing loss (Daniel, 2007; Holte, 2003; Kenna, 2004). The exact sound level that produces hearing loss is unknown.

Pathology

Disorders of hearing are categorized according to the location of the defect. Conductive or middle ear hearing loss results from interference with transmission of sound to or by the middle ear. It is the most common of all types of hearing loss and most frequently is a result of recurrent serous otitis media.

Conductive hearing impairment mainly involves interference with the loudness of sound.

Sensorineural hearing loss involves damage to the inner ear structures or the auditory nerve. The most common causes are congenital defects of inner ear structures and consequences of acquired conditions, such as kernicterus, infection, administration of ototoxic drugs, or exposure to excessive noise. Sensorineural hearing loss results in distortion of sound and problems in auditory discrimination. Although the child hears some of everything going on around him or her, the sounds are distorted, which severely affects discrimination and comprehension.

Mixed conductive-sensorineural hearing loss results from interference with transmission of sound in the middle ear and along neural pathways. It frequently results from recurrent otitis media and its complications.

Central auditory imperception includes all hearing losses for which defects in the conductive or sensorineural structures are not demonstrated. They are usually divided into organic and functional losses. In the organic type of central auditory imperception, the defect involves the reception of auditory stimuli along the central pathways and the processing of the message into meaningful communication. Examples are aphasia, the inability to express ideas in written or verbal form; agnosia, the inability to interpret sound correctly; and dysacusis, difficulty in processing details of sound or in discriminating among sounds. The functional type of hearing loss has no organic lesion to explain a central auditory loss. A functional hearing loss may occur in conversion disorder (an unconscious withdrawal from hearing to block remembrance of a traumatic event).

Symptom Severity

Hearing impairment is expressed in terms of the decibel (dB), a unit of loudness (Table 24-4). It is measured at various sound frequencies, such as 500, 1000, and 2000 cycles/sec, the critical listening range for speech. Hearing impairment can be classified according to hearing level (the individual's hearing threshold as measured by an audiometer) and the degree of symptom severity as it affects speech (Table 24-5). These classifications offer only general guidelines regarding the effect of the impairment on any individual child, because children differ greatly in their ability to use residual hearing.

Therapeutic Management

Treatment of hearing loss depends on the cause and type of hearing impairment. Many conductive hearing defects respond to medical or surgical treatment, such as antibiotic therapeutic management. When conductive loss is permanent, hearing can be improved with the use of a hearing aid to amplify sound.

Treatment for sensorineural hearing loss is much less satisfactory. Because the defect is not one of sound intensity, hearing aids are of less value in this type of defect. The use of cochlear implants (surgically implanted prosthetic devices) provides a sensation of hearing for children with severe to profound hearing loss (Hayes, Geers, Treiman, et al, 2009; Zeng and Liu, 2006). Children with sensorineural hearing loss have damage to the tiny hair cells lining the cochlea or to nerve cells that transmit auditory stimuli to the brain. Therefore hearing aids often provide little benefit, because even amplified sounds cannot be processed as a result of damage to the inner ear. A cochlear implant bypasses the damage and directly stimulates undamaged auditory nerve fibers that transmit signals to the brain, where they can be perceived as sound. Technologic refinements have produced multichannel cochlear implants that stimulate the auditory nerve at multiple locations. This produces improved processing of different frequencies represented in speech sounds so the individual can better understand and develop oral speech (Hayes, Geers, Treiman, et al, 2009; Winters, Collett, and Myers, 2005). Implantation of cochlear devices as early as possible in children with congenital or prelingual hearing impairment appears to facilitate development of speech (Haensel, Engelke, Ottenjann, et al, 2005; Hayes, Geers, Treiman, et al, 2009; Winters, Collett, and Myers, 2005).

TABLE 24-4	INTENSITY OF SOUNDS EXPRESSED IN DECIBELS
DECIBELS	**REPRESENTATIVE SOUNDS**
0	Softest sound normal ear can hear
10	Heartbeat, rustling of leaves
20	Whisper at 1.5 m (5 ft)
30-45	Normal conversation
60	Noise in average restaurant
70-80	Street noises
80	Loud radio in home
90-100	Train
120	Thunder, rock music
140	Jet plane during departure
>140	Pain threshold

TABLE 24-5	CLASSIFICATION OF HEARING LOSS BASED ON SYMPTOM SEVERITY
DEGREE OF LOSS— HEARING LEVEL (dB)	**EFFECT**
Slight—16-25	Has difficulty hearing faint or distant speech
	Usually is unaware of hearing difficulty
	Likely to achieve in school but may have problems
	No speech defects
Mild to moderate—26-55	May have speech difficulties
	Understands face-to-face conversational speech at 3-5 ft
Moderately severe— 56-70	Unable to understand conversational speech unless loud
	Considerable difficulty with group or classroom discussion
	Requires special speech training
Severe—71-90	May hear a loud voice if nearby
	May be able to identify loud environmental noises
	Can distinguish vowels but not most consonants
	Requires speech training
Profound—91	May hear only loud sounds
	Requires extensive speech training

Nursing Care Management

Assess for Hearing Concerns

Assessment of children for hearing impairment is a critical nursing responsibility. Identification of a hearing loss within the first 3 to 6 months of life is essential to facilitate language and educational development for children with hearing impairments (Bradham and Bess, 2004; Kenna, 2004; Tierney and Brown, 2008). Assessment involves (1) identifying those children who by virtue of their history are at risk (Box 24-7), (2) observing for behaviors that indicate a hearing loss, and (3) screening all children for auditory function. This discussion focuses on the development and behavior associated with hearing impairment. There is controversy regarding which children should be assessed and when they should be assessed. The Joint Committee on Infant Hearing (2000) issued guidelines on auditory screening of newborns and infants to detect early hearing loss and implement intervention programs.

Infancy. At birth the nurse can observe the neonate's response to auditory stimuli as evidenced by the startle reflex, head turning, eye blinking, and cessation of body movement. The intensity of the infant's response may vary, depending on the state of alertness. However, a consistent absence of a reaction should lead to suspicion of hearing loss. Other clinical manifestations of hearing impairment in the infant are summarized in Box 24-8.

Childhood. The child who is profoundly hearing impaired is much more likely to have the condition diagnosed during infancy than is the child who is less severely affected. If the defect is not detected during early childhood, the likelihood is that it will be discovered after entry into school, when the child has difficulty in learning. Unfortunately, some children with hearing impairments are erroneously placed in special classes for students with learning disabilities or CI. Therefore it is essential that the nurse suspect a hearing impairment in any child who demonstrates the behaviors listed in Box 24-8.

Of primary importance is the effect of hearing impairment on speech development. A child with a mild conductive hearing loss may speak fairly clearly but in a loud, monotone voice. A child with a sensorineural defect usually has difficulty in articulation. For example, inability to hear higher frequencies may lead the child to pronounce the word *spoon* as *poon.* Children with articulation problems need to have their hearing tested.

! NURSING ALERT

Stress to parents the importance of storing batteries for hearing aids in a safe location out of reach of children and of teaching children not to remove the battery from the hearing aid (or supervising young children when they do so). Battery ingestion requires immediate emergency management.

! NURSING ALERT

When parents express concern about their child's hearing and speech development, refer the child for a hearing evaluation. Absence of well-formed syllables *(da, na, yaya)* by 11 months of age should result in immediate referral.

BOX 24-7 RISK CRITERIA FOR SENSORINEURAL HEARING IMPAIRMENT IN YOUNG CHILDREN

Neonates (Birth to 28 Days)

Family history of congenital or delayed-onset childhood sensorineural impairment

Congenital infection known or suspected to be associated with sensorineural hearing impairment, such as toxoplasmosis, syphilis, rubella, and cytomegalovirus or herpes infection

Craniofacial anomalies, including morphologic abnormalities of the pinna and ear canal, absent philtrum, low hairline

Birth weight less than 1500 g (3.3 lb)

Hyperbilirubinemia at a level exceeding indication for exchange transfusion

Administration of ototoxic medications, including but not limited to the aminoglycosides, for more than 5 days (e.g., gentamicin, tobramycin, kanamycin, streptomycin) and use of loop diuretics in combination with aminoglycosides

Bacterial meningitis

Severe depression at birth, which may include infants with Apgar scores of 0 to 3 at 5 minutes and those who fail to initiate spontaneous respiration by 10 minutes or those with hypotonia persisting to 2 hours of age

Mechanical ventilation for 10 days or longer (e.g., persistent pulmonary hypertension)

Stigmata or other findings associated with a syndrome known to include sensorineural hearing loss (e.g., Waardenburg or Usher syndrome)

Maternal prenatal alcohol abuse

Infants (29 Days to 2 Years)

Parent or caregiver concern regarding hearing, speech, language, and/or developmental delay

Bacterial meningitis

Neonatal risk factors that may be associated with progressive sensorineural hearing loss (e.g., cytomegalovirus infection, prolonged mechanical ventilation, and inherited disorders)

Head trauma, especially with either longitudinal or transverse fracture of the temporal bone

Stigmata or other findings associated with syndromes known to include sensorineural hearing loss (e.g., Waardenburg or Usher syndrome)

Administration of ototoxic medications, including but not limited to the aminoglycosides, for more than 5 days (e.g., gentamicin, tobramycin, kanamycin, streptomycin) and use of loop diuretics in combination with aminoglycosides

Neurodegenerative disorders such as neurofibromatosis, myoclonic epilepsy, Werdnig-Hoffmann disease, Tay-Sachs disease, Niemann-Pick disease, any metachromatic leukodystrophy, or any infantile demyelinating neuropathy

Childhood infectious diseases known to be associated with sensorineural hearing loss (e.g., mumps, measles)

From American Speech-Language Hearing Association: Joint Committee on Infant Hearing 1990 position statement, *ASHA* 33(Suppl 5):3-6, 1991.

Promote the Communication Process

The nurse's initial role in rehabilitation is to encourage the family to participate in an auditory training program.* Rehabilitation training provides assistance in learning appropriate methods for improving communication, such as use of

---

*Home training correspondence programs are sponsored by the John Tracy Clinic, 806 W. Adams Blvd., Los Angeles, CA 90007; 213-748-5481, 800-522-4582; fax: 213-749-1651; TTY: 213-747-2924; **www. johntracyclinic.org.**

BOX 24-8   CLINICAL MANIFESTATIONS OF HEARING IMPAIRMENT

Infants

Lack of startle or blink reflex to a loud sound
Failure to be awakened by loud environmental noises
Failure to localize a source of sound by 6 months of age
Absence of babble or inflections in voice by age 7 months
General indifference to sound
Lack of response to the spoken word; failure to follow verbal directions
Response to loud noises as opposed to the voice

Children

Use of gestures rather than verbalization to express desires, especially after age 15 months
Failure to develop intelligible speech by age 24 months
Monotone speech quality, unintelligible speech, lessened laughter
Vocal play, head banging, or foot stamping for vibratory sensation
Yelling or screeching to express pleasure, annoyance (tantrums), or need
Asking to have statements repeated or answering them incorrectly
Greater response to facial expression and gestures than to verbal explanation
Avoidance of social interaction; frequent puzzlement and unhappiness in such situations; preference for playing alone
Inquiring, sometimes confused facial expression
Suspicious alertness, sometimes interpreted as paranoia, alternating with cooperation
Frequent stubbornness because of lack of comprehension
Irritability at not making self understood
Shy, timid, and withdrawn behavior
Frequent appearance of being "dreamy," "in a world of his or her own," or markedly inattentive

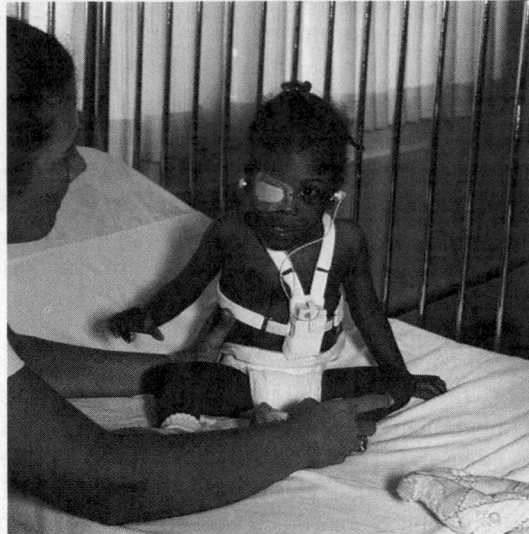

Fig. 24-7 On-the-body hearing aids are convenient for young children, such as this child with severe bilateral hearing loss. Note eye patch for strabismus.

hearing aids, lipreading, sign language, and speech and language therapy.

Hearing Aids. Nurses, especially those who care for hearing impaired children who are hospitalized, should be familiar with the types of hearing aids and their basic care and handling.* Types of aids include those worn in or behind the ear, models that are incorporated into an eyeglass frame, and types worn on the body with a wire connection to the ear (Fig. 24-7). One of the most common problems with a hearing aid is acoustic feedback, an annoying whistling usually caused by improper fit of the ear mold. Sometimes the whistling may be at a frequency that the child cannot hear but that is annoying to others. In this case, if children are old enough, they are told of the noise and asked to readjust the aid.

> **NURSING TIP** To reduce or eliminate whistling from a hearing aid, try removing and reinserting the aid, making certain that no hair is caught between the ear mold and canal; cleaning the ear mold or ear; or lowering the volume of the aid.

As children grow older, they may be self-conscious about the device. Make every effort to ensure that the aid is inconspicuous, such as by styling the hair appropriately to cover behind-the-ear or in-the-ear models, and providing attractive frames

*Information about hearing aids is available from the International Hearing Society, 16880 Middlebelt Road, Suite 4, Livonia, MI 48154; 734-522-7200, fax: 734-522-0200; http://ihsinfo.org.

for glasses with connected hearing aids. Give children responsibility for the care of the device as soon as they are able, since fostering independence is a primary goal of rehabilitation.

Lipreading. Although the child may become an expert at lipreading, only about 40% of spoken words are understood, and less if the speaker has an accent, mustache, or beard. Exaggerating pronunciation or speaking in an altered rhythm further lessens comprehension. Parents can help the child understand the spoken word by using the suggestions in the Nursing Care Guidelines box. The child learns to supplement the spoken word through sensitivity to visual cues, primarily body language and facial expression (e.g., tightening of the lips, muscle tension, and eye contact).

NURSING CARE GUIDELINES

Facilitating Lipreading

- Attract child's attention before speaking; use light touch to signal speaker's presence.
- Stand close to child.
- Face child directly or move to a 45-degree angle.
- Stand still; do not walk back and forth or turn away to point or look elsewhere.
- Establish eye contact and show interest.
- Speak at eye level and with good lighting on speaker's face.
- Be certain nothing interferes with speech patterns, such as chewing food or gum.
- Speak clearly and at a slow and even rate.
- Use facial expression to assist in conveying messages.
- Keep sentences short.
- Rephrase message if child does not understand the words.

Cued Speech. The cued speech method of communication is an adjunct to straight lipreading. It uses hand signals to help the hearing impaired child distinguish between words that look alike when formed by the lips (e.g., *mat, bat*). It is most commonly employed with hearing impaired children who are using speech rather than those who are nonverbal.

Sign Language. Sign language, such as American Sign Language (ASL) or British Sign Language (BSL), is a visual-gestural language that uses hand signals that roughly correspond to specific words and concepts in the English language. Encourage family members to learn signing, since using or watching hands requires much less concentration than lipreading or talking. Also, a symbol method enables some hearing impaired children to learn more and to learn faster.

Speech and Language Therapy. The most formidable task in the education of a child with profound hearing impairment is learning to speak. Speech is learned through a multisensory approach, using visual, tactile, kinesthetic, and auditory stimulation. Because the usual mechanism for learning language (imitation and reinforcement) is not available to the hearing impaired child, systematic formal education is required. Encourage parents to participate fully in the learning process.

Additional Aids. Everyday activities present problems for older children with hearing impairment. For example, they may not be able to hear the telephone, doorbell, or alarm clock. Several commercial devices are available to help them adjust to these dilemmas. Flashing lights can be attached to a telephone or doorbell to signal its ringing. Trained hearing ear dogs can assist hearing impaired individuals by alerting them to sounds such as someone approaching, a moving car, a signal to wake up, or a child's cry. Special teletypewriters (TTY) or telecommunications devices (TDD) help hearing impaired people communicate with each other over the telephone; the typed message is conveyed via the telephone lines and displayed on a small screen.*

Any audiovisual medium presents dilemmas for these children, who can see the picture but cannot hear the message. With closed captioning, however, a special decoding device is attached to the television, and the audio portion of a program is translated into subtitles that appear on the screen.

As children learn to compensate for their lack of hearing, they become extremely sensitive to visual and vibratory changes. They often know when another person wishes to talk to them because the person will walk close by but not pass. They learn to be alert to the approach of other people by seeing their shadows or feeling the vibrations of their footsteps. They are acutely aware of facial expressions and may comprehend the unspoken word more quickly than the spoken word.

Socialization. Socialization is extremely important to the child's development. If children attend a special school for the hearing impaired, they are able to socialize with peers in that setting. Classmates become a potential source of close friendships because they communicate more easily among themselves. Encourage parents to promote these relationships whenever possible.

Children with a hearing impairment may need special help in school or social activities. For those children wearing hearing aids, keep background noise to a minimum. Because many of these children are able to attend regular classes, the teacher may need assistance in adapting methods of teaching for the child's benefit. The school nurse is often in an optimum position to emphasize methods of facilitated communication, such as lipreading (see Nursing Care Guidelines box, p. 926). Because group projects and audiovisual teaching aids may hinder the hearing impaired child's learning, carefully evaluate the use of these educational methods.

In a group setting, it is helpful for the other members to sit in a semicircle in front of the hearing impaired child. Because one of the difficulties in following a group discussion is that the hearing impaired child is unaware of who will speak next, someone should point out each speaker. Speakers can also be given numbers, or their names can be written down as each person talks. If one person writes down the main topic of the discussion, the child is able to follow lipreading more closely. Such practices can increase the child's ability to participate in sports, in group projects, and in clubs such as scouts.

Support the Child and Family

Once the diagnosis of hearing impairment is made, parents may need extensive support to adjust to the shock of learning about their child's disability and an opportunity to realize the extent of the hearing loss. If the hearing loss occurs during childhood, the child also requires sensitive, supportive care during the long and often difficult adjustment to this sensory loss. Early rehabilitation is one of the best strategies for fostering adjustment. Progress in learning communication may not always coincide with emotional adjustment, however. Depression or anger is common, and such feelings are a normal part of the grieving process. Parent support groups are often helpful because other parents have dealt with the same issues and can offer practical advice and emotional support.† (See Chapter 22 for an extensive discussion of the emotional support of the child and family.)

Care for the Child During Hospitalization

The needs of the hospitalized child with a hearing impairment are the same as those of any other child, but the disability presents special challenges to the nurse (see Critical Thinking Exercise). For example, verbal explanations must be supplemented using tactile and visual aids, such as books or actual demonstration and practice. Children's understanding of the explanation needs to be constantly reassessed. If their verbal skills are poorly developed, they can answer questions through drawing, writing, or gesturing. For example, if the nurse is attempting to clarify where a spinal tap is done, ask the child to point to where the procedure will be done on the body. Because hearing impaired children often need more time to grasp the full meaning of an explanation, the nurse needs to be patient, allowing ample time for understanding.

When communicating with the child, the nurse should use the same principles as those outlined for facilitating lipreading. Ideally nurses without foreign accents should be assigned to

---

*Directory listings stating "TDD or TTY only" before a telephone number indicate that regular telephone use is not possible; "TDD or TTY and voice" indicates that both TDD-TTY users and speaking-hearing people can use the telephone number. Additional information is available from the National Captioning Institute, 3725 Concord Pkwy., Suite 100, Chantilly, VA 20151; voice/TTY: 703-917-7600; fax: 703-917-9853; www.ncicap.org.

†The Alexander Graham Bell Association for the Deaf and Hard of Hearing has a free resource kit designed for parents of infants or toddlers newly identified as deaf and hard-of-hearing. The kit is available by contacting the office at www.oraldeafed.org/info/agbell.html.

? CRITICAL THINKING EXERCISE

Hearing Impairment

Four-year-old Jason has a severe congenital hearing impairment. Jason has been admitted to the outpatient surgery postanesthesia care unit (PACU) after a herniorrhaphy and regional block. As he emerges from anesthesia, he becomes more and more agitated.

1. Evidence—Is there sufficient evidence to draw conclusions about Jason's increasing agitation after surgery?
2. Assumptions—Describe an underlying assumption about each of the following:
   a. Severe congenital hearing impairment in a preschool child
   b. Preschooler with severe congenital hearing impairment recovering in the PACU after surgery
   c. Preschooler with severe congenital hearing impairment recovering from herniorrhaphy and after regional block.
3. What priorities for nursing care should be established for Jason?
4. Does the evidence support your nursing intervention?

care for the child. The child's hearing aid is checked to ensure that it is working properly. If it is necessary to awaken the child at night, the nurse should gently shake the child or turn on the hearing aid before waking the child. The nurse should always make certain that the child can see him or her before any procedures, even routine ones such as changing a diaper or regulating an infusion. It is important to remember that the child may not be aware of the nurse's presence until alerted through visual or tactile cues.

Ideally parents should room with the child. However, the nurse must convey to them that this is not done for the nurse's convenience but for the child's benefit. Although the parents' aid can be enlisted in familiarizing the child with the hospital and explaining procedures, the nurse should also talk directly to the youngster, encouraging expression of feelings about the experience. If the child's speech is difficult to understand, try to become familiar with his or her pronunciation of words. Parents often can help by explaining the child's usual speech habits. Nonverbal communication devices that employ pictures or words to which the child can point are also available. The nurse can also make boards by drawing pictures or writing on cardboard the words representing common needs, such as parent, food, water, and toilet.

The nurse has a special role as child advocate for the hearing impaired and is in a strategic position to alert other health care team members and other patients to the child's special needs regarding communication. For example, the nurse should accompany other practitioners on visits to the child's room to ensure that they speak to the child and that the child understands what is said. Not infrequently, caregivers forget that the child has the ability to perceive and learn despite a hearing loss, and consequently they communicate only with the parents. As a result, the child's needs and feelings remain unrecognized and unaddressed.

Because children with hearing impairment may have difficulty forming social relationships with other children, introduce the child to roommates and encourage them to play. The hospital setting can provide growth-promoting opportunities for social relationships. With the assistance of a child life specialist, the child can learn new recreational activities, experiment with group games, and engage in therapeutic play. Playing with puppets or dollhouses, role playing with dress-up clothes, building with a hammer and nails, finger painting, playing with syringes, and participating in water play can help the child express feelings that previously were suppressed.

Assist in Measures to Prevent Hearing Impairment

A primary nursing role is prevention of hearing loss. Because the most common cause of impaired hearing is chronic otitis media, it is essential to institute appropriate measures to treat existing infections and prevent recurrences. (See Chapter 32.) Children with a history of ear or respiratory tract infections or any other condition known to increase the risk of hearing impairment should receive periodic auditory testing.

To prevent the causes of hearing loss that begin prenatally and perinatally, pregnant women need counseling regarding the necessity for early prenatal care, including genetic counseling regarding known familial disorders; avoidance of all ototoxic drugs, especially during the first trimester; testing to rule out syphilis, rubella, and blood incompatibility; medical management of maternal diabetes; strict control of alcoholism; and adequate dietary intake. Stress the need for routine immunization during childhood to eliminate the possibility of acquired sensorineural loss from rubella, mumps, or measles (encephalitis).

Exposure to excessive noise pollution is a well-established cause of sensorineural hearing loss. The nurse should routinely assess the possibility of environmental noise pollution and advise children and parents of the potential danger. When individuals engage in activities associated with high-intensity noise, such as model airplane flying, target shooting, or snowmobiling, they should wear ear protection such as earmuffs or earplugs—not ordinary dry cotton, although any protection is better than none. Even common household equipment, such as lawn mowers and power vacuum cleaners, can be harmful.

! NURSING ALERT

Suspect hazardous noise if the listener experiences (1) difficulty in communication while hearing the sound, (2) ringing in the ears (tinnitus) after exposure to the sound, or (3) muffled hearing after leaving the sound.

VISUAL IMPAIRMENT

Visual impairment is a common problem during childhood. In North America the prevalence of serious visual impairment in the pediatric population is estimated to be between 30 and 64 children per 100,000 population. Visual impairment such as refractive error, amblyopia, strabismus, and astigmatism affects 5% to 10% of all preschoolers (Tingley, 2007). Early detection and prompt treatment of ocular disorders in children are important to avoid lifelong visual impairment. The nurse's role is one of assessment, detection, prevention, referral, and, in some instances, rehabilitation.

Definition and Classification

Visual impairment has many causes and may be due to multiple defects affecting any structure or function along the visual pathways (Olitsky, Hug, and Smith, 2007a). **Legal blindness** is defined as a visual acuity of 20/200 or lower or a visual field of

20 degrees or less in the better eye. **Partial sight** is defined as a visual acuity of better than 20/200 but worse than 20/70 in the better eye with correction. These children can generally use normal-sized print, since near vision is nearly always better than distance vision. **Visual impairment** is a general term that includes both these categories. Children who are visually impaired, including those who are legally blind, often have considerable useful vision and are able to use printed material, such as large-print books, as their major method of learning. It is important to keep in mind that legal blindness is not a medical diagnosis but a legal definition. Educational and governmental agencies in the United States use the legal definition of blindness to determine tax status, eligibility for entrance into special schools, and eligibility for financial aid and other benefits.

Etiology

A number of genetic and prenatal or postnatal conditions can cause visual impairment. These include perinatal infections (herpes, chlamydial infection, gonorrhea, rubella, syphilis, or toxoplasmosis); retinopathy of prematurity; trauma; postnatal infections (meningitis); and disorders such as sickle cell disease, juvenile rheumatoid arthritis, Tay-Sachs disease, albinism, and retinoblastoma. In many instances, such as with refractive errors, the cause of the defect is unknown.

Refractive errors are the most common type of visual disorder in children. The term **refraction** means bending and refers to the bending of light rays as they pass through the lens of the eye. Normally light rays enter the lens and fall directly on the retina. However, in refractive disorders the light rays fall either in front of the retina (myopia) or beyond it (hyperopia). Other eye problems, such as strabismus, may or may not include refractive errors, but they are important because, if untreated, they result in visual impairment from amblyopia. Box 24-9 summarizes these along with other, less frequent visual disorders. In addition to these disorders, other visual problems can result from infection or trauma.

Trauma

Trauma is a common cause of visual impairment in children. Injuries to the eyeball and adnexa (supporting or accessory structures, such as eyelids, conjunctiva, and lacrimal glands)

BOX 24-9   TYPES OF VISUAL IMPAIRMENT

Refractive Errors

Myopia
Nearsightedness—Ability to see objects clearly at close range but not at a
 distance

Pathophysiology
Results when eyeball is elongated, which causes image to fall in front of retina

Clinical Manifestations
Excessive eye rubbing
Head tilt or forward head thrust
Difficulty reading or doing other close work
Reading with books held close to eyes
Writing or coloring with head close to table
Clumsiness; walking into objects
Blinking more than is usual or irritability when doing close work
Inability to see objects clearly
Poor performance in school, especially in subjects that require demonstration,
 such as arithmetic
Dizziness
Headaches
Nausea after doing close work

Treatment
Corrected with biconcave lenses that focus rays on retina
May be corrected with laser surgery

Hyperopia
Farsightedness—Ability to see objects at a distance but not at close range

Pathophysiology
Results when eyeball is too short, which causes image to focus beyond retina

Clinical Manifestations
Because of accommodative ability, child can usually see objects at all ranges
Most children normally hyperopic until about 7 years of age

Treatment
When required, corrected with convex lenses that focus rays on retina
May be corrected with laser surgery

Astigmatism
Unequal curvatures in refractive apparatus

Pathophysiology
Results from unequal curvatures in cornea or lens that cause light rays to bend
 in different directions

Clinical Manifestations
Depend on severity of refractive error in each eye
Possible clinical manifestations of myopia

Treatment
Corrected with special lenses that compensate for refractive errors
May be corrected with laser surgery

Anisometropia
Different refractive strength in each eye

Pathophysiology
May lead to amblyopia as weaker eye is used less

Clinical Manifestations
Depend on severity of refractive error in each eye
Possible clinical manifestations of myopia

Treatment
Treated with corrective lenses, preferably contact lenses, to improve vision in
 each eye so they work as a unit
May be corrected with laser surgery

Amblyopia
Lazy eye—Reduced visual acuity in one eye

Pathophysiology
Results when one eye does not receive sufficient stimulation
Each retina receives different images, which results in diplopia (double vision)
Brain accommodates by suppressing less intense image
Visual cortex eventually does not respond to visual stimulation, with loss of
 vision in that eye

Clinical Manifestations
Poor vision in affected eye

Continued

BOX 24-9 TYPES OF VISUAL IMPAIRMENT—cont'd

Amblyopia—cont'd

Treatment

Preventable if treatment of primary visual defect, such as anisometropia or strabismus, begins before 6 years of age

Strabismus

"Squint" or cross-eye—Malalignment of eyes
Esotropia—Inward deviation of eye
Exotropia—Outward deviation of eye

Pathophysiology

May result from muscle imbalance or paralysis, poor vision, or congenital defect
Because visual axes are not parallel, brain receives two images, and amblyopia can result

Clinical Manifestations

Squinting of eyelids together or frowning
Difficulty in focusing from one distance to another
Inaccurate judgment in picking up objects
Inability to see print or moving objects clearly
Closing of one eye to see
Tilting of head to one side
If combined with refractive errors, any of the manifestations listed for refractive errors
Diplopia
Photophobia
Dizziness
Headaches
Crossed eyes

Treatment

Depends on cause of strabismus
May involve occlusion therapy (patching stronger eye) or surgery to increase visual stimulation to weaker eye
Early diagnosis essential to prevent vision loss

Cataracts

Opacity of crystalline lens

Pathophysiology

Prevents light rays from entering eye and refracting on retina

Clinical Manifestations

Gradual decrease in ability to see objects clearly
Possible loss of peripheral vision
Nystagmus (with complete blindness)
Gray opacities of lens
Strabismus
Absence of red reflex

Treatment

Requires surgery to remove cloudy lens and replace it (with intraocular lens implant, removable contact lens, prescription glasses)
Must be treated early to prevent visual impairment from amblyopia

Glaucoma

Increased intraocular pressure

Pathophysiology

Congenital type results from defective development of some component related to flow of aqueous humor
Increased pressure on optic nerve causes eventual atrophy and visual impairment

Clinical Manifestations

Loss of peripheral vision; mostly seen in acquired types
Possible bumping into objects not directly in front
Perception of halos around objects
Possible complaint of mild pain or discomfort (severe pain, nausea, vomiting, if sudden rise in pressure)
Eye redness
Excessive tearing (epiphora)
Photophobia
Spasmodic winking (blepharospasm)
Corneal haziness
Enlarged eyeball (buphthalmos)

Treatment

Requires surgical treatment (goniotomy) to open outflow tracts
May require more than one procedure

---

can be classified as penetrating or nonpenetrating. Penetrating wounds are most often caused by sharp instruments, such as sticks, knives, or scissors; propulsive objects, such as firecrackers, guns, bows and arrows, or slingshots; or a blunt object. Devastating eye injuries have been caused by the popular gas-propulsion paintball guns and air-powered BB guns, used primarily by boys 11 to 15 years of age (Michaud and American Academy of Pediatrics, 2004; Listman, 2004; Olitsky, Hug, and Smith, 2007b). Nonpenetrating injuries may result from foreign objects in the eyes, lacerations, a blow from a blunt object (in baseball, softball, basketball, or racquet sports) or a fist, or thermal or chemical burns.

Treatment is directed toward preventing further ocular damage and is primarily the responsibility of the ophthalmologist. It involves adequate examination of the injured eye (with the child sedated or anesthetized in cases of severe injury); appropriate immediate intervention, such as removal of the foreign body or suturing of the laceration; and prevention of complications, such as administration of antibiotics or steroids and complete bed rest to allow the eye to heal and blood to reabsorb (see Emergency Treatment box). The prognosis varies depending on the type of injury. It is usually guarded in all cases of penetrating wounds because of the high risk of serious complications.

Infections

Infections of the adnexa and the structures of the eyeball or globe are not infrequent in children. The most common eye infection is conjunctivitis. (See Chapter 16.) Treatment is usually with ophthalmic antibiotics. Severe infections may require systemic antibiotic therapy. Steroids are used cautiously because they exacerbate viral infections such as herpes simplex, increasing the risk of damage to the involved structures.

Nursing Care Management

Nursing care of visually impaired children is a specialized area requiring additional training in vision testing and habilitation. However, general measures that focus on assessment, prevention, and rehabilitation of the child with visual impairment are every nurse's responsibility. In addition, nurses may have to care for a visually impaired child who is hospitalized and must know how to best meet the child's and family's special needs.

✚ EMERGENCY TREATMENT

Eye Injuries

Foreign Object

Examine eye for presence of a foreign body (evert upper lid to examine upper eye).

Remove a freely movable object with pointed corner of gauze pad lightly moistened with water.

Do not irrigate eye or attempt to remove a penetrating object (see later).

Caution child against rubbing eye.

Chemical Burns

Irrigate eye copiously with tap water for 20 minutes.

Evert upper lid to flush thoroughly.

Hold child's head with eye under tap of running lukewarm water.

Take to emergency department.

Have child rest with eyes closed.

Keep room darkened.

Ultraviolet Burns

If skin is burned, patch both eyes (make sure lids are completely closed); secure dressing with Kling bandages wrapped around head rather than with tape.

Have child rest with eyes closed.

Refer to an ophthalmologist.

Hematoma ("Black Eye")

Use flashlight to check for gross hyphema (hemorrhage into anterior chamber; visible fluid meniscus across iris; more easily seen in light-colored than in brown eyes).

Apply ice for first 24 hours to reduce swelling if no hyphema is present.

Refer to an ophthalmologist immediately if hyphema is present.

Have child rest with eyes closed.

Penetrating Injuries

Take child to emergency department.

Never remove an object that has penetrated eye.

Follow strict aseptic technique in examining eye.

Observe for:

- Aqueous or vitreous leaks (fluid leaking from point of penetration)
- Hyphema
- Shape and equality of pupils, reaction to light
- Prolapsed iris (not perfectly circular)

Apply Fox shield if available (not regular eye patch) and apply patch over unaffected eye to prevent bilateral movement.

Maintain bed rest with child in 30-degree Fowler position.

Caution child against rubbing eye.

Refer to ophthalmologist.

Assess for Visual Concerns

Assessment of children for visual impairment is a critical nursing responsibility. Discovery of a visual impairment as early as possible is essential to prevent social, physical, and psychologic damage to the child. Assessment involves (1) identifying those children who by virtue of their history are at risk; (2) observing for behaviors that indicate a vision loss; and (3) screening all children for visual acuity and signs of other ocular disorders, such as strabismus. Clinical manifestations of various types of visual problems are listed in Box 24-9. Chapter 6 discusses vision testing.

Infancy. At birth the nurse should observe the neonate's response to visual stimuli, such as following a light or object and cessation of body movement. The intensity of the response may vary, depending on the infant's state of alertness.

Of special importance in detecting visual impairment during infancy are parental concerns regarding visual responsiveness in their child. Their concerns, such as lack of eye contact from the infant, must be taken seriously. During infancy the child should be tested for strabismus. Lack of binocularity after 4 months of age is considered abnormal and must be treated to prevent amblyopia.

❗ NURSING ALERT

Suspect visual impairment in an infant who does not react to light and in a child of any age if parents express concern.

Childhood. Because the most common visual impairment during childhood is refractive error, testing for visual acuity is essential. The school nurse usually assumes major responsibility for vision screening in schoolchildren. In addition to assessing for refractive errors, the nurse should be aware of signs and symptoms that indicate other ocular problems. If the family is given a referral requesting further eye testing, the school nurse is responsible for follow-up concerning the recommendation.

Support the Child and Family

Learning that their child is visually impaired or only partially sighted precipitates an immense crisis for families. Of all types of disabilities, many people fear loss of sight the most. Vision is involved in almost every activity of daily living. Parents need support during the initial phase of learning about the diagnosis and help to gain a realistic understanding of their child's abilities. Encourage the family to investigate appropriate early intervention and educational programs for their child as soon as possible. Sources of information include state commissions for the blind; local schools for the blind; and the American Foundation for the Blind,* National Federation of the Blind,† National Association for Parents of Children with Visual Impairments,‡ National Association for Visually Handicapped,§ and American Council of the Blind.‖

With newly acquired visual impairment, children need a great deal of support to help them adjust to the disability. They are usually frightened and confused by the sudden or progressive loss of sight and benefit from an environment that provides security and familiarity.

Promote Parent-Child Attachment

A crucial time in the life of a visually impaired infant is when the infant and its parents are getting acquainted with each other. Pleasurable patterns of interaction between the infant and

---

*Two Penn Plaza, Suite 1102, New York, NY 10121; 212-502-7600, 800-232-5463; fax: 212-502-7777; www.afb.org.

†200 E. Wells St., Baltimore, MD 21230; 410-659-9314, fax: 410-685-5653; www.nfb.org.

‡PO Box 317, Watertown, MA 02471; 617-972-7441, 800-562-6265; fax: 617-972-7444; www.spedex.com/napvi.

§22 W. 21st St., 6th Floor, New York, NY 10010; 212-889-3141; fax: 212-727-2931; www.navh.org.

‖2200 Wilson Blvd., Suite 650, Arlington, VA 22201; 202-467-5081, 800-424-8666; fax: 202-465-5085; www.acb.org. In Canada contact CNIB, 1929 Bayview Ave., Toronto, Ontario M4G 3E8, Canada; 800-563-2642; fax: 416-480-7700; www.cnib.ca.

parents may be lacking if there is not enough reciprocity. For example, if a parent gazes fondly at the infant's face and seeks eye contact but the infant fails to respond because he or she cannot see the parent, a troubled cycle of responses may occur. The nurse can help parents learn to look for other cues that indicate the infant is responding to them, for example, blinking of the eyelids; acceleration or slowing of the activity level; change in respiratory patterns, such as faster or slower breathing when the parents come near; and production of throaty sounds by the infant when they speak to the infant. In time parents learn that the infant has unique ways of relating to them. Encourage them to show affection using nonvisual methods, such as talking or reading, cuddling, and walking the child.

Promote the Child's Optimum Development

Promoting the child's optimum development requires rehabilitation in a number of important areas. These include learning self-help skills and appropriate communication techniques to become independent. Although nurses may not be directly involved in such programs, they can provide direction and guidance to families regarding the availability of programs and the importance of promoting these activities in their child.

Development and Independence. Motor development depends on sight almost as much as verbal communication depends on hearing. Encourage parents to expose the infant with any sight to as many visual-motor experiences as possible from earliest infancy, such as by having the infant sit supported in an infant seat or swing and providing opportunities for holding up the head, sitting unsupported, reaching for objects, and crawling.

Despite visual impairment, a child can become independent in all aspects of self-care. The same principles used for promoting independence in sighted children apply, with additional emphasis given to nonvisual cues. For example, the child may need help in dressing, such as special arrangement of clothing for style coordination and Braille tags to distinguish colors and prints.

The visually impaired child also must learn to become independent in navigation. The two main techniques are the tapping method (use of a cane to survey the environment for direction and to avoid obstacles) and the use of guides, such as a human sighted guide or a dog guide (e.g., a Seeing Eye dog). Partially sighted children may benefit from ocular aids, such as a monocular telescope.

Play and Socialization. Visually impaired children do not learn to play automatically. Because they cannot imitate others or actively explore the environment as sighted children do, they depend much more on others to stimulate them and teach them how to play. Parents need help in selecting appropriate play materials, especially those that encourage fine and gross motor development and stimulate the senses of hearing, touch, and smell. Toys with educational value, such as dolls with various clothing closures, are especially useful.

Visually impaired children have the same needs for socialization as sighted children. Because they have little difficulty learning verbal skills, they are able to communicate with age-mates and participate in suitable activities. The nurse discusses with parents opportunities for socialization outside of the home, especially regular preschools. The trend is to include these children with sighted children to help them adjust to the outside world to promote eventual independence.

To compensate for inadequate stimulation, these children may develop self-stimulatory activities such as body rocking, finger flicking, or arm twirling. Discourage such habits because they delay the child's social acceptance. Behavior modification is often successful in reducing or eliminating the self-stimulatory activities.

Education. The main obstacle to learning is the child's total dependence on nonvisual cues. Although the child can learn via verbal lecturing, he or she is unable to read the written word or to write without special education. Therefore the child must rely on Braille, a system that uses raised dots to represent each letter and number. The child can read the Braille with the fingers and can write a message using a small typewriter-like device called a braillewriter. However, this type of communication is not useful for communicating with others unless they read Braille. A more portable system for written communication is the use of a Braille slate and stylus or a microcassette tape recorder. A recorder is especially helpful for leaving messages for others and for taking notes during classroom lectures. For mathematic calculations, portable calculators with voice synthesizers are available.*

Records and tapes are significant sources of reading material other than Braille books, which are large and cumbersome. The Library of Congress† has talking books, Braille books, and a special records program; these materials are available at many local and state libraries and directly from the Library of Congress. The talking book machine and tape player are provided at no cost to families, and there is no postage fee for returning the materials. Recording for the Blind and Dyslexic‡ also provides texts and tapes of books, which are helpful for secondary and college students who are visually impaired.

Learning to use a regular typewriter is another means of writing but has the disadvantage that the visually impaired person is unable to check the accuracy of the typing. Computers eliminate this drawback; a home computer with a voice synthesizer can speak each letter or word that has been typed.

The child with partial sight benefits from specialized visual aids that produce a magnified retinal image. The basic methods are accommodative techniques, such as bringing the object closer; devices such as special plus lenses, handheld and stand magnifiers, telescopes, and video projection systems; and the use of large-print materials. Special equipment is available to enlarge print. Information about services for the partially sighted is available from the National Association for Visually Handicapped and the American Foundation for the Blind. Children with diminished vision often prefer to do close work

---

*A catalog of numerous products for people with vision problems is available from Lighthouse International, 111 E. 59th St., New York, NY 10022-1202; 212-821-9200, 800-829-0500; fax: 212-821-9707; TTY: 212-821-9713; www.lighthouse.org.

†National Library Service for the Blind and Physically Handicapped, Library of Congress, 1291 Taylor St., NW, Washington, DC 20011; 202-707-5100, 888-657-7323; fax: 202-707-0712; TDD: 202-707-0744; www.loc.gov/nls. (State listings of libraries for visually impaired and physically handicapped readers, as well as other reference circulars, are available from this office.)

‡20 Roszel Road, Princeton, NJ 08540; 800-221-4792; www.rfbd.org.

without their glasses and compensate by bringing the object very near to their eyes. This should be allowed. The exception is the child with vision in only one eye, who should always wear glasses for protection. The National Federation of the Blind* has information on job opportunities for the visually impaired.

Care for the Child During Hospitalization

Because nurses are more likely to care for children who are hospitalized for procedures that involve temporary loss of vision, the following discussion concentrates primarily on the needs of such children. The nursing care objectives in either situation are to (1) reassure the child and family throughout every phase of treatment, (2) orient the child to the surroundings, (3) provide a safe environment, and (4) encourage independence. Whenever possible, the same nurse should care for the child to ensure consistency in the approach. These same principles also apply to caring for any visually impaired child who requires hospitalization.

When sighted children temporarily lose their vision, almost every aspect of the environment becomes bewildering and frightening. They often rely on nonvisual senses for help in adjusting to the visual impairment without the benefit of any special training. Nurses have a major role in minimizing the effects of temporary loss of vision. They need to talk to the child about everything that is occurring, emphasizing aspects of procedures that are felt or heard. They should always identify themselves as soon as they enter the room and before they approach the child. Because unfamiliar sounds are especially frightening, these are explained. Encourage parents to room with their child and participate in the child's care. A familiar object, such as a teddy bear or doll, from home will help lessen the strangeness of the hospital. As soon as the child is able to be out of bed, orient him or her to the immediate surroundings. If the child is able to see on admission, take this opportunity to point out significant aspects of the room. Encourage the child to practice ambulation with the eyes closed to become accustomed to this experience.

The room is arranged with safety in mind. For example, place a stool or chair next to the bed to help the child climb into and out of bed. The furniture is always placed in the same position to prevent collisions. Remind cleaning personnel of the need to keep the room in order. If the child has difficulty navigating by feeling the walls, attach a rope from the bed to the point of destination, such as the bathroom. Attention to details such as well-fitting slippers and robes that do not hang on the floor is important to prevent tripping. Unlike the child who is visually impaired, these children are not familiar with navigating with a cane.

Encourage the child to be independent in self-care activities, especially if the visual loss may be prolonged or potentially permanent. For example, during bathing, the nurse sets up all the equipment and encourages the child to participate. At mealtime the nurse explains where each food item is on the tray, opens any special containers, and prepares cereal or toast, but encourages the child in self-feeding. Favorite finger foods, such as sandwiches, hamburgers, hot dogs, or pizza, may be good

selections. Praise the child for efforts at being cooperative and independent. Any improvements made in self-care, no matter how small, are stressed.

Provide appropriate recreational activities; a child life specialist, if available, can help with planning. Because children with temporary visual loss have a wide variety of play experiences to draw on, they are encouraged to select activities. For example, if they like to read, they may enjoy listening to books on tape or having someone read to them. If they prefer manual activity, they may appreciate playing with clay or building blocks or feeling different textures and naming them. Simple board and card games can be played if the child has a "seeing partner" or if the opponent helps with the game. Children should have familiar toys from home to play with, since familiar items are more easily manipulated than new ones. If parents wish to bring presents, they should be objects that stimulate hearing and touch, such as a radio, music box, or stuffed animal.

Occasionally children who are visual impaired come to the hospital for procedures to restore their vision. Although this is an extremely happy time, intervention is also required to help these children adjust to sight. They need an opportunity to take in all that they see. They should not be bombarded with visual stimuli. They may need to concentrate on people's faces or their own to become accustomed to this experience. They often need to talk about what they see and to compare the visual images with their mental ones. These children may also go through a period of depression, which must be respected and supported. Encourage them to discuss how it feels to see, especially seeing themselves.

Newly sighted children also need time to adjust to the ability to engage in activities that were impossible before. For example, they may prefer to use Braille to read, rather than learning a new visual approach, because of familiarity with the touch system. Eventually, as they learn to recognize letters and numbers, they will integrate these new skills into reading and writing. However, parents and teachers must be careful not to push them before they are ready. This principle applies to social relationships and physical activities as well as to learning situations.

Assist in Measures to Prevent Visual Impairment

An essential nursing goal is to prevent visual impairment. This involves many of the same interventions discussed under hearing impairment: (1) prenatal screening for pregnant women at risk, such as those with rubella or syphilis infection and family histories of genetic disorders associated with visual loss; (2) adequate prenatal and perinatal care to prevent prematurity and iatrogenic damage from excessive administration of oxygen; (3) periodic screening of all children, especially newborns through preschoolers, for congenital and acquired visual impairments caused by refractive errors, strabismus, and other disorders; (4) rubella immunization of all children; and (5) safety counseling regarding the common causes of ocular trauma. Safety counseling should include instruction regarding safe practices when working with, playing with, or carrying objects such as scissors, knives, and balls.

> **! NURSING ALERT**
>
> A helmet with a face mask should be required for children playing baseball, hockey, or football.

---

*For contact information, see footnote, p. 931.

After detection of eye problems, the nurse should encourage the family to prevent further ocular damage by undertaking corrective treatment. For the child with strabismus, this often necessitates occlusion patching of the stronger eye. Compliance with the procedure is greatest during the early preschool years. It is more difficult to encourage young school-age children to wear the occlusive patch because the poor visual acuity of the uncovered weaker eye interferes with schoolwork and the patch sets them apart from their peers. In school they benefit from being positioned favorably (closer to the chalkboard or primary instructional area) and being allowed extra time to read or complete an assignment. If treatment of the eye disorder requires instillation of ophthalmic medication, teach the family the correct procedure. (See Chapter 27.)

Children who need glasses to correct refractive errors need time to adjust to wearing these. Young children, who often pull glasses off, may benefit from the use of temporal pieces that wrap around the ears or an elastic strap attached to the frames and around the back of the head to hold the glasses on securely. Once children appreciate the value of clear vision, they are more likely to wear the corrective lenses.

Glasses should not interfere with activity. Special protective guards are available to prevent accidental injury during contact sports, and all corrective lenses should be made from safety glass, which is shatterproof. Often corrective lenses improve visual acuity so dramatically that children are able to compete more effectively in sports. This in itself is a tremendous inducement to continue wearing glasses.

Contact lenses are a popular alternative to conventional glasses. Several types are available, such as gas-permeable and soft lenses, which may be designed for daily or extended wear. Contact lenses offer several advantages over glasses, such as greater visual acuity, total corrected field of vision, convenience (especially with the extended-wear type), and optimum cosmetic benefit. Unfortunately, they are usually more expensive and require much more care than glasses, including considerable practice to learn techniques for insertion and removal. If they are prescribed, the nurse can be helpful in teaching parents or older children how to care for the lenses.

Because trauma is the leading cause of visual impairment, the nurse has the major responsibility for preventing further eye injury until the specific treatment is instituted. The major principles to follow when caring for an eye injury are outlined in the Emergency Treatment box, p. 931. Because patients with a serious eye injury fear visual loss, the nurse should stay with the child and family to provide support and reassurance.

HEARING-VISUAL IMPAIRMENT

The most traumatic sensory impairment is loss of both sight and hearing. Historically, one of the chief causes of visual and hearing impairment was congenital rubella syndrome, but immunization has decreased its incidence. Other cases usually occur when one congenital sensory impairment is combined with an acquired impairment, such as congenital visual impairment and acquired hearing deficit from meningitis, or congenital hearing impairment and acquired visual loss from an eye injury. Most children with multisensory impairments have

some residual hearing and vision to supplement the senses of touch, smell, and taste.

Combined auditory and visual impairments have profound effects on the child's development. They interfere with the normal sequence of physical, intellectual, and psychosocial growth. Although the child often achieves the usual motor milestones, they are delayed. Children only learn communication with specialized training. Finger spelling is one desirable method often taught to these children. Words are spelled letter by letter into the hearing-visually impaired child's hand, and the child spells out ideas to the other person. Another type of tactile communication is the Tadoma method, in which the child places a hand over the speaker's face and neck to monitor facial movements associated with speech production. Some children with residual hearing or vision impairment can learn to speak. Whenever possible, encourage speech because it allows communication with individuals not familiar with the preceding approaches.

Programs for these children vary. The John Tracy Clinic* offers a home correspondence course for parents, and the American Foundation for the Blind,† Helen Keller Services for the Blind,‡ Perkins School for the Blind,§ and Junior Blind of America‖ provide publications and various special services. The Library of Congress National Library Service for the Blind and Physically Handicapped¶ publishes a reference circular titled *Deaf-Blindness: National Resources and Organizations.*

Nursing Care Management

One of the major concerns of families with children who are hearing and visually impaired is helping them establish communication. The nurse is in a vital position to help parents with this goal. Because infants may not coo, laugh, or make directed eye movements, they are limited in the cues they can send and receive. Therefore initiating and maintaining communication is the caregiver's responsibility. The nurse discusses with parents behaviors that signal the infant's recognition of them, such as quieting behavior, blinking, and change in respiration. Encourage the parents to find ways of increasing stimulation for the child, especially cues that help the child identify each parent. For example, each person involved with the child should choose something that only he or she does, such as a kiss on the forehead or a stroke on the cheek. In this way the infant learns to discriminate among people in the environment.

Provide as many sensory experiences as possible, such as placing children in different positions during the day in relation to light and providing variation in stimuli so that they will be motivated to move toward, reach, touch, and explore the environment. Changing position also encourages muscle development and movement patterns. Bring sounds near and make them interesting to these children. For example, they can par-

---

*For contact information, see footnote, p. 925.
†For contact information, see footnote, p. 931.
‡141 Middleneck Road, Sands Point, NY 11050; voice/TTY: 516-944-8900; fax: 516-944-7302 (also regional offices); **www.helenkeller.org**.
§175 N. Beacon St., Watertown, MA 02472; 617-924-3434; fax: 617-926-2027; **www.perkins.org**.
‖5300 Angeles Vista Blvd., Los Angeles, CA 90043; 323-295-4555, 800-352-2290; fax: 323-296-0424; **www.juniorblind.org**.
¶For contact information see footnote, p. 932.

ticipate in hearing by placing the hand on a radio or on a person's throat. Consistent tactile cues should be associated with a change of position and activities so that the movement is experienced as a positive, nonthreatening experience.

Children who are hearing and visually impaired need secure, safe experiences while learning to walk and gain confidence. Once ambulatory, they need help in exploring the environment on a gradual, planned basis. After they succeed in becoming well oriented to the environment, they are ready for a plan of locomotion. Ambulation with a sighted guide, trailing (movement directed by touching objects, such as the wall), and cane walking are three methods. An individually planned mobility program is based on the child's age, needs, and functional status and is shared with the child's therapist, teachers, parents, and siblings.

The future prospects for hearing and visually impaired children are at best unpredictable. Sometimes congenital hearing and visual impairment is accompanied by other physical or neurologic handicaps, which further lessen the child's learning potential. The most favorable prognosis is for children with acquired hearing and visual impairments and few, if any, associated disabilities. Their learning capacity is greatly potentiated by their developmental progress before the sensory impairments and the assistance of a trained companion. Although total independence, including gainful vocational training, is the goal, some hearing and visually impaired children are unable to develop to this level. They may require lifelong parental or residential care. The nurse working with such families helps them deal with future goals for the child, including possible alternatives to home care during the parents' advancing years.

COMMUNICATION IMPAIRMENT

GENERAL CONCEPTS

Communication impairment is a broad term that refers to the inability to (1) receive or process symbol systems for the spoken word, (2) represent concepts or symbol systems, or (3) transmit and use symbol systems. In cases of severe communication impairment, the child may need other symbol systems, such as nonverbal methods (e.g., gestures, sign language, Braille), to substitute for the spoken word.

Because of the complexity of communication, various classification systems are available, and there is no universal agreement on one system. Basically a communication impairment may occur in language, speech, or hearing or any combination of these. The problems encountered when hearing is affected are discussed earlier in this chapter. Language primarily refers to the symbol system used to convey thoughts or feelings to others. The two major types are **receptive language**, or understanding the spoken word, and **expressive language**, or speaking verbal symbols. Speech is the oral production of language, including articulation of sounds, rhythm, and tone. Pragmatics involves the rules for the use of language (including nonverbal communication), as in social contexts.

Delayed development of language and speech is the most common symptom of developmental disability in children. Speech problems are more prevalent than language disorders, and both impairments decline as children grow older.

Communication impairment often occurs in conjunction with impairment in other developmental realms. In the absence of other affected domains, the term *developmental language disorder* may be used.

Etiology

The most common cause of communication impairment is CI, followed by hearing impairment. Other causes include (1) CNS dysfunction or injury, such as learning disabilities or traumatic brain injury; (2) autism; (3) childhood schizophrenia; (4) organic problems, such as cerebral palsy, cleft palate, vocal cord injury, and paralysis or foreshortening of the soft palate and uvula; and (5) some genetic disorders, such as cri du chat syndrome and Gilles de la Tourette syndrome. In some instances, such as in stuttering, the cause is unknown or speculative.

Language Impairment

Language disorders include impairment in:
- Assigning meaning to words (vocabulary)
- Organizing words into sentences
- Altering word forms to indicate tense, possession, and plurality

Examples of language disorders are failure to develop vocabulary at the expected age; a reduced vocabulary for age; use of poor sentence structure, such as "Me see dog"; or omission of words from a sentence, such as "Me fun." Such short or "telegraphic" phrases are normal during the first 2 years but should be replaced by more complete statements during the preschool years. Clinical manifestations of language disorders are listed in Box 24-10.

Speech Impairment

Speech impairments include differences from the norm in articulation, fluency, and voice production. Articulation errors are speech sounds that a child makes incorrectly or inappropriately. For example, the child may tend to distort or substitute a few consonants or blends, especially those that are learned last (s, l,

---

BOX 24-10   CLINICAL MANIFESTATIONS OF LANGUAGE DISORDERS

Assigning Meaning to Words
Failure to utter first words before second birthday
Vocabulary size that is reduced for age or fails to show steady increase
Difficulty in describing characteristics of objects, although child may be able to name them
Infrequent use of modifier words (adjectives or adverbs)
Excessive use of jargon past 18 months

Organizing Words into Sentences
Failure to utter first sentences before third birthday
Use of short and incomplete sentences
Tendency to omit words (articles, prepositions)
Misuse of *be, do,* and *can* verb forms
Difficulty understanding and producing questions
Plateauing at an early developmental level; use of easy speech patterns

Altering Word Forms
Omission of endings for plurals and tenses
Inappropriate use of plurals and tense endings
Inaccurate use of possession words

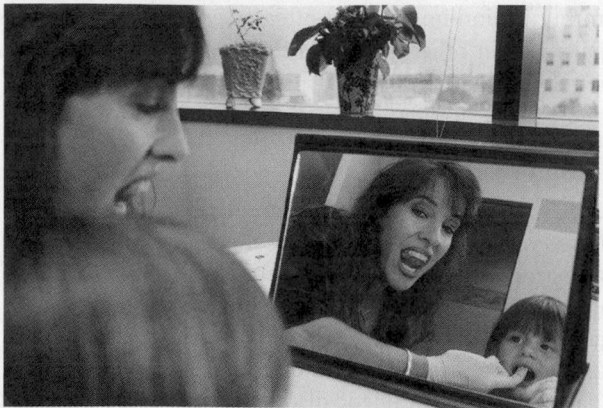

Fig. 24-8 Using visual and tactile cues, the clinician demonstrates tongue placement for production of the *L* sound. (Courtesy Paul Vincent Kuntz, Texas Children's Hospital, Houston.)

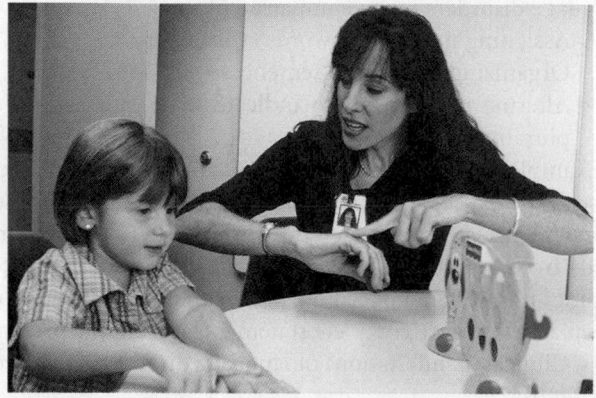

Fig. 24-9 Child practices a gestural cue to elicit sustained airflow for the *S* sound. (Courtesy Paul Vincent Kuntz, Texas Children's Hospital, Houston.)

r, and *th),* or the child may omit many consonants, usually at the ends of words, and substitute the letters *t, d, k,* or *y* for them (Figs. 24-8 and 24-9).

Dysfluencies, or rhythm disorders, usually consist of repetitions of sounds, words, or phrases. One of the most common and potentially serious dysfluencies is stuttering. Stuttering is dysfluent speech characterized by tense repetition of sounds or complete blockage of sounds or words. A stutter is sometimes referred to as a block when no sound comes out when the person tries to speak.

Voice production disorders are characterized by deviations in pitch, loudness, or voice quality. Clinical manifestations of speech disorders are given in Box 24-11.

NONSPEECH COMMUNICATION

Many individuals who have severe disabilities, such as CI or multiple physical impairments, comprehend language but are unable to speak. Consequently, they benefit from communication methods that employ nonverbal symbols, such as sign language. Besides the use of hand or body gestures, numerous other communication systems exist. For example, Blissymbolics is a highly stylized system of graphic symbols that represent words, ideas, and concepts. Although education is required to use Blissymbols, no reading skill is needed. These symbols or

---

BOX 24-11 CLINICAL MANIFESTATIONS OF SPEECH DISORDERS

Dysfluency (Stuttering)
Disturbance in normal fluency and time patterning of speech (inappropriate for individual's age), characterized by frequent occurrences of one or more of the following:
- Sound and syllable repetitions
- Sound prolongations
- Interjections
- Broken words (e.g., pauses within a word)
- Audible or silent blocking (filled or unfilled pauses in speech)
- Circumlocutions (word substitutions to avoid problematic words)
- Production of words with an excess of physical tension
- Monosyllabic whole-word repetitions (e.g., "I-I-I see him")

Disturbance in fluency that interferes with academic or occupational achievement or with social communication

If a speech-motor or sensory deficit is present, speech difficulties in excess of those usually associated with these problems

Articulation Deficiency
Lack of intelligibility of conversational speech by age 3 years
Omission of consonants at beginning of words by age 3 years and at end of words by age 4 years
Persisting articulation faults after age 7 years
Omission of a sound where one should occur
Distortion of a sound
Substitution of an incorrect sound for a correct one

Voice Disorders
Deviations in pitch (too high or too low, especially for age and sex); monotone speech
Deviations in loudness
Deviations in quality (hypernasality or hyponasality)

---

other self-explanatory graphics are usually arranged on a board, and the person points to the symbol(s) to convey a message; more sophisticated devices employ voice synthesizers that "speak" the symbol's meaning. For children with physical limitations that prevent fine hand movements, numerous devices are available that facilitate isolating a symbol. Nonverbal communication systems allowing individuals with severe communication disorders to lead much more meaningful lives; many children are able to learn more and learn faster.* The situated approach is a shift from an emphasis on correcting the disabilities to supporting those with disabilities so they can achieve more. The goals of a situated approach are to increase opportunities for these children to participate in everyday life activities.

AUTISM SPECTRUM DISORDERS (AUTISM)

Autism spectrum disorders (ASDs) are complex neurodevelopmental disorders of unknown etiology with a genetic basis. ASD is manifested during early childhood, primarily from 18 to 36 months of age. It occurs in 6.6 to 6.7 in 1000 children or 58.7 in 10,000; is about four times more common in males than in

---

*Information about communication aids for children is available from Crestwood Communication Aids, Inc., PO Box 090107, Milwaukee, WI 53209-0107; 414-351-0311; fax: 414-446-9255; e-mail: crest-comm@aol.com; www.communicationaids.com.

females (although females are more severely affected); and is not related to socioeconomic level, race, or parenting style (Johnson, 2008; Twedell, 2008a; Shah, Dalton, and Boris, 2007). ASD encompasses autistic disorder, Asperger syndrome, and pervasive developmental disorder–not otherwise specified; these impairments range from mild to severe (Johnson, 2008).

Etiology

The cause of ASD is unknown. However, considerable evidence supports multiple biologic causes. Individuals with ASD may have abnormal electroencephalograms, epileptic seizures, delayed development of hand dominance, persistence of primitive reflexes, metabolic abnormalities (elevated blood serotonin levels), and hypoplasia of the vermis of the cerebellum (the part of the brain involved in regulating motion and some aspects of memory).

There is also strong evidence for a genetic basis that in twins is consistent with an autosomal recessive pattern of inheritance. There is a high concordance (60% to 90%) for monozygotic (identical) twins and less than 5% concordance for dizygotic (nonidentical) twins. In addition, between 5% and 16% of males with ASD test positive for the fragile X chromosome (American Academy of Pediatrics, 2001b, Schaefer and Lutz, 2006).

There is a relatively high risk of recurrence of ASD in families with one affected child (American Academy of Pediatrics, 2001b, Schaefer and Lutz, 2006; Shah, Dalton, and Boris, 2007). Although multiple genes have been suggested as possible caus-

ative factors in ASD, no specific gene for the disorder has been identified (Dawson, 2007; Muhle, Trentacoste, and Rapin, 2004). Researchers are studying the *MET* gene, located in the area of chromosome 7, which encodes a receptor tyrosine kinase functions in both brain development and gastrointestinal repair (Twedell, 2008b). The *MET* gene appears to be dysregulated in many children with ASD, and the disrupted *MET* signaling may contribute to increased risk of developing ASD (Bates, 2009; Campbell, Buie, Winter, et al, 2009). There is a need for future prospective research regarding the genetic association with ASD.

Contrary to some reports, ASD does not appear to be caused by thimerosal-containing vaccines nor the measles-mumps-rubella vaccine (Muhle, Trentacoste, and Rapin, 2004; Shah, Dalton, and Boris, 2007) (see Evidence-Based Practice box). ASD has been reported in association with a number of conditions such as fragile X syndrome, tuberous sclerosis, metabolic disorders, fetal rubella syndrome, *Haemophilus influenzae* meningitis, and structural brain anomalies (Dawson, 2007; Muhle, Trentacoste, and Rapin, 2004). Retrospective studies have tied ASD to certain perinatal events; a higher incidence of maternal uterine bleeding during pregnancy, lower incidence of maternal vaginal infections during pregnancy, decreased maternal use of contraceptives, and higher incidence of neonatal hyperbilirubinemia were found to be associated with ASD (Muhle, Trentacoste, and Rapin, 2004). These same researchers, however, urge caution in interpreting these findings.

EVIDENCE-BASED PRACTICE

Thimerosal-Containing Vaccines and Autism Spectrum Disorders

ASK THE QUESTION

Is the incidence of autism spectrum disorders (ASDs) and/or other neurodevelopmental disorders increased in children receiving vaccines containing thimerosal?

SEARCH FOR THE EVIDENCE

Search strategies
Search selection criteria included English language, publication within the past 15 years, research-based articles (level 3 or lower), and child populations.

Databases used
PubMed, Cochrane Collaboration, MDConsult, Vaccine Adverse Events Reporting System (VAERS) database, American Academy of Pediatrics, Autism Research Institute

CRITICALLY ANALYZE THE EVIDENCE

GRADE criteria: Evidence quality strong; recommendation strong (Guyatt, Oxman, Vist, et al, 2008)

- Researchers from the Cochrane Vaccines Field conducted a systematic review of 139 identified studies to assess the evidence of effectiveness and unintended effects associated with the trivalent measles, mumps, and rubella (MMR) on healthy patients up to 15 years of age. Of the 139 identified studies, 31 studies were included in the review and all were published by 2004. No credible evidence of an involvement of MMR with either autism or Crohn disease was found. The impact of mass MMR immunization on the elimination of the diseases has been demonstrated worldwide (Demicheli, Jefferson, Rivetti, et al, 2005).

- Parker, Schwartz, Todd, and colleagues (2004) conducted a systematic critical review of original epidemiologic and pharmacokinetic studies to evaluate quality of evidence that suggests a potential association between thimerosal-containing vaccines and ASDs. Of the 12 publications evaluated, the preponderance of the 10 epidemiologic studies did not support a link between the thimerosal-containing vaccines and ASDs. The two pharmacokinetic studies suggested the half-life of ethylmercury is significantly short, which makes an association with ASDs less likely. The epidemiologic studies that supported a link demonstrated significant design flaws that invalidated the conclusions. The evidence reviewed indicated no association between thimerosal-containing vaccines and ASDs.

- A case-control study of vaccinated children ages 10 to 12 years in the United Kingdom compared 98 children with ASDs with two control groups consisting of 52 special educational need children without ASDs and 90 typically developing children to test measles involvement in the pathogenesis of ASDs. The children were tested for measles virus or raised serum antibody titers after receiving MMR vaccination. No difference was detected in measles antibody or in measles virus in the ASD cases compared with controls, regardless of the number of MMR doses. No association between measles vaccination and ASD was shown (Baird, Pickles, Simonoff, et al, 2007).

- A cohort study of 467,450 children in Denmark compared the risk of ASDs in children vaccinated with thimerosal-containing vaccines to that in children vaccinated with a thimerosal-free formulation of the same vaccine. Results found no relationship between childhood vaccination with thimerosal-containing vaccines and the development of ASDs (Hviid, Stellfeld, Wohlfahrt, et al, 2003).

Continued

EVIDENCE-BASED PRACTICE—cont'd

Thimerosal-Containing Vaccines and Autism Spectrum Disorders

CRITICALLY ANALYZE THE EVIDENCE—cont'd

- A longitudinal study monitored more than 14,000 children born in 1991 or 1992 in the United Kingdom. The mercury exposure from thimerosal-containing vaccines was recorded and calculated at ages 3, 4, and 6 months and compared to cognitive and behavioral-developmental assessments performed from 6 to 91 months of age. Researchers found no evidence that early exposure to thimerosal had any deleterious effect on neurologic or psychologic outcome (Heron, Golding, and the ALSPAC Study Team, 2004).

- Between 1985 and 1989 and again during the late 1990s, Stehr-Green, Tull, Stellfeld, and colleagues (2003) compared the incidence and prevalence of autism-like disorders in California, Sweden, and Denmark. Findings indicated that the incidence and prevalence of autism-like disorders began to rise from 1985 to 1989 and increased in incidence until the early 1990s. In the United States the thimerosal level in vaccines increased throughout the 1990s, whereas in Sweden and Denmark the already low thimerosal level in the vaccines steadily decreased in the 1980s and was virtually eliminated from all vaccines in the early 1990s. This study concludes that an increased exposure to thimerosal-containing vaccines does not correlate with the increased rates of autism in young children observed in Sweden and Denmark.

- Madsen, Lauritsen, Pedersen, and colleagues (2003) studied 956 children diagnosed with autism from 1971 to 2000 and showed that the incidence was stable until 1990 with increased rates thereafter, in spite of the decreased amount of thimerosal used from 1970 to 1992. The rise in the incidence of autism continued even in children born after discontinuation of the use of thimerosal-containing vaccines in Denmark in 1992.

- In 2004 the Institute of Medicine (IOM) reconsidered the hypothesis that vaccines are associated causally with autism. The IOM completed an extensive review of the evidence and rejected the hypothesis that there is a causal relationship between thimerosal-containing vaccines and autism. The IOM review concluded that there is no link between exposure to thimerosal and autism (McCormick, Bayer, Berg, et al, 2004).

- In 2001 the IOM completed an extensive review of the evidence and concluded that there was inadequate information to either accept or reject a causal relationship between thimerosal exposure from childhood vaccines and the onset of autism. The IOM supported the effort to remove thimerosal from vaccines to reduce any mercury exposure to infants and children (Stration, Gable, Shetty, et al, 2001).

APPLY THE EVIDENCE: NURSING IMPLICATIONS

Decisions about the total elimination of thimerosal (even traces) from vaccines must balance the potential benefit of no exposure to mercury against the risks of decreased vaccine coverage due to higher cost of the thimerosal-free vaccine, the risks of sepsis due to the potential bacterial contamination of the preservative-free formulations, and the risk of exposure to alternative preservatives that might replace the thimerosal preservative.

Thimerosal as a preservative has been removed or reduced to trace amounts in all vaccines routinely administered to children, except influenza vaccine, in the United States. The maximum total exposure during the first 6 months of life is less than 3 mcg of mercury. Based on guidelines established by the FDA and other government monitoring agencies, no children will be exposed to excessive mercury from childhood vaccines regardless of whether they receive influenza vaccine that contains thimerosal as a preservative (**www.fda.gov/BiologicsBloodVaccines/SafetyAvailability/VaccineSafety/UCM096228**). The best available scientific evidence to date supports that there is no link between vaccines containing thimerosal and autism or other neurodevelopmental disorders.

References

Baird A, Pickles A, Simonoff E, et al: Measles vaccination and antibody response in autism spectrum disorders, *Arch Dis Child* 93:832-837, 2007.

Demicheli V, Jefferson T, Rivetti A, et al: Vaccines for measles, mumps and rubella in children, *Cochrane Database Syst Rev* (4):CD004407.DOI:10.1002/14651858.CD004407.PUB2, 2005.

Guyatt GH, Oxman AD, Vist GE, et al: GRADE: an emerging consensus on rating quality of evidence and strength of recommendations, *BMJ* 336:924-926, 2008.

Heron J, Golding J, ALSPAC Study Team: Thimerosal exposure in infants and developmental disorders: a prospective cohort study in the United Kingdom does not support a causal association, *Pediatrics* 114(3):577-583, 2004.

Hviid A, Stellfeld M, Wohlfahrt J, et al: Association between thimerosal-containing vaccine and autism, *JAMA* 290(13):1763-1766, 2003.

Madsen KM, Lauritsen MB, Pedersen CB, et al: Thimerosal and the occurrence of autism: negative ecological evidence from Danish population-based data, *Pediatrics* 112(3):604-606, 2003.

McCormick M, Bayer R, Berg A, et al: *Report of the Institute of Medicine Immunization Safety Review: vaccines and autism*, Washington, DC, 2004, National Academy Press.

Parker SK, Schwartz B, Todd J, et al: Thimerosal-containing vaccines and autistic spectrum disorder: a critical review of published original data, *Pediatrics* 114(3):793-804, 2004.

Stehr-Green P, Tull P, Stellfeld M, et al: Autism and thimerosal-containing vaccines: lack of consistent evidence for an association, *Am J Prev Med* 25(2):101-106, 2003.

Stration K, Gable A, Shetty P, et al: *Report of the Institute of Medicine Immunization Safety Review: thimerosal-containing vaccines and neurodevelopmental disorders*, Washington, DC, 2001, National Academy Press.

Clinical Manifestations and Diagnostic Evaluation

Children with ASD demonstrate core deficits primarily in social interactions, communication, and behavior. Impaired social interaction is one of the hallmarks of ASD (Twedell, 2008a; Shah, Dalton, and Boris, 2007). Social interaction deficits may include early abnormal eye contact, failure to smile, failure to orient to name, lack of imitation, lack of interactive play, and lack of gesture use such as pointing and waving (Johnson, 2008; Shah, Dalton, and Boris, 2007).

Communicative impairment has been a common presenting sign in young children diagnosed with ASD. Communicative impairment may range from absent to delayed speech to an atypical language such as humming or grunting for extended periods, laughing inappropriately, or use of echolalia (echoing another's speech). Autism regression is when the ASD child seems to develop normally then regresses suddenly; this is a red flag that has been frequently displayed in expressive language (Johnson, 2008). Approximately 25% to 30% of ASD children develop autistic regression between 18 and 21 months (Johnson, 2008). Any child who does not display such language skills as babbling or gesturing by 12 months, a single word by 16 months, and two-word phrases by 24 months is recommended for immediate hearing and language evaluation.

Behavior impairments range from mild to severe and include unusual stereotypies and repetitive, impulsive, restrictive (having a narrow range of interest), and obsessive behavioral patterns (Johnson, 2008; Twedell, 2008a). Repetitive, impulsive stereotypies such as rocking, flapping hands, head nodding, spinning, twirling, and self-injurious behaviors (e.g., self-biting, head banging) are common signs of ASD (Twedell, 2008a; Shah, Dalton, and Boris, 2007). Box 24-12 describes diagnostic criteria for ASD according to the American Psychiatric Association's DSM-IV-TR. The majority of children with ASD have some degree of CI, with scores typically in the range of

BOX 24-12 DIAGNOSTIC CRITERIA FOR AUTISM SPECTRUM DISORDERS

A. A total of six (or more) items from (1), (2), and (3), with at least two from (1), and one each from (2) and (3):
  (1) Qualitative impairment in social interaction, as manifested by at least two of the following:
    (a) Marked impairment in the use of multiple nonverbal behaviors such as eye-to-eye gaze, facial expression, body postures, and gestures to regulate social interaction
    (b) Failure to develop peer relationships appropriate to developmental level
    (c) A lack of spontaneous seeking to share enjoyment, interests, or achievements with other people (e.g., by a lack of showing, bringing, or pointing out objects of interest)
    (d) Lack of social or emotional reciprocity
  (2) Qualitative impairments in communication as manifested by at least one of the following:
    (a) Delay in, or total lack of, the development of spoken language (not accompanied by an attempt to compensate through alternative modes of communication such as gesture or mime)
    (b) In individuals with adequate speech, marked impairment in the ability to initiate or sustain a conversation with others
    (c) Stereotyped and repetitive use of language or idiosyncratic language
    (d) Lack of varied, spontaneous make-believe play or social imitative play appropriate to developmental level
  (3) Restricted repetitive and stereotyped patterns of behavior, interests, and activities, as manifested by at least one of the following:
    (a) Encompassing preoccupation with one or more stereotyped and restricted patterns of interest that is abnormal either in intensity or focus
    (b) Apparently inflexible adherence to specific, nonfunctional routines or rituals
    (c) Stereotyped and repetitive motor mannerisms (e.g., hand or finger flapping or twisting, or complex whole-body movements)
    (d) Persistent preoccupation with parts of objects
B. Delays or abnormal functioning in at least one of the following areas, with onset before age 3 years: (1) social interaction, (2) language as used in social communication, or (3) symbolic or imaginative play
C. The disturbance is not better accounted for by Rett disorder or childhood disintegrative disorder

From American Psychiatric Association: *Diagnostic and statistical manual of mental disorders (DSM-IV-TR)*, ed 4, text rev, Washington, DC, 2000, The Association.

moderate to severe CI. Despite their relatively moderate to severe disability, some children with ASD (known as savants) excel in particular areas, such as art, music, memory, mathematics, or perceptual skills such as puzzle building.

NURSING TIP Claims of beneficial results from the use of secretin, a peptide hormone that stimulates pancreatic secretion, have not been substantiated by scientific study (Shah, Dalton, and Boris, 2007; Williams, Wray, and Wheeler, 2005.*

*Additional information on secretin may be found by contacting the Autism Society, 4340 East-West Hwy., Suite 350, Bethesda, MD 20814; 301-657-0881, 800-328-8476; www. autism-society.org.

Early recognition, referral, diagnosis, and intensive early intervention tend to improve outcomes for children with ASD. Unfortunately, a diagnosis often is not made until 2 to 3 years after symptoms are first recognized and based on diagnostic criteria of DSM-IV-TR. Combined communicative impairment, social delays, and regression in communication or social milestones are important early red flags for ASD and should prompt an immediate evaluation. Several screening tools have been developed to aid in early detection of ASD in young children (Shah, Dalton, and Boris, 2007). The Checklist for Autism in Toddlers (CHAT) combines parent responses with direct observation of 18- to 24-month-old toddlers, with the modified CHAT parent questionnaire evaluating the 16- to 48-month-old (Shah, Dalton, and Boris, 2007). The Pervasive Developmental Disorders Screening Test measures various aspects of language, social skills, pretend play, attachment, sensory responses, and motor stereotypes in children 18 to 48 months of age (Shah, Dalton, and Boris, 2007). With early diagnosis of ASD, the provider can assist in enrolling the child in appropriate intervention programs that benefit the child, the family, and future schools and society (Diggle and McConachie, 2002; Johnson, 2008; Twedell, 2008b). If the results of the screening are negative, make an additional appointment within a month to monitor the child's progress and to address any parental or provider concerns (Johnson, 2008).

Prognosis

Even though ASD is usually a severely disabling condition, some children improve with acquisition of language skills and communication with others (Bloom-DiCicco, Lord, Zwaigenbaum, et al, 2006). Some ultimately achieve independence, but most require lifelong adult supervision. Aggravation of psychiatric symptoms occurs in about half of children during adolescence, with girls having a tendency for continued deterioration. However, early diagnosis and intervention improve outcomes, empower families, decrease the need for special education services in later years, and increase the child's chance for independence and gainful employment as an adult, especially if there are no coexisting cognitive deficits (Johnson, 2008). A better prognosis is associated with higher intelligence, functional speech, and less behavioral impairment (Shah, Dalton, and Boris, 2007).

Nursing Care Management

Therapeutic intervention for the child with ASD is a specialized area involving professionals with advanced training. Although there is no cure for ASD, numerous therapies have been used. The most promising results have been achieved through highly structured and intensive behavior modification programs. In general, the objective in treatment is to provide positive reinforcement, increase social awareness of others, teach verbal communication skills, and decrease unacceptable behavior. Providing a structured routine for the child to follow is key in the management of ASD.

When children with ASD are hospitalized, the parents are essential to planning care and ideally should stay with the child as much as possible. Nurses should recognize that not all children with ASD are the same, and each requires individual assessment and treatment. Decreasing stimulation by placing the child in a private room, avoiding extraneous auditory and visual distraction, and encouraging the parents to bring in possessions to which the child is attached may lessen the disruptiveness of hospitalization. Because physical contact often upsets these children, minimum holding and eye contact may be necessary to avoid behavioral outbursts. Take care when performing procedures on, administering medicine to, or feeding these children because they may be fussy eaters who willfully starve themselves or gag to prevent eating, or indiscriminate hoarders who swallow any available edible or inedible item, such as a thermometer. Eating habits of ASD children may be particularly problematic for families and may involve food refusal accompanied by mineral deficiencies, mouthing of objects, consumption of nonedibles, and smelling and throwing of food (Belschner, 2007; Caronna, Augustyn, and Zuckerman, 2007).

Children with ASD need to be introduced slowly to new situations, and visits with staff caregivers should be short whenever possible. Because these children have difficulty organizing their behavior and redirecting their energy, they need to be told directly what to do. Communication should be at the child's developmental level, brief, and concrete.

Family Support

ASD, as with so many other chronic conditions, involves the entire family and often becomes a "family disease." Nurses can help alleviate the guilt and shame often associated with this disorder by stressing what is known from a biologic standpoint, as well as how little is known about the cause of ASD. It is imperative to help parents understand that they are not the cause of the child's condition.

Parents need expert counseling early in the course of the disorder and should be referred to the Autism Society. The society provides information on education, treatment programs and techniques, and facilities such as camps and group homes. There is also sibling and family member support on the Autism Society website.* Other helpful resources for parents of children with ASD are the local and state departments of mental health and developmental disabilities. These agencies provide important programs for autistic children and in-school programs throughout the United States.

As much as possible, encourage the family to care for the child in the home. With the help of family support programs in many states, families are often able to provide home care and assist with the educational services the child needs. As the child approaches adulthood and parents become older, the family may require assistance in locating a long-term placement facility. (See Chapter 22.)

NURSING CARE OF CHILDREN WITH COMMUNICATION IMPAIRMENT

Prevention

The primary intervention for communication disorders is prevention. Much of prevention directly relates to factors that predispose children to language and speech impairment, namely, CI and hearing deficits. Infants at risk for either condition (see Boxes 24-1 and 24-7) should be referred for audiologic evaluation within the first 3 to 6 months of life so that audiologic and speech therapy can be initiated immediately when required.

Prevention also involves early recognition of children at risk for language delays and timely intervention to promote adequate language development. Nurses are often able to provide education for families that help them foster the child's communication skills.

Stuttering is one area in which prevention of communication impairment through appropriate parental guidance is particularly important. This hesitancy or dysfluency in speech pattern is a normal characteristic of language development during the preschool years. It occurs because children know what they want to say but hesitate or repeat words or sounds as they try to find the vocabulary to express themselves. Eventually their language skills parallel their other abilities, and speech becomes fluent.

When parents or other significant persons place undue stress on the child with this pattern of dysfluency, however, an abnormal speech pattern may result. Chances for reversal of stuttering are good until about 5 years of age. Therefore prevention must begin early. The nurse discusses with parents the normal dysfluencies in children's speech. When stuttering does occur, advise parents to use the suggestions given in the Family-Centered Care box to avoid inadvertently reinforcing the dysfluent pattern. If the parent is excessively concerned or the child is frustrated and struggling, the child is referred for speech and language evaluation.†

👪 FAMILY-CENTERED CARE

Stuttering in Young Children

To Be Encouraged

Viewing hesitancy and dysfluency as a normal part of speech development

Giving the child plenty of time and the impression that you are not rushed or in a hurry

Looking directly at the child while he or she is talking; being patient and never ridiculing or criticizing

Setting a good example by speaking clearly and articulating well

Identifying situations when stuttering increases and avoiding them or ignoring the hesitancy

Minimizing stress, such as talking at the child's eye level; avoiding frequent questioning; and preventing interruptions while the child is speaking

Capitalizing on periods of fluent speech with positive reinforcement, such as singing songs or repeating nursery rhymes

To Be Avoided

Practicing the natural tendency to finish the sentence for the child by supplying the word when the child has a block

Telling the child to stop and start over, to think before speaking, or to take it easy and go slowly

Showing great concern for, embarrassment at, or disapproval of hesitancy

Doing anything that emphasizes stuttering and calls the child's attention to speech skills

Promising a reward for proper speech

❗ NURSING ALERT

Dysfluency must be arrested before the child develops an awareness or anticipation of the difficulty and begins to mistrust his or her speech skills.

---

†Information on sources of assistance is available from the Stuttering Foundation of America, 3100 Walnut Grove Road, Suite 603, PO Box 11749, Memphis, TN 38111-0749; 901-452-7343, 800-992-9392; fax: 901-452-3931; e-mail: info@stutteringhelp.org; www.stuttersfa.org.

*See footnote p. 939.

TABLE 24-6	NORMAL SPEECH AND LANGUAGE DEVELOPMENT DURING EARLY CHILDHOOD	
AGE (yr)	**SPEECH DEVELOPMENT**	**SPEECH INTELLIGIBILITY**
1	Says two or three words with meaning Imitates sounds of animals Omits most final and some initial consonants	Usually no more than 25% intelligible to unfamiliar listener Height of unintelligible jargon at age 18 mo
2	Uses two- or three-word phrases Has vocabulary of about 300 words Uses *I, me,* and *you* Articulation lags behind vocabulary	50% intelligible in context
3	Says four- or five-word sentences Has vocabulary of about 900 words Uses *who, what,* and *where* in asking questions Uses plurals, pronouns, and prepositions Often repeats and hesitates	75% intelligible
4-5	Has vocabulary of about 1500-2100 words Able to use most grammatical forms correctly, such as past tense of verb with *yesterday* Uses complete sentences with nouns, verbs, prepositions, adjectives, adverbs, and conjunctions	100% intelligible at age 4 yr, although some sounds are still imperfect
5-6	Has vocabulary of 3000 words Comprehends *if, because,* and *why* Masters most sounds; still distorts *s, z, sh, ch,* and *j*	

Assessment

Communication disorders can occur at any age but are most often found during childhood. The preschool period is considered critical to language development and therefore is a prime age for assessment and intervention. Failure to detect communication disorders during early childhood affects the development of social relationships and emotional interactions, increases difficulty in developing academic skills, and lessens the chances for successful correction of deficient skills.

Assessment of abnormalities requires knowledge of normal speech and language development. Awareness of when children achieve given milestones enables nurses to distinguish when specific communication characteristics are expected and when they are considered deviations (Table 24-6). Nurses must also be aware of clinical manifestations of speech and language impairment (see Boxes 24-10 and 24-11) and cognitive or hearing deficits (see Boxes 24-2 and 24-8 and Cognitive Impairment, p. 908).

Three methods are available for assessing speech and language development. Direct observation necessitates spontaneous language interaction between the child and the nurse. Suggestions for initiating conversation include showing the child an object and asking the child to describe it. The word-imitative procedure may also be used by having the child repeat sentences or words. This approach is valid because children are not able to reproduce statements using correct grammatical forms that they have not previously learned to use. Whenever possible, the child's conversation should be tape-recorded for serial documentation of progressive speech and language development and further evaluation by or consultation with a speech and language therapist.

Indirect assessment relies on parental information obtained by taking a history. Key questions that help identify problems in language or speech are listed in the Nursing Care Guidelines box. Information obtained from the history is critically important, and parental concerns must be taken seriously. However, caution must also be exercised in evaluating parental comments. Parents may be unaware of the child's difficulties because of lack of comparison with normal language development. Also, they may not realize the degree of unintelligibility of the child's speech because of their familiarity with the child's approximation of words. Conversely, parents may have unrealistic expectations regarding verbal development and may exaggerate the degree of dysfluency, misarticulation, or delays in word usage.

Consequently, screening tests are an important component of objective measurement of speech development. The Denver Articulation Screening Exam (DASE) employs the word-imitative procedure and is one of the most frequently used tests. The child repeats 22 words but pronounces 30 different sound elements. The raw score, or the number of correctly pronounced sounds, is then compared with the percentile rank for children in that age-group. The examiner must be careful to evaluate the specific sound rather than the quality of the entire word. For beginning examiners, it is helpful to validate the final score by comparing the results with those obtained by a different examiner, ideally a speech therapist. The child is also scored on intelligibility using one of four possible categories: (1) easy to understand, (2) understandable half of the time, (3) not understandable, or (4) cannot evaluate. The DASE is a reliable, effective screening tool because it requires only 10 minutes for the examiner to administer and is designed to discriminate between significant speech delay and normal variations in the acquisition of speech sounds. It also detects common abnormal physical conditions such as hyponasality, hypernasality, tongue thrust, and lateral lisp.

The Early Language Milestone Scale, Second Edition (ELM Scale-2), is a standardized screening instrument for assessing language development in children younger than 3 years of age. The test focuses on expressive, receptive, and visual language, and the revised form includes intelligibility (Coplan, Contello, Cunningham, et al, 1998; Simms and Schum, 2007). The ELM Scale-2 relies primarily on the parent's report, with occasional

NURSING CARE GUIDELINES

Assessing Communication Impairment

Key Questions for Language Disorders

How old was your child when he (or she) began to speak his (or her) first words?

How old was your child when he (or she) began to put words into sentences?

Does your child have difficulty in learning new vocabulary words?

Does your child omit words from sentences (i.e., do sentences sound telegraphic?) or use short or incomplete sentences?

Does your child have trouble with grammar, such as the verbs *is, am, are, was,* and *were?*

Can your child follow two or three directions given at once?

Do you have to repeat directions or questions?

Does your child respond appropriately to questions?

Does your child ask questions beginning with *who, what, where,* and *why?*

Does it seem that your child has made little or no progress in speech and language in the last 6 to 12 months?

Key Questions for Speech Impairment

Does your child ever stammer or repeat sounds or words?

Does your child seem anxious or frustrated when trying to express an idea?

Have you noticed certain behaviors, such as blinking the eyes, jerking the head, or attempting to rephrase thoughts with different words, when your child stammers?

What do you do when any of these occurs?

Does it seem like your child uses *t, d, k,* or *g* in place of most other consonants when speaking?

Does your child omit sounds from words or replace the correct consonant with another one (such as *wabbit* for *rabbit*)?

Do you have any difficulty understanding your child's speech? How much of it is intelligible?

Has anyone else ever remarked about having difficulty in understanding your child?

Has there been any recent change in the sound of your child's voice?

 NURSING CARE GUIDELINES

Indications for Referral Regarding Communication Impairment

Age 2 Years

Failure to speak any meaningful words spontaneously

Consistent use of gestures rather than vocalizations

Difficulty in following verbal directions

Failure to respond consistently to sound

Age 3 Years

Speech that is largely unintelligible

Failure to use sentences of three or more words

Omission of initial consonants

Frequent omission of final consonants

Use of vowels rather than consonants

Age 5 Years

Stuttering or any other type of dysfluency

Noticeably impaired sentence structure

Substitution of easily produced sounds for more difficult ones

Omission of word endings (e.g., plurals, tenses of verbs)

School Age

Poor voice quality (monotonous, loud, or barely audible)

Vocal pitch inappropriate for age

Distortions, omissions, or substitutions of sounds after age 7 years

Connected speech characterized by use of unusual confusions or reversals

General

Signs suggesting hearing impairment (see Boxes 24-7 and 24-8)

Indication that the child is embarrassed or disturbed by his or her speech

FAMILY-CENTERED CARE

Helping a Child Learn Language

Provide listening opportunities:
- Select a small group of words connected to a specific activity (e.g., say "open" each time a door is opened).
- Repeat the word with the activity several times, then repeat the word but wait for the child to initiate the activity.

Choose vocabulary that is useful, easy to pronounce, and understandable to the child.

Encourage vocabulary development by having the child say the word rather than gesture before fulfilling a request (e.g., expect the child to say all or part of the word *drink* before giving a beverage).

Speak at a level slightly above the child's level (e.g., if the child speaks two words, use three- or four-word phrases).

Replace questions with statements about an observed activity (e.g., rather than asking, "What's that?" say, "Look at the kitty").

Reinforce the child's attempt to use language with verbal praise and affection.

direct testing of the child, and takes 1 to 4 minutes to administer.

A number of other tests are available to screen children for impaired language development. The Denver II, a revision of the Denver Developmental Screening Test, includes an expanded section on language items, and delays in that area provide an early indication that those children require further evaluation. (See Chapter 6.) For children ages 2 to adults age 90 years and older, the Peabody Picture Vocabulary Test-4 is a useful screening instrument to measure receptive (hearing) vocabulary for verbal ability, giftedness, and CI in English-speaking individuals (Dunn and Dunn, 2007).

Referral

After assessment and detection of language or speech problems, the nurse can assist the family in deciding on an appropriate referral. Waiting and watching for progression of symptoms is often to the detriment of the child's future development. Because children normally vary greatly in their development of verbal skills, the nurse needs guidelines for determining what is abnormal development. The Nursing Care Guidelines box lists recommended general criteria for referring children for specialized audiologic and language evaluations. Information regarding available services for language, speech, and hearing is available from the American Speech-Language-Hearing Association*

and the Council for Exceptional Children† (see footnotes on pp. 925-927 for organizations devoted to hearing impairment).

Education

When a child has delayed language development, it is important to try to structure the parents' communication to expand the

---

*2200 Research Blvd., Rockville, MD 20850-3289; 800-638-8255; TTY: 301-296-5650; fax: 301-296-8580; www.asha.org.

†Council for Exceptional Children, 1110 N. Glebe Road, Suite 300, Arlington, VA 22201-5704;, 888-232-7733; fax: 703-264-9494; TTY: 866-915-5000; www.cec.sped.org.

child's language, including acquisition of new words, new sentence constructions, and rules of grammar. The underlying principle is not to overwhelm children with words so that they learn more vocabulary, but to plan what will be said to them, what responses will be expected, and how they will be reinforced. The Family-Centered Care box presents suggestions to help parents foster their child's attainment of language skills.

Parents should also be aware that children learn language through imitation. Therefore serving as role models by speaking clearly, fluently, and with proper grammar is essential to children's mastery of language and speech. Parents need guidance regarding normal language and speech development so that they expect neither too little nor too much from their child.

KEY POINTS

- The AAIDD defines CI or intellectual disability as significantly subaverage intellectual functioning that exists concurrently in two or more adaptive skill areas (communication, self-care, home living, social skills, leisure, health and safety, self-direction, functional academics, use of community resources, and work) and is manifested before age 18 years.
- Diagnosis of CI is based on standard developmental tests and an accurate history, and no child is too young to be assessed.
- Causes of severe CI are primarily genetic, biochemical, and infectious. Mild CI is associated primarily with familial, social, and environmental causes, whereas severe CI is more likely to be associated with specific syndromes.
- Prevention of CI focuses on support for the premature neonate and other high-risk newborns; rubella immunization; genetic counseling; the importance of adequate nutrition; and maternal education regarding chemical, genetic, and infectious risks.
- Education of children with CI emphasizes development of sensory and verbal discrimination, improvement of short-term memory, motivation, and technologic support.
- Promotion of optimum development can be achieved through family guidance regarding play, communication, discipline, socialization, and sexuality.
- Down syndrome, a chromosomal abnormality, is characterized by mild to moderate CI, distinctive physical features, slowed social development, congenital anomalies, sensory problems, and diminished growth and sexual development.
- Fragile X syndrome is characterized by CI and phenotypic findings mostly in affected males. It is considered the most common hereditary form of CI or intellectual disability and the second most common genetic cause after Down syndrome.
- Hearing disorders may be classified according to the location of the defect as conductive, sensorineural, mixed conductive-sensorineural, or central auditory.
- Prevention of hearing impairment includes treatment of infection, newborn auditory screening and auditory testing,

immunization, pregnancy and genetic counseling, and reduction of noise pollution.
- Rehabilitation for hearing impairment involves the provision of hearing aids, instruction in lipreading and sign language, speech therapy, promotion of socialization for the child, and parental education and support.
- Common causes of visual impairment in childhood are refractive errors, amblyopia, strabismus, cataracts, glaucoma, trauma, and infections.
- Prevention of visual impairment focuses on prenatal screening, prenatal and perinatal care, periodic vision screening, immunization, and safety counseling.
- Nursing goals in visual rehabilitation include helping the family and child adjust to the child's visual impairment, promoting parent-child attachment, fostering optimum development and independence, providing for play and socialization, and identifying educational facilities.
- For the child undergoing ocular surgery, nursing care is aimed at reassuring the child and family throughout treatment, orienting the child to the surroundings, providing a safe environment, and encouraging independence.
- *Communication impairment* is a broad term that refers to the inability to (1) receive or process symbol systems for the spoken word, (2) represent concepts or symbol systems, or (3) transmit and use symbol systems. In cases of severe communication impairment, other symbol systems, such as nonverbal methods (e.g., gestures, sign language, Braille), may be needed to substitute for the spoken word.
- The most common cause of communication impairment is CI, followed by hearing impairment.
- The primary preventive intervention for communication disorders is the early identification of children who are at risk for language delays and the promotion of adequate language development.
- ASDs are complex neurodevelopmental disorders of unknown etiology with a genetic basis.

ANSWERS TO CRITICAL THINKING EXERCISES

Diagnosis of Down Syndrome

1. **Yes.** Parents with three other children are shocked to be told that their newborn has Down syndrome.
2. **a.** Melissa is a developmentally delayed newborn who requires time-consuming care.
   b. Melissa will develop a variety of medical problems causing a huge economic expense.
   c. Melissa will always require parent and/or sibling supervision and care.

3. The first priority is to allow the parents to express their feelings of grief, anger, sadness, and guilt regarding the birth of a cognitively impaired child. Demonstrate acceptance of the child, since parents are sensitive to professionals' attitude.
4. **Yes.** The parents' response suggests unexpressed feelings of anger, loss, sadness, and confusion.

Hearing Impairment

1. **Yes.** Jason is severely hearing impaired and recovering in an unfamiliar environment after a surgical procedure. Jason's

recovery in an unfamiliar environment with monitors, an intravenous line, and other equipment may create fear, anxiety, and agitation.

2. **a.** Jason's inability to hear and communicate promotes frustration and fear.

b. Jason's increasing agitation may be due to not having his hearing aids.

c. Jason, who is recovering from regional block for herniorrhaphy, is unable to clearly verbalize or use sign language to express his needs.

3. The first priority is to establish communication with Jason by directly facing him to facilitate lip reading, touching him to get his attention, and correctly placing his hearing aids if available. Determine his usual means of communicating and encourage expression of feelings and questions regarding the environment, equipment, and procedures. Explain procedures before performing them, using gestures, objects, or pictures, and speak slowly and clearly. Allow ample time for the child to show understanding of explanations. Decrease environmental noise. Listen closely as the child speaks, and focus on his pronunciation of words.

4. **Yes.** Jason's behavior does not suggest the transitory confusion associated with the initial emergence from anesthesia. Rather, it suggests that he became increasingly frustrated as he became aware of his environment because of the inability to communicate his desires and feelings. Although pain is a possibility and needs to be evaluated, regional blocks are typically given during surgery to keep children comfortable until after they are discharged.

REFERENCES

American Academy of Pediatrics, Committee on Sports Medicine and Fitness: Protective eyewear for young athletes, *Pediatrics* 113(3):619-622, 2004.

American Academy of Pediatrics, Committee on Genetics: Health supervision for children with Down syndrome, *Pediatrics* 107(2):442-449, 2001a.

American Academy of Pediatrics, Committee on Children with Disabilities: The pediatrician's role in the diagnosis and management of autistic spectrum disorder in children, *Pediatrics* 107(5):1221-1226, 2001b.

American Academy of Pediatrics, Committee on Children with Disabilities: Provision of educationally-related services for children and adolescents with chronic diseases and disabling conditions, *Pediatrics* 105(2):448-451, 2000.

American Psychiatric Association: *Diagnostic and statistical manual of mental disorders (DSM-IV-TR),* ed 4, text rev, Washington, DC, 2000, The Association.

Bailey DB Jr, Beskow LM, Davis AM, et al: Changing perspectives on the benefits of newborn screening, *Ment Retard Dev Disabil Res Rev* 12(4):270-279, 2006.

Bates B: Risk of GI disorders increased with autism, *Pediatric News* 43(3):15, 2009.

Belschner RA: Stop, assess and motivate: the SAM approach to autism spectrum disorders, *Am J Nurse Pract* 11(4):43-50, 2007.

Bernstein D: Congenital heart disease. In Kliegman RM, Behrman RE, Jenson HB, et al, editors: *Nelson textbook of pediatrics,* ed 18, Philadelphia, 2007, Saunders.

Bloom-DiCicco E, Lord C, Zwaigenbaum I, et al: The development neurobiology of autism spectrum disorder, *J Neurosci* 26(26):6897-6906, 2006.

Bradham TS, Bess FH: The pediatrician's guide to hearing loss identification and management, *Infect Dis Child* 17(12):6, 10, 11, 2004.

Caronna EB, Augustyn M, Zuckerman B: Revisiting parental concerns in the age of autism spectrum disorders, *Arch Pediatr Adolesc Med* 161:406-407, 2007.

Campbell DB, Buie TM, Winter H, et al: Distinct genetic risk based on association of *MET* in families with co-occurring autism and gastrointestinal conditions, *Pediatrics* 123:1018-1024, 2009.

Chiu S, Wegelin JA, Blank J, et al: Early acceleration of head circumference in children with fragile X syndrome and autism, *J Dev Behav Pediatr* 28(1):31-35, 2007.

Coplan J, Contello KA, Cunningham CK, et al: Early language development in children exposed to or infected with human immunodeficiency virus, *Pediatrics* 102(1):e8, 1998.

Cunningham M, Cox EO, Committee on Practice and Ambulatory Medicine, et al: Hearing assessment in infants and children: recommendations beyond neonatal screening, *Pediatrics* 111(2):436-440, 2003.

Daniel E: Noise and hearing loss: a review, *J Sch Health* 77(5):225-231, 2007.

Dawson G: Despite major challenges, autism research continues to offer hope, *Arch Pediatr Adolesc Med* 161:411-412, 2007.

Descartes M, Carroll AJ: Cytogenetics. In Kliegman RM, Behrman RE, Jenson HB, et al, editors: *Nelson textbook of pediatrics,* ed 18, Philadelphia, 2007, Saunders.

Diggle TTJ, McConachie HHR: Parent-mediated early intervention for young children with autism spectrum disorder, Cochrane Database Syst Rev (2):DOI:10.1002/14651858. CD003496, 2002.

Dunn L, Dunn L: *The Peabody Picture Vocabulary Test,* ed 4, Bloomington, Minn, 2007, NCS Pearson.

Eastgate G: Sex, consent and intellectual disability, *Austral Fam Physician* 34(3):163-166, 2005.

Goodlin-Jones BL, Tassone F, Gane LW, et al: Autistic spectrum disorder and the fragile X permutation, *J Dev Behav Pediatr* 25(6):392-398, 2004.

Grech V: An overview and update regarding medical problems in Down syndrome, *Indian J Pediatr* 68:863-866, 2001.

Gregg RB, Wiorek MA, Arvedson JC: Pediatric audiology: a review, *Pediatr Rev* 25(7): 224-234, 2004.

Haddad J: Hearing loss. In Kliegman RM, Behrman RE, Jenson HB, et al, editors: *Nelson textbook of Pediatrics,* ed 18, Philadelphia, 2007, Saunders.

Haensel J, Engelke J, Ottenjann W, et al: Long-term results of cochlear implantation in children, *Otolaryngol Head Neck Surg* 132(3):456-458, 2005.

Hagerman RJ, Berry-Kravis E, Kaufmann WE, et al: Advances in the treatment of fragile X syndrome, *Pediatrics* 123:378-390, 2009.

Hall JG: Chromosomal clinical abnormalities. In Kliegman RM, Behrman RE, Jenson HB, et al, editors: *Nelson textbook of pediatrics,* ed 18, Philadelphia, 2007, Saunders.

Hartway S: Family teaching toolbox, *Adv Neonatal Care* 9(1):31-33, 2009a.

Hartway S: A parent's guide to the genetics of Down syndrome, *Adv Neonatal Care* 9(1):27-30, 2009b.

Hatton DD, Sideris J, Skinner M, et al: Autistic behavior in children with fragile X syndrome: prevalence, stability, and the impact of FMRP, *Am J Med Genet A* 140A(17):1804-1813, 2006.

Hayes H, Geers A, Treiman R, et al: Receptive vocabulary development in deaf children with cochlear implants: achievement in an intensive auditory-oral educational setting, *Ear Hearing* 30:128-135, 2009.

Holte L: Early childhood hearing loss: a frequently overlooked cause of speech and language delay, *Pediatr Ann* 32(7):461-465, 2003.

Johnson CP: Recognition of autism before age 2 years, *Pediatr Rev* 29(3):86-96, 2008.

Johnson CP, Kastner TA, American Academy of Pediatrics, Committee/Section on Children with Disabilities: Helping families raise children with special health care needs at home, *Pediatrics* 115(2):507-511, 2005.

Johnson CP, Walker WO: Mental retardation management and prognosis, *Pediatr Rev* 27(7):249-256, 2006.

Joint Committee on Infant Hearing: Year 2000 position statement: principles and guidelines for early hearing detection and intervention programs, *Pediatrics* 106(4):798-817, 2000.

Kenna MA: Medical management of childhood hearing loss, *Pediatr Ann* 33(12):822-832, 2004.

Lambros KM, Leslie LK: Management of the child with a learning disorder, *Pediatr Ann* 34(4):274-287, 2005.

Listman DA: Paintball injuries in children: more than meets the eye, *Pediatrics* 113(1):15-18, 2004.

McCoy SW, Bowman A, Smith-Blockley J, et al: Harris Infant Neuromotor Test: comparison of US and Canadian normative data and examination of concurrent validity with the ages and stages questionnaire, *Phys Ther* 89(2):173-180, 2009.

Menon V, Leroux J, White CD, et al: Frontostriatal deficits in fragile X syndrome: relation to FMR1 gene expression, *Proc Natl Acad Sci USA* 101(10):3615-3620, 2004.

Michaud LJ, American Academy of Pediatrics, Committee on Children with Disabilities: Prescribing therapy services for children with motor disabilities, *Pediatrics* 113(6):1836-1838, 2004.

Muhle R, Trentacoste SV, Rapin I: The genetics of autism, *Pediatrics* 113(5):e472-e486, 2004.

Murray E: Self-harm among adolescents with developmental disabilities: what are they trying to tell us? *J Psychosoc Nurs* 41(11):37-45, 2003.

National Down Syndrome Society: *About Down syndrome,* New York, 2009a, The Society, available at www.ndss.org/index.php?option=com_content&view=article&id=54&Itemid=74 (accessed March 16, 2009).

National Down Syndrome Society: *Education, development and community life,* New York, 2009b, The Society, available at www.ndss.org/index.php?option=com_content&view=article&id=56&Itemid=81 (accessed March 16, 2009).

National Down Syndrome Society: *Incidences and maternal age,* New York, 2009c, The Society, available at www.ndss.org/index.php?option=com_content&view=article&id=61&Itemid=78 (accessed March 16, 2009).

National Down Syndrome Society: *Questions and answers about Down syndrome,* New York, 2009d, The Society, available at www.ndss.org/index.php?option=com_content&view=article&id=55&Itemid=75 (accessed March 16, 2009).

National Fragile X Foundation: *Genetics home reference,* 2009, available at http://ghr.nlm.nih.gov/handbook (accessed March 16, 2009).

Olitsky SE, Hug D, Smith LP: Disorders of vision. In Kliegman RM, Behrman RE, Jenson HB, et al, editors: *Nelson textbook of pediatrics,* ed 18, Philadelphia, 2007a, Saunders.

Olitsky SE, Hug D, Smith LP: Injuries to the eye. In Kliegman RM, Behrman RE, Jenson HB, et al, editors: *Nelson textbook of pediatrics,* ed 18, Philadelphia, 2007b, Saunders.

Pueschel SM: The child with Down syndrome. In Levine MD, Carey WB, Crocker AC, editors: *Developmental-behavioral pediatrics,* ed 3, Philadelphia, 1999, Saunders.

Ranweiler R: Assessment and care of the newborn with Down syndrome, *Adv Neonatal Care* 9(1):17-24, 2009.

Rapaport R: Disorders of the gonads. In Kliegman RM, Behrman RE, Jenson HB, et al, editors: *Nelson textbook of pediatrics,* ed 18, Philadelphia, 2007, Saunders.

Rehm RS, Bradley JF: Social interactions at school of children who are medically fragile and developmentally delayed, *J Pediatr Nurs* 21(4):299-307, 2006.

Rittey CD: Learning difficulties: what the neurologist needs to know, *J Neurol Neurosurg Psychiatry* 74(Suppl 1):i30-i36, 2003.

Roberts JE, Mirrett P, Burchinal M: Receptive and expressive communication development of young males with fragile X syndrome, *Am J Ment Retard* 106(3):216-230, 2001.

Schaefer GB, Lutz RE: Diagnostic yield in the clinical genetic evaluation of autism spectrum disorders, *Genet Med* 8(9):549-556, 2006.

Schalock RL, Luckasson RA, Shogren KA, et al: The renaming of mental retardation: understanding the change to the term intellectual disability, *Intellect Devel Dis* 45(2):116-124, 2007.

Shah PE, Dalton R, Boris NW: Pervasive developmental disorders and childhood psychosis. In Kliegman RM, Behrman RE, Jenson HB, et al, editors: *Nelson textbook of pediatrics,* ed 18, Philadelphia, 2007, Saunders.

Shapiro BK, Batshaw ML: Mental retardation (intellectual disability). In Kliegman RM, Behrman RE, Jenson HB, et al, editors: *Nelson textbook of pediatrics,* ed 18, Philadelphia, 2007, Saunders.

Silber T, Batshaw ML: Ethical dilemmas in the treatment of children with disabilities, *Pediatr Ann* 33(11):752-761, 2004.

Simms MD, Schum RL: Language development and communication disorders. In Kliegman RM, Behrman RE, Jenson HB, et al, editors: *Nelson textbook of pediatrics,* ed 18, Philadelphia, 2007, Saunders.

Smith RJH, Bale JF, White KR: Sensorineural hearing loss in children, *Lancet* 365:879-890, 2005.

Tassone F, Pan R, Amiri K, et al: A rapid polymerase chain reaction–based screening method for identification of all expanded alleles of the fragile X (*FMRI*) gene in newborn and high-risk populations, *J Mol Diagn* 10(1):43-49, 2008.

Thompson GH: The neck. In Kliegman RM, Behrman RE, Jenson HB, et al, editors: *Nelson textbook of pediatrics,* ed 18, Philadelphia, 2007, Saunders.

Tierney CD, Brown PJ: Development of children who have hearing impairment, *Pediatr Rev* 29(12):e72-e73, 2008.

Tingley DH: Vision screening essentials: screening today for eye disorders in the pediatric patient, *Pediatr Rev* 28(2):54-61, 2007.

Twedell D: Autism, part I, Deficits, prevalence, symptoms, and environmental factors, *J Contin Educ Nurs* 39(2): 55-56, 2008a.

Twedell D: Autism, part II, Genetics, diagnosis, and treatment, *J Contin Educ Nurs* 39(3):102-103, 2008b.

Wehmeyer ML, Buntinx WHE, Lachapelle Y, et al: The intellectual disability construct and its relation to human functioning, *Intellect Devel Dis* 46(4):311-318, 2008.

Wiesner GL, Cassidy SB, Grimes SJ, et al: Clinical consult: developmental delay/fragile X syndrome, *Prim Care* 31:621-625, 2004.

Williams KJ, Wray JJ, Wheeler DM: Intravenous secretin for autism spectrum disorder, *Cochrane Database Syst Rev* (3):CD003495. DOI:10.1002/14651858.CD003495.pub2, 2005.

Winters NC, Collett BR, Myers KM: Ten-year review of rating scales, part VII, Scales assessing functional impairment, *J Am Acad Child Adolesc Psychiatry* 44(4):309-338, 2005.

Wiseman FK, Alford KA, Tybulewicz VLJ, et al: Down syndrome: recent progress and future prospects, *Human Molec Genet* 18(1):R75-R83, 2009.

Zeng FG, Liu S: Speech perception in individuals with auditory neuropathy. *J Speech Lang Hearing Res* 49:367-380, 2006.

CHAPTER
25

Family-Centered Home Care

David Wilson

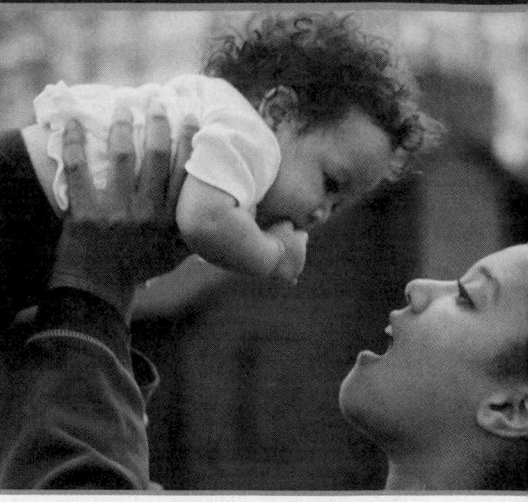

GENERAL CONCEPTS OF HOME CARE

Home care nursing has become a routine option for the pediatric patient in today's health care environment. Advances in medical technology have produced a large population of children with a variety of health care needs. The growing demand for home care services came in part as the result of increasing health costs of institutionalized care. More important, home-based health care recognizes the family's valuable contribution to the child's overall health in his or her natural environment. Many children with special health care needs may be cared for in the home setting once their medical condition has stabilized. Although there is limited evidence on the ability of home care to reduce hospital admissions and emergency department visits, home care programs lead to greater parent satisfaction, improved quality of life, and a reduction in length of hospital stay (Cooper, Wheeler, Woolfenden, et al, 2006).

Nursing education has also shifted to incorporate a broader focus on community and home health nursing. Nurses wishing to work in the home care setting must develop pertinent skills for this challenging subspecialty.

Home care is not a new concept in pediatrics. Over time the term has referred to parents caring for mildly ill children at home, nursing home visits after children are discharged from the hospital, hospice care, and care at home for children with more serious chronic illness and dependence on medical technology. As discussed in this chapter, home care refers to care provided for children with simple or complex health care needs and their families in their places of residence for the purpose of promoting, maintaining, or restoring health or for maximizing the level of independence while minimizing the effects of disability and illness, including terminal illness.

Home care differs from hospice care, which is a program of palliative and supportive care services that provides physical, psychologic, social, and spiritual care for dying persons, their families, and other loved ones. Hospice services are available both in the home and in inpatient settings and are discussed more fully in Chapter 23. Consider end-of-life care and planning for any child with a terminal diagnosis. Some patients may be admitted for end-of-life home care services before being ready for admission to hospice services. Many hospice programs have admission criteria that do not permit therapies such as intravenous antibiotics, total parenteral nutrition, or enteral feedings that the family may wish to continue. It is therefore important to discuss the type of care the family wishes for the child early in discharge planning to clarify expectations for home care.

Rice (2006) emphasizes the relationship-centered nature of home care that has a holistic rather than technologic focus. As such, nursing interventions in the home may involve the entire household and incorporate health teaching along with psychologic, spiritual, physical, and spiritual care.

HOME CARE TRENDS

Numerous factors have influenced the shift toward home-based health care. Providing high-quality home health care for children generally requires parental desire and ability, professional assistance, and community preparedness. A natural family environment optimizes growth and development when stress is minimized and support is maximized.

Advances in medical technology have resulted in increased survival for children with congenital and acquired illnesses. Preterm infants or children who are ventilator dependent were once cared for indefinitely in an intensive care unit or long-term care facility. These children are now able to live with their families in their own home (Feudtner, Villareale, Morray, et al, 2005). Safe and effective noninvasive ventilation modes and airway clearance devices and methods have also increased the home care of children with neuromuscular diseases. The survival of such children into adulthood has been enhanced by improvements in antibiotic therapy, evidence-based practices, more effective airway clearance techniques, and greater portability of technologic devices that were once impossible to transport into the home environment.

Children with cancer, kidney disorders, cystic fibrosis, spina bifida, cardiac and respiratory disorders, gastrointestinal disorders, neurodegenerative diseases, and human immunodeficiency virus (HIV) infection may have ongoing health care needs as a result of the disease, its treatment, or side effects of treatment (Balaguer and Gonzalez de Dios, 2008; Magrabi, Lovell, Henry, et al, 2005; Davis, 2006; Stevens, McKeever, Law, et al, 2006). Parents frequently face ongoing stressors after a child's hospitalization for diagnosis and treatment. Subsequent needs may include reinforcing teachings about the disease process, addressing the child's physical care needs, providing emotional support during this change in parental role, and teaching in a low-stress environment. Home-based nutrition programs are useful, safe, and well tolerated in children. There is sufficient evidence that these programs provide a better quality of life, decrease cost of therapy, and improve survival (DiBaise and Scolapio, 2007; Daveluy, Guimber, Uhlen, et al, 2006; Howard, 2006).

Improving the quality of life for both the child and the family is one of the driving forces in the efforts to move technology-dependent children from the hospital to the home setting. The concept of normalization describes the process whereby families of children with chronic illness over time begin to perceive the child and their family life as normal (Knafl and Deatrick, 2002). This has important implications for pediatric home care nurses in relation to the assessment of family function and understanding of family dynamics. The normalized family tends to be more flexible with treatments and incorporates the child with a disability or illness into the routines of daily living (Knafl and Deatrick, 2002).

The cost of care is an important factor in the health care delivery system today. Shorter inpatient stays are a reaction in part to the overwhelming cost of lengthy hospitalizations. Children either are not admitted to the hospital at all or are returned home as soon as possible after their illness. Home-based nursing care has decreased the length of hospital stays (Cooper, Wheeler, Woolfenden, et al, 2006). Shifting the financial burden from acute care to home care agencies is an attractive alternative to third-party reimbursers. Likewise, a portion of the financial burden is shifted to the family. The family may be forced to absorb the costs of certain medications, supplies, transportation, shelter, utilities, food, laundry, housekeeping, and a portion of the nursing care. Over time the care of chronically ill children can cause a financial burden to the family. Families may use up lifetime insurance benefits quickly, the primary caregiver may be unable to work, and many costs of health care are simply not covered by other means (Martinson, Widmer, and Portillo, 2002).

The American Academy of Pediatrics (2006) has issued statements supporting home health care of children by their families and urges policy makers, insurers, and government bodies to provide adequate coverage for children who require home health and for those who provide their care. Wilson, Moskowitz, Acree, and colleagues (2005) evaluated the cost of care for children with HIV being cared for at home; the cost of home care for these children was $9300 annually, whereas for children with other chronic illnesses requiring home care the annual cost was $25,900. The researchers further suggest that paid care only accounted for approximately 8% to 16% of the total care time and that informal care by relatives and other caregivers in the home represent a significant benefit not only to the child but also to society.

Home health care of children, however, is not restricted to children with chronic health care needs. Short-term intermittent therapies such as phototherapy, apnea monitoring, chemotherapy, and intravenous antibiotic administration may be successfully provided in a home setting rather than in an acute care setting. One study found that home care nurses providing asthma education to families of children hospitalized for an asthma exacerbation increased the family's and caregiver's knowledge about asthma symptoms, triggers, and management (Navaie-Waliser, Misener, Mersman, et al, 2004). A number of strategies can be implemented in the home setting to reduce the triggers that cause acute asthma exacerbations and often result in hospitalization. (See Asthma, Chapter 32.)

With the increased demand for nurses in home care and pervasive short supply, increasing attention has focused on the role of the family caregiver in providing home care. A recent survey by the National Alliance for Caregiving (2009) revealed that 30% of U.S. households have a person being cared for by another family member; this represents care above and beyond the daily routine care of the family household.

Sullivan-Bolyai, Sadler, Knafl, and colleagues (2003) explored the literature on adult and pediatric family caregivers' responsibilities in the care of a family member who has a chronic illness. Their review of the literature revealed four family-related caregiving responsibilities adapted from the adult literature that may be applied to children's caregivers as well:

- Managing the illness (providing daily hands-on care, monitoring the child's medical condition, and educating others to care for the child)
- Identifying, accessing, and coordinating resources (locating appropriate resources in the community to meet the child's needs and the needs of the family as the child's caregiver)
- Maintaining the family unit (continuing to nurture the family unit—siblings' needs, husband-wife relationships, and household maintenance)
- Maintaining self (grieving the loss of the healthy child; balancing caregiver responsibilities with own physical, emotional, mental, and personal needs; recognizing stressors and potential caregiver burnout)

The researchers developed a multifaceted list of parent caregiving management responsibilities and associated activities that the home care nurse may use to facilitate discussions with parents and families regarding caregiving in the home and its unique requirements (Sullivan-Bolyai, Knafl, Sadler, et al, 2004). Nurses can use the results of this research to better understand the responsibilities facing the caregiving family and assist in finding resources to provide the family some respite from caring for the child to care for each other and maintain self and family integrity.

The American Academy of Pediatrics supports the philosophy of permanency planning, wherein children with special health care needs obtain permanent family placement and ongoing relationship with caring adults (Johnson, Kastner, and American Academy of Pediatrics, 2005). Within this framework the child's home environment with the child's family is perceived as the best place for the child to be reared. Should the family be unable to support the child because of poor resources or family structure, options include extended family members, birth family plus an unrelated family sharing parental responsibilities, or two unrelated families sharing parental responsibilities. In addition, adoptive families may participate in care of the child with special health care needs. The American Academy of Pediatrics further stresses the importance of providing the child's family with adequate resources and support to promote family well-being (Johnson, Kastner, and American Academy of Pediatrics, 2005).

Respite care for caregivers of children with special care needs has been slow in its development and availability, although respite care centers are now common for adults. Such care for ventilator-dependent children and those with skilled technologic care requirements is lacking throughout the United States. Respite care provides temporary relief to parents and allows a break from the responsibilities of caring for the child

on a daily basis. Nurses can play an important role in advocating for the provision of high-quality respite care so families and caregivers can maintain appropriate family function, care for themselves, and continue to care for the child as necessary (Parra, 2003).

EFFECTIVE HOME CARE

Providing home-based care for children gives the nurse an opportunity to assess and interact with the family in its environment. This assessment can provide the health care team with valuable information about safety, support systems, nutrition, parental ability, and actual health care practices. This valuable information will inform future decisions for individualized care and realistic outcomes (Thompson, 2000).

Pediatric home care nurses have two distinct areas of implementation of care. Nurses who perform intermittent skilled nursing visits may see many different types and numbers of patients each day. These nurses typically have a caseload assigned to them and accept responsibility for implementing the care plan. This mode of nursing care is the most commonly used today as a result of personnel shortages and decreased reimbursement. Most home visits now focus on helping the patient and caregiver achieve independence with care in the home, including home care by therapists, home infusion teaching by nurses, and care management, rather than direct provision of physical care.

Nurses who perform private-duty nursing or block nursing are usually assigned individual patients, and they remain in the home for a predetermined time (e.g., 8- or 12-hour blocks). The care plan is implemented over the course of the time in the home.

Required nursing skills depend on patient need, parental ability, complexity of family, and the home environment. In both types of home care, the pediatric nurse is responsible for assessing the patient and family and evaluating the appropriateness of the care plan (Petit de Mange, 1998) (Box 25-1).

A major issue in providing home care in this era is the nursing shortage. Agencies and families are facing much more difficulty in staffing required home care services; thus more and more of the home care must be carried out by family members or other caregivers. According to some experts, the lack of pediatric training in some nursing programs, increased acuity of home care patients, and increased pay for nurses working in acute care settings have contributed to a greater than ever nursing shortage in pediatric home health care (Page, 2001). Greater demand for home care due to an increasing elder population, in combination with the effects of a nursing shortage, negatively affects home health care more than other health care areas, according to some experts (Carter, 2009). An increasing trend, resulting from the nursing shortage and limitations in reimbursement, is providing short-term treatment for patients in nonhospital ambulatory settings (such as ambulatory infusion centers).

Consideration of the caregiver's willingness, ability, and limitations are of utmost importance when assessing the appropriateness of the care plan. It is vital to ensure that patients and families have adequate back-up support and access to resources such as social services. An increasing concern in pediatric home

BOX 25-1   INTERMITTENT SKILLED NURSING

Health Care Need

Child at risk—Parental substance abuse, growth failure, social or family situation potentially detrimental to child's well-being

Chronically ill, but medically stable child with multiple care needs

Skilled procedures—Regularly scheduled injections or infusions, ostomy care, dressing changes, phototherapy

Reinforcement of home care teaching; evaluation of caregiver's skills

Technology-dependent child (e.g., ventilator or tracheostomy, home total parenteral nutrition, or enteral feedings by pump)

Chronically ill child with multiple skilled nursing needs

Intervention

Regularly scheduled visits to assess patient status, evaluate home environment, teach care provider skills, determine status of growth and development, set goals with family for positive health outcomes

As-needed home visits during illness exacerbation to assess physical status and determine appropriate intervention

Assistance with transportation of child to ambulatory center or practitioner's office for evaluation and diagnostic services

Regular visits of limited duration to perform skilled nursing intervention, assess parental ability and desire to perform procedure, teach procedure technique, supervise parental performance of procedure

Assessment of patient status; evaluation of safety of home environment; teaching, evaluation, and reinforcement of caregiver skills; determination of status of growth and development; goal setting with family for positive health outcomes

BOX 25-2   SERVICES THAT SUPPORT EFFECTIVE HOME CARE

- Adequate family training and preparation
- Primary care physician willing to oversee medical aspects of home care
- Professional caregivers trained in relevant nursing and communication skills
- Developmental intervention (e.g., physical, occupational, and speech therapy; early intervention)
- Appropriately designed and well-maintained equipment
- Supportive therapies (e.g., respiratory therapy, parenteral therapy, nutritional support)
- Adequate social and psychologic support services
- High-quality respite care
- Appropriate home renovation
- Telephone service in the home
- Appropriate transportation
- Appropriate locally available emergency facilities
- Competent case management services
- Safe home environment (electricity, refrigeration, cleanliness)

Data from Office of Technology Assessment, Congress of the United States: *Technology dependent children: hospital v. home care—a technical memorandum*, OTA-TM-H-38, Washington, DC, 1987, US Government Printing Office; and Bakewell-Sachs S, Porth S: Discharge planning and home care of the technology-dependent infant, *J Obstet Gynecol Neonat Nurs* 24(1):77-83, 1995.

BOX 25-3   CHARACTERISTICS OF A HIGH-QUALITY PEDIATRIC HOME CARE AGENCY

- Fully trained pediatric staff to provide for all aspects of care (nursing, rehabilitation therapies, pharmacy, dietitian, social work, home medical equipment)
- Prompt, responsive staff with 24-hour availability
- Family-centered care
- Comprehensive continuing education programs
- Certification of local, state, and federal regulatory agencies
- Accreditation by The Joint Commission or Community Health Accreditation Program

Data from Dittbrenner H: Pediatric home care as a viable new service, *Caring* 18(2):12-15, 1999; and Lovejoy D: *Making the transition to home health nursing: a practical guide*, New York, 1997, Springer Publishing.

health care is obtaining a managing practitioner. Declining reimbursement and short hospital stays have increased patients' rapid movement through the continuum of care. For example, a patient may be seen in the emergency department or neonatal intensive care unit, and then discharged to home care without ever seeing a primary care physician. It is therefore imperative that the provision of care for home patients involve multidisciplinary cooperation and communication among health care workers.

From technology dependence to pain management to wound care, pediatric nurses are appropriate professionals to meet a child's health care needs at home. High-quality interdisciplinary care can have a significant, positive impact on family coping and child outcomes (Box 25-2) (Betz, 2000).

DISCHARGE PLANNING AND SELECTION OF A HOME CARE AGENCY

Identifying appropriate local community resources is critical to a successful transfer to home care (Box 25-3). The ultimate goal of discharge planning is for the family to become familiar with the child's needs and to be competent in providing that care. A discharge plan should include emergency management and provision of social and emotional support. General guidelines for discharge that allow for family individuality provide for ideal outcomes.

The American Academy of Pediatrics (Johnson, Kastner, and American Academy of Pediatrics, 2005) emphasizes that the goal for a home health care program for infants, children, or adolescents with chronic conditions or disabilities is the provision of community-based, culturally effective, comprehensive, and cost-effective health care within a nurturing home

environment that maximizes the capabilities of the individual and minimizes the effects of the disabilities.

> **NURSING TIP** If home care equipment is different from hospital equipment, have the portable equipment delivered to the hospital to allow family use before discharge.

Much of the success of home care, particularly for the child who is dependent on medical technology or who has complex medical problems, depends on careful planning and preparation. General principles of discharge planning and the transition to home care are presented in Chapter 26. Discharge planning must begin early; should be based on criteria of child and family readiness; must be a multidisciplinary process, including representatives from acute care facilities, home care, and community settings; and must involve the family.

BOX 25-4	EXAMPLE OF PREDISCHARGE ASSESSMENT FOR TECHNOLOGY-DEPENDENT INFANT

The Child's Family

Identification and training of primary caretakers

Identification and training of caretakers for respite and emergency care

Parent employment status while caring for child at home

Family financial picture, especially if one parent must stop working

Sibling preparation

Availability of psychosocial support services

Technical Equipment and Supplies for the Home

Home care company's availability and experience

Home care company's coordination of services with local health care provider and others

Twenty-four-hour availability and coverage for unexpected situations

Community Nursing and Support Services

Availability, training, and experience

Adequacy of number of personnel to meet needs

Additional training of staff, if needed

Twenty-four-hour availability of ambulance services

Physical Environment of the Home

Adequacy of space for equipment and supplies

Heavy equipment (e.g., ventilator, oxygen tanks, compressor) accessibility

Layout of home (e.g., number of floors, stairways, room accessibility, room sizes)

Location and layout of bedrooms

Adequacy of apartment building elevator and fire escape

Telephone access

Type of transportation family uses

Possibility of modifying living space to minimize invasiveness of technology without isolating child

Adequacy of heating and cooling systems

Adequacy of electrical system to accommodate equipment

Infection control measures

Emergency Plan

Identification and training of those involved

Written implementation plan: who, what, where, when, how (include telephone numbers)

Notification of utility companies for priority repairs and maintenance

Notification of emergency medical unit (911)

Emergency drill

Primary Care Provider

Identification of local primary provider or pediatrician who is able to assume direct care responsibility and coordinate other care providers

Inclusion of local provider in discharge planning

Needs of local provider before child's discharge

Alternate provider if primary is unavailable

From Bakewell-Sachs S, Porth S: Discharge planning and home care of the technology-dependent infant, *J Obstet Gynecol Neonat Nurs* 24(1):77-83, 1995.

BOX 25-5	CRITICAL HOME CARE REFERRAL INFORMATION

- Scheduled medications
- Durable medical equipment
- Medical supplies
- Transportation needs
- Adaptive equipment
- Rehabilitation therapies (occupational, physical, and speech therapy)
- Psychologic counseling
- Social work referral
- Nursing care
- Respite plans
- Key family members
- Demographic information
- Reimbursement information

Modified from Townsend JL: Assessment of the child and family. In Votroubek WL, Townsend JL, editors: *Pediatric home care*, ed 2, Gaithersburg, Md, 1997, Aspen.

educational and developmental services, respite care, and emergency plans

- Emergency care and transport plan
- Financial arrangements
- Infection control practices
- Plan for follow-up medical care (designated medical home)

Creative financial planning, including negotiating arrangements with the insurance company, health maintenance or managed care organization, and public programs, may be required.

Early involvement of the home care agency in the discharge planning process promotes continuity of care and a smooth transition from hospital to home (Box 25-5). Before discharge, a general plan, sometimes called an individualized home care plan, should be developed with multidisciplinary input. This care plan should address the range of needs identified as part of the comprehensive predischarge assessment.

One method of providing home care instructions is with video recordings. Once the family masters the procedures, consider recording their performance on video. Visual learning is most helpful for people who cannot read or who are not fluent in English.

The plans for transition from hospital to home should include family members (ideally two persons) both learning and demonstrating all aspects of the child's care in the hospital. An in-hospital trial period, during which parents provide total care for the child, is generally beneficial. The home care nurse plays an important role in assessing this experience with the family. A predischarge home visit offers the home care nurse the opportunity to meet the family and help them assess their own preparedness and that of the home environment. It also helps them to discuss plans for arranging the child's equipment at home (Fig. 25-1), reinforce prior discharge teaching, and implement any additional teaching that is necessary (American Academy of Pediatrics, 2008).

A comprehensive discharge plan includes the care plan, specific written instructions to facilitate continuity, and detailed information about home care outcomes.

Predischarge assessment (Box 25-4) and planning should include:

- The child's medical, nursing, educational, and other therapeutic needs (respiratory, pharmaceutical)
- Family members' (including siblings') education and training, coping skills, and adjustment needs (including transportation of equipment and child)
- Community readiness in areas such as availability of equipment, appropriate nursing and other personnel,

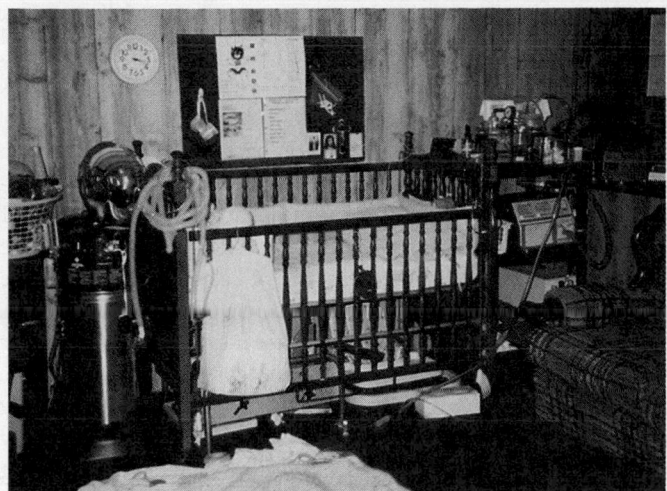

Fig. 25-1 An essential aspect of preparation for home care is the arrangement of equipment and supplies.

CARE COORDINATION (CASE MANAGEMENT)

Traditional definitions of case management generally focus on cost control, attainment of desired clinical outcomes, and the monitoring and evaluation of care provided. However, for optimum home care of the child who is technology dependent, case management (or care coordination) should be viewed more broadly.

Changes in health care over the past three decades have not only improved survival and decreased morbidity among children with special health care needs, but have also heralded higher costs for health care and services provided. As a result, insurance companies have focused on reducing services to contain costs. The advent of managed care and fee-for-service reimbursement has changed the outlook for families desiring to have the child in the home. Often services are provided by multiple organizations and multiple vendors with different missions and lack of consistent single systems linking home health care. In addition, eligibility criteria for receiving funding and services are complex and vary from one state to another. As a result, coordination of home care can be challenging, frustrating, and complicated for the family (American Academy of Pediatrics, 2005).

The concept of care coordination is to link children with special home health care needs (and their families) to services and resources in a coordinated effort to provide the child with optimum care (American Academy of Pediatrics, 2005). Care coordination has several purposes. Its primary goal is ensuring continuity for the child and family across hospital, home, educational, therapeutic, and other settings. Other goals involve facilitating timely access to services and enhancing child and family well-being (Lindeke, Leonard, Presler, et al, 2002). Care should be coordinated among multiple providers to reduce the complexity of care for the child, reduce fragmentation of care, prevent duplication of services, and decrease the burden of care for the family. Case managers from a number of agencies may be involved in the patient's care, which may add to the parents' confusion. The home care nurse may assume the role of care coordinator and should make efforts to coordinate all case managers for meetings with the family to minimize confusion and prevent duplication. Lindeke, Leonard, Presler, and colleagues (2002) proposed

> **BOX 25-6** **CARE COORDINATION FOR CHILDREN WITH SPECIAL HEALTH CARE NEEDS**
>
> - Facilitate timely access to services and resources.
> - Promote continuity of care.
> - Provide family support and enhance family well-being.
> - Improve health, developmental, educational, vocational, psychosocial, and functional outcomes.
> - Maximize efficient, effective use of resources.

Modified from Presler B: Care coordination for children with special health care needs, *Orthop Nurs* 17(25 Suppl):45-51, 1998.

that the ideal situation is when the family serves as lead care coordinator within the context of family-centered care. Care coordination should ensure that the child's medical, nursing, and health maintenance needs, as well as financial issues, psychosocial concerns, and educational needs of the child and family, are addressed (American Academy of Pediatrics, 2005).

Care coordination is most effective if a single person works with the family to accomplish the many tasks and responsibilities involved (Box 25-6). The nurse case manager should have a minimum of a baccalaureate degree in nursing and 3 years' experience (American Nurses Association, 1998). The nurse case manager should be knowledgeable about community resources, including (Thompson, 2000):

- Primary, secondary, and tertiary health care services
- Speech, language, hearing, and vision resources
- Respite care services
- Financial assistance programs
- Parent groups
- Advocacy groups
- Local, state, and federal public officials
- Transportation services
- Private-sector individuals with an interest in children with disabilities

With a greater focus on outcomes of home health care, the nurse case manager has to be resourceful and skilled in communication at a number of levels (Rice, 2006). A valuable tool for nurse case managers is the care path, which is a multidisciplinary care plan aimed at measuring the quality of patient care outcomes derived from standardized patient outcomes. The care path evaluates the quality of patient care with respect to cost-effectiveness and timeliness. (For samples of home care clinical care paths, see Rice, 2006.) Care paths may also be used to help nurses and other health care workers learn home care. Nurses should share care paths with the family members involved in patient care to provide direction and help the family see the eventual goals of care (Rice, 2006).

Although professionals must always see part of their role as ensuring that integrated, coordinated care is provided, care coordination should promote the family's role as primary decision maker and enhance the family's capability to meet the special needs of the child and the family unit. Families may choose to be involved to varying degrees in coordinating their child's care. Many parents take on increasing responsibility for care coordination over time. Encourage and support families in this role. Home care nurses and case managers should be aware that the termination of private-duty or home care nursing can be a difficult transition for which families may need preparation. A gradual reduction in services provided allows patients and families to adjust favorably to the changes. Care coordination by office-based nurses for children and youth with special health care needs decreased emergency department visits and periodic office visits, thus significantly decreasing the cost of health care; increased health care costs were associated with more physician-dependent care coordination activities among such children (Antonelli, Stille, and Antonelli, 2008).

ROLE OF THE NURSE, TRAINING, AND STANDARDS OF CARE

The home care nurse must share a level of technical expertise with the critical care nurse while being able to adapt equipment, procedures, and the nursing process to the home setting. (See Chapters 27, 28, and 31 and many citations in the references for specific technical skills that may be required in home care practice.) The need for technical expertise must be matched by knowledge of child development and the ability to work creatively with the child who is challenged by chronic illness and technology dependence. When practicing in the home, the home care nurse must be comfortable making independent nursing judgments and problem solving with no immediate assistance. At the same time the nurse must have excellent interpersonal skills, an ability to work with other professionals and the family, and, most important, respect for family autonomy. Patient outcomes are more readily achieved with a balance of nursing skills that demonstrate clinical excellence; adaptability; accountability; and the ability to develop positive relationships with patients, families, and practitioners (Petit de Mange, 1998) (Box 25-7).

When working with a home care agency, nurses should expect to receive patient placements appropriate to their expertise. They should also expect to receive orientation to the skills and knowledge base of the home care nursing specialty and subsequent continuing education to develop as expert practitioners. The minimum initial orientation should include the individual patient's care plan and equipment needs; the agency's policies and procedures, including procedures for addressing any problems that may occur when care is provided in the home; legal liability issues; and documentation procedures. The orientation should place strong emphasis on issues specific to home care. For example, the nursing care plan should be based on information obtained about the environment, family dynamics, and health-related behaviors. The multidisciplinary care path may assist nurses, technicians, other health care providers involved in the child's care, and the family, serving as a focal point for achievement of patient and family outcomes.

Reimbursement-driven documentation in home care differs from documentation practices in the hospital setting. Increasingly, documentation must be written in specific ways to qualify for reimbursement.

Supervision of practice, including occasional site visits by a nursing supervisor, should be provided. Mentoring or precepting is ideal. Because of the unique practice environment of home care nurses, it is important for an agency to facilitate sharing among peers to decrease work-related stress, increase job satisfaction, and support high-quality patient care.

Nurses in pediatric home health face increasing demands for providing high-quality care with fewer resources to achieve positive patient outcomes. In doing so, the nurse often must rely on delegation skills to adequately ensure the patient and family receive the necessary care. Delegation often involves assigning nursing tasks to other health care workers (Timm, 2003).

Public or private home care agencies that participate in the Medicare or Medicaid programs must be certified by a federally designated state certification body and abide by federal and state regulations. Additionally, the American Nurses Association has developed standards of nursing practice for public health and home care nurses (American Nurses Association, 2007a, 2007b). Generalist and clinical specialist certification in both home health and community health is offered by the American Nurses Credentialing Center,* a subsidiary of American Nurses Association. The Hospice and Palliative Nurses Association offers certification in hospice nursing. Despite important differences between pediatric and adult care in the home, as of this writing no national standards specific to pediatric home care practice have been developed. Nursing practice in pediatric home care should be guided by published guidelines, textbooks, peer-reviewed articles, and written standards of care for pediatric patients. Professional nursing organizations such as Infusion Nurses Society, National Association of Neonatal Nurses, Society of Pediatric Nurses, Association of Pediatric Hematology/Oncology Nurses, National Association of Pediatric Nurse Practitioners, and others have published standards of care that apply to pediatric home health nursing practice (Box 25-8). In 2009 the National Consensus Project for Quality Palliative Care published the second edition of *Clinical Practice Guidelines for Quality Palliative Care*, available at www.nationalconsensusproject.org/guideline.pdf. These guidelines provide a description of palliative care services that includes children and their families.

A quality improvement program is an important component of an effective home care agency. Evidence-based practice is rapidly becoming an important aspect of home health care, as is benchmarking, in which the product or practice (in this case, patient outcome) is compared with other agencies' outcomes and practices to determine best practice; this allows agencies to see how they measure in comparison to other similar agencies (Wilson, 2003; Yoder-Wise, 2007). The OASIS (Outcome and Assessment Information Set), as part of Medicare, has been established for adults in home health care; however, as of this writing no such data exist for children younger than age 18 years. As a part of OASIS, home health care quality measures

---

BOX 25-7	QUALITIES OF A PEDIATRIC HOME CARE NURSE

- Demonstrates flexibility in skills and case management
- Recognizes that the nurse is a guest in the home
- Respects family culture and adapts appropriately
- Works as an interdisciplinary team member
- Demonstrates expertise in pediatric care (assessment and technical skills)
- Possesses and uses effective communication skills

---

*8515 Georgia Ave., Suite 400, Silver Spring, MD 20910-3492; 800-284-2378; www.nursecredentialing.org.

BOX 25-8 SELECTED RESOURCES FOR HOME CARE

American Academy of Pediatrics
141 Northwest Point Blvd.
Elk Grove Village, IL 60007
847-434-4000
Fax: 847-434-8000
www.aap.org

Association of Maternal and Child Health Programs
2030 M St., NW, Suite 350
Washington, DC 20036
202-775-0436
Fax: 202-775-0061
www.amchp.org

Children's Hospice International
1101 King St., Suite 360
Alexandria, VA 22314
800-2-4-CHILD, 703-684-0330
www.chionline.org

Father's Network
Kindering Center, 16120 N.E. Eighth St.
Bellevue, WA 98008-3937
425-653-4286
www.fathersnetwork.org

National Association for Home Care and Hospice
228 Seventh St., SE
Washington, DC 20003
202-547-7424
Fax: 202-547-3540
www.nahc.org

National Dissemination Center for Children with Disabilities
1825 Connecticut Ave., NW, Suite 700
Washington, DC 20009
Voice/TTY: 800-695-0285, 202-884-8200
Fax: 202-884-8441
www.nichcy.org

National Hospice and Palliative Care Organization
1731 King St., Suite 100
Alexandria, VA 22314
703-837-1500
www.nhpco.org/templates/1/homepage.cfm

Pediatric Home Care Association of America
Division of National Association for Home Care and Hospice (see contact information above); special feature on website is peds@home, an electronic newsletter

PediatricNursing.com
Health resources for parents
www.pediatricnursing.com/parents

Sibling Support Project
www.siblingsupport.org

have been established to measure patient care outcomes for Medicare reimbursement purposes. Other certification and licensing organizations that may oversee and regulate practice in home health include The Joint Commission, Centers for Medicare and Medicaid Services, Occupational Safety and Health Administration, and Community Health Accreditation Program. The Health Insurance Portability and Accountability Act of 1996 guidelines affect the manner in which patient records are handled in home health care to ensure patient confidentiality (Wilson, 2004).

FAMILY-CENTERED HOME CARE

Technology dependence, chronic illness, and complex care requirements cross social, cultural, spiritual, and economic boundaries. Regardless of a family's background, the nurse must respect family values in the provision of home care services. *The home is the family's domain,* and the child is at home because the family's central role is to nurture and raise the child. The ultimate responsibility for managing the child's health, developmental, and emotional needs lies with the family. Roush and Cox (2000) developed a framework for helping the home health care nurse understand the significance of the home to the family. The three central concepts of the model are:

1. Home as familiar—the environment where one is comfortable and at ease because of the familiarity with living arrangements and routines of home
2. Home as center—the location of everyday experiences related to time, space, and one's social life
3. Home as protector—the preservation of privacy, safety, and identity in the environment of the home

The home care nurse must respect and encourage the family's central role in care of the child and must collaborate with the family in efforts to care for the child. Family-centered nursing practice is essential in the home setting. Family-centered care has become the acknowledged standard of care for children with special health care needs (Johnson, 2000).

The philosophic basis for family-centered practice is the recognition that the family is the constant in the child's life, whereas the service systems and personnel within those systems fluctuate. Professionals working with families of children with complex chronic problems must respect the family's central, caring role; their knowledge; and their particular and unique expertise. Families have the most intimate knowledge of the child's strengths and abilities, the challenges of providing care, and the abilities and needs of other family members (Newton, 2000). Believing that no one knows the child better than the family is critical to the success of any health care plan.

DIVERSITY IN HOME CARE

Respect for varied family structures and for racial, ethnic, cultural, and socioeconomic diversity among families is essential in home care. Home care nurses work in close relationship with family members throughout the course of an illness (see Family-Centered Care box). The nurse must assess and respect the family's background and lifestyle choices. Pay particular attention to communication. The meaning of the words used and the way in which they are said may affect various cultural groups in different ways. Take volume of speech and language style into consideration as part of a family cultural assessment.

NURSING TIP One should not assume that everyone who speaks English can read the language. Color-coded medication bottles, written schedules, and pillboxes or oral syringes may aid compliance with prescription administration. Pictures or special symbols may be helpful when providing instructions for procedures and medication administration.

FAMILY-CENTERED CARE

Developing Relationships with Culturally Diverse Families

I work in the inner city, and my home care patients come from a variety of racial and ethnic backgrounds. I am Caucasian, from Australia. Often, when I first visit a family, there is an initial coolness or apprehension toward me. This is understandable because I am a stranger, and perhaps families think I'll judge them in one way or another. By the end of the first visit, however, there is usually a smile as I leave. By the second visit they often greet me with a smile at the door; and by the third visit we usually have a friendship, trust, and an ease of communication.

If I'm working on a case for an extended time, I use a holistic nursing approach. This involves being aware of how the child's illness affects the entire family. As I listen over many weeks to their fears and questions, and often as I share faith perspectives, a bond begins to form. I find it a privilege to share in their joys and their pain, and I feel rewarded by the trust that they invest in me.

Julie Edgerton, RN
Home Care Nurse
Children's National Medical Center
Washington, DC

The home care nurse must also pay particular attention to nonverbal communication. Body language, eye contact, and degree of physical contact have different meanings within a particular culture.

Families may also differ in their cultural view of children, health care, childrearing practices, illness, and its causes and meaning. The family's health care practices and beliefs may influence the level of investment a family makes in the child's care. The family's religion or spirituality also can have a major influence on a family's response to the child's special health care needs. Some families look for spiritual meaning and purpose for the illness. Other families may choose to reject past religious ties. In some cultures, religion and beliefs about health care and illness are closely intertwined (McEvoy, 2003); thus it is important that home care nurses assess the relationship between culture, religion, and the family's beliefs about the child's illness (see Community Focus box).

COMMUNITY FOCUS

Spiritual Assessment

The mnemonic BELIEF was developed by McEvoy (2003) for pediatric nurses to initiate discussions with parents and children about their faith or religious values and beliefs. The components of the assessment tool are:

Belief system
Ethics or values
Lifestyle
Involvement in a spiritual community (church, synagogue, mosque)
Education
Future events

The tool may be used to develop a culturally sensitive dialogue regarding spiritual matters and practices that affect the child and family.

A variety of cultural assessment tools are available (Andrews and Boyle, 2007; Giger and Davidhizar, 2002). The home care nurse, aware that personal values drive behavior, needs to learn about the family's culture, ask questions without implying judgment, interpret the mainstream medical culture for the family,

and help families design interventions that meet their preferences. When possible, use culture-specific teaching materials. In the United States there is an increased emphasis on health care workers becoming culturally competent to better understand and effectively deliver holistic care to the patient populations they serve (National Center for Cultural Competence, 2002) (see Complementary and Alternative Therapy box).

COMPLEMENTARY AND ALTERNATIVE THERAPY

Use of Complementary and Alternative Medicine in Children

A wide variety of complementary and alternative medicine (CAM) strategies are used in the home setting by adults. In such settings, use of CAM by the children is also common. Prayer, herbal remedies, acupuncture, massage, meditation, breathing, and music and art therapy are but a sample of the variety of therapies used in North American households (Rice, 2006).

Respect for family diversity and an awareness of the family's stages of development and of adjustment to a child's illness assist the home care nurse in recognizing and promoting family strengths and in respecting various coping mechanisms. Labels such as *dysfunctional, difficult,* and *noncompliant* can reinforce negative expectations and shape the behaviors of both parents and professionals. On the other hand, identifying, emphasizing, and building on family strengths and coping mechanisms are strategies that promote a central goal in nursing care of the child and family: family empowerment. The home care nurse working with families should remain flexible and open minded because new family strengths may emerge over time and coping mechanisms may wax and wane with the stresses of caring for a child with serious or multiple problems.

PARENT-PROFESSIONAL COLLABORATION

Family-centered nursing practice is built on a foundation of parent-professional collaboration, which represents a shift from the traditional unidirectional relationships between health care providers and families. The Collaborative Family Healthcare Coalition has developed core competencies for professionals collaborating with families (McDaniel and Campbell, 1996). Collaborative caring allows the nurse and family to work together and share outcomes in a deep and meaningful way. This approach, essential in the home care setting, is characterized by the following (Kellett and Mannion, 1999):

- Encouraging activities to develop self-confidence and self-esteem
- Displaying increased awareness of and respect for family caregivers
- Recognizing that families vary in defining their role
- Demonstrating an ability to understand the family's approach to caregiving
- Sharing perspectives, not just tasks and functions
- Supporting family in their primary, irreplaceable role as caregiver
- Exchanging expertise in providing care to the child
- Assisting family in recognizing their contributions as worthwhile

- Identifying strengths and resources of child and family
- Negotiating options, priorities, and preferences
- Assisting with coping by allowing family to find meaning in caring for child at home

Communication with the family should not be intrusive. There is no need to collect information from the family that can be obtained from the child's records. The nurse should explain to the family the reason for questions, particularly those that the family may perceive as intrusive, and should tell families who will have access to the information. The nurse must also assure families that they have a right to expect confidentiality in regard to the data collected. When working in the home, the nurse must respect the privacy of family communications that may be overheard.

Communication with family members should include sharing with the family, in a supportive manner, complete and unbiased information about all aspects of the child's condition and care. Parents often feel overwhelming frustration when trying to obtain accurate information about their child's illness and its management. Parents want information given slowly and repeated as necessary over time; they want explanations in terms they can understand; and they want the opportunity to ask questions, which should be answered in a straightforward manner. Stating "I don't know" or "I'll find out" is better than pretending to know or giving excuses. Unfortunately, the home care nurse may become a source of added stress on the caregiver or family when the nurse displays unprofessional attitudes or fails to show proper respect for the family's knowledge of the child's needs and care (Harrigan, Ratliffe, Patrinos, et al, 2002).

Nurses can make plans with the parents to gather relevant information when necessary (Newton, 2000). Nurses should share information with families in a way that has meaning in their cultural context. Many parents report a preference for interactions with professionals who communicate empathy and concern (Harrigan, Ratliffe, Patrinos, et al, 2002). Families vary in the amount of information they prefer regarding their child's status.

Home care nurses should restrict their communications with other professionals to clinically relevant information about the family.

On occasion, parents and nurses may disagree about proper procedures for the child's care. Nurses should respect parental preferences in any situation that does not pose danger or risk for the child (see Family-Centered Care box). If parents wish to alter a treatment plan that is part of medical orders, the nurse should ask that they negotiate the change with the practitioner because the nurse must follow the written medical orders. If they cannot resolve disagreements, contact a home care supervisor or case manager (care coordinator) to assist with problem solving. Increasingly, home care agencies are developing ethics committees and policies for managing difficult situations such as treatment refusal (see Critical Thinking Exercise).

A tool that might be helpful to the pediatric home care nurse is the Caregiver Strain Index, a 13-item assessment designed to ascertain caregiver stress and subsequently develop appropriate strategies for individual and family coping (Sullivan, 2003). For further information on conflict resolution, see Askew, Williams, Rachel, and colleagues (2008).

FAMILY-CENTERED CARE
Knowledgeable Parents

It is not unusual for parents, particularly those whose children have chronic illnesses or complex care regimens, to be more knowledgeable about their child's condition than a nurse who is assigned to the child's care. This can be disconcerting for both the parents and the nurse. It is important to remember and reinforce that, regardless of the condition, parents will always know more about their child than the professional caring for the child. The nurse and parents can set goals for care in an atmosphere of mutual respect. If the parents' goal is respite from prolonged caregiving, they are less likely to want to give long explanations about the child's care, and it may be more appropriate for the nurse to seek assistance from an experienced peer. If the parents wish to maintain maximum participation in care delivery, the nurse and the parents can negotiate the collaboration.

When teaching parents to perform complex chronic care regimens at home, advise them to expect to know more about their child's care than professionals who may come to assist them, whether that be home health, hospital, or outpatient personnel. At the same time, assure them that various professionals, experienced in working with a multitude of families, will have a scientific knowledge base and a wealth of options for addressing and solving care problems.

Teresa L. Hall, MS, RN
Hathaway Children's Services
Sylmar, California

CRITICAL THINKING EXERCISE
Family-Centered Home Care and Conflicts

A family wants to begin oral feeding of their 3-year-old daughter, Sarah, who is ventilator dependent, has a tracheostomy, and is being tube fed through a skin-level gastrostomy feeding tube. The mother, who is Sarah's primary caretaker, is adamant about starting oral feedings so Sarah can be more like other children her age. One day the mother asks you, the nurse case manager overseeing the child's home care, to feed Sarah baby food by mouth to see how she tolerates the feeding. The child is alert and sociable yet cannot communicate her wishes except through crying and whining. She has a seizure disorder and has had several episodes of aspiration pneumonia since birth. Sarah appears to have a considerable amount of tongue thrusting and lots of oral mucus that must be suctioned frequently to prevent aspiration; her cough reflex is compromised and usually only elicited with tracheal suctioning.

1. Evidence—Is there sufficient evidence to draw any conclusions about the issue of feeding Sarah at this time?
2. Assumptions—Describe some underlying assumptions about the following:
   a. Sarah's readiness for oral feedings
   b. Sarah's ability to tolerate oral feedings
   c. The mother's request for Sarah to start oral feedings
3. What implications and priorities for nursing care may be drawn at this time?
4. Does the evidence objectively support your argument (conclusion)?

In addition to maintaining a sense of control over their child's care, families need to control their home and personal lives. For this reason, nurses should discuss "house rules" with the family and address issues such as the physical environment, private areas in the home, responsibility for maintaining the child's environment, and interactions with siblings (see Nursing Care Guidelines box).

Home care nursing encourages a close and rewarding relationship with the family. One of the most important aspects of

NURSING CARE GUIDELINES
Negotiating "House Rules" for Home Care

House Rules

Parking—Specify where the nurse should park and any community regulations.

Access—Specify where the nurse enters the home. Is knocking preferred or ringing the bell?

Personal belongings—Where does the nurse store own coat, boots, etc.? Does the family prefer slippers to shoes in the home?

Meals—Where can the nurse store own food? NOTE: This is important given the cultural diversity of families.

Radio and television—Identify preferences regarding usage. Remember, this may help nurses remain awake at night.

Patient room—The nurse is responsible for the child's immediate environment. Maintaining a clean working area and cleaning up the room at the end of the shift is the nurse's responsibility.

Telephone—Agency policy may dictate that all personal calls be limited to brief periods. Clarify expectations regarding mobile phone use in the home setting by the nurse. NOTE: Many nurses do need to check in with home at some interval during the evening but this practice should not interfere with the nurse's responsibility to the child and family in her or his care.

Visitors—Identify who may enter the home when the parents are away (e.g., child's friends or grandparents). A list of names should be available.

Privacy—Describe what parts of the home are off limits to the nurse and at what times.

Child

Routine—Specify times for playtime, bathtime, and bedtime. To what extent does the parent want to participate in these routines?

Mealtime—Specify where the family wants the child fed; if tube fed, specify a preference as to how and where it is done.

Clothing—Identify who picks out the child's clothes. Identify where the laundry is and who is responsible for washing the sick child's clothing.

Discipline—Discuss specific guidelines for discipline.

Homework—Discuss when it should be done and who is responsible for ensuring it is completed.

Siblings

Discipline—Establish guidelines regarding how parents should be informed of siblings' conflicts and how discipline should be handled. NOTE: Parents or another caregiver must be in the home when siblings are home.

Patient care—Be specific regarding how children can help with the child's care. Discuss any concerns regarding behavior that may compromise the child's or siblings' safety.

Nursing

Parental notification—Specify what information the family wishes to be aware of immediately and what can wait until they are home.

Limits of responsibility—Specify duties the nurse may not perform, such as transporting the child to care facilities or baby-sitting the child or siblings not under the nurse's care.

Environment—Discuss the need to have adequate lighting and a comfortable working area.

Modified from Klug R: Clarifying roles and expectations in home care, *Pediatr Nurs* 19(4):375, 1993.

? CRITICAL THINKING EXERCISE
Maintaining Therapeutic Boundaries

As the home care nurse who has been working with a 4-year-old ventilator-dependent child, Derek, weekly for about 5 months, you are aware that the parents have become increasingly argumentative with each other. Most of the arguments are about whether Mr. Jones helps enough with the child's care and the house cleaning. Mr. Jones works full time at one job, then supplements the family income by working at a part-time job every weekend. Ms. Jones complains to you about her husband's lack of involvement with the child and his care. Derek requires constant care, and the family has many expenses related to his physical care; the child is severely developmentally impaired and is not expected to improve significantly despite numerous medical interventions. He is the only child, although Ms. Jones stated at one time they wanted to have many children.

1. Evidence—Is there sufficient evidence to draw any conclusions about the family situation at this time?
2. Assumptions—Describe some underlying assumptions about:
   a. Home care of the child with a chronic, terminal condition (see p. 953)
   b. Impact of the chronic condition, child's prognosis, and required care on the parents
   c. Status of the marriage relationship between Mr. and Ms. Jones
3. What implications and priorities for nursing care may be drawn at this time?
4. Does the evidence objectively support your argument (conclusion)?

BOX 25-9 SAMPLE FAMILY ASSESSMENT QUESTIONS

- What are the child's and family's experiences and expectations of disease or illness?
- How does that affect the current situation?
- Is the current coping status a reflection of a new condition, the same chronic condition, or a new phase in a chronic condition?
- How can the nurse address family needs and promote health among all family members?
- What specific nursing interventions will facilitate a healthy response to child and family limitations caused by the illness?

Modified from Gedaly-Duff V, Heims ML: Family child health nursing. In Hanson SMH, Boyd ST, editors: *Family health care nursing*, Philadelphia, 1996, FA Davis.

this relationship is maintaining professional boundaries and a therapeutic role that is supportive of the client and family but does not cross the line of nursing professionalism (Wright, 2006) (see Critical Thinking Exercise).

THE NURSING PROCESS

The most recent American Nurses Association (2007a) standards for home health care nursing practice include six standards of practice, which are the components of the nursing process: assessment, diagnosis, outcomes identification, planning, implementation, and evaluation (Gorski, 2008). In the home the family is a partner in each step of the nursing process. Assessment should address family strengths and resources, as well as the child's health status (Box 25-9).* (See Box 6-8.) The principles of communication discussed previously guide data collection. The nurse shares observations neutrally, without value judgment, and in a way that preserves the family's own role in decision making.

All information gathered as part of the assessment process is shared with the family. The nurse should recognize that the

---

*Self-report instruments to help families identify concerns, priorities, resources, and sources of support include Family Needs Survey, which is available from FPG Child Development Institute, University of North Carolina at Chapel Hill, CB 8180, Chapel Hill, NC 27599; 919-966-2622; or can be downloaded from www.fpg.unc.edu.

family's perception of their most important need will generally guide their behavior and consume their attention and energy. Family priorities should guide the planning process.

> **NURSING TIP** At each visit physically handle and look at all medications. Check them against the medical orders and read the labels. There may be discrepancies, duplications, or changes between hospitalizations or follow-up visits. Clarify medication purpose, effect, and dosages for the family.

The nurse should outline both short- and long-term goals, and the child, family, and professionals involved should agree on them. The care plan should integrate various disciplines that may be involved with the child to eliminate duplication and coordinate and consolidate care requirements. Cross-training of professionals and a multidisciplinary mode of treatment is also useful when a child has multiple and complex care requirements. For example, certain physical or occupational therapy routines may be incorporated into the child's morning nursing procedures, or speech therapy interventions may be conducted by the parent or nurse around eating times so that the entire day is not occupied by procedures. A written schedule of daily routines should be developed and followed by all caregivers. Ratcliff (2007) stresses the importance of the written care plan for the ventilator-dependent child in the home to ensure that the care being given is consistent; written instructions regarding the frequency of equipment cleaning, chest physiotherapy, and reused versus discarded supplies assist in providing consistent care.

Goals of care and achievement of established outcomes are supported by intervention strategies that reflect normalization (see Chapter 22) and the interests and abilities of the child and family. Nurses can help the family explore a range of alternative strategies, services, and resources so that the family can choose the best match for their situation.

Family participation in evaluating a home care plan can occur on several levels. Families and care providers should regularly review the goals of care and update the care plan as required. The nurse can ask the family open-ended questions at regular intervals to assess their opinions on the effectiveness of care. As part of the evaluation process, acknowledge families for their successes and accomplishments. Finally, give families an opportunity to evaluate individual home care nurses, the home care agency, and other service providers periodically. The evaluation should address the nurse's knowledge, skills, and respect for the family's choices. The agency should use these evaluations to improve quality of care (see Family-Centered Care box).

Technologic trends that influence the nursing process in home care include the use of laptop computers (notebooks) to document the home visit and mobile telephones and other small hand-held computers that store large amounts of data, including addresses, appointments, patient tracking systems, textbooks, and pharmacologic databases (Lewis and Sommers, 2003). Internet and e-mail services, which increase patient-practitioner accessibility and communication, and telemedicine or telehealth, which has various features, including electronic systems that can transmit physiologic data directly to the practitioner via the telephone, also influence the nursing process

(Cady, Kelly, and Finkelstein, 2008; Vasquez, 2008). Telephone triage has become standard in many health care institutions, and standards for pediatric triage have been published elsewhere. Concerns with the increasing use of technology in health care are cost, governmental regulations and patient care standards, liability and malpractice issues, ethics, and confidentiality matters (Rice, 2006). In addition, the use of any technology raises concerns regarding the nurse-patient relationship (high tech–low touch) and the nurse's role.

PROMOTION OF OPTIMUM DEVELOPMENT, SELF-CARE, AND EDUCATION

There is little question that living at home offers most children with complex medical problems great social and emotional advantages over living in the hospital or other institutional setting. However, in infancy and throughout the developmental stages, a child's medical condition and dependence on medical technology can place constraints on and pose challenges to normal development. For example, the child may have lengthy and repeated hospitalizations; developmental regression can occur in response to stress; fatigue may result from an underlying pathologic condition, the exacerbation of an illness, or medication side effects; and equipment requirements may impede mobility, exploration, and independence. The challenge of providing support for normal development in a child who is chronically ill and technology dependent is to maximize the opportunities for developmentally appropriate experiences while respecting the limits of the medical condition and the equipment requirements.

Home care plans are designed to promote optimum child development through assessment, planning, and referrals and through interventions that address normalization issues and self-care (Box 25-10). General principles for a family-centered assessment and planning process are addressed earlier in this

BOX 25-10 INCORPORATING DEVELOPMENTAL SUPPORT INTO THE HOME CARE PLAN

Example: 6-month-old infant with a history of 24-week prematurity; currently using cardiorespiratory monitor, oxygen via nasal cannula, and nasogastric feeding tube

Outcome Criteria

Age-appropriate growth—developmental activities promoted with normal parameters achieved

Absence of growth and development deficits for age within limits imposed by illness

Intervention

Assess growth and development with the Denver II Developmental Assessment (see Appendix A).

Reassess growth and development every 4 weeks.

Provide consistent caregiver.

Instruct parents in normal growth and development for child's age, reasons for delay, and anticipated outcomes.

Inform parents of age-related play and other activities that enhance growth and development and provide stimulation.

Consult with physical, occupational, and speech therapists to incorporate recommendations in daily routines.

Provide visual, auditory, and tactile stimulation, including mobiles with or without color, music, toys, books, television.

Hold, rock, pat, and talk to child.

Data from Klijanowicz AS: Care of high-risk infant. In Votroubek WL, Townsend JL, editors: *Pediatric home care*, ed 2, Gaithersburg, Md, 1997, Aspen; and Jaffe M: *Pediatric nursing care plans*, ed 2, Englewood, Col, 1998, Skidmore-Roth.

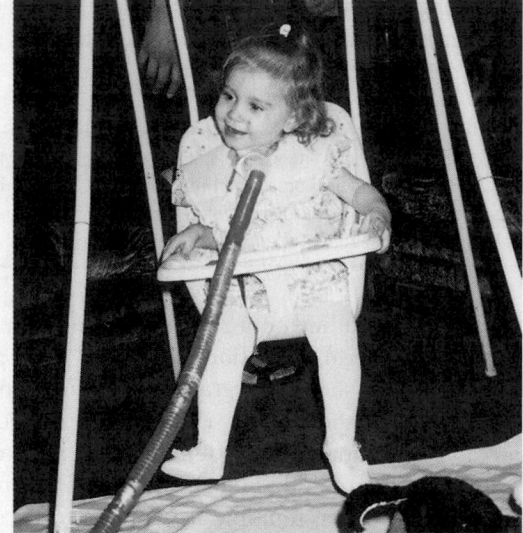

Fig. 25-2 The use of lengthy tubing facilitates a child's freedom of movement.

chapter and are also applied in developmental assessment and planning.

Some parents may not pursue early developmental intervention because they do not believe their child needs the services. In this case professionals need to explain the child's developmental needs in ways that are meaningful from the parents' own cultural and socioeconomic perspectives. Only then can parents make truly informed decisions. Once parents have been fully informed of the child's condition, likely developmental sequelae, and the expected benefits of intervention, developmental goals outlined by the child and family should guide planning and intervention.

Several principles underlie the appropriate developmental intervention plans for children with complex medical problems. First, understanding a child's medical condition ensures that the nurse and family can plan to maximize developmental opportunities at times when the child has the most energy and endurance, while noting stress signals that determine the child's tolerance for type, intensity, and duration of activity. Second, plans for developmental support must be flexible and tailored to the individual child's abilities, interests, and needs. Third, familiarity with the child's medical equipment facilitates the planning of creative ways to meet the child's developmental needs. For example, the use of lengthy oxygen tubing allows the active toddler freedom of movement during the day (Fig. 25-2), portable equipment of any type facilitates family outings, and mounting a ventilator to a wheelchair allows the school-age child and adolescent greater independence.

Chapter 22 discusses the impact of chronic illness on development. Behaviors that the nurse may observe in children receiving home care that need to be addressed include:

Infants—Crying, withdrawal, detachment, inability to achieve developmental milestones

Toddlers—Inactivity; sadness; screaming; regressive behavior; delays in motor, speech, social skills

Preschoolers—Temper tantrums, refusal to comply with routines, refusal to eat or participate in self-care

School-age children—Expression of loneliness, boredom, isolation, depression, or worry about school absences; altered physical growth

Adolescents—Dependency, uncooperativeness, withdrawal, fear of loss of peer status or acceptance at school, altered image

Promoting coping and capability can reduce stress and contribute to mental health and self-esteem in a child with a chronic illness. The extent to which a child is involved in his or her own care depends on many factors, including parental comfort and support and the child's developmental age, level of interest, and physical ability. Self-care, both in activities of daily living and in regard to the medical condition, is important. The goal for self-care in activities of daily living should be attaining age-appropriate competence. Some modifications in the environment, the medical equipment, or the techniques for daily activities may be required to promote and support self-care. Effective teaching for self-care focuses on the child's own level of conceptual understanding. The nurse can enhance teaching through the use of dolls, other models and diagrams, simple explanations, and repetition.

Educational planning is important for the child who has a chronic medical condition. Federal laws ensure that all children receive a public education. Before age 3 years, children with developmental delays are eligible for an early intervention program. The child can receive rehabilitation therapies as appropriate (physical, occupational, or speech therapy). After age 3 years, the local school system is responsible for providing this education. Some children may be eligible for special education preschools. The home care nurse should refer the family to local educational programs.

Each family is entitled to an individualized family service plan (IFSP), or individualized care plan, to help ensure early intervention. All states in the United States provide agencies that develop IFSPs; each state's plan can easily be accessed on the Internet by entering the term *individualized* (or *individual*) *family service plan* in an Internet search engine such as Yahoo or Google. The IFSP provides the child with a disability, from birth to age 3 years, with a plan for integrating early intervention and rehabilitation, based on the child's and family's needs.

When a child requiring special medical care is to be placed in an educational setting, the parents, child, school health coordinator, educational evaluation team, and education and administrative staff should meet to determine safe and appropriate placement and the necessary services and personnel to enable the child to attend school in the least restrictive environment. Training of education staff and caregivers is essential to ensuring the child's safety in the educational setting.* Special assistance can also be beneficial in reintegrating previously schooled children, such as those with cancer, into the school setting. The home care nurse may need to assist parents in developing the skills necessary to advocate effectively for their child in the educational system.

SAFETY ISSUES IN THE HOME

Safety is an important consideration in pediatric home care, and the nurse should include this in the home care plan.

> **NURSING TIP** Arrangements should be made to ensure that, in case of emergencies, the family has adequate methods of communicating (e.g., telephone) with properly trained emergency medical personnel. A cellular phone may be used in place of a local telephone, but it is advisable to check with the local emergency facilities regarding policies for cell phone use and emergency 911 calls.

The telephone and electric companies (if the use of medical equipment requires electricity) must be notified to place the family on a priority service list. In this way the family will learn of any anticipated interruptions in service and will receive priority in reinstatement of interrupted services. Prior contact with rescue squad and local emergency facility personnel can help ensure prompt and appropriate interventions if required. This is especially important if the family lives in a rural location that may not be familiar to local emergency responders. It is recommended that a map be given local authorities with key landmarks and intersections for rapid access to the home.

Before hospital discharge, develop and review emergency protocols with the parents and professional caregivers. Once an emergency plan is developed with the family, it is helpful to print this up and have it in a central location for easy access and referral. The emergency plan should include assigned responsibilities (family members). In the case of a technology-dependent child, it may be helpful to have a fire drill evacuation on occasion to work out any problems in the system. Performing the skill rather than just discussing the actions may help participants in time of emergency recall the steps involved. Post cardiopulmonary resuscitation guidelines, if appropriate, near the child's bedside or in another accessible location. Place a list of emergency telephone numbers near each home phone and include the numbers of the rescue squad, emergency department, managing physician(s), nursing agency, and equipment vendor(s) or providers. Additional issues to consider are advance directives and out-of-hospital do-not-resuscitate orders (may vary by state), as indicated. If the patient and family desire an advance directive to be enforced, specific guidelines must be followed and could potentially prevent undesired lifesaving measures for children with terminal illnesses.

Infection control in the home setting should not be overlooked. Although the child may be exposed to fewer organisms than in the acute care setting, it is still important to maintain "clean" and "dirty" areas to protect the child, family members, and caregivers. Needle and sharps disposal should be a priority in home care (see Community Focus box). The home health care agency should have in place policies and procedures for infection control in relation to disposal of contaminated dressings and sharps for the protection of its employees. Impenetrable needle disposal containers should be available for the protection of those in the household and the community. Hand hygiene is the cornerstone of infection control, and the nurse and family should identify appropriate areas and items in the home setting for hand hygiene to be carried out with ease. Personal protective equipment may be required in some cases; these items should be available to the caretakers as well as the nurse. Some medical equipment may be washed with an appropriate disinfectant and reused to decrease cost of care; however, appropriate infection control practices should not be compromised to save money.

> ### 🏠 COMMUNITY FOCUS
>
> #### *Safe Disposal of Needles and Lancets*
>
> The growing number of persons being cared for in homes setting has increased the amount of medical waste that communities must properly dispose of to prevent accidental needlesticks and the spread of diseases such as hepatitis and human immunodeficiency virus. Many states have programs to assist with the disposal of sharps such as needles and lancets to prevent environmental contamination and accidental mishaps involving needle exposures. Contact one of the resources listed below to obtain further information about needle disposal in your state or discuss the proper disposal of sharp medical equipment with your health professional.
>
> If your state or community does not have programs for safe needle disposal, an option is to place sharps such as needles or lancets in a rigid container such as a bleach bottle or aluminum coffee can. Place the lid on the container to prevent accidental needle exposure. Once the container is about three-quarters full and ready to be discarded, you may add to it a liquid mixture such as cement or plaster to harden the contents and prevent needle exposure. Special devices that break off the needle into a rigid container are also available in some communities.
>
> Additional information is available at Coalition for Safe Community Needle Disposal, 800-643-1643, **www.safeneedledisposal.org**; and Environmental Protection Agency, **www.epa.gov/osw/nonhaz/industrial/medical/disposal.htm**.

---

*A thorough discussion of training issues, content, and guidelines for care in the school are provided in Porter S, Bierle T, Haynie M, et al, editors: *Children and youth assisted by medical technology in educational settings: guidelines for care*, ed 2, Baltimore, 1997, Paul H. Brookes.

Another aspect of safety relates to the provision of care by appropriately trained individuals. Family members should receive thorough training in the child's care requirements and have the opportunity to demonstrate knowledge and confidence before hospital discharge. Children with complex medical care needs are often admitted to an acute care center for nonmedical reasons, including parents' lack of training and inability to care for a child with complex medical needs (Schanwald, 2005). One study found that although technology-dependent children cared for in the home received adequate care, the time demands of such care had negative effects on the caregiver's school, employment, and social life; a shortage of skilled caregivers often leads to disrupted sleep patterns and increased stress (Heaton, Noyes, Sloper, et al, 2005). Professional staff caring for the child should have the appropriate background and training for the child's particular care needs (Boroughs and Dougherty, 2009). Because of the child's body size, special skill and caution are required in the performance of procedures (e.g., gastrostomy feedings, tracheostomy suctioning) and in monitoring the use of equipment (e.g., ventilator settings, intravenous flow rates, and total fluid volumes) (see Chapters 27, 28, and 31) (Fig. 25-3).

The activity level and curiosity of young children raise additional safety considerations in the provision of home care. All medications, needles, syringes, and contaminated materials must be securely stored well out of the reach of curious hands. Make arrangements for the disposal of sharp items or contaminated materials with the home health agency. Pay special attention to childproofing the control panels on ventilators, pumps, monitors, and other equipment. The use of clear plastic tape, covers, or panels to cover control knobs or buttons reduces the risk of accidental changes in settings. Much of the medical equipment now in use has special lock-out capabilities to prevent someone from accidentally altering settings. Keep electrical cords short and out of reach, and use safety covers on any open outlets. Unplug equipment when not in use, and store any wires (e.g., lead wires for an apnea monitor) out of reach. (See Chapter 13 for use of apnea monitors in the home.)

Care at night poses other safety concerns. Parents or other caregivers need to be able to clearly hear monitor, ventilator, or pump alarms at night. They can use an inexpensive intercom system or baby monitor. Take steps to prevent accidental strangulation by apnea, oximeter, or cardiac monitor wires or lengthy intravenous tubing during sleep.

> **NURSING TIP** Coiling extra tubing and taping it at the exit site, as well as running wires or tubes out the bottoms of pajamas or the back of one-piece pajamas, are precautions against strangulation.

Safe transportation is a vital concern. Wheelchairs and other medical equipment must be properly secured to the vehicle, including vans and buses. Appropriate child restraints must be used. If necessary, an extra adult should be present to monitor the child while in transit. Information on car seat safety and transportation for children with special needs is available from Riley Hospital for Children at 800-KID-N-CAR. See also American Academy of Pediatrics (1999) reference for guidelines for wheelchairs in cars, supine car seats, and equipment transportation. The American Academy of Pediatrics (Bull, Engle, and American Academy of Pediatrics, 2009) has recently issued new guidelines for the safe transportation of preterm and low-birth-weight infants as well.

FAMILY-TO-FAMILY SUPPORT

Family-to-family support networks can be an important source of emotional and instrumental support and empowerment for families of children with chronic health problems. (See Establishing a Support System, Chapter 22.) Family-to-family support does not replace professional sources of support but rather is a unique resource that promotes family strengths through shared experience.

Families will most likely experience increased emotional stress as the result of living with and caring for a child with special needs. Parents and families of technology-dependent children reported that they felt isolated from the community when caring for the child in the home; the parents believed the community as a whole was not supportive of the child's needs, suggesting that the child's life was not worth maintaining. The families reported an overall theme in their lives of living daily with distress and enrichment (Carnevale, Alexander, Davis, et al, 2006).

Identifying meaningful sources of support can make a difference in coping abilities. Montagnino and Mauricio (2004) surveyed a group of mothers who were providing home care for children with a tracheostomy and gastrostomy. The researchers found that the mothers experienced significant anxiety, and social interaction within and outside the family was disrupted as a result of the child's condition. The authors recommended that families of children with special health care needs network with other parents in similar conditions through online and local support groups to prevent social disruption and maintain a sense of family normalcy despite the child's condition.

Baum (2004) surveyed caregivers of children with special health care needs about the value of an Internet parent support group. The researcher used stress and coping theory as a guide for measuring perceived satisfaction and a number of other characteristics. The survey indicated that parents were satisfied with the information obtained through the Internet support

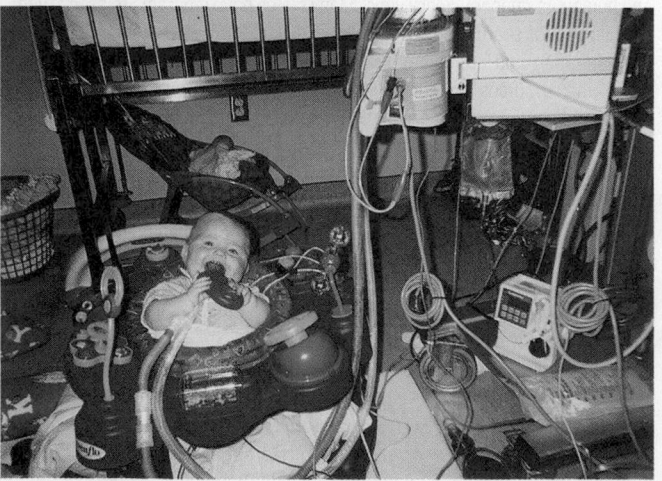

Fig. 25-3 Child with a tracheostomy being managed at home.

group, and improved caregiver-child relationship was the strongest outcome factor. The author suggests that undesirable results may also be obtained via such an Internet group and that the quality of such support groups should be carefully evaluated by those involved.

The nurse can assist the family in increasing their involvement in community social networks. For example, a referral to a parent support group may meet an individual family's needs. The nurse should inform the parents of the group's goals so that the family can determine whether they might benefit from this connection. In addition, informal support networks can be extremely beneficial. A link to a family in the same or a similar situation allows the sharing of common experiences. This in itself may decrease the sense of isolation and provide a connection with someone who can really identify with family struggles.

Positive outcomes can include understanding, empathizing, problem solving, or just talking to someone who will listen.

The nurse should remember that the needs of each family member differ. The care plan should acknowledge each family member's needs (mother, father, siblings, grandparents). Peer support for school-age children and adolescents with complex care needs may be beneficial. These connections can include letter writing, e-mails, telephone calls, or specialty camping programs (Johnson, Ravert, and Everton, 2001). Most school-age children and adolescents just want to be accepted by their peers and fit in as a part of the group. Same-age peers may at first be distant to children with disabilities, but this is likely out of fear and lack of understanding. Helping others see that they have the same dreams, desires, goals, and interests promotes group cohesiveness and understanding.

KEY POINTS

- Effective home care depends on many factors, including the child's medical stability; the family's willingness, training, and ability to accommodate the child's care requirements; and professional, financial, and community support.
- Comprehensive, multidisciplinary discharge planning should begin early and should include the family and a home care coordinator in addition to hospital personnel.
- Thorough education and training of the family or primary caregiver can ease the transition to home.
- Care coordination ensures continuity of care, prevents duplication of services, and reduces fragmentation of services. The family may assume responsibility for varying degrees of care coordination over time.
- The home care nurse must possess a high level of technical expertise while being able to adapt equipment, procedures, and the nursing process to the home setting.
- Federal standards apply to agencies that participate in Medicare or Medicaid; standards of practice by the American Nurses Association and other professional nursing organizations can guide nurses in the home setting.
- Family-centered nursing practice is applied in the home setting; respect diversity in family structures, cultural backgrounds, strengths, and coping mechanisms.

- Collaborative relationships between parents and home care providers are characterized by communication, dialogue, active listening, awareness and acceptance of differences, and negotiation.
- The nursing process is adapted to involve the family in each step and to preserve the family's central role in decision making.
- House rules agreed on by the nurse, child, and family allow the family to maintain a feeling of control over their own environment when professionals are present.
- Individualized home care plans are designed to promote optimum development of the child and to focus on normalization, the impact of the child's medical condition and technologic requirements on development, self-care, and educational needs.
- Safety in the provision of home care services involves emergency preparations and protocols, appropriate training of family and home care personnel, and the safe use and childproofing of medical equipment.
- Family-to-family support networks can provide emotional and instrumental support and encourage family empowerment.

ANSWERS TO CRITICAL THINKING EXERCISES

Family-Centered Home Care and Conflicts

1. **Yes.** There is sufficient evidence to arrive at some possible conclusions (see p. 953).
2. **a.** Sarah demonstrates tongue thrusting, which is common in healthy children from birth to 4 or 5 months and in children who have little experience with oral feedings and oral stimulation. This indicates she may not be ready for oral feedings; an assessment by a speech-language pathologist would be helpful. (See Feeding Resistance, Chapter 10.)
  b. Given Sarah's history and assessment data, there are risks, primarily choking and aspiration, involved in starting oral feedings.
  c. The mother's request is not unusual. Parents want the best for their children despite handicaps that often set them apart from other peers. Although it may seem complicated

to engage in communication, negotiation, and consultation over the seemingly simple issue of giving baby food to a 3-year-old, many issues must be considered. The family appears to have legitimate reasons for wanting their daughter started on baby foods. The nurse should further explore reasons for wanting the child to be fed orally. They may believe that health care providers have overlooked this aspect of normal development. They may be attempting to assist their daughter in achieving age-appropriate skills and may also want their daughter to participate in family mealtimes. These are legitimate, commendable goals, and the family should be supported in making such choices for their child.

3. A child who is 3 years old and has not been fed orally will benefit from an oral-motor assessment by an occupational therapist/speech language pathologist (OT/SLP) to explore

the possibility of starting minimum oral feedings. Specific plans with incremental steps to reduce oral-motor defensiveness and improve the ability to accept foods orally should precede feeding. Nutritional consultation may also be important as feeding plans shift from gastrostomy to oral feedings. The nurse and the family should continue to discuss the issue, plan for consultations and evaluations related to the child's oral-motor progress, and thereby arrange to meet the family's goals of oral feeding in safer incremental steps. Communication between the nurse and the family may also lead to other approaches to normalizing mealtimes for Sarah and her family. After the OT/SLP has completed the assessment, specific short- and long-term goals for modified oral feedings may be developed, involving the family in such discussions. In addition, the family should be made aware of potential problems with oral feedings, including aspiration pneumonia or airway obstruction with further respiratory compromise.

4. **Yes.** The evidence supports implementing this care plan. The nurse should not dismiss the parents' request for oral feedings, yet should not acquiesce to their request without assessing the situation, developing conclusions based on the assessment, and implementing an appropriate care plan that may be evaluated by the outcomes. It would not be appropriate to begin oral feedings without first consulting an OT/SLP regarding Sarah's oral-motor abilities.

Maintaining Therapeutic Boundaries

1. **Yes.** There is sufficient evidence to arrive at some conclusions regarding the situation.

2. **a.** Home care of any person, especially a child with a chronic debilitating condition, is stressful on any family, regardless of its stability and resources. The seeming lack of coping skills and decreased financial resources make the stress worse. It is not unusual for stress and conflict to surround the child's care, especially if one parent seems to be less involved in the daily care. The needs of the primary caretaker, Ms. Jones in this instance, are not being met, and she is expressing that frustration to the nurse, who perhaps is perceived as an ally in the situation.

   b. The impact of a chronic condition on parents can be devastating and lead to misunderstandings, competition over the child's care, and neglect of the feelings of one's partner. Because the child's prognosis is poor, this can exacerbate feelings of frustration, anger, helplessness, fatigue, and conflict among parents. Parents may feel guilty about their feelings toward the child. On one hand, they may love and care for the child; on the other hand, the presence of a child with a chronic condition with poor prognosis who requires constant physical care may engender a desire to see an end to the situation with the child's death. These ambivalent feelings are not unusual in parents, and there may also be gender differences in how feelings over such conditions are expressed. Unmet expectations are a source of conflict among parents with a child who is sick; expectations of each other's role in the family setting may have suffered with the loss of the "perfect" child. These feelings may last for months or even years without an appropriate resolution if adequate resources for resolution are not provided.

   c. The status of the marriage appears to be strained at this time; however, there is not sufficient evidence to draw a simple conclusion without further exploration (assessment). This may be the way each parent deals with crisis situations—the mother fusses and complains, and the father withdraws by going to work and being less involved. Some anticipatory grieving may be occurring, but this needs to be explored by health care persons who can be objective and properly evaluate the marriage status.

3. The concept of therapeutic boundaries supports the idea that they are not rigid and fixed. The home care nurse must be responsive to the relationship preferred by the family and the style with which the family operates. Individual roles change according to the expectations that person has about her or his role and the particular situation. In this case it would be appropriate for the nurse to mention that home care can be stressful for a family, indicate that referrals for counseling may be provided if desired by the parents, and listen and reflect with Ms. Jones about her feelings. Exploring issues such as an additional home care aide to help take care of Derek might be appropriate; this would enable Ms. Jones to take a break from his care and have time to herself. Additional financial aid may be explored by a qualified case manager or social worker so Mr. Jones would not have to work as much away from home. It is important to explore the couple's feelings regarding Derek's condition and care and their role in providing for him, as well as their relationship to each other. It is not unusual for families in crisis to become so involved in the care of the child that they forget what their marriage and relationship is about. If one or both parties do not desire counseling by another professional, perhaps other avenues such as family support groups could be explored as an option. No matter what your opinion, it would be inappropriate to agree with Ms. Jones that her husband is not helping enough with the child's care. Such an action implies a judgment that is outside the nurse's role and undermines rather than supports the family system. Families in crisis often require professional assistance in the form of counseling to explore coping skills and help involve appropriate community resources.

4. Some preliminary evidence supports the argument that professional help is warranted in this situation. In addition, as the feelings of Mr. and Ms. Jones are explored, additional evidence may arise that alters the course of action proposed.

REFERENCES

American Academy of Pediatrics: Hospital discharge of the high-risk neonate, *Pediatrics* 122(5):1119-1126, 2008.

American Academy of Pediatrics: Financing of pediatric home health care, *Pediatrics* 118(2): 834-838, 2006.

American Academy of Pediatrics: Care coordination in the medical home: integrating health and related systems of care for children with special health care needs, *Pediatrics* 116(5):1238-1244, 2005.

American Academy of Pediatrics: Transporting children with special health care needs, *Pediatrics* 104(4):988-992, 1999.

American Nurses Association: *Home health nursing scope and standards of practice*, Washington, DC, 2007a, The Association.

American Nurses Association: *Public health nursing scope and standards of practice,* Washington, DC, 2007b, The Association.

American Nurses Association: *Nursing case management,* Washington, DC, 1998, The Association.

Andrews MM, Boyle JS, editors: *Transcultural concepts in nursing care,* ed 5, Philadelphia, 2007, Lippincott.

Antonelli RC, Stille CJ, Antonelli DM: Care coordination for children and youth with special health care needs: a descriptive, multisite study of activities, personnel, costs, and outcomes, *Pediatrics* 122(1): e209-e216, 2008.

Askew R, Williams PR, Rachel M, et al: Resolving conflict in the home care setting, *Home Healthcare Nurse* 26(10):589-593, 2008.

Balaguer A, Gonzalez de Dios J: Home intravenous antibiotics for cystic fibrosis, *Cochrane Database Syst Rev* 16(3):CD001917, 2008.

Baum LS: Internet parent support groups for primary caregivers of a child with special health care needs, *Pediatr Nurs* 30(5):381-388, 401, 2004.

Betz CL: Children and youth in out-of home placements: nursing care opportunities for pediatric nurses, *J Pediatr Nurs* 15(1):1-2, 2000.

Boroughs D, Dougherty JA: Care of technology-dependent children in the home, *Home Healthcare Nurse* 27(1):37-42, 2009.

Bull MJ, Engle WA, American Academy of Pediatrics, Committee on Injury, Violence, and Poison Prevention and Committee on Fetus and Newborn: Safe transportation of preterm and low birth weight infants at hospital discharge, *Pediatrics* 123(5):1424-1429, 2009.

Cady R, Kelly A, Finkelstein S: Home telehealth for children with special healthcare needs, *J Telemed Telecare* 14(4):173-177, 2008.

Carnevale FA, Alexander E, Davis M, et al: Daily living with distress and enrichment: the moral experience of families with ventilator-assisted children at home, *Pediatrics* 117(1):e48-e60, 2006.

Carter A: Nursing shortage predicted to be hardest on home healthcare, *Home Healthcare Nurse* 27(3):198, 2009.

Cooper C, Wheeler DM, Woolfenden SR, et al: Specialist home-based nursing services for children with acute and chronic illnesses, *Cochrane Database Syst Rev* 18(4):CD004383, 2006.

Daveluy W, Guimber D, Uhlen S, et al: Dramatic changes in home-based enteral nutrition practices in children during an 11-year period, *J Pediatr Gastroenterol Nurs* 43(2):240-244, 2006.

Davis C: Safe on the home watch, *Nurs Stand* 20(34):20-22, 2006.

DiBaise JK, Scolapio JS: Home parenteral and enteral nutrition, *Gastroenterol Clin North Am* 36(1):123-144, 2007.

Feudtner C, Villareale V, Morray NL, et al: Technology-dependence among patients discharged from a children's hospital: a retrospective cohort study, *BMC Pediatrics* 5(8):1-8, 2005.

Giger JN, Davidhizar R: The Giger and Davidhizar Transcultural Assessment Model, *J Transcult Nurs* 13(3):185-188, 2002.

Gorski L: Implementing home health standards in clinical practice: an overview of the updated standards, *Home Healthcare Nurse* 26(5):308-316, 2008.

Harrigan RC, Ratliffe C, Patrinos ME, et al: Medically fragile children: an integrative review of the literature and recommendations for future research, *Issues Compr Pediatr Nurs* 25(1):1-20, 2002.

Heaton J, Noyes J, Sloper P, et al: Families' experiences of caring for technology-dependent children: a temporal perspective, *Health Soc Care Community* 13(5):441-450, 2005.

Howard L: Home parenteral nutrition: survival, cost, and quality of life, *Gastroenterology* 130(2 Suppl 1):S52-S59, 2006.

Johnson BH: Family-centered care: facing the new millennium: interview by Elizabeth Ahmann, *Pediatr Nurs* 26(1):87-90, 2000.

Johnson CP, Kastner TA, American Academy of Pediatrics, Committee on Children with Disabilities: Helping families raise children with special health care needs at home, *Pediatrics* 115(2):507-511, 2005.

Johnson KB, Ravert RD, Everton A: Hopkins Teen Central: assessment of an internet-based support system for children with cystic fibrosis, *Pediatrics* 107(2):e24, 2001.

Kellett UM, Mannion J: Meaning in caring: reconceptualizing the nurse–family carer relationship in community practice, *J Adv Nurs* 29(3):697-703, 1999.

Knafl KA, Deatrick JA: The challenges of normalization for families of children with chronic conditions, *Pediatr Nurs* 28(1):49-53, 56, 2002.

Lewis JA, Sommers CO: Personal data assistants: using new technology to enhance nursing practice, *MCN* 28(2):66-71, 2003.

Lindeke LL, Leonard BJ, Presler B, et al: Family-centered care coordination for children with special needs across multiple settings, *J Pediatr Health Care* 16(6):290-297, 2002.

Magrabi F, Lovell NH, Henry RL, et al: Designing home telecare: a case study in monitoring cystic fibrosis, *Telemed J e-Health* 11(6):707-719, 2005.

Martinson IM, Widmer AG, Portillo C: *Home healthcare nursing,* ed 2, Philadelphia, 2002, Saunders.

McDaniel SH, Campbell TL: Training for collaborative family healthcare, *Fam Syst Health* 14(2):147-150, 1996.

McEvoy M: Culture and spirituality as an integrated concept in pediatric care, *MCN* 28(1):39-43, 2003.

Montagnino BA, Mauricio RV: The child with a tracheostomy and gastrostomy: parental stress and coping in the home—a pilot study, *Pediatr Nurs* 30(5):373-380, 401, 2004.

National Alliance for Caregiving: The Evercare Survey of the economic downturn and its impact on family caregiving, Bethesda, Md, 2009, The Alliance, available at www.caregiving.org/data/EVC_Caregivers_Economy_Report%20FINAL_4-28-09.pdf (accessed February 20, 2010).

National Center for Cultural Competence: Developing cultural competence in health care settings, *Pediatr Nurs* 28(2):133-137, 2002.

Navaie-Waliser M, Misener M, Mersman C, et al: Evaluating the needs of children with asthma in home care: the vital role of nurses as caregivers and educators, *Pub Health Nurs* 21(4):306-315, 2004.

Newton MS: Family-centered care: current realities in parent participation, *Pediatr Nurs* 26(2):164-168, 2000.

Page DR: Pediatric home care: nursing the shortage, *Caring* 20(6):46-47, 2001.

Parra MM: Nursing and respite care services for ventilator-assisted children, *Caring* 22(5):6-9, 2003.

Petit de Mange EA: Pediatric considerations in homecare, *Crit Care Nurs Clin North Am* 10(3):339-346, 1998.

Ratcliff JD: Home health admission and care of a pediatric ventilator-dependent client, *Home Healthcare Nurse* 25(1):34-40, 2007.

Rice R: Case management and leadership strategies in home care. In Rice R, editor: *Home care nursing practice: concepts and application,* ed 4, St Louis, 2006, Mosby.

Roush CV, Cox JE: The meaning of home: how it shapes the practice of home and hospice care, *Home Healthcare Nurse* 18(6):388-394, 2000.

Schanwald PR: Gaps in pediatric care, *Caring* 25(9):20-25, 2005.

Stevens B, McKeever P, Law MP, et al: Children receiving chemotherapy at home: perceptions of children and parents, *J Pediatr Oncol Nurs* 23(5):276-285, 2006.

Sullivan T: Caregiver Strain Index, *Home Healthcare Nurse* 21(3):197-198, 2003.

Sullivan-Bolyai S, Knafl K, Sadler L, et al: Great expectations: a position description for parents as caregivers, part II, *Pediatr Nurs* 30(1):52-56, 2004.

Sullivan-Bolyai S, Sadler L, Knafl K, et al: Great expectations: a position description for parents as caregivers, part I, *Pediatr Nurs* 29(6):457-460, 2003.

Thompson J: Pediatric assessment in the home, *Home Healthcare Nurs* 18(10):639-646, 2000.

Timm S: Effectively delegating nursing activities in home care, *Home Healthcare Nurse* 21(4):260-265, 2003.

Vasquez MS: Down to the fundamentals of telehealth and home healthcare nursing, *Home Healthcare Nurse* 26(5):280-287, 2008.

Wilson A: Understanding benchmarks, *Home Healthcare Nurse* 21(2):102-107, 2003.

Wilson H: HIPAA: the big picture for home care and hospice, *Home Health Care Manage Pract* 16(2):127-137, 2004.

Wilson L, Moskowitz T, Acree M, et al: The economic burden of home health for children with HIV and other chronic illnesses, *Am J Pub Health* 95(8):1445-1452, 2005.

Wright LD: Professional boundaries in home care, *Home Healthcare Nurse* 24(10):672-675, 2006.

Yoder-Wise P: *Leading and managing in nursing,* ed 4, St Louis, 2007, Mosby.

Family-Centered Care of the Child During Illness and Hospitalization

Jennifer Sanders

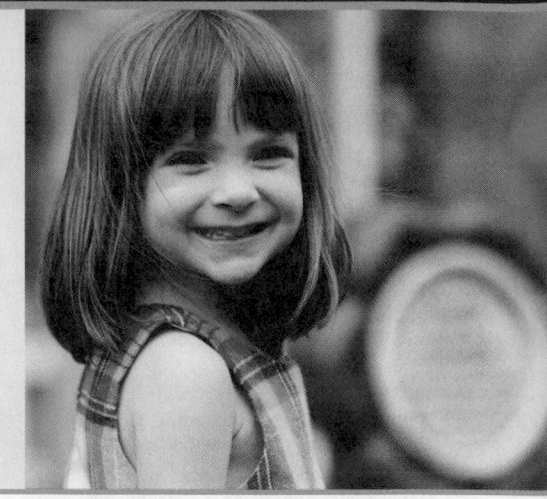

evolve WEBSITE

RELATED TOPICS

CHAPTER OUTLINE

WHAT IS FAMILY-CENTERED CARE?

The theory of family-centered care began to materialize in health care in the late 1960s, as physicians realized the necessity of meeting patient's psychosocial and developmental needs, as well as including families in care. Now the American Academy of Pediatrics (2003) defines family-centered care as "an approach to health care that shapes health care policies, programs, facility design, and day-to-day interactions among patients, families, physicians, and other health care professionals." Proponents of family-centered care believe that collaboration must exist between patients, family members, physicians, nurses, and all members of the health care team in order to reach desired outcomes for the patient. In addition, the Institute for Family-Centered Care acknowledges that families are "essential to patients' health and well-being and are allies for quality and safety within the health care system" (Conway, Johnson, Edgman-Levitan, et al, 2006). The family-centered care movement gained further momentum due to a report from the Institute of Medicine (2001) titled "Crossing the Quality Chasm: A New Health System for the 21st Century," which calls for changes in the health care environment to improve patient safety and quality of care. In this report, the Institute of Medicine called for increased involvement of patients in their own health care decisions, better communication to patients regarding treatment options, and care that is respectful of patient preferences and values.

Nursing professionals should engage patients and families in the care planning and decision-making process. Inherent in nursing philosophy is the idea that nurses nurture patients and form a partnership with parents or families. This collaboration leads to nurses and parents working together to treat the child holistically, thus meeting all of his or her needs. As a partner in care, nurses are challenged to incorporate family and child preferences to decrease stress, minimize the negative effects of hospitalization, maximize the benefits of hospitalization, ensure adequate discharge planning and preparation, and provide overall comfort and support.

STRESSORS OF HOSPITALIZATION AND CHILDREN'S REACTIONS

Often illness and hospitalization are the first crises children must face. Especially during the early years, children are particularly vulnerable to the crises of illness and hospitalization because (1) stress represents a change from the usual state of health and environmental routine and (2) children have a limited number of coping mechanisms to resolve stressors. Major stressors of hospitalization include separation from parents and loved ones; fear of the unknown; loss of control and autonomy; bodily injury resulting in discomfort, pain, and mutilation; and the fear of death. Children's developmental age; previous experience with illness, separation, or hospitalization; their innate and acquired coping skills; the seriousness of the diagnosis; and the support system available influence their reaction to these crises.

SEPARATION ANXIETY

The major stress from middle infancy throughout the preschool years, especially for children ages 16 to 30 months, is separation anxiety, also called anaclitic depression. Box 26-1 summarizes

---

BOX 26-1 MANIFESTATIONS OF SEPARATION ANXIETY IN YOUNG CHILDREN

Phase of Protest
Behaviors Observed During Later Infancy
Cries
Screams
Searches for parent with eyes
Clings to parent
Avoids and rejects contact with strangers

Additional Behaviors Observed During Toddlerhood
Verbally attacks strangers (e.g., "Go away")
Physically attacks strangers (e.g., kicks, bites, hits, pinches)
Attempts to escape to find parent
Attempts to physically force parent to stay
Behaviors possibly lasting from hours to days
Protests, such as crying, often continuous, ceasing only with physical exhaustion
Increased protests precipitated by approach of stranger

Phase of Despair
Inactive
Withdrawn from others
Depressed, sad
Uninterested in environment
Uncommunicative
Regresses to earlier behavior (e.g., thumb sucking, bed-wetting, use of pacifier, use of bottle)
Behaviors lasting for variable length of time
Child's physical condition deteriorating from refusal to eat, drink, or move

Phase of Detachment
Shows increased interest in surroundings
Interacts with strangers or familiar caregivers
Forms new but superficial relationships
Appears happy
Detachment occurring usually after prolonged separation from parent; rarely seen in hospitalized children
Behaviors representative of a superficial adjustment to loss

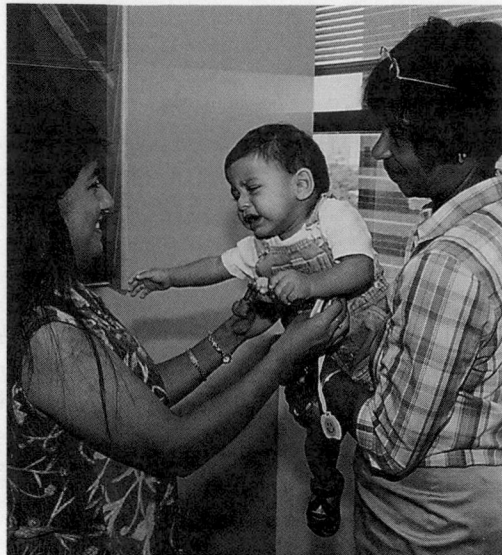

Fig. 26-1 In the protest phase of separation anxiety, children cry loudly and are inconsolable in their grief for the parent. (Courtesy James DeLeon, Texas Children's Hospital, Houston.)

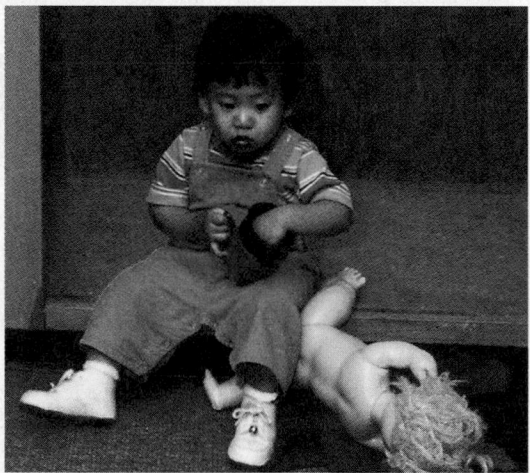

Fig. 26-2 During the despair phase of separation anxiety, children are sad, lonely, and uninterested in play or food.

the principal behavioral responses of these children to the three phases of separation anxiety.

During the phase of protest, children react aggressively to separation from the parent. They cry and scream for their parents, refuse the attention of anyone else, and are inconsolable in their grief (Fig. 26-1). They may continue this behavior for a few hours to several days. Some children may protest continuously, ceasing only from physical exhaustion. If a stranger approaches them, children initially protest even louder. During the phase of despair, the crying stops and depression is evident. The child is much less active, is uninterested in play or food, and withdraws from others. The child looks sad, lonely, isolated, and apathetic (Fig. 26-2).

During the third phase, detachment, or denial, the child appears to have finally adjusted to the loss. The child becomes more interested in the surroundings, plays with others, and seems to form new relationships. In this phase, care givers and health care professionals often think the child has adjusted to hospitalization. However, this behavior is a result of resignation and is not a sign of contentment. The child detaches from the parent in an effort to escape the emotional pain of desiring the parent's presence. The child copes by forming shallow relationships with others, becoming increasingly self-centered, and attaching primary importance to material objects. This is the most serious phase because reversal of the potential adverse effects is less likely to occur once detachment is established. However, if separations imposed by hospitalization are temporary, they do not cause prolonged parental absences that lead to detachment. In addition, considerable evidence suggests that, even with stresses such as separation, permanent ill effects are rare.

Although progression to detachment is uncommon, the initial phases of separation anxiety are frequently observed even with brief separations from either parent. Without understanding the meaning of each stage of behavior, health team members may erroneously label the behaviors as positive or negative. In the phase of protest, they may view the loud crying as "bad" behavior. Because the protesting increases if a stranger approaches, staff may interpret the reaction as evidence of their need to stay away. During the quiet, withdrawn phase of despair, they regard the child as finally "settling in" to the new surroundings and see the detachment behaviors as proof of a "good adjustment." The faster a child reaches this stage, the more likely it is that health care providers will regard the child as the ideal patient.

If parents cannot remain with their child throughout the hospitalization, children may exhibit a variety of responses to parental presence or visitation. During the protest phase, children do not outwardly appear happy to see their parents and may even cry louder than they did before the visit began. Depressed children may protest when parents visit or completely reject their parents' company. Other children may cling to their parents to force their continued presence. In the phase of detachment, children respond no differently to their parents than to any other person. Due to these negative responses and reactions, uninformed observers may think that parental visitation is disturbing the child's adjustment and feel justified in restricting visitation.

Seeing these reactions to hospitalization is distressing to parents, who may be unaware of their meaning. Because of their child's behaviors, parents may see their absence as beneficial to the child's adjustment and recovery. They may respond to the child's behavior by staying for short periods, decreasing the frequency of visits, or deceiving the child when it is time to leave. The result is a destructive cycle of misunderstanding and unmet needs.

Early Childhood

Separation anxiety is the greatest stress imposed by hospitalization during early childhood. If separation is avoided or decreased, young children have a tremendous capacity to withstand any other stress. In this age-group, the typical reactions just described are seen. However, children in the toddler stage demonstrate more goal-directed behaviors. For example, they may verbally plead for their parents to stay and physically attempt to secure or find them. They may demonstrate displeasure on the parents' return or departure by having temper tantrums; refusing to comply with the usual routines of mealtime, bedtime, or toileting; or regressing to more primitive levels of development. Temper tantrums, bed-wetting, or other behaviors may also be explained as expressions of anger or can be a physiologic response to stress.

Because preschoolers are much more secure interpersonally than toddlers, they can tolerate brief periods of separation from their parents and are more inclined to develop substitute trust in other significant adults. The stress of illness, however, usually renders them less able to cope with separation. As a result, they manifest many of the behaviors of separation anxiety, although the protest behaviors are more subtle and passive than those seen in younger children. Preschoolers may demonstrate separation anxiety by refusing to eat, having difficulty sleeping, crying quietly for their parents, continually asking when they will visit, or withdrawing from others. They may express anger indirectly by breaking their toys, hitting other children, or refusing to cooperate during usual self-care activities. Nurses need to be sensitive to these less obvious signs of separation anxiety in order to intervene appropriately.

Later Childhood

Previous research, usually based on adult recollections, indicated that the family does not play as important a role for school-age children as it does during the toddler and preschool years. However, in a qualitative study of children ages 5 to 9 years, children described hospitalization in stories that focused on being alone and feeling scared, mad, or sad. These children also described the need for protection and companionship while hospitalized (Wilson, Megel, Enenbach, et al, 2010).

Although school-age children are better able to cope with separation in general, the stress and often accompanying regression imposed by illness or hospitalization may increase their need for parental security and guidance. This is particularly true for young school-age children who have only recently left the safety of the home and are struggling with the crisis of school adjustment. Middle and late school-age children may react more to the separation from their usual activities and peers than to absence of their parents. These children have a high level of physical and mental activity that frequently finds no suitable outlets in the hospital environment. Even when they dislike school, they admit to missing its routine and associated activities and worry that they will not be able to compete or "fit in" with their classmates on returning to school. Feelings of loneliness, boredom, isolation, and depression are common. Such reactions may occur more as a result of separation than from concern over the illness, treatment, or hospital setting.

School-age children may need and desire parental guidance or support from other adult figures, but be unable or unwilling to ask for it. Because the goal of attaining independence is so important in this age-group, they are reluctant to seek help directly for fear that they will appear weak, childish, or dependent. Cultural expectations to "act like a man" or to "be brave and strong" bear heavily on these children, especially boys, who tend to react to stress with stoicism, withdrawal, or passive acceptance. Often the need to express hostility, anger, or other negative feelings finds alternate outlets, such as irritability and aggression toward parents, withdrawal from hospital personnel, inability to relate to peers, rejection of siblings, or subsequent problems in school.

For adolescents, separation from home and parents may be difficult. However, loss of peer-group contact may be a severe emotional threat because of loss of group status, inability to exert group control or leadership, and loss of group acceptance. Deviations within peer groups are poorly tolerated, and although members may express concern for the adolescent's illness or need for hospitalization, they continue their group activities, quickly filling the gap of the absent member. During the temporary separation from their usual group, ill adolescents may benefit from group associations with other hospitalized teenagers.

LOSS OF CONTROL

The amount of perceived control that children have in the hospital environment directly influences the amount of stress imposed by hospitalization. Lack of control increases the perception of threat and can affect children's coping skills. Many hospital situations decrease the amount of control a child feels. Although the usual sensory stimulations are lacking, the additional hospital stimuli of sight, sound, and smell may be overwhelming. Without an insight into the type of environment conducive to children's optimum growth, the hospital experience can at best temporarily slow development and at worst permanently retard it. Because the needs of children vary greatly depending on their age, the major areas of loss of control in terms of physical restriction, altered routine or rituals, and dependency are discussed for each age-group.

Infants

Infants are developing the most important attribute of a healthy personality, trust. Trust is established through consistent, loving care by a nurturing person. Infants attempt to control their environment through emotional expressions, such as crying or smiling. In the hospital setting, cues may be missed or misinterpreted, and routines may be established to meet the hospital staff's needs instead of the infant's needs. Inconsistent care and deviations from the infant's daily routine may lead to mistrust and a decreased sense of control.

Toddlers

Toddlers are striving for autonomy, and this goal is evident in most of their behaviors: motor skills, play, interpersonal relationships, activities of daily living, and communication. When their egocentric pleasures meet with obstacles, toddlers react with negativism, especially temper tantrums. Any restriction or limitation of movement, such as the simple act of laying toddlers on their backs, can cause forceful resistance and noncompliance.

Loss of control also results from altered routines and rituals. Toddlers rely on the consistency and familiarity of daily rituals to provide a measure of stability and control in their life. The experience of hospitalization or illness severely limits their sense of expectation and predictability, since practically every detail of the hospital environment differs from that of home.

Toddlers' main areas for rituals include eating, sleeping, bathing, toileting, and play. When the routines are disrupted, difficulties can occur in any or all of these areas. The principal reaction to such change is regression. For example, when mealtime and food choices differ from those at home, toddlers often refuse to eat, demand a bottle, or request that others feed them. Although regression to earlier forms of behavior may seem to increase toddlers' security and comfort, in reality it is threatening for them to relinquish their most recently acquired achievements.

Enforced dependency is a chief characteristic of the sick role and accounts for the numerous instances of toddler negativism. For example, rigid schedules, altered caregiving activities, unfamiliar surroundings, separation from parents, and medical procedures take over toddlers' control over their world. Although most toddlers initially react negatively and aggressively to such dependency, prolonged loss of autonomy may result in passive withdrawal from interpersonal relationships and regression in all areas of development. Therefore the effects of the sick role are most severe in instances of chronic, long-term illnesses or in families that foster the sick role despite the child's improved state of health.

Preschoolers

Preschoolers also suffer from loss of control caused by physical restriction, altered routines, and enforced dependency. However, their specific cognitive abilities, which make them feel all powerful, also make them feel out of control. This loss of control in the context of their sense of self-power is a critical factor influencing their perception of and reaction to separation, pain, illness, and hospitalization.

Preschoolers' egocentric and magical thinking limits their ability to understand events because they view all experiences from their own self-referenced perspective. Without adequate preparation for unfamiliar settings or experiences, preschoolers' fantasy explanations are usually more exaggerated, bizarre, and frightening than the facts. One typical fantasy to explain the reason for illness or hospitalization is that it represents punishment for real or imagined misdeeds. In response to such thinking the child usually feels shame, guilt, and fear.

Preschoolers' preoperational thinking means that they understand explanations only in terms of real events. Verbal instructions are often inadequate because of their inability to abstract and synthesize beyond what their senses tell them. When combined with their egocentric and magical thinking, this characteristic may lead them to interpret messages according to their particular past experiences. Even with the best preparation for a procedure, they may misconstrue the details.

Transductive reasoning implies that preschoolers deduce from the particular to the particular, rather than from the specific to the general, or vice versa. For example, if preschoolers' concept of nurses is that they inflict pain, preschoolers will think that every nurse or caregiver will also inflict pain.

School-Age Children

Because of their striving for independence and productivity, school-age children are particularly vulnerable to events that may lessen their feeling of control and power. In particular, their loss of control may stem from altered family roles; physical disability; and fears of death, abandonment, or permanent injury. Loss of peer acceptance, lack of productivity, and inability to cope with stress according to perceived cultural expectations can also reduce their feelings of control.

Because of the nature of the patient role, many routine hospital activities take priority over individual power and identity. For these children, dependent activities such as enforced bed rest, use of a bedpan, inability to choose meals, lack of privacy, help with a bath, or transport by a wheelchair or stretcher can be a direct threat to their security. Although all these procedures seem routine and inconsequential, they allow no freedom of choice to children who want to "act grown-up." However, when children are allowed to exert a measure of control, regardless of how limited it may be, they generally respond well to any procedure. For example, some of the most cooperative, satisfied, and contented patients are school-age children who help make their beds, choose their schedule of activities, and assist in procedures. An increased sense of control usually results from a feeling of usefulness and productivity.

In addition to the hospital environment, illness may also cause a feeling of loss of control. One of the most significant problems of children in this age-group is boredom. When physical or enforced limitations curtail their usual abilities to care for themselves or to engage in favorite activities, school-age children generally respond with depression, hostility, or frustration. Keeping a normally active child confined to a small hospital room or on bed rest is difficult. However, emphasizing areas of control and capitalizing on quiet activities, particularly hobbies such as building models or playing appropriate video and computer games, promote their adjustment to physical restriction.

Adolescents

Adolescents' struggle for independence, self-assertion, and liberation centers on the quest for personal identity. Anything that interferes with this poses a threat to their sense of identity and results in a loss of control. Illness, which limits one's physical abilities, and hospitalization, which separates one from usual support systems, constitutes major situational crises (see Family-Centered Care box).

The patient role fosters dependency and depersonalization. Adolescents may react to dependency with rejection, uncooperativeness, or withdrawal. They may respond to depersonalization with self-assertion, anger, or frustration. Regardless of which response they manifest, hospital personnel often regard them as difficult, unmanageable patients. Parents may not be a source of help, since these behaviors further isolate them from understanding the adolescent. Although peers may visit, they may not be able to offer the type of support and guidance needed. Sick adolescents often voluntarily isolate themselves from age-mates until they think they can compete on an equal basis and meet group expectations. As a result, ill adolescents may be left with virtually no support system.

Loss of control also occurs for many of the reasons discussed for school-age children. However, adolescents are more sensitive than younger children to potential instances of loss of control and dependency. For example, both groups seek information about their physical status and rely heavily on anticipatory preparation to decrease fear and anxiety. Adolescents, however, react not only to information supplied them, but also to the means by which it is conveyed. They may feel threatened by others who relate facts in a condescending manner. Adolescents want to know that others can relate to them on

An Adolescent's Reflections on Hospitalization

July 1997 will always be a significant date to me. It was a time when my life took an unexpected turn. I was diagnosed with osteosarcoma, a type of bone cancer. I was 14 years old at the time. I knew cancer was not a good thing, but I knew nothing else about it.

After the doctors verified that I had cancer, it was time to talk about treatment. At first I thought that I would only need to have surgery and then I could go back to my normal life in a few weeks. When the doctors discussed treatment with me, I realized it wasn't going to be that easy. Looking back, I think I was not fully aware of what I was dealing with. The doctors talked about chemotherapy; surgery; and many possible side effects such as hearing loss, heart damage, nausea, vomiting, and hair loss.

The first chemotherapy was awful. I couldn't stop vomiting. I received methotrexate, cisplatin, and doxorubicin. Those medicines cause a lot of nausea and vomiting. The doctors and nurses tried giving me all sorts of medicines for nausea, but nothing seemed to work. Some of the medicines made me sleepy. Anything was better than feeling sick and throwing up. From then on, I knew what to expect the next time and all the times after that.

The chemotherapy also caused many mouth sores, so many that on the few times I felt like eating, I couldn't because of the mouth sores. Sometimes the mouthwashes I was given worked and I didn't get that many sores, but sometimes I forgot to use them. It always helped when the nurses reminded me.

When I went home, I wasn't there for too long. I would be home for about 2 days and then I would have to go back to the hospital. I would start to dehydrate from not eating or drinking enough, or I would develop a fever. I didn't like being hospitalized for a long time because I couldn't spend much time at home with my family. I practically felt like I lived in the hospital; I felt trapped and incarcerated being there. It was hard and depressing to be in the hospital for so long. The only good thing about feeling like I lived in the hospital was that I also felt as if I had a second family there.

The nurses and doctors were great. Diane and Julie were two of my favorite daytime nurses; they would always cheer me up and keep me company. Tiffany and Carrie were two of my favorite night nurses. When I wasn't sleepy, they would talk or play a game with me. All the nurses helped me feel better and made me forget about everything else for a while.

Modified from Fuentes S: Looking back, looking forward, *J Pediatr Oncol Nurs* 17(3):188-190, 2000.

their own level. This necessitates a careful assessment of their intellectual abilities, previous knowledge, and present needs. It may also require the nurse to learn the adolescent's language.

BODILY INJURY AND PAIN

Fears of bodily injury and pain are prevalent among children. The consequences of these fears can be far-reaching. Adults who experience more medical fear and pain in childhood are more fearful of medical pain as adults and tend to avoid medical care (Justus, Wyles, Wilson, et al, 2006; Brewer, Gleditsch, Syblik, et al, 2006).

In caring for children, nurses must appreciate their concerns about bodily harm and the reactions to pain at different developmental periods. Table 26-1 summarizes developmental considerations related to children's understanding of illness and pain.

Infants

Newborns and infants undergo a significant number of painful events related to hospitalization. These can include blood draws, lumbar punctures, urinary catheterization, and intrave-

TABLE 26-1	CHILDREN'S DEVELOPMENTAL CONCEPTS OF ILLNESS AND PAIN
CONCEPT OF ILLNESS*	**CONCEPT OF PAIN†**
Preoperational Thought (2-7 Yr)	
Phenomenism—Perceives an external, unrelated, concrete phenomenon as cause of illness (e.g., "being sick because you don't feel well")	Relates to pain primarily as physical, concrete experience
	Thinks in terms of magical disappearance of pain
Contagion—Perceives cause of illness as proximity between two events that occurs by "magic" (e.g., "getting a cold because you are near someone who has a cold")	May view pain as punishment for wrongdoing
	Tends to hold someone accountable for own pain and may strike out at person
Concrete Operational Thought (7-10 Yr)	
Contamination—Perceives cause as person, object, or action external to child that is "bad" or "harmful" to the body (e.g., "getting a cold because you didn't wear a hat")	Relates to pain physically (e.g., headache, stomachache)
	Is able to perceive psychologic pain (e.g., someone dying)
Internalization—Perceives illness as having external cause but as being located inside the body (e.g., "getting a cold by breathing in air and bacteria")	Fears bodily harm and annihilation (body destruction and death)
	May view pain as punishment for wrongdoing
Formal Operational Thought (≥13 Yr)	
Physiologic—Perceives cause as malfunctioning or nonfunctioning organ or process; can explain illness in sequence of events	Is able to give reason for pain (e.g., fell and hit nerve)
	Perceives several types of psychologic pain
Psychophysiologic—Realizes that psychologic actions and attitudes affect health and illness	Has limited life experiences to cope with pain as adult might cope despite mature understanding of pain
	Fears losing control during painful experience

*From Bibace R, Walsh ME: Development of children's concepts of illness, *Pediatrics* 66(6):912-917, 1980.
†From Hurley A, Whelan EG: Cognitive development and children's perception of pain, *Pediatr Nurs* 14(1):21-24, 1988.

nous (IV) line insertions. The infant's response to pain varies markedly in measures of distress, especially initial cry and heart rate, which may decrease in some infants. The most consistent indicator of distress is a facial expression of discomfort (Fig. 26-3). Infants may express pain physically by actions such as squirming or flailing (Franck, Greenberg, and Stevens, 2000). Some infants may cry loudly after the procedure, whereas a gentle hug may calm others easily. It is important to recognize and respect such early signs of individuality and to realize that children who react less intensely may still be experiencing significant discomfort.

Infants younger than 6 months of age seem to have no obvious memory of previous painful experiences and may react to a potentially stressful situation with less apprehension and fear than older children. Research has found that infants have stored memories of acute pain experiences (such as repeated heelsticks) and react in subsequent painful events with

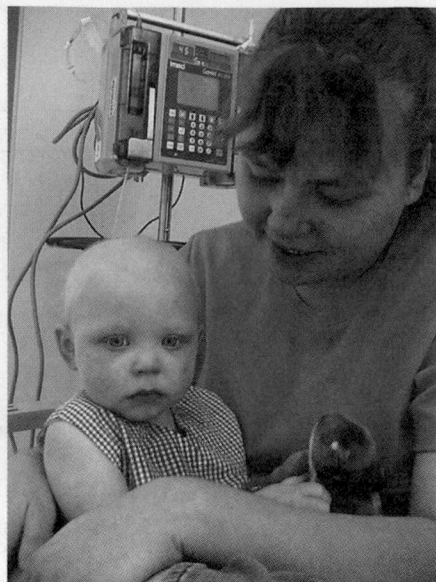

Fig. 26-3 Facial expressions reflect distress and are consistent behavioral indicators of pain in infants. (Courtesy E. Jacob, Texas Children's Hospital, Houston.)

heightened responses to pain (Taddio, Shah, Gilbert-MacLeod, et al, 2002; Taddio and Katz, 2005). There is also evidence that repeated painful procedures can alter brain structure and behavioral and hormonal response to pain (American Academy of Pediatrics, 2000; Anand and Scalzo, 2000).

After 6 months of age, children's response to pain is influenced by their memory of prior painful experiences and the emotional reaction of parents during the procedure. Older infants react intensely with physical resistance and uncooperativeness. They may refuse to lie still, attempt to push the person away, or try to escape with whatever motor activity they have achieved. Distraction does little to lessen their immediate reaction to pain, and anticipatory preparation, such as showing them the equipment, tends to increase their fear and resistance.

Toddlers

Toddlers' concept of body image, particularly the definition of body boundaries, is poorly developed. Intrusive experiences, such as examining the ears or mouth or taking a rectal temperature, produce anxiety. Toddlers may react to such painless procedures as intensely as they do to painful ones.

Toddlers' reactions to pain are similar to those seen during infancy, except that the variables influencing the individual response are highly complex and varied. Memory, physical restraint, separation from the parent or guardian, emotional reactions of others, and lack of preparation partially determine the intensity of the behavioral response. In general, children in this age-group continue to react with intense emotional upset and physical resistance to any actual or perceived painful experience. Behaviors indicating pain include grimacing; clenching the teeth or lips; opening the eyes wide; rocking; rubbing; and aggressiveness, such as biting, kicking, hitting, or running away. Unlike adults, who usually decrease their activity when in pain, young children typically become restless and overactive; frequently this response is not recognized as a consequence of pain.

By the end of this age period, toddlers usually are able to communicate about their pain. Although they have not developed the ability to describe the type or intensity of the pain, they usually are able to localize it by pointing to a specific area.

Preschoolers

Concepts of illness begin during the preschool period and are influenced by the cognitive abilities of the preoperational stage. Preschoolers differentiate poorly between themselves and the external world. Their thinking is focused on externally perceived events, and causality is based on the proximity of two events. Consequently, children define illness according to what they are told or are given external evidence of, such as "You are sick because you have a fever." The cause of illness is a concrete action the child does or fails to do, such as "catching a stomach virus because you don't wash your hands." Consequently, illness implies a degree of responsibility and self-blame. Another explanation may be based on contagion, that is, the proximity of two objects or persons causes the illness (e.g., "A person gets a cold when someone else with a cold gets near him").

The psychosexual conflicts of children in this age-group make them vulnerable to threats of bodily injury. Intrusive procedures, whether painful or painless, are threatening to preschoolers, whose concept of body integrity is still poorly developed. Preschoolers may react to an injection with as much concern for withdrawal of the needle as for the actual pain. They fear that the intrusion or puncture will not close and that their "insides" will leak out.

Concerns of mutilation are paramount during this age period. Loss of any body part is threatening, but preschool boys' fears of castration complicate their understanding of surgical or medical procedures associated with the genital area, such as circumcision, repair of hypospadias or epispadias, cystoscopy, or catheterization. Their limited comprehension of body functioning also increases their difficulty in understanding how or why body parts are "fixed." For example, telling preschoolers that their tonsils are to be removed may be interpreted as "taking out their voice." Preschoolers understand words such as *dye, cut off, take out,* or *draw* (as in "draw some blood"), and using these words can lead to confusion and fear. (See Communicating with Children, Chapter 6.)

Reactions to pain tend to be similar to those seen during toddlerhood, although some differences become apparent. For example, preschoolers respond more favorably to preparatory interventions, such as explanation and distraction, than younger children. Physical and verbal aggression is more specific and goal directed. Instead of showing total body resistance, preschoolers may push the offending person away, try to secure the equipment, or attempt to lock themselves in a safe place. Much more thought is evident in their plan of attack or escape.

Verbal expression in particular demonstrates their advanced development in response to stress. They may verbally abuse the attacker by stating, "Go away" or "I hate you." They may also use the more cunning approach of trying to persuade the person to delay the intended activity. A common plea is "I have to go to the bathroom." Some statements are not only attempts to avoid the event but also evidence of children's perceptions about the experience.

School-Age Children

Fears of the physical nature of the illness surface at this time. School-age children may be less concerned with pain than with disability, uncertain recovery, or possible death. Because of their developing cognitive abilities, school-age children are aware of the significance of different illnesses, the indispensability of certain body parts, potential hazards in treatment, lifelong consequences of permanent injury or loss of function, and the meaning of death. A major concern of hospitalized school-age children is their fear of being told that something is wrong with them. They generally take an active interest in their health or illness. Even those children who rarely ask questions usually accumulate detailed information on their condition by attentively listening to all that is said around them. They request factual information and quickly perceive lies or half-truths. Seeking information tends to be one way they maintain a sense of control despite the stress and uncertainty of illness.

School-age children define illness by a set of multiple concrete symptoms, such as signs of a cold, and view the cause as primarily germs or bacteria. The germs have a powerful, almost magical quality, so that in the child's mind, illness can be prevented by avoiding people with the germs. They also believe in the idea of contamination, which is similar to that seen in the younger age-group. For example, the illness occurs because of physical contact or because the child engaged in a harmful action and became contaminated. Consequently, feelings of self-blame and guilt may be associated with the reason for becoming ill.

School-age children begin to show concern for the potential beneficial and hazardous effects of procedures. Besides wanting to know if a procedure will hurt, they want to know what it is for, how it will make them well, and what injury or harm could result. For example, these children fear the actual procedure of anesthesia. Unlike preschoolers, who fear the mask and the strange surroundings, school-age children fear what might happen while they are asleep, whether they will wake up, and whether they might die. Preadolescents also worry about the procedure itself, particularly one that will result in visible changes in body appearance.

Intrusive procedures, such as routine physical examination of the ears, nose, mouth, and throat, are generally well tolerated. However, concerns for privacy become increasingly significant. Although school-age children may cooperate during examination of, or procedures performed on, the genital area, it is usually stressful for them, especially for preadolescents who are beginning pubertal changes. Nurses who respect children's need for privacy can provide them with assurance and support.

By the age of 9 or 10, most school-age children show less fright or overt resistance to pain than younger children. They generally have learned passive methods of dealing with discomfort, such as holding rigidly still, clenching their fists or teeth, or trying to act brave. If they display signs of overt resistance, such as biting, kicking, pulling away, trying to escape, crying, or plea bargaining, they may deny such reactions later, especially to their peers, for fear of embarrassment.

School-age children verbally communicate about their pain in respect to its location, intensity, and description. Unlike younger children, who may have difficulty choosing words to describe pain, children 8 years and older (like adults) use a wide variety of words and phrases, such as *hurting, sore, burning, stinging,* and *aching* (Franck, Greenberg, and Stevens, 2000).

School-age children also use words as a means of controlling their reactions to pain. For example, these children may ask the nurse to talk to them during a procedure. Some prefer to participate in a procedure, whereas others choose to distance themselves by not looking at what is happening. Most appreciate an explanation of the procedure and seem less fearful when they know what to expect. Others try to gain control by attempting to postpone the event. A typical request is, "Start the IV when I am finished with this." Although the ability to make decisions does increase their sense of control, unlimited procrastination and bargaining result in heightened anxiety. When choices are allowed, such as which arm for the IV line, it is best to structure the number of options and to limit the number of procrastination or bargaining techniques. Nurses must also exercise caution when asking the child to make choices to ensure that the choice can be honored.

Similar to their more passive acceptance of pain is their nondirective request for support or help. School-age children rarely initiate a conversation about their feelings or ask someone to stay with them during a lonely or stressful period. Their visible composure, calmness, and acceptance often mask their inner longing for support. It is especially important to be aware of nonverbal clues, such as a serious facial expression, a half-hearted reply of "I am fine," silence, lack of activity, or social isolation, as signs of the need for help. Usually when someone identifies the unspoken messages and offers support, they readily accept it.

Adolescents

Although the development of body image begins early in life, its relevance is paramount during adolescence. Injury, pain, disability, and death are viewed primarily in terms of how each affects adolescents' views of themselves in the present. Any change that differentiates the adolescent from peers is regarded as a major tragedy. For example, chronic diseases such as diabetes mellitus often present a more difficult adjustment period for children in this age-group than for younger children because of the necessary changes in lifestyle. Conversely, serious, even life-threatening illnesses that entail no visible bodily changes or physical restrictions may have less immediate significance for the adolescent. Therefore the nature of bodily injury may be more important in terms of adolescents' perception of the illness than its actual degree of severity.

Adolescents' rapidly changing body image during pubertal development often makes them feel insecure about their bodies. Illness, medical or surgical intervention, and hospitalization increase their existing concerns for normalcy. They may respond to such events by asking numerous questions, withdrawing, rejecting others, or questioning the adequacy of care. Frequently their fear for loss of control and body image change is demonstrated as overconfidence.

Because of the development of secondary sexual characteristics, adolescents are concerned about privacy. Lack of respect for this need can cause greater stress than physical pain. In addition, adolescents look for signs that indicate they are developing normally and according to acceptable standards. When

---

BOX 26-2	POSTHOSPITAL BEHAVIORS IN CHILDREN

Young Children
Initial aloofness toward parents; may last from a few minutes (most common) to a few days
Tendency to cling to parents
Demanding parents' attention
Vigorously opposing any separation (e.g., staying at preschool or with a baby-sitter)
New fears (e.g., nightmares)
Resistance to going to bed, night waking
Withdrawal and shyness
Hyperactivity
Temper tantrums
Food finickiness
Attachment to blanket or toy
Regression in newly learned skills (e.g., toileting)

Older Children
Emotional coldness, followed by intense, demanding dependence on parents
Anger toward parents
Jealousy toward others (e.g., siblings)

BOX 26-3	RISK FACTORS THAT INCREASE CHILDREN'S VULNERABILITY TO THE STRESSES OF HOSPITALIZATION

- "Difficult" temperament (See also Temperament, Chapter 12.)
- Lack of fit between child and parent
- Age (especially between 6 months and 5 years)
- Male gender
- Below-average intelligence
- Multiple and continuing stresses (e.g., frequent hospitalizations)

---

illness occurs, they fear that growth may be retarded, leaving them behind their peers. Although they may not voice this concern, they may demonstrate it by carefully observing others' reactions to them.

Adolescents typically react to pain with much self-control. Physical resistance and aggression are unusual at this age, unless the adolescents are unprepared for a procedure. As with older school-age children, they are concerned with remaining composed and feel embarrassed and ashamed of losing control. They are able to describe their pain experience and to use the pain assessment tools developed for adults. However, they may be reluctant to disclose their pain, requiring the nurse to listen closely and observe physical indications, such as limited movement, excessive quiet, or irritability. Adolescents may also believe that the nurse knows how they feel; thus they may see no need to ask for analgesia.

EFFECTS OF HOSPITALIZATION ON THE CHILD

Children may react to the stresses of hospitalization before admission, during hospitalization, and after discharge (Box 26-2). A child's conception of illness is even more important than age and intellectual maturity in predicting the level of adjustment before hospitalization. This may or may not be affected by the duration of the condition or prior hospitalizations. Therefore nurses should avoid making incorrect assumptions regarding the illness concepts of children with prior medical experience.

Individual Risk Factors

A number of risk factors make some children more vulnerable than others to the stresses of hospitalization (Box 26-3). Because separation is such an important issue surrounding hospitalization for young children, children who are active and have a strong will tend to fare better when hospitalized than youngsters who are passive. Nurses should be alert to children who

passively accept all changes and requests, since these children may need more support than the "oppositional" child.

The stressors of hospitalization may cause young children to experience short- and long-term negative outcomes. Adverse outcomes may be related to the length and number of admissions, multiple invasive procedures, and parents' anxiety. Common responses include regression, separation anxiety, apathy, fears, and sleep disturbances, especially for children younger than 7 years of age (Melnyk, 2000). Supportive practices, such as family-centered care, frequent family visits, and mothers who know exactly how they can be involved in their child's care, may lessen the detrimental effects of hospitalization. Research also indicates that the child's pain experience determines how the child will experience the overall hospitalization. Consequently, nurses should attempt to identify children who are at risk for poor coping outcomes (Small, 2002).

Changes in the Pediatric Population

Children are hospitalized for different reasons today than two decades ago. Despite the growing trend toward shortened hospital stays and outpatient surgery, a greater percentage of the children hospitalized today have more serious and complex problems than those hospitalized in the past. Many of these children are medically fragile newborns and children with severe injuries or disabilities who survived because of incredible technologic advances, yet were left with chronic or disabling conditions that require frequent and lengthy hospital stays. The nature of their conditions increases the likelihood that this group of children will experience more invasive and traumatic procedures while they are hospitalized. These factors make them more vulnerable to the emotional consequences of hospitalization and result in their needs being significantly different from those of short-term patients. (See Chapter 22 for further discussion on children with special needs.) The majority of these children are infants and toddlers, the age-group most vulnerable to the effects of hospitalization.

Concern in recent years has focused on the increasing length of hospitalization because of complex medical and nursing care, elusive diagnoses, and complicated psychosocial issues. Without special attention devoted to meeting the child's psychosocial and developmental needs in the hospital environment, the damaging consequences of prolonged hospitalization may be severe.

Beneficial Effects of Hospitalization

Although hospitalization can be and usually is stressful for children, it can also be beneficial. The most obvious benefit is the recovery from illness, but hospitalization also can present an opportunity for children to master stress and feel competent in their coping abilities. The hospital environment can provide children with new socialization experiences that can broaden their interpersonal relationships. The psychologic benefits need to be considered and maximized during hospitalization. Appropriate nursing strategies to achieve this goal are presented later in this chapter.

STRESSORS AND REACTIONS OF THE FAMILY OF THE CHILD WHO IS HOSPITALIZED

PARENTAL REACTIONS

The crisis of childhood illness and hospitalization is a major source of stress and anxiety for every member of the nuclear family. Parents' reactions to their child's illness depend on a variety of factors. Although one cannot predict which factors are most likely to influence their response, a number of variables have been identified (Box 26-4).

Fear, anxiety, and frustration are common feelings expressed by parents. Fear and anxiety may be related to the seriousness of the illness and the type of medical procedures involved. Anxiety is frequently related to the trauma and pain inflicted on the child from the various procedures. Parents may question why they and their child have to go through this experience, as well as the purpose of pain and suffering (Feudtner, Haney, and Dimmers, 2003). Frustration is often related to lack of information about procedures and treatments, unfamiliarity with hospital rules and regulations, unfriendly staff, or fear of asking questions. Nurses can alleviate much frustration in the pediatric unit by making parents aware of what to expect and what is expected of them, encouraging them to participate in their child's care, and treating them as the most significant contributors to the child's total health.

Parents eventually may react with some degree of depression. Mothers often comment on their feeling of physical and mental exhaustion after all the other family members have adapted to the crisis. Parents may also worry about and miss their other children, who may be left in the care of family, friends, or neighbors. Other reasons for anxiety and depression are related to concerns for the child's future well-being, including negative effects produced by the hospitalization and any subsequent financial burden incurred.

BOX 26-4	FACTORS AFFECTING PARENTS' REACTIONS TO THEIR CHILD'S ILLNESS

- Seriousness of the threat to the child
- Previous experience with illness or hospitalization
- Medical procedures involved in diagnosis and treatment
- Available support systems
- Personal ego strengths
- Previous coping abilities
- Additional stresses on the family system
- Cultural and religious beliefs
- Communication patterns among family members

In a retrospective database survey of more than 50,000 parents of a hospitalized child, parents identified seven priorities from their perspective to improve the care of the hospitalized child (Miceli and Clark, 2005). The parents' highest priority was to improve staff's sensitivity to the disruption and inconvenience of the child being hospitalized. Additional leading suggestions included improving the degree to which hospital staff address the family's emotional and spiritual needs during the child's hospitalization, improving staff's response when parents express concerns or voice complaints during the child's stay, including parents in decisions regarding treatments, improving visitor (family) accommodations and comfort, providing information about nearby services and lodging facilities for family members, and improving staff concerns to make the child's stay as restful and comfortable as possible. In each of the seven categories the researchers provide additional issues parents raised in relation to the primary theme.

Studies highlight the need for family-centered nursing care that considers the effects of hospitalization on the child and the parents (Miceli and Clark, 2005; Stratton, 2004; Feudtner, Haney, and Dimmers, 2003). Hospital staff members must continually assess the parents' need for information and reassurance. Although the child's care may take precedence over parents' needs, nurses must make every effort to improve parent coping to optimize patient outcomes. By maintaining sensitivity to the family's needs, the nurse can become equal partners with parents in the child's care.

SIBLING REACTIONS

Siblings' reactions to a sister's or brother's illness or hospitalization are discussed in Chapters 22 and 23 and differ little when a child has an acute illness. Siblings may experience loneliness, fears, and worry. Siblings frequently fear acquiring the illness of their ill sibling. Behavioral reactions include anger, resentment, jealousy, and guilt. Various factors have been identified that influence the siblings' reactions to the child's hospitalization. Although these factors are similar to those seen when a child has a chronic illness, Craft (1993) reported that the following factors are related specifically to the hospital experience and have been found to increase the effects on the sibling:

- Being younger and experiencing many changes
- Being cared for outside the home by care providers who are not relatives
- Receiving little information about their ill brother or sister
- Perceiving their parents as treating them differently compared with before their sibling's hospitalization

Parents are often unaware of the effect on siblings of a sick child's hospitalization and of the benefit of simple interventions to minimize such effects, such as explicit explanations about the illness and provisions for the siblings to remain at home. Sibling visitation is advocated and is usually advantageous. However, unless siblings are prepared for what they may see, their visits may confuse them, leaving room for greater anxiety and worry when they are home, away from their hospitalized brother or sister. Siblings need to be given developmentally appropriate information about their sibling's illness or injury and be given an opportunity to ask questions.

ALTERED FAMILY ROLES

In addition to the effects of separation on family roles, loss of the parent and sibling roles may affect each family member differently. One of the most common reactions of parents is intensified attention toward the sick child. The other siblings may regard this as unfair and interpret the parents' attitude toward them as rejection and abandonment. Although such responses are usually unconscious and unintended, they place unique burdens on ill children. For example, the ill child may feel obligated to play the sick role to meet parents' expectations, especially in the case of children who have had limited physical ability and regain normal health status, such as following corrective heart surgery. Parents also may have difficulty perceiving the child's recovery and therefore continue the pattern of overprotection and indulgent attention.

Ill children may also feel jealousy and resentment from siblings. Because of their singular position in the family, they may be denied the companionship of their brothers and sisters. Rivalry tends to be greatest with the sibling who is nearest the ill child's age. Without an understanding of the interpersonal dynamics between siblings, parents are likely to blame the well children for antisocial behavior. Illness may also result in a child's loss of status within either the family or peer group. For example, illness in the oldest child may temporarily terminate special privileges as "big" brother or sister.

NURSING CARE OF THE CHILD WHO IS HOSPITALIZED

Children and their families require competent and sensitive care to minimize the potential negative effects of hospitalization and also to promote positive benefits from the experience. Interventions should focus on (1) eliminating or minimizing the stressors of separation, loss of control, and bodily injury and pain for children; and (2) providing specific supportive strategies for family members, such as fostering family relationships and providing information.

Initiate a family assessment using the guidelines in Box 26-7. Assess the parents and other immediate family members for coping and for special assistance needs (e.g., temporary child care for siblings, lodging, meals, and transportation to and from hospital).

PREVENTING OR MINIMIZING SEPARATION

A primary nursing goal is to prevent separation, particularly in children under 5 years of age. Hospitals no longer consider parents "visitors" and welcome their presence at all times throughout the child's hospitalization. Many hospitals have adopted a philosophy of family-centered care, which recognizes the integral role of the family in a child's life and acknowledges the family as an essential part of the child's care and illness experience. In the broadest sense, the family is considered to be partners in the care of the child (Smith and Conant Rees, 2000). Emphasis is placed on providing services that demonstrate the value of collaboration between the health care provider, the child, and the family. Many hospitals provide a chair or bed for at least one person per child, unit kitchen privileges, and other amenities that create a welcoming atmosphere for parents. Still, the parents' own schedules may prevent them from being present. In such instances, strategies to minimize the effects of separation must be implemented.

Parent Participation

Although some health facilities provide special accommodations for parents, the concept of family-centered care can be instituted anywhere. The first requirement is the staff's positive attitude toward parents. A negative attitude toward parent participation can create barriers to collaborative working relationships (Smith and Conant Rees, 2000). Unfortunately, although nurses often express explicit support for the concept of family-centered care, some of their practices and beliefs suggest otherwise (Newton, 2000).

Hospital staff who genuinely appreciate the importance of continued parent-child attachment foster an environment that encourages parents to be active caregivers. When nurses include parents in the care planning and ensure them that they are contributing to the child's recovery, parents are more inclined to remain with their child and have more emotional reserves to support themselves and the child through the crisis. An empowerment model of helping allows the nurse to focus on parents' strengths and to seek ways to promote growth and family functioning (Fig. 26-4). Strategies such as bedside reporting that allow parents to be involved in the discussion of the child's current status are moving health care settings closer to family-centered care (Anderson and Mangino, 2006). Liaison nursing roles in tertiary care settings are also focused on improving communication between parents and health care providers (Caffin, Linton, and Pellegrini, 2007).

Parents may display different and varied needs regarding involvement in their child's care. Not all parents feel comfortable assuming responsibility, and they may be under such great emotional stress that they need a temporary reprieve from caregiving activities. Others may feel insecure in participating in specialized care. On the other hand, some parents may feel a

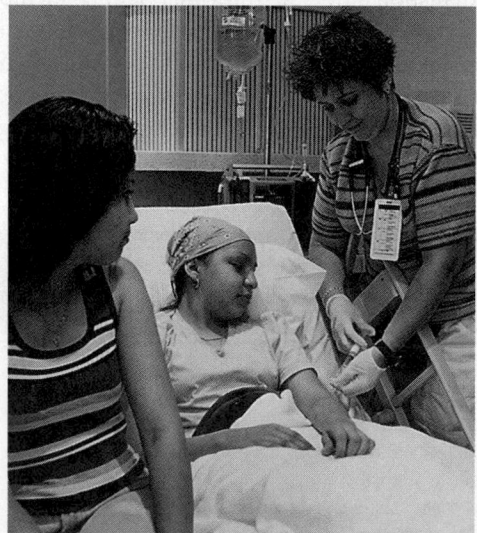

Fig. 26-4 Family presence during hospitalization, including during procedures, provides emotional support. (Courtesy Paul Vincent Kuntz, Texas Children's Hospital, Houston.)

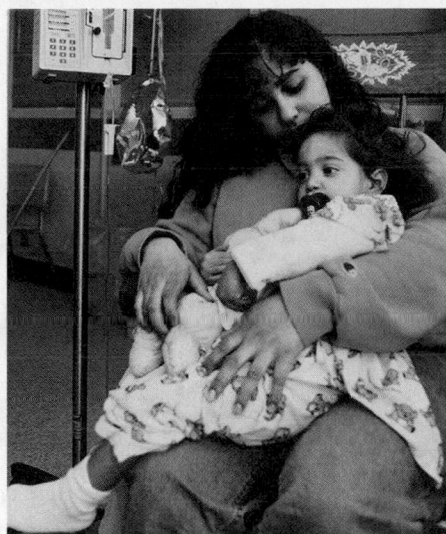

Fig. 26-5 Despite changing lifestyles and gender roles, mothers tend to be the usual family caregiver and spend more time at the hospital than fathers.

need to control their child's care and wish to be involved in every way possible. Individual assessment of each parent's preferred involvement is necessary to prevent the effects of separation while supporting parents' needs. Because the mother tends to be the usual family caregiver, she may spend more time in the hospital than the father (Fig. 26-5). Fathers need to be included in the care plan and respected for their parental role. For some fathers, the child's hospitalization may represent an opportunity to alter their usual caregiving role and increase their involvement. In single-parent families the caregiver may not be a parent but an extended family member, such as a grandparent or aunt. Parents and other family members should be prepared and supported for the roles they choose.

One of the potential problems with continuous parent visitation is that the parent often neglects the need for sleep, nutrition, and relaxation. The sleeping accommodations may be limited to a chair, and sleep is disrupted by nursing procedures. After a few days, parents may become exhausted but feel obligated to stay at their child's bedside. Encouraging them to leave for brief periods, arranging for sleeping quarters on the unit but outside the child's room, and planning a schedule of alternating visitation with the other parent or with a family member can minimize the stresses for the parent.

All too often, nurses respond to parental participation by abandoning their patient responsibilities. Nurses need to restructure their roles to complement and augment the parents' caregiving functions and to promote family health (Hopia, Tomlinson, Paavilainen, et al, 2005). Even in units structured to promote care by parents, parents frequently feel anxiety in their caregiving responsibilities. Those more involved in direct care may feel greater anxiety than those less involved. A moderate amount of visitation and participation may be optimum for many. Nursing assistance should always be available to these families.

Strategies to Minimize the Effects of Separation

When separation cannot be prevented, the nurse can employ numerous strategies to minimize the effects of temporary separation on children. Ideally, a primary nurse is assigned to meet the child's needs. The nurse should obtain a thorough, detailed history that specifically identifies the child's daily routine (see Box 26-7, p. 988). Usual daily activities such as meal preparation and method of feeding help establish a complementary schedule of caregiving practices. It also helps the parents feel as though they are participating in the child's care but through another person. A consistent staff member can also keep the family informed of the child's condition and support the family's concerns and priorities.

The nurse caring for the child must be aware of the child's separation behaviors. As discussed earlier, phases of protest and despair are normal. The child is allowed to cry. Even if the child rejects strangers, the nurse provides support through physical presence. This includes spending time being physically close to the child, using a quiet tone of voice, appropriate words, eye contact, and touch in ways that establish rapport and communicate empathy. If detachment behaviors are evident, the nurse maintains the child's contact with the parents by frequently talking with them; encouraging the child to remember them; and stressing the significance of their visits, telephone calls, or letters.

Separation may be equally difficult for parents, especially when they do not understand the behaviors of separation anxiety. To avoid the immediate protest, parents may sneak out or lie to the child about leaving. As a result, the child does not learn to associate absence with a guaranteed return because there is an element of uncertainty. Helping parents recognize that separation behaviors are normal and expected can decrease anxiety and may ease their fears about leaving the child. Explaining to parents how the child reacts after they leave may also be helpful. Many parents think the child cries for hours after they leave, whereas in reality the child may cry for a few minutes but then settle down when comforted by someone else.

Toddlers and preschoolers have a limited concept of time. Time is measured in associations, such as "eating dinner when daddy comes home." Therefore, when helping parents with their fears of separation, nurses need to suggest ways of explaining leaving and returning. For example, if parents must leave to go to work or to make meals for the other family members, they should tell the hospitalized child the reason for leaving. They also need to convey the expected time of return in terms of anticipated events. For example, if the parents return in the morning, they can tell the child that they will see him or her "when it's time for breakfast" or "when [a favorite program] is on television."

The young child's ability to tolerate parental absence is limited. Therefore parental visits should be frequent. For example, it is better for parents to visit three times a day for short periods than once a day for an extended time. This may necessitate that each parent visit at different times to lessen the length of separation. When parents cannot visit, the presence of other significant people may comfort the child (Fig. 26-6).

If parents leave after the child is asleep, they still need to communicate their absence. The parents of a 5-year-old boy solved this problem by devising a sign; on one side they drew a picture of a telephone and on the other a hamburger. Before they left, they turned the sign to the appropriate side to tell the child when he awoke that they were out using the telephone or eating.

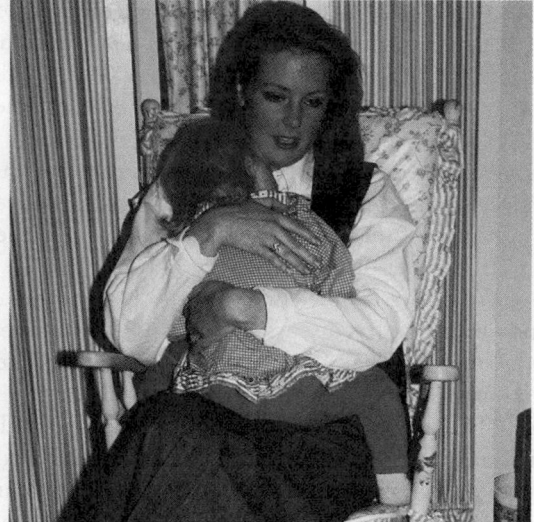

Fig. 26-6 When parents cannot visit, other significant persons can provide comfort to the hospitalized child.

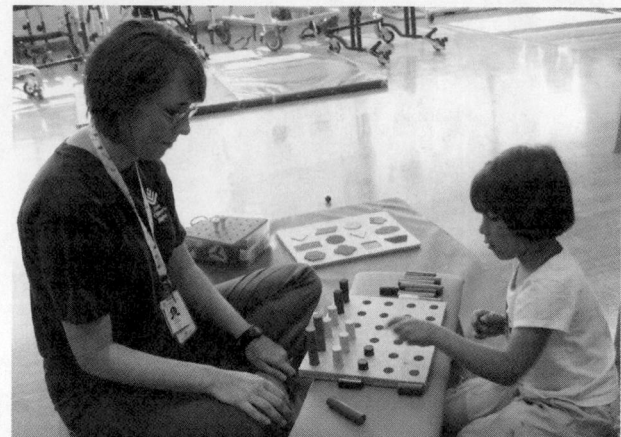

Fig. 26-7 For extended hospitalizations, children enjoy having projects to occupy time. (Courtesy E. Jacob, Texas Children's Hospital, Houston.)

For older children who know how to tell time, it is helpful to give them a clock or watch. However, these children have the same needs for honesty from their parents regarding visiting schedules. Because peer groups are also important, adolescents often appreciate planning visiting hours to provide them with some private time for friends. Many hospitals today also offer Internet connectivity, which allows older children and adolescents to remain in contact with family members and peers via e-mail or social networking sites.

Familiar surroundings also increase the child's adjustment to separation. If parents cannot stay with the child, they should leave favorite articles from home, such as a blanket, toy, bottle, feeding utensil, or article of clothing. Because young children associate such objects with significant people, they gain comfort and reassurance from these possessions. They make the association that, if the parent left this, the parent will surely return. Other mementos of home include photographs and recordings of family members reading a story, singing a song, or relating events at home. Some units allow pets to visit, which can be a special event for a child and can have therapeutic benefits.

Older children also appreciate familiar articles from home, particularly photographs, a favorite toy or game, and their own pajamas. The importance of treasured objects for school-age children may be overlooked or criticized. However, approximately half of school-age children have a special object to which they formed an attachment in early childhood. This is a normal and healthy phenomenon. Therefore such treasured or transitional objects can help even older children feel more comfortable in a strange environment.

The sights and sounds in the hospital that are commonplace for the nurse can be strange, frightening, and confusing for children. It is important for the nurse to try to evaluate stimuli in the environment from the child's point of view (considering also what the child may see or hear happening to other patients) and to make every effort to protect the child from frightening and unfamiliar sights, sounds, and equipment. The nurse should offer explanations or prepare the child for those experiences that are unavoidable. Combining familiar or comforting sights with the unfamiliar can relieve much of the harshness of medical care.

> **NURSING TIP** Soften medical equipment (e.g., use decorations to transform an IV pump into a friendly animal) to create a pleasant and more familiar environment for children.

Helping children maintain their usual contacts also minimizes the effects of separation imposed by hospitalization. This includes continuing school lessons during the illness and confinement, visiting with friends either directly or through e-mail, and participating in stimulating projects whenever possible (Fig. 26-7). For extended hospitalizations, youngsters enjoy personalizing the hospital room to make it "home" by decorating the walls with posters and cards and rearranging the furniture (when possible).

MINIMIZING LOSS OF CONTROL AND AUTONOMY

Feelings of loss of control result from separation, physical restriction, changed routines, enforced dependency, magical thinking, and altered roles within the family or peer group. Although some of these cannot be prevented, most can be minimized through individualized nursing care.

Promoting Freedom of Movement

Younger children react most strenuously to any type of physical restriction or immobilization. Although some restraint may be necessary, such as temporarily immobilizing an extremity for maintenance of an IV line, most physical restriction can be avoided if the nurse gains the child's cooperation.

For young children, particularly infants and toddlers, preserving parent-child contact is the best means of decreasing the need for or stress of restraint. For example, the nurse can perform almost the entire physical examination with the child in a parent's lap, with the parent hugging the child for procedures such as otoscopy. For painful procedures the nurse assesses the parents' preferences for assisting, observing, or waiting outside the room.

Environmental factors may restrict movement. Keeping children in cribs or playpens may not represent immobilization in the strictest sense, but it certainly limits sensory stimulation. Increasing mobility by transporting children in carriages, wheelchairs, carts, or wagons provides them with a sense of freedom.

In some cases physical restraint or isolation is necessary. Whenever possible, remove restraints to allow the child some period of supervised freedom, such as during baths or visits from parents. When restraints or isolation cannot be discontinued, such as with severe burns, the environment can be altered to increase sensory freedom. Moving the bed toward the door or window; opening window shades; providing musical, visual, or tactile toys; and increasing interpersonal contact can substitute mental mobility for the limitations of physical movement.

Maintaining the Child's Routine

Altered daily schedules and loss of rituals are particularly stressful for toddlers and early preschoolers and may increase separation anxiety. As stated previously, the nursing admission history provides a baseline for planning care around the child's usual home activities.

Children's response to loss of routine and ritualism is often demonstrated in problems with activities such as eating, sleeping, dressing, bathing, toileting, and social interaction. Although some regression is expected, sensitivity to the child's special needs can minimize the negative effects. For example, loss of appetite and marked food preferences are common in children who are ill or hospitalized. In addition, the food selections on hospital menus may differ greatly from preferred cultural or ethnic food preparation. Encouraging the child to eat is often a challenge, yet it is an essential nursing responsibility. Chapter 27 discusses suggestions for feeding sick children.

A frequently neglected aspect of altered routines is the change in the child's daily activities. A nonhospitalized child's day, especially during the school years, is structured with specific times for eating, dressing, going to school, playing, and sleeping. However, this time structure vanishes when the child is hospitalized. Although the nurses have a set schedule, the child is frequently unaware of it. Many children obtain significantly less sleep in the hospital than at home, primarily because sleep is delayed and then ends early due to hospital routines. Not only are hours of sleep disrupted, but waking hours are spent in passive activities. For example, few institutions impose any restrictions on the amount of time children spend watching television, which tends to be considerably more time than they spend watching at home.

One technique that can minimize the disruption in the child's routine is establishing a daily schedule. This approach is most suitable for the noncritically ill school-age and adolescent child who has mastered the concept of time. It involves scheduling the child's day to include all necessary activities that are important to patient care procedures, activities of daily living, mealtimes, and medications. Together, the nurse, parent, and child plan a daily schedule with times and activities written down, with blocks of free time available for playroom activities, hobbies, and television viewing (Fig. 26-8). The child is given a copy of the schedule and a clock. For lengthy hospitalizations,

Eric's Daily Schedule			
7:30 AM	– Breakfast, morning bath	3:00 PM	– Tutor (M, W, F)
			– Study time (T, Th)
9:00	– Medications, dressing change	4:00	– Physical therapy
		5:30	– Dinner
11:00	– Physical therapy	9:00	– Medications, dressing change
12:00 PM	– Lunch	9:15	– Bedtime

Fig. 26-8 A daily schedule helps normalize the hospital environment and increases the child's sense of control.

a calendar may be constructed identifying special events such as favorite television programs, visits by friends or relatives, events in the playroom, holidays or birthdays, and any expected changes in treatment (e.g., "beginning physical therapy in 2 days").

> **NURSING TIP** Ask the young child to select or draw pictures or symbols to represent daily or weekly fun activities (e.g., favorite TV programs, family visits, playroom times). Next to the child's representation, draw a clock face with the hands of the clock depicting the time each event will occur. Have the child compare the clock on the schedule with a clock or watch in the room. When the two match, the child knows that it is time for a favorite activity and exactly what that activity is.

Encouraging Independence

The dependent role of being hospitalized imposes feelings of loss on older children. Principal interventions should focus on respect for individuality and the opportunity for decision making. Although these sound simple, their efficacy depends on nurses who are flexible and tolerant. It is also important to empower the patient and not be threatened by a sense of lessened control.

Fostering children's control involves helping them maintain independence and promoting self-care. **Self-care** refers to the practice of activities that individuals initiate and perform on their own behalf to maintain life, health, and well-being (Orem, 2001). Although self-care is limited by the child's age and physical condition, most children beyond infancy can perform some activities with little or no help. Whenever possible, encourage these activities in the hospital. Other approaches include structuring time and allowing the child to jointly plan care, wear street clothes, make choices in food selections and bedtime, continue school activities, and room with an appropriate agemate. For example, adolescents generally prefer a roommate their own age and, ideally, quarters separate from the pediatric unit.

Promoting Understanding

Loss of control can occur both from feelings of having too little influence on one's destiny and from sensing overwhelming control or power over fate. Although preschoolers' cognitive abilities predispose them most to creative thinking and delusions of power, all children are vulnerable to misinterpreting causes for stresses such as illness and hospitalization.

Most children feel more in control when they know what to expect, since this reduces the element of fear. Providing anticipatory preparation and information helps greatly to lessen stress and prevent misunderstanding. (See Preparation for Diagnostic and Therapeutic Procedures, Chapter 27.)

Informing children of their rights while hospitalized fosters greater understanding and may relieve some of the feelings of powerlessness they experience. Standards used to accredit hospitals recommend that hospitals providing services to children have a hospital-wide policy on the rights and responsibilities of these patients and of their parents or guardians (Joint Commission on Accreditation of Healthcare Organizations, 2004). Present information regarding patient rights to children and their families during the admission process.

PREVENTING OR MINIMIZING FEAR OF BODILY INJURY

Beyond early infancy all children fear bodily injury either from mutilation, intrusion, body image change, disability, or death. In general, preparation of children for painful procedures decreases their fears. Manipulating procedural techniques for children in each age-group also minimizes fear of bodily injury. For example, since toddlers and young preschoolers are traumatized by insertion of a rectal thermometer, axillary or tympanic electronic temperature probes can be effectively substituted. Whenever procedures are performed on young children, the most supportive intervention is to do them as quickly as possible and maintain parent-child contact.

Because of the toddler's and preschooler's poorly defined body boundaries, the use of bandages may be particularly helpful. For example, telling children that the bleeding will stop after the needle is removed does little to relieve their fears, whereas applying a Band-Aid usually reassures them. The size of bandages is also significant to children in this age-group. The larger the bandage, the more importance is attached to the wound. Successively smaller surgical dressings are one way they measure healing and improvement. Removing a dressing may cause them concern for their well-being.

In children who fear mutilation of body parts, repeatedly stressing the reason for a procedure and evaluating their understanding are essential to minimize fear. For example, explaining cast removal to preschoolers may seem simple enough, but the child's comprehension of the details may vary considerably. Asking them to draw a picture of what they think will happen provides substantial evidence of how they perceive events.

Children may fear bodily injury from a great variety of sources. Diagnostic imaging machines, strange equipment for examinations, unfamiliar rooms, or awkward positions can be perceived as potentially hazardous. In addition, thoughts and actions can be imagined sources of bodily damage. Therefore it is important to investigate imagined reasons for illness. Children may fear revealing such thoughts, and techniques such as drawing or doll play may help reveal their misconceptions.

Older children fear bodily injury of both internal and external origins. For example, school-age children are aware of the heart's significance and may fear an actual procedure involving the heart as much as the pain, the stitches, and the possible scar.

Adolescents may express concern for the surgery but be much more anxious over the resulting scar. An appreciation of each child's special concerns helps nurses focus on critical areas when preparing patients for procedures or explaining the disease processes.

Children can grasp information only if it is presented on or close to their level of cognitive development. This necessitates an awareness of the words used to describe events or processes. For example, young children told that they are going to have a CAT scan may wonder, "Will there be cats? Or something that scratches?" It is clearer to describe the procedure in simple terms and explain what the letters of the common name stand for.

When children are upset about their illness, the nurse can change their perception by (1) providing a somewhat different and less negative account of the disease or (2) offering an explanation that is characteristic of the next stage of cognitive development. An example of the first strategy is reassuring a preschool child who, after a tonsillectomy, fears that another sore throat means a second operation. Explaining that once tonsils are "fixed," they do not need fixing again can help relieve the fear. An example of the second strategy is to explain that germs made the tonsils sick and even though germs can cause another sore throat, they cannot cause the tonsils to ever be sick again. This higher-level explanation is based on the school-age child's concept of germs as a cause of disease.

PROVIDING DEVELOPMENTALLY APPROPRIATE ACTIVITIES

A primary goal of nursing care for the child who is hospitalized is to minimize threats to the child's development. Many strategies (e.g., minimizing separation) have been discussed and may be all that the short-term patient requires. However, children who experience prolonged or repeated hospitalization are at greater risk for developmental delay or regression. The nurse who provides opportunities for the child to participate in developmentally appropriate activities further normalizes the child's environment and helps reduce interference with the child's ongoing development. (See Normalization, Chapter 22.)

Child life specialists are health care professionals with extensive knowledge of child growth and development and the special psychosocial needs of children who are hospitalized and their families (Box 26-5). They help prepare children for hospitalization, surgery, and procedures. Although all members of the health care team share these responsibilities, this is the primary role of the child life specialist. A collaborative effort between the nurse, child life specialist, and other members of the child's health care team will help ensure the best possible hospital experience for the child and family (American Academy of Pediatrics, 2000).

USING PLAY AND EXPRESSIVE ACTIVITIES TO MINIMIZE STRESS

Play is one of the most important aspects of a child's life and one of the most effective tools for managing stress. Because illness and hospitalization constitute crises in the child's life and often involve overwhelming stresses, acting out fears and anxi-

BOX 26-5 CHILD LIFE PROGRAMS*

The inclusion of child life programs in pediatric settings has become widely accepted and advocated by organizations such as the American Academy of Pediatrics (2006) and the National Association of Children's Hospitals and Related Institutions (1996). An American Academy of Pediatrics (2006) statement describes child life programs as "the standard in pediatric settings to address the psychosocial concerns that accompany hospitalization and other health care experiences." National Association of Children's Hospitals and Related Institutions (1996) has stated that provision of such services is a quality benchmark of an integrated child health delivery system.

Although the structure of a program may vary depending on the size of the pediatric facility, the patient population, and the availability of ancillary services, the two primary program objectives for child life are consistent: (1) to reduce the stress and anxiety related to the hospitalization or health care–related experiences and (2) to promote normal growth and development in the health care setting and at home (Thompson and Stanford, 1981; Thompson, 2009).

With expertise in child development, child life specialists promote effective coping and adjustment during potentially stressful situations through play, psychologic preparation, education, and support. Child life specialists collaborate with other members of the health care team to develop a care plan. As members of the interdisciplinary health care team, child life specialists identify the patient's perception and current understanding of the anticipated health care experience, with the goal of enhancing the child's coping and adjustment.†

Child life programs are typically staffed by certified child life specialists (CCLSs) and may also include child life assistants, creative arts therapists (such as music or art), other therapists, play therapists, librarians, and volunteers. A CCLS has a minimum of a bachelor's degree in child life, child development, or closely related field; has completed a clinical internship with a minimum of 480 hours under the supervision of a CCLS; and has successfully completed the Child Life Professional Certification Examination.

Child Life Services

Play and psychologic preparation are the primary tools used by child life specialists while providing direct patient care. Play is considered the cornerstone of child life practice and is adapted to each child's developmental needs (American Academy of Pediatrics, 2006). Although there are many different types of play, child-directed medical play is a primary modality facilitated by the child life specialist to help the child cope (Gaynard, Wolfer, Goldberger, et al, 1990; American Academy of Pediatrics, 2006). This type of play provides an opportunity for the child to manipulate medical equipment and possibly role play procedures or treatments on dolls; it is not, however, used to prepare a patient for a procedure.

A child's response to medical play can provide child life specialists and other members of the interdisciplinary health care team with information regarding the child's concerns, misconceptions, and current understanding of medical events. Therapeutic play, another type of play often associated with health care settings, is also child directed and refers to specialized activities that are developmentally supportive and facilitate the emotional well-being of pediatric patients. Children engage in this type of play when they attempt to master a developmental milestone or a stressful event, like hospitalization.†

Child life specialists prepare children psychologically for medical procedures and events to increase their sense of mastery, reduce anxiety, and plan and rehearse coping strategies. Psychologic preparation is adult directed and is defined as a "process of communicating accurate and developmentally appropriate information, identifying potential stressors, as well as planning and practicing coping strategies" (American Academy of Pediatrics, 2006). Psychologic preparation is also linked to a specific goal in the child's care plan.†

In addition to play and psychologic preparation, other direct patient care activities provided by child life specialists include sibling and family support, bereavement activities, and developmentally appropriate diagnosis teaching. In conjunction with direct patient care, child life services consist of consultation within and outside the hospital environment; supervision of students, volunteers, and others; education of other care providers, parents, and students; advocacy; and environmental planning.

*By Quinn Franklin.
†For more information see Evidence-Based Practice statements on the Child Life Council's website, **www.childlife.org**.

BOX 26-6 FUNCTIONS OF PLAY IN THE HOSPITAL

- Provides diversion and relaxation
- Helps the child feel more secure in a strange environment
- Lessens the stress of separation and feelings of homesickness
- Provides a means for release of tension and expression of feelings
- Encourages interaction and development of positive attitudes toward others
- Provides an expressive outlet for creative ideas and interests
- Provides a means for accomplishing therapeutic goals (See Use of Play in Procedures, Chapter 27.)
- Places the child in active role, providing an opportunity to make choices and be in control

eties gives the child a means to cope with these stresses. Children who play are coping positively; children who cannot play are waiting, testing, holding back, or making some inner decisions about the setting.

Play is essential to children's mental, emotional, and social well-being. As with their developmental needs, the need for play does not stop when children are ill or when they enter the hospital. On the contrary, play in the hospital serves many functions (Box 26-6). Of all hospital facilities, no room probably does more to alleviate the stressors of hospitalization than the playroom. In this room children temporarily distance themselves from the fears of separation, loss of control, and bodily injury. They can work through their feelings in a non-threatening, comfortable atmosphere and in the manner most natural for them. They also know that the boundaries of this room are safe from intrusive or painful procedures, strange faces, and probing questions. The playroom becomes a sanctuary of peace and safety in an otherwise frightening environment (see Critical Thinking Exercise).

Engaging in play activities puts children in charge, removing them for a time from the usual passive role of recipients of a constant stream of procedures and hospital routines. In the hospital environment most decisions are made for the child, but play and other expressive activities offer the child much-needed opportunities to make choices. Even if a child chooses not to participate in a particular activity, the nurse has offered the child a choice, perhaps one of but a few real choices the child has had that day.

Children who are ill and hospitalized typically have lower energy levels than healthy children. Therefore children may not appear enthusiastic about an activity even when they are enjoying the experience. Rather than assuming otherwise, the nurse can observe for subtle signs—such as a fleeting smile or

? CRITICAL THINKING EXERCISE

Playroom and Hospital Procedures

Hannah, a 7-year-old with cystic fibrosis, has been hospitalized numerous times with complications from the condition. She is playing Candyland with her brother, sister, and several other children in the playroom on the pediatric unit. A pediatric phlebotomist enters the playroom and says, "Hannah, I need to take some blood. I can see that you are playing a game, so I'll just do it while you play. It will just take a minute." Hannah nods her head indicating that she agrees to let the phlebotomist draw the blood at this time. The playroom is usually off-limits for invasive procedures. As Hannah's nurse, you are aware that her physician, Dr. Lung, wants the results of the laboratory studies as soon as possible to make a decision about her course of therapy.

1. Evidence—Is there sufficient evidence to draw any conclusions about this situation at this time?
2. Assumptions—What are some underlying assumptions about the following?
   a. Children and painful procedures such as venipuncture
   b. The function of play in a hospitalized child
   c. The priority in performing the procedure
   d. Implications of performing the procedure in the playroom
3. What implications and priorities for nursing care can be drawn at this time (i.e., What will you do?)?
4. Does the evidence objectively support your argument (conclusion)?

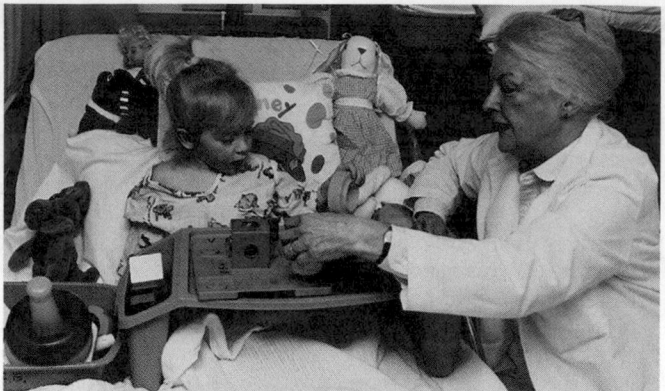

Fig. 26-9 Play materials for children in the hospital need to be appropriate for their age, interests, and limitations.

intense concentration—or simply ask children if they are enjoying themselves.

Children in various age-groups require different types of play facilities. Infants and toddlers need maximum safety, whereas school-age children and adolescents benefit most from group activities. Providing space for special needs of children in each age-group can be difficult in institutions where space is limited, but innovative solutions can ensure practical answers. Structure playroom schedules to allow one age-group at a time; for example, adolescents can use the facility in the evening when younger children are asleep. Older children can also congregate in one patient's room and listen to music, play games, or just talk. If the location of the session rotates each evening, older children can look forward to arranging or setting up for the activities.

> **NURSING TIP** When adolescents must share a common activity room with younger patients, referring to the area as the "activity room" rather than the "playroom" may entice them to visit the room and participate in activities. Ideally, adolescents should have their own space.

Diversional Activities

Almost any form of play can be used for diversion and recreation, but the activity should be selected on the basis of the child's age, interests, and limitations (Fig. 26-9). Children do not necessarily need special direction for using play materials. All they require are the materials with which to work and adult approval and supervision to help keep their natural enthusiasm or expression of feelings from getting out of control. Young children enjoy a variety of small, colorful toys they can play with in bed or in their room or more elaborate play equipment, such as playhouses, sandboxes, rhythm instruments, and large boxes and blocks, that may be a part of the hospital playroom.

Games that can be played alone or with another child or an adult are popular with older children, as are puzzles; reading material; quiet individual activities such as sewing, stringing beads, and weaving; and Tinker-Toys, Lego blocks, and other building materials. Assembling models is an excellent pastime, and developmentally appropriate books are of infinite value to the child. Having someone read aloud provides hours of pleasure and is of special value to the child who has limited energy to expend in play.

Computers with access to the Internet are popular features in hospital playrooms and offer a window to the world for hospitalized children. A child can talk electronically with others and share experiences or even join a virtual support group. Today's technology also provides the opportunity for children to explore every imaginable interest. As with television and other types of electronic entertainment, parents and nurses should monitor both the content and the time that a child spends engaging in these activities to avoid their becoming a substitute for social interaction or therapeutic play.

When supervising play for children who are ill or convalescing, it is best to select activities that are simpler than would normally be chosen according to the child's developmental level. Children may not have the energy to cope with more challenging activities. Other limitations also influence the type of activities. Special consideration must be given to the child who has limited movement, has a restricted extremity, or is isolated. Toys for children on isolation must be disposable or be disinfected after use. For this reason stuffed animals are not recommended for use as community toys on a hospital unit.

Toys

Parents of hospitalized children often ask nurses about the types of toys that would be best to bring for their child. Most want to bring new ones to cheer and comfort the child and assuage their guilt regarding the child's need for hospitalization. The nurse should tell the parents that, although wanting to provide these things for their child is natural, it is often better to wait to bring new things, especially for younger children. Small children need the comfort and reassurance of familiar things, such as the stuffed animal the child hugs for comfort and takes to bed at night. These are a link with home and the world outside the hospital. The nurse is responsible for assessing the safety of the toys brought to the child.

Large numbers of toys often confuse and frustrate a small child. A few small, well-chosen toys are usually preferred to one large, expensive one. Children who are hospitalized for an extended time benefit from changes. Rather than a confusing accumulation of toys, replace older toys periodically as interest wanes.

> **NURSING TIP** Have parents provide the child with a shoe box, a small suitcase, or a backpack for easy storage to prevent small items from becoming lost in the sheets or under the bed.

A highly successful diversion for a child who is hospitalized for a long time is a box with small, inexpensive, and brightly wrapped items with a different day of the week printed on the outside. The child will eagerly anticipate the time for opening each one. When the parents know when their next visit will be, they can provide the number of packages that corresponds to the days between visits. In this way the child knows that the diminishing packages also represent the anticipated visit from the parent.

Expressive Activities

Play provides one of the best opportunities for encouraging emotional expression, including the safe release of anger and hostility. Nondirective play that allows children freedom for expression can be therapeutic. Therapeutic play, however, should not be confused with the psychologic technique of play therapy. Play therapy is reserved for use by trained and qualified therapists who use the technique as an interpretative method with emotionally disturbed children. Therapeutic play, on the other hand, is an effective nondirective modality for helping children deal with their concerns and fears; at the same time, it often helps the nurse gain insights into their needs and feelings.

Tension release can be facilitated through almost any activity. With younger ambulatory children, large-muscle activity, such as the use of tricycles and wagons, is especially beneficial. Much aggression can be safely directed into games and activities that involve pounding and throwing. Beanbags are often thrown at a target or open receptacle with surprising vigor and hostility. A pounding board is employed with enthusiasm by young children; clay and play dough are beneficial at any age.

Creative Expression

Although all children derive physical, social, emotional, and cognitive benefits from engaging in art or other creative activities, children's need for such activities increases when they are hospitalized. Drawing and painting are excellent media for expression (Fig. 26-10). Children are more at ease expressing their thoughts and feelings through art than through words. The child needs only the raw materials, such as crayons and paper. Children usually require little direction for self-expression; however, older children may be given some direction in what to paint or draw. Groups of children can enjoy this creative activity either working individually or collaborating on a group project such as a mural painted on a long piece of paper.

Although interpretation of children's drawing requires special training, observing changes in a series of the child's drawings over time can be helpful in assessing psychosocial adjustment and coping. The nurse can use children's drawings, stories, poetry, and other products of creative expression as a springboard for discussion of thoughts, fears, and understanding of concepts or events. A child's drawing before surgery or chemotherapy, for example, will often reveal unvoiced concerns about mutilation, body changes, and loss of self-control.

Holidays provide stimulus and direction for unlimited creative projects. Making pictures and decorations for their rooms gives the children a sense of pride and accomplishment. This is especially beneficial for immobilized and isolated children. Making gifts or decorations for someone at home helps maintain interpersonal ties.

Dramatic Play

Dramatic play is a well-recognized technique for emotional release, allowing children to reenact frightening or puzzling hospital experiences. Through use of puppets and replicas or actual hospital equipment, children can act out the situations that are a part of their hospital experience (Fig. 26-11). Dramatic play enables children to learn about procedures and events that

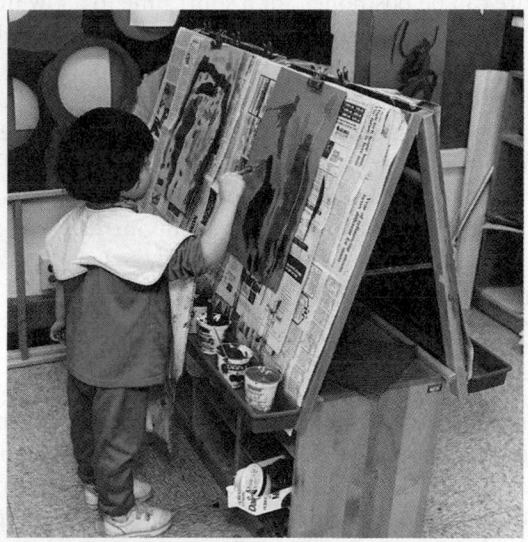

Fig. 26-10 Drawing and painting are excellent media for expression.

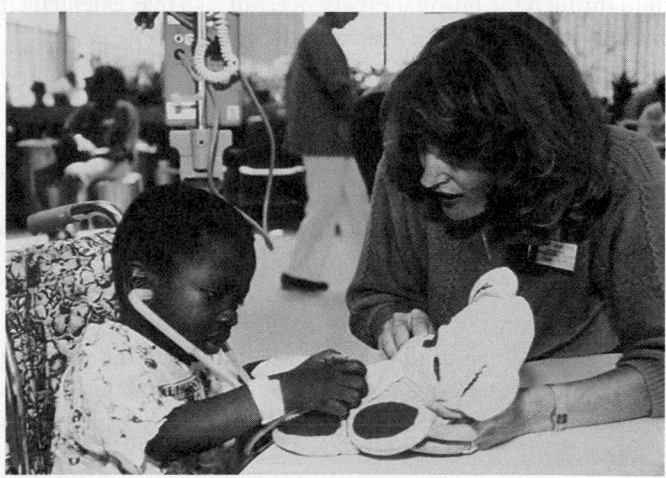

Fig. 26-11 Playing with miniature hospital equipment allows children to explore feelings and concerns and achieve mastery over hospital situations. (Courtesy St. Louis Children's Hospital.)

are of concern to them and to assume the roles of the adults in the hospital environment.

Puppets are particularly effective for communicating with children. Most young children view them as peers and readily communicate with them. Children will tell the puppet feelings that they would hesitate to express to adults. Puppets dressed to represent figures in the child's environment (e.g., a physician, nurse, child patient, therapist, and members of the child's own family) are especially useful. Small, appropriately attired dolls are also effective in encouraging the child to play out situations, although puppets are usually best for direct conversation.

> **NURSING TIP** Make a simple puppet using a large handkerchief. Place some cotton balls in the center of the cloth and wrap a rubber band over the handkerchief and cotton balls to form a "head." Place the head over the index finger so that the rubber band secures it to the finger. Let the cloth drape over the front and back of the hand. The cloth forms four parts of the puppet: the index finger controls the head, the thumb and other fingers are the arms, and the draped cloth is the body. Decorate the head by drawing features on it.

Playing must accommodate medical needs, but at times a procedure can be postponed for a short time to allow the child to complete a special activity. Playing also must consider any limitations imposed by the child's condition. For example, small children may eat paste and other creative media; therefore a child who is allergic to wheat should not be given finger paint made from wallpaper paste or play dough made with flour. A child with restricted salt intake should not play with modeling dough, since salt is one of its major components.*

MAXIMIZING POTENTIAL BENEFITS OF HOSPITALIZATION

Fostering Parent-Child Relationships

The crisis of illness or hospitalization can mobilize parents into more acute awareness of their child's needs. For example, hospitalization provides opportunities for parents to learn more about their child's growth and development. When parents understand children's usual reactions to stress, such as regression or aggression, they not only are better able to support the child through the hospital experience, but also may extend their insight into childrearing practices after discharge.

Difficulties in parent-child relationships that may result in feeding problems, negative behavior, and enuresis may decrease during hospitalization. The temporary cessation of such problems sometimes alerts parents to the role they may be playing in propagating the negative behavior. With assistance from health professionals, parents can restructure ways of relating to their children to foster more positive behavior.

On occasion, hospitalization may represent a temporary reprieve or refuge from a disturbed home. Typically, abused or neglected children's dramatic physical and social improvement during hospitalization is proof of the growth potential of this experience. Hospitalized children temporarily are able to seek support, reassurance, and security from new relationships, particularly with nurses and hospitalized peers.

Providing Educational Opportunities

School is an integral part of the school-age child's and adolescent's development. Accreditation standards for hospitals consider access to appropriate educational services when a child's treatment requires a significant absence from school (Joint Commission on Accreditation of Healthcare Organizations, 2004). The nurse can encourage children to resume schoolwork as quickly as their condition permits, help them schedule and protect a selected time for studies, and help the family coordinate hospital educational services with their children's schools. Children should have the opportunity to continue to progress through art and music classes, as well as their academic subjects.

Hospitalization also presents an excellent opportunity for children and other family members to learn more about their bodies, each other, and the health professions. For example, during a child's admission for a diabetic crisis, the child may learn about the disease. The parents may also learn about the child's needs for independence, normalcy, and appropriate limits. Each of them may find a new support system in the hospital staff.

Promoting Self-Mastery

The experience of facing a crisis such as illness or hospitalization, coping successfully with it, and maturing as a result of it constitutes an opportunity for self-mastery. Younger children have the chance to test out fantasy versus reality. They realize that they were not abandoned, mutilated, or punished. In fact, they were loved, cared for, and treated with respect for their individual concerns. It is not unusual for children who have undergone hospitalization or surgery to tell others that "it was nothing" or to proudly display their scars or bandages. For older children, hospitalization may represent an opportunity for decision making, independence, and self-reliance. They are proud of having survived the experience and may feel a genuine self-respect for their achievements. Nurses can facilitate such feelings of self-mastery by emphasizing aspects of personal competence in the child and not acknowledging uncooperative or negative behavior.

Providing Socialization

Hospitalization may offer children a special opportunity for social acceptance. Lonely, asocial, and even delinquent children find a sympathetic environment in the hospital. Children who have physical disabilities or are different in some other way from their peers may find an accepting social peer group. Although this does not always spontaneously occur, nurses can structure the environment to foster a supportive child group. For example, judicious selection of a roommate can help children gain a new friend and learn more about themselves. Forming relationships with significant members of the health care team, such as the physician, nurse, child life specialist, or social worker, can greatly enhance the child's adjustment in many areas of life.

Parents may also encounter a new social group in other parents who have similar problems. They meet while in the

---

*Information about art materials can be obtained from the Glassell School of Art, 5101 Montrose Blvd., Houston, TX 77006; 713-639-7500.

hospital or clinic and discuss their children's illnesses and treatment. Nurses can capitalize on this informal gathering by encouraging parents to discuss collectively their concerns and feelings. They can also refer parents to organized parent groups or can solicit the help and support of parents of recovered hospitalized patients. It is important that nurses emphasize that each child responds differently to certain aspects of the disease or treatment and that parents should clarify with a nurse or physician any questions or concerns raised in discussions with other parents. (See discussion of parent-to-parent support in Chapter 22.)

SUPPORTING FAMILY MEMBERS

Family-centered care is the focus of pediatric care because nursing care of children is not optimum unless the family as a whole is the designated patient. (See Family-Centered Care, Chapter 1.) Family-centered care supports the family by establishing the priority of their values and needs, developing collaborative relationships, and empowering the family unit (Lewandowski and Tesler, 2003).

Providing emotional support for family members involves the willingness to be present and listen to parents' verbal and nonverbal messages. Sometimes the nurse does not give support directly. For example, the nurse may offer to stay with the child to allow the parents time alone or may discuss with other family members the parents' need for relief. Extended family and friends may want to help but do not know how. The nurse can suggest baby-sitting, preparing meals, cleaning the house, doing laundry, or transporting the siblings to school and activities as ways to lessen the parents' responsibilities. An ongoing parent support group held on the pediatric unit has also proved effective in helping parents share emotions and concerns related to hospitalization.

The clergy may also provide support. Parents with religious beliefs may appreciate the counsel of a clergy member, but because of their stress they may not have sufficient energy to initiate the contact. Nurses can be supportive by assessing spiritual needs, arranging for clergy to visit, and respecting and upholding parents' religious beliefs (Feudtner, Haney, and Dimmers, 2003).

Support involves acceptance of cultural, socioeconomic, and ethnic values. For example, various ethnic groups define health and illness differently. For some, disorders that have few outward manifestations of illness, such as diabetes or cardiac problems, are not viewed as a sickness. Consequently, following a prescribed treatment may seem unnecessary. Nurses who appreciate the influences of culture are more likely to intervene therapeutically. (See Chapter 2 for an extensive discussion of cultural and religious influences on health care.)

Parents may need help in accepting their own feelings toward the ill child. If given the opportunity, parents often disclose their feelings of loss of control, anger, and guilt. They often resist admitting to such feelings because they expect others to disapprove of behavior that is less than perfect.

Providing Information

One of the most important nursing interventions is to provide information regarding (1) the disease, its treatment, and prognosis; (2) the child's emotional and physical reaction to illness and hospitalization; and (3) the probable emotional reactions of family members to the crisis.

For many families the child's illness is their first contact with hospitalization. Often parents are not prepared for the child's behavioral reactions to hospitalization, such as separation anxiety, regression, aggression, and hostility. Providing the parents with information about these normal and expected behaviors can decrease the parents' stress during the hospital admission. The family is equally unfamiliar with hospital rules, which often adds to their confusion and anxiety. Therefore the family needs clear explanations about what to expect and what is expected of them. Nurses can also help family members become more adept at seeking information about their child's condition by asking questions that elicit meaningful information (see Nursing Care Guidelines box). In giving information, nurses need to be alert to information overload. Repetition can be helpful.

NURSING CARE GUIDELINES

Helping Families Elicit Information

- Find out what the family wants to know.
- Teach them to avoid general questions, such as "Why is my child sick?"
- Help them prepare specific questions, such as "What is causing my child's pain?" or "What does this drug do?"
- Encourage the use of short and open-ended questions.
- Have the family write down the questions, preferably in a diary or journal that is kept in an accessible area, such as a pocket, to have available when needed.
- Encourage the family to speak up when they do not understand an answer and to ask to have it explained in clearer or simpler language.
- Have the family repeat the information to be certain they understand it and record unfamiliar terms.

Modified from Norris L: Coaching the question, *Nursing 86* 16(5):100, 1986.

Parents also need to be aware of the effects of illness on the family and strategies that prevent negative changes. Specifically, parents should keep the family informed and communicating as much as possible. They should treat all the children as equally and as normally as before the illness. Discipline, which initially may be lessened for the ill child, should be continued to provide a measure of security and predictability. When ill children know that their parents expect certain standards of conduct from them, they feel certain they will recover. When all limits are removed, they fear that something catastrophic will happen.

Helping parents understand and accept the meaning of post-hospitalization behaviors in the sick child is necessary for them to tolerate and support such behaviors. Consequently, the nurse should warn them of the common reactions following discharge. Parents who do not expect such reactions may misinterpret them as evidence of the child's "being spoiled" and demand perfect behavior at a time when the child is still reacting to the stress of illness and hospitalization. If the behaviors, especially the demand for attention, are dealt with in a supportive manner, most children are able to relinquish them and assume precrisis levels of functioning.

Nurses should also prepare parents for some of the common reactions of siblings to the ill child—particularly anger, jealousy, and resentment. Older siblings may deny such reactions because they provoke guilt. However, everyone needs outlets for emotions, and the repressed feelings may surface as problems in school or with peers, as psychosomatic illnesses, or in delinquent behavior.

Probably one of the most neglected areas involves giving information to siblings. Age frequently becomes the primary factor that leads to an awareness of this need, since older children may begin to ask questions or request explanations. However, even in this situation the information may be seriously inadequate. Children in every age-group deserve some explanation of the child's illness or hospitalization, preferably appropriate written information for older children. Although the exact wording may differ, the answer should focus on the following concerns: (1) Will I get sick and have to go to the hospital? (2) Did I cause the illness? (for actual or imagined reasons), and (3) Will my parents abandon me if my brother or sister does not recover? By addressing these three questions, parents or nurses can minimize the siblings' fears of illness, guilt, and abandonment.

Nursing approaches with siblings can be direct or indirect. Direct services might include (1) incorporating siblings into hospital admission programs; (2) liberalizing visiting regulations; (3) extending parent participation programs to include sibling involvement, such as through family dining or group play sessions; and (4) developing programs designed specifically for siblings, such as group sessions to discuss their concerns or posthospital discharge visits to evaluate the siblings' adjustment. Older siblings may not wish to attend a group; the nurse can be available for casual talks or for a tour, which may encourage the youngster to talk or ask questions (Lewandowski and Tesler, 2003).

Indirect services (which can be influenced by any existing nursing role) involve helping parents understand, cope with, and support the siblings' reactions to the experience. Siblings do best with as little disruption in their lives as possible. Other interventions include helping well siblings maintain contact with the child who is hospitalized through telephone calls, recordings, letters, or postcards (see Family-Centered Care box).

PREPARATION FOR HOSPITALIZATION

The rationale for preparing children for the hospital experience and related procedures is based on the principle that fear of the unknown exceeds fear of the known. Therefore decreasing the elements of the unknown results in less fear. When children do not have paralyzing fears to cope with, they can direct their energies toward dealing with the other unavoidable stresses of hospitalization and benefit optimally from the growth potential of the experience.

For children past infancy and early toddlerhood, in-hospital or home preparation for hospitalization reduces their stress. Even when children are too young to benefit from direct preparation, parents benefit from prehospital counseling to lessen their fears and thus increase their ability to support the child psychologically. Prehospital counseling has two major goals:

1. To make the hospital less strange and frightening to parents and children

FAMILY-CENTERED CARE

How Parents Can Support Siblings During Hospitalization

- Trade off staying at the hospital with spouse or have a parent surrogate who knows the siblings well stay in the home.
- Offer information about the child's condition to young siblings, as well as older siblings; respect the sibling who avoids information as a means of coping with the situation.
- Arrange for children to visit their brother or sister in the hospital if possible.
- Encourage phone visits and mail between brothers and sisters; provide children with phone numbers, writing supplies, and stamps.
- Help each sibling identify an extended family member or friend to be their support person and provide extra attention during parental absence.
- Make or buy inexpensive toys or trinkets for siblings, one gift for each day the child will be hospitalized.
- Wrap each gift separately and place in a basket or box at each child's bedside.
- Instruct siblings to open one gift each night at bedtime and to remember that he or she is in the parent's thoughts.
- If the child's condition is stable and distance is not prohibitive, plan a special time at home with the siblings or have a spouse or another relative or friend bring the children to meet the parents at a restaurant or other location near the hospital.
- Have extended family members or friends schedule a visit to the child in hospital during parental absence.
- Arrange a pass for the child to leave the hospital to join the family if the child's condition permits it.

Modified from Craft M, Craft J: Perceived changes in siblings of hospitalized children: a comparison of sibling and parent reports, *Child Health Care* 18(1):42-48, 1989; and Rollins J: *Brothers and sisters: a discussion guide for families*, Landover, Md, 1992, Epilepsy Foundation of America.

2. To establish a positive atmosphere and trusting relationship with hospital staff and family members

Although preparation may create stress for children initially, eventually the process results in greater trust in parents and staff, increased integration of information, and greater ability to cooperate and participate in treatment.

GUIDELINES IN PREPARING FOR HOSPITALIZATION

Although preparation for hospitalization is a common practice, no universal standard or program is advocated in both general and children's hospitals. Some hospital admission programs focus on group preparation before actual admission, whereas others prepare each child either before or the day of admission. The preparation process may include tours, puppet shows, or therapeutic play with toy or real medical equipment (Justus, Wyles, Wilson, et al, 2006). Other strategies for preparation include books, photograph albums, videos, or films; or it may be a simple description of the major aspects of a hospital stay. Ono, Oikawa, Hirabayashi, and colleagues (2008) developed a customized picture book that included a story of the operation day and the hospital stay plus a guidebook for parents. They found that the picture book played an important role in parent and child education at the time of day surgery.

The primary audience of most hospital preparation programs is children and families who are experiencing an initial hospitalization. Subsequent readmissions, however, may also be stressful and anxiety provoking. Children's fear and fantasies may not subside with repeated hospital stays but may intensify. Also, concerns change as children develop and grow. Older children need preparation as well, although the type of program needs to be individualized and may differ from the following guidelines for planning prehospital tours for groups or individual families who have not yet experienced hospital admission.

Ideally, preparatory procedures should be:
- Planned by hospital staff before the child's admission to the hospital
- Appropriately designed for each child's developmental age
- Sufficiently individualized to account for different children's previous experience with hospitalization, present reason for admission, and available support system

Child life programs have become the standard in pediatric settings to address the psychosocial concerns precipitated by hospitalization and other health care experiences. Child life programs facilitate coping and the adjustment of children and families by presenting developmentally appropriate information about events and procedures, providing therapeutic play experiences, and establishing therapeutic relationships with children and parents to encourage and support family involvement in the children's care (American Academy of Pediatrics, 2000). (In addition to the following discussion, the reader should review Preparation for Diagnostic and Therapeutic Procedures, Chapter 27.)

Group Size and Timing of Preparation

If group preparation is used, group size should be small (about 10 children) to provide individualized attention and facilitate discussion. If tours are arranged for each child, the parents and possibly the well siblings should be included.

Because standardized programs cannot adequately meet the needs of the full age range of pediatric patients, some hospitals have developed preparation programs that target a specific age-group, such as toddlers or adolescents. The length of the session should be suited to the children's attention span: the younger the child, the shorter the program. The optimum approach is one that is individualized for each child and family.

Setting of the Tour

The hospital tour should avoid any frightening aspects of the environment and should typically include an inpatient room, the playroom (a highlight of the tour), the parents' waiting room, the nurses' station, and other special areas such as the group dining room. Other areas that may be visited are the radiology department and laboratory area, the preoperative area, and the recovery room. Different hospitals may tailor this tour to include special rooms, such as the "OR playroom," where children and parents first go before anesthesia induction is administered. Children who are undergoing serious surgery requiring special postoperative care may be taken to visit the intensive care unit (ICU). Children scheduled for special tests, such as cardiac catheterization or cystoscopy, are sometimes shown these areas. Young children may respond better to shorter tours that concentrate on the areas of most concern,

such as the pediatric unit, playroom, and recovery room. In any case, throughout the tour, the nurse (or other guide) must be alert to signs of concern or fear in the children. Strange noises, sights, sounds, and smells that are routine to hospital personnel can be frightening to children.

Preparatory Materials

The most suitable type of presentation for children includes a variety of preparatory materials, including films, lecture, demonstration, and play. The following discussion explores some of the typical methods used in preparing children for elective surgery.

A puppet show may reenact the basic steps of hospitalization: admission procedures, preparation for surgery, the operating and recovery rooms, and postsurgical treatment. Each scene focuses on concrete actions and models to familiarize family members with what will occur. The puppets talk about children's common fears: pain, anesthesia, and parent separation. Although the sophistication of the materials varies, the basic characters should include a puppet family (mother, father, and child) and hospital staff (physician, nurse) that are ethnically representative of the patient and hospital population. For example, both African-American and Caucasian dolls are required in many areas. Hospital equipment includes mask, cap, gloves, gown, IV equipment, syringes, thermometer, blood pressure machine, stethoscope, scale, oxygen mask, suture removal set, bandages, bed, and sheets. If children are routinely admitted for diagnostic evaluations, miniature replicas of equipment (e.g., diagnostic imaging machines) or slides may be used as visual aids. The use of scaled-down models is especially beneficial for young children, who may be frightened by the actual proportions of some equipment. However, the intent of what is conveyed greatly surpasses the sophistication of the materials used.

Opportunity for Discussion

Any type of preparatory program needs to provide ample opportunity for discussion both before and after the tour. During the tour, encourage family members to ask questions and to familiarize themselves with the environment by sitting on a bed, using the electric bed controls, riding in a wheelchair, or handling the equipment in the special rooms. Ideally, the tour should also be an opportunity for meeting the child's primary nurse. Although this is not always possible because of staffing schedules, the nursing staff should be introduced to the children by name. Introducing them to one specific nurse, such as the head nurse, clinical specialist, or nurse practitioner, helps them feel more comfortable in knowing who is available for questions or concerns during the hospital stay.

After the tour a question-and-answer period should be held in which the nurse is a participant. Sometimes the group is reticent about asking questions. In this case the nurse can stimulate discussion by posing a question to the audience or inviting the children to see and touch the puppets and equipment. Allowing children to play with the equipment and having them draw pictures about what they observed are excellent methods of evaluating the learning process and clarifying any misconceptions. The parents should also be encouraged to contact the appropriate provider before admission if questions or concerns arise.

Skill—Admitting a Child to the Health Care System

Prehospital Counseling by Parents

In many situations the preparation of children for hospitalization is left up to parents. Parents may abandon this responsibility for a variety of reasons. For example, they sometimes think the child is too young to understand or is better off not knowing beforehand. Often they are unable to prepare the child because of their own lack of knowledge and understanding.

Professionals can help parents prepare their children by adequately informing them of the specific details of hospitalization and related procedures, through both direct discussion and written material. Nurses working with these parents should also assess their level of anxiety regarding the impending hospitalization. A parent who is at ease will convey that feeling to the child.

HOSPITAL ADMISSION PROCEDURE

The preparation that children require on the day of admission depends on their prehospital counseling. If they have been prepared in a formalized program, they usually know what to expect in terms of initial medical procedures, inpatient facilities, and nursing staff. However, prehospital counseling does not preclude the need for support during procedures such as drawing blood, x-ray tests, or physical examination. For example, undressing young children before they feel comfortable in their new surroundings can be upsetting. Causing needless anxiety and fear during admission may adversely affect the nurse's establishment of trust with these children. Therefore nursing assistance during the admission procedure is vital, regardless of how well prepared any child is for the hospitalization. In addition, spending this time with the child gives the nurse an opportunity to evaluate understanding of subsequent procedures, such as surgery (Fig. 26-12). The usual admission procedures for children are outlined in the Nursing Care Guidelines box.

Nursing Admission History

The nursing admission history refers to a systematic collection of data about the child and family that allows the nurse to plan individualized care. The nursing admission history presented in Box 26-7 facilitates the formulation of nursing diagnoses. (See Nursing Diagnosis, Chapter 1.) One of the main purposes of the history is to assess the child's usual health habits at home to promote a more normal environment in the hospital. Therefore questions related to activities of daily living are a major part of the assessment. The questions under the health perception–health management pattern are directed toward evaluation of the child's preparation for hospitalization and are key factors in determining whether additional preparation is needed.

As with any history form, the questions are only guidelines; for optimum communication, nurses should ask these questions as a part of conversation, not as a direct questionnaire. Answers to questions that are broad and nonspecific, such as "What does your child know about this hospitalization?" need to be followed by more specific questions, such as "Tell me what you told him." Children may respond to questions regarding

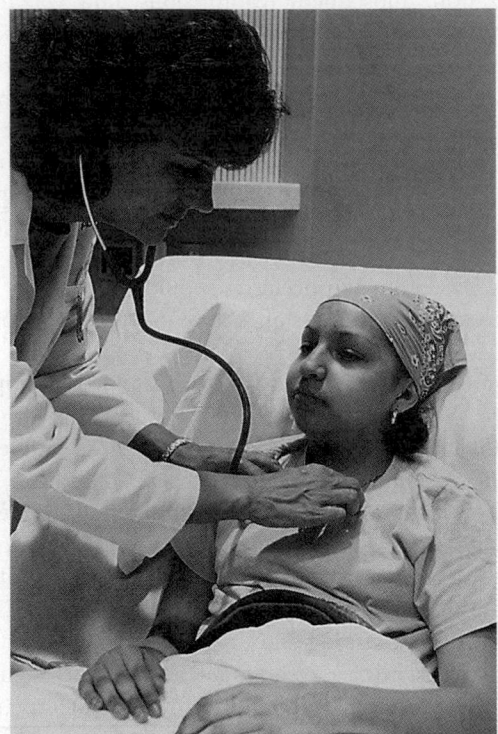

Fig. 26-12 The initial admission procedures may be coordinated by a nurse practitioner who examines the child on admission. (Courtesy Paul Vincent Kuntz, Texas Children's Hospital, Houston.)

their knowledge of hospitalization with statements such as "I don't know why I am here." Although this may be correct, frequently they have been given some explanation concerning the reason for hospitalization. Such an answer may mean that the explanation was inadequate, their anxiety blocked the recall, or they are testing out the explanation by prompting the nurse to supply additional information.

The nurse should also inquire about the use of any complementary or alternative medicine (CAM) practices. Results from the 2007 National Health Interview Survey found that approximately one in nine children (11.8%) used CAM in the past 12 months (Barnes, Bloom, and Nahin, 2009). The most commonly used therapies were nonvitamin, nonmineral, natural products (3.9%) and chiropractic or osteopathic manipulation (2.8%). Children whose parent used CAM were almost five times as likely (23.9%) to use CAM as children whose parent did not use CAM (5.1%). See the Complementary and Alternative Therapy box for other examples of CAM (see also Critical Thinking Exercise and Box 26-7).

Once the nurse has collected data as part of the nursing admission history, they must be applied to the nursing process and communicated to other staff. It makes little sense to assess a child's home routine if none of this knowledge is integrated into the care plan. Most nursing units have provisions for care plans in which specific information about the child's habits and needs are recorded.

Physical Assessment

Although physical examinations by practitioners are a required part of the admission procedure, nurses should also use the valuable information gained from physical assessments in their

NURSING CARE GUIDELINES

Supporting the Child and Family During Hospital Admission

Preadmission

Assign a room based on developmental age, seriousness of diagnosis, communicability of illness, and projected length of stay.

Prepare roommate(s) for the arrival of a new patient; when children are too young to benefit from this consideration, prepare parents.

Prepare room for child and family, with admission forms and equipment nearby.

Admission

Introduce primary nurse to child and family.

Orient child and family to inpatient facilities, especially to assigned room and unit; emphasize positive areas of pediatric unit:
- Room—Explain call light, bed controls, television; show bathroom, telephone.
- Unit—Direct to playroom, desk, activity room, dining area, other areas.

Introduce family to roommate and his or her parents.

Apply identification band to child's wrist, ankle, or both (if not already done).

Explain hospital regulations and schedules (e.g., visiting hours, mealtimes, bedtime, limitations); give written information if available.

Perform nursing admission history. (See Box 26-7.)

Take vital signs, blood pressure, height, and weight.

Obtain specimens as needed, and order required laboratory studies.

Support child and perform or assist practitioner with physical examination (for purposes of nursing assessment).

Emergency Admission

Lengthy preparatory admission procedures are often impossible and inappropriate for emergency situations.

Unless an emergency is life threatening, children need to participate in their care to maintain a sense of control.

Focus on essential components of admission counseling, including:
- Appropriate introduction to the family
- Use of child's name, not terms such as "honey" or "dear"
- Determination of child's age and some judgment about developmental age (if the child is of school age, asking about the grade level to obtain some evidence of concurrent intellectual ability)
- Information about child's general state of health, any problems that may interfere with medical treatment (e.g., sensitivity to medication), and previous hospitalizations or surgeries
- Information about the chief complaint from both the parents and the child

Admission to Intensive Care Unit

Prepare child and parents for elective intensive care unit (ICU) admission, such as for postoperative care after cardiac surgery.

Prepare child and parents for unanticipated ICU admission by focusing primarily on the sensory aspects of the experience and on usual family concerns (e.g., persons in charge of child's care, schedule for visiting, area where family can stay).

Prepare parents regarding child's appearance and behavior when they first visit child in ICU.

Accompany family to bedside to provide emotional support and answer questions.

Prepare siblings for their visit; plan length of time for sibling visitation; monitor siblings' reactions during visit to prevent them from becoming overwhelmed.

Encourage parents to stay with their child:
- If visiting hours are limited, allow flexibility in schedule to accommodate parental needs.
- Give family members a written schedule of visiting times.
- If visiting hours are liberal, be aware of family members' needs and suggest periodic breaks.

Assure family they can call the unit any time.

Prepare parents for expected role changes, and identify ways for parents to participate in child's care without overwhelming them with responsibilities:
- Help with bath or feeding.
- Touch and talk to child.
- Help with procedures.

Provide information about child's condition in developmentally appropriate language:
- Repeat information often.
- Seek clarification of understanding.
- During bedside conferences, interpret information for family members and child or, if appropriate, conduct report outside room.

Prepare child for procedures, even if this involves explanation while procedure is performed.

Assess and manage pain; recognize that a child who cannot talk, such as an infant or child in a coma or on a ventilator, can be in pain.

Establish a routine that maintains some similarity to daily events in child's life whenever possible:
- Organize care during normal waking hours.
- Keep regular bedtime schedules, including quiet times when television or radio is lowered or turned off.
- Provide uninterrupted sleep cycles (60 minutes for infant, 90 minutes for older child).
- Close and open drapes and dim lights to allow for day-night differentiation.
- Place curtain around bed for privacy as needed.
- Orient child to day and time; have clock or calendar in easy view for older children.

Schedule a time when child is left undisturbed (e.g., during naps, visit with family, playtime, or favorite program).

Provide opportunities for play.

Reduce stimulation in environment:
- Refrain from loud talking or laughing.
- Keep equipment noise to a minimum.
- Turn alarms as low as safely possible.
- Perform treatments requiring equipment at one time.
- Turn off bedside equipment that is not in use, such as suction and oxygen.
- Avoid loud, abrupt noises.

---

planning of care. (See Chapter 6.) Subjecting children to two separate examinations is unnecessary if the nurse and other practitioners cooperate during the procedure. For example, the nurse can also use the opportunity to observe the child's body for any bruises, rashes, signs of neglect, deformities, or physical limitations. Collaboration also prevents the often frustrating and needless waste of the family's time in repeating histories and examinations, especially when the child has a chronic condition that requires many hospitalizations.

The nurse should listen to the heart and lungs or do other target assessments pertinent to the illness or reason for hospi-

talization. It is impossible to evaluate improvement in respiratory function in a child admitted with pulmonary disease unless baseline data are available with which to compare subsequent findings.

Placing the Child

Room assignments are usually made before the child is admitted to the pediatric unit. The minimum considerations for room assignment are age, sex, and nature of the illness. Ideally, however, room selection should be based on a variety of developmental and psychobiologic needs. Determining compatible

BOX 26-7 NURSING ADMISSION HISTORY ACCORDING TO FUNCTIONAL HEALTH PATTERNS*

Health Perception–Health Management Pattern

Why has your child been admitted?

How has your child's general health been?

What does your child know about this hospitalization?

- Ask the child why he or she came to the hospital.
- If answer is "for an operation or for tests," ask the child to tell you what will happen before, during, and after the operation or tests.

Has your child ever been in the hospital before?

- How was that hospital experience?
- What things were important to you and your child during that hospitalization? How can we be most helpful now?

What medications does your child take at home?

- Why are they given?
- When are they given?
- How are they given (if a liquid, with a spoon; if a tablet, swallowed with water; or other)?
- Does your child have any trouble taking medication? If so, what helps?
- Is your child allergic to any medications, food, or natural products such as latex?

What, if any, forms of alternative or complementary medicine are being used?

Nutrition-Metabolic Pattern

What are the family's usual mealtimes?

Do family members eat together or at separate times?

What are your child's favorite foods, beverages, and snacks?

- Average amounts consumed or usual size portions
- Special cultural practices, such as family eating only ethnic food

What foods and beverages does your child dislike?

What are your child's feeding habits (bottle, cup, spoon, eats by self, needs assistance, any special devices)?

How does your child like the food served (warmed, cold, one item at a time)?

How would you describe your child's usual appetite (hearty eater, picky eater)?

Has being sick affected your child's appetite?

Are there any known or suspected food allergies? Is your child on a special diet?

Are there any feeding problems (excessive fussiness, spitting up, colic); any dental or gum problems that affect feeding?

What do you do for these problems?

Elimination Pattern

What are your child's toilet habits (diaper, toilet trained [day only or day and night], use of word to communicate urination or defecation, potty chair, regular toilet, other routines)?

What is your child's usual pattern of elimination (bowel movements)?

Do you have any concerns about elimination (bed-wetting, constipation, diarrhea)?

What do you do for these problems?

Does your child sweat a lot?

Sleep-Rest Pattern

What is your child's usual hour of bedtime and awakening?

What is your child's schedule for naps; length of naps?

Is there a special routine before sleeping (bottle, drink of water, bedtime story, nightlight, favorite blanket or toy, prayers)?

Is there a special routine during sleep time, such as waking to go to the bathroom?

What type of bed does your child sleep in?

What are the home sleeping arrangements (alone or with others, such as a sibling, parent, other person)?

What is your child's favorite sleeping position?

Are there any sleeping problems (falling asleep, waking during night, nightmares, sleep walking)?

Are there any problems awakening and getting ready in the morning?

What do you do for these problems?

Activity-Exercise Pattern

What is your child's schedule during the day (preschool, daycare center, regular school, extracurricular activities)?

What are your child's favorite activities or toys (both active and quiet)?

What is your child's usual television viewing schedule at home?

What are your child's favorite programs?

Are there any TV restrictions?

Does your child have any illness or disabilities that limit activity? If so, how?

What are your child's usual habits and schedule for bathing (bath in tub or shower, sponge bath, shampoo)?

What are your child's dental habits (brushing, flossing, fluoride supplements or rinses, favorite toothpaste); schedule of daily dental care?

Does your child need help with dressing or grooming?

Are there any problems with the above (dislike of or refusal to bathe, shampoo hair, or brush teeth)?

What do you do for these problems?

Are there special devices that your child requires help in managing (eyeglasses, contact lenses, hearing aid, orthodontic appliances, artificial elimination appliances, orthopedic devices)?

NOTE: Use the following code to assess functional self-care level for feeding, bathing/hygiene, dressing/grooming, toileting:

0—Full self-care

I—Requires use of equipment or device

II—Requires assistance or supervision from another person

III—Requires assistance or supervision from another person and equipment or device

IV—Is dependent and does not participate

Cognitive-Perceptual Pattern

Does your child have any hearing difficulty?

- Does the child use a hearing aid?
- Have myringotomy tubes been placed in your child's ears?

Does your child have any vision problems?

- Does the child wear glasses or contact lenses?

Does your child have any learning difficulties?

What is the child's grade in school?

Self-Perception–Self-Concept Pattern

How would you describe your child (e.g., shy, friendly, quiet, talkative, serious, playful, stubborn, easygoing)?

What makes your child angry, annoyed, anxious, or sad? What helps?

How does your child act when annoyed or upset?

What have been your child's experiences with and reactions to temporary separation from you (parent)?

Does your child have any fears (places, objects, animals, people, situations)? How do you handle them?

Do you think your child's illness has changed the way he or she thinks about self (e.g., shy, embarrassed, less competitive with friends, stays at home more)?

Role-Relationship Pattern

Does your child have a favorite nickname?

What are the names of other family members or others who live in the home (relatives, friends, pets)?

Who usually takes care of your child during the day or night (especially if other than parent, such as baby-sitter, relative)?

Which members of your family or extended family participate in childrearing and health decisions? To what extent?

What are the parents' occupation and work schedules?

Are there any special family considerations (adoption, foster child, stepparent, divorce, single parent)?

Have any major changes in the family occurred lately (death, divorce, separation, birth of a sibling, loss of a job, financial strain, mother beginning a career, other)? Describe child's reaction.

---

*The focus of the admission history is the child's psychosocial environment. Most of the questions are worded in terms of parental responses. Depending on the child's age, they should be addressed directly to the child when appropriate.

BOX 26-7   NURSING ADMISSION HISTORY ACCORDING TO FHPs—cont'd

Who are your child's play companions or social groups (peers, younger or older children, adults, prefers to be alone)?

Do things generally go well for your child in school or with friends?

Does your child use "security" objects at home (pacifier, thumb, bottle, blanket, stuffed animal or doll)? Did you bring any of these to the hospital?

How do you handle discipline problems at home? Are these methods always effective?

Does your child have any condition that interferes with communication? If so, what are your suggestions for communicating with your child?

Will your child's hospitalization affect the family's financial support or care of other family members (e.g., other children)?

What concerns do you have about your child's illness and hospitalization?

Who will be staying with your child while hospitalized?

How can we contact you or a close family member outside the hospital?

Sexuality-Reproductive Pattern
(Answer questions that apply to the child's age-group.)

Has your child begun puberty (developing physical sexual characteristics, menstruation)? Have you or your child had any concerns?

Does your daughter know how to do breast self-examination?

Does your son know how to do testicular self-examination?

How have you approached topics of sexuality with your child?

Do you think you might need help with some topics?

Has your child's illness affected the way he or she feels about being a boy or a girl? If so, how?

Do you have any concerns about your child's behaviors, such as masturbation, asking many questions or talking about sex, not respecting others' privacy, or wanting too much privacy?

Initiate a conversation about an adolescent's sexual concerns with open-ended to more direct questions and using the terms *friends* or *partners* rather than *girlfriend* or *boyfriend*:
- Tell me about your social life.
- Who are your closest friends? (If one friend is identified, could ask more about that relationship, such as how much time they spend together, how

serious they are about each other, if the relationship is going the way the teenager hoped.)
- Consider asking about dating and sexual issues, such as the teenager's views on sex education, "going steady," "living together," or premarital sex.
- Which friends would you like to have visit in the hospital?

Coping–Stress Tolerance Pattern
(Answer questions that apply to the child's age-group.)

What does your child do when tired or upset?
- If upset, does your child want a special person or object? If so, explain.

If your child has temper tantrums, what causes them and how do you handle them?

Whom does your child talk to when worried about something?

How does your child usually handle problems or disappointments?

Have there been any big changes or problems in your family recently? How did you handle them?

Has your child ever had a problem with drugs of abuse or alcohol or tried suicide?

Value-Belief Pattern

Do you practice organized religion?

How is religion or faith important in your child's life?

What religious practices would you like continued in the hospital (e.g., prayers before meals or bedtime; visit by minister, priest, or rabbi; prayer group)?

What religious practices do you follow that affect childrearing and health practice (e.g., fasting, herbal remedies)?

What do you believe caused your child's illness or condition?

When illness or injury occurs, do you use any herbs, medicines, healer, rituals, or ceremonies?

What are your family's prior health care experiences?

What are your concerns with this health care system?

What do you do when your child is sick? What person do you go to first?

What generation immigrant are you (first, second, third)?

What languages does your child speak or understand? What languages do you and other family members speak or understand?

With whom do you discuss child-related concerns or problems?

 COMPLEMENTARY AND ALTERNATIVE THERAPY

Medicine Practices and Examples

Nutrition, diet, and lifestyle or behavioral health changes—Macrobiotics, megavitamins, diets, lifestyle modification, health risk reduction or health education, wellness

Mind-body control therapies—Biofeedback, relaxation, prayer therapy, guided imagery, hypnotherapy, music or sound therapy,* education therapy

Traditional and ethnomedicine therapies—Acupuncture, ayurvedic medicine, herbal medicine, homeopathic medicine, Native American medicine, natural products, traditional Asian medicine

Structural manipulation and energetic therapies—Acupressure, chiropractic medicine, massage, reflexology, rolfing, therapeutic touch, Qi Gong

Pharmacologic and biologic therapies—Antioxidants, cell treatment, chelation therapy, metabolic therapy, oxidizing agents

Bioelectromagnetic therapies—Diagnostic and therapeutic application of electromagnetic fields (e.g., transcranial electrostimulation, neuromagnetic stimulation, electroacupuncture)

*An excellent resource for providing environmental stimulation with music is Froehlich M: *Music therapy with hospitalized children*, Cherry Hill, NJ, 1996, Jeffrey Books.

 CRITICAL THINKING EXERCISE

Complementary and Alternative Medicine

Maria, a 10-year-old Hispanic girl, has had severe nosebleeds. She is admitted to the hospital for a complete workup in an attempt to determine the cause. Her parents and grandparents have gathered around her bed. When you enter her room to begin admitting procedures, you notice an unusual scent. Maria's mother is rubbing the contents from an unfamiliar bottle of liquid on Maria. Meanwhile, the grandmother is rubbing Maria's head. She is startled at your entry and drops something on the floor near your feet. You bend over to pick it up and discover that it is a penny.

1. Evidence—Is there sufficient evidence to draw any conclusions?
2. Assumptions—What are some underlying assumptions that may be drawn from the data about the following?
   a. Complementary or alternative medical remedies
   b. The role of ethnic or folk remedies in modern health care practice
   c. The nurse's role in cases where alternative (versus traditional Western) medicine is practiced
3. What implications and priorities for nursing care can be drawn at this time?
4. Does the evidence objectively support your argument (conclusion)?

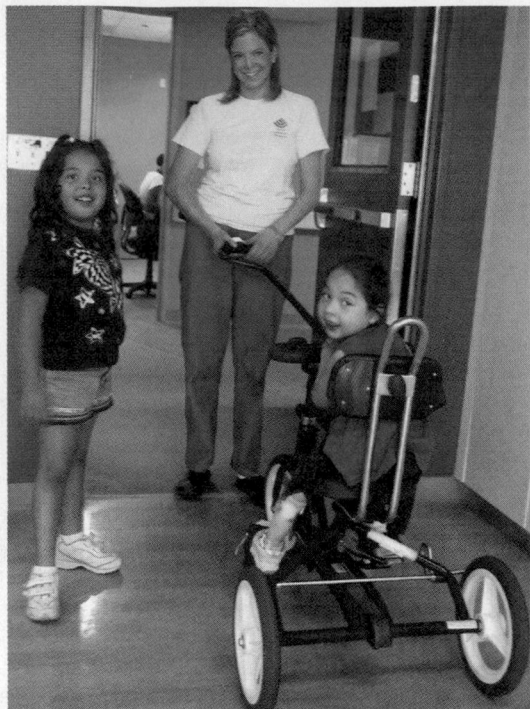

Fig. 26-13 Placing children of the same age-group and with similar types of illness near each other on the unit is both psychologically and medically advantageous. (Courtesy E. Jacob, Texas Children's Hospital, Houston.)

roommates, both for the children and for parents, greatly influences satisfaction with the hospital experience.

Although no absolute rules govern room selection, in general, placing children of the same age-group and with similar types of illness in the same room is both psychologically and medically advantageous (Fig. 26-13). However, there are many exceptions. For example, a child in traction may be therapeutic for another child confined to bed because of a serious illness. A child who is independent despite physical disabilities may help another child with limitations and the parents achieve deeper insight and acceptance of the disorder.

Adolescent Unit

To meet the unique needs of adolescents, hospitals have developed special units that provide privacy, increased socialization, and appropriate activities. Typically these units are set apart from the general pediatric facility so that the teenagers do not share space with younger children, who are often perceived as a threat to their maturity. These units also provide more flexible routines and activities, such as more group activity, provisions to leave the adolescent unit temporarily, and access to the items important to teenagers—telephones, computers, compact disc players, DVD players, video game systems, and televisions. Because adolescents' food habits are rarely limited to three meals a day, a supply of snacks should be available. One of the most important benefits of these units is increased socialization with peers. In addition, many staff members enjoy working with this age-group and are well suited to establishing the trust that is essential for communication.

Despite the advantages of adolescent units, all young people require preparation for the experience. They need orientation to the unit, introduction to staff and other patients, and an atmos-

phere of warmth and welcome. Just as teenagers form cliques in normal social relationships, this also occurs in the hospital. Staff must be aware of exclusiveness of group membership, especially when new patients are admitted. Scheduled and supervised group meetings are effective in preventing feelings of "nonbelonging" and in facilitating introductions and new friendships. They also provide an excellent opportunity for discussions about typical adolescent concerns (e.g., sexuality, drugs, alcohol, parental relations) and special illness-related concerns of adolescents (e.g., peer rejection for being different).

NURSING CARE DURING SPECIAL HOSPITAL SITUATIONS

In addition to a general pediatric unit, children may be admitted to special facilities, such as an ambulatory/outpatient setting, an isolation room, or intensive care.

Ambulatory/Outpatient Setting

The ambulatory/outpatient setting provides needed medical services for the child without an overnight admission. Among the benefits of ambulatory/outpatient care are (1) minimization of the stressors of hospitalization, especially separation from the family; (2) reduced risk of infection; and (3) cost savings. Admission to the ambulatory/outpatient hospital setting usually is for surgical or diagnostic procedures, such as insertion of myringotomy tubes, hernia repair, adenoidectomy, tonsillectomy, cystoscopy, or bronchoscopy. In addition, improved outpatient care and treatment of chronic conditions have resulted in the need for fewer overnight hospitalizations.

In the ambulatory/outpatient setting, adequate preparation is particularly challenging. Ideally, the child and parents should receive preadmission preparation, including a tour of the facility and a review of the day's events. Parents need information in advance to help prepare the child and themselves for surgery and enable them to care for the child at home after the procedure. Parents also appreciate suggestions for items to bring for the child's trip home, such as blankets or stuffed animals. When preadmission preparation is not possible, allow time on the day of the procedure for children to become acquainted with their surroundings and for nurses to assess, plan, and implement appropriate teaching.

Waiting is practically inevitable in ambulatory/outpatient settings. Families often report waiting to be the most stressful part of the hospitalization experience. Providing a pager allows the family (and in many instances, the child) to leave the area and then be paged to return when needed. The need for creating a welcoming environment for children and families often may be overlooked in the ambulatory/outpatient setting, particularly in day surgery centers or settings that are not exclusively focused on pediatric patients. Toys, books, and other play materials should be available to children while they wait.

Explicit discharge instructions are important after outpatient surgery (see Family-Centered Care box). Parents need guidelines on when to call their practitioner regarding a change in the child's condition. A telephone follow-up system allows nurses to check on the child's progress within 48 to 72 hours after discharge. It provides an opportunity for the nurse to review discharge information and answer questions.

FAMILY-CENTERED CARE

Discharge from Ambulatory Settings

1. Before beginning, explain that all instructions will also be presented in writing for the family to refer to later.
2. Provide an overview of the typical trajectory (expected pattern) of recovery.
3. Discuss expected progression of the child's activity level during the post-discharge period (e.g., "Mary will probably sleep for the rest of the day, feel tired most of tomorrow, but be back to her usual activities the next day").
4. Explain which activities the child is allowed and what is not permitted (e.g., bed rest, bathing).
5. Discuss dietary restrictions, being specific and giving examples of "clear fluids" or what is meant by a "full liquid diet."
6. Discuss nausea and vomiting, if applicable, explaining how much is "normal" and what to do if more occurs (e.g., "Juan may be sick to his stomach and vomit. This is normal. However, if he vomits more than three times, please call us at this number right away.").
7. Discuss fever and the comfort measures to use, explaining how much fever is considered "normal," and specifically what to do if the child goes beyond the range.
8. Explain the amount, location, and kind of pain or discomfort the child may experience.
   - Give any prescribed medication before leaving the facility.
   - Send a pain scale home with the family. (See Table 7-2.)
   - Explain how much pain and discomfort is "normal" and what to do if the child surpasses that level or if pain management interventions are unsuccessful.
   - Discuss pain management, including dosage for pain medications and details in writing on how to administer them.
   - Describe appropriate nonpharmacologic comfort measures, such as holding, rocking, or distraction techniques.
9. Provide written information about each medication that the child will be taking at home.
   - Review the details, including dosage, route, and side effects.
   - Demonstrate how to administer medications, if necessary (e.g., how to use suppositories).
10. Make certain the family has all the equipment and supplies (e.g., gauze and tape for dressing changes) they will need at home.
11. Discuss complications that may occur and the steps to take if they do.
12. Ensure that appropriate measures are in place for safe transport home.
    - Remind family to use a seat belt or car seat for the child.
    - Determine whether there will be one person whose sole responsibility is helping ensure the child's safety and comfort during transport.
    - Discuss measures the driver may need to take if this is impossible (e.g., be certain a basin is within the child's reach should vomiting occur; take a route that permits slower traffic and has places along the roadside to stop if necessary).
    - Determine the availability of a blanket, pillow, and cup with a cap and straw for the child's use in the car.
    - Provide a basin or plastic bag in case of vomiting.
    - Suggest the parent bring the child an extra change of clothing and towel(s) in case of vomiting.
13. Provide 24-hour emergency phone numbers for the family to call.
14. Explain that the family will be contacted to follow up on the child but that they should not hesitate to call if concerns arise before then.
15. Ask the family and child, if appropriate, if they have any questions, and problem solve with family members to meet any needs.

NURSING TIP Help the family prepare for transportation home by suggesting they:
- Have a blanket and pillow in the car. (Always use the car safety system.)
- Take a basin or plastic bag in case of vomiting.
- Use a cup with a cap and straw for the child to drink fluids.
- Give any prescribed pain medication before leaving facility.

Isolation

Admission to an isolation room increases all the stressors typically associated with hospitalization. There is further separation from familiar persons; additional loss of control; and added environmental changes, such as sensory deprivation and the strange appearance of visitors. Isolation also affects orientation to time and place. These stressors are compounded by children's limited understanding of isolation. Preschool children have difficulty understanding the rationale for isolation because they cannot comprehend the cause-and-effect relationship between germs and illness. They are likely to view isolation as punishment. Older children understand the causality better but still require information to decrease fantasizing or misinterpretation.

When a child is placed in isolation, preparation is essential for the child to feel in control. With young children, the best approach is a simple explanation, such as "You need to be in this room to help you get better. This is a special place to make all the germs go away. The germs made you sick, and you could not help that."

All children, but especially younger ones, need preparation in terms of what they will see, hear, or feel in isolation. Therefore the nurse should show them the mask, gloves, and gown and encourage them to "dress up" in them. Playing with the strange apparel lessens the fear of seeing "ghostlike" people walk into the room. Before entering the room, nurses and other health personnel should introduce themselves and let the child see their face before donning a mask. In this way the child associates them with tangible features and gains a sense of familiarity in an otherwise strange and lonely environment.

When the child's condition improves, provide appropriate play activities to minimize boredom, stimulate the senses, provide a real or perceived sense of movement, orient the child to time and place, provide social interaction, and reduce depersonalization. For example, the environment can be manipulated to increase sensory freedom by moving the bed toward the door or window. Opening window shades; providing musical, visual, or tactile toys; and increasing interpersonal contact can substitute mental mobility for the limitations of physical movement. Rather than dwelling on the negative aspects of isolation, encourage the child to view this experience as challenging and positive. For example, the nurse can help the child look at isolation as a method of keeping others out and letting only special people in. Children often think of intriguing signs for their doors, such as "Enter at your own risk." These signs also encourage people "on the outside" to talk with the child about the ominous greeting.

Emergency Admission

One of the most traumatic hospital experiences for the child and parents is an emergency admission. A sudden illness or injury leaves little time for preparation and explanation. Sometimes the emergency admission is compounded by admission to an ICU or the need for immediate surgery. However, even in those instances requiring only outpatient treatment, the child is exposed to a strange, frightening environment and to experiences that may elicit fear or cause pain. Thus every medical emergency requires psychologic intervention to reduce the fear and anxiety frequently associated with the experience. Child life specialists are essential to provide teaching and support in these situations.

There is often a wide discrepancy between what constitutes a medically defined emergency and a client-defined emergency. A growing concern is the use of major emergency departments for routine primary care health visits. To offset overcrowding in emergency departments, many facilities have minor emergency units or pediatric minor emergency units for after-hours health care. Telephone triage for minor illnesses for patients is also emerging as a health care delivery mode to distinguish illnesses such as common cold from true life-threatening conditions that require immediate practitioner attention and intervention. Other factors contributing to the overuse of emergency departments (as opposed to the primary practitioner's office) include the increasing number of uninsured persons and households where both parents work full time and cannot afford to take off during the daytime to take the sick child to a practitioner.

In pediatric populations, most visits are for respiratory tract infections, skin conditions, gastrointestinal disorders, and trauma. The most common reason parents give for bringing the child to the emergency department is concern about the illness worsening. However, practitioners may not consider the progressive symptoms as necessitating immediate or emergency care. One of the nurse's primary goals is to assess the parents' perception of the event and their reasons for considering it serious or life threatening.

Lengthy preparatory admission procedures are often inappropriate for emergency situations. In such instances, nurses must focus their nursing interventions on the essential components of admission counseling (see Nursing Care Guidelines box, p. 987) and complete the process as soon as the child's condition is stabilized.

Unless an emergency is life threatening, children need to participate in their care to maintain a sense of control. Because emergency departments are frequently hectic, staff has a tendency to rush through procedures to save time. However, the extra few minutes needed to allow children to participate may save many more minutes of useless resistance and uncooperativeness during subsequent procedures. Other supportive measures include ensuring privacy, accepting various emotional responses to fear or pain, preserving parent-child contact, explaining all events before or as they occur, and remaining calm.

At times, because of the child's physical condition, little or no preparatory counseling for emergency hospitalization can be done. In such situations, counseling after the event has therapeutic value. The process involves evaluating children's thoughts regarding admission and related procedures. It is similar to precounseling techniques; however, instead of supplying information, the nurse listens to the child's explanations. Projective techniques such as drawing, doll play, or storytelling are especially effective. The nurse then bases additional teaching on what has already been learned.

Intensive Care Unit

Admission to an ICU can be traumatic for both the child and parents (Fig. 26-14). The nature and severity of the illness, the

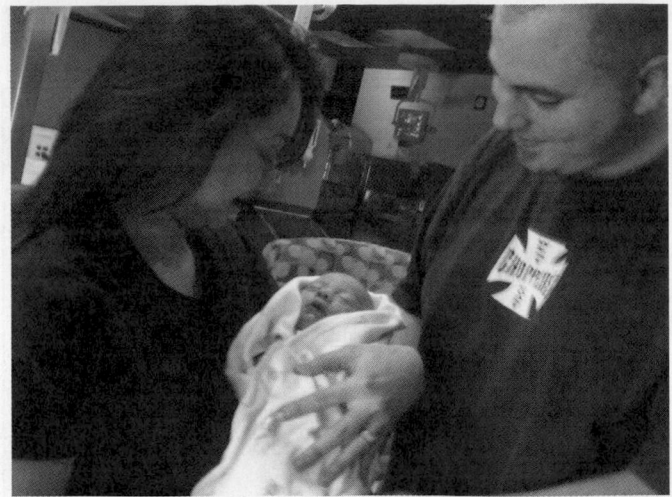

Fig. 26-14 Parents should be encouraged to be actively involved when their infant is critically ill and requires care in an intensive care unit. (Courtesy E. Jacob, Texas Children's Hospital, Houston.)

circumstances surrounding the admission, and the highly technologic, unfamiliar environment are major factors, especially for parents. Parents experience significantly more stress when the admission is unexpected rather than expected. Nurses can assist with coping by asking parents to identify stressors and implement appropriate interventions. Assessment should be repeated periodically to account for changes in perceptions over time. The use of daily patient goal sheets has been successful in improving communication among health care providers caring for children in the ICU (Agarwal, Frankel, Tourner, et al, 2008; Phipps and Thomas, 2007). By clearly defining daily patient care goals, health care providers believed that care was improved.

In a qualitative study of 19 parents of 10 children in the ICU, parents reported that they wanted nurses to nurture the child in ICU as the family would (Harbaugh, Tomlinson, and Kirschbaum, 2004). Nurse behaviors that exemplified affection, caring, watching, and protecting were perceived as helpful in decreasing stress and maintaining the family unit during the crisis of hospitalization. Nurse behaviors perceived as not helpful to the family included giving care without appearing to care, separating parents from the child, excluding parents from decision making, and communicating poorly with parents.

The family's emotional needs are paramount when a child is admitted to an ICU. Although the same interventions discussed earlier for separation anxiety, loss of control, and bodily injury and pain apply here, additional interventions may also benefit the family and child (see Nursing Care Guidelines box, p. 987, and Family-Centered Care box). Critical care must be family centered.

Critically ill children become the focus of the parents' lives, and the parents' need for information regarding their child is paramount. They want to know if their child will live and, if so, whether the child will be the same as before. They need to know why various interventions are being done for the child, that the child is being treated for pain or is comfortable, and that the child may be able to hear them even though the child is not awake.

FAMILY-CENTERED CARE

Artists as Partners in Care

A teenage boy with a rare genetic disorder, having made steady progress after awakening from a coma, relapsed and seemed depressed. When told that a musician was visiting the pediatric intensive care unit, he immediately perked up and asked to have his room lights turned on. He whispered endless song requests to the musician. Family members and staff were treated to some of his first smiles in days; his biggest came when the musician held his hand and guided it across the guitar strings while they sang "Born to Be Wild" together at the boy's request. His dad was misty eyed as he thanked the musician for the visit.

A few weeks later the boy's condition worsened and he again lapsed into a coma. There was nothing more to be done. His parents began the necessary preparations to take their son home to die.

We continued to visit our friend and his family, offering a song or a story or just to say hello. I hold a vivid picture of our final visit. We stood around the boy's bed with his parents singing together songs they remembered from their youth, from more carefree times. Song and laughter filled the boy's room.

Perhaps the boy heard his parents' laughter and knew then that they would be okay. He died a few days later on the morning he was to have been discharged.

Judy Rollins, MS, RN
Washington, DC

Modified from Rollins J: *Placed in our keeping*, 1995, Unpublished.

When an ICU admission is planned (e.g., postoperative care after cardiac surgery), the child and parents should be prepared for the admission. Some units advocate a tour, whereas others use picture books of the unit to familiarize the family with the environment and usual equipment. Nurses can use dolls to demonstrate the equipment, types of tubes, and dressings that the child may have.

A major stressor for parents of a child in the ICU is the child's appearance (Latour, van Goudoever, and Hazelzet, 2008). When parents first visit the child in the ICU, they need preparation about the appearance of the child. Ideally, the nurse should accompany the family to the bedside to provide emotional support and answer any questions. If siblings visit, they need the same preparation as parents. Whether they should visit soon after the child is admitted or after the child's condition has stabilized is controversial. Early visiting minimizes the opportunity for siblings to fantasize about the experience and imagine the situation is worse than it actually is. However, early visiting may be frightening, especially when the patient is in pain or unresponsive and attached to numerous tubes and equipment. If there is a concern that the child may not survive the illness, however, an early visit may be the only option. The length of time for sibling visitation should be planned ahead and monitored during the visit to prevent the well child from becoming overwhelmed.

Children admitted to the ICU need their parents' comfort and security, and nurses should encourage parents to stay with their child. If visiting hours are limited, the schedule should be flexible to accommodate parental needs. Family members should be given a schedule of the visiting times permitted and assured that they can call the unit at any time. With liberalization of visiting hours, many parents think they must stay with their child. Nurses need to be sensitive to parental needs, suggesting periodic respites from the stressful ICU environment.

Because altered parental roles are a major stress for parents, nurses need to implement interventions to minimize this concern, such as (1) educating and preparing parents for the expected role changes; (2) identifying ways in which parents can continue to fulfill parenting functions, such as helping with the bath or feeding, touching, and talking to the child; and (3) determining new roles, such as helping with procedures. Information sharing can increase parents' sense of control and responsibility, but facts must be conveyed simply and repeated often, with care taken to avoid overwhelming family members. Because medical jargon is used frequently in a complex environment such as the ICU, unfamiliar terms need to be clarified and simpler terms substituted. (See Nursing Care Guidelines boxes under Psychologic Preparation, Chapter 27.)

As in emergency admissions, there is a tendency in the ICU to perform procedures quickly and without attention to the child's preparational needs. Therefore nurses need to remember the special concerns about bodily injury of children in each age-group. Explaining each procedure, altering it whenever possible to decrease the child's fears, and supporting the child are essential. Giving children an object that symbolizes their coping, such as a "hero badge" or an "ICU diploma," provides a positive memento of an otherwise stressful experience. Depending on the numerous procedures performed on the child and the nature of the illness, pain management needs to receive a high priority.

Of particular importance in decreasing fear is ensuring that discussions that do not directly include the family are held where the child and family cannot overhear them. Casual conversation in the nursing station or in the halls can often be overheard and taken out of context. When discussions are held at the bedside, it is easy to forget the patient and make remarks that are misunderstood. Usually a quiet reminder of how frightened the child can become from listening to these discussions is sufficient. If bedside conferences are necessary, the nurse interprets them for family members in words they can comprehend.

Extensive monitoring makes a usual day-night cycle difficult in an ICU. However, some schedule should be established that is similar to daily events in the child's life. These include organizing care during normal waking hours; keeping regular bedtime schedules, including quiet times when televisions and radios are lowered or turned off; closing and opening drapes as appropriate; dimming lights; placing a curtain around the bed for privacy and decreased stimulation; and having clocks or calendars in easy view for older children. In particular, staff members must realize the need for quiet and refrain from loud talking or laughing. Equipment noise should be kept to a minimum by turning alarms as low as safely possible, scheduling nursing care in blocks of time to minimize interruptions, turning off bedside equipment not in use (e.g., suction, oxygen), and avoiding loud, abrupt noises. Such measures can reduce the sensory overload and the sleep deprivation commonly associated with ICU admissions.

Provide play opportunities for every child. Although children who are critically ill may be unable to initiate spontaneous play, others (e.g., nurse, social worker, child life specialist, parent, sibling) can structure play interactions in which children watch and direct the person who plays for them.

Despite the stresses normally associated with ICU admission, a special security develops from being carefully monitored and receiving individualized care. Therefore planning for transition to the regular unit is essential and should include (1) assignment of a primary nurse on the regular unit who visits before the transfer; (2) continued visits by the ICU staff to assess the child's and parents' adjustment and to act as a temporary liaison with the nursing staff; (3) explanation of the differences between the two units and the rationale for the change to less intense monitoring of the child's physical condition; and (4) selection of an appropriate room, such as one close to the nursing station, and a compatible roommate. In one study of parents whose children were being transferred from the ICU to the regular pediatric unit, parents who received a transfer preparation letter and verbal explanation of the process had significantly lower anxiety scores than parents who did not receive this information (Bouve, Roozmus, and Giordano, 1999).

DISCHARGE PLANNING AND HOME CARE

Most hospitalizations necessitate some type of discharge planning. Often this involves education of the family for continued care and follow-up in the home. Depending on the diagnosis, this may be relatively simple or complex. With the current concern for cost containment and recognition of children's emotional needs, home care for children with technologically complex care, such as ventilators, has become increasingly common. Preparing the family for home care demands a high degree of competence in planning and implementing discharge instruction. (See Chapter 25.) Adequate preparation for optimal home care includes an interdisciplinary approach, with all members of the health care team working together with the patient and family.

Nurses are often key individuals in initiating the discharge process and collaborating with others in planning and implementation. Although it is not possible to discuss all the details needed for effective discharge planning and home care, this section presents a brief overview of the more critical aspects. More specific details are discussed throughout the text for conditions such as home apnea monitoring, tracheostomy care, or total parenteral nutrition, and numerous sources of information exist in the literature.

Assessment

Discharge planning for home care must begin with an assessment of the family's desires and capability in assuming care responsibilities. Ideally, at least two individuals should be committed to learning the skills needed for home care. The family should participate in a thorough assessment of their needs and the home environment to ensure that their emotional and physical resources are sufficient to manage the tasks of home care. (For a discussion of family and home assessment strategies, see Chapters 22 and 25.) In addition to adequate family resources, an investigation of community services is needed to ensure that appropriate support agencies are available, such as emergency facilities, respite care, home health agencies, and equipment vendors. To coordinate the immense task of assessment and to plan implementation, a discharge planning coordinator should be appointed early in the process.

Planning

Ideally, preparation for hospital discharge and home care begins during the admission assessment with the establishment of short- and long-term goals. These goals are concerned with the child's physical needs and the psychologic needs of the child and family. For children who require complex care, discharge planning focuses on obtaining appropriate equipment and health care personnel for the home and on the skills that parents or children are expected to continue at home. In planning appropriate teaching, nurses need to assess (1) the actual and perceived complexity of the skill, (2) the parents' or child's ability to learn the skill, and (3) the parents' or child's previous or present experience with such procedures. (See Compliance, Chapter 27, for guidelines for effective teaching.)

The teaching plan should incorporate levels of learning, such as observing, participating with assistance, and a return demonstration of the skill. Each skill should be divided into discrete steps, and each step taught to the family member. Return demonstration of the skill should be requested before introducing new skills. A record of teaching and performance provides an efficient checklist for evaluation. Before leaving the hospital, all families should receive detailed written instructions about home care and telephone numbers should they require assistance.

Transitional Care

Once the family is competent in performing required skills, they should be given responsibility for the care. Whenever possible, the family should have a transition or trial period to assume care with minimum supervision. This may be arranged on the unit, during a home pass, or in a facility (e.g., a motel or Ronald McDonald House) near the hospital. Some programs incorporate a hospital trial into their discharge criteria, necessitating that the family successfully manage this phase before discharge to home. Such transitions provide a safe practice period for the family, with assistance readily available when needed, and are especially valuable when the family lives far from the hospital.

Evaluation and Continuing Support

Evaluation is a critical part of any discharge plan and assumes even more importance in home care of children with complex needs. Factors to consider in home care planning include need for subsequent hospitalization, child's developmental and physical progress, effects of home care on the family, actual versus expected use of resources by the family and home care team, and financial costs and savings.

In most instances parents need only simple instructions and understanding of follow-up care. However, the often overwhelming care assumed by some families necessitates continued professional support after discharge. A follow-up home visit or telephone call gives the nurse an opportunity to individualize care and provide information in perhaps a less stressful learning environment than the hospital; this may be coordinated with home health care providers for a smooth transition to home. Appropriate referrals and resources may include visiting nurse or home health agencies, private nurse services, the school system, physical therapist, mental health counselor, social worker, and various community agencies, including special organizations. Sharing the important issues surrounding the child's and family's needs is essential. Referral summaries should be concise, specific, and factual. When numerous support services are involved, periodic collaboration among the professionals (interdisciplinary conferences) and the family is an excellent strategy to ensure efficient implementation and comprehensive delivery of services.

KEY POINTS

- Children are particularly vulnerable to the stresses of illness and hospitalization because stress represents a change from the usual state of health and routine and because they possess limited coping mechanisms.

- The three phases of separation anxiety are protest, despair, and detachment.

- Feelings of loss of control are caused by unfamiliar environmental stimuli, physical restriction, altered routine, and dependency.

- Fear of pain may be manifested in the following ways: infants—facial expressions, body movements; toddlers—intense emotional upset, physical resistance; preschoolers—aggression, verbal expression, dependency; school-age children—precise verbalization of pain, passive requests for support or help, procrastination technique; adolescents—self-control, irritability, limited movement.

- Because of their separation from significant people, children who are hospitalized may lack the opportunity to form new attachments in the strange environment and may exhibit negative behaviors after discharge.

- Family reactions are influenced by the seriousness of illness, experience with illness or hospitalization, diagnostic or therapeutic procedures, available support systems, personal ego strengths, coping abilities, additional stresses, cultural and religious beliefs, and family communication patterns.

- The following factors increase the negative effects of a brother's or sister's illness or hospitalization on siblings: fear of contracting the illness, their age, a close relationship with the ill sibling, substitute child care, minimum explanation of the illness, and perceived changes in parenting.

- Nursing care of children who are hospitalized is aimed at preventing or minimizing separation, decreasing loss of control, minimizing bodily injury and pain, using play and other expressive activities to lessen stress, maximizing potential benefits of hospitalization, and supporting family members.

- The child life specialist plays an important role in using play and other expressive activities as effective tools in minimizing stress.

- The nurse can maximize potential benefits of hospitalization by fostering parent-child relations, providing educational opportunities, promoting self-mastery, and encouraging socialization.

- Supporting family members involves listening to parents' verbal and nonverbal messages; providing social and spiritual support; accepting cultural, socioeconomic, and ethnic values; and giving information to families and siblings.

- The major goals of prehospital counseling are to make the hospital less strange and frightening to parents and children and to establish a positive atmosphere and trusting relationships with staff and family members.

- In preparing families for hospitalization, the nurse should consider small group size and timing of the event, setting of the tour, inclusion of preparatory materials, time for discussion, and prehospital counseling for parents.

- Emergency admission or admission to an ambulatory/outpatient setting, isolation room, or ICU requires additional intervention strategies to meet the child's and family's needs.

ANSWERS TO CRITICAL THINKING EXERCISES

Playroom and Hospital Procedures

1. There is sufficient evidence regarding this incident to draw some conclusions.

2. **a.** Regardless of how minor a procedure such as a venipuncture may seem to an adult health care worker, it represents a major threat to a child. One must consider the child's age, illness, developmental level, and previous experiences with venipuncture.

   b. Play is an important function of childhood whether the child is sick or well. Through play children may act out fears, concerns, anger, and other emotions that they may not feel comfortable expressing to adults in a confrontational manner. Play is an important part of the hospitalized child's life, and it is a vehicle for promoting optimum development.

   c. It is important to have the blood drawn so Dr. Lung may plan a therapeutic regimen; however, there appears to have been no advance preparation of the child's skin to minimize or prevent pain from the procedure. Regardless of the phlebotomist's skill in performing the procedure, it is also important to consider that the negative repercussions of performing the procedure at this point may outweigh the benefits.

   d. All staff on the pediatric floor must agree about respecting the child's personal space in the playroom and must adhere to unit policies or rules so that respect is maintained.

Failure to respect the child's space may engender further fear in other children who perceive that the playroom is not a safe place after all when certain procedures need to be done. The fear of having other procedures performed in the playroom may prevent children from going there to participate in therapeutic and interactive play.

3. It is important to maintain a fair balance between therapeutic management of illness and childhood recreation. It would be appropriate in this situation to intervene and ask the phlebotomist to return in 30 minutes to an hour and indicate that the child will be ready for the venipuncture in the treatment room at that time. It is important to stress that the playroom is off-limits for procedures. It would be appropriate to discuss this plan with Hannah, indicating that the procedure will be performed at the designated time. It is also important to explore pain management issues with Hannah and her parent: does she usually use EMLA (lidocaine-prilocaine) or another topical remedy to prevent pain at the site? If so, it will be necessary to make such arrangements in advance, possibly now, so her pain is managed appropriately. As the nurse, it is appropriate to discuss a delay in obtaining the laboratory results with Dr. Lung and the reasons for the delay. Medical and nursing staff on the pediatric floor must communicate effectively. Should this arrangement not suit Dr. Lung's time frame for accomplishing certain tasks, one might suggest a trade-off. The nurse could draw the blood in the treatment room once preparations are made and Hannah agrees to a time. Remember, however, that school-age children are prone to bargain for more time to delay or prevent the event, since it is painful. One must be gently firm about the agreed-on time of the procedure and not allow further delays.

Even if one accepts the conclusion that it is okay with Hannah to have blood drawn in the playroom, it is important to consider the possible negative implications for the other children in the room, who may be confused about even a simple procedure (e.g., checking blood pressure) or the sanctuary status of the playroom. Proceeding with the blood draw in the playroom would violate the child's trust about what adult health care workers say regarding the purpose of the playroom as a sanctuary from painful procedures. Such action would likely result in less cooperation from the children who are present and may also make other parents who are present, or who hear about the incident, wonder about the staff's sincerity. Interrupting the children's game is not necessary, since this does not represent a life-threatening situation.

4. Yes. There is sufficient evidence to support these decisions and the plan of action.

Complementary and Alternative Medicine

1. There is limited evidence to draw certain conclusions without obtaining more data from the parents. It would be appropriate to gather more information before jumping to any major conclusions at this time.

2. **a.** Complementary and alternative medicine (CAM) is more common in U.S. households than previously reported. Much of the concern surrounding complementary therapies, especially in children, is the lack of sufficient data regarding their effectiveness, benefit, and potential harm that may occur as a result of such treatments. In some cases CAM therapies may counteract certain medications or the effects of prescribed therapies. It has become more common for practitioners in emergency medicine to encounter patients who are taking CAM therapy in addition to prescription medications or treatments for conditions such as eczema, asthma, colds, and upper respiratory tract problems.

b. Folk remedies are common among certain ethnic groups and subgroups in the United States. Many are based on traditional family remedies that have been proved neither effective nor harmful. However, a few remedies could be potentially harmful, especially to children, by counteracting the effects of prescribed treatments that are known to be effective; some remedies' ingredients may be toxic to children.

c. The nurse's role in such cases is to gather sufficient data from the family about the practice, discuss the treatment (CAM) in a nonjudgmental manner, and be cognizant of the effects of the treatment on the child's current health status and potential effects on other medical treatment regimens.

3. Give the family their penny and open a dialogue about the traditional practice they are using. Gather additional information in a nonjudgmental manner; the discussion should center on the family's traditional beliefs regarding the practices, the prescribed medical regimen, and whether there is conflict or potential for harm. There is no need to stop the treatment unless potential harm to the child may occur. A discussion with the primary practitioner regarding the use of CAM for Maria should ensue, followed by a discussion with the entire family if necessary.

The contents of the bottle will likely be revealed during the discussion with the family. It is important to respect the family's wishes regarding traditional folk or CAM rituals, yet remain mindful of potential harmful effects on the child. It is not likely that telling the family to stop the ritual will have much success, since these beliefs are deeply ingrained into cultural, religious, and medical practice; the family may continue the ritual at home on discharge and further disregard other instructions for care should the nursing and medical staff adopt a confrontational approach. The important concept for the staff and family to focus on is the ultimate well-being of the child.

What you have probably observed is Santeria, the African-Caribbean religion that was brought to the New World by slaves from West Africa. It is common among immigrants from Cuba, Puerto Rico, Brazil, and Santo Domingo; a majority of Latin immigrants will probably have contact with Santeria sometime in their lives.

4. As yet, there is insufficient evidence to indicate that harm is being done by the CAM ritual. Further data need to be gathered and then a decision made about further discussion of the CAM practice.

REFERENCES

Agarwal S, Frankel L, Tourner S, et al: Improving communication in a pediatric intensive care unit using daily patient goal sheets, *J Crit Care* 23(2):227-235, 2008.

American Academy of Pediatrics, Committee on Hospital Care: Child life services, *Pediatrics* 118(4):1757-1763, 2006.

American Academy of Pediatrics: Family centered care and the pediatrician's role policy statement, *Pediatrics* 112(5):691-696, 2003.

American Academy of Pediatrics, Committee on Hospital Care: Child life services, *Pediatrics* 106(5):1156-1159, 2000.

Anand KJ, Scalzo FM: Can adverse neonatal experiences alter brain development and subsequent behavior? *Biol Neonate* 77(2):69-82, 2000.

Anderson CD, Mangino RR: Nurse shift report: who says you can't talk in front of the patient? *Nurs Adm Q* 30(2):112-122, 2006.

Barnes PM, Bloom B, Nahin RL: Complementary and alternative medicine use among adults and children: United States 2007. *Natl Health Stat Report* 10(12):1-23, 2009.

Bouve LR, Roozmus CL, Giordano P: Preparing parents for their child's transfer from the PICU to the pediatric floor, *Appl Nurs Res* 12(3):114-120, 1999.

Brewer S, Gleditsch SL, Syblik D, et al: Pediatric anxiety: child life intervention in day surgery, *J Pediatr Nurs* 21(1):13-22, 2006.

Caffin CL, Linton S, Pellegrini J: Introduction of a liaison nurse role in a tertiary paediatric ICU, *Intensive Crit Care Nurs* 23(4):226-233, 2007.

Conway J, Johnson BH, Edgman-Levitan S, et al: Partnering with patients and families to design a patient- and family-centered health care system: a roadmap for the future—a work in progress, Institute for Family-Centered Care and Institute for Healthcare Improvement, available at www.familycenteredcare.org/pdf/Roadmap.pdf (accessed June 26, 2009), 2006.

Craft MJ: Siblings of hospitalized children: assessment and intervention, *J Pediatr Nurs* 8(5):289-297, 1993.

Feudtner C, Haney J, Dimmers MA: Spiritual care needs of hospitalized children and their families: a national survey of pastoral care providers' perceptions, *Pediatrics* 111(1):e67-e72, 2003.

Franck LS, Greenberg CS, Stevens B: Pain assessment in infants and children, *Pediatr Clin North Am* 47:487-512, 2000.

Gaynard L, Wolfer J, Goldberger J, et al: *Psychosocial care of children in hospitals,* Bethesda, Md, 1990, Association for the Care of Children's Health.

Harbaugh BL, Tomlinson PS, Kirschbaum M: Parents' perceptions of nurses' caregiving behaviors in the pediatric intensive care unit, *Issues Compr Pediatr Nurs* 27(3):163-177, 2004.

Hopia H, Tomlinson PS, Paavilainen E, et al: Child in hospital: family experiences and expectations of how nurses can promote family health, *J Clin Nurs* 14(2):212-222, 2005.

Institute of Medicine, Committee on Quality of Healthcare in America: *Crossing the quality chasm: a new health system for the 21st century,* Washington, DC, 2001, National Academy Press.

Joint Commission on Accreditation of Healthcare Organizations: *Comprehensive accreditation manual for hospitals,* Oakbrook Terrace, Ill, 2004, The Commission.

Justus R, Wyles D, Wilson J, et al: Preparing children and families for surgery: Mount Sinai's multidisciplinary perspective, *Pediatr Nurs* 32(1):35-43, 2006.

Latour JM, van Goudoever JB, Hazelzet JA: Parent satisfaction in the pediatric ICU, *Pediatr Clin North Am* 55(3):779-790, 2008.

Lewandowski LA, Tesler MD: *Family-centered care: putting it into action,* Washington, DC, 2003, American Nurses Association.

Melnyk BM: Intervention studies involving parents of hospitalized young children: an analysis of the past and future recommendations, *J Pediatr Nurs* 15(1):4-13, 2000.

Miceli PJ, Clark PA: Your patient—my child: seven priorities for improving pediatric care from the parent's perspective, *J Nurs Care Qual* 20(1):43-53, 2005.

National Association of Children's Hospitals and Related Institutions: *Pediatric excellence in healthcare delivery systems,* 1996, available at www.childrenshospitals.net/AM/Template.cfm?Section=Search3&section=Reports1&template=/CM/ContentDisplay.cfm&ContentFileID=7629 (accessed July 27, 2009).

Newton MS: Family-centered care: current realities in parent participation, *Pediatr Nurs* 26(2):164-168, 2000.

Ono S, Oikawa I, Hirabayashi Y, et al: Preparation of a picture book to support parents and autonomy in preschool children facing day surgery, *Pediatr Nurs* 34(1):82-83, 88, 2008.

Orem D: *Nursing concepts of practice,* ed 6, St Louis, 2001, Elsevier.

Phipps LM, Thomas NJ: Hepatitis C: the use of a daily goals sheet to improve communication in the paediatric intensive care unit, *Intensive Crit Care Nurs* 23(5):264-271, 2007.

Small L: Early predictors of poor coping outcomes in children following intensive care hospitalization and stressful medical encounters, *Pediatr Nurs* 28(4):393-401, 2002.

Smith T, Conant Rees HL: Making family-centered care a reality, *Semin Nurs Manage* 8(3):136-142, 2000.

Stratton KM: Parents' experiences of their child's care during hospitalization, *J Cult Divers* 11(1):4-11, 2004.

Taddio A, Katz J: The effects of early pain experience in neonates on pain responses in infancy and childhood, *Pediatr Drugs* 7(4):245-257, 2005.

Taddio A, Shah V, Gilbert-MacLeod C, et al: Conditioning and hyperalgesia in newborns exposed to repeated heel lances, *JAMA* 288(7):857-861, 2002.

Thompson R: *The handbook of child life: A guide for pediatric psychosocial care,* Springfield, Ill, 2009, Charles C Thomas.

Thompson R, Stanford G: *Child life in hospitals: Theory and practice,* Springfield, Ill, 1981, Charles C Thomas.

Wilson ME, Megel ME, Enenbach L, et al: The voices of children: stories about hospitalization, *J Pediatr Health Care* 24(2):95-102, 2010.

Pediatric Variations of Nursing Interventions

Terri L. Brown

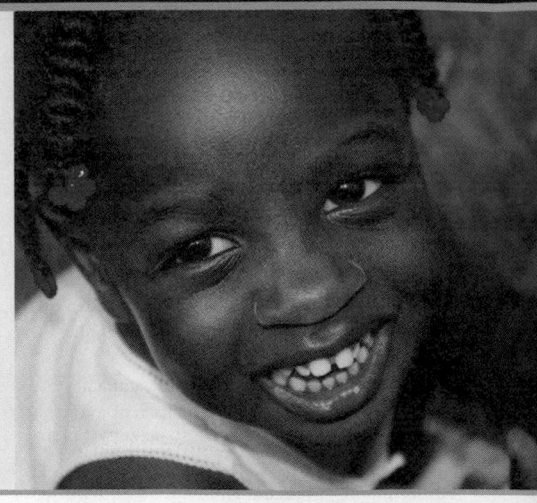

℮volve WEBSITE

RELATED TOPICS

CHAPTER OUTLINE

Many aspects of the nursing role encompass safe implementation of procedures with emphasis on comfort and support. An evidence-based approach to care provides nursing interventions with a foundation on which to build quality care. Throughout this chapter Evidence-Based Practice boxes provide the basis for pediatric nurses to promote excellence in direct patient care.

GENERAL CONCEPTS RELATED TO PEDIATRIC PROCEDURES

INFORMED CONSENT

Before undergoing any invasive procedure, the patient or the patient's legal surrogate must receive sufficient information on which to make an informed health care decision. **Informed consent** should include the expected care or treatment; potential risks, benefits, and alternatives; and what might happen if the patient chooses not to consent. To obtain valid informed consent, health care providers must meet the following three conditions:

1. The person must be capable of giving consent; he or she must be over the age of majority (usually age 18 years) and must be considered competent (i.e., possessing the mental capacity to make choices and understand their consequences).
2. The person must receive the information needed to make an intelligent decision.
3. The person must act voluntarily when exercising freedom of choice without force, fraud, deceit, duress, or other forms of constraint or coercion.

The patient has the right to accept or refuse any health care. If a patient is treated without consent, the hospital or health care provider may be charged with assault and held liable for damages.

Requirements for Obtaining Informed Consent

Written informed consent of the parent or legal guardian is usually required for medical or surgical treatment of a minor, including many diagnostic procedures. One universal consent is not sufficient. Separate informed permissions must be obtained for each surgical or diagnostic procedure, including:

- Major surgery
- Minor surgery (e.g., cutdown, biopsy, dental extraction, suturing a laceration [especially one that may have a cosmetic effect], removal of a cyst, closed reduction of a fracture)
- Diagnostic tests with an element of risk (e.g., bronchoscopy, angiography, lumbar puncture, cardiac catheterization, bone marrow aspiration)
- Medical treatments with an element of risk (e.g., blood transfusion, thoracentesis or paracentesis, radiotherapy)

Other situations that require patient or parental consent include:

- Photographs for medical, educational, or public use
- Removal of the child from the health care institution against medical advice
- Postmortem examinations, except in unexplained deaths, such as sudden infant death, violent death, or suspected suicide
- Release of medical information

Decision making involving the care of older children and adolescents should include the patient's **assent** (if feasible), as well the parent's consent. Assent means the child or adolescent has been informed about the proposed treatment, procedure, or research and is willing to permit a health care provider to perform it. Assent should include:

- Helping the patient achieve a developmentally appropriate awareness of the nature of his or her condition
- Telling the patient what he or she can expect
- Making a clinical assessment of the patient's understanding
- Soliciting an expression of the patient's willingness to accept the proposed procedure

Health care providers should use multiple methods to provide information, including age-appropriate methods (e.g., videos, peer discussion, diagrams, and written materials). The nurse should provide an assent form for the child to sign, and the child should keep a copy. By including the child in the decision-making process and gaining his or her acceptance, staff members demonstrate respect for the child. Assent is not a legal requirement but an ethical one to protect the rights of children.

Eligibility for Giving Informed Consent
Informed Consent of Parents or Legal Guardians

Parents have full responsibility for the care and rearing of their minor children, including legal control over them. As long as children are minors, their parents or legal guardians are required to give informed consent before medical treatment is rendered or any procedure is performed. If the parents are married to each other, consent from only one parent is required for nonurgent pediatric care. If the parents are divorced, consent usually rests with the parent who has legal custody (Berger and American Academy of Pediatrics Committee on Medical Liability, 2003). Parents also have a right to withdraw consent later.

Evidence of Consent

Regulations on obtaining informed consent vary from state to state, and policies differ at each health care facility. It is the physician's legal responsibility to explain the procedure, risks, benefits, and alternatives. The nurse witnesses the patient's, parent's, or legal guardian's signature on the consent form and may reinforce what the patient has been told. A signed consent form is the legal document that signifies that the process of informed consent has occurred. If parents are unavailable to sign consent forms, verbal consent may be obtained via the telephone in the presence of two witnesses. Both witnesses record that informed consent was given and by whom. Their signatures indicate that they witnessed the verbal consent.

Informed Consent of Mature and Emancipated Minors

State laws differ with regard to the age of majority, the age at which a person is considered to have all the legal rights and responsibilities of an adult. In most states, 18 is the age of majority. Competent adults can give informed consent on their own behalf. An emancipated minor is one who is legally under the age of majority but is recognized as having the legal capacity of an adult under circumstances prescribed by state law, such as pregnancy, marriage, high school graduation, independent living, or military service.

Treatment Without Parental Consent

Exceptions to requiring parental consent before treating minor children occur in situations in which children need urgent medical or surgical treatment and a parent is not readily available to give consent or refuses to give consent. For example, a child may be brought to an emergency department accompanied by a grandparent, child care provider, teacher, or others. In the absence of parents or legal guardians, persons in charge of the child may be given permission by the parents to give informed consent by proxy. In emergencies, including danger to life or the possibility of permanent injury, appropriate care should not be withheld or delayed because of problems obtaining consent (Berger and American Academy of Pediatrics Committee on Medical Liability, 2003; American Academy of Pediatrics, 2003). The nurse should document any efforts made to obtain consent.

Refusal to give consent can occur when the treatment, such as blood transfusions, conflicts with the parents' religious beliefs. All states recognize such exceptions and have statutory procedures to permit treatment if the life or health of such a minor is in jeopardy or if delayed treatment would create a risk to the minor's health. Evaluation for child abuse or neglect can occur without parental consent and without notification to the state before evaluation in most states.

Adolescents, Consent, and Confidentiality

The Health Insurance Portability and Accountability Act of 1996 (HIPAA) was passed to help protect and safeguard the security and confidentiality of a person's health information. Because adolescents are not yet adults, parents have the right to make most decisions on their behalf and receive information. Adolescents, however, are more likely to seek care in a setting in which they believe their privacy will be maintained. All 50 states have enacted legislation that entitles adolescents to consent to treatment, without the parents' knowledge, to one or more "medically emancipated" conditions such as sexually transmitted infections, mental health services, alcohol and drug dependency, pregnancy, and contraceptive advice (Anderson, Schaechter, and Brosco, 2005; Tillett, 2005; American Academy of Pediatrics, 2003). Consent to abortion is controversial, and statues vary widely by state. State law preempts HIPAA regardless of whether that law prohibits, mandates, or allows discretion about a disclosure.

Informed Consent and Parental Right to the Child's Medical Chart

Some state statutes give parents the unrestricted right to a copy of children's medical records. In states without statues, the best practice is to allow parents to review or have a copy of minors' charts under reasonable circumstances. Practitioners should avoid restrictive requirements such as review permitted only in the presence of a clinician. Rather, an appropriate practitioner should be available to answer any questions that parents may have during their reviews.

PREPARATION FOR DIAGNOSTIC AND THERAPEUTIC PROCEDURES

Technologic advances and changes in health care have resulted in more pediatric procedures being performed in a variety of settings. Many procedures are both stressful and painful experiences. For most procedures the focus of care is psychologic preparation of the child and family. However, some procedures require the administration of sedatives and analgesics.

Psychologic Preparation

Preparing children for procedures decreases their anxiety, promotes their cooperation, supports their coping skills and may teach them new ones, and facilitates a feeling of mastery in experiencing a potentially stressful event. Many institutions have developed preadmission teaching programs designed to educate the pediatric patient and family by offering hands-on experience with hospital equipment, the procedure performed, and departments they will visit. Preparatory methods may be formal, such as group preparation for hospitalization. Most preparation strategies are informal, focus on providing information about the experience, and are directed at stressful or painful procedures. The most effective preparation includes the provision of sensory-procedural information and helping the child develop coping skills, such as imagery, distraction, or relaxation.

The Nursing Care Guidelines boxes describe general guidelines for preparing children for procedures, along with age-specific guidelines that consider children's developmental needs and cognitive abilities. In addition to these suggestions, nurses should consider the child's temperament, existing coping strategies, and previous experiences in individualizing the preparatory process. Children who are distractible and highly active or those who are "slow to warm up" may need individualized sessions—shorter for the active child or more slowly paced for the shy child. Youngsters who tend to cope well may need more emphasis on using their present skills, whereas those who appear to cope less adequately can benefit from more time devoted to simple coping strategies, such as relaxing, breathing, counting, squeezing a hand, or singing. Children with previous health-related experiences still need preparation for repeat or new procedures; however, the nurse must assess what they know, correct misconceptions, supply new information, and introduce new coping skills as indicated by their previous reactions. Especially for painful procedures, the most effective preparation includes providing sensory-procedural information and helping the child develop coping skills, such as imagery or relaxation (see Nursing Care Guidelines box).

NURSING TIP Prepare a basket, toy chest, or cart to keep near the treatment area. Items ideal for the basket include a Slinky; a sparkling "magic" wand (sealed, acrylic tube partially filled with liquid and suspended metallic confetti); a soft foam ball; bubble solution; party blowers; pop-up books with foldout, three-dimensional scenes; real medical equipment, such as a syringe, adhesive bandages, and alcohol packets; toy medical supplies or a toy medical kit; marking pens; a note pad; and stickers. Have the child choose an item to help distract and relax during a procedure. After the procedure, allow the child to choose a small gift, such as a sticker, or to play with items, such as medical equipment.

Children differ in their "information-seeking dimension." Some actively ask for information about the intended procedure, whereas others characteristically avoid information. Parents can often guide nurses in deciding how much information is enough for the child, since parents know whether the child is typically inquisitive or satisfied with short answers. Asking older children their preferences about the amount of explanation is also important.

The exact timing of the preparation for a procedure varies with the child's age and the type of procedure. No exact guidelines govern timing, but in general the younger the child, the closer the explanation should be to the actual procedure to prevent undue fantasizing and worrying. With complex procedures, more time may be needed for assimilation of information, especially with older children. For example, the explanation for an injection can immediately precede the procedure for all ages, but preparation for surgery may begin the day before for

---

NURSING CARE GUIDELINES
Preparing Children for Procedures

- Determine details of exact procedure to be performed.
- Review parents' and child's present understanding.
- Base teaching on developmental age and existing knowledge.
- Incorporate parents in the teaching if they desire, especially if they plan to participate in care.
- Inform parents of their supportive role during procedure, such as standing near child's head or in child's line of vision and talking softly to child, as well as typical responses of children undergoing the procedure.
- Allow for ample discussion to prevent information overload and ensure adequate feedback.
- Use concrete, not abstract, terms and visual aids to describe procedure. For example, use a simple line drawing of a boy or girl and mark the body part that will be involved in the procedure. Use nonthreatening but realistic models.*
- Emphasize that no other body part will be involved.
- If the body part is associated with a specific function, stress the change or noninvolvement of that ability (e.g., after tonsillectomy, child can still speak).
- Use words and sentence length appropriate to child's level of understanding (a rule of thumb for the number of words in a child's sentence is equal to their age in years plus 1).
- Avoid words and phrases with dual meanings (see Nursing Care Guidelines box, p. 1004) unless child understands such words.
- Clarify all unfamiliar words (e.g., "Anesthesia is a *special* sleep").
- Emphasize sensory aspects of procedure—what child will feel, see, hear, smell, and touch and what child can do during procedure (e.g., lie still, count out loud, squeeze a hand, hug a doll).
- Allow child to practice those procedures that will require cooperation (e.g., turning, deep breathing, using an incentive spirometry).
- Introduce anxiety-inducing information last (e.g., starting an intravenous line).
- Be honest with child about unpleasant aspects of a procedure but avoid creating undue concern. When discussing that a procedure may be uncomfortable, state that it feels differently to different people.
- Emphasize end of procedure and any pleasurable events afterward (e.g., going home, seeing parents).
- Stress positive benefits of procedure (e.g., "After your tonsils are fixed, you won't have as many sore throats").
- Provide a positive ending, praising efforts at cooperation and coping.

*Soft-sculptured dolls and customized adapters and overlays for preparing children and families about procedures and as teaching models for technical care are available from Legacy Products, Inc., 508 S. Green St., PO Box 267, Cambridge City, IN 47327; 800-238-7951; e-mail: info@legacyproductsinc.com; **www.legacyproductsinc.com**.

---

young children and a few days before for older children, although the nurse should elicit the older children's preferences. (See Preparation for Hospitalization, Chapter 26.)

Establish Trust and Provide Support

The nurse who has spent time with and established a positive relationship with a child usually finds it easier to gain cooperation. If the relationship is based on trust, the child will associate the nurse with caregiving activities that give comfort and pleasure most of the time, rather than discomfort and stress. If the nurse does not know the child, it is best for the nurse to be introduced by another staff person whom the child trusts. The first visit with the child should not include any painful procedure and ideally should focus on the child first and then on an explanation of the procedure.

NURSING CARE GUIDELINES

Age-Specific Preparation of Children for Procedures Based on Developmental Characteristics

Infant—Developing Trust and Sensorimotor Thought
Attachment to Parent
Involve parent in procedure if desired.*
Keep parent in infant's line of vision.
If parent is unable to be with infant, place familiar object with infant (e.g., stuffed toy).

Stranger Anxiety
Have usual caregivers perform or assist with procedure.*
Make advances slowly and in nonthreatening manner.
Limit number of strangers entering room during procedure.*

Sensorimotor Phase of Learning
During procedure use sensory soothing measures (e.g., stroking skin, talking softly, giving pacifier).
Use analgesics (e.g., topical anesthetic, intravenous opioid) to control discomfort.*
Cuddle and hug infant after stressful procedure; encourage parent to comfort infant.

Increased Muscle Control
Expect older infants to resist.
Restrain adequately.
Keep harmful objects out of reach.

Memory for Past Experiences
Realize that older infants may associate objects, places, or persons with prior painful experiences and will cry and resist at the sight of them.
Keep frightening objects out of view.*
Perform painful procedures in a separate room, not in crib (or bed).*
Use nonintrusive procedures whenever possible (e.g., axillary or tympanic temperatures, oral medications).*

Imitation of Gestures
Model desired behavior (e.g., opening mouth).

Toddler—Developing Autonomy and Sensorimotor to Preoperational Thought
Use same approaches as for infant, plus the following.

Egocentric Thought
Explain procedure in relation to what child will see, hear, taste, smell, and feel.
Emphasize those aspects of procedure that require cooperation (e.g., lying still).
Tell child it's okay to cry, yell, or use other means to express discomfort verbally.

Negative Behavior
Expect treatments to be resisted; child may try to run away.
Use firm, direct approach.
Ignore temper tantrums.
Use distraction techniques (e.g., singing a song *with* a child).
Restrain adequately.

Animism
Keep frightening objects out of view (young children believe objects have lifelike qualities and can harm them).

Limited Language Skills
Communicate using gestures or demonstrations.
Use a few simple terms familiar to child.
Give child one direction at a time (e.g., "Lie down," then "Hold my hand").
Use small replicas of equipment; allow child to handle equipment.
Use play; demonstrate on doll but avoid child's favorite doll, since child may think doll is really "feeling" procedure.
Prepare parents separately to avoid child's misinterpreting words.

Limited Concept of Time
Prepare child shortly or immediately before procedure.
Keep teaching sessions short (about 5 to 10 minutes).
Have preparations completed before involving child in procedure.
Have extra equipment nearby (e.g., alcohol swabs, new needle, adhesive bandages) to avoid delays.
Tell child when procedure is completed.

Striving for Independence
Allow choices whenever possible but realize that child may still be resistant and negative.
Allow child to participate in care and to help whenever possible (e.g., drink medicine from a cup, hold a dressing).

Preschooler—Developing Initiative and Preoperational Thought
Egocentric
Explain procedure in simple terms and in relation to how it affects child (as with toddler, stress sensory aspects).
Demonstrate use of equipment.
Allow child to play with miniature or actual equipment.
Encourage "playing out" experience on a doll both before and after procedure to clarify misconceptions.
Use neutral words to describe the procedure (see Nursing Care Guidelines box, p. 1004).

Increased Language Skills
Use verbal explanation but avoid overestimating child's comprehension of words.
Encourage child to verbalize ideas and feelings.

Limited Concept of Time and Frustration Tolerance
Implement same approaches as for toddler but may plan longer teaching session (10 to 15 minutes); may divide information into more than one session.

Illness and Hospitalization Viewed as Punishment
Clarify why each procedure is performed; a child will find it difficult to understand how medicine can make him or her feel better and can taste bad at the same time.
Ask child thoughts regarding why a procedure is performed.
State directly that procedures are never a form of punishment.

Animism
Keep equipment out of sight, except when shown to or used on child.

Fears of Bodily Harm, Intrusion, and Castration
Point out on drawing, doll, or child where procedure is performed.
Emphasize that no other body part will be involved.
Use nonintrusive procedures whenever possible (e.g., axillary temperatures, oral medication).
Apply an adhesive bandage over puncture site.
Encourage parental presence.
Realize that procedures involving genitalia provoke anxiety.
Allow child to wear underpants with gown.
Explain unfamiliar situations, especially noises or lights.

Striving for Initiative
Involve child in care whenever possible (e.g., hold equipment, remove dressing).
Give choices whenever possible but avoid excessive delays.
Praise child for helping and attempting to cooperate; never shame child for lack of cooperation.

School-Age Child—Developing Industry and Concrete Thought
Increased Language Skills; Interest in Acquiring Knowledge
Explain procedures using correct scientific and medical terminology.
Explain procedure using simple diagrams and photographs.
Discuss why procedure is necessary; concepts of illness and bodily functions are often vague

NURSING CARE GUIDELINES—cont'd

Age-Specific Preparation of Children for Procedures Based on Developmental Characteristics

Explain function and operation of equipment in concrete terms.

Allow child to manipulate equipment; use doll or another person as model to practice using equipment whenever possible (doll play may be considered childish by older school-age child).

Allow time before and after procedure for questions and discussion.

Improved Concept of Time

Plan for longer teaching sessions (about 20 minutes).

Prepare up to 1 day in advance of procedure to allow for processing of information.

Increased Self-Control

Gain child's cooperation.

Tell child what is expected.

Suggest several ways of maintaining control the child may select from (e.g., deep breathing, relaxation, counting).

Striving for Industry

Allow responsibility for simple tasks (e.g., collecting specimens).

Include child in decision making (e.g., time of day to perform procedure, preferred site).

Encourage active participation (e.g., removing dressings, handling equipment, opening packages).

Developing Relationships with Peers

Prepare two or more children for same procedure or encourage one to help prepare another.

Provide privacy from peers during procedure to maintain self-esteem.

Adolescent—Developing Identity and Abstract Thought

Increasing Abstract Thought and Reasoning

Discuss why procedure is necessary or beneficial.

Explain long-term consequences of procedures; include information about body systems working together.

Realize adolescent may fear death, disability, or other potential risks.

Encourage questioning regarding fears, options, and alternatives.

Consciousness of Appearance

Provide privacy; describe how the body will be covered and what will be exposed.

Discuss how procedure may affect appearance (e.g., scar) and what can be done to minimize it.

Emphasize any physical benefits of procedure.

Concern More with Present Than with Future

Realize that immediate effects of procedure are more significant than future benefits.

Striving for Independence

Involve adolescent in decision making and planning (e.g., time, place, individuals present during procedure, clothing, whether they will watch procedure).

Impose as few restrictions as possible.

Explore what coping strategies have worked in the past; they may need suggestions of various techniques.

Accept regression to more childish methods of coping.

Realize that adolescent may have difficulty accepting new authority figures and may resist complying with procedures.

Developing Peer Relationships and Group Identity

Same as for school-age child but assumes even greater significance.

Allow adolescents to talk with other adolescents who have had the same procedure.

*Applies to any age.

Parental Presence and Support

Children need support during procedures, and for young children the greatest source of support is the parents. They represent security, protection, safety, and comfort. Several studies have reported a positive impact on parental distress and satisfaction and no difference in technical complications when parents remain with children (Piira, Sugiura, Champion, et al, 2005). Controversy exists regarding the role parents should assume during the procedure, especially if discomfort is involved. (See Evidence-Based Practice box, Family Presence During Resuscitation of a Child, Chapter 31.) Several professional associations support the option of family presence during invasive procedures (Emergency Nurses Association, 2005; American Association of Critical Care Nurses, 2006; American Academy of Pediatrics, American College of Emergency Physicians, O'Malley, et al, 2006). The nurse should assess the parents' preferences for assisting, observing, or waiting outside the room, as well as the child's preference for parental presence. Respect the child's and parents' choices. Give parents who wish to stay appropriate explanation about the procedure and coach them about where to sit or stand and what to say or do to help the child through the procedure. Support parents who do not want to be present in their decision and encourage them to remain close by so that they can be available to support the child immediately after the procedure. Parents should also know that someone will be with their child to provide support. Ideally, this person should inform the parents after the procedure about how the child did.

Provide an Explanation

Age-appropriate explanations are one of the most widely used interventions for reducing anxiety in children undergoing procedures. Before performing a procedure, explain what is to be done and what is expected of the child. The explanation should be short, simple, and appropriate to the child's level of comprehension. Long explanations may increase anxiety in a young child. When explaining the procedure to parents with the child present, the nurse uses language appropriate to the child, since unfamiliar words can be misunderstood (see Nursing Care Guidelines box). If the parents need additional preparation, this is done in an area away from the child. Teaching sessions are planned at times most conducive to the child's learning (e.g., after a rest period) and for the usual span of attention.

Special equipment is not necessary for preparing a child, but for young children who cannot yet think conceptually, using objects to supplement verbal explanation is important. Allowing children to handle actual items that will be used in their care, such as a stethoscope, sphygmomanometer, or oxygen mask, helps them develop familiarity with these items and reduces the fear often associated with their use. Miniature versions of hospital items such as gurneys and x-ray

NURSING CARE GUIDELINES

Selecting Nonthreatening Words or Phrases

WORDS AND PHRASES TO AVOID	SUGGESTED SUBSTITUTIONS
Shot, bee sting, stick	Medicine under the skin
Organ	Special place in body
Test	To see how (specify body part) is working
Incision, cut	Special opening
Edema	Puffiness
Stretcher, gurney	Rolling bed, bed on wheels
Stool	Child's usual term
Dye	Special medicine
Pain	Hurt, discomfort, "owie," "boo-boo," sore, achy, scratchy
Deaden	Numb, make sleepy
Fix	Make better
Take (as in "take your temperature")	See how warm you are
Take (as in "take your blood pressure")	Check your pressure; hug your arm
Put to sleep, anesthesia	Special sleep so you won't feel anything
Catheter	Tube
Monitor	Television screen
Electrodes	Stickers, ticklers
Specimen	Sample

and intravenous (IV) equipment can be used to explain what the children can expect and permit them to safely experience situations that are unfamiliar and potentially frightening. Written and illustrated materials are also valuable aids to preparation.*

> **NURSING TIP** Use photographs of children in different areas of the hospital (e.g., radiology department, operating room) to give children a more realistic idea of equipment they may encounter.

Physical Preparation

One area of special concern is the administration of appropriate sedation and analgesia before stressful procedures. Chapter 7 describes sedative medications used for procedures.

Performance of the Procedure

Supportive care continues during the procedure and can be a major factor in a child's ability to cooperate. Ideally, the same nurse who explains the procedure should perform or assist with the procedure. Before beginning, all equipment is assembled and the room is readied to prevent unnecessary delays and

*Preparatory materials include *Going to the Hospital* and *Going to the Doctor*, available from Family Communications, 4802 Fifth Ave., Pittsburgh, PA 15213; 412-687-2990; www.fci.org; *Hospital Friends*, available from Centering Corporation, 7230 Maple St., Omaha, NE 68134; 866-218-0101; www.centering.org. Other resources include *Berenstein Bears Go to the Doctor* and *Berenstein Bears Visit the Dentist* (New York, Random House).

> **NURSING TIP** To avoid a delay during a procedure, have extra supplies handy. For example, have tape, bandages, alcohol swabs, and an extra needle when performing an injection or venipuncture.

interruptions that increase the child's anxiety. Minimizing the number of people present during the procedure also can decrease a child's anxiety.

To promote long-term coping and adjustment, give special consideration to the patient's age, coping skills, and procedure to be performed in determining where a procedure will occur. Treatment rooms should be used for procedures requiring sedation, such as bone marrow aspirates and lumbar punctures in younger children. Traumatic procedures should never be performed in "safe" areas, such as the playroom. If the procedure is lengthy, avoid conversation that could be misinterpreted by the child. As the procedure is nearing completion, the nurse should inform the child that it is almost over in language the child understands.

Expect Success

Nurses who approach children with confidence and who convey the impression that they expect to be successful are less likely to encounter difficulty. It is best to approach a child as though cooperation is expected. Children sense anxiety and uncertainty in an adult and respond by striking out or actively resisting. Although it is not possible to eliminate such behavior in every child, a firm approach with a positive attitude tends to convey a feeling of security to most children.

Involve the Child

Involving children helps to gain their cooperation. Permitting choices gives them some measure of control. However, a choice is given only in situations in which one is available. Asking children, "Do you want to take your medicine now?" leads them to believe they have an option and provides them the opportunity to legitimately refuse or delay the medication. This places the nurse in an awkward, if not impossible, position. It is much better to state firmly, "It's time to drink your medicine now." Children usually like to make choices, but the choice must be one that they do indeed have (e.g., "It's time for your medicine. Do you want to drink it plain or with a little water?").

Many children respond to tactics that appeal to their maturity or courage. This also gives them a sense of participation and achievement. For example, preschool children will be proud that they can hold the dressing during the procedure or remove the tape. The same is true for the school-age child, who often cooperates with minimal resistance.

Provide Distraction

Distraction is a powerful coping strategy during painful procedures (Uman, Chambers, McGrath, et al, 2006). It is accomplished by focusing the child's attention on something other than the procedure. Singing favorite songs, listening to music with a headset, counting aloud, or blowing bubbles to "blow the hurt away" are effective techniques. (For other nonpharmacologic interventions, see Chapter 7.)

Allow Expression of Feelings

The child should be allowed to express feelings of anger, anxiety, fear, frustration, or any other emotion. It is natural for children to strike out in frustration or to try to avoid stress-provoking situations. The child needs to know that it is all right to cry. Behavior is children's primary means of communication and coping and should be permitted unless it inflicts harm on them or those caring for them.

Postprocedural Support

After the procedure the child continues to need reassurance that he or she performed well and is accepted and loved. If the parents did not participate, the child is united with them as soon as possible so that they can provide comfort.

Encourage Expression of Feelings

Planned activity after the procedure is helpful in encouraging constructive expression of feelings. For verbal children, reviewing the details of the procedure can clarify misconceptions and garner feedback for improving the nurse's preparatory strategies. Play is an excellent activity for all children. Infants and young children should have the opportunity for gross motor movement. Older children are able to vent their anger and frustration in acceptable pounding or throwing activities. Play-Doh is a remarkably versatile medium for pounding and shaping. Dramatic play provides an outlet for anger and places the child in a position of control, in contrast to the position of helplessness in the real situation. Puppets also allow the child to communicate feelings in a nonthreatening way. One of the most effective interventions is therapeutic play, which includes well-supervised activities such as permitting the child to give an injection to a doll or stuffed toy to reduce the stress of injections (Fig. 27-1).

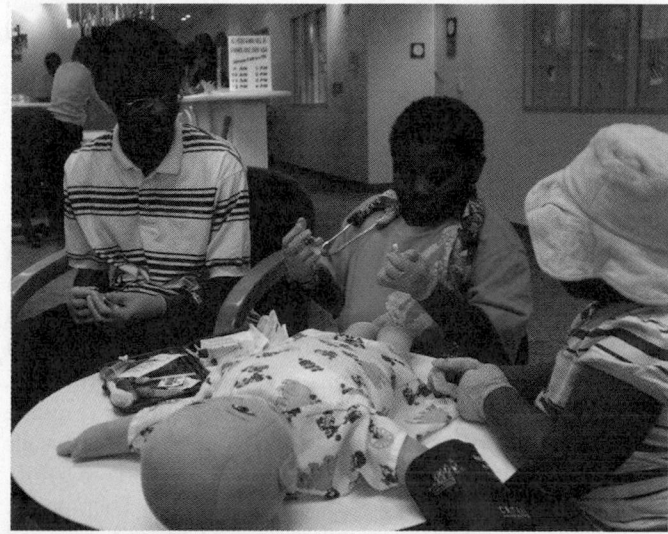

Fig. 27-1 Playing with medical objects provides children with the opportunity to play out fears and concerns with supervision by a nurse or child life specialist.

Positive Reinforcement

Children need to hear from adults that they did the best they could in the situation—no matter how they behaved. It is important for children to know that their worth is not being judged on the basis of their behavior in a stressful situation. Reward systems, such as earning stars, stickers, or a badge of courage, are appealing to children.

Returning to the child a short while after the procedure helps the nurse strengthen a supportive relationship. Relating with the child in a relaxed and nonstressful period allows him or her to see the nurse not only as someone associated with stressful situations but as someone with whom to share pleasurable experiences.

Use of Play in Procedures

The use of play is an integral part of relationships with children. As such, its value in specific situations is discussed throughout this book, such as in Chapter 26 in relation to hospitalization. Many institutions have elaborate and well-organized play areas and programs under the direction of child life specialists. Other institutions have limited facilities. No matter what the institution provides for children, nurses can include play activities as part of nursing care. Play can be used to teach, express feelings, or achieve a therapeutic goal. Consequently, it should be included in preparing children for and encouraging their cooperation during procedures. Play sessions after procedures can be structured, such as directed toward needle play, or general, with a wide variety of equipment available for children to play with.

Routine procedures such as measuring blood pressure and oral administration of medication may be of concern to children. Box 27-1 describes suggestions for incorporating play into nursing procedures and activities for the hospitalized child that facilitate learning and adjustment to a new situation.

SURGICAL PROCEDURES

Preoperative Care

Children experiencing surgical procedures require both psychologic and physical preparation. An important concern is restriction of food and fluids before surgery to avoid aspiration during anesthesia. Infants require special attention to fluid needs. They should not be without oral fluids for an extended period preoperatively to avoid glycogen depletion and dehydration. Table 27-1 contains current preoperative fasting guidelines.

In general, psychologic preparation is similar to that discussed earlier for any procedure and employs many of the same techniques used in preparing a child for hospitalization, such as films, books, brochures, play, and tours. (See Chapter 26.) Stress points before and after surgery include the admission process, blood tests, injection of preoperative medication (if

BOX 27-1   PLAY ACTIVITIES FOR SPECIFIC PROCEDURES

Fluid Intake

Make ice pops using child's favorite juice.

Cut gelatin into fun shapes.

Make a game out of taking a sip when turning page of a book or in games such as Simon Says.

Use small medicine cups; decorate the cups.

Color water with food coloring or powdered drink mix.

Have a tea party; pour at a small table.

Let child fill a syringe and squirt it into mouth or use it to fill small decorated cups.

Cut straws in half and place in a small container (much easier for child to suck liquid).

Use a "crazy" straw.

Make a "progress poster"; give rewards for drinking a predetermined quantity.

Deep Breathing

Blow bubbles with a bubble blower.

Blow bubbles with a straw (no soap).

Blow on a pinwheel, feather, whistle, harmonica, balloon, party blower.

Practice band instruments.

Have a blowing contest using balloons,* boats, cotton balls, feathers, marbles, Ping-Pong balls, pieces of paper; blow such objects on a table top over a goal line, over water, through an obstacle course, up in the air, against an opponent, or up and down a string.

Suck paper or cloth from one container to another using a straw.

Dramatize stories such as "I'll huff and puff and blow your house down" from the Three Little Pigs.

Do straw-blowing painting.

Take a deep breath and "blow out the candles" on a birthday cake.

Use a little paint brush to "paint" nails with water and blow nails dry.

Range of Motion and Use of Extremities

Throw beanbags at a fixed or movable target or throw wadded-up paper into a wastebasket.

Touch or kick Mylar balloons held or hung in different positions (if child is in traction, hang balloon from a trapeze).

Play "tickle toes"; have the child wiggle them on request.

Play Twister game or Simon Says.

Play pretend and guessing games (e.g., imitate a bird, butterfly, horse).

Have tricycle or wheelchair races in safe area.

Play kickball or throw ball with a soft foam ball in a safe area.

Position bed so that child must turn to view television or doorway.

Climb wall with fingers like a "spider."

Pretend to teach aerobic dancing or exercises; encourage parents to participate.

Encourage swimming if feasible.

Play videogames or pinball (fine motor movement).

Play hide and seek: hide toy somewhere in bed (or room if ambulatory) and have child find it using specified hand or foot.

Provide clay to mold with fingers.

Paint or draw on large sheets of paper placed on floor or wall.

Encourage combing own hair; play "beauty shop" with "customer" in different positions.

Soaks

Play with small toys or objects (cups, syringes, soap dishes) in water.

Wash dolls or toys.

Pick up marbles or pennies* from bottom of bath container.

Make designs with coins on bottom of container.

Pretend a boat is a submarine by keeping it immersed.

Read to child during soaks; sing with child; or play game, such as cards, checkers, or other board game (if both hands are immersed, move board pieces for child).

Sitz bath: give child something to listen to (music, stories) or look at (View-Master, book).

Punch holes in bottom of plastic cup, fill with water, and let it "rain" on child.

Injections

Let child handle syringe, vial, and alcohol swab, and give an injection to doll or stuffed animal.

Use syringes to decorate cookies with frosting, squirt paint, or target shoot into a container.

Draw a "magic circle" on area before injection; draw smiling face in circle after injection, but avoid drawing on puncture site.

Allow child to have a "collection" of syringes (without needles); make "wild" creative objects with syringes.

If multiple injections or venipunctures are planned, make a "progress poster"; give rewards for predetermined number of injections.

Have child count to 10 or 15 during injection.

Ambulation

Give child something to push:
- Toddler: push-pull toy
- School-age child: wagon or a doll in a stroller or wheelchair
- Adolescent: decorated intravenous stand

Have a parade; make hats, drums, etc.

Extending Environment (e.g., for Patients in Traction)

Make bed into a pirate ship or airplane with decorations.

Put up mirrors so patient can see around room.

Move bed frequently to playroom, hallway, or outside.

*Small objects such as marbles or coins, as well as gloves or balloons, are unsafe for young children because of possible aspiration. Latex products also carry the risk of an allergic reaction.

---

prescribed), transport to the operating room, the mask on the face during induction, and the stay in the postanesthesia care unit (PACU). Wearing a hospital gown without the security of underpants or pajama bottoms can also be traumatic. Therefore these articles of clothing should be allowed to be worn into the operating room and removed after induction of anesthesia. Children are at higher risk of ineffective response to anesthesia due to higher anxiety associated with stranger anxiety (infants), separation anxiety (toddlers and preschoolers), and fear of injury or death (adolescents) (Romino, Keatley, Secrest, et al, 2005).

Psychologic intervention consisting of systematic preparation, rehearsal of the forthcoming events, and supportive care at each of these points has shown to be more effective than a single-session preparation or consistent supportive care without systematic preparation and rehearsal (Kain, Caldwell-Andrews, Mayes, et al, 2007). A family-centered preoperative preparation program may consist of a tour of the perioperative areas with short explanations of the events 5 to 7 days before surgery, a video to take home and review a couple of times with additional explanations and demonstrations of perioperative processes, a mask to take home and practice with, pamphlets to guide parents on supporting children during induction, phone calls to coach parents on preparing children 1 or 2 days before surgery, and toys and supplies in the holding area. Therapeutic play is an effective strategy in preparing children, and increased familiarity with medical procedures decreases anxiety (Li, Lopez, and Lee, 2007).

TABLE 27-1	FASTING RECOMMENDATIONS TO REDUCE THE RISK OF PULMONARY ASPIRATION*	
INGESTED MATERIAL	**MINIMUM FASTING PERIOD (hr)†**	
Clear liquids‡	>2	
Breast milk	4	
Infant formula	6	
Nonhuman milk§	6	
Light meal¶	6	

From American Society of Anesthesiologists: Practice guidelines for preoperative fasting and the use of pharmacologic agents to reduce the risk of pulmonary aspiration: application to healthy patients undergoing elective procedures, *Anesthesiology* 90(3):896-905, 1999.
*These recommendations apply to healthy patients who are undergoing elective procedures. They are not intended for women in labor. Following the guidelines does not guarantee complete gastric emptying has occurred.
†Fasting periods noted in chart apply to all ages.
‡Examples of clear liquids include water, fruit juices without pulp, carbonated beverages, clear tea, and black coffee.
§Because nonhuman milk is similar to solids in gastric emptying time, the amount ingested must be considered when determining appropriate fasting period.
¶Light meal typically consists of toast and clear liquids. Meals that include fried or fatty foods or meat may prolong gastric emptying time. Both amount and type of foods ingested must be considered when determining appropriate fasting period.

Parental Presence

Some institutions support parental presence during induction of anesthesia (see Fig. 27-2 and Research Focus box). Appropriate education is essential to help parents understand the stages of anesthesia, what to expect, and how to support their child. When parents choose not to or are not allowed to attend the induction, leaving a favorite possession with the child and uniting the child and parents as soon as possible after surgery (preferably in the PACU) are important interventions. During surgery the family should have a designated place to wait and should be kept informed of the child's progress. They also should know where and when they can visit the child after surgery.

RESEARCH FOCUS

Parent Presence During Anesthesia Induction

According to research conducted by Kain, Caldwell-Andrews, Mayes, and colleagues (2007), benefits of well-prepared children and parents along with parental presence during induction of anesthesia include reduced anxiety for children and parents, lower doses of postoperative analgesia, lower incidence of severe emergence delirium symptoms, and shorter discharge time for short procedures. Other studies have not universally supported these benefits. Concern exists regarding the appropriateness of this practice for all parents. Some parents may become upset by the rapid succession of induction events, by observing their child becoming limp, and by leaving the child in the care of strangers. Even though some parents may become anxious, most control their anxiety, do not disrupt the induction, and support the child (Munro and D'Errico, 2000). Parents who are anxious before surgery tend to become even more anxious after the induction, whereas the reverse is true of parents with little anxiety.

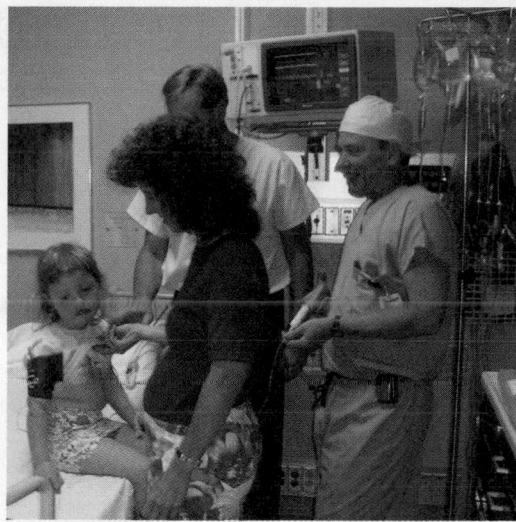

Fig. 27-2 Parental presence during induction of anesthesia can minimize the child's and parents' anxiety during the preoperative period.

Preoperative Sedation

Historically the most upsetting event for children has been the preoperative injection. An increasing number of anesthesiologists use preoperative sedative premedication, usually midazolam (Versed), and parental presence for children undergoing surgery (Kain, Caldwell-Andrews, Krivutza, et al, 2004).

The goals for using preoperative medications include (1) anxiety reduction, (2) amnesia, (3) sedation, (4) antiemetic effect, and (5) reduction of secretions (Manworren and Fledderman, 2000). (Chapter 7 includes an extensive discussion of pain management strategies for children undergoing surgery.) When drugs are administered, they should be delivered atraumatically via oral or IV routes. Numerous preanesthetic drug regimens are used with children, and no consensus exists on the optimal method. Midazolam provides excellent preoperative anxiety reduction, amnesia, and sedation. It is popular because of its short duration, predictable onset, and rare occurrence of respiratory depression. Oral transmucosal fentanyl (OTFC, or Fentanyl Oralet) is available as a sweetened lozenge on a plastic stick. When first approved, this appeared to be an excellent, atraumatic route of administration. However, nausea and vomiting, respiratory depression, and the need for more intensive monitoring and observation than with other oral sedatives have limited its popularity (Klein, Diekema, Paris, et al, 2002). If children have no preoperative pain, are well prepared psychologically for surgery, and have their parents nearby, however, preoperative medication may be unnecessary.

Anesthesia induction of the pediatric patient is commonly accomplished by administering inhalation agents in combination with nitrous oxide and oxygen by mask. Children may fear induction of anesthesia by mask. Practices that can minimize anxiety related to inhalation anesthesia are (1) disguising the unpleasant odor of anesthetic gases by applying a pleasant-smelling substance on the mask; (2) using a transparent plastic mask rather than an opaque black mask and gradually bringing it toward the face; (3) directing a stream of gas toward the child's face from the bare tube until the child becomes drowsy, then using the mask; (4) allowing the child to sit up rather than

TABLE 27-2   POTENTIAL CAUSES OF POSTOPERATIVE VITAL SIGN ALTERATIONS IN CHILDREN

ALTERATION	POTENTIAL CAUSE	COMMENTS
Heart Rate		
Increase	Decreased perfusion (shock)	Heart rate may increase to maintain cardiac output.
	Elevated temperature	
	Pain	
	Respiratory distress (early)	
	Medications (atropine, morphine, epinephrine)	
	Hypoxia	
Decrease	Vagal stimulation	Bradycardia is of more concern in young child than tachycardia.
	Increased intracranial pressure	
	Respiratory distress (late)	
	Medications (neostigmine [Prostigmin])	
Respiratory Rate		
Increase	Respiratory distress	Body responds to respiratory distress primarily by increasing rate.
	Fluid volume excess	
	Hypothermia	
	Elevated temperature	
	Pain	
Decrease	Anesthetics, opioids	Decreased respiratory rate from opioids may be compensated for
	Pain	by increased depth of respiration.
Blood Pressure		
Increase	Excess intravascular volume	This is serious in premature infants because it increases risk of
	Increased intracranial pressure	intraventricular hemorrhage.
	Carbon dioxide retention	
	Pain	
	Medication (ketamine, epinephrine)	
Decrease	Vasodilating anesthetic agents (halothane, isoflurane, enflurane)	Decreased blood pressure is late sign of shock because of
	Opioids (e.g., morphine)	elasticity and constriction of vessels to maintain cardiac output.
Temperature		
Increase	Shock (late sign)	Fever associated with infection usually occurs later than fever of
	Infection	noninfectious origin. Absence of fever does not rule out
	Environmental causes (warm room, excess coverings)	infection, especially in infants.
	Malignant hyperthermia	Malignant hyperthermia requires immediate treatment.
Decrease	Vasodilating anesthetic agents (halothane, isoflurane, enflurane)	Neonates are especially susceptible to hypothermia, with serious
	Muscle relaxants	or fatal consequences.
	Environmental causes (cool room)	
	Infusion of cool fluids or blood	

From Smith DP: *Comprehensive child and family nursing skills,* St Louis, 1991, Mosby.

lie down for anesthesia induction; and (5) allowing preoperative play with a mask and a doll or manikin.

Postoperative Care

Various psychologic and physical interventions and observations help prevent or minimize possible unpleasant effects from anesthesia and the surgical procedure. Although the incidence of serious postoperative complications in healthy children undergoing surgery is less than 1% (Maxwell and Yaster, 2000), continuous monitoring of the child's cardiopulmonary status is essential during the immediate postoperative period. Postanesthesia complications such as airway obstruction, postextubation croup, laryngospasm, and bronchospasm make maintaining a patent airway and maximum ventilation critical.

Monitoring the patient's oxygen saturation and providing supplemental oxygen as needed, maintaining body temperature, and promoting fluid and electrolyte balance are important aspects of immediate postoperative care. Vital signs are continuously monitored, and each vital sign is evaluated in terms of side effects from anesthesia, shock, or respiratory compromise (Table 27-2).

A change in vital signs that demands immediate attention in the perioperative period is caused by malignant hyperthermia (MH), a potentially fatal pharmacogenetic disorder involving a defective calcium channel in the sarcoplasmic reticulum membrane. In susceptible children, inhaled anesthetics (e.g., halothane, sevoflurane, desflurane) and the muscle relaxant succinylcholine trigger the disorder, producing hypermetabolism. Symptoms of MH include hypercarbia (increasing end-tidal carbon dioxide), elevated temperature, tachycardia, tachypnea, acidosis, muscle rigidity, and rhabdomyolysis (Rosenberg, Davis, and James, 2007). A family or previous history of sudden high fever associated with a surgical procedure and myotonia increase the risk for MH. Children who have successfully undergone prior surgery without adverse effects may still be considered susceptible.

Treatment of MH includes immediate discontinuation of the triggering agent, hyperventilation with 100% oxygen, and

NURSING CARE GUIDELINES

Postoperative Care

Ensure that preparations are made to receive child:
- Bed or crib is ready.
- Intravenous pumps and poles, suction apparatus, and oxygen flow meter are at bedside.

Obtain baseline information:
- Take vital signs, including blood pressure; keep blood pressure cuff in place and deflated to lessen disturbance to child.
- Take and record vital signs more frequently if any value fluctuates.
- Inspect operative area.
  —Check dressing if present.
  —Outline any bleeding area on dressing or cast with pen.
  —Reinforce, but do not remove, loose dressing.
  —Observe areas below surgical site for blood that may have drained toward bed.
  —Assess for bleeding and other symptoms in areas not covered with a dressing, such as throat after tonsillectomy.
- Assess skin color and characteristics.
- Assess level of consciousness and activity.

Notify physician of any irregularities in child's condition.
Assess for evidence of pain. (See Pain Assessment, Chapter 7.)
Review surgeon's orders after completing initial assessment, and check that any preoperative orders, such as seizure or cardiac medications, have been reordered and can be given by available routes (oral preparations may be contraindicated).
Monitor vital signs as ordered and more often if indicated.
Check dressings for bleeding or other abnormalities.
Check bowel sounds.
Observe for signs of shock, abdominal distention, and bleeding.
Assess for bladder distention.
Observe for signs of dehydration.
Detect presence of infection:
- Take vital signs every 2 to 4 hours, as ordered.
- Collect or request needed specimens.
- Inspect wound for signs of infection—redness, swelling, heat, pain, and purulent drainage.

IV dantrolene sodium. If the child is hyperthermic, initiate cooling measures such as ice packs to the groin, axillae, and neck and iced nasogastric lavage. The surgery may be discontinued, or if it is emergent, it may be continued with a different anesthetic agent. The patient should be transferred to an intensive care unit for at least 36 hours and is closely monitored for stabilization of vital signs, metabolic state, and possible recurrence of symptoms.

Managing pain is a major nursing responsibility after surgery. The nurse should assess pain frequently and administers analgesics to provide comfort and facilitate cooperation with postoperative care such as ambulation and deep breathing. Opioids are the most commonly used analgesics. Routinely scheduled IV analgesics, patient-controlled analgesia, and epidural infusions, rather than as-needed orders, provide excellent analgesia in postoperative pediatric patients.

Because respiratory tract infections are a potential complication of anesthesia, make every effort to aerate the lungs and remove secretions. The lungs are auscultated regularly to identify abnormal sounds or any areas of diminished or absent breath sounds. To prevent pneumonia, encourage respiratory movement with incentive spirometers or other motivating activities (see Box 27-1). If these measures are presented as games, the child is more likely to comply. The child's position is changed every 2 hours, and deep breathing is encouraged.

> **NURSING TIP** Because deep breathing is usually painful after surgery, be certain the child has received analgesics. Have the child splint the operative site (depending on its location) by hugging a small pillow or a favorite stuffed animal.

During the recovery period, spend some time with the child to assess his or her perceptions of surgery. Play, drawing, and storytelling are excellent methods of discovering the child's thoughts. With such information the nurse can support or correct the child's perceptions and boost his or her self-esteem for having endured a stressful procedure.

Many pediatric patients are discharged shortly after surgery. Preparation for discharge begins with the preadmission preparation visit. The nurse should discuss instructions for postoperative care and review them throughout the perioperative visit. After discharge, the nursing staff often makes phone calls to check the patient's status. Patient education and compliance with discharge instructions can also be assessed during these phone calls (Barnes, 2000) (see Nursing Care Guidelines box).

COMPLIANCE

Compliance, also termed *adherence*, refers to the extent to which the patient's behavior coincides with the prescribed regimen in terms of taking medication, following diets, or executing other lifestyle changes. In developing strategies to improve compliance, the nurse must first assess level of compliance. Because many children are too young to assume partial or total responsibility for their care, parents are usually primarily responsible for home management.

Factors relating to the care setting are important in ensuring compliance and should be considered in planning strategies to improve compliance. Basically, any aspect of the health care setting that increases the family's satisfaction with the physical setting and the relationship with the practitioner positively influences adherence to the treatment regimen. However, the more complex, expensive, inconvenient, and disruptive the treatment protocol, the less likely the family is to comply. During long-term conditions that involve multiple treatments and considerable rearrangement of lifestyle, compliance is severely affected.

Although it is helpful to know those factors that influence compliance, assessment must include more direct measurement techniques. A number of methods exist, each with advantages and disadvantages. The most successful approach includes a combination of at least two of the following methods:

Clinical judgment—This is subject to bias and inaccuracy unless the nurse carefully evaluates the criteria used in assessment.

Self-reporting—Most people overestimate their compliance by about 20%, even when they admit to lapses.

Direct observation—This is difficult to employ outside the health care setting and awareness of being observed frequently affects performance.

Monitoring appointments—Keeping appointments indirectly indicates compliance with the prescribed care.

Monitoring therapeutic response—Few treatments yield directly measurable results (e.g., decreased blood pressure, weight loss); record on a graph or chart.

Pill counts—The nurse counts the number of pills remaining in the original container and compares the number missing with the number of times the medication should have been taken. Although this is a simple method, families may forget to bring the container or deliberately alter the number of pills to avoid detection. This method is also poorly suited to liquid medication. Another technique is the use of pill container caps that record every opening as a presumptive dose.

Chemical assay—For certain drugs, such as digoxin, measurement of plasma drug levels provides information on the amount of drug recently ingested. However, this method is expensive, indicates only short-term compliance, and requires precise timing of the assay for accurate results.

Compliance Strategies

Strategies to improve compliance involve interventions that encourage families to follow the prescribed treatment regimen. Some evidence suggests that higher levels of self-esteem and increased autonomy favorably affect adolescent compliance (Kyngas, Kroll, and Duffy, 2000). However, family factors are important, and characteristics associated with good compliance include family support, family reminders, good communication, and expectations for successful completion of the therapeutic regimen. No one approach is always successful, and the best results occur when at least two strategies are employed.

Organizational strategies involve the care setting and the therapeutic plan. This may involve increasing the frequency of appointments, designating a primary practitioner, reducing the cost of medication by prescribing generic brands, reducing the treatment's disruption of the family's lifestyle, and using "cues" to minimize forgetting. Numerous devices are available commercially or can be improvised for cueing, such as pill dispensers; watches with alarms; charts to record completed therapy; messages on the refrigerator or morning coffee pot; and treatment schedules that incorporate the treatment plan into the daily routine, such as physical therapy after the evening bath.

The nurse instructs the family about the treatment plan. Although education is an important factor in enhancing compliance and patients who are more knowledgeable about their condition are more likely to comply, education alone does not ensure compliant behavior. The nurse should incorporate teaching principles known to enhance understanding and retention of material. Written materials are essential, especially in any regimen requiring multiple or complex treatments, and they need to be understandable to the average individual, who reads at about the fourth-grade level. Involvement of the immediate and extended family (e.g., grandparents) in education sessions may enhance compliance.

Treatment strategies relate to the child's refusal or inability to take the prescribed medication. The family may also have difficulty following a prescribed treatment regimen. They may remember and understand the instructions but may not be able to give the medicine as prescribed. Assess the reason for refusal. For example, the child may not be able to swallow pills. In this case, perhaps pills could be crushed or a liquid medication substituted (always review medication to ensure that crushing is acceptable before giving this instruction).

Assess the treatment and medication schedule to determine whether it is reasonable for a home situation. Although an every-6-hour or every-8-hour schedule is reasonable for hospitals, a parent would have difficulty getting up once or twice nightly. Instead the patient could take a medication during the day at times that would be easy to remember.

Behavioral strategies are designed to modify behavior directly. There are several effective strategies that the nurse can use with children to encourage the desired behavior. Positive reinforcement is one strategy that strengthens the behavior. One example of this is the child earning stars or tokens, which can be exchanged for a special privilege or gift. At times, however, disciplinary techniques, such as time-out for young children or withholding privileges for older children, may be needed to improve compliance.

> **NURSING TIP** To encourage a child to perform a treatment (e.g., soaking a foot) for a certain period, ask the child to soak during a favorite television show, including commercials. This technique also helps evaluate compliance by asking the child what show was watched.

GENERAL HYGIENE AND CARE

MAINTAINING HEALTHY SKIN

Maintaining an IV line, removing a dressing, positioning a child in bed, changing a diaper, using electrodes, or using restraints have the potential to contribute to skin injury. Skin care must go beyond the daily bath and become a part of each nursing intervention. General guidelines for skin care are listed in the Nursing Care Guidelines box. (Specific guidelines for skin care of neonates are provided in Chapter 10 under Skin Care.)

Assessment of the skin is easiest to accomplish during the bath. Examine for early signs of injury. Risk factors include impaired mobility, protein malnutrition, edema, incontinence, sensory loss, anemia, infection, failure to turn the patient, and intubation. Critically ill children are at higher risk of pressure ulcers and skin breakdown, since they often have several risk factors combined. The incidence in these children has been reported as high as 27% (Curley, Quigley, and Lin, 2003). Identification of risk factors helps to determine those children who need a more thorough skin assessment. Several risk assessment scales are available for use in pediatrics, such as the Braden Q Scale (Curley, Razmus, Roberts, et al, 2003) and the Glamorgan Scale (Willock, Baharestani, and Anthony, 2009).

NURSING CARE GUIDELINES

Skin Care

- Cleanse skin with mild nonalkaline soap or soap-free cleaning agents for routine bathing.
- Provide daily cleansing of eyes, oral and diaper or perineal areas, and any areas of skin breakdown.
- Apply moisturizing agents during or immediately after bathing; cleanse skin of old cream before adding a new layer.
- Use minimum amount of tape and adhesives. On very sensitive skin, use a protective, pectin-based or hydrocolloid skin barrier between skin and tape or adhesives.
- Use water or adhesive remover (if skin is not fragile) when removing tape or adhesives.
- Place pectin-based or hydrocolloid skin barriers directly over excoriated skin. Leave barrier undisturbed until it begins to peel off, or for 5 to 7 days. With wet, oozing excoriations, place a small amount of stoma powder on site, remove excess powder, and apply skin barrier. Hold barrier in place for several minutes to allow barrier to soften and mold to skin surface.
- Alternate electrode placement and thoroughly assess skin underneath electrodes at least every 24 hours. Alcohol-free skin sealant under leads protects skin from epidermal stripping.
- Be certain fingers or toes are visible whenever extremity is used for intravenous (IV) or arterial line.
- Keep skin dry (may apply absorbent powder, e.g., cornstarch) and use soft, smooth bed linen and clothes.
- Use a draw sheet to move a child in bed or onto a stretcher; do not drag the child from under the arms.
- Identify children who are at risk for skin breakdown before it occurs. Employ measures such as pressure-reducing or pressure-relieving devices (e.g., mattress overlays, low air loss bed, gel pillows).
- Do not massage reddened bony prominences, since this can cause deep tissue damage; provide pressure relief to those areas instead.
- Keep skin free of excess moisture (e.g., urine or fecal incontinence, wound drainage, excessive perspiration).
- Routinely assess the child's nutritional status. A child who is NPO (nothing by mouth) for several days and is receiving only IV fluid is nutritionally at risk, which can also affect the skin's ability to maintain its integrity. Consider parenteral nutrition.

Assessment should occur within 24 hours of admission to identify pressure ulcers and wounds that occurred before admission. Pressure ulcers in children typically occur on the occiput, ears, sacrum, and scapula (Amlung, Miller, and Bosley, 2001), whereas the heels and sacrum are common sites in adults.

When capillary blood flow is interrupted by pressure, the blood flows back into the tissue when the pressure is relieved. As the body attempts to reoxygenate the area, a bright red flush appears. This reactive hyperemia, or flush, is the earliest sign of tissue compromise and pressure-related ischemia. If pressure is prolonged, reactive hyperemia will not be sufficient to revitalize ischemic tissue. Pressure ulcers in hospitalized children are uncommon, with reported rates of 1% to 13% (Noonan, Quigley, and Curley, 2006). Risk factors associated with pressure ulcers in pediatric ICU patients include edema, length of stay, increasing positive end-expiratory pressure, lack of turning, use of a specialty bed in the turning mode, and weight loss (McCord, McElvain, Sachdeva, et al, 2004). Medical devices such as pulse oximeter probes, bilevel and continuous positive airway pressure masks, oxygen cannulas, orthotics, and casts can also cause pressure ulcers.

Pressure ulcers are staged to classify the amount of tissue damage that has occurred.* Necrotic tissue must be removed so that the tissue depth can accurately be assessed (Box 27-2). Accurate documentation of redness or obvious skin breakdown is essential. Color, size (diameter and depth), location, presence of sinus tracts, odor, exudate, and response to treatment are observed and recorded at least daily. (For treatment of wounds, see Chapter 18.)

Pressure ulcers can develop when the pressure on the skin and underlying tissues is greater than the capillary closing pressure, causing capillary occlusion. If the pressure remains unrelieved, vessels can collapse, resulting in tissue anoxia and cellular death. Pressure ulcers most often occur over bony prominences. These lesions are usually very deep (stage IV), extending into subcutaneous tissue or even more deeply into muscle, tendon, or bone.

A pressure reduction device reduces pressure but does not prevent pressure from causing capillary closure; therefore turning and repositioning are always included when using these devices. Most of these items are overlays that are placed on top of the regular mattress. A pressure-relief device maintains pressure below that which would cause capillary closure. These devices are usually high-technology beds that are used for patients who have multiple problems and cannot be turned effectively.

Friction and shear contribute to pressure ulcers. Friction occurs when the surface of the skin rubs against another surface, such as bed sheets. The skin may have the appearance of an abrasion. The skin damage is usually limited to the epidermal and upper layers. It most often occurs over the elbows, heels, or occiput. Prevention of friction injury includes the use of customized splinting over infants' heels; gel pillows under the head of infants and toddlers; moisturizing agents; transparent dressings over susceptible areas; and soft, smooth bed linens and clothing (Baharestani and Ratliff, 2007). By itself, friction does not cause tissue necrosis, but when it acts with gravity, it results in shear injury.

Shear is the result of the force of gravity pushing down on the body and friction of the body against a surface, such as the bed or chair. For example, when a patient is in the semi-Fowler position and begins to slide to the foot of the bed, the skin over the sacral area remains in the same place because of the resistance of the bed surface. The blood vessels in the area are stretched and may cause small-vessel thrombosis and tissue death (Bryant and Doughty, 2000). Prevention of shear injury includes using lift sheets when repositioning a patient, elevating the bed no more than 30 degrees for short periods, and using the knee gatch to interrupt the pull of gravity on the body toward the foot of the bed.

Epidermal stripping results when the epidermis is unintentionally removed when tape is removed. These lesions are usually shallow and irregularly shaped. Babies are at increased risk for epidermal injury. Prevention includes using no tape when possible, securing dressings with laced binders

---

*Staging of pressure ulcers and guidelines for prevention and management of pressure ulcers are available from the National Pressure Ulcer Advisory Panel, http://npuap.org.

BOX 27-2 PRESSURE ULCER STAGES

Suspected Deep Tissue Injury
Purple or maroon localized area of discolored intact skin or blood-filled blister due to damage of underlying soft tissue from pressure and/or shear. The area may be preceded by tissue that is painful, firm, mushy, boggy, warmer or cooler as compared to adjacent tissue.
Further description—Deep tissue injury may be difficult to detect in individuals with dark skin tones. Evolution may include a thin blister over a dark wound bed. The wound may further evolve and become covered by thin eschar. Evolution may be rapid, exposing additional layers of tissue even with optimal treatment.

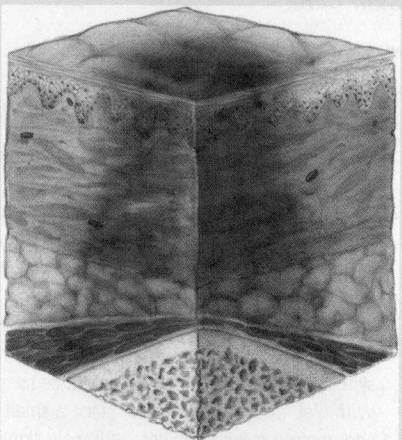

Stage I
Intact skin with nonblanchable redness of a localized area, usually over a bony prominence. Darkly pigmented skin may not have visible blanching; its color may differ from the surrounding area.
Further description—The area may be painful, firm, soft, warmer or cooler as compared to adjacent tissue. Stage I may be difficult to detect in individuals with dark skin tones. May indicate "at risk" persons (a heralding sign of risk).

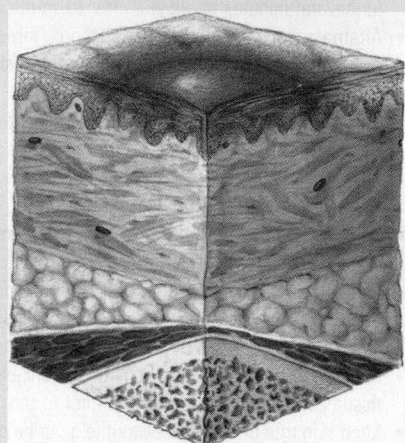

Stage II
Partial thickness loss of dermis presenting as a shallow open ulcer with a red pink wound bed, without slough. May also present as an intact or open/ruptured serum-filled blister.
Further description—Presents as a shiny or dry shallow ulcer without slough or bruising.* This stage should not be used to describe skin tears, tape burns, perineal dermatitis, maceration, or excoriation.

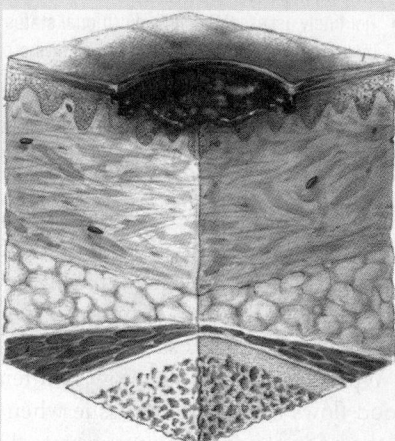

Stage III
Full thickness tissue loss. Subcutaneous fat may be visible but bone, tendon, and muscle are not exposed. Slough may be present but does not obscure the depth of tissue loss. May include undermining and tunneling.
Further description—The depth of a stage III pressure ulcer varies by anatomical location. The bridge of the nose, ear, occiput, and malleolus do not have subcutaneous tissue, and stage III ulcers can be shallow. In contrast, areas of significant adiposity can develop extremely deep stage III pressure ulcers. Bone or tendon is not visible or directly palpable.

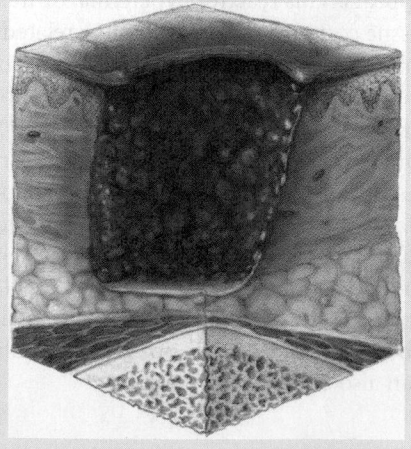

BOX 27-2   PRESSURE ULCER STAGES—cont'd

Stage IV

Full-thickness tissue loss with exposed bone, tendon, or muscle. Slough or eschar may be present on some parts of the wound bed. Often include undermining and tunneling.

Further description—The depth of a stage IV pressure ulcer varies by anatomical location. The bridge of the nose, ear, occiput, and malleolus do not have subcutaneous tissue, and these ulcers can be shallow. Stage IV ulcers can extend into muscle and/or supporting structures (e.g., fascia, tendon, or joint capsule), making osteomyelitis possible. Exposed bone or tendon is visible or directly palpable.

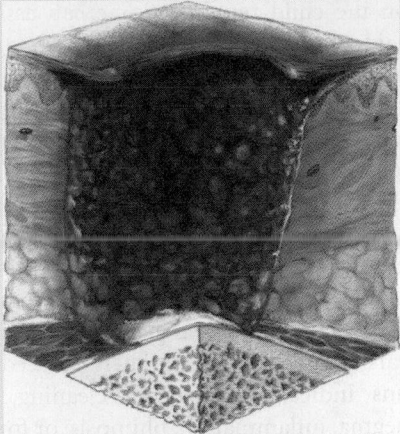

Unstageable

Full-thickness tissue loss in which the base of the ulcer is covered by slough (yellow, tan, gray, green, or brown) and/or eschar (tan, brown, or black) in the wound bed.

Further description—Until enough slough and/or eschar is removed to expose the base of the wound, the true depth, and therefore stage, cannot be determined. Stable (dry, adherent, intact without erythema or fluctuance) eschar on the heels serves as "the body's natural (biological) cover" and should not be removed.

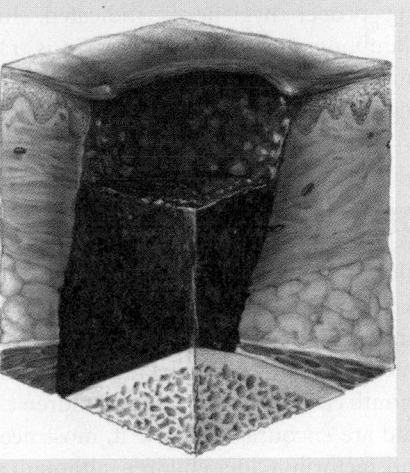

From the National Pressure Ulcer Advisory Panel, 2007. Reprinted with permission. Reproduction of the National Pressure Ulcer Advisory Panel (NPUAP) materials in this document does not imply endorsement by the NPUAP of any products, organizations, companies, or any statements made by any organization or company.

For more information, contact **www.npuap.org** or 202-521-6789.

*Bruising indicates suspected deep tissue injury.

(Montgomery straps) or stretchy netting (Spandage or stockinette). Using porous or low-tack tapes (e.g., Medipore, paper, hydrogel), using alcohol-free skin sealants (No Sting Barrier Film), or picture framing wounds with hydrocolloid or wafer barriers (e.g., DuoDERM, Coloplast, Stomahesive) and then taping on top of the barrier also will reduce epidermal stripping.

Tape is placed so that there is no tension, traction, or wrinkles on the skin. To remove tape, slowly peel the tape away while stabilizing the underlying skin. Adhesive remover may be used to break the adhesive bond but may be drying to the skin. Avoid adhesive removers in preterm neonates, since absorption rates vary and toxicity may occur. Remove the adhesive with water to prevent absorption and irritation. Wetting the tape with water or alcohol-based foam hand cleansers may facilitate removal.

Chemical factors can also lead to skin damage. Fecal incontinence, especially when mixed with urine; wound drainage; or gastric drainage around gastrostomy tubes can erode the epidermis. The skin can quickly progress from redness to denudement if exposure continues. Moisture barriers, gentle cleansing as soon after exposure as possible, and skin barriers can be used to prevent damage caused by chemical factors. In addition, foam dressings that wick moisture away from the skin are helpful around gastrostomy tubes and tracheostomy sites.

BATHING

Most infants and children can be bathed in a basin at the bedside or on the bed, in a standard bathtub or shower. For infants and young children confined to bed, use the towel method. Immerse two towels in a dilute soap solution and wring them damp. With the child lying supine on a dry towel, place one damp towel on top of the child and use it to gently clean the body. Discard this towel, and dry the child and turn him or her prone. Repeat the procedure using the second damp towel. Commercially available bath cloths may also be used.

Infants and small children are never left unattended in a bathtub, and infants who are unable to sit alone are securely held with one hand during the bath. The nurse securely supports the infant's head with one hand, or grasps the infant's farther arm while the head rests comfortably on the nurse's arm. Children who are able to sit without assistance need only close supervision and a pad placed in the bottom of the tub to prevent slipping and loss of balance.

School-age children and adolescents may shower or bathe. Nurses need to use judgment regarding the amount of supervision the child requires. Some can assume this responsibility unaided, whereas others need someone in constant attendance. Children with cognitive impairments, physical limitations such as severe anemia or leg deformities, or suicidal or psychotic problems (who may commit bodily harm) require close supervision.

Areas that require special attention are ears, between skinfolds, neck, back, and genital area. The genital area should be carefully cleansed and dried, with particular care given to skinfolds. In uncircumcised boys, usually those over 3 years of age, the foreskin should be gently retracted, the exposed surfaces cleansed, and the foreskin then replaced. If the condition of the glans indicates inadequate cleaning, such as accumulated smegma, inflammation, phimosis, or foreskin adhesions, teaching proper hygiene is indicated. In the Vietnamese and Cambodian cultures the foreskin is traditionally not retracted until adulthood. Older children have a tendency to avoid cleaning the genitalia; therefore they may need a gentle reminder.

ORAL HYGIENE

Mouth care is an integral part of daily hygiene and should be continued in the hospital. For some young children, this is their first introduction to the use of a toothbrush. Infants and debilitated children require the nurse or a family member to perform mouth care. Although young children can manage a toothbrush and are encouraged to use it, most need assistance to perform satisfactorily. Older children, although capable of brushing and flossing without assistance, sometimes need to be reminded.

HAIR CARE

Children should have their hair brushed and combed at least once daily. The hair is styled for comfort and in a manner pleasing to the child and parents. The hair should not be cut without parental permission, although clipping hair to provide access to a scalp vein for IV insertion may be necessary.

If children are hospitalized for more than a few days, the hair may need shampooing. With infants, the hair may be washed during the daily bath or less frequently. For most children, washing the hair and scalp once or twice weekly is sufficient unless there is an indication for more frequent washing, such as following a high fever and profuse sweating. Adolescents normally have increased oily sebaceous secretions that require frequent hair care and more frequent shampoos.

Almost any child can be transported to an accessible sink for shampooing. Those who are unable to be transported can receive a shampoo in their beds with adequate protection, specially adapted equipment or positioning, or dry shampoo caps. When necessary, a shampoo basin may be used or the child may be positioned near the edge of the bed, towels placed under the shoulders, a large plastic garbage bag draped at the edge of the bed with one open end under the shoulders, and the hair placed inside the opening. The other end is opened and placed in a collection container. Water can be transported in a basin.

> **NURSING TIP** For a convenient source of water, fill an empty enema bag with warm water, hang the bag from an IV pole, and use the clamp on the bag's tubing to adjust the flow of water.

For the child with curly hair, most standard combs are inadequate and may cause hair breakage and discomfort. Use a special comb with widely spaced teeth. It is also much easier to comb the hair after shampooing when it is wet. Use a special hair dressing or pomade, which usually has a coconut oil base. Rub the preparation on the hands and then transfer it to the hair to make it more pliable and manageable. Consult the child's parents regarding the preparation to use on the child's hair and ask if they can provide some for use during the child's hospitalization. Petroleum jelly should not be used. If braiding or plaiting the hair, weave it loosely while the hair is damp. The hair tightens as it dries, which could result in tension folliculitis.

FEEDING THE SICK CHILD

Loss of appetite is a symptom common to most childhood illnesses. Because an acute illness is usually short, the nutritional state is seldom compromised. Urging food on the sick child may precipitate nausea and vomiting. In most cases children can usually determine their own need for food.

Refusing to eat may also be one way children can exert power and control in an otherwise helpless situation. For young children, loss of appetite may be related to depression caused by separation from their parents. Parents' concern with eating can intensify the problem. Forcing a child to eat meets with rebellion and reinforces the behavior as a control mechanism. Encourage parents to relax any pressure during an acute illness. Although it is best to provide high-quality nutritious foods, the child may desire foods and liquids that contain mostly empty or nonnutritional calories. Some well-tolerated foods include gelatin, diluted clear soups, carbonated drinks, flavored ice pops, dry toast, and crackers. Even though these substances are not nutritious, they can provide necessary fluid and calories.

Dehydration is always a hazard when children have a fever or anorexia, especially when accompanied by vomiting or diarrhea. Fluids should not be forced, and the child is not awakened to take fluids. Forcing fluids may create the same difficulties as urging the child to eat unwanted food. Gentle persuasion with preferred beverages will usually meet with success. Using play techniques can also be effective (see Nursing Care Guidelines box).

An understanding of children's feeding habits can also increase food consumption. For example, if children are given all their food at one time, they generally eat the dessert first. Likewise, if they are presented with large portions, they often push the food away because the amount overwhelms them. If young children are not supervised during mealtime, they tend to play with the food rather than eat it. Therefore nurses should present food in the usual order, such as soup first, followed by small portions of meat, potatoes, and vegetables, and ending with dessert. The principles of conservation can also be used to increase food consumption. (See Cognitive Development, Chapter 15.)

NURSING CARE GUIDELINES

Feeding the Sick Child

Take a dietary history (see Chapter 6) and use information to make eating time as much like home as possible.

Encourage parents or other family members to feed child or to be present at mealtimes.

Make mealtimes pleasant; avoid any procedures immediately before or after eating; make certain child is rested and pain free.

Serve small, frequent meals rather than three large meals, or serve three meals and nutritious between-meal snacks.

Provide finger foods for young children.

Involve children in food selection and preparation whenever possible.

Serve small portions, and serve each course separately, such as soup first; followed by meat, potatoes, and vegetables; and ending with dessert. With young children, camouflage size of food by cutting meat thicker so that less appears on plate or by folding a cheese slice in half. Offer second helpings.

Ensure a variety of foods, textures, and colors.

Provide food selections that are favorites of most children, such as peanut butter and jelly sandwiches, hot dogs, hamburgers, macaroni and cheese, pizza, spaghetti, tacos, fried chicken, corn, and fruit yogurt.

Avoid foods that are highly seasoned, have strong odors, or are all mixed together, unless typical of cultural practices.

Provide fluid selections that are favorites of most children, such as fruit punch, cola, ginger ale, sweetened tea, flavored ice pops, sherbet, ice cream, milk, milkshakes, pudding, gelatin, clear broth, or creamed soups.

Offer nutritious snacks, such as frozen yogurt or pudding, ice cream, oatmeal or peanut butter cookies, hot cocoa, cheese slices, pieces of raw vegetable or fruit, and dried fruit or cereal.

Make food attractive and different; for example:
- Serve a "picnic lunch" in a paper bag.
- Pack food in a Chinese take-out container; decorate container.
- Put a "face" or a "flower" on a hamburger or sandwich with pieces of vegetable.
- Use a cookie cutter to shape a sandwich.
- Serve pudding, yogurt, or juice frozen as an ice pop.
- Make Slurpies or snow cones by pouring flavored syrup on crushed ice.
- Add food coloring to water or milk.
- Serve fluids through brightly colored or unusually shaped straws.
- Make "bowtie" sandwiches by cutting them in triangles and placing two points together.
- Slice sandwiches into "fingers."
- Grate mounds of cheese.
- Cut apples horizontally to make circles.
- Put a banana on a hot dog bun and spread with peanut butter.
- Break uncooked spaghetti into toothpick lengths and skewer cheese, cold meat, vegetables, or fruit chunks.

Praise children for what they do eat.

Do not punish children for not eating by removing their dessert or putting them to bed.

Once the child is feeling better, appetite usually begins to improve. It is best to take advantage of any hungry period by serving high-quality foods and snacks. If the child still refuses to eat, offer nutritious fluids, such as prepared breakfast drinks. Parents can help by bringing in food items from home, especially if the family's cultural eating habits differ from the hospital food. A clinical dietitian may be consulted for alternative food choices.

When children are placed on special diets, such as clear liquids after surgery or during episodes of diarrhea, assessment of their intake and readiness to advance to more complex foods is essential.

Regardless of the type of diet, charting the amount consumed is an important nursing responsibility. Descriptions need to be detailed and accurate, such as "4 oz of orange juice, one pancake, and 8 oz of milk." Comments such as "ate well" or "ate poorly" are inadequate. Charting the percentage of the meal eaten is also inadequate unless food is measured before serving.

If parents are involved in the child's care, encourage them to keep a list of everything eaten. Using a premeasured cup for fluids ensures a more accurate estimate of intake. A comparison of the intake at each meal can isolate food deficiencies, such as insufficient intake of meat or vegetables. Behaviors associated with mealtime also identify possible factors influencing appetite. For example, the observation, "Child eats well when with other children but plays with food if left alone in room," helps the nurse plan mealtime activities that stimulate the child's appetite.

Although sick children's appetites may be poor and not characteristic of their home eating habits, the hospital stay provides numerous opportunities for nurses to assess the family's

knowledge of good nutrition and to implement teaching as needed to improve nutritional intake.

CONTROLLING ELEVATED TEMPERATURES

An elevated temperature, most frequently from fever but occasionally caused by hyperthermia, is one of the most common symptoms of illness in children. This manifestation is a great concern to parents. To facilitate an understanding of fever, the following terms are defined:

Set point—The temperature around which body temperature is regulated by a thermostat-like mechanism in the hypothalamus

Fever (hyperpyrexia)—An elevation in set point such that body temperature is regulated at a higher level; may be arbitrarily defined as temperature above 38° C (100.4° F)

Hyperthermia—Body temperature exceeding the set point, which usually results from the body or external conditions creating more heat than the body can eliminate, such as in heat stroke, aspirin toxicity, seizures, or hyperthyroidism

Body temperature is regulated by a thermostat-like mechanism in the hypothalamus. (See Chapter 6.) This mechanism receives input from centrally and peripherally located receptors. When temperature changes occur, these receptors relay the information to the thermostat, which either increases or decreases heat production to maintain a constant set point temperature. However, during an infection, pyrogenic substances cause an increase in the body's normal set point, a process that is mediated by prostaglandins. Consequently, the hypothalamus increases heat production until the core temperature reaches the new set point.

During the fever (febrile) state, shivering and vasoconstriction generate and conserve heat during the chill phase of fever, raising central temperatures to the level of the new set point. The temperature reaches a plateau when it stabilizes in the higher range. When the temperature is greater than the set point or when the pyrogen is no longer present, a crisis, or defervescence, of the temperature occurs.

Most fevers in children are of brief duration with limited consequences and are viral in origin. When fever is caused by bacteria, endotoxins are produced that activate the inflammatory process and produce fever (Rote, Huether, and McCance, 2000). Fever has physiologic benefits: increased white blood cell activity, interferon production and effectiveness, and antibody production and enhancement of some antibiotic effects (Considine and Brennan, 2007). Contrary to popular belief, neither the rise in temperature nor its response to antipyretics indicates the severity or etiology of the infection, which casts doubt on the value of using fever as a diagnostic or prognostic indicator.

Therapeutic Management

Treatment of elevated temperature depends on whether it is due to a fever or hyperthermia. Because the set point is normal in hyperthermia but increased in fever, different approaches must be used to lower body temperature successfully.

Fever

The principal reason for treating fever is the relief of discomfort. Relief measures include pharmacologic and environmental intervention. The most effective intervention is the use of antipyretics to lower the set point.

Antipyretics include acetaminophen, aspirin, and nonsteroidal antiinflammatory drugs (NSAIDs). Acetaminophen is the preferred drug. Aspirin should not be given to children because of its association in children with influenza virus or chickenpox and Reye syndrome. One nonprescription NSAID, ibuprofen, is approved for fever reduction in children as young as 6 months of age (Table 27-3). Dosage is based on the initial temperature level: 5 mg/kg of body weight for temperatures less than 39.2° C (102.6° F) or 10 mg/kg for temperatures greater than 39.2° C. The recommended dosage for pain is 10 mg/kg every 6 to 8 hours, and the recommended maximum daily dose for pain and fever is 40 mg/kg. The duration of fever reduction is generally 6 to 8 hours and is longer with the higher dose.

The recommended doses of acetaminophen are listed in Table 27-4. Acetaminophen should be given every 4 hours, but no more than five times in 24 hours. Because body temperature normally decreases at night, three or four doses in 24 hours will control most fevers. The temperature is usually retaken 30 minutes after the antipyretic is given to assess its effect but should not be repeatedly measured. The child's level of discomfort is the best indication for continued treatment.

The nurse can use environmental measures to reduce fever if they are tolerated by the child and if they do not induce shivering. Shivering is the body's way of maintaining the elevated set point by producing heat. Compensatory shivering greatly increases metabolic requirements above those already caused by the fever.

TABLE 27-3	DOSE RECOMMENDATIONS FOR IBUPROFEN (CHILDREN'S MOTRIN)*			
WEIGHT (lb [kg])	AGE	ORAL DROPS (50 mg/1.25 ml)	SUSPENSION (100 mg/5 ml)	CAPLETS (100 mg)
12-17 (5.4-7.7)	6-11 mo	1 dropper (1.25 ml)	—	—
18-23 (8.2-10.4)	12-23 mo	1½ droppers (1.875 ml)	—	—
24-35 (10.9-15.9)	2-3 yr	—	1 tsp (5 ml)	—
36-47 (16.3-21.3)	4-5 yr	—	1½ tsp (7.5 ml)	—
48-59 (21.8-26.8)	6-8 yr	—	2 tsp (10 ml)	2
60-71 (27.2-32.2)	9-10 yr	—	2½ tsp (12.5 ml)	2½
72-95 (32.7-43.1)	11 yr	—	3 tsp (15 ml)	3

Modified from McNeil Consumer Healthcare: *Motrin*, 2010, available at www.motrin.com (accessed March 5, 2010).
*Dosages based on fever <39.2° C (102.6° F) and a dose of 5 mg/kg. For fever ≥39.2° C, may use 10 mg/kg. Doses administered every 6-8 hr. Another nonprescription ibuprofen is Children's Advil.

TABLE 27-4	DOSE RECOMMENDATIONS FOR ACETAMINOPHEN (TYLENOL)*					
WEIGHT (lb [kg])	AGE	DOSE (mg)	CONCENTRATED TYLENOL INFANT DROPS (80 mg/0.8 ml)	CHILDREN'S TYLENOL SUSPENSION (160 mg/5 ml)	CHILDREN'S TYLENOL MELTAWAY TABLETS (80 mg/tablet)	JR. TYLENOL MELTAWAY TABLETS (160 mg/tablet)
6-11 (2.8-5)	<3 mo	40	½ dropper (0.4 ml)	—	—	—
12-17 (5.4-7.7)	4-11 mo	80	1 dropper (0.8 ml)	—	—	—
18-23 (8.2-10.4)	12-23 mo	120	1½ droppers (1.2 ml)	—	—	—
24-35 (10.9-15.9)	2-3 yr	160	2 droppers (1.6 ml)	1 tsp (5 ml)	2 tablets	—
36-47 (16.3-21.3)	4-5 yr	240	—	1½ tsp (7.5 ml)	3 tablets	—
48-59 (21.8-26.8)	6-8 yr	320	—	2 tsp (10 ml)	4 tablets	2 tablets
60-71 (27.2-32.2)	9-10 yr	400	—	2½ tsp (12.5 ml)	5 tablets	2½ tablets
72-95 (32.7-43.1)	11 yr	480	—	3 tsp (15 ml)	6 tablets	3 tablets
96 (43.5)	≥12 yr	640	—	—	—	4 tablets

*Doses should be administered 4-5 times daily but should not exceed 5 doses in 24 hr.

Traditional cooling measures, such as wearing minimum clothing, exposing the skin to air, reducing room temperature, increasing air circulation, and applying cool, moist compresses to the skin (e.g., the forehead), are effective if employed approximately 1 hour after an antipyretic is given so that the set point is lowered. Cooling procedures such as sponging or tepid baths are ineffective in treating febrile children (these measures are effective for hyperthermia) either when used alone or in combination with antipyretics, and they cause considerable discomfort (Axelrod, 2000).

Seizures associated with a fever occur in 3% to 4% of all children, usually in those between 6 months and 6 years of age. About 30% of children have subsequent febrile seizures; a younger age at onset and a family history of febrile seizures are associated with increased incidence of recurring episodes. There is little evidence to support the use of antipyretic drugs or anticonvulsants to prevent a second febrile seizure; nursing intervention should focus on ways to provide care and comfort during a febrile illness. Simple febrile seizures lasting less than 10 minutes do not cause brain damage or other debilitating effects (Jones and Jacobsen, 2007; Sadleir and Scheffer, 2007). (See Febrile Seizures, Chapter 37.)

Hyperthermia

Unlike in fever, antipyretics are of no value in hyperthermia because the set point is already normal. Consequently, cooling measures are used. Cool applications to the skin help reduce the core temperature. Cooled blood from the skin surface is conducted to inner organs and tissues, and warm blood is circulated to the surface, where it is cooled and recirculated. The surface blood vessels dilate as the body attempts to dissipate heat to the environment and facilitate this cooling process.

Commercial cooling devices, such as cooling blankets or mattresses, are available to reduce body temperature. Place the patient on the bed and cover with a sheet or lightweight blanket. Frequent temperature monitoring is essential to prevent excessive cooling of the body.

Traditionally, cool compresses decrease high temperature. For tepid tub baths, it is usually best to start with warm water and gradually add cool water until the desired water temperature of 37° C (98.6° F) is reached to acclimate the child to the lower water temperature. Generally the temperature of the water only has to be 1° C (or 2° F) less than the child's temperature to be effective. The child is placed directly in the tub of tepid water for 15 to 20 minutes while water is gently squeezed from a washcloth over the back and chest or gently sprayed over the body from a sprayer. In the bed or crib, cool washcloths or towels are used, exposing only one area of the body at a time. Continue sponging for approximately 20 minutes.

After the tub or sponge bath, the child is dried and dressed in lightweight pajamas, a nightgown, or a diaper and placed in a dry bed. The child is dried by gently rubbing the skin surface with a towel to stimulate circulation. The temperature is retaken 30 minutes after the tub or sponge bath. The tub or sponge bath should not be continued or restarted until the skin surface is warm or if the child feels chilled. Chilling causes vasoconstriction, which defeats the purpose of the cool applications. In this condition, little blood is carried to the skin surface; the blood remains primarily in the viscera to become heated.

Whether a temperature elevation in the critically ill child is caused by fever or hyperthermia, it should be treated aggressively. The metabolic rate increases 10% for every 1° C increase in temperature and three to five times during shivering, thus increasing oxygen, fluid, and caloric requirements. If the child's cardiovascular or neurologic system is already compromised, these increased needs are especially hazardous. In all children with an elevated temperature, attention to adequate hydration is essential. Most children's needs can be met through additional oral fluids.

FAMILY TEACHING AND HOME CARE

Fever is one of the most common problems for which parents seek health care. High levels of parental anxiety (fever phobia) surrounding potential complications of fever such as seizures and dehydration are prevalent and can result in overusing antipyretics (Purssell, 2008). Parents need to know that sponging is indicated for elevated temperatures from hyperthermia rather than fever and that ice water and alcohol are inappropriate, potentially dangerous solutions (Axelrod, 2000). Parents should know how to take the child's temperature, how to read the thermometer accurately, and when to seek professional care (see Family-Centered Care box). Some of the newer temperature-measuring devices, such as plastic strip or digital thermometers, may be better suited for home use. (See Temperature, Chapter 6.) If the use of acetaminophen or ibuprofen is indicated, the parents need instructions in administering the drug. Emphasize accuracy in both the amount of drug given and the time intervals at which the drug is administered. Along with reduced activity, encourage small, frequent sips of clear liquids. Dress the child in light clothing; use a light blanket for children who are cold or shivering (Walsh and Edwards, 2006).

FAMILY-CENTERED CARE
The Child with Fever

Call Office Immediately If:
Your child is younger than 2 months old.
The fever is over 40.6° C (105° F).
Your child looks or acts very sick: stiff neck, persistent vomiting, purplish spots on skin, confusion, trouble breathing after you have cleaned his nose, or inability to be comforted.

Call Within 24 Hours If:
The fever is between 40° and 40.6° C (104° and 105° F), especially if your child is younger than 2 years old.
Your child has had a fever for more than 24 hours without an obvious cause or location of infection.
Your child has had a fever for more than 3 days.
Your child has burning or pain with urination.
Your child has a history of febrile seizures.
The fever went away for more than 24 hours and then returned.
You have other concerns or questions.

Modified from Schmitt BD: *Instructions for pediatric patients*, ed 2, Philadelphia, 1999, Saunders.

SAFETY

Safety is an essential component of any patient's care, but children have special characteristics that require an even greater concern for safety. Because small children in the hospital are separated from their usual environment and do not possess the capacity for abstract thinking and reasoning, it is the responsibility of everyone who comes in contact with them to maintain protective measures throughout their hospital stay. Nurses need to understand the age level at which each child is operating and plan for safety accordingly.

Identification bands are particularly important for children. Infants and unconscious patients are unable to tell or respond to their names. Toddlers may answer to any name or to a nickname only. Older children may exchange places, give an erroneous name, or choose not to respond to their own names as a joke, unaware of the hazards of such practices.

ENVIRONMENTAL FACTORS

All the environmental safety measures for the protection of adults apply to children, including good illumination, floors clear of fluid or objects that might contribute to falls, and nonskid surfaces in showers and tubs. All staff members should be familiar with the area-specific fire plan. Elevators and stairways should be made safe.

All windows should be secured. Blind and curtain cords should be out of reach with split cords to prevent strangulation. Pacifiers should not be tied around the neck or attached to an infant by string.

Electrical equipment should be in good working order and used only by personnel familiar with its use. It should not be in contact with moisture or situated near tubs. Electrical outlets should have covers to prevent burns in small children, whose exploratory activities may extend to inserting objects into the small openings.

Staff members should practice proper care and disposal of small objects such as syringe caps, needle covers, and temperature probes. Staff also must carefully check bathwater before placing the child in it and never leave children alone in a bathtub. Infants are helpless in water, and small children (and some older ones) may turn on the hot water faucet and be severely burned.

Furniture is safest when it is scaled to the child's proportions, is sturdy, and is well balanced to prevent its being easily tipped over. A special hazard for children is the danger of entrapment under an electronically controlled bed when it is activated to descend. Infants and small children must be securely strapped into infant seats, feeding chairs, and strollers. Baby walkers should not be used because they provide access to hazards, resulting in burns, falls, and poisonings. Infants; young children; and those who are weak, paralyzed, agitated, confused, sedated, or cognitively impaired are never left unattended on treatment tables, on scales, or in treatment areas. Even premature infants are capable of surprising mobility; therefore portholes in incubators must be securely fastened when not in use.

Crib sides are kept up and fastened securely unless an adult is at the bedside. It is safer to leave crib sides up, regardless of the child's ability to get out and even when the crib is unoccupied, to remove the temptation to climb in. Anyone attending an infant or small child in a crib with the sides down should never turn away without maintaining hand contact with the

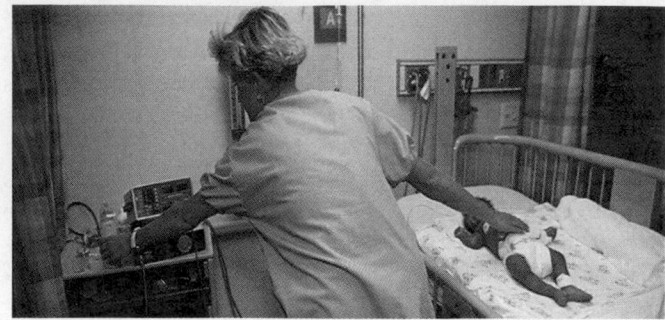

Fig. 27-3 The nurse maintains hand contact when her back is turned.

child, that is, keeping one hand on the child's back or abdomen to prevent rolling, crawling, or jumping from the open crib (Fig. 27-3). A child who is likely to climb over the sides of the crib is safest when placed in a specially constructed crib with a cover over the top. (See Injury Prevention, Chapter 12.)

The safest sleeping position to prevent sudden infant death syndrome is wholly supine (American Association of Pediatrics, 2005). No pillows should be placed in a young infant's crib while the infant is sleeping.

Toys

Toys play a vital role in the everyday life of children, and they are no less important in the hospital setting. Nurses are responsible for assessing the safety of toys brought to the hospital by well-meaning parents and friends. Toys should be appropriate to the child's age, condition, and treatment. For example, if the child is receiving oxygen, electrical or friction toys or equipment are not safe, since sparks can cause oxygen to ignite. Inspect toys to ensure they are nonallergenic, washable, and unbreakable and that they have no small, removable parts that can be aspirated or swallowed or can otherwise inflict injury on a child. All objects within reach of children younger than 3 years should pass the choke tube test. A toilet paper roll is a handy guide. If a toy or object fits into the cylinder (items <$1\frac{1}{4}$ inches across or balls <$1\frac{3}{4}$ inches in diameter), it is a potential choking danger to the child. Latex balloons pose a serious threat to children of all ages. If the balloon breaks, a child may put a piece of the latex in his or her mouth. If it is aspirated or swallowed, the latex piece is difficult to remove, resulting in choking. Latex balloons should never be permitted in the hospital setting.

Preventing Falls

Falls prevention begins with identification of children most at risk for falls. Pediatric hospitals use various methods to identify a child's risk of falls (Child Health Corporation of America, 2009). Once a risk assessment is performed, multiple interventions are needed to minimize pediatric patients' risk of falling, including education of patient, family, and staff.

To identify children at risk of falling, perform a fall risk assessment on patients on admission and throughout hospitalization. Risk factors for hospitalized children include:

- Medication effects—Postanesthesia or sedation; analgesics or narcotics, especially in those who have never had narcotics in the past and in whom effects are unknown
- Altered mental status—Secondary to seizures, brain tumors, or medications

- Altered or limited mobility—Reduced skill at ambulation secondary to developmental age, disease process, tubes, drains, casts, splints, or other appliances; new to ambulation with assistive devices such as walkers or crutches
- Postoperative children—Risk of hypotension or syncope secondary to large blood loss, a heart condition, or extended bed rest
- History of falls
- Infants or toddlers in cribs with side rails down or on the daybed with family members

Once children at risk of falls have been identified, alert other staff members by posting signs on the door and at the bedside, applying a special colored armband labeled "Fall Precautions," labeling the chart with a sticker, or documenting information on the chart.

Prevention of falls requires alterations in the environment, including:
- Keep bed in lowest position, breaks locked, and side rails up.
- Place call bell within reach.
- Ensure that all necessary and desired items are within reach (e.g., water, glasses, tissues, snacks).
- Offer toileting on a regular basis, especially if patient is taking diuretics or laxatives.
- Keep lights on at all times, including dim lights while sleeping.
- Lock wheelchairs before transferring patients.
- Ensure that patient has appropriate size gown and nonskid footwear. Do not allow gowns or ties to drag on the floor during ambulation.
- Keep floor clean and free of clutter. Post "wet floor" sign if floor is wet.
- Ensure that patient has glasses on if he or she normally wears them.

Preventing falls also relies on age-appropriate education of patients. Assist the child with ambulation even though he or she may have ambulated well before hospitalization. Patients who have been lying in bed need to get up slowly, sitting on the side of the bed before standing.

The nurse also needs to educate family members:
- Call the nursing staff for assistance, and do not allow patients to get up independently.
- Keep the side rails of the crib or bed up whenever patient is in the crib or bed.
- Do not leave infants on the daybed; put them in the crib with the side rails up.
- When all family members need to leave the bedside, notify staff and ensure the patient is in the bed or crib with side rails up and call bell within reach (if appropriate).

INFECTION CONTROL

According to the Centers for Disease Control and Prevention, approximately 2 million patients each year develop nosocomial (hospital-acquired) infections. These infections occur when there is interaction among patients, health care personnel, equipment, and bacteria (Quality, Equipment Hold Keys to Infection Control, 2006). Nosocomial infections are preventable if caregivers practice meticulous cleaning and disposal techniques.

Standard Precautions synthesize the major features of Universal (blood and body fluid) Precautions (designed to reduce the risk of transmission of blood-borne pathogens) and body substance isolation (designed to reduce the risk of transmission of pathogens from moist body substances). Standard Precautions involve the use of barrier protection, such as gloves, goggles, gown, or mask, to prevent contamination from (1) blood; (2) all body fluids, secretions, and excretions except sweat, regardless of whether they contain visible blood; (3) nonintact skin; and (4) mucous membranes. Standard Precautions are designed for the care of all patients to reduce the risk of transmission of microorganisms from both recognized and unrecognized sources of infection.

Transmission-Based Precautions are designed for patients with documented or suspected infection or colonization (presence of microorganisms in or on patient but without clinical signs and symptoms of infection) with highly transmissible or epidemiologically important pathogens for which additional precautions beyond Standard Precautions are needed to interrupt transmission in hospitals. There are three types of Transmission-Based Precautions: Airborne Precautions, Droplet Precautions, and Contact Precautions. They may be combined for diseases that have multiple routes of transmission (Box 27-3). They are to be used in addition to Standard Precautions.

Airborne Precautions reduce the risk of airborne transmission of infectious agents. Airborne transmission occurs by dissemination of either airborne droplet nuclei (small-particle residue [≤5 mm] of evaporated droplets that may remain suspended in the air for long periods) or dust particles containing the infectious agent. Microorganisms carried in this manner can be dispersed widely by air currents and may become inhaled by or deposited on a susceptible host within the same room or over a longer distance from the source patient, depending on environmental factors. Special air handling and ventilation are required to prevent airborne transmission. Airborne Precautions apply to patients with known or suspected infection with pathogens transmitted by the airborne route such as measles, varicella, and tuberculosis.

Droplet Precautions reduce the risk of droplet transmission of infectious agents. Droplet transmission involves contact of the conjunctivae or the mucous membranes of the nose or mouth of a susceptible person with large-particle droplets (>5 mm) containing microorganisms generated from a person who has a clinical disease or who is a carrier of the microorganism. Droplets are generated from the source person primarily during coughing, sneezing, or talking and during procedures such as suctioning and bronchoscopy. Transmission requires close contact between source and recipient persons, since droplets do not remain suspended in the air and generally travel only short distances, usually 3 feet or less, through the air. Because droplets do not remain suspended in the air, special air handling and ventilation are not required to prevent droplet transmission. Droplet Precautions apply to any patient with known or suspected infection with pathogens that can be transmitted by infectious droplets (see Box 27-3).

BOX 27-3 TYPES OF PRECAUTIONS AND PATIENTS REQUIRING THEM

Standard Precautions for Prevention of Transmission of Pathogens
Use Standard Precautions for the care of all patients.

Airborne Precautions
In addition to Standard Precautions, use Airborne Precautions for patients known or suspected to have serious illnesses transmitted by airborne droplet nuclei. Examples of such illnesses include measles, varicella (including disseminated zoster), and tuberculosis.

Droplet Precautions
In addition to Standard Precautions, use Droplet Precautions for patients known or suspected to have serious illnesses transmitted by large particle droplets. Examples of such illnesses include:
- Invasive *Haemophilus influenzae* type b disease, including meningitis, pneumonia, epiglottitis, and sepsis
- Invasive *Neisseria meningitidis* disease, including meningitis, pneumonia, and sepsis
- Other serious bacterial respiratory tract infections spread by droplet transmission, including diphtheria (pharyngeal), mycoplasmal pneumonia, pertussis, pneumonic plague, streptococcal pharyngitis, pneumonia, or scarlet fever in infants and young children
- Serious viral infections spread by droplet transmission, including adenovirus, influenza, mumps, parvovirus B19, and rubella

Contact Precautions
In addition to Standard Precautions, use Contact Precautions for patients known or suspected to have serious illnesses easily transmitted by direct patient contact or by contact with items in the patient's environment. Examples of such illnesses include:
- Gastrointestinal, respiratory, skin, or wound infections or colonization with multidrug-resistant bacteria judged by the infection control program, based on current state, regional, or national recommendations, to be of special clinical and epidemiologic significance
- Enteric infections with a low infectious dose or prolonged environmental survival, including *Clostridium difficile*; for diapered or incontinent patients: enterohemorrhagic *Escherichia coli* O157:H7, *Shigella* organisms, hepatitis A, or rotavirus
- Respiratory syncytial virus, parainfluenza virus, or enteroviral infections in infants and young children.
- Skin infections that are highly contagious or that may occur on dry skin, including diphtheria (cutaneous), herpes simplex virus (neonatal or mucocutaneous), impetigo, major (noncontained) abscesses, cellulitis or decubitus, pediculosis, scabies, staphylococcal furunculosis in infants and young children, zoster (disseminated or in the immunocompromised host)
- Viral or hemorrhagic conjunctivitis
- Viral hemorrhagic infections (Ebola, Lassa, or Marburg)

Modified from Garner JS: Guidelines for isolation precautions in hospitals, *Infect Control Hosp Epidemiol* 17(1):66, 1996.

Contact Precautions reduce the risk of transmission of microorganisms by direct or indirect contact. Direct-contact transmission involves skin-to-skin contact and physical transfer of microorganisms to a susceptible host from an infected or colonized person, such as occurs when turning or bathing patients. Direct-contact transmission also can occur between two patients (e.g., by hand contact). Indirect contact transmission involves contact of a susceptible host with a contaminated intermediate object, usually inanimate, in the patient's environment. Contact Precautions apply to specified patients known

---

! NURSING ALERT

The most common piece of medical equipment, the stethoscope, can be a potent source of harmful microorganisms and nosocomial infections.

or suspected to be infected or colonized with microorganisms that can be transmitted by direct or indirect contact.

Nurses caring for young children are frequently in contact with body substances, especially urine, feces, and vomitus. Nurses need to exercise judgment concerning those situations when gloves, gowns, or masks are necessary. For example, wear gloves and possibly gowns for changing diapers when there are loose or explosive stools. Otherwise, the plastic lining of disposable diapers provides a sufficient barrier between the hands and body substances.

Antimicrobial-resistant organisms are causing increasing numbers of nosocomial infections. In hospitals, patients are the most significant sources of methicillin-resistant *Staphylococcus aureus*, and the main mode of transmission is patient to patient via the hands of a health care provider (Eaton, 2005; Quality, Equipment Hold Keys to Infection Control, 2006). Hand washing is the most critical infection control practice.

During feedings, wear gowns if the child is likely to vomit or spit up, which often occurs during burping. When wearing gloves, wash the hands thoroughly after removing the gloves, since gloves fail to provide complete protection. The absence of visible leaks does not indicate that gloves are intact.

Another essential practice of infection control is that all needles (uncapped and unbroken) are disposed of in a rigid, puncture-resistant container located near the site of use. Consequently, these containers are installed in patients' rooms. Since children are naturally curious, extra attention is needed in selecting a suitable type of container and a location that prevents access to the discarded needles (Fig. 27-4). The use of needleless systems allows secure syringe or IV tubing

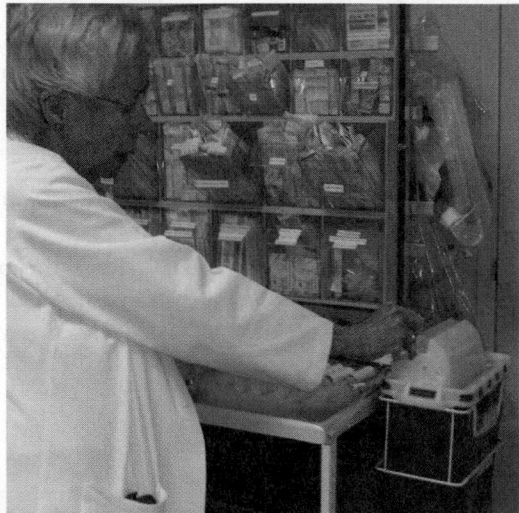

Fig. 27-4 To prevent needlestick injuries, used needles (and other sharp instruments) are not capped or broken and are disposed of in rigid, puncture-resistant container located near site of use. Note placement of container to prevent children's access to contents.

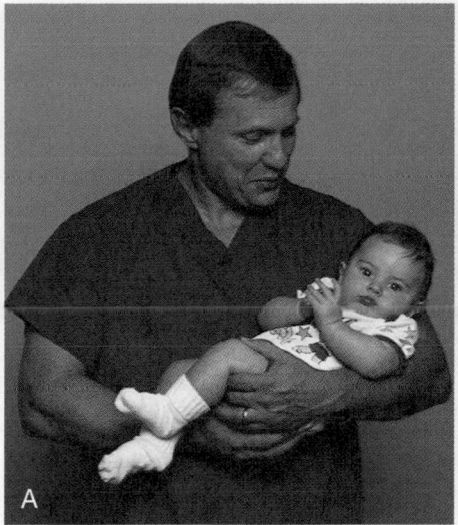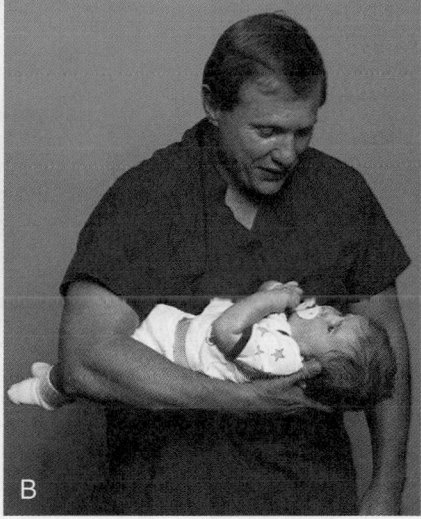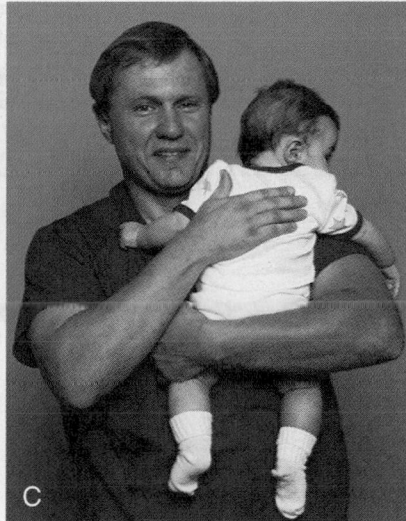

Fig. 27-5 Transporting infants. **A,** Infant's thigh firmly grasped in nurse's hand. **B,** Football hold. **C,** Back supported.

attachment to vascular access devices without the risk of needlestick injury to the child or nurse.

TRANSPORTING INFANTS AND CHILDREN

Infants and children need to be transported within the unit and to areas outside the pediatric unit. Infants and small children can be carried for short distances within the unit, but for more extended trips the child should be securely transported in a suitable conveyance.

Small infants can be held or carried in the horizontal position with the back supported and the thigh grasped firmly by the carrying arm (Fig. 27-5, *A*). In the football hold, the infant is carried on the nurse's arm with the head supported by the hand and the body held securely between the nurse's body and elbow (Fig. 27-5, *B*). Both of these holds leave the nurse's other arm free for activity. The infant also can be held in the upright position with the buttocks on the nurse's forearm and the front of the body resting against the nurse's chest. The infant's head and shoulders are supported by the nurse's other arm in case the infant moves suddenly (Fig. 27-5, *C*). Older infants are able to hold their heads erect but are still subject to sudden movements.

The method of transporting children depends on their age, condition, and destination. Older children are safe in wheelchairs or on stretchers. Younger children can be transported in their crib, on a stretcher, in a wagon with raised sides, or in a wheelchair with a safety belt. Stretchers should be equipped with high sides and a safety belt, both of which are secured during transport.

Special care is needed in transporting critically ill patients in the hospital. Critically ill children should always be transported on a stretcher or bed (rather than carried) by at least two staff members with monitoring continued during transport. A blood pressure monitor (or standard blood pressure cuff), pulse oximeter, and cardiac monitor/defibrillator should accompany every patient (Warren, Fromm, Orr, et al, 2004). Airway equipment and emergency medications should accompany the patient.

RESTRAINING METHODS AND THERAPEUTIC HOLDING

The Joint Commission (2001) defines restraint as "any method, physical or mechanical, which restricts a person's movement, physical activity, or normal access to his or her body." Before initiating restraints, the nurse completes a comprehensive assessment of the patient to determine whether the need for a restraint outweighs the risk of not using one. Restraints can result in loss of dignity, violation of patient rights, psychologic harm, physical harm, and even death. Consider alternative methods first and document them in the patient's record. The nurse is responsible for selecting the least restrictive type of restraint (Table 27-5). Using less restrictive restraints is often possible by gaining the cooperation of the child and parents.

The two types of restraints used with children are classified as medical-surgical and behavioral restraints. When a standard or protocol states that immobilization is required 100% of the time as a part of the procedure or postprocedural care process, the restraint device is considered a part of routine care. For example, the postoperative use of elbow restraints after a cleft lip repair, if written in the protocol or standard of care and used for 100% of patients, would not fall under The Joint Commission or Centers for Medicare and Medicaid Services mandates concerning restraints.

Medical-surgical restraints are used for children with an artificial airway or airway adjunct for delivery of oxygen, indwelling catheters, tubes, drains, lines, pacemaker wires, or suture sites. The medical-surgical restraint is used to ensure that safe care is given to the patient. The potential risks of the restraint are offset by the potential benefit of providing safer care. Medical-surgical restraints may be instituted for any of the following reasons:

- Risk for interruption of therapy used to maintain oxygenation or airway patency
- Risk of harm if indwelling catheter, tube, drain, line, pacemaker wire, or sutures are removed, dislodged, or ruptured

TABLE 27-5	RESTRAINING CHILDREN: LESS RESTRICTIVE TO MORE RESTRICTIVE TECHNIQUES					
TECHNIQUE OR DEVICE	**LESS RESTRICTIVE TO MORE RESTRICTIVE**					
Extremities						
Sleeves	X					
Hand mitts, mittens	X					
Stockinette		X				
Elbows (no-no's)			X			
Arm board				X		
1-2 Limbs					X	
3-4 Limbs						X
Chest and Body						
Belts, safety belts	X					
Posey vest, safety jacket			X			
Mummy restraint						X
Papoose board						X
Environment						
Side rails			X			
Crib tops			X			
Seclusion						X
Other						
Chemical				X		

Adapted from Selekman J, Snyder B: Uses of and alternatives to restraints in pediatric settings, *AACN Clinical Issues* 7(4):603-610, 1996.

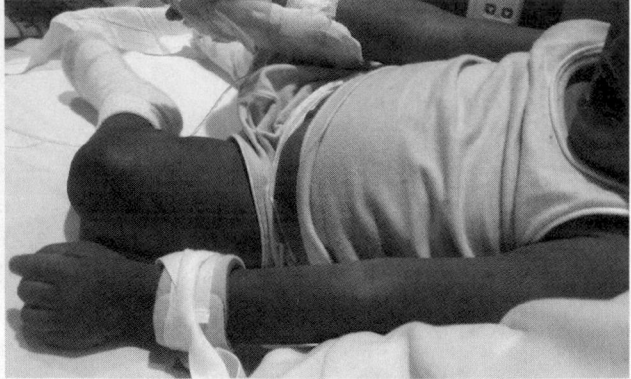

Fig. 27-6 Soft wrist restraints on young child. Wrist restraints must be padded and loose enough to prevent undue pressure, constriction, or tissue injury; and the extremity must be observed frequently for signs of irritation or impaired circulation.

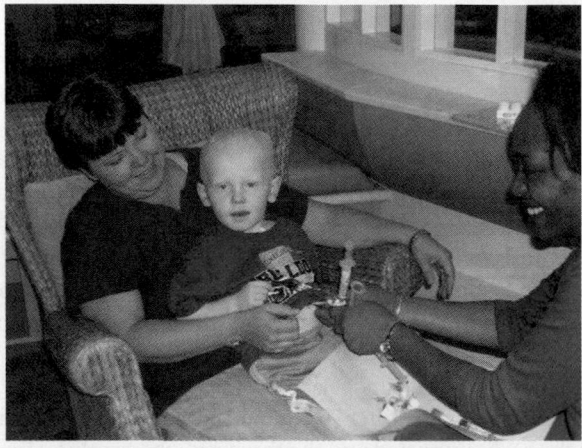

Fig. 27-7 Therapeutic holding by parent.

• Patient confusion, agitation, unconsciousness, or developmental inability to understand direct requests or instructions

Medical-surgical restraints can be initiated by an individual order or by protocol; the use of the protocol must be authorized by an individual order. The order for continued use of restraints must be renewed each day. Patients are monitored at least every 2 hours.

Behavioral restraints are limited to situations with a significant risk of patients physically harming themselves or others because of behavioral reasons and when nonphysical interventions are not effective. Before initiating a behavioral restraint, the nurse should assess the patient's mental, behavioral, and physical status to determine the cause for the child's potentially harmful behavior. If behavioral restraints are indicated, a collaborative approach involving the patient (if appropriate), the family, and the health care team should be used. An order must be obtained as soon as possible, but no longer than 1 hour after the initiation of behavioral restraints. Behavioral restraints for children must be reordered every 1 to 2 hours, based on age. A licensed independent practitioner must conduct an in-person evaluation within 1 hour and again every 4 hours until restraints are discontinued. Children in behavioral restraints must be *continuously* observed and assessed every 15 minutes. Assessment components include signs of injury associated with applying restraint, nutrition and hydration, circulation and range-of-motion of extremities, vital signs, hygiene and elimination, physical and psychologic status and comfort, and readiness for discontinuation of restraint. The nurse must use clinical judg-

ment in setting a schedule for when each of these parameters needs to be evaluated because every parameter must be assessed during each 15-minute physical assessment.

Restraints with ties must be secured to the bed or crib frame, not the side rails. Suggestions for increasing safety and comfort while the child is in a restraint include leaving one finger breadth between skin and the device (Fig. 27-6) and tying knots that allow for quick release. The nurse can also increase safety by ensuring the restraint does not tighten as the child moves and decreasing wrinkles or bulges in the restraint. Placing jacket restraints over an article of clothing; placing limb restraints below waist level, below knee level, or distal to the IV; and tucking in dangling straps also increase safety and comfort.

An alternative approach for temporary restraint is therapeutic holding. **Therapeutic holding** is the use of a secure, comfortable, temporary holding position that provides close physical contact with the parent or caregiver for 30 minutes or less (Fig. 27-7). The use of restraints can often be avoided with adequate preparation of the child; parental or staff supervision of the child; or adequate protection of a vulnerable site, such as an infusion device. The nurse needs to assess the child's development, mental status, potential to hurt others or self, and safety. The nurse should carefully consider alternative measures to using restraints. Some examples of alternative measures include bringing a child to the nurses' station for continuous

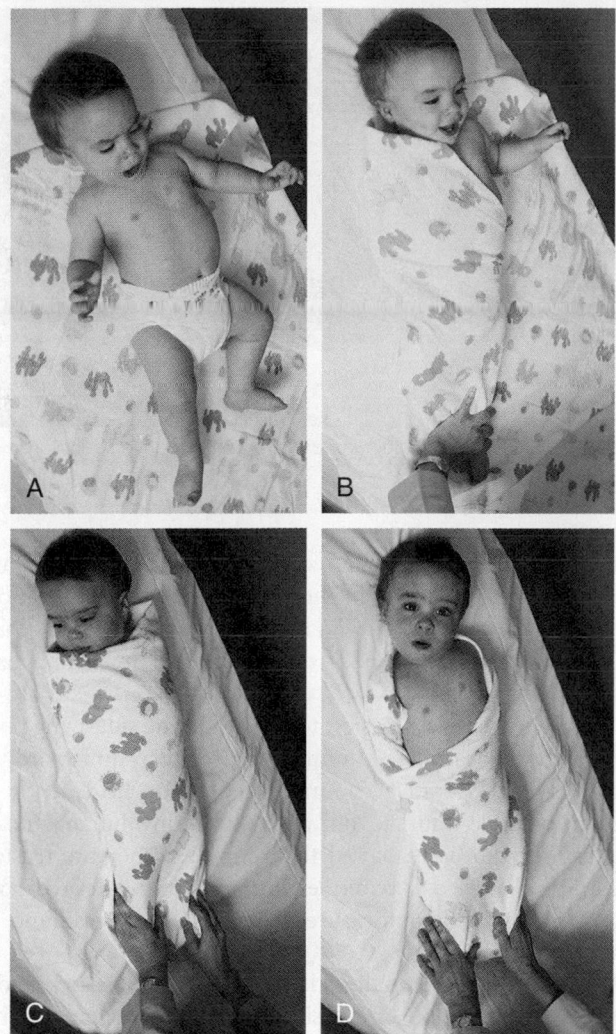

Fig. 27-8 Application of mummy restraint. **A,** Infant placed on folded corner of blanket. **B,** One corner of blanket brought across body and secured beneath body. **C,** Second corner brought across body and secured, and lower corner folded and tucked or pinned in place. **D,** Modified mummy restraint with chest uncovered.

observation, providing diversional activities, or encouraging the participation of the parents.

Mummy Restraint or Swaddle

When an infant or small child requires short-term restraint for examination or treatment that involves the head and neck (e.g., venipuncture, throat examination, gavage feeding), a papoose board with straps or a mummy wrap effectively controls the child's movements. A blanket or sheet is opened on the bed or crib with one corner folded to the center. The infant is placed on the blanket with shoulders at the fold and feet toward the opposite corner (Fig. 27-8, *A*). With the infant's right arm straight down against the body, the right side of the blanket is pulled firmly across the infant's right shoulder and chest and secured beneath the left side of the body (Fig. 27-8, *B*). The left arm is placed straight against the infant's side, and the left side of the blanket is brought across the shoulder and chest and locked beneath the body on the right side (Fig. 27-8, *C*). The lower corner is folded and brought over the body and tucked or fastened securely with safety pins. Safety pins can be used to fasten the blanket in place at any step in the process.

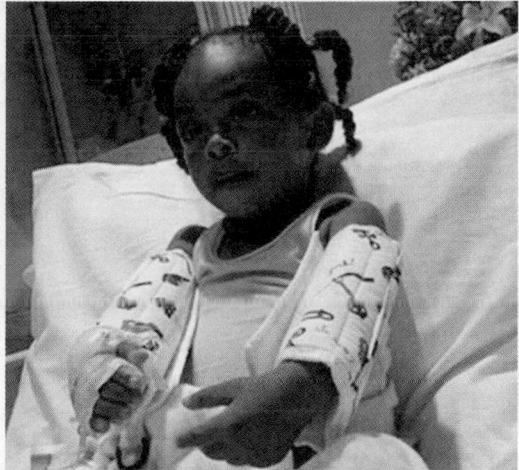

Fig. 27-9 The most common form of elbow restraint consists of a firm material that is padded and reaches comfortably from just below axilla to wrist.

To modify the mummy restraint for chest examination, bring the folded edge of the blanket over each arm and under the back, and then fold the loose edge over and secure it at a point below the chest to allow visualization and access to the chest (Fig. 27-8, *D*).

Jacket Restraint

A jacket restraint is sometimes used to keep the child safe in various chairs. The jacket is put on the child with the ties in back so that the child is unable to manipulate them. The jacket restraint is also useful as a means for maintaining the child in a desired horizontal position. The long tapes, secured to the understructure of the crib, keep the child inside the crib.

Arm and Leg Restraints

Occasionally the nurse needs to restrain one or more extremities or limit their motion. Several commercial restraining devices are available, including disposable wrist and ankle restraints. Restraints must be appropriate to the child's size and padded to prevent undue pressure, constriction, or tissue injury; and the extremity must be observed frequently for signs of irritation or impaired circulation. The ends of the restraints are never tied to the side rails, since lowering the rail will disturb the extremity, frequently with a jerk that may hurt or injure the child.

Elbow Restraint

Sometimes it is important to prevent the child from reaching the head or face (e.g., after lip surgery or when a scalp vein infusion is in place or to prevent scratching in skin disorders). Elbow restraints fashioned from a variety of materials function well (Fig. 27-9). Commercial elbow restraints are available. An improvised form of elbow restraint consists of a piece of muslin long enough to reach comfortably from just below the axilla to the wrist, with a number of vertical pockets into which tongue depressors are inserted. The restraint is wrapped around the arm and secured with tapes or pins. It may be necessary to pin the top of the restraint to the undershirt sleeve to prevent the restraint from slipping.

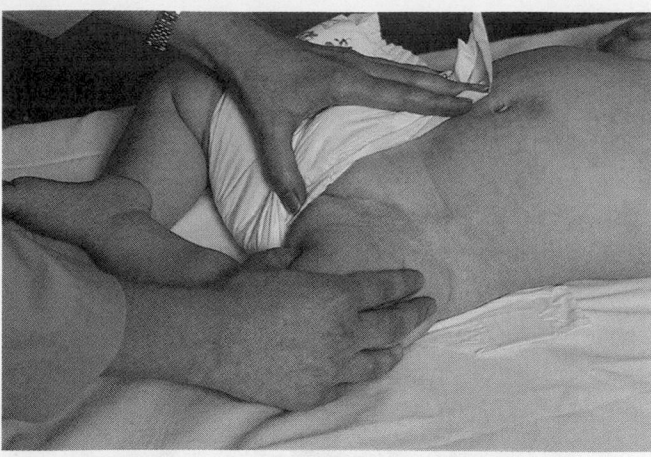

Fig. 27-10 Positioning infant for femoral venipuncture.

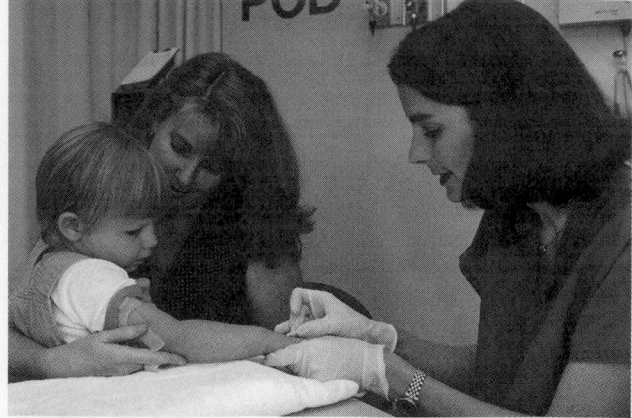

Fig. 27-11 Therapeutic holding of child for extremity venipuncture with parental assistance.

POSITIONING FOR PROCEDURES

Infants and small children are unable to cooperate for many procedures. Therefore the nurse is responsible for minimizing their movement and discomfort with proper positioning. Older children usually need only minimal, if any, restraint. Careful explanation and preparation beforehand and support and simple guidance during the procedure are usually sufficient. For painful procedures the child should receive adequate analgesia and sedation to minimize pain and the need for excessive restraint. For local anesthesia, use buffered lidocaine to reduce the stinging sensation or a topical anesthetic. (See Pain Management, Chapter 7.)

FEMORAL VENIPUNCTURE

The nurse places the child supine with the legs in a frog position to provide extensive exposure of the groin area. The infant's legs can be effectively controlled by the nurse's forearms and hands (Fig. 27-10). Only the side used for the venipuncture is uncovered so that the practitioner is protected should the child urinate during the procedure. Apply pressure to the site to prevent oozing from the site.

EXTREMITY VENIPUNCTURE

The most common sites of venipuncture are the veins of the extremities, especially the arm and hand. A convenient position is to place the child in the parent's (or assistant's) lap, with the child facing the parent and in the straddle position. Next, place the child's arm for venipuncture on a firm surface, such as a treatment table. The nurse can partially stabilize the child's outstretched arm and have the parent hug the child's upper body, preventing movement; the nurse can then use the parent's arm to immobilize the venipuncture site. This type of restraint also comforts the child because of the close body contact and allows each person to maintain eye contact (Fig. 27-11).

LUMBAR PUNCTURE

Pediatric lumbar puncture (LP) sets contain smaller spinal needles, but sometimes the practitioner will specify a different size or type of needle. The technique for LP in infants and children is similar to that in the adult, although modifications are suggested in neonates, who have less distress in a side-lying position with modified neck extension than in flexion or a sitting position.

Children are usually easiest to control in the side-lying position, with the head flexed and the knees drawn up toward the chest. Even cooperative children need to be held gently to prevent possible trauma from unexpected, involuntary movement. They can be reassured that, although they are trusted, holding will serve as a reminder to maintain the desired position. It also provides a measure of support and reassurance to them.

The child is placed on the side with the back close to the edge of the examining table on the side from which the practitioner is working. Maintain the child's spine in a flexed position by holding the child with one arm behind the neck and the other behind the thighs (Fig. 27-12, *A*). The flexed position enlarges the spaces between the lumbar vertebrae, which facilitates access to the spinal fluid space. It is helpful to wrap the legs before positioning to decrease leg movement.

An alternate position used with small infants and some older children is the sitting position. The child is placed with the buttocks at the edge of the table and with the neck flexed so that the chin rests on the child's chest or the nurse's shoulder. The nurse's hands immobilize the infant's arms and legs (Fig. 27-12, *B*).

> **! NURSING ALERT**
>
> The sitting position may interfere with chest expansion and diaphragm excursion, and in infants the soft, pliable trachea may collapse. Therefore observe the child for difficulty with breathing.

Specimens and spinal fluid pressure are obtained, measured, and sent for analysis in the same manner as for the adult patient. Take vital signs as ordered, and observe the child for any changes in level of consciousness, motor activity, or other neurologic signs. Post-LP headache may occur and is related to postural changes; this is less severe when the child lies flat. Headache is seen much less frequently in young children than in adolescents.

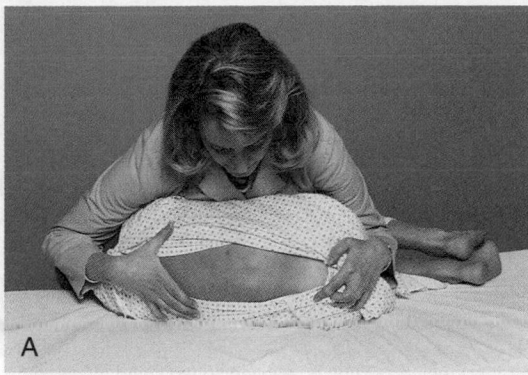

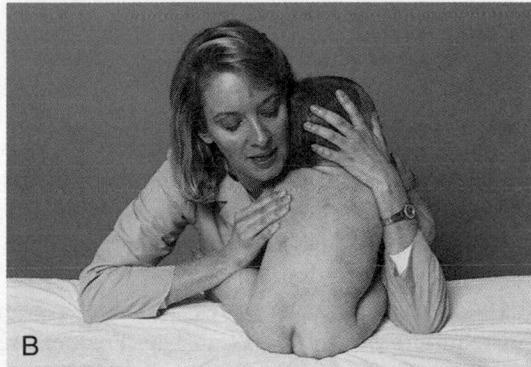

Fig. 27-12 A, Side-lying position for lumbar puncture. **B,** Infant sitting position allows flexion of lumbar spine.

BONE MARROW ASPIRATION OR BIOPSY

The position for a bone marrow aspiration or biopsy depends on the chosen site. In children the posterior or anterior iliac crest is most frequently used, although in infants the tibia may be selected because it is easy to access the site and hold the child.

If the posterior iliac crest is used, the child is positioned prone. Sometimes a small pillow or folded blanket is placed under the hips to facilitate obtaining the bone marrow specimen. Children should receive adequate analgesia or anesthesia to relieve pain. If the child might awaken, he or she may need to be held, preferably by two people—one person to immobilize the upper body and a second person to immobilize the lower extremities.

COLLECTION OF SPECIMENS

Many of the specimens needed for diagnostic examination of children are collected in much the same way as they are for adults. Older children are able to cooperate if given proper instruction regarding what is expected of them. Infants and small children, however, are unable to follow directions or control body functions sufficiently to help in collecting some specimens.

URINE SPECIMENS

Older children and adolescents can use a bedpan or urinal or can be trusted to follow directions for collection in the bathroom. However, they may have special needs. School-age children are cooperative but curious. They are concerned about the reasons behind things and are likely to ask questions regarding the disposition of their specimen and what one expects to discover from it. Self-conscious adolescents may be reluctant to carry a specimen through a hallway or waiting room and appreciate a paper bag for disguising the container. The presence of menses may be an embarrassment or a concern to teenage girls; therefore it is a good idea to ask them about this and make adjustments as necessary. The specimen can be delayed or a notation made on the laboratory slip to explain the presence of red blood cells.

Preschoolers and toddlers are usually unable to void on request. It is often best to offer them water or other liquids that they enjoy and wait about 30 minutes until they are ready to void voluntarily.

> **NURSING TIP** In infants wipe the abdomen with an alcohol pad and fan it dry; the cooling effect often causes voiding within 2 minutes. Apply pressure over the suprapubic area or stroke the paraspinal muscles (along the spine) to elicit the Perez reflex; in infants 4 to 6 months of age, this reflex causes crying, extension of the back, flexion of the extremities, and urination.

Children will better understand what is expected if the nurse uses familiar terms, such as "pee-pee," "wee-wee," or "tinkle." Some have difficulty voiding in an unfamiliar receptacle. Potty chairs or a potty hat placed on the toilet is usually satisfactory. Toddlers who have recently acquired bladder control may be especially reluctant, since they undoubtedly have been admonished for "going" in places other than those approved by parents. Enlisting the parents' help usually leads to success. For infants and toddlers who are not toilet trained, special urine collection bags with self-adhering material around the opening at the point of attachment are used. To prepare the infant, the genitalia, perineum, and surrounding skin are washed and dried thoroughly, since the adhesive will not stick to a moist, powdered, or oily skin surface. The collection bag is easiest to apply if attached first to the perineum, progressing to the symphysis pubis (Fig. 27-13). With girls the perineum is stretched taut during application to ensure a leakproof fit. With boys the penis and sometimes the scrotum are placed inside the bag. The adhesive portion of the bag must be firmly applied to the skin all around the genital area to avoid leakage. For low-birth-weight infants, small bags with adhesive that is gentle to the skin are available.* The diaper is carefully replaced. The bag is checked frequently and removed as soon as the specimen is available, since the moist bag may become loosened on an active child. For some types of urine testing, such as specific gravity, ketones, glucose, and protein, the nurse can aspirate urine directly from the diaper. If the urine is not tested within 30 minutes, the specimen is refrigerated or placed in a sterile container with a preservative.

Urine obtained from disposable diapers can be tested accurately for glucose, ketones, protein, blood, and urea. Super-absorbent disposable diapers may absorb all urine and may also produce a false crystalluria. Specific gravity measurements are accurate for up to 4 hours provided that the disposable diapers

*Available from Hollister, Inc., 2000 Hollister Drive, Libertyville, IL 60048; 888-740-8999; **www.hollister.com**.

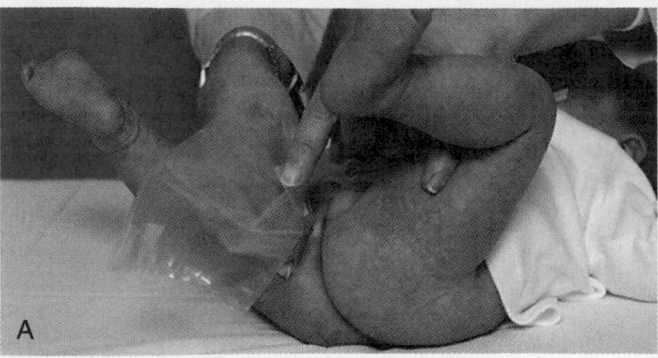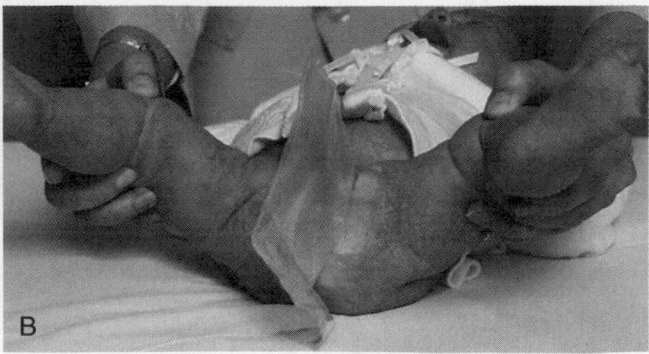

Fig. 27-13 Application of urine collection bag. **A,** On female infants, adhesive portion is applied to exposed and dried perineum first. **B,** Bag adheres firmly around perineal area to prevent urine leakage.

> **NURSING TIP** When using a urine collection bag, cut a small slit in the diaper and pull the bag through to allow room for urine to collect and to facilitate checking on the contents. To obtain small amounts of urine, use a syringe without a needle to aspirate urine directly from the diaper. If diapers with absorbent gelling material that trap urine are used, place a small gauze dressing, some cotton balls, or a urine collection device inside the diaper to collect urine and aspirate the urine with a syringe.

are kept folded. Urine samples collected by the cotton ball method were accurate for pH and specific gravity and were atraumatic to the skin of newborns (Burke, 1995).

At times parents may be asked to bring a urine sample to a health care facility for examination, especially when infants are unable to void during an outpatient visit. In this instance parents need instructions on applying the collection device and storing the specimen. Ideally, the specimen should be brought to the designated place as soon as possible. If there is a delay, the sample should be refrigerated and the lapsed time reported to the examiner.

Clean-Catch Specimens

Clean-catch specimen traditionally refers to a urine sample obtained for culture after the urethral meatus is cleaned and the first few milliliters of urine are voided (midstream specimen). In females the perineum is wiped with an antiseptic-soaked cotton ball or pad from front to back at least three times, using a new cotton ball or pad each time. In males the tip of the penis is cleansed. The area may be wiped with sterile water to prevent accidental contamination of the urine with a solution that may destroy pathogens.

Twenty-Four-Hour Collection

For a 24-hour collection, collection bags are required in infants and small children. Older children require special instruction about notifying someone when they need to void or have a bowel movement so that urine can be collected separately and is not discarded. Some older school-age children and adolescents can take responsibility for collection of their own 24-hour specimens and can keep output records and transfer each voiding to the 24-hour collection container.

The collection period always starts and ends with an empty bladder. At the time the collection begins, instruct the child to

void and discard the specimen. All urine voided in the subsequent 24 hours is saved in a container with a preservative or is placed on ice. Twenty-four hours from the time the precollection specimen was discarded, the child is again instructed to void, the specimen is added to the container, and the entire collection is taken to the laboratory.

Infants and small children who are bagged for 24-hour urine collection require a special collection bag. Frequent removal and replacement of adhesive collection devices can produce skin irritation. A thin coating of sealant, such as Skin-Prep, applied to the skin helps to protect it and aids adhesion (unless its use is contraindicated, such as in a premature infant or a child with irritated skin). Plastic collection bags with collection tubes attached are ideal when the container must be left in place for a time. These can be connected to a collecting device or emptied periodically by aspiration with a syringe. When such devices are not available, a regular bag with a feeding tube inserted through a puncture hole at the top of the bag serves as a satisfactory substitute. However, take care to empty the bag as soon as the infant urinates to prevent leakage and loss of contents. An indwelling catheter may also be placed for the collection period.

Bladder Catheterization and Other Techniques

Bladder catheterization or suprapubic aspiration is employed when a specimen is urgently needed or a child is unable to void or otherwise provide an adequate specimen. In young infants less than 3 months of age who are febrile, urine specimens should be collected by bladder catheterization (McGillivray, Mok, Mulrooney, et al, 2008). (See Evidence-Based Practice box in Chapter 30, p. 1146.) The American Academy of Pediatrics recommends that urine collected by the bag can be used to determine whether it is necessary to obtain a catheterized urine specimen for culture (Wald, 2005).

Preparation for catheterization includes instruction on pelvic muscle relaxation whenever possible. The toddler, preschooler, or younger child should blow on a pinwheel and press the hips against the bed or procedure table during catheterization to relax the pelvic and periurethral muscles. The nurse describes the location and function of the pelvic muscles briefly to the older child or adolescent. The patient then contracts and relaxes the pelvic muscles, and the relaxation procedure is repeated during catheter insertion. If the patient vigorously contracts the pelvic muscles when the catheter reaches the striated sphincter (proximal urethra in boys and midurethra in girls), catheter insertion is temporarily stopped. The catheter is neither removed nor advanced; instead, the child is helped to press the hips against the bed or examining table and relax the pelvic muscles. The catheter is then gently advanced into the bladder (Gray, 1996).

Catheterization is a sterile procedure, and Standard Precautions for body substance protection should be followed. When placing a catheter to obtain a sterile urine specimen or to check for residual urine, the nurse may use a sterile feeding tube if an appropriately sized catheter is unavailable. If the catheter is to remain in place, a Foley catheter is used. Table 27-6 gives guidelines for choosing the appropriate-size catheter and length of insertion. The supplies needed for this procedure include sterile gloves, sterile lubricant anesthetic, the appropriate-size catheter, povidone-iodine (Betadine) swabs or an alternative cleansing agent and 4 × 4-inch gauze squares, a sterile drape, and a syringe with sterile water if a Foley catheter is used. Test the balloon of the Foley catheter by injecting sterile water before catheter insertion.

Adolescent boys and children with a history of urethral surgery may be catheterized with a coudé-tipped catheter. The child with myelodysplasia or one who has been identified as being sensitive or allergic to latex is catheterized with a catheter manufactured from an alternative material. When an indwelling catheter is indicated for urinary drainage, a lubricious-coated or silicone catheter is selected because these materials produce less irritation of the urethral mucosa compared with a Silastic or latex catheter when the catheter is left in place for more than 72 hours.

A 2% lidocaine lubricant with applicator is assembled according to the manufacturer's instructions, and several drops of the lubricant are placed at the meatus. The child is advised that the lubricant is used to reduce any discomfort associated with inserting the catheter and that introduction of the catheter into the urethra will produce a sensation of pressure and a desire to urinate (Gray, 1996) (see Evidence-Based Practice box).

TABLE 27-6	STRAIGHT CATHETER OR FOLEY CATHETER*	
	SIZE (LENGTH OF INSERTION [cm]) FOR GIRLS	SIZE (LENGTH OF INSERTION [cm]) FOR BOYS
Term neonate	5-6 (5)	5-6 (6)
Infant–3 yr	5-8 (5)	5-8 (6)
4-8 yr	8 (5-6)	8 (6-9)
8 yr–prepubertal	10-12 (6-8)	8-10 (10-15)
Pubertal	12-14 (6-8)	12-14 (13-18)

*Foley catheters are approximately 1 French size larger because of circumference of balloon. Example: 10 French Foley = approximately 12 French calibration.

EVIDENCE-BASED PRACTICE

The Use of Lidocaine Lubricant for Urethral Catheterization

ASK THE QUESTION

In children does a lidocaine lubricant decrease the pain associated with urethral catheterization?

SEARCH FOR THE EVIDENCE

Search strategies

Search selection criteria included English language publications, research-based studies, and review articles on use of the lidocaine lubricant before urethral catheterization.

Databases used

Cochrane Collaboration, PubMed, MD Consult, BestBETs, American Academy of Pediatrics

CRITICALLY ANALYZE THE EVIDENCE

GRADE criteria: Evidence quality moderate; recommendation weak (Guyatt, Oxman, Vist, et al, 2008)

- Smith and Adams (1998) surveyed 46 children's hospitals to determine the existence of standardized practice guidelines for urethral catheter insertion in children. Only 54% of the institutions had a written policy providing guidelines for the procedure, and practices had wide variations.
- Gray (1996) published a review of strategies to minimize distress associated with urethral catheterization in children and supported intraurethral instillation of a local anesthetic that contains 2% lidocaine before catheter insertion.
- One prospective, double-blind, placebo-controlled trial evaluated the use of lidocaine lubricant for discomfort in 20 children before urethral catheterization. Lidocaine lubricant instilled into the urethra significantly reduced pain and distress during urethral catheterization (Gerard, Cooper, Duethman, et al, 2003).
- A placebo-controlled, double-blind, randomized controlled trial of 115 children less than 2 years of age found no significant difference when 2% lidocaine gel was compared to a nonanesthetic lubricant. The lubricant was applied to the genital mucosa for 2 to 3 minutes and liberally applied to the catheter, but not instilled into the urethra (Vaughn, Paton, Bush, et al, 2005).

APPLY THE EVIDENCE: NURSING IMPLICATIONS

- Although only one published research study was found to support the use of anesthetic before urethral catheterization, the study found significant reductions in procedural pain. Several publications support its effectiveness in clinical practice.
- When possible, transurethral instillation of 2% lidocaine gel before urethral catheterization may be considered.

References

Gerard LL, Cooper CS, Duethman KS, et al: Effectiveness of lidocaine lubricant for discomfort during pediatric urethral catheterization, *J Urol* 170:564-567, 2003.

Gray M: Atraumatic urethral catheterization of children, *Pediatr Nurs* 22(4):306-310, 1996.

Guyatt GH, Oxman AD, Vist GE, et al: GRADE: an emerging consensus on rating quality of evidence and strength of recommendations, *BMJ* 336:924-926, 2008.

Smith AB, Adams LL: Insertion of indwelling urethral catheters in infants and children: a survey of current nursing practice, *Pediatr Nurs* 24(3):229-234, 1998.

Vaughn H, Paton EA, Bush A, et al: Does lidocaine gel alleviate the pain of bladder catheterization in young children? A randomized, controlled trial, *Pediatrics* 116(4):917-920, 2005.

In male patients, grasp the penis with the nondominant hand and retract the foreskin. In uncircumcised newborns and infants, the foreskin may be adhered to the shaft; use care when retracting. If the penis is pendulous, place a sterile drape under the penis. Using the sterile hand, swab the glans and meatus three times with povidone-iodine. Gently introduce the tip of the lidocaine jelly applicator into the urethra 1 to 2 cm (0.4 to 0.8 inch) so that the lubricant flows only into the urethra; insert 5 to 10 ml 2% lidocaine lubricant into the urethra and hold in place for 2 to 3 minutes by gently squeezing the distal penis. Lubricate the catheter and insert into the urethra while gently stretching the penis and lifting it to a 90-degree angle to the body. Resistance may occur when the catheter meets the urethral sphincter. Ask the patient to inhale deeply and advance the catheter. Do not force a catheter that does not easily enter the meatus, particularly if the child has had corrective surgery. For indwelling catheters, once urine is obtained, advance the catheter to the hub, inflate the balloon with sterile water, pull it back gently to test inflation, and connect it to the closed drainage system. Cleanse the glans and meatus and replace retracted foreskin. If blood is seen at any time during the procedure, discontinue the procedure and notify the practitioner.

In female patients, place a sterile drape under the buttocks. Use the nondominant hand to gently separate and pull up the labia minora to visualize the meatus. Swab the meatus from front to back three times, using a different povidone-iodine swab each time. Place 1 to 2 ml 2% lidocaine lubricant on the periurethral mucosa, and insert the lubricant 1 to 2 ml into the urethral meatus. Delay catheterization for 2 to 3 minutes to maximize absorption of the anesthetic into the periurethral and intraurethral mucosa. Add lubricant to the catheter, and gently insert it into the urethra until urine returns; then advance the catheter an additional 2.5 to 5 cm (1 to 2 inches). When using an indwelling Foley catheter, inflate the balloon with sterile water and gently pull back, then connect to a closed drainage system. Cleanse the meatus and labia (see Cultural Competence box). Because the use of lidocaine jelly can increase the volume of intraurethral lubricant, urine return may not be as rapid as when minimal lubrication is used.

⊕ CULTURAL COMPETENCE

Bladder Catheterization

Parents may be upset when their child is catheterized. Aside from the trauma the child experiences, some parents may fear that the procedure affects the daughter's virginity. To correct this misconception, the family may benefit from a detailed explanation of the genitourinary anatomy, preferably with a model that shows the separate vaginal and urethral openings. The nurse can also indicate that catheterization has no effect on virginity.

Suprapubic aspiration is mainly used when the bladder cannot be accessed through the urethra (such as with some congenital urologic birth defects) or to reduce the risk of contamination that may be present when passing a catheter. With the advent of small catheters (5 and 6 French straight catheters), the need for suprapubic aspiration has decreased. Access to the bladder via the urethra has a much higher success rate than suprapubic aspiration, where success depends on the practi-

tioner's skill at assessing the location of the bladder and the amount of urine in the bladder.

Suprapubic aspiration involves aspirating bladder contents by inserting a 20- or 21-gauge needle in the midline approximately 1 cm (0.4 inch) above the symphysis pubis and directed vertically downward. The nurse prepares the skin as for any needle insertion, and the bladder should contain an adequate volume of urine. This can be assumed if the infant has not voided for at least 1 hour or the bladder can be palpated above the symphysis pubis. This technique is useful for obtaining sterile specimens from young infants, since the bladder is an abdominal organ and is easily accessed. Suprapubic aspiration is painful, and therefore pain management during the procedure is important (see Atraumatic Care box).

ATRAUMATIC CARE

Bladder Catheterization or Suprapubic Aspiration

- Use distraction to help the child relax (blowing bubbles, deep breathing, singing a song).
- Use lidocaine jelly to anesthetize the area before insertion of the catheter. EMLA cream (a eutectic mix of lidocaine and prilocaine) or LMX cream (lidocaine) may lessen an infant's discomfort as the needle passes through the skin for suprapubic aspiration, but care should be taken that the site is thoroughly cleaned and prepped before the procedure.
- Children often become agitated at being restrained for either procedure. Use comfort measures through touch and voice, both during and after the procedure, to help reduce the child's distress.

STOOL SPECIMENS

Stool specimens are frequently collected from children to identify parasites and other organisms that cause diarrhea, to assess gastrointestinal function, and to check for occult (hidden) blood. Ideally, stool should be collected without contamination with urine, but in children wearing diapers, this is difficult unless a urine bag is applied. Children who are toilet trained should urinate first, flush the toilet, and then defecate into the toilet or a bedpan (preferably one that is placed on the toilet to avoid embarrassment) or a commercial potty hat.

NURSING TIP To obtain a stool specimen, place plastic wrap over the toilet bowl before defecation. Use a tongue depressor or disposable spoon or knife to collect the stool.

Stool specimens should be large enough to obtain an ample sampling, not merely a fecal fragment. Specimens are placed in an appropriate container, which is covered and labeled. If several specimens are needed, mark the containers with the date and time and keep them in a specimen refrigerator. Exercise care in handling the specimen because of the risk of contamination.

BLOOD SPECIMENS

Whether the specimen is collected by the nurse or by others, the nurse is responsible for making certain that specimens, such as serial examinations and fasting specimens, are collected on time and that the proper equipment is available. Collecting, transporting, and storing specimens can have a major impact on laboratory results.

Venous blood samples can be obtained by venipuncture or by aspiration from a peripheral or central access device. Withdrawing blood specimens through peripheral lock devices in small peripheral veins has varying degrees of success. Although it avoids an additional venipuncture for the child, attempting to aspirate blood from the peripheral lock may shorten the life of the device. However, the nurse can use central lines to withdraw blood samples (see Fig. 27-14, Evidence-Based Practice box, and Atraumatic Care box). When using an IV infusion site for specimen collection, consider the type of fluid being infused. For example, a specimen collected for glucose determination would be inaccurate if removed from a

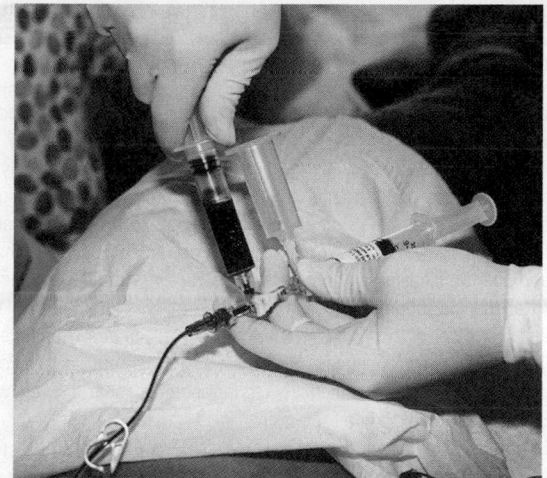

Fig. 27-14 Drawing blood from a central line.

EVIDENCE-BASED PRACTICE
Joy Hesselgrave

Obtaining Blood Specimens from Central Venous Catheters in Children

ASK THE QUESTION

In children, do blood specimens obtained from central venous catheters using the discard, reinfusion, or push-pull method yield more accurate samples?

SEARCH FOR THE EVIDENCE

Search strategies

Search selection criteria included English language research-based publications on pediatric blood specimen collection from central venous access.

Databases used

National Guideline Clearinghouse (AHRQ), Cochrane Collaboration, Joanna Briggs Institute, PubMed, TRIP Database Plus, MD Consult, PedsCCM, BestBETs

CRITICALLY ANALYZE THE EVIDENCE

GRADE criteria: Evidence quality very low; recommendation weak (Guyatt, Oxman, Vist, et al, 2008)

Limited scientific research exists that describes the optimal method for drawing blood samples from central venous access devices (VADs) in the pediatric patient.

A convenience sample of paired specimens compared blood drawn from central lines via push-pull method and discard method on 28 pediatric patients 6 months to 12 years of age. Of the 438 pairs of measurements that were compared, 420, or 95.9%, were within limits of agreement for hemograms, electrolytes, and glucose. The push-pull method eliminates loss of blood and decreases the amount of times the central line is accessed (Barton, Chase, Latham, et al, 2004).

Forty-two nonneutropenic pediatric patients ages 2 to 20 years were randomly assigned to one of two syringe-handling methods for blood sampling. The discard specimen, routinely reinfused, was collected using the usual clean procedure and an exaggerated unclean alternative procedure. Neither the sterile specimens nor the unclean specimens grew organisms, thus suggesting that the reinfusion of the blood specimen would be safe. This study did not evaluate for clots in the discard specimen (Hinds, Wentz, Hughes, et al, 1991).

Thirty bone marrow transplant units were surveyed to evaluate how blood samples were drawn from central VADs. The average patient age was 5 to 16 years old. Seventy-five percent of the units used the discard method, with the volume of discard ranging from 0.5 to 10 ml and an average of 4 to 6 ml. Fourteen percent used the reinfusion method, and 11% used the push-pull or mixing method (Keller, 1994).

The Infusion Nurses Society (2006) recommends that the discard method be used when drawing blood samples from central VADs. The discard volume should be 1.5 to 2 times the fill volume of the central VAD.

Frey (2003) summarizes evidence for the practice of all three blood sampling methods. The discard method is most widely reported, with disadvantages including blood loss, blood exposure risk for clinicians, and the potential to mistake the discard specimen for the blood sample. The reinfusion method does not deplete blood volume but risks blood exposure for clinicians and has the potential for reinfusing a contaminated specimen or clots in the discard volume. The push-pull or mixing method demonstrates accuracy for studies other than coagulation and drug levels and reduces blood loss and clinician exposure risk.

APPLY THE EVIDENCE: NURSING IMPLICATIONS

- There is limited pediatric research that clearly supports any particular central line blood sampling method as being superior. All three methods yield accurate results and appear safe. The discard method is the most frequently reported in the literature and benchmarking. However, if there is a concern about blood volume, the push-pull or reinfusion method should be considered.
- Attach a syringe or stopcock depending on specimen method selected, to the injection cap, not directly to the catheter hub. The injection cap at the catheter hub should be removed only if blood cultures are drawn.

References

Barton S, Chase T, Latham B, et al: Comparing two methods to obtain blood specimens from pediatric central venous catheters, *J Pediatr Oncol Nurs* 21(6):320-326, 2004.

Frey M: Drawing blood samples from vascular access devices, *J Infus Nurs* 26(5):285-293, 2003.

Guyatt GH, Oxman AD, Vist GE, et al: GRADE: an emerging consensus on rating quality of evidence and strength of recommendations, *BMJ* 336:924-926, 2008.

Hinds PS, Wentz T, Hughes W, et al: An investigation of the safety of the blood reinfusion step used with tunneled venous access devices in children with cancer, *J Pediatr Oncol Nurs* 8(4):59-64, 1991.

Infusion Nurses Society: *Policies and procedures for infusion nursing*, ed 3, South Norwood, Mass, 2006, The Society.

Keller CA: Methods of drawing blood samples through central venous catheters in pediatric patients undergoing bone marrow transplant: results of a national survey, *Oncol Nurs Forum* 21(5):879-884, 1994.

ATRAUMATIC CARE

Guidelines for Skin and Vessel Punctures

To reduce the pain associated with heel, finger, venous, or arterial punctures:

- Apply EMLA (a eutectic mix of lidocaine and prilocaine) topically over the site if time permits (≥60 minutes). LMX cream (lidocaine) also may be used and requires a shorter application time (30 minutes). To remove the transparent dressing atraumatically, grasp opposite sides of the film and pull the sides away from each other to stretch and loosen the film. After the film begins to loosen, grasp the other two sides of the film and pull. Use iontophoresis (Numby Stuff) over the site if time permits (8 to 20 minutes, depending on the amount of current), a vapocoolant spray, or buffered lidocaine (injected intradermally near the vein with a 30-gauge needle) to numb the skin.
- Use nonpharmacologic methods of pain and anxiety control (e.g., ask child to take a deep breath when the needle is inserted and again when the needle is withdrawn, to exhale a large breath or blow bubbles to "blow hurt away," or to count slowly and then faster and louder if pain is felt).
- Keep all equipment out of sight until used.
- Enlist parents' presence or assistance if they wish.
- Restrain child *only as needed* to perform the procedure safely; use therapeutic holding (p. 1022).
- Allow the skin preparation to dry completely before penetrating the skin.
- Use the smallest-gauge needle (e.g., 25 gauge) that permits free flow of blood; a 27-gauge needle can be used for obtaining 1 to 1.5 ml of blood and for prominent veins (needle length is only 1.25 cm [0.5 inch]).
- If possible, avoid putting an intravenous (IV) line in the dominant hand or the hand the child uses to suck the thumb.
- Use an automatic lancet device for precise puncture depth of the finger or heel; press the device lightly against the skin; avoid steadying the finger against a hard surface.
- Have a "two-try" only policy to reduce excessive insertion attempts— two operators each have two insertion attempts. ⊖ If insertion is not successful after four punctures, consider alternative venous access, such as a peripherally inserted central catheter (PICC); have a policy for identifying children with difficult access and appropriate interventions (e.g., most experienced operator for the first attempt, use transilluminator or ultrasound for insertion guidance).

For Multiple Blood Samples

Use an intermittent infusion device (saline lock) to collect additional samples from an existing IV line; consider PICC lines early, not as a last resort.

Coordinate care to allow several tests to be performed on one blood sample using micromethods of testing.

Anticipate tests (e.g., drug levels, chemistry, immunoglobulin levels) and ask the laboratory to save blood for additional testing.

For Heel Lancing in Newborns

Heel lancing has shown to be more painful than venipuncture (Shah and Ohlsson, 2007); consider venipuncture when the amount of blood from the heel would require much squeezing (e.g., genetic screening tests).

The effectiveness of EMLA is controversial, although application of 0.5 g for 30 minutes four times a day in preterm infants was found to be safe (Essink-Tebbes, Wuis, Liem, et al, 1999).

Place diapered newborn against mother's bare chest in skin-to-skin contact 10 to 15 minutes before and during heel lance (Gray, Watt, and Blass, 2000).

During the procedure, administer sucrose and encourage the newborn to suck a pacifier. When commercially manufactured 24% sucrose solution is unavailable, add 1 tsp of table sugar to 4 tsp of sterile water. Use this solution to coat the pacifier or administer 2 ml to the tongue 2 minutes before the procedure. (See Evidence-Based Practice Box, Reduction of Minor Procedural Pain in Infants, Chapter 7.)

One study found that breastfeeding during a neonatal heel lance was more effective than sucrose in reducing pain (Codipietro, Ceccarelli, and Ponzone, 2008).

catheter through which glucose-containing solution was being administered.

The needed specimens are quickly collected, and pressure is applied to the puncture site with dry gauze until bleeding stops. The arm should be extended, not flexed, while pressure is applied for a few minutes after venipuncture in the antecubital fossa to reduce bruising. The nurse then covers the site with an adhesive bandage. In young children, adhesive bandages pose an aspiration hazard, so avoid using them or remove the adhesive bandage as soon as the bleeding stops. Applying warm compresses to ecchymotic areas increases circulation, helps remove extravasated blood, and decreases pain.

Arterial blood samples are sometimes needed for blood gas measurement, although noninvasive techniques, such as transcutaneous oxygen monitoring and pulse oximetry, are used frequently. Arterial samples may be obtained by arterial puncture using the radial, brachial, or femoral arteries, or from indwelling arterial catheters. Assess adequate circulation before arterial puncture by observing capillary refill or performing the Allen test, a procedure that assesses the circulation of the radial, ulnar, or brachial arteries. (See Blood Gas Determination, Chapter 31.) Because unclotted blood is required, use only heparinized collection tubes or syringes. In addition, no air bubbles should enter the tube because they can alter blood gas concentration. Crying, fear, and agitation affect blood gas values; therefore make every effort to comfort the child. Pack the blood samples in ice to reduce blood cell metabolism and take it to the laboratory immediately.

NURSING TIP To obtain a blood specimen from a central venous line or peripheral lock when the infusion solution may interfere with the test results, first aspirate a quantity of blood equal to the volume of fluid in the catheter and discard; then aspirate the blood sample. For a blood culture, use the first sample of blood, since organisms are most likely to collect within the catheter itself.

Take capillary blood samples from children by finger stick. A common method for taking peripheral blood samples from infants younger than 6 months of age is by a heel stick. Before the blood sample is taken, warm the heel for 3 minutes and cleanse the area with alcohol. Holding the infant's foot firmly with the free hand, the nurse then punctures the heel with an automatic lancet device. An automatic device delivers a more precise puncture depth and is less painful than using a lance (Vertanen, Fellman, Brommels, et al, 2001). A surgical blade of any kind is contraindicated. An example of a safe device is the BD Quickheel Safety Lancet. The Tenderfoot Preemie device* was compared with the Monolet lancet and was found to be safer than the lancet and required fewer heel punctures, less collection time, and lower recollection rates (Kellam, Sacks, Wailer, et al, 2001). Shepherd, Glenesk, Niven, and colleagues (2005) reported the Tenderfoot device was more effective and safer than a lancet for newborn screening tests. Although obtaining capillary blood gases is a common practice, these measures may not accurately reflect arterial values.

---

*The Tenderfoot Preemie device is manufactured by ITC, Edison, NJ; www.itcmed.com/tenderfoot.shtml.

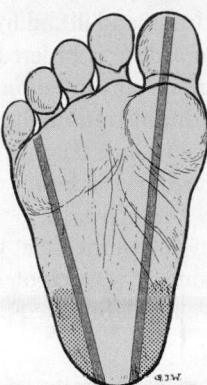

Fig. 27-15 Puncture site *(colored stippled area)* on sole of infant's foot.

The most serious complications of infant heel puncture are necrotizing osteochondritis from lancet penetration of the underlying calcaneus bone, infection, and abscess of the heel. To avoid osteochondritis, the puncture should be no deeper than 2 mm and should be made at the outer aspect of the heel. The boundaries of the calcaneus can be marked by an imaginary line extending posteriorly from a point between the fourth and fifth toes and running parallel with the lateral aspect of the heel and another line extending posteriorly from the middle of the great toe and running parallel with the medial aspect of the heel (Fig. 27-15). Repeated trauma to the walking surface of the heel can cause fibrosis and scarring that may interfere with locomotion.

No matter how or by whom the specimen is collected, children, even some older ones, fear the loss of their blood. This is particularly true for children whose condition requires frequent blood specimens. They mistakenly believe that blood removed from their body is a threat to their lives. Explaining to them that their body continuously produces blood provides them a measure of reassurance. When the blood is drawn, a comment such as, "Just look how red it is. You're really making a lot of nice red blood," confirms this information and affords them an opportunity to express their concern. An adhesive bandage gives them added assurance that the vital fluids will not leak out through the puncture site.

Children also dislike the discomfort associated with venous, arterial, or capillary punctures. Children have identified these procedures as the ones most frequently causing pain during hospitalization and an arterial puncture as being one of the most painful of all procedures experienced. Toddlers are most distressed by venipuncture, followed by school-age children and then adolescents. Consequently, nurses need to institute pain reduction techniques to lessen the discomfort of these procedures. (See Pain Management, Chapter 7.)

RESPIRATORY SECRETION SPECIMENS

Collection of sputum or nasal discharge is sometimes required for diagnosis of respiratory infections, especially tuberculosis and respiratory syncytial virus (RSV). Older children and adolescents are able to cough as directed and supply sputum specimens when given proper directions. The nurse must make it clear to them that a coughed specimen, not mucus cleared from the throat, is needed. It is helpful to demonstrate a deep cough. Infants and small children are unable to follow directions to cough and will swallow any sputum produced; therefore gastric

washings (lavage) may be used to collect a sputum specimen. Sometimes a satisfactory specimen can be obtained using a suction device such as a mucus trap if the catheter is inserted into the trachea and the cough reflex elicited. A catheter inserted into the back of the throat is not sufficient. For children with a tracheostomy, a specimen is easily aspirated from the trachea or major bronchi by attaching a collecting device to the suction apparatus.

Nasal washings are usually obtained to diagnose an infection of RSV. The child is placed supine, and 1 to 3 ml of sterile normal saline is instilled with a sterile syringe (without needle) into one nostril. The contents are aspirated using a small, sterile bulb syringe and are placed in a sterile container. Another method uses a syringe with 5 cm (2 inches) of 18- to 20-gauge tubing. The saline is quickly instilled and then aspirated to recover the nasal specimen. To prevent any additional discomfort, all of the equipment should be ready before beginning the procedure.

Other respiratory secretion collection methods include nasopharyngeal swabs to diagnose *Bordetella pertussis* and throat cultures. The nurse swabs both the tonsils and the posterior pharynx when obtaining a throat culture. The swab stick is inserted into the culture tube. Some culture kits require squeezing an ampule to release the culture medium.

ADMINISTRATION OF MEDICATION

DETERMINATION OF DRUG DOSAGE

Nurses must have an understanding of the safe dosage of medications they administer to children, as well as the expected action, possible side effects, and signs of toxicity. Unlike with adult medications, there are few standardized pediatric dosage ranges, and with a few exceptions, drugs are prepared and packaged in average adult-dosage strengths.

Factors related to growth and maturation significantly alter an individual's capacity to metabolize and excrete drugs. Immaturity or defects in any of the important processes of absorption, distribution, biotransformation, or excretion can significantly alter the effects of a drug. Newborn and premature infants with immature enzyme systems in the liver (where most drugs are broken down and detoxified), lower plasma concentrations of protein for binding with drugs, and immaturely functioning kidneys (where most drugs are excreted) are particularly vulnerable to the harmful effects of drugs. Beyond the newborn period, many drugs are metabolized more rapidly by the liver, necessitating larger doses or more frequent administration. This is particularly important in pain control, when the dosage of analgesics may need to be increased or the interval between doses decreased.

Various formulas involving age, weight, and body surface area (BSA) as the basis for calculations have been devised to determine children's drug dosages. Because the administration of medication is a nursing responsibility, nurses need to have not only knowledge of drug action and patient responses, but also resources for estimating safe dosages for children. Children's dosages are most often expressed in units of measure per body weight (mg/kg). Some medications, such as chemotherapy, are more precisely dosed using BSA. The ratio of BSA to weight varies inversely with length; therefore the infant who is shorter and weighs less than an older child or adult has relatively more BSA than would be expected from the weight. BSA is based on the West nomogram and is easily determined using conversion programs widely available on the Internet.

Checking Dosage

Administering the correct dosage of a drug is a shared responsibility between the practitioner who orders the drug and the nurse who carries out that order. Children react with unex-

pected severity to some drugs, and ill children may be especially sensitive to drugs. When a dose is ordered that is outside the usual range or when there is some question regarding the preparation or the route of administration, the nurse should check with the prescribing practitioner before proceeding with the administration, since the nurse is legally liable for any drug administered.

Even when it has been determined that the dosage is correct for a particular child, many drugs are potentially hazardous or lethal. Most facilities have regulations requiring specified drugs

---

EVIDENCE-BASED PRACTICE   *Shelly Nalbone*

Medication Safety and Insulin Therapy

ASK THE QUESTION

What practices decrease the number of errors in children receiving insulin therapy?

SEARCH FOR THE EVIDENCE

Search strategies

Search selection criteria included English language publications, research-based studies, and pediatric populations.

Databases used

National Guideline Clearinghouse (AHRQ), Cochrane Collaboration, PubMed, CINAHL, University of Michigan Evidence-Based Pediatrics, Micromedex, EMBASE, ProQuest, TRIP Database, Medscape, RxMed, STAT!Ref, RxKinetics

CRITICALLY ANALYZE THE EVIDENCE

GRADE criteria: Evidence quality very low; recommendation strong (Guyatt, Oxman, Vist, et al, 2008)

The American Society of Health-System Pharmacists (2006) conducted a review of all relevant literature and evidence-based reviews on insulin therapy focusing on safety and patient outcomes in the hospital setting. Practice recommendations included preprinted order sets or computerized order entry and ongoing and annual training.

A quality improvement project to reduce medication errors and assess a standardized protocol for supplemental sliding scale insulin (SSI) in nonintensive care units was described by Donihi, DeVita, and Korytkowski (2006). Before implementation, more than 20 different types of SSI were used. The number of prescribing errors found on chart review 1 year after implementation was reduced from 10.3 to 1.2 per 100 SSI days. Authors recommend preprinted standardized SSI protocols and intense, ongoing education for direct patient care providers.

Ragone and Lando (2002) evaluated sources of errors and stated that, with the advent of new insulin analogs and premixed insulin combinations, the potential for errors in insulin therapy has increased. Errors have occurred when health care workers have mistaken rapid-acting insulin (Humalog) for glargine at bedtime. Inappropriate use of the proper insulin syringe has also led to errors. Excessive heat, inappropriate labeling of vials after opening, and improper handling of insulin pens can affect the efficacy of insulin. Staff education leads to decreased errors and improved patient outcomes.

Heatlie (2003) found in a qualitative study that long delays existed in the dosing of insulin after blood glucose was obtained. Recommendations included preprinted insulin order forms, increased nursing education surrounding diabetes management, and implementation of a 1-hour time limit from blood glucose specimen to insulin administration.

Davis, Harwood, Midgett, and colleagues (2005) described the safety and efficacy of insulin therapy in intermediate care units. They reviewed staffing patterns, order trends, and past errors. Intense educational offerings were developed and implemented. Three months of data collection revealed 275 correct insulin drip rate calculations out of a possible 276. Audit results indicated that insulin therapy could be safely managed with a 1:5 to 1:6 nurse/patient ratio with proper nursing education.

Cohen, Robinson, and Mandrack (2003) identified methods to increase the safety of medication administration, including preprinted medication orders, the use of "smart pumps" for medication administration, and routine double checking by two licensed nurses when administering high-alert medications such as insulin.

APPLY THE EVIDENCE: NURSING IMPLICATIONS

- Preprinted order sets or computerized order entry for insulin therapy should be used in hospital settings.
- SSI should be administered with a set of standardized protocols for hospitals, and use should be minimized.
- Staff education should be ongoing.
- Direct care provider education should be performed annually and be readily available for just-in-time training.
- Processes should be implemented to include annual education and competency validation for all involved staff.
- Patients receiving insulin therapy should be limited to designated areas of the hospital where staff have received appropriate training and development.
- Well-defined policies should be in place to support appropriate patient placement, safe and effective medication administration, strict insulin management, and judicious documentation.

References

American Society of Health-System Pharmacists: *Professional practice recommendations for safe use of insulin in hospitals*, Bethesda, Md, 2006, Inpatient Care Practitioners.

Cohen H, Robinson E, Mandrack M: Getting to the root of medication errors, *Nursing* 33(9):36-46, 2003.

Davis E, Harwood K, Midgett L, et al: Implementation of a new intravenous insulin method in intermediate-care units in hospitalized patients, *Diabetes Educ* 31(6):818-823, 2005.

Donihi A, DeVita M, Korytkowski M: Use of a standardized protocol to decrease medication errors and adverse events related to sliding scale insulin, *Qual Saf Health Care* 15:89-91, 2006.

Guyatt GH, Oxman AD, Vist GE, et al: GRADE: an emerging consensus on rating quality of evidence and strength of recommendations, *BMJ* 336:924-926, 2008.

Heatlie J: Reducing insulin medication errors: evaluation of a quality improvement initiative, *J Nurs Staff Dev* 19(2):92-98, 2003.

Ragone M, Lando H: Errors of insulin commission? *Clin Diabetes* 20(4):221-222, 2002.

to be double-checked by another nurse before giving them to the child. Among drugs that require such safeguards are anti-arrhythmics, anticoagulants, chemotherapeutic agents, and insulin. Others frequently included are epinephrine, opioids, and sedatives. Even if this precaution is not mandatory, nurses are wise to take such precautions. Errors in decimal point placement may occur and may result in a tenfold or greater dosage error. See the Evidence-Based Practice box for additional information about medication safety and insulin therapy.

Identification

Before the administration of any medication, the child must be correctly identified using two identifiers (e.g., name and medical record number or birth date). With the infant, young child, or nonverbal child, the parent or guardian (if present) can verify the child's identity. After verbal verification of the child's identity (by the parent, guardian, or child), the identification band should be verified using two identifiers. Bedside computers to scan the ID bracelet for electronic record updating may also be used.

Preparing Parents

Nearly all parents have given some type of medication to their child and can describe the approaches they have found successful. In some cases it is less traumatic for the child if a parent gives the medication, provided that the nurse prepares the medication and supervises its administration. Children being given daily medications at home are accustomed to the parent's functioning in this capacity and are less likely to fuss than if a stranger administers the medication. Individual decisions need to be made regarding parental presence and participation, such as holding the child during injections. (See Parent Participation, Chapter 26, p. 974.)

Preparing the Child

Every child requires psychologic preparation for parenteral administration of medication and supportive care during the procedure (see p. 1000). Even if children have received several injections, they rarely become accustomed to the discomfort and have as much right as any other child to understanding and patience from those giving the injection.

ORAL ADMINISTRATION

The oral route is preferred for administering medications to children because of the ease of administration. Most are dissolved or suspended in liquid preparations. Although some children are able to swallow or chew solid medications at an early age, solid preparations are not recommended for young children because of the danger of aspiration.

Most pediatric medications come in palatable and colorful preparations for added ease of administration. Some have a slightly unpleasant aftertaste, but most children swallow these liquids with little if any resistance. The nurse can taste a minute amount of an oral preparation to see whether it is palatable or bitter. Complaints of dislike from the child can be accepted and the taste camouflaged whenever possible. Most pediatric units have preparations available for this purpose (see Atraumatic Care box).

Preparation

The devices available to measure medicines are not always sufficiently accurate for measuring the small amounts needed in pediatric nursing practice (Fig. 27-16). Molded plastic cups offer reasonable accuracy in measuring moderate doses of liquids; paper cups, on the other hand, are likely to have irregularly shaped or crumpled bottoms and retain considerable amounts of thick medication. Measures less than 1 tsp are impossible to determine accurately with a medicine cup.

The teaspoon is an inaccurate measuring device and is subject to error. Teaspoons vary greatly in capacity, and different persons using the same spoon will pour different amounts. Therefore measure a drug ordered in teaspoons in milliliters; the established standard is 5 ml/tsp. A convenient hollow-handled medicine spoon is available to accurately measure and administer the drug (see Fig. 27-16, *A*).

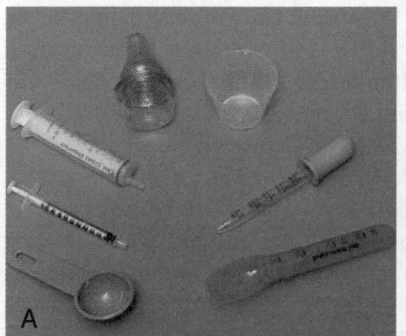
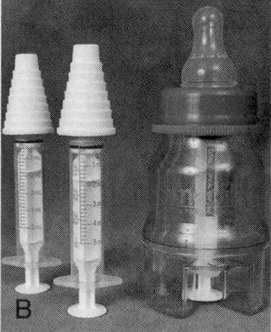

Fig. 27-16 A, Acceptable devices for measuring and administering oral medication to children *(clockwise from bottom left:* measuring spoon, plastic syringes, calibrated nipple, plastic medicine cup, calibrated dropper, hollow-handled medicine spoon. **B,** Medibottle used to deliver oral medication via a syringe. **(B,** Courtesy Paul Vincent Kuntz, Texas Children's Hospital, Houston.)

Household *measuring* spoons can also be used when other devices are not available. A device called the Medibottle has shown to be more effective in delivering oral medication to infants than the oral syringe (Kraus, Stohlmeyer, Hannon, et al, 2001) (see Fig. 27-16, *B*).

Another unreliable device for measuring liquids is the dropper, which varies to a greater extent than the teaspoon or measuring cup. The volume of a drop varies according to the viscosity (thickness) of the liquid measured. Viscous fluids produce much larger drops than thin liquids. Many medications are supplied with caps or droppers designed for measuring each specific preparation. These are accurate when used to measure that specific medication but are not reliable for measuring other liquids. Emptying dropper contents into a medicine cup invites additional error. Because some of the liquid clings to the sides of the cup, a significant amount of the drug can be lost.

The most accurate means for measuring small amounts of medication is the plastic disposable syringe, especially the tuberculin syringe for volumes less than 1 ml. Not only does the syringe provide a reliable measure, but it also serves as a convenient means for transporting and administering the medication. The medication can be placed directly into the child's mouth from the syringe.

Young children and some older children have difficulty swallowing tablets or pills. Because a number of drugs are not available in pediatric preparations, the tablet needs to be crushed before it can be given to these children. Commercial devices* are available, or simple methods can be employed for crushing tablets. Not all drugs can be crushed (e.g., medication with an enteric or protective coating or formulated for slow release).

The nurse can teach children who must take solid oral medication for an extended period to swallow tablets or capsules. Training sessions include using verbal instruction, demonstration, reinforcement for swallowing progressively larger candy or capsules, no attention for inappropriate behavior, and gradual withdrawal of guidance once children can swallow their medication.

Because pediatric doses often require dividing adult preparations of medication, the nurse may be faced with the dilemma of accurate dosage. With tablets, only those that are scored can be halved or quartered accurately. If the medication is soluble, the tablet or contents of a capsule can be mixed in a small, premeasured amount of liquid and the appropriate portion given. For example, if half a dose is required, the tablet is dissolved in 5 ml of water, and 2.5 ml is given.

Administration

Although administering liquids to infants is relatively easy, the nurse must take care to prevent aspiration. While holding the infant in a semireclining position, place the medication in the mouth from a spoon, plastic cup, dropper, or syringe (without needle). It is best to place the dropper or syringe along the side of the infant's tongue, and administer the liquid slowly in small amounts, waiting for the child to swallow between deposits.

> **NURSING TIP** In infants up to 11 months of age and children with neurologic impairments, blowing a small puff of air in the face frequently elicits a swallow reflex.

Medicine cups can be used effectively for older infants who are able to drink from a cup. Because of the natural outward tongue thrust in infancy, medications may need to be retrieved from the lips or chin and refed. Allowing the infant to suck the medication that has been placed in an empty nipple or inserting the syringe or dropper into the side of the mouth, parallel to the nipple, while the infant nurses are other convenient methods for giving liquid medications to infants. Medication is not added to the infant's formula feeding because the child may subsequently refuse the formula. Dispose of any plastic covers that may be on the ends of syringes as these covers are choking hazards.

The young child who refuses to cooperate or resists consistently despite explanation and encouragement may require mild physical coercion. If so, it is carried out quickly and carefully. Make every effort to determine why the child resists, and explain the reasons for the coercion in such a way that the child knows it is being carried out for his or her well-being and is not a form of punishment. There is always a risk in using even mild forceful techniques. A crying child can aspirate a medication, particularly when lying on the back. If the nurse holds the child in the lap with the child's right arm behind the nurse, the left hand firmly grasped by the nurse's left hand, and the head securely cradled between the nurse's arm and body, the medication can be slowly poured into the mouth (Fig. 27-17).

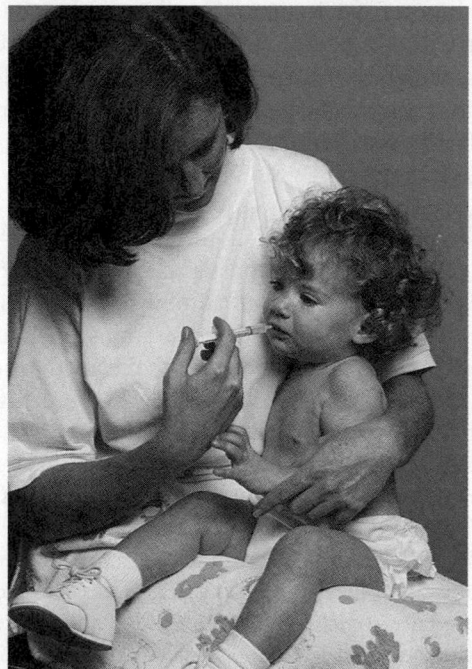

Fig. 27-17 Nurse partially restrains child for easy and comfortable administration of oral medication.

---

*Several styles of pill crushers are available from Trademark Medical, 449 Sovereign Court, St. Louis, MO 63011; 800-325-9044; www.trademarkmedical.com.

INTRAMUSCULAR ADMINISTRATION

Selecting the Syringe and Needle

The volume of medication prescribed for small children and the small amount of tissue available for injection necessitate selection of a syringe that can measure small amounts of solution. For volumes less than 1 ml, the tuberculin syringe, calibrated in 0.01-ml increments, is appropriate. Minute doses may require the use of a 0.5-ml, low-dose syringe. These syringes, along with specially constructed needles, minimize the possibility of inadvertently administering incorrect amounts of a drug because of dead space, which allows fluid to remain in the syringe and needle after the plunger is pushed completely forward. A minimum of 0.2 ml of solution remains in a standard needle hub; therefore, when very small amounts of two drugs are combined in the syringe, such as mixtures of insulin, the ratio of the two drugs can be altered significantly. Measures that minimize the effect of dead space are (1) when two drugs are combined in the syringe, always draw them up in the same order to maintain a consistent ratio between the drugs; (2) use the same brand of syringe (dead space may vary between brands); and (3) use one-piece syringe units (needle permanently attached to the syringe).

Dead space is also an important factor to consider when injecting medication, since flushing the syringe with an air bubble adds an additional amount of medication to the prescribed dose. This can be hazardous when very small amounts of a drug are given. Consequently, flushing is not recommended, especially when less than 1 ml of medication is given. Syringes are calibrated to deliver a prescribed drug dose, and the amount of medication left in the hub and needle is not part of the syringe barrel calibrations. Certain drugs such as iron dextran and diphtheria and tetanus toxoid may cause irritation when tracked into the subcutaneous tissue. The Z-track method is recommended for use in infants and children rather than an air bubble. Changing the needle after withdrawing the fluid from the vial is another technique to minimize tracking.

The needle length must be sufficient to penetrate the subcutaneous tissue and deposit the medication into the body of the muscle. A summary of the evidence evaluating needle length for intramuscular (IM) injections is found in Chapter 12, pp. 507-508. The needle gauge should be as small as possible to deliver the fluid safely. Smaller-diameter (25- to 30-gauge) needles cause the least discomfort, but larger gauges are needed for viscous medication and prevention of accidental bending of longer needles.

Determining the Site

Factors to consider when selecting a site for an IM injection on an infant or child include:

- The amount and character of the medication to be injected
- The amount and general condition of the muscle mass
- The frequency or number of injections to be given during the course of treatment
- The type of medication being given
- Factors that may impede access to or cause contamination of the site
- The child's ability to assume the required position safely

Older children and adolescents usually pose few problems in selecting a suitable site for IM injections, but infants, with their small and underdeveloped muscles, have fewer available sites. It is sometimes difficult to assess the amount of fluid that can be safely injected into a single site. Usually 1 ml is the maximum volume that should be administered in a single site to small children and older infants. The muscles of small infants may not tolerate more than 0.5 ml. As the child approaches adult size, the nurse can use volumes approaching those given to adults. However, the larger the amount of solution, the larger the muscle at the injection site must be.

Injections must be placed in muscles large enough to accommodate the medication, while avoiding major nerves and blood vessels. The preferred site for infants is the vastus lateralis (Table 27-7). The ventrogluteal site is relatively free of major nerves and blood vessels, is a relatively large muscle with less subcutaneous tissue than the dorsal site, has well-defined landmarks for safe site location, and is easily accessible in several positions. These advantages make it a preferred site over the dorsogluteal muscle and challenge the recommendation that the ventrogluteal site not be used until children are walking.

Cook and Murtagh's (2006) research into IM injection sites in children indicates that the ventrogluteal site has not been associated with complications and is the preferred site in children of all ages (see Table 27-7). In clinical practice this site has been safely used in children as young as newborns. The deltoid muscle, a small muscle near the axillary and radial nerves, can be used for small volumes of fluid in children as young as 18 months of age. Its advantages are less pain and fewer side effects from the injectate (as observed with immunizations), compared with the vastus lateralis. Table 27-7 summarizes the three major injection sites and illustrates the location of the preferred IM injection sites for children.

Administration

⊜ Although injections that are executed with care seldom cause trauma to the child, there have been reports of serious disability related to IM injections in children. Repeated use of a single site has been associated with fibrosis of the muscle with subsequent muscle contracture. Injections close to large nerves, such as the sciatic nerve, have been responsible for permanent disability, especially when potentially neurotoxic drugs are administered. There are several reports of tissue damage from penicillin. One of the difficulties in administering the opaque preparations, such as penicillin G (Bicillin), is that aspirated blood cannot be detected at the bottom of the syringe, thus increasing the risk of injecting into a blood vessel. When such drugs are injected, use great care in locating the correct site. When aspirating, the nurse should look for blood at the top of the syringe near the plunger, since blood may be drawn up through the column of penicillin. One study of IM injection techniques revealed that the straighter the path of needle insertion (e.g., 90-degree angle), the less displacement and shear to tissue, causing less discomfort (Katsma and Smith, 1997) (see Table 27-7).

A reported potential hazard with medication in glass ampules is the presence of glass particles in the ampule after the container is broken. When the medication is withdrawn into the syringe, the glass particles are also withdrawn and subsequently

TABLE 27-7 INTRAMUSCULAR INJECTION SITES IN CHILDREN

SITE	DISCUSSION
Vastus Lateralis 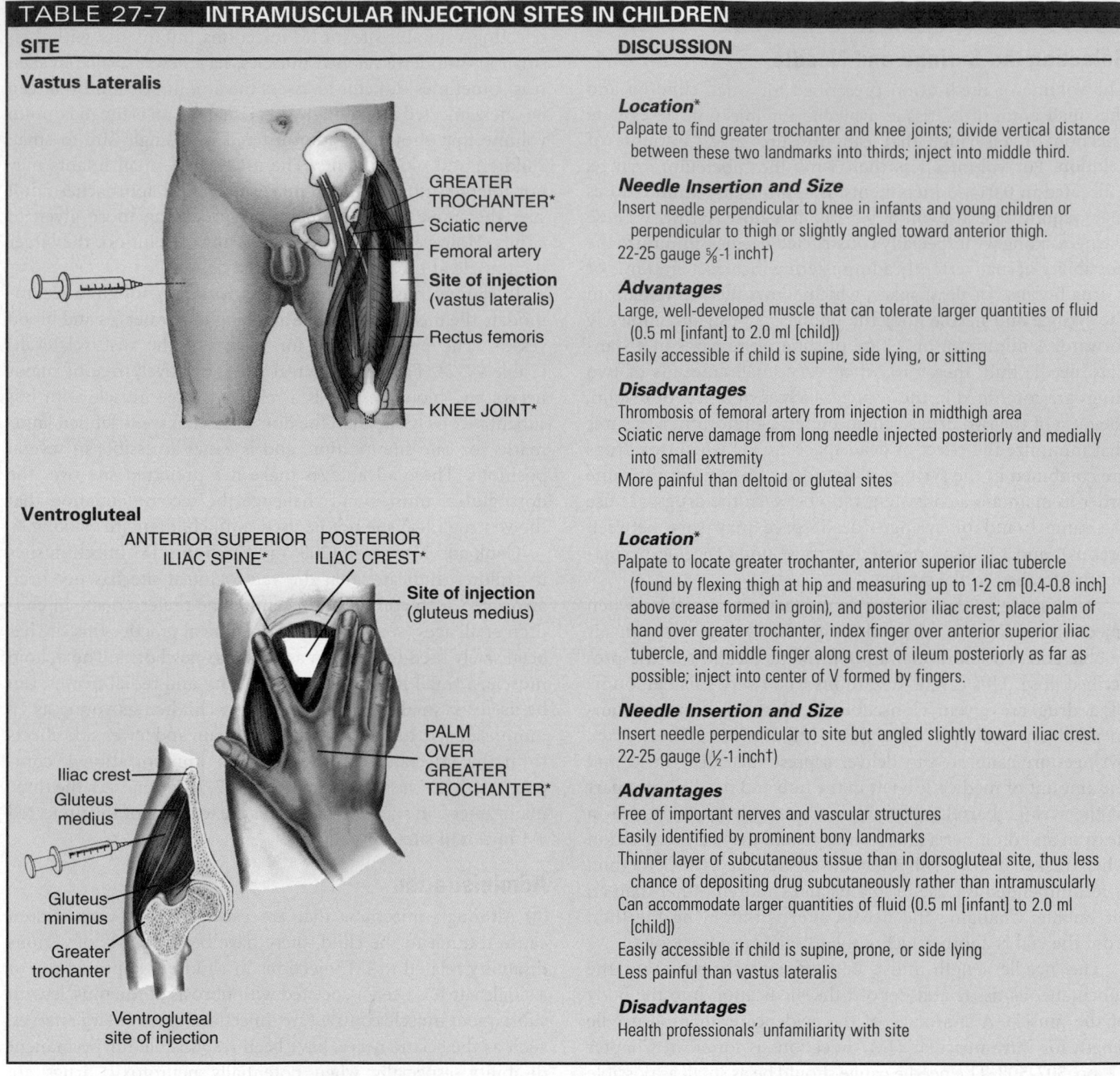	**Location*** Palpate to find greater trochanter and knee joints; divide vertical distance between these two landmarks into thirds; inject into middle third. **Needle Insertion and Size** Insert needle perpendicular to knee in infants and young children or perpendicular to thigh or slightly angled toward anterior thigh. 22-25 gauge ⅝-1 inch†) **Advantages** Large, well-developed muscle that can tolerate larger quantities of fluid (0.5 ml [infant] to 2.0 ml [child]) Easily accessible if child is supine, side lying, or sitting **Disadvantages** Thrombosis of femoral artery from injection in midthigh area Sciatic nerve damage from long needle injected posteriorly and medially into small extremity More painful than deltoid or gluteal sites
Ventrogluteal	**Location*** Palpate to locate greater trochanter, anterior superior iliac tubercle (found by flexing thigh at hip and measuring up to 1-2 cm [0.4-0.8 inch] above crease formed in groin), and posterior iliac crest; place palm of hand over greater trochanter, index finger over anterior superior iliac tubercle, and middle finger along crest of ileum posteriorly as far as possible; inject into center of V formed by fingers. **Needle Insertion and Size** Insert needle perpendicular to site but angled slightly toward iliac crest. 22-25 gauge (½-1 inch†) **Advantages** Free of important nerves and vascular structures Easily identified by prominent bony landmarks Thinner layer of subcutaneous tissue than in dorsogluteal site, thus less chance of depositing drug subcutaneously rather than intramuscularly Can accommodate larger quantities of fluid (0.5 ml [infant] to 2.0 ml [child]) Easily accessible if child is supine, prone, or side lying Less painful than vastus lateralis **Disadvantages** Health professionals' unfamiliarity with site

Labels in Vastus Lateralis figure: GREATER TROCHANTER*, Sciatic nerve, Femoral artery, Site of injection (vastus lateralis), Rectus femoris, KNEE JOINT*

Labels in Ventrogluteal figure: ANTERIOR SUPERIOR ILIAC SPINE*, POSTERIOR ILIAC CREST*, Site of injection (gluteus medius), PALM OVER GREATER TROCHANTER*, Iliac crest, Gluteus medius, Gluteus minimus, Greater trochanter, Ventrogluteal site of injection

injected into the patient. As a precaution, medication from glass ampules is only drawn through a needle with a filter.

Most children are unpredictable, and few are totally cooperative when receiving an injection. Even children who appear to be relaxed and constrained can lose control under the stress of the procedure. It is advisable to have someone available to help hold the child if needed. Because children often jerk or pull away unexpectedly, the nurse should carry an extra needle to exchange for the contaminated one so that the delay is minimal. The child, even a small one, is told that he or she is receiving an injection (preferably using a phrase such as "putting the medicine under the skin"), and then the procedure is carried out as quickly and skillfully as possible to avoid prolonging the stressful experience. Invasive procedures such as injections are especially anxiety provoking in young children, who may associate any assault to the "behind" with punishment. Because

injections are painful, the nurse should employ excellent injection techniques and effective pain reduction measures to reduce discomfort (see Nursing Care Guidelines box).

Small infants offer little resistance to injections. Although they squirm and may be difficult to hold in position, they can usually be restrained without assistance. A larger infant's body can be securely restrained between the nurse's arm and body. To inject into the body of a muscle, the nurse firmly grasps the muscle mass between the thumb and fingers to isolate and stabilize the site (Fig. 27-18). However, in obese children it is preferable to first spread the skin with the thumb and index finger to displace subcutaneous tissue and then grasp the muscle deeply on each side.

If medication is given around the clock, the nurse must wake the child. Although it may seem easier to surprise the sleeping child and do it quickly, this can cause the child to fear going

TABLE 27-7   INTRAMUSCULAR INJECTION SITES IN CHILDREN—cont'd

SITE	DISCUSSION
Deltoid 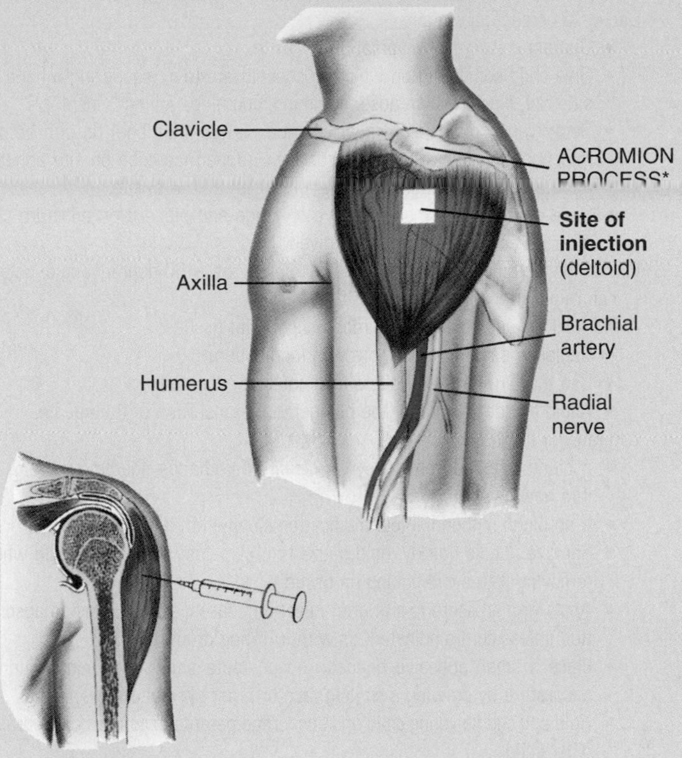 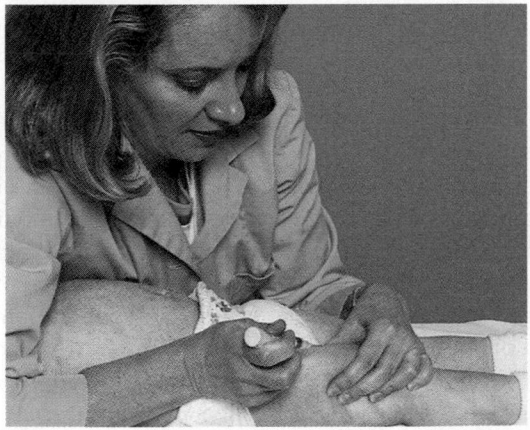 Clavicle — ACROMION PROCESS* — Site of injection (deltoid) — Axilla — Brachial artery — Humerus — Radial nerve	**Location*** Locate acromion process; inject only into upper third of muscle that begins about two finger breadths below acromion. **Needle Insertion and Size** Insert needle perpendicular to site but angled slightly toward shoulder. 22-25 gauge (½-1 inch) **Advantages** Faster absorption rates than gluteal sites Easily accessible with minimal removal of clothing Less pain and fewer local side effects from vaccines when compared with vastus lateralis **Disadvantages** Small muscle mass; only limited amounts of drug can be injected (0.5-1.0 ml) Small margins of safety with possible damage to radial nerve and axillary nerve (not shown, lies under deltoid at head of humerus)

*Locations are indicated by asterisks on illustrations.

†Research has shown that a 1-inch needle is needed for adequate muscle penetration in infants 4 mo old and possibly in infants as young as 2 mo (Cook and Murtagh, 2002).

Fig. 27-18 Holding small child for intramuscular injection. Note how nurse isolates and stabilizes muscle.

back to sleep. When awakened first, children will know that nothing will be done to them unless they are forewarned. The Nursing Care Guidelines box summarizes administration techniques that maximize safety and minimize the discomfort often associated with injections.

A needleless injection system (e.g., Biojector) delivers IM or subcutaneous injections without the use of a needle and eliminates the risk of accidental needle puncture. This needle-free injection system uses a carbon dioxide cartridge to power the delivery of medication through the skin. Although it is not painless, it may reduce pain and the anxiety of seeing the needle.

SUBCUTANEOUS AND INTRADERMAL ADMINISTRATION

Subcutaneous and intradermal injections are frequently administered to children, but the technique differs little from the method used with adults. Examples of subcutaneous injections include insulin, hormone replacement, allergy desensitization, and some vaccines. Tuberculin testing, local anesthesia, and allergy testing are examples of frequently administered intradermal injections.

Techniques to minimize the pain associated with these injections include changing the needle if it pierced a rubber stopper on a vial, using 26- to 30-gauge needles (only to inject the solution), and injecting small volumes (<0.5 ml). The angle of the needle for the subcutaneous injection is typically 90 degrees. In children with little subcutaneous tissue, some practitioners insert the needle at a 45-degree angle. However, the benefit of using the 45-degree angle rather than the 90-degree angle remains controversial.

Although subcutaneous injections can be given anywhere there is subcutaneous tissue, common sites include the center third of the lateral aspect of the upper arm, the abdomen, and the center third of the anterior thigh. Some practitioners believe it is not necessary to aspirate before injecting subcutaneously; for example, this is an accepted practice in the administration of insulin. Automatic injector devices do not aspirate before injecting.

NURSING CARE GUIDELINES

Intramuscular Administration of Medication

Check child's identification.

Apply EMLA (a eutectic mix of lidocaine and prilocaine) or LMX cream (lidocaine) topically over site if time permits. (See Pain Management, Chapter 7.)

Prepare medication.

- Select appropriately sized needle and syringe.
- If withdrawing medication from an ampule, use a needle equipped with a filter that removes glass particles; then use a new, nonfilter needle for injection.
- Maximum volume to be administered in a single site is 1 ml for older infants and small children.
- Have medication at room temperature before injection.

Determine site of injection (see Table 27-7); make certain that muscle is large enough to accommodate volume and type of medication.

- For infants and small or debilitated children, use the vastus lateralis or ventrogluteal muscles; the dorsogluteal muscle is insufficiently developed to be a safe site for infants and small children.

Obtain sufficient help in restraining child.

Explain briefly what is to be done and, if appropriate, what child can do to help.

Expose injection area for unobstructed view of landmarks.

Select a site where skin is free of irritation and danger of infection; palpate for and avoid sensitive or hardened areas.

With multiple injections, rotate sites.

Place child in a lying or sitting position; child is not allowed to stand because landmarks are more difficult to assess, restraint is more difficult, and the child may faint and fall.

- Ventrogluteal—on side with upper leg flexed and placed in front of lower leg.
- Vastus lateralis—supine, lying on side, or sitting.

Use a new, sharp needle (not one that has pierced rubber stopper on vial) with smallest diameter that permits free flow of the medication.

Grasp muscle firmly between thumb and fingers to isolate and stabilize muscle for deposition of drug in its deepest part; in obese children, spread skin with thumb and index finger to displace subcutaneous tissue and grasp muscle deeply on each side.

Allow skin preparation to dry completely before penetrating skin.

Decrease perception of pain.

- Distract child with conversation.
- Give child something on which to concentrate (e.g., squeezing a hand or side rail, pinching own nose, humming, counting, yelling "Ouch!").
- Spray vapocoolant (e.g., ethyl chloride or fluorimethane) on site before injection, or place a cold compress or wrapped ice cube on site about a minute before injection, or apply cold to contralateral site.
- Have child hold a small adhesive bandage and place it on puncture site after intramuscular injection is given.

Insert needle quickly, using a dartlike motion at a 90-degree angle unless contraindicated.

Avoid tracking any medication through superficial tissues:

- Replace needle after withdrawing medication.
- Use the Z-track or air-bubble technique as indicated.
- Avoid any depression of the plunger during insertion of the needle.

Aspirate for blood.

- If blood is found, remove syringe from site, change needle, and reinsert into new location.
- If no blood is found, inject medication slowly into a relaxed muscle.
- Remove needle quickly; hold gauze firmly against skin near needle when removing it to avoid pulling on tissue.
- Apply firm pressure to site after injection; massage site to hasten absorption unless contraindicated, as with irritating drugs.
- Place a small adhesive bandage on puncture site; with young children decorate it by drawing a smiling face or other symbol of acceptance.
- Hold and cuddle young child and encourage parents to comfort child; praise older child.
- Allow expression of feelings.

Discard syringe and uncapped, uncut needle in puncture-resistant container located near site of use.

Record time of injection, drug, dose, and injection site.

When giving an intradermal injection into the volar surface of the forearm, the nurse should avoid the medial side of the arm, where the skin is more sensitive.

> **NURSING TIP** Families often need to learn injection techniques to administer medications, such as insulin, at home. Begin teaching as early as possible to allow the family the maximum amount of practice time.

INTRAVENOUS ADMINISTRATION

The IV route for administering medications is frequently used in pediatric therapy. For some drugs it is the only effective route. This method is used for giving drugs to children who:

- Have poor absorption as a result of diarrhea, vomiting, or dehydration
- Need a high serum concentration of a drug
- Have resistant infections that require parenteral medication over an extended time
- Need continuous pain relief
- Require emergency treatment

Chapter 28 discusses insertion sites and observation of the IV infusion under Parenteral Fluid Therapy and Venous Access

Devices. The nurse needs to consider several factors in relation to IV medication. When a drug is administered intravenously, the effect is almost instantaneous and further control is limited. Most drugs for IV administration require a specified minimum dilution and/or rate of flow, and many are highly irritating or toxic to tissues outside the vascular system. In addition to the precautions and nursing observations commonly related to IV therapy, factors to consider when preparing and administering drugs to infants and children by the IV route include:

- Amount of drug to be administered
- Minimum dilution of drug and whether child is fluid restricted
- Type of solution in which drug can be diluted
- Length of time over which drug can be safely administered
- Rate limitations of child, vascular system, and infusion equipment
- Time that this or another drug is to be administered
- Compatibility of all drugs that child is receiving intravenously
- Compatibility with infusion fluids

Before any IV infusion, check the site of insertion for patency. Never administer medications with blood products. Only one antibiotic should be administered at a time. Extra fluids needed to administer IV medications can be problematic for infants and fluid-restricted children. Syringe pumps are often used to deliver IV medication because they minimize fluid requirements and more precisely deliver small volumes of medication compared with large-volume infusion pumps. Regardless of the technique, the nurse must know the minimum dilutions for safe administration of IV medications to infants and children.

Several methods of venous access are available and include the peripheral lock device, central venous catheters, and implanted infusion ports. (See Venous Access Devices, Chapter 28.)

NASOGASTRIC, OROGASTRIC, OR GASTROSTOMY ADMINISTRATION

When a child has an indwelling feeding tube or a gastrostomy, oral medications are usually given via that route. An advantage of this method is the ability to administer oral medications around the clock without disturbing the child. A disadvantage is the risk of occluding, or clogging, the tube, especially when giving viscous solutions through small-bore feeding tubes. The most important preventive measure is adequate flushing after the medication is instilled (see Nursing Care Guidelines box).

 NURSING CARE GUIDELINES

Nasogastric, Orogastric, or Gastrostomy Medication Administration in Children

Use elixir or suspension (rather than tablet) preparations of medication whenever possible.

Dilute viscous medication or syrup with a small amount of water if possible.

If administering tablets, crush tablet to a fine powder and dissolve drug in a small amount of warm water.

Never crush enteric-coated or sustained-release tablets or capsules.

Avoid oily medications because they tend to cling to side of tube.

Do not mix medication with enteral formula unless fluid is restricted. If adding a drug:
- Check with pharmacist for compatibility.
- Shake formula well and observe for any physical reaction (e.g., separation, precipitation).
- Label formula container with name of medication, dosage, date, and time infusion started.

Have medication at room temperature.

Measure medication in a calibrated cup or syringe.

Check for correct placement of nasogastric or orogastric tube (see Nursing Care Guidelines box, p. 1044).

Attach syringe (with adaptable tip but without plunger) to tube.

Pour medication into syringe.

Unclamp tube and allow medication to flow by gravity.

Adjust height of container to achieve desired flow rate (e.g., increase height for faster flow).

As soon as syringe is empty, pour in water to flush tubing.
- Amount of water depends on length and gauge of tubing.
- Determine amount before administering any medication by using a syringe to fill completely an unused nasogastric or orogastric tube with water. Amount of flush solution is usually 1.5 times this volume.
- With certain drug preparations (e.g., suspensions) more fluid may be needed.

If administering more than one drug at the same time, flush tube between each medication with clear water.

Clamp tube after flushing, unless tube is left open.

RECTAL ADMINISTRATION

The rectal route for administration is less reliable but sometimes used when the oral route is difficult or contraindicated. It is also used when oral preparations are unsuitable to control vomiting. Some of the drugs available in suppository form are acetaminophen, aspirin, sedatives, analgesics (morphine), and antiemetics. The difficulty in using the rectal route is that, unless the rectum is empty at the time of insertion, the absorption of the drug may be delayed, diminished, or prevented by the presence of feces. Sometimes the drug is later evacuated, securely surrounded by stool.

Remove the wrapping on the suppository, and lubricate the suppository with water-soluble jelly or warm water. Rectal suppositories are traditionally inserted with the apex (pointed end) foremost. Reverse contractions or the pressure gradient of the anal canal may help the suppository slip higher into the canal. Using a glove or finger cot, quickly but gently insert the suppository into the rectum, beyond both of the rectal sphincters. Then hold the buttocks together firmly to relieve pressure on the anal sphincter until the urge to expel the suppository has passed, which occurs within 5 to 10 minutes. Sometimes the amount of drug ordered is less than the dose available. The irregular shape of most suppositories makes the process of dividing them into a desired dose difficult if not dangerous. If it must be halved, it should be cut lengthwise. However, there is no guarantee that the drug is evenly dispersed throughout the petrolatum base.

If medication is administered via a retention enema, the same procedure is used. Drugs given by enema are diluted in the smallest amount of solution possible to minimize the likelihood of being evacuated.

OPTIC, OTIC, AND NASAL ADMINISTRATION

There are few differences in administering eye, ear, and nose medication to children and to adults. The major difficulty is in gaining children's cooperation. Older children need only explanation and direction. Although the administration of optic, otic, and nasal medication is not painful, these drugs can cause unpleasant sensations, which can be eliminated with various techniques.

To instill eye medication, place the child supine or sitting with the head extended and ask the child to look up. Use one hand to pull the lower lid downward; the hand that holds the dropper rests on the head so that it may move synchronously with the child's head, thus reducing the possibility of trauma to a struggling child or dropping medication on the face (Fig. 27-19). When the lower lid is pulled down, a small conjunctival sac is formed; apply the solution or ointment to this area, rather than directly on the eyeball. Another effective technique is to pull the lower lid down and out to form a cup effect, into which the medication is dropped. Gently close the lids to prevent expression of the medication. Wipe excess medication from the inner canthus outward to prevent contamination to the contralateral eye.

Instilling eye drops in infants can be difficult because they often clench the lids tightly closed. One approach is to place the drops in the nasal corner where the lids meet. The medication

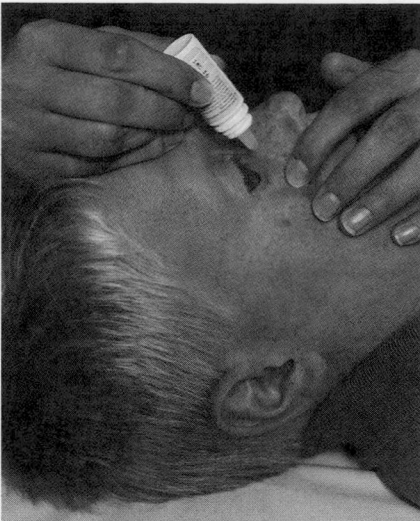

Fig. 27-19 Administering eye drops.

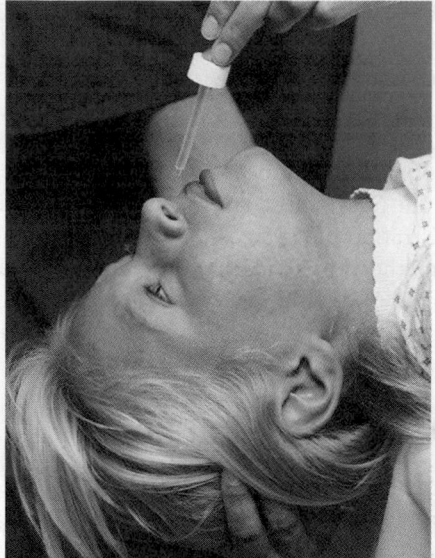

Fig. 27-20 Proper position for instilling nose drops.

NURSING TIP To reduce unpleasant sensations when administering medications:

Eye—Apply finger pressure to the lacrimal punctum at the inner aspect of the lid for 1 minute to prevent drainage of medication to the nasopharynx and the unpleasant "tasting" of the drug.

Ear—Allow medications stored in the refrigerator to warm to room temperature before instillation.

Nose—Position the child with the head hyperextended to prevent strangling sensations caused by medication trickling into the throat rather than up into the nasal passages.

---

pools in this area, and when the child opens the lids, the medication flows onto the conjunctiva. For young children, playing a game can be helpful, such as instructing the child to keep the eyes closed to the count of three and then open them, at which time the drops are quickly instilled. Ointment can be applied by gently pulling down the lower lid and placing the ointment in the lower conjunctival sac.

NURSING TIP If both eye ointment and drops are ordered, give drops first, wait 3 minutes, and then apply the ointment to allow each drug to work. When possible, administer eye ointments before bedtime or naptime, since the child's vision will be blurred temporarily.

Ear drops are instilled with the child in the prone or supine position and the head turned to the appropriate side. For children younger than 3 years of age, the external auditory canal is straightened by gently pulling the pinna downward and straight back. The pinna is pulled upward and back in children older than 3 years of age (see Fig. 6-24). To place the drops deep into the ear canal without contaminating the tip of the dropper, place a disposable ear speculum in the canal and administer the drops through the speculum. After instillation, the child should remain lying on the unaffected side for a few minutes. Gentle massage of the area immediately anterior to the ear facilitates the entry of drops into the ear canal. The use of cotton pledgets prevents medication from flowing out of the external canal.

However, they should be loose enough to allow any discharge to exit from the ear. Premoistening the cotton with a few drops of medication prevents the wicking action from absorbing the medication instilled in the ear.

Nose drops are instilled in the same manner as in the adult patient. Unpleasant sensations associated with medicated nose drops are minimized when care is taken to position the child with the head extended well over the edge of the bed or pillow (Fig. 27-20). Depending on size, infants can be positioned in the football hold (see Fig. 27-5, *B*); in the nurse's arm with the head extended and stabilized between the nurse's body and elbow, and the arms and hands immobilized with the nurse's hands; or with the head extended over the edge of the bed or a pillow. After instillation of the drops, the child should remain in position for 1 minute to allow the drops to come in contact with the nasal surfaces. Insert nasal spray dispensers into the naris vertically and then angle them to avoid trauma to the septum and to direct medication toward the inferior turbinate.

FAMILY TEACHING AND HOME CARE

The nurse usually assumes responsibility for preparing families to administer medications at home. The family should understand why the child is receiving the medication and the effects that might be expected, as well as the amount, frequency, and length of time the drug is to be administered. Instruction should be carried out in an unhurried, relaxed manner, preferably in an area away from a busy ward or office.

Instruct the caregiver carefully regarding the correct dosage. Some persons have difficulty understanding medical terminology, and just because they nod or otherwise indicate they understand, the nurse should not assume that the message is clear. It is important to ascertain their interpretation of a teaspoon, for example, and to be certain they have acceptable devices for measuring the drug. If the drug is packaged with a dropper, syringe, or plastic cup, the nurse should show or mark the point on the device that indicates the prescribed dose and demonstrate how the dose is drawn up into a dropper or syringe, measured, and the bubbles eliminated. If the nurse has any doubts about the parent's ability to administer the correct dose, the parent should give a return demonstration. This is essential when the drug has potentially serious consequences from incorrect dosage, such as insulin or digoxin, or when more complex administration is required, such as parenteral injections. When teaching a parent to give an injection, the nurse must allot adequate time for instruction and practice.

Home modifications are often necessary because the availability of equipment or assistance can differ from the hospital setting. For example, the parent may need guidance in devising methods that allow one person to hold the child and safely give the drug.

The nurse should clarify with parents the time that the drug

NURSING TIP To administer oral, nasal, or optic medication when only one person is available to hold the child, use the following procedure:
- Place child supine on a flat surface (bed, couch, floor).
- Sit facing child so that child's head is between operator's thighs and child's arms are under operator's legs.
- Place lower legs over child's legs to restrain lower body, if necessary.
- To administer oral medication, place a small pillow under child's head to reduce risk of aspiration.
- To administer nasal medication, place a small pillow under child's shoulders to aid flow of liquid through nasal passages.

---

is to be administered. For instance, when a drug is prescribed in association with meals, the number of meals that the family is accustomed to eating influences the amount of drug the child receives. Does the family have meals twice a day or five times a day? When a drug is to be given several times during the day, together the nurse and parents can work out a schedule that accommodates the family's routine. This is particularly significant if a drug must be given at equal intervals throughout a 24-hour period. For example, telling parents that the child needs 1 tsp of medicine four times a day is subject to misinterpretation, since the parents may routinely schedule the doses at incorrect times. Instead, a preplanned schedule based on 6-hour intervals should be set up with the number of days required for the therapeutic dosage listed. Modification should also be made to accommodate sleep schedules. Written instructions should accompany all drug prescriptions.

NURSING TIP If parents have difficulty reading or understanding English, use colors to convey instructions. For example, mark each drug with a color and place the appropriate color on a calendar chart or on a drawing of a clock to identify when the drug needs to be given. If a liquid medication and syringe are used, also mark the syringe at the place the plunger needs to be with color-coded tape.

ALTERNATIVE FEEDING TECHNIQUES

Some children are unable to take nourishment by mouth because of anomalies of the throat, esophagus, or bowel; impaired swallowing capacity; severe debilitation; respiratory distress; or unconsciousness. These children are frequently fed by way of a tube inserted orally or nasally into the stomach (oro-

gastric or nasogastric gavage) or duodenum-jejunum (enteral gavage) or by a tube inserted directly into the stomach (gastrostomy) or jejunum (jejunostomy). Such feedings may be intermittent or by continuous drip. Feeding resistance, a problem that may result from any long-term feeding method that bypasses the mouth, is discussed in Chapter 10. During gavage or gastrostomy feedings, infants are given a pacifier. Nonnutritive sucking has several advantages, such as increased weight gain and decreased crying. However, only pacifiers with a safe design can be used to prevent the possibility of aspiration. Using improvised pacifiers made from bottle nipples is not a safe practice.

When a child is concurrently receiving continuous-drip gastric or enteral feedings and parenteral (IV) therapy, the potential exists for inadvertent administration of the enteral formula through the circulatory system. The possibility for error increases when the parenteral solution is a fat emulsion, a milky-appearing substance. Safeguards to prevent this potentially serious error include:

- Use a separate, specifically designed enteral feeding pump mounted on a separate pole for continuous-feeding solutions.
- Label all tubing of continuous enteral feeding with brightly colored tape or labels.
- Use specifically designed continuous-feeding bags to contain the solutions instead of parenteral equipment, such as a burette.
- Whenever access or connections are made, trace the tubing all the way from the patient to the bag to ensure the correct tubing source is selecting.

GAVAGE FEEDING

Infants and children can be fed simply and safely by a tube passed into the stomach through either the nares or the mouth. The tube can be left in place or inserted and removed with each feeding. In older children it is usually less traumatic to tape the tube securely in place between feedings. When this alternative is used, the tube should be removed and replaced with a new tube according to hospital policy, specific orders, and the type of tube used. Meticulous hand washing is practiced during the procedure to prevent bacterial contamination of the feeding, especially during continuous-drip feedings.

Preparations

The equipment needed for gavage feeding includes:
- A suitable tube selected according to the child's size, the viscosity of the solution being fed, and anticipated duration of treatment.
- A receptacle for the fluid. For small amounts a 10- to 30-ml syringe barrel or Asepto syringe is satisfactory; for larger amounts a 60-ml syringe with a catheter tip is more convenient.
- A 10-ml barrel syringe to aspirate stomach contents after the tube has been placed.
- Water or water-soluble lubricant to lubricate the tube. Sterile water is used for infants.
- Paper or nonallergenic tape to mark the tube and to attach the tube to the infant's or child's cheek (and nose, if placed through the nares).

- pH paper to determine the correct placement in the stomach.
- The solution for feeding.

Not all feeding tubes are the same. Polyethylene and polyvinylchloride types lose their flexibility and need to be replaced frequently, usually every 3 or 4 days. Polyurethane and silicone tubes remain flexible so that they can remain in place up to 30 days. Advantages of small-bore tubes include reduced incidence of pharyngitis, otitis media, aspiration, and discomfort. Disadvantages include difficulty during insertion (may require a stylet or metal guide wire), collapse of the tube during aspiration of gastric contents to test for correct placement, dislodgment during forceful coughing, migration out of position, knotting, occlusion, and unsuitability for thick feedings.

Procedure

Infants are easier to control if they are first wrapped in a mummy restraint (see Fig. 27-8). Even tiny infants with random movements can grasp and dislodge the tube. Preterm infants do not ordinarily require restraint, but, if they do, a small blanket folded across the chest and secured beneath the shoulders is usually sufficient. Be careful so that breathing is not compromised.

Whenever possible, the infant should be held and provided with a means for nonnutritive sucking during the procedure to associate the comfort of physical contact with the feeding. When this is not possible, gavage feeding is carried out with the infant or child on the back or toward the right side and the head and chest elevated. Feeding the child in a sitting position helps maintain placement of the tube in the lowest position, thus increasing the likelihood of correct placement in the stomach.

Although the most accurate method for testing tube placement is radiography, this practice is not always possible before each feeding (see Research Focus box). Research indicates that bedside assessment of gastrointestinal aspirate color and pH is useful in predicting feeding tube placement (see Evidence-Based Practice box). If doubt exists regarding correct placement, consult the practitioner. The Nursing Care Guidelines box describes the procedure for gavage feeding.

In a survey of 113 level II and III nurseries, 98% of the nurseries measured from the nose or mouth to the earlobe and then to the xiphoid process to calculate the length of the feeding tube for placement in preterm infants. For very low–birth-weight infants, daily weight can be used to predict insertion length. Until more definitive data are available, no method that results in a shorter distance than these methods should be used.

GASTROSTOMY FEEDING

Feeding by way of gastrostomy, or G tube, is often used for children in whom passage of a tube through the mouth, pharynx, esophagus, and cardiac sphincter of the stomach is contraindicated or impossible. It is also used to avoid the constant irritation of a nasogastric tube in children who require tube feeding over an extended period. A gastrostomy tube may be placed with the child under general anesthesia or percutaneously using an endoscope with the patient sedated and under local anesthesia (percutaneous endoscopic gastrostomy [PEG]). The tube is inserted through the abdominal wall into the

stomach about midway along the greater curvature and secured by a purse-string suture. The stomach is anchored to the peritoneum at the operative site. The tube used can be a Foley, wing-tip, or mushroom catheter. Immediately after surgery the catheter may be left open and attached to gravity drainage for 24 hours or more.

Direct postoperative care of the wound site toward prevention of infection and irritation. Cleanse the area at least daily or as often as needed to keep the area free of drainage. After

RESEARCH FOCUS

Nasogastric and Orogastric Tube Length

Studies evaluating nasogastric (NG) and orogastric (OG) tube length in infants and children found that age-specific methods for predicting the distance based on height is a more accurate estimate of internal distance to the stomach (Beckstrand, Ellett, and McDaniel, 2007; Klasner, Luke, and Scalzo, 2002). The morphologic measure most commonly used by clinicians, nose-ear-xiphoid distance is often too short to locate the entire tube pore span in the stomach. However, the nose-ear–midxiphoid umbilicus span approached the accuracy of the age-specific prediction equations and is easier to use in a clinical setting. The best option is to adapt the nose-ear–midxiphoid umbilicus measurement for NG/OG tube length (Fig. 27-21, A). (See Nursing Care Guidelines box, p. 1044, and Atraumatic Care box.)

Ellett and Beckstrand (1999) found significant tube placement errors (43.5%) in a study of 39 hospitalized children. Children who were comatose or semicomatose, were inactive, had swallowing difficulty, or had Argyle tubes experienced increased tube placement errors. Findings supported the effectiveness of radiographs in documenting tube placement.

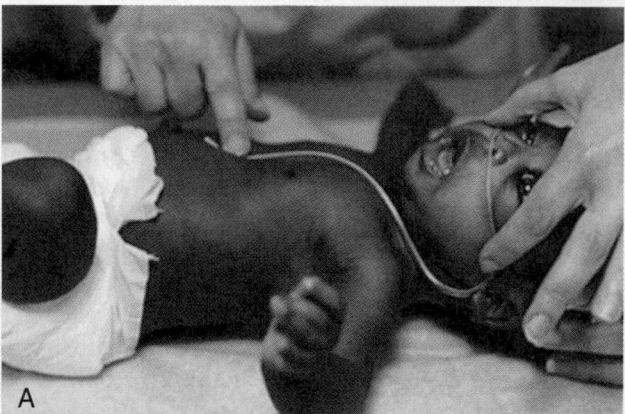

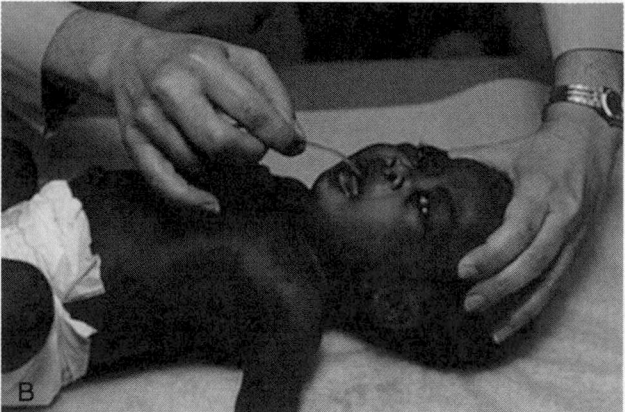

Fig. 27-21 Gavage feeding. **A,** Measuring tube for orogastric feeding from tip of nose to earlobe and to midpoint between end of xiphoid process and umbilicus. **B,** Inserting tube.

Assessing Correct Placement of Nasogastric or Orogastric Tubes in Children

ASK THE QUESTIONS

What is the most reliable method of predicting correct nasogastric (NG) or orogastric (OG) tube placement in infants and children? What steps should be taken when pH testing does not confirm NG/OG correct placement? What pediatric conditions decrease the reliability of gastric pH assessment? How frequently should NG/OG tube placement be verified during intermittent and continuous feedings? What is the most effective method for obtaining NG/OG aspirate for pH testing?

SEARCH FOR THE EVIDENCE

Search strategies

Search selection criteria included English language research studies published in the past 20 years on NG placement verification in infants and children 0 to 18 years old.

Databases used

Cochrane Collaboration, Agency for Healthcare Research and Quality, PubMed, CINAHL, Up-To-Date, Trip, BestBETs, American Academy of Pediatrics, American Association of Critical-Care Nurses, National Patient Safety Agency–United Kingdom, Association of Women's Health, Obstetric and Neonatal Nurses, National Association of Neonatal Nurses, The Joint Commission

CRITICALLY ANALYZE THE EVIDENCE

GRADE criteria: Evidence quality low; recommendation strong (Guyatt, Oxman, Vist, et al, 2008)

Placement verification

Observation methods should be combined to confirm tube placement (Ellett, 2004, 2006; Ellett, Croffie, Cohen, et al, 2005; Metheny, Schnelker, McGinnis, et al, 2005; Huffman, Piper, Jarczyk, et al, 2004; Metheny and Stewart, 2002).

pH and color

Placement should be determined at the bedside by aspirating fluid to examine color and testing the pH. If the pH is less than 5, then the tube can be presumed to be in the stomach. Gastric aspirate is grassy green, clear and colorless, or cloudy white (residual formula). Postpyloric tube aspirate usually appears golden yellow, yellow-brown, or greenish brown with a pH greater than 6.

Tube marking

Once the tube is in place, use an indelible pen to mark the point or document the centimeter marking where the tube exits the nose or mouth. Compare the marked point on the tube with each NG tube placement evaluation.

Physical symptoms

Observe for respiratory symptoms (coughing, cyanosis, dyspnea), restlessness and irritability, pallor, mottling, severe discomfort, hoarseness, weak cry, and inability to cry. Assessing the patient's physical symptoms remains the most essential component of ensuring the tube is properly positioned.

When pH does not confirm placement

There is controversy as to whether a chest x-ray study (CXR) should be obtained if the pH is greater than 5 to verify proper placement. However, this is often unnecessary if a careful evaluation is completed. If the pH is over 5, then continue the assessment of tube placement: evaluate the NG/OG tube marking and the child's physical symptoms. Evaluate current medications that may be interfering with gastric pH. Determine whether a recent x-ray exists to use as a reference. A risk assessment guideline should be established that provides clear decision points on whether a CXR should be ordered (Wilkes-Holmes, 2006; Richardson, Branowicki, Zeidman-Rogers, et al, 2006; Huffman, Piper, Jarczyk, et al, 2004).

Conditions that decrease the reliability of gastric pH assessment

Gastric fluid volume in infants is small, and obtaining aspirate can be difficult. Newborns have a transient raised gastric pH from swallowing amniotic fluid. Preterm infants have a reduced ability to produce gastric acid. The benefit of using pH assessment is obvious: if an aspirate can be obtained, a pH less than 5 will exclude 100% of placements in the lung and 93.9% of placements in the small intestine (Ellett, 2004). Researchers are currently evaluating gastric pH in neonatal intensive care unit settings and are finding that, although it is difficult to gain aspirate, the pH is almost always less than 5 in neonates who have been NPO (taking nothing by mouth) for 2 to 3 hours between bolus feedings and less than 6 for those on continuous feedings.

Administration of acid-inhibiting medications and H_2 receptor blockers elevates gastric pH and decreases acid secretion. Researchers support the use of pH testing with a cutoff of 5.9 to 6.0 to assess NG/OG tubes in patients receiving acid-inhibitors and H_2 receptor blockers (Khair, 2005; Metheny, Stewart, Smith, et al, 1999; Metheny, Reed, and Wiersema, 1993). Three studies were specific to children (Ellett, Croffie, Cohen, et al, 2005; Westhus, 2004; Gharpure, Meert, Sarnaik, et al, 2000).

Frequency of placement verification

Tube placement should be verified on insertion, before intermittent feeds and medication administration, during continuous feeds (frequency not evaluated), and whenever there is concern regarding tube placement.

- Intermittent feedings should have pH, color and tube marking assessment *before* each feeding. If pH is greater than 5, wait 30 minutes to 1 hour for gastric pH to reduce and then retest (Ellett, 2005; Stevenson, 2005).
- For continuous feedings, ensure the tube marking is unchanged; assess pH; if it is less than 6, it is an appropriate cutoff for patients on continuous feeding regimens (Metheny and Stewart, 2002; Metheny and Titler, 2001). Frequency of assessment is not addressed in these studies.

APPLY THE EVIDENCE: NURSING IMPLICATIONS

To obtain NG/OG aspirate for pH testing:

- Aspirate 0.2 to 1 ml of fluid using a 10-ml syringe.
- If unable to obtain aspirate, reposition patient on one side, then the other, and inject 1 to 2 ml of air into the tube using a 10-ml syringe; then try to aspirate fluid again.
- If still unable to obtain aspirate, advance the tube 1 cm and try again.
- Inject 1 to 2 ml of air again, then try again to aspirate fluid.

Continued

EVIDENCE-BASED PRACTICE—cont'd

Assessing Correct Placement of Nasogastric or Orogastric Tubes in Children

References

Ellett M: Important facts about intestinal feeding tube placement, *Gastroenterol Nurs* 29(2):112-124, 2006.

Ellett M: What I know about methods of correctly placing gastric tubes in adults and children, *Gastroenterol Nurs* 27(6):253-259, 2004.

Ellett M, Croffie JM, Cohen MD, et al: Gastric tube placement in young children, *Clin Nurs Res* 14(3):238-252, 2005.

Gharpure V, Meert KL, Sarnaik AP, et al: Indicators of postpyloric feeding tube placement in children, *Crit Care Med* 28(8):2962-2966, 2000.

Guyatt GH, Oxman AD, Vist GE, et al: GRADE: an emerging consensus on rating quality of evidence and strength of recommendations, *BMJ* 336:924-926, 2008.

Huffman S, Piper P, Jarczyk KS, et al: Methods to confirm feeding tube placement: application of research in practice, *Pediatr Nurs* 30(1):10-13, 2004.

Khair J: Guidelines for testing the placing of nasogastric tubes, *Nurs Times* 101(20):26-27, 2005.

Metheny N, Reed L, Wiersema L, et al: Effectiveness of pH measurements in predicting feeding tube placement: an update, *Nurs Res* 42(6):324-331, 1993.

Metheny NA, Schnelker R, McGinnis J, et al: Indicators of tube site during feedings, *J Neurosci Nurs* 37(6):320, 2005.

Metheny NA, Stewart BJ: Testing feeding tube placement during continuous tube feedings, *Appl Nurs Res* 15(4):254-258, 2002.

Metheny NA, Stewart BJ, Smith L, et al: pH and concentration of bilirubin in feeding tube aspirates as predictors of tube placement, *Nurs Res* 48(4):189-197, 1999.

Metheny NA, Titler MG: Assessing placement of feeding tubes, *AJN* 101(5):36-45, 2001.

Richardson DS, Branowicki PA, Zeidman-Rogers L, et al: An evidence-based approach to nasogastric tube management: special considerations, *J Pediatr Nurs* 5(21): 388-393, 2006.

Stevenson E: *How to confirm the correct position of naso and orogastric feeding tubes in babies under the care of neonatal units*, London, 2005, National Patient Safety Agency.

Westhus N: Methods to test feeding tube placement in children, *Am J MCN* 29(5):282-287, 2004.

Wilkes-Holmes C: Safe placement of nasogastric tubes in children, *Paediatr Nurs* 18(9):14-17, 2006.

 NURSING CARE GUIDELINES

Nasogastric Tube Feedings in Children

Place child supine with head slightly hyperflexed or in a sniffing position (nose pointed toward ceiling).

Measure the tube for approximate length of insertion, and mark the point with a small piece of tape.

Insert a tube that has been lubricated with sterile water or water-soluble lubricant through either the mouth or one of the nares to the predetermined mark. Because most young infants are obligatory nose breathers, insertion through the mouth causes less distress and helps stimulate sucking. In older infants and children the tube is passed through the nose and alternated between nostrils. An indwelling tube is almost always placed through the nose.

- When using the nose, slip the tube along the base of the nose and direct it straight back toward the occiput.
- When entering through the mouth, direct the tube toward the back of the throat (see Fig. 27-21, *B*).
- If the child is able to swallow on command, synchronize passing the tube with swallowing.

Confirm placement (see Evidence-Based Practice box, p. 1043).

Stabilize the tube by holding or taping it to the cheek, not to the forehead, because of possible damage to the nostril. To maintain correct placement, measure and record the amount of tubing extending from the nose or mouth to the distal port when the tube is first positioned. Recheck this measurement before each feeding.

Warm the formula to room temperature. Do not microwave! Pour formula into the barrel of the syringe attached to the feeding tube. To start the flow, give a gentle push with the plunger, but then remove the plunger and allow the fluid to flow into the stomach by gravity. The rate of flow should not exceed 5 ml every 5 to 10 minutes in premature and very small infants and 10 ml/min in older infants and children to prevent nausea and regurgitation. The rate is determined by the diameter of the tubing and the height of the reservoir containing the feeding and is regulated by adjusting the height of the syringe. A usual feeding may take 15 to 30 minutes to complete.

Flush the tube with sterile water (1 or 2 ml for small tubes to 5 to 15 ml or more for large ones), or see discussion of flushing for administering medication through nasogastric tubes in the Nursing Care Guidelines box, p. 1039, to clear it of formula.

Cap or clamp indwelling tubes to prevent loss of feeding.

- If the tube is to be removed, first pinch it firmly to prevent escape of fluid as the tube is withdrawn. Withdraw the tube quickly.

Position the child with the head elevated 30 to 45 degrees or on the right side for 30 to 60 minutes in the same manner as after any infant feeding to minimize the possibility of regurgitation and aspiration. If the child's condition permits, bubble the youngster after the feeding.

Record the feeding, including the type and amount of residual, the type and amount of formula, and how it was tolerated.

- For most infant feedings, any amount of residual fluid aspirated from the stomach is refed to prevent electrolyte imbalance, and the amount is subtracted from the prescribed amount of feeding. For example, if the infant is to receive 30 ml and 10 ml is aspirated from the stomach before the feeding, the 10 ml of aspirated stomach contents is refed along with 20 ml of feeding. Another method can be used in children. If residual fluid is more than one fourth of the last feeding, return the aspirate and recheck in 30 to 60 minutes. When residual fluid is less than one fourth of the last feeding, give the scheduled feeding. If large amounts of aspirated fluid persist and the child is due for another feeding, notify the practitioner.

---

healing, meticulous care is needed to keep the area surrounding the tube clean and dry to prevent excoriation and infection. Daily applications of antibiotic ointment or other preparations may be prescribed to aid in healing and prevent irritation (see p. 1049). Exercise care to prevent excessive pull on the catheter that might cause widening of the opening and subsequent leakage of highly irritating gastric juices. Secure the tube to the abdomen, leaving a small loop of tubing at the exit site to prevent tension on the site (see Evidence-Based Practice box).

Granulation tissue may grow around a gastrostomy site (Fig. 27-22). This moist, beefy red tissue is not a sign of infection. However, if it continues to grow, the excess moisture can irritate the surrounding skin.

For children receiving long-term gastrostomy feeding, a skin-level device (e.g., MIC-KEY, Bard Button) offers several advantages. The small, flexible silicone device protrudes slightly from the abdomen, is cosmetically pleasing, affords increased comfort and mobility to the child, is easy to care for, and is fully immersible in water. The one-way valve at the proximal end minimizes reflux and eliminates the need for clamping. However, the skin-level device requires a well-established gastrostomy site and is more expensive than the conventional tube.

EVIDENCE-BASED PRACTICE

Caterina Nicole Landry, Andrea J. Harrison,
Mary Hershey Pascual, and Barbara Montagnino

Skin Care: Prevention and Management of Gastrostomy Button and Gastrostomy Tube Breakdown

ASK THE QUESTION

In children with skin breakdown around the gastrostomy device (tube or skin-level button), what are the recommended interventions for management of skin issues?

SEARCH FOR THE EVIDENCE

Search strategies

Search selection criteria included English language publications on children and adults published on gastrostomy, care practice guidelines, and manufacturer product information.

Databases used

Cochrane Collaboration Database, Joanna Briggs Institute, Proquest, PubMed, Scopus, National Guideline Clearinghouse (AHRQ), SUMSearch, CINAHL, Wound Ostomy and Continence Nurses Society, American Pediatric Surgical Nurses Association, patient and family listservs

CRITICALLY ANALYZE THE EVIDENCE

GRADE criteria: Evidence quality very low; recommendation strong (Guyatt, Oxman, Vist, et al, 2008)

Skin care of the gastrostomy tube

Routine skin care around the gastrostomy tube (G tube) is key in reducing risk of infection and preventing skin breakdown. Most authors recommend cleaning with mild soap and water and keeping skin dry. Historically, hydrogen peroxide has been used around the stoma; however, this practice may be detrimental to skin and actually contribute to the complication of peristomal hypergranulation.

- The American Pediatric Surgical Nurses Association (2006) recommends cleaning the skin around the gastrostomy twice daily and as needed with warm soap and water and keeping the area dry. It is important to remove crusted areas around the G tube. Diluted half strength hydrogen peroxide may be used to clean for the first 2 weeks.
- The Wound Ostomy and Continence Nurses Society (2008) clinical guidelines identify the use of hydrogen peroxide as one of the possible causes of hypergranulation tissue. The guidelines recommend routine assessment of the site and keeping the skin around the G tube dry to prevent complications.
- McClave and Neff (2006) suggest cleaning the skin around the G tube with mild antibacterial soap and water. The use of hydrogen peroxide is discouraged because it is corrosive to the skin and leads to excessive drying of the tissue. Prompt treatment of skin irritation is vital in preventing further skin breakdown.
- Borkowski (2004, 2005) discourages the use of hydrogen peroxide because it can cause skin irritation and may be cytotoxic, disrupting wound healing. The author recommends gently cleaning the skin with water and patting dry, since aggressive cleaning around the G tube may also interfere with the healing process.
- Product information by the manufacturer of MIC-KEY (Kimberly-Clark, 2006) advises cleaning the skin around the G button with soap and water using a soft cotton tip applicator or washcloth. The document recommends inspecting the skin daily and reporting any complications to a health care provider.

Skin barriers

Although a small amount of leakage around the G tube is to be expected, excessive drainage or leakage can result in skin breakdown. Many products are available to protect the skin from leakage around the G tube. Some products protect the skin from moisture; others assist with the healing process and prevent further damage.

- The Wound Ostomy and Continence Nurses Society (2008) clinical guidelines recommend the use of barrier ointments such as zinc oxide and nonalcohol skin barrier film to control leakage. If skin irritation is present, the guidelines recommend adding absorptive powders and skin barrier wafers to help manage leakage and promote healing.
- Borkowski (2004, 2005) uses protective barriers such as zinc oxide and petrolatum to provide skin protection. For maceration around the stoma, the use of a solid skin barrier (pectin-based wafer Stomahesive) to provide an environment for protection and healing of the skin is recommended.

Stabilization

In long G tubes, stabilization is important to prevent accidental dislodgment and migration and to minimize irritation. Maintaining correct position is essential in preventing potential complications. Low-profile devices avoid these complications. Long tubes can be stabilized by commercial securing devices or other anchoring techniques.

- The Wound Ostomy and Continence Nurses Society (2008) recommends that the stabilizer be placed on the skin without excessive tension and pulling. If a long tube is not stabilized, it can increase the risk for infection, cause hyperplasia, and lead to skin breakdown.
- In three patients with peristomal irritation due to G tube mobility, Borkowski (2004) successfully managed two patients by applying a stabilization method to the G tube. In the third patient, despite the author's recommendation, the family refused to stabilize the G tube and preferred to treat the irritation with protective barrier ointments only. This finding illustrates the need to individualize care. There was no follow-up reported in the article regarding the success of the family's methods.
- McClave and Neff (2006) reported on their experience with percutaneous endoscopic gastrostomy (PEG) tubes. PEG tubes have increased risk for mobility and migration, which leads to ulceration and enlargement of the stoma. This can be prevented by stabilizing the tube.
- Crawley-Coha (2004) strongly recommends the use of stabilizing techniques to promote healing postoperatively and prevent dislodgment. In active children, the use of additional products such as elastic wraps and flexible dressings to immobilize the gastrostomy device is recommended.

Hypergranulation

The development of hypergranulation tissue is a common problem often occurring within a week of G tube placement. Granulation tissue is triggered by the body's reaction to the G tube as a foreign body. As stated previously, hypergranulation is aggravated by tube instability, skin irritation due to moisture, and the use of hydrogen peroxide.

- In a longitudinal study of 40 children with G tubes, granulation tissue occurred two times more often in children with long tube devices than those who had skin level devices (Thorne, Radford, Onyskiw, et al, 1998).
- In a prospective study of eight patients, granulation tissue was the complication that prompted the most hospital and physician visits. Granulation tissue affected five patients (63%). Although families and caregivers were educated about the potential complications, this did not eliminate unscheduled health care contacts (Crosby and Duerksen, 2007).

Continued

Skin Care: Prevention and Management of Gastrostomy Button and Gastrostomy Tube Breakdown

Hypergranulation—cont'd

- Borkowski (2004, 2005) recommends the use of triamcinolone (0.5% to 0.1%) cream as a less painful alternative to the traditional silver nitrate sticks. Polyurethane foam may be used to absorb moisture and keep the skin dry to prevent further breakdown. One 2 × 2 gauze may be placed to create a snug fit for an ill-fitting low-profile device and assist with keeping the skin dry. Stabilization of the tube is a priority to prevent the development of hypergranulation.
- In the experience of Crawley-Coha (2004), hypergranulation tissue can occur regardless of type of G tube placed and method of stabilization used. Treatment options include the application of silver nitrate, sharp débridement, and topical steroids. This author used triamcinolone cream (0.5%) three times a day with great success for the previous 6 years. In some patients, polyurethane foam dressing is also used to manage hypergranulation tissue.
- The Wound Ostomy and Continence Nurses Society (2008) clinical guidelines recommend managing hypergranulation by stabilizing the tube, keeping the peristomal area dry by applying polyurethane foam, and using triamcinolone (0.5%) three times a day. Silver nitrate may also be used for hypergranulation.

Individualizing care

When teaching a family about the management of their child's G tube and its associated complications, it is important to individualize teaching to meet the family's needs.

- Borkowski (2004) acknowledges when children with G tube develop complications despite family education on alternative management options, families may have chosen to continue to use familiar techniques. The care plan for managing complications should consider the child's developmental age, activity level, and parental preferences.
- Crawley-Coha (2004) recommends providing parents with individualized written instructions before discharge. Ongoing support should be provided by the child's medical team. To assist with transition to the home information on support groups for patients with G tubes may be offered (e.g., Oley Foundation, **www.oley.org**).

APPLY THE EVIDENCE: NURSING IMPLICATIONS

1. Use mild soap and water to clean peristomal area.
2. If skin irritation or breakdown is noted, use appropriate skin barriers:
   - Zinc oxide–based ointment, petrolatum-based ointment, or nonalcohol skin barrier for prevention or treatment of breakdown
   - Solid pectin-based wafer for maceration
3. Stabilize long G tube using one of the three methods: commercial stabilization device, polyurethane foam, or the H tape method.
4. Request order for triamcinolone cream for short-term treatment of hypergranulation.
5. Individualize skin care management.

References

American Pediatric Surgical Nurses Association: Gastrostomy, 2006. Available at http://data.memberclicks.com/site/aps/GASTROSTOMY.doc. Accessed December 17, 2008.

Borkowski S: G tube care: managing hypergranulation tissue, *Nursing* 35(8):24, 2005.

Borkowski S: Similar gastrostomy peristomal skin irritations in three pediatric patients, *J Wound Ostomy Contin Nurs* 31(4):201-206, 2004.

Crawley-Coha T: A practical guide for the management of pediatric gastrostomy tubes based on 14 year experience, *J Wound Ostomy Contin Nurs* 31(4):193-200, 2004.

Crosby J, Duerksen D: A prospective study of tube- and feeding-related complications in patients receiving long-term home enteral nutrition, *J Parenter Enter Nutr* 31(4):274-277, 2007.

Guyatt GH, Oxman AD, Vist GE, et al: GRADE: an emerging consensus on rating quality of evidence and strength of recommendations, *BMJ* 336:924-926, 2008.

Kimberly-Clark: *MIC-KEY: low profile gastrostomy feeding tube—your guide to proper care,* 2006. Available at http://kchealthcare.com/docs/R8201B%20MIC-KEY%20Care%20guide%20English.pdf. Accessed December 10, 2008.

McClave S, Neff R: Care and long-term maintenance of percutaneous endoscopic gastrostomy tubes [electronic version], *J Parenter Enter Nutr* 30(1):S27-S38, 2006.

Thorne S, Radford J, Onyskiw J, et al: A comparative longitudinal study of gastrostomy devices in children [electronic version], *West J Nurs Res* 20(2):145-165, 1998.

Wound Ostomy and Continence Nurses Society: *Management of gastrostomy tube complications for the pediatric and adult patient,* 2008. Available at www.wocn.org/WOCN_Library. Accessed December 2, 2008.

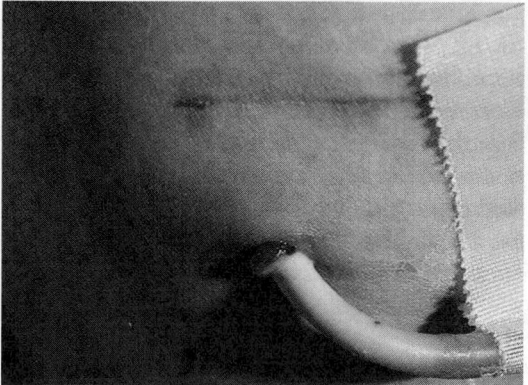

Fig. 27-22 Appearance of healthy granulation tissue around stoma.

In addition, the valve may become clogged. When functioning, the valve prevents air from escaping; therefore the child may require frequent bubbling. With some devices, during feedings the child must remain fairly still because the tubing easily disconnects from the opening if the child moves. With other devices, extension tubing can be securely attached to the opening (Fig. 27-23). The feeding is instilled at the other end of the tubing in a manner similar to that for a regular gastrostomy. The extension tubing may also have a separate medication port. Both the feeding and the medication ports have plugs attached. Some skin-level devices require a special tube to be able to decompress the stomach (to check residual or decompress air).

Feeding of water, formula, or pureed foods is carried out in the same manner and rate as for gavage feeding. A mechanical pump may be used to regulate the volume and rate of feeding. After feedings the infant or child is positioned on the right side or in the Fowler position, and the tube may be clamped or left open and suspended between feedings, depending on the child's condition. A clamped tube allows more mobility but is only appropriate if the child can tolerate intermittent feedings without vomiting or prolonged backup of feeding into the tube. Sometimes a Y tube is used to allow for simultaneous

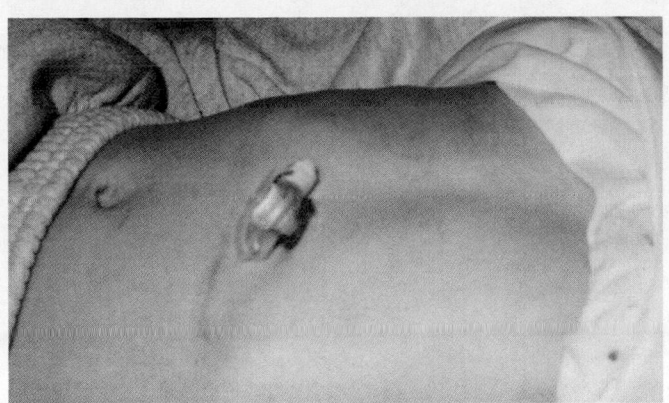

Fig. 27-23 Child with skin-level gastrostomy device (MIC-KEY), which provides for secure attachment of extension tubing to gastrostomy opening.

decompression during feeding. If a Foley catheter is used as the gastrostomy tube, apply very slight tension. The tube is securely taped to maintain the balloon at the gastrostomy opening and prevent leakage of gastric contents and the tube's progression toward the pyloric sphincter, where it may occlude the stomach outlet. As a precaution, the length of the tube is measured postoperatively and then remeasured each shift to be certain it has not slipped. The nurse can make a mark above the skin level to further ensure its placement. When the gastrostomy tube is no longer needed, it is removed; the skin opening usually closes spontaneously by contracture.

NASODUODENAL AND NASOJEJUNAL TUBES

Children at high risk for regurgitation or aspiration such as those with gastroparesis, mechanical ventilation, or brain injuries may require placement of a postpyloric feeding tube. A trained practitioner inserts the nasoduodenal or nasojejunal tube because of the risk of misplacement and potential for perforation in tubes requiring a stylet. Accurate placement is verified by radiography. Small-bore tubes may easily clog. Flush tube when feeding is interrupted, before and after medication administration, and routinely every 4 hours or as directed by institutional policy. Tube replacement should be considered monthly to ensure optimal tube patency. Continuous feedings are delivered by mechanical pump to regulate volume and rate. Bolus feeds are contraindicated. Tube displacement is suspected in the child showing signs of feeding intolerance such as vomiting. Stop feedings and notify the practitioner.

TOTAL PARENTERAL NUTRITION

Total parenteral nutrition (TPN) provides for the total nutritional needs of infants or children whose lives are threatened because feeding by way of the gastrointestinal tract is impossible, inadequate, or hazardous.

TPN therapy involves IV infusion of highly concentrated solutions of protein, glucose, and other nutrients. The solution is infused through conventional tubing with a special filter attached to remove particulate matter or microorganisms that may have contaminated the solution. The highly concentrated solutions require infusion into a vessel with sufficient volume and turbulence to allow for rapid dilution. The wide-diameter

vessels selected are the superior vena cava and innominate or intrathoracic subclavian veins approached by way of the external or internal jugular veins. The highly irritating nature of concentrated glucose precludes the use of the small peripheral veins in most instances. However, dilute glucose-protein hydrolysates that are appropriate for infusing into peripheral veins are being used with increasing frequency. When peripheral veins are used, intralipid becomes the major calorie source. For long-term alimentation, central venous catheters are usually used.

The major nursing responsibilities are the same as for any IV therapy: control of sepsis, monitoring of the infusion rate, and assessment of the patient. The TPN solution must be prepared under rigid aseptic conditions, which is best accomplished by specially trained technicians. Specially trained nurses should change the solution and tubing and redress the infusion using meticulous aseptic precautions. In some institutions this may be a nursing responsibility. If so, the procedure is carried out according to hospital protocol.

The infusion is maintained at a constant rate by means of an infusion pump to ensure the proper concentrations of glucose and amino acids. Accurate calculation of the rate is required to deliver a measured amount in a given length of time. Because alterations in flow rate are relatively common, the drip should be checked frequently to ensure an even, continuous infusion. The TPN infusion rate should not be increased or decreased without the practitioner being informed, since alterations can cause hyperglycemia or hypoglycemia.

General assessments, such as vital signs, input and output measurements, and checking results of laboratory tests, facilitate early detection of infection or fluid and electrolyte imbalance. Additional amounts of potassium and sodium chloride are often required in hyperalimentation; therefore observation for signs of potassium or sodium deficit or excess is part of nursing care. This is rarely a problem except in children with reduced renal function or metabolic defects. Hyperglycemia may occur during the first day or two as the child adapts to the high-glucose load of the hyperalimentation solution. Although hyperglycemia occurs infrequently, insulin may be required to help the body adjust. When this occurs, nursing responsibilities include blood glucose testing. To prevent hypoglycemia when the hyperalimentation is disconnected, the rate of the infusion and the amount of insulin are decreased gradually.

FAMILY TEACHING AND HOME CARE

When alternative feedings are needed for an extended period, the family needs to learn how to feed the child with a nasogastric, gastrostomy, or TPN feeding regimen. The same principles apply as discussed earlier in this chapter for compliance, especially in terms of education, and in Chapter 26 for discharge planning and home care. Plan ample time for the family to learn and perform the procedures under supervision before they assume full responsibility for the child's care. Refer the family to community agencies that provide support and practical assistance. The Oley Foundation* is a nonprofit research

*214 Hun Memorial, MC-28, Albany Medical Center, Albany, NY 12208; 800-776-OLEY; www.oley.org.

Evidence-Based Practice—Central Venous Catheter Site Care

and education organization that assists persons receiving enteral nutrition and home TPN.

PROCEDURES RELATED TO ELIMINATION

ENEMA

The procedure for giving an enema to an infant or child does not differ essentially from that for an adult, except for the type and amount of fluid administered and the distance for inserting the tube into the rectum (Table 27-8). Depending on the volume, use a syringe with rubber tubing, an enema bottle, or an enema bag.

An isotonic solution is used in children. Plain water is not used because, being hypotonic, it can cause rapid fluid shift and fluid overload. The Fleet enema (pediatric or adult sized) is not advised for children because of the harsh action of its ingredients (sodium biphosphate and sodium phosphate). Commercial enemas can be dangerous to patients with megacolon and to dehydrated or azotemic children. The osmotic effect of the Fleet enema may produce diarrhea, which can lead to metabolic acidosis. Other potential complications are extreme hyperphosphatemia, hypernatremia, and hypocalcemia, which may lead to neuromuscular irritability and coma (Walton, Thomas, Aly, et al, 2000).

> **NURSING TIP** If prepared saline is not available, the nurse can make some by adding 1 tsp table salt to 500 ml (1 pint) of tap water.

Because infants and young children are unable to retain the solution after it is administered, the buttocks must be held together for a short time to retain the fluid. The enema is administered and expelled while the child is lying with the buttocks over the bedpan and with the head and back supported by pillows. Older children are ordinarily able to hold the solution if they understand what to do and if they are not expected to hold it for too long. The nurse should have the bedpan handy or, for the ambulatory child, ensure that the bathroom is available before beginning the procedure. An enema is an intrusive procedure and thus threatening to the preschool child; therefore a careful explanation is especially important to ease possible fear.

A preoperative bowel preparation solution given orally or through a nasogastric tube is increasingly being used instead of an enema. The polyethylene glycol–electrolyte lavage solution (GoLYTELY) mechanically flushes the bowel without significant absorption, thereby avoiding potential fluid and electrolyte imbalances. NuLYTELY, a modification of GoLYTELY, has the

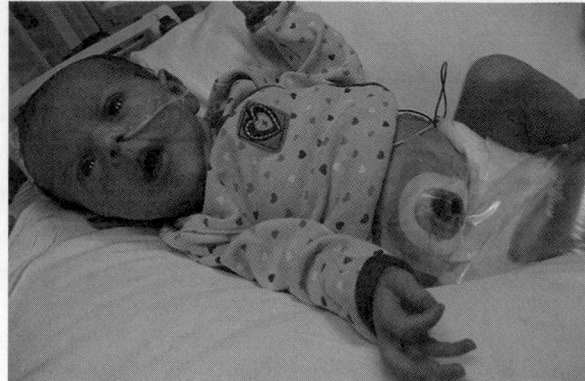

Fig. 27-24 Infant with ostomy and pouch.

same therapeutic advantages as GoLYTELY and was developed to improve on the taste. Another effective oral cathartic is magnesium citrate solution.

OSTOMIES

Children may require stomas for various health problems. The most frequent causes in the infant are necrotizing enterocolitis and imperforate anus and, less often, Hirschsprung disease. In the older child the most frequent causes are inflammatory bowel disease, especially Crohn disease (regional enteritis), and ureterostomies for distal ureter or bladder defects.

Care and management of ostomies in the older child differ little from the care of ostomies in the adult patient. The major emphasis in pediatric care is preparing the child for the procedure and teaching care of the ostomy to the child and family. The basic principles of preparation are the same as for any procedure (see p. 1000). Simple, straightforward language is most effective, together with the use of illustrations and a replica model (e.g., drawing a picture of a child with a stoma on the abdomen and explaining it as "another opening where bowel movements [or any other term the child uses] will come out"). At another time the nurse can draw a pouch over the opening to demonstrate how the contents are collected. Using a doll to demonstrate the process is an excellent teaching strategy, and special books are available.

Children with ileostomies are fitted immediately after surgery with an appliance to protect the skin from the proteolytic enzymes in the liquid stool. Infants may not be fitted with a pouch in the immediate postoperative period. When stomal drainage is minimal, as is often the case in small or preterm infants, a gauze dressing will suffice. Give your parents a choice of caring for the colostomy with or without an appliance. Pediatric appliances are available in a variety of sizes to ensure an adequate fit.*

Ostomy equipment consists of a one- or two-piece system with a hypoallergenic skin barrier to maintain peristomal skin integrity (Fig. 27-24). The pouch should be large enough to contain a moderate amount of stool and flatus but not so large as to overwhelm the infant or child. A backing helps minimize

---

*Parents may find the following pamphlets helpful: *A Parent's Guide to Necrotizing Enterocolitis* or *Parent's Guide to Ostomy Care for Children*, available from ConvaTec (**www.convatec.com**).

TABLE 27-8	ADMINISTRATION OF ENEMAS TO CHILDREN	
AGE	**AMOUNT (ml)**	**INSERTION DISTANCE**
Infant	120-240	2.5 cm (1 inch)
2-4 yr	240-360	5 cm (2 inch)
4-10 yr	360-480	7.5 cm (3 inch)
11 yr	480-720	10 cm (4 inch)

the risk of skin breakdown from moisture trapped between the skin and pouch. Avoid small clips or rubber bands to prevent choking in the young child.

Protection of the peristomal skin is a major aspect of stoma care. Well-fitting appliances are important to prevent leakage of contents. Before applying the appliance, prepare the skin with a skin sealant that is allowed to dry. Then apply stoma paste around the base of the stoma or to the back of the wafer. The sealant and paste work together to prevent peristomal skin breakdown.

In infants with a colostomy left unpouched, skin care is similar to that of any diapered child. However, protect the peristomal skin with a barrier substance (e.g., zinc oxide ointment [Sensi-Care] or a mixture of zinc oxide ointment and stoma powder [Stomahesive]). A diaper larger than the one usually worn may be needed to extend upward over the stoma and absorb drainage. If the skin becomes inflamed, denuded, or infected, the care is similar to the interventions used for diaper dermatitis. (See Chapter 13.) A zinc-based product helps protect healthy skin, heal excoriated skin, and minimize pain associated with skin breakdown. The skin protectant adheres to denuded, weeping skin. The nurse can apply zinc-based products over topical antifungal and antibacterial agents if infection is present. No-sting barrier film is a skin sealant that has no alcohol base and can be used on open skin without stinging.

With young children, preventing them from pulling off the pouch is also an important consideration. One-piece outfits keep exploring hands from reaching the pouch, and the loose waist avoids any pressure on the appliance. Keeping the child occupied with toys during the pouch change is also helpful. As children mature, encourage their participation in ostomy care. Even preschoolers can assist by holding supplies, pulling paper backings from the appliance, and helping clean the stoma area. Toilet training for bladder control needs to begin at the appropriate time, as for any other child.

Older children and adolescents should eventually have total responsibility for ostomy care just as they would for usual bowel function. During adolescence, concerns for body image and the ostomy's impact on intimacy and sexuality emerge. The nurse should stress to teenagers that the presence of a stoma need not interfere with their activities. These youngsters can choose which ostomy equipment is best suited to their needs. Attractively designed and decorated pouch covers are well liked by teenagers.

Children with familial adenomatous polyposis may require a colectomy with ileoanal reservoir to prevent or treat carcinoma of the colon. Peristomal skin care for these children is particularly challenging because of increased liquid stools, increased digestive enzymes that may cause skin breakdown, and the stoma being at skin level rather than raised. Additional care with this condition includes close monitoring of fluid and electrolyte status and increased incidence of bowel obstruction.

An enterostomal therapy nurse specialist is an important member of the health care team and will have additional suggestions and assistance with skin care information and ostomy pouching options. The nurse can obtain further information by contacting the Wound, Ostomy and Continence Nurses Society.*

FAMILY TEACHING AND HOME CARE

Because these children are almost always discharged with a functioning colostomy, preparation of the family should begin as early as possible in the hospital. The nurse instructs the family in the application of the device (if used), care of the skin, and appropriate action in case skin problems develop. Early evidence of skin breakdown or stomal complications, such as ribbonlike stools, excessive diarrhea, bleeding, prolapse, or failure to pass flatus or stool, is brought to the attention of the physician, nurse, or stoma specialist. The same principles are applied as discussed earlier in this chapter for compliance, especially in terms of education, and in Chapter 26 for discharge planning and home care.

---

*888-224-9626; www.wocn.org.

▌ KEY POINTS

- Informed consent is valid when the person is capable of giving consent (is over the age of majority and is competent), is supplied with information needed to make an intelligent decision, and acts voluntarily when exercising freedom of choice.
- Informed consent is needed for major surgery, minor surgery, and diagnostic tests and medical treatments with an element of risk.
- The major principles in psychologic preparation of the child for surgery are to establish trust, provide support, and give an explanation in easy-to-understand terms.
- Preparation for procedures should be based on developmental characteristics of the child and family, emphasizing the importance of the parents' role.
- Most parents and children want to be together during stressful procedures and should be offered this opportunity, with guidance on how the parent can comfort the child.

- The use of play activities to provide teaching about necessary nursing and medical interventions is an effective tool for use with children.
- In the performance of a procedure, the nurse should expect success, involve the child when possible in the procedure, provide distraction, and allow for expression of feelings.
- Proper positioning of infants and small children for procedures is essential to minimize movement and discomfort.
- In giving postprocedural support, the nurse should encourage children to express their feelings and praise them for completion of the procedure.
- Stressful times before and after surgery that produce anxiety in children are admission, blood tests, injection of preoperative medication (if used), transportation to the operating room, and return from the PACU.
- Assessment of compliance entails measuring factors that affect compliance through clinical judgment, self-reporting,

- direct observation, monitoring of appointments and therapeutic response, pill counts, and chemical assay.
- Compliance strategies may be classified as organizational, educational, and behavioral.
- Knowledge of the ill child's eating habits and favorite foods can help in maintaining adequate nutrition.
- Skin care is essential to prevent skin breakdown.
- Control of fever may be accomplished by administration of antipyretics; hyperthermia is controlled by environmental means (minimum clothing, increased air circulation, hypothermia mattress, or cool compresses).
- Infection control is based on two systems. Standard Precautions provide protection when the infected person is undiagnosed. Transmission-Based Precautions add extra interventions for patients diagnosed with or suspected of having an infection.

- Ensuring safety in the hospital setting is a major concern and can be achieved through environmental measures, infection control measures, limit setting, and safe transportation.
- Restraints are used cautiously and require a medical order. Therapeutic hugging can avoid the use of restraints.
- Factors that affect drug dosage determination are growth and maturation, difficulty in evaluating drug response, and BSA.
- Family teaching regarding medication administration includes telling parents why the child is receiving the drug; its possible effects; and the amount, frequency, and length of time the drug is to be administered.
- Alternative forms of feeding include gavage feeding, gastrostomy feeding, and TPN.
- In the care of children with ostomies, nurses play an important role in family support and instruction in care of the stoma site.

REFERENCES

American Academy of Pediatrics: Consent for emergency medical services for children and adolescents, *Pediatrics* 111(3):703-706, 2003.

American Academy of Pediatrics, Task Force on Sudden Infant Death Syndrome: The changing concept of sudden infant death syndrome: diagnostic coding shifts, controversies regarding the sleeping environment, and new variables to consider in reducing risk, *Pediatrics* 116(5):1245-1255, 2005.

American Academy of Pediatrics, Committee on Pediatric Emergency Medicine, American College of Emergency Physicians, Pediatric Emergency Medicine Committee, O'Malley P, et al: Patient- and family-centered care and the role of the emergency physician providing care to a child in the emergency department, *Pediatrics* 118(5):2242-2244, 2006.

American Association of Critical Care Nurses: Practice alert: Family presence during CPR and invasive procedures, 2006. Available at www.aacn.org. Accessed July 7, 2009.

Amlung SR, Miller WL, Bosley LM: The 1999 national pressure ulcer prevalence survey: a benchmarking approach, *Adv Skin Wound Care* 14:297-301, 2001.

Anderson SL, Schaechter J, Brosco JP: Adolescent patients and their confidentiality: staying within legal bounds, *Contemp Pediatr* 22(7):54, 2005.

Axelrod P: External cooling in the management of fever, *Clin Infect Dis* 31(Suppl 5):S224-S229, 2000.

Baharestani MM, Ratliff CR: Pressure ulcers in neonates and children: an NPUAP white paper, *Adv Skin Wound Care* 20(4):208-220, 2007.

Barnes S: Not a social event: the follow-up phone call, *J Perianesth Nurs* 14(4):223-255, 2000.

Beckstrand J, Ellett MLC, McDaniel A: Predicting internal distance to the stomach for positioning NG and OG feeding tubes in children, *J Adv Nurs* 59(3):274-289, 2007.

Berger JE, American Academy of Pediatrics Committee on Medical Liability: Consent by proxy for nonurgent pediatric care, *Pediatrics* 112(5):1186-1195, 2003.

Bryant RA, Doughty D, editors: *Acute and chronic wounds: nursing management,* ed 2, St Louis, 2000, Mosby.

Burke N: Alternative methods for newborn urine sample collection, *Pediatr Nurs* 21(6):546-549, 1995.

Child Health Corporation of America: Pediatric falls: state of the science, *Pediatr Nurs* 35(4):227-231, 2009.

Codipietro L, Ceccarelli M, Ponzone A: Breastfeeding or oral sucrose solution in term neonates receiving heel lance: a randomized, controlled trial, *Pediatrics* 122(3):e716-e721, 2008.

Considine J, Brennan D: Effect of an evidence-based education programme on ED discharge advice for febrile children, *J Clin Nurs* 16:1687-1694, 2007.

Cook IF, Murtagh J: Ventrogluteal area—a suitable site for intramuscular vaccination of infants and toddlers, *Vaccine* 24(13):2403-2408, 2006.

Cook IF, Murtagh J: Needle length required for intramuscular vaccination of infants and toddlers: an ultrasonographic study, *Aust Fam Physician* 31(3):295-297, 2002.

Curley MAG, Quigley SM, Lin M: Pressure ulcers in pediatric intensive care: incidence and associated factors, *Pediatr Crit Care Med* 4:284-290, 2003.

Curley MAQ, Razmus IS, Roberts KE, et al: Predicting pressure ulcer risk in pediatric patients: the Braden Q scale, *Nurs Res* 52:22-33, 2003.

Eaton L: Hand washing is more important than cleaner wards in controlling MRSA, *BMJ* 330(7497):922, 2005.

Ellett ML, Beckstrand J: Examination of gavage tube placement in children, *J Soc Pediatr Nurs* 4(2):51-60, 1999.

Emergency Nurses Association: Family presence at the bedside during invasive procedures and resuscitation, 2005. Available at www.ena.org. Accessed July 7, 2009.

Essink-Tebbes CM, Wuis EW, Liem KD, et al: Safety of lidocaine-prilocaine cream application four times a day in premature neonates: a pilot study, *Eur J Pediatr* 158(5):421-423, 1999.

Gray L, Watt L, Blass EM: Skin-to-skin contact is analgesic in healthy newborns, *Pediatrics* 105(1):110-111, 2000. Available at www.pediatrics.org/cgi/content/full/105/1/E14. Accessed June 10, 2009.

Gray M: Atraumatic urethral catheterization of children, *Pediatr Nurs* 22(4):306-310, 1996.

Joint Commission on Accreditation of Healthcare Organizations: *Comprehensive accreditation manual for hospitals: restraint and seclusion standards,* TX7.1-TX7.5.5, Oakbrook Terrace, Ill, 2001, The Commission.

Jones T, Jacobsen SJ: Childhood febrile seizures: overview and implications, *Intl J Med Sci* 4(2):110-114, 2007.

Kain ZN, Caldwell-Andrews AA, Krivutza DM, et al: Trends in the practice of parental presence during induction of anesthesia and the use of preoperative sedative premedication in the United States, 1995-2002: results of a follow-up national survey, *Anesth Analg* 98(5):1252-1259, 2004.

Kain ZN, Caldwell-Andrews AA, Mayes LC, et al: Family-centered preparation for surgery improves perioperative outcomes in children, *Anesthesiology* 106(1):65-74, 2007.

Katsma D, Smith G: Analysis of needle path during intramuscular injection, *Nurs Res* 46(5):288-292, 1997.

Kellam B, Sacks LM, Wailer JL, et al: Tenderfoot Preemie vs a manual lancet: a clinical evaluation, *Neonatal Netw* 20(7):31-36, 2001.

Klasner AE, Luke DA, Scalzo AJ: Pediatric orogastric and nasogastric tubes: a new formula evaluated, *Ann Emerg Med* 39(3):268-272, 2002.

Klein EJ, Diekema DS, Paris CA, et al: A randomized, clinical trial of oral midazolam plus placebo versus oral midazolam plus oral transmucosal fentanyl for sedation during laceration repair, *Pediatrics* 109(5):894-897, 2002.

Kraus D, Stohlmeyer LA, Hannon DR, et al: Effectiveness and infant acceptance of the Rx Medibottle versus the oral syringe, *Pharmacotherapy* 21(4):416-423, 2001.

Kyngas H, Kroll T, Duffy M: Compliance in adolescents with chronic diseases: a review, *J Adolesc Health* 26:379-388, 2000.

Li HCW, Lopez V, Lee TLI: Psychoeducational preparation of children for surgery: the importance of parental involvement, *Patient Educ Counsel* 65:34-41, 2007.

Manworren R, Fledderman M: Preparation of the child and family for surgery. In Wise BV, McKenna C, Garvin G, et al, editors: *Nursing care of the general pediatric surgical patient,* Gaithersburg, Md, 2000, Aspen.

Maxwell LG, Yaster M: Perioperative management issues in pediatric patients, *Anesthesiol Clin North Am* 18(3):601-632, 2000.

McCord S, McElvain V, Sachdeva R, et al: Risk factors associated with pressure ulcers in the pediatric intensive care unit, *J Wound Ostomy Continence Nurs* 31(4):179-183, 2004.

McGillivray D, Mok E, Mulrooney E, et al: A head-to-head comparison: "clean-void" bag versus catheter urinalysis in the diagnosis of urinary tract infection in young children, *J Pediatr* 147(4), 451-456, 2008.

Munro H, D'Errico FC: Parental involvement in perioperative anesthetic management, *J Perianesth Nurs* 15(6):397-400, 2000.

Noonan C, Quigley S, Curley MAQ: Skin integrity in hospitalized infants and children: a prevalence survey, *J Pediatr Nurs* 21(6):445-453, 2006.

Piira T, Sugiura T, Champion GD, et al: The role of parental presence in the context of children's medical procedures: a systematic review, *Child Care Health Devel* 31(2):233-243, 2005.

Purssell E: Parental fever phobia and its evolutionary correlates, *J Clin Nurs* 18:210-218, 2008.

Quality, equipment hold keys to infection control, *ED Manage* 18(2):19-21, 2006.

Rosenberg H, Davis M, James D: Malignant hyperthermia, *Orphanet J Rare Dis* 2:21, 2007.

Romino SL, Keatley VM, Secrest J, et al: Parental presence during anesthesia induction in children, *AORN J* 81(4):780-792, 2005.

Rote N, Huether S, McCance K: Infections and alterations in immunity and inflammation. In Huether S, McCance K, editors: *Understanding pathophysiology,* ed 2, St Louis, 2000, Mosby.

Sadleir LG, & Scheffer IE: Febrile seizures, *BMJ* 334:307-311, 2007.

Shah V, Ohlsson A: Venepuncture versus heel lance for blood sampling in term neonates, *Cochrane Database Syst Rev* (4):CD001452, 2007.

Shepherd AJ, Glenesk A, Niven CA, et al: A Scottish study of heel-prick blood sampling in newborn babies, *Midwifery* 22(2):158-168, 2005.

Tillett J: Adolescents and informed consent: ethical and legal issues, *J Perinat Neonat Nurs* 19(2):112-121, 2005.

Uman LS, Chambers CT, McGrath PJ, et al: Psychological interventions for needle-related procedural pain and distress in children and adolescents, *Cochrane Database Syst Rev* (4):CD005179.DOI:10.1002/14651858. CD005179.pub2, 2006.

Vertanen H, Fellman V, Brommels M, et al: An automatic incision device for obtaining blood samples from the heels of the preterm infants causes less damage than a conventional manual lancet, *Arch Dis Child Fetal Neonatal Educ* 84:F53-F55, 2001.

Wald ER: To bag or not to bag, *J Pediatr* 174(4):418-419, 2005.

Walsh A, Edwards H: Management of childhood fever by parents: literature review, *J Adv Nurs* 54(2):217-222, 2006.

Walton DM, Thomas DC, Aly HZ, et al: Morbid hypocalcemia associated with phosphate enema in a 6-week-old infant, *Pediatrics* 106:e37, 2000.

Warren J, Fromm RE Jr, Orr RA, et al: Guidelines for the inter- and intrahospital transport of critically ill patients, *Crit Care Med* 32(1):256-262, 2004.

Willock J, Baharestani M, Anthony D: The development of the Glamorgan paediatric pressure ulcer risk assessment scale, *J Wound Care* 18(1):17-21, 2009.

CHAPTER

28

Balance and Imbalance of Body Fluids

David Wilson

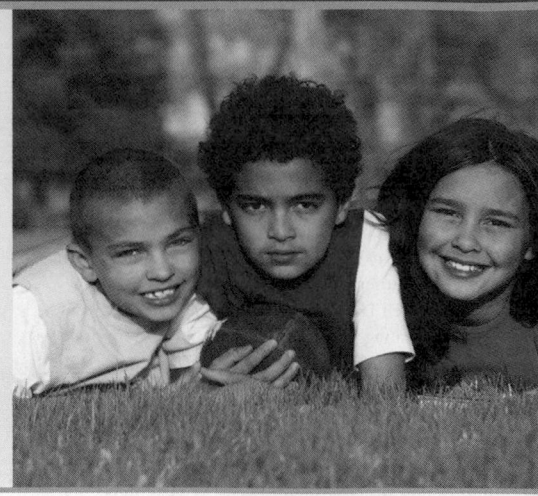

CHAPTER OUTLINE

▌DISTRIBUTION OF BODY FLUIDS

The distribution of body fluids, or total body water (TBW), involves the presence of intracellular fluid (ICF) and extracellular fluid (ECF). Water is the major constituent of body tissues,

and the TBW in an individual ranges from 45% (in late adolescence) to 75% (in term newborn) of total body weight.

The ICF refers to the fluid contained within the cells, whereas the ECF is the fluid outside the cells. The ECF is further broken down into several components: intravascular (contained within the blood vessels), interstitial (surrounding the cell; the location of most ECF), and transcellular (contained within specialized body cavities such as cerebrospinal, synovial, and pleural fluid). In the newborn about 50% of the body fluid is contained within the ECF, whereas 30% of the toddler's body fluid is contained within the ECF.

Body water is important in body function not only because of its abundance but also because it is the medium in which body solutes are dissolved and all metabolic reactions take place. Because even small alterations in fluid composition affect these metabolic processes, precise regulation of the volume and composition of the fluid is essential. In healthy individuals, body water remains singularly constant, but marked alterations in either its volume or distribution, which occur in many disease states, can produce severely damaging physiologic consequences.

WATER BALANCE

Under normal conditions the amount of water ingested closely approximates the amount of urine excreted in a 24-hour period, and the water in food and from oxidation approximates the amount lost in feces and through evaporation. In this way, the body maintains equilibrium.

Mechanisms of Fluid Movement

Water is retained in the body in a relatively constant amount and, with few exceptions, is freely exchangeable among all body fluid compartments. The proximity of the extravascular compartment to the cells allows for continuous change in volume and distribution of fluids, largely determined by solutes (especially sodium) and physical forces (Fig. 28-1). Transport mechanisms are the basis for all activity within the cells, and because the cells have limited ability to store materials, movement in and out of cells must be rapid. Internal control mechanisms are responsible for distribution and maintenance of fluid balance (Box 28-1).

Maintaining Water Balance

Maintenance water requirement is the volume of water needed to replace obligatory fluid loss such as that from insensible water loss (through the skin and respiratory tract), evaporative water loss, and losses through urine and stool formation. The amount and type of these losses may be altered by disease states such as fever (with increased sweating), diarrhea, gastric suction, and pooling of body fluids in a body space (often referred to as *third spacing*).

Nurses should be alert for altered fluid requirements in various conditions:

Increased requirements:
- Fever (add 12% per rise of 1° C)
- Vomiting, diarrhea
- High-output kidney failure
- Diabetes insipidus
- Diabetic ketoacidosis
- Burns
- Shock
- Tachypnea
- Radiant warmer (preterm infant)
- Phototherapy (infants)
- Postoperative bowel surgery (gastroschisis, omphalocele)

Decreased requirements:
- Congestive heart failure
- Syndrome of inappropriate antidiuretic hormone
- Mechanical ventilation
- After surgery
- Oliguric renal failure
- Increased intracranial pressure

Basal maintenance calculations for required body water are based on the body's requirements for water in a normometabolic state, at rest; estimated fluid requirements are then increased or decreased from these parameters based on increased or decreased water losses, such as with elevated body temperature or congestive heart failure. Daily maintenance fluid requirements are listed in Table 28-1.

Maintenance fluids contain both water and electrolytes and can be estimated from the child's age, body weight, degree of activity, and body temperature. Basal metabolic rate (BMR) is derived from standard tables and adjusted for the child's activity, temperature, and disease state. For example, for afebrile patients at rest, the maintenance water requirement is approximately 100 ml for each 100 kcal expended. Children with fluid losses or other alterations require adjustment of these basic needs to accommodate abnormal losses of both water and electrolytes as a result of a disease state. For example, insensible losses increase when basal expenditure increases by fever or hypermetabolic states. Hypometabolic states, such as hypothyroidism and hypothermia, decrease the BMR.

Changes in Fluid Volume Related to Growth

The percentage of TBW varies among individuals and in adults and older children is related primarily to the amount of body fat. Consequently, females, who have more body fat than males, and obese persons tend to have less water content in relation to weight.

The fetus is composed primarily of water, with little tissue substance. As the organism grows and develops, a progressive decrease occurs in TBW, with the fastest rate of decline taking place during fetal life. The changes in water content and distribution that occur with age reflect the changes that take place in the relative amounts of bone, muscle, and fat making up the body. At maturity the percentage of TBW is somewhat higher in the male than in the female and is probably a result of the differences in body composition, particularly fat and muscle content (Fig. 28-2).

Another important aspect of growth change as it corresponds to water distribution is related to the ICF and ECF compartments. In the fetus and prematurely born infant, the largest proportion of body water is contained in the ECF compartment. As growth and development proceed, the proportion within this fluid compartment decreases as the ICF and cell solids increase. The ECF diminishes rapidly from approximately 40% of body weight at birth to less than 30% at 1 year of age. The different effects on males and females become apparent at puberty.

Water Balance in Infants

Because of several characteristics, infants and young children have a greater need for water and are more vulnerable to alterations in fluid and electrolyte balance. Compared with older children and adults, they have a greater fluid intake and output

PATHOPHYSIOLOGY REVIEW

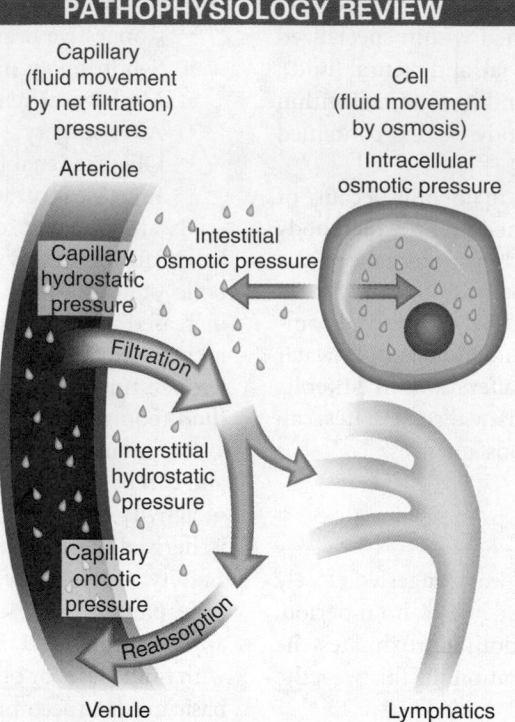

Arterial Capillary Pressures		Venous Capillary Pressures	
Capillary hydrostatic pressure	35 mm Hg	Capillary hydrostatic pressure	18 mm Hg
Interstitial fluid hydrostatic pressure	2 mm Hg	Interstitial fluid hydrostatic pressure	1 mm Hg
Net hydrostatic pressure	**33 mm Hg**	**Net hydrostatic pressure**	**17 mm Hg**
Capillary oncotic pressure	24 mm Hg	Capillary oncotic pressure	25 mm Hg
Interstitial fluid oncotic pressure	0 mm Hg	Interstitial fluid oncotic pressure	0 mm Hg
Net oncotic pressure	**24 mm Hg**	**Net oncotic pressure**	**25 mm Hg**
Net filtration pressure	+9 mm Hg	Net filtration pressure	−8 mm Hg

Fig. 28-1 Capillary filtration forces. Water, electrolytes, and small molecules exchange freely between the vascular compartment and the interstitial space at the site of capillaries and small venules. The rate and amount of exchange are driven by the physical forces of hydrostatic and oncotic pressures and the permeability and surface area of the capillary membranes. The two opposing hydrostatic pressures are capillary hydrostatic pressure and interstitial hydrostatic pressure. The two opposing oncotic pressures are capillary oncotic pressure and interstitial oncotic pressure. The *forces that favor filtration* from the capillary are capillary hydrostatic pressure and interstitial oncotic pressure, and the *forces that oppose filtration* are capillary oncotic pressure and interstitial hydrostatic pressure. The sum of their effects is known as *net filtration pressure*. In the example of normal exchange above, a small amount of fluid moves to the lymph vessels, which accounts for the net filtration difference between the arterial and venous ends of the capillary. (From McCance K, Huether S: *Pathophysiology: the biological basis for disease in adults and children*, ed 6, St Louis, 2010, Mosby.)

relative to size. Water and electrolyte disturbances occur more frequently and more rapidly, and children adjust less promptly to these alterations.

The fluid compartments in the infant vary significantly from those in the adult, primarily because of an expanded extracellular compartment. The ECF compartment constitutes more than half of the TBW at birth and has a greater relative content of extracellular sodium and chloride. The infant loses a large amount of fluid in the first few days after birth and still maintains a larger amount of ECF than the adult until about 2 to 3 years of age. This contributes to greater and more rapid water loss during this age period.

Fluid losses create compartment deficits that reflect the duration of dehydration. In general, approximately 60% of fluid is lost from the ECF, and the remaining 40% comes from the ICF. The amount of fluid lost from the ECF increases with acute illness and decreases with chronic loss.

Fluid losses may be divided into insensible, urinary, and fecal losses and vary with the patient's age. Approximately two thirds of insensible losses occur through the skin, and the remaining one third is lost through the respiratory tract. Environmental heat and humidity, skin integrity, body temperature, and respiratory rate all influence insensible fluid loss. Infants and children have a much greater tendency to become

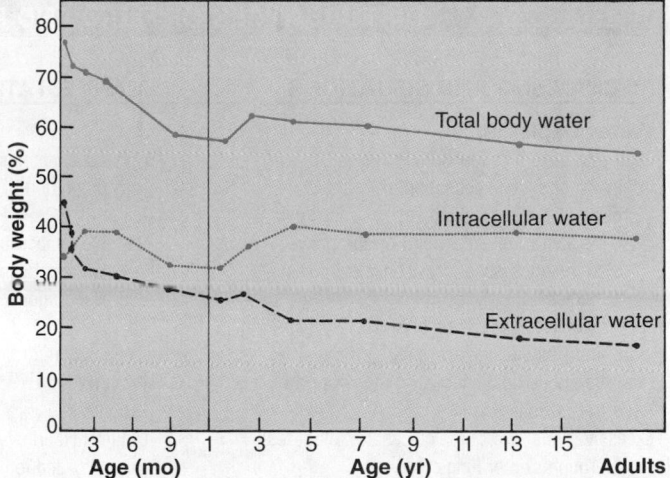

Fig. 28-2 Changes in total body water, intracellular water, and extracellular water in percentages of body weight. (Based on data from Friis-Hansen B: Body water compartments in children: changes during growth and related changes in body composition, *Pediatrics* 28:169-181, 1961.)

TABLE 28-1   DAILY MAINTENANCE FLUID REQUIREMENTS*

BODY WEIGHT	AMOUNT OF FLUID PER DAY
1-10 kg	100 ml/kg
11-20 kg	1000 ml plus 50 ml/kg for each kg >10 kg
>20 kg	1500 ml plus 20 ml/kg for each kg >20 kg

*Not appropriate for neonatal use.

highly febrile than do adults. Fever increases insensible water loss by approximately 7 ml/kg/24 hr for each 1° F rise in temperature above 37.2° C (99° F). Fever and increased surface area relative to volume both contribute to greater insensible fluid losses in young patients.

Body Surface Area

The infant's relatively greater body surface area (BSA) allows larger quantities of fluid to be lost through the skin. It is estimated that the BSA of the premature neonate is five times more, and that of the newborn is two or three times more, than that of the older child or adult. The proportionately longer gastrointestinal tract in infancy is also a source of relatively greater fluid loss, especially from diarrhea.

Metabolic Rate

The rate of metabolism in infancy is significantly higher than in adulthood because of the larger BSA in relation to the mass of active tissue. Consequently, infants have a greater production of metabolic wastes that the kidneys must excrete. Any condition that increases metabolism causes greater heat production, with its concomitant insensible fluid loss and an increased need for water for excretion. The BMR in infants and children is higher to support cellular and tissue growth.

Kidney Function

The infant's kidneys are functionally immature at birth and are therefore inefficient in excreting waste products of metabolism. Of particular importance for fluid balance is the inability of the infant's kidneys to concentrate or dilute urine, to conserve or excrete sodium, or to acidify urine. Therefore the infant is less able to handle large quantities of solute-free water than is the older child and is more likely to become dehydrated when given concentrated formulas or overhydrated when given excessive free water or dilute formula.

Fluid Requirements

As a result of these characteristics, infants ingest and excrete a greater amount of fluid per kilogram of body weight than do older children. Because electrolytes are excreted with water and the infant has limited ability for conservation, maintenance requirements include both water and electrolytes. The daily exchange of ECF in the infant is much greater than that of older children, which leaves the infant little fluid volume reserve in dehydrated states. Fluid requirements depend on hydration status, size, environmental factors, and underlying disease.

DISTURBANCES OF FLUID AND ELECTROLYTE BALANCE

Disturbances of fluids and their solute concentration are closely interrelated. Alterations in fluid volume affect the electrolyte component, and changes in electrolyte concentration influence fluid movement. Because intracellular water and electrolytes move to and from the ECF compartment, any imbalance in the ICF is reflected by an imbalance in the ECF. Disturbances in the ECF involve either an excess or a deficit of fluid or electrolytes. Of these, fluid loss occurs more frequently.

Depletion of ECF, usually caused by gastroenteritis, is one of the most common problems encountered in infants and children. (See Chapter 29.) Until modern techniques for fluid replacement were perfected, gastroenteritis was one of the chief causes of infant mortality. Fluid and electrolyte problems related to specific diseases and their management are discussed throughout the book where appropriate. The major fluid disturbances, their usual causes, and clinical manifestations are listed in Table 28-2; the most common fluid disturbances, dehydration and edema, are elaborated further in the following sections. Problems of fluid and electrolyte disturbance always

TABLE 28-2   DISTURBANCES OF FLUID AND ELECTROLYTE BALANCE

MECHANISMS AND SITUATIONS	MANIFESTATIONS	MANAGEMENT AND NURSING CARE
Water Depletion Failure to absorb or reabsorb water Complete or sudden cessation of intake or prolonged diminished intake: • Neglect of intake by self or caregiver—confused, psychotic, unconscious, or helpless • Loss from gastrointestinal tract—vomiting, diarrhea, nasogastric suction, fistula Disturbed body fluid chemistry: inappropriate ADH secretion Excessive renal excretion: glycosuria (diabetes) Loss through skin or lungs: • Excessive perspiration or evaporation—febrile states, hyperventilation, increased ambient temperature, increased activity (basal metabolic rate) • Impaired skin integrity—transudate from injuries • Hemorrhage Iatrogenic: • Overzealous use of diuretics • Improper perioperative fluid replacement • Use of radiant warmer or phototherapy	General symptoms dependent to some extent on proportion of electrolytes lost with water Thirst Variable temperature—increased (infection) Dry skin and mucous membranes Poor skin turgor Poor perfusion (decreased pulse, slowed capillary refill time) Weight loss Fatigue Diminished urinary output Irritability and lethargy Tachycardia Tachypnea Altered level of consciousness, disorientation Laboratory findings: • High urine specific gravity • Increased hematocrit • Variable serum electrolytes • Variable urine volume • Increased blood urea nitrogen • Increased serum osmolality	Provide replacement of fluid losses commensurate with volume depletion. Provide maintenance fluids and electrolytes. Determine and correct cause of water depletion. Measure fluid intake and output. Monitor vital signs. Monitor urine specific gravity. Monitor body weight. Monitor serum electrolytes.
Water Excess Water intake in excess of output: • Excessive oral intake • Hypotonic fluid overload • Plain water enemas Failure to excrete water in presence of normal intake: • Kidney disease • Congestive heart failure • Malnutrition	Edema: • Generalized • Pulmonary (moist rales or crackles) • Intracutaneous (noted especially in loose areolar tissue) Elevated venous pressure Hepatomegaly Slow, bounding pulse Weight gain Lethargy Increased spinal fluid pressure Central nervous system manifestations (seizures, coma) Laboratory findings: • Low urine specific gravity • Decreased serum electrolytes • Decreased hematocrit • Variable urine volume	Limit fluid intake. Administer diuretics. Monitor vital signs. Monitor neurologic signs as necessary. Determine and treat cause of water excess. Analyze laboratory electrolyte measurements frequently. Implement seizure precautions.
Sodium Depletion (Hyponatremia) Prolonged low-sodium diet Decreased sodium intake Fever Excess sweating Increased water intake without electrolytes Tachypnea (infants) Cystic fibrosis Burns and wounds Vomiting, diarrhea, nasogastric suction, fistulas Adrenal insufficiency Renal disease Diabetic ketoacidosis (DKA) Malnutrition	Associated with water loss: • Same as with water loss—dehydration, weakness, dizziness, nausea, abdominal cramps, apprehension • Mild—apathy, weakness, nausea, weak pulse • Moderate—decreased blood pressure, lethargy Laboratory findings: • Sodium concentration <130 mEq/L (may be normal if volume loss) • Urine specific gravity depends on water deficit or excess	Determine and treat cause of sodium deficit. Administer IV fluids with appropriate saline concentration. Monitor fluid intake and output.

ADH, Antidiuretic hormone; *ECG*, electrocardiogram; *IV*, intravenous.

TABLE 28-2   DISTURBANCES OF FLUID AND ELECTROLYTE BALANCE—cont'd

MECHANISMS AND SITUATIONS	MANIFESTATIONS	MANAGEMENT AND NURSING CARE
Sodium Excess (Hypernatremia) High salt intake—enteral or IV Renal disease Fever Insufficient breast milk intake in neonate (dehydration hypernatremia) High insensible water loss: • Increased temperature • Increased humidity • Hyperventilation • Diabetes insipidus • Hyperglycemia	Intense thirst Dry, sticky mucous membranes Flushed skin Temperature possibly increased Hoarseness Oliguria Nausea and vomiting Possible progression to disorientation, convulsions, muscle twitching, nuchal rigidity, lethargy at rest, hyperirritability when aroused Laboratory findings: • Serum sodium concentration ≥ 150 mEq/L • High plasma volume • Alkalosis	Determine and treat cause of sodium excess. Administer IV fluids as prescribed. Measure fluid intake and output. Monitor laboratory data. Monitor neurologic status. Ensure adequate intake of breast milk and provide lactation assistance with new mother-baby pair before hospital discharge.
Potassium Depletion (Hypokalemia) Starvation Clinical conditions associated with poor food intake Malabsorption IV fluid without added potassium Gastrointestinal losses—diarrhea, vomiting, fistulas, nasogastric suction Diuresis Administration of diuretics Administration of corticosteroids Diuretic phase of nephrotic syndrome Healing stage of burns Potassium-losing nephritis Hyperglycemic diuresis (e.g., diabetes mellitus) Familial periodic paralysis IV administration of insulin in DKA Alkalosis	Muscle weakness, cramping, stiffness, paralysis, hyporeflexia Hypotension Cardiac arrhythmias, gallop rhythm Tachycardia or bradycardia Ileus Apathy, drowsiness Irritability Fatigue Laboratory findings: • Decreased serum potassium concentration ≤ 3.5 mEq/L • Abnormal ECG—notched or flattened T waves, decreased ST segment, premature ventricular contractions	Determine and treat cause of potassium deficit. Monitor vital signs, including ECG. Administer supplemental potassium. Assess for adequate renal output before administration. For IV replacement, administer potassium slowly. Always monitor ECG for IV bolus potassium replacement. For oral intake, offer high-potassium fluids and foods. Evaluate acid-base status.
Potassium Excess (Hyperkalemia) Renal disease Renal failure Adrenal insufficiency (Addison disease) Associated with metabolic acidosis Too rapid administration of IV potassium chloride Transfusion with old donor blood Severe dehydration Crushing injuries Burns Hemolysis Dehydration Potassium-sparing diuretics Increased intake of potassium (e.g., salt substitutes)	Muscle weakness, flaccid paralysis Twitching Hyperreflexia Bradycardia Ventricular fibrillation and cardiac arrest Oliguria Apnea—respiratory arrest Laboratory findings: • High serum potassium concentration ≥ 5.5 mEq/L • Variable urine volume • Flat P wave on ECG, peaked T waves, widened QRS complex, increased PR interval	Determine and treat cause of potassium excess. Monitor vital signs, including ECG. Administer exchange resin, if prescribed. Administer IV fluids as prescribed. Administer IV insulin (if ordered) to facilitate movement of potassium into cells. Monitor potassium levels. Evaluate acid-base status.

Continued

involve both water and electrolytes; therefore replacement includes administration of both, calculated on the basis of ongoing processes and laboratory serum electrolyte values.

In problems that involve alterations in the amount and composition of body fluid compartments, nurses consider many factors when planning management (Box 28-2). The following discussion is concerned with the general concepts of two common fluid volume disturbances, dehydration and edema,

which are features of a variety of conditions. Specific disorders are discussed in Chapters 29 and 30 and elsewhere in the book where appropriate.

DEHYDRATION

Dehydration is a common body fluid disturbance encountered in the nursing care of infants and children; it occurs

TABLE 28-2	DISTURBANCES OF FLUID AND ELECTROLYTE BALANCE—cont'd	
MECHANISMS AND SITUATIONS	**MANIFESTATIONS**	**MANAGEMENT AND NURSING CARE**
Calcium Depletion (Hypocalcemia)		
Inadequate dietary calcium	Neuromuscular irritability	Determine and treat cause of calcium deficit.
Vitamin D deficiency	Tingling of nose, ears, fingertips, toes	Administer calcium supplements as prescribed; administer IV slowly.
Rapid transit through gastrointestinal tract	Tetany	Monitor IV site; calcium may cause vascular irritation.
Advanced renal insufficiency	Laryngospasm	
Administration of diuretics	Generalized convulsions	
Hypoparathyroidism	May be changes in clotting	Monitor serum calcium, vitamin D, and parathyroid levels.
Alkalosis	Positive Chvostek and Trousseau signs	Monitor serum protein levels.
Calcium trapped in diseased tissues	Hypotension	Avoid cow's milk in infants younger than 12 months.
Increased serum protein (albumin)	Cardiac arrest	
Cow's milk—tetany of the newborn (inappropriate calcium/phosphorus ratio in whole milk for newborn)	Laboratory findings: • Decreased serum calcium concentration (8.8-10.8 mEq/L) or increased serum protein levels	
Exchange transfusion with citrated blood	• Prolonged QT interval	
Inadequate parenteral administration in diseased status		
Calcium Excess (Hypercalcemia)		
Acidosis	Constipation	Determine and treat cause of calcium excess.
Prolonged immobilization	Weakness, fatigue	Monitor serum calcium levels.
Conditions associated with increased bone catabolism	Nausea, vomiting	Monitor ECG.
Hypoproteinemia	Anorexia	
Kidney disease	Dry mouth (thirst)	
Hypervitaminosis D	Muscle hypotonicity	
Hyperparathyroidism	Bradycardia or cardiac arrest	
Hyperthyroidism	Increased calcium concentration in urine, causing formation of kidney stones	
Excessive IV or oral administration	Laboratory findings: • Increased serum calcium levels or decreased serum protein levels	
	• Prolonged QRS complex or PR interval, shortened QT interval	

ADH, Antidiuretic hormone; *ECG*, electrocardiogram; *IV*, intravenous.

BOX 28-2	AREAS OF CONCERN IN PLANNING MANAGEMENT OF FLUID PROBLEMS

- Volume of body fluids (i.e., water content of the patient)
- Osmolality of the body fluids, which affects the distribution of body water among the various compartments
- Hydrogen ion status (i.e., whether there has been a disturbance in the pH of body fluids or a disturbance in the homeostatic mechanisms that maintain the pH)
- Electrolyte deficits from cells and extracellular water
- Disturbances in the equilibrium between the mineral skeleton and body fluids
- Length of time alteration in fluid status has existed

❗ NURSING ALERT

In a child with a history of fluid loss and potential or actual dehydration, gear nursing assessment toward the possibility of impending shock.

In early dehydration (during the first 2 days), fluid loss is derived from both the ECF and the ICF because the increased osmolality of the diminished ECF volume causes fluid from the ICF compartment to move into the ECF compartment. As dehydration becomes chronic, the cellular losses become greater.

Types of Dehydration

Because sodium is the primary osmotic force that controls fluid movement between the major fluid compartments, dehydration is often described according to plasma sodium concentrations (i.e., isonatremic, hyponatremic, or hypernatremic). Other osmotic forces, however, such as glucose in diabetic ketoacidosis and protein in nephrotic syndrome, may also play a dominant role. Consequently, dehydration is conventionally classified as isotonic, hypotonic, or hypertonic.

Isotonic (isosmotic or isonatremic) dehydration occurs in conditions in which electrolyte and water deficits are present in

whenever the total output of fluid exceeds the total intake, regardless of the underlying cause. Although dehydration can result from lack of oral intake (especially in elevated environmental temperatures), more often it is a result of abnormal losses, such as those that occur in vomiting or diarrhea, when oral intake only partially compensates for the abnormal losses. Other significant causes of dehydration are diabetic ketoacidosis and extensive burns.

approximately balanced proportions. This is the primary form of dehydration occurring in children. The observable fluid losses are not necessarily isotonic, but losses from other avenues make adjustments so that the sum of all losses, or the net loss, is isotonic. Because no osmotic force is present to cause a redistribution of water between the ICF and ECF, the major loss is sustained from the ECF compartment. This significantly reduces the plasma volume and thus the circulating blood volume, with its effect on the skin, muscles, and kidneys. Shock is the greatest threat to life in isotonic dehydration, and the child with isotonic dehydration displays symptoms characteristic of hypovolemic shock. Plasma sodium remains within normal limits, between 130 and 150 mEq/L (Huether, 2010).

Hypotonic (hyposmotic or hyponatremic) dehydration occurs when the electrolyte deficit exceeds the water deficit. Because ICF is more concentrated than ECF in hypotonic dehydration, water transfers from the ECF to the ICF to establish osmotic equilibrium. This movement further increases the ECF volume loss, and shock is a frequent result. Because there is a greater proportional loss of ECF in hypotonic dehydration, the physical signs tend to be more severe with smaller fluid losses than in isotonic or hypertonic dehydration. Plasma sodium concentrations are typically less than 130 mEq/L (Huether, 2010).

Hypertonic (hyperosmotic or hypernatremic) dehydration results from water loss in excess of electrolyte loss and is usually caused by a proportionately larger loss of water or a larger intake of electrolytes. This type of dehydration is the most dangerous and requires much more specific fluid therapy. This sometimes occurs in infants with diarrhea who are given fluids by mouth that contain large amounts of solute or in children receiving high-protein nasogastric tube feedings that place an excessive solute load on the kidneys. In hypertonic dehydration, fluid shifts from the lesser concentration of the ICF to the ECF. Plasma sodium concentration is greater than 150 mEq/L (Huether, 2010).

Because the ECF volume is proportionally larger, hypertonic dehydration consists of a greater degree of water loss for the same intensity of physical signs. Shock is less apparent in hypotonic dehydration. However, neurologic disturbances, such as seizures, are more likely to occur. Cerebral changes are serious and may result in permanent damage. These include disturbance of consciousness, poor ability to focus attention, lethargy, increased muscle tone with hyperreflexia, and hyperirritability to stimuli (tactile, auditory, bright lights).

Degree of Dehydration

Diagnosis of the type and degree of dehydration is necessary to develop an effective plan of therapy. The degree of dehydration has been described as a percentage of body weight dehydrated: mild—less than 3% in older children or less than 5% in infants; moderate—5% to 10% in infants and 3% to 6% in older children; and severe—more than 10% in infants and more than 6% in older children (Greenbaum, 2007). Water constitutes only 60% to 70% of the infant's weight. However, adipose tissue contains little water and is highly variable in individual infants and children. A more accurate means of describing dehydration is to reflect acute loss (time frame of ≤48 hours) in milliliters per kilogram of body weight. For example, a loss of 50 ml/kg is

TABLE 28-3	EVALUATING EXTENT OF DEHYDRATION		
CLINICAL SIGNS	**LEVEL OF DEHYDRATION**		
	MILD	**MODERATE**	**SEVERE**
Weight loss— infants	3%-5%	6%-9%	≥10%
Weight loss— children	3%-4%	6%-8%	10%
Pulse	Normal	Slightly increased	Very increased
Respiratory rate	Normal	Slight tachypnea (rapid)	Hyperpnea (deep and rapid)
Blood pressure	Normal	Normal to orthostatic (>10 mm Hg change)	Orthostatic to shock
Behavior	Normal	Irritable, more thirsty	Hyperirritable to lethargic
Thirst	Slight	Moderate	Intense
Mucous membranes*	Normal	Dry	Parched
Tears	Present	Decreased	Absent, sunken eyes
Anterior fontanel	Normal	Normal to sunken	Sunken
External jugular vein	Visible when supine	Not visible except with supraclavicular pressure	Not visible even with supraclavicular pressure
Skin*	Capillary refill >2 sec	Slowed capillary refill (2-4 sec [decreased turgor])	Very delayed capillary refill (>4 sec) and tenting; skin cool, acrocyanotic or mottled
Urine specific gravity	>1.020	>1.020; oliguria	Oliguria or anuria

Data from Jospe N, Forbes G: Fluids and electrolytes—clinical aspects, *Pediatr Rev* 17(11):395-403, 1996; and Steiner MJ, DeWalt DA, Byerly JS: Is this child dehydrated? *JAMA* 291(22): 2746-2754, 2004.
*These signs are less prominent in patients who have hypernatremia.

considered to be a mild fluid loss, whereas a loss of 100 ml/kg produces severe dehydration.

Clinical signs provide clues to the extent of dehydration (Table 28-3). The earliest detectable sign is usually tachycardia, followed by dry skin and mucous membranes, sunken fontanels, signs of circulatory failure (coolness and mottling of extremities), loss of skin elasticity, and prolonged capillary filling time (see Table 28-4 for clinical manifestations of dehydration and Fig. 28-3 for signs of dehydration).

Compensatory mechanisms attempt to maintain fluid volume by adjusting to these losses. Interstitial fluid moves into the vascular compartment to maintain the blood volume in response to hemoconcentration and hypovolemia, and vasoconstriction of peripheral arterioles helps maintain pumping pressure. When fluid losses exceed the body's ability to sustain blood volume and blood pressure, circulation is seriously compromised and the blood pressure falls. This results in tissue hypoxia with accumulation of lactic acid, pyruvate, and other acid metabolites, which contribute to the development of metabolic acidosis.

TABLE 28-4	CLINICAL MANIFESTATIONS OF DEHYDRATION		
MANIFESTATION	**ISOTONIC (LOSS OF WATER AND SALT)**	**HYPOTONIC (LOSS OF SALT IN EXCESS OF WATER)**	**HYPERTONIC (LOSS OF WATER IN EXCESS OF SALT)**
Skin			
Color	Gray	Gray	Gray
Temperature	Cold	Cold	Cold or hot
Turgor	Poor	Very poor	Fair
Feel	Dry	Clammy	Thickened, doughy
Mucous membranes	Dry	Slightly moist	Parched
Tearing and salivation	Absent	Absent	Absent
Eyeball	Sunken	Sunken	Sunken
Fontanel	Sunken	Sunken	Sunken
Body temperature	Subnormal or elevated	Subnormal or elevated	Subnormal or elevated
Pulse	Rapid	Very rapid	Moderately rapid
Respirations	Rapid	Rapid	Rapid
Behavior	Irritable to lethargic	Lethargic or comatose; convulsions	Marked lethargy with extreme hyperirritability on stimulation

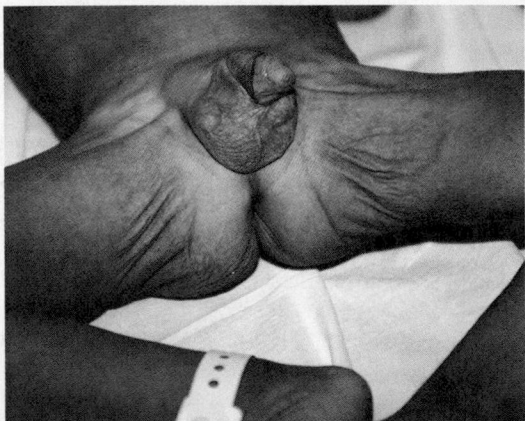

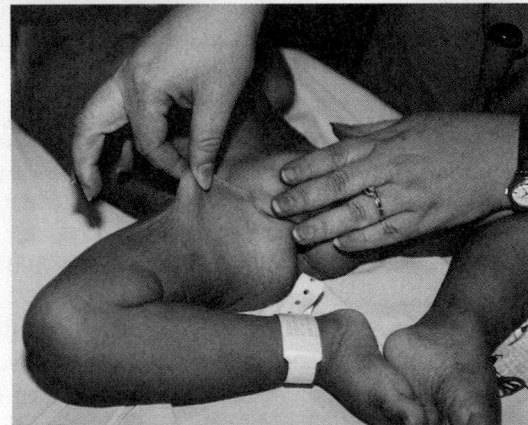

Fig. 28-3 Loss of skin elasticity because of dehydration.

Renal compensation is impaired by reduced blood flow through the kidneys, and little urine is formed. Increased serum osmolality stimulates the secretion of antidiuretic hormone (ADH) to conserve fluid and initiates the renin-angiotensin mechanisms in the kidney, causing further vasoconstriction. Aldosterone is released to promote sodium retention and conserve water in the kidneys. If dehydration increases in severity, urine formation is greatly diminished and metabolites and hydrogen ions that are normally excreted by this route are retained.

Shock, a common manifestation of severe depletion of ECF volume, is preceded by tachycardia and signs of poor perfusion and tissue oxygenation (by pulse oximeter readings). Peripheral circulation is poor as a result of reduced blood volume; therefore the skin is cool and mottled, with decreased capillary filling after blanching. Impaired kidney circulation often leads to oliguria and azotemia. Although low blood pressure may accompany other symptoms of shock, in infants and young children it is usually a late sign and may herald the onset of cardiovascular collapse.

Diagnostic Evaluation

To initiate a therapeutic plan, several factors must be determined:

- The degree of dehydration based on physical assessment
- The type of dehydration based on the pathophysiology of the specific illness responsible for the dehydrated state
- Specific physical signs other than general signs
- Initial plasma sodium concentrations
- Serum bicarbonate concentration
- Any associated electrolyte (especially serum potassium) and acid-base imbalances (as indicated).

Initial and regular, ongoing evaluations assess the patient's progress toward equilibrium and the effectiveness of therapy.

In the examination of an infant or younger child, one of the most important determinants of the extent of dehydration is the weight, since this can assist in determining the percentage of total body fluid lost; however, since the preillness weight is often unknown, clinical manifestations must be evaluated (see Research Focus box). Important clinical manifestations include changing sensorium (irritability to lethargy); decreased response to stimuli; integumentary changes (decreased elasticity and turgor); prolonged capillary refill; increased heart rate; sunken eyes; and, in infants, sunken fontanels. Using multiple

◢ **RESEARCH FOCUS**

Pediatric Dehydration

In a review of 13 articles related to pediatric dehydration, the best three individual examination signs for assessing dehydration were prolonged capillary refill time (>2 seconds), abnormal skin turgor, and abnormal respiratory pattern (Emond, 2009; Steiner, DeWalt, and Byerly, 2004).

predictors increases the sensitivity of assessing the fluid deficit, and early studies have shown a reasonably high degree of agreement between experienced observers in assessment of the level of dehydration. Objective signs of dehydration are present at a fluid deficit of less than 5%.

Laboratory data are said to be useful only when results are significantly abnormal (Emond, 2009). Urine specific gravity, urine ketones, and urinary output during rehydration are reportedly unreliable assessments for determining dehydration in children (Steiner, Nager, and Wang, 2007).

Therapeutic Management

Medical management is directed at correcting the fluid imbalance and treating the underlying cause. When the child is alert, awake, and not in danger, correction of dehydration may be attempted with oral fluid administration. Most cases of dehydration are mild and can be managed at home by this method. Several commercial rehydration fluids are available for use (see Table 29-2). Oral rehydration management consists of replacement of fluid loss over 4 to 6 hours, replacement of continuing losses, and provision for maintenance fluid requirements. In general, the mildly dehydrated child may be given 50 ml/kg of oral rehydration solution (ORS), whereas the child with moderate dehydration may be given 100 ml/kg of ORS. The child with fluid losses from diarrhea may be given 10 ml/kg for each stool (Greenbaum, 2007). Amounts and rates are determined from body weight and severity of dehydration and are increased if rehydration is incomplete or if excess losses continue, until the child is well hydrated and the basic problem is under control.

The child may not be thirsty even though dehydrated and may refuse oral fluids initially for fear of continued emesis (if occurring) or because of decreased strength, oral stomatitis, or thrush. In such children rehydration may proceed by administering 2 to 5 ml of ORS by a syringe or small medication cup every 2 to 3 minutes until the child is able to tolerate larger amounts; if the child has emesis, administering small amounts (5 to 10 ml) of ORS every 5 minutes or so may help overcome fluid deficit, and the emesis will often lessen over time (Greenbaum, 2007). Oral administration of ondansetron (Zofran) to children with acute gastroenteritis and vomiting may reduce emesis and increase time to oral rehydration, thus preventing intravenous (IV) therapy (DeCamp, Byerly, Doshi, et al, 2008; Freedman, Adler, Seshadri, et al, 2006; Roslund, Hepps, and McQuillen, 2008). Oral rehydration therapy (ORT) is effective for treating mild or moderate dehydration in children, is less expensive, and involves fewer complications than therapy (American Academy of Pediatrics, 2009; Spandorfer, Alessandrini, Joffe, et al, 2005). (See Diarrhea, Chapter 29, for a complete discussion of fluid replacement therapy for dehydration.)

NURSING TIP Enhance the flavor of an ORS such as Pedialyte (unflavored) by adding a teaspoon of unsweetened powder Kool-Aid to each 60 to 90 ml of ORS. Older children may take a small Popsicle orally instead of fluids that require drinking. Many commercially available Popsicles are relatively inexpensive, contain small amounts of sucrose, and contain approximately 40 to 50 ml of fluid. Frozen oral hydration may be accepted by some children when conventional ORS is rejected (see Family-Centered Care box).

FAMILY-CENTERED CARE

Recipe for Home WHO Oral Rehydration Solution

The World Health Organization has developed a home recipe for an oral rehydration solution that provides carbohydrate as 20 g/L glucose, 90 mEq/L sodium, 20 mEq/L potassium, 80 mEq/L chloride, 30 mEq/L citrate, 2.5 cal/fl oz, and an osmolality of 310 mOsm/kg. The recipe is:

- 3.5 g (½ tsp) table salt
- 1.5 g (1¼ tsp) potassium chloride or potassium salt
- 2.5 g (½ tsp) baking soda
- 20 g (2 tbsp) glucose or 8 tsp sugar

Add the above ingredients together in 1 L of water.

Adapted from Centers for Disease Control and Prevention: Prevention of specific infectious diseases: traveler's diarrhea. In Arguin PM, Kozarsky PE, Navin AW, editors: *Health information for international travel 2005-2006*, Atlanta, 2005, US Department of Health and Human Services, Public Health Service.

QUALITY PATIENT OUTCOMES: Fluid Volume Deficit
- Moist mucous membranes
- Sodium and potassium WNL
- Voiding (>1 ml/kg/hr)
- Capillary refill of 2 seconds or less
- Skin turgor brisk
- Fluid I&O balanced

Parenteral Fluid Therapy

Parenteral fluid therapy is initiated whenever the child is unable to ingest sufficient amounts of fluid and electrolytes to (1) meet ongoing daily physiologic losses, (2) replace previous deficits, and (3) replace ongoing abnormal losses. Patients who usually require IV fluids are those with severe dehydration, those with uncontrollable vomiting, those who are unable to drink for any reason (e.g., extreme fatigue, coma), or those with severe gastric distention.

Because dehydration constitutes a great threat to life, the first priority is the restoration of circulation by rapid expansion of the ECF volume to treat or prevent shock. IV administration of fluid begins immediately, although the exact nature of the dehydration and the serum electrolyte values are not known. The solution selected is based on what is known regarding the probable type and cause of the dehydration. This usually involves an isotonic solution such as 0.9% sodium chloride or lactated Ringer, both of which are close to the body's serum osmolality of 285 to 300 mOsm/kg and do not contain dextrose (which is contraindicated in the early treatment stages of diabetic ketoacidosis).

Parenteral rehydration therapy has three phases. The initial therapy is used to expand ECF volume quickly and to improve circulatory and renal function (Greenbaum, 2007). During initial therapy, an isotonic electrolyte solution is used at a rate of 20 ml/kg, given as an IV bolus over 20 minutes and repeated as necessary after assessment of the child's response to therapy (Ford, 2009; Friedman, 2009). Subsequent therapy is used to replace deficits, meet maintenance water and electrolyte requirements, and catch up with ongoing losses. Water and sodium requirements for the deficit, maintenance, and ongoing losses are calculated at 8-hour intervals, taking into consideration the amount of fluids given with the initial boluses and the amount administered during the first 24-hour period. With improved circulation during this phase, water and electrolyte deficits can be evaluated, and acid-base status can be corrected either directly through the administration of fluids or indirectly through improved renal function. Potassium is withheld until kidney function is restored and assessed and circulation has improved.

The final phase of therapy allows the patient to return to normal and begin oral feedings, with a gradual correction of total body deficits. The potassium loss in ICF is replaced slowly by way of the ECF. The body fat and protein stores are replaced through diet. If the child is unable to eat or if feeding aggravates a chronic condition, IV maintenance fluids are provided.

Although the initial phase of fluid replacement is rapid in both isotonic and hypotonic dehydration, it is contraindicated in hypertonic dehydration because of the risk of water intoxication, especially in the brain cells, specifically the central pontine cells. Central pontine myelinolysis may occur with an overcorrection of fluid deficit and an overly rapid correction of serum sodium concentration (Greenbaum, 2007). There is an apparent lag time for sodium to reach a steady state when diffusing in and out of brain cells, whereas water diffuses almost instantaneously. Consequently, rapid administration of fluid will cause equally rapid diffusion of water into the dehydrated brain cells, causing marked cerebral edema. Because ECF volume is maintained relatively well in hypertonic as opposed to the other types of dehydration, shock is not a usual manifestation.

WATER INTOXICATION

Water intoxication, or water overload, is observed less often than dehydration. However, it is important that nurses and others who care for children be alert to this possibility in certain situations. Children who ingest excessive amounts of electrolyte-free water develop a concurrent decrease in serum sodium accompanied by central nervous system (CNS) symptoms. There is a large urinary output and, because water moves into the brain more rapidly than sodium moves out, the child may also exhibit irritability, somnolence, headache, vomiting, diarrhea, or generalized seizures. The affected child usually appears well hydrated but may be edematous or even dehydrated.

Fluid intoxication can occur during acute IV water overloading, too rapid dialysis, tap water enemas, feeding of incorrectly mixed formula, or excess water ingestion, or with too rapid reduction of glucose levels in diabetic ketoacidosis (Metheny, 2000; Greenbaum, 2007). Patients with CNS infections occasionally retain excessive amounts of water. Administration of inappropriate hypotonic solutions (e.g., 0.45% sodium chloride) may cause a rapid reduction in sodium and result in symptoms of water overload.

Infants are especially vulnerable to fluid overload. Their thirst mechanism is not well developed; therefore they are unable to "turn off" fluid intake appropriately. A decreased glomerular filtration rate does not allow for repeated excretion of a water load, and ADH levels may not be maximally reduced. Consequently, infants are unable to excrete a water overload effectively.

Administration of inappropriately prepared formula is one of the more common causes of water intoxication in infants (Greenbaum, 2007; Metheny, 2000). Families who cannot afford to buy enough formula may dilute the formula to increase the volume or even substitute water for the formula. A family may run out of formula and dilute the remaining amount to make it last until they are able to purchase more. In addition, water is sometimes used for pacification. Water intoxication can also occur in infants who receive overly vigorous hydration during a febrile illness.

A number of clinicians have reported water intoxication in infants after swimming lessons (Fann, 1998; Metheny, 2000). Although they hold their breath, some infants apparently swallow a large amount of water during repeated submersion. Anticipatory guidance to parents should include a discussion of swimming instruction and advice to stop a lesson if the child swallows unusual amounts of water or exhibit any symptoms of hyponatremia.

EDEMA

Edema represents an abnormal accumulation of fluid within the interstitial tissue and subsequent tissue expansion and develops when a defect in the normal cardiovascular circulation or a failure in the lymphatic drainage to remove the increased amounts occurs. The processes responsible for fluid removal include venous hydrostatic pressure, oncotic pressure of intravascular and interstitial spaces, an intact semipermeable capillary wall, tissue tension, and lymphatic flow.

Mechanisms of Edema Formation

A defect of any of the homeostatic mechanisms maintaining fluid balance can cause accumulation of interstitial fluid. Disequilibrium results from anything that (1) alters the retention of sodium, such as renal disease or hormonal influences; (2) affects the formation or destruction of plasma proteins, such as starvation or liver disease; or (3) alters membrane permeability, such as minimal change nephrotic syndrome or trauma.

Edema may be localized to a small or large area, such as that occurring in urticaria, infection, and pulmonary congestion, or it can be generalized, as in the hypoproteinemia of the nephrotic syndrome and starvation. A severe, generalized accumulation of great amounts of fluid in all body tissues is termed anasarca.

Increased Venous Pressure

The colloidal osmotic pressure of the plasma proteins draws fluid back into the vascular system as long as this force is greater than the venous hydrostatic pressure. However, when the venous pressure increases, fluid tends to be retained in the interstitial spaces. This can occur when an individual remains in the same position for a long time, such as swollen ankles and feet after standing or sitting for long periods. Constrictive dressings or restraints applied too tightly to extremities will obstruct venous return, increase venous and capillary pressure, and cause edema. The most graphic pathologic illustrations are pulmonary edema caused by pulmonary circulation overload in cardiac defects with a left-to-right shunt and ascites caused by portal hypertension. Edema from any cause is increased in dependent areas because of this added factor of increased venous hydrostatic pressure and the gravitational effects in these areas.

Capillary Permeability

Damage to capillary walls or alteration in their permeability permits exudation of plasma protein into the interstitial space. Most often this occurs as local edema, such as that manifested in inflammatory and hypersensitivity reactions. Capillary damage from burns allows extensive exudation of protein-rich fluid into the interstitial spaces to compound edema formation.

Diminished Plasma Proteins

A fall in plasma protein levels hampers the osmotic pull back into the vessels. Consequently, fluid remains in the interstitial spaces. Although other factors play a role, such as hydrostatic pressure of both the arterial vascular system and the tissues and sodium concentration, significantly low protein levels (<4.5 mg/dl) are associated with edema. Examples of this are the massive albumin losses of the minimal change nephrotic syndrome, diminished serum protein from insufficient dietary protein, and (sometimes) hemodilution of plasma proteins from IV fluid administration in chronic dehydration.

Lymphatic Obstruction

Obstruction of lymph flow creates edema high in protein content. This occurs infrequently in childhood but can result from trauma to the lymphatic glands or from removal of lymph nodes.

Tissue Tension

Tissue hydrostatic pressure is ordinarily of little consequence. However, it plays a significant role in determining distribution of edema fluid in certain pathologic conditions. Loose tissues allow a greater amount of fluid accumulation than tissues that are tightly bound by dense fibrous bands in which tissue pressure rapidly increases to limit further extravasation of fluid. Edema appears earlier and more readily in loose structures such as those in the periorbital and genital tissues. The alveolar structure of lung tissue is probably a contributing factor in pulmonary edema, as well as in increased hydrostatic pressure in the pulmonary vessels.

Other Factors in Edema Formation

Any factor that causes sodium retention by the kidneys will produce or augment edema formation. This includes stimulation of the renin-angiotensin-aldosterone mechanisms for sodium reabsorption created by the diminished plasma volume in edema, which resulted from primary causes. The salt-retaining property of steroids is responsible for the edema associated with their administration.

Several types of edema exist, all of which can provide a palpable swelling of the interstitial space that is either localized or generalized. These include:

- Peripheral edema, or localized or generalized palpable swelling of the interstitial space
- Ascites, or the accumulation of fluid in the abdominal cavity (usually associated with renal or liver abnormalities)
- Pulmonary edema, which occurs when interstitial volume increases
- Cerebral edema, which is a particularly threatening form of edema caused by trauma, infection, or other etiologic factors, including vascular overload or injudicious IV administration of hypotonic solutions

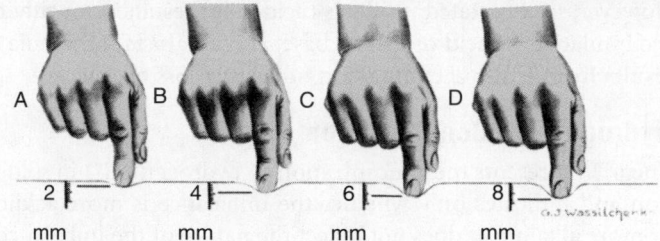

Fig. 28-4 Assessment of pitting edema. **A,** +1. **B,** +2. **C,** +3. **D,** +4. (From Lowdermilk DL, Perry SE: *Maternity and women's health care,* ed 9, St Louis, 2007, Mosby.)

- Overall fluid gain, especially seen in patients with kidney disease

Assessment

Generalized edema resulting from any of the above types is manifested by swelling in the extremities, face, perineum, and torso. Loss of normal skin creases may be assessed. Daily weights are more sensitive indicators of water gain or loss and should be obtained. Abdominal girth measurement changes may also be an indicator of edema in children. Pitting edema may occur and can be assessed by pressing the fingertip against a bony prominence for 5 seconds. If the tissue rebounds immediately on removing the finger, the patient does not have pitting edema. A quick way to determine the severity is to measure the degree of pitting edema (Fig. 28-4).

Therapeutic Management

The primary goal in the management of edema is treatment of the underlying disease process, which is discussed elsewhere in relation to the specific disorder. However, an essential aspect in the management of any fluid overload is early recognition, in which nurses play a vital role. The management of edema is discussed throughout the text with specific conditions.

> **QUALITY PATIENT OUTCOMES: Fluid Volume Excess**
> - Fluid I&O balanced
> - No edema
> - No weight gain
> - No respiratory distress related to fluid volume excess

DISTURBANCES OF ACID-BASE BALANCE

The body's ability to regulate acid-base status is one of the most crucial physiologic functions. Many disease states, such as diarrhea, vomiting, or febrile conditions, are complicated by disturbances in the acid-base balance, which are often more hazardous to the child's survival than the primary disease process. Sometimes simply providing adequate hydration, replacing electrolytes, and correcting acid-base disturbances are all that is needed to sustain an infant or child until the primary disorder has stabilized.

ACID-BASE IMBALANCE

A disturbance of acid-base equilibrium in the direction of acidosis or alkalosis may come about in a variety of ways.

However, simply stated, acidosis (acidemia) results from either accumulation of acid or loss of base, and alkalosis (alkalemia) results from either accumulation of base or loss of acid.

Hydrogen Ion Concentration

The pH represents the concentration of hydrogen (H^+) in solution and indicates only whether the imbalance is more acidic or more alkaline. It does not reflect the nature of the imbalance (i.e., whether it is of metabolic or respiratory origin). Body metabolism affects primarily the base bicarbonate (HCO_3^-); therefore alterations in the concentration of bicarbonate are termed *metabolic disturbances of acid-base balance*. Also, because the amount of carbon dioxide (CO_2) exhaled through the lungs affects the carbonic acid (H_2CO_3), changes in carbonic acid concentration are referred to as *respiratory disturbances*. Consequently, the simple disturbances (those with a single primary cause) are categorized as metabolic acidosis or alkalosis and respiratory acidosis or alkalosis (Greenbaum, 2007).

It is also significant that the major signs and symptoms of hydrogen ion imbalances (acidosis and alkalosis) reflect CNS involvement. Depression of the CNS, manifested by lethargy, diminished mental capacity, delirium, stupor, and coma, is observed in acidosis of either metabolic or respiratory origin. On the other hand, alkalosis produces clinical manifestations of nervous system stimulation and excitement, including overexcitability, nervousness, tingling sensations, and tetany that may progress to seizures. Persons with epilepsy are particularly susceptible to seizures, which can be precipitated by hyperventilation.

It is also important to note that eventually all body systems become dysfunctional if the "normal" limits of pH are violated for long. The extent and severity of signs and symptoms depend on the length of time the imbalance has existed and the magnitude or degree of the deviation from normal. A rapid, severe imbalance will seriously compromise the compensatory mechanisms to the point where it is incompatible with life, whereas the body will be able to compensate adequately for a mild, gradual distortion and produce few if any observable signs or symptoms.

Compensatory Mechanisms

Respiratory regulation in acid-base balance involves carbon dioxide regulation; that is, the rate and depth of alveolar ventilation determine the concentration of carbon dioxide that is eliminated or retained. Renal processes, however, involve the regulation of bicarbonate via reabsorption, regeneration, and secretion of hydrogen ions. When the fundamental acid-base ratio is altered for any reason, the body attempts to correct the deviation. In a simple disturbance, a single primary factor affects one component of the acid-base pair and is usually accompanied by a compensatory or secondary change in the component that is not primarily affected. For example, increased formation of metabolic acid rapidly reduces the bicarbonate in the formation of carbonic acid. The respiratory mechanism immediately attempts to compensate for the imbalance by eliminating the carbonic acid through exhaled carbon dioxide and water. The imbalance is corrected when the kidneys excrete hydrogen and ammonium ions in exchange for reabsorbed sodium bicarbonate.

TABLE 28-5	PRIMARY AND COMPENSATORY ACID-BASE CHANGES					
	PRIMARY DISTURBANCE			**COMPENSATIONS**		
	pH	Pco_2	HCO_3^-	pH	Pco_2	HCO_3^-
Metabolic acidosis	↓	N	↓	↑-N	↓	↓
Metabolic alkalosis	↑	N	↑	↓-N	↑	↑
Respiratory acidosis	↓	↑	N	↑-N	↑	↑
Respiratory alkalosis	↑	↓	N	↓-N	↓	↓

HCO_3^-, Bicarbonate; *N*, normal; ↑-*N*, increase toward normal; ↓-*N*, decrease toward normal; Pco_2, carbon dioxide partial pressure; *pH*, measure of the acidity or alkalinity of a solution.

When the secondary changes (the hyperventilation and renal excretion of hydrogen ions in the preceding example) succeed in preventing a distortion of the acid-base ratio and the pH is restored to normal, the disturbance is described as **compensated**. The **uncompensated** state exists when there is no compensatory effect and the pH remains uncorrected. The imbalance is said to be corrected when physiologic mechanisms fully correct the primary abnormality. *Mixed* acid-base imbalances may also occur in diseases states, and the patient will manifest two simultaneous acid-base imbalances rather than a single imbalance. It is not within the scope of this text to discuss the many variations of mixed acid-base imbalances; the reader is referred to other published sources for such material (Huether, 2010; Curley and Moloney-Harmon, 2001) (see also Table 28-5).

Laboratory Measurements

Several laboratory tests are employed to assess the nature and extent of acid-base disturbances. The importance of these data is readily apparent when a clinical observation such as hyperventilation can represent either the primary factor in respiratory alkalosis or a secondary or compensatory factor in metabolic acidosis. The laboratory tests of value in the assessment of acid-base status are outlined in Table 28-6. To determine the acid-base status, three variables—the respiratory component (Pco_2), the metabolic component (arterial bicarbonate or serum carbon dioxide [HCO_3^-]), and the serum pH—must be determined. In addition, the anion gap (AG) may be useful in determining the cause and extent of metabolic acidosis; therefore serum chemistry is obtained as well. Measurement of any two variables (Pco_2, pH, HCO_3^-) will allow computation of the third using the Henderson-Hasselbach equation. A summary of relationships between these and other variables is outlined in Table 28-7.

Associated Disturbances in Acid-Base Balance

Physiologic functions of the body take place optimally when the pH is maintained within a normal range. The disequilibrium created by moderately altered pH can produce disordered func-

TABLE 28-6 LABORATORY TESTS EMPLOYED IN ASSESSMENT OF ACID-BASE STATUS

ABBREVIATION	TEST	NORMAL VALUES*	DESCRIPTION
pH	Partial pressure of hydrogen	Birth: 7.11-7.36 1 day: 7.29-7.45 Child: 7.35-7.45	Expression of hydrogen ion concentration
P_{CO_2}	Partial pressure of carbon dioxide or carbon dioxide tension	Newborn: 27-40 mm Hg Infant: 27-41 mm Hg Girls: 32-45 mm Hg Boys: 35-48 mm Hg	Measure of carbon dioxide tension; reflects carbonic acid (H_2CO_3) concentrations of plasma
HCO_3^- (serum) arterial	Carbon dioxide content or carbon dioxide combining power	Infant: 21-28 mEq/ml Thereafter: 22-26 mEq/ml	Concentration of base bicarbonate
BE	Base excess (whole blood)	Newborn: −2 to −10 Infant: −1 to −7 Child: +2 to −4 Thereafter: +3 to −3	Used to express extent of deviation from normal buffer base concentration; indicates quantity of blood buffers remaining after hydrogen ion is buffered
AG	Anion gap; using chemistry profile and serum bicarbonate	10-12,† (4-11*)	Reflects difference between measured cation sodium and anions (also measured) of chloride and bicarbonate

*Data from Kliegman RM, Behrman RE, Jenson HB, et al, editors: *Nelson textbook of pediatrics,* ed 18, Philadelphia, 2007, Saunders.
†Huether SE: The cellular environment: fluids and electrolytes, acids and bases. In McCance KL, Huether SE, Brashers VL, et al, editors: *Pathophysiology: the biologic basis for disease in adults and children,* ed 6, St Louis, 2010, Mosby.

TABLE 28-7 SUMMARY OF SIMPLE ACID-BASE DISTURBANCES (PARTIALLY COMPENSATED)

DISTURBANCE	PLASMA pH	PLASMA P_{CO_2}	PLASMA HCO_3^-
Respiratory acidosis	↓	↑	↑
Respiratory alkalosis	↑	↓	↓
Metabolic acidosis	↓	↓	↓
Metabolic alkalosis	↑	↑	↑

tion of physiologic and enzyme systems, but great divergences are incompatible with life. In addition, electrolyte shifts that take place in response to changes in pH alter the electrolyte concentration in the fluid compartments to disturb the normal concentrations. For example, cell membrane permeability is affected by changes in pH. A lowered pH allows potassium (K^+) to move from the ICF to the ECF. Serum potassium levels increase with acidosis and decrease with alkalosis.

Serum Potassium
One of the disturbances that complicate both fluid losses and acid-base imbalance is an alteration of potassium levels. During dehydration, fluid moves out of the ICF compartment into the ECF compartment in an attempt to balance the fluid losses. In doing so, potassium also moves out, creating a total body potassium depletion. Because renal function is drastically reduced in dehydration, normal excretion of potassium does not take place. This causes elevated serum levels that can produce all the signs and symptoms of hyperkalemia. During rapid rehydration therapy for gastrointestinal losses and diabetic ketoacidosis, the ECF potassium moves back into the ICF compartment, thereby posing the risk of hypokalemia unless there is an anticipated replacement. However, potassium is not replaced until the ICF is sufficient to restore adequate renal function.

Serum Calcium
Disturbed ECF calcium (Ca^{++}) levels may occur in various types of dehydration. Usually the disturbance is in the form of reduced serum calcium levels, especially where there is a concomitant potassium loss. Although hypocalcemia is a common finding, it rarely reaches a point of tetany in current practice, which includes adequate replacement of potassium losses. Immediate effects of calcium imbalance associated with acidosis or alkalosis are tetany of metabolic alkalosis; long-term effects of chronic acidosis are related to bone resorption from renal disturbances.

Oxygen Combination
The capacity of oxygen to combine with hemoglobin is also affected by changes in pH. The affinity of hemoglobin for oxygen decreases with a decrease in pH so that, in a state of acidosis, less oxygen will be picked up by the hemoglobin as blood travels through the lungs. However, oxygen is more easily released to the tissues when the pH is lowered. The opposite effects operate during an increase in pH.

Blood Flow
Changes in pH alter blood flow in various areas. Pulmonary circulation constricts in acidosis, whereas decreased pH (acidosis) causes vasodilation in systemic vessels. This has distinct implications when caring for the newborn infant who is experiencing difficulty in making an effective cardiopulmonary transition to extrauterine life. (See Persistent Pulmonary Hypertension of the Newborn, Chapter 10.)

RESPIRATORY ACIDOSIS
Respiratory acidosis results from diminished or inadequate pulmonary ventilation that causes an elevation in plasma P_{CO_2} and thus an increased concentration of dissolved carbonic acid, which leads to elevated carbonic acid and hydrogen ion concentration. Conditions that produce respiratory acidosis can originate at three levels in the respiratory system and result in inadequate gas exchange (Box 28-3).

Compensation is mediated through the kidneys, which are stimulated to conserve and thus increase the plasma bicarbonate concentration and to excrete hydrogen ions. Laboratory findings in respiratory acidosis include elevated plasma bicarbonate concentration.

The treatment of respiratory acidosis is aimed at correcting the underlying cause and improving gas exchange at the alveolar level to provide more efficient removal of carbon dioxide. Oxygen therapy is usually indicated, as well as mechanical ventilation as the condition warrants. Administration of buffers such as sodium bicarbonate to reduce hydrogen ion concentration is usually not indicated, since it can result in fluid volume excess by causing an osmolar fluid shift from the blood to the intravascular space, which would only further compromise respiratory function and aggravate the acidosis. In children with chronic metabolic acidosis, oral sodium bicarbonate may be administered (Greenbaum, 2007). IV sodium bicarbonate may be administered in acute cases of metabolic acidosis as a bolus push or titrated in a continuous infusion solution. However, the administration of IV sodium bicarbonate may be harmful and cause more problems, especially in neonates, prompting some clinicians to advocate for the cessation of this practice in neonatal resuscitation (Aschner and Poland, 2008). In preterm infants rapid volume expansion with sodium bicarbonate may increase intravascular volume with subsequent periventricular hemorrhage. Any patient receiving IV sodium bicarbonate is at risk for hypernatremia if sodium intake from other sources is not carefully monitored. Because sodium bicarbonate produces carbon dioxide as it is metabolized, patients who are not being effectively ventilated may actually develop a more severe respiratory acidosis as P_{CO_2} accumulates.

RESPIRATORY ALKALOSIS

Conversely, respiratory alkalosis is caused by a primary increase in the rate and depth of pulmonary ventilation, resulting in unusually large amounts of carbon dioxide being exhaled, or "blown off." This reduces the plasma P_{CO_2} and raises the pH. Metabolic compensation for a respiratory alkalosis, usually performed by the kidneys, is more gradual and may occur over a period of days; thus the pH and the bicarbonate level may remain normal (Greenbaum, 2007). Box 28-4 lists conditions that stimulate the respiratory center to produce hyperventilation.

A frequent cause of hyperventilation in children is voluntary hyperventilation before underwater swimming. The condition may also be seen in children with an anxiety attack and subsequent hyperventilation. It is also a consideration in the care of persons having mechanical ventilation, extracorporeal membrane oxygenation (ECMO), and hemodialysis (Greenbaum, 2007). Incorrectly set mechanical ventilators can cause respiratory rates and tidal volumes in excess of physiologic needs.

Compensation of respiratory alkalosis takes place in the kidneys and consists of excretion of carbonic acid in association with sodium (Na^+) and potassium to conserve hydrogen. Laboratory findings include elevated plasma pH (>7.45), depressed plasma carbonic acid concentration (<23 mEq/L in older children, <20 mEq/L in young children), and lowered P_{CO_2} (<35 mm Hg).

Treatment of respiratory alkalosis consists of correction of the underlying cause and prevention of lost anions and the associated potassium deficit. Rebreathing carbon dioxide slows respirations and provides rapid relief, as does oxygen therapy.

METABOLIC ACIDOSIS

Metabolic acidosis is a lowered plasma pH caused by any process that reduces the bicarbonate concentration. Metabolic acidosis can be produced by the gain of nonvolatile acids or the loss of bicarbonate. Strong acid is gained, and bicarbonate is lost by several specific mechanisms and routes (Box 28-5).

Compensation of metabolic acidosis is respiratory, with alveolar hyperventilation occurring immediately as the decrease in pH is sensed by the respiratory center. Strong acids are immediately buffered to generate the weaker carbonic acid, which the respiratory system attempts to eliminate through increased alveolar ventilation. In this respiratory effort the breathing is deep and rapid—the Kussmaul or air-hunger type of respirations. Bicarbonate conservation and excretion by the kidneys is a slower mechanism. Laboratory findings of uncompensated metabolic acidosis include lowered plasma pH (<7.35) and diminished plasma bicarbonate concentration.

The plasma AG may be helpful in the evaluation of patients with metabolic acidosis. The AG reflects the difference between the measured cation sodium and the anions (also measured) of chloride and bicarbonate (Greenbaum, 2007). Two diagnostic groups exist: those with a normal AG or those with an increased (high) AG. The formula for calculating the anion gap is as follows:

$$AG = [Na^+] - [Cl^-] - [HCO_3^-]$$

BOX 28-5   METABOLIC ACIDOSIS

Strong acid is gained by:
- Gain of exogenous acid (e.g., ammonium chloride) by ingestion or infusion (e.g., salicylates, methanol, ethylene glycol)
- Incomplete oxidation of fatty acids, which occurs in conditions such as diabetic ketoacidosis, starvation (including patients receiving nothing by mouth for therapeutic purposes)
- Incomplete oxidation of carbohydrate that produces large amounts of lactic acid as a result of primary lactic acidosis (rare) or secondary to tissue hypoxia from excessive exercise, serious trauma, or severe infection
- Inability of the renal system to excrete the normal, ongoing volume of inorganic acid metabolites, which results from the azotemic acidosis of advanced kidney failure, renal tubular acidosis, and potassium-sparing diuretics

Base bicarbonate is lost by:
- Losses from the gastrointestinal tract—secretions distal to the pyloric sphincter containing large amounts of bicarbonate, which may be lost during conditions that produce diarrhea or vomiting, fistula drainage, and suction
- Losses as a result of inappropriate bicarbonate excretion in the kidneys because of renal tubular acidosis

BOX 28-6   METABOLIC ALKALOSIS

Loss of acid can result from the following:
- In children the most common cause of hydrogen ion depletion is loss of hydrochloric acid (HCl) incident to hypertrophic pyloric stenosis. The infant produces large amounts of HCl, which is vomited with repeated feedings. HCl is also lost in gastric tube drainage.
- Less often, hydrogen ions are lost through the kidneys in diuretic therapy, potassium depletion, or administration of adrenocortical hormones.

A gain in base is usually iatrogenic and relatively uncommon in children but can result from:
- Gain of exogenous bicarbonate from ingestion or infusion
- Oxidation of salts or organic acid from infusion or ingestion of lactate, citrate, or acetate

The normal AG is 4 to 11 mEq/L (Greenbaum, 2007). With a high AG there is an increase in the number of unmeasured ions (potassium, magnesium, calcium); conditions with a high AG include diabetic ketoacidosis, other ketoacidoses (starvation [e.g., disordered eating], alcoholic ketoacidosis), lactic acidosis, kidney failure (may also be mixed high and normal), some inborn errors of metabolism, and poisonings (ethylene glycol intoxication, salicylate intoxication, methyl alcohol intoxication). Diarrhea, renal tubular acidosis, acetazolamide ingestion, biliary or pancreatic fistulas, and excessive administration of isotonic saline or ammonium chloride are examples of conditions that are seen with a normal AG (Metheny, 2000; Greenbaum, 2007). In mild cases of metabolic acidosis and with certain conditions, the AG is not as helpful as other laboratory determinations and a comprehensive history and physical examination (Greenbaum, 2007).

Treatment is directed at correcting the basic deficit and replacing the excessive losses of bicarbonate with sodium or potassium bicarbonate or sodium lactate.

METABOLIC ALKALOSIS

Metabolic alkalosis is represented by an elevated plasma pH that occurs when there is a reduction in hydrogen ion concentration and an excess of bicarbonate. This can be caused by a gain in base or a loss of acid (Box 28-6).

Compensation in metabolic alkalosis theoretically should be respiratory; however, such compensation is irregular and unpredictable. In addition, renal correction is complicated by losses of sodium, potassium, and chloride, which are lost in conditions such as hypertrophic pyloric stenosis through vomiting. The kidneys attempt to conserve the sodium and potassium concentration at the expense of hydrogen concentration and acid-base balance. Laboratory findings include elevated urine pH, elevated plasma pH, elevated plasma bicarbonate, and, if in conjunction with chloride deficit, reduced chloride concentration. Treatment of metabolic alkalosis is aimed at preventing further losses of acid and replacing lost electrolytes.

NURSING RESPONSIBILITIES IN FLUID AND ELECTROLYTE DISTURBANCES

Nursing observation and intervention are essential to the detection and therapeutic management of disturbances in fluid and electrolyte balance. Imbalances may be precipitated by a variety of circumstances, and the balance may be so precarious, especially in newborns and infants, that changes can take place in a very short time. Therefore an important nursing responsibility is anticipation and perceptive observation for any signs of imbalance, particularly in those situations and conditions in which imbalance is likely to occur. Conditions in which changes can develop with surprising rapidity in young children include diarrhea; vomiting; sweating; fever; disorders such as type 1 diabetes, renal disease, and cardiac anomalies; administration of certain drugs such as diuretics and steroids; and trauma, such as major surgery, burns, and other extensive injury. Preterm infants with respiratory distress syndrome and other pulmonary conditions may exhibit acid-base imbalances. In such infants compensatory mechanisms are immature, and the child may not survive without prompt intervention. (See also Chapter 10.)

Nurses must be comfortable with equipment used to deliver fluids to infants and children and be familiar with the information and techniques for physical assessment of each age-group. An understanding of normal serum chemistry levels provides additional data on which to base assessments and interventions and to validate observations. Data that are helpful in assessment related to fluid and electrolyte balance include the proposed treatment plan, including medications and fluid therapies, laboratory reports, history of illness, and records of fluid intake and output (I&O). An important nursing role is teaching parents to recognize early signs of dehydration.

ASSESSMENT

Whether the child is at home, in the practitioner's office or clinic, or in the hospital, nursing assessment is an essential part of the nursing care plan. The assessment of suspected or potential fluid and electrolyte disturbance begins with the observation of general appearance. Ill children usually have drawn expressions, have dry mucous membranes and lips, and "look sick." Loss of appetite is one of the first behaviors observed in most childhood illnesses, and the infant's or child's activity level is diminished from baseline or usual activities. The cry of an ill infant is less vigorous, often whining, and higher pitched than usual. The child is irritable, seeks the parent's comfort and attention, and displays purposeless movements and inappropriate responses to people and familiar objects. In some cases the child may not protest advances by the health care worker and procedures such as taking vital signs or starting an IV infusion. These are signs that the child truly feels bad and that the condition is serious and immediate intervention is necessary. As the child's illness and level of dehydration become more severe, irritability progresses to lethargy and even unconsciousness.

History

The nurse can obtain much of the information regarding the child's behavior from the parent or primary caregiver. In addition to initial observations, a good history is extremely valuable to the assessment. The amount and type of fluid I&O (especially abnormal output) are important. An accurate estimate of fluid losses is beyond the capacity of history givers, but rough estimates of excessive fluid losses or diminished output can usually be obtained from information such as the number and consistency of stools the child has passed in the past 24 hours, the number of times the child voided, and the type and amount of food and fluid ingested or vomited. For an infant, ask about the number of wet diapers in the past 24 hours. Parents frequently omit this information from their discussion with the health professional. They tell how much has been taken but not how much was excreted unless asked specifically. Having the parents estimate the amount of urine in the diaper at each void is of little value because of the absorbent diaper material, which pulls fluids away from the child's skin.

Both the type and the amount of intake provide valuable information. The quality and quantity can be determined—is intake sustained, excessive, or curtailed? Loss early in diarrheal illness progresses rapidly, and the water losses can exceed sodium losses, leading to hypernatremia. Hypernatremic dehydration indicates a significant interference with water intake. Also important is a history of normal or increased intake of an unusual fluid, such as one containing sucrose, tea, juice, athletic hydration fluid (e.g., Gatorade), an alternative home remedy fluid, or other solute-containing fluids, which can contribute to hyponatremic dehydration in the face of abnormal losses.

A history of gradual weight gain and observations of any puffiness, especially in areas with less dense tissues (periorbital, scrotal), or "clothes fitting tighter" offer early clues to edema. A history of excessive water intake, especially when associated with diminished output, is important in assessing edema and water intoxication.

Clinical Observations

Fever and infection can also produce tachycardia, the earliest manifestation of dehydration. Therefore these are considered in the assessment of dehydration. Dry skin and mucous membranes (oral) usually appear early. A sunken fontanel is a useful observation if the status of the fontanel is known when the infant is healthy. Signs of circulatory failure usually indicate severe dehydration, since compensatory mechanisms are able to sustain blood pressure in the low normal range for some time. Loss of skin elasticity, generally manifested in children less than 2 years of age, is measured by the time it takes for pinched abdominal skin to recoil. This sign is also observed in undernourished children. Also, in hypertonic dehydration the skin has a smooth, velvety feel before it develops disturbed elasticity.

Assess capillary filling time by pinching a toe or a thumb or lightly pressing the abdominal skin and estimating the time it takes for the blood to return. Capillary filling time in mild dehydration is less than 2 seconds, increasing to more than 4 seconds in severe dehydration. The technique is effective in children of all ages. However, it can be altered in the presence of heart failure, which affects circulation time, and hypertonic dehydration, in which fluid loss is primarily intracellular. Additional clinical signs observed in children with dehydration include cool mottled extremities, sunken eyes, tachypnea, and changes in sensorium.

When caring for the ill child, assess vital signs as often as every 15 to 30 minutes, and record weight frequently during the initial phase of therapy. It is important to use the same scale each time the child is weighed and to predetermine the weight of any equipment or devices that must remain attached during the weighing process, including arm boards, and any clothing the child might be wearing. Take routine weights at the same time each day.

Intake and Output Measurement

One of the nurse's most important roles in fluid and electrolyte disturbance is related to I&O. Accurate measurements are essential to the assessment of fluid balance. Measurements from all sources—including gastrointestinal and parenteral I&O from urine, stools, vomitus, fistulas, nasogastric suction, sweat, and drainage from wounds—must be taken into consideration. Although the practitioner usually indicates when I&O are to be recorded, it is a nursing responsibility to keep an accurate I&O record on certain children, including those:

- Receiving IV therapy
- Who underwent major surgery
- With severe thermal burns or injuries
- With renal disease or damage
- With congestive heart failure
- With dehydration
- With diabetes mellitus
- With oliguria
- Receiving diuretic therapy
- Receiving corticosteroid therapy
- In respiratory distress
- With chronic lung disease

NURSING TIP 1 g wet diaper weight = 1 ml urine.

NURSING TIP In infants with diapers, weigh all the dry diapers to be used for that child and note in a colored indelible marker the dry weight of the diaper to be used; when there is fluid (urine or liquid stool) in the diaper, the amount of output can be approximated by subtracting the weight of the dry diaper from the weighed amount of the wet diaper.

Infants or small children who are unable to use a bedpan or those who have bowel movements with every voiding will require the application of a collecting device. (See Urine Specimens, Chapter 27.) Collecting bags may not be suitable for all infants (e.g., preterm and other infants whose fragile skin does not tolerate some types of self-adhesive appliances). If collecting bags are not used, wet diapers or pads are carefully weighed to ascertain the amount of fluid lost. This includes liquid stool, urine, vomitus, and other losses. The volume of fluid in milliliters is approximately equivalent to the weight of the fluid measured in grams. The specific gravity as a measure of osmolality is determined with a refractometer or urine dipsticks and assists in assessing the degree of hydration.

Disadvantages of the weighed diaper method of fluid measurement include (1) inability to differentiate one type of loss from another because of admixture (liquid stool versus urine); (2) loss of urine or liquid stool from leakage or evaporation, especially if the infant is under a radiant warmer; and (3) additional fluid in the diaper (superabsorbent disposable type) from absorption of atmospheric moisture (high-humidity incubators). Evaporative losses render measurements inaccurate unless the diaper is weighed and measured for specific gravity at least every 30 minutes when critical values are needed. Evaporative losses are greater in very low–birth-weight and extremely low–birth-weight infants, those under radiant warmers, and those being treated with phototherapy. However, research indicates that accurate specific gravity measurements can be made for up to 2 hours on urine obtained from a diaper that has been removed from an infant, folded, and stored in a utility room (Kee and Paulanka, 2000; Metheny, 2000).

It is important to measure and record all intake, oral and parenteral, as well as output from all sources, including urine, stool, emesis, drainage tubes, fistulas, and wounds from which appreciable amounts of fluid are lost. At home, advise parents to observe the number of times and how much the child voids. The newborn may be expected to void at least once in the first 24 hours, two or three times in the second 24 hours of life, three or four times in the third and fourth days of life, and a minimum of five or six times by the fifth and sixth days; if intake is adequate, the infant 5 to 6 days old and older may be expected to have a minimum of six to eight voidings per day (American Academy of Pediatrics, 2009). Infants younger than 1 year of age may void every 1 to 2 hours; toddlers urinate approximately every 3 hours. As children get older, they void less frequently. Instruct the parents to notify the nurse or clinician if the child appears to be voiding an insufficient amount or persistently losing fluid through vomiting or diarrhea.

ORAL FLUID INTAKE

Under ordinary circumstances an adequate oral intake is no problem in children who are able to respond to thirst cues. Hydration becomes a nursing problem when infants or children are unable to take in fluids by mouth because of illness or because fatigue or discomfort makes them reluctant to swallow. Children with elevated temperatures, continued gastrointestinal losses, labile type 1 diabetes, or cystic fibrosis are especially prone to dehydration. Occasionally dehydration caused by

inadequate breast milk intake has been observed in breast-fed infants in the first few weeks of life.

ORT is recommended for mild to moderate dehydration. An ORS containing 75 to 90 mMol sodium and 111 to 139 mMol glucose (e.g., World Health Organization solution, Pedialyte RS, Rehydralyte) is most commonly recommended for the first 4 to 6 hours. If this is tolerated, then oral fluids containing 30 to 60 mMol sodium and 111 to 139 mMol glucose (e.g., Pedialyte, Lytren, Resol, Infalyte) can be given for the next 18 to 24 hours at a dose of 45 to 60 ml/kg (1 to 2 oz) divided into frequent feedings consisting of 90 to 120 ml (3 to 4 oz) for young children. Older children can be given 30 to 60 ml (1 to 2 oz) every hour.

The American Academy of Pediatrics (2009) does not advocate withholding food and fluids for 24 hours after the onset of diarrhea, or administering the BRAT diet (bananas, rice, applesauce, and toast), which is low in protein and electrolytes and high in carbohydrates. Breast-fed infants should continue breast-feeding, provided that milk supply is adequate for hydration; once the older infant or child has successfully achieved rehydration, he or she may consume a regular diet, avoiding fat (no French fries!!), high sugar drinks, soda, Jell-O, or rice water (American Academy of Pediatrics, 2009; Wade, 2010). Flavored frozen Popsicles that are low in sucrose (≤5%) may be offered; these often contain 30 to 45 ml of fluid and are enticing to the child who is being rehydrated. Encourage the child to eat as little as desired and, after a given trial period, offer a second Popsicle. An antiemetic such as ondansetron (also available in oral dissolving tablet) may be given (as ordered), then followed in 20 to 30 minutes with an oral fluid challenge (the Popsicle). A lactation specialist should be consulted for assistance if ineffective latch-on in the breast-fed infant is part of the intake problem.

Persuading a reluctant child to drink fluids can be a nursing challenge and is not uncommon in the care of infants and children. Older children often respond to the challenge of meeting a specific goal for fluid intake (or deprivation) and can be active participants in planning an intake schedule. Contracts and rewards are effective strategies. However, young children require more creative tactics. Suggestions for encouraging children to drink fluids are discussed in Chapter 27. (See Chapter 27 for a discussion of nasogastric alimentation.)

The Child Who Is NPO

Infants or children who are unable or not permitted to take fluids by mouth (NPO) have special needs. To ensure that they do not receive fluids, place a sign in some obvious place, such as over their beds or pinned to their shirts, to alert others to the NPO status. Remove fluids from the bedside to reduce the temptation.

Oral hygiene, a part of routine hygienic care, is especially important when fluids are restricted or withheld. (See Chapter 27.) For young children who cannot brush their teeth or rinse their mouth without swallowing fluid, clean the mouth and teeth and keep it moist by swabbing with saline-moistened gauze. Judicious administration of ice chips provides moist, cool relief (if permitted by the practitioner). To meet the need to suck, provide infants a safe commercial pacifier.

The child on restricted fluids provides an equal challenge. Having fluids limited is often more difficult for the child than being NPO, especially when IV fluids are also eliminated. To make certain the child does not drink the entire amount allowed early in the day, the daily allotment is calculated to provide fluids at periodic intervals throughout the child's waking hours. Serving the fluids in small containers gives the illusion of larger servings. No extra liquid is left at the bedside.

PARENTERAL FLUID THERAPY

Intravenous Infusion

Before beginning an IV infusion, the nurse performs several preparatory activities. All needed equipment is gathered so that the operator can proceed without interruption. More important, the child and the family must be prepared for this stressful procedure.

Solution and Equipment

The composition of the IV solution is based on patient history and the diagnosis, or the type of fluid volume deficit being treated, and is selected on the basis of tonicity (osmolarity) and electrolyte content. A solution that is isotonic has the same osmolality, or tonicity, as body fluids such as plasma. A hypertonic solution is one that has a greater concentration of solutes than plasma; a hypotonic solution has a lower concentration. Examples of isotonic solutions are 0.9% normal saline solutions, lactated Ringer solution, and 5% dextrose in water; 10% glucose in water is a hypertonic solution; plain water (without electrolytes) and a solution with 0.2% sodium are hypotonic solutions. Although it is larger, one molecule of glucose has only half the osmolality of one molecule of sodium chloride (NaCl) because the sodium chloride ionizes in solution into two particles, the sodium and the chloride ions. Thus one molecule of sodium chloride exerts twice the osmotic pressure of one molecule of glucose.

Most common pediatric maintenance solutions include a combination of dextrose (usually 5% or 10%) and sodium chloride (usually 0.22% to 0.45%). The hypotonic solution is necessary for children, since their daily turnover of free water exceeds that of adults. Because infants and young children are subject to rapid fluid shifts, any IV solution given to them should contain at least 0.2% sodium chloride to prevent brain edema, a disorder to which they are susceptible if given plain water. Glucose is rapidly metabolized; therefore the osmolality of 5% glucose is further diminished.

To avoid infusing too much of the IV solution, the volume of the solution container should be based on the child's age, size, and 24-hour volume needs. For infants and small children it is best to place 3 to 4 hours of required maintenance IV solution in a small container such as a graded buretrol to avoid fluid overload in the event of equipment failure (runaway infusion). Solution containers (usually a plastic bag) containing 250 to 500 ml are commonly used in infants and small children, as opposed to the 1000-ml containers used in adolescents and adults.

For most IV infusions in children, an over-the-needle 24- to 22-gauge catheter may be used if therapy will last less than 5 days. The smallest gauge and shortest length catheter that will accommodate the prescribed therapy should be chosen for the placement of a peripheral IV (PIV) line. The length of the catheter may be directly related to infection or embolus formation—the shorter the catheter, the fewer the complications. The gauge of the catheter should maintain adequate flow of the infusate into the cannulated vein while allowing adequate blood flow around the catheter walls to promote proper hemodilution of the infusate. Because stainless steel needles tend to dislodge and infiltrate more frequently than catheters, limit the use of these to short-term or single-dose administration.

The goal of IV therapy is to deliver the prescribed fluids or medications without complications. Determining the best catheter for the patient early in the therapy provides the best chance of avoiding catheter-related complications. As the length of therapy increases, explore decisions regarding the type of infusion device (short peripheral, midline, peripherally inserted central catheter [PICC], or central venous catheter).

The Infusion Nurses Society (2006) supports the use of chlorhexidine gluconate, or, povidone-iodine, as preferred antiseptics for cleaning the site before initiating a PIV. Several clinical trials in adults have demonstrated enhanced skin antisepsis when using chlorhexidine-containing products (Crosby and Mares, 2001; Milstone, Passaretti, and Perl, 2008). A number of published studies have demonstrated that 2% aqueous chlorhexidine is superior to 10% povidone-iodine and alcohol-based products for preventing catheter-related bacteremia in children (Kline, 2005). U.S. Food and Drug Administration approval for patients above the age of 2 months has led to the introduction of one such product, ChloraPrep. It is a sterile applicator composed of 2% chlorhexidine gluconate and 70% isopropyl alcohol. Researchers have demonstrated the safety and efficacy of 0.5% chlorhexidine scrub versus povidone-iodine as a skin disinfectant in a neonatal intensive care unit (Linder, Prince, Barzilai, et al, 2004). Chlorhexidine gluconate appears to be a safe and effective skin antiseptic solution for central venous catheter site care in children; however, several researchers (Carson, 2004; Lee and Johnston, 2005) point to conflicting evidence with regards to the most effective concentration of chlorhexidine (2% or 0.5 %) for preventing central venous catheter–related bloodstream infection in children, and the overall safety of the antiseptic solution in neonates and preterm infants has yet to be established.

Suggested equipment for starting a PIV includes:
- Gloves (if latex, check for patient latex sensitivity)
- Skin antiseptic (chlorhexidine, alcohol, or povidone-iodine)
- Buffered lidocaine, LMX4 (4% liposomal lidocaine), or EMLA (a eutectic mix of lidocaine and prilocaine) to anesthetize the area
- A tourniquet (again, check for patient latex sensitivity)
- Rolled towels or small blankets for maintaining position of head or extremity
- Tape (or dressing and bacteriostatic ointment as required by hospital policy)
- Sterile transparent occlusive dressing
- A T or J connector (an extension tube that decreases tension and movement of the catheter hub at the site, provides a port for piggyback medications, and makes changing the dressing and tubing easier)

- Blood collection tubes and syringes for collecting blood (blood samples should be collected at the time of IV insertion whenever possible to avoid an additional needlestick)
- Prefilled normal saline syringes to test patency of IV site before attaching the IV fluids
- A protection device to protect the IV site after insertion

The prescribed solution is flushed or primed through the T or J connector (if blood samples will not be collected), tubing, filter, and infusion pump in advance, ready to connect to the catheter hub after insertion of the IV catheter. A sharps container should be within reach if the IV catheter needle does not retract into a safety shield after the catheter is in place.

NURSING TIP Applying the tourniquet over a piece of clothing or wrapping the area with a washcloth before applying the tourniquet will reduce the pain caused by pressure or pinching of the tourniquet. A small tourniquet "belt" is also available, which reduces pinching of the skin.

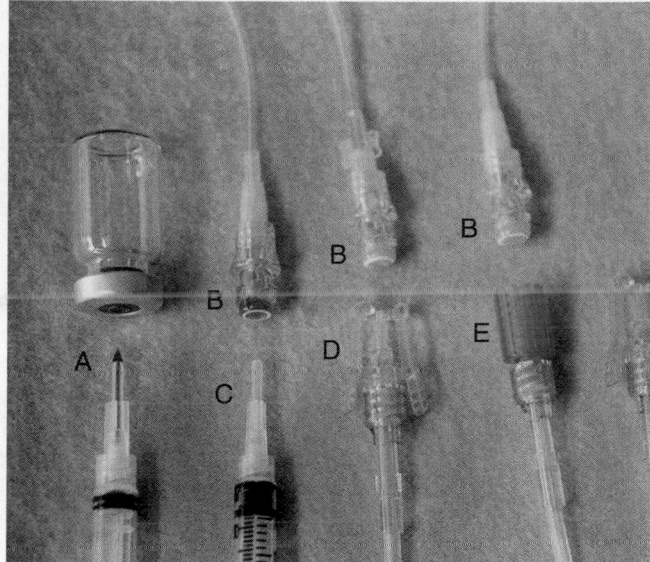

Fig. 28-5 Interlink intravenous access systems. **A,** Blue spike syringe. **B,** Preslit injection port (needleless). **C,** Blunt plastic cannula syringe. **D,** Lever lock cannula. **E,** Threaded lock cannula.

Safety Catheters and Needleless Systems

One of the main causes for change in IV therapy is the concern about needlestick injuries. To provide safer care for the patient and health care worker, and to comply with Occupational Safety and Health Administration standards and the Needlestick Safety and Prevention Act of 2001 (Regulation 1910.1030; available at www.osha.gov), manufacturers have developed safety catheters and needleless IV systems (Marini, Giangregorio, and Kraskinski, 2004).

Over-the-needle IV catheters with hollow-bore needles carry a high risk for transmission of blood-borne pathogens from needlestick injuries (Whitby, McLaws, and Slater, 2008). A number of safety catheters are currently used to prevent accidental needlesticks with over-the-needle IV catheters (Marini, Giangregorio, and Kraskinski, 2004). Needleless IV systems, which are designed to prevent needlestick injuries during administration of IV push medications and IV piggyback medications, may vary from manufacturer to manufacturer, but the concept is essentially the same. Some needleless systems are universal, whereas others require complete use of the entire IV delivery system for compatibility. Needleless IV systems rely on prepierced septa that are accessed by blunted plastic cannulas or systems that use valves that open and close a fluid path when activated by insertion of a syringe.

Blunt plastic cannulas and preslit injection port sites found in Interlink IV access systems (Fig. 28-5) eliminate the need for steel needles and conventional injection port sites but remain accessible to hypodermic needle use or access, a drawback except in emergent situations. Systems that do not permit needle access enhance safety by preventing health care workers from attempting to use needles; however, such systems are limited by the lack of needle access (interchangeability between needleless and needle insertion systems), especially in emergency situations. A syringe with a blue spike is available to access a single-dose vial (see Fig. 28-5, *A*). The preslit injection port sites are identified by a white ring surrounding the port; this ring alerts users that the system is needleless (see Fig. 28-5, *B*). Syringes are available with the blunt plastic cannula for accessing these sites (see Fig. 28-5, *C*). A lever lock (see Fig. 28-5, *D*) or threaded lock cannula (see Fig. 28-5, *E*) attaches to an IV line, IV Y site, or peripheral intermittent infusion device. A preslit universal vial adapter (not pictured) provides access to standard multiple-dose vials, and syringe cannulas are then used to access the adapter.

Infusion Pumps

Several modifications are made in equipment used for IV infusion for children. A gravity drainage apparatus for children is much the same as that for adults except that it is designed to deliver a reduced drop size (60 drops/ml) and contains a calibrated volume control chamber (e.g., a buretrol or soluset) that regulates the amount of fluid that can be infused. A microdropper facilitates calculation of flow rate, since a prescribed number of milliliters per hour equals the number of drops per minute. For example, if the solution is to infuse at a rate of 30 ml/hr, the infusion is regulated to deliver 30 drops/min.

A variety of infusion pumps are available. The IV solution is refillable from the bag, bottle, or soluset above or contained in a syringe pump to minimize the possibility of overloading the circulation. Infusion pumps are recommended in infants and small children because they can accurately infuse fluids (especially the syringe pumps, which infuse very small amounts of fluids) and accurately provide the prescribed amount of IV solution. It is an important nursing responsibility to understand and follow manufacturer's directions for use, calculate the amount to be infused in a given time, set the infusion rate, and monitor the apparatus frequently (at least every 1 to 2 hours) to make certain that the desired rate is maintained, the integrity of the system remains intact, the site remains intact (free of redness, edema, infiltration, or irritation), and the infusion does not stop.

Continuous infusion pumps, although convenient and efficient, are not without risks. Overreliance on the machine's accuracy can cause either too much or too little fluid to be infused; therefore its use does not eliminate careful periodic assessment by the nurse. Excess pressure can build up if the machine is set at a rate faster than the vein is able to accommodate (or continues to pump when the needle or cannula is out of the vessel lumen). This is especially true in very small infants. Regardless of the device used, a thorough understanding of the apparatus is essential for safe fluid administration.

Intraosseous Infusion

Situations may occur in which rapid establishment of systemic access is vital and venous access is complicated by peripheral circulatory collapse, hypovolemic shock (secondary to vomiting or diarrhea, burns, or trauma), cardiopulmonary arrest, or other conditions (de Caen, Reis, and Bhutta, 2008). It is recommended that intraosseous access be obtained if venous access cannot be readily achieved in a pediatric resuscitation (de Caen, Reis, and Bhutta, 2008; Hazinski, Zaritsky, Nadkarni, et al, 2002). Intraosseous infusion provides a rapid, safe, and lifesaving alternate route for administration of fluids and medications until intravascular access is possible, especially in children 6 years old or younger. Health care providers, including physicians, nurses, and paramedics, can secure intraosseous cannulation within 30 to 60 seconds. Some hospitals recommend pediatric advanced life support training before performing this procedure. This procedure is usually reserved for children who are unconscious or for those receiving analgesia, since the procedure is painful. Local anesthesia should be used for a semiconscious patient.

A large-bore rigid needle such as a bone marrow aspiration needle (e.g., Jamshidi) or an intraosseous needle (e.g., Cook) is inserted into the medullary cavity of a long bone. The anteromedial aspect of the tibia—1 to 3 cm (0.4 to 1.2 inch) below the tibial tuberosity—is the preferred site for children of all ages because it is flat and has a large marrow cavity. In newborns the distal third of the femur may be used. The distal tibia is an alternative site.

Observe the extremity closely for swelling or oozing of fluid at the insertion site. Give particular attention to the dependent tissue of the leg. Extravasation of fluid from the bone marrow may be hidden under the leg. Check for swelling of the entire lower leg when the intraosseous bone marrow needle is in the tibia or ankle, and check the entire upper leg when the intraosseous needle is in the femur. Compartment syndrome has resulted from an infiltrated intraosseous line. Other complications, although rare, include fractures, skin necrosis, osteomyelitis, and cellulitis (de Caen, Reis, and Bhutta, 2008; Fiorito, Mirza, Doran, et al, 2005).

Once the bone marrow needle is in place, the needle should stand alone and feel secure. Tape and gauze are used to secure the needle to the leg. Gauze should be built up around the needle to provide support and prevent trauma or dislodgment. Drugs may be pushed and fluids delivered via an infusion pump. The intraosseous line may be discontinued after IV access has been achieved.

Preparing the Child and Parents

Children of any age are anxious and fearful of injections, and unless the IV infusion is implemented as an emergency procedure, there will be time to prepare them. (See Preparation for Diagnostic and Therapeutic Procedures, Chapter 27.) Many children have never undergone the procedure, and those who have will remember the experience. Using an age-appropriate developmental approach, the nurse can ask them what they think about the procedure and why it is needed for them specifically. Children's perceptions of the anticipated experience reveal any misconceptions that need to be clarified and help the nurse prepare them for what to expect. In addition, children's observations provide some insight into how to cope with their reactions during the insertion procedure and throughout the course of the IV therapy. For children who have repeated venipunctures, it is helpful to ask them or their parents which vein has been successfully accessed in the past.

Play, always an excellent stress reduction technique, can be employed during the preparation process. Allowing children to handle the equipment and to "start" an IV infusion on a toy animal or doll helps familiarize them with the frightening aspects of the procedure. In some instances it may be helpful to introduce a child to another child who is coping well in the same situation.

It is best to arrange for a quiet, private setting for the child during the insertion. Avoid "safe places," such as the playroom or the child's hospital room when possible. The assurance of privacy relieves the child of some anxieties concerning loss of control in front of others. It also avoids subjecting other children to the potentially stress-provoking scene. Provide the child with some distracting activity, such as those described for injections, and perhaps allow them to "help" by holding supplies such as a gauze square, helping to clean the site with an antiseptic, and assisting in taping the site after the procedure.

Children usually cooperate better and feel more in command if they are allowed to sit up during the process, although this may not be possible even in some older, normally cooperative children. Toddlers and young children can be held on a parent's lap, with the child's legs tucked between the parent's legs, and the child's arm (not being used for the venipuncture) behind the parent. A hug should both restrain the child and provide comfort. The torso of the patient is held against the parent with the same hug. It is a mistake to assume that children will not lose control even after they promise to cooperate. It is wise to have ample assistance available in the event that a child cannot control anxiety. The child need not be restrained until necessary, but the assistant should be prepared to grasp a child gently but firmly during the insertion. Explaining to children what is being done during each step of the procedure and how they can participate helps obtain their cooperation and reduce their stress. Make every effort to reduce the pain of the needle insertion (see Atraumatic Care box).

Inform parents about the procedure, including the reasons for the procedure, how long the catheter must remain in place, and what they can expect during and after the insertion. Offer them the option of remaining with their child or leaving. Encourage parents who remain to kiss, hug, and distract the child during the procedure.

The Procedure

The site selected for PIV infusion depends on accessibility and convenience. Although it is possible to use any accessible vein in older children, consider the child's developmental, cognitive,

ATRAUMATIC CARE

Venipuncture

To minimize or prevent the pain of the needle puncture for an intravenous (IV) line (or blood sample or implanted port access), apply EMLA (a eutectic mix of lidocaine and prilocaine) (use 0.5 to 1 g per site; see manufacturers' recommendations for repeated dosing) to the site 60 minutes before the procedure. Cover at least two sites in case the first attempt is not successful. Although some evidence indicates that EMLA causes minor vasoconstriction, no well-controlled studies support this concern. LMX4 (formerly Ela-Max), a 4% lidocaine cream, may also be used as a topical anesthetic before venipuncture or for accessing an implanted port. LMX4 does not require a dressing except for safety purposes, and the anesthetic has been reported to be active within 30 minutes of application; no vasoconstriction is reported with this topical preparation (Wong, 2003; Weise and Nahata, 2005). Ametop gel (4% tetracaine) is a topical anesthetic available in Canada and Europe; the gel works within 30 to 45 minutes (Ellis, Sharp, Newhook, et al, 2004).

Another option for pain management is the use of intradermal buffered lidocaine, which may be more appropriate for older children, since a needle-stick is required for application (usually a 30-gauge needle is used) (Luhmann, Hurt, Shootman, et al, 2004), or Numby Stuff (Doellman, 2003). (See Pain Management, Chapter 7.)

A needless system has been used to deliver powdered lidocaine to the skin in older children for venipuncture; the J-tip delivers 1% buffered lidocaine, which numbs the skin within 1 to 3 minutes (Jimenez, Bradford, Seidel, et al, 2006; Spanos, Booth, Koenig, et al, 2008; Zempsky, 2008).

Vapocoolant spray provides transient skin anesthesia within seconds of application; this method was effective at reducing pain in children ages 6 to 12 years undergoing IV cannulation (Farion, Splinter, Newhook, et al, 2008).

A 24% solution of oral sucrose (0.5 to 2 ml) may be given with a syringe to preterm infants (>32 weeks of gestation) and full-term infants 2 minutes before the procedure; allow the infant to suck on a pacifier during venipuncture and administer the oral sucrose solution at least two more times (during and after the procedure). Oral sucrose decreases procedural pain in neonates (Stevens, Taddio, Ohlsson, et al, 1997; Taddio, Shah, Hancock, et al, 2008; Thompson, 2005). Additional nonpharmacologic interventions for infants include swaddling and containment. (See also the Atraumatic Care box, Heel Punctures, in Chapter 8.)

Nonpharmacologic measures such as distraction, guided imagery, relaxation, massage, and modeling may also be used to decrease the psychologic anxiety of venipuncture in children (Doellman, 2003). A combination of pharmacologic and nonpharmacologic measures helps to decrease the pain of venipuncture in infants and children.

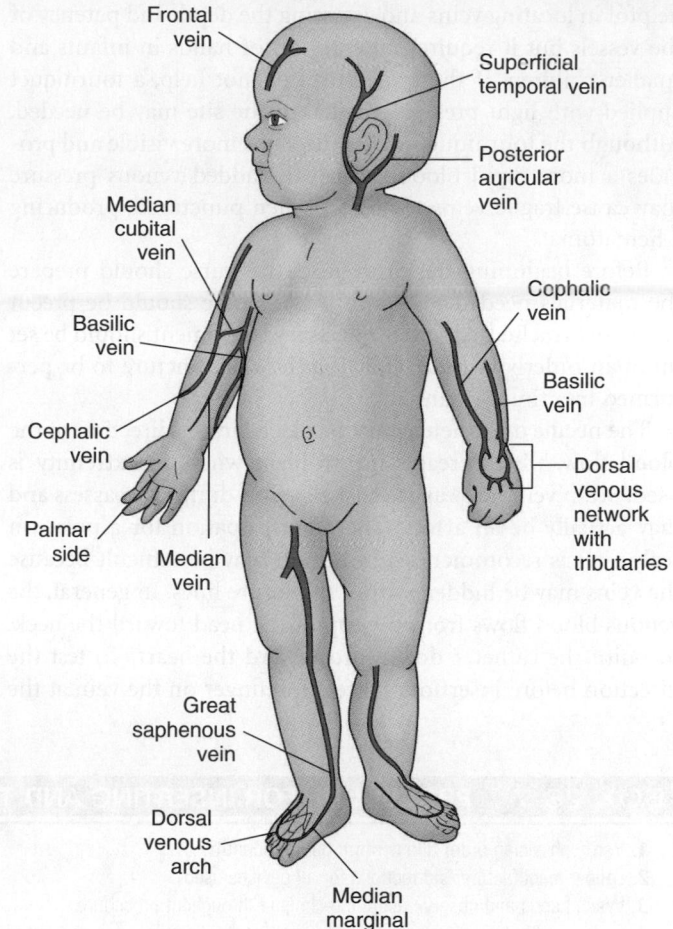

Fig. 28-6 Preferred sites for venous access in infants.

and mobility needs when selecting a site. Whenever possible, it is best to avoid the child's favored hand to reduce the disability related to the procedure. Choose a site that restricts the child's movements as little as possible; a site over a joint in an extremity is avoided as much as possible. An older child can help select the site and thereby maintain some measure of control.

For veins in the extremities, it is best to start with the most distal sites. If the vein is damaged, using distal sites initially preserves access to the vein in proximal sites. A scalp vein or a superficial vein of the wrist may also be used if larger veins are not accessible (Fig. 28-6). Avoid arteries for PIV therapy.

Most infants have one or two possible IV sites on each hand, arm, and foot and four to eight sites on the scalp. Because insertion is easy, scalp veins are sometimes used for IV therapy in infants less than 9 months of age but should be used only when attempts at other sites have failed. The temporal and forehead areas are suitable and do not interfere with side-to-side head movements. The use of a scalp vein site may require removing hair around the site to better visualize the vein and provide a

smoother surface on which to tape the tubing. Clipping off a portion of the infant's hair is upsetting to parents; therefore always tell them what to expect and reassure them that the hair will grow in again rapidly (save the hair, since parents often wish to keep it). Remove as little hair as possible directly over the insertion site and taping surface. To avoid microabrasions, do not shave the site, which increases the potential for introduction of microorganisms into the vascular system (Infusion Nurses Society, 2006). A rubber band slipped onto the head from brow to occiput will usually suffice as a tourniquet, although if the vessel is visible, a tourniquet may not be necessary in some infants.

An assistant should carefully restrain the extremity or head to facilitate venipuncture and minimize trauma from the child's inadvertent movement. (See Chapter 27 for additional restraining methods.) For a scalp site it is helpful to visualize the way in which the needle will be secured after insertion.

Locating an extremity vein may be difficult because the veins are smaller and children have a significant amount of subcutaneous fat. When veins are not readily visible, applying a warm compress to the site, running warm water over the extremity, or holding the limb in a dependent position below body level will help fill the veins for better visualization. Gentle tapping sometimes causes the veins to stand out. A flashlight held against the skin below the intended site sometimes assists in locating vessels. A commercial vein transilluminator is often helpful in locating veins and assessing the depth and patency of the vessels but it requires an extra set of hands in infants and smaller children. If these measures do not help, a tourniquet applied with light pressure medial to the site may be needed. Although the tourniquet makes the veins more visible and provides a more rapid blood return, the added venous pressure may cause fragile veins to "blow" when punctured, producing a hematoma.

Before beginning the procedure, the nurse should prepare the materials needed to secure the IV. Tape should be precut and easily reached. All other necessary equipment should be set up in an orderly fashion, allowing the venipuncture to be performed in a timely manner.

The needle or catheter must be placed in the direction of the blood flow, which creates no problem when an extremity is used. Scalp veins are easy to visualize but difficult to assess and may actually be an artery. Therefore palpation for a pulse on scalp sites is recommended but again may be difficult because the veins may be hidden within the suture lines. In general, the venous blood flows from the top of the head toward the neck, so point the catheter downward toward the heart. To test the direction before insertion, place a forefinger on the vein at the site chosen for venipuncture. While gently pressing the vein, use a second finger to "strip" the vein in the direction of the top of the head. Release the pressure from the second finger. If the vein fills distal to the compressing finger, the direction of flow is toward the stationary finger.

Securing a Peripheral Intravenous Line

To maintain the integrity of the IV line, adequate protection of the site is required (Box 28-7). Firmly secure the catheter hub at the puncture site with a transparent dressing or clear, nonallergenic tape. Transparent dressings are ideal because the insertion site is easy to observe. Use minimum tape at the puncture site and on about 2.5 to 5 cm (1 to 2 inches) of skin beyond the site to avoid obscuring the insertion site for early detection of infiltration.

! NURSING ALERT

Avoid opaque covering; however, if any type of opaque covering is used to secure the IV line, the insertion site and extremity distal to the site should be visible to detect an infiltration. If these sites are not visible, the nurse must check them frequently to detect problems early.

BOX 28-7   PROCEDURE FOR INSERTING AND TAPING A PERIPHERAL INTRAVENOUS CATHETER

1. Verify physician order and confirm patient identity.
2. Follow manufacturer's directions for all devices used.
3. Wash hands and observe aseptic technique throughout procedure.
4. Choose catheter insertion site and an alternative site in case the initial attempt is unsuccessful.
5. Prepare insertion site by applying with friction an antiseptic solution in a circular motion, working from the center of the insertion site to the exterior edge, approximately 5 cm (2 inches). Allow solution to dry completely, but do not blow dry, blot dry, or fan the area.
6. Don nonsterile gloves.
7. Apply tourniquet when site is ready for catheter insertion.
8. Stretch the skin taut downward below the point of insertion, upward above the site of insertion, or from underneath level with the point of insertion. This technique helps stabilize veins that roll or move away from the catheter as attempts are made to enter the vein.
9. Inspect catheter, looking for damage (e.g., bent stylet, shavings on the catheter, or frayed catheter tip [follow employer's policy for reporting defective devices]). If stylet and catheter are intact, break the seal between the two (if recommended by manufacturer) by gently twisting the two pieces and separating them a minuscule amount. This allows easy advancement of the catheter from the stylet after entering the vein.
10. Insert catheter through the skin, bevel up, at a 15- to 30-degree angle and enter the vein. This direct approach is best for large veins and enters the skin and vein in one step. The indirect approach for smaller veins enables the catheter to enter the vein from the side. It is sometimes helpful with short veins to start the catheter below the intended site and advance through the superficial layers of skin so that the advancement of the catheter in the vein is a shorter distance.
11. Watch for blood return in the flashback chamber. Some 22- and 24-gauge catheters provide visualization of the flashback within the catheter so immediate vein entrance is recognized before the needle punctures the back of the vessel or goes through the other side of the vessel.
12. Once the flashback is seen, lower the angle between the skin and catheter to 15 degrees. Advance the catheter another 0.16 to 0.3 cm ($\frac{1}{16}$ to $\frac{1}{8}$ inch) to ensure that both the metal stylet and catheter are inside the vein. Look closely at the intravenous (IV) catheter before inserting it and notice that the stylet tip is slightly longer than the catheter. It is necessary to have both

pieces inside the vein before advancing the catheter. Holding the stylet steady, push the catheter off the stylet and into the vein until the catheter hub is situated against the skin at the insertion site. Activate safety mechanism if necessary (some safety catheters are passive and activate automatically), remove the stylet, and discard into sharps container. Apply pressure to catheter within the vein to prevent backflow of blood before attaching extension tubing.

13. Connect the extension tubing and reinforce connection with a junction securement device (Luer-Lok, clasping device, threaded device) to prevent accidental disconnection and subsequent air embolism or blood loss.
14. Collect blood if ordered. Remove the tourniquet. Flush the IV line with normal saline to check for patency (ease of flushing fluid and lack of resistance while flushing), complaints of pain, or swelling to the site. If line flushes easily, proceed to secure the catheter to the skin.
15. Place transparent dressing across catheter hub, up to but not including the junction securement device, and surrounding skin.
16. Further secure the catheter to the skin using tape or adhesive securement devices (also known as adhesive anchors). Follow manufacturer's directions for adhesive anchors.
17. Place a $\frac{1}{4}$- to $\frac{1}{2}$-inch strip of clear tape across the width of the transparent dressing and the catheter hub but avoid the insertion site. This will serve as an anchor tape strip, and all other tape will be affixed to this strip (tape-on-tape method). This strip will not compromise the transparent dressing properties or interfere with visual inspection of the catheter-skin insertion site.
18. To stabilize the catheter and junction securement device, attach 1 to $1\frac{1}{2}$ inches of clear tape that is $\frac{1}{4}$ to $\frac{1}{2}$ inch wide, adhesive side up, to the underneath side of the catheter hub and junction securement device at their connection. Wrap the ends of the tape around the connections and meet on top to form a V shape (sometimes referred to as a chevron); secure the overlapping ends onto the anchor tape strip.
19. Loop the IV tubing away from the catheter hub and toward the IV fluid source. Secure the looped tubing with a piece of tape on the anchor tape strip.
20. Secure a commercial protective device over the catheter hub and looped tubing. Bending one corner of the tape over and onto itself provides a free tab to lift the tape easily for site visualization.

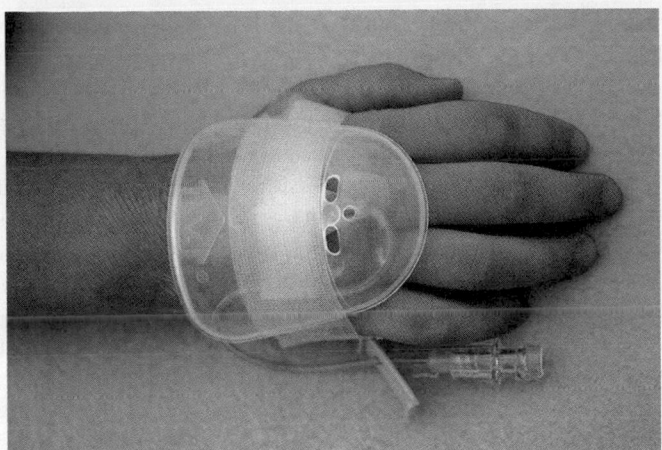

Fig. 28-7 I.V. House used to protect intravenous site.

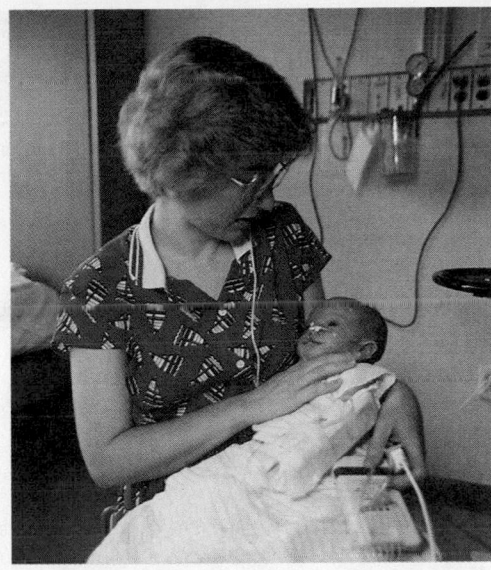

Fig. 28-8 Intravenous infusion, as well as other equipment, does not prevent infant from being picked up and cuddled.

Apply a sterile dressing such as a transparent semipermeable membrane directly over the catheter insertion site to protect the infusion site (Infusion Nurses Society, 2006). Consider easy access to the IV site for frequent (hourly) assessments (Infusion Nurses Society, 2006). Improvised plastic cups that are cut in half with the ridged edges covered with tape should not be used, since they have injured patients. A commercial site protector, I.V. House, is available in different sizes (Fig. 28-7). Its ventilation holes prevent moisture from accumulating under the dome. This device is designed to protect the IV site and allows for visibility of the site. The device also minimizes use of padded boards, splints, or other restraints and tape and maintains skin integrity. The connector tubing or extension tubing can be looped to make it small enough to fit under the protective cover to prevent accidental snagging of the catheter. It is important to safely secure the IV tubing to prevent infants and children from becoming entangled in the tubing or from accidentally pulling the catheter or needle out. This securement also eliminates movement of the catheter hub at the insertion site (mechanical manipulation). Apply a colorful and interesting sticker to the protective device to add a positive note to the procedure.

Finger or toe areas are left unoccluded by dressings or tape to allow for assessment of circulation. The thumb should not be immobilized because of the danger of contractures with limited movement later on. An extremity should never be encircled with tape, since this may impede necessary blood flow to and from the extremity. The use of roll gauze, self-adhering stretch bandages, and Ace bandages can cause the same constriction and hide signs of infiltration.

Traditionally, padded boards or splints were used to partially immobilize the IV site. When metal needles were inserted into the vein, padded boards or splints and restraints were appropriate to prevent the sharp end from puncturing the vessel, especially at a joint. With the more recent use of soft, pliable catheters, arm or leg boards may not be necessary and have several disadvantages. They obscure the IV site, can constrict the extremity, may excoriate the underlying tissue and promote infection, can cause joint contracture, restrict useful movement of the extremity, and are uncomfortable. Unfortunately, no research has been conducted to demonstrate their proposed benefit of increasing dwell time (patency of the IV line).

Adequate taping and protection with a commercial device should eliminate the need for padded boards in most circumstances. A number of elbow restraint or protective arm restraint devices are available that prevent the child from bending the arm or pulling at the IV site on the arm; these are made of cloth and a semi-rigid mold with Velcro straps or ties so the device may be adjusted to the child's limb size and does not impair circulation. (See Chapter 27.) Older children who are alert and cooperative can usually be trusted to protect the IV site.

Immobilization is intolerable to the naturally active child, and the nurse should make every effort to reduce the use of restraints. To relieve the stress of immobilization, frequent removal of the restraints (if used at all) allows the child to move the extremities. Whenever possible, the infant or child is held and cuddled to help meet emotional needs during this trying time (Fig. 28-8). Range-of-motion exercises are employed for infants and children who are too ill or unable to move their extremities, but others should be encouraged to move their arms and legs. Most infants or small children instinctively move their extremities when released. If not, a toy or other stimulus can provide incentive.

Appropriate documentation of the procedure, type of cannula used, patient tolerance, and status of the skin site is an important nursing intervention (Box 28-8).

Removal of a Peripheral Intravenous Line

When it comes time to discontinue an IV infusion, many children are distressed by the thought of catheter removal. Therefore they need a careful explanation of the process and suggestions for helping. Encouraging children to remove or help remove the tape from the site provides them with a measure of control and often fosters their cooperation. The procedure consists of turning off any pump apparatus, occluding the IV tubing, removing the tape, pulling the catheter out of the vessel in the opposite direction of insertion, and exerting firm pressure at the site after the catheter is removed until bleeding stops. (It is painful to apply pressure on the catheter while pulling it out.) Place a small dry dressing (adhesive bandage strip) over the

---

BOX 28-8   DOCUMENTATION OF A PERIPHERAL INTRAVENOUS CATHETER

The entire procedure for inserting and taping a peripheral intravenous (IV) catheter should be documented in the patient's medical record. Important information includes the following:

IV Insertion Documentation
Normally part of the patient's medical record:
- Date and time of insertion; name or initials of clinician inserting IV
- Manufacturer, gauge, and length of catheter
- Site of insertion (e.g., "right ankle," or more specifically "right saphenous vein")
- Number of attempts (e.g., "24 gauge, 1 inch, Insyte initiated in right saphenous vein in first attempt," or "24 gauge, 1 inch, Insyte initiated in right saphenous vein after one unsuccessful attempt to left saphenous vein")
- Name of blood samples drawn and sent to laboratory, if applicable
- Activation of junction securement devices (Luer-Lok) and explanation of taping (e.g., "IV catheter secured with transparent dressing and Transpore tape")
- Appearance of site (e.g., "Site is soft without redness or edema, flushes easily")
- Flushing solution, amount used
- Connection to IV solution, naming the fluid and amount in the bag
- Tolerance of procedure; describe specific behaviors displayed by the patient or use quotations (e.g., "Patient cried during insertion but quieted easily and fell asleep in mom's arms after procedure," or "Patient stated, 'That hurt but it feels better now'")

IV Site Documentation
Can be noted on a piece of tape at the site:
- Date, time, gauge and length of catheter, and initials of nurse initiating

IV Fluid Documentation
Frequently written on an IV flow sheet:
- Date and time of fluid initiation
- Type and volume of bag hung (e.g., "500-ml bag of normal saline")
- Type of delivery system used and rate of infusion (e.g., "IV connected to Baxter pump and infusing at a rate of 25 ml/hr")
- Any additives, type and dose, in the primary solution (e.g., "potassium chloride 10 mEq/L")

Ongoing IV Site Assessment
Follow hospital's policy, but assessment recommended at least every 1 to 2 hours (can be documented in medical record or on the IV flow sheet):
- Appearance (e.g., "Site is soft without redness or edema" [any protective device needs to be lifted to see the entire site])
- Any patient comments regarding IV

Discontinuation of IV Therapy
Can be documented in medical record:
- Reason for discontinuing IV (e.g., end of therapy, infiltration, or accidentally removed)
- Integrity of device, including length and condition of catheter
- Appearance of site
- Dressing applied
- Patient tolerance; again direct quotations from patient best (age appropriate)

---

may occur. To remove transparent dressings (e.g., OpSite or Tegaderm), pull the opposing edges parallel to the skin to loosen the bond. If a catheter was used for the IV infusion, inspect the tip to make certain the catheter is intact and no portion remains in the vein.

Removal of the IV line, especially the tape, is another painful and frightening experience for the child. Consider the child's age, developmental and neurologic status, and predictability (how the child responds to painful treatments) when determining the need for assistance to maintain safety with this procedure. Manual removal of tape is the preferred method. Only if absolutely necessary should a small cut be made in the tape, using bandage scissors, to facilitate its removal. Before cutting the tape:

- Ensure that all digits are visible.
- Remove any barrier that hinders visibility, such as a protective covering.
- Protect the child's skin and digits by sliding own finger(s) between the tape and the child's skin so that the scissors do not touch the patient.
- Cut the tape on the medial aspect (thumb side) of the extremity.

Complications

The same precautions regarding maintenance of asepsis, prevention of infection, and observation for infiltration are carried out with patients of any age. However, infiltration is often more difficult to detect in infants and small children than in adults. The increased amount of subcutaneous fat and the amount of tape used to secure the catheter hub obscure the signs of early infiltration. When the fluid appears to be infusing too slowly or ceases, the usual assessment for obstruction within the apparatus (i.e., kinks; screw clamps; shutoff valve; and positioning interference, such as a bent elbow or wrist) often locates the difficulty. When these actions fail to detect the problem, it may be necessary to carefully remove some of the tape and other material that obscure a clear view of the venipuncture site. Examine dependent areas, such as the palm and undersides of the extremity or the occiput and behind the ears.

Whenever possible, place the IV infusion in an extremity to which the identification band (or bracelet) is not attached. Serious circulatory impairment can result from infiltrated solution distal to the band, which acts as a tourniquet preventing adequate venous return. To check for return blood flow through the catheter, lower the solution bag below the level of the infusion site. A good blood return, or lack thereof, is not always an indicator of infiltration in small infants. Flushing the catheter and observing the site for discoloration (i.e., blanching or redness), pain, tenderness, and edema or noting any exudate or drainage and increase in skin or basal temperatures is an appropriate assessment of the IV site. If the tubing is connected to an infusion pump, it must be removed from the pump before lowering.

IV therapy in pediatrics tends to be difficult to maintain because of mechanical and physical factors that tend to shorten dwell times. Such factors include vascular trauma resulting from PIV device selection (gauge and length of the catheter), the insertion site, the catheter dwell time, the size of the vessel, vessel fragility, and pressure of the infusion pump (determined

puncture site. The use of adhesive removal pads can decrease the pain of tape removal, but the skin should be washed off after use to avoid irritation. An adhesive removal agent should be used with caution in some preterm infants and children with compromised skin because absorption is variable and toxicity

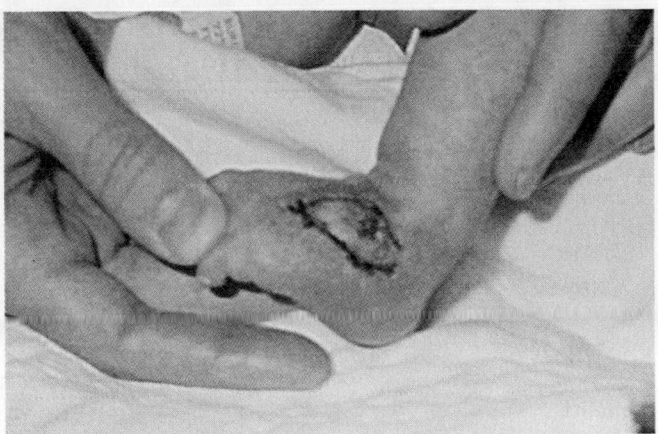

Fig. 28-9 Intravenous infiltration in an infant's foot.

in PSI, or pounds per square inch). Different infusion pumps have preset pressures for infusion, delivery, and occlusion; therefore the pump's occlusion alarm is not entirely reliable for detecting infiltration. The patient's activity level, operator skill and insertion technique, forceful administration of boluses of fluid, type of infusion solution, antibiotics and other medications being infused, and infusion of irritants or vesicants through a small vessel are also factors. These factors cause infiltration and extravasation injuries, which are reported with relative frequency (Fig. 28-9).

Infiltration is defined as inadvertent administration of a nonvesicant parenteral solution or medication into surrounding tissue as a result of catheter dislodgment (Infusion Nurses Society, 2006). **Extravasation** is defined as inadvertent administration of vesicant solution or medication into surrounding tissue as a result of catheter dislodgment (Infusion Nurses Society, 2006). A vesicant or sclerosing agent causes varying degrees of cellular damage when even minute amounts escape into surrounding tissue. A scale that provides a uniform standard for measuring the degree of infiltration is available from the Infusion Nurses Society*; the characteristics of infiltration include the degree of skin discoloration, blanching, edema, the amount of pain, and warmth or coolness of the area (Infusion Nurses Society, 2006).

Phlebitis, or inflammation of the vessel wall, may also develop in children who require IV therapy. Lamagna and MacPhee (2004) describe three types of phlebitis: mechanical (caused by rapid infusion rate, manipulation of the IV), chemical (caused by medications such as nafcillin, amphotericin B), and bacterial (caused by staphylococcal organisms). The initial sign of phlebitis is erythema (redness) at the insertion site. Pain may or may not be present (Lamagna and MacPhee, 2004).

Standardized IV site assessment tools, such as the one used at Children's Hospital of Boston, assist in detection of infiltration, extravasation, and phlebitis in children so early intervention can prevent vessel and skin damage (Lamagna and MacPhee, 2004). Treatment of an infiltration or extravasation varies according to the type of infusate (see Nursing Care Guidelines box).

*315 Norwood Park South, Norwood, MA 02062; 781-440-9408; www.ins1.org.

NURSING CARE GUIDELINES

Peripheral Intravenous Infiltration or Extravasation

When an infiltration or extravasation is observed (signs include erythema, pain, edema, blanching, streaking on the skin along the vein, and darkened area at the insertion site), immediately stop the infusion, elevate the extremity, notify the practitioner, and initiate the ordered treatment as soon as possible. Dry heat may be applied, except if the infused solution is sclerosing. Remove the intravenous line only when it is no longer needed (e.g., after infusing an antidote).

The following guidelines should be considered when starting a pediatric PIV:

- Avoid reinserting a stylet into the catheter. This can damage the catheter and cause catheter fragment embolus.
- If IV insertion is unsuccessful, obtain a new catheter for the subsequent attempts.
- Some parents count the number of times the catheter is moved in, out, and around the area of insertion while trying to locate the vein (probing) as sticks their child receives as opposed to counting the number of IV insertion attempts. Limit the amount of probing because it is painful.
- When setting up the supplies for the IV insertion, use caution in determining where to affix the precut tape. Keep in mind that the precut tape should be affixed to a clean surface.

PIV catheters are the most commonly used intravascular devices. Heavy cutaneous colonization of the insertion site is the single most important predictor of catheter-related infection with all types of short-term, percutaneously inserted catheters. Phlebitis, largely a mechanical rather than infectious process, remains the most important complication associated with the use of peripheral venous catheters (see Community Focus box).

COMMUNITY FOCUS

Preventing Intravenous Site Infections

With the increasing use of intravenous (IV) therapy in the community, preventing infection is essential. The most effective ways to prevent infection of an IV site are to wash hands between each patient, wear gloves when inserting an IV catheter, closely monitor the date of IV placement, and inspect the insertion site and physical condition of the IV dressing (if dressing used).

Proper education of the patient and family regarding signs and symptoms of an infected site can help prevent infections from going unnoticed. When an IV infusion continues for several days, the tubing and solution administration set is changed at regular intervals according to hospital policy or at least every 72 hours for a continuous infusion and at least every 24 hours for an intermittent infusion (Infusion Nurses Society, 2006). Gillies, O'Riordan, Wallen, and colleagues (2004) recommend changing IV administration solution sets and tubing every 72 hours to decrease the probability of infection. Lipid-containing parenteral nutrition (PN) fluids such as three-in-one solutions should be changed after 24 hours (Gillies, O'Riordan, Wallen, et al, 2005; Infusion Nurses Society, 2006), whereas a 12-hour limit is recommended for pure intralipid infusions (O'Grady, Alexander, Dellinger, et al, 2002). The dressing can be left in place for the duration of the IV infusion unless the integrity has been compromised. To ensure that the solution and IV equipment is changed regularly, it is labeled with the date and time that the new bag and tubing are attached. Any signs of inflammation, such as redness or pain, are reported immediately. This usually requires removing the infusion and restarting it at another site or administering the medication by another route.

Prevention of insertion site infection can be decreased by strict adherence to the following guidelines:

- Practice good hand washing before starting an IV infusion.
- Cleanse the skin with an appropriate antiseptic before catheter insertion.
- When cleansing the insertion site, use a circular motion starting from the center and working outward.
- Allow the antiseptic to dry for 30 to 60 seconds before inserting the catheter.
- Avoid palpating the insertion site after the skin has been cleansed with the antiseptic.

VENOUS ACCESS DEVICES

Venous access devices (VADs) have several different characteristics. The practitioner has to consider the best type of catheter for the individual patient's needs. Factors that can influence the decision include the reason for placement of the catheter (diagnosis), patient age, length of therapy, risk to the patient in placement of the catheter, and availability of resources to assist the family in maintaining the catheter.

Central catheters can be categorized in three types:
1. Short-term or nontunneled catheters (subclavian, femoral, and jugular)
2. PICCs (Box 28-9)
3. Long-term, tunneled catheters and implanted ports (Table 28-8)

Short-term or nontunneled catheters are used in acute care, emergency, and intensive care units. These catheters are made of polyurethane and are placed in large veins such as the subclavian, femoral, or jugular. Take a chest radiograph to verify placement of the catheter tip before administration of fluids or medications. The other types are discussed in the following sections.

Peripheral Intermittent Infusion Device

The peripheral lock, also known as an intermittent infusion device or saline or heparin lock, is an alternative for a keep-open infusion when extended access to a vein is required without the need for continuous fluid. It is most frequently employed for intermittent infusion of medication into a peripheral venous route. A short, flexible catheter is used as the lock device, and a site is selected where there will be minimum movement, such as the forearm. The catheter is inserted and secured in the same

---

BOX 28-9 PERIPHERALLY INSERTED CENTRAL CATHETERS

Description
Made of Silastic or polyurethane material
Single or double lumen available
Inserted into antecubital fossa and passed through basilic or cephalic vein into superior vena cava (SVC)
Positioning of tip in SVC maximizes hemodilution and reduces likelihood of vessel wall damage, phlebitis, or thrombus formation
Can be placed as "midline" catheter, also known as a halfway catheter, ending near axillary vein (not suitable for total parenteral nutrition, hyperosmolar solutions, or vesicant chemotherapy)

Benefits
Do not require operating room placement
Can be inserted by specially trained registered nurses
Can use small insertion needles
Fast placement
Sepsis rates of 2% or less

Care Considerations
Sometimes difficult to thread into SVC
Reports of resistance to removal
Not suitable for rapid fluid replacement because of small lumen size
Five- to 10-ml syringe used for flushing to prevent catheter wall rupture

---

manner as any IV infusion device, but the hub on the proximal end is occluded with a stopper or injection cap.

The type of device used may vary, and the care and use of the peripheral lock are carried out according to the specific protocol of the institution or unit. However, the general concept is the same. The catheter remains in place and is flushed with saline or heparin (1 : 10 units/ml) after infusion of the medication. The flush solution prevents blood from clotting in the device between infusions. Because heparin is incompatible with many drugs, the peripheral lock must also be flushed with saline before and after administering medication. There are conflicting data regarding the use of saline flush versus a heparinized saline flush and the dwell time of peripheral locks in children (see Evidence-Based Practice box). Some children are discharged with a peripheral lock in place in order to continue receiving medications without hospitalization; this is usually reserved for children who require medications on a short-term basis and are referred to a home-based infusion company. Those with chronic illnesses who require repeated blood sampling or medications, long-term chemotherapy, or frequent hyperalimentation or antibiotic therapy are best managed with a long-term central VAD.

There is controversy concerning the need to flush with heparin in any VAD, peripheral or central. A more important issue is the technique of flushing. The use of the turbulent-flow flush has proven successful in preventing clot formation in the device. It is described as the forward flushing motion on the syringe with a flush-stop-flush-stop technique. This causes a swirling and vigorous fluid movement that clears the catheter better than the continuous flush motion most commonly used. This procedure is combined with the positive pressure technique. As the flush is completed, hold the syringe stopper down, clamp the catheter, then remove the syringe. This prevents blood from backing into the tip of the catheter.

TABLE 28-8 COMPARISON OF LONG-TERM CENTRAL VENOUS ACCESS DEVICES

DESCRIPTION	BENEFITS	CARE CONSIDERATIONS
Tunneled Catheter (e.g., Hickman or Broviac Catheter)		
Silicone, radiopaque, flexible catheter with open ends 1 or 2 Dacron cuffs or VitaCuffs (biosynthetic material impregnated with silver ions) on catheter(s) enhances tissue ingrowth May have >1 lumen	Reduced risk of bacterial migration after tissue adheres to cuff Easy to use for self-administered infusions Removal requires pulling catheter from site (nonsurgical procedure)	Requires daily heparin flushes Must be clamped or have clamp nearby at all times Must keep exit site dry Heavy activity restricted until tissue adheres to cuff Water sports may be restricted (risk of infection) Risk of infection still present Protrudes outside body, susceptible to damage from sharp instruments and may be pulled out; may affect body image More difficult to repair Patient and family must learn catheter care
Groshong Catheter		
Clear, flexible, silicone, radiopaque catheter with closed tip and 2-way valve at proximal end Dacron or VitaCuff on catheter enhances tissue ingrowth May have >1 lumen	Reduced time and cost for maintenance care; no heparin flushes needed Reduced catheter damage; no clamping needed because of 2-way valve Increased patient safety because of minimum potential for blood backflow or air embolism Reduced risk of bacterial migration after tissue adheres to cuff Easily repaired Easy to use for self-administered intravenous infusions	Requires weekly irrigation with normal saline Must keep exit site dry Heavy activity restricted until tissue adheres to cuff Water sports may be restricted (risk of infection) Risk of infection still present Protrudes outside body; susceptible to damage from sharp instruments and may be pulled out; can affect body image Patient and family must learn catheter care
Implanted Ports (Port-a-Cath, Infusaport, Mediport, NorPort, Groshong Port)		
Totally implantable metal or plastic device that consists of self-sealing injection port with top or side access with preconnected or attachable silicone catheter that is placed in large blood vessel	Reduced risk of infection Placed completely under skin, so much less likely to be pulled out or damaged No maintenance care and reduced cost for family Heparinized monthly and after each infusion to maintain patency (Groshong port requires only saline flush) No limitations on regular physical activity, including swimming Dressing only needed when port accessed with Huber needle that is not removed No or only slight change in body appearance (slight bulge on chest)	Must pierce skin for access; pain with insertion of needle; can use local anesthetic (EMLA [lidocaine and prilocaine], LMX4 [4% liposomal lidocaine], or intradermal buffered lidocaine before accessing port) Special noncoring needle (Huber) with straight or angled design used to inject into port Skin preparation needed before injection Difficult to manipulate for self-administered infusions Catheter may dislodge from port, especially if child "plays" with port site (twiddler syndrome) Vigorous contact sports generally not allowed Removal requires surgical procedure

EVIDENCE-BASED PRACTICE

Normal Saline or Heparinized Saline Flush Solution in Pediatric Intravenous Lines

ASK THE QUESTION

Is there a significant difference in the longevity of intravenous (IV) intermittent infusion locks in children when normal saline (NS) is used as a flush instead a heparinized saline (HS) solution?

SEARCH FOR THE EVIDENCE

Search strategies
Selection criteria included evidence during the years 1992 to 2008 with the following terms: saline versus heparin intermittent flush, children's heparin lock flush, heparin lock patency, peripheral venous catheter in children.

Databases used
CINAHL, PubMed

CRITICALLY ANALYZE THE EVIDENCE

GRADE criteria: Evidence quality moderate; recommendation strong (Guyatt, Oxman, Vist, et al, 2008)
- A systematic Cochrane Review by Shah, Ng, and Sinha (2005) revealed 10 studies that were randomized or quasi-randomized trials of HS administration versus NS, placebo, or no treatment in neonates. The authors of the review concluded that the heterogeneity among the studies, variability in methodologic quality and clinical details, and variability in reporting outcomes resulted in no strong evidence regarding the effectiveness and safety of heparin in prolonging catheter life in neonates.
- No significant statistical difference was found between HS and NS flushes for maintaining catheter patency in children (Hanrahan, Kleiber, and Fagan, 1994; Kotter, 1996; Schultz, Drew, and Hewitt, 2002; Hanrahan, Kleiber, and Berends, 2000; Heilskov, Kleiber, Johnson, et al, 1998; Mok, Kwong, and Chan, 2007).

CRITICALLY ANALYZE THE EVIDENCE—cont'd

- Several studies reported increased incidence of pain or erythema with HS flushing of infusion devices (Hanrahan, Kleiber, and Fagan, 1994; Robertson, 1994; Nelson and Graves, 1998; McMullen, Fioravanti, Pollack, et al, 1993).
- Several studies found increased patency and/or longer dwell times with HS solutions versus NS in 24-gauge catheters (Mudge, Forcier, and Slattery, 1998; Danek and Noris, 1992; Beecroft, Bossert, Chung, et al, 1997; Gyr, Burroughs, Smith, et al, 1995; Hanrahan, Kleiber, and Berends, 2000; Tripathi, Kaushik, and Singh, 2008).
- Younger children and preterm neonates with lower gestational ages were associated with shorter patency of IV catheters (Paisley, Stamper, Brown, et al, 1997; Robertson, 1994; McMullen, Fioravanti, Pollack, et al, 1993; Tripathi, Kaushik, and Singh, 2008).
- Infusion devices flushed with NS lasted longer than those flushed with HS (Nelson and Graves, 1998; Le Duc, 1997; Goldberg, Sankaran, Givelichian, et al, 1999).
- When measured and reported, length of time between flushing peripheral devices affected dwell time (Crews, Gnann, Rice, et al, 1997; Gyr, Burroughs, Smith, et al, 1995).
- None of the studies cited anticoagulation-associated complications with HS, which is a concern in preterm neonates, who are at higher risk for development of clotting problems as a result of heparin (Klenner, Fusch, Rakow, et al, 2003).
- The American Society of Hospital Pharmacists (ASHP) 2006 Position Statement asserts that 0.9% sodium chloride injection is safe for maintaining patency of peripheral locks in adults and children over age 12 years (ASHP Commission on Therapeutics, 2006).
- The 2006 Infusion Nurses Society policy manual indicates that either preservative-free heparin or preservative-free 0.9% sodium chloride may be used to flush a peripheral IV; however, the appendix includes a notation that catheter patency may be maintained by flushing with saline when converting from continuous to intermittent use.

APPLY THE EVIDENCE: NURSING IMPLICATIONS

- Further research is still needed with larger samples of children, especially preterm neonates, using small-gauge catheters (24 gauge) and other gauge catheters, flushed with NS and HS as intermittent infusion devices only (no continuous infusions); variables to be considered include catheter dwell time; medications administered; period between regular flushing and flushing associated with medication administration; pain, erythema, or other localized complications; concentration and amount of heparin solutions used; flush method (positive pressure technique versus no specific technique); reason for IV device removal; and complications associated with either solution.
- NS is a safe alternative to HS flush in infants and children with intermittent IV locks larger than 24 gauge; smaller neonates may benefit from HS flush (longer dwell time), but the evidence is inconclusive for all weight ranges and gestational ages.

References

ASHP Commission on Therapeutics: ASHP therapeutic position statement on the institutional use of 0.9% sodium chloride injection to maintain patency of peripheral indwelling intermittent infusion devices, *Am J Health Syst Pharm* 63(13):1273-1275, 2006.

Beecroft PC, Bossert E, Chung K, et al: Intravenous lock patency in children: dilute heparin versus saline, *J Pediatr Pharm Practice* 2(4):211-223, 1997.

Crews BE, Gnann KK, Rice MH, et al: Effects of varying intervals between heparin flushes on pediatric catheter longevity, *Pediatr Nurs* 23(1):87-91, 1997.

Danek GD, Noris EM: Pediatric IV catheters: efficacy of saline flush, *Pediatr Nurs* 18(2):111-113, 1992.

Goldberg M, Sankaran R, Givelichian L, et al: Maintaining patency of peripheral intermittent infusion devices with heparinized saline and saline: a randomized double blind controlled trial in neonatal intensive care and a review of literature, *Neonat Intensive Care* 12(1):18-22, 1999.

Guyatt GH, Oxman AD, Vist GE, et al: GRADE: an emerging consensus on rating quality of evidence and strength of recommendations, *BMJ* 336:924-926, 2008.

Gyr P, Burroughs T, Smith K, et al: Double blind comparison of heparin and saline flush solutions in maintenance of peripheral infusion devices, *Pediatr Nurs* 21(4):383-389, 1995.

Hanrahan KS, Kleiber C, Berends S: Saline for peripheral intravenous locks in neonates: evaluating a change in practice, *Neonat Netw* 19(2):19-24, 2000.

Hanrahan KS, Kleiber C, Fagan C: Evaluation of saline for IV locks in children, *Pediatr Nurs* 20(6):549-552, 1994.

Heilskov J, Kleiber C, Johnson K, et al: A randomized trial of heparin and saline for maintaining intravenous locks in neonates, *J Soc Pediatr Nurs* 3(3):111-116, 1998.

Infusion Nurses Society: Policies and procedures for infusion nursing, ed 3, Norwood, Mass, 2006, The Society.

Klenner AF, Fusch C, Rakow A, et al: Benefit and risk of heparin for maintaining peripheral venous catheters in neonates: a placebo-controlled trial, *J Pediatr* 143(6):741-745, 2003.

Kotter RW: Heparin vs. saline for intermittent intravenous device maintenance in neonates, *Neonat Netw* 15(6):43-47, 1996.

Le Duc K: Efficacy of normal saline solution versus heparin solution for maintaining patency of peripheral intravenous catheters in children, *J Emerg Nurs* 23(4):306-309, 1997.

McMullen A, Fioravanti ID, Pollack D, et al: Heparinized saline or normal saline as a flush solution in intermittent intravenous lines in infants and children, *MCN* 18(2):78-85, 1993.

Mok E, Kwong TK, Chan ME: A randomized controlled trial for maintaining peripheral intravenous lock in children, *Int J Nurs Pract* 13(1):33-45, 2007.

Mudge B, Forcier D, Slattery MJ: Patency of 24-gauge peripheral intermittent infusion devices: a comparison of heparin and saline flush solutions, *Pediatr Nurs* 24(2):142-149, 1998.

Nelson TJ, Graves SM: 0.9% Sodium chloride injection with and without heparin for maintaining peripheral indwelling intermittent infusion devices in infants, *Am J Heath Syst Pharm* 55:570-573, 1998.

Paisley MK, Stamper M, Brown T, et al: The use of heparin and normal saline flushes in neonatal intravenous catheters, *J Pediatr Nurs* 23(5):521-527, 1997.

Robertson J: Intermittent intravenous therapy: a comparison of two flushing solutions, *Contemp Nurs* 3(4):174-179, 1994.

Schultz AA, Drew D, Hewitt H: Comparison of normal saline and heparinized saline for patency of IV locks in neonates, *Appl Nurs Res* 15(1):28-34, 2002.

Shah PS, Ng E, Sinha AK: Heparin for prolonging peripheral intravenous catheter use in neonates, *Cochrane Database Syst Rev* (4):CD002774, 2005.

Tripathi S, Kaushik V, Singh V: Peripheral IVs: factors affecting complications and patency—a randomized controlled trial, *J Infus Nurs* 31(3):182-188, 2008.

Peripherally Inserted Central Catheters

PICCs can be used for short-term to moderate-length therapy (see Box 28-9). These catheters consist of silicone or polymer material and are placed by specially trained nurses (Gamulka, Mendoza, and Connolly, 2005). The most common insertion site is the antecubital area using the median, cephalic, or basilic vein. The catheter is threaded either with or without a guide wire into the superior vena cava. The modified Seldinger technique is often used with ultrasonography to access very small veins in infants and children (Mickler, 2008). PICCs are sometimes inserted a shorter length; this is often referred to as a "midline" catheter. The insertion length of the midline catheter is usually somewhere between the insertion site and the axilla; in some cases the midline catheter may be placed in a scalp vein and threaded into the external jugular vein (Petit, 2006). The midline has an average dwell time of 6 to 10 days in neonates (Petit, 2006). Centrally placed catheter tips are associated with fewer complications (phlebitis, occlusion, leaking) than noncentrally placed catheters (Racadio, Doellman, Johnson, et al, 2001).

If the catheter is threaded midline, total parenteral nutrition (TPN) should not be administered, because the high concentration of glucose irritates the vessel; it should be infused through a central catheter.

> **! NURSING ALERT**
>
> Most PICC lines are not sutured, so care is needed when changing the dressing.

The decision to insert a PICC needs to be made before several attempts at IV insertions are done. In one center PICC lines were inserted in children undergoing operative procedures. The PICCs were inserted in the operating room in pediatric patients under general anesthesia whose hospital stay was expected to be at least 4 days; when compared with similar patients undergoing surgery and with only a PIV, children in the PICC group experienced fewer needlesticks for blood draws and failed PIV complications postoperatively. The cost of PICC insertion was higher than PIV, but satisfaction was greater and complications were lower (Schwengel, McGready, Berenholtz, et al, 2004). Once the antecubital veins have been punctured repeatedly, they are not considered candidates for this type of catheter. Because this catheter is the least costly VAD and has a lower risk of complications than other central VADs, it is an excellent choice for many pediatric patients. This catheter is also usually inserted in the unit's treatment room.

PICC lines may be used for blood draws, although there is often a greater number of occlusions with blood draws (Knue, Doellman, Rabin, et al, 2005).

PICCs can create problems with removal. Causes for resistance in removal include infectious processes, fibrin formation, and endothelial thrombosis. Methods to free the catheter include gentle traction to the catheter, taping the catheter to create tension on the line, and warm soaks to the site. Aggressive pulling of the catheter is contraindicated.

Long-Term Central Venous Access Devices

Long-term central VADs include tunneled catheters (Broviac, Hickman, or Groshong) and implanted infusion ports (see Table 28-8). They may have single, double, or triple lumens. Several lumens (multilumen catheters) allow more than one therapy to be administered at the same time. Reasons to use multilumen catheters include repeated blood sampling, TPN infusion, administration of blood products or infusion of large quantities or concentrations of fluids, administration of incompatible drugs or fluids at the same time (through different lumens), and central venous pressure monitoring.

With the patient under local or general anesthesia, the long-term catheter of choice is placed with aseptic technique. A vein, such as the jugular or subclavian, is entered through a small cutdown site, and the catheter is threaded to the junction of the superior vena cava and right atrium, confirmed by radiography with fluoroscopic dye injection, and then sutured in place. To stabilize the catheter and reduce the risk of infection, the remainder is tunneled beneath the skin to exit through a small incision at a convenient location on the anterior aspect of the chest or upper abdomen (Fig. 28-10, *A* and *B*). One or two Dacron cuffs or VitaCuffs on the catheter remain in the subcutaneous tunnel; as tissue adheres to the cuff, the cuff provides a barrier to infection. The cutdown site is surgically closed, the catheter is sutured to the skin at the exit site, and a sterile dressing is applied. A radiograph is taken to ascertain the location of the catheter before instillation of fluids. With any of the central venous catheters, medications are easily instilled through the injection cap. Maintenance of the catheter includes dressing changes, flushing to maintain patency, and prevention of occlusion or dislodgment.

> **! NURSING ALERT**
>
> A safety rule of thumb when working with tunneled catheters, PICCs, and PIVs is to avoid the use of *any* scissors around the tubing or dressing. Removal is best accomplished using fingers and much patience. In the event that a tunneled catheter such as a Broviac is accidentally cut, use a padded clamp and clamp the catheter proximal to the exit site to avoid blood loss. Repair kits are available, which may save the catheter and avoid further surgery to replace a cut catheter.

Children may benefit from an implanted port, which consist of a small, circular "port of entry" that is placed under the skin (while the patient is under local or general anesthesia) over a bony prominence to provide a stable surface, usually under the distal third of the clavicle (Fig. 28-10, *C* and *D*). A tunnel is created from the port to the point where the catheter enters a central vein leading to the entrance to the right atrium. Medication or other solution is injected with a special Huber needle (a 90-degree angled needle) through the skin into the port. The device can remain situated indefinitely and may be placed in small infants as well as older children and adolescents.

With the implanted device, palpate the port for placement and stabilize it with the thumb and index finger. Cleanse the overlying skin, and use only special noncoring Huber needles to pierce the port's diaphragm on the top or side, depending on the style. A special infusion set with a Huber needle and extension tubing with Luer connection can be used to access the port when blood work or infusion therapy (chemotherapy or blood product administration) is required. A small gauze pad is placed under the horizontal portion of the protruding needle and a transparent dressing is placed over the protruding needle and gauze for stabilization and infection control. In small, curious children the tubing may be tunneled under a cotton shirt or one-piece suit and out the leg or back to prevent the child from pulling on the port tubing.

With the port accessed, the injection procedure is the same as for the venous catheters. To prevent infection, use meticulous aseptic technique anytime the devices are accessed, including instillation of heparin or saline to prevent clotting. Protocols are established in most centers for periodic flushing with normal saline and heparin solution (amount and frequency). Maintenance includes intermittent flushing to prevent clotting and a dressing change if the Huber needle is left in place for long periods (>1 week). There should be a protocol stating that the Huber needle needs to be changed at established intervals, usually 5 to 7 days. Advantages to the port include cosmetic

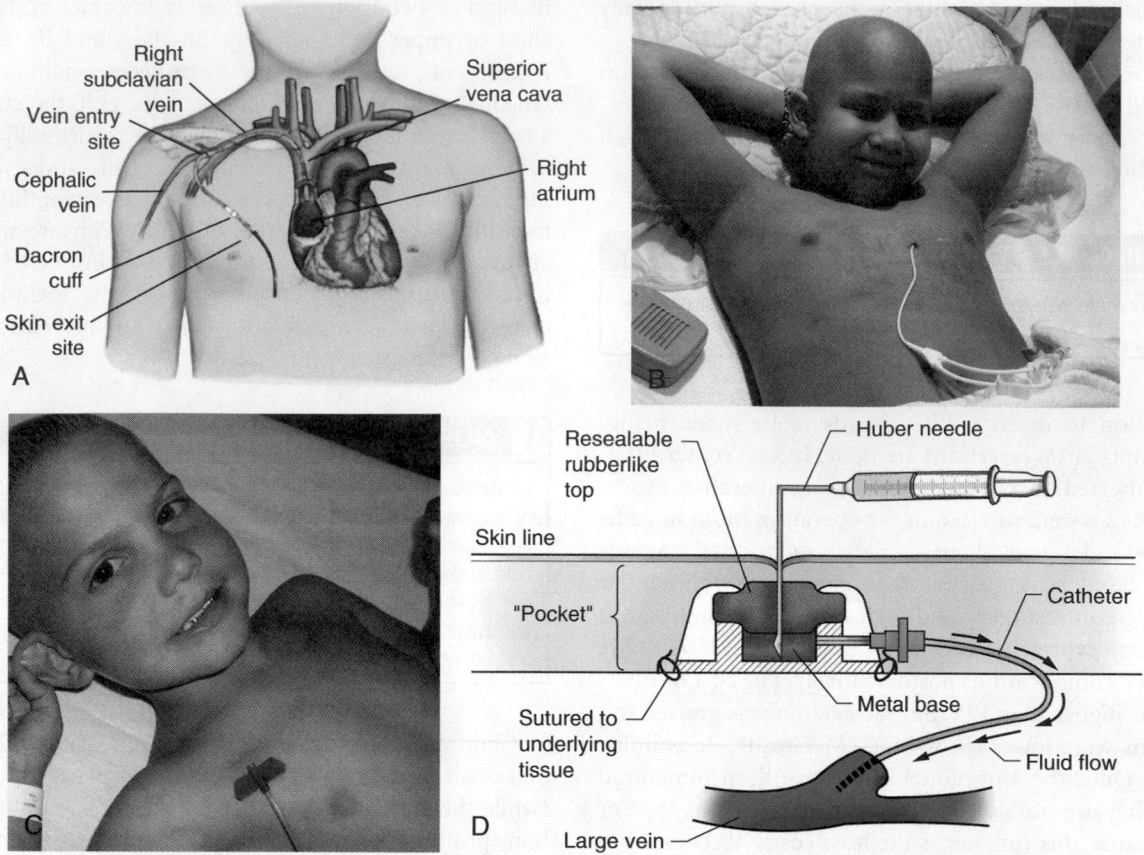

Fig. 28-10 Venous access devices. **A,** External central venous catheter insertion and exit site. **B,** Child with external central venous catheter (dressing removed for photo). **C,** Child with implanted port with Huber needle in place. (NOTE: Dressing usually covers needle insertion site; removed for photo only.) **D,** Side view of implanted port.

appearance, which may be important for older school-aged children and adolescents, and relatively easy access for blood work and fluid and medication administration. When the port must be accessed with a Huber needle, apply a topical anesthetic such as EMLA or LMX4 before the procedure to reduce the pain of penetrating the skin with the Huber needle (see Atraumatic Care box, p. 1073).

Chapter 10 discusses umbilical artery and venous catheters used in neonates.

Complications

Central venous line bacteremia can be of major concern in a child. The mean incidence of catheter-related bloodstream infection in children varies in the literature, but it averages around 3% to 7% with an estimated cost of $9000 to $46,000 per episode (Kline, 2005). Centrally placed catheters are associated with fewer complications than are peripherally placed catheters (Racadio, Doellman, Johnson, et al, 2001).

Catheter-related bloodstream infections have a significant impact on the duration of the catheter and cost of care. Studies have shown that the following practices result in a decrease in catheter-related bloodstream infections (Krein, Hofer, Kowalski, et al, 2007; Morgan and Thomas, 2007; Smith, 2008):

- Using maximum barrier techniques during insertion
- Practicing good hand washing
- Performing skin antisepsis with 2% chlorhexidine
- Using antimicrobial-impregnated catheter
- Promptly removing catheters when not in use

Guidelines for prevention, diagnosis, and management of intravascular catheter–related infections are available from the Infectious Diseases Society of America (Mermel, Allon, Bouza, et al, 2009).

Line connections should have a Luer-Lok connection device or be wrapped with tape to prevent accidental disconnection. The nurse should minimize the number of line accesses for blood withdrawal or medication administration. Central line dressing protocols should be developed, and nurses experienced in dressing change techniques should be responsible for line care. Family teaching must include how to care for the line, what to do if the line becomes disconnected or broken, and how to flush the line using aseptic technique.

Catheter-related central venous thrombosis and catheter occlusion can also be serious problems in children (McCloskey, 2002). Approximately 60% of all catheter-related occlusions occur as a result of thrombus formation (Fisher, Deffenbaugh, Poole, et al, 2004). Small thrombi at the tip of the catheter can usually be prevented with regular heparin flushes (Table 28-9) and, if present, lysed with a thrombolytic solution. The most common drug used to treat catheter-related thrombi is alteplase, a tissue plasminogen activator, which initiates fibrinolysis and clot dissolution. Alteplase has been demonstrated to be safe and effective for treating catheter-related occlusions in children (Blaney, Shen, Kerner, et al, 2006; Fisher, Deffenbaugh, Poole, et al, 2004; Kerner, Garcia-Careaga, Fisher, et al, 2006; Shen, Li, Murdock, et al, 2003). Written protocols should be available for the administration of alteplase for cath-

TABLE 28-9	HEPARIN FLUSH GUIDELINES			
	INTERMITTENT		**DORMANT**	
	≤2 yr OR ≤24-GAUGE CATHETER	**>2 yr**	**≤2 yr OR ≤24-GAUGE CATHETER**	**>2 yr**
Children				
Peripheral lines (Heplock)	10 units/ml; 1 ml heparin after medications or q 8 hr	5 ml normal saline after medications or q 8 h	10 units/ml; 1 ml heparin q 8 hr	5 ml normal saline q 8 hr
External central line (nonimplanted, tunneled, or peripherally inserted central catheter [PICC])	10 units/ml; 3 ml heparin after medications		10 units/ml; 3 ml heparin every day	100 units/ml; 3 ml heparin every day
Midline	10 units/ml; 3 ml heparin in 5-ml syringe after medications or q 8 hr		10 units/ml; 3 ml heparin in 5-ml syringe q 8 hr	
Arterial and central venous pressure continuous monitored lines	Heparin, 2 units/ml, in 55-ml syringes run at 1 ml/hr		N/A	
Neonates and Infants				
Peripheral lines (Heplock)	2 units/ml; 2 ml heparin to check for line patency and between medications or TPN known to be incompatible		2 units/ml; 2 ml heparin q 8 hr	
Percutaneous central catheter (PICC)	2 units/ml in 20-ml syringe run at 0.2 ml/hr		N/A	
Surgically placed central venous catheter (CVC) ≤5 French	2 units/ml; 2 ml heparin to check for line patency and between medications or TPN known to be compatible		2 units/ml; 2 ml heparin q 8 hr	
Surgically placed CVC >5 French	2 units/ml; 3 ml heparin to check for line patency and between medications or TPN known to be compatible		2 units/ml; 3 ml heparin q 8 hr	

Adapted from Texas Children's Hospital: *Heparin flush guidelines,* Houston, 2002, The Hospital.
N/A, Not applicable; *TPN,* total parenteral nutrition.

eter occlusion in children in health care institutions and home care.

Catheter occlusion may be partial, in which case fluid can be flushed into the device, or complete, in which case fluid or blood can be neither withdrawn nor flushed through the catheter (McCloskey, 2002). A fibrin sheath may form over the inner tip of the catheter within the vessel; the catheter may flush easily, but when attempts to withdraw fluid or blood are made, the sheath falls over the tip of the catheter, thus precluding withdrawal of blood or fluid (McCloskey, 2002). Larger thrombi outside of the catheter may require removal and anticoagulant therapy. A central venous thrombosis may also develop as the catheter brushes against the vessel wall, prompting thrombus formation, which may lead to superior vena cava syndrome (McCloskey, 2002). Symptoms of large thrombi include signs of superior vena cava occlusion, such as facial swelling and cyanosis, distended neck veins, blurred vision, vertigo, and swelling of the upper arm.

Complications associated with indwelling ports include port migration and difficulty accessing the port; the latter problem may occur if the Huber needle is not long enough to penetrate the subcutaneous skin.

Parent and Child Teaching

Regardless of which catheter is used, teach the child and family the care and management of the device with practice under supervision. It can be frightening to both child and parents to know that the catheter tip is situated near the heart. They need reassurance that with reasonable care they will do no harm to the apparatus. It is often useful to introduce the family to other children and families who are using central venous catheters successfully and with whom they can share concerns and helpful tips regarding care and management. This sharing is especially valuable for teenage patients. Because teenagers usually have a positive attitude toward use of the catheter, it is beneficial for them to share their experiences with adolescents who face the prospects of catheter placement.

Parents of children who engage in outside activities, go to school, or are otherwise under the supervision of another adult should inform the teacher, school nurse, coach, and baby-sitter about the presence of the central venous catheter. Vigorous contact sports, such as football, soccer, and hockey, are generally not allowed. Provide a written information sheet concerning the VAD, including its purpose, pertinent facts about any restrictions for the child, and directions related to management of the device, for their reference. The nurse or the parents should teach grandparents and other family members who care for the child the care and management of the catheter.

Procedures and published standards for catheter care vary widely among organizations, and there is no evidence that one method is superior. For example, some advocate covering the healed catheter site with a dressing; others do not. All companies that manufacture central catheters have patient and professional teaching kits. The user should become thoroughly familiar with the specific device selected for use.

The catheter is not a deterrent to most routine daily activities, including showers or tub bathing. However, the practitioner is consulted before activities such as swimming or physical contact sports are attempted. Swimming is usually prohibited but may be allowed in certain situations. If the exit site is healed and the cuff adheres to the tissue, place a transparent dressing over the catheter and exit site. Swimming may be permitted for a limited time, such as 1 hour or less, in a chlorinated pool. Most contact sports are prohibited because of the possibility of the catheter being hit or pulled. A protective vest can prevent active children from accidentally dislodging the catheter.

> **NURSING TIP** A pocket sewn on the inside of a T-shirt provides a place in which to coil the catheter line while the child is at play if a dressing is not used.

Family members need to know the signs of infection and an occluded catheter. Signs of a localized infection are redness, swelling, and pain at the vein entry site. Bacteremia is a serious complication that produces fever, chills, general malaise, and an ill appearance. Prevent uncapping by taping the cap securely to the catheter and the clamped line to the dressing. Prevent leaks by using a smooth-edged or padded clamp. Caution parents to keep scissors away from the child to prevent accidental cutting of the catheter. If the catheter leaks, they are instructed to tape it above the leak (between the leak and the entry site on the skin) and then clamp the catheter at the taped site. The child should be taken to the practitioner as soon as possible to prevent infection, blood loss, or clotting following a catheter leak.

> **! NURSING ALERT**
>
> If a central venous catheter is accidentally removed, apply pressure to the entry site to the vein, not the exit site on the skin.

TOTAL PARENTERAL NUTRITION AND TOTAL NUTRIENT ADMIXTURE

TPN, also known as IV alimentation, provides for the nutritional needs of infants or children who cannot consume an adequate amount of nutrients to support physical growth, positive nitrogen balance, and water and electrolyte homeostasis. Parenteral nutrition (PN) is defined by the American Society for Parenteral and Enteral Nutrition as any PN delivered into a large diameter vessel such as the subclavian vein (Teitelbaum, Guenter, Howell, et al, 2005). Total nutrient admixture (TNA) refers to the PN formula with carbohydrates, lipids, amino acids, vitamins, minerals, water, trace elements, and other additives in a single container (Teitelbaum, Guenter, Howell, et al, 2005). TNA may also be referred to as a three-in-one admixture, trimix, or all-in-one parenteral admixture. In many instances TPN may refer to a dextrose and amino acid solution with lipids piggybacked into the administration setup.

The following discussion on TPN encompasses TNA as well. Although the terms are not always synonymous in a clinical context, the complications and assessments are often the same for both TPN and TNA.

Common conditions for which TPN is used therapeutically include chronic intestinal obstruction from peritoneal sepsis or adhesions, extensive bowel resections with necrotizing enterocolitis, and conditions such as gastroschisis or large omphalocele that prevent optimum bowel functioning soon after surgery. TPN is also used for bowel fistulas; inadequate intestinal length with subsequent malabsorption; chronic, nonremitting, severe diarrhea; extensive body burns; and abdominal tumors treated by surgery, irradiation, and chemotherapy. TPN may also be initiated prophylactically when prolonged starvation is expected. Since the advent of PN in the 1960s, it has been recognized that prolonged periods of gut starvation (NPO) cause alterations in the gastrointestinal mucosa that affect the ability to absorb nutrients effectively once the gut has healed from surgical resection or manipulation. Therefore providers make attempts to resume some type of trophic feedings to minimize intestinal mucosal atrophy.

PN therapy involves IV infusion of solutions of protein, glucose, electrolytes, microminerals, and other nutrients on a short-term basis. Lipid emulsion is often initiated after a few days (although the time is variable depending on patient status) of PN to prevent **essential fatty acid deficiency**; lipids may be initially added as a piggyback infusion to the PN to ascertain tolerance and to avoid changing out the entire PN admixture if further changes in the solution are required. The alimentation solution is infused through conventional tubing with a special filter attached to remove particulate matter or microorganisms that may have contaminated the solution. The solution of glucose, lipids, amino acids, at times insulin, and other nutrients can be mixed together in a bag and delivered through an infusion pump. The solutions require infusion into a vessel with sufficient volume to allow for rapid dilution to minimize phlebitis and irritation. The wide-diameter vessels selected are the superior vena cava and innominate or intrathoracic subclavian veins approached by way of the external or internal jugular veins. In some situations the inferior vena cava from a femoral vein serves as an alternative route.

Central VADs are ideal for long-term and home parenteral nutrition (HPN). The TNA solution is prepared under sterile conditions, usually under a laminar-flow hood in a pharmacy equipped to appropriately mix the required ingredients on a daily basis. The IV tubing and administration set is likewise assembled under a laminar hood as a single unit to prevent contamination and minimize bacterial growth. Because concentrated glucose and protein solutions are optimum breeding sources for bacterial growth, take special care to connect the administration set and tubing to the patient's VAD using strict aseptic technique and to avoid adding other solutions or medications to the bag once it leaves the pharmacy.

Assessment of tolerance to TPN includes those tests performed for patients receiving parenteral fluids and who have a VAD. These include serum and urine chemistry and electrolyte profile, liver function tests, triglycerides, albumin, renal function, and body weight and height measurements. Hyperglycemia and hypoglycemia are common complications of TPN or TNA therapy until the child adjusts to the glucose load when high glucose solutions are used. The nurse is alert for signs and symptoms of hypoglycemia or hyperglycemia, and bedside glucose monitoring is instituted as necessary. Insulin is often added to the TNA to promote glucose utilization at the cellular level and growth; therefore monitoring for serum glucose levels is important. Hyperglycemia may cause an osmotic diuresis and increased loss of body fluid with subsequent fluid, electrolyte, and glucose imbalances for which the nurse should be vigilant. Once the child's condition stabilizes, the TNA is adjusted according to metabolic needs to promote growth and maintain a positive nitrogen balance, in addition to fluid and electrolyte homeostasis.

Children on full TPN programs may receive TPN either on a 24-hour basis or according to a plan established so the child receives the infusion at night (over 8 to 12 hours) while asleep to minimize disruption of daily activities such as school. Cycling TPN also allows the liver to rest for a period and is believed to prevent TPN-induced liver damage (Hwang, Lue, and Chen, 2000). However, evidence demonstrating significantly improved liver function with cyclic TPN in children is inconclusive (Jensen, Goldin, Koopmeiners, et al, 2009; Shulman and Phillips, 2003). In some cases the child may take regular fluids throughout the day for maintenance purposes and therefore is not dependent on the infusion for maintenance of electrolyte balance (depending on the nature of the illness). A plan may be established wherein the child may take small amounts of oral fluids or even small amounts of specific kinds of solid foods as tolerated during the day to provide a normal mealtime atmosphere. TPN may be combined with an enteral feeding program, as gastrointestinal tolerance allows, so the child is not totally dependent on TPN.

If prolonged nonoral feedings are required, the infant is allowed nonnutritive sucking to meet those needs. A consultation with a feeding specialist may be helpful so the child does not experience an aversion to foods fed orally when these are eventually implemented.

Because many children are treated with TPN regimens for long periods, it is especially important to be attuned to the child's growth and development needs. An individualized developmental care program is initiated as early as feasible to prevent developmental delays. (See Developmental Outcome, Chapter 10.) Delays in the areas of gross motor and language skills observed in infants receiving long-term PN (>3 months) may be caused by reduced mobility and social interaction.

Complications

Complications from TPN and TNA are numerous, and a major nursing responsibility is to prevent these when possible and to be alert to signs of their development. Complications are either (1) related to the infusate (metabolic complications); or (2) mechanical complications related to the indwelling catheter, the administration set, or the infusion pump.

Metabolic complications are associated with the infant's or child's capacity for the various components of the TNA or TPN solution. Excessive intake of any of the components will create an imbalance, such as hyperglycemia, azotemia, acid-base disorders, anemia, bone demineralization, vitamin and mineral deficiencies, hyperosmotic dehydration and coma, fluid overload, and a variety of electrolyte imbalances.

Liver disease is the most important gastrointestinal complication in pediatric populations. The cause is obscure, but liver disease appears to be more prevalent in preterm infants who were begun on TPN at an early age. In general, the lower the birth weight and gestational age, the higher the incidence of TPN-associated cholestasis; approximately 50% of infants weighing less than 1000 g develop TPN-associated cholestasis (Xanthakos and Balistreri, 2007). Affected infants develop cholestasis, hepatocellular necrosis, and, in advanced disease, cirrhosis or hepatic failure. Manifestations are often insidious and include hepatomegaly; jaundice; and elevated serum aminotransferase, bilirubin, and alkaline phosphatase levels, which become evident approximately 2 weeks after initiation of TPN (Xanthakos and Balistreri, 2007). In the low-birth-weight infant on TPN, onset of jaundice may overlap the phase of neonatal jaundice; therefore fractionated serum bilirubin measurements are recommended (Xanthakos and Balistreri, 2007). TPN-associated cholestasis is less common in older children. Cholelithiasis is an uncommon but possible occurrence in pediatric patients. Therefore children receiving TNA should be assessed periodically for signs and symptoms of cholelithiasis or cholecystitis.

Mechanical complications include catheter-related complications such as those involving catheter placement: pneumothorax, hemothorax, perforation, catheter dislodgment, and thrombus formation. However, the major complication associated with the catheter is infection: infection at the catheter entrance site, catheter "seeding" sepsis, venous thrombosis with infection and embolization, and endocarditis.

Pediatric TPN solution generally has a higher concentration of calcium and phosphorus, which makes some solutions more susceptible to precipitation. In the event of observed precipitation, stop the infusion and disconnect the container and tubing from the child; notify the practitioner so that a replacement infusion of dextrose can be started to prevent hypoglycemia. Other additives, including electrolytes, may need to be added depending on the child's status and the contents of the original solution. The nurse should take the original solution to the originating pharmacy for analysis.

Home Parenteral Nutrition

Some children require TPN over an extended period, often weeks, months, or even years. For many children, HPN is an alternative to long-term hospitalization. The child must be one who is unable to maintain adequate enteral alimentation, has no medical problems requiring hospitalization, has a parent who is able to manage the home care (or is an older child who can participate in his or her own care), and has the potential to benefit from the treatment.

Before a home care program can be implemented, a thorough assessment is made of the family and the home situation. The parents must be capable of performing the technical aspects of the procedure and be able to adapt to the changes inherent in the home program. Psychosocial readiness of the family; family support systems; and practical considerations are investigated, including availability of a pharmacy to prepare the parenteral alimentation solution, a practitioner to handle day-to-day emergency needs, and a cooperating insurance company or agency (because of the exorbitant cost of maintaining long-term parenteral feeding). In many areas home health care agencies are able to assume the major management of HPN for families; however, a shortage of skilled nursing staff and decreased third-party reimbursement often require a family member to assume major responsibility for the child's home care. (See also Family-Centered Home Care, Chapter 25.)

The major nursing responsibilities for the child and family with HPN include assurance that the proper solution is infusing, proper maintenance of the VAD, prevention of sepsis and other mechanical complications, monitoring of infusion rate, and assessment of the patient's tolerance to the solution. In most cases a family member may assume responsibility for starting (hanging) and monitoring the infusion. The TPN or TNA solution is prepared under sterile conditions, usually in a hospital pharmacy or home health agency pharmacy, and then is distributed to the primary caretaker by a home health aide or family member. Teach family members how to maintain the child's VAD, including dressing changes and routine flushing as required, and how to evaluate the progress of the infusion. In most cases the infusion is delivered by an infusion pump to prevent too rapid an infusion, which may cause fluid and electrolyte problems. HPN complications include those listed above for long-term TPN: infection (catheter-related sepsis), exit site infection, catheter occlusion, catheter tears, thrombosis, fluid and electrolyte imbalance, and liver dysfunction (Howard and Ashley, 2003).

In a study of adult and pediatric patients on HPN, Howard and Ashley (2003) found that the single most important factor influencing the outcome of home TPN was the patient's primary diagnosis. Mortality and morbidity for patients with cancer was much greater than for those with bowel disorders such as obstruction and Crohn disease.

Colomb, Dabbas-Tyan, Taupin, and colleagues (2007) also noted that most children on HPN with primary digestive disease survived if early referral occurred; survival probabilities in the study at 2, 5, 10, and 15 years were 97%, 89%, 81%, and 72%, respectively. In this study the primary diagnosis strongly influenced the outcome and survival rate of the child on HPN. Johnson and Sexton (2006) noted that HPN was associated with fewer catheter infections than hospital PN; however, HPN was associated with more physical and psychologic stress for families. Social isolation, depression, and loneliness were identified in children and families with HPN.

An important goal with HPN is the normalization of the child to optimize ability to perform activities of daily living and promote a healthy lifestyle in anticipation of the day when TPN or TNA is no longer required. (See also Chapter 25.) One study found that the quality of life for children and their families on HPN was not significantly different from that of a reference group of healthy children without HPN (Gottrand, Staszewski, Colomb, et al, 2005). The researchers concluded that children on HPN developed appropriate coping skills; parents of children on HPN, especially parents of infants, had lower quality-of-life scores than controls, and adolescents on HPN had quality-of-life scores similar to those of controls, except for those with ileostomy, who scored lower on quality-of-life issues.

Before beginning HPN, the parents are prepared for taking over the child's total care. Teaching may occur in the hospital or at home, depending on the policies of insurance companies and the home health care agency monitoring the family. The

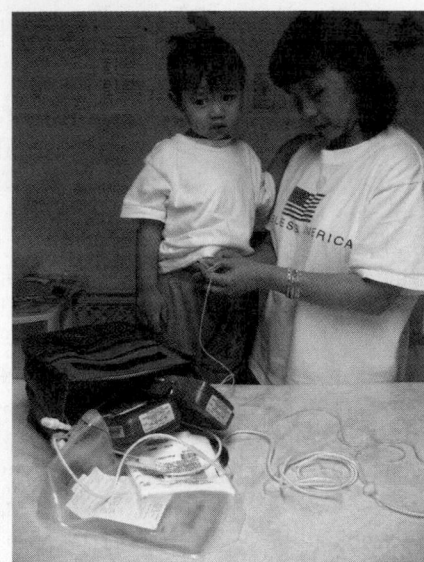

Fig. 28-11 Home total parenteral nutrition requires modifications in lifestyle and adjustments in activities for child and family.

parents assume full responsibility for the child's care, with help being readily available when needed.

The emotional and economic benefits of this approach are readily apparent. The familiar environment and the atmosphere of normality are enormously therapeutic, and the stress of separation is avoided. With multidisciplinary support from health professionals, a home care program can be the ideal alternative to hospitalization for a capable, motivated family of a child who requires TNA.

Encourage the family to make the home life as normal as possible for the child within the limits imposed by the therapy. For example, having the infant or child at the table during mealtimes and including the child in family activities contribute to a normal family atmosphere. Activity restrictions often depend on the child's illness, the type of VAD, and period of HPN (continuous versus intermittent), but the provider should promote normalization of all allowed activities (Fig. 28-11). Allow infants and toddlers to crawl and pull up to a standing position to promote optimum development. The length of tubing can be adjusted to accommodate such activities. Running the tubing under a one-piece clothing outfit and out the back often encourages ambulation. At times the nurse must give the parents permission to allow the child to play because they may be frightened by the tubing and VAD setup. Once the parents or caregivers becomes familiar with the usual complications of mobility, they are resourceful at adapting the clothing and home environment to allow the child to play with minimum restrictions. It is also important to make certain the child's dental care is not neglected.

The family is referred to community agencies that provide support and practical assistance. The Oley Foundation,* a non-profit research and education organization, maintains a national registry of persons receiving HPN and publishes a bimonthly newsletter for consumers, families, clinicians, and home care services.

---

*214 Hun Memorial, MC-28, Albany Medical Center, Albany, NY 12208-3478; 800-776-6539 (in United States and Canada), 518-262-5079 (in other countries); www.oley.org.

KEY POINTS

- Water distribution and maintenance are determined by solutes, physical forces, internal control mechanisms, and boundary organs through which external exchanges occur.
- Infants are subject to fluid depletion because of their relatively greater surface area, their high rate of metabolism, and their immature kidney function.
- Management of fluid volume disturbances focuses on volume of body fluids, osmolality, hydrogen ion status, electrolyte deficits, and disturbances in mineral skeleton and body fluid equilibrium.
- Fluid disturbances experienced by children are dehydration, water intoxication, and edema.
- Dehydration may be classified as isotonic, hypotonic, or hypertonic.
- Parenteral fluid therapy is initiated to meet ongoing daily physiologic losses, restore previous deficits, and replace ongoing abnormal losses.
- Fluid gains or losses from the interstitial spaces depend on venous hydrostatic pressure, colloidal osmotic pressure, semipermeable capillary wall, tissue tension, and lymphatic flow.
- Edema formation is caused by increased venous pressure, capillary permeability, diminished plasma proteins, lymphatic obstruction, or decreased tissue tension.
- Disturbances in acid-base balance are respiratory acidosis, respiratory alkalosis, metabolic acidosis, and metabolic alkalosis.
- Respiratory acidosis may result from factors that depress the respiratory center, affect the lungs, or interfere with the bellows action of the chest wall.
- Respiratory alkalosis results primarily from CNS stimulation.
- Metabolic acidosis is a lowered plasma pH caused by any process that reduces base bicarbonate concentration or increases metabolic acid formation.
- Metabolic alkalosis is an elevated plasma pH that occurs when there is a reduction of hydrogen ion concentration or an excess of base bicarbonate.
- Nursing assessment of fluid and electrolyte disturbances entails observation of general appearance, vital signs, daily weights, I&O measurement, and review of relevant laboratory results.
- Long-term venous access is accomplished by intermittent IV devices; central venous catheters, including short-term (subclavian, femoral, and jugular), short-term to moderate-term (PICCs), and long-term (tunneled) catheters and ports; or implanted ports.
- PN provides for total nutritional needs when feeding via the gastrointestinal tract is impossible, inadequate, or hazardous.
- Before initiating HPN, the nurse assesses the parents' ability to perform the procedure, existence of family support systems, availability of nearby pharmacies, and insurance coverage.

REFERENCES

American Academy of Pediatrics: *Pediatric nutrition handbook,* ed 6, Elk Grove Village, Ill, 2009, The Academy.

Aschner JL, Poland RL: Sodium bicarbonate: basically useless therapy, *Pediatrics* 122(4):831-835, 2008.

Blaney M, Shen V, Kerner JA, et al: Alteplase for the treatment of central venous catheter occlusion in children: results of a prospective, open-label, single-arm study (the Cathflo Activase Pediatric Study), *J Vasc Interv Radiol* 17(11 Pt 1):1745-1751, 2006.

Carson SM: Chlorhexidine versus povidone-iodine for central venous catheter site care in children, *J Pediatr Nurs* 19(1):74-80, 2004.

Colomb V, Dabbas-Tyan M, Taupin P, et al: Long-term outcome of children receiving home parenteral nutrition: a 20-year single-center experience in 302 patients, *J Pediatr Gastroenterol Nutr* 44(3):347-353, 2007.

Crosby CT, Mares A: Skin antisepsis: past, present, and future, *J Vasc Access Devices* 6(1):26-31, 2001.

Curley MAQ, Moloney-Harmon PA: *Critical care nursing of infants and children,* ed 2, Philadelphia, 2001, Saunders.

de Caen AR, Reis A, Bhutta A: Vascular access and drug therapy in pediatric resuscitation, *Pediatr Clin North Am* 55(4):909-927, 2008.

DeCamp LR, Byerly JS, Doshi N, et al: Use of antiemetic agents in acute gastroenteritis: a systematic review and meta-analysis, *Arch Pediatr Adolesc Med* 162(9):858-865, 2008.

Doellman D: Pharmacologic versus nonpharmacologic techniques in reducing venipuncture psychological trauma in pediatric patients, *J Infusion Nurs* 26(2):103-109, 2003.

Ellis JA, Sharp D, Newhook K, et al: Selling comfort: a survey of interventions for needle procedures in a pediatric hospital, *Pain Manage Nurs* 5(4):144-152, 2004.

Emond S: Dehydration in infants and young children, *Ann Emerg Med* 53(3):395-397, 2009.

Fann B: Fluid and electrolyte balance in the pediatric patient, *J Intraven Nurs* 21(3):153-159, 1998.

Farion KJ, Splinter KL, Newhook K, et al: The effect of vapocoolant spray on pain due to intravenous cannulation in children: a randomized controlled trial, *CMAJ* 179(1):31-36, 2008.

Fiorito BA, Mirza F, Doran TM, et al: Intraosseous access in the setting of pediatric critical care transport, *Pediatr Crit Care Med* 6(1):50-53, 2005.

Fisher AA, Deffenbaugh C, Poole R, et al: The use of alteplase for restoring patency to occluded central venous access devices in infants and children, *J Infusion Nurs* 27(3):171-174, 2004.

Ford DM: Fluid, electrolyte, and acid-base disorders. In Hay WW, Levin MJ, Sondheimer JM, et al, editors: *Current diagnosis and treatment,* ed 19, Philadelphia, 2009, McGraw Hill.

Freedman SB, Adler M, Seshadri R, et al: Oral ondansetron for gastroenteritis in a pediatric emergency department, *N Engl J Med* 354(16):1698-1705, 2006.

Friedman A: Fluid and electrolyte therapy: a primer, *Pediatr Nephrol,* May 15, 2009, E-pub ahead of print.

Gamulka B, Mendoza C, Connolly B: Evaluation of a unique, nurse-inserted, peripherally inserted central catheter program, *Pediatrics* 115(6):1602-1606, 2005.

Gillies D, O'Riordan L, Wallen M, et al: Optimal timing for intravenous administration set replacement, *Cochrane Database Syst Rev* 19(4): CD003588, 2005.

Gillies D, O'Riordan L, Wallen M, et al: Timing of intravenous administration set changes: a systematic review, *Infect Control Hosp Epidemiol* 25(3):240-250, 2004.

Gottrand F, Staszewski P, Colomb V, et al: Satisfaction in different life domains in children receiving home parenteral nutrition and their families, *J Pediatr* 146(6):793-797, 2005.

Greenbaum LA: Pathophysiology of body fluids and fluid therapy. In Behrman RE, Kliegman RM, Jenson HB, editors: *Nelson textbook of pediatrics,* ed 18, Philadelphia, 2007, Saunders.

Hazinsky MF, Zaritsky AL, Nadkarni VM, et al: *PALS provider manual*, Dallas, 2002, American Heart Association.

Howard L, Ashley C: Management of complications in patients receiving home parenteral nutrition, *Gastroenterology* 124(6):1651-1661, 2003.

Huether SE: The cellular environment: fluids and electrolytes, acids and bases. In McCance KL, Huether SE, Brashers VL, et al, editors: *Pathophysiology: the biologic basis for disease in adults and children,* ed 6, St Louis, 2010, Mosby.

Hwang TL, Lue MC, Chen LL: Early use of cyclic TPN prevents further deteriorations of liver functions for the TPN patients with impaired liver function, *Hepatogastroenterology* 47(35): 1347-1350, 2000.

Infusion Nurses Society: *Policies and procedures for infusion nursing,* ed 3, Norwood, Mass, 2006, The Society.

Jensen AR, Goldin AB, Koopmeiners JS, et al: The association of cyclic parenteral nutrition and decreased incidence of cholestatic liver disease in patients with gastroschisis, *J Pediatr Surg* 44(1):183-189, 2009.

Jimenez N, Bradford H, Seidel KD, et al: A comparison of a needle-free injection system for local anesthesia versus EMLA for intravenous catheter insertion in the pediatric patient, *Anesth Analg* 102(2):411-414, 2006.

Johnson T, Sexton E: Managing children and adolescents on parenteral nutrition: challenges for the nutritional support team, *Proc Nutr Soc* 65(3):217-221, 2006.

Kee J, Paulanka B: *Handbook of fluid, electrolyte and acid-base imbalances,* Albany, NY, 2000, Delmar.

Kerner JA, Garcia-Careaga MG, Fisher AA, et al: Treatment of catheter occlusion in pediatric patients, *J Parenter Enteral Nutr* 30(Suppl 1): S73-S81, 2006.

Kline AM: Pediatric catheter-related bloodstream infections: latest strategies to decrease risk, *AACN Clin Issues* 16(2):185-198, 2005.

Knue M, Doellman D, Rabin K, et al: The efficacy and safety of blood sampling through peripherally inserted central catheters devices in children, *J Infus Nurs* 28(1):30-35, 2005.

Krein SL, Hofer TP, Kowalski CP, et al: Use of central venous catheter–related bloodstream infection prevention practices by US hospitals, *Mayo Clin Proc* 82(6):672-678, 2007.

Lamagna P, MacPhee M: Phlebitis and infiltration: troubleshooting pediatric peripheral IVs, *Nurse Week* (Heartland ed) 5(4):20, 26, 28, 2004.

Lee OK, Johnston L: A systematic review for effective management of central venous catheters and catheter sites in acute care paediatric patients, *Worldviews Evid Based Nurs* 2(1):4-13, 2005.

Linder N, Prince S, Barzilai A, et al: Disinfection with 10% povidone-iodine versus 0.5% chlorhexidine gluconate in 70% isopropanol in the neonatal intensive care unit, *Acta Paediatr* 93(2):205-210, 2004.

Luhmann J, Hurt S, Shootman M, et al: A comparison of buffered lidocaine versus Ela-Max before peripheral intravenous catheter insertions in children, *Pediatrics* 113(3 Pt 1):e217-e220, 2004.

Marini MA, Giangregorio M, Kraskinski JC: Complying with the Occupational Safety and Health Administration's bloodborne pathogen standard: implementing needleless systems and intravenous safety devices, *Pediatr Emerg Care* 20(3):209-214, 2004.

McCloskey DJ: Catheter-related thrombosis in pediatrics, *Pediatr Nurs* 28(2):97-105, 2002.

Mermel LA, Allon M, Bouza E, et al: Clinical practice guidelines for the diagnosis and management of intravascular catheter-related infection: 2009 update by the Infectious Diseases Society of America, *Clin Infect Dis* 49:1-45, 2009, available at www.cdc.gov/publiccomments/comments/guidelines-for-the-prevention-of-intravascular-catheter-related-infections/1862.ashx (accessed March 8, 2010).

Metheny N: *Fluid and electrolyte balance,* ed 4, Philadelphia, 2000, Lippincott.

Mickler PA: Neonatal and pediatric perspectives in PICC placement, *J Infusion Nurs* 31(5):282-285, 2008.

Milstone AM, Passaretti CL, Perl TM: Chlorhexidine: expanding the armamentarium for infection control and prevention, *Clin Infect Dis* 46(2):274-281, 2008.

Morgan LM, Thomas DJ: Implementing evidence-based nursing practice in the pediatric intensive care unit, *J Infus Nurs* 30(2):105-112, 2007.

O'Grady NP, Alexander M, Dellinger EP, et al: Guidelines for the prevention of intravascular catheter-related infections, *MMWR* 51(RR10):1-26, 2002.

Petit J: Fostering a new era of vascular access device selections in neonates, *Newborn Infant Nurs Rev* 6(4):186-192, 2006.

Racadio JM, Doellman DA, Johnson ND, et al: Pediatric peripherally inserted central catheters: complication rates related to catheter tip location, *Pediatrics* 107(2):e28, 2001.

Roslund G, Hepps TS, McQuillen KK: The role of oral ondansetron in children with vomiting as a result of acute gastritis/gastroenteritis who have failed oral rehydration therapy: a randomized controlled trial, *Ann Emerg Med* 52(1):22-29, 2008.

Schwengel DA, McGready J, Berenholtz SM, et al: Peripherally inserted central catheters: a randomized, controlled, prospective trial in pediatric surgical patients, *Anesthesiol Analg* 99(4):1038-1043, 2004.

Shen V, Li X, Murdock M, et al: Recombinant tissue plasminogen activator (alteplase) for restoration of function to occluded central venous catheters in pediatric patients, *J Pediatr Hematol Oncol* 25(1):38-45, 2003.

Shulman RJ, Phillips S: Parenteral nutrition in infants and children, *J Pediatr Gastroent Nutr* 36(5):587-607, 2003.

Smith MJ: Catheter-related bloodstream infections in children, *Am J Infect Control* 36(10):S173:e1-e3, 2008.

Spandorfer PR, Alessandrini EA, Joffe MD, et al: Oral versus intravenous rehydration of moderately dehydrated children: a randomized, controlled trial, *Pediatrics* 115(2):295-301, 2005.

Spanos S, Booth R, Koenig H, et al: Jet injection of 1% buffered lidocaine versus topical ELA-Max for anesthesia before peripheral intravenous catheterization in children: a randomized controlled trial, *Pediatr Emerg Care* 24(8):511-515, 2008.

Steiner MJ, DeWalt D, Byerly JS: Is this child dehydrated? *JAMA* 291(22):2746-2754, 2004.

Steiner MJ, Nager AL, Wang VJ: Urine specific gravity and other urinary indices: inaccurate tests for dehydration, *Pediatr Emerg Care* 23(5):298-303, 2007.

Stevens B, Taddio A, Ohlsson A, et al: The efficacy of sucrose for relieving procedural pain in neonates: a systematic review and meta-analysis, *Acta Paediatr* 86(8):837-842, 1997.

Taddio A, Shah V, Hancock R, et al: Effectiveness of sucrose analgesia in newborns undergoing painful medical procedures, *CMAJ* 179(1)37-43, 2008.

Teitelbaum D, Guenter P, Howell WH, et al: Definition of terms, style, and conventions used in ASPEN guidelines and standards, *Nutr Clin Pract* 20(2):281-285, 2005.

Thompson DG: Utilizing an oral sucrose solution to minimize neonatal pain, *JSPN* 10(1):3-10, 2005.

Wade G: Fluid problems in infants and children. In Kee JL, Paulanka BJ, Polek C, editors: *Handbook of fluid, electrolytes, and acid-base imbalance,* ed 3, Clifton Park, NY, 2010, Delmar, Cengage Learning.

Weise KL, Nahata MC: EMLA for painful procedures in infants, *J Pediatr Healthcare* 19(1):42-47, 2005.

Whitby M, McLaws ML, Slater K: Needlestick injuries in a major teaching hospital: the worthwhile effect of hospital-wide replacement of conventional hollow-bore needles, *Am J Infect Control* 36(3):180-186, 2008.

Wong DL: Topical anesthetics: two products for pain relief during minor procedures, *AJN* 103(6):42-45, 2003.

Xanthakos SA, Balistreri WF: Liver disease associated with systemic disorders. In Kliegman RM, Behrman RE, Jenson HB, et al, editors: *Nelson textbook of pediatrics,* ed 18, Philadelphia, 2007, Saunders.

Zempsky WT: Pharmacologic approaches for reducing venous access pain in children, *Pediatrics* 122(Suppl 3):S140-S153, 2008.

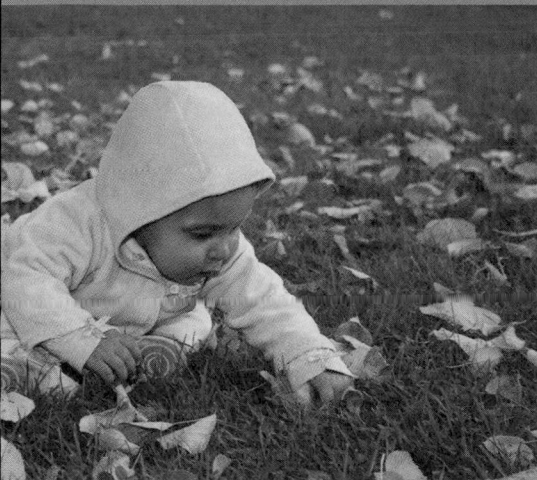

Conditions That Produce Fluid and Electrolyte Imbalance

Rose Ann Urdiales Baker, Mary A. Mondozzi,
and Marilyn J. Hockenberry

ⓔvolve WEBSITE

http://evolve.elsevier.com/wong/ncic
Animation
  Burns in Children
  Capillary Leak
Case Studies
  Acute Diarrhea (Gastroenteritis)
  Burns
  Dehydration and Diarrhea
Critical Thinking Exercise
  Shock
Key Points Audio Summaries
NCLEX Review Questions
Nursing Care Plans
  The Child with Acute Diarrhea
  The Child with Burns
  The Child in Shock (Cardiovascular Failure)
Spanish/English Translations
WebLinks

RELATED TOPICS

The Child with Cardiovascular Dysfunction, **Ch. 34**
The Child with Gastrointestinal Dysfunction, **Ch. 33**
Diaper Dermatitis, **Ch. 13**
Disorders Affecting the Skin, **Ch. 18**
Family-Centered Care of the Child During Illness and
  Hospitalization, **Ch. 26**
Family-Centered Care of the Child with Chronic Illness or
  Disability, **Ch. 22**
Family-Centered Home Care, **Ch. 25**
Injury Prevention: Infant, **Ch. 12**; Toddler, **Ch. 14**; School-Age
  Child, **Ch. 17**
Intestinal Parasitic Diseases, **Ch. 16**
Pain Assessment and Pain Management, **Ch. 7**

CHAPTER OUTLINE

GASTROINTESTINAL DISORDERS

DIARRHEA

Diarrhea is a symptom that results from disorders involving digestive, absorptive, and secretory functions. Diarrhea is caused by abnormal intestinal water and electrolyte transport.

Worldwide, there are an estimated 1.3 billion episodes of diarrhea each year. Approximately 24% of all deaths in children living in developing countries are related to diarrhea and dehydration. Most children living in developed countries have mild forms of gastroenteritis. However, in the United States, approximately 200,000 children younger than age 5 are hospitalized and approximately 200 children younger than 5 years die of

---

BOX 29-1 **CONSEQUENCES OF FLUID AND ELECTROLYTE LOSS**

Dehydration
Voluminous losses of fluid in frequent, watery stools
Losses when there is also vomiting
Reduced fluid intake resulting from nausea or anorexia
Increased insensible losses from fever, hyperpnea, and, sometimes, high environmental temperature
Continued (although diminished) obligatory renal losses

Electrolyte Imbalance
Losses of sodium, chloride, potassium, and, in some cases, bicarbonate
Inadequate replacement of electrolytes when hypotonic or hypertonic solutions are used

Metabolic Acidosis
Increased absorption of short-chain fatty acids produced in the colon from bacterial fermentation of unabsorbed dietary carbohydrates
Accumulation of lactic acid from tissue hypoxia secondary to hypovolemia
Loss of bicarbonate in stools
Ketosis from fat metabolism when glycogen stores are depleted in untreated diarrheal dehydration or inadequate carbohydrate intake; may result in malnutrition

---

BOX 29-2 **CAUSES OF ACUTE DIARRHEA**

Infection and Parasitic Infestation
Bacteria—*Salmonella, Shigella, Campylobacter, Escherichia coli, Yersinia, Aeromonas, Clostridium difficile, Staphylococcus aureus*
Viruses—Rotavirus, Norwalk virus, small and round viruses, adenovirus, pestivirus, astrovirus, calicivirus, parvovirus
Parasites—*Giardia lamblia, Cryptosporidium, Isospora belli, Microsporidia, Strongyloides, Entamoeba histolytica*

Associated Conditions
Upper respiratory tract infections
Urinary tract infections
Otitis media

Dietary Causes
Overfeeding
Introduction of new foods
Reinstituting milk too soon after diarrheal episode
Osmotic diarrhea from excess sugar in formula or juice
Excessive ingestion of sorbitol or fructose

Medications
Antibiotics
Laxatives

Toxic Causes
Ingestion of:
• Heavy metals (arsenic, lead, mercury)
• Organic phosphates

Functional Causes
Irritable bowel syndrome

Other Causes
Pseudomembranous enterocolitis
Hirschsprung enterocolitis

---

diarrhea and dehydration each year (Malek, Curns, Holman, et al, 2006; Staat, 2006).

Diarrhea is caused by abnormal intestinal water and electrolyte transport. The transport of fluid and electrolytes in the developing gastrointestinal (GI) tract is related to the child's age. The intestinal mucosa of the young infant is more permeable to water than that of an older child. Therefore in young infants with increased intestinal luminal osmolality caused by diarrhea, more fluid and electrolytes are lost than in older children (Box 29-1). Diarrhea results from several pathophysiologic processes.

Types of Diarrhea

Diarrheal disturbances involve the stomach and intestines (gastroenteritis), the small intestine (enteritis), the colon (colitis), or the colon and intestines (enterocolitis). Diarrhea is classified as acute or chronic.

Acute diarrhea, a leading cause of illness in children younger than 5 years of age, is defined as a sudden increase in frequency and a change in consistency of stools, often caused by an infectious agent in the GI tract (Box 29-2). It may be associated with upper respiratory or urinary tract infections, antibiotic therapy, or laxative use. Acute diarrhea is usually self-limited (<14 days' duration) and subsides without specific treatment if dehydration does not occur. Acute infectious diarrhea (infectious gastroenteritis) is caused by a variety of viral, bacterial, and parasitic pathogens (Table 29-1).

Chronic diarrhea is an increase in stool frequency and increased water content with a duration of more than 14 days. It is often caused by chronic conditions such as malabsorption syndromes, inflammatory bowel disease (IBD), immunodeficiency, food allergy, lactose intolerance, or chronic nonspecific diarrhea, or as a result of inadequate management of acute diarrhea.

Intractable diarrhea of infancy is a syndrome that occurs in the first few months of life, persists for longer than 2 weeks with no recognized pathogens, and is refractory to treatment. The most common cause is acute infectious diarrhea that was not managed adequately.

Chronic nonspecific diarrhea (CNSD), also known as irritable colon of childhood and toddlers' diarrhea, is a common cause of chronic diarrhea in children 6 to 54 months of age. These children have loose stools, often with undigested food particles, and diarrhea greater than 2 weeks' duration. Children with CNSD grow normally and have no evidence of malnutrition, no blood in their stool, and no enteric infection. Research has linked poor dietary habits and food sensitivities to chronic diarrhea. The excessive intake of juices and artificial sweeteners such as sorbitol, a substance found in many commercially prepared beverages and foods, may be a factor. Box 29-3 lists other factors that predispose patients to chronic diarrhea.

Etiology

Most pathogens that cause diarrhea are spread by the fecal-oral route through contaminated food or water or are spread from person to person where there is close contact (e.g., daycare centers). Lack of clean water, crowding, poor hygiene, nutritional deficiency, and poor sanitation are major risk factors, especially for bacterial or parasitic pathogens. Infants are often more susceptible to frequent and severe bouts of diarrhea because their immune system has not been exposed to many pathogens and has not acquired protective antibodies (Box 29-4). Worldwide, the most common causes of acute gastroenteritis are infectious agents, viruses, bacteria, and parasites. In

TABLE 29-1 INFECTIOUS CAUSES OF ACUTE DIARRHEA

AGENTS	PATHOLOGY	CHARACTERISTICS	COMMENTS
Viral			
Rotavirus Incubation—48 hr Diagnosis—EIA	Fecal-oral transmission 7 groups (A-G)—Most group A virus replicates in mature villus epithelial cells of small intestine; leads to (1) imbalance in ratio of intestinal fluid absorption to secretion and (2) malabsorption of complex carbohydrates	Mild to moderate fever Vomiting followed by onset of watery stools Fever and vomiting generally abate in approximately 2 days, but diarrhea persists 5-7 days	Most common cause of diarrhea in children <5 yr of age; infants 6-12 mo most vulnerable; affects all ages; usually milder in children >3 yr of age Immunocompromised children at greater risk for complications. Peak occurrences in winter months Important cause of nosocomial infections
Norwalk-like organisms Also called caliciviruses Incubation—12-48 hr Diagnosis—EIA	Fecal-oral; contaminated water Pathology similar to that of rotavirus; affects villus epithelial cells of small intestine, leading to (1) imbalance in ratio of intestinal fluid absorption to secretion and (2) malabsorption of complex carbohydrates	Abdominal cramps, nausea, vomiting, malaise, low-grade fever, watery diarrhea without blood; duration 2-3 days; tends to resemble so-called food poisoning symptoms with nausea predominating	Affects all ages Multiple strains often named for the location of outbreak (e.g., Norwalk, Sapporo, Snow Mountain, Montgomery)
Bacterial			
Escherichia coli Incubation—3-4 days; variable depending on strain Diagnosis—Sorbitol MacConkey (SMAC) agar positive for blood, but fecal leukocytes absent or rare	*E. coli* strains produce diarrhea as result of enterotoxin production, adherence, or invasion (enterotoxigenic-producing *E. coli*, enterohemorrhagic *E. coli*, enteroaggregative *E. coli*)	Watery diarrhea 1-2 days, then severe abdominal cramping and bloody diarrhea Can progress to hemolytic uremic syndrome	Food-borne pathogen Traveler's diarrhea Highest incidence in summer Cause of nursery epidemics Symptomatic treatment Antibiotics may worsen course Avoid antimotility agents and opioids
***Salmonella* groups** (nontyphoidal) Gram-negative rods, nonencapsulated nonsporulating Incubation—6-72 hr Diagnosis—Gram stain, stool culture	Invasion of mucosa in the small and large intestine, edema of the lamina propria, focal acute inflammation with disruption of the mucosa and microabscesses	Nausea, vomiting, colicky abdominal pain, bloody diarrhea, fever; symptoms variable (mild to severe) May have headache and cerebral manifestations (e.g., drowsiness, confusion, meningismus, seizures) Infants may be afebrile and nontoxic May result in life-threatening septicemia and meningitis Nausea and vomiting typically of short duration; diarrhea may persist as long as 2-3 wk Typically shed virus for average of 5 wk; cases reported up to 1 yr	Incidence highest in warm months (July-November); food-borne outbreaks common Usually transmitted person to person but may transmit via undercooked meats or poultry; about half the cases caused by poultry and poultry products In children, related to pets (e.g., dogs, cats, hamsters, turtles) Communicable as long as organisms are excreted Antibiotics not recommended in uncomplicated cases Antimotility agents also not recommended—prolong transit time and carrier state Incidence decreasing over past 10 yr
Salmonella typhi Produces enteric fever—systemic syndrome Incubation—usually 7-14 days but could be 3-30 days depending on size of inoculum Diagnosis—positive blood cultures; also sometimes positive stool and urine cultures Late stage—positive bone marrow culture	Bloodstream invasion; after ingestion, organism attaches to microvilli of ileal brush borders and bacteria invade the intestinal epithelium via Peyer patches Next, organism is transported to intestinal lymph nodes and enters bloodstream via thoracic ducts, and circulating organism reaches reticuloendothelial cells, causing bacteremia	Manifestations dependent on age Abdominal pain, diarrhea, nausea, vomiting, high fever, lethargy Must be treated with antibiotics	Incidence much lower in developed countries; about 400 cases/yr in United States; 65% of U.S. cases acquired via international cases Ingestion of foods and water contaminated with human feces is most common mode of transmission Congenital and intrapartum transmission possible Three vaccines available
***Shigella* groups** Gram-negative nonmotile anaerobic bacilli Incubation—1-7 days Diagnosis—stool culture loaded with polymorphonuclear leukocytes	Enterotoxins—invades the epithelium with superficial mucosal ulcerations	Children appear sick Symptoms begin with fever, fatigue, anorexia Crampy abdominal pain preceding watery or bloody diarrhea Symptoms usually subside in 5-10 days	Most cases in children younger than 9 yr, with about a third of cases in children ages 1-4 wk Antibiotics shorten illness and lower mortality All patients at risk for dehydration Acute symptoms may persist for ≥1 wk Antidiarrheal medications not recommended, since they may predispose patient to toxic megacolon

CNS, Central nervous system; *EIA*, enzyme immunoassay; *ELISA*, enzyme-linked immunosorbent assay; *GI*, gastrointestinal.

Continued

TABLE 29-1   INFECTIOUS CAUSES OF ACUTE DIARRHEA—cont'd

AGENTS	PATHOLOGY	CHARACTERISTICS	COMMENTS
Yersinia enterocolitis Incubation—dose dependent, 1-3 wk Diagnosis—stool culture, ELISA Patients have leukocytosis, elevated sedimentation rate	Pathology poorly understood; possibly caused by production of enterotoxin	Mucoid diarrhea, sometimes bloody; abdominal pain suggestive of appendicitis; fever, vomiting	Seen more frequently in the winter months Transmitted by pets and food Antibiotics usually do not alter the clinical course in uncomplicated cases; antibiotics used in complicated infections and compromised hosts
Campylobacter jejuni Microaerophilic, motile, gram-negative bacilli Incubation—1-7 days Ability to cause illness appears dose related Diagnosis—stool culture, sometimes blood culture Commonly found in GI tract of wild or domestic animals	Not fully understood, possibly (1) adherence to intestinal mucosa by toxin, (2) invasion of the mucosa in the terminal ileum and colon, (3) translocation in which the organisms penetrate the mucosa and replicate in the lamina propria	Fever, abdominal pain, diarrhea that can be bloody, vomiting Watery, profuse, foul-smelling diarrhea Clinically like infection by *Salmonella* or *Shigella* organisms Fecal-oral transmission	Most infections in humans relate to consumption of contaminated foods or water, such as undercooked meats, particularly chicken Also acquired from contaminated household pets (e.g., dogs, cats, hamsters) Bimodal peaks in infants <1 yr and again at ages 15-29 yr Antibiotics do not prolong the carriage of bacteria and may eliminate organism more quickly Erythromycin is the drug of choice Antimotility agents not recommended because they tend to prolong symptoms
Vibrio cholerae Gram-negative, motile, curved bacillus living in bodies of salt water Incubation—1-3 days Diagnosis—stool culture	Enters via oral route in contaminated food or water; if survives acid stomach environment, travels to the small intestine, adheres to the mucosa, and produces toxin	Onset abrupt; vomiting, watery diarrhea without cramping or tenesmus Dehydration can occur quickly	More prevalent in developing countries Rehydration most important treatment Antibiotics can shorten diarrhea Despite continued efforts, still no vaccine
Clostridium difficile Gram-positive anaerobic bacillus with the ability to produce spores Diagnosis—by detecting *C. difficile* toxin in stool culture	Produces two important toxins (A and B) Toxin binds to the enterocyte surface receptor, resulting in alteration permeability, protein synthesis, and direct cytotoxicity	Mostly mild watery diarrhea lasting a few days Some prolonged diarrhea and illness May cause pseudomembranous colitis Some individuals extremely ill with high fever, leukocytosis, hypoalbuminemia	Associated with alteration of normal intestinal flora by antibiotics Adults tend to have more severe symptoms than children Treatment with antibiotics (metronidazole) in mildly to moderately symptomatic patients; for nonresponders, give vancomycin Resistant strains have developed Relapse common
Clostridium perfringens Anaerobic, gram-positive, spore-producing bacilli Incubation—8-24 hr	Toxins produced in the intestine after ingestion of organism	Acute onset—watery diarrhea, crampy abdominal pain Fever, nausea, and vomiting are rare Duration of illness usually 24 hr	Transmitted by contaminated food products, most often meats and poultry Usually self-limiting and medical intervention not needed Oral rehydration usually sufficient Antibiotics serve no purpose and should not be used
Clostridium botulinum Gram-positive anaerobic spore-producing bacilli Incubation—12-26 hr (range, 6 hr–8 days) Diagnosis—To detect toxin, submit blood and stool culture to special laboratory (usually state health department)	Botulism caused by binding of toxin to the neuromuscular junction	Clinical presentation related to age and the strain of the botulism GI—abdominal pain, cramping, and diarrhea Other strains—respiratory compromise, CNS symptoms	Transmitted in contaminated food products Can be acquired via wound infection Treatment is supportive care and neutralization of the toxin
Staphylococcus organisms Gram-positive nonmotile, aerobic or facultative anaerobic bacteria Incubation—generally short, 1-8 hr Diagnosis—identify organism in food, blood, pus, aspirate	Direct tissue invasion and production of toxin	Clinical presentation dependent on site of entry In food poisoning, profuse diarrhea, nausea, and vomiting	Transmitted in inadequately cooked or refrigerated foods Self-limiting Symptomatic treatment

CNS, Central nervous system; *EIA,* enzyme immunoassay; *ELISA,* enzyme-linked immunosorbent assay; *GI,* gastrointestinal.

BOX 29-3 FACTORS THAT PREDISPOSE TO DIARRHEA

Age—As a rule, the younger the child, the greater the susceptibility and the more severe the diarrhea. Diarrhea occurs more commonly in infancy, is a lesser threat in early childhood, and usually constitutes only a minor problem in older children.

Impaired health—Malnourished or immunocompromised children are more susceptible and tend to have more severe diarrhea.

Environment—Diarrhea occurs with greater frequency where there is crowding, substandard sanitation, poor facilities for preparation and refrigeration of food, and generally inadequate health care education. The frequency of diarrhea in infancy is closely related to the ingestion of contaminated milk; breast-fed infants have a lower incidence of diarrhea.

BOX 29-4 CAUSES OF CHRONIC DIARRHEA*

Malabsorptive Causes
Celiac disease
Pancreatic insufficiency (cystic fibrosis, chronic pancreatitis, Shwachman syndrome)
Short-bowel syndrome
Lactose intolerance
Congenital enzyme deficiency (sucrase-isomaltase deficiency)

Allergic Causes
Allergic gastroenteropathy
Eosinophilic gastroenteritis

Immunodeficiency
Acquired hypoglobulinemia
Wiskott-Aldrich syndrome
Agammaglobulinemia
Severe combined immunodeficiency disease
Thymic hypoplasia
Selective immunoglobulin A deficiency
Human immunodeficiency virus or acquired immunodeficiency syndrome

Inflammatory Bowel Disease
Ulcerative colitis
Crohn disease

Endocrine Causes
Hyperthyroidism
Congenital adrenal hyperplasia
Addison disease

Motility Disorders
Hirschsprung disease
Intestinal pseudoobstruction

Parasitic Infestations
Ascaris organisms
Giardia organisms

Other Causes
Radiation enteritis
Protein-losing enteropathy (Ménétrier disease, intestinal lymphangiectasia)
Abdominal tumors

*See Chapter 33 for a discussion of chronic gastrointestinal disorders.

developed nations, viruses, primarily rotavirus, cause 70% to 80% of infectious diarrhea.

Rotavirus is the most important cause of serious gastroenteritis among children and a significant nosocomial (hospital-acquired) pathogen, accounting for 55,000 to 70,000 hospitalizations annually (Committee on Infectious Diseases, 2007; Centers for Disease Control and Prevention, 2008; Staat,

2006). Rotavirus disease is most severe in children 3 to 24 months of age. Children younger than 3 months of age have some protection from the disease because of maternally acquired antibodies. Approximately 25% of severe cases of rotavirus occur in older children (Coffin, 2001).

Salmonella, Shigella, and *Campylobacter* organisms are the most frequently isolated bacterial pathogens. *Salmonella* infection has the highest occurrence in infants; *Giardia* and *Shigella* infections have the highest incidence among toddlers. *Shigella* infection is uncommon in the United States, accounting for less than 5% of diarrheal illnesses in infants and toddlers. *Campylobacter* infection has a bimodal presentation (highest in children less than 12 months of age with a second rise in incidence at ages 15 to 19 years). *Giardia* and *Cryptosporidium* organisms are parasites. *Giardia* infection represents 15% of nondysenteric illness in the United States; *Cryptosporidium* infection is often associated with outbreaks in young children in daycare centers. *Plesiomonas* and *Yersinia* are also parasites that are frequently responsible for causing diarrhea that lasts more than 10 days in a previously healthy adolescent. (See also Intestinal Parasitic Diseases, Chapter 16.)

Antibiotic administration is frequently associated with diarrhea because antibiotics alter the normal intestinal flora, resulting in an overgrowth of other bacteria such as *Clostridium difficile.* Antibiotic-associated diarrhea can also be caused by *Salmonella* organisms, *Clostridium porringers* type A, and *Staphylococcus aureus* pathogens (Jabbar and Wright, 2003).

Pathophysiology

Invasion of the GI tract by pathogens results in increased intestinal secretion as a result of enterotoxins, cytotoxic mediators, or decreased intestinal absorption secondary to intestinal damage or inflammation. Enteric pathogens attach to the mucosal cells and form a cuplike pedestal on which the bacteria rest. The pathogenesis of the diarrhea depends on whether the organism remains attached to the cell surface, resulting in a secretory toxin (noninvasive, toxin-producing, noninflammatory type diarrhea), or penetrates the mucosa (systemic diarrhea). Noninflammatory diarrhea is the most common diarrheal illness, resulting from the action of enterotoxin that is released after attachment to the mucosa. The most serious and immediate physiologic disturbances associated with severe diarrheal disease are (1) dehydration, (2) acid-base imbalance with acidosis, and (3) shock that occurs when dehydration progresses to the point that circulatory status is seriously impaired.

Diagnostic Evaluation

Evaluation of the child with acute gastroenteritis begins with a careful history that seeks to discover the possible cause of diarrhea, to assess the severity of symptoms and the risk of complications, and to elicit information about current symptoms indicating other treatable illnesses that could be causing the diarrhea. The history should include questions about recent travel, exposure to untreated drinking or washing water sources, contact with animals or birds, daycare center attendance, recent treatment with antibiotics, or recent diet changes. History questions should also explore the presence of other symptoms such as fever and vomiting, frequency and character of stools (e.g., watery, bloody), urinary output, dietary habits, and recent food intake.

Extensive laboratory evaluation is not indicated in children who have uncomplicated diarrhea and no evidence of dehydration, since most diarrheal illnesses are self-limiting. Laboratory tests are indicated for children who are severely dehydrated and receiving intravenous (IV) therapy. Watery, explosive stools suggest glucose intolerance; foul-smelling, greasy, bulky stools suggest fat malabsorption. Diarrhea that develops after the introduction of cow's milk, fruits, or cereal may be related to enzyme deficiency or protein intolerance. Neutrophils or red blood cells in the stool indicate bacterial gastroenteritis or IBD. The presence of eosinophils suggests protein intolerance or parasitic infection. Perform stool cultures only when blood, mucus, or polymorphonuclear leukocytes are present in the stool, when symptoms are severe, when there is a history of travel to a developing country, and when a specific pathogen is suspected. Gross blood or occult blood may indicate pathogens such as *Shigella, Campylobacter,* or hemorrhagic *Escherichia coli* strains. Providers may use an enzyme-linked immunosorbent assay (ELISA) to confirm the presence of rotavirus or *Giardia* organisms. If there is a history of recent antibiotic use, test the stool for *C. difficile* toxin. When bacterial and viral cultures are negative and when diarrhea persists for more than a few days, examine stools for ova and parasites. A stool specimen with a pH of less than 6 and the presence of reducing substances may indicate carbohydrate malabsorption or secondary lactase deficiency. Stool electrolyte measurements may help identify children with secretory diarrhea.

Determine urine specific gravity if dehydration is suspected. Obtain a complete blood count, serum electrolytes, creatinine, and blood urea nitrogen (BUN) in the child who requires hospitalization. The hemoglobin, hematocrit, creatinine, and BUN levels are usually elevated in acute diarrhea and should normalize with rehydration.

Therapeutic Management

The major goals in the management of acute diarrhea include (1) assessment of fluid and electrolyte imbalance, (2) rehydration, (3) maintenance fluid therapy, and (4) reintroduction of an adequate diet. Treat infants and children with acute diarrhea and dehydration first with **oral rehydration therapy (ORT)**. ORT is one of the major worldwide health care advances. It is more effective, safer, less painful, and less costly than IV rehydration. The American Academy of Pediatrics, World Health Organization, and Centers for Disease Control and Prevention all recommend ORT as the treatment of choice for most cases of dehydration caused by diarrhea (Centers for Disease Control and Prevention, 2003) (Box 29-5). **Oral rehydration solutions (ORSs)** enhance and promote the reabsorption of sodium and water. These solutions greatly reduce vomiting, volume loss from diarrhea, and the duration of the illness. ORSs, including reduced osmolarity ORS, are available in the United States as commercially prepared solutions and are successful in treating the majority of infants with dehydration (Table 29-2). Guidelines for rehydration recommended by the American Academy of Pediatrics are given in Table 29-3.

QUALITY PATIENT OUTCOMES: Diarrhea
- Adequate hydration maintained during illness
- Appropriate diagnostic tests performed
- Antibiotics given only if appropriate
- No repeat visits to the emergency department or pediatrician during the course of the illness
- No tissue breakdown
- Normal elimination returns

After rehydration, ORS may be used during maintenance fluid therapy by alternating the solution with a low-sodium fluid such as water, breast milk, lactose-free formula, or half-strength lactose-containing formula. In older children ORS can be given and a regular diet continued. Ongoing stool losses should be replaced on a 1:1 basis with ORS. If the stool volume is not known, approximately 10 ml/kg (4 to 8 oz) of ORS should be given for each diarrheal stool.

Solutions for oral hydration are useful in most cases of dehydration, and vomiting is not a contraindication. Give a child who is vomiting an ORS at frequent intervals and in small amounts. For young children the caregiver may give the fluid with a spoon or small syringe in 5- to 10-ml increments every 1 to 5 minutes. An ORS may also be given via nasogastric or

---

BOX 29-5   MODEL FOR REHYDRATION

- Rehydration solution should consist of 75 to 90 mEq of sodium per liter.
- Give 40 to 50 ml/kg of rehydration solution over 4 hours.
- Replacement and maintenance solution should consist of 40 to 60 mEq of sodium per liter.
- Reevaluate the need for further rehydration; initiate maintenance therapy using maintenance formulations, with daily volumes not to exceed 150 ml/kg/day.
- In children with diarrhea without significant dehydration, the maintenance phase may be initiated without the need for rehydration solution.
- If additional fluids are needed, use low-salt fluids such as breast milk or water.

Modified from Centers for Disease Control and Prevention: Managing acute gastroenteritis among children: oral rehydration, maintenance, and nutritional therapy, *MMWR* 52(RR-16):1-16, 2003.

TABLE 29-2	COMPOSITION OF SOME ORAL REHYDRATION SOLUTIONS				
FORMULA	Na (mEq/L)	K (mEq/L)	CL (mEq/L)	BASE (mEq/L)	GLUCOSE (g/L)
Pedialyte (Abbott)*	45	20	35	30 (citrate)	25
Rehydralyte (Abbott)	75	20	65	30 (citrate)	25
Infalyte (Mead Johnson)	50	25	45	34 (citrate)	30
World Health Organization†	90	20	80	30 (bicarbonate)	20

Cl, Chloride; *K,* potassium; *Na,* sodium.
*Note that many generic products are available with compositions identical to Pedialyte.
†Must be reconstituted with 1 L water.

TABLE 29-3	TREATMENT OF ACUTE DIARRHEA			
DEGREE OF DEHYDRATION	SIGNS AND SYMPTOMS	REHYDRATION THERAPY*	REPLACEMENT OF STOOL LOSSES	MAINTENANCE THERAPY
Mild (5%-6%)	Increased thirst Slightly dry buccal mucous membranes	ORS, 50 ml/kg within 4 hr	ORS, 10 ml/kg (for infants) or 150-250 ml at a time (for older children) for each diarrheal stool	Breast-feeding, if established, should continue; give regular infant formula if tolerated. If lactose intolerance suspected, give undiluted lactose-free formula (or half-strength lactose-containing formula for brief period only); infants and children who receive solid food should continue their usual diet.
Moderate (7%-9%)	Loss of skin turgor, dry buccal mucous membranes, sunken eyes, sunken fontanel	ORS, 100 ml/kg within 4 hr	Same as above	
Severe (>9%)	Signs of moderate dehydration plus 1 of following: rapid thready pulse, cyanosis, rapid breathing, lethargy, coma	Intravenous fluids (Ringer lactate), 40 ml/kg/hr until pulse and state of consciousness return to normal; then 50-100 ml/kg or ORS	Same as above	

ORS, Oral rehydration solution.

*If no signs of dehydration are present, rehydration therapy is not necessary. Proceed with maintenance therapy and replacement of stool losses.

gastrostomy tube infusion. Infants without clinical signs of dehydration do not need ORT. They should, however, receive the same fluids recommended for infants with signs of dehydration in the maintenance phase and for ongoing stool losses. The use of probiotics reduces the risk of antibiotic-associated diarrhea in children by 56% (Szajewska, Ruszcynski, and Radzikowski, 2006).

> **! NURSING ALERT**
>
> Encouraging intake of clear fluids by mouth, such as fruit juices, carbonated soft drinks, and gelatin, does not help diarrhea. These fluids usually have a high carbohydrate content, a very low electrolyte content, and a high osmolality. Have patients avoid caffeinated soda because caffeine is a mild diuretic and may lead to increased loss of water and sodium. Chicken or beef broth is not given because it contains excessive sodium and inadequate carbohydrate. A BRAT diet (bananas, rice, applesauce, and toast or tea) is contraindicated for the child and especially for the infant with acute diarrhea, since this diet has little nutritional value (low in energy and protein), is high in carbohydrates, and is low in electrolytes (Centers for Disease Control and Prevention, 2003).

Early reintroduction of nutrients is desirable and is gaining more widespread acceptance. Continued feeding or early reintroduction of a normal diet has no adverse effects and actually lessens the severity and duration of the illness and improves weight gain when compared with the gradual reintroduction of foods (Zangwill, 2006). Infants who are breast-feeding should continue to do so, and ORS should be used to replace ongoing losses in these infants. Formula-fed infants should resume their formula; if it is not tolerated, a lactose-free formula may be used for a few days. In older children a regular diet, including milk, can generally be offered after rehydration has been achieved. In toddlers there is no contraindication to continuing soft or pureed foods. A diet of easily digestible foods such as cereals, cooked vegetables, and meats is adequate for the older child.

In cases of severe dehydration and shock, IV fluids are initiated whenever the child is unable to ingest sufficient amounts of fluid and electrolytes to (1) meet ongoing daily physiologic losses, (2) replace previous deficits, and (3) replace ongoing abnormal losses. Patients who usually require IV fluids are those with severe dehydration, those with uncontrollable vomiting, those who are unable to drink for any reason (e.g., extreme fatigue, coma), and those with severe gastric distention.

Select the IV solution on the basis of what is known regarding the probable type and cause of the dehydration. The type of fluid normally used is a saline solution containing 5% dextrose in water. Sodium bicarbonate may be added, since acidosis is usually associated with severe dehydration. Although the initial phase of fluid replacement is rapid in both isotonic and hypotonic dehydration, rapid replacement is contraindicated in hypertonic dehydration because of the risk of water intoxication, especially in the brain cells.

After the severe effects of dehydration are under control, begin specific diagnostic and therapeutic measures to detect and treat the cause of the diarrhea. Because of the self-limiting nature of vomiting and its tendency to improve when dehydration is corrected, the use of antiemetic agents is not recommended. The use of antibiotic therapy in children with acute gastroenteritis is controversial. Antibiotics may shorten the course of some diarrheal illnesses (e.g., those caused by *Shigella* organisms). However, most bacterial diarrheas are self-limiting, and the diarrhea often resolves before the causative organism can be determined. Antibiotics may prolong the carrier period for bacteria such as *Salmonella*. Antibiotics may be considered, however, in patients with immunosuppression, severe symptoms, or persistent disease or in patients who have had transplantation (Jabbar and Wright, 2003). (See Intestinal Parasitic Diseases, Chapter 16.)

Nursing Care Management

The management of most cases of acute diarrhea takes place in the home with education of the caregiver. Teach caregivers to monitor for signs of dehydration (especially the number of wet diapers or voidings) and the amount of fluids taken by mouth, and to assess the frequency and amount of stool losses (see Nursing Care Plan). Education relating to ORT, including the administration of maintenance fluids and replacement of ongoing losses, is important (see Critical Thinking Exercise). ORS should be administered in small quantities at frequent intervals. Vomiting is not a contraindication to ORT

◎ **NURSING CARE PLAN**

The Child with Acute Diarrhea

NURSING DIAGNOSIS	EXPECTED PATIENT OUTCOMES	NURSING INTERVENTIONS	RATIONALE
Deficient Fluid Volume related to diarrhea (gastrointestinal [GI]) losses, inadequate intake	Child will exhibit signs of adequate hydration.	Administer oral rehydration solutions (ORSs) for both rehydration and replacement of stool losses (see Table 29-2).	To rehydrate and replace stool losses
Child's/Family's Defining Characteristics (Subjective and Objective Data)	**The Following NOC Concepts Apply to These Outcomes**	Give ORS frequently (every 5-10 minutes) in small amounts (1-2 tsp), especially if child is vomiting (vomiting, unless severe, is not a contraindication to using ORS).	To prevent vomiting when large amounts of fluid are given at once
Dry mucous membranes	Nutritional Status: Food and Fluid Intake		
Loss of skin turgor	Weight Control	Administer and monitor intravenous (IV) fluids as prescribed (for severe dehydration and vomiting).	To treat severe dehydration and vomiting
Sunken eyes, sunken fontanel	Hydration		
Rapid, thready pulse; rapid breathing; lethargy		Administer antimicrobial agents as prescribed to treat specific pathogens causing excessive GI losses.	To treat specific identified pathogens causing excessive GI losses
Weakness		After rehydration, offer child regular diet as tolerated.	To reduce number of stools and weight loss and shorten duration of illness through early reintroduction of normal diet
		Alternate ORS with a low-sodium fluid such as water, breast milk, lactose-free formula, or half-strength lactose-containing formula for maintenance fluid therapy (see Table 29-3).	To provide maintenance fluid therapy
		Maintain strict record of fluid intake and output (urine, stool, and emesis).	To evaluate effectiveness of intervention
		Monitor urine specific gravity every 8 hours or as indicated to assess hydration.	To assess hydration status
		Weigh child daily.	To assess hydration status and observe for weight loss
		Assess vital signs, including temperature, skin turgor, mucous membranes, and mental status every 4 hours or as indicated.	To assess hydration status
		Administer antipyretics for fever.	To reduce fever and maintain comfort
		Discourage intake of (clear) fluids such as fruit juices, carbonated soft drinks, and gelatin (these fluids usually are high in carbohydrates, are low in electrolytes, and have a high osmolality); gelatin may be given once the child is rehydrated.	To provide fluids high in carbohydrates, low in electrolytes, and with a high osmolality
		Instruct family in providing appropriate therapy, monitoring intake and output, and assessing for signs of dehydration to ensure optimum results and improve compliance with the therapeutic regimen.	To ensure optimum results and improve compliance with the therapeutic regimen
		The Following NIC Concepts Apply to These Interventions	
		Nutrition Therapy	
		Nutritional Counseling	
		Nutritional Monitoring	
		Fluid Management	
		Fever Treatment	
		Diarrhea Management	

NURSING CARE PLAN—cont'd

The Child with Acute Diarrhea

NURSING DIAGNOSIS	EXPECTED PATIENT OUTCOMES	NURSING INTERVENTIONS	RATIONALE
Risk for Infection related to microorganisms invading GI tract	Child will not exhibit signs of GI infection.	Implement enteric isolation or other hospital infection control practices, including appropriate disposal of stool and laundry and appropriate handling of specimens.	To reduce risk of spreading infection
Child's/Family's Defining Characteristics (Subjective and Objective Data)	Infection will not spread systemically or to others.	Maintain frequent and careful hand washing.	To reduce risk of spreading infection
Loose stools	**The Following NOC Concept Applies to These Outcomes**	Use superabsorbent disposable diapers.	To contain feces and decrease chance of diaper dermatitis
Fever	Infection Status		
Lethargy		Obtain stool sample for cultures, ova, and parasites, as prescribed.	To identify organism causing illness
Decreased appetite		Attempt to keep infants and small children from placing hands to mouth and eyes (and objects in diaper area).	To reduce risk of spreading infection
Vomiting			
Stomach pain		Teach children, when possible, protective measures such as hand washing after using toilet.	To reduce risk of spreading infection
		Instruct family members and visitors in isolation practices, especially hand washing.	To reduce risk of spreading infection
		The Following NIC Concepts Apply to These Interventions Communicable Disease Management Environmental Management Skin Surveillance	

NURSING DIAGNOSIS	EXPECTED PATIENT OUTCOMES	NURSING INTERVENTIONS	RATIONALE
Impaired Skin Integrity related to irritation caused by frequent, loose stools	Child will have no evidence of skin breakdown.	Change diaper frequently.	To keep skin clean and dry
Child's/Family's Defining Characteristics (Subjective and Objective Data)	**The Following NOC Concepts Apply to These Outcomes**	Cleanse buttocks gently with bland, nonalkaline soap and water or immerse child in a bath for gentle cleansing.	To eliminate bacteria in diarrheal stools, which are highly irritating to skin
Excoriated skin	Tissue Integrity	Apply barrier ointment such as zinc oxide to area.	To protect skin from irritation
Skin breakdown	Wound Healing	Expose slightly reddened intact skin to air whenever possible.	To promote healing
Pain		Avoid using commercial baby wipes containing alcohol on excoriated skin.	To avoid stinging
		Observe buttocks and perineum for infection.	To initiate appropriate therapy
		Apply appropriate antifungal medication if infection is present.	To treat fungal infection of skin
		The Following NIC Concepts Apply to These Interventions Infection Control Infection Protection Skin Care: Topical Treatments Medication Administration: Skin Skin Surveillance Teaching: Procedure/Treatment	

unless it is severe. Information concerning the introduction of a normal diet is essential. Parents need to know that a slightly higher stool output initially occurs with continuation of a normal diet and with ongoing replacement of stool losses. The benefits of a better nutritional outcome with fewer complications and a shorter duration of illness outweigh the potential increase in stool frequency. Address parents' concerns to ensure adherence to the treatment plan.

If the child with acute diarrhea and dehydration is hospitalized, the nurse must obtain an accurate weight and carefully monitor intake and output. The child may be placed on parenteral fluid therapy with nothing by mouth for 12 to 48 hours. Monitoring the IV infusion is an important nursing function. The nurse must ensure that the correct fluid and electrolyte concentration is infused, that the flow rate is adjusted to deliver the desired volume in a given time, and that the IV site is maintained.

Accurate measurement of output is essential to determine whether renal blood flow is sufficient to permit the addition of potassium to the IV fluids. The nurse is responsible for examination of stools and collection of specimens for laboratory examination. (See Collection of Specimens, Chapter 27.) Take

❓ CRITICAL THINKING EXERCISE

Diarrhea

A mother brings her 8-month-old infant, Mary, to the primary care clinic. The mother reports that Mary has had a "cold" for about 2 days, and this morning she began to vomit and has had diarrhea for the past 8 hours. The mother states that Mary is still breast-feeding, but that she is not taking as much fluid as usual and she is having three times as many stools as usual (the stools are watery). When the nurse practitioner examines Mary, she notes that her temperature is 38° C (100.4° F), her pulse and blood pressure are in the normal range, her mucous membranes are moist, and she has tears when she cries. The nurse practitioner also notes that Mary's weight has not changed from what it was when she was seen in the clinic 2 weeks ago for her well-child visit. What interventions should the nurse practitioner include in her initial management of Mary?

1. Evidence—Is there sufficient evidence for the nurse practitioner to draw any conclusions for her initial plan of management?
2. Assumptions—Describe some underlying assumptions about the following:
   a. Clinical manifestations of various levels of dehydration
   b. Management of acute diarrhea
   c. Breast-feeding and the management of acute diarrhea
   d. Use of antidiarrheal medications for acute diarrhea
3. What nursing interventions should the nurse practitioner implement at this time?
4. Does the evidence support your conclusion?

care when obtaining and transporting stools to prevent possible spread of infection. Use a clean tongue depressor to obtain specimens for laboratory examination or as an applicator for transfer to a culture medium. Transport stool specimens to the laboratory in appropriate containers and media according to hospital policy.

Diarrheal stools are highly irritating to the skin, and extra care is necessary to protect the skin of the diaper region from excoriation. (See Diaper Dermatitis, Chapter 13.) Avoid taking temperatures rectally because they stimulate the bowel, increasing passage of stool.

Support for the child and family involves the same care and consideration given all hospitalized children. (See Chapter 26.) Keep parents informed of the child's progress and instruct them in the use of frequent and proper hand washing and the disposal of soiled diapers, clothes, and bed linen. Everyone caring for the child must be aware of "clean" areas and "dirty" areas, especially in the hospital, where the sink in the child's room is used for many purposes. Discard soiled diapers and linen in receptacles close to the bedside. To remind caregivers to keep diapers and other soiled articles away from clean areas, place signs identifying "clean" (e.g., bed table) and "dirty" (e.g., sink, bathroom) areas. List the articles that may be stored in each area on these signs.

Prevention

The best intervention for diarrhea is prevention. The fecal-oral route spreads most infections, and parents need information about preventive measures such as personal hygiene, protection of the water supply from contamination, and careful food preparation.

Meticulous attention to perianal hygiene, disposal of soiled diapers, proper hand washing, and isolation of infected persons

also minimizes the transmission of infection. (See Infection Control, Chapter 27.)

Parents need information about preventing diarrhea while traveling. Caution them against giving their children adult medications that are used to prevent traveler's diarrhea. Until vaccines or other prophylactic measures are safe for children, the best measure during travel to areas where water may be contaminated is to allow children to drink only bottled water and carbonated beverages (from the container through a straw supplied from home). Children should also avoid tap water, ice, unpasteurized dairy products, raw vegetables, unpeeled fruits, meats, and seafood.

❗ NURSING ALERT

To reduce the risk of bacteria transmitted via food, encourage parents to:
- Quickly freeze or refrigerate all ground meat and other perishable foods.
- Never thaw food on the counter or let it sit out of the refrigerator for more than 2 hours.
- Wash hands, utensils, and work areas with hot, soapy water after contact with raw meat to keep bacteria from spreading.
- Check ground meat with a fork to make certain no pink is showing before taking a bite.
- Cook all dishes made with ground meat until brown or gray inside or to an internal temperature of 71° C (160° F).

VOMITING

Vomiting is the forceful ejection of gastric contents through the mouth. It is a well-defined, complex, coordinated process that is under central nervous system control and is usually accompanied by nausea and retching. In contrast, regurgitation is a simpler, more passive, and effortless phenomenon. Vomiting has many causes, including acute infectious diseases, increased intracranial pressure (ICP), toxic ingestions, food intolerances and allergies, mechanical obstruction of the GI tract, metabolic disorders, and psychogenic problems (Acker, 2002). Vomiting is common in childhood, is usually self-limiting, and requires no specific treatment. However, complications can occur in children, including dehydration and electrolyte disturbances, malnutrition, aspiration, and Mallory-Weiss syndrome (small tears in the distal esophageal mucosa).

Etiology

The child's age, pattern of vomiting, and duration of symptoms help determine the cause. For example, chronic and intermittent episodes of vomiting may indicate malrotation, whereas vomiting on a specific day at the same time before school is not likely to be a result of organic disease. The color and consistency of the emesis vary according to the cause. Green, bilious vomiting suggests bowel obstruction. Curdled stomach contents, mucus, or fatty foods that are vomited several hours after ingestion suggest poor gastric emptying or high intestinal obstruction. Gastric irritation by certain medicines, foods, or toxic substances may cause vomiting.

Associated symptoms also help identify the cause. Fever and diarrhea accompanying vomiting suggest an infection. Constipation associated with vomiting suggests an anatomic or functional obstruction. Localized abdominal pain and vomiting often occur with appendicitis, pancreatitis, or peptic ulcer disease. A change in the level of consciousness or a headache associated with vomiting indicates a central nervous system or metabolic disorder. Forceful vomiting is associated with pyloric stenosis.

Pathophysiology

The act of vomiting, including nausea and retching, is under control of the central nervous system. Two areas of the medulla are involved as the vomiting center. The medullary center is also activated by impulses from a second center, the chemoreceptor trigger zone, which is located in the floor of the fourth ventricle (Box 29-6). Nausea is a sensation that may be induced by visceral, labyrinthine (inner ear), or emotional stimuli. It is characterized by the desire to vomit, with discomfort felt in the throat or abdomen. Nausea is often associated with autonomic symptoms such as salivation, pallor, sweating, and tachycardia. Retching may occur with or without vomiting. Retching involves a series of spasmodic movements during inspiration, creating a negative intrathoracic pressure, and contraction of the abdominal muscles. Projectile vomiting is preceded and accompanied by vigorous peristaltic waves.

Vomiting is a well-recognized response to psychologic stress. During stress, adrenaline levels rise and may stimulate the chemoreceptor trigger zone. Nausea and vomiting are likely a protective mechanism to remove toxins from the system. Vomiting may follow GI infection or toxic ingestion, or it can be a learned behavioral response.

Cyclic vomiting syndrome is a rare disorder characterized by bouts of vomiting that can last from hours to several days (McRonald and Fleisher, 2005). The cause of this syndrome is unknown (Bullard and Page, 2005).

Diagnostic Evaluation

The diagnostic evaluation includes a thorough history and physical examination. The description of the vomitus; relationship to meals or specific foods; behavior; and presence of pain, constipation, diarrhea, or jaundice are important components of the history. Physical examination should include an assessment of the hydration status and an abdominal examination.

Further evaluation may include analysis of urine for protein or blood, serum electrolytes, and radiographic studies. A plain radiograph of the chest or abdomen or ultrasonography may reveal anatomic abnormalities. Brain scans are used to detect tumors. Endoscopy of the upper GI tract may be a valuable diagnostic procedure if the provider suspects esophagitis. A psychiatric evaluation may be indicated if cyclic vomiting, anorexia nervosa, bulimia, or self-poisoning is present. Self-induced vomiting and rumination may be a self-stimulation or gratification activity.

Therapeutic Management

Direct the management of vomiting toward detection and treatment of the cause of the vomiting and prevention of complications such as dehydration and malnutrition. Vomiting is often a symptom of a common infectious illness that is self-limiting and resolves with no specific treatment. Further investigation is indicated if there is dehydration, progressively severe vomiting, or persistent vomiting for more than 24 hours, or if the history and physical examination fail to suggest a diagnosis. If vomiting leads to dehydration, oral rehydration or parenteral fluids may be required.

Antiemetic drugs may be indicated when the vomiting can be anticipated, is of limited duration, and has a known cause. Limited adverse effects are rare with antiemetic use for vomiting in children (Li, DiGiuseppe, and Christakis, 2003). Antiemetic drugs may block the receptors in the chemoreceptor trigger zone (ondansetron [Zofran] or trimethobenzamide [Tigan]), enhance gastroduodenal peristalsis (metoclopramide [Reglan]), or compete for H_1-receptor sites (promethazine [Phenergan]). For children who are prone to motion sickness, it is often helpful to administer an appropriate dose of dimenhydrinate (Dramamine) before a trip (see Evidence-Based Practice box).

Nursing Care Management

The major emphasis of nursing care of the vomiting infant or child is on observation and reporting of vomiting behavior and associated symptoms and on the implementation of measures to reduce the vomiting. Accurate assessment of the type of vomiting, appearance of the vomitus, and the child's behavior in association with the vomiting greatly aids in establishing a diagnosis of disorders that have vomiting as a clinical feature.

The cause of the vomiting determines the nursing intervention. When the vomiting is a manifestation of improper feeding methods, establishing proper techniques through teaching and example ordinarily corrects the situation. If the vomiting is a probable sign of GI obstruction, the nurse usually withholds food or implements special feeding techniques. When vomiting is related to concurrent infection, dietary indiscretion, or emotional factors, direct efforts toward maintaining hydration or preventing dehydration.

The thirst mechanism is the most sensitive guide to fluid needs, and ad libitum administration of a glucose-electrolyte solution to an alert child restores water and electrolytes satisfactorily. It is important to include carbohydrates to spare body protein and to avoid ketosis resulting from exhaustion of glycogen stores. Small, frequent feedings of fluids or foods are preferable and more effective. Once vomiting has abated, offer more liberal amounts of fluids, followed by gradual resumption of the regular diet.

EVIDENCE-BASED PRACTICE

Use of Antiemetics in Children with Acute Gastroenteritis

ASK THE QUESTION

In children with acute gastroenteritis (AGE), should antiemetics be used?

SEARCH FOR THE EVIDENCE

Search strategies

Search criteria included English-language publications within the past 2 years (2006 to 2008), research-based articles (level 3 or lower) on children with AGE.

Databases used

PubMed/Medline, CINAHL, Cochrane, Google Scholar, UpToDate, National Guideline Clearinghouse (AHRQ), American Academy of Pediatrics, Cincinnati Children's Hospital Medical Center, University of Michigan, Emory University School of Medicine, Canadian Medical Association, Scottish Intercollegiate Guidelines Network, New Zealand Guideline Group, National Institute of Health and Clinical Excellence, European Society for Paediatric Gastroenterology, Hepatology, and Nutrition, Joanna Briggs Institute

CRITICALLY ANALYZE THE EVIDENCE

GRADE criteria: Evidence quality moderate; recommendation strong (Guyatt, Oxman, Vist, et al, 2008)

A review of the literature revealed four studies evaluating the use of antiemetics in the treatment of children with AGE. Findings from the studies support the use of an antiemetic in children with AGE who are vomiting.

- A systematic review consisting of 11 studies (6 of which were randomized controlled trials [RCTs]) examined the use of antiemetics (e.g., ondansetron [Zofran], domperidone, trimethobenzamide, pyrilamine-pentobarbital, metoclopramide, dexamethasone, promethazine) and whether or not they reduced vomiting and decreased the need for further intervention in children with AGE without causing significant adverse effects. A meta-analysis was conducted using the data from the RCTs (N = 745, age range: 1 month to 22 years). These results showed that ondansetron therapy decreases the risk of persistent vomiting, the use of intravenous fluid, and hospital admissions in children with vomiting due to AGE in comparison to a control group. However, diarrheal episodes increased in three of the RCTs (DeCamp, Byerley, Doshi, et al, 2008).
- Alhashimi, Alhashimi, and Fedorowicz (2006) included three RCTs in their systematic review and evaluated the effectiveness of antiemetics on gastroenteritis-induced vomiting in children and adolescents (N = 396, age < 18 years). Results indicated that ondansetron may reduce the amount of acute vomiting and reduce the number of children who required intravenous rehydration and hospital admission for AGE.
- In a meta-analysis conducted by Szajewska, Gieruszczak-Bialek, and Dylag (2007) ondansetron was effective in reducing the need for intravenous rehydration. Four RCTs were included with a sample size of 490 children who were vomiting as a result of AGE.
- Similarly, Roslund, Hepps, and McQuillen (2008) found that children who receive oral ondansetron were more likely to tolerate oral rehydration, less likely to receive intravenous hydration, and less like to be admitted to a hospital in comparison to children who did not receive ondansetron. These authors conducted a double-blind, placebo-controlled RCT studying children with acute gastritis or gastroenteritis who had failed oral rehydration therapy. A total of 106 children were studied, ranging from 1 to 10 years old.

APPLY THE EVIDENCE: NURSING IMPLICATIONS

Ondansetron reduces the amount and duration of vomiting and should be used for children with AGE who are seen with vomiting. The number of children requiring intravenous rehydration and hospital admission for AGE is also reduced with administration of antiemetics.

References

Alhashimi D, Alhashimi H, Fedorowicz Z: Antiemetics for reducing vomiting related to acute gastroenteritis in children and adolescents, *Cochrane Database Syst Rev* (4):CD005506. DOI:10.1002/14651858. CD005506.pub3, 2006.

DeCamp LR, Byerley JS, Doshi N, et al: Use of antiemetic agents in acute gastroenteritis: a systematic review and meta-analysis, *Arch Pediatr Adolesc Med* 162(9):858-865, 2008.

Guyatt GH, Oxman AD, Vist GE, et al: GRADE: an emerging consensus on rating quality of evidence and strength of recommendations, *BMJ* 336:924-926, 2008.

Roslund G, Hepps T, McQuillen K: The role of oral ondansetron in children with vomiting as a result of acute gastritis/gastroenteritis who have failed oral rehydration therapy: a randomized controlled trial, *Ann Emerg Med* 52(1):22-29, 2008.

Szajewska H, Gieruszczak-Bialek D, Dylag M: Meta-analysis: ondansetron for vomiting in acute gastroenteritis, *Aliment Pharmacol Ther* 25:393-400, 2007.

Position the infant or child who is vomiting to prevent aspiration and observe him or her for evidence of dehydration. It is important to emphasize the need for the child to brush the teeth or rinse the mouth after vomiting to dilute the hydrochloric acid that comes in contact with the teeth. Carefully monitor fluid and electrolyte status to avoid the possibility of electrolyte imbalance.

SHOCK STATES

SHOCK

Shock, or circulatory failure, is a complex clinical syndrome characterized by tissue perfusion that is inadequate to meet the metabolic demands of the body, which results in cellular dysfunction and eventual organ failure. Although the causes are different, the physiologic consequences are the same: hypotension, tissue hypoxia, and metabolic acidosis.

Etiology

The most common type of circulatory failure in children is **hypovolemic shock**, which follows a reduction in circulating blood volume related to blood loss (e.g., trauma, major bleeding), plasma losses (e.g., burns, peritonitis), or extracellular fluid losses (e.g., diarrhea, dehydration) beyond the child's physiologic ability to compensate. **Cardiogenic shock** results from impaired cardiac muscle function that leads to decreased cardiac output. It is uncommon in children but may be seen after cardiac surgery and in children with acute dysrhythmias, congestive heart failure, or cardiomyopathy. **Distributive shock**, or vasogenic shock, results from a vascular abnormality that produces maldistribution of blood supply throughout the body. This term includes (1) neurogenic shock, characterized by massive vasodilation resulting from the loss of sympathetic nervous system tone, which can occur with spinal cord injuries; (2) anaphylactic shock, which is characterized by a hypersensitivity reaction that causes massive vasodilation and capillary leak and may occur with drug or latex allergy, insect stings, or blood transfusion; and (3) septic shock, characterized by a decreased cardiac output and derangements in the peripheral circulation in response to a severe, overwhelming infection. Obstructive shock may resemble hypovolemic shock but is caused by cardiac tamponade, tension pneumothorax, ductal-dependent congenital heart lesions, or massive pulmonary embolism. The types of shock are described in Box 29-7 (Ralston, Hazinski, Zaritsky, et al, 2006).

Pathophysiology

The circulatory system of the healthy child is able to transport oxygen and nutrients to meet the essential needs of body tissues and can respond to increased demands resulting from an elevated metabolic rate. The cardiac output and distribution to the various body tissues can change rapidly in response to intrinsic (myocardial and intravascular) or extrinsic (neuronal) control mechanisms. In shock states these mechanisms are altered or challenged.

Reduced blood flow, as in hypovolemic shock, causes diminished venous return to the heart, low central venous pressure (CVP), low cardiac output, and hypotension. The reduced intravascular volume triggers a chain of compensatory mechanisms. Fluid is mobilized from the extracellular compartment. Vasomotor centers in the medulla are signaled, causing depressed vagal activity and increased sympathetic activity, which increase the force and rate of cardiac contraction and constrict the arterioles and veins, thereby increasing peripheral vascular resistance.

Simultaneously the lowered blood volume also leads to the release of large amounts of catecholamines, antidiuretic hormone, adrenocorticosteroids, and aldosterone in an effort to conserve body fluids. The catecholamines augment the vasomotor activity to produce vasoconstriction and reduce blood flow to the skin, kidneys, muscles, and splanchnic viscera in order to shunt the available blood to the brain and heart. Consequently, the skin feels cold and clammy, there is poor capillary filling, and glomerular filtration and urinary output are significantly reduced.

Impaired perfusion to the peripheral tissues also produces metabolic alterations. Oxygen depletion causes the cells to revert to anaerobic glycolytic metabolism, forming pyruvic acid; pyruvic acid is then converted to lactic acid, producing lactic acidosis. The acidosis places an extra burden on the lungs as they attempt to compensate for the metabolic acidosis by increasing the respiratory rate. Impaired cellular uptake and metabolism of glucose create an early, transient hyperglycemia. When plasma fluid is lost, hemoconcentration and diminished blood flow increase the viscosity of the blood and further impair perfusion.

Prolonged vasoconstriction results in fatigue, and the release of vasodilator substances such as histamine leads to vasodilation. Venules, which are less sensitive to vasodilator substances, remain constricted for a time. This causes massive pooling in

the capillary and venular beds and transudation of plasma fluid into the tissues, which further depletes blood volume.

Complications of shock create further hazards. Central nervous system hypoperfusion may eventually lead to cerebral edema, cortical infarction, or intraventricular hemorrhage. Renal hypoperfusion causes renal ischemia with possible tubular or glomerular necrosis and renal vein thrombosis. Reduced blood flow to the lungs can interfere with surfactant secretion and result in shock lung or acute respiratory distress syndrome (ARDS). ARDS is characterized by sudden

---

BOX 29-7 **TYPES OF SHOCK**

Hypovolemic Shock
Characteristics
Reduction in size of vascular compartment
Falling blood pressure
Poor capillary filling
Low central venous pressure

Most Common Causes
Blood loss (hemorrhagic shock)—Trauma, gastrointestinal bleeding, intracranial hemorrhage
Plasma loss—Increased capillary permeability associated with sepsis and acidosis, hypoproteinemia, burns, peritonitis
Extracellular fluid loss—Vomiting, diarrhea, glycosuric diuresis, sunstroke

Distributive Shock
Characteristics
Reduction in peripheral vascular resistance
Profound inadequacies in tissue perfusion
Increased venous capacity and pooling
Acute reduction in return blood flow to the heart
Diminished cardiac output

Most Common Causes
Anaphylaxis (anaphylactic shock)—Extreme allergy or hypersensitivity to a foreign substance
Sepsis (septic shock, bacteremic shock, endotoxic shock)—Overwhelming sepsis and circulating bacterial toxins
Loss of neuronal control (neurogenic shock)—Interruption of neuronal transmission (spinal cord injury)
Myocardial depression and peripheral dilation—Exposure to anesthesia or ingestion of barbiturates, tranquilizers, narcotics, antihypertensive agents, or ganglionic blocking agents

Cardiogenic Shock
Characteristic
Decreased cardiac output

Most Common Causes
Following surgery for congenital heart disease
Primary pump failure—Myocarditis, myocardial trauma, biochemical derangements, congestive heart failure
Dysrhythmias—Paroxysmal atrial tachycardia, atrioventricular block, ventricular dysrhythmias; secondary to myocarditis or biochemical abnormalities

Obstructive Shock
Characteristics
Elevated central venous pressure and venous congestion with poor perfusion

Most Common Causes
Cardiac tamponade
Tension pneumothorax
Ductal-dependent congenital heart lesions
Massive pulmonary embolism

From Ralston M, Hazinski MF, Zaritsky AL, et al, editors: *Pediatric life support*, Dallas, 2006, American Heart Association.

pulmonary congestion and atelectasis with formation of a hyaline membrane. (See Chapter 32.) GI tract bleeding and perforation are always a possibility following splanchnic ischemia and necrosis of intestinal mucosa. Metabolic complications of shock may include hypoglycemia, hypocalcemia, and other electrolyte disturbances.

Shock syndromes characterized by vascular abnormalities (distributive shock) have a somewhat different pathophysiologic pattern of hemodynamic collapse. In neurogenic shock, the sympathetic nervous system mechanisms that maintain vascular tone are interrupted, causing reduced vascular resistance and peripheral pooling of blood; with this increased vascular capacity there is loss of effective circulating blood volume. Septic shock produces a hyperdynamic state in which there is often an elevated plasma volume and reduced peripheral resistance that lead to widespread vasodilation. In many cases there is a high cardiac output caused by the vasodilation in infected tissues and elsewhere, plus a high metabolic rate resulting from the elevated body temperature. Degenerating tissues cause aggregation of red blood cells and sludging of the blood. Development of disseminated intravascular coagulation, triggered by either the degenerating tissue or bacterial toxins, consumes the clotting factors and produces widespread hemorrhages. (See Chapter 35.)

Clinical Manifestations

Shock can be regarded as a form of compensation for circulatory failure and, because of its progressive nature, can be divided into three stages or phases: compensated, decompensated, and irreversible. At all stages the principal differentiating signs are the (1) degree of tachycardia and perfusion to extremities, (2) level of consciousness, and (3) blood pressure (BP). Additional signs or modifications of these more universal signs may be present depending on the type and cause of the shock.

Compensated Shock

When vital organ function is maintained by intrinsic mechanisms and the child's ability to compensate is effective, cardiac output and systemic arterial BP are usually normal or increased. However, blood flow is generally uneven or maldistributed in the microcirculation. Early clinical signs are subtle and include apprehension, irritability, normal BP, narrowing pulse pressure, thirst, pallor, and diminished urinary output.

> **! NURSING ALERT**
>
> Unexplained mild tachycardia and a decrease in perfusion of the hands and feet are differentiating features of compensated shock.

Decompensated Shock

As shock progresses, perfusion in the microcirculation becomes marginal despite compensatory adjustments, and the signs are more obvious and indicate early decompensation. These signs are tachypnea; moderate metabolic acidosis; oliguria; and cool, pale extremities with decreased skin turgor and poor capillary filling. The outcomes of circulatory failure that progress beyond the limits of compensation are tissue hypoxia, metabolic acidosis, and eventual dysfunction of all organ systems.

> **! NURSING ALERT**
>
> In decompensated shock, tachycardia is pronounced; BP is maintained, but pulse pressure (difference between systolic and diastolic BP) becomes narrowed. There is poor capillary filling, and the child exhibits confusion, sleepiness, and decreased responsiveness.

Irreversible Shock

Irreversible, or terminal, shock implies damage to vital organs (e.g., the heart or brain) of such magnitude that the entire system is disrupted regardless of therapeutic intervention. There is pronounced systemic vasoconstriction and hypoxia of visceral and cutaneous circulations with hypotension, acidosis, lethargy or coma, and oliguria or anuria. The child is totally obtunded. A thready and weak pulse, hypotension, periodic breathing or apnea, anuria, and stupor or coma are signs of impending cardiopulmonary arrest. Death occurs even if cardiovascular measurements return to normal levels with therapy.

Diagnostic Evaluation

The nurse can discern the cause of shock from the history and physical examination. The extent of the shock is determined by measurement of vital signs, including CVP and capillary filling. Laboratory tests that assist in assessment are blood gas measurements, pH, and sometimes liver function tests. Coagulation status (prothrombin time, partial thromboplastin time, platelet count, fibrinogen, fibrin) is evaluated when there is evidence of bleeding, such as oozing from a venipuncture site, bleeding from any orifice, petechiae, or purpura. Cultures of blood and other sites are indicated when there is a high suspicion of sepsis. Perform renal function tests when impaired renal function is evident.

Therapeutic Management

⊖ Treatment of shock consists of three major thrusts: (1) ventilation, (2) fluid administration, and (3) improvement of the pumping action of the heart (vasopressor support). The first priority is to establish an airway and administer oxygen. Once the airway is ensured, circulatory stabilization is the major concern. Placement of one or more multilumen central lines, preferably above the diaphragm (to deliver drugs closer to the heart and limit tissue injury from caustic medications), is a priority in shock (Jindal, Hollenberg, and Dellinger, 2000). These lines are needed for rapid volume replacement, administration of vasoactive drugs, and hemodynamic monitoring. An alternative is rapid surgical cutdown cannulation of the saphenous vein. The vein is anatomically accessible, can accommodate the volumes of fluid needed, and is situated where it does not interfere with any necessary resuscitation procedures. Another effective emergency method is intraosseous administration of fluids. (See Chapter 28.)

Ventilatory Support

The lung is the organ most sensitive to shock. The decrease in or redistribution of blood flow to respiratory muscles plus the increased work of breathing can rapidly lead to respiratory failure. Critically ill patients are unable to maintain an adequate airway. To place the lung at rest and improve ventilation, endotracheal intubation is initiated early with positive-pressure ventilation and supplemental oxygen. Blood gases, oxygen saturation (using pulse oximetry), and pH are monitored frequently.

Increased extravascular lung water caused by edema—both hydrostatic and permeable—contributes to the development of respiratory complications. Hydrostatic edema occurs from the elevation of pulmonary microvascular pressure as a result of left ventricular dysfunction; permeable edema occurs when damage to alveolar cell and pulmonary capillary epithelium causes fluid to leak into the interstitial space, resulting in ARDS. (See Chapter 32.) Direct therapy toward maintaining normal arterial blood gas measurements, normal acid-base balance, and circulation. Make efforts to remove fluid and prevent its accumulation by increasing oncotic pressure and decreasing microvascular hydrostatic pressure. Promote elevated oncotic pressure by diuresis with furosemide or mannitol, colloid administration, or both.

Cardiac Support

In many cases rapid restoration of blood volume is the main therapy needed in the resuscitation of the child in shock. An isotonic crystalloid solution (normal saline or lactated Ringer's solution) is usually the first choice for fluid replacement. Crystalloid is given in IV boluses of 10 to 20 ml/kg over 10 to 15 minutes and repeated as necessary. The child's response is assessed after each bolus. An increase in BP and a decrease in heart rate indicate successful resuscitation. An increased cardiac output results in improved capillary circulation and skin color. Colloids (protein-containing fluids) are often administered to children in shock; albumin is the most common. Because albumin is a protein solution, it remains in the vascular space much longer than crystalloid fluids. A smaller volume of albumin can be given to increase intravascular volume and support cardiac output; with crystalloid fluids, a larger volume is needed to achieve the same effect. In general, because of the infectious risks, blood is administered only in situations of known blood loss, active bleeding, or markedly decreased hematocrit. Fresh-frozen plasma is used to correct coagulopathies, not as volume replacement.

For the critically ill child with shock and multisystem organ dysfunction, more aggressive monitoring is necessary. Central venous measurements of right atrial pressure or pulmonary wedge pressure help guide fluid therapy. In children with persistent shock, place a Swan-Ganz catheter for more accurate monitoring. Determination of arterial blood gases, hematocrit, serum electrolytes, glucose, and calcium concentrations provides additional information concerning composition of circulating blood. Correction of acidosis, hypoxemia, and any metabolic derangements is mandatory.

Vasopressor Support

Temporary pharmacologic support may be required to enhance myocardial contractility, reverse metabolic or respiratory acidosis, and maintain arterial pressure. The principal agents used to improve cardiac output and circulation are the exogenous catecholamines, administered by constant infusion pump. Dopamine is the preferred drug in most situations because it also improves renal perfusion. Other agents (e.g., dobutamine,

⚡ **DRUG ALERT**

Vasodilators

> Vasodilator medications are often used in combination with vasopressors. Common vasodilators are nitroprusside, inamrinone, and hydralazine. It is important that the patient have adequate circulating blood volume before administering vasodilators.

isoproterenol, epinephrine) may be used to improve cardiac output, depending on the situation.

Metabolic acidosis is usually corrected with adequate tissue perfusion and improved renal function. This is accomplished with adequate ventilatory support, including oxygen, and restoration of blood volume and peripheral circulation. Sodium bicarbonate may also be administered to correct acidosis resulting from shock. It should be given in small boluses that are diluted to avoid acute changes in osmolality. The major complications of bicarbonate administration are sodium overload and hyperosmolality.

Calcium chloride may be administered to improve cardiac function and to offset the reduced ionized calcium associated with large amounts of albumin, whole blood, or fresh-frozen plasma. Diuretics, such as furosemide (Lasix), cause a reduction in ventricular filling pressures without changing cardiac output or heart rate and promote sodium and water excretion by the kidney in cases in which pulmonary congestion is a problem.

Other Therapies

Peritoneal dialysis may be necessary if hyperkalemia, acidosis, hypervolemia, or altered mental status occurs. Nutritional support is provided by both enteral and parenteral routes. Prevention of infection is a primary concern because host resistance is depressed in patients in shock. Other complicating disorders, such as disseminated intravascular coagulation and GI problems (e.g., paralytic ileus, stress ulceration), are managed appropriately. The intraaortic balloon pump may be used for a child with low cardiac output who is refractory to conventional medical management. Extracorporeal membrane oxygenation, where available, is used occasionally as a last resort.

Nursing Care Management

The child in shock requires observation and care, preferably in an intensive care environment. The initial action in caring for the child in shock is ensuring adequate tissue oxygenation (see Emergency Treatment box). The nurse should be prepared to administer oxygen by the appropriate route and to assist with any indicated intubation and ventilation procedures. Other procedures and activities that require immediate attention are establishing an IV line, estimating body weight (for calculating drug dosages), obtaining baseline vital signs, placing an indwelling urinary catheter, obtaining blood gas and other measurements, and administering medications as indicated.

The child is best positioned flat with the legs elevated. Hypotensive patients show no benefit from the traditional Trendelenburg position. Head-down positioning tends to increase ICP, decrease diaphragmatic excursion and lung volume, and decrease venous return to the heart because of the altered thoracic pressure. Elevating the lower extremities

✚ EMERGENCY TREATMENT

Shock

Ventilation
Establish airway; be prepared for intubation.
Administer oxygen, usually 100% by mask.

Fluid Administration
Restore blood or fluid volume as ordered.

Cardiovascular Support
Administer vasopressors (epinephrine 1:1000, 0.01 mg/kg subcutaneously; maximum dose of 0.5 mg; may repeat if needed).

General Support
Keep child flat with legs raised above level of heart.
Keep child warm and calm.

QUALITY PATIENT OUTCOMES: Shock
- Oxygen content of blood optimized
- Cardiac output improved
- Oxygen demand reduced
- Metabolic abnormalities corrected
- Type of shock identified and treated

❗ NURSING ALERT

When shock is a likely complication, the child is observed carefully for early signs, such as irritability, unexplained increase in heart rate, thirst, pallor, or diminished urinary output. The appearance of any of these signs requires further evaluation and initiation of therapy.

---

decreases pooling in the extremities, thereby returning blood supply to the heart.

The nurse's responsibilities are to monitor vital signs (BP in particular); monitor intake and output; and perform a general assessment of the level of consciousness, circulatory perfusion, and parenteral infusion sites. The nurse titrates IV medications according to patient responses and obtains vital signs every 15 minutes during the critical periods and thereafter as needed. Measure urinary output hourly, and monitor blood gases, hematocrit, pH, and electrolytes frequently to assess the child's status and the efficacy of therapy. Apnea and cardiac monitors are attached and monitored continuously. Oxygen saturation monitors provide continuous measurement of oxygenation. In the initial stages of acute shock, care of the child often requires more than one nurse because of all the activities that must be carried out simultaneously.

Family Support

Throughout the intense activity, do not overlook the parents. A member of the staff, such as a nurse, social worker, or clergy, may be called to provide comfort and support. If the family is not at the hospital, someone should contact them at frequent intervals to inform them about what is being done and whether there is any improvement. Ideally, someone should remain with the parents to serve as a liaison between them and the intensive care team. However, this is not always feasible in such a critical situation. As soon as possible, the parents should be allowed to see the child.

BOX 29-8 DEFINITIONS OF SYSTEMIC INFLAMMATORY RESPONSE SYNDROME, INFECTION, SEPSIS, AND SEVERE SEPSIS

Systemic inflammatory response syndrome (SIRS)—The presence of at least two of the following four criteria, one of which must be abnormal temperature or leukocyte count:
1. Core temperature of more than 38.5° C (101.3° F) or less than 36° C (96.8° F).
2. Tachycardia, defined as a mean heart rate more than 2 SD above normal for age in the absence of external stimulus, chronic drugs, or painful stimuli; or otherwise unexplained persistent elevation over a 30-minute to 4-hour period; or, for children less than 1 year old: bradycardia, defined as a mean heart rate less than the 10th percentile for age in the absence of external vagal stimulus, beta-blocker drugs, or congenital heart disease; or otherwise unexplained persistent depression over a half-hour period.
3. Mean respiratory rate more than 2 SD above normal for age or mechanical ventilation for an acute process not related to underlying neuromuscular disease or the receipt of general anesthesia.
4. Leukocyte count elevated or depressed for age (not secondary to chemotherapy-induced leukopenia) or more than 10% immature neutrophils.

Infection—A suspected or proven (by positive culture, tissue stain, or polymerase chain reaction test) infection caused by any pathogen; or a clinical syndrome associated with a high probability of infection. Evidence of infection includes positive findings on clinical examination, imaging, or laboratory tests (e.g., white blood cells in a normally sterile body fluid, perforated viscus, chest radiograph consistent with pneumonia, petechial or purpuric rash, or purpura fulminans).

Sepsis—SIRS in the presence of or as a result of suspected or proven infection.

Severe sepsis—Sepsis plus cardiovascular organ dysfunction or acute respiratory distress syndrome; or two or more other organ dysfunctions.

Modified from Goldstein B, Giroir B, Randolph A: International pediatric sepsis consensus conference: definitions for sepsis and organ dysfunction in pediatrics, *Pediatr Crit Care Med* 6(1):2-8, 2005; used with permission.

SEPTIC SHOCK

Sepsis and septic shock are caused by an infectious organism (Maar, 2004). Normally an infection triggers an inflammatory response in a local area, which results in vasodilation, increased capillary permeability, and eventually elimination of the infectious agent. The widespread activation and systemic release of inflammatory mediators is called the systemic inflammatory response syndrome (SIRS) (Goldstein, Giroir, and Randolf, 2005). Box 29-8 provides the exact definitions for SIRS, infection, sepsis, and severe sepsis. SIRS can occur in response to both infectious and noninfectious (e.g., trauma, burns) causes. When caused by infection, it is called *sepsis*. Septic shock is sepsis with organ dysfunction and hypotension. Most of the physiologic effects of shock occur because the exaggerated immune response triggers more than 30 different mediators, which results in diffuse vasodilation, increased capillary permeability, and maldistribution of blood flow. This impairs oxygen and nutrient delivery to the cells, resulting in cellular dysfunction. If the process continues, multiple organ dysfunction occurs and may result in death. Table 29-4 includes the age-specific vital signs and laboratory values reflective of septic shock in children.

TABLE 29-4	AGE-SPECIFIC VITAL SIGNS AND LABORATORY VARIABLES IN SEPTIC SHOCK*				
	HEART RATE (beats/min)		RESPIRATORY RATE (breaths/min)	LEUKOCYTE COUNT (leukocytes × 10³/mm³)	SYSTOLIC BLOOD PRESSURE (mm Hg)
AGE-GROUP	TACHYCARDIA	BRADYCARDIA			
0 days–1 wk	>180	<100	>50	>34	<65
1 wk–1 mo	>180	<100	>40	>19.5 or <5	<75
1 mo–1 yr	>180	<90	>34	>17.5 or <5	<100
2-5 yr	>140	N/A	>22	>15.5 or <6	<94
6-12 yr	>130	N/A	>8	>13.50 or <4.5	<105
13-<18 yr	>110	N/A	>4	>11 or <4.5	<117

From Goldstein B, Giroir B, Randolph A: International pediatric sepsis consensus conference: definitions for sepsis and organ dysfunction in pediatrics, *Pediatr Crit Care Med* 6(1):2-8, 2005; used with permission.

N/A, Not applicable.

*Lower values for heart rate, leukocyte count, and systolic blood pressure are for 5th percentile, and upper values for heart rate, respiratory rate, or leukocyte count are for 95th percentile.

The incidence of septic shock is increasing in adults and children (Arnal and Stein, 2003), possibly as a result of greater numbers of immunosuppressed patients, more widespread use of invasive devices in the seriously ill, increased awareness of the diagnosis, and a growing number of resistant microorganisms.

Three stages have been identified in septic shock. In early septic shock the patient has chills, fever, and vasodilation with increased cardiac output, which results in warm, flushed skin that reflects vascular tone abnormalities and hyperdynamic, warm, or hyperdynamic-compensated responses. BP and urinary output are normal. The patient has the best chance for survival in this stage. The second stage—the normodynamic, cool, or hyperdynamic-decompensated stage—lasts only a few hours. The skin is cool, but pulses and BP are still normal. Urinary output diminishes, and the mental state becomes depressed. With advancing disease, certain signs of circulatory decompensation that deteriorate to signs of circulatory collapse are indistinguishable from late shock of any cause. In the hypodynamic, or cold, stage of shock, cardiovascular function progressively deteriorates, even with aggressive therapy. The patient has hypothermia, cold extremities, weak pulses, hypotension, and oliguria or anuria. Patients are severely lethargic or comatose. Multiorgan failure is common. This is the most dangerous stage of shock.

Management of septic shock involves measures to provide hemodynamic stability and adequate oxygenation to the tissues and the use of antimicrobials to treat the infectious organism (Brierley, Choong, Cornell, et al, 2008; Dellinger, Levy, Carlet, et al, 2008). As with other forms of shock, hemodynamic stability is achieved with fluid volume resuscitation and inotropic agents as needed (Table 29-5). Providing adequate oxygenation often requires intubation and mechanical ventilation, supplemental oxygen, sedation, and paralysis to decrease the work of breathing. Septic shock involves activation of complement proteins that promote clumping of the granulocytes in the lung. The granulocytes can release chemicals that can cause direct lung injury to the pulmonary capillary endothelium. This causes a fluid leak into the alveoli, which causes stiff, noncompliant lungs. Disseminated intravascular coagulation and multiorgan dysfunction may also occur and require prompt assessment and management.

Nursing Care Management

Early identification of the symptoms of septic shock is critical to patient survival. A high index of suspicion is required in all critically ill patients who are at greater risk for sepsis because of multiple invasive lines and devices, poor nutrition, and impaired immune function. Subtle alterations in tissue perfusion and unexplained tachypnea and tachycardia often are early warning signs. Identification of the infectious agent and prompt treatment are also critical to patient survival. Patients should receive broad-spectrum antibiotics, and the nurse should remove the site of infection if possible (e.g., drain abscesses, remove indwelling lines). Manage patients in an intensive care unit, in which continuous monitoring and sophisticated cardiac and respiratory support are available. Multidisciplinary collaboration is essential in managing these critically ill patients.

> **! NURSING ALERT**
>
> To aid in early identification and management, nurses caring for children at risk for septic shock should be alert to early signs: fever, tachycardia, and tachypnea.

ANAPHYLAXIS

Anaphylaxis is the acute clinical syndrome resulting from the interaction of an allergen and a patient who is hypersensitive. This antigen-antibody (immunoglobulin E [IgE]) reaction stimulates the release of chemical substances, primarily histamine, from mast cells (Bohlke, Davis, DeStefano, et al, 2004). Histamine release causes vasodilation and increases capillary permeability, allowing fluid to leak into the interstitial space. Severe reactions are immediate; are often life threatening; and often involve multiple systems, primarily the cardiovascular, respiratory, GI, and integumentary systems. Exposure to the antigen can be through ingestion, inhalation, skin contact, or injection (Bohlke, Davis, DeStefano, et al, 2004). The most common allergens are listed in Box 29-9.

Prevention of a reaction is the primary goal. Preventing exposure is more easily accomplished in children known to be at risk, including those with (1) a history of a previous allergic

TABLE 29-5 PEDIATRIC SEPTIC SHOCK GOAL-DIRECTED THERAPY

PHYSIOLOGIC PARAMETER	THERAPEUTIC GOAL	MONITORING METHOD	MANIPULATION

Tissue perfusion	Capillary refill: <2 sec
	Mean arterial pressure:
	  65-70 mm Hg
	Urinary output: >0.5 ml/kg/hr
	CVP: 8-12 mm Hg
		Capillary refill
		Mean arterial pressure
		Urinary output
		CVP
			Fluids (crystalloids, colloids): 20 ml/kg
			  bolus; 40-60 ml/kg in 1st hr
			Sympathomimetics: dopamine (1st line),
			  norepinephrine or epinephrine (2nd line)
			Vasodilators: nitroprusside

Oxygenation	O_2 saturation: >93% Central venous O_2 saturation: >70% Hemoglobin within normal range for age Hematocrit: 30% O_2 extraction: 0.3-0.6 Serum lactate: <2 mmol/L	O_2 saturation Central venous O_2 saturation Hemoglobin concentration Hematocrit Arterial blood gases O_2 extraction: $(CaO_2 - Cvo_2)/CaO_2$ Serum lactate	Fio_2 PEEP Mean arterial pressure Transfusion (blood, PRBC) if hemoglobin <10 mg/dl

Urinary output and renal perfusion	Urinary output: >0.5 ml/kg/hr	Urinary output
		Creatinine clearance
		BUN
			Continuous renal replacement therapy:
			  CVVHD at 10% fluid overload or acute
			  renal failure
			Dialysis

Metabolic and nutritional support	Glucose: 80-110 mg/dl
	iCa++: 1.14-1.29
	Positive nitrogen balance
		Serum glucose
		Serum iCa++
		Healing of wounds and overall status
		Weight
		Albumin-prealbumin, total protein,
		  albumin/globulin ratio
		Indirect calorimetry
			Dextrose
			Insulin
			iCa++
			Enteral feeding
			Total parenteral nutrition
			Micronutrients: vitamins (vitamin K),
			  minerals

Adrenal support	Prevention of adrenal insufficiency and refractory hypotension	Cortisol level Blood pressure Therapeutic trial	Hydrocortisone

From Arnal LE, Stein F: Pediatric septic shock, *Semin Pediatr Infect Dis* 14(2):165-172, 2003; used with permission.
BUN, Blood urea nitrogen; *CVP,* central venous pressure; *CVVHD,* continuous venovenous hemofiltration/dialysis; *iCa++,* serum ionized calcium; *PEEP,* positive end-expiratory pressure; *PRBC,* packed red blood cells.

BOX 29-9 COMMON ALLERGENS ASSOCIATED WITH ANAPHYLAXIS

Drugs and Medical Products
Antibiotics (penicillin, cephalosporins, tetracycline, aminoglycosides, streptomycin, amphotericin B)
Analgesics (aspirin, indomethacin, phenylbutazone)
Local anesthetics (lidocaine, procaine, bupivacaine, tetracaine)
Chemotherapeutic agents (bleomycin, cisplatin, carboplatin, l-asparaginase, etoposide)
Antiepileptic drugs
Diagnostic contrast media (sulfobromophthalein sodium dye, dehydrocholic acid [Decholin], iodinated contrast media, iopanoic acid [Telepaque])
Latex (gloves, catheters) (See Latex Allergy, Chapter 11.)
Blood products

Foods
Milk and milk products
Nuts and seeds
Legumes (peanuts, soybeans, beans, lentils)
Eggs
Seafood (fish, shellfish)
Wheat
Citrus fruits, strawberries
Chocolate

Venoms
Hymenopteran (bee, yellow jacket, hornet, wasp, fire ant)
Snake
Jellyfish
Spider

Biologic Agents
Allergen extracts
Antisera (snake, tetanus, diphtheria)
Enzymes
Hormones
Immunoglobulin (gamma globulin, blood, plasma)

reaction to a specific antigen, (2) a history of allergy (atopy), (3) a history of severe reactions in immediate family members, and (4) a reaction to a skin test (although skin tests are not available for all allergens).

Pathophysiology

An anaphylactic reaction occurs as a result of an interaction between an allergen and preexisting specific IgE. When the antigen enters the circulatory system, a generalized reaction rapidly occurs. Vasoactive amines (principally histamine or histamine-like substances) are released from mast cells and cause vasodilation, bronchoconstriction, and increased capillary permeability. Consequently, there is increased venous capacity and pooling, reduced arterial pressure, and rapid loss of fluid into interstitial spaces, causing a marked decrease in venous return to the heart.

BOX 29-10   POSSIBLE MANIFESTATIONS OF ANAPHYLACTIC REACTION

Cardiovascular
Tachycardia
Dysrhythmia
Hypotension
Relative hypovolemia

Respiratory
Rhinitis (sneezing, nasal itching, rhinorrhea)
Laryngeal edema (stridor)
Bronchospasm (cough, wheezing)

Gastrointestinal
Nausea and vomiting
Abdominal pain
Diarrhea

Cutaneous (Skin)*
Diffuse flushing, feeling of warmth
Urticaria (itching of skin and raised rash [hives])
Angioedema (periorbital, perioral)

Central Nervous System, Other
Sense of impending doom*
Sometimes loss of consciousness*
Headache*
Seizures

*Early signs.

Clinical Manifestations

The onset of clinical symptoms usually occurs within seconds or minutes of exposure to the antigen. The rapidity of the reaction is directly related to its intensity—the sooner the onset, the more severe the reaction. However, the onset may be delayed for as long as 2 hours. Typically the reaction is preceded by one or more prodromal signs and symptoms, including vague complaints of uneasiness or impending doom, restlessness, irritability, severe anxiety, headache, dizziness, paresthesia, and disorientation. The patient may lose consciousness. Cutaneous signs are the most common initial sign, and the child may complain of feeling warm. Angioedema is most noticeable in the eyelids, lips, tongue, hands, feet, and genitalia. As outlined in Box 29-10, any or all of several reactions may affect one or more organ systems.

Bronchiolar constriction often follows cutaneous manifestations. Bronchiolar constriction causes a narrowing of the airway, dilated pulmonary circulation produces pulmonary edema and hemorrhages, and there is often life-threatening laryngeal edema. Shock occurs as a result of mediator-induced vasodilation and sudden inadequacy of the circulation. Hypovolemia is further enhanced by increased capillary permeability and loss of intravascular fluid into the interstitial space. Laryngeal edema, with its acute upper airway obstruction and related hypovolemic shock, carries a more ominous prognosis.

Therapeutic Management

Successful outcome of anaphylactic reactions depends on rapid recognition of their severity and prompt treatment (Liberman and Teach, 2008). The goals of treatment are providing ventila-

tion, restoring adequate circulation, and preventing further exposure by identifying and removing the cause when possible.

⚡ DRUG ALERT

Epinephrine

Epinephrine is the first line of therapy, and administration should never be delayed. As in any shock state, the airway is the first concern. The most important drug is aqueous epinephrine 1 : 1000. The dose is 0.01 ml/kg to a maximum of 0.5 mg administered subcutaneously. If the IV route is accessible, epinephrine 1 : 10,000 is used (0.1 ml/kg). Usually a single dose is effective, but additional doses are given if needed.

Observe the child for at least 6 hours because late deterioration may occur. Other routes of epinephrine administration are intramuscular and via an airway, either nebulized or by injection through an endotracheal tube. Strongly consider additional interventions such as fluid resuscitation, beta-agonists, antihistamines, and corticosteroids.

Position and monitor the child in the same way as for any shock patient. If this is the initial anaphylactic reaction, it is especially important to identify the allergen and implement measures to prevent any future reaction. The patient should carry medical identification at all times. Desensitization may be recommended in certain cases.

The nurse can manage a mild cutaneous reaction with no evidence of respiratory distress or cardiovascular compromise with antihistamines, such as diphenhydramine (Benadryl) and epinephrine. Moderate or severe distress presents a life-threatening emergency and requires immediate intervention. Severely unresponsive patients are transferred to hospital intensive care units when possible.

Nursing Care Management

The major nursing responsibility in anaphylaxis is anticipating which children are likely to develop a reaction, recognizing the early signs, and intervening appropriately. When an anaphylactic reaction is suspected, nursing responsibilities include immediate intervention and preparation for medical therapy. The nurse will need help and should notify the practitioner, but must not leave the patient. The child is placed in a head-elevated position (unless contraindicated by hypotension) to facilitate breathing, and oxygen is administered. If the child is not breathing, cardiopulmonary resuscitation is initiated.

QUALITY PATIENT OUTCOMES: Anaphylaxis
- Early recognition of symptoms
- Airway patency maintained
- Adequate circulation restored and maintained
- Further exposure to allergic agent prevented

If the cause can be determined, implement measures to slow the spread of the offending substance. For example, discontinue an IV medication or dye infusion. If an IV infusion line is not in place, establish one immediately, and monitor the flow rate carefully. Monitor vital signs every 15 minutes, and measure urinary output at regular intervals. Administer medications as prescribed, with regular assessment to monitor their effectiveness and to detect side effects of the medication and fluid overload.

To prevent an anaphylactic reaction, parents are always asked about possible allergic responses to foods, medications, products such as latex, and environmental conditions. (See Nursing Care Guidelines box, p. 408) These are displayed prominently on the patient's chart. Note the specific allergen and the type and severity of the reaction. Parents are excellent historians, especially when the child has displayed a dramatic reaction to a substance. Drugs, including related drugs (e.g., penicillin and nafcillin), that have produced a previous reaction are never given.

! NURSING ALERT

Families should always inform other caregivers (e.g., daycare staff) and school personnel, especially the school nurse, of their children's allergies. These individuals should be prepared to respond immediately to a severe reaction.

The child and the parents need as much reassurance as can be provided without giving false hope. Keep them informed of the child's progress, the reasons for the therapies, and what they can reasonably expect. This is a frightening experience and one that the family will remember and make every effort to prevent from recurring. The use of a convenient and visible method of conveying medical information, such as a bracelet or necklace, is encouraged. For the child who is allergic to insect venom, prescribe the family an emergency kit to be kept with the child at all times (e.g., EpiPen or EpiPen Jr Auto-Injector). Teach both the family and the child, if the child is old enough and is likely to be away from the family (e.g., at school), how to use the equipment. (See Chapter 27.)

TOXIC SHOCK SYNDROME

Toxic shock syndrome (TSS) is a relatively rare condition caused by the toxins produced by the *Staphylococcus* bacteria. First described in 1978, TSS can cause acute multisystem organ failure and a clinical picture that resembles septic shock. TSS became well known in 1980 because of the striking relationship between the disease and tampon use (Nakase, 2000). An aggressive health education campaign about the dangers of prolonged tampon use and a change in the chemical composition of tampons have markedly reduced the incidence of TSS in menstruating women. Cases of TSS have also been reported in men, older women, and children.

Pathophysiology

Evidence from several sources suggests that TSS occurs secondary to infection with phage group 1 *S. aureus* (Chuang, Huang, and Lin, 2005). The organism is believed to produce an epidermal toxin, but the precise mode of transmission is not known.

In approximately half the cases, TSS is seen in menstruating women and is usually associated with tampon use. The tampon may carry the organism from the fingers or vulva into the vagina during insertion, may traumatize the vaginal wall, or may provide a favorable environment for growth of the organism. TSS has also been associated with other bacterial infections, such as sinusitis or pneumonia, catheter site infections, skin infections, postoperative wound infections, and infection related to foreign bodies such as nasal packing or contraceptive diaphragms (Chuang, Huang, and Lin, 2005).

Clinical Manifestations

The sudden development of high fever, vomiting and diarrhea, profound hypotension, shock, oliguria, and an erythematous macular rash with subsequent desquamation are characteristic manifestations of TSS. Other manifestations include headache, blurred vision, purulent conjunctivitis, abdominal guarding, and purulent vaginal discharge.

Complications of TSS include respiratory distress, cardiac dysfunction, hematologic changes (particularly disseminated intravascular coagulation), and abnormal liver function. Impaired perfusion to the extremities may become severe, with eventual necrosis and loss of extremities.

Diagnostic Evaluation

The diagnosis is established on the basis of criteria in the TSS case definition of the Centers for Disease Control and Prevention (Box 29-11). A history of tampon use contributes to the diagnosis. Laboratory tests may include cultures from blood, vagina, cervix, and discharge from any suspected source of infection. Other laboratory tests are those that facilitate the management of shock.

Therapeutic Management

The management of TSS is the same as management of shock of any cause. Because the disease is highly varied in intensity, direct therapy toward supportive care in mild cases

---

BOX 29-11   DIAGNOSTIC CRITERIA OF TOXIC SHOCK SYNDROME

Major diagnostic criteria:
- Fever of 38.9° C (102° F) or higher
- Presence of diffuse macular erythroderma
- Desquamation, particularly of palms and soles, 1 to 2 weeks after onset of illness
- Hypotension, defined as a systolic blood pressure of 90 mm Hg or less for adults and below the 5th percentile for children younger than 16 years of age; or an orthostatic drop in diastolic blood pressure of 15 mm Hg or more with a change from lying to sitting; or orthostatic syncope; or orthostatic dizziness
- Involvement of three or more of the following organ systems: gastrointestinal, muscular, mucous membrane, renal, hepatic, hematologic, and central nervous system

Toxic shock syndrome is probable when four of the five major criteria are fulfilled.

In addition, if blood and cerebrospinal fluid cultures are obtained, they must be negative for any organisms other than *Staphylococcus aureus*. Serologic tests for Rocky Mountain spotted fever, leptospirosis, and measles also must be negative.

Modified from American Academy of Pediatrics, Committee on Infectious Diseases, Pickering L, editor: *2009 Red book: report of the Committee on Infectious Diseases*, ed 28, Elk Grove Village, Ill, 2009, The Academy.

to hospitalization and intensive care in severe cases. Appropriate parenteral antibiotics are usually administered after cultures are obtained. Preventing complications of impaired circulation demands constant observation and immediate therapeutic intervention for hypotension, pulmonary dysfunction, acidosis, hematologic changes, and renal impairment.

Nursing Care Management

Nursing care and observation of the acutely ill patient are the same as those described for shock of any cause. Because the disease is relatively rare, direct the major nursing efforts toward prevention. The association between TSS and the use of tampons provides some direction for education. Teach adolescent girls who use tampons general hygiene measures, such as hand washing before insertion of the tampon and not using a tampon that has been dropped or otherwise soiled. Insert tampons carefully to avoid vaginal abrasion. Also it is wise to modify their use. For example, use tampons intermittently during the menstrual cycle, alternating with sanitary napkins—perhaps using napkins at the night, when at home during the day, and when flow is light. Advise young girls not to use superabsorbent tampons and not to leave any tampon in the body for more than 4 to 6 hours.

! NURSING ALERT

Patients who use tampons need to understand that they should remove the tampon and consult their health care professional if they develop a sudden high fever, vomiting, diarrhea, muscle pain, dizziness, fainting or near-fainting when standing up, or a rash that resembles a sunburn.

▌BURNS

OVERVIEW

⊜ Burn injuries are usually attributed to extreme heat sources but may also result from exposure to cold, chemicals, electricity, or radiation. Most burns are relatively minor and do not require definitive medical treatment. However, burns involving a large body surface area, critical body parts, or the geriatric or pediatric population often benefit from treatment in specialized burn centers. The American Burn Association (2006) has established criteria to guide decisions regarding the severity of injury and the need for transfer for specialized care.

Epidemiology and Etiology

Burn injuries represent one of the most severe traumas a body can sustain. Ongoing efforts toward education, burn prevention, safer home and work environments, and new methods of firefighting have significantly decreased burn injuries. The death rate from fire and flame injury among children 14 years of age and under declined by 68% from 1987 to 2005. Fire and burns are the fourth leading cause of unintentional injury–related death among children 14 years of age and under. Children, particularly those 5 years of age and under, are at greatest risk from home fire death and injury, having a death rate of nearly twice the national average (Safe Kids Worldwide, 2008, 2009).

Another source of burn injury is nonaccidental injury due to maltreatment. Such injuries most commonly occur to children 3 years of age and younger. Maltreated children are most likely to live in poverty-level households headed by a young, single parent who has two or more children. Thirty percent of children suffering recurrent burn injury are eventually mortally injured (Robert, Blakeney, and Herndon, 2007). Scald burns are the most common injury, followed by contact burns. Suspect abuse if there is a burn distribution inconsistent with the reported incident, a delay in seeking treatment, and a history of family instability and inability to deal with stress in crisis situations. Laws now exist in all states requiring health care workers to report suspected child abuse.

The use of alternative heating devices such as kerosene heaters and wood-burning stoves has increased the risk of contact burns in all age-groups. Most contact burns result from the lack of shielding to prevent contact with hot surfaces. Flame burns involving flammable liquids such as gasoline account for approximately 30% of injuries seen in the pediatric population, especially in children over 8 years of age. The ignition of clothing is the second leading cause of burn injury. In the past, girls were more susceptible, but the incidence has decreased significantly and clothing ignition deaths have decreased as clothing styles have changed; such injuries are now rare among children, with little overall gender difference. From 1975, when it was mandated for sleep wear in sizes from 0 to 6x to successfully pass a standard flame test, until 1999 when that law was repealed, the percentage of clothing burns caused by sleep wear in children ages 0 to 12 decreased from 55% to 27%. Sleep wear–related burns are being closely monitored to assess the effect of deregulation of sleep wear garments on related burns (Pruitt, Wolf, and Mason, 2007).

Children playing with matches or other ignition devices account for 1 in 10 residential fire deaths. Boys 2 to 5 years of age have the highest rate of nonfatal burns, and children younger than 9 years old cause fire-related death and injury due to child play fires (Pruitt, Wolf, and Mason, 2007). Careless smoking is associated with the majority of fatal house fires and is the most common cause of residential fire deaths. The use of alternative heating sources is another common cause of house fires. The source of ignition is often a combustible material stored near the device, the buildup of creosote in the chimney, spillage of fuel, or use of the wrong fuel. Many of these fires result in multiple deaths and injuries, especially in rural areas. The majority of fatal house fires occur during the cold winter months, most commonly in the Eastern part of the United States from December through February. The single most important element in the decrease in fire-related deaths seen since 1978 is the use of smoke detectors.

The majority of burns result from contact with thermal agents such as a flame, hot surfaces, or hot liquids. Electrical injuries caused by household current have the greatest incidence in young children, who insert conductive objects into electrical outlets or bite or suck on connected electrical cords in sockets (Pruitt, Wolf, and Mason, 2007). They occur most commonly during the spring and summer months and are also associated with risk-taking behaviors in young boys. Direct contact with high-or low-voltage current and lightning strikes are the most frequent mechanism of injury. The resistance of the tissue and the path of the electric current are responsible for the damage incurred. Electric current travels through the body on the path of least resistance—tissue, fluid, blood vessels, and nerves. A more localized burn is produced if skin resistance is high at the area of contact, whereas a more systemic pattern of injury is produced if the skin resistance is low. Often compared to a crush injury, serious electrical trauma results from current passing through vital organs, muscle compartments, and nerve or vascular pathways. Loss of limbs, cardiac fibrillation, respiratory collapse, and burns are common after exposure to electrical energy.

Chemical burns can cause extensive injury. The severity of injury is related to the chemical agent (acid, alkali, or organic compound) and the duration of contact. The mechanism of injury differs from that in other burns in that there is a chemical disruption and alteration of the physical properties of the exposed body area. Noxious agents exist in many cleaning products commonly found in the home. In addition to concern for localized damage, the potential for systemic toxicity must also be addressed. Of particular concern are the exposure of the eyes to chemical agents and the ingestion of caustic substances.

Although radiation injuries are rare, the most common sources in pediatrics are related to radiation exposure from medical therapies and ultraviolet light.

The causative agent in all burns has important implications for the treatment and prognosis of the pediatric patient. The nurse uses knowledge of the pathophysiologic processes of each type of injury in assessing the trauma and in planning, implementing, and evaluating care. Psychosocial issues are also important considerations in planning for the optimum long-term outcome.

BURN WOUND CHARACTERISTICS

The child's physiologic responses, therapy, prognosis, and physical disposition are directly related to the amount of tissue destroyed; therefore the severity of the burn injury is assessed on the basis of the percentage of body surface area burned and the depth of the burn. Also important in determining the seriousness of injury are the location of the wounds, the child's age and general health, the causative agent, respiratory involvement, and concomitant injuries.

Extent of Injury

The extent of the burn is expressed as a percentage of total body surface area (TBSA) injured. The child has different body proportions than the adult, resulting in inaccurate estimation of injury if the standard adult rule of nines is used. The proportions of the child's trunk and arms are roughly the same as those of the adult. However, the infant's head and neck make up 18% of the TBSA, and each lower extremity accounts for 14% of the TBSA. A modified rule of nines for the pediatric population proposes that for each year of life after age 2 years, 1% is deducted from the head and 0.5% is added to each leg (Helvig, 1993). It is generally more efficient to use any of a variety of charts designed to assign body proportions to children of different ages (Fig. 29-1).

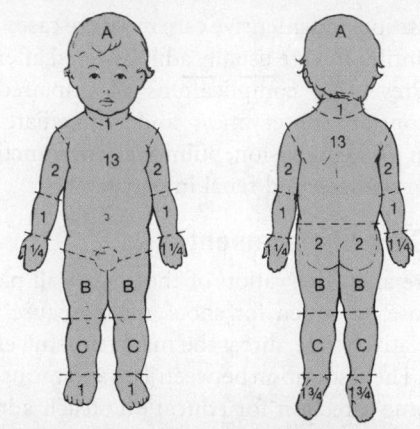

RELATIVE PERCENTAGES OF AREAS AFFECTED BY GROWTH

AREA	BIRTH	AGE 1 YR	AGE 5 YR
A = ½ of head	9½	8½	6½
B = ½ of one thigh	2¾	3¼	4
C = ½ of one leg	2½	2½	2¾

A

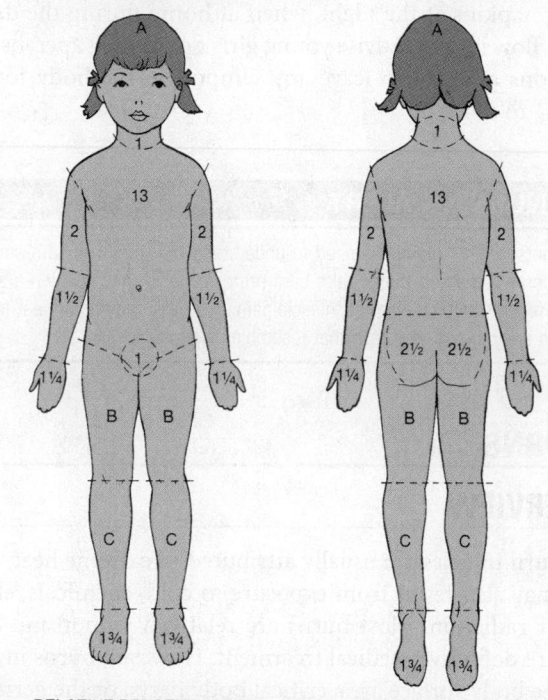

RELATIVE PERCENTAGES OF AREAS AFFECTED BY GROWTH

AREA	AGE 10 YR	AGE 15 YR	ADULT
A = ½ of head	5½	4½	3½
B = ½ of one thigh	4½	4½	4¾
C = ½ of one leg	3	3¼	3½

B

Fig. 29-1 Charts for estimation of distribution of burns in children. **A,** Children from birth to age 5 years. **B,** Older children.

Depth of Injury

A thermal injury is a three-dimensional wound and is also assessed in relation to the depth of injury. Traditionally the terms *first, second, third,* and *fourth degree* have been used to describe the depth of tissue injury. However, with the current emphasis on wound healing, this traditional terminology is being replaced by more descriptive terms related to the extent of destruction to the epithelializing elements of the skin. In general, first-degree burns are classified as superficial, and

			WOUND APPEARANCE	WOUND SENSATION	COURSE OF HEALING
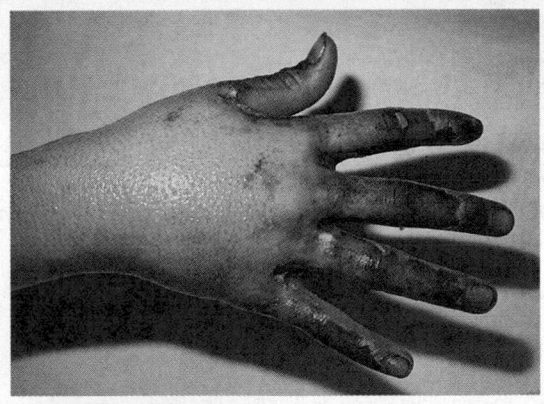	PARTIAL-THICKNESS BURN	1st-degree	Epidermis remains intact and without blisters Erythema; skin blanches with pressure	Painful	Discomfort lasts 48-72 hours. Desquamation occurs in 3-7 days.
		2nd-degree	Wet, shiny, weeping surface Blisters Wound blanches with pressure	Painful Very sensitive to touch, air currents	Superficial partial-thickness burn heals in <21 days. Deep partial-thickness burn requires >21 days for healing. Healing rates vary with burn depth and presence/absence of infection.
	FULL-THICKNESS BURN	3rd-degree	Color variable (i.e., deep red, white, black, brown) Surface dry Thrombosed vessels visible No blanching	Insensate (↓ pinprick sensation)	Autografting is required for healing.
		4th-degree	Color variable Charring visible in deepest areas Extremity movement limited	Insensate	Amputation of extremities is likely. Autografting is required for healing.

Labels on diagram: EPIDERMIS — Sweat duct, Capillary; Sebaceous gland, Nerve endings; DERMIS — Hair follicle; Sweat gland, Fat, Blood vessels; Bone

Fig. 29-2 Classification of burn depth according to depth of injury. (From Black JM: *Medical-surgical nursing: clinical management for positive outcomes*, ed 8, Philadelphia, 2008, Saunders.)

second-degree burns as partial-thickness. Third- and fourth-degree wounds are classified as full-thickness wounds. Partial-thickness wounds are further classified as superficial or deep in relation to the time required for healing to occur and the functional and cosmetic results anticipated. Because both terminologies are often used interchangeably, they are both presented in Fig. 29-2, which describes the characteristics of burn wounds.

Superficial (first-degree) burns are usually of minor significance. There is often a latent period followed by erythema due to vasodilation. Tissue damage is minimum, the protective functions of the skin remain intact, and systemic effects are rare. Pain is the predominant symptom, and blisters do not form. The dead epidermis sloughs and is replaced by regenerating keratinocytes within 3 or 4 days without scarring (Pham, Gibran, and Heimbach, 2007). The burning sensation and pain usually resolve in 48 to 72 hours, and in 3 to 6 days the damaged epithelium peels off in small scales or sheets (Carrougher, 1998). A mild sunburn is an example of a superficial first-degree burn.

Partial-thickness (second-degree) injuries involve the epidermis and varying degrees of the dermis. These wounds are painful, moist, red, and blistered. Superficial partial-thickness burns involve the epidermis and part of the dermis. Dermal elements are intact, and the wound should heal in approximately 14 days with variable amounts of scarring. The wound is extremely sensitive to temperature changes, exposure to air, and light touch. Although classified as second-degree or partial-thickness burns, deep dermal burns resemble full-thickness injuries in many respects. Sweat glands and hair follicles remain intact. The burn may appear mottled, with pink, red, or waxy white areas exhibiting blisters and edema formation (Fig. 29-3). Systemic effects are similar to those encountered with full-

Fig. 29-3 Deep partial-thickness burn.

thickness burns. Although these wounds heal spontaneously in approximately 21 days, they do so with extensive scarring.

Full-thickness (third-degree) burns are serious injuries that involve the entire epidermis and dermis and extend into subcutaneous tissue. Thrombosed vessels can be seen beneath the surface of the wound, and nerve endings, sweat glands, and hair follicles are destroyed. The burn varies in color from red to tan, waxy white, brown, or black and is distinguished by a dry, leathery appearance (Fig. 29-4). Normally, full-thickness burns lack sensation in the area of injury because of the destruction of nerve endings. However, most full-thickness burns have superficial and partial-thickness burned areas at the periphery of the burn, where nerve endings are intact and exposed. Also, excised eschar and donor sites cause exposed nerve fibers. Finally, as peripheral fibers regenerate, painful sensation returns. Consequently, children often experience severe pain related to the size and depth of the burn. Full-thickness wounds are not capable of reepithelialization and require surgical excision and grafting to close the wound.

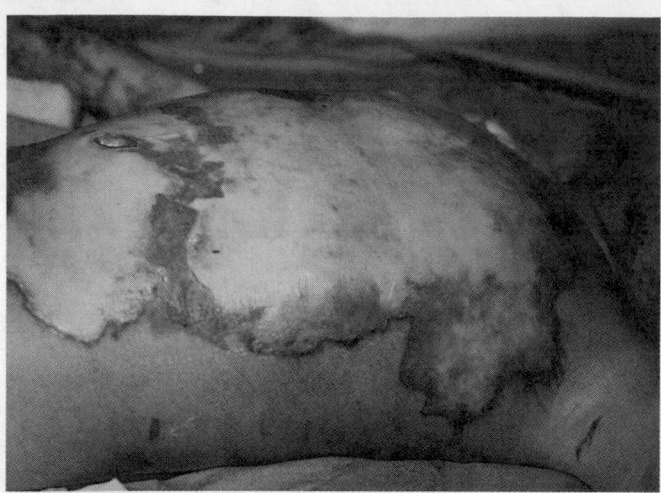

Fig. 29-4 Full-thickness thermal injury.

TABLE 29-6	**SEVERITY GRADING SYSTEM ADOPTED BY AMERICAN BURN ASSOCIATION**		
	MINOR*	**MODERATE**	**MAJOR**
Partial-thickness burns	<10% of total body surface area (TBSA)	10%-20% of TBSA	>20% of TBSA
Full-thickness burns			All
Treatment	Usually outpatient; may require 1- to 2-day admission	Admission to hospital, preferably one with expertise in burn care	Admission to burn center

From Vaccaro P, Trofino RB: Care of the patient with minor to moderate burns. In Trofino RB, editor: *Nursing care of the burn-injured patient*, Philadelphia, 1991, FA Davis.
*Minor burns exclude any burn involving the face, hands, feet, perineum, or crossing joints; electrical burns; any injury complicated by inhalation injury or concomitant trauma; and children with psychosocial factors affecting the injury.

Fourth-degree burns are also full-thickness injuries and involve underlying structures such as muscle, fascia, and bone. The wound appears dull and dry, and ligaments, tendons, and bone may be exposed.

Severity of Injury

Burns are classified as major, moderate, or minor, which is useful in determining the patient's disposition for treatment. Burn patients can usually be distinguished as (1) those with a major burn injury, who require the services and facilities of a specialized burn center; (2) those with a moderate burn, who may be treated in a hospital with expertise in burn care; and (3) those with minor injuries, who can be treated on an outpatient basis (Table 29-6). The severity of the injury depends on the extent and depth of the burn, the causative agent, the body area involved, the patient's age, and concomitant injuries and illnesses.

The nurse makes initial assessment of the extent of skin damage by observation and simple diagnostic techniques. The extent of body surface area involvement is readily calculated, and the appearance of the wound provides clues as to whether the injury involves the full thickness of the skin or only a portion of the skin layers. Touching injured surfaces to test for blanching and capillary refill indicates whether circulation to the area is intact.

It is important to consider the cause of injury and the duration of contact with the burning agent. In general, the more intense the heat source and the longer the contact, the deeper the resulting injury. Hot liquids may result in partial-thickness burns, whereas full-thickness injuries are associated with flame burns. This may vary with the child's age. Very young children are likely to sustain deeper injuries because of the thin nature of infant skin. This makes estimation of burn depth difficult in young children, especially after scald injuries. Inflicted injuries tend to be more severe than accidental burns because contact with the burning agent is prolonged. Electrical injuries may also be difficult to assess initially. Visible tissue destruction may appear minimum, and damage to underlying structures may not be evident. The circumstances of the burn may also suggest the presence of associated injuries.

Certain areas of the body carry a higher risk of complications and therefore require specialized care. Burns of the hands and feet and across joints may not necessarily involve a large body surface area, but injury and scar formation may interfere with normal growth and development. Specialized care is required to preserve maximum function. Burns to the face and neck, along with a history of the injury occurring in an enclosed space, raise a high index of suspicion of inhalation injury. In addition, airway compromise and hypoxia may result from edema formation and pulmonary injury. Damage to the delicate cartilage of the nose and ears results in facial deformities. Facial burns may involve the eyes and have long-term consequences for vision. Perineal burns are prone to infection and maceration in all patients, especially in young children who are not toilet trained. Scar bands and contractures in the perineal area may interfere with hygiene and mobility.

Children younger than 2 years of age have a significantly higher mortality rate than older children with burns of a similar magnitude. The infant has minimum protein stores, which are rapidly depleted during burn shock; an immature immune response, which increases the risk of infection and sepsis; and a greater amount of body water in proportion to size that is intolerant of rapid fluid shifts. In addition, the child has not achieved mature renal function. This negatively affects the ability to retain sodium and water. These considerations, combined with the previously discussed fragility of the skin in the very young, increase the severity of injury.

Many patients sustaining thermal injuries may also suffer associated trauma. The circumstances of the accident may offer clues to related trauma. Children involved in house fires may have jumped from a window, sustaining fractures. Motor vehicle accidents and electrical injuries often result in concomitant injuries. Any suspicion of child abuse should alert the health care team to rule out other injuries.

PATHOPHYSIOLOGY

A burn injury represents a catastrophic insult that involves all organ systems. Understanding the pathophysiology

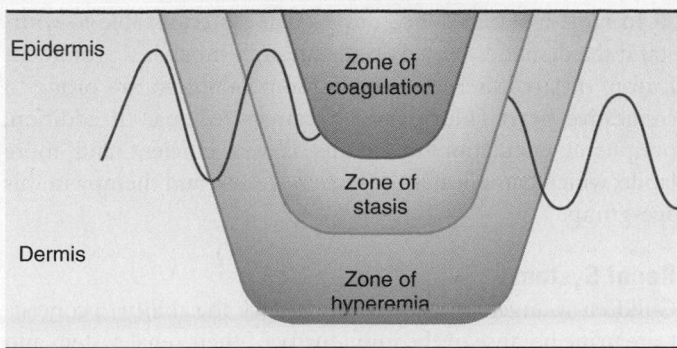

Fig. 29-5 Zones of injury in burn. (From Townsend CM: *Sabiston textbook of surgery*, ed 18, Philadelphia, 2007, Saunders.)

BOX 29-12 ZONES OF BURN INJURY

Zone of coagulation (necrosis)—Area beneath obviously destroyed tissue. Capillary flow has ceased and tissue destruction is irreversible; tissue is dead.

Zone of stasis—Area beneath and surrounding zone of coagulation; markedly reduced capillary flow; tissue severely damaged from heat but not coagulated. Tissue in this zone can be saved with prevention of further injury and with adequate perfusion.

Zone of hyperemia—Area metabolically active; displays usual response to tissue injury.

---

underlying thermal trauma is essential to provide appropriate nursing care to the pediatric burn victim.

Local Response

Damage to human skin by heat results in two types of injury: an immediate direct cellular response and a delayed response caused by dermal ischemia. Irreversible cellular damage from protein denaturation occurs at temperatures exceeding 45° C (113° F). Three zones of injury demonstrate the evolution of local tissue damage (Fig. 29-5). The unstable area of injured cells, which may survive under ideal conditions, is designated the zone of stasis. Progressive injury caused by dermal ischemia may occur in this zone (Box 29-12).

Edema Formation

Thermal injury to the vessels in the two outer zones results in increased capillary permeability. At the same time, vasodilation causes an increase in hydrostatic pressure within the capillaries. The increased hydrostatic pressure, combined with the increased capillary permeability, causes loss of water, protein, and electrolytes from the circulating volume into the interstitial spaces.

To understand the physiologic mechanism of the formation of burn edema, an understanding of the microvascular fluid balance is necessary. Burn injury not only causes edema at the site, but extravasated and sequestered fluid and protein also enters nonburned tissue. The directly injured cells have a damaged cell membrane that leads to an increase in sodium and potassium shift, resulting in cell swelling. Intracellular water and sodium increase. This process not only occurs in injured cells, but also with those that are not directly heat injured. Edema develops when the rate of fluid being filtered from the microvessels exceeds that of the lymph flow. The amount of

edema depends on the type and extent of burn injury (Kramer, Lund, and Beckman, 2007).

Fluid Loss

Fluid transport across the microcirculatory wall in normal and pathologic states is quantitatively described by the Landis-Starling equation. This equation describes the physical forces and physiologic mechanisms that govern fluid transfer between vascular and extravascular compartments. Normal capillary barriers that separate the intravascular and interstitial compartments are disrupted, which results in severe depletion of plasma volume and an increase in extracellular fluid. Clinically this is manifested as hypovolemia (Warden, 2007).

Circulatory Status

Significant circulatory alterations take place in the zone of stasis located around the dead coagulated tissue. Heated red blood cells become spherical. These heat-damaged cells, together with hemoconcentration from fluid shifts, depressed cardiac output, and tissue edema, reduce the blood flow in the burned area, resulting in capillary stasis. Thrombi develop, which further impedes circulation and produces tissue ischemia and necrosis. Hyperviscosity and impaired blood flow are attributed to the release of substances such as thromboplastin and clot-activating factors from damaged cells. These substances cause the production of microemboli, platelet adhesion and aggregation, and increased pain and edema. Circulation in the area around partial-thickness wounds ceases immediately after injury but is usually restored within 24 to 48 hours. In full-thickness burns, however, the vascular supply is completely occluded, and no appreciable circulation is reestablished until granulation takes place at the interface between burned and unburned skin.

Tissue Repair

With reasonable care, superficial partial-thickness injuries heal spontaneously and uneventfully through the generative capacity of the stratum germinativum and epithelial cells of the lining of skin appendages. The wound should heal in approximately 14 days with minimum scarring.

Deep partial-thickness burns heal more slowly by regeneration from the epithelial lining of skin appendages, sweat glands, and hair follicles. A thin epithelial covering develops in 25 to 35 days, but this type of burn may require several months to heal. Scarring is common. Infection, trauma, or severe hypothermia easily converts a partial-thickness wound to a full-thickness injury, especially in the normally thinner skin of young children. Fluid loss and metabolic consequences may be considerable.

Cell destruction by coagulation necrosis occurs in full-thickness burns. Dead tissue and exudate convert to a thick, leathery eschar in 48 to 72 hours; the eschar liquefies and begins to separate in 12 to 21 days if not surgically excised. This process is a result of autolysis, leukocyte digestion, and disintegration of collagen fibers. The dead avascular tissue provides an ideal environment for bacterial growth. If tissue is not grafted, new granulation tissue forms on the wound bed. The wound heals slowly by proliferation from the edges, with a high risk of infection and severe scarring. Full-thickness burns result in severe edema with fluid and electrolyte shifts and extensive metabolic changes.

Systemic Responses

Cardiovascular System

The immediate postburn period is marked by dramatic alterations in circulation, known as burn shock. A precipitous drop in cardiac output precedes any change in circulating blood or plasma volumes. This initial decrease in cardiac output (approximately 50% of normal resting values) is attributed to a circulating myocardial depressant factor that is associated with severe burn injury and directly affects the contractility of the heart muscle. As a result of fluid losses through denuded skin, increased capillary permeability, and vasodilation, the circulating volume decreases rapidly; cardiac output is reduced even further, usually leveling off at approximately 20% of normal resting values. After adequate fluid resuscitation, cardiac output spontaneously returns to normal in 24 to 36 hours. If fluid is not replaced, cardiac output continues to decrease, resulting in inadequate perfusion, organ dysfunction, and ultimately death.

Capillary permeability with leakage of fluid takes place both in uninjured areas and in the burn wound. Together with the shrinkage of drying eschar, severe edema caused by the rapid fluid shift to the interstitial spaces may produce a tourniquet effect, resulting in compartment syndrome. Compartments are composed of groups of muscles in the extremities and are surrounded by fibrous tissue. The inability of the fascia to expand in the presence of massive edema increases the pressure in the compartment, compromising circulation and entrapping nerves. Treatment is required during the acute phase and consists of surgical incision of the burned tissue (escharotomy) to restore distal circulation. If the escharotomy is not sufficient, an incision of the muscle sheath (fasciotomy) is performed (Fig. 29-6).

Edema fluid accumulates rapidly in the first 18 hours after injury and reaches a maximum in approximately 48 hours. Capillary permeability returns to normal, and fluid is reabsorbed, chiefly by way of the lymphatics. Reabsorption usually proceeds at the rate of fluid accumulation, although it may persist longer. Redistribution of fluid is often complex and unpredictable and is marked by diuresis.

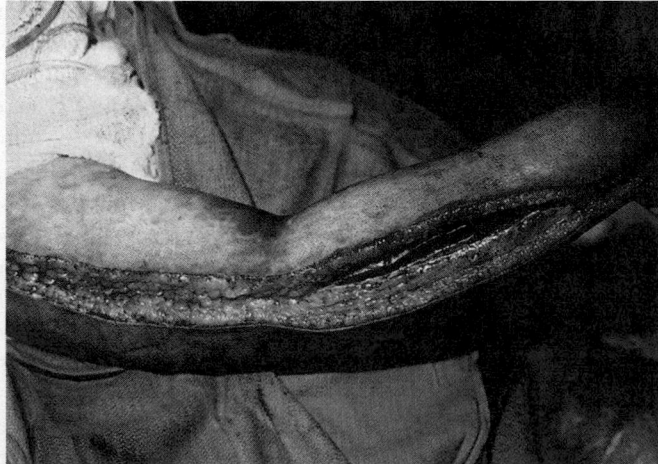

Fig. 29-6 Escharotomy and fasciotomy in severely burned arm.

In most children the cardiovascular system is able to withstand the demands placed on it, although shock is a prominent feature of large thermal injuries. Some children are prone to congestive heart failure and pulmonary edema. In addition, peripheral circulation in infants is less efficient and more labile, which complicates the burn response and therapy in this age-group.

Renal System

Children younger than 2 years of age lack the ability to concentrate urine because of the immaturity of their renal system and are therefore at an increased risk for dehydration. In addition, the child has a relatively larger TBSA in relation to weight than an adult. These issues, combined with limited physiologic reserves, increase the fluid requirements for children during burn shock resuscitation and in compensating for evaporative water losses (Warden, 1992). Loss of fluid from the intravascular compartment causes renal vasoconstriction that in turn leads to reduced renal plasma flow and depressed glomerular filtration. When adequate fluids are provided, the glomerular filtration rate returns to normal, and by the third or fourth postburn day, urinary output increases as edema fluid is mobilized and eliminated. In the first few days oliguria is more commonly the result of inadequate fluid replacement than of acute renal failure. If the child does not respond to treatment or if there is inadequate fluid resuscitation, acute renal failure may develop, with significant kidney damage.

BUN and creatinine levels are elevated as a result of tissue breakdown, decreased circulating volume, and oliguria. Hematuria may also be evident from the hemolysis of red blood cells, and oliguria may develop as a consequence of the increased pigment load. Myoglobinuria is especially common after extensive electrical injury. Cell destruction releases large amounts of myoglobin, which occludes the kidney tubules and places the victim of electrical trauma at high risk for renal failure.

Gastrointestinal System

The GI system has been recognized as a target of systemic shock. After a burn injury, blood flow decreases to the GI system by one third even though cardiac output is maintained by resuscitation fluids. Ischemia results and can produce ulcer formation, enterocolitis (severe enough to cause full-thickness necrosis), and even intestinal perforation. Poor perfusion to the kidney and the liver can ensue, resulting in organ dysfunction. The GI tract functions as a barrier to contain GI bacteria within it. Disruption of the GI mucosal integrity is possibly a focus for sepsis in the burn patient. The exact mechanism by which bacteria and their products pass through the GI barrier is not clear. Both intracellular and transcellular processes may be involved. These consequences can be profound, and translocating whole bacteria can be a direct source of sepsis (Sheridan and Tompkins, 2007b).

With the placement of a nasogastric tube, gastric decompression empties the stomach to control aspiration of gastric contents until motility is reestablished. Take care to observe for signs of aspiration of gastric contents into the lung as a result of incompetence of the gastroesophageal junction. With GI function intact, enteral feedings with a nasogastric tube are begun immediately after acute resuscitation (Andrews, 1994).

Metabolism

The greatly accelerated metabolic rate in burn patients is supported by protein and lipid catabolism. The child has limited glycogen stores to provide energy, which therefore accelerates the protein and lipid breakdown. No other disease state produces as great a hypermetabolism as the burn injury. Therefore the child is vulnerable to prolonged starvation (Lee and Herndon, 2007). When the burn injury is extensive (>50% of TBSA), energy needs may approach twice the predicted basal requirements.

The stress of injury places high demands on the body. Stress-invoked glycogen breakdown depletes the energy stores in 12 to 24 hours, after which the body resorts to glyconeogenesis for high-energy needs. Blood glucose levels may be elevated as a result of insulin resistance. Rapid protein breakdown and muscle wasting occur if sufficient protein replacement is not provided.

Body temperature reflects the net balance between heat production and heat loss. As a result of the accelerated metabolism, children with burn injuries typically exhibit an elevated body temperature, even in the absence of infection. The thermoregulatory response is activated and results in an elevation of core body temperature. Burn injured patients strive for a core body temperature of about 38° C (100.4° F). Low or "normal" temperature may indicate overwhelming sepsis, or a fatigued physiologic capability to maintain temperature, and should be viewed with concern. Routine methods of heat conservation after a major burn injury are inadequate because of excessive heat loss through evaporation and convection (Saffle and Graves, 2007). Heat is lost as a result of the energy-consuming process of water evaporation from the damaged skin surface. The body tries to raise the core and skin temperature to offset heat losses secondary to evaporation through the burn eschar (Norbury and Herndon, 2007). Infants and young children are especially vulnerable because of the large surface area relative to metabolically active tissue. Burning destroys a lipid layer and converts skin that is normally impermeable to water to a state that transmits water vapor at least four times as rapidly as unburned skin. In partial-thickness burns this loss is greatest on the day of injury; in full-thickness burns it rises slowly at first and rapidly increases to reach a peak approximately the fourth day after the burn. Evaporative losses continue until partial-thickness wounds are healed and full-thickness burns are grafted. Therefore body stores of energy are rapidly depleted unless sufficient replacement is provided or losses are reduced.

Medications that affect metabolic rate may be used to prevent loss of body protein stores, thus protecting immunity, wound healing, muscle integrity, and organ function. Oxandrolone is an anabolic steroid that works to maintain and restore muscle mass, increase weight gain, and promote wound healing. Supplements of essential amino acids such as glutamine and arginine provide an anticatabolic effect, support wound healing, indirectly preserve lean body mass, improve immune function, and provide an antioxidant quality (Demling, 2005).

Neuroendocrine System

As a response to stress of any origin, the hypothalamic-hypophyseal mechanism restores equilibrium by secreting trophic hormones, which stimulate various target organs of the neuroendocrine system. Adrenal activity is markedly increased. The medulla responds by secreting additional amounts of the catecholamines epinephrine and norepinephrine. Adrenocortical hormones reach a peak immediately after injury and remain elevated for some time. Aldosterone secretion and a release of antidiuretic hormone are sustained at a high level throughout hospitalization. Despite this increased adrenal activity, adrenal insufficiency is a rare complication.

Anemia and Metabolic Acidosis

The hematocrit is initially elevated because of hemoconcentration resulting from fluid shifts to the interstitial spaces and red blood cell destruction. In addition, a reduced red blood cell half-life results from increased cell fragility. A significant loss of circulating red blood cell mass is predominantly associated with major burns.

Most burn patients exhibit some degree of metabolic acidosis as a result of the disruption of the body's buffering action because of the fluid shift to the extravascular spaces and the altered concentrations of potassium, sodium, chloride, and bicarbonate ions. Reduced blood volume and cardiac output result in diminished perfusion and tissue hypoxia, with a shift to anaerobic metabolism. The resultant formation of metabolic acids is usually sufficiently compensated by respiratory mechanisms. Renal compensatory activities are impaired by the decreased blood flow.

Growth and Development

Children may demonstrate postburn growth retardation. Regular height and extremity assessment are necessary to detect subtle deformities until development is normalized (see Research Focus box). *Contractures can develop & may not be able to utilize this limb.*

🔳 RESEARCH FOCUS

Children with Major Burn Injuries

Children who have sustained major burn injuries have shown severe growth delays in height and weight. This growth lag lasted as long as 3 years postburn for some children before a return to normal growth velocity (Suman, Przkora, Blakeney, et al, 2007). Children with major burn injuries may also demonstrate reduced bone mass and may develop bone remodeling. The effects of bone remodeling are profound and long lasting. Studies involving children with major burns revealed persistent decreased bone formation from biopsies of the iliac crest and cross-sectional studies (Klein, Przkora, and Herndon, 2007).

Complications

Thermally injured children are subject to a number of serious complications, both from the wound and from systemic alterations resulting from the injury. The immediate threat to life is related to airway compromise and profound shock. During healing, infection—both local and systemic sepsis—is the primary complication. Mortality associated with thermal trauma in children increases with the severity of injury and decreases as age advances. In children older than 3 years, the mortality rate is similar to that of adults. Below this age, the rate of survival from the burn and its associated complications lessens considerably.

Pulmonary System

The impact of thermal injury on pulmonary function includes a full range of respiratory dysfunctions, including inhalation injury, aspiration of gastric contents, bacterial pneumonia, pulmonary edema and insufficiency, and emboli. In every age and burn size category, pneumonia is one of the most common infections in burn patients and is associated with high risk of mortality (Murphey, Sherwood, and Toliver-Kinsky, 2007).

Inhalation injuries result from trauma to the tracheobronchial tree after inhalation of the heated gases and toxic chemicals produced during combustion. Although direct thermal injury to the upper airway may occur, heat damage below the vocal cords is rare. Inspired heated air is cooled in the upper airway before reaching the trachea. Reflex closure of the cords and laryngeal spasm prevent full inhalation. Evidence of direct thermal injury to the upper airway includes burns of the face and lips, singed nasal hairs, and laryngeal edema. Clinical manifestation may be delayed as long as 24 to 48 hours. Wheezing, increasing secretions, hoarseness, wet rales, and carbonaceous secretions are signs of respiratory tract involvement. Upper airway obstruction is often associated with burn shock and fluid resuscitation. In such situations endotracheal intubation may be necessary to preserve a patent airway.

Suspect inhalation of carbon monoxide when the injury has occurred in an enclosed space. (See Smoke Inhalation Injury, Chapter 32, for a discussion of carbon monoxide inhalation.) Inhalation of other products of combustion, such as smoke and toxic chemicals, can produce varying degrees of pulmonary damage. Smoke from burning wood is extremely irritating; burning plastic materials, especially polyvinyl chloride, release smoke with gases containing chlorine, sulfuric acid, and cyanide. Respiratory injury is manifested by mucosal erythema and edema followed by sloughing of the mucosa. A mucopurulent membrane replaces the mucosal lining and seriously compromises respiration and ventilation.

A common etiologic factor in respiratory failure in the pediatric population is bacterial pneumonia, which may be secondary to airway injury or contamination from intubation or may be acquired through hematogenous spread of bacteria. Early in the postburn period the largest percentage of pulmonary infections result from nosocomial exposure, immobility, and abdominal distention. The hematogenous variety occurs later and is related to the septic burn wound or other foci, such as phlebitis at the site of an invasive IV line. A less common complication is pulmonary edema resulting from fluid overload or ARDS in association with gram-negative sepsis. (See Chapter 32.) This syndrome results from pulmonary capillary damage and leakage of fluid into the interstitial spaces of the lung. A loss of compliance and interference with oxygenation are the consequences of pulmonary insufficiency in conjunction with systemic sepsis.

Deep burns, especially those circling the thorax, may cause restriction of chest excursion as a result of edema and inelastic eschar formation. Young children are particularly at risk because of the pliability of the skeletal structure. Hypoxia is relieved by an escharotomy of longitudinal incisions along the anterior axillary lines combined with a transverse incision at the costal level. This procedure allows expansion of the chest wall to facilitate ventilation.

Wound Sepsis

Sepsis is a critical problem in the treatment of burns and is an ever-present threat after the shock phase. Initially, burn wounds are relatively pathogen free unless contaminated with potentially infectious material such as dirt or polluted water. However, dead tissue and exudate provide a fertile field for bacterial growth. On approximately the third postburn day, early colonization of the wound surface by a preponderance of gram-positive organisms (primarily staphylococci) changes to predominantly gram-negative opportunistic organisms, particularly *Pseudomonas aeruginosa*. By the fifth postburn day, bacterial invasion is well underway beneath the surface of the burn wound.

Characteristics of the burn wound contribute to the proliferation of pathogenic organisms. Vascular supply to full-thickness burns is occluded immediately, and no appreciable blood is supplied to the area for approximately 3 weeks after the injury. In partial-thickness wounds the circulation to the injured area is suspended for 24 to 48 hours; circulation is then restored unless infection supervenes. Thrombosis from bacterial invasion will impair circulation sufficiently to convert partial-thickness wounds to full-thickness injuries. These large amounts of nonviable tissue also provide an excellent medium for the growth of microorganisms.

Occlusion of the local blood supply impairs the delivery of both humoral and cellular defense mechanisms to the burned area. Initially there is a decrease in inflammatory and phagocytic cells to the wound, but the number of phagocytes gradually increases until they are present in abundance by the third postburn week, when granulation tissue is forming. Granulation tissue, with its rich blood supply, affords increasing resistance to infection. Organisms are normally a part of skin flora; therefore cultures with an organism concentration of 105/g of tissue have been arbitrarily chosen as the level of burn wound invasion.

The microflora present at any institution are influenced by the treatment modalities and choice of antibiotics. During the past 30 years there has been a reduction in the percentage of specific bacteria and fungi recovered from burn wounds. This reduction reflects improvements in patient management, nutritional support, aggressive excision and grafting of wounds, and topical antimicrobial therapy. Sepsis, in burn injury, is a major complication and a significant factor in morbidity and mortality (Sherwood and Traber, 2007).

> **! NURSING ALERT**
>
> Disorientation in the burned patient is one of the first signs of overwhelming sepsis. A spiking fever and diminished bowel sounds accompanied by paralytic ileus occur and progressively increase over 48 to 72 hours, after which the temperature falls to subnormal limits. At this time the wound deteriorates, the white blood cell count is depressed, and septic shock becomes manifest.

Gastrointestinal System

GI dysfunction is common after burn injury as evidenced by feeding intolerance; mucosa ulceration; and bleeding, particularly in the stomach and duodenum. Within 72 hours of a major burn injury a significant number of patients may develop mucosal changes. This may progress to ulceration with septic episodes and hypoxemia. Potential causes of stress ulcers in burn patients are (1) mucosal ischemia, (2) increased acid production, (3) increased acid back-diffusion, (4) energy depletion, (5) bile reflux, and (6) direct mucosal injury with placement of intraluminal tubes.

Enteral feeding is one of the most important means of providing nutrition and has led to a decrease in mortality. Early enteral feeding often prevents some of these potential complications. Aggressive fluid resuscitation aids in maintaining adequate mucosal blood flow. Antacid and H_2 receptor antagonist therapy can effectively prevent ulceration of the stomach and duodenum.

Ileus is also a common complication after a burn injury. Sepsis, electrolyte imbalance, narcotics, and renal failure are common causes. Patients experience abdominal distention and pain. Early enteral feeding again can assist in avoiding intestinal complications (Beierle and Chung, 2007).

Central Nervous System

Burn encephalopathy, as characterized by lethargy, withdrawal, or coma, occurs in children. Symptoms such as delirium and transient psychosis occur rarely among children under the age of 10 years. In such cases, electroencephalograms typically reveal diffuse, nonspecific, slow waves. In most cases burn encephalopathy can be attributed to hypoxemia, hyponatremia, hypovolemia, septicemia, and drug administration. Hallucinations are uncommon, but when they do occur, stress is the most likely cause, followed by pain and various medications. These symptoms, though short lived, are upsetting to the family and treatment team.

Proper treatment must first address organic causes of delirium or encephalopathy. The nurse must stabilize vital signs and normalize blood chemistries, glucose, and oxygenation. Sepsis must be ruled out and pain addressed. Then psychotropic medications may be administered (Thomas, Meyer, and Blakeney, 2007). There is usually full neurologic recovery, even with prolonged and serious manifestations.

THERAPEUTIC MANAGEMENT

Emergency Care

The initial management of the burn patient begins at the scene of injury. The first priority is to stop the burning process. The child should then be transported immediately to the nearest medical facility for definitive treatment and evaluation for transfer to a burn center. The child and the family will be extremely frightened and anxious; sensitivity to their emotional state provides reassurance during the transport process.

Stop the Burning Process

The chief aim of rescue in flame burns is to smother the fire, not fan it. Children tend to panic and run, which serves only to spread the flames and make assistance more difficult. Place the injured child in a horizontal position and rolled in a blanket, rug, or similar article, taking care to not cover the head and face because of the danger of inhaling toxic fumes. If nothing is available, the victim should lie down, cover the mouth with the hands, and roll over slowly to extinguish the flames. Remaining

in the vertical position may cause the hair to ignite or may lead to the inhalation of flames, heat, or smoke.

Major burns with large amounts of denuded skin should briefly be cooled with a single application of tepid water. Heat is rapidly lost from burned areas, and additional cooling leads to a drop in core body temperature and potential circulatory collapse. Continuous wet dressings or the application of ice promotes vasoconstriction because of cooling, resulting in impaired circulation to the burned area and increased tissue damage. Chemical burns present special circumstances and require flushing with copious amounts of water during transport to a medical facility. The use of neutralizing agents on the skin is contraindicated because a chemical reaction is initiated and further injury may result. If the chemical is in powder form, the addition of water may spread the caustic agent. The powder should be brushed off if possible. If the chemical burn produces a blister, it is advisable to open the blister with a sterile object to remove any chemical present.

Remove burned clothing to prevent further damage from smoldering fabric and hot beads of melted synthetic materials. Also remove jewelry to eliminate the transfer of heat from the metal and constriction from edema formation. These steps also provide better access to the wound and preclude more painful removal later on.

Assess the Victim's Condition

As soon as the flames are extinguished, assess the victim's condition. Airway, breathing, and circulation are the priority concerns. Cardiopulmonary and cerebral emergencies are always a consideration after trauma. Cardiopulmonary complications may result from exposure to electric current, inhalation of toxic fumes and smoke, hypovolemia, and shock. Institute emergency measures as appropriate.

Cover the Burn

Cover the burn wound with a clean dry cloth to prevent contamination and alleviate pain by eliminating air contact. Cover the child who has extensive burns to prevent hypothermia. No attempt should be made to treat the burn. The application of topical ointments, oils, or other home remedies is contraindicated.

Transport the Child to Medical Aid

Do not give the child with an extensive burn anything by mouth to avoid aspiration in the presence of paralytic ileus and upper airway edema and to prevent water intoxication. The child is transported to the nearest medical facility. If this cannot be accomplished within a relatively short time, establish IV access if possible with a large-bore catheter. Oxygen, if available, is administered at 100%. Give a report of the initial assessment and any interventions implemented to the medical facility assuming responsibility for the child's care.

Provide Reassurance

Providing reassurance and psychologic support to both the family and the child helps immeasurably during postinjury crisis. Reducing anxiety helps conserve the energy needed to cope with the physiologic and emotional stress of a traumatic injury.

Management of Minor Burns

Treatment of burns classified as minor can usually be managed adequately on an outpatient basis when the caregiver is reliable and able to carry out instructions for care and observation. Patients with less than optimum circumstances may require close follow-up to ensure compliance with the treatment program.

Cleanse the wound with mild soap and tepid water. Débridement of the wound includes removal of any embedded debris, chemicals, and devitalized tissue. Removal of intact blisters remains controversial. Some authorities argue that blisters provide a barrier against infection; others maintain that blister fluid is an effective medium for the growth of microorganisms (Smith, 2000). Most practitioners favor covering the wound with an antimicrobial ointment to reduce the risk of infection and provide some pain relief. The dressing consists of a fine-mesh gauze placed over the ointment and a light wrap of gauze dressing that avoids interference with movement. This helps keep the wound clean and protect it from trauma. Instruct the caregiver to wash the wound, reapply the dressing, and return the child to the office or clinic as directed for wound observation. The frequency of dressing changes can vary from every other day to twice a day.

Other practitioners prefer an occlusive dressing, such as a hydrocolloid, which is placed over the wound after cleansing. This method eliminates the discomfort associated with frequent dressing changes but impairs visualization of the wound surface.

If there is a high probability of infection or other complications or if there is doubt about the ability to carry out instructions, direct the parents to return daily for dressing changes and inspection, or a nurse may be assigned to make a home visit for that purpose. Frequent removal of the dressing is an effective mode of débridement. Soaking the dressing in tepid water before removal helps loosen the dressing and debris and reduces discomfort. Burns of the face and ears are usually treated by an open method (Carrougher, 1998). The wound is washed and débrided in the same manner, and a thin film of antimicrobial ointment is applied twice a day.

Obtain a tetanus history on admission. Tetanus prophylaxis is administered if there is no history of immunization or if more than 5 years have passed since the last immunization. Administration of antibiotics for minor burns is controversial. A mild analgesic such as acetaminophen is usually sufficient to relieve discomfort; the antipyretic effect of the drug also alleviates the sensation of heat.

Most minor burns heal without difficulty, but hospitalization is indicated if the wound margin becomes erythematous, gross purulence is noted, or the child develops evidence of systemic reaction (e.g., fever or tachycardia). Evaluate the child for functional impairment, and instruct the caregiver in the exercise and ambulation program. After wound healing, an evaluation of scar maturation and range of motion will indicate any need for further therapy.

Management of Major Burns

When a child with extensive burns is admitted to the hospital for treatment, a variety of assessments are conducted and therapies initiated. Of these, the priority concerns include the estab-

---

BOX 29-13   MAJOR BURN MANAGEMENT

- Ascertain the adequacy of the airway, and provide oxygen, intubation, and ventilatory support as indicated.
- Insert a large-bore intravenous (IV) line, preferably through unburned skin, to deliver fluids at a sufficiently rapid rate to effect resuscitation.
- Remove clothing and jewelry, and examine for secondary trauma.
- Evaluate the burn wound, and determine the extent and depth of injury.
- Obtain an admission weight.
- Calculate fluid requirements, and establish the appropriate regimen.
- Insert a nasogastric tube to empty stomach contents and maintain gastric decompression.
- Insert an indwelling Foley catheter to obtain specimens and monitor hourly output.
- Provide IV medication for control of pain and anxiety only after adequate oxygenation is ensured and fluid resuscitation is initiated.
- Obtain baseline laboratory studies.
- Perform escharotomy or fasciotomy to the chest and extremities for constricting circumferential eschar, elevated compartment pressures, or impaired circulation.
- Apply topical antimicrobials and dressings to the burn wounds.
- Obtain a history regarding the injury and other pertinent data.
- Administer appropriate tetanus prophylaxis.
- Prophylactic antibiotic administration is not recommended.

---

lishment and maintenance of an adequate airway, initiation of fluid administration, and evaluation and treatment of the wound. Although the order of implementation may vary from institution to institution, a number of procedures and activities are generally initiated on admission. Some are carried out simultaneously (Box 29-13).

Other therapies, including nutritional support, positioning and splinting to prevent contractures, treatment of anemia and hypoproteinemia, psychosocial support, and rehabilitative aspects of burn management, are initiated as appropriate throughout the course of treatment.

Establishment of an Adequate Airway

The first priority of care is airway maintenance. Thermal injuries to the face, nares, and upper torso; a history of injury in an enclosed space; an examination of the oral and nasal membranes that reveals edema, hyperemia, and blisters; and evidence of trauma to the upper respiratory passages all suggest inhalation of noxious agents or respiratory burns. If there is evidence of respiratory involvement, administer 100% oxygen and determine blood gas values, including carbon monoxide levels.

If the child exhibits changes in sensorium, air hunger, or other signs of respiratory distress, insert an endotracheal tube to maintain the airway. When severe edema of the face and neck is anticipated, perform intubation before swelling makes it difficult or impossible. A controlled intubation is preferred to an emergency procedure. Intubation allows for the delivery of humidified oxygen, the removal of secretions from respiratory passages, and the provision of ventilatory support.

Treatment may include bronchodilators (e.g., albuterol) to reduce bronchospasm. Bronchopulmonary hygiene to prevent atelectasis and pooling of secretions reduces the risk of pneumonia. Therapies include percussion and postural drainage, frequent position changes, and suctioning to remove secretions.

Placing the child in a semi-Fowler position with high-flow oxygen and maximum humidity is often sufficient to relieve bronchospasm produced by trauma to the bronchial mucosa.

When full-thickness burns encircle the chest, constricting eschar may limit chest wall excursion. The child becomes increasingly difficult to ventilate. Escharotomy of the chest relieves this pressure and improves ventilation.

Fluid Replacement Therapy

The objectives of fluid therapy are compensation for water and sodium losses to the traumatized area and the interstitial spaces, replenishment of sodium deficits, restoration of circulating volume, provision of adequate perfusion, correction of acidosis, and improvement of renal function. Initiate treatment for burn shock in children with burns in excess of 15% to 20% of TBSA.

Types of fluid and electrolyte therapy in the first 24 hours after injury remain controversial. Lactated Ringer solution appears to be the most common resuscitation fluid currently used. Proponents of crystalloids alone for resuscitation report that other solutions, specifically colloids, are no better and certainly more expensive than crystalloids for maintaining intravascular volume after burn injury. The most common reason for not using colloids is that even large proteins leak from the capillary after burn injury (Warden, 2007).

The composition of the fluid administered varies with the philosophy of the individual practitioner and may consist of an isotonic saline solution, a near-isotonic solution, or even a hypertonic saline solution. Children's decreased tolerance to hypertonic solutions may result in hypernatremia, hyperosmolality, and intracellular dehydration. Many formulas have been proposed as guidelines for fluid administration after burn injury. Perhaps the most commonly employed regimen is the Parkland formula. It is important to remember that any formula used during resuscitation serves only as a guideline; individual adjustments must be made based on the patient's response to therapy. Fluid replacement is maintained at a rate that provides an hourly urinary output of 30 ml in older children and 1 to 2 ml/kg in children weighing less than 30 kg (66 lb). Other parameters monitored during fluid resuscitation include vital signs, capillary refill, and sensorium.

Some common reasons for patients to require fluids well in excess of the calculated volume include underestimation of burn size (particularly in pediatric patients), pulmonary injury that sequesters resuscitation fluid in the lung, electrical injury with greater tissue destruction than is visible, and delay in the initiation of fluid resuscitation (Smith, 2000). Irreversible burn shock that persists despite aggressive fluid resuscitation remains a significant cause of death in the immediate postburn period. Exchange transfusion consisting of the replacement of circulating volume by banked whole blood provides a therapeutic modality that may benefit the patient who fails to respond to conventional resuscitation. Inflammatory response factors, thought to be important in burn shock, are removed, thus lowering the concentration present in the body, restoring capillary integrity, and substantially reducing fluid requirements.

After the initial 24 to 48 hours, the capillary seal is restored. Fluid requirements decrease to a constant that persists until wound coverage is achieved. Colloid solutions such as albumin or plasma are useful to maintain plasma volume. Fluid balance may continue to be a problem throughout the course of treatment; especially during periods of increased evaporative loss from the burn wound. Approximately 48 to 72 hours after injury, interstitial fluid returns to the vascular compartment and diuresis occurs to eliminate excess fluids. During this phase, increasing intake to match urinary output can result in circulatory overload.

Nutrition

For 2 or 3 days immediately after injury, burn patients experience a hypometabolic phase when their metabolic rate and cardiac output decrease. Following this phase patients experience a hypermetabolic phase. This hypermetabolism is characterized by a hyperdynamic circulatory response with increased body temperature, oxygen and glucose consumption, carbon dioxide production, glycogenolysis, proteolysis, and lipolysis. This response begins on the fifth postburn day and continues up to 9 months after the burn, causing erosion of lean body mass, muscle weakness, immunodepression, and poor wound healing (Norbury and Herndon, 2007). This hypermetabolism is thought to slow wound healing, prolong generalized weakness, lead to loss of lean body mass, and increase morbidity (Lee and Herndon, 2007). Nutritional support, particularly through enteral feedings, recently has become more aggressive. The continuity of these feedings is important.

Some burn patients are able to eat. Encourage a high-protein, high-calorie diet as soon as possible after resolution of paralytic ileus. However, many have poor appetites and are unable to meet energy requirements solely by oral feeding. Most children with burns in excess of 25% TBSA require supplementation with tube feeding. An absence of bowel sounds does not preclude enteral nutrition. Because the small bowel maintains motility and absorptive capabilities, the placement of a small-bore feeding tube into the duodenum allows for the safe delivery of enteral nutrition during periods of paralytic ileus associated with trauma, sepsis, and anesthesia. A nasogastric tube that decompresses the stomach protects the patient from aspiration.

Use of total parenteral nutrition (TPN) has now been essentially replaced by enteral nutrition for both theoretical and practical reasons. Enteral nutrition directly nourishes the bowel mucosa with nutrients (e.g., glutamine). Small amounts of these nutrients within the bowel lumen stimulate the function of intestinal cells and normal mucosa function. This may help preserve normal blood supply to the intestines. Maintaining intestinal integrity may reduce bacterial translocation and sepsis, as well as preserve immune function. Along with the hazards of central venous access, TPN appears to be associated with increased secretion of tumor necrosis factor and other proinflammatory mediators (Saffle and Graves, 2007).

Specific guidelines for vitamin and micronutrient supplementation for the burn patient have not been established.

! NURSING ALERT

Capillary refill, alterations in sensorium, and urinary output are the most reliable indicators for assessing the adequacy of fluid resuscitation in burned children. BP can remain normotensive even in a state of hypovolemia.

Limited research has been done on the homeostasis of vitamins and trace elements after burn injury (Klein, Przkora, and Herndon, 2007).

Medication

Antibiotics are usually not administered prophylactically. The administration of systemic antibiotics to control wound colonization is not indicated, since decreased circulation to the injured area prevents delivery of the medication to areas of deepest injury. Surveillance cultures and monitoring of the clinical course provide the most reliable indicators of developing infection. Appropriate antibiotics can then be instituted to treat the identified organism. Group B streptococci cultured from the throat or wounds are particularly destructive to grafted tissue. Do not overlook otitis media as a source of fever in the pediatric population.

Some form of sedation and analgesia is required in the care of burned children (Henry and Foster, 2000). During the initial resuscitation period, IV administration of narcotics, along with anxiolytics, is required for baseline and procedural pain management. Morphine, fentanyl (Sublimaze), and midazolam (Versed) are the most commonly used agents (Kahana, 2003). (See Pain Management, Chapter 7.)

Anesthetic agents such as nitrous oxide, propofol, and ketamine also are used to control procedural pain. A major drawback with nitrous oxide is that staff is exposed to the gas because it is self-administered by the patient. Propofol is a nonbarbiturate hypnotic agent without analgesic activity. It also causes depressed respiratory drive, loss of airway reflexes, and hypertension. Propofol must be given in doses large enough to cause loss of consciousness to prevent response to painful procedures. Ketamine may preserve airway reflex; however, side effects may be noted such as production of copious upper airway secretions, tachycardia, and hypertension. Ketamine can produce postadministration hallucinations, particularly in adolescent boys. Repeated use may produce tolerance, so increased doses are required over time. To avoid volatile anesthetics, a combination of midazolam and fentanyl can be given intravenously (Meyer, Patterson, Jaco, et al, 2007).

⚡ DRUG ALERT

Entonox

Entonox is a useful short-term analgesic mixture of gases in a fixed ratio of 50% nitrous oxide and 50% oxygen. Initiation of action is approximately 1 minute, with a peak effect reached in 3 to 5 minutes. It is eliminated from the body, mostly via the lungs, within 2 to 5 minutes. Entonox is useful for alleviating anxiety and raising the threshold of pain during procedures. The child must be able to follow instructions and may self-administer the gas with assistance. No treatment should last longer than 30 minutes, and the nurse should monitor the child continuously during the procedure. Side effects of nitrous oxide administration may include excitability, nausea, or vomiting. It is not recommended for children who are sedated, hypotensive, unconscious, pregnant, or intoxicated or for those with head or chest injuries (Selbst, 2003).

Management of the Burn Wound

After the initial period of shock and restoration of fluid balance, the primary concern is the burn wound. The primary goal for burn wound management is to close the wound as soon as possible (Gordon and Marvin, 2007). The objectives of wound management include prevention of infection, removal of devitalized tissue, and closure of the wound. The application of dressings and topical antimicrobial therapy reduce pain by minimizing air exposure.

Primary Excision

In children with large, full-thickness burn wounds, excision is performed as soon as the patient is hemodynamically stable after initial resuscitation. Because the burn wound is precipitating the exaggerated physiologic response, many associated complications do not resolve until the eschar is excised and the wound is closed. One of the most effective therapies for decreasing mortality from major burn injuries is the early excision of the burn wound and its coverage by various techniques (Barrow and Herndon, 2007).

Wound Hygiene

Hydrotherapy is used to cleanse the wound and assist with separating eschar. There are variances from institution to institution on the particular method, but the common approach is to cleanse and débride once or twice a day. Hydrotherapy helps cleanse not only the wound but the entire body and also aids in maintenance of range of motion. Partial-thickness wounds require débridement of devitalized tissue to promote healing. Débridement is very painful and requires some type of analgesia before the procedure. The water acts to loosen and remove sloughing tissue, exudate, and topical medications. Mesh gauze entraps the exudative slough and is readily removed during hydrotherapy (Fig. 29-7). Any loose tissue is carefully trimmed away before the wound is redressed (Fig. 29-8).

Wound Dressings

Daily dressing changes of the burn wound are recommended to allow for inspection and cleansing of the wound. Dressing changes offer an opportunity to meticulously observe the burn for infection. The volume of draining and the physical condition of the dressing also dictate frequency of dressing change. Often wound dressings become saturated, soiled, or disheveled, indicating that additional dressing changes may be required (Hartford and Kealey, 2007).

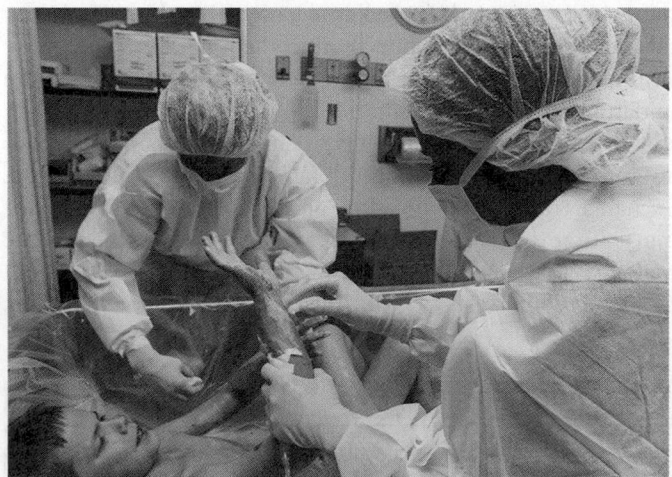

Fig. 29-7 Removal of dressing during hydrotherapy. (Courtesy CR Boeckman Regional Burn Center, Akron, Ohio.)

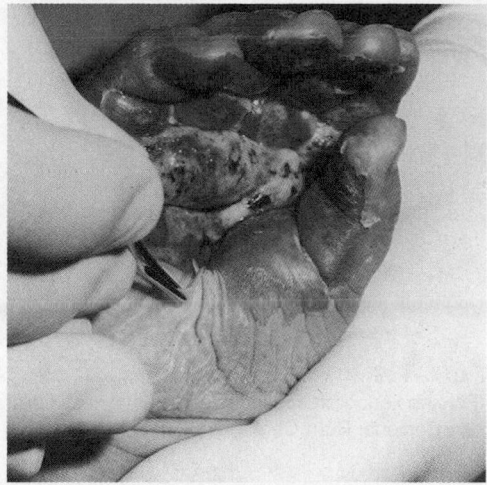

Fig. 29-8 Dead skin and debris are carefully trimmed away before dressing is applied. (Courtesy CR Boeckman Regional Burn Center, Akron, Ohio.)

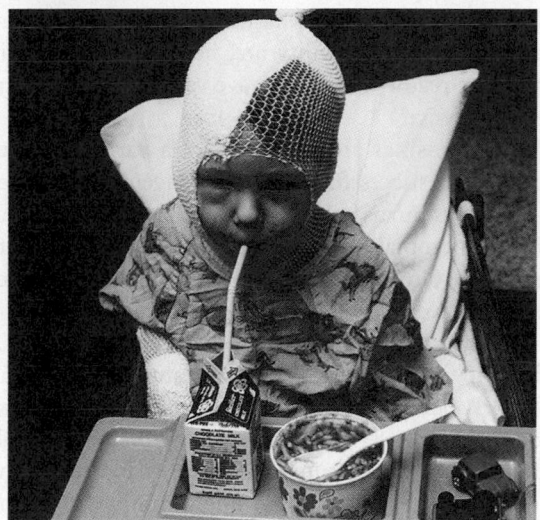

Fig. 29-9 Burn wound covered with gauze dressings and secured with tubular elastic netting. (Courtesy CR Boeckman Regional Burn Center, Akron, Ohio.)

BOX 29-14 METHODS OF BURN WOUND MANAGEMENT

Exposure—Wounds are left open to air; crust forms on partial-thickness wounds, and eschar forms on full-thickness burns.

Open—Topical antimicrobial agent is applied directly to the wound surface, and the wound is left uncovered.

Modified—Antimicrobial is applied directly or impregnated into thin gauze and applied to the wound; gauze or net secures the area (see Fig. 29-10).

Occlusive—Antimicrobial is impregnated in gauze or applied directly to the wound; multiple layers of bulky gauze are placed over the primary layer and secured with gauze or net. Occlusive methods may impede joint movement due to bulky gauze wraps. Advantages include reduction of evaporative heat loss from the wound, comfort, and protection.

Topical Antimicrobial Agents

Several methods are used for covering the burn wound (Box 29-14 and Fig. 29-9). All meet the objective of preparation for permanent wound coverage, and all use some type of topical agent. Before the development of effective topical agents for

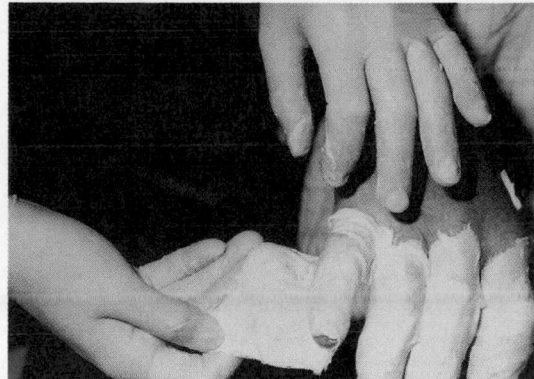

Fig. 29-10 Gauze impregnated with ointment applied to burn wound. Note how each finger is wrapped separately. (Courtesy CR Boeckman Regional Burn Center, Akron, Ohio.)

reducing the incidence of invasive organisms, wound sepsis was the major cause of mortality from burn injury. The goal is to minimize wound colonization. A variety of specific agents are available, including silver sulfadiazine (Thermazene), mafenide acetate (Sulfamylon), and bacitracin. Topical agents do not eliminate organisms from the wound but can effectively inhibit bacterial growth. To be effective, a topical application must be nontoxic, capable of diffusing through eschar, harmless to viable tissue, inexpensive, and easy to apply. It should not encourage the development of resistant strains of bacteria and should produce minimum electrolyte derangement.

Some topical agents are packaged and prepared on a fine-mesh gauze, which allows ease of application (Fig. 29-10). The gauze provides necessary protection for the wound, maximizes patient comfort, increases the rate of healing, reduces the necessity for frequent dressing changes, and is cost-effective. Examples include a nanocrystalline film of pure silver (Acticoat and Silverlon) and a hydrofiber with ionic silver (Aquacel Ag). Most often these gauzes are used on superficial second-degree burns, on donor sites, and for graft care, except for Acticoat, which can also be used for full-thickness wounds (Bessey, 2007).

Temporary Skin Substitute

Permanent coverage of extensive burns is a prolonged process that requires repeated operations for débridement and grafting. Temporary skin substitutes provide transient physiologic wound closure, thereby helping control pain, absorb wound exudates, and prevent wound desiccation (Sheridan and Tompkins, 2007a). Temporary skin substitutes markedly reduce pain and facilitate movement of joints to retain range of motion.

Allograft (homograft) skin comes from human cadavers and is processed by commercial skin banks (Box 29-15). These skin banks screen donors for communicable diseases and track the skin much like blood transfusions. Allograft skin is particularly useful in the coverage of surgically excised, deep partial-thickness and full-thickness wounds in extensive burns when available donor sites are limited. Severe immunosuppression occurs in massively burned children, and the allograft becomes adherent (Fig. 29-11). The allograft can remain in place until suitable donor sites become available. Typically rejection occurs approximately 14 days after application. The use of an allograft is

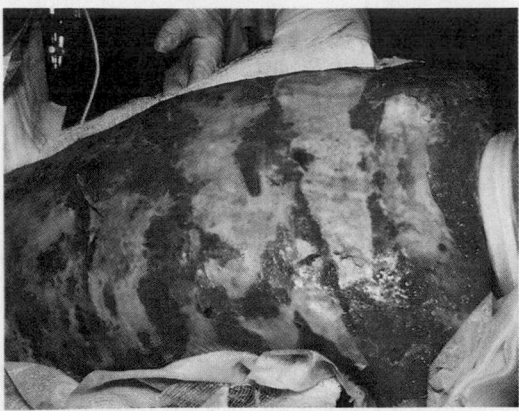

Fig. 29-11 Adherent allograft applied to excised full-thickness wound.

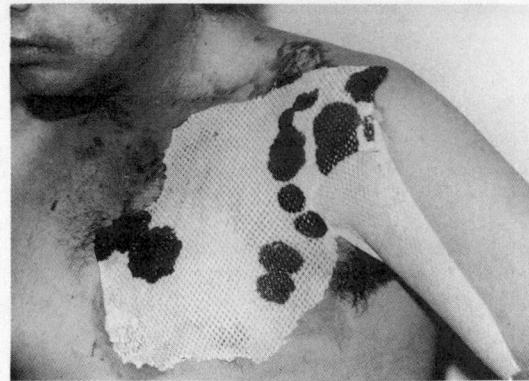

Fig. 29-12 Porcine xenograft applied to partial-thickness burn. (Courtesy CR Boeckman Regional Burn Center, Akron, Ohio.)

BOX 29-15 TYPES OF SKIN GRAFTS

Temporary Grafts

Allografts (homografts)—Skin that is obtained from genetically different members of the same species who are free of disease

Xenografts (heterografts)—Skin that is obtained from members of a different species, primarily pigskin

Permanent Grafts

Autografts—Tissue obtained from undamaged areas of the patient's own body

Isografts—Histocompatible tissue obtained from genetically identical individuals

Methods of Applying Split-Thickness Grafts

Sheet graft—A sheet of skin, removed from the donor site, is placed intact over the recipient site and sutured in place (see Fig. 29-14).

Mesh graft—A sheet of skin is removed from the donor site and passed through a mesher, which produces tiny slits in the skin. The meshing allows the expansion of the skin to cover $1\frac{1}{2}$ to 9 times the area of the sheet graft (see Fig. 29-15).

---

limited by the availability of tissue banks and the supply of suitable donors.

Although various animal skins have been used for many years to provide temporary coverage of wounds, only porcine xenograft is widely used today. Porcine xenograft does not vascularize, but it will adhere to a clean superficial burn and provide excellent pain control while the burn heals (Sheridan and Tompkins, 2007a). Pigskin dressings are replaced daily or every 2 or 3 days. They are particularly effective in children with partial-thickness scald burns of the hands and face because they allow relatively pain-free movement, which reduces contracture formation and has the added benefit of improving appetite and morale (Fig. 29-12).

When applied early to a superficial partial-thickness injury, biologic dressings appear to accelerate wound healing. They create an environment at the wound surface that is conducive to epithelial growth; this is in contrast to topical antimicrobial agents, which may slow epithelialization. Biologic dressings must be applied to clean wounds. If the dressing covers areas of heavy microbial contamination, infection occurs beneath the dressing. In the case of partial-thickness burns, such an infection may convert the wound to a full-thickness injury. It is important to observe the wound daily for any signs of an infectious process.

Synthetic Skin Coverings

A number of satisfactory skin substitutes are available for the management of partial-thickness burn wounds. Ideally, the dressing should provide many of the properties of human skin: adherence, elasticity, durability, and hemostasis. Synthetic skin substitutes are readily available, have varied shelf lives, and are relatively expensive.

Synthetic dressings are composed of a variety of materials and can be used successfully in the management of superficial partial-thickness burns and donor sites. These dressings do not contain antimicrobial properties. Examples include a pertrolatum dressing (Xeroform), synthetic silicone meshed products (Biobrane), a hydrocolloid dressing (DuoDERM), and transparent adhesive films (OpSite and Tegaderm) (Bessey, 2007). As with biologic dressings, it is important that the wound be free of debris before applying the dressing. Body temperature elevation or evidence of purulence, erythema, or cellulitis around the wound edges may indicate that the wound has become infected beneath the dressing. Prompt discontinuance of the synthetic dressing is indicated. All synthetic dressings are reputed to hasten wound healing and reduce discomfort.

Artificial Skin

Integra, a biologic two-layer product that allows the dermis to regenerate, has significantly improved burn wound healing and decreased scar formation. It is applied to partial- and full-thickness burns. The inner layer is porous woven fiber made of a pure form of collagen (a fibrous protein taken from animal tendons and cartilage) and other materials designed to induce better regeneration of the patient's normal tissue. The outer layer is a soft silicone membrane that holds moisture for 2 to 3 weeks. The silicone layer is peeled off after the dermis is formed. The application of artificial skin does not replace the grafting procedure, but it prepares the burn wound to accept an ultrathin autograft. Advantages include faster healing of the burn wound when integrity of the dermis is restored, faster healing of donor sites with the use of ultrathin grafts, and restoration of sweat glands and hair follicles. A disadvantage is its high cost.

Permanent Skin Coverings

Permanent coverage of deep partial- and full-thickness burns is usually accomplished with a split-thickness skin graft. This graft consists of the epidermis and a portion of the dermis removed

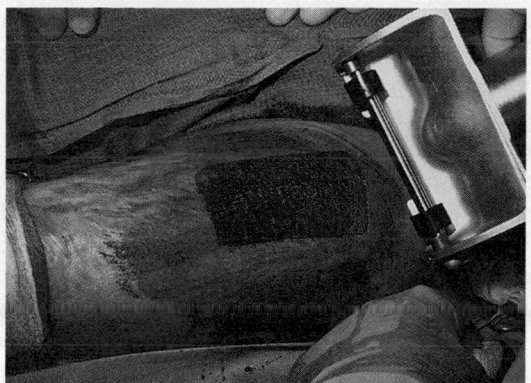

Fig. 29-13 Removal of split-thickness skin graft with a dermatome.

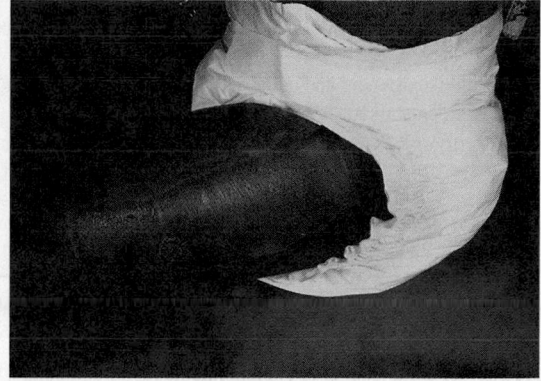

Fig. 29-16 Healed donor site.

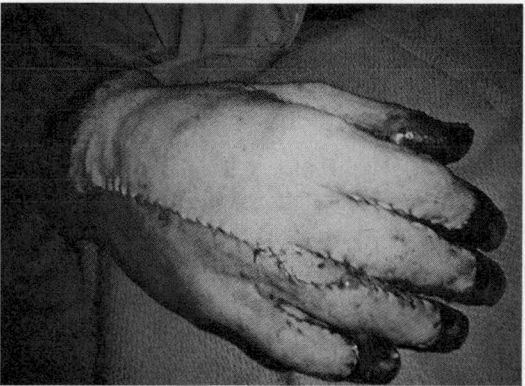

Fig. 29-14 Sheet graft.

BOX 29-16 REQUIREMENTS FOR A SUCCESSFUL GRAFT

- Sufficient nourishment until the new blood supply is established from the base of the recipient bed
- Primary tissue contact (i.e., actual contact between the surface of the graft and a recipient bed that is free of bacteria and necrotic skin)
- Avoidance of bleeding, hematoma formation, and fluid accumulation beneath the graft
- Prevention of infection
- Prevention of mechanical trauma

Until blood supply to the grafted skin is established, it is nourished by osmotic interchange with the recipient bed. Wound healing occurs as the area releases fibrin, which attaches the graft to the bed. The fibrin is infiltrated by leukocytes, fibroblasts, and the capillary buds of the granulation tissue. This process begins within hours of grafting, and vascularization is established after 3 days. Within 2 weeks the graft is attached to the recipient bed by connective tissue.

The donor site is dressed with synthetic wound coverings or fine-mesh gauze until the dressing separates at 10 to 14 days, when the wound is healed. Dressings are not changed on donor sites to avoid damage to newly healed, delicate epithelium. Healed donor sites are available for reharvesting in patients with extensive burns and limited undamaged skin (Fig. 29-16). The quality of skin from donor sites is decreased when multiple grafts are taken.

Cultured Epithelium

For more than 20 years it has been possible to culture vast numbers of epithelial cells from a small skin biopsy, and this has led to the widespread use of cultured epithelial grafts to cover burns. Colonies of epithelial cells expand into broad sheets of undifferentiated epithelial cells. The resulting sheets are attached to a petrolatum gauze carrier to ease handling. Many of the imperfections associated with epithelial cell wound closure may be attributed to the lack of dermis. Despite scattered cases, application of cultured epithelial grafts onto artificial skin has not been proven effective (Sheridan and Tompkins, 2007a). High cost is a disadvantage of using both applications.

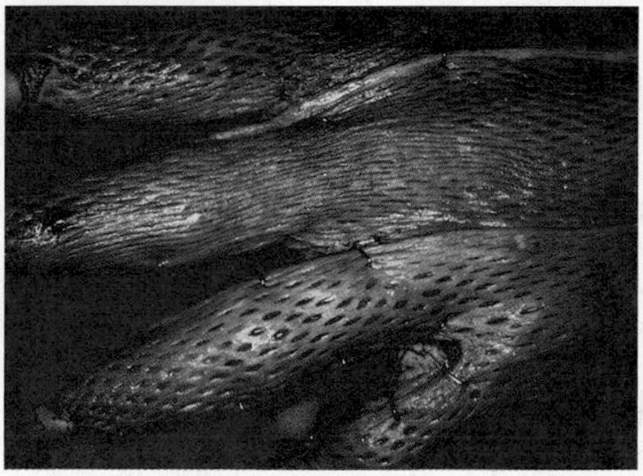

Fig. 29-15 Mesh graft.

from an intact area of skin by a special instrument: the dermatome (Fig. 29-13). If all the wounds cannot be grafted at once, there are priority areas for coverage: the face, hands, joint surfaces, and neck. These preferential sites are chosen to hasten healing, establish function, and improve the patient's sense of well-being.

With extensive burns it is often difficult to find enough viable skin to cover the wounds; therefore available donor sites are used to the best advantage by special techniques. Box 29-15 describes the various types of split-thickness skin grafts. Sheet grafts (Fig. 29-14) are used in areas where cosmetic results are most visible; mesh grafts (Fig. 29-15) result in a less desirable cosmetic and functional outcome. Requirements for the successful vascularization of any graft are listed in Box 29-16.

> **QUALITY PATIENT OUTCOMES: Acute Management of Burns**
> - Stable body temperature.
> - Adequate fluid replacement and urinary output.
> - Adequate nutrition and reduction of metabolic losses.
> - No evidence of acute complications.
> - Pain controlled.
> - Evidence of wound healing.
> - No evidence of contractures.
> - Adequate emotional support.

NURSING CARE MANAGEMENT

Nursing care of the pediatric burn patient represents a challenge to the nurse's knowledge of anatomy and physiology, the behavioral sciences, and pathophysiology. Patient outcome after thermal injury is the result of the collaboration of a professional multidisciplinary team using a family-centered care approach. In addition to providing nursing care, the nurse coordinates the efforts of a multidisciplinary burn team (Henry and Foster, 2000).

Because the care of burned children encompasses such a broad range of skills and foci, it has been divided into segments that correspond with the major phases of burn treatment. The acute phase, also referred to as the emergent or resuscitative phase, involves the first 24 to 48 hours. The management phase extends from the completion of adequate resuscitation through wound coverage. The rehabilitative phase begins once the majority of the wounds have healed and rehabilitation becomes the predominant focus of the care plan. This phase continues until all reconstructive procedures and corrective measures have been accomplished and often extends over a period of months or years.

Acute Phase

The primary emphasis during the emergent phase is the treatment of burn shock and management of pulmonary status. Monitoring vital signs, output, fluid infusion, and respiratory parameters are ongoing activities in the hours immediately after injury. IV infusion begins immediately and is regulated to maintain a urinary output of at least 1 to 2 ml/kg in children weighing less than 30 kg (66 lb). Expect an output of 30 to 50 ml/hr in children weighing more than 30 kg. Urinary output and specific gravity, vital signs, laboratory data, and objective signs of adequate hydration guide the rate of fluid administration.

> **! NURSING ALERT**
>
> Early indicators for the adequacy of hydration are level of consciousness and capillary refill.

The nurse observes patients for changes in all parameters. They require constant observation and assessment, with special attention given to signs of respiratory, cardiac, and renal complications. Alterations in electrolyte balance can produce clinical symptoms of confusion, weakness, cardiac irregularities,

and seizures. Changes in respiratory function and gas exchange are reflected clinically by restlessness, irritability, increased work of breathing, and alterations in blood gas values. The loss of the skin's protective function exposes burned children to an increased risk of hypothermia.

Care of the burn wound is secondary to the more critical problems of respiratory and cardiac failure. When transfer to a special burn care facility is anticipated, it is important to cover the wounds with clean sheets and wrap the child in blankets to maintain body temperature during transfer. The burn wound can be evaluated and dressed after arrival at the burn center. If no burn unit is available, the wound is cleansed and dressed in the emergency department. Many burn units maintain a pictorial record of the wound to record progress and for legal purposes, especially in cases of suspected child maltreatment. The burn wound is treated according to the protocol of the specific burn facility. The burn team implements infection control procedures and ensures that staff and visitors comply with established protocols to prevent cross-contamination in the burn unit.

Throughout the acute phase of care, do not overlook the psychosocial needs of the children and their families. The child is frightened, uncomfortable, and often confused. Children may be isolated from familiar persons and surroundings, and the often overwhelming physical needs at this time are the primary focus of the staff and parents. In addition to feeling concern for their child, the parents experience guilt, which is related to the fact they did not or could not protect their child. Consistency in the information presented and the attitude of the staff creates a sense of familiarity and stability during the emergent phase.

Management and Rehabilitative Phases

After the patient's condition is stabilized, the management phase begins. The multidisciplinary team concentrates on preventing wound infections, closing the wound as quickly as possible, and managing the numerous complications that may occur. Although the rehabilitative phase begins when permanent wound closure has been achieved, rehabilitation issues are identified on admission and are included in the care plan throughout the hospital course (see Nursing Care Plan).

The management phase of burn care involves intensive nursing care, which is often difficult for the patient, family, and nursing staff. Except for minor burn injuries, care should take place in a burn unit and involve a variety of disciplines, such as physical therapy, nutrition, social services, and respiratory care.

Comfort Management

The severe pain of the wound and resultant therapies, the anxiety generated by these experiences, sleep deprivation, itching related to wound healing, and the conscious and unconscious interpretations of traumatic events contribute to the psychologic reactions and behaviors commonly observed in children with burns. It is important to assess the individual experiences and needs of the burn-injured child. A common myth in pediatrics is that children do not feel pain as intensely as adults do. What may be more accurate is that children do not always express their pain in the same way as adults. Children may display pain through behaviors of fear, anxiety,

◎ NURSING CARE PLAN

The Child with Burns: Management and Rehabilitative Stages

NURSING DIAGNOSIS	EXPECTED PATIENT OUTCOMES	NURSING INTERVENTIONS	RATIONALE
Risk for Ineffective Thermoregulation related to heat loss and disruption of skin's defense mechanisms to maintain body temperature	Child will maintain optimum therm-oregulation as evidenced by (normal) body temperatures ranging from 37° to 38.1° C (98.6° to 100.5° F).	Assess skin for coolness, color changes, and capillary refill (acrocya-nosis, nail bed color, and mottling).	To identify vascular accommodation of heat loss
Child's/Family's Defining Characteristics <u>(Subjective and Objective Data)</u>	**The Following NOC Concept Applies to These Outcomes** Thermoregulation	Monitor vital signs, especially temperature.	To identify significant trends in tem-perature fluctuation
Changes in skin temperature, capil-lary refill, and color		Observe for chilling and shivering.	To evaluate signs of heat loss and provide comfort
Chilling and shivering		Avoid exposure to cold stress proce-dures (limit wound hygiene time; cover the head of a child younger than 6 months of age; cover the child and use a warm blanket or warming devices).	To maintain stable body temperature and prevent body heat loss
Changes in temperature from cold exposure		Maintain ambient room temperature at 30° to 33° C (86° to 91° F).	To maintain stable body temperature and prevent body heat loss
		The Following NIC Concepts Apply to These Interventions Hypothermia Treatment Vital Signs Monitoring Environmental Management Fluid Monitoring Fever Management	

NURSING DIAGNOSIS	EXPECTED PATIENT OUTCOMES	NURSING INTERVENTIONS	RATIONALE
Deficient Fluid Volume related to normal fluid loss from tissues sec-ondary to burn insult	Child will maintain adequate fluid hydration status during the acute postburn period.	Administer crystalloid or colloid fluid per protocol, monitoring effect and maintaining intravenous line.	To replace fluid loss related to burn injury
Child's/Family's Defining Characteristics <u>(Subjective and Objective Data)</u>	**The Following NOC Concepts Apply to These Outcomes** Electrolyte and Acid-Base Balance Fluid Balance	Assess fluid replacement status: observe for changes in vital signs, mental status, and urinary output.	To recognize appropriate fluid balance
Decreased skin turgor		Monitor daily weights.	To evaluate status of fluid retention or excess fluid loss and possible diuresis
Increased pulse			
Decreased urinary output		Observe and monitor hemodynamic parameters for changes in stability related to hypovolemia or fluid overload.	To detect change in blood pressure, which is a late sign of shock
Decreased circulation status		Monitor laboratory results.	To identify fluid and electrolyte imbalance
		Monitor for tissue edema.	To implement therapies to reestab-lish intravascular protein and pre-vent further tissue damage
		Administer potassium-rich or potas-sium-restricted fluids or foods if child is hypokalemic or hyperkalemic.	To supplement intravenous therapy as needed to maintain electrolyte balance and prevent sequelae from alteration in potassium balance
		The Following NIC Concepts Apply to These Interventions Acid-Base Management Acid-Base Monitoring Electrolyte Monitoring Fluid Monitoring Hemodynamic Regulation Intravenous Therapy Laboratory Data Interpretation Vital Sign Monitoring	

Continued

NURSING CARE PLAN—cont'd

The Child with Burns: Management and Rehabilitative Stages

NURSING DIAGNOSIS	EXPECTED PATIENT OUTCOMES	NURSING INTERVENTIONS	RATIONALE
Impaired Skin Integrity related to thermal injury **Child's/Family's Defining Characteristics (Subjective and Objective Data)** Inflammation at burn site, redness, and swelling Lack of granulation of burned tissues; no evidence of epithelialization Child scratching or picking at wound, causing redness and irritation at the site	Child will show evidence of wound healing. Wounds will heal without evidence of damage or inflammation. **The Following NOC Concepts Apply to These Outcomes** Tissue Integrity: Skin and Mucous Membranes Wound Healing	Shave hair to a 2-inch margin from the wound and area immediately surrounding the burn. Thoroughly cleanse the wound and surrounding skin and débride devitalized tissue. Keep child from scratching and picking at the wound. • Keep fingernails clean and clipped short. • Apply socks to hands if necessary; elbow restraints as needed. • Administer antipruritic medications. • Provide distraction appropriate to child's age. Maintain care in handling the wound. Offer high-calorie, high-protein meals and snacks. Maintain sterile technique with dressing changes. Administer supplementary vitamins and minerals (vitamins A, B, C; iron; and zinc). Pad burned ears. Monitor for signs and symptoms of wound infection. Wrap fingers and toes separately. Place child on pressure-sensitive mattress if prolonged bed rest. Monitor skin at pressure points. **The Following NIC Concepts Apply to These Interventions** Infection Control Medication Administration Skin Care: Topical Treatments Skin Surveillance Wound Care Infection Protection Splinting Wound Irrigation	To remove a reservoir for infection To decrease the risk of infection and promote healing To prevent infection and prevent impaired tissue healing To avoid damaging epithelializing and granulating tissues To supplement protein and calorie requirements caused by increased metabolism and catabolism To prevent infection, which can delay wound healing and convert partial-thickness wounds to full-thickness wounds To facilitate wound healing and tissue epithelialization To prevent tissue necrosis caused by minimum blood flow to cartilage To ensure prompt recognition and treatment To avoid tissue adherence from prolonged contact To prevent pressure point skin breakdown and further tissue damage
NURSING DIAGNOSIS	EXPECTED PATIENT OUTCOMES	NURSING INTERVENTIONS	RATIONALE
Impaired Physical Mobility (specify level) related to pain, impaired joint movement, scar formation **Child's/Family's Defining Characteristics (Subjective and Objective Data)** Limited and/or restricted movement in joint or muscle	Child will achieve optimum physical functioning (mobility). **The Following NOC Concepts Apply to These Outcomes** Joint Movement: Active Mobility Level Transfer Performance	Carry out range-of-motion exercises. Administer pain medication (analgesia) 30 to 45 minutes before physical therapy. Encourage mobility if child is able to move extremities. Have child walk as soon as feasible. Splint involved joints in extension at night and during rest periods. Encourage and promote self-help activities. Encourage participation in activities of daily living and play activities. **The Following NIC Concepts Apply to These Interventions** Body Mechanics Promotion Energy Management Exercise Promotion: Strength Training Exercise Therapy: Joint Mobility	To maintain optimum joint and muscle function To minimize or eliminate pain from mobilization of tight skin at joints To make child more likely to cooperate and be mobile To decrease the adverse effects of prolonged immobilization on body systems To minimize contracture formation To increase mobility and positive self-esteem To incorporate exercise into enjoyable events

⊚ NURSING CARE PLAN—cont'd

The Child with Burns: Management and Rehabilitative Stages

NURSING DIAGNOSIS	EXPECTED PATIENT OUTCOMES	NURSING INTERVENTIONS	RATIONALE
Pain related to skin trauma, therapies	Child will experience reduction of pain to a level acceptable to the child.	Assess needs for medication.	To minimize intense pain caused by burns
Child's/Family's Defining Characteristics (Subjective and Objective Data)		Recognize that burn pain is often overwhelming, engulfing, and irrepressible.	To provide adequate pain interventions for overwhelming pain
	The Following NOC Concepts Apply to These Outcomes	Position in extension position.	To minimize pain resulting from exercising to regain extension
Pain on movement	Comfort Control	Implement passive and active exercise.	To minimize contracture formation
Pain associated with treatment	Pain: Disruptive Effects	Reduce skin irritation by bed linens, other items as applicable.	To prevent increased pain
Irritation at burn site	Pain Control	Administer medication for pruritus after therapy and treatments.	To provide comfort
Pain on extension of joint		Touch or stroke unburned areas.	To provide physical contact and comfort
		Employ appropriate nonpharmacologic measures in pain reduction techniques.	To provide comfort and reduce pain
		Promote control and predictability during painful procedures.	To minimize pain and anxiety
		Anticipate need for pain medication and administer before onset of severe pain at regular intervals.	To prevent pain recurrence
		The Following NIC Concepts Apply to These Interventions	
		Analgesic Administration	
		Positioning	
		Presence	
		Pain Management	
		Relaxation Therapy	
		Sleep Enhancement	
		Coping Enhancement	

agitation, anger, aggression, tantrums, depression, withdrawal, and regression.

How the child's experience of pain from the burn injury and anxiety from the hospitalization are managed has lasting psychologic effects. A careful nursing history that includes the child's past experiences with pain and ways that caregivers successfully handled those events may provide clues to the control of current pain. Caregiver involvement is especially important for a child (Lee and Herndon, 2007). Interventions may include medications (including IV morphine and short-term anesthetics such as propofol or ketamine), relaxation techniques, distraction therapy, cutaneous stimulation by touching, and family participation. Nonpharmacologic therapies may be used as adjuncts in the treatment of pain. In young children, distraction and imagery work well (Kahana, 2003; Henry and Foster, 2000).

To reduce the anxiety associated with an unfamiliar environment and frightening treatments, it is important to offer thorough, age-appropriate explanations to the child before procedures. Compounding the pain is the child's interpretation of it and of the procedure; this is closely related to the child's developmental level. Children often feel anger, guilt, and depression; as in all illnesses, they may also exhibit regressive behavior. When children appear to accept pain with little or no response, psychologic consultation is in order.

Care of the Burn Wound

The nurse has a major responsibility for cleansing, débriding, and applying topical medications and dressings to the burn wound. Because dressing removal is a painful procedure, children should receive adequate analgesia before the scheduled dressing change. The nurse should administer medication so that the drug's peak effect coincides with the procedure. Children who have an understanding of the procedure to be performed and some perceived control demonstrate less maladaptive behavior. Children respond well to participating in decisions and the actual procedure as their condition allows.

With some children, nonpharmacologic interventions are effective means of coping with pain. Distraction therapy, deep breathing, and relaxation techniques may facilitate the procedure. Most children also benefit from parental participation. Medical play is often effective in helping the younger child gain some mastery over the procedure. Incorporate those techniques that work best for the individual patient into the care plan and consistently implement them during the dressing change procedure.

Outer dressings are removed; any dressings that have adhered to the wound are easier to remove by applying tepid water. Loose or easily detached tissue is also débrided during the cleansing process. Encourage children to participate in dressing removal. Giving them something constructive to do helps them focus on something other than the procedure. In dressing the wound, it is important that all areas be clean, that medication be amply applied, and that no two burned surfaces touch each other (e.g., fingers or toes, or ears touching the side of the head). If touching, the burned surfaces will heal together, causing deformity or dysfunction.

Topical medications are applied directly to the wound with a clean gloved hand or impregnated into fine-mesh gauze before application. Then apply dressings to assist in exudate absorption, wound débridement, and increased patient comfort. All dressings applied circumferentially should be wrapped in a distal-to-proximal manner. Apply the dressing with sufficient tension to remain in place without impairing circulation or limiting motion. A stable dressing is especially important when the child is ambulatory.

Burns that involve the eyelids require special care to prevent corneal ulceration. No solution other than saline should come in contact with the eyes during the cleansing process. Avoid vigorous débridement in this area of thin, delicate tissue. Assess the patient throughout the healing process for the ability to close the eyes. Inability to close the eyes because of contracture formation, administration of paralytic agents, or corneal burns requires instilling ophthalmic ointment and covering the eyes with a patch to prevent further corneal damage (Achauer and Adair, 2000).

Universal Precautions, including the use of protective garb and barrier techniques, should be followed when caring for all patients with thermal injuries. Frequent hand and forearm washing is the single most important element of the infection control program. Implement strict policies for cleaning the environment and patient care equipment to minimize the risk of cross-contamination. All visitors and members of other departments should be oriented to the infection control policies, including the importance of hand and forearm washing and use of protective garb. Screen all visitors for infection and contagious diseases before patient contact.

Nutrition

Oral feedings are common unless the child is intubated or paralytic ileus persists. Because children often lack an appetite, the nursing staff must provide a great deal of encouragement, help, and patience. Consultation between the parents and dietitian helps determine food preferences. Include children who are old enough to participate in meal planning.

Nourishing snacks are provided between scheduled meals. Painful procedures should not be scheduled around meals; most children are too physically exhausted and emotionally upset to eat at this time. Many children eat better in an atmosphere more nearly like what they are accustomed to at home. When their condition allows, children enjoy sitting at a table for meals and interacting with other children.

Children who require enteral supplementation by tube feeding must be monitored on an ongoing basis for intolerance and tube malposition. The nurse should monitor and record any indications of abdominal distention, diarrhea, or electrolyte and metabolic derangement. Accurate documentation of oral, parenteral, and enteral nutritional intake is essential to evaluate the adequacy of nutritional support.

Prevention of Complications: Acute Care

The maintenance of body temperature is important to the child with burns. Reduction of heat loss is imperative to decrease energy demands and evaporative water loss. Ambient temperatures and humidity should be maintained at 28° to 33° C (82.4° to 91.4° F) and 80%, respectively, to control heat loss (Lee and Herndon, 2007). Large areas of the body should not be exposed simultaneously during dressing changes. Warmed solutions, linens, occlusive dressings, heat shields, a radiant warmer, and warming blankets assist in preventing hypothermia. The optimum environment for the child with burns can be uncomfortable for persons attending the child.

The chief danger during acute care is infection—wound infection, generalized sepsis, or bacterial pneumonia. The burn wound should be assessed for changes indicative of wound infection, which include conversion of a partial-thickness to a full-thickness burn injury, early eschar separation, subeschar hemorrhage, degeneration of granulation tissue, discoloration of unburned skin at the wound margins, or green discoloration of subcutaneous fat (indicative of *Pseudomonas* and other gram-negative organisms). In addition to the signs of developing wound infection, the child with systemic sepsis may have a core temperature of more than 38.5° C (101.3° F) or less than 36° C (96.8° F), tachycardia, tachypnea, and leukocytosis or leukopenia. Tachycardia and tachypnea are common presenting symptoms in many pediatric diseases. Children with septic shock often maintain a normal BP until they are severely ill. Shock may occur long before hypotension in children. It is a sign of late and decompensated shock. Meticulous assessment should include signs of decreased perfusion (including decreased peripheral pulses), altered alertness, prolonged capillary refill (2 seconds), mottled or cool extremities, or decreased urinary output (Goldstein, Giroir, and Randolph, 2005).

Children are reluctant to move when doing so causes pain, and they are likely to assume a position of comfort. Unfortunately, the most comfortable position is often one that encourages the formation of contractures and loss of function. Ongoing efforts to prevent contractures include the positioning and splinting of involved extremities in extension, active and passive physical therapy, and the encouragement of spontaneous movement when feasible. In addition to maintenance of proper body alignment, frequent position changes are important to improve bronchopulmonary hygiene and capillary perfusion to common pressure areas. Low–air loss beds are beneficial for the morbidly obese or for children with posterior grafts. Areas of particular concern for pressure area development in the pediatric population are the posterior scalp, heels, and areas exposed to mechanical irritation from splints and dressings.

Prevention of Complications: Long-Term Care

The rehabilitative phase of care begins once wound coverage has been achieved. Scar formation becomes a major problem as burn wounds heal (Fig. 29-17). The scar tissue is metabolically active and highly vascular; collagen is deposited in an undefined pattern. Contractile properties of the scar tissue can result in disabling contractures, deformity, and disfigurement. As long as the scar is raised, red, and firm, it is considered active (Fig. 29-18). Hypertrophic scarring typically reaches a peak approximately 4 to 6 months after wound healing, and most scars mature or become inactive in 1 to 2 years. The mature scar is characterized by pigmented color, flattening, and increased suppleness of the tissue (Fig. 29-19).

Uniform pressure applied to the scar decreases the blood supply and forces the collagen into a more normal alignment.

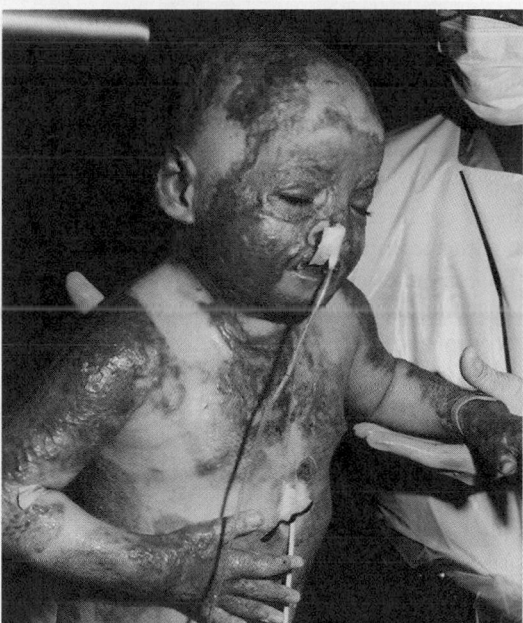

Fig. 29-17 Extensive scars from flame burn. (Courtesy CR Boeckman Regional Burn Center, Akron, Ohio.)

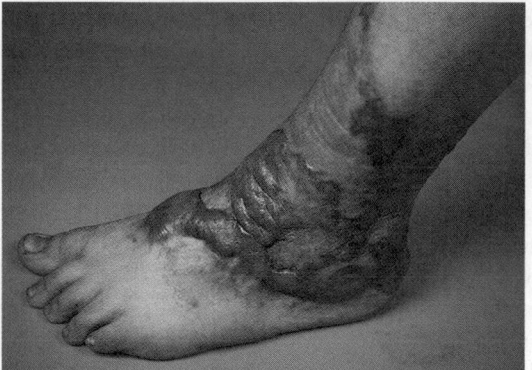

Fig. 29-18 Hypertrophic immature scar.

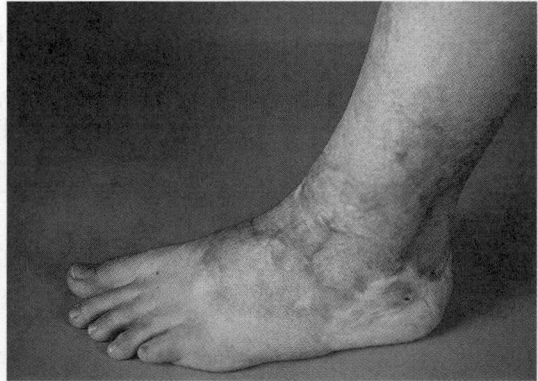

Fig. 29-19 Flat, mature scar after pressure.

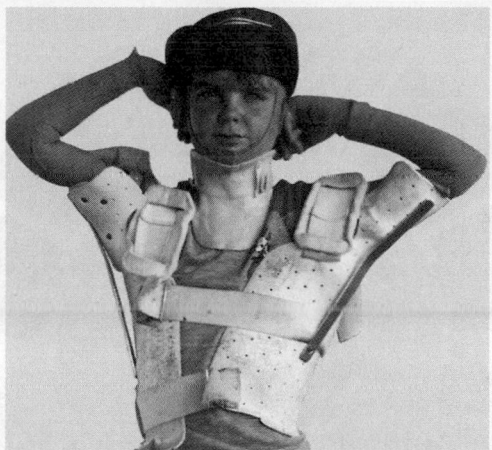

Fig. 29-20 Child in elasticized (Jobst) garment and "airplane" splints.

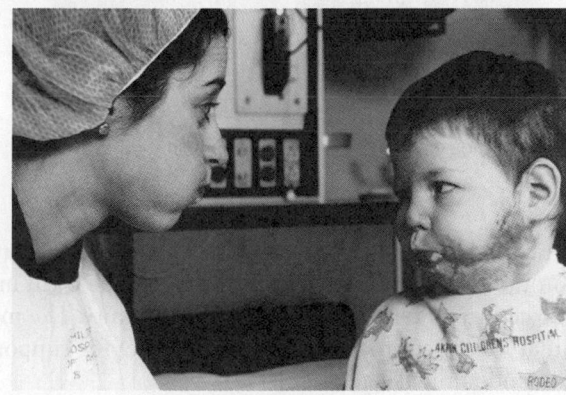

Fig. 29-21 Daily physical therapy to prevent contracture deformity is continued at home or in an outpatient setting. Note how nurse encourages child to imitate her facial action. (Courtesy CR Boeckman Regional Burn Center, Akron, Ohio.)

When pressure is removed, blood supply to the scar is immediately increased; therefore periods without pressure should be brief to avoid nourishment of the hypertrophic tissue. Continuous pressure to areas of scarring can be achieved by elastic bandages or commercially available pressure garments. Because these custom-made garments are often worn for months, revision may be required as the child grows. It is much easier to prevent scarring and contracture of the wound than to resolve an existing problem. Splints and appliances may also be necessary until wound maturation occurs (Fig. 29-20). Part of outpatient and home care often includes the continuation of regular physical therapy (Fig. 29-21).

Scar tissue has certain significant properties, particularly for growing children. Intense itching occurs in healing burn wounds and scar tissue until the scar is no longer active. Itching is usually treated with hydroxyzine (Atarax) or diphenhydramine and frequent applications of a moisturizer, such as Eucerin, cocoa butter, or Nivea. Massage therapy during the application of moisturizers is also beneficial to stretch scar tissue and help prevent contracture. Scar tissue has no sweat glands, and children with extensive scarring may experience difficulty during hot weather. Alert caregivers to this possibility and make sure they are prepared to institute alternate methods of cooling when necessary.

Scar tissue does not grow and expand like normal tissue, which may create difficulties, especially in functional areas such as the hands and over joints. Additional surgery is sometimes required to allow independent functioning in daily activities, to improve cosmetic appearance, or to restore anatomic integrity. Reconstructive surgery employs various techniques, including local or distant flaps, full- or partial-thickness grafts, tissue expanders, or pedicle flaps.

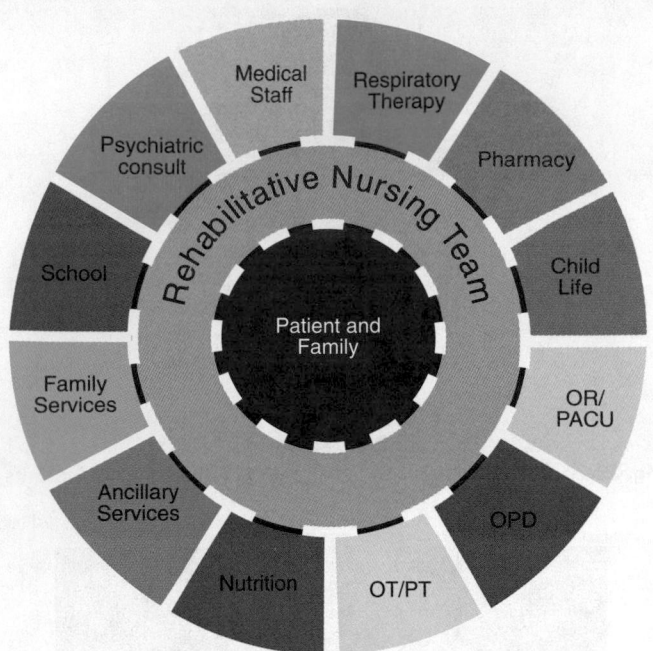

Fig. 29-22 Multidisciplinary approach to rehabilitation of pediatric burn patient.

The nursing activities in the rehabilitative phase of treatment focus on the child's and family's adaptation to the burn injury and their ability to reintegrate into the community. The multidisciplinary team approach remains the model for support of the child and family (Fig. 29-22).

The psychologic pain and impact of severe burn injury are as intense as the physical trauma. The impact of severe burns taxes the capabilities at all ages. Very young children, who suffer acutely from separation anxiety, and adolescents, who are developing an identity, are probably the most affected psychologically. Toddlers cannot understand why the parents they love and who have protected them can leave them in such a frightening and unfamiliar place. Adolescents, in the process of achieving independence from the family, find themselves in a dependent role with a damaged body. Being different from others at a time when conformity with peers is so important is difficult to accept.

Anticipation of the return to school can be overwhelming and frightening. It is essential that health care professionals recognize the importance of preparing teachers and classmates for the child's return. Provide teachers with information to assist the child and family and to promote the child's optimum adjustment. Hospital-sponsored school reentry programs use a variety of methods to provide education and information about the implications of the injury, the garments and appliances, and the need for support and acceptance. Telephone calls, videotapes, information packets, and visits by members of the health care team offer opportunities to help with reintegration into the school environment—a focal point of the child's life.

Psychosocial Support of the Child

Children should begin early to do as much for themselves as possible and to be active participants in their care. Loss of control and perceived helplessness may result in acting-out behaviors. Nurses should be sensitive to these feelings and allow the child the opportunity for choices and decision making as the condition allows. At the same time, it is important to set boundaries and establish a daily schedule to provide a sense of predictability, security, and control. During illness, children regress to a previous developmental level that allows them to deal with stress. As children begin to participate in their care, they gain in confidence and self-esteem. Fears and anxieties diminish with accomplishment and self-confidence. If the child demonstrates nonadherence in the rehabilitative phase, initiate a behavior modification program to promote or reward the child's accomplishment in care.

Select and encourage activities on the basis of each child's developmental level and interest. Quiet activities such as reading, coloring, and games are always appropriate. Critically ill children enjoy tapes and stories, even though they may not be able to actively participate in play. Television is a satisfactory diversion but should not replace contact with others. Play that encourages the expression of anger, frustration, and guilt is especially therapeutic. Medical play is a valuable tool to teach children what to expect and their role in the treatment process. School-age children benefit by continuing study activities as they are able.

Children need to feel they look nice. The burns, dressings, and medical equipment do little to foster a positive self-image. Small things, such as careful hair combing, a bright ribbon or pajamas, a pretty blanket, or colorful stickers will help them feel better about themselves and feel worthwhile to others.

Children need to know that their injury and the treatments are not punishment for real or imagined transgressions and that the nurse understands their fear, anger, and discomfort. They also need body contact. This is often difficult to arrange for the child with massive burns; stroking areas of unburned skin is comforting. Even older children enjoy sitting on the nurse's or parent's lap and being cuddled and hugged. This can be a reward or a comfort in times of stress, but most of all it is a natural part of childhood.

Psychosocial Support of the Family

There is a growing recognition that trauma affects not only the victim but also those closest to the child. Severe trauma challenges the belief that the world is safe and predictable. Parents and other family members are concerned about the child's survival, recovery, and future potential. Recognizing and respecting each family's strengths, differences, and methods of coping allows the nurse to respond to their unique needs by implementing a family-centered approach to care. It is the family, particularly the parents, who are the most significant persons in the child's life.

As in any emergency situation, all attention is focused on the child, and the parents feel powerless and ineffectual. Most parents feel overwhelming guilt, whether or not the guilt is justified. They feel responsible for the injury. These feelings may have a negative effect on the child's rehabilitation. For example, parents may indulge the child and allow poor behavior that affects physical and emotional recovery.

Nurses have the opportunity to assist parents in coping with the stresses of the child's illness and with their own feelings of guilt and helplessness. The parents need to be informed of the child's progress and assisted in coping with their feelings while providing support to their child. The nurse can help them understand that it is not selfish to look after themselves and their own needs to better meet the needs of their child. Definitive professional help may be needed for parents whose response to the injury is severe or whose response to stress is manifested in destructive behavior.

The parents are members of the multidisciplinary team and participate in the development of the care plan. It is important to address their input to consider all aspects of the physical, emotional, social, and cultural factors affecting the child and family and to establish a realistic home therapy program. The family's willingness to assume responsibility for care and their ability to implement the therapeutic regimen are assessed. Explore home, school, and other environmental factors with the family, as well as financial concerns and available community resources. The nurse can then develop a specific care plan, with an anticipated follow-up program.

Caring for the Caregiver

Burn care is a complex and demanding specialty. Nurses who choose this field reap many rewards and endure many stresses. Ongoing support from peers, the multidisciplinary team, and nursing management is important to assist burn nurses in caring for themselves so they can continue to render high-quality care to their patients.

Prevention of Burn Injury

Burn prevention is the responsibility of all members of the community. Nurses have an obligation to participate in educational efforts directed at parents, children, and others regarding the prevention of burn injuries and fire-related deaths. The best cure is prevention.

Infants and toddlers are most commonly injured by hot liquids in the kitchen and bathroom. These injuries often occur as a result of inadequate supervision of this curious and energetic age-group. Target prevention efforts at parents and other caregivers; education includes the importance of adequate supervision and the establishment of safe play areas in the home. Hot liquids should be kept out of reach; tablecloths and dangling appliance cords are often pulled by toddlers, spilling hot grease and liquids on them. Electrical cords and outlets represent a potential risk to small children, who may chew on accessible cords and insert objects into outlets.

Since 1974, the Consumer Product Safety Commission has recommended a reduction of hot water heater thermostats to a maximum of 49° C (120° F). This recommendation has been supported by utility companies, burn treatment centers, medical personnel, and others interested in public safety. However, many hot water heaters remain set at levels well above the safe level. Small children are especially at risk for scald injuries from hot tap water because of their decreased reaction time and agility, their curiosity, and the thermal sensitivity of their skin (Fig. 29-23). Educate caregivers about never leaving a child in a bath without adult supervision. Caregiver should also test the water before placing a child in the tub or shower.

Microwave ovens, although perceived by many as safer than conventional ovens and stoves, heat foods and liquids to high temperatures that can result in burns from spills, splashes, and the release of steam (Box 29-17).

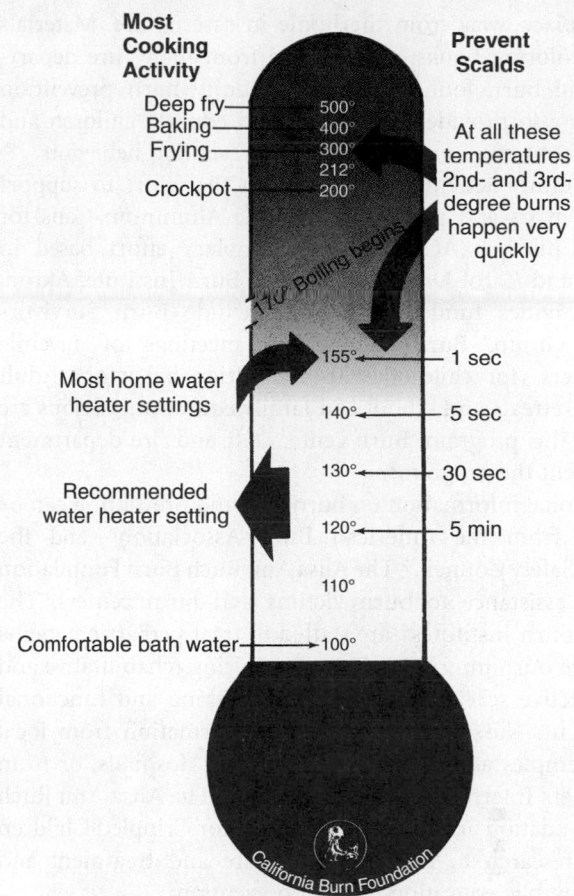

NOTE: Microwave cooking presents special hazards. Fillings in doughnuts, pies, tarts, etc., become superheated (600° or more) and may explode when moved.

Fig. 29-23 Temperatures associated with common burn injuries in the home. All temperatures given in Fahrenheit. NOTE: Most authorities recommend that water heaters be kept at the lowest safe setting of 120° F (49° C). (Courtesy California Burn Foundation, Canoga Park, Calif.)

BOX 29-17 MICROWAVE SAFETY

- Place microwave ovens at a safe height (but higher than children's faces) and within easy reach to avoid spills.
- Never heat baby formula or milk in a plastic bottle liner because it may burst.
- Before adding a cold liquid to a liquid heated in the microwave, insert a spoon to prevent bubbling over of the hot liquid.
- For food heated in containers, puncture plastic wrap, use vented lids, or wait 1 minute before removing a sealed covering, then lift the covering from the corner farthest away from face or arm.

As children mature, risk-taking behaviors increase. Matches and lighters are dangerous in the hands of the young. In 2006 alone, an estimated 14,500 structural fires were reported to U.S. fire departments as a result of children playing with fire (National Fire Protection Association, 2009). Adults must remember to keep potentially hazardous items out of the reach of children; a lighter, like a match, is a tool for adult use.

Education related to fire safety and survival should begin with the very young. They can practice "stop, drop, and roll" to extinguish a fire and the fire escape route, including a safe meeting place away from the home in case of fire. Materials such as coloring books are available from many fire departments and burn foundations. Community burn prevention programs also provide opportunities to educate children and parents about fire, burn hazards, and prevention behaviors.

Community activities are helpful in the effort to support burn survivors and prevent burns. The Aluminum Cans for Burned Children (ACBC) is an exemplary effort based in the Paul and Carol David Foundation Burn Institute, Akron, Ohio. Activities funded by ACBC include Burn Survivors Support Group, Burn Camp, and meetings of Juvenile Firestoppers (for children with fire-setting behavior). Adult weekend retreats and school and family education sessions are a part of this program. Burn center staff and fire department staff present the programs.

Additional information on burn care and prevention can be obtained from the American Burn Association* and the National Safety Council.† The Alisa Ann Ruch Burn Foundation provides assistance to burn victims and burn centers. The Shriners Burn Institutes‡ are staffed to treat pediatric patients after acute burn injuries and those requiring rehabilitative and reconstructive services as a result of scarring and functional impairment. Nurses can also obtain information from local Shrine Temples and Clubs, from Shriners Hospitals, or from the Shriners International Headquarters.§ The Alisa Ann Ruch Burn Foundation and Shriners Hospitals for Crippled Children support research to improve burn care and treatment and promote public education in burn prevention.

FUTURE RESEARCH NEEDS

Many advances in burn prevention have reduced the occurrence of burn injury. Early excision and grafting of the burn wound, with control of infection, have improved survival rates for burn injury. Areas for future research include the rate of wound healing, characteristics of the healed wound, support techniques for inhalation injury, the effect of hypothermia immediately after burn injury, nursing interventions that promote healing of donor sites and skin grafts, and the most effective wound-cleansing protocol. Evidence for improvement of burn nursing care is best organized with research findings (Carrougher, 1998). Evidence-based practice integrates nurse's clinical expertise with the best methods. It helps structure how to make accurate and timely decisions for care of the patient (Gordon and Marvin, 2007).

---

*625 North Michigan Ave., Suite 2550, Chicago, IL 60611; 312-642-9260; fax: 312-642-9130; e-mail: info@ameriburn.org; www.ameriburn.org.

†1121 Spring Lake Drive, Itasca, IL 60143-3201; 630-285-1121, e-mail: info@nsc.org; www.nsc.org.

‡2501 W. Burbank Blvd., Suite 201, Burbank, CA 91505; 800-242-BURN; www.aarbf.org.

§2900 Rocky Point Drive, Tampa, FL 33607; Shriners International Headquarters website: www.shrinershq.org; Shriners Hospitals for Children website: www.shriners.com/Hospitals/_Hospitals_for_Children.

▮ KEY POINTS

- GI disorders of childhood that commonly cause fluid depletion and electrolyte disturbance are diarrhea and vomiting.
- The four general mechanisms of diarrhea are secretory, cytotoxic, osmotic, and dysenteric diarrhea.
- The treatment for acute diarrhea consists primarily of oral rehydration and provision of an adequate diet.
- Burns are caused by thermal, electrical, chemical, or radioactive agents.
- The severity of burn injury is assessed on the basis of the percentage of TBSA burned, depth, location, age, etiologic agent, concomitant injuries, and general health.
- Emergency measures for severe burns include stopping the burning process; assessing for airway, breathing, and circula-

tion; covering the burn; transporting the child to the hospital; and providing reassurance to the child and family.
- Management of minor burns consists of facilitating wound healing, relieving pain and discomfort, and preventing complications.
- Management of major burn injuries involves facilitating wound healing, relieving pain and discomfort, replacing destroyed skin, preventing or treating complications, and providing rehabilitation.
- Active participation by the child and family is important in the care of the child with burn trauma.

▮ ANSWERS TO CRITICAL THINKING EXERCISE

Diarrhea

1. **Yes,** there are sufficient data for the nurse practitioner to arrive at some conclusions.
2. a. See Table 28-3, p. 1059, Evaluating Extent of Dehydration, and note the criteria for mild dehydration.
   b. Infants and children with mild dehydration are managed with oral rehydration therapy and early reintroduction of an adequate diet. In cases of severe dehydration, or when infants and children have uncontrollable vomiting, intravenous fluids are used in the management of acute diarrhea.

c. Breast-feeding generally can be continued in mild dehydration.
   d. Antidiarrheal medications are not recommended for the treatment of acute infectious diarrhea. These medications have adverse effects such as slowed motility and can prolong the illness.
3. At present, Mary meets all the criteria for mild dehydration. It is highly probable that she has acute infectious diarrhea because her mother noted that she has had a "cold" for several days and she is vomiting, has diarrhea, and has an

elevated temperature. The priority for nursing care at this time is to provide rehydration via an oral rehydration solution (ORS). ORS is an effective, safe, and cost-effective way to treat mild dehydration. The nurse practitioner should instruct the mother to give Mary ORS at frequent intervals and in small amounts. The mother should also be instructed to continue with breast-feeding and normal feedings. Early reintroduction of normal nutrients is desirable in cases of mild dehydration; delayed introduction of food may be harmful and can prolong the illness. Mary's mother should also be told to avoid the use of antidiarrheal medications.

4. **Yes,** the evidence supports this initial plan of management.

REFERENCES

Achauer BM, Adair SR: Acute and reconstructive management of the burned eyelid, *Clin Plast Surg* 27(1):87-96, 2000.

Acker ME: Vomiting in children, *Adv Nurse Pract* 10(1):51-56, 68, 2002.

American Burn Association: *Guidelines for the operation of burn centers,* Chicago, 2006, The Association, available at www.ameriburn.org/Chapter14.pdf (accessed March 11, 2010).

Andrews DA: Management of the burned child, *Prob Gen Surg* 11(4):662-665, 1994.

Arnal LE, Stein F: Pediatric septic shock: why has mortality decreased? The utility of goal-directed therapy, *Semin Pediatr Infect Dis* 14(2):165-172, 2003.

Barrow RE, Herndon DN: History of the treatment of burns. In Herndon DN, editor: *Total burn care,* Philadelphia, 2007, Saunders.

Beierle EA, Chung DH: Surgical management of complications of burn injury. In Herndon DN, editor: *Total burn care,* Philadelphia, 2007, Saunders.

Bessey PQ: Wound care. In Herndon DN, editor: *Total burn care,* Philadelphia, 2007, Saunders.

Bohlke K, Davis RL, DeStefano F, et al: Epidemiology of anaphylaxis among children and adolescents enrolled in a health maintenance organization, *J Allergy Clin Immunol* 113(3):536-542, 2004.

Brierley J, Choong K, Cornell T, et al: 2007 American College of Critical Care Medicine clinical practice parameters for hemodynamic support of pediatric and neonatal septic shock, *Crit Care Med* Nov 28, 2008 (Epub).

Bullard J, Page NE: Cyclic vomiting syndrome: a disease in disguise, *Pediatr Nurs* 31(1):27-29, 2005.

Carrougher G: *Burn care and therapy,* St Louis, 1998, Mosby.

Centers for Disease Control and Prevention: Delayed onset and diminished magnitude of rotavirus activity—United States, November 2007–May 2008. *MMWR* 57(25):697-700, 2008.

Centers for Disease Control and Prevention: Managing acute gastroenteritis among children: oral rehydration, maintenance, and nutritional therapy. *MMWR* 52(RR-16):1-16, 2003.

Chuang YY, Huang YC, Lin TY: Toxic shock syndrome in children: epidemiology, pathogenesis, and management (review), *Paediatr Drugs* 7(1):11-25, 2005.

Coffin SE: Future vaccines: recent advances and future prospects, *Primary Care* 28(4):869-887, 2001.

Committee on Infectious Diseases: Prevention of rotavirus disease: guidelines for use of rotavirus vaccine, *Pediatrics* 119(1):171-182, 2007.

Dellinger RP, Levy MM, Carlet JM, et al: Surviving sepsis campaign: international guidelines for management of severe sepsis and septic shock: 2008, *Crit Care Med* 36(1):296-327, 2008.

Demling RH: The role of anabolic hormones for wound healing in catabolic states, *J Burns Wounds* 4:e2, 2005.

Goldstein B, Giroir B, Randolph A: International pediatric sepsis consensus conference: definitions for sepsis and organ dysfunction in pediatrics, *Pediatr Crit Care Med* 6(1):2-8, 2005.

Gordon M, Marvin J: Burn nursing. In Herndon DN, editor: *Total burn care,* Philadelphia, 2007, Saunders.

Hartford CE, Kealey GP: Care of outpatient burns. In Herndon DN, editor: *Total burn care,* Philadelphia, 2007, Saunders.

Helvig E: Pediatric burn injuries, *AACN Clin Issues* 4(2):433-442, 1993.

Henry DB, Foster RL: Burn pain management in children, *Pediatr Clin North Am* 47(3):681-698, 2000.

Jabbar A, Wright RA: Gastroenteritis and antibiotic-associated diarrhea, *Primary Care* 30(1):63-80, 2003.

Jindal N, Hollenberg SM, Dellinger RP: Pharmacologic issues in the management of septic shock, *Crit Care Clin* 16(2):233-249, 2000.

Kahana MD: Burn pain management: avoiding the "private nightmare." In Schechter N, Berde C, Yaster M, editors: *Pain in infants, children, and adolescents,* Baltimore, 2003, Williams & Wilkins.

Klein GL, Przkora R, Herndon DN: Vitamin and trace element homeostasis following severe burn injury. In Herndon DN, editor: *Total burn care,* Philadelphia, 2007, Saunders.

Kramer GC, Lund T, Beckman OK: Pathophysiology of burn shock and burn edema. In Herndon DN, editor: *Total burn care,* Philadelphia, 2007, Saunders.

Lee JO, Herndon DN: The pediatric burned patient. In Herndon DN, editor: *Total burn care,* Philadelphia, 2007, Saunders.

Li ST, DiGiuseppe DL, Christakis DA: Antiemetic use for acute gastroenteritis in children, *Arch Pediatr Adolesc Med* 157(5):475-479, 2003.

Liberman DB, Teach SJ: Management of anaphylaxis in children, *Pediatr Emerg Care* 24(12):867-869, 2008.

Maar SP: Emergency care in pediatric septic shock, *Pediatr Emerg Care* 20(9):617-624, 2004.

Malek MA, Curns AT, Holman RC, et al: Diarrhea- and rotavirus-associated hospitalizations among children less than 5 years of age: United States, 1997 and 2000, *Pediatrics* 117(6):1887-1892, 2006.

McRonald FE, Fleisher DR: Anticipatory nausea in cyclical vomiting, *BMC Pediatr* 5(1):3, 2005.

Meyer WJ, Patterson DR, Jaco M, et al: Management of pain and other discomforts in burned patients. In Herndon DN, editor: *Total burn care,* Philadelphia, 2007, Saunders.

Murphey ED, Sherwood ER, Toliver-Kinsky T: The immunological response and strategies for intervention. In Herndon DN, editor: *Total burn care,* Philadelphia, 2007, Saunders.

Nakase J: Update on emerging infections from the Centers for Disease Control and Prevention, *Ann Emerg Med* 36(3):268-270, 2000.

National Fire Protection Association: *Children playing with fire,* 2009, available at www.nfpa.org/categoryList.asp?categoryID=281&URL=Research%20&%Reports/Fact%20sheets/Children%20and%20fire (accessed March 11, 2010).

Norbury WB, Herndon DN: Modulation of the hypermetabolic response after burn. In Herndon DN, editor: *Total burn care,* Philadelphia, 2007, Saunders.

Pham TN, Gibran NS, Heimbach DM: Evaluation of the burn wound: management decisions. In Herndon DN, editor: *Total burn care,* Philadelphia, 2007, Saunders.

Pruitt BA, Wolf SE, Mason AD: Epidemiological, demographic, and outcome characteristics of burn injury. In Herndon DN, editor: *Total burn care,* Philadelphia, 2007, Saunders.

Ralston M, Hazinski MF, Zaritsky AL, et al editors: *Pediatric life support.* Dallas, 2006, American Heart Association.

Robert R, Blakeney P, Herndon DN: Maltreatment by burning. In Herndon DN, editor: *Total burn care,* Philadelphia, 2007, Saunders.

Safe Kids Worldwide: *Fire safety,* Washington, DC, 2009, The Company, available at www.usa.safekids.org (accessed March 11, 2010).

Safe Kids Worldwide: *Report to the nation: trends in unintentional childhood injury mortality and parental views on child safety,* Washington DC, 2008, National Safe Kids Campaign.

Saffle JR, Graves C: Nutritional support of the burned patient. In Herndon DN, editor: *Total burn care,* Philadelphia, 2007, Saunders.

Selbst SM: Sedation and analgesia in the ER department. In Schechter N, Berde C, Yaster M, editors: *Pain in infants, children, and adolescents,* Baltimore, 2003, Williams & Wilkins.

Sheridan RL, Tompkins RG: Alternative wound coverings. In Herndon DN, editor: *Total burn care,* Philadelphia, 2007a, Saunders.

Sheridan RL, Tompkins RG: Etiology and prevention of multisystem organ failure. In Herndon DN, editor: *Total burn care,* Philadelphia, 2007b, Saunders.

Sherwood ER, Traber DL: The systemic inflammatory response syndrome. In Herndon DN, editor: *Total burn care,* Philadelphia, 2007, Saunders.

Smith ML: Pediatric burns: management of thermal, electrical, and chemical burns and burn-like dermatologic conditions, *Pediatr Ann* 29(6):367-378, 2000.

Staat MA: What is the disease burden associated with rotavirus? In: *The management and prevention of rotavirus,* Thorofare, NJ, 2006, Vindico Medical Education.

Suman OE, Przkora R, Blakeney P, et al: Mitigation of the burn-induced hypermetabolic response during convalescence. In Herndon DN, editor: *Total burn care,* Philadelphia, 2007, Saunders.

Szajewska H, Ruszcynski M, Radzikowski A: Probiotics in the prevention of antibiotic-associated diarrhea in children: a meta-analysis of randomized controlled trials, *J Pediatr* 149(3):367-372, 2006.

Thomas CR, Meyer WJ, Blakeney PE: Psychiatric disorders associated with burn injury. In Herndon DN, editor: *Total burn care,* Philadelphia, 2007, Saunders.

Warden GD: Fluid resuscitation and early management. In Herndon DN, editor: *Total burn care,* Philadelphia, 2007, Saunders.

Warden GD: Burn shock resuscitation, *World J Surg* 1(1):16-32, 1992.

Zangwill KM: Protecting against rotavirus disease and its complications. In: *The management and prevention of rotavirus,* Thorofare, NJ, 2006, Vindico Medical Education.

The Child with Renal Dysfunction

Barbara Montagnino and Patricia A. Ring

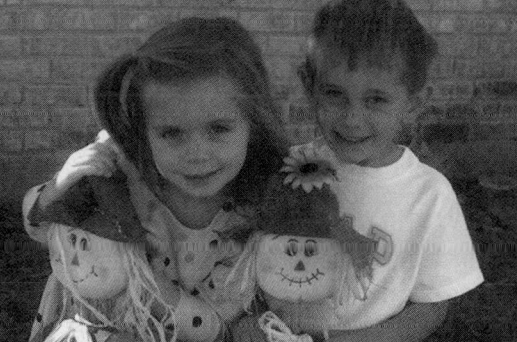

RENAL STRUCTURE AND FUNCTION

The kidney's primary responsibility is to maintain the composition and volume of the body fluids in equilibrium. To maintain this constant internal environment, the kidney must respond appropriately to alterations in the internal environment caused by variations in dietary intake and extrarenal losses of water and solutes. This is accomplished by the formation of urine (the product of glomerular filtration), tubular reabsorption, and tubular secretion. **Reabsorption** is the transport of a substance from the tubular lumen to the blood in surrounding vessels. **Secretion** is transport in the opposite direction (i.e., from the blood to the lumen). These processes are either active or passive.

Excretion is the elimination of a substance from the body, in this case urine.

A secondary function of the kidney is the production of certain humoral substances. One such substance is an enzyme, erythropoietin-stimulating factor (or erythrogenin), which acts on a plasma globulin to form erythropoietin, which in turn stimulates erythropoiesis in the bone marrow. Its production increases in the presence of hypoxia and androgens. Few red blood cells form in the absence of erythropoietin, which accounts somewhat for the anemia associated with advanced kidney disease. The kidney also secretes another enzyme, renin, in response to reduced blood volume, decreased blood pressure, or increased secretion of catecholamines. Renin stimulates the production of the angiotensins, which produce arteriolar constriction and an elevation in blood pressure and stimulate the production of aldosterone by the adrenal cortex.

RENAL PHYSIOLOGY

The structural and functional unit of the kidney is the **nephron**, which contains a complex system of tubules, arterioles, venules, and capillaries (Fig. 30-1, *A*). The nephron consists of the Bowman capsule, which encloses a tuft of capillaries and is joined successively to the proximal convoluted tubule, the loop of Henle, the distal convoluted tubule, and the straight or collecting duct (Fig. 30-1, *B*). Collecting tubules join larger ducts, and all the larger collecting ducts of one renal pyramid join to form a single duct that opens into a minor calyx. A number of calyces empty into one of several major calyces that converge into the renal pelvis. The renal pelvis narrows after it leaves the kidney and forms what then becomes a ureter, through which urine drains into the urinary bladder.

The blood supply to the kidneys constitutes approximately one fifth of the total cardiac output; therefore profuse bleeding can accompany renal trauma. Because interstitial tissue is sparse, individual nephrons with their blood vessel component are closely packed together. A sizable afferent arteriole, which separates into capillary loops that constitute the glomerular tuft, supplies each nephron. Blood leaves by a smaller efferent arteriole. From there the efferent arterioles branch into a peritubular capillary network and hairpin loops called the vasa recta, which parallel the loops of Henle and collecting ducts. The total surface area of the renal capillaries is approximately equal to the total surface area of the tubules.

The Bowman capsule is composed of two cellular layers that separate the blood from the glomerular filtrate: the capillary endothelium and a layer of tubular epithelial lining cells.

PATHOPHYSIOLOGY REVIEW

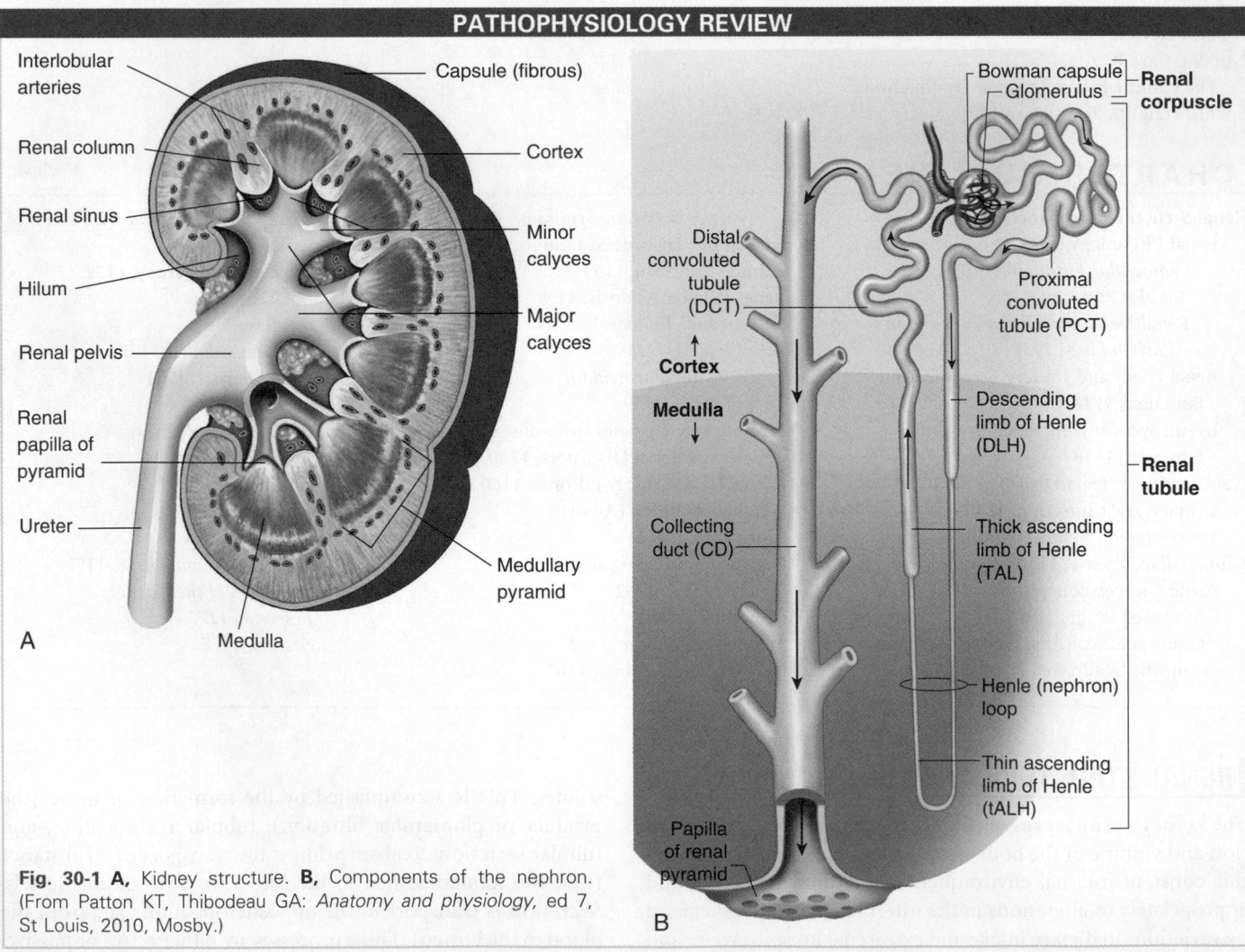

Fig. 30-1 A, Kidney structure. **B,** Components of the nephron. (From Patton KT, Thibodeau GA: *Anatomy and physiology,* ed 7, St Louis, 2010, Mosby.)

Situated between these layers is the basal lamina, or basement membrane. This glomerular membrane is permeable because the capillary endothelium is fenestrated with pores, or fenestrae. Also, the outer surface of the glomerular epithelium consists of fingerlike projections (pseudopodia, or podocytes), which cover the entire surface to form slits called slit pores. The basement membrane has no visible openings but behaves as though it contains pores or channels. Consequently, the glomerular filtrate (which has essentially the same composition as plasma except for the large protein molecules and cellular elements) passes through these three layers at a rapid rate. The structure of these layers becomes altered in kidney disease.

Glomerular Filtration

Filtration through the glomerular capillaries is governed by the same mechanism as filtration across other capillaries in the body (i.e., the size of the capillary bed, the permeability of the capillaries, and the hydrostatic and osmotic pressure gradients across the capillaries). The filtration capacity of the glomerulus is the product of permeability of the glomerular capillaries and three pressure forces: glomerular hydrostatic pressure, colloidal osmotic (oncotic) pressure (COP), and intracapsular pressure.

Blood enters the nephron at a substantial pressure. This hydrostatic pressure forces plasma fluid and solutes through the capillary membrane and into the unit's collecting apparatus. As this filtrate travels through the renal tubules, water and solutes are selectively reabsorbed back into the vascular compartment. That which is not reabsorbed is excreted as urine. Filtration takes place as long as hydrostatic pressure within the glomerular capillaries exceeds the opposing COP of the plasma proteins. If the pressure becomes equal through decreased hydrostatic pressure or decreased COP, no further filtration takes place. In a state of dehydration, more water is reabsorbed; when water intake is increased, more is excreted as urine. In conditions that produce osmotic diuresis (i.e., when large solutes, such as glucose, are filtered through the capillaries in such excessive amounts that they cannot be reabsorbed), the osmotic attraction of the solute causes less water to be reabsorbed, resulting in water being excreted in the urine with the solute.

Tubular Function

The function of the renal tubules is to modify the glomerular filtrate. Tubular cells may add more of a substance to the filtrate (tubular secretion), remove some or all of a substance from the filtrate (tubular reabsorption), or both. The reabsorption is selective and discriminating for substances essential to body processes and equilibrium, whereas nonessential substances are eliminated as waste. The substances are secreted or reabsorbed in the tubules by osmosis, passive movement down a chemical or electric gradient, or are actively transported against these gradients. These processes operate throughout the length of the tubules, but there are variations in the types, amounts, and mechanisms by which substances are secreted or reabsorbed in the different tubular segments. The cellular characteristics of each segment are largely responsible for these variations (see Fig. 30-1).

Active transport mechanisms move vital substances both inward and outward from the tubular filtrate. For example, the proximal tubule reabsorbs essential substances such as glucose, amino acids, and sodium ions and returns them directly to the blood. Active transport mechanisms here, as elsewhere, have a limited capacity, or threshold, for moving the solute. When the maximum of the transport mechanism is reached, no more substance is reabsorbed, and the remainder is excreted in the urine. For example, when blood glucose concentrations exceed their transport capacity, the surplus remains in the filtrate to be excreted in the urine (glycosuria). When two substances share a common transport mechanism, the first substance may be blocked by the addition of a second substance (selective inhibition). The effect of many therapeutic agents (e.g., diuretics) depends on this process.

Electrolytes are moved by both active transport and diffusion; the transport of certain electrolytes, particularly sodium, has important effects on other substances. For example, sodium is actively transported from all parts of the nephron. The movement of sodium ions produces both an electric and an osmotic gradient, which causes chloride ions and water to diffuse from the tubules in an effort to establish equilibrium. This is the obligatory water reabsorption in the kidneys. There is a limit to the concentration gradient against which sodium can be transported out; therefore, when larger than normal amounts of sodium ions remain in the tubules, water is obliged to remain with the sodium.

Under normal conditions the kidneys are able to adjust the urine and solute excretion in response to the requirements for body water and electrolyte balance. They are able to excrete or conserve both water and most electrolytes in addition to excreting the end products of protein metabolism, principally urea. The volume of urine excreted by the kidneys in a given period depends on the water balance (including intravascular filtration pressure), the quantity of solutes presented to the kidneys, and the capacity of the kidneys to dilute or concentrate the filtrate.

Renal Development and Function in Early Infancy

Development of the kidney begins within the first weeks of embryonic life but is not completed until about the end of the first year after birth. The nephrons increase in number throughout gestation and reach their full complement by birth. However, at this point they are immature and less efficient than at later ages. Many of the tubular sections are not fully formed, and the glomeruli enlarge considerably after birth.

Glomerular filtration and absorption are relatively low in the infant and do not reach adult values until between 1 and 2 years of age. This appears to be related to a barrier imposed by more cuboidal-shaped glomerular epithelial cells and higher afferent arteriole resistance. Consequently, the newborn is unable to dispose of excess water and solutes rapidly or efficiently.

The tubular length of nephrons is highly variable. Glomerular size is less variable. The juxtaglomerular nephrons show more advanced development than the cortical nephrons. The loop of Henle (the site of the urine-concentrating mechanism) is short in the newborn, which reduces the ability to reabsorb sodium and water and therefore produces very dilute urine; however, the newborn pituitary gland secretes adequate amounts of antidiuretic hormone. The length of tubules gradually increases until concentrating ability reaches adult levels by approximately the third month of life. Urea synthesis and excretion are slower during this time, and the newborn retains large quantities of nitrogen and essential electrolytes to meet the needs for growth in the first weeks of life. Consequently, the excretory burden is minimized. The lower concentration of urea, the principal end product of nitrogen metabolism, also reduces concentrating capacity because it contributes to the concentration mechanism.

Other characteristics of the newborn's kidneys result in renal function that differs from that of older children and adults. Because of some as yet undetermined cause, newborn infants are unable to excrete a water load at rates similar to those of older persons. Hydrogen ion excretion is reduced, acid secretion is lower for the first year of life, and plasma bicarbonate levels are low. Because of these inadequacies of the kidney and because of less efficient blood buffers, the newborn is more liable to develop severe metabolic acidosis. Sodium excretion is reduced in the immediate newborn period, and the kidneys are less able to adapt to sodium deficiencies and excesses. For example, an isotonic saline infusion may produce edema because of impaired ability to eliminate excess. Conversely, inadequate reabsorption of sodium from the tubules may increase sodium losses in disorders such as vomiting or diarrhea. Moreover, infants have a diminished capacity to reabsorb glucose and, during the first few days, to produce ammonium ions.

The kidney functions during fetal life and produces urine that contributes to the amniotic fluid volume. The 24-hour urine volume is low at birth, rapidly increases in the neonatal period, and steadily increases with normal growth. (See Appendix C.) The kidneys continue to grow in size until body growth is complete in adolescence.

RENAL PELVIS AND URETERS: STRUCTURE AND FUNCTION*

The renal pelvis is a funnel-shaped structure that originates at the major calyces and terminates in the funnel-shaped ureteropelvic junction. The ureter is a thin mucomuscular tube that extends from the ureteropelvic to the ureterovesical junction in the base of the bladder. Three areas—the ureteropelvic junction, the ureterovesical junction, and the segment nearest the sacroiliac junction—are particularly narrow and prone to obstruction when a solid body (such as a urinary calculus ["stone"]) passes.

The principal function of the renal pelvis and ureter is the transport of urine from the kidney to the bladder. Urine is moved via a process called **peristalsis**, whereby muscular movements originating in the renal pelvis propel a bolus of urine toward the urinary bladder for storage and eventual evacuation when the child urinates. The renal pelvis stores only a relatively small volume of urine (approximately 15 ml in adults) before a contraction is triggered that pushes the urine toward the bladder. The forward movement of urine from the kidney to the bladder is called **efflux**, whereas abnormal (or backward) urine movement is termed **reflux**. Aside from mechanical

stretching, neurogenic and hormonal factors modulate ureteral peristalsis.

The ureterovesical junction joins the ureters and bladder. It is made up of three principal components: the lowest segment of the ureter, the trigone muscle, and the adjacent bladder wall. The ureters allow the passage of urine from the upper urinary tracts while preventing regurgitation of urine from the bladder to the ureters. During bladder filling, intravesical pressure remains relatively low and the detrusor muscle remains in a relaxed state. A peristaltic contraction of the ureter propels urine into the bladder. During micturition, the intravesical pressure rises as the detrusor muscle contracts; this raises the potential for harmful reflux into the upper urinary tracts. Several mechanisms in the normal ureterovesical junction act together to prevent reflux. The terminal (intravesical) ureteral segment tunnels through the bladder wall at an oblique angle. During bladder contraction, tension in the detrusor muscle squeezes the intravesical ureter closed. The trigone muscle that surrounds the ureteral orifice of the terminal ureter enhances this process. In addition, the longitudinally arranged muscle of the intravesical ureter contracts, providing further resistance to reflux. Anatomic defects of the ureterovesical junction, such as lateral displacement of the ureter or reduced length of the intravesical ureter, predispose the child to primary reflux. In children with normal anatomy, voiding dysfunction associated with infections and high bladder pressures predisposes them to secondary reflux (Sillen, 2008).

URETHROVESICAL UNIT: STRUCTURE AND FUNCTION*

The urethrovesical unit consists of the bladder, urethra, and pelvic muscles; it is also called the lower urinary tract. The urinary bladder is a muscle-lined sac that stores and empties itself of urine. In the infant the bladder lies entirely in the abdomen. The bladder assumes its place in the true pelvis shortly before puberty. This change in position is due to the maturation of the pelvic bone rather than migration of the bladder and urethra.

The bladder has two inlets (the ureteral orifices) and a single outlet (the urethral orifice). The base of the bladder is a relatively fixed, triangular area consisting of the bladder neck and trigone. In contrast, the body of the bladder is distensible, changing from a tetrahedron (four-sided shape) when relatively empty to a nearly spherical shape as the bladder fills.

One of the four layers of the bladder wall consists of smooth muscle bundles that promote bladder evacuation via micturition. Collectively this muscular tunic is called the **detrusor**. The muscular tunic of the bladder wall also contains **collagen**, a tough, nonelastic substance that maintains the integrity of the bladder wall while also preventing overdistention. Certain pathologic factors, including denervation of the bladder and obstruction of the outlet, may cause an overabundance of collagen in the detrusor muscle. This causes a loss of bladder compliance (distensibility), abnormally high filling pressures, and trabeculation of the bladder wall.

The urethra is a mucomuscular tube that connects the external meatus and the bladder. The male urethra originates at the bladder neck, piercing the prostate and pelvic floor before tun-

*Mikel Gray, PhD, CUNP, CCCN, FAAN, originally wrote these sections.

neling through the posterior portion of the penis and terminating at the glans penis. The proximal portion of the urethra comprises the sphincter mechanism, whereas the distal portion serves as a conduit for the passage of urine or semen. The urethral meatus is a vertical slit located at the summit of the glans penis.

The female urethra follows a relatively short, straight course compared with the male. It originates at the bladder base and terminates at an external meatus located immediately superior to (in front of) the vaginal orifice. The distal two thirds of the female urethra are fused with the vaginal wall.

The primary responsibilities of the bladder are to store urine manufactured by the kidneys and to evacuate this urine at regular intervals via the process of micturition. During infancy the bladder is expected to empty spontaneously; by the fourth year of life (or earlier) the child is expected to gain control of detrusor and urethral sphincter function. Control of the urethrovesical unit is referred to as urinary continence. Continent individuals are expected to hold their urine for at least 2 hours while awake. During sleeping hours they may arise once to urinate, although many children and young adults sleep for 8 hours or more without interruption. Three factors—anatomic integrity of the lower urinary tract, detrusor control, and competence of the urethral sphincter mechanism—must function normally for an individual to achieve and maintain continence.

Detrusor control requires successful integration of neurologic structures in the brain, spinal cord, and peripheral nervous systems. The brain influences bladder function via its inhibitory role on detrusor contractions. The stable detrusor contracts only when its owner gives permission. Several areas of the brain act together to control detrusor stability. A pathologic condition of one of these areas is known to produce detrusor instability, or the loss of control over detrusor contractions.

The spinal cord influences lower urinary tract function because it transmits messages between the brain and the target organ. Two areas in the spinal cord are particularly significant. The thoracolumbar cord (spinal levels T10-L2) influences bladder and urethral sphincter function. Sympathetic impulses from the brain travel to the bladder body and smooth muscle of the urethra, causing relaxation of the detrusor muscle and contraction of urethral smooth muscle. This combination of actions promotes bladder filling and storage of urine. The sacral spinal cord (spinal segments S2-S4) influences the bladder muscle, promoting micturition. Parasympathetic impulses travel from these nuclei, causing contraction of the detrusor muscle and indirectly promoting relaxation of smooth muscle in the urethra.

Two peripheral nerve plexuses directly influence control of the detrusor muscle. The pelvic plexus provides parasympathetic innervation to the bladder and urethra, and the inferior hypogastric plexus provides sympathetic innervation (Sugarman, 2000).

The final mechanism responsible for the attainment and maintenance of continence is the urethral sphincter mechanism. Traditionally two sphincters are described. The internal sphincter consists of the smooth muscle of the bladder and proximal urethra, and the external sphincter consists of the periurethral striated muscle. However, it is better to describe a single mechanism consisting of elements of compression and elements of tension.

Elements of compression are necessary for the urethra to form a watertight seal between episodes of urination. The softness (collapsibility) of the urethral wall is important for continence, particularly when a catheter alters urethral integrity. The mucus produced by the epithelium further enhances the watertight seal of the urethra. The mucus reduces surface tension, promoting collapse of the walls and sealing the microscopic fissures against urinary leakage.

The vascular cushion also acts as an element of compression (in addition to producing tension), contributing to urethral closure during physical stress. The vascular cushion, or network of the arterioles, venules, and arteriovenous communications in the urethra, promotes urethral compression by transmitting pressure from the muscles surrounding the urethra and those intrinsic to its walls. The vascular cushion contributes to urethral closure pressure because it is filled with an incompressible fluid that has its own intrinsic pressure.

The elements of tension in the urethral sphincter mechanism consist of the vascular cushion, intrinsic smooth and skeletal muscles, and periurethral striated muscle. These muscles are specially innervated to maintain the tension needed for urethral closure between episodes of micturition and to provide an extra measure of urethral tension, which is needed when significant physical exertion stresses sphincter closure. The pelvic muscles receive somatic innervation, which allows voluntary interruption of the urinary stream and provides added protection against precipitous rises in abdominal pressure.

Clinical Manifestations

As in most disorders of childhood, the incidence and type of kidney or urinary tract dysfunction change with the child's age and maturation. In addition, the presenting complaints and their significance vary with maturation. For example, a complaint of enuresis has greater significance at age 8 years than at age 4. In the newborn, urinary tract disorders are associated with a number of obvious malformations of other body systems, including the curious and unexplained but frequent association between malformed or low-set ears and urinary tract anomalies. Important signs and symptoms that suggest possible renal or genitourinary tract disease in children at different ages are outlined in Box 30-1.

Many clinical manifestations are common to a variety of childhood disorders, but their presence is an indication to obtain further information from the patient history, family history, and laboratory studies as part of a complete physical examination. Radiographic studies and renal biopsy can be used to further evaluate suspected kidney disease.

Laboratory Tests

Both urine and blood studies contribute vital information for the detection of renal problems. The single most important test is probably routine urinalysis. Specific urine and blood tests provide additional information.

Glomerular filtration rate is a measure of the amount of plasma from which a given substance is totally cleared in 1 minute. Clearance is calculated from the ratio of substance excreted to the concentration of that substance in the plasma.

BOX 30-1   SIGNS AND SYMPTOMS OF URINARY TRACT DISORDERS OR DISEASE

Neonatal Period (Birth to 1 Month)
Poor feeding
Vomiting
Failure to gain weight
Rapid respiration (acidosis)
Respiratory distress
Spontaneous pneumothorax or pneumomediastinum
Frequent urination
Screaming on urination
Poor urinary stream
Jaundice
Seizures
Dehydration
Other anomalies or stigmata
Enlarged kidneys or bladder

Infancy (1 to 24 Months)
Poor feeding
Vomiting
Failure to gain weight
Excessive thirst
Frequent urination
Straining or screaming on urination
Foul-smelling urine
Pallor
Fever
Persistent diaper rash
Seizures (with or without fever)
Dehydration
Enlarged kidneys or bladder

Childhood (2 to 14 Years)
Poor appetite
Vomiting
Growth failure
Excessive thirst
Enuresis, incontinence, frequent urination
Painful urination
Swelling of face
Seizures
Pallor
Fatigue
Blood in urine
Abdominal or back pain
Edema
Hypertension
Tetany

A number of substances can be used, but the most useful clinical estimation of glomerular filtration is the clearance of creatinine, an end product of protein metabolism in muscle and a substance that is freely filtered by the glomerulus and secreted by renal tubular cells. The production and secretion of creatinine remain relatively constant from day to day, and its appearance in the urine is determined by the serum level. When the collection is complete and accurately timed, the results are fairly reliable and compare favorably with clearance of other substances (e.g., insulin) that require special equipment and long immobilization of the child to evaluate.

Any significant degree of renal disease can diminish the glomerular filtration rate, but renal vascular disease and diseases of the glomerulus have the most immediate effect. The nurse's responsibility in this test is collection of urine, usually a 12- or 24-hour specimen.

Table 30-1 outlines the major urine and blood tests. Radiologic and other tests of urinary system function are described in Table 30-2. Blood tests of renal function are outlined in Table 30-3.

Nursing Care Management

Nursing responsibilities in the assessment of renal disorders and diseases begins with observation of the child for any manifestations that might indicate dysfunction. The most significant ongoing assessments in children with renal conditions are accurate measurement and recording of weight, intake and output, and blood pressure. (See Chapter 6.) These assessments are necessary not only for children with known renal dysfunction but also for those children at risk for developing renal complications (e.g., children in shock, postoperative patients).

In addition to the general manifestations of renal conditions (see Box 30-1), many conditions have specific characteristics that distinguish them from other disorders. These are discussed as appropriate throughout the chapter.

The nurse is generally responsible for preparing infants, children, and parents for tests and collection of urine and (sometimes) blood specimens. (See Preparation for Diagnostic and Therapeutic Procedures, and Collection of Specimens, Chapter 27.) Nurses observe the characteristics of the urine collected, often perform any of a number of tests on urine specimens (e.g., urine specific gravity, protein, blood, glucose, ketones), and assist with more complex diagnostic tests (e.g., radiography, cystoscopy). Nurses must be familiar with significant laboratory tests, their implications, and preprocedural care.

⚡ DRUG ALERT

Fleet Enemas

Use of Fleet enemas in children with acute or chronic renal failure is potentially lethal because of hyperphosphatemia. Requests for Fleet enemas in this situation should not be implemented without careful investigation.

GENITOURINARY TRACT DISORDERS

URINARY TRACT INFECTION

Urinary tract infection (UTI) is a clinical condition that may involve the urethra and bladder (lower urinary tract) and the ureters, renal pelvis, calyces, and renal parenchyma (upper urinary tract). Because it is often impossible to localize the infection, the broad designation *UTI* is applied to the presence of significant numbers of microorganisms anywhere within the urinary tract (except the distal third of the urethra, which is usually colonized with bacteria).

Infection of the urinary tract may be present with or without clinical symptoms. As a result, the site of infection is often difficult to pinpoint with accuracy. The various terms used to describe urinary tract disorders are defined in Box 30-2.

The peak incidence of UTI not caused by structural anomalies occurs between 2 and 6 years of age. Except for the neonatal

TABLE 30-1	URINE TESTS OF RENAL FUNCTION		
TEST	**NORMAL RANGE**	**DEVIATIONS**	**SIGNIFICANCE OF DEVIATIONS**
Physical Tests			
Volume	Age related	Polyuria	Osmotic factors (urinary glucose level in diabetes mellitus)
	Newborn: 30-60 ml	Oliguria	Retention caused by obstructive disease
	Children: Bladder capacity (oz) = Age (yr) + 2		Inadequate bladder emptying caused by neurogenic bladder or obstructive disorder
		Anuria	Obstruction of urinary tract; acute renal failure
Specific gravity	With normal fluid intake: 1.016-1.022	High	Dehydration
			Presence of protein or glucose
	Newborn: 1.001-1.020		Presence of radiopaque contrast medium after radiologic examinations
	Others: 1.001-1.030	Low	Excessive fluid intake
			Distal tubular dysfunction
			Insufficient antidiuretic hormone
			Diuresis
		Fixed at 1.010	Chronic glomerular disease
Osmolality	Newborn: 50-600 mOsm/L	High or low	Same as for specific gravity
	Thereafter: 50-1400 mOsm/L		More sensitive index than specific gravity
Appearance	Clear pale yellow to deep gold	Cloudy	Contains sediment
		Cloudy reddish pink to reddish brown	Blood from trauma or disease
			Myoglobin after severe muscle destruction
		Light	Dilute
		Dark	Concentrated
		Red	Trauma
Chemical Tests			
pH	Newborn: 5-7	Weak acid or neutral	If associated with metabolic acidosis, suggests tubular acidosis
	Thereafter: 4.8-7.8		If associated with metabolic alkalosis, suggests potassium deficiency
	Average: 6		Urinary tract infection
		Alkaline	Metabolic alkalosis
Protein level	Absent	Present	Abnormal glomerular permeability (e.g., glomerular disease, changes in blood pressure)
			Most kidney disease
			Orthostatic in some individuals
Glucose level	Absent	Present	Diabetes mellitus
			Infusion of concentrated glucose-containing fluids
			Glomerulonephritis
			Impaired tubular reabsorption
Ketone levels	Absent	Present	Conditions of acute metabolic demand (stress)
			Diabetic ketoacidosis
Leukocyte esterase	Absent	Present	Can identify both lysed and intact white blood cells via enzyme detection
Nitrites	Absent	Present	Most species of bacteria convert nitrates to nitrites in the urine
Microscopic Tests			
White blood cell count	<1-2	>5 polymorphonuclear leukocytes/field	Urinary tract inflammatory process
		Lymphocytes	Allograft rejection
			Malignancy
Red blood cell count	<1-2	4-6/field in centrifuged specimen	Trauma
			Stones
			Glomerular injury
			Infection
			Neoplasms
Presence of bacteria	Absent to a few	>100,000 organisms/ml in centrifuged specimen	Urinary tract infection
Presence of casts	Occasional	Granular casts	Tubular or glomerular disorders
			Degenerative process in advanced renal disease
		Cellular casts	Pyelonephritis
		• White blood cell	Glomerulonephritis
		• Red blood cell	Proteinuria; usually transient
		Hyaline casts	

TABLE 30-2 RADIOLOGIC AND OTHER TESTS OF URINARY SYSTEM FUNCTION

TEST	PROCEDURE	PURPOSE	COMMENTS AND NURSING RESPONSIBILITIES
Urine culture and sensitivity	Collection of sterile specimen	Determines presence of pathogens and drugs to which they are sensitive	This test does not require specific parental permission. Send specimen to laboratory immediately after collection. Catheterization, clean-catch, or suprapubic specimen is used.
Renal or bladder ultrasound	Transmission of ultrasonic waves through renal parenchyma, along ureteral course, and over bladder	Allows visualization of renal parenchyma, renal pelvis without exposure to external beam radiation or radioactive isotopes. Visualization of dilated ureters and bladder wall also possible	Noninvasive procedure
Testicular (scrotal) ultrasound	Transmission of ultrasonic waves through scrotal contents and testis	Allows visualization of scrotal contents, including testis. Testicular ultrasound used to identify masses, and Doppler-enhanced ultrasound used to differentiate hyperemia of epididymoorchitis from ischemia of torsion	Noninvasive procedure
Scout film	Flat plate x-ray film of abdomen and pelvis for kidney, ureters, bladder (KUB)	Detects and establishes renal outlines, presence of calculi, or opaque foreign bodies in bladder	Prepare child as for routine x-ray film.
Voiding cystourethrography	Contrast medium injected into bladder through urethral catheter until bladder is full; films taken before, during, and after voiding	Visualizes bladder outline and urethra, reveals reflux of urine into ureters, and shows complications of bladder emptying	Prepare child for catheterization.
Radionuclide (nuclear) cystogram	Radionuclide-containing fluid injected through urethral catheter until bladder is full; images generated before, during, and after voiding	Alternative to voiding cystourethrography in children with allergy to intravesical contrast material. Allows evaluation of reflux, although visualization of anatomic details is relatively poor	Prepare child for catheterization. Reassure patient and parents that allergic response to contrast materials is avoided by use of radionuclide.
Radioisotope imaging studies	Contrast medium injected intravenously; computer analysis to measure uptake or washout (excretion) for analysis of organ function	DTPA radioisotope used to measure glomerular filtration rate; estimate of differential renal function and renal washout to determine presence and location of upper urinary tract obstruction. DMSA radioisotope to visualize renal scars and differential renal function; ureters and bladder not visualized. MAG3 radioisotope combines features of DTPA (evaluation of upper urinary tract obstruction) with features of DMSA radioisotope (differential renal function)	Insert or assist with insertion of intravenous infusion. Monitor intravenous infusion. Urethral catheterization may accompany DTPA radioisotope scan; prepare child for catheterization when indicated.
Intravenous pyelography (IVP) (intravenous urogram; excretory urogram)	Intravenous injection of a contrast medium. Medium secreted and concentrated by tubules. X-ray films made 5, 10, and 15 min after injection; delayed films (30, 60 min, etc.) obtained if obstruction suspected	Defines urinary tract. Provides information about integrity of kidneys, ureters, and bladder. Retroperitoneal masses visualized when they shift position of ureters	Prepare child for test: Infants <2 yr of age—No solid food, omit one bottle on morning of examination; studies should be performed early to avoid withholding of fluids. Children ages 2-14 yr—Give cathartic evening before examination, nothing orally after midnight, enema (Fleet [see Drug Alert, p. 1140] or soapsuds) morning of examination.
Computed tomography (CT)	Narrow-beam x-rays and computer analysis providing precise reconstruction of area	Visualizes vertical or horizontal cross section of kidney. Especially valuable to distinguish tumors and cysts	Noncontrast scan is noninvasive. Contrast-enhanced CT scan preparation is similar to that for IVP.
Cystoscopy	Direct visualization of bladder and lower urinary tract through small scope inserted via urethra	Investigation of bladder and lower tract lesions; visualizes urethral openings, bladder wall, trigone, and urethra	Give nothing orally after midnight. Carry out preoperative preparations.
Retrograde pyelography	Contrast medium injected through urethral catheter	Visualizes pelvic calyces, ureters, and bladder	Prepare child for cystoscopy.

TABLE 30-2 RADIOLOGIC AND OTHER TESTS OF URINARY SYSTEM FUNCTION—cont'd

TEST	PROCEDURE	PURPOSE	COMMENTS AND NURSING RESPONSIBILITIES
Renal angiography	Contrast medium injected directly into renal artery via catheter placed in femoral artery (or umbilical artery in newborn) and advanced to renal artery	Visualizes renal vascular system, especially for renal arterial stenosis	Give cathartic if ordered. Give preoperative medication if ordered Observe for reaction to contrast medium. Monitor vital signs after procedure.
Whitaker perfusion test	Injection of contrast material through renal pelvis and ureters Pressures measured in renal pelvis and urinary bladder	Determine presence of obstruction causing upper urinary tract dilation	Prepare child for insertion of spinal needle or perfusion catheter in renal pelvis (anesthetic often required).
Renal biopsy	Removal of kidney tissue by open or percutaneous technique for study by light, electron, or immunofluorescent microscopy	Yields histologic and microscopic information about glomeruli and tubules; helps distinguish between types of nephritic syndromes Distinguishes other renal disorders	Give nothing orally 4-6 hr before test. Premedicate child as ordered. Prepare setup for procedure. Assist with procedure. Take vital signs. Apply pressure to area with pressure dressing and, if feasible, a sandbag. Have child on bed rest for 24 hr. Observe for abdominal pain, tenderness. Monitor intake and output; surgical incision may be required in infants.
Urodynamics	Set of tests to measure bladder filling, storage, and evacuation functions: Uroflowmetry—Test to determine efficiency of urination Cystometrogram—Graphic comparison of bladder pressure as function of volume Voiding pressure study—Comparison of detrusor contraction pressure, sphincter electromyelogram, and urinary flow	Determine characteristic of voiding dysfunction Used to identify type (cause) of incontinence or urinary retention Especially valuable for voiding dysfunction complicated by urinary tract infection, urinary retention, or neurogenic bladder dysfunction	Prepare child for catheterization. Insertion of rectal tube will produce feelings of rectal fullness or pressure. Insertion of needles may be required for sphincter electromyography.

DMSA, Dimercaptosuccinic acid; *DTPA,* diethylenetriamine pentaacetic acid; *MAG3,* mertiatide.

TABLE 30-3 BLOOD TESTS OF RENAL FUNCTION

TEST	NORMAL RANGE (mg/dl)	DEVIATIONS	SIGNIFICANCE OF DEVIATIONS
Blood urea nitrogen (BUN)	Newborn: 4-18 Infant, child: 5-18	Elevated	Renal disease—acute or chronic (the higher the BUN, the more severe the disease) Increased protein catabolism Dehydration Hemorrhage High protein intake Corticosteroid therapy
Uric acid	Child: 2.0-5.5	Increased	Severe renal disease
Creatinine	Infant: 0.2-0.4 Child: 0.3-0.7 Adolescent: 0.5-1.0	Increased	Severe renal impairment

BOX 30-2 CLASSIFICATIONS OF URINARY TRACT INFECTIONS OR INFLAMMATIONS

Bacteriuria—Presence of bacteria in the urine

Asymptomatic bacteriuria—Significant bacteriuria with no evidence of clinical infection (usually defined as >100,000 colony-forming units/mm^3)

Symptomatic bacteriuria—Bacteriuria accompanied by physical signs of urinary infection (dysuria, suprapubic discomfort, hematuria, fever)

Recurrent urinary tract infection (UTI)—Repeated episode of bacteriuria or symptomatic UTI

Persistent UTI—Persistence of bacteriuria despite antibiotic treatment

Febrile UTI—Bacteriuria accompanied by fever and other physical signs of UTI; presence of a fever typically implies pyelonephritis

Cystitis—Inflammation of the bladder

Urethritis—Inflammation of the urethra

Pyelonephritis—Inflammation of the upper urinary tract and kidneys

Urosepsis—Febrile UTI coexisting with systemic signs of bacterial illness; blood culture reveals presence of urinary pathogen

period, females have a 10 to 30 times greater risk for developing UTI than males. It is estimated that 5% to 6% of girls will have had at least one episode of bacteriuria between the time they enter first grade and graduate from high school. The likelihood of recurrence is 50% or greater in girls; the recurrence rate is lower in boys (Mingin, Hinds, Nguyen, et al, 2004).

Approximately, 20% to 25% of children with a negative radiologic evaluation have recurrent UTI (Mingin, Hinds, Nguyen, et al, 2004; Bratslavsky, Feustel, Aslan, et al, 2004). UTI in newborns differs in some respects from infections occurring in older children. In the neonatal age-group, boys with UTIs outnumber girls. At all ages asymptomatic bacteriuria is more common than symptomatic disease. An increased incidence of UTI is observed in adolescents, especially those with evidence of sexual activity.

Etiology

A variety of organisms can be responsible for UTI. *Escherichia coli* (80% of cases) and other gram-negative enteric organisms are most commonly implicated; all are common to the anal, perineal, and perianal region. Other organisms associated with UTI include *Proteus, Pseudomonas, Klebsiella, Staphylococcus aureus, Haemophilus*, and coagulase-negative staphylococci. A number of factors contribute to the development of UTI, including anatomic, physical, and chemical conditions or properties of the host's urinary tract.

Anatomic and Physical Factors

The structure of the lower urinary tract is believed to account for the increased incidence of bacteriuria in females. The short urethra, which measures approximately 2 cm (0.75 inch) in young girls and 4 cm (1.5 inches) in mature women, provides a ready pathway for invasion of organisms. In addition, the closure of the urethra at the end of micturition may return contaminated bacteria to the bladder.

The longer male urethra (as long as 20 cm [8 inches] in an adult) and the antibacterial properties of prostatic secretions inhibit the entry and growth of pathogens. The presence or absence of the foreskin contributes to the differences in UTI rates in infants. Infant girls had a 5% incidence of developing a UTI, whereas UTI rates were 21% in uncircumcised infant boys and only 2% in circumcised infant boys (Zorc, Levine, Platt, et al, 2005; Shaikh, Morone, Bost, et al, 2008). The presence of a foreskin is associated with a preputial colonization of uropathic bacteria that can ascend the urethra easily (Balat, Karakok, Guler, et al, 2008). The incidence of renal scarring is greatest in patients whose first infection occurs during infancy.

The single most important host factor influencing the occurrence of UTI is urinary stasis. Ordinarily urine is sterile, but at 37° C (98.6° F) it provides an excellent culture medium. Under normal conditions the act of completely and repeatedly emptying the bladder flushes away any organisms before they have an opportunity to multiply and invade surrounding tissue. However, urine that remains in the bladder allows bacteria from the urethra to rapidly become established in the rich medium.

Incomplete bladder emptying (stasis) may result from reflux (see p. 1138 for a discussion of reflux), anatomic abnormalities (especially those involving the ureters), or extrinsic ureteral or

---

BOX 30-3 SYMPTOMS OF DYSFUNCTIONAL VOIDING

- Urinary tract infection without fever
- Changes in urinary frequency
- Constipation
- Squatting or holding to stay dry
- Daytime or nighttime wetting
- Straining to void
- Urgency to void

Modified from Plachter NB, Schulman SL, Canning DA: Identification and management of urinary tract infection in the preschool child, *J Pediatr Health Care* 13(6 Pt 1):268-272, 1999.

---

bladder compression. The pressure of overdistention within the bladder may increase the risk of infection by decreasing host resistance, probably as a result of lessened blood flow to the mucosa. This often occurs in a neurogenic bladder or as a consequence of voluntarily holding back urine despite the urge to void.

Urinary stasis may also occur because of dysfunctional voiding. Dysfunctional voiding refers to an abnormality in either the storage or emptying phase of micturition and is associated with urgency, frequency, incontinence, UTI, and secondary vesicoureteral reflux (VUR) (Berry, 2005). Children may also exhibit bowel elimination symptoms such as constipation (Plachter, Schulman, and Canning, 1999) (Box 30-3).

Extrinsic factors that may be responsible for functional bladder neck obstruction are pregnancy and chronic and intermittent constipation. In both conditions the full uterus or rectum displaces the bladder and posterior urethra in the fixed and limited space of the bony pelvis, causing obstruction, incomplete micturition, and urinary stasis. Treating constipation and administering antibiotic therapy for UTI reduces the recurrence of infection. Failure to relieve the fecal retention in spite of adequate treatment of the UTI may result in recurrence.

Other extrinsic factors that can contribute to UTI include catheters, especially short-term indwelling catheters, and administration of antimicrobial agents. Antimicrobials alter the host's normal perineal flora, allowing easier colonization of uropathogens. Tight clothing or diapers, poor hygiene, and local inflammation, such as from vaginitis, masturbation, or pinworm infestation, may also increase the risk of ascending infection. The essential oils in bubble baths and shampoos can irritate the urethra of both boys and girls, causing painful and frequent urination. Therefore bubble baths are discouraged. There is no evidence that plain tub baths increase the risk of UTI, but infections have been related to the use of hot tub or whirlpool baths. Sexual intercourse may produce transient bacteriuria in females and is associated with an increased risk of UTI.

Altered Urine and Bladder Chemistry

Several mechanical and chemical characteristics of the urinary tract promote urine sterility. Adequate fluid intake promotes urinary transport and lowers the concentration of pathogens (and nutrients) in the urine. Diuresis also enhances the antibacterial properties of the renal medulla, probably as a result of increased blood flow, which hastens leukocytosis; diuresis promotes the mechanical removal of pathogens (see Research Focus box).

Pathophysiology

After invasion by bacteria, the first line of defense in the lower urinary tract is complete evacuation by voiding. Inflammation in the bladder and urethral walls is apparent within 30 minutes of invasion by a bacterial pathogen. Polymorphonuclear leukocytes rapidly migrate to the bladder wall, which becomes completely injected within 2 hours. Complete evacuation of the bladder is particularly important for the eradication of bacteria from the urine. Urination not only removes bacteria and associated toxins contained in the urine, it also allows more efficient destruction of the bacteria remaining on the thin film of urine that is closely adherent to the vesical wall.

Recurrent infection of the urinary bladder predisposes the individual to transient episodes of VUR. After resolution of the infection the reflux is not detectable on voiding cystourethrography (VCUG). Although it is known that certain adherent bacteria promote urinary system dilation, the relationship between bladder wall inflammation and ureterovesical junction competence remains unclear (Wein, Kavoussi, Norvick, et al, 2006).

Clinical Manifestations

The clinical manifestations of UTIs depend on the child's age. In newborn infants and children less than 2 years of age the signs are characteristically nonspecific. They more nearly resemble gastrointestinal tract disorders: failure to thrive, feeding problems, vomiting, diarrhea, abdominal distention, and jaundice. Newborns may have fever, hypothermia, or sepsis. Other evidence includes frequent or infrequent voiding, constant squirming and irritability, strong-smelling urine, and an abnormal stream. A persistent diaper rash is also a helpful clue.

The classic symptoms of UTI are often observed in children more than 2 years of age. These include enuresis or daytime incontinence in the child who has been toilet trained, fever, strong- or foul-smelling urine, increased frequency of urination, dysuria, or urgency. The children may also complain of abdominal pain or costovertebral angle tenderness (flank pain). Some patients are seen with hematuria. Some preschoolers may vomit. Infants and young boys frequently develop obstructive uropathy, which is characterized by dribbling of urine, straining with urination, or a decrease in the force and size of the urinary stream. High fever and chills accompanied by flank pain, severe abdominal pain, and leukocytosis suggest pyelonephritis. However, flank pain and tenderness may be the only indication of pyelonephritis on physical examination.

Manifestations in adolescents are more specific. Symptoms of lower tract infections include frequency and painful urination of a small amount of turbulent urine that may be grossly bloody. Fever is usually absent. Upper tract infection is characterized by fever; chills; flank pain; and lower tract symptoms, which may appear 1 or 2 days after the upper tract symptoms.

Many UTIs in children are asymptomatic or atypical in clinical presentation, and many complaints may be unrelated to the urinary tract. Many are treated as respiratory or gastrointestinal tract infections. It is important to identify these children so treatment can be initiated. Significant scarring can occur, especially in infants and young children.

Diagnostic Evaluation

The diagnosis of UTI depends on a high degree of suspicion, evaluation of the history and physical examination, and urinalysis and culture. Urine with a possible infection appears cloudy, hazy, or thick with noticeable strands of mucus and pus; it also smells fishy and unpleasant, even when fresh. A presumptive UTI diagnosis can be made on the basis of microscopic examination of the urine, which often reveals pyuria (5 to 8 white blood cells/ml of uncentrifuged urine) and the presence of at least one bacterium in a Gram stain. However, a normal urinalysis may also be present in conditions of asymptomatic bacteriuria.

Detection of bacteria in a urine culture confirms the diagnosis of UTI, but urine collection is often difficult, especially in infants and small children. (See Collection of Specimens, Chapter 27.) Several factors may alter a urine specimen. Contamination of a specimen by organisms from sources other than the urine is the most common cause of false-positive results. Bag urine specimens are commonly contaminated by perineal and perianal flora and are usually considered inadequate for a definitive diagnosis. The American Academy of Pediatrics recommends collecting urine by the bag to determine whether it is necessary to obtain a catheterized urine specimen for culture (Wald, 2005).

> **NURSING TIP** Clean-catch urine specimen collection from a young girl is easier when the child sits on the toilet facing the tank. In this position the child (especially the toddler) is more stable and relaxed. The labia are naturally separated, decreasing the likelihood of contamination. This position is also useful for older girls who perform clean, intermittent self-catheterization.

EVIDENCE-BASED PRACTICE *Ashley R. Breland*

Urinary Specimen Collection in Children with Suspected Urinary Tract Infection

ASK THE QUESTION

In infants or children with a possible urinary tract infection (UTI), what is the preferred method for collecting a urine specimen?

SEARCH FOR THE EVIDENCE

Search strategies

Search criteria included English-language publications within the past 10 years, research-based articles on infants or children with signs or symptoms of UTI.

Databases used

Cochrane Collaboration, Joanna Briggs Institute, National Guideline Clearinghouse (AHRQ), PubMed

CRITICALLY ANALYZE THE EVIDENCE

GRADE criteria: Evidence quality moderate; recommendation strong (Guyatt, Oxman, Vist, et al, 2008)

A review of the literature revealed two studies evaluating specimen collection techniques in infants and children. Findings from the pediatric studies revealed that suprapubic aspiration of urine was the gold standard for urine collection. This is a highly invasive and costly method used exclusively in infants and children. Evidence supported collection of urine specimens from infants via urinary catheterization. For children who are toilet-trained, specimens may be collected via clean-catch technique. Collection via urine bag is useful for screening but does not provide a high-quality specimen for culture because of contamination.

- An observational study of 3066 infants less than 93 days old evaluated specimen collection via urinary catheterization compared with a urine bag. Results showed that bag specimens sent for urine culture were more likely to have two organisms, nonpathogenic bacteria, and ambiguous results. Although parents prefer the urine bag method of specimen collection, culture results are more accurate when specimens are collected via urinary catheterization (Schroeder, Newman, Wasserman, et al, 2005).
- McGillivray, Mok, Mulrooney, and colleagues (2008) compared sensitivity and specificity of specimens collected via "clean-void" bag technique versus specimens collected via urinary catheterization to diagnose UTIs. The authors concluded that urine samples should be collected via catheterization in infants less than 90 days old due to low sensitivity of bag specimens. Bag specimens are an acceptable method of collecting urine to screen for UTI but can miss up to 12% of UTIs.

APPLY THE EVIDENCE: NURSING IMPLICATIONS

- Urine specimens should be collected via catheterization technique in non-toilet-trained infants or children. In older children samples for urinalysis should be obtained by the least invasive route, such as midstream clean catch.
- The perineum should be prepped before collection of urine via mid-stream, clean-catch technique to reduce the incidence of contamination.
- If a urine specimen is to be sent for culture, the specimen should be collected via urinary catheterization.

References

Guyatt GH, Oxman AD, Vist GE, et al: GRADE: an emerging consensus on rating quality of evidence and strength of recommendations, *BMJ* 336:924-926, 2008.

McGillivray D, Mok E, Mulrooney E, et al: A head-to-head comparison: "clean-void" bag versus catheter urinalysis in the diagnosis of urinary tract infection in young children, *J Pediatr* 147(4):451-456, 2008.

Schroeder AR, Newman TB, Wasserman RC, et al: Choice of urine collection methods for the diagnosis of urinary tract infection in young, febrile infants, *Arch Pediatr Adolesc Med* 159(10):915-922, 2005.

Unless the specimen is a first morning sample, a recent high fluid intake may indicate a falsely low organism count. Therefore do not encourage children to drink large volumes of water in an attempt to obtain a specimen quickly.

The most accurate tests of bacterial content are suprapubic aspiration (for children <2 years of age) and properly performed bladder catheterization (as long as the first few milliliters are excluded from collection). Care of a urine specimen obtained for culture is an important nursing responsibility related to diagnosis. The specimen should be taken to the laboratory for culture immediately. If culture is delayed, place the sample in a refrigerator for up to 24 hours, but storage can result in a loss of formed elements, such as blood cells and casts (Froom, Bieganiec, Ehrenrich, et al, 2000) (see Evidence-Based Practice box).

NURSING TIP For best results, wash the perineal area thoroughly before applying the urine collection bag, and promptly remove the bag as soon as voiding occurs. Leaving the device in situ for more than 1 hour is more likely to yield a contaminated urine specimen (Li, Ma, and Wong, 2002).

Tests to detect bacteriuria are being used with increased frequency in UTI screening. The plastic dipstick and agar-coated slide tests are quick and inexpensive methods for detecting infection before obtaining final culture results. The presence of nitrites on dipstick analysis of urine has been shown to have a predictive value of as much as 100% (identifies infected urine) (Raymond and Sauvestre, 1998). The absence of nitrites and leukocyte esterase in combination has been shown to have 92% negative predictive value (identifies uninfected urine) (Raymond and Sauvestre, 1998) (see Table 30-1). The agar-coated slides have a positive predictive value (identify infected urine) of 96% and negative predictive value (identify uninfected urine) of 99.8% (Colodner and Keness, 2000). These test results are used to initiate treatment of UTI while culture results are pending. It is important to remember that some organisms that cause UTI are non–nitrite producing (e.g., *Pseudomonas* organisms).

Localization of the infection site may involve more specific tests, including ureteral catheterization, bladder washout procedures, and radioisotope renography. Other tests, such as ultrasonography, VCUG, intravenous pyelography, and dimercaptosuccinic acid (DMSA) scan, may be performed after the infection subsides to identify anatomic abnormalities contributing to the development of infection and existing kidney changes from a recurrent infection.

TABLE 30-4	COMMON SIDE EFFECTS OF URINARY ANTIINFECTIVE AGENTS	
DRUG	**SIDE EFFECTS**	**NURSING INTERVENTIONS**
Trimethoprim-sulfamethoxazole (Bactrim, Septra)	Rash, urticaria, photosensitivity, nausea, bone marrow depression (long term use)	Maintain adequate fluid intake. Advise parents and child to use sunscreen. Perform complete blood count every 3 mo (long-term use).
Amoxicillin (Amoxil, Polymox, Trimox)	Nausea, vomiting, diarrhea	Refrigerate suspension; discard suspension after 14 days.
Nitrofurantoin (Macrodantin, Furadantin)	Nausea, pneumonitis or pulmonary fibrosis (long-term use)	Administer with food or milk.
Cephalexin (Keflex)	Nausea, diarrhea	Administer with food or milk.
Carbenicillin (Geocillin, Geopen)	Nausea, diarrhea, urticaria	Take tablets with juice to mask foul taste. Do not administer if child is allergic to penicillin.
Ceftazidime (Fortaz)	Renal toxicity	Keep child well hydrated.
Gentamicin (Garamycin)	Renal toxicity, ototoxicity	Monitor urinary output, blood urea nitrogen, creatinine. Monitor serum levels, especially in infants.

Therapeutic Management

The objectives of treatment of children with UTI are to (1) eliminate the current infection, (2) identify contributing factors to reduce the risk of recurrence, (3) prevent urosepsis, and (4) preserve renal function (American Academy of Pediatrics, 1999). Antibiotic therapy depends on laboratory culture and sensitivity tests. Nonetheless, empiric therapy on the basis of the child's history and presenting symptoms may be necessary when fever or systemic illness complicates UTI. Common antiinfective agents used for UTI include the penicillins, sulfonamide (including trimethoprim-sulfamethoxazole), the cephalosporins, nitrofurantoin, and the tetracyclines. All antibiotics may cause side effects or prove ineffective because of bacterial resistance (Table 30-4).

Children with suspected pyelonephritis and fever are admitted to the hospital and given appropriate antibiotics intravenously for a minimum of 48 hours. Blood and urine cultures are obtained on admission and after therapy. Urine cultures are usually repeated at monthly intervals for 3 months and at 3-month intervals for another 6 months.

Renal scarring can develop during the initial infection, especially in younger children. Therefore some practitioners believe that the first UTI in childhood necessitates radiologic evaluation, regardless of the patient's age and sex. The standard assessment of UTI with renal ultrasound and VCUG is now being reconsidered. Instead the "top-down" approach of early DMSA renal scanning to identify acute pyelonephritis and renal injury is often recommended (Tseng, Lin, Lo, et al, 2007; Hardy and Austin, 2008). Children with a negative DMSA scan during their first UTI rarely have VUR. Negative DMSA results could

reduce the need for children to undergo the often traumatic VCUG (Tseng, Lin, Lo, et al, 2007; Hardy and Austin, 2008).

Anatomic defects such as primary reflux or bladder neck obstruction may require surgical correction to prevent recurrent infection or may indicate the need for prophylactic antibiotics and careful follow-up monitoring. Follow-up study is an important component of medical management, since the relapse rate is high and recurrent infection tends to occur 1 to 2 months after termination of treatment. The aim of therapy and careful follow-up in such cases is to prevent morbidity and reduce the chance of renal scarring.

Prognosis

With prompt and adequate treatment at the time of diagnosis, the long-term prognosis for UTIs is usually excellent. The hazard of progressive renal injury is greatest when infection occurs in young children (especially <2 years of age) and is associated with congenital renal malformations and reflux. Therefore early diagnosis of children at risk is particularly important during infancy and toddlerhood.

QUALITY PATIENT OUTCOMES: Urinary Tract Infections
- Treatment based on culture and sensitivity
- Renal function maintained
- Appropriate diagnosis of renal abnormalities

Nursing Care Management

Objectives of nursing care include identification of children with UTI and education of parents and children regarding prevention and treatment of infection. Aside from the influence of renal abnormalities, girls between the ages of 2 and 6 years are in general a high-risk group. Because they are not a captive population, mass screening is difficult. However, the annual health examination should include a routine urinalysis. In addition, nurses should instruct parents to observe regularly for clues that suggest UTI. Unfortunately, the signs of UTI are not as evident as those of upper respiratory tract infection. Therefore many cases go undetected because no one thought to investigate this common problem.

! NURSING ALERT

A child who exhibits the following should be evaluated for UTI:
- Incontinence in a toilet-trained child
- Strong-smelling urine
- Frequency or urgency

NURSING TIP To detect UTI in infants and toddlers, check the diaper every half hour; frequent observations increase the opportunity for observing the stream for such findings as straining or fretting before voiding begins, signs of discomfort before and during urination, intermittent starting and stopping of the stream, and frequent dripping of small amounts of urine.

Because infants and young children are unable to express their feelings and sensations verbally, it is difficult to detect any discomfort they may be experiencing from dysuria. A careful history regarding voiding habits, stooling pattern, and episodes of unexplained irritability may assist in detecting less obvious cases of UTI. Encourage parents to observe for specific clues of UTI in suspected cases (see Critical Thinking Exercise).

❓ CRITICAL THINKING EXERCISE

Urinary Tract Infection and Constipation

During your assessment of Ginger, a 4-year-old admitted to the hospital for a severe urinary tract infection (UTI), her mother tells you that Ginger has bowel movements every third or fourth day. They are usually large, hard-formed stools, and Ginger sometimes has trouble evacuating the stool.

1. Evidence—Is there sufficient evidence to draw conclusion about Ginger's UTI and constipation?
2. Assumptions—Describe an underlying assumption about each of the following:
   a. UTIs and females
   b. Normal bowel patterns for 4-year-old children
   c. Association between UTIs and constipation
3. What priorities for nursing care should be established for Ginger?
4. Does the evidence support your nursing intervention?

Collecting an appropriate specimen is essential when the nurse suspects infection. It is the nurse's responsibility to take every precaution to obtain acceptable, clean-voided specimens in order to avoid using other collecting procedures except when absolutely indicated.

Other tests are often performed to detect anatomic defects. Prepare children for these tests as appropriate for their age. Children who are old enough to understand need an explanation of the procedure, its purpose, and what they will experience. (See Preparation for Diagnostic and Therapeutic Procedures, Chapter 27.) Sometimes a simple description of the urinary system is helpful. For children under 3 to 4 years of age, the nurse can explain the procedure using a doll. For those who are older, a simple drawing of the bladder, urethra, ureters, and kidneys makes the explanation more understandable. Especially with preschool children, the nurse must clarify that the urinary tract is separate from any sexual function and that the test is for a problem that they did not cause. It is not uncommon for children to associate blame for perceived wrongdoing (e.g., masturbation) or unacceptable thoughts with the reason for the illness or tests.

Children may be treated as outpatients to avoid overnight separation from home. In such cases be careful not to overlook the need for adequate preparation. If surgery is subsequently indicated, the children will have an understanding of these procedures, which helps decrease fear and anxiety regarding more extensive medical-surgical intervention.

Because antiinfective drugs are indicated in the treatment of UTI, the nurse teaches the patient and parents the appropriate dosage and scheduling and provides suggestions for administration of the agent. Certain drugs are available in liquid form; others are available only in capsule or pill form. In general, capsules are separated and pills are crushed, with their contents mixed into a small volume of food or chilled liquid to mask a disagreeable taste. A simple suggestion is to introduce a medicine in divided doses and mixed with a flavored gelatin in an ice cube tray. Children tolerate other medications best with a small portion of partially frozen grape or apple juice.

Encourage adequate fluid intake for the prevention and treatment of UTI, since bacterial eradication from the urinary tract is partially dependent on urine flow and voiding frequency (Dacher and Savoye-Collet, 2004; Wilde and Brasch, 2008). It is recommended that a person drink 100 ml/kg, or approximately 50 ml/lb of body weight, daily. The patient should primarily drink clear liquids. Have children avoid caffeinated or carbonated beverages because of their potentially irritative effect on the bladder mucosa. The child who is febrile and unable to drink liquids is given intravenous (IV) hydration until the fever resolves and oral liquids are tolerated.

Prevention

Prevention is the most important goal in both primary and recurrent infection. Most preventive measures are simple, ordinary hygienic habits that should be a routine part of daily care. Investigate any signs of intestinal parasites (e.g., scratching between the legs and around the anal area) and treat them appropriately. Advise sexually active adolescent girls to urinate as soon as possible after intercourse to flush out bacteria introduced during sex play. Also teach parents and older children health practices that prevent UTI (see Nursing Care Guidelines box).

📋 NURSING CARE GUIDELINES

Prevention of Urinary Tract Infection

FACTORS PREDISPOSING TO DEVELOPMENT	MEASURES OF PREVENTION
Short female urethra close to vagina and anus	Perineal hygiene—wipe from front to back. Avoid tight clothing or diapers; wear cotton panties rather than nylon.
Incomplete emptying (reflux) and overdistention of bladder	Check for vaginitis or pinworms, especially if child scratches between legs. Avoid "holding" urine; encourage child to void frequently, especially before a long trip or other circumstances in which toilet facilities are not available. Empty bladder completely with each void. Avoid straining at stool.
Concentrated and alkaline urine	Encourage generous fluid intake. Acidify urine with a diet high in animal protein.
Constipation	Increase dietary fiber and fluid. Use stool softener as needed.

Children who experience recurrent febrile UTIs or recurrent infections complicated by VUR may be given a suppressive or prophylactic antibiotic for a period of months or several years. The medication is commonly administered once a day; the patient and parents are advised to give the antibiotic before sleep because this represents the longest period without voiding. A sulfonamide-trimethoprim, nitrofurantoin, or cephalosporin is often used for antibiotic prophylaxis.

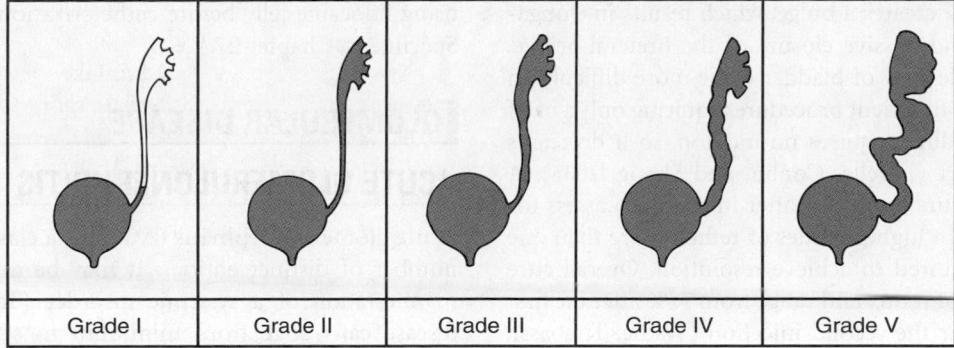

| Grade I | Grade II | Grade III | Grade IV | Grade V |

Fig. 30-2 Grades of reflux. (From Retik AB, Cukier J, editors: *Pediatric urology*, Baltimore, 1987, Williams & Wilkins.)

VESICOURETERAL REFLUX

VUR refers to the retrograde flow of bladder urine into the ureters. Reflux increases the chance for and perpetuates febrile UTI because with each void urine is swept up the ureters and then allowed to empty after voiding. Therefore the residual urine from the ureters remains in the bladder until the next void. The International Classification System describes the degree of reflux from the bladder into upper genitourinary tract structures (Fig. 30-2).

Primary reflux results from a congenital anomaly that affects the ureterovesical junction. Ectopic or orthotopic implantation of the ureter, abnormal tunneling of the intramural ureteral segment, and defects in the configuration of the ureter orifice are associated with primary reflux. Primary reflux has a significant familial pattern; the incidence of reflux in siblings of affected children has been reported as 36%. Moreover, screening should occur early, since siblings evaluated after 2 years of age had twice the risk of already having renal damage as detected by renal scan (Houle, Cheikhelard, Barrieras, et al, 2004). Although reflux occurs more often in females, siblings of both genders should be screened. One study found affected brothers of male children with reflux had a higher grade of reflux and were more likely to have renal scarring than female siblings (Pirker, Mohanan, Colhoun, et al, 2006) Screening for reflux in siblings through 72 months of age is recommended to prevent renal damage, which can occur in the absence of symptomatic UTI.

Secondary reflux occurs as a result of an acquired condition such as UTI or obstruction. UTI can produce transient reflux. Neuropathic bladder dysfunction, particularly when poor bladder compliance coexists with bladder outlet obstruction, may produce secondary reflux as urine seeks to escape the high pressures of the lower urinary tract. Obstruction may also be due to renal stones, strictures, or tumors affecting the urinary tract. Children who routinely "hold in" urine (dysfunctional voiding) may ultimately develop secondary reflux (Dacher and Savoye-Collet, 2004; Berry, 2005).

Reflux with infection is the most common cause of pyelonephritis in children. Refluxed urine ascending into the collecting tubules of the nephrons allows the microorganisms to gain access to the renal parenchyma, initiating renal scarring. The shape of renal papillae and the angle of entry of the collecting ducts change with advancing age, making intrarenal reflux difficult. Therefore most renal scars associated with reflux occur at a young age and are present at the time of diagnosis; few develop after 5 to 6 years of age. Between 30% and 60% of children with VUR have evidence of renal scarring, and scarring is almost always found in association with reflux. Careful routine follow-up care is a critical part of management of children with UTIs; children with reflux as documented by VCUG are assessed repeatedly during ensuing years.

Therapeutic Management

In most cases of VUR, conservative, nonoperative therapy is effective in controlling infection. There is a high incidence of spontaneous resolution over time—approximately 20% to 30% for each 2-year period throughout childhood. An 80% probability of remission may occur in grades I and II reflux when managed medically (Koff, 1997). Therapy consists of continuous low-dose antibacterial therapy with frequent urine cultures, which can usually be performed at home by the dip slide or dipstick methods. This long-term therapy requires medical supervision and reliable, cooperative parents. Surgical correction of reflux may be required for grades IV and V reflux. Grade III is managed conservatively unless there are complications.

The major indications for surgical intervention include significant anatomic abnormality at the ureterovesical junction, recurrent UTIs, high grades of VUR, noncompliance with medical therapy, intolerance to antibiotics, and VUR after puberty in females. Antireflux surgery consists of reimplantation of the ureters.

Renal ultrasonography is performed 1 month postoperatively to check for ureteral obstruction. If there is no obstruction, antibiotic therapy is discontinued. A renal ultrasound and VCUG are recommended 6 months after surgery. Because of the anxiety experienced by some children undergoing catheterization for cystography and the high success rate of antireflux surgical procedures, some practitioners may omit VCUG at this time. Two years after surgery, the child is seen for a final renal ultrasound to assess renal growth.

For some children with less severe reflux, a minimally invasive endoscopic option (subtrigonal injection, or STING) for the treatment of VUR is an attractive alternative to years of daily antibiotics or surgical intervention. During cystoscopy, the surgeon locates the affected ureter and injects a gel-like bulking agent—dextranomer–hyaluronic acid copolymer (Deflux)—into the mucous membrane where the ureter enters the bladder.

This injected material creates a bulge, which results in elongation of the tunnel and passive closure of the ureteral orifice, making the retrograde flow of bladder urine more difficult. In addition to being an outpatient procedure requiring only a brief anesthetic, the procedure requires no incision, so it decreases the child's discomfort (Lavelle, Conlin, and Skoog, 2005). A follow-up VCUG occurs 3 months after injection to assess for correction of reflux. In higher grades of reflux, more than one injection may be required to achieve resolution. Overall cure rates relate to degree of reflux and range from 77% after the first injection to 96% after the second injection (Wadie, Tirabassi, Courtney, et al, 2007; Cerwinka, Scherz, and Kirsch, 2008).

Nursing Care Management

The primary nursing goal in children receiving medical therapy is encouraging compliance. Emphasize the importance of maintaining the medical regimen to parents and older children. The medications prescribed are usually well tolerated by children, but parents may need help encouraging children to take the medication. The methods described in Chapter 27 provide some guidelines for administration and encouraging compliance. The importance of hygiene and a frequent voiding schedule are also discussed.

Because siblings are at risk for VUR, nurses should encourage parents to have their other children screened using renal ultrasonography and cystography. All children require age-appropriate preparation for the tests. Atraumatic care includes using lidocaine jelly before catheterization. (See Collection of Specimens, Chapter 27.)

GLOMERULAR DISEASE

ACUTE GLOMERULONEPHRITIS

Acute glomerulonephritis (AGN) as a classification includes a number of distinct entities. It may be a primary event or a manifestation of a systemic disorder (Table 30-5), and the disease can range from minimum to severe. The common features include oliguria, edema, hypertension and circulatory congestion, hematuria, and proteinuria. Most cases are post-infectious and have been associated with pneumococcal, streptococcal, and viral infections. All postinfectious diseases are presumed to result from immune complex formation and glomerular deposition, and the clinical presentations may be indistinguishable. Postinfectious glomerulonephritis exhibits a better clinical course than other acute proliferative glomerulonephritis (Ozaltin, Besbas, Bakkaloglu, et al, 2005).

Acute poststreptococcal glomerulonephritis (APSGN) is the most common of the noninfectious renal diseases in childhood and the one for which a cause can be established in the majority of cases. APSGN can occur at any age but primarily affects early school-age children, with a peak age of onset of 6 to 7 years (Hahn, Knox, and Forman, 2005). It is uncommon in children younger than 2 years of age.

TABLE 30-5	RENAL INVOLVEMENT ASSOCIATED WITH SYSTEMIC DISEASE PROCESS		
DISEASE	**MECHANISM**	**RENAL MANIFESTATION**	**COMMENTS**
Systemic lupus erythematosus (SLE)	Deposition of autoantibody-antigen complexes in kidney	Variable degrees of hematuria and proteinuria More severe—Nephrotic syndrome, hypertension, renal insufficiency	Responsive to corticosteroid and antimetabolite therapy Renal failure most common cause of death from SLE Rare before adolescence but may occur in school-age children
Anaphylactoid (Schönlein-Henoch) purpura	Deposition of immunoglobulin (primarily IgA) in the glomerular mesangium	Hematuria (gross or microscopic) Less common—Edema, hypertension Nephrotic syndrome with oliguria and hypertension, indicating severe involvement Rarely—Acute renal failure	Renal involvement in 20%-70% of cases Renal involvement most serious manifestation of the disease More common in children >6 yr old Responsive to corticosteroid therapy Management similar to that for persistent glomerulonephritis
Sickle cell disease	Infarction of renal vessels by sickle cells (especially medullary) Results in decreased circulation in vasa recta and impaired sodium and chloride ion reabsorption in collecting ducts	Hematuria Nephrotic syndrome Defective urine concentration Progressive glomerulonephritis	Irreversible with increasing age Severe urinary tract infections with bacteremia not uncommon
Polyarteritis nodosa	Fibroid necrosis of arterial walls Large vessels—Patchy renal infarction Microscopic vessels—Necrotizing glomerulitis	Proteinuria Hematuria Severe hypertension	Kidney involvement of secondary importance in infancy
Bacterial endocarditis	Focal or diffuse, immune-complex deposition related to chronic bacteremia Some embolization of glomeruli by bacteria and fibrin from endocardial vegetations	Proteinuria Hematuria	Renal involvement seen in approximately 50% of cases Renal involvement seldom of major significance
Prolonged bacteremia (infected atrioventricular shunts)	Immune-complex deposition with exudation and cellular proliferation	Variable degrees of persistent nephrotic syndrome	Vigorous antibiotic therapy or removal of infected shunt required

IgA, Immunoglobulin A.

Etiology

It is now generally accepted that APSGN is an immune-complex disease (i.e., a reaction that occurs as a by-product of an antecedent streptococcal infection with certain strains of the group A β-hemolytic streptococci). Most streptococcal infections do not cause APSGN. A latent period of 10 to 14 days occurs between the streptococcal infection of the throat or skin and the onset of clinical manifestations. The peak incidence of disease corresponds to the incidence of streptococcal infections. Disease secondary to streptococcal pharyngitis is more common in the winter or spring. However, when associated with pyoderma (principally impetigo), it may be more prevalent in later summer or early fall, especially in warmer climates. Multiple cases tend to occur in families. Second attacks are rare.

Pathophysiology

The mechanism by which the reaction takes place is still speculative. The most popular proposal to explain the pathologic process is that the streptococcal infection is followed by the release of a membranelike material from the specific organism into the circulation. Because it is antigenic, antibodies are formed and an immune-complex reaction occurs after the appropriate period. These immune complexes become trapped in the glomerular capillary loop.

The kidney itself appears normal or moderately enlarged, but microscopic examination reveals a diffuse proliferative and exudative process. Glomerular capillary loops are almost obliterated by swelling, and infiltration with polymorphonuclear leukocytes adds to the appearance of increased cellularity. Consequently, the glomeruli appear dense and lobulated. Examination with the electron microscope reveals discrete nodules or "humps" in the basement membrane, which are identified as deposits of immune complexes. These deposits are not evident after approximately 6 weeks.

Endothelial cell proliferation and edema occlude the capillary lumen of affected glomeruli, and the afferent arteriole is probably constricted by vasospasm, both of which significantly reduce the glomerular filtration rate. This occurs without a proportional decrease in renal blood flow and results in a reduced capacity to form filtrate from the glomerular plasma flow. Vascular and tubular changes are mild and nonspecific; therefore tubular function is less severely impaired.

The decreased filtration of plasma results in an excessive accumulation of water and retention of sodium. These cause expanded plasma and interstitial fluid volumes that lead to circulatory congestion and edema. It is unclear whether a decreased glomerular filtration rate, increased capillary permeability, or vascular spasm is responsible for these various manifestations. The cause of the hypertension associated with AGN is also unexplained. Plasma renin activity is low during the acute phase, but hypervolemia may be a factor.

Clinical Manifestations

Typically, affected children are in good health until they experience the antecedent infection. In some instances there is no history of an infection, or it is described as only a mild cold. The onset of nephritis appears after an average latent period of approximately 10 days. Because the child appears well during this time, parents may not recognize the association.

Initial signs of nephrotic reaction include puffiness of the face, especially around the eyes (periorbital edema); anorexia; and the passage of cola-colored urine. The edema is more prominent in the face in the morning but spreads during the day to involve the extremities and abdomen. The edema is only moderate and may not be appreciated by someone unfamiliar with the child's normal appearance. The urine is cloudy, smoky brown, or what parents describe as resembling tea or cola, and it is severely reduced in volume.

! NURSING ALERT

Evaluate a child who exhibits the following for possible AGN:
- Periorbital edema, which parents may report is worse in the morning
- Loss of appetite
- Decreased urinary output
- Cola- or tea-colored urine
- Antecedent streptococcal infection

The child is pale, irritable, and lethargic and appears unwell but seldom expresses specific complaints. Older children may complain of headaches, abdominal discomfort, and dysuria. On examination there is usually a mild to moderate elevation in blood pressure compared with normal values for age. Occasionally a child will have an onset with severe symptoms such as seizures from hypertensive encephalopathy, pulmonary and circulatory congestion, or hematuria in the absence of hypertension and edema. Table 30-6 compares APSGN and minimal change nephrotic syndrome (MCNS).

Clinical Course

The acute edematous phase of glomerulonephritis usually persists from 4 to 10 days but may persist for 2 or 3 weeks, during which time the child remains listless, anorexic, and apathetic. The weight fluctuates, the urine remains smoky brown, and the blood pressure may suddenly reach dangerously high levels at any time during this phase.

The first sign of improvement is a small increase in urinary output with a corresponding decrease in body weight. With diuresis the child begins to feel better, the appetite improves, and the blood pressure decreases to normal with the reduction of edema. Gross hematuria diminishes, in part because of dilution of the red blood cells in the more dilute urine, but microscopic hematuria may persist for weeks or months. Blood urea nitrogen (BUN) and creatinine levels decrease during diuresis and usually return to normal. A slight to moderate proteinuria may persist for several weeks.

Prognosis

Almost all children correctly diagnosed as having APSGN recover completely, and specific immunity is conferred so that subsequent recurrences are uncommon (Kasahara, Hayakawa, Okubo, et al, 2001). Deaths from complications still occur but fortunately are rare. A few of these children may develop chronic disease, but many of these cases are believed to be (probably) different glomerular diseases misdiagnosed as poststreptococcal disease.

	TABLE 30-6	COMPARISON OF POSTSTREPTOCOCCAL GLOMERULONEPHRITIS AND NEPHROTIC SYNDROME	
MANIFESTATIONS	**ACUTE POSTSTREPTOCOCCAL GLOMERULONEPHRITIS**	**MINIMAL CHANGE NEPHROTIC SYNDROME**
Streptococcal antibody titers	Elevated	Normal
Blood pressure	Elevated	Normal or decreased
Edema	Primarily periorbital and peripheral	Generalized, severe
Circulatory congestion	Common	Absent
Proteinuria	Mild to moderate	Massive
Hematuria	Gross or microscopic	Microscopic or none
Red blood cell casts	Present	Absent
Azotemia	Present	Absent
Serum potassium levels	Normal or increased	Normal
Serum protein levels	Minimum reduction	Markedly decreased
Serum lipid levels	Normal	Elevated
Peak age at onset (yr)	5-7	2-3

Complications

The major complications that may develop during the acute phase of glomerulonephritis are hypertensive encephalopathy, acute cardiac decompensation, and acute renal failure (ARF). Normally, cerebral blood flow responds to acute arterial hypertension by vasoconstriction. However, acute and severe hypertension may cause this protective autoregulation of cerebral blood flow to fail, leading to hyperperfusion of the brain and cerebral edema. The premonitory signs of encephalopathy are headache, dizziness, abdominal discomfort, and vomiting. If the condition progresses, there may be transient loss of vision or hemiparesis, disorientation, and generalized tonic-clonic seizures.

Hypervolemia, not cardiac failure, causes cardiac decompensation during the acute edematous phase of nephritis. However, signs of circulatory congestion are evident. The heart is enlarged, and increased pulmonary vascular markings are evident on x-ray examination. Increased pulmonary capillary permeability is also believed to be an important factor in the development of pulmonary edema.

ARF with persistent oliguria or anuria is an uncommon complication but one that requires an appropriate treatment regimen.

Diagnostic Evaluation

Urinalysis during the acute phase characteristically shows hematuria, proteinuria, and increased specific gravity. The specific gravity is moderately elevated and seldom exceeds 1.020. Proteinuria generally parallels the hematuria but is not the massive proteinuria seen in nephrotic syndrome. Gross discoloration of urine reflects its red blood cell and hemoglobin content. Microscopic examination of the sediment shows many red blood cells, leukocytes, epithelial cells, and granular and red blood cell casts. Bacteria are not seen, and urine cultures are negative.

Unless the disease has progressed to renal failure, the blood examination reveals normal electrolyte (sodium, potassium, and chloride ions) and carbon dioxide levels. Azotemia resulting from impaired glomerular filtration is reflected in elevated BUN and creatinine levels in at least 50% of cases.

When proteinuria is heavy, there may be changes associated with nephrotic syndrome (i.e., transient hypoproteinemia and hyperlipidemia).

Cultures of the pharynx are positive for streptococci in only a few cases, and the numbers are not significantly greater than the normal carrier incidence in many communities. Positive cultures help establish a diagnosis. Cultures should be obtained from other household members, and persons positive for group A streptococci should receive a course of antistreptococcal therapy.

Serologic tests are needed for diagnosis. Antibody responses to the extracellular products of the streptococci provide indirect evidence of previous streptococcal infection. These include antistreptolysin O (ASO), antistreptokinase (ASKase), antihyaluronidase (AHase), antideoxyribonuclease B (ADNase-B), and antinicotyladenine dinucleotidase (ANADase). The ASO titer is the most familiar and readily available test for streptococcal antibodies. ASO appears in the serum approximately 10 days after the initial infection; however, there is no correlation between the degree of elevation and the severity or prognosis of the glomerulonephritis. It is a useful diagnostic tool when nephritis follows a pharyngeal infection but is of less value after pyoderma. An ASO titer of 250 Todd units or higher is of diagnostic significance, as is a rising titer in two samples taken 1 week apart. More consistent and reliable antibody tests following streptococcal skin infections are elevated AHase and ADNase-B titers.

Of more importance for clinical serologic diagnosis is measurement of the serum complement level (C3). Serum C3 level is decreased initially but returns to normal 8 to 10 weeks after onset of the glomerulonephritis. Other studies include a chest x-ray examination, which shows characteristic generalized cardiac enlargement, pulmonary congestion, and pleural effusion during the edematous phase of acute disease. Renal biopsy for diagnostic purposes is seldom required but may be useful in the diagnosis of atypical cases.

Therapeutic Management

No specific treatment is available for AGN, but recovery is spontaneous and uneventful in most cases. Management consists of general supportive measures and early recognition and treatment of complications. Children who have normal blood pressure and a satisfactory urinary output can generally be treated at home. Those with substantial edema, hypertension, gross hematuria, or significant oliguria are often hospitalized because of the unpredictability of complications. Short hospitalization is the rule in uncomplicated cases; prolonged hospitalization is required only for children with severely impaired renal function.

General Measures

Bed rest is no longer recommended during the acute phase because ambulation does not seem to have an adverse effect on the course of the disease once the gross hematuria, edema, hypertension, and azotemia have ceased. Because they are generally listless and experience fatigue and malaise, most children voluntarily restrict their activities during the most active phase of the disease.

Fluid Balance

Regular measurement of vital signs, body weight, and intake and output is essential to monitor the disease's progress and detect complications that may appear at any time during the course of the disease. A record of daily weight is the most useful means to assess fluid balance and should be kept for children treated at home and for those who are hospitalized. Sodium and water restriction is useful when the output is significantly reduced (<2 to 3 dl/24 hr). In these children the water allowed is equivalent to the calculated insensible loss plus the volume of urine excreted.

Diuretics are of limited value when severe renal failure is present, since little sodium reaches the distal tubules as a result of the reduced filtration rate. However, when renal failure is not severe, diuretic therapy (usually furosemide [Lasix]) is helpful if significant edema and fluid overload are present. Rarely, children with AGN develop ARF with oliguria that significantly alters the fluid and electrolyte balance. These children require careful management that may include peritoneal dialysis (PD) or hemodialysis.

Loss of glomerular filtration in children with severe forms of APSGN may produce electrolyte imbalances, especially hyperkalemia, acidosis, hypocalcemia, and hyperphosphatemia. Management of these electrolyte disturbances is described under Acute Renal Failure.

Hypertension

Acute hypertension must be anticipated and identified early. Blood pressure measurements are taken every 4 to 6 hours. Significant but not severe hypertension is controlled with loop diuretics. Other antihypertensive drugs, such as calcium channel blockers, beta blockers, or angiotensin-converting enzyme inhibitors, may be needed in severe cases. Seizure activity associated with hypertensive encephalopathy requires anticonvulsant therapy and antihypertensive agents (see Renal Failure, p. 1162, for management of severe hypertension).

Nutrition

Dietary restrictions depend on the stage and severity of the disease, especially the extent of edema. A regular diet is permit-

ted in uncomplicated cases, but sodium intake is usually limited (no salt is added to foods). Moderate sodium restriction is usually instituted for children with hypertension or edema. Foods with substantial amounts of potassium are generally restricted during the period of oliguria. Protein restriction is reserved only for children with severe azotemia resulting from prolonged oliguria. The loss of appetite associated with the disease usually limits the protein intake sufficiently.

Antibiotics

Antibiotic therapy is indicated only for those children with evidence of persistent streptococcal infections. Antibiotics do not alter the course of the disease but are often recommended to prevent transmission of nephritogenic streptococci to other family members. Authorities are divided on the use of prophylactic antimicrobials for other family members.

Nursing Care Management

Nursing care of the child with glomerulonephritis involves careful assessment of the disease status, with regular monitoring of vital signs (including frequent measurement of blood pressure), fluid balance, and behavior. Vital signs provide clues to the severity of the disease and early signs of complications. The nurse carefully measures them and records and reports any abnormalities. The nurse notes the volume and character of urine and weighs the child daily. Assessment of the child's appearance for signs of cerebral complications is an important nursing function because the severity of the acute phase is variable and unpredictable. The child with edema, hypertension, and gross hematuria may be subject to complications, and anticipatory preparations are included in the Nursing Care Plan on p. 1171.

For most children a regular diet is allowed but should contain no added salt. Foods high in sodium and salted treats are eliminated, and the nurse should advise parents and friends against bringing items such as potato chips or pretzels. However, the total amount of salt ingested is usually less than prescribed because of poor appetite. Fluid restriction, if prescribed, is more difficult; the amount permitted should be evenly divided throughout the waking hours and served in small cups to give the illusion of larger servings. Meal preparation and service require special attention because the child has a poor appetite and is indifferent to meals during the acute phase. Collaboration with parents and the dietitian and special consideration for food preferences will facilitate meal planning.

During the acute phase children are generally content to lie in bed. As they begin to feel better and their symptoms subside, they will want to be up and about. Activities should be planned to allow for frequent rest periods and avoidance of fatigue.

Children with mild edema and no hypertension, as well as convalescent children being treated at home, need follow-up care. Parents are instructed regarding general measures, including activity, diet, and prevention of infection. Strenuous activity is usually restricted until there is no evidence of proteinuria or macroscopic hematuria. Health supervision is continued with weekly, followed by monthly, visits for evaluation and urinalysis. Parent education and support in preparation for discharge and home care include education in home management and the need for follow-up care and health supervision.

CHRONIC OR PROGRESSIVE GLOMERULONEPHRITIS

The majority of cases of renal glomerular disease are AGN, MCNS, and glomerulonephritis associated with systemic diseases. These pose relatively few problems of diagnosis, and their natural course is fairly predictable. A few cases present a prolonged course and a poor ultimate prognosis. They are a rather heterogeneous group and are defined by correlating the clinical manifestations, pathologic conditions, and natural course of the individual diseases.

Chronic glomerulonephritis (CGN) describes a variety of different disease processes that may be distinguished from each other by renal biopsy. These include membranoproliferative glomerulonephritis, membranous glomerulonephritis, focal segmental glomerulosclerosis, and immunoglobulin A nephropathy. In CGN tissue damage and progression to fibrosis are related to the immune response that brings about inflammation, failure to activate glomerular repair, and excessive fibrogenic activity (Coppo and Amore, 2004). *Rapidly progressive glomerulonephritis* is the term used to describe an acute illness with severe, acute onset that causes rapidly progressive deterioration of renal function in weeks to months. Renal biopsy of these patients shows a variety of diseases with the common feature of greater than 50% glomerular crescents found in the biopsy section.

Pathophysiology

In most cases of CGN, immunologic mechanisms can be implicated either through direct attack on the kidney or secondary to the accumulation of immune complexes in the glomerular filter or fibrin deposition from previously damaged glomeruli. Either can contribute to further glomerular damage and can initiate chronic changes in the glomerular structure (Coppo and Amore, 2004). In many cases there is no history of an acute glomerular disease. In other cases CGN may represent one of a succession of exacerbations of a preexisting disease. CGN that is not associated with other diseases may go undetected for years and be relatively asymptomatic until kidney destruction produces marked reduction in renal function. Consequently, the disease is more common in adolescents than in younger children. Renal insufficiency with all its manifestations occurs as the ultimate event.

Clinical Manifestations

The clinical manifestations and laboratory findings reflect deteriorating renal function. Nephrotic syndrome often develops. Hypertension, edema, proteinuria, cardiac failure, dyspnea, osteodystrophy, and anemia are common manifestations of progressive disease.

Diagnostic Evaluation

Laboratory findings may include proteinuria, with casts and red and white blood cells. Elevated BUN, creatinine, and uric acid levels are evidence of failing renal function. Electrolyte alterations include metabolic acidosis, elevated potassium, elevated phosphorus, and decreased calcium levels. The renal insufficiency may extend from 5 to 15 years and even longer, or rapid deterioration may progress to end-stage renal disease (ESRD).

Therapeutic Management

Early in the course of the disease, treatment is appropriate to the underlying disease and is largely symptomatic in most cases. Directs nursing efforts toward providing optimum conditions for the child's physical, psychologic, and social development. As few restrictions as feasible are imposed, and the child is allowed to live as normal a life as possible for as long as possible. Some forms of CGN are treated with corticosteroids or cytotoxic agents. Marked hypertension is controlled with antihypertensive agents, and anemia may require recombinant erythropoietin and iron supplements. Ultimately, dialysis and transplantation may be needed to restore relatively good health; however, these alternatives are reserved until renal failure is far advanced. (See Chronic Renal Failure, p. 1167, for more detailed management of specific problems.) Children with rapidly progressive glomerulonephritis are usually referred to a center specializing in renal disease.

Nursing Care Management

The problems of CGN and those encountered in chronic renal insufficiency from any cause are discussed under Chronic Renal Failure.

NEPHROTIC SYNDROME

Nephrotic syndrome is the most common presentation of glomerular injury in children. It is defined as massive proteinuria, hypoalbuminemia, hyperlipidemia, and edema, but the disorder is a clinical manifestation of a large number of distinct glomerular disorders in which increased glomerular permeability to plasma protein results in massive urinary protein loss (Bagga and Mantan, 2005). After a description of the three major forms of nephrotic syndrome, the remainder of the discussion is devoted to minimal change disease.

Types of Nephrotic Syndrome

Nephrotic syndrome can be classified as primary, when the syndrome is restricted to glomerular injury, or secondary, when it develops as part of a systemic illness. Although it may have several different histologic variations, the most common form of the primary disease is MCNS. A congenital form is also recognized.

Minimal Change Nephrotic Syndrome

Approximately 80% of cases of nephrotic syndrome in children result from MCNS. MCNS can be seen at any age but is predominantly a disease of the preschool child. The disease is rare in children younger than 6 months of age, uncommon in infants younger than 1 year of age, and unusual after the age of 8 years. The incidence of the disease in North America is approximately 2 to 7 per 100,000 children per year, and males outnumber females 2:1. In adolescence the ratio is 1:1.

The cause of MCNS (also known as idiopathic nephrosis, minimal lesion nephrosis, nil disease, childhood nephrosis, lipoid nephrosis, or uncomplicated nephrosis) remains obscure. A nonspecific illness, usually a viral upper respiratory tract infection, often precedes the manifestations by 4 to 8 days but is considered to be a precipitating factor rather than a cause.

Secondary Nephrotic Syndrome

Nephrotic syndrome may occur after or in association with glomerular damage of known or presumed cause. Prominent among causes of glomerular damage is AGN or CGN. Less commonly, secondary nephrotic syndrome occurs during the course of collagen vascular diseases (such as disseminated lupus erythematosus and anaphylactoid purpura) or as a result of toxicity to drugs (such as trimethadione and heavy metals), stings, or venom. Nephrotic syndrome is the major presenting symptom of renal disease in pediatric patients with acquired immunodeficiency syndrome. Diverse, rare causes are sickle cell disease, hepatitis, malaria, cyanotic heart disease, tuberculosis, infected ventriculojugular shunts, renal vein thrombosis, or malignancies.

Congenital Nephrotic Syndrome

The hereditary form of nephrotic syndrome is caused by a recessive gene on an autosome. Infants who have nephrotic syndrome are small for gestational age, and proteinuria and edema manifest early. The disease does not respond to the usual therapy, and death in the first year or 2 of life is the rule if the infant does not receive dialysis or a successful kidney transplant.

Pathophysiology

The pathogenesis of MCNS is not completely understood. A metabolic, biochemical, or physiochemical disturbance in the basement membrane of the glomeruli may lead to increased permeability to protein, but the causes and mechanisms are only speculative.

The glomerular membrane, which is normally impermeable to albumin and other large proteins, becomes permeable to proteins, especially albumin, which leak through the membrane and are lost in urine (hyperalbuminuria). This reduces the serum albumin level (hypoalbuminemia), which decreases the COP in the capillaries (Bagga and Mantan, 2005). As a result, the hydrostatic pressure exceeds the pull of the COP, and fluid accumulates in the interstitial spaces and body cavities, particularly the abdominal cavity (ascites). The shift of fluid from the plasma to the interstitial spaces reduces the vascular fluid volume (hypovolemia), which in turn stimulates the renin-angiotensin system and the secretion of antidiuretic hormone and aldosterone. Tubular reabsorption of sodium and water increases in an attempt to increase intravascular volume. The elevation of serum cholesterol, phospholipids, and triglycerides is not fully understood. The sequence of events in nephrotic syndrome is diagrammed in Fig. 30-3.

Clinical Manifestations

A previously well child begins to gain weight, which progresses insidiously over a period of days or weeks. Puffiness of the face, especially around the eyes, is apparent on arising in the morning but subsides during the day, when swelling of the abdomen and lower extremities is more prominent. The generalized edema

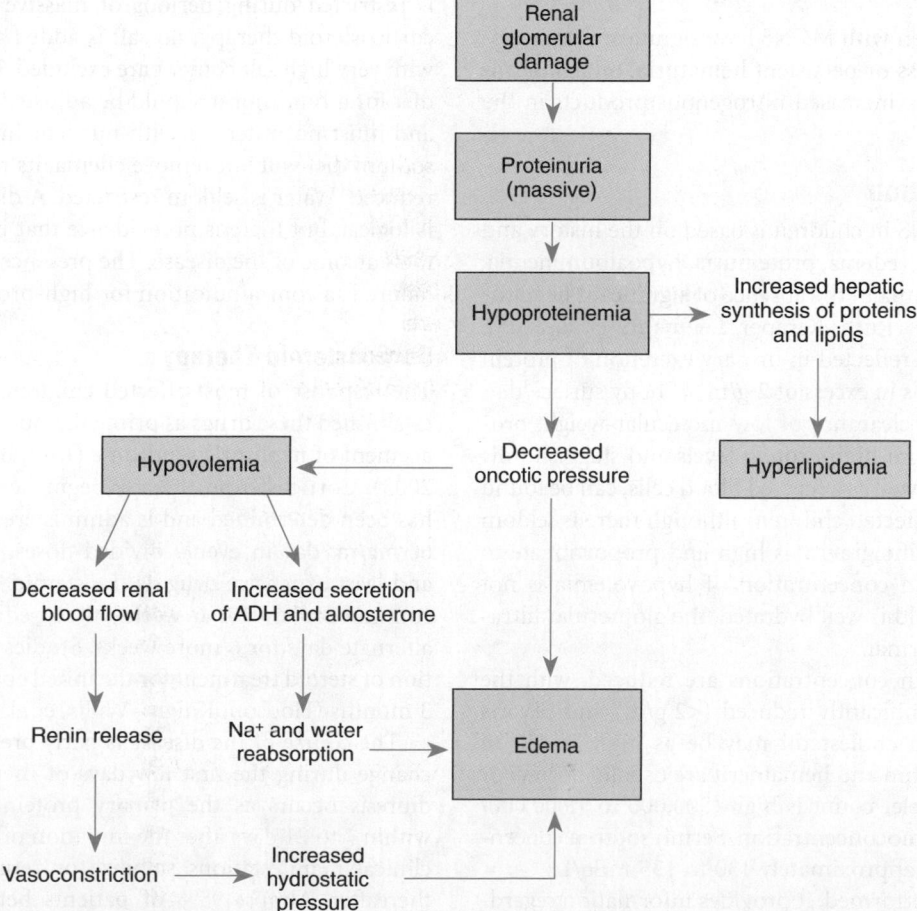

Fig. 30-3 Sequence of events in nephrotic syndrome. *ADH,* Antidiuretic hormone.

may develop so slowly that parents consider it a sign of healthy growth. Although an acute infection may precipitate severe generalized edema (anasarca), the usual course is one of progressive weight gain until either a rapid or a gradual increase in edema prompts the family to seek medical evaluation. Usually present are periorbital edema, abdominal swelling from ascites, and labial or scrotal swelling. Edema of the intestinal mucosa may cause diarrhea, loss of appetite, and poor intestinal absorption. The volume of urine is decreased, and it appears darkly opalescent and frothy.

The child often has extreme skin pallor and may experience skin breakdown during periods of severe edema. The child is irritable and may be more easily fatigued or lethargic but does not appear seriously ill. Weight loss from poor appetite and loss of protein is not uncommon, although it is often obscured by edema. Changes in the nails appear as white (Muehrcke) lines parallel to the lunula, which are caused by prolonged hypoalbuminemia. The blood pressure is usually normal or slightly decreased. The child is more susceptible to infection, especially cellulitis, pneumonia, peritonitis, or sepsis.

⚠ NURSING ALERT

Evaluate a child who exhibits the following for the possibility of nephrotic syndrome:
- Periorbital, gonadal, or lower extremity edema
- Weight gain greater than that expected based on previous pattern
- Decreased urinary output
- Pallor, fatigue

In rare cases children with MCNS have significant or persistent hypertension, gross or persistent hematuria, or significant or persistent azotemia (increased nitrogenous products in the blood).

Diagnostic Evaluation

The diagnosis of MCNS in children is based on the history and clinical manifestations (edema, proteinuria, hypoalbuminemia, and hypercholesterolemia in the absence of significant hematuria and hypertension) (Ruth, Kemper, Leumann, et al, 2005). Massive proteinuria is reflected in urinary excretion of protein that often reaches levels in excess of 2 g/m² of body surface/day, with relatively greater clearance of low-molecular-weight proteins. Hyaline casts from high protein levels and sluggish flow and oval fat bodies, as well as a few red blood cells, can be found in the urine of most affected children, although there is seldom gross hematuria. Specific gravity is high and proportionate to the amount of protein concentration. If hypovolemia is not significant and the child is well hydrated, the glomerular filtration rate is usually normal.

Total serum protein concentrations are reduced, with the albumin fractions significantly reduced (<2 g/dl) and plasma lipids elevated. Serum cholesterol may be as high as 450 to 1500 mg/dl. Hemoglobin and hematocrit are usually normal or elevated, and the platelet count is high (500,000 to 1,000,000/mm³) as a result of hemoconcentration. Serum sodium concentration is usually low, approximately 130 to 135 mEq/L.

If renal biopsy is performed, it provides information regarding the glomerular status and type of nephrotic syndrome, the likely response to drugs, and the probable course of the disease. Under the microscope the foot processes of the basement membrane appear fused. The major focuses in differential diagnosis are to establish the edema as renal in origin and to distinguish MCNS from other glomerulopathies with nephrotic syndrome as a manifestation.

Therapeutic Management

Medical management consists of both general and specific measures. The primary objective is to reduce the excretion of urinary protein and maintain protein-free urine. Additional objectives include prevention or treatment of acute infection, control of edema, establishment of good nutrition, and readjustment of any disturbed metabolic processes. Children with severe symptoms may be hospitalized for assessment and observation for evidence of infection, response to therapy, and parental education.

General Measures

General treatment is principally supportive. During the edema phase the child is often limited to quiet activities, but activity is not restricted during remission. Children can be remarkably active; there is no evidence that restriction affects the ultimate outcome. Acute and intercurrent infections are treated with appropriate antibiotics, and providers make efforts to minimize the risk of infection.

Diet

The child in remission maintains a regular diet. However, salt is restricted during periods of massive edema and while on corticosteroid therapy; no salt is added at the table, and foods with very high salt content are excluded. The child tolerates this diet for a time, but it should be adjusted to the child's appetite and must not interfere with nutrient intake. Although a low-sodium diet will not remove edema, its rate of increase may be reduced. Water is seldom restricted. A diet generous in protein is logical, but there is no evidence that it is beneficial or alters the outcome of the disease. The presence of azotemia and renal failure is a contraindication for high-protein intake.

Corticosteroid Therapy

The response of most affected children to corticosteroids has established these drugs as prime therapeutic agents in the management of nephrotic syndrome (Kim, Bellew, Silverstein, et al, 2005). Corticosteroid therapy begins as soon as the diagnosis has been determined and is administered orally in a dosage of 60 mg/m²/day in evenly divided doses. Prednisone, the safest and least expensive drug, is the steroid of choice. The drug is continued daily for 6 weeks, then reduced to 40 mg/m² on alternate days for 6 more weeks. Studies suggest that the duration of steroid treatment for the initial episode should be at least 3 months (Hodson, Knight, Willis, et al, 2004).

The course of the disease is fairly predictable. There is little change during the first few days of therapy. In most patients diuresis occurs as the urinary protein excretion diminishes within 7 to 21 days after the initiation of steroid therapy. Other clinical manifestations stabilize or return to normal shortly thereafter. Almost 95% of patients between 1 and 10 years of age who have satisfactory laboratory measurements of C3 complement and a renal clearance of immunoglobulin G, as well as no hypertension, hematuria, or renal insufficiency, will have complete resolution of proteinuria with therapy. If the child has not responded to therapy within 28 days of daily steroid administration, the likelihood of subsequent response diminishes rapidly.

Children with MCNS are often described according to their response to corticosteroid therapy (Box 30-4). Children with MCNS typically relapse one to three times per year. Steroid-dependent children tend to have frequent relapses over many years and receive large amounts of steroids, which results in cushingoid features and may cause growth retardation. They also require supportive treatment (diuretics, diet). Steroid-resistant children are thought to have a high risk of developing chronic renal failure (CRF) (Kim, Bellew, Silverstein, et al, 2005).

⚡ DRUG ALERT

Steroids

Children who require frequent courses of steroid therapy are highly susceptible to complications of steroids, such as growth retardation, behavior changes, cataracts, increased appetite, obesity, hypertension, gastrointestinal bleeding, bone demineralization, infections, and hyperglycemia. Children who do not respond to steroid therapy, those who have frequent relapses, and those in whom the side effects threaten their growth and general health may be considered for a course of therapy using other immunosuppressant medications.

Immunosuppressant Therapy

It is possible to reduce the relapse rate and induce long-term remission in children with frequent relapsing or steroid-resistant nephrotic syndrome with administration of an oral alkylating agent, usually cyclophosphamide (Cytoxan) or chlorambucil. Prolonged courses of cyclosporin and levamisole reduce the risk of relapse in children compared with corticosteroids alone (Durkan, Hodson, Willis, et al, 2005). The drugs share many characteristics, and the response to oral alkylating agents appears to depend on dose, duration of therapy, age, and duration of the disease.

The nurse must consider significant side effects of cyclophosphamide and discuss them with parents of children for whom this drug is contemplated. Anticipate leukopenia, and

remember that cyclophosphamide may cause azoospermia with potential sterility in males treated for more than 2 to 3 months and may cause variable effects on gonadal function in females.

Diuretics

One characteristic of the edema of nephrotic syndrome is its usual lack of responsiveness to diuretic agents. However, loop diuretics, usually furosemide in combination with metolazone, are sometimes useful in cases in which edema interferes with respiration or there is hypotension, hyponatremia, or skin breakdown. In addition, plasma expanders such as salt-poor human albumin may be administered to severely edematous children requiring prompt control; however, they must be administered frequently because the glomeruli are readily permeable to albumin in the acute stage.

Prognosis

The prognosis for ultimate recovery in most cases is good. MCNS is a self-limiting disease, and in children who respond to steroid therapy the tendency to relapse decreases with time. With early detection and prompt implementation of therapy to eradicate proteinuria, progressive basement membrane damage is minimized so that renal function is usually normal or near normal when the tendency for relapses is past. It is estimated that approximately 80% of affected children have this favorable prognosis, although half the children have relapses even after 5 years, and 20% after 10 years (Bagga and Mantan, 2005).

QUALITY PATIENT OUTCOMES: Nephrotic Syndrome
- Protein-free urine
- Acute infections prevented
- Edema absent or minimal
- Nutrition maintained
- Metabolic abnormalities controlled

Nursing Care Management

Daily monitoring of intake and output is an important nursing function. Strict and accurate measurement is essential but may be difficult in very young children. In these cases the nurse can measure for output by methods such as weighing diapers. Other methods of monitoring progress include examination of the urine for albumin, daily weight, and measurement of abdominal girth. Assessment of edema such as increased or decreased swelling around the eyes and dependent areas, the degree of pitting (if noted), and the color and texture of the skin are part of nursing care. The nurse monitors vital signs to detect any early signs of complications such as shock or an infectious process.

In children hospitalized with MCNS, elevating edematous parts may be helpful to shift fluid to more comfortable distributions, but diuresis with medications and salt and water restriction to remove edema fluid are the best therapy. Areas that are particularly edematous, such as the scrotum, abdomen, and legs, may require support. Clean skin surfaces and separate them with clothing, cotton, or antiseptic powder to prevent intertrigo.

Because these children are particularly vulnerable to upper respiratory tract infection, protect them from contact with infected roommates, family, or visitors. Spontaneous peritonitis can occur secondary to migration of intestinal bacteria across the bowel wall and into the peritoneum. Monitor vital signs to detect any early signs of an infectious process.

Loss of appetite that accompanies active nephrosis creates a perplexing problem for nurses. During this time the combined efforts of the nurse, dietitian, parents, and child are necessary to formulate a nutritionally adequate and attractive diet. Salt and fluids are restricted during the edema phase. Make every effort to serve attractive meals with a minimum of fuss, but it usually requires a little creativity to get the child to eat. Games, rewards, and special treats often help, but each child is unique; trial and error may be necessary to arrive at a successful strategy. Also, the same strategy may not work consistently. (See Feeding the Sick Child, Chapter 27.)

As the edema subsides, children are allowed increased fluids. Suitable recreational and diversional activities are also an important part of their care. Once the edema fluid has been lost, children resume their usual activities without problems. Irritability and mood swings accompanying the disease process and steroid therapy are not unusual manifestations in these children and create an additional challenge to the nurse and the family.

Family Support and Home Care

Most children are treated at home during relapses. Teach parents to detect signs of relapse and to notify the health care provider if they occur. Home care is preferred unless the edema and proteinuria are severe. Instruct parents in urine testing for albumin, administration of medications, and general care. Urine is usually tested daily while the child is receiving medicine for nephrotic syndrome or if the child has an illness, and twice a week during remission. Salt is restricted to no additional salt during relapse and steroid therapy, but a regular diet is suitable for the child in remission. Instruct parents regarding avoiding contact with infected playmates, but the child is permitted to attend school. It is important for parents of children on corticosteroid therapy to be aware of the common side effects of steroid therapy (e.g., rounding of the face, increased appetite, behavior changes, abdominal distention, and hirsutism) and to distinguish some of these from the edema formation of the disease. Reassure parents that the symptoms will disappear gradually after discontinuation of the drug. The child should receive close medical or nursing observation to detect unusual but more serious side effects (see Critical Thinking Exercise).

The prolonged course of the relapsing form of nephrotic syndrome is taxing to both the child and the family. In the worst cases of frequent remissions and exacerbations with periodic disruption of family life by hospitalization, a severe strain is placed on the child and the family, both psychologically and financially. Parents of children with frequent relapses poorly responsive to medications need reassurance regarding this characteristic of the disease so they do not become discouraged. At the same time, impress on them the importance of long-term care to gain their cooperation. A satisfactory response is more likely when relapses are detected and therapy is instituted early, and remissions are prolonged when instructions are carried out faithfully. For example, one child had an exacerbation when his

mother reduced the dosage of his drug because it was so expensive.

Social isolation is a problem for these children. Isolation is related to frequent hospitalization or confinement during relapse, the risk of infection that may precipitate an exacerbation, lack of energy, and the child's reluctance to face friends at home or school because of the changes in appearance resulting from the disease or the medication. Both parents and child need someone to listen to their complaints, to assist them in coping with both short- and long-term problems associated with the disease, and to find solutions to their problems. Continuous support of the child and family is one of the major nursing considerations.

▌ RENAL TUBULAR DISORDERS

Disorders of renal tubular function include a variety of conditions involving one or more abnormalities in specific mechanisms of tubular transport or reabsorption, although initially glomerular function is normal or comparatively less impaired (Roth and Chan, 2001). Eventually more widespread kidney destruction with renal failure may occur. In some cases the dysfunction has little, if any, effect on renal function. These disorders may be permanent or transient and may originate as primary defects or arise as a secondary effect of metabolic disease or exogenous toxins. Renal tubular disorders may be congenital (usually displaying characteristic patterns of genetic transmission), appear without evidence of hereditary transmission, or be acquired as a result of known or unknown causes.

? CRITICAL THINKING EXERCISE

Nephrotic Syndrome

Reese is an 8-year-old boy with relapsing nephrotic syndrome who has become steroid dependent. During your initial assessment in the outpatient clinic you identify the following: (1) weight has increased 2 kg (4.4 lb) in the past 2 weeks; (2) blood pressure is 100/70 mm Hg; (3) mother reports that Reese is not urinating very much, and she does not know how much he has been drinking; (4) while you are measuring Reese's abdominal girth, he guards his abdomen and complains of stomachache; and (5) his temperature is 38° C (100.4° F) orally. You should first do which of the following correct actions?

1. Examine Reese's abdomen while eliciting a thorough history of illness symptoms for the past 24 hours from his mother.
2. Elicit a 24-hour recall of food and fluid intake from Reese and his mother together.
3. Obtain a clean-catch urine specimen. Divide the specimen so that you can perform a dipstick analysis immediately and retain the rest of the specimen for possible urinalysis and culture after consultation with the primary health practitioner.
4. Explore the mother's understanding of Reese's illness and its relationship to his current condition to begin outlining your teaching plan for this family.

Questions

1. Evidence—Are there sufficient data to support your answer?
2. Assumptions—Describe some underlying assumptions about the following:
   a. Peritonitis in children with nephrotic syndrome
   b. Infection in a child on corticosteroid therapy
3. What are the priorities for discharge planning at this time?
4. Does the evidence support your conclusion?

Unlike the classic manifestations of glomerular diseases, edema and hypertension are absent and the BUN level and routine urinalysis are usually normal. Tubular proteinuria may be demonstrated. Manifestations of tubular disorders are primarily metabolic disturbances or deficiencies, such as failure to thrive, metabolic bone disease, or persistent acidosis. The variety of these disorders is extensive, and the incidence is rare.

TUBULAR FUNCTION

The function of the proximal tubules is the reabsorption of substances from the glomerular filtrate, including sodium, potassium, chloride, bicarbonate, glucose, phosphate, and amino acids (Roth and Chan, 2001). A number of disorders feature impairment of reabsorption of one or more filtrate constituents, and most involve defects in the transport mechanisms for these substances. Impaired tubular reabsorption of any specific substance causes that substance to appear in the urine, sometimes with reduced levels in the blood. Examples include bicarbonate and phosphate.

The primary functions of the distal renal tubules are acidification of urine; potassium secretion; and selective and differential reabsorption of sodium, chloride, and water, which determines the final urinary concentration. Because the contribution of the distal tubule to urine composition depends in part on the volume and composition of the filtrate from the proximal tubule, the net contribution of the distal tubule is related to proximal tubular function and glomerular filtration.

RENAL TUBULAR ACIDOSIS

Renal tubular acidosis is a syndrome of sustained metabolic acidosis in which there is impaired reabsorption of bicarbonate or excretion of net hydrogen ion but in which glomerular function is normal or comparatively less impaired. On the basis of underlying pathophysiology, renal tubular acidosis is divided into proximal renal tubular acidosis and distal renal tubular acidosis. Proximal renal tubular acidosis results from a defect in bicarbonate reabsorption, whereas distal renal tubular acidosis results from inability to establish an adequate gradient of pH between blood and tubular fluid.

Proximal Tubular Acidosis (Type II)

Impaired bicarbonate reabsorption in the proximal tubule causes proximal tubular acidosis. It may occur as an isolated defect (primary); however, more often it appears in association with other proximal tubular disorders (secondary). As a result of a depressed renal threshold, bicarbonate reabsorption in the proximal tubule is incomplete, causing the plasma concentration of bicarbonate to stabilize at a lower level than normal. This results in a hyperchloremic metabolic acidosis. There is no impairment of distal tubular integrity or, in most cases, of the distal acidifying mechanism.

A more complex abnormality in the proximal tubules is Fanconi syndrome, in which transport mechanisms are damaged by the accumulation of toxic metabolites or the tubular epithelium is damaged by heavy metals such as lead, cadmium, or platinum. Fanconi syndrome can be part of a number of hereditary diseases, be acquired, or be idiopathic

(with a cause that is not identifiable). The major clinical manifestation and presenting symptom of Fanconi syndrome is growth failure. Tachypnea from hyperchloremic metabolic acidosis is also evident. Dehydration, vomiting, episodic fever, nephrolithiasis secondary to hypercalciuria, muscle weakness or paralysis as a result of hypokalemia, and episodes of severe life-threatening acidemia (sometimes triggered by a concurrent infection) may also be seen. Complications are rare. The disorder appears to be transient and resolves spontaneously in time.

Distal Tubular Acidosis (Type I)

Distal tubular acidosis is caused by the kidney's inability to establish a normal pH gradient between tubular cells and tubular contents. Its most characteristic feature is the inability to produce a urinary pH below 6.0 despite the presence of severe metabolic acidosis (Watanabe, 2005).

Distal renal tubular acidosis may occur as a primary, isolated defect or in association with other diseases or disorders. Most secondary causes are rare. The primary disorder is usually considered to be a hereditary defect with a variable degree of expression and a greater penetrance in females. After the age of 2 years the child usually has growth failure, often with a history of vomiting, polyuria, dehydration, anorexia, and failure to thrive. Evidence of bone demineralization may be present, along with the occasional formation of urinary calculi (urolithiasis) in older children.

The inability to secrete hydrogen ions causes an accumulation of the ions in the body, which soon depletes the available hydrogen buffer and produces a sustained acidosis. Acidosis slows normal somatic growth, and demineralization of bone occurs as bone salts are mobilized to buffer the excessive hydrogen ions. Increased serum levels of both calcium and phosphorus contribute to the development of stones within the renal system. Both sodium and potassium are secreted in larger amounts. Serum potassium levels are depleted as the distal tubules excrete large amounts of potassium ions in an attempt to conserve sodium because hydrogen ions are unable to participate in the exchange. Hyponatremia stimulates increased aldosterone secretion, which further aggravates the hypokalemia. With the depletion of bicarbonate ions, more chloride is reabsorbed in the proximal tubule to create a hyperchloremia.

Prognosis

The primary disorder is usually permanent. However, secondary effects on growth and stone formation can be avoided with early diagnosis and therapy. When the disorder occurs as a secondary complication and renal damage is prevented, the prognosis is good.

Therapeutic Management

Treatment of both proximal and distal disorders consists of the administration of sufficient bicarbonate or citrate to balance metabolically produced hydrogen ions; to maintain the plasma bicarbonate level within normal range; and to correct associated electrolyte disorders, especially hypokalemia. Proximal disorders require large volumes of bicarbonate to compensate for urinary losses; in distal disorders the alkali required to maintain a normal plasma concentration is low. Most authorities favor a mixture of sodium and potassium bicarbonate (or citrate) to prevent deficiencies of either cation. The citrate solutions (Bicitra, Polycitra, or Shohl solution) are usually more easily tolerated than bicarbonate solutions. Shohl solution is effective but has the disadvantage of requiring preparation by a pharmacist.

Nursing Care Management

Nursing goals include recognizing the possibility of renal tubular acidosis in children who fail to thrive or who display other symptoms suggestive of the disorders and referring these children for medical evaluation. Helping parents understand the importance of adhering to the medication plan as a long-term goal is essential. (See Compliance and Administration of Medication, Chapter 27.) Children who must continue the medication indefinitely need to learn the importance of taking the medications as soon as they are old enough to assume responsibility for their own care.

NEPHROGENIC DIABETES INSIPIDUS

Nephrogenic diabetes insipidus (NDI) is the major disorder associated with a defect in the ability to concentrate urine. In this disorder the distal tubules and collecting ducts are insensitive to the action of antidiuretic hormone or its exogenous counterpart, vasopressin. Although several inheritance patterns have been identified, more than 90% of patients have an X-linked defect of the vasopressin receptor (Knoers and Monnens, 2004). The disease is more variable in female carriers of the defective gene, who may exhibit only a mild defect in urine-concentrating ability. The differential diagnosis for NDI should include chronic obstructive renal disorders, sickle cell disease, renal tuberculosis, and other renal disorders that may cause high urinary output with failure of the kidney to respond to vasopressin.

Clinical Manifestations and Diagnostic Evaluation

NDI is manifested in the newborn period by vomiting, unexplained fever, failure to thrive, and severe recurrent dehydration with hypernatremia. The passage of copious amounts of dilute urine, which produces severe dehydration and hypoelectrolytemia, is a serious threat to life during this period and may be responsible for the high incidence of cognitive impairment and motor retardation found in affected persons. Growth retardation is probably related to diminished food intake and poor general health because of uncontrolled polydipsia. Diagnosis is suspected on the basis of the patient and family history and confirmed by a urine osmolality value consistently below that of plasma. Lack of response to vasopressin administration rules out other causes.

Therapeutic Management

Therapy involves provision of adequate volumes of water to compensate for urinary losses and minimize urine output through diet and medication (Dell and Avner, 2007). As a result of an insatiable thirst, most of the child's time is spent drinking and voiding, with little time for activity and stimulation. These children may go to great lengths to satisfy their thirst. A low-sodium, low-solute diet and the use of chlorothiazide or ethacrynic acid diuretics to increase the reabsorption of sodium and

water in the proximal tubule help to reduce the amount of tubular fluid delivered to the distal tubules and to diminish the volume of water excreted. Urinary output may be reduced when nonsteroidal antiinflammatory drugs (NSAIDs) are administered in conjunction with chlorothiazide. Supplemental potassium may be required to prevent hypokalemia as a result of thiazide therapy. Normal growth and a normal life span are possible if the disease is recognized early and treatment is instituted and maintained.

Nursing Care Management

Nursing goals for children with NDI and their families are to recognize signs of the disorder early and assist them in coping with the long-term inconvenience of the continual thirst and elimination problems. Families need to learn to administer medications and help with diet planning for those on sodium restriction and needing supplemental potassium. The problem of ensuring adequate hydration is lifelong, and families need to adapt to away-from-home fluid needs and avoid activities that contribute to dehydration when fluids may not be available. Genetic counseling is recommended.

MISCELLANEOUS RENAL DISORDERS

HEMOLYTIC UREMIC SYNDROME

Hemolytic uremic syndrome (HUS) is an acute renal disease characterized by a triad of manifestations: ARF, hemolytic anemia, and thrombocytopenia (Caprioli, Peng, and Remuzzi, 2005). HUS occurs primarily in infants and small children between the ages of 6 months and 3 years. It has been recognized predominantly in Caucasians and, although it occurs worldwide, is more prevalent in South Africa, Argentina, and the west coasts of North and South America. HUS represents one of the main causes of ARF in early childhood (Kliegman, Behrman, Jenson, et al, 2007).

Etiology

In the majority of cases of HUS no causative agents have been identified, although recent theories implicate genetic factors, prostacyclin deficiency, neuraminidase and agglutination, endotoxins (especially *Shigella* endotoxin), antithrombin III deficiency, deficiency of antioxidants, and reduced platelet aggregation. The appearance of the disease has been associated with *Rickettsia* organisms; viruses such as coxsackievirus, echovirus, and adenovirus; *E. coli*; pneumococci; *Shigella* organisms; and *Salmonella* organisms and may represent an unusual response to these infections. HUS caused by enteric infection of the *E. coli* O157:H7 serotype is the most prevalent pathogen in the United States and Europe, with about 70,000 cases and 60 deaths occurring annually (Bell, Griffin, Lozano, et al, 1997; Caprioli, Peng, and Remuzzi, 2005). Occurrences have been traced to undercooked meat, especially ground beef; unpasteurized apple juice; alfalfa sprouts; and public pools.

The disease usually follows an acute gastrointestinal or upper respiratory tract infection and tends to occur in scattered outbreaks in small geographic areas. HUS is clinically and pathologically similar to thrombocytopenic purpura, except for the hypertension associated with HUS.

Pathophysiology

The primary site of injury appears to be the endothelial lining of the small glomerular arterioles, but other organs and tissues may be involved (e.g., the liver, brain, heart, pancreatic islet cells, and muscles). The endothelium becomes swollen and occluded with the deposition of platelets and fibrin clots (intravascular coagulation). Red blood cells are damaged as they move through the partially occluded blood vessels. The spleen removes these fragmented red blood cells, causing acute hemolytic anemia. Fibrinolytic action on the precipitated fibrin causes these fibrin-split products to appear in the serum and urine. The characteristic thrombocytopenia is produced by the platelet aggregation within damaged blood vessels or the damage and removal of platelets.

Clinical Manifestations

The disease occurs after a prodromal period during which there is an episode of diarrhea and vomiting. Less often the preceding illness is an upper respiratory tract infection or, occasionally, varicella, measles, or a UTI.

The hemolytic process persists for several days to 2 weeks. During this time the child is anorexic, irritable, and lethargic. There is marked and rapid onset of pallor accompanied by hemorrhagic manifestations such as bruising, purpura, or rectal bleeding. Severely affected patients are anuric and often hypertensive. Seizures and stupor suggest central nervous system involvement, and there may be signs of acute heart failure. Mild cases demonstrate anemia, thrombocytopenia, and azotemia; urinary output may be reduced or increased.

Diagnostic Evaluation

The triad of anemia, thrombocytopenia, and renal failure is sufficient for diagnosis. Proteinuria, hematuria, and urinary casts are evidence of renal involvement; BUN and serum creatinine levels are elevated. A low hemoglobin and hematocrit and a high reticulocyte count confirm the hemolytic nature of the anemia.

Therapeutic Management

In general, providers direct treatment toward control of the complications and hematologic manifestations of renal failure (Siegler and Oakes, 2005). The initial supportive measures for most children are those used in managing renal failure: fluid replacement (calculated with great care), treatment of hypertension, and correction of acidosis and electrolyte disorders (Siegler and Oakes, 2005). The most consistently effective treatment is early hemodialysis, PD, or continuous hemofiltration, which is instituted in any child who has been anuric for 24 hours or who demonstrates oliguria with uremia or hypertension and seizures. Blood transfusions with fresh, washed packed cells are administered for severe anemia but are used with caution to prevent circulatory overload from added volume.

Once vomiting and diarrhea have resolved, the child is restarted on enteral nutrition. Sometimes parenteral nutrition is required for children with severe, persistent colitis and for those in whom tissue catabolism is marked. There is no substantial evidence that heparin, corticosteroids, or fibrinolytic agents are beneficial, and in some instances they may aggravate the condition. The usefulness of plasma infusion for treatment of HUS is currently being studied; it may be useful in selected cases.

Prognosis

With prompt treatment the recovery rate is approximately 95%, but residual renal impairment ranges from 10% to 50%. Death is usually caused by residual renal impairment or central nervous system injury.

Nursing Care Management

Nursing care is the same as that provided in ARF and, for children with continued impairment, includes management of chronic disease. Because of the sudden and life-threatening nature of the disorder in a previously well child, parents are often ill prepared for the impact of hospitalization and treatment. Therefore support and understanding are especially important aspects of care.

> **! NURSING ALERT**
>
> To prevent infection from contaminated meat, the internal temperature of the food, such as hamburger, should be at least 74° C (165° F). Cooking the ground beef until no pink color is seen may not be sufficient to kill the bacteria. Therefore a meat thermometer is needed to ensure a safe product. Discourage parents from giving children unpasteurized apple juice and unwashed raw vegetables. Also discourage the use of antimotility drugs for diarrhea.

FAMILIAL NEPHRITIS (ALPORT SYNDROME)

The syndrome of chronic hereditary glomerulopathy consists of hematuria, high-frequency sensorineural deafness, ocular disorders, and CRF (Anker, Amemann, and Neumann, 2003). The disease appears to be inherited as an autosomal dominant trait, which suggests a possible X-linked dominant trait, although rare male-to-male transmission does occur. Alport syndrome is uncommon but not rare and accounts for a significant percentage of persistent glomerular disease in childhood.

The clinical manifestations are indistinguishable from those of mild acute nephritis. Initial symptoms include hematuria, proteinuria, malaise, and mild edema. Onset of gross hematuria may be associated with an acute respiratory tract infection. The average age of onset is 6 years, but the condition may be noted in infancy. It begins slowly and progresses until uncontrollable renal failure develops in adolescence or early adulthood. There is usually a positive family history. Most untreated boys develop severe symptoms, whereas affected girls generally have a milder disease and a normal life expectancy.

Treatment is symptomatic and supportive. Dialysis and kidney transplantation are ultimate therapeutic measures for ESRD. Hearing loss and ocular disorders should receive appropriate attention, and families should be counseled regarding the genetic implications of the disease.

UNEXPLAINED PROTEINURIA

Often apparently healthy children with no suggestion of renal disease demonstrate proteinuria on routine urinalysis. The percentage of children with unexplained proteinuria ranges from

1% at 6 years of age to 11% at puberty, reaching a maximum prevalence at age 13 in girls and age 16 in boys.

Unexplained proteinuria can be categorized as (1) transient (inconstant); (2) persistent; or (3) orthostatic, or postural. Transient proteinuria is a common finding with no known cause but sometimes increases with febrile illness, exercise, cold, or emotions. Persistent proteinuria usually signifies renal disease. Orthostatic proteinuria is seen in 3% to 5% of adolescents and young adults; although proteinuria is evident in both the recumbent and the erect position, it is quantitatively and qualitatively greater in the erect position. The cause is unknown, but minor glomerular changes occur in many instances. The condition is benign and generally resolves over time.

In cases of unexplained proteinuria, it is important to confirm or exclude renal disease with appropriate diagnostic tests. Repeated examination for proteinuria, an orthostatic test, urine culture, and (if proteinuria is persistent) more definitive tests—including 24-hour protein excretion, renal ultrasound, and renal scan—are indicated.

RENAL TRAUMA

Serious injuries of the genitourinary tract are not uncommon in the pediatric age-group, with a peak incidence between ages 10 and 20 years. Despite their relatively protected location, the kidneys are among the organs most often injured in children. However, the kidneys in children are more mobile than they are in adults, and the outer borders are less well protected. They are separated from the skin surface by only 2 to 3 cm (0.75 to 1.2 inches) in young children.

Most injuries are of the nonpenetrating or blunt type and usually involve falls, athletic injuries, and motor vehicle accidents. Cycling is the most common cause of sports-related kidney injury, causing more than three times more kidney injuries than football (Grinsell, Showalter, Gordon, et al, 2006). Penetrating trauma (e.g., gunshot or stab wound) is much less common in children. Many children have preexisting renal abnormalities, particularly congenital anomalies associated with mild to moderate hydronephrosis, that were unrecognized before the injury.

Suspect renal injury in children who complain of flank pain, and often have abrasions or contusions on the overlying skin. Hematuria is consistently present, but the amount of blood in the urine is not a reliable indicator of the seriousness of the injury. Many relatively insignificant injuries are associated with grossly bloody urine, whereas some of the most severe injuries are found in children with only microscopic hematuria (Box 30-5).

Renal rupture involves the actual splitting open of the kidney capsule, causing extravasation of blood or a mixture of blood and urine into the surrounding retroperitoneal space. Renal vascular injury, although unusual, requires immediate recognition and surgical intervention. Because the volume-per-minute blood flow through the kidney is greater (25% of cardiac output) than to any other abdominal organ, injury to the kidney may result in a rapid loss of blood.

Active children may or may not have a history of unusual trauma. Abdominal or flank pain and tenderness are caused by bleeding around the kidney and may or may not be associated

---

BOX 30-5   CLASSIFICATION OF RENAL INJURY

Grade I—Renal contusion or subcapsular hematoma; gross or microscopic hematuria
Grade II—Parenchymal laceration <1.0 cm deep; nonexpanding perirenal hematoma
Grade III—Parenchymal laceration >1.0 cm deep; no urinary extravasation
Grade IV—Laceration extending from parenchyma into collecting system and/or injury to main renal artery or vein
Grade V—Shattered kidney; thrombosis of main renal artery

Modified from Moore EE, Shackford SR, Pachter HL, et al: Organ injury scaling: spleen, liver, and kidney, *J Trauma* 29(12):1664-1666, 1989.

---

with fever. Clots passing down the ureter may cause pain similar to that of renal colic, and dysuria is common. Patients with more severe injuries may complain of nausea or abdominal pain. There may be a palpable abdominal mass caused by loss of blood or urine into the retroperitoneum. The fibrous capsule enclosing the kidney prevents expansion of a hematoma; therefore exsanguination and shock are seldom observed, even in severe renal trauma.

Diagnosis is made on the basis of intravenous pyelography, angiography, or retrograde pyelography. Unsuspected hydronephrosis often is first detected as a result of traumatic injury.

Therapeutic Management

Severe injury requires close observation in the hospital intensive care unit and blood replacement if there is severe internal or external bleeding. In most cases bleeding subsides spontaneously. Surgical exploration is indicated if there are multiple injuries, extravasation of blood around the kidneys, or disruption of the major vessels or the collecting system. Children with less severe injuries, such as contusions only, are placed on bed rest. They should remain on bed rest for 3 days after cessation of gross bleeding, since the substance released from injured renal tissue (urinary urokinase) has strongly fibrinolytic properties that may precipitate serious bleeding. The prognosis depends on the nature and extent of the injury.

Nursing Care Management

Nursing management is directed toward recognizing and assisting in the diagnosis of renal injury. Care of both the child and the family is primarily supportive. The nurse implements all the concepts related to emergency hospitalization and care. (See Chapter 26.) Postsurgical care, if indicated, is the same as for any other surgical patient. Recommendations for children with a solitary kidney participating in sports are varied. Each child should be individually assessed and advised on the need for protective equipment before engaging in contact, collision, or limited contact activities (Rice and Council on Sports Medicine and Fitness, 2008).

RENAL FAILURE

Renal failure is the inability of the kidneys to excrete waste material, concentrate urine, and conserve electrolytes. The disorder can be acute or chronic and affects most of the systems in the body. Two terms that are often used in relation to renal failure need some clarification: azotemia is the accumulation of nitrogenous waste within the blood, whereas uremia is a more advanced condition in which retention of nitrogenous products produces toxic symptoms. Azotemia is not life threatening, whereas uremia is a serious condition that often involves other body systems.

ACUTE RENAL FAILURE

ARF is said to exist when the kidneys suddenly are unable to appropriately regulate the volume and composition of urine in response to food and fluid intake and the needs of the organism. The principal feature is oligoanuria* associated with azotemia, acidosis, and diverse electrolyte disturbances. ARF is not common in childhood, but the outcome depends on the cause, associated findings, and prompt recognition and treatment.

Etiology

ARF can develop as a result of a large number of related or unrelated clinical conditions: poor renal perfusion; acute renal injury; or the final expression of chronic, irreversible renal disease. The most common cause in children is transient renal failure resulting from dehydration or other causes of poor perfusion that respond to restoration of fluid volume. Causes of ARF are usually classified as prerenal, intrinsic renal, and postrenal. Severe or longstanding prerenal or postrenal causes can produce severe secondary renal damage.

Prerenal Causes

Prerenal causes of ARF are most common in children and are always related to the reduction of renal perfusion in an anatomically and physiologically normal kidney and collecting system. Dehydration secondary to diarrheal disease or persistent vomiting is the most common cause of prerenal failure in infants and children. Surgical shock and trauma (including burns) are also common causes. Hypovolemia and decreased renal perfusion cause a decreased glomerular filtration rate and stimulate the secretion of renin, aldosterone, and antidiuretic hormone, which further diminish urine flow. Extended and severe hypoperfusion (secondary to procedures such as cardiac surgery) can produce cortical or tubular necrosis; however, when medical care is available, this is seldom allowed to occur. In general, the azotemia that accompanies this type of renal failure is rapidly reversible with prompt attention to expansion of the extracellular fluid volume. Prerenal failure is often difficult to distinguish from tubular or cortical necrosis. Renal artery stenosis, altered peripheral vascular resistance related to sepsis, and hepatorenal syndrome are less common causes.

Intrinsic Renal Causes

Intrinsic renal causes of ARF constitute the largest group that requires extended management. These include diseases and nephrotoxic agents that damage the glomeruli, tubules, or renal vasculature. Glomerular disease is the most common cause of glomerular damage, whereas tubular destruction is more often

caused by ischemia or nephrotoxins. Vascular damage is an uncommon cause of renal failure in childhood. The type and extent of damage determine the degree and duration of renal insufficiency, and it is difficult to predict in any given case whether acute necrosis will develop.

Postrenal Causes

ARF resulting from obstructive uropathy is uncommon in children except during the first year of life. Relief of the obstruction can restore renal function. The degree of recovery depends on the duration of the renal failure.

Pathophysiology

ARF is usually reversible, but the deviations of physiologic function can be extreme, and mortality in the pediatric age-group is still high. There is severe reduction in the glomerular filtration rate, an elevated BUN level, and decreased tubular reabsorption of sodium from the proximal tubule. Consequently, there is increased concentration of sodium in the distal tubule, which causes stimulation of the renin mechanism. The local action of angiotensin causes vasoconstriction of the afferent arteriole, which further reduces glomerular filtration and prevents urinary losses of sodium. There is a significant reduction in renal blood flow.

The pathologic conditions that produce ARF caused by glomerulonephritis, HUS, and other renal disorders are discussed in relation to those disease processes. The necrotic processes within the nephron can be cortical, tubular, or both.

Cortical Necrosis

Complete cortical necrosis usually results from severe ischemia, infection, or intravascular coagulation and represents a severe, irreversible cause of ARF. In the pediatric age-group this occurs as a fatal event, most commonly during the neonatal period as a result of hypoxia and shock. When cortical destruction is incomplete, some recovery of renal function may occur. Intravascular coagulation is believed to play a significant role as an intermediate factor in the development of ARF, especially in cases related to sepsis.

Tubular Necrosis

Damage to the renal tubules can be broadly classified as (1) secondary to renal ischemia and (2) associated with the ingestion or inhalation of substances toxic to the kidneys. Renal tubules are particularly vulnerable to a wide variety of toxic agents that produce vasoconstriction and to focal patches of ischemia that cause a uniform necrosis of the tubular epithelium down to, but not including, the basement membrane. A lesion produced by sustained reduction in renal blood flow also involves the basement membrane, which may become fragmented and ruptured to the extent that the continuity of tubular structure is disrupted. The lesions may affect any segment of the tubules, appearing at irregular intervals along with normal segments throughout the kidney.

Reepithelialization in the areas with intact basement membrane heals tubular lesions. Such healing is unable to take place in areas in which the basement membrane has been disrupted; connective tissue grows through the ruptured membrane, thus preventing reestablishment of tubular integrity. Individual cells

---

*The definition of oligoanuria varies extensively in the literature—from 1.8 to 4 dl/m²/24 hr.

within the nephron, but not the entire nephron, are capable of regeneration.

Clinical Course

The clinical course of the child with ARF is variable and depends on the cause. In reversible ARF there is a period of severe oliguria, or a low-output phase, followed by an abrupt onset of diuresis, or a high-output phase; this phase is followed by a gradual return to, or toward, normal urine volumes. The length of the oliguric phase in older children and adolescents is 10 to 14 days but is highly variable at all ages. It tends to be shorter (3 to 5 days) in infants, children, and milder cases. The onset of the diuretic phase appears unexpectedly, and over several days it proceeds in stepwise fashion from very low to above-normal urine volumes. During the oliguric phase, manifestations of uremia are present but may also be accompanied by other clinical disorders that make assessment difficult, such as infection, anoxia, and shock.

Clinical Manifestations

In many instances of ARF the infant or child is already critically ill with the precipitating disorder, and the explanation for development of oliguria may or may not be readily apparent. The underlying illness often overshadows the renal failure and often assumes the priority of care (e.g., the patient who is in shock from endotoxemia, the infant who is severely dehydrated from gastroenteritis, or a child who is subject to seizures as a result of hypertensive encephalopathy associated with AGN).

The prime manifestation of ARF is oliguria, generally a urinary output of less than 1 ml/kg/hr. Anuria (no urinary output in 24 hours) is uncommon except in obstructive disorders. Other symptoms related to ARF include edema, drowsiness, circulatory congestion, and cardiac arrhythmia from hyperkalemia. Seizures may be caused by hyponatremia or hypocalcemia and tachypnea from metabolic acidosis. With continued oliguria, biochemical abnormalities can develop rapidly, and circulatory and central nervous system manifestations appear.

Diagnostic Evaluation

When a previously well child develops ARF without obvious cause, a careful history is obtained to reveal symptoms that may be related to glomerulonephritis; obstructive uropathy; or exposure to nephrotoxic chemicals, such as ingestion of heavy metals or inhalation of carbon tetrachloride or other organic solvents or drugs (e.g., methicillin, sulfonamides, NSAIDs, neomycin, polymyxin, and kanamycin). Laboratory data reflect the kidney dysfunction—hyperkalemia, hyponatremia, metabolic acidosis, hypocalcemia, anemia, or azotemia (Table 30-7).

Therapeutic Management

The most effective management of ARF is prevention. The development of ARF is a known risk in certain situations. This should be anticipated and recognized, and adequate therapy should be implemented (e.g., fluid therapy for children with hypovolemia in conditions such as dehydration, burns, and hemorrhage). Nephrotoxic drugs should be used with caution or avoided in children with renal disease, and all personnel should be knowledgeable about precautions related to their

TABLE 30-7	LABORATORY FINDINGS ASSOCIATED WITH ACUTE RENAL FAILURE	
CLINICAL PROBLEM	**MECHANISM**	**CLINICAL CONSIDERATIONS**
Azotemia	Ongoing protein catabolism	Lower rate of production in neonates and persons with depleted protein stores
Elevated blood urea nitrogen levels	Significantly decreased excretion	Increased in situations involving large amounts of necrotic tissue or extravasated blood
Elevated plasma creatinine levels	Continued production Significantly decreased excretion	Production less affected by other factors
		More sensitive measure of intensity of azotemia
		Low in neonate because of small muscle mass relative to size
Metabolic acidosis	Continued endogenous acid production Significantly decreased excretion Depletion of extracellular and intracellular fluid buffers	Compensatory hyperventilation Opisthonos Major threat to life
Hyponatremia	Dilution of extracellular fluid Decreased excretion of water	May develop cerebral signs
Hyperkalemia	Ongoing protein catabolism Decreased excretion compounded by metabolic acidosis	Most important electrolyte to be considered in acute renal failure
		May contribute to cardiac arrhythmia
		With electrocardiogram changes, major threat to life
		Loss may be from gastrointestinal tract
Hypocalcemia	Associated with metabolic acidosis and hyperphosphatemia	During alkali therapy, may cause tetany

administration. For example, a generous fluid intake is needed for children receiving antimetabolite drugs and after radiotherapy.

The treatment of ARF is directed toward (1) treatment of the underlying cause, (2) management of the complications of renal failure, and (3) provision of supportive therapy within the constraints imposed by the renal failure. Treatment of poor perfusion resulting from dehydration consists of volume restoration as described in the treatment of dehydration. (See Chapter 28.) If oliguria persists after restoration of fluid volume or if the renal failure is caused by intrinsic renal damage, the physiologic and biochemical abnormalities that have resulted from kidney dysfunction must be corrected or controlled. Central venous pressure monitoring is usually implemented.

Initially a Foley catheter is inserted to rule out urine retention, to collect available urine for electrolytes and analysis, and to monitor the results of diuretic administration. The catheter may or may not be removed. Some clinicians believe that it serves little purpose during the oliguric phase and predisposes the patient to bladder infection prefer collection bags for measuring urinary output. Others maintain a catheter for hourly urine measurements.

Oliguria

When a child has persistent oliguria in the presence of adequate hydration and no lower tract obstruction, mannitol, furosemide, or both may be administered rapidly as a test to provoke a flow of urine. When glomerular function is intact, the administration of these substances will behave as nonreabsorbable solute in the tubular fluid to evoke an osmotic diuresis. The presence of mannitol in tubular fluid and the obligatory water that follows it also serve to dilute the concentration of any nephrotoxin that may be present in the tubules to below toxic levels. The furosemide blocks reabsorption of tubular filtrate. If urine flow is generated to the extent of 6 to 10 ml/kg of body weight in 1 to 3 hours, the initial dosage is reduced and continued, if needed, to sustain the flow. If no urine is produced within 2 hours after the single dose, the drugs are not repeated, and an oliguric regimen is instituted to control water balance and other abnormalities.

Fluid and Calories

The amount of exogenous water provided should not exceed the amount needed to maintain zero water balance. It is calculated on the basis of estimated endogenous water formation and losses from sensible (primarily gastrointestinal) and insensible sources. No allotment is calculated for urine as long as oliguria persists.

The child with ARF has a tendency to develop water intoxication and hyponatremia, both of which make it difficult to provide calories in sufficient amounts to meet the child's needs and reduce tissue catabolism, metabolic acidosis, hyperkalemia, and uremia. If the child is able to tolerate oral foods, concentrated food sources high in carbohydrates and fat but low in protein, potassium, and sodium may be provided. However, many children have functional disturbances of the gastrointestinal tract, such as nausea and vomiting. Therefore the IV route is generally preferred, and nourishment usually consists of essential amino acids or a combination of essential and nonessential amino acids administered by the central venous route.

Control of water balance in these patients requires careful monitoring of feedback information, such as accurate intake and output, body weight, and electrolyte measurements. In general, during the oliguric phase, no sodium, chloride, or potassium is given unless there are other large, ongoing losses. Regular measurement of plasma electrolytes, pH, BUN, and creatinine levels is required to assess the adequacy of fluid therapy and to anticipate complications that require specific treatment.

Hyperkalemia

An elevated serum potassium level is the most immediate threat to the life of the child with ARF. Potassium ions are not being excreted, while at the same time the release of potassium from cells is accelerated by acidosis, stress, and tissue breakdown in cases associated with internal bleeding or trauma. Because cardiac arrhythmia and cardiac arrest may result, electrocardio-

grams (ECGs) and serum potassium ion levels are monitored regularly. Hyperkalemia can be minimized and sometimes avoided by eliminating potassium from all food and fluids, by reducing tissue catabolism, and by correcting acidosis.

> **! NURSING ALERT**
>
> Any of the following signs of hyperkalemia constitute an emergency and should be reported immediately:
> - Serum potassium concentrations in excess of 7 mEq/L
> - Presence of ECG abnormalities, such as loss of P wave, prolonged RS complex, depressed ST segment, tall and tented T waves, bradycardia, or heart block

Several measures are available to reduce the serum potassium concentration, and the priority of implementation is usually based on the rapidity with which the measures are effective. Temporary measures that produce a rapid but transient effect as follows:

- Calcium gluconate, 0.5 ml/kg, administered intravenously over 2 to 4 minutes with continuous ECG monitoring, exerts a protective effect on cardiac conduction.
- Sodium bicarbonate, 2 to 3 mEq/kg, administered intravenously over 30 to 60 minutes, elevates the serum pH to cause a transient shift of extracellular fluid potassium into the intracellular fluid. However, there is risk of hypocalcemia, tetany, and fluid overload.
- Glucose, 50%, and insulin, 1 unit/kg, administered intravenously, accelerate glycogen synthesis, causing glucose and potassium to move into the cells. Insulin facilitates the entry of glucose into cells.

These effects produce only transient protection by redistributing existing potassium stores; they do not remove potassium from the body. However, they provide relief while more definitive but slower-acting measures are being implemented. Potassium can be removed by either of two methods:

1. Administration of a cation exchange resin such as sodium polystyrene sulfonate (Kayexalate), 1 g/kg, administered orally or rectally, to bind potassium and remove it from the body. This requires time to be effective, and a sodium ion is exchanged for each potassium ion. This increased sodium concentration adds to the body fluids, which may contribute to fluid overload, hypertension, and cardiac failure.
2. Dialysis or continuous hemofiltration (see p. 1176). Hemodialysis is efficient but requires specialized facilities. PD is simpler and can be carried out in almost any hospital setting. Indications for dialysis in ARF are continued oliguria associated with any of the following:
   - Severe, persistent acidosis
   - Inability to reduce serum potassium levels to a safe range with other methods
   - Clinical uremic syndrome consisting of nausea and vomiting, drowsiness, and progression to coma
   - Circulatory overload, hypertension, and evidence of cardiac failure

A popular philosophy is to institute renal replacement therapy (see p. 1172) after 24 to 48 hours of oliguria, regardless of other symptoms. Supporters of this approach believe that early intervention is associated with reduced morbidity and mortality and permits improved nutrition with relaxed diet restrictions. The combination of renal replacement therapy and nutrition tends to reduce the complications of ARF.

Hypertension

Hypertension is a common and serious complication of ARF, and blood pressure determinations are taken every 4 to 6 hours to detect it early. The most common cause of hypertension in ARF is overexpansion of the extracellular fluid and plasma volume together with activation of the renin-angiotensin system. The goal of therapy is to prevent hypertensive encephalopathy and avoid overtaxing the cardiovascular system.

When there is a threat of encephalopathy, labetalol (a beta and alpha blocker) may be administered intravenously as bolus infusions or a continuous drip. Sodium nitroprusside may be given but requires close monitoring. For less urgent situations, hydralazine, clonidine, or verapamil may be given intravenously. Oral drugs used for acute hypertension include nifedipine, captopril, minoxidil, hydralazine, propranolol, or furosemide.

Other Complications

Other complications that may occur with ARF are anemia, seizures and coma, cardiac failure, and pulmonary edema. Anemia is commonly associated with ARF, but transfusion is not recommended unless the hemoglobin level drops below 6 g/dl. Transfusions consist of fresh, packed red blood cells given slowly to reduce the likelihood of increasing blood volume, hypertension, and hyperkalemia.

Seizures occur often when renal failure progresses to uremia and are also related to hypertension, hyponatremia, and hypocalcemia. Treatment is directed toward the specific cause when known. More obscure causes are managed with antiepileptic drugs.

Cardiac failure with pulmonary edema is almost always associated with hypervolemia. Treatment is directed toward reduction of fluid volume, with water and sodium restriction and administration of diuretics. Digitalis is ineffective and can be hazardous.

Diuretic, or High-Output, Phase

When the output begins to increase, either spontaneously or in response to diuretic therapy, monitor the intake of fluid, potassium, and sodium, and provide adequate replacement to prevent depletion and its consequences. In some cases the high-output phase is mild and lasts only a few days; in others enormous amounts of electrolyte-rich urine are passed.

Prognosis

The prognosis of ARF depends largely on the nature and severity of the causative factor or precipitating event and the promptness and competence of management. The mortality rate is less than 20%. The outcome is least favorable in children with rapidly progressive nephritis and cortical necrosis. Children in whom ARF is a result of HUS or AGN may recover completely, but residual renal impairment or hypertension is more often the rule. Complete recovery is usually expected in children whose renal failure is a result of dehydration, nephrotoxins, or ischemia. ARF following cardiac surgery has a less favorable prognosis. It is often impossible to assess the extent of recovery for several months.

QUALITY PATIENT OUTCOMES: Acute Renal Failure
- Underlying cause of ARF identified and treated
- Water balance maintained
- Hypertension controlled
- Electrolyte balance maintained
- Diet maintains calories while minimizing tissue catabolism, metabolic acidosis, hyperkalemia, and uremia

---

Nursing Care Management

Nursing care of the infant or child with ARF involves addressing the underlying cause plus carefully observing and managing the renal status. The major goal is reestablishment of renal function (with emphasis on providing an adequate caloric intake to minimize reduction of protein stores); prevention of complications; and monitoring of fluid balance, laboratory data, and physical manifestations. The probability of dialysis or continuous hemofiltration is high, and the nurse must anticipate the availability of the necessary equipment. Because the child requires intensive observation and often specialized equipment, the usual disposition is admission to an intensive care unit where equipment and trained personnel are available.

The major nursing tasks in the care of the infant or child with ARF are monitoring and assessing fluid and electrolyte balance. Limiting fluid intake requires ingenuity on the part of caregivers to cope with the child who is thirsty. One strategy involves rationing the daily intake with small amounts of fluid served in containers that give the impression of larger volumes. Older children who understand the rationale of fluid limits can help determine how their daily ration should be distributed.

Meeting nutritional needs is sometimes a problem because the child may be nauseated and because getting the child to eat concentrated foods without fluids may be difficult. When nourishment is provided by the IV route, careful monitoring is essential to prevent fluid overload. This can become a major challenge in the face of nutritional requirements and administration of IV medications. The IV drugs being used may be nephrotoxic, which can require a specified volume of solution for delivery. In some instances blood products must also be delivered. Preventing fluid overload while delivering medications and calories requires concerted collaboration. In addition, nursing measures such as maintaining an optimum thermal environment, reducing any elevation of body temperature, and reducing restlessness and anxiety are used to decrease the rate of tissue catabolism.

The nurse must be continually alert for behavior changes that indicate the onset of complications. Infection from reduced resistance, anemia, and general morbidity is a constant threat. Fluid overload and electrolyte disturbances can precipitate cardiovascular complications such as hypertension and cardiac failure. Fluid and electrolyte imbalances, acidosis, and accumulation of nitrogenous waste products can produce neurologic involvement manifested by coma, seizures, or alterations in sensorium.

Although children with ARF are usually quite ill and voluntarily diminish their activity, infants may become restless and irritable, and children are often anxious and frightened. Frequent, painful, and stress-producing treatments and tests must be performed. A supportive, empathetic nurse can provide comfort and stability in a threatening and unnatural environment.

Family Support

Providing support and reassurance to parents is among the major nursing responsibilities. The seriousness and emergency nature of ARF are stressful to parents, and most feel some degree of guilt regarding the child's condition, especially when the illness is the result of ingestion of a toxic substance, dehydration, or a genetic disease. They need reassurance and an empathetic listener. They also need to be kept informed of the child's progress and provided explanations regarding the therapeutic regimen. The equipment and the child's behavior are sometimes frightening and anxiety provoking. Nurses can do much to help parents comprehend and deal with the stresses of the situation.

CHRONIC RENAL FAILURE

The kidneys are able to maintain the chemical composition of fluids within normal limits until more than 50% of functional renal capacity is destroyed by disease or injury. Chronic renal failure or insufficiency begins when the diseased kidneys can no longer maintain the normal chemical structure of body fluids under normal conditions (Groothoff, 2005). Progressive deterioration over months or years produces a variety of clinical and biochemical disturbances that conclude in the clinical syndrome known as uremia. The final stage of CRF, ESRD, is irreversible. Treatment with dialysis or transplantation is required when the glomerular filtration rate decreases below 10% to 15% of normal. The pattern of renal dysfunction is remarkably uniform no matter what disease process initiates the advanced disease.

Etiology

A variety of diseases and disorders can result in CRF. The most common causes of CRF before age 5 years are congenital renal and urinary tract malformations (particularly renal hypoplasia and dysplasia and obstructive uropathy) and VUR. Glomerular and hereditary renal disease predominate in children 5 to 15 years of age. The glomerular diseases that most commonly lead to CRF are chronic pyelonephritis, CGN, and glomerulonephropathy associated with systemic diseases such as anaphylactoid purpura and lupus erythematosus. Hereditary nephritis, congenital nephrotic syndrome, Alport syndrome, polycystic kidney, and several other hereditary disorders result in renal failure in childhood. Renal vascular disorders such as HUS, vascular thrombosis, or cortical necrosis are less common causes.

Pathophysiology

Early in the course of progressive nephron destruction, the child remains asymptomatic with only minimum biochemical abnormalities. Unless its presence is detected in the process of routine assessment, signs and symptoms that indicate advanced renal damage often emerge only late in the course of the disease. Midway in the disease process, as increasing numbers of nephrons are totally destroyed and most others are damaged to varying degrees, the few that remain intact are hypertrophied but functional. These few normal nephrons are able to make sufficient adjustments to stresses to maintain reasonable degrees of fluid and electrolyte balance. Definitive biochemical examination at this time reveals restricted tolerance to excesses or restrictions. As the disease progresses to the end stage because of severe reduction in the number of functioning nephrons, the kidneys are no longer able to maintain fluid and electrolyte balance, and the features of the uremic syndrome appear.

The following sections briefly summarize the pathophysiology of specific biochemical abnormalities.

Retention of Waste Products

A moderate decrease in renal function is not associated with a rise in fasting BUN concentration. With progressive nephron destruction and diminished function, the serum level of these end products of protein metabolism increases. However, the BUN level is affected by protein intake, whereas the creatinine concentration depends on muscle mass; therefore creatinine is a more reliable index of renal failure.

Water and Sodium Retention

The damaged kidneys are able to maintain sodium and water balance under normal circumstances, although the few remaining functional nephrons are required to increase their rate of filtration and reabsorption in proportion to their numbers. The limitations of this capacity become apparent under stress. The nature of abnormalities in adjustment depends on the underlying renal disease. Infants and small children with kidney dysplasia or urinary obstructive disease tend to excrete large volumes of dilute urine low in sodium content. Children with glomerular disease tend to retain both sodium and water as a result of a greater reduction of glomerular filtration than of tubular reabsorption. Children with defective sodium reabsorption from tubular disease tend to lose sodium with a corresponding osmotic water loss. Consequently, sodium excesses may cause edema and hypertension, whereas sodium deprivation can result in hypovolemia and circulatory failure. Only in ESRD is markedly reduced glomerular filtration inadequate to handle normal amounts of sodium and water. Retention of these substances leads to edema and vascular congestion.

Hyperkalemia

Dangerous hyperkalemia is uncommon in CRF until the end stage. However, the kidneys are unable to adjust readily to increased ingestion of potassium, and they require a longer period to rid the body of this excess.

Acidosis

A sustained metabolic acidosis is characteristic of CRF; it results from the damaged kidney's inability to excrete a normal load of metabolic acids generated by normal metabolic processes. There is reduced capacity of the distal tubules to produce ammonia and impaired reabsorption of bicarbonate. Despite continuous hydrogen ion retention and bicarbonate loss, the

---

BOX 30-6 FACTORS RELATED TO BONE DEMINERALIZATION IN CHRONIC RENAL FAILURE

- In a state of acidosis there is dissolution of the alkaline salts of bone, which serve as buffers, and the release of phosphorus and calcium into the bloodstream.
- Reduced glomerular filtration and excretion of inorganic phosphate lead to an elevation of plasma phosphate with a concomitant decrease in serum calcium.
- Decreased serum calcium concentration stimulates the secretion of parathyroid hormone, which results in reabsorption of calcium from bones. Under normal circumstances parathyroid hormone inhibits the tubular reabsorption of phosphates.
- Diseased kidneys are unable to complete the synthesis of vitamin D to its most active form, 1,25-dihydroxycholecalciferol, which is necessary for the absorption of calcium from the gastrointestinal tract and deposition of calcium in bone. This acquired resistance to vitamin D decreases calcium absorption, permits retention of phosphorus, and contributes to secondary hyperparathyroidism.

BOX 30-7 CAUSES OF ANEMIA IN CHRONIC RENAL FAILURE

- Shortened life span of red blood cells caused by some extracorpuscular factor associated with the uremic state
- Impaired red blood cell production resulting from decreased production of erythropoietin
- Blood loss related to increased tendency to bleed, associated with a prolonged bleeding time, probably related to impaired platelet function and laboratory blood samples
- Hyperparathyroidism
- Hypersplenism, which may be related to silicone deposition (from dialysis blood lines) and granuloma formation in the spleen
- Diseases related to hemolytic anemia, such as systemic lupus erythematosus and sickle cell disease

---

plasma pH is maintained at a level compatible with life by other buffering mechanisms, particularly the bone salt (see the following sections).

Calcium and Phosphorus Disturbances

One of the distressing features of CRF is its effect on calcium and phosphorus homeostasis. Profound and complex disturbances in the metabolism of these substances result in significant bone demineralization and impaired growth. This appears to be related to several factors (Box 30-6). These complex disturbances in calcium, phosphorus, and bone metabolism produce growth arrest or delay; bone pain; and deformities known as renal osteodystrophy, sometimes called renal rickets, because the disorganization of bone growth and demineralization are similar to that caused by vitamin D–resistant rickets.

Anemia

A consistent feature of chronic renal insufficiency is anemia, which appears to result from several factors (Box 30-7).

Growth Disturbance

One of the most striking effects of CRF in childhood, and one that can have profound psychologic and social consequences

---

BOX 30-8 PROBABLE CAUSES OF GROWTH FAILURE IN CHRONIC RENAL FAILURE

- Renal osteodystrophy
- Poor nutrition associated with dietary restrictions (especially protein) and loss of appetite
- Biochemical abnormalities associated with renal failure, such as sustained acidosis or renal sodium wasting
- Hypertension
- Corticosteroid treatment
- Tissue resistance to growth hormone
- Trace mineral and vitamin deficiencies

---

for the developing child, is delayed growth. The cause is poorly understood but may be related to nutritional and biochemical factors (Box 30-8).

Sexual maturation may be delayed or may not occur in children with CRF, and secondary amenorrhea commonly develops in girls past puberty. CRF can also cause sexual dysfunction by creating imbalances in gonadal hormone levels. Decreased testosterone levels impair spermatogenesis in males; decreased estrogen, luteinizing hormone, and progesterone cause anovulation and menstrual irregularities (usually amenorrhea) in females. Autonomic neuropathy and anemia are also factors that can alter sexual function.

Other Disturbances

Children with CRF are more susceptible to infection, especially pneumonia, UTI, and septicemia, although the reason for this is not entirely clear. Hyperventilation, a manifestation of the respiratory compensatory mechanism for metabolic acidosis, and pulmonary edema may contribute to upper respiratory tract infection. These children become extraordinarily sensitive to changes in vascular volume that may cause, in addition to pulmonary overload, cerebral symptoms and circulatory manifestations such as hypertension and cardiac failure.

Numerous neurologic manifestations appear with advanced renal failure, although no specific toxin or biochemical defect has been identified. However, disturbances in enzyme function, disturbances in water and electrolyte balance, altered calcium ion concentration, hypertension, and accumulation of various "uremic toxins" have been implicated.

Clinical Manifestations

The first evidence of difficulty is usually loss of normal energy and increased fatigue on exertion. For example, the child may prefer quiet, passive activities rather than participation in more active games and outdoor play. The child is usually somewhat pale, but the change is often so subtle that it may not be evident to parents or others. Blood pressure is sometimes elevated. Growth is affected early in the development of CRF, and falling behind on the growth chart is often the first measurable sign.

Other manifestations may appear as the disease progresses. The child does not eat as well (especially breakfast), shows less interest in normal activities such as schoolwork or play, and has a decreased or increased urinary output and a compensatory intake of fluid. For example, a child who has achieved bladder control may wet the bed at night. Pallor becomes more evident as the skin develops a characteristic sallow, muddy appearance as a result of anemia and deposition of urochrome pigment in the skin. The child may complain of headache, muscle cramps, and nausea. Other signs and symptoms include weight loss, facial puffiness, malaise, bone or joint pain, growth retardation, dryness or itching of the skin, bruised skin, and sometimes sensory or motor loss. Amenorrhea is common in adolescent girls.

Therapy is generally initiated before the appearance of the uremic syndrome, although on some occasions the symptoms may be observed. Manifestations of untreated uremia reflect the progressive nature of the homeostatic disturbances and general toxicity. Gastrointestinal symptoms include loss of appetite, nausea, and vomiting. Bleeding tendencies are apparent in bruises, bloody diarrheal stools, stomatitis, and bleeding from the lips and mouth. There is intractable itching, probably related to hyperparathyroidism. Deposits of urea crystals may appear on the skin as uremic frost but are seldom seen because of the availability of dialysis and transplantation (Springhouse, 2008). There may be an unpleasant uremic odor to the breath. Respirations become deeper as a result of metabolic acidosis, and circulatory overload is manifested by hypertension, congestive heart failure, and pulmonary edema. Progressive confusion, dulling of the sensorium, and ultimately coma are signs of neurologic involvement. Other signs may include tremors, muscular twitching, and seizures.

Diagnostic Evaluation

The diagnosis of CRF is usually suspected on the basis of any of a number of clinical manifestations, a history of prior renal disease, or biochemical findings. The onset is usually gradual, and the initial signs and symptoms are vague and nonspecific. Laboratory and other diagnostic tools and tests are of value in assessing the extent of renal damage, biochemical disturbances, and related physical dysfunction. Often they can help establish the nature of the underlying disease and differentiate between other disease processes and the pathologic consequences of renal dysfunction.

Therapeutic Management

The multiple complications of CRF are managed according to medical protocols such as the National Kidney Foundation Kidney Disease Outcomes Quality Initiative evidence-based clinical practice guidelines (**www.kidney.org/professionals/ KDOQI**). The goals of management are to promote effective renal function, maintain body fluid and electrolyte balance within acceptable limits, treat systemic complications, and promote as active and normal a life as possible for the child for as long as possible. This becomes increasingly difficult as the disease progresses toward its inevitable end. Therapeutic measures designed to relieve one manifestation may negatively affect another. For example, antihypertensive agents may further impair renal function.

Activity

Allow children unrestricted activity and to set their own limits regarding rest and extent of exertion. Encourage them to attend school. When the effort is too great, home tutoring is arranged.

Diet

Regulation of diet has been seen as the most effective means, short of dialysis, for reducing the quantity of materials that require renal excretion. The goal of the diet in renal failure is to provide sufficient calories and protein for growth while minimizing the excretory demands made on the kidney, to limit metabolic bone disease (osteodystrophy), and to minimize fluid and electrolyte disturbances. Dietary protein intake is limited to the recommended dietary allowance (RDA) for the child's age. Restriction of protein intake below the RDA is believed to negatively affect growth and neurodevelopment. Dietary phosphorus may need to be restricted. Remember that any attempt to restrict dietary intake in children potentially restricts caloric intake and can limit growth.

Protein in the diet should include foods of high biologic value. When given with meals, substances that bind phosphorus in the intestines prevent its absorption and allow a more liberal intake of phosphorus-containing protein. Sodium and water are not usually limited unless there is evidence of edema or hypertension.

Potassium is not restricted as long as creatinine clearance remains at acceptable limits (30 to 35 ml/min). However, restrictions are instituted for patients with oliguria or anuria. Restrictions of any or all of these minerals may be imposed in later stages or at any time in which factors cause abnormal serum concentrations.

Because of modified dietary intake, altered metabolism, and poor appetite, some dietary supplementation is usually needed. Because fat-soluble vitamins can accumulate in patients with CRF, vitamins A, E, and K are not supplemented beyond normal dietary intake. An active form of vitamin D is prescribed, and water-soluble vitamin supplementation may be required if the diet is inadequate. Other dietary needs are discussed in relation to osteodystrophy and anemia. Dietary management of the child with renal failure is a difficult and complex problem that necessitates collaboration with a registered dietitian who is knowledgeable about pediatric nutrition and the impact of renal failure.

Osteodystrophy

Measures directed at prevention or correction of the calcium/phosphorus imbalance are reduction of dietary phosphorus, administration of a phosphorus-binding agent, provision of supplemental calcium, control of acidosis, and administration of an active form of vitamin D.

The reduction of protein and milk intake can control dietary phosphorus. Oral administration of phosphorus-binding agents, which combine with the phosphorus to decrease gastrointestinal absorption and thus the serum levels of phosphate, can further reduce phosphorus levels. Calcium carbonate preparations can be used as phosphorus binders. These medications act as (1) phosphate binders, (2) calcium supplements, and (3) alkalizing agents. Calcium carbonate preparations can be given with meals to bind phosphorus if the child is hyperphosphatemic or mildly hypocalcemic. If given 1 to 2 hours after meals, they act as calcium supplements for children with stable phosphorus but low calcium levels. Calcium acetate can also be used. Aluminum hydroxide gels are effective phosphorus binders but have been shown to cause aluminum loading when used in children with renal failure. Aluminum intoxication leads to altered sensorium, an inability to talk, ataxia, seizures, and severe bone disease.

When serum phosphate levels are within a normal range, appropriate therapy with an active form of vitamin D is instituted. These drugs are administered to increase the absorption of calcium through the gastrointestinal tract and include dihydrotachysterol (Hytakerol) or calcitriol (Rocaltrol). The serum calcium level is monitored weekly during periods when the drugs are being changed or regulated. Parathyroid hormone levels are measured every 2 to 3 months.

Osseous deformities that result from renal osteodystrophy, especially those related to ambulation, are troublesome and require correction if they occur. Careful attention to the management of osteodystrophy and bone growth can prevent deformities in some children.

Acidosis

Pharmacologic treatment of acidosis is initiated early in children who have chronic renal insufficiency. In addition to reducing the formation of metabolic acids by decreasing the dietary intake of protein, alkalizing agents such as sodium bicarbonate or a combination of sodium and potassium citrate (Bicitra, Polycitra, or Shohl solution) alleviate acidosis. Correction of acidosis is best attempted after calcium levels are elevated, since rapid correction may precipitate tetany in a hypocalcemic child.

Anemia

Because the anemia associated with renal failure is related to decreased production of erythropoietin, it usually cannot be successfully managed with hematinic agents. Provide sufficient sources of folic acid and iron in the diet, although this is difficult when protein sources are restricted. Inadequate intake and iron losses that may occur are managed by supplemental iron, usually ferrous sulfate. Providing adequate sources of ascorbic acid at the same time that iron-rich foods or supplements are given enhances the absorption.

The medication recombinant human erythropoietin (r-HuEPO) corrects anemia (improving energy level and general well-being) and eliminates the need for frequent blood transfusions in patients with CRF. To support the formation of new red blood cells before r-HuEPO therapy, iron stores must be adequate. Iron supplements are required in conjunction with r-HuEPO.

Hypertension

Hypertension of advanced renal disease may be managed initially by cautious use of a low-sodium diet, fluid restriction, and perhaps diuretics such as thiazides or furosemide. Strict restriction of sodium intake may be necessary in patients with oliguria. Severe hypertension may require the combination of a beta blocker and a vasodilator (propranolol and hydralazine). Other drugs that may be used include nifedipine, atenolol, minoxidil, prazosin, captopril, or labetalol, either singly or in combinations.

Growth Retardation

One major consequence of CRF is growth retardation. Children with onset of renal failure earlier in life have more severe growth impairment than those diagnosed later (Gorman, Fivush, and Frankenfield, 2005). These children grow poorly both before and after initiation of dialysis. In addition to a number of metabolic abnormalities, depletion of body protein is characteristic of children with CRF. The use of recombinant human growth hormone has shown marked acceleration in growth velocity in children with growth retardation secondary to CRF (Gorman, Fivush, and Frankenfield, 2005).

Miscellaneous Complications

Intercurrent infections are treated with appropriate antimicrobials at the first sign of infection. Most of these drugs are excreted through the kidneys; therefore the dosage is usually reduced in proportion to the decrease in renal function, and the interval between doses is extended in these children to avoid possible toxic effects from accumulation. Any drug eliminated through the kidneys is administered with caution. Serum levels of ototoxic or nephrotoxic drugs (e.g., aminoglycosides or vancomycin) are assessed regularly to ensure a safe, nontoxic level.

Dental defects are common in children with chronic kidney disease; the earlier the onset of the disease, the more severe the dental manifestations. These defects include hypoplasia, hypomineralization, tooth discoloration, alteration in the size and shape of teeth, malocclusion (secondary to deficient skeletal growth), ulcerative stomatitis, occasional oral hematomas, and an increase in calcific deposits around the teeth. Regular dental care is especially important in these children. Other nondental complications are treated symptomatically (e.g., chlorpromazine [Thorazine] or prochlorperazine [Compazine] is given for nausea, antiepileptics are given for seizures, and diphenhydramine [Benadryl] is given for pruritus). Once evidence of ESRD appears, the disease runs its relentless course and terminates in death in a few weeks unless waste products and toxins are removed from body fluids by dialysis or kidney transplantation. Since the adaptation of these techniques for infants and small children, the outlook for these patients has improved remarkably. In cases in which the patient has other serious illnesses or organ system failures and aggressive care is considered futile, the appropriate end-of-life recommendation may be for palliative care and comfort measures only.

QUALITY PATIENT OUTCOMES: Chronic Renal Failure
- Sufficient calories and protein for growth maintained
- Excretory demands made on the kidney are limited
- Metabolic bone disease (osteodystrophy) minimal
- Fluid and electrolyte disturbances managed
- Hypertension managed
- Growth retardation treated

Nursing Care Management

The child with CRF has a life maintained by drugs and artificial means, and the multiple stresses placed on these children and their families are often overwhelming. The unrelenting course of the disease process is one of progressive deterioration. There is no means by which to prevent the irreversible progress of renal insufficiency, nor is there any known cure. As the affected child progresses from renal insufficiency to uremia and then to dialysis and transplantation with intense therapy, the need for

◉ NURSING CARE PLAN

The Child with Chronic Renal Failure

NURSING DIAGNOSIS	EXPECTED PATIENT OUTCOMES	NURSING INTERVENTIONS	RATIONALE
Risk for Injury related to accumulated electrolytes and waste products	The child will exhibit no evidence of waste product accumulation.	Assist with renal dialysis.	To maintain renal excretory function
Child's/Family's Defining Characteristics (Subjective and Objective Data)	**The Following NOC Concept Applies to This Outcome** Risk Control	Administer sodium polystyrene sulfonate (Kayexalate).	To reduce serum potassium levels
Excesses in potassium, sodium, and phosphorus		Provide diet low in potassium, sodium, and phosphorus.	To reduce excretory demand on kidneys
Evidence of hyperkalemia, hyperphosphatemia, uremia		Observe for evidence of accumulated waste products.	To ensure prompt treatment
Excess blood urea nitrogen		Increase water intake.	To increase waste excretion by kidneys
		The Following NIC Concepts Apply to These Interventions Risk Identification Medication Administration Surveillance Teaching: Individual	

NURSING DIAGNOSIS	EXPECTED PATIENT OUTCOMES	NURSING INTERVENTIONS	RATIONALE
Altered Nutrition: Less Than Body Requirements related to restricted diet	The child will consume an adequate amount of appropriate foods. The child will show no evidence of deficiencies or weight loss.	Provide dietary instructions for foods that reduce excretory demands on kidney and provide sufficient calories and protein for growth.	To encourage appropriate diet, which can reduce kidney demands
Child's/Family's Defining Characteristics (Subjective and Objective Data)	**The Following NOC Concepts Apply to These Outcomes** Nutritional Status: Nutrient Intake	Limit phosphorus, salt, and potassium as prescribed.	To prevent mineral excess
Weight loss, inadequate growth Poor nutritional intake	Nutritional Status: Food and Fluid Intake Weight Control	Encourage intake of carbohydrates and foods high in calcium.	To provide calories for growth and calcium to prevent bone demineralization
		Arrange for renal dietitian to meet with family to review allowable foods and assist in dietary planning.	To provide family with understanding of the child's dietary needs
		Help hemodialysis patient to fill out menu requests for meals.	To promote appropriate food choice decisions
		The Following NIC Concepts Apply to These Interventions Nutritional Therapy Prescribed Diet Vital Signs Monitoring Fluid Management Nutrition Management Nutrition Therapy Nutritional Monitoring	

supportive nursing care is also intensified. Team effort is more important than ever and involves coordination of personnel from medicine, nursing, social services, child life, physical and occupational therapy, dietetics, and psychologic or psychiatric specialties (see Nursing Care Plan).

Progressive disease places a number of stresses on the child and family. There is a continuing need for repeated examinations that often entail painful procedures, side effects, and frequent hospitalizations. Diet therapy can become progressively more restrictive and intense, and parents may need help in learning to select appropriate foods, read labels carefully for sodium and potassium content, and modify meals to accommodate the child's special needs. The child is required to take a variety of medications. Compliance is difficult when long-term therapies are involved. Ever present in all aspects of the treatment regimen is the agonizing realization that, without treatment, death is inevitable.

ESRD presents the same nonspecific stresses on child and family as any other chronic or life-threatening illness. (See Chapters 22 and 23.) The reactions and adaptation of the child and family depend on the child's age and developmental stage, the family's cultural and socioeconomic background, the quality of the interpersonal relationships of family members, and the communication patterns within the family. In general, the problems observed and the emotional responses to the stress of the illness are influenced less by the nature of the illness than by the family relationships and personalities (see Family-Centered Care box).

One of the first and most noticeable changes is the alteration in physical appearance—fluctuations in weight, anemia, and failure to grow. Children must adjust to the fact that they will always be different from their peers in some ways. They will be shorter, often more tired, and unable to participate in all the activities that are attractive to young people. Children who have had diversion procedures, dialysis, and other surgeries or who urinate into a bag need to learn positive coping strategies for the alterations in their body image and for the questions and potential teasing of peers. It is not unusual for children with chronic conditions to exhibit behavioral regression. This is particularly so for children with renal failure because their appearance is often of a child much younger than their chronologic age.

School is often difficult for these children. Frequent absences for illnesses, evaluations, or treatments disrupt the educational process and socialization. Teachers and school systems are not always sympathetic to the rights and needs of a child with a chronic illness (e.g., the right to equal education and the need for flexibility and special help at times), which places an additional burden on the parents.

In some families illness and stressful experiences act as a unifying force; in other families stress aggravates preexisting problems and contributes to family disharmony. The relentless nature of the disease and its therapies not only places physical and emotional stresses on the family but is also a chronic drain on the family finances. Insurance rarely covers the full cost of the multiple hospitalizations and outpatient expenses. The federal Medicare program, for which most children qualify, funds ESRD care. However, there are many hidden costs, such as transportation to special treatment centers, meals, and sometimes lodging away from home. Some private foundations, churches, and community groups provide temporary assistance, and nurses should become familiar with those in the area of their practice that can offer financial and educational services to these families. For example, the National Kidney Foundation* and numerous other agencies provide services and information for families, including pamphlets and descriptive literature. Particularly useful are booklets written for children with renal disease.

Certain specific stresses related to ESRD and its treatment are predictable. When it first becomes apparent that kidney failure is inevitable, both the child and the parents experience

BOX 30-9   PROCESSES OF FLUID AND ELECTROLYTE MOVEMENT

Osmosis—Passive movement of water from a solution of lower concentration to a solution of higher concentration of particles
Diffusion—Random movement of particles from an area of greater concentration to an area of lower concentration
Ultrafiltration—Process by which plasma water is removed because of a pressure gradient between the blood and dialysate compartments

depression and anxiety. Acceptance is particularly difficult if renal failure progresses rapidly after the diagnosis. Children, and especially parents, usually express denial and disbelief. Denial can also develop when progression to ESRD has been prolonged and both the child and the parents come to believe it will never occur.

Once the renal failure is established and the symptoms become progressively more distressing, parents usually perceive the initiation of hemodialysis or kidney transplantation as a positive experience. After the initial concerns of implementing the treatment, the child begins to feel better, and parental anxiety is relieved for a time.

RENAL REPLACEMENT THERAPY

Technologic advances in the care of children with ARF and CRF provide several renal replacement therapies for maintaining excretory function in acute disease and for prolonging life in those with ESRD. The primary modalities are hemodialysis, PD, hemofiltration, and transplantation.

Dialysis is the process of separating colloids and crystalline substances in solution by the difference in their rate of diffusion through a semipermeable membrane. This movement across the membrane is accomplished by three processes: osmosis, diffusion, and ultrafiltration (Box 30-9). Methods of dialysis currently available for clinical management of renal failure are:

- Hemodialysis, in which blood is circulated outside the body through artificial cellophane membranes that permit a similar passage of water and solutes
- PD, wherein the abdominal cavity acts as a semipermeable membrane through which water and solutes of small molecular size move by osmosis and diffusion according to their respective concentrations on either side of the membrane
- Hemofiltration, in which blood filtrate is circulated outside the body by hydrostatic pressure exerted across a semipermeable membrane and replaced (simultaneously) by electrolyte solution

The choice of whether to use hemodialysis, PD, or hemofiltration depends on the nature of the renal failure (acute versus chronic) and the cause of the renal failure. For chronic dialysis, family lifestyles and preferences are considered in choice of treatment. Hemodialysis is more efficient than PD but is technically more difficult in infants and very young children. In these children hemofiltration may be a viable substitute for dialysis. As a rule, dialysis is reserved for children who are in end-stage renal failure, since it requires creation of an access and special equipment. It may be used acutely for conditions such as severe metabolic acidosis, accidental poisoning, chronic heart failure with fluid overload, hyperkalemia, severe hypernatremia, severe hyperphosphatemia, and tumor lysis syndrome.

The absolute indications for dialysis are life-threatening electrolyte abnormalities; severe volume overload; and bilateral neoplastic disease or bilateral nephrectomies performed for various reasons, including intractable hypertension. Although each child is assessed on an individual basis, indications for instituting dialysis in CRF are biochemical abnormalities, including elevated BUN, acidosis, severe hyperphosphatemia, and elevated potassium. Other indications include deteriorating central nervous system function or congestive heart failure that is unresponsive to other therapy. Growth failure, severe osteodystrophy, insufficient caloric intake, and an inability to carry out normal activities are sometimes criteria for dialysis.

Most children show rapid clinical improvement with the implementation of dialysis, although it is directly related to the duration of uremia before dialysis and the extent to which dietary regulations are followed. Growth rate and skeletal maturation improve, but recovery of normal growth is uncommon. In many cases sexual development, although delayed, has progressed to completion.

HEMODIALYSIS

Hemodialysis is the preferred dialytic method for children with acute conditions such as life-threatening hyperkalemia or poisoning with dialyzable compounds. Protein loss is less extensive than with PD. However, hemodialysis is technically difficult in small children less than 20 kg (44 lb) because their delicately balanced cardiovascular dynamics may be upset by the rapid changes in blood volume and systemic blood pressure that may occur with this method. In addition, it may be difficult to place vascular access for hemodialysis in small children.

Hemodialysis is the preferred form of dialysis for certain family situations in which any one person is unable to take the time and responsibility to perform the procedures at home. It is best suited to children who live close to the dialysis center, since they must come to the center as often as three or more times a week for treatments. Children who are not good candidates for PD because of family noncompliance, recurrent peritoneal infections, or unstable living conditions are treated with hemodialysis.

Procedure

Hemodialysis requires special dialysis equipment—the hemodialyzer, or so-called artificial kidney (Figs. 30-4 and 30-5). Hemodialyzers are available in two forms: parallel flow (plate) and hollow fiber. Hollow fiber dialyzers are preferable for children because their blood compartment is rigid and available in relatively small volumes. Pediatric dialysis can be safely carried out when the total dialysis circuit volume does not exceed 10% of the child's estimated blood volume.

Hemodialysis also requires one of three means of blood access: grafts, fistulas, or external access devices. An arteriovenous fistula is an access in which a vein and artery are connected surgically. The preferred site is the radial artery and a forearm vein. The creation of a subcutaneous (internal) arteriovenous fistula by anastomosing a segment of the radial artery and bra-

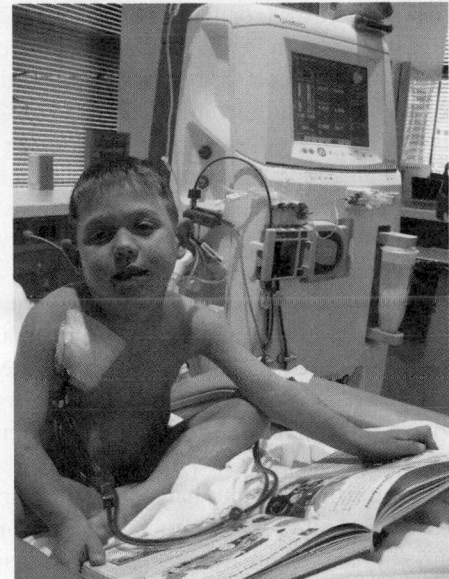

Fig. 30-4 Diversional activities help lessen the boredom children can experience during hemodialysis.

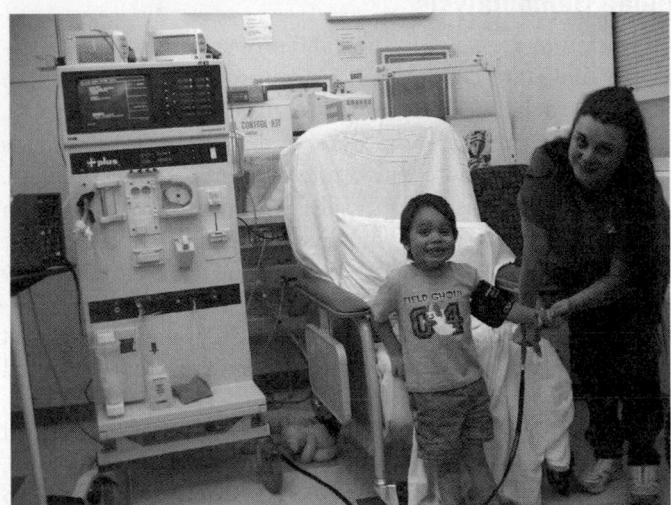

Fig. 30-5 Young child receiving hemodialysis.

chiocephalic vein produces dilation and thickening of the superficial vessels of the forearm to provide easy access for repeated venipuncture. Fewer complications and less restriction of activity are observed with the use of a fistula. If vessels are inadequate for an autogenous fistula, a synthetic graft may be placed in the arm or thigh with either a loop or straight configuration. Both the graft and the fistula require needle insertion at each dialysis. For short-term external vascular access, percutaneous catheters are inserted in the femoral or internal jugular veins, even in very small children. Avoid subclavian access because of the potential complication of stenosis. For long-term external vascular access, cuffed, dual-lumen (single-lumen for infants) catheters can be surgically placed similarly to other central venous access devices. They are ready to be used immediately, and do not require needles.

Various hemodialysis schedules are used, but most centers recommend dialysis three times a week for 3 to 5 hours, depending on the child's size. The length of a hemodialysis treatment, the blood flow rate, and dialyzer characteristics contribute to adequacy of treatment. Current target levels for adequacy are a urea reduction ratio of 65% or higher or a Kt/V (Clearance × Time/Volume) of 1.4 or higher. For a complete description of the highly specialized process of hemodialysis, see the numerous references available on this topic.

Dietary limitations are necessary in chronic dialysis to avoid biochemical complications. Fluid and sodium are restricted to prevent fluid overload and its associated symptoms of hypertension, cerebral manifestations, and congestive heart failure. Potassium is restricted to prevent complications related to hyperkalemia; phosphorus restriction helps prevent parathyroid hyperactivity and its attendant risk of abnormal calcification in soft tissues. Adequate protein intake is necessary to maximize growth potential. Fluid limitations are determined by residual urinary output and the need to limit intradialytic weight gain.

Seizures during or after hemodialysis are now uncommon. With the current practice of hemodialysis, cerebral edema caused by alterations in osmolality in the brain when the BUN level is lowered rapidly (associated with dialysis disequilibrium syndrome) is rare.

Home Hemodialysis

With appropriate cannulization and proper training and education of both the child and the parents, hemodialysis can be performed at home. Time spent in transportation is eliminated, the environment is more pleasant and secure, and the child is able to assume a more active role in the treatment program. Home hemodialysis is especially advantageous for children waiting for a transplant who live a great distance from the dialysis center or for children who have had one or more kidney transplant failures.

Home hemodialysis units are available to some children, and the preparation and management are similar to those required for hemodialysis in the hospital (Geary, Piva, Tyrrell, et al, 2005). The patient is equipped with a dialysis unit that is used with the vascular access established for outpatient dialysis. Parents of children on home hemodialysis must know how to operate the equipment, connect the unit to the vascular access, and assess the child's status. Home hemodialysis is more prevalent in sparsely populated regions of the country.

Nursing Care Management

Initiating a hemodialysis regimen is a traumatic and anxiety-provoking experience for most children. After surgery for implantation of the graft, fistula, or long-term external access device, the initial experience with the hemodialysis machine and its implication can be frightening. They need reassurance about the preparations for dialysis and the conduct of the treatment. They are anxious about repeated venipunctures (with implanted shunts and for blood chemistries) and about the sight of their blood leaving their body and entering the machine (see Atraumatic Care box). The child's physiologic response to the treatment (e.g., nausea and vomiting, cramps, or seizures) can also cause anxiety. These are usually individual responses related to the child's overall well-being and degree of compliance with the total medical regimen. Once the initial fear of the machine has been resolved, the nurse can help children develop strategies for dealing with restricted activity and movement for the duration of each treatment (see Fig. 30-5).

With their increased need for independence and their urge for rebellion, adolescents may not adapt as well. They resent dependency on a machine, parents, professional staff, and an unrelenting therapy program. Depression, hostility, or both are common in adolescents undergoing hemodialysis. The adverse consequences of the disease include the need for diet restrictions, limitations in physical activity (resulting from lack of energy, frequent illnesses, and specific restrictions related to access), and the sense of being different from other children. Withdrawal from peers and social isolation are the rule, and noncompliance with the therapeutic regimen is not uncommon.

Body changes related to the disease process, such as growth retardation, skin color changes, and lack of sexual maturation, are stress provoking. Dietary restrictions are particularly burdensome for both children and parents. Children feel deprived when unable to eat foods previously enjoyed and unrestricted for other family members. Consequently, failure to cooperate is not uncommon. Diet restrictions are interpreted as punishment; because they may not be able to fully understand the purpose of the restrictions, some will sneak forbidden food items at every opportunity. Allowing children, especially adolescents, maximum participation in and responsibility for their own treatment program is helpful. The extent of adherence and adjustment depends on the personalities of the involved persons, the quality of their relationships, and their coping mechanisms.

After weeks, months, or years of hemodialysis, the parents and the child feel anxiety associated with the prognosis and continued pressures of the treatment. The relentless need for treatment interferes with family plans and activities, including school. Graft and fistula problems are a common source of aggravation. Most families and children on hemodialysis look to kidney transplantation as a desirable alternative to long-term treatment.

PERITONEAL DIALYSIS

For acute conditions, PD is quick, relatively easy to learn, and safe to perform and requires minimum equipment and specially trained nurses. PD is a slow, gentle process, which decreases the stress on body organs that can occur with the rapid chemical and volume changes of hemodialysis. The procedure is indicated for neonates, children with severe cardiovascular disease, or those who are poor risks for vascular access.

Chronic PD is the preferred form of dialysis for children and parents who are independent; families who live a long distance from the medical center; infants; school-age children; and adolescents, who prefer fewer dietary restrictions and a gentler form of dialysis. Chronic PD is most often performed at home.

Contraindications for the use of PD include recent abdominal surgery or peritoneal adhesions and scarring. A higher rate of infection (peritonitis) is observed with this modality.

Procedure

In acute situations PD catheter insertion may be accomplished at the bedside; catheters for long-term use are placed surgically in the operating room with the patient under anesthesia. A catheter is inserted through the anterior abdominal wall, and the catheter cuff is sutured into place. Chronic PD catheters are tunneled through a subcutaneous tract before exiting the skin in a manner similar to implantation of central venous access devices. At the time of dialysis a commercially prepared dialysis solution is allowed to flow by gravity through the catheter and into the peritoneal cavity, where it remains while equilibrium between plasma and dialysis fluid takes place. Approximately 30 to 50 ml/kg, or 1100 ml/m^2, of dialysis solution is instilled at each cycle. The fluid is then allowed to flow by gravity drainage into a receptacle, and fresh dialysis solution is again instilled.

In PD each pass or cycle is characterized by inflow time, dwell time, and drain time. The length of each portion of the cycle is part of the dialysis prescription. The dwell time varies according to the goals of the treatment (i.e., removal of water, solute, electrolyte, or all of these) (Schroder, 2005). The procedure is usually continued until renal function is restored, waste products are reduced, or (in prolonged need) the patient is switched to a form of chronic PD—continuous ambulatory peritoneal dialysis (CAPD) or continuous cycling peritoneal dialysis (CCPD). An acute PD catheter may remain in place for several weeks provided that aseptic technique is adhered to by all who enter the system.

Home Dialysis

The development of satisfactory methods for CAPD and its alternative, CCPD, has provided additional means for managing ESRD at home. In both methods commercially available sterile dialysis solution is instilled into the peritoneal cavity through the surgically implanted indwelling catheter. The warmed solution is allowed to enter the peritoneal cavity by gravity and remains a variable length of time according to the procedure used. Dialysis solution is infused and dialysate drained through a single catheter.

In CAPD the dialysis solution is instilled and the line is clamped off and worn attached to the abdomen or thigh or even placed in a pocket. Manufacturers offer a variety of disconnect devices (e.g., Y set), all of which minimize the connectivity and amount of tubing the patient carries between exchanges. The solution remains in the peritoneum for 4 to 6 hours. The dialysate is then drained via gravity into a bag. Another warmed bag is infused, and the process is repeated so that there is fluid in the abdomen continuously. The procedure is performed a minimum of three times during the day and once at night. For an active child CAPD has proved to be a satisfactory alternative to hemodialysis.

CCPD is a modification of CAPD and intermittent PD. The dialysis exchange is usually performed at night using a PD machine that warms the dialysis fluid and automates the cycles of inflow of dialysis fluid and outflow of dialysate. As with CAPD, the CCPD system is opened during the day, but only twice as opposed to multiple times. Nighttime dialysis allows the child more freedom during the day and relieves parents of the need to perform multiple exchanges.

The care and management of the procedure are the responsibility of the parents of young children. Older children and adolescents are able to carry out the procedure themselves, thus providing them with some control and less dependency. This is especially important for adolescents.

Complications

CAPD and CCPD are currently considered the methods of choice for most children who require dialysis because they are easier to initiate and maintain than hemodialysis. Peritonitis is the major complication of home PD. The patients are treated intraperitoneally with antibiotics, and some may require catheter replacement. Although the risk of infection is continuously present, most practitioners believe it is not great enough to discourage the use of these methods.

However, other complications have been noted in patients on home PD. Tunnel infections are evidenced by swelling, warmth, and tenderness along the subcutaneous catheter tract; such infections are managed with administration of antibiotics or catheter replacement. Peritoneal leaks and ventral hernias caused by the sustained intraabdominal pressure that develops within the peritoneum have also been found in a significant number of children. Few of these patients respond to a reduction in dialysis solution volume, and many require surgical intervention.

> **! NURSING ALERT**
>
> Observe for changes in the color of the dialysis solution draining from the child. The solution should be straw colored and clear. If the color is pink, bright yellow, or brown, or if the solution is cloudy, notify the practitioner immediately.

Nursing Care Management

The availability of home dialysis has offered a greater degree of freedom for persons undergoing long-term dialysis. It eliminates the need for a residence convenient to a dialysis unit and for frequent trips to the unit, except for monthly evaluations. The nurse is responsible for teaching the family. Education focuses on (1) the disease, its implications, and the therapeutic plan; (2) the possible psychologic effects of the disease and the treatment; and (3) the technical aspects of the procedure.

The family must learn how to take vital signs before and after the dialysis and how to interpret the significance of blood pressure and temperature variations. They need to know how to vary the composition of the dialysis solution to compensate for variations in the vital signs and to maintain an accurate record of all aspects of the treatment.

Parents of the young child using CAPD need to learn how to exchange bags and manage the procedure at home. Even newborn infants are able to benefit from PD. Older children can learn to take responsibility for their own treatments as much as possible. Encourage the family to ask questions throughout the preparation time, including those that clarify anatomy and physiology, mechanical functioning, and side effects of the disease and the treatment. The PD schedule is outlined to meet the individual needs of the patient and family. Most schedules are arranged for uninterrupted sleep at night and coordination of the dialysis with school and other activities. The nurse discusses diet, medication, and activity and explores feelings about the entire therapeutic program with the child and family.

Infection is the greatest hazard of PD; therefore instruct the family to contact the appropriate persons at the earliest evidence of peritonitis. In most instances peritonitis can be controlled with antibiotics. Unfortunately, there is a high incidence of peritonitis, and repeated infections may necessitate replacement of the catheter or its removal and abandonment of the peritoneum as an access route.

The importance of emotional and material support cannot be overemphasized. The National Kidney Foundation, mentioned previously, provides a number of services and information for families of children with renal disease. A relatively new organization, the American Association of Kidney Patients,* has been organized to promote the interest and welfare of kidney patients. It provides education and support for patients and public education regarding all areas of kidney disease.

CONTINUOUS VENOVENOUS HEMOFILTRATION

A third type of "dialysis" or renal replacement therapy used primarily in acute care settings is continuous venovenous hemofiltration (CVVH). This type of therapy uses specialized equipment (hemofilter, blood pump, tubing connected to a vascular access) to ultrafiltrate blood continuously at a very slow rate. With this procedure, fluid balance may be achieved within 24 to 48 hours after initiation. Continuous venovenous hemodialysis (CVVHD) is used to remove excess fluid from patients with severe oliguric fluid overload.

CVVHD is an ideal form of renal replacement therapy for children with fluid overload from surgical procedures (e.g., cardiovascular surgery) who do not have severe biochemical abnormalities. It is commonly used for critically ill children who require volume-expanding fluids such as hyperalimentation solution, albumin, or packed red cells. It creates space for the infusion of these replacement solutions in fluid-sensitive patients. CVVHD has proved to be a highly successful alternative form of dialysis for critically ill children who might not survive the rapid volume changes that occur with hemodialysis and PD.

TRANSPLANTATION

Kidney transplantation is the preferred means of renal replacement therapy in the pediatric age-group. Although PD and hemodialysis are life preserving and are able to be carried out in the home in a large number of cases, neither method is compatible with a normal lifestyle. Transplantation, on the other hand, offers the opportunity for a relatively normal life.

*3505 E. Frontage Road, Suite 315, Tampa, FL 33607; 800-749-2257; www.aakp.org.

Kidneys for transplant are available from two sources: (1) a living related donor, usually a parent, grandparent, or sibling; or (2) a deceased donor, wherein the family of a dead or brain-dead patient consents to donation of a healthy kidney. The criteria for selection of kidney recipients are liberal, but uniform criteria have not been established among the various centers that specialize in the procedure. In general, there is no limit to age. In some cases a person's mental status (e.g., emotional instability or nonadherence to drug therapy) may be reason to defer transplantation until the recipient's psychoemotional status improves and it is reasonable to assume that the recipient will carry out the posttransplant regimen (see Family-Centered Care box).

FAMILY-CENTERED CARE
Medical Care Rationing

The criteria for selection of renal transplant recipients sometimes create dilemmas for professionals. In most cases the decision is simply a matter for the transplant team and the family to resolve for the benefit of the child involved. However, in some situations the solution is less clear, especially in view of the scarcity of donor kidneys and the expense of the procedure. The matter creates more questions than answers.

For example, should a child without a severe mental or physical disability take priority over one with these disabilities? Should financial responsibility be a consideration? Some youngsters with kidney transplants have discontinued their medications, thereby either causing damage to their kidney or losing the graft. Should these youngsters receive a second transplant? Should very young children whose families have proved unreliable in adhering to a therapeutic regimen be given a transplant when the success of the graft depends on following a prescribed therapeutic plan? Are young, single, adolescent mothers likely to be less adherent in following the prescribed medical regimen? Can persons on limited incomes manage to acquire the costly medications? If not, should the government subsidize payment?

What solutions to these dilemmas are available, and how do providers justify decisions? Should hospital ethics committees make the decisions?

Children who have ESRD secondary to uncontrolled malignancy must be cancer free for a specified time before transplantation (in remission for 2 years with patient off chemotherapy). Generalized infection must be eradicated before attempted transplantation, and the recipient should have adequate bladder capacity. Some children may have bladder augmentation or other genitourinary surgery as preparation for transplantation. Children with abnormal urinary tracts may be subject to more posttransplant urologic complications and infection than they would otherwise be.

Procedure

The kidney graft is placed in the extraperitoneal space, usually the anterior iliac fossa; the renal artery is anastomosed to the internal iliac or hypogastric artery; the renal vein is anastomosed to the hypogastric vein; and the ureter is implanted into the bladder or anastomosed to the recipient's ureter. Small children receiving a large donor kidney may require placement within the abdomen with vessel anastomoses to the aorta and inferior vena cava. Unless there is medical contraindication, the recipient's failed kidneys are left in place. Severe hypertension, neoplasm, large and continuous protein losses, and persistent severe VUR are the usual reasons for nephrectomy.

The primary goal in transplantation is the long-term survival of the grafted tissue. The means by which this is attempted include (1) securing tissues that are antigenically similar to that of the recipient and (2) suppressing the recipient's immune mechanism.

Selection of Donor Tissue

The source of a donor kidney is either a live person or a deceased donor. The closer the genetic relationship between the donor and recipient, the better the possibility of long-term survival. The only truly compatible tissue match is that between identical twin siblings. The next best possible match is a sibling, then a parent or grandparent. In some states the use of siblings is impossible until the possible donor is of age to give consent for removal of a kidney. Unrelated donors are least likely to be compatible. Careful immunologic studies are carried out to determine the donor whose kidney is least likely to be rejected by the recipient.

Suppression of the Immune Response

After the best possible tissue match is obtained for a transplant, the survival time can be significantly lengthened by suppressing the recipient's immune response. The immunosuppressant therapy of choice in kidney transplantation is corticosteroids (prednisone) in conjunction with cyclosporine and azathioprine. Other therapies include antilymphocyte globulin or monoclonal antibodies, administered intravenously for 14 days either for induction or rescue from rejection.

The administration of these drugs is not without hazard. The major problem encountered with nonspecific immunosuppression is that it not only suppresses the immune response to the grafted tissue but also suppresses the body's capacity to respond to other antigenic stimuli. Consequently, the child is vulnerable to overwhelming infections.

Prednisone is an immunosuppressant and antiinflammatory agent that acts to stabilize cell walls, reduce migration of white blood cells into the inflamed area, and inhibit deposition of fibrin and collagen. It also depresses T cells, B cells, and phagocytes. A number of complications from corticosteroid therapy are cause for concern. Interference with linear growth has led many centers to use alternate-day administration in an effort to improve growth rates and to decrease other long-term side effects such as cataracts, fluid and sodium retention, hypertension, gastric ulcer, and obesity. Researchers are studying steroid free and early steroid withdrawal treatment protocols with the goal of minimizing side effects without compromising graft survival (Miller and Brennan, 2009).

Cyclosporine is a powerful immunosuppressant that acts to decrease the production of T cells. The side effects of this drug are hypertension, which may appear within several days of transplant; hirsutism; and nephrotoxicity. Serum blood levels determine maintenance doses of cyclosporine. After the initial IV therapy immediately after the transplant, the drug is administered orally. When the liquid form is used, each center has specific instructions for administering cyclosporine. The concerns are that the complete dose will be taken and absorption of the medication will be maximized.

Azathioprine, another immunosuppressant, interferes with cellular protein synthesis. The problem related to the toxic effect of azathioprine is mainly neutropenia, which is usually managed by reduced dosage. (See Chapter 36 for a discussion of immunosuppressive therapy and related nursing care.)

Rejection

Rejection of a transplanted kidney is the most common cause of transplant failure. Rejection can be one of three types: hyperacute, acute, or chronic. Hyperacute rejection is irreversible, develops immediately or within a few hours after revascularization, and is related to circulating antibodies preformed in the recipient against the donor tissue antigens.

Acute rejection usually occurs between the first few days and months after transplantation but may occur years later, especially if the patient becomes poorly compliant with immunosuppressant medications. Both biochemical and clinical abnormalities are evidence of rejection. The most common finding is fever, which is usually accompanied by swelling and tenderness over the graft, hypertension, and diminished urinary output. A severe reaction may cause oliguria. Increases in serum BUN and creatinine levels are laboratory evidence of decreased transplant function. Most acute rejection episodes respond to IV administration of methylprednisolone sodium succinate (Solu-Medrol), antilymphocyte globulin, or monoclonal antibodies.

> **! NURSING ALERT**
>
> The child with a kidney transplant who exhibits any of the following should be evaluated immediately for possible rejection:
> - Fever
> - Swelling and tenderness over graft area
> - Diminished urinary output
> - Elevated blood pressure
> - Elevated serum creatinine

Slow, gradual deterioration of renal function that typically begins 6 months or more after transplantation characterizes chronic rejection. Elevated serum creatinine, proteinuria, or hematuria are all signs of rejection. In addition, the rejection may have symptomatology indistinguishable from that of the original kidney disease. No present therapy can halt the process, which inevitably leads to loss of the implanted kidney.

Prognosis

The overall graft survival rate for kidneys at 1, 3, and 5 years is 96%, 91%, and 86% from living donors and 94%, 81%, and 80% from deceased donors, according to the annual report of the North American Pediatric Renal Trials and Collaborative Studies (2008). Predictors of graft survival for children include age at transplantation, pretransplantation dialysis, early rejection, and race. Malignancies, infection, and hypertension are the most life-threatening problems after transplantation (Groothoff, 2005). Long-term graft survival is not guaranteed, and many children require a second or third transplant. Successful kidney transplantation does improve rehabilitation of children with CRF, both educationally and psychologically.

Nursing Care Management

The possibility of kidney transplantation often comes as a hope for relief from the rigors of dialysis or the restriction of a conservative management regimen. Most children and families respond well to a kidney transplant. Children with successful kidney transplants are usually able to resume life activities similar to those of their unaffected peers. The rehabilitation of children with kidney transplants is influenced primarily by their pattern of functioning before becoming ill. It is important to remember that transplantation is a treatment that has a far less negative impact on the child's normal life activities than dialysis. However, stresses remain for the child and family in relation to the uncertainty of the future, the child's health and well-being, social isolation, and financial burdens.

A variety of serious emotional and psychologic conflicts may arise as a consequence of donor selection, including ambivalence of donors faced with surgery and relinquishing a kidney, feelings of guilt if one should prove to be unacceptable as a donor, and the emotional impact of having a live relative–donated kidney rejected by the recipient. This especially can result in guilt feelings when a parent is the donor.

The child recipient responds in various ways to a kidney transplant. The concept of having a foreign body, especially a deceased donor kidney, inside their own body is sometimes disturbing to children. They often speculate about the age, sex, personality, and physical characteristics of the donor. They may fear that the kidney will wear out if it came from an older person. Some children are distressed to find that their donor kidney came from a person of the opposite sex. Corticosteroid therapy, necessary in kidney transplants, creates undesirable side effects (e.g., growth failure, obesity, characteristics of Cushing syndrome [see Fig. 38-5], acne, and hirsutism) that are often a source of emotional and social problems for older children. Gum hyperplasia, brittle fingernails, and hair breaking can also occur.

⚡ DRUG ALERT

Medication Noncompliance After Kidney Transplant

The most common reason for poor medication adherence in childhood kidney transplant recipients is dislike of undesirable side effects. The cosmetic implications of the side effects can be overwhelming, especially to adolescent girls. Deliberate discontinuation of the drugs is most common in teenage girls. Problems with adherence are also commonly seen in children from poorly communicating families who are not supportive. (See Compliance, Chapter 27.)

Working with children and their families during the various stages of renal failure, dialysis, and transplantation is a difficult and challenging experience. Nurses must become familiar with the family; assess family strengths, weaknesses, and coping mechanisms; and be prepared to provide intensive support and guidance during the prolonged experience. The child and family need help accepting what is happening to them. They also need help in following the nurse's anticipatory guidance regarding predictable stresses and in dealing constructively with the physical, emotional, and financial burdens that are an ongoing part of this prolonged disability.

▐ KEY POINTS

- The main function of the kidney is to maintain the composition and volume of body fluids in equilibrium. Common inflammatory disorders of the genitourinary tract include UTI, nephrotic syndrome, and AGN.
- Management of UTIs is directed at eliminating infection, detecting and correcting functional or anatomic abnormalities, preventing recurrences, and preserving renal function.
- VUR is the retrograde flow of bladder urine into the ureters.
- Common features of AGN are oliguria, edema, hypertension, circulatory congestion, hematuria, and proteinuria.
- Therapeutic management of AGN involves maintenance of fluid balance and treatment of hypertension.
- Nephrotic syndrome is characterized by increased glomerular permeability to protein.
- Management of nephrotic syndrome is aimed at reducing excretion of protein, reducing or preventing fluid retention by tissues, and preventing infection and other complications. These are accomplished through dietary control, use of diuretics, corticosteroid therapy, and immunosuppressant therapy.
- Primary functions of the renal tubules are acidification of urine; potassium secretion; and selective and differential reabsorption of sodium, chloride, water, and other substances.
- The most common renal tubular disorders are renal tubular acidosis and NDI.
- Management of HUS is aimed at control of hematologic manifestations and complications of renal failure.
- In ARF management is directed at determining treatment of the underlying cause, managing the complications of renal failure, and providing supportive therapy.
- Abnormalities in CRF are waste product retention, water and sodium retention, hyperkalemia, acidosis, calcium and phosphorus disturbance, anemia, hypertension, and growth disturbances.
- When the child needs home dialysis, the nurse educates the family about the disease, its implications, the therapeutic plan, possible psychologic effects of the disease, and the treatment and technical aspects of the procedure.
- The major concerns in kidney transplantation are tissue matching, prevention of rejection, and psychologic concerns involving self-image as related to possible body changes resulting from the effects of corticosteroid therapy.

ANSWERS TO CRITICAL THINKING EXERCISES

Urinary Tract Infection and Constipation

1. **Yes.** Ginger's mother reports a history of constipation with large, hard-formed stools occurring only every 3 or 4 days. Ginger was diagnosed with a UTI severe enough to be admitted to the hospital.

2. **a.** The structure of the lower urinary tract is believed to account for the increased incidence of bacteriuria in females.
b. A history of hard, large stools occurring every 3 or 4 days is not a normal elimination pattern for 4-year-old children.
c. The presence of a large stool mass within the colon is likely to cause pressure on the bladder and urethra and not allow the bladder to empty completely. Stasis of the urine can lead to infection.

3. The first priority at this time is to begin treatment for the UTI. Ginger's diet and fluid intake should be evaluated and a plan developed to prevent constipation in the future.

4. Yes. Ginger's history reflects chronic problems with constipation that must be addressed.

Nephrotic Syndrome

1. **Yes.** The best response is 1. One of the complications of severe nephrotic syndrome is peritonitis. A careful abdominal examination and thorough history can provide important information.

2. **a.** Peritonitis can occur secondary to migration of intestinal bacteria across the bowel wall and into the protein-rich acidic fluid.
b. Infection is a constant source of danger to edematous children and those receiving corticosteroid therapy.

3. The fever and abdominal pain are the first priority. Actions 3 and 4 must be addressed, along with evaluation of the current stress level in the home, after the fever and pain have been addressed. Although his weight gain and reduced urinary output are major concerns, they are secondary to peritonitis. Obtaining a urine specimen for dipstick analysis is part of the initial assessment for Reese.

4. **Yes.** Children who are on steroid therapy are highly susceptible to complications of steroids. Infection is a major concern, and any child with fever and the other symptoms that Reese is currently exhibiting warrants a complete evaluation for peritonitis.

REFERENCES

American Academy of Pediatrics, Committee on Quality Improvement, Subcommittee on Urinary Tract Infections: Practice parameters: the diagnosis, treatment and evaluation of the initial urinary tract infection in febrile infants and young children, *Pediatrics* 103(4):843-853, 1999.

Anker MC, Amemann J, Neumann K: Alport syndrome with diffuse leiomyomatosis, *Am J Med Genet A* 119(3):381-385, 2003.

Bagga A, Mantan M: Nephrotic syndrome in children, *Indian J Med Res* 122(1):13-28, 2005.

Balat A, Karakok M, Guler E, et al: Local defense systems in the prepuce, *Scand J Urol Nephrol* 42:63-65, 2008.

Bell BP, Griffin PM, Lozano P, et al: Predictors of hemolytic uremic syndrome in children during a large outbreak of *Escherichia coli* O157-H7 infections, *Pediatrics* 100(1):127, 1997; available at www.pediatrics.org/cgi/content/full/100/1/e12 (accessed January 22, 2009).

Berry A: Helping children with dysfunctional voiding, *Urol Nurs* 25(3):193-201, 2005.

Bratslavsky G, Feustel PJ, Aslan AR, et al: Recurrence risk in infants with urinary tract infections and a negative radiographic evaluation, *J Urol* 172(4 Pt 2):1610-1613, 2004.

Caprioli J, Peng L, Remuzzi G: The hemolytic uremic syndromes, *Curr Opin Crit Care* 11(5):487-492, 2005.

Cerwinka WH, Scherz HC, Kirsch AJ: Endoscopic treatment of vesicoureteral reflux with dextranomer/hyaluronic acid in children, *Adv Urol*, 2008, doi: 10.1155/2008/513854.

Colodner R, Keness Y: Evaluation of DipStreak containing CNA-MacConkey agar: a new bedside urine culture device, *Isr Med Assoc J* 2(7):563-565, 2000.

Coppo R, Amore A: New perspectives in treatment of glomerulonephritis, *Pediatr Nephrol* 19(3):256-265, 2004.

Dacher JN, Savoye-Collet C: Urinary tract infection and functional bladder sphincter disorders in children, *Eur Radiol* 14(Suppl 4):L101-L106, 2004.

Dell KMR, Avner ED: Nephrogenic diabetes insipidus. In Kliegman RM, Behrman RE, Jenson HB, et al, editors: *Nelson textbook of pediatrics*, ed 18, Philadelphia, 2007, Saunders.

Durkan A, Hodson EM, Willis NS, et al: Non-corticosteroid treatment of nephrotic syndrome in children, *Cochrane Database Syst Rev* (2):CD002290, 2005.

Froom P, Bieganiec B, Ehrenrich Z, et al: Stability of common analytes in urine refrigerated for 24 hours before automated analysis by test strips, *Clin Chem* 46(9):1384-1386, 2000.

Geary DF, Piva E, Tyrrell J, et al: Home nocturnal hemodialysis in children, *J Pediatr* 147(3):383-387, 2005.

Gorman G, Fivush B, Frankenfield D: Short stature and growth hormone use in pediatric hemodialysis patients, *J Pediatr Nephrol* 20(12):794-800, 2005.

Grinsell MM, Showalter S, Gordon KA, et al: Single kidney and sports participation: perception versus reality, *Pediatrics* 118(3):1019-1027, 2006.

Groothoff JW: Long-term outcomes of children with end-stage renal disease, *Pediatr Nephrol* 20(7):849-853, 2005.

Hahn RG, Knox LM, Forman TA: Evaluation of poststreptococcal illness, *Am Fam Physician* 71(10):1949-1954, 2005.

Hardy RD, Austin JC: DMSA renal scans and the top-down approach to urinary tract infection, *Pediatr Infect Dis J* 27(5):476-477, 2008.

Hodson M, Knight JF, Willis NS, et al: Corticosteroid therapy for nephrotic syndrome in children, *Cochrane Database Syst Rev* (2):CD001533, 2004.

Houle AM, Cheikhelard A, Barrieras D, et al: Impact of early screening for reflux in siblings on the detection of renal damage, *BJU Int* 94(1):123-125, 2004.

Jepson RG, Craig JC: A systematic review of the evidence for cranberries and blueberries in UTI prevention, *Mol Nutr Food Res* 51(6):738-745, 2007.

Kasahara T, Hayakawa H, Okubo S, et al: Prognosis of acute poststreptococcal glomerulonephritis (APSGN) is excellent in children, when adequately diagnosed, *Pediatr Int* 43(4):364-367, 2001.

Kim JS, Bellew CA, Silverstein DM, et al: High incidence of initial and late steroid resistance in childhood nephrotic syndrome, *Kidney Int* 68(3):1275-1281, 2005.

Kliegman RM, Behrman RE, Jenson HB, et al: Hemolytic-uremic syndrome. In Kliegman RM, Behrman RE, Jenson HB, et al, editors: *Nelson textbook of pediatrics*, ed 18, Philadelphia, 2007, Saunders Elsevier.

Knoers NV, Monnens LA: Nephrogenic diabetes insipidus. In Avner ED, Harmon WE, Niaudet P, editors, *Pediatric nephrology*, ed 5, Philadelphia, 2004, Lippincott Williams & Wilkins.

Koff SA: Non-neuropathic vesicourethral dysfunction in children. In O'Donnel B, Koff SA, editors: *Pediatric urology*, Oxford, 1997, Butterworth-Heinemann.

Lavelle MT, Conlin MJ, Skoog SJ: Subureteral injection of Deflux for correction of reflux: analysis of factors predicting success, *Urology* 65(3):564-567, 2005.

Li PS, Ma LC, Wong SN: Is bag urine culture useful in monitoring urinary tract infection in infants? *J Paediatr Child Health* 38(4):377-381, 2002.

Miller BW, Brennan, DC: Withdrawal or avoidance of glucocorticoids after renal transplantation, *UpToDate* 2009, available at www.uptodate.com (accessed March 30, 2010).

Mingin GC, Hinds A, Nguyen HT, et al: Children with a febrile urinary tract infection and a negative radiologic workup: factors predictive of recurrence, *Urology* 63(3):562-565, 2004.

North American Pediatric Renal Trials and Collaborative Studies: *2008 Annual report*, 2008, available at http://web.emmes.com/study/ped/annlrept/annlrept.html (accessed March 30, 2010).

Ozaltin F, Besbas N, Bakkaloglu A, et al: Apoptosis and proliferation in childhood acute proliferative glomerulonephritis, *Pediatr Nephrol* 20(11):1572-1577, 2005.

Pirker ME, Mohanan N, Colhoun E, et al: Familial vesicoureteral reflux: influence of sex on prevalence and expression, *J Urol* 176(4 Pt 2):1776-1780, 2006.

Plachter NB, Schulman SL, Canning DA: Identification and management of urinary

tract infection in the preschool child, *J Pediatr Health Care* 13(6 Pt 1):268-272, 1999.

Raymond J, Sauvestre C: Microbiological diagnosis of urinary tract infections in the child: importance of rapid tests, *Arch Paediatr* 5(Suppl 3):260S-265S, 1998.

Raz R, Chazan B, Dan M: Cranberry juice and urinary tract infection, *Clin Infect Dis* 38(10):1413-1419, 2004.

Rice SG, Council on Sports Medicine and Fitness: Medical conditions affecting sports participation, *Pediatrics* 121(4):841-848, 2008.

Roth KS, Chan JC: Renal tubular acidosis: a new look at an old problem, *Clin Pediatr* 40(10):533-543, 2001.

Ruth EM, Kemper MH, Leumann EP, et al: Children with steroid-sensitive nephrotic syndrome come of age: long term outcome, *J Pediatr* 147(2):202-207, 2005.

Schlager TA, Anderson S, Trudell J, et al: Effect of cranberry juice on bacteriuria in children with neurogenic bladder receiving intermittent catheterization, *J Pediatr* 135(6):698-702, 1999.

Schroder CS: How to increase adequacy of peritoneal dialysis in children? *Peri Dial Int* 24(S3):S135-S136, 2005.

Shaikh N, Morone NE, Bost JE, et al: Prevalence of urinary tract infection in childhood: a meta-analysis, *Pediatr Inf Dis J* 27(4):302-308, 2008.

Siegler R, Oakes R: Hemolytic uremic syndrome: pathogenesis, treatment, and outcome, *Curr Opin Pediatr* 17(2):200-204, 2005.

Sillen U: Bladder dysfunction and vesicoureteral reflux, *Adv Urol* 2008, doi:10.1155/2008/815472.

Springhouse: Uremic frost. In: *Professional guide to signs and symptoms*, ed 5, Philadelphia, 2008, Lippincott Williams & Wilkins.

Sugarman RA: Structure and function of the neurologic system. In Huether SE, McCance KL, editors: *Understanding pathophysiology*, ed 2, St Louis, 2000, Mosby.

Tseng MH, Lin WJ, Lo WT, et al: Does a normal DMSA obviate the performance of voiding cystourethrography in evaluation of young children after their first urinary tract infection? *J Pediatr* 150:96-99, 2007.

Wadie GM, Tirabassi MV, Courtney RA, et al: The deflux procedure reduces the incidence of urinary tract infections in patients with vesicoureteral reflux, *J Laparoendosc Adv Surg Tech A* 17(3):353-359, 2007.

Wald ER: To bag or not to bag, *J Pediatr* 174(4):418-419, 2005.

Watanabe T: Proximal renal tubular dysfunction in primary distal renal tubular acidosis, *Pediatr Nephrol* 20(1):86-88, 2005.

Wein AJ, Kavoussi LR, Norvick AC, et al: *Campbell-Walsh urology*, ed 9, Philadelphia, 2006, Saunders.

Wilde MH, Brasch J: A pilot study of self-monitoring urine flow in people with long-term urinary catheters, *Res Nurs* 31:490-500, 2008.

Zorc JJ, Levine DA, Platt SL, et al: Clinical and demographic factors associated with urinary tract infection in young febrile infants, *Pediatrics* 116(3):644-648, 2005.

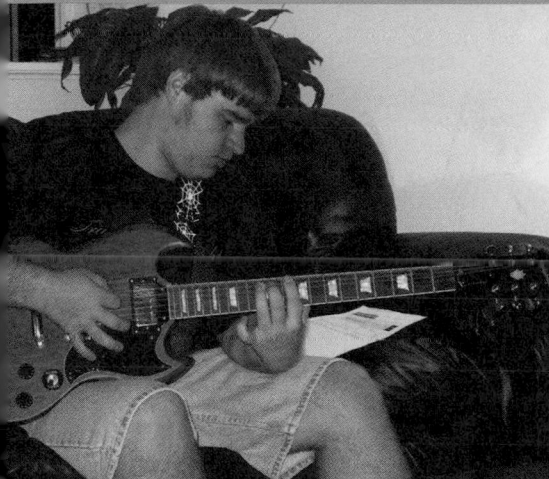

The Child with Disturbance of Oxygen and Carbon Dioxide Exchange

David Wilson

RESPIRATORY TRACT STRUCTURE AND FUNCTION

Disorders of the respiratory tract occur frequently in infancy and childhood. Anatomically, several factors influence the manner in which children, particularly infants, respond to respiratory disturbances.

The respiratory tract consists of many complex structures. The primary function of these structures is to distribute air and exchange gases so that cells are supplied with oxygen (O_2) for body metabolism while carbon dioxide (CO_2), the volatile product of metabolism, is removed. The nose, pharynx, larynx, trachea, bronchi, and lungs are structures of the respiratory system through which gases enter the body. The circulatory system distributes gases to and from the millions of cells throughout the body. All the structures of the respiratory system, except the minute air sacs (alveoli) of the lung tissue, function in air distribution. It is within the alveoli that gas exchange takes place.

STRUCTURE

The thoracic cavity, located in the bony framework provided by the ribs, vertebrae, and sternum, consists of three major sections: the three-lobed lung on the right; the two-lobed lung on the left; and the mediastinum, or the space between the lungs. The mediastinum contains the esophagus, trachea, large blood vessels, and heart. Smooth parietal pleura line the entire thoracic cavity and adhere to the ribs and superior surface of the diaphragm. Each lung is encased in a separate visceral pleural sac that, when inflated, lies against the parietal pleura. Normally the two pleural membranes are separated by only enough fluid to lubricate the surface for painless movement during filling and emptying of the lungs. In disease states this space may contain air (pneumothorax), fluid (pleural effusion), serum (hydrothorax), blood (hemothorax), or pus (pyothorax, also known as empyema). Inflammation of the pleura causes the painful friction of pleurisy during respiratory movements.

Chest

The chest has a relatively round configuration at birth but changes gradually to one that is more or less flattened in the anteroposterior (front-to-back) diameter in adulthood. In some lung diseases, chronic overinflation causes changes in these measurements. For example, in severe obstructive lung disease (e.g., asthma, cystic fibrosis) the anteroposterior measurement approaches the transverse (side-to-side) measurement to produce the so-called barrel chest. Periodic measurements provide clues to the course of the lung disease or the efficacy of therapy. Increased size indicates progressive obstructive lung disease.

The elliptic shape of the ribs and the angle at which they are attached to the spine allow the thorax to change size during respiration. Contraction of the intercostal muscles lifts the ribs from a downward angle to a more horizontal angle, which increases both the anteroposterior and the lateral dimensions of the chest (Fig. 31-1, *A*). This also changes the diameter of the bronchi; the diameter increases during inspiration and decreases during expiration, an important factor when the bronchi are narrowed as a result of obstruction or inflammation. Contraction and relaxation of the diaphragm cause the chest cavity to lengthen and shorten, which also increases the volume of the chest cavity during inspiration. Normal expiration is passive, although contraction of the internal intercostal muscles pulls the rib cage downward, and contraction of the abdominal muscles forces the diaphragm upward to actively decrease the chest size. (See Fig. 6-30.)

An adult's ribs articulate with the vertebrae and sternum from a downward and lateral angle. During inspiration the

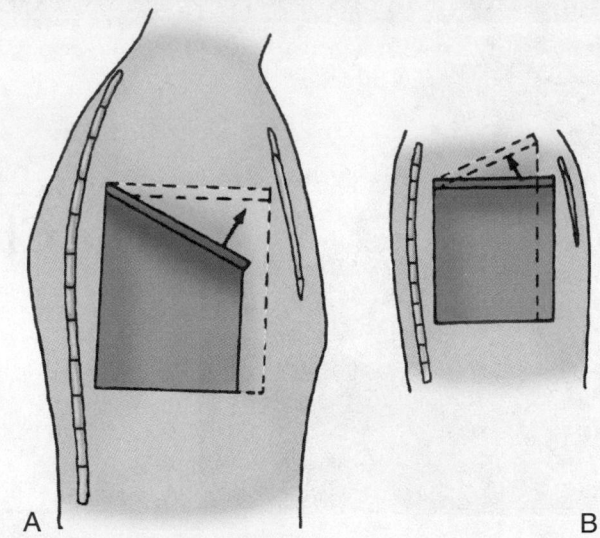

Fig. 31-1 Mechanisms of respiratory excursion. **A,** Downward and lateral position of rib in adult and expansion of lung capacity on thoracic inspiration. **B,** More horizontal position of rib in infant and decreased expansion of lung capacity on thoracic inspiration.

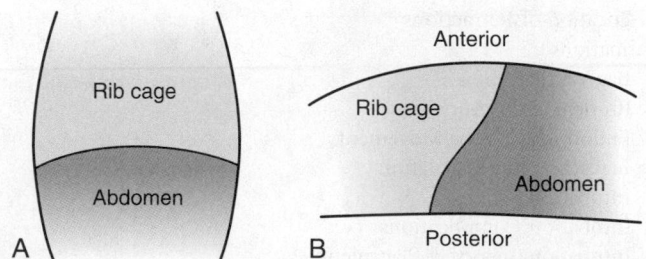

Fig. 31-2 Relationship of diaphragm and abdominal contents in upright **(A)** and supine **(B)** positions.

respiratory muscles contract and the thorax enlarges. In the newborn infant, however, the ribs articulate with the spine at a horizontal rather than a downward slope; consequently, during inspiration the diameter of the chest decreases (Fig. 31-1, *B*). The infant relies almost entirely on diaphragmatic-abdominal breathing. During inspiration the diaphragm is forced downward, increasing the available space for lung expansion; the intercostal muscles serve primarily as stabilizing forces. Respiration is facilitated by the processes of (1) **compliance**, the elastic property of lung tissue that allows it to expand and recoil; and (2) **resistance**, which affects the amount of flow through the airways (see p. 1185).

Variations occur in lung volume relative to posture. In the upright position the evenly distributed weight of the abdominal contents contributes to uniform application of negative intrathoracic pressure. However, in the supine position the abdominal contents apply weight caudally to create a nonuniform distribution of positive pressure to the diaphragm. Consequently, lung volume is increased in the upright position and decreased in the supine position. In addition, the mechanical attachment of the diaphragm to the rib cage is such that contraction elevates the rib cage in the upright position but in the supine position tends to pull in the rib cage (Fig. 31-2).

In the newborn the diaphragm is attached higher in front. Therefore this already stretched diaphragm is unable to contract as far or as forcefully as that of the older infant or child. Young infants are also less able to withstand diaphragmatic fatigue because of fewer energy-producing components. Abdominal distention from gas or fluid can impede diaphragmatic excursion significantly.

Airways

The rigid nasal structures, which are lined with ciliated mucous membranes, serve as passageways for air, warming and moistening air, filtering its impurities, and destroying microorganisms that come in contact with immune defenses in the mucosa. In infancy the nasal passages are narrow, and infants are primarily nose breathers. Any factor that decreases the size of the nasal passages and increases airway resistance, such as nasal mucosal swelling and mucus accumulation, hampers breathing and feeding.

The **upper airway** (oronasopharynx, pharynx, larynx, and upper part of the trachea) is shared by both the respiratory and the alimentary tracts, and many of the muscles in this area participate in several complex acts. However, the sequence of airway muscle activation is different in breathing and swallowing. The upper airway dilates during inspiration and constricts during exhalation. During some activities these dimensions are modified. For example, inspiration is short during crying, coughing, and sneezing, but with crying the larynx and pharynx dilate. The net result of swallowing is closure of the upper airway with interruption of airflow. Consequently, the timing and magnitude of muscle activation have important implications for airway size and patency.

The pharynx is a passageway for the entry and exit of air, and it plays a role in phonation by helping to produce vowel sounds. The pharynx contains the palatine and lingual tonsils, which are involved in infection control.

The larynx, situated at the upper end of the trachea, is made of a rigid circular framework of cartilage and contains the epi-

glottis and glottis (vocal cords). These structures prevent solids or liquids from entering the airway during swallowing, and the vibrations of the vocal cords produce voice sounds. In infancy the glottis is located more cephalad (toward the head) than in later childhood, and the laryngeal reflexes are active. The epiglottis is longer and projects farther posteriorly in infants. The narrowest portion of the larynx is at the level of the cricoid cartilage. In the infant and young child the ciliated columnar epithelium below the vocal cords is loosely bound with areolar connective tissue and is therefore more susceptible to edema formation. Swelling of the glottis and epiglottis produces hoarseness and often life-threatening obstruction of this portion of the airway.

The **lower airway** is made up of the lower trachea, mainstem bronchi, segmental bronchi, subsegmental bronchioles, terminal bronchioles, and alveoli. The trachea, which is composed of smooth muscle supported by C-shaped rings of cartilage, ensures an open airway to the bronchi and lungs. The trachea divides at the carina into two primary bronchi. The right one is situated slightly more vertical than the left, which causes aspirated objects to lodge more frequently in the right bronchus. Each bronchus enters the lung on its respective side, where it divides into secondary bronchi that continue to branch and divide into progressively smaller bronchioles. The entire bronchial tree is lined with mucous membrane and is composed of spiral smooth muscle supported by rings of cartilage. As the bronchioles become smaller, the cartilaginous rings become increasingly irregular and then disappear completely in the smallest bronchioles, the walls of which consist of only a single layer of cells (Fig. 31-3). There is a range of 23 to 26 levels of branches divided into two categories: the conducting airways and the terminal respiratory units. These branch levels are called *generations*.

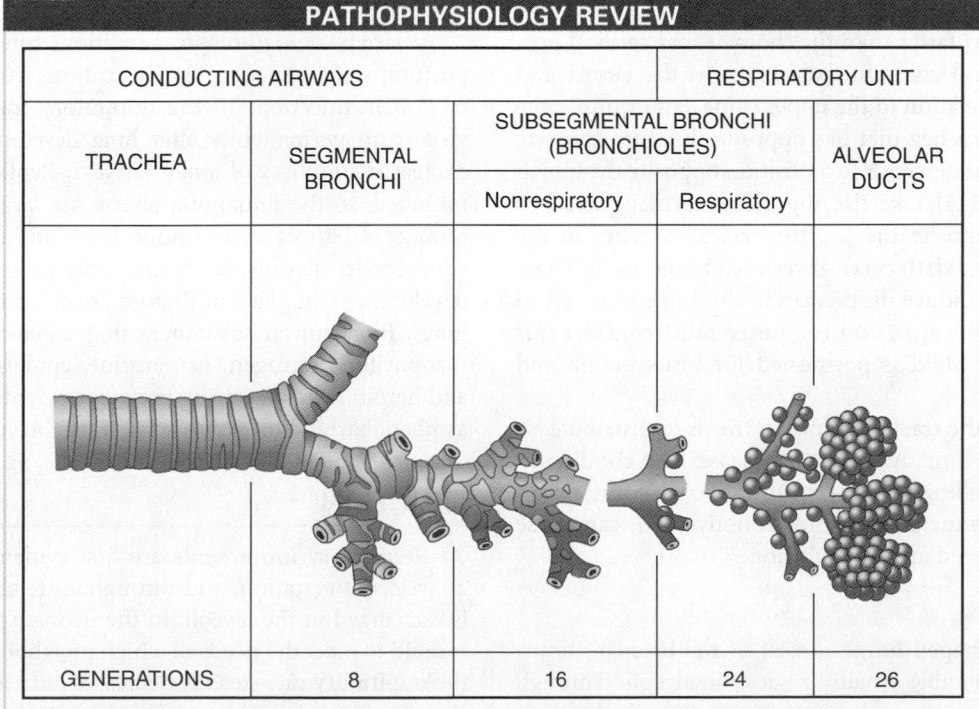

PATHOPHYSIOLOGY REVIEW

CONDUCTING AIRWAYS				RESPIRATORY UNIT
TRACHEA	SEGMENTAL BRONCHI	SUBSEGMENTAL BRONCHI (BRONCHIOLES)		ALVEOLAR DUCTS
		Nonrespiratory	Respiratory	
GENERATIONS	8	16	24	26

Fig. 31-3 Structures of the lower airway. (Redrawn from Thompson JM, McFarland GK, Hirsch JE, et al: *Mosby's clinical nursing,* ed 5, St Louis, 2002, Mosby.)

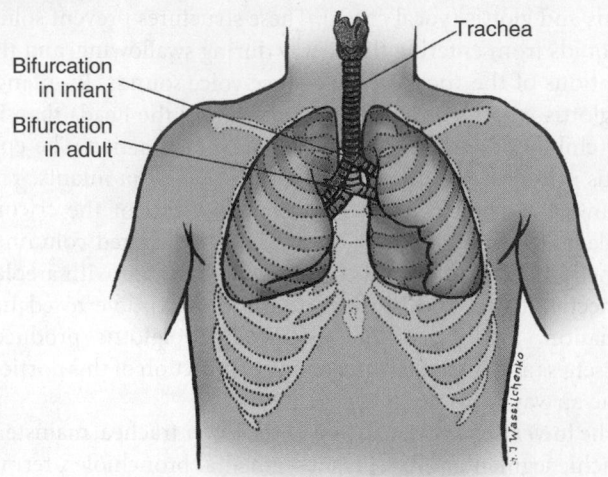

Fig. 31-4 Difference in level of bifurcation of trachea in the infant and adult.

All the structures are subject to obstruction from edema or foreign objects, but the degree of obstruction from constriction of smooth muscle differs. The diameter of the relatively rigid upper airway is less subject to constriction than the lower airway structures, which contain little cartilaginous support. The highly reactive bronchiolar smooth muscle of the lower airway structures can cause life-threatening obstruction during bronchospasm. The airway cartilage in young infants is soft and compressible; therefore the intrathoracic airways are highly reactive to stimuli, such as vagal nerve stimulation.

The airways of the newborn have little smooth muscle, but in children 4 to 5 months of age they contain sufficient muscle to cause narrowing in response to irritating stimuli. By 1 year of age, smooth muscle development and reactivity are comparable to those in the adult. Growth of the respiratory system follows the general growth curve during the early weeks of life, but the airways grow faster than the thoracic and cervical portions of the vertebral column. Consequently, the larynx and trachea descend in relation to the upper spine. For example, the bifurcation of the trachea that lies opposite the third thoracic vertebra in the infant descends to a position opposite the fourth in adulthood (Fig. 31-4). Likewise, the cricoid cartilage descends from a position opposite the fourth cervical vertebra in the infant to opposite the sixth cervical vertebra in the adult. These anatomic changes produce differences in the angle of access to the trachea at various ages, and the nurse must consider this when the infant or child is positioned for resuscitation and airway clearance.

The function of the tracheobronchial tree is to distribute air to the alveoli of the lung. A variety of diseases and conditions, such as mucosal swelling, muscular contraction, and mechanical obstruction by mucus or a foreign body (FB), can cause localized or generalized airway occlusion.

Respiratory Units

The two cone-shaped lungs consist of the bronchi; bronchioles; and innumerable small air sacs, or alveoli. Through these thin-walled sacs, gas exchange occurs by simple diffusion between the inspired air and the bloodstream. The amount of gas exchanged depends on many factors, including the amount and composition of air inhaled, thickness of the alveolar wall, adequacy of circulation to the alveoli, and substances within the alveoli that either prevent their inflation (e.g., surface-active surfactant) or prevent gas exchange (e.g., fluids).

With age, changes take place in the air passages that increase the respiratory surface area. The major changes are in the number and size of alveoli and in the increased branching of terminal bronchioles. Although the number of conducting airways is complete early in fetal life, the air sacs are shallow with wide necks and have few shared walls, or septa, at birth. This promotes patency but limits surface area for gas exchange. The alveoli are large with thick septa that have little elastic recoil (not unlike the emphysemic lung). During the first year, bronchioles continue to branch, and the globular alveoli formed earlier in the terminal units rapidly increase in number with each generation. These alveoli partition and divide existing alveoli to form smaller lobular units separated by thinner septa, thus enlarging the area available for gas exchange.

Alveoli increase steadily in number, but it is unclear when septal division ceases and an increase in size begins. It appears to occur sometime during middle childhood, although evidence indicates that an increase in the number of alveoli for each terminal airway takes place at puberty. Approximately nine times more alveoli are present at age 12 years than at birth. In later stages of growth the structures lengthen and enlarge. In addition, collateral pathways of ventilation develop, including pores through alveolar walls and possibly pathways between bronchioles.

All these factors have significant implications for respiratory disorders in children. Infants and young children have less alveolar surface area for gas exchange, the narrowly branching peripheral airways become easily obstructed, and lack of collateral pathways inhibits ventilation beyond obstructed units. Consequently, young children are subject to obstruction and atelectasis, especially as a result of repeated infection.

A variety of pathologic conditions affect lung growth. A postural defect such as kyphoscoliosis reduces the number of alveoli. Infections of the respiratory tract (e.g., coxsackievirus) can permanently alter lung development, resulting in decreased numbers of small airways. Replication of alveoli is inhibited, so the remaining alveoli are large but decreased in number. Changes in hormone levels influence lung growth. Glucocorticosteroids, thyroxine, and prolactin enhance lung development, but lack of thyroid hormone results in immature lungs. Biochemical substances that enhance lung growth are theophylline, estrogen, isoxsuprine, epidermal growth factor, and heroin injected during pregnancy. Some medications such as phenobarbital or excess insulin inhibit lung growth.

FUNCTION

Respiratory movements are first evident at approximately 20 weeks of gestation, and throughout fetal life amniotic fluid is exchanged in the alveoli. In the neonate the respiratory rate is rapid to meet the needs of a high metabolism. During growth the respiratory rate steadily decreases until it levels off at maturity. (See inside back cover.) The volume of air inhaled increases with the growth of the lungs and is closely related to body size. In addition, a qualitative difference exists in expired air at different ages. During growth the amount of oxygen in the expired air gradually decreases and the amount of carbon dioxide increases.

Ventilation, the exchange of gases in the lung, results from changes in pressure gradients created by changes in the size of the thoracic cavity. Contraction of the diaphragm and external intercostal muscles increases the size of the thorax and decreases the intrathoracic pressure. As a result, air moves from the atmosphere, which has a higher pressure, into the lungs, which have a lower pressure. The principles of artificial or mechanical ventilation are based on this concept. Mechanical (artificial) respiratory devices increase the pressure entering the air passages (positive pressure breathing devices) or lower the pressure around the body (negative pressure ventilator).

The two primary forces that affect the mechanics of breathing are compliance and resistance; conditions that either increase or decrease these two forces are listed in Box 31-1. Compliance is a measure of chest wall and lung distensibility. It represents the relative ease with which the chest and lungs expand with increasing volume and then collapse away from the pleural wall with decreasing volume (elastic recoil). The two major factors determining compliance are (1) alveolar surface tension, which is lowered by surfactant, a lipoprotein at the air-fluid interface that allows alveolar expansion and prevents alveolar collapse; and (2) elastic recoil, the tendency of the lungs to return to the resting state after inspiration (a passive process that requires no muscular effort). Other factors influencing compliance include the degree of tissue hydration, lung blood volume, surface forces at the air-fluid interface, and chest or

lung tissue pathologic state (e.g., fibers of elastin or collagen). Factors that interfere with compliance and recoil increase the work of breathing.

Compliance is normally high in the newborn and infant because of a more pliant (flexible) rib cage. This greater compliance causes the rib cage to be easily distorted with increased negative pressure in the pleural cavity or when factors inhibit the stabilizing action of the intercostal muscles. As the child grows, chest wall compliance decreases and elastic recoil increases; therefore ventilation becomes progressively more efficient. In pathologic states an increase in compliance indicates that the lungs or chest wall is abnormally easy to inflate and has lost some elastic recoil, such as in asthma. A decrease in compliance indicates that the lungs or chest wall is abnormally stiff or difficult to inflate, such as in respiratory distress syndrome (McCance and Huether, 2010).

Any condition that decreases or increases compliance or increases airway resistance results in increased work of breathing (increased respiratory rate, retractions, nasal flaring). When respiratory muscle fatigue develops, respiratory failure will occur.

Resistance is determined primarily by airway size. The body must overcome three sources of resistance during breathing: tissue resistance in the chest wall (about 20% resistance); tissue resistance in the lungs (about 15% resistance); and, most important, flow resistance in the airways (which often increases with respiratory disease). The four factors determining resistance are flow rate velocity, gas viscosity, length of airway, and airway diameter. If any of the first three variables increases, resistance to airflow also increases. If airway diameter decreases, resistance increases exponentially.

The small diameter of children's airways increases the potential risk of any condition that reduces airway size. Fig. 31-5 illustrates the difference that airway size plays in older children's and infants' responses to airway compromise.

The diameter of the airways and thus the airflow are determined by the balance of forces that tend to widen or narrow the airways. One of these is neural regulation of bronchial smooth muscles mediated through autonomic nerves. Sympathetic impulses relax the airways; parasympathetic impulses constrict them. Reflex constriction occurs in response to irritating inhalants such as dust, smoke, or sulfur dioxide; arterial hypoxemia and hypercapnia; cold air; and some drugs, such as acetylcholine and histamine. Other factors that alter airway size are peribronchial pressure, which tends to narrow the airways, and intraluminal pressure, which tends to keep the airways open. For example, forced expiration causes increased peribronchial pressure and hence narrowing of the airways; a positive pressure breathing apparatus increases intraluminal pressure, keeping the airways open.

Gas Exchange

Gases in the blood are measured by the partial pressures (tensions) of the individual gases and are expressed in millimeters of mercury. With oxygen therapy it is important to understand the relationship between the concentration of the inspired gas and the partial pressure of that gas in the arteries (Pao_2). Inspired oxygen is expressed as the fraction of inspired oxygen (Fio_2), with 1.0 indicating 100% oxygen, 0.5 indicating 50%

Newborn

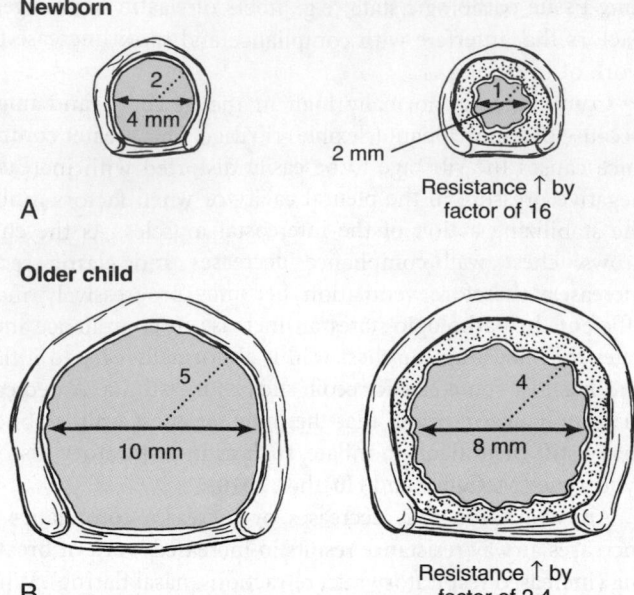

Older child

A

Resistance ↑ by factor of 16

B

Resistance ↑ by factor of 2.4

Fig. 31-5 Effects of 1 mm of circumferential edema in small neonate and older child. **A,** Neonate possesses a larynx approximately 4 mm in diameter and 2 mm in radius. If 1 mm of circumferential edema develops, it will halve the airway radius and increase resistance to air flow by a factor of 16. **B,** Older child possesses a larynx approximately 10 mm in diameter and 5 mm in radius. The 1 mm of circumferential edema will reduce the radius by 20% (from 5 mm to 4 mm) and increase resistance to air flow by a factor of 2.4. (From Hazinski MF, editor: *Nursing care of the critically ill child*, ed 2, St Louis, 1992, Mosby.)

oxygen, and so on. Patients breathing room air have an FiO_2 of 0.21 because ambient air contains 21% oxygen.

Ambient air is composed of 21% oxygen, trace amounts of carbon dioxide, and 79% nitrogen (N). Water vapor (H_2O) also exerts pressure. The water vapor does not change with the barometric pressure (P_B) but exerts a constant pressure of 47 mm Hg when the gas is fully saturated at body temperature. Each gas contributes to the total barometric pressure as follows:

$$P_B = P_{O_2} + P_{CO_2} + P_{N_2} = P_{H_2O}$$

At sea level, the total pressure of gases in the atmosphere and the blood (P_B) is always equal to 760 mm Hg.

The significance of inspired gases lies in the FiO_2 and the pressure it exerts (PiO_2). At sea level this can be calculated as follows:

$$PiO_2 = FiO_2 \times (P_B - P_{H_2O})$$
$$PiO_2 = 0.21 \times (760 - 47)$$
$$PiO_2 = 0.21 \times 713$$
$$PiO_2 = 150 \text{ mm Hg}$$

When the FiO_2 increases (e.g., to 50%), the pressure exerted also increases:

$$PiO_2 = 0.50 \times (760 - 47)$$
$$PiO_2 = 0.50 \times 713$$
$$PiO_2 = 356.5 \text{ mm Hg}$$

As the inspired gas travels down the airway and reaches the alveoli, the pressure drops as carbon dioxide is added to the mixture. Ambient air contains only traces of carbon dioxide. As

BOX 31-2   FACTORS AFFECTING GAS DIFFUSION IN ALVEOLI

Pressure gradient between alveolar air and capillary blood—For gases to diffuse across this gradient, the gas molecules must pass through the barrier of liquid surfactant lining the alveolus. Disease can greatly increase this barrier, thus interfering with the diffusion process.

Alveolar ventilation, or amount of air that reaches the alveoli—Any obstruction to air passing from the upper airways through the bronchi to the alveoli decreases the volume of air available for diffusion. Minute ventilation is the amount of air inhaled in a normal breath (tidal volume) multiplied by the respiratory rate. Factors affecting the respiratory rate or tidal volume may decrease the amount of air available for diffusion.

Relationship between amount of alveolar air and alveolar perfusion—Factors that decrease the amount of alveolar perfusion increase the ventilation/perfusion ratio. Factors or disease states that increase or decrease the amount of alveolar air also create a ventilation/perfusion mismatch and abnormal levels of PO_2 or PCO_2 in the blood.

the gas diffuses from the capillary blood to the alveoli, however, the amount and pressure of carbon dioxide in the alveoli increase to the carbon dioxide levels in the venous blood (approximately 40 mm Hg). By subtracting the PCO_2 from the PiO_2, one can determine the alveolar oxygen pressure (PAO_2). The $PACO_2$ is first divided by 0.8. This correlation factor, or respiratory quotient (RQ), is used to calculate the ratio of oxygen absorbed to carbon dioxide eliminated. The alveolar pressure can then be expressed as:

$$PAO_2 = PiO_2 - (PACO_2 \div 0.8)$$
$$PAO_2 = 150 - (40 \div 0.8)$$
$$PAO_2 = 150 - 50$$
$$PAO_2 = 100 \text{ mm Hg}$$

Because normal venous PO_2 is approximately 40 mm Hg, a gradient is created when the PAO_2 is 100 mm Hg and diffusion occurs between the alveoli and capillary blood. When the patient's PAO_2 decreases, the FiO_2 can be raised to increase the PAO_2, thereby increasing the gradient for diffusion. Because carbon dioxide is more soluble than oxygen, it diffuses 21 times faster; therefore diffusion of carbon dioxide from the blood to the alveoli is not impaired. The amount of oxygen that diffuses into the blood and the amount of carbon dioxide removed by the lungs depend on several factors (Box 31-2).

Oxygen and Carbon Dioxide Transport

Once oxygen has diffused from the alveolus to the pulmonary capillary, it is transported throughout the body in two ways. A small amount (PaO_2) is transported as a solute dissolved in the plasma and the water of red blood cells. A larger portion (40 to 70 times as much) is carried by hemoglobin as oxyhemoglobin. Because each gram of hemoglobin can combine with 1.34 ml of oxygen, the transport capacity is largely determined by the amount of hemoglobin present. Thus children with severe anemia tend to be fatigued and breathe more rapidly. In addition, increasing the amount of oxygen delivered to the alveoli can increase the amount carried by the blood only in relation to the amount of hemoglobin present. For example, at a PaO_2 of 100 mm Hg, hemoglobin is 97.5% saturated. Hemoglobin saturation is commonly termed *arterial oxygen saturation* (SaO_2)

or *oxyhemoglobin saturation*. The nonlinear relationship between the Pao_2 and the Sao_2 is described by the oxyhemoglobin dissociation curve (see Fig. 31-10).

Carbon dioxide is carried in the blood in a number of ways. A small amount ($Paco_2$) is transported dissolved in the plasma and the water of red blood cells. A large amount (more than half) hydrates to form carbonic acid, which dissociates and is carried as bicarbonate and hydrogen ions. The remaining carbon dioxide combines with certain plasma proteins and hemoglobin. The association of carbon dioxide with hemoglobin is accelerated by an increasing $Paco_2$ and a decreasing Pao_2 and is decreased by the opposite conditions. The diffusion of carbon dioxide into the alveoli is very rapid. Thus the equilibrium between the $Paco_2$ of the pulmonary capillaries and the alveoli is achieved promptly. Transport between blood and tissue cells is accomplished down a diffusion gradient, just as it is between the blood and the alveoli.

Regulation of Respiration

The mechanisms that control respiration are divided into two categories: (1) a neural system that maintains a coordinated, rhythmic respiratory cycle and regulates the depth of respiration; and (2) a chemical system that regulates alveolar ventilation and maintains normal blood gas pressures.

Neural control in the respiratory center is located in three areas: a pneumotaxic center, which modulates the respiratory frequency and depth; an apneustic center, which produces an inspiratory spasm and is modulated by the pneumotaxic and medullary centers and by vagal afferent impulses; and the medullary respiratory centers, both inspiratory and expiratory, which regulate the rhythmicity of respirations. Impulses from other areas also affect the respiratory centers. Proprioceptive vagal impulses in the lung parenchyma are sensitive to stretching. When lungs become stretched, impulses are transmitted by the vagus nerve to the respiratory center, which inhibits further inflation and prevents overdistention (the Hering-Breuer reflex). The cerebral cortex also helps control respirations by voluntary inhibition or acceleration of the rate and depth of respirations. Reflex apnea can result from sudden painful stimulation, sudden cold stimulation, and stimulation to the larynx or pharynx (the choking reflex, which serves to prevent aspiration).

Chemical control is mediated by specialized structures—central chemoreceptors, located in the medulla, and peripheral chemoreceptors, located in the great vessels—that respond to changes in pH, Pco_2, and Po_2. Peripheral chemoreceptors of greatest physiologic importance are the carotid bodies, located at the division of the common carotid artery into its external and internal branches, and the aortic bodies that lie between the ascending aorta and the pulmonary artery. Carbon dioxide and hydrogen ions control respiration by acting directly on the respiratory center; the peripheral chemoreceptors respond to changes in Po_2. Thus an increase in ventilation can result from either (1) stimulation of the respiratory center by an increased $Paco_2$ or pH; or (2) a decreased Pao_2, which stimulates the carotid and aortic bodies. These bodies then transmit signals to the brain to excite the respiratory center.

The lungs also have an important role in acid-base balance. Less rapid than the chemical buffers, the respiratory mechanism begins to act within 1 to 3 minutes to make adjustments in pH by eliminating or retaining carbon dioxide. When the levels of carbon dioxide are altered sufficiently, the respiratory centers in the brain respond by either increasing or decreasing the rate and depth of respiration. For example, when the pH of the blood drops, as from increased exercise, a compensatory increase in respirations rids the body of the carbon dioxide derived from carbonic acid, which is formed from buffered acid metabolites. Carbon dioxide buildup from breath holding produces the same response, again increasing the carbonic acid and reducing the serum pH. Therefore the lungs serve as compensatory organs in metabolic disturbances and respond quite rapidly.

Defenses of the Respiratory Tract

The respiratory tract has several anatomic and biochemical characteristics that provide natural defenses against the many biologic and inanimate agents that can damage respiratory tissues. Intact defenses help repel and resist the impact of injurious agents; factors that reduce the integrity of these mechanisms increase the vulnerability of these tissues to invasion and disease. Respiratory tract defenses include:

Lymphoid tissues—Faucial, lingual, and pharyngeal tonsils (adenoids) and other pharyngeal lymphoid tissues form a protective circle around the entrance to the respiratory tract. These help localize and contain invading organisms so they can be destroyed by the body's humoral defense mechanisms.

Mucous blanket—The epithelium of the respiratory tract secretes sticky mucus to which airborne organisms adhere.

Ciliary action—The mucus secreted by the columnar epithelium of the respiratory tract is kept flowing, carrying microorganisms and other foreign agents away from the lungs to be coughed or swallowed.

Epiglottis—The epiglottis and the epiglottis reflex protect the respiratory tract from invading material, including infectious exudate from the upper tract, and prevent such material from being aspirated into the lower tract.

Cough—The expulsive force of the cough reflex propels foreign material out of the lower tract.

Position changes—Changes in body position encourage drainage of tracheobronchial passages.

Lymphatics—Lymphatics draining the terminal bronchi and bronchioles remove invading organisms, which are filtered and destroyed in the regional lymph nodes.

Humoral defenses—Organisms and other foreign material are removed or destroyed by phagocytes, enzymes, and immunoglobulins, especially immunoglobulin A, secreted by the bronchial epithelium.

Some children have conditions (e.g., chronic asthma, cystic fibrosis, and the various immunodeficiency disorders) that predispose them to infection as a result of interference with the efficiency of these mechanisms. Frequent, intense exposure to organisms that accompany conditions of crowding or continual exposure to irritating substances in the air results in breakdown of healthy defenses. Concurrent illness, malnutrition, or fatigue reduces the efficiency of natural defenses. Drying of the mucous membranes also inhibits the activity of humoral defenses, such as immunoglobulins.

ASSESSMENT OF RESPIRATORY FUNCTION

PHYSICAL ASSESSMENT

Information about the child's respiratory status is obtained from observations of physical signs and behavior. However, to make a useful assessment, the nurse must know what to look for and how to interpret findings. (See Physical Examination: Chest, Chapter 6.) Auscultation of the lung fields is helpful in identifying specific pathologic conditions and in assessing the child's responses to treatment. Auscultation is essential when determining airway patency. Palpation and percussion provide information regarding areas of pain and tissue density. Chapter 6 describes breath sounds and their terminology.

Respiration

Assess the configuration of the chest and the pattern of respiratory movement, including rate, regularity, symmetry of movements, depth, effort expended in respiration, and use of accessory muscles of respiration. To determine deviations, the nurse must know the normal type and rate of respiration in relation to the child's size and age. (See inside back cover.) Respirations (ventilations) are best determined when the child is sleeping or quietly awake.

Tachypnea (rapid respirations) often occurs with anxiety, elevated temperature, severe anemia, and metabolic acidosis. It may also be associated with respiratory alkalosis caused by psychoneurosis and with central nervous system (CNS) disturbances. By observing changes in respiratory rate, the nurse can follow and evaluate the progress of disorders that contribute to low compliance, such as the pneumonias, pulmonary edema, and pleural effusion.

Alterations in the depth of respirations—too deep (hyperpnea) or too shallow (hypopnea)—are recognized as abnormal only in the extremes. Hyperpnea is noted with fever, severe anemia, respiratory alkalosis associated with psychosis, CNS disturbances, and respiratory acidosis that accompanies disorders such as diabetic ketoacidosis or diarrhea. Hypoventilation may occur with metabolic alkalosis in conditions such as hypertrophic pyloric stenosis and respiratory acidosis that accompanies diaphragmatic paralysis or CNS depression. Hypoventilation in preterm infants may occur as a result of pulmonary immaturity, absence of adequate substrate to support respiratory muscle activity, neurologic insult, and neurologic immaturity. Children with neuromuscular diseases such as spinal muscular atrophy may also exhibit hypoventilation. Congenital central hypoventilation syndrome, or Ondine curse, is a rare CNS defect in which respiratory failure occurs as a result of the respiratory system's failure to respond to increasing carbon dioxide levels; this condition has been known to occur in children with Hirschsprung disease and is often manifested on the first day of life (Haddad, 2007).

Associated Observations

Retractions, or a sinking in of soft tissues relative to the cartilaginous and bony thorax, may occur in some pulmonary disorders. In disease states (particularly in severe airway obstruction), retractions become extreme. Subcostal retraction, observed anteriorly at the lower costal margins, indicates a flattened diaphragm because it not only lowers the floor of the thorax, but also pulls on the rib cage in response to a greater than normal decrease in intrathoracic pressure. In severe airway obstruction, retractions extend to the supraclavicular areas and the suprasternal notch (Fig. 31-6).

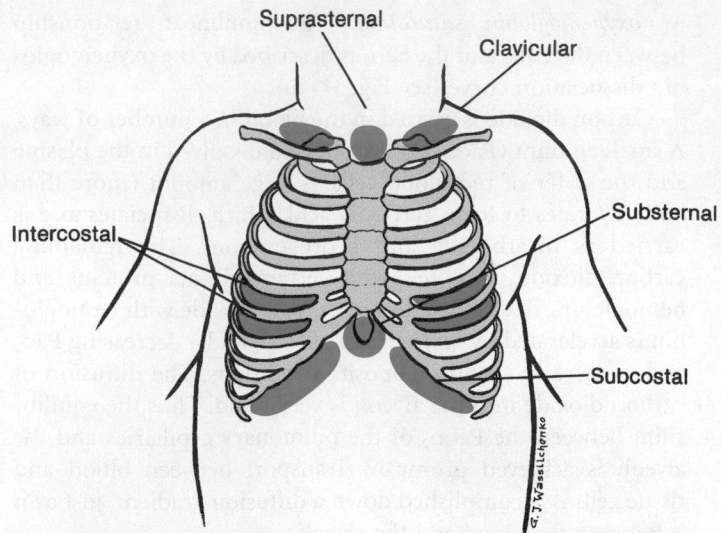

Fig. 31-6 Location of retractions.

Nasal flaring is a sign of respiratory distress and a significant finding in an infant. The enlargement of the nostrils helps reduce nasal resistance and maintains airway patency. Nasal flaring may be intermittent or continuous and should be described as minimum or marked.

Head bobbing in a sleeping or exhausted infant is a sign of dyspnea. The head, supported on the caregiver's arm only at the suboccipital area, bobs forward with each inspiration. This is caused by neck flexion resulting from contraction of the scalene and sternocleidomastoid muscles. Noisy breathing such as "snoring" is frequently associated with hypertrophied adenoidal tissue, choanal obstruction, polyps, or an FB in the nasal passages.

Stridor, which is a high-pitched, noisy respiration, is usually an indication of narrowing of the upper airway, either as a result of edema and inflammation, or in association with an upper airway obstruction, often from mucus secretions or possibly from a foreign object. Stridor may be inspiratory or expiratory. Common causes in children include croup, epiglottitis, FB, or tracheitis (Boat and Green, 2007).

Grunting is frequently a sign of pain in older children, suggesting acute pneumonia or pleural involvement. It is also observed in pulmonary edema and is a characteristic of respiratory distress in newborns and infants. It is the body's attempt at more efficient respirations. Grunting serves to increase end-respiratory pressure and thus prolong the period of oxygen and carbon dioxide exchange across the alveolocapillary membrane.

Wheezing is a continuous musical sound originating from vibrations in narrowed airways (Watts and Goodman, 2007). Wheezing is primarily heard on expiration and may be either polyphonic (with widespread narrowing of the airways [e.g., asthma]), or monophonic (single-pitched sound produced in the larger airways [e.g., tracheomalacia]). Infants may have wheezing as a result of increased airway resistance and a compliant chest wall; there is evidence that inflammatory mediators such as histamines, leukotrienes, and interleukins may also contribute to wheezing in infants (Watts and Goodman, 2007). Older children often have wheezing with a lower respiratory tract infection as a result of inflammation, bronchospasm, and accumulated secretions, all of which serve to narrow the airways and produce the characteristic wheezing sound.

Color changes of the skin, especially mottling, pallor, and cyanosis, are important. Except for the peripheral bluish discoloration (acrocyanosis) resulting from circulatory stasis in the newborn or the mottling or peripheral cyanosis resulting from a cool environment, mottling and cyanosis are significant and usually indicate cardiopulmonary disease.

Chest pain may be a complaint of older children and may have a variety of causes, both pulmonary and nonpulmonary. It may be caused by disease of any of the chest structures—esophagus, pericardium, diaphragm, pleura, or chest wall. Parietal pleural pain is usually localized over the affected area and is aggravated by respiratory movements. The pain of diaphragmatic pleural irritation may be referred to the base of the neck posteriorly and anteriorly or to the abdomen. Most pleural pain is related to respiration; therefore respiratory movements are shallow and rapid and may be accompanied by grunting, especially in the younger patient.

Clubbing, or proliferation of tissue about the terminal phalanges, accompanies a variety of conditions, frequently those associated with chronic hypoxia, primarily cardiac defects, and chronic pulmonary disease (e.g., cystic fibrosis). Although clubbing often worsens with lung disease, it does not accurately reflect disease progression. The degree of clubbing depends on the extent to which the nail base is lifted on the dorsal surface of the phalanx by the tissue proliferation. The greater the angle formed above the finger or toe at the skin-nail junction, the more pronounced the clubbing, especially when there is a decided curvature to the nail (Fig. 31-7).

Cough is often associated with respiratory disease, although it may suggest other disorders (Box 31-3). It serves as a protective mechanism and an indicator of irritation. A cough can be initiated voluntarily but is usually a result of a complex reflex consisting of three components: afferent nerve fibers, the cough center, and efferent nerve fibers. The respiratory epithelium contains afferent receptors that are sensitive to mechanical or chemical stimuli. These receptors are concentrated in the areas of the larynx, the carina, and the bifurcations of the large and medium-sized bronchi. When a stimulus is applied to these areas, impulses are transmitted via the vagus nerve to the cough center in the brainstem. Efferent impulses travel via the vagus, phrenic, and spinal motor nerves to the larynx, intercostal muscles, diaphragm, abdominal muscles, and pelvic floor. An inspiratory gasp and closure of the glottis are followed by contraction of muscles in the chest wall, diaphragm, abdomen, and pelvic floor. The resulting compression and increase in pleural, alveolar, and subglottic pressure cause a sudden opening of the glottis and immediate release of trapped air at extremely rapid expiratory flow rates, which forces undesirable material from the respiratory tract.

Inflammation or infection in the upper or lower respiratory tract may produce coughing. Some types of cough are characteristic of specific diseases. For example, a severe cough is associated with measles and cystic fibrosis, and the paroxysmal cough accompanied by an inspiratory "whoop" is typical of pertussis in small children. A brassy, nonproductive cough is part of the symptomatology of croup and FB aspiration. Because there are no cough receptors in the alveoli, a cough may be absent in a child with pneumonia in the early stages of the disease but is a common feature during active pneumonia and recovery. The nurse assesses a cough according to the features listed in Box 31-4.

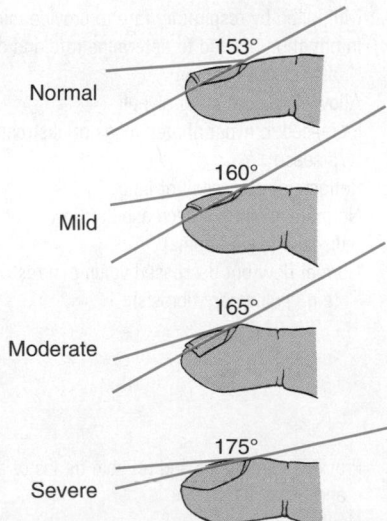

Fig. 31-7 Stages of clubbing. Degree of angle formed above finger at skin-nail junction indicates extent of clubbing. Angle greater than 160 degrees and decided curvature of nail are good criteria for presence of clubbing. (Modified from Waring WW: The history and physical examination. In Chernick V, editor: *Kendig's disorders of the respiratory tract in children*, ed 6, Philadelphia, 1998, Saunders.)

BOX 31-3 CAUSES OF COUGH

Inflammatory disorders
- Asthma
- Infection—viral or bacterial

Lung disease
- Cystic fibrosis
- Bronchiolitis/respiratory syncytial virus
- Retained foreign body
- Congenital malformations (e.g., tracheomalacia)
- Other

Focal or anatomic lesions
Psychogenic or habit cough
Postnasal drip or sinusitis
Allergic rhinitis (hay fever) with postnasal drainage
Bacterial bronchitis
Gastroesophageal reflux disease

BOX 31-4 COUGH ASSESSMENT

Onset and duration
Age of child
Type—Dry, hacking, moist or wet, barking, brassy, paroxysmal (a sudden attack, outburst, or intensification of symptoms)
Progress—Better, worse, unchanged, persistent
Pattern—Daytime, nighttime, both, different intensity with time or activity
Associated symptoms—Sore throat, dyspnea, pain and its location
Secretions—Sputum presence, consistency, color, frequency, evidence of swallowing sputum, postnasal drip

DIAGNOSTIC PROCEDURES

Several procedures are available for assessing respiratory function and diagnosing respiratory disease. All these procedures require preparation and support of the child and the family to ensure cooperation and accurate results (see Family-Centered Care box). These procedures not only are useful in diagnosis, but also provide information that guides nursing interventions,

FAMILY-CENTERED CARE

Preparing the Family for Procedures and Equipment

When Janet was 4 weeks old, she was hospitalized suddenly with pneumonia and was admitted to the pediatric intensive care unit. Janet was attached to several monitors, was receiving oxygen, and had a small device on her toe that gave off a little red light. Janet was our first baby, and to see her with all this equipment was frightening. I was not prepared for any of it. However, a wonderful nurse who was taking care of Janet explained the reason for the oxygen and told me that the mysterious red light was called a pulse oximeter. The nurse said that this device measured the amount of oxygen Janet had in her blood. The nurse also told me what the numbers should be to indicate that Janet had a normal amount of oxygen in her blood. I could see that the oxygen Janet was getting kept the amount of oxygen in the normal range. Once the nurse had told me all this, I was much more relaxed and could concentrate on talking to Janet and breast-feeding her. This nurse's explanation meant so much to me. I wish I could tell every nurse just how important it is to keep explaining all the procedures and equipment to parents.

Janet's mother

such as positioning, use of supplemental oxygen, and monitoring oxygenation and respiratory status.

Pulmonary Function Tests

Noninvasive pulmonary mechanics are often measured at the bedside of infants and children with the use of pneumotachography or spirometry. However, information obtained limits diagnosis because the same functional abnormality may occur in different diseases. These tests are useful to evaluate the severity and course of a disease and to study the effects of treatment (Table 31-1 and Fig. 31-8).

Radiology and Other Diagnostic Procedures

Radiography is used frequently in diagnostic evaluation of children (Table 31-2). Although no definitive information exists on the effects of low-dose radiation, providers take action to protect vulnerable areas from possible damage. When possible, technicians and others try to prevent unnecessary exposure of the child (and nursing personnel), and they protect the more radiosensitive areas. Careful protection of the patient's immature gonads with lead shields is essential. Other sensitive areas are the thyroid gland, ocular lens, and bone marrow.

Although nurses have limited control over the length, frequency, and correct application of the x-ray beam, they can make certain that the infant or child receives proper protection from possible hazards. Lead shields, correctly placed and consistently applied to areas not needed for diagnostic purposes,

TABLE 31-1   PULMONARY FUNCTION TESTS USED IN CHILDREN

TEST	MEASUREMENT	SIGNIFICANCE
Forced vital capacity (FVC) (peak flow)	Maximum amount of air that can be expired after maximum inspiration	Reduced in obesity Reduced in obstructive airway disease Normal in restrictive disease
Forced expiratory volume in 1 (FEV$_1$) or 3 (FEV$_3$) sec	Amount of air that can be forced from lungs after maximum inspiration in 1 and 3 sec	Normally 80% of FVC in 1 sec Reduced in obstructive disease Is single best measure of airway function
Tidal volume (TV or V$_T$)	Amount of air inhaled and exhaled during any respiratory cycle	Multiplied by respiratory rate to provide minute volume Information needed to determine rate and depth of artificial ventilation
Functional residual volume (FRV); functional residual capacity (FRC)	Volume of air remaining in lungs after passive expiration	Allows for aeration of alveoli Increased in hyperinflated lungs of obstructive lung disease
Dynamic compliance	Relationship between change in volume and pressure difference	Reflects elastic recoil of lung Normal volume but decreased airflow in obstructive disease (e.g., asthma) Normal flow but decreased volume in restrictive disease (e.g., pulmonary fibrosis)
Pulmonary resistance	Changes in pressure with changes in flow on inspiration and expiration	
Work of breathing	Total work expended moving lung and chest	
Respiratory time constancy	Time for proximal and alveolar airway pressure to equilibrate	
Transcutaneous oxygen/carbon dioxide monitoring (TCM)	Skin electrodes heated and applied to well-perfused areas of trunk; measurements in mm Hg	Provides continuous and reliable trends of arterial O$_2$ and CO$_2$ Noninvasive
Pulse oximetry	Photometric measurement of oxygen saturation (SaO$_2$) Measurements in percentages	Provides continuous noninvasive measurements of hemoglobin saturation
FEV$_1$/FVC or FEV$_3$/FVC	Percentage of maximum inspiration that is expired in 1 or 3 sec	Normally 95% of FVC in 3 sec Reduced in obstructive disease

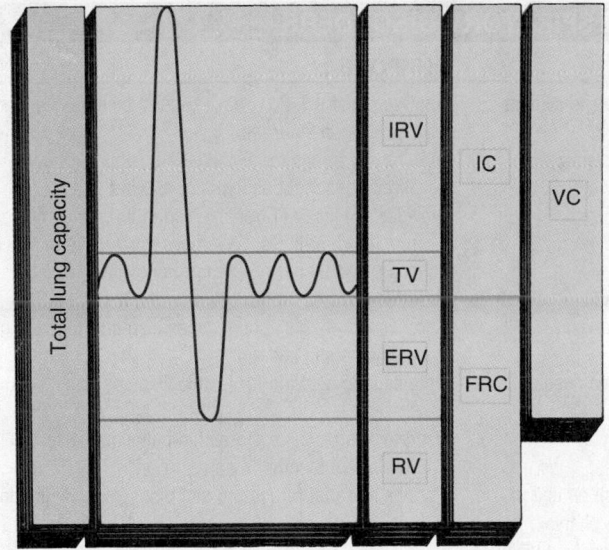

Fig. 31-8 Divisions of total lung capacity. Total lung capacity (TLC) is maximum amount of air contained in lungs. TLC is divided into four primary volumes: *IRV*, inspiratory reserve volume; *TV*, tidal volume; *ERV*, expiratory reserve volume; and *RV*, residual volume. Capacities are combinations of two or more lung volumes. These include inspiratory capacity *(IC)*, functional residual capacity *(FRC)*, and vital capacity *(VC)*. (From Shapiro BA, Harrison RA, Walton R: *Clinical application of blood gases*, ed 3, St Louis, 1982, Mosby.)

are essential. Play and modification of methodology effectively reduce the trauma sometimes associated with the procedure and gain the child's cooperation. Nurses, regardless of age and pregnancy status, should use protective equipment to guard against unnecessary radiation exposure during diagnostic examinations.

Several other procedures are used to diagnose lung disorders (Table 31-3). Most require specialized equipment and skills. All require preparation of the child.

Blood Gas Determination

Blood gas measurements are sensitive indicators of change in respiratory status in acutely ill patients (Table 31-4). They provide valuable information regarding lung function, lung adequacy, and tissue perfusion and are essential for monitoring conditions involving hypoxemia, carbon dioxide retention, and pH. For the acutely ill patient, this information also guides decisions regarding therapeutic interventions, such as adjusting mechanical ventilator settings, modifying chest physiotherapy (CPT), administering oxygen, or positioning the child for maximum ventilation. Both invasive and noninvasive methods are available (see Atraumatic Care box).

Pulse oximetry provides a continuous or intermittent noninvasive method of determining oxygen saturation (Sao_2).

TABLE 31-2	RADIOLOGIC EXAMINATIONS		
TEST	**DESCRIPTION**	**PURPOSE**	**COMMENT**
Radiography	Pictures obtained by passing x rays through body and recording them on sensitized film	Produces images of internal structures of chest, including air-filled lungs, airways, vascular markings, heart, and great vessels	Requires preparation, cooperation, and immobilization of child
Fluoroscopy	Projection of electronically intensified image on viewing screen	Used primarily to study diaphragmatic excursion and respiratory motion of lungs	Requires preparation and immobilization of child
		Examination of contrast-filled esophagus to outline mediastinal abnormalities	
Bronchography	Contrast medium instilled directly into bronchial tree through opaque catheter inserted via orotracheal tube	Valuable to demonstrate and inspect bronchiectasis	Carried out with child under general anesthesia or sedation
		Detects distal bronchial obstruction	Used less frequently than other examinations
		Detects malformations	Requires preparation of child for anesthesia
Barium (contrast solution) swallow	Esophagus outlined when barium solution or contrast is swallowed	Esophageal displacement defining mediastinal masses	Valuable adjunct for diagnosis
			Performed under fluoroscope
		Detects swallowing disorders and malformations (e.g., gastroesophageal reflux, tracheoesophageal fistula)	Requires preparation of child for procedure
Angiography	Injection of dye to produce image of pulmonary vasculature	Investigation of pulmonary vascular anomalies and pulmonary hypertension	Performed with child under general anesthesia
			Requires preparation of child for anesthesia
Computed tomography (CT)	Sequence of x rays, each representing a cross section or "cut" through lung tissue at different depth	Useful in identifying presence of calcium or cavity within a lesion, hilar adenopathy, mediastinal masses, or abnormalities	Usually reserved for children old enough to suspend respiration voluntarily
			Requires preparation of child for procedure
Magnetic resonance imaging (MRI)	Use of large magnet and radio waves to produce two- or three-dimensional image	Clearly identifies soft tissues	Requires cooperation or sedation of child
			Requires preparation of child for procedure or anesthesia
Radioisotope scanning	Intravenous injection of albumin labeled with radioisotopes or inhalation of radioactive aerosols or xenon gas, followed by radiation scanning	Delineates defects in pulmonary arterial perfusion and diseased areas of lungs	Requires cooperation or sedation of child
		Detects location of aspirated foreign body	Requires preparation of child for procedure
Ultrasonography	Transmission of sound waves through chest	Identifies opacification	Limited use in diagnosis of respiratory disorders
			Requires preparation of child for anesthesia depending on age and ability to hold still

TABLE 31-3   DIAGNOSTIC PROCEDURES USED IN RESPIRATORY DISORDERS

PROCEDURE	DESCRIPTION	PURPOSE
Arterial blood gas	Blood obtained from an artery with a needle and syringe	Analyze blood pH, Pco_2, base excess, bicarbonate, and blood oxygen saturation
Tracheal aspiration	Sputum obtained by direct aspiration from trachea	Obtains secretions for examination, culture
Bronchoscopy	Direct observation of tracheobronchial tree via bronchoscope	Localizes abnormalities in major airways Provides access to (1) remove aspirated foreign bodies from major airways, (2) remove obstructive mucous plugs, and (3) perform bronchial lavage
Capnography	Measures carbon dioxide during inhalation and exhalation cycle and produces a graph of carbon dioxide concentration over time	Provides end-tidal carbon dioxide levels to determine trends and identify shunts; may also be used during anesthesia and sedation
Lung puncture	Needle aspiration of lung fluid via syringe and needle through intercostal space	Obtains lung aspirate for histologic study or culture
Lung biopsy	Removal of lung tissue via open thoracotomy or closed-needle procedures	Used for diagnosis of protracted pulmonary disease unexplained by other means
Brush biopsy	Material for biopsy obtained with nylon brush on end of wire passed through tube placed via nose, pharynx, trachea, and airways (via fluoroscope) to involved lung segment	Obtains material for culture and histologic examination
Percutaneous transtracheal aspiration	Needle and catheter aspiration of tracheal secretions through thyroid cartilage	Obtains secretions for laboratory examination and culture

TABLE 31-4   BLOOD GAS ANALYSIS

COMPONENT	DEFINITION	NORMAL VALUE*	ACIDOSIS	ALKALOSIS
pH	Indicates acid-base status of body	Adult: 7.35-7.45 Child: 7.39	<7.35 indicates excess of acid	>7.45 indicates excess of base
Pco_2	Pressure exerted by dissolved carbon dioxide in blood Under control of lungs Respiratory component	Adult: 35-45 mm Hg Child: 37 mm Hg	>45 mm Hg Causes—Obstructive lung disease, hypoventilation of any cause	<35 mm Hg Causes—Hypoxia, pulmonary embolism, hyperventilation of any cause
Bicarbonate (HCO_3)	Buffers effect of acid in blood Under control of kidneys Metabolic component	Adult: 22-26 mEq/L Child: 22 mEq/L	<22 mEq/L Causes—Diarrhea, lactic acidosis, renal failure, shock, therapy with acetazolamide, diabetic ketoacidosis, drainage of pancreatic juice	>26 mEq/L Causes—Fluid loss from upper gastrointestinal tract, diuretics, corticosteroid therapy
Base excess (BE)	Reflects status of all bases in blood	Adult: ±2 Child: ±3	More negative	More positive
Po_2	Pressure exerted by dissolved oxygen in blood Indicates effectiveness of oxygenation by lungs	Adult: 90-110 mm Hg Child: 96 mm Hg	<80 mm Hg; hypoxia Causes—Obstructive lung disease, high carbon dioxide levels, low Fio_2, hypoventilation	>100 mm Hg; hyperoxygenation Causes—High Fio_2, hyperventilation

Modified from Custer JW, Rau RE, editors, Johns Hopkins Hospital Department of Pediatrics: *The Harriet Lane handbook,* ed 18, St Louis, 2009, Mosby.
*Values for child are for those ages 7-19 yr.
NOTE: The Sao_2 printed with blood gas reports cannot be used as a standard to confirm oximetry readings. Blood gas analyzers provide only approximate blood oxygen saturations based on calculations using measured blood gases, pH, and Pao_2.

ATRAUMATIC CARE

Blood Gas Monitoring

For continuous monitoring of blood gases, noninvasive measurements are used whenever possible. Oximetry should be used before arterial punctures are performed when information about oxygen saturation is sufficient to evaluate the child's condition.

A sensor composed of a light-emitting diode (LED) and a photodetector is placed in opposition around a foot, hand, finger, toe, or earlobe, with the LED placed on top of the nail when digits are used (Fig. 31-9). The diode emits red and infrared lights that pass through the skin to the photodetector. The photodetector measures the amount of each type of light absorbed by functional hemoglobins (those capable of carrying oxygen). Hemoglobin saturated with oxygen (oxyhemoglobin) absorbs more infrared light than does hemoglobin not saturated with oxygen (deoxyhemoglobin). A microprocessor determines the difference between absorption of the red and

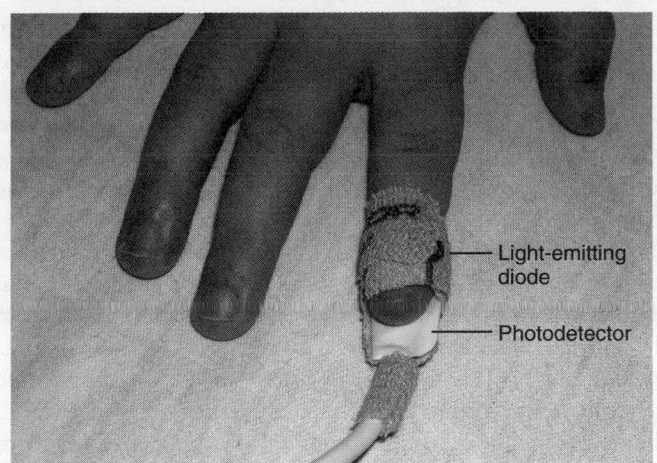

Fig. 31-9 Oximeter sensor on right second finger. Note that sensor is positioned with light-emitting diode opposite photodetector.

- Light-emitting diode
- Photodetector

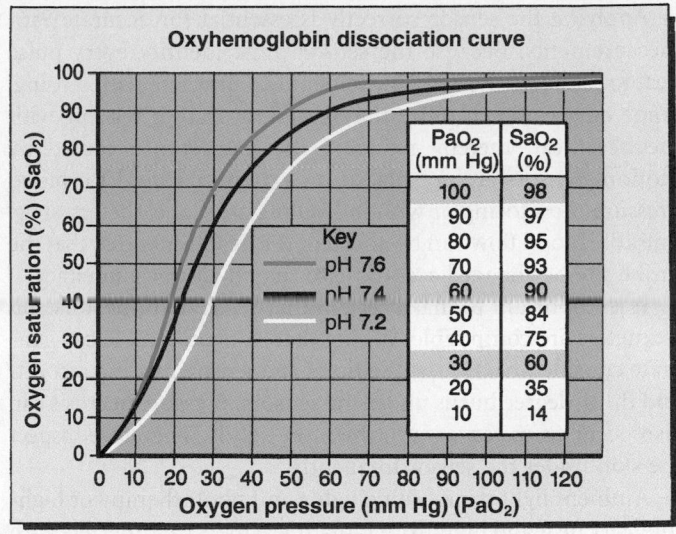

Fig. 31-10 Oxyhemoglobin dissociation curve. Changes in affinity of hemoglobin for oxygen shift the position of oxyhemoglobin dissociation curve. Standard curve *(black):* Assumes normal pH (7.4), temperature, and PCO_2 levels. Shift to left *(blue):* Increased oxygen affinity of hemoglobin: increased pH, decreased temperature and PCO_2. Shift to right *(white):* Decreased oxygen affinity of hemoglobin: decreased pH, increased temperature and PCO_2.

NURSING TIP A quick formula for calculating correlation of Pao_2 with Sao_2 is the 30-60, 60-90 rule. Assuming a normal pH, $Paco_2$, and body temperature, this rule can apply:

When Pao_2 = 30, Sao_2 = 60; when Pao_2 = 60, Sao_2 = 90

---

infrared light. The percentage of the total normal hemoglobin that is oxygenated is displayed on a monitor.

Pulsatile blood flow is the primary physiologic factor that influences accuracy of the pulse oximeter. In most infants with continuous pulse oximetry monitoring, the nurse must change the electrode site at least every 3 to 4 hours to prevent pressure necrosis (in infants with poor perfusion or disrupted skin integrity). In infants with poor perfusion and temperature problems such as hypothermia or sensitive skin, the probe may need more frequent changing. In an active or crying infant motion artifact may make the reading more difficult to obtain.

Another noninvasive method is transcutaneous monitoring (TCM), which provides continuous monitoring of transcutaneous partial pressure of oxygen in arterial blood ($tcPao_2$) and, with some devices, of carbon dioxide in arterial blood ($tcPaco_2$). An electrode is attached to the warmed skin to facilitate arterialization of cutaneous capillaries. The site of the electrode must be changed every 3 to 4 hours (or more frequently according to skin status) to avoid burning the skin, and the machine must be calibrated with every site change. This monitoring is used frequently in neonatal intensive care units, but it may not reflect an accurate Pao_2 in infants with impaired local circulation.

The Pao_2 can be correlated with the Sao_2 by means of the oxyhemoglobin dissociation curve (Fig. 31-10), although changes in Pao_2 do not cause identical (linear) changes in Sao_2. The curve represents the relationship between Pao_2 (measured in the blood) and Sao_2 (measured by the pulse oximeter). As seen on the graph, when the Pao_2 is 60 mm Hg, the Sao_2 is 90%. Increasing the Pao_2 above this point does not significantly increase Sao_2 or greatly improve oxygen delivery to the tissues. At this point, further increases in the Pao_2 will only increase the dissolved oxygen in the blood and will not, under normal conditions, contribute significantly to the arterial oxygen content. On the lower part of the curve, however, even small changes in the Pao_2 produce large changes in saturation. This is an advantage at the tissue level, especially in low oxygen states (hypoxia) because a small decrease in Pao_2 will cause a relatively large unloading of oxygen to the tissues.

Oximetry is insensitive to hyperoxia because hemoglobin approaches 100% saturation for all Pao_2 readings above approx-

imately 100 mm Hg, which is a potentially dangerous situation for the preterm infant at risk for developing oxidative stress. Oxidative stress may lead to complications such as bronchopulmonary dysplasia and retinopathy of prematurity. (See Chapter 10.) Therefore the preterm infant being monitored with oximetry should have a range of upper limits identified, such as 89% to 93%, and a protocol should be established for decreasing oxygen when saturations are high.

Several factors affect the degree to which oxygen combines with hemoglobin. A shift of the curve to the left causes an increased affinity of hemoglobin for oxygen, but the oxygen is not easily released to the tissues. This represents an increase in the Sao_2 if it is measured against the same Pao_2 of the normal oxyhemoglobin dissociation curve. This left shift can be caused by an increase in blood pH or a decrease in $Paco_2$ or body temperature.

A shift of the curve to the right causes a decreased affinity of hemoglobin for oxygen but improved oxygen release to the tissues. This represents a lower Sao_2 if measured against the same Pao_2 of the normal oxyhemoglobin dissociation curve. This rightward shift can be caused by a decrease in blood pH or an increase in $Paco_2$ or body temperature.

Oximetry offers several advantages over TCM. Oximetry (1) does not require heating the skin, thus reducing the risk of burns; (2) eliminates a delay period for transducer equilibration; and (3) maintains an accurate measurement regardless of the patient's age or skin characteristics or the presence of lung disease.

Applying the sensor correctly is essential for accurate Sao_2 measurements. Because the sensor must identify every pulse beat to calculate the Sao_2, movement can interfere with sensing. Some devices synchronize the oxygen saturation reading with the heartbeat, thereby reducing the interference caused by motion. Sensors are not placed on extremities used for blood pressure monitoring or with indwelling arterial catheters, since pulsatile blood flow can be affected. It is recommended that the probe site be changed according to manufacturer guidelines.

It is important to make certain that sensory connectors and oximeters are compatible. Wiring that is incompatible can generate considerable heat at the tip of the sensor, causing second- and third-degree burns under the sensors. Pressure necrosis can also occur from sensors attached too tightly. Therefore inspect the skin under the sensor frequently.

Ambient light from ceiling lights and phototherapy or high-intensity heat and light from radiant warmers can interfere with readings. Therefore cover the sensor to block these light sources. Intravenous dyes; green, purple, or black nail polish; nonopaque synthetic nails; and possibly ink used for footprinting can also cause inaccurate Sao_2 measurements. The nurse should remove the dyes or, in the case of porcelain nails, use a different area used for the sensor. Skin color, thickness, and edema do not affect the readings. Elevated levels of carboxyhemoglobin, methemoglobin, and fetal hemoglobin affect the accuracy of the device because it can only distinguish between oxyhemoglobin and deoxyhemoglobin; therefore the child with carbon monoxide poisoning may have a normal Sao_2 reading but an abnormal (low) Pao_2.

NURSING TIP

For the infant—Secure the sensor to the great toe and tape the wire to the sole of the foot (or use a commercial holder that fastens with a self-adhering closure). Placing a snugly fitting sock over the foot may help anchor the device, but check the site frequently for color, temperature, and pulses.

For the child—Secure the sensor to the index finger and tape the wire to the back of the hand. Use self-adhering Ace type of wrap (e.g., Coban) around the finger or hand to further secure the sensor and wire. For the child with compromised skin, check the site periodically for color, temperature, and pulses.

Arterial blood gas (ABG) sampling helps to evaluate gas exchange and oxygenation and may be performed on blood from an artery or a capillary. Historically, some controversy surrounds the collection of "arterialized" capillary blood for blood gas measurements. However, many believe it to be a safe, convenient, and relatively accurate method, and that capillary blood gas (CBG) can accurately reflect the arterial pH and Pco_2 in most pediatric disease states (Yildizdas, Yapicioglu, Yilmaz, et al, 2004; Bilan, Behbahan, and Khosroshahi, 2008). The blood samples are obtained by a heel stick after dilation of the vascular bed by warming. The first drop of blood is discarded, and subsequent blood is collected directly into heparinized capillary tubes held in a horizontal position.

ABG samples may also be obtained through an indwelling arterial catheter or by arterial puncture. The sites most commonly used for arterial puncture include the radial, dorsalis pedis, posterior tibial, and femoral arteries. A catheter may also be placed in the neonate's umbilical artery for ABG sampling. The femoral artery is the last choice because hemorrhage and hematomas are difficult to control in this area and the risk for limb ischemia is high if the femoral artery is damaged (Curley and Moloney-Harmon, 2001). Risks of arterial puncture include pain, artery damage, decreased perfusion to the extremity distal to the puncture site, thrombosis, and hemorrhage (see Atraumatic Care box). Before a radial artery puncture, perform the Allen test to assess adequacy of the collateral circulation. To perform the test, elevate the extremity distal to the puncture site and blanch it by squeezing gently (such as making a fist). The two arteries supplying blood flow to the extremity (such as the radial and ulnar arteries in the wrist) are then occluded. Lower the extremity, and remove pressure from one artery (such as the ulnar). If color returns to the blanched extremity in less than 5 seconds, this indicates collateral circulation.

ATRAUMATIC CARE

Arterial Blood Punctures

Arterial blood punctures are painful. Buffered lidocaine, a local anesthetic, may be administered intradermally immediately over the artery to minimize discomfort during the blood-drawing procedure. However, small volumes of the anesthetic should be used because large volumes can produce arterial spasm (Zander and Hazinski, 1992). EMLA (a eutectic mix of lidocaine and prilocaine) or LMX4 (4% lidocaine), both topical anesthetics, can be applied (EMLA 1 hour before procedure under an occlusive dressing and LMX4 15 to 30 minutes before procedure; dressing is optional for LMX4).

An accurate ABG or CBG requires unclotted whole or capillary blood; therefore use a heparinized syringe or capillary tube to draw blood samples. Do not allow air bubbles to enter the sample, since air alters the blood gas concentration. Many institutions use prepackaged ABG sampling kits, which allow air-free samples to be drawn without the need for heparin dilutions. The amount collected depends on the child's size. Depending on the laboratory facilities, as little as 0.1 ml may be sufficient in small infants. After obtaining the blood sample, pack it in ice to reduce blood cell metabolism and have it taken to the laboratory immediately for analysis. Table 31-4 lists normal ABG and pH measurements on room air at sea level for adults and children 7 to 19 years of age.

Although ABG values are similar for children and adults, newborns can have slightly lower values and still be considered normal. For example, normal pH values for a newborn range from 7.26 to 7.29, the average Pao_2 is 70 mm Hg, the average $Paco_2$ is 33 mm Hg, and the average bicarbonate is 20 mEq/L.

ABG values also depend on the concentration of oxygen the child is breathing. The arterial Po_2 should rise in proportion to the oxygen concentration being inhaled. Therefore, when evaluating ABG values, consider the following: the percentage of oxygen administered (if any), the child's body temperature (as little as 1° F can alter the blood gas values 5% to 8%), and the presence of anxiety (if children hyperventilate, carbon dioxide is exhaled) or crying (can cause breath holding, resulting in decreased Pao_2).

The significance of ABG determination is related primarily to the relationships among the following three parameters: pH,

TABLE 31-5	ADVANTAGES AND DISADVANTAGES OF VARIOUS OXYGEN-DELIVERY SYSTEMS	
SYSTEMS	**ADVANTAGES**	**DISADVANTAGES**
Oxygen mask	Various sizes available; delivers higher oxygen concentration than cannula Able to provide a predictable concentration of oxygen (with Venturi mask) whether child breathes through nose or mouth	Skin irritation Possibility child has fear of mask or suffocation Accumulation of moisture on face Possibility of aspiration of vomitus Difficulty in controlling precise oxygen delivery concentration
Nasal cannula	Provides low-moderate oxygen concentration (22%-40%) Child able to eat and talk while getting oxygen Possibility of more complete observation of child because nose and mouth remain unobstructed	Must have patent nasal passages May cause abdominal distention and discomfort or vomiting Difficulty controlling oxygen concentrations if child breathes through mouth Inability to provide mist if desired
Oxygen tent (rarely used)	Achievement of lower oxygen concentrations ($FiO_2 \leq 0.3$-0.5) Child able to receive increased inspired oxygen concentrations even while eating	Necessity for right fit around bed to prevent leakage of gas Cool and wet tent environment Poor access to patient; inspired oxygen levels fall when tent is entered
Oxygen hood	Achievement of high oxygen concentrations ($FiO_2 < 1.00$) Free access to patient's chest for assessment	High humidity environment Need to remove patient for feeding and care

Modified from Hazinski MF, editor: *Nursing care of the critically ill child,* ed 2, St Louis, 1992, Mosby.

PO_2, and PCO_2. (See Acid-Base Imbalance, Chapter 28.) Any change in a blood gas value must be compared with the other values and with previous readings, as well as with the child's clinical appearance and behavior, medical history, and associated physiologic factors.

Clinical indications for blood gas analysis include changes in pulse oximetry, color (e.g., mottling, pallor, cyanosis, or duskiness), depth or rate of respirations (e.g., shallow and rapid), behavior or sensorium, and vital signs. Blood gas analysis is also used to determine adequacy of treatment and optimal ventilator settings in infants and children on supplemental oxygen and noninvasive and invasive mechanical ventilation. The nurse may or may not obtain the blood sample by arterial puncture, depending on the institution's policies. In any event, nurses must understand the results of blood gas analyses because these results provide essential information to guide nursing interventions (e.g., changing the position, performing suction, administering prescribed drugs, or notifying the practitioner).

One approach to determine a simple acid-base disturbance:

- Evaluate the pH to determine whether acidosis or alkalosis is present.
- Evaluate the PCO_2 to determine whether the imbalance is respiratory.
- Evaluate the bicarbonate levels to determine whether the imbalance is metabolic.

In a patient with a mixed acid-base disorder, compensatory factors (renal, pulmonary, or both) have been set in motion to equilibrate the blood pH. (See Acid-Base Imbalance, Chapter 28.)

RESPIRATORY THERAPY

OXYGEN THERAPY

The indication for administration of oxygen is hypoxemia (reduced blood oxygenation). Oxygen is delivered by mask,

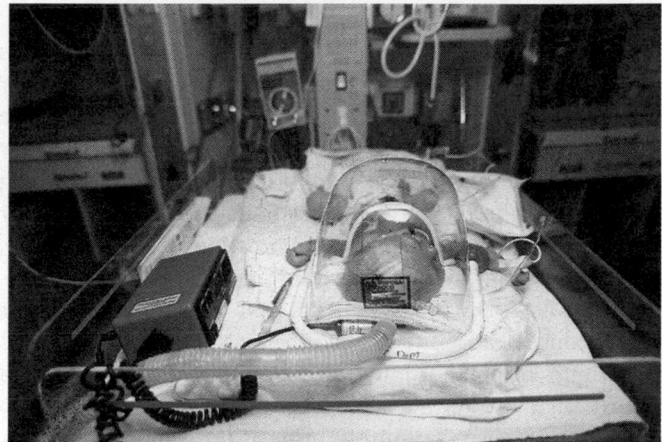

Fig. 31-11 Oxygen administered to infant by means of plastic hood. Note oxygen analyzer (blue machine).

nasal cannula, tent, hood, face tent, or ventilator (Table 31-5). The mode of delivery is selected on the basis of the concentration needed and the child's ability to cooperate in its use. The concentration of oxygen delivered should be regulated according to the individual child's needs. There are hazards related to its use; therefore continue oxygen only as long as needed and at the prescribed amount. Because medical-grade oxygen from piped systems or tanks is anhydrous, humidification of the gas before administration to the patient is essential.

Oxygen therapy is frequently administered in the hospital, although increasing numbers of children are receiving oxygen in the home. It is the responsibility of the nurse or respiratory care practitioner to ensure uninterrupted delivery of the appropriate oxygen concentration and to monitor the child's response to the therapy.

Oxygen Administration

Oxygen delivered to infants is well tolerated by using a plastic hood (Fig. 31-11). Low and high concentrations of oxygen can be easily maintained in this head hood, and most nursing procedures can continue without interrupting the oxygen delivery.

At least 4 to 5 L/min of flow is necessary to maintain oxygen concentrations and remove the exhaled carbon dioxide.

The humidified oxygen should not be blown directly into the face of an infant in a hood. Cold fluid or air applied to the face stimulates receptors that trigger the diving reflex, which causes bradycardia and shunting of blood from peripheral to central circulation. The oxygen hood should not rub against the infant's neck, chin, or shoulder.

Older infants and children can use a nasal cannula or prongs. Nasal cannula may also be used for lower concentrations of oxygen for infants and children who do not require high oxygen concentrations; the cannula has two soft prongs, which are inserted into the nares, providing flow into the nasopharynx. Skin care of the nasal alae is important to prevent breakdown.

Oxygen masks are available in pediatric sizes. The simple oxygen mask fits over the patient's nose and oxygen is delivered as the child breathes. The simple oxygen mask is used for short-term oxygen therapy, and it should be used at oxygen flow rates greater than 5 to 6 L/min to minimize carbon dioxide rebreathing. The simple mask has side holes to permit room air to enter into the mask to be mixed with oxygen. Signs of carbon dioxide rebreathing include somnolence, dizziness, headache, tingling, and eventually unconsciousness. A partial rebreathing mask is similar to the simple mask in that the plastic reservoir fits over the child's face; the partial rebreather has a reservoir at the base of the mask that receives expired air and fresh gas so lower oxygen flow rates (<4 L/min) can be used. The nonrebreathing mask is similar to the partial rebreathing mask, but the former has a one-way valve that limits rebreathing carbon dioxide. Another valve on the nonrebreathing mask's reservoir ensures that room air is not mixed with oxygen, thus providing higher oxygen concentrations (provided the mask fits correctly).

At times the child or infant may become quite agitated with the use of a mask, and a blow-by method may be used to provide low oxygen concentrations (<30%), humidification, or aerosolized medication. The blow by can be made with any oxygen tubing, corrugated tubing, or a mask held approximately 2 to 3 inches from the child's nose and mouth. It is recognized that this method is not the optimal choice of oxygen delivery.

Face masks may not be well tolerated by children, since the fit must be snug to the face to ensure adequate oxygen delivery. A face tent or bucket is often better tolerated, since this soft piece of plastic sits beneath the child's chin and allows for the direction of oxygen up to the area of the mouth and nose without having the mouth and nose enclosed by plastic (Curley and Moloney-Harmon, 2001).

Historically the oxygen tent (often referred to as a croup tent) was used as a satisfactory means for oxygen administration in older infants and some small children; however, these are rarely used in developed countries. A tent does not require any device to come into direct contact with the face, but the concentration of oxygen within the tent is difficult to control and to maintain above 30% to 50%. A major difficulty with the use of the tent is keeping the tent closed so that oxygen concentration is maintained; the humidification also presents a problem as the linens and child's clothing becomes saturated quite easily and must be changed often. Closely monitor the child's temperature in an oxygen tent.

Oxygen Toxicity

Oxygen is essential to life and a valuable therapeutic aid. Prolonged exposure to high oxygen tensions, however, can damage lung tissue. Although the exact pathogenesis of the pulmonary changes is unclear, evidence indicates damage to lung capillaries, which causes diffuse microhemorrhagic changes, diminished mucus flow, inactivation of surfactant, and altered ciliary function. The result of these changes is a gradual impairment of alveolar ventilation.

Atelectasis may occur as a result of the "washing out" of nitrogen from the alveoli by the high concentrations of oxygen. This is more likely to occur in persons with low tidal volume and retention of mucus or other secretions.

Oxygen-induced carbon dioxide narcosis is a physiologic hazard of oxygen therapy that may occur in persons with chronic pulmonary disease. It is rare in children, except those with cystic fibrosis. These children have chronic alveolar hypoventilation with a concomitant chronic carbon dioxide retention and hypoxemia. The respiratory center has adapted to the continuously higher $Paco_2$ levels, and therefore hypoxia becomes the more powerful stimulus to respiration. When the Pao_2 is elevated during oxygen administration, the hypoxic drive is removed, causing progressive hypoventilation and increased $Paco_2$ levels, and the child rapidly becomes unconscious. Carbon dioxide narcosis can also be induced by the administration of sedation in these patients.

Other suspected toxic effects of oxygen include changes in the renal tubules, sympathoadrenal medullary stimulation precipitating neurogenic seizures, and an increased rate of destruction of red blood cells. In extremely preterm infants the risk of retinopathy of prematurity is a major concern in oxygen administration, although the exact correlation between the two is unclear. (See Chapter 10.)

AEROSOL THERAPY

Aerosol therapy can be effective in depositing medication directly into the airway. However, the value of aerosolized water, or "mist therapy," is controversial. Continuous administration of mist, or aerosolized water, often viewed as a traditional and helpful remedy, is not a treatment of choice for most inflammatory conditions of the airways. The exception is the child with mild viral croup, who might benefit from cool-mist therapy, including a walk outside in the cool, humid night air. The effectiveness of this practice, however, has also been questioned. Mist therapy may not help the child with reactive airway disease and croup because humidity may worsen the bronchospasm.

This route of administration can be useful in avoiding the systemic side effects of certain drugs and in reducing the amount of drug necessary to achieve the desired effect. Bronchodilators, steroids, and antibiotics, suspended in particulate form, can be inhaled so that the medication reaches the small airways. Aerosol therapy is particularly challenging in children who are too young to cooperate with controlling the rate and depth of breathing. Administration of this therapy requires skill, patience, and creativity.

Medications can be aerosolized or nebulized with air or with oxygen-enriched gas. Hand-held nebulizers are common. The medicated mist is discharged into a small plastic mask, which the child holds over the nose; for older children the mouthpiece may be used instead of the mask. (See Fig. 32-12.) To avoid particle deposition in the nose and pharynx, instruct the child to take slow, deep breaths through an open mouth during treatment. For home or school, use an air compressor–driven nebulizer to force air through the liquid medication to form the aerosol. Compact, portable units can be obtained or rented from health equipment companies.

The metered dose inhaler (MDI) is a self-contained, hand-held device that allows for intermittent delivery of a specified amount of medication. (See Fig. 32-11.) Many bronchodilators are available in this form and are used successfully by children with asthma or cystic fibrosis. (See Chapter 32.) For children less than 5 or 6 years of age or children who have difficulty learning to use an MDI, a spacer device or holding chamber attached to the MDI can help coordinate breathing and aerosol delivery. The spacer allows the aerosolized particles to remain in suspension for a longer time. The MDI should be attached to a spacer when an inhaled corticosteroid is administered to prevent yeast infections in the mouth if the child is too young to rinse the mouth after the treatment. Dry powder inhalers such as the Rotahaler and Turbuhaler are also commonly used for inhaled medications.

A major nursing responsibility during aerosol therapy is to assess the effectiveness of the treatment, the patient's tolerance of the procedure, and the patient's ability to perform the procedure and use equipment correctly. Assess breath sounds, work of breathing, and pulse oximetry readings before and after treatments. Young children who become upset with a mask held close to the face may become fatigued from fighting the procedure and may appear worse during and immediately after the therapy. It may be necessary to spend a few minutes calming the child after the therapy and allowing vital signs to return to baseline levels to accurately assess changes in breath sounds and work of breathing. Alternatively, if the child's condition permits, the end of a 1-inch wide tubing (using a 6-inch pigtail) may be used to administer aerosol therapy (similar to blow-by oxygen administration).

BRONCHIAL (POSTURAL) DRAINAGE

Bronchial drainage is indicated whenever excessive fluid or mucus in the bronchi is not removed by normal ciliary activity and cough. Positioning the child to take maximum advantage of gravity facilitates removal of secretions. Postural drainage can be effective in children with chronic pulmonary illness characterized by thick mucus secretions, such as cystic fibrosis. Postural drainage may be used in combination with percussion, which serves to facilitate the loosening of secretions in the lower airways.

Postural drainage is carried out three or four times daily (or as necessary) and is more effective when it follows other respiratory therapy, such as bronchodilator or nebulized medication. Bronchial drainage is generally performed before meals (or 1 to 1½ hours after meals) to minimize the chance of vomiting and is repeated at bedtime. The duration of treatment depends on the child's condition and tolerance—usually 20 to 30 minutes. Several positions facilitate drainage from all major lung segments (Fig. 31-12); all positions are not used at each session.

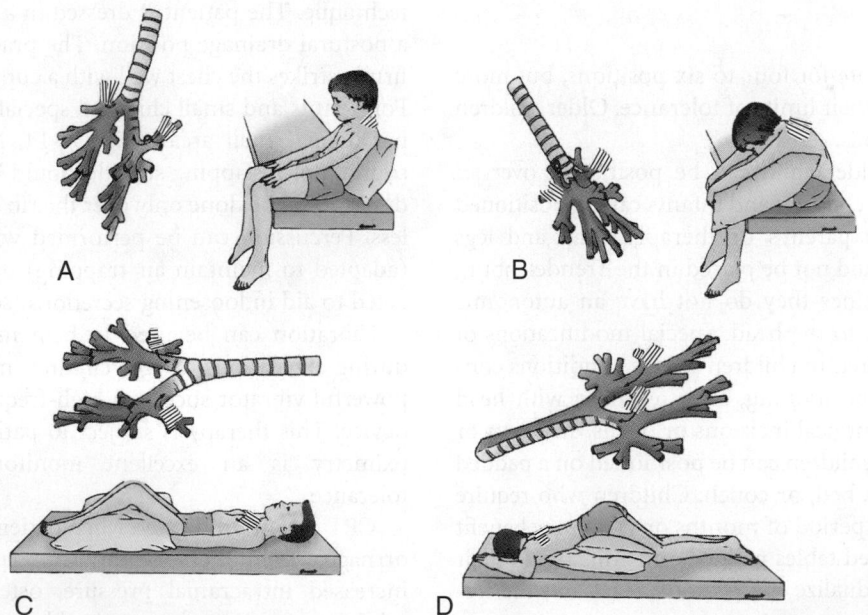

Fig. 31-12 Bronchial drainage positions for all major lung segments of child. For each position, model of tracheobronchial tree is projected beside child to show segmental bronchus *(striped)* being drained and pathway of secretions out of bronchus. Drainage platform is horizontal. Striped area on child's chest or back indicates area to be cupped or vibrated by therapist. **A,** Apical segment of right upper lobe and apical subsegment of apical-posterior segment of left upper lobe. **B,** Posterior segment of right upper lobe and posterior subsegment of apical-posterior segment of left upper lobe. **C,** Anterior segments of both upper lobes. Child should be rotated slightly away from side being drained. **D,** Superior segments of both lower lobes. (Modified from Chernick V, editor: *Kendig's disorders of the respiratory tract of children,* ed 6, Philadelphia, 1998, Saunders.)

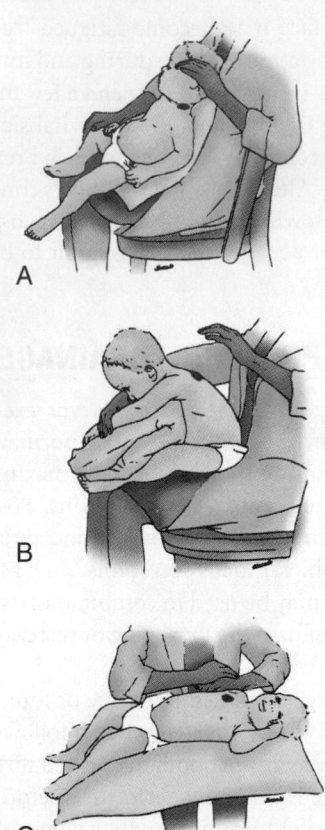

Fig. 31-13 Bronchial drainage positions for all major lung segments of infant. Procedure is most easily carried out in therapist's lap. Therapist's hand indicates area *(solid red)* to be cupped or vibrated. **A,** Apical segment of left upper lobe. **B,** Anterior segment of left upper lobe. **C,** Posterior basal segment of right lower lobe. (Modified from Cystic Fibrosis Foundation: *Infant segmental bronchial drainage*, Rockville, Md, n.d., The Foundation.)

Children usually cooperate for four to six positions, but more than six tends to exceed their limits of tolerance. Older children can tolerate longer periods.

In the hospital an older child can be positioned over an elevated knee rest. Small children and infants can be positioned with pillows or on the parent's or therapist's lap and legs (Fig. 31-13). Infants should not be placed in the Trendelenburg (head-down) position, since they do not have an autonomic regulation of blood flow to the head. Special modifications of the techniques are required in children whose conditions contraindicate head-down positioning, such as those with head injuries, some types of surgical incisions or burns, and casts or traction. At home small children can be positioned on a padded slant board, parent's lap, bed, or couch. Children who require postural drainage over a period of months or years may benefit from specially constructed tables padded and adjusted to their individual needs. Individualize the position used and the frequency and duration of treatment.

Chest Physiotherapy

CPT usually refers to the use of postural drainage in combination with adjunctive techniques that are thought to enhance the clearance of mucus from the airway. These are often referred to as *airway clearance techniques*. These techniques include manual or mechanical percussion, vibration, and squeezing of the chest;

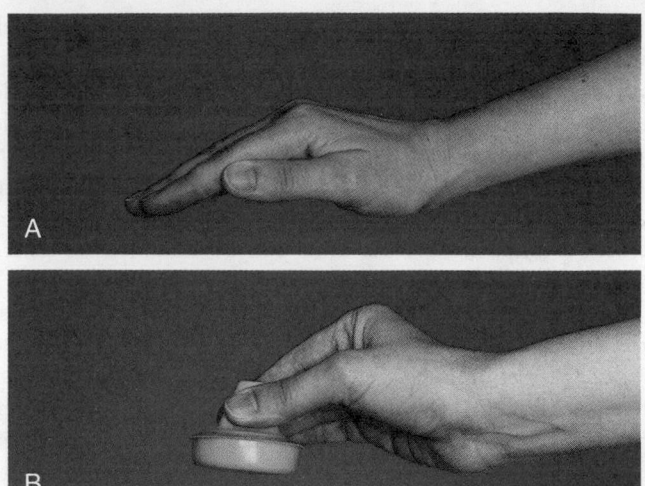

Fig. 31-14 A, Cupped hand position for percussion. **B,** Device for infant percussion.

cough; forceful expiration (exhalation) or huffing; and breathing exercises. Special mechanical devices (e.g., vest-type percussors) are also currently used to perform CPT in children with chronic pulmonary illness such as cystic fibrosis (see p. 1280). Additional methods include the flutter device (see p. 1284), Acapella, and intrapulmonary percussive ventilation (Marks, 2008). Postural drainage in combination with forced expiration has been beneficial.

Common techniques used in association with postural drainage include manual percussion of the chest wall and percussion with mechanical devices such as a high-frequency hand-held chest compression device. Nurses may be responsible for this procedure, and they should become skilled in the technique. The patient is dressed in a light shirt and placed in a postural drainage position. The practitioner then gently but firmly strikes the chest wall with a cupped hand (Fig. 31-14, *A*). For infants and small children, special devices are available for percussing small areas (Fig. 31-14, *B*). A "popping," hollow sound, not a slapping sound, should be the result. The procedure should be done only over the rib cage and should be painless. Percussion can be performed with a soft, circular mask (adapted to maintain air trapping) or a percussion cup marketed to aid in loosening secretions (see Fig. 31-14, *B*).

Vibration can be used to help move secretions cephalad during exhalations. Larger children may benefit from a more powerful vibrator such as a high-frequency chest compression device. This therapy is subject to patient tolerance, and pulse oximetry is an excellent monitoring tool for therapy tolerance.

CPT is contraindicated when patients have pulmonary hemorrhage, pulmonary embolism, end-stage renal disease, increased intracranial pressure, osteogenesis imperfecta, or minimum cardiac reserves. Avoid the head-down positions in children with gastroesophageal reflux (Marks, 2008). McIlwaine (2007) notes that the head-down position is detrimental and should not be used; Naylor, McLean, Chow, and colleagues (2006) also recommend that the head-down position be used infrequently because of an increase in cardiovascular adverse effects. Guidelines for performing CPT are given in the Nursing Care Guidelines box.

NURSING CARE GUIDELINES

Performing Chest Physiotherapy

- Chest physiotherapy should be used for patients who have increased sputum production. It is probably of no value to the uncomplicated postoperative patient or the patient with pneumonia.
- Forced expiration combined with postural drainage is more effective than cough alone.
- Appropriate use of bronchodilators before chest physiotherapy will enhance mucus clearance.

Squeezing is sometimes useful while the child is in the drainage position. Direct the child to take a deep breath and then exhale through the mouth rapidly and as completely as possible. The depth of the expiratory effort is increased by brief, firm pressure from the practitioner's hands compressing the sides of the chest. This decreases the volume of the tracheobronchial tree and facilitates the expression of secretions. Inspiration after the activity often stimulates a deep, productive cough. Another technique to force exhalation is to use abdominal thrusts in conjunction with a MAC device (see discussion below).

Encourage deep breathing when the child is relaxed and in the desired position for drainage. Direct the child to take several deep breaths using diaphragmatic breathing. The use of deep breathing enlarges the tracheobronchial tree, enabling air to circulate around and through secretions that are not affected by usual tidal volumes. Exhalations after these deep breaths often carry secretions and may stimulate a cough. Other methods that can be employed to stimulate deep breathing are the use of incentive spirometers and incorporation of play that extends the expiratory time and increases expiratory pressure. For example, play may include blowing pinwheel toys, moving small items by blowing through a straw, blowing cotton balls or a Ping-Pong ball on a table, preventing a tissue from falling by blowing it against a wall, blowing up balloons (under supervision), singing loudly (especially songs with a lot of words between breaths), or blowing soap bubbles.

With or without stimulation, encourage children to cough, not to suppress a cough, and not to waste strength and energy with repeated weak and ineffective coughs. One or two hard coughs after a deep breath are more efficient. Because many children have difficulty coughing when in a dependent position, have them sit up while they cough. Having the child hug a stuffed toy or a small pillow offers comfort, as well as physical support, during coughing. As an alternative, reinforce the child's efforts by encircling the chest with your hands and compressing the sides of the lower chest in synchrony with the cough. This is less fatiguing and increases the effectiveness of the cough efforts.

Mechanical-assisted cough (MAC) devices are available for children with acute or chronic pulmonary disease and neuromuscular disease to assist in clearing the airway when the cough reflex is ineffective or diminished. These devices may be used with CPT to enhance the removal of mucus from the airways. The mechanical cough insufflator-exsufflator (MIE) has been evaluated and found to be safe and effective in the daily management of respiratory function (Fauroux, Guillemot, Aubertin, et al, 2008; Homnick, 2007). The MIE delivers positive inspiratory pressures at a set rate, followed by negative pressure exsufflation coordinated with the patient's own breathing rhythm. The exsufflation is designed to mimic a cough reflex so mucus can be effectively cleared. Airway suctioning after exsufflation is accomplished as necessary to clear the airways. In children the MIE may be connected directly to a tracheostomy or used with a mouthpiece or face mask.

Breathing and postural exercises are useful techniques with motivated children and children with kyphoscoliosis, cystic fibrosis, asthma, and bronchiectasis. Breathing exercises are part of a total therapy program and are more convenient when performed in association with bronchial drainage.

The goals of breathing exercises are to (1) develop more effective diaphragmatic and lower intercostal breathing; (2) relax all muscles, especially those of the upper chest, shoulder girdle, and neck; and (3) attain correct posture. The number and type of exercises depend on the child's age, motivation, and strength and the type and extent of the physiologic disturbance. Select breathing exercises to meet the specific child's needs. The most important exercises are diaphragmatic breathing and side bending, with emphasis on abdominal expansion and lateral expansion.

MECHANICAL VENTILATION

If a child's respiratory status is deteriorating and the respiratory effort is excessive or inadequate, mechanically assisted ventilation may become necessary (Box 31-5).

A variety of methods are available for controlling or assisting ventilation. Temporary assistance can be provided by a hand-operated self-inflating ventilation bag with a mask and a nonreturnable valve to prevent rebreathing, commonly referred to as a bag and valve mask (BVM). With the mask placed on the nose and mouth, the bag is rhythmically compressed, forcing gas from the bag into the patient's airways. The self-inflating bag is equipped with a reservoir to deliver a high percentage of oxygen. To avoid barotrauma, self-inflating bags should have a preset (or adjustable) pop-off valve that allows maximum peak inspiratory pressure of 30 to 35 cm H_2O (Curley and Moloney-Harmon, 2001).

Another type of bag used for manual ventilation is the flow-inflating Mapleson bag. This anesthesia bag inflates only if a

---

BOX 31-5   INDICATIONS FOR MECHANICAL VENTILATION

Progressive hypoxia, despite oxygen therapy, measured by decreasing oxygen saturations or blood gas analysis (high $Paco_2$ and low pH)

Inadequate ventilation caused by:
- Apnea
- Central nervous system injury or infection
- Alveolar hypoventilation
- Respiratory muscle weakness
- Medication toxicity
- Infectious pathologic condition
- Foreign body obstruction

Excessive work of breathing, manifested by retractions, tachypnea, decreasing oxygen saturation, abnormal respiratory patterns

Inadequate respiratory effort

Hyperventilation for treatment of increased intracranial pressure

continuous flow of oxygen is available. The bag is commonly used in the operating room or intensive care unit and requires trained personnel to use it. Regardless of the type of manual ventilation bag used, establish an open airway by correct positioning with the patient's chin directed forward and the neck extended to the "sniffing" position. It is important not to hyperextend an infant's neck, since this can occlude the airway.

Several types of noninvasive positive pressure ventilation (NPPV) devices can support pediatric patients who have respiratory difficulties in acute, chronic, and home settings. NPPV does not require endotracheal (ET) intubation or a tracheostomy, but the ventilation is instead delivered via a nasal or oral mask attached to a ventilation system. Three types of NPPV can be delivered: (1) continuous positive airway pressure (CPAP), (2) intermittent positive pressure breathing (IPPB), and (3) bilevel positive airway pressure (BiPAP). CPAP provides a constant flow of positive pressure to prevent collapse of the alveoli. IPPB is a type of CPAP used intermittently to deliver aerosol medications. BiPAP provides constant positive pressure at two different pressure settings—one for inspiration and one for expiration. BiPAP has been used for pediatric patients with obstructive sleep apnea, tracheomalacia, diaphragm paralysis, progressive neuromuscular disorders, cystic fibrosis, and asthma (Curley and Moloney-Harmon, 2001). Noninvasive ventilation modes such as BiPAP are used frequently in children with neuromuscular disease to maintain adequate ventilation, especially during sleep, and are said to have prolonged life expectancy in many children (Kennedy and Martin, 2009).

Negative pressure ventilators create a subatmospheric pressure around the chest wall and create negative abdominal pressure, which allows the diaphragm to distend and pull air into the chest. Negative pressure ventilators come in many forms: the cuirass, the iron lung, and raincoats or ventilator suits. This form of ventilation can be used continuously or intermittently (at night or during naptime) to allow rest for patients with neuromuscular disease.

For acute respiratory support, mechanical ventilation replaces the function of the diaphragm and thoracic chest wall muscles. For the delivery of positive pressure ventilation by a ventilator, the patient will have an ET tube or a tracheostomy. Positive pressure ventilation inflates the lungs by creating pressure at the airway opening that is greater than the intraalveolar pressure. This results in improved gas distribution within the lung because of re-recruitment or reopening of partially collapsed lung segments. The overall effect is improvement of gas exchange.

Ventilators are usually classified according to the factors that regulate cycling. The method by which inspiration is terminated can be categorized as pressure cycled, volume cycled, or time cycled (Box 31-6). High-frequency ventilation uses a rapid cycling rate and delivers small tidal volumes with each cycle. Different high-frequency ventilation techniques include high-frequency oscillation ventilation, high-frequency positive pressure ventilation, high-frequency flow interruption, and high-frequency jet ventilation. With each high-frequency ventilation strategy, lung volume is held relatively constant, the cycle of inflation and deflation associated with conventional ventilation is reduced, and gas exchange is maintained with a

> ### BOX 31-6   TYPES OF VENTILATORS
>
> **Pressure-cycled ventilator**—Terminates the respiratory cycle when a preset inspiratory pressure is reached. Volume differs greatly, depending on the flow rate of the delivery of gas. The lung's compliance affects the tidal volume even though the pressure remains constant.
> **Volume-cycled ventilator**—Terminates respiration when a preset volume (tidal volume) is delivered. The lung's compliance and resistance change the pressure needed to deliver the preset volume.
> **Time-cycled ventilator**—Terminates inspiration when a preset time is reached. Tidal volume is greatly affected by the compliance of the ventilator tubing, lung compliance and resistance, and flow rate of the delivered gas. The duration of the inspiratory pressure is affected by the preset inspiratory time and the flow rate of the delivered gas.

lower incidence of lung injury (Curley and Moloney-Harmon, 2001).

Research is ongoing to support the benefits of numerous ventilation strategies in the pediatric population. The PALISI Network (Pediatric Acute Lung Injury and Sepsis Investigators; http://pedsccm.org/PALISI_network.php) is a collaborative group of investigators who study ways to optimize ventilation strategies in pediatric patients.

Critically ill children on mechanical ventilation are at risk for acquisition of ventilator-associated pneumonia (VAP). Evidence-based guidelines for the prevention of VAP have been published elsewhere (Centers for Disease Control and Prevention, 2004). Recommendations for nurses working with mechanically ventilated patients include appropriate hand hygiene measures; wearing gloves to handle respiratory secretions or contaminated objects; elevating the head of the bed 30 to 45 degrees; and routine oral hygiene, which includes oropharyngeal suctioning of secretions (Centers for Disease Control and Prevention, 2004).

An invasive technique to provide respiratory support is extracorporeal membrane oxygenation (ECMO). ECMO is a form of cardiopulmonary bypass that provides both pulmonary and cardiac support using an external oxygenation device and a pump. (See Chapter 10.)

Increasing attention is being paid to *lung protective strategies*, which are aimed at decreasing the effects of high distending pressures, lung barotrauma, and associated problems such as acute lung injury and bronchopulmonary dysplasia. Lung protective strategies include the use of permissive hypercapnia and ventilation with low inspiratory tidal volume pressure (Rogovik and Goldman, 2008).

> ### ! NURSING ALERT
>
> Patients requiring mechanical ventilation should always have a self-inflating ventilation bag with a reservoir at the bedside. When the patient's condition or the mechanical ventilator's operation is in doubt, use the ventilation bag.

Nursing Care Management

The regulation and maintenance of mechanical ventilators are often the responsibility of respiratory care practitioners. However, the nurse should understand the function of the ventilator and how to detect signs of malfunction and deviations from the desired settings. The nursing process in the care of the pediatric patient on mechanical ventilation involves baseline and continuous respiratory assessment and provision of optimum ventilation through interventions such as preventing accidental or unplanned extubation; positioning for optimum ventilation and comfort; suctioning the airway only as necessary; monitoring for potential side effects of mechanical ventilation (e.g., pneumothorax); preventing infection; ensuring that adequate humidification is provided; and providing support, comfort, and reassurance to the child and the family. It is important to help the family understand why the intubated child cannot speak when an ET tube is in place. The nurse can enhance the family's role in providing emotional support to the child by allowing family involvement in the child's care. With mechanical ventilation, nutrition and hydration needs must be met with either gastrostomy feedings or parenteral nutrition. (See Chapter 10 for assisted and controlled ventilation in the neonate.)

> **! NURSING ALERT**
>
> The use of a mechanical ventilator does not guarantee that the child is being ventilated effectively. Therefore nursing assessment of respiratory status and oxygenation is essential.

Nursing assessment of the child requiring mechanical ventilation focuses on physical examination, vital signs, response to treatment, pulmonary status, oxygenation, comfort, airway patency (e.g., obstruction or unplanned extubation and dislodgment), laboratory analysis (ABGs), and pulse oximetry. All infants and children who are intubated and on mechanical ventilation should be placed on a cardiorespiratory monitor.

When an infant or child is intubated, medications are usually administered for achieving a successful, atraumatic intubation and decreasing the child's anxiety. Because pain and agitation are often difficult to distinguish in children, it is important that nurses assess and treat agitation in the ventilated infant and child to decrease the potential for self-harm, maximize the effects of the therapy (oxygenation of tissues), and prevent self-extubation (Brinker, 2004). *Rapid sequence intubation* (RSI) is commonly performed in pediatric (and some neonatal) patients to induce an unconscious, neuromuscular blocked condition to avoid the use of positive pressure ventilation and the risk of possible aspiration (Bottor, 2009). Atropine, fentanyl, and vecuronium or rocuronium are drugs commonly used during RSI. In neonates endotracheal intubation is often a stressful event, and hypoxia and pain are commonly associated with routine intubation; RSI in neonates may serve to prevent such adverse events (Bottor, 2009).

Objective assessment tools to measure anxiety in intubated children should guide medication administration; the Comfort scale has been used in critically ill ventilated patients (Brinker, 2004). Medications used for sedation in children on mechanical ventilation include opioids (fentanyl and morphine), benzodiazepines (midazolam [Versed] and lorazepam [Ativan]), and neuromuscular blockade agents (pancuronium, vecuronium, and rocuronium). Propofol may be used short term in intubated children. Prolonged use of sedating agents may cause withdrawal, physical dependence, and tolerance, and plans should be implemented to counteract untoward effects, especially during the weaning process (Brinker, 2004).

Other important criteria to assess include nutritional status, intake and output (urinary output should be at least 2 ml/kg/hr for the infant and younger child and 1 ml/kg/hr for the older child), and skin integrity (especially around the face and lips for the child with an ET tube, and around the neck and stoma for the child with a tracheostomy). In some cases there is an increase in the amount of oral or nasal secretions, which requires appropriate perioral skin care. The child's lips and mouth may be dry and uncomfortable; therefore provision of oral care and moisture is important to decrease discomfort.

Weaning the patient from a ventilator involves gradual physical and psychologic withdrawal from dependence on the mechanical device. Criteria for beginning the weaning process vary with the primary disease.

If the intubated child is receiving nasogastric feedings and is at risk for aspiration, feedings are usually stopped a few hours before extubation. Steroids may be administered before the extubation to control laryngeal edema. The child should remain on a cardiorespiratory monitor, and resuscitation and reintubation equipment must be available at the bedside.

CPT and suctioning are ordinarily performed just before tube removal, and cool mist or a noninvasive form of oxygen delivery (nasal cannula, face mask) is initiated immediately after extubation. The nurse monitors the child for respiratory distress and observes adequacy of oxygenation through ABG measurements or pulse oximetry. The most common complications after extubation are airway edema and pain, fatigue, and atelectasis. Stridor results from airway edema and often responds to nebulized racemic epinephrine. This can be given several times to reduce airway swelling and avoid reintubation.

Endotracheal Airways

An artificial airway is commonly used in association with artificial ventilation and in children with upper airway obstruction (Box 31-7). ET intubation can be accomplished by the nasal (nasotracheal), oral (orotracheal), or direct tracheal (tracheostomy) routes. Oral intubation is usually the method of choice for emergency situations, but for prolonged intubation a nasotracheal tube is often used. Nasotracheal intubation facilitates oral hygiene and provides more stable fixation, which reduces the complication of tracheal erosion and the danger of accidental extubation. Nasotracheal intubation also allows for age-appropriate oral development such as learning to suck on a pacifier. This normal development decreases the possibility

> **BOX 31-7   INDICATIONS FOR POSSIBLE ENDOTRACHEAL INTUBATION**
>
> - Airway obstruction
> - Respiratory arrest
> - Neuromuscular compromise or paralysis
> - Inadequate ventilation
> - Hypoxemia despite supplemental oxygen
> - Pulmonary lavage; instillation of medications
> - Respiratory acidosis
> - Need for mechanical ventilation for any reason

Animation—Intubation

Animation—Intubation in Infant

Animation—Intubation, Incorrect Placement

that the patient will develop oral aversions and perhaps even later feeding difficulties as a result of being intubated. One potential disadvantage of nasal intubation is erosion of the nasal septum; therefore meticulous skin care and monitoring for skin breakdown are essential.

Use only uncuffed ET tubes in children less than 8 years of age (Curley and Moloney-Harmon, 2001). Although infants have been successfully maintained on ET tubes for longer periods, tracheostomy is usually considered in some infants and older children who require intubation for an extended period. However, infants may experience complications as a result of prolonged intubation, including tracheomalacia. Therefore it is not uncommon to attempt early weaning. Prolonged mechanical ventilation in infants has also been associated with the development of bronchopulmonary dysplasia, or chronic lung disease.

> **NURSING TIP** The nurse can determine the size of an ET tube in three ways:
> 1. Using patient length and the Broselow resuscitation tape
> 2. ET tube size = (Age [yr] + 16) ÷ 4
> 3. "Pinky" rule: the diameter of a child's pinky finger is approximately the size of the trachea

The decision to change from an ET tube to a tracheostomy is made on an individual basis. The tracheostomy allows the child to speak (by temporarily occluding the opening with a special speaking device) and eat and also facilitates clearing of secretions. Suctioning an ET tube is carried out with the same care as suctioning a tracheostomy.

The practice of instilling sterile saline in the ET tube or tracheostomy before suctioning is still common in many intensive care units. However, the routine use of saline is not recommend because of increased incidence of oxygen desaturation, increased intracranial pressure, increased arterial blood pressure, and nosocomial infection (Ridling, Martin, Bratton, et al, 2003; Celik and Kanan, 2006; Morrow and Argent, 2008; Gardner and Shirland, 2009). The conclusions drawn from neonatal and adult studies are that routinely instilling saline is not supported by research. A review of 14 studies contends that normal saline (NS) does not liquefy or thin out thick secretions in the endotracheal tube; the researchers pointed out that sputum recovery with NS instillation was minimal and did not outweigh the adverse effects of routine NS instillation (Halm and Krisko-Hagel, 2008). Policies about instillation of sterile saline while suctioning vary among institutions (see Evidence-Based Practice box). Evidence-based guidelines for ET suctioning in neonates and infants have been published elsewhere (Gardner and Shirland, 2009).

Complications

The most severe complication related to immediate intubation is hypoxia with accompanying bradycardia. Closely monitor patients during intubation attempts, and if hypoxia occurs, discontinue the procedure until vital signs are stable. Ventilation with BVM and oxygen is reinstituted. Other complications include aspiration; trauma to the mouth, teeth, and trachea; epistaxis; creation of air leaks; and vagal-mediated

changes in vital signs. The most common sequela of intubation is a sore throat, which disappears within 48 to 72 hours without therapy, although a humidified atmosphere is beneficial. Other complications include traumatic laryngitis, infection, glottic edema, and mucosal lesions of the larynx secondary to pressure exerted by the rigid ET tube. The most severe sequela of intubation is subglottic stenosis secondary to fibrosis.

TRACHEOSTOMY

Tracheotomy is a surgical opening in the trachea between the second and fourth tracheal rings (Fig. 31-15). The tracheostomy tube is inserted through the exterior tracheal stoma into the trachea to provide an airway. Congenital or acquired structural defects, such as subglottic stenosis, tracheomalacia, and vocal cord paralysis, account for many long-term tracheostomies. A tracheotomy may be necessary in an emergency situation for epiglottitis, croup, or FB aspiration. These tracheostomies usually remain in place for a short time. An infant or child requiring long-term ventilatory support may also have a tracheostomy.

Pediatric tracheostomy tubes are usually made of plastic or Silastic (Fig. 31-16). The most common types are the Hollinger,

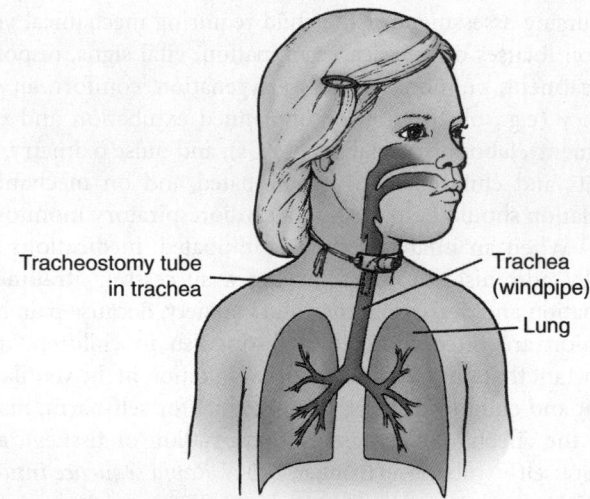

Fig. 31-15 Tracheostomy tube in trachea and securely tied with cloth tape.

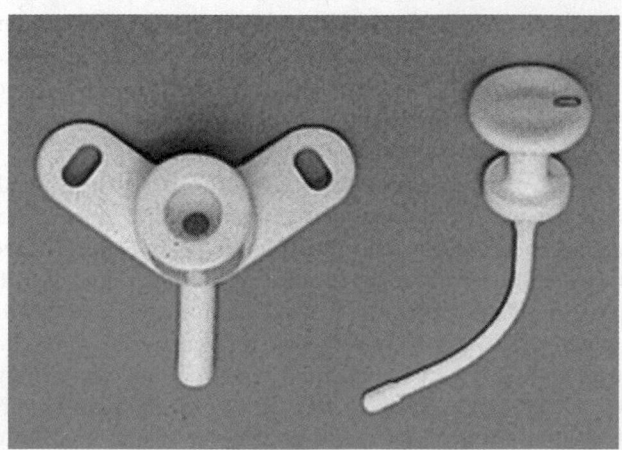

Fig. 31-16 Silastic pediatric tracheostomy tube and obturator.

EVIDENCE-BASED PRACTICE

Normal Saline Instillation Before Endotracheal or Tracheostomy Suctioning—Helpful or Harmful?

ASK THE QUESTION

In intubated children and those with tracheostomy, is normal saline (NS) instillation before suctioning helpful or harmful?

SEARCH FOR THE EVIDENCE

Search strategies
All English-language literature from 1980 to 2009 was searched.

Databases used
PubMed, Cochrane Collaboration, MDConsult, BestBETs, PedsCCM

CRITICALLY ANALYZE THE EVIDENCE

GRADE criteria: Evidence quality moderate; recommendation strong (Guyatt, Oxman, Vist, et al, 2008)

- Instillation of NS before endotracheal (ET) tube suctioning has been used for years to loosen and dilute secretion, lubricate the suction catheter, and promote cough. In recent years the possible adverse effects of this procedure have been explored. Adult studies have found decreased oxygen saturation, increased frequency of nosocomial pneumonia, and increased intracranial pressure after instillation of NS before suctioning (O'Neal, Grap, Thompson, et al, 2001; Kinlock, 1999; Hagler and Traver, 1994; Reynolds, Hoffman, Schlichtig, et al, 1990; Ackerman, 1993; Ackerman and Gugerty, 1990; Bostick and Wendelgass, 1987).
- Two of the first research studies evaluating the effect of NS instillation before suctioning in neonates found no deleterious effects. Shorten, Byrne, and Jones (1991) found no significant differences in oxygenation, heart rate, or blood pressure before or after suctioning in a group of 27 intubated neonates.
- In a second study of nine neonates acting as their own controls, no adverse effects on lung mechanics were found after NS instillation and suctioning (Beeram and Dhanireddy, 1992).
- A study evaluating the effects of NS instillation before suctioning in children found results similar to those in the previously published adult studies. Ridling, Martin, and Bratton (2003) evaluated the effects of NS instillation before suctioning in a group of 24 critically ill children, ages 10 weeks to 14 years (level 1 evidence). A total of 104 suctioning episodes were analyzed. Children experienced significantly greater oxygen desaturation after suctioning if NS was instilled.
- The American Thoracic Society's (2005) official position statement on the care of children with tracheostomies now states that NS should not be instilled before suctioning.
- Gardner and Shirland (2009) evaluated 10 studies on the effects of instilling NS in intubated neonates and concluded that the evidence does not support routine instillation of NS; however, the evidence indicating adverse effect of NS instillation is abundant.
- Morrow and Argent (2008) suggest that despite evidence indicating the detriment of the use of saline for suctioning in adults, evidence is lacking in the pediatric population. They conclude, however, that saline should not be routinely used for suctioning infants and children.

APPLY THE EVIDENCE: NURSING IMPLICATIONS

Studies support the contention that the adverse effects of NS instillation before suctioning in children are similar to those found for adults. This technique causes a significant reduction in oxygen saturation that can last up to 2 minutes after suctioning. The evidence does not support the use of NS instillation before ET suctioning in children.

References

Ackerman MH: The effect of saline lavage prior to suctioning, *Am J Crit Care* 2(4):326-330, 1993.

Ackerman MH, Gugerty B: The effect of normal saline bolus instillation in artificial airways, *J Soc Otorhinolaryngol Head Neck Surg* 8:14-17, 1990.

American Thoracic Society: *Care of the child with a chronic tracheostomy*, 2005, available at www.thoracic.org/sections/publications/statements/pages/respiratory-disease-pediatric/childtrach1-12.html (accessed April 17, 2006).

Beeram MR, Dhanireddy R: Effects of saline instillation during tracheal suction on lung mechanics in newborn infants, *J Perinatol* 12(2):120-123, 1992.

Bostick J, Wendelgass ST: Normal saline instillation as part of the suctioning procedure: effects of Pao₂ and amount of secretions, *Heart Lung* 16(5):532-537, 1987.

Gardner DL, Shirland L: Evidence-based guideline for suctioning the intubated neonate and infant, *Neonat Netw* 28(5):281-302, 2009.

Guyatt GH, Oxman AD, Vist GE, et al: GRADE: an emerging consensus on rating quality of evidence and strength of recommendations, *BMJ* 336:924-926, 2008.

Hagler DA, Traver GA: Endotracheal saline and suction catheters: sources of lower airway contamination, *Am J Crit Care* 3(6):444-447, 1994.

Kinlock D: Instillation of normal saline during endotracheal suctioning: effects on mixed venous oxygen saturation, *Am J Crit Care* 8(4):231-240, 1999.

Morrow BM, Argent AC: A comprehensive review of pediatric endotracheal suctioning: effects, indications, and clinical practice, *Pediatr Crit Care Med* 9(5):465-477, 2008.

O'Neal PV, Grap MJ, Thompson C, et al: Level of dyspnoea experienced in mechanically ventilated adults with and without saline instillation prior to endotracheal suctioning, *Intensive Crit Care Nurs* 17(6):356-363, 2001.

Reynolds P, Hoffman LA, Schlichtig R, et al: Effects of normal saline instillation on secretion volume, dynamic compliance, and oxygen saturation (abstract), *Am Rev Respir Dis* 141:A574, 1990.

Ridling DA, Martin LD, Bratton SL: Endotracheal suctioning with or without instillation of isotonic sodium chloride in critically ill children, *Am J Crit Care* 12(3):212-219, 2003.

Shorten DR, Byrne PJ, Jones RL: Infant responses to saline instillations and endotracheal suctioning, *J Obstet Gynecol Neonatal Nurs* 20(6):464-469, 1991.

Jackson, Aberdeen, and Shiley tubes. These tubes are constructed with a more acute angle than adult tubes, and they soften at body temperature, conforming to the contours of the trachea. Because these materials resist the formation of crusted respiratory secretions, they are made without an inner cannula.

Tracheostomy Care

Before the tracheotomy is performed, it is important to prepare the child and family. Teaching before the procedure should include the child (if age appropriate), family, and other primary caregivers. It should address the child's appearance with a tracheostomy, the communication method to be used after the procedure, and postoperative procedures. If time permits, medical play or hands-on experience with tracheostomy supplies and a tour of the pediatric intensive care unit are helpful to decrease anxiety.

The child returns from the operating room with the tracheostomy tube in place and long sutures (stay sutures) taped to the chest. These sutures are attached to the tracheal rings and can be used to hold the stoma open in the event of accidental decannulation. In approximately 5 days a tract is formed in the trachea, subcutaneous tissue, and skin, at which time the stay sutures are no longer required. The nurse should tell the child that removal of the stay sutures is not painful.

Children who have undergone a tracheotomy must be closely monitored for complications such as hemorrhage, edema, aspiration, accidental decannulation, tube obstruction, and the entrance of free air into the pleural cavity. Nursing care focuses on maintaining a patent airway, facilitating the removal of secretions, providing humidified air or oxygen, offering comfort care, cleansing the stoma, monitoring the child's ability to swallow, and teaching while simultaneously preventing complications.

Because the child may be unable to signal for help, direct observation of the child and the use of respiratory and cardiac monitors are essential. Perform respiratory assessments (including breath sounds and work of breathing, vital signs, pulse oximetry, tightness of the tracheostomy ties, and the type and amount of secretions) every 15 minutes until the patient is stable and then every 1 to 2 hours for the first 24 hours. Perform assessments thereafter every 2 to 4 hours or more frequently if needed.

> ### ⚠ NURSING ALERT
>
> Large amounts of bloody secretions in a child with a tracheostomy tube are uncommon and should be considered a sign of hemorrhage. Notify the practitioner immediately if this occurs.

Position the child with the head of the bed raised, or in the position most comfortable to the child. Suction catheters, the suction source, gloves, sterile saline, sterile gauze for wiping away secretions, scissors, an extra tracheostomy tube of the same size with ties already attached, another tracheostomy tube one size smaller, and the obturator are kept at the bedside. Provide a source of humidification, since the normal humidification and filtering functions of the airway have been bypassed. Intravenous fluids ensure adequate hydration until the child is able to swallow sufficient amounts of fluids.

Suctioning

The airway must remain patent and may require frequent suctioning during the first few hours after a tracheotomy to remove mucous plugs and excessive secretions. However, although it is necessary to prevent obstruction of the airway, suctioning is not without inherent risks, including atelectasis, hypoxemia, trauma, infection, bronchospasm, and increased mucus production (Ireton, 2007). Ireton (2007) emphasizes the importance of evidence-based practice for effective and safe tracheostomy suctioning in children. However, suctioning is often based on tradition rather than evidence and further research is needed to clarify best practice.

Proper vacuum pressure and suction catheter size are important to prevent atelectasis and decrease hypoxia from the suctioning procedure. Vacuum pressure should range from 60 to 100 mm Hg for infants and children and from 40 to 60 mm Hg

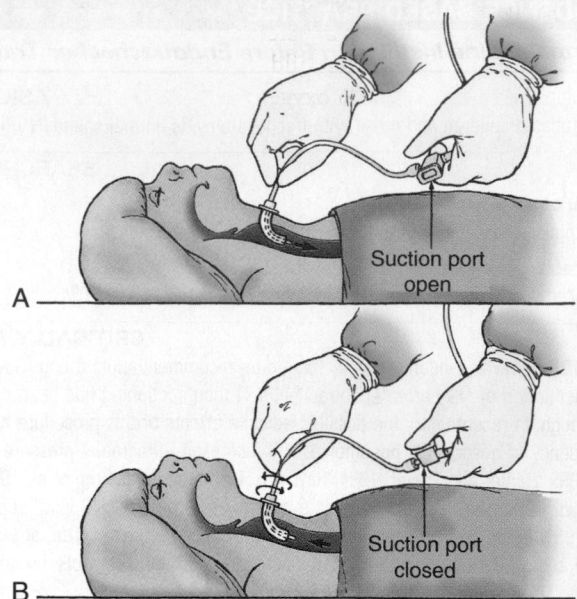

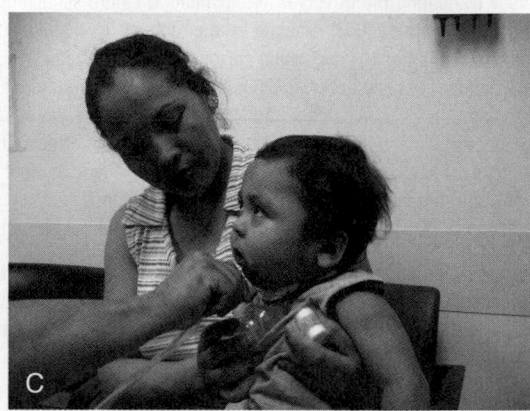

Fig. 31-17 Tracheostomy suctioning. **A,** Insertion, port open. **B,** Withdrawal, port occluded. Note that catheter is inserted just slightly beyond end of tracheostomy tube. **C,** Closed tracheal suctioning of child's tracheostomy.

for preterm infants. Unless secretions are thick and tenacious, the lower range of negative pressure is recommended. Tracheal suction catheters are available in a variety of sizes. The catheter selected should have a diameter one half the diameter of the tracheostomy tube. If the catheter is too large, it can block the airway and cause atelectasis and hypoxemia. The catheter is constructed with a side port so that the catheter is introduced without suction and removed while simultaneous intermittent suction is applied by covering the port with the thumb (Fig. 31-17). Catheters with three holes (versus a single hole) are recommended to decrease inflammatory reactions (Ireton, 2007). The catheter is inserted just slightly beyond the end (0.5 cm) of the tracheostomy tube to prevent tracheal edema and inflammation; the use of a premeasured suction catheter is recommended to avoid deep suctioning. Routine instillation of NS for suctioning is not recommended (Ireton, 2007; Morrow and Argent, 2008).

Counting one–one thousand, two–one thousand, three–one thousand, and so on while suctioning is a simple means for monitoring the time. For infants it is recommended that the suction time be limited to less than 5 seconds, whereas for children suctioning for less than 10 seconds is recommended (Ireton, 2007). Without a safeguard, the airway may be obstructed for too long. The child may be hyperoxygenated and hyperventilated with 100% oxygen before and after suctioning (using a BVM or increasing the Fio_2 ventilator setting) to prevent hypoxia. However, these practices vary somewhat throughout the nation (Paul-Allen and Ostrow, 2000; Sole, Byers, Ludy, et al, 2003), and some recommend hyperoxygenation only if the child is on 40% oxygen or has not tolerated suctioning for brief periods without significant desaturations (Ireton, 2007).

Closed tracheal suctioning systems that allow for uninterrupted oxygen delivery may also be used. In a closed suctioning system a suction catheter is directly attached to the ventilator tubing. This system has several advantages. First, there is no need to disconnect the patient from the ventilator, which allows for better oxygenation. Second, the suction catheter is enclosed in a plastic sheath, which reduces the risk of the caregiver's exposure to the patient's secretions. Morrow and Argent (2008) indicate there is currently no strong evidence to support closed- or open-system suctioning.

> **! NURSING ALERT**
>
> Suctioning is carried out only as often as needed to keep the tube patent. Signs of mucus partially occluding the airway include an increased heart rate, a rise in respiratory effort, a drop in oxygen saturation, cyanosis, or an increase in the positive inspiratory pressure on the ventilator.

The child is allowed to rest for 30 to 60 seconds after each aspiration to allow oxygen saturation to return to normal. Then, the process is repeated until the trachea is clear. Suctioning should be limited to about three aspirations in one period. Oximetry is an effective feedback tool to monitor suctioning and prevent hypoxia.

In the acute care setting, aseptic technique is used during care of the tracheostomy. Secondary infection is a major concern because the air entering the lower airway bypasses the natural defenses of the upper airway. Standard Precautions are recommended, and the nurse should wear gloves during suctioning procedure, although a sterile glove is needed only on the hand touching the catheter. It is recommended that the nurse follows the institution protocols for the use of nonsterile and sterile gloves during suctioning. Use a new sterile suction catheter and sterile gloves each time in the acute care setting. In the home care setting nonsterile gloves may be worn, and the suction catheter may be rinsed with water internally and cleansed with alcohol on the external surface (Sherman, Davis, Albamonte-Petrick, et al, 2000).

Nursing Care Management

The tracheostomy stoma requires daily care. Assessments of the stoma area include observations for signs of infection and breakdown of the skin. Keep the skin clean and dry, and gently remove secretions around the stoma with warm soap and water or saline. Do not use hydrogen peroxide with sterling silver tracheostomy tubes because it tends to pit and stain the silver surface. Peroxide is no longer recommended for stoma care but

may be used to clean secretions or crusts that are adhered to the trach tube flanges. The nurse should be aware of wet tracheostomy dressings, which can predispose the peristomal area to skin breakdown. Several products are available to prevent or treat excoriation. The Allevyn tracheostomy dressing is a hydrophilic sponge with a polyurethane back that is highly absorptive. Other possible barriers to help maintain skin integrity include the use of hydrocolloid wafers (e.g., DuoDERM CGF, Hollister Restore, Mepilex Lite) under the tracheostomy flanges and extrathin hydrocolloid wafers under the chin (see Research Focus box).

> **⟨⟩ RESEARCH FOCUS**
>
> ### Skin and Wound Cleansers
>
> An in vitro study determined that hydrogen peroxide, modified Dakin solution, and 10% povidone were the most toxic agents when applied to keratinocytes. Dial antibacterial soap and Ivory Liqui-Gel were the most toxic to fibroblasts. The solutions with least measured toxicity to fibroblasts were saline, SAF-Clens, and Shur-Clens. Biolex, Shur-Clens, and Techni-Care were the least toxic agents to keratinocytes. Keratinocytes and fibroblasts are necessary for the repair of cutaneous tissue. The researchers suggest that skin cleansing agents be used with caution on wounds and healing tissue (Wilson, Mills, Prather, et al, 2005).

Myers (2008) states there are abundant data indicating that agents such as povidone-iodine, Dakin solution, and hydrogen peroxide are cytotoxic to living cells, even when diluted. Therefore, until there are sufficient data to indicate otherwise, the practice of using hydrogen peroxide on tracheostomy stoma is no longer recommended.

Tracheostomy ties made of a durable, nonfraying material hold the tracheostomy tube in place. The ties are changed daily and when soiled. Ties fastened with self-adhering Velcro closures are available and are commonly used. These devices are made of a soft, cushioning, slightly stretchy, and comfortable material. They are increasingly popular because of their ease of use and ability to maintain better skin integrity. If Velcro ties are not available, cotton ties can be looped through the tracheostomy flanges and tied snugly in a triple knot at the side of the neck before the soiled ties are cut and removed. The ties should be tight enough to allow just a fingertip to be inserted between the ties and the neck (Fig. 31-18). It is easier to ensure a snug

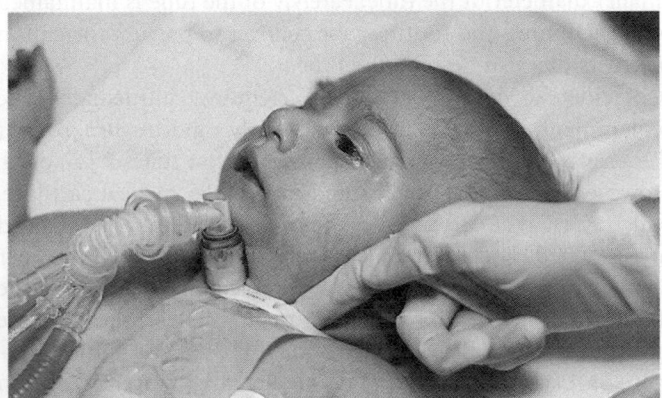

Fig. 31-18 Tracheostomy ties are snug but allow one finger to be inserted.

fit if the child's head is flexed rather than extended while the ties are being secured. Routine tracheostomy tube changes are usually carried out weekly after a tract has been formed to minimize formation of granulation tissue. The first change is usually performed by the surgeon. Subsequent changes are performed by the nurse and, if the child is discharged home with the tracheostomy, by either a parent or a visiting nurse. Ideally, two caregivers participate in the procedure to assist with positioning the child.

The tracheostomy tube is changed using strict aseptic technique. A gown and eye protection should be worn to change the tracheostomy. Sterile gloves may be worn for insertion of the sterile trach tube, but clean gloves may be used for trach tubes that are cleansed and reused. Tube changes should occur before meals or 2 hours after the last meal. Continuous feedings should be turned off at least an hour before a tube change. Prepare the new tube by inserting the obturator and attaching new ties. Suction the child as necessary before the procedure to minimize secretions, then restrain and position the child with the neck slightly extended. One caregiver removes the old ties and removes the tube from the stoma. Insert the new tube gently into the stoma (using a downward and forward motion that follows the curve of the trachea), remove the obturator, and secure the ties. Assess the adequacy of ventilation after a tube change because the tube can be inserted into the soft tissue surrounding the trachea. Therefore carefully monitor breath sounds and respiratory effort.

Supplemental oxygen is always delivered with a humidification system to prevent drying of the respiratory mucosa. Humidification of room air for an established tracheostomy can be intermittent if secretions remain thin enough to be coughed or suctioned from the tracheostomy. Direct humidification via tracheostomy collar can be provided during naps and at night so that the child is able to be up and around unencumbered during much of the day. Room humidifiers are also used successfully.

The inner cannula, if used, should be removed with each suctioning, cleaned with sterile saline and pipe cleaners to remove crusted material, dried thoroughly, and reinserted.

Emergency Care: Tube Occlusion and Accidental Decannulation

Occlusion of the tracheostomy tube is life threatening. Infants and children are at greater risk than adults because of the smaller diameter of the tube. Patency of the tube is maintained with suctioning and routine tube changes to prevent formation of crusts that can occlude the tube.

Accidental decannulation also requires immediate tube replacement. Some children have a fairly rigid trachea, so that the airway remains partially open when the tube is removed. However, others have malformed or flexible tracheal cartilage, which causes the airway to collapse when the tube is removed or dislodged. Because many infants and children with upper airway problems have little airway reserve, if replacement of the dislodged tube is impossible, insert a smaller tube. Provide ventilation with a BVM to the stoma if the child is apneic. Bag-valve-stoma ventilation can be challenging, since it is often difficult to attain a good seal between the mask and the stoma. If these ventilations are ineffective (as evidenced by minimum chest movement with breaths or other signs of ineffective breathing such as cyanosis or decreased pulse oximetry readings), the stoma can be occluded with the gloved finger of one provider while another provider does BVM ventilation to the patient's mouth and nose. If the stoma cannot be cannulated with another tracheostomy tube, oral intubation should be performed.

Decannulation

The tracheostomy tube is removed as soon as it is no longer needed. Airway problems of short duration (e.g., FB obstruction) usually allow early removal, but some conditions (e.g., tracheomalacia, tracheostenosis, vocal cord paralysis) may require that the tracheostomy tube remain in place indefinitely.

Opinions differ regarding the best means for removing the tube, especially after lengthy intubation. The usual procedure may take up to several months to wean or "downsize" the child to the smallest possible tracheostomy tube. Once this has been accomplished and the child's respiratory status is unimpaired for 24 hours, the tube is occluded, and then removed within the next 24 hours. A small bandage is usually placed over the open stoma, which will close within a short time. The procedure is carried out in a clinical setting where continuous observation is available and emergency reintubation can be accomplished without delay, if necessary. After successful decannulation, the child remains under close observation for an additional period.

Home Care of the Child with a Tracheostomy

The early return of the infant or child with a tracheostomy to a home setting can reduce developmental delays or social handicaps related to prolonged hospitalization. Placement in the home also allows for reestablishment of routines and a regular schedule of normal activities. Physical, occupational, and speech therapy continues in the home setting. Nursing care may also be continued in the home through private-duty care or by routine, frequent nursing visits.

Preparing the family to care for the child with a tracheostomy at home is multifaceted (see Family-Centered Care box). Teaching sessions should be short, and written material must accompany instructions to reinforce what is taught. The family must be able to demonstrate tracheostomy care before the child is discharged from the hospital. Home-based care of a tracheostomy includes suctioning the tracheostomy; cleaning the stoma; changing the tracheostomy ties; changing the tracheostomy tube; adapting the home environment; and recognizing warning signs of obstruction, infection, or a worsening condition.

To prepare for any emergency, the family must learn infant or child cardiopulmonary resuscitation (CPR). The local utility company and local emergency medical service (EMS) should be notified of the child's condition and the equipment used in the home. Prior notification allows for a quick response if help is needed.

The home should have all the necessary equipment before the child arrives. Supplies include sterile saline; a portable suction machine (and a DeLee suction trap); connecting tubing for suction; suction catheters; tracheostomy dressings; twill tape or self-adhering tracheostomy ties; pipe cleaners or a tracheostomy brush; an extra tracheostomy tube; a BVM; and a

Lack of Privacy: Children with Respiratory Problems in Home Care

Currently, many children with chronic respiratory problems are discharged home on apnea monitors, on oxygen, or with a tracheostomy or ventilator assistance. When a child is on an apnea monitor, the family may need to make only a few adjustments in their routines to accommodate this need. However, when a child has a tracheostomy or requires ventilator assistance, many family routines may need to be changed. In particular, the family needs to give up some privacy to accommodate many different people coming into the home. Nurses, equipment vendors, respiratory therapists, rehabilitation therapists, and social workers all may need to visit frequently. One mother of a child in home care counted 25 different health-related professionals who came to her home in a single day. All these intrusions seriously limit privacy and tax the family's coping strategies. Many mothers of children in home care state that no one prepared them for the constant interruptions in daily routines, the continuous demands on their time, the loss of family leisure time, and the need to interact with so many different people. Nurses who work with families of children in home care because of respiratory problems need to provide information concerning the changes the family can anticipate in their everyday routines, the stress these changes can produce, the need for respite care, and the benefits of support groups in providing emotional support.

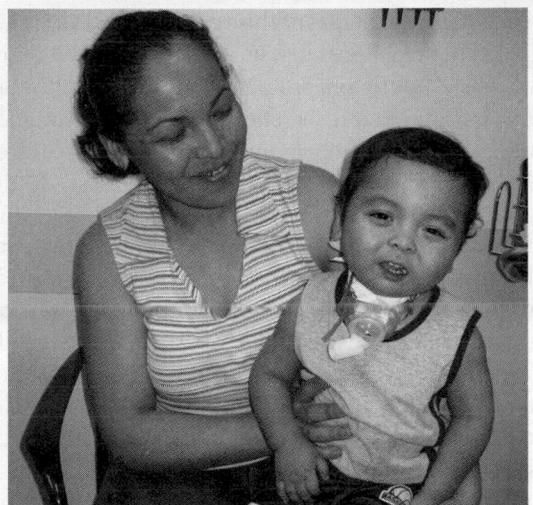

Fig. 31-19 Child with a tracheostomy.

cool mist humidifier. Many children receive oxygen at home, so this too must be in place. Finally, an apnea monitor or pulse oximeter may be needed in some situations.

Encourage the family to take the child out of the home for routine outings. Two people should always be present when traveling because the child may need attention while riding in the car or at the destination. In addition to routine child care supplies, the family should always bring the portable suction machine, suction catheters, gloves, and an extra tracheostomy tube.

Management of the Tracheostomy

Clean technique and thorough, strict hand washing are taught for suctioning, cleaning the tracheostomy site, and changing the tracheostomy tube. After initial use, the catheter is rinsed with sterile water and then stored between uses in a clean cup or jar once it has dried sufficiently. The catheter may be used and cleansed appropriately as long as it remains intact and secretions can be visualized in the catheter.

Skin at the tracheostomy site is assessed for areas of breakdown or drainage. The area can be cleansed with an antibacterial soap and water.

Encourage the family to avoid frequently suctioning the child because this increases mucus production and irritates the mucosal lining. The care provider should be alert to changes in the child's secretions regarding the amount, color, or viscosity. Awareness of these changes can prompt early medical interventions if necessary.

The family must be able to remove a plugged, clogged, or obstructed tracheostomy tube and replace it with a clean one. This situation can result in life-threatening circumstances. Older children and adolescents should be taught to care for their tracheostomies. The child should be encouraged to assume as much of his or her care as is developmentally appropriate. Independence is enhanced as the child takes responsibility for tracheostomy care.

Home Environment

Changes in the home environment may be necessary before bringing the child home. Toys, blankets, clothing, and pets that shed fine hair or lint, as well as aerosols, powders, dust, and smoke, should be avoided. Fine particles from any of these items can accumulate in the tracheostomy tube and obstruct the airway. Toys that have small removable parts (that could be placed in the tracheostomy tube) should also be eliminated.

Clothing should have a loose-fitting collar that does not cover the tracheostomy tube opening (Fig. 31-19). When the child is outside, the artificial nose or a thin cloth such as a bandanna or face mask can be placed loosely over the tracheostomy tube to prevent cold air, dust, dirt, or sand from entering the tube. The child can be bathed in a tub filled with shallow water, although it is important to ensure that no water or soap enters the tracheostomy tube. If this does occur, the tracheostomy should be suctioned immediately. Older children may shower if they are able to tolerate plugging the tube while under the shower spray.

Vocalization

The life of a child with a tracheostomy should be normalized. After the child returns home, the family should establish routines that allow the child to renew skills and enhance childhood development. Verbalization and speaking are major tasks that are often overlooked. Vocalization for the child with a tracheostomy has recently become a reality. Several tracheostomy speaking valves have been created to aid in the development of uninterrupted speech without the necessity of finger occlusion. When the speaking valve is used, air enters through the tracheostomy but is expelled over the vocal cords and through the mouth and nose. This creates a more normal passage of air through the upper airway.

A speaking valve offers many benefits. The child develops an improved self-image, since the tracheostomy can be disguised and finger occlusion for speech is not needed. The ability to swallow improves, because pressure can now accumulate as a result of the decreased amount of air released from the tracheostomy. This also allows for the creation of back pressure into the lungs. The lungs then remain open for improved gas exchange. Other advantages of this redirection of air by a speaking valve into the upper airway include improved senses of smell and taste. Secretion production is decreased because of normal evaporation, and secretions can now be coughed into the mouth, decreasing the amount of suctioning required.

Several speaking valves are available. The Passy-Muir valve is a one-way valve that attaches to the hub of all types and sizes of tracheostomies. The Passy-Muir valve will not function properly without an air leak around the tracheostomy tube and is contraindicated if there is no air leak around the tube or there is an upper airway obstruction (Kaut, Turcott, and Lavery, 1996). Therefore a cuffed tracheostomy tube must be fully deflated when using the Passy-Muir valve. If the cuff is not deflated and the Passy-Muir valve is attached, the patient will lose his or her airway. This valve can be used in infants and in children who are ventilator assisted (Engleman and Turnage-Carrier, 1997).

Two types of speaking valves are available for adolescents and adults. The first, the Kistner valve—a part of all Kistner tracheostomy tubes—is made of thin, soft plastic and does not protrude into the trachea. (Jackson metal tracheostomy tubes can also be used with a Kistner valve.) The second type is the Tucker valve, which is built into the inner cannula as a one-way leaflet. The leaflet opens on inspiration to allow air in and closes on expiration to force air into the upper airway. The Tucker valve inner cannula can be used with Tucker tracheostomy tubes sizes 4 to 9 and with Jackson tracheostomy tubes sizes 4 to 8. Tucker valves can only be used with sterling silver tracheostomy tubes.

Tracheostomy speaking valves are inappropriate for use in children who require an inflated cuff tracheostomy; who have a laryngectomy, severe tracheostenosis, or copious or excessive secretions; or who are unconscious or seriously ill.

Socialization

School-age children can be in a regular classroom environment and participate in school activities as their physical abilities allow. They should be encouraged to interact with their peers to facilitate development of socialization skills. Participation in ability-appropriate extracurricular activities is also advocated.

Many children with tracheostomies benefit from attending summer camps for children with tracheostomies who may or may not be ventilator dependent. Camping environments provide the child with independent living and a normal camping experience. Some camping sites allow the family to vacation together yet provide special care and assistance for the child with a tracheostomy.

RESPIRATORY EMERGENCY

RESPIRATORY FAILURE

An inadequate supply of oxygen results in blood hypoxemia and tissue hypoxia; inadequate carbon dioxide removal causes hypercapnia. Often both gases may be insufficiently exchanged. In general, the term **respiratory insufficiency** is applied to two conditions: (1) when there is increased work of breathing but gas exchange function remains near normal, and (2) when normal blood gas tensions cannot be maintained and hypox-

emia and acidosis develop secondary to carbon dioxide retention.

Respiratory failure is the inability of the respiratory apparatus to maintain adequate gas exchange. This process involves pulmonary dysfunction that generally results in impaired alveolar-capillary gas exchange, which can lead to hypoxemia or hypercapnia. **Respiratory arrest** is the cessation of respiration. Respiratory failure is the most common cause of cardiopulmonary arrest in children (Rotta and Wiryawan, 2003).

Apnea is generally defined as cessation of breathing for more than 20 seconds or for a shorter period when associated with hypoxemia or bradycardia (Dudell and Stoll, 2007). Apnea can be (1) central, in which both airflow and chest wall movement are absent; (2) obstructive, in which airflow is absent but chest wall motion is present; and (3) mixed, in which both central and obstructive components are present.

Effective pulmonary gas exchange requires clear airways, normal lungs and chest wall, and adequate pulmonary circulation. Anything that affects these functions or their relationships can compromise respiration.

Respiratory dysfunction may have an abrupt or an insidious onset. Respiratory failure can occur as an emergency situation or may be preceded by gradual and progressive deterioration of respiratory function. Most clinical manifestations are nonspecific and are affected by variations among individual patients and differences in the severity and duration of inadequate gas exchange.

The diagnosis of respiratory failure is determined by the combined application of three sources of information:

1. Presence or history of a condition that might predispose to respiratory failure
2. Observation of respiratory failure
3. Measurement of ABGs

Conditions That Predispose to Respiratory Failure

Respiratory disorders are classified according to three dominant functional abnormalities, although all three types may be present in the disease. In obstructive lung disease there is increased resistance to airflow in either the upper or the lower respiratory tract. Obstruction can result from anomalies (tracheomalacia, choanal atresia, vocal paralysis), aspiration (meconium, mucus, vomitus, FB), infection (epiglottitis, pneumonia, pertussis, severe tonsillitis), tumors (hemangioma, cystic hygroma), anaphylaxis, and laryngospasm from local irritation (intubation, drowning, aspiration).

In restrictive lung disease, impaired lung expansion results from loss of lung volume, decreased distensibility, or chest wall disturbance. Causes of pulmonary restriction include respiratory distress syndrome, pneumonia, cystic fibrosis, pneumothorax, pulmonary edema, pleural effusion, near drowning, congenital diaphragmatic hernia, abdominal distention, muscular dystrophy, paralytic conditions (poliomyelitis, botulism), and severe structural obstructions such as severe scoliosis.

In primary inefficient gas transfer there is insufficient alveolar ventilation for carbon dioxide removal or impaired oxygenation of pulmonary capillary blood as a result of dysfunction of the respiratory control mechanism or a diffusion defect. Causes of respiratory center depression include cerebral trauma (birth injuries); intracranial tumors; CNS infection (meningitis, encephalitis, sepsis); overdose with barbiturates, opioids, or benzodiazepines (diazepam [Valium] or midazolam); severe asphyxia (hypercapnia, hypoxemia); and tetanus. Pulmonary diffusion defects include pulmonary edema, fibrosis, embolism, or hypertension; collagen disorders; *Pneumocystis carinii* pneumonia; anemia; and hemorrhage.

Recognition of Respiratory Failure

Respiratory failure that occurs as a result of acute obstruction of a major airway or cardiac arrest is sudden and readily apparent. Gradual and more covert development of signs and symptoms is less easily recognized. Insufficient alveolar ventilation from any cause ultimately leads to hypoxemia and hypercapnia. However, in some situations severe respiratory distress may be present without significant carbon dioxide retention, and hypoxemia may occur without clinically detectable cyanosis. Therefore evaluation of respiratory adequacy is based on both clinical assessment and laboratory studies. Nursing observation and judgment are vital to successful management of respiratory failure. Nurses must be able to assess a situation and initiate appropriate action within moments.

Unless respiratory arrest occurs suddenly, signs of hypoxemia and hypercapnia are usually subtle in their development, becoming more obvious as respiratory failure progresses. The unknowing observer may attribute early signs such as mood changes and restlessness to other causes, and some signs can be altered by other factors. Clinical manifestations of respiratory failure are listed in Box 31-8.

In clinical situations in which impaired ventilation can be anticipated or clinical manifestations indicate impending hypoxemia, serial measurements of blood gases should be obtained and monitored to detect impending respiratory failure, and therapy should be implemented before respiratory acidosis becomes extreme.

NURSING CARE MANAGEMENT

The interventions used in the management of respiratory failure are often dramatic, requiring special skills, and are frequently emergency procedures. If respiratory arrest occurs, the primary objectives are to recognize the situation and immediately initiate resuscitative measures, such as opening the airway and positioning, administering supplemental oxygen and positive pressure ventilation, suctioning, performing CPR, or intubating if the child's status continues to deteriorate. When the situation is not an arrest, the suspicion of respiratory failure is confirmed by assessment, and the severity is defined by capillary or arterial blood gas analysis. Interventions such as administering supplemental oxygen, opening the airway, positioning, stimulation, suctioning, and early intubation may avert an arrest. When severity is established, an attempt is made to determine the underlying cause by thorough evaluation.

Treatment of respiratory dysfunction involves both specific and nonspecific therapy. Specific therapies are directed toward reversal of the causative factors. However, nonspecific measures are necessary to maintain oxygenation and enhance carbon dioxide removal until specific methods take effect. The major reasons for implementing nonspecific treatments are (1) unknown etiology, (2) lack of specific treatment for a known

> ### BOX 31-8   CLINICAL MANIFESTATIONS OF RESPIRATORY FAILURE
>
> **Cardinal Signs**
> Restlessness
> Tachypnea
> Tachycardia
> Diaphoresis
>
> **Early But Less Obvious Signs**
> Mood changes, such as euphoria or depression
> Headache
> Altered depth and pattern of respirations (increased work of breathing)
> Hypertension
> Exertional dyspnea
> Anorexia
> Increased cardiac output and urinary output
> Central nervous system symptoms (decreased efficiency, impaired judgment, anxiety, confusion, restlessness, irritability, depressed level of consciousness)
> Nasal flaring
> Retractions
> Expiratory grunting
> Wheezing or prolonged expiration
>
> **Signs of More Severe Hypoxia**
> Hypotension or hypertension
> Depressed respirations
> Dimness of vision
> Bradycardia
> Somnolence
> Cyanosis, peripheral or central
> Stupor
> Coma
> Dyspnea

cause, (3) lack of time for a specific treatment to take effect, and (4) need for specialized personnel or equipment for specific treatment.

The principles of management are to (1) maintain ventilation and maximize oxygen delivery, (2) correct hypoxemia and hypercapnia, (3) treat the underlying cause, (4) minimize extrapulmonary organ failure, (5) apply specific and nonspecific therapy to control oxygen demands, and (6) anticipate complications. Monitoring the patient's condition is critical.

Observation and Monitoring

The nurse monitors the child to anticipate respiratory failure, determine a course of action, and assess the patient's response to treatment. If close, continuous monitoring is required, the child is transferred to a pediatric intensive care unit. The child is kept as comfortable as possible, and observation is geared toward general appearance, responsiveness, pulse oximetry, and vital signs. The child is positioned to allow maximum lung expansion and comfort, such as sitting upright or leaning forward (depending on respiratory status).

Prone positioning improves oxygenation and lung mechanics in adult patients with acute lung injury and acute respiratory distress syndrome. A multicenter pediatric trial for prone positioning showed it to be ineffective in improving oxygenation in acute lung injury or acute respiratory distress syndrome (Curley, Hibberd, Fineman, et al, 2005). At this point, the only

---

BOX 31-9   NURSING OBSERVATIONS FOR THE CHILD WITH RESPIRATORY FAILURE

Observation of respiratory effort or distress—Nasal flaring, grunting, gasping, retractions, agonal respirations

Observation of diaphragmatic movement, lung expansion, and use of accessory muscles—Depth, symmetry, inspiration/expiration ratio

Auscultation of chest to assess:

- Breath sounds—presence, intensity, quality, symmetry
- Abnormal sounds—stridor, wheezes, crackles, rhonchi, increase or decrease in sounds
- Endotracheal tube placement and need for suction

Visual inspection of skin color, capillary refill

Observation of activity level and level of consciousness

---

indications for its use are in the case of bronchial compression by the heart or the need to augment secretion clearance. The nurse monitors the child's cardiac and respiratory status by observation and by electronic means. However, no monitoring equipment can replace conscientious nursing observations (Box 31-9), which should focus primarily on the child's airway, oxygenation, ventilation, and tissue perfusion.

Because one goal of therapy is to control the body's oxygen demands, assessments of fever and pain should be frequent. Both conditions (as well as cold stress) can dramatically increase oxygen requirements, especially in younger children, and therefore increase respiratory effort. Measure oxygenation by the use of pulse oximetry or blood gas monitoring.

Family Support

Children who are in respiratory distress often relax after an airway is established and their respiratory effort is assisted. However, they are anxious and frightened when they are unable to communicate; therefore it is important to effectively manage the child's anxiety. This may be accomplished initially with mild sedation until the child's ventilatory status has improved.

It is often frightening for young children to discover they are unable to make vocal sounds, including crying. It is also stressful to parents to watch their child's inability to vocalize and helplessness. It is important to talk to children and reassure them that their voices will return when the breathing tube (ET tube or tracheostomy) is removed.

Parents have many concerns relative to ET tubes and ventilators. Before intubation, the nurse should discuss with them the reasons for the decision to implement the therapy, the expected results, and the approximate length of time it will remain in place. Parents are often concerned about the (often) life-threatening implications generated by the need for the procedure and the possible long-term effects on the child, both physiologic and psychologic. They are also concerned about the long-term residual effects on the brain and on the child's psychologic status. Parents who must face the possibility of caring for the child with a tracheostomy or a home ventilator have additional worries regarding their ability to assume this responsibility (see p. 1206).

For families whose child has had a respiratory arrest, support focuses on keeping the family informed of the child's status and helping them cope with a near-death experience or an actual death. (See Chapter 23.) Knowing that their child requires CPR is a frightening and often overwhelming experience for parents. Uncertainty regarding outcome—both mortality and morbidity—is a primary concern. Traditionally family members have not been allowed to be present during resuscitation efforts (see Evidence-Based Practice box).

Nurses can serve as the family's advocate by either being present with them or making certain a support person, such as a clergy member, is present. After the child's recovery or death, the family needs continued support and thorough medical information regarding lifesaving measures, the prognosis if the child survives, and the cause of death if the child dies.

CARDIOPULMONARY RESUSCITATION

Cardiac arrest in the pediatric population is less often of cardiac origin than a result of prolonged hypoxemia secondary to inadequate oxygenation, ventilation, and circulation (shock). Some causes include injuries, suffocation (e.g., FB aspiration), smoke inhalation, anaphylaxis, apparent life-threatening event, and infection. In small infants the small size of the airway may easily be compromised by improper positioning with the chin resting on the chest. This is easy to remedy by positioning the infant with the chin elevated (but not hyperextended) so the airway is open. This is common in newborns or infants who are not positioned properly in an infant seat or car restraint seat.

Respiratory arrest is associated with a better survival rate than cardiac arrest. Recent studies indicate that infants survived out-of-hospital cardiac arrest (including survival to hospital discharge) at a rate similar to that of adults—3.3% for infants and 4.5 % for adults. However, older children and adolescents survived out-of-hospital cardiac arrest at higher rates—9.1% and 8.9%, respectively (Atkins, Everson-Stewart, Sears, et al, 2009). Ventricular fibrillation, previously believed to be rare in children, occurred in 25% of patients with in-hospital pediatric cardiac arrest and 7% of those with out-of-hospital pediatric cardiac arrest (Topjian, Nadkarni, and Berg, 2009). Studies demonstrated that more males required resuscitation in pre-hospital settings, and the overall survival rate was approximately 9% (Young, Gausche-Hill, McClung, et al, 2004).

Complete apnea signals the need for rapid and vigorous action to prevent cardiac arrest. In such situations nurses must be prepared to initiate action immediately. In the hospital, emergency equipment should be readily available in areas in which respiratory arrest might take place, and the status of this resuscitation equipment should be checked at least once daily. Regardless of the cause of the arrest, basic procedures are carried out and modified somewhat according to the child's size.

Outside the hospital the first action in an emergency is to quickly assess the extent of any injury and determine whether the child is unconscious. A child who is struggling to breathe but conscious should be transported immediately to an advanced life support (ALS) facility, allowing the child to maintain whatever position affords the most comfort. Attempting to transport a child by personal vehicle wastes valuable time in obtaining help. Transport by EMS is recommended. Services in larger communities can institute ALS immediately or en route to a medical facility.

EVIDENCE-BASED PRACTICE

Family Presence During Resuscitation of a Child

ASK THE QUESTION

Is family presence at the resuscitation of a child perceived by the family as a positive event?

SEARCH FOR THE EVIDENCE

Search strategies

The English-language literature between 1994 and 2009 was searched to obtain information regarding the presence of family members during the resuscitation of a child family member.

Databases used

PubMed, CINAHL, professional organization websites

CRITICALLY ANALYZE THE EVIDENCE

GRADE criteria: Evidence quality moderate; recommendation strong (Moreland, 2005)

- A number of studies in adult patients indicate that family presence during invasive procedures and resuscitation alleviates the family's anger about being separated from the patient during a crisis, reduces their anxiety, eliminates doubts about what was done to help the patient, facilitates the grieving process, increases the perception of the patient as an individual and increases respect for the patient, lessens the family's feelings of helplessness, allows closure and a chance to say good-bye, facilitates a relationship between the medical staff and family through increased communication, and helps family understand the gravity or severity of the patient's condition (Mangurten, Scott, Guzzetta, et al, 2006; Meyers, Eichhorn, Guzzetta, et al, 2000; Powers and Rubenstein, 1999; Sacchetti, Lichenstein, Caraccio, et al, 1996; Eichhorn, Meyers, Mitchell, et al, 1996; Tucker, 2002). In many cases family members expressed that it was their right to be present when a family member receives emergent treatment or resuscitation.
- Interviews with 39 English-speaking family members and 96 health care providers who were present in the emergency department (ED) during invasive procedures or cardiopulmonary resuscitation (CPR) revealed that their presence at the procedure was helpful and that they would do it again (Meyers, Eichhorn, Guzzetta, et al, 2000). Ninety-six percent of the nurses and 79% of the attending physicians supported family presence and thought it should be continued at the hospital. Eighty percent of family members said they wanted to be at the patient's side during an ED visit that involved resuscitation. The sample consisted mostly of adult patients with a mean age of 44.5 (±23.1) years.
- In a survey of parents with children admitted to the ED for invasive procedures and possibly CPR, family members responded favorably to being present if the child was conscious (less favorably if child was unconscious) on admission to the ED, and 83% of the respondents expressed a desire to be present if the child was likely to die (Boie, Moore, Brummett, et al, 1999). The survey consisted of five case scenarios with increasing levels of invasiveness, and the parents were asked whether they would want to be present at the family member's bedside during the procedure.
- Tinsley, Hill, Shah, et al (2008) conducted 40 interviews of guardians or parents who were present during the child's resuscitation in a PICU. Seventy-one percent of the parents and guardians surveyed felt their presence during the resuscitation comforted the child, whereas 67% of the parents and guardians expressed that their presence helped them adjust to the loss of the child. This study is unique in that all of the children resuscitated died 6 months before the interview.
- Professional organizations support the presence of family members during CPR. The Emergency Nurses Association (2001) has developed national guidelines for family presence during invasive procedures and CPR. These guidelines include recommendations for assessing family members to determine whether family presence is appropriate and the use of a family facilitator (e.g., nurse, child life specialist, social worker, or chaplain) who remains with the family during resuscitation to answer questions, clarify information, and offer comfort.
- The American Heart Association (2005) recommends that providers offer families the option to remain with the loved one during resuscitation. Likewise, the PALS [pediatric advanced life support] Provider Manual (Hazinski, Zaritsky, Nadkarni, et al, 2002) supports the presence of family during the child's CPR with the presence of a family support facilitator. A sample protocol to prepare and support family presence, based on the recommendations of the Association for the Care of Children's Health, can be found in a publication by Meyers, Eichhorn, Guzzetta, and colleagues (2000).
- Some studies addressed health care workers' attitudes about family presence during resuscitation of a child (Sanford, Pugh, and Warren, 2002). Health care workers' attitudes about family presence during resuscitation vary considerably. Sixty percent of the health care workers (nurses and physicians) surveyed said they felt comfortable performing resuscitation procedures with a family member present; no distinction was made between adult or child patient (Mangurten, Scott, Guzzetta, et al, 2005). ED staff with previous experience in having family members present during pediatric resuscitation favored the practice, whereas the staff without prior exposure to family presence were against the practice (Sacchetti, Caraccio, Leva, et al, 2000). Tsai (2002) asserted that most physicians and nurses do not favor family members' presence during resuscitation procedures, and in a survey of pediatricians, nurses, and residents, 65% said they would not allow family presence during pediatric CPR (O'Brien, Creamer, Hill, et al, 2002). Dudley, Hansen, Furnival, and colleagues (2009) found that family presence in the ED did not delay time to CT scan or the resuscitation procedure itself for pediatric patients requiring trauma resuscitation.
- Two critical reviews examined the presence of family members during resuscitation. Moreland's 2005 review of 23 studies on family presence during resuscitation and invasive procedures emphasizes the differing aspects of each study reviewed; mixed research methodologies make it difficult to draw conclusions for the general population, and most were based on sample interviews and questionnaires after the event. Moreland concludes that further research is needed to evaluate the long-term effects of family presence on family members and health care providers. Nibert and Ondrejka (2005) concluded that there is no research supporting the exclusion of family from resuscitation events, that many clinician beliefs and practices on the topic are not evidence based, and that families want to be consulted regarding their presence during the resuscitation of a child.

SUMMARY OF FINDINGS

- The studies reviewed included information regarding family presence during invasive procedures and resuscitation, not solely pediatric resuscitation.
- Only one of these studies evaluated the responses of family members actually present during a pediatric resuscitation in the ED (Dudley, Hansen, Furnival, et al, 2009) but the goal of the study was to evaluate the effect of family presence on the procedure itself; therefore minimal family opinions were obtained.
- Most of the studies published to date did not address the issue of family presence during resuscitation in areas other than the ED (general pediatric floor, post-anesthesia care unit, PICU, outpatient settings). Three studies identified family presence in the PICU as being important for invasive procedures and end-of-life decisions but did not address family presence during resuscitation and subsequent reactions to the event (Anderson, McCall, Leversha, et al, 1994; Meyer, Burns, Griffith, et al, 2002; Powers and Rubenstein, 1999).

Continued

Family Presence During Resuscitation of a Child

SUMMARY OF FINDINGS—cont'd

- Studies addressed the reactions and opinions of the health care workers regarding family presence during the resuscitative event. Health care worker beliefs and opinions for or against the practice of family presence during resuscitation were not a significant part of this review.
- There is no evidence to support excluding family members during a child's resuscitation unless a facilitator is unavailable to communicate with the family during the process.
- Further research is needed to validate the effects of family presence in childhood resuscitation events.

APPLY THE EVIDENCE: NURSING IMPLICATIONS

- The presence of family at the resuscitation of a child can be beneficial provided that a facilitator is present to communicate with the family.
- Giving the family the option of being present during a pediatric resuscitation may help the family be a part of the decision making process and help achieve closure in the event of the child's death.
- Health care workers should encourage family presence during resuscitation when appropriate.
- Protocols for family presence during resuscitation should be developed and implemented in institutions where children and families are served.

References

American Heart Association: 2005 American Heart Association guidelines for cardiopulmonary resuscitation and emergency cardiovascular care, *Circulation* 112(24, Suppl I):IV-166, 2005.

Anderson B, McCall E, Leversha A, et al: A review of children's dying in a paediatric intensive care unit, *New Zealand Med J* 107(985):345-347, 1994.

Boie T, Moore GP, Brummett C, et al: Do parents want to be present during invasive procedures performed on their children in the emergency department? A survey of 400 parents, *Ann Emerg Med* 34(1):70-74, 1999.

Dudley NC, Hansen KW, Furnival RA, et al: The effect of family presence on the efficacy of pediatric trauma resuscitations, *Ann Emerg Med* 53(6):777-784, 2009.

Eichhorn DJ, Meyers TA, Mitchell TG, et al: Opening the doors: family presence during resuscitation, *J Cardiovasc Nurs* 10(4):59-70, 1996.

Emergency Nurses Association: *Position statement: family presence at the bedside during invasive procedures and resuscitation*, 2001, available at www.ena.org/about/position (accessed June 2005).

Hazinski MF, Zaritsky AL, Nadkarni VM, et al: *PALS provider manual*, Dallas, 2002, American Heart Association.

Mangurten J, Scott SH, Guzzetta CE, et al: Effects of family presence during resuscitation and invasive procedures in a pediatric emergency department, *J Emerg Nurs* 32(3):225-233, 2006.

Mangurten JA, Scott SH, Guzzetta CE, et al: Family presence: making room, *AJN* 105(5):40-48, 2005.

Meyer EC, Burns JP, Griffith JL, et al: Parental perspectives on end-of-life care in the pediatric intensive care unit, *Crit Care Med* 30(1):226-231, 2002.

Meyers TA, Eichhorn DJ, Guzzetta CE, et al: Family presence during invasive procedures and resuscitation, *Am J Nurs* 100(2):32-42, 2000.

Moreland P: Family presence during invasive procedures and resuscitation in the emergency department: a review of the literature, *J Emerg Nurs* 31(1):58-72, 2005.

Nibert L, Ondrejka D: Family presence during pediatric resuscitation: an integrative review of evidence-based practice, *J Pediatr Nurs* 20(2):145-147, 2005.

O'Brien M, Creamer KM, Hill EE, et al: Tolerance of family presence during pediatric cardiopulmonary resuscitation: a snapshot of military and civilian pediatricians, nurses, and residents, *Pediatr Emerg Care* 18(6):409-413, 2002.

Powers KS, Rubenstein JS: Family presence during invasive procedures in the pediatric intensive care unit: a prospective study, *Arch Pediatr Adolesc Med* 153(9):955-958, 1999.

Sacchetti A, Caraccio C, Leva E, et al: Acceptance of family member presence during pediatric resuscitations in the emergency department: effects of personal experiences, *Pediatr Emerg Care* 16(2):85-87, 2000.

Sacchetti A, Lichenstein R, Caraccio CA, et al: Family member presence during pediatric emergency department procedures, *Pediatr Emerg Care* 12(4):268-271, 1996.

Sanford M, Pugh D, Warren NA: Family presence during CPR: new decisions in the twenty-first century, *Crit Care Nurs Q* 25(2):61-66, 2002.

Tinsley C, Hill B, Shah J, et al: Experience of families during cardiopulmonary resuscitation in a pediatric intensive care unit, *Pediatrics* 122(4):e799-e804, 2008.

Tsai E: Should family members be present during cardiopulmonary resuscitation? *N Engl J Med* 346(13):1019-1021, 2002.

Tucker T: Family presence during resuscitation, *Crit Care Clin North Am* 14(2):177-185, 2002.

An unconscious child is managed with care to prevent additional trauma if a head or spinal cord injury has been sustained. The circumstances in which the child is found offer clues to a possible injury. For example, a child who has been thrown from a bicycle or has fallen from a tree is more likely to have sustained trauma than a child who is discovered in bed. The child should not be moved unless there is a life-threatening condition such as a fire; if moved, the victim must be appropriately immobilized with spinal and cervical immobilization devices.

Resuscitation Procedure

The American Heart Association (2005) implemented several changes in CPR guidelines that incorporate the use of the automatic external defibrillator (AED) as part of the treatment of cardiorespiratory arrest in children 1 year of age and older. The 2005 guidelines state that AEDs can be safely and effectively used in children ages 1 to 8 years; however, there are insufficient data to support or refute the use of AEDs in children younger than 1 year old. Appropriate-sized pediatric pads must be used for small children. Health care providers are advised to

give children 1 year and older a defibrillatory shock after providing approximately five cycles of CPR (approximately 2 minutes of cycles of 30 compressions and two ventilations by the lone rescuer), provided the AED is sensitive to pediatric rhythms, the device is capable of delivering a pediatric dosage of 2 joules/kg, and a shockable rhythm (usually ventricular fibrillation) is present. In a hospital situation, where weight-based defibrillation dosing is possible, manual defibrillation is the mode of choice instead of AED. When using an AED, health care providers are advised to give adults and children older than 8 years a defibrillatory shock within 5 minutes of collapse outside the hospital and within 3 minutes in the hospital.

Changes in resuscitation procedure for the lay rescuer are discussed in the following section. The sequence of CPR steps for the health care provider is discussed in both the text and Fig. 31-20.

If two rescuers are present, one rescuer should begin CPR while the second rescuer activates the EMS system by calling 911 and obtaining an AED. Pediatric rescuers provide five cycles of basic life support (approximately 2 minutes) before

Maneuver	Adult **Lay rescuer:** ≥8 yr **HCP:** Adolescent and older	Child **Lay rescuer:** 1–8 yr **HCP:** 1 yr to adolescence	Infant **Infant** <1 yr of age
Activate Emergency response Number (1 rescuer)	Activate when victim found unresponsive. **HCP:** If asphyxial arrest likely, call after 5 cycles (2 min) of CPR.	Activate after performing 5 cycles of CPR. For sudden, witnessed collapse, activate after verifying that victim unresponsive.	
Airway	Head tilt–chin lift (**HCP:** suspected trauma, use jaw thrust)		
Breaths Initial	2 breaths at 1 sec/breath	2 effective breaths at 1 sec/breath	
HCP: Rescue breathing without chest compressions	10-12 breaths/min (approximately 1 breath every 5-6 sec)	12-20 breaths/min (approximately 1 breath every 3-5 sec)	
HCP: Rescue breaths for CPR with advanced airway	8-10 breaths/min (approximately 1 breath every 6-8 sec)		
Foreign-body airway obstruction	Abdominal thrusts		Back slaps and chest thrusts
Circulation **HCP:** Pulse check (≤10 sec)	Carotid (**HCP** can use femoral in child)		Brachial or femoral
Compression landmarks	Center of chest, between nipples		Just below nipple line
Compression method Push hard and fast Allow complete recoil	**2 Hands:** Heel of 1 hand, other hand on top	**2 Hands:** Heel of 1 hand with second on top *or* **1 Hand:** Heel of 1 hand only	**1 Rescuer:** 2 fingers **HCP, 2 rescuers:** 2 thumb-encircling hands
Compression depth	1½-2 inches	Approximately ⅓-½ the depth of the chest	
Compression rate	Approximately 100/min		
Compression-ventilation ratio	30:2 (1 or 2 rescuers)	30:2 (1 rescuer) **HCP:** 15:2 (2 rescuers)	
Defibrillation (AED)	Use adult pads. Do not use child pads/child system. **HCP:** For out-of-hospital response, may provide 5 cycles/2 min of CPR before shock if response >4-5 min and arrest not witnessed.	**HCP:** Use AED as soon as available for sudden collapse and in-hospital. **All:** Use after 5 cycles of CPR (out-of-hospital). If available, use child pads/child system for child 1-8 yr. If pads/system not available, use adult AED pads.	No recommendation for infants <1 yr of age.

Fig. 31-20 Summary of basic life support maneuvers for infants, children, and adults (newborn-neonatal information not included). *CPR,* Cardiopulmonary resuscitation; *HCP,* maneuvers used only by health care provider; *AED,* automated external defibrillator. (From American Heart Association: 2005 American Heart Association guidelines for cardiopulmonary resuscitation and emergency cardiovascular care, *Circulation* 112[24 Suppl 1]:IV-166, 2005.)

activating EMS; each cycle consists of 30 chest compressions and two ventilations. Because pediatric arrests are most commonly caused by respiratory arrest, maintaining ventilation is primary.

Open the Airway

For effective CPR, place the victim on the back on a firm, flat surface, using appropriate precautions. With loss of consciousness the tongue, which is attached to the lower jaw, relaxes and falls back, obstructing the airway. To open the airway, the lay rescuer positions the head with a head tilt–chin lift maneuver. Health professionals should open the airway using either a head tilt–chin lift or jaw thrust maneuver. A head tilt is accomplished by placing one hand on the victim's forehead and applying firm, backward pressure with the palm to tilt the head back. Place the fingers of the free hand under the bony portion of the lower jaw near the chin to lift and bring the chin forward (chin lift). This supports the jaw and helps tilt the head back (Fig. 31-21).

The jaw thrust is accomplished by grasping the angles of the victim's lower jaw and lifting with both hands, one on each side, displacing the mandible upward and outward. *The jaw thrust is recommended for use only by health care workers.* In suspected neck injuries, use the jaw thrust method while the cervical spine

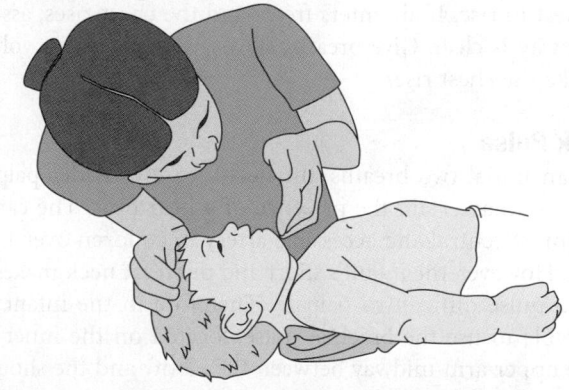

Fig. 31-21 Open airway using the head tilt–chin lift maneuver, and check breathing.

is completely immobilized. After a patent airway is restored by removal of foreign material and secretions (if indicated), if the child is not breathing, continue maintenance of the airway and initiate rescue breathing.

Give Breaths

To ventilate the lungs in the infant (from birth to 1 year of age), place the BVM or operator's mouth in such a way that both the

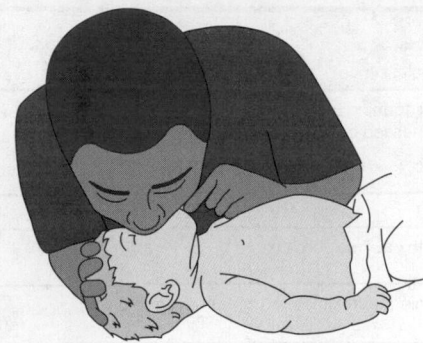

Fig. 31-22 Mouth-to-mouth and nose breathing for infant.

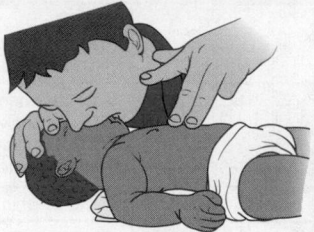

Fig. 31-24 Combining chest compressions with breathing in infant.

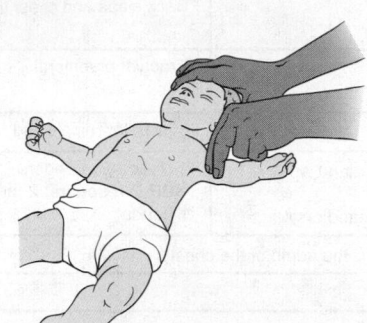

Fig. 31-23 Locating brachial pulse in infant.

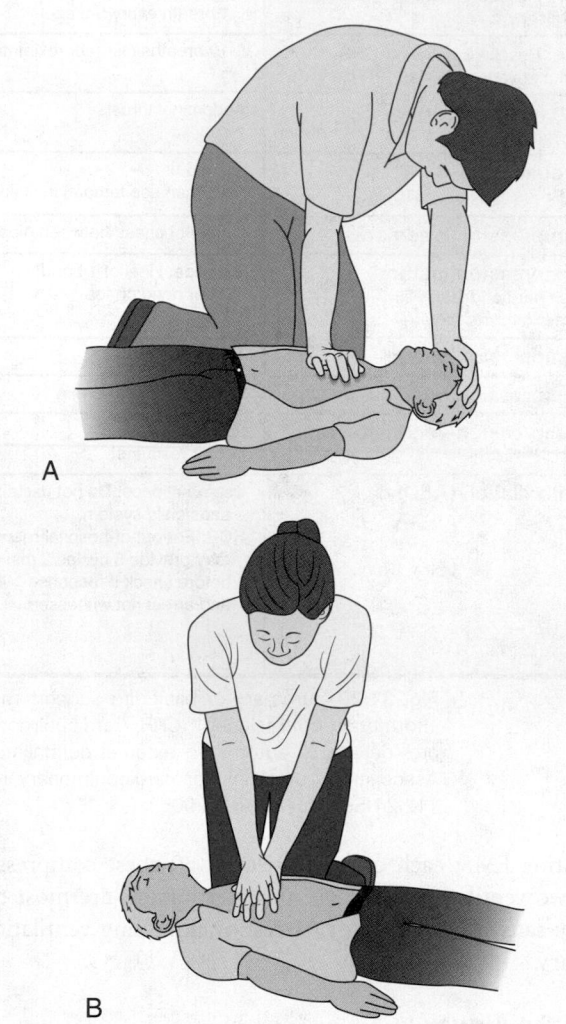

A

B

Fig. 31-25 Chest compressions in child: one hand for smaller child **(A)** and two hands for larger child **(B)**.

mouth and the nostrils are covered (Fig. 31-22). Children over 1 year of age are ventilated through the mouth while the nostrils are firmly pinched for airtight contact.

The volume of air in an infant's lungs is small, and the air passages are considerably smaller, with resistance to flow potentially higher than in adults. The rescuer should deliver small puffs of air and assess the rise of the chest to ensure that over-inflation does not occur. A gentle rise of the chest is a sufficient indicator of adequate inflation.

The correct volume for each breath is the volume that causes the chest to rise. If air enters freely and the chest rises, assume the airway is clear. Give breaths slowly with sufficient volume to make the chest rise.

Check Pulse

After an initial two breaths, the health care provider palpates the pulse to ascertain the presence of a heartbeat. The carotid is the most central and accessible artery in children over 1 year of age. However, the infant's short and often fat neck makes the carotid pulse difficult to palpate. Therefore in the infant it is preferable to use the brachial pulse, located on the inner side of the upper arm midway between the elbow and the shoulder (Fig. 31-23). Absence of a carotid or brachial pulse is considered sufficient indication to begin external cardiac massage. *Lay rescuers are not taught to check the pulse but are taught to look for signs of circulation (e.g., normal breathing, coughing, or air movement) in response to rescue breaths.*

Perform Chest Compression

External chest compression consists of serial, rhythmic compressions of the chest to maintain circulation to vital organs until the child achieves spontaneous vital signs or ALS can be provided. *Chest compressions are always interspersed with venti-*

lation of the lungs. For optimal compressions it is essential that the child's spine be supported on a firm surface during compressions of the sternum and that sternal pressure is forceful but not traumatic. For a small infant the hard surface can be the rescuer's hand or forearm, with the palm supporting the infant's back. Position the child's head for optimum airway opening using the head tilt–chin lift maneuver. It is essential to prevent overextension of the head of small infants because this tends to close the flexible trachea.

Place the fingers for compression in infants at a point on the lower sternum just below the intersection of the sternum and an imaginary line drawn between the nipples (Fig. 31-24). Apply compressions on the child 1 to 8 years of age to the lower half of the sternum (Fig. 31-25). Sternal compression to infants is applied with two fingers on the sternum, exerting a firm downward thrust; chest compression for children is applied with the heel of one hand or two hands, depending on the child's size. Current American Heart Association (2005) guidelines include the addition of the two-thumb technique for chest compressions for infants when two health care providers are present. In the two-thumb technique, one of the two rescuers places both thumbs side by side over the lower half of the infant's sternum; the remaining fingers encircle the infant's chest and support the back. The two-thumb technique is not taught to lay rescuers and is not practical for the health care provider working alone.

Adapt the depth of compression to the child's size. The location, rate, and depth for children older than 8 years of age are the same as for adults.

Lone-rescuer CPR is continued at the ratio of two breaths to 30 compressions for all ages until signs of recovery appear. These signs include palpable peripheral pulses, return of pupils to normal size, the disappearance of mottling and cyanosis, and possibly return of spontaneous respiration. When two rescuers are present, they should deliver two breaths to each 15 compressions. According to the new guidelines (American Heart Association, 2005), the lay rescuer is not taught two-rescuer CPR. An update to these guidelines is anticipated in 2011.

Administer Medications

Medications are an important adjunct to CPR, especially cardiac arrest, and are used during and after resuscitation in children. Medications are used to (1) correct hypoxemia, (2) increase perfusion pressure during chest compression, (3) stimulate spontaneous or more forceful myocardial contraction, (4) accelerate cardiac rate, (5) correct metabolic acidosis, and (6) suppress ventricular ectopy. Appropriate fluid therapy is initiated immediately in the hospital or by EMS personnel during transport. (See Parenteral Fluid Therapy, Chapter 28; and Shock, Chapter 29.) A complete supply of emergency medications is kept and maintained in all EMS vehicles and on all hospital units. The supply is checked on a regular basis (usually once on each 8- or 12-hour shift). Table 31-6 lists resuscitation medications.

When administering drugs during CPR (or a "code"), use a saline flush between medications to prevent drug interactions.

Document all drugs, dosages, and the time and route of administration.

AIRWAY OBSTRUCTION

Attempts at clearing the airway should be considered for (1) children in whom aspiration of an FB is witnessed or strongly suspected; and (2) unconscious, nonbreathing children whose airways remain obstructed despite the usual maneuvers to open them. When aspiration is strongly suspected, encourage the child to continue coughing as long as the cough remains forceful.

In a conscious choking child, attempt to relieve the obstruction only if:

- The child is unable to make any sounds.
- The cough becomes ineffective.
- There is increasing respiratory difficulty with stridor.

> **! NURSING ALERT**
>
> Avoid blind finger sweeps in infants and children under 8 years old.

Infants

A combination of back blows (over the spine between the shoulder blades) and chest thrusts (on the sternum, in the same location as for chest compressions) is recommended to relieve the FB obstruction in infants (Fig. 31-26). Place a choking infant face down over the rescuer's arm with the head supported and lower than the trunk. For additional support the rescuer should support the arm firmly against the thigh. Deliver up to five quick, sharp, back blows between the infant's shoulder blades with the heel of the rescuer's hand. Use less force than would be applied to an adult. After delivery of the back blows, place the free hand flat on the infant's back so that the infant is "sandwiched" between the two hands, making certain the neck and chin are well supported. While maintaining support with the infant's head lower than the trunk, turn the infant and place the infant supine on the rescuer's thigh, and apply up to five quick downward chest thrusts in rapid succession in the same location as external chest compressions described for CPR. Continue back blows and chest thrusts until the object is removed or the infant becomes unconscious.

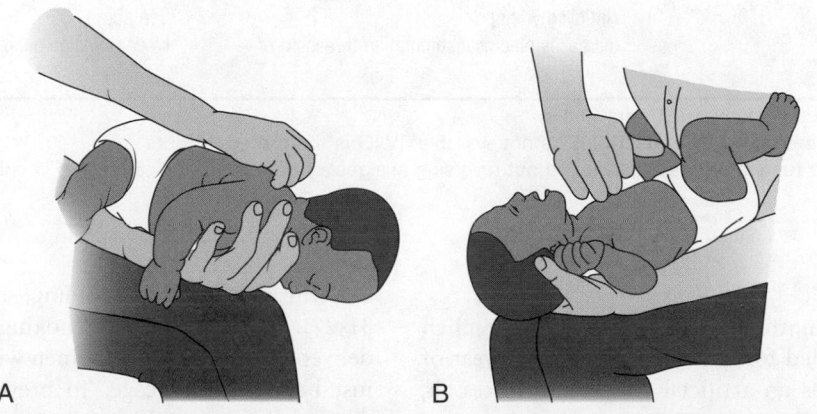

Fig. 31-26 Relief of foreign body obstruction in infant. **A,** Back blows. **B,** Chest thrusts.

TABLE 31-6   DRUGS FOR PEDIATRIC CARDIOPULMONARY RESUSCITATION

DRUG AND DOSE	ACTION	IMPLICATION
Epinephrine HCl* IV/IO: 0.01 mg/kg (1:10,000) Repeat doses: 0.01 mg/kg (1:10,000) Endotracheal tube (ET): 0.1 mg/kg (1:1000)	Adrenergic Acts on both alpha- and beta-receptor sites, especially heart and vascular and other smooth muscle	Most useful drug in cardiac arrest Disappears rapidly from bloodstream after injection; instill 5 ml saline after ET administration May produce renal vessel constriction and decreased urine formation
Sodium bicarbonate IV/IO: 1 mEq/kg dose Newborn: 0.5 mEq/ml (4.2%)	Alkalinizer Buffers pH	Infuse slowly and only when ventilation is adequate; flush with saline before and after administration Do not mix with catecholamines or calcium
Atropine sulfate* 0.02 mg/kg/dose Minimum dose: 0.1 mg Maximum single dose: infants and children, 0.5 mg; adolescents, 1 mg	Anticholinergic-parasympatholytic Increases cardiac output, heart rate by blocking vagal stimulation in heart	Used to treat bradycardia after ventilatory assessment Always provide adequate ventilation and monitor oxygen saturation Produces pupillary dilation, which constricts with light
Calcium chloride 10% 20 mg/kg IV/IO 0.2 mg/kg/dose q 10 min	Electrolyte replacement Needed for maintenance of normal cardiac contractility	Used only for hypocalcemia, calcium blocker overdose, hyperkalemia, or hypermagnesemia Administer slowly; very sclerosing; administer in central vein Incompatible with phosphate solutions
Lidocaine HCl* 1 mg/kg/dose	Antidysrhythmic Inhibits nerve impulses from sensory nerves	Used for ventricular arrhythmias only
Amiodarone IV: 5 mg/kg over 30 min followed by continuous infusion Start at 5 mcg/kg/min May increase to maximum 10 mcg/kg/min	Antidysrhythmic agent Inhibits adrenergic stimulation; prolongs action potential and refractory period in myocardial tissues; decreased atrioventricular (AV) conduction and sinus node function	Recommended as first choice for shock-refractory ventricular tachycardia Contraindicated in severe sinus node dysfunction, marked sinus bradycardia, second- and third-degree AV block Monitor ECG and blood pressure
Adenosine 0.1-0.2 mg/kg as a rapid IV bolus Maximum single initial dose: 6-12 mg (given over 1-2 sec) May repeat administration: double initial dose (maximum dose = 12 mg) Follow with ≥5 ml normal saline flush	Antidysrhythmic, for supraventricular tachycardia Causes temporary block through AV node and interrupts reentry circuits	Administer by rapid IV push followed by saline flush May cause transient bradycardia
Naloxone (Narcan)* 0.1 mg/kg/dose† May repeat q 2-3 min	Reverses respiratory arrest caused by excessive opiate administration	Evaluate level of pain after administration because analgesic effects of opioids are reversed with large doses of naloxone
Magnesium sulfate 25-50 mg/kg IV/IO Maximum: 2 g	Inhibits calcium channels and causes smooth muscle relaxation	Given by rapid IV infusion for suspected hypomagnesemia Have calcium gluconate (IV) available as antidote
Infusions		
Epinephrine HCl infusion 0.05 mcg/kg/min	Adrenergic See above	Titrated to desired hemodynamic effect
Dopamine HCl infusion 2 mcg/kg/min	Agonist Acts on alpha receptors, causing vasoconstriction Increases cardiac output	Titrated to desired hemodynamic response
Dobutamine HCl infusion 2 mcg/kg/min	Adrenergic direct-acting β₂-agonist Increases contractility and heart rate	Titrated to desired hemodynamic response Little vasoconstriction, even at high rates
Lidocaine HCl infusion 20-50 mcg/kg/min	Antidysrhythmic Increases electrical stimulation threshold of ventricle	See above Lower infusion dose used in shock

ECG, Electrocardiogram; *IO*, intraosseous; *IV*, intravenous.
*These drugs may be administered via ET tube if IV/IO is not available; IV/IO is the preferred route.
†Dose of naloxone to reverse respiratory depression without reversing analgesia from opioids is 0.5 mcg/kg in children <40 kg (88 lb) (American Pain Society, 1999).

Children

A series of subdiaphragmatic abdominal thrusts (Heimlich maneuver) is recommended for children older than 1 year of age. The maneuver creates an artificial cough that forces air, and with it the FB, out of the airway. The procedure is carried out with the child in a standing, sitting, or lying position (Fig. 31-27). In the conscious choking child, upward thrusts are delivered to the upper abdomen with the fisted hand at a point just below the rib cage. To prevent damage to the internal organs, the rescuer's hands should not touch the xiphoid

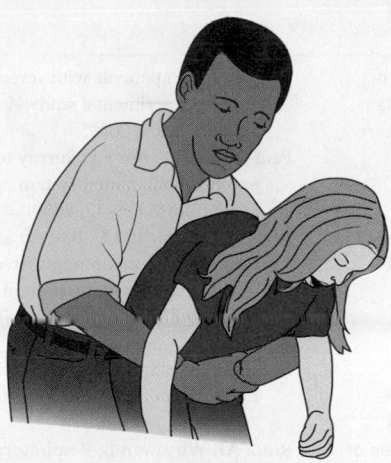

Fig. 31-27 Abdominal thrusts in standing child for relief of foreign body obstruction.

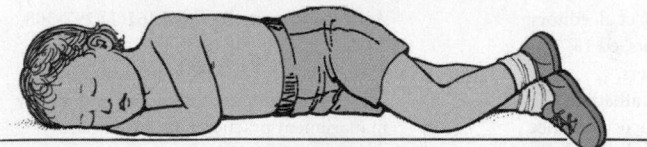

Fig. 31-28 Recovery position for child after respiratory emergency.

process of the sternum or the lower margins of the ribs. Repeat up to five thrusts in rapid succession until the FB is expelled.

It is neither necessary nor desirable to squeeze or compress the arms during the procedure. It is not a punch or a bear hug. The child may vomit after relief of the obstruction and should be positioned to prevent aspiration. After breathing is restored, the child should receive medical attention and be assessed for complications.

The success of the technique is primarily a result of the obstruction occurring at the end of a maximum respiration. The victim is most likely to choke on food during inspiration; therefore the tidal volume plus expiratory reserve volume is present in the lungs. When pressure is exerted on the diaphragm by the maneuver, the food bolus is ejected with considerable force by this trapped air.

If the victim is breathing or resumes effective breathing after emergency interventions, place in the recovery position: move the head, shoulders, and torso simultaneously and turn onto the side. The leg not in contact with the ground may be bent and the knee moved forward to stabilize the victim (Fig. 31-28). Do not move the victim in any way if trauma is suspected, and do not place the child in the recovery position if rescue breathing or CPR is required.

KEY POINTS

- The major functions of the respiratory tract are to distribute air and exchange gases to supply cells with oxygen and to remove carbon dioxide.
- Several anatomic features predispose infants and young children to airway obstruction and atelectasis: they have less alveolar surface for gas exchange, narrowly branching peripheral airways become easily obstructed, and lack of collateral pathways inhibits ventilation beyond obstructed units.
- Gas exchange depends on the amount and composition of gases inhaled, thickness of the alveolar wall, adequacy of circulation to the alveoli, and substances within the alveoli that prevent their inflation or gas exchange.
- The amount of oxygen that diffuses into the blood depends on a pressure gradient between alveolar air and capillary blood, the total functional surface area of the alveolocapillary membrane, minute volume, and alveolar ventilation.
- Defense mechanisms of the respiratory tract include the lymphatic system, mucus secretions, ciliary action, epiglottis, cough reflex, tracheobronchial dynamics, body position changes, and humoral defenses.
- Complete assessment of respiratory function involves a detailed history, physical examination, pulmonary function tests, radiography, and blood gas determination.
- Pulse oximetry is a noninvasive method of determining the oxygen saturation in the blood. One limitation of the technology is that it does not identify dangerously high oxygen levels.
- Improvement in respiratory function may be accomplished with measures such as oxygen therapy, positioning, humidification, aerosol therapy, and artificial ventilation.
- Always humidify oxygen when administering it to children.

- CPT is useful for patients with increased sputum production but is contraindicated for some.
- Implications for possible intubation include airway obstruction, respiratory arrest, neuromuscular compromise or paralysis, and hypoxemia.
- Respiratory failure is the inability of the respiratory system to maintain adequate oxygenation of the blood, with or without carbon dioxide retention.
- Management of respiratory failure is to provide oxygen, maintain ventilation, apply appropriate therapy, and anticipate complications.
- ET and tracheostomy suctioning involves premeasured insertion of the catheter, application of suction for 3 or 4 seconds when withdrawing the catheter, and supplemental oxygen before and after suctioning.
- Occlusion of the ET and tracheostomy tube is life threatening; therefore equipment for replacing a tube must always be available.
- Pediatric CPR includes five cycles (about 2 minutes) of ventilations (two) and compressions (30) before summoning emergency help.
- Automatic external defibrillators are safe to use in children 1 year and older in an arrest situation where there is no pulse.
- Choking and respiratory failure are respiratory emergencies that require immediate intervention.
- Use abdominal thrusts in children in whom FB obstruction is witnessed or strongly suspected. Use a combination of back blows and chest thrusts for infants with FB obstruction.
- In a conscious choking child, make attempts to relieve the obstruction only if the child is unable to make any sounds, the cough becomes ineffective, or the child has increasing respiratory difficulty with stridor.

REFERENCES

American Heart Association: 2005 American Heart Association guidelines for cardiopulmonary resuscitation and emergency cardiovascular care, *Circulation* 112 (24 Suppl 1):IV-166, 2005.

American Pain Society: *Principles of analgesic use in the treatment of acute pain and chronic cancer pain*, ed 4, Skokie, Ill, 1999, The Society.

Atkins DL, Everson-Stewart S, Sears GK, et al: Epidemiology and outcome from out-of-hospital cardiac arrest in children: the resuscitation Outcomes Consortium Epistry–Cardiac Arrest, *Circulation* 119(11):1484-1491, 2009.

Bilan N, Behbahan AG, Khosroshahi AJ: Validity of venous blood gas analysis for diagnosis of acid-base imbalance in children admitted to paediatric intensive care unit, *World J Pediatr* 4(2):114-117, 2008.

Boat TF, Green TP: Chronic or recurrent respiratory symptoms. In Behrman RE, Kliegman RM, Jenson HB, et al, editors: *Nelson textbook of pediatrics*, ed 18, Philadelphia, 2007, Saunders.

Bottor LT: Rapid sequence intubation in the neonate, *Adv Neonat Care* 9(3):111-117, 2009.

Brinker D: Sedation and comfort issues in the ventilated infant and child, *Crit Care Nurs Clin North Am* 16:365-377, 2004.

Celik SA, Kanan N: A current conflict: use of isotonic sodium chloride solution on endotracheal suctioning in critically ill patients, *Dimens Crit Care Nurs* 25(1):11-14, 2006.

Centers for Disease Control and Prevention: Guidelines for preventing health-care-associated pneumonia, 2003, *MMWR Recomm Rep* 53(RR03):1-36, 2004.

Curley MA, Hibberd PL, Fineman LD, et al: Effect of prone positioning on clinical outcomes in children with acute lung injury: a randomized controlled trial, *JAMA* 294(2):248-250, 2005.

Curley MAQ, Moloney-Harmon PA: *Critical care nursing of infants and children*, ed 2, Philadelphia, 2001, Saunders.

Dudell GG, Stoll BJ: Respiratory tract disorders. In Kliegman RM, Behrman RE, Jenson HB, et al, editors: *Nelson textbook of pediatrics*, ed 18, Philadelphia, 2007, Saunders.

Engleman SG, Turnage-Carrier C: Tolerance of the Passy-Muir speaking valve™ in infants and children less than 2 years of age, *Pediatr Nurs* 23:571-573, 1997.

Fauroux B, Guillemot N, Aubertin G, et al: Physiologic benefits of mechanical insufflations-exsufflation in children with neuromuscular diseases, *Chest* 133(1):161-168, 2008.

Gardner DL, Shirland L: Evidence-based guideline for suctioning the intubated neonate and infant, *Neonat Netw* 28(5):281-302, 2009.

Halm MA, Krisko-Hagel K: Instilling normal saline with suctioning: beneficial technique or potentially harmful sacred cow? *Am J Crit Care* 17(5):469-472, 2008.

Haddad GG: Congenital central hypoventilation syndrome (Ondine curse). In Behrman RE, Kliegman RM, Jenson HB, et al, editors: *Nelson textbook of pediatrics*, ed 18, Philadelphia, 2007, Saunders.

Homnick DN: Mechanical insufflations-exsufflation for airway mucus clearance, *Respir Care* 52(10):1296-1305, 2007.

Ireton J: Tracheostomy suction: a protocol for practice, *Paediatr Nurs* 19(10):14-18, 2007.

Kaut K, Turcott JC, Lavery M: Passy-Muir speaking valve, *Dimens Crit Care Nurs* 15:298-306, 1996.

Kennedy JD, Martin AJ: Chronic respiratory failure and neuromuscular disease, *Pediatr Clin North Am* 56(1):261-273, 2009.

Marks JH: Pulmonary care of children and adolescents with developmental disabilities, *Pediatr Clin North Am* 55(6):1299-1314, 2008.

McCance KL, Huether SE: *Pathophysiology: the biological basis for disease in adults and children*, ed 6, St Louis, 2010, Mosby.

McIlwaine M: Chest physical therapy breathing techniques and exercise in children with CF, *Paediatr Respir Rev* 8(1):8-16, 2007.

Morrow BM, Argent AC: A comprehensive review of pediatric endotracheal suctioning: effects, indications, and clinical practice, *Pediatr Crit Care Med* 9(5):465-477, 2008.

Myers BA: *Wound management*, Upper Saddle River, NJ, 2008, Pearson/Prentice Hall.

Naylor JM, McLean A, Chow CM, et al: A modified postural drainage position produces less cardiovascular stress than a head-down position in patients with severe heart disease: a quasi-experimental study, *Aust J Physiother* 52(3):201-209, 2006.

Paul-Allen J, Ostrow CL: Survey of nursing practices with closed-system suctioning, *Am J Crit Care* 9(1):9-17, 2000.

Ridling DA, Martin LD, Bratton SL, et al: Endotracheal suctioning with or without instillation of isotonic sodium chloride in critically ill children, *Am J Crit Care* 12(3):212-219, 2003.

Rogovik A, Goldman R: Permissive hypercapnia, *Emerg Med Clin North Am* 26(4):941-952, 2008.

Rotta AT, Wiryawan B: Respiratory emergencies in children, *Respir Care* 48(3):248-260, 2003.

Sherman JM, Davis S, Albamonte-Petrick S, et al: Care of the child with a tracheostomy: official statement of the American Thoracic Society, *Am J Respir Crit Care Med* 161(1):297-308, 2000.

Sole ML, Byers JF, Ludy JE, et al: A multisite survey of suctioning techniques and airway management practices, *Am J Crit Care* 12(3):220-230, 2003.

Topjian AA, Nadkarni VM, Berg RA: Cardiopulmonary resuscitation in children, *Curr Opin Crit Care* 15(3):203-208, 2009.

Watts KD, Goodman DM: Wheezing, bronchiolitis, and bronchitis. In Behrman RE, Kliegman RM, Jenson HB, et al, editors: *Nelson textbook of pediatrics*, ed 18, Philadelphia, 2007, Saunders.

Wilson JR, Mills JG, Prather ID, et al: A toxicity index of skin and wound cleansers used on in vitro fibroblasts and keratinocytes, *Adv Skin Wound Care* 18(7):373-378, 2005.

Yildizdas D, Yapicioglu H, Yilmaz HL, et al: Correlation of simultaneously obtained capillary, venous, and arterial blood gases of patients in a paediatric intensive care unit, *Arch Dis Child* 89(2):176-180, 2004.

Young KD, Gausche-Hill M, McClung CD, et al: A prospective, population-based study of the epidemiology and outcome of out-of-hospital pediatric cardiopulmonary arrest, *Pediatrics* 114(1):157-164, 2004.

Zander J, Hazinski MF: Pulmonary disorders. In Hazinski MF, editor: *Nursing care of the critically ill child*, ed 2, St Louis, 1992, Mosby.

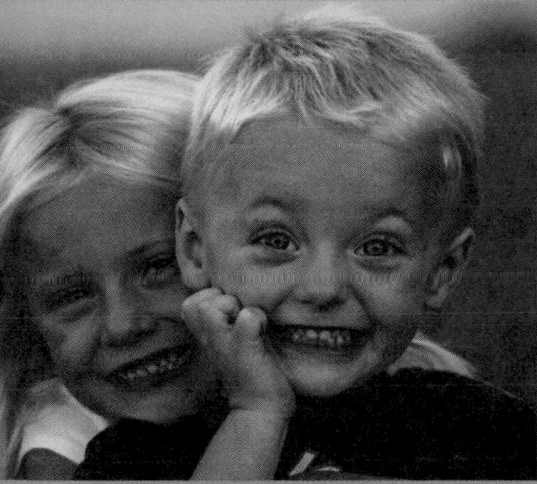

The Child with Respiratory Dysfunction

David Wilson

CHAPTER OUTLINE

GENERAL ASPECTS OF RESPIRATORY TRACT INFECTIONS

Infections of the respiratory tract are described according to the areas of involvement. The upper respiratory tract, or upper airway, consists of the oronasopharynx, pharynx, larynx, and upper part of the trachea. The lower respiratory tract consists of the bronchi, bronchioles, and alveoli. The bronchi and bronchioles are the reactive portion of the lower respiratory tract, since they have smooth muscle content and the ability to constrict. Respiratory tract infections spread from one structure to another because of the contiguous nature of the mucous membrane lining the entire tract. Consequently, infections of the respiratory tract involve several areas rather than a single structure, although the effect on one may predominate in any given illness.

ETIOLOGY AND CHARACTERISTICS

Respiratory tract infections account for the majority of acute illnesses in children. The age of the child, season, living conditions, and preexisting medical problems influence the cause and course of these infections.

Infectious Agents

The respiratory tract is subject to a wide variety of infective organisms. Most infections are caused by viruses, particularly respiratory syncytial virus (RSV) and the parainfluenza viruses. Other agents involved in primary or secondary invasion include group A β-hemolytic streptococci (GABHS), staphylococci, *Haemophilus influenzae*, *Chlamydia trachomatis*, *Mycoplasma* organisms, and pneumococci.

Age

Healthy full-term infants under age 3 months are presumed to have a lower infection rate because of the protective function of maternal antibodies. The infection rate increases from age 3 to 6 months, the period between the disappearance of maternal antibodies and the infant's own antibody production. The viral infection rate continues to remain high during the toddler and preschool years. By the time the child reaches 5 years of age, viral respiratory tract infections are less frequent, but the incidence of *Mycoplasma pneumoniae* and GABHS infections increases. The amount of lymphoid tissue increases throughout middle childhood, and repeated exposure to organisms confers increasing immunity as children grow older.

Some viral agents produce a mild illness in older children but cause severe lower respiratory tract illness or croup in infants. For example, pertussis causes a relatively harmless tracheobronchitis in childhood but is a serious disease in infancy.

Size

Anatomic differences influence the response to respiratory tract infections. The diameter of the airways is smaller in young children and subject to considerable narrowing from edematous mucous membranes and increased production of secretions. (See Fig. 31-5.) In addition, the distance between structures within the tract is shorter in the young child. Therefore organisms move more rapidly down the respiratory tract for more extensive involvement. The relatively short and open eustachian tube in infants and young children allows pathogens easy access to the middle ear.

Resistance

The ability to resist invading organisms depends on several factors. Deficiencies of the immune system place the child at risk for infection. Other conditions that decrease resistance are malnutrition, anemia, fatigue, and chilling of the body. Conditions that weaken defenses of the respiratory tract and predispose a child to infection include allergies (e.g., allergic rhinitis), bronchopulmonary dysplasia (chronic lung disease), asthma, cardiac anomalies that cause pulmonary congestion, and cystic fibrosis (CF). Daycare attendance, especially if the caregivers smoke, also increases the likelihood of infection.

Seasonal Variations

The most common respiratory tract pathogens appear in epidemics during the winter and spring months, but mycoplasmal infections occur more often in autumn and early winter. Infection-related asthma (e.g., asthmatic bronchitis) occurs more frequently during cold weather. Winter and spring are typically RSV season, or the time when children are indoors in close contact and more likely to spread the disease to each other.

CLINICAL MANIFESTATIONS

Infants and young children, especially those between 6 months and 3 years of age, react more severely to acute respiratory tract infection than do older children. Young children display a number of generalized signs and symptoms and local manifestations that differ from those seen in older children and adults. Signs and symptoms associated with respiratory tract illnesses are outlined in Box 32-1. See Box 32-2 for components for assessing respiratory function.

BOX 32-1   SIGNS AND SYMPTOMS ASSOCIATED WITH RESPIRATORY TRACT INFECTIONS IN INFANTS AND SMALL CHILDREN

Fever

May be absent in neonates (≤28 days)

Greatest at ages 6 months to 3 years

Temperature may reach 39.5° to 40.5° C (103° to 105° F) even with mild infections

Often appears as first sign of infection

May leave child listless and irritable or somewhat euphoric and more active than normal temporarily; leads some children to talk with unaccustomed rapidity

Tendency to develop high temperatures with infection in certain families

May precipitate febrile seizures (See Chapter 37.)

Febrile seizures uncommon after 3 or 4 years of age

Meningismus

Meningeal signs without infection of the meninges

Occurs with abrupt onset of fever

Accompanied by:
- Headache
- Pain and stiffness in the back and neck
- Presence of Kernig and Brudzinski signs

Subsides as the temperature drops

Anorexia

Common with most childhood illnesses

Frequently the initial evidence of illness

Persists to a greater or lesser degree throughout febrile stage of illness; often extends into convalescence

Vomiting

Occurs readily in small children with illness

A clue to the onset of infection

May precede other signs by several hours

Usually short lived but may persist during the illness

Is frequent cause of dehydration

Diarrhea

Usually mild, transient diarrhea, but may become severe

Often accompanies viral respiratory tract infections

Abdominal Pain

Common complaint

Sometimes indistinguishable from pain of appendicitis in older child

May be caused by mesenteric lymphadenitis

May represent referred pain (e.g., chest pain associated with pneumonia)

May be related to muscle spasms from vomiting, especially in nervous, tense children

Nasal Blockage

Small nasal passages of infants easily blocked by mucosal swelling and exudation

Can interfere with respiration and feeding in infants

May contribute to the development of otitis media and sinusitis

Nasal Discharge

Common feature

May be thin and watery (rhinorrhea) or thick and purulent

Depends on the type and stage of infection

Associated with itching

May irritate upper lip and skin surrounding the nose

Cough

Common feature

May be evident only during the acute phase

May persist several months after a disease

Respiratory Sounds

Sounds associated with respiratory disease:
- Cough
- Hoarseness
- Grunting
- Stridor
- Wheezing

Findings on auscultation:
- Wheezing
- Crackles
- Absence of air movement

Sore Throat

Frequent complaint of older children

Young children (unable to describe symptoms) may not complain even when highly inflamed

Increased drooling noted by parents

Refusal by child to take oral fluids or solids

BOX 32-2   COMPONENTS FOR ASSESSING RESPIRATORY FUNCTION

Pattern of Respirations

Rate—Rapid (tachypnea), normal, or slow for the particular child

Depth—Normal depth, too shallow (hypopnea), too deep (hyperpnea); usually estimated from the amplitude of thoracic and abdominal excursion (age dependent)

Ease—Effortless, labored (dyspnea), orthopnea, associated with intercostal or substernal retractions (inspiratory "sinking in" of soft tissues in relation to the cartilaginous and bony thorax), pulsus paradoxus (blood pressure falling with inspiration and rising with expiration), nasal flaring, head bobbing (head of sleeping child with suboccipital area supported on caregiver's forearm bobbing forward in synchrony with each inspiration), grunting, or wheezing

Labored breathing—Continuous, intermittent, becoming steadily worse, sudden onset, at rest or on exertion, associated with wheezing, grunting, associated with chest pain

Rhythm—Variation in rate and depth of respirations

Other Observations

Evidence of infection—Check for elevated temperature; enlarged cervical lymph nodes; inflamed mucous membranes; and purulent discharges from the nose, ears, or lungs (sputum).

Cough—Observe the characteristics of the cough (if present): when the cough is heard (e.g., night only, on arising), the nature of the cough (paroxysmal with or without wheeze, "croupy" or "brassy"), frequency of the cough, association with swallowing or other activity, character of the cough (moist or dry), productivity.

Wheeze—Note whether it is expiratory or inspiratory, high pitched or musical, prolonged, slowly progressive or sudden, associated with labored breathing.

Cyanosis—Note distribution (peripheral, perioral, facial, trunk as well as face), degree, duration, association with activity.

Chest pain—Older children may complain of this. Note location and circumstances: localized or generalized; referred to base of neck or abdomen; dull or sharp; deep or superficial; associated with rapid, shallow respirations or grunting.

Sputum—Older children may provide sputum sample by coughing, whereas young children may need use of bulb suction or gastric lavage in early morning to provide a sample. Note volume, color, viscosity, and odor.

Bad breath—May be associated with some throat and lung infections.

NURSING CARE OF THE CHILD WITH A RESPIRATORY TRACT INFECTION

Assessment

Assessment of the respiratory system follows the guidelines described in Chapter 6 (for nose, mouth and throat, chest, and lungs). The assessment should include heart rate, respiratory rate, depth and rhythm, and hydration status. In addition to these, special attention is given to the observations outlined in Box 32-1, the components in Box 32-2, and assessment of the following:

- Respiratory effort (respiratory rate, accessory muscle use, retractions, nasal flaring)
- Oxygenation (pulse oximetry, color)
- Body temperature
- Child's activity level
- Child's level of comfort

> **! NURSING ALERT**
>
> A noninvasive pulse oximeter (oxygen saturation) measurement should be performed on *all* children as part of the routine physical assessment.

The nursing care of the child with a respiratory tract infection follows established guidelines based on the child's and family's individualized needs (see Nursing Care Plan).

Ease Respiratory Efforts

Many acute respiratory tract infections are mild and cause few symptoms. Although children may feel uncomfortable and have a stuffy nose and some mucosal swelling, acute respiratory distress occurs infrequently. The interventions described here are usually sufficient to relieve minor discomfort and ease respiratory efforts. However, children with croup or epiglottitis may develop sufficient swelling to obstruct the airway. These children may require hospitalization for observation and therapy.

Warm or cool mist is a common therapeutic measure for symptomatic relief of respiratory discomfort. The moisture soothes inflamed membranes and is beneficial when there is hoarseness or laryngeal involvement. Mist tents have been used in the hospital for humidifying the air and relieving discomfort but are seldom used in developed countries. The use of steam vaporizers in the home is often discouraged because of the hazards related to their use and limited evidence to support their efficacy. Shallow pans with wide surface areas for evaporation increase humidity, but parents should place them where they do not pose a safety hazard.

A time-honored method (but not evidence based) of producing steam is the shower. Running a shower of hot water into the empty bathtub or open shower stall with the bathroom door closed produces a quick source of steam. Keeping a child in this environment for 10 to 15 minutes may help ease respiratory efforts. A small child can sit on the lap of a parent or other adult. Older children can sit in the bathroom under the supervision of an adult.

Promote Rest

Children who have an acute febrile illness should be encouraged to rest and engage in quiet activities. Most children are self-limiting when febrile and increase activity as the fever subsides. Often children are more likely to stay quiet if they are allowed to lie quietly on a couch where they can watch television or participate in a quiet activity such as coloring or reading a book.

Promote Comfort

Older children are usually able to manage nasal secretions with little difficulty. Instruct parents in the correct administration of nose drops and throat gargles, if ordered. For very young infants, who normally breathe through their noses, an infant nasal aspirator or a rubber ear syringe is helpful in removing nasal secretions before feeding. This practice, in addition to instillation of saline nose drops, may clear nasal passages and promote feeding.

For older children who can tolerate decongestants, vasoconstrictive nose drops may be administered 15 to 20 minutes before feeding and at bedtime. Two drops are instilled, and, because this shrinks only the anterior mucous membranes, two more drops are instilled 5 to 10 minutes later. Phenylephrine (Neo-Synephrine) 0.25% and ephedrine 1% are frequently prescribed. Older cooperative children often prefer nasal sprays. They learn to compress the plastic container at the moment of inspiration. Spray bottles and bottles of nose drops should be used only for one child and only for one illness, since they become easily contaminated with bacteria. To avoid rebound congestion, nose drops or sprays should not be administered for more than 3 days.

> **NURSING TIP** To prevent cross-contamination with nose drops, draw about 0.25 ml of nose spray solution into a clean tuberculin syringe. Inject a small amount of the nose spray solution into the child's nostrils using the blunt syringe.

Hot or cold applications sometimes provide relief for children with painful cervical adenitis. An ice bag or heating pad applied to the neck decreases the discomfort, but safety precautions must be observed to prevent burns. The ice bag or heating device must be covered, and the heating pad should not be set at high ranges.

Prevent Spread of Infection

Careful hand washing is carried out when caring for children with respiratory tract infections. Children and families should use a tissue or their hand to cover their nose and mouth when they cough or sneeze, dispose of the tissues properly, and wash their hands. Used tissues should be immediately thrown into the wastebasket, not allowed to accumulate in a pile. Children with respiratory tract infections should not share drinking cups, washcloths, or towels.

To decrease contamination with respiratory viruses, wash hands frequently and do not touch eyes or nose with hands.

Parents should try to remove affected children from contact with other children. Parents should also keep affected children out of school or daycare settings to prevent the spread of infection. Ideally, ill children should be isolated in a separate room at the first sign of illness. This may be a problem when living arrangements are crowded and the family has several children. An effort should be made to teach well children to stay away

NURSING CARE PLAN

The Child with Acute Respiratory Tract Infection

NURSING DIAGNOSIS	EXPECTED PATIENT OUTCOMES	NURSING INTERVENTIONS	RATIONALE
Ineffective Breathing Pattern related to inflammatory process	Child's respirations will be nonlabored.	Position child for maximum ventilatory efficiency and airway patency.	To allow increased chest expansion
Child's/Family's Defining Characteristics (Subjective and Objective Data)	**The Following NOC Concept Applies to These Outcomes**	Position child to facilitate drainage of secretions.	To maintain patent airway and prevent airway obstruction
Use of accessory muscles to breathe	Respiratory Status: Airway Patency, Ventilation	Provide humidified oxygen as necessary.	To improve oxygenation
Dyspnea		Monitor oxygenation status, including vital signs, for changes in condition.	To determine need for additional interventions
Shortness of breath		Suction airway (nose, trachea) as necessary.	To remove secretions and maintain airway patency
Nasal flaring			
Altered chest excursion		Provide gentle chest percussion and chest physiotherapy (CPT) as necessary.	To facilitate secretion removal
Assumption of three-point (tripod) position		Encourage deep breathing and cough (as age appropriate) after CPT	To remove secretions
Respiratory rate outside normal parameter for child's age (increased or decreased rate)		Administer bronchodilator medications.	To promote bronchodilation and improve ventilation
		Administer antiinflammatory medications.	To decrease airway inflammation
		Administer antibiotics (if bacterial).	To decrease inflammatory response
		The Following NIC Concepts Apply to These Interventions	
		Aspiration Precautions	
		Positioning	
		Respiratory Monitoring Surveillance	
		Oxygen Therapy	
		Airway Suctioning	
		Vital Signs Monitoring	
		Cough Enhancement	

NURSING DIAGNOSIS	EXPECTED PATIENT OUTCOMES	NURSING INTERVENTIONS	RATIONALE
Ineffective Airway Clearance related to inflammation, mechanical obstruction, increased secretions	Child's airways will remain patent.	Position child to facilitate drainage of secretions.	To prevent airway obstruction
Child's/Family's Defining Characteristics (Subjective and Objective Data)	**The Following NOC Concepts Apply to These Outcomes**	Perform CPT.	To loosen and remove secretions
	Aspiration Control	Suction airway as necessary.	To remove secretions
Dyspnea	Airway Patency	Provide humidified oxygen.	To moisten secretions and prevent airway drying
Difficulty vocalizing			
Orthopnea		Assist with coughing (as developmentally or age appropriate).	To remove secretions
Adventitious breath sounds (crackles, wheezing, rhonchi)		Avoid throat examination if epiglottitis is suspected.	To prevent airway compromise
Cough ineffective or absent			
Restlessness		Assure child (as appropriate) all measures will be taken to ensure adequate airway is maintained.	To allay anxiety
Changes in respiratory rate and rhythm		Implement comfort measures such as allowing parental presence, parental holding, favorite blanket or stuffed animal at side; explain all procedures beforehand.	To reduce anxiety and decrease effects of medical therapy, including hospitalization if required
		The Following NIC Concepts Apply to These Interventions	
		Cough Enhancement	
		Positioning	
		Chest Physiotherapy	
		Vital Signs Monitoring	
		Anxiety Reduction	

Continued

from ill children, to wash their hands frequently, and to avoid eating or drinking from the same utensils or cups.

Reduce Temperature

If the child has a significantly elevated temperature, controlling the fever is important. The parent should know how to take a child's temperature and read the thermometer accurately. Nurses should not assume that all parents can read a thermometer; those who cannot require instruction.

If the practitioner has prescribed an antipyretic such as ibuprofen or acetaminophen (Tylenol), parents may need help administering the drug. Most parents can read the label and

NURSING CARE PLAN—cont'd

The Child with Acute Respiratory Tract Infection

NURSING DIAGNOSIS	EXPECTED PATIENT OUTCOMES	NURSING INTERVENTIONS	RATIONALE
Risk for Injury related to presence (only as indicated) of infective organisms	Child will remain free from complications of infection.	Maintain aseptic environment using sterile suction equipment and technique. Implement and practice Standard Precautions. Implement Contact and Airborne Precautions as necessary.	To prevent spread of infectious organisms in child and family
Child's/Family's Defining Characteristics (Subjective and Objective Data)	**The Following NOC Concept Applies to These Outcomes** Risk Control	Obtain (secretion, tissue, or blood) specimen as indicated.	To identify infective organism
Tissue hypoxia Abnormal blood profile People or provider (nosocomial agents)		Encourage child and family contacts to practice frequent hand washing and avoid hand-to-eye and hand-to-mouth contact.	To prevent spread of infection
Mode of transport Developmental age		Teach child (as age appropriate) and family how to decrease spread of organisms through coughing and other secretions (e.g., by covering mouth when coughing; disposing of secretions to avoid cross-contamination).	To prevent spread of infection
		Administer antibiotic or antiviral medications.	To treat infection source
		Administer fever reduction medication(s) as appropriate.	To promote comfort if fever is present
		Monitor and assess for signs and symptoms of secondary complications: hypoxia, skin breakdown, poor nutrient and fluid intake, increased work of breathing, deteriorating cardiorespiratory status.	To implement therapy for prevention of secondary complications
		The Following NIC Concepts Apply to These Interventions Risk Identification Environmental Management Infection Control Parent Education	

NURSING DIAGNOSIS	EXPECTED PATIENT OUTCOMES	NURSING INTERVENTIONS	RATIONALE
Interrupted Family Processes related to child's illness, hospitalization, and medical or therapeutic regimen	Family will demonstrate ability to cope with child's illness.	Allow family to remain with child. Promote family-centered care.	To decrease effects of separation
Child's/Family's Defining Characteristics (Subjective and Objective Data)	**The Following NOC Concepts Apply to These Outcomes** Family Functioning	Explain procedures and therapeutic regimen to family. Keep family informed of child's status.	To provide accurate information regarding therapy and child's condition
Communication patterns Participation in decision making Availability for emotional support	Family Normalization Parenting	Encourage family involvement in child's care. Provide support and referral for continued support as necessary.	To promote family sense of control and involvement in care
Expressions of conflict within family Patterns and rituals		**The Following NIC Concepts Apply to These Interventions** Caregiver Support Family Support Coping Enhancement Emotional Support Financial Resource Assistance	

calculate the desired dose, but some may require careful instruction. It is important to emphasize accuracy in both the amount of drug given and the time intervals for drug administration to avoid cumulative effects. *Parents should also be cautious of over-the-counter combination "cold" remedies, since these often include acetaminophen.* Careful calculation of both the acetaminophen given separately and the acetaminophen in combination medications is necessary to avoid an overdose. To reduce the temperature and minimize the chances of dehydra-

tion, encourage cool liquids. (See Controlling Elevated Temperatures, Chapter 27.)

Promote Hydration

Dehydration is a potential complication when children have respiratory tract infections and are febrile or anorexic, especially when vomiting or diarrhea is present. Infants are especially prone to fluid and electrolyte deficits when they have a respiratory illness because a rapid respiratory rate that accompanies such illnesses precludes adequate fluid intake. In addition, the presence of fever increases the total body fluid turnover in infants. If the infant has nasal secretions, this further prevents adequate respiratory effort by blocking the narrow nasal passages when the infant reclines to bottle- or breast-feed and ceases the compensatory mouth breathing effort, thus causing the child to limit intake of fluids. Parents can encourage adequate fluid intake by offering small amounts of favorite fluids (clear liquids if vomiting) at frequent intervals. High-calorie liquids, such as colas, fruit juice drinks, water flavored and sweetened with corn syrup, or similar drinks, help prevent catabolism and dehydration but should be avoided if diarrhea is present. Oral rehydration solutions, such as Infalyte or Pedialyte, are beneficial for infants, and drinks such as sports drinks or those containing electrolytes are appropriate for older children. Fluids should not be forced, and children should not be awakened to take fluids unless the practitioner advises it. Forcing fluids may create the same difficulties as urging unwanted food (discussed below). Gentle persuasion with preferred beverages is usually successful. (See Chapter 28 for instructions on oral hydration.)

For infants who are breast- or bottle-feeding and who have a respiratory illness and secretions, encourage the parent to instill nasal saline drops and suction the passages with a bulb syringe before the feeding. This should alleviate some of the congestion and allow infants to nurse effectively.

To assess their child's level of hydration (see Chapter 28), advise parents to observe the frequency of voiding and to notify the nurse or practitioner if there is insufficient voiding.

> **NURSING TIP** Counting the number of wet diapers in a 24-hour period is a satisfactory method of assessing output in infants and toddlers who are not acutely ill. Otherwise urinary output should be approximately 1 ml/kg/hr in a child who weighs less than 30 kg (66 lb) and 30 ml/hr for children 30 kg and larger.

Provide Nutrition

Loss of appetite is characteristic of children with acute infections, and in most cases children can be permitted to determine their own need for food. Urging foods on anorexic children may precipitate nausea and vomiting and cause an aversion to feeding that can extend into the convalescent period and beyond. Many children show no decrease in appetite, and others respond well to foods such as gelatin, Popsicles, soup, and puddings. (See Feeding the Sick Child, Chapter 27.)

Provide Family Support and Home Care

Young children with respiratory tract infections are irritable and difficult to comfort. Therefore the family needs support, encouragement, and practical suggestions concerning comfort measures and administration of medication.

In addition to antipyretics and nose drops, the child may require antibiotic therapy. Parents of children receiving oral antibiotics need to understand the importance of administering the drug regularly and continuing it for the prescribed length of time, regardless of whether the child appears ill.

Also caution parents against giving the child any medications that are not approved by the health practitioner. Adverse effects have occurred in children who have received preparations intended for adults (e.g., some long-acting nose drops and dextromethorphan cough squares [mistaken for candy]). Caution parents about giving the child unprescribed antibiotics left over from a previous illness. Self-medication with unprescribed antibiotics can produce serious side effects, and the likelihood of adverse reactions is increased when medications are administered to children without consulting the practitioner. (See Chapter 27 for administration of medications and teaching parents.)

UPPER RESPIRATORY TRACT INFECTIONS

ACUTE VIRAL NASOPHARYNGITIS

A number of viruses, usually rhinoviruses, RSV, adenovirus, influenza virus, and parainfluenza virus, cause acute nasopharyngitis (the equivalent of the common cold).

Clinical Manifestations

Symptoms of nasopharyngitis are more severe in infants and children than in adults. Fever is common, especially in young children. Older children have low-grade fevers, which appear early in the illness. In children 3 months to 3 years, fevers occur suddenly and are associated with irritability, restlessness, decreased appetite and fluid intake, and decreased activity. Nasal inflammation may lead to obstruction of passages, producing open-mouth breathing. Vomiting and diarrhea may also be present.

The initial symptoms in older children are dryness and irritation of nasal passages and the pharynx, followed by sneezing, chilly sensations, muscular aches, an irritating nasal discharge, and sometimes cough. Nasal inflammation may lead to obstruction. Continual wiping away of secretions causes skin irritation to nares.

The disease is self-limiting and usually resolves within 4 to 10 days without complications. Occasionally fever recurs and a child (particularly an infant) might experience otitis media (OM), usually early or after the initial phase of nasopharyngitis is past. Pneumonia is less frequent but may be observed in some infants.

Therapeutic Management

Children with nasopharyngitis are managed at home. There is no specific treatment, and effective vaccines are not available. Antipyretics are prescribed for mild fever and discomfort. (See Chapter 27 for management of fever.) Rest is recommended until the child is free of fever for at least 1 day. Decongestants may be prescribed for children over 5 years of age to shrink swollen nasal passages. The decongestants that exert their effect by vasoconstriction are usually less effective when taken orally than when applied topically as nose drops. Because these drugs affect all vascular beds, they should be given with caution to children with diabetes.

Cough suppressants containing dextromethorphan may be prescribed for a dry, hacking cough. Some preparations contain up to 22% alcohol. They should not be administered to young children continuously and must be stored securely away from children.

Recent concerns regarding serious side effects of cough and cold preparations in young children, particularly infants, and lack of convincing evidence that such medications are effective in reducing symptoms, has prompted recommendations by health experts to carefully evaluate the benefits and risks of recommending such preparations for children under 6 years of age (Ryan, Brewer, and Small, 2008).

Antihistamines are largely ineffective in treatment of nasopharyngitis. These drugs have a weak atropine-like effect that dries secretions, but they can cause drowsiness or, paradoxically, have a stimulatory effect on children. There is no support for the usefulness of expectorants, and antibiotics are usually not indicated.

⚡ DRUG ALERT

Over-the-Counter Cold Preparations

Over-the-counter cold preparation such as pseudoephedrine and some antihistamines are not appropriate for the treatment of the common cold in infants and toddlers; these may cause serious side effects in such children and have been associated with death in infants (Rimsza and Newberry, 2008; Ryan, Brewer, and Small, 2008). Advise parents to consult the primary care physician before using these drugs in infants and toddlers.

Prevention

Nasopharyngitis is so widespread in the general population that it is impossible to prevent. Children are more susceptible to colds because they have not yet developed resistance to many types of viruses. Very young infants are subject to relatively serious complications; therefore they should be protected from exposure.

Nursing Care Management

A cold is often the parents' first introduction to an illness in their infants. Most discomfort of nasopharyngitis is related to the nasal obstruction, especially in small infants. Elevating the head of the bed or crib mattress assists with drainage of secretions; suctioning and vaporization may also provide relief. Saline nose drops and gentle suction with a bulb syringe, particularly before feeding, are useful.

Maintaining adequate fluid intake is essential during any infectious process. Although a child's appetite for solid foods is usually diminished for several days, it is important to offer favorite fluids to prevent dehydration. Fluids can be cool or warm, depending on individual preference.

Because nasopharyngitis is spread from secretions, the best means for prevention is avoiding contact with affected persons. This goal is difficult when large numbers of people are confined in a small area for a long time, such as daycare centers and classrooms. Family members with a cold should try to "keep it to themselves" by carefully disposing of tissues and not sharing towels, glasses, or eating utensils. They should also cover the mouth and nose with tissues when coughing or sneezing; and wash hands thoroughly after nose blowing or sneezing. The most frequent carriers of infection are the human hands, which deposit viruses on doorknobs, faucets, and other everyday objects. Children should wash their hands thoroughly before putting them near their nose, mouth, or eyes.

BOX 32-3 EARLY EVIDENCE OF RESPIRATORY COMPLICATIONS

Parents are instructed to notify the health professional if they note any of the following:
- Evidence of earache (see p. 1232)
- Respirations faster than 50 to 60 beats/min
- Fever over 38.3° C (101° F)
- Listlessness
- Increasing irritability with or without fever
- Persistent cough for 2 days or more
- Wheezing
- Crying
- Refusal to eat
- Restlessness and poor sleep patterns

Modified from National Association of Pediatric Nurse Associates and Practitioners: *Baby's first cold*, New York, 1989, Winthrop Consumer Products. Copies available from National Association of Nurse Practitioners, 20 Brace Road, Suite 200, Cherry Hill, NJ 08034; 856-857-9700; e-mail: info@napnap.org; **www.napnap.org**.

Family Support

Support and reassurance are important elements of care for families of young children with recurrent upper respiratory tract infections (URIs). Because URIs are so frequent in children less than 3 years of age, families may feel they are on an endless roller coaster of illness. Reassure them that frequent colds are a normal part of childhood and that by 5 years of age, most children will have developed immunity to many viruses. Parents who work outside the home should expect to take time off to care for ill children during the fall and winter months. If the children are cared for routinely in daycare centers, the infection rate will be higher than if they are cared for in the home. Parents should know the signs of respiratory complications and should notify a health professional if any signs of complications appear or if the child does not improve within 2 or 3 days (Box 32-3).

ACUTE STREPTOCOCCAL PHARYNGITIS

GABHS infection of the upper airway (strep throat) is not in itself a serious disease, but affected children are at risk for serious sequelae: acute rheumatic fever, an inflammatory disease of the heart, joints, and central nervous system (see Chapter 34); and acute glomerulonephritis, an acute kidney infection (see Chapter 30). Permanent damage can result from these sequelae, especially acute rheumatic fever. GABHS may also cause skin manifestations including, impetigo and pyoderma.

Scarlet fever may also occur as a result of a strain of group A streptococcus. The clinical manifestations of scarlet fever include pharyngitis and a characteristic erythematous sandpaper-like rash; otherwise scarlet fever shares the same clinical manifestations as those mentioned for GABHS, and treatment and sequelae are the same. Severe scarlet fever is rarely seen in the United States.

Clinical Manifestations

GABHS infection is generally a relatively brief illness that varies in severity from subclinical (no symptoms) to severe toxicity.

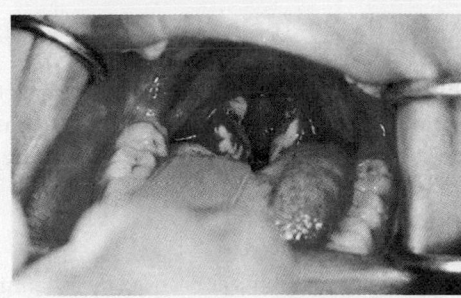

Fig. 32-1 Tonsillitis and pharyngitis. (Courtesy Dr. Edward L. Applebaum, Head, Department of Otolaryngology, University of Illinois Medical Center, Chicago.)

The onset is often abrupt and characterized by pharyngitis, headache, fever, and abdominal pain. The tonsils and pharynx may be inflamed and covered with exudate (50% to 80% of cases) (Fig. 32-1), which usually appears by the second day of illness. However, streptococcal infections should be suspected in children over the age of 2 years who have pharyngitis even if no exudate is present.

Anterior cervical lymphadenopathy (30% to 50% of cases) usually occurs early, and the nodes are often tender. Pain can be relatively mild to severe enough to make swallowing difficult. Clinical manifestations usually subside in 3 to 5 days unless complicated by sinusitis or parapharyngeal, peritonsillar, or retropharyngeal abscess. Nonsuppurative complications may appear after the onset of GABHS—acute nephritis in about 10 days and rheumatic fever in an average of 18 days.

Children who are GABHS carriers may have a positive throat culture but often experience a coincidental viral illness. Although antibiotic administration is not indicated for most GABHS carriers, some conditions require antibiotic therapy; these are published in the American Academy of Pediatrics (2009b) *Red Book*. Transmission to others from a carrier is reportedly minimal.

Diagnostic Evaluation

Although 80% to 90% of all cases of acute pharyngitis are viral, a throat culture should be performed to rule out GABHS. Because some children normally harbor streptococci in their throats, a positive culture is not always conclusive evidence of active disease. Most streptococcal infections are short-term illnesses, and antibody (antistreptolysin O) responses appear later than symptoms and are useful only for retrospective diagnosis.

Rapid identification of GABHS with diagnostic test kits is possible in the office or clinic setting. However, because these kits have questionable sensitivity, they are not yet considered a substitute for culture, and a confirmatory throat culture is recommended in patients who have a negative test result with a rapid diagnostic test kit (American Academy of Pediatrics, 2009b).

Therapeutic Management

If streptococcal sore throat infection is present, oral penicillin is prescribed in a dose sufficient to control the acute local manifestations and to maintain an adequate level for at least 10 days to eliminate organisms that might remain to initiate rheumatic fever symptoms. Penicillin does not prevent the development

of acute glomerulonephritis in susceptible children. However, it may prevent the spread of a nephrogenic strain of GABHS to others in the family. Penicillin usually produces a prompt response within 24 hours. Some patients require retreatment if the organism is not eradicated.

Intramuscular (IM) penicillin G benzathine is also an appropriate therapy. This drug ensures adequate blood concentrations and avoids the problem of compliance, yet it is painful. Some preparations contain penicillin G procaine as well to decrease the pain. Oral erythromycin is indicated for children allergic to penicillin. Other drugs that have been used to treat GABHS pharyngitis include clarithromycin, azithromycin and clindamycin, oral cephalosporins, amoxicillin, and amoxicillin with clavulanic acid (American Academy of Pediatrics, 2009b).

Nursing Care Management

The nurse often obtains a throat swab for culture and instructs the parents about administering penicillin and analgesics as prescribed. Some children may prefer quiet activities during the acute phase of the illness, whereas others may limit activity only if the temperature is elevated. Cold or warm compresses to the neck may provide relief. In children old enough to cooperate, warm saline gargles offer some relief of throat discomfort. Pain may interfere with oral intake, and the child should not be forced to eat. Instead encourage cool liquids or ice chips, which are usually more acceptable than solids.

Special emphasis is placed on correctly administering oral medication and completing the course of antibiotic therapy. (See Administration of Medication, and Compliance, Chapter 27.) If an antibiotic injection is required, it must be administered deep into a large muscle mass (e.g., the vastus lateralis or ventrogluteal muscle). Parents need to be aware of the residual tenderness. Local applications of heat are helpful in relieving discomfort. (For other atraumatic strategies to reduce injection pain, such as application over the site of EMLA [a eutectic mix of lidocaine and prilocaine] $2\frac{1}{2}$ hours before the injection or LMX4 [lidocaine 4%] 30 minutes beforehand, see Administration of Medication: Intramuscular Administration, Chapter 27.)

⚡ DRUG ALERT

Administration of Procaine or Benzathine Penicillin

Never administer penicillin G procaine or penicillin G benzathine suspensions intravenously; they may cause embolism or toxic reaction with ensuing death in minutes. Instead, administer these medications deep into the muscle tissue to decrease localized reactions and pain.

Prevention

No immunization is available for prevention of streptococcal disease. The organism is spread by close contact with affected persons—direct projection of large droplets or physical transfer of respiratory secretions containing the organism. Spread of infection is common in families, classrooms, and daycare centers. Children with streptococcal infection are noninfectious to others 24 hours after initiation of antibiotic therapy. It is generally recommended that children not return to school or daycare until they have been taking antibiotics for a full 24-hour period.

Nurses should remind children with a streptococcal throat infection to discard their toothbrush and replace it with a new one after they have been taking antibiotics for 24 hours.

It is important to know when the organism is epidemic in the community so that families can be alert for symptoms. Directors of daycare centers and school officials should share infectious disease information with parents. Obtaining throat cultures from children who are close family contacts of patients with streptococcal infection is advised.

TONSILLITIS

The tonsils are masses of lymphoid tissue located in the pharyngeal cavity. The tonsils filter and protect the respiratory and alimentary tracts from invasion by pathogenic organisms. They also play a role in antibody formation. Although the size of tonsils varies, children generally have larger tonsils than adolescents or adults. This difference is thought to be a protective mechanism, since young children are especially susceptible to URIs.

Pathophysiology

Several pairs of tonsils are part of a mass of lymphoid tissue encircling the nasopharynx and oropharynx, known as the Waldeyer tonsillar ring (Fig. 32-2). The palatine, or faucial, tonsils are located on either side of the oropharynx, behind and below the pillars of the fauces (opening from the mouth). A surface of the palatine tonsils is usually visible during oral examination. The palatine tonsils are those removed during tonsillectomy. The pharyngeal tonsils, also known as the adenoids, are located above the palatine tonsils on the posterior wall of the nasopharynx. Their proximity to the nares and eustachian tubes causes difficulties in instances of inflammation. The lingual tonsils are located at the base of the tongue. The tubal tonsils, found near the posterior nasopharyngeal opening of the eustachian tubes, are not part of the Waldeyer tonsillar ring.

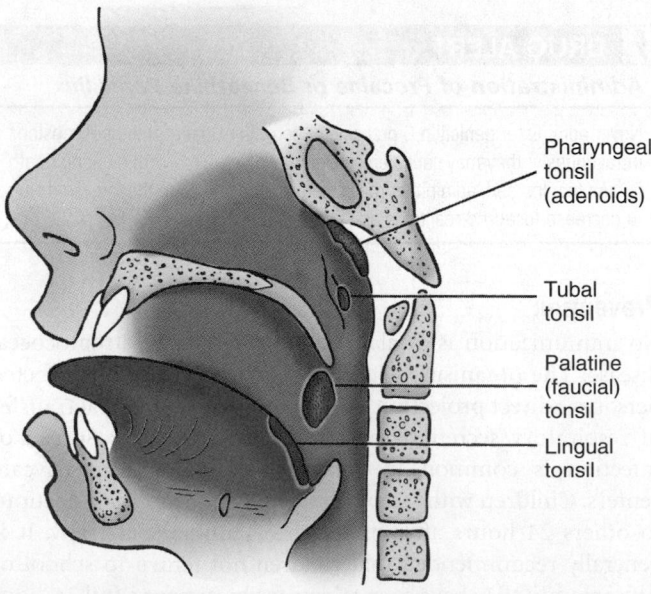

Fig. 32-2 Location of various tonsillar masses.

Etiology

Tonsillitis often occurs with pharyngitis. Because of the abundant lymphoid tissue and the frequency of URIs, tonsillitis is a common cause of illness in young children. The causative agent may be viral or bacterial.

Clinical Manifestations

The manifestations of tonsillitis are caused by inflammation. As the palatine tonsils enlarge from edema, they may meet in the midline (kissing tonsils), obstructing the passage of air or food. The child has difficulty swallowing and breathing. When enlargement of the adenoids occurs, the space behind the posterior nares may become blocked, making it difficult or impossible for air to pass from the nose to the throat. As a result, the child breathes through the mouth.

If mouth breathing is continuous, the mucous membranes of the oropharynx become dry and irritated. There may be an offensive mouth odor and impaired senses of taste and smell. Because air cannot be trapped for proper speech sounds, the voice has a nasal and muffled quality. A persistent cough is also common. Because of the proximity of the adenoids to the eustachian tubes, this passageway is frequently blocked by swollen adenoids, interfering with normal drainage and frequently resulting in OM or difficulty hearing.

Therapeutic Management
Medical Treatment

Because the illness is self-limiting, treatment of viral pharyngitis is symptomatic. Throat cultures positive for GABHS infection require antibiotic treatment. It is important to differentiate between viral and streptococcal infection in febrile exudative tonsillitis. Because the majority of infections are of viral origin, early rapid tests can eliminate unnecessary antibiotic administration.

Surgical Treatment

Surgical treatment of chronic tonsillitis is controversial. Except in documented cases of recurrent, frequent streptococcal infection or a history of development of a peritonsillar abscess, tonsillectomy is not indicated in the child who has recurrent pharyngitis.

Tonsillectomy (surgical removal of the palatine tonsils) may be indicated for massive hypertrophy that results in difficulty breathing or eating. Absolute indications are malignancy and obstruction of the airway that result in cor pulmonale. Adenoidectomy (the surgical removal of the adenoids) is recommended for children who have hypertrophied adenoids that obstruct nasal breathing; additional indications for adenoidectomy include recurrent adenoiditis and sinusitis, OM with effusion, airway obstruction and subsequent sleep-disordered breathing, and recurrent rhinorrhea (Benninger and Walner, 2007). The American Academy of Otolaryngology–Head and Neck Surgery (2000) lists a number of indications for tonsillectomy, one of which is three or more infections of the tonsils or adenoids per year despite adequate medical therapy. For some children the effectiveness of tonsillectomy or adenoidectomy is modest and may not justify the risk of surgery. In practice, most primary care providers rely on individualized decision making and do not subscribe to an absolute set of eligibility criteria for these surgical procedures (Paradise, Blucstone, Colborn, et al, 2002) (see Research Focus box).

🔍 RESEARCH FOCUS

Adenotonsillectomy for Recurrent Sore Throat

A recent Cochrane review (Burton and Glasziou, 2009) concluded there was a modest benefit to adenotonsillectomy in children with recurrent sore throat; others have reached similar conclusions (Blakley and Magit, 2009).

Contraindications to either tonsillectomy or adenoidectomy are (1) cleft palate, since both tonsils help minimize escape of air during speech; (2) acute infections at the time of surgery because the locally inflamed tissues increase the risk of bleeding; and (3) uncontrolled systemic diseases or blood dyscrasias.

Generally, removal of the tonsils should not occur until after 3 or 4 years of age because of the problem of excessive blood loss in young children and the possibility of regrowth or hypertrophy of lymphoid tissue. The tubal and lingual tonsils often enlarge to compensate for the lost lymphoid tissue, resulting in continued pharyngeal and eustachian tube obstruction.

Nursing Care Management

Nursing care of the child with tonsillitis involves providing comfort and minimizing activities or interventions that precipitate bleeding. A soft to liquid diet is generally preferred. A cool-mist vaporizer keeps the mucous membranes moist during periods of mouth breathing. Warm saltwater gargles, throat lozenges, and analgesic-antipyretic drugs such as acetaminophen are useful to promote comfort. Often opioids are needed to reduce pain for the child to drink. Combination nonopioid and opioid elixirs such as acetaminophen with codeine or with hydrocodone (Lortab) relieve pain and should be given routinely every 4 hours.

If surgery is needed, the child requires the same psychologic preparation and physical care as for any procedure. (See Chapters 26 and 27.) The following discussion focuses on specific nursing care for tonsillectomy and adenoidectomy (T&A), although both procedures may not be performed.

The nurse takes a complete history, with special notation of any bleeding tendencies because the operative site is highly vascular. Baseline vital signs are important for postoperative monitoring and observation. Signs of any URI are noted and reported, and bleeding and clotting times may be obtained with the usual laboratory work requests. During physical assessment the presence of any loose teeth is noted. (See Surgical Procedures, Chapter 27.)

After the surgery, until they are fully awake, children are placed on the abdomen or side to facilitate drainage of secretions. Suctioning is performed carefully to avoid trauma to the oropharynx. When alert, children may prefer sitting up, although they should remain in bed for the remainder of the day. They are discouraged from coughing frequently, clearing their throat, blowing their nose, or any activities that could aggravate the operative site.

Some secretions, particularly dried blood from surgery, are common. Inspect all secretions and vomitus for evidence of fresh bleeding (some blood-tinged mucus is expected). Dark brown (old) blood is usually present in the emesis, as well as in the nose and between the teeth. If parents are not prepared for this, they may be frightened at a time when they need to be calm and reassuring.

The throat is very sore after surgery. An ice collar may provide relief, but many children find it bothersome and refuse to use it. Most children experience moderate pain after a T&A and need pain medication for at least the first 24 hours. Analgesics may need to be given intravenously to avoid the oral route. Because pain is continuous, analgesics should be administered at regular intervals. Local anesthetics, such as tetracaine lollipops or ice pops, and antiemetics, such as ondansetron (Zofran) may be administered postoperatively. (See Pain Management, Chapter 7.)

Food and fluid are restricted until children are fully alert with no signs of hemorrhage. Cool water, crushed ice, flavored ice pops, or diluted fruit juice is given, and fluids with a red or brown color are avoided to distinguish fresh or old blood in emesis from the ingested liquid. Straws should be avoided, since these may damage the surgical site and cause subsequent bleeding. Citrus juice may cause discomfort and is usually poorly tolerated. Milk, ice cream, or pudding is not usually offered until clear fluids are retained because milk products coat the mouth and throat, causing the child to clear the throat, which may initiate bleeding.

Children often begin soft foods, particularly gelatin, cooked fruits, sherbet, soup, and mashed potatoes, on the first or second postoperative day or as the child tolerates feeding. The pain from surgery often inhibits intake, reinforcing the need for adequate pain control.

❗ NURSING ALERT

The most obvious early sign of bleeding is the child's continuous swallowing of the trickling blood. While the child is sleeping, note the frequency of swallowing. If continuous bleeding is suspected, notify the surgeon immediately.

Postoperative hemorrhage is unusual but can occur. The nurse observes the throat directly for evidence of bleeding, using a good source of light and, if necessary, carefully inserting a tongue depressor. Other signs of hemorrhage are tachycardia, pallor, frequent clearing of the throat or swallowing by a younger child, and vomiting of bright red blood. Restlessness, an indication of hemorrhage, may be difficult to differentiate from general discomfort after surgery. Decreasing blood pressure is a much later sign of shock. A cream-colored membrane is often visible on the tonsillar bed postoperatively; reassure parents this is an expected finding.

Surgery may be required to cauterize or ligate a bleeding vessel. Airway obstruction may also occur as a result of edema or accumulated secretions and is indicated by signs of respiratory distress, such as stridor, drooling, restlessness, agitation, increasing respiratory rate, and progressive cyanosis. Suction equipment and oxygen should be available after tonsillectomy.

Family Support and Home Care

Discharge instructions include (1) avoiding foods that are irritating or highly seasoned, (2) avoiding the use of gargles or vigorous toothbrushing, (3) discouraging the child from coughing or clearing the throat or putting objects in the mouth, (4) using analgesics or an ice collar for pain, and (5) limiting activity to decrease the potential for bleeding. Hemorrhage may occur up to 10 days after surgery as a result of tissue sloughing from the healing process. Any sign of bleeding warrants immediate medical attention. Objectionable mouth odor and slight ear pain with a low-grade fever are common for a few days postoperatively. However, persistent severe earache, fever, or cough requires medical evaluation. Most children are ready to resume normal activity within 1 to 2 weeks after the operation.

Most children are admitted to a same-day surgery or ambulatory surgery unit and discharged home after a recovery period. T&A often represents the first hospitalization experience for the child and family. Because the surgery is usually an elective procedure, there is ample opportunity to prepare both children and parents for this event. Both need reassurance about what to expect at the time of admission, before and after surgery, and at discharge. Children are informed about postoperative discomfort and reassured that they will be able to talk. Some children believe the procedure will immediately "make the throat all better" and are dismayed to find that it still hurts after the surgery.

INFECTIOUS MONONUCLEOSIS

Infectious mononucleosis is an acute, self-limiting infectious disease that is common among young people under 25 years of age. The disease is characterized by an increase in the mononuclear elements of the blood and by symptoms of an infectious process. The course is usually mild but occasionally can be severe or, rarely, accompanied by serious complications.

Etiology and Pathophysiology

The herpeslike Epstein-Barr virus is the principal cause of infectious mononucleosis. It appears in both sporadic and epidemic forms, but the sporadic cases are more common. The virus is believed to be transmitted by direct contact with oral secretions, blood transfusion, or transplantation. It is mildly contagious, and the period of communicability is unknown. There is evidence that the virus is spread through sexual contact, especially when multiple partners are involved (Rimsza and Kirk, 2005). The incubation period after exposure in adolescents is estimated to be 30 to 50 days (American Academy of Pediatrics, 2009b).

Clinical Manifestations

Symptoms of infectious mononucleosis appear anywhere from 10 days to 6 weeks after exposure and may be acute or insidious. The common presenting symptoms vary greatly in type, severity, and duration. The characteristics of the disease are malaise, sore throat, and fever with generalized lymphadenopathy and splenomegaly that may persist for several months. Often the symptoms appear insidiously with fatigue, lack of energy, and

sore throat. The child's chief complaint is difficulty in maintaining the usual level of activity. This is often attributed to lack of sleep or a URI. In many instances the manifestations never arouse enough concern to bring the affected individual to medical attention. The clinical manifestations of infectious mononucleosis are usually less severe (often subclinical or unapparent) and the recovery phase is shorter in younger children than in older children and young adults. Many young children do not develop all the expected clinical and laboratory findings. Often a complication is the only or the presenting symptom.

A skin rash that involves a discrete macular eruption (most prominent over the trunk) is present in some cases and is often associated with the administration of ampicillin or amoxicillin. Other symptoms include headache, epistaxis, and a severe sore throat. The tonsils may be enlarged, reddened, and sometimes covered with a diphtheria-like membrane. In some cases airway compromise may occur with tonsillar swelling, requiring careful airway management, corticosteroids, humidified air, and intravenous (IV) hydration (Jenson, 2007). In about half the cases the spleen is enlarged. Splenic hemorrhage or rupture may occur but is usually related to trauma (Jenson, 2007). The extensive mononuclear infiltration produces symptoms related to any body tissue, and the clinical picture can resemble that of many conditions, including neurologic manifestations and cardiac involvement.

Diagnostic Evaluation

The diagnosis is established on the basis of clinical manifestations, increase in atypical leukocytes in a peripheral blood smear, and a positive heterophil agglutination test. Differential diagnosis depends on the clinical symptoms present. For example, the pharyngitis may simulate symptoms of diphtheria and streptococcal pharyngitis. Lymphadenopathy, fever, malaise, central nervous system manifestations, and skin eruptions may be similar to symptoms seen in a variety of conditions. The leukocyte count may be normal or low, but usually lymphocytic leukocytosis develops.

The heterophil antibody test determines the extent to which the patient's serum will agglutinate sheep red blood cells. In infectious mononucleosis a titer of 1:160 is considered diagnostic, although a rising titer during the earlier stages is the best indicator. Because young children have a lower rate of heterophil antibody responses, the diagnosis may be overlooked in this group.

The spot test (Monospot) is a slide test of high specificity for the diagnosis of infectious mononucleosis. It is rapid, sensitive, inexpensive, and easy to perform, and it has the advantage that it can detect significant agglutinins at lower levels, thus permitting earlier diagnosis. Blood is usually obtained for the test by finger puncture and is placed on special paper. If the blood agglutinates, forming fragments or clumps, the test is positive for the infection.

Therapeutic Management

No specific treatment exists for infectious mononucleosis. Common symptoms are ordinarily relieved by simple remedies. A mild analgesic is usually sufficient to relieve the bothersome symptoms of headache, fever, and malaise. Bed rest is encouraged for fatigue but is not imposed for any specified time. Affected children and adolescents should regulate activities according to their own tolerance unless complicating factors are present. If the spleen is enlarged, children should avoid activities in which they might receive a blow to the abdomen or chest.

A short course of corticosteroids may assist in decreasing some of the complications (e.g., airway obstruction) of the illness. Administration of ampicillin or amoxicillin frequently precipitates a maculopapular rash in affected persons (80% of cases); therefore their use is contraindicated. Gargles; hot drinks; analgesic or anesthetic troches; or analgesics, including opioids, can relieve a sore throat. Although corticosteroids have been used to treat respiratory distress from tonsillar hypertrophy, hemolytic anemia, thrombocytopenia, and neurologic complications, the routine use of steroids is not recommended (American Academy of Pediatrics, 2009b).

Prognosis

The course of infectious mononucleosis is self-limiting and usually uncomplicated. Contrary to popular belief, mononucleosis is not necessarily a difficult, prolonged, or disabling disease, and the prognosis is generally good. Acute symptoms usually disappear within 7 to 10 days, and the persistent fatigue subsides within 2 to 4 weeks. A number of affected children or adolescents may need to restrict activities for 2 to 3 months; the disease rarely extends for longer periods.

Complications are uncommon but can be serious and require appropriate management. Neurologic complications occur in some outbreaks and vary in severity and outcome. These include seizures; ataxia; and perceptual distortions of shapes, spatial relationships, and sizes. Other complications include pneumonitis, myocarditis, hemolytic anemia, thrombocytopenia, and ruptured spleen. Rarely Reye syndrome or Guillain-Barré syndrome may develop following the acute phase of the illness (Jenson, 2007). Some evidence indicates a depressed cellular immune reactivity during the course of the disease and for some time afterward. Thus it is best to avoid live vaccines until several months after recovery.

Nursing Care Management

Direct nursing responsibilities toward providing comfort measures to relieve the symptoms and toward helping affected children and adolescents and their families determine appropriate activities for the stage of the disease and their interests. Airway assessment for impending obstruction during the acute phase of the illness is imperative. The adolescent with infectious mononucleosis may not be able to swallow secretions and may be in considerable pain. The child or adolescent is encouraged to increase clear fluid intake and decrease solid foods that may exacerbate the pain. In addition, the nurse should encourage the administration of age-appropriate antipyretics and encourage the affected individual to curtail activities that are strenuous until splenomegaly is resolved. Pain medications in elixir form such as acetaminophen with codeine or hydrocodone may be required during the acute phase so the adolescent can swallow liquids. Make every effort to prevent a secondary infection by counseling the adolescent to limit exposure to persons outside the family, especially during the acute phase of illness.

! NURSING ALERT

Advise the family to seek medical evaluation of the child or adolescent if:
- Breathing becomes difficult.
- Severe abdominal pain develops.
- Sore throat pain is so severe that the child is unable to eat or drink.
- Respiratory stridor is observed.

INFLUENZA

Three of the orthomyxoviruses, which are antigenically distinct, cause the influenza, or "flu": types A and B, which cause epidemic disease, and type C, which is unimportant epidemiologically. The viruses undergo significant changes from time to time. Major changes that occur at intervals of usually 5 to 10 years are called antigenic shift; minor variations within the same subtypes, antigenic drift, occur almost annually. Consequently, antigenic drift can alter the virus sufficiently to result in susceptibility of individuals to a type for which they were previously immunized or infected.

The disease is spread from one individual to another by direct contact (large-droplet infection) or by articles recently contaminated by nasopharyngeal secretions. There is no predilection for a specific age-group, but attack rates are highest in young children who have not had previous contact with a strain. It is frequently most severe in infants and older adults. During epidemics, infection among school-age children is believed to be a major source of transmission in a community. Influenza is more common during the winter months.

The disease has a 1- to 4-day incubation period, and affected persons are most infectious for 24 hours before and after the onset of symptoms. The virus has a peculiar affinity for epithelial cells of the respiratory tract mucosa, where it destroys ciliated epithelium with metaplastic hyperplasia of the tracheal and bronchial epithelium with associated edema. The alveoli may also become distended with a hyaline-like material. The viruses can be isolated from nasopharyngeal secretions early after the onset of infection, and serologic tests identify the type by complement fixation or the subgroups by hemagglutination inhibition.

H1N1 (swine flu) is a subtype of influenza type A. The current pandemic of H1N1 caused significant morbidity and mortality, particularly in Mexico and the United States. The signs and symptoms of H1N1 flu are the same as those mentioned below for influenza. A pandemic is defined by the World Health Organization as the spread of a new disease to which the population has little or no immunity and that spreads rapidly from human to human. In response to the 2009 H1N1 pandemic, the World Health Organization (2009) recommends that those infected with the virus be given either oseltamivir (Tamiflu) or zanamivir; a few isolated cases of H1N1 flu resistant to oseltamivir have been reported, but these are not believed to represent a significant threat. In the United States there are two vaccinations for H1N1: a live attenuated H1N1 influenza virus (LAIV) vaccine given intranasally, and an inactivated influenza (H1N1) monovalent vaccine given intramuscularly (Centers for Disease Control and Prevention, 2009b). Targeted candidates to receive the first supplies of vaccine available included pregnant women, persons ages 6 months to 24 years, health care and emergency workers, persons living with or providing care for infants less than 6 months of age, and persons ages 25 to 64 years who have medical conditions that place them at higher risk for influenza-related complications (Centers for Disease Control and Prevention, 2009b). The most updated information on the status of this disease may be found at the Centers for Disease Control and Prevention and World Health Organization websites: www.cdc.gov and www.who.int/csr/disease/swineflu/en/index.html.

Clinical Manifestations

The manifestations of influenza may be subclinical, mild, moderate, or severe. In most cases the throat and nasal mucosa are dry, and there is a dry cough and a tendency toward hoarseness. A sudden onset of fever and chills is accompanied by flushed face, photophobia, myalgia, hyperesthesia, and sometimes prostration. Subglottal croup is common, especially in infants. The symptoms last 4 or 5 days. Complications include severe viral pneumonia (often hemorrhagic); encephalitis; and secondary bacterial infections, such as OM, sinusitis, or pneumonia.

Therapeutic Management

Uncomplicated influenza in children usually requires only symptomatic treatment: acetaminophen or ibuprofen for fever and sufficient fluids to maintain hydration. Amantadine hydrochloride (Symmetrel) has been effective in reducing symptoms associated with type A disease if administered within 24 to 48 hours after their onset; the symptoms associated with influenza are reportedly shortened by 24 hours but the drug does not "cure" the disease. It is ineffective against type B or C influenza or other viral diseases. It should not be given to children under 1 year of age but is recommended for unvaccinated high-risk children. Since early 2006, however, there has been an increase in influenza strains resistant to amantadine, and thus the neuraminidase inhibitors oseltamivir and zanamivir have been recommended for influenza treatment (American Academy of Pediatrics, 2009b). A small number of influenza strains are resistant to oseltamivir.

Zanamivir and rimantadine have been approved for the treatment of flu symptoms in children under 18 years of age. Both medications must also be started within 48 hours of symptom onset. Zanamivir is an inhaled medication effective for type A and B influenza. The drug is taken twice daily for 5 days and is administered by a specially designed oral inhaler (Diskhaler). Zanamivir cannot be used for children less than 7 years of age except for specific prophylaxis indications in children ages 5 years and above (US Food and Drug Administration, 2009). Zanamivir is recommended for persons ages 7 years and above who have been exposed to H1N1 in 2009. A fourth drug, oseltamivir, is a neuroaminidase inhibitor that may be administered orally for 5 days to children over 3 months (and adults) to decrease the flu symptoms. As with other antiviral drugs, this must be taken within 2 days of the onset of symptoms. It is effective for types A and B influenza (American Academy of Pediatrics, 2009b). Bronchospasm and a decline in lung function can occur when zanamivir is used in patients with underlying airway disease such as asthma or chronic obstructive pulmonary disease. Rimantadine is effective only for type A

virus; this drug is taken orally in tablet or syrup twice daily for 7 days. Rimantadine cannot be used for children less than 1 year of age. Children with influenza (or other similar viruses) should not receive aspirin because of its possible link with Reye syndrome.

Prevention

The influenza vaccine is now recommended annually for children 6 months to 18 years (completed). Influenza vaccine (trivalent inactivated influenza vaccine [TIV]) may be given to any healthy children 6 months old and older. The vaccine may be given simultaneously with other vaccines but at a separate site. TIV is administered yearly because different strains of influenza are used each year in the manufacture of the vaccine.

LAIV is an acceptable alternative to the IM trivalent vaccine in specific age-groups. Either TIV or LAIV may be given to healthy, nonpregnant persons ages 2 to 49 years (American Academy of Pediatrics, 2009b). Yearly influenza vaccine should be administered to children ages 6 to 59 months with medical conditions that place them at risk for influenza-related complications (including asthma, cardiac disease, human immunodeficiency virus [HIV], diabetes, and sickle cell disease) and to health care workers. (See Immunizations, Chapter 12.)

Nursing Care Management

Nursing care is the same as for any child with a URI, including helping the family implement measures to relieve symptoms. The greatest danger to affected children is development of a secondary infection. Prolonged fever or appearance of fever during early convalescence is a sign of secondary bacterial infection and should be reported to the practitioner for antibiotic therapy. In addition to the measures mentioned previously, nursing care of the child with influenza includes educating the parents regarding the prevention of the spread of the disease to other individuals, especially those who are at higher risk for complications, and educating the parents about the use of anti-influenza medications. Parents are informed about the nature of antiviral drugs in regards to symptom management. Parents may also ask the practitioner to prescribe an antibiotic for the influenza, not understanding that these are ineffective against viral infections; indiscriminate use of antibiotics may lead to increased resistance to common antibiotics. The nurse should also educate parents regarding yearly influenza immunization and its effectiveness at decreasing morbidity among children.

OTITIS MEDIA

OM is one of the most prevalent illnesses of early childhood. Its incidence is highest in the winter months. Many cases of bacterial OM are preceded by a viral respiratory tract infection. The two viruses most likely to precipitate OM are RSV and influenza. Most episodes of acute otitis media (AOM) occur in the first 24 months of life, but the incidence decreases with age, except for a small increase at age 5 or 6 years when children enter school. OM occurs infrequently in children older than 7 years of age. Preschool-age boys are affected more frequently than preschool-age girls. Children who have siblings or parents with a history of chronic OM have a higher incidence of OM. Out-of-home daycare is a significant risk factor for OM.

Children living in households with many members (especially smokers) are more likely to have OM than those living with fewer persons. Passive smoking increases the risk of persistent middle ear effusion by enhancing attachment of the pathogens that cause otitis to the respiratory epithelium in the middle ear space, prolonging the inflammatory response, and impeding drainage through the eustachian tube (American Academy of Pediatrics, 2004a). Family socioeconomic status and extent of exposure to other children are the two most important identifiable risk factors for the occurrence of OM (American Academy of Pediatrics 2004a; Kershner, 2007).

OM has been defined in a variety of ways. The standard terminology is given in Box 32-4, and AOM and OM with effusion (OME) guidelines have been published (American Academy of Pediatrics, 2004a, 2004b).

Etiology

AOM is frequently caused by *Streptococcus pneumoniae*, *H. influenzae*, and *Moraxella catarrhalis*. The two viruses most likely to precipitate OM are RSV and influenza, although the adenoviruses, metapneumoviruses, and rhinoviruses also cause a significant number of URIs and OM. The etiology of the noninfectious type is unknown, although it is frequently the result of blocked eustachian tubes from the edema of URIs, allergic rhinitis, or hypertrophic adenoids. Chronic OM is frequently an extension of an acute episode.

A relationship has been observed between the incidence of OM and infant feeding methods. Infants fed breast milk have a lower incidence of OM compared with formula-fed infants. Breast-feeding may protect infants against respiratory viruses and allergy because it contains secretory immunoglobulin A, which limits the exposure of the eustachian tube and middle ear mucosa to microbial pathogens and foreign proteins. Reflux of milk up the eustachian tubes is less likely in breast-fed infants because of the semivertical positioning during breast-feeding compared with bottle-feeding.

Pathophysiology

OM is primarily a result of a dysfunctioning eustachian tube. The eustachian tube is part of a contiguous system composed of the nares, nasopharynx, eustachian tube, middle ear, and mastoid antrum and air cells. Eustachian tubes have three functions relative to the middle ear: (1) protection of the middle ear from nasopharyngeal secretions, (2) drainage of secretions produced in the middle ear into the nasopharynx, and (3) ventilation of the middle ear to equalize air pressure within the middle ear and atmospheric pressure in the external ear canal and replenishment of oxygen that has been absorbed.

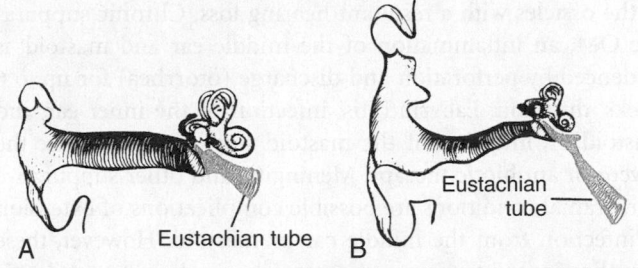

Fig. 32-3 Comparison of anatomic position of eustachian tube in a child **(A)** and an adult **(B)**. Eustachian tube is shorter, wider, straighter, and more horizontal in a child than in an adult.

Mechanical or functional obstruction of the eustachian tube causes accumulation of secretions in the middle ear. Infection or allergy can cause intrinsic obstruction. Extrinsic obstruction is usually a result of enlarged adenoids or nasopharyngeal tumors. Persistent collapse of the tube during swallowing can cause functional obstruction associated with decreased stiffness or an inefficient opening mechanism. Eustachian tube obstruction results in negative middle ear pressure and, if persistent, produces a transudative middle ear effusion. Sustained negative pressure and impaired ciliary transport within the tube inhibit drainage. When the passage is not totally obstructed, contamination of the middle ear can take place by reflux, aspiration, or insufflation during crying, sneezing, nose blowing, and swallowing when the nose is obstructed.

Several factors predispose infants and young children to development of OM (Box 32-5 and Fig. 32-3).

Complications

The consequences of prolonged middle ear disorders can be either functional or structural. The principal functional consequence is hearing loss, although loss in most children is conductive in nature and mild in severity. The causes of hearing loss are negative middle ear pressure, effusion in the middle ear, or structural damage to the tympanic membrane. However, the most feared consequence of hearing loss is its adverse effect on development of speech, language, and cognition. Children who have prolonged periods of middle ear effusion perform less well on speech and language tests than those who have few or no middle ear diseases.

Structural complications or sequelae involve primarily the tympanic membrane. Tympanic membrane retraction or retraction pockets occur in areas of low tensile strength or atrophic segments of the drum head when continued negative middle ear pressure draws the tympanic membrane inward. This retraction may result in impaired sound transmission, perforation of the thinned-out areas, or infection in the pockets and, later, cholesteatoma.

Tympanosclerosis (eardrum scarring) is the deposition of hyaline material into the fibrous layer of the tympanic membrane. It often occurs in children with inflammatory middle ear disease or those with repeated tympanoplasty tube placement. Eardrum perforation is a common complication in AOM and often accompanies chronic disease. Persistent perforation is a complication of tympanostomy tube placement. Surgery is required to close some perforations.

Adhesive OM (glue ear) is a thickening of the mucous membrane by proliferation of fibrous tissue that can cause fixation of the ossicles with a resultant hearing loss. Chronic suppurative OM, an inflammation of the middle ear and mastoid, is evidenced by perforation and discharge (otorrhea) for up to 6 weeks' duration. Labyrinthitis, infection of the inner ear, and mastoiditis, infection of the mastoid sinus, are rare since the advent of antibiotic therapy. Meningitis and other suppurative intracranial conditions are possible complications of extension of infection from the middle ear or mastoid. However, these complications occur infrequently when adequate antibiotic therapy is implemented.

Cholesteatoma is the least common but most potentially dangerous sequela of OME. A cholesteatoma forms when the keratinizing, stratified, squamous epithelial cell lining desquamates to form scales that accumulate within the middle ear space. As it enlarges, the cholesteatoma erodes all structures it encounters, especially bone, destroying the ossicles and gaining entry to the inner ear and meninges. Clinical signs are a foul-smelling, grayish yellow discharge; sometimes pain; and permanent, progressive hearing loss. Treatment is surgical excision of the entire cholesteatoma.

Clinical Manifestations

As purulent fluid accumulates in the small space of the middle ear chamber, pain results from the pressure on surrounding structures. Infants become irritable and indicate their discomfort by holding or pulling at their ears and rolling their head from side to side. Young children usually verbally complain of the pain. A temperature as high as 40° C (104° F) is common, and postauricular and cervical lymph glands may be enlarged. Rhinorrhea, vomiting, diarrhea, and signs of concurrent respiratory tract or pharyngeal infection may also be present. Loss of appetite typically occurs, and sucking or chewing tends to aggravate the pain. In children with OME, exudate accumulates and pressure increases, with the potential for tympanic membrane rupture.

As a result of rupture, there is immediate relief of pain, a gradual decrease in temperature, and the presence of purulent discharge in the external auditory canal.

Severe pain or fever is usually absent in OME, and the child may not appear ill. Instead there is a feeling of "fullness" in the ear, a popping sensation during swallowing, and a feeling of "motion" in the ear if air is present above the level of fluid. Because chronic serous OM is the most frequent cause of conductive hearing loss in young children, audiometry may reveal deficient hearing.

Diagnostic Evaluation

Careful assessment of tympanic membrane mobility with a pneumatic otoscope is essential to differentiate AOM from OME (American Academy of Pediatrics, 2004a). If an accumulation of cerumen prevents adequate visualization of the tympanic membrane, the cerumen should be removed before inspection of the membrane. A diagnosis of AOM is made if visual inspection of the tympanic membrane reveals a purulent, discolored effusion and a bulging or full, opacified, or very reddened immobile membrane. Some practitioners also consider the presence of acute onset of less than 48 hours of ear pain with the preceding criteria to be a diagnostic factor in AOM (Powers, 2007). An immobile tympanic membrane or an orange-discolored membrane indicates OME. Clinical symptoms of otitis are also helpful in making the diagnosis. In AOM, symptoms such as acute ear pain, fever, and a bulging yellow or red tympanic membrane are usually present. In OME these symptoms may be absent, and other nonspecific symptoms such as rhinitis, cough, or diarrhea are often present.

Several tests provide an assessment of mobility of the tympanic membrane. Chapter 6, under Ears, discusses pneumatic otoscopy and tympanometry. Acoustic reflectometry measures the level of sound transmitted and reflected from the middle ear to a microphone located in a probe tip placed against the ear canal opening and directed toward the tympanic membrane. The information provides a measure of canal length and presence of effusion. The greater the cancellation of transmitted sound by reflected sound, the greater the probability of middle ear effusion.

Therapeutic Management: Acute Otitis Media

Treatment for AOM is one of the most common reasons for antibiotic use in the ambulatory setting. However, recent concerns about drug-resistant *S. pneumoniae* and other drug-resistant strains have led infectious disease authorities to recommend careful and judicious use of antibiotics for treatment of this illness. Current literature indicates that waiting up to 72 hours for spontaneous resolution is safe and appropriate management of AOM in healthy infants over 6 months and children (American Academy of Pediatrics, 2004a; Bhetwal and McConaghy, 2007). Furthermore some reviews of the treatment of AOM reveal no clear evidence that antibiotics improve outcomes in children younger than 2 years of age with uncomplicated AOM. However, the watchful waiting approach is not recommended for children younger than 2 years who have persistent acute symptoms of fever and severe ear pain (Kershner, 2007). In addition, all cases of AOM in infants younger than 6 months of age should be treated with antibiotics because of the infant's immature immune system and the potential for infection with bacteria other than the three most common organisms found in older infants and children with AOM.

When antibiotics are necessary, oral amoxicillin in high doses (80 to 90 mg/kg/day, divided twice daily) is the treatment of choice for initial episodes of AOM in children who have not received antibiotics within the past month (American Academy of Pediatrics, 2004a; Bhetwal and McConaghy, 2007; Pichichero and Casey, 2005). The recommendation for the duration of antibiotic therapy is 10 days for severe AOM; for children with mild to moderate disease and those who are 6 years and older, a 5- to 7-day course is adequate (American Academy of Pediatrics, 2009b).

Second-line antibiotics used to treat OM include amoxicillin-clavulanate (Augmentin); azithromycin; and cephalosporins such as cefdinir, cefuroxime, and cefpodoxime. IM ceftriaxone is used if the causative organism is a highly resistant pneumococcus or if there is noncompliance with the therapy. An important consideration with the use of single-dose IM injections is the pain involved in this therapy. One strategy to minimize pain at the injection site is to reconstitute the cephalosporin with 1% lidocaine (without epinephrine). The use of steroids, decongestants, and antihistamines to treat AOM is not recommended.

Supportive care or symptomatic treatment of AOM includes treating the fever and pain. For fever or discomfort associated with OM, analgesic-antipyretic drugs such as acetaminophen or ibuprofen (ibuprofen only if >6 months of age) may be given. Topical pain relief is recommended by external application of heat or cold, or the practitioner may prescribe topical pain relief drops such as benzocaine drops. Antibiotic ear drops have no value in treating AOM.

Children with AOM should be seen after antibiotic therapy is complete to evaluate the effectiveness of the treatment and to identify potential complications, such as effusion or hearing impairment.

Myringotomy, a surgical incision of the eardrum, may be necessary to alleviate the severe pain of AOM. A myringotomy is also performed to drain infected middle ear fluid in the presence of complications (mastoiditis, labyrinthitis, or facial paralysis) or to allow purulent middle ear fluid to drain into the ear canal for culture. A minimally invasive laser-assisted myringotomy procedure may be performed in outpatient settings. These procedures should only be performed by ear, nose, and throat (ENT) specialists.

Therapeutic Management: Recurrent Otitis Media

Therapy for recurrent AOM has included chemoprophylaxis with long-term antibiotic therapy, immunotherapy, and surgery. Children receiving long-term antibiotic therapy should be evaluated once a month to detect any evidence of effusion. Any acute infection during prophylaxis is treated with an alternate antibiotic regimen.

Tympanostomy tube placement and adenoidectomy are surgical procedures that may be done to treat recurrent OM. Tympanostomy tubes are pressure-equalizer (PE) tubes or grommets that facilitate continued drainage of fluid and allow ventilation of the middle ear. Adenoidectomy is not recommended for treatment of AOM and is performed only in children with recurrent AOM or chronic OME with postnasal obstruction, adenoiditis, or chronic sinusitis.

Therapeutic Management: Otitis Media with Effusion

In some children, residual middle ear effusions remain after episodes of AOM. Management options for OM with residual effusion include observation, antibiotics alone, or a combination of antibiotic and corticosteroid therapy. Antibiotics are not required for initial treatment of OME but may be indicated for children with persistent effusion for more than 3 months (American Academy of Pediatrics, 2004a). It has been estimated that avoiding unnecessary treatment of OME with antibiotics would save millions of courses of antibiotics each year (American Academy of Pediatrics, 2004a).

Some children have fluid that persists in the middle ear for weeks or months. OME is frequently associated with mild to moderate hearing impairment. The major goal of therapy is to establish and maintain an aerated middle ear that is free of fluid with a normal mucosa and ultimately to achieve normal hearing.

Placement of tympanostomy tubes is recommended after a total of 4 to 6 months of bilateral effusion with a bilateral hearing deficit (American Academy of Pediatrics, 2004b). This therapy allows for mechanical drainage of the fluid, which promotes healing of the membrane and prevents scar formation and loss of elasticity. The primary objective is to allow the eustachian tube a period of recovery while the surgically placed tube performs its functions. The surgery is relatively benign; however, sometimes the tubes become plugged and they often require reinsertion. Complications of repeated or long-term tube placement are tympanosclerosis, localized or diffuse atrophy of the membrane, persistent perforation, or, rarely, cholesteatoma. Myringotomy with or without insertion of PE tubes should *not* be performed for initial management of OME, but may be recommended for children who have recurrent episodes of OME with a long cumulative duration. A Cochrane review concluded that tympanostomy tubes had a significant effect on decreasing the incidence of AOM in the first 6 months after insertion (McDonald, Langston Hewer, and Nunez, 2008).

Tonsillectomy, either alone or with adenoidectomy, is not considered an effective treatment of OME (American Academy of Pediatrics, 2004b). According to guidelines published by the Agency for Healthcare Research and Quality,* steroids are not recommended for treatment of OME in children of any age.

Prevention

Routine immunization with the pneumococcal conjugate vaccine PCV 7 (Prevnar) has reduced the incidence of AOM in some infants and children (American Academy of Pediatrics, 2009b). In 2010 the FDA approved a new conjugate vaccine, Prevnar 13, which replaces Prevnar. The vaccine is administered as a four-dose series beginning at 2 months of age; infants and children who have started the series with Prevnar may complete the series with Prevnar 13 (Centers for Disease Control and Prevention, 2010).

Parents can reduce risk factors for AOM by breast-feeding infants for at least the first 6 months of life, avoiding propping the bottle, decreasing or discontinuing pacifier use after 6 months, and preventing exposure to tobacco smoke (American Academy of Pediatrics, 2004a).

Prognosis

Most cases of OM resolve eventually. However, hearing loss, typically conductive, is a common complication of OM. The

---

*A parent guide (94-0624) and more detailed clinical practice guidelines (94-0620) are available in English and Spanish from AHRQ Publications Clearinghouse, OME/AAP, PO Box 8547, Silver Spring, MD 20907; 800-358-9295; www.ahrq.gov.

degree of hearing loss can vary from none to severe. Although conductive hearing loss is most often associated with OM, sensorineural hearing loss may also be present, especially in severe forms of chronic or recurrent OM, because of the passage of toxic products from fluids into the cochlea through the tympanic membrane. The longer the fluid is present, the greater the sensorineural hearing loss. Children who are prone to OM should be referred to a pediatric otolaryngologist and possibly a pediatric allergist for identification and treatment of the cause of their eustachian tube dysfunction. They should also be referred to a speech and language pathologist for primary prevention counseling. In addition, the child should ideally be monitored by an audiologist to evaluate the adequacy of hearing.

Nursing Care Management

Nursing objectives for the child with AOM include (1) relieving pain, (2) facilitating drainage when possible, (3) preventing complications or recurrence, (4) educating the family in care of the child, and (5) providing emotional support to the child and family.

Analgesics are helpful to reduce severe earache. High fever, particularly in infants, should be reduced with antipyretic drugs. An advantage of using ibuprofen rather than acetaminophen is its longer duration of action (about 6 hours), especially for nighttime comfort. Ibuprofen is only indicated for those over 6 months of age. For more severe pain, the Centers for Disease Control and Prevention and American Academy of Pediatrics guidelines recommend a stronger analgesic such as codeine. The application of heat may reduce pain in some children but may aggravate discomfort in others. Local heat should be placed over the ear while the child lies on the affected side. This position also facilitates drainage of the exudate if the eardrum has ruptured or if myringotomy was performed.

If the ear is draining, the external canal may be cleaned with sterile cotton swabs or pledgets coupled with topical antibiotic treatment. If ear wicks or lightly rolled sterile gauze packs are placed in the ear after surgical treatment, they should be loose enough to allow accumulated drainage to flow out of the ear; otherwise the infection may be transferred to the mastoid process. Parents should keep these wicks dry during shampoos or baths. Occasionally drainage is so profuse that the pinna and surrounding skin become excoriated from exudate. Frequent cleansing and application of various moisture barriers (e.g., Aloe Vesta Protective Ointment, Proshield Plus Skin Protectant), zinc oxide, or petrolatum jelly (e.g., Vaseline) can prevent this.

Parents require anticipatory guidance regarding temporary hearing loss that accompanies OM. For example, they may need to speak louder, at closer proximity, and while facing the child. They are reminded that the child is not ignoring them. The child may not be able to localize where a sound is coming from because awareness and understanding of speech are reduced either unilaterally or bilaterally, depending on the degree of hearing deficit. The schoolteacher may also need to place the child closer to the front of the class if hearing has been impaired or if the teacher believes the child is not hearing all of the information being given in class. The family should also be aware of possible behavioral changes with hearing loss, including inattentiveness to or lack of awareness of environmental sounds; requests for repetition in conversation or mishearing of content; softer or louder voice than usual; poor attention span and fidgety behavior when in a group listening situation (e.g., classroom); aggressiveness and low frustration tolerance because of frequent communication breakdowns; and impaired speech and language skills. Persistent difficulty in hearing beyond the acute stage should be evaluated.

Preventing recurrence requires adequate parent education regarding antibiotic therapy. Because the symptoms of pain and fever usually subside within 24 to 48 hours, nurses must emphasize that, although the child may appear well, the infection is not completely eradicated until all the prescribed medication is taken. It is important to stress the potential complications of OM, especially hearing loss, which can be prevented with adequate treatment and follow-up care. (See Administration of Medication, and Compliance, Chapter 27.)

Tympanostomy tubes may allow water to enter the middle ear, but recommendations for earplugs are inconsistent. Research indicates that swimming without earplugs poses a slightly increased risk of infection (Goldstein, Mandel, Kurs-Lasky, et al, 2005). Moreover, lake water is contaminated, and wearing earplugs while swimming in a lake prevents total flooding of the external canal. Parents should keep bathwater and shampoo water out of the ear, if possible, since soap reduces the surface tension of water and facilitates entry through the tube. Parents should be aware of the appearance of a grommet (usually a tiny, white, plastic spool-shaped tube) so they can recognize it if it falls out. They are reassured that this is normal and requires no immediate intervention, although they should notify the practitioner.

Parents sometimes ask about preventing ear discomfort in their infants during ascent or descent of an airplane. During ascent, air in the middle ear expands, but decompression takes place through a normal eustachian tube. If the tissues are congested with a URI, the passage of air may be blocked. A nasal mucosa–shrinking spray or oral decongestant before the trip may be helpful. During descent, the air within the middle ear decreases as atmospheric pressure increases. Swallowing is the simplest and most effective method for inflating the middle ear on descent; therefore feeding or offering a pacifier to infants during descent is beneficial.

Reducing the chances of OM is possible with simple measures, such as sitting or holding an infant upright for feedings. Propping bottles is discouraged to avoid pooling of milk while the child is in the supine position and to encourage human contact during feeding. Eliminating tobacco smoke and known allergens is also recommended. Forceful nose blowing during a URI is discouraged to avoid forcing organisms to ascend through the eustachian tube. Early detection of middle ear effusion is essential in prevention of complications. Infants and preschool children should be screened for effusion, and all schoolchildren, especially those with learning disabilities, should be tested for middle ear effusion. Frequent audiologic evaluations, medical consultation, and education of parents and children are advised when middle ear effusion is detected.

OTITIS EXTERNA

Infections of the external ear result from normal ear flora (*Staphylococcus epidermidis* and *Corynebacterium* organisms) that assume pathogenic characteristics under conditions of excessive wetness or dryness. Ordinarily the external ear canal is protected by a waxy, water-repellent coating composed of highly viscid secretions of the sebaceous glands and the watery, pigmented secretions of apocrine glands in combination with exfoliated surface cells. Inflammation occurs when this environment is altered by swimming, bathing, or increased environmental humidity; by infection, dermatoses, or insufficient cerumen; or by trauma from a foreign body (FB) or a finger.

Secondary invasion of foreign pathogens also occurs. In addition to the resident flora, the offending agents can be *Pseudomonas aeruginosa* (most common), *Enterobacter aerogenes*, *Proteus mirabilis*, *Klebsiella pneumoniae*, streptococci, and fungi such as *Candida* and *Aspergillus* organisms. The ear canal becomes irritated, and maceration takes place.

The predominant symptom of external ear infection, or swimmer's ear, is ear pain accentuated by manipulation of the pinna, especially pressure on the tragus. The pain often appears to be out of proportion to the degree of inflammation. Conductive hearing loss may be present as a result of the edema, secretions, and accumulation of debris within the canal. Edema, erythema, a cheesy green-blue-gray discharge, and tenderness appear as the infection progresses. The external canal may be so tender and swollen that visualization is difficult. There may be fever. In advanced cases the pain is intense, constant, and aggravated by jaw motion or ear manipulation.

Therapeutic objectives include relief of pain, edema, and itching and restoration of normal flora, cerumen, and canal epithelium. Analgesics are prescribed for pain. Debris is removed with gentle suction and wisps of cotton on metal cotton carriers. Otic preparations containing neomycin with either colistin or polymyxin and corticosteroids are instilled in the canal. A gauze wick may be inserted if edema is present to facilitate the medication reaching the site of inflammation. The wick is removed after swelling and pain have subsided, but the drops are continued for at least 3 days after relief of pain. The best management for external ear inflammation is prevention.

Nursing Care Management

Nurses can teach parents or patients simple steps to prevent recurrent infections. Children should limit their stay in the water to less than an hour, if possible, and ears should dry completely (1 to 2 hours) before entering the water again. The ear canal can also be dried with a small tuft of cotton (not a swab). Placing a combination of white vinegar and rubbing alcohol (50:50) in both ear canals on arising, at bedtime, and at the end of each swim is effective in preventing recurrence. A 2% acetic acid solution may also be used. The solution should remain in the canal for 5 minutes. Caution children not to pick at the ears with a pencil, cotton swab, bobby pin, or other object, which can injure or infect the ear canal.

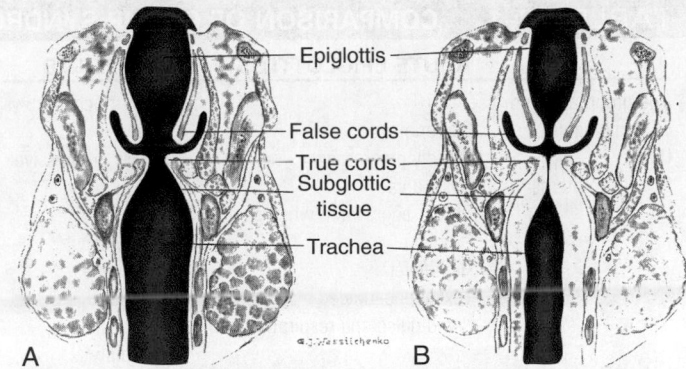

Fig. 32-4 A, Normal larynx. **B,** Obstruction and narrowing resulting from edema of croup.

> **NURSING TIP** In an older child (usually >3 years), to keep the ear dry, pull the auricle up and out to straighten the canal, then use a conventional hair dryer, set on low or no heat, held at a distance of 18 to 24 inches for 30 seconds, three times a day.

CROUP SYNDROMES

Croup is a general term applied to a group of symptoms characterized by hoarseness, a resonant cough described as "barking" or "brassy" (croupy), varying degrees of inspiratory stridor, and varying degrees of respiratory distress resulting from swelling or obstruction in the region of the larynx. Acute infections of the larynx are of greater importance in infants and small children than they are in older children because of the increased incidence in children in this age-group and the smaller diameter of the airway, which renders it subject to significantly greater narrowing with the same degree of inflammation (Fig. 32-4). With widespread immunization programs aimed at preventing *H. influenzae* type b, most cases of croup in the United States are attributed to viruses, namely parainfluenza virus, influenza types A and B, adenovirus, RSV, and measles (Roosevelt, 2007).

Croup is a common respiratory disease of childhood and occurs more often in boys than in girls. The number of croup cases increases in the late autumn through early winter months and occurs primarily in children 6 months to 3 years of age. Hospitalization may be necessary for some children with croup, and a small percentage of hospitalized children require intubation.

Croup syndromes affect to varying degrees the larynx, trachea, and bronchi. However, laryngeal involvement often dominates the clinical picture because of the severe effects on the voice and breathing. Croup syndromes are usually described according to the primary anatomic area affected (i.e., epiglottitis [or supraglottitis], laryngitis, laryngotracheobronchitis [LTB], and tracheitis). In general, LTB tends to occur in very young children, whereas epiglottitis is more characteristic of older children. Table 32-1 gives a comparison of croup syndromes.

Because croup is one of the most benign conditions causing upper airway obstruction, it is vitally important to correctly identify it and distinguish the type of croup syndrome or

TABLE 32-1	COMPARISON OF CROUP SYNDROMES			
	ACUTE EPIGLOTTITIS	**ACUTE LTB**	**ACUTE SPASMODIC LARYNGITIS**	**ACUTE TRACHEITIS**
Age-group affected	2-5 yr	Infant or child <5 yr	1-3 yr	1 mo–6 yr
Etiologic agent	Bacterial	Viral	Viral with allergic component	Viral with allergic component
Onset	Rapidly progressive	Slowly progressive	Sudden; at night	Moderately progressive
Major symptoms	Dysphagia	URI	URI	URI
	Stridor aggravated when supine	Stridor	Croupy cough	Croupy cough
	Drooling	Brassy cough	Stridor	Purulent secretions
	High fever	Hoarseness	Hoarseness	High fever
	Toxic appearance	Dyspnea	Dyspnea	No response to LTB therapy
	Rapid pulse and respirations	Restlessness	Restlessness	
		Irritability	Symptoms awakening child	
		Low-grade fever	Symptoms disappearing during day	
		Nontoxic appearance	Tendency to recur	
Treatment	Airway protection	Racemic epinephrine	Cool mist	Antibiotics
	Racemic epinephrine	Corticosteroids		Fluids
	Corticosteroids	Fluids		
	Fluids	Reassurance		
	Reassurance			

LTB, Laryngotracheobronchitis; *URI,* upper respiratory tract infection.

condition (i.e., spasmodic croup or LTB as opposed to a potentially life-threatening condition such as epiglottitis, bacterial tracheitis, FB aspiration, or a peritonsillar abscess). The key differences between LTB and epiglottitis are the absence of cough, the presence of dysphagia, and the high degree of toxicity in children with epiglottitis. Children with epiglottitis usually look worse than they sound, in contrast to children with LTB, who sound worse than they look (see Critical Thinking Exercise).

> ### ❓ CRITICAL THINKING EXERCISE
> **Croup Syndrome**
>
> Kim, a 4-year-old, is admitted to the emergency department with a sore throat, pain on swallowing, drooling, and a fever of 39° C (102.2° F). She looks ill, is agitated, and prefers to sit up and lean over. What nursing interventions should the nurse implement in this situation?
> 1. Evidence—Is there sufficient evidence to draw any conclusions about Kim's condition at this time?
> 2. Assumptions—Describe some underlying assumptions about each of the following:
>   a. Epiglottitis in children
>   b. Symptoms of epiglottitis
>   c. Precautions to be taken when a child has suspected epiglottitis
>   d. Immediate nursing interventions when caring for a child with epiglottitis
> 3. What priorities for nursing care can be drawn at this time?
> 4. Does the evidence objectively support your argument (conclusion)?

ACUTE EPIGLOTTITIS

Acute epiglottitis, or acute supraglottitis, is a serious obstructive inflammatory process that occurs principally in children between 2 and 5 years of age but can occur from infancy to adulthood. The disorder is a medical emergency and requires immediate medical attention. The obstruction is supraglottic, as opposed to the subglottic obstruction of laryngitis. LTB and epiglottitis do not occur together.

Clinical Manifestations

The onset of epiglottitis is abrupt, less often preceded by cold symptoms and more often by a sore throat. It can rapidly progress to severe respiratory distress. The child usually goes to bed asymptomatic to awaken later complaining of sore throat and pain on swallowing. The child has a fever and appears sicker than clinical findings suggest. The child insists on sitting upright and leaning forward (tripod position), with the chin thrust out, mouth open, and tongue protruding. Drooling of saliva is common because of the difficulty or pain on swallowing and excessive secretions.

> ### ❗ NURSING ALERT
> Three clinical observations that are predictive of epiglottitis are absence of spontaneous cough, presence of drooling, and agitation.

The child is irritable and extremely restless and has an apprehensive and frightened expression. The voice is thick and muffled, with a froglike croaking sound on inspiration. The child is not hoarse. Suprasternal and substernal retractions may be visible. The child seldom struggles to breathe, and slow, quiet breathing provides better air exchange. The sallow color of mild hypoxia may progress to frank cyanosis if treatment is delayed. The throat is red and inflamed, and a distinctive, large, cherry red, edematous epiglottis is visible on careful throat inspection. Throat inspection should only be performed when emergency resuscitation personnel and equipment are available.

Therapeutic Management

Epiglottitis may develop suddenly, with respiratory obstruction appearing rapidly. Progressive obstruction leads to hypoxia, hypercapnia, and acidosis followed by decreased muscular tone; reduced level of consciousness; and, when obstruction becomes more or less complete, sudden death. A presumptive diagnosis of epiglottitis constitutes an emergency.

The child is best transported while sitting in a parent's lap to reduce distress. Examination of the throat with a tongue depressor is contraindicated until experienced personnel and equipment are at hand in the event that the examination precipitates further or complete obstruction. Immediate intubation or tracheotomy may need to be performed.

When a lateral neck radiograph of the soft tissues is indicated, the same experienced personnel should accompany the child to the radiology department. For a young child who is likely to become more agitated by the procedure, it is preferable that the child not be transported but remain on the parent's lap in the examination area during portable radiology.

Nasotracheal intubation or tracheotomy is usually considered for the child with epiglottitis with severe respiratory distress. It is recommended that the intubation or tracheotomy and any invasive procedure, such as starting an IV infusion, be performed in an area where emergency airway maintenance can be easily and quickly accomplished. Humidified oxygen is administered as necessary either via mask in older children or as blow-by in younger children to avoid further agitation. Whether or not there is an artificial airway, the child requires intensive observation by experienced personnel. The epiglottal swelling usually decreases after 24 hours of antibiotic therapy, and the epiglottis is near normal by the third day.

Children with suspected bacterial epiglottitis are given antibiotics intravenously, followed by oral administration to complete a 7- to 10-day course. The use of corticosteroids for reducing edema may be beneficial during the early hours of treatment. Most intubated children have a course of corticosteroids for 24 hours before extubation.

Prevention

The American Academy of Pediatrics (2009b) recommends that all children, beginning at 2 months of age, receive the *H. influenzae* type b conjugate vaccine. Since administration of the vaccine has become a routine part of the immunization schedule, the incidence of epiglottitis has declined. Patients now tend to be older and have disease caused by viral agents. (See Immunizations, Chapter 12.)

Nursing Care Management

Epiglottitis is a serious and frightening disease for the child, family, and health professionals. It is important to act quickly but calmly and provide support without unduly increasing anxiety. The child is allowed to remain in the position that provides the most comfort and security, and parents are reassured that everything possible is being done to obtain relief for their child.

> **⚠ NURSING ALERT**
>
> Nurses who suspect epiglottitis should not attempt to visualize the epiglottis directly with a tongue depressor or take a throat culture but should have the child seen by the primary care provider immediately. Resuscitation equipment and suction should be immediately available and ready at the child's bedside.

Acute care of the child is the same as that described for the child with acute respiratory distress and artificial airways in Chapter 31. Continuous monitoring of respiratory status, including pulse oximetry (or blood gases if the patient is intubated), is part of nursing observations, and the IV infusion is maintained. (See Chapter 28.)

ACUTE LARYNGITIS

Acute infectious laryngitis is a common illness in older children and adolescents. Infants and smaller children experience more generalized involvement. (See next section on LTB.) Viruses are the usual causative agents, and the principal complaint is hoarseness, which may be accompanied by other upper respiratory symptoms (e.g., coryza, sore throat, nasal congestion) and systemic manifestations (e.g., fever, headache, myalgia, malaise). Other complaints vary with the infecting virus. For example, adenoviruses and influenza viruses are responsible for more systemic involvement; parainfluenza virus, rhinoviruses, and RSV cause more mild illness.

Therapeutic and Nursing Care Management

The disease is almost always self-limiting without long-term sequelae. Treatment is supportive with fluids and humidified air.

ACUTE LARYNGOTRACHEOBRONCHITIS

LTB is the most common type of croup experienced by children admitted for hospitalization and primarily affects children less than 5 years of age. Organisms responsible for LTB are the parainfluenza virus type 1, followed by parainfluenza virus types 3 and 2, RSV, influenza types A and B, measles and *M. pneumoniae*. The illness is usually preceded by a URI, which gradually descends to adjacent structures. It is characterized by the gradual onset of low-grade fever, and the parents often report that the child went to bed and later awoke with a barky, brassy cough and at times inspiratory stridor. Symptoms are typically worse at night, and agitation and crying tend to exacerbate the symptoms.

Inflammation of the mucosa lining the larynx and trachea causes a narrowing of the airway. When the airway is significantly narrowed, the child struggles to inhale air past the obstruction and into the lungs, producing the characteristic inspiratory stridor and suprasternal retractions. Other classic manifestations include cough and hoarseness. Respiratory distress in infants and toddlers may be manifested by nasal flaring, intercostal retractions, tachypnea, and continuous stridor. The typical child with LTB is a toddler who develops the classic barking or seal-like cough and acute stridor after several days of coryza. The degree of respiratory distress varies; hypoxia and decreased oxygen saturations are observed primarily when complete airway obstruction is imminent. Radiographs are not helpful in establishing the diagnosis of LTB.

Therapeutic Management

The major objective in medical management of infectious LTB is maintaining an airway and providing for adequate respiratory exchange. Children with mild croup (no stridor at rest) are managed at home. Parents need to learn the signs of respiratory distress so that they can call professional help if needed. Children whose symptoms progressively get worse should receive medical attention.

Cool mist provides relief for most children, although there is no substantial evidence to its efficacy. A cool-air vaporizer can be used at home. In the hospital mist may be provided with a face mask or as blow-by. Controversy surrounds the use of mist therapy to treat croup. Studies have failed to demonstrate any improvement in subglottic edema with mist therapy (Moore and Little, 2006).

The cool-temperature therapy modalities assist by constricting edematous blood vessels. In the home environment, suggestions to provide cool air include taking the child outside to breathe in cool night air, using a cold-water vaporizer or humidifier, standing in front of the open freezer, and taking the child to a cool basement or garage. Although these are often recommended, there is no evidence to unconditionally support their use.

Nebulized epinephrine (racemic epinephrine) is now used in children with croup that is not alleviated with cool mist. The α-adrenergic effects cause mucosal vasoconstriction and subsequent decreased subglottic edema. The onset of action is rapid. Peak effect is observed in less than 2 hours. Additional doses may be administered every 20 to 30 minutes as needed. Close observation of patients receiving nebulized racemic epinephrine is critical to detect the reappearance of symptoms, monitor the response to therapy, and note any deterioration in respiratory status. There is evidence that use of L-epinephrine is just as effective as racemic epinephrine but without the side effects of tachycardia and hypertension (Roosevelt, 2007). The patient who has received racemic epinephrine for croup should be observed for 2 to 3 hours for any visible signs of respiratory distress.

The use of corticosteroids is beneficial because the antiinflammatory effects decrease subglottic edema. Oral steroids are effective in the treatment of croup. IM dexamethasone may be given to children who are unable to tolerate oral dosing. Nebulized budesonide may be administered in conjunction with IM dexamethasone. A single dose of oral corticosteroid has shown to decrease hospitalizations and the need for multiple racemic epinephrine treatments in children with mild croup (Roosevelt, 2007). The onset of action is clinically detectable as early as 6 hours after administration, with continued improvement over a period of 12 to 24 hours.

In severe cases of LTB the administration of a mixture of helium and oxygen (heliox) may reduce the work of breathing and relieve the airway obstruction. Because helium has a lower density than room air, it forms a respirable gas (with oxygen) that reduces airway turbulence. The use of heliox, however, has not proved to be more effective than standard treatments and is currently not recommended as a standard management for croup (Myers, 2006; Vorwek and Coats, 2008).

It is essential to allow children with mild croup to continue to drink beverages they like and to encourage parents to use comforting measures with their child (e.g., holding, rocking,

> **! NURSING ALERT**
>
> Children with severe respiratory distress (traditionally, a respiratory rate >60 breaths/min for infants) should not be given anything by mouth to prevent aspiration and increased work of breathing.

walking, singing). If the child is unable to take oral fluids, IV fluid therapy may be indicated.

Nursing Care Management

The most important nursing function in the care of children with LTB is continuous, vigilant observation and accurate assessment of respiratory status. Cardiac, respiratory, and pulse oximetry monitoring supplement visual observations. Changes in therapy are frequently based on nurses' observations and assessment of a child's status, response to therapy, and tolerance of procedures. The trend away from early intubation of children with LTB emphasizes the importance of nursing observation and the ability to recognize impending respiratory failure so that intubation can be implemented without delay. Intubation equipment and bag and valve mask equipment should be readily accessible and taken with the child during transport to other areas (e.g., pediatric intensive care if intubation and further observation are required).

> **! NURSING ALERT**
>
> Early signs of impending airway obstruction include increased pulse and respiratory rate; substernal, suprasternal, and intercostal retractions; nasal flaring; and increased restlessness.

To conserve energy, children are given every opportunity to rest. Infants or small children find that being placed on a face mask, coughing, having laryngeal spasms, and needing IV therapy are additional sources of distress. Infants and small children prefer sitting upright, and most want to be held. Children need the security of the parent's presence. Because crying increases respiratory distress and hypoxia, the nurse needs to assess a child's individual tolerance for these therapies. An extremely fussy child may do better when held in the parent's lap with cool mist directed toward the child's face.

The rapid progression of croup, the alarming sound of the cough and stridor, and the child's apprehensive behavior and ill appearance combine to create a frightening experience for the parents. They need reassurance regarding the child's progress and an explanation of treatments. The family should be allowed to remain with the child as much as possible, especially when this decreases the child's distress.

Fortunately, as the crisis subsides and the child responds to therapy, breathing becomes easier and recovery is generally prompt. Home care after discharge includes continued humidity, adequate hydration, and nourishment. Encourage parents to ask questions about home care and preparation for discharge.

ACUTE SPASMODIC LARYNGITIS

Acute spasmodic laryngitis (spasmodic croup, "midnight croup," or "twilight croup") is distinct from laryngitis and LTB and characterized by paroxysmal attacks of laryngeal obstruction that occur chiefly at night. Signs of inflammation are absent or mild, and there is often a history of previous attacks lasting for 2 to 5 days followed by uneventful recovery. It usually affects children ages 1 to 3 years. Some children appear to be predisposed to the condition; allergy and psychogenic factors contribute to some cases.

The child goes to bed well or with some mild respiratory symptoms but awakes suddenly with characteristic barking, metallic cough; hoarseness; noisy inspirations; and restlessness. The child appears anxious and frightened. Excitement can aggravate dyspnea. However, there is no fever, the attack subsides in a few hours, and the child appears well the next day with the exception of slight hoarseness.

Therapeutic and Nursing Care Management

Children with spasmodic croup are managed at home. Cool mist is recommended for the child's room. Warm mist provided by steam from hot running water in a closed bathroom may be helpful. Humidification may help, but warm temperatures will not relieve the constriction. Sometimes sudden exposure to cold air relieves the spasm (as when the child is taken out into the night air to see the practitioner). Parents are usually advised to have the child sleep in humidified air until the cough has subsided to prevent subsequent episodes. Children with moderately severe symptoms may be hospitalized for observation and therapy with cool mist and racemic epinephrine, as for LTB. Patients may respond to corticosteroid therapy. The disease is usually self-limiting.

BACTERIAL TRACHEITIS

Bacterial tracheitis, an infection of the mucosa of the upper trachea, is a distinct entity with features of both croup and epiglottitis. The disease is more common in children younger than 3 years and may be a serious cause of airway obstruction—severe enough to cause respiratory arrest. It is believed to be a complication of LTB, and although *Staphylococcus aureus* is the

most frequent organism responsible, *M. catarrhalis*, *S. pneumoniae*, and *H. influenzae* have also been implicated.

Many of the manifestations of bacterial tracheitis are similar to those of LTB but are unresponsive to LTB therapy. There is a history of previous URI with croupy cough, stridor unaffected by position, toxicity, absence of drooling, and high fever. A prominent manifestation is the production of thick, purulent tracheal secretions. Respiratory difficulties are secondary to these copious secretions. Children with this condition may develop a life-threatening upper airway obstruction, respiratory failure, acute respiratory distress syndrome (ARDS), and multiple organ dysfunction (Hopkins, Lahiri, Salerno, et al, 2006).

Therapeutic and Nursing Care Management

Bacterial tracheitis requires vigorous management with antipyretics and antibiotics. Many children require endotracheal intubation and mechanical ventilation; patients are closely monitored for impending respiratory failure if not intubated. Early recognition to prevent life-threatening airway obstruction is essential.

INFECTIONS OF THE LOWER AIRWAYS

The reactive portion of the lower respiratory tract includes the bronchi and bronchioles in children. Cartilaginous support of the large airways is not fully developed until adolescence. Consequently, the smooth muscle in these structures represents a major factor in constriction of the airway, particularly in the bronchioles, that portion that extends from the bronchi to the alveoli.

Table 32-2 compares some of the major features of bronchial and bronchiolar infections.

TABLE 32-2	COMPARISON OF CONDITIONS AFFECTING THE BRONCHI		
	ASTHMA*	**BRONCHITIS**	**BRONCHIOLITIS**
Description	Exaggerated response of bronchi to a trigger such as URI, dander, cold air, exercise Bronchospasm, exudation, and edema of bronchi	Usually occurs in association with URI Seldom an isolated entity	Most common infectious disease of lower airways Maximum obstructive impact at bronchiolar level
Age-group affected	Infancy to adolescence	First 4 yr of life	Usually children 2-12 mo of age; rare after age 2 yr
Etiologic agents	Most often viruses such as RSV in infants but may be any of a variety of URI pathogens	Usually viral Other agents (e.g., bacteria, fungi, allergic disorders, airborne irritants) can trigger symptoms	Peak incidence approximately age 6 mo Viruses, predominantly RSV; also adenoviruses, parainfluenza viruses, human meta-pneumovirus, and *Mycoplasma pneumoniae*
Predominant characteristics	Wheezing, cough	Persistent dry, hacking cough (worse at night), becoming productive in 2-3 days	Labored respirations, poor feeding, cough, tachypnea, retractions, flaring nares, emphysema, increased nasal mucus, wheezing, may have fever
Treatment	Inhaled corticosteroids, bronchodilators, leukotriene modifiers, allergen, and control of triggers	Cough suppressants if needed	Provide supplemental oxygen if saturations ≤90%; bronchodilators (optional) Suction nasopharynx Ensure adequate fluid intake Maintain adequate oxygenation

RSV, Respiratory syncytial virus; *URI*, upper respiratory tract infection.
*See Asthma, p. 1263.

BRONCHITIS

Bronchitis (sometimes referred to as tracheobronchitis) is an inflammation of the large airways (trachea and bronchi), which is frequently associated with a URI. Viral agents are the primary cause of the disease, although *M. pneumoniae* is a common cause in children older than 6 years of age. The condition is characterized by a dry, hacking, and nonproductive cough that is worse at night and becomes productive in 2 or 3 days.

Bronchitis is a mild, self-limiting disease that requires only symptomatic treatment, including analgesics, antipyretics, and humidity. Cough suppressants may be useful to allow rest but can interfere with clearance of secretions. Most patients recover uneventfully in 5 to 10 days.

RESPIRATORY SYNCYTIAL VIRUS AND BRONCHIOLITIS

Bronchiolitis is an acute viral infection with maximum effect at the bronchiolar level. The infection occurs primarily in winter and spring. Although most cases of bronchiolitis are caused by RSV, adenoviruses and parainfluenza viruses are also implicated; recently, human meta-pneumovirus has also been associated with bronchiolitis in children. By age 3 years most children have been infected at least once. Reinfection with RSV may occur in as many as three fourths of affected children in the second year of life; the antibody response to the virus is inadequate to protect against subsequent reinfection (Robinson, 2008). RSV affects males more than females, it occurs less frequently in breast-fed infants, and it has a higher rate in children in crowded living conditions (Goodman, 2007). RSV infection is the most frequent cause of hospitalization in children less than 1 year old. In addition, severe RSV infections in the first year of life represent a significant risk factor for the development of asthma up to age 13 (Chávez-Bueno, Mejías, Jafri, et al, 2005). The precise link between RSV and asthma is unknown, but genetic predisposition to inflammation has been suggested (Mailaparambil, Grychtol, and Heinzmann, 2009; Thomsen, van der Sluis, Stensballe, et al, 2009). RSV infection may also occur in children older than 1 year who have a chronic or serious disabling illness and in preterm infants. Hospitalization may occur in 1% to 3% of infants with RSV infection (Mcintosh, 2007). It is important to note that not all infants and children with RSV will develop a lower respiratory tract infection (Goodman, 2007).

Etiology

RSV is a paramyxovirus containing a single strand of ribonucleic acid and is related to parainfluenza virus. RSV strains have two major subgroups: A (the more virulent) and B. More children develop bronchiolitis and pneumonia from RSV subgroup A infections than from subgroup B infections during major outbreaks. The disease usually begins in the fall, reaches a peak during the winter, and then decreases during the spring. In tropical regions, peaks of activity are less pronounced, and outbreaks tend to occur in rainy seasons.

Pathophysiology

RSV affects the epithelial cells of the respiratory tract. The ciliated cells swell, protrude into the lumen, and lose their cilia. RSV produces a fusion of the infected cell membrane with cell membranes of adjacent epithelial cells, thus forming a giant cell with multiple nuclei. At the cellular level this fusion results in multinucleated masses of protoplasm, or syncytia.

The bronchiolar mucosa swells, and lumina are subsequently filled with mucus and exudate. The walls of the bronchi and bronchioles are infiltrated with inflammatory cells, and peribronchiolar interstitial pneumonitis is usually present. Because luminal epithelial cells are shed into the bronchioles when they die, the lumina are frequently obstructed, particularly on expiration. The varying degrees of obstruction produced in small air passages lead to hyperinflation, obstructive emphysema resulting from partial obstruction, and patchy areas of atelectasis. Dilation of bronchial passages on inspiration allows sufficient space for intake of air, but narrowing of the passages on expiration prevents air from leaving the lungs. Thus air is trapped distal to the obstruction and causes progressive overinflation (emphysema).

Transmission

The transmission of RSV is predominantly through direct contact with respiratory secretions, mainly as a result of inoculation from hand to eye, nose, or other mucous membranes. It can also occur by direct inoculation by large-particle aerosols or by self-inoculation from contaminated fomites (Mcintosh, 2007). RSV in secretions can survive for hours on countertops, gloves, paper tissues, and cloth, and for half an hour on skin; it remains infectious when transferred from hands or objects. There is no documentation of distant spread of RSV by small-particle aerosols (airborne transmission).

Clinical Manifestations

The younger the infant, the greater the likelihood that severe lower respiratory tract disease requiring hospitalization will occur. The peak incidence for RSV is 2 to 7 months of age, but reinfection with RSV is common at all ages, with the highest rates being reported in children who attend a daycare center. The severity of RSV tends to diminish with age and repeated infections.

The illness usually begins with a URI after an incubation of about 5 to 8 days. Symptoms such as rhinorrhea and low-grade fever often appear first. OM and conjunctivitis may also be present. In time a cough may develop. If the disease progresses, it becomes a lower respiratory tract infection and manifests typical symptoms (Box 32-6). Infants may have several days of URI symptoms or no symptoms except slight lethargy, poor feeding, or irritability.

Once the lower airway is involved, classic manifestations include signs of altered air exchange, such as wheezing, retractions, crackles, dyspnea, tachypnea, and diminished breath sounds. Pneumonia may occur in conjunction with RSV bronchiolitis. Apnea is a complication of bronchiolitis and is more common in term infants less than 1 month old, in preterm infants with a postconceptual age less than 48 weeks, and in

BOX 32-6 SIGNS AND SYMPTOMS OF RESPIRATORY SYNCYTIAL VIRUS

Initial
Rhinorrhea
Pharyngitis
Coughing, sneezing
Wheezing
Possible ear or eye infection
Intermittent fever

With Progression of Illness
Increased coughing and wheezing
Fever
Tachypnea and retractions
Refusal to nurse or bottle feed
Copious secretions

Severe Illness
Tachypnea >70 breaths/min
Listlessness
Apneic spells
Poor air exchange; poor breath sounds
Cyanosis

infants with a previous history of apnea (Seiden and Scarfone, 2009).

Diagnostic Evaluation

Because RSV infection may be manifested as a URI, it is often difficult to identify the specific etiologic agent by clinical criteria alone. The most difficult distinction is between RSV and asthma, since both conditions involve the lower airway and have similar symptoms.

Identification has been simplified by the development of tests done on nasal or nasopharyngeal secretions, using either rapid immunofluorescent antibody–direct fluorescent antibody staining (DFA) or enzyme-linked immunosorbent assay (ELISA) techniques for RSV antigen detection. The more traditional viral culture is becoming obsolete, since it takes several days to get a result. Other simultaneous infections may occur with RSV. The infant should be carefully evaluated for the presence of urinary tract infection, meningitis, and bacteremia; antibiotics are prescribed for a coexisting bacterial infection (Sorce, 2009).

Therapeutic Management

Uncomplicated cases of bronchiolitis are treated symptomatically with supplemental oxygen as required, adequate fluid intake, airway maintenance, and medications. Most children with bronchiolitis can be managed at home. Hospitalization is usually recommended for children with respiratory distress or those who cannot maintain adequate hydration. Other reasons for hospitalization include complicating conditions, such as underlying lung or heart disease (e.g., prematurity), or caregiver inability to provide adequate care during illness. The child who is tachypneic or apneic, has marked retractions, seems listless, or has a history of poor fluid intake should be admitted. Pneumonia and electrolyte imbalance are commonly seen in infants who are hospitalized with RSV infection.

The American Academy of Pediatrics practice parameter (2006) recommends the use of supplemental oxygen if the infant fails to maintain a consistent oxygen saturation of at least 90% after nasal suctioning and repositioning. Routine chest physiotherapy (CPT) is not recommended; infants with abundant nasal secretions benefit from periodic suctioning. Fluids by mouth may be contraindicated because of tachypnea, weakness, and fatigue. Therefore IV fluids are preferred until the acute stage of the disease has passed. Nasogastric fluids may be required if the infant is unable to tolerate oral fluids and a peripheral IV is difficult to establish.

Clinical assessments, noninvasive oxygen monitoring, and in severe cases, blood gas values guide therapy. Medical therapy for bronchiolitis is primarily supportive and aimed at decreasing airway hyperresonance and inflammation and promoting adequate fluid intake. Bronchodilators may provide short-term benefits, yet overall significant improvement in the child's condition is not always appreciable. A short acting β-agonist bronchodilator may be given as a test dose initially; if no improvement occurs, the medication is discontinued. Approximately 50% of infants with RSV lower airway infection and obstruction respond to a short acting β-agonist. Some centers use racemic epinephrine to produce modest improvement in ventilation status. The use of 3% nebulized (hypertonic) saline is associated with an increase in mucociliary clearance in children with RSV (Sorce, 2009) and has shown to be effective in treating RSV in a few small studies (Seiden and Scarfone, 2009).

The use of systemic corticosteroids is controversial but may be used in some centers. Antibiotics are not part of the treatment of RSV unless there is a coexisting bacterial infection such as OM (American Academy of Pediatrics, 2006). Additional treatment recommendations in the American Academy of Pediatrics practice guideline (2006) are to encourage breast-feeding; avoid passive tobacco smoke exposure; and promote preventive measures, including hand washing and the administration of palivizumab (Synagis) to high-risk infants.

Ribavirin, an antiviral agent (synthetic nucleoside analog), is the only specific therapy approved for hospitalized children. However, use of this drug in infants with RSV is controversial because of concerns about the high cost, aerosol route of administration, potential toxic effects among exposed health care personnel, and conflicting results of efficacy trials (American Academy of Pediatrics, 2006; Chávez-Bueno, Mejías, Jafri, et al, 2005; Ventre and Randolph, 2007).

The only product available in the United States for prevention of RSV is palivizumab, a monoclonal antibody, which is given monthly in an IM injection. According to the American Academy of Pediatrics practice guideline (2006), candidates for palivizumab include infants born before 32 weeks of gestation who required medical therapy such as supplemental oxygen or mechanical ventilation. Infants and children younger than 2 years of age with bronchopulmonary dysplasia who have received medical therapy (supplemental oxygen, bronchodilator, diuretic, or corticosteroid therapy) for the condition within 6 months before the anticipated RSV season may benefit from palivizumab prophylaxis. Children with more severe bronchopulmonary dysplasia may benefit from palivizumab prophylaxis for two RSV seasons. Children with severe immunodeficiencies (e.g., severe combined immunodeficiency or acquired immunodeficiency syndrome) may also benefit from prophylaxis. Infants and children younger than 2 years of age with hemodynamically significant congenital heart disease benefit from five monthly IM injections of palivizumab. Prophylaxis for RSV should be initiated at the onset of the RSV season and terminated at the end of the season (November to March). Additional age and condition recommendations are outlined in the American Academy of Pediatrics practice guideline (2006). At the time of this writing, RSV prophylaxis is only available for this subset of infants; other children may be at risk for acquiring the illness but do not qualify for palivizumab prophylaxis, which costs approximately $725 per dose. In addition, some children acquire the illness despite palivizumab prophylaxis (Sorce, 2009).

A second-generation monoclonal antibody, motavizumab, is currently undergoing phase III clinical trials; this drug is reported to be more effective in the prevention of RSV than palivizumab (DeVincenzo, 2008).

⚡ DRUG ALERT

Palivizumab Administration

> The lyophilized powder form of palivizumab should be administered within 6 hours of being reconstituted with sterile water because it is preservative free. A new liquid form of the drug may be available for future use.

QUALITY PATIENT OUTCOMES: Bronchiolitis
- Room air or O_2 sat ≥90%
- Respiratory rate ≤60 breaths/min
- Adequate PO intake

Nursing Care Management

Children admitted to the hospital with suspected RSV infection may need separate rooms or rooms with other RSV-infected children. Use Contact and Standard Precautions, including hand washing, not touching the nasal mucosa or conjunctiva, and using gloves and gowns when entering the patient's room. Other isolation procedures of potential benefit are those aimed at diminishing the number of hospital personnel, visitors, and uninfected children in contact with the child. In some cases visitors, especially children, may be screened for illness before being allowed to visit high-risk infants. Another measure is to make patient assignments so that nurses assigned to children with RSV are not caring for other patients who are considered high risk.

Infants with RSV often have copious nasal secretions, making breathing and nursing or bottle-feeding difficult. This engenders concerns that the child will lose weight or stop breast-feeding altogether. Encourage breast-feeding mothers to pump their milk and store appropriately for later use. (See Chapter 8.) Parents should learn how to instill normal saline drops into the nares and suction the mucus with a bulb syringe before feedings and before bedtime so the child may eat and rest better; unfortunately no medications appropriate for infants can help

with these symptoms. To address the issue of decreased fluid intake, parents may offer small amounts of clear fluids, 5 to 10 ml at a time, with a medication syringe every 10 minutes or so. Infants may cough or vomit as the secretions settle in the stomach and make them prone to emesis of such secretions.

The nurse aims additional interventions at monitoring oxygenation with pulse oximetry, ensuring bronchodilator therapy is optimized by using a small mask for delivery (versus blow-by), monitoring IV fluids administered, monitoring fever and administering antipyretics, and providing information for the parent regarding the infant's status. Inform the parents that the infant's cough may persist for a few weeks.

The critically ill infant with RSV usually is placed in the pediatric intensive care unit for continuous monitoring of respiratory status, cardiac output, and maintenance of adequate systemic pressure. IV fluids, antibiotics, mechanical ventilation, and inotropes are often required in the unstable child. Parents and family members need emotional support and information regarding the child's status during this crisis.

The unpredictability of the infant's individual response to the disease compounds parental anxiety when they hear about children who had serious morbidity or died from RSV. However, in most cases the infant recovers quickly from the disease and resumes normal daily activities, including fluid intake. Such infants are at risk for further episodes of wheezing that may or may not involve an RSV infection. Reinfection with the virus may occur in the same season, but subsequent infections are not as severe as the first.

PNEUMONIA

Pneumonia, an inflammation of the pulmonary parenchyma, is common in childhood, occurring more frequently in infancy and early childhood. Clinically, pneumonia may occur either as a primary disease or as a complication of another illness.

Pneumonia can be classified according to morphology, etiologic agent, or clinical form. Although morphologic classification is typically used (Box 32-7), the most useful classification is based on the etiologic agent (i.e., viral, bacterial, mycoplasmal, or aspiration of foreign substances) (Box 32-8). The causative agent is usually introduced into the lungs through inhalation or from the bloodstream. Pneumonia may be caused by histomycosis, coccidioidomycosis, and other fungi. Other terms that describe pneumonias are hemorrhagic, fibrinous, and necrotizing. Pneumonitis is a localized acute inflammation of the lung without the toxemia associated with lobar pneumonia.

BOX 32-7   TYPES OF PNEUMONIA

Lobar pneumonia—All or a large segment of one or more pulmonary lobes is involved. When both lungs are affected, it is known as *bilateral* or *double pneumonia.*

Bronchopneumonia—Begins in the terminal bronchioles, which become clogged with mucopurulent exudate to form consolidated patches in nearby lobules; also called *lobular pneumonia.*

Interstitial pneumonia—Inflammatory process more or less confined within the alveolar walls (interstitium) and the peribronchial and interlobular tissues.

BOX 32-8   ORGANISMS CAUSING PNEUMONIA IN CHILDREN

Neonates—Group B streptococci, gram-negative enteric bacteria, cytomegalovirus, *Ureaplasma urealyticum*, *Listeria monocytogenes*, *Chlamydia trachomatis*

Infants—Respiratory syncytial virus (RSV), parainfluenza virus, influenza virus, adenovirus, metapneumovirus, *Streptococcus pneumoniae*, *Haemophilus influenzae*, *Mycoplasma pneumoniae*, *Mycobacterium tuberculosis*

Preschool children—RSV, parainfluenza virus, influenza virus, adenovirus, metapneumovirus, *S. pneumoniae*, *H. influenzae*, *M. pneumoniae*, *M. tuberculosis*

School-age children—*M. pneumoniae*, *Chlamydia pneumoniae*, *M. tuberculosis*, and respiratory viruses

Data from Ranganathan SC, Sonnappa S: Pneumonia and others respiratory infections, *Pediatr Clin North Am* 56(1):135-156, 2009.

The clinical manifestations of pneumonia vary depending on the etiologic agent, the child's age, the child's systemic reaction to the infection, the extent of the lesions, and the degree of bronchial and bronchiolar obstruction. The clinical history, the child's age, the general health history, the physical examination, radiography, and the laboratory examination can help identify the etiologic agent.

VIRAL PNEUMONIA

Viral pneumonias occur more frequently than bacterial pneumonias and are seen in children of all age-groups. They are often associated with viral URIs, and the pathologic changes involve interstitial pneumonitis with inflammation of the mucosa and the walls of bronchi and bronchioles. Viruses that cause pneumonia include RSV in infants and parainfluenza, influenza, human meta-pneumovirus, and adenovirus in older children. There are few clinical symptoms to distinguish between the responsible organisms, and only laboratory examination can differentiate between specific viruses.

Clinical Manifestations

The onset may be acute or insidious, and symptoms vary from mild fever, slight cough, and malaise to high fever, severe cough, and fatigue. Early in the illness, the cough is likely to be unproductive or productive of small amounts of whitish sputum. Breath sounds may include a few wheezes or fine crackles. Radiography reveals diffuse or patchy infiltration with a peribronchial distribution.

Therapeutic and Nursing Care Management

The prognosis is generally good, although viral infections of the respiratory tract render the affected child more susceptible to secondary bacterial invasion. Treatment is usually symptomatic and includes measures to promote oxygenation and comfort, such as oxygen administration, CPT and postural drainage, antipyretics for fever management, fluid intake, and family support. Although some authorities recommend antimicrobial therapy in the hope of reducing or preventing secondary bacterial infection, it is usually reserved for children in whom the presence of such infection is demonstrated by appropriate cultures.

PRIMARY ATYPICAL PNEUMONIA

Atypical pneumonia refers to pneumonia that is caused by pathogens other than the traditionally most common and readily cultured bacteria (e.g., *S. pneumoniae*). In the category of atypical pneumonias, *M. pneumoniae* and *Chlamydia pneumoniae* are the most common causes of community-acquired pneumonia in children 5 years old or older (Rafei and Lichenstein, 2006). It occurs principally in the fall and winter months and is more prevalent in crowded living conditions.

Clinical Manifestations

The onset may be sudden or insidious and is usually accompanied by general systemic symptoms, including fever, chills (in older children), headache, malaise, anorexia, and muscle pain (myalgia). These symptoms are followed by rhinitis; sore throat; and a dry, hacking cough. The cough, initially nonproductive, produces seromucoid sputum that later becomes mucopurulent or blood streaked. The degree of fever varies widely, from several days to 2 weeks. Dyspnea occurs infrequently.

Radiographic examination reveals evidence of pneumonia before physical signs are apparent. There may be fine crepitant crackles over various areas of the lung fields, but consolidation is usually not demonstrated. The pathologic process consists of interstitial round cell infiltration and edema of alveolar septa and varying distribution of areas of inflammation, necrosis, and ulceration of the mucosal lining of bronchi and bronchioles. Areas of consolidation and emphysema are present.

Therapeutic and Nursing Care Management

Most affected persons recover from acute illness in 7 to 10 days with symptomatic treatment, followed by a week of convalescence. Hospitalization is rarely necessary.

BACTERIAL PNEUMONIA

Bacterial pneumonia is often a serious infection. The pathogenetic mechanisms involved are often aspiration or hematogenous dissemination. The cause varies depending on the child's age, underlying illness, and degree of immunosuppression or immunocompetence.

Etiology and Epidemiology

S. pneumoniae is the most common bacterial pathogen responsible for community-acquired pneumonia in both children and adults (Rafei and Lichenstein, 2006). Other bacteria that cause pneumonia in children are group A streptococci, *S. aureus*, *M. catarrhalis*, *M. pneumoniae*, and *C. pneumoniae*.

Beyond the neonatal period, bacterial pneumonias display distinct clinical patterns that facilitate their differentiation from other forms of pneumonia. The onset of illness is abrupt and generally follows a viral infection that disturbs the natural defense mechanisms of the upper respiratory tract. In the 3-month to 5-year age-group, *S. pneumoniae*, *M. catarrhalis*, and group A streptococci are common causes. *H. influenzae* type b is causing fewer infections because of the Hib vaccine. *S. aureus* pneumonia is also now rarely seen in infants and toddlers.

Fever—Usually quite high
Respiratory signs
- Cough: unproductive to productive with whitish sputum
- Tachypnea
- Breath sounds: rhonchi or fine crackles
- Dullness with percussion
- Chest pain
- Retractions
- Nasal flaring
- Pallor to cyanosis (depends on severity)

Chest x-ray—Diffuse or patchy infiltration, with peribronchial distribution
Behavior—Irritable, restless, lethargic
Gastrointestinal signs—Anorexia, vomiting, diarrhea, abdominal pain

Clinical Manifestations

The child with bacterial pneumonia usually appears ill. Symptoms include fever, malaise, rapid and shallow respirations, cough, and chest pain. The older child may complain of headache, chills, abdominal pain, chest pain, or meningeal symptoms (**meningism**) (Box 32-9). Respiratory distress may or may not be present. In some cases the only finding is an increased respiratory rate. The pain of pneumonia may be referred to the abdomen and confused with appendicitis.

Infants and young children develop more severe symptoms than older children. Cyanosis and apnea are common, and the parent may report the infant's activity and eating pattern was decreased for a few days. Additional clinical manifestations in infants include abrupt fever, vomiting, diarrhea, and abdominal distention (Sectish and Prober, 2007). Because pneumonia in newborns carries a high morbidity and mortality rate, suspect bacterial infection in all neonates with respiratory symptoms.

Initially, the cough is usually hacking and nonproductive, and breath sounds are diminished or heard as scattered crackles. When consolidation is present, breath sounds may be tubular in quality with no adventitious noises. As the infection resolves, coarse crackles and wheezing are heard, and the cough becomes productive with purulent sputum.

Staphylococcal pneumonia is rare but particularly progressive and must be treated aggressively. The onset is rapid, with rapid deterioration. Conjunctivitis and furuncles are signs of a probable staphylococcal infection.

Diagnostic Evaluation

The key to a preliminary diagnosis is finding pulmonary infiltrates on radiographic examination, usually revealing lobar consolidation and, in some severe cases, pleural effusion. Laboratory studies include Gram stain and culture of sputum in older children, nasopharyngeal specimens, blood cultures, and lung aspiration and biopsy. The white blood cell count may be elevated, but it may be normal for infants with staphylococcal disease. Children with streptococcal disease usually have an elevated antistreptolysin O titer. The infant or child with recurrent pneumonia should be further evaluated for CF or an immunodeficiency disease. Diagnostic evaluation should include ruling out aspiration pneumonia as a potential cause.

Therapeutic Management

Antimicrobial therapy has significantly reduced the morbidity and mortality from bacterial pneumonia. Oral amoxicillin is widely used for outpatient management of infants and children younger than 5 years of age. Patients incompletely immunized against *H. influenzae* should receive amoxicillin-clavulanate or a second-generation cephalosporin (cefuroxime, cefadroxil). Erythromycin is the drug of choice for older children and adolescents because of its activity against *M. pneumoniae*. In the hospital, medications are given parenterally for rapid action and maximum effect. IV cefuroxime, cefotaxime, and ceftriaxone are considered the primary antibacterial agents for bacterial pneumonia in the hospitalized child (Sectish and Prober, 2007). Parenteral or oral erythromycin should be added for children older than 5 years of age until *M. pneumoniae* is ruled out. CPT with postural drainage may be helpful in clearing secretions in some cases.

Most older children with pneumonia can be treated at home, especially if the condition is recognized and treatment initiated early. Antibiotic therapy, rest, liberal oral intake of fluid, and administration of antipyretics for fever are the principal therapeutic measures. Hospitalization is indicated when **pleural effusion** or **empyema** accompanies the disease, when compliance with therapy is estimated to be poor, in infants less than 1 month old, and when there are chronic illnesses such as congenital heart disease or bronchopulmonary dysplasia (Rafei and Lichenstein, 2006). Pneumonia in the infant or young child may also require hospitalization because the course of illness is variable and complications are more common in very young patients. In addition, IV fluid administration is frequently necessary, and oxygen may be required if the child is in respiratory distress.

Prognosis

The prognosis for pneumonia is generally good, with rapid recovery when it is recognized and treated early. The course of staphylococcal pneumonia is generally prolonged. The prognosis varies with the length of the illness before treatment, although early recognition and treatment are usually beneficial.

Prevention

The use of the pneumococcal conjugate vaccine (PCV 13; Prevnar 13) is recommended for infants and children younger than 23 months to be administered at 2, 4, 6, and between 12 and 15 months. The four-dose series may be completed with Prevnar 13 if PCV 7 was given for any of the previous doses, as long as a total of four doses are administered. Prevnar 13 is also recommended for children aged 60 to 71 months with underlying medical conditions who are at high risk for the development of pneumococcal disease or complications (Centers for Disease Control and Prevention, 2010). Studies have demonstrated a decrease in pneumococcal pneumonia in children younger than 24 months. (See Immunizations, Chapter 12.)

Complications

At present the classic features and clinical course of pneumonia are rarely seen because of early and vigorous antibiotic and supportive therapy. However, some children, especially infants,

PATHOPHYSIOLOGY REVIEW

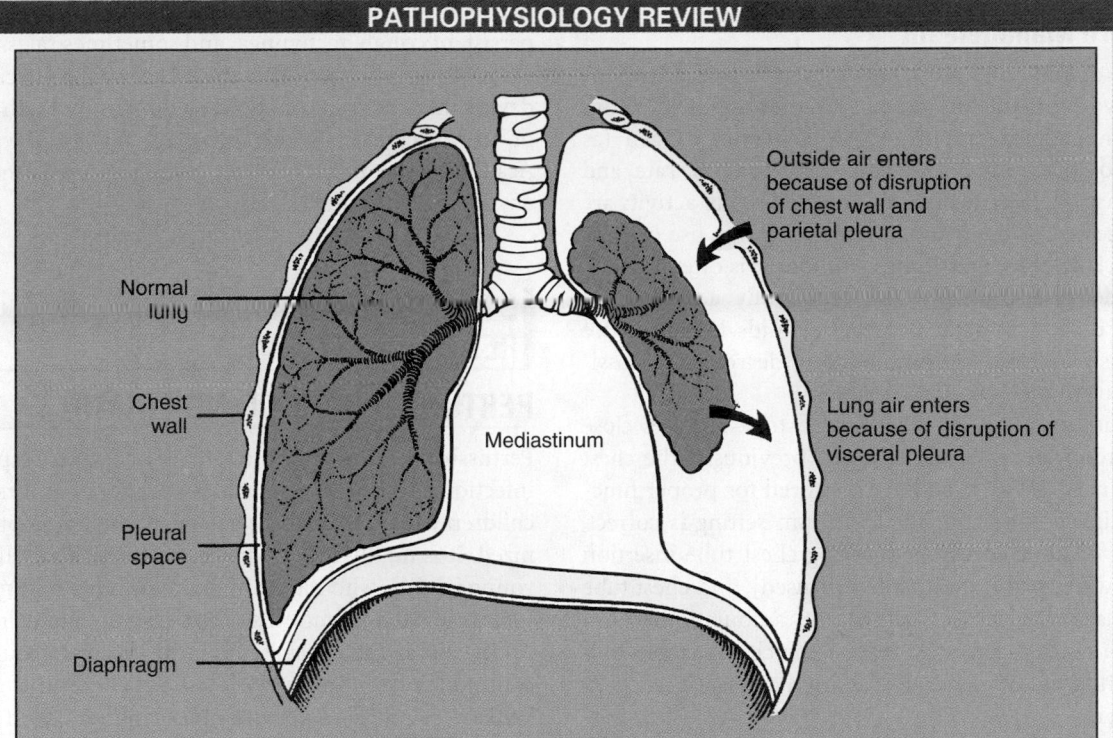

Normal lung

Chest wall

Pleural space

Diaphragm

Mediastinum

Outside air enters because of disruption of chest wall and parietal pleura

Lung air enters because of disruption of visceral pleura

Fig. 32-5 Pneumothorax. Air in the pleural space causes the lung to collapse around the hilus and may push mediastinal contents (heart and great vessels) toward the other lung. (From McCance KL, Huether SE: *Pathophysiology: the biological basis for disease in adults and children,* ed 6, St Louis, 2010, Mosby.)

BOX 32-10 PNEUMOTHORAX

Pneumothorax occurs when air accumulates in the pleural space; this air increases intrapleural pressure, making it more difficult to expand the affected lung. This leads to the clinical manifestations of dyspnea, chest pain and often back pain, labored respirations, tachycardia, and decreased oxygen saturation. In neonates and infants on mechanical ventilation the first clinical signs of a pneumothorax are oxygen desaturation and hypotension. The three major types of pneumothorax are tension, spontaneous, and traumatic. The definitive diagnosis of pneumothorax is a chest radiograph. The emergent treatment involves needle aspiration of the air within the pleural space; subsequently a chest tube to closed drainage is usually inserted to prevent the reaccumulation of air.

Pleural effusion occurs when there is an excessive accumulation of fluid in the pleural space. The diagnosis is made by chest radiograph, and the treatment involves evacuation of the fluid by needle aspiration followed by insertion of a chest tube to closed drainage.

---

with staphylococcal pneumonia develop empyema, pyopneumothorax, or tension pneumothorax (Fig. 32-5). AOM and pleural effusion are common in children with pneumococcal pneumonia (Box 32-10).

When fluid is either suspected or identified by radiograph in the pleural cavity, a needle aspiration or thoracentesis is performed. Nonpurulent effusions do not require surgical drainage.

Continuous closed chest drainage may be instituted with a complicated pleural effusion. Closed drainage is continued until drainage fluid is free of pathogens, which rarely requires more than 5 to 7 days. Additional therapies for empyema may involve the instillation of antibiotic into the pleural space via the chest tube, instillation of intrapleural fibrinolytics such as urokinase or streptokinase, or video-assisted thoracoscopy (Ranganathan and Sonnappa, 2009; Bergelson, Shah, and Zaouitis, 2008).

Thoracentesis

Dyspnea resulting from pressure from fluid accumulation in the pleural cavity requires removal by thoracentesis. Thoracentesis is also performed to obtain fluid for culture or to instill antibiotics directly into the pleural cavity. Nursing responsibilities include obtaining and setting up equipment, preparing the child physically and psychologically, monitoring the sedated child's vital signs during the procedure and recovery, and assisting with the procedure. If continuous closed chest drainage is anticipated, this equipment should also be available. Procedural sedation may be performed using a number of drugs singly or in combination (ketamine, propofol, fentanyl, morphine, midazolam) to provide adequate anxiolysis and analgesia (Meredith, O'Keefe, and Galwankar, 2008). Additional nursing responsibilities include documenting the patient's tolerance of procedure and managing pain after the procedure.

In addition, the nurse makes the child comfortable and records observations and physical and emotional responses, the amount and description of the fluid obtained, and any medication instilled. Specimens are sent to the laboratory for culture. Continuous closed chest drainage is managed according to the same protocol as for the child with a thoracotomy. (See Chapter 34.)

Nursing Care Management

Nursing care of the child with pneumonia is primarily supportive and symptomatic but necessitates thorough respiratory assessment and administration of supplemental oxygen (as required) and antibiotics. The child's respiratory rate and status, oxygenation, general disposition, and level of activity are frequently assessed. If the cough is disturbing, the use of antitussives, especially before rest times and meals, is often helpful. To prevent dehydration, fluids are frequently administered intravenously during the acute phase. Oral fluids, if allowed, are given cautiously to avoid aspiration and to decrease the possibility of aggravating a fatiguing cough.

Nursing care of the child with a chest tube requires close attention to respiratory status, as noted previously; the chest tube and drainage device used are monitored for proper function (i.e., drainage is not impeded, vacuum setting is correct, tubing is free of kinks, dressing covering chest tube insertion site is intact, water seal is maintained [if used], and chest tube remains in place). Movement in bed and ambulation with a chest tube are encouraged according to the child's respiratory status, but children often require a mild analgesic such as acetaminophen.

If needed, supplemental oxygen may be administered by nasal cannula; newborns may receive oxygen via a plastic hood. Children are usually more comfortable in a semierect position but should be allowed to determine the position of comfort. Control fever by cooling the environment and administering antipyretic drugs as prescribed. Temperature is monitored regularly to detect a rise that might trigger a febrile seizure.

Monitor vital signs and oxygenation to assess the progress of the disease and to detect early signs of complications. Children with ineffectual cough or those with difficulty handling secretions, especially infants, require suctioning to maintain a patent airway. A simple bulb suction syringe is usually sufficient for clearing the nares and nasopharynx of infants, but mechanical suction should be readily available if needed. Older children can usually handle secretions without assistance. Postural drainage and CPT are generally prescribed every 4 hours or more often, depending on the child's condition.

The hospitalized child may be apprehensive, and the treatments and tests are frightening and stress producing. It is important to involve the entire family in the care as appropriate and to encourage questions and facilitate effective communication. Reducing the child's anxiety, apprehension, and psychologic distress leads to relaxation and decreased respiratory efforts. Easing respiratory efforts further reduces the child's apprehension. Encouraging the presence of the caregiver provides the child with a source of comfort and support.

CHLAMYDIAL PNEUMONIA

C. trachomatis, an intracellular microorganism similar to gram-negative bacteria, is responsible for one of the most common sexually transmitted infections. Newborn infants acquire pulmonary infection from their mothers via ascending infection just before or in the process of birth.

Chlamydial pneumonia is usually an afebrile illness that occurs between 2 and 19 weeks after delivery (American Academy of Pediatrics, 2009b). It is also characterized by a persistent cough, tachypnea, and sometimes rales. Radiographs show nonspecific abnormalities. Oral azithromycin given for 5 days is the treatment of choice; alternatively erythromycin base or ethylsuccinate is administered for 14 days (American Academy of Pediatrics, 2009b). Nursing care is the same as for any infant with pneumonia.

OTHER INFECTIONS OF THE RESPIRATORY TRACT

PERTUSSIS (WHOOPING COUGH)

Pertussis, or whooping cough, is an acute respiratory tract infection caused by *Bordetella pertussis* that occurs primarily in children younger than 4 years of age who have not been immunized. It is highly contagious and is particularly threatening in young infants, who have a higher morbidity and mortality rate. Infants less than 6 months of age may not come in to the practitioner with the typical cough; in this age-group, apnea is a common presenting manifestation (American Academy of Pediatrics, 2009b). Likewise older children often manifest the disease with a persistent cough and the absence of the characteristic whoop. (See Table 16-1 for signs, symptoms, and management of pertussis.) The incidence is highest in the spring and summer months, and a single attack confers lifetime immunity.

The resurgence of pertussis in the United States, particularly among children 10 years old and older, has prompted concerns over the long-term effects of the pertussis vaccine. Consequently a new booster vaccine for pertussis has been approved for children. Boostrix contains acellular pertussis, diphtheria toxoid, and tetanus toxoid and is indicated as a booster for children ages 10 to 18 years (American Academy of Pediatrics, 2009b); one additional acellular pertussis vaccine (Adacel) has now been approved for persons ages 11 to 64 years. (See also Immunizations, Chapter 12.) Parapertussis (*Bordetella parapertussis*) causes pertussis but cases are milder than those caused by *B. pertussis*; parapertussis is more common in Eastern and Western Europe than in the United States (Long, 2007).

TUBERCULOSIS

Since 1993 the incidence of tuberculosis (TB) has steadily declined significantly in the United States, yet it remains high in certain populations. According to the Centers for Disease Control and Prevention (2009a), preliminary data from 2008 show the lowest rate of TB since 1953—4.2 cases per 100,000 population. The rate of TB among foreign-born immigrants was 10 times higher than those with the United States as country of origin. In recent years, foreign-born children have accounted for more than one fourth of newly diagnosed cases of TB in children 14 years of age or younger in the United States (American Academy of Pediatrics, 2009b). Four states—Florida, New York, Texas, and California—combined accounted for more than 50% of all cases of TB reported in 2008 (Centers for Disease Control and Prevention, 2009a). TB is a significant factor in the mortality of persons infected with HIV. Global estimates show that approximately 2 million persons, including 500,000 children, die each year from TB disease (Ranganathan and Sonnappa, 2009).

Etiology

TB is caused by *Mycobacterium tuberculosis*, an acid-fast bacillus not readily decolorized by acids after staining. Children are susceptible to the human *(M. tuberculosis)* and the bovine *(Mycobacterium bovis)* organisms. In parts of the world where TB in cattle is not controlled or milk is not pasteurized, the bovine type is a common source of infection.

Although the causative agent for TB is the tubercle bacillus, other factors influence the degree to which the organism produces an altered state in the host. These include heredity (resistance to the infection may be genetically transmitted), gender (higher rates in adolescent girls), age (lower resistance in infants, higher incidence during adolescence), stress (emotional or physical), nutritional state, and intercurrent infection (especially HIV, measles, and pertussis). Children with HIV infection have an increased incidence of TB disease, and all children with TB should be tested for HIV (Box 32-11).

Pathophysiology

The source of infection in children is usually an infected member of the household or any frequent visitor to the household, such as a baby-sitter or domestic worker. Transmission

---

BOX 32-11   FACTORS AFFECTING RESISTANCE TO TUBERCULOSIS

Heredity
No evidence of hereditary tendency
Evidence that resistance to infection may be genetically transmitted

Sex
Early years: no sex differences in incidence
Later childhood and adolescence: morbidity and mortality higher in girls than in boys

Age
Diminished resistance to infection in infancy
- Delay in development of acquired immunity
- Diminished capacity to resist extension of infective process
Increased tendency to develop disease during puberty and adolescence
- New infection superimposed on a previous one
- Increased contacts
- Indigenous reinfection stimulated by metabolic changes or suboptimum diets during a period of rapid growth

Stress States
Temporary stressful circumstances (e.g., injury or illness, undernutrition, emotional distress, chronic fatigue) increasing susceptibility to infection
Increased secretion of adrenal steroids suppressing protective inflammatory response and permitting infection to spread
Therapeutic administration of corticosteroids (similar effect)

Nutrition
Active disease inversely proportional to state of nutrition
Excellent nutrition essential to young children's recovery from disease

Intercurrent Infection
Infectious diseases (especially human immunodeficiency virus, measles, pertussis) activating latent tuberculosis
Noncompliance with therapy

---

of *M. tuberculosis* occurs when the child inhales microdroplets (usually 1 to 5 mm in size) into the respiratory tract after someone has coughed or sneezed. Although the lung is the most frequent portal of entry in humans, the organism *M. bovis* can be ingested via infected milk (unpasteurized milk or fresh cheese). When the *M. tuberculosis* droplet is inhaled, it passes down the bronchial tree, implants in either a bronchiole or alveolus, and starts to multiply. *M. bovis* typically causes cervical lymphadenitis, meningitis, and intestinal TB disease and is more common in adults and children from countries where *M. bovis* is prevalent (American Academy of Pediatrics, 2009b).

Epithelial cells surround and encapsulate the multiplying bacilli in an attempt to wall off the invading organisms, thus forming the typical tubercle. During the inflammatory process, some bacilli leave the focal area and are carried to the regional lymph nodes that drain the area; as a result, the child develops a fever. Radiographic examinations may be positive if such tests are performed when the child is known to have been exposed. The tuberculin skin test is positive.

Extension of the primary lesion at the original site causes progressive tissue destruction as it spreads within the lung, discharges material from foci to other areas of the lungs (e.g., bronchi or pleura), or produces pneumonia. Erosion of blood vessels by the primary lesion can cause widespread dissemination of the tubercle bacillus to near and distant sites (miliary TB). Organisms deposited in the upper lung zones, bones, kidneys, and brain may find favorable environments for growth, but organs and tissue such as bone marrow, liver, and spleen appear to inhibit multiplication of the bacilli.

Extrapulmonary TB may be manifested as superior lymphadenitis, meningitis, or osteoarthritis and may appear in the middle ear and mastoid and on the skin (American Academy of Pediatrics, 2009b; Feja and Saiman, 2005). With the exception of meningitis, treatment for extrapulmonary TB may be the same drug regimen as for pulmonary TB. Renal TB is rare in children but may occur in adolescents.

For children not immunosuppressed or immunocompromised, a strong cell-mediated immune response provides specific immunity that usually limits further multiplication of the bacilli. These children remain asymptomatic, and the lesions usually heal. TB infection is manifested by a positive skin test only. In a small percentage of persons with newly acquired TB, replication of the organism continues and TB disease occurs, as evidenced by a positive chest radiograph, positive sputum culture, and signs of disease.

Clinical Manifestations

Clinical manifestations of pulmonary TB in children are extremely variable. The disease may be asymptomatic or produce a broad range of symptoms, including general responses such as fever, malaise, anorexia, and weight loss or more specific symptoms related to the site of infection (e.g., lungs, bone, brain, kidneys). Lung disease may or may not include cough (which progresses slowly over weeks to months), aching pain and tightness in the chest, and (rarely) hemoptysis.

As increasing amounts of lung tissue become involved, the respiratory rate increases, the lung on the affected side does not expand as well as the other, auscultation reveals diminished breath sounds and crackles, and there is dullness to percussion. In children (usually infants) who are unable to contain the spread of infection, the fever persists; the generalized symptoms are manifest; and the patient develops pallor, anemia, weakness, and weight loss.

Diagnostic Evaluation

Diagnosis is based on information derived from physical examination, history, reaction to a tuberculin test, organism cultures, and radiographic examinations. In addition, it must be determined if the lesion is in the active, quiescent, or healed stage.

History

Symptoms generally do not contribute significantly to a diagnosis. A history of possible contact with a person known to be infected or subsequently found to be infected is helpful. All contacts of an affected child are examined for the disease.

Tuberculin Test

The tuberculin skin test (TST) is the most important indicator of whether a child has been infected with the tubercle bacillus. The standard dose of purified protein derivative (PPD) is 5 tuberculin units in 0.1 ml of solution, which is administered using a 27-gauge needle and a 1-ml syringe intradermally into the volar aspect of the forearm. Creation of a visible wheal is crucial to accurate testing. A primary infection initiates a hypersensitivity reaction to the protein fraction of the tubercle bacillus, which can be detected 2 to 10 weeks after the infection. In the past, multiple puncture tests such as the tine test were used, but these tests have significant problems and are no longer recommended (Selekman, 2006).

The American Academy of Pediatrics (2009b) has recommended a change in TB screening procedures. It no longer recommends universal testing of all children for TB. Now a targeted testing method is used, wherein only children and adolescents at high risk for contracting the disease and those patients at risk for progression to TB disease are screened. A risk factor questionnaire has been developed to facilitate screening pediatric populations at high risk. Factors included on the questionnaire include a close association with persons having latent TB infection (LTBI) or active disease, foreign birth, or foreign travel (Pediatric Tuberculosis Collaborative Group, 2004; the entire questionnaire is available at this reference). Recommendations for TB skin testing of children are given in Box 32-12.

The QuantiFERON-TB Gold and T-SPOT TB are tests of interferon quantification (interferon gamma release assay [IGRA]) used in the diagnosis of TB in adults; however, their use in children is limited, especially in those under 5 years of age. The IGRA tests may be helpful in confirming the presence of TB disease in a child who has received BCG (bacille Calmette-Guérin, a vaccine containing bovine bacilli with reduced virulence) and has a borderline positive or negative TST (American Academy of Pediatrics, 2009b; Ranganathan and Sonnappa, 2009).

The tuberculin is injected intradermally with the bevel of the needle pointing upward. A wheal 6 to 10 mm in diameter should form between the layers of the skin when the solution is injected properly. If the wheal does not form, the procedure

---

BOX 32-12   TUBERCULIN SKIN TEST (TST) RECOMMENDATIONS FOR INFANTS, CHILDREN, AND ADOLESCENTS*

Children for Whom Immediate TST Is Indicated

Contacts of persons with confirmed or suspected contagious tuberculosis (contact investigation)

Children with radiographic or clinical findings suggesting tuberculosis disease

Children immigrating from endemic countries (e.g., Asia, Middle East, Africa, Latin America)

Children with travel histories to endemic countries or significant contact with indigenous persons from such countries

Children Who Should Have Annual TST†

Children infected with human immunodeficiency virus (HIV)

Incarcerated adolescents

Children Who Some Experts Recommend Should Be Tested Every 2 to 3 Years†

Children with ongoing exposure to the following people: HIV-infected people, homeless people, residents of nursing homes, institutionalized adolescents or adults, users of illicit drugs, incarcerated adolescents or adults, or migrant farm workers; foster children with exposure to adults in the preceding high-risk groups are included

Children Who Some Experts Recommend Should Be Considered for TST at 4 to 6 and 11 to 16 Years

Children whose parents immigrated (with unknown TST status) from regions of the world with high prevalence of tuberculosis; continued potential exposure by travel to the endemic areas, or household contact with persons from the endemic areas (with unknown TST status) should be an indication for repeat TST

Children at Increased Risk for Progression of Infection to Disease

Children with other medical risk factors, including diabetes mellitus, chronic renal failure, malnutrition, and congenital or acquired immunodeficiencies, deserve special consideration. Without recent exposure, these people are not at increased risk of acquiring tuberculosis infection. Underlying immunodeficiencies associated with these conditions theoretically would enhance the possibility for progression to severe disease. Initial histories of potential exposure to tuberculosis should be included for all of these patients. If these histories or local epidemiologic factors suggest a possibility of exposure, immediate and periodic TST should be considered. An initial TST should be performed before initiation of immunosuppressive therapy, including prolonged steroid administration, for any child with an underlying condition that necessitates immunosuppressive therapy.

From American Academy of Pediatrics, Committee on Infectious Diseases, Pickering L, editor: *2009 Red book: report of the Committee on Infectious Diseases,* ed 28, Elk Grove Village, Ill, 2009, The Academy.
*Bacille Calmette-Guérin (BCG) immunization is not a contraindication to TST.
†Initial TST is done at the time of diagnosis or circumstance, beginning at 3 months of age.

---

is repeated. The volar or dorsal surface of the forearm is the usual injection site. The reaction to the skin test is determined in 48 to 72 hours; reactions occurring after 72 hours should be measured and considered the result. The size of the transverse diameter of induration, not the erythema, is measured. The diameter transverse to the long axis of the forearm is the only one standardized for measurement purposes (American Academy of Pediatrics, 2009b).

Guidelines for interpreting the TST are listed in Box 32-13. The American Academy of Pediatrics (2009b) and the Pediatric

BOX 32-13   DEFINITION OF POSITIVE TUBERCULIN SKIN TESTING RESULTS IN INFANTS, CHILDREN, AND ADOLESCENTS*

Induration ≥5 mm

Children in close contact with known or suspected contagious cases of tuberculosis disease

Children suspected to have tuberculosis disease:
- Findings on chest x-ray film consistent with active or previously active tuberculosis
- Clinical evidence of tuberculosis disease†

Children receiving immunosuppressive therapy‡ or who have immunosuppressive conditions, including human immunodeficiency virus (HIV) infection

Induration ≥10 mm

Children at increased risk of disseminated disease:
- Those younger than 4 years of age
- Those with other medical risk conditions, including Hodgkin disease, lymphoma, diabetes mellitus, chronic renal failure, or malnutrition

Children with increased risk of exposure to tuberculosis disease:
- Those born, or whose parents were born, in high-prevalence (TB) regions of the world
- Those frequently exposed to adults who are HIV-infected, homeless, users of illicit drugs, residents of nursing homes, incarcerated or institutionalized, or migrant farm workers
- Those who travel to high-prevalence regions of the world

Induration ≥15 mm

Children 4 years of age or older without any risk factors

From American Academy of Pediatrics, Committee on Infectious Diseases, Pickering L, editor: *2009 Red book: report of the Committee on Infectious Diseases,* ed 28, Elk Grove Village, Ill, 2009, The Academy.
*These definitions apply regardless of previous Bacille Calmette-Guérin (BCG) immunization; erythema at tuberculin skin test (TST) site does not indicate a positive test result. TSTs should be read 48 to 72 hours after placement.
†Evidence by physical examination or laboratory assessment that would include tuberculosis in the working differential diagnosis (e.g., meningitis).
‡Including immunosuppressive doses of corticosteroids.

BOX 32-14   CIRCUMSTANCES PRODUCING FALSE-NEGATIVE REACTIONS TO TUBERCULIN TESTS

Tuberculin reaction suppressed by:
- Intercurrent diseases (e.g., viral diseases such as measles, rubella, influenza, mumps, varicella, and probably others [about 4 weeks])
- Live-virus vaccines (e.g., measles, mumps, and rubella vaccines [about 4 weeks])
- Corticosteroids and other immunosuppressive agents
- Cellular immunodeficiency disease
- Severe malnutrition
- Malignancies (leukemia, lymphoma, Hodgkin disease)

Testing before the body develops a sensitivity to the protein fraction of the tubercle bacillus (e.g., newborn or child younger than 2 years)

Use of outdated testing material; mixture that has been prepared for too long or has been exposed to sunlight

Faulty technique (e.g., deep injection, no wheal formed, improper measurement of solution, or leaking of solution from a defective or loosely fitting syringe)

Overwhelming tuberculosis infections; end-stage and terminal miliary disease

Improper reading (interpretation of results)

Early tuberculosis infection (<12 weeks)

Tuberculosis Collaborative Group (2004) recommend that TST results be read only by a health care professional.

A positive TST reaction indicates that the person has been infected and has developed sensitivity to the protein of the tubercle bacillus; it does not, however, confirm the presence of active disease. Once individuals react positively, they will always react positively. A positive reaction in a previously negative reactor indicates that the person has been infected since the last test.

A negative reaction does not exclude the presence of LTBI or active disease. Children with immunosuppression, concurrent viral infection (e.g., measles, varicella, influenza), HIV, disseminated TB disease, and recent TB infection may have decreased TST reactivity. Several factors can produce false-negative results (Box 32-14). Tuberculin testing should not be carried out at the same time as measles immunization. Viral interference from the measles vaccine may cause a false-negative reaction. Prompt radiographic evaluation of all children with a positive TST is recommended.

A finding of LTBI indicates infection in a person who has a positive TST, no physical findings of disease, and normal chest radiograph findings. The American Academy of Pediatrics (2009b) states that a diagnosis of LTBI or TB disease in a young child represents a public health sentinel event indicating recent transmission of the *M. tuberculosis* organism. The term *tuberculosis disease* is used when a child has clinical symptoms or radiographic manifestations caused by the *M. tuberculosis* organism.

Bacteriologic Examination

A definitive diagnosis is made by demonstrating the presence of mycobacteria in culture. The organism is identified from microscopic examination of properly prepared and stained smears from early-morning gastric washings or from sputum, pleural fluid, urine, spinal fluid, draining lymph nodes, and other body fluids. Induced sputum and gastric lavage sputum specimens are often obtained for culture from children who are unable to expectorate a sputum specimen.

Radiographic Studies

Radiographic examinations may be done, but the lesions of numerous chronic intrathoracic diseases resemble tuberculous lesions. Therefore radiographic examinations are used to supplement other diagnostic methods.

Therapeutic Management

Medical management of tuberculous lesions in children consists of adequate nutrition, antimicrobial therapy, general supportive measures, prevention of unnecessary exposure to other infections that further compromise the body's defenses, prevention of reinfection, and sometimes surgical procedures.

A child with LTBI is treated with antimicrobial drugs to decrease the risk of acquiring active TB disease in the years following the initial acquisition and to reduce the lifelong chance of developing TB disease (Ranganathan and Sonnappa, 2009). The recommended drug regimen for LTBI in children and adolescents includes a daily dose of isoniazid (INH) for 9 months or alternatively two or three times per week with directly observed therapy (DOT) (Pediatric Tuberculosis Collaborative Group, 2004). Rifampin (daily for 6 months) may be used to treat children or adolescents who are INH resistant. The Pediatric Tuberculosis Collaborative Group (2004) does not recommend treatment for children or adolescents who have positive tuberculin test results but who have no risk factors.

For the child with clinically active TB, the goal is to achieve sterilization of the tuberculous lesion. The American Academy of Pediatrics (2009b) recommends a 6-month regimen consisting of INH, rifampin, ethambutol, and pyrazinamide (PZA) given daily for the first 2 months, followed by INH and rifampin given two or three times a week by DOT for the remaining 4 months. Alternative treatment regimens may be used when managed by a TB specialist. DOT decreases the rates of relapse, treatment failures, and drug resistance and is recommended for treatment of children and adolescents with TB in the United States.

DOT means that a health care worker or other responsible, mutually agreed-on individual is present when medications are administered to the patient. If the reliability of self-administration of medications is in doubt, directly observed, twice-weekly therapy must be administered by a health care professional.

Infection with *M. bovis* may be treated with the same four-drug regimen as TB disease, although *M. bovis* may be resistant to PZA, in which case an appropriate substitute should be used.

When drug resistance is suspected, either ethambutol or an aminoglycoside is added to the therapeutic regimen until drug susceptibility results are available. Therapy should always include at least four drugs initially and be continued for at least 9 months. INH, rifampin, and PZA, usually with ethambutol or an aminoglycoside, should be given for at least the first 2 months. The three-drug regimen can be used after drug-resistant disease is excluded. Optimum therapy for TB in children with HIV infection has not been established, and consultation with a specialist is advised. Any child diagnosed with TB disease should also be tested for HIV (American Academy of Pediatrics, 2009b). It is not within the scope of this text to outline the treatment regimen for multiple drug–resistant and extensively drug–resistant TB.

Surgical procedures may be required to remove the source of infection in tissues that are inaccessible to antimicrobial therapy or that are destroyed by the disease. Orthopedic procedures for correction of bone deformities, bronchoscopy for removal of a tuberculous granulomatous polyp, or resection of a portion of a diseased lung may also be performed.

Prognosis

Most children recover from primary TB infection and may be unaware of its presence. However, very young children have a higher incidence of disseminated disease. It is a serious disease during the first 2 years of life, during adolescence, and in children infected with HIV. Except in cases of tuberculous meningitis, death seldom occurs in treated children. Antibiotic therapy has decreased mortality and hematogenous spread from primary lesions.

Prevention

The only certain means to prevent TB is to avoid contact with the tubercle bacillus. Maintaining an optimum state of health with adequate nutrition and avoiding debilitating infections promote natural resistance but do not prevent infection.

Pasteurization of milk and routine testing and elimination of diseased cattle have helped reduce the incidence of bovine TB. Infants and children should be given only pasteurized milk from TB-free cattle.

A source of concern is that the infected child or family members may spread the disease when visiting in the hospital. Most children with TB need not be isolated and can be hospitalized on an open unit if they are receiving chemotherapy. Children and adolescents with infectious pulmonary TB (i.e., those whose sputum smears show acid-fast bacilli) should be on Isolation Precautions until effective chemotherapy has been initiated, their sputum smears show a diminishing number of organisms, and their cough is improving. Masks are indicated only when the child is coughing and does not reliably cover his or her mouth. Gowns are indicated only if needed to prevent gross contamination of clothing. Family members should be managed with Airborne Precautions when visiting until they are demonstrated not to have infectious TB.

Limited immunity can be produced by administration of BCG. The freshly prepared vaccine, injected intradermally, produces definite although incomplete protection against TB (ranging from 0% to 80%). In most instances, positive tuberculin reactions develop after inoculation. BCG vaccination is not generally recommended for use in the United States. However, it may be recommended for long-term protection of infants and children with negative TST who are not infected with HIV and who (1) are at high risk for continuing exposure to persons with infectious pulmonary TB or (2) are continuously exposed to persons with TB who have bacilli resistant to both INH and rifampin (American Academy of Pediatrics, 2009b).

Nursing Care Management

Hospitalization for TB is seldom necessary in the United States. Only children with the more serious forms of the disease are placed in the hospital. The major nursing care of children with TB involves nurses in ambulatory settings: outpatient departments, schools, and public health agencies.

Asymptomatic children can lead an essentially unrestricted life. They can and should attend school (or daycare), but older children are restricted from vigorous activities such as competitive games and contact sports during the active stage of primary TB. They should be protected from stresses, including parental anxieties, overprotection, and pressures regarding nutritional intake. They should also continue the regular immunization schedule and maintain optimum health with proper diet, adequate rest, and avoidance of infection.

Nurses assume several roles in management of the disease, including helping the family understand the rationale for diagnostic procedures, assisting with radiographic examinations, performing skin tests, and obtaining specimens for laboratory examination. Skin tests must be carried out correctly to obtain accurate results (see previous discussion on Tuberculin Test).

Sputum specimens are difficult or impossible to obtain from an infant or young child because they swallow any mucus coughed from the lower respiratory tract. The best means for obtaining material for smears or culture is by gastric washing (i.e., aspiration of lavaged contents from the fasting stomach with a nasogastric tube). The procedure is carried out and the specimen obtained early in the morning before the customary breakfast time. In some cases an induced sputum specimen may be obtained by administering aerosolized normal saline for 10 to 15 minutes, followed by CPT and suctioning of the nasopharynx for sputum collection.

Ambulatory Care

Nursing supervision of the child at home involves teaching the parents and child about the disease and its ramifications. Historically the disease has been regarded with fear, and numerous misconceptions need to be addressed. Reducing parental anxieties helps them deal with the illness more constructively and collaborate more effectively in planning the child's continued care. Because the success of therapy depends on compliance with drug therapy, instruct the parents regarding the importance of giving the medication as often and as long as it is ordered. (See Compliance, Chapter 27.) Promoting optimum general health and preventing intercurrent infections and reinfections with the tubercle bacillus are important. The American Lung Association has excellent patient education materials.*

Case Finding

Case finding and follow-up of known contacts are important nursing responsibilities. Every case of TB identified in the community involves nurses in follow-up of known contacts—individuals from whom the affected person may have acquired the disease and persons who may have been exposed to the diseased individual. Early diagnosis affords a means for early protection or treatment and prevents further spread of the disease.

RESPIRATORY DISTURBANCE CAUSED BY NONINFECTIOUS IRRITANTS

FOREIGN BODY INGESTION AND ASPIRATION

Small children characteristically explore objects with their hands and mouth and are prone to place FBs into the air passages (nose and mouth). They also place objects such as beads, paper clips, plastic toys, small magnets, or food items in the nose, which can easily be aspirated into the trachea. Small items may also be placed into the external ear canal; small rocks and pebbles appear to be a favorite item for boys, whereas girls prefer colorful beads.

When such objects are placed into the nose or mouth, they can be aspirated into the airway, causing subsequent obstruction. Ingestion or aspiration of an FB can occur at any age but is most common in older infants and children ages 1 to 3 years. Severity depends on the location, type of object aspirated, and extent of obstruction. For example, dry vegetable matter, such as a seed, nut, piece of carrot, or popcorn, that does not dissolve and that may swell when moistened creates a particularly difficult problem. The high fat content of potato chips and peanuts

*1301 Pennsylvania Ave., NW, Washington, DC 20004; 202-785-3355, 800-548-8252; www.lungusa.org.

may cause the added risk of lipoid pneumonia. "Fun foods" such as hard candy and hot dog wieners are among the worst offenders. Offending foods, in the order of frequency of aspiration, are hot dog, round candy, peanut or other nut, grape, cookie or biscuit, other meat, carrot, apple, peas, and peanut butter. Round foods are the most frequent offenders. The first four items together make up more than 40% of all aspirated food items. Other items include plastic or glass beads, button or disk batteries, and coins. Objects such as small lithium or cadmium batteries may cause esophageal or tracheal corrosion.

A sharp or irritating object produces irritation and edema. A round, pliable object that does not readily break apart is more likely to occlude an airway than an object with a different shape. A small object may cause little if any pathologic change, whereas an object of sufficient size to obstruct a passage can produce various changes, including atelectasis, emphysema, inflammation, and abscess.

Pathophysiology

Most inhaled FBs lodge in a mainstem or lobar bronchus, a few find their way into more distal portions of the lung field, and the remaining FBs lodge in the trachea. The site is determined by the object's size, weight, and configuration. For example, heavy objects such as bullets, coins, and nails are more likely to drop into the dependent portions of the tracheobronchial tree. The object may remain in the same location or move in the airway. It can be coughed from a smaller to a larger airway and reaspirated in a different passage—or it might be ejected forcefully into the mouth and subsequently swallowed.

Signs of obstruction caused by an FB in a bronchus are explained by the same mechanisms that control the flow of fluids in pipes (Fig. 32-6). During normal respiration the caliber of bronchi and bronchioles becomes larger during inspiration and smaller during expiration. When a small object partially obstructs a passage, air passes around the obstruction during both inspiration and expiration (bypass valve). In this type of obstruction a wheeze is heard. A somewhat larger obstruction will allow air to enter the distal portion when bronchioles enlarge during inspiration, but when they diminish in caliber during expiration, the lumen becomes occluded and air becomes trapped distal to the obstruction (check valve). This type of obstruction produces obstructive hyperinflation. When there is complete blockage of the bronchus by an FB or by the FB and swollen mucosa, air is unable to move in either direction (stop valve), and the air distal to the obstruction is absorbed, leaving an area of obstruction atelectasis. The right bronchus, with its shorter length and straighter angle, is the usual site of bronchial obstruction.

Clinical Manifestations

Initially, an FB in the air passages produces choking, gagging, or coughing, but symptoms depend on the site of obstruction and on the interval between aspiration and presentation. Up to half of all children with FB ingestion may be asymptomatic (Uyemura, 2005). Laryngotracheal obstruction most commonly causes dyspnea, cough, stridor, and hoarseness because of a decreased air entry. Cyanosis may also occur if the obstruction becomes worse. Bronchial obstruction usually produces

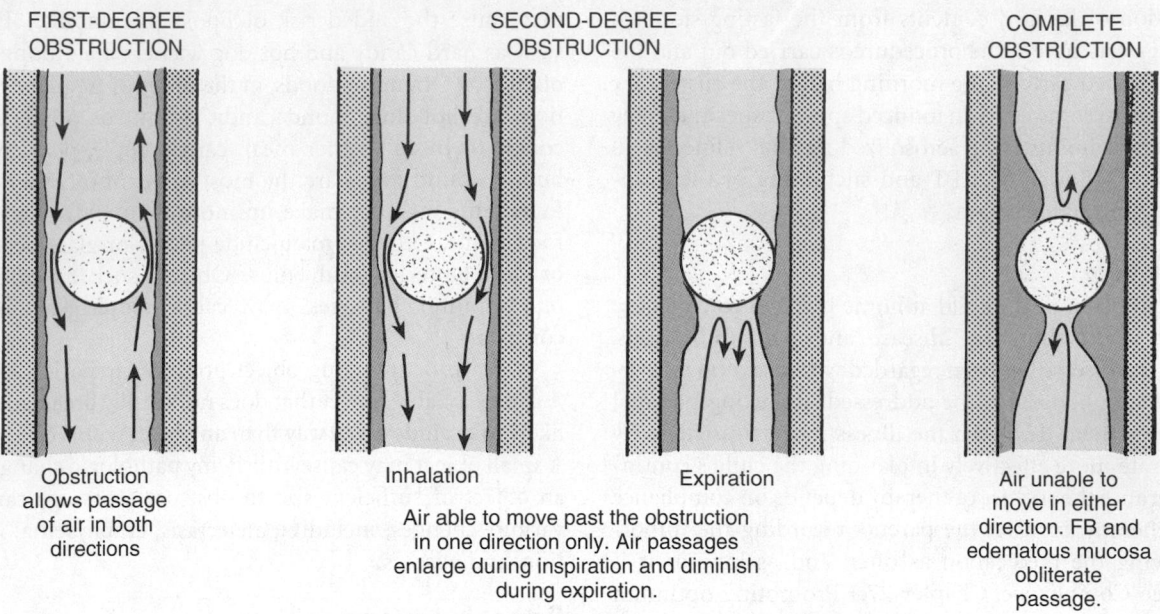

| FIRST-DEGREE OBSTRUCTION | SECOND-DEGREE OBSTRUCTION | | COMPLETE OBSTRUCTION |

Obstruction allows passage of air in both directions

Inhalation

Expiration

Air able to move past the obstruction in one direction only. Air passages enlarge during inspiration and diminish during expiration.

Air unable to move in either direction. FB and edematous mucosa obliterate passage.

Fig. 32-6 Mechanisms of airway obstruction by foreign body *(FB)*.

cough (frequently paroxysmal), wheezing, asymmetric breath sounds, decreased airway entry, and dyspnea.

If the obstruction progresses, the child's face may become livid, and sometimes the child becomes unconscious and dies of asphyxiation if the object is not removed. If obstruction is partial, hours, days, or even weeks may pass without symptoms after the initial period. Secondary symptoms are related to the anatomic area in which the FB is lodged and are usually caused by a persistent respiratory tract infection located distal to the obstruction. A history of recurrent intractable pneumonia is reason to consider an FB in an airway. Often, by the time secondary symptoms appear, the parents have forgotten the initial episode of coughing and gagging. The most common symptoms observed in children brought to medical attention are stridor, wheezing, sternal retraction, and cough. When an object is lodged in the larynx, the child is unable to speak or breathe.

Diagnostic Evaluation

The diagnosis of FB obstruction is usually suspected on the basis of the history and physical signs. Radiographic examination reveals opaque FBs but is of limited value in localizing vegetable matter and some plastic items. Bronchoscopy is required for a definitive diagnosis of objects in the larynx and trachea. Fluoroscopic examination is valuable in detecting FBs in the bronchi.

On fluoroscopy a check-valve–obstructed lung remains expanded, the diaphragm remains low and fixed on the obstructed side, and the heart and mediastinum shift to the unobstructed side during expiration. In a stop-valve obstruction the heart and mediastinum are drawn to the obstructed side and remain there during both inspiration and expiration. The diaphragm on the obstructed side remains high, whereas that on the unobstructed side moves normally.

The mainstay of diagnosis and management of foreign bodies is endoscopy. If there is doubt about the presence of an FB, endoscopy can be diagnostic and therapeutic. When endoscopy is used to remove an FB, the procedure should be performed by an endoscopist who is experienced and comfortable in caring for children. The endoscopist should also have access to state-of-the-art endoscopy equipment and should perform the procedure in a setting that can accommodate any complication or emergency.

Therapeutic Management

FB aspiration may result in life-threatening airway obstruction, especially in infants because of the small diameters of their airways. Current recommendations for the emergency treatment of the choking child include the use of abdominal thrusts for children over 1 year of age and back blows and chest thrusts for children less than 1 year of age. (See Cardiopulmonary Resuscitation, Chapter 31.) An FB is rarely coughed up spontaneously; therefore it must be removed by endoscopy. Removal of the FB must be done as soon as possible, since the progressive local inflammatory process triggered by the foreign material hampers removal. In addition, a chemical pneumonia soon develops and vegetable matter begins to macerate within a few days, further complicating its removal.

Nursing Care Management

A major role of nurses is to recognize the signs of FB aspiration and implement immediate measures to relieve the obstruction. All persons working with children should be prepared to deal effectively with aspiration of an FB. Choking on food or other material should not be fatal. Two simple procedures—back blows and the abdominal thrust, which can be used by both health professionals and laypersons—can save lives. It is the nurse's obligation to learn these techniques and teach them to parents and other groups. (See Figs. 31-26 and 31-27.) To aid a child who is choking, nurses need to recognize the signs of distress. Not every child who gags or coughs while eating is truly choking.

Prevention

Small children should not be allowed access to small objects that they might place in their nose or mouth. Anticipatory guidance for parents of small children is essential. Nurses are in a position to teach prevention in a variety of settings (see Community Focus box). They can educate parents singly or in groups about hazards of aspiration in relation to the developmental level of their children and encourage them to teach their children safety. Caution parents about behaviors that their children might imitate (e.g., holding foreign objects, such as pins, nails, and toothpicks, in their lips or mouth). (Chapters 12 and 14 discuss prevention based on the child's age.)

🏠 COMMUNITY FOCUS

Foreign Body Aspiration

Everyone who has contact with young children between the ages of 9 months and 3 years should be on guard for potential situations in which these children could aspirate small pieces of food, toys, or other objects. In general, pediatric nurses should teach parents about the dangers of aspiration and how to keep their children safe. In addition, pediatric nurses are in an excellent position to educate ancillary health personnel, daycare providers, and baby-sitters. In the school setting, nurses should also be alert to situations in which younger siblings might be at risk for aspiration of small objects found in the school. Nurses can become more active in their communities by alerting toy manufacturers of potentially unsafe toys and games.

BOX 32-15   CONDITIONS THAT INCREASE RISK OF ASPIRATION

Altered Level of Consciousness
Central nervous system injury or disease (e.g., meningitis, seizures, paralysis, trauma, poisoning, toxic ingestion)
Sedation
General anesthesia
Cardiopulmonary resuscitation

Dysphagia
Esophageal dysmotility
Neurologic deficit
Gastroesophageal reflux

Mechanical Disruption of Defensive Barriers
Endotracheal tube
Tracheostomy
Cleft lip/palate
Feeding tube (orogastric or nasogastric)

Persistent Vomiting
Gastrointestinal infection
Chemotherapy
Postanesthesia

Modified from Hazinski MF, editor: *Nursing care of the critically ill child*, ed 2, St Louis, 1992, Mosby.

FOREIGN BODY IN THE NOSE

Children sometimes place foreign objects, such as food (peanuts are a favorite), crayons, small plastic toys, pieces of plastic, beans, beads, erasers, wads of paper, round peas, and small stones, into their nose. An FB is suspected when there is unilateral nasal discharge that is foul smelling, local obstruction with sneezing, mild discomfort, and (rarely) pain. The irritation produces local mucosal swelling if the items increase in size as they absorb moisture (hygroscopic). Signs of obstruction and discomfort may increase with time. Infection usually follows, as evidenced by foul breath and a purulent or bloody discharge from one nostril.

Although the object is usually situated anteriorly, unskilled attempts at removal may move it further posteriorly. Removal should occur as soon as possible to prevent the risk of aspiration and local tissue necrosis. Removal usually occurs easily with either forceps or suction. In some cases mild sedation may be necessary.

ASPIRATION PNEUMONIA

Aspiration pneumonia occurs when food, secretions, inert materials, volatile compounds, or liquids enter the lung and cause inflammation and a chemical pneumonitis. Many conditions increase the risk of aspiration (Box 32-15). Aspiration of fluid or food substances is particularly hazardous in the child who has difficulty swallowing or is unable to swallow because of paralysis, weakness, debility, congenital anomalies such as cleft palate or tracheoesophageal fistula, or absent cough reflex (unconsciousness) or who is force fed, especially while crying or breathing rapidly.

Clinical signs of the aspiration of oral secretions may not be distinguishable from other forms of acute bacterial pneumonia. For example, if vegetable matter has been aspirated, manifestations may not appear for several weeks after the event. Classic symptoms include an increasing cough or fever with foul-smelling sputum, deteriorating chest radiographs, and other signs of lower airway involvement. These deviations may persist for weeks, however, while the child starts to feel better.

Hydrocarbon Pneumonia

Children frequently develop pneumonia secondary to the ingestion of various forms of hydrocarbons, such as kerosene, gasoline, solvents, lighter fluid, furniture polish, and mineral oil. Petroleum distillates are generally impure substances contaminated with heavy metals or other toxic chemicals that cause systemic, as well as local, effects. Many hydrocarbons are made from petroleum and are found in the home or garage.

Hydrocarbons are usually packaged in attractive containers, and some have a pleasant aroma; consequently, they are frequently ingested accidentally by young children. On average, children swallow less than 30 ml (often about 3 to 4 ml). They begin coughing severely and swallow no more. Although central nervous system abnormalities, gastrointestinal irritation, cardiomyopathy, and renal toxicity can occur, the most serious complication is pneumonitis.

Distillates that have high volatility (evaporate quickly), decreased viscosity (thinner solution), and low surface tension are more likely to be aspirated and produce respiratory complications. Decreased viscosity enhances penetration into distal airways. Lower surface tension facilitates spread over a larger area of lung surface. Consequently, ingestion of lighter fluid, kerosene, or gasoline is more likely to cause a pathologic condition than substances that have high viscosity (e.g., petroleum jelly, tar, or lubricating oil).

Pathogenesis

The severity of the lung injury depends on the pH of the aspirated material, the presence of bacteria, and the volatility and viscosity of the substance. Irritation from aspiration during swallowing, vomiting, or gastric lavage may also cause pulmonary involvement. Pathologic changes include signs of inflammation (edema, hyperemia, infiltration of polymorphonuclear cells); vascular thrombosis and hemorrhage; and necrosis of bronchial, bronchiolar, and alveolar tissues. Other reactions are bronchospasm, atelectasis, emphysema, pulmonary hemorrhage, necrosis, surfactant impairment, and pulmonary edema. Even in small amounts, hydrocarbons spread over the surface of tissues and the lungs and interfere with gas exchange. Aspiration of inert fluids may not produce a chemical or bacterial pneumonia, but these fluids can decrease lung compliance and cause hypoxemia.

Clinical Manifestations

Acid aspiration may produce immediate pulmonary symptoms that worsen over the first 24 hours. Coughing and vomiting, which occur almost immediately after ingestion, contribute to the aspiration. Central nervous system symptoms include agitation, restlessness, confusion, drowsiness, and coma. The temperature is elevated (37.8° to 40° C [100° to 104° F]). (See Ingestion of Injurious Agents, Chapter 16.)

After swallowing, coughing, and choking, the child becomes short of breath, and older children complain of dyspnea. There are varying degrees of cyanosis, tachycardia, tachypnea, nasal flaring, and retractions. Intercostal retractions, grunting, cough, and fever may appear within 30 minutes or be delayed for a few hours. Localized areas of dullness are felt on percussion, and moderately intense wheezes and crackles are heard. Severe injury causes hemoptysis, pulmonary edema, severe cyanosis, and death within 24 hours of aspiration.

Therapeutic Management

Inducing the child to vomit is contraindicated because of the renewed danger of aspiration. Hydrocarbons are readily absorbed by the gastrointestinal tract and excreted by the lungs. Bronchitis or pneumonia usually develops early (within the first 24 hours) but may be delayed. Recovery from pulmonary involvement occurs in most instances despite a severe clinical course. Death is generally the result of hepatic failure complicated by pulmonary factors. Treatment is the same as for any lower respiratory tract inflammation and consists of high humidity, supplemental oxygen, hydration, and treatment of any secondary infection. Endotracheal intubation may be required if the child develops respiratory failure.

Lipoid Pneumonia

Oily substances aspirated into the respiratory passages initially cause an interstitial proliferative inflammation that may include an exudative pneumonia. The next stage involves a diffuse, chronic, proliferative fibrosis that is often complicated by acute bronchopneumonia. The final stage features multiple localized nodules or tumorlike paraffinomas. There are no characteristic manifestations. Cough is usually present, and dyspnea occurs in severe cases. Secondary bronchopneumonia is common. The outcome depends on the extent of pulmonary damage, the general condition of the infant or child, and discontinuation of the oily inhalation. No specific treatment exists.

Powder Inhalation

A significant number of infants suffer talcum powder aspiration. Commercial talcum powder is predominantly a mixture of talc (hydrous magnesium silicate) and other silicates. Severe respiratory distress occurs immediately as a result of an inflammatory reaction in small bronchioles initiated by deep inhalation of the extremely light powder. (See Chapter 12 for further discussion of powder inhalation.)

Nursing Care Management

Care of the child with aspiration pneumonia is the same as that described for the child with pneumonia from other causes. However, the major focus of nursing care is on *prevention* of aspiration. Proper feeding techniques should be carried out for weak, debilitated, and uncooperative children, and measures should be taken to prevent aspiration of any material that might enter the nasopharynx. Nasogastric tubes used for feedings are checked before the initiation of bolus feedings; continuous nasogastric tube feedings are also evaluated periodically for proper tube placement. Children who are at risk for swallowing difficulties as a result of illness, physical debilitation, anesthesia, or sedation are kept NPO (nothing by mouth) until they can properly swallow fluids effectively. The child who is at risk for vomiting and incapable of protecting the airway should be positioned in a side-lying recovery position. (See Fig. 31-28.)

Oily nose drops and oil-based vitamin preparations are not appropriate for infants and small children. Solvents, lighter fluid, and other hydrocarbon substances should be kept away from older infants and small children, who are likely to put anything in their mouth and who may be attracted by the slightly sweet smell.

Talcum powder should not be used. If used, careful application (placing it on the caregiver's hand and then on the child's skin) and proper storage are essential.

ACUTE RESPIRATORY DISTRESS SYNDROME AND ACUTE LUNG INJURY

ARDS occurs in children and adults and has been associated with clinical conditions and injuries such as sepsis, trauma, viral pneumonia, fat emboli, drug overdose, reperfusion injury after lung transplantation, smoke inhalation, and near-drowning. ARDS is characterized by respiratory distress and hypoxemia that occur within 72 hours of a serious injury or surgery in a person with previously normal lungs. ALI is said to involve a spectrum of inflammatory disease responses to a precipitating event, with ARDS being the more severe form of ALI (Frye, 2005; Randolph, 2009).

ARDS and ALI cause acute respiratory failure and account for significant morbidity and mortality in critically ill patients. Acute pulmonary inflammation with alveolar capillary membrane destruction results in significant hypoxemia, and mechanical ventilation is often required. ARDS is the most severe in the spectrum of illnesses in relation to the degree of hypoxemia. Hypoxemia is expressed as the ratio of partial pressure of oxygen (Pao_2) to fraction of inspired oxygen (Fio_2), or P/F ratio, with the P/F ratio for ALI being 300 or less and the P/F ratio for ARDS being 200 or less. Both ALI and ARDS demonstrate radiographic evidence of bilateral alveolar infiltrates without evidence of left-sided heart failure (Rice and Bernard, 2006).

The hallmark of ARDS is increased permeability of the alveolocapillary membrane that results in pulmonary edema. During the acute phase of ARDS, the alveolocapillary membrane is damaged, with an increasing pulmonary capillary permeability and resulting interstitial edema. Later stages are characterized by pneumocyte and fibrin infiltration of the alveoli, with the start of either the healing process or fibrosis. When fibrosis occurs, the child may demonstrate respiratory distress and the need for mechanical ventilation. In ARDS the lungs become stiff as a result of surfactant inactivation, gas diffusion is impaired, and eventually bronchiolar mucosal swelling and congestive atelectasis occur. The net effect is decreased functional residual capacity, pulmonary hypertension, and increased intrapulmonary right-to-left shunting of pulmonary blood flow. Surfactant secretion is reduced, and the atelectasis and fluid-filled alveoli provide an excellent medium for bacterial growth (Fig. 32-7).

The criteria for diagnosis of ARDS in children are an acute antecedent illness or injury, acute respiratory distress or failure, severe arterial hypoxemia (see above) unresponsive to oxygen therapy alone, no evidence of left atrial hypertension, and diffuse bilateral infiltrates evidenced on chest radiography (Randolph, 2009). The child with ARDS may first demonstrate only symptoms caused by an injury or infection, but as the condition deteriorates, hyperventilation, tachypnea, increasing respiratory effort, cyanosis, and decreasing oxygen saturation occur. In one study severe sepsis with pneumonia as the primary infection focus was the leading cause of ALI (Zimmerman, Akhtar, Caldwell, et al, 2009).

Therapeutic Management

Treatment involves supportive measures such as maintenance of adequate oxygenation and pulmonary perfusion, treatment of infection (or the precipitating cause), maintenance of adequate cardiac output and vascular volume, hydration, adequate nutritional support, comfort measures, prevention of complications such as gastrointestinal ulceration and aspiration, and psychologic support. Prone positioning may be used to improve oxygenation, but studies have not demonstrated prone positioning to decrease the total number of days on mechanical ventilation; in addition this requires close communication and coordination among the health care team (Curley, Hibberd, Fineman, et al, 2005; Frye, 2005). Definitive therapy is directed toward improvement of oxygenation. The use of endotracheal intubation, positive end-expiratory pressure, and low tidal volume may be required to ensure maximum oxygen delivery by increasing functional residual capacity, reducing intrapulmonary shunting, and reducing pulmonary fluid. Ventilation with low tidal volume (6 ml/kg of ideal body weight) has been associated with lower mortality rates in children with ALI (Albuali, Singh, Fraser, et al, 2007; Hanson and Flori, 2006).

Additional supportive strategies in the treatment of ARDS in children include the use of permissive hypercapnia, inhaled nitric oxide, exogenous surfactant administration, high-frequency ventilation, partial liquid ventilation, and extracorporeal life support (extracorporeal membrane oxygenation, or ECMO). Exogenous surfactant therapy has increased oxygenation status in infants and children with ARDS-ALI and decreased disease severity (Willson, Chess, and Notter, 2008). Once the underlying cause is identified, specific treatment (e.g., antibiotics for infection) is initiated.

Prognosis

In spite of advances in understanding and treating ARDS-ALI, childhood mortality rates of 18% to 49% have been reported (Albuali, Singh, Fraser, et al, 2007; Randolph, 2009), and prolonged respiratory failure requiring an average of 10 to 16 days on mechanical ventilation is common (Randolph, 2009). The precipitating disorder influences the outcome. The worst prognosis is associated with profound hypoxemia, uncontrolled sepsis, bone marrow transplantation, cancer, and multisystem involvement with hepatic failure. Children who recover may have persistent cough and exertional dyspnea.

Nursing Care Management

The child with ARDS is cared for in intensive care during the acute stages of illness. Nursing care involves close monitoring of oxygenation and respiratory status, cardiac output, perfusion, fluid and electrolyte balance, and renal function (urinary output). Blood gas analysis and pulse oximetry are important evaluation tools. Parenteral and enteral nutritional support is often required because of the length of the acute phase of the illness. Medications are administered to reduce pulmonary fluid, decrease pulmonary hypertension, and treat the underlying cause (e.g., antibiotics for sepsis). Nursing management also includes managing pain, monitoring the effects of the numerous parenteral fluids and drugs used to stabilize the child, and monitoring for changes in the child's hemodynamic status. Most children with ARDS require invasive monitoring via a central venous line and possibly a pulmonary artery catheter to monitor oxygenation and administer medications. The nursing

PATHOPHYSIOLOGY REVIEW

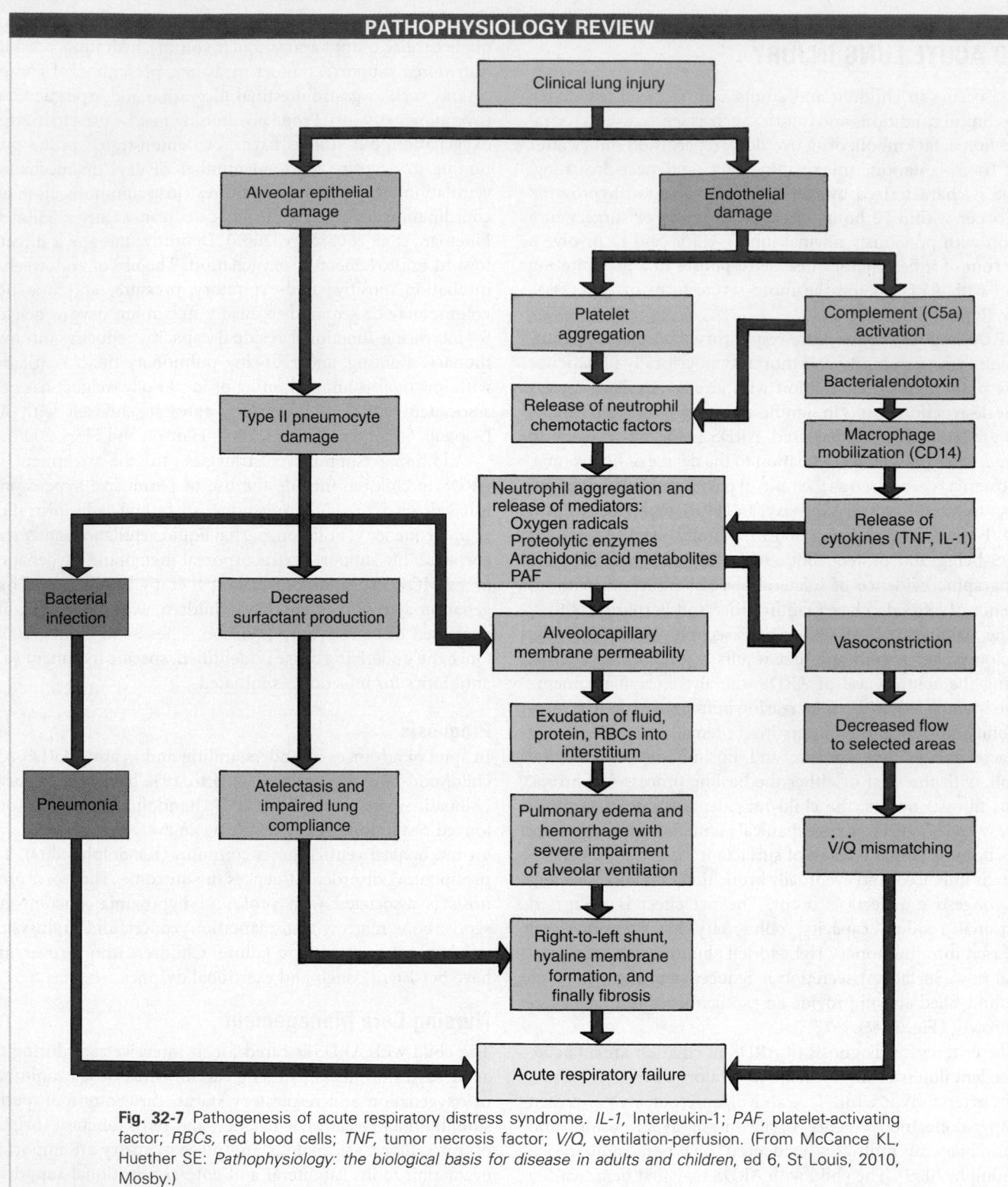

Fig. 32-7 Pathogenesis of acute respiratory distress syndrome. *IL-1,* Interleukin-1; *PAF,* platelet-activating factor; *RBCs,* red blood cells; *TNF,* tumor necrosis factor; *V̇/Q̇,* ventilation-perfusion. (From McCance KL, Huether SE: *Pathophysiology: the biological basis for disease in adults and children,* ed 6, St Louis, 2010, Mosby.)

care of the child with ARDS also involves close observation of skin condition and prevention of breakdown, passive range of motion for prevention of muscle atrophy and contractures, and nutritional support.

Respiratory distress is a frightening situation for both the child and the parents, and attention to their psychologic needs is a major element in the care of these children. The child is often sedated during the acute phase of the illness, and weaning from sedation requires close monitoring for anxiety reduction

and comfort. Because the mortality rate of ARDS is high, keep the family informed of the child's status, progression through the various stages of the illness, and, as appropriate, the possibility of death. (See Chapter 23.)

SMOKE INHALATION INJURY

A number of noxious substances that may be inhaled are toxic to humans. They are primarily products of incomplete combustion and cause more deaths from fires than flame injuries do. The severity of the injury depends on the nature of the substances generated by the material being burned, whether the victim is confined in a closed space, and the duration of contact with the smoke.

General Aspects

Possible inhalation injury is suspected when there is a history of flames in a closed space, whether or not burns are present. Sooty material around the nose or in the sputum; singed nasal hairs; or mucosal burns of the nose, lips, mouth, or throat are all signs that the affected person requires observation for possible pulmonary injury from inhalants. A hoarse voice and cough are further evidence of airway involvement, and increased inspiratory and expiratory stridor indicates severe damage to the upper passages. Signs of respiratory distress also include tachypnea; tachycardia; and diminished or abnormal breath sounds, including crackles and wheezes.

Three distinct syndromes of pulmonary complications may occur in the child suffering from inhalation injury: (1) early carbon monoxide poisoning, airway obstruction, and pulmonary edema; (2) ARDS occurring at 24 to 48 hours, or later in some cases; and (3) late complications of bronchopneumonia, and pulmonary emboli (Antoon and Donovan, 2007). Strangulation may also occur from the cervical eschar secondary to a severe burn.

Smoke inhalation causes three different types of injury: heat, local chemical, and systemic.

Heat Injury

Heat causes thermal injury to the upper airway, but because air has low specific heat, the injury goes no farther than the upper airway. Reflex closure of the glottis prevents injury to the lower airway. Heat may reach the middle airway occasionally, but it rarely penetrates to the lungs.

Chemical Injury

The combustion of materials such as clothing, furniture, and floor coverings can generate a wide variety of gases. Acids, alkalis, and their precursors in smoke can produce chemical burns. These substances can be carried deep into the respiratory tract, including the lower respiratory tract, in the form of insoluble gases. Soluble gases tend to dissolve in the upper respiratory tract.

Synthetic materials are especially toxic, producing gases such as oxides of sulfur and nitrogen, acetaldehyde, formaldehyde, hydrocyanic acid, and chlorine. Heated plastics are the source of extremely toxic vapors, including chlorine and hydrochloric acid from polyvinylchloride, and hydrocarbons, aldehydes, ketones, and acids from polyethylene. Irritant gases such as nitrous oxide or carbon dioxide combine with water in the lungs to form corrosive acids. Aldehydes cause denaturation of proteins, cellular damage, and edema of pulmonary tissues. Chemical burns to the airways are similar to burns on the skin, except they are painless because the tracheobronchial tree is relatively insensitive to pain.

Inhalation of small amounts of noxious irritants produces alveolar and bronchiolar damage that can lead to obstructive bronchiolitis. Severe exposure causes further injury, including alveolocapillary damage with hemorrhage, necrotizing bronchiolitis, and inhibited secretion of surfactant, with resultant atelectasis.

Systemic Injury

Gases that are nontoxic to the airways (e.g., carbon monoxide, hydrogen cyanide) can cause injury and death by interfering with or inhibiting cellular respiration. Carbon monoxide is a colorless, odorless gas with an affinity for hemoglobin 230 times greater than that of oxygen. When carbon monoxide enters the bloodstream, it readily binds with hemoglobin to form carboxyhcmoglobin (COHb). Because carbon monoxide combines more readily and is released less readily than oxygen, very low levels of tissue oxygen must be reached before appreciable amounts of oxygen are released from the hemoglobin. Therefore tissue hypoxia reaches dangerous levels before oxygen is available to meet tissue needs.

> ### ! NURSING ALERT
>
> With carbon monoxide poisoning, the oxygen saturation (Sao_2) obtained by pulse oximetry will be normal because the device measures only oxygenated and deoxygenated hemoglobin; it does not measure dysfunctional hemoglobin, such as COHb.

Accidental carbon monoxide poisoning is most often a result of exposure to fumes from heaters or smoke from structural fires, although poorly ventilated recreational vehicles with improperly operated or maintained gas lamps or stoves and cooking in underventilated areas with charcoal grills or hibachis are also frequent causes. Intentional carbon monoxide poisoning may occur in an attempted suicide in the vehicle parked in a closed garage for a long period. Accidental carbon monoxide poisoning may also occur in a vehicle with inadequate vented exhaust which leaks into the vehicle's passenger (or closed truck bed) compartment. Carbon monoxide is produced by incomplete combustion of carbon or carbonaceous material, such as wood or charcoal.

The signs and symptoms of carbon monoxide poisoning are secondary to tissue hypoxia and vary with the level of COHb. Mild manifestations include headache, visual disturbances, irritability, and nausea, whereas more severe intoxication causes confusion, hallucinations, ataxia, and coma. Carbon monoxide may increase cerebral blood flow, increase cerebral capillary permeability, and increase cerebrospinal fluid pressure, all of which contribute to the central nervous system signs observed. The bright, cherry red lips and skin often described are less common than pallor and cyanosis.

Therapeutic Management

The treatment of children with smoke toxicity is largely symptomatic. The most widely accepted treatment is placing the child on humidified 100% oxygen as quickly as possible and monitoring for signs of respiratory distress and impending failure. Blood gases are drawn to determine baseline arterial blood gases and COHb levels. Arterial oxygen partial pressure may be within normal limits unless there is marked respiratory depression. If carbon monoxide poisoning is confirmed, 100%

oxygen is continued until COHb levels fall to the nontoxic range of about 10%.

Respiratory distress may occur early in the course of smoke inhalation as a result of hypoxia, or patients who are breathing well on admission may suddenly develop respiratory distress. Therefore endotracheal intubation equipment should be readily available. Transient edema of the airways can occur at any level in the tracheobronchial tree. Assessment and localization of the obstruction should be accomplished before severe swelling of the head, neck, or oropharynx occurs. Intubation is often necessary when (1) severe burns in the area of the nose, mouth, and face increase the likelihood of developing oropharyngeal edema and obstruction; (2) vocal cord edema causes obstruction; (3) the patient has difficulty handling secretions; and (4) progressive respiratory distress requires artificial ventilation. Controversy surrounds tracheotomy, but many prefer this procedure when the obstruction is proximal to the larynx and reserve nasotracheal intubation for lower tract involvement.

Pulmonary care may be facilitated by bronchodilators, inhaled corticosteroids, humidification, and CPT to enhance the removal of necrotic material, minimize bronchoconstriction, and avoid atelectasis. Bronchoscopy may be needed to clear heavy secretions.

Carbon monoxide is excreted primarily through the lungs. Treatment of carbon monoxide intoxication with 100% oxygen via nonrebreathing face mask reduces the COHb level by one half in 40 to 60 minutes. Hyperbaric oxygen may be required for severe carbon monoxide poisoning (COHb level >25% in children) (Rodgers, Condurache, Reed, et al, 2007).

Nursing Care Management

Nursing care of the child with inhalation injury is the same as that for any child with respiratory distress. The initial goal is to maintain a patent airway and effective ventilation status; endotracheal intubation may be required early depending on the patient's respiratory status and the progression of airway and pulmonary edema. (See also Respiratory Failure, Chapter 31.) In the acute phase take vital signs, oxygenation, work of breathing, and other respiratory assessments frequently, and carefully observe and maintain the pulmonary status. The administration of nebulized bronchodilators, humidified oxygen, and inhaled corticosteroids is often part of the nursing care if a respiratory specialist is not available. CPT is also an important part of the therapeutic program. IV fluids are often required to maintain adequate hydration if the patient's respiratory status is deteriorating. Fluid requirements for children experiencing inhalation injury are greater than for those with surface burns alone. However, one concern is the development of pulmonary edema; therefore accurate monitoring of intake and output is essential. For the patient requiring mechanical ventilation, the nurse monitors respiratory status and ensures airway patency is maintained. Such patients may be mildly sedated initially; once they are alert, the nurse reassures the patients of the temporary nature of the inability to speak, effectively manages any pain they are experiencing, and implements comfort measures.

In addition to the observation and management of the physical aspects of inhalation injury, the nurse also deals with the psychologic needs of a frightened child and distraught parents.

Parents need support; reassurance; and information about their child's condition, treatment, and progress.

ENVIRONMENTAL TOBACCO SMOKE EXPOSURE

Numerous investigations indicate that parental smoking is an important cause of morbidity in children. Children exposed to passive or environmental tobacco smoke have an increased number of respiratory illnesses, increased respiratory symptoms (e.g., cough, sputum, and wheezing), and reduced performance on pulmonary function tests (PFTs). AOM and OME are also increased in children who have smoking parents. Indoor exposure to environmental tobacco smoke has been linked to asthma in children (Morkjaroenpong, Rand, Butz, et al, 2002). Among children with asthma, there is an association between parental cigarette smoking and asthma exacerbations, trips to the emergency department, medication use, and impaired recovery after hospitalization for acute asthma. Children exposed to second-hand smoke experience more wheezing episodes as infants. Maternal cigarette smoking is associated with increased respiratory symptoms and illnesses in children; decreased fetal growth; increased deliveries of low-birth-weight, preterm, and stillborn infants; and a greater incidence of sudden infant death syndrome (SIDS). Antenatal maternal smoking has emerged as a significant risk factor for SIDS (American Academy of Pediatrics, 2005). The risk for diagnosis of early-onset asthma in the first 3 years of life is associated with in utero exposure to maternal smoking; grand-maternal smoking was also associated with an increased risk of early-onset asthma in the grandchild even if the mother did not smoke during pregnancy (Li, Langholz, Salam, et al, 2005). Exposure to tobacco smoke during childhood may also contribute to the development of bronchopulmonary dysplasia in the adult.

State, federal, and local governments have enacted legislation prohibiting smoking in public and work places. Children experience more second-hand smoke exposure in the home setting than anywhere else. The impact of tobacco smoke also contributes to an increase in childhood deaths attributed to residential fires in households where adults smoke. The financial impact of second-hand smoke exposure is significant. The Centers for Disease Control and Prevention (2008) estimates that from 2001 to 2004 the average annual smoking-attributable health care expenditures were $96 billion.

Recently concern has grown regarding third-hand tobacco exposure—the tobacco toxins that remain in the environment long after the smoker has stopped smoking. Such toxins may be found in elevators, cars, and homes and on clothing. The 2006 surgeon general's report concluded there is no risk-free level of tobacco exposure because of the residual effects of the chemical toxins in tobacco (Surgeon General Report, 2006). The effect of such chemicals on the developing child's brain are under evaluation.

The amount of passive smoke exposure in infants and children is directly related to the presence of smoking parents and the number of smokers in a household. Past studies that have measured passive smoke exposure have analyzed the amount of cotinine in a child's urine (Winkelstein, Tarzian, and

Wood, 1997; Olivieri, Bodini, Peroni, et al, 2006). Cotinine, a by-product of nicotine, is considered a valid biochemical marker for environmental smoke exposure. Urinary cotinine levels are increased in children who live in homes with smokers, and these levels increase proportionally with the number of smokers in the home. Cotinine levels have also been used to document exposure to passive smoke in the fetus and newborn.

Nursing Care Management

Passive smoke exposure during childhood may also contribute to the development of bronchopulmonary dysplasia in adulthood, and some have attributed infertility in adults to exposure to second-hand smoke as children. Nurses and other health care professionals need to include assessments of passive smoke exposure in all children, especially those with respiratory illnesses. In families where smokers refuse to quit, house rules should be established for reducing smoke in the child's environment. Nurses should also inform caregivers of the health hazards of children's exposure to tobacco smoke*; set an example for children and families; and become advocates for "no smoking" ordinances in public places, prohibition of advertising tobacco products in the media, and inclusion of health warnings of sidestream smoke on tobacco products. Nurses also have an important role in offering tobacco smoking cessation counseling and in teaching such classes in the community at large. The role of the nurse in promoting smoking cessation among adolescents is discussed in Chapter 21.

LONG-TERM RESPIRATORY DYSFUNCTION

ALLERGIC RHINITIS

Allergic rhinitis affects as many as 20% to 40% of the pediatric population (Ahmad and Zacharek, 2008) and is associated with numerous airway disorders, including asthma, OME, and chronic sinusitis. Seasonal allergic rhinitis (also known as hay fever) usually follows a spring-fall pattern and is caused by tree, grass, and weed pollens. Seasonal allergic rhinitis usually does not develop until the individual has been sensitized by two or more pollen seasons. Year-round or perennial allergic rhinitis is more common and is triggered by household inhaled allergens such as feathers, household dust, animal dander, air pollutants, and molds. Peak incidence for allergic rhinitis is in the adolescent and postadolescent age-groups, but younger children are also affected. The risk for allergic rhinitis is increased in children exposed to tobacco smoke and is also associated with early feeding of milk and foods in early infancy (Milgrom and Leung, 2007). Allergic rhinitis may be further classified as seasonal allergic rhinitis (SAR) and perennial allergic rhinitis (PAR). SAR has a cyclic, well-defined course, and PAR causes year-round symptoms (Ahmad and Zacharek, 2008; Milgrom and Leung, 2007).

Pathophysiology

Allergic rhinitis requires two conditions: a familial predisposition to develop allergy and exposure of a sensitized person to the allergen. Inhalants in the form of microscopic airborne particles (e.g., pollens, mold, animal danders, and environmental dusts) enter the upper respiratory tract with inhalation and bind to submucosal mast cells in the respiratory tract epithelium.

In the allergic child, symptoms are mediated by immunoglobulin E (IgE), which is produced by the child's B lymphocytes. The IgE molecules on the cell surfaces trigger the rapid release of mast cell mediators (e.g., histamine, prostaglandins, and leukotrienes), as well as the slower synthesis of cell interactive compounds called cytokines; this action is often called the early-phase response, which occurs about 10 to 30 minutes after allergen exposure (Ahmad and Zacharek, 2008; Milgrom and Leung, 2007). Histamine, a potent vasodilator, acts directly on local receptors to produce vasodilation, mucosal edema, and increased production of mucus. The cytokines summon cells to the area and are responsible for the slower late-phase allergic reaction of inflammation and destruction of the mucosal surface, which progresses to chronic nasal obstruction. The late phase response typically occurs 4 to 8 hours after antigen exposure as a result of the migration of neutrophils, basophils, eosinophils, macrophages, and T lymphocytes into the nasal mucosa (Ahmad and Zacharek, 2008). Repeated exposure of these sensitized membranes to specific aeroallergens results in clinical allergic disease.

Clinical Manifestations

Children who have allergic rhinitis have a history of watery rhinorrhea, nasal obstruction, sneezing, or nasal pruritus. Symptoms may be chronic, recurrent, or acute and include itching of the nose, eyes, palate, pharynx, and conjunctiva. The nasal stuffiness sometimes progresses to partial or total obstruction of airflow, and mucus secretion with postnasal drainage can occur. Nasal itching is troublesome, and the affected child attempts to alleviate the symptoms by rubbing the nose—the "allergic salute" (Fig. 32-8). Other symptoms include snoring

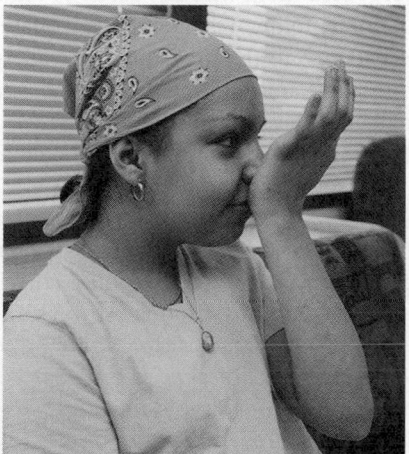

Fig. 32-8 "Allergic salute." (Courtesy Paul Vincent Kuntz, Texas Children's Hospital, Houston.)

---

*For a copy of the Environmental Protection Agency report *Respiratory Health Effects of Passive Smoking*, visit http://cfpub.epa.gov/ncea/CFM/recordisplay.cfm?deid=2835.

during sleep, fatigue, malaise, and poor school performance. Frequently children have an associated URI.

On physical examination, children may display dark circles beneath their eyes, or "allergic shiners," secondary to obstruction of normal outflow from regional lymphatics and veins. If the nasal obstruction is severe, the child becomes an obligate mouth breather and is seen with an open mouth, or "allergic gape." Facial findings include a horizontal nasal crease across the lower third of the nose caused by frequent rubbing induced by the nasal pruritus, and Dennie lines, or extra wrinkles below the lower eyelids. The child may develop facial tics and mannerisms in an attempt to avoid scratching the nose. Examination of the child's nose often reveals a pale, boggy nasal mucosa with enlarged nasal turbinates.

Symptoms that appear during peak symptom periods include tearing and soreness of the eyes and gelatinous conjunctival discharge in the morning, irritability, fatigue, depression, and loss of appetite.

When the nurse suspects allergic rhinitis, it is important to obtain information regarding clinical signs of related disorders, including middle ear disease, ear pain, delayed speech or language development, chronic cough, wheezing, exercise intolerance, eczema, or urticaria. It is also important to ask about any family history of allergies and to obtain information about specific triggers or environmental changes that may have precipitated an episode of rhinitis, such as seasonal pollens, pets, cigarette smoking, or the use of a woodburning stove for cooking or as a heat source. Chronic rhinitis with significant nasal obstruction can lead to various abnormalities in growth and in physical, psychosocial, and intellectual development.

Diagnostic Evaluation

Diagnosis of allergic rhinitis is based on a thorough history and physical examination. Because allergic rhinitis is often associated with atopic dermatitis or asthma, examination of the skin and chest is indicated. Diagnostic tests include a nasal smear to determine the number of eosinophils in the nasal secretions, blood examination for total IgE and elevated eosinophils, skin tests, and various challenge tests.

Skin testing is a useful adjunct in establishing a definitive diagnosis for allergic rhinitis. Skin testing involves the injection of specific allergens and should be performed by a practitioner trained in allergy treatment who has access to reliable reagents, experience in interpreting results, and adequate facilities to treat adverse reactions to the procedure. The allergenic extract is introduced into the epidermis by (1) scratch, prick, or puncture; (2) a single intradermal injection of a dilute concentration of specific allergen; or (3) serial dilution (threefold or tenfold) injections to determine the end point of reactivity. After a suitable time (10 to 30 seconds), the size of the resultant wheal and flare reaction is measured to assess the patient's sensitivity. The magnitude of the wheal and flare response correlates roughly with the severity of symptoms produced by natural exposure to the same allergen. However, a positive skin test does not always indicate the presence of clinical reactivity. Before skin testing occurs, the patient should withhold medications such as montelukast (Singulair) (1 day) and antihistamines (5 to 7 days for second generation and 3 or 4 days for first generation) to prevent false-negative results (Milgrom and Leung, 2007).

Skin testing and immunotherapy (see discussion below) are generally safe procedures, but they are not without risk. Severe and even fatal reactions can occur within a short time, depending on the type of extract used and individual sensitivity.

> **! NURSING ALERT**
>
> The onset of a reaction is often insidious. Mild initial symptoms may include local pruritus, pallor, flushing, cyanosis, shortness of breath, dyspnea, cough, malaise, or abdominal pain. Later developments include hypotension, airway obstruction, chest pain, ventricular fibrillation, and loss of consciousness.

Therapeutic Management

Therapy is directed toward avoidance of offending allergens and the use of medication and immunotherapy (hyposensitization or desensitization). Avoidance measures involve removing allergens from the environment and are usually effective for allergy to foods, drugs, and animals. If a patient is unable to avoid allergens, symptoms can be controlled with medication, but treatment should be individualized. Antihistamines and nasal corticosteroids are the first-line drugs used for allergic rhinitis.

Antihistamines are effective in treating sneezing, rhinorrhea, and nasal itching. Antihistamines act by inhibiting the effects of histamine by binding to H_1 receptors. Classic first-generation antihistamines such as diphenhydramine (Benadryl) and chlorpheniramine (Chlor-Trimeton) are effective but may produce undesirable side effects such as sedation, restlessness, dry mouth, urinary retention, constipation, and impaired school performance. The newer second-generation antihistamines such as loratadine (Claritin) and cetirizine hydrochloride (Zyrtec) are approved for use in children 6 months of age and older (Milgrom and Leung, 2007; Hagemann, 2005). Fexofenadine hydrochloride (Allegra) is approved for children 6 years of age and older. Azelastine is a topically active antihistamine available in nasal spray for children over 5 years old. These drugs are nonsedating and have few cardiovascular adverse effects.

If nasal obstruction is a prominent feature, children may use α-adrenergic decongestants, such as pseudoephedrine, in combination with an antihistamine to relieve nasal stuffiness. Nasal or oral administration of a decongestant often provides symptomatic relief. Take caution, however, with long-term use because of rebound effects (return of symptoms) and habituation (lessened effectiveness). Other side effects of these drugs include nervousness, insomnia, and tachycardia.

Topical nasal corticosteroids (beclomethasone [Vancenase and Beconase], flunisolide [Nasalide], fluticasone [Flovent], triamcinolone [Nasacort], mometasone [Nasonex], and budesonide [Rhinocort or Pulmicort]) are safe, effective alternatives to the use of cromolyn sodium and can be used effectively on a short-term basis during periods of exacerbation. Side effects are minimal, with occasional nasal irritation and epistaxis. Inhaled corticosteroids are administered with the nasal tip pointing away from the nasal septum (cartilage). Experts have expressed concerns in relation to possible decreased linear growth in children who take intranasal corticosteroids. To date, studies have not conclusively demonstrated growth failure, yet the American Academy of Allergy, Asthma and Immunology suggests taking height measurements every 6 months in children receiving long-term inhaled corticosteroids (Hagemann, 2005).

Cromolyn sodium is used prophylactically on a regular basis and is effective in preventing both the early and the late responses to antigen. Its usefulness is limited by the fact that it must be taken four to six times a day, a schedule that is difficult to maintain in children. Ipratropium bromide (Atrovent), available as a nasal spray, may be used for serious rhinorrhea but should be limited to 3 to 5 days per month (Milgrom and Leung, 2007).

The leukotriene modifier montelukast has been approved for children 2 years and older in the management of seasonal allergic rhinitis. It is approved for patients 6 months or older with perennial allergic rhinitis. In adults and adolescents the drug has been effective in decreasing symptoms, but there are no studies of their effects in younger children with allergic rhinitis. This class of drugs inhibits mucosal edema and mucus production and decreases bronchoconstriction.

⚡ DRUG ALERT

Montelukast

In June 2009 the U.S. Food and Drug Administration (FDA) issued a warning regarding cases of neuropsychiatric side effects in children taking the leukotriene modifier montelukast. Adverse effects include agitation, aggression, anxiety, hallucinations, depression, insomnia, and suicidal thoughts.

Immunotherapy may be necessary if drug therapy and avoidance of allergens are ineffective in controlling symptoms or if drugs evoke undesirable side effects. Before immunotherapy is begun, a positive skin test reaction to the allergen should be confirmed. Immunotherapy involves a series of injections with extracts of the specific allergens that cause symptoms for the child. Initially treatment is given weekly with dilute exposures, and the tolerated dosage is then gradually increased. This process takes about 4 to 8 months to complete, and then maintenance treatment is continued every 3 to 4 weeks for 3 to 5 years. Infants under 1 year rarely mount an appropriate response to allergens. Immunotherapy is most effective in reducing symptoms caused by seasonal pollen-related allergy. Sublingual immunotherapy has been used successfully in Europe; a portion of the allergen is placed under the tongue and symptom relief is achieved in 2 years (Ahmad and Zacharek, 2008).

Nursing Care Management

An important aspect in nursing care of the child with allergic rhinitis is to counsel the parents and patient about the causes of the condition, or triggers, and assist in the implementation of steps to avoid the triggers. Environmental modification in the home is important (see Allergen Control, p. 1268). Nurses can also help by recognizing rhinitis and referring children for diagnosis and therapy.

Another important aspect of caring for the child with allergic rhinitis is preparation for skin tests and immunotherapy injections. These procedures are a source of stress for many children. Young children, in particular, cannot understand how uncomfortable injections that must be given regularly over a long period will make them feel better. All children who receive skin tests need an explanation of the procedure, and many children benefit from strategies that minimize trauma (see Atraumatic Care box).

ATRAUMATIC CARE

Reducing Pain of Allergy Skin Tests and "Allergy Shots"

To help allay children's fears of skin tests, give them a careful and thorough explanation of what is to be done and how many "pricks" are involved (usually a series of eight on each site, for a total of 30 tests). Very young anxious patients may benefit from one prick on the arm to demonstrate how it feels. The skin is pierced with a stylet rather than a regular needle and syringe, then a drop of allergen is placed on the site. Another helpful distraction is to have the child count off the number of pricks with the nurse. For intradermal skin injections, EMLA (a eutectic mix of lidocaine and prilocaine) or LMX4 (lidocaine 4%), both topical anesthetics, reduce or eliminate pain without altering test results.

NURSING TIP To distinguish allergies from colds, be aware that:
- Allergies occur repeatedly and are often seasonal.
- Allergies are seldom accompanied by fever.
- Allergies often involve itching in the eyes and nose.
- Allergies usually trigger constant and consistent bouts of sneezing.
- Allergies are often accompanied by ear and eye problems.

Children with allergic rhinitis and their family members need specific and detailed information relating to their medications. In the case of seasonal rhinitis, antihistamines or topical antiinflammatory medications are often started approximately 2 weeks before the allergy season begins. Phone or mailed reminders to families to start their medications are helpful in preventing lower respiratory tract complications of allergic rhinitis. In addition, some nasal sprays may not reach their maximum effect or improve symptoms until a week after they are started. First-generation antihistamines that have sedation as a side effect should not be given to teenagers who are driving, and children should be cautioned to avoid hazardous activities such as bicycling or skating if drowsiness occurs; these are often best taken at night to minimize daytime drowsiness. School nurses, teachers, and parents should monitor children receiving sedating antihistamines for any changes in learning or intellectual functioning in school. Follow-up monitoring is essential to be sure that children or their parents do not exceed the correct dosage and that they follow correct administration procedures, especially with inhaled medications (see pp. 1269 and 1278).

ASTHMA

Asthma is a chronic inflammatory disorder of the airways in which many cells (mast cells, eosinophils, and T lymphocytes) play a role. In susceptible children, inflammation causes recurrent episodes of wheezing, breathlessness, chest tightness, and cough, especially at night or in the early morning. These asthma episodes are associated with airflow limitation or obstruction that is reversible either spontaneously or with treatment. The inflammation also causes an increase in bronchial hyperresponsiveness to a variety of stimuli (National Asthma Education and Prevention Program, 2007). Recognition of the importance of inflammation has made the use of antiinflammatory agents, especially inhaled steroids, a key component in the treatment of asthma.

Childhood asthma may be manifested in two primary types: (1) recurrent wheezing in early childhood which is usually precipitated by a viral respiratory tract infection (e.g., RSV); and (2) chronic asthma associated with allergy persisting into later childhood and often adulthood. A third type of childhood asthma is associated with girls who develop obesity and early-onset puberty (by 11 years of age) (Liu, Covar, Spahn, et al, 2007). *Cough-variant asthma* is a term used to describe a type of asthma in which a chronic cough is the predominant symptom; wheeze and dyspnea are usually absent. Cough-variant asthma may be treated with inhaled bronchodilators and inhaled corticosteroids (Abouzgheib, Pratter, and Bartter, 2007).

Based on the symptom indicators of disease severity, asthma is classified into four categories: intermittent, mild persistent, moderate persistent, and severe persistent. The intermittent category has the least number of symptoms; symptoms increase in frequency or intensity until the last category of severe persistent asthma (Box 32-16). These categories provide a stepwise approach to the pharmacologic management, environmental control, and educational interventions needed for each category (National Asthma Education and Prevention Program, 2007). For example, if control of asthma is not maintained at one level or step, pharmacologic therapy for the next step up should be considered. If control is adequate at one step, a gradual stepwise reduction in therapy may be possible. The stepwise approach is a guide to assist clinical decision making, but it is not a specific prescription. Therapy and management should be reviewed every 1 to 6 months and should be individualized to the patient. In addition to pharmacologic management, environmental control and educational interventions are essential at each step (National Asthma Education and Prevention Program, 2007).

A new component of the asthma severity classification system includes the domains of impairment and risk for each category; these categories emphasize the multifaceted aspect of the disease for consideration of the effects of symptoms on present quality of life and functional capacity and the future risk of adverse events (National Asthma Education and Prevention Program, 2007).

Asthma prevalence, morbidity, and mortality are increasing in the United States, especially among African-Americans (Linzer, 2007). These increases may result from worsening air pollution, poor access to medical care, or underdiagnosis and undertreatment. Asthma is the most common chronic disease of childhood, the primary cause of school absences, and the third leading cause of hospitalizations in children under the age of 15. Although the onset of asthma may occur at any age, 80% to 90% of children have their first symptoms before 4 or 5 years of age. Boys are affected more frequently than girls until adolescence, when the trend reverses.

Studies of children with asthma indicate that allergy influences both the persistence and the severity of the disease. In fact, **atopy**, or the genetic predisposition for the development

---

BOX 32-16 ASTHMA SEVERITY CLASSIFICATION IN CHILDREN: AGES 0 TO 11*

Step 5 or 6: Severe Persistent Asthma
Continual symptoms throughout the day
Frequent nighttime symptoms
Peak expiratory flow (PEF): <60%
Forced expiratory volume in 1 second (FEV_1): <75% of predicted value
Interference with normal activity: Extremely limited
Use of short-acting β-agonist for symptom control: Several times a day

Step 3 or 4: Moderate Persistent Asthma
Daily symptoms
Nighttime symptoms three or four times a month (ages 0 to 4); more than once per week but not nightly (ages 5 to 11)
PEF: 60% to 80% of predicted value
FEV_1: 75% to 80%
PEF variability: >30%
Interference with normal activity: Some limitation
Use of short-acting β-agonist for symptom control: Daily

Step 2: Mild Persistent Asthma
Symptoms more than two times a week, but less than one time a day
Nighttime symptoms: One or two times a month (ages 0 to 4); three or four times a month (ages 5 to 11)
PEF or FEV_1: ≥80% of predicted value
PEF variability: 20% to 30%
Interference with normal activity: Minor limitation
Use of short-acting β-agonist for symptom control: More than 2 days a week but not daily

Step 1: Intermittent Asthma
Symptoms less than 2 days a week
Nighttime symptoms (awakenings): None (ages 0 to 4); less than two times a month (ages 5 to 11)
PEF or FEV_1: ≥80% of predicted value
PEF variability: <20%
Interference with normal activity: None
Use of short-acting β-agonist for symptom control: Less than 2 days a week

From National Asthma Education and Prevention Program: *Guidelines for the diagnosis and management of asthma: summary report 2007,* available at www.nhlbi.nih.gov/guidelines/asthma/index.htm (accessed August 22, 2009).
*The presence of one clinical feature of severity is sufficient to place a patient in that category. An individual should be assigned to the most severe grade in which any feature occurs. The characteristics in this table are general and may overlap because asthma is highly variable. An individual's classification may change over time. Risk factors for each category are not presented in this table. See the original table referenced above for additional classification data. Asthma treatment should not be based on this table.

---

of an IgE-mediated response to common aeroallergens, is the strongest identifiable predisposing factor for developing asthma (National Asthma Education and Prevention Program, 2007). Although allergens play an important role in asthma, 20% to 40% of children with asthma have no evidence of allergic disease. The allergic reaction in the airways is significant for two reasons: (1) it can cause an immediate reaction, with obstruction; and (2) it can precipitate a late bronchial obstructive reaction several hours after the initial exposure. This delayed bronchial response is associated with an increase in the airway hyperresponsiveness to nonimmunologic stimuli and can persist for several weeks or more after a single allergen exposure.

BOX 32-17   TRIGGERS TENDING TO PRECIPITATE OR AGGRAVATE ASTHMATIC EXACERBATIONS

Allergens:
    Outdoor—Trees, shrubs, weeds, grasses, molds, pollens, air pollution, spores
    Indoor—Dust or dust mites, mold, cockroach antigen
    Irritants—Tobacco smoke, wood smoke, odors, sprays
Exposure to occupational chemicals
Exercise
Cold air
Changes in weather or temperature
Environmental change—Moving to new home, starting new school, etc.
Colds and infections
Animals—Cats, dogs, rodents, horses
Medications—Aspirin, nonsteroidal antiinflammatory drugs, antibiotics, beta blockers
Strong emotions—Fear, anger, laughing, crying
Conditions—Gastroesophageal reflux, tracheoesophageal fistula
Food additives—Sulfite preservatives
Foods—Nuts, milk and dairy products
Endocrine factors—Menses, pregnancy, thyroid disease

In addition to allergens, other substances and conditions can serve as triggers that may exacerbate asthma (Box 32-17). Asthma is a complex disorder involving biochemical, genetic, immunologic, environmental, infectious, endocrine, and psychologic factors. Evidence shows that viral respiratory tract infections may have a significant role in the development and expression of asthma (National Asthma Education and Prevention Program, 2007).

Risk factors for asthma include:

- Age
- Atopy
- Heredity
- Gender
- Mother under age 20 years
- Smoking (maternal and grandmaternal)
- Ethnicity (African-Americans at greatest risk)
- Previous life-threatening attacks
- Lack of access to medical care
- Psychologic and psychosocial problems

There is additional evidence of a genetic component to asthma primarily in linkages to allergic and inflammatory genes on chromosome 5 (Liu, Covar, Spahn, et al, 2007).

Pathophysiology

There is general agreement that inflammation contributes to heightened airway reactivity in asthma. Multiple mechanisms contribute to airway inflammation, involving a number of different pathways. It is unlikely that asthma is caused by either a single cell or a single inflammatory mediator. Rather, it appears that asthma results from complex interactions among inflammatory cells, mediators, and the cells and tissues present in the airways (Fig. 32-9) (National Asthma Education and Prevention Program, 2007). However, recognition of the importance of inflammation has made the use of antiinflammatory agents a key component of asthma therapy.

Another important component of asthma is bronchospasm and obstruction. The mechanisms responsible for the obstructive symptoms in asthma (Fig. 32-10) include (1) inflammatory response to stimuli; (2) airway edema and accumulation and secretion of mucus; and (3) spasm of the smooth muscle of the bronchi and bronchioles, which decreases the caliber of the bronchioles.

Bronchial constriction is a normal reaction to foreign stimuli, but in the child with asthma it is abnormally severe, producing impaired respiratory function. The smooth muscle arranged in spiral bundles around the airway causes narrowing and shortening of the airway, which significantly increases airway resistance to airflow. Determine airflow by the size of the airway lumen, degree of bronchial wall edema, mucus production, smooth muscle contraction, and muscle hypertrophy.

Because the bronchi normally dilate and elongate during inspiration and contract and shorten on expiration, the respiratory difficulty is more pronounced during the expiratory phase of respiration.

Increased resistance in the airway causes forced expiration through the narrowed lumen. The volume of air trapped in the lungs increases as airways are functionally closed at a point between the alveoli and the lobar bronchi. This trapping of gas forces the individual to breathe at higher and higher lung volumes. Consequently, the person with asthma fights to inspire sufficient air. This expenditure of effort for breathing causes fatigue, decreased respiratory effectiveness, and increased oxygen consumption. The inspiration occurring at higher lung volumes hyperinflates the alveoli and reduces the effectiveness of the cough. As the severity of obstruction increases, there is reduced alveolar ventilation with carbon dioxide retention, hypoxemia, respiratory acidosis, and eventually respiratory failure.

Chronic inflammation may also cause permanent damage (airway remodeling) to airway structures; this remodeling cannot be prevented by and is not responsive to current treatments (National Asthma Education and Prevention Program, 2007).

Exacerbations are episodes of progressively worsening shortness of breath, cough, wheezing, or chest tightness or some combination of these changes. A decrease in expiratory airflow is also characteristic. Airways narrow because of bronchospasm, mucosal edema, and mucous plugging, with air being trapped behind occluded or narrowed airways. Functional residual capacity rises because the child is breathing close to total lung capacity; hyperinflation enables the child to keep the airways open and permits gas exchange to occur. Hypoxemia can occur during such episodes because of the mismatching of ventilation and perfusion. This is seen with increasing carbon dioxide tension and decreasing oxygen tension levels.

Many children with asthma exhibit an allergic component. Allergy is the strongest epidemiologic risk factor for chronic asthma morbidity and mortality. Many substances in the environment can induce an asthmatic response, but the most significant are those that are antigenic (i.e., that evoke the immune response). The antigen (or foreign substance) is deposited on the respiratory mucosa, where lysozymes immediately digest its outer coating, releasing fragments of foreign protein that initiate the immune sequence. The antibody (immunoglobulin)

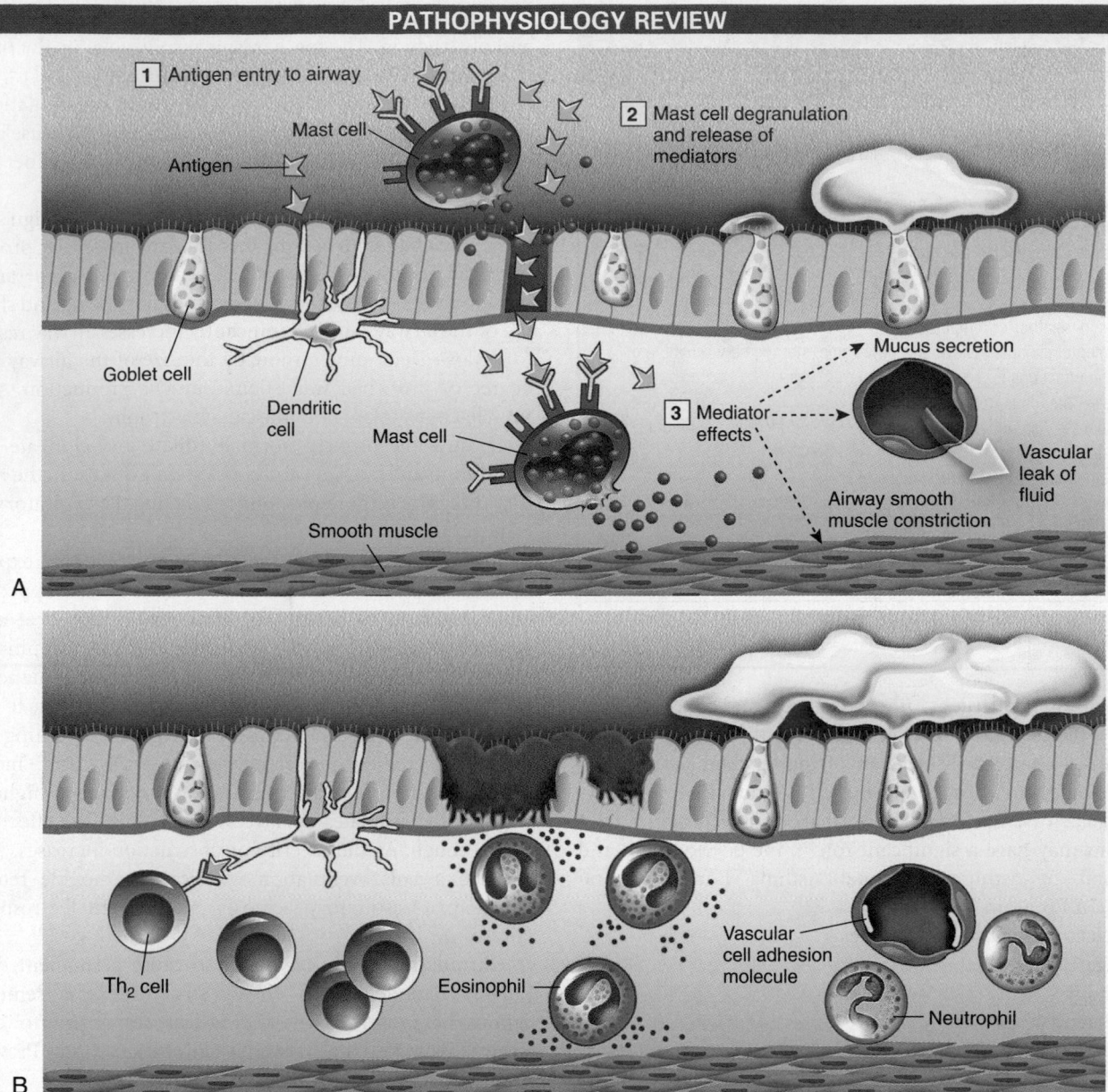

Fig. 32-9 Asthmatic responses. **A,** In the early asthmatic response, inhaled antigen *(1)* binds to preformed immunoglobulin E (IgE) on mast cells. Mast cells degranulate *(2)* and release mediators such as histamine, leukotrienes, prostaglandin D_2, platelet-activating factor, and others. Acute inflammation opens intercellular tight junctions, allowing antigen to penetrate and activate submucosal mast cells. Secreted mediators *(3)* induce active bronchospasm, edema, and mucus secretion. Inflammatory responses are set in motion by chemotactic factors and upregulation of adhesion molecules (not shown). At the same time, as shown on the left, antigen may be received by dendritic cells that process and later present it, either in regional lymph nodes to naive (Th_o) T lymphocytes or locally to memory Th_2 cells in the airway mucosa (see **B**). **B,** In the late asthmatic response areas of epithelial damage are caused at least in part by toxicity of eosinophil products (major basic protein, eosinophilic cationic protein, eosinophil-derived neurotoxin, and eosinophil peroxidase). Many inflammatory cells have been recruited by chemokines and upregulation of vascular cell adhesion molecules. Local T lymphocytes display a predominant Th_2 cytokine profile. They produce interleukin-4 (IL-4) and IL-13, which promote switching of B cells to favor IgE production, and IL-3, IL-5, and granulocyte-macrophage colony–stimulating factor, which encourage eosinophil differentiation and survival. (From McCance KL, Huether SE: *Pathophysiology: the biological basis for disease in adults and children,* ed 6, St Louis, 2010, Mosby.)

most active in allergic disorders, including asthma, is IgE, located primarily in skin and mucous membranes

IgE mediates the immediate hypersensitive reaction in the bronchial mucosa that leads to specific tissue binding. IgE attaches to surfaces of mast cells and basophils, where it reacts with the specific antigen to which they have developed a bonding capacity. Antigenic substances trigger an immediate hypersensitivity reaction with subsequent release of chemical mediators from mast cells and basophils: histamine; leukotrienes; platelet-activating factor; and other substances, including prostaglandins, serotonin, and various kinins. The major effects of the mediators in the airways are increased permeability of the blood vessels, contraction of smooth muscle, and stimulation of mucus secretion.

PATHOPHYSIOLOGY REVIEW

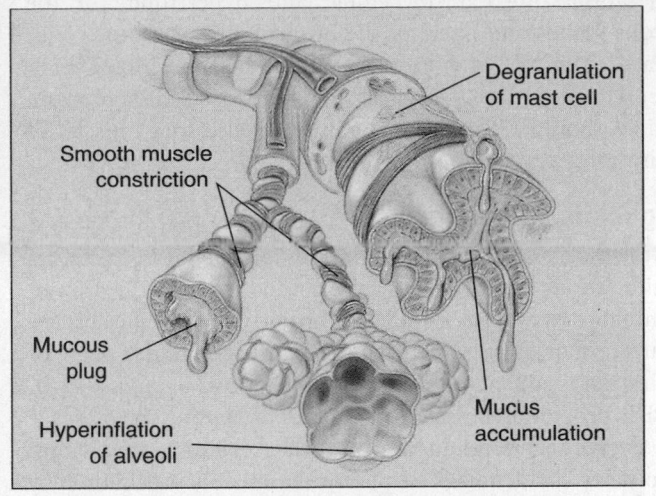

Fig. 32-10 Airway obstruction caused by asthma. **A,** The normal lung. **B,** Bronchial asthma: thick mucus, mucosal edema, and smooth muscle spasm causing obstruction of small airways; breathing becomes labored and expiration is difficult. (Modified from Des Jardins T, Burton GG: *Clinical manifestations and assessment of respiratory disease,* ed 3, St Louis, 1995, Mosby.)

Clinical Manifestations

The classic manifestations of asthma are dyspnea, wheezing, and coughing. However, children may experience symptoms that range from acute episodes of shortness of breath, wheezing, and cough followed by a quiet period to a relatively continuous pattern of chronic symptoms that fluctuate in severity. Older children may complain of chest tightness and an intermittent generalized chest pain. An attack may develop gradually or appear abruptly and may be preceded by a URI. Symptoms are often worse at night. The child's age is often a significant factor, since the first attack frequently occurs between ages 3 and 8 years. In infancy an attack usually follows a respiratory tract infection. Bronchoconstriction in response to an allergen can have an immediate, histamine type of pattern or a late response with airway hypersensitivity lasting for days, weeks, or months. A second wave of symptoms can occur 6 to 8 hours after the initial antigen exposure.

Children may experience a prodromal itching localized at the front of the neck or over the upper part of the back. An asthmatic episode usually begins with children feeling uncomfortable or irritable and increasingly restless. They may also complain of having a headache, feeling tired, or feeling tightness in the chest. Respiratory symptoms include a hacking, paroxysmal, irritative, and nonproductive cough caused by bronchial edema. Accumulated secretions, acting as an FB, stimulate the cough. As the secretions become more profuse, the cough becomes rattling and productive of frothy, clear, gelatinous sputum. Bronchial spasm and mucosal edema reduce the size of the bronchial lumen, and the bronchi may be occluded by mucous plugs.

A common symptom of asthma is coughing in the absence of respiratory tract infection, especially at night. This may disrupt sleep, leading to excessive fatigue during the day and poor school performance. Wheezing may be mild or discernible only on auscultation at the end of expiration, or severe enough to be audible.

Younger children have a tendency to assume the tripod sitting position, whereas older children have a tendency to sit upright with shoulders hunched over, hands on the bed or chair, and arms braced to facilitate the use of accessory muscles of respiration. The child speaks with short, panting, broken phrases. Infants and small children are restless, irritable, and unable to be comforted.

Infants may display supraclavicular, intercostal, suprasternal, subcostal, and sternal retractions. However, clinical symptoms of asthma may be less obvious in infancy. Because infants have a more pliant (flexible) chest, a prolonged expiratory phase may not be easy to observe. Wheezing, a characteristic symptom often associated with asthma, may occur in infants with respiratory tract infections, cardiac defects, and aspiration pneumonia.

Examination of the chest reveals hyperresonance on percussion. Breath sounds are coarse and loud, with sonorous crackles throughout the lung fields. Expiration is prolonged. Coarse rhonchi can be heard, as well as generalized inspiratory and expiratory wheezing that becomes more high pitched as obstruction progresses. With minimum obstruction, wheezing may be mild (discernible only on auscultation at the end of expiration) or even absent.

With severe spasm or obstruction, breath sounds and crackles may be inaudible. Cough is ineffective despite repeated hacking maneuvers. This represents a lack of air movement and may be misinterpreted as improvement by unknowing examiners.

! NURSING ALERT

Shortness of breath with air movement in the chest restricted to the point of absent breath sounds accompanied by a sudden rise in respiratory rate is an ominous sign indicating ventilatory failure and imminent asphyxia.

Children with chronic asthma develop generalized vascularization, mucosal thickening, and hypertrophy of the mucous glands and fibers of the bronchial musculature. With repeated episodes the thoracic cavity becomes fixed in a hyperaerated state (barrel chest), with a depressed diaphragm, elevated shoulders, and increased use of accessory muscles of respiration.

Diagnostic Evaluation

The diagnosis is determined primarily on the basis of clinical manifestations, history, physical examination, and to a lesser extent laboratory tests. Generally, chronic cough in the absence of infection or diffuse wheezing during the expiratory phase of respiration is sufficient to establish a diagnosis.

PFTs provide an objective method of evaluating the presence and degree of lung disease and the response to therapy. Spirometry can generally be performed reliably on children by the age of 5 or 6 years and includes either the traditional and simple mechanical spirometer often used in clinics, offices, and the home or new computerized versions. The National Asthma Education and Prevention Program (2007) recommends that spirometry testing be done at the time of initial assessment of asthma, after treatment is initiated and symptoms have stabilized, and at least every 1 to 2 years to assess the maintenance of airway function.

Bronchoprovocation testing (i.e., direct exposure of the mucous membranes to a suspected antigen in increasing concentrations) helps to identify inhaled allergens. Exposure to methacholine, histamine, or cold or dry air may be performed to assess airway responsiveness or reactivity. Exercise challenges may be used to identify children with exercise-induced bronchospasm (EIB) (Liu, Covar, Spahn, et al, 2007). Although these tests are highly specific and sensitive, they place the child at risk for an asthmatic episode and should be done under close observation in a qualified laboratory or clinic.

Skin testing is useful in identifying specific allergens, and those obtained by the puncture technique correlate better than intracutaneous tests with symptoms and measurements of specific IgE antibody. It is recommended that all patients with year-round asthma symptoms be tested with skin tests or laboratory blood analysis to determine sensitization to perennial allergens (e.g., house dust mites, cats, dogs, cockroaches, molds, and fungus) (National Asthma Education and Prevention Program, 2007).

In addition to these tests, other important tests include laboratory tests (complete blood count with differential) and chest radiographs. The complete blood count may show a slight elevation in the white blood cell count during acute asthma, but elevations to more than 12,000/mm³ or an increased percentage of band cells may indicate respiratory tract infection. On the other hand, the presence of eosinophilia greater than 500/mm³ tends to suggest an allergic or inflammatory disorder.

Frontal and lateral radiographs show infiltrates and hyperexpansion of the airways, with the anteroposterior diameter on physical examination indicating an increased diameter (suggestive of barrel chest). Additional diagnostic tests for conditions such as gastroesophageal reflux may be carried out to determine whether they may contribute to asthma symptoms. Radiography may assist in ruling out a respiratory tract infection.

Therapeutic Management: General

The overall goals of asthma management are to maintain normal activity levels, maintain normal pulmonary function, prevent chronic symptoms and recurrent exacerbations, provide optimal drug therapy with minimal or no adverse effects, and assist the child in living as normal and happy a life as possible. This includes facilitating the child's social adjustments in the family, school, and community and normal participation in recreational activities and sports. To accomplish these goals, several treatment principles need to be followed (National Asthma Education and Prevention Program, 2007):

- A continuous care approach with regular visits (at least every 1 to 6 months) to the health care provider is necessary to control symptoms and prevent exacerbations.
- Prevention of exacerbations includes avoiding triggers, avoiding allergens, and using medications as needed.
- Therapy includes efforts to reduce underlying inflammation and relieve or prevent symptomatic airway narrowing.
- Therapy includes patient education, environmental control, pharmacologic management, and the use of objective measures to monitor the severity of disease and guide the course of therapy.

Allergen Control

Nonpharmacologic therapy is aimed at the prevention and reduction of exposure to airborne allergens and irritants. House dust mites and other components of house dust are frequent agents identified in children allergic to inhalants. The cockroach, another common household inhabitant, is an important allergen in many locations. Exterminating live cockroaches, carefully cleaning kitchen floors and cabinets, putting food away after eating, and taking trash out in the evening are essential measures to control cockroaches. The mouse allergen is the most recent allergen to be identified in the homes of inner-city children with asthma. The role of cat and dog dander in allergen-induced asthma has also been studied. Sensitized persons should carefully evaluate having such pets in the household; there are inconclusive data on cat dander, but there is some evidence that dog dander either has no effect or may be protective (Sharma, Hansel, Matsui, et al, 2007). Additional sources of pollutants include ozone, particulate matter produced by tobacco smoke, wood-burning stoves, pesticides, lead, mold spores, nitrogen dioxide, and sulfur dioxide; these are believed to contribute to asthma morbidity in children and should be avoided or minimized (Diette, McCormack, Hansel, et al, 2008). Exposure to tobacco smoke is a significant contributing factor in the development of asthma in infants and small children (Sharma, Hansel, Matsui, et al, 2007).

Skin testing can identify specific allergens. Steps are then taken to eliminate or avoid them. Often, simply removing the offending environmental allergens or irritants (e.g., removing carpeting from the home of a child sensitive to mold and dust particles) decreases the frequency of asthma episodes. Dehumidifiers or air conditioners control nonspecific factors, such as extremes of temperature, that trigger an episode. Avoiding known outdoor allergens such as tree, grass, and weed pollen when these are high may reduce asthma exacerbations as well. Additional suggestions include:

- Cover pillows and mattresses with plastic covers.
- Avoid using feather- or down-filled pillows and mattresses.
- Keep child indoors while lawn is being mowed, bushes and trees are being trimmed, or pollen count is high.
- Keep windows and doors closed during pollen season; use air conditioner if possible or go to places that are air conditioned, such as libraries and shopping malls, when the weather is hot.
- Wet-mop bare floors weekly; wet-dust and clean child's room weekly; child should not be present during cleaning activities.
- Limit or prevent child's exposure to tobacco and wood smoke; do not allow cigarette smoking in the house or car; select daycare centers, play areas, and shopping malls that are smoke free.
- Use air conditioners with a high-efficiency particulate air [HEPA] filters.
- Use indoor air purifier with HEPA filter.

Despite the proven association between the incidence of asthma and exposure to these residential hazards, little evidence-based research demonstrates an overall reduction in symptoms, even with significant interventions aimed at environmental (housing) modifications such as removal of carpeting, cleaning, and extermination (Sandel, Phelan, Wright, et al, 2004; Sharma, Hansel, Matsui, et al, 2007) (see Complementary and Alternative Therapy box).

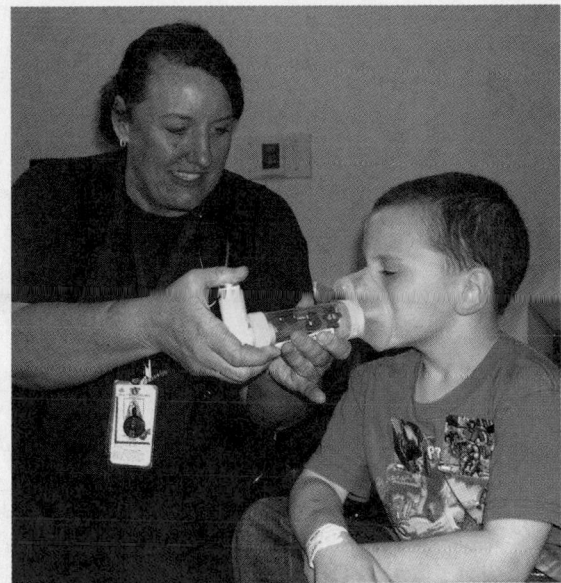

Fig. 32-11 Child using metered-dose inhaler with aerochamber and face mask.

COMPLEMENTARY AND ALTERNATIVE THERAPY

Herbal Treatment of Asthma

Herbs and plants are often used by adults and children to treat asthma; however, the safety and effectiveness of such therapies has been controversial. A recent Cochrane review of 27 studies evaluated the effects of 21 herbs taken by adults and children for asthma. Two studies reported positive outcomes for change in forced expiratory volume in 1 second (FEV$_1$), and one study reported negative effects. The authors concluded that the effects of herbal treatments for asthma in children and adults was hampered by the lack of consistency in reporting outcomes (Arnold, Clark, Lassersson, et al, 2009).

Drug Therapy

Pharmacologic therapy is used to prevent and control asthma symptoms, reduce the frequency and severity of asthma exacerbations, and reverse airflow obstruction. A stepwise approach is recommended based on the severity of the child's asthma. Because inflammation is considered an early and persistent feature of asthma, therapy is directed toward long-term suppression of inflammation.

Asthma medications are categorized into two general classes: long-term control medications (preventive medications) to achieve and maintain control of inflammation, and quick-relief medications (rescue medications) to treat symptoms and exacerbations (National Asthma Education and Prevention Program, 2007).

Quick-relief and long-term medications are often used in combination. Inhaled corticosteroids, cromolyn sodium and nedocromil, long-acting β_2-agonists, methylxanthines, and leukotriene modifiers are used as long-term control medications. Short-acting β_2-agonists, anticholinergics, and systemic corticosteroids are used as quick-relief (or rescue) medications. Bronchodilators that relax bronchial smooth muscle and dilate the airways include β_2-agonists, methylxanthines, and anticholinergics that can be used as both quick-relief and long-term medications.

Many asthma medications are given by inhalation with a nebulizer or a **metered-dose inhaler (MDI)**. The MDI should always be attached to a spacer when an inhaled corticosteroid is administered to prevent yeast infections in the mouth. Spacers are also important for children who have difficulty coordinating or learning proper inhalation technique (Pongracic, 2003). The spacer and holder can be equipped with a mask or a mouthpiece (Fig. 32-11) (see Family-Centered Care box, p. 1278). Pharmaceutical companies are currently mandated to produce inhalers that do not contain chlorofluorocarbons (CFCs) as the propellant because CFCs have been linked to damage and depletion of the earth's ozone level. An alternative propellant to the CFCs is hydrofluoroalkanes; the advantages include delivery of more fine particles and less oral deposition. Several currently available CFC-free MDI devices use dry powder (and also called dry powder inhalers [DPIs]); these include the Diskus inhaler and the Turbuhaler. These devices are breath activated, and the child needs to inhale as quickly and deeply as possible to use them effectively. The Diskhaler and Aerosolizer are similar, but with the Aerosolizer the medication must be loaded into the inhaler before use. Infants and young children who have difficulty using MDIs or other inhalers can receive their asthma medications via a **hand-held nebulizer** (Fig. 32-12). When this device is used, the medication is mixed with saline (also available in premixed form) and nebulized with compressed air. Children should breathe normally with the mouth open to provide a direct route to the trachea.

Corticosteroids are antiinflammatory drugs used to treat reversible airflow obstruction and control symptoms and reduce bronchial hyperresponsiveness in chronic asthma. A

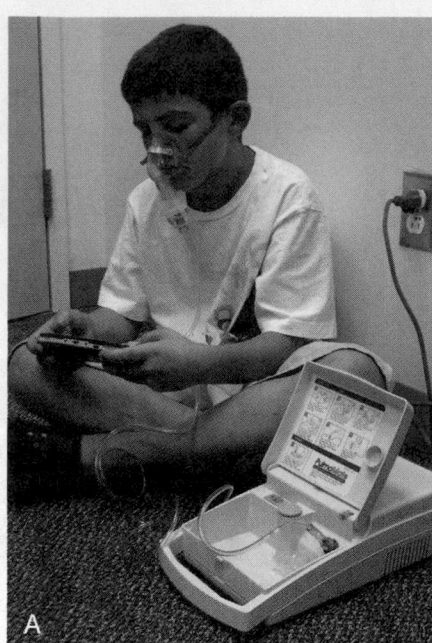
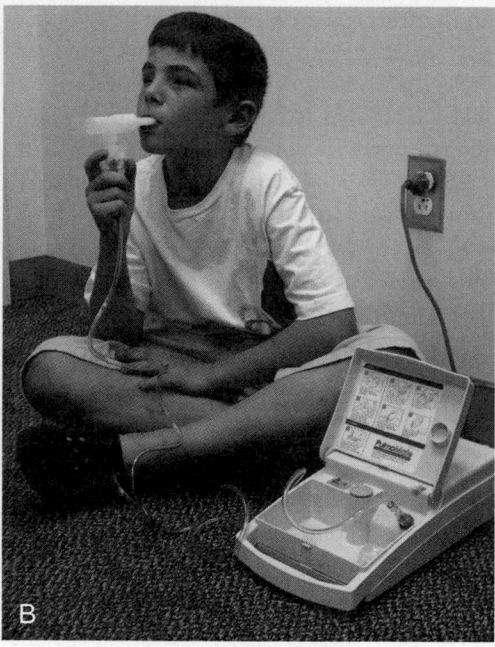

Fig 32-12 Child with asthma may take a nebulized aerosol treatment with **(A)** a mask or **(B)** mouthpiece. (Courtesy Texas Children's Hospital, Houston.)

major change in the last two revisions of the National Asthma Education and Prevention Program guidelines (2007) is the recommendation that inhaled corticosteroids be used as first-line therapy in children over 5 years of age. Clinical studies of corticosteroids have indicated significant improvement of all asthma parameters, including decreases in symptoms, emergency visits, and medication requirements (National Asthma Education and Prevention Program, 2007).

Corticosteroids may be administered parenterally, orally, or by inhalation. Oral medications are metabolized slowly, with an onset of action up to 3 hours after administration and peak effectiveness occurring within 6 to 12 hours. Oral systemic steroids may be given for short periods (e.g., 3- or 10-day "bursts") to gain prompt control of inadequately controlled persistent asthma or to manage severe persistent asthma. These drugs should be given in the lowest effective dose. They have few side effects (cough, dysphonia, and oral thrush), and there is strong evidence that they improve the long-term outcomes for children of all ages with mild or moderate persistent asthma. Evidence from clinical trials that monitored children for 6 years indicates that the use of inhaled corticosteroids at recommended dosages does not have long-term significant effects on growth, bone mineral density, ocular toxicity, or suppression of the adrenal-pituitary axis (National Asthma Education and Prevention Program, 2007). However, primary care providers should frequently monitor (at least every 3 to 6 months) the growth of children and adolescents taking corticosteroids to assess the systemic effects of these drugs and make appropriate reductions in dosages or changes to other types of asthma therapy when necessary. The inhaled corticosteroids include budesonide and fluticasone.

Cromolyn sodium is a nonsteroidal antiinflammatory drug (NSAID) for asthma. It stabilizes mast cell membranes; inhibits activation and release of mediators from eosinophil and epithelial cells; and inhibits the acute airway narrowing after exposure to exercise, cold dry air, and sulfur dioxide. There is no way to reliably predict whether a child will respond to the drug. Cromolyn sodium has minimal side effects (occasional coughing on inhalation of the powder formulation) and may be given via nebulizer or MDI. **Nedocromil sodium** inhibits the bronchoconstrictor response to inhaled antigens and inhibits the activity of and release of histamine, leukotrienes, and prostaglandins from inflammatory cells associated with asthma. The drug has few side effects and is used for maintenance therapy in asthma. The drug is not effective for reversal of acute exacerbations and is not used in children under 5 years of age

β-Adrenergic agonists (short acting) (primarily albuterol, levalbuterol [Xopenex], and terbutaline) are used for treatment of acute exacerbations and for the prevention of EIB. These drugs bind with the β-receptors on the smooth muscle of airways, where they activate adenylate cyclase and convert adenosine monophosphate (AMP) to cyclic AMP (cAMP). The increased cAMP enhances binding of intracellular calcium to the cell membrane, reducing the availability of calcium and thus allowing smooth muscle to relax. Other effects of the drug help stabilize mast cells to prevent release of mediators. Most β-adrenergics used in asthma therapy affect predominantly the $β_2$-receptors, which help eliminate bronchospasm. $β_1$-Adrenergic effects such as increased heart rate and gastrointestinal disturbances have been minimized. These drugs can be given via inhalation or as oral or parenteral preparations. The inhaled drug has a more rapid onset of action than the oral form. Inhalation also reduces troublesome systemic side effects: irritability, tremor, nervousness, and insomnia. Levalbuterol reportedly causes fewer side effects; however, its overall effectiveness in childhood asthma is controversial (Linzer, 2007). The 2007 National Asthma Education and Prevention Program guidelines recommend the addition of a long-acting $β_2$-agonist to a low- or medium-dose inhaled corticosteroid to improve lung function and asthma symptoms and decrease the need for a short-acting β_2-agonist. This combination may actually allow the practitioner to lower the corticosteroid dose and manage asthma symptoms just as effectively. Inhaled β-adrenergic agents should not be taken more than three or four times daily for acute symptoms without medical supervision. A continuous nebulization therapy with a short-acting β_2-agonist may be used in the acute setting with an acute exacerbation.

Salmeterol (Serevent) is a long-acting β_2-agonist (bronchodilator) that is used twice a day (no more frequently than every 12 hours). This drug is added to antiinflammatory therapy and used for long-term prevention of symptoms, especially nighttime symptoms, and EIB. Salmeterol is not used in children younger than 12 years of age.

⚡ DRUG ALERT

Salmeterol

Salmeterol is *never* used to treat acute symptoms or exacerbations.

Theophylline was used for decades to relieve symptoms and prevent asthma attacks; however, it is now used primarily in the emergency department when the child is not responding to maximal therapy (Linzer, 2007). Therapeutic levels should be obtained with this drug because it has a narrow therapeutic window.

Leukotrienes are mediators of inflammation that cause increases in airway hyperresponsiveness. Leukotriene modifiers (such as zafirlukast [Accolate] and montelukast sodium) block inflammatory and bronchospasm effects. These drugs are not used to treat acute episodes but are given orally in combination with β-agonists and steroids to provide long-term control and prevent symptoms in mild persistent asthma. Montelukast is approved for children 12 months old and older, whereas zafirlukast is approved for children 7 years and older.

Anticholinergics (atropine and ipratropium) help relieve acute bronchospasm. However, these drugs have adverse side effects that include drying of respiratory secretions, blurred vision, and cardiac and central nervous system stimulation. The primary anticholinergic drug used is ipratropium, which does not cross the blood-brain barrier and therefore elicits no central nervous system effects (as does atropine). Ipratropium, when used in combination with albuterol, has been effective during acute severe asthma in significantly improving lung function and reducing hospitalizations in children coming to the emergency department (Liu, Covar, Spahn, et al, 2007).

A fairly new asthma drug, omalizumab (Xolair), is a **monoclonal antibody** that blocks the binding of IgE to mast cells. Blocking this interaction eventually inhibits the inflammation that is associated with asthma. Because many patients with asthma are atopic and possess specific IgE antibodies to allergens responsible for airway inflammation, this drug is a promising adjunct to the treatment of asthma. It has been approved for use in children 12 years and older. The drug is administered once or twice a month by subcutaneous injection. Efficacy of omalizumab is not immediate, and clinical trials report that response to the drug was not evident before 12 weeks (Strunk and Bloomberg, 2006). Clinical trials of the drug indicate that it can be an effective therapy for patients with symptomatic

moderate to severe allergic asthma that is poorly controlled with inhaled corticosteroids. However, it is expensive (Courtney, McCarter, and Pollart, 2005), and there have been reported cases of severe anaphylactic reactions. In early 2007 the FDA added a "black box warning" to the drug, which highlights the risk of anaphylaxis.

Some children with severe asthma and a history of severe life-threatening episodes may need a primary care practitioner prescription for an EpiPen (subcutaneous injectable epinephrine) (Liu, Covar, Spahn, et al, 2007).

Magnesium sulfate, a potent muscle relaxant that acts to decrease inflammation and improves pulmonary function and peak flow rate, may be used in pediatric patients treated in the emergency department with moderate to severe asthma. The drug is administered intravenously at 25 to 75 mg/kg (Liu, Covar, Spahn, et al, 2007).

Chest Physiotherapy

CPT includes breathing exercises and physical training. These therapies help produce physical and mental relaxation, improve posture, strengthen respiratory musculature, and develop more efficient patterns of breathing. For the motivated child, breathing exercises and controlled breathing help prevent overinflation and improve efficiency of the cough. However, CPT is not recommended during acute, uncomplicated exacerbations of asthma (National Asthma Education and Prevention Program, 2007) (see Bronchial [Postural] Drainage, Chapter 31).

Hyposensitization

The role of hyposensitization in childhood asthma is somewhat controversial. In the past, immunotherapy was used for seasonal allergies and when single substances were identified as the offending allergen. It is not recommended for allergens that can be eliminated, such as foods, drugs, and animal dander.

The National Asthma Education and Prevention Program guidelines (2007) recommend immunotherapy for asthma patients in the following situations:

- When there is evidence of a relationship between asthma symptoms and unavoidable exposure to an allergen to which the patient is sensitive
- When symptoms occur all year or at least during a major portion of the year
- When symptom control is difficult with drug therapy because multiple medications are required, the patient is not responsive to available drugs, or the patient refuses to take the medications

Injection therapy is usually limited to clinically significant allergens. The initial dose of the offending allergen(s), based on the size of the skin reaction, is injected subcutaneously. The amount is increased at weekly intervals until a maximum tolerance is reached, after which a maintenance dose is given at 4-week intervals. This may be extended to 5- or 6-week intervals during the off-season for seasonal allergens. Successful treatment is continued for a minimum of 3 years and then stopped. If no symptoms appear, acquired immunity is assumed; if symptoms recur, treatment begins again. Hyposensitization injections should be administered only with emergency equipment and medications readily available in the event of an anaphylactic reaction.

TABLE 32-3 ESTIMATING SEVERITY OF ASTHMA EXACERBATIONS				
SIGN AND SYMPTOM ASSESSMENT	MILD	MODERATE	SEVERE	RESPIRATORY ARREST IMMINENT
Breathless	While walking Can lie down	While at rest (infant: softer, shorter cry; difficulty feeding) Prefers sitting	While at rest (infant: stops feeding) Sits upright	
Talks in	Sentences	Phrases	Words	
Alertness	May be agitated	Usually agitated	Usually agitated	Drowsy or confused
Respiratory rate	Increased	Increased	Often >30 breaths/min	
Accessory muscle used; suprasternal retractions	Usually not present	Commonly present	Usually present	Paradoxic thoracoabdominal movement
Wheeze	Moderate, often only end expiratory	Loud, throughout exhalation	Usually loud throughout inhalation and exhalation	Absence of wheeze
Pulse (beats/min)	<100	100-120	>120	Bradycardia
Pulsus paradoxus	Absent <10 mm Hg	May be present 10-25 mm HG	Often present 20-40 mm Hg (child)	Absence suggests respiratory muscle fatigue
PEF (percent predicted or percentile personal best)	≥70%	~40%-69% or response lasts <2 hr	50%	<25% PEF testing may not be needed in severe attacks
Oxygen saturation (SaO$_2$), (on air) at sea level	>95%	90%-95%	<90%	
PaO$_2$ (on air)	Normal	≥60 mm Hg	<60 mm Hg; possible cyanosis	
PaCO$_2$	<42 mm Hg	<42 mm Hg	≥42 mm Hg; possible respiratory failure	

From National Asthma Education and Prevention Program: *Expert Panel Report 3: Guidelines for diagnosis and management of asthma,* Bethesda, Md, 2007, National Heart, Lung, and Blood Institute, National Institutes of Health.
NOTE: Hypoventilation develops more rapidly in children than adults or adolescent.
PEF, Peak expiratory flow.

Exercise and Exercise-Induced Bronchospasm

EIB is an acute, reversible, usually self-terminating airway obstruction that develops during or after vigorous activity, reaches its peak 5 to 10 minutes after stopping the activity, and usually stops in another 20 to 30 minutes. Patients with EIB have cough, shortness of breath, chest pain or tightness, wheezing, and endurance problems during exercise, but an exercise challenge test in a laboratory is necessary to make the diagnosis.

The problem occurs rarely in activities that require short bursts of energy (e.g., baseball, sprints, gymnastics, skiing) and more common in those that involve endurance exercise (e.g., soccer, basketball, distance running). Swimming is well tolerated by children with EIB because they are breathing air fully saturated with moisture and because of the type of breathing required in swimming.

Children with asthma are often excluded from exercise by parents, teachers, and practitioners, as well as by the children themselves, because they are reluctant to provoke an attack. However, this practice can seriously hamper peer interaction and physical health. Exercise is advantageous for children with asthma, and most children can participate in activities at school and in sports with minimal difficulty, provided their asthma is under control. Evaluate participation on an individual basis. Appropriate prophylactic treatment with β-adrenergic agents or cromolyn sodium before exercise usually permits full participation in strenuous exertion.

Therapeutic Management: Specific

Children with asthma have exacerbations at varying intervals, with severity ranging from wheezing to life-threatening status asthmaticus (Table 32-3). Protocols have been developed for treating the child experiencing an asthmatic episode at home or in the emergency department (National Asthma Education and Prevention Program, 2007).

Successful home management of acute asthma begins before symptoms develop. All patients and family members should learn how to monitor symptoms to recognize early signs of deterioration. Children with moderate to severe persistent asthma and those with a history of severe exacerbations should learn how to monitor their peak flow rate to assess the severity of the exacerbation and the response to therapy. All children should be given a written action plan to follow in the event of symptoms or an exacerbation. This plan should include information on how to adjust medications in response to signs, symptoms, and peak flow measurements and when to seek medical help. School-age children should have a written action plan that is appropriate for the school setting.

Status Asthmaticus

Status asthmaticus is a medical emergency that can result in respiratory failure and death if unrecognized and untreated. Children who continue to display respiratory distress despite vigorous therapeutic measures, especially the use of sympathomimetics (e.g., albuterol, epinephrine), are in status asthmaticus. The condition may develop gradually or rapidly, often coincident with complicating conditions, such as pneumonia or a respiratory virus, which can influence the duration and treatment of the exacerbation.

Therapy for status asthmaticus is aimed at improving ventilation, decreasing airway resistance and relieving bronchospasm, correcting dehydration and acidosis, allaying child and

---

! NURSING ALERT

The child with asthma who sweats profusely, remains sitting upright, and refuses to lie down is in severe respiratory distress. Also, the child who suddenly becomes agitated, or the agitated child who suddenly becomes quiet, may be seriously hypoxic and requires immediate intervention.

---

parent anxiety related to the severity of the event, and treating any concurrent infection. Humidified oxygen is recommended and should be given to maintain an oxygen saturation greater than 90%. Inhaled aerosolized short-acting β_2-agonists are recommended for all patients. Three treatments of β_2-agonists spaced 20 to 30 minutes apart are usually given as initial therapy, and continuous administration of β_2-agonists may be initiated. A systemic corticosteroid (oral, IV, or IM) may also be given to decrease the effects of inflammation. An anticholinergic such as ipratropium bromide may be added to the aerosolized solution of the β_2-agonist. Anticholinergics have resulted in additional bronchodilation in patients with severe airflow obstruction. An IV infusion is often initiated to provide a means for hydration and to administer medications. Correction of dehydration, acidosis, hypoxia, and electrolyte disturbance is guided by frequent determination of arterial pH, blood gases, and serum electrolytes.

Additional therapies in acute asthma attacks include the use of IV magnesium sulfate, a potent muscle relaxant that decreases inflammation and improves pulmonary function and peak flow rate among pediatric patients treated in the emergency department with moderate to severe asthma. Heliox may be administered to decrease airway resistance and thereby decrease the work of breathing; it can be delivered via a nonrebreathing face mask from premixed tanks, which may be blended in a stand-alone unit or within a ventilator. It may be used in acute exacerbations as an adjunct to β_2-agonist and IV corticosteroid therapy to improve pulmonary function until the two latter medications have time to take full effect in decreasing bronchospasm; the effects of heliox are usually seen within 20 minutes of administration, whereas other drugs may take longer to exert the desired effect. Ketamine, a dissociative anesthetic, is believed to cause smooth muscle relaxation and decrease airway resistance caused by severe bronchospasm in acute asthma (Linzer, 2007); it may be administered as an adjunct to other therapies mentioned previously.

Antibiotics should not be used to treat acute asthma attacks except when a bacterial infection resulting from another condition such as pneumonia or sinusitis is present (National Asthma Education and Prevention Program, 2007).

A child suspected of having status asthmaticus is usually seen in the emergency department and is often admitted to a pediatric intensive care unit for close observation and continuous cardiorespiratory monitoring. A key component in the prevention of morbidity is helping the child, parents, teachers, coaches, and other adults recognize features of deteriorating respiratory status, use the correct rescue drugs effectively, and immediately place the child with deteriorating respiratory status into the care of trained health care professionals instead of waiting to see if the asthma gets better on its own. The child going into early status asthmaticus is no different from the adult who is having an acute myocardial infarction in terms of needing trained medical assistance before the condition deteriorates to irreversible respiratory failure and possible death. Community education regarding asthma recognition and management is an important component of nursing care.

Prognosis

According to recent Centers for Disease Control and Prevention (2009c) data, 9.1% of U.S. children ages birth to 17 years, or 6.7 million children, were reported to have asthma. Although deaths from asthma have been relatively uncommon since the 1980s, the rate of death from asthma increased steadily in the United States until it peaked in the mid-1990s. Asthma-related deaths decreased between 1996 and 2005 by approximately 3.9% per year (Akinbami, Moorman, Garbe, et al, 2009). Data for the year 2008 indicate a significant increase in asthma symptoms, emergency department visits, and hospitalization among boys from birth to 4 years of age. Mortality and morbidity for asthma are especially high among African-American children, whose hospitalization and death rates are three times higher than those of Caucasian and Hispanic children (Liu, Covar, Spahn, et al, 2007). Most asthma deaths in children occur in the home, school, or community before lifesaving medical care can be administered.

The outlook for children with asthma varies widely. Some children's asthma symptoms may improve at puberty, but up to two thirds of children with asthma continue to have symptoms through puberty and into adulthood. The prognosis for control or disappearance of symptoms varies in children from those who have rare and infrequent attacks to those who are constantly wheezing or are subject to status asthmaticus. In general, when symptoms are severe and numerous, when symptoms have been present for a long time, and when there is a family history of allergy, there is a greater likelihood of a poor prognosis. Risk factors that may predict persistence of symptoms into childhood (from infancy) include atopy, male gender, exposure to environmental tobacco, and maternal history of asthma. Many children who outgrow their exacerbations continue to have airway hyperresponsiveness and cough as adults. Furthermore, airway hyperresponsiveness in adults appears to be associated with decreased lung function.

The adolescent age-group appears to be the most vulnerable, with the greatest increase in mortality from the condition occurring in children 10 to 14 years of age. No reliable data exist to explain this increase. Factors that have been postulated include exposure of atopic persons to more allergens (particularly in large urban centers), change in severity of the disease, abuse of drug therapy (toxicity), failure of families and practitioners to recognize the severity of asthma, and psychologic factors such as denial and refusal to accept the disease.

Risk factors for asthma deaths include early onset, frequent attacks, difficult-to-manage disease, adolescence, history of respiratory failure, psychologic problems (refusal to take medications), dependency on or misuse of asthma drugs (high use), presence of physical stigmata (barrel chest, intercostal retractions), and abnormal PFTs.

Nursing Care Management
Acute Asthma Care

Children who are admitted to the hospital with acute asthma are ill, anxious, and uncomfortable. The progression or resolution of status asthmaticus is variable. Continual observation and assessment are essential (see Nursing Care Plan).

When β$_2$-agonists and corticosteroids are given, the child is monitored closely and continuously for relief of respiratory distress and signs of side effects (tachycardia, restlessness, irritability, hyperactivity). Although food may not be well tolerated in the acute phase, the child may avoid upset stomach associated with β-agonists by taking small amounts of a food, such as a few crackers, once the respiratory status has stabilized

NURSING CARE PLAN

The Child with Acute Asthma Exacerbation

NURSING DIAGNOSIS	EXPECTED PATIENT OUTCOMES	NURSING INTERVENTIONS	RATIONALE
Ineffective Airway Clearance related to inflammation and constriction (spasm) of the bronchial tree	Child will exhibit effective ventilatory capacity (specify). Child will breathe easily, without dyspnea.	Allow child to assume position of comfort (tripod or other).	To promote maximum ventilatory function
		Administer oxygen by face mask to maintain oxygen saturation above 90%.	To enhance oxygenation of tissues
Child's Defining Characteristics (Subjective and Objective Data)	**The Following NOC Concepts Apply to These Outcomes** Airway Patency Asthma Control Anxiety Control	Provide reassurance that symptoms will be managed and air hunger will subside.	To decrease anxiety related to hypoxia
Dyspnea		Administer rescue medications (as prescribed) (National Asthma Education and Prevention Program, 2007):	To open constricted airways and allow air exchange
Diminished breath sounds (air movement)		• Inhaled β$_2$-agonist by metered-dose inhaler or aerosolized nebulization (up to three treatments in first 60 minutes), OR	To enhance tissue oxygenation
Adventitious breath sounds (wheezing)		• Inhaled high-dose β$_2$-agonist (albuterol) and anticholinergic (ipratropium bromide [as age appropriate]) in nebulized form with oxygen (as necessary to keep saturation >90%)	
Difficulty vocalizing Changes in respiratory rate and rhythm		• Oral corticosteroid	
(Related Factors) Allergen exposure		Assess child's response to rescue medications	To determine need for more aggressive interventions
Allergic airway Respiratory tract infection		Administer rescue medications ordered as appropriate every 60 minutes until optimum response is obtained.	To control asthma symptoms
		Observe for exacerbation of asthma symptoms.	To prevent recurrence of acute episode
		Encourage small amounts of clear oral fluids.	To maintain hydration
		For severe, unresponsive exacerbation, initiate peripheral intravenous line.	To maintain hydration and administer medications
		Titrate or wean oxygen concentration according to patient's response to rescue medications (based on work of breathing and oxygen saturation).	To prevent hyperoxemia
		Collaboratively evaluate cause of asthma exacerbation and treat if infection.	To prevent recurrence
		Provide discharge instructions for continued control of asthma symptoms.	To educate for management of symptoms and prevention of exacerbations
		• Review home medication use.	
		• Review written action plan for asthma symptom control.	To provide sense of control
		• Review signs and symptoms requiring immediate medical attention.	To enhance self-esteem
		• Control or eradicate allergens, irritants, and other precipitating factors.	
		• Follow up with practitioner.	
		The Following NIC Concepts Apply to These Interventions Positioning Anxiety Reduction Vital Signs Monitoring Surveillance Medication Administration: Inhalation, Oral Administration Infection Control Fluid Management Fever Treatment	

somewhat. Pulse oximetry is monitored along with rate and depth of breathing, auscultation of air movement, adventitious sounds, and any signs of respiratory distress (e.g., nasal flaring, tachypnea, retractions). The child on supplemental oxygen requires intermittent or continuous oxygenation monitoring depending on severity of respiratory compromise and initial oxygenation status. The child in status asthmaticus should be placed on continuous cardiorespiratory (including blood pressure) and pulse oximetry monitoring.

IV access is usually initiated once the child has been placed on oxygen. The child may respond well to topical pain management for the procedure. Oral fluid intake may be limited during the acute phase; IV fluid replacement may be required to provide adequate tissue hydration. Endotracheal intubation equipment should be readily available. Medications administered intravenously are monitored for their desired effect and for any untoward effects.

Children with acute asthma are apprehensive and anxious, and they often hyperventilate as a result of the anxiety. Calm coaching to increase depth and slow rate of respirations while administering oxygen with a simple mask may alleviate the child's fears. The calm, efficient presence of a nurse helps reassure the child that he or she is safe and will be cared for during this stressful period. Assure children that they will not be left alone and that their parents are allowed to remain with them.

Parents need reassurance and want to be informed of their child's condition and therapies. They may believe that they have in some way contributed to the child's condition or could have prevented the episode. Reassurance regarding their efforts expended on the child's behalf and their parenting capabilities can help alleviate their stress. Efforts to reduce parental apprehension also reduce the child's distress. Anxiety is easily communicated to the child from parents and members of the staff.

General Care

The nursing care of the child with asthma begins with a review of the child's health history; the home, school, and play environment; parent and child attitudes about the child's condition; and a comprehensive physical assessment with focus on the respiratory system. Nursing care of children with asthma involves both acute and long-term care. Nurses who are involved with children in the home, hospital, school, outpatient clinic, or practitioner's office play an important role in helping children and their families learn to live with the condition. The disease can be managed so that it does not require hospitalization or interfere with family life, physical activity, or school attendance. The nursing process in the care of the child with asthma is outlined in the Nursing Care Plan.

Physical assessment of asthma involves the same observations and techniques described in Chapter 6. In addition, the nurse notes and evaluates physical characteristics of chronic respiratory involvement, including chest configuration (e.g., barrel chest), posturing (tripod), and type of breathing. A history of the current and previous episodes and precipitating factors or events provides important information.

Nurses may perform a variety of functions in asthma care, including asthma education in the primary care setting and in schools and other community settings, care of the child with asthma in the acute care setting, ambulatory care, and intensive care. Nurses also obtain information on how asthma affects the child's everyday activities and self-concept, the child's and family's adherence to the prescribed therapy, and their personal treatment goals. Make every effort to build a partnership between the child and family and the health care team. Communication is an essential part of this partnership, and health care providers should routinely assess the effectiveness of patient-provider communication. In particular, assess the child's and family's satisfaction with asthma control and with the quality of care. The nurse should also assess their perception of the severity of the disease and their level of social support.

One of the major emphases of nursing care is outpatient management by the family. Parents are taught how to avoid allergens (especially tobacco smoke), recognize and respond to symptoms of bronchospasm, maintain health and prevent complications, and promote normal activities. The child's asthma action plan should be reviewed periodically at least every 6 months in children with moderate to severe disease; precipitating factors, illness management, and medication use should be discussed. The nurse should determine any cultural or ethnic beliefs or practices that influence self-management and that may necessitate modifications in educational approaches to meet the family's needs.

Avoid Allergens

One goal of asthma management is avoidance of an exacerbation. Parents need to know how to avoid allergens that precipitate asthma episodes. The nurse assists the parent in modifying the environment to reduce contact with the offending allergen(s). Caution the parents to avoid exposing a sensitive child to excessive cold, wind, or other extremes of weather; smoke; sprays; or other irritants. Parents should also eliminate from the diet any foods known to provoke symptoms.

Approximately 2% to 6% of children with asthma are sensitive to aspirin; therefore nurses should caution parents to use other analgesic-antipyretic drugs for discomfort or fever and to read package labeling. Although aspirin is rarely given to children in the United States, salicylate compounds are in other common medicines such as Pepto-Bismol. Children with aspirin-induced asthma may also be sensitive to NSAIDs and tartrazine (yellow dye number 5, a common food coloring).

Teach parents to avoid administering aspirin to *any* child because of its association with Reye syndrome unless specifically recommended by and under the supervision of a health practitioner. Acetaminophen is safe for children and is the analgesic of choice.

Relieve Bronchospasm

Teach parents and older children to recognize early signs and symptoms of an impending attack so that it can be controlled before symptoms become distressing. Most children can recognize prodromal symptoms well before an attack (about 6 hours) and implement preventive therapy. Objective signs that parents may observe include rhinorrhea, cough, low-grade fever, irritability, itching (especially in front of the neck and chest), apathy, anxiety, sleep disturbance, abdominal discomfort, and loss of appetite.

The **peak expiratory flow rate (PEFR)** measures the maximum flow of air that can be forcefully exhaled in 1 second.

NURSING CARE PLAN

The Child with Asthma

NURSING DIAGNOSIS	EXPECTED PATIENT OUTCOMES	NURSING INTERVENTIONS	RATIONALE
Risk for Suffocation related to interaction between individual and triggering factors (allergens, respiratory tract infection, exercise, irritants, emotions, temperature changes) **Child's/Family's Defining Characteristics (Subjective and Objective Data)** Wheezing Dry cough Labored respirations Dyspnea Intercostal retractions Complaints of tightness in chest, shortness of breath Bronchial inflammation and airway constriction	Child will have adequate airway exchange. Family and child will assume responsibility for asthma symptom management. **The Following NOC Concepts Apply to These Outcomes** Asthma Control Anxiety Control Child Development	Assist child and family in recognizing factors such as allergens, irritants, temperature changes, and upper respiratory tract infections that trigger asthma symptoms. Assist child (according to developmental age) and family in recognizing early signs of an asthmatic episode (use peak expiratory flow meter [PEFM]). Educate child and family in the use of inhaled corticosteroids and bronchodilator. Educate child and family regarding proper use of rescue medications in case of disease exacerbation. Educate child and family regarding the proper use of metered-dose inhaler with spacer, aerosolized nebulizer, and PEFM (know child's personal best). **The Following NIC Concepts Apply to These Interventions** Respiratory Monitoring Administering Inhaled Medications Risk Identification Family Integrity Promotion Energy Management Coping Enhancement Environmental Management	To avoid asthma exacerbations and initiate appropriate treatment To control symptoms with medication To control symptoms and minimize shortness of breath To prevent illness exacerbations and hospitalization; to prevent side effects from improper use of certain asthma drugs To help child and family effectively manage asthma symptoms independently

NURSING DIAGNOSIS	EXPECTED PATIENT OUTCOMES	NURSING INTERVENTIONS	RATIONALE
Interrupted Family Processes related to child with a chronic illness **Child's/Family's Defining Characteristics (Subjective and Objective Data)** Anxiety Disruptive family interactions with child and members Family conflicts Inadequate child support Child's health status ignored Family ignoring other members' needs for those of the child with asthma	Family will cope with effects of the disease. Family will provide child an appropriate protective environment. **The Following NOC Concepts Apply to These Outcomes** Family Support Family Normalization	Provide family and child (as age appropriate) with explanations about the disease and management. Cooperate with family to develop a written action plan for asthma management. Discuss facilitators and barriers to effective asthma management. Encourage family and child (as age appropriate) to discuss the impact of the illness on the family's lifestyle. Evaluate family resources for asthma management in relation to: • Access to health care • Medication availability in home and school (or daycare, as appropriate) • Allergen exposure control and eradication **The Following NIC Concepts Apply to These Interventions** Emotional Support Anticipatory Guidance Family Involvement Promotion Financial Resource Assistance Decision-Making Support Mutual Goal Setting	To provide adequate information To provide realistic expectations To provide family and child a sense of control To assist family members in understanding their role as being vital in the management of asthma To provide opportunity to verbalize frustrations and challenges of having a child with a chronic illness To enhance family's ability to cope with child's chronic illness

Additional nursing diagnoses that apply include Ineffective Airway Clearance, Risk for Deficient Fluid Volume, and Risk for Ineffective Infant Feeding Pattern.

PEFR is measured in liters per minute using a peak expiratory flow meter (PEFM). Three zones of measurement are typically used to interpret PEFR. The zone system is patterned after a traffic light to make the categories easy to understand and remember (see Nursing Care Guidelines box). Each child needs to establish his or her personal best value. A personal best value should be established during a 2- to 3-week period when the child's asthma is stable. During this period the child records the PEFR at least twice a day. After the personal best value has been established, the child's current PEFR on any occasion can be compared with the personal best value. PEFR monitoring can be used for short-term monitoring, managing exacerbations, and daily long-term monitoring.

NURSING CARE GUIDELINES

*Interpreting Peak Expiratory Flow Rates**

- Green (80% to 100% of personal best) signals all clear. Asthma is under reasonably good control. No symptoms are present, and the routine treatment plan for maintaining control can be followed.
- Yellow (50% to 79% of personal best) signals caution. Asthma is not well controlled. An acute exacerbation may be present. Maintenance therapy may need to be increased. Call the practitioner if the child stays in this zone.
- Red (below 50% of personal best) signals a medical alert. Severe airway narrowing may be occurring. A short-acting bronchodilator should be administered. Notify the practitioner if the peak expiratory flow rate does not return immediately and stay in yellow or green zone.

*These zones are guidelines only. Specific zones and management should be individualized for each child.

Because measurement of PEFR depends on effort and technique, children need instructions, demonstrations, and frequent reviews of technique (see Family-Centered Care box). Each individual child's PEFR varies according to age, height, sex, and race.

A variety of easy-to-use, inexpensive PEFMs are available for use in the home and at school to assess changes in pulmonary function. In general, children 5 years of age and older are able to use a PEFM successfully. However, young children need to be supervised while they are learning to use their PEFM, and their technique should be checked frequently to ensure it is correct. Children should use the same PEFM over time, and they should bring it for use at every follow-up visit. Using the same brand of meter is recommended because different brands can give significantly different values. The use of a PEFM provides objective monitoring regarding the severity of asthma and can decrease asthma episodes, health care visits, and missed school days (Burkhart, Rayens, Revelette, et al, 2007).

Children who use a nebulizer, MDI, Diskus, or Turbuhaler to deliver drugs need to learn how to use the device correctly. The MDI device delivers medication directly to the airways; therefore the child needs to learn to breathe slowly and deeply for better distribution to narrowed airways (see Family-Centered Care box).

Young children and those who are unable to manipulate the MDI or hold their breath for 10 seconds should use a spacer. In infants and small children a mask may be used to facilitate

FAMILY-CENTERED CARE

Use of a Peak Expiratory Flow Meter

1. Before each use, make certain the sliding marker or arrow on the peak expiratory flow meter is at the bottom of the numbered scale.
2. Stand up straight.
3. Remove gum or any food from the mouth.
4. Close your lips tightly around the mouthpiece. Be certain to keep your tongue away from the mouthpiece.
5. Blow out as hard and as quickly as you can, a "fast, hard puff."
6. Note the number by the marker on the numbered scale.
7. Repeat entire routine three times, but wait at least 30 seconds between each routine.
8. Record the highest of the three readings, not the average.
9. Measure your peak expiratory flow rate (PEFR) close to the same time and same way each day (e.g., morning and evening; before and 15 minutes after taking medication).
10. Keep a record of your PEFRs.

delivery of the medication. These devices allow the parent or child to deliver the medication from the MDI into the spacer, from which the child then inhales the medication while taking slow steady breaths. Spacers also prevent yeast infections in the mouth when corticosteroids are inhaled via an MDI.

The nurse also needs to caution the child and parents about the adverse effects of prescribed drugs and the dangers of overuse of β_2-agonists. They should know that it is important to use these drugs when needed but not indiscriminately or as a substitute for avoiding the symptom-provoking allergen. Caution parents against purchasing over-the-counter preparations because these medications can place the children at risk for increased dosage of a drug and toxicity.

The family should obtain a PEFM and learn to use this device to monitor the child's asthma. A written asthma action plan that includes the three peak flow meter zones and the child's asthma medications may be obtained from the child's primary care provider (Fig. 32-13). A home asthma action plan may reduce the risk of asthma death by 70% (Liu, Covar, Spahn, et al, 2007). Medications used for asthma exacerbations are also included in the asthma plan. This action plan should be used to make decisions about asthma management at home and at school. The nurse may assist the child and family in preparing this plan, emphasizing that they, and not the health professionals, determine the success of the plan.

Teach parents how to read labels on prepared foods and snacks to determine the presence of allergens.

Maintain Health and Prevent Complications

The child should be protected from a respiratory tract infection that can trigger an attack or aggravate the asthmatic state, especially in young children whose airways are mechanically smaller and more reactive. Annual influenza vaccinations are recommended for children with persistent asthma (American Academy of Pediatrics, 2009b). Equipment used for the child, such as nebulizers, must be kept absolutely clean to decrease the chances of contamination with bacteria and fungi.

Teach and encourage breathing exercises and controlled breathing for motivated children, and provide information concerning activities that promote diaphragmatic breathing,

FAMILY-CENTERED CARE

Use of a Metered-Dose Inhaler

Steps for Checking How Much Medicine Is in the Canister

1. If the canister is new, it is full.
2. If the canister has been used repeatedly, it might be empty. (Check product label to see how many inhalations should be in each canister.)
3. The most accurate way to determine how many doses remain in a metered-dose inhaler (MDI) is to count and record each dose as it is used.
4. Many dry powder inhalers have a dose-counting device or dose indicator on the canister to let you know when the canister is empty.
5. Placing dry powder inhalers or MDIs with hydrofluoroalkanes in water will destroy these inhalers.

Steps for Using the Inhaler with Mouthpiece

1. Remove the cap and hold inhaler upright.
2. Shake the inhaler.
3. Attach spacer, as appropriate.
4. Tilt the head back slightly and breathe out slowly.
5. With the inhaler in an upright position, insert the mouthpiece:
   a. About 3 to 4 cm (1 to 1½ inches) from the mouth or
   b. Into the mouth, forming an airtight seal between the lips and the mouthpiece
6. At the end of a normal expiration, depress the top of the inhaler canister firmly to release the medication (into the mouth), and breathe in slowly (about 3 to 5 seconds). Relax the pressure on the top of the canister.
7. Hold the breath for at least 5 to 10 seconds to allow the aerosol medication to reach deeply into the lungs.
8. Remove the inhaler and breathe out slowly through the nose.
9. Wait 1 minute between puffs (if an additional puff is needed) when using a bronchodilator.

NOTE: Inhaled dry powder such as budesonide (Pulmicort) requires a different inhalation technique. To use a dry powder inhaler, the base of the device is turned until a click is heard. It is important to close the mouth tightly around the mouthpiece of the inhaler and inhale rapidly.

Steps for Using the Inhaler with an Aerochamber

(see Fig. 32-11)

1. Remove the cap and hold inhaler upright.
2. Shake the inhaler.
3. Attach aerochamber.
4. With the inhaler in an upright position, insert the mouthpiece into the back of the aerochamber.
5. Apply aerochamber mask to child's face and make sure there is a good seal.
6. Have child breathe slow regular breaths. Depress the top of the inhaler canister firmly to release the medication (into the aerochamber), as the child breathes slowly in and out. Relax the pressure on the top of the canister.
7. Hold the aerochamber in place over the child's face until six breaths have been taken. Give one puff at a time.
8. Remove the inhaler and aerochamber.
9. Wait 1 minute between puffs (if an additional puff is needed) when using a bronchodilator.

Common Problems for Children Using Inhalers

- Child refuses or resists treatment.
- Inhalation is too rapid.
- Child is unable to coordinate the spray with inhalation.
- Breath is not held long enough after inhalation.

Modified from Nurses' Asthma Education Working Group: *Nurses: partners in asthma care,* NIH Pub No 95-3308, Bethesda, Md, 1995, National Heart, Lung, and Blood Institute, National Institutes of Health.

side expansion, and improved mobility of the chest wall. Play techniques that can be used for younger children to extend their expiratory time and increase expiratory pressure include blowing cotton balls or a Ping-Pong ball on a table, blowing a pinwheel, blowing bubbles, or preventing a tissue from falling by blowing it against the wall.

Promote Self-Care and Normalization

Self-care and asthma self-management programs are important in helping the child and family cope with asthma. Most asthma self-management programs for children convey several principles. First, asthma is a common disease that can be controlled with appropriate drug therapy, environmental control, education, and management skills. Second, it is much easier to prevent than to treat an asthma episode; adherence to a therapeutic program is necessary to prevent exacerbations. Third, children with asthma can live full and active lives.

Asthma camps provide an opportunity for children with asthma to engage in physical activity while learning about their disease in a controlled environment with their peers and health professionals. Children who attend asthma camps often demonstrate improved asthma self-management skills.

Self-contained programs and brochures for patient education are available from the Asthma and Allergy Foundation of America* and the American Lung Association.† The National Heart, Lung, and Blood Institute‡ provides educational materials for asthma education in the school setting and also copies of the *Guidelines for the Diagnosis and Management of Asthma* for the practitioner (National Asthma Education and Prevention Program, 2007). Another publication designed for health care practitioners, *Pediatric Asthma: Promoting Best Practice,* can be obtained from the American Academy of Allergy Asthma and Immunology.§

Child and Family Support

The nurse working with children with asthma can provide support in a number of ways. Many children voice frustration because their exacerbations interfere with their daily activities and social lives. They need education about what to do to prevent an asthma episode. These children also need reassurance from the health team that they can learn to control and cope with their asthma and live a normal life. Be aware of children, especially adolescents, who demonstrate signs of depression and may not comply with therapy as a means of passive suicide.

Children in disruptive family situations (divorce, separation, violence, custodial battles) may disregard daily asthma medication regimen or may be at higher risk as a result of neglect by adults who are in charge of their care. Adolescents struggling with a sense of identity and body image often regard asthma as

*8201 Corporate Drive, Suite 1000, Landover, MD 20785; 800-727-8462; www.aafa.org.
†1301 Pennsylvania Ave., NW, Washington, DC 20004; 202-785-3355, 800-548-8252; www.lungusa.org.
‡NHLBI Health Information Center, PO Box 30105, Bethesda, MD 20824-0105; 301-592-8573; fax: 240-629-3246; www.nhlbi.nih.gov.
§555 E. Wells St., Suite 1100, Milwaukee, WI 53202; 414-272-6071; http://aaaai.org.

Asthma Medicine Plan

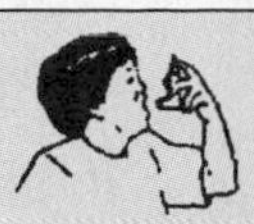

You can use the colors of a traffic light to help learn about your asthma medicines.

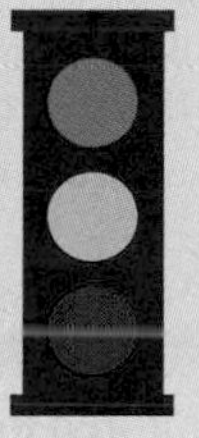

1. **Green** means **Go.**
   Use preventive medicine.

2. **Yellow** means **Caution.**
   Use quick-relief medicine.

3. **Red** means **Stop.**
   Get help from a doctor.

Name: _____

Doctor: _____ Date: _____

Phone for doctor or clinic: _____

Emergency contact phone and name: _____

1. Green — Go

- Breathing is good
- No cough or wheeze
- Can work and play

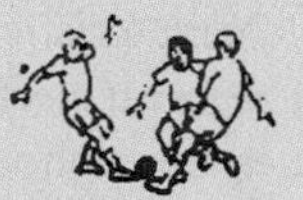

Peak flow number
_____ to _____

Personal best peak flow _____

Use preventive medicine.

Medicine	How much to take	When to take it

5 to 60 minutes before exercise, use this medicine:
_____

2. Yellow — Caution

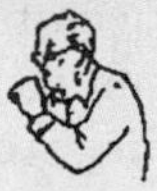

Cough 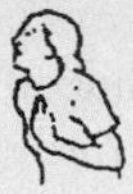   Wheeze 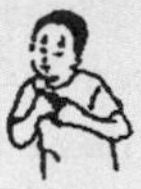   Tight chest

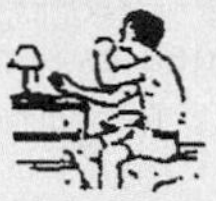

Wake up at night

Peak flow number
_____ to _____
(50 to 80% of my best peak flow)

Take quick-relief medicine to keep an asthma attack from getting bad

Medicine	How much to take	When to take it
(short-acting beta$_2$ agonist)		

If symptoms return to Green Zone after 1 hour of taking above quick-relief medication, take_____ (medicine) and _____ (medicine).

If symptoms **do not** return to Green Zone after 1 hour of taking the quick-relief medication, take_____ (medicine) and add _____ (medicine).
     (short-acting beta$_2$ agonist)   (oral steroid)

Call your doctor if symptoms do not improve within_____ hours after taking the oral steroid or if your symptoms are in the Red Zone.

3. Red — Stop — Danger

- Medicine is not helping
- Breathing is hard and fast
- Nose opens wide
- Can't walk
- Ribs show
- Can't talk well

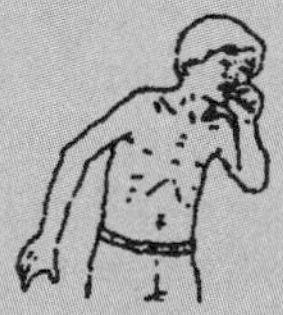

Peak flow number
_____ to _____
(50% or less of personal best)

Get help from a doctor now!
Take these medicines until you talk with the doctor.

Medicine	How much to take	When to take it
(short-acting beta$_2$ agonist)		
(oral steroid)		

Go to the emergency department immediately or call the ambulance if you cannot reach your doctor and you are still in the Red Zone after 15 minutes.

These signs signal **DANGER:**
- Difficulty walking or breathing
- Mental confusion
- Fingernails or lips are blue

Call the ambulance.

Fig 32-13 Asthma action plan. (Redrawn from the National Asthma Education and Prevention Program, National Heart, Lung and Blood Institute: *Asthma management and prevention: global initiative for asthma.* NIH Publication No. 96-3659A, Washington, DC, 1995, National Institutes of Health.)

a condition that will "go away," especially if there is a time lapse between symptoms, and may abandon the therapeutic regimen. In some cases adolescents find themselves in charge of other siblings in blended family situations and may ignore their own health needs. Referral for counseling and guidance is appropriate when the child's or adolescent's life is potentially in danger and the therapeutic regimen for asthma is abandoned due to other crises.

The short- and long-term adaptation of children with asthma often depends on the family's acceptance of the disorder. The task of living day-to-day with affected children involves the entire family. There are periodic crises and the ever-present threat of a crisis, requiring parental vigilance; sleepless nights; frequent trips to the physician, emergency department, or hospital; and often overwhelming medical expenses. Throughout these stresses, encourage parents to promote as normal a life as possible for their children.

CYSTIC FIBROSIS

CF is a condition characterized by exocrine (or mucus-producing) gland dysfunction that produces multisystem involvement. CF is the most common lethal genetic illness among Caucasian children, adolescents, and young adults. It is estimated that 1 in 29 Caucasians in the United States is a symptom-free carrier. More than 95% of the documented cases of CF occur in Caucasians (1 in 3500 live births); the incidence in other ethnic groups varies, affecting African-Americans in 1 in 15,000 live births, and Asian-Americans in 1 in 31,000 life births (Boat and Acton, 2007; Strausbaugh and Davis, 2007).

Etiology

CF is inherited as an autosomal recessive trait. The affected child inherits the defective gene from both parents, with an overall incidence of 1:4. The mutated gene responsible for CF is located on the long arm of chromosome 7. This gene codes a protein of 1480 amino acids called the cystic fibrosis transmembrane regulator (CFTR). The CFTR protein is related to a family of membrane-bound glycoproteins. The glycoproteins constitute a cAMP-activated chloride channel and also regulate other chloride and sodium channels at the surfaces of the epithelial cells.

Functional expression of the CF defect reduces the ability of the epithelial cells in the airways and pancreas to transport chloride. Abnormal transport of sodium and chloride across the epithelium leads to increased viscosity of airway mucus, abnormal mucociliary clearance, and lung disease. The severity of lung disease and presence of hepatic disease cannot be predicted by genotype, which suggests a major environmentally acquired component of organ system dysfunction or another gene that modifies the CF phenotype (Boat and Acton, 2007).

The ΔF508 gene mutation is the most common alteration found in CF. It occurs in 70% of all known CF chromosomes and is closely related to pancreatic insufficiency. Most of the remaining cases of CF are explained by more than 1500 other mutations. CFTR may be divided into six classes based on the type of defect. Individuals in the first three classes have more severe pulmonary disease and pancreatic insufficiency, whereas those in classes 4 and 5 have milder pulmonary symptoms and better weight gain. However, the researchers emphasize that even within each class there is substantial phenotype variability (McKone, Emerson, Edwards, et al, 2003; Strausbaugh and Davis, 2007).

Pathophysiology

With the discovery of the *CFTR* gene, research is continuing to determine its multisystem effects on the body. Several unrelated clinical features characterize CF: increased viscosity of mucous gland secretions, a striking elevation of sweat electrolytes, an increase in several organic and enzymatic constituents of saliva, and abnormalities in autonomic nervous system function. Although both sodium and chloride are affected, the defect appears to be primarily a result of abnormal chloride movement; the CFTR appears to function as a chloride channel.

Children with CF demonstrate decreased pancreatic secretion of bicarbonate and chloride and an increase in sodium and chloride in both saliva and sweat. This last characteristic is the basis for the sweat chloride diagnostic test. The sweat electrolyte abnormality is present from birth, continues throughout life, and is unrelated to the severity of the disease or the extent to which other organs are involved. The sodium and chloride content of sweat in 98% to 99% of children with CF is two to five times greater than that of the controls.

The primary factor, and the one responsible for many of the clinical manifestations of the disease, is mechanical obstruction caused by the increased viscosity of mucous gland secretions (Fig. 32-14). Instead of forming a thin, freely flowing secretion, the mucous glands produce a thick, heavy mucoprotein that accumulates and dilates them. Small passages in organs such as the pancreas and bronchioles become obstructed as secretions precipitate or coagulate to form concretions in glands and ducts.

Because of the increased viscosity of bronchial mucus, there is greater resistance to ciliary action (probably secondary to infection and ciliary destruction); a slower flow rate of mucus; and incomplete expectoration, which also contributes to the mucus obstruction. This retained mucus serves as an excellent medium for bacterial growth. Reduced oxygen–carbon dioxide exchange causes variable degrees of hypoxia, hypercapnia, and acidosis. In severe, progressive lung involvement, compression of pulmonary blood vessels and progressive lung dysfunction frequently lead to pulmonary hypertension, cor pulmonale, respiratory failure, and death.

Pulmonary complications are present in almost all children with CF, but the onset and extent of involvement are variable. Symptoms are produced by stagnation of mucus in the airways, with eventual bacterial colonization leading to destruction of lung tissue. The abnormally viscous and tenacious secretions are difficult to expectorate and gradually obstruct the bronchi and bronchioles, causing scattered areas of bronchiectasis, atelectasis, and hyperinflation.

The most common pathogens are *P. aeruginosa, Burkholderia cepacia, S. aureus, H. influenzae, Escherichia coli,* and *K. pneumoniae.* The pseudomonal strains are particularly pathogenic for children with CF because in most patients the alveolar macrophages cannot destroy *Pseudomonas* organisms. The pseudomonal strains also quickly develop resistance to most medications by developing mucoid strains, and once a person with CF is colonized with these organisms, they are difficult to eradicate. *B. cepacia* is especially worrisome, since this organ-

Critical Thinking Exercise—Cystic Fibrosis Inheritance Risks

Case Study—Cystic Fibrosis

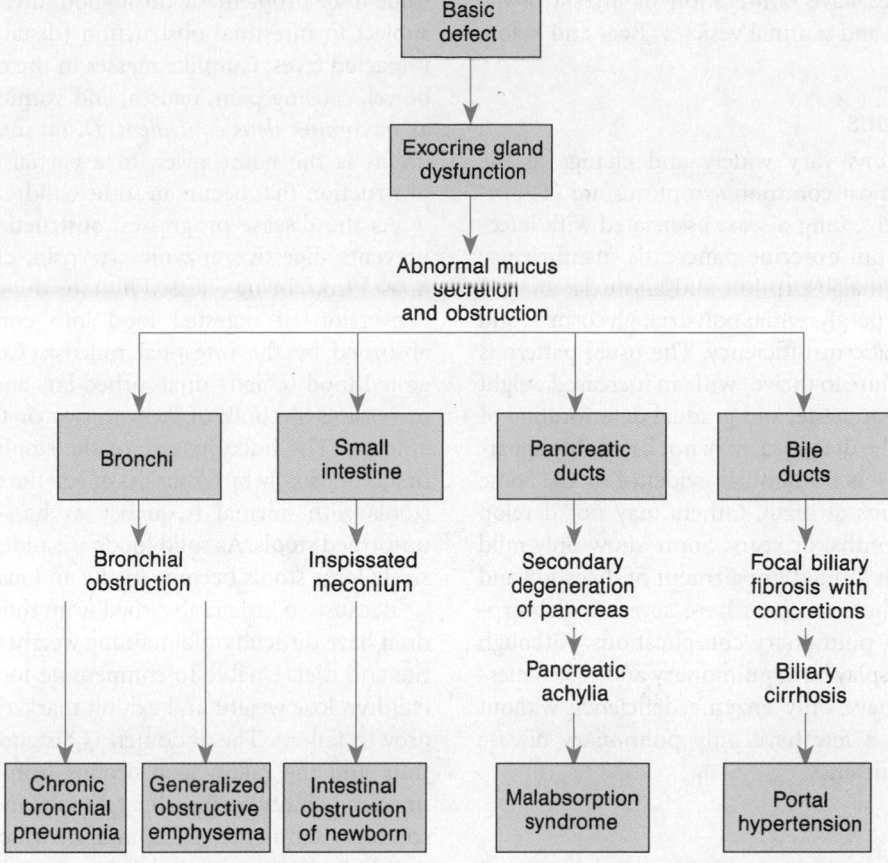

Fig. 32-14 Various effects of exocrine gland dysfunction in cystic fibrosis.

ism is extremely virulent, produces bacteremia, and has been associated with rapid pulmonary function deterioration and death in a significant number of CF patients (Boat and Acton, 2007).

P. aeruginosa infection is not specific for CF but occurs much more frequently in CF than in other diseases characterized by chronic airway obstruction. The patient develops multiple antibodies to the bacteria, which are ineffective in controlling infection; the host is able to tolerate large concentrations of bacteria without overt evidence of worsening.

Gradual progression of pulmonary disease follows chronic infection. Bronchial epithelium is destroyed, and infection spreads to peribronchial tissues, resulting in weakening of bronchial walls and peribronchial fibrosis. The pattern is chronic, progressive fibrosis with decreased oxygen–carbon dioxide exchange and a concurrent alteration in pulmonary vasculature. Chronic hypoxemia causes contraction and hypertrophy of medial muscle fibers in pulmonary arteries and arterioles, leading to pulmonary hypertension and eventual cor pulmonale. Pneumothorax may occur when peripheral bullae rupture; hemoptysis can occur with the erosion of bronchial arteries into a bronchus.

The paranasal sinuses are often filled with secretions and inflammatory products. Nasal and sinus polyps are common, sometimes resulting in bone erosion (Boat and Acton, 2007). Treatment for chronic sinusitis may involve oral antibiotics, decongestants, nasal saline lavage, and nasal corticosteroids.

The extent of gastrointestinal involvement varies. In the pancreas of many patients, thick secretions block the ducts, leading to cystic dilations of the acini (small lobes of the gland),

which then undergo degeneration and progressive diffuse fibrosis. This event prevents essential pancreatic enzymes from reaching the duodenum, which causes marked impairment in the digestion and absorption of nutrients, particularly fats, proteins, and, to a lesser degree, carbohydrates. Disturbed absorption is reflected in excessive stool fat (steatorrhea) and protein (azotorrhea).

The endocrine function of the pancreas often remains unchanged because the islets of Langerhans are normal but may decrease in number as pancreatic fibrosis progresses. The incidence of diabetes mellitus (cystic fibrosis–related diabetes [CFRD]) is greater in CF children than in the general population (Balinsky and Zhu, 2004), which may be caused by changes in pancreatic architecture and diminished blood supply over time. Consequently, with increased survival, and primarily in adolescents and adults, type 1 diabetes is becoming a more frequent finding. There is no relationship between the progression of pulmonary disease and the development of diabetes mellitus in CF.

In the liver, focal biliary obstruction and fibrosis are common and become more extensive with time, eventually giving rise to a distinctive type of multilobular biliary cirrhosis. Some children develop extensive liver involvement with fatty infiltration despite adequate nutrition. The gallbladder is small and contains a firm, gelatinous material that also fills the cystic duct. Findings similar to those in the pancreas are found in the salivary glands and contribute to a dry mouth and susceptibility to infection as a result of interference with salivation.

The glands of the uterine cervix are often filled with mucus, and copious amounts of mucus may block the cervical canal.

More than 95% of males have obliteration or atresia of the epididymis, vas deferens, and seminal vesicles (Boat and Acton, 2007).

Clinical Manifestations

The clinical manifestations vary widely and change as the disease progresses. The most common symptoms are (1) progressive chronic obstructive lung disease associated with infection; (2) maldigestion from exocrine pancreatic insufficiency; (3) growth failure from malabsorption and anorexia; and (4) diabetes symptoms of hyperglycemia, polyuria, glycosuria, and weight loss from pancreatic insufficiency. The usual pattern is one of growth failure (failure to thrive) with an increased weight loss despite an increased appetite, and gradual deterioration of the respiratory system. The diagnosis may not be readily apparent, especially when there is no familial evidence of CF. Some children display symptoms at birth. Others may not develop symptoms for weeks, months, or years. Some show only mild forms of the disease, with limited impairment of digestion and respiratory problems, whereas others have severe malabsorption and life-threatening pulmonary complications. Although most affected children display both pulmonary and gastrointestinal symptoms, a few have only enzyme deficiency without pulmonary disease, and a few have only pulmonary disease without pancreatic insufficiency.

Respiratory Tract

Initial pulmonary manifestations are often wheezing respirations and a dry, nonproductive cough. Eventually diffuse bronchial and bronchiolar obstruction leads to irregular aeration with progressive pulmonary disturbance and secondary infection. The most prominent and constant feature of pulmonary involvement is chronic cough. Dyspnea increases, the cough often becomes paroxysmal, and the mucoid impactions within the small air passages cause a generalized obstructive hyperinflation and patchy areas of atelectasis.

Progressive pulmonary involvement with hyperaeration of functioning alveoli produces the overinflated, barrel-shaped chest in which the anteroposterior diameter approaches the lateral diameter. Bronchiectatic cysts and subpleural blebs in the upper lobes occur in advanced disease and may rupture, causing pneumothorax (Boat and Acton, 2007). When ventilation and subsequent diffusion and gas exchange are significantly impaired, cyanosis and clubbing of the fingers and toes may occur. The child or adolescent has repeated episodes of bronchitis and bronchopneumonia and is subject to chronic nasal congestion, rhinitis, chronic sinusitis, and nasal polyps. The incidence of ENT surgeries is higher in this group of children when compared with the general population.

Gastrointestinal Tract

The earliest postnatal manifestation of CF is meconium ileus, which occurs in 15% to 20% of newborns with the disease (Boat and Acton, 2007). Thick, puttylike, tenacious, mucilaginous meconium blocks the lumen of the small intestine, usually at or near the ileocecal valve, which gives rise to signs of intestinal obstruction, including abdominal distention, vomiting, failure to pass stools, and rapid development of dehydration with associated electrolyte imbalance. Thick intestinal secretions continue to be problematic throughout life. Children of all ages are subject to intestinal obstruction (distal ileum) from heavy or impacted feces. Gumlike masses in the cecum can obstruct the bowel, causing pain, nausea, and vomiting. This is referred to as *meconium ileus equivalent. Distal intestinal obstruction syndrome* is the name given to a partial or complete intestinal obstruction that occurs in some children with CF.

As the disease progresses, obstruction of pancreatic ducts prevents digestive enzymes (trypsin, chymotrypsin, amylase, lipase) from being released into the duodenum, which prevents conversion of ingested food into compounds that can be absorbed by the intestinal mucosa. Consequently, the undigested food (chiefly unabsorbed fats and proteins) is excreted, increasing the bulk of feces to two or three times the normal amount. The bulky nature of the stools may go unnoticed at first, but usually by 6 months of age the child passes large, loose stools with normal frequency or has chronic diarrhea with unformed stools. As solid foods are added to the diet, the excessively large stools become frothy and extremely foul smelling.

Because so little is absorbed from the intestine, affected children have difficulty maintaining weight despite a healthy appetite and diet. Unable to compensate for the fecal losses, many children lose weight and exhibit marked wasting of tissues and growth failure. The abdomen is distended, the extremities are thin, and the sallow skin droops from wasted buttocks. The impaired ability to absorb fats results in a deficiency of the fat-soluble vitamins A, D, E, and K, which may cause bleeding problems if vitamin K deficiency is significant. Anemia is a common complication. Growth failure may be an initial diagnosis in young children with previously undiagnosed CF. Many older children with CF have an increased prevalence of gastroesophageal reflux.

Another common gastrointestinal complication is prolapse of the rectum, which occurs in infancy and early childhood and is related to large, bulky stools; malnutrition; and increased intraabdominal pressure secondary to paroxysmal cough. Appendicitis, intussusception, and volvulus may also occur more frequently in children with CF (Hazle, 2010).

Reproductive System

Delayed puberty in girls with CF is common even when their nutritional and clinical status is good. CF affects the reproductive systems of both males and females. Females with CF have normal fallopian tubes and ovaries. Fertility can be inhibited by highly viscous cervical secretions, which act as a plug, blocking sperm entry. Women with CF who become pregnant have an increased incidence of premature labor and delivery and low birth weight in the infant. Favorable nutritional status and pulmonary function are positively correlated with favorable pregnancy outcomes. Most adult men (approximately 95%) with CF are sterile, which may be caused by blockage of the vas deferens with abnormal secretions or by failure of normal development of the wolffian duct structures (vas deferens, epididymis, and seminal vesicles), resulting in decreased or absent sperm production.

Integumentary System

The consistent finding of abnormally high sodium and chloride concentrations in the sweat is a unique characteristic of CF.

Parents frequently observe that their infants taste "salty" when they kiss them. The chloride channel defect in sweat glands prevents reabsorption of sodium and chloride, which leaves the affected person at risk for abnormal salt loss, dehydration, and hypochloremic and hyponatremic alkalosis during hyperthermic conditions. This is especially important to the infant because of limited fluid stores and the potential for inadequate sodium intake with most commercially prepared infant formulas.

The disease is sometimes expressed in other ways (e.g., hyponatremia caused by massive losses through sweat, especially in high environmental temperatures or febrile episodes). Infants with CF who have growth failure frequently demonstrate hypoalbuminemia resulting from diminished absorption of protein, which in severe cases causes generalized edema.

Diagnostic Evaluation

Traditionally the diagnosis of CF was based on a positive sweat chloride test, absence of pancreatic enzymes, radiography, chronic obstructive pulmonary disease, and family history. Newer diagnostic methods make it possible to diagnose CF early in infancy so therapies can be implemented to increase the child's overall survival and quality of life. In addition to the sweat chloride test and factors listed previously, diagnosis may be confirmed by any one of the following: newborn screening, deoxyribonucleic acid (DNA) identification of mutant genes, and abnormal nasal potential difference measurement.

The quantitative sweat chloride test (pilocarpine iontophoresis) involves stimulating the production of sweat with a special device (involving stimulation with 3-mA electric current), collecting the sweat on filter paper, and measuring the sweat electrolytes. The quantitative analysis requires a sufficient volume of sweat (>75 mg). Two separate samples are collected to ensure the reliability of the test. Normally sweat chloride content is less than 40 mEq/L, with a mean of 18 mEq/L. A chloride concentration greater than 60 mEq/L is diagnostic of CF; in infants younger than 3 months a sweat chloride concentration greater than 40 mEq/L is highly suggestive of CF. In some situations DNA testing may be substituted for the sweat test. The presence of a mutation known to cause CF on each *CFTR* gene predicts with a high degree of certainty that the individual has CF; however, multiple *CFTR* mutations may also be present and detected with DNA assay.

Chest radiography reveals characteristic patchy atelectasis and obstructive emphysema. PFTs are sensitive indices of lung function, providing evidence of abnormal small airway function in CF. Other diagnostic tools that may aid in diagnosis include stool fat or enzyme analysis. Stool analysis requires a 72-hour sample with accurate recording of food intake during that time. Radiographs, including barium enema, are used for diagnosis of meconium ileus.

In some cases CF may go undiagnosed until the child is older and is seen with clinical manifestations that previously were not acute. Ten percent of new CF diagnoses made in 2007 were in children over 10 years old (Cystic Fibrosis Foundation, 2009a).

Screening

Universal newborn screening for CF has been proposed yet remains controversial, since many states lack the resources for such screening programs. In 2009 all but two states offered some type of CF newborn screening (National Newborn Screening and Genetics Resource Center, 2009). The Centers for Disease Control and Prevention (2004) emphatically recommends newborn screening for CF. In one study infants with early diagnosed CF had asymptomatic lung disease and bacterial infection (*S. aureus* and *P. aeruginosa*). Children who were identified and treated early in infancy with aggressive nutritional support had improved height and weight well into adolescence (Sly, Brennan, Gangell, et al, 2009).

The newborn screening test consists of an immunoreactive trypsinogen (IRT) analysis performed on a dried spot of blood, which may be followed by direct analysis of DNA for the presence of the $\Delta F508$ mutation or other mutations on the same dried blood spot. Benefits of early screening and detection include earlier nutritional intervention and preservation of lung function for identified infants (Farrell, Rosenstein, White, et al, 2007; Linnane, Hall, Nolan, et al, 2008; Southern, Merelle, Dankert-Roelse, et al, 2009). Perceived disadvantages to early screening include the parental anxiety false-positive results may generate. Although the technology is available to conduct carrier screening for the general population, this issue remains controversial, and widespread implementation of carrier screening programs is not recommended. An in utero diagnosis of CF is also possible based on detection of two CF mutations in the fetus.

Therapeutic Management

Improved survival among patients with CF during the past two decades is attributable largely to antibiotic therapy and improved nutritional management. Goals of CF therapy are to (1) prevent or minimize pulmonary complications, (2) ensure adequate nutrition for growth, (3) encourage appropriate physical activity, and (4) promote a reasonable quality of life for the child and family. To attain these goals, health care providers use a multidisciplinary system approach to treatment. Current research and modern technologies are exploring methods to attack the genetic defect. For example, a number of clinical trials are underway to examine the feasibility of correcting the underlying genetic defect using gene therapy. Evidence-based guidelines for the management of infants with CF have recently been published elsewhere (Borowitz, Robinson, Rosenfeld, et al, 2009).

Management of Pulmonary Problems

Direct management of pulmonary problems toward prevention and treatment of pulmonary infection by improving ventilation, removing mucopurulent secretions, and administering antimicrobial agents. Many children develop respiratory symptoms by 3 years of age. The large amounts and viscosity of respiratory secretions in children with CF contribute to the likelihood of respiratory tract infections. Recurrent pulmonary infections in the child with CF result in greater the damage to the airways; small airways are destroyed, causing bronchiectasis.

The most common pathogens responsible for pulmonary infections are *P. aeruginosa*, *B. cepacia*, *S. aureus*, *H. influenzae*, *E. coli*, and *K. pneumoniae*. *P. aeruginosa* and *B. cepacia* are particularly pathogenic for children with CF, and infections with these organisms are difficult to clear. In addition, children with CF who are chronically colonized with these organisms have poorer survival rates than children who are not colonized (Boat and Acton, 2007). Colonization and infection with methicillin-resistant *S. aureus* (MRSA) has recently emerged as a critical factor in lung infection and pulmonary function in patients with CF. Patients with MRSA required longer hospitalization and multiple antibiotic regimens (Ren, Morgan, Konstan, et al, 2007). Fungal colonization with *Candida* or *Aspergillus* organisms in the respiratory tract is also common in CF patients.

Airway Clearance Therapy

Prevention of pulmonary infection involves a daily routine of CPT to maintain pulmonary hygiene. (See Chapter 31.) CPT is usually performed on average twice daily (on rising and in the evening) and more frequently if needed, especially during pulmonary infection. The **Flutter mucus clearance device** is a small, hand-held plastic pipe with a stainless-steel ball on the inside that facilitates removal of mucus (Fig. 32-15). It has the advantages of increasing sputum expectoration and being used without assistance. Hand-held percussors and mechanical percussors may be used to loosen secretions. Another method to clear mucus is high-frequency chest compression, in which the child temporarily wears a mechanical vest device that provides high-frequency chest wall oscillation. Some children and adolescents with an implantable port may experience localized pain with the vest.

Patients with CF have been found to regress when conventional CPT is discontinued. Therefore, although it is time consuming for the child and family, *CPT remains the cornerstone of pulmonary therapy.* Forced expiration, or "huffing," with the glottis partially closed helps move secretions from the small airways so that subsequent coughing can move secretions forcefully from the large airways. This maneuver enhances the pulmonary function of patients with CF. Autogenic drainage involves a variety of breathing techniques, which the older child can use to force mucus in lower lobes up into the airways so it can be successfully expelled. Another mucus-clearing technique involves use of a positive expiratory pressure mask; this technique involves breathing into a mask attached to a one-way

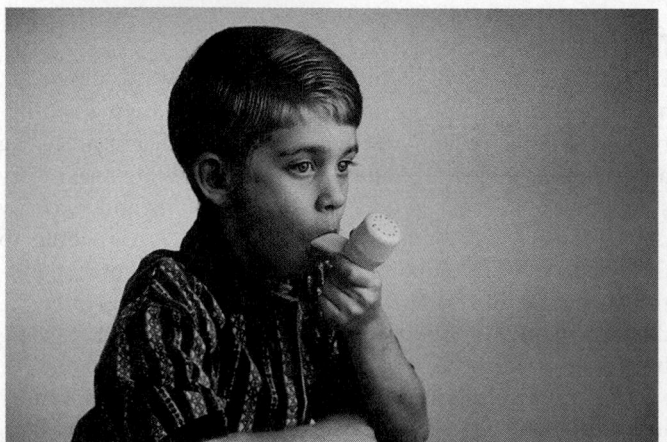

Fig. 32-15 Child using Flutter mucus clearance device. (Courtesy Scandipharm, Inc.)

valve, which creates resistance—as the patient exhales, the airway is kept open by the pressure and mucus is forced into the upper airway for expulsion.

Bronchodilator medication delivered in an aerosol opens bronchi for easier expectoration and is administered before CPT when the patient exhibits evidence of reactive airway disease or wheezing. Another aerosolized medication is recombinant human deoxyribonuclease (DNase, known generically as dornase alfa [Pulmozyme]), which decreases the viscosity of mucus. It is well tolerated and has no major adverse effects; minor reactions are voice alterations and laryngitis. This medication, given once or twice daily via nebulization, has resulted in improvements in spirometry, PFTs, dyspnea scores, and perceptions of well-being and has reduced the viscosity of sputum (Redding, 2009). Nebulized hypertonic saline (6% to 7%) has been shown to be effective in improving airway hydration and increases mucus clearance in patients with CF; this treatment, however, causes bronchospasm and may not be recommended for patients with severe disease (Redding, 2009; Rowe and Clancy, 2006). Clinical trials are in progress to examine the effects of inhaled dry powdered mannitol for improving mucociliary clearance in CF by rehydrating the airway (Minasian, Wallis, Metcalfe, et al, 2008).

Physical exercise is an important adjunct to daily CPT. Exercise stimulates mucus excretion and provides a sense of well-being and increased self-esteem. Any aerobic exercise that the patient enjoys should be encouraged. The ultimate aim of exercise is to increase lung vital capacity, remove secretions, increase pulmonary blood flow, and maintain healthy lung tissue for effective ventilation.

Colonization with *P. aeruginosa* and *B. cepacia* signals progressive involvement. Although the bacteria are impossible to eradicate, they can be successfully controlled. Inhaled antibiotics are administered as a prophylactic measure in some centers, but once the organisms have become established, antibiotic therapy is most effective when given intravenously. Patients with CF metabolize antibiotics more rapidly than normal; therefore drug dosage is often higher than would be expected. Depending on its sensitivity, *P. aeruginosa* is usually treated with aminoglycosides in combination with antipseudomonal β-lactam antibiotics (ticarcillin, piperacillin, ceftazidime). Antibiotic treatment of *B. cepacia* should be based on susceptibility and synergy testing. The duration of therapy depends on the patient's response, measured by clinical indicators, including cough, fatigue, and exercise intolerance, in addition to tests such as PFTs, chest radiography, and oxygen and carbon dioxide measurements.

Pulmonary infections are treated as soon as they are recognized. In CF patients characteristic signs of pulmonary infection—fever, tachypnea, and chest pain—may be absent. Therefore a careful history and physical examination are essential. The presence of anorexia, weight loss, and decreased activity alert the practitioner to pulmonary infection and the need for an antibiotic regimen (Boat and Acton, 2007). Aerosolized antibiotics such as tobramycin, ticarcillin, and gentamicin are beneficial for patients with frequent pulmonary exacerbations (Redding, 2009). These medications are usually administered by jet or ultrasonic nebulizers after CPT is performed. This type of delivery system allows for direct antimicrobial application with little systemic absorption. It is not uncommon for the hospitalized child with CF to be placed on as many as two or three antibiotics and one antifungal medication to treat coexisting pulmonary infections.

IV antibiotics may be administered at home as an alternative to hospitalization. The use of peripherally inserted central catheters (PICCs) for the administration of antibiotics in children with CF is a viable option with limited complications and fewer needle punctures to obtain blood specimens and to maintain often lengthy treatment with parenteral antibiotics (Tolomeo and Mackey, 2003). Alternatively, an implanted port offers the advantage of access for blood draws and antibiotic infusion. Patients may receive antibiotic therapy at home and continue daily activities with minimum disruptions. However, when pulmonary function does not improve with outpatient management, hospitalization may be recommended for continued antibiotic therapy and vigorous CPT and postural drainage. Oxygen administration is used for children with acute episodes but must be used cautiously because many children with CF have chronic carbon dioxide retention, and the unsupervised use of oxygen can be harmful. (See Oxygen Therapy, Chapter 31.) With repeated infection and inflammation, bronchial cysts and emphysema may develop. These cysts may rupture, resulting in a pneumothorax (see Box 32-10).

> ### ! NURSING ALERT
>
> Signs of a pneumothorax are usually nonspecific and include tachypnea, tachycardia, dyspnea, pallor, and cyanosis. A subtle drop in oxygen saturation (measured by pulse oximetry) may be an early sign of pneumothorax.

Blood streaking of the sputum is usually associated with increased pulmonary infection and often requires no specific treatment. Hemoptysis greater than 250 ml/24 hr for the older child (less for a younger child) indicates a potentially life-threatening event and needs to be treated immediately. Sometimes bleeding can be controlled with bed rest, IV antibiotics, replacement of acute blood loss, IV conjugated estrogens (Premarin) or vasopressin (Pitressin), and correction of any coagulation defects with vitamin K or fresh frozen plasma. If hemoptysis persists, the site of bleeding should be localized via bronchoscopy and cauterized or embolized.

Children and adolescents with CF should be given the age-appropriate immunizations, including the annual influenza virus vaccine. The trivalent inactivated influenza virus vaccine is appropriate for such individuals.

Treatment of nasal polyps includes intranasal corticosteroids, oral antihistamines, and decongestants. If these measures are ineffective, surgical interventions may be necessary.

Because pulmonary damage in patients with CF is believed to be caused by the inflammatory process that occurs with frequent infections, the use of corticosteroids has been studied; however, treatment with corticosteroids found only a modest efficacy and numerous side effects, including linear growth restriction, glucose tolerance abnormalities, and cataract formation (Boat and Acton, 2007). Antiinflammatory medications such as the NSAID ibuprofen have shown significant benefits particularly in younger patients with mild disease (Boat and Acton, 2007). Long-term daily ibuprofen given in a dose sufficient to achieve a peak plasma concentration between 50 and 100 mcg/ml has been shown to slow the rate of decline in pulmonary function and to decrease the need for IV antibiotics in young patients with mild pulmonary involvement Although this therapy is generally well tolerated, careful monitoring for adverse effects (gastrointestinal bleeding) is essential (Boat and Acton, 2007).

Lung transplantation is a final therapeutic option for many CF patients with severe disease. Heart-lung and double-lung procedures have been successfully performed in children with advanced pulmonary vascular disease and hypoxia; however, whether such procedures significantly improve quality of life and survival rates in children with CF is debated in the current literature. Some experts state that infections such as *B. cepacia* represent a negative factor for long-term survival after transplant (Kotloff, 2009; Liou, Adler, Cox, et al, 2007). Data show that 5-year survival in adults with CF and without *B. cepacia* is less than 50% (Kotloff, 2009). The obstacles surrounding this technique are availability of donated organs; complications from surgery; and recurrence of pulmonary infections and obstructive bronchiolitis, which decreases transplanted lung function. Living-donor lobar transplantation is an alternative to cadaveric transplantation for those who might otherwise succumb to pulmonary and cardiac failure while waiting for a transplant (Goldberg and Deykin, 2007).

Management of Gastrointestinal Problems

The principal treatment for pancreatic insufficiency is replacement of pancreatic enzymes, which are administered with meals and snacks to ensure that digestive enzymes are mixed with food in the duodenum. Enteric-coated products prevent the neutralization of enzymes by gastric acids, thus allowing activation to occur in the alkaline environment of the small bowel. The amount of enzymes depends on the severity of the insufficiency, the child's response to enzyme replacement, and the practitioner's philosophy. Usually one to five capsules are administered with a meal, and fewer are taken with snacks. Capsules can be swallowed whole or taken apart, and the contents sprinkled on a small amount of food to be taken at the beginning of the meal. The amount of enzyme is adjusted to achieve normal growth and a decrease in the number of stools to one or two per day. Pancreatic enzymes should be taken within 30 minutes of eating. The enteric-coated beads should not be chewed or crushed, since destroying the enteric coating can lead to inactivation of the enzymes and excoriation of oral mucosa. The powder form should be used cautiously because inhalation of the powder may precipitate acute bronchospasm. Enzymes are mixed into cereal or fruit such as applesauce for small children.

One issue of concern with pancreatic enzymes is that generic enzymes are not considered adequate and only proprietary enzymes should be given to children with CF (Stallings, Stark, Robinson, et al, 2008). Because the uptake of fat-soluble vitamins is decreased, water-miscible forms of these vitamins (A, D, E, and K) are given, along with multivitamins and the pancreatic enzymes. When high-fat foods are eaten, the child is encouraged to add extra enzymes.

Children with CF require a well-balanced, high-protein, high-caloric diet, with unrestricted fat (because of the impaired intestinal absorption). Improved nutrition in children with CF has been associated positively with improved lung function. To meet his or her energy requirements, the patient with minimal pulmonary disease must consume 5% to 10% more than the recommended dietary allowance (RDA); for those with severe lung disease energy requirements may be as high as 20% to 50% or more of the RDA (American Academy of Pediatrics, 2009a). A group of experts recently recommended that children and adolescents with CF 2 to 20 years of age have an energy intake of 110% to 200% of standards for healthy persons (Stallings, Stark, Robinson, et al, 2008). Regular nutritional monitoring should be a standard part of the medical care of the child with CF and should occur every 3 to 4 months (American Academy of Pediatrics, 2009a). Breast-feeding with enzyme supplementation should be continued whenever possible and, when necessary, supplemented with a higher-calorie-per-ounce (e.g., 24 kcal/oz) formula. For formula-fed infants, commercial cow's milk–based formulas may be adequate to achieve desired growth, but additional caloric intake may be required. In older children with CF three daily meals and three snacks are recommended to meet energy and growth requirements (American Academy of Pediatrics, 2009a).

Growth failure despite adequate nutritional support may indicate deterioration of pulmonary status. Data indicate that better forced expiratory volume in 1 second (FEV_1) status (≥80%) strongly correlates with body mass index percentiles above 50th percentile; therefore the target weight for children with CF 2 to 20 years old should be ideally maintained above the 50th percentile (Stallings, Stark, Robinson, et al, 2008). A persistent weight loss over 6 months to 1 year or persistent malnutrition requires aggressive nutritional therapy to prevent declining pulmonary and general physical health status (American Academy of Pediatrics, 2009a). Patients with CF may experience frequent anorexia as a result of the copious amounts of mucus produced and expectorated, persistent cough, effect of medications, fatigue, and sleep disruption. They may be placed on nighttime (or continuous) supplemental gastrostomy feedings or parenteral alimentation in an effort to build up nutritional reserves if there has been a history of inability to maintain weight. Enzyme supplement is encouraged with gastrostomy feedings; these may be given at the initiation of the infusion, at bedtime, and at the conclusion of the feeding infusion (American Academy of Pediatrics, 2009a).

Meconium ileus and meconium ileus equivalent, or total or partial intestinal obstruction, can occur at any age. Constipation is often the result of a combination of malabsorption (either from inadequate pancreatic enzyme dosage or a failure to take the enzymes), decreased intestinal motility, and abnormally viscous intestinal secretions. These problems usually do not require surgical interventions and may be treated with GoLYTELY or Colyte (osmotic solutions given orally or by nasogastric tube), other laxatives, stool softeners, or rectal administration of diatrizoate meglumine (Gastrografin).

Rectal prolapse occurs in a small number of children with CF. The first episode of rectal prolapse is frightening to both parents and child. Its reduction usually requires immediate guidance and intervention, which is managed by simply guiding the rectum back into place with a gloved, lubricated finger with the child lying on her or his side. Further management usually involves attempting to decrease the bulk of daily stools through pancreatic enzyme replacement.

Children with CF often experience transient or chronic gastroesophageal reflux, which should be treated with the appropriate histamine-receptor antagonist and gastrointestinal motility drug, dietary modifications, and an upright position after feedings or meals (Hazle, 2010).

Management of Endocrine Problems

The management of CFRD is critical in the therapeutic treatment of the child with CF. CFRD presents a combination of insulin resistance and insulin deficiency, with unstable glucose homeostasis in the presence of acute lung infection and treatment. Children with CFRD require close monitoring of blood glucose, administration of oral glucose-lowering agents or insulin injections, and diet and exercise management; children with CF may be at increased risk for glucose management problems as a result of decreased nutrient absorption, anorexia, and severity of pulmonary illness. The prevalence of CFRD increases with age, and there is increased morbidity and mortality among children with CFRD compared to those without (Strausbaugh and Davis, 2007). Microvascular complications such as retinopathy and nephropathy may occur in children and adolescents with CFRD (Schwarzenberg, Thomas, Olsen, et al, 2007). However, ketoacidosis is reported to be rare in individuals with CFRD (Boat and Acton, 2007).

Bone health is of concern in children and adults with CF. The pancreatic insufficiency of CF and chronic steroid use present potential risks for less than optimum bone growth in such children. Assessment of bone health by history and bone mass density evaluation should be considered in assessing the child's (≥8 years old) health status to detect and prevent osteoporosis or osteopenia (Borowitz, Baker, and Stallings, 2002).

The administration of growth hormone (somatropin [Nutropin]) is being investigated as a nutritional adjunct in children with CF to achieve optimum growth; one small study sample suggests an improvement in CF clinical status (Hardin, Rice, Ahn, et al, 2005). One randomized study indicates that the drug is well tolerated but does not result in short-term improvement of FEV in CF patients (Schnabel, Grasemann, Staab, et al, 2007).

Prognosis

In 1966 the median life expectancy for individuals with CF was 7.5 years. The median survival age for the CF patient in 2008 was 37.4 years, and approximately 45% of all patients with CF are 18 years old and older (Cystic Fibrosis Foundation, 2009b).

Lung, heart, pancreas, and liver transplantation have increased survival rates among some CF patients. Heart-lung and double-lung procedures have been successfully performed in children with advanced pulmonary vascular disease and hypoxia. In 2008 estimates of 5-year survival after transplantation were approximately 60% (Hazle, 2010). The obstacles surrounding this technique are availability of donated organs; complications from surgery; pulmonary infections; and recurrence of obstructive bronchiolitis, which decreases transplanted lung function.

Despite considerable progress and a recent surge in new treatment modalities, CF remains a progressive and incurable disease. The pulmonary involvement ultimately determines the patient's outcome because pancreatic enzyme deficiency is less of a problem if adequate nutrition is ensured. With advances in technology, parents and adolescents are challenged to set future goals that may include college, careers, social relationships, and marriage. Concurrently they are faced with increasing morbidity and higher rates of CF complications as they grow older.

Nursing Care Management

Assessment of the child with CF involves comprehensive assessment of all affected systems with special focus on pulmonary and gastrointestinal systems. Pulmonary assessment is the same as that described for asthma, with special attention to lung sounds, observation of cough, and evidence of decreased activity or fatigue. Gastrointestinal assessment primarily involves observing the frequency and nature of the stools and abdominal distention. The observer is also alert to evidence of growth failure (e.g., weight loss, muscle wasting, pallor, anorexia, decreased activity [from baseline norm]). Family members are interviewed to determine the child's eating and eliminating habits and confirm a history of frequent respiratory tract infections or bowel obstruction in infancy.

The nurse assesses the newborn for feeding and stooling patterns, which may indicate a potential problem such as meconium ileus. The nurse also participates in diagnostic testing such as the initial newborn screening, IRT, DNA analysis, or sweat chloride test.

Parents are often anxious and puzzled about the diagnostic tests and the possible implications of the test results. They need careful explanations of the disease, how it might affect their family, and what they can do to provide the best possible care for their child. It is crucial to involve the parents in the follow-up for early diagnostic testing; the neonate may require several follow-up visits in the first few weeks of life if initial test results are not conclusive.

The uncertainty, fear, and initial shock associated with the diagnosis are overwhelming to parents. They must face the impact of the chronic, life-threatening nature of the disease and the prospect of intensive treatment, for which they must assume a major part of the responsibility and for which they are ill prepared. They often fear that they will be unable to provide the care the child needs.

Hospital Care

Most patients with CF require hospitalization only for treatment of pulmonary infection, uncontrolled diabetes, or a coexisting medical problem that cannot be treated on an outpatient basis. Therefore, when patients with CF are hospitalized, implement Standard Precautions with meticulous hand washing to decrease the nosocomial spread of organisms to the CF patient and between hospitalized CF patients (especially when MRSA is prevalent). Contact Precautions may be required for specific infections.

When the child with CF is hospitalized for diagnosis or treatment of pulmonary complications, aerosol therapy, chest percussion therapy, and postural drainage are instituted or continued. Respiratory therapists often initiate, supervise, and provide these treatments; however, it is the nurse's responsibility to monitor the patient's tolerance to the procedure and evaluate its effectiveness in relation to treatment goals. The nurse may at times administer aerosol therapy, perform CPT, assist with airway clearance interventions such as the mechanical vest, and teach breathing exercises. CPT should not be performed before or immediately after meals. Planning CPT so that it does not coincide with meals is difficult in the hospital situation but is essential to the effectiveness of this treatment.

Administer supplemental oxygen therapy to the child with mild or moderate respiratory distress, and assess the child's tolerance to the procedure. Noninvasive pulse oximetry provides valuable data about the patient's oxygenation status, but nursing assessments, including observation of respiratory pattern, work of breathing, and lung auscultation, are vital.

One of the nursing challenges in the care of the child with CF is encouraging compliance with the therapeutic medication regimen, which often involves a significant number of medications; pancreatic enzymes; vitamins A, D, E, and K; oral antifungals for *Candida* infection; antihistamines; antiinflammatory agents; and oral antibiotics. This may be overwhelming to the child. Factor in multiple inhaled bronchodilators, CPT and aerosol treatments, blood glucose monitoring and insulin administration, various other medications, and increased mucus production during the acute phase, and it is not uncommon for the child with CF to rebel and be noncompliant with this regimen.

Gentle coaxing, positive reinforcement, and frank negotiation may be required to enlist cooperation for effective medication compliance. The child's sleep is disrupted frequently by hospital routines; therefore nursing care should be flexible enough to allow him or her some quiet time without affecting vital care. In some cases a daily schedule of events, including medication administration, CPT, aerosolized therapy, and dressing changes, may need to be mutually developed with the child, nurses, and physician so that the child feels he or she has some control of the care.

The diet for the child with CF represents another challenge; careful planning with a pediatric dietitian and the child's input may help decrease the loss of appetite and weight loss that are often part of the condition. Patients with CF, especially adolescents, enjoy foods brought from home or an occasional fast food of choice (provided these meet therapeutic requirements). Children in the early stages of CF often have a good appetite. With infection and increased lung involvement, their appetite diminishes, and eventually it becomes a challenge to tempt failing appetites. Age-appropriate nutrition education with specific nutritional goals for CF patients may increase compliance with prescribed enzyme therapy and nutritional supplements (Pitts, Flack, and Goodfellow, 2008).

When dietary intake fails to meet the child's needs for growth, enteral feedings or supplements may be considered (Borowitz, Baker, and Stallings, 2002). These feedings may be administered via gastrostomy tube during the night to minimize the disruption of daily activities, including school. Additional pancreatic enzymes are required with supplemental feedings to obtain best results. A skin-level feeding gastrostomy affords the child few activity restrictions and minimum disruption of body image in comparison to a nasogastric tube or conventional gastrostomy tube. The child and parents are encouraged to perceive this therapy not as a last-ditch effort but as an adjunct therapy to maintain optimum growth and prevent excessive weight loss (Borowitz, Baker, and Stallings, 2002). In some cases adolescents are taught to insert a nasogastric tube for nighttime supplemental feedings; the tube may then be removed in the morning.

The child needs support during the many treatments and tests that are a part of the hospitalization. IV fluids, IV antibiotics and antifungals, and blood tests are almost always a part of the acute care treatment, and the child soon associates hospitalization with these stress-provoking procedures.

Providing support to both the child and the family is essential. The progressive nature of the disease makes each illness requiring hospitalization a potentially life-threatening event. Skilled nursing care and sympathetic attention to the emotional needs of the child and family help them cope with the stresses associated with repeated respiratory tract infections and hospitalizations.

The child or adolescent who is immobilized as a result of CF requires the same care and attention as the child with immobility from any other chronic or acute illness, including skin care, bowel management, passive range of motion, and positioning.

Home Care

Most children and adolescents with CF can be managed at home. The goals of care include normalization and daily activities, including school and peer involvement. The care plan should be flexible so that family activities are disrupted as little as possible. Parents may initially require assistance finding and contacting durable medical equipment companies that provide home care equipment. They also need opportunities to learn how to use the equipment and to solve problems they may encounter while delivering therapy at home. The many aspects of home care for the child with CF are similar to those of home care for other children. (See Chapter 25.)

Patients and family members need education about the preferred diet of nutritious meals with tolerated fat, increased protein and carbohydrate, and the administration of pancreatic enzymes. For infants and young children, the enzymes can be mixed with pureed fruit such as applesauce and fed with a spoon. Capsules are usually suitable for older children. It is important to stress to parents that the enzymes, in the amount regulated to the child's needs, should be administered at the beginning of all meals and snacks.

One of the most important aspects of educating parents for home care is teaching techniques for airway clearance (CPT, mechanical vest, forced expiration) and breathing exercises. The success of a therapy program depends on conscientious performance of these treatments regularly as prescribed. The number of times these therapies are performed each day is determined on an individual basis, and often parents readily learn to adjust the number and intensity of the treatments to the child's needs. For pulmonary infection, home IV antibiotics may be prescribed. Home IV care may be preferred for willing and competent families, since it reduces tension and usually brings a sense of belonging to the family members; however, this option depends on a number of factors, including availability of an agency with adequate staff to perform multiple daily home antibiotic infusions. With use of the venous access devices such as PICC lines and implanted ports, the parents and child learn the technique of direct administration into the IV line. Around-the-clock administration may be difficult for families and requires certain adjustments such as waking at least once during the night to give the drug.

For the child or adolescent with chronic sinusitis, daily nasal lavage with sterile normal saline may be helpful. Caution parents to avoid commercial saline preparations with benzyl alcohol, since these may burn the nasal mucosa (Manning, 2005). A dental jet irrigator may be used or a bulb syringe to inject the saline into the paranasal sinuses; slightly tilt the child's head back for instillation, then have the child lean forward to drain the saline into an emesis basin or the bathroom sink. Adolescents need instruction on performing this procedure themselves.

Families also need information about medications and possible side effects. If a child is receiving ibuprofen, serum drug levels need to be monitored closely to establish therapeutic dosages, and observations for side effects such as gastrointestinal irritation are essential.

Children and adolescents with CF should receive routine primary care with special attention to diet, growth and development, and immunizations. Primary care providers should be alert to any weight loss or flattening in the growth curve associated with loss of appetite, which could indicate a pulmonary exacerbation in children with CF (Hazle, 2010). In addition to all the recommended routine immunizations, CF patients should be immunized against influenza starting at age 6 months and followed by an annual booster (American Academy of Pediatrics, 2009b). Anticipatory guidance concerning issues of discipline, how to incorporate aspects of the treatment regimen into the school environment, and delayed pubertal development are also important considerations for the primary care provider.

Home palliative care for the child or adolescent with CF who is in the terminal stages may be carried out with the assistance of hospice. (See Chapter 23.)

The nurse can assist the family in contacting resources that provide help to families with affected children. Various special child health services, many local clinics, private agencies, service clubs, and other community groups offer equipment and medications either free or at reduced rates. The Cystic Fibrosis Foundation* has chapters throughout the United States to provide education and services to families and professionals.

---

*6931 Arlington Road, 2nd floor, Bethesda, MD 20814-3205; 301-951-4422 or 800-344-4422; www.cff.org. In Canada: Canadian Cystic Fibrosis Foundation, 2221 Yonge St., Suite 601, Toronto, Ontario M4S 2B4; www.cysticfibrosis.ca. Two excellent publications available from the Cystic Fibrosis Foundation are *What Everyone Should Know About Cystic Fibrosis*, and *Cystic Fibrosis: A Summary of Symptoms, Diagnosis, and Treatment*. For information about specialized medications, especially dornase alfa, and equipment for CF and other pulmonary diseases, contact Cystic Fibrosis Pharmacy, HHCS Health Group, 3901 E. Colonial Drive, Orlando, FL 32803; 888-307-4427; www.cfpharmacy.com.

Family Support

The most challenging aspect of providing care for the family of a child or adolescent with CF is meeting the emotional needs of the child and family. The diagnosis, treatment, and prognosis for CF are often associated with many problems and frustrations. The diagnosis can evoke feelings of guilt and self-recrimination in parents.

The long-range problems for an infant, child, or adolescent with CF are those encountered in any chronic illness. (See Chapter 22.) Both the child and the family must make many adjustments, the success of which depends on their ability to cope and also on the quality and quantity of support they receive from outside sources. Combined efforts of a variety of health professionals are needed to provide the most comprehensive services to families. It is often the nurse who assesses the home situation, organizes and coordinates these services, and collects the data needed to evaluate the effectiveness of the services.

The persistent need for treatment several times a day places tremendous strain on the family. When the child is young, a family member must perform postural drainage and CPT. Children often balk at these treatments, and the parents are in the position of insisting on adherence. The stress and anxiety related to this routine may produce feelings of resentment in both the child and the family members. When possible, occasional trusted respite care should be available to allow parents to leave the situation for short periods without undue anxiety about the child's welfare.

The affected child or adolescent may become resentful about the disease, its relentless routine of therapy, and the necessary restrictions it places on activities and relationships. The child's activities are interrupted or built around treatments, medications, and diet. This imposes hardships and influences his or her quality of life. The nurse should encourage the child to attend school and join age-appropriate peer groups to live as normally and productively as possible. Sports are often an important part of the child's and adolescent's life; interaction with peers is a valuable life experience, especially to adolescents. The child or adolescent with CF should be encouraged to participate in sports activities as much as physical and pulmonary health allows. Exercise is encouraged to increase pulmonary vital capacity, promote muscle development, and enhance cardiovascular function.

Depression, anxiety, and disturbed self-image may occur in children and adolescents with CF; young adults with severe symptoms may be especially prone to depression as they face the poor prognosis and the reality of unmet life expectations and goals. Nurses should monitor adolescents with CF for signs of eating disturbances. One study found that 24% of the adolescents in the study group had eating disturbance, but most did not fit the criteria for anorexia or bulimia (Bryon, Shearer, and Davies, 2008). One study found that psychologic problems, including depression and anxiety, increased in adult CF patients with disease progression (Shanmugam, Bhutani, Khan, et al, 2007).

As the disease progresses, however, family stress should be expected, and the patient may become angry and noncompliant. It is important for the nurse to recognize the family's changing needs and the grief they may experience as the CF worsens. Families should be made aware of resources for counseling. Patients need to be guided into activities that enable them to express anger, sorrow, and fear without guilt.

Transition to Adulthood

As life expectancy continues to rise for children and adolescents with CF, issues related to marriage, sexuality, childbearing, and career choice become more pressing. Males must be informed at some point that they will often be unable to produce offspring. It is important that the distinction be made between sterility and impotence. Normal sexual relationships can be expected. Female patients may be able to bear children but should be informed of the possible harmful effects on the respiratory system created by the burden of pregnancy. They also need to know that their children will be carriers of the CF gene; therefore genetic counseling for those planning on having children is essential. Adolescent females should be offered counseling concerning the use of oral contraceptives and other contraceptive options (Hazle, 2010).

Adolescents with CF should take personal ownership and management of the illness to maximize their life's potential. Many adolescents and young persons with the illness enroll in college or vocational and technical training school and complete degrees by either distance learning or attending a local school. Young people should set life goals and live normal lives to the extent their illness allows. Adolescents who have had lung transplantation are encouraged to continue taking antirejection medications even though they may feel as though their respiratory status has improved to the point that these medications are no longer necessary.

Life as an independent adult should be encouraged for children with CF. From the time that children can take partial responsibility for their own care (e.g., CPT and taking enzymes), independence and accountability should be fostered. Although the prognosis for these children has improved, many will need continued support as they cope with the demands of surviving with CF.

Anticipatory grieving and other aspects related to care of a child with a terminal illness are also part of nursing care. For example, it is important to prepare the child and family members for end-of-life decisions and care. Families may need information about specific interventions such as hospice and treatments for pain and dyspnea. (See Chapter 23.)

OBSTRUCTIVE SLEEP APNEA SYNDROME

Pediatric obstructive sleep-disordered breathing reportedly affects between 10% and 12% of children ages 2 to 8 years; obstructive sleep may occur in as many as 2% of all children (Benninger and Walner, 2007). However, Au and Li (2009) suggest that the true prevalence of obstructive sleep apnea syndrome (OSAS) is between 1% and 4%. Obstructive sleep-disordered breathing is said to form a continuum of respiratory conditions that are exacerbated during sleep and, if left untreated, may result in significant morbidity (Au and Li, 2009). Sleep-disordered breathing problems in this spectrum range from partial obstruction of the upper airway to continuous episodes of complete upper airway obstruction, with the most severe form being OSAS (Benninger and Walner, 2007).

Obstructive sleep apnea is defined by the American Thoracic Society (1996) as a disorder of breathing during sleep with prolonged partial upper airway obstruction and/or complete obstruction that disrupts normal respiration during sleep and normal sleep patterns. The American Academy of Pediatrics (2002) published a clinical practice guideline for the diagnosis and management of OSAS in children; this discussion focuses only on obstructive sleep apnea syndrome as defined by the academy (2002).

Adenotonsillar hypertrophy has been postulated to be the main cause of OSAS, but some have suggested there may also be an impaired central nervous system response to mechanical stimulation of the respiratory system because many children without tonsils and adenoids continue to have OSAS (Au and Li, 2009). OSAS in children is a distinctly separate condition from OSAS in adults with regard to etiology, clinical manifestations, and treatment (Au and Li, 2009).

Common symptoms of OSAS include nightly snoring, interrupted or disturbed sleep patterns, enuresis, and daytime neurobehavioral problems (American Academy of Pediatrics, 2002; Chan, Edman, and Koltai, 2004). OSAS is to be distinguished from primary snoring, which is snoring without obstructive apnea, frequent sleep arousals, or abnormalities in gas exchange (American Academy of Pediatrics, 2002). Interestingly, children with OSAS do not exhibit daytime sleepiness as do adults; the exception may be obese children (Chan, Edman, and Koltai, 2004). If left untreated, OSAS may result in complications such as growth failure, cor pulmonale, hypertension, poor attention span, hyperactivity, behavioral problems, attention deficit hyperactivity disorder, and death.

The diagnosis of OSAS is made by an overnight sleep study (polysomnography), which provides evidence of sleep disturbance, respiratory pauses, and changes in oxygenation. The six-channel polysomnography can be performed in children of all ages with videotaping or audiotaping, and abbreviated (versus full-night sleep study) polysomnography may be useful; however, this latter method does not predict the severity of OSAS (American Academy of Pediatrics, 2002). Polysomnography can distinguish between OSAS and primary snoring (Owens, 2007).

A common treatment for OSAS in children is T&A (adenotonsillectomy), provided there is evidence of adenotonsillar hypertrophy (Benninger and Walner, 2007; Owens, 2007). Cure rates following adenotonsillectomy are reported to range between 75% and 100% in normal healthy children (Owens, 2007). Complications of these surgical interventions are discussed previously in this chapter. Continuous positive airway pressure (CPAP) and bilevel (cycles between high and low pressure) positive airway pressure (BiPAP) may be helpful in older children with OSAS whose condition persists after surgical intervention. CPAP is a long-term therapy with frequent assessments to evaluate the required amount of pressure and the overall effectiveness of the intervention.

Surgical interventions such as tracheotomy or mandibular distraction may be required for children with craniofacial syndromes such as Goldenhar, Pierre Robin, Apert, and Crouzon, in which there is partial or complete upper airway obstruction (Chan, Edman, and Koltai, 2004; Owens, 2007).

Nursing care of the child with OSAS involves early detection by observation of the infant's or child's sleep patterns and active participation in the diagnostic polysomnography. Important nursing roles are inserting the pH probe into the esophagus, ensuring accurate placement by radiography, and monitoring the sleep study and the patient's response to diagnostic therapy. Counseling families of children with OSAS may involve dietary counseling for exercise programs and weight management, use of the CPAP or BiPAP equipment, and direct postoperative care after the surgical intervention of tonsillectomy or adenoidectomy. The nurse can be instrumental in helping the child and family cope with the chronic illness diagnosis should intervention such as CPAP or BiPAP be required.

KEY POINTS

- Acute infection of the respiratory tract is the most common cause of illness in infancy and childhood.
- The incidence and severity of respiratory tract infections are influenced by the infectious agent involved, the child's age, and the child's natural defenses.
- Symptoms of respiratory tract infections include fever, anorexia, vomiting, abdominal pain, nasal blockage and discharge, wheezing, cough, adventitious respiratory sounds, and sore throat.
- Common respiratory tract infections of childhood include acute nasopharyngitis, acute pharyngitis, influenza, tonsillitis, and OM.
- Severe bleeding from the tonsil site can occur within 6 hours to 5 to 10 days after tonsillectomy.
- Factors that predispose children to OM are the shape and position of eustachian tubes, undeveloped cartilage lining, abundant pharyngeal lymphoid tissue, immature humoral defense mechanisms, exposure to tobacco smoke, and the recumbent position (in infants) for feeding.

- The most common URIs are categorized as croup syndromes, which include acute LTBI, acute spasmodic laryngitis, and acute epiglottitis.
- Epiglottitis is a medical emergency and is characterized by fever, anxious appearance, stridor, and difficulty swallowing.
- The primary nursing function in the care of children with croup is observation for signs of respiratory (airway) compromise and relief of anxiety.
- Lower airway conditions constitute the majority of respiratory problems in children and are usually viral in nature (excluding FB aspiration).
- Common infections of the lower airway include bacterial tracheitis, asthmatic bronchitis, bronchitis, bronchiolitis, and pneumonia.
- Pneumonias are generally classified either by site (lobar, bronchial, or interstitial) or by etiologic agent (viral, bacterial, mycoplasmal, or associated with FBs).
- Management of uncomplicated bronchiolitis and viral pneumonia is symptomatic in otherwise healthy infants.

- In TB, resistance to the bacillus can be altered by heredity, gender, age, stress states, poor nutrition, intercurrent infection, and noncompliance with therapy.
- Signs of choking include inability to speak, color change, and decreased level of activity.
- Inhaled objects are rarely coughed up spontaneously; therefore they must be removed by direct bronchoscopy or laryngoscopy.
- Inducing a child to vomit is contraindicated in the event of hydrocarbon ingestion because of the danger of hydrocarbon aspiration.
- Asthma is the leading cause of chronic illness in children.
- General therapeutic management of asthma includes allergen control, drug therapy, exercise, and sometimes hyposensitization.
- Support for the family of the child with asthma includes education about the disease and its therapy and facilitation of self-management.
- CF is the most frequently occurring inherited disease of Caucasian children and is transmitted by an autosomal recessive gene located on chromosome 7.
- Diagnosis of CF may be based on a number of criteria, including family history, absence of pancreatic enzymes, chronic pulmonary involvement, laboratory identification of CF mutations, positive newborn screening test, and abnormally high sweat chloride concentration (pilocarpine test [or sweat test]).

ANSWERS TO CRITICAL THINKING EXERCISE

Croup Syndrome

1. **Yes,** there are sufficient data to arrive at a possible conclusion in this situation.
2. **a.** Epiglottitis is a serious obstructive inflammatory process that occurs in children 2 to 5 years of age.
   b. Symptoms of epiglottitis include throat pain, restlessness, drooling, and a desire to sit upright and lean forward.
   c. Because epiglottitis can quickly progress to severe respiratory distress, the nurse should not examine the child's throat with a tongue depressor or take a throat culture until the child is examined by a practitioner.

d. Nursing interventions for the child with epiglottitis include monitoring the child's respiratory status, allowing the child to remain in the position that is most comfortable, having an artificial airway (e.g., tracheotomy) and emergency equipment available, and assisting with insertion of an intravenous line and administration of antibiotics.
3. The suspicion of epiglottitis constitutes an emergency. The priority for nursing care at this time is to maintain the child's airway.
4. **Yes,** the evidence supports the conclusion.

REFERENCES

Abouzgheib W, Pratter M, Bartter T: Cough and asthma, *Curr Opin Pulm Med* 13(1):44-48, 2007.

Ahmad N, Zacharek MA: Allergic rhinitis and rhinosinusitis, *Otolaryngol Clin North Am* 41(2):267-281, 2008.

Akinbami LJ, Moorman JE, Garbe PL, et al: Status of childhood asthma in the United States, 1980-2007, *Pediatrics* 123(Suppl 3):S131-S145, 2009.

Albuali WH, Singh RN, Fraser DD, et al: Have changes in ventilation practice improved outcome in children with acute lung injury? *Pediatr Crit Care Med* 8(4):324-330, 2007.

American Academy of Otolaryngology–Head and Neck Surgery: 2000 Clinical indicators compendium, *Bulletin* 19:6, 2000.

American Academy of Pediatrics: *Handbook of pediatric nutrition*, ed 6, Elk Grove Village, IL, 2009a, The Academy.

American Academy of Pediatrics, Committee on Infectious Diseases, Pickering L, editor: *2009 Red book: report of the Committee on Infectious Diseases*, ed 28, Elk Grove Village, Ill, 2009b, The Academy.

American Academy of Pediatrics: Clinical practice guideline: diagnosis and management of bronchiolitis, *Pediatrics* 118(4):1774-1793, 2006.

American Academy of Pediatrics: The changing concept of sudden infant death syndrome: diagnostic coding shifts, controversies

regarding the sleeping environment, and new variables to consider in reducing risk, *Pediatrics* 116(5):1245-1255, 2005.

American Academy of Pediatrics: Clinical practice guidelines: diagnosis and management of acute otitis media, *Pediatrics* 113(5):1451-1465, 2004a.

American Academy of Pediatrics: Clinical practice guidelines: otitis media with effusion, *Pediatrics* 113(5):1412-1429, 2004b.

American Academy of Pediatrics: Clinical practice guideline: diagnosis and management of childhood obstructive sleep apnea syndrome, *Pediatrics* 109(4):704-712, 2002.

American Thoracic Society: Standards and indications for cardiopulmonary sleep studies in children, *Am J Respir Crit Care Med* 153(2):866-878, 1996.

Antoon AY, Donovan MK: Burn injuries. In Kliegman RM, Behrman RE, Jenson HB, et al, editors: *Nelson textbook of pediatrics*, ed 18, Philadelphia, 2007, Saunders.

Arnold E, Clark CE, Lassersson TJ, et al: Herbal interventions for chronic asthma in adults and children, *Cochrane Database Syst Rev* (3):CD005989, 2009.

Au CT, Li AM: Obstructive sleep breathing disorders, *Pediatr Clin North Am* 56(1):243-259, 2009.

Balinsky W, Zhu CW: Pediatric cystic fibrosis: evaluating costs and genetic testing, *J Pediatr Health Care* 18:30-34, 2004.

Benninger M, Walner D: Obstructive sleep-disordered breathing in children, *Clin Cornerstone* 9(Suppl 1):S6-S12, 2007.

Bergelson JM, Shah SS, Zaouitis TE, editors: *Pediatric infectious diseases: the requisites in pediatrics*, Philadelphia, 2008, Mosby.

Bhetwal N, McConaghy JR: The evaluation and treatment of children with acute otitis media, *Primary Care* 34(1):59-70, 2007.

Blakley BW, Magit AE: The role of tonsillectomy in reducing recurrent pharyngitis: a systematic review, *Otolaryngol Head Neck Surg* 140(3):291-297, 2009.

Boat TF, Acton JD: Cystic fibrosis. In Kliegman RM, Behrman RE, Jenson HB, et al, editors: *Nelson textbook of pediatrics*, ed 18, Philadelphia, 2007, Saunders.

Borowitz D, Baker RD, Stallings V: Consensus report on nutrition for pediatric patients with cystic fibrosis, *J Pediatr Gastroenterol Nutr* 35(3):246-259, 2002.

Borowitz D, Robinson KA, Rosenfeld M, et al: Cystic Fibrosis Foundation evidence-based guidelines for management of infants with cystic fibrosis, *J Pediatrics* 155(Suppl 6):S73-S93, 2009.

Bryon M, Shearer J, Davies H: Eating disorders and disturbance in children and adolescents with cystic fibrosis, *Child Health Care* 37(1):67-77, 2008.

Burkhart PV, Rayens MK, Revelette WR, et al: Improved health outcomes with peak flow monitoring for children with asthma, *J Asthma* 44(2):137-142, 2007.

Burton MJ, Glasziou PP: Tonsillectomy or adeno-tonsillectomy versus non-surgical treatment for chronic/recurrent acute tonsillitis, *Cochrane Database Syst Rev* (1): CD001802, 2009.

Centers for Disease Control and Prevention: Licensure of a 13-valent pneumococcal conjugate vaccine (PCV13) and recommendations for use among children— Advisory Committee on Immunization Practices (ACIP), 2010, *MMWR Weekly* 59(09):258-261, 2010.

Centers for Disease Control and Prevention: Trends in tuberculosis—United States, 2008, *MMWR* 58(10):249-253, 2009a.

Centers for Disease Control and Prevention: Use of influenza A (H1N1) 2009 monovalent vaccine: recommendations of the Advisory Committee on Immunization Practices (ACIP), 2009, *MMWR Recomm Rep* 58(RR10):1-8, 2009b.

Centers for Disease Control and Prevention: Summary health statistics for U.S. children: National Health Interview Survey, 2008, *Vital Health Stat 10* 244:1-78, 2009c.

Centers for Disease Control and Prevention: Smoking-attributable mortality, years of potential life lost, and productivity losses— United States, 2000-2004, *MMWR* 57(45):1226-1228, 2008.

Centers for Disease Control and Prevention: Newborn screening for cystic fibrosis, *MMWR Recomm Rep* 53(RR13):1-36, 2004.

Chan J, Edman JC, Koltai PJ: Obstructive sleep apnea in children, *Am Fam Physician* 69(5):1147-1154, 1159-1160, 2004.

Chávez-Bueno S, Mejías A, Jafri H, et al: Respiratory syncytial virus: old challenges and new approaches, *Pediatr Ann* 34(1):62-68, 2005.

Courtney AU, McCarter DF, Pollart SM: Childhood asthma: treatment update, *Am Fam Physician* 71(10):1959-1968, 2005.

Curley M, Hibberd PL, Fineman LD, et al: Effect of prone positioning on clinical outcomes in children with acute lung injury: a randomized controlled trial, *JAMA* 294(2):229-237, 2005.

Cystic Fibrosis Foundation: *Patient registry: annual data report, 2008*, Bethesda, Md, 2009a, Cystic Fibrosis Foundation, available at www.cff.org/UploadedFiles/research/ ClinicalResearch/2008-Patient-Registry-Report.pdf (accessed March 28, 2010).

Cystic Fibrosis Foundation: *Frequently asked questions*, Bethesda, Md, 2009b, The Foundation, available at www.cff.org/ AboutCF/Faqs (accessed July 23, 2009).

DeVincenzo J: Passive antibody prophylaxis for RSV, *Pediatr Infect Dis J* 27(1):69-70, 2008.

Diette GB, McCormack MC, Hansel NN, et al: Environmental issues in managing asthma, *Respir Care* 53(5):602-615, 2008.

Farrell PM, Rosenstein BJ, White TB, et al: Evidence on improved outcomes with early diagnosis of cystic fibrosis through neonatal screening: enough is enough! *J Pediatr* 147(Suppl 3):S30-S36, 2007.

Feja K, Saiman L: Tuberculosis in children, *Clin Chest Med* 26(2):295-312, 2005.

Frye AD: Acute lung injury and acute respiratory distress syndrome in the pediatric patient, *Crit Care Nurs Clin North Am* 17(4):311-318, 2005.

Goldberg HJ, Deykin A: Advances in lung transplantation for patients who have cystic fibrosis, *Clin Chest Med* 28(2):445-457, 2007.

Goldstein NA, Mandel EM, Kurs-Lasky M, et al: Water precautions and tympanostomy tubes: a randomized, controlled trial, *Laryngoscope* 115(2):324-330, 2005.

Goodman D: Wheezing, bronchiolitis, and bronchitis. In Kliegman RM, Behrman RE, Jenson HB, et al, editors: *Nelson textbook of pediatrics*, ed 18, Philadelphia, 2007, Saunders.

Hagemann TM: Pediatric allergic rhinitis drug therapy, *J Pediatr Health Care* 19(4):238-244, 2005.

Hanson JH, Flori H: Application of the acute respiratory distress syndrome network low-tidal volume strategy to pediatric acute lung injury, *Respir Care Clin North Am* 12(3):349-357, 2006.

Hardin DS, Rice J, Ahn C, et al: Growth hormone treatment enhances nutrition and growth in children with cystic fibrosis receiving enteral nutrition, *J Pediatr* 146(3):324-328, 2005.

Hazle LA: Cystic fibrosis. In Allen PJ, Vessey JA, Schapiro NA, editors, *Primary care of the child with a chronic condition*, ed 5, St Louis, 2010, Mosby.

Hopkins A, Lahiri T, Salerno R, et al: Changing epidemiology of life-threatening upper airway infections: the reemergence of bacterial tracheitis, *Pediatrics* 118(4):1418-1421, 2006.

Jenson H: Epstein-Barr virus. In Kliegman RM, Behrman RE, Jenson HB, et al, editors: *Nelson textbook of pediatrics*, ed 18, Philadelphia, 2007, Saunders.

Kershner, JE: Otitis media. In Kliegman RM, Behrman RE, Jenson HB, et al, editors: *Nelson textbook of pediatrics*, ed 18, Philadelphia, 2007, Saunders.

Kotloff RM: Does lung transplantation confer a survival benefit? *Curr Opin Organ Transplant* 14(5):499-503, 2009.

Li YF, Langholz B, Salam MT, et al: Maternal and grandmaternal smoking patterns are associated with early childhood asthma, *Chest* 127(4):1232-1241, 2005.

Linnane BM, Hall GL, Nolan G, et al: Lung function in infants with cystic fibrosis diagnosed by newborn screening, *Am J Respir Crit Care Med* 178(12):1239-1244, 2008.

Linzer JF: Review of asthma: pathophysiology and current treatment options, *Clin Pediatr Emerg Med* 8(2):87-95, 2007.

Liou TG, Adler FR, Cox DR, et al: Lung transplantation and survival in children with cystic fibrosis, *N Engl J Med* 357(21):2143-2152, 2007.

Liu AH, Covar RA, Spahn JD, et al: Childhood asthma. In Kliegman RM, Behrman RE, Jenson HB, et al, editors: *Nelson textbook of pediatrics*, ed 18, Philadelphia, 2007, Saunders.

Long SS: Pertussis (*Bordetella pertussis* and *Bordetella parapertussis*). In Kliegman RM, Behrman RE, Jenson HB, et al, editors: *Nelson*

textbook of pediatrics, ed 18, Philadelphia, 2007, Saunders.

Mailaparambil B, Grychtol R, Heinzmann A: Respiratory syncytial virus bronchiolitis and asthma: insights from recent studies and implications for therapy, *Inflamm Allergy Drug Targets* 8(3):202-207, 2009.

Manning S: Medical management of nasosinus infection and inflammatory disease. In Cummings CW, Flint PW, Haughey BH, et al, editors, *Otolaryngology: Head and neck surgery*, ed 4, Philadelphia, 2005, Mosby.

McDonald S, Langston Hewer CD, Nunez DA: Grommets (ventilation tubes) for recurrent acute otitis media in children, *Cochrane Database Syst Rev* (4):CD004741, 2008.

Mcintosh K: Respiratory syncytial virus. In Kliegman RM, Behrman RE, Jenson HB, et al, editors: *Nelson textbook of pediatrics*, ed 18, Philadelphia, 2007, Saunders.

McKone EF, Emerson SS, Edwards KL, et al: Effect of genotype on phenotype and mortality in cystic fibrosis: a retrospective cohort study, *Lancet* 361(9370):1671-1676, 2003.

Meredith JR, O'Keefe KP, Galwankar S: Pediatric procedural sedation and analgesia, *J Emerg Trauma Shock* 1(2):88-96, 2008.

Milgrom H, Leung DYM: Allergic rhinitis. In Kliegman RM, Behrman RE, Jenson HB, et al, editors: *Nelson textbook of pediatrics*, ed 18, Philadelphia, 2007, Saunders.

Minasian C, Wallis C, Metcalfe C, et al: Bronchial provocation testing with dry powder mannitol in children with cystic fibrosis, *Pediatr Pulmonol* 43(11):1078-1084, 2008.

Moore M, Little P: Humidified air inhalation for treating croup, *Cochrane Database Syst Rev* 19(3):CD002870, 2006.

Morkjaroenpong V, Rand CS, Butz AM, et al: Environmental tobacco smoke exposure and nocturnal symptoms among inner-city children with asthma, *J Allergy Clin Immunol* 110(1):147-153, 2002.

Myers TR: Use of heliox in children, *Respir Care* 51(6):619-631, 2006.

National Asthma Education and Prevention Program: *Expert Panel Report 3: guidelines for the diagnosis and management of asthma*, Bethesda, Md, 2007, National Heart Lung and Blood Institute, National Institutes of Health, available at www.nhlbi.nih.gov/guidelines/ asthma/01_front.pdf (accessed March 2010).

National Newborn Screening and Genetics Resource Center: National newborn screening status report, NNSGRC, Austin, TX, 2009, available at http://genes-r-us.uthscsa.edu/ nbsdisorders.pdf (accessed April 26, 2009).

Olivieri M, Bodini A, Peroni DG, et al: Passive smoking in asthmatic children: effect of "smoke-free house" measured by urinary cotinine levels, *Allergy Asthma Proc* 27(4):350-353, 2006.

Owens JA: Sleep medicine. In Kliegman RM, Behrman RE, Jenson HB, et al, editors: *Nelson textbook of pediatrics*, ed 18, Philadelphia, 2007, Saunders.

Paradise JL, Bluestone CD, Colborn DK, et al: Tonsillectomy and adenotonsillectomy for recurrent throat infection in moderately affected children, *Pediatrics* 110:7-15, 2002.

Pediatric Tuberculosis Collaborative Group: Targeted tuberculin skin testing and treatment of latent tuberculosis infection in children and adolescents, *Pediatrics* 114(Suppl 4):1175-1201, 2004.

Pichichero ME, Casey JR: Acute otitis media: making sense of recent guidelines on antimicrobial treatment, *J Fam Pract* 54(4):313-322, 2005.

Pitts J, Flack J, Goodfellow J: Improving nutrition in the cystic fibrosis patient, *J Pediatr Health Care* 22(2):137-140, 2008.

Pongracic JA: Asthma delivery devices: age-appropriate use, *Pediatr Ann* 32(1):50-54, 2003.

Powers JH: Diagnosis and treatment of acute otitis media: evaluating the evidence, *Infect Dis Clin North Am* 21(2):409-426, 2007.

Rafei K, Lichenstein R: Airway infectious disease emergencies, *Pediatr Clin North Am* 53(2):215-242, 2006.

Ranganathan SC, Sonnappa S: Pneumonia and other respiratory infections, *Pediatr Clin North Am* 56(1):135-156, 2009.

Randolph AG: Management of acute lung injury and acute respiratory distress syndrome in children, *Crit Care Med* 37(8):2448-2454, 2009.

Redding GJ: Bronchiectasis in children, *Pediatr Clin North Am* 56(1):157-171, 2009.

Ren CL, Morgan WJ, Konstan MW, et al: Presence of methicillin-resistant *Staphylococcus aureus* in respiratory cultures from cystic fibrosis patients is associated with lower lung function, *Pediatr Pulmonol* 42(6):513-518, 2007.

Rice TW, Bernard GR: Acute lung injury and the acute respiratory distress syndrome: challenges in clinical trial testing, *Clin Chest Med* 27(4):733-754, 2006.

Rimsza ME, Kirk GM: Common medical problems of the college student, *Pediatr Clin North Am* 52(1):vii, 9-24, 2005.

Rimsza ME, Newberry S: Unexpected infant deaths associated with use of cough and cold medications, *Pediatrics* 122(2):e318-e322, 2008.

Robinson RF: Impact of respiratory syncytial virus in the United States, *Am J Syst Pharm* 65(Suppl 8):S3-S6, 2008.

Rodgers GC, Condurache T, Reed MD, et al: Poisonings. In Kliegman RM, Behrman RE, Jenson HB, et al, editors: *Nelson textbook of pediatrics*, ed 18, Philadelphia, 2007, Saunders.

Roosevelt GE: Acute inflammatory upper airway obstruction. In Kliegman RM, Behrman RE,

Jenson HB, et al, editors: *Nelson textbook of pediatrics*, ed 18, Philadelphia, 2007, Saunders.

Rowe SM, Clancy JP: Advances in cystic fibrosis therapies, *Curr Opin Pediatr* 18(6):604-613, 2006.

Ryan T, Brewer M, Small L: Over-the-counter cough and cold medication use in young children, *Pediatr Nurs* 34(2):174-180, 184, 2008.

Sandel M, Phelan K, Wright R, et al: The effects of housing interventions on child health, *Pediatr Ann* 33(7):475-481, 2004.

Schnabel D, Grasemann C, Staab D, et al: A multicenter, randomized, double-blind, placebo-controlled trial to evaluate the metabolic and respiratory effects of growth hormone in children with cystic fibrosis, *Pediatrics* 119(6):e1230-e1238, 2007.

Schwarzenberg SJ, Thomas W, Olsen TW, et al: Microvascular complications in cystic fibrosis–related diabetes, *Diabetes Care* 30(5):1056-1061, 2007.

Sectish TC, Prober CG: Pneumonia. In Kliegman RM, Behrman RE, Jenson HB, et al, editors: *Nelson textbook of pediatrics*, ed 18, Philadelphia, 2007, Saunders.

Seiden JA, Scarfone RJ: Bronchiolitis: an evidence-based approach to management, *Clin Pediatr Emerg Med* 10(2):75-81, 2009.

Selekman J: Changes in the screening for tuberculosis in children, *Pediatr Nurs* 32(1):73-75, 2006.

Shanmugam G, Bhutani S, Khan DA, et al: Psychiatric considerations in pulmonary disease, *Psychiatr Clin North Am* 30(4):761-780, 2007.

Sharma HP, Hansel NN, Matsui E, et al: Indoor environmental influences on children's asthma, *Pediatr Clin North Am* 54(1):103-120, 2007.

Sly PD, Brennan S, Gangell C, et al: Lung disease at diagnosis in infants with cystic fibrosis detected by newborn screening, *Am J Respir Crit Care Med* 180(2):146-152, 2009.

Sorce LR: Respiratory syncytial virus: from primary care to critical care, *J Pediatr Health Care* 23(2):101-108, 2009.

Southern KW, Merelle MM, Dankert-Roelse JE, et al: Newborn screening for cystic fibrosis, *Cochrane Database Syst Rev* (1):CD001402, 2009.

Stallings VA, Stark LJ, Robinson KA, et al: Evidence-based practice recommendations for nutrition-related management of children and adults with cystic fibrosis and pancreatic insufficiency: results of a systematic review, *J Am Diet Assoc* 108(5):832-839, 2008.

Strausbaugh SD, Davis PB: Cystic fibrosis: a review of epidemiology and pathobiology, *Clin Chest Med* 28(2):279-288, 2007.

Strunk RC, Bloomberg GR: Omalizumab for asthma, *N Engl J Med* 354(25):2689-2695, 2006.

Surgeon General Report: *The health consequences of involuntary exposure to tobacco smoke: a report of the surgeon general*, Washington, DC, 2006, US Department of Health and Human Services, Office of the Surgeon General.

Thomsen SF, van der Sluis S, Stensballe LG, et al: Exploring the association between severe respiratory syncytial virus infection and asthma: a registry-based twin study, *Am J Respir Care Med* 179(12):1091-1097, 2009.

Tolomeo C, Mackey W: Peripherally inserted central catheters (PICCs) in the CF population: one center's experience, *Pediatr Nurs* 29(5):355-359, 2003.

US Food and Drug Administration: *Zanamivir fact sheet for health care providers*, Washington, DC, 2009, The Administration, available at www.fda.gov/downloads/Drugs/DrugSafety/InformationbyDrugClass/UCM143858.pdf (accessed July 18, 2009).

Uyemura MC: Foreign body ingestion in children, *Am Fam Physician* 72(2):287-291, 2005.

Ventre K, Randolph AG: Ribavirin for respiratory syncytial virus infection of the lower respiratory tract in infants and young children, *Cochrane Database Syst Rev* 24(1):CD000181, 2007.

Vorwek C, Coats TJ: Use of helium-oxygen mixture in the treatment of croup: a systematic review, *Emerg Med J* 25(9):547-550, 2008.

Willson DF, Chess PR, Notter RH: Surfactant for pediatric acute lung injury, *Pediatr Clin North Am* 55(3):545-575, 2008.

Winkelstein ML, Tarzian A, Wood RA: Parental smoking behavior and passive smoke exposure in children with asthma, *Ann Allergy Asthma Immunol* 78(4):419-423, 1997.

World Health Organization: *Use of antiviral drugs against influenza A (H1N1)*, World Health Organization Global Alert and Response (GAR), Geneva, May 2009, The Organization, available at www.who.int/csr/disease/swineflu/frequently_asked_questions/swineflu_faq_antivirals/en/index.html (accessed July 20, 2009).

Zimmerman JJ, Akhtar SR, Caldwell E, et al: Incidence and outcomes of acute pediatric lung injury, *Pediatrics* 124(1):87-95, 2009.

The Child with Gastrointestinal Dysfunction

Marilyn J. Hockenberry

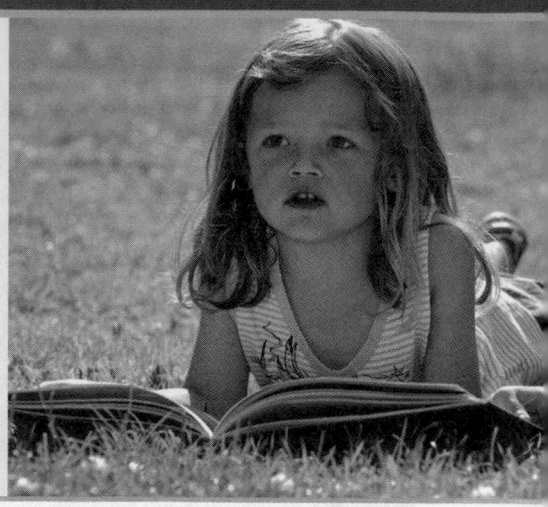

CHAPTER OUTLINE

GASTROINTESTINAL STRUCTURE AND FUNCTION

The primary function of the gastrointestinal (GI) tract is the digestion and absorption of nutrients. The GI tract also has secretory, barrier, endocrine, and immunologic functions (Box 33-1). The extensive surface area of the GI tract and its digestive function represent the major means of exchange between the human organism and the environment. Thus any dysfunction of the GI tract can cause significant problems with the exchange of fluids, electrolytes, and nutrients.

DEVELOPMENT OF THE GASTROINTESTINAL TRACT

The development of the GI tract (from mouth to anus) occurs in several stages from conception through birth. The GI tract may be divided into three parts in intrauterine life: foregut (esophagus, stomach, and proximal duodenum), midgut (distal duodenum, jejunum, ileum, cecum, and proximal colon), and hindgut (distal colon and rectum). The salivary glands, liver, gallbladder, and pancreas are outgrowths of the foregut and midgut.

The esophagus develops from the foregut and can be identified by 4 weeks of gestation. It elongates rapidly after the fourth week to a length of approximately 10 cm (4 inches) at term. The stomach also develops from the primitive foregut and can be identified by the fourth week of gestation. It continues to develop in the second trimester. From the fifth week of gestation until term, the intestine lengthens a thousandfold.

The third trimester is the period of most extensive and rapid growth of the gut. At full term, the small intestine is approximately 250 to 300 cm (98 to 118 inches) and will grow to approximately 2 to 4 m (6.5 to 13 feet) in the adult. The large intestine develops from the midgut and the hindgut and is approximately 30 to 50 cm (12 to 20 inches) at term.

During pregnancy the fetus receives nutrients via the placenta. At birth the full-term infant is capable of adaptation to extrauterine nutrition. This adaptation process includes coordinated sucking and swallowing, efficient gastric emptying and intestinal motility, regulation of digestive secretions and enzymes, efficient digestion and absorption, and excretion of waste products. The infant's capacity to adapt to enteral nutrition depends on the gestational age at birth and the type of nutrients to which the GI tract is exposed.

BOX 33-1 FUNCTIONS OF THE GASTROINTESTINAL TRACT

- Process and absorb nutrients necessary to maintain metabolic processes and to support growth and development.
- Perform an excretory function for both digestive residue and other waste products that pour into the intestine from the blood or are excreted in the bile.
- Provide detoxification while other routes of elimination (kidneys, liver, skin) are still immature.
- Participate in maintaining fluid and electrolyte balance in infancy.
- Serve a lymphoid function by providing a barrier to bacteria, viruses, parasites. The liver also processes antigens and produces immunoglobulins.

Movement of nutrients through the GI tract occurs as a result of contraction of the intestinal smooth muscles. A combination of myogenic, neural, and neuroendocrine input during fasting and digestion regulates GI movement. By 26 weeks of gestation, uncoordinated contractions occur, but gastric emptying is slow. By 36 weeks of gestation, motility is similar to that of the full-term infant, and coordinated sucking and swallowing allow preterm infants to feed orally. Intestinal motility improves with gestational age, but it is not known whether the introduction of enteral feeding initiates coordinated motor activity. **Meconium,** a thick greenish black material consisting of epithelial cells, digestive tract secretions, and residue of swallowed amniotic fluid, is normally expelled from the intestine shortly after birth and provides evidence of patency of the GI tract.

At term the mechanical functions of digestion are relatively immature. Swallowing is an automatic reflex action for the first 3 months, and the infant has no voluntary control of swallowing until the striated muscles in the throat establish their cerebral connections. This begins at approximately 6 weeks of age. By 6 months the infant is capable of swallowing, holding food in the mouth, or spitting it out at will. The mechanism of sucking is also a reflexive activity in the newborn, and the muscular action of the tongue has a typical forward thrust. With neural and muscular development, the infant gradually acquires the ability to perform the coordinated muscular action typical of the adult type of swallowing. (See Chapter 12.) The eruption of the primary teeth facilitates chewing. The timing of dietary changes closely parallels these progressive developmental capabilities. First foods are those that require merely swallowing; these are followed by foods that need no mastication and finally those that require biting and chewing.

The stomach, which lies horizontally, is round until the child is approximately 2 years of age. It then gradually elongates until approximately 7 years of age, when it assumes the shape and anatomic position of the adult stomach. This anatomic placement of the stomach in infancy influences positioning practices during and after feeding. (See Chapter 8.) At birth the stomach capacity is small, but it increases rapidly with age.

The frequency and character of stools are affected by the rate of peristalsis and the nature of ingested food. The frequent, yellow stools of the neonate gradually assume a more adult regularity and character in the infant. When compared with the older child, the capacity of the infant's stomach is smaller, but the emptying time is faster. Both the stomach capacity and the emptying time have implications for the amount and frequency of feedings during infancy.

The secretory cells of the GI tract are believed to be functional at birth. However, because most of the digestive enzymes depend on a specific pH, their efficiency may be impaired. The newborn produces only small amounts of saliva, which contain the starch-splitting enzyme amylase. Therefore its primary purpose at this time is to moisten the mouth and throat. By the end of the second year, the salivary glands have increased in size about five times to reach their full size and function.

DIGESTION

Three processes—digestion, absorption, and metabolism—are necessary for the body to convert nutrients into forms it can use. Nutrients are composed of six major substances: carbohydrates, proteins, fats, vitamins, minerals, and water. Digestion is the initial preparation of food for use by the body. Two basic activities are involved: mechanical or muscular activity producing GI motility (movement) and chemical or enzymatic activity resulting from GI secretions.

Mechanical digestion occurs through a series of neuromuscular actions that move and mix food along the GI tract at a rate suitable for digestion and absorption. Three types of muscles in the stomach and intestines contribute to this motility: (1) circular muscles churn and mix food particles; (2) longitudinal muscles propel the food mass; and (3) sphincter muscles (the lower esophageal, pyloric, ileocecal, and anal sphincters) control passage of the food mass to the next segment. The nervous system regulates these muscular actions. The intramural plexus forms the complex network of nerves within the GI wall that control smooth muscle contractions.

Chemical digestion involves five types of GI secretions: (1) enzymes (specific actions on degradation of nutrients), (2) hormones (stimulate or inhibit GI secretions), (3) hydrochloric acid (produces the pH necessary for the activity of specific enzymes), (4) mucus (lubricates and protects the GI tract), and (5) water and electrolytes (transport nutrients for digestion and absorption). Numerous cells and glands produce these secretions. The cells that secrete mucus and GI hormones are found primarily in the mucosa of the stomach and small intestine. The salivary glands and pancreas secrete enzymes, the gastric glands secrete enzymes and hydrochloric acid, and the liver secretes bile.

Mechanical and chemical digestion begins in the mouth. Biting and chewing mix food with saliva and reduce the food into a bolus. The saliva moistens the food to aid in swallowing. Salivary amylase begins the process of digestion of complex carbohydrates, or starches.

The next phase of digestion is swallowing, or deglutition. Safe swallowing requires coordination of the oral and pharyngeal phases of swallowing to prevent food material from entering the airway. The coordination of swallowing is controlled by the interaction of the cranial nerves and the muscles of the mouth, pharynx, and esophagus. The oral phase of swallowing is voluntary. The pharyngeal phase is involuntary and consists of elevation of the palate, uvula, and larynx, followed by a peristaltic wave. The upper esophageal sphincter (UES) then relaxes to allow passage of the bolus into the esophagus. Peristalsis (wavelike movements that squeeze food along the entire length of the alimentary tract) moves the food through the esophagus, and the lower esophageal sphincter (LES) relaxes to allow the food to enter the stomach.

Once a bolus of food has entered the stomach, the LES contracts to prevent food from refluxing (returning) into the esophagus. The stomach stores, mixes, and empties the food during digestion. The gastric glands secrete enzymes, hydrochloric acid, and mucus, which mix with the food to continue the process of digestion. The enzyme pepsin, formed from pepsinogen, begins the breakdown of whole proteins into polypeptides. Hydrochloric acid, secreted by the parietal cells, aids in the digestion of proteins. The hormone gastrin is released in the stomach in response to food. Gastrin stimulates the parietal cells to produce more hydrochloric acid. When the pH is very

low, a feedback mechanism stops secretion of gastrin to prevent excessive acid formation. The mucus serves primarily to form a protective barrier between the acid and the gastric mucosa.

Partially digested food and watery secretions (chyme) are delivered to the small intestine. Up to this time, most of the digestion has been mechanical. The major part of chemical digestion, as well as several types of movement that aid in mechanical digestion, occurs in the small intestine. The small intestine secretes a large number of enzymes, each of which is specific for one of the fundamental types of nutrients. The mucosa of the small intestine secretes disaccharidases (maltase, lactase, and sucrase) that convert maltose, lactose, and sucrose to monosaccharides (glucose, fructose, and galactose). Aminopeptidase and dipeptidase convert polypeptides to smaller peptides and amino acids.

Secretions from the liver and pancreas complete the process of chemical digestion. The pancreas produces insulin (a hormone necessary for the metabolism of carbohydrates, fats, and proteins) and several enzymes that digest nutrients. Amylase converts starch to disaccharides. Trypsin and chymotrypsin convert proteins and polypeptides to smaller polypeptides. Lipase converts fats to glycerides and fatty acids. These pancreatic enzymes become active only after the inactive forms are secreted into the small intestine. For example, the enzyme enterokinase, secreted by the intestinal mucosal glands, is necessary for trypsinogen to be converted into trypsin. Otherwise, activated enzymes would digest the pancreas and pancreatic duct.

Another important aid in digestion and absorption in the small intestine is bile. Bile is produced in the liver and stored by the gallbladder. When fat enters the small intestine, the hormone cholecystokinin, which stimulates the gallbladder to release bile, is secreted by the intestinal mucosal glands. Bile, an emulsifying agent for fats that facilitates the digestion of fats by lipase, is necessary for the absorption of the fat-soluble vitamins A, D, E, and K. Absence of bile causes increased amounts of ingested fat to appear in the feces (steatorrhea), as well as a deficiency of these vitamins.

ABSORPTION

After digestion of the food is complete, the simplified nutrient end products—monosaccharides (glucose, fructose, and galactose) from carbohydrates, fatty acids and glycerides from fats, and small peptides and amino acids from proteins—are ready for absorption. Vitamins and minerals are also released as a result of digestion. Water and electrolytes contribute to the fluid food mass that is finally absorbed.

The principal site for absorption of nutrients in the GI tract is the small intestine. The wall of the GI tract consists of folds and projections that are progressively smaller (Fig. 33-1). These mucosal folds, villi, and microvilli increase the inner surface area approximately 600 times over the outer serosa, yielding an extremely large surface for absorption.

The mucosal folds are elevated folds along the mucosa. The villi can be seen by light microscope and are small, fingerlike projections covering the mucosal folds. The villi increase the surface area further. Each villus has a vascular supply, including venous and arterial capillaries and lacteals (lymphatic vessels in

PATHOPHYSIOLOGY REVIEW

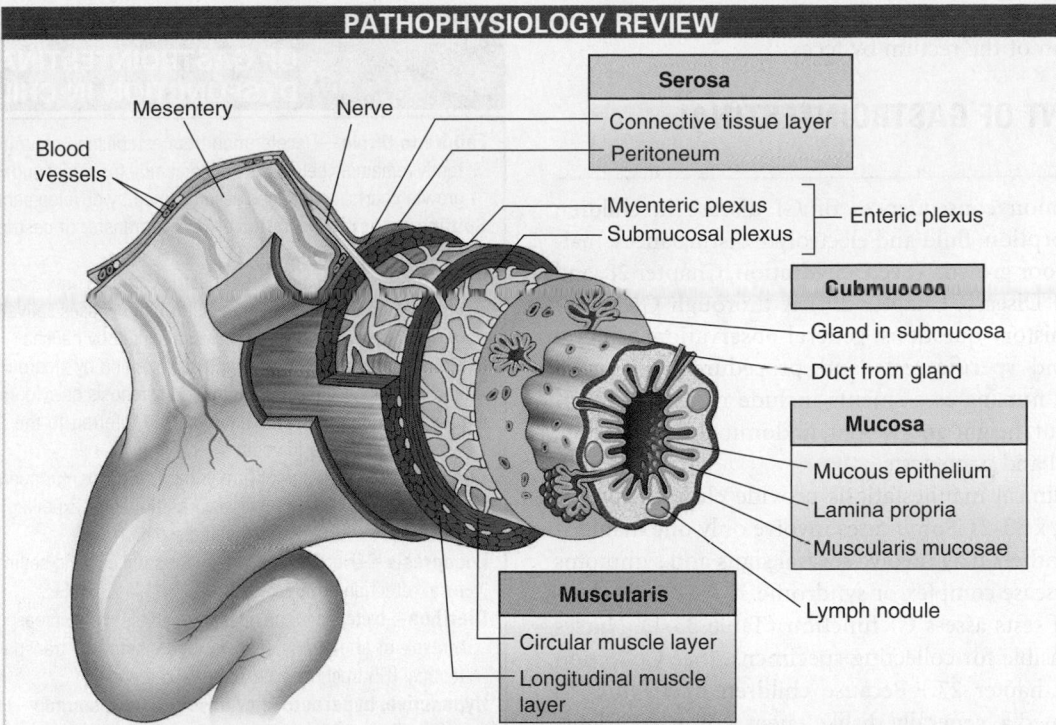

Fig. 33-1 Wall of the gastrointestinal (GI) tract. The wall of the GI tract is made up of four layers with a network of nerves between the layers. Shown here is a generalized diagram of a segment of the GI tract. Note that the serosa is continuous with a fold of serous membrane called a *mesentery*. Note also that digestive glands may empty their products into the lumen of the GI tract by way of ducts. (From Patton KT, Thibodeau GA: *Anatomy and physiology*, ed 7, St Louis, 2010, Mosby.)

the small intestine that contain the substance chyle). The microvilli, numerous minute projections on the surface of each villus (visible by electron microscope), form the brush border.

The small intestine has several mechanisms of absorption, including passive diffusion, carrier-mediated diffusion, active energy-driven transport, and engulfment. Passive diffusion (osmosis) occurs across the epithelial membrane in the direction from higher concentration to lower concentration. Carrier-mediated diffusion occurs as molecules are carried across the epithelial cells of microvilli by a molecule that serves as a vehicle. Large molecules must be combined with a smaller molecule to pass from a greater pressure gradient to a lesser one. For example, vitamin B_{12} requires intrinsic factor to be carried into the intestinal circulation.

In active energy-driven transport, nutrients require energy to be absorbed and to cross the intestinal epithelial membrane. This mechanism is referred to as a *pump*. The pump transports molecules across the membrane by means of energy supplied by the cell's metabolism. The sodium pump, which transports glucose, is an example of this mechanism.

Engulfment, or pinocytosis, is the process that allows large macromolecules to be absorbed by the epithelial cells of the villi. The epithelial cell engulfs the macromolecule and opens to allow the particle to enter the interior of the cell. The particle then enters the capillary blood. This mechanism transports some whole proteins and fat droplets.

After absorption by these mechanisms, the end products of carbohydrates and proteins are absorbed into the intestinal capillaries and enter the portal blood circulation of the liver, where further metabolic conversion occurs. The transfer of the end products of fat digestion is unique in that the fat molecules pass between the cells of the intestinal mucosa and into the lacteals of the villi. From there, they enter the larger lymph vessels and then the portal blood flow at the thoracic duct. Exceptions include the medium- and short-chain fatty acids, which can be absorbed directly into the blood circulation of the villi. Most of the fats commonly consumed are long-chain fatty acids, however, which are transported by way of the lacteals.

Fat-soluble vitamins are absorbed with digested fats in the presence of bile. Water-soluble vitamins, vitamin B complex, and vitamin C are absorbed in the small intestine. Absorption of vitamin B_{12} takes place only in the ileum. The majority of water and electrolyte absorption also takes place in the small intestine.

The large intestine completes the process of absorption and functions primarily to absorb sodium and additional water. The remainder of the products of digestion passes into the large intestine through the ileocecal valve. The muscular activity of the large intestine propels the mass forward. Most of the water and sodium is absorbed into the bloodstream in the proximal half of the colon. The colonic bacteria synthesize vitamin K, vitamin B_{12}, and some of the vitamin B complex. Bacteria also affect the color and odor of the stool and gas formation. The odor is primarily caused by products of bacterial action and depends on the type of colonic flora and ingested food. (Defects in digestion or absorption notably alter the odor and appearance of feces.) Color is the result of bilirubin end products converted by bacteria to urobilinogen and then oxidized to urobilin (stercobilin). The feces that are excreted consist of undigested residue, water, bacteria, and mucus. Defecation occurs when the internal and external anal sphincters relax following distention of the rectum by feces.

ASSESSMENT OF GASTROINTESTINAL FUNCTION

The most common consequences of GI disease in children include malabsorption, fluid and electrolyte disturbances, malnutrition, and poor growth. (See Dehydration, Chapter 28, and Acute Diarrheal Disease, Chapter 29.) A thorough GI assessment includes history questions, general observations, clinical examination, and specific tests and procedures. The most important basic nursing assessments include measurement of intake and output, height and weight, abdominal examination, and simple stool and urine tests.

Numerous clinical manifestations provide clues to specific GI problems (Box 33-2). Some cases involve only one manifestation, whereas others may involve several signs and symptoms as part of the disease complex or syndrome.

A number of tests assess GI function (Table 33-1). Nurses are often responsible for collecting specimens. (See Collection of Specimens, Chapter 27.) Because children may refuse to drink contrast media, generally dislike enemas, and are frightened by unfamiliar equipment, they need preparation for procedures and collection of specimens. (See Preparation for Diagnostic and Therapeutic Procedures, Chapter 27.)

INGESTION OF FOREIGN SUBSTANCES

Children are prone to ingesting foreign substances because they frequently put their hands or other objects or substances in their mouth. Infants and small children in particular instinctively explore items with the mouth. Older children often place items in their mouth and accidentally swallow them. Rarely, a child deliberately swallows unusual objects or substances. Hands come into contact with dirt and contaminated objects that may contain lead, bacteria, or parasites. (See Chapter 16.)

PICA

Pica is an eating disorder characterized by the compulsive and excessive ingestion of both food and nonfood substances. Food picas include the excessive eating of ordinary foods or unprepared food substances, such as coffee grounds or uncooked cereals. Nonfood picas include the ingestion of substances such as clay, soil, stones, laundry starch, paint chips, ice, hair, paper, rubber, and feces. Pica is more common in children, women (especially during pregnancy), individuals who have autism or cognitive impairment, and those with anemia or chronic renal failure. In some cultures pica is an accepted practice based on the presumed nutritional or therapeutic properties or on religious or superstitious beliefs.

There are several theories on the cause of pica, including psychologic theories (compulsive neurosis) and nutritional theories (craving caused by a nutrient deficiency). Pica is clearly associated with both iron and zinc deficiencies, although controversy exists regarding whether pica is the cause or the result of the deficiency. Pica has also been reported as the presenting symptom in children with celiac disease thought to be caused

Critical Thinking Exercise—Ingestion of a Foreign Body

> ### BOX 33-2 CLINICAL MANIFESTATIONS OF GASTROINTESTINAL DYSFUNCTION IN CHILDREN
>
> **Failure to thrive**—Deceleration from established growth pattern or consistently remaining below the 5th percentile for height and weight on standard growth charts; sometimes accompanied by developmental delays
>
> **Spitting up or regurgitation**—Passive transfer of gastric contents into the esophagus or mouth
>
> **Vomiting**—Forceful ejection of gastric contents; involves a complex process under central nervous system control that causes salivation, pallor, sweating, and tachycardia; usually accompanied by nausea
>
> **Projectile vomiting**—Vomiting accompanied by vigorous peristaltic waves and typically associated with pyloric stenosis or pylorospasm
>
> **Nausea**—Unpleasant sensation vaguely referred to the throat or abdomen with an inclination to vomit
>
> **Constipation**—Passage of firm or hard stools or infrequent passage of stool with associated symptoms such as difficulty expelling the stools, blood-streaked stools, and abdominal discomfort
>
> **Encopresis**—Overflow of incontinent stool causing soiling; often caused by fecal retention or impaction
>
> **Diarrhea**—Increase in the number of stools with increased water content as a result of alterations of water and electrolyte transport by the gastrointestinal (GI) tract; may be acute or chronic
>
> **Hypoactive, hyperactive, or absent bowel sounds**—Evidence of intestinal motility problems that may be caused by inflammation or obstruction
>
> **Abdominal distention**—Protuberant contour of the abdomen that may be caused by delayed gastric emptying, accumulation of gas or stool, inflammation, or obstruction
>
> **Abdominal pain**—Pain associated with the abdomen that may be localized or diffuse, acute or chronic; often caused by inflammation, obstruction, or hemorrhage
>
> **Gastrointestinal bleeding**—Bleeding from an upper or lower GI source; may be acute or chronic
>
> **Hematemesis**—Vomiting of bright red blood or denatured blood that results from bleeding in the upper GI tract or from swallowed blood from the nose or oropharynx
>
> **Hematochezia**—Passage of bright red blood per rectum, usually indicating lower GI tract bleeding
>
> **Melena**—Passage of dark-colored, tarry stools caused by denatured blood, suggesting upper GI tract bleeding or bleeding from the right colon
>
> **Jaundice**—Yellow coloration of the skin and sclerae associated with liver dysfunction
>
> **Dysphagia**—Difficulty swallowing caused by abnormalities in the neuromuscular function of the pharynx or upper esophageal sphincter or by disorders of the esophagus
>
> **Dysfunctional swallowing**—Impaired swallowing resulting from central nervous system defects or structural defects of the oral cavity, pharynx, or esophagus; can cause feeding problems or aspiration
>
> **Fever**—Common manifestation of illness in children with GI disorders; usually associated with dehydration, infection, or inflammation

by iron deficiency. Pica for dirt (geophagia) is the principal risk factor for visceral larva migrans (a common parasite in children and adults).

In some instances pica is relatively harmless. However, when the ingested substance contains a toxic ingredient (e.g., lead in paint), the consequences can be serious. Surgical complications, such as intestinal obstruction, perforation, inflammation, or hemorrhage, can result.

The nurse can detect pica by the history, physical examination, and radiologic studies. However, it is often unrecognized, and children may deny any unusual eating behaviors. The nurse

TABLE 33-1	GASTROINTESTINAL DIAGNOSTIC PROCEDURES		
TEST	**DESCRIPTION**	**PURPOSE**	**COMMENTS**
Stool examination	Gross, microscopic, and chemical examination of stool specimen	To detect normal and abnormal constituents	Explain process for collecting samples. Fresh specimen is optimum.
Ova and parasites (O&P)	Microscopic examination of stool contents for parasites or their eggs	To aid in diagnosis of parasitic infections	Requires several fresh specimens placed in special preservative. Obtaining three samples improves probability of detection of organism.
Bacterial culture	Sample contents grown on culture medium	To detect bacterial pathogens in stool	Fresh specimen is important to improve probability of detection of organism. Serologic tests determine presence of bacterial toxins.
Stool assay for vital pathogens	ELISA (enzyme-linked immunosorbent assay)	To detect viral pathogens in stool	Standard ELISA test is available for detection of rotavirus and adenovirus.
Giardia antigen	ELISA	To detect presence of Giardia organisms	This is more sensitive than single stool for O&P.
Quantitative fat	Detection of abnormal quantities of fat in stool	To aid in diagnosis of pancreatic insufficiency or malabsorption by measuring stool-reducing substances	This requires 72-hr collection of stool and simultaneous food intake record. Instruct patient to consume >50 g of fat.
Reducing substances	Unabsorbed sugars measured in stool (glucose, fructose, lactose, galactose, and pentose)	To detect elevated levels of reducing substances in stool, which are abnormal and suggest carbohydrate malabsorption	This requires random fresh stool specimen delivered immediately to laboratory. Fermentation by bacteria can give false low if stool is not tested immediately.
pH	Stool pH <5 suggestive of carbohydrate malabsorption; colonic bacterial fermentation produces short-chain fatty acids, which lower stool pH	To detect carbohydrate malabsorption	Obtain random fresh stool and refrigerate. Avoid barium procedures and laxatives before study. These can alter test results.
Occult blood guaiac test	Stool smeared on guaiac-impregnated paper, and 2 drops of developing solution added to reverse side; blue color indicates hemoglobin	To detect presence of blood in stool	This is an easily and quickly measured screening test. Small amounts of blood (e.g., from bleeding mouth, gums, nose) may give positive results.
***Helicobacter pylori* Testing**			
Serology test	Blood test for antibody to H. pylori (anti-HgIgG)	To assess for exposure to H. pylori	This test does not determine whether infection is acute or chronic.
C urea breath test	Collection of breath after ingestion of isotopic urea with either carbon 14 or carbon 13; measures labeled carbon dioxide in expired air	To determine if there is active infection with H. pylori in the stomach	This is one of most accurate methods to determine H. pylori infection in children ages 2 or older. Carbon 13 is nonradioactive (preferred), and carbon 14 has low level of radioactivity.
Urease test	Biopsy of stomach, which is stained and placed in Christensen urea medium, which turns color in presence of H. pylori	To determine presence of H. pylori in stomach	Sample must be obtained during endoscopy.
Pancreatic function	Pancreatic secretions collected via duodenal tube under stimulated conditions and analyzed for water, ions, and enzymes. Serial samples collected	To determine functional secretory capacity of pancreas	Patient takes nothing by mouth (NPO) before procedure. Prepare family and child for study. This is invasive and expensive test.
Radiography			
Plain films	Anteroposterior and lateral radiographs of abdomen and pelvis	To detect foreign body or mass, reveal bowel gas patterns, and detect obstruction or perforation in GI tract	Prepare family and child for study. No special physical preparation is required.
Contrast studies—upper GI and lower GI series	Radiopaque media (barium or water-soluble contrast) or air swallowed or administered as enema	To assess structure and function of GI tract and to detect luminal defects, or masses	Barium enema sometimes requires cleansing enemas and oral cathartics before procedure. Contrast material may be given by nasogastric (NG) or gastrostomy tube. Contrast enemas may reduce intussusception. Prepare family and child for swallowing contrast media, NG tube insertion, or enema. Encourage fluids after procedure.

GER, Gastroesophageal reflux; *GI*, Gastrointestinal.

Continued

TABLE 33-1	**GASTROINTESTINAL DIAGNOSTIC PROCEDURES—cont'd**		
TEST	**DESCRIPTION**	**PURPOSE**	**COMMENTS**
Radiography—cont'd			
Ultrasonography (sonography)	Measures and records reflection of pulsed or continuous high-frequency sound waves	To locate, measure, and delineate abdominal organs	Prepare family and child for study. This is noninvasive, with no radiation involved. Doppler studies demonstrate presence and direction of blood flow; often require intravenous (IV) contrast material.
Computed tomography (CT)	Pinpoint x ray directed on horizontal or vertical plane to provide series of "cuts" or "slices" that are fed into computer and assembled in image displays on video screen and transferred to permanent record	To visualize horizontal and vertical cross section of abdomen at any axis To distinguish density of various tissue structure of organs To detect blunt trauma to internal organs and masses	Prepare family and child for study. CT is usually noninvasive, but may require oral or IV contrast material and may require sedation.
Magnetic resonance imaging (MRI)	Images formed by reemission of radio signals by atomic nuclei stimulated in magnetic field	To visualize internal body structures in any plane; permits soft tissue discrimination unavailable with many techniques	Prepare family and child for procedure. MRI is usually noninvasive, but may require oral or IV contrast material. MRI may require sedation for lengthy procedure. Patient remains NPO 3-4 hr before study; patient is immobilized, and test takes long time. MRI does not expose patient to ionizing radiation. No magnetic material can be present in scanner.
Manometry			
Esophagus	Multilumen catheter inserted into esophagus, and water perfusion or solid state sensed by transducer and recorded	To evaluate dysphagia, esophageal spasm, achalasia, dysmotility	Teach and prepare child and family before procedure. Patient remains NPO 6-8 hr before procedure. Patient cooperation is required.
Rectal	Records reflex responses of anal sphincter to transient distention of rectal balloon	To measure sphincter function, especially to screen for constipation and Hirschsprung disease	Teach and prepare child and family before procedure. Administer enema to clear rectum before procedure.
Biopsy			
Liver	Removal of small piece of living tissue for microscopic examination by needle or surgically General sedation or local anesthesia used	To evaluate for biliary obstruction, hepatitis, metabolic disease To assess response to treatment interventions	Teach and prepare patient and family before procedure. Preliminary laboratory studies are needed. Liver biopsy is contraindicated with prolonged bleeding or clotting times, anemia, infection, or obstructive jaundice.
Esophagus, stomach, intestine	Small sample of mucosal tissue taken for microscopic evaluation	To evaluate for infection, inflammation, mucosal abnormalities	Teach and prepare patient and family before procedure. This biopsy requires conscious or general sedation. It is usually obtained with endoscopy.
Endoscopy			
Upper GI, colonoscopy, flexible sigmoidoscopy, anoscopy	Endoscope introduced into area to be examined Endoscope has flexible-tip light source and aspiration and instrument channel	To directly visualize GI tract to evaluate abnormalities, detect lesions, obtain biopsies To perform therapeutic procedures—polypectomies, removal of foreign bodies, sclerotherapy of esophageal varices, placement of feeding tubes or percutaneous catheters	Teach and prepare patient and family before procedure. Patient remains NPO 4-8 hr before procedure. Lower GI requires bowel cleansing. Patient requires conscious or general sedation.
Esophageal pH monitoring	Probe that measures pH placed through nose into distal esophagus and records pH over time	To determine frequency and duration of gastric acid refluxed into the esophagus (GER) To establish association between patient symptoms (pain, apnea, failure to thrive, asthma, wheezing, hoarseness) and acid reflux	Teach and prepare patient and family before procedure. This is usually done over 24-hr period, along with events diary to determine association or relation between symptoms and acid/GER. Patient remains NPO 4 hr before tube is passed; discontinue antacids and other medications 24 hr–7 days (omeprazole) before study.

TABLE 33-1	GASTROINTESTINAL DIAGNOSTIC PROCEDURES—cont'd		
TEST	**DESCRIPTION**	**PURPOSE**	**COMMENTS**
Breath hydrogen test	Noninvasive study to assess for carbohydrate intolerance Hydrogen generated in colon by bacterial fermentation of undigested carbohydrates and then absorbed into blood, where it diffuses into expired air via lungs	To evaluate for bacterial overgrowth, lactase or sucrase-isomaltase deficiency To evaluate for malabsorption or bacterial overgrowth by detecting rise in expired hydrogen after oral loading with specific carbohydrate	Teach and prepare patient and family before procedure. Patient remains NPO 12 hr before test. Previous nights' dinner should consist of meat, rice, and water; avoid other starches. Antibiotics may reduce hydrogen levels.
D-Xylose absorption test	D-Xylose solution administered orally; serum levels of D-xylose measured at 30, 60, 90, and 120 min Urine collected for total of 5 hr to measure D-xylose excretion	To evaluate absorptive capacity of small intestinal mucosa To diagnose small-bowel malabsorption caused by celiac disease	Teach and prepare patient and family before procedure. Patient remains NPO 4-8 hr before test. Test is used less often, largely replaced by endoscopic biopsies to evaluate for villous atrophy.
Hepatobiliary scintigraphy	Nuclear medicine study Radiopharmaceutical administered intravenously, then sequential images of liver, biliary system, and bowel obtained	To evaluate conditions of liver and biliary tract abnormalities and gallbladder disease To aid in diagnosis and monitoring of these conditions, such as biliary atresia	Prepare family and child for study. Images may be obtained for up to 24 hr if excretion is delayed.

GER, Gastroesophageal reflux; *GI*, Gastrointestinal.

should consider pica when children known to be at risk for this condition develop abdominal pain, other GI symptoms, or anemia. Children exhibiting signs of this disorder should be evaluated, and if a potentially harmful substance is involved, it should be removed from the child's environment. Nursing education regarding the dangers of pica, especially lead, and assistance in helping families remove the substance are important. (See Chapter 16.)

FOREIGN BODIES

Foreign body ingestions are most common in infants and children between the ages of 6 months and 3 years, and are the leading cause of accidental death in children less than 6 years of age (Hollinger, 2007). Annually 300 children die in the United States from choking, and approximately 85% of these are younger than 3 years. The peak incidence is between the ages of 1 and 2 years. Boys are twice as likely as girls to aspirate, and children with neurologic problems are at greatest risk. Coins, peanuts, nuts, vegetables, metal or plastic objects, and bones are the most frequently aspirated items.

Where the foreign bodies are retained depends on the GI tract's size, shape, diameter, and motility. Foreign bodies tend to become impacted at normally narrow sites of the GI tract. Pathologic narrowing of the intestine or intestinal stomas can also be a cause of foreign body obstruction. Foreign bodies in the stomach or intestine usually pass on their own. However, if they do become impacted, it generally occurs at the ileocecal valve, and sometimes at the pylorus, duodenum, or appendix. The most common anatomic sites in the esophagus are (1) the thoracic inlet (upper third of the esophagus), at the border of the cricopharyngeal muscle (UES); (2) the point where the esophagus crosses the aortic arch in the midesophagus; and (3) the LES (Gilger, 2003).

Signs and Symptoms

A history of choking followed by an acute episode of coughing is the most common presentation of foreign body ingestion (Lea, Nawaf, Yoav, et al, 2005). Initial signs and symptoms also may include dyspnea and wheezing. Aspirated foreign bodies that lodge in the larynx or trachea cause stridor. When these are in the large bronchi, crepitations and wheezes can be found. Wheezes and crepitations can be heard in both lungs, but unilateral findings have a higher specificity for foreign body aspiration (Kadmon, Stern, Bron-Harlev, et al, 2008).

Other symptoms may be those that are common with GI complaints in general (e.g., dysphagia, excessive drooling, poor feeding, vomiting, gagging, anorexia, neck or throat pain, sensation of a foreign object, and refusal to eat or drink).

Complications

Less than 1% of esophageal bodies cause a significant problem. However, serious problems that can occur include mediastinitis, pleural effusion, pneumothorax, and lung abscess. Foreign bodies are generally classified as sharp or dull, pointed or blunt, and toxic or nontoxic.

Food bolus foreign bodies should be immediately removed if the child is in severe distress and unable to swallow secretions. Disc batteries are a medical emergency if they are lodged in the esophagus because, if both poles of the battery come in contact with the flat wall of the esophagus, it may result in liquefaction, necrosis, and perforation. However, if the battery passes into the stomach, it will generally pass without incident. Sharp objects (straight pins, needles, straightened paper clips) need to be removed if lodged in the esophagus. If they pass into the stomach, they generally will pass out of the body, but there is a 35% risk of complications.

Diagnostic Evaluation

As mentioned, there may be no signs or symptoms, but some children come to the physician for evaluation because of problems. The nurse should perform a complete history and physical examination. Assess the airway and breathing first. Findings on the chest evaluation might include inspiratory stridor or expiratory wheezing. Findings on an abdominal examination could be small bowel obstruction or perforation. The physical examination might demonstrate swelling, erythema, or crepitus suggestive of esophageal perforation.

Assessment often involves radiologic evaluation. A plain x-ray film of the neck, chest, and abdomen may be ordered. Biplane radiographic studies identify radiopaque esophageal foreign bodies. Flat objects such as coins may be visible in the coronal plane. Objects in the trachea generally orient into the sagittal plane and are easiest to see in the lateral projection. Hand-held metal detectors have been used to detect coins. Endoscopy should be done in patients with symptoms suggestive of obstruction even if the radiographic evidence is negative.

Therapeutic Management

Intervention is urgent when a child has sharp objects, magnets, or disc batteries lodged in the esophagus because of the risk of perforation or acid burns (Kiger, Brenkert, and Losek, 2008). Urgent intervention is also important any time the airway is compromised. If the child is asymptomatic and the foreign body does not carry an emergent risk, it is reasonable to wait 24 hours to see if it will pass. Foreign objects should not be allowed to remain in the esophagus for more than 24 hours because of the potential for complications such as erosion, perforation, or formation of fistulas.

Flexible endoscopy allows direct visualization of the esophagus, stomach, and duodenum. It is the best approach for removing a foreign object. It involves passing a narrow tube with a camera on the end through the mouth into the esophagus, stomach, and duodenum with the patient under sedation. The foreign object can be detected and removed. Rigid endoscopy is used to remove impacted sharp objects at the level of the hypopharynx and cricopharyngeal muscle.

Another technique that has been used is bougienage (Uyemura, 2005). This involves passing a dilator to push objects into the stomach. The drawback is this method does not allow inspection of the esophagus to assess for injury or damage, and it increases the risk of perforation of the esophagus.

Another method involves passing a Foley catheter into the esophagus, inflating it distal to the obstruction, and then withdrawing it (Uyemura, 2005). Again there is a risk of airway obstruction and an inability to directly visualize the esophagus.

Coins have been removed using the penny pincher technique, which involves passing grasping forceps through a nasogastric (NG) tube using fluoroscopic guidance. This is an improvement over the Foley technique because it allows for direct control of the object, but again it does not permit inspection of the esophagus.

Important variables in the application of treatment guidelines include the type of foreign object, its location in the GI tract, and whether the patient is symptomatic. Of all foreign bodies that reach the stomach, 80% to 90% pass spontaneously, 10% to 20% require endoscopic removal, and 1% requires surgery (Byrne, 1999). The progress of a foreign body may be followed radiographically. Examine all stools to detect the passage of the object. The child should be fed the usual diet. Sharp objects such as long pins or chicken or fish bones should be removed endoscopically rather than risk perforation by allowing them to pass spontaneously (Byrne, 1999). Endoscopic or surgical intervention should be implemented if the object fails to progress through the GI tract (Uyemura, 2005).

Nursing Care Management

The primary nursing intervention is prevention of foreign body ingestion through family teaching. All children who are old enough to understand are taught not to put anything in their mouth except food. Infants and young children who cannot follow such advice must have their environment protected.

Prevention includes supervision and ongoing education as the child matures. Any small items, diaper pins, or sharp objects are placed out of the area where an infant is usually cared for, plays, or sleeps. As the infant becomes more mobile, the environment is inspected carefully for hazardous objects. Any potentially dangerous items are placed out of reach of a young child or discarded where they cannot be retrieved easily. Toys are carefully examined for small or removable parts that could be accidentally ingested. If infants and small children wear earrings, the earrings should have screw backs to prevent them from falling off. Infants and small children who wear other jewelry should be carefully supervised. Infants or young children should not be allowed to play with marbles, coins, or objects with small batteries.

Once an object is swallowed, parents need guidelines on seeking treatment (see Emergency Treatment box). When no treatment is advised and the object is left to pass spontaneously, parents should examine all stools for verification that the object has passed safely through the GI tract, usually within 3 or 4 days. For children in diapers, this is easily accomplished by squeezing the stool between the diaper to locate the object. For toilet-trained children a piece of plastic wrap placed across the

---

✚ EMERGENCY TREATMENT

Foreign Body Ingestion

Seek medical treatment immediately if:
- Any sharp or large object or a battery was ingested.
- There are signs that the object may have been aspirated (i.e., coughing, choking, inability to speak, or difficulty breathing). (See Chapter 31 for emergency treatment of acute airway obstruction.)
- There are signs of GI perforation (i.e., chest or abdominal pain; evidence of bleeding in vomitus, stool, hematocrit, or vital signs).
- There are signs that the object may be lodged in the esophagus (i.e., increased salivation, drooling, gagging, or difficulty swallowing).
- There are signs that the object may be lodged in the pharynx (i.e., discomfort in the throat or chest—more likely with a fish or chicken bone or large piece of meat).

Seek medical advice even if the object is smooth and small (usually less than the size of a nickel).

If no treatment is advised, check the stool for passage of the object; do not give laxatives.

toilet bowl to collect the stool makes it easier to examine the feces. A tongue blade or similar disposable object may be needed to break up the stool for inspection.

DISORDERS OF MOTILITY

CONSTIPATION

Constipation is a symptom, not a disease. It is defined as a decrease in bowel movement frequency or trouble defecating for more than 2 weeks (Philichi, 2008). Constipation is an alteration in the frequency, consistency, or ease of passing stool. Parents often define constipation as passing less than three stools per week. It may also be defined as painful bowel movements, which are often blood streaked or include the retention of stool, with or without soiling, even with a stool frequency of more than three stools per week (Loening-Baucke and Pashankar, 2006). The frequency of bowel movements, however, is not considered a diagnostic criterion because it varies widely among children. Having extremely long intervals between defecation is obstipation. Constipation with fecal soiling is encopresis.

Constipation may arise secondary to a variety of organic disorders or in association with a wide range of systemic disorders. Structural disorders of the intestine, such as strictures, ectopic anus, and Hirschsprung disease (HD), may be associated with constipation. Systemic disorders associated with constipation include hypothyroidism, hypercalcemia resulting from hyperparathyroidism or vitamin D excess, and chronic lead poisoning. Constipation is also associated with drugs such as antacids, diuretics, antiepileptics, antihistamines, opioids, and iron supplementation. Spinal cord lesions may be associated with loss of rectal tone and sensation. Affected children are prone to chronic fecal retention and overflow incontinence.

The majority of children have idiopathic or functional constipation, since no underlying cause can be identified. Chronic constipation may occur as a result of environmental or psychosocial factors, or a combination of both. Transient illness, withholding and avoidance secondary to painful or negative experiences with stooling, and dietary intake with decreased fluid and fiber all play a role in the etiology of constipation.

Infancy

The onset of constipation frequently occurs during infancy and may result from organic causes such as HD, hypothyroidism, and strictures. It is important to differentiate these conditions from functional constipation. Constipation in infancy is often related to dietary practices. It is less common in breast-fed infants, who have softer stools than bottle-fed infants. Breast-fed infants may also have decreased stools because of more complete use of breast milk with little residue. When constipation occurs with a change from human milk or modified cow's milk to whole cow's milk, simple measures such as adding or increasing the amount of cereal, vegetables, and fruit in the infant's diet usually correct the problem. When a bottle-fed infant passes a hard stool that results in an anal fissure, stool-withholding behaviors may develop in response to pain on defecation (see Critical Thinking Exercise).

Childhood

Most constipation in early childhood is due to environmental changes or normal development when a child begins to attain control over bodily functions. A child who has experienced discomfort during bowel movements may deliberately try to withhold stool. Over time, the rectum accommodates to the accumulation of stool, and the urge to defecate passes. When the bowel contents are ultimately evacuated, the accumulated feces are passed with pain, thus reinforcing the desire to withhold stool.

Constipation in school-age children may represent an ongoing problem or a first-time event. The onset of constipation at this age is often the result of environmental changes, stresses, and changes in toileting patterns. A common cause of new-onset constipation at school entry is fear of using the school bathrooms, which are noted for their lack of privacy. Early and hurried departure for school immediately after breakfast may also impede bathroom use.

Therapeutic Management

Treatment of constipation depends on the cause and duration of symptoms. A complete history and physical examination are essential to determine appropriate management (Tobias, Mason, Lutkenhoff, et al, 2008). Meconium plugs are often evacuated after digital examination. It may be necessary to facilitate passage of the obstruction by irrigation with a hypertonic solution or water-soluble enema such as diatrizoate meglumine (Gastrografin) or diatrizoate sodium (Hypaque). If the constipation is due to HD, surgical treatment may include resection of the intestine and saline irrigations.

Management of the infant should include education of the parents concerning normal bowel habits. Short, transient periods of constipation usually require no intervention. Mild constipation usually resolves as solid food is introduced in the diet. Stool softeners such as malt extract or lactulose may be used for hard stools or anal fissures. The persistent use of rectal stimulation with thermometers or cotton-tipped applicators is

Critical Thinking Exercise—Constipation

BOX 33-3 TREATMENT FOR ORGANIC CAUSES OF CONSTIPATION

Phase I: Clean Out and Disimpaction (3 to 5 Days)
Oral clean-out method preferred for children older than 4 years
- High-dose mineral oil
- Polyethylene glycol
- Magnesium hydroxide

Enema clean-out
- Milk and molasses
- Normal saline solution
- Microlax, mineral oil, or hypertonic phosphate

Nasogastric lavage (hospitalization)
- Polyethylene glycol electrolyte solution

Phase 2: Maintenance (6 to 12 Months)
Oral laxatives
- Polyethylene glycol
- Mineral oil
- Lactulose
- Magnesium hydroxide

High-fiber diet
Increased fluid intake
Behavioral training

Phase 3: Weaning
Gradual tapering of laxatives
Continue high-fiber diet, fluid intake, behavior modification

Adapted from Tobias N, Mason D, Lutkenhoff M, et al: Management principles of organic causes of childhood constipation, *J Pediatr Health Care* 22(1):12-23, 2008.

discouraged because these methods often result in anal fissures and increased pain that may trigger stool withholding.

The management of simple constipation consists of a plan to promote regular bowel movements. Often this is as simple as changing the diet to provide more fiber and fluids, eliminating foods known to be constipating, and establishing a bowel routine that allows for regular passage of stool. Stool-softening agents such as docusate or lactulose may also be helpful. Polyethylene glycol (PEG) 3350 without electrolytes (MiraLax) is a chemically inert polymer that has been introduced as a new laxative in recent years. Children tolerate it well because it can be mixed in a beverage of choice (Loening-Baucke and Pashankar, 2006). If other symptoms such as vomiting, abdominal distention, or pain and evidence of growth failure are associated with the constipation, investigate the condition further.

Management of chronic constipation requires an organized approach. It is important for families to realize that it usually requires at least 6 to 12 months of treatment to be effective (Tobias, Mason, Lutkenhoff, et al, 2008). The goals for management include restoring regular evacuation of stool, shrinking the distended rectum to its normal size, and promoting a regular toileting routine. This requires a combination of therapies and should include bowel cleansing, maintenance therapy to prevent stool retention, modification of diet, bowel habit training, and behavioral modification (Box 33-3).

⚡ DRUG ALERT

Mineral Oil

Mineral oil must be given carefully to avoid the risk of aspiration. It should not be used in children younger than 1 year (Philichi, 2008).

After the impaction is removed, maintenance therapy often lasting for 6 to 12 months is necessary to promote easy passage of stool and to prevent stool retention. Maintenance therapy includes mineral oil, stool softeners, and laxatives. Stool softeners are often ineffective for severe constipation; laxative therapy may be necessary to return the rectum to its normal size. Polyethylene glycol is a more favorable constipation intervention than lactulose (Dupont, Leluyer, Maamri, et al, 2005). Polyethylene glycol increases fluid in the colon. The additional volume of fluid stimulates the urge to defecate.

Changes in the diet may be helpful but are usually not effective alone. A recent study comparing a liquid yogurt fiber mixture to lactulose in 147 children revealed comparable results in the treatment of constipation (Kokke, Scholtens, Alles, et al, 2008). Encouraging the intake of fiber ultimately helps maintain regular elimination once the rectum returns to normal size and the laxatives are tapered. Effective counseling is an essential element of the treatment plan for children with chronic constipation. Explain normal bowel function, the purpose of interventions, and the need for persistence to the child and family.

Retraining therapy involves habit training, reinforcement for sitting on the toilet and defecating, and emotional support. Parents should establish a regular toilet time once or twice a day, preferably after a meal. A reasonable amount of time (5 to 10 minutes) should be spent attempting to defecate completely. Biofeedback may be indicated as a form of behavior modification and as a means to teach children to relax the anal sphincter during defecation.

Nursing Care Management

Unfortunately, constipation tends to be self-perpetuating. A child who has difficulty or discomfort when attempting to evacuate the bowels has a tendency to retain the bowel contents, and thus constipation becomes a chronic problem. Nursing assessment begins with a history of bowel habits; diet; events that may be associated with the onset of constipation; drugs or other substances that the child may be taking; and the consistency, color, frequency, and other characteristics of the stool. If there is no evidence of a pathologic condition that requires further investigation, the nurse's major task is to educate the parents regarding normal stool patterns and to participate in the education and treatment of the child.

Dietary modifications are helpful in preventing constipation. Fiber is an important part of the diet. Parents benefit from guidance about foods high in fiber (Box 33-4) and ways to promote healthy food choices in children. If bran is added to the diet, creative ways to disguise the consistency, such as adding it to cereal, peanut butter, mashed potatoes, fruit shakes, and baked goods, are helpful. Beans are often found in Mexican dishes children enjoy and can be added to soups, salads, and stews. Beyond the age when foreign body aspiration is a hazard, a good source of fiber is corn and popcorn.

Parents need reassurance concerning the prognosis for establishing normal bowel habits. Many parents are concerned about constipation and view the condition as dangerous. Families need thorough instructions about the treatment plan. If the child needs enemas or medication, give the family the appropriate instructions. It is important to discuss attitudes and expectations regarding toilet habits and the treatment plan.

BOX 33-4   HIGH-FIBER FOODS

Bread, Grains
Whole-grain bread or rolls
Whole-grain cereals
Bran
Pancakes, waffles, and muffins with fruit or bran
Unrefined (brown) rice

Vegetables
Raw vegetables, especially broccoli, cabbage, carrots, cauliflower, celery, lettuce, and spinach
Cooked vegetables, such as those listed above, and asparagus, beans, Brussels sprouts, corn, potatoes, rhubarb, squash, string beans, and turnips

Fruits
Prunes, raisins, or other dried fruits
Raw fruits, especially those with skins or seeds, other than ripe banana or avocado

Miscellaneous
Legumes (beans), popcorn, nuts, seeds
High-fiber snack bars

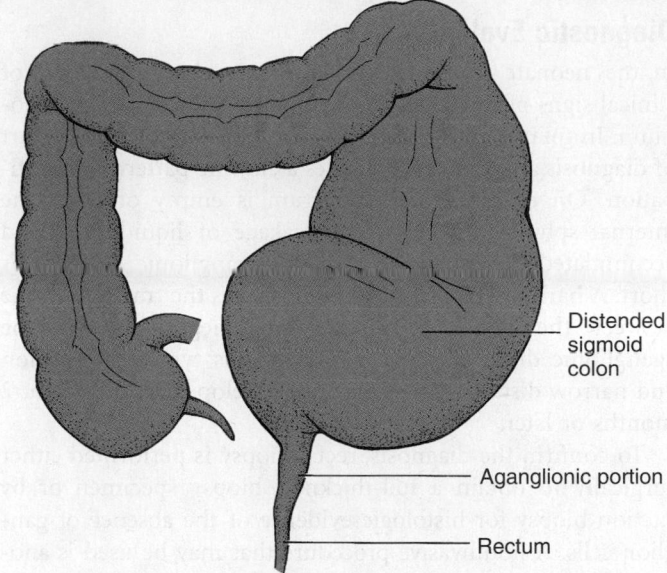

Fig. 33-2 Hirschsprung disease.

HIRSCHSPRUNG DISEASE (CONGENITAL AGANGLIONIC MEGACOLON)

HD is a congenital anomaly that results in mechanical obstruction from inadequate motility of part of the intestine. It accounts for about one fourth of all cases of neonatal intestinal obstruction. The incidence is 1 in 5000 live births. It is four times more common in males than in females and follows a familial pattern in a small number of cases. Mutations in the *RET* protooncogene have been found in 17% to 38% of children with short-segment HD and in 70% to 80% of those with long-segment involvement (Dasgupta and Langer, 2004). In more than 80% of cases the aganglionosis is restricted to the internal sphincter, rectum, and a few centimeters of the sigmoid colon and is termed *short-segment disease* (Theocharatos and Kenny, 2008).

Pathophysiology

The pathology of HD relates to the absence of ganglion cells in the affected areas of the intestine, resulting in a loss of the rectosphincteric reflex and an abnormal microenvironment of the cells of the affected intestine (Theocharatos and Kenny, 2008). The term *congenital aganglionic megacolon* describes the primary defect, which is the absence of ganglion cells in the myenteric plexus of Auerbach and the submucosal plexus of Meissner (Fig. 33-2).

The absence of ganglion cells in the affected bowel results in a lack of enteric nervous system stimulation, which decreases the internal sphincter's ability to relax. Unopposed sympathetic stimulation of the intestine results in increased intestinal tone. In addition to the contraction of the abnormal bowel and the resulting lack of peristalsis, there is a loss of the rectosphincteric reflex. Normally when a stool bolus enters the rectum, the internal sphincter relaxes and the stool is evacuated. In HD, the internal sphincter does not relax. In most cases the aganglionic segment includes the rectum and some portion of the distal colon. However, the entire colon or part of the small intestine

BOX 33-5   CLINICAL MANIFESTATIONS OF HIRSCHSPRUNG DISEASE

Newborn Period
Failure to pass meconium within 24 to 48 hours after birth
Refusal to feed
Bilious vomiting
Abdominal distention

Infancy
Failure to thrive
Constipation
Abdominal distention
Episodes of diarrhea and vomiting
Signs of enterocolitis
  • Explosive, watery diarrhea
  • Fever
  • Appears significantly ill

Childhood
Constipation
Ribbonlike, foul-smelling stools
Abdominal distention
Visible peristalsis
Easily palpable fecal mass
Undernourished, anemic appearance

may be involved. Occasionally, skip segments or total intestinal aganglionosis may occur.

Clinical Manifestations

Most children with HD are diagnosed in the first few months of life. Clinical manifestations vary according to the age when symptoms are recognized and the presence of complications, such as enterocolitis (Box 33-5). A neonate usually is seen with distended abdomen, feeding intolerance with bilious vomiting, and delay in the passage of meconium. Typically, 95% of normal term infants pass meconium in the first 24 hours of life, whereas less than 10% of infants with HD do so. In older children, a careful history is helpful.

Diagnostic Evaluation

In the neonate the diagnosis is suspected on the basis of clinical signs of intestinal obstruction or failure to pass meconium. In infants and children the history is an important part of diagnosis and typically includes a chronic pattern of constipation. On examination the rectum is empty of feces, the internal sphincter is tight, and leakage of liquid stool and accumulated gas may occur if the aganglionic segment is short. A barium enema often demonstrates the transition zone between the dilated proximal colon (megacolon) and the aganglionic distal segment. However, this typical megacolon and narrow distal segment may not develop until the age of 2 months or later.

To confirm the diagnosis, rectal biopsy is performed either surgically to obtain a full-thickness biopsy specimen or by suction biopsy for histologic evidence of the absence of ganglion cells. A noninvasive procedure that may be used is anorectal manometry, in which a catheter with a balloon attached is inserted into the rectum. The test records the reflex pressure response of the internal anal sphincter to distention of the balloon. A normal response is relaxation of the internal sphincter followed by a contraction of the external sphincter. In HD the external sphincter contracts normally but the internal sphincter fails to relax.

Therapeutic Management

The majority of children with HD require surgery rather than medical therapy with frequent enemas (Levitt, Martin, Olesevich, et al, 2009). Once the child is stabilized with fluid and electrolyte replacement, if needed, surgery is performed, with a high rate of success. Surgical management consists primarily of the removal of the aganglionic portion of the bowel to relieve obstruction, restore normal motility, and preserve the function of the external anal sphincter. The transanal Soave endorectal pull-through procedure is often performed and consists of pulling the end of the normal bowel through the muscular sleeve of the rectum, from which the aganglionic mucosa has been removed (Huang, Zheng, and Xiao, 2008). With earlier diagnosis the proximal bowel may not be extremely distended, thus allowing for a primary pull-through or one-stage procedure and eliminating the need for a temporary colostomy. Simpler operations, such as an anorectal myomectomy, may be indicated in very short–segment disease.

After the pull-through procedure, anal stricture and incontinence may occur and require further therapy, including dilations or bowel retraining therapy. Constipation and fecal incontinence are chronic problems in a significant proportion of patients after surgical correction for HD (Levitt, Martin, Olesevich, et al, 2009). As these children grow older, this can significantly affect their quality of life (Mills, Konkin, Milner, et al, 2008).

Nursing Care Management

The nursing concerns depend on the child's age and the type of treatment. If the disorder is diagnosed during the neonatal period, the main objectives are (1) to help the parents adjust to a congenital defect in their child, (2) to foster infant-parent bonding, (3) to prepare them for the medical-surgical intervention, and (4) to assist them in colostomy care after discharge.

Preoperative Care

The child's preoperative care depends on the age and clinical condition. A child who is malnourished may not be able to withstand surgery until his or her physical status improves. Often this involves symptomatic treatment with enemas; a low-fiber, high-calorie, and high-protein diet; and in severe situations the use of total parenteral nutrition (TPN).

Physical preoperative preparation includes the same measures that are common to any surgery. (See Surgical Procedures, Chapter 27.) In the newborn, whose bowel is sterile, no additional preparation is necessary. However, in other children, preparation for the pull-through procedure involves emptying the bowel with repeated saline enemas and decreasing bacterial flora with oral or systemic antibiotics and colonic irrigations using antibiotic solution. Enterocolitis is the most serious complication of HD. Emergency preoperative care includes frequent monitoring of vital signs and blood pressure for signs of shock; monitoring fluid and electrolyte replacements, as well as plasma or other blood derivatives; and observing for symptoms of bowel perforation, such as fever, increasing abdominal distention, vomiting, increased tenderness, irritability, dyspnea, and cyanosis.

Because progressive distention of the abdomen is a serious sign, the nurse measures abdominal circumference with a paper tape measure, usually at the level of the umbilicus or at the widest part of the abdomen. The nurse marks the point of measurement with a pen to ensure reliability of subsequent measurements. Abdominal measurement can be obtained with the vital sign measurements and is recorded in serial order so that any change is obvious (see Atraumatic Care box).

ATRAUMATIC CARE

Abdominal Circumference Measurements

To reduce any stress to the acutely ill child when frequent measurements of abdominal circumference are needed, leave the tape measure in place beneath the child. Measure the abdomen at the same time that vital signs are taken to avoid disturbing the child more than necessary.

The child's age dictates the type and extent of psychologic preparation. Because a colostomy is usually performed, the child who is of preschool age is told about the procedure in concrete terms with the use of visual aids. (See Chapter 27.) It is important to time explanations appropriately to prevent the anxiety and confusion that could result from too much information. It is also important to stress to parents and older children that the colostomy for HD is temporary, unless so much bowel is involved that a permanent ileostomy must be performed. In most instances the extent of bowel resection is known before surgery, although the nurse should be aware of cases when doubt exists concerning repair. Remember that although a temporary colostomy is favorable in terms of future health and adjustment, it requires additional surgery, which may be stressful to parents and children.

Postoperative Care

Postoperative care is the same as that for any child or infant with abdominal surgery. (See Surgical Procedures, Chapter 27.) When a colostomy is part of the corrective procedure, stomal care is a major nursing task. (See Ostomies, Chapter 27.) To prevent contamination of an infant's abdominal wound with urine, pin the diaper below the dressing. Sometimes a Foley catheter is used in the immediate postoperative period to divert the flow of urine away from the abdomen.

Discharge Care

After surgery, parents need instruction concerning colostomy care. Even a preschooler can be included in the care by handing articles to the parent, rolling up the colostomy pouch after it is emptied, or applying barrier preparations to the surrounding skin. Although the diagnosis of HD is less frequent in school-age children or adolescents, children this age can often be involved in colostomy care to the point of total responsibility.

Some institutions and communities have enterostomal therapists who provide expert assistance in planning home care. If families require financial assistance and psychologic support, referral to a social worker, home health care agency, or community health nurse provides continuity of care.

GASTROESOPHAGEAL REFLUX

Gastroesophageal reflux (GER) is defined as the transfer of gastric contents into the esophagus. This phenomenon is physiologic, occurring throughout the day, most frequently after meals and at night; therefore it is important to differentiate GER from gastroesophageal reflux disease (GERD). GERD represents symptoms or tissue damage that result from GER. Approximately 50% of infants less than 2 months old are reported to have GER (Suwandhi, Ton, and Schwarz, 2006). This "physiologic" GER usually resolves spontaneously by 1 year of age. GER becomes a disease when complications such as failure to thrive, bleeding, or dysphagia develop.

Certain conditions predispose children to a high prevalence of GERD, including neurologic impairment, hiatal hernia, repaired esophageal atresia, and morbid obesity (Suwandhi, Ton, and Schwarz, 2006). Sandifer syndrome is an uncommon condition, usually occurring in young children, characterized by repetitive stretching and arching of the head and neck that can be mistaken for a seizure. This maneuver likely represents a physiologic neuromuscular response attempting to prevent acid refluxate from reaching the upper portion of the esophagus (Cavataio and Guandalini, 2005).

Infants who are prone to develop GER include premature infants and infants with bronchopulmonary dysplasia. Children who have had tracheoesophageal or esophageal atresia repairs, neurologic disorders, scoliosis, asthma, cystic fibrosis, or cerebral palsy are also prone to develop GER.

Clinical Manifestations

During infancy the most common clinical manifestation of GER is passive regurgitation or emesis. Recurrent vomiting occurs in 50% of infants in the first 3 months of life, 67% of 4-month-olds, and 5% of 10- to 12-month-old infants (Rudolph, Mazur, Liptak, et al, 2001). Vomiting generally resolves spon-

---

BOX 33-6 CLINICAL MANIFESTATIONS AND COMPLICATIONS OF GASTROESOPHAGEAL REFLUX

Symptoms in Infants
Spitting up, regurgitation, vomiting (may be forceful)
Excessive crying, irritability, arching of the back, stiffening
Weight loss, failure to thrive
Respiratory problems (cough, wheeze, stridor, gagging, choking with feedings)
Hematemesis
Apnea or apparent life-threatening event

Symptoms in Children
Heartburn
Abdominal pain
Noncardiac chest pain
Chronic cough
Dysphagia
Nocturnal asthma
Recurrent pneumonia

Complications
Esophagitis
Esophageal stricture
Laryngitis
Recurrent pneumonia
Anemia
Barrett esophagus

Adapted from Rudolph CD, Mazur LJ, Liptak GS, et al: Guidelines for evaluation and treatment of gastroesophageal reflux in infants and children: recommendations of the North American Society for Pediatric Gastroenterology and Nutrition, *J Pediatr Gastroenterol Nutr* 32(Suppl 2): S1-S31, 2001.

---

taneously in most of these infants. Clinical manifestations of gastroesophageal reflux are listed in Box 33-6. GER is one of the causes of apparent life-threatening events and has also been associated with chronic respiratory disorders, including reactive airways disease, recurrent stridor, chronic cough, and recurrent pneumonia in infants. Esophagitis can also cause discomfort in the chest area, which may be manifested as unusual irritability or poor intake of nutrients. Poor weight gain and poor growth may occur in a child with an insufficient intake of nutrients or with a large amount of regurgitation.

For preschool children GER may occur with intermittent vomiting. Older children tend to initially come to the physician with a more adultlike pattern of heartburn, regurgitation, and reswallowing. GERD may cause severe inflammation, chronic blood loss with anemia and hematemesis, hypoproteinemia, or melena. If the inflammation goes untreated, scarring and strictures may form. Barrett mucosa, another potential finding in the presence of chronic inflammation, is characterized by changes in the distal esophageal mucosa with metaplastic potentially malignant epithelium.

GER is common in children with asthma, but recurrent pneumonia caused by GER is uncommon except in children with neurologic impairments. Hoarseness has also been associated with GER in children.

Diagnostic Evaluation

The history and physical examination are usually sufficiently reliable to establish the diagnosis of GER. However, the upper

GI series is helpful in evaluating the presence of anatomic abnormalities (e.g., pyloric stenosis, malrotation, annular pancreas, hiatal hernia, esophageal stricture). The 24-hour intraesophageal pH monitoring study is the gold standard in the diagnosis of GER (Suwandhi, Ton, and Schwarz, 2006). Endoscopy with biopsy may be helpful to assess the presence and severity of esophagitis, strictures, and Barrett esophagus and to exclude other disorders such as Crohn disease (CD). Scintigraphy detects radioactive substances in the esophagus after a feeding of the compound and assesses gastric emptying. It can differentiate between aspiration of gastric contents from reflux and aspiration from poor oropharyngeal muscle coordination.

Therapeutic Management

Therapeutic management of GER depends on its severity. No therapy is needed for the infant who is thriving and has no respiratory complications. Avoidance of certain foods that exacerbate acid reflux (e.g., caffeine, citrus, tomatoes, alcohol, peppermint, spicy or fried foods) can improve mild GER symptoms. Lifestyle modifications in children (e.g., weight control if indicated; small, more frequent meals) and feeding maneuvers in infants (e.g., thickened feedings, upright positioning) can help as well. Twenty research trials involving 771 children found thickened feeds reduced the regurgitation severity (Craig, Hanlon-Dearman, Sinclair, et al, 2004). Thickened feeding has a significant effect on the reduction of regurgitation frequency and amount in otherwise healthy infants. However, the occurrence of acid GER was not reduced (Wenzi, Schneider, Scheele, et al, 2003).

Feedings thickened with 1 tsp to 1 tbsp of rice cereal per ounce of formula may be recommended. This may benefit infants who are underweight as a result of GERD. Constant NG feedings may be necessary for the infant with severe reflux and failure to thrive until surgery can be performed. Elevating the head of the bed did not have any effect on GER symptoms in the Cochrane systematic review of 20 research trials (Craig, Hanlon-Dearman, Sinclair, et al, 2004). Prone positioning of infants also decreases episodes of GER but is recommended only with extreme caution when the risk of GERD complications exceeds the risk of sudden infant death syndrome (Cavataio and Guandalini, 2005). The American Academy of Pediatrics continues to recommend supine positioning for sleep. (See Chapter 11.)

Pharmacologic therapy may be used to treat infants and children with GERD. Both H_2-receptor antagonists (cimetidine [Tagamet], ranitidine [Zantac], or famotidine [Pepcid]) and proton pump inhibitors (PPIs; esomeprazole [Nexium], lansoprazole [Prevacid], omeprazole [Prilosec], pantoprazole [Protonix], and rabeprazole [Aciphex]) reduce gastric hydrochloric acid secretion and may stimulate some increase in LES tone. Use of available prokinetic drugs (e.g., bethanechol [Urecholine] and metoclopramide) remains controversial. Careful analyses of published data have failed to demonstrate clinical efficacy in modifying the natural history or therapeutic outcomes of GER in childhood (Suwandhi, Ton, and Schwarz, 2006).

Surgical management of GER is reserved for children with severe complications such as recurrent aspiration pneumonia,

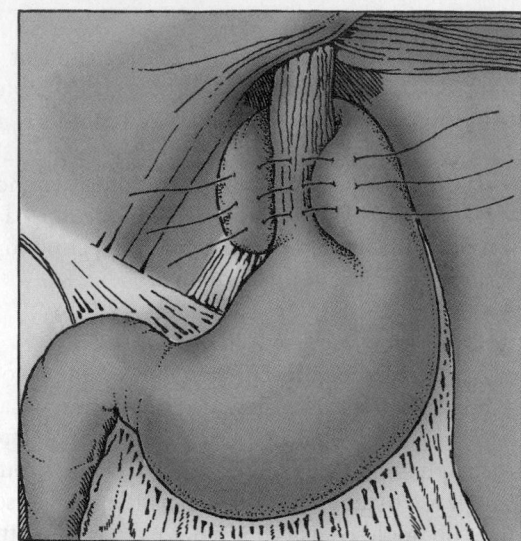

Fig. 33-3 Nissen fundoplication sutures passing through esophageal musculature. (Redrawn from Campbell A, Ferrara B: Toupet partial fundoplication, *AORN J* 57:671-679, 1993.)

apnea, severe esophagitis, or failure to thrive, and for children who have failed to respond to medical therapy. The Nissen fundoplication (Fig. 33-3) is the most common surgical procedure (Christian and Buyske, 2005). This surgery involves passage of the gastric fundus behind the esophagus to encircle the distal esophagus. Complications following fundoplication include breakdown of the wrap, small bowel obstruction, gasbloat syndrome, infection, retching, and dumping syndrome (Rudolph, Mazur, Liptak, et al, 2001).

Prognosis

The majority of infants with GER have a mild problem that generally improves by 12 to 18 months of age and requires only conservative lifestyle changes or medical therapy. If GER is severe and remains unsuccessfully treated, multiple complications can occur. Esophageal strictures caused by persistent esophagitis with scarring are one of the most significant complications. Recurrent respiratory distress with aspiration pneumonia, another serious complication, is an indication for surgery. Failure to thrive caused by GER can often be managed with medical therapy and nutritional support.

QUALITY PATIENT OUTCOMES: Gastroesophageal Reflux
- Adequate weight gain
- Limited spitting up or vomiting
- Good sleep habits
- No recurrent pneumonias

Nursing Care Management

Nursing care is directed at (1) identifying children with symptoms suggestive of GER; (2) educating parents regarding home care, including feeding, positioning, and medications when indicated; and (3) caring for the child undergoing surgical intervention. For the majority of infants, parental reassurance of the benign nature of the condition and its relationship to physiologic maturity is the most important intervention. To help parents cope with the inconvenience of dealing with a child who spits up or regurgitates frequently, simple tips such as using bibs and protective clothes during feeding and prone positioning when holding the infant after feeding are beneficial.

It is important to educate and reassure parents about positioning. In the past, recommendations encouraged upright positioning during sleeping for both infants and older children. The supine position for sleeping continues to be recommended by the American Academy of Pediatrics (2005). Parents should not place infants on their sides as an alternative to fully supine sleeping, and avoidance of soft bedding and soft objects in the bed is important. Rescheduling of the family's routine may be required to accommodate more frequent feeding times. If parents thicken formula with cereal, they should also enlarge the nipple opening for easier sucking. Usually breast-feeding may continue, and the mother may provide more frequent feeding times or express the milk for thickening with rice cereal. Parents should avoid feeding the child spicy foods or any foods that they find aggravate symptoms in general, and avoid caffeine, chocolate, tobacco smoke, and alcohol when breast-feeding. Other practical advice includes advising the parents to avoid vigorous play after feedings and to avoid feeding just before bedtime.

When regurgitation is severe and growth is a problem, continuous NG tube feedings may decrease the amount of emesis and provide constant buffering of gastric acid. Special preparation of caregivers is required when this type of nutritional therapy is indicated.

The nurse can support the family by providing information about all aspects of treatment. Parents often require specific information about the medications given for GER. PPIs are most effective when administered 30 minutes before breakfast so that the peak plasma concentrations occur with mealtime. If they are given twice a day, the second best time for administration is 30 minutes before the evening meal. Parents need to be reassured because it takes several days of administration to achieve a steady state of acid suppression. They may not see the results that they expect right away. A number of new formulations available in PPIs allow for more efficient administration. Some preparations are available in dissolvable pills. There are powder and granule preparations as well. Many pharmacies will compound the medication in a liquid form for administration.

Postoperative nursing care after the Nissen fundoplication is similar to that for other types of abdominal surgery. (See Chapter 27.) Gastric decompression by an NG tube or gastrostomy must be maintained to avoid distention in the immediate postoperative period. Usually the NG tube should not be replaced by the nurse if it is accidentally removed because of the risk of injury to the operative site. When postoperative ileus resolves, the NG tube is removed or the gastrostomy tube is elevated in preparation for feeding. If bolus feedings are initiated through the gastrostomy, the tube may need to remain vented for several days or longer to avoid gastric distention from swallowed air. Edema surrounding the surgical site and a tight gastric wrap may prohibit the infant from expelling air through the esophagus. Some infants benefit from clamping of the tube for increasingly longer intervals until they are able to tolerate continuous clamping between feedings. During this time, if the infant displays increasing irritability and evidence of cramping, some relief may be provided by venting the tube.

Preparation for Home Care

If medical management is prescribed or surgery is performed, nursing responsibilities include educating caregivers about administering drugs at home, special feeding regimens or formula preparation, gastrostomy care, and postoperative care. (See Chapter 27.) After surgery, reflux is completely controlled in most cases, with these children attaining normal health and growth. If a gastrostomy tube is inserted during surgery, it may be removed after several months unless nutritional supplementation is needed. In severe cases of bloating or dumping syndrome, continuous tube feedings may be better tolerated. Caregivers should be aware of potential postoperative problems, such as difficulty vomiting, bloating symptoms, or discomfort with large solid-food meals, and seek guidance from their health care provider as needed.

IRRITABLE BOWEL SYNDROME

Irritable bowel syndrome (IBS) is one of the most common adult problems treated by gastroenterologists. Recently IBS has been identified as a cause of recurrent abdominal pain in 4% to 25% of school-age children (Huertas-Ceballos, Logan, Bennett, et al, 2009). (See Recurrent Abdominal Pain, Chapter 18.) IBS is classified as a functional GI disorder. As with other forms of recurrent abdominal pain, the symptoms should be present either recurrently or constantly over a 3-month period (Huertas-Ceballos, Logan, Bennett, et al, 2009). Children with IBS often have alternating diarrhea and constipation, flatulence, bloating or a feeling of abdominal distention, lower abdominal pain, a feeling of urgency when needing to defecate, and a feeling of incomplete evacuation of the bowel. IBS also has psychosocial effects.

The cause of IBS is not clear, but it is believed to involve a combination of motor, autonomic, and psychologic factors. Children with IBS are evaluated to rule out organic causes for their symptoms such as inflammatory bowel disease (IBD), lactose intolerance, and parasitic infections. Many children with symptoms appear active and healthy and have normal growth.

Therapeutic Management

The long-range goal of treatment is development of regular bowel habits and relief of symptoms. A Cochrane systematic review found weak evidence of any medication benefits for children with IBS (Huertas-Ceballos, Logan, Bennett, et al, 2009). A 2009 Cochrane systematic review found no high-quality evidence on the effectiveness of any dietary interventions that included fiber supplements, lactose free-diets, or lactobacillus supplementation for children with IBS (Huertas-Ceballos, Logan, Bennett, et al, 2009).

Nursing Care Management

The primary nursing goal is family support and education. The disorder is stressful to children and parents. The nurse can help by providing support and reassurance that, although the symptoms are difficult to deal with, the disorder is not generally a threat to the child's health (see Community Focus box).

🏠 COMMUNITY FOCUS
Irritable Bowel Syndrome

Parents, school nurses, and teachers frequently interact with children and adolescents who complain of abdominal pain. Complaints of abdominal pain can lead to interruption of activities and absence from school. Those caring for children should be aware of this symptom complex and become skilled in the identification of its manifestations. If the student has other worrisome features, such as weight loss, rectal bleeding, or significant fatigue, further diagnostic evaluation may be necessary. However, many students with uncomplicated abdominal pain and irritable bowel syndrome benefit from reassurance, diet counseling, and stress management. Parents, school nurses, and teachers should also remember that helping adolescents learn to cope with life events may influence their anxiety and depression and ultimately reduce the symptoms of abdominal pain and irritable bowel syndrome.

BOX 33-7   CLINICAL MANIFESTATIONS OF APPENDICITIS

- Right lower quadrant abdominal pain
- Fever
- Rigid abdomen
- Decreased or absent bowel sounds
- Vomiting (typically follows onset of pain)
- Constipation or diarrhea
- Anorexia
- Tachycardia, rapid shallow breathing
- Pallor
- Lethargy
- Irritability
- Stooped posture

INFLAMMATORY CONDITIONS

ACUTE APPENDICITIS

Appendicitis, inflammation of the **vermiform appendix** (blind sac at the end of the cecum), is the most common cause of emergency abdominal surgery in childhood. In the United States, 60,000 to 80,000 cases are diagnosed each year. The average age of children with appendicitis is 10 years, with boys and girls equally affected before puberty. Classically, the first symptom of appendicitis is periumbilical pain, followed by nausea, right lower quadrant pain, and later vomiting with fever (Kwok, Kim, and Gorelick, 2004). Perforation of the appendix can occur within approximately 48 hours of the initial complaint of pain. At the time of initial presentation, about one third of all cases involve an already perforated appendix. Complications from appendiceal perforation include major abscess, phlegmon, enterocutaneous fistula, peritonitis, and partial bowel obstruction (Kwok, Kim, and Gorelick, 2004). A **phlegmon** is an acute suppurative inflammation of subcutaneous connective tissue that spreads.

Etiology

The cause of appendicitis is obstruction of the lumen of the appendix, usually by hardened fecal material (fecalith). Swollen lymphoid tissue, frequently occurring after a viral infection, can also obstruct the appendix. Another rare cause of obstruction is a parasite such as *Enterobius vermicularis*, or pinworms, which can obstruct the appendiceal lumen.

Pathophysiology

With acute obstruction, the outflow of mucus secretions is blocked and pressure builds within the lumen, resulting in compression of blood vessels. The resulting ischemia is followed by ulceration of the epithelial lining and bacterial invasion. Subsequent necrosis causes perforation or rupture with fecal and bacterial contamination of the peritoneal cavity. The resulting inflammation spreads rapidly throughout the abdomen (**peritonitis**), especially in young children, who are unable to localize infection. Progressive peritoneal inflammation results in functional intestinal obstruction of the small bowel (**ileus**) because intense GI reflexes severely inhibit bowel motility. Because the peritoneum represents a major portion of total body surface, the loss of extracellular fluid to the peritoneal cavity leads to electrolyte imbalance and hypovolemic shock.

Clinical Manifestations

The first symptom of appendicitis is usually colicky, cramping, abdominal pain located around the umbilicus (Box 33-7). **Referred pain** is the term used for this vague periumbilical localization. The midgut shares the same T10 dermatome, so pain is often perceived to be coming from this area. Generally, this pain progresses and becomes constant. The most important physical finding is focal abdominal tenderness. As the inflammation progresses to involve the serosa of the appendix and the peritoneum of the abdominal wall, the pain may shift to the right lower quadrant. The McBurney point, located two thirds the distance along a line between the umbilicus and the anterosuperior iliac spine, is the most common point of tenderness. Localized peritoneal signs may occur with gentle percussion or maneuvers such as heel strike or shaking the bed. Another helpful finding is Rovsing sign, tenderness in the right lower quadrant that occurs during palpation or percussion of other abdominal quadrants (Colvin, Bachur, and Kharbanda, 2007). Rebound tenderness—pain on deep palpation with sudden release—may be present, but is not a finding specific to appendicitis (Ceydeli, Lavotshkin, Yu, et al, 2006). Nausea, vomiting, and anorexia typically occur after the pain starts. Diarrhea, as well as other common signs of childhood illness such as upper respiratory tract congestion, poor feeding, lethargy, or irritability, may accompany appendicitis.

The child may not be able to walk well and may complain of pain in the right hip caused by inflammation in the psoas or iliopsoas muscles. Low-grade fever (>38° C [100.4° F]) may be present but occurs in only about 55% of all patients. The absence of fever does not exclude appendicitis. Temperature elevations of 38.8° to 39.4° C (102° to 103° F) can occur after perforation; however, very high fevers (>39.4° C [103° F]) are uncommon (Ceydeli, Lavotshkin, Yu, et al, 2006). Because of the great variability in the presentation and location of appendicitis, any child with focal tenderness, regardless of the location, should be considered to potentially have acute appendicitis (see Community Focus box).

COMMUNITY FOCUS

Acute Appendicitis

Abdominal pain is a common complaint among school-age children, but in some cases it may indicate acute appendicitis. School nurses and nurse practitioners in school-based clinics should become familiar with the "typical" pattern of symptoms in acute appendicitis and how to assess and evaluate an acute abdomen. School nurses also need to impress on teachers and coaches the importance of early referral to the health suite for further assessment. Early referral to the health suite and an alert school nurse or nurse practitioner may make the difference between an uncomplicated appendectomy and a delayed diagnosis of a perforated appendix with peritonitis.

! NURSING ALERT

Signs of peritonitis in addition to fever usually include sudden relief from pain after perforation; subsequent increase in pain, which is usually diffuse and accompanied by rigid guarding of the abdomen; progressive abdominal distention; tachycardia; rapid, shallow breathing as the child refrains from using abdominal muscles; pallor; chills; irritability; and restlessness.

Diagnostic Evaluation

Diagnosis is not always straightforward. Fever, vomiting, abdominal pain, and an elevated white blood count are associated with appendicitis but are also seen in IBD, pelvic inflammatory disease, gastroenteritis, urinary tract infection, right lower lobe pneumonia, mesenteric adenitis, Meckel diverticulum, and intussusception. Prolonged symptoms and delayed diagnosis often occur in younger children, in whom the risk of perforation is greatest because of their inability to verbalize their complaints.

The diagnosis is based primarily on the history and physical examination (see Box 33-7). Pain, the cardinal feature, is initially generalized (usually periumbilical). However, it usually descends to the lower right quadrant. The most intense site of pain may be at McBurney point. Rebound tenderness is not a reliable sign and is extremely painful to the child. Referred pain, elicited by light percussion around the perimeter of the abdomen, indicates peritoneal irritation. Movement, such as riding over bumps in an automobile or gurney, aggravates the pain. In addition to pain, significant clinical manifestations include fever, a change in behavior, anorexia, and vomiting.

Laboratory studies usually include a complete blood count (CBC); urinalysis (to rule out a urinary tract infection); and, in adolescent females, serum human chorionic gonadotropin (to rule out an ectopic pregnancy). A white blood cell count greater than 10,000/mm^3 and a C-reactive protein (CRP) are common but are not necessarily specific for appendicitis. An elevated percentage of bands (often referred to as "a shift to the left") may indicate an inflammatory process. CRP is an acute-phase reactant that rises within 12 hours of the onset of infection.

Computed tomography (CT) scan has become the imaging technique of choice, although ultrasound may also be helpful in diagnosing appendicitis. A CT scan is considered positive in the presence of enlarged appendiceal diameter; appendiceal wall thickening; and periappendiceal inflammatory changes, including fat streaks, phlegmon, fluid collection, and extraluminal gas (Kaiser, Frenchner, and Jorulf, 2002).

Therapeutic Management

The treatment for appendicitis before perforation is surgical removal of the appendix (appendectomy). Usually antibiotics are administered preoperatively. Intravenous (IV) fluids and electrolytes are often required before surgery, especially if the child is dehydrated as a result of the marked anorexia characteristic of appendicitis.

The operation is usually performed through a right lower quadrant incision (open appendectomy). Laparoscopic surgery is increasingly being used to treat nonperforated acute appendicitis in pediatric patients. Three cannulas are inserted in the abdomen: one in the umbilicus, one in the left lower abdominal quadrant, and one in the suprapubic area. A small telescope is inserted through the left lower quadrant cannula, and an endoscopic stapler is inserted through the umbilical cannula. The appendix is ligated with the stapler and removed through the umbilical cannula. Advantages of laparoscopic appendectomy include reduced time in surgery and under anesthesia and also reduced risk of postoperative wound infection (Bensard, Hendrickson, Fyffe, et al, 2009).

Ruptured Appendix

Management of the child diagnosed with peritonitis caused by a ruptured appendix often begins preoperatively with IV administration of fluid and electrolytes, systemic antibiotics, and NG suction. Postoperative management includes IV fluids, continued administration of antibiotics, and NG suction for abdominal decompression until intestinal activity returns. Sometimes surgeons close the wound after irrigation of the peritoneal cavity. Other times, they leave the wound open (delayed closure) to prevent wound infection.

The treatment of a localized perforation with an appendiceal abscess is controversial. Some surgeons prefer to treat these children with antibiotics and IV fluids and allow the abscess to drain spontaneously. An elective appendectomy is then performed 2 to 3 months later.

Prognosis

Complications are uncommon after a simple appendectomy, and recovery is usually rapid and complete. The mortality rate from perforating appendicitis has improved from nearly certain death a century ago to 1% or less at the present time (Strahlman, 2001). Complications, however, including wound infection and intraabdominal abscess, are not uncommon. Early recognition of the illness is important to prevent complications.

QUALITY PATIENT OUTCOMES: Appendicitis

- Early recognition of signs and symptoms of appendicitis
- No readmission for postoperative complications within 5 days
- Appropriate use of antibiotic therapy
- No complications (e.g., negative appendectomy, abscess, wound infection)
- Appropriate laboratory orders and diagnostic x-ray studies ordered

! NURSING ALERT

In any instance in which severe abdominal pain is observed, the nurse must be aware of the danger of administering laxatives or enemas. Such measures stimulate bowel motility and increase the risk of perforation.

Nursing Care Management

Because successful treatment of appendicitis is based on prompt recognition of the disorder, a primary nursing objective is to assist in establishing a diagnosis. Because abdominal pain is a common childhood complaint, the nurse needs to make some preliminary assessment of the severity of the pain. (See Chapter 7.) One of the most reliable estimates is the degree of change in behavior. A child who stays home from school and voluntarily lies down or refuses to play is much more likely to have considerable pain than a child who is absent from school but plays contentedly at home. The younger, nonverbal child may assume a rigid, side-lying position with the knees flexed and have decreased range of motion of the right hip. For nurses involved in primary ambulatory care, the responsibility of recognizing a possible case of appendicitis and prompt medical or surgical referral is particularly important. The importance of a detailed history and thorough abdominal examination cannot be overemphasized. Palpating the abdomen should be delayed until all other assessments have been made. Instruct the child to point with one finger to the site of the abdominal pain. Rebound tenderness may be present but is not always a sufficiently reliable test in children. Light palpation will satisfactorily elicit pain without causing excessive trauma (see Atraumatic Care box). Chapter 6 discusses other techniques for assessment of the abdomen.

ATRAUMATIC CARE

Palpating the Abdomen for Abdominal Pain

⊖ Because children associate the stethoscope with listening, use the bell piece for initial palpation of the abdomen for tenderness. Children usually endure pressure from the stethoscope that they would not tolerate from a probing hand. Follow with manual palpation, using a gentle touch without lifting the hand from the abdomen while observing the child's face for signs of discomfort, such as a grimace and watchful eyes on the examination of the abdomen.

Ask the child with mild pain to lift the heels and drop them to the floor two or three times, to hop on one foot, or to "puff out" or "pull in" the abdomen to check for tenderness without more painful probing.

Physical preparation of the child with appendicitis is similar to that for any child undergoing surgery. (See Chapter 27.) In situations in which medical treatment is required to correct problems associated with peritonitis, the nurse must anticipate procedures and set up equipment as quickly as possible to avoid any delay in preparing the child for surgery. Psychologic preparation of the child and parents is similar to that used in other emergency situations. (See Chapter 27.)

Postoperative Care

Postoperative care for the nonperforated appendix is the same as for most abdominal operations. Care of the child with a ruptured appendix and peritonitis is more complex. The child may need to remain in the hospital for several days or may be discharged with home care services to provide IV antibiotics and dressing changes.

Postoperatively the child is maintained on IV fluids and antibiotics and is allowed nothing by mouth (NPO). The child

also remains on low, intermittent gastric decompression until there is evidence of return of intestinal motility. Listening for bowel sounds and observing for other signs of bowel activity (such as passage of stool) are part of the routine assessment.

A drain may be placed in the wound during surgery, and frequent dressing changes with meticulous skin care are essential to prevent excoriation of the surgery area. If the wound is left open, moist dressings (usually saline-soaked gauze) and wound irrigations with antibacterial solution are used to provide an optimum healing environment.

Pain management is an essential part of the child's care. Not only is the incision painful, but the repeated dressing changes and irrigations also cause considerable distress. Because pain is continuous during the first few postoperative days, analgesics are given regularly to control pain. Procedures are performed when the analgesics are at peak effect. (See Pain Assessment, Pain Management, Chapter 7.)

Psychosocial care after surgery is also important. Sudden, acute illnesses cause unique stress, since there is little time for preparation or planning. Parents and older children need an opportunity to express their feelings and concerns regarding the events surrounding the illness and hospitalization. The nurse can provide important education and psychosocial support to promote adequate coping, with alleviation of anxiety for both the child and the family (see Nursing Care Plan).

MECKEL DIVERTICULUM

Meckel diverticulum is a remnant of the fetal omphalomesenteric duct, which connects the yolk sac with the primitive midgut during fetal life (Olson, Kim, and Donnelly, 2009). Normally the structure is obliterated by the seventh to eighth week of gestation, when the placenta replaces the yolk sac as the source of nutrition for the fetus. Failure of obliteration may result in an omphalomesenteric fistula (a fibrous band connecting the small intestine to the umbilicus), known as Meckel diverticulum.

Meckel diverticulum is a true diverticulum because it arises from the antimesenteric border of the small intestine and includes all layers of the intestinal wall. The position of the diverticulum varies, but it is usually found within 40 to 50 cm (16 to 20 inches) of the ileocecal valve.

Meckel diverticulum is the most common congenital malformation of the GI tract and is present in 2% to 4% of the population, with more frequent occurrence in boys than girls (Menezes, Tareen, Saeed, et al, 2008). Often it exists without ever causing symptoms.

Pathophysiology

Bleeding, obstruction, or inflammation causes the symptomatic complications of Meckel diverticulum. Gastric mucosa is the most common ectopic tissue found in a Meckel diverticulum. Bleeding, which is the most common problem in children, is caused by peptic ulceration or perforation because of the unbuffered acidic secretion. Several mechanisms may cause obstruction (Olson, Kim, and Donnelly, 2009). Intussusception may be led by Meckel diverticulum. Obstruction may also be caused by entanglement of the small intestine around a fibrous cord, by trapping of a loop of intestine under the band, by

NURSING CARE PLAN

The Child with Appendicitis

NURSING DIAGNOSIS	EXPECTED PATIENT OUTCOMES	NURSING INTERVENTIONS	RATIONALE
Acute Pain related to inflamed appendix **Child's/Family's Defining Characteristics** (Subjective and Objective Data) Crying Guarding abdomen Limited movement Withdrawal Refusal to eat or drink Fever Increased pulse	The child will have no pain or pain will be reduced to a level acceptable to child. **The Following NOC Concepts Apply to These Outcomes** Comfort Level Pain Control Pain: Disruptive Effects	Allow child to choose position most comfortable (usually legs flexed). Provide small pillow for abdomen. Administer analgesia per orders. **The Following NIC Concepts Apply to These Interventions** Analgesic Administration Positioning Presence Coping Enhancement Pain Management	To promote the most comfortable position To splint the abdomen To provide pain relief

NURSING DIAGNOSIS	EXPECTED PATIENT OUTCOMES	NURSING INTERVENTIONS	RATIONALE
Risk for Deficient Fluid Volume related to decreased intake and losses secondary to loss of appetite, vomiting **Child's/Family's Defining Characteristics** (Subjective and Objective Data) Dry mucous membranes Loss of skin turgor Sunken eyes, sunken fontanel Rapid thready pulse, rapid breathing Lethargy	Child will receive sufficient fluids to replace losses. Child will exhibit signs of adequate hydration (specify). **The Following NOC Concepts Apply to These Outcomes** Electrolyte and Acid-Base Balance Fluid Balance	Maintain nothing by mouth (NPO) status. Maintain integrity of infusion site for intravenous (IV) fluids. Administer IV fluids and electrolytes as prescribed. Monitor intake and output. **The Following NIC Concepts Apply to These Interventions** Acid-Base Monitoring Electrolyte Monitoring Fluid Monitoring Fluid Management IV Therapy Laboratory Data Interpretation Vital Signs Monitoring	To minimize losses through vomiting and minimize abdominal distention To infuse fluids and electrolytes To replace losses To assess hydration

NURSING DIAGNOSIS	EXPECTED PATIENT OUTCOMES	NURSING INTERVENTIONS	RATIONALE
Delayed Surgical Recovery related to the absence of bowel motility **Child's/Family's Defining Characteristics** (Subjective and Objective Data) Abdominal distention Nausea and vomiting Absence of bowel sounds Abdominal tenderness No passage of stools	Child will not experience abdominal distention or vomiting caused by delayed bowel mobility. **The Following NOC Concept Applies to These Interventions** Immobility Consequences: Physiological	Maintain NPO status in early postoperative period. Maintain nasogastric tube decompression. Assess abdomen for distention, tenderness, and presence of bowel sounds. Monitor passage of flatus and stool. **The Following NIC Concepts Apply to These Interventions** Bowel Management Flatulence Reduction Positioning	To prevent abdominal distention and vomiting To rest bowel until motility returns To assess presence of peristalsis To assess for an indicator of bowel motility

incarceration within a hernia sac, or by volvulus of the intestinal segment containing the diverticulum. Diverticulitis occurs when peptic ulceration or obstruction leads to inflammation.

Clinical Manifestations

Signs and symptoms are based on the specific pathologic process, such as inflammation, bleeding, or intestinal obstruction (Box 33-8). The most common clinical presentation is rectal bleeding caused by ulceration at the junction of the ectopic gastric mucosa and normal ileal mucosa. The bleeding is usually painless and may be dramatic and occur as bright red or currant jelly–like stools, or it may occur intermittently and appear as tarry stools. The bleeding may be significant enough to cause hypotension. Obstruction occurs more often in adults, but volvulus and intussusception are common obstructive symptoms in children with Meckel diverticulum.

Diagnostic Evaluation

Diagnosis is usually based on the history, physical examination, and radiographic studies. Meckel diverticulum is often a diagnostic challenge. Radionucleotide scintigraphy (Meckel scan) is most often used, but is less reliable in the presence of bleeding (Menezes, Tareen, Saeed, et al, 2008). CT scan, wireless capsule endoscopy, and mesenteric angiography may be used to investigate complications of Meckel diverticulum (Thurley, Halliday, Somers, et al, 2009). Laboratory studies are usually part of the general workup to rule out any bleeding disorder and to evaluate the severity of the anemia.

Therapeutic Management

The standard treatment for symptomatic Meckel diverticulum is surgical removal. In instances in which severe hemorrhage increases the surgical risk, medical intervention to correct hypovolemic shock (e.g., blood replacement, IV fluids, and oxygen) may be necessary. In diverticulitis, antibiotics may be used preoperatively to control infection. If intestinal obstruc-

tion has occurred, appropriate preoperative measures are used to correct fluid and electrolyte imbalances and prevent abdominal distention.

Prognosis

If Meckel diverticulum is diagnosed and treated early, full recovery is likely. The mortality rate of untreated Meckel diverticulum ranges from 2.5% to 15%. The serious complications of untreated Meckel diverticulum include GI hemorrhage and bowel obstruction.

Nursing Care Management

Nursing objectives are the same as for any child undergoing surgery. (See Chapter 27.) When intestinal bleeding is present, specific preoperative considerations include (1) frequent monitoring of vital signs and blood pressure, (2) keeping the child on bed rest, and (3) recording the approximate amount of blood lost in stools.

Postoperatively the child requires IV fluids and an NG tube for decompression and evacuation of gastric secretions. Because the onset of illness is usually rapid, psychologic support is important, as in other acute conditions, such as appendicitis. It is important to remember that massive rectal bleeding is usually traumatic to both the child and the parents and may significantly affect their emotional reaction to hospitalization and surgery.

INFLAMMATORY BOWEL DISEASE

IBD should not be confused with IBS. *IBD* is a term used to refer to two major forms of chronic intestinal inflammation: CD and ulcerative colitis (UC). CD and UC have similar epidemiologic, immunologic, and clinical features, but they are distinct disorders.

In addition to GI symptoms, both CD and UC are characterized by extraintestinal and systemic inflammatory responses. Exacerbations and remissions without complete resolution are also characteristics of IBD. Growth failure, particularly common in CD, is an important problem unique to the pediatric population. CD is also more disabling, has more serious complications, and is often less amenable to medical and surgical treatment than is UC. Because UC is confined to the colon, theoretically it may be cured by a colectomy.

The prevalence of IBD is between 12 and 40 per 100,000 persons, with 25% of these individuals being diagnosed before 20 years of age (Wong, Clark, Garnett, et al, 2009). Over the past 30 years the incidence of CD has risen, while the incidence of UC in children has remained stable. Children 6 to 17 years of age with CD appear to have a more complicated disease course compared with that of 0- to 5-year-old children (Gupta, Bostrom, Kirschner, et al, 2008).

Etiology

Despite decades of research, the etiology of IBD is not completely understood, and there is no known cure. There is evidence to indicate a multifactorial etiology. Research is focused on theories of defective immunoregulation of the inflammatory response to bacteria or viruses in the GI tract in individuals with a genetic predisposition (Silbermintz and Markowitz, 2006). In CD the chronic immune process is characterized by a T helper 1 cytokine profile, whereas in UC the response is more humoral and mediated by T helper 2 cells (Silbermintz and Markowitz, 2006).

Development of IBD has a genetic influence. Several IBD susceptibility genes have now been identified through family and twin studies (Sauer and Kugathasan, 2010). Family-based genetic studies have linked chromosome 6 in UC and the NOD2 gene in CD (Sauer and Kugathasan, 2010).

Pathophysiology

The inflammation found with UC is limited to the colon and rectum, with the distal colon and rectum the most severely affected. Inflammation affects the mucosa and submucosa and involves continuous segments along the length of the bowel with varying degrees of ulceration, bleeding, and edema. Thickening of the bowel wall and fibrosis are unusual, but longstanding disease can result in shortening of the colon and strictures. Extraintestinal manifestations are less common in UC than in CD. Toxic megacolon is the most dangerous form of severe colitis.

The chronic inflammatory process of CD involves any part of the GI tract from the mouth to the anus but most often affects the terminal ileum. The disease involves all layers of the bowel wall (transmural) in a discontinuous fashion, meaning that between areas of intact mucosa, there are areas of affected mucosa (skip lesions). The inflammation may result in ulcerations; fibrosis; adhesions; stiffening of the bowel wall; stricture formation; and fistulas to other loops of bowel, bladder, vagina, or skin.

Clinical Signs and Symptoms

Children with UC may experience mild, moderate, or severe symptoms, depending on the extent of mucosal inflammation and systemic symptoms. Most include bloody diarrhea or occult fecal blood, abdominal pain, and varying degrees of systemic manifestations and growth abnormalities (Beattie, Croft, Fell, et al, 2006; Leichtner and Higuchi, 2004). One of the earliest signs of UC may be growth failure with decreased linear growth velocity (Beattie, Croft, Fell, et al, 2006). Growth failure is most likely a result of chronic poor dietary intake caused by anorexia related to GI symptoms. UC often manifests with the insidious onset of diarrhea, possibly with hematochezia, and usually without fever or weight loss. The course of the disease may remain mild with intermittent exacerbations. Some children and adolescents are seen with grossly bloody diarrhea, cramps, urgency with defecation, mild anemia, fever, anorexia, weight loss, and moderate signs of systemic illness. Severe UC is characterized by frequent bloody stools, abdominal pain, significant anemia, fever, and weight loss. Extraintestinal manifestations are less common in UC than in CD and may precede colitis. The erythrocyte sedimentation rate (ESR) may be elevated, indicating a systemic response to an inflammatory process. Enlarged lymph nodes (lymphadenopathy), arthritis, and the skin lesions of erythema nodosum may be present.

Common presenting manifestations of CD include diarrhea, abdominal pain with cramps, fever, and weight loss. Mild GI symptoms, poor growth, and extraintestinal manifestations may be present for several years before overt GI symptoms are present. Both malabsorption and anorexia are factors that contribute to the growth problems that are prevalent in CD. The effects of UC and CD are listed in Fig. 33-4.

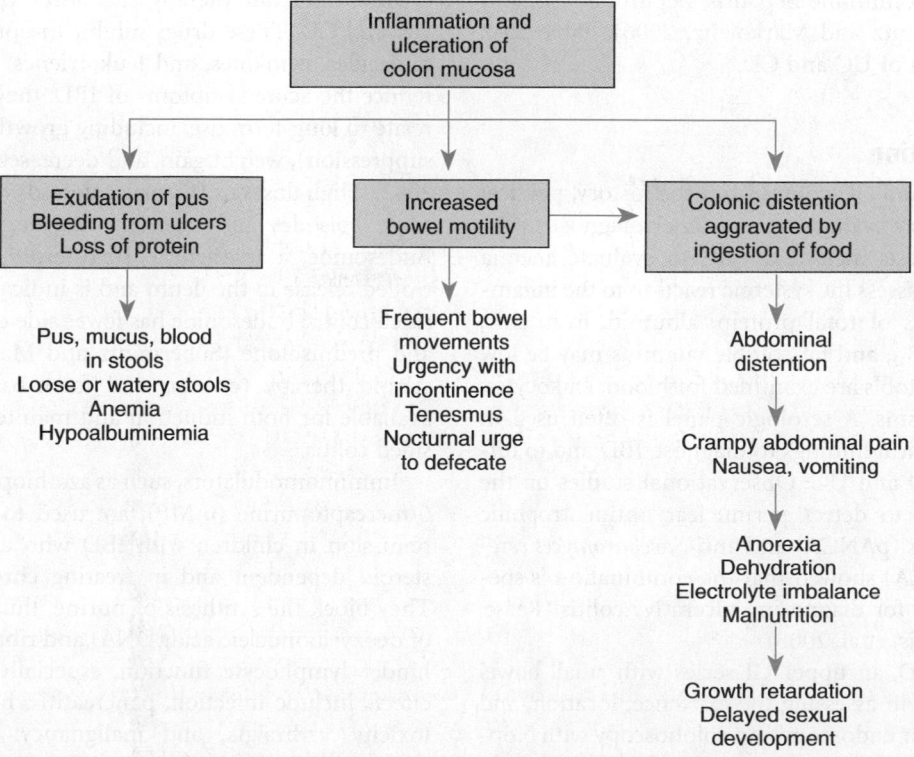

Fig. 33-4 Effects of ulcerative colitis or Crohn disease.

TABLE 33-2	CLINICAL MANIFESTATIONS OF INFLAMMATORY BOWEL DISEASES	
CHARACTERISTICS	**ULCERATIVE COLITIS**	**CROHN DISEASE**
Rectal bleeding	Common	Uncommon
Diarrhea	Often severe	Moderate to severe
Pain	Less frequent	Common
Anorexia	Mild or moderate	May be severe
Weight loss	Moderate	May be severe
Growth retardation	Usually mild	May be severe
Anal and perianal lesions	Rare	Common
Fistulas and strictures	Rare	Common
Rashes	Mild	Mild
Joint pain	Mild to moderate	Mild to moderate

Children with CD have multiple risk factors for impaired bone accrual, including poor growth, delayed maturation, malnutrition, decreased activity, chronic inflammation, and steroid therapy (Dubner, Shults, Baldassano, et al, 2009). Growth delay persists in many children with CD following diagnosis, despite improved disease activity (Pfefferkorn, Burke, Griffiths, et al, 2009).

The disease process can also involve the colon, causing diarrhea, cramps, and urgency with defecation. Signs of colitis, such as gross rectal bleeding or stool with occult blood, are similar to those seen in UC. Perianal disease, including skin tags, abscesses, fissures, and fistulas, is a feature of CD. Extraintestinal manifestations include erythema nodosum, pyoderma gangrenosum, arthralgia and arthritis, uveitis and episcleritis, sclerosing cholangitis, autoimmune hepatitis, nephrolithiasis, and pneumonitis (Silbermintz and Markowitz, 2006). Table 33-2 provides a comparison of UC and CD.

Diagnostic Evaluation

The diagnosis of UC and CD comes from the history, physical examination, laboratory evaluation, and other diagnostic procedures. Laboratory tests include a CBC to evaluate anemia and an ESR or CRP to assess the systemic reaction to the inflammatory process. Levels of total protein, albumin, iron, zinc, magnesium, vitamin B_{12}, and fat-soluble vitamins may be low in children with CD. Stools are examined for blood, leukocytes, and infectious organisms. A serologic panel is often used in combination with clinical findings to diagnose IBD and to differentiate between CD and UC. Observational studies on the utility of blood tests to detect perinuclear antineutrophilic cytoplasmic antibodies (pANCA) and anti-*Saccharomyces cerevisiae* antibodies (ASCA) showed that the combination is specific, but not sensitive for diagnosing ulcerative colitis (Reese, Constantinides, Simillis, et al, 2006).

In patients with CD, an upper GI series with small bowel follow-through assists in assessing the existence, location, and extent of disease. Upper endoscopy and colonoscopy with biopsies are an integral part of diagnosing IBD (Langan, Gotsch, Krafczyk, et al, 2007). Endoscopy allows direct visualization of the surface of the GI tract so that the extent of inflammation and narrowing can be evaluated. CT and ultrasound also may be used to identify bowel wall inflammation, intraabdominal abscesses, and fistulas. CD lesions may pierce the walls of the small intestine and colon, creating tracts called fistulas between the intestine and adjacent structures such as the bladder, anus, vagina, or skin.

Therapeutic Management

The natural history of the disease continues to be unpredictable and characterized by recurrent flare-ups that can severely impair patients' physical and social functioning (Vernier-Massouille, Balde, Salleron, et al, 2008). The goals of therapy are to (1) control the inflammatory process to reduce or eliminate the symptoms, (2) obtain long-term remission, (3) promote normal growth and development, and (4) allow as normal a lifestyle as possible. Treatment is individualized and managed according to the type and the severity of the disease, its location, and the response to therapy.

Medical Treatment

The goal of any treatment regimen is first to induce remission of acute symptoms and then to maintain remission over time. 5-Aminosalicylates (5-ASAs) are effective in the induction and maintenance of remission in mild to moderate UC. Mesalamine, olsalazine, and balsalazide are now preferred over sulfasalazine because of reduced side effects (headache, nausea, vomiting, neutropenia, and oligospermia). Suppository and enema preparations of mesalamine are used to treat left-sided colitis. These drugs decrease inflammation by inhibiting prostaglandin synthesis. 5-ASAs can be used to induce remission in mild CD. Corticosteroids, such as prednisone and prednisolone, are indicated in induction therapy in children with moderate to severe UC and CD. These drugs inhibit the production of adhesion molecules, cytokines, and leukotrienes. Although these drugs reduce the acute symptoms of IBD, they have side effects that relate to long-term use, including growth suppression (adrenal suppression), weight gain, and decreased bone density (Baron, 2002). High doses of IV corticosteroids may be administered in acute episodes and tapered according to clinical response. Budesonide, a synthetic corticosteroid, is designed for controlled release in the ileum and is indicated for ileal and right-sided colitis; budesonide has fewer side effects than prednisone and prednisolone (Silbermintz and Markowitz, 2006). Rectal steroid therapy (enemas and foam-based preparations) are available for both induction and maintenance therapy in left-sided colitis.

Immunomodulators, such as azathioprine and its metabolite 6-mercaptopurine (6-MP), are used to induce and maintain remission in children with IBD who are steroid resistant or steroid dependent and in treating chronic draining fistulas. They block the synthesis of purine, thus inhibiting the ability of deoxyribonucleic acid (DNA) and ribonucleic acid (RNA) to hinder lymphocyte function, especially that of T cells. Side effects include infection, pancreatitis, hepatitis, bone marrow toxicity, arthralgia, and malignancy. Methotrexate is also useful in inducing and maintaining remission in CD patients unresponsive to standard therapies. Cyclosporine and tacrolimus have both been effective in inducing remission in severe steroid-dependent UC. 6-MP or azathioprine is then used to maintain remission. Patients on immunomodulating medications require regular monitoring of their CBC and differential to assess for changes that reflect suppression of the immune system, since many of the side effects can be prevented or managed by dose reduction or discontinuation of medication.

Antibiotics, such as metronidazole and ciprofloxacin, may be used as an adjunctive therapy to treat complications such as perianal disease or small bowel bacterial overgrowth in CD. Side effects of these drugs are peripheral neuropathy, nausea, and a metallic taste.

Biologic therapies act to regulate inflammatory and antiinflammatory cytokines. With the emergence of the biologic agents, specifically the use of antitumor necrosis factor-α (TNF-α) agents, progress has been made in targeting specific pathogenetic mechanisms and achieving a more prolonged clinical response (Ricart, García-Bosch, Ordás, et al, 2008; Hyams and Markowitz, 2005). TNF-α is believed to influence active inflammation.

Nutritional Support

Nutritional support is important in the treatment of IBD. Growth failure is a common serious complication, especially in CD. Growth failure is characterized by weight loss, alteration in body composition, retarded height, and delayed sexual maturation. Malnutrition causes the growth failure, and its etiology is multifactorial. Malnutrition occurs as a result of inadequate dietary intake, excessive GI losses, malabsorption, drug-nutrient interaction, and increased nutritional requirements. Inadequate dietary intake occurs with anorexia and episodes of increased disease activity. Excessive loss of nutrients (protein, blood, electrolytes, and minerals) occurs secondary to intestinal inflammation and diarrhea. Carbohydrate, lactose, fat, vitamin, and mineral malabsorption, as well as vitamin B_{12} and folic acid deficiencies, occur with disease episodes and with drug administration and when the terminal ileum is resected. Finally, nutritional requirements are increased with inflammation, fever, fistulas, and periods of rapid growth (e.g., adolescence).

The goals of nutritional support include (1) correction of nutrient deficits and replacement of ongoing losses, (2) provision of adequate energy and protein for healing, and (3) provision of adequate nutrients to promote normal growth. Nutritional support includes both enteral and parenteral nutrition. A well-balanced, high-protein, high-calorie diet is recommended for children whose symptoms do not prohibit an adequate oral intake. There is little evidence that avoiding specific foods influences the severity of the disease. Supplementation with multivitamins, iron, and folic acid is recommended.

Special enteral formulas, given either by mouth or continuous NG infusion (often at night), may be required. Elemental formulas are completely absorbed in the small intestine with almost no residue. A diet consisting only of elemental formula not only improves nutritional status but also induces disease remission, either without steroids or with a diminished dosage of steroids required. An elemental diet is a safe and potentially effective primary therapy for patients with CD. Unfortunately, remission is not sustained when NG feedings are discontinued unless maintenance medications are added to the treatment regimen.

TPN has also improved nutritional status in patients with IBD. Short-term remissions have been achieved after TPN, although complete bowel rest has not reduced inflammation or added to the benefits of improved nutrition by TPN. Nutritional support is less likely to induce a remission in UC than in CD. Improvement of nutritional status is important, however, in preventing deterioration of the patient's health status and in preparing the patient for surgery.

Surgical Treatment

Surgery is indicated for UC when medical and nutritional therapies fail to prevent complications. Surgical options include a subtotal colectomy and ileostomy that leaves a rectal stump as a blind pouch. A reservoir pouch is created in the configuration of a J or S to help improve continence postoperatively. An ileoanal pull-through preserves the normal pathway for defecation. Pouchitis, an inflammation of the surgically created pouch, is the most common late complication of this procedure and had been reported to occur in up to 50% of cases. In many cases UC can be cured with a total colectomy.

Surgery may be required in children with CD when complications cannot be controlled by medical and nutritional therapy. Segmental intestinal resections are performed for small bowel obstructions, strictures, or fistulas. Partial colonic resection is not curative, and the disease often recurs.

Prognosis

IBD is a chronic disease. Relatively long periods of quiescent disease may follow exacerbations. The outcome is influenced by the regions and severity of involvement, as well as by appropriate therapeutic management. Malnutrition, growth failure, and bleeding are serious complications. The overall prognosis for UC is good.

The development of colorectal cancer (CRC) is a long-term complication of IBD. In UC, the cumulative incidence of CRC is 2.5% after 20 years, increasing to 10.8% after 30 years (Rutter, Saunders, Wilkinson, et al, 2006). Surveillance colonoscopy with multiple biopsies should begin approximately 10 years after diagnosis of UC or Crohn colitis and continue every 1 to 2 years (Rubin and Kavitt, 2006). Removal of the diseased colon prevents development of CRC. In CD, however, surgical removal of the affected colon does not prevent cancer from developing elsewhere in the GI tract.

Nursing Care Management

The nursing considerations in the management of IBD extend beyond the immediate period of hospitalization. These interventions involve continued guidance of families in terms of (1) managing diet; (2) coping with factors that increase stress and emotional lability; (3) adjusting to a disease of remissions and exacerbations; and (4) when indicated, preparing the child and parents for the possibility of diversionary bowel surgery.

Because nutritional support is an essential part of therapy, encouraging the anorexic child to consume sufficient quantities of food is often a challenge. Successful interventions include involving the child in meal planning; encouraging small, frequent meals or snacks rather than three large meals a day; serving meals around medication schedules when diarrhea, mouth pain, and intestinal spasm are controlled; and preparing high-protein, high-calorie foods such as eggnog, milkshakes, cream soups, puddings, or custard (if lactose is tolerated). (See Feeding the Sick Child, Chapter 27.) Using bran or a high-fiber diet for active IBD is questionable. Bran, even in small amounts, has been shown to worsen the patient's condition. Occasionally the occurrence of aphthous stomatitis further complicates adherence to dietary management. Mouth care before eating and the selection of bland foods help relieve the discomfort of mouth sores.

When NG feedings or TPN is indicated, nurses play an important role in explaining the purpose and the expected outcomes of this therapy. The nurse should acknowledge the anxieties of the child and family members and give them adequate time to demonstrate the skills necessary to continue the therapy at home if needed (see Critical Thinking Exercise).

The importance of continued drug therapy despite remission of symptoms must be stressed to the child and family members. Failure to adhere to the pharmacologic regimen can result in exacerbation of the disease. (See Compliance, Chapter 27.) Unfortunately, exacerbation of IBD can occur even if the child and family are compliant with the treatment regimen; this is difficult for the child and family to cope with.

? CRITICAL THINKING EXERCISE

Inflammatory Bowel Disease

Susan, a 13-year-old girl, was admitted to the hospital because of bloody diarrhea, abdominal pain, and weight loss. After a thorough evaluation, including laboratory tests, radiographic studies, and gastrointestinal endoscopy procedures, the diagnosis of Crohn disease (CD) was made. Medical treatment, including corticosteroid drugs and nutritional support, was implemented during this hospitalization.

Susan has improved considerably and is to be discharged home this week. Enteral formula administered by continuous nighttime nasogastric (NG) tube infusion will be continued at home, and both Susan and her family are eager to learn how to perform these feedings. You are the nurse responsible for Susan's discharge planning. Which interventions relating to these feedings should you include in Susan's preparations for discharge?

1. Evidence—Are there sufficient data to formulate any specific interventions for discharge?
2. Assumptions—Describe some underlying assumptions about:
   a. The goals of nutritional support for children with CD
   b. Teaching required by an adolescent or family member who is administering NG tube feedings at home
   c. Psychosocial issues related to CD
3. What are the priorities for discharge planning at this time?
4. Does the evidence support your conclusion?

Family Support

The nurse should attend to the emotional components of the disease and assess any sources of stress. Frequently, the nurse can help children adjust to problems of growth retardation, delayed sexual maturation, dietary restrictions, feelings of being "different" or "sickly," inability to compete with peers, and necessary absence from school during exacerbations of the illness.

If a permanent colectomy-ileostomy is required, the nurse can teach the child and family how to care for the ileostomy. The nurse can also emphasize the positive aspects of the surgery, particularly accelerated growth and sexual development, permanent recovery, the eliminated risk of colonic cancer in UC, and the normality of life despite bowel diversion. Introducing the child and parents to other ostomy patients, especially those who are the same age, is effective in fostering eventual acceptance. Whenever possible, offer continent ostomies as options to the child, although they are not performed in all centers in the United States.

Because of the chronic and often life-long nature of the disease, families benefit from the educational services provided by organizations such as the Crohn's and Colitis Foundation of America (CCFA).* If diversionary bowel surgery is indicated, United Ostomy Associations of America† and the Wound, Ostomy and Continence Nurses Society‡ are available to assist with ileostomy care and provide important psychologic support through their self-help groups. Adolescents often benefit by participating in peer-support groups, which are sponsored by the CCFA.

PEPTIC ULCER DISEASE

Peptic ulcers may be classified as acute or chronic, and peptic ulcer disease (PUD) is a chronic condition that affects the stomach or duodenum. Ulcers are described as gastric or duodenal and as primary or secondary. A **gastric ulcer** involves the mucosa of the stomach; a **duodenal ulcer** involves the pylorus or duodenum. Most **primary ulcers** occur in the absence of a predisposing factor and tend to be chronic, occurring more frequently in the duodenum. **Stress ulcers** result from the stress of a severe underlying disease or injury (e.g., severe burns, sepsis, increased intracranial pressure, severe trauma, multisystem organ failure) and are more frequently acute and gastric.

About 1.7% of children in general pediatric practices have PUD, and the disease represents about 3.4% per 10,000 pediatric hospital admissions. Primary ulcers are more common in children older than 6 years, and stress ulcers are more common in infants younger than 6 months. Except for very young chil-

---

*386 Park Ave. S., 17th Floor, New York, NY 10016; 800-932-2423; www.ccfa.org. In Canada: Crohn's and Colitis Foundation of Canada, www.ccfc.ca.

†PO Box 66, Fairview, TN 37062-0066; 800-826-0826; www.uoaa.org. In Canada: United Ostomy Association of Canada, 344 Bloor St. W., Suite 501, Toronto, Ontario M5S 3A7; 416-595-5452; fax: 416-595-9924; www.ostomycanada.ca.

‡1500 Commerce Pkwy., Suite C, Mt. Laurel, NJ 08054; 888-224-9626; www.wocn.org.

dren, the incidence is two to three times greater in boys than in girls.

Etiology

The exact cause of PUD is unknown, although infectious, genetic, and environmental factors are important. There is an increased familial incidence, and the disease is increased in persons with blood group O.

There is a significant relationship between the bacterium *Helicobacter pylori* and ulcers. *H. pylori* is a microaerophilic, gram-negative, slow-growing, spiral-shaped, and flagellated bacterium known to colonize the gastric mucosa in about half of the population of the world (Sung, Kuipers, and El-Serag, 2009). *H. pylori* synthesizes the enzyme urease, which hydrolyses urea to form ammonia and carbon dioxide. Ammonia then absorbs acid to form ammonium, thus raising the gastric pH. *H. pylori* may cause ulcers by weakening the gastric mucosal barrier and allowing acid to damage the mucosa. It is believed that it is acquired via the fecal-oral route, and this hypothesis is supported by finding viable *H. pylori* in feces.

In addition to ulcerogenic drugs, both alcohol and smoking contribute to ulcer formation. There is no conclusive evidence to implicate particular foods, such as caffeine-containing beverages or spicy foods, but polyunsaturated fats and fiber may play a role in ulcer formation. Psychologic factors may play a role in the development of PUD, and stressful life events, dependency, passiveness, and hostility have all been implicated as contributing factors.

Pathophysiology

Most likely, the pathologic condition is due to an imbalance between the destructive (cytotoxic) factors and defensive (cytoprotective) factors in the GI tract. The toxic mechanisms include acid, pepsin, medications such as aspirin and nonsteroidal antiinflammatory drugs (NSAIDs), bile acids, and infection with *H. pylori*. The defensive factors include the mucus layer, local bicarbonate secretion, epithelial cell renewal, and mucosal blood flow. Prostaglandins play a role in mucosal defense because they stimulate both mucus and alkali secretion. The primary mechanism that prevents the development of peptic ulcer is the secretion of mucus by the epithelial and mucus glands throughout the stomach. The thick mucus layer acts to diffuse acid from the lumen to the gastric mucosal surface, thus protecting the gastric epithelium. The stomach and the duodenum produce bicarbonate, decreasing acidity on the epithelial cells and thereby minimizing the effects of the low pH (Chelimsky and Czinn, 2001). When abnormalities in the protective barrier exist, the mucosa is vulnerable to damage by acid and pepsin. Exogenous factors, such as aspirin and NSAIDs, cause gastric ulcers by inhibition of prostaglandin synthesis.

Zollinger-Ellison syndrome may occur in children who have multiple, large, or recurrent ulcers. This syndrome is characterized by hypersecretion of gastric acid, intractable ulcer disease, and intestinal malabsorption caused by a gastrin-secreting tumor of the pancreas. The pathogenesis, manifestations, and complications of PUD are outlined in Fig. 33-5.

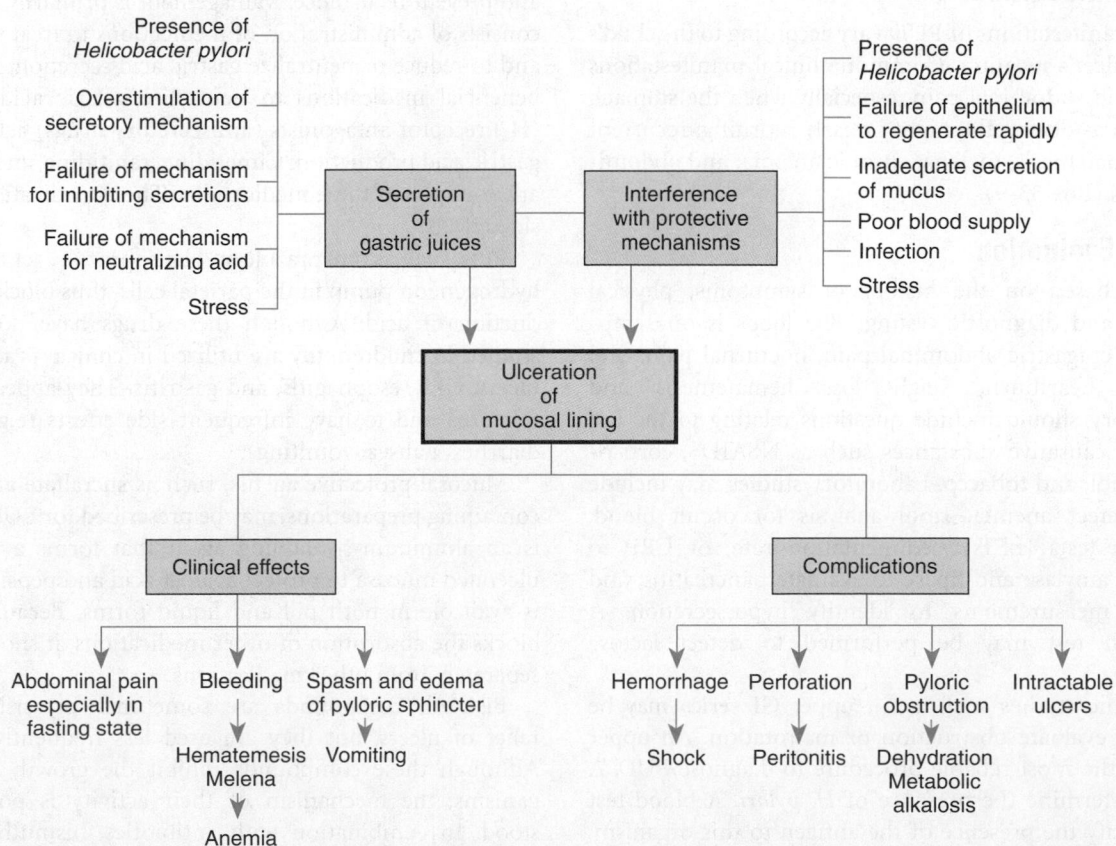

Fig. 33-5 Possible causes and effects of peptic ulcer.

Clinical Manifestations

The clinical manifestations of PUD vary according to the child's age and the ulcer's location. Common clinical manifestations include chronic abdominal pain, especially when the stomach is empty, such as during the night or early morning; recurrent vomiting; hematemesis; melena; chronic anemia; and abdominal tenderness (Box 33-9).

Diagnostic Evaluation

Diagnosis is based on the history of symptoms, physical examination, and diagnostic testing. The focus is on symptoms such as epigastric abdominal pain, nocturnal pain, oral regurgitation, heartburn, weight loss, hematemesis, and melena. History should include questions relating to the use of potentially causative substances such as NSAIDS, corticosteroids, alcohol, and tobacco. Laboratory studies may include a CBC to detect anemia, stool analysis for occult blood, liver function tests (LFTs), sedimentation rate, or CRP to evaluate IBD; amylase and lipase to evaluate pancreatitis; and gastric acid measurements to identify hypersecretion. A lactose breath test may be performed to detect lactose intolerance.

Radiographic studies such as an upper GI series may be performed to evaluate obstruction or malrotation. An upper endoscopy is the most reliable procedure to diagnose PUD. A biopsy can determine the presence of *H. pylori*. A blood test can also identify the presence of the antigen to this organism.

The ^{13}C urea breath test measures bacterial colonization in the gastric mucosa. This test is used to screen for *H. pylori* in adults and children. Polyclonal and monoclonal stool antigen tests are an accurate, noninvasive method both for the initial diagnosis of *H. pylori* and for the confirmation of its eradication after treatment (Gisbert, de la Morena, and Abraira, 2006).

Diagnosis is based on the history (pattern of pain) and physical examination. Frequently a history of epigastric and periumbilical pain accompanies PUD. However, children often find it difficult to describe the location of their pain and frequently indicate the location by moving their hand in a circular movement all around the stomach area. Asking the child to take one finger and point to the area where it hurts the most often helps to identify the location of the pain. Pain may also be elicited during the examination with palpation. Routine laboratory studies to diagnose PUD include a CBC with differential, ESR, blood chemistry studies, urinalysis, and stool analysis to identify anemia or inflammation and to rule out infection. A ^{13}C urea breath test is often performed to determine the presence of antibodies to *H. pylori*. An upper GI series is rarely helpful in identifying ulcers in children; fiberoptic endoscopy is the most reliable way to detect PUD in children. Direct visualization of the gastric and duodenal mucosa with biopsy to determine the presence of *H. pylori* is the most commonly used and effective way to arrive at the diagnosis.

Therapeutic Management

The major goals of therapy for children with PUD are to relieve discomfort, promote healing, prevent complications, and prevent recurrence. Management is primarily medical and consists of administration of medications to treat the infection and to reduce or neutralize gastric acid secretion. Antacids are beneficial medications to neutralize gastric acid. Histamine (H$_2$) receptor antagonists (antisecretory drugs) act to suppress gastric acid production. Cimetidine, ranitidine, and famotidine are examples of these medications. These medications have few side effects.

PPIs, such as omeprazole and lansoprazole, act to inhibit the hydrogen ion pump in the parietal cells, thus blocking the production of acid. Although these drugs have not been well studied in children, thy are utilized in clinical practice to treat ulcers, GER, esophagitis, and gastritis. They appear to be well tolerated and to have infrequent side effects (e.g., headache, diarrhea, nausea, vomiting).

Mucosal protective agents, such as sucralfate and bismuth-containing preparations, may be prescribed for PUD. Sucralfate is an aluminum-containing agent that forms a barrier over ulcerated mucosa to protect against acid and pepsin. Sucralfate is available in both pill and liquid forms. Because sucralfate blocks the absorption of other medications, it should be given separately from other medications.

Bismuth compounds are sometimes prescribed for the relief of ulcers, but they are used less frequently than PPIs. Although these compounds inhibit the growth of microorganisms, the mechanism of their activity is poorly understood. In combination with antibiotics, bismuth is effective against *H. pylori*. Although concern has been expressed about the use of bismuth salts in children because of potential side effects, none of these side effects has been reported when these compounds have been used in the treatment of *H. pylori* infection.

Triple-drug therapy is the standard first-line treatment regimen for *H. pylori* (O'Connor, Gisbert, and O'Morain, 2009). Combination therapy has demonstrated 90% effectiveness in eradication of *H. pylori* when compared with antibiotic monotherapy. Examples of drug combinations used in triple therapy are (1) bismuth, clarithromycin, and metronidazole; (2) lansoprazole, amoxicillin, and clarithromycin; and (3) metronidazole, clarithromycin, and omeprazole. The benefits on the use of probiotics as an adjunct to treatment remain unclear, with conflicting literature on their effect on eradication and minimizing side effects (O'Connor, Gisbert, and O'Morain, 2009).

Common side effects of medications include diarrhea, nausea, and vomiting. In addition to medications, the child with PUD should have a nutritious diet and avoid caffeine. Warn adolescents about gastric irritation associated with alcohol use and smoking.

Children with an acute ulcer who have developed complications, such as massive hemorrhage, require emergency care. The administration of IV fluids, blood, or plasma depends on the amount of blood loss. Replacement with whole blood or packed cells may be necessary for significant loss.

Surgical intervention may be required for complications such as hemorrhage, perforation, or gastric outlet obstruction. Ligation of the source of bleeding or closure of a perforation is performed. A vagotomy and pyloroplasty may be indicated in children with recurring ulcers despite aggressive medical treatment.

Prognosis

The long-term prognosis for PUD is variable. Many ulcers are successfully treated with medical therapy; however, primary duodenal peptic ulcers often recur. Complications such as GI bleeding can occur and extend into adult life. The effect of maintenance drug therapy on long-term morbidity remains to be established with further studies.

Nursing Care Management

The primary nursing goal is to promote healing of the ulcer through compliance with the medication regimen. If an analgesic-antipyretic is needed, acetaminophen, not aspirin or NSAIDs, is used. Critically ill neonates, infants, and children in intensive care units should receive H_2 blockers to prevent stress ulcers.

⚡ **DRUG ALERT**

H_2 Blockers

Critically ill children receiving IV H_2 blockers should have their gastric pH values checked at frequent intervals.

For nonhospitalized children with chronic illnesses, consider the role stress plays. In children, many ulcers occur secondary to other conditions, and the nurse should be aware of family and environmental conditions that may aggravate or precipitate ulcers. Children may benefit from psychologic counseling and from learning how to cope constructively with stress.

OBSTRUCTIVE DISORDERS

Obstruction in the GI tract occurs when the passage of nutrients and secretions is impeded by a constricted or occluded lumen, or when there is impaired motility (paralytic ileus). Obstructions may be congenital or acquired. Congenital obstructions, such as esophageal or intestinal atresias and malrotation, usually appear in the neonatal period. (See Chapter 11.) Obstruction in the GI tract from many causes is characterized by similar signs and symptoms, although the progression may vary greatly.

Usually, acute intestinal obstruction is characterized by abdominal pain, nausea, vomiting, abdominal distention, and a change in stooling patterns (Box 33-10). Pain is caused by intermittent muscular contractions proximal to the obstruction as the bowel attempts to move luminal contents along the normal path. It may also be due to severe abdominal distention, which results from accumulation of gas and fluid above the level of the obstruction. As abdominal distention progresses, the abdomen may become extremely tender, rigid, and firm.

When abdominal contents continue to accumulate, nausea and vomiting occur. Vomiting of gastric contents is often the first sign of a high obstruction, such as obstruction of the pylorus, and vomiting of bile-stained material is a sign of obstruction of the small intestine. Persistent vomiting can lead to dehydration and electrolyte disturbances. Constipation

---

BOX 33-10 CLINICAL MANIFESTATIONS OF MECHANICAL (PARALYTIC) INTESTINAL OBSTRUCTION

Colicky abdominal pain—From peristalsis attempting to overcome the obstruction

Abdominal distention—As a result of accumulation of gas and fluid above the level of the obstruction

Vomiting—Often the earliest sign of a high obstruction; a later sign of lower obstruction (may be bilious or feculent)

Constipation and obstipation—Early signs of low obstructions; later signs of higher obstructions

Dehydration—From losses of large quantities of fluid and electrolytes into the intestine

Rigid and boardlike abdomen—From increased distention

Bowel sounds—Gradually diminish and cease

Respiratory distress—Occurs as the diaphragm is pushed up into the pleural cavity

Shock—Caused by plasma volume diminishing as fluids and electrolytes are lost from the bloodstream into the intestinal lumen

Sepsis—Caused by bacterial proliferation with invasion into the circulation

and obstipation (prolonged absence of defecation) are early signs of low obstructions and later signs of higher obstructions. In acute conditions such as intussusception, the clinical manifestations are apparent within a few hours of the onset of the disorder. In other conditions such as pyloric stenosis the signs and symptoms may have a more gradual onset. Bowel sounds may initially be hyperactive, then diminish or cease. Respiratory distress may occur when the diaphragm is pushed up into the pleural cavity as a result of severe abdominal distention.

HYPERTROPHIC PYLORIC STENOSIS

Hypertrophic pyloric stenosis (HPS) occurs when the circumferential muscle of the pyloric sphincter becomes thickened, resulting in elongation and narrowing of the pyloric canal. This produces an outlet obstruction and compensatory dilation, hypertrophy, and hyperperistalsis of the stomach. This condition usually develops in the first few weeks of life, causing projectile vomiting, dehydration, metabolic alkalosis, and failure to thrive. The precise etiology of HPS is not known. It is more common in first-born children, and boys are affected five times more frequently than girls. HPS is seen less frequently in African-American infants than in Caucasian infants. It is more likely to affect full-term infants than premature ones. Inheritance is polygenic, with an increased risk in the siblings and offspring of affected persons. The greatest risk of recurrence (20%) is in the first-born boy of a mother who was affected (Milla, 2004).

Pathophysiology

The circular muscle of the pylorus thickens as a result of hypertrophy. This produces severe narrowing of the pyloric canal between the stomach and the duodenum. Consequently, the lumen at this point is partially obstructed. Over time the size of the opening is reduced, and the partial obstruction may progress to complete obstruction. The hypertrophied pylorus may be palpable as an olivelike mass in the upper abdomen (Fig. 33-6).

Pyloric stenosis is not a congenital disorder. Evidence suggests that local innervation may be involved in the pathogenesis. In most cases this is an isolated lesion; however, it may be associated with intestinal malrotation, esophageal and duodenal atresia, and anorectal anomalies.

Clinical Manifestations

Infants with HPS have nonbilious vomiting in the early stages (Box 33-11). The vomiting may be projectile and progressive, becoming brown in later stages if gastritis develops. Vomiting usually begins at 3 weeks of age but can start as early as 1 week and as late as 5 months. Initially the infant is hungry and irritable, but prolonged vomiting may lead to dehydration, weight loss, and failure to thrive. Gastric peristalsis may be visible on examination, and the olive-shaped mass in the epigastrium just to the right of the umbilicus may be palpated (see Fig. 33-6, *A*).

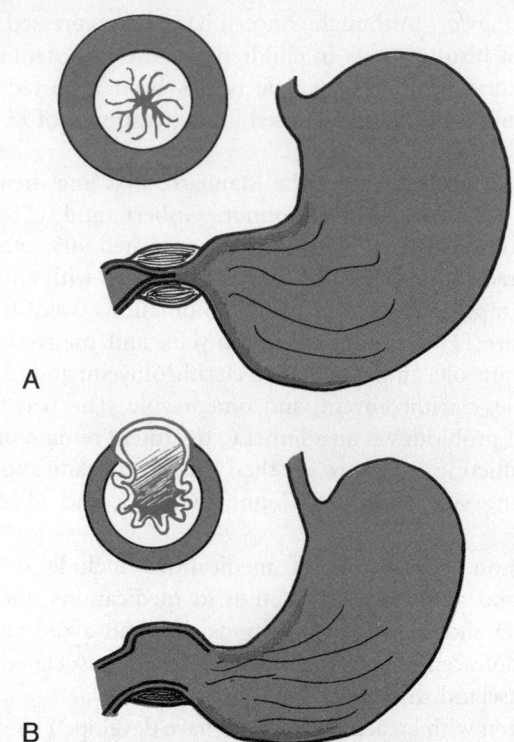

Fig. 33-6 Hypertrophic pyloric stenosis. **A,** Enlarged muscular tumor nearly obliterates pyloric canal. **B,** Longitudinal surgical division of muscle down to submucosa establishes adequate passageway.

BOX 33-11   CLINICAL MANIFESTATIONS OF HYPERTROPHIC PYLORIC STENOSIS

Projectile vomiting
- May be ejected 3 to 4 feet from the child when in a side-lying position, 1 foot or more when in a back-lying position
- Usually occurs shortly after a feeding, but may not occur for several hours
- May follow each feeding or appear intermittently
- Nonbilious vomitus that may be blood tinged

Infant hungry, avid nurser; eagerly accepts a second feeding after vomiting episode

No evidence of pain or discomfort except that of chronic hunger

Weight loss

Signs of dehydration

Distended upper abdomen

Readily palpable olive-shaped tumor in the epigastrium just to the right of the umbilicus

Visible gastric peristaltic waves that move from left to right across the epigastrium

---

Diagnostic Evaluation

The diagnosis of HPS is often made after the history and physical examination. The olivelike mass is most easily palpated when the stomach is empty, the infant is quiet, and the abdominal muscles are relaxed. If the diagnosis is inconclusive from the history and physical examination, ultrasonography will demonstrate an elongated mass surrounding a long pyloric canal. If ultrasonography does not demonstrate a hypertrophied pylorus, upper GI radiography should be done to rule out other causes of vomiting.

Laboratory findings reflect the metabolic alterations created by severe depletion of both water and electrolytes from extensive and prolonged vomiting. There are decreased serum levels of both sodium and potassium, although these may be masked by the hemoconcentration from extracellular fluid depletion. Of greater diagnostic value are a decrease in serum chloride levels and increases in pH and bicarbonate (carbon dioxide content), indicative of metabolic alkalosis. The blood urea nitrogen will be elevated as evidence of dehydration.

Therapeutic Management

Surgical relief of the pyloric obstruction by pyloromyotomy is the standard therapy for this disorder. Preoperatively the infant must be rehydrated and metabolic alkalosis corrected with parenteral fluid and electrolyte administration. Replacement fluid therapy usually delays surgery for 24 to 48 hours. The stomach is decompressed with an NG tube. In infants with no evidence of fluid and electrolyte imbalance, surgery is performed without delay.

The surgical procedure is often performed by laparoscope and consists of a longitudinal incision through the circular muscle fibers of the pylorus down to, but not including, the submucosa (pyloromyotomy, sometimes called Fredet-Ramstedt procedure) (see Fig. 33-6, *B*). The procedure has a high success rate. The use of a small incision for the laparoscope may result in a shorter surgical time, more rapid postoperative feeding, and shorter hospital stay (van der Bilt, Kramer, van der Zee, et al, 2004).

Feedings are usually begun 4 to 6 hours postoperatively, beginning with small, frequent feedings of glucose, water, or electrolyte solution. If clear fluids are retained, about 24 hours after surgery formula is started in the same small increments. The amount and the interval between feedings are gradually increased until a full feeding schedule is reinstated, which usually takes about 48 hours.

Prognosis

The prognosis is excellent, and the mortality rate is low. Approximately 15% of infants with HPS also have GER (Milla, 2004).

Nursing Care Management

Nursing care involves primarily observation for clinical features that help establish the diagnosis, careful regulation of fluid therapy, and reestablishment of normal feeding patterns. Nurses must be alert to signs of HPS in infants and refer them for medical evaluation. Consider the possibility of HPS in the very young infant who appears alert but fails to gain weight and has a history of vomiting after meals. Base assessment on observation of eating behaviors, evidence of characteristic clinical manifestations, hydration, and nutritional status.

Preoperatively the emphasis is on restoring hydration and electrolyte balance. The infant is kept NPO and given IV fluids of glucose and electrolytes based on serum electrolyte values—usually sodium chloride solution with added potassium (when there is adequate urinary output). Careful monitoring of the IV fluids and strict monitoring of intake, output, and urine specific

gravity are important. Record accurate description of any vomiting and the number and character of stools.

Observations include assessment of vital signs, particularly those that indicate fluid or electrolyte imbalances. These infants are especially prone to metabolic alkalosis from loss of hydrogen ions and depletion of potassium, sodium, and chloride, all of which are contained in gastric secretions. Assess the skin and mucous membranes for alterations in hydration status; daily weights provide added clues to water gain or loss. (See Chapter 28 for manifestations of fluid and electrolyte disturbances.)

When stomach decompression and gastric lavage are part of preoperative management, the nurse is responsible for ensuring that the NG tube is patent and functioning properly and that the type and amount of NG drainage is recorded. General hygienic care, with particular attention to the skin and mouth in dehydrated infants, is important. Protection from infection is essential because infants with impaired nutritional status are more susceptible to infection than normal newborns.

Encourage parents to visit and become involved in the child's care. Most parents need support and reassurance that the condition is caused by a structural problem and is not a reflection of their parenting skills and capacities.

Postoperative Care

Postoperative vomiting is not uncommon, and most infants, even with successful surgery, exhibit some vomiting during the first 24 to 48 hours. IV fluids are administered until the infant is taking and retaining adequate amounts by mouth. Much of the same care that was instituted before surgery is continued postoperatively, including observation of vital signs, monitoring of IV fluids, and careful monitoring of intake and output. In addition, the infant is observed for responses to the stress of surgery and for evidence of pain. Appropriate analgesics should be given around the clock, since pain is continuous.

The NG tube may be maintained after surgery for a short time. Feedings are usually instituted within 24 hours postoperatively, beginning with clear liquids containing glucose and electrolytes. They are offered in small quantities at frequent intervals. If the infant has been breast-fed, breast milk, expressed by the mother, may be given by bottle when the infant is able to tolerate feedings, or the mother is instructed to limit nursing time and gradually increase the time to previous patterns. Supervision of feedings is an important part of postoperative care. Observe the operative site for any drainage or signs of inflammation. Poorly nourished infants may have problems with wound healing.

INTUSSUSCEPTION

Intussusception is the most common cause of intestinal obstruction in children between the ages of 3 months and 3 years (Waseem and Rosenberg, 2008). Intussusception is more common in males than in females and is more common in children with cystic fibrosis. Although specific intestinal lesions occur in a small percentage of the children, generally the cause is not known. More than 90% of intussusceptions do not have a pathologic lead point, such as a polyp, lymphoma, or Meckel diverticulum. The idiopathic cases may be caused by hypertrophy of intestinal lymphoid tissue secondary to viral infection.

PATHOPHYSIOLOGY REVIEW

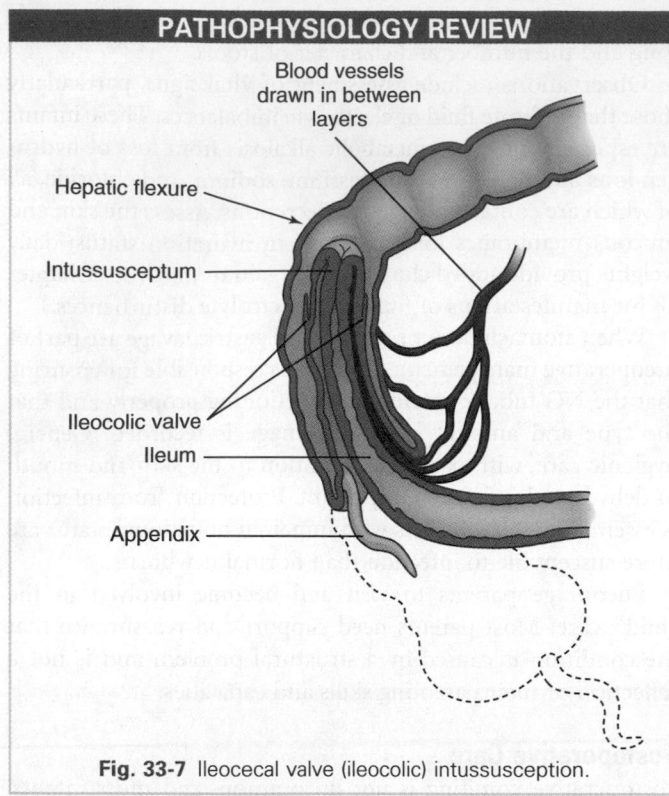

Fig. 33-7 Ileocecal valve (ileocolic) intussusception.

Pathophysiology

Intussusception occurs when a proximal segment of the bowel telescopes into a more distal segment, pulling the mesentery with it. The mesentery is compressed and angled, resulting in lymphatic and venous obstruction. As the edema from the obstruction increases, pressure within the area of intussusception increases. When the pressure equals the arterial pressure, arterial blood flow stops, resulting in ischemia and the pouring of mucus into the intestine. Venous engorgement also leads to leaking of blood and mucus into the intestinal lumen, forming the classic currant jelly–like stools (Wyllie, 2007). The most common site is the ileocecal valve (ileocolic), where the ileum invaginates into the cecum and then further into the colon (Fig. 33-7). Other forms include ileoileal (one part of the ileum invaginates into another section of the ileum) and colocolic (one part of the colon invaginates into another area of the colon) intussusceptions, usually in the area of the hepatic or splenic flexure or at some point along the transverse colon.

Clinical Manifestations

Intussusception usually manifests with the sudden onset of crampy abdominal pain, inconsolable crying, and a drawing up of the knees to the chest in an otherwise healthy child (Box 33-12). Between episodes the child appears normal. As the obstruction progresses, bilious vomiting may occur and lethargy increases. The classic triad of intussusception symptoms (abdominal pain, abdominal mass, bloody stools) is present in only 29% to 33% of children (Huppertz, Soriano-Gaabarro, Grimprel, et al, 2006). With atypical cases, lethargy may be the primary symptom. If the distal bowel remains distended, necrosis and perforation are possible.

BOX 33-12 CLINICAL MANIFESTATIONS OF INTUSSUSCEPTION

- Sudden acute abdominal pain
- Child screaming and drawing the knees onto the chest
- Child appearing normal and comfortable between episodes of pain
- Vomiting
- Lethargy
- Passage of red, currant jelly–like stools (stool mixed with blood and mucus)
- Tender, distended abdomen
- Palpable sausage-shaped mass in upper right quadrant
- Empty lower right quadrant (Dance sign)
- Eventual fever, prostration, and other signs of peritonitis

⚠ NURSING ALERT

The classic signs and symptoms of intussusception may not be present; a more chronic picture may occur, characterized by diarrhea, anorexia, weight loss, occasional vomiting, and periodic pain. The older child may have pain without other signs or symptoms. Because this condition is potentially life threatening, be aware of such signs and closely observe and refer these children for further medical investigation.

Diagnostic Evaluation

Frequently the diagnosis can be made on subjective findings alone. However, definitive diagnosis is based on a barium enema, which clearly demonstrates the obstruction to the flow of barium. Initially an abdominal radiograph is obtained to detect intraperitoneal air from a bowel perforation, which would contraindicate a barium enema. A rectal examination reveals mucus, blood, and occasionally a low intussusception itself.

Therapeutic Management

Conservative treatment consists of radiologist-guided pneumoenema (air enema) with or without water-soluble contrast or ultrasound-guided hydrostatic (saline) enema, the advantage of the latter being that no ionizing radiation is needed (Huppertz, Soriano-Gaabarro, Grimprel, et al, 2006). Recurrence of intussusception after conservative treatment is rare. Herwig, Brenkert, and Losek (2009) found hospitalized children needed minimal interventions after undergoing enema-reduced intussusception.

IV fluids, NG decompression, and antibiotic therapy may be used before hydrostatic reduction is attempted. If these procedures are not successful, the child may require surgical intervention. Surgery involves manually reducing the invagination and, when indicated, resecting any nonviable intestine.

Prognosis

Nonoperative reduction is successful in approximately 80% of cases (Huppertz, Soriano-Gaabarro, Grimprel, et al, 2006). Surgery is required for patients in whom the contrast enema is unsuccessful. With early diagnosis and treatment, serious complications and death are uncommon.

Nursing Care Management

The nurse can help establish a diagnosis by listening to the parent's description of the child's physical and behavioral symptoms. It is not unusual for parents to state that they thought something was seriously wrong before others shared their concerns. The description of the child's severe colicky abdominal pain combined with vomiting is a significant sign of intussusception.

As soon as a possible diagnosis of intussusception is made, the nurse prepares the parents for the immediate need for hospitalization, the nonsurgical technique of hydrostatic reduction, and the possibility of surgery. It is important to explain the basic defect of intussusception. The nurse can easily demonstrate this by creating a model of the defect. Use the example of a telescoping rod, or push the end of a finger on a rubber glove back into itself. Then demonstrate the principle of reduction by hydrostatic pressure by filling the glove with water, which pushes the "finger" into a fully extended position.

Physical care of the child does not differ from that for any child undergoing abdominal surgery. Even though nonsurgical intervention may be successful, the usual preoperative procedures, such as maintenance of NPO status, routine laboratory testing (CBC and urinalysis), signed parental consent, and preanesthetic sedation, are performed. For the child with signs of electrolyte imbalance, hemorrhage, or peritonitis, additional preparation, such as replacement fluids, whole blood or plasma, and NG suctioning, may be needed. Before surgery the nurse monitors all stools.

! NURSING ALERT

Passage of a normal brown stool usually indicates that the intussusception has reduced itself. This is immediately reported to the practitioner, who may choose to alter the diagnostic and therapeutic care plan.

Postprocedural care includes observations of vital signs, blood pressure, intact sutures and dressing, and the return of bowel sounds. After spontaneous or hydrostatic reduction, the nurse observes for passage of water-soluble contrast material (if used) and the stool patterns, since the intussusception may recur. Children may be admitted to the hospital or monitored on an outpatient basis. A recurrence of intussusception is treated with the conservative reduction techniques described above, but a laparotomy is considered for multiple recurrences.

Because hospitalization may be the child's first separation from the parents, it is important to preserve the parent-child relationship by encouraging rooming-in or extended visiting. It may be the parents' first experience with hospitalization, necessitating their preparation for procedures such as IV therapy, frequent vital sign and blood pressure monitoring, dressings, and NPO. Because of the rapidity of the onset, diagnosis, and treatment, parents may feel stunned or numb. They may ask few questions, or they may constantly make inquiries, sometimes the same ones several times. Because of the circumstances surrounding this condition, be accepting and understanding of the parents' reactions.

MALROTATION AND VOLVULUS

Malrotation of the intestine occurs as a result of the abnormal rotation of the intestine around the superior mesenteric artery during embryologic development. Malrotation may manifest in utero or may be asymptomatic throughout life. Infants may have intermittent bilious vomiting, recurrent abdominal pain, distention, or lower GI bleeding. Malrotation is the most serious type of intestinal obstruction because, if the intestine undergoes complete volvulus (the intestine twisting around itself), compromise of the blood supply will result in intestinal necrosis, peritonitis, perforation, and death.

Diagnostic Evaluation

It is imperative that malrotation and volvulus be diagnosed promptly and surgical treatment instituted quickly. An upper GI series is the definitive procedure to diagnose this condition.

Therapeutic Management

Surgery is indicated to remove the affected area. Because of the extensive nature of some lesions, short-bowel syndrome (SBS) is a postoperative complication.

Nursing Care Management

Preoperatively the nursing care is the same as that provided to an infant or child with intestinal obstruction. Postoperatively the nursing care is similar to that provided to the infant or child who has undergone abdominal surgery.

MALABSORPTION SYNDROMES

Chronic diarrhea and malabsorption of nutrients characterize malabsorption syndromes. An important complication of malabsorption syndromes in children is failure to thrive. Most cases are classified according to the location of the supposed anatomic or biochemical defect. The term celiac disease is often used to describe a symptom complex with four characteristics: (1) steatorrhea (fatty, foul, frothy, bulky stools), (2) general malnutrition, (3) abdominal distention, and (4) secondary vitamin deficiencies.

Digestive defects are conditions in which the enzymes necessary for digestion are diminished or absent, such as (1) cystic fibrosis, in which pancreatic enzymes are absent; (2) biliary or liver disease, in which bile flow is affected; or (3) lactase deficiency, in which there is congenital or secondary lactose intolerance.

Absorptive defects are conditions in which the intestinal mucosal transport system is impaired. This may occur because of a primary defect (e.g., celiac disease) or secondary to inflammatory disease of the bowel that results in impaired absorption because bowel motility is accelerated (e.g., UC). Obstructive disorders (e.g., HD) also cause secondary malabsorption from enterocolitis.

Anatomic defects, such as extensive resection of the bowel or SBS, affect digestion by decreasing the transit time of substances and affect absorption by severely compromising the absorptive surface.

CELIAC DISEASE (GLUTEN-SENSITIVE ENTEROPATHY)

Celiac disease, also known as gluten-induced enteropathy, gluten-sensitive enteropathy, and celiac sprue, is a permanent intestinal intolerance to dietary wheat gliadin and related proteins that produces mucosal lesions in genetically susceptible individuals (Dieterich, Esslinger, and Schuppan, 2003). It is second only to cystic fibrosis as a cause of malabsorption in children.

The incidence is variable and has been reported in 1 in 3000 to 1 in 4000 people. The disease is seen more frequently in Europe than in the United States. It is more prevalent in women than men and is rarely reported in Asians or African-Americans. Although the exact cause is unknown, it is now generally accepted that celiac disease is an immunologically mediated small intestine enteropathy. The mucosal lesions contain features that suggest both humoral and cell-mediated immunologic overstimulation.

Pathophysiology

Celiac disease is characterized by villous atrophy in the small bowel in response to the protein gluten (Maki and Lohi, 2004). Gluten is found in wheat, barley, rye, and oat grains. When individuals are unable to digest the gliadin component of gluten, an accumulation of a toxic substance that is damaging to the mucosal cells occurs. Damage to the mucosa of the small intestine leads to villous atrophy, hyperplasia of the crypts, and infiltration of the epithelial cells with lymphocytes. Villous atrophy leads to malabsorption due to the reduced absorptive surface area (see Fig. 33-1 and the discussion of absorption on p. 1296).

Clinical Manifestations

Symptoms of celiac disease appear when solid foods such as beans and pasta are introduced in the child's diet between the ages of 1 and 5 years (Box 33-13). There is usually an interval of several months between the introduction of gluten into the diet and the onset of symptoms. Intestinal symptoms are common in children diagnosed within the first 2 years of life.

BOX 33-13 CLINICAL MANIFESTATIONS OF CELIAC DISEASE

Impaired Fat Absorption
Steatorrhea (excessively large, pale, oily, frothy stools)
Exceedingly foul-smelling stools

Impaired Nutrient Absorption
Malnutrition
Muscle wasting (especially prominent in legs and buttocks)
Anemia
Anorexia
Abdominal distention

Behavioral Changes
Irritability
Uncooperativeness
Apathy

Celiac Crisis*
Acute, severe episodes of profuse watery diarrhea and vomiting
May be precipitated by:
- Infections (especially gastrointestinal)
- Prolonged fluid and electrolyte depletion
- Emotional disturbance

*In very young children.

Other symptoms include failure to thrive, chronic diarrhea, abdominal distention, muscle wasting, anorexia, and irritability. (See Critical Thinking Exercise on Inflammatory Bowel Disease.)

Diagnostic Evaluation

The diagnosis of celiac disease is based on a biopsy of the small intestine demonstrating the characteristic changes of mucosal inflammation, crypt hyperplasia, and villous atrophy (Dieterich, Esslinger, and Schuppan, 2003).

Therapeutic Management

Treatment of celiac disease consists primarily of dietary management. Although a gluten-free diet is prescribed, it is difficult to remove every source of this protein. Some patients are able to tolerate restricted amounts of gluten. Because gluten occurs mainly in the grains of wheat and rye, but also in smaller quantities in barley and oats, these four foods are eliminated. Corn, rice, and millet are substitute grain foods.

Children with untreated celiac disease may have lactose intolerance, especially if their mucosal lesions are extensive. Lactose intolerance usually improves as the mucosa heals with gluten withdrawal. Specific nutritional deficiencies, such as iron, folic acid, and fat-soluble vitamin deficiencies, are treated with appropriate supplements.

Prognosis

Celiac disease is a chronic disease; its severity varies greatly among children. The most severe symptoms usually occur in early childhood and again in adult life. Most children who comply with dietary management are healthy and remain free of symptoms and complications. Strict dietary avoidance of gluten may minimize the risk of developing lymphoma, especially of the small intestine, one of the most serious complications of the disease.

Nursing Care Management

The main nursing consideration is helping the child adhere to the dietary regimen. Considerable time is involved in explaining the disease process to the child and parents, the specific role of gluten in aggravating the disorder, and those foods that must be restricted. It is difficult to maintain a diet indefinitely when the child has no symptoms and temporary transgressions result in no difficulties. However, the majority of individuals who relax their diet will experience a relapse of their disease and possibly exhibit growth retardation, anemia, or osteomalacia. There is also the risk of developing malignant lymphoma of the small intestine or other GI malignancies.

Although the chief source of gluten is cereal and baked goods, grains are frequently added to processed foods as thickeners or fillers. To compound the difficulty, gluten is added to many foods as hydrolyzed vegetable protein, which is derived from cereal grains. The nurse must advise parents of the necessity of reading all label ingredients carefully to avoid hidden sources of gluten.

Many of children's favorite foods contain gluten, including bread, cake, cookies, crackers, donuts, pies, spaghetti, pizza, prepared soups, some processed ice cream, many types of chocolate candy, milk preparations such as malts, hot dogs, luncheon meats, meat gravy, and some prepared hamburgers. Many of these products can be eliminated from the infant's or young child's diet fairly easily, but monitoring the diet of the school-age child or adolescent is more difficult. Luncheon preparation away from home is particularly difficult, since bread, luncheon meats, and instant soups are not allowed. For families on restricted food budgets, the diet adds an additional financial burden because many inexpensive or convenient foods cannot be used.

In addition to restricting gluten, other dietary alterations may be necessary. For example, in some children who have more severe mucosal damage, the digestion of disaccharides is impaired, especially in relation to lactose. Therefore these children often need a temporarily lactose-free diet, which necessitates eliminating all milk products. In general, dietary management includes a diet high in calories and proteins, with simple carbohydrates such as fruits and vegetables, but low in fats. Because the bowel is inflamed as a result of the pathologic processes in absorption, the child must avoid high-fiber foods, such as nuts, raisins, raw vegetables, and raw fruits with skin, until inflammation has subsided.

It is important to stress long-range complications and to remind parents of the child's physical status before dietary treatment and the dramatic improvement after treatment. The nurse can be instrumental in allowing the child to express concerns and frustration while focusing on ways in which the child can still feel normal. Encourage the child and parents to find new recipes using suitable ingredients, such as Mexican or Chinese dishes that use corn or rice. Consult a nutritionist to provide children and their families with detailed dietary instructions and education.*

Several resources are available to assist children and parents in all aspects of coping with celiac disease. The Celiac Sprue Association/United States of America† provides support and guidance to families and supplies educational materials concerning a gluten-free diet, food sources, recipes, and travel information.

SHORT-BOWEL SYNDROME

SBS is a malabsorptive disorder that occurs as a result of decreased mucosal surface area, usually because of extensive resection of the small intestine. Malabsorption may be exacerbated by other factors, such as bacterial overgrowth and dysmotility. The most common causes of SBS in children are necrotizing enterocolitis, volvulus, jejunal atresias, and gastroschisis. Other causes include midgut volvulus and diffuse small bowel CD in older children. Less frequent causes include trauma to the GI tract and total colonic aganglionosis with extension into the small bowel.

*A booklet, *Pointers for Parents: Coping with Celiac Sprue,* provides information on shopping, cooking, and living with an affected child and is available from the Clinical Dietetics Department, Children's Memorial Hospital, 2300 Children's Plaza, Chicago, IL 60614; 773-880-4793.
†PO Box 31700, Omaha, NE 68131-0700; 877-CSA-4CSA or 402-558-0600; www.csaceliacs.org. In Canada: Canadian Celiac Association, 5170 Dixie Road, Suite 204, Mississauga, Ontario, Canada, L4W 1E3; 905-507-6208; www.celiac.ca.

The definition of SBS includes two important findings: (1) decreased intestinal surface area for absorption of fluid, electrolytes, and nutrients; and (2) a need for parenteral nutrition (PN) (Goday, 2009). The prognosis for infants with SBS has improved dramatically in the past 20 to 30 years as a result of advances in PN and enteral feeding.

Therapeutic Management

The goals of therapy for infants and children with SBS include (1) preserve as much length of bowel as possible during surgery; (2) maintain optimum nutritional status, growth, and development while intestinal adaptation occurs; (3) stimulate intestinal adaptation with enteral feeding; and (4) minimize complications related to the disease process and therapy (Goday, 2009).

Nutritional Support

Nutritional support is the long-term focus of care for children with SBS (Sadlier, 2008). The initial phase of therapy includes PN as the primary source of nutrition. The second phase is the introduction of enteral feeding, which usually begins as soon as possible after surgery. Elemental formulas containing glucose, sucrose and glucose polymers, hydrolyzed proteins, and medium-chain triglycerides facilitate absorption. Usually these formulas are given by continuous infusion through an NG or gastrostomy tube. As the enteral feedings are advanced, the PN solution is decreased in terms of calories, amount of fluid, and total hours of infusion per day.

The final phase of nutritional support occurs when growth and development are sustained exclusively by enteral feedings. When PN is discontinued, there is a risk of nutritional deficiency secondary to malabsorption of fat-soluble vitamins (A, D, E, K) and trace minerals (iron, selenium, zinc). Obtain serum vitamin and mineral levels, and require enteral supplementation of vitamins and minerals. Pharmacologic agents have been used to reduce secretory losses. H_2 blockers, PPIs, and octreotide inhibit gastric or pancreatic secretion. Cholestyramine is often prescribed to improve diarrhea that is associated with bile salt malabsorption. Growth factors have also been used to hasten adaptation and to enhance mucosal growth, but these uses are still experimental.

Numerous complications are associated with SBS and long-term PN. Infectious, metabolic, and technical complications can occur. Catheter sepsis can occur after improper care of the catheter. The GI tract can also be a source of microbial seeding of the catheter. Bowel atrophy may foster increased intestinal permeability of bacteria. A lack of adequate sites for central lines may become a significant problem for the child in need of long-term PN. Hepatic dysfunction, hepatomegaly with abnormal LFTs, and cholestasis may also occur (Diamond, Sterescu, Pencharz, et al, 2009).

Bacterial overgrowth is likely to occur when the ileocecal valve is absent or when stasis exists as a result of a partial obstruction or a dilated segment of bowel with poor motility. Alternating cycles of broad-spectrum antibiotics are used to reduce bacterial overgrowth. This treatment may also decrease the risk of bacterial translocation and subsequent central venous catheter infections. Other complications of bacterial overgrowth and malabsorption include metabolic acidosis and gastric hypersecretion.

Many surgical interventions, including intestinal valves, tapering enteroplasty or stricturoplasty, intestinal lengthening, and interposed segments, have been used to slow intestinal transit, reduce bacterial overgrowth, or increase mucosal surface area. Intestinal transplantation has been performed successfully in children. Only children with a permanent dependence on PN or severe complications of long-term PN are candidates for transplantation.

Prognosis

The prognosis for infants with SBS has improved with advances in PN and with the understanding of the importance of intraluminal nutrition. Improved surgical techniques for the management of therapy-related problems and the development of more specific immunosuppressive medications for transplantation have all contributed to improved management. The prognosis depends in part on the length of the residual small intestine. An intact ileocecal valve also improves the prognosis. Infants and children with SBS die from PN-related problems, such as fulminant sepsis or severe PN cholestasis.

Nursing Care Management

The most important components of nursing care are administration and monitoring of nutritional therapy. During PN therapy, take care to minimize the risk of complications related to the central venous access device (i.e., catheter infections, occlusions, dislodgment, or accidental removal). Care of the enteral feeding tubes and monitoring of enteral feeding tolerance are also important nursing responsibilities (see Critical Thinking Exercise).

❓ CRITICAL THINKING EXERCISE

Short-Bowel Syndrome

The parents of a 2-year-old boy with short-bowel syndrome (SBS) call their health care professional to report that their child has passed many more stools than usual with an increased watery consistency in the past 24 hours. He also has a fever of 39° C (102.2° F) and has vomited several times. The boy is admitted to the hospital. During the initial period of nursing assessment, which of the following would you monitor?

1. Stool pH, urine pH, vital signs
2. Vital signs, weight, urine specific gravity, intake and output
3. Vital signs, stool-reducing substances, stool culture
4. Urine specific gravity, stool for blood, electrolytes

Questions

1. Evidence—Are there sufficient data to support your decision?
2. Assumptions—Describe some underlying assumptions about the following:
   a. Description of SBS
   b. Risk factors associated with chronic malabsorption disorders
   c. Other assessment parameters
3. What are the priorities for this child at this time?
4. Does the evidence support your conclusion?

When hospitalization is prolonged, the child's developmental and emotional needs must be met. This often requires special planning to promote normal family adjustment and adaptation of the hospital routines. Chapter 26 discusses care of the hospitalized child.

Many infants with SBS have an intestinal ostomy performed at the time of the initial bowel resection. Routine ostomy care is another important nursing responsibility. Since infants and children with SBS have chronic diarrhea, perineal skin irritation is often a problem after ostomy closure. Frequent diaper changes, gentle perineal cleansing, and protective skin ointments help prevent skin breakdown. (See Diaper Dermatitis, Chapter 13.)

When hospitalization is prolonged, the child's developmental and emotional needs must be part of the care plan. This often requires special efforts to promote normal family adaptation to hospital routines. It may be months to years before the child no longer requires specialized nutritional support. Family members require psychosocial support and education to cope successfully with SBS.

Home Care

When long-term PN is required, preparation of the family for home care of the child is a major nursing responsibility. Preparation for home nutritional support begins as early as possible to prevent lengthy hospitalizations with subsequent problems such as developmental delays and family stresses. Many infants and children can be successfully cared for at home with enteral and parenteral nutrition if the family is thoroughly prepared and provided with adequate support services. Most families benefit from home nursing care to assist with and supervise therapy. Nurses can advocate, on behalf of patients and families, for necessary services and supplies for home care. Careful follow-up care by a multidisciplinary nutritional support service is essential. Most home health agencies now provide portable enteral and parenteral equipment, which enables the child and family to maintain a more normal and active lifestyle.

GASTROINTESTINAL BLEEDING

GI bleeding in infants and children is an uncommon but potentially serious problem (Gilger, 2004). Most actual or apparent instances of GI bleeding cause great anxiety for the parents or caregivers. Blood may be vomited or passed per rectum, but the origin of the blood may not be the GI tract. In the newborn, swallowed maternal blood at the time of delivery may account for some episodes of apparent GI bleeding. A bleeding site on the nipple of a nursing mother may lead to heme-positive stools in the breast-fed infant. Finally, blood can be swallowed during epistaxis and then passed as hematemesis or melena.

Once it has been established that the cause of bleeding is from a source in the GI tract, further investigation for the source and cause is undertaken. Upper GI bleeding comes from above the ligament of Treitz, which is attached to the duodenum at its junction with the jejunum. Lower GI bleeding comes from a source distal to the ligament of Treitz. Diagnostic studies such as endoscopy, scintigraphy, and angiography have improved the ability to localize the site of bleeding.

Etiology

The esophagus is a common site of upper GI bleeding. Esophagitis caused by GER may lead to chronic and often occult blood loss. Esophageal varices secondary to portal hypertension may cause massive bleeding. Peptic inflammation (gastritis and duodenitis) or ulceration is the most common cause of upper GI bleeding in children. Hemorrhagic gastritis may occur in the newborn infant after a difficult delivery or asphyxia. In this circumstance gastric perforation is a serious complication that requires emergent treatment. Less common causes of upper GI bleeding include bleeding disorders, vascular malformations, GI duplications, Mallory-Weiss syndrome (an esophageal tear caused by protracted vomiting), and hematobilia (bleeding into biliary passages).

In lower GI bleeding, small amounts of bright red blood in the stool of a healthy child may be due to an anal fissure. Colonic polyps are another cause of passage of bright red blood per rectum in toddlers and older children. Bleeding associated with diarrhea may indicate a serious problem. Enteric infections remain the leading cause, but the nurse should consider necrotizing enterocolitis, hemolytic uremic syndrome, IBD, and food allergy. Other causes are intussusception with the passage of blood per rectum (see p. 1323) or Meckel diverticulum with the painless passage of currant jelly–like stools (see p. 1312).

Pathophysiology

The GI tract has an extensive surface area and a rich vascular supply. Bleeding can occur anywhere along the GI tract from a vein, artery, or vascular malformation. In an otherwise healthy newborn infant, hemophilia or inherited coagulation-factor deficits are rarely accompanied by bleeding unless other conditions are superimposed (Gilger, 2004). Children with liver disease may also have deficient coagulation factors because of poor synthesis and malabsorption of vitamin K, which is a risk factor for GI bleeding.

Portal hypertension may lead to GI bleeding because the formation of portosystemic shunts can result in dilated venous channels in vulnerable locations such as the esophagus and stomach. These dilated venous channels (varices) may bleed, causing severe GI hemorrhage.

Diagnostic Evaluation

The diagnosis of GI bleeding is often made on the basis of the history and physical examination. Hematemesis is the vomiting of bright red blood or denatured blood that looks like coffee grounds, usually representing an upper GI source of bleeding. Hematochezia is the passage of bright red blood per rectum, indicating lower GI bleeding. This blood may precede or follow a bowel movement or be mixed with or coat the stool. Bright red blood that coats the stool may be due to a hard bowel movement, hemorrhoids, or anal fissures. Blood mixed with stool indicates a bleeding source proximal to the rectum. Blood passed alone after a bowel movement is most likely due to bleeding in the perianal or rectal area, possibly caused by a polyp. Blood with mucus in the stool indicates an inflammatory or infectious condition, and currant jelly–like stools indicate vascular compromise, such as intussusception. Melena is the passage of black, tarry stools that contain denatured (digested) blood and suggests an upper GI source of bleeding. Occasionally, bright red blood may be passed per rectum from an upper GI source of bleeding when the bleeding is massive. It is important to test emesis or stool for occult blood to differentiate true

bleeding from the ingestion of food containing food coloring. In older children, false-positive stool tests for occult blood can also occur with the ingestion of red meats and iron preparations.

Laboratory studies are determined on the basis of the history and physical examination. In many instances, a CBC with platelet quantification, prothrombin, partial thromboplastin, and coagulation studies will be done. Children who have acute illness, fever, and joint pain in addition to GI bleeding need an ESR and stool studies with culture to evaluate for enteric pathogens, ova and parasites, and *Clostridium difficile*. When IBD is suspected, a metabolic panel to determine total protein and albumin may be added to a CBC, ESR, and LFTs. The child with massive painless rectal bleeding may require a nuclear medicine scan to rule out Meckel diverticulum. If there is evidence of portal hypertension or chronic liver disease, LFTs, liver imaging studies, and a liver biopsy may be necessary. A barium enema is performed if intussusception is suspected.

Imaging studies help differentiate among several suspected diagnoses. CT of the sinuses helps localize bleeding that is coming from the nasopharynx or sinuses. A chest radiograph may distinguish hemoptysis related to cystic fibrosis, bronchiectasis, or other chronic lung conditions from hematemesis. Angiography can be used to identify the source of bleeding and to allow embolization or vasopressin infusion for treatment. Endoscopy is the diagnostic method chosen when the source of bleeding is thought to be secondary to gastritis, esophagitis, PUD, colitis, or polyps. Endoscopic examinations also permit visualization of the intestinal mucosa and collection of biopsy specimens and cultures.

Therapeutic Management

Treatment of GI bleeding in children depends on its severity and cause. The first step in management of acute GI bleeding is to assess the magnitude of blood loss and restore the child's hemodynamic stability. Severe bleeding necessitates hospitalization. IV fluids (normal saline or lactated Ringer solution) are administered rapidly. Oxygen therapy is indicated if the bleeding is severe. Transfusion of blood products may be required if the blood loss is significant, and any existing coagulopathy should be corrected.

Upper GI mucosal lesions are usually treated with H_2 receptor antagonists (cimetidine, ranitidine, or famotidine) or PPIs (omeprazole or lansoprazole) and antacids to reduce acidity and promote mucosal healing. Variceal hemorrhage can be treated with peripheral vasopressin infusion and endoscopic sclerotherapy to hasten tissue fibrosis. Balloon tamponade to place pressure on the bleeding area may be performed as a temporary measure until endoscopic sclerotherapy can be done.

Therapy for lower GI bleeding is directed toward the primary underlying condition. The treatment may include medical or surgical management. Surgery may be required if the bleeding is severe despite aggressive medical intervention.

Nursing Care Management

The infant or child with acute and severe GI bleeding requires emergency care. Initial management includes assessment of the magnitude of bleeding and hemodynamic status and assistance with resuscitation efforts (see Critical Thinking Exercise).

? CRITICAL THINKING EXERCISE

Hematemesis

A 6-month-old infant is seen in the emergency department. The parents brought the infant to the hospital because he spit up formula with blood streaks. In the emergency department the infant has tachypnea, tachycardia, and a fever of 39° C (102.2° F). A chest x-ray film shows pneumonia. The infant is admitted to the hospital to receive antibiotics and for observation. Several hours after admission to the inpatient unit, the mother calls the nurse when the infant vomits a large amount of bright red blood. The infant is pale and lethargic. Which of the following should *not* be included in the initial nursing actions?

1. Call for assistance and estimate the amount of blood loss.
2. Obtain vital signs and monitor capillary refill, skin color, and behavior.
3. Prepare to pass a nasogastric tube, obtain blood for laboratory analyses, and start an intravenous line.
4. Test stool for blood (Hematest or Hemoccult).

Questions

1. Evidence—Are there sufficient data to support your decision?
2. Assumptions—Describe some underlying assumptions about the following:
   a. Hematemesis in an infant
   b. The diagnosis of hematemesis
3. What are the priorities for this child at this time?
4. What are the nursing actions that need to be implemented?

! NURSING ALERT

Monitor closely for signs of shock: restlessness; increased respiratory and heart rate; poor capillary refill; pallor; cool, clammy extremities; and decreased blood pressure (a late sign). Call for assistance immediately if these signs are observed.

Administer oxygen, and make certain suction equipment is available. An IV catheter should be inserted and preparation made for the administration of IV fluids, usually normal saline or lactated Ringer solution. Draw blood for laboratory analysis, including hemoglobin, hematocrit, blood urea nitrogen, creatinine, coagulation studies, and type and crossmatch. The nurse should be prepared to insert an NG tube to help locate the site of bleeding and to lavage the stomach with normal saline at room temperature if upper GI bleeding is suspected. Avoid taking rectal temperatures to prevent further irritation or damage to the rectal mucosa of a child suspected of having rectal bleeding or fissures. After the child is stabilized, ongoing monitoring in an intensive care setting may be indicated.

In cases of mild or chronic bleeding, there is more time for a thorough history and diagnostic evaluation, often in an outpatient setting. Important nursing responsibilities include assisting with the history and physical examination, diagnostic procedures, and education regarding the therapeutic plan.

The parents or caregivers of a child with GI bleeding may be extremely anxious and panic stricken. They need reassurance that most instances of bleeding are self-limiting and can be treated successfully. In life-threatening situations, special emotional support is required. Keep the family informed about the source, cause, and treatment of the bleeding.

HEPATIC DISORDERS

The liver is an active, vital organ whose functions can be divided into several groups: (1) vascular functions of storing and filtering blood; (2) secretory function of producing bile; (3) metabolism of carbohydrate, protein, and fat; (4) synthesis of blood-clotting components and storage of iron and vitamins (A, D, B_{12}, and K); and (5) detoxification and excretion of certain drugs and metabolic substances. Many disorders, including biliary atresia, hepatitis, and cirrhosis, can cause liver dysfunction in children. (See Chapter 11.)

ACUTE HEPATITIS

Hepatitis is an acute or chronic inflammation of the liver that can result from several different causes. One cause is infection. Many types of hepatitis are caused by viruses such as the hepatitis viruses, Epstein-Barr virus (EBV), cytomegalovirus (CMV), and the human immunodeficiency virus (HIV). Other causes of hepatitis are nonviral (abscess, amebiasis), autoimmune, metabolic, chemical, neoplastic, anatomic (choledochal duct cyst and biliary atresia), hemodynamic (shock, congestive heart failure), and idiopathic (sclerosing cholangitis and Reye syndrome).

Etiology

The majority (90%) of cases of viral hepatitis are caused by six viruses:

1. Hepatitis A virus (HAV)
2. Hepatitis B virus (HBV)
3. Hepatitis C virus (HCV)
4. Hepatitis D virus (HDV)
5. Hepatitis E virus (HEV)
6. Hepatitis G virus (HGV)

In earlier resources the HCV, HDV, HEV, and HGV infections were characterized as non-A, non-B; most of these non-A, non-B infections were caused by HCV (Castiglia, 1996, 2001). In addition, CMV, EBV, and herpes simplex virus may occasionally cause hepatitis. The clinical symptoms of these viruses are similar. Epidemiologic features and serologic testing are used to differentiate the causes. Table 33-3 compares the features of HAV, HBV, and HCV.

Hepatitis A incidence in the United States has declined 92%, from 12.0 cases per 100,000 population in 1995 to 1.0 case per 100,000 population in 2007, the lowest rate ever recorded. Declines were greatest among children and in those states where routine vaccination of children was recommended beginning in 1999 (Daniels, Grytdal, Wasley, et al, 2009). The virus is spread directly or indirectly by the fecal-oral route by either ingestion of contaminated foods, direct exposure to infected fecal material, or close contact with an infected person. The virus is particularly prevalent in developing countries with poor living conditions, inadequate sanitation, crowding, and poor personal hygiene practices. The spread of HAV has been associ-

TABLE 33-3   COMPARISON OF HEPATITIS TYPES A, B, AND C

CHARACTERISTICS	TYPE A	TYPE B	TYPE C
Incubation period	15-50 days, average 25-30 days	45-160 days, average 120 days	14-180 days, average 45 days
Period of communicability	Believed to be latter half of incubation period to first week after onset of clinical illness	Variable Virus in blood or other body fluids during late incubation period and acute stage of disease; may persist in carrier state for years to lifetime	Begins before onset of symptoms May persist in carrier state for years
Mode of transmission	Principal route—fecal-oral Rarely—parenteral	Principal route—parenteral Less frequent route—oral, sexual, any body fluid Perinatal transfer—transplacental blood (last trimester), at delivery, or during breast-feeding, especially if mother has cracked nipples	Principal route—parenteral Nonparenteral spread possible
Clinical features			
Onset	Usually rapid, acute	More insidious	Usually insidious
Fever	Common and early	Less frequent	Less frequent
Anorexia	Common	Mild to moderate	Mild to moderate
Nausea and vomiting	Common	Sometimes present	Mild to moderate
Rash	Rare	Common	Sometimes present
Arthralgia	Rare	Common	Rare
Pruritus	Rare	Sometimes present	Sometimes present
Jaundice	Present (many cases anicteric)	Present	Present
Immunity	Present after one attack; no crossover to type B or C	Present after one attack; no crossover to type A or C	Present after one attack; no crossover to type A or B
Carrier state	No	Yes	No
Chronic infection	No	Yes	No
Prophylaxis			
Immune globulin (IG)	Passive immunity Successful, especially in early incubation period and preexposure prophylaxis	Passive immunity Inconsistent benefits; probably of no use	Not currently recommended by Centers for Disease Control and Prevention
HAV vaccine	Two inactivated vaccines administered to all children ages 12-23 mo: Havrix and Vaqta; given in a 2-dose schedule (6 mo between doses)		
HBV immune globulin (HBIG)	No benefit	Postexposure protection possible if given immediately after definite exposure	No benefit
HBV vaccine		Provides active immunity Universal vaccination recommended for all newborns	
Mortality	0.1%-0.2%	0.5%-2.0% in uncomplicated cases; may be higher in complicated cases	1%-2% in uncomplicated cases; may be higher in complicated cases

HAV, Hepatitis A virus; *HBV,* hepatitis B virus.

ated with improper food handling and high-risk areas such as households with infected persons, residential centers for the disabled, and daycare centers. The average incubation period is about 4 weeks, with a range of 15 to 50 days. Fecal shedding of the virus can occur for 2 to 3 weeks before and for a week after the onset of jaundice. During this time, although the individual is asymptomatic, the virus is most likely to be transmitted. Infants with HAV infection are likely to be asymptomatic (anicteric hepatitis). Children often have diarrhea, and their symptoms are frequently attributed to gastroenteritis. Only 1 in 12 young children develops jaundice. Most adults develop clinical signs with icteric hepatitis. The prognosis of HAV infection is usually good, and complications are rare.

Hepatitis B can be an acute or chronic infection, ranging from an asymptomatic, limited infection to fatal, fulminant (rapid and severe) hepatitis (Yuen and Lai, 2001). There are no

environmental or animal reservoirs for HBV. Humans are the main source of infections. HBV may be transmitted parenterally, percutaneously, or transmucosally. Hepatitis B surface antigen (HBsAg) has been found in all body fluids, including feces, bile, breast milk, sweat, tears, vaginal secretions, and urine, but only blood, semen, and saliva have been found to contain infectious HBV particles. HBV infection from human bites has been documented, but transmission from feces has not. Hepatitis B has been acquired after blood transfusion, but the likelihood of this has been reduced through blood product–screening procedures. Adults whose occupations are associated with considerable exposure to blood or blood products, such as health care workers, are at an increased risk of contracting HBV.

Most HBV infection in children is acquired perinatally. Transmission from mother to infant during the perinatal period (i.e., blood exposure during delivery) results in chronic infection in 70% to 90% of infants if the mother is positive for HBsAg and HBeAg (Tran, 2009; American Academy of Pediatrics, 2009). Perinatal infection occurs during the birthing process when the infant comes in contact with maternal body fluids, most likely blood. It is still not known if the virus enters the infant via mucosal membranes, intestinal tract, or skin abrasions. HBsAg has been detected in breast milk, but it is not clear whether HBV infection is transmitted through ingested breast milk or from swallowed maternal blood from injured nipples (Tran, 2009). Infants and children who are not infected during the perinatal period remain at high risk for acquiring person-to-person transmission from their mother during the first 5 years of life.

HBV infection occurs in children and adolescents in specific high-risk groups: (1) individuals with hemophilia or other disorders who have received multiple transfusions, (2) children and adolescents involved in IV drug abuse, (3) institutionalized children, (4) preschool children in endemic areas, and (5) individuals engaged in heterosexual activity or sexual activity with homosexual males. The incubation period for HBV infection ranges from 45 to 160 days with an average of 120 days (American Academy of Pediatrics, 2009). HBV infection can cause a carrier state and lead to chronic hepatitis with eventual cirrhosis or hepatocellular carcinoma in adulthood.

Hepatitis C (HCV) is transmitted parenterally through exposure to blood and blood products from HCV-infected persons (Bonkovsky and Mehata, 2001). Recent improvements in donor screening and inactivation procedures for blood products such as the factor concentrates used for hemophilia patients have significantly reduced the risk of transmission through blood products. The mechanism of nonparenteral or nonpercutaneous transmission of HCV is uncertain. Sexual transmission among monogamous couples and among family contacts is uncommon. Maternal coinfection with HIV has been associated with increased risk of perinatal transmission of HCV and may depend on the HCV genotype and the serum titer of maternal HCV-RNA. All persons with HCV antibody or HCV-RNA in their blood are considered to be infectious (American Academy of Pediatrics, 2009).

The clinical course is variable. The incubation period for HCV ranges from 14 to 180 days, with an average of 45 days. The natural history of the disease in children is not well defined. Some children may be asymptomatic, but hepatitis C can become a chronic condition and can cause cirrhosis and hepatocellular carcinoma. About 60% to 70% of individuals infected with HCV develop chronic disease. Infection with HCV is the leading reason for liver transplantation in the United States (America Academy of Pediatrics, 2009).

Hepatitis D occurs in children already infected with HBV. HDV is a defective RNA virus that requires the helper function of HBV. The incubation period is from 2 to 8 weeks. Both acute and chronic forms of hepatitis D tend to be more severe than hepatitis B and can lead to cirrhosis. HDV infection occurs mostly in drug abusers, individuals with hemophilia, and persons immigrating from endemic areas.

Hepatitis E is enterically transmitted non-A, non-B hepatitis. Transmission may occur through the fecal-oral route or from contaminated water. The incubation period is 2 to 9 weeks. This illness is uncommon in children, does not cause chronic liver disease, is not a chronic condition, and has no carrier state. However, it can be a devastating disease among pregnant women, with an unusually high case-fatality rate.

HGV is blood borne but can also be transmitted by organ transplantation. High-risk groups include transfusion recipients, IV drug users, and individuals infected with HCV. Individuals with the virus are often asymptomatic, and most infections are chronic. The incubation period is unknown.

Pathophysiology

Pathologic changes occur primarily in the parenchymal cells of the liver and result in variable degrees of swelling; infiltration of liver cells by mononuclear cells; and subsequent degeneration, necrosis, and fibrosis. Structural changes within the hepatocyte account for altered liver functions, such as impaired bile excretion, elevated transaminase levels, and decreased albumin synthesis. The disorder may be self-limiting, with regeneration of liver cells without scarring, leading to a complete recovery. However, some forms of hepatitis do not result in complete return of liver function. These include fulminant hepatitis, which is characterized by a severe, acute course with massive destruction of the liver tissue causing liver failure and high mortality within 1 to 2 weeks, and subacute or chronic active hepatitis, which is characterized by progressive liver destruction, uncertain regeneration, scarring, and potential cirrhosis.

The progression of liver disease is characterized pathologically by four stages: (1) stage one is characterized by mononuclear inflammatory cells surrounding small bile ducts, (2) in stage two there is proliferation of small bile ductules, (3) stage three is characterized by fibrosis or scarring, and (4) stage four is cirrhosis.

Clinical Manifestations

The clinical manifestations and course of uncomplicated acute viral hepatitis are similar for most of the hepatitis viruses. Usually the prodromal, or anicteric, phase (absence of jaundice) lasts 5 to 7 days. Anorexia, malaise, lethargy, and easy fatigability are the most common symptoms. Fever may be present, especially in adolescents. Nausea, vomiting, and epigastric or right upper quadrant abdominal pain or tenderness may occur. Arthralgia and skin rashes may occur and are more likely in children with hepatitis B than those with hepatitis A. The transaminases, rather than the bilirubin, will often be elevated in acute hepatitis, and hepatomegaly may be present. Some mild cases of acute viral hepatitis do not cause symptoms or can be mistaken for influenza.

In young children most of the prodromal symptoms disappear with the onset of jaundice, or the icteric phase. Many children with acute viral hepatitis, however, never develop jaundice. If jaundice occurs, it is often accompanied by dark urine and pale stools. Pruritus may accompany jaundice and can be bothersome for children.

Children with chronic active hepatitis may be asymptomatic but more commonly have nonspecific symptoms of malaise, fatigue, lethargy, weight loss, or vague abdominal pain. Hepatomegaly may be present, and the transaminases are often very high, with mild to severe hyperbilirubinemia.

Fulminant hepatitis is due primarily to HBV or HCV. Many children with fulminant hepatitis develop characteristic clinical symptoms and rapidly develop manifestations of liver failure, including encephalopathy, coagulation defects, ascites, deepening jaundice, and increasing white blood cell count. Changes in mental status or personality indicate impending liver failure. Although children with acute hepatitis may have hepatomegaly, a rapid decrease in the size of the liver (indicating loss of tissue due to necrosis) is a serious sign of fulminant hepatitis. Complications of fulminant hepatitis include GI bleeding, sepsis, renal failure, and disseminated coagulopathy.

Diagnostic Evaluation

Diagnosis is based on the history; physical examination; and serologic markers for hepatitis A, B, and C. No LFT is specific for hepatitis, but serum aspartate and serum aminotransferase levels are markedly elevated. Serum bilirubin levels peak 5 to 10 days after clinical jaundice appears. Histologic evidence from liver biopsy may be required to establish the diagnosis and to assess the severity of the liver disease. Serologic markers indicate the antibodies or antigens formed in response to the specific virus and confirm the diagnosis. Serum immunologic tests are not available to detect HAV antigen, but there are two HAV antibody tests: anti-HAV immunoglobulin G (IgG) and immunoglobulin M (IgM). Anti-HAV antibodies are present at the onset of the disease and persist for life. A positive anti-HAV antibody test indicates the following: acute infection, immunity from past infection, passive antibody acquisition (e.g., from transfusion, serum immunoglobulin infusion), or immunization. To diagnose an acute or recent HAV infection, a positive anti-HAV IgM test that is present with the onset of the disease and that persists for only 2 or 3 days is required.

Diagnosis of hepatitis B is confirmed by the detection of various hepatitis virus antigens and the antibodies that are produced in response to the infection. These antibodies and antigens and their significance include:

HBsAg—Hepatitis B surface antigen (found on the surface of the virus), indicating ongoing infection or carrier state

Anti-HBs—Antibody to surface antigen HbsAg, indicating resolving or past infection

HBcAg—Hepatitis B core antigen (found on the inner core of the virus), detected only in the liver

Anti-HBc—Antibody to core antigen HbcAg, indicating ongoing or past infection

HBeAg—Hepatitis Be antigen (another component of the HBV core), indicating active infection

Anti-HBe—Antibody to HbeAg, indicating resolving or past infection

IgM anti-HBc—IgM antibody to core antigen

Tests are available for detection of all the HBV antigens and antibodies except HBcAg. HBsAg is detectable during acute infection. Presence of HBsAg indicates that the individual has been infected with the hepatitis virus. If the infection is self-limiting, HBsAg disappears in most patients before serum anti-HBs can be detected (termed the *window phase of infection*). IgM anti-HBc is highly specific in establishing the diagnosis of acute infection, as well as during the window phase in older children and adults. However, IgM anti-HBc usually is not present in perinatal HBV infection (American Academy of Pediatrics, 2009). Neonatal infection is most likely to occur in infants born to mothers who are HbeAg positive. In contrast, hepatitis B is much less likely to occur in infants whose mothers are HbsAg positive but HbeAg negative and who have antibodies to HBeAg (Chang, 2004).

Clinical improvement is usually associated with a decrease in or disappearance of these antigens, followed by the appearance of their antibodies. For example, anti-HBc of the IgM class often occurs early in the disease, followed by a rise in anti-HBc of the IgG class. Because the antibodies persist indefinitely, they are used to identify the carrier state (individuals with HBV who have no clinical disease but are able to transmit the organism). Persons with chronic HBV infection have circulating HBsAg and anti-HBc, and on rare occasions anti-HBsAg is present. Both anti-HBs and anti-HBc are detected in persons with resolved infection, but anti-HBs alone is present in individuals who have been immunized with the HBV vaccine.

HCV-RNA is the earliest serologic marker for HCV. HCV-RNA can be detected during the incubation period before symptoms of HCV disease are expressed. A positive HCV-RNA indicates active infection, and persistence of HCV-RNA indicates chronic infection. A negative test correlates with resolution of the disease. HCV-RNA is also used to determine patient response to antiviral therapy for HCV.

The history of all patients should include questions to seek evidence of (1) contact with a person known to have hepatitis, especially a family member; (2) unsafe sanitation practices, such as contaminated drinking water; (3) ingestion of certain foods, such as clams or oysters (especially from polluted water); (4) multiple blood transfusions; (5) ingestion of hepatotoxic drugs, such as salicylates, sulfonamides, antineoplastic agents, acetaminophen, and anticonvulsants; and (6) parenteral administration of illicit drugs or sexual contact with a person who uses these drugs.

Therapeutic Management

Treatment options for viral hepatitis are limited. The goals of management include early detection, support and monitoring of the disease, recognition of chronic liver disease, and prevention of spread of the disease. No specific effective therapy for either acute or chronic hepatitis B or hepatitis C exists. Special high-protein, high-carbohydrate, low-fat diets are generally not of value. The use of corticosteroids alone or with immunosuppressive drugs is not advocated in the treatment of chronic viral hepatitis. However, steroids have been used to treat chronic autoimmune hepatitis. Hospitalization is required in the event of coagulopathy or fulminant hepatitis. Human interferon-α has been used in the treatment of chronic hepatitis B and C in adults and is being used to treat these infections in children. Therapy for hepatitis depends on the severity of inflammation and the cause of the disorder.

A number of antiviral medications are being used currently to treat HBV and HCV (Degertekin and Lok, 2009). Telbivudine is more potent than lamivudine but is associated with a high rate of antiviral resistance compared with entecavir or tenofovir. Combined therapy with lamivudine and adefovir reduces the rate of antiviral resistance compared with lamivudine monotherapy. Individualizing dose and duration of pegylated interferon and ribavirin according to on-treatment virologic response may improve sustained virologic response rates. Several specifically targeted antiviral therapies, notably protease and polymerase inhibitors, are promising but must be used in combination with pegylated interferon and ribavirin. These agents have multiple side effects, and patients require regular monitoring and support. Many products are under current investigation in clinical trials, largely with adult patients.

Prevention

Proper hand washing and Standard Precautions prevent the spread of viral hepatitis. Prophylactic use of standard immune globulin is effective in preventing hepatitis A in situations of preexposure (such as anticipated travel to areas where HAV is prevalent) or within 2 weeks of exposure.

Hepatitis B immune globulin (HBIG) is effective in preventing HBV infection after one-time exposures such as accidental needle punctures or other contact of contaminated material with mucous membranes and should be given to newborns whose mothers are HbsAg positive. HBIG is prepared from plasma that contains high titers of antibodies against HBV. HBIG should be given within 72 hours of exposure.

Vaccines have been developed to prevent HAV and HBV infection (see Table 33-3). HBV vaccination is recommended for all newborns and for high-risk groups. HAV is recommended for infants starting at 12 months. (See Immunizations, Chapter 12.) In addition, the American Academy of Pediatrics (2009) recommends universal immunization of all adolescents with the HBV vaccine. Because HDV cannot be transmitted in the absence of HBV infection, it is possible to prevent HDV infection by preventing HBV infection. The U.S. Public Health Service recommends that individuals who received an IV immune globulin preparation called Gammagard between April 1, 1993, and February 23, 1994, be screened for HCV infection and tested for aminotransferase concentrations and for the anti-HCV globulin. Routine serologic testing for anti-HCV of children born to women previously identified as being infected with HCV is also recommended (American Academy of Pediatrics, 2009).

Prognosis

The prognosis for children with hepatitis is variable and depends on the type of virus and the child's age and immunocompetence. Hepatitis A and E are usually mild, brief illnesses with no carrier state. Hepatitis B can cause a wide spectrum of acute and chronic illness. Infants are more likely than older children to develop chronic hepatitis. Hepatocellular carcinoma during adulthood is a potentially fatal complication of chronic HBV infection. Hepatitis C frequently becomes chronic, and cirrhosis may develop in these children. Limited data concerning hepatitis G suggest that the rate of progression to cirrhosis with this virus may be very low. The highest mortality occurs in hepatitis D. Viral hepatitis causes approximately 50% of the cases of fulminant hepatic failure. The mechanism by which fulminant hepatic failure occurs is not well understood, and survival varies.

Nursing Care Management

Nursing objectives depend largely on the severity of the hepatitis, the medical treatment, and factors influencing the control

and transmission of the disease. Because children with mild viral hepatitis are frequently cared for at home, it is often the nurse's responsibility to explain any medical therapies and infection control measures. When further assistance is needed for parents to comply with instructions, a public health nursing referral is necessary.

QUALITY PATIENT OUTCOMES: Hepatitis
- Increased awareness of hepatitis A and B vaccination
- Reduced spread of infection
- Minimal complications
- Inproved quality of life in cases of chronic hepatitis

Encourage a well-balanced diet and a schedule of rest and activity adjusted to the child's condition. Because the child with HAV is not infectious within a week after the onset of jaundice, the child may feel well enough to resume school shortly thereafter. Caution parents about administering any medication to the child, since normal doses of many drugs may become dangerous because of the liver's inability to detoxify and excrete them.

Standard Precautions are followed when children are hospitalized. However, these children are not usually isolated in a separate room unless they are fecally incontinent or their toys and other personal items are likely to become contaminated with feces. Discourage children from sharing their toys. (See Infection Control, Chapter 27.)

Hand washing is the single most effective measure in prevention and control of hepatitis in any setting. (For a discussion of preventive measures in the daycare center, see Chapter 15; see also Infection Control, Chapter 27.) Parents and children need an explanation of the usual ways in which HAV (fecal-oral route) and HBV (parenteral route) are spread. Parents should also be aware of the recommendation for universal vaccination against HBV for newborns and adolescents. (See Chapter 12.)

In young people with HBV infection who have a known or suspected history of illicit drug use, the nurse has the responsibility of helping them realize the associated dangers of drug abuse, stressing the parenteral mode of transmission of hepatitis, and encouraging them to seek counseling through a drug program.

CIRRHOSIS

Cirrhosis occurs as an end stage of many chronic liver diseases, including biliary atresia and chronic hepatitis. Infectious, autoimmune, or toxic factors and chronic diseases such as hemophilia and cystic fibrosis can cause severe liver damage. A cirrhotic liver is irreversibly damaged.

Pathophysiology

Cirrhosis occurs as a result of hepatocyte injury with necrosis, fibrosis, regeneration, and eventual degeneration. The diminished parenchymal cell mass causes regeneration of tissue with nodular areas of proliferating hepatocytes that stretch the surrounding connective tissue. Hepatocytes respond to injury with deposition of collagen that forms fibrous connective tissue. This scar tissue and nodular areas of regeneration impair the intrahepatic blood flow. Ongoing necrosis and self-perpetuation of this pathologic process are the result of cirrhosis.

Failure of hepatocellular function and portal hypertension occur and often lead to complications, including ascites, severe cholestasis, encephalopathy (hepatic coma), and GI bleeding.

Clinical Manifestations

Clinical manifestations of cirrhosis include jaundice, poor growth, anorexia, muscle weakness, and lethargy. Ascites, edema, GI bleeding, anemia, and abdominal pain may be present in children with impaired intrahepatic blood flow. Pulmonary function may be impaired because of pressure against the diaphragm due to hepatosplenomegaly and ascites. Dyspnea and cyanosis may occur, especially on exertion. Intrapulmonary arteriovenous shunts may develop, which can also cause hypoxemia. Spider angiomas and prominent blood vessels on the upper torso are often present.

Diagnostic Evaluation

The diagnosis of cirrhosis is based on (1) the history, especially in regard to prior liver disease, such as hepatitis; (2) physical examination, particularly hepatosplenomegaly or a sudden decrease in liver size; (3) laboratory evaluation, especially LFTs, such as bilirubin and aminotransferases, ammonia, albumin, cholesterol, and prothrombin time; and (4) liver biopsy for characteristic changes. Doppler ultrasonography of the liver and spleen is useful to confirm ascites, to evaluate the blood flow through the liver and spleen, and to determine the patency and size of the portal vein if liver transplantation is considered.

> **⚠ NURSING ALERT**
>
> The most common complication from percutaneous liver biopsy is internal bleeding. Monitor vital signs and laboratory values, especially hematocrit, for evidence of hemorrhage and shock.

Therapeutic Management

Unfortunately, there is no successful treatment to arrest the progression of cirrhosis. The goals of management include monitoring liver function and managing specific complications such as esophageal varices and malnutrition. Assessment of the child's degree of liver dysfunction is important so that the child can be evaluated for transplantation at the appropriate time.

Liver transplantation has improved the prognosis substantially for many children with cirrhosis. The combination of new immunosuppressive medications and new surgical techniques has resulted in 90% 1-year survival rates in many large hospital centers. The policy governing the allocation of livers for transplantation by the United Network for Organ Sharing allows patients with acute fulminant liver failure, plus those with failed liver grafts and the sickest pediatric patients, to be placed at the top of the network's transplantation lists (Ott, 1997). Although this change has benefited many pediatric patients, the shortage of available donors for children continues to dictate transplantation decisions, and many children continue to die while waiting for a suitable donor. (See Biliary Atresia, Chapter 11.)

Nutritional support is an important therapy for children with cirrhosis and malnutrition. Supplements of fat-soluble vitamins are often required, and mineral supplements may be indicated. In some instances aggressive nutritional support in the form of continuous tube feedings or PN may be necessary.

Esophageal and gastric varices are a life-threatening complication of portal hypertension. Acute hemorrhage is managed with IV fluids, blood products, vasopressin, and gastric lavage. Balloon tamponade with a Sengstaken-Blakemore tube may be indicated. Endoscopic sclerotherapy and endoscopic banding ligation are also effective therapies for esophageal and gastric varices.

Ascites can be managed by sodium restriction and diuretics. Severe ascites with respiratory compromise can be managed with administration of albumin or by paracentesis.

Although the full mechanism of hepatic encephalopathy is unknown, failure of the damaged liver to remove endogenous toxins, such as ammonia, plays a role. Treatment is directed at limiting the ammonia formation and absorption that occur in the bowel, especially with the drugs neomycin and lactulose. Because ammonia is formed in the bowel by the action of bacteria on ingested protein, neomycin reduces the number of intestinal bacteria so less ammonia is produced. The fermentation of lactulose by colonic bacteria produces short-chain fatty acids, which lower the colonic pH, thereby inhibiting bacterial metabolism. This decreases the formation of ammonia from bacterial metabolism of protein.

Prognosis

The success of liver transplantation has revolutionized the approach to liver cirrhosis. Liver failure and cirrhosis are indications for transplantation. Careful monitoring of the child's condition and quality of life are necessary to evaluate the need for and timing of transplantation.

Nursing Care Management

Several factors influence nursing care of the child with cirrhosis, including the cause of the cirrhosis, the severity of complications, and the prognosis. The prognosis is often poor unless successful liver transplantation occurs. Therefore nursing care of this child is similar to that for any child with a life-threatening illness. (See Chapter 23.) Hospitalization is required when complications such as hemorrhage, severe malnutrition, or hepatic failure occur. Nursing assessments are directed at monitoring the child's condition, and interventions are aimed at treatment of specific complications. If liver transplantation is an option, the family needs support and assistance to cope (see Family-Centered Care box).

> **👪 FAMILY-CENTERED CARE**
>
> **End-Stage Liver Disease**
>
> In many cases the child with liver disease and the family must cope with an uncertain progression of the disease. The only hope for long-term survival may be liver transplantation. Transplantation can be successful, but the waiting period may be long, since there are many more children in need of organs than there are donors. The procedure is expensive and is only performed at designated medical centers, which are often far from the family's home. The nurse should recognize the unique stresses of coping with end-stage liver disease and waiting for transplantation, and should offer support and assistance to the family in coping with these stressors. The assistance of social workers and support from other parents can also be beneficial.

KEY POINTS

- The essential functions of the GI system are to process and absorb nutrients necessary to maintain metabolic processes and support growth and development, to perform excretory functions, to provide detoxification, to maintain fluid and electrolyte balance, and to serve a lymphoid function.
- Digestion is the catabolism of foodstuffs (water, vitamins, minerals, carbohydrates, proteins, and fats) from their original complex form to simple, assimilable nutrients.
- The small intestine is the principal absorptive site in the GI system.
- Most ingested foreign bodies pass through the alimentary tract without difficulty. Those lodged in the esophagus or objects with sharp edges require further evaluation.
- Constipation is managed with diet changes and laxative therapy in an organized program to promote regular bowel habits.
- HD requires surgical removal of aganglionic segments of bowel.
- Nursing care of GER is aimed primarily at instructing caregivers regarding home care feeding and positioning, and caring for the child undergoing surgical intervention.
- Although the cause of appendicitis is poorly understood, it is typically a result of obstruction of the lumen, usually by a fecalith. Common signs and symptoms are colicky abdominal pain, guarding of the abdomen, and fever.
- Meckel diverticulum is a congenital malformation of the GI tract characterized by bloody stools.
- IBD refers to UC and CD. Chronic diarrhea and growth abnormalities are common features.
- Management of IBD includes nutritional support, sulfasalazine, corticosteroids or other immunosuppressive drugs, antibiotics, and general supportive therapy. Current research is focused on drugs that block the inflammatory response. Surgical removal of inflamed bowel may be necessary.

- Peptic ulcers are poorly understood, but contributing factors include interference with the normal protective mechanisms of the mucosal lining and the presence of *H. pylori*.
- General signs of GI obstruction include abdominal pain, nausea and vomiting, abdominal distention, and a decline in the amount of stool excreted.
- HPS is characterized by projectile vomiting without loss of appetite, dehydration, and metabolic alkalosis. Therapy is surgical pyloromyotomy.
- Intussusception is a common cause of intestinal obstruction during infancy. Treatment is either nonsurgical hydrostatic reduction or surgical reduction.
- Malabsorption syndromes are disorders associated with some degree of impaired digestion or absorption. They include digestive defects, absorptive defects, and anatomic defects.
- The prognosis for children with SBS improved dramatically as a result of advances in parenteral and enteral nutritional support, which is the primary therapy for this condition. Home care is important in improving these children's quality of life.
- Celiac disease is characterized by intolerance for gluten. The nurse's major role is to help the parents and child adhere to diet therapy.
- GI bleeding may be from the upper or lower GI tract. Initial management should include assessment of the magnitude of bleeding and restoration of hemodynamic stability.
- Viral hepatitis is caused by six types of virus: HAV, HBV, HCV, HDV, HEV, and HGV.
- HAV is spread by a fecal-oral route, whereas HBV and HCV viruses are transmitted primarily by the parenteral route. The single most effective measure in prevention and control of hepatitis in any setting is hand washing.
- Universal immunization against HBV is recommended for all newborns.
- Liver transplantation offers hope to children with end-stage liver disease.

ANSWERS TO CRITICAL THINKING EXERCISES

Constipation

1. **Yes,** there is sufficient evidence to arrive at some conclusions for an initial plan of management.
2. **a.** Constipation in infancy can be caused by medical conditions such as Hirschsprung disease, hypothyroidism, or strictures, or it can be simple functional constipation.
   b. In infancy, changes in dietary practices such as a change from human milk to cow's milk may precipitate functional constipation.
   c. Functional constipation is usually treated by dietary modifications such as increasing the amount of carbohydrate, fruit, or vegetables in the infant's diet.
3. Initially, the nurse practitioner can tell Harry's mother that functional constipation may occur with changes in the diet (e.g., the change from breast-feeding 6 weeks ago to bottle-feeding of cow's milk–based formula). The nurse practitioner can recommend that Harry's mother slowly introduce

cereal and prune juice into Harry's diet. Cereal and one or two offerings of fruit juice each day may help to prevent further constipation. Often, simple measures such as the introduction of solid foods or other dietary modifications help to remedy functional constipation.
4. The initial data seem to point to the conclusion that Harry has functional constipation. However, the one episode of diarrhea and the two episodes of passage of ribbonlike stools do not usually occur with functional constipation.

Inflammatory Bowel Disease

1. **Yes,** there are sufficient data to arrive at some conclusions about what to include in Susan's discharge planning.
2. **a.** The goals of nutritional support for a patient with CD include (1) correction of nutrient deficits and replacement of ongoing losses, (2) provision of adequate energy and protein for healing, and (3) provision of adequate nutrients to support normal growth.

b. See discussion on gavage feeding, Chapter 27, p. 1041.

c. Adolescents who are diagnosed with CD must adjust to the fact that they have a chronic illness that is characterized by remissions and exacerbations. CD may affect their activities of daily living, their social interactions with peers, and their ability to attend school. An important goal of therapy for adolescents with CD is to allow them to have as normal a lifestyle as possible.

3. The most immediate priority for discharge is to teach Susan and her family how to insert the NG tube, how to administer the feedings, how to obtain the supplies needed for the tube feedings at home, and how to observe for any untoward effects of the NG feedings. As Susan's discharge nurse, you should have Susan and another family member insert the NG tube, demonstrate how to check the placement of the NG tube, and show how to start and stop the feedings while Susan is in the hospital. You also need to arrange for the appropriate vendors to deliver the feeding tube supplies and feeding pump to Susan's home before discharge. While doing all this teaching, you should also be alert to any questions or anxieties that Susan or her family members may express.

4. Yes. Susan is to receive nighttime NG tube infusions at home, and her family has expressed a desire to perform this procedure at home. Therefore this discharge teaching is needed and required.

Short-Bowel Syndrome

1. Yes. The best response is answer 2. Dehydration and electrolyte disturbances are common with diarrhea. Important initial nursing interventions include assessment of the child's hydration status, including vital signs, weight, urine specific gravity, and intake and output.

2. a. SBS is a malabsorptive disorder that occurs as a result of decreased mucosal surface area, usually because of extensive resection of the small intestine.

b. Children with SBS are at risk for dehydration and electrolyte imbalance with acute episodes of diarrhea contributing to dehydration.

c. Laboratory analyses, including serum electrolytes, blood urea nitrogen, and creatinine, will also be necessary to guide the fluid and electrolyte therapy. Stool samples may need to be obtained to detect bacterial or viral pathogens.

3. Prevention of dehydration and electrolyte disturbances are priorities for this child. Temperature management also is important.

4. Children with chronic malabsorption may have severe diarrhea and are particularly susceptible to dehydration and electrolyte imbalance with an acute episode of illness such as infectious gastroenteritis.

Hematemesis

1. Yes. The best response is 4. Because this infant has acute severe gastrointestinal (GI) bleeding, immediate nursing actions include an assessment of hemodynamic status for possible shock (option 2). The infant should not be left unattended, and the nurse should immediately call for assistance because further vomiting and potential aspiration may occur.

2. a. Hematemesis in an infant can indicate GI bleeding and can quickly lead to shock. Immediate assessment of the child's hemodynamic state should be completed.

b. The diagnosis of GI bleeding is often made on the basis of the history and physical examination. Hematemesis is the vomiting of bright red blood, usually representing an upper GI source of bleeding.

3. Treatment of GI bleeding in children depends on its severity and cause. The first step in management of acute GI bleeding is to restore the child's hemodynamic stability and assess the magnitude of blood loss.

4. Severe bleeding necessitates immediate attention. Intravenous fluids (normal saline or lactated Ringer solution) are administered rapidly. Oxygen therapy is indicated if the bleeding is severe. Transfusion of blood products may be required if the blood loss is significant, and any existing coagulopathy should be corrected. The nurse should also anticipate that an NG tube will be inserted to lavage the stomach and monitor for further bleeding. A correct conclusion is that blood will need to be drawn for laboratory studies, including hemoglobin, hematocrit, platelet count, white blood cell count, and a type and crossmatch for potential transfusion.

REFERENCES

American Academy of Pediatrics, Committee on Infectious Diseases, Pickering L, editor: *Red book: report of the Committee on Infectious Diseases*, ed 28, Elk Grove Village, Ill, 2009, The Academy.

American Academy of Pediatrics, Task Force on Sudden Infant Death Syndrome: The changing concept of sudden infant death syndrome: diagnostic coding shifts, controversies regarding the sleep environment and new variables to consider in reducing risk, *Pediatrics* 116(5):1245-1255, 2005.

Baron ML: Crohn disease in children: this chronic illness can be painful and isolating, but new treatments may help, *Am J Nurs* 102(10):26-34, 2002.

Beattie RM, Croft NM, Fell JM, et al: Inflammatory bowel disease, *Arch Dis Child* 91(5):426-432, 2006.

Bensard DD, Hendrickson RJ, Fyffe CJ, et al: Early discharge following laparoscopic appendectomy in children utilizing an evidence-based clinical pathway, *J Laparoendosc Adv Surg Tech A* 19(Suppl 1):S81-S86, 2009.

Bonkovsky HL, Mehata S: Hepatitis C: a review and update, *J Am Acad Dermatol* 44(2):159-182, 2001.

Byrne WJ: Foreign bodies. In Wyllie R, Hyams JS, editors: *Pediatric gastrointestinal disease: physiology, diagnosis, management*, ed 2, Philadelphia, 1999, Saunders.

Castiglia PT: Constipation in children, *J Pediatr Health Care* 14(4):200-202, 2001.

Castiglia PT: Hepatitis in children, *J Pediatr Health Care* 10(6):286-288, 1996.

Cavataio F, Guandalini S: Gastroesophageal reflux. In Guandalini S, editor: *Essential pediatric gastroenterology and nutrition*, New York, 2005, McGraw-Hill.

Ceydeli A, Lavotshkin S, Yu J, et al: When should we order a CT scan and when should we rely on the results to diagnose an acute appendicitis? *Curr Surg* 63(6):464-468, 2006.

Chang M: Postnatal infections. In Walker WA, Goulet O, Kleinman RE, et al, editors: *Pediatric gastrointestinal disease: pathophysiology, diagnosis, management*, ed 4, Hamilton, Ontario, Canada, 2004, Decker.

Chelimsky G, Czinn S: Peptic ulcer disease in children, *Pediatr Rev* 22(10):349-355, 2001.

Christian DJ, Buyske J: Current status of antireflux surgery, *Surg Clin North Am* 85(5):931-947, 2005.

Colvin JM, Bachur R, Kharbanda A: The presentation of appendicitis in preadolescent children, *Pediatr Emerg Care* 23(12):849-855, 2007.

Craig WR, Hanlon-Dearman A, Sinclair C, et al: Metoclopramide, thickened feedings, and positioning for gastroesophageal reflux in children under two years, *Cochrane Database Syst Rev* (3):CD003502. DOI:10.1002/14651858.CD003502.pub2, 2004.

Daniels D, Grytdal S, Wasley A, et al: Surveillance for acute viral hepatitis—United States, 2007, *MMWR Surveill Summ* 58(3):1-27, 2009.

Dasgupta R, Langer JC: Hirschsprung disease, *Curr Probl Surg* 41(12):942-988, 2004.

Degertekin B, Lok AS: Update on viral hepatitis: 2008, *Curr Opin Gastroenterol* 25(3):180-185, 2009.

Diamond IR, Sterescu A, Pencharz PB, et al: Changing the paradigm: omegaven for the treatment of liver failure in pediatric short bowel syndrome, *J Pediatr Gastroenterol Nutr* 48(2):209-215, 2009.

Dieterich W, Esslinger B, Schuppan D: Pathomechanisms in celiac disease, *Int Arch Allergy Immunol* 132(2):98-108, 2003.

Dubner SE, Shults J, Baldassano RN, et al: Longitudinal assessment of bone density and structure in an incident cohort of children with Crohn's disease, *Gastroenterology* 136(1):123-130, 2009.

Dupont C, Leluyer B, Maamri N, et al: Double-blind randomized evaluation of clinical and biological tolerance of polyethylene glycol 4000 versus lactulose in constipated children, *J Pediatr Gastroenterol Nutr* 41(5):625-633, 2005.

Gilger MA: Gastrointestinal bleeding. In Walker WA, Goulet O, Kleinman RE, et al, editors: *Pediatric gastrointestinal disease: pathophysiology, diagnosis, management*, ed 4, Hamilton, Ontario, Canada, 2004, Decker.

Gilger MA: Foreign bodies of the esophagus in children, *Up To Date Online*, 2003, available at www.utdol.com/utd/content/topic.do?topicKey=pedigast/2334&type=P&selectedTitle=2~5 (accessed June 3, 2009).

Gisbert JP, de la Morena F, Abraira V: Accuracy of monoclonal stool antigen test for the diagnosis of *H. pylori* infection: a systematic review and meta-analysis, *Am J Gastroenterol* 101(8):1921-1930, 2006.

Goday PS: Short bowel syndrome: how short is too short? *Clin Perinatol* 36(1):101-110, 2009.

Gupta N, Bostrom AG, Kirschner BS, et al: Presentation and disease course in early-compared to later-onset pediatric Crohn's disease, *Am J Gastroenterol* 103(8):2092-2098, 2008.

Herwig K, Brenkert T, Losek JD: Enema-reduced intussusception management: is hospitalization necessary? *Pediatr Emerg Care* 25(2):74-77, 2009.

Hollinger LD: Foreign bodies of the airway. In Kliegman R, Behrman R, Jenson H, et al, editors: *Nelson textbook of pediatrics*, ed 18, Philadelphia, 2007, Saunders.

Huang Y, Zheng S, Xiao X: A follow-up study on postoperative function after a transanal Soave 1-stage endorectal pull-through procedure for Hirschsprung's disease, *J Pediatr Surg* 43(9):1691-1695, 2008.

Huertas-Ceballos A, Logan S, Bennett S, et al: Dietary interventions for recurrent abdominal pain (RAP) and irritable bowel syndrome (IBS) in childhood. *Cochrane Database Syst Rev* (1):CD003019. DOI: 10.1002/14651858.CD003019.pub3. 2009.

Huppertz H-I, Soriano-Gaabarro M, Grimprel E, et al: Intussusception among young children in Europe, *Pediatr Infect Dis J* 25(1):S22-S29, 2006.

Hyams JS, Markowitz JR: Can we alter the natural history of Crohn disease in children? *J Pediatr Gastroenterol Nutr* 40(3):262-272, 2005.

Kadmon G, Stern Y, Bron-Harlev E, et al: Computerized scoring system for the diagnosis of foreign body aspiration in children, *Ann Otol Rhinol Laryngol* 117(11):839-843, 2008.

Kaiser S, Frenchner B, Jorulf HK: Suspected appendicitis in children: US and CT—a prospective randomized study, *Radiology* 223(3):633-638, 2002.

Kiger JR, Brenkert TE, Losek JD: Nasal foreign body removal in children, *Pediatr Emerg Care* 24(11):785-789, 2008.

Kokke FT, Scholtens PA, Alles MS, et al: A dietary fiber mixture versus lactulose in the treatment of childhood constipation: A double-blind randomized controlled trial, *J Pediatr Gastroenterol Nutr* 47(5):592-597, 2008.

Kwok MY, Kim MK, Gorelick MH: Evidence-based approach to the diagnosis of appendicitis in children, *Pediatr Emerg Care* 20(10):690-698, 2004.

Langan RC, Gotsch PB, Krafczyk MA, et al: Ulcerative Colitis: Diagnosis and treatment, *Am Fam Physician* 76:1323-1330, 2007.

Lea E, Nawaf H, Yoav T, et al: Diagnostic evaluation of foreign body aspiration in children: A prospective study. *J Pediatr Surg* 40:1122-1127, 2005.

Leichtner AM, Higuchi L: Ulcerative colitis. In Walker WA, Goulet O, Kleinman RE, et al, editors: *Pediatric gastrointestinal disease: pathophysiology, diagnosis, management*, ed 4, Hamilton, Ontario, Canada, 2004, Decker.

Levitt MA, Martin CA, Olesevich M, et al: Hirschsprung disease and fecal incontinence: Diagnostic and management strategies, *J Pediatr Surg* 44(1):271-277, 2009.

Loening-Baucke V, Pashankar DS: A randomized, prospective, comparison study of polyethylene glycol 3350 without electrolytes and milk of magnesia for children with constipation and fecal incontinence, *Pediatrics* 118(2):528-535, 2006.

Maki M, Lohi O: Celiac disease. In Walker WA, Goulet O, Kleinman RE, et al, editors: *Pediatric gastrointestinal disease: pathophysiology, diagnosis, management*, ed 4, Hamilton, Ontario, Canada, 2004, Decker.

Menezes M, Tareen F, Saeed A, et al: Symptomatic Meckel's diverticulum in children: a 16-year review, *Pediatr Surg Int* 24(5):575-577, 2008.

Milla P: Motor disorders including pyloric stenosis. In Walker WA, Goulet O, Kleinman RE, et al, editors: *Pediatric gastrointestinal disease: pathophysiology, diagnosis, management*, ed 4, Hamilton, Ontario, Canada, 2004, Decker.

Mills JLA, Konkin DE, Milner R, et al: Long-term bowel function and quality of life in children with Hirschsprung's disease, *J Pediatr Surg* 43(5):899-905, 2008.

O'Connor A, Gisbert J, O'Morain C: Treatment of *Helicobacter pylori* infection, *Helicobacter* 14(Suppl 1):46-51, 2009.

Olson DE, Kim YW, Donnelly LF: CT findings in children with Meckel diverticulum, *Pediatr Radiol* 39(7):659-663, 2009.

Ott BB: Changes in liver transplantation policy, *Pediatr Nurs* 23(2):167-168, 1997.

Pfefferkorn M, Burke G, Griffiths A, et al: Growth abnormalities persist in newly diagnosed children with Crohn disease despite current treatment paradigms, *J Pediatr Gastroenterol Nutr* 48(2):168-174, 2009.

Philichi L: When the going gets tough: pediatric constipation and encopresis, *Gastroenterol Nurs* 31(2):121-130, 2008.

Reese GE, Constantinides VA, Simillis C, et al: Diagnostic precision of anti–*Saccharomyces cerevisiae* antibodies and perinuclear antineutrophil cytoplasmic antibodies in inflammatory bowel disease, *Am J Gastroenterol* 101:2410-2422, 2006.

Ricart E, García-Bosch O, Ordás I, et al: Are we giving biologics too late? The case for early versus late use, *World J Gastroenterol* 14(36):5523-5527, 2008.

Rubin DT, Kavitt RT: Surveillance for cancer and dysplasia in inflammatory bowel disease, *Gastroenterol Clin North Am* 35(3):581-604, 2006.

Rudolph CD, Mazur LJ, Liptak BS, et al: Guidelines for evaluation and treatment of gastroesophageal reflux in infants and children: recommendations of the North American Society for Pediatric Gastroenterology and Nutrition, *J Pediatr Gastroenterol Nutr* 32(Suppl 2):S1-S31, 2001.

Rutter MD, Saunders BP, Wilkinson KH, et al: Thirty-year analysis of colonoscopic surveillance program for neoplasia in ulcerative colitis, *Gastroenterology* 130(4):1030-1038, 2006.

Sadlier C: Intestinal failure and long-term parenteral nutrition in children, *Paediatr Nurs* 20(10):37-43, 2008.

Sauer CG, Kugathasan S: Pediatric inflammatory bowel disease: highlighting pediatric differences in IBD, *Med Clin North Am* 94(1):35-52, 2010.

Silbermintz A, Markowitz J: Inflammatory bowel diseases, *Pediatr Ann* 35(4):268-274, 2006.

Strahlman RS: Appendicitis. In Hoekelman RA, Adam H, Nelson N, et al, editors: *Primary pediatric care*, ed 4, St Louis, 2001, Mosby.

Sung JJ, Kuipers EJ, El-Serag HB: Systematic review: The global incidence and prevalence of peptic ulcer disease, *Aliment Pharmacol Ther* 29(9):938-946, 2009.

Suwandhi E, Ton MN, Schwarz SM: Gastroesophageal reflux in infancy and childhood, *Pediatr Ann* 35(4):259-266, 2006.

Theocharatos S, Kenny SE: Hirschsprung's disease: Current management and prospects for transplantation of enteric nervous system progenitor cells, *Early Hum Dev* 84(12):801-804, 2008.

Thurley PD, Halliday KE, Somers JM, et al: Radiological features of Meckel's diverticulum and its complications, *Clin Radiol* 64(2):109-118, 2009.

Tobias N, Mason D, Lutkenhoff M, et al: Management principles of organic causes of childhood constipation, *J Pediatr Health Care* 22(1):12-23, 2008.

Tran TT: Management of hepatitis B in pregnancy: weighing the options, *Cleve Clin J Med* 76(Suppl 3):S25-S29, 2009.

Uyemura MC: Foreign body ingestion in children, *Am Fam Physician* 72(2):287-291, 2005.

van der Bilt JD, Kramer WL, van der Zee DC, et al: Laparoscopic pyloromyotomy for hypertrophic pyloric stenosis: Impact of experience on the results of 182 cases, *Surg Endosc* 18(6):907-909, 2004.

Vernier-Massouille G, Balde M, Salleron J, et al: Natural history of pediatric Crohn's disease: a population-based cohort study, *Gastroenterology* 135(4):1106-1113, 2008.

Waseem M, Rosenberg HK: Intussusception, *Pediatr Emerg Care* 24(11):793-800, 2008.

Wenzi TG, Schneider S, Scheele F, et al: Effects of thickened feeding on gastroesophageal reflux in infants: A placebo-controlled crossover study using intraluminal impedance, *Pediatr* 111(4 Pt 1):2355-2359, 2003.

Wong AP, Clark AL, Garnett EA, et al: Use of complementary medicine in pediatric patients with inflammatory bowel disease: results from a multicenter survey, *J Pediatr Gastroenterol Nutr* 48(1):55-60, 2009.

Wyllie R: Ileus, adhesions, intussusception, and closed-loop obstruction. In Kliegman R, Behrman R, Jenson H, et al, editors: *Nelson textbook of pediatrics*, ed 18, Philadelphia, 2007, Saunders.

Yuen MF, Lai CL: Treatment of chronic hepatitis B, *Lancet Infect Dis* 1(4):383-393, 2001.

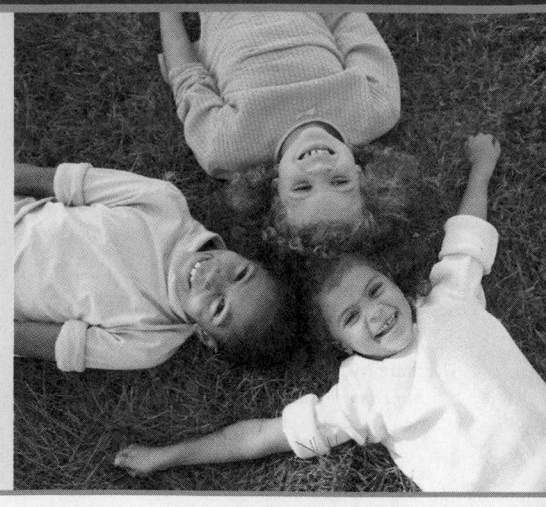

evolve WEBSITE

RELATED TOPICS

CHAPTER OUTLINE

CARDIAC STRUCTURE AND FUNCTION

Cardiovascular disorders in children are divided into two major groups: congenital cardiac defects and acquired heart disorders. Congenital heart defects are anatomic abnormalities present at birth that result in abnormal cardiac function. The clinical consequences of congenital heart defects fall into two broad categories: heart failure (HF) and hypoxemia. *Acquired cardiac disorders* refer to disease processes or abnormalities that occur after birth and can be seen in the normal heart or in the presence of congenital heart defects. They result from various factors, including infection, autoimmune responses, environmental factors, and familial tendencies.

Understanding the effects of congenital and acquired heart defects requires knowledge of the normal heart's structure and function, including embryologic development, fetal circulation, and the changes that occur with postnatal growth. Basic cardiac physiology is presented in this section; altered hemodynamics are discussed on p. 1350.

CARDIAC DEVELOPMENT AND FUNCTION

The heart is a muscular four-chambered organ whose primary purpose is to pump blood throughout the body. It is located slightly to the left of the sternum in the space between the two pleural cavities, called the mediastinum. The main mass of the heart is formed by the muscular tissue, the myocardium. Lining the inner surface of the myocardium is the endocardium, a thin layer of endothelial tissue. The heart also has its own special covering, a double-walled membrane called the pericardium. Between the two layers is a slight space (pericardial space), which is filled with a few drops of serous fluid (pericardial fluid). These layers provide for frictionless movement of the heart muscle.

The interior of the heart is divided into four chambers. The two upper chambers are called atria; the two bottom chambers are called ventricles. The atria are divided into the right atrium (RA) and the left atrium (LA) by the atrial septum. The ventricles are divided into the right ventricle (RV) and the left ventricle (LV) by the ventricular septum. Located within the heart are four valves, whose main function is to prevent the backflow of blood. The tricuspid valve, so named because it has three leaflets, or cusps, of endocardial tissue projecting into the ventricles, is located between the RA and the RV. The mitral valve has two leaflets and is located between the LA and the LV. Together these two valves are often termed atrioventricular (AV) valves. The valve leaflets are attached to the heart muscle

by several cordlike structures called chordae tendineae. The semilunar valves are located in the pulmonary artery (pulmonic valve) and the aorta (aortic valve). Heart sounds (S_1 and S_2) are related to the vibrations that result during closing of these valves. (See Chapter 6.)

Embryologic Development

The heart and other components of the circulatory system (blood, blood vessels, lymph) begin to develop from the mesoderm during the fourth week of gestation and are completely formed by the eighth week. Cardiac development progresses with the embryo's increasing nutritional needs.

During the third week, two endocardial tubes fuse to become the heart tube. As the tube elongates, it begins to coil to the right (dextro- or D-looping). This looping occurs by approximately the twenty-eighth day, when the heart begins to beat. Concentrations of mesenchymal cells enlarge and cause their lining (endocardium) to bulge into the heart lumen. These internal bulges are called *endocardial cushions* and eventually merge to divide the heart chambers.

The developing heart tube bulges until it finally lies in the pericardial cavity. The tube remains attached to the pericardium at its cephalic and caudal ends but is free at the midsection. During the fifth week the midcardiac tube grows rapidly and assumes a characteristic convoluted shape with identifiable structures. These structures ultimately give rise to the heart chambers and great vessels and include (1) a common atrium; (2) a common ventricle; (3) the bulbus cordis, which eventually helps form the outflow tracts of the ventricles; (4) the sinus venosus, which develops into the inferior and superior vena cava and coronary sinus; and (5) the truncus arteriosus, which divides into the pulmonary artery and aorta and also gives rise to the aortic arch.

The formation of the heart's internal structures, particularly the cardiac septa (partitions), takes place almost simultaneously. The atrial septum is formed by the growth of both the septum primum and the septum secundum at about the fourth week of fetal development. Overlapping of the septum primum and septum secundum before fusion results in a temporary flap opening known as the foramen ovale.

The ventricular septum develops from the joining of the muscular and membranous ventricular septa during the fourth to eighth weeks of growth. The muscular septum develops when the right and left ventricular chambers fuse, whereas the membranous septum develops out of an intricate growth of the endocardial cushions, conal cushions, and conotruncal septum (Fig. 34-1). Congenital defects may result if disturbances occur in the formation of various structures during this partitioning process.

Fetal Circulation

The characteristics of fetal circulation ensure that the most vital organs and tissues receive the maximum concentration of oxygenated blood. The fetal brain requires the highest oxygen concentration. The lungs are essentially nonfunctional, and the liver is only partially functional. Therefore the fetus needs less blood in these organs during fetal life.

Blood carrying oxygen and nutritive materials from the placenta enters the fetal system through the umbilicus via the large umbilical vein (Fig. 34-2, *A*). The blood then travels to the liver, where it divides. Part of the blood enters the portal and hepatic circulation of the liver, and the remainder travels directly to the inferior vena cava (IVC) by way of the ductus venosus. Because

of the higher pressure of blood entering the RA from the IVC, it is directed in a straight pathway across the RA and through the foramen ovale to the LA. In this way the better-oxygenated blood enters the LA and LV to be pumped through the aorta to the head and upper extremities. Blood from the head and upper extremities entering the RA from the superior vena cava (SVC) is directed downward through the tricuspid valve into the RV. From there it is pumped through the pulmonary artery, where the major portion is shunted to the descending aorta via the ductus arteriosus. A small amount flows to and from the non-functioning fetal lungs. Blood is returned to the placenta from the descending aorta through the two umbilical arteries.

Before birth, the high pulmonary vascular resistance created by the collapsed fetal lung causes greater pressures in the right side of the heart and the pulmonary artery. At the same time, the free-flowing placental circulation and the ductus arteriosus produce a low systemic vascular resistance in the remainder of the fetal vascular system. With the clamping of the umbilical cord and the expansion of the lungs at birth, the hemodynamics of the fetal vascular system undergoes pronounced and abrupt changes. These changes are the direct result of cessation of the placental blood flow and the beginning of lung respiration. Chapter 8 discusses the changes occurring at birth, and Fig. 34-2, *B*, shows the circulatory changes in the heart.

Postnatal Development

In infancy the size of the heart in relation to total body size is larger, and the heart occupies a larger space within the mediastinum. The ventricular walls are more or less equal in thickness at birth. With the postnatal rise in systemic vascular resistance, the LV walls become thicker than the walls of the RV, and the pressures on the left side of the heart rise.

Right-sided pressures decrease because the RV is pumping blood to the low-pressure pulmonary bed. An increase in heart

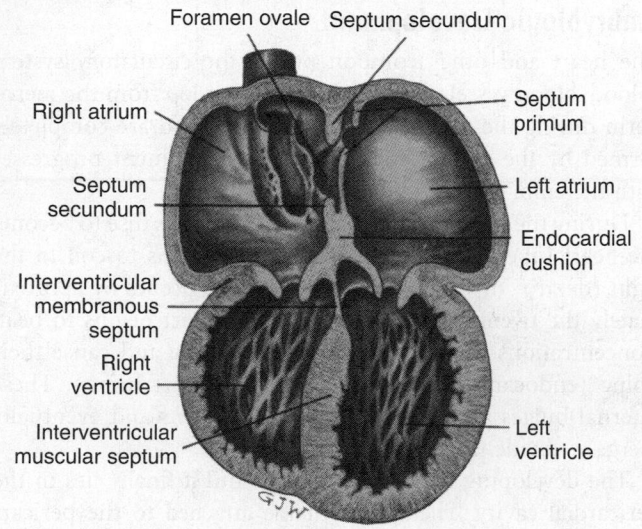

Fig. 34-1 Septal development of the heart.

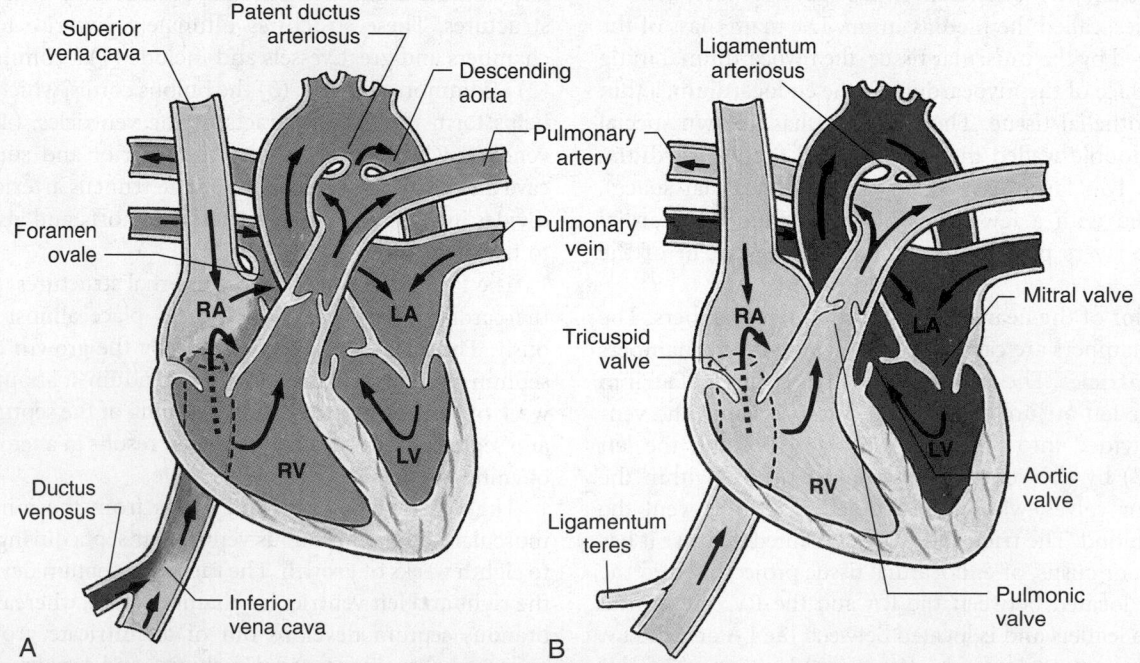

Fig. 34-2 Changes in circulation at birth. **A,** Prenatal circulation. **B,** Postnatal circulation. *Arrows* indicate direction of blood flow. Although four pulmonary veins enter the LA, for simplicity this diagram shows only two. *RA,* Right atrium; *LA,* left atrium; *RV,* right ventricle; *LV,* left ventricle.

size accompanies the adolescent growth spurt, with a resulting increase in blood pressure (BP) and decrease in heart rate. The heart rate at any age shows an inverse relationship to body size. (See inside back cover.)

The arteries and veins elongate to keep pace with expanding body dimensions, and the vessel walls thicken to cope with the increased pressure. The systolic BP after birth is low, reflecting the weaker LV of the neonate. With the developing strength and power of the left side of the heart, the systolic pressure rises rather sharply during the first 6 weeks and continues to rise but at a much slower rate until shortly before puberty, at which point it rises rapidly to adult levels. (See inside back cover.)

Postnatal Circulation

Once the cardiorespiratory system adjusts to the changes necessary to support extrauterine life, the circulation through the heart assumes a pathway that allows for oxygenation of blood by the lungs and delivery of oxygenated blood to the systemic circulation. Blood returning from the body via the SVC and IVC is received in the RA. It flows to the RV through the tricuspid valve. The RV pumps the blood through the pulmonic valve into the pulmonary artery and then to the lungs, where

the blood becomes saturated with oxygen. The blood is then returned from the lungs via the pulmonary veins into the LA, where it flows through the mitral valve to the LV, and finally through the aortic valve to the aorta and into the systemic circulation (see Fig. 34-2, *B*).

Arteries are thicker-walled blood vessels with thin muscular layers that carry highly oxygenated blood away from the heart to the capillary bed, which supplies oxygen and nutrients to the tissues. Veins are thin-walled blood vessels that return desaturated blood to the heart. The arterial system provides resistance to blood flow to maintain BP and circulation. The venous system acts as a collecting system and a reservoir to accommodate changes in circulating blood volume. Both work together to provide equilibrium and maintain BP.

The heart muscle receives its blood supply through the coronary circulation. The right and left coronary arteries, which arise above the aortic valve, supply all of the myocardium. The heart is the first organ to receive blood with each heartbeat; the brain is next. These two organs depend most on adequate oxygen levels for normal function. Coronary veins collect the blood and return it to the RA directly or through the coronary sinus, which drains into the RA. The flow of blood throughout the systemic circulatory system is shown in Fig. 34-3.

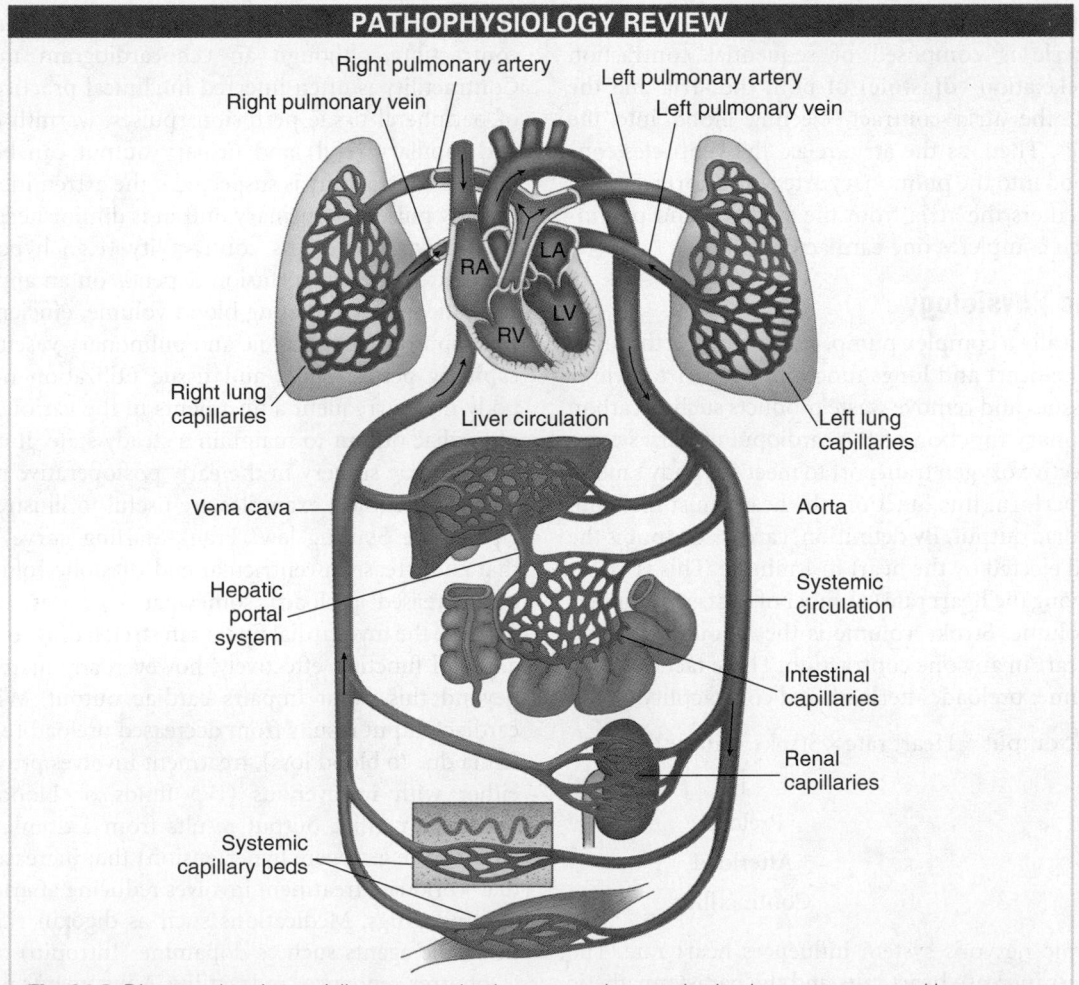

PATHOPHYSIOLOGY REVIEW

Fig. 34-3 Diagram showing serially connected pulmonary and systemic circulatory systems and how to trace the flow of blood. Right heart chambers propel unoxygenated blood through the pulmonary circulation, and the left side of the heart propels oxygenated blood through the systemic circulation. See Fig. 34-2 for abbreviations. (From McCance KL, Huether SE: *Pathophysiology: the biological basis for disease in adults and children*, ed 6, St Louis, 2010, Mosby.)

Conduction System

To maintain an orderly and effective pumping action, the heart has a specialized electrical conduction system. Electrical impulses generated within the heart initiate the mechanical contraction that leads to the circulation of blood. Although all myocardial cells are capable of developing an action potential and depolarizing without external stimulation, certain specialized cells make up the heart's normal conduction system. These structures include the following:

Sinoatrial (SA) node, located within the RA wall near the opening of the SVC

AV node, also located within the RA but near the lower end of the septum

AV bundle (bundle of His), which extends from the AV node along each side of the interventricular septum and then divides into right and left bundle branches

Purkinje fibers, which extend from the AV bundle into the walls of the ventricles

The SA node is normally the heart's pacemaker and initiates an impulse. The impulse spreads from the SA node throughout the atria to cause depolarization. As the atria depolarize, impulses spread to the AV node to conduct to the ventricles. The AV node is the major pathway by which the impulses from the atria can be transmitted to the ventricles. The impulses then spread to the AV bundle and Purkinje fibers to cause simultaneous depolarization of the ventricles.

A cardiac cycle is composed of sequential contraction (systole) and relaxation (diastole) of both the atria and the ventricles. First, the atria contract, ejecting blood into the relaxed ventricles. Then, as the atria relax, the ventricles contract to eject blood into the pulmonary artery and aorta. During diastole, blood enters the atria from the systemic and pulmonary veins, which completes one cardiac cycle.

Basic Cardiac Physiology

The heart is basically a complex pump, ejecting blood throughout the body. The heart and lungs function together to deliver oxygen to the tissues and remove waste products such as carbon dioxide. The primary function of the cardiopulmonary system is to provide effective oxygen transport to meet the body's metabolic needs. To perform this function, the heart must maintain an adequate cardiac output. By definition, **cardiac output** is the volume of blood ejected by the heart in 1 minute. This is calculated by multiplying the heart rate (number of beats per minute) by the stroke volume. Stroke volume is the amount of blood ejected by the heart in any one contraction. Three factors influence stroke volume: preload, afterload, and contractility.

$$\text{Cardiac output} = \text{Heart rate} \times \text{Stroke volume}$$

$$\uparrow$$

Preload

Afterload

Contractility

The autonomic nervous system influences heart rate. The sympathetic fibers increase heart rate, and the parasympathetic fibers, acting through the vagus nerve, decrease heart rate. Levels of circulating catecholamines and other hormones also influence heart rate. Generally, an increase in heart rate increases

cardiac output, and a decrease or irregularity in heart rate (bradycardia, dysrhythmia) impairs cardiac output. However, a very fast heart rate shortens diastole and impairs coronary artery perfusion, which causes eventual impairment of cardiac muscle function.

In simple terms, **preload** is the volume of blood returning to the heart, or the circulating blood volume. In physiologic terms, preload refers to myocardial fiber length. If the amount of blood delivered to the heart increases, then the myocardial fibers lengthen, and a greater amount of blood is pumped out of the heart. The circulating blood volume is easiest to assess clinically using the central venous pressure (CVP).

Afterload refers to the resistance against which the ventricles must pump when ejecting blood (ventricular ejection). Conditions that make it more difficult for the heart to pump blood forward into the circulation (e.g., severe hypertension) increase the afterload. Afterload is determined by several complex factors, primarily the relative resistances of the systemic circulation (systemic vascular resistance) and the pulmonary circulation (pulmonary vascular resistance). Clinically, in the absence of hemodynamic monitoring, measurement of arterial BP gives some indication of afterload. Higher BP indicates greater afterload.

Contractility refers to the efficiency of myocardial fiber shortening, or the ability of the cardiac muscle to act as an efficient pump. There is no simple bedside technique to assess contractility, although an echocardiogram may be useful. Contractility is often inferred in clinical practice. Assessments of peripheral tissue perfusion (pulses, warmth of extremities, and capillary refill) and urinary output can be helpful. Decreased contractility is suspected if the extremities are cool with thready pulses and urinary output is diminished. Certain states are known to depress contractility (e.g., hypoxia, acidosis). Adequate systemic perfusion depends on an appropriate heart rate, adequate circulating blood volume, efficient pump function, appropriate systemic and pulmonary vascular resistances, capillary permeability, and tissue utilization of oxygen. The body makes frequent adjustments in the various determinants of cardiac output to maintain a steady state. It often decreases after cardiac surgery in the early postoperative period.

Several clinical examples are useful to illustrate these principles. The Starling law (Frank-Starling curve) demonstrates that an increase in ventricular end-diastolic volume (caused by an increased preload) somewhat increases stroke volume. Because the myocardial fibers can stretch only to a certain point and still function effectively, however, any increase in volume beyond this point impairs cardiac output. When decreased cardiac output results from decreased preload (e.g., in hypovolemia due to blood loss), treatment involves providing volume, either with intravenous (IV) fluids or blood products. If decreased cardiac output results from a dramatic increase in afterload (e.g., severe hypertension) that increases the myocardial workload, treatment involves reducing afterload with vasodilating drugs. Medications such as digoxin (Lanoxin) or IV inotropic agents such as dopamine (Intropin) or dobutamine (Dobutrex) enhance contractility. Adjustments in heart rate are the most common response to changes in cardiac output. The heart rate is slowest during sleep and can more than double with strenuous physical exercise.

ASSESSMENT OF CARDIAC FUNCTION

History

Taking an accurate health history is an important first step in assessing an infant or child for possible heart disease. Parents may have specific concerns, such as poor feeding or fast breathing in their infant or the inability of their 7-year-old to keep up with his friends on the soccer field. Other parents may not realize that their child has a medical problem; the child may always have been pale and a fussy baby.

Asking details about the mother's health history, pregnancy, and birth history are important in assessing infants. Mothers with chronic health conditions, such as diabetes or lupus erythematosus, are more likely to have infants with heart disease. Some medications, such as phenytoin (Dilantin), are teratogenic to the fetus. Maternal alcohol use or illicit drug use increases the risk of congenital heart defects. Exposure to infection, such as rubella, early in pregnancy may result in congenital anomalies. Infants with low birth weight because of intrauterine growth restriction are more likely to have congenital anomalies. High-birth-weight infants, often offspring of diabetic mothers, also have an increased incidence of heart disease.

A detailed family history is also important. There is an increased incidence of congenital cardiac defects if either parent or a sibling has a heart defect. Some diseases, such as Marfan syndrome and hypertrophic cardiomyopathy, are hereditary. A family history of frequent fetal loss, sudden infant death, and sudden death in adults may indicate heart disease. Congenital heart defects occur in many disorders such as Down syndrome and Turner syndrome.

The health history of an infant should include details about feeding patterns, weight gain, and development. Feeding difficulties accompanied by fatigue, rapid breathing, and sweating with feeds and poor weight gain are common in infants with heart disease. Discuss the incidence of respiratory infections and breathing problems. Report the onset and frequency of color changes, particularly cyanosis.

With older children and adolescents, history taking should include questions about exercise tolerance and activities, edema and respiratory problems, chest pain, palpitations, and neurologic problems such as fainting or headaches. Recent infections or toxic exposures may precede the development of heart diseases such as cardiomyopathy or rheumatic fever.

In all patients, a review of all other health problems and the presence of other congenital anomalies is important. All medications taken, including over-the-counter medications and herbal supplements, should be reviewed, since prolonged or incorrect use of many medications can cause cardiac symptoms.

Physical Examination

Assessment of vital signs is helpful in screening patients for diseases of the cardiovascular system. A normal pulse rate varies with age. The younger the patient, the faster the rate. A heart rate that is abnormally fast (**tachycardia**) or abnormally slow (**bradycardia**) may indicate cardiac disease. It is important to note that an acceleration of the heart rate with inspiration is normal. A fast respiratory rate (**tachypnea**) may indicate HF. Hypertension is diagnosed by serial BP measurements.

Differences in BP between the upper and lower extremities may indicate coarctation of the aorta (see Box 34-5).

> ### ! NURSING ALERT
>
> A systolic BP difference between the upper and lower extremities with upper extremity hypertension and bounding pulses in the arms and reduced pulses in the legs is suggestive of coarctation of the aorta (Beekman, 2008).

Several aspects of physical examination may yield evidence of heart disease. (See Chapter 6 for a general discussion of physical assessment of the heart.) During inspection perform a general assessment of skin color (particularly the presence of cyanosis), position of comfort, and overall nutritional status. During palpation establish the point of maximum intensity and the apical impulse, because they may offer clues to the position of the heart. Note the presence of a thrill, a soft vibration over the heart that reflects the transmitted sound of a heart murmur. Assess the quality of chest activity ("active precordium"), quality and symmetry of all pulses, warmth of extremities, and presence or absence of edema. Locating the hepatic and splenic borders for evidence of organ enlargement is also important.

Auscultation of heart sounds begins with assessment of heart rate and rhythm. The normal heart sounds S_1 and S_2 are auscultated, and the normal physiologic splitting of S_2 is noted. This splitting is caused by the normal closure of the aortic valve before the pulmonic valve. The presence of additional heart sounds, such as a gallop or a murmur, is noted. Auscultation of lung sounds, in particular crackles, wheezing, grunting, or decreased or absent breath sounds in some areas, is also important in the assessment of cardiovascular disease.

Murmurs are heart sounds that reflect the flow of blood within the heart. They may occur in either systole or diastole or in both (a continuous murmur). They may reflect blood flow through a normal heart (particularly during periods of increased cardiac output such as fever, anemia, or rapid growth) or indicate abnormalities within the heart or the great arteries. (See Chapter 6 for a more detailed discussion of heart murmurs.) About 80% of children have an innocent murmur of one type at some point during childhood (Park, 2008). Innocent murmurs are present in infants and children with normal cardiac anatomy and heart function.

TESTS OF CARDIAC FUNCTION

A variety of invasive and noninvasive tests may be employed in the diagnosis of heart disease. Table 34-1 briefly outlines cardiac diagnostic procedures. The more frequently conducted tests are described here.

Radiologic Imaging

A chest x-ray examination is the most frequently ordered radiologic test for children with suspected cardiac problems. A chest film provides a permanent record of (1) the heart's size and configuration, its chambers, and the great vessels; and (2) the pattern of blood flow, especially in pulmonary vessels. Fluoroscopy is used mainly in conjunction with cardiac catheterization.

Animation—Heart Sounds

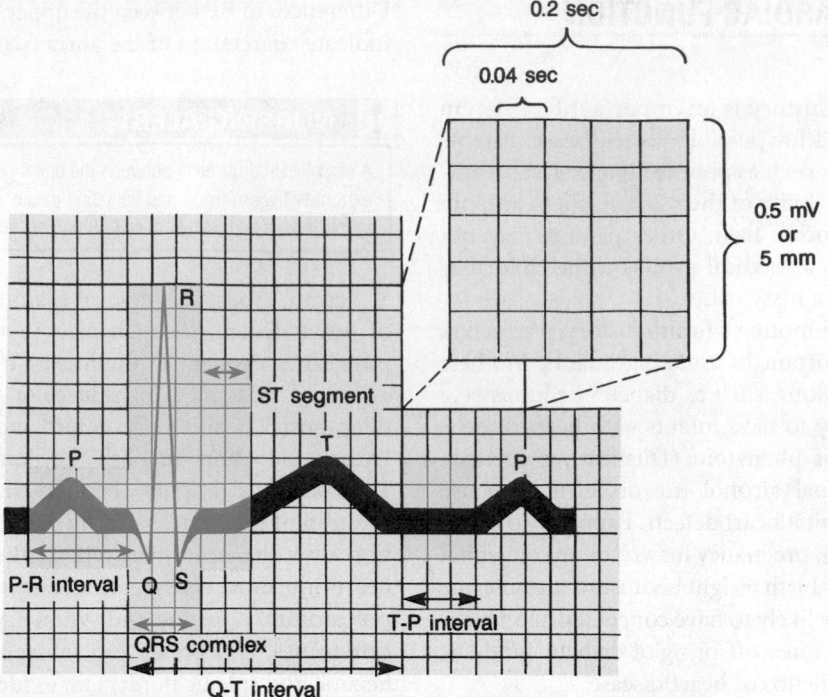

Fig. 34-4 Normal electrocardiogram pattern. Inset *(upper right)* shows conventional time and voltage or amplitude (height) calibrations.

TABLE 34-1	PROCEDURES FOR CARDIAC DIAGNOSIS
PROCEDURE	**DESCRIPTION**
Chest radiography (x-ray)	Provides information on heart size and pulmonary blood flow patterns
Electrocardiography (ECG)	Graphic measure of electrical activity of heart
Holter monitoring	24-hr continuous ECG recording used to assess dysrhythmias
Echocardiography	Uses high-frequency sound waves obtained by a transducer to produce an image of cardiac structures
Transthoracic	Done with transducer on chest
M-mode	Provides one-dimensional graphic view to estimate ventricular size and function
Two-dimensional	Provides real-time, cross-sectional views of heart to identify cardiac structures and cardiac anatomy
Doppler	Shows blood flow patterns and pressure gradients across structures
Fetal	Images fetal heart in utero
Transesophageal	Uses transducer placed in esophagus behind heart to obtain images of posterior heart structures or improve views in patients with poor images from chest approach
Cardiac catheterization	Uses radiopaque catheters placed in a peripheral blood vessel and advanced into heart to measure pressures and oxygen levels in heart chambers and visualize heart structures and blood flow patterns
Hemodynamics	Measures pressures and oxygen saturations in heart chambers
Angiography	Involves injection of contrast material to illuminate heart structures and blood flow patterns
Biopsy	Employs special catheter to remove tiny samples of heart muscle for microscopic evaluation; used in assessing infection, inflammation, or muscle dysfunction disorders and to evaluate for rejection after heart transplantation
Electrophysiologic study	Employs special catheters with electrodes to record electrical activity from within heart; used to diagnose rhythm disturbances
Exercise stress test	Monitors heart rate, blood pressure, ECG, and oxygen consumption at rest and during progressive exercise on a treadmill or bicycle
Cardiac magnetic resonance imaging	Noninvasive imaging technique; allows evaluation of vascular anatomy outside of heart (e.g., coarctation of the aorta, vascular rings) and estimation of ventricular mass and volume

Electrocardiography

Electrocardiography measures the electrical activity of the heart and records it on graph paper in the electrocardiogram (ECG). This allows the evaluation of the sequence and magnitude of the electrical impulses generated by the heart (Fig. 34-4). The normal ECG consists of:

P wave—Represents the spread of the impulse over the atria (atrial depolarization). The sinus node's electrical activity is not represented in the ECG.

P-R interval—Represents the time that elapses from the beginning of atrial depolarization to the beginning of ventricular depolarization. It is termed P-R instead of P-Q because the Q wave is frequently absent.

QRS complex—Represents ventricular depolarization. It is actually composed of three separate waves—the Q, the R, and the S—that result from the currents generated when the ventricles depolarize before their contraction.

T wave—Represents ventricular repolarization.

Q-T interval—Represents ventricular depolarization and repolarization. This interval varies with heart rate; the faster the rate, the shorter the Q-T interval. Therefore in children this interval is normally shorter than in adults.

ST segment—Represents the time that the ventricles are in the absolute refractory period, the period between ventricular depolarization and repolarization.

Information supplied by an ECG includes heart rate and rhythm and indications of conduction abnormalities, muscular damage (ischemia), hypertrophy, electrolyte imbalance, effects of various drugs, and pericardial disease. The ECG gives no direct information about the mechanical performance of the heart as a pump.

Special uses of the ECG include (1) continuous ambulatory monitoring, which employs a Holter monitor, a transistorized tape recorder attached to chest leads; and (2) exercise stress testing, in which the ECG is monitored during controlled exercise, usually on a treadmill.

An ECG is taken by placing leads or electrodes on the skin to transmit electrical impulses back to a recording machine. Usually the electrodes are attached to the extremities and chest with an adhesive, such as hydrogel, or with a suction bulb. An electrolyte lubricant is placed between the skin and the lead to increase conductivity. Chest leads must be positioned correctly, since even minor misplacement can cause considerable inaccuracy in the recording. The standard adult ECG is measured using 12 leads (six limb leads and six chest leads). The standard pediatric ECG is measured using 15 leads, with leads added on the right side of the chest and on the left lateral chest area. Although all ECG testing is painless, the leads can be frightening. Children old enough to understand benefit from an explanation of the procedure. The child must remain still for the standard ECG; infants and young children may be more cooperative if they can rest in the parent's lap during the procedure.

Bedside ECG cardiac monitoring is commonly used in pediatrics, especially in the care of children with heart disease. The bedside monitor provides valuable information about heart rate and rhythm through a graphic display of the ECG tracing and a digital display. An alarm can be set with parameters matched to individual patient requirements and will sound if the heart rate is above or below the set parameters. Gelfoam electrodes are commonly used and are placed on the right side of the chest (above the level of the heart) and on the left side of the chest; a ground electrode is placed on the abdomen (Fig. 34-5). Electrodes should be changed every 1 or 2 days because they irritate the skin. Bedside monitors are an adjunct to patient care and should never be substituted for direct assessment and auscultation of heart sounds. The nurse should assess the patient, not the monitor.

Holter recording is often used when a child is having daily symptoms of a potential arrhythmia. The Holter monitor records the heart rhythm continuously for 24 to 72 hours, using electrodes that are attached to the child's chest. The rhythm is recorded with a cassette tape and then sent to a pediatric cardiologist to interpret. Also instruct the child and the parents to keep a diary of activities so that any correlation between activity and any rhythm event may be interpreted (Park, 2008).

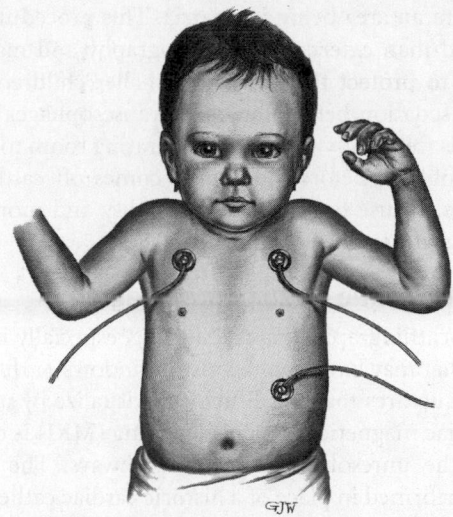

Fig. 34-5 Electrode placement for standard chest lead II in cardiac monitoring.

Echocardiography

Echocardiography is one of the most frequently used procedures for detecting cardiac dysfunction in children. Recent improvements in echocardiographic techniques have made it possible to confirm the diagnosis of many congenital heart defects without resorting to cardiac catheterization as in the past. Many defects can now be diagnosed prenatally with fetal echocardiography, and the number of infants diagnosed with heart defects in utero is rising.

Echocardiography involves the use of ultra-high-frequency sound waves to produce an image of the heart's structure. A transducer placed directly on the chest wall delivers repetitive pulses of ultrasound and processes the returned signals (echoes).

There are two types of transthoracic echocardiography. Motion-mode (M-mode) echocardiography provides a one-dimensional view of the heart and is useful in determining its size, the presence or absence of structures, and their relationship to one another. Two-dimensional (2-D), or cross-sectional, echocardiography provides information about spatial relationships between structures. Pulse, or continuous Doppler, echocardiography is primarily a velocity-sensing system and is generally used with 2-D "echo" to provide information about volume flow rate. Depending on the type of test, the nurse can obtain information regarding the integrity of septa, chamber size, and position and contractility. The nurse can also obtain information about the presence, position, size, and function of the valves, velocity of blood flow, and relationship between and size of the great vessels.

Although the test is noninvasive, painless, and associated with no known side effects, it can be stressful for children. The child must lie quietly in the standard echocardiographic positions; crying, nursing, or sitting up often leads to diagnostic errors or omissions. Therefore infants and young children may need a mild sedative (see Preoperative Sedation, p. 1007); older children benefit from psychologic preparation for the test. The distraction of a videotape is often helpful.

Transesophageal echocardiography can provide information in cases in which it is difficult to obtain information using the transthoracic approach. A transducer is passed into the esophagus to an area behind the atria. This procedure is more complicated than external echocardiography and may require intubation to protect the airway of smaller children. Patients require IV sedation before this test. Transesophageal echocardiography is frequently used in the operating room to assess for residual problems before the patient comes off cardiopulmonary bypass. Its use has reduced morbidity and mortality following surgical repair (Smallhorn, 2002).

Cardiac Magnetic Resonance Imaging

When echocardiography may be limiting, especially in the case of a child that may have poor acoustic windows or difficult and complex structures that are difficult to visualize by ultrasound alone, cardiac magnetic resonance imaging (MRI) is often used to define the unresolved anatomic pathways. The MRI can often be performed in place of a historic cardiac catheterization to obtain true three-dimensional angiography (Wood, 2006). In today's practice, cardiac MRI is increasingly used in conjunction with other imaging modalities for assessment of cardiac anatomy, measurement of blood flow, and evaluation of myocardial perfusion and viability (Prakash, Powell, Krishnamurthy, et al, 2004). Although MRI is noninvasive, children under the age of 7 often require anesthesia, deep sedation, or conscious sedation. The patient's developmental age and maturity are often the primary consideration in these choices, but length of the anticipated procedure and previous experience with such procedures should be considered (Geva and Van der Velde, 2006).

Cardiac Catheterization

The most invasive diagnostic procedure is cardiac catheterization, in which a radiopaque catheter is inserted through a peripheral blood vessel into the heart. It is usually combined with angiography (angiocardiography), in which a radiopaque contrast material is injected through the catheter and into the circulation. Cardiac catheterization provides information regarding:

- Oxygen saturation of blood within the chambers and great vessels
- Pressure changes within these structures
- Cardiac output or stroke volume (the amount of blood pumped out of the LV into the aorta with each contraction)
- Anatomic abnormalities, such as septal defects or obstruction to flow

Cardiac catheterization may be performed for diagnostic, interventional, or electrophysiologic purposes. The two main types of diagnostic cardiac catheterization are (1) right-sided, or venous, catheterization, in which the catheter is introduced from a vein into the RA; and (2) left-sided, or arterial, catheterization, in which the catheter is threaded by way of a systemic artery retrograde into the aorta and LV, or from a right-sided approach across the LA by means of a septal puncture or through an existing abnormal septal opening. In children the most common method is right-sided catheterization, since septal defects permit entry into the left side of the heart. The number of diagnostic catheterizations is decreasing as improvements in echocardiography and other noninvasive imaging methods allow more accurate diagnosis.

The catheter is usually introduced through a percutaneous puncture into the femoral vein (the catheter is threaded over a guide wire inserted through a large-bore needle). Rarely, a cutdown procedure is needed to gain access to the vein. This approach is associated with an increased risk of infection, hemorrhage, and obstruction. Once the vessel is entered, the catheter is guided through the heart with the aid of fluoroscopy. As the tubing is advanced, the child may feel pressure at the insertion site and vasospasm (fluttering) of the small vessels. Once the catheter is within the heart, blood samples and pressure readings are taken for analysis. Then contrast material may be injected and films taken of the dilution and circulation of the material. As the contrast medium is administered, the child may experience warmth, nausea, vomiting, restlessness, or headache.

Interventional cardiac catheterization is the use of a catheter to treat heart disease, such as use of a balloon catheter to dilate narrowed valves and vessels and catheter delivery of devices to close some simple defects. It has rapidly expanded in the last 20 years as new techniques, devices, and applications have been developed. It has replaced surgical treatment for some congenital heart defects, such as isolated valvular pulmonary artery stenosis, and has become an alternate therapy for others, such as patent ductus arteriosus, some atrial septal defects, and some types of ventricular septal defects. Complications are more common during interventional catheterizations and include balloon or device damage to vessels or valves and damage to structures due to thrombus or embolization (Lock, 2006).

Electrophysiologic studies are increasingly being used to evaluate and treat dysrhythmias. Diagnostic electrophysiologic catheterization employs catheters with tiny electrodes that record the heart's electrical impulses directly from the conduction system. Interventional electrophysiologic catheterization uses radiofrequency ablation to destroy accessory pathways, which cause some tachydysrhythmias.

Nursing Care Management

Cardiac catheterization has become a routine procedure and may be done on an outpatient basis. Catheterization is not without risks, however, especially in neonates and seriously ill infants and children. Possible complications include acute hemorrhage from the entry site (more likely with interventional procedures because larger catheters are used), low-grade fever, nausea, vomiting, loss of a pulse in the catheterized extremity (usually transient, resulting from a clot, hematoma, or intimal tear), and transient dysrhythmias (generally catheter induced). Therefore it is essential that the nurse employ good nursing judgment and physical assessment before and after the procedure.

Preprocedural Care. A complete nursing assessment is necessary to ensure the safety of the procedure and minimize complications. This assessment should include an accurate measurement of height (essential to correct catheter selection) and weight. Obtaining a history of allergic reactions is important, since some of the contrast agents are iodine based. Specific attention to signs and symptoms of infection is crucial. Severe diaper rash may be a reason to cancel the procedure if femoral access is required. Because assessment of pedal pulses is important after catheterization, the nurse should assess and mark

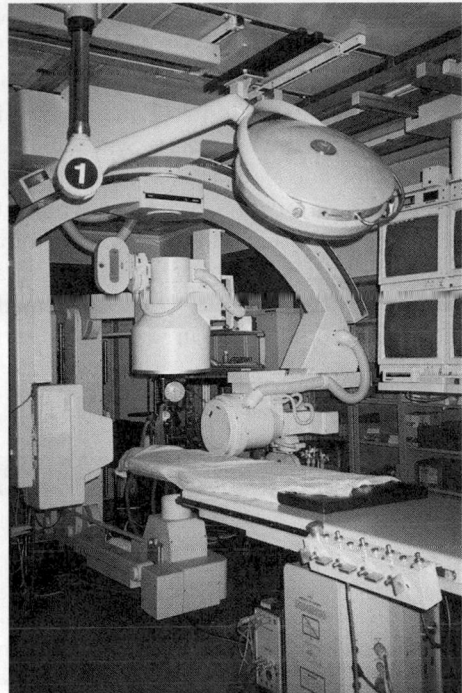

Fig. 34-6 Cardiac catheterization laboratory.

pulse locations (dorsalis pedis, posterior tibial) before the child goes to the catheterization room. Clearly document the presence and quality of pulses in both feet. Also record baseline oxygen saturation in children with cyanosis.

Preparing the child for the procedure is the joint responsibility of the physician, nurse, and parents. School-age children and adolescents benefit from a description of the catheterization laboratory (Fig. 34-6) and a chronologic explanation of the procedure emphasizing what they will see, feel, and hear. Preparation materials such as picture books or videotapes or tours of the catheterization laboratory may be helpful. Preparation should be geared to the child's developmental level. (See further discussion on p. 1376 and in Chapter 27.) The child's caregivers often benefit from the same explanations. Additional information, such as the expected length of the catheterization procedure, description of the child's appearance after catheterization, and usual postprocedural care, should be outlined.

Methods of sedation vary among institutions and may include oral or IV medications. (See Preoperative Sedation, p. 1007.) General anesthesia is usually unnecessary except in selected interventional procedures. Typically the child is allowed nothing by mouth (NPO) before catheterization, although polycythemic infants and children may require IV fluids to prevent dehydration, and neonates may need dextrose solution for up to 2 hours before the procedure to prevent hypoglycemia. Usually the morning dose of all oral medications is withheld, although this is clarified beforehand with the practitioner.

Postprocedural Care. Patients may recover from the catheterization procedure in a recovery unit or in their hospital rooms. Some may require care in the intensive care unit (ICU). Patients are usually placed on a cardiac monitor and a pulse oximeter for the first few hours after catheterization.

The most important nursing responsibility is observation of the following for signs of complications:

- Pulses, especially below the catheterization site, for equality and symmetry (Pulse distal to the site may be weaker for the first few hours after catheterization but should gradually increase in strength.)
- Temperature and color of the affected extremity, since coolness or blanching may indicate arterial obstruction
- Vital signs, which may be taken as frequently as every 15 minutes, with special emphasis on the heart rate, which is counted for 1 full minute for evidence of dysrhythmias or bradycardia
- BP, especially for hypotension, which may indicate hemorrhage from cardiac perforation or bleeding at the site of initial catheterization
- Dressing, for evidence of bleeding or hematoma formation in the femoral or antecubital area
- Fluid intake, both IV and oral, to ensure adequate hydration (Blood loss in the catheterization laboratory, the child's preprocedure NPO status, and diuretic actions of contrast material used during the procedure put the child at risk for hypovolemia and dehydration.)

Infants are particularly at risk for hypoglycemia. They should receive dextrose-containing IV fluids, and blood glucose levels should be checked.

> **! NURSING ALERT**
>
> If bleeding occurs, direct continuous pressure is applied 2.5 cm (1 inch) above the percutaneous skin site to localize pressure over the vessel puncture.

Depending on hospital policy, the child may remain in bed with the affected extremity maintained straight for 4 to 6 hours after venous catheterization and 6 to 8 hours after arterial catheterization to facilitate healing of the cannulated vessel. If younger children have difficulty complying, they can be held in the parent's lap with the leg maintained in the correct position. The child's usual diet can be resumed as soon as tolerated, beginning with sips of clear liquids and advancing as the condition allows it. Generally there is only slight discomfort at the percutaneous site. Acetaminophen (Tylenol), with or without codeine, or ibuprofen, can be given for pain. The catheterization site is covered with an occlusive waterproof pressure dressing (usually a foam tape dressing tightly applied) to prevent bleeding and contamination that could cause infection. The dressing is left on until the next day. Home care instructions are listed in the Family-Centered Care box.

CONGENITAL HEART DISEASE

The incidence of congenital heart disease (CHD) in children is approximately 5 to 8 in 1000 live births (Park, 2008). About 2 to 3 in 1000 infants are symptomatic during the first year of life with significant heart disease that requires treatment (Hoffman and Kaplan, 2002). CHD is the major cause of death (other than prematurity) in the first year of life. Although there are more than 35 well-recognized defects, the most common heart anomaly is ventricular septal defect (Box 34-1).

FAMILY-CENTERED CARE

After Cardiac Catheterization

- Remove pressure dressing the day after catheterization. Cover site with an adhesive bandage strip for several days. Put a new bandage on every day for the next 2 days.
- Keep site clean and dry. Avoid tub baths for the first 3 days; older children may shower the first day after catheterization.
- Observe site for redness, swelling, drainage, and bleeding. Monitor the child for fever. Observe the catheter leg for coolness. Notify practitioner if these occur.
- The child should avoid strenuous exercise for several days but may attend school.
- The child can resume regular diet without restrictions.
- Use acetaminophen or ibuprofen for pain.
- Keep follow-up appointments per practitioner's instruction.

Modified from Children's Hospital (Boston) Cardiovascular Program, 2009.

BOX 34-1 STATISTICS ON CONGENITAL CARDIOVASCULAR DEFECTS

A total of 3531 people in the United States died from congenital cardiovascular defects in 2005. At least 15 types of cardiovascular defects are recognized, with many additional anatomic variations.

Thousands of babies are born each year with cardiovascular defects. Of these:

- 4% to 10% have atrioventricular septal defects.
- 8% to 11% have coarctation of the aorta.
- 9% to 14% have tetralogy of Fallot.
- 10% to 11% have transposition of the great arteries.
- 14% to 16% have ventricular septal defects.
- 4% to 8% have hypoplastic left heart syndrome.

About 650,000 to 1,300,000 Americans with cardiovascular defects are alive today.

In 2006 death rates per 100,000 adults for congenital cardiovascular defects were 1.3 for white males, 1.7 for black males, 1.0 for white females, and 1.3 for black females.

Death rates for infants (<1 year) were 36.5 per 100,000 white infants and 52.2 per 100,000 black infants.

From 1996 to 2006 death rates for congenital cardiovascular defects declined 33.3%, while the actual number of deaths declined 26.7%.

From American Heart Association, *Congenital cardiovascular defects: statistics*, 2007, available at **www.americanheart.org/presenter.jhtml?identifier=4576** (accessed March 29, 2010).

The exact cause of most congenital cardiac defects is unknown. Most are thought to be a result of multiple factors—a complex interaction of genetic and environmental influences. The tremendous amount of information being discovered through molecular biology and the Human Genome Project will likely increase our understanding of the genetic causes of congenital heart defects.

Some risk factors are known to be associated with increased incidence of congenital heart defects. Maternal risk factors include chronic illnesses such as diabetes or poorly controlled phenylketonuria, alcohol consumption, and exposure to environmental toxins and infections. Family history of a cardiac defect in a parent or sibling increases the likelihood of a cardiac anomaly. The risk of CHD increases if a first-degree relative (parent or sibling) is affected. The familial risk is higher with left-sided obstructive lesions.

Congenital heart anomalies are often associated with chromosomal abnormalities, specific syndromes, or congenital defects in other body systems (see Research Focus box). Down syndrome (trisomy 21) and trisomy 13 and 18 are highly correlated with congenital heart defects. Syndromes associated with heart defects include Noonan syndrome (pulmonic valve anomalies and cardiomyopathy), Williams syndrome (aortic and pulmonic stenosis), and Holt-Oram syndrome (upper limb anomalies and atrial septal defect). Extracardiac defects such as tracheoesophageal fistula, renal abnormalities, and diaphragmatic hernia are seen in association with heart anomalies.

RESEARCH FOCUS

DiGeorge Syndrome

DiGeorge syndrome is a genetic disorder that presents with multiple health complications, commonly cardiac defects. Recent research in gene mapping has identified deletion of part of chromosome 22 (22q11) in patients with DiGeorge syndrome, velocardiofacial syndrome, and conotruncal anomaly face syndrome. The features of these syndromes include congenital cardiac defects, soft palate abnormalities, dysmorphic facial features, and speech and developmental delays. In addition, mild immunologic abnormalities of T cells, absence or hypoplasia of the thymus, and parathyroid abnormalities resulting in hypocalcemia are seen with DiGeorge syndrome. Commonly associated cardiac defects are interrupted aortic arch, truncus arteriosus, tetralogy of Fallot, and posterior malaligned ventricular septal defects. These congenital defects occur in 75% to 80% of patients with a 22q11 deletion (Goldmuntz and Lin, 2008).

ALTERED HEMODYNAMICS

If the physiology of heart defects is to be understood, the role of pressure gradients, flow, and resistance within the circulation must be reviewed. Blood flows because of pressure gradients in different parts of the body and because of the heart's pumping action. Like any fluid, blood flows from an area of high pressure to one of low pressure and takes the path of least resistance. The rate of flow is directly proportional to the pressure gradient (i.e., the higher the pressure gradient, the greater the rate of flow) and inversely proportional to the resistance (i.e., the higher the resistance, the lower the rate of flow). However, increased resistance does not always decrease flow. If the proximal cardiac chamber can increase the driving pressure proportionally, flow can remain unchanged.

Normally the pressure on the right side of the heart is lower than that on the left side, and the resistance in the pulmonary circulation is less than that in the systemic circulation. Likewise, vessels entering or exiting these chambers have corresponding pressures (e.g., lower pressure in the pulmonary artery and higher pressure in the aorta). Therefore, if an abnormal connection exists between the heart chambers, such as a septal defect, blood flows from an area of higher pressure (left side) to one of lower pressure (right side). This directional flow of blood is termed a *left-to-right shunt*. If the opening is small, the amount of blood shunted to the atrium or ventricle may be minimal.

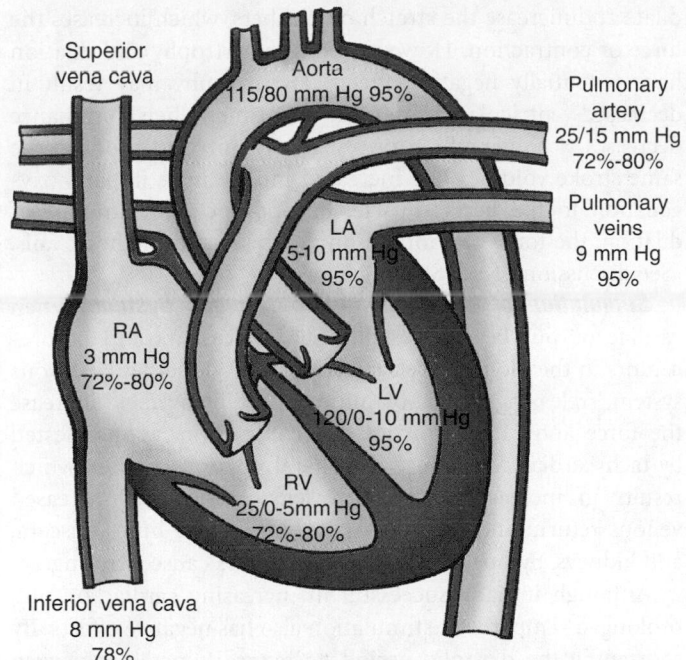

Fig. 34-7 Normal chamber pressures (mm Hg) and oxygen saturations (SaO₂) in cardiac chambers and great arteries. For simplicity, only two of the four pulmonary veins are shown. See Fig. 34-2 for abbreviations.

An understanding of saturations within the heart is also helpful in understanding CHD. The blood returning to the heart via the great veins (the SVC and the IVC) should have the lowest oxygen saturation because the tissues should have extracted oxygen, leaving the venous blood desaturated. Saturations in the RA, RV, and pulmonary artery should be equal. Blood returning from the lungs to the heart through the pulmonary veins should be fully saturated, the most oxygen-rich blood in the body. Saturations on the left side of the heart should all be equal, with fully saturated blood entering the aorta and first supplying the heart muscle through the coronary arteries and then supplying the brain (Fig. 34-7). Normally, saturated blood circulates separately from desaturated blood. Depending on the type of defect, saturated and desaturated blood may be mixed. The amount of mixed blood that reaches the systemic circulation is a significant feature of several cardiac anomalies, and varying degrees of hypoxemia and cyanosis result.

CLINICAL CONSEQUENCES OF CONGENITAL HEART DISEASE

Depending on the severity of the cardiac defect and the altered hemodynamics, two principal clinical consequences can occur: HF and hypoxemia. Defects that result in left-to-right shunting of blood cause symptoms of HF. Defects that result in decreased pulmonary blood flow cause cyanosis. The conditions can occur alone or together. Pulmonary hypertension, an uncommon condition, may occur as a result of congenital heart defects and is included in this section, although some cases may occur from unknown causes. Nursing care plays a critical role in the early identification and supportive management of these conditions.

HEART FAILURE

HF is the inability of the heart to pump an adequate amount of blood to the systemic circulation at normal filling pressures to meet the body's metabolic demands. Causes of HF can be classified in terms of the following changes:

- Volume overload, especially with left-to-right shunts that may cause the RV to hypertrophy to compensate for the additional blood volume
- Pressure overload, primarily resulting from obstructive lesions, such as valvular stenosis or coarctation of the aorta
- Decreased contractility, primarily decreased contractility of the myocardium, caused by factors such as cardiomyopathy or myocardial ischemia from severe anemia or asphyxia; heart block; acidemia; and low levels of potassium, glucose, calcium, or magnesium
- High cardiac output demands, in which the body's need for oxygenated blood exceeds the heart's cardiac output (even though the volume may be normal), such as in sepsis, hyperthyroidism, and severe anemia

The etiology of heart failure varies according to the age of onset; HF occurs in children with both CHD and normal cardiac structure (Box 34-2). HF occurs most frequently secondary to congenital heart defects in which structural abnormalities result in an increased volume load or increased pressure load on the ventricles. For example, septal defects can cause large left-to-right shunts, which result in a volume load on the RV. Obstruction to flow out of the LV, such as narrowing of the aorta (coarctation of the aorta), can cause increased pressure inside the ventricle. HF can also be a result of an excessive workload on a normal myocardium. Myocardial failure, in which the contractility of the heart muscle is impaired, can result from cardiomyopathy, drugs, electrolyte imbalances, dysrhythmias, and other causes. Diseases in other organ systems, particularly the lungs, also can cause HF. Obstructive changes in the lungs result in increased pulmonary vascular resistance, which increases the RV workload. In time, the right side of the heart has difficulty pumping blood forward to the lungs, becomes dilated, and hypertrophies; then signs and symptoms of right-sided heart failure are seen. *Cor pulmonale* is the term for HF resulting from obstructive lung diseases such as cystic fibrosis or bronchopulmonary dysplasia.

Pathophysiology

Theoretically, heart failure may be divided into two types: right-sided failure and left-sided failure. In right-sided failure, RV function is reduced. RV end-diastolic pressure rises, causing increased CVP and systemic venous engorgement. Systemic venous hypertension causes hepatomegaly and may cause edema in the extremities. In left-sided failure, LV dysfunction occurs and LV end-diastolic pressure rises; the result is increased pressure in the LA and also in the pulmonary veins. The lungs become congested with blood, which leads to elevated pulmonary pressures and pulmonary edema.

Although each type of heart failure produces different signs and symptoms, clinically it is unusual to observe solely right- or left-sided failure in children. Because each side of the heart

BOX 34-2 ETIOLOGIES OF HEART FAILURE BY AGE

Neonate or Infant
Normal Cardiac Structure
Anemia
Dysrhythmias
Cardiomyopathy
Electrolyte imbalances
Endocrinopathies
Extracardiac shunts
Hypertension
Hypoxic-ischemic events
Kawasaki disease
Sepsis

Congenital Heart Disease
Obstruction to flow out of the left ventricle (aortic stenosis, coarctation of the aorta)
Obstruction to flow into the left ventricle (mitral stenosis)
Pulmonary vein stenosis
Total anomalous pulmonary venous connection
Systemic ventricular volume overload (aortic or mitral valve regurgitation, patent ductus arteriosus, atrioventricular canal defect, ventricular septal defect)
Single ventricle
Truncus arteriosus

Child or Adolescent
Normal Cardiac Structure
Anemia
Dysrhythmias
Cardiomyopathy
Hypertension
Inherited
Kawasaki disease
Medications
Myocarditis
Renal failure
Other noncardiac diseases (e.g., muscular dystrophy, cystic fibrosis)

Congenital Heart Disease
Aortic regurgitation
Mitral regurgitation
Mitral stenosis
Pulmonary vein stenosis
Failed palliation procedures

Adapted from Margossian R: Contemporary management of pediatric heart failure, *Expert Rev Cardiovasc Ther* 6(2):187-197, 2008.

depends on adequate functioning of the other side, failure of one chamber causes a reciprocal change in the opposite chamber.

Compensatory Mechanisms

The heart initially tries to meet the body's demand for increased cardiac output through several compensatory mechanisms called the cardiac reserve. These include hypertrophy and dilation of the cardiac muscle and stimulation of the sympathetic nervous system (Fig. 34-8).

Hypertrophy and Dilation of the Cardiac Muscle. In response to the need to increase cardiac output, the cardiac muscle hypertrophies, developing greater tension. It is able to generate increased pressure within the ventricle, pumping blood out of the heart at a higher pressure. Also, the cardiac muscle can dilate and increase the stretch of its fibers, which increases the force of contraction. However, both hypertrophy and dilation have potentially negative effects. Hypertrophy may result in decreased ventricular compliance over time. When compliance decreases, a higher filling pressure is required to produce the same stroke volume. The increased muscle mass impairs oxygenation to the heart muscle. Beyond a certain amount of dilation, the force of contraction decreases and the heart fails. (See discussion of the Starling law, p. 1344.)

Stimulation of the Sympathetic Nervous System. When cardiac output begins to fall, stretch receptors and baroreceptors in the blood vessels stimulate the sympathetic nervous system, releasing catecholamines. Catecholamines increase the force and rate of myocardial contraction, as manifested by tachycardia. They cause peripheral vasoconstriction, which results in increased systemic vascular resistance; increased venous return; and reduced blood flow to the limbs, viscera, and kidneys. Sympathetic cholinergic fibers cause sweating.

Although initially successful in increasing cardiac output, prolonged sympathetic stimulation also has negative effects. By shortening the diastolic period, tachycardia increases oxygen consumption by the heart muscle, eliminates the heart's resting phase, and impairs coronary artery perfusion. A continued increase in systemic vascular resistance increases the afterload on the heart muscle, which requires extra work by the heart muscle and reduces systemic blood flow.

The renal system is particularly sensitive to reductions in blood flow and renal perfusion, which activate the renin-angiotensin-aldosterone mechanism. Renin-angiotensin secretion causes vasoconstriction and leads to an increase in aldosterone secretion, which causes retention of salt and water. Retention of salt and water causes an increase in preload. Although at first helpful to the failing heart, the sodium and water retention becomes excessive, resulting in signs of systemic venous congestion and fluid overload.

Clinical Manifestations

As the capacity of the compensatory mechanisms is exceeded, the child exhibits signs of HF because of decreased myocardial contraction, increased preload, and increased afterload. The signs and symptoms of HF can be divided into three groups: (1) impaired myocardial function, (2) pulmonary congestion, and (3) systemic venous congestion (Box 34-3). Because these hemodynamic changes occur from different causes and at differing times, the clinical presentation may vary among children.

Impaired Myocardial Function

One of the earliest signs of HF is tachycardia (sleeping heart rate >160 beats/min in infants) as a direct result of sympathetic stimulation. Heart rate is elevated even during rest but becomes extremely rapid with the slightest exertion. Ventricular dilation and excess preload result in extra heart sounds S_3 and S_4, referred to as gallop rhythm. Diaphoresis often occurs, especially on the head during exertion. Children are easily fatigued, have poor exercise tolerance, and are often irritable. Decreased cardiac output results in poor perfusion, manifested by cold extremities, weak pulses, slow capillary refill, low BP, and mottled skin. Extreme pallor or duskiness is an ominous sign.

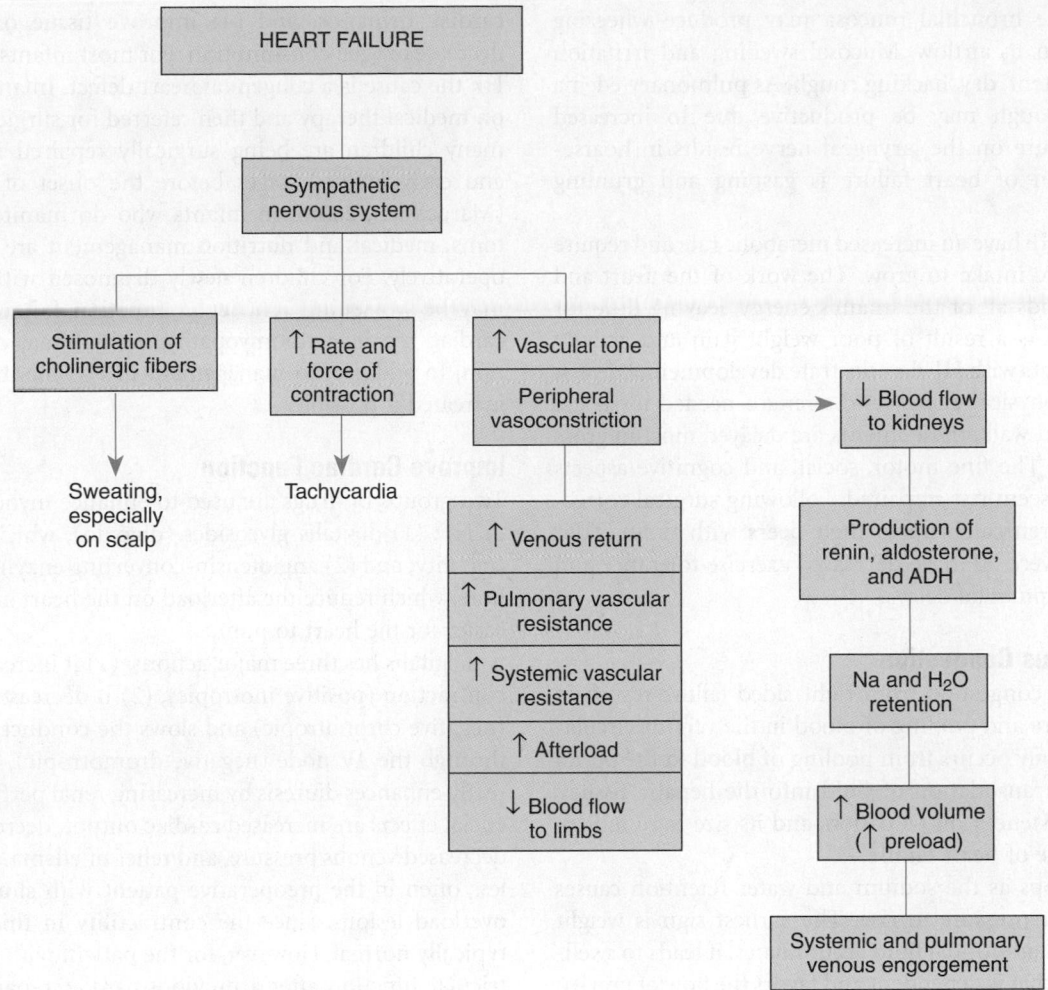

Fig. 34-8 Pathophysiology of heart failure. *ADH*, Antidiuretic hormone.

BOX 34-3   CLINICAL MANIFESTATIONS OF HEART FAILURE

Impaired Myocardial Function
Tachycardia
Sweating (inappropriate)
Decreased urinary output
Fatigue
Weakness
Restlessness
Anorexia
Pale, cool extremities
Weak peripheral pulses
Decreased blood pressure
Gallop rhythm
Cardiomegaly

Pulmonary Congestion
Tachypnea
Dyspnea
Retractions (infants)
Flaring nares
Exercise intolerance
Orthopnea
Cough, hoarseness
Cyanosis
Wheezing
Grunting

Systemic Venous Congestion
Weight gain
Hepatomegaly
Peripheral edema, especially periorbital
Ascites
Neck vein distention (children)

Pulmonary Congestion

Tachypnea (respiratory rate >60 breaths/min in infants) occurs in response to decreased lung compliance (ability to expand). Tachypnea can lead to hypoxemia because oxygen does not reach the alveoli for gas exchange in adequate amounts with fast breathing rates. Mild cyanosis results from impaired gas exchange and is relieved by oxygen administration. Dyspnea is caused by a decrease in the distensibility of the lungs. Inability to feed with resultant poor weight gain is primarily a result of tachypnea and dyspnea on exertion. Costal retractions occur as the pliable chest wall in the infant is drawn inward during attempts to ventilate the noncompliant lungs. Initially dyspnea may be evident only on exertion, but it may progress to the point that even slight activity results in labored breathing. In infants dyspnea at rest is a prominent sign and may be accompanied by flaring nares.

As the LV fails, blood volume and pressure increase in the LA, pulmonary veins, and lungs. Eventually the pulmonary capillary pressure exceeds the plasma osmotic pressure, which forces fluid into the interstitial space and finally causes pulmonary edema. Increased interstitial lung water also decreases the compliance of the lungs and increases the work of breathing.

Orthopnea (dyspnea in the recumbent position) is caused by increased blood flow to the heart and lungs from the extremities. It is relieved by sitting up, since then blood pools in the lower extremities, which decreases venous return. In addition, this position decreases pressure from the abdominal organs on the diaphragm. In infants orthopnea may be evident in the inability to lie supine and the desire to be held upright.

Edema of the bronchial mucosa may produce wheezing from obstruction to airflow. Mucosal swelling and irritation result in a persistent, dry, hacking cough. As pulmonary edema increases, the cough may be productive due to increased secretions. Pressure on the laryngeal nerve results in hoarseness. A late sign of heart failure is gasping and grunting respirations.

Infants with HF have an increased metabolic rate and require additional caloric intake to grow. The work of the heart and breathing demands all of the infant's energy, leaving little for normal activity. As a result of poor weight gain and activity intolerance, infants with HF demonstrate developmental delays. Because of the physical energy and strength needed to sit up, pull to stand, and walk, these infants are delayed most in gross motor activities. The fine motor, social, and cognitive aspects of development seem less impaired. Following surgical correction, most children catch up to their peers with time. Older children with severe HF have decreased exercise tolerance and persistent developmental delays.

Systemic Venous Congestion

Systemic venous congestion from right-sided failure results in increased pressure and pooling of blood in the venous circulation. Hepatomegaly occurs from pooling of blood in the portal circulation and transudation of fluid into the hepatic tissues. The liver may be tender on palpation, and its size is an indication of the course of heart failure.

Edema develops as the sodium and water retention causes systemic vascular pressure to rise. The earliest sign is weight gain. However, as additional fluid accumulates, it leads to swelling of soft tissue that is dependent and favors the flow of gravity, such as the sacral area and scrotum (when recumbent) and loose periorbital tissues. In infants edema is usually generalized and difficult to detect. Gross fluid accumulation may produce ascites and pleural effusions.

Distended neck and peripheral veins result from consistently elevated CVP. Normally neck and hand veins collapse when the head or hands are raised above the level of the heart, because the blood drains by gravity back to the heart. When the venous pressure is high, however, it slows venous return, which causes the veins to remain distended. Distended neck veins are difficult to detect in the short, fat necks of infants and are usually observed only in older children.

Diagnostic Evaluation

Diagnosis is made on the basis of clinical symptoms such as tachypnea and tachycardia at rest, dyspnea, retractions, activity intolerance (especially during feeding in infants), weight gain caused by fluid retention, and hepatomegaly. A chest x-ray film demonstrates cardiomegaly and increased pulmonary vascular markings due to increased pulmonary blood flow. Signs of ventricular hypertrophy appear on the ECG. Echocardiography is performed to determine the cause of HF, such as a congenital heart defect or poor ventricular function.

Therapeutic Management

The goals of treatment are to (1) improve cardiac function (increase contractility and decrease afterload), (2) remove accumulated fluid and sodium (decrease preload), (3) decrease cardiac demands, and (4) improve tissue oxygenation and decrease oxygen consumption. For most infants diagnosed with HF the cause is a congenital heart defect. Infants are stabilized on medical therapy and then referred for surgical repair. Today many children are being surgically repaired in the neonatal and early infancy stages before the onset of HF symptoms (Margossian, 2008). In infants who do manifest these symptoms, medical and nutrition management are optimized preoperatively. For children newly diagnosed with HF the cause may be worsening ventricular function following a previous cardiac repair, cardiomyopathy, arrhythmia, or other condition. In addition to management of HF, the underlying cause is treated if possible.

Improve Cardiac Function

Two groups of drugs are used to enhance myocardial function in HF: (1) digitalis glycosides (digoxin), which improve contractility; and (2) angiotensin-converting enzyme (ACE) inhibitors, which reduce the afterload on the heart and thus make it easier for the heart to pump.

Digitalis has three major actions: (1) it increases the force of contraction (positive inotropic), (2) it decreases the heart rate (negative chronotropic) and slows the conduction of impulses through the AV node (negative dromotropic), and (3) it indirectly enhances diuresis by increasing renal perfusion. The beneficial effects are increased cardiac output, decreased heart size, decreased venous pressure, and relief of edema. Digoxin is used less often in the preoperative patient with shunt and volume overload lesions, since the contractility in this population is typically normal. However, for the patient with worsening ventricular function after a previous cardiac repair, digoxin continues to be used in conjunction with ACE inhibitors, diuretics, and beta blockers.

In pediatrics, digoxin is used because of its rapid onset of action and decreased risk of toxicity as a result of its relatively short half-life (1½ days) compared with other digitalis preparations. It is available as an elixir (50 mcg/ml) for oral administration or in a parenteral preparation (0.1 mg/ml). For infants the dosage is often calculated in micrograms (1000 mcg = 1 mg). Because digoxin has a very narrow margin of safety, the dosage must be calculated exactly. Premature infants are more sensitive to digoxin and require smaller dosages because their impaired renal excretion causes the drug to accumulate in the blood faster than in full-term infants and children.

Treatment involves administration of a digitalizing dose, given intravenously or orally in divided doses over 24 hours to bring the child's serum digoxin level into the therapeutic range. A maintenance dose, usually one eighth of the digitalizing dose, is given orally twice a day to maintain blood levels (Table 34-2).

Digoxin is the only oral inotropic agent generally available for infants and children, although other oral inotropic agents are being used in clinical trials in adults. For patients with severe HF, IV inotropic agents such as dopamine or milrinone are used to improve contractility. They are generally given in ICU settings.

Another group of drugs used in the treatment of HF, the ACE inhibitors, inhibits the normal function of the renin-angiotensin system in the kidney. The production of renin

TABLE 34-2	ORAL DIGOXIN DOSAGE IN INFANTS AND CHILDREN*	
AGE	**TOTAL DIGITALIZING DOSE†**	**DAILY MAINTENANCE DOSE‡**
Premature infant	20	5
Full-term infant	30	8-10
<2 yr	40-50	10-12
>2 yr	30	8-10

*Dosage in mcg/kg of body weight.
†Total dose given in several divided doses over 12-24 hr.
‡Maintenance dose given in two divided doses.

triggers the production of angiotensin I and angiotensin II, which cause vasoconstriction and aldosterone secretion. The ACE inhibitors block the conversion of angiotensin I to angiotensin II so that, instead of vasoconstriction, vasodilation occurs. Vasodilation results in decreased pulmonary and systemic vascular resistance, decreased BP, a reduction in afterload, and decreased RA and LA pressures. It also reduces the secretion of aldosterone, which reduces preload by preventing volume expansion from fluid retention and decreases the risk of hypokalemia. Renal blood flow is improved, which enhances diuresis.

ACE inhibitors are employed frequently in pediatrics, but their use in children has not been extensively studied. Common medications in this class are captopril (Capoten), given three times a day; enalapril (Vasotec), given twice a day; and lisinopril, given once daily. The principal side effects of ACE inhibitors are hypotension, renal dysfunction, and cough. Captopril may also have some immune-based side effects, including fever and allergic reactions. Because enalapril has the same principal side effects but fewer immune-based side effects, patients may be switched from one preparation to the other (see Box 34-12) (Phillips and Somers, 2000).

⚡ DRUG ALERT

ACE Inhibitors

Because ACE inhibitors also block the action of aldosterone, the addition of potassium supplements or spironolactone (Aldactone) to the drug regimen of patients taking diuretics is usually not needed and may cause hyperkalemia.

Beta blockers, specifically metoprolol and carvedilol (Coreg), are the newest medications to be added to the treatment of some children with chronic HF. The α- and β-adrenergic receptors are blocked, causing decreased heart rate, decreased BP, and vasodilation. In addition, beta blockers have antiarrhythmic effects, coronary artery vasodilatory effects, and negative chronotropic effects (Moffett and Chang, 2006). Carvedilol has been shown to decrease morbidity and mortality in some adults with heart failure and is being used selectively in children. When added to standard heart failure therapy, it improved symptoms and LV function in a recent multicenter study (Bruns, Chrisant, Lamour, et al, 2001). Side effects included dizziness, headache, and hypotension.

Cardiac resynchronization therapy (CRT) using biventricular pacing is an effective treatment in adult patients with heart failure and is beginning to be applied in the pediatric population. With pharmacologic therapies discussed above, CRT has the potential to improve cardiac function in this group of patients. The causes for heart failure in the young are more varied and often include patients with a single ventricle, making CRT more challenging. Initial studies of CRT in this population demonstrate improved outcomes in those with adequate follow-up (Cecchin, Frangini, Brown, et al, 2009; Dubin, Janousek, Rhee, et al, 2005).

Remove Accumulated Fluid and Sodium

Treatment to remove accumulated fluid and sodium consists of administration of diuretics, possible fluid restriction, and possible sodium restriction. Diuretics are the mainstay of therapy to eliminate excess water and salt and to prevent reaccumulation. The most commonly used agents are listed in Table 34-3. Because furosemide (Lasix) and the thiazides cause loss of potassium, the child receives potassium supplements and rich dietary sources of the electrolyte (see Evidence-Based Practice box).

❗ NURSING ALERT

A fall in the serum potassium level enhances the effects of digoxin, increasing the risk of digoxin toxicity. Increased serum potassium levels diminish digoxin's effect. Therefore serum potassium levels (normal range, 3.5 to 5.5 mmol/L) must be carefully monitored.

Fluid restriction may be required in the acute stages of HF and must be carefully calculated to avoid dehydrating the child, especially if cyanotic CHD and significant polycythemia are present. Infants rarely need fluid restriction, since HF makes feeding so difficult that they struggle to take maintenance fluids.

Sodium-restricted diets are used less often in children than in adults to control HF because of their potential negative effects on the child's appetite and ultimate growth. If salt intake is restricted, the diet usually focuses on avoiding additional table salt and highly salted foods. Low-salt formulas are available but are used infrequently, since infants need a normal sodium source to offset the sodium depletion of chronic diuretic therapy. Most infant formulas have slightly more sodium than does breast milk.

Decrease Cardiac Demands

To lessen the workload on the heart, metabolic needs are minimized by (1) providing a neutral thermal environment to prevent cold stress in infants, (2) treating any existing infections, (3) reducing the effort of breathing (by placement in semi-Fowler position), (4) using medication to sedate an irritable child, and (5) providing for rest and decreasing environmental stimuli.

Improve Tissue Oxygenation

All the preceding measures serve to increase tissue oxygenation, either by improving myocardial function or by lessening tissue

TABLE 34-3 DIURETICS USED IN HEART FAILURE

ACTIONS	COMMENTS	NURSING CARE MANAGEMENT
Furosemide (Lasix)		
Blocks reabsorption of sodium and water in proximal renal tubule and interferes with reabsorption of sodium in the loop of Henle and in the most proximal portion of distal tubule	Drug of choice in severe heart failure Causes excretion of chloride and potassium (hypokalemia may precipitate digitalis toxicity)	Begin to record output as soon as drug is given. Observe for dehydration caused by profound diuresis. Observe for side effects (nausea and vomiting, diarrhea, ototoxicity, hypokalemia, dermatitis, postural hypotension). Encourage consumption of foods high in potassium and/or give potassium supplements. Monitor chloride and acid-base balance with long-term therapy. Observe for signs of digoxin toxicity.
Chlorothiazide (Diuril)		
Acts directly on distal tubules to decrease sodium, water, potassium, chloride, and bicarbonate absorption	Less frequently used drug Causes hypokalemia, acidosis in large doses	Observe for side effects (nausea, weakness, dizziness, paresthesia, muscle cramps, skin eruptions, hypokalemia, acidosis). Encourage consumption of foods high in potassium and/or give potassium supplements.
Spironolactone (Aldactone)		
Blocks action of aldosterone, which promotes retention of sodium and excretion of potassium	Weak diuretic Has potassium-sparing effect; frequently used with thiazides, furosemide Poorly absorbed from gastrointestinal tract Takes several days to achieve maximum actions	Observe for side effects (skin rash, drowsiness, ataxia, hyperkalemia). Do not administer potassium supplements.

EVIDENCE-BASED PRACTICE

Ashley R. Breland

Diuretics in Children with Acute Heart Failure

ASK THE QUESTION

In children with acute heart failure are loop diuretics an effective part of treatment?

SEARCH FOR THE EVIDENCE

Search strategies

Search criteria included English-language publications, research-based articles on infants and children with acute heart failure who received loop diuretics.

Databases used

Cochrane Collaboration, Joanna Briggs Institute, National Guideline Clearinghouse (AHRQ), PubMed

CRITICALLY ANALYZE THE EVIDENCE

GRADE criteria: Evidence quality moderate; recommendation strong (Guyatt, Oxman, Vist, et al, 2008)

A review of the literature revealed one meta-analysis and one observational study. The meta-analysis and observational study were conducted in the adult population.

The meta-analysis included 14 randomized control trials (seven were placebo controlled, and seven compared loop diuretics to other agents such as angiotensin-converting enzyme inhibitors and digoxin). In the placebo-controlled trials, mortality and the incidence of worsening heart failure were lower in patients treated with diuretics. Exercise capacity was increased in those who received diuretics in addition to active control (Faris, Flather, Purcell, et al, 2006).

In the observational study, investigators analyzed changes in cardiac output and pulmonary wedge pressures in 13 patients with heart failure. Diuresis increased stroke volume and decreased pulmonary wedge pressure, mean blood pressure, and systemic vascular resistance. Diuresis improved performance and reduced afterload (Wilson, Reichek, Dunkman, et al, 1981).

APPLY THE EVIDENCE: NURSING IMPLICATIONS

- The use of diuretics in patients with heart failure is necessary for symptom management. If symptoms are moderate to severe, the medication may be given intravenously.
- Response to an intravenous dose of diuretic should occur within 1 hour of administration.
- Frequent assessment of cardiac and respiratory systems is needed to evaluate effectiveness of medication.
- Children with chronic heart failure are likely to receive regular doses of diuretic as a part of their home management plan. Patients and caregivers need to understand dose regimen, medication action, and side effects.

References

Faris RF, Flather M, Purcell H, et al: Diuretics for heart failure, *Cochrane Database Syst Rev* 2006, Jan 25(1):CD003838.

Guyatt GH, Oxman AD, Vist GE, et al: GRADE: an emerging consensus on rating quality of evidence and strength of recommendations, *BMJ* 336:924-926, 2008.

Wilson JR, Reichek N, Dunkman WB, et al: Effect of diuresis on the performance of the failing left ventricle in man, *Am J Med* 70:234-239, 1981.

oxygen demands. In addition, supplemental cool humidified oxygen may be administered to increase the amount of available oxygen during inspiration. Oxygen administration is especially helpful in patients with pulmonary edema, intercurrent respiratory tract infections, and increased pulmonary vascular resistance (oxygen is a vasodilator that decreases pulmonary vascular resistance).

> **! NURSING ALERT**
>
> Oxygen is a drug and is administered only with an appropriate order.

An oxygen hood, face tent, or nasal cannula is used to deliver supplemental oxygen. Nasal cannulas are ideal for long-term oxygen administration because the child can be ambulatory and can easily eat and drink. Cool humidification is necessary to counteract the drying effect of oxygen. The amount of cool humidity is carefully regulated to prevent chilling.

Nursing Care Management

Infants or children with HF may be acutely ill, and some may require intensive care until their symptoms improve. Expert nursing care is essential to reduce the cardiac demands that strain the failing heart muscle (see Nursing Care Plan, p. 1360). During this time the child and family require emotional support; for some children severe HF represents end-stage cardiac disease.

Although the objectives of nursing care are the same, interventions for infants are different from those for older children.

> **QUALITY PATIENT OUTCOMES: Heart Failure**
> - Adequate cardiac output
> - Decreased cardiac demands
> - Improved respiratory function
> - No evidence of fluid excess
> - Adequate support and education

Assist in Measures to Improve Cardiac Function

The nurse's responsibility in administering digoxin includes calculating and giving the correct dosage and observing for signs of toxicity. The child's apical pulse is always checked before administering digoxin. As a rule, the drug is not given if the pulse is below 90 to 110 beats/min in infants and young children or below 70 beats/min in older children (the cutoff point for adults is 60 beats/min). However, because the pulse rate varies in children in different age-groups, the written drug order should specify at what heart rate the drug is withheld. The nurse should also use judgment in evaluating the pulse rate. If it is significantly lower than the previous recording, the dose should be withheld until the practitioner is notified.

The apical rate is measured because a pulse deficit (radial pulse rate lower than apical) may be present with decreased cardiac output. The pulse is auscultated for 1 full minute to evaluate alterations in rhythm. If the child is monitored by ECG, a rhythm strip is obtained and attached to the chart for rate and rhythm analysis, such as abnormal lengthening of the P-R interval (>50% increase over the predigitalization interval) and dysrhythmias.

Digoxin is a potentially dangerous drug because the margin of safety between therapeutic, toxic, and lethal doses is very narrow. Many toxic responses are extensions of its therapeutic effects. Therefore the nurse must be vigilant for signs of toxicity when administering digoxin. The most common signs of digoxin toxicity in infants and children are bradycardia (although other dysrhythmias may occur), anorexia, nausea, and vomiting. Although vomiting should alert the nurse to observe for other evidence of cardiac toxicity, one episode of vomiting does not warrant cessation of the drug, since vomiting from other causes frequently occurs, especially in infants. Vomiting associated with digoxin toxicity is often unrelated to feedings, and infants are usually less interested in feeding and show a recent decrease in oral intake. When in doubt regarding what caused the vomiting and whether another dose of digoxin should be given, the nurse should seek the practitioner's advice before administering the next dose. When concerned about possible digoxin toxicity, the nurse should check the digoxin drug level.

> **⚡ DRUG ALERT**
> *Digoxin Toxicity*
>
> Therapeutic serum digoxin levels range from 0.8 to 2 mcg/L. Observe for signs of toxicity, especially bradycardia and vomiting.

Other extracardiac signs of toxicity are neurologic and visual disturbances, which are extremely difficult to identify in children and consequently are of little value in assessing toxicity in infants.

Because digoxin toxicity can occur from accidental overdose, great care must be taken in properly calculating and measuring the dosage. When converting milligrams to micrograms to milliliters, the nurse carefully checks the placement of the decimal point, since an error causes a significant change in dosage. For example, 0.1 mg is 10 times the dosage of 0.01 mg.

> **⚡ DRUG ALERT**
> *Digoxin Dosing*
>
> Infants rarely receive more than 1 ml (50 mcg, or 0.05 mg) in one dose; a higher dose is an immediate warning of a dosage error. To ensure safety, compare the calculation with that of another staff member before giving digoxin.

If digoxin toxicity occurs, especially as a result of a drug overdose, withhold all subsequent doses. The nurse monitors the child closely for dysrhythmias, which are treated appropriately if they occur. Digoxin immune Fab fragments are used as an antidote to digoxin in cases of severe digitalis toxicity. Because of the long half-life of digoxin (18 to 35 hours in infants and children with normal renal function; longer in those with renal impairment and in premature infants and adults), it may be several days before the blood level returns to normal (Taketomo, Hodding, and Kraus, 2009).

These same principles are taught to parents in preparation for the child's discharge, although the correct dose in milliliters is usually specified on the container, which reduces potential errors in calculation. The nurse observes the parent measuring the elixir in the dropper and stresses that the level mark is the meniscus of the fluid observed at eye level. Other instructions for administering digoxin are listed in the Family-Centered Care box. Nurses should also advise parents of the signs of digoxin toxicity.

👪 FAMILY-CENTERED CARE

Administering Digoxin

- Give digoxin at regular intervals, usually every 12 hours, such as at 8 AM and 8 PM.
- Administer the drug carefully by slowly directing it to the side and back of the mouth.
- Do not mix the drug with foods or other fluids, since refusal to consume these would result in inaccurate intake of the drug.
- If the child has teeth, give water after administering the drug; whenever possible, brush the teeth to prevent tooth decay from the sweetened liquid.
- If a dose is missed, do not give an extra dose or increase the dose. Stay on the same medication schedule.
- If the child vomits, do not give a second dose.
- If more than two consecutive doses have been missed, notify the physician or other designated practitioner.
- Frequent vomiting, poor feeding, or slow heart rate can be signs of digoxin toxicity; if they occur, contact the physician.
- If the child becomes ill, notify the physician or other designated practitioner immediately.
- Keep digoxin in a safe place, preferably in a locked cabinet.
- In case of accidental overdose of digoxin, call the nearest poison control center immediately.

Reduce Afterload

For patients receiving ACE inhibitors for afterload reduction, the nurse should carefully monitor BP before and after dose administration, observe for symptoms of hypotension, and notify the practitioner if BP is low. Monitor serum electrolyte levels. Because ACE inhibitors also block the action of aldosterone, they act as potassium-sparing agents. Most patients do not need potassium supplements or spironolactone while receiving these medications. Numerous medications affecting the kidney can potentiate renal dysfunction, so children taking multiple diuretics along with an ACE inhibitor require careful assessment.

Decrease Cardiac Demands

The infant requires rest and conservation of energy for feeding. Make every effort to organize nursing activities to allow for uninterrupted periods of sleep. Whenever possible, encourage parents to stay with their infant to provide the holding, rocking, and cuddling that help children sleep more soundly. To minimize disturbing the infant, changing bed linen and complete bathing are done only when necessary. Plan feeding to accommodate the infant's sleep and wake patterns. The child is fed when hungry, such as when sucking on fists, rather than when crying for a bottle, since the stress of crying exhausts the limited energy supply. Because infants with HF tire easily and may sleep through feedings, smaller feedings every 3 hours may be helpful. Gavage feedings may be instituted to provide adequate nutrition and allow the infant to rest.

Make every effort to minimize unnecessary stress. With infants this primarily involves preserving the parent-child relationship and meeting the infant's needs to reduce frustration. Older children need an explanation of what is happening to them to decrease anxiety about their illness and necessary treatments, such as cardiac monitoring, oxygen administration, and medications. Outlining a plan for the day, preparing the child for tests and procedures, providing quiet activities, and providing adequate rest periods are all helpful interventions with older children. Some infants and children require sedation during the acute phase of illness to allow them to rest.

Carefully monitor temperature for hyperthermia (a sign of infection) or hypothermia (loss of heat to ambient air). Report fevers, since infection must be treated promptly. Fever increases oxygen demands and is poorly tolerated. If body temperature is low, keep the child warm with additional blankets or a radiant heater. Maintaining body temperature is important for children who are receiving cool, humidified oxygen and for children who tend to be diaphoretic, losing heat via evaporation.

Prevent skin breakdown from edema with frequent change of position and the use of pressure-relieving or pressure-reducing mattresses or beds. The skin, especially over the sacrum, is checked for evidence of redness from pressure.

Reduce Respiratory Distress

Careful assessment, positioning, and oxygen administration can reduce respiratory distress. Respirations are counted for 1 full minute during a resting state. Any evidence of increased respiratory distress is reported, since this may indicate worsening heart failure.

Position infants to encourage maximum chest expansion, with the head of the bed elevated. They should sit up in an infant seat or be held at a 45-degree angle. Children prefer to sleep on several pillows and remain in a semi-Fowler or high Fowler position during waking hours. Shirts and diapers are pinned loosely to allow maximum chest expansion. Safety restraints, such as those used with infant seats, are applied low on the abdomen and loosely enough to provide safety and maximum expansion.

The infant or child is often given humidified supplemental oxygen via an oxygen hood or tent, nasal cannula, or mask. The child's response to oxygen therapy is carefully evaluated by noting the respiratory rate; ease of respiration; color; and especially oxygen saturations, as measured by oximetry.

Respiratory tract infections can exacerbate HF and should be appropriately treated and prevented if possible. The child should be protected from persons with respiratory tract infections and should have a noninfectious roommate. Practice good hand-washing technique before and after caring for any hospitalized child. Antibiotics may be given to combat respiratory tract infection. The nurse ensures that the drug is given at equal intervals over a 24-hour period to maintain high blood levels of the antibiotic.

Maintain Nutritional Status

Meeting the nutritional needs of infants with HF or serious cardiac defects is a nursing challenge. The metabolic rate of these infants is greater because of poor cardiac function and increased heart and respiratory rates. Their caloric needs are greater than those of the average infant because of their increased metabolic rate, yet fatigue limits their ability to take in adequate calories. Feeding a fragile infant with serious CHD is similar to exercise in an adult, and the infant often does not have the energy or cardiac reserve to do extra work. The nurse seeks measures to enable the infant to feed easily without excess fatigue and to increase the caloric density of the formula.

The infant should be well rested before feeding and fed soon after awakening so as not to expend energy on crying. A 3-hour feeding schedule works well for many infants. (Feeding every 2 hours does not provide enough rest between feedings, and a 4-hour schedule requires an increased volume of feeding, which many infants are unable to take.) The feeding schedule should be individualized to the infant's needs. Use of a soft preemie nipple or a regular nipple slit to enlarge the opening decreases the energy expenditure of the infant while sucking. Infants should be well supported and fed in a semiupright position. The infant may need to rest frequently and may need to have the jaw and cheeks stroked to encourage sucking. Generally, giving an infant about a half hour to complete a feeding is reasonable. Prolonging the feeding time can exhaust the infant and decrease the rest period between feedings.

Infants with feeding difficulties are often gavage fed using a nasogastric tube to supplement oral feedings and ensure adequate caloric intake. If they are stressed and fatigued, in respiratory distress, or tachypneic at 80 to 100 breaths/min, oral feedings may be withheld and all nutrition given by gavage feedings. Gavage feedings are usually a temporary measure until the infant's medical status improves and nutritional needs can be met through oral feedings. Some infants with severe HF, neurologic deficits, or significant gastroesophageal reflux may need placement of a gastrostomy tube to allow adequate nutrition.

The caloric density of formulas is frequently increased by concentration and then the addition of Polycose (or, less commonly, corn oil or medium-chain triglycerides oil). Infant formulas provide 20 kcal/oz, and the use of additives can increase the calories to 30 kcal/oz or more. This allows the infant to obtain more calories despite intake of a smaller volume of formula. The caloric density of the formula must be increased slowly (by 2 kcal/oz/day) to prevent diarrhea or formula intolerance. Encourage breast-feeding mothers to provide the infant with alternating feedings of breast milk and high-calorie formula. Some lactating mothers prefer to feed the child expressed breast milk that has been fortified with Similac or Enfamil powder, Polycose, or corn oil to increase caloric intake. A supplemental nurser may also be helpful. A diet plan specific to the individual infant's needs is calculated and prescribed by the nutritionist in collaboration with the other health care personnel. The nurse needs to reinforce this information with the parents as necessary.

Assist in Measures to Promote Fluid Loss

When diuretics are given, the nurse records fluid intake and output and monitors body weight at the same time each day to evaluate the benefit of the drug. Because profound diuresis may cause dehydration and electrolyte imbalance (loss of sodium, potassium, chloride, bicarbonate), the nurse observes for signs indicating either complication, as well as signs and symptoms suggesting reactions to the drugs. Give diuretics early in the day to children who are toilet trained to avoid the need to urinate at night. If potassium-losing diuretics are given, the nurse encourages consumption of foods high in potassium, such as bananas, oranges, whole grains, legumes, and leafy vegetables, and administers prescribed supplements.

> **! NURSING ALERT**
>
> Observe for signs of hypokalemia (muscle weakness, hypotension, dysrhythmias, tachycardia or bradycardia, irritability, drowsiness) or hyperkalemia (muscle weakness, twitching, bradycardia, ventricular fibrillation, oliguria, apnea) from supplement overdose.

Fluid restriction is rarely necessary in infants because of their difficulty in feeding. However, if fluids are restricted, the nurse plans fluid intake schedules for a 24-hour period, allowing for administration of most fluids during waking hours. With toddlers and preschoolers it is psychologically advantageous to give small amounts of liquid in small cups so that the containers appear full. Suitable containers are decorated medicine cups, small paper cups, doll-sized teacups, and measuring cups. It is also important to avoid leaving extra fluids at the bedside, since older children may help themselves to additional servings. Placing them in charge of recording fluid intake will help gain their cooperation.

If salt intake is to be limited, the nurse discusses food sources of sodium with the family and discourages their bringing salt-containing treats to the child. At mealtime check the child's tray to make sure the appropriate diet is provided.

Support the Child and Family

HF is a serious complication of heart disease. Parents and older children are usually acutely aware of the critical nature of the condition. Because stress places additional demands on cardiac function, the nurse should focus on reducing anxiety through anticipatory preparation, frequent communication with the parents regarding the child's progress, and constant reassurance that everything possible is being done.

Home care involves many of the same interventions discussed later under Plan for Discharge and Home Care (see p. 1381). The nurse teaches the family about the medications that need to be administered and alerts them to the signs of worsening HF that require medical attention, such as increased sweating, decreased urinary output (noted in fewer wet diapers or infrequent use of the toilet), or poor feeding. Compliance can be a major issue, since patients are often prescribed multiple medications, and the medication regimen can change frequently. Facilitate the family's adherence to the medication schedule by adapting the schedule to their usual home routines, avoiding medication administration at night, making it as simple as possible, and providing charts or visual aids to help them remember when to give medications. (See Chapter 27.) Written instructions regarding correct administration of digitalis (digoxin) are essential (see Family-Centered Care box, p. 1358), including an explanation regarding signs of toxicity.

If HF is the end stage of a severe heart defect, the nurse cares for the child the same as for any child who is terminally ill, using the principles discussed in Chapter 23 (see Nursing Care Plan).

HYPOXEMIA

Hypoxemia refers to an arterial oxygen tension (or pressure, Pao_2) that is lower than normal and can be identified by measuring arterial oxygen saturation (Sao_2) or Pao_2 to detect decreased levels. Hypoxia is a reduction in tissue oxygenation that is caused by low Sao_2 and Pao_2 and results in impaired cellular processes. Cyanosis is a blue discoloration of the mucous membranes, skin, and nail beds of the child with reduced oxygen saturation. It results from the presence of deoxygenated hemoglobin (hemoglobin not bound to oxygen) at a concentration of 5 g/dl of blood or more. Cyanosis is usually apparent when Sao_2 is 85% or lower. Determination of cyanosis is subjective. Its appearance can vary depending on skin pigment, quality of light, color of the room, and clothing worn by the child. The presence of cyanosis may not accurately reflect arterial hypoxemia, since both Sao_2 and the amount of circulating hemoglobin are involved. Children with severe anemia may

---

◎ NURSING CARE PLAN

The Child with Heart Failure

NURSING DIAGNOSIS	EXPECTED PATIENT OUTCOMES	NURSING INTERVENTIONS	RATIONALE
Decreased Cardiac Output related to structural defect, myocardial dysfunction, altered hemodynamics	Child will have adequate cardiac output as evidenced by: • Heart rate within acceptable range (state specific range) • Respiratory rate within acceptable range (state specific range) • Skin warm to touch	Assess and record heart rate, respiratory rate, blood pressure, and any signs or symptoms of decreased cardiac output (listed under defining characteristics) every 2 to 4 hours and as necessary.	To detect change in vital signs and child's physical status that reflect altered cardiac output
Child's/Family's Defining Characteristics **(Subjective and Objective Data)** Tachycardia Tachypnea Ineffective peripheral circulation, cool extremities Hypotension Rapid, weak peripheral pulses Prolonged capillary refill, longer than 2 or 3 seconds Narrow pulse pressure Distended neck veins in older children Cardiomegaly revealed on chest radiograph Gallop rhythm Edema Rapid weight gain Feeding difficulty Irritability	• Strong and equal peripheral pulses • Blood pressure normal for age • Brisk capillary refill within 2 or 3 seconds • Lack of distended neck veins • Normal sinus rhythm • Lack of edema • Adequate urinary output (state specific; 1-2 ml/kg/hr) • Age-appropriate weight gain on standardized growth curve • Successful feeding Child and/or family will be able to state at least four characteristics of heart failure such as: • Rapid heart rate • Fast breathing • Cool extremities • Puffiness (edema) • Fussiness • Decreased appetite Child and/or family will be able to state knowledge of care regarding: • Medication administration • Head elevated positioning • Sufficient rest periods • Monitoring of intake and output • When to contact health care provider	Administer cardiac drugs on schedule. Assess and record any side effects or any signs and symptoms of toxicity. Follow hospital protocol for administration. Keep accurate record of intake and output. Weigh child or infant on same scale at same time of day as previously. Document results and compare to previous weight. Administer diuretics on schedule. Assess and record effectiveness and any side effects noted. Elevate head of bed at a 30- to 45-degree angle. Offer small, frequent feedings to infant's or child's tolerance. Organize nursing care to allow child or infant uninterrupted rest. Educate child and family about characteristics of HF. Assess and record teaching session. Educate child and family about care such as medication administration. Assess and record results and family's participation in care.	To avoid dangers inherent in failure to administer cardiac drugs as prescribed and to perform careful assessment before administration To detect heart failure (HF), which causes decreased urinary output To monitor for weight increases, which may indicate excess fluid accumulation To eliminate excess water and salt, since fluid retention commonly occurs with HF To promotes maximum chest expansion To increase caloric intake and compensate for fatigue during feeding and increased metabolic rate due to poor cardiac function To allow adequate rest, since poor cardiac output decreases energy level and lowers tolerance to activity To promote measures to improve cardiac function and decrease demands To promote safety and minimize medication side effects
	The Following NOC Concepts Apply to These Outcomes Cardiac Pump Effectiveness Knowledge: Illness Care Tissue Perfusion: Cardiac	**The Following NIC Concepts Apply to These Interventions** Cardiac Care Fluid Management Medication Administration Positioning Parent/Child Education Vital Signs Monitoring	

NURSING CARE PLAN—cont'd
The Child with Heart Failure

NURSING DIAGNOSIS	EXPECTED PATIENT OUTCOMES	NURSING INTERVENTIONS	RATIONALE
Ineffective Breathing Pattern related to pulmonary congestion, decreased cardiac output	Child will have effective breathing pattern as evidenced by:	Assess and record respiratory rate, breath sounds, and any signs or symptoms of ineffective pattern (listed under characteristics) every 2 to 4 hr and as needed.	To detect indicators of worsening HF
Child's/Family's Defining Characteristics (Subjective and Objective Data)	• Respiratory rate within acceptable range (state specific range) • Clear and equal breath sounds bilaterally, anteriorly, and posteriorly	Administer humidified oxygen in correct amount and route of delivery. Record percent of oxygen and route of delivery.	To reduce respiratory distress by easing respiratory effort
Tachypnea Dyspnea Retractions Crackles Shortness of breath Cyanosis Pallor Mottling Nasal flaring Grunting Head bobbing Cough Use of accessory muscles Activity intolerance	• Pink or tan color • Absence of nasal flaring, retractions, cough, and head bobbing • Unlabored breath sounds • Tolerance of activities appropriate for age Child and/or family will be able to state four characteristics of ineffective breathing pattern such as: • Color change from pink or tan to pale, dusky, or blue • Fast breathing • Change in amount and/or characteristics of secretions • Retractions, head bobbing • Ineffective cough • Decreased or altered activity level Child and/or family will be able to state knowledge of care regarding: • Positioning to facilitate respiratory effort • Oxygen administration • When to contact health care provider	Assess and record child's response to therapy. Keep head of bed elevated at a 30- to 45-degree angle. Suction if child has ineffective cough or is unable to manage secretions. Assess and record amount and characteristics of secretions. Assess and record oxygen saturation every 2 to 4 hours and as needed. Educate child and family about characteristics of ineffective breathing pattern. Assess and record results. Educate child and family about care. Assess and record results and family participation in care.	To promote maximum chest expansion To maintain patent airway to promote respiratory expansion To evaluate pulmonary effectiveness To promote measures to improve breathing effort To provide parent education that can promote measures to improve breathing effort
	The Following NOC Concepts Apply to These Outcomes Activity Tolerance Knowledge: Illness Care Respiratory Status: Gas Exchange Tissue Perfusion: Pulmonary	**The Following NIC Concepts Apply to These Interventions** Airway Management Airway Suctioning Chest Physiotherapy Family Involvement Promotion Health Education	

not be cyanotic despite severe hypoxemia, since the hemoglobin level may be too low to produce the characteristic blue color. Conversely, patients with polycythemia may appear cyanotic despite a near-normal Pao$_2$.

Altered Hemodynamics

Heart defects that cause hypoxemia and cyanosis are those that allow desaturated venous blood (blue blood) to enter the systemic circulation without passing through the lungs. Three types of defect cause cyanosis in infants. The first involves severe obstruction to pulmonary blood flow and blood shunting from the right side to the left side of the heart, or right-to-left shunting. Tetralogy of Fallot is the most common example. The second is mixing of arterial and venous blood within the chambers of the heart itself; a single ventricle is an example. The third defect, transposition of the great arteries, presents a unique situation in which the pulmonary and systemic circulations are parallel rather than in sequence. Fully oxygenated

blood returns to the lungs, and desaturated blood returns to the body. Newborns with transposition of the great arteries depend on intracardiac mixing from a patent foramen ovale, septal defect, or ductus arteriosus to allow oxygenation.

Infants and children with some complex cardiac anomalies can be both hypoxemic and cyanotic and have symptoms of HF. Defects resulting in one functional ventricle, hypoplastic left heart syndrome, and transposition of the great arteries with a ventricular septal defect are examples.

Clinical Manifestations

Over time, two physiologic changes occur in the body in response to chronic hypoxemia: polycythemia and clubbing. Persistent hypoxemia stimulates erythropoiesis, which results in polycythemia, an increased number of red blood cells. Theoretically a greater number of red blood cells increase the oxygen-carrying capacity of the blood. However, this increased red blood cell formation may result in anemia if iron is not

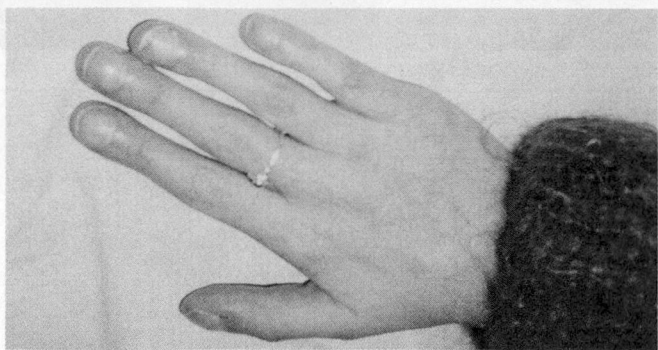

Fig. 34-9 Clubbing of the fingers.

readily available for the formation of hemoglobin. In addition, polycythemia increases the viscosity of the blood, and platelets and other coagulation factors tend to be crowded out. These hematologic changes increase the likelihood of postoperative bleeding. Clubbing, a thickening and flattening of the tips of the fingers and toes, is thought to occur because of chronic tissue hypoxemia and polycythemia (Fig. 34-9).

Infants with mild hypoxemia may be asymptomatic except for cyanosis and exhibit near-normal growth and development. Those with more severe hypoxemia may exhibit fatigue with feeding, poor weight gain, tachypnea, and dyspnea. Flaccidity is usually a sign of severe cardiovascular compromise. Children who are cyanotic from birth are generally smaller than their peers, exhibit poor weight gain, have dyspnea on exertion, fatigue easily, and have poor exercise tolerance.

Severe hypoxemia resulting in tissue hypoxia is manifested by clinical deterioration and signs of poor perfusion. The infant is pale and dusky with increased cyanosis; cool to the touch with diminished pulses; and lethargic with signs of respiratory distress, including hyperpnea and gasping respirations. Tissue hypoxia causes metabolic acidosis, which leads to hyperventilation and a rapidly worsening clinical course unless prompt treatment is instituted.

Hypercyanotic spells, also referred to as *blue spells* or *tet spells* because they are often seen in infants with tetralogy of Fallot, may occur in any child whose heart defect includes obstruction to pulmonary blood flow and communication between the ventricles (see Fig. 34-12). The infant becomes acutely cyanotic and hyperpneic because when sudden infundibular spasms decreases pulmonary blood flow and increases right-to-left shunting (the proposed mechanism in tetralogy of Fallot). This then leads to hypoxia. With other anomalies, an increase in oxygen requirements, which the infant is unable to meet, may cause a spell. Hypoxia causes acidosis, which further increases pulmonary vascular resistance; this, in turn, further decreases pulmonary blood flow. Thus a vicious cycle ensues. Spells, rarely seen before 2 months of age, occur most frequently in the first year of life and more often in the morning, and they may be preceded by feeding, crying, or defecation. Because profound hypoxemia causes cerebral hypoxia, hypercyanotic spells require prompt assessment and treatment to prevent brain damage or possibly death.

Patients with persistent right-to-left shunts as a result of CHD are at risk for significant neurologic complications. Polycythemia and the resultant increased viscosity of the blood

increase the risk of thromboembolic events. Small blood clots in the venous system reach the right side of the heart and can enter the systemic circulation and travel to the brain through the right-to-left shunt. The presence of poor ventricular function and atrial arrhythmias further increases the risk of cerebrovascular accidents (CVAs), or strokes. More common in patients with severe cyanosis, thromboembolic events may occur spontaneously but often follow an acute febrile illness; a hypoxic spell; cardiac catheterization; or cardiac surgery, including the Fontan procedure with fenestration (see Box 34-6).

Patients who are cyanotic, especially those with systemic-to-pulmonary shunts, are at increased risk of bacterial endocarditis (BE; infective) (see p. 1382).

Negative developmental consequences, particularly in the area of motor and cognitive development, may occur from chronic hypoxemia. Fifty percent of postnatal brain growth takes place in the first year of life, so chronic hypoxemia, poor growth, and poor nutrition during this period can have significant adverse effects. In addition, the risks of CVA; periods of profound cyanosis and hypoxia during hypercyanotic spells; and multiple surgeries, hospitalizations, and cardiac catheterizations significantly increase the possibility of neurologic insult resulting in developmental delays, a danger that increases with each year of life. The desire to minimize these risks is an important factor in the trend toward early corrective surgical repair of cyanotic defects in infancy.

Diagnostic Evaluation

Cyanosis in the newborn can be a result of cardiac, pulmonary, metabolic, or hematologic disease, although cardiac and pulmonary causes occur most often. To distinguish between the two, a hyperoxia test may be helpful. The infant is placed in a 100% oxygen environment, and blood parameters are monitored. A Pao_2 of 100 mm Hg or higher suggests lung disease, and a Pao_2 lower than 100 mm Hg suggests cardiac disease (the problem is related to inadequate perfusion of the pulmonary bed) (Park, 2008). An accurate history, a chest radiograph (demonstrating reduced pulmonary blood flow), and especially an echocardiogram contribute to the diagnosis of cyanotic heart disease.

Therapeutic Management

Newborns generally exhibit cyanosis within the first few days of life as the ductus arteriosus, which provided pulmonary blood flow, begins to close. Prostaglandin E_1, which causes vasodilation and smooth muscle relaxation and thus increases dilation and patency of the ductus arteriosus, is administered intravenously to reestablish pulmonary blood flow. The use of prostaglandins has been lifesaving for infants with ductus-dependent cardiac defects. The increase in oxygenation allows the infant's condition to be stabilized and a complete diagnostic evaluation to be performed before further treatment is needed.

Hypercyanotic spells occur suddenly, and prompt recognition and treatment are essential. In the hospital setting, spells are often seen during blood drawing or IV line insertion, when the child is highly agitated, or following cardiac catheterization. Treatment of a hypercyanotic spell is outlined in the Nursing

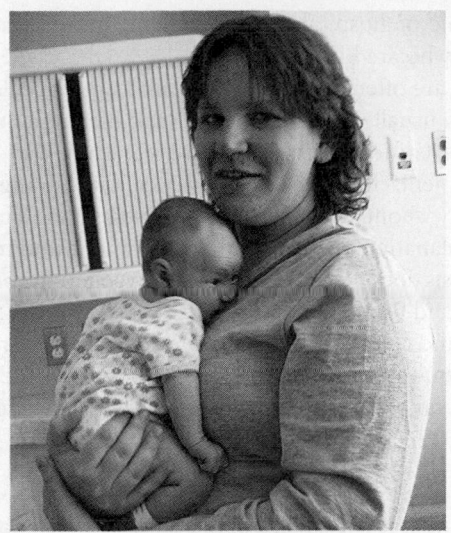

Fig 34-10 Infant held in the knee-chest position.

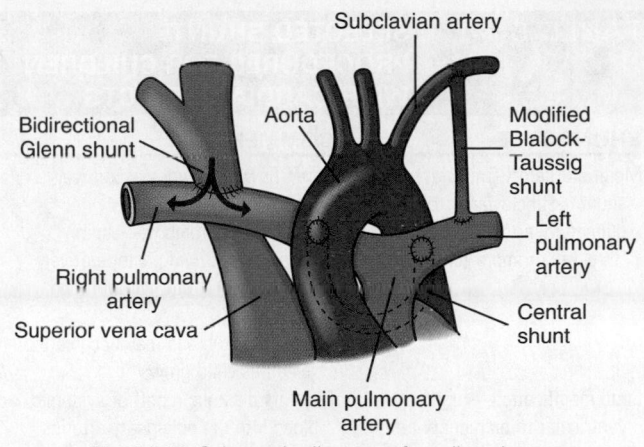

Fig. 34-11 Schematic diagram of cardiac shunts.

Care Guidelines box. Placing an infant in the knee-chest position reduces the venous return from the legs (which is desaturated) and increases systemic vascular resistance, which diverts more blood into the pulmonary artery (Fig. 34-10). Morphine, administered subcutaneously or through an existing IV line, is helpful in reducing infundibular spasm. A spell may indicate the need for prompt surgical treatment. In rare cases, propranolol (Inderal) may be given in the interim to prevent infundibular spasm.

NURSING CARE GUIDELINES

Treating Hypercyanotic Spells

- Place infant in knee-chest position (see Fig. 34-10).
- Employ calm, comforting approach.
- Administer 100% oxygen by face mask.
- Give morphine subcutaneously or through existing intravenous line.
- Begin intravenous fluid replacement and volume expansion, if needed.
- Repeat morphine administration.

The cyanotic infant or child is well hydrated to keep the hematocrit and blood viscosity within acceptable limits to reduce the risk of CVA. Fevers are carefully evaluated, since bacteremia can result in bacterial endocarditis. Monitor the infant closely for anemia because of the risk of CVAs and the reduced arterial oxygen-carrying capacity that occurs. Iron supplementation and possibly blood transfusion are used as needed. Older children and adolescents may require serial phlebotomy to reduce blood viscosity and minimize the risk of CVA. The goal is to reduce the hematocrit to approximately 60% by removing small aliquots of blood and replacing blood with normal saline or other IV solutions to maintain intravascular volume. This procedure is a temporary measure but may relieve symptoms of dyspnea, headache, and malaise for short periods and can be repeated every 1 or 2 months if polycythemia is severe.

Respiratory tract infections or reduced pulmonary function from any cause can worsen hypoxemia in the cyanotic child. Aggressive pulmonary hygiene, chest physiotherapy, adminis-

tration of antibiotics, and use of oxygen to improve arterial saturations are important interventions.

Palliative Surgery

Severely hypoxemic newborns with cardiac defects not initially amenable to corrective repair may undergo a palliative surgical procedure to establish a shunt. The shunt serves the same purpose as the ductus arteriosus: to increase blood flow to the lungs through a systemic artery–to–pulmonary artery connection. Currently, a modified Blalock-Taussig operation, in which a Gore-Tex or Impra tube graft is placed to create a communication between the right or left subclavian artery and the pulmonary artery on the same side, is the preferred procedure. The original Blalock-Taussig shunt procedure directly anastomosed the subclavian artery to the pulmonary artery to provide pulmonary blood flow and was the first operation devised for patients with cyanotic heart disease. Because of the higher resistance in the systemic circulation, blood flows from the subclavian artery to the pulmonary artery and to the lungs for oxygenation. The small diameter of the subclavian artery and the shunt (often 3.5 or 4 mm) automatically restricts the volume of blood flow to the pulmonary artery, which prevents severe pulmonary overcirculation and HF. Table 34-4 outlines the most commonly performed shunt procedures today (Fig. 34-11). Corrective surgical repair is always preferred to a palliative shunt procedure if it can be performed at low risk. Corrective techniques are described in the discussion of the particular cardiac defect.

After a shunt procedure, assess the infant for signs of increased or decreased pulmonary blood flow. If the shunt is too small or has narrowed, the newborn may remain severely hypoxemic, with oxygen saturations below 70%. Surgical revision of the shunt or placement of an additional shunt may be needed. More often, the shunt is too large and the pulmonary blood flow may be excessive, resulting in signs and symptoms of HF and oxygen saturations above 85%. The infant may require digoxin and diuretic therapy (see discussion of HF). Most surgeons place infants on low-dose aspirin therapy for several months to prevent platelet aggregation and subsequent narrowing of the shunt. Acute cyanosis and signs of tissue hypoxia may occur if the shunt is occluded and pulmonary blood flow is severely limited; shunt occlusion is a medical

TABLE 34-4	SELECTED SHUNT PROCEDURES FOR CHILDREN WITH CARDIAC DEFECTS
SHUNT TYPE	**COMMENTS**
Modified Blalock-Taussig shunt—Subclavian artery to pulmonary artery using Gore-Tex or Impra tube graft	Shunt flow sometimes excessive, requiring use of diuretics Possibility of thrombosis; aspirin usually prescribed postoperatively Easy to ligate at time of definitive correction Shunt size fixed and may become too small as child grows
Sano modification—Right ventricular to pulmonary artery conduit using Gore-Tex	Prevents diastolic runoff of systemic blood into the pulmonary arteries Provides a higher diastolic blood pressure and seemingly better coronary perfusion Used in place of the Modified Blalock-Taussig shunt in the Norwood procedure
Central shunt—Ascending aorta to main pulmonary artery using Gore-Tex graft	Length of shunt acts to restrict blood flow; symptoms of heart failure may occur; diuretic therapy may be required Uncommon; used when modified Blalock-Taussig shunt cannot be used Easy to insert and remove at time of repair Possibility of thrombosis; aspirin usually prescribed postoperatively
Bidirectional Glenn shunt (cavopulmonary anastomosis)—Superior vena cava to side of right pulmonary artery; blood flow to both lungs	Done as a second shunt; often used as a staging step to a Fontan procedure Can be incorporated into eventual modified Fontan procedure Relieves severe cyanosis and decreases volume overload on ventricle Carries risk of embolic events (mixing defect); aspirin often prescribed Pulmonary arteriovenous fistulas may occur months or years later, causing desaturation (uncommon finding)

emergency. The presence of prosthetic material puts patients at risk for infective (bacterial) endocarditis.

Nursing Care Management

The general appearance of infants and children with significant cyanosis poses unique concerns. Blue lips and fingernails are obvious signs of the hidden cardiac defect. Clubbing and small, thin stature in older children further indicate severe heart disease. Body image concerns are important. These children are often teased about their appearance and singled out as different. Adolescents are especially concerned about their body image, and cyanosis can become a particular issue for them. Many children, when asked what surgery will do, reply, "Make me pink." Their joy and excitement after surgery are evident when they see their pink fingers. Accentuating the normal and positive and being careful not to call attention to their cyanosis are helpful interventions. Meeting other children who are cyanotic

in the clinic or hospital reassures them that they are not the only ones who are blue.

Parents are often fearful of their child's bluish color because cyanosis is usually associated with lack of oxygen and severe illness (see Critical Thinking Exercise). They also must deal with comments from relatives, friends, and strangers in the community about their child's abnormal color. They need a simple explanation of hypoxemia and cyanosis and reassurance that cyanosis does not imply a lack of oxygen to the brain. Their questions and fears need to be addressed in a calm, supportive manner, and positive aspects of their child's growth and development must be emphasized. Teach parents the treatment for hypercyanotic spells. (See Nursing Care Guidelines box, p. 1363.)

❓ CRITICAL THINKING EXERCISE

Hypercyanotic Spell

A 4-month-old infant known to have tetralogy of Fallot is seen in the emergency department because of a 2-day history of diarrhea, low-grade fever, and poor oral intake. When blood tests are obtained, he becomes acutely cyanotic with rapid shallow respirations.

1. Evidence—Is there sufficient evidence to draw conclusions about this infant's condition?
2. Assumptions—Describe an underlying assumption about each of the following:
   a. Symptoms associated with tetralogy of Fallot
   b. Diarrhea, low-grade fever, and poor oral intake in a 4-month-old infant
   c. Acute cyanotic episodes in a 4-month-old infant
3. What priorities for nursing care should be established for this infant?
4. Does the evidence support your nursing interventions?

Dehydration must be prevented in hypoxemic children because it increases the risk of CVAs. Fluid status is carefully monitored through accurate intake and output and daily weight measurements. Maintenance fluid therapy is the minimum requirement; supplemental fluids should be readily available, and gavage feeding or IV hydration is given to children unable to take in adequate fluids orally. Fever, vomiting, and diarrhea can cause dehydration and require prompt treatment. Instruct parents in the importance of adequate fluid intake and measures to prevent dehydration. An oral electrolyte solution such as Pedialyte should be available at home in the event that the infant is unable to tolerate the usual formula. The practitioner should be notified of fever, vomiting, diarrhea, or other problems.

Preventive measures and accurate assessment of respiratory infection are important nursing considerations. Any compromise in pulmonary function increases the infant's hypoxemia. Good hand washing and protection from individuals with an obvious respiratory tract infection are important. Aggressive pulmonary hygiene, treatment with antibiotics or antiviral agents as indicated, and delivery of supplemental oxygen to decrease hypoxemia are necessary measures. Infants may need to be gavage fed or given parenteral nutrition if respiratory distress prevents oral feeding.

CLASSIFICATION OF CONGENITAL HEART DEFECTS

Congenital heart defects have been classified into several categories. Traditionally a physical characteristic, cyanosis, has been used as the distinguishing feature, so that the anomalies have been divided into acyanotic and cyanotic defects. In clinical practice this system is problematic, since children with acyanotic defects may develop cyanosis. Also, more often, those with cyanotic defects may be pink and have more clinical signs of HF. Because of the complexity of many defects and the variability of their clinical manifestations, the cyanotic-acyanotic classification system has proven to be inadequate and misleading.

A more useful classification system is based on hemodynamic characteristics, or movements involved in the circulation of blood. The defining characteristic is blood flow patterns: (1) increased pulmonary blood flow; (2) decreased pulmonary blood flow; (3) obstruction to blood flow out of the heart; and (4) mixed blood flow, in which saturated and desaturated blood mix within the heart or great arteries. Fig. 34-12 outlines both classification systems.

With the hemodynamic classification system, the clinical manifestations of each group are more uniform and predictable. Defects that allow blood flow from the high-pressure left side of the heart to the lower-pressure right side (left-to-right shunt) result in increased pulmonary blood flow and cause HF. Obstructive defects impede blood flow out of the ventricles; obstruction on the left side of the heart results in HF, whereas severe obstruction on the right side causes cyanosis. Defects that cause decreased pulmonary blood flow result in cyanosis. Mixed lesions present a variable clinical picture based on the degree of mixing and amount of pulmonary blood flow; hypoxemia (with or without cyanosis) and HF usually occur together. (For more detailed explanations, see discussions of specific defects later in this chapter.)

More than 35 types of congenital heart defect have been identified, and some patients have multiple defects. Although some defects are common and fairly uniform, like atrial septal defects or pulmonic stenosis, others are uncommon and highly variable, like single-ventricle anomalies. In a review by Hoffman and Kaplan (2002), defects are categorized as mild, moderate, or severe. Mild defects are found in the largest number of patients, many of who are asymptomatic and may not require treatment. Mild defects include small patent ductus arteriosus, small ventricular septal defects, and mild pulmonic stenosis. Moderate defects include mild aortic stenosis, moderate pulmonic stenosis, coarctation of the aorta, atrial septal defects, and ventricular septal defects. Most patients with moderate defects are symptomatic during childhood and require treatment. Severe defects include all cyanotic heart disease and other complex defects such as AV canal, critical aortic stenosis, critical coarctation of the aorta, and complex ventricular septal defects. Most patients with these defects are identified during the newborn period or early infancy, are severely ill, and require surgical treatment. The clinical presentation and management of the most common defects are outlined in the following sections and in Boxes 34-4 to 34-7.

The outcomes of surgical treatment for patients with moderate to severe disease are variable. Patient risk factors for increased morbidity and mortality include prematurity or low birth weight, a genetic syndrome, multiple cardiac defects, a noncardiac congenital anomaly, and age at the time of surgery (neonates are a higher-risk group). For example, aortic stenosis and coarctation presenting in the first week of life are more severe and carry a higher mortality than if they manifest at 1 year of age. Outcomes for surgical repair of similar congenital heart defects also vary among treatment centers. The most recent mortality rates and statistics on incidence of CHD from the American Heart Association are found in Box 34-1. Individual center results may be better or worse than those listed. In general, the outcomes of surgical procedures have steadily improved, with mortality rates for many severe defects

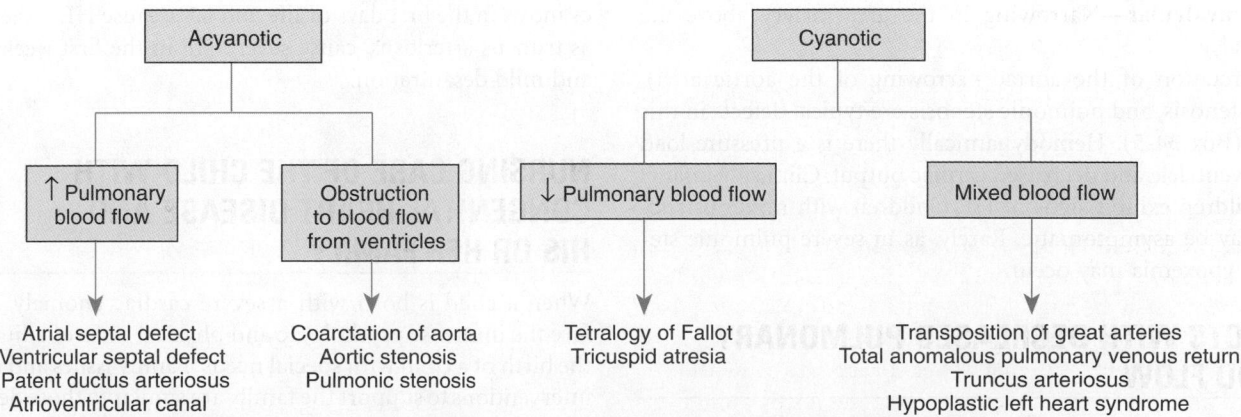

Fig. 34-12 Comparison of acyanotic-cyanotic and hemodynamic classification systems for congenital heart disease.

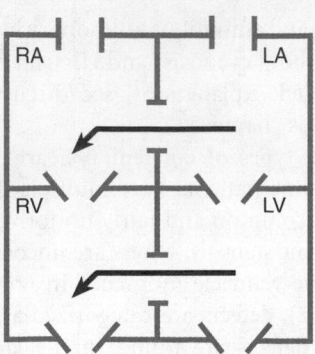

Fig. 34-13 Hemodynamics in defects with increased pulmonary blood flow. See Fig. 34-2 for abbreviations.

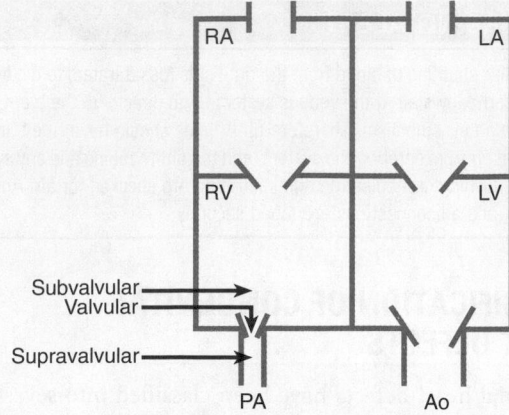

Fig. 34-14 Obstruction to ventricular ejection can occur at the valvular level (shown), below the valve (subvalvular), or above the valve (supravalvular). Pulmonic stenosis is shown here. *Ao,* Aorta; *PA,* pulmonary artery. See Fig. 34-2 for other abbreviations.

below 10%, and the incidence of complications and length of hospital stay have declined.

DEFECTS WITH INCREASED PULMONARY BLOOD FLOW

In cardiac defects with increased pulmonary blood flow, intracardiac communications along the septum or an abnormal connection between the great arteries allows blood to flow from the high-pressure left side of the heart to the lower-pressure right side of the heart (Fig. 34-13). Increased blood volume on the right side of the heart increases pulmonary blood flow at the expense of systemic blood flow. Clinically patients demonstrate signs and symptoms of HF. Atrial and ventricular septal defects and patent ductus arteriosus are typical anomalies in this group (Box 34-4).

OBSTRUCTIVE DEFECTS

Obstructive defects are those in which blood exiting the heart meets an area of anatomic narrowing (stenosis), which causes obstruction to blood flow. The pressure in the ventricle and in the great artery before the obstruction is increased, and the pressure in the area beyond the obstruction is decreased. The location of the narrowing is usually near the valve (Fig. 34-14):

Valvular—Narrowing at the site of the valve itself

Subvalvular—Narrowing in the ventricle below the valve (also referred to as the *ventricular outflow tract*)

Supravalvular—Narrowing in the great artery above the valve

Coarctation of the aorta (narrowing of the aortic arch), aortic stenosis, and pulmonic stenosis are typical defects in this group (Box 34-5). Hemodynamically there is a pressure load on the ventricle and decreased cardiac output. Clinically infants and children exhibit signs of HF. Children with mild obstruction may be asymptomatic. Rarely, as in severe pulmonic stenosis, hypoxemia may occur.

DEFECTS WITH DECREASED PULMONARY BLOOD FLOW

In defects with decreased pulmonary blood flow, there is obstruction of pulmonary blood flow and an anatomic defect (atrial septal defect or ventricular septal defect) between the right and left sides of the heart (Fig. 34-15). Because blood has difficulty exiting the right side of the heart via the pulmonary artery, pressure on the right side increases, exceeding left-side pressure. This allows desaturated blood to shunt right to left, which causes desaturation in the left side of the heart and in the systemic circulation. Clinically these patients are hypoxemic and usually appear cyanotic. Tetralogy of Fallot and tricuspid atresia are the more common defects in this group (Box 34-6).

MIXED DEFECTS

Many complex cardiac anomalies are classified together in the mixed category (Box 34-7), since survival in the postnatal period depends on mixing of blood from the pulmonary and systemic circulations within the heart chambers. Hemodynamically, fully saturated systemic blood mixes with the desaturated pulmonary blood, which causes a relative desaturation of the systemic blood. Pulmonary congestion occurs because the differences in pulmonary artery pressure and aortic pressure favor pulmonary blood flow. Cardiac output decreases because of a volume load on the ventricle. Clinically these patients have a variable picture that combines some degree of desaturation (although cyanosis is not always visible) and signs of HF. Some defects, such as transposition of the great arteries, cause severe cyanosis in the first days of life and later cause HF. Others, such as truncus arteriosus, cause severe HF in the first weeks of life and mild desaturation.

NURSING CARE OF THE CHILD WITH CONGENITAL HEART DISEASE AND HIS OR HER FAMILY

When a child is born with a severe cardiac anomaly, parents face the immense psychologic and physical tasks of adjusting to the birth of a child with special needs. Family issues and nursing interventions to support the family are similar to those described in Chapters 11 and 22. The following discussion concerns primarily (1) interactions with the family of an infant who has a serious heart defect and requires home care before definitive

BOX 34-4 DEFECTS WITH INCREASED PULMONARY BLOOD FLOW

Atrial Septal Defect

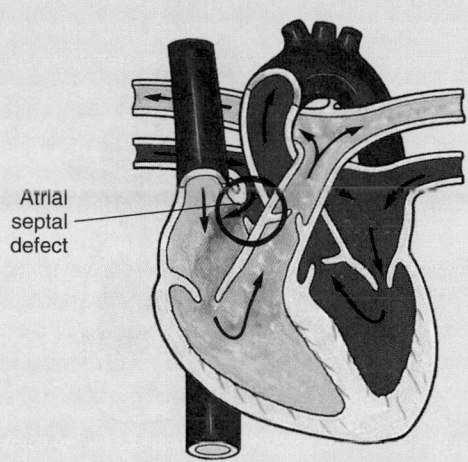

Atrial septal defect

Ventricular Septal Defect

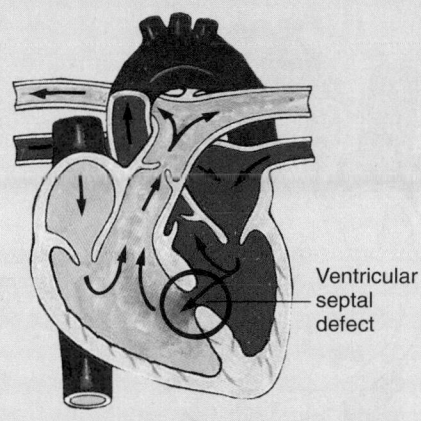

Ventricular septal defect

Description—Abnormal opening between the atria, allowing blood from the higher-pressure left atrium to flow into the lower-pressure right atrium. There are three types of atrial septal defect (ASD):

Ostium primum (ASD 1)—Opening at lower end of septum; may be associated with mitral valve abnormalities

Ostium secundum (ASD 2)—Opening near center of septum

Sinus venosus defect—Opening near junction of superior vena cava and right atrium; may be associated with partial anomalous pulmonary venous connection

Pathophysiology—Because left atrial pressure slightly exceeds right atrial pressure, blood flows from the left to the right atrium, causing an increased flow of oxygenated blood into the right side of the heart. Despite the low pressure difference, a high rate of flow can still occur because of low pulmonary vascular resistance and the greater distensibility of the right atrium, which further reduces flow resistance. This volume is well tolerated by the right ventricle because it is delivered under much lower pressure than with a ventricular septal defect. Although there is right atrial and ventricular enlargement, cardiac failure is unusual in an uncomplicated ASD. Pulmonary vascular changes usually occur only after several decades if the defect is left unrepaired.

Clinical manifestations—Patients may be asymptomatic. They may develop heart failure (HF), particularly in the third or fourth decade of life if the ASD goes undiagnosed, as the pulmonary artery pressure then begins to rise. There is a characteristic murmur. Patients are at risk for atrial dysrhythmias (probably caused by atrial enlargement and stretching of conduction fibers) and pulmonary vascular obstructive disease and emboli formation later in life from chronically increased pulmonary blood flow.

Surgical treatment—Surgical patch closure (pericardial patch or Dacron patch) is done for moderate to large defects. Open repair with cardiopulmonary bypass is usually performed before school age. In addition, the sinus venosus defect requires patch placement, so the anomalous right pulmonary venous return is directed to the left atrium with a baffle. The ASD 1 type may require mitral valve repair or, rarely, replacement of the mitral valve.

Nonsurgical treatment—ASD 2 closure with a device during cardiac catheterization is becoming commonplace and can be done as an outpatient procedure. The Amplatzer septal occluder is most commonly used. Smaller defects that have a rim around them for attachment of the device can be closed with a device; large, irregular defects without a rim require surgical closure. Successful closure in appropriately selected patients yields results similar to surgery but involves shorter hospital stays and fewer complications. Patients receive low-dose aspirin for 6 months (Rome and Kreutzer, 2004).

Prognosis—Operative mortality is very low (<1%). The presence of moderate or severe pulmonary hypertension has a marked adverse effect on survival of patients over 24 years of age at the time of operation (Porter and Edwards, 2008).

Description—Abnormal opening between the right and left ventricles. May be classified according to location: membranous (accounting for 80%) or muscular. May vary in size from a small pinhole to absence of the septum, which results in a common ventricle. Ventricular septal defects (VSDs) are frequently associated with other defects, such as pulmonic stenosis, transposition of the great vessels, patent ductus arteriosus, atrial defects, and coarctation of the aorta. Many VSDs (20% to 60%) close spontaneously. Spontaneous closure is most likely to occur during the first year of life in children having small or moderate defects.

Pathophysiology—Because of the higher pressure within the left ventricle and because the systemic arterial circulation offers more resistance than the pulmonary circulation, blood flows through the defect into the pulmonary artery. The increased blood volume is pumped into the lungs, which may eventually result in increased pulmonary vascular resistance. Increased pressure in the right ventricle as a result of left-to-right shunting and pulmonary resistance causes the muscle to hypertrophy. If the right ventricle is unable to accommodate the increased workload, the right atrium may also enlarge as it attempts to overcome the resistance offered by incomplete right ventricular emptying.

Clinical manifestations—HF is common. There is a characteristic murmur.

Surgical treatment

Palliative—Pulmonary artery banding (placement of a band around the main pulmonary artery to decrease pulmonary blood flow) may be done in infants with multiple muscular VSDs or complex anatomy. Improvements in surgical techniques and postoperative care make complete repair in infancy the preferred approach.

Complete repair (procedure of choice)—Small defects are repaired with sutures. Large defects usually require sewing a knitted Dacron patch over the opening. Cardiopulmonary bypass is used for both procedures. The approach for the repair is generally through the right atrium and the tricuspid valve. Postoperative complications include residual VSD and conduction disturbances.

Nonsurgical treatment—Catheter closure of muscular, postoperative, or fenestrated defects is also widely used in centers nationwide. Device closures of VSDs carry more risk than with ASDs. Knauth, Lock, Perry, and colleagues (2004) reviewed a 13-year experience at Children's Hospital, Boston, with patients undergoing transcatheter device closure of unrepaired congenital or postoperative residual VSDs. Adverse events were common, occurring in 90% of patients; most had hemodynamic instability associated with device positioning. Although these adverse events are common, they were manageable and did not outweigh the benefits.

Prognosis—Risks depend on the location of the defect, the number of defects, and the presence of other associated cardiac defects. Single membranous defects are associated with low mortality (<2%); multiple muscular defects can carry a higher risk (Jacobs, Mavroudis, Jacobs, et al, 2004).

Continued

BOX 34-4   DEFECTS WITH INCREASED PULMONARY BLOOD FLOW—cont'd

Atrioventricular Canal Defect

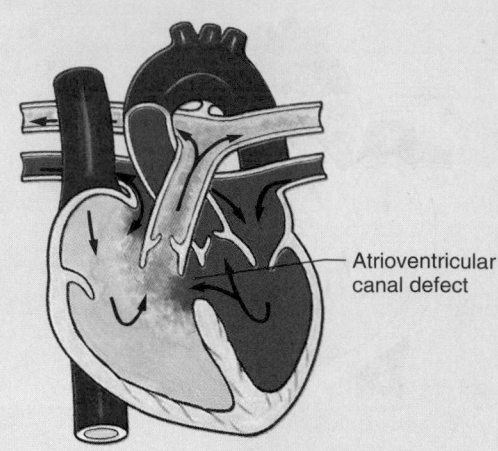

Atrioventricular canal defect

Description—Incomplete fusion of the endocardial cushions. Consists of a low ASD that is continuous with a high VSD and clefts of the mitral and tricuspid valves, which creates a large central atrioventricular (AV) valve that allows blood to flow between all four chambers of the heart. The directions and pathways of flow are determined by pulmonary and systemic resistance, left and right ventricular pressures, and the compliance of each chamber, although flow is generally from left to right. It is the most common cardiac defect in children with Down syndrome.

Pathophysiology—The alterations in hemodynamics depend on the severity of the defect and the child's pulmonary vascular resistance. Immediately after birth, while the newborn's pulmonary vascular resistance is high, there is minimum shunting of blood through the defect. Once this resistance falls, left-to-right shunting occurs and pulmonary blood flow increases. The resultant pulmonary vascular engorgement predisposes the child to development of HF.

Clinical manifestations—Patients usually have moderate to severe HF. There is a characteristic murmur. There may be mild cyanosis that increases with crying. Patients are at high risk for developing pulmonary vascular obstructive disease.

Surgical treatment

Palliative—Pulmonary artery banding is occasionally done in small infants with severe symptoms. Complete repair in infancy is most common.

Complete repair—Surgical repair consists of patch closure of the septal defects and reconstruction of the AV valve tissue (either repair of the mitral valve cleft or fashioning of two AV valves). Postoperative complications include heart block, HF, mitral regurgitation, dysrhythmias, and pulmonary hypertension.

Prognosis—Operative mortality is less than 5% (Jacobs, Mavroudis, Jacobs, et al, 2004). A potential later problem is mitral regurgitation, which may require valve replacement.

⊖ Patent Ductus Arteriosus

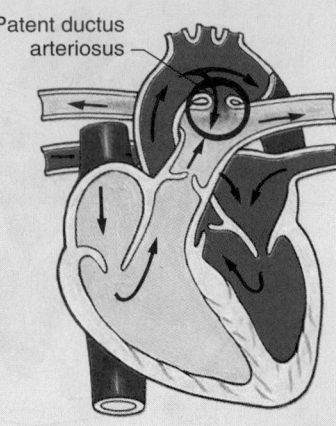

Patent ductus arteriosus

Description—Failure of the fetal ductus arteriosus (artery connecting the aorta and pulmonary artery) to close within the first weeks of life. The continued patency of this vessel allows blood to flow from the higher-pressure aorta to the lower-pressure pulmonary artery, which causes a left-to-right shunt.

Pathophysiology—The hemodynamic consequences of patent ductus arteriosus (PDA) depend on the size of the ductus and the pulmonary vascular resistance. At birth the resistance in the pulmonary and systemic circulations is almost identical, so that the resistance in the aorta and pulmonary artery is equalized. As the systemic pressure comes to exceed the pulmonary pressure, blood begins to shunt from the aorta across the duct to the pulmonary artery (left-to-right shunt). The additional blood is recirculated through the lungs and returned to the left atrium and left ventricle. The effect of this altered circulation is increased workload on the left side of the heart, increased pulmonary vascular congestion and possibly resistance, and potentially increased right ventricular pressure and hypertrophy.

Clinical manifestations—Patients may be asymptomatic or show signs of HF. There is a characteristic machinery-like murmur. A widened pulse pressure and bounding pulses result from runoff of blood from the aorta to the pulmonary artery. Patients are at risk for infective endocarditis and pulmonary vascular obstructive disease in later life from chronic excessive pulmonary blood flow.

Medical management—Administration of indomethacin (prostaglandin inhibitor) has proved successful in closing a patent ductus in premature infants and some newborns.

Surgical treatment—Surgical division or ligation of the patent vessel is performed via a left thoracotomy. In video-assisted thoracoscopic surgery, a thoracoscope and instruments are inserted through three small incisions on the left side of the chest to place a clip on the ductus. The technique is used in some centers and eliminates the need for a thoracotomy, thereby speeding postoperative recovery.

Nonsurgical treatment—Coils to occlude the PDA are placed in the catheterization laboratory in many centers. Premature or small infants (with small-diameter femoral arteries) and patients with large or unusual PDAs may require surgery.

Prognosis—Both surgical and nonsurgical procedures can be done at low risk with less than 1% mortality. PDA closure in very premature infants has a higher mortality rate because of the additional significant medical problems.

---

repair, and (2) preparation and care of the child and family when invasive procedures (catheterization and surgery) are performed. For nursing care related to the child with hypoxemia and HF, the reader should refer to earlier discussions of these topics.

Nursing care of the child with a congenital heart defect begins as soon as the diagnosis is suspected. Prenatal diagnosis of congenital heart defects is becoming increasingly frequent. New demands are being placed on nurses to counsel and support families as they prepare for the birth of these infants.

BOX 34-5   OBSTRUCTIVE DEFECTS

Coarctation of the Aorta

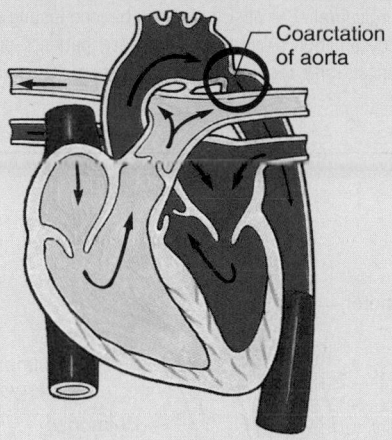

Coarctation of aorta

Description—Localized narrowing near the insertion of the ductus arteriosus, which results in increased pressure proximal to the defect (head and upper extremities) and decreased pressure distal to the obstruction (body and lower extremities).

Pathophysiology—The effect of a narrowing within the aorta is increased pressure proximal to the defect (upper extremities) and decreased pressure distal to it (lower extremities).

Clinical manifestations—There may be high blood pressure and bounding pulses in the arms, weak or absent femoral pulses, and cool lower extremities with lower blood pressure. There are signs of heart failure (HF) in infants. In infants with critical coarctation, the hemodynamic condition may deteriorate rapidly with severe acidosis and hypotension. Mechanical ventilation and inotropic support are often necessary before surgery. Older children may experience dizziness, headaches, fainting, and epistaxis resulting from hypertension. Patients are at risk for hypertension, ruptured aorta, aortic aneurysm, and stroke.

Surgical treatment—Surgical repair is the treatment of choice for infants younger than 6 months of age and for patients with long-segment stenosis or complex anatomy; surgery may be performed for all patients with coarctation. Repair is by resection of the coarcted portion with an end-to-end anastomosis of the aorta or enlargement of the constricted section using a graft of prosthetic material or a portion of the left subclavian artery. Because this defect is outside the heart and pericardium, cardiopulmonary bypass is not required, and a thoracotomy incision is used. Postoperative hypertension is treated with intravenous sodium nitroprusside, esmolol, or milrinone followed by oral medications, such as angiotensin-converting enzyme inhibitors or beta blockers. Residual permanent hypertension after repair of coarctation of the aorta (COA) seems to be related to age and time of repair. To prevent both hypertension at rest and exercise-provoked systemic hypertension after repair, elective surgery for COA is advised within the first 2 years of life. There is increased risk of recurrence in patients who underwent surgical repair as infants (Beekman, 2008). Percutaneous balloon angioplasty techniques have proved to be very effective in relieving residual postoperative coarctation gradients.

Nonsurgical treatment—Balloon angioplasty is a primary intervention for COA in older infants and children. In adolescents, stents may be placed in the aorta to maintain patency. The goal of the procedure is to achieve a reduction in gradient to less than 10%, or more than 90% relief of obstruction angiographically. Dilation and/or stent implantation for native or recurrent coarctation seems to immediately relieve obstruction in more than 90% of cases (Holzer, Chisolm, Hill, et al, 2008).

Prognosis—Mortality is less than 5% in patients with isolated coarctation; risk is increased in infants with other complex cardiac defects (Jacobs, Mavroudis, Jacobs, et al, 2004).

Aortic Stenosis

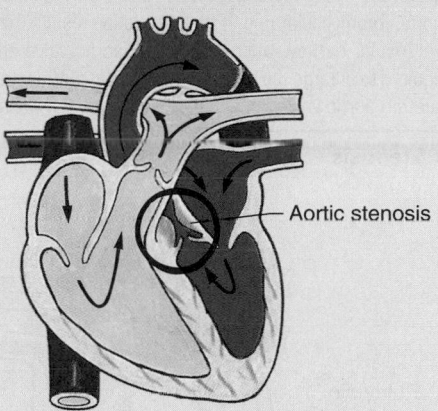

Aortic stenosis

Description—Narrowing or stricture of the aortic valve, causing resistance to blood flow in the left ventricle, decreased cardiac output, left ventricular hypertrophy, and pulmonary vascular congestion. The prominent anatomic consequence of aortic stenosis (AS) is hypertrophy of the left ventricular wall. Left ventricular hypertrophy also interferes with coronary artery perfusion and may result in myocardial infarction or scarring of the papillary muscles of the left ventricle. Valvular stenosis, the most common type, is usually caused by malformed cusps that result in a bicuspid rather than tricuspid valve or fusion of the cusps. Subvalvular stenosis is a stricture caused by a fibrous ring below a normal valve; supravalvular stenosis occurs infrequently. Valvular AS is a serious defect because (1) the obstruction tends to be progressive; (2) sudden episodes of myocardial ischemia, or low cardiac output, can result in sudden death; and (3) surgical repair rarely results in a normal valve. This is one of the rare instances in which strenuous physical activity may be curtailed because of the cardiac condition.

Pathophysiology—A stricture in the aortic outflow tract causes resistance to ejection of blood from the left ventricle. The extra workload on the left ventricle causes hypertrophy. If left ventricular failure develops, left atrial pressure will increase; this causes increased pressure in the pulmonary veins, which results in pulmonary vascular congestion (pulmonary edema).

Clinical manifestations—Newborns with critical AS demonstrate signs of decreased cardiac output with faint pulses, hypotension, tachycardia, and poor feeding. Children show signs of exercise intolerance, chest pain, and dizziness when standing for a long period. There is a characteristic murmur. Patients are at risk for infective endocarditis, coronary insufficiency, and ventricular dysfunction.

Valvular Aortic Stenosis

Surgical treatment—Aortic valvotomy is performed under inflow occlusion. Used rarely, since balloon dilation in the catheterization laboratory is the first-line procedure. Newborns with critical AS and small left-sided structures may undergo a stage 1 Norwood procedure (see Hypoplastic Left Heart Syndrome, Box 34-7).

Prognosis—Aortic valve replacement is a viable treatment option and may lead to normalization of left ventricular size and function (Arnold, Ley-Zaporozhan, Ley, et al, 2008). However, aortic valvotomy remains a palliative procedure, and approximately 25% of patients require additional surgery within 10 years for recurrent stenosis. A valve replacement may be required at the second procedure. An aortic homograft with a valve may also be used (extended aortic root replacement), or the pulmonic valve may be moved to the aortic position and replaced with a homograft valve (Ross procedure).

Nonsurgical treatment—The narrowed valve is dilated using balloon angioplasty in the catheterization laboratory. This procedure is usually the first intervention.

Prognosis—Complications include aortic insufficiency or valvular regurgitation, tearing of the valve leaflets, and loss of pulse in the catheterized limb.

Continued

BOX 34-5 OBSTRUCTIVE DEFECTS—cont'd

Aortic Stenosis—cont'd
⊜ *Subvalvular Aortic Stenosis*
Surgical treatment—Procedure may involve incising a membrane if one exists or cutting the fibromuscular ring. If the obstruction results from narrowing of the left ventricular outflow tract and a small aortic valve annulus, a patch may be required to enlarge the entire left ventricular outflow tract and annulus and replace the aortic valve, an approach known as the Konno procedure.

Prognosis—Surgical relief of obstruction can be long lasting without aortic or mitral valve dysfunction. About 20% of these patients develop recurrent subaortic stenosis and require additional surgery (Schneider and Moore, 2008).

Pulmonic Stenosis

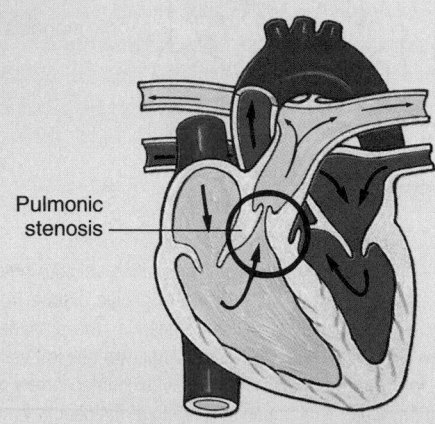

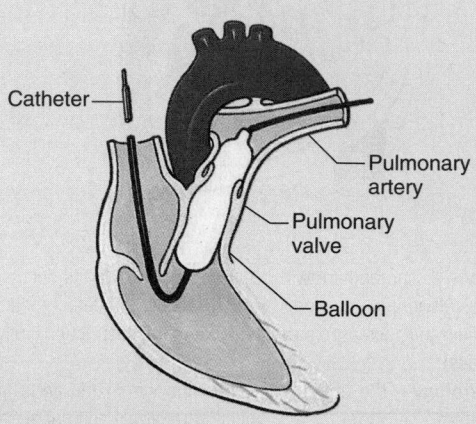

Description—Narrowing at the entrance to the pulmonary artery. Resistance to blood flow causes right ventricular hypertrophy and decreased pulmonary blood flow. Pulmonary atresia is the extreme form of pulmonic stenosis (PS) in that there is total fusion of the commissures and no blood flows to the lungs. The right ventricle may be hypoplastic.

Pathophysiology—When PS is present, resistance to blood flow causes right ventricular hypertrophy. If right ventricular failure develops, right atrial pressure increases, and this may result in reopening of the foramen ovale, shunting of unoxygenated blood into the left atrium, and systemic cyanosis. If PS is severe, HF occurs, and systemic venous engorgement is noted. An associated defect such as a patent ductus arteriosus partially compensates for the obstruction by shunting blood from the aorta to the pulmonary artery and into the lungs.

Clinical manifestations—Patients may be asymptomatic; some have mild cyanosis or HF. Progressive narrowing causes increased symptoms. Newborns with severe narrowing are cyanotic. There is a characteristic murmur. Cardiomegaly is evident on chest radiographic films. Patients are at risk for infective endocarditis.

Surgical treatment—In infants, transventricular (closed) valvotomy (Brock procedure). In children, pulmonary valvotomy with cardiopulmonary bypass. Need for surgical treatment is rare with widespread use of balloon angioplasty techniques.

Nonsurgical treatment—Balloon angioplasty in the cardiac catheterization laboratory to dilate the valve. A catheter is inserted across the stenotic pulmonic valve into the pulmonary artery, and a balloon at the end of the catheter is inflated and rapidly passed through the narrowed opening. (See figure below, left.) The procedure is associated with few complications and has proved to be highly effective. It is the treatment of choice for discrete PS in most centers and can be done safely in neonates.

Prognosis—Risk is low for both surgical and nonsurgical procedures; mortality is low, slightly higher in neonates. Both balloon dilation and surgical valvotomy leave the pulmonic valve incompetent because they involve opening the fused valve leaflets; however, these patients are clinically asymptomatic. Long-term problems with restenosis or valve incompetence may occur.

QUALITY PATIENT OUTCOMES: Congenital Heart Disease
- Improved cardiac function
- Prevention of fluid and sodium overload
- Decreased cardiac demands
- Improved oxygenation
- Reduced respiratory distress

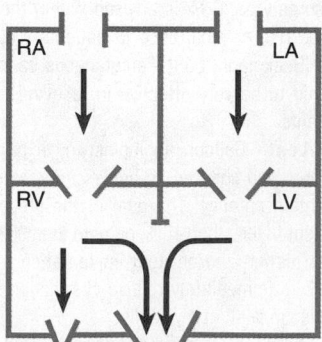

Fig. 34-15 Hemodynamic defects with decreased pulmonary blood flow. See Fig. 34-2 for abbreviations.

Help the Family Adjust to the Disorder

Once parents learn of the heart defect, they are initially in a period of shock, followed by high anxiety, especially fear of the child's death. This reaction may occur soon after the child's birth or at a later period. Whatever its timing, the family needs a period of grief before assimilating the meaning of the defect.

BOX 34-6 DEFECTS WITH DECREASED PULMONARY BLOOD FLOW

Tetralogy of Fallot

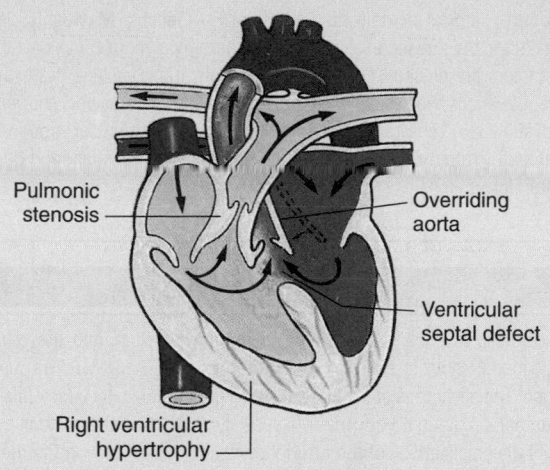

Pulmonic stenosis

Overriding aorta

Ventricular septal defect

Right ventricular hypertrophy

Description—The classic form includes four defects: (1) ventricular septal defect (VSD), (2) pulmonic stenosis, (3) overriding aorta, and (4) right ventricular hypertrophy.

Pathophysiology—The alteration in hemodynamics varies widely, depending primarily on the degree of pulmonic stenosis, but also on the size of the VSD and the pulmonary and systemic resistance to flow. Because the VSD is usually large, pressures may be equal in the right and left ventricles. Therefore the shunt direction depends on the difference between pulmonary and systemic vascular resistance. If pulmonary vascular resistance is higher than systemic resistance, the shunt is from right to left. If systemic resistance is higher than pulmonary resistance, the shunt is from left to right. Pulmonic stenosis decreases blood flow to the lungs and consequently the amount of oxygenated blood that returns to the left side of the heart. Depending on the position of the aorta, blood from both ventricles may be distributed systemically.

Clinical manifestations—Some infants may be acutely cyanotic at birth; others have mild cyanosis that progresses over the first year of life as the pulmonic stenosis worsens. There is a characteristic murmur. There may be acute episodes of cyanosis and hypoxia, called *blue spells* or *tet spells* (see p. 1362). Anoxic spells occur when the infant's oxygen requirements exceed the blood supply, usually during crying or after feeding. Patients are at risk for emboli, seizures, and loss of consciousness or sudden death following an anoxic spell.

Surgical treatment

Palliative shunt—In infants who cannot undergo primary repair, a palliative procedure to increase pulmonary blood flow and increase oxygen saturation may be performed. The preferred procedure is a modified Blalock-Taussig shunt operation, which provides blood flow to the pulmonary arteries from the left or right subclavian artery via a tube graft (see Table 34-4). In general, however, shunts are avoided because they may result in pulmonary artery distortion.

Complete repair—Elective repair is usually performed in the first year of life. Indications for repair include increasing cyanosis and the development of hypercyanotic spells. Complete repair involves closure of the VSD and resection of the infundibular stenosis, with placement of a pericardial patch to enlarge the right ventricular outflow tract. In some repairs, the patch may extend across the pulmonic valve annulus (transannular patch), making the pulmonic valve incompetent. The procedure requires a median sternotomy and the use of cardiopulmonary bypass.

Prognosis—The operative mortality for total correction of tetralogy of Fallot is less than 3% (Jacobs, Mavroudis, Jacobs, et al, 2004). With improved surgical techniques there is a lower incidence of dysrhythmias and sudden death; surgical heart block is rare. Heart failure may occur postoperatively.

Tricuspid Atresia

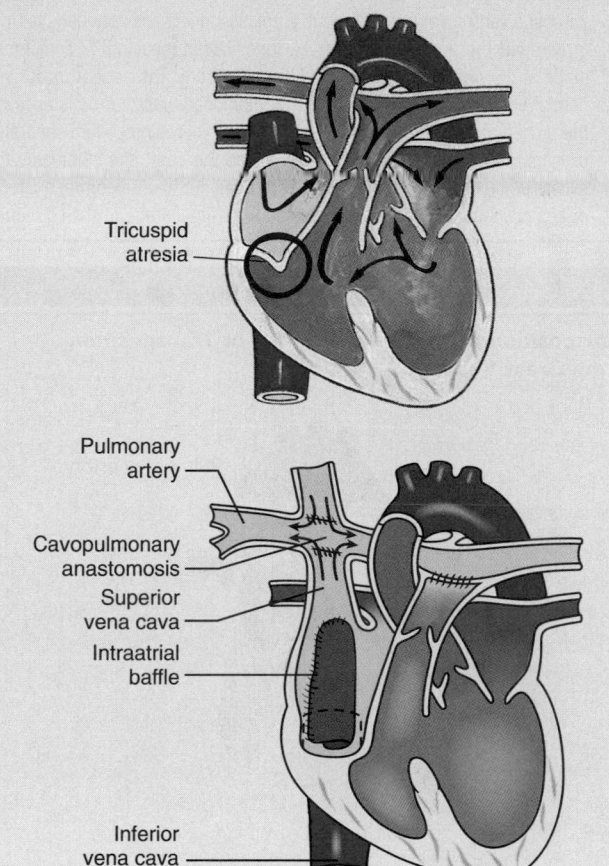

Tricuspid atresia

Pulmonary artery

Cavopulmonary anastomosis

Superior vena cava

Intraatrial baffle

Inferior vena cava

Description—The tricuspid valve fails to develop; consequently there is no communication from the right atrium to the right ventricle. Blood flows through an atrial septal defect (ASD) or a patent foramen ovale to the left side of the heart and through a VSD to the right ventricle and out to the lungs. The condition is often associated with pulmonic stenosis and transposition of the great arteries. There is complete mixing of unoxygenated and oxygenated blood in the left side of the heart, which results in systemic desaturation, and varying amounts of pulmonary obstruction, which causes decreased pulmonary blood flow.

Pathophysiology—At birth the presence of a patent foramen ovale (or other atrial septal opening) is required to permit blood flow across the septum into the left atrium; the patent ductus arteriosus allows blood flow to the pulmonary artery into the lungs for oxygenation. A VSD allows a modest amount of blood to enter the right ventricle and pulmonary artery for oxygenation. Pulmonary blood flow usually is diminished.

Clinical manifestations—Cyanosis is usually seen in the newborn period. There may be tachycardia and dyspnea. Older children have signs of chronic hypoxemia with clubbing.

Therapeutic management—For the neonate whose pulmonary blood flow depends on the patency of the ductus arteriosus, a continuous infusion of prostaglandin E_1 is started at 0.1 mg/kg of body weight/min until surgical intervention can be arranged.

Surgical treatment—Palliative treatment is the placement of a shunt (pulmonary–to–systemic artery anastomosis) to increase blood flow to the lungs. If the ASD is small, an atrial septostomy is performed during cardiac catheterization. Some children have increased pulmonary blood flow and require pulmonary artery banding to lessen the volume of blood to the lungs. A bidirectional Glenn shunt (cavopulmonary anastomosis) may be performed at 4 to 9 months as a second stage.

Continued

BOX 34-6   DEFECTS WITH DECREASED PULMONARY BLOOD FLOW—cont'd

Tricuspid Atresia—cont'd

Modified Fontan procedure—Systemic venous return is directed to the lungs without a ventricular pump through surgical connections between the right atrium and the pulmonary artery. A fenestration (opening) is sometimes made in the right atrial baffle to relieve pressure. The patient must have normal ventricular function and a low pulmonary vascular resistance for the procedure to be successful. The modified Fontan procedure separates oxygenated and unoxygenated blood inside the heart and eliminates the excess volume load on the ventricle but does not restore normal anatomy or hemodynamics. This operation is also the final stage in the correction

of many complex defects with a functional single ventricle, including hypoplastic left heart syndrome.

Prognosis—Surgical mortality is less than 5% (Jacobs, Mavroudis, Jacobs, et al, 2004); the rate increases when the anatomy is more complex and other risk factors are present. Postoperative complications include dysrhythmias, systemic venous hypertension, pleural and pericardial effusions, and ventricular dysfunction. Long-term concerns are the development of protein-losing enteropathy, atrial dysrhythmias, late ventricular dysfunction, and developmental delays.

BOX 34-7   MIXED DEFECTS

Transposition of the Great Arteries or Transposition of the Great Vessels

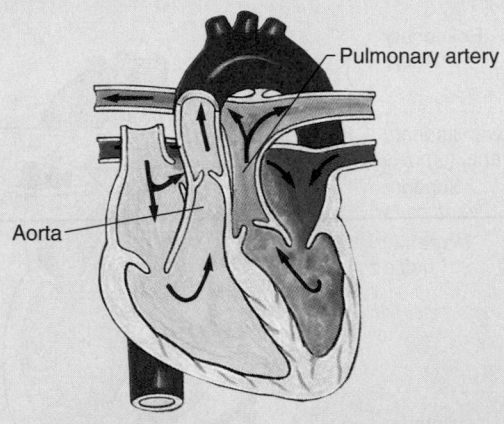

Description—The pulmonary artery leaves the left ventricle, and the aorta exits from the right ventricle, with no communication between the systemic and pulmonary circulations.

Pathophysiology—Associated defects such as septal defects or patent ductus arteriosus must be present to permit blood to enter the systemic circulation or the pulmonary circulation for mixing of saturated and desaturated blood. The most common defect associated with transposition of the great arteries (TGA) is a patent foramen ovale. At birth there is also a patent ductus arteriosus, although in most instances this closes after the neonatal period. Another associated defect may be a ventricular septal defect (VSD). The presence of a VSD increases the risk of heart failure (HF), because it permits blood to flow from the right to the left ventricle, into the pulmonary artery, and finally to the lungs. However, it also produces high pulmonary blood flow under high pressure, which can result in high pulmonary vascular resistance.

Clinical manifestations—Depend on the type and size of the associated defects. Newborns with minimum communication are severely cyanotic and have depressed function at birth. Those with large septal defects or a patent ductus arteriosus may be less cyanotic but have symptoms of HF. Heart sounds vary according to the type of defect present. Cardiomegaly is usually evident a few weeks after birth.

Therapeutic management (to provide intracardiac mixing)—Intravenous prostaglandin E_1 may be administered to keep the ductus arteriosus open to temporarily increase blood mixing and provide an oxygen saturation of 75% or to maintain cardiac output. During cardiac catheterization or under echocardiographic guidance, a balloon atrial septostomy (Rashkind procedure) may also be performed to increase mixing by opening the atrial septum.

Surgical treatment—An arterial switch procedure is the procedure of choice performed in the first weeks of life. It involves transecting the great arteries and anastomosing the main pulmonary artery to the proximal aorta (just above the aortic valve) and anastomosing the ascending aorta to the proximal pulmonary artery. The coronary arteries are switched from the proximal aorta to the proximal pulmonary artery to create a new aorta. Reimplantation of

the coronary arteries is critical to the infant's survival, and they must be reattached without torsion or kinking to provide the heart with its supply of oxygen. The advantage of the arterial switch procedure is the reestablishment of normal circulation, with the left ventricle acting as the systemic pump. Potential complications of the arterial switch include narrowing at the great artery anastomoses and coronary artery insufficiency.

Intraatrial baffle repairs—Intraatrial baffle repairs are rarely performed, although many adolescents and adults survive today with repairs that were done more than 15 years ago. An intraatrial baffle is created to divert venous blood to the mitral valve and pulmonary venous blood to the tricuspid valve using the patient's atrial septum (Senning procedure) or a prosthetic material (Mustard procedure). A disadvantage is the continuing role of the right ventricle as the systemic pump and the late development of right ventricular failure and rhythm disturbances. Other potential postoperative complications include loss of normal sinus rhythm, baffle leaks, and ventricular dysfunction.

Rastelli procedure—This procedure is the operative choice in infants with TGA, VSD, and severe pulmonic stenosis. It involves closure of the VSD with a baffle, so that left ventricular blood is directed through the VSD into the aorta. The pulmonic valve is then closed, and a conduit is placed from the right ventricle to the pulmonary artery to create a physiologically normal circulation. Unfortunately, this procedure requires multiple conduit replacements as the child grows.

Prognosis—Operative mortality is less than 2% (Jacobs, Mavroudis, Jacobs, et al, 2004). Potential long-term problems include suprapulmonic stenosis and neoaorta dilation and regurgitation.

Total Anomalous Pulmonary Venous Connection

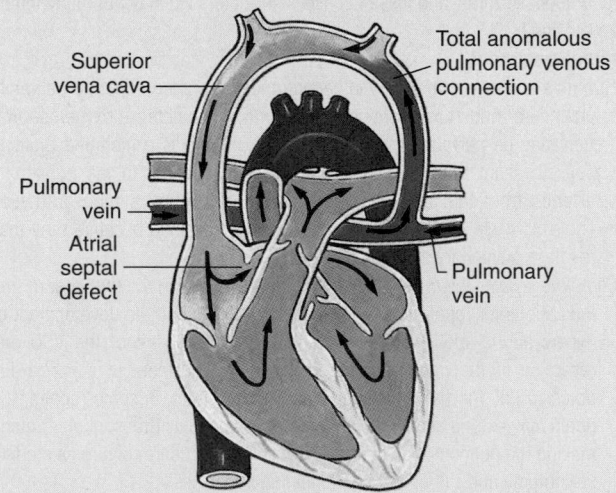

Description—Rare defect characterized by failure of the pulmonary veins to join the left atrium. Instead, the pulmonary veins are abnormally connected to the systemic venous circuit via the right atrium or various veins draining toward the right atrium, such as the superior vena cava. The abnormal

BOX 34-7   MIXED DEFECTS—cont'd

Total Anomalous Pulmonary Venous Connection—cont'd

attachment results in mixed blood's being returned to the right atrium and shunted from the right to the left through an atrial septal defect (ASD). Total anomalous pulmonary venous connection (TAPVC; also called *total anomalous pulmonary venous return* or *total anomalous pulmonary venous drainage*) is classified according to the pulmonary venous point of attachment as follows:

Supracardiac—Attachment above the diaphragm, such as to the superior vena cava (most common form) (see Fig. 34-11)

Cardiac—Direct attachment to the heart, such as to the right atrium or coronary sinus

Infradiaphragmatic—Attachment below the diaphragm, such as to the inferior vena cava (most severe form)

Pathophysiology—The right atrium receives all the blood that normally would flow into the left atrium. As a result, the right side of the heart hypertrophies, whereas the left side, especially the left atrium, may remain small. An associated ASD or patent foramen ovale allows systemic venous blood to shunt from the higher-pressure right atrium to the left atrium and into the left side of the heart. As a result, the oxygen saturation of the blood in both sides of the heart (and ultimately in the systemic arterial circulation) is the same. If the pulmonary blood flow is large, pulmonary venous return is also large, and the amount of saturated blood is relatively high. However, if there is obstruction to pulmonary venous drainage, pulmonary venous return is impeded, pulmonary venous pressure rises, and pulmonary interstitial edema develops and eventually contributes to HF. Infradiaphragmatic TAPVC is often associated with obstruction to pulmonary venous drainage and is a surgical emergency.

Clinical manifestations—Most infants develop cyanosis early in life. The degree of cyanosis is inversely related to the amount of pulmonary blood flow—the more pulmonary blood, the less cyanosis. Children with unobstructed TAPVC may be asymptomatic until pulmonary vascular resistance decreases during infancy, increasing pulmonary blood flow, with resulting signs of HF. Cyanosis becomes worse with pulmonary vein obstruction; once obstruction occurs, the infant's condition usually deteriorates rapidly. Without intervention, cardiac failure progresses to death.

Surgical treatment—Corrective repair is performed in early infancy. The surgical approach varies with the anatomic defect. In general, however, the common pulmonary vein is anastomosed to the back of the left atrium, the ASD is closed, and the anomalous pulmonary venous connection is ligated. The cardiac type is most easily repaired; the infradiaphragmatic type carries the highest morbidity and mortality because of the higher incidence of pulmonary vein obstruction. Potential postoperative complications include reobstruction; bleeding; dysrhythmias, particularly heart block; pulmonary artery hypertension; and persistent heart failure.

Prognosis—Mortality for all types is less than 10% (Jacobs, Mavroudis, Jacobs, et al, 2004) and is lowest for the cardiac type; morbidity increases with the presence of pulmonary vein obstruction.

Truncus Arteriosus

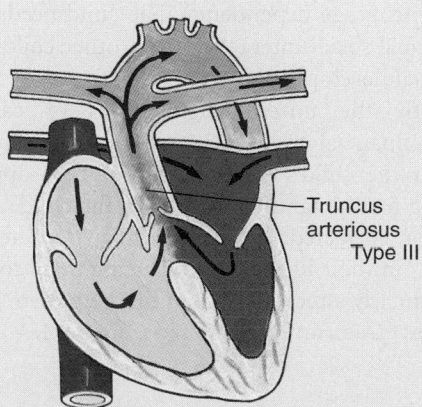

Truncus arteriosus Type III

Description—Failure of normal septation and division of the embryonic bulbar trunk into the pulmonary artery and the aorta, which results in development of a single vessel that overrides both ventricles. Blood from both ventricles mixes in the common great artery, which leads to desaturation and hypoxemia. Blood ejected from the heart flows preferentially to the lower-pressure pulmonary arteries, so that pulmonary blood flow is increased and systemic blood flow is reduced. There are three types:

Type I—A single pulmonary trunk arises near the base of the truncus and divides into the left and right pulmonary arteries.

Type II—The left and right pulmonary arteries arise separately but in close proximity and at the same level from the back of the truncus.

Type III—The pulmonary arteries arise independently from the sides of the truncus.

Pathophysiology—Blood ejected from the left and right ventricles enters the common trunk, so that pulmonary and systemic circulations are mixed. Blood flow is distributed to the pulmonary and systemic circulations according to the relative resistances of each system. The amount of pulmonary blood flow depends on the size of the pulmonary arteries and the pulmonary vascular resistance. Generally, resistance to pulmonary blood flow is less than systemic vascular resistance, which results in preferential blood flow to the lungs. Pulmonary vascular disease develops at an early age in patients with truncus arteriosus.

Clinical manifestations—Most infants are symptomatic with moderate to severe HF and variable cyanosis, poor growth, and activity intolerance. There is a characteristic murmur. Thirty-five percent of patients have 22q11 deletions (Goldmuntz and Lin, 2008).

Surgical treatment—Early repair is performed in the first month of life. It involves closing the VSD so that the truncus arteriosus receives the outflow from the left ventricle, and excising the pulmonary arteries from the aorta and attaching them to the right ventricle by means of a homograft. Currently homografts (segments of cadaver aorta and pulmonary artery that are treated with antibiotics and cryopreserved) are preferred over synthetic conduits to establish continuity between the right ventricle and pulmonary artery. Homografts are more flexible and easier to use during the procedure and appear less prone to obstruction. Postoperative complications include persistent heart failure, bleeding, pulmonary artery hypertension, dysrhythmias, and residual VSD. Because conduits are not living tissue, they will not grow along with the child and may also become narrowed with calcifications. One or more conduit replacements will be needed in childhood.

Prognosis—Mortality is greater than 10%; future operations are required to replace the conduits.

Hypoplastic Left Heart Syndrome (HLHS)

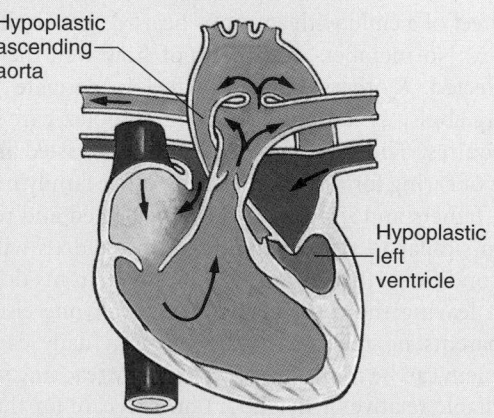

Hypoplastic ascending aorta

Hypoplastic left ventricle

Description—Underdevelopment of the left side of the heart, resulting in a hypoplastic left ventricle and aortic atresia. Most blood from the left atrium flows across the patent foramen ovale to the right atrium, to the right ventricle, and out the pulmonary artery. The descending aorta receives blood from the patent ductus arteriosus supplying systemic blood flow.

Continued

BOX 34-7   MIXED DEFECTS—cont'd

Hypoplastic Left Heart Syndrome—cont'd

Pathophysiology—An ASD or patent foramen ovale allows saturated blood from the left atrium to mix with desaturated blood from the right atrium and to flow through the right ventricle and out into the pulmonary artery. From the pulmonary artery, the blood flows both to the lungs and through the ductus arteriosus into the aorta and out to the body. The amount of blood flow to the pulmonary and systemic circulations depends on the relationship between the pulmonary and systemic vascular resistances. The coronary and cerebral vessels receive blood by retrograde flow through the hypoplastic ascending aorta.

Clinical manifestations—There is mild cyanosis and signs of HF until the patent ductus arteriosus closes, then progressive deterioration with cyanosis and decreased cardiac output, leading to cardiovascular collapse. The condition is usually fatal in the first months of life without intervention.

Therapeutic management—Neonates require stabilization with mechanical ventilation and inotropic support preoperatively. A prostaglandin E_1 infusion is needed to maintain ductal patency and ensure adequate systemic blood flow.

Surgical treatment—Multiple-stage approach is used. The first stage is a Norwood procedure, which involves an anastomosis of the main pulmonary artery to the aorta to create a new aorta, shunting to provide pulmonary blood flow (usually with a modified Blalock-Taussig shunt), and creation of a large ASD. Postoperative complications include imbalance of systemic and pulmonary blood flow, bleeding, low cardiac output, and persistent heart failure. A new modification of the first-stage repair is the use of a right ventricle–to–pulmonary artery homograft conduit instead of a shunt to supply pulmonary

blood flow. The second stage is often a bidirectional Glenn shunt procedure (see Fig 34-11) or a hemi-Fontan operation. Both involve anastomosing the superior vena cava to the right pulmonary artery so superior vena cava flow bypasses the right atrium and flows directly to the lungs. The procedure is usually done at 3 to 6 months of age to relieve cyanosis and reduce the volume load on the right ventricle. The final repair is a modified Fontan procedure. (See Tricuspid Atresia, Box 34-6.)

Transplantation—Heart transplantation in the newborn period is another option for these infants. Problems include the shortage of newborn organ donors, risk of rejection, long-term problems with chronic immunosuppression, and infection (see Heart Transplantation, p. 1403).

Prognosis—For the first-stage surgical repair, mortality rates range from 5% to 30% (Tweddell, Hoffman, Ghanayem, et al, 2008). Improved outcomes have been associated with early diagnosis and repair and increased monitoring in the hospital and at home (Tweddell, Hoffman, Ghanayem, et al, 2008). Because of this, there has been increased use nationwide of a home monitoring program, in which the infant and the caregiver are discharged with a pulse oximeter and home scale. Parents or caregivers are instructed to maintain a diary and are given specific criteria of when to notify their cardiac team: saturation below 75% or above 90%, acute weight loss of 30 g or more, failure to gain at least 20 g during a 3-day period, or enteral intake below 100 mL/kg/day (Tweddell, Hoffman, Ghanayem, et al, 2008). Long-term problems with repair include worsening ventricular function, tricuspid regurgitation, recurrent aortic arch narrowing, dysrhythmias, and developmental delays. There is a risk of mortality between surgical procedures. The mortality for the later two operations is less than 5%.

Unfortunately, the demands for medical treatment may not allow this, necessitating that the parents be informed of the condition to give informed consent for diagnostic and therapeutic procedures. The nurse can be instrumental in supporting parents in their loss, assessing their level of understanding, supplying information as needed, and helping other members of the health team understand the parents' reactions.

Severely ill newborns usually remain in the hospital. The nurse can promote parent-infant attachment by encouraging parents to hold, touch, and look at their child and by providing time and privacy to the parents to spend with their newborn. (See Chapter 10 for suggestions for promoting attachment between parents and their hospitalized newborn.)

The effect of a child with a serious heart defect on the family is complex. No members, regardless of how well they adjust, are unaffected. Mothers frequently feel inadequate in their mothering ability because of the more complex care such an infant requires. They may be constantly exhausted from the pressures of caring for this child and the other family members. Likewise, fathers and siblings may feel neglected and resentful, a reaction similar to that in families with children with other chronic conditions. (See Chapter 22.) Often parents do not feel confident leaving the child in the care of anyone else, which affords parents no relief from the constant daily caregiving. This problem can be minimized by gradually teaching someone else (a reliable relative or neighbor) how to care for the child.

The need to maintain discipline and set consistent limits can be difficult for parents. A study by Uzark and Jones (2003) found higher levels of stress in parents of children with heart disease, particularly with regard to limit setting and discipline. Behavior modification techniques using either concrete rewards (e.g., a favorite food) or social reinforcement (e.g., approval)

can be effective. However, these techniques are most beneficial if used before the child learns to control the family. Therefore guiding parents toward the need for discipline while the child is in infancy is necessary to prevent later problems.

Another problem that may develop within family relationships is overdependency on the part of the child. This is often a result of parental fear that the child may die and overcompensation through what has been termed *benevolent overreaction*. (See Chapter 22.) Research has shown no correlation between the severity of the child's heart defect and maternal anxiety or parental stress (Morelius, Lundh, and Nelson, 2002). The best approach to dealing with this dilemma is prevention. Parents need guidance to recognize the eventual hazards of continuing dependency and protectiveness as the child grows older, and the nurse can assist parents in learning ways to foster optimum development. Unless parents have help to see what activities the child can do, they may focus on physical limitations and encourage dependency. The child needs opportunities for normal social interaction with other children to foster normal social development.

Frequently the unremitting stresses of care—physical exhaustion, financial costs, emotional upset, fear of death, and concern for the child's future—are not fully appreciated by those caring for the family. Even when the child's condition is stabilized or corrected, the family may need to make new adjustments in their lifestyle. Introducing them to other families with similarly affected children can help them adjust to the daily stresses* (see Family-Centered Care box).

---

*Some local affiliates of the American Heart Association have organized parent groups.

FAMILY-CENTERED CARE

The Diagnosis of Heart Disease

Remember, we don't have your experience. We don't see children every day who have heart disease. We would have been upset finding out our child had to have his tonsils out. How could we ever be prepared for this? Please remember, we only know people who have trivial heart murmurs. How could we ever expect this to happen? And to us, this is the worst problem we've ever heard of.

We still fear most what we don't know and understand. Be honest with us. If you don't know either, tell us. But at least don't leave us wondering about what you know and we don't. Not knowing anything really can be worse than knowing something bad. Be honest, but don't strip us of hope. …

Please, remember we are trying to learn complex information in a moment of time. And trying to learn it in a context of great pain and emotional investment. This is our lives you're talking about. Please be thorough, but keep it simple. Tell us again, maybe even again and again, when we can hear better.

From Schrey C, Schrey M: A parent's perspective: our needs and our message, *Crit Care Nurs Clin North Am* 6(1):113-119, 1994.

Educate the Family About the Disorder

Once parents are ready to hear about their child's heart condition, it is essential that they receive a clear explanation based on their level of understanding. A review of normal cardiac anatomy is helpful before explaining the anatomic defect. A simple diagram, pictures, or a model of the heart can be most helpful in visualizing the heart and the congenital defect. Parents appreciate receiving written information about the specific condition.* Health care professionals should take advantage of subsequent encounters with the family to assess parental understanding of the condition and clarify information as needed.

Different health personnel may convey the same information using different diagrams and medical terms. To prevent this from becoming a problem, the same type of diagram should be used by all, and the parents should write down any unclear terms or ask for clarification. Sometimes it is helpful to provide the family with a glossary of frequently used words for reference.

Parents often use multiple resources to obtain information about their child's heart defect. Increasingly, families are using the Internet as a source of information. Locating information can be easy with helpful information located at national organizations and large parent support groups.† Parents also find

support through contacts with other parents and parent groups. It is important for parents to realize that not all websites offer medically accurate information and that information from other parents may not be applicable to their own situation. Some children with rare, complex heart defects require individualized treatment plans, and general information on the Internet or in books may not apply to them. Parents should talk to their health care team, in particular their cardiologist, about information they have received from other sources.

The nurse must give information to the child in a manner that is appropriate to the child's developmental age. As the child matures, the level of information is revised to match the child's new cognitive level. Preschoolers need basic information about what they will experience more than what is actually occurring physiologically. School-age children benefit from a concrete explanation of the defect. Preadolescents and adolescents often appreciate a more detailed description of how the defect affects their heart. Children of all ages need to be able to express their feelings concerning the diagnosis.

Help the Family Manage the Illness at Home

Parents are the child's principal caregivers and need to develop a positive, supportive working relationship with the health care team. Because most children spend the majority of their time at home with episodic trips to the hospital, parents manage their child's illness on a daily basis. They monitor for signs of illness, give medications and treatments, bring their child to appointments, work with a variety of caregivers, and alert the team to problems. Successful relationships are a partnership between parents and caregivers that is built on mutual trust and respect. Good communication between the family, the cardiology specialists, and the primary care practitioner is essential. As children reach adolescence, they begin to take a larger role in managing their illness and making decisions about their care.

Parents should be aware of the symptoms of their child's cardiac condition and signs of worsening clinical status. Parents should know how to contact their child's cardiologist at all times and know what to do in an emergency. Parents of children who may develop HF should be familiar with the symptoms (see p. 1352) and know when to contact the practitioner. Parents of children with cyanosis should be informed about fluid management and hypercyanotic spells (see p. 1362). Parents should have an information sheet with their child's diagnosis, significant treatments such as surgical procedures, allergies, other health care problems, current medications, and health care providers' contact numbers available in case of emergencies and to share with other caregivers such as teachers, baby-sitters, or daycare providers.

The family also needs to be knowledgeable regarding the therapeutic management of the disorder and the role that surgery, other procedures, medications, and a healthy lifestyle play in maintaining good health. Medications play a critical role in the management of some cardiac conditions such as arrhythmias and severe HF, in anticoagulation after implantation of artificial valves, and in antirejection treatment after heart transplantation. Some patients must take multiple medications daily for life. Many medications can be dangerous if taken incorrectly and require close monitoring. Teach parents the

---

*American Heart Association, 7272 Greenville Ave., Dallas, TX 75231; 800-242-8721; www.americanheart.org; Kids with Heart National Association for Children's Heart Disorders, PO Box 12504, Green Bay, WI 54307; 800-538-5390; http://kidswithheart.org; Little Hearts, Inc., PO Box 171, Cromwell, CT 06416; 860-635-0006, 866-435-4673; www.littlehearts.org.

†Congenital Heart Information Network, http://tchin.org; Pediheart Organization, www.pediheart.org/parents; Heart Rhythm Society (information on arrhythmias), www.hrsonline.org; Adult Congenital Heart Association, www.achaheart.org; Congenital Heart Defects, www.congenitalheartdefects.com; Children's Heart Foundation, www.childrensheartfoundation.com. Many major medical centers that perform pediatric heart surgery also have information on their websites.

correct procedure for giving medications and caution them to keep them in a safe area to prevent accidental ingestion (see Family-Centered Care box, p. 1358).

Another area of parental concern is the child's level of physical activity. Most children do not need to restrict activity, and the best approach is to treat the child normally and allow self-limited activity. Exceptions primarily involve strenuous recreational and competitive sports in children with specific cardiac problems. Discuss activities and exercise restrictions with the child's cardiologist. Avoid deliberately attempting to prevent crying because it can establish a maladaptive parental pattern of relating to the infant.

Infants and children with CHD require good nutrition. Breast-feeding should be possible for many infants with CHD. Countering a common misconception that breast-feeding would not be possible for these infants because they would get tired or exhibit poor growth, Barbas and Kelleher (2004) found that breast-feeding could be successful with adequate support and education of the mother. Providing adequate nutrition to infants with HF or complex congenital defects is especially difficult due to their high caloric requirements and inability to suck effectively because of fatigue and tachypnea. Instructing parents in feeding methods that decrease the work of the infant and giving high-calorie formula are important interventions (see p. 1359 for a discussion on feeding the infant with HF).

Children with severe cardiac defects are often anorexic. Encouraging them to eat can be a tremendous challenge. Because of the parents' concern over eating, children learn early to manipulate parents through eating, such as making unrealistic demands for foods that are not available. The nurse advises parents of this potential problem, since prevention yields greater success than intervention. For example, give the child a choice of available high-nutrient foods. Chapter 27 provides suggestions for encouraging sick children to eat.

Infants with heart disease should be immunized according to the current guidelines. Immunization schedules may need to be modified around times of acute illness or surgical procedures (Smith, 2001). Infants and children younger than 2 years of age with unrepaired heart defects, cyanotic lesions, pulmonary hypertension, or a history of prematurity should receive the vaccine for respiratory syncytial virus (RSV) monthly during RSV season (November to April in North America) to prevent RSV infection (American Academy of Pediatrics, 2009). Use of the RSV vaccine palivizumab has been shown to reduce hospitalization due to RSV infection in infants and young children with hemodynamically significant CHD (Feltes, Cabalka, Meissner, et al, 2003). (See Chapter 32.)

Infants and children who have serious heart disease are at risk for developmental delays and there is growing interest in characterizing these outcomes (see Research Focus box). Multiple factors can influence neurodevelopmental outcomes, including genetics (chromosomal abnormalities and microdeletions), family background (parental intelligence quotient [IQ] and socioeconomic status), preoperative factors (including prematurity, cyanosis, shock), intraoperative factors (use of cardiopulmonary bypass, deep hypothermic circulatory arrest), and postoperative factors (hemodynamic instability, hypoxia, acidosis, cardiac arrest, stroke, ischemic events).

◢ RESEARCH FOCUS

Congenital Heart Disease and Cognitive Development

Research in the past decade has begun to identify specific risk factors and common developmental concerns for congenital heart disease. Bellinger, Wypij, duPlessis, and colleagues (2003) found an association between longer periods of deep hypothermic circulatory arrest (a cardiopulmonary bypass technique commonly used in infants needing complex repairs) and the presence of postoperative seizures, delayed motor development, and a downward trend in full-scale intelligence quotient (IQ). At 8 years of age, more than a third of the study patients had received remedial services in school. Shillingford, Glanzman, Ittenbach, and colleagues (2008) also found that a significant proportion of children with complex congenital heart disease were at risk for inattention and hyperactivity, and nearly half were using remedial school services. In another longitudinal study, Limperopoulos, Majnemer, Shevell, and colleagues (2002) found that preoperative and early postoperative neurologic status, microcephaly, type of cardiac lesion, length of deep hypothermic circulatory arrest, age at surgery, and length of intensive care unit stay were predictors of developmental disability.

Recent efforts to limit the time of deep hypothermic circulatory arrest and provide better neuroprotection during surgery on infants may improve outcomes in the future. Although most children with serious heart disease are within the normal range for IQ, there is a higher incidence of neurodevelopmental deficits—specifically deficits in speech and language, fine motor skills, and cognitive processes—in children who have undergone heart surgery than in the normal population (Majnemer and Limperopoulos, 1999). Severe neurologic problems such as cerebral palsy, epilepsy, and cognitive impairment are uncommon.

Prepare the Child and Family for Invasive Procedures

Chapter 27 provides an extensive discussion of the principles for preparing children for invasive procedures. In 2003 the American Heart Association published a scientific statement, "Recommendations for Preparing Children and Adolescents for Invasive Cardiac Procedures" (LeRoy, Elixson, O'Brien, et al, 2003), that addresses issues specific to the child with heart disease. The reader is referred to these resources for a complete review of the topic. The following discussion highlights some important aspects of preparation for cardiac catheterization and cardiac surgery.

The expected outcomes for preprocedure preparation include reducing anxiety, improving patient cooperation with procedures, enhancing recovery, developing trust with caregivers, and improving long-term emotional and behavioral adjustment following procedures (LeRoy, Elixson, O'Brien, et al, 2003). Important factors to consider in planning preparation strategies are the child's cognitive developmental level, the child's previous hospital experiences, the child's temperament and coping style, the timing of the preparation, and the involvement of the parents. The most beneficial preparation strategies usually combine information giving and training in coping skills such as conscious breathing exercises, distraction techniques, guided imagery, and other behavioral interventions.

Handling preoperative and precatheterization workups on an outpatient basis is common for most elective procedures. Children are then admitted on the morning of the procedure. Preprocedure teaching is often done in the clinic setting or at home, and a tour of the ICU and the inpatient facilities may be added. Children of different ages and developmental levels require different amounts of information and different approaches. Young children should be prepared close in time to the event; older children and adolescents may benefit from teaching several weeks in advance. Include parents in the preparation session to support their child and learn about upcoming events.

The preoperative or precatheterization preparation should include information on the environment, equipment, and procedures that the child will encounter during and following the procedure. The nurse can use many educational techniques, such as verbal and written information, hospital tours, preoperative classes, and picture books or videos. Information about what the child will see, hear, and feel should be included, especially for older children and adolescents. Some of the sensory experiences of being in an ICU or catheterization laboratory include sights (monitors, many people, lots of equipment), sounds (beeping noises, alarms, voices), and sensations (lines and dressings, tape, feelings of discomfort, thirst). Familiar aspects of the environment, like BP cuffs, stethoscopes, or oximeter probes, are reviewed, and new equipment such as monitors, IV lines, and oxygen masks are described. Comforting aspects of the environment are emphasized, such as play areas, chairs for parents, and televisions. Many patients who will be sedated during catheterization or receive narcotic pain relievers after surgery will have minimal recall of that period and will not need detailed information about the equipment or procedures used. Information should be specific to the planned procedure for each patient.

Discuss ways the child can cope with the experience and be helped to recover. For young children, bringing a familiar stuffed animal or comfort object with them will help relieve anxiety, whereas for older children bringing a music player with headphones and favorite recordings to the catheterization laboratory will help distract them during the procedure. Topics to discuss regarding recovery after catheterization include the need to lie still to prevent bleeding at the catheter site, progression of the diet, pain control measures, and monitoring methods. Review the importance of ambulation, coughing and deep breathing, and drinking and eating after surgery, and describe pain management and monitoring routines. Review simple coping strategies for use during painful procedures, including distraction techniques such as counting, blowing, singing, or telling stories.

Children and their families should have a choice about an ICU tour. Exposure to the ICU environment can actually increase anxiety in some children, particularly young children, those with previous hospital experiences, and those who are highly anxious (LeRoy, Elixson, O'Brien, et al, 2003). If a visit to the recovery room and ICU is planned, it should take place when there is minimal activity in the area, when the parents can accompany the child, and when the child is well rested. Usually the day before the procedure is ample time to allow the child to ask questions and to prevent undue fantasizing about the experience. Protect the child from frightening sights in the unit. Equipment that will not be in view postoperatively, such as equipment located behind or below the bed, needs less attention. The child and parents are encouraged to ask questions and to explore further any equipment in the room, but they should not be pushed to assimilate more information than they are able.

Preoperative physical care differs little, if any, from that provided for any other surgery and is discussed in Chapter 27. Assure the child that the parents will be there when the child wakes up. Also allow the parents to accompany the child as far as possible to the operating suite. (See Evidence-Based Practice box, p. 1211.) After all of the equipment and procedures have been explained, it is important to talk about "getting well" and going home.

Provide Postoperative Care

Immediate postoperative care is usually provided by specially trained nurses in the ICU. Performing many of the procedures, such as arterial pressure and CVP monitoring and observations related to vital functions, requires advanced educational training (the reader should refer to critical care texts for further information). However, nurses caring for the child before surgery and during the convalescent period need to be familiar with the major principles of care.

Observe Vital Signs and Arterial and Venous Pressures

Record vital signs frequently, including BP, until the child's condition is stable. The heart rate and respirations are counted for 1 full minute, compared with the values on the ECG monitor, and recorded with activity. The heart rate is normally increased after surgery. The nurse observes cardiac rhythm and notifies the practitioner of any changes in regularity. Dysrhythmias may occur postoperatively secondary to administration of anesthetics, acid-base and electrolyte imbalance, hypoxia, surgical intervention, or trauma to conduction pathways.

At least hourly, auscultate the lungs for breath sounds. Diminished or absent breath sounds may indicate an area of atelectasis, pleural effusion, or pneumothorax. All such cases require further assessment. Auscultation guides the nurse's selective use of postural drainage and percussion to those pulmonary lobes most in need. It also allows a more objective evaluation of effective ventilation.

Temperature changes are typical during the early postoperative period. Hypothermia is expected immediately after surgery due to hypothermia procedures, effects of anesthesia, and loss of body heat to the cool environment. During this period the child is kept warm to prevent additional heat loss. Infants may be placed under radiant heat warmers. During the next 24 to 48 hours the body temperature may rise to 37.8° C (100° F) or slightly higher as part of the inflammatory response to tissue trauma. After this period an elevated temperature is most likely a sign of infection and warrants immediate investigation for probable cause.

Intraarterial monitoring of BP is almost always done following open-heart surgery. Residual vasoconstriction after cardiopulmonary bypass makes indirect BP readings less reliable, and intraarterial monitoring permits continuous rather than intermittent observation. A catheter is passed into the radial artery or the dorsalis pedis or posterior tibial artery, and the other end is attached to an electronic monitoring system, which provides a continuous recording of the BP. The intraarterial line is maintained with a low-rate, constant infusion of heparinized saline to prevent clotting. Continuous BP readings are compared with those taken indirectly using a sphygmomanometer or oscillometric device (Dinamap). A discrepancy between the two may indicate a change in peripheral vascular resistance, a malfunction in the electronic device, or human error in using the wrong-size BP cuff. The nurse also observes for potential complications of intraarterial monitoring, such as arterial thrombosis, infection, air emboli, or blood loss through the catheter. Prevention of each of these hazards is similar to care for any other type of infusion line.

The intraarterial line is maintained with a low-rate, constant infusion of heparinized saline to prevent clotting. The amount of irrigant is recorded as intake fluid. The dressing at the site is changed daily.

Several IV lines are inserted preoperatively: a peripheral IV to give fluids and medications and a CVP line that is usually inserted in a large vessel in the neck. Intracardiac monitoring lines are placed intraoperatively in the RA, LA, or pulmonary artery. Intracardiac lines allow assessment of pressures inside the cardiac chambers, which give vital information on blood volume, cardiac output, ventricular function, pulmonary artery pressures, and responses to drug therapy in the immediate postoperative period. The RA and CVP lines may also be used to infuse fluids and medications. LA lines and pulmonary artery lines are used with more complex repairs. Intracardiac lines are used only in the ICU, although CVP lines may remain for use as a central IV line outside the ICU. All lines must be cared for using strict aseptic technique to prevent infection. Patients must be carefully assessed for bleeding at the time of line removal. See critical care texts for a more complete discussion of intracardiac lines.

Maintain Respiratory Status

Infants usually require mechanical ventilation in the immediate postoperative period. Children may be extubated in the operating room or in the first few postoperative hours, especially if cardiopulmonary bypass was not required. When weaning and extubation are completed, oxygen is delivered by mask, hood, or nasal cannula and is humidified to prevent drying of mucosa. Encourage the child to turn and deep breathe at least hourly. Every means is employed to enhance ventilation and decrease pain, such as splinting of the operative site and use of analgesics.

Suctioning is performed only as needed and is done carefully to avoid vagal stimulation (which can trigger cardiac dysrhythmias) and laryngospasm, especially in infants. Suctioning is intermittent and is maintained for no more than 5 seconds to prevent depleting the oxygen supply. Supplemental oxygen is administered with a manual resuscitation bag before and after the procedure to prevent hypoxia. The heart rate is monitored after suctioning to detect changes in rhythm or rate, especially bradycardia. The child should always be positioned facing the nurse to permit assessment of the child's color and tolerance of the procedure.

> **! NURSING ALERT**
>
> During suctioning, observe for signs and symptoms of respiratory distress, such as tachypnea, use of accessory muscles for breathing, and restlessness.

Chest tubes may be inserted into the pleural or mediastinal space during surgery or in the immediate postoperative period to remove secretions and air and allow reexpansion of the lung. The chest tube is attached to a disposable water-seal drainage system. The underwater drainage prevents air from traveling up the tube into the pleural space and causing pneumothorax. Nursing considerations include (1) do not interrupt water-seal drainage unless the chest tube is clamped, (2) check for tube patency (fluctuation in the water-seal chamber), and (3) maintain sterility.

Check drainage hourly for color and quantity. Immediately postoperatively the drainage may be bright red, but afterward it should be serous. The largest volume of drainage occurs in the first 12 to 24 hours, and drainage is greater after extensive heart surgery.

> **! NURSING ALERT**
>
> Chest tube drainage of more than 3 ml/kg/hr for more than 3 consecutive hours or 5 to 10 ml/kg in any 1 hour is excessive and may indicate postoperative hemorrhage. Notify the surgeon immediately, since cardiac tamponade can develop rapidly and is life threatening.

Chest radiographs are taken when the tubes are inserted to check their location and after they are removed to evaluate the inflation of the lungs. Chest tubes are usually removed on the first to third postoperative day when drainage has diminished.

Removal of chest tubes can be an uncomfortable, frightening experience (see Atraumatic Care box). Warn children that they will feel a sharp, momentary pain. After the suture is cut, the tubes are quickly pulled out at the end of full inspiration in the extubated patient to prevent intake of air into the pleural cavity. (In the intubated patient, the tubes are pulled out on inspiration, since the lungs are stented open with the positive pressure ventilation.) A purse-string suture (placed when the tubes were inserted) is pulled tight to close the opening. A petrolatum-covered gauze dressing is immediately applied over the wound and securely taped to the skin on all four sides so that an airtight seal is formed. The dressing is checked for signs of drainage. It is removed the next day. Breath sounds are auscultated, since pneumothorax is a possible complication of chest tube removal. A chest x-ray film is usually obtained after removal to assess for pneumothorax or pleural effusion.

> **ATRAUMATIC CARE**
>
> **Chest Tube Removal**
>
> Intravenous analgesics such as morphine sulfate (0.1 mg/kg), often in combination with midazolam (Versed), may be given before the procedure. Oral analgesics and sedatives have also been used.

Provide Maximum Rest

After heart surgery maximum rest should be provided to decrease the workload of the heart and promote healing. Nursing care is planned according to the child's usual activity and sleep patterns. The simplest way to ensure individualized, efficient, high-quality care is to plan at the beginning of the shift the nursing procedures to be done. Identify periods of rest. Share the schedule with parents to allow them to visit at the most advantageous times, such as after a rest period when no special treatments are anticipated.

Provide Comfort

Heart surgery is both painful and frightening for children, and providing comfort is a primary nursing concern. Several incisions are used for heart surgery. A median sternotomy following the sternum down the center of the chest is most common. A ministernotomy opens the lower sternum. A thoracotomy incision is most uncomfortable because it goes through muscle tissue. It allows access to the side of the chest through an incision that runs from under the arm around the back to the scapula.

Adequate pain control decreases postoperative complications such as atelectasis, pneumonia, and deep vein thrombosis by improving coughing and ambulation. Pain level is now considered the fifth vital sign. Many pain assessment tools are available for infants and children of different ages. (See Pain Assessment, Chapter 7.)

Continuous IV infusion of opioids, particularly morphine and fentanyl, is a safe and effective method of pain control. Patient-controlled analgesia may be used with children old enough to understand the concept (Macfadyen and Buckmaster, 1999). Epidural morphine is another option. Children receiving opioid infusions for a prolonged period are weaned slowly from the medication to prevent withdrawal symptoms. Nonsteroidal antiinflammatory drugs (NSAIDs) such as IV ketorolac (Toradol) or oral ibuprofen may be used to provide relief of moderate postoperative pain.

Most patients need IV analgesics for pain control during the 24- to 48-hour postoperative period. After lines and tubes have been removed and when patients are tolerating oral fluids, pain may be controlled with oral narcotics such as codeine or oxycodone, often combined with acetaminophen or an oral NSAID such as ibuprofen, or with acetaminophen alone. As noted earlier, thoracotomy incisions are usually more painful than sternotomies because the incision is through muscle. Higgins, Turley, Harr, and colleagues (1999) have found that round-the-clock use of acetaminophen or ibuprofen to augment narcotics is advantageous in providing pain relief after heart surgery. Acetaminophen or ibuprofen alone is usually adequate for pain control after discharge. (See Pain Management, Chapter 7.)

In addition to providing pharmacologic pain control, make every effort to minimize the discomfort of procedures by other means, such as by placing a firm pillow or favorite stuffed animal against the chest incision during coughing and performing treatments after pain medication is given, preferably at a time that coincides with the drug's peak effect. Employ nonpharmacologic measures to lessen the perception of pain, and encourage parents to comfort their child as much as possible. (See Pain Management, Chapter 7.)

Monitor Fluids

Intake and output of all fluids must be accurately calculated. Intake is primarily IV fluids; however, the nurse also needs to keep a record of fluid used to flush the arterial and CVP lines or to dilute medications. Monitoring of output includes hourly recordings of urine (usually a Foley catheter is inserted and attached to a closed collecting device), drainage from chest and nasogastric tubes, and blood drawn for analysis. Urine is analyzed for specific gravity to evaluate the kidneys' concentrating ability and to assess the body's degree of hydration. Renal failure is a potential risk from a transient period of low cardiac output.

> **! NURSING ALERT**
>
> The signs of renal failure are decreased urinary output (<1 ml/kg/hr) and elevated levels of blood urea nitrogen and serum creatinine.

During open-heart surgery, the cardiopulmonary pump is primed with a large volume of fluid (usually electrolyte solution), which may greatly dilute the patient's blood. The large amount of fluid also diffuses into the interstitial spaces, causing total-body edema and pulmonary edema. Patients return from the operating room with fluid overload. Fluids are restricted to less than maintenance level during the first postoperative day, and drugs are used to promote diuresis. A return to maintenance fluid levels then occurs over the next few days as patients resume normal nutrition. Electrolyte levels are closely monitored because electrolyte imbalances, especially hypokalemia, are a common result of diuresis and fluid shifts, and electrolytes may need replacement.

Fluid requirements are based on the child's weight and body surface area. The child is weighed daily, preferably in the morning, using the same scale and in similar clothing. The child is usually given nothing by mouth for the first 24 hours. Oral fluids are usually withheld until the child is extubated. Patients begin taking clear liquids when bowel sounds are heard and advance slowly to a regular diet. Nausea and vomiting are common in the first few days after surgery, likely a side effect of anesthesia and analgesics. Providing adequate nutrition, ideally by oral intake, becomes important by the fourth or fifth postoperative day. Consider nasogastric tube feedings or parenteral nutrition for patients who are unable to tolerate oral feedings.

Plan for Progressive Activity

Fatigue and weakness are common after heart surgery. However, moderate activity is essential to prevent pulmonary and vascular complications. Initially, turning, coughing, and deep breathing are sufficient to promote respiratory expansion. Passive range-of-motion exercises, especially to the lower extremities, are instituted to prevent venous stasis.

A progressive schedule of ambulation and activity is planned, based on the child's preoperative activity patterns and postoperative cardiovascular and pulmonary function. Provide the child with toys to encourage movement. It is important to plan the activity at times when the child is well rested, is comfortable (usually has had analgesic medication), and is not scheduled for any strenuous procedure or treatment immediately afterward.

Ambulation is initiated early, usually by the second postoperative day, after extubation and when many lines and tubes have been removed. Patients progress from sitting on the edge of the bed and dangling the legs to standing up and to sitting in a chair while being assisted and assessed by the nursing staff.

Carefully monitor the heart rate and respirations to assess the degree of cardiac demand imposed by each activity. Tachycardia, dyspnea, cyanosis, desaturation, progressive fatigue, or dysrhythmias indicate the need to limit further energy expenditure. After ambulation a rest period is scheduled.

Observe for Complications of Heart Surgery

Several complications can occur after heart surgery, most of which are related to open-heart surgery and the use of cardiopulmonary bypass. Many of the procedures discussed in the preceding paragraphs are aimed at preventing these problems. Only those that have not already been discussed are included here. A serious complication, infective endocarditis (bacterial), is discussed on p. 1382.

Cardiac Changes. Preoperatively the workload of the heart is increased because of the abnormal hemodynamics caused by the congenital defect. In the initial postoperative period the heart is under increased stress because of the effects of surgery and the use of the heart-lung machine. In some cases cardiac function can actually be worse in the early postoperative period despite repair of the congenital defect. HF, hypoxia, low cardiac output, dysrhythmias, and tamponade are all potential postoperative problems.

HF may occur postoperatively because of excessive pulmonary blood flow or fluid overload (see p. 1354 for assessment and management of HF). Hypoxia may occur because of inadequate pulmonary blood flow or because of respiratory problems. Rapid assessment of the causes of hypoxia and appropriate interventions to improve ventilation and perfusion are vital, since hypoxia can rapidly lead to acidosis, which can impair ventricular function.

Low cardiac output syndrome and decreased peripheral perfusion can occur from hypothermia or inability of the LV to maintain systemic circulation. It affects up to 25% of infants and young children after cardiac surgery (Hoffman, Wernovsky, Atz, et al, 2003). The most important signs of adequate peripheral perfusion are rapid capillary refill, good skin color, warm extremities, and strong pulses. Indications of low cardiac output are similar to signs of shock (i.e., decreased BP, decreased pulse pressure, cool extremities, metabolic acidosis, and oliguria). Low cardiac output states are aggressively treated with IV inotropic medications such as dopamine, dobutamine, and milrinone. Milrinone, widely used in pediatrics, has also been shown to prevent low cardiac output syndrome (Hoffman, Wernovsky, Atz, et al, 2003). If maximum medical therapy is failing, cardiac assist methods such as extracorporeal membrane oxygenation or a ventricular assist device may be used in some centers under certain circumstances. Mortality is higher than 50% for patients who require mechanical support. Patients who have recovery of ventricular function within 2 to 3 days and have a short period of support have the best outcomes (Craig, Smith, and Fineman, 2001).

Dysrhythmias are common in the early postoperative period and can result from electrolyte imbalance, especially hypokalemia, and surgical intervention to the septum or myocardium. The heart rate and rhythm are carefully monitored by observing the ECG pattern and by counting the apical pulse for 1 full minute. In some children, a faster than normal rate may be required to maintain an adequate cardiac output

in the postoperative period, and a slower than normal rhythm can impair cardiac output. Epicardial pacing wires may be inserted during surgery for managing cardiac dysrhythmias postoperatively.

Cardiac tamponade is compression of the heart by blood and other effusion (clots) in the pericardial sac, which severely restricts the normal heart movement. Signs include rising and equalizing RA and LA filling pressures, narrowing pulse pressure, tachycardia, dyspnea, apprehension, and an abrupt stop to chest tube drainage from mediastinal tubes. The nurse immediately reports any evidence of this potentially fatal complication. An echocardiogram confirms the diagnosis. Treatment consists of prompt pericardiocentesis to remove the blood or fluid. If active hemorrhage and coagulopathy are present, steps are taken to enhance blood clotting.

Pulmonary Changes. Areas of atelectasis are common immediately after surgery as a result of deflation of the lung during cardiopulmonary bypass. Other pulmonary complications include pneumothorax, especially caused by faulty chest tubes; pulmonary edema from increased pulmonary blood flow or heart failure; and pleural effusion caused by persistent venous congestion. Signs of pneumothorax are persistent decreased breath sounds, sudden dyspnea, tachycardia, rapid shallow respirations, cyanosis, and sometimes sharp chest pain. Signs of pulmonary edema are tachypnea, rales, wheezing, moist dyspneic respirations, tachycardia, cyanosis, and restlessness. Signs and symptoms of pleural effusions include increased respiratory rate, vomiting, decreased breath sounds, fatigue, irritability, and decreased oxygen saturation. Chest radiography is important in the accurate diagnosis of pulmonary complications and is done frequently postoperatively.

Neurologic Changes. Neurologic complications such as seizures, strokes, cerebral edema, and hypoxic or ischemic brain injury are uncommon after open-heart surgery but can be devastating when they occur. Nurses are alert to the possibility of neurologic symptoms and perform ongoing neurologic assessments, including evaluation of the equality of strength and reflexes in both extremities for evidence of paralysis; pupil size, equality, reaction to light, and accommodation; and the child's orientation to the environment. The nurse also observes for focal or generalized seizure activity. Any evidence of cerebral damage is reported immediately. Further neurologic evaluation and management are needed for all abnormalities.

Seizures are the most common neurologic condition, seen most often in infants. Longer periods of deep hypothermic cardiopulmonary bypass (>40 minutes), sometimes needed in complex repairs on neonates, have been associated with an increased risk of seizure activity and later developmental delays (Wypij, Newberger, Rappaport, et al, 2003). Significant improvements in cardiopulmonary bypass techniques, arterial filters, and equipment and a better understanding of neuroprotection during heart surgery have resulted in a reduced incidence of seizures, movement disorders, and coma (Menasche, duPlessis, Wessel, et al, 2002).

Infection. All patients are at risk for infections postoperatively; especially vulnerable are infants, those with poor cardiac function, and those who require multiple invasive lines and procedures for a prolonged period. Prophylactic antibiotics are given for the first 1 or 2 days. All dressings are applied and changed using aseptic technique. Good hand washing, careful use of aseptic technique when placing and accessing lines, and close attention to surgical wounds are all important to prevent infection. Monitor patients closely for fever and signs of infection. Monitor all IV sites for signs of infection or phlebitis. Appropriate treatment is instituted if an infection is identified.

Hematologic Changes. While passing through the heart-lung machine, blood is exposed to substantial trauma because of mechanical action and direct contact with oxygen, foreign substances, and massive doses of anticoagulants. The result of mechanical trauma is red blood cell hemolysis and potential renal tubular necrosis. Heparinization of the blood during extracorporeal circulation can result in clotting abnormalities from decreased thrombin and prothrombin levels, decreased levels of platelets, and altered platelet aggregation.

Hemolysis of red blood cells leads to blood loss and anemia, which may require packed red blood cell transfusion. The nurse monitors results of complete blood counts to identify the severity of the hemolysis. All urine is tested for blood. If transfusions are required, the child is closely observed for signs of reaction and fluid overload. (See Table 35-2.) The need to measure urinary output hourly has already been discussed.

Because blood-clotting mechanisms are affected, signs of hemorrhage, especially bleeding from the chest tubes and a fall in arterial and venous pressures, are important observations. Hemorrhage is more likely to occur in patients who undergo repair of cyanotic heart defects because of the associated physiologic thrombocytopenia.

Normally the filter and bubble trap on the heart-lung machine remove air emboli, tiny clots, fat debris, and organisms from the arterialized (oxygenated) blood before its return to the body. However, the entry of impure blood into the systemic circulation can cause fat embolism, thromboembolism, and infection anywhere in the body and, most important, in the brain.

Postpericardiotomy Syndrome. The postpericardiotomy syndrome of fever, leukocytosis, pericardial friction rub, or pericardial and pleural effusion can occur anytime the pericardium is opened, either in the immediate postoperative period or after surgery, typically around day 7 to 21. The cause is unknown, although etiologic theories include viral infection, autoimmune response to myocardial tissue, and a reaction to blood in the pericardium. The syndrome is self-limiting and is treated with rest, salicylates, NSAIDs, and sometimes steroids. Pericardiocentesis or pleurocentesis may be needed to treat large effusions.

Provide Emotional Support

Children may become depressed after surgery. This is thought to be caused by preoperative anxiety, postoperative psychologic and physiologic stress, and sensory overstimulation. Typically the child's disposition improves on leaving the ICU. (See Chapter 26.)

Children may also be angry and uncooperative after surgery as a response to the physical pain and to the loss of control imposed by the surgery and treatments. They need an opportunity to express feelings, either verbally or through activity. Nurses can praise children for their efforts to cooperate and

should refrain from expecting too much courage or bravery. Children often regress in their behavior during the stress of surgery and hospitalization. Children also may express feelings of anger or rejection toward parents. The nurse must reassure parents that this is normal and that with continued support the anger will subside.

The nurse can support the parents by being available to provide information and explaining all the procedures to them. The first few postoperative days are particularly difficult because parents see their child in pain and realize the potential risks from surgery. They often are overwhelmed by the physical environment of the ICU and feel useless because they can do so little for their child. The nurse can minimize such feelings by including parents in caregiving activities and comfort and play activities; by providing information about the child's condition; and by being sensitive to their emotional and physical needs. The importance of their presence in making the child feel more secure is stressed, even if they do not provide physical care.

Plan for Discharge and Home Care

Assessment of discharge needs should begin at admission so parents and health care providers have ample time to plan for a safe discharge and arrange for necessary equipment and supports. The family needs verbal and written instructions on medication, nutrition, activity restrictions, wound care, pain management, and signs and symptoms of infection or complications. Other discussion topics may include return to school and work, special medication teaching for warfarin (Coumadin) or other drugs that require detailed home management, and infective endocarditis (subacute bacterial endocarditis [SBE]) prophylaxis. Referrals to community agencies may be necessary to assist parents in the transition from hospital to home and to reinforce the teaching (see Family-Centered Care box).

FAMILY-CENTERED CARE

Topics to Include in Discharge Teaching After Cardiac Surgery

- Medication teaching (for digoxin, see p. 1358)
- Activity restrictions
- Diet and nutrition
- Wound care (include dressings if any, suture removal, bathing)
- Infective endocarditis (bacterial) prophylaxis (see p. 1383)
- Follow-up appointments (cardiologist, primary care provider)
- Contact information for community agencies as needed (visiting nurse service, early developmental intervention)
- Circumstances in which to call practitioner; signs and symptoms of postoperative problems
- Review of cardiac defect and surgical repair

The parents also need clear instructions on when to seek medical care for complications and how to contact the health care provider. Follow-up with the cardiologist, usually within 2 weeks, and with the primary care provider is also arranged before discharge. Encourage parents to keep an updated summary of their child's diagnosis, surgical procedures, allergies, medications, health care providers with contact information, and other health problems readily available for emergencies and to share this summary with school personnel, baby-sitters, and others. Appropriate medical identification, such as a MedicAlert bracelet, is indicated for children with a pacemaker or a heart transplant and for those receiving anticoagulation therapy or antidysrhythmic medication.

The nurse also discusses common behavior disturbances that may occur after discharge, such as nightmares, sleep disturbances, separation anxiety, and overdependence. A supportive, consistent response is essential to allow the child to overcome the surgical experience. The child may work out feelings and fears through therapeutic play, and this should be encouraged.

Although surgical correction of heart defects has improved dramatically, it is still not possible to totally repair many complex anomalies. Some repairs require several operations over a period of years. For many children, repeat procedures are required to replace conduits or valves or to manage complications such as restenosis. Consequently, the long-term prognosis is uncertain, and full recovery is not always possible. For these families, close medical follow-up and continued emotional support are essential.

ACQUIRED CARDIOVASCULAR DISORDERS

Acquired cardiac disorders include disease processes or abnormalities that occur after birth and can be seen in the otherwise normal heart or in the presence of congenital heart defects. They occur for a variety of reasons, including infection, autoimmune response, environmental factors, and familial tendencies. Nursing care often plays a critical role in the identification and supportive management of these cardiovascular disorders.

BACTERIAL (INFECTIVE) ENDOCARDITIS

BE or SBE is now commonly referred to as infective endocarditis (IE). IE is an infection of the valves and inner lining of the heart, which can potentially damage or destroy the heart valves with high morbidity and mortality for affected patients. Although IE can occur without underlying heart disease, it most often is a sequela of bacteremia in children with acquired or congenital anomalies of the heart or great vessels. It especially affects children who have undergone surgery to repair or palliate complex cyanotic heart defects, valvular abnormalities, prosthetic valves, conduits, ventricular septal defects, patent ductus arteriosus, tetralogy of Fallot, or sequelae of rheumatic heart disease with valve involvement. Children with indwelling catheters are also at risk. Endocarditis can also occur without any known risk factors, commonly affecting the mitral or aortic valve. The incidence of IE appears to have increased in the pediatric and neonatal population, most likely due to improved survival among children at risk for BE (those with congenital heart defects and hospitalized infants) (Ferrieri, Gewitz, Gerber, et al, 2002).

The most common causative agents are *Streptococcus viridans* and *Staphylococcus aureus*. Gram-negative bacteria, enterococcus and fungi such as *Candida albicans* are also causes of IE (Wilson, Taubert, Gewitz, et al, 2007).

The presentation of IE varies among individuals. Signs and symptoms may include fever, malaise, a new murmur, and the findings of vegetations (verrucae) on echocardiography. Positive blood cultures are present in most patients; however, endocarditis can also be present despite negative blood cultures, especially if antibiotics have already been given.

Pathophysiology

The microorganisms in IE usually grow on a section of the endocardium that has been subjected to abnormal blood streaming and turbulence, such as occurs when blood flow is restricted by an anatomic narrowing or forced through an abnormal opening. Growth may also begin where the abnormal jet of blood strikes the opposing endocardium, causing thickening of the lining or damage to the valvular endothelium. Changes in the endocardium predispose it to the deposition of platelets and fibrin and ultimately make the area susceptible to the growth of invading organisms.

Organisms may enter the bloodstream from any site of localized infection. Transient bacteremia also occurs with trauma to mucosal surfaces encountered in normal daily activities (brushing, flossing gums, chewing, etc.). The microorganisms grow on the endocardium, forming vegetations. The lesion may grow to invade adjacent tissues, such as aortic and mitral valves and myocardium, and may break off and embolize elsewhere, especially in the spleen, kidney, central nervous system, lung, skin, and mucous membranes.

Clinical Manifestations

The onset of symptoms is usually insidious, with unexplained low-grade, intermittent fever. Other common nonspecific symptoms are malaise, myalgias, arthralgias, headache, diaphoresis, and weight loss (Day, Gauvreau, Shulman, et al, 2009). Sometimes, children can manifest IE more acutely with high fevers and rapidly declining health, requiring immediate hospitalization and treatment.

A new murmur or a change in a previously existing one is frequently found as a result of damage to valves or perforation of the myocardium. Another finding, especially in those with prolonged illness, is splenomegaly. Other signs that result from embolus formation elsewhere in the body include splinter hemorrhages (thin black lines) under the nails, Osler nodes (red, painful intradermal nodes with white centers found on the pads of the phalanges), Janeway spots (painless hemorrhagic areas on the palms and soles), and petechiae on the oral mucous membranes, although these signs are less common in children than in adults. Neonates may have feeding difficulties, respiratory distress, tachycardia, HF, or symptoms of septicemia (Ferrieri, Gewitz, Gerber, et al, 2002).

Diagnostic Evaluation

A combination of laboratory and other findings may support the diagnosis of IE, such as ECG changes (AV block), anemia, an elevated erythrocyte sedimentation rate, leukocytosis, microscopic hematuria, and radiographic evidence of cardiomegaly. Definitive diagnosis can be made after growth of the organism and identification of the causative agent in the blood. Several blood specimens (three are recommended) are drawn for culturing to rule out contamination during venipuncture and dilution. Strict sterile technique is practiced in obtaining cultures to avoid contamination. As soon as an organism is isolated, sensitivity studies are done to determine appropriate antibiotic therapy. Vegetation formation and myocardial abscess may be visualized on 2-D echocardiography. Transesophageal echocardiography is used in patients with unsatisfactory transthoracic echo windows. Echocardiographic findings include new or increasing valvular insufficiency, vegetations, and abscesses. A diagnosis of culture-negative endocarditis is made when the patient has echocardiographic or clinical evidence of IE but no organism can be cultured (Ferrieri, 2002).

The Duke criteria are guidelines for the diagnosis of IE in adults and are useful in the diagnosis of childhood endocarditis as well. These criteria divide signs and symptoms into major and minor criteria. The two major criteria are positive blood culture results and echocardiographic evidence of endocardial involvement (vegetations or new valvular regurgitation); minor criteria include fever, predisposing risk factors, and vascular and immunologic signs (Durack, Lukes, and Bright, 1994).

Therapeutic Management

Treatment for IE includes the administration of high-dose antibiotics given intravenously for 2 to 8 weeks to completely eradicate the infecting microorganism (Taubert and Gewitz, 2008). Infectious disease specialists should be consulted to assist in determining the appropriate regimen for each patient. Blood cultures are performed periodically to evaluate the response to antibiotic therapy. In cases in which antibiotic therapy is unsuccessful, HF develops, valvular obstruction is present, or recurrent systemic emboli occur, surgical intervention is warranted.

Early medical treatment for IE is successful in many patients. However, cases diagnosed late; those caused by antibiotic-resistant organisms or fungi; or those that involve HF, embolic events, or significant valvular dysfunction carry a higher mortality rate and may necessitate surgical intervention. Death is most often caused by HF, myocardial infarction from coronary emboli, or cardiac perforation. Nonfatal complications result from embolism to other structures, especially to the central nervous system (causing hemiplegia, aphasia, meningitis, convulsions), kidney (resulting in hematuria, proteinuria), spleen, and bowel.

Prevention of Endocarditis

The American Heart Association has established new guidelines for the prevention of IE (Wilson, Taubert, Gewitz, et al, 2007). The new guidelines no longer recommend antibiotic prophylaxis for all patients with CHD. The data reviewed in the recent AHA statement conclude that antibiotic prophylaxis prevents only a small percentage of the cases of IE and that the risk of widespread use of antibiotics exceeds the potential benefit. The majority of cases of IE occur randomly rather than in association with a particular procedure. Therefore the new guidelines now recommend antibiotic prophylaxis only in those patients with the highest risk of adverse outcomes if they get IE (Wilson, Taubert, Gewitz, et al, 2007). High-risk patients are defined as those patients with cardiac conditions listed in Box 34-8.

Prevention in these high-risk patients involves administration of prophylactic antibiotic therapy 1 hour before dental procedures (Table 34-5). If a patient is taking an antibiotic for another reason, it is recommended that they wait 10 days after antibiotics are completed to have a dental procedure so that

---

BOX 34-8   HIGH-RISK PATIENTS FOR ENDOCARDITIS

Artificial heart valves
Previous diagnosis of infective endocarditis
Congenital heart disease (CHD), including only*:
- Unrepaired cyanotic CHD, including palliative shunts and conduits
- Repaired CHD using prosthetic material or device during the first 6 months after the procedure (including surgical or catheterization placement of these materials)
- Residual defects after CHD repair at the site or adjacent to the site of a prosthetic patch or prosthetic device (inhibiting endothelialization)
Cardiac transplantation recipients with cardiac valvulopathy

Adapted from Wilson W, Taubert KA, Gewitz M, et al: Prevention of bacterial endocarditis: guidelines from the American Heart Association, *Circulation* 116(15):1736-1754, 2007.
*Other than these high-risk patients, antibiotic prophylaxis is no longer routinely recommended.

TABLE 34-5   DENTAL PROPHYLAXIS REGIMENS FOR PATIENTS AT HIGH RISK FOR INFECTIVE ENDOCARDITIS

SITUATION	AGENT	REGIMEN—SINGLE DOSE 30-60 MIN BEFORE PROCEDURE
Oral	Amoxicillin	50 mg/kg
Unable to take oral medication	Ampicillin *OR*	50 mg/kg IM or IV
	Cefazolin or ceftriaxone	50 mg/kg IM or IV
Allergic to penicillins or ampicillin—oral	Cephalexin*† *OR*	50 m/kg
	Clindamycin or	20 mg/kg
	Azithromycin or Clarithromycin	15 mg/kg
Allergic to penicillins or ampicillin and unable to take oral medication	Cefazolin or ceftriaxone† *OR*	50 mg/kg IM or IV
	Clindamycin	20 mg/kg IM or IV

Modified from Wilson W, Taubert KA, Gewitz M, et al: Prevention of infective endocarditis: guidelines from the American Heart Association, *Circulation* 116(15):1736-1754, 2007.
IM, Intramuscular; *IV,* intravenous.
*Or other first- or second-generation oral cephalosporin in equivalent adult or pediatric dosage.
†Cephalosporins should not be used in an individual with a history of anaphylaxis, angioedema, or urticaria with penicillins or ampicillin.

---

normal flora can regenerate. If a patient requires chronic antibiotic therapy, a different antibiotic should be used for prophylaxis. Additional procedures that require prophylaxis (only in this high-risk group) include invasive procedures of the respiratory tract and procedures on infected skin or musculoskeletal tissue. Antibiotic prophylaxis is no longer recommended for gastrointestinal-genitourinary procedures. Maintenance of excellent oral hygiene is still of utmost importance, especially in children with CHD.

Nursing Care Management

The objective of nursing care is to counsel parents of high-risk children concerning the need for prophylactic antibiotic therapy before procedures such as dental work. The family's regular dentist should be advised of existing cardiac problems in the child as an added precaution to ensure preventive treatment in appropriate patients. These children should also maintain the highest level of oral health to reduce the chance of bacteremia from oral infections. (See also discussion on dental care in Chapter 14.)

QUALITY PATIENT OUTCOMES: Bacterial (Infective) Endocarditis
- Prevention in high-risk patients with antibiotic prophylaxis
- Early recognition and treatment

Parents should also have a high index of suspicion regarding potential infections. Without unduly alarming them, the nurse should educate patients and families to bring unexplained fever, weight loss, or change in behavior (lethargy, malaise, anorexia) to the practitioner's attention. Such symptoms should not be self-diagnosed as a cold or flu, and children at risk (e.g., those with CHD) should have blood drawn for culture if they have a fever without an obvious source. Early diagnosis and treatment are important in preventing further cardiac damage, embolic complications, and growth of resistant organisms.

Treatment of endocarditis requires long-term parenteral antibiotics. In some cases IV antibiotics may be administered at home via a peripherally inserted central catheter, with nursing supervision for part of the treatment course. Nursing goals during this period include (1) preparation of the child for IV infusion, usually with an intermittent-infusion device, and performance of several venipunctures to draw blood for culture and laboratory values; (2) observation for side effects of antibiotics, especially inflammation along venipuncture sites along with assessments of renal function; (3) observation for complications, including embolism and HF; and (4) education regarding the importance of follow-up visits for cardiac evaluation, echocardiographic monitoring, and blood culturing.

RHEUMATIC FEVER

Rheumatic fever (RF) is a poorly understood inflammatory disease that occurs after pharyngitis caused by group A β-hemolytic streptococci (GABHS). It is a self-limiting illness that involves the joints, skin, brain, serous surfaces, and heart. Cardiac valve damage (referred to as *rheumatic heart disease*) is the most significant complication of RF (World Health Organization, 2004; Bitar, Hayek, Obeid, et al, 2000). In developed countries RF and rheumatic heart disease have become uncommon, probably as a result of antibacterial control of streptococcal infection, successful treatment of rheumatic heart disease, and a change in the organism itself. However, RF remains a devastating problem in developing (third world) countries and is more likely to recur in this setting. It has also reappeared in some parts of the United States (Gentles, Colan, Wilson, et al, 2001).

Etiology

Strong evidence supports a relationship between upper respiratory tract infection with GABHS and subsequent development of RF (usually within 2 to 6 weeks). In almost all cases of RF a previous infection with GABHS can be documented by laboratory evidence of rising antibody titers. Diagnosis and treatment of GABHS infection prevents RF.

Pathophysiology and Clinical Manifestations

The principal manifestations of RF are observed in the heart, joints, skin, and central nervous system. Inflammatory hemorrhagic bullous lesions, called *Aschoff bodies,* are formed, which cause swelling, fragmentation, and alterations in the connective tissue. Aschoff bodies are found in virtually all patients with clinical rheumatic activity. These lesions occur in the heart, blood vessels, brain, and serous surfaces of the joints and pleura.

The major cardiac manifestation of RF is carditis involving the endocardium, pericardium, and myocardium. In the acute illness, clinical signs and symptoms reflect valvulitis, myocarditis, and pericarditis. Clinically, rheumatic carditis is most commonly associated with the mitral valve. The presence of an apical systolic murmur reflecting mitral regurgitation is a common clinical finding in acute rheumatic carditis. This murmur is a long, high-pitched, blowing murmur that begins with the first heart sound (S_1) and continues throughout systole. Other murmurs in the acute phase may reflect aortic regurgitation. In addition, myocarditis produces tachycardia that is out of proportion to the degree of fever, especially during rest or sleep. Signs and symptoms of HF may result, and chest radiographic examination may demonstrate cardiomegaly. Signs and symptoms of pericarditis include muffled heart sounds because of pericardial effusion. In addition, the patient may demonstrate a pericardial friction rub and complain of chest pain. Pericardial effusions can be documented by echocardiography. Patients with mitral or aortic valve involvement may experience progressive valvular damage as time passes. Carditis is the only manifestation that can lead to permanent damage (Narula, Chandrasekhar, Rahimtoola, et al, 1999).

The second major manifestation is polyarthritis caused by edema, inflammation, and effusions in joint tissue. The arthritis is reversible and migratory, favoring large joints such as the knees, elbows, hips, shoulders, and wrists. The affected joint is swollen, hot, red, and exquisitely painful for 1 or 2 days, after which a different joint is affected. Joint manifestations usually accompany the acute febrile period, most often in the first 1 to 2 weeks; however, they can persist for 4 weeks in untreated patients.

The third major manifestation is erythema marginatum. This is a distinct erythematous macule with a clear center and wavy, well-demarcated border. This transitory, nonpruritic rash is most often found on the trunk and proximal portion of the extremities.

The fourth major manifestation is the development of subcutaneous nodules, which are small (0.5- to 1-cm), nontender swellings that persist indefinitely after the onset of the disease and gradually resolve with no resulting damage. They are rare but may be found in crops over bony prominences such as the feet, hands, elbows, scalp, scapulae, and vertebrae.

The last major manifestation, which reflects central nervous system involvement, is chorea, referred to as *St. Vitus dance* or *Sydenham chorea.* Chorea is characterized by sudden, aimless, irregular movements of the extremities, involuntary facial grimaces, speech disturbances, emotional lability, and muscle weakness that can be profound. It is usually exaggerated by anxiety and attempts at deliberate fine motor activity and is relieved by rest, especially sleep. Chorea is seen almost exclusively in children, with a higher incidence in females (World Health Organization, 2004). The time course of symptoms of chorea are variable, but 75% of patients recover in 6 months.

In addition to these major manifestations, minor manifestations that may support the diagnosis include arthralgia and fever, which may be low grade and which often spikes in the late afternoon. Laboratory findings reflect an inflammatory process. Other vague signs and symptoms include unexplained epistaxis, abdominal pain that may be severe enough to simulate appendicitis, weakness, fatigue, pallor, anorexia, and weight loss.

Diagnostic Evaluation

No single symptom or laboratory test can provide a definitive diagnosis of RF. Rather, the diagnosis is based on a set of guidelines by the American Heart Association (Dajani, Ayoub, Bierman, et al, 1993). These guidelines are designed to aid in the diagnosis only of the initial episode of RF (Ferrieri, 2002) (Box 34-9). Clinical and laboratory findings are divided into major and minor manifestations; evidence of recent streptococcal infection is present in the majority of instances.

Although the majority of patients with RF meet these criteria, in three circumstances exceptions are allowed. In patients who have chorea as the only symptom and in patients who are seen late with continued carditis, the late diagnosis may preclude the presence of supporting manifestations and laboratory findings. Finally, a recurrence of RF in a patient with a previous history of the disorder may not fulfill the standard Jones criteria. However, if a single major or several minor manifestations

are seen in a patient who has a history of prior disease along with evidence of recent GABHS infection, the diagnosis may be made without strict adherence to the criteria.

Streptolysin O (O because it is oxygen labile) is a streptococcal extracellular product that produces lysis of the red blood cell. Antistreptolysin O (ASLO) titers measure the concentration of antibodies formed in the blood against this product. Normally the titers begin to rise about 7 days after onset of the infection and reach maximum levels in 4 to 6 weeks. Therefore a rising titer demonstrated by at least two ASLO tests is the most reliable evidence of recent streptococcal infection. Normal values are between 0 and 120 Todd units. Elevations over 333 Todd units indicate recent streptococcal infection in children.

Therapeutic Management

The goals of management include (1) eradication of GABHS (primary prevention), (2) prevention of permanent cardiac damage, (3) palliation of the other symptoms, and (4) prevention of recurrences (secondary prevention) (Gerber, Baltimore, Eaton, et al, 2009).

Penicillin (oral or intramuscular injections) remains the drug of choice, with macrolides or cephalosporins as a substitute in penicillin-sensitive children. Initial therapy includes a full 10-day course of penicillin or an alternative antibiotic.

Children who have had acute RF are susceptible to recurrent RF for the rest of their lives, and therefore prophylactic treatment against RF recurrence is started immediately after the initial course of antibiotics is complete. Secondary prevention involves monthly intramuscular injections of benzathine penicillin G, two daily oral doses of penicillin V, or one daily dose of sulfadiazine-sulfisoxazole or erythromycin. The duration of long-term prophylaxis varies and depends on whether the child has had cardiac involvement (Table 34-6).

The use of SBE prophylaxis should follow the recent American Heart Association guidelines that recommend prophylaxis only for very-high-risk patients. Therefore SBE prophylaxis is no longer recommended for patients with RF unless they have had a valve replacement. (Wilson, Taubert, Gewitz, et al, 2007).

Salicylates are used to reduce fever and discomfort and to control the inflammatory process, especially in the joints. Patients with arthritis from RF are generally responsive to

---

BOX 34-9   GUIDELINES FOR DIAGNOSING INITIAL ATTACK OF RHEUMATIC FEVER (JONES CRITERIA, 1992 UPDATE)*

Major Manifestations
Carditis
Polyarthritis
Chorea
Erythema marginatum
Subcutaneous nodules

Minor Manifestations
Clinical findings
Arthralgia
Fever
Laboratory findings: elevated values for acute-phase reactants
 • Erythrocyte sedimentation rate
 • C-reactive protein level

Supporting Evidence of Antecedent Group A Streptococcal Infection
Positive results on throat specimen culture or rapid streptococcal antigen test
Elevated or rising streptococcal antibody titer

From Guidelines for the diagnosis of rheumatic fever: Jones criteria, 1992 update, *JAMA* 268(15):2070, 1992.
*If supported by evidence of preceding group A streptococcal infection, the presence of two major manifestations or of one major and two minor manifestations indicates a high probability of acute rheumatic fever.

TABLE 34-6   SUGGESTED DURATION OF SECONDARY PROPHYLAXIS FOR RHEUMATIC FEVER

CATEGORY OF PATIENT	DURATION OF PROPHYLAXIS
No proven carditis	For 5 yr after the last attack, or until 21 yr of age (whichever is longer)
Carditis (but no residual heart disease; no valvular disease)	For 10 yr after the last attack, or until 21 yr of age (whichever is longer)
Carditis and residual heart disease (ongoing valvular disease)	For 10 yr or until 40 yr old (whichever is longer); sometimes lifelong prophylaxis (see guidelines for indications)

Modified from Gerber MA, Baltimore RS, Taubert KA, et al: Prevention of rheumatic fever and diagnosis and treatment of acute streptococcal pharyngitis; a scientific statement from the AHA, *Circulation* 119:1541-1551, 2009.

salicylate therapy; however, salicylates should not be administered before diagnosis, since their use may mask the polyarthritis. Administration of prednisone may be indicated in some patients with heart failure. Neither salicylates nor prednisone has been shown to affect cardiac sequelae. Traditionally, bed rest or at least limited activity has been recommended during the acute illness.

Patients who have symptoms of heart failure due to significant valvular heart disease require medical therapy for their HF. They are also at risk for atrial fibrillation and embolic complications. Surgery may be indicated in this group of patients and may include valve repair or valve replacement.

Nursing Care Management

The objectives of nursing care for the child with RF are to (1) encourage compliance with drug regimens, (2) facilitate recovery from the illness, (3) provide emotional support, and (4) prevent recurrence of the disease. Because compliance is a major concern in long-term drug therapy, make every effort to encourage adherence to the therapeutic plan. (See Compliance, Chapter 27.) When compliance is poor, monthly injections may be substituted for daily oral administration of antibiotics, and children need preparation for this often dreaded procedure.

Interventions during home care are primarily concerned with providing rest and adequate nutrition. Usually, once the febrile stage is over, children can resume moderate activity and their appetite improves. If carditis is present, the family must be aware of any activity restrictions and may need help choosing less strenuous activities for the child.

QUALITY PATIENT OUTCOMES: Rheumatic Fever
- GABHS tonsillopharyngitis identified and treated
- Early recognition and treatment to prevent cardiac valve damage
- Recurrence prevented with prophylaxis compliance

One of the most disturbing and frustrating manifestations of the disease is chorea. The onset is gradual and may occur weeks to months after the illness, sometimes even in children who have not been diagnosed with RF. It may be mistaken for nervousness, clumsiness, behavioral changes, inattentiveness, and learning disability. It is usually a source of great frustration to the child because the movements, incoordination, and weakness severely limit physical skill. The child needs an opportunity to verbalize feelings. Of utmost importance is stressing to parents and schoolteachers that the movements are involuntary and sudden, that the chorea is transitory, and that all manifestations eventually disappear.

Nurses also have a role in prevention, primarily in screening school-age children for sore throats that may be caused by GABHS. This may involve actively participating in throat culture screening programs or referring children with a possible streptococcal infection for testing.

KAWASAKI DISEASE (MUCOCUTANEOUS LYMPH NODE SYNDROME)

Kawasaki disease (KD) is an acute systemic vasculitis of unknown cause. The illness is self-limiting and resolves in 6 to 8 weeks. Without treatment, however, approximately 20% to 25% of children develop cardiac sequelae. Damage to the blood vessels that supply the heart muscle (the coronary arteries) and damage to the heart muscle itself can occur. The most common sequela is ectasia (dilation) of the coronary arteries, or coronary artery aneurysm formation. Infants younger than 1 year of age are at the greatest risk for heart involvement. Children older than 5 years of age are also at increased risk of developing coronary sequelae, perhaps because KD is often not suspected in older children, which may lead to delayed diagnosis and treatment. KD has become a leading cause of acquired heart disease in children in the United States.

KD is seen in children of most racial and ethnic backgrounds. The incidence rate is estimated at 112 cases per 100,000 children under 5 years of age. KD occurs 1.5 to 1.7 times more frequently in males than in females, and 76% of affected children are younger than 5 years of age, with peak incidence in the toddler age-group (Holman, Curns, Belay, et al, 2003).

The etiology of KD remains unconfirmed. Although KD is not spread by person-to-person contact, several factors support an infectious cause. KD is often seen in geographic and seasonal outbreaks, with most cases reported in the late winter and early spring. KD is also a pediatric illness, which suggests the development of passive immunity. Because an etiologic agent has not been found, some experts believe that the illness may represent a final common pathway for more than one potential agent. Some recent studies have focused on genetics, trying to ascertain why some children are more likely to get KD than others (i.e., the possibility that the illness represents a final common pathway in a genetically susceptible host).

Pathophysiology

KD involves widespread inflammation of the small and medium-sized blood vessels (Connor and McCance, 2000), with the coronary arteries being the most susceptible to damage. During the acute stage of the illness there is progressive inflammation of the small vessels (capillaries, venules, arterioles) along with pancarditis. This inflammation is reflected in the clinical signs and symptoms and in laboratory test results. Inflammatory markers (C-reactive protein level and erythrocyte sedimentation rate) are elevated in the acute illness. The vasculitis progresses to the medium-sized muscular arteries, potentially damaging the walls of the vessels and leading to the formation of coronary artery aneurysms in some children. Initial evidence of enlargement of the coronary arteries by echocardiogram can be detected as early as day 7 of illness. Affected vessels continue to enlarge for several weeks and generally reach their largest diameter approximately 4 to 6 weeks from the onset of fever. Longer duration of fever (most likely reflecting the severity of inflammation) is strongly associated with the development of aneurysms. Aneurysms of the peripheral vessels (axillary, brachial, iliac, cervical, and renal arteries) can occur, although this is rare and usually is seen only in children who also have giant coronary aneurysms (>8 mm). In the acute phase, myocarditis (inflammation of the myocardium) is common. Decreased LV function may be evident on echocardiogram; however, the majority of children do not have clinical signs of heart failure. Ventricular function usually improves after the administration of IV immune globulin (IVIG).

Occasionally, however, a child will be seen with severe ventricular dysfunction and/or cardiogenic shock. The systemic inflammation gradually subsides and eventually ceases with normalization of inflammatory markers 6 to 8 weeks from the onset of fever.

Over time, aneurysmal vessels try to heal through multiplication of cells in the vessels in an attempt to restore a "normal" lumen diameter. This process is called myointimal proliferation. The smaller the dilation, the more likely that the vessel will regress to a normal size. However, even if the lumen size is restored, the affected vessel may not be completely normal. The walls of these vessels are thicker and may be subject to scarring and calcification, especially at the distal ends of the aneurysm in patients with large aneurysms.

Almost all of the morbidity and morality resulting from KD are due to cardiac complications and mainly occur in patients who have giant aneurysms (≥8 mm). Coronary thrombosis may result from sluggish blood flow in a dilated or aneurysmal vessel. Over the years, stenosis and scarring may also lead to impeded blood flow, which can result in myocardial ischemia or infarction.

Clinical Manifestations

The course of KD can be divided into three phases: acute, subacute, and convalescent. The acute phase begins with an abrupt onset of high fever that is unresponsive to antibiotics and antipyretics. Over the next week or so, the diagnostic symptoms become evident. The bulbar conjunctivae of the eyes become reddened, with clearing around the iris (limbal sparing). The eyes are generally dry, without significant drainage. Inflammation of the pharynx and the oral mucosa develops, with red, cracked lips and the characteristic "strawberry tongue" (the normal coating of the tongue sloughs off, leaving the large papillae exposed, so that the tongue resembles a strawberry). The rash of KD differs from child to child but is never vesicular and is most often accentuated in the perineum. Often the area affected by the rash may desquamate. In addition, the child's hands and feet become edematous, and the palms and soles become erythematous. The child may have cervical lymphadenopathy (a single node ≥1.5 cm). The node is not usually very tender or red. To meet "classic" criteria, children have prolonged fever (≥4 days) along with four out of five of the diagnostic criteria. During the acute stage, the child is typically very irritable and inconsolable. This behavior may continue for several weeks. Approximately one third of patients develop a temporary arthritis beginning in the small joints. Cardiac manifestations during this period include myocarditis with resultant potential ECG changes, decreased LV function, pericardial effusion, and mitral regurgitation. Generally, these findings are subclinical, but occasionally children with poor function are seen with symptoms of cardiogenic shock. On physical examination, the child may be tachycardic with a gallop rhythm. The coronary arteries may begin to show enlargement during this phase.

The subacute phase begins with resolution of the fever and lasts until all outward clinical signs of KD have disappeared. If changes in the coronary arteries occur, some enlargement or dilation is generally evident by echocardiography during the second week of illness. Damaged vessels can continue to enlarge and reach their maximum diameter approximately 4 to 6 weeks

from the onset of illness. Thrombocytosis and hypercoagulability in a child with expanding aneurysms and disrupted blood flow place him or her at risk for coronary thrombosis. During the subacute period, the child may develop periungual desquamation (peeling that begins under the fingertips and toes) of the hands and feet. Arthritis may be evident during this phase and can affect the larger weight-bearing joints. Irritability persists during this period.

In the convalescent phase the clinical signs of KD have mostly resolved, but the laboratory values are still abnormal. The erythrocyte sedimentation rate and C-reactive protein level may remain elevated, which reflects lingering inflammation. Thrombocytosis may still be present. Arthritis may continue into this stage, and coronary complications may remain a concern as coronary dimensions peak 4 to 6 weeks from the onset of illness. This phase is complete when all blood values return to normal (6 to 8 weeks after onset). At the end of this stage, parents report that the child appears to have returned to normal in terms of temperament, energy, and appetite.

Cardiac Involvement

The most serious complication of KD is the development of coronary artery aneurysms and the potential for myocardial infarction in children with aneurysm formation. Myocardial ischemia can result from thrombotic occlusion or stenotic occlusion of a coronary aneurysm. The groups at highest risk for thrombus formation are children with "giant" aneurysms (>8 mm in diameter). Symptoms of acute myocardial infarction in young children can be subtle and may include abdominal pain, vomiting, restlessness, inconsolable crying, pallor, and shock. Complaints of actual chest pain or pressure are more typical in older children (Kato, Ichinose, and Kawasaki, 1986).

Diagnostic Evaluation

Currently no specific diagnostic test exists for KD. Therefore the diagnosis is established on the basis of clinical findings and associated laboratory results. The criteria in Box 34-10 should be used as guidelines. Many children with KD do not meet standard diagnostic criteria, and infants often have an incomplete presentation. It is therefore important to consider KD as a possible diagnosis in any infant or child with prolonged elevated temperature that is unresponsive to antibiotics and is not attributable to another cause. The American Heart Association recently published guidelines that include a diagnostic algorithm to guide the evaluation and treatment of patients with incomplete symptoms who have prolonged fever or other features of KD (Fig. 34-16).

Associated laboratory findings, when combined with clinical data, can be helpful in making the diagnosis. The typical child with KD is anemic and has a leukocytosis with a "shift to the left" (increased immature white blood cells) during the acute phase. Thrombocytosis with hypercoagulability becomes evident in the subacute phase and peaks approximately 3 weeks after the onset of fever. An elevated erythrocyte sedimentation rate and C-reactive protein level reflect ongoing inflammation and generally persist for 6 to 8 weeks. The erythrocyte sedimentation rate can be further elevated by the administration of IVIG; therefore it is better to measure C-reactive protein level as an indicator of inflammation. Microscopic urinalysis reveals a sterile pyuria with mononuclear cells that will not be evident with a regular dipstick test, since the white blood cells are not polymorphonuclear neutrophils. Transient elevation of liver enzymes may occur during the acute phase, reflecting inflammation of the liver. Examination of cerebrospinal fluid may show aseptic meningitis (presence of inflammatory cells). Albumin levels may be lower than normal.

Echocardiograms are used to monitor myocardial and coronary artery status. Obtain a baseline echocardiogram at the time of diagnosis for comparison with future studies and to evaluate ventricular and valvular function. Common findings on echocardiogram during the acute phase include pericardial effusions, mitral regurgitation, and decreased ventricular function. Follow-up echocardiograms should be performed at approximately 2 weeks after onset and again at 6 to 8 weeks from the onset of fever to determine the diameter of the coronary arteries and to assess LV contractility and valvular function. More frequent studies to assess coronary dimensions may be indicated in patients who have continued fever, those who require retreatment with IVIG, and those with coronary dilation on baseline or other studies.

Therapeutic Management

The current treatment of KD includes high-dose IVIG along with salicylate therapy. High-dose IVIG has been shown to reduce the duration of fever and the incidence of coronary artery abnormalities when given within the first 10 days of illness and optimally within the first 7 days. A single large infusion of 2 g/kg over 8 to 12 hours is recommended (Newburger, Takahashi, Gerber, et al, 2004).

Aspirin is given initially in an antiinflammatory dosage (80 to 100 mg/kg/day in divided doses every 6 hours) to control fever and symptoms of inflammation. The duration of therapy varies among institutions. Once fever has subsided and the child has been afebrile for 48 to 72 hours, the aspirin dosage is generally decreased to an antiplatelet dosage (3 to 5 mg/kg/day). Low-dose aspirin therapy is continued in patients without echocardiographic evidence of coronary abnormalities until the platelet count has returned to normal (6 to 8 weeks). If the child develops coronary abnormalities, low-dose (antiplatelet) salicylate therapy is continued indefinitely. Additional anticoagulation therapy, such as clopidogrel or warfarin administration, may be indicated in children with coronary enlargement. Children with giant aneurysms (>8 mm), who are at the greatest risk for morbidity and mortality, are usually maintained on warfarin and aspirin (Newburger, Takahashi, Gerber, et al, 2004). International normalized ratio (INR) levels are maintained at 2.0 to 3.0 in these patients.

Prognosis

Most children with KD recover fully after treatment. When cardiovascular complications occur, however, serious morbidity may result. Death occurs rarely (<0.1% to 0.2%) and is almost always a result of ischemia caused by coronary thrombosis or stenosis. Children with coronary abnormalities are followed closely. Long-term testing may include periodic ECGs, echocardiography, stress testing (stress echoes and/or myocardial perfusion scans) at rest and during exercise, and cardiac MRI, depending on individual risk and the availability of various testing modalities at the individual centers (Newburger, Takahashi, Gerber, et al, 2004; Baker and Newburger, 2008). Although echocardiography is sensitive in visualizing coronary dilation, it does not detect stenoses of the coronary arteries. Cardiac catheterization of the coronary arteries remains the gold standard and may be performed in children who still have significant abnormalities after 1 year and in situations in which myocardial ischemia is suspected from the results of noninvasive testing. A rare sequela of KD can be sensorineural hearing loss. If decreased hearing is suspected, the child should undergo audiologic testing.

Children without coronary artery aneurysms have now been followed for more than 30 years in Japan and the United States and do not show an increased incidence of premature heart disease. However, both coronary and peripheral arteries may be stiffer than normal, even in individuals who did not suffer obvious coronary artery dilation. For this reason it is especially important that children who have had KD have as few other risk factors for coronary disease as possible. Cholesterol levels and BP should be monitored, and these children should be encouraged to lead a heart-healthy lifestyle in terms of diet, exercise, and avoidance of smoking.

Nursing Care Management

The nursing care of children with KD is challenging. Inpatient care focuses on symptomatic relief, emotional support, diagnostic assistance, medication administration, and education of the child and family.

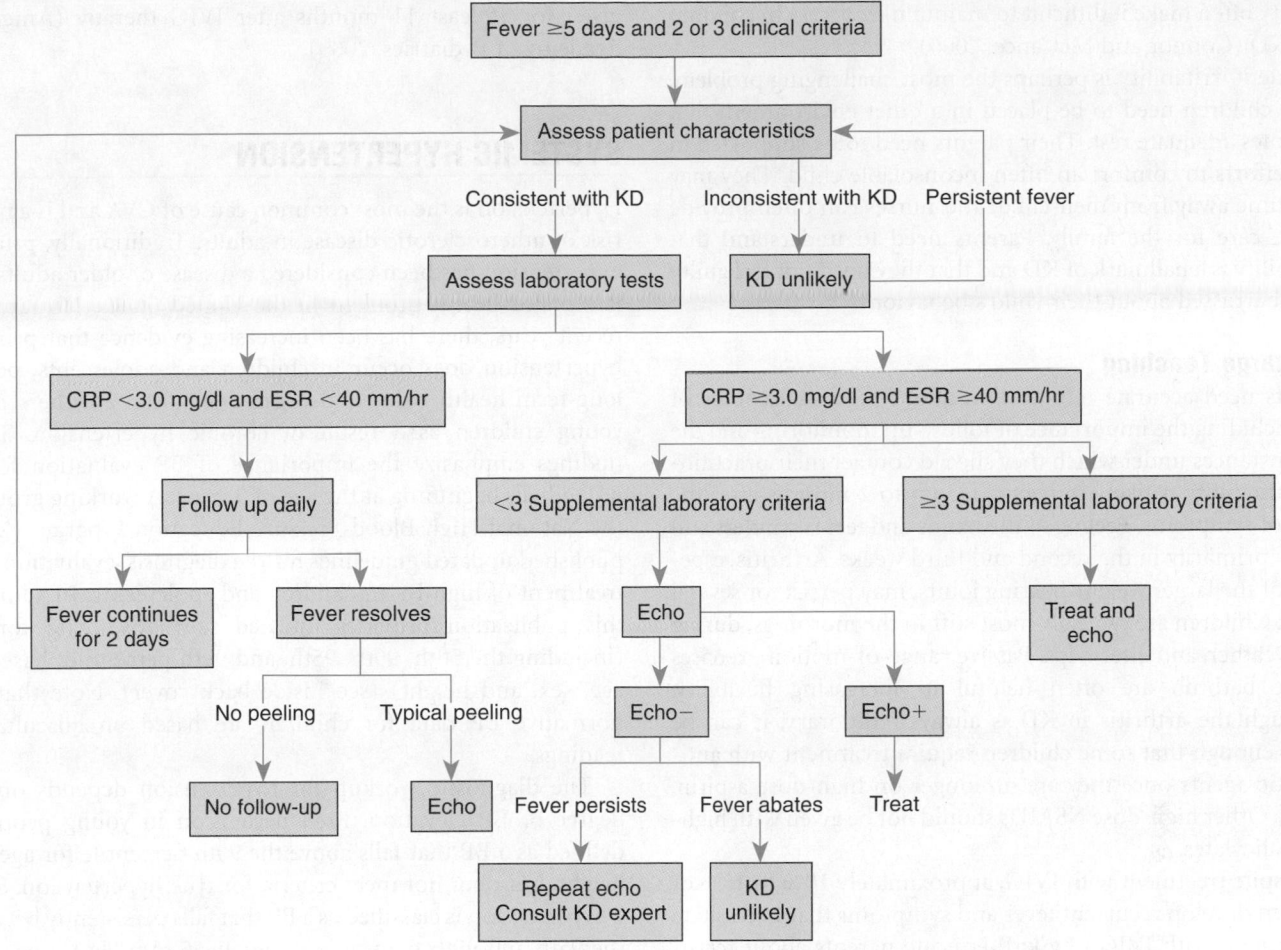

Fig. 34-16 Algorithm for evaluation of suspected incomplete Kawasaki disease *(KD)*. *CRP,* C-reactive protein; *echo,* echocardiography; *ESR,* erythrocyte sedimentation rate. (From Newburger JW, Takahashi M, Gerber MA, et al: Diagnosis, treatment, and long-term management of Kawasaki disease: a statement for health professionals from the Committee on Rheumatic Fever, Endocarditis, and Kawasaki Disease, Council on Cardiovascular Disease in the Young, American Heart Association, *Circulation* 110(17):2747-2771, 2004.)

QUALITY PATIENT OUTCOMES: Kawasaki Disease
- Early diagnosis and treatment
- Prevention of cardiovascular complications

In the initial phase of illness, the nurse must monitor the child's cardiac status carefully. Intake and output and daily weight measurements are recorded. Although the child may be reluctant to eat and therefore may be partially dehydrated, fluids need to be administered with care because of the usual finding of myocarditis. Assess the child frequently for signs of HF, including decreased urinary output, gallop rhythm, tachycardia, and respiratory distress. Cardiac monitoring is suggested in the following cases: before the initial ECG and echocardiogram are recorded and shown to be normal, during the infusion of IVIG (because of the large fluid load), in children younger than 1 year of age, and in any child with cardiac symptoms. Sedation is generally required before echocardiography in children younger than 2½ to 3 years of age, since the child must remain still for up to 1 hour to obtain adequate visualization of the coronary arteries and cardiac structures and function.

Nursing care focuses primarily on symptomatic relief. To minimize skin discomfort, application of cool cloths and unscented lotions and use of soft, loose clothing are helpful. During the acute phase, mouth care, including application of lubricating ointment to the lips, is important for the mucosal inflammation. Offer clear liquids and soft foods and monitor temperature carefully. It is important to document temperature just before aspirin administration, since fever reflects ongoing inflammation and may indicate the need for further treatment. If the temperature is very high, acetaminophen may be given in addition to high-dose aspirin. (See Controlling Elevated Temperatures, Chapter 27.) If arthritis develops, passive range-of-motion exercise may be indicated and can be done most easily during the child's bath.

The administration of IVIG should follow the same guidelines as for administration of any blood product, with frequent monitoring of vital signs. Patients must be watched for allergic reactions. (See Table 35-2.) The nurse must monitor cardiac status because of the large fluid volume being administered to patients who may have subclinical myocarditis or diminished LV function. Check patency of the IV line because extravasation can result in tissue damage. Hypercoagulability and venous fragility often make it difficult to maintain IV access in children with KD (Connor and McCance, 2000).

Patient irritability is perhaps the most challenging problem. These children need to be placed in a quiet environment that promotes adequate rest. Their parents need to be supported in their efforts to comfort an often inconsolable child. They may need time away from their child, and nurses can often provide respite care for the family. Parents need to understand that irritability is a hallmark of KD and that they need not feel guilty or embarrassed about their child's behavior.

Discharge Teaching

Parents need accurate information about the usual course of KD, including the importance of follow-up monitoring and the circumstances under which they should contact their practitioner. Irritability is likely to persist for up to 2 months after the onset of symptoms. Peeling of the hands and feet is painless and occurs primarily in the second and third weeks. Arthritis, especially of the larger weight-bearing joints, may persist for several weeks. Children are typically most stiff in the mornings, during cold weather, and after naps. Passive range-of-motion exercises in the bathtub are often helpful in increasing flexibility. Although the arthritis in KD is always temporary, it can be severe enough that some children require treatment with antiarthritic agents once they are no longer on high-dose aspirin. (NOTE: Other high-dose NSAIDs should not be given with high-dose salicylates.)

Despite treatment with IVIG, approximately 10% to 15% of children develop recurrent fever and symptoms that necessitate retreatment with IVIG (2 g/kg). Educate parents about recrudescent illness after discharge. Persistent or recrudescent fever 48 hours after the initiation of IVIG infusion would prompt reevaluation and probably retreatment with IVIG. Instruct the parents to take the child's temperature daily after discharge and to contact their physician or practitioner if there is any increase in temperature.

Also instruct parents about the administration of salicylates and, if the child is receiving high dosages, make them aware of the signs of aspirin toxicity: ringing in the ears (tinnitus), headache, dizziness, and confusion. The main side effect of low-dose aspirin is easy bruising. In addition, stop the aspirin and notify the practitioner if the child is exposed to chickenpox or influenza because of the drug's possible association with Reye syndrome.

All parents should understand the unlikely but real possibility of myocardial infarction and the signs and symptoms of cardiac ischemia in a child. At the time of hospital discharge, the final cardiac sequelae are generally not fully known, since changes in the coronary arteries occur over the first 4 to 6 weeks after the onset of KD. In addition, parents of children with known severe coronary artery sequelae should know cardiopulmonary resuscitation. Finally, children with coronary abnormalities may require indefinite antiplatelet therapy with low-dose aspirin or other anticoagulants. In such cases children should avoid contact sports and have yearly influenza vaccines. The administration of measles-mumps-rubella vaccine should be delayed for 11 months after the administration of IVIG because the body might not produce the appropriate number of antibodies. In addition, the varicella vaccine should not be given for at least 11 months after IVIG therapy (American Academy of Pediatrics, 2009).

SYSTEMIC HYPERTENSION

Hypertension is the most common cause of CVA and is a major risk of atherosclerotic disease in adults. Traditionally, primary hypertension has been considered a disease of older adults and is a major health problem in the United States. However, in recent years, there has been increasing evidence that primary hypertension does occur in children and adolescents, posing long-term health risks. End-organ effects can also be seen in young children as a result of chronic hypertension. These findings emphasize the importance of BP evaluation for all individuals beginning at the age of 3 years. A working group of the National High Blood Pressure Education Program (2004) published updated guidelines for the diagnosis, evaluation, and treatment of high BP in children and adolescents. In addition, this publication provides updated normative data for BP (including the 50th, 90th, 95th, and 99th percentiles based on age, sex, and height) (see inside back cover). Note that the normative BP data for children are based on auscultatory readings.

The diagnostic workup for hypertension depends on the degree of BP elevation. Prehypertension in young people is defined as a BP that falls above the 90th percentile for age and height, but does not meet criteria for true hypertension. Stage 1 hypertension is classified as a BP that falls persistently between the 95th and 99th percentile value plus 5 mm Hg for age, sex, and height. Stage 2 hypertension is defined as a BP that is persistently at or above the 99th percentile value plus 5 mm Hg for age, sex, and height. White-coat hypertension is diagnosed when the patient's BP is higher that the 90th percentile in the clinician's office but falls within the normal range outside of this setting.

Etiology

Hypertension in young children, compared to older adolescents and adults, more commonly is secondary to a structural abnormality or an underlying pathologic process, although the results of screening programs of relatively healthy children have challenged this view. The most common cause of secondary hypertension in young children is renal disease, followed by cardiovascular, endocrine, and some neurologic disorders. As a rule, the younger the child and the more severe the hypertension, the more likely it is to be secondary. The conditions associated with secondary hypertension in children and adolescents are listed in Box 34-11.

The causes of primary hypertension are undetermined. There is evidence that both genetic and environmental factors play a role. The incidence of hypertension is greater in children with a family history of hypertension. African-Americans have a higher incidence of hypertension than Caucasians. In the African-American population hypertension develops earlier and is frequently more severe. Environmental factors that contribute to the risk of developing hypertension include obesity; salt ingestion; smoking; lead exposure; medications, including certain stimulant drugs; and stress.

BOX 34-11   CONDITIONS ASSOCIATED WITH SECONDARY HYPERTENSION IN CHILDREN

Renal Disorders

Congenital defects
- Polycystic kidney, ectopic kidney, horseshoe kidney
- Obstructive anomalies
- Hydronephrosis

Renal tumor
- Wilms tumor
- Renovascular tumor

Abnormalities of renal arteries

Renal vein thrombosis

Acquired disorders
- Glomerulonephritis (acute or chronic)
- Pyelonephritis
- Nephritis associated with collagen disease

Cardiovascular Disease

Coarctation of aorta

Arteriovenous fistula

Patent ductus arteriosus

Aortic or mitral insufficiency

Metabolic and Endocrine Diseases

Adrenal tumors
- Adenoma
- Pheochromocytoma
- Neuroblastoma

Cushing syndrome

Adrenogenital syndrome

Hyperthyroidism

Aldosteronism

Hypercalcemia

Diabetes mellitus

Neurologic Disorders

Space-occupying lesions of the cranium (increased intracranial pressure)
- Tumors, cysts, hematoma
- Cerebral edema
- Encephalitis (including Guillain-Barré and Reye syndromes)

Miscellaneous Causes

Drugs (corticosteroids, oral contraceptives, pressor agents, amphetamines)

Burns

Genitourinary surgery

Trauma (e.g., stretching of femoral nerve with leg traction)

Insect bites (e.g., scorpion)

Intravascular overload (blood, fluid)

Hypernatremia

Toxemia of pregnancy

Heavy metal poisoning

Clinical Manifestations

Although the clinical manifestations associated with hypertension depend largely on the underlying cause, some observations can provide clues to the practitioner that an elevated BP may be a factor. Adolescents and older children with hypertension may complain of frequent headaches, dizziness, or changes in vision. In infants or young children who cannot communicate symptoms, observation of behavior provides clues, although gross behavioral changes may not be apparent until complications are present. Parents of infants and small children who have been treated for hypertension report that their child had previously been irritable and often indulged in an abnormal degree of head banging or rubbing.

Diagnostic Evaluation

It is clear from the increasing numbers of cases of hypertension and prehypertension being identified in children and adolescents that a BP determination should be a routine part of annual assessment in all children older than 3 years of age. Measure BP in children of any age if they are diagnosed as having or are suspected of having coarctation of the aorta, unexplained heart failure, unexplained heart murmurs, prematurity, unexplained seizures or other neurologic signs, an abdominal mass or masses, edema, ascites, evidence of renal failure, hypernatremia, failure to thrive, possible obstructive sleep apnea, respiratory distress, hyperlipidemia, or unexplained headaches. Because hypertension is strongly associated with obesity, a BMI should be calculated for each child at the routine physical examination.

Before a diagnosis of hypertension is made, measure BP in the sitting position on at least three separate occasions. To obtain an accurate reading, take care to quiet the child or relax the adolescent while the measurement is recorded to avoid false readings caused by excitement. The chief cause of falsely elevated BP readings is the use of improperly fitting, narrow cuffs. Therefore attention to correct measurement technique is essential. (See Blood Pressure, Chapter 6.) Note that a child who is large for his or her age may normally have a higher BP than a child who is of average size. Document upper and lower extremity BP when hypertension is suspected, along with the presence of femoral pulses. Twenty-four-hour BP (ambulatory BP [AMBP]) monitoring devices detect changes in pressure throughout the day and night, and thus may give a more realistic picture. These devices are especially helpful in diagnosing white-coat hypertension and are most easily used with older children or adolescents, who are able to tolerate being attached to an ambulatory monitor. The child or parent should keep a log during AMBP monitoring to document level of activity or, at a minimum, sleep and waking times. AMBP monitors should document readings at least hourly and ideally more often. Evaluation of the child with high BP is aimed at assessment of lifestyle and additional risk factors, detection of potential secondary causes, and documentation of the presence or absence of end-organ effects. Table 34-7 outlines the recommended workup for children with BP over the 90th percentile (National High Blood Pressure Education Program Working Group, 2004).

Take a careful medical history of the child or adolescent, including additional medical problems and current medications, drug use, or smoking. In addition, obtain a thorough family history to screen for other relatives with hypertension or other cardiovascular risk factors. In children with documented hypertension or prehypertension, initial laboratory data are also obtained.

The extent of additional testing depends on the degree of BP elevation. Diagnostic testing may include urinalysis, urine culture, renal function studies such as a creatinine and blood urea nitrogen levels, a lipid profile, fasting glucose level, complete blood count, and electrolyte levels. Additional laboratory data may include urine and blood catecholamine, renin, and

TABLE 34-7   CHILDHOOD HYPERTENSION EVALUATION

DIAGNOSTIC PROCEDURES OR TESTS	RATIONALE	CHILDREN AT RISK
History, including sleep history, family history, risk factors, diet, and habits such as smoking and drinking alcohol; physical examination	Help to focus further evaluation	Children with blood pressure (BP) persistently ≥95th percentile
Complete blood count	Identify anemia, consistent with chronic renal disease	Children with BP persistently ≥95th percentile
Blood urea nitrogen, creatinine, electrolyte levels, urinalysis, and urine culture	Identify renal disease and chronic pyelonephritis	Children with BP persistently ≥95th percentile
Fasting lipid panel, fasting glucose level	Identify hyperlipidemia, metabolic abnormalities	Overweight children with BP at 90th-94th percentile; children with BP ≥95th percentile; family history of hypertension or cardiovascular disease; children with chronic renal disease
Renal ultrasonography	Identify renal scar, congenital anomaly, or disparate renal size	Children with BP persistently ≥95th percentile
Polysomnography	Identify sleep disorder associated with hypertension	Children with history of loud, frequent snoring
Drug screen	Identify substances that cause hypertension	Children with history suggestive of possible contribution by substances or drugs
Echocardiography	Identify left ventricular hypertrophy and provides other indicators of cardiac movement	Children with comorbid risk factors* and BP at 90th-94th percentile; all children with BP ≥95th percentile
Retinal examination	Identify retinal vascular changes	Children with comorbid risk factors* and BP at 90th-94th percentile; all children with BP ≥95th percentile
Additional Evaluation as Indicated		
Plasma renin level	Identify low renin level, which suggests mineralocorticoid-related disease	Young children with stage 1 hypertension and all children or adolescents with stage 2 hypertension Children with positive family history of severe hypertension
Renovascular imaging • Isotopic scintigraphy (renal scan) • Magnetic resonance angiography • Duplex Doppler flow studies • 3-Dimensional computed tomography • Arteriography: digital subtraction or classic	Identify renovascular disease	Young children with stage 1 hypertension and all children or adolescents with stage 2 hypertension
Ambulatory BP monitoring	Identify white-coat hypertension, abnormal diurnal BP pattern, BP load	Children in whom white-coat hypertension is suspected and those for whom other information on BP pattern is needed
Plasma and urine catecholamine levels	Identify catecholamine-mediated hypertension	Young children with stage 1 hypertension and all children or adolescents with stage 2 hypertension
Plasma and urine steroid levels	Identify steroid-mediated hypertension	Young children with stage 1 hypertension and all children or adolescents with stage 2 hypertension

Modified from National High Blood Pressure Education Program Working Group on High Blood Pressure in Children and Adolescents: The fourth report on the diagnosis, evaluation, and treatment of high blood pressure in children and adolescents, *Pediatrics* 114(2):555-576, 2004.
*Comorbid risk factors include diabetes mellitus and kidney disease.

aldosterone levels. In children who have significant hypertension, secondary causes should be investigated thoroughly. A renal ultrasonographic scan provides a first-line screen for renovascular hypertension or other renal disease (e.g., polycystic kidneys). Additional renovascular imaging may include a 99mTc dimercaptosuccinic acid (DMSA) scan (to rule out scarring) and/or a renal CT angiogram. Echocardiography is indicated in patients with BPs over the 90th percentile to assess LV hypertrophy. A finding that the child's LV mass is higher than normal would support the presence of chronically elevated BP, since heart muscle thickens in response to chronic hypertension. A retinal examination may provide additional information about end-organ effects.

Therapeutic Management

Therapy for secondary hypertension involves diagnosis and treatment of the underlying cause. In those cases amenable to surgical repair, the nature of the condition, the type of surgery, and the child's age are all important considerations. Children or adolescents with consistently elevated BP readings from no known cause (primary hypertension) or those with secondary hypertension not amenable to surgical correction may be treated with a combination of nonpharmacologic and pharmacologic interventions.

Dietary practices and lifestyle changes are important in the control of hypertension both for children and for adults and should be instituted first, except in severe cases.

Because obesity and hypertension are closely related, a weight reduction program is recommended for overweight youngsters. In salt-sensitive children, high salt intake increases the risk of hypertension for those genetically predisposed and aggravates existing hypertension unless salt intake is limited. Regular aerobic exercise augments weight reduction and alone has been shown to normalize BP. The exercise regimen is individualized to the child's interest. It is helpful to quantify how much time is spent doing sedentary activities (e.g., watching television, using the computer, playing video games) compared with how much time daily is spent in aerobic activities. Stress reduction strategies may be beneficial and include biofeedback and relaxation. Smoking should be avoided.

Drug therapy is initiated with caution in children. Because the long-term effects of antihypertensive agents on children are not known, drug treatment of asymptomatic children with mild or borderline hypertension is not recommended. Antihypertensive drug therapy is indicated for treating those patients who have significant elevations of BP despite nonpharmacologic intervention. This includes children and adolescents with symptomatic hypertension; those with secondary hypertension; those with end-organ evidence of hypertension (e.g., increased LV mass); and those who have significant additional risk factors, such as diabetes (National High Blood Pressure Education Program Working Group, 2004).

The National High Blood Pressure Education Program Working Group on High Blood Pressure in Children and Adolescents (2004) recommends beginning pharmacologic therapy with one drug and adding other agents only if control is not obtained. The goal of therapy is to reduce BP levels below the 95th percentile. If additional risk factors (e.g., diabetes or renal disease) are present, however, BP values should ideally be reduced to less than the 90th percentile.

The oral antihypertensive drugs used most often in children are the ACE inhibitors (lisinopril, captopril, and enalapril), beta blockers (propranolol, atenolol [Tenormin]), calcium channel blockers (amlodipine [Norvasc]), angiotensin receptor blockers (losartan [Cozaar]), and diuretics (hydrochlorothiazide [HydroDIURIL]), to mention a few.

⚡ DRUG ALERT

Beta Blockers and ACE Inhibitors

Beta blockers can cause lipid abnormalities or mood disturbances such as depression in some children. In addition, ACE inhibitors and angiotensin receptor blockers are teratogenic and therefore should not be used by teenage girls who are at risk of becoming pregnant.

Pharmacologic intervention is tailored to meet the needs of the individual child and is determined by the hypotensive effect produced and the appearance of any side effects. For example, ACE inhibitors and angiotensin receptor blockers have been effective in children with diabetes or certain renal diagnoses, whereas beta blockers and calcium channel blockers are often used by children with a history of migraine headaches (National High Blood Pressure Education Program Working Group, 2004). The goal is to achieve a normotensive state throughout the day without accompanying side effects. For many antihy-

pertensive drugs, minimal data are available regarding side effects in children. Therefore consider any behavioral or physical changes that occur after institution of therapy a possible effect, and revise therapy as needed.

Nursing Care Management

The nurse is a valuable link in the delivery of health care for hypertension in the pediatric age-group. Active in detection, diagnosis, and therapy in any setting—hospital, school, clinic, private office, public health service, and private practice—nurses are frequently the primary contact in well-child care and follow-up clinics. They are often the liaison between the family and the health care services.

QUALITY PATIENT OUTCOMES: Hypertension
- Underlying cause of hypertension identified
- Blood pressure control maintained
- Dietary practices and lifestyle changes effectively used to control hypertension
- Compliance with medication regimen, if prescribed

A BP measurement should be part of the routine assessment of children over the age of 3 years and in younger children who have risk factors for hypertension. In carrying out the procedure, it is important for the nurse to use the correct cuff size. Any questionable reading is repeated. Ideally, BP should be assessed with the child in the sitting position with both feet on the floor. The right arm should be used for consistency in measurements. In addition, initial comparisons should be made between the upper and lower extremities.

Nursing counseling and guidance of affected children is a challenge. Education aimed at understanding hypertension and its implications over the life span is essential in promoting patient and family compliance with both nonpharmacologic and pharmacologic therapies. (See Compliance, Chapter 27.)

Home BP measurement can facilitate surveillance in youngsters with chronic hypertension and can document the effectiveness of therapy. A family member can be instructed in how to take and record accurate BP measurements, which can decrease the number of trips to a health care facility. This individual needs to understand when to contact the practitioner regarding elevated values. When this option is not feasible, the school nurse can often be a valuable resource in monitoring BP.

The nurse plays an important role in assessing individual families and providing targeted information regarding nonpharmacologic modes of intervention, such as diet, weight loss, smoking cessation, and exercise programs. If extensive dietary counseling is required, the child should be referred to a registered dietitian with expertise in working with children and adolescents. Exercise regimens should be individualized. Schoolchildren and young adolescents generally prefer team sports rather than individual training, which they may view as a burden rather than an enjoyable activity. If peers and family members can participate in any of the management strategies, the child is more likely to comply with the plan.

If drug therapy is prescribed, the nurse needs to provide information to the family regarding the reasons for drug therapy, how the drug works, frequency of BP monitoring, and

---

BOX 34-12 ANTIHYPERTENSIVE DRUGS COMMONLY USED IN THE TREATMENT OF PEDIATRIC HYPERTENSION, WITH NURSING INTERVENTIONS*

Angiotensin-Converting Enzyme Inhibitors
Action—Act primarily by interfering with the production of angiotensin II, a potent vasoconstrictor

Captopril (Capoten)
Monitor blood pressure and pulse.
Instruct to take 1 hour before meals to increase absorption.
Instruct to report any evidence of infection.
Advise to avoid rapid position changes (can initially cause dizziness).

Enalapril (Vasotec)
Monitor blood pressure and pulse (may cause hypotension).
Instruct to report any swelling of face or lips and difficulty breathing (may rarely cause laryngeal edema).
Instruct to report any evidence of infection.
Advise not to use potassium supplements (can increase serum levels).

Lisinopril (Zestril, Prinivil)
Longer half-life; can be administered in a single daily dose.
May cause hypotension, dizziness.
Monitor levels of electrolytes, blood urea nitrogen, creatinine (can increase serum levels).

Beta Blockers
Actions—Block response to beta stimulation; depress renin output

Propranolol (Inderal)
Monitor pulse and blood pressures (can cause bradycardia and hypotension).
Instruct to take with meals.
Advise that drug may cause fatigue, a decrease in exercise tolerance, weakness, and cold extremities.
Warn males of possible impotence.

Atenolol (Tenormin)
Monitor pulse and blood pressures (can cause bradycardia and hypotension).
Advise that drug can be given once a day.
Instruct not to discontinue abruptly (needs to be withdrawn over a 2-week period).

Calcium Channel Blockers
Actions—Decrease the force of contraction of the myocardium.

Amlodipine (Norvasc)
May cause tachycardia, peripheral edema, flushing, dizziness, or headache.
Do no discontinue suddenly.

Vasodilators
Actions—Act on vascular smooth muscle; thought to produce their effects by direct action on blood vessels to cause arterial vasodilation

Hydralazine (Apresoline)
Instruct to take with meals.
Advise that drug may cause drowsiness and that caution should be used in operating machinery or doing other hazardous activity.
Instruct to report if sore throat, fever, muscle and joint aches, or skin rash develops.

Angiotensin Receptor Blocker
Losartan (Cozaar)
Contraindicated in pregnancy.
Check serum potassium and creatinine levels.
Not used in children with decreased creatinine clearance.

Diuretics
See Table 34-3.

*For all drugs, instruct child or adolescent (and family) that (1) child should rise slowly from a horizontal position and avoid sudden position changes, (2) drug should be taken as prescribed, and (3) practitioner should be notified if unpleasant side effects occur but drug should not be discontinued.

---

possible side effects of the medication (Box 34-12). Explain that the drug needs to be taken consistently to achieve any prolonged control of BP. Stress the need for follow-up, especially because antihypertensive therapy can sometimes be safely discontinued if BP remains under control over time.

Learning needs vary greatly depending on developmental levels and individual differences. Some children and families require a great deal of support, education, and guidance, whereas others need only education and periodic follow-up. A positive approach is essential; negative feedback will only alienate the family. Exploring the reasons for difficulty in compliance can often provide realistic alternatives. Continued education, support, and reinforcement for positive behavior are major nursing responsibilities.

HYPERLIPIDEMIA (HYPERCHOLESTEROLEMIA)

Hyperlipidemia is a general term for excessive lipids (fat and fatlike substances); hypercholesterolemia refers to excessive cholesterol in the blood (Cook, 2009). High lipid or cholesterol levels play an important role in producing atherosclerosis (buildup of fatty plaques in the arteries), which eventually can lead to coronary artery disease (CAD), the leading cause of morbidity and mortality in the adult population in the United

States (Box 34-13). The risk of premature CAD has been shown to increase with elevated plasma concentrations of total cholesterol and low-density lipoprotein (LDL) cholesterol and with low levels of high-density lipoprotein (HDL) cholesterol. Interventions that decrease LDL levels and increase HDL levels have been shown to lower the risk for CAD. In addition to abnormal cholesterol levels, risk factors for CAD include:

- Positive family history of elevated cholesterol or early heart disease
- Cigarette smoking
- Diabetes (type 1 or 2)
- Obesity
- Hypertension

Research over the past four decades indicates that a presymptomatic phase of atherosclerosis begins in childhood with the development of fatty streaks evident on autopsies of children who died of noncardiac causes (Kavey, Allada, Daniels, et al, 2007). The extent of atherosclerosis is positively associated with the number of adult risk factors such as obesity, cholesterol abnormalities, and hypertension. These data continue to support early screening and management of lipid levels to identify children with risk factors for cardiovascular disease and provide early intervention (lifestyle modifications and/or medications).

BOX 34-13 WHAT IS CHOLESTEROL?

Cholesterol, a fatlike steroid alcohol, is part of the lipoprotein complex in plasma that is essential for cellular metabolism. Triglycerides, natural fats synthesized from carbohydrates, are used for energy. Both are major lipids transported on lipoproteins, a combination of lipids and proteins, which include the following:

Chylomicrons—Produced in the intestine in response to the intake of dietary fat. These are the principal transporters of dietary fat (triglycerides) from the intestine to the blood and ultimately to the fatty tissue. Chylomicrons are usually not present in the blood after a 12- to 14-hour fast.

Very-low-density lipoproteins (VLDLs)—Contain high concentrations of triglycerides, moderate concentrations of cholesterol, and little protein.

Low-density lipoproteins (LDLs)—Contain low concentrations of triglycerides, high levels of cholesterol, and moderate levels of protein. The end product of VLDL synthesis, LDLs are the major carriers of cholesterol to the cells. Cells use cholesterol for synthesis of membranes and steroid production. Elevated levels of circulating LDL are a strong risk factor for cardiovascular disease.

High-density lipoproteins (HDLs)—Contain very low concentrations of triglycerides, relatively little cholesterol, and high levels of protein. HDLs transport free cholesterol to the liver for secretion in the bile. High levels of HDL are thought to protect against cardiovascular disease, whereas low levels of HDLs are considered an independent risk factor.

The cholesterol profile includes the following:

Total cholesterol = LDL + HDL + VLDL

Levels of total cholesterol, triglycerides, and HDL cholesterol are measured directly via a blood test. In the fasting state, LDL concentration is calculated using the following formula:

LDL = Total cholesterol − [HDL + (Triglycerides/5)]

A calculated LDL is considered accurate as long as the fasting triglyceride level is below 350 to 400 mg/dl. If triglycerides are higher than this, LDL cholesterol can be measured directly using a more specialized test.

In addition to the risk factors noted above, children are considered to be at high risk for atherosclerosis because of coexisting health problems such as:

- Chronic inflammatory diseases
- Cancer
- Transplantation
- CHD
- A history of KD

Lifestyle habits, including diet, exercise patterns, and smoking—all known to be potential risk factors for cardiovascular disease—are normally established at a young age. Risk factor modification and lipid-lowering measures in adults are known to decrease the incidence of CAD. There is increasing evidence that modification of risk factors earlier in life will have a positive effect on the likelihood of atherosclerosis in adult life.

Diagnostic Evaluation and Screening

Diagnosis of hyperlipidemia is based on analysis of blood. A blood specimen for determination of a full lipid profile should be drawn after a 12-hour fast. Total cholesterol and HDL cholesterol values obtained at any time in the nonfasting state are also accurate. It is important to note that lipid values can be affected by febrile illnesses and therefore lipids should not be drawn within 3 weeks of a febrile illness. Average lipid values vary by age and gender, with HDL values decreasing in boys as they go through puberty. Children are considered to have elevated total cholesterol if their total cholesterol value is more than 200 mg/dl and/or their LDL cholesterol value is more than 130 mg/dl. Some providers recommend using age- and gender-specific cutpoints.

Screening of children for hypercholesterolemia remains controversial. Consistent with previous recommendations, current guidelines continue to recommend a two-pronged strategy, providing complementary approaches: (1) a population approach that aims to lower the average levels of blood cholesterol among all American children through population-wide changes in nutrient intake and eating patterns, and (2) an individualized approach based on selective screening (see Evidence-Based Practice box). First presented by the National Cholesterol Education Panel in 1992, selective screening of individuals thought to be at high risk was recommended by the American Academy of Pediatrics in their 2008 statement (Daniels, Greer, and the Committee on Nutrition, 2008). Children more than 2 years old should be screened if they have a first- or second-degree relative with lipid abnormalities or with early cardiovascular disease (<55 years in a man or <65 years in a woman). In addition, perform screening in children with individual risk factors (see Box 34-2). The major change in the recent guidelines is that a full fasting profile is now recommended as the initial screen in children with familial or individual risk factors, including obesity. In addition, the American Academy of Pediatrics endorses screening for children with an unknown family history and those who have disease-state risk factors, such as diabetes (Daniels, Greer, and the Committee on Nutrition, 2008). Individualized treatment for these patients includes lifestyle modification and possibly lipid-lowering medication in the most severely affected.

Therapeutic Management

Treatment of high cholesterol levels in children begins with lifestyle modification. The American Heart Association and the American Academy of Pediatrics recommend a heart-healthy diet for all American children, with dietary counseling recommended for those children with known elevated cholesterol values (Daniels, Greer, and the Committee on Nutrition, 2008). A heart-healthy diet focuses on a balanced intake for children over 2 years old, favoring low-fat dairy products, avoiding *trans* fats, and reducing sweetened beverages. The recommended diet is rich in fruits and vegetables and whole grains. In addition, children with abnormal LDL cholesterol levels should reduce saturated fat intake to 7% of total calories and dietary cholesterol intake to less than 200 mg/day.

Research supports the benefit of diets low in saturated fats and *trans* fats and higher in monounsaturated fats (such as those found in olive and canola oil). It is important to provide accurate dietary information to families. Food labeling is confusing. Without counseling, patients tend to replace foods high in fat with foods low in fat but high in simple sugars; this can raise triglyceride values, decreasing the effectiveness of nutritional interventions and providing wasted calories.

Current thinking favors a Mediterranean-type diet, based on whole grains, fruits, and vegetables. In addition, this diet allows the use of monounsaturated fats, such as olive oil and canola oil, which have beneficial effects on HDL cholesterol values.

EVIDENCE-BASED PRACTICE

Cholesterol Screening for Children

ASK THE QUESTION

Should cholesterol screening be performed in children?

SEARCH FOR THE EVIDENCE

Search strategies

Selection criteria included English-language publications, research-based articles (level 3 or lower), infant and child populations.

Databases used

PubMed, Cochrane Collaboration, MD Consult, Joanna Briggs Institute, National Guidelines Clearinghouse (AHRQ), TRIP Database Plus, PedsCCM, BestBETs

CRITICALLY ANALYZE THE EVIDENCE

GRADE criteria: Evidence quality moderate; recommendation strong (Guyatt, Oxman, Vist, et al, 2008)

The rationale for lipid screening and management in children is evolving now that lipid levels have been followed from childhood into adulthood. Children who have cholesterol levels in the upper percentiles seem to have an increased risk of remaining in the upper percentiles into adulthood (Nicklas, von Duvillard, and Berenson, 2002). The more severely affected children are generally the ones targeted for dietary and possibly pharmacologic intervention. On the other hand, children in the lower percentiles are unlikely to have high cholesterol levels as adults.

Cholesterol levels in childhood appear to be a major population predictor for adult cholesterol levels. Cholesterol screening can begin in children over the age of 2 when risk factors like family history are present. The precursors of atherosclerosis are present in young people. Findings from autopsy studies of young people who have died of accidents and injuries have shown that the atherosclerotic process begins early in life (Enos, Holmes, and Beyer, 1953; Strong, Malcom, McMahan, et al, 1999). Furthermore, the extent of atherosclerosis is related to the presence and degree of cardiovascular risk factors in adults (Berenson, Srinivasan, Bao, et al, 1998).

Many experts favor selective screening because high blood cholesterol levels aggregate in families as a result of shared genetic and environmental factors (American Academy of Pediatrics, 2008). In addition, the most severely affected children generally come from families in which there is a high incidence of early heart disease.

APPLY THE EVIDENCE: NURSING IMPLICATIONS

Current recommendations include selective screening of children over the age of 2 years who have a sibling, parent, or grandparent with an elevated cholesterol level of 240 mg/dl or higher. In addition, children should be screened if they have a first- or second-degree relative with early atherosclerotic disease (stroke, myocardial infarction, sudden cardiac death, angina, or peripheral vascular disease). Screening should also be done if the child has any individual risk factors such as diabetes, hypertension, obesity, a history of Kawasaki disease, or nephrotic syndrome. Screening should include a fasting lipid profile in these patients. Lastly, cholesterol screening should be performed if the child's genetic family history is unknown.

References

American Academy of Pediatrics: Lipid screening and cardiovascular health in childhood, *Pediatrics* 122:198-208, 2008.

Berenson GS, Srinivasan SR, Bao W, et al: Association between multiple cardiovascular risk factors and atherosclerosis in children and young adults, *N Engl J Med* 338(23):1650-1656, 1998.

Enos WF, Holmes RH, Beyer J: Coronary disease among United States soldiers killed in action in Korea, *JAMA* 152(12):1090-1093, 1953.

Guyatt GH, Oxman AD, Vist GE, et al: GRADE: an emerging consensus on rating quality of evidence and strength of recommendations, *BMJ* 336:924-926, 2008.

Nicklas TA, von Duvillard SP, Berenson GS: Tracking of serum lipids and lipoproteins from childhood to dyslipidemia in adults: the Bogalusa Heart Study, *Int J Sports Med* 23(Suppl 1):S39-S43, 2002.

Strong JP, Malcom GT, McMahan CA, et al: Prevalence and extent of atherosclerosis in adolescents and young adults: implications for prevention from the Pathobiological Determinants of Atherosclerosis in Youth Study, *JAMA* 281(8):727-735, 1999.

The use of these fats also makes the diet more realistic and helps keep children satiated. Dietary recommendations can be confusing, and individualized guidelines should be provided by a certified nutritionist or dietitian with expertise in lipid management.

If the child's BMI is elevated, weight management should be addressed. In addition to food choice, portion size may also be an issue for these children. Increased physical exercise should be encouraged (ideally 45 minutes to 1 hour, 5 days a week) and is critical to the success of a weight-loss program. Population recommendations meant to decrease cardiovascular risk have been in place for almost two decades, yet unfortunately the incidence of childhood obesity in this country has tripled during the last 25 years (de Ferranti and Ludwig, 2008). Education and programs aimed at decreasing this trend and increasing heart-healthy living (e.g., diet, exercise, avoidance of smoking) are extremely important to decrease cardiovascular risk for the next generation. Assessment of BMI, education,

referral to weight-loss programs if indicated, and follow-up should be an integral part of every well-child visit.

Dietary changes alone can decrease LDL values 10% to 15%; however, it is likely that children with severe genetic hypercholesterolemia will require lipid-lowering medication in addition to lifestyle modification. Lipid-lowering drugs used in children and teenagers include bile acid–resin binders such as cholestyramine (Questran) and colestipol (Colestid), hydroxymethylglutaryl–coenzyme A (HMG-CoA) reductase inhibitors (statins such as atorvastatin, simvastatin, pravastatin). Nicotinic acid can help raise HDL cholesterol but is rarely used in pediatrics because of symptoms of flushing and documentation of elevated liver transaminases.

The American Academy of Pediatrics guidelines (Daniels, Greer, and the Committee on Nutrition, 2008; McCrindle, Urbina, Dennison, et al, 2007) lowered the recommended age for initiation of lipid-lowering medication, including statins, to children as young as 8 years old in patients with:

- LDL cholesterol greater than 190 mg/dl in patients without a positive history of early heart disease
- LDL cholesterol greater than 160 mg/dl with a positive family history or two risk factors
- LDL cholesterol greater than 130 mg/dl in patients with diabetes

---

⚡ DRUG ALERT

Statins

In clinical practice, statins are used for children severely affected with particularly adverse family histories. The tendency is to allow a progression through puberty, particularly for young girls. The target level for LDL cholesterol is less than 130 mg/dl, and optimally less than 100 mg/dl. Certain individual risk factors, such as diabetes, hypertension, or a history of coronary artery aneurysms from KD, all lower the threshold for pharmacologic intervention.

Bile acid–resin binders act by binding bile acids in the intestinal lumen. Because they are not absorbed by the intestine, they are not thought to produce systemic toxicity and are generally safe for children. Cholestyramine and colestipol are both powders that are mixed with water or juice just before ingestion. Many patients cannot tolerate resin binders because they have a gritty texture and do not dissolve completely in water. Side effects may include constipation, abdominal pain, gastrointestinal bloating, flatulence, and nausea. The average dosage for a child is 4 g three times daily or 6 g twice daily. Colesevelam (Welchol) comes in a pill form (625 mg/tablets); the effective dosage is two or three tablets taken twice a day.

Patients who take resin binders should take one multivitamin supplement daily, since bile acid–binding agents may interfere with the absorption of fat-soluble vitamins. Since they can interfere with absorption of other medications, any other medications should be given at least 1 hour before or 6 hours after the bile acid–binding agent is ingested. The results of a complete blood count; chloride and folate levels; and serum concentrations of vitamins A, D, and E should be evaluated yearly.

HMG-CoA reductase inhibitors (statins) continue to be the most effective medication for lipid lowering and are the first-line treatment for adults. Statins are being used more commonly in children and adolescents, especially those with severe familial dyslipidemia. Statin medications are most effective if taken in the evening. Because statins are metabolized by the liver, baseline liver function tests (alanine aminotransferase, aspartate aminotransferase) results, as well as creatine kinase levels, are obtained before the initiation of therapy. These tests, along with a fasting lipid profile, are repeated at approximately 4 weeks and 8 weeks after the initiation of therapy and with any dosage changes. Once the patient is taking a stable dosage, laboratory tests are repeated at 6-month intervals. In addition to elevation of liver transaminase levels, other potentially serious side effects include rhabdomyolysis, which can cause renal failure. Rhabdomyolysis has been reported rarely in adult patients. Instruct patients to discontinue the medication and contact their clinician if they experience the new onset of muscle aches or dark brown urine. In addition, female patients need to be educated that statins are considered teratogenic and cannot be taken during pregnancy. Oral contraceptives may be given in conjunction with lipid-lowering medication; however, they may increase lipid values, potentially necessitating modification of the statin dosage.

A relatively new drug, ezetimibe, works by inhibiting cholesterol absorption. It lowers LDL levels by preventing intestinal uptake of dietary and biliary cholesterol. Recommended use is in combination therapy with a statin, further lowering LDL values. This medication is currently approved for children older than 10 years of age with extremely severe hyperlipidemia. However, clinical trials have shown inconclusive evidence regarding this drug's clinical benefit. Several large clinical trials are in process, and more information should be available in the next few years.

Nursing Care Management

Nurses play an important role in the screening, education, and support of children with hyperlipidemia and their families. When a child is referred to a lipid clinic, it is essential that the family be adequately prepared for the first visit. Generally, the parents are asked to keep a dietary history for the child before this visit. Sometimes they need to complete a questionnaire regarding the child's normal dietary habits over the preceding year. Families are instructed to keep their child fasting for at least 12 hours before screening. Therefore it is important to schedule the blood test early in the morning and to arrange for nourishment immediately thereafter. At the visit, a complete individual and family health history is taken. The family history should include both biologic parents and all first-degree relatives. Questions are asked about early heart disease, hypertension, CVAs, sudden death, hyperlipidemia, diabetes, metabolic syndrome, and endocrine abnormalities. Nurses may also uncover risk factors when obtaining a health history for other purposes. It is therefore important that nurses be familiar with current screening practices and with available resources for children with positive family histories.

Parents and extended families should be informed about cholesterol and hyperlipidemia. This education should include a brief introduction to the different lipoprotein categories, including cholesterol, HDL, LDL, and triglycerides. Also, review behavioral risk factors for heart disease, such as smoking and lack of exercise. For management to be effective, parents and older children need to understand the rationale for dietary and pharmacologic intervention in the prevention of future cardiovascular disease.

Nutritional education is part of the treatment of any child or teenager with high cholesterol and ideally should be provided by a nutritionist with expertise in lipid disorders. Dietary compliance may become an issue of control and a source of great stress for many families, particularly for teenagers. Children with high cholesterol levels should not be viewed as having a disease. Instead, emphasize the positive aspects of healthy eating, regular exercise, and avoidance of smoking. Encourage basic dietary changes for the whole family, so that the affected child is not singled out. The focus is positive, with emphasis on making healthy dietary choices, such as substituting chicken and fish for hot dogs and hamburgers and substituting frozen yogurt for ice cream (Box 34-14). Cultural differences must be considered and recommendations

BOX 34-14 AMERICAN HEART ASSOCIATION DIETARY RECOMMENDATIONS FOR INFANTS, CHILDREN, AND ADOLESCENTS TO PROMOTE CARDIOVASCULAR HEALTH

Infancy

Breast-feeding is ideal nutrition and sufficient to support optimal growth and development for approximately the first 4 to 6 months after birth. Try to maintain breast-feeding for 12 months. Transition to other sources of nutrients should begin at approximately 4 to 6 months of age to ensure sufficient micronutrients in the diet.

Delay the introduction of 100% juice until at least 6 months of age and limit to no more than 4 to 6 oz/day. Juice should be fed only from a cup, not a bottle.

Do not overfeed infants and young children. Children should not be forced to finish meals if not hungry because they often vary caloric intake from meal to meal.

Introduce healthy foods and continue offering if initially refused. Do not introduce foods without overall nutritional value simply to provide calories.

Eating Pattern for Families*

Energy (calories) should be adequate to support growth and development and to reach or maintain desirable body weight.

Eat foods low in saturated fat, *trans* fat, cholesterol, salt (sodium), and added sugars.

Keep total fat intake between 30% and 35% of calories for children 2 to 3 years of age and between 25% and 35% of calories for children and adolescents 4 to 18 years of age, with most fats coming from sources of polyunsaturated and monounsaturated fatty acids, such as fish, nuts, and vegetable oils.

Choose a variety of foods to get enough carbohydrates, protein, and other nutrients.

Eat only enough calories to maintain a healthy weight for height and build. Be physically active for at least 60 minutes a day.

Serve whole grain breads and cereals rather than refined grain products. Look for "whole grain" as the first ingredient on the food label and make at least half of grain servings whole grain. Recommended grain intake ranges from 2 oz/day for a 1-year-old to 7 oz/day for a 14- to 18-year-old boy.

Serve a variety of fruits and vegetables daily, while limiting juice intake. Each meal should contain at least one fruit or vegetable. Children's recommended fruit intake ranges from 1 cup/day between ages 1 and 3 years to 2 cups/day for a 14- to 18-year-old boy. Recommended vegetable intake ranges from ¾ cup/day at age 1 year to 3 cups/day for a 14- to 18-year-old boy.

Introduce and regularly serve fish as an entrée. Avoid commercially fried fish.

Serve nonfat and low-fat dairy foods. From ages 1 to 8 years, children need 2 cups of milk or its equivalent each day. Children ages 9 to 18 years need 3 cups.

Don't overfeed. Estimated calories needed by children range from 900/day for a 1-year-old to 1800/day for a 14- to 18-year-old girl and 2200/day for a 14- to 18-year-old boy.

*This eating pattern supports a child's normal growth and development. It provides enough total energy and meets or exceeds the recommended dietary allowances for all nutrients for children and adolescents, including iron and calcium.

individualized. For example, it is more realistic to suggest frying food in a monounsaturated oil such as canola oil than to forbid frying food altogether in families in which this is common practice. Emphasize substitution rather than elimination. Visual aids (e.g., test tubes depicting the amount of fat in a hot dog) are often helpful, especially for children. Diets should be flexible and individually tailored by a nutritionist experienced in combining recommendations that meet both the nutritional demands of the growing child and lipid modifications. Encourage parents to participate in dietary and educational sessions, ask questions, and share ideas and experiences.

Parents often feel guilty about the hereditary component of hyperlipidemia. Many of these same parents believe they have failed if diet alone is not making a significant difference in their child's lipid profile. They are reassured that a dietary approach alone is often not sufficient, especially for children with values higher than the 95th percentile.

Parents of children who require pharmacologic therapy must understand the purpose, dosage, and possible side effects of the various drugs. Medication schedules should remain flexible and should not interfere with the child's daily activities. As an example, children of elementary school age may have better compliance if they take a resin-binding agent (e.g., cholestyramine, colestipol) twice a day (i.e., before school and at night) rather than the standard three times a day. Follow-up phone calls by the nurse between visits allow parents to discuss their concerns and ask any questions that have arisen.

! NURSING ALERT

The recommendations for fat intake for the general population are intended for children over 2 years of age. Children under the age of 2 require a higher percentage of calories from fat. However, recent studies have supported the safety of low-fat dairy products in younger children. Therefore low-fat dairy products are appropriate for children less than 1 year old who are obese or who have additional cardiovascular risk factors, as long as adequate sources of monounsaturated and polyunsaturated fats are maintained (Daniels, Greer, and the Committee on Nutrition, 2008).

CARDIAC DYSRHYTHMIAS

Dysrhythmias, or abnormal heart rhythms, can occur in children with structurally normal hearts, as features of some congenital heart defects, and in patients following surgical repair of congenital heart defects. They occur in patients with cardiomyopathy and cardiac tumors. They can occur secondary to metabolic and electrolyte imbalances. Childhood dysrhythmias can have a genetic or familial etiology. Dysrhythmias can be classified in several ways, such as by heart rate characteristics (bradycardia and tachycardia) or by the origin of the dysrhythmia in the atria or ventricles. Most are due to abnormalities in impulse generation in the RA or to abnormalities in the conduction pathways.

Some dysrhythmias are well tolerated and self-limiting. Others may cause decreased cardiac output with associated symptoms. Some dysrhythmias can cause sudden death. Treatment depends on the cause of the dysrhythmia and its severity. Underlying causes are treated if possible (as with electrolyte imbalances). Some dysrhythmias (such as bradycardia caused by congenital heart block) are well tolerated and may not require treatment for many years. Others may require medications, radiofrequency ablation, or pacemaker placement. Some can be difficult to treat and require multiple therapies.

Many advances have been made in the diagnosis and treatment of pediatric dysrhythmias. Improvements in technology have allowed better diagnosis, the development of ablation techniques, and the expansion of pacemaker capabilities. New antidysrhythmic medications have proven safe and effective in children. Radiofrequency ablation has offered a cure for some dysrhythmias. Pediatric electrophysiology has become a highly specialized field, and the student is referred to more detailed sources for an in-depth discussion. The following sections describe diagnostic studies and provide a general discussion of the most common tachycardia (supraventricular tachycardia) and the most common bradycardia (complete heart block) that require treatment in the pediatric population.

Diagnostic Evaluation

Before diagnosing an infant or child with an abnormal heart rate, nurses must be familiar with the standards for normal heart rate in the particular age-group. (See inside back cover.) Heart rate patterns considered normal for a particular child can vary tremendously. An initial nursing responsibility is recognition of an abnormal heartbeat, either in rate or in rhythm. When a dysrhythmia is suspected, the apical rate is counted for 1 full minute and compared with the radial rate, which may be lower because not all of the apical beats are felt. Consistently high or low heart rates should be regarded as suspicious. Accurate nursing assessment is essential. The patient should be placed on a cardiac monitor with recording capabilities. A 12-lead ECG yields more information than the monitor recording and should be taken as soon as possible. Recent advances in bedside telemetry allow storage of ECG tracings for later analysis.

Several advances in the diagnosis of cardiac dysrhythmias have greatly improved the understanding and treatment of these conditions in children. The basic diagnostic procedure is the ECG, including 24-hour Holter monitoring. However, more definitive procedures include both noninvasive and invasive techniques.

Electrophysiologic cardiac catheterization allows identification of conduction disturbances and immediate investigation of drugs that may control the dysrhythmia. Electrode catheters are introduced intravenously and directed toward the right side of the heart. The heart is then selectively stimulated to induce dysrhythmias. Once a dysrhythmia occurs, different antidysrhythmic drugs are administered intravenously to monitor which pharmacologic agent is most successful in terminating the dysrhythmia.

Another procedure that may be employed is transesophageal recording. An electrode catheter is passed to the lower esophagus and, when in position at a point proximal to the heart, is used to stimulate and record dysrhythmias.

The onset and diagnosis of a cardiac dysrhythmia are frightening experiences for parents and older children. Sometimes the dysrhythmia rapidly leads to heart failure and a medical crisis. In this situation parents need much support to express their feelings and to understand the diagnosis and its treatment. Often parents and children have an unspoken fear of potential death even if the dysrhythmia is benign, and repeated explanations are needed to relieve anxiety.

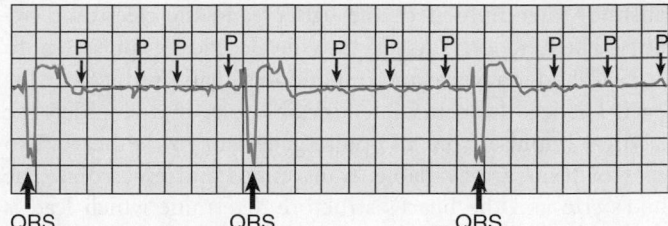

Fig. 34-17 Complete heart block. Note slow rhythm and several P waves not followed by a QRS complex.

Bradydysrhythmias

Sinus bradycardia in children can be due to the influence of the autonomic nervous system, as with hypervagal tone, or can be in response to hypoxia and hypotension. Once the infant receives adequate oxygenation and any acidosis is eliminated, the heart rate often returns to baseline. Sinus bradycardias are also known to develop after atrial repairs involving atrial suture lines such as in the Fontan procedure.

Complete AV block is also referred to as *complete heart block* (Fig. 34-17). This can be either congenital (occurring in children with structurally normal hearts) or acquired after surgery to repair cardiac defects. AV blocks are most often related to edema around the conduction system and resolve without treatment. Temporary epicardial wires are placed in most patients at surgery; if a rhythm disturbance occurs, temporary pacing can be employed. Just before discharge the health practitioner removes the wires by pulling slowly and deliberately down on them from the site of insertion.

A permanent pacemaker may be needed in some children, such as those with postsurgical AV block or, less frequently, congenital AV block. The pacemaker takes over or assists in the heart's conduction function. The surgical implantation of a pacemaker is usually a low-risk procedure. Once the wire has been introduced, a small incision is made and a pocket is formed under the muscle to house and protect the generator. The generator is placed under the abdominal muscle in infants and young children and in the upper chest below the clavicle in older children and adolescents. Depending on patient size and cardiac anatomy, some pacemakers can be placed transvenously in the catheterization laboratory, rather than in the operating room. Continuous ECG monitoring is necessary during the recovery phase to assess pacemaker function. The nurse should be aware of the programmed rate and expected individual generator variations. A baseline ECG and chest x-ray film are obtained for future comparison. The pacemaker pocket site is monitored for signs of infection. Analgesics are given for pain.

Pacemaker functions have become dramatically more sophisticated; pacemakers can control heart rate according to activity, cardiac output, and respirations. In addition, some models can be programmed for overdrive pacing or cardioversion when the generator detects accelerated rates beyond established normal values.

When a pacemaker is implanted, the education of the parents and child includes an explanation of the device, a description of the component parts, an explanation of the surgical procedure, and discharge teaching. The pacemaker is made up of two basic parts: the pulse generator and the lead. The pulse generator is composed of the battery and the electronic circuitry. The function is to produce the electrical impulse sent to the heart and to receive and respond to signals produced by the heart. The lead is an insulated, flexible wire that conducts the electrical impulse from the pulse generator to the heart. Two types of leads are available: transvenous and epicardial. The child's size and the heart's structure determine which lead is more appropriate. Transvenous leads are inserted into a large vein, often the subclavian, and advanced into the right side of the heart. Placement is secured by engaging a small corkscrew or fishhook attachment at the end of the lead into the endocardium. Epicardial leads are attached directly to the epicardial layer of the heart. Parents should be aware of which type of lead is in place in their child.

Discharge teaching includes information about the signs and symptoms of infection, general wound care, and activity restrictions. Parents, and patients if they are old enough, should learn to take the pulse and should know the settings of the pacemaker. If the patient's low rate is set at 80 beats/min and the heart rate is only 68 beats/min, there is a possible problem with the pacemaker that needs to be investigated. Instructions for telephone transmission of ECG readings are also given. Telephone connections can be used to transmit ECG data and also to monitor battery life and pacemaker function. The pacemaker generator has to be replaced periodically because of battery depletion. Children with pacemakers should wear a medical alert device, and their parents should have a paper identification card with specific pacer data in case of an emergency. Cardiopulmonary resuscitation instruction is suggested for parents.

Tachydysrhythmias

Sinus tachycardia (abnormally fast heart rate) secondary to fever, anxiety, pain, anemia, dehydration, or any other etiologic factor requiring increased cardiac output should be ruled out first before diagnosing it as pathologic. Supraventricular tachycardia (SVT), the most common tachydysrhythmia found in children, refers to a rapid regular heart rate of 200 to 300 beats/min (Fig. 34-18). As many as 1 in 250 children experiences SVT (Schlente, Boramanand, and Funk, 2008). The rapid rhythm originates in the atria. The onset and termination of SVT are abrupt. The QRS complex is usually narrow (in contrast with ventricular tachycardia, in which the QRS complexes are typically wide), and the P waves are often absent. Infants and

young children with SVT may be unable to compensate for the rapid heart rate, and the clinical course can progress to HF. Important signs in the infant and young child are poor feeding, extreme irritability, and pallor. Children may experience palpitations, dizziness, chest pain, and diaphoresis.

Ventricular tachycardias are rare in children and are not discussed here.

The treatment of SVT depends on the degree of compromise imposed by the dysrhythmia. In some instances, vagal maneuvers, such as applying ice to the face, massaging the carotid artery (on one side of the neck only), or having an older child perform a Valsalva maneuver (e.g., exhaling against a closed glottis, blowing on the thumb as if it were a trumpet for 30 to 60 seconds), can reverse the SVT. When vagal maneuvers fail, adenosine may be used to end the episode of SVT by impairing AV node conduction. IV adenosine is the first-line pharmacologic measure for termination of SVT in infants and children in the emergency setting (Dixon, Foster, Wyllie, et al, 2005). Adenosine must be given by rapid IV push with a saline bolus immediately following the drug. Incrementally increasing doses given about 2 minutes apart may be needed. The desired effect usually occurs in 10 to 20 seconds.

Traditional first-line medical management of chronic SVT includes digoxin. If the infant or child is minimally symptomatic, digitalization can be initiated, with careful monitoring of vital signs and patient response to the intervention. More aggressive pharmacologic treatment with medications such as propranolol or amiodarone may be needed for those with more severe symptoms or recurrence of SVT while digoxin is being taken.

If cardiac output is significantly compromised or signs of HF exist, esophageal overdrive pacing or synchronized cardioversion can be employed in the intensive care setting. Transesophageal atrial overdrive pacing is accomplished through placement of a protected lead into the esophagus, behind the LA of the heart. The lead is then attached to a stimulator capable of pacing at very rapid rates to interrupt the tachydysrhythmia. Synchronized cardioversion is the timed delivery of a preset amount of energy through the chest wall in an attempt to reestablish an organized rhythm. Sedation is needed for both procedures. Cardioversion should never be performed on a conscious patient.

Radiofrequency ablation has become first-line therapy for some types of SVT. The procedure is done in the cardiac catheterization laboratory and begins with mapping of the conduction system to identify the dysrhythmia focus. A catheter delivering radiofrequency current is directed at the site, and the identified area is heated to destroy the tissue in the area. Success rates vary between 60% and 90% depending on the type of SVT (LeRoy, 2001). A successful ablation is curative, and antidysrhythmic medications can be discontinued.

A newer procedure, cryoablation, is also used in treatment of SVT. Liquid nitrous oxide is used to cool a catheter to subfreezing temperatures, which then destroys the tissue of target by freezing. This procedure takes pace in the cardiac electrophysiology catheterization laboratory. This method allows reversible cooling so that the electrophysiologist can test an area first before freezing it to a point where a permanent lesion is formed (Chun and Van Hare, 2004).

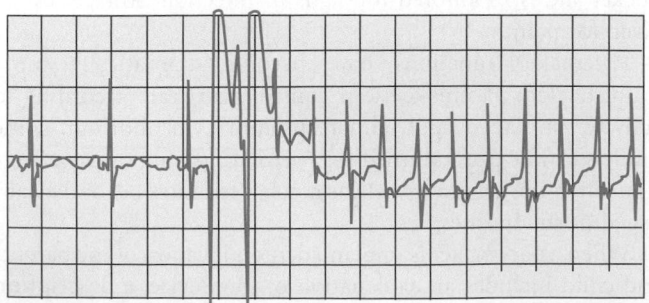

Fig. 34-18 Supraventricular tachycardia (SVT). Note normal sinus rhythm (three PQRST complexes) on the left and abrupt onset of a very fast rhythm (SVT) on the right.

Preparation is similar to that for cardiac catheterization and other electrophysiologic studies. The risks and benefits of ablation need to be reviewed. These are lengthy procedures, often 6 to 8 hours, and sedation or general anesthesia is required. Postprocedure care is similar to that for cardiac catheterization (see p. 1349) with the addition of careful dysrhythmia monitoring. Patients and their families often have great hope for a cure and are disappointed if the ablation is unsuccessful.

A primary focus of nursing care is education of the family regarding the symptoms of SVT and the treatment. SVT may occur again despite therapy. After the first episode of SVT, parents should learn to take a radial pulse for 1 full minute. If medication is prescribed, instructions regarding accurate dosage and the importance of administering the correct dose at specified intervals are stressed (see Critical Thinking Exercise).

❓ CRITICAL THINKING EXERCISE

The Infant with a Tachydysrhythmia

You are working in the emergency department when a father comes through the doors, carrying his 1-month-old crying infant. The infant is awake and very irritable. Father reports that the infant has not been feeding well for the past 6 hours, and dad has noticed sweating (diaphoresis) with attempted feeds. No history of fever noted. Further assessment reveals a diaphoretic infant, crying, with a respiratory rate of 60, BP 60/40 mm Hg, and a heart rate that is too fast to count by auscultation. When the infant is attached to the cardiorespiratory monitor, heart rate is 220 beats/min, nonvariable, with an oxygen saturation of 97%. Capillary refill time is slightly prolonged at 3 seconds, and femoral pulses are palpable, but weak.

1. Evidence—Is there sufficient evidence to draw conclusions about this infant?
2. Assumptions—Describe an underlying assumption about each of the following:
   a. Symptoms associated with heart failure
   b. An infant less than 3 months with poor feeding
   c. Tachydysrhythmias in infants
3. What priorities for nursing care should be established?
4. Does the evidence support your nursing interventions?

PULMONARY ARTERY HYPERTENSION

Pulmonary artery hypertension (PAH) refers to a group of rare conditions that result in an elevation of pulmonary artery pressure. Generally, these abnormalities result in remodeling of the pulmonary circulation, characterized by occlusion of the lumen in medium and small pulmonary arteries due to cellular proliferation (Michelakis, Wilkins, and Rabinovitch, 2008). These disorders can occur in children and adults and are poorly understood. Until recently they had no treatment beyond supportive care. There is now evidence of a genetic basis for some cases of PAH; some mutations localized to chromosome 2 have been identified in about half of patients with familial PAH (Lane, Machado, Pauciulo, et al, 2000).

PAH is a progressive, eventually fatal disease for which there is no known cure. It can be difficult to diagnose in the early stages. Often when patients become symptomatic and a diagnosis is made, their disease progresses rapidly, treatment is unsuccessful, and death occurs within several years. Significant new information about the disease process, genetic links, diagnosis, and treatment has recently been learned. Recent therapeutic advances, including use of endothelial receptor antagonists and vasodilator therapy with nitric oxide and prostacyclin (epoprostenol), have improved the outlook for this group of patients. Improvements in quality of life, exercise capacity, hemodynamics, and long-term survival have been seen with treatment.

Pulmonary hypertensive diseases have been classified into five categories: (1) pulmonary arterial hypertension, including idiopathic PAH, familial PAH, and PAH related to risk factors or associated conditions, including collagen vascular disease, congenital systemic-to-pulmonary shunts, and human immunodeficiency virus infection; (2) pulmonary venous hypertension (often related to left-sided heart disease); (3) PAH associated with hypoxemia; (4) PAH related to chronic thrombotic or embolic disease; and (5) PAH due to miscellaneous causes (Simonneau, Galie, Rubin, et al, 2004).

Congenital heart defects with a large left-to-right shunt (such as in ventricular septal defect, patent ductus arteriosus, or complete AV canal), which cause increased pulmonary blood flow, may result in pulmonary hypertension. If these defects are not repaired early, the high pulmonary flow will cause changes in the pulmonary artery vessels and the vessels will lose their elasticity. This causes increased resistance in the pulmonary bed and results in eventual right-sided heart failure because the heart cannot pump against the greater resistance. The flow of blood becomes right to left, and cyanosis is seen. This is known as Eisenmenger syndrome. Because of surgical repair of these defects early in life, this occurs infrequently now.

The diagnostic workup is extensive, and diagnostic guidelines have been developed to guide clinicians (Barst, McGoon, Torbicki, et al, 2004; McGoon, Gutterman, Steen, et al, 2004). Detection of PAH can be difficult. It may be diagnosed when symptoms arise, through screening of patients at risk, or as an incidental finding. Initial evaluation involves physical examination, chest radiography, ECG, and echocardiography. An extensive workup is needed to better characterize the causes, associated factors, hemodynamics, and disease severity and includes evaluation of cardiac and pulmonary function, coagulation tests, collagen vascular evaluation, and other studies. Right-sided cardiac catheterization is essential to evaluate the degree of pulmonary hypertension and the response to vasodilator therapy. Oxygen, nitric oxide, and prostacyclin may all be used during the catheterization to assess the ability of various therapies to reduce pulmonary artery pressure. Exercise capacity, as assessed by the 6-minute walk test, is predictive of disease severity.

Clinical Manifestations

The clinical manifestations include dyspnea with exercise, chest pain, and syncope. Dyspnea is the most common symptom and is caused by impaired oxygen delivery. Chest pain is the result of coronary ischemia in the RV from severe hypertrophy. Syncope reflects a limited cardiac output leading to decreased cerebral blood flow. Right-sided heart dysfunction is steadily progressive as the pulmonary vessels become obstructed and the pulmonary artery pressure increases. The RV hypertrophies to attempt to maintain a normal cardiac output. With time and continued increases in pulmonary vascular resistance, the cardiac output decreases. When signs of right-sided heart failure with systemic venous congestion and edema are evident, the prognosis is poor.

Therapeutic Management

Although no cure is known, several therapies have shown promise in slowing the progression of the disease and improving quality of life. In general, situations that may exacerbate the disease and cause hypoxia are avoided. Exercise prescriptions are specific to each patient. Patients should avoid high altitudes because of the relative hypoxia, and some patients have moved to sea level to slow the progress of the disease. Supplemental oxygen is commonly used to relieve hypoxia, especially at night while sleeping. Patients with PAH are at risk for thromboembolic events. Anticoagulation therapy has been shown to increase survival in adults. Many patients are treated with warfarin to prevent pulmonary embolism, which can be fatal. Digoxin and diuretics are often used to treat right-sided heart failure.

A number of new drug treatments have been used in this patient population in the past decade and have shown promise in improving both quality of life and survival. Medications are often used in combination, and different drugs are used at different stages of illness. Current research efforts are expanding the understanding of the disease and offering new treatments. Several medications are in clinical trials. Evidence-based guidelines for medical therapy and reviews of therapies in clinical trials have been outlined (Badesch, Abman, Ahearn, et al, 2004; Galie, Seeger, Naeije, et al, 2004).

For patients who respond to vasodilator drug testing during cardiac catheterization, oral calcium channel blockers have been successful and are the treatment of choice. Some patients eventually become nonresponders and then need another therapy. For patients who are nonresponders in vasodilator testing, bosentan, an endothelin-receptor antagonist, is available; it reduces pulmonary artery pressure and resistance and is safe and well tolerated in children (Barst, Ivy, Dingemanse, et al, 2003). It has been used in combination with IV prostacyclin.

Continuous IV prostacyclin has been used with success in children who did not respond to a trial of vasodilation during catheterization. The drug imitates a natural prostacyclin that dilates smooth muscle. It also prevents thrombus formation. It is given by a continuous IV infusion through an indwelling catheter with a portable battery-operated pump. It has been shown to improve exercise capacity and survival.

Nitric oxide is an endothelium-derived relaxing factor. When inhaled, it can relax pulmonary vascular smooth muscle. It is short acting and is inactivated by contact with hemoglobin in the capillary bed. It is a selective pulmonary vasodilator with minimal hemodynamic side effects. Nitric oxide has been used most often in the ICU to manage acute pulmonary hypertensive crisis after congenital cardiac surgery or for diagnostic purposes in the cardiac catheterization laboratory.

Lung transplantation may be another treatment option for children, primarily those with severe disease. Patients with PAH and Eisenmenger syndrome have had a higher early mortality after lung transplantation than other lung transplant patients. Bilateral lung transplantation is the procedure of choice (Doyle, McCrory, Channick, et al, 2004).

As new information is learned and new drugs and new combination therapies are tested and evaluated, the management of patients with PAH will continue to evolve.

Nursing Care Management

The diagnosis of PAH is devastating for the child and family. There is no known cure, and the treatments require significant lifestyle changes and commitment on the part of patient and family to make them successful. Anxiety, depression, and fear of the future are common. Patients and families require extensive education about the disease and its management. They need emotional support to cope with a poor prognosis and make decisions about treatment options.

The medical treatment is complex and involves different medications and therapies. Families are often referred to a specialized center that has experience in the management of PAH. This may involve travel far from home with associated emotional and financial hardships. The patient and family must cope with the symptoms of the disease and the side effects of the treatment. Dealing with a continuous IV infusion or continuous oxygen administration requires a major adjustment in lifestyle to accommodate the therapy. The prostacyclin infusion cannot be interrupted at any time, since symptoms can worsen and cause acute pulmonary hypertensive crisis, which can be fatal. Backup systems must be in place at all times. The patient and family must make a commitment to adhere to a complex regimen of preparing the infusion, maintaining the equipment, and maintaining sterility of the central line. Treatments are expensive, so insurance coverage and financial issues are critical. Nurses have an important role in preparing families to perform these complex therapies. Discharge planning involves many team members and outside agencies. The nurse has a pivotal role in coordinating the child's care in the hospital and the transition to home.

CARDIOMYOPATHY

Cardiomyopathy refers to abnormalities of the myocardium in which the cardiac muscles' ability to contract is impaired. Cardiomyopathies are relatively rare in children. Possible causes include familial or genetic factors, infection, deficiency states, metabolic abnormalities, and collagen vascular diseases. Most cardiomyopathies in children are considered primary or idiopathic disorders, in which the cause is unknown and the cardiac dysfunction is not associated with systemic disease. Abnormalities of the cardiac myocyte and essential cellular functions underlie the clinical manifestations of organ dysfunction. Some of the known causes of secondary cardiomyopathy are toxicity from anthracyclines (e.g., the antineoplastic agents doxorubicin [Adriamycin] and daunomycin), hemochromatosis (from excessive iron storage), Duchenne muscular dystrophy, KD, collagen diseases, and thyroid dysfunction.

Cardiomyopathies can be divided into three broad clinical categories according to the type of abnormal structure and dysfunction present: dilated cardiomyopathy, hypertrophic cardiomyopathy, and restrictive cardiomyopathy. Dilated cardiomyopathy is characterized by ventricular dilation and greatly decreased contractility, which result in symptoms of HF. This is the most common type of cardiomyopathy in children. Its cause is often unknown, although carnitine and selenium deficiency, metabolic diseases, drug toxicities, dysrhythmias, and infection causing myocarditis should be considered. A specific syndrome or genetic abnormality was diagnosed in 27% of children in the Pediatric Cardiomyopathy Registry (Lipshultz, Sleeper, Towbin, et al, 2003). The clinical findings are of HF with tachycardia, dyspnea, hepatosplenomegaly, fatigue, and poor growth. Dysrhythmias may be present and may be more difficult to control with worsening heart failure. Chest radiography demonstrates cardiomegaly and congested lung fields. The echocardiogram demonstrates poor ventricular contractility, dilated LV, and reduced shortening and ejection fraction. Cardiac catheterization with endomyocardial biopsy is usually performed for diagnosis and identification of a possible infectious cause. In one review, mortality of patients with dilated cardiomyopathy was 13% at 2 years (Lipshultz, Sleeper, Towbin, et al, 2003).

Hypertrophic cardiomyopathy is characterized by an increase in heart muscle mass without an increase in cavity size. It usually occurs in the LV and is associated with abnormal diastolic filling. Mutations of eight genes that encode proteins of the cardiac sarcomere have been identified. The expression of clinical disease varies greatly among patients. Infants of diabetic mothers may have a hypertrophic cardiomyopathy that resolves with time. Clinical symptoms usually appear in the school-age period or adolescence and may include anginal chest pain, dysrhythmias, and syncope. Sudden death is possible. One recent study confirmed that unexplained syncope in the childhood age-group (<18 years of age) with known hypertrophic cardiomyopathy had a 60% cumulative risk of sudden death within 5 years of the syncopal event (Spirito, Autore, Rapezzi, et al, 2009). Presentation in infancy includes signs of HF and carries a poor prognosis. Chest radiography shows a mildly enlarged heart. The ECG demonstrates LV hypertrophy, often with ST-T changes. The echocardiogram is most helpful and demonstrates asymmetric septal hypertrophy and an increase in LV wall thickness, with a small LV cavity.

Restrictive cardiomyopathy, rare in children, involves a restriction to ventricular filling caused by endocardial or myocardial disease or both. RA or LA enlargement or both, apparent on the ECG, are often seen. The chest radiograph shows an enlarged heart. The echocardiogram reveals atrial dilation. Systolic function, the ability of the heart to squeeze, is often normal or mildly impaired, whereas diastolic function, the ability of the heart to relax, is very abnormal. Patients are at risk for embolic events and the development of pulmonary hypertension. Symptoms are those of HF (see p. 1352).

Therapeutic Management

Treatment is directed at correcting the underlying cause whenever feasible. In most affected children, however, this is not possible, and treatment is aimed at managing HF (see p. 1354) and dysrhythmias. Administration of digoxin and diuretics and aggressive use of afterload-reduction agents have been found to be helpful in managing symptoms in those with dilated cardiomyopathy. The use of beta blockers, specifically carvedilol, is limited in pediatric patients, but one study reported improvement in symptoms in some patients (Bruns, Chrisant, Lamour, et al, 2001). Practice guidelines for the management of heart

failure in children have been outlined and provide an in-depth review of available therapies (Rosenthal, Chrisant, Edens, et al, 2004). Digoxin and inotropic agents are usually not helpful in the other forms of cardiomyopathy because increasing the force of contraction may exacerbate the muscular obstruction and actually impair ventricular ejection. Beta blockers such as propranolol or calcium channel blockers such as verapamil (Calan) have been used to reduce LV outflow obstruction and improve diastolic filling in those with hypertrophic cardiomyopathy.

Careful monitoring and treatment of dysrhythmias are essential. The placement of an implantable defibrillator should be considered for patients at high risk of sudden death due to ventricular arrhythmias. Anticoagulants may be given to reduce the risk of thromboembolism, a complication of the sluggish circulation through the heart. For worsening heart failure and signs of poor perfusion, severely ill children may benefit from mechanical ventilation, oxygen administration, IV inotropic support, and IV administration of afterload-reduction agents such as milrinone. Mechanical support devices such as extracorporeal membrane oxygenation or LV assist devices may be used in patients with progressive decline in cardiac status. Extracorporeal membrane oxygenation is employed primarily for infants and younger patients. Its use is limited to several weeks or less because of complications such as bleeding and infection. Ventricular assist devices, currently available for older children and adolescents, can be used for longer periods. Risks include infection and embolic complications. Both devices can be used as a bridge to heart transplantation to allow more time to wait for a donor organ. Heart transplantation may be a treatment option for patients who have worsening symptoms despite maximum medical therapy (see below).

Nursing Care Management

Because of the poor prognosis for many children with cardiomyopathy, nursing care is consistent with that for any child with a life-threatening disorder. (See Chapter 23.) One of the most difficult adjustments for the child may be the realization of failing health and the need for restricted activity, especially if the child is a normally active youngster. Include the child in decisions regarding activity and allow him or her to discuss feelings, particularly if the disease follows a progressive and fatal course. Once symptoms of HF or dysrhythmias develop, implement the same nursing care as discussed on pp. 1354-1360. If cardiac transplantation is being considered, the child and family have great needs in terms of psychologic preparation and postoperative care. The nurse plays an important role in assessing the family's understanding of the procedure and long-term consequences. Children of school age and older should be fully informed to give their assent to the procedure. (See Informed Consent, Chapter 27.)

HEART TRANSPLANTATION

Heart transplantation has become a treatment option for infants and children with worsening heart failure and a limited life expectancy despite maximum medical and surgical management. Indications for cardiac transplantation in children are cardiomyopathy and end-stage CHD. It is also an option for patients with some forms of complex congenital cardiac defects such as hypoplastic left heart syndrome for whom conventional surgical approaches have a high mortality.

The heart transplant procedure may be orthotopic or heterotopic. Orthotopic heart transplantation refers to removal of the recipient's own heart and implantation of a new heart from a donor who has experienced brain death but whose heart is healthy. The donor and recipient are matched by weight and blood type. In heterotopic heart transplantation, the recipient's own heart is left in place and a new heart is implanted to act as an additional pump or "piggyback" heart; this type of transplantation is rarely done in children.

Before transplantation, potential recipients undergo a careful cardiac evaluation to determine whether any other medical or surgical options could improve the patient's cardiac status. Other organ systems are assessed to identify problems that might preclude or increase the risk of transplantation. A psychosocial evaluation of the patient and family is done to assess family function, support systems, and ability to comply with the complex medical regimen after the transplant. Support services to help the family successfully care for their child are provided when possible. Parents and older adolescents need extensive education about the risks and benefits of transplantation so that they can make an informed decision.

Patients are listed on a national computer network organized by the United Network for Organ Sharing (2001) to match donors and recipients. (See Organ or Tissue Donation and Autopsy, Chapter 23.) Although the total number of pediatric candidates on the waiting list has steadily increased from 1739 in 1997 to 2124 candidates in 2006, the number of pediatric candidates has been steady with 106 active on the waiting list by the end of 2006, according to the Scientific Registry of Transplant Recipients (2007). The 1-year survival rate for pediatric heart recipients increased with increasing age from 81% for those less than 1 year old to 91% for 11- to 17-year-olds.

Waiting list mortality remains high, particularly in the smallest children. Recent progress in suitable ventricular assist devices for use in children as a bridge to transplantation has made outcomes to survival for cardiac transplantation more successful (Blume, Naftel, Bastardi, et al, 2006). A multicenter study using the U.S. Scientific Registry of Transplant Recipients was recently conducted (Almond, Thiagarajian, Piercy, et al, 2009). Among 3098 children listed for a heart transplant between 1999 and 2006, the median age was 2 years. Sixty percent of patients were listed as top status (30% ventilated and 18% on supportive measures), and of those children, 17% died, 63% received transplants, 8% recovered, and 12% remained listed. These numbers indicate that waiting time in the United States remains high in the current era, and high-risk groups in these categories could benefit from emerging cardiac assist devices, such as extracorporeal membrane oxygenation and ventricular assist devices.

The posttransplantation course is complex. Although heart function is greatly improved or normal after transplantation, the risk of rejection is serious. The leading cause of death in the first 3 years after heart transplantation is rejection, with the greatest risk in the first 6 months (Blume, 2003). Rejection of the heart is diagnosed primarily by endomyocardial biopsy in older children. Serial echocardiograms are often used in infants and young children to reduce the need for invasive biopsies.

Immunosuppressants must be taken for life and have many systemic side effects. Triple drug therapy for immunosuppression with a calcineurin inhibitor (cyclosporine or tacrolimus), steroids, and azathioprine is most commonly used in pediatric patients, although mycophenolate mofetil is being used more frequently and replacing azathioprine. Steroid dosages are progressively lowered in the first year, and the drugs may be discontinued in some patients.

Infection is always a risk. Potential long-term problems that may limit survival include chronic rejection, which causes CAD; renal dysfunction and hypertension resulting from cyclosporine administration; lymphoma; and infection. CAD is the leading cause of death among late survivors of heart transplantation (Boucek, Edwards, Keck, et al, 2004). In the short term, after successful transplantation, children are able to return to full participation in age-appropriate activities and appear to adapt well to their new lifestyle. Transplantation is not a cure, because patients must live with the lifetime consequences of chronic immunosuppression.

NURSING CARE MANAGEMENT

Nursing care following transplantation is complex, demanding careful attention to both the physical needs of the child and the emotional needs of the child and family. Successfully caring for a child after heart transplantation requires the expertise and dedication of many members of the health care team. Nurses play vital roles in assessment, coordination of care, psychosocial support, and patient and family education. The nurse must monitor the heart transplant recipient carefully for signs of rejection, infection, and the side effects of the immunosuppressant medications. Optimizing long-term health includes managing cholesterol levels, participating in routine exercise, refraining from smoking, aggressively controlling BP, and optimizing bone health (Blume, 2003). The nurse also needs to assess the patient and family's psychosocial well-being to identify issues such as increased family stress, depression, substance abuse, and school problems. Noncompliance with an intense medication regimen, especially during adolescence, can lead to serious medical problems and can be fatal. Some patients and families need psychiatric support, and many patients need supportive services for learning problems. Chapter 30 discusses immunosuppressants and their nursing implications in relation to renal transplantation. Chapter 36 reviews care of the immunosuppressed child. Chapter 23 presents psychosocial concerns and appropriate interventions for the child with a life-threatening disorder.

The first 6 months to 1 year after transplantation are most intense, since the risk of complications is greatest and the patient and family are adjusting to a new lifestyle. Parents of heart transplant recipients also have a high incidence of posttraumatic stress symptoms, and the transplant team should routinely assess the parent or caretaker's psychologic functioning (Farley, DeMaso, D'Angelo, et al, 2007). The health care team monitors patients closely, with frequent visits and laboratory tests. Care is usually shared between local health care providers and the transplant center. Many patients are able to return to school and other age-appropriate activities within 2 to 3 months after the transplant.

KEY POINTS

- CHD is the most common form of cardiac disease in children and the most common congenital anomaly.
- The most common tests used in assessing cardiac function are radiography, ECG, echocardiography, and cardiac catheterization.
- Cardiac catheterization procedures can be divided into three groups: (1) diagnostic procedures, including angiography, that measure pressures and saturations to establish a cardiac diagnosis; (2) interventional procedures, in which catheters or balloon devices are used to correct cardiac defects; and (3) electrophysiologic procedures for diagnosis and treatment of dysrhythmias.
- Cardiac catheterization provides important information about oxygen saturation of blood within the chambers and great vessels, pressure changes, changes in cardiac output or stroke volume, and anatomic abnormalities.
- Several prenatal factors may increase the child's risk for CHD: maternal rubella during pregnancy, maternal alcoholism, and maternal type 1 diabetes.
- Congenital heart defects can be divided into four main groups, as determined by hemodynamic patterns: (1) defects that result in increased pulmonary blood flow, (2) obstructive defects, (3) defects that result in decreased pulmonary blood flow, and (4) mixed defects.
- Cardiac output is determined by the interaction of several factors: preload, afterload, contractility, and heart rate.
- Clinical consequences of congenital heart defects include HF and hypoxemia. A child can have both hypoxemia and HF, although usually they occur independently.
- Clinical manifestations of HF are impaired myocardial function (tachycardia, cardiomegaly), pulmonary congestion (dyspnea, tachypnea, orthopnea, cyanosis), and systemic congestion (hepatosplenomegaly, edema, distended veins).
- Nursing measures in the care of a child with HF are to assist in improving cardiac function, decrease cardiac demands, reduce respiratory distress, maintain nutritional status, promote fluid loss, and provide family support.
- Clinical manifestations of hypoxemia are cyanosis, polycythemia, clubbing, and delayed growth and development. The child is at increased risk for hypercyanotic spells, CVAs, and BE.
- Caring for the child with CHD and the family requires helping them adjust to the disorder and cope with the effects of the defect and fostering growth-promoting family relationships.
- Preoperative care of the child with a congenital defect involves introducing the child and family to the hospital and preparing them for preoperative and postoperative procedures.
- Provision of postoperative care includes observing vital signs and arterial and venous pressures, maintaining respiratory status, allowing maximum rest, providing comfort, monitoring fluids, planning for progressive activities, giving emotional support, observing for complications of surgery, and planning for discharge and home care.
- Acquired cardiovascular disorders include IE, RF, KD, systemic hypertension, hyperlipidemia, cardiomyopathy, and cardiac dysrhythmias.
- Prevention of BE in certain children with CHD involves administration of prophylactic antibiotics when specific procedures are performed.
- Acute RF is a systemic inflammatory disease that can damage the cardiac valves and is associated with previous GABHS infection. Its incidence has increased in some areas of the United States.
- KD is an extensive inflammation of small vessels and capillaries that may progress to involve the coronary arteries, causing aneurysm formation. The administration of IVIG is an important aspect of treatment.
- Education of children with hypertension and their families focuses on drug therapy, diet control, and appropriate exercise.
- Cholesterol screening in children is controversial; currently children with known risk factors for hyperlipidemia are screened and treated as needed. The influence of childhood cholesterol levels on later development of CAD is under investigation.
- Cardiomyopathy, or abnormality of the myocardium, is a serious and often fatal disorder. Heart transplantation may offer more favorable options for some children than drug therapy or other treatment regimens.
- Common dysrhythmias in children include slow rhythms (bradycardias, heart block) and fast rhythms (sinus tachycardia, SVT).
- Heart transplantation may benefit infants and children with cardiomyopathy and complex congenital heart defects resulting in severe ventricular dysfunction.

ANSWERS TO CRITICAL THINKING EXERCISES

Hypercyanotic Spell

1. **Yes.** The patient has a history of tetralogy of Fallot, which is associated with acute episodes of cyanosis and hypoxia. Hypercyanotic episodes occur suddenly and are common with crying.

2. **a.** Infants with tetralogy of Fallot may be acutely cyanotic at birth; others have mild cyanosis that progresses over the first year of life as pulmonic stenosis worsens.

b. Symptoms of diarrhea, low-grade fever, and poor oral intake can be indicative of an acute infection in a young child. However, the hypercyanotic spell requires immediate attention.

c. Acute cyanotic spells, called *blue spells* or *tet spells,* can occur suddenly when the infant's oxygen requirements exceed oxygen availability. This may occur during crying or after feeding.

3. The priorities are to immediately calm the infant, place in the knee-chest position, administer blow-by oxygen, and call for assistance.

4. **Yes.** The infant is having a hypercyanotic spell, and the first actions should be to calm the infant, place in the knee-chest position, and give supplemental oxygen. A hypercyanotic spell will likely worsen without immediate intervention, so prompt action is needed. If the nurse fails to accept the conclusions, negative implications may result, since a severe hypercyanotic spell may require intravenous medications, hydration, and resuscitative measures to stabilize the infant.

The Infant with a Tachydysrhythmia

1. **Yes.** The infant has a history of poor feeding and irritability and has an abnormally fast heart rate that is nonvariable, consistent with supraventricular tachycardia (SVT).

    a. Clinical manifestations of heart failure include irritability, tachypnea, poor feeding, and pallor.

    b. Because the infant is less than 3 months old, an accurate temperature should be taken because of the infant's increased risk for infection, which can also correlate with poor feeding and irritability. Newborns are at increased risk for meningitis and other community-acquired infections (both viral and bacterial) and has not been immunized against common organisms that could otherwise be tolerated in an older child.

    c. SVT is the most common arrhythmia in the pediatric population and is characterized by a consistent heart rate over 200 beats/min. The QRS complex is narrow, and there is no variation in the rate.

3. The nurse should immediately ensure that respiratory status is closely observed and that the infant maintains stable oxygen saturations at more than 95%. Oxygen therapy should be administered if there is any compromise in perfusion (as in this case). Blood pressure should be monitored closely. A practitioner should immediately be notified, since infants can tolerate SVT for 6 hours, but then may rapidly deteriorate. If no intravenous (IV) access is readily accessible, a bag of ice may be placed on the infant's face or on the diaper region (femoral area) for 15 to 20 seconds to stimulate the vagal-dive reflex. Continuous cardiorespiratory monitoring should be in place. The practitioner, after IV access is obtained, may order adenosine if the infant remains in SVT.

4. **Yes.** The infant is in SVT and, following basic life support protocol, airway and respiratory management are the priority. In the case of stable SVT, vagal maneuvers and adenosine are the first line in management. If those interventions are unsuccessful, electrical cardioversion may be performed, only in the presence of an experienced practitioner.

REFERENCES

Almond C, Thiagarajian RR, Piercy GE, et al: Waiting list mortality among children listed for heart transplantation in the United States, *Circulation* 119:717-727, 2009.

American Academy of Pediatrics, Pickering L, editor: *2009 Red book: report of the Committee on Infectious Diseases*, ed 28, Elk Grove Village, Ill, 2009, The Academy.

Arnold R, Ley-Zaporozhan J, Ley S, et al: Outcome after mechanical aortic valve replacement in children and young adults, *Ann Thorac Surg* 85(2):604-610, 2008.

Badesch DB, Abman SH, Ahearn GS, et al: Medical therapy for pulmonary arterial hypertension, *Chest* 126(Suppl):35S-62S, 2004.

Baker AL, Newburger JW: Kawasaki disease, *Circulation* 118:e110-e112, 2008.

Barbas KH, Kelleher DK: Breastfeeding success among infants with congenital heart disease, *Pediatr Nurs* 30:285-289, 2004.

Barst RJ, Ivy D, Dingemanse J, et al: Pharmacokinetics, safety, and efficacy of bosentan in pediatric patients with pulmonary artery hypertension, *Clin Pharmacol Ther* 73:372-382, 2003.

Barst RJ, McGoon M, Torbicki A, et al: Diagnosis and differential assessment of pulmonary artery hypertension, *JACC* 43(12, Suppl S):40S-48S, 2004.

Beekman RH: Coarctation of the aorta. In Allen HD, Driscoll DJ, Shaddy RE, et al, editors: *Moss and Adams' heart disease in infants, children, and adolescents*, ed 7, Philadelphia, 2008, Lippincott Williams & Wilkins.

Bellinger DC, Wypij D, duPlessis AJ, et al: Neurodevelopmental status at eight years in

children with dextro-transposition of the great arteries: the Boston Circulatory Arrest Trial, *J Thorac Cardiovasc Surg* 126:1385-1396, 2003.

Bitar FF, Hayek P, Obeid M, et al: Rheumatic fever in children: a 15-year experience in a developing country, *Pediatr Cardiol* 21(2):119-122, 2000.

Blume ED: Current status of heart transplantation in children: update 2003, *Pediatr Clin North Am* 50:1375-1391, 2003.

Blume ED, Naftel DC, Bastardi HJ, et al: Outcomes of children bridged to heart transplantation with ventricular assist devices: A multi-institutional study, *Circulation* 113:2313-2319, 2006.

Boucek MM, Edwards LB, Keck BM, et al: The Registry of the International Society for Heart and Lung Transplantation: seventh official pediatric report—2004, *J Heart Lung Transplant* 23:933-947, 2004.

Bruns LA, Chrisant MK, Lamour JM, et al: Carvedilol as therapy in pediatric heart failure: an initial multicenter experience, *J Pediatr* 138:505-511, 2001.

Cecchin F, Frangini PA, Brown DW, et al: Cardiac resynchronization therapy (and multisite pacing) in pediatrics and congenital heart disease: five years experience in a single institution, *J Cardiovasc Electrophysiol* 20(1):58-65, 2009.

Chun TUH, Van Hare GH: Advances in the approach to treatment of supraventricular tachycardia in the pediatric population, *Curr Cardiol Rep* 6:322-326, 2004.

Connor J, McCance K: Alterations of cardiovascular function. In Huether S,

McCance K, editors: *Understanding pathophysiology*, ed 2, St Louis, 2000, Mosby.

Cook S: Hypercholesterolemia Among Children: When Is It High, and When Is It Really High? *Circulation* 119:1075-1077, 2009.

Craig J, Smith JB, Fineman LD: Tissue perfusion. In Curley MAQ, Moloney-Harmon P, editors: *Critical care nursing of infants and children*, ed 2, Philadelphia, 2001, Saunders.

Dajani AS, Ayoub E, Bierman FZ, et al: Guidelines for the diagnosis of rheumatic fever: Jones criteria, updated 1992, *Circulation* 87:302-307, 1993.

Daniels SR, Greer FR, the Committee on Nutrition: Lipid Screening and Cardiovascular Health in Childhood, *Pediatrics* 122:198-208, 2008.

Day MD, Gauvreau K, Shulman S, et al: Characteristics of children hospitalized with infective endocarditis, *Circulation* 119(6):865-870, 2009.

de Ferranti S, Ludwig DS: Storm over statins: the controversy surrounding pharmacologic treatment of children, *N Engl J Med* 359(13):1309-1312, 2008.

Dixon J, Foster K, Wyllie J, et al: Guidelines and adenosine dosing in supraventricular tachycardia, *Arch Child Dis* 90:1190-1191, 2005.

Doyle RL, McCrory D, Channick RN, et al: Surgical treatments/interventions for pulmonary arterial hypertension: ACCP evidence-based clinical practice guidelines, *Chest* 126(Suppl):63S-72S, 2004.

Dubin AM, Janousek J, Rhee E, et al: Resynchronization therapy in pediatric and congenital heart disease patients, *JACC* 46(12):2277-2283, 2005.

Durack DT, Lukes AS, Bright DK: New criteria for diagnosis of infective endocarditis: utilization of specific echocardiographic findings, Duke Endocarditis Service, *Am J Med* 96:200-209, 1994.

Farley LM, DeMaso DR, D'Angelo E, et al: Parenting stress and parental post-traumatic stress disorder in families after pediatric heart transplantation, *J Heart Lung Transplant* 2:120-126, 2007.

Feltes TF, Cabalka AK, Meissner HC, et al: Palivizumab prophylaxis reduces hospitalization due to respiratory syncytial virus in young children with hemodynamically significant congenital heart disease, *J Pediatr* 143:532-540, 2003.

Ferrieri P: Jones Criteria Working Group: proceedings of the Jones Criteria Workshop, *Circulation* 106:2521-2523, 2002.

Ferrieri P, Gewitz MH, Gerber MA, et al: Unique features of infective endocarditis in childhood, *Circulation* 105(17):2115-2126, 2002.

Galie N, Seeger W, Naeije R, et al: Comparative analysis of clinical trials and evidence-based treatment algorithm in pulmonary arterial hypertension, *JACC* 43(Suppl):81S-88S, 2004.

Gentles T, Colan SD, Wilson NJ, et al: Left ventricular mechanics during and after acute rheumatic fever: contractile dysfunction is closely related to valve regurgitation, *JACC* 37(1):201-207, 2001.

Gerber MA, Baltimore RS, Eaton CB, et al: Prevention of rheumatic fever and diagnosis and treatment of acute streptococcal pharyngitis: a scientific statement from the American Heart Association, *Circulation* 119:1541-1551, 2009.

Geva T, Van der Velde ME: Imaging techniques: echocardiography, magnetic resonance imaging and computerized tomography. In Keane JF, Lock J, Fyler DF, editors: *Nadas' pediatric cardiology*, ed 2, Philadelphia, 2006, Saunders.

Goldmuntz E, Lin A: Genetics of Congenital Heart Defects. In Allen HD, Driscoll DJ, Shaddy RE, et al, editors: *Moss and Adams' heart disease in infants, children, and adolescents*, ed 7, Philadelphia, 2008, Lippincott Wiliams & Wilkins.

Higgins SS, Turley KM, Harr J, et al: Prescription and administration of around the clock analgesics in postoperative pediatric cardiovascular surgery patients, *Prog Cardiovasc Nurs* 14:19-24, 1999.

Hoffman JIE, Kaplan S: The incidence of congenital heart disease, *JACC* 39:1890-1900, 2002.

Hoffman TM, Wernovsky G, Atz AM, et al: Efficacy and safety of milrinone in preventing low cardiac output syndrome in infants and children after corrective surgery for congenital heart disease, *Circulation* 107:996-1002, 2003.

Holman RC, Curns AT, Belay ED, et al: Kawasaki syndrome hospitalizations in the United States, 1997 and 2000, *Pediatrics* 112(3 pt 1):495-501, 2003.

Holzer RJ, Chisolm JL, Hill SL, et al: Stenting complex aortic arch obstructions, *Catheter Cardiovasc Interv* 71(3):375-382, 2008.

Jacobs JP, Mavroudis C, Jacobs ML, et al: Lessons learned from the data analysis of the second harvest (1998-2001) of the Society of Thoracis Surgeons (STS) Congenital Heart Surgery Database, *Eur J Cardiothroac Surg* 26(1):18-37, 2004.

Kato H, Ichinose E, Kawasaki T: Myocardial infarction in Kawasaki disease: clinical analysis in 195 cases, *J Pediatr* 108(6):923-927, 1986.

Kavey RW, Allada V, Daniels SR, et al: Cardiovascular risk reduction in high-risk pediatric patients: a scientific statement from the American Heart Association Expert Panel on Population and Prevention Science; the Councils on Cardiovascular Disease in the Young, Epidemiology and Prevention, Nutrition, Physical Activity and Metabolism, High Blood Pressure Research, Cardiovascular Nursing, and the Kidney in Heart Disease; and the Interdisciplinary Working Group on Quality of Care and Outcomes Research: endorsed by the American Academy of Pediatrics, *Circulation* 114:2710-2738, 2007.

Knauth AL, Lock JE, Perry SB, et al: Transcatheter device closure of congenital and postoperative residual ventricular septal defects, *Circulation* 110(5):501-507, 2004.

Lane KB, Machado RD, Pauciulo MW, et al: Heterozygous germline mutations in BMPR2 encoding a TGF-beta receptor, causing familial primary pulmonary hypertension: the International PPH Consortium, *Nat Genet* 26:81-84, 2000.

LeRoy SS: Clinical dysrhythmias after surgical repair of congenital heart disease, *AACN Clin Issues* 12:87-99, 2001.

LeRoy S, Elixson EM, O'Brien P, et al: Recommendations for preparing children and adolescents for invasive cardiac procedures: AHA scientific statement, *Circulation* 108:2550-2564, 2003.

Limperopoulos C, Majnemer A, Shevell MI, et al: Predictors of developmental disabilities after open heart surgery in young children with congenital heart defects, *J Pediatr* 141:51-58, 2002.

Lipshultz SE, Sleeper LA, Towbin JA, et al: The incidence of pediatric cardiomyopathy in two regions of the United States, *N Engl J Med* 348:1647-1655, 2003.

Lock JE: Cardiac catheterization. In Keane JF, Lock J, Fyler DF, editors: *Nadas' pediatric cardiology*, ed 2, Philadelphia, 2006, Saunders.

Macfadyen AJ, Buckmaster MA: Pain management in the PICU, *Crit Care Clin* 15:185-200, 1999.

Majnemer A, Limperopoulos C: Developmental progress of children with congenital heart defects requiring open heart surgery, *Semin Pediatr Neurol* 6:12-19, 1999.

Margossian R: Contemporary management of pediatric heart failure, *Expert Rev Cardiovasc Ther* 6(2):187-197, 2008.

McCrindle VW, Urbina EM, Dennison BA, et al: Drug therapy of high-risk lipid abnormalities in children and adolescents: a scientific statement from the American Heart Association Atherosclerosis, Hypertension, and Obesity in Young Committee, Council of Cardiovascular Disease in the Young, with the Council of Cardiovascular Nursing, *Circulation* 115:1948, 2007.

McGoon M, Gutterman D, Steen V, et al: Screening, early detection, and diagnosis of pulmonary arterial hypertension: ACCP evidence-based clinical practice guidelines, *Chest* 126(Suppl):14S-34S, 2004.

Menasche CC, duPlessis AJ, Wessel DL, et al: Current incidence of acute neurological complications after open heart operations in children, *Ann Thorac Surg* 73:1752-1758, 2002.

Michelakis ED, Wilkins MR, Rabinovitch M: Emerging concepts and translational priorities in pulmonary arterial hypertension, *Circulation* 118:1486-1495, 2008.

Moffett BS, Chang AC: Future pharmacologic agents for treatment of heart failure in children, *Pediatr Cardiol* 27:533-551, 2006.

Morelius E, Lundh U, Nelson N: Parental stress in relation to the severity of congenital heart disease in the offspring, *Pediatr Nurs* 28:28-34, 2002.

Narula J, Chandrasekhar Y, Rahimtoola S, et al: Diagnosis of acute rheumatic carditis, *Circulation* 100:1576-1581, 1999.

National High Blood Pressure Education Program Working Group on High Blood Pressure in Children and Adolescents: The fourth report on the diagnosis, evaluation, and treatment of high blood pressure in children and adolescents, *Pediatrics* 114(2):555-576, 2004.

Newburger JW, Takahashi M, Gerber MA, et al: Diagnosis, treatment, and long-term management of Kawasaki disease: a statement for health professionals from the Committee on Rheumatic Fever, Endocarditis, and Kawasaki Disease, Council on Cardiovascular Disease in the Young, American Heart Association, *Circulation* 110(17):2747-2771, 2004.

Park MK: *Pediatric cardiology handbook*, ed 5, Philadelphia, 2008, Mosby.

Phillips BG, Somers VK: *Drug information handbook for cardiology 2000-2001*, Cleveland, 2000, Lexi-Comp.

Porter CJ, Edwards WD: Atrial septal defects. In Allen HD, Driscoll DJ, Shaddy RE, et al, editors: *Moss and Adams' heart disease in infants, children, and adolescents*, ed 7, Philadelphia, 2008, Lippincott Wiliams & Wilkins.

Prakash A, Powell AJ, Krishnamurthy R, et al: Magnetic resonance imaging evaluation of myocardial perfusion and viability in congenital and acquired pediatric heart disease, *Am J Cardiol* 93:657, 2004.

Rome JJ, Kreutzer J: Pediatric interventional catheterization: reasonable expectations and outcomes, *Pediatr Clin North Am* 51:1589-1610, 2004.

Rosenthal D, Chrisant MR, Edens E, et al: International Society for Heart and Lung Transplantation: practice guidelines for management of heart failure in children, *J Heart Lung Transplant* 23:1313-1333, 2004.

Schlente EA, Boramanand N, Funk MF: Supraventricular tachycardia in the pediatric primary care setting: age-related presentation, diagnosis, and management, *J Pediatr Healthcare* 22(5):289-299, 2008.

Schneider DJ, Moore JW: Aortic stenosis. In Allen HD, Driscoll DJ, Shaddy RE, et al, editors: *Moss and Adams' heart disease in infants, children, and adolescents*, ed 7, Philadelphia, 2008, Lippincott Williams & Wilkins.

Scientific Registry of Transplant Recipients: 2007 Annual Report of the US Organ Procurement and Transplantation Network and the Scientific Registry of the Transplant Recipients: transplant data 1998-2006, US Department of Health and Human Services, Health Resources and Services Administration, Healthcare Systems Bureau, Division of Transplantation, 2007, Rockville, Md.

Shillingford AJ, Glanzman MM, Ittenbach RF, et al: Inattention, hyperactivity, and school performance in a population of school-age children with complex congenital heart disease, *Pediatrics* 121:e759-e767, 2008.

Simonneau G, Galie N, Rubin LJ, et al: Clinical classification of pulmonary hypertension, *JACC* 43(12 Suppl S):5S-12S, 2004.

Smallhorn JF: Intraoperative transesophageal echocardiography in congenital heart disease, *Echocardiography* 119:709-723, 2002.

Smith PA: Primary care in children with congenital heart disease, *J Pediatr Nurs* 16:308-319, 2001.

Spirito P, Autore C, Rapezzi C, et al: Syncope and risk of sudden death in hypertrophic cardiomyopathy, *Circulation* 1109:1703-1710, 2009.

Taketomo C, Hodding J, Kraus D: *Pediatric dosage handbook*, ed 16, Hudson, Ohio, 2009, Lexi-Comp.

Taubert KA, Gewitz M: Infective endocarditis. In Allen HD, Driscoll DJ, Shaddy RE, et al, editors: *Moss and Adams' heart disease in infants, children, and adolescents*, ed 7, Philadelphia, 2008, Lippincott Williams & Wilkins.

Tweddell JS, Hoffman GM, Ghanayem NS, et al: Hypoplastic left heart syndrome. In Allen HD, Driscoll DJ, Shaddy RE, et al, editors: *Moss and Adams' hearth disease in infants, children, and adolescents*, ed 7, Philadelphia, 2008, Lippincott Williams & Wilkins.

United Network for Organ Sharing: *UNOS scientific registry annual report*, Richmond, Va, 2001, The Network.

Uzark K, Jones K: Parenting stress and children with heart disease, *J Pediatr Health Care* 17:163-168, 2003.

Wilson W, Taubert KA, Gewitz M, et al: Prevention of infective endocarditis: guidelines from the American Heart Association, *Circulation* 116(15):1736-1754, 2007.

Wood J: Anatomical assessment of congenital heart disease, *J Cardovasc Magnetic Resonance* 8:595-606, 2006.

World Health Organization: *Rheumatic fever and rheumatic heart disease: report of a WHO Expert Consultation*, Tech Rep Series no 923, Geneva, 2004, The Organization.

Wypij D, Newberger JW, Rappaport LA, et al: The effect of duration of deep hypothermic circulatory arrest in infant heart surgery on late neurodevelopment: the Boston Circulatory Arrest Trial, *J Thorac Cardiovasc Surg* 126:1397-1403, 2003.

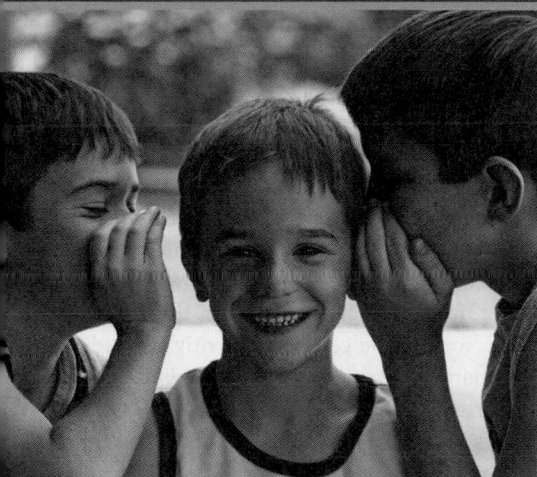

The Child with Hematologic or Immunologic Dysfunction

Rosalind Bryant

evolve WEBSITE

Animations
  Hemophilia A
  Platelets and Blood Clotting
  Sickle Cell Anemia
Case Study
  Sickle Cell Anemia
Critical Thinking Case Studies
  Idiopathic Thrombocytopenic Purpura
  Iron Deficiency Anemia
Critical Thinking Exercises
  Bleeding
  HIV Testing in Children
Key Points Audio Summaries
NCLEX Review Questions
Nursing Care Plans
  The Child with Anemia
  The Child with Sickle Cell Disease
Spanish/English Translations
WebLinks

RELATED TOPICS

CHAPTER OUTLINE

THE HEMATOLOGIC SYSTEM AND ITS FUNCTION

ORIGIN OF FORMED ELEMENTS

Blood is composed of a fluid portion called plasma and a cellular portion known as the formed elements of the blood. The two components are approximately equal in volume. Plasma is about 90% water and 10% solutes. The principal solutes are albumin, electrolytes, and proteins. Among the proteins are clotting factors, globulins, circulating antibodies, and fibrinogen. The cellular elements sequentially develop into mature red blood cells (RBCs, erythrocytes), white blood cells (WBCs, leukocytes), and platelets (thrombocytes) (Fig. 35-1).

The major hematopoietic (blood-forming) organs of the body are the red bone marrow (myeloid tissue) and the lymphatic system, which consists of lymph (fluid), lymphatic vessels, and lymphoid structures (the lymph nodes, spleen, thymus, and tonsils). Although the lymphatic system plays an important role in regulating blood cells, the lymph vessels and fluids do not produce cells. The lymph nodes regulate the manufacture of WBCs. The spleen and liver are the primary organs for hematopoiesis in the young fetus and for cell removal in postnatal life. Macrophages (formerly called *reticular cells*) are cells of mesodermal origin that are widely dispersed in the lining of the vascular and lymph channels. Macrophages form a network and are capable of phagocytosis (ingestion and digestion of foreign substances); formation of immune bodies; and differentiation into other cells, such as hemocytoblasts, myeloblasts, and lymphoblasts.

All of the formed elements of the blood, except to some extent the agranulocytes, are produced in myeloid tissue during postnatal life. During embryonic development the mesenchyme, spleen, liver, thymus, and yolk sac serve as additional sites of blood cell formation. In individuals with certain blood disorders these sites, particularly the spleen, can be stimulated to produce blood cells and constitute extramedullary hematopoiesis. In infants and young children all of the bone contains red marrow (so-called because of its color from the formation of erythrocytes), but as bone growth ceases near the end of adolescence, only the ribs, sternum, vertebrae, and pelvis continue to produce blood cells. The remainder of the bone marrow becomes yellow from deposition of fat. However, in conditions of increased demand for blood cells, the yellow marrow can revert to red marrow and become another hematopoietic source.

Although the progressive development of each blood cell is fairly well delineated, there is considerable controversy regarding the origin of the blood cell. One of the most widely held theories (monophyletic theory) is that each blood cell originates from a primordial (primitive) cell called a blast, or totipotential stem cell, which has the ability to self-replicate and transform into all the blood components.

The second-generation stem cell, called the pluripotent stem cell, is committed to produce erythroblast, myeloblast, monoblast, lymphoblast, or megakaryoblast (see Fig. 35-1). The blast cells sequentially develop into mature RBCs (erythrocytes), WBCs (leukocytes), platelets (thrombocytes), and other cells (such as mast cells and macrophages) (see Fig. 35-1).

Red Blood Cells (Erythrocytes)

The erythrocyte is formed from the hemocytoblast in the red bone marrow. As illustrated in Fig. 35-1, the pluripotential stem cell forms the proerythroblast. The initial cell of this series has a deep blue–staining (basophilic) cytoplasm and therefore is called a basophilic erythroblast. The chief change in the erythroblast is accumulation of hemoglobin in the cytoplasm. As the basophilic material decreases and the amount of hemoglobin increases, the cell comes to be called a polychromatic erythroblast, which describes its mixture of staining properties. At the same time that the nucleus decreases in size, the basophilic material disappears, so that the cell is uniformly stained by eosin dye—hence the name *orthochromatic erythroblast,* or *normoblast.* Finally, the normoblast completely loses its nucleus by a process of extrusion as it squeezes through the pores of the membrane into the capillary. Because of the loss of its nucleus, the cell caves in on both sides, which gives the mature erythrocyte its characteristic appearance as a biconcave disk. During each of these stages the different cells continue to undergo mitosis so that increasingly greater numbers of cells are produced. Because the mature RBC does not have a nucleus, it is unable to multiply.

The reticulocyte is the last stage of development before the mature erythrocyte. Reticulocytes are slightly larger than erythrocytes, and their presence indicates active RBC production (erythropoiesis). Ordinarily the total proportion of circulating reticulocytes is between 0.5% and 1.5%. The reticulocyte, or "retic," count is a simple laboratory test frequently used to indirectly analyze hematopoiesis.

Regulation of Erythrocyte Production

The usual life span of the mature erythrocyte is 120 days. Apparently, as RBCs grow old, their membranes become fragile and eventually rupture. The contents of the cell fragment as they circulate through the blood vessels and are phagocytized by the macrophages in the spleen, liver, and bone marrow. The hemoglobin is broken down into the iron-containing pigment hemosiderin and the bile pigments biliverdin and bilirubin. Most of the iron is reused by the bone marrow for production of new RBCs or stored in the liver and other tissues for future use. The bile pigments are excreted by the liver in bile.

Normally there is a homeostatic balance between RBC production and destruction. This balance ensures adequate tissue oxygenation and a blood viscosity that allows the blood to flow freely through the vessels. The basic regulator of erythrocyte production is tissue oxygenation and renal production of erythropoietin (also called erythropoietic stimulating factor). In states of tissue hypoxia, the kidney releases erythropoietin into the bloodstream. As a result the bone marrow is stimulated to produce new RBCs. The major activity seems to be an increase in both maturation rate and mitosis at all stages of erythrocyte production, but primarily at the stem cell level.

During this rapid increase in RBC production, the circulating erythrocytes may not be totally mature. Consequently the number of reticulocytes may increase dramatically (as high as 30% or more of the total RBC count). Even normoblasts or nucleated RBCs may appear in the blood. A failure of this rise in erythrocyte and reticulocyte count to occur may indicate bone marrow failure.

PATHOPHYSIOLOGY REVIEW

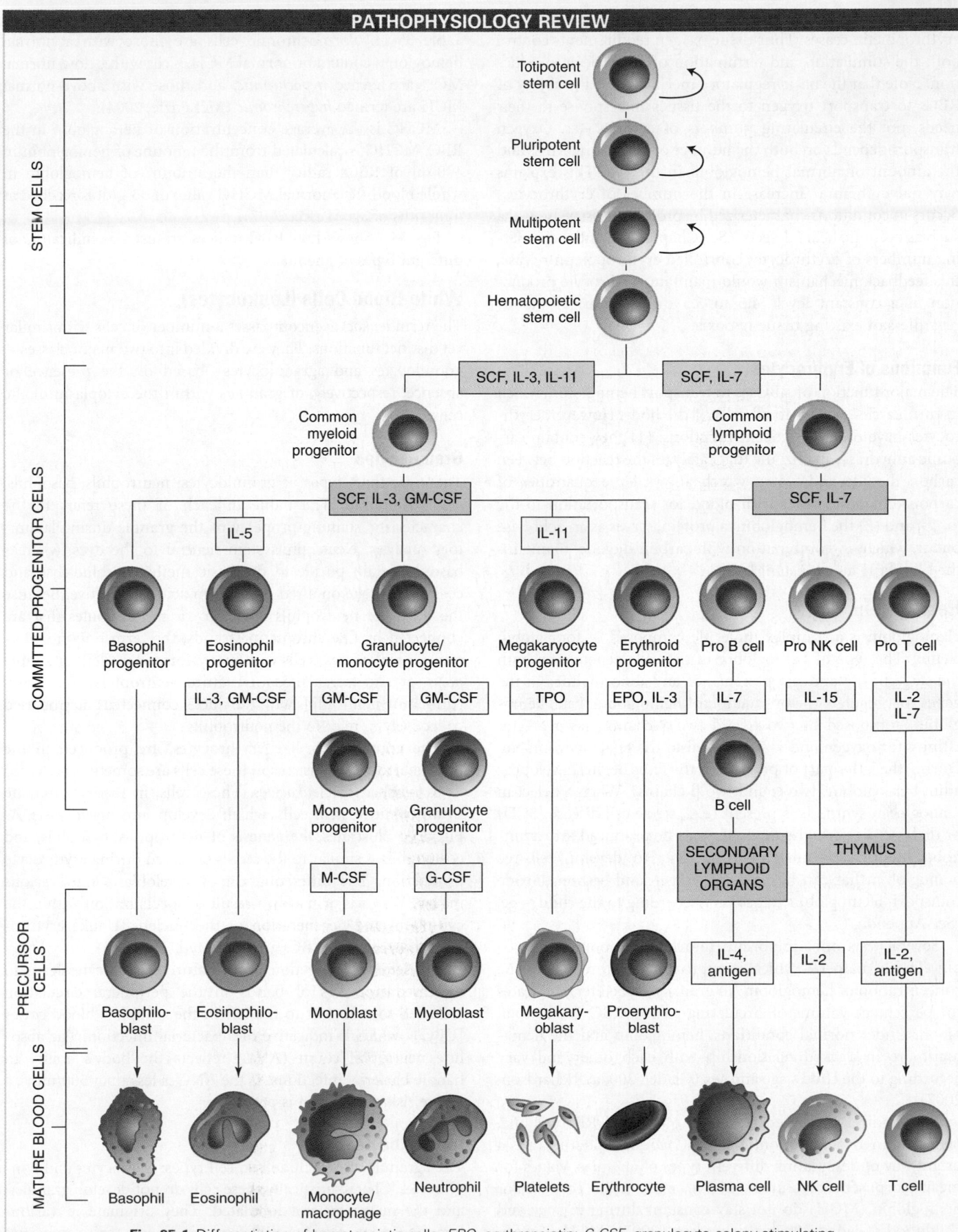

Fig. 35-1 Differentiation of hematopoietic cells. *EPO*, erythropoietin; *G-CSF*, granulocyte colony-stimulating factor; *GM-CSF*, granulocyte-macrophage colony-stimulating factor; *IL*, interleukin; *M-CSF*, macrophage colony-stimulating factor; *NK*, natural killer; *SCF*, stem cell factor; *TPO*, thrombopoietin. (From McCance KL, Huether SE: *Pathophysiology: the biological basis for disease in adults and children*, ed 6, St Louis, 2010, Mosby.)

Once tissue oxygenation is adequate, the production of erythropoietin ceases. Thus tissue oxygen requirements control both the stimulation and termination of erythrocyte production. Note that the basic regulatory mechanism is the ability of RBCs to transport oxygen to the tissues in response to their needs, not the circulating numbers of erythrocytes. Oxygen transport depends on both the number of circulating RBCs and the amount of normal hemoglobin in the cell. This explains why polycythemia (increase in the number of erythrocytes) occurs in conditions characterized by prolonged tissue hypoxia, such as cyanotic heart defects. (See Chapter 34.) If the circulating numbers of erythrocytes controlled erythropoietin release, this feedback mechanism would maintain erythrocyte production at a constant level (4.5 to 5.5 million/mm^3 of blood) regardless of existing tissue hypoxia.

Functions of Erythrocytes

The major function of RBCs is to transport hemoglobin, which in turn carries oxygen to all cells of the body. However, erythrocytes have other significant functions: (1) they contain carbonic anhydrase, an enzyme that catalyzes the reaction between carbon dioxide and water, which allows large quantities of carbon dioxide to react with blood for transportation to the lungs; and (2) the hemoglobin, a protein, serves as an acid-base buffer, which, in combination with carbon dioxide, maintains the blood pH at a constant level.

Hemoglobin

Hemoglobin is a complex molecule composed of four globin chains. The type of hemoglobin in the cells depends on both the stage of life and the presence of any abnormalities in the genes that regulate the production of hemoglobin. Fetal hemoglobin, composed of two α and two γ chains, has a greater affinity for oxygen and is best suited to the fetal environment. During the latter part of pregnancy, the fetus begins developing adult hemoglobin (two α and two β chains). When a defect in hemoglobin synthesis is present (e.g., sickle cell disease [SCD] or thalassemia), fetal hemoglobin may be produced into adulthood. Research is currently underway to develop cell-free hemoglobin that can be used for oxygen and carbon dioxide transport. Hemoglobin values vary according to the child's age. (See Appendix C.)

Several tests offer important information about hemoglobin. The hematocrit, which is approximately three times the concentration of hemoglobin (in grams per deciliter), indicates the percentage volume of circulating packed RBCs in the total blood. Under normal conditions, hemoglobin and the hematocrit are in a fixed relationship with each other and vary according to the child's age and sex (Glader, 2007a; Richardson, 2007).

RBC indices are based on ratios of packed RBC volume, hemoglobin concentration, and RBC count, and they are a useful way of designating different types of anemias. Values for mean corpuscular volume (MCV) and mean corpuscular hemoglobin (MCH) do not stay constant during infancy and childhood (Glader, 2007b; Richardson, 2007). MCH concentration (MCHC) values, however, are more constant.

MCV is the average (mean) volume or size of a single RBC. The normal range for RBCs is given in Table 35-1.

MCH is the average weight of hemoglobin in each RBC (see Table 35-1). Normochromic cells are those with a normal hemoglobin content or normal MCH. Cells with below-normal MCH are termed *hypochromic,* and those with above-normal MCH are termed *hyperchromic* (McKenzie, 2004).

MCHC is the average concentration of hemoglobin in the RBC. MCHC is calculated from the amount of hemoglobin in 100 ml of RBCs rather than the amount of hemoglobin in whole blood. The normal MCHC value of 33 g/dl is reached at 6 months of age (Pesce, 2007).

Fig. 35-2 shows how RBC indices are used as indicators of different types of anemia.

White Blood Cells (Leukocytes)

The term *leukocyte* encompasses a number of cells with similar yet distinct functions. They are divided into two major classes—granulocytes and agranulocytes—based on the presence or absence, respectively, of granules within the cytoplasm of the cells.

Granulocytes

There are three types of granulocytes: neutrophils, basophils, and eosinophils. The name of each of these refers to the characteristic staining property of the granule during laboratory analysis. Neutrophils stain neutral to the dyes, whereas basophils stain purple to the basic methylene blue dye, and eosinophils take on a red color from acidic eosin dye. Because the nuclei of neutrophils have two or more lobules that are connected by fine chromatin strands, the term polymorphonuclear leukocytes (cells with many-formed nuclei), or simply *polys,* or *segs* (segmented or mature neutrophils) and *bands* (immature neutrophils with the nuclei connected) may be used collectively to refer to the neutrophils.

The granulocytes, like erythrocytes, are produced in the bone marrow. For this reason these cells are sometimes referred to as *myelogenous leukocytes.* These cells, in theory, originate from primitive stem cells, which develop into myeloblasts. As Fig. 35-1 illustrates, the genesis of neutrophils, basophils, and eosinophils is similar to the stages observed during erythrocyte production. The differentiation of myeloblasts into various mature WBCs is primarily a result of specialization within the cytoplasm and degeneration of the nucleus. Unlike erythrocytes, however, all WBCs are nucleated.

Accelerated production of immature granulocytes leads to increased numbers of bands in the peripheral circulation (referred to as a shift to the left in the complete blood count [CBC]), which is indicative of a bacterial infection. The absolute neutrophil count (ANC) reflects the body's ability to handle bacterial infections. If the ANC is less than 500/mm^3, a severe risk of infection is present.

Agranulocytes

The agranulocytes include two cell types: monocytes and lymphocytes. Characteristically these cells do not develop granules, and the nuclei are not lobulated. They originate in various lymphogenous organs, and for this reason are sometimes referred to as lymphogenous leukocytes. However, because stem cells and reticular cells are capable of differentiating into monocytes or lymphocytes, the origin of these cells is frequently

TABLE 35-1   TESTS PERFORMED AS PART OF A COMPLETE BLOOD COUNT

TEST (AVERAGE VALUE)*	DESCRIPTION, COMMENTS
Red blood cell (RBC) count (4.5-5.5 million/mm³)	Number of RBCs/mm³ of blood
	Indirectly estimates Hgb content of blood
	Reflects function of bone marrow
Hemoglobin (Hgb) determination (11.5-15.5 g/dl)	Amount of Hgb (g)/dl of whole blood
	Total blood Hgb primarily depends on number of circulating RBCs but also on amount of Hgb in each cell
Hematocrit (Hct) (35%-45%)	Percent volume of packed RBCs in whole blood
	Indirectly measures Hgb content
	Is approximately three times Hgb content
RBC indices	
Mean corpuscular volume (MCV) (77-95 fl)	Average or mean volume (size) of a single RBC
	MCV values are expressed as femtoliters (fl) or cubic microns (mm³)
Mean corpuscular hemoglobin (MCH) (25-33 pg/cell)	Average or mean quantity (weight) of Hgb in a single RBC
	MCH values are expressed as picograms (pg) or micromicrograms (mmcg)
Mean corpuscular hemoglobin concentration (MCHC) (31%-37% Hgb [g]/dl RBC)	Average concentration of Hgb in a single RBC
	MCHC values are expressed as percent Hgb (g)/cell or Hgb (g)/dl RBC
	MCV and MCH depend on accurate counts of RBCs, whereas MCHC does not; therefore, MCHC is often more reliable
	All indices depend on average cell measurements and do not show individual RBC variations (anisocytosis)
RBC volume distribution width (RDW) (13.4% ± 1.2%)	Average size of RBCs
	Differentiates some types of anemia
Reticulocyte count (0.5%-1.5% erythrocytes)	Percent reticulocytes in RBCs
	Index of production of mature RBCs by bone marrow
	Decreased count indicates depressed bone marrow function
	Increased count indicates erythrogenesis in response to some stimulus
	When reticulocyte count is extremely high, other forms of immature RBCs (normoblasts, even erythroblasts) may be present
	Indirectly estimates hypochromic anemia
	Usually elevated in patients with chronic hemolytic anemia
White blood cell (WBC) count (4.5-13.5 × 10³ cells/mm³)	Number of WBCs/mm³ of blood
	Total number of WBCs less important than differential count
Differential WBC count	Inspection and quantification of WBC types present in peripheral blood
	Values are expressed as percentages; to obtain absolute number of any type of WBC, multiply its respective percentage by total number of WBCs
Neutrophils (polys) (54%-62%) (3-5.8 × 10³ cells/mm³)	Primary defense in bacterial infection; capable of phagocytizing and killing bacteria
Bands (3%-5%) (0.15-0.4 × 10³ cells/mm³)	Immature neutrophil
	Increased numbers in bacterial infection
	Also capable of phagocytosis and killing
Eosinophils (1%-3%) (0.05-0.25 × 10³ cells/mm³)	Named for their staining characteristics with eosin dye
	Increased in allergic disorders, parasitic diseases, certain neoplasms, and other diseases
Basophils (0.075%) (0.015-0.030 × 10³ cells/mm³)	Named for their characteristic basophilic stippling
	Contain histamine, heparin, and serotonin; believed to cause increased blood flow to injured tissues while preventing excessive clotting
Lymphocytes (25%-33%) (1.5-3.0 × 10³ cells/mm³)	Involved in development of antibody and delayed hypersensitivity
Monocytes (3%-7%)	Large phagocytic cells that are involved in early stage of inflammatory reaction
Absolute neutrophil count (ANC) (>1000/mm³)	Percent neutrophils/bands times WBC count
	Indicates body's capability to handle bacterial infections
Platelet count (150-400 × 10³/mm³)	Number of platelets/mm³ of blood
	Cellular fragments that are necessary for clotting to occur
Stained peripheral blood smear	Visual estimation of amount of Hgb in RBCs and overall size, shape, and structure of RBCs
	Various staining properties of RBC structures may be evidence of immature forms of erythrocytes
	Shows variation in size and shape of RBCs: microcytic, macrocytic, poikilocytic (variable shapes)

*See Appendix C for normal values according to ages.

designated as the *lymphomyeloid complex,* which includes bone marrow, lymph nodes, spleen, liver, thymus, subepithelial lymphoid tissue (tonsils, vermiform appendix, and intestinal lymphoid tissues), and connective tissues (mesenchymal cells of the reticuloendothelial system).

The monocytes follow the same sequence of development from the stem cell as the granulocytes (see Fig. 35-1). The monocytes in turn have the ability to exit the vessels and develop into macrophages, large cells that are highly effective phagocytes. Kupffer cells are macrophages located in the liver.

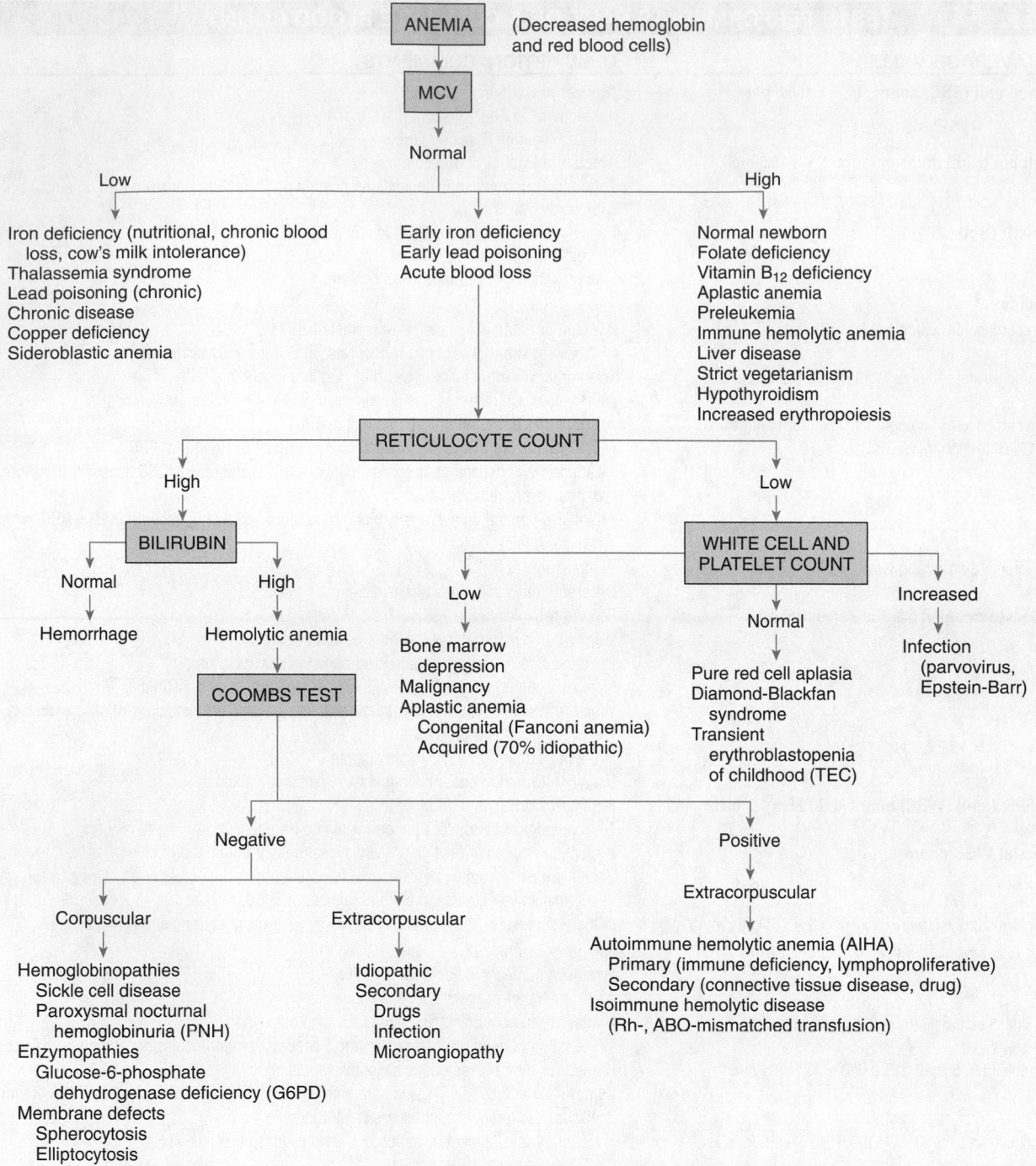

Fig. 35-2 Approach to the diagnosis of anemia by mean corpuscular volume *(MCV)* and reticulocyte count. (Modified from Lanzkowsky P: *Manual of pediatric hematology and oncology,* New York, 2005, Churchill Livingstone; Glader B: The anemias. In Kliegman RM, Jenson HB, Behrman RE, et al, editors: *Nelson textbook of pediatrics,* ed 18, Philadelphia, 2007, Saunders; and McKenzie SB: Introduction to anemia. In McKenzie SB, editor: *Clinical laboratory hematology,* Upper Saddle River, NJ, 2004, Pearson, Prentice Hall.)

Histiocytes are macrophages in the connective tissue. These names are remnants of the old reticular endothelial system designations.

Lymphocytopoiesis (lymphocyte formation) takes place anywhere in the lymphomyeloid complex. Lymphocytes develop from blast (stem) cells (see Fig. 35-1). The lymphocyte has the potential to develop into other cells, such as T cells or B cells (see p. 1410).

Regulation of Leukocyte Production

The exact life span of the leukocytes is not as clearly defined as that of the erythrocytes, since they exist in the circulation primarily for transport to extravascular areas, where they reside in reservoirs or where they are needed to resist infection. Therefore their survival rate is described in terms of three phases: (1) the hematopoietic phase, extending from the development of the blast cell to the delivery of the mature leukocyte into the circulation; (2) the intravascular phase, the period within the circulation; and (3) the extravascular phase, the time spent in the viscera or tissues.

Granulocytes have a half-life of 6 to 8 hours in the blood and, after entering the tissues, die over a period of 4 to 5 days. Agranulocytes live for an extended period because they remain in inflamed tissue areas longer than the granulocytes. Monocytes wander back and forth between the blood and tissues and are capable of becoming macrophages; their half-life in the blood is 8 to 10 hours, but their half-life in the tissue is 60 to 90 days.

The regulation of leukocytes is based on the body's need for them. Tissue damage from bacterial or viral agents promotes leukocyte circulation and production. However, **leukocytosis** (increase in leukocytes) results from tissue destruction from almost any source, such as hemorrhage, neoplastic disease, toxicity, operative procedures, chemical and thermal injury, and tissue ischemia.

The leukocytes probably die as a result of their activity at the site of injury and are phagocytized by other newly formed WBCs. Effective control of the inflammatory process with subsequent tissue recovery most likely results in feedback to the bone marrow and causes lymphogenous organs to cease increased production of WBCs.

Functions of Leukocytes

Although all of the leukocytes play some role in the immune process, each of the WBCs has a specific role. Neutrophils and monocytes are effective phagocytes and as a result are primarily involved in inflammatory reactions. **Neutrophilia** (increased numbers of neutrophils) is most evident in an acute inflammation, whereas **monocytosis** (increased numbers of monocytes) is more evident in chronic conditions. The reason is that, as the affected area becomes acidic from tissue necrosis, neutrophils, which prefer a neutral environment, become less efficient, and monocytes, which become macrophages, become more powerful. These cells also increase in number during chronic inflammation. The other functions of lymphocytes in terms of the immune process are discussed on p. 1451.

The function of eosinophils is still not completely known. They seem to have parasiticidal properties because they can selectively destroy parasites. They may also function in the immediate type of allergic or anaphylactic hypersensitivity reaction, since **eosinophilia** (increased numbers of eosinophils) is well documented in such conditions. Eosinophils also are thought to release a substance called profibrinolysin, which, when activated to form fibrinolysin, digests fibrin and thereby helps dissolve a clot.

The function of basophils is also not completely understood, although **basophilia** (increased numbers of basophils) occurs during the healing phase of inflammation and during prolonged inflammation. Basophils in the blood exit the vessels and become mast cells in the tissue. They are responsible for histamine release, which results in increased permeability of the vessels to allow WBCs to exit the vessels at the site of injury.

Platelets

Platelets are actually small fragments of megakaryocytes. They are smaller than blood cells, do not possess a cellular structure, and consist of a clear substance containing granules. Platelets originate from part of the myelogenous group of WBCs (see Fig. 35-1). Platelets are formed when the megakaryocytic membrane invaginates, fuses within the cell to separate the cytoplasm, and then fragments.

Regulation of Platelet Production

The life span of platelets is estimated as 8 to 10 days. Apparently the body regulates platelet levels to maintain a fairly constant level (between 150,000 and 400,000/mm^3). Platelet production is probably regulated by a hormone, thrombopoietin, but the source and mode of action of this substance are unknown. Old platelets are most likely removed by the liver and spleen.

Function of Platelets

The term **thrombocyte** means "clot" (*thrombo*) and "cell" (*cyte*) and accurately describes the main function of platelets. When there is a break in the continuity of a blood vessel, the platelets, which are normally flat and round or oval, come in contact with the wet vessel surface and dramatically change their shape to become swollen spheres with long, irregular projections called pseudopodia (false feet). As a result, the platelets begin to adhere to the wet endothelium and to each other. The first platelets at the site of injury release substances that attract other thrombocytes to the area. This causes a layering of platelets, which eventually forms a plug. This plug is large enough to partially or totally occlude the opening in the vessel wall but small enough to allow blood flow to continue unimpaired through the vessel.

In small vessel tears the platelet plug is sufficient to produce hemostasis, and additional blood coagulation is not necessary. When platelet counts are low, however, these numerous small ruptures, which occur continually in the body as a result of general functioning, are not repaired. Consequently, small hemorrhagic areas called **petechiae** form under the skin. They are similar in appearance to reddish freckles or tiny spider webs.

Platelets also influence hemostasis by releasing a substance called serotonin at the site of injury. Serotonin is a vasoconstrictor that produces vascular spasm to decrease the blood flow to the injured area.

ASSESSMENT OF HEMATOLOGIC FUNCTION

Several tests assess hematologic function, and additional procedures can identify the cause of the dysfunction. The following discussion is limited to a description of the most common and one of the most valuable tests, the CBC. Other procedures, such as those related to iron, coagulation, and immune status, are discussed throughout the chapter as appropriate.

The CBC consists of the following determinations: RBC count, WBC count, hematocrit, hemoglobin level, differential WBC count, RBC indices (MCV, MCH, and MCHC), and peripheral smear. Additional tests may be included, such as the reticulocyte count, RBC volume distribution width, and platelet count. Table 35-1 describes each of these. Most of the determinations can be performed on a small quantity of blood (micromethod), and values are computed automatically. The nurse should be familiar with the significance of the findings from the CBC (see Table 35-1) and should be aware of the normal values for age. (See Appendix C.)

The history and physical examination are essential to the identification of hematologic dysfunction, and the nurse is often the first person to suspect a problem based on information from these sources. Comments by the parent regarding the child's lack of energy, food diary showing decreased sources of iron, frequent infections, and bleeding that is difficult to control offer clues to the more common disorders affecting the blood. A careful physical appraisal can reveal findings such as persistent fatigue, pallor, petechiae, or bruising that may indicate minor or serious hematologic conditions. Nurses need to be aware of the clinical manifestations of blood diseases to assist in recognizing symptoms and establishing a diagnosis.

RED BLOOD CELL DISORDERS

ANEMIA

Anemia is a reduction in RBCs mass and/or hemoglobin concentration compared with normal values for age (Brugnara, Oski, and Nathan, 2009; Glader, 2007a). The anemias are the most common hematologic disorders of infancy and childhood and are not diseases but manifestations of underlying pathologic processes (see Fig. 35-2).

Classification

The anemias can be classified using two basic approaches: (1) etiology as manifested by erythrocyte or hemoglobin depletion; and (2) morphology, the characteristic changes in RBC size, shape, and color (Box 35-1).

Although the morphologic classification is useful in the laboratory evaluation of anemia, the etiology provides direction for planning nursing care. For example, anemia with reduced hemoglobin concentration may be caused by a dietary depletion of iron, and the principal intervention is replenishing iron stores.

The main causes of anemia are (1) inadequate production of RBCs or RBC components, (2) increased destruction of RBCs, and (3) excessive loss of RBCs through hemorrhage. Each of these factors affects the amount of hemoglobin that is available to carry oxygen to the cells (see Box 35-1). Therefore the classification is based on the various conditions that can result from any of these physiologic changes.

Pathophysiology and Clinical Manifestations

The basic physiologic defect caused by anemia is a decrease in the oxygen-carrying capacity of blood and consequently a reduction in the amount of oxygen available to the cells. When the anemia has developed slowly, the child usually adapts to the declining hemoglobin level. Most children seem to have a remarkable ability to function well despite low levels of hemoglobin. Also, compensatory mechanisms such as a shift in the oxyhemoglobin dissociation curve may delay the development of any obvious signs (see p. 1193).

When the hemoglobin level falls sufficiently to produce clinical manifestations, the signs and symptoms (e.g., weakness, fatigue, and a waxy pallor in severe anemia) are due to tissue hypoxia (Box 35-2). Cyanosis, which results from an increased quantity of deoxygenated hemoglobin in arterial blood, is typi-

cally not evident. Anemia is caused by decreased levels of hemoglobin or RBCs, not inadequate oxygen saturation of existing hemoglobin.

Central nervous system manifestations include headache, dizziness, lightheadedness, irritability, slowed thought processes, decreased attention span, apathy, and depression. Growth retardation resulting from decreased cellular metabolism, and coexisting anorexia is a common finding in chronic severe anemia. It is frequently accompanied by delayed sexual maturation in the older child.

The effects of anemia on the circulatory system can be profound. A reduction in hemoglobin concentration that results in decreased oxygen-carrying capacity of the blood is associated with a compensatory increase in heart rate and cardiac output (see Box 35-2). Initially this greater cardiac output compensates

---

BOX 35-1   RED BLOOD CELL MORPHOLOGY

Size (Cell Size)
Variation in red blood cell (RBC) sizes (anisocytosis)
- Normocytes (normal cell size)
- Microcytes (smaller than normal cell size)
- Macrocytes (larger than normal cell size)

Shape (Cell Shape)
Variation in RBC shapes (poikilocytosis)
- Spherocytes (globular cells)
- Drepanocytes (sickle-shaped cells)
- Numerous other irregularly shaped cells

Color (Staining Characteristics)
Variation in hemoglobin concentration in the RBC
- Normochromic (sufficient or normal amount of hemoglobin per RBC)
- Hypochromic (reduced amount of hemoglobin per RBC)
- Hyperchromic (increased amount of hemoglobin per RBC)

BOX 35-2   SIGNS AND SYMPTOMS OF ANEMIA

Decreased Red Blood Cell Production
Pallor
Tachycardia
Fatigue, headache
Muscle weakness
Systolic heart murmur
Frontal bossing

Increased Red Blood Cell Destruction
Icteric sclera, jaundice
Fatigue, headache
Tachycardia
Dark urine
Splenomegaly
Hepatomegaly
Low blood pressure (late sign of shock)

Increased Red Blood Cell Loss
Pallor
Fatigue, headache
Muscle weakness
Cool skin
Tachycardia
Decreased peripheral pulses

for the lower oxygen-carrying capacity of the blood, since blood replenished with oxygen returns to the tissues at a faster than normal rate. The increased circulation and turbulence within the heart may produce a heart murmur. Because the cardiac workload increases during exercise, infection, or emotional stress, cardiac failure may occur.

Acute or chronic hemorrhage results in loss of plasma and all formed elements of the blood. After acute hemorrhage the body replaces plasma within 1 to 3 days, maintaining blood volume. However, this results in a low concentration of RBCs, which are gradually replaced within 3 to 4 weeks. During this period there is usually a normocytic normochromic anemia, provided that iron stores are sufficient for hemoglobin synthesis.

In chronic blood loss the actual number of RBCs may be normal because of continuous replacement. However, insufficient iron is available to form hemoglobin as quickly as it is lost. As a result, erythrocytes are usually microcytic and hypochromic.

Routine Screening

The Put Prevention into Practice program developed for the U.S. Public Health Service cites the following recommendations of major authorities (US Department of Health and Human Services, 2009):

American Academy of Family Physicians and U.S. Preventive Services Task Force—All children should be screened for anemia once during infancy.

American Academy of Pediatrics—Hemoglobin concentration or hematocrit should be measured once during infancy (between 9 and 12 months), early childhood (between 1 and 5 years), late childhood (between 5 and 12 years), and adolescence (between 14 and 20 years).

Canadian Task Force on the Periodic Health Examination—Hemoglobin concentration screening should be performed on children at high risk for iron deficiency anemia: preterm infants, infants born of a multiple pregnancy or to an iron deficient woman, and children in low socioeconomic groups.

Diagnostic Evaluation

In general, anemia may be suspected from findings on the history and physical examination, such as lack of energy, easy fatigability, and pallor. Unless the anemia is severe, however, the first clue to the disorder may be alterations in the CBC, such as decreased numbers of RBCs, and decreased hemoglobin and hematocrit levels. Although anemia is sometimes defined as a hemoglobin level below 10 or 11 g/dl, this arbitrary cutoff is inappropriate for all children, since hemoglobin levels normally vary with age. (See Appendix C.)

Various findings of the CBC are also significant, such as increased reticulocyte levels, which indicate the body's response to an increased demand for RBCs. A peripheral smear may demonstrate significant changes in the shape of RBCs, such as sickled cells. Tests to measure the amount of hemoglobin in a single cell are helpful in determining the cause of the anemia (see Table 35-1 and p. 1412). Sometimes a bone marrow aspiration may be necessary to evaluate the body's ability to produce normal cells. For example, in leukemia the bone marrow is hyperplastic (producing increased numbers of cells), whereas in aplastic anemia the bone marrow is hypoplastic (producing decreased numbers of cells) or aplastic (producing no cells).

Tests for hematologic function do not always reflect the immediate changes occurring in the blood. For example, in acute massive hemorrhage the hemoglobin and hematocrit values may not be reliable, since the plasma volume may not increase for several hours. Without the hemodilution caused by the reexpansion of the vascular space, the hemoglobin and hematocrit may be close to normal, and the RBC loss may not be apparent. Consequently, assessing the quantity of blood loss in a seriously ill child may be difficult. The estimated volume of blood loss must be analyzed in conjunction with the child's total blood volume to determine the percentage of blood loss. Blood specimens obtained from central lines may more accurately reflect the patient's status than specimens obtained from an extremity because of the vasoconstriction of the peripheral vasculature. Decreased blood pressure changes are a late sign because of the compensatory mechanisms.

Therapeutic Management

The objective of medical management is to reverse the anemia by treating the underlying cause. In nutritional anemias the specific deficiency is corrected. In blood loss from acute hemorrhage, RBC transfusion may be given. In patients with severe anemia, supportive medical care may include oxygen therapy, bed rest, and replacement of intravascular volume with intravenous (IV) fluids. In addition to these general measures, the nurse may implement more specific interventions depending on the cause. The next sections discuss these interventions.

Nursing Care Management

The physical examination yields valuable evidence regarding the severity of the anemia and some indication of its possible cause (see Fig. 35-2 and Box 35-2). In interviewing the family, the nurse stresses the following areas: (1) nutrition, especially if the child is lactose intolerant or has inadequate intake of iron; (2) past history of chronic, recurrent infection; (3) eating habits, particularly pica (consumption of nonnutritive substances such as dirt, starch, lead-based paint chips, paper); (4) bowel habits and presence of frank blood in stools or black, tarry stools as a result of chronic blood loss; and (5) familial history of hereditary diseases, such as SCD or thalassemia.

The nurse should also be aware of the importance of taking a thorough history to obtain pertinent information that may aid in identifying the cause of the anemia. For example, statements such as "The baby drinks lots of milk" or "My teenager is on a liquid or vegetarian diet" are clues to possible iron deficiency.

Prepare the Child and Family for Laboratory Tests

Several blood tests may be ordered sequentially. Therefore the child may undergo multiple finger or heel sticks or venipunctures. These invasive procedures need not be painful with the application of a topical anesthetic known as EMLA (a eutectic mixture of local anesthetics) or LMX (lidocaine) cream.

The nurse is responsible for preparing the child for the tests by (1) explaining the significance of each test, particularly why the tests are not all done at one time; (2) encouraging parents or another supportive person to be with the child during the procedure; and (3) allowing the child to try out with the equipment on a doll or participate in the actual procedure (e.g., by holding the Band-Aid).

Older children may appreciate the opportunity to observe the blood cells under a microscope or in photographs. This is especially important if a serious blood disorder, such as leukemia, is suspected, since it serves as a foundation for explaining the pathophysiology of the disorder.

Bone marrow aspiration is not a routine hematologic test but is essential for definitive diagnosis of the leukemias, lymphomas, and certain anemias. (Chapter 27 presents information on preparing the child.)

NURSING TIP Suggested explanations to use in teaching children about blood components are:

Red blood cells—Carry the oxygen you breathe from your lungs to all parts of your body

White blood cells—Help keep germs from causing infection

Platelets—Small parts of cells that help make bleeding stop by forming a clot (scab) over the hurt area

Plasma—The liquid portion of blood; has clotting factors that help make bleeding stop

---

Decrease Tissue Oxygen Needs

Because the basic pathology in anemia is a decrease in the oxygen-carrying capacity of the RBCs, an important nursing responsibility is to minimize tissue oxygen needs by continual assessment of the child's energy level. In most instances of anemia this is not necessary, but when it is, the nurse must implement several important interventions. These same interventions apply to any child with a nursing diagnosis of fatigue or activity intolerance.

⚠ NURSING ALERT

Signs of exertion include tachycardia, palpitations, tachypnea, dyspnea, hyperpnea, dizziness, lightheadedness, diaphoresis, and change in skin color. The child looks fatigued (sagging, limp posture; slow, strained movements; inability to tolerate additional activity; difficulty sucking in infants).

Assess the child's level of tolerance for activities of daily living and play, and make adjustments to allow as much self-care as possible without undue exertion. During periods of rest the nurse measures vital signs and observes behavior to establish a baseline of nonexertion energy expenditure. During periods of activity the nurse repeats these measurements and observations to compare them with resting values.

Once a baseline of physical tolerance has been established, the nurse anticipates which activities will be physically taxing, such as dressing, feeding, or getting out of bed, and allows for conservation of energy by assisting the child as needed. Because dependency can be threatening, however, allow the child as much control in the environment as possible. For example, a child with severe anemia may be unable to walk to the bathroom but may be able to use a bedside commode or be transported in a wheelchair to the lavatory rather than having to use a bedpan. Scheduling activities throughout the day with planned rest periods in between maximizes the child's energy potential without causing undue exertion. Anticipate and implement necessary safety measures (e.g., staying with the child when the child is out of bed and raising side rails when the child is in the bed to prevent falls).

Plan diversional activities that promote rest but prevent boredom and withdrawal. Because short attention span, irritability, and restlessness are common in anemia and increase stress demands on the body, plan appropriate activities such as:

- Listening to music, using a tape recorder
- Watching television or playing video games
- Reading or listening to stories or comics
- Continuing a favorite hobby, such as stamp collecting
- Coloring or drawing
- Playing board and card games
- Being wheeled in a carriage or chair

Choosing the appropriate roommate, such as a child of similar age with a diagnosis that also requires restricted activity, is another helpful intervention.

If infants or young children are hospitalized, consider the importance of preventing separation from parents. Crying and fretfulness place greater stress demands on the body, which increase oxygen needs. Parents may need help in understanding the importance of their presence and the basis for their child's mood changes.

Prevent Complications

Children with anemia are prone to infection because tissue hypoxia causes cellular dysfunction and the disturbed metabolic processes weaken the host's defenses against foreign agents. Infection also worsens the anemia by increasing metabolic needs and, in instances of chronic infection, also interferes with erythropoiesis and shortens the survival time of RBCs. Take all of the usual precautions to prevent infection, such as practicing thorough hand washing, selecting an appropriate room in a noninfectious area, restricting the presence of visitors or hospital personnel with active infection, and maintaining adequate nutrition. The nurse also observes for signs of infection, particularly temperature elevation and leukocytosis. However, an elevated WBC count sometimes occurs in anemia without the presence of systemic or local infection.

Drawing multiple blood samples may present a problem with cumulative blood loss and necessitate blood replacement. This situation occurs most often in infants with severe anemia. To prevent this situation, blood may be withdrawn through a continuous IV line and replaced after the exact amount needed has been tested and discarded. As a precaution, keep a record of the volume of blood withdrawn. Using micromethods of testing whenever possible minimizes the amount of blood required for the test. The nurse needs to observe for cumulative effects of blood loss, particularly signs of shock and increased hypoxia, and to explain to parents the necessity for taking multiple blood samples and the reason for blood replacement.

The main complication of anemia is cardiac decompensation, which can result from excessive demands on the heart due to increased metabolic needs or cardiac overload. The nurse needs to observe for signs and symptoms of heart failure such as tachycardia, dyspnea, rales, moist respirations, cough, and sweating. Obviously, preventing heart failure by minimizing hypoxia and closely monitoring IV infusions is of first priority. Packed RBCs are usually administered to prevent circulatory hypervolemia. When blood transfusions are required in severe anemia to increase the hemoglobin level, follow all of the usual precautions for administering blood and observe for signs of transfusion reactions (Table 35-2).

BLOOD TRANSFUSION THERAPY

Technologic advances in blood banking and transfusion medicine allow the administration of only the blood component needed by the child, such as packed RBCs in anemia or platelets for bleeding disorders (Table 35-3). Regardless of the blood component administered, the nurse must be aware of the possibility of transfusion reactions.

Although hemolytic reactions are rare, ABO incompatibility remains the most common cause of death from blood transfusion, and human error is usually responsible (e.g., administration of blood of the wrong type to the patient or mislabeling of a blood product) (Bell, 2007; Stainsby, Jones, Wells, et al, 2008). Blood is usually matched between the donor and recipient for blood group (A, B, AB, or O) and Rh factor (positive or negative). However, AB-type RBCs can be transfused into individuals with blood types A, B, and AB, and Rh-negative RBCs can be given to Rh-positive individuals. (See Chapter 9 for a discussion of blood groups and ABO and Rh incompatibility.)

When blood is mismatched, the A or B antiagglutinin is mixed with RBCs containing A or B agglutinogens, respectively, and **agglutination** (clumping) of the RBCs occurs. The agglutinins, which are bivalent, attach themselves to two different erythrocytes at the same time, causing the cells to clump together and clog small blood vessels. Over a few hours to days, the entrapped cells degenerate and hemolyze, liberating excessive quantities of hemoglobin into the circulation. The eventual hemolysis of large numbers of RBCs decreases the blood volume, which causes circulatory failure and shock. Treatment is aimed at replacing lost blood and using plasma volume expanders.

Acute kidney shutdown and eventual renal failure are the result of renal vasoconstriction caused by antigen-antibody complexes derived from the RBC surface. The greatly reduced blood flow leads to complete renal failure and death within 7 to 12 days. Treatment involves promoting diuresis with rapid administration of dilute IV fluids and diuretics such as furosemide and mannitol, and alkalinizing body fluids, which renders hemoglobin more soluble.

Another consequence of hemolysis is the release of large quantities of phospholipids, which are capable of stimulating disseminated intravascular coagulation (DIC) (see p. 1448). As a result, the plasma is depleted of the coagulation factors needed to prevent hemorrhage. Without treatment with heparin to prevent the coagulation and with blood components to initiate clotting, death from generalized hemorrhage can occur.

In addition to the nursing precautions and responsibilities outlined in Table 35-2, some other general guidelines that apply to all transfusions are:

- Take vital signs, including blood pressure, before administering blood to establish baseline data for intratransfu-

sion and posttransfusion comparison; 15 minutes after initiation; hourly while blood is infusing; and on completion of the transfusion.
- Check the blood type and group of the recipient against the donor's, regardless of the blood product used.
- Administer the first 50 ml of blood or initial 20% of volume (whichever is smaller) slowly and stay with the child.
- Administer with normal saline in a piggyback setup or have normal saline available.
- Administer blood through an appropriate filter to eliminate particles in the blood and prevent the precipitation of formed elements; gently shake the container frequently.
- Use blood within 30 minutes of its arrival from the blood bank. If it is not used, return it to the blood bank; do not store it in a regular unit refrigerator.
- Infuse a unit of blood (or the specified amount) within 4 hours. If the infusion will exceed this time, divide the blood into appropriate-size quantities by the blood bank, with the unused portion refrigerated under controlled conditions.
- If a reaction of any type is suspected, take vital signs, stop the transfusion, maintain a patent IV line with normal saline and new tubing, notify the practitioner, and do not restart the transfusion until the child's condition has been medically evaluated.

Blood is usually administered to children by infusion pump; therefore the usual precautions and management related to pumps apply. When the blood infusion begins with a standard transfusion set, the filter chamber is filled to allow the total filter to be used. The drip chamber is partially filled with blood to permit counting of the drops. When the flow rate is adjusted, remember that blood administration sets do not use microdrops (60 drops/ml) but regular drops (usually 10 or 15 drops/ml). The nurse must consider this when calculating the flow rate.

Oxygen may be administered to provide optimum environmental conditions for hemoglobin saturation. Oxygen administration is of limited value, however, because each gram of hemoglobin is able to carry a limited amount of the gas. In addition, prolonged use of supplemental oxygen can decrease erythropoiesis. Therefore monitor the child closely for evidence of decreasing benefit from oxygen. One of the first signs of hypoxia is restlessness.

ANEMIA CAUSED BY NUTRITIONAL DEFICIENCIES

IRON DEFICIENCY ANEMIA

Anemia caused by an inadequate supply or loss of iron is the most prevalent nutritional disorder in the United States and the most preventable mineral disturbance. Without the intake of iron-fortified formula and cereals, term infants tend to develop iron deficiency, both with and without anemia, between 9 and 24 months of age (Andrews, Ullrich, and Fleming, 2009; Glader, 2007b). Adolescents are also at risk for iron deficiency

TABLE 35-2	NURSING CARE OF THE CHILD RECEIVING BLOOD TRANSFUSIONS	
COMPLICATION	**SIGNS AND SYMPTOMS**	**PRECAUTIONS AND NURSING RESPONSIBILITIES**
Immediate Reactions		
Hemolytic reactions Most severe type, but rare Incompatible blood Incompatibility in multiple transfusions	Sudden severe headache Chills Shaking Fever Pain at needle site and along venous tract Nausea and vomiting Sensation of tightness in chest Red or black urine Flank pain Progressive signs of shock or renal failure	Identify donor and recipient blood types and groups before transfusion is begun; verify with another nurse or practitioner. Transfuse blood slowly for first 15-20 min and/or initial 20% of blood volume; remain with patient. Stop transfusion immediately in event signs or symptoms occur, maintain patent intravenous line, and notify practitioner. Save donor blood to recrossmatch with patient's blood. Monitor for evidence of shock. Insert urinary catheter and monitor hourly outputs. Send sample of patient's blood and urine to laboratory for presence of hemoglobin (indicates intravascular hemolysis). Observe for signs of hemorrhage resulting from disseminated intravascular coagulation. Support medical therapies to reverse shock.
Febrile reactions Leukocyte or platelet antibodies Plasma protein antibodies	Fever Chills	May give acetaminophen for prophylaxis. Leukocyte-poor red blood cells (RBCs) are less likely to cause reaction. Stop transfusion immediately; report to practitioner for evaluation.
Allergic reactions Recipient reaction to allergens in donor's blood	Urticaria Pruritus Flushing Asthmatic wheezing Laryngeal edema	Give antihistamines for prophylaxis to children with tendency to allergic reactions. Stop transfusion immediately. Administer epinephrine for wheezing or anaphylactic reaction.
Circulatory overload Too rapid transfusion (even a small quantity) Transfusion of excessive quantity of blood (even slowly)	Precordial pain Dyspnea Rales Cyanosis Dry cough Distended neck veins Hypertension	Transfuse blood slowly. Prevent overload by using packed RBCs or administering divided amounts of blood. Use infusion pump to regulate and maintain flow rate. Stop transfusion immediately if signs of overload. Place child upright with feet in dependent position to increase venous resistance.
Air emboli May occur when blood is transfused under pressure	Sudden difficulty in breathing Sharp pain in chest Apprehension	Normalize pressure before container is empty when infusing blood under pressure. Clear tubing of air by aspirating air with syringe at nearest Y connector if air is observed in tubing; disconnect tubing and allow blood to flow until air has escaped only if a Y connector is not available.
Hypothermia	Chills Low temperature Irregular heart rate Possible cardiac arrest	Allow blood to warm at room temperature (<1 hr). Use approved mechanical blood warmer or electric warming coil to warm blood rapidly; never use microwave oven. Take temperature if patient complains of chills; if subnormal, stop transfusion.
Electrolyte disturbances Hyperkalemia (in massive transfusions or in patients with renal problems)	Nausea, diarrhea Muscular weakness Flaccid paralysis Paresthesia of extremities Bradycardia Apprehension Cardiac arrest	Use washed RBCs or fresh blood if patient is at risk.
Delayed Reactions		
Transmission of infection Hepatitis Human immunodeficiency virus (HIV) infection Malaria Syphilis Other bacterial or viral infection	Signs of infection (e.g., jaundice) Toxic reaction—High fever, severe headache or substernal pain, hypotension, intense flushing, vomiting or diarrhea	Blood is tested for antibodies to HIV, hepatitis C virus, and hepatitis B core antigen; in addition, blood is tested for hepatitis B surface antigen and alanine aminotransferase, and a serologic test is performed for syphilis. Units that test positive are destroyed. Individuals at risk for carrying certain viruses are deterred from donation. Report any sign of infection and, if it occurs during transfusion, stop transfusion immediately, send sample for culture and sensitivity testing, and notify practitioner.
Alloimmunization Antibody formation Occurs in patients receiving multiple transfusions	Increased risk of hemolytic, febrile, and allergic reactions	Use limited number of donors. Observe carefully for signs of reactions.
Delayed hemolytic reaction	Destruction of RBCs and fever 5-10 days after transfusion	Observe for posttransfusion anemia and decreasing benefit from successive transfusion.

TABLE 35-3   NURSING ADMINISTRATION OF BLOOD COMPONENTS

COMPONENT AND INDICATIONS	DOSAGE	NURSING ADMINISTRATION
Packed red blood cells (PRBCs) Symptomatic anemia Renal or liver disease Hemolysis Decreased erythropoiesis Splenic or liver sequestration	Volume packed RBCs = Weight (kg) × Change in hematocrit (Hct) desired	1. Assess for PRBC reaction (e.g., pruritus, rash, cough, fever). 2. Regulate infusion rate using microaggregate filter via infusion pump to 5 ml/kg/hr over 2-4 hr (usual rate). Do not use the tubing to infuse more than 1 unit of blood. 3. Monitor vital signs before transfusion, 15 min after initiation, hourly during transfusion, and on completion of transfusion.
Whole blood (rarely used) Acute massive blood loss	Volume of whole blood = Weight (kg) × Change in Hct desired × 2	4. Do not refrigerate blood in the nursing unit. Use only the blood bank refrigerator. 5. Ensure that each unit is infused ≤4 hr. If a longer infusion time is needed, the unit must be divided in the blood bank. 6. Do not infuse solutions other than normal saline in the line with RBCs.
Fresh frozen plasma (FFP) Deficiencies of plasma clotting factors in bleeding patients (e.g., disseminated intravascular coagulation [DIC]); liver failure; vitamin K deficiency with bleeding; or replacement of antithrombin III (ATIII), protein C, or protein S	10-15 ml/kg (use within 6-24 hr of thawing)	1. Assess for FFP reaction (e.g., pain, bleeding, swelling). 2. Regulate infusion rate using microaggregate filter to 20 ml/min over 1-2 hr q 12-24 hr until hemorrhage stops. 3. Monitor prothrombin time (PT) and partial thromboplastin time (PPT) before and after FFP infusion. 4. Monitor levels of other coagulation factors (e.g., fibrinogen, fibrin split products, D-dimer, ATIII, protein C, and protein S).
Platelets (plt) Active hemorrhage, DIC Thrombocytopenia with bleeding or if indicated by clinical status	1 unit/10 kg or 6 unit/m² intravenously (IV)	1. Assess for plt reaction (e.g., pruritus, rash, fever, bleeding). 2. Regulate infusion rate using 170-mm microaggregate filter to 10 ml/kg/hr, IV push or over 1 hr or as fast as patient can tolerate. 3. Monitor vital signs before transfusion, 15 min after initiation, and at the end of infusion. 4. Obtain postplatelet count 60 min–24 hr after infusion.
Granulocytes (rarely used) As adjunct with other measures in treatment of severe infections in the septic neonate or high-risk patient (e.g., proven bacterial infection in severely neutropenic patient unresponsive to antibiotic therapy)	10-15 ml/kg IV usually daily × 4 days	1. Assess for granulocyte reaction (e.g., chills, rash, dyspnea). 2. Monitor vital signs before transfusion, 15 min after initiation, and at the end of transfusion. 3. Premedicate 1 hr before transfusion, usually with antihistamines, acetaminophen, or steroids. 4. Infuse at slow rate (2-4 hr) using 170-mm blood filter within a 24-hr period. 5. Minimum of 4-6 hr between amphotericin B and granulocyte infusion recommended.
Factor VIII (plasma derived or recombinant) Hemophilia A Acquired factor VIII deficiency	1 unit/kg IV of factor VIII = 2% of factor activity 35-50 units/kg IV of factor VIII q 12-24 hr	1. Assess adverse reaction (e.g., hives, itchy wheals with redness, tightness in chest, wheezing, low blood pressure, or dyspnea). Notify health care provider immediately if symptoms are present. 2. Use reconstituted factor within 3 hr of mixing. 3. Inject reconstituted factor intravenously over 2-5 min.
Factor IX (plasma derived or recombinant) Hemophilia B	1 unit/kg of factor IX = 1% of factor activity 30-50 units/kg IV q 24 hr	
FEIBA (factor eight inhibitor bypass activity), plasma derived Hemophilia A or B with inhibitors (antibodies)	75-100 units/kg IV q 8-24 hr (maximum dose 200 units/kg/day)	
Factor VIIa (recombinant) Hemophilia A or B with inhibitors	90 mcg/kg IV q 2 hr (35-120 mcg/kg dosage range)	
Cryoprecipitate (CRYO) (rarely used) Control bleeding in patients with DIC Hypofibrinogenemia	4 bags CRYO/10 kg IV	1. Assess CRYO reaction (e.g., rash, bleeding). 2. Monitor closely PT/PPT and levels of fibrinogen, fibrinogen split products, D-dimer. 3. Use a filter needle to draw up and administer within 15-30 min.

because of their rapid growth rate, menses, poor eating habits, obesity, and strenuous activities (Andrews, Ullrich, and Fleming, 2009; Glader, 2007a; Nead, Halterman, Kaczorowski, et al, 2004). The decline in the prevalence of iron deficiency anemia in the United States over the past several decades may be due to the initiation of the U.S. Special Supplemental Food Program and the American Academy of Pediatrics' promotion of formula for the first year of life (Altucher, Rasmussen,

Barden, et al, 2005; Andrews, Ullrich, and Fleming, 2009). The promotion of iron supplement in the exclusively breast-fed infant, introduction of iron-fortified infant formula and cereal, weaning from the bottle by 1 year of age, limiting intake of cow's milk to 16 to 24 oz/day, and delayed introduction of cow's milk into the diet have all contributed to the decreased incidence of iron deficiency anemia in infants and young children (Andrews, Ullrich, and Fleming, 2009; Glader, 2007b;

BOX 35-3   CAUSES OF IRON DEFICIENCY ANEMIA

Inadequate Supply of Iron
Deficient dietary intake
- Rapid growth rate
- Excessive milk intake, delayed addition of solid foods
- Poor general eating habits
- Exclusive breast-feeding of infant after 6 months of age

Inadequate iron stores at birth
- Low birth weight, prematurity, multiple births
- Severe iron deficiency in mother (hemoglobin level <9 g/dl)
- Fetal blood loss at or before delivery

Impaired Iron Absorption
Presence of iron inhibitors
- Phytates, phosphates, or oxalates
- Gastric alkalinity

Malabsorption disorders
- Lactose intolerance
- Inflammatory bowel disease

Chronic diarrhea

Blood Loss
Acute or chronic hemorrhage
Parasitic infestation

Excessive Demands for Iron Required for Growth
Prematurity
Adolescence
Pregnancy

Richardson, 2007). However, iron deficiency still occurs in infants, children, adolescents, and child-bearing women of all races and ethnic groups (Andrews, Ullrich, and Fleming, 2009; Glader, 2007b; Richardson, 2007; White, 2005) and continues to be a significant health problem.

Etiology

Iron deficiency anemia can be caused by any number of factors that decrease the supply of iron, impair its absorption, increase the body's need for iron, or affect the synthesis of hemoglobin (Box 35-3). Although the clinical manifestations and diagnostic evaluation are similar regardless of the cause, the therapeutic and nursing care management depends on the specific reason for the iron deficiency. The following discussion is limited to iron deficiency anemia resulting from inadequate iron in the diet.

At birth the full-term infant has approximately a 0.5 g supply of iron, and an average of 0.8 mg of iron must be absorbed each day during the first 15 years of life (Glader, 2007b). During the last trimester of pregnancy, iron is transferred from the mother to the fetus at the rate of 4 mg/day. Most of the iron is stored in the circulating hemoglobin of the erythrocytes, and the remainder is deposited in the liver, spleen, and bone marrow. Maternally derived iron stores are adequate for the first 5 to 6 months in the full-term infant but for only about 2 to 3 months in premature infants or infants of multiple births. If dietary sources of iron are not supplied to meet the infant's growth demands after depletion of fetal iron stores, iron deficiency anemia results. Physiologic anemia should not be confused with iron deficiency anemia resulting from nutritional causes.

Vegetarian diets, popular among teenage girls, have been associated with nutritional deficiencies. Some infants and toddlers who have been fed inappropriate vegetarian diets have had severe protein-energy malnutrition, as well as deficiencies of iron, vitamin B_{12}, and vitamin D. Unrefined cereals contain substances that modify the absorption of minerals such as zinc, calcium, and iron. Individuals consuming strict vegetarian diets that include a large amount of unrefined cereals could be at a greater risk of rickets, vitamin B_{12} and folate deficiency, and iron deficiency anemia (Hubbard, 2004; Renda and Fischer, 2009).

Pathophysiology

Iron is required for the production of hemoglobin. One molecule of hemoglobin consists of protein (globin) combined with four molecules of a pigmented compound (heme). Each molecule of heme contains one atom of iron. When iron stores are deficient, the production of hemoglobin is reduced. Consequently, the main effect of iron deficiency is decreased hemoglobin level and reduced oxygen-carrying capacity of the blood.

Clinical Manifestations

The clinical manifestations are directly attributable to the reduction in the amount of oxygen available to the tissues and resemble those seen in any type of anemia. Usually the signs are insidious and obscure, and the severity is directly related to the duration of the dietary deficiency.

Although infants with iron deficiency anemia tend to be underweight, many are overweight because of excessive milk ingestion (known as *milk baby*). These children become anemic for two reasons: (1) milk, a poor source of iron, is given almost to the exclusion of solid foods; and (2) increased fecal loss of blood occurs in 50% of iron deficient infants fed cow's milk. This asymptomatic loss of hemoglobin causes iron deficiency (Glader, 2007b; Richardson, 2007). Although chubby, these infants are pale (sometimes porcelain-like), usually demonstrate poor muscle development, and are prone to infection.

Although the mechanism is unknown, iron deficiency anemia enhances the leakage of plasma proteins, which causes edema; retarded growth; and decreased serum concentration of the proteins albumin, gamma globulin, and transferrin (a protein that binds iron and transports it through the plasma). Other manifestations of iron deficiency include irritability, tachycardia, fatigue, glossitis, angular stomatitis, and koilonychia (concave or "spoon" fingernails). The association between iron deficiency anemia and impaired neurocognitive function (attention span, alertness, and learning) in both infants and adolescents has been well established, but the mechanism by which iron deficiency anemia impairs neurologic function is unknown (Akman, Cebecci, Okur, et al, 2004; Andrews, Ullrich, and Fleming, 2009; Glader, 2007b).

Diagnostic Evaluation

Laboratory tests that measure or describe hemoglobin, the morphologic changes in the RBC, and iron concentration are usually performed (see Table 35-1). The RBC count may be normal, borderline, or moderately reduced in the child with iron deficiency anemia. Typically the nearly normal number of erythrocytes is strikingly out of proportion to the low hemoglobin concentration. RBCs are typically small (microcytic), so that MCV is decreased (see Box 35-1). For infants 1 year of age, an MCV below 70 femtoliters (fl) is considered diagnostic. In children from 1 to 10 years of age, an MCV value of 70 fl plus the child's age in years is a quick calculation of the lower limit of normal.

The reticulocyte count is usually normal or slightly reduced because of decreased stores of iron (see Table 35-1). However, in severe anemia, when tissue hypoxia elicits an erythropoietic response, the reticulocyte count may be elevated to 3% or 4%. The level of erythrocyte protoporphyrin, the immediate precursor of heme, becomes elevated in RBCs whenever heme synthesis is disturbed.

In terms of differential diagnosis, a stool analysis for occult blood (guaiac test) is commonly performed to confirm or rule out the possibility of chronic fecal blood loss, especially from milk intolerance or structural anomalies such as diverticulitis.

Iron Studies

In addition to tests that indirectly indicate the level of iron by revealing the effects of iron deficiency on the RBCs, several other tests are usually performed that more directly measure the amount of circulating iron. The serum iron concentration (SIC) is the amount of circulating iron and is normally about 70 mcg/dl in infants and slightly higher in older children. Lower limits of SIC vary not only with age but also with the time of day; they are highest in the morning, when the test should be performed.

The **total iron-binding capacity (TIBC)** is the amount of transferrin (iron-binding globulin), which is necessary for the transport of iron in the bloodstream. When combined with transferrin, the iron is loosely bound to the globulin molecule so that it can be released easily to tissue cells anywhere in the body. In iron deficiency anemia TIBC is elevated above the normal range of 350 mcg/dl (6 months to 2 years) or 450 mcg/dl (children >2 years and adults). The elevated TIBC represents the body's compensatory mechanism to absorb more iron from exogenous sources than normally during states of deficiency. Transferrin saturation is calculated by dividing the SIC by the TIBC and multiplying the result by 100 to express the value as a percentage. A transferrin saturation of 10% suggests anemia.

These biochemical test (ferritin, TIBC, SIC) are acute phase reactants, which means in an inflammatory setting a positive acute phase reactant may overestimate iron stores (Andrews, Ullrich, and Fleming, 2009; Glader, 2007b). Other tests not affected by inflammation that are available in some clinical laboratories are the serum transferring receptor (elevated in iron deficiency) and reticulocyte hemoglobin content, which has been used to accurately assess iron status in adults (Andrews, Ullrich, and Fleming, 2009; Glader, 2007b).

Therapeutic Management

Prevention is the primary goal and is achieved through optimum nutrition and appropriate iron supplementation. In infants, the following guidelines are recommended to prevent iron deficiency (American Academy of Pediatrics, 1999; Glader, 2007a)

- Use only breast milk or iron-fortified formula (containing 7 to 12 mg/L for full-term infants and 15 mg/L for preterm infants of iron) for the first 12 months.

- Iron supplementation of 1 mg/kg/day should be provided by 4 to 6 months of age in full-term infants and 2 mg/kg/day by 2 months of age in preterm infants.
- Administer iron drops at a dosage of 2 to 3 mg/kg/day to a maximum of 15 mg/day of elemental iron to breast-fed preterm infants after 2 months of age, and give iron-fortified infant cereal when solid foods are introduced.
- Limit the amount of formula to no more than 1 L/day to encourage intake of iron-rich solid foods.

Once the diagnosis of iron deficiency anemia is made, therapeutic management focuses on increasing the amount of supplemental iron the child receives. This usually occurs through dietary counseling and the administration of oral iron supplements. In formula-fed infants the most convenient and best sources of supplemental iron are iron-fortified commercial formula and iron-fortified infant cereal (Glader, 2007b; Mabry-Hernandez, 2009). Iron-fortified formula provides a relatively constant and predictable amount of iron and is not associated with an increased incidence of gastrointestinal symptoms, such as colic, diarrhea, or constipation. Infants younger than 12 months of age should not be given fresh cow's milk to decrease the possibility of gastrointestinal blood loss from intolerance to the milk protein.

Addition of iron-rich foods to the diet may not provide sufficient supplemental quantities of the mineral. Oral supplements of ferrous iron are given because this form is more readily absorbed than ferric iron and results in higher hemoglobin levels. Ingested iron is absorbed largely from the duodenum, and absorption is facilitated by an acid environment. Children normally absorb an average of 10% to 20% of the iron in oral supplements, but during periods of iron deficiency they absorb an additional 5% to 10%. Oral iron supplementation is prescribed as 3 to 6 mg of elemental iron per kilogram per day. Lower dosages of iron are associated with fewer side effects. Ideally the daily dose of iron should be given in two or three divided doses between meals. Side effects of oral iron therapy include nausea, gastric irritation, diarrhea or constipation, and anorexia, but these occur infrequently, especially in infants. If the iron produces vomiting and diarrhea, it should be administered with meals and in gradually increasing doses.

The response to oral iron therapy is reflected in a peak increase in the reticulocyte count by the fifth to the tenth day of administration. Following the reticulocyte rise, the hemoglobin and hematocrit levels and RBC count increase. The hemoglobin level rises as much as 0.5 g/dl/24 hr; therefore a substantial increase should occur by the end of 1 month (Glader, 2007b; Richardson, 2007).

If the hemoglobin level is very low or if the level fails to rise after 1 month of oral therapy, it is important to assess whether the iron is being administered correctly. Parenteral iron administration is painful; expensive; and occasionally associated with regional lymphadenopathy, transient arthralgias, or serious allergic reaction (Andrews, Ullrich, and Fleming, 2009; Glader, 2007b). Therefore parenteral iron administration is reserved for children who have iron malabsorption or chronic hemoglobinuria. The Z-track method of intramuscular injection must be used to minimize staining of the skin, and careful observation is required because of the risk of anaphylaxis. Transfusions are indicated for the most severe anemia and in cases of serious infection, cardiac dysfunction, or surgical emergency when anesthesia is required. Packed RBCs (2 to 3 ml/kg), not whole blood, are used to minimize the chance of circulatory overload. Supplemental oxygen is administered when tissue hypoxia is severe.

Next to iron deficiency, folate deficiency is the most common micronutrient deficiency (Watkins, Whitehead, and Rosenblatt, 2009). Causes of folate deficiency include inadequate diet, overcooking of vegetables with loss of folates, and malabsorption. The deficiency is treated with adequate prepared and intake of folate-enrich foods and/or 1 mg of folate daily (Watkins, Whitehead, and Rosenblatt, 2009). As macrocytic anemias, both folate and vitamin B_{12} deficiencies result in defective ribonucleic acid (RNA) and deoxyribonucleic acid (DNA) synthesis (Kaferle and Strzoda, 2009).

Vitamin B_{12} deficiency commonly develops when the gastric mucosa fails to secrete sufficient intrinsic factor, which is essential for absorption of vitamin B_{12}. Deprived of vitamin B_{12}, the bone marrow produces fewer but macrocytic RBCs. The erythrocytes are usually immature and, because of their extremely fragile cell membranes, are rapidly destroyed during circulation. Treatment initially involves the administration of 100 mcg or higher dose of vitamin B_{12} parenteral therapy for several days, followed by injections of 500 or 1000 mcg of vitamin B_{12} every 1 to 2 months. Researchers compared oral and parenteral vitamin B_{12} therapy and found that they yielded comparable benefits (Bolarman, Kadikoylu, Yukselen, et al, 2003; Butler, Vidal-Alaball, Cannings-John, et al, 2006).

Prognosis

Prognosis for a child with iron deficiency anemia, folate deficiency, or vitamin B_{12} deficiency is very good. However, there is evidence that if the anemia is severe and longstanding, then diminished cognitive function, behavioral changes, delayed infant growth and development, decreased exercise tolerance, and impaired immune function may develop (Andrews, Ullrich, and Fleming, 2009; Richardson, 2007).

Nursing Care Management

A primary nursing objective is to prevent nutritional anemia through family education. Nurses need to be aware of recommendations regarding iron supplementation during infancy and appropriate sources of dietary iron. The nurse should encourage parents to limit the quantity of milk, to use iron-fortified infant formulas, and to introduce solid foods. This may be difficult when parents believe milk is best for the infant and equate the resultant weight gain with "healthiness." Although milk is an excellent food, it is deficient in iron, vitamin C, zinc, and fluoride. Sources of each of these nutrients and the role they play in preventing deficiencies need to be discussed with the family, especially the person responsible for feeding the infant. For example, the mother may have less decision-making power regarding feeding than the grandmother who cares for the child.

Also stress that overweight is not synonymous with good health. If the infant has obvious signs of anemia, such as pallor, listlessness, frequent infections, and muscular weakness, point these out as evidence of suboptimum health. In some instances it is helpful to chart the hemoglobin or hematocrit values

to visually impress on parents the change in iron levels. Often, increased blood values correspond to improved physical status and reinforce the benefit of dietary or oral iron supplementation.

QUALITY PATIENT OUTCOMES: Iron Deficiency Anemia
- Early recognition of signs and symptoms of iron deficiency anemia
- Appropriate quantity of milk, use of iron-fortified infant formula, and introduction of solid foods
- Adherence to oral iron supplement and appropriate administration
- Hemoglobin increase within 1 month and anemia resolved within 6 months

---

Instructing parents regarding proper administration of oral iron supplements is an essential nursing responsibility. Several factors, such as stomach acidity, affect the absorption of iron (see Box 13-1).

⚡ DRUG ALERT

Iron Supplements

Ideally iron supplements are administered in two divided doses between meals, when the presence of free hydrochloric acid is greatest, and are accompanied by a citrus fruit or juice, which helps reduce iron to its most soluble state.

An adequate dosage of oral iron turns the stools a tarry green or black color. The nurse advises parents of this normally expected change and inquires about its occurrence on follow-up visits. Absence of the greenish black stool may be a clue to poor compliance. If compliance is an issue, make every effort to institute strategies to improve adherence to the medication regimen, such as administering the drug once a day at the most convenient time. (See Compliance, Chapter 27.)

! NURSING ALERT

Because iron ingested in excessive quantities is toxic, even fatal, parents should keep no more than a 1-month supply in the home and store it safely away from the reach of children.

Oral iron supplements are available in liquid or tablet form. Liquid preparations may temporarily stain the teeth. If possible, take the medication through a straw or give it through a syringe or medicine dropper placed toward the back of the mouth. Brushing the teeth after administration of the drug lessens the discoloration.

Counseling families whose children are anemic is often a difficult and challenging task. Meal planning must be based on the family's budget, cultural pattern, and food preferences (see Cultural Competence box). Often this requires more than a brief discussion with the mother or usual caregiver about foods high in iron (see Table 13-2). For teaching to be effective, the nurse may need to offer recipes, assist in planning a shopping list, and investigate food prices for economy. Because the physical effects of anemia are insidious, parents may not consider their child ill and consequently may view the medication and diet changes as unnecessary. Stressing the physical and behavioral improvements and what effect the improved diet will have on all family members may encourage parents to adhere to the treatment plan.

🌐 CULTURAL COMPETENCE
Tea Drinking and Nonheme Iron Absorption

In cultures in which tea is drunk as a common beverage, administer iron with some other liquid because the tannins in tea form an insoluble complex with nonheme iron that is from foods other than meat. In addition, the phytates in legumes and maize and the phenolic compounds in herbal teas may adversely affect the uptake of iron (Diaz, Rosado, Allen, et al, 2003). There is clear evidence to show that tea drinking limits the absorption of nonheme iron whereas ascorbic acid enhances iron absorption (Nelson and Poulter, 2004; Thankachan, Walczyk, Muthayya, et al, 2008).

Diet education of teenagers is difficult, especially because teenage girls are particularly prone to following weight-reduction diets. Emphasizing the effect of anemia on appearance (pallor) and energy level (difficulty maintaining popular activities) may be useful. (See Table 13-2 and Mineral Disturbances, Chapter 13, for sources of iron-rich foods.)

ANEMIAS CAUSED BY INCREASED DESTRUCTION OF RED BLOOD CELLS

Excessive destruction or hemolysis of erythrocytes can occur from a defect in the RBC (intracorpuscular defect) that shortens the life span of the cell so that production cannot keep pace with destruction. In sickle cell anemia and thalassemia, erythrocyte life spans are decreased because of a hemoglobin defect, whereas in spherocytosis erythrocyte life span is decreased due to a defective red cell membrane. Extracorpuscular factors are those conditions that cause hemolysis in otherwise normal RBCs. A classic example is blood group incompatibility, such as hemolytic disease of the newborn or incompatibility secondary to mismatched blood transfusion. Damage to a normal red cell may be caused by toxic drugs, burns, poisonings (such as from lead), infections (such as malaria), and splenic sequestration (hypersplenism).

HEREDITARY SPHEROCYTOSIS

Hereditary spherocytosis (HS), a common hemolytic disorder, is caused by a defect in the proteins that form the RBC membrane (Grace and Lux, 2009; Segel, 2007). It occurs in most ethnic groups, but is primarily prevalent in persons of northern European heritage with a reported incidence of 1 in 5000 (Grace and Lux, 2009; Segel, 2007).

The condition is transmitted in an autosomal dominant pattern. However, 25% of cases are thought to represent new mutations or inheritance through an autosomal recessive mode or autosomal dominant mode with reduced penetrance (Segel, 2007; Shah and Vega, 2004). The affected cells have a smaller surface area relative to their volume than normal RBCs, so that they become inflexible spheres known as **spherocytes**. The

inflexibility of these cells makes it difficult for them to circulate through the spleen and leads to their early destruction.

Clinical manifestations vary widely and include anemia (usually mild), splenomegaly (usually modest and does not correlate with the severity of disease), and jaundice (most often scleral icterus). HS frequently manifests in the first 24 hours of the newborn's life as severe hyperbilirubinemia. Folic acid supplementation should be given to these children to prevent deficiency due to the rapid cell turnover. Laboratory findings include hemoglobin level between 7 and 10 g/dl, reticulocyte count of 3% to 15% (inversely correlated with hemoglobin level), and an increase in osmotic fragility.

Aplastic crisis, which results in a sudden cessation of RBC production by the bone marrow, is a serious complication. Hemoglobin and hematocrit values drop rapidly, which results in severe anemia. Transfusion support may be needed, and close monitoring of the child's cardiovascular status is necessary.

Splenectomy, a treatment for HS, is generally reserved for children older than 5 years of age with symptomatic anemia. The splenectomy corrects the hemolysis but not the RBC defect. Occasionally splenectomy is performed in children younger than 5 years of age who are severely anemic and are showing signs of failure to thrive. Children who are scheduled to undergo a splenectomy should be evaluated for the presence of gallstones before surgery. If gallstones are present, a cholecystectomy is performed at the time of splenectomy.

Because of the risk of life-threatening bacterial infection after splenectomy, these children are immunized with the pneumococcal, meningococcal, and *Haemophilus influenzae* type b vaccines before surgery and receive prophylactic penicillin for several years after splenectomy. Instruct parents in the importance of seeking immediate medical attention if their child develops a fever of 38.3° C (101° F) or higher as a common sign of infection or postsplenectomy sepsis (Grace and Lux, 2009; Lanzkowsky, 2005; Shah and Vega, 2004). Given the lifelong increased risk of severe infection and thromboembolic complications in splenectomized children, partial splenectomy has been investigated for selected patients with HS with the goal of decreasing hemolysis while maintaining splenic phagocytic function (Grace and Lux, 2009; Segel, 2007).

SICKLE CELL ANEMIA

Sickle cell anemia (SCA) is one of a group of diseases collectively termed **hemoglobinopathies** in which normal adult hemoglobin (hemoglobin A [HgbA]) is partly or completely replaced by abnormal sickle hemoglobin (HgbS). SCD refers to a group of hereditary disorders, all of which are related to the presence of HgbS. Although the name *SCD* is sometimes used to refer to SCA, this usage is incorrect. The correct terms for SCA are *HgbSS disease* and *homozygous sickle cell disease*. In the United States the most common forms of SCD are:

SCA—The homozygous form of the disease (HgbSS), in which valine, an amino acid, is substituted for glutamic acid at the sixth position of the β chain.

Sickle cell C disease—A heterozygous variant of SCD (HgbSC), characterized by the presence of both HgbS and hemoglobin C (HgbC), in which lysine is substituted for glutamic acid at the sixth position of the β chain.

Sickle thalassemia disease—A combination of sickle cell trait and β-thalassemia trait. In the β⁺ (beta plus) form some normal adult hemoglobin can still be produced. In the β⁰ (beta zero) form there is no ability to produce normal adult hemoglobin.

Of the SCDs, SCA is the most common form in African-Americans in the United States, followed by sickle cell C disease and sickle β-thalassemia. Numerous other sickle syndromes exist in which HgbS is paired with rare mutant globins.

SCD is one of the most common genetic diseases worldwide, affecting approximately 90,000 Americans; those of other nationalities, such as Africans, Hispanics, Italians, Greeks, Iranians, and Turks; and individuals of Arab, Caribbean, and Asian Indian descent. The incidence of the disease varies in different geographic locations. Among African-Americans, the incidence of sickle cell trait is about 8%, whereas among inhabitants of West Africa the frequency of sickle cell trait is reportedly as high as 40%. The high incidence of sickle cell trait in these individuals is believed to be a selective protection against death from malaria caused by endemic *Plasmodium falciparum* infection (Driscoll, 2007). The physiologic basis for the influence of malaria on the sickle gene (so-called balanced polymorphism) is not well understood (Heeney and Dover, 2009).

Mode of Transmission

The gene that determines the production of HgbS is situated on an autosome. When both parents have sickle cell trait, there is a 25% chance with each pregnancy of producing an offspring with SCA. In the United States it is estimated that 1 in 12 African-Americans carries the trait; therefore the risk of two African-American parents having a child with the disease is 0.7%. Other forms of SCD occur through the union of two individuals who carry the heterozygous form of hemoglobin variants.

Basic Defect

The basic defect responsible for the sickling of erythrocytes is contained in the globin fraction of hemoglobin, which is composed of 574 amino acids. Under conditions of dehydration, acidosis, hypoxia, and temperature elevation, the relatively insoluble HgbS changes its molecular structure to form long, slender crystals. These filamentous crystals cause distortion of the cell membrane, so that the cell changes from a pliable disk to a crescent- or sickle-shaped RBC. The filamentous forms are associated with much greater viscosity than those with the normal holly leaf structure of HgbA.

In most instances the sickling response is reversible under conditions of adequate oxygenation and hydration. During this time the RBCs are indistinguishable from normal erythrocytes on peripheral examination. RBCs with HgbS can sickle and unsickle under appropriate conditions. After repeated cycles of sickling and unsickling, the RBCs become irreversibly sickled.

Although the defect is inherited, the sickling phenomenon is usually not apparent until later in infancy because of the presence of fetal hemoglobin (HgbF). HgbF is composed of two α and two γ polypeptide chains. At 32 weeks of gestation, the production of β and δ chains begins. These combine with α chains to form the major adult hemoglobins: HgbA (two α and two β chains) and HgbA₂ (two α and two δ chains). The

newborn with SCD is generally asymptomatic because of the protective effect of HgbF (60% to 80%), but this rapidly decreases during the first year, so that the child is at risk for sickle cell–related complications (Heeney and Dover, 2009; Driscoll, 2007).

Sickle Cell Trait

Persons with sickle cell trait have the same basic defect, but only about 35% to 45% of the total hemoglobin is HgbS. The remainder is HgbA. Normally these individuals are asymptomatic. Although complications are rare, they have been described in individuals with sickle cell trait. Nonpainful gross hematuria is the major complication, seen primarily in the teenage and adult years. Under conditions of extreme or prolonged deoxygenation, such as riding in a nonpressurized aircraft or undergoing military training, splenic sequestration with profound anemia can occur, resulting in death.

Pathophysiology and Clinical Manifestations

The clinical manifestations of SCA are primarily the result of (1) obstruction caused by the sickled RBCs' adhesion to vascular endothelium accompanied by inflammatory process and (2) increased RBC destruction. The entanglement and enmeshing of rigid sickle-shaped cells block the microcirculation, causing vasoocclusion (Fig. 35-3). The resultant absence of blood flow to adjacent tissues causes local hypoxia, which leads to tissue ischemia and infarction (cellular death) (Box 35-4). The sickle cell adhesion to the vascular endothelium actually sets in motion the abnormal adhesion-inflammation–increased adhesion of the sickling cycle (Redding-Lallinger and Knoll, 2006). Most of the complications seen in SCA can be traced to this cycle and its impact on various organs of the body (Fig. 35-4).

Initially the spleen may become enlarged from congestion and engorgement with sickled cells. This repeated insult to the splenic sinuses results in infarction. The functioning cells are gradually replaced by fibrotic tissue until, by the age of 5 years, the spleen has decreased in size and has been totally replaced by a fibrous mass (functional asplenia). Without the spleen to filter bacteria and to promote the release of large numbers of phagocytic cells, these individuals are highly susceptible to infection.

The liver is also altered in form and function. Liver failure and necrosis are the result of severe impairment of hepatic blood flow from anemia and capillary obstruction. Moderate hepatomegaly is common by age 1 and usually persists throughout childhood and early adulthood. The rapid destruction of RBCs often results in the development of pigmented gallstones. Obstruction of the common bile duct by gallstones is uncommon; therefore cholecystectomy is generally not recommended for asymptomatic patients. If recurrent episodes of right upper abdominal pain occur, cholecystectomy may be indicated.

Kidney abnormalities are probably the result of the same cycle of congestion of glomerular capillaries and tubular arterioles with sickle cells and hemosiderin, tissue necrosis, and eventual scarring. The principal results of kidney ischemia are hematuria, inability to concentrate urine, enuresis, and occasionally nephrotic syndrome.

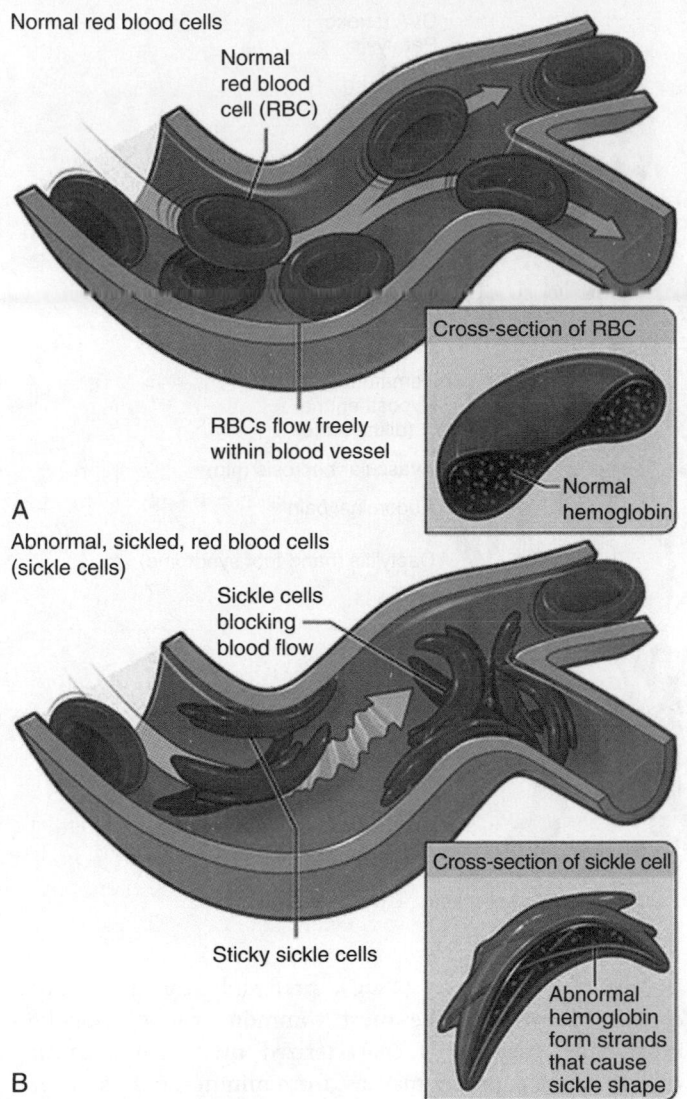

Normal red blood cells

Normal red blood cell (RBC)

RBCs flow freely within blood vessel

A

Abnormal, sickled, red blood cells (sickle cells)

Cross-section of RBC

Normal hemoglobin

Sickle cells blocking blood flow

Sticky sickle cells

Cross-section of sickle cell

Abnormal hemoglobin form strands that cause sickle shape

B

Fig. 35-3 A, Normal red blood cells *(RBCs)* flowing freely in a blood vessel. The inset image shows a cross-section of a normal red blood cell with normal hemoglobin. **B,** Abnormal, sickled red blood cells clumping and blocking blood flow in a blood vessel. (Other cells also may play a role in this clumping process.) The inset image shows a cross-section of a sickle cell with abnormal hemoglobin. (From National Heart, Lung, and Blood Institute: *What is sickle cell anemia?* Bethesda Md, August 2008, National Institutes of Health.)

Bone changes include hyperplasia and congestion of the bone marrow, which result in osteoporosis, widening of the medullary spaces, and thinning of the cortices. As a result of the weakening of bone, especially in the lumbar and thoracic regions, skeletal deformities, particularly lordosis and kyphosis, may occur. Because of chronic hypoxia, the bone becomes susceptible to osteomyelitis, frequently from *Salmonella* organisms. Aseptic necrosis of the femoral head from chronic ischemia is an occasional problem.

Changes in the central nervous system are primarily vascular and result from the same cyclic reaction of occlusion, ischemia, and infarction. Stroke, or cerebrovascular accident, is a major complication that occurs in approximately 11% of children with SCD by the age of 20 years and can result in permanent paralysis or death (DeBaun and Vichinsky, 2007; Driscoll, 2007). Any number of neurologic symptoms can indicate a

---

BOX 35-4   CLINICAL MANIFESTATIONS OF SICKLE CELL ANEMIA

General
Possible growth retardation
Chronic anemia (hemoglobin level of 6 to 9 g/dl)
Possible delayed sexual maturation
Marked susceptibility to sepsis

Vasoocclusive Crisis
Pain in area(s) of involvement
Manifestations related to ischemia of involved areas:
  Extremities—Painful swelling of hands and feet (sickle cell dactylitis, or hand-foot syndrome), painful joints
  Abdomen—Severe pain resembling acute surgical condition
  Cerebrum—Stroke, visual disturbances
  Chest—Symptoms resembling pneumonia, protracted episodes of pulmonary disease
  Liver—Obstructive jaundice, hepatic coma
  Kidney—Hematuria
  Genitals—Priapism (painful penile erection)

Sequestration Crisis
Pooling of large amounts of blood
  • Hepatomegaly
  • Splenomegaly
  • Circulatory collapse

Effects of Chronic Vasoocclusive Phenomena
Heart—Cardiomegaly, systolic murmurs
Lungs—Altered pulmonary function, susceptibility to infections, pulmonary insufficiency
Kidneys—Inability to concentrate urine, enuresis, progressive renal failure
Liver—Hepatomegaly, cirrhosis, intrahepatic cholestasis
Spleen—Splenomegaly, susceptibility to infection, functional reduction in splenic activity progressing to autosplenectomy
Eyes—Intraocular abnormalities with visual disturbances, sometimes progressive retinal detachment and blindness
Extremities—Avascular necrosis of hip or shoulder; skeletal deformities, especially lordosis and kyphosis; chronic leg ulcers; susceptibility to osteomyelitis
Central nervous system—Hemiparesis, seizures

---

minor cerebral insult, such as headache, aphasia, weakness, convulsions, visual disturbances, or unilateral hemiplegia. Loss of vision is usually the result of progressive retinopathy and retinal detachment. Cognitive impairment from SCA without any overt signs of neurologic injury is known as silent cerebral infarct (Driscoll, 2007; Buchanan, DeBaun, Quinn, et al, 2004). Silent cerebral infarct occurs in 22% of children with SCA and is defined as an abnormality on magnetic resonance imaging (Driscoll, 2007; Steen, Fineberg-Buchner, Hankins, et al, 2005; Buchanan, DeBaun, Quinn, et al, 2004).

Heart problems are mainly attributable to the stress of chronic anemia, which can eventually result in decompensation and failure. Cardiomegaly is visualized on chest radiographic examination, and a systolic flow murmur is frequently present as a consequence of the anemia. An echocardiogram shows cardiomegaly, septal hypertrophy, and impaired contractility (Heeney and Dover, 2009; Lanzkowsky, 2005).

With the formation of sickled erythrocytes, mechanical fragility increases, which decreases the life span of the RBC. Hemolysis occurs both during intravascular circulation and as

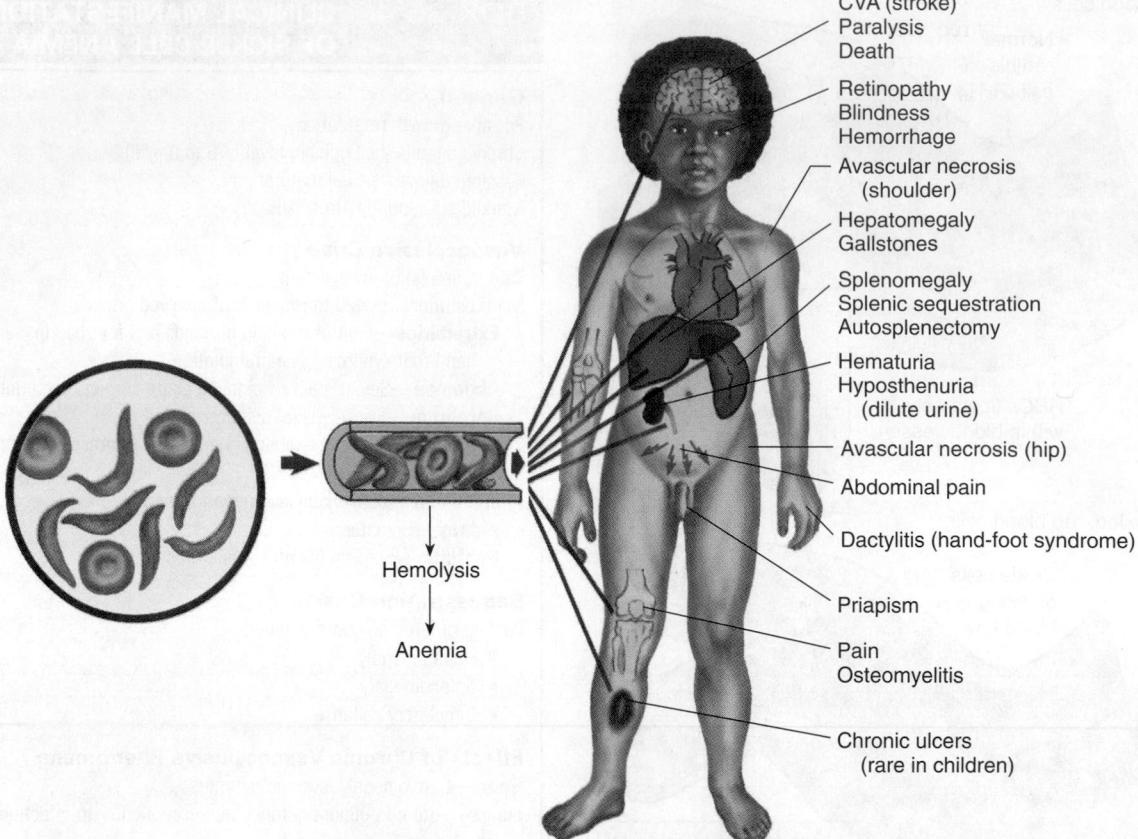

CVA (stroke)
Paralysis
Death

Retinopathy
Blindness
Hemorrhage

Avascular necrosis
(shoulder)

Hepatomegaly
Gallstones

Splenomegaly
Splenic sequestration
Autosplenectomy

Hematuria
Hyposthenuria
(dilute urine)

Avascular necrosis (hip)

Abdominal pain

Dactylitis (hand-foot syndrome)

Priapism

Pain
Osteomyelitis

Chronic ulcers
(rare in children)

Hemolysis

Anemia

Fig. 35-4 Effects of sickled red blood cells on circulation with related complications. *CVA*, Cerebrovascular accident.

a result of stagnation of sickled cells in the congested spleen (see Fig. 35-3). Although the body attempts to compensate through stimulated erythropoietic activity, as evidenced by a hyperplastic bone marrow, the rate of destruction exceeds the rate of production. A normocytic normochromic anemia results. With increased hemolysis, hemosiderosis (increased storage of iron) is present in the liver, spleen, bone marrow, kidneys, and lymph nodes (see Box 35-4).

Other Signs and Symptoms

In addition to the effects of sickling on various organ structures, the child with SCA may have a variety of complaints such as exercise intolerance, anorexia, jaundiced sclera, and gallstones. Chronic leg ulcers are common in adolescents and adults and are thought to be a result of decreased circulation due to vasoocclusion and tissue ischemia. Other generalized effects include retardation of growth in both height and weight, delayed sexual maturation, and decreased fertility. When the child reaches adulthood, full sexual development and adult height are usually achieved.

Sickle Cell Crises

The clinical manifestations of SCA vary markedly in severity and frequency. The most acute symptoms of the disease occur during periods of exacerbation called crises. There are several types of episodic crisis: vasoocclusive, acute splenic sequestration, aplastic, hyperhemolytic, stroke, chest syndrome, and infection related. The crises may occur individually or concomitantly with one or more other crises.

Vasoocclusive crisis (VOC), preferably called a *painful episode* or *event,* is the most common type of non–life-threatening crisis. It is characterized by ischemia causing mild to severe pain that may last from minutes to days. A child experiencing a VOC alone may have localized or generalized pain, acute abdominal pain from visceral hypoxia or gallstones, priapism (an unwanted painful penile erection), and arthralgia. The pain is often migratory with the presence of a low-grade fever.

VOCs can result in a variety of skeletal problems. One of the more frequent is hand-and-foot syndrome (dactylitis), which occurs primarily in young children ages 6 months to 2 years. It is caused by infarction of short tubular bones and is characterized by pain and swelling of the soft tissue over the hands and feet. It usually resolves spontaneously within a couple of days to weeks. Localized swelling over joints with arthralgia can occur from erythrostasis with sickle cells.

Sequestration crisis is caused by the pooling of large quantities of blood, usually in the spleen and infrequently in the liver, which causes a decrease in blood volume and ultimately shock. The splenic crisis may be acute or chronic. The chronic manifestation is termed hypersplenism. The acute form occurs most commonly in children between 2 months and 5 years of age and may result in death from profound anemia and cardiovascular collapse. Splenic sequestration has occurred in older children and adolescents with sickle cell C disease or sickle β-thalassemia.

Aplastic crisis is diminished RBC production, usually triggered by infection with a virus (especially the human parvovirus) or other organism. When it is superimposed on the rapid destruction of RBCs, a profound anemia results. Packed RBC transfusion is occasionally required in children exhibiting signs and symptoms of congestive heart failure.

Megaloblastic anemia is attributed to an excessive nutritional need for folic acid and/or vitamin B_{12} during periods of pronounced erythropoiesis. Because infection is not always antecedent to aplastic or hypoplastic crises, it is possible that folic acid deficiency is a causative agent.

Hyperhemolytic crisis is an accelerated rate of RBC destruction characterized by anemia, jaundice, and reticulocytosis. This complication frequently suggests other coexisting conditions, such as viral illness; transfusion reactions to alloantibodies; or glucose-6-phosphate dehydrogenase (G6PD) deficiency, which is also common in African-Americans.

A cerebrovascular accident is a sudden and severe complication, often with no related illnesses. Sickled cells block the major blood vessels in the brain, which results in cerebral infarction causing variable degrees of neurologic impairment. Repeat strokes causing progressively greater brain damage occur in approximately 70% of children who have already experienced one stroke and do not receive monthly transfusions (Heeney and Dover, 2009). The mortality rate for untreated children is approximately 20% (Heeney and Dover, 2009).

Another serious complication is acute chest syndrome, which is clinically similar to pneumonia. It is the presence of a new pulmonary infiltrate associated with chest pain, fever, cough, tachypnea, wheezing, and hypoxia (Driscoll, 2007; Heeney and Dover, 2009). Researchers believe that a VOC or infection results in sickling in the small blood vessels of the lungs, with ensuing occlusion, stasis, and anemia. Repeated episodes of chest syndrome may cause restrictive lung disease and pulmonary hypertension.

Overwhelming infection, especially with *Streptococcus pneumoniae* and *H. influenzae* type b as a result of defective splenic function, is the major cause of death in children with SCD under the age of 5 years. Repeated insults on the splenic sinuses by sickled cells result in impaired filtration and function, which allows the development of septicemia and possibly subsequent death.

Diagnostic Evaluation

Although SCA has been reported during the neonatal period and early part of infancy, it may not be recognized until the toddler or preschool period, during a crisis precipitated by an acute upper respiratory tract or gastrointestinal infection. However, early diagnosis (before 3 months of age) facilitates initiation of appropriate interventions to minimize complications. Several specific tests detect abnormal hemoglobin in the homozygous or heterozygous form of the disease.

Examination of a stained blood smear may reveal a few sickled RBCs. Because the erythrocyte assumes its normal discoid shape under adequate oxygenation, however, no sickled cells may be present even in the homozygous form of the disease. Whenever sickle cells are found, diagnostic test results are usually positive for SCA, not sickle cell trait.

For screening purposes the sickle turbidity test (Sickledex) is performed on anticoagulated blood, which is mixed with a special solution. Because HgbS is normally much less soluble than HgbA or HgbF (as well as other variants), when it is com-

bined with this solution, it forms a cloudy or turbid mixture. All other forms of hemoglobin result in a clear suspension. This test is a reliable screening method that uses blood from a finger or heel stick and yields accurate results in 3 minutes. If the test result is positive, however, hemoglobin electrophoresis is necessary to distinguish between those children with the trait and those children with the disease.

In hemoglobin electrophoresis, the blood is specially prepared and separated into various hemoglobins by high-voltage electrophoresis. The resulting pattern of the separated peptides as it appears on paper is referred to as *fingerprinting* of the protein. This test is accurate, rapid, and specific for detecting the homozygous and heterozygous forms of the disease, as well as the percentages of the various hemoglobins.

Screening of Newborns

Screening for SCD in the newborn period can identify children with hemoglobinopathies. Screening of newborns for SCD is performed in the majority of states, the District of Columbia, Puerto Rico, and the Virgin Islands (Driscoll, 2007; Pack-Mabien and Haynes, 2009). It provides early identification of these children before complications develop. Early diagnosis facilitates parental education regarding the importance of immunizations, penicillin prophylaxis, detection of splenomegaly, and the need to report fever and increasing pallor, all of which may be lifesaving (DeBaun and Vichinsky, 2007; Heeney and Dover, 2009).

The death rate from splenic sequestration and septicemia has decreased. Teach parents to palpate the child's spleen and seek medical attention at the first sign of complications (DeBaun and Vichinsky, 2007; Heeney and Dover, 2009; Pack-Mabien and Haynes, 2009). Penicillin prophylaxis is started by 2 months of age, and parents are instructed to seek medical attention if their child develops a fever of 38.3° C (101° F) or higher (see Evidence-Based Practice box).

Therapeutic Management

The aims of therapy are (1) to prevent the sickling phenomenon, which is responsible for the pathologic sequelae; and (2) to treat the medical emergency of sickle cell crisis. The successful achievement of these aims depends on prompt nursing interventions and medical therapies, child and family preventive measures, and innovative treatment interventions.

Three general forms of treatment are available: supportive-symptomatic, specific, and curative. Hydroxyurea is the only effective drug approved by the U.S. Food and Drug Administration (FDA) to reduce the incidence of recurrent severe painful episodes and acute chest syndrome by increasing the concentration of HgbF and ultimately to reduce complications (DeBaun and Vichinsky, 2007; Pack-Mabien and Haynes, 2009). Recent research is investigating the use of hydroxyurea to prevent stroke (Gulbis, Haberman, DuFour, et al, 2005; Heeney and Ware, 2008). Hematopoietic stem cell transplantation (HSCT) is the only potential for cure of SCD with a high risk of neurologic complications (DeBaun and Vichinsky, 2007; Driscoll, 2007).

Medical management of a crisis is directed at supportive, symptomatic, and specific treatments. The main objectives are to provide (1) bed rest to minimize energy expenditure and to

Case Study—Sickle Cell Anemia

EVIDENCE-BASED PRACTICE

Sickle Cell Anemia and Penicillin Prophylaxis

ASK THE QUESTION

In children with sickle cell anemia does prophylaxis with penicillin reduce the risk of pneumococcal infection?

SEARCH FOR THE EVIDENCE

Search strategies

Search selection criteria included English-language publications within the past 25 years, research-based articles (level 3 or lower), and child populations.

Databases used

PubMed, Cochrane Collaboration, MD Consult

CRITICALLY ANALYZE THE EVIDENCE

GRADE criteria: Strong evidence, strong recommendation (Guyatt, Oxman, Vist, et al, 2008)

Hirst and Owusu-Ofori (2009) conducted an updated systematic Cochrane review of three trials that showed a reduced rate of infection in children with sickle cell disease receiving penicillin preventively. Two trials looked at whether treatment was effective. The third trial continued one of the early trials and looked at when it was safe to stop treatment. Adverse drug effects were rare and minor. Researchers found that penicillin given preventively reduces the rate of pneumococcal infections in children with sickle cell disease under 5 years old.

Researchers combined the clinical experiences of three sickle cell programs in the eastern United States in an attempt to determine the age and disease-specific risk of *Streptococcus pneumoniae* bacteremia and meningitis in children with SCD at a time when penicillin prophylaxis was routine (Hord, Byrd, Stowe, et al, 2002). Forty-seven pneumococcal infections (44 bacteremia, 3 meningitis) among 40 patients with SCD were observed. Most children who developed infections were reportedly taking prophylactic penicillin and received pneumococcal vaccine (Pneumovax) at age 24 months. The observed severe pneumococcal infection rate in HgbSS children younger than 5 years was less than that reported before penicillin prophylaxis in this specific population.

Administration of oral prophylactic penicillin was compared to the 14-valent pneumococcal vaccine in preventing pneumococcal infection in 242 children between the ages of 6 months and 3 years with homozygous sickle cell disease (John, Ramlal, Jackson, et al, 1984). In the first 5 years of the trial, there were 11 pneumococcal infections in the pneumococcal vaccine group and higher infection rates in those given the vaccine before 1 year of age. No pneumococcal isolates were found in the group receiving penicillin, although four pneumococcal isolates were found in this group within 1 year of stopping the penicillin prophylaxis at age 3 years. This study supported the use of penicillin prophylaxis to prevent pneumococcal infection in children younger than 3 years of age.

In a multicenter, randomized, double-blind, placebo-controlled clinical trial, 105 children received penicillin twice daily; a control group of 110 children received a placebo twice daily (Gaston, Verter, Woods, et al, 1986). The trial was terminated 8 months early when an 84% reduction in the incidence of pneumococcal infections was observed in the group treated with penicillin compared with the placebo group. There were no deaths in the penicillin group, but three deaths from infection occurred in the placebo group. Researchers stressed the importance of screening children during the neonatal period and prescribing prophylactic penicillin to decrease the morbidity and mortality associated with pneumococcal infection.

Zarkowsky, Gallagher, Gill, and colleagues (1986) conducted a retrospective analysis of 178 episodes of bacteremia in children with sickle hemoglobinopathies that occurred during 13,771 patient-years of follow-up ($N = 3451$). The predominant pathogen in patients younger than 6 years of age was *S. pneumoniae* (66%), and gram-negative organisms were responsible for 50% of the bacteremias in patients 6 years and older. The incidence of pneumococcal bacteremia in children with sickle cell anemia younger than 3 years of age was 6.1 events per 100 patient-years. The results of this study supported prophylactic administration of penicillin for prevention of pneumococcal bacteremia in children younger than 3 years of age.

A cohort study of 315 patients with homozygous sickle cell disease who lived in Jamaica was conducted between June 1973 and December 1981 (Lee, Thomas, Cupidore, et al, 1995). The patients were divided into three groups to determine whether interventions such as penicillin prophylaxis, parental education in early diagnosis of acute splenic sequestration, and close monitoring in a sickle cell clinic improved survival. A significant decline in deaths from acute splenic sequestration and pneumococcal septicemia and meningitis was found. The research indicated that early detection of sickle cell disease and prophylactic measures could significantly reduce deaths associated with homozygous sickle cell disease.

Riddington and Owusu-Ofori (2002) conducted a systematic review of randomized controlled trials evaluating the effectiveness of prophylactic antibiotic administration in preventing pneumococcal infection in children with sickle cell disease. The review of published research found that penicillin prophylaxis significantly reduced the risk of pneumococcal infection in children with homozygous sickle cell disease with minimal adverse reactions.

APPLY THE EVIDENCE: NURSING IMPLICATIONS

- The evidence demonstrated that penicillin prophylaxis significantly reduces the risk of pneumococcal infection in children with sickle cell anemia.
- The epidemiologic studies strongly suggest that all children with sickle cell anemia should be started on prophylactic penicillin at 2 months of age.
- Nurse should instruct parents and children with sickle cell anemia in the importance of taking the prophylactic penicillin twice daily and seeking medical attention immediately for acute illness, especially if the temperature exceeds 38.3° C (101° F), regardless of the use of prophylaxis.

References

Gaston MH, Verter JI, Woods G, et al: Prophylaxis with oral penicillin in children with sickle cell anemia: a randomized trial, *N Engl J Med* 314(25):1593-1599, 1986.

Guyatt GH, Oxman AD, Vist GE, et al: GRADE: an emerging consensus on rating quality of evidence and strength of recommendations, *BMJ* 336:924-926, 2008.

Hirst C, Owusu-Ofori S: Prophylactic antibiotics for preventing pneumococcal infection in children with sickle cell disease, *Cochrane Syst Rev* 3:CD003427, 2009.

Hord J, Byrd R, Stowe L, et al: *Streptococcus pneumoniae* sepsis and meningitis during the penicillin prophylaxis era in children with sickle cell disease, *J Pediatr Hematol Oncol* 24(6):470-472, 2002.

John AB, Ramlal A, Jackson H, et al: Prevention of pneumococcal infection in children with homozygous sickle cell disease, *BMJ* 288(6430):1567-1570, 1984.

Lee A, Thomas P, Cupidore L, et al: Improved survival in homozygous sickle cell disease: lessons from cohort study, *BMJ* 311(7020):1600-1602, 1995.

Riddington C, Owusu-Ofori S: *Prophylactic antibiotics for preventing pneumococcal infection in children with sickle cell disease*, 2002, available at www.cochrane.org/reviews/en/ab003427.html (accessed August 19, 2005).

Zarkowsky HS, Gallagher D, Gill FM, et al: Bacteremia in sickle hemoglobinopathies, *J Pediatr* 109(4):579-585, 1986.

improve oxygen utilization; (2) hydration through oral and IV therapy; (3) electrolyte replacement, since hypoxia results in metabolic acidosis, which also promotes sickling; (4) analgesia for severe pain from vasoocclusion (see pp. 1432-1433); (5) blood replacement to treat anemia and to reduce the viscosity of the sickled blood; and (6) antibiotic therapy to treat any existing infection.

Administration of pneumococcal, *H. influenzae* type b, and meningococcal vaccines is recommended for these children because of their susceptibility to infection from functional asplenia. (See Immunizations, Chapter 12.) Oral penicillin prophylaxis is recommended by 2 months of age to reduce the chance of pneumococcal sepsis (see Evidence-Based Practice box, p. 1430). The nurse assumes an important role in helping the family comply with a medication regimen and seek medical attention immediately when the child has a fever of 38.3° C (101° F) or higher, an increase in spleen size, or severe pallor (Akinyanju, Otaigbe, and Ibidapo, 2005; Driscoll, 2007; Pack-Mabien and Haynes, 2009).

Oxygen therapy is of little therapeutic value unless the patient is hypoxic (Heeney and Dover, 2009). Oxygen administration is usually not effective in reversing sickling or reducing pain because the oxygen is not able to reach the enmeshed sickled RBCs through the clogged vessels (Chiocca, 1996; Perkins, 2001). In addition, prolonged administration of oxygen can depress bone marrow activity, which further aggravates the anemia (Khoury and Grimsley, 1995).

The use of blood transfusions is another important component of care. An RBC transfusion is used in aplastic, hyperhemolytic, and splenic sequestration crises; in stroke prevention; and before general surgery. Exchange transfusion is a successful, rapid method of reducing the number of circulating sickle cells and therefore slowing down the vicious circle of hypoxia, tissue ischemia, and injury. It is used in acute chest syndrome and after a stroke to prevent recurrence and further tissue damage. Routine transfusions to maintain the hemoglobin value between 9 and 10 g/dl in children with central nervous system disease can minimize the chances of further neurologic problems. In the event of major surgery, exchange or partial exchange transfusions may be given preoperatively to prevent anoxia and suppress the formation of new sickle cells. A simple packed RBC transfusion to raise the hemoglobin value to 10 g/dl, as well as maintenance hydration preoperatively and postoperatively, is sufficient to prevent sickling complications secondary to anesthesia (DeBaun and Vichinsky, 2007; Heeney and Dover, 2009; Vichinsky, Haberkern, Neumayr, et al, 1995). However, sickle cell patients with a higher surgical risk, which may include a history of pulmonary disease, previous acute chest syndrome, stroke, or multiple hospitalizations, should undergo exchange transfusion or multiple simple transfusions to reduce the chance of SCD complications by decreasing the level of HgbS to less than 30%.

Multiple transfusions carry the risk of transmission of viral infection, hyperviscosity, transfusion reactions, alloimmunization, and hemosiderosis (Hankins, Jeng, Harris, et al, 2005; Heeney and Dover, 2009). To reduce iron overload, chelation therapy may be started (see p. 1438). Historically, deferoxamine (Desferal), as an effective parenteral chelator, was administered at 30 to 40 mg/kg over 8 to 10 hours for 5 or 6 nights per week. Deferoxamine is now used either alone or in combination with an oral chelator. Deferasirox (approved by the FDA in 2004) and deferiprone (not been approved by the FDA, but approved in more than 40 other countries) are two new oral iron chelators used worldwide alone or in combination with deferoxamine (Cunningham, Sankaran, Nathan, et al, 2009).

The appropriate time for beginning treatment is controversial, but chelation is often initiated when the ferritin level is higher than 1000 ng/ml or after a year or more of three or four weekly transfusions. Because the ferritin level is also an acute phase reactant, it is recognized as an ineffective or inaccurate test to determine iron overload (DeBaun and Vichinsky, 2007; Olivieri, 1999). In contrast, testing of a liver biopsy specimen allows an accurate and direct measurement of iron concentration but is not without risk of hemorrhage, infection, and discomfort (Cunningham, Sankaran, Nathan, et al, 2009; Olivieri, 1999). Emerging noninvasive alternatives for liver biopsy based on the magnetic properties of iron are known as *magnetic susceptometry* and *superconducting quantum interference devices*. Both devices provide an accurate measurement of hepatic iron (Brown, Subramony, May, et al, 2009; DeBaun and Vichinsky, 2007). However, neither of these specialized devices is readily available to the majority of centers.

Children with HgbSS disease and HgbS-β⁰-thalassemia have the highest risk of stroke and should be monitored with transcranial Doppler ultrasonography (TCD) (Driscoll, 2007; Heeney and Dover, 2009). TCD is a cost-effective, noninvasive ultrasound technique that screens for stroke risk in children who have SCD. TCD is performed yearly on children with SCD from 2 to 16 years of age and measures the intracranial vascular flow within the large cerebral arteries (Bulas, 2005; DeBaun and Vichinsky, 2007; Platt, 2006). The recommended treatment for children with confirmed abnormal TCD findings is chronic transfusion therapy (DeBaun and Vichinsky, 2007; Armstrong-Wells, Grimes, Sidney, et al, 2009). Multiple transfusions carry the risk of transmission of viral infection, hyperviscosity, transfusion reactions, alloimmunization, and hemosiderosis, which must be discussed with the parents or legal guardian before the initiation of a transfusion program.

In children with recurrent life-threatening splenic sequestration, splenectomy may be a lifesaving measure. However, the spleen usually atrophies on its own through progressive fibrotic changes (functional asplenia) by 6 years of age in children with SCA. Surgical splenectomy or autosplenectomy has several benefits because the spleen is the major site of sickling, sequestration, and destruction of RBCs.

Prognosis

The prognosis varies, but most patients live into their fifth decade. The greatest risk is usually in children younger than 5 years of age, and the majority of deaths in these children are caused by overwhelming infection. As the child grows older, however, the crises usually become less severe and less frequent, although death in early adulthood is not uncommon. Consequently SCA is a chronic illness with a potentially terminal outcome. Physical and sexual maturation are delayed in adolescents with SCA. Although adults achieve normal height, weight, and sexual function, the delay may present problems to the adolescent (Heeney and Dover, 2009; Redding-Lallinger, and Knoll, 2006). In some young people chronic pain becomes a significant problem. HSCT offers a curative approach for some children with SCD with an event-free survival of 95% (Driscoll, 2007; Haining, Duncan, and Lehmann, 2009).

Children and adolescents younger than 16 years of age who have severe complications (stroke, recurrent acute chest syndrome, or refractory pain) and have a human leukocyte antigen (HLA)–matched donor available are the best candidates for transplantation (DeBaun and Vichinsky, 2007; Haining, Duncan, and Lehmann, 2009). Eventually, improved survival with other HSCT modalities, such as umbilical cord blood transplantation, haploidentical transplants, and nonmyeloablative conditioning regimens, may augment sibling donor protocols and widen the availability of HSCT as a potential cure to SCD patients (Driscoll, 2007).

Nursing Care Management

Many nurses are involved in SCA screening programs to identify persons with the abnormal hemoglobin so that therapy can be implemented for homozygotes and genetic counseling provided for heterozygotes. The nurse should seek medical attention immediately for young children who exhibit any of the signs previously described and whose families belong to a racial or geographic group know to be at risk for SCD.

QUALITY PATIENT OUTCOMES: Sickle Cell Disease
- Early recognition of signs and symptoms of sickle cell anemia
- Tissue deoxygenation minimized
- Sickle cell crisis prevented or quickly managed
- Pain appropriately managed
- Stroke prevented
- Prophylactic penicillin regimen followed
- Hypoxia prevented when surgery is necessary
- Pneumococcal, *H. influenzae* type b, and meningococcal vaccines administered

---

Assessment of the child in sickle cell crisis includes all areas and systems that can be affected by circulatory obstruction, including vital signs; neurologic signs; vision; hearing; and the respiratory, gastrointestinal, renal, and musculoskeletal systems. It is also important to identify the location and intensity of pain.

Minimize Tissue Deoxygenation

Anything that increases cellular metabolism also results in tissue hypoxia. For the child, minimization of tissue deoxygenation includes (1) taking frequent rest breaks during physical activities; (2) avoiding contact sports if the spleen is enlarged, because rupture will cause massive internal hemorrhage; (3) avoiding environments with low oxygen concentration, such as high altitudes or nonpressurized airplane flights; and (4) avoiding known sources of infection. If the child has even a mild infection, the parents must seek medical attention at once.

Promote Hydration

The nurse emphasizes the importance of adequate hydration to prevent sickling and delay the vasoocclusion and hypoxia-ischemia cycle. The nurse calculates the child's fluid requirements (approximately 1600 ml/m²/day), which is the minimum daily fluid intake. The nurse also assesses the child's usual fluid consumption to evaluate its adequacy and makes adjustments

based on this knowledge. It is not sufficient to advise parents to "force fluids" or "encourage drinking." They need specific instructions on how many glasses or bottles of fluid are required. Many foods are also a source of fluid, particularly soups, popsicles, yogurt, ice cream, sherbet, gelatin, and puddings.

Encourage children to drink by giving them a special cup, thermos, or water bottle with a straw from which to drink throughout the day. The nurse advises parents to take advantage of times of thirst, such as on awakening or after playing; to serve frequent small portions; and to leave the cup within easy reach for self-service. Flavored ice pops and crushed ice "slurpies" are sources of fluid commonly accepted by children.

Because the kidneys' ability to concentrate urine is impaired, the child is especially prone to dehydration. Dilute urine or urine of low specific gravity is no longer a valid sign of adequate hydration. Parents should observe for other indications of fluid loss, such as dry mucous membranes, dry diapers, weight loss, and a sunken fontanel in infants. In addition, without the ability to conserve water by concentrating urine, the child is prone to dehydration from environmental factors, particularly overheating. The nurse alerts parents to the need for the child to wear proper indoor and outdoor clothing and avoid excessive exposure to the sun.

Increased fluid intake combined with impaired kidney function result in the problem of enuresis. Parents who are unaware of this fact frequently employ the usual measures to discourage bed-wetting, such as limiting fluids at night, and may resort to punishment and shaming to force bladder control. The nurse discusses this problem with the parents, stressing that the child's ability to concentrate urine is impaired. Reminding the child to urinate frequently during the day is helpful, and waking the child during the night may prove beneficial if the child's sleep patterns are not disturbed. Parents who are toilet training their toddlers should be aware of the more frequent pattern of urination and increased difficulty in learning control. Enuresis is treated as a complication of the disease to alleviate parental pressure on the child and to prevent any fluid restriction.

Minimize Crises

Because infection is the major cause of death due to the body's inability to resist infection, the nurse stresses to parents the importance of adequate nutrition, frequent medical supervision, proper hand washing, and isolation from known sources of infection. Keep in mind that children also need to live a normal life. Overprotection can be as devastating emotionally as an infection is physically. Parents need to be aware of the need to seek prompt medical care at the first sign of any infection.

Teach the family the signs and symptoms of crises and advise them to seek medical attention immediately when any are present. Teaching parents spleen palpation for earlier detection of splenic sequestration can reduce mortality from this serious complication.

Promote Supportive Therapies

The success of many of the medical therapies relies heavily on nursing implementation. Management of pain is an especially difficult problem and often involves experimenting with various analgesics, including opioids, and various schedules before relief is achieved. Unfortunately, these children tend to be undermedicated, which results in "clock watching" and demands for additional doses sooner than might be expected. Often this incorrectly raises suspicion of drug addiction, when in fact the problem is one of inadequate pain control (see Family-Centered Care box). In choosing and scheduling analgesics, the goal is prevention of pain.

Pain is the most common and debilitating symptom experienced by patients with SCD (Driscoll, 2007; Shaiova and Wallenstein, 2004) (see Fig. 35-4). Beyer (2000) found that 15 of 21 children with SCD who were receiving IV pain medication for a painful crisis continued to report moderate to severe pain. Recommendations for continuous adjustment of analgesics were emphasized in this study.

The chronic nature of this pain can greatly affect the child's development. A multidisciplinary approach is best for its management. When mild to moderate pain is reported, acetaminophen (Tylenol) or ibuprofen is initially used. If acetaminophen or ibuprofen alone is not effective, codeine can be added. The dosages of the drugs are titrated (adjusted) to a therapeutic level. Opioids such as immediate- and sustained-release morphine, oxycodone, hydromorphone, and methadone are administered parenterally or orally for severe pain and are given around the clock. Patient-controlled analgesia (PCA) has been used successfully for sickle cell–related pain. PCA reinforces the patient's role and responsibility in managing the pain and provides flexibility, since pain may vary in severity over time. If PCA devices are not available or delayed in set-up, a recent study reported intranasal diamorphine was safely combined with oral morphine to manage initial sickle cell pain in most pediatric cases until commencement of IV opiates (Telfer, Lahoz, Ali, et al, 2009).

Medication given by mouth can be as effective as IV medication when equianalgesic dosages are prescribed.

The nurse should combine any pain management program with psychologic support to help the child deal with the depression, anxiety, and fear that accompany the disease. This includes regular visits with the child to discuss his or her concerns during the hospitalization and positive reinforcement of adaptive coping skills, such as successful methods of dealing with the pain and compliance with treatment prescriptions. To reduce the negative connotation associated with the term *crisis*, it is best to say "pain episode."

Frequently heat to the affected area is soothing. Cold compresses are not applied to the area because doing so enhances vasoconstriction and occlusion. Bed rest is usually well tolerated during a crisis, although the actual rest obtained depends a great deal on pain alleviation and the use of organized schedules of nursing care. Although the objective of bed rest is to minimize oxygen consumption, some activity, particularly passive range-of-motion exercises, is beneficial to promote circulation. Usually the best course is to let children determine their activity tolerance.

If blood transfusions or exchange transfusions are given, the nurse has the responsibility of observing for signs of transfusion reaction (see Table 35-2). Because hypervolemia from too rapid transfusion can increase the workload of the heart, the nurse also must be alert to signs of cardiac failure.

In splenic sequestration, gently measure the size of the spleen, since increasing splenomegaly is an ominous sign. A decrease in the size of the spleen denotes response to therapy. The nurse also closely monitors vital signs and blood pressure to detect impending shock. Anemia is typically not a presenting complication in VOCs but is a critical problem in other types of crisis. The nurse monitors for evidence of increasing anemia and institutes appropriate nursing intervention.

Oxygen administration is not beneficial in vasoocclusive episodes unless hypoxemia is present (Heeney and Dover, 2009). It does not reverse sickled RBCs, and if used in a non-hypoxic patient, it decreases erythropoiesis (Vichinsky and Styles, 1996). Because prolonged oxygen therapy can aggravate the anemia, report any signs of lack of therapeutic benefit, such as restlessness, increased pallor, and continued pain.

Record intake, especially of IV fluids, and output. The child's weight should be taken on admission, since it serves as a baseline for evaluating hydration. Because diuresis can result in electrolyte loss, the nurse observes for signs of hypokalemia and should be familiar with normal serum electrolyte values to report changes. Nurses also need to be aware of the signs of chest syndrome and stroke, both potentially fatal complications (see Nursing Alert, p. 1434).

Decrease Surgical Risks

The main surgical risk is hypoxia from anesthesia. However, emotional stress, the demands of wound healing, and infection potentially increase the sickling phenomenon, both in children with the disease and in those with the trait. The primary nursing objectives are to minimize each of these threats preoperatively and postoperatively by keeping the child well hydrated, preparing the child psychologically, and preventing infection.

Encourage Screening and Genetic Counseling

Screening is recommended during the neonatal period, since early diagnosis allows earlier, more prevention-oriented treatment, such as prophylactic antibiotic therapy and parent education about potential complications. The advantages of trait identification lie in selective reproduction of offspring not afflicted with HgbS. Alternate methods of childbearing include artificial insemination, adoption, and abortion of affected fetuses. However, for some these alternatives are unacceptable.

To be effective, combine screening with genetic counseling and long-term follow-up. The nurse can be instrumental in such programs by conducting parent education sessions, providing follow-up for the family in the home, disseminating correct information about the disease and trait to the community, and rendering support to parents of children newly diagnosed with the trait or the disease. A primary consideration in genetic counseling is informing parents of the 25% chance with each pregnancy of having a child with the disease when both parents carry the trait. (See Chapter 5.)

> **NURSING TIP** One simple yet graphic way of illustrating the difference between normal discoid RBCs and sickle cells is to roll round or oval objects, such as marbles, through a tube to demonstrate normal blood cell circulation and then roll pointed objects such as screws or jacks through the tube. The effect of sickling and clumping of the pointed objects is especially noticeable at a bend or slight narrowing of the tube. This same idea can be expanded to discuss the importance of increased fluid in keeping the pointed objects suspended away from each other to prevent concentration.

Prenatal diagnosis is possible through amniocentesis or fetoscopy and fetal blood sampling during the sixteenth week of gestation. Analysis of amniotic cells for a DNA fragment associated with the gene responsible for sickled β-globulin chain synthesis can be performed as early as the twelfth week with chorionic sampling. In the event the fetus is affected, the decision regarding termination of the pregnancy should be left to the couple.

Explain the Disease

Because SCA may be recognized when the child is a toddler, most of the nurse's counseling is directed at the parents. The nurse explains to parents the basic effect of tissue hypoxia on RBCs and the effect of sickling on the circulation (see Fig. 35-3). Taking time to establish a sound basis of understanding regarding why certain measures are beneficial to the child encourages parents to practice them.*†

---

*Sickle Cell Disease Association of America, Inc., 231 E. Baltimore St., Suite 800, Baltimore, MD 21202; 410-528-1555, 800-421-8453; fax: 410-528-1495; e-mail: scdaa@sicklecelldisease.org; www.sicklecelldisease.org; Sickle Cell Information Center, PO Box 109, Grady Memorial Hospital, 80 Jesse Hill Jr. Drive SE, Atlanta, GA 30303; 404-616-3572; fax: 404-616-5998; e-mail: aplatt@emory.edu; www.scinfo.org; National Heart, Lung, and Blood Institute Health Information Center, PO Box 30105, Bethesda, MD 20824-0105; 301-592-8573; TTY: 240-629-3255; fax: 240-629-3246; www.nhlbi.nih.gov. *Guideline for the Management of Acute and Chronic Pain in Sickle-Cell Disease* is available from the American Pain Society, 4700 W. Lake Ave., Glenview, IL 60025-1485; 847-375-4715; fax: 866-572-2654; e-mail: info@ampainsoc.org, www.ampainsoc.org.

†A video, *Sickle Cell Is More Than Pain Management—Student Manual,* is available from maxiSHARE, PO Box 2041, Milwaukee, WI 53201; 800-444-7747; fax: 414-266-1540; www.maxishare.com.

The nurse advises the parents to inform all treating practitioners of the child's condition. The use of a medical identification bracelet is another way of ensuring awareness of the disease. Some people view such identification as "negative labeling." The nurse can stress the benefits of displaying this information, especially in emergencies when anesthesia may be required.

> **! NURSING ALERT**
>
> Report signs of the following immediately:
> Acute chest syndrome
> - Severe chest pain, back, or abdominal pain
> - Fever of 38.3° C (101° F) or higher
> - Cough
> - Dyspnea, tachypnea
> - Retractions
> - Declining oxygen saturation (by oximetry)
>
> Stroke
> - Severe, unrelieved headaches
> - Severe vomiting
> - Jerking or twitching of the face, legs, or arms
> - Seizures
> - Strange, abnormal behavior
> - Inability to move an arm or a leg
> - Stagger or an unsteady walk
> - Stutter or slurred speech
> - Weakness in the hands, feet, or legs
> - Changes in vision

Support the Family

Families need the opportunity to discuss their feelings regarding transmitting a potentially fatal, chronic illness to their child. Some parents are able to cope with this fact; some feel great guilt and remorse for giving their child the disease, whereas others regret not knowing that they carried the trait. For many parents decision making regarding subsequent pregnancies is fraught with doubt and ambivalence.

Because of the widely publicized prognosis for children with SCA, many parents express their fear of death. The prognosis varies; with early diagnosis and treatment these children are living longer. The predictors of a severe course of SCA are a low hemoglobin level (approximately 7 g/dl), dactylitis or painful episode, and elevated WBC count exhibited before the age of 24 months (DeBaun and Vichinsky, 2007; Miller, Sleeper, Pegelow, et al, 2000). The nurse should care for the family as for any family with a child who has a chronic and life-threatening illness, and give some consideration to the siblings' reactions, the stress on the marital relationship, and the childrearing attitudes displayed toward the child (see Nursing Care Plan). (See Chapters 22 and 23.)

β-THALASSEMIA

Worldwide, thalassemia is a common genetic disorder affecting as many as 15 million people (Yalsh, 2009). The term *thalassemia* comes from the Greek word *thalassa,* meaning "sea," and is applied to a variety of inherited blood disorders characterized by deficiencies in the rate of production of specific globin chains in hemoglobin. The name appropriately refers to people

◎ NURSING CARE PLAN

The Child with Sickle Cell Anemia

NURSING DIAGNOSIS	EXPECTED PATIENT OUTCOMES	NURSING INTERVENTIONS	RATIONALE
Risk for Injury related to abnormal hemoglobin level, decreased ambient oxygen level **Child's/Family's Defining Characteristics (Subjective and Objective Data)** Shortness of breath, dyspnea Fatigue, headache, pallor Icteric sclera or jaundice Systolic murmur, cyanosis, increased pulse rate	Child will avoid situations that reduce tissue oxygenation and allow for adequate tissue oxygenation. **The Following NOC Concept Applies to This Outcome** Risk Control	Explain measures to minimize complications related to physical exertion and emotional stress. Prevent infection. Advise to avoid low-oxygen environments (e.g., high altitudes, nonpressurized airplane flights). **The Following NIC Concepts Apply to These Interventions** Health Education Behavior Modification	To avoid additional tissue oxygen needs To reduce risk for infection due to reduced tissue oxygenation To prevent a decrease in oxygenation

NURSING DIAGNOSIS	EXPECTED PATIENT OUTCOMES	NURSING INTERVENTIONS	RATIONALE
Deficient Fluid volume **Child's/Family's Defining Characteristics (Subjective and Objective Data)** Dry mucous membranes Loss of skin turgor Sunken eyes No or diminished tears Sunken fontanel Dark urine Rapid, thready pulse Rapid breathing Lethargy, weakness	Child will take adequate amounts of fluids and show no signs of dehydration. **The Following NOC Concepts Apply to These Outcomes** Fluid Balance Electrolyte and Acid/Base Balance	Calculate recommended daily fluid intake (1600 ml/m^2/day) and base child's fluid requirements on this amount. Increase fluid intake above minimum requirements during physical exercise or emotional stress and during a crisis. Give parents written instructions regarding specific quantity of fluid required daily. Encourage child to drink. Stress importance of avoiding overheating. Teach family signs of dehydration. **The Following NIC Concepts Apply to These Interventions** Fluid Management Fluid/Electrolyte Management	To ensure adequate hydration To compensate for additional fluid needs To encourage compliance To ensure adequate hydration To minimize fluid loss To avoid delay in rehydration therapy

NURSING DIAGNOSIS	EXPECTED PATIENT OUTCOMES	NURSING INTERVENTIONS	RATIONALE
Acute Pain related to tissue anoxia (vasoocclusive crisis) **Child's/Family's Defining Characteristics (Subjective and Objective Data)** Pain can be in any location in the body; can be rapid in onset and severe, may be localized or generalized Low-grade fever may be present Localized swelling over joints with arthralgia can occur	Child will experience no or minimal pain. **The Following NOC Concepts Apply to These Outcomes** Comfort Level Pain Control	Discuss preventive schedule of medication around the clock with parents. Encourage high level of fluid intake. Recognize that various analgesics, including opioids and medication schedules, may need to be tried. Reassure child and family that analgesics, including opioids, are medically indicated, that high doses may be needed, and that children rarely become addicted. Apply heat to or massage affected area. Avoid applying cold compresses. Instruct parents to seek medical attention immediately for sudden, persistent headache; weakness on one side of the body; sudden gait or speech problems; or altered mental status. **The Following NIC Concepts Apply to These Interventions** Medication Management Pain Management Patient-Controlled Analgesia Assistance	To prevent pain To ensure hydration To ensure satisfactory pain relief To avoid needless suffering because of unfounded fears To prevent vasoconstriction that may enhance sickling To prevent vasoconstriction that may enhance sickling To prevent progressive central nervous system (CNS) damage through recognition of acute CNS events

Continued

⊚ **NURSING CARE PLAN—cont'd**

The Child with Sickle Cell Anemia

NURSING DIAGNOSIS	EXPECTED PATIENT OUTCOMES	NURSING INTERVENTIONS	RATIONALE
Risk for Infection **Child's/Family's Defining Characteristics (Subjective and Objective Data)** Fever, chills, pain, redness Lethargy, increased pallor, listlessness, irritability Increased pulse and respiration rates History of prior sepsis	Child will remain free of infection. **The Following NOC Concept Applies to This Outcome** Infection Severity	Stress importance of adequate nutrition; routine immunizations, including pneumococcal and meningococcal vaccinations; protection from known sources of infection; and frequent health evaluation and regularly scheduled comprehensive evaluation. Report any signs of infection immediately. Promote compliance with prophylactic antibiotic therapy Instruct parents regarding signs and symptoms of splenic sequestration and regular palpation of the spleen. **The Following NIC Concepts Apply to These Interventions** Environmental Management Communicable Disease Management Medication Prescribing Medication Administration Medication Management	To encourage preventive measures and decrease risk for infection exposure To avoid delay in treatment To prevent and treat infection To enable early recognition of splenic sequestration crisis
NURSING DIAGNOSIS	EXPECTED PATIENT OUTCOMES	NURSING INTERVENTIONS	RATIONALE
Deficient Knowledge related to understanding of sickle cell disease and its management **Child's/Family's Defining Characteristics (Subjective and Objective Data)** Lack of understanding Inability to identify signs and symptoms of painful crises Inability to follow disease management guidelines Difficulty describing treatment plan Improper medication administration	Child and family will demonstrate understanding of the disease, its cause, and its treatment. **The Following NOC Concepts Apply to These Outcomes** Family Coping Knowledge: Illness Care	Teach family and children characteristics of basic genetic defect and measures to minimize complications. Stress importance of informing significant health personnel of child's disease. Explain signs of developing complications such as fever, pallor, respiratory distress, persistent headaches, and pain. Reinforce basic information regarding trait transmission and refer to genetic counseling services. Teach parents to be an advocate for their child. Educate the school and teachers regarding the cause of sickle cell disease and measures to avoid complications within the classroom. Stress with educators the need to provide tutorials and to allow child time to make up schoolwork during medical absences. **The Following NIC Concepts Apply to These Interventions** Teaching: Disease Process Teaching: Prescribed Medication	To minimize complications of sickling To provide support and prevent complications To ensure prompt and appropriate treatment To allow for informed decision making To provide support and prevent complications To provide support and prevent complications To provide support and prevent complications

living near the Mediterranean Sea, namely, Italians, Greeks, and Syrians, or to their descendants. Evidence suggests that the high incidence of the disorder among these groups is a result of selective advantage of the trait in protecting against malaria, as is postulated for SCD. The disorder has a wide geographic distribution, however, probably as a result of genetic migration through intermarriages or possibly as a result of spontaneous mutation.

The thalassemias are classified according to the hemoglobin chain affected and the amount of the globin chain that is synthesized. The two major categories are α-thalassemia and

β-thalassemia. Thalassemia is seen in various population groups, such as Asians, Africans, and inhabitants of the Mediterranean and Middle Eastern regions, and the majority of births of affected individuals occur in these groups (Cohen, Galanello, Rennell, et al, 2004; Cunningham, 2008).

β-Thalassemia is the most common of the thalassemias and occurs in four forms: two heterozygous forms, *thalassemia minor* (generally an asymptomatic silent carrier state) and *thalassemia trait* (which produces a mild microcytic anemia); *thalassemia intermedia*, which may involve either homozygous or heterozygous abnormalities and is manifested as splenomegaly

BOX 35-5 CLINICAL MANIFESTATIONS OF β-THALASSEMIA

Anemia (Before Diagnosis)
Pallor
Unexplained fever
Poor feeding
Enlarged spleen or liver

Progressive Anemia
Signs of chronic hypoxia
Headache
Precordial and bone pain
Decreased exercise tolerance
Listlessness
Anorexia

Other Features
Small stature
Delayed sexual maturation
Bronzed, freckled complexion (if not receiving chelation therapy)

Bone Changes (Older Children If Untreated)
Enlarged head
Prominent frontal and parietal bosses
Prominent malar eminences
Flat or depressed bridge of the nose
Enlarged maxilla
Protrusion of the lip and upper central incisors and eventual malocclusion
Generalized osteoporosis

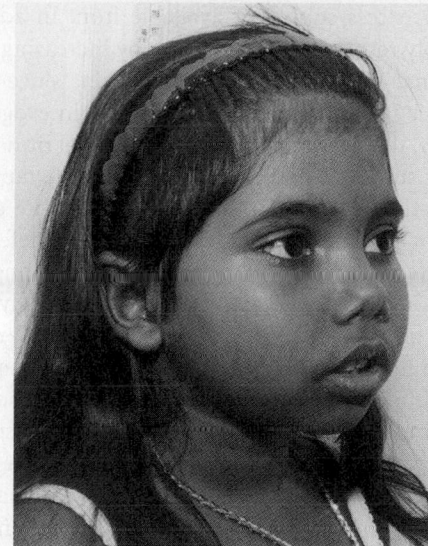

Fig. 35-5 A young girl with β-thalassemia demonstrating mild frontal bossing of the right forehead and mild maxillary prominence. (Courtesy James DeLeon, Texas Children's Hospital, Houston.)

and moderate to severe anemia; and a homozygous form, *thalassemia major* (also known as Cooley anemia), which results in a severe anemia that is not compatible with life without transfusion support.

Mode of Transmission

Thalassemia is an autosomal recessive disorder with varying expressivity. Both parents must be carriers to produce a child with β-thalassemia major. The typical mode of transmission is between parents who are heterozygous for thalassemia.

Pathophysiology and Clinical Manifestations

Normal postnatal HgbA is composed of two α and two β polypeptide chains. In β-thalassemia there is a partial or complete deficiency in the synthesis of the β chain of the hemoglobin molecule. Consequently there is a compensatory increase in the synthesis of α chain, and γ-chain production remains activated, which results in formation of defective hemoglobin. This unbalanced polypeptide unit is unstable; when it disintegrates, it damages the RBCs, which causes severe anemia. To compensate for the hemolytic process, an overabundance of erythrocytes is formed unless transfusion therapy suppresses the bone marrow. Excess iron from packed RBC transfusions and from the rapid destruction of defective cells is stored in various organs (hemosiderosis).

The onset of clinical manifestations in thalassemia major may be insidious and not recognized until late infancy or early toddlerhood (Box 35-5). The clinical effects of thalassemia major are primarily attributable to (1) defective synthesis of HgbA, (2) structurally impaired RBCs, and (3) the shortened life span of the erythrocyte. The major consequences of thalas-

semia are caused by the pathologic condition, resultant chronic hypoxia, and iron overload from the supportive treatment of multiple blood supplements (Fig. 35-5 and Box 35-5).

Anemia results from the body's inability to maintain a level of erythropoiesis commensurate with hemolysis. The bone marrow compensates by producing large numbers of immature cells, such as normoblasts and erythroblasts; large cells that are extremely thin and form bizarre shapes; and target cells, which have abnormal staining properties. As a result of the excessive production of abnormal RBCs, their life span is severely shortened.

Aplastic crises after infection, folic acid deficiencies from the demands of bone marrow hyperplasia, and progressive hemolysis from repeated blood transfusions all worsen anemia. The spleen becomes greatly enlarged as a result of extramedullary hematopoiesis, rapid destruction of the defective erythrocytes, and, rarely, progressive fibrosis from hemochromatosis. Splenomegaly may progress until the organ's very size interferes with the function of other abdominal organs and respiratory expansion.

With progressive anemia, signs of chronic hypoxia—namely, headache, irritability, precordial and bone pain, decreased exercise tolerance, listlessness, and anorexia—may develop. Another common symptom in these children is frequent epistaxis, although the exact reason is unknown. Hyperuricemia and gout from rapid cellular catabolism also occur.

Hemosiderosis refers to excess iron storage in various tissues of the body, especially the spleen, liver, lymph glands, heart, and pancreas, but without associated tissue injury. **Hemochromatosis** refers to excess iron storage that results in cellular damage. It is not known how iron storage causes tissue destruction. Chronic hypoxia is believed to be an important contributing factor.

In thalassemia, excess of hemosiderin, the iron-containing pigment from the breakdown of hemoglobin, results from decreased hemoglobin synthesis and increased hemolysis of transfused erythrocytes. Decreased production of hemoglobin results in an excess supply of available iron. In addition, the body probably responds to the anemia by increasing the rate of gastrointestinal absorption of dietary iron, since ineffective erythropoiesis is a potent controlling factor in exogenous iron use. However, the primary source of additional iron is from the hemolysis of supplemental erythrocytes and the rapid destruction of defective RBCs. With the prophylactic use of deferoxamine and/or oral chelators (deferiprone and deferasirox) to minimize excess iron storage, the characteristic changes in body structures from hemochromatosis have been greatly reduced.

Retarded growth and, especially, delayed sexual maturation are common findings. There is evidence that both may also be caused by pituitary failure, although the exact reasons for this are unclear, but the impaired growth is probably also related to hemochromatosis. It is possible that the endocrine glands are extremely sensitive to iron toxicity and that even small amounts of deposited iron can produce organ dysfunction. Children with severe disease usually exhibit significant growth retardation. The development of secondary sexual characteristics is delayed or absent in many adolescents (Cunningham, Sankaran, Nathan, et al, 2009).

Diagnostic Evaluation

Hematologic studies reveal characteristic changes in the RBCs (e.g., microcytosis, hypochromia, anisocytosis, poikilocytosis, target cells, and basophilic stippling of various stages). Low hemoglobin and hematocrit levels often occur in severe anemia, although they are typically less pronounced than the reduction in the RBC count because of the proliferation of immature erythrocytes.

Hemoglobin electrophoresis confirms the diagnosis and is helpful in distinguishing the type and severity of the thalassemia because it analyzes the quantity and kind of hemoglobin variants found in the blood. In β-thalassemia, levels of HgbF and $HgbA_2$ (a type of normal adult hemoglobin) are elevated because neither depends on β chain polypeptides for synthesis.

Therapeutic Management

The objective of supportive therapy is to maintain sufficient hemoglobin levels to prevent bone marrow expansion and bony deformities and to provide sufficient RBCs to support growth and normal physical activity. Transfusions are the foundation of medical management, with a goal of maintaining the hemoglobin level above 9.5 g/dl, an aim that may require transfusions as often as every 3 weeks. The advantages of this therapy include (1) improved physical and psychologic well-being because of the ability to participate in normal activities, (2) decreased cardiomegaly and hepatosplenomegaly, (3) fewer bone changes, (4) normal or near-normal growth and development until puberty, and (5) fewer infections.

One of the potential complications of frequent blood transfusions is iron overload (hemosiderosis). Because the body has no effective means of eliminating the excess iron, the mineral is deposited in body tissues. To minimize the development of hemosiderosis and hemochromatosis, deferoxamine, an iron-chelating agent, is given with oral supplements of vitamin C. Vitamin C should be given only to patients who are ascorbate depleted and only while deferoxamine is being administered.

Administration of vitamin C significantly augments iron excretion in response to deferoxamine, particularly in patients with vitamin C deficiency (Cunningham, Sankaran, Nathan, et al, 2009). As postulated, vitamin C may delay the conversion of ferritin to hemosiderin, which allows more iron to remain in chelatable form.

Deferoxamine is given intravenously or subcutaneously at home via a portable infusion pump over a period of 8 to 10 hours (usually during sleep) for 5 to 7 days a week. Significant liver fibrosis, cardiac dysfunction and growth impairment may be prevented if chelation therapy is adequate during childhood (Cunningham, Sankaran, Nathan, et al, 2009). Therefore adherence to an intensive schedule is required for substantial chelation therapy. The availability of oral chelators (deferiprone and deferasirox) is a major advance in the care of patient undergoing long-term transfusion therapy. Deferasirox was approved by the FDA in 2004 for the treatment of patients 2 years and older with chronic iron overload secondary to recurrent blood transfusions (Cunningham, Sankaran, Nathan, et al, 2009; Raphael, Bernhardt, Mahoney, et al, 2009). A daily dose of 20 to 30 mg/kg of deferasirox is generally well tolerated, with mild gastrointestinal events and rash as common toxicities (Cohen, Glimm, and Porter, 2008). Deferiprone is currently available only on a compassionate-use basis in the United States (Neufeld, 2008).

⚡ DRUG ALERT

Chelation

New strategies for chelation, such as combination parenteral and oral chelation therapy and organ-targeted chelation, may soon have a considerable impact on the quality of life of patients with thalassemia (Cohen, Galanello, Rennell, et al, 2004; Naithani, Chandra, and Sharma, 2005; Cunningham, Sankaran, Nathan, et al, 2009).

New methods to assess cardiac and liver iron overload using magnetic resonance imaging have recently been developed (Cohen, Galanello, Rennell, et al, 2004; Hankins and Aygun, 2009).

In some children with severe splenomegaly who require repeated transfusions, a splenectomy may be necessary to decrease the disabling effects of abdominal pressure and to increase the life span of supplemental RBCs. Over time the spleen may accelerate the rate of RBC destruction and therefore increase transfusion requirements. After a splenectomy children generally require fewer transfusions, although the basic defect in hemoglobin synthesis remains unaffected. A major postsplenectomy complication is severe and overwhelming infection. Therefore these children are often on prophylactic antibiotics with close medical supervision for many years and should receive the pneumococcal and meningococcal vaccines in addition to regularly scheduled immunizations. (See Immunizations, Chapter 12.)

Prognosis

Most children treated with blood transfusions and early chelation therapy survive well into adulthood (Cunningham, Sankaran, Nathan, et al, 2009). The most common causes of death are heart disease, postsplenectomy sepsis, and multiorgan failure secondary to hemochromatosis (Cunningham, Sankaran, Nathan, et al, 2009). A curative treatment for some children is HSCT. (See Chapter 36.) Children younger than 16 years of age who undergo allogeneic HSCT have a high rate of complication-free survival; approximately 80% of these children are cured (Lucarelli and Gaziev, 2008). An experimental approach for correction of thalassemia through the introduction of new genetic material into pluripotent stem cells is ongoing but continues to have shortcomings (Cunningham, Sankaran, Nathan, et al, 2009; Ye, Chang, Lin, et al, 2009).

Nursing Care Management

The objectives of nursing care are to (1) promote compliance with transfusion and chelation therapy, (2) assist the child in coping with the anxiety-provoking treatments and the effects of the illness, (3) foster the child's and family's adjustment to a chronic illness, and (4) observe for complications of multiple blood transfusions. Basic to each of these goals is explaining to parents and older children the defect responsible for the disorder, its effect on RBCs, and the potential effects of untreated hemosiderosis (such as delayed growth and maturation and heart disease). Because this condition is prevalent among families of Mediterranean descent, the nurse also inquires about the family's previous knowledge about thalassemia. All families with a child with thalassemia should be tested for the trait and referred for genetic counseling.

Support the Family

As with any chronic illness, the family's needs must be met for optimum adjustment to the stresses imposed by the disorder. (See Chapter 22.) Sources of information for the family are the Cooley's Anemia Foundation* and the Thalassemia Action Group.* Genetic counseling for the parents and fertile offspring is mandatory, and both prenatal diagnosis using amniocentesis or fetal blood sampling and screening for thalassemia trait are available. There has been a marked decline in the number of new cases of thalassemia worldwide. This may be a result of education and testing of parents.

Assist in Coping with the Effects of the Disorder

Body image alterations, decreased growth, and sexual immaturity are frequently difficult adjustment problems for older children. These children feel different from their peers, and the delayed sexual development is a major issue for the maturing adolescent with an improved life expectancy. Adolescents need an opportunity to express their thoughts and feelings about these complex issues. They can learn grooming measures that make them appear more sexually mature, such as wearing up-to-date clothing, adopting new hairstyles, and wearing well-applied makeup. Children with the characteristic bone changes may benefit from surgery or use of orthodontic appliances to improve facial structure.

With frequent transfusion therapy there is less restriction on physical activity because of severe anemia, and the nurse should encourage these children to pursue activities that they are able

*330 Seventh Ave., No. 900, New York, NY 10001; 800-522-7222; fax: 212-279-5999; e-mail: info@cooleysanemia.org; **www.thalassemia. org.**

to tolerate. The frequency of treatment, however, can interfere with a normal lifestyle. To minimize disruptions and improve cooperation, the nurse can help arrange for blood transfusions and medical supervision at times that interfere least with the child's regular activities, especially school.

ANEMIAS CAUSED BY IMPAIRED OR DECREASED PRODUCTION OF RED BLOOD CELLS

Impaired or decreased production of RBCs can occur as a result of either bone marrow failure or deficiency of essential nutrients. Bone marrow failure may be caused by (1) replacement of bone marrow by fibrous tissue or by neoplastic cells, as in leukemia; (2) depression of marrow activity by irradiation, chemicals, or drugs; and (3) interference with bone marrow activity caused by systemic disorders such as severe infection, chronic renal disease, widespread malignancy (without marrow infiltration), collagen diseases, or hypothyroidism. When depression of the hematologic system is extensive, aplastic anemia develops.

The reason systemic disorders affect erythrocyte production varies according to the condition. For example, in severe chronic infection there is evidence that depression of erythropoiesis is caused by a defect in the conversion of protoporphyrin into hemoglobin. In addition, there is some degree of hemolysis, although the exact mechanism is not known.

APLASTIC ANEMIA

Aplastic anemia refers to a condition in which production of all formed elements of the blood is simultaneously depressed. The peripheral blood smear demonstrates pancytopenia or the triad of profound anemia, leukopenia, and thrombocytopenia. Hypoplastic anemia is characterized by a profound depression of RBC formation but normal or slightly decreased production of WBCs and platelets. One type of hypoplastic anemia is pure RBC aplasia, which can be congenital or acquired. The acquired defect in erythropoiesis is an autoimmune condition that occurs mostly in adults (Brodsky and Jones, 2005; Young, Calado, and Scheinberg, 2006). The congenital condition (Diamond-Blackfan syndrome) is marked by complete or almost complete absence of all cells of the erythroid series with normal production of the other myeloid cells. Its treatment, which consists of transfusions, splenectomy, and administration of corticosteroids, is similar to that for other diseases that result in profound anemia, such as the thalassemias. The prognosis varies, although long-term survival is possible. The principal causes of death are cardiac failure, hepatitis from transfusion therapy, and sepsis. Hemosiderosis and hemochromatosis (see p. 1437) also affect vital tissues necessary for survival.

Aplastic anemia can be primary (congenital, or present at birth) or secondary (acquired). The best-known congenital disorder of which aplastic anemia is an outstanding feature is Fanconi syndrome, a rare hereditary disorder that is characterized by pancytopenia, hypoplasia of the bone marrow, and patchy brown discoloration of the skin due to the deposition of melanin. It is associated with multiple congenital anomalies of the musculoskeletal and genitourinary systems. The syndrome appears to be inherited as an autosomal recessive trait with varying penetrance; therefore affected siblings may demonstrate different combinations of defects.

Several factors contribute to the development of acquired hypoplastic anemia, including suppressed erythropoiesis from multiple-transfusion therapy; hemolytic syndromes (such as SCA); and autoimmune or allergic states. Box 35-6 lists the most common causes of acquired aplastic anemia. The following discussion focuses on acquired severe aplastic anemia, which carries a poorer prognosis and follows a more rapidly fatal course than the primary types.

Diagnostic Evaluation

The onset of clinical manifestations, which include anemia, leukopenia, and decreased platelet count, is usually insidious, not unlike that seen in leukemia. Definitive diagnosis is made by examination of bone marrow aspirates, which demonstrate the conversion of red bone marrow to yellow, fatty bone marrow.

Therapeutic Management

The objectives of treatment are based on the recognition that the underlying disease process is failure of the bone marrow to carry out its hematopoietic functions. Therefore therapy is directed at restoring function to the marrow and involves two main approaches: (1) immunosuppressive therapy to counter the presumed immunologic responses that prolong aplasia, and (2) replacement of the bone marrow through transplantation. Bone marrow transplantation is the treatment of choice for severe aplastic anemia when a suitable donor exists.

Immunosuppressive therapy is an alternative first-line treatment for children with acquired aplastic anemia who do not have a matched sibling bone marrow donor (Pongtanakul, Das, Charpentier, et al, 2008). These strategies are based on the use of antilymphocyte globulin and antithymocyte globulin (ATG). The two products are similar; therefore the terms are used interchangeably here.

The use of immunosuppressive therapy, including cyclosporin A (CSA) and ATG, with the addition of human recombinant granulocyte or granulocyte-macrophage colony-stimulating factor (G-CSF or GM-CSF) and methylprednisolone (to prevent ATG serum sickness), has greatly improved the prognosis for patients with aplastic anemia. The rationale for using ATG is the possibility that aplastic anemia may be a result of autoimmunity.

In children who fail to respond to therapy with ATG, CSA, and growth factors, success has been achieved using high-dose cyclophosphamide as an effective immunosuppressive agent. Androgens may be used with ATG to stimulate erythropoiesis if the aplastic anemia is nonresponsive to initial therapies.

HSCT should be considered early in the course of the disease if a compatible donor can be found. Transplantation is more successful if performed before multiple transfusions have sensitized the child to leukocyte and HLA antigens. Children who are eligible for transplantation should be transferred to one of the medical centers that specialize in this procedure. Many different preparative regimens are available, and all aim to decrease the rate of graft-versus-host disease. All regimens include immunosuppressive therapy, and some also include irradiation (either total body or thoracoabdominal). Patients who have received a large number of transfusions before bone marrow transplantation have a higher rejection rate and lower survival rate (Marsh, 2005; Young, Calado, and Scheinberg, 2006). With the use of immunosuppressive therapy and HLA-identical sibling donor, the allogeneic bone marrow transplantation offers 90% chance of long-term survival (Hord, 2007; Trigg, 2004; Marsh, 2005).

Nursing Care Management

The care of the child with aplastic anemia is similar to the care of the child with leukemia (i.e., preparing the family for the diagnostic and therapeutic procedures, preventing complications from the severe pancytopenia, and emotionally supporting the family regarding the potentially fatal outcome). (See Chapters 23 and 36.) Because each of these nursing care interventions has been covered elsewhere, only the interventions specific to aplastic anemia are presented here. (Chapter 36 discusses bone marrow transplantation.)

Because growth factors are usually given subcutaneously over several days, an anesthetic cream, EMLA, may be used to minimize pain at the injection site. Because chemotherapeutic agents may be used, many of the common reactions to these drugs, such as nausea and vomiting, alopecia, and mucosal ulceration, may be encountered. In addition, the oral area mucosa may have extensive ecchymotic areas from thrombocytopenia that require meticulous mouth care to prevent breakdown, bleeding, and infection. Fortunately, these lesions, which look painful, cause little or no discomfort. Local anesthetics are not necessary, but anorexia is still a consequence because of the edematous nature of the lesions. Liquid, bland, and soft diets are usually tolerated best. (See Feeding the Sick Child, Chapter 27.)

DEFECTS IN HEMOSTASIS

Hemostasis is the process that stops bleeding when a blood vessel is injured. Vascular and plasma clotting factors, as well as platelets, are required. A complex system of clotting, anticlotting, and clot breakdown (**fibrinolysis**) mechanisms exists in equilibrium to ensure clot formation only in the presence of blood vessel injury and to limit the clotting process to the site of vessel wall injury. Dysfunction in these systems leads to bleeding or abnormal clotting.

MECHANISMS INVOLVED IN NORMAL HEMOSTASIS

Understanding the role that factor deficiencies play in promoting bleeding tendencies requires a review of the normal coagulation process of the blood. Although the coagulation process is complex, clotting depends on three main elements: vascular events, platelets, and clotting factors.

Vascular Events

At the time and site of injury, several events occur to initiate hemostasis: local vasoconstriction, compression of the blood vessels by extravasated blood, and release of von Willebrand factor by endothelial walls. Collagen present in exposed subendothelial cells acts as a site for platelet adhesion.

Platelets

Normally the platelets do not adhere to each other or to normal endothelium. However, at the time a blood vessel is injured, the following events take place: Platelet adhesion occurs at the site of the injury, providing a plug. The platelets change shape, develop pseudopods, and release a variety of chemicals to stimulate vasoconstriction and vessel repair and to activate and recruit more platelets to the injury site. Receptor sites are located on the platelets for fibrinogen and other adhesive proteins, which cause the platelets to stick together (**aggregation**). As the membranes of the platelets change, the phospholipids necessary for blood coagulation are exposed so that fibrin, which secures the platelet plugs to the site, can be produced. Finally, the clot compresses and is secured to the injury.

Defects in platelets and clotting factors are the most common causes of bleeding during childhood. The following

TABLE 35-4	BLOOD-CLOTTING FACTORS
FACTOR NUMBER	**SYNONYMS**
I	Fibrinogen
II	Prothrombin
III	Platelet factor 3, thromboplastin
IV	Calcium
V	Labile factor, proaccelerin, Ac globulin
VII	Serum prothrombin conversion accelerator (SPCA), proconvertin, stable factor
VIII	Antihemophilic factor (AHF)
IX	Plasma thromboplastin component (PTC), Christmas factor
X	Stuart-Prower factor
XI	Plasma thromboplastin antecedent (PTA)
XII	Hageman factor
XIII	Fibrin-stabilizing factor (FSF)
KAL	Prekallikrein, Fletcher factor
HMK	High-molecular-weight kininogen, Fitzgerald factor

discussion focuses on the major conditions that require nursing intervention.

Clotting Factors

The clotting factors (Table 35-4 and Fig. 35-6) are activated in sequence to develop a fibrin clot. Two mechanisms exist that can generate prothrombin to produce thrombin:

1. **Intrinsic pathway**—Factor XII, high-molecular-weight kininogen (HMK, Fitzgerald factor), and prekallikrein (KAL, Fletcher factor) react on a negatively charged surface (contact activation reaction) to activate factor XI (PTA, plasma thromboplastin antecedent). The partial thromboplastin time measures abnormalities in the intrinsic pathway (abnormalities in factors I, II, V, VIII, IX, X, XII, HMK, and KAL).
2. **Extrinsic pathway**—A lipoprotein tissue factor stimulates activation of factor VII. The prothrombin time measures abnormalities of the extrinsic pathway (abnormalities in factors I, II, V, VII, and X).

Table 35-5 presents laboratory tests to assess hemostasis.

HEMOPHILIA

The term *hemophilia* refers to a group of bleeding disorders resulting from congenital deficiency of specific coagulation proteins (Montgomery, Gill, and Di Paola, 2009; Sharathkumar and Pipe, 2008). Although the symptomatology is similar regardless of which clotting factor is deficient, the identification of specific factor deficiencies has allowed definitive treatment with replacement agents.

In about 80% of all cases of hemophilia, the inheritance pattern is demonstrated as X-linked recessive. (See Chapter 5.) The two most common forms of the disorder are factor VIII deficiency (hemophilia A, or classic hemophilia) and factor IX deficiency (hemophilia B, or Christmas disease), with prevalence in the general population of approximately 1 in 5000 and 1 in 50,000, respectively (Brown, 2005; Sharathkumar and Pipe, 2008). The following discussion is primarily concerned with

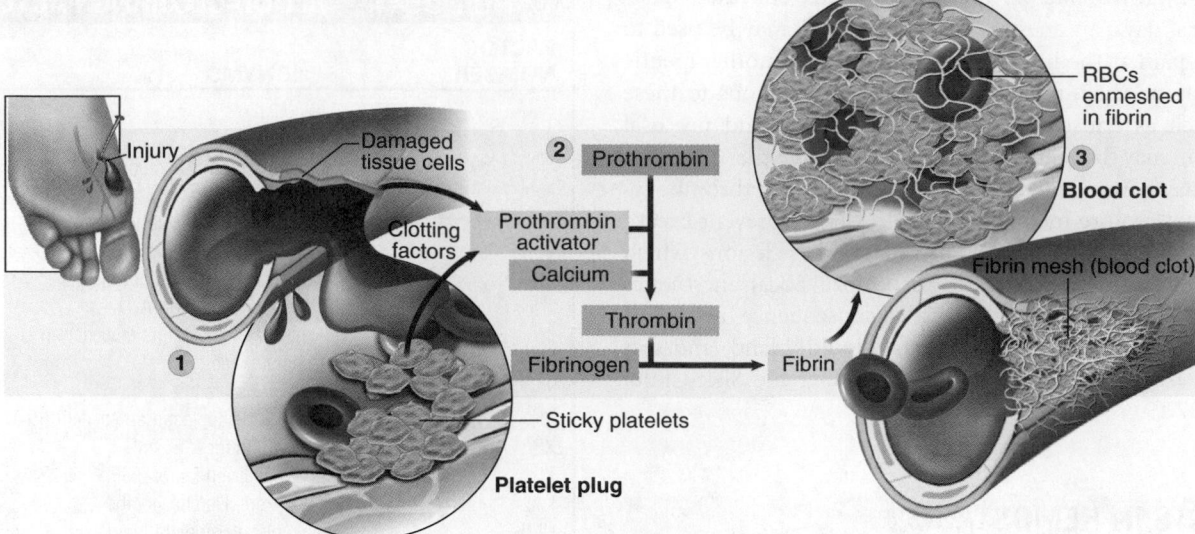

Fig. 35-6 Blood clotting. The extremely complex clotting mechanism can be distilled into three basic steps: *(1)* release of clotting factors from both injured tissue cells and sticky platelets at the injury site (which form a temporary platelet plug); *(2)* series of chemical reactions that eventually result in the formation of thrombin; and *(3)* formation of fibrin and trapping of red blood cells *(RBCs)* to form a clot. (From Thibodeau GA, Patton KT: *The human body in health and disease*, ed 5, St Louis, Mosby, 2010.)

TABLE 35-5   LABORATORY TESTS TO ASSESS HEMOSTASIS*

TEST	DESCRIPTION	COMMENTS
Platelet Function		
Platelet function analyzer (PFA 100)	Measures platelet function and interaction with von Willebrand factor. Has replaced bleeding time in some centers	Results are altered with intake of NSAIDs, anticoagulants, ASA, or ASA-containing products
Bleeding time	Measures time it takes for bleeding from small superficial wound to cease	Function depends on platelet aggregation and vasoconstriction; two common methods used are Ivy (incision made on the forearm) and Duke (incision made on the earlobe)
Tourniquet test	Measures platelet function and capillary fragility; pressure applied to forearm with tourniquet for 5-10 min	Normal response is absence of petechiae or <10 petechiae. Abnormal in platelet and connective tissue disorders
Clot retraction test	Measures degree to which clot shrinks and expresses serum	Depends on platelet function
Blood Clotting Mechanisms		
Whole blood clotting time	Measures time it takes for clot to form *within* blood	Prolonged clotting time indicates problem in thrombin-to-fibrin phase or in any factor in intrinsic clotting mechanism; difficult test to standardize; therefore often unreliable results
Prothrombin time (PT)	Measures activity of prothrombin and factors necessary for its conversion to thrombin and fibrinogen	Actually measures not prothrombin levels but activity; because it bypasses intrinsic-extrinsic mechanism, detects deficiencies of factors V, VII, X, and fibrinogen as well as prothrombin
Partial thromboplastin time (PPT)	Similar to PT but measures activity of thromboplastin, which depends on intrinsic clotting factors	Specific for factor deficiencies, except factor VII, which results in a normal PTT but prolonged PT
Thromboplastin generation test	Measures blood's ability to generate thromboplastin	Allows for determination of specific factor deficiencies, especially distinguishing between factors VII and IX
Prothrombin consumption test	Indirectly measures thromboplastin generation and prothrombin response	Normally, as blood clots, prothrombin is converted to thrombin so that serum is depleted of prothrombin; if thromboplastin is decreased (as a result of extrinsic factor deficiencies), not all prothrombin will be converted and removed from serum
Fibrinogen level	Directly measures fibrinogen levels in blood	Not dependent on phase I or II deficiencies

ASA, Acetylsalicylic acid; *NSAIDs,* nonsteroidal antiinflammatory drugs.
*Normal values are listed in Appendix C.

factor VIII deficiency, which accounts for about 80% of all cases.

Modes of Transmission

Hemophilia is transmitted as an X-linked recessive disorder; however, only about 60% of affected children have a positive family history for the disease. Up to one third of all hemophilia cases may be caused by a gene mutation. The most frequent pattern of transmission is through the union of an unaffected male with a trait-carrier female. Because the treatment of persons with hemophilia has improved, the results of a union between an affected male and a normal female or a carrier female must also be considered. For example, the chances are equal (i.e., 1 in 4) that an offspring of an affected male and a carrier female will be an affected son, an affected daughter, a carrier daughter, or a normal son. Such parentage is one of the few ways in which a female inherits the disorder. Female carriers may have low levels of factor VIII and be symptomatic.

Pathophysiology and Clinical Manifestations

The basic defect of hemophilia A is a deficiency of factor VIII (antihemophilic factor). Factor VIII is produced by the liver and is necessary for the formation of thromboplastin in phase I of blood coagulation. The less factor VIII found in the blood, the more severe the disease.

A major feature of hemophilia is that its expression varies markedly with regard to the degree of bleeding severity. Hemophilia is generally classified into three groups according to the severity of the factor deficiency; 60% to 70% of children with hemophilia demonstrate the severe form of the disorder (Table 35-6).

The effect of hemophilia is prolonged bleeding anywhere from or in the body. With severe factor deficiencies, hemorrhage can occur as a result of minor trauma, such as after circumcision, during loss of deciduous teeth, or as a result of a slight fall or bruise. In children with less severe deficiencies, however, the bleeding tendency may not be noted until the onset of walking.

Subcutaneous and intramuscular hemorrhages are common. Hemarthrosis, which refers to bleeding into the joint cavities, especially the knees, elbows, and ankles, is the most frequent form of internal bleeding. Bony changes and crippling deformities occur after repeated bleeding episodes over several years. Early signs of hemarthrosis are a feeling of stiffness, tingling, or ache in the affected joint, followed by a decrease in the ability to move the joint. Obvious signs and symptoms are warmth, redness, swelling, and severe pain with considerable loss of movement. Spontaneous hematuria is not uncommon. Epistaxis may occur but is not as frequent as other kinds of hemorrhage. Petechiae are uncommon in persons with hemophilia because repair of small hemorrhages depends on platelet function, not on blood-clotting mechanisms.

Bleeding into the tissue can occur anywhere but is serious if it occurs in the neck, mouth, or thorax because the airway can become obstructed. Intracranial hemorrhage can have fatal consequences and is one of the major causes of death. Hemorrhage anywhere along the gastrointestinal tract can lead to anemia, and bleeding into the retroperitoneal cavity is especially hazardous because of the large space for blood to accumulate. Hematomas in the spinal cord can cause paralysis.

Diagnostic Evaluation

The diagnosis is usually made from a history of bleeding episodes, evidence of X-linked inheritance (only one third of cases are new mutations), and laboratory findings. To understand the significance of various tests of hemostasis, it is helpful to recall the usual mechanisms to control bleeding (i.e., the function of platelets and clotting factors). The results of tests that measure platelet function, such as the bleeding time, are all normal in persons with hemophilia, whereas the results of tests that assess clotting factor function may be abnormal (see Table 35-5). The tests specific for hemophilia include factor VIII and IX assays, procedures normally done by specialized laboratories. Other tests are those that depend on specific factors for a reaction to occur, especially the partial thromboplastin time. Carrier detection is possible in classic hemophilia using DNA testing and is an important consideration in families in which female offspring may have inherited the trait.

Therapeutic Management

The primary therapy for hemophilia is replacement of the missing clotting factor. The products currently available are factor VIII concentrates, either produced through genetic engineering (recombinant form) or derived from pooled plasma, which are reconstituted with sterile water immediately before use. A synthetic form of vasopressin, 1-deamino-8-D-arginine vasopressin (DDAVP), is the treatment of choice in mild hemophilia and von Willebrand disease (vWD) (types I and IIA only) if the child shows an appropriate response. After DDAVP administration a threefold to fourfold rise in factor VIII activity should occur. Because the goal is to raise the factor VIII level at least 30%, patients with moderate factor VIII deficiency do not benefit. In addition, various therapies are employed when bleeding occurs or is anticipated (Table 35-7).

TABLE 35-6	CLINICAL SEVERITY OF HEMOPHILIA	
CLINICAL SEVERITY	**FACTOR VIII ACTIVITY**	**BLEEDING TENDENCY**
Severe	<1%	Spontaneous bleeding without trauma
Moderate	1%-5%	Bleeding with trauma
Mild	>5%-40%	Bleeding with severe trauma or surgery

⚡ DRUG ALERT

Cryoprecipitate

Cryoprecipitate is no longer recommended for use in treating factor VIII deficiency. Since the availability of highly purified factor VIII concentrate (monoclonal) in 1988 and the licensing of recombinant factor VIII concentrate in 1992 (marketed not as a blood product but as a drug), the National Hemophilia Foundation has advised practitioners to use only these products. Cryoprecipitate cannot be treated to safely eliminate hepatitis or human immunodeficiency virus (HIV).

Animation—Hemophilia A

TABLE 35-7	ADJUNCT THERAPIES FOR HEMOPHILIA A
SITE OF BLEED	**TREATMENT**
Joint	Rest, ice, elevation
	Splint, elastic wrap, crutches
	Physical therapy
Soft tissue	Ice, elevation
	Splint or elastic wrap
Muscle	Rest, ice, elevation
	Splint, elastic wrap, crutches
	Physical therapy
	Complete bed rest for iliopsoas muscle bleed
Mucous membrane (e.g., nose, mouth)	Pressure to nares (for nosebleed)
	Topical antifibrinolytic agent (ε-aminocaproic acid)
	Nasal pack (sometimes necessary)

Aggressive factor concentrate replacement therapy is initiated to prevent chronic crippling effects from joint bleeding. If replacement therapy begins immediately, local measures such as ice applications and splinting are seldom needed. Other drugs may be included in the therapy plan, depending on the source of the hemorrhage. Corticosteroids are given for hematuria, acute hemarthrosis, and chronic synovitis. It is recommended that patients with hemophilia avoid aspirin and nonsteroidal antiinflammatory drugs (NSAIDs) because they inhibit platelet function (Scott and Montgomery, 2007). However, NSAIDs such as ibuprofen are effective in relieving pain caused by synovitis and are occasionally used with caution (Curry, 2004). Oral use of ε-aminocaproic acid (EACA, Amicar) prevents clot destruction. Its use is limited to mouth trauma or surgery with a dose of factor concentrate given first. The child may rinse the mouth with this medication and then swallow it.

A regular program of exercise and physical therapy is an important aspect of management. If started early and continued throughout adulthood, planned, individualized physical activity strengthens muscles around joints and may decrease the number of spontaneous bleeding episodes.

❗ NURSING ALERT

Passive range-of-motion exercises should never be part of an exercise regimen after an acute episode because the joint capsule could easily be stretched and bleeding could recur. Active range-of-motion exercises are best so that the patient can gauge his or her own pain tolerance.

Treatment without delay results in more rapid recovery and a decreased likelihood of complications; therefore most children are treated at home. The family should learn how to perform venipuncture and how to administer factor VIII to children over 2 to 3 years of age. The child learns the procedure for self-administration at 8 to 12 years of age. Home treatment is highly successful, and the rewards, in addition to the immediacy, are less disruption of family life, fewer school or work days missed, and enhancement of the child's self-esteem and independence.

Prophylactic therapy is periodic factor replacement for children with severe hemophilia to prevent bleeding complications, including arthropathy and spontaneous and life-threatening bleeding events (Scott and Montgomery, 2007; Sharathkumar and Pipe, 2008; Montgomery, Gill, and Di Paola, 2009). Primary prophylaxis in patients with severe hemophilia has been practiced for many years in developed countries and has proved to be effective in preventing naturopathy. In primary prophylaxis, factor VIII concentrate is infused on a regular basis before the onset of joint damage. Secondary prophylaxis involves the infusion of factor VIII concentrate on a regular basis after the child experiences his or her first joint bleed. The infusions are given every other day or three times a week for several weeks to promote healing. Episodic factor replacement may be a cost-effective alternative to primary prophylaxis, but prophylaxis decreases the development of joint disease compared to on-demand treatment (Manco-Johnson, Abshire, Shapiro, et al, 2007). However, prompt appropriate treatment of hemorrhage and prophylactic therapy are key to excellent care and prevention of long-term morbidity in patients with hemophilia (Montgomery, Gill, and Di Paola, 2009).

Prognosis

The progress made in hemophilia care over the years has been striking. The advent of home infusion therapy coupled with recent advances in producing safer and more effective factor concentrates has revolutionized the treatment and management of hemophilia (Montgomery, Gill, and Di Paola, 2009). Early recognition of joint and muscle bleeds is emphasized, since immediate adequate treatment with clotting factor is possible using home infusion therapy. Early treatment has significantly reduced the morbidity formerly associated with hemophilia. The availability of comprehensive hemophilia treatment centers offers the child with hemophilia and the family a coordinated multidisciplinary approach to meeting their needs and improving the child's health and well-being.

Although there is no cure for hemophilia, its symptoms can be controlled and its potentially crippling deformities markedly reduced or even avoided. Today many children with hemophilia function with minimal or no joint damage. They have an average life expectancy and are normal in every aspect but one: they have a tendency to bleed, which is a significant inconvenience but not necessarily a life-threatening event.

Unfortunately, those individuals with hemophilia who were treated before the development of current purification techniques for factor VIII concentrate (between 1979 and 1985) may have been exposed to HIV. It is estimated that more than 50% of these patients seroconverted to HIV-positive status, and 30% developed acquired immunodeficiency syndrome (AIDS) (Butler, Schultz, Forsberg, et al, 2003). Individuals with hemophilia diagnosed since the 1990s and treated with recombinant factor products are at virtually no risk for developing HIV infection from treatment. Recombinant factor VIII and factor IX products that are devoid of human protein materials have become the treatment of choice for children and previously untreated hemophilia patients (Brown, 2005; Montgomery, Gill, and Di Paola, 2009).

Gene therapy may prove to be a treatment option in the future. Techniques are under development to introduce the factor VIII or IX genes into hepatocytes, fibroblasts, and endothelial cells using adeno-associated viral vectors (National

Hemophilia Foundation and American Red Cross, 2005; Nienhuis, 2008). The scientific community remains undaunted in its attempt to make gene-addition therapy a twenty-first century reality for patients with hemophilia A and B. Gene therapy is expected to be available in the next 5 to 10 years, but many problems remain, including selection of both appropriate vectors and the appropriate cell in which to express the gene (Montgomery, Gill, and Di Paola, 2009).

Nursing Care Management

The earlier a bleeding episode is recognized, the more effectively it can be treated. Signs that indicate internal bleeding are especially important to recognize. Children are aware of internal bleeding and are reliable in telling the examiner the location of an internal bleed. In addition, the nurse maintains a high level of suspicion when a child with hemophilia shows signs such as headache; slurred speech; loss of consciousness (from cerebral bleeding); and black, tarry stools (from gastrointestinal bleeding).

QUALITY PATIENT OUTCOMES: Hemophilia
- Early recognition of signs and symptoms of hemophilia
- Bleeding episodes prevented
- Bleeding episodes treated early with factor replacement
- Adherence to prophylactic factor replacement program when indicated
- Hemarthrosis prevented when possible with limited joint damage
- Exercise program and physical therapy ongoing

Prevent Bleeding

The goal of prevention of bleeding episodes involves decreasing the risk of injury. Measures are geared mostly toward encouraging appropriate exercises to strengthen muscles and joints and to allow age-appropriate activity. During infancy and toddlerhood the normal acquisition of motor skills creates innumerable opportunities for falls, bruises, and minor wounds. Restraining the child from mastering motor development can bring more serious long-term problems than allowing the behavior. However, the environment should be made as safe as possible, with close supervision maintained during playtime to minimize incidental injuries.

For older children the family usually needs assistance in preparing the child for school. A nurse who knows the family can assist in discussing the situation with the school nurse and in joint planning of an appropriate activity schedule. Because almost all individuals with hemophilia are boys, the physical limitations with regard to active sports may require a difficult adjustment, and activity restrictions must be tempered with sensitivity to the child's emotional and physical needs. Children should always use appropriate safety equipment. Children and adolescents with severe hemophilia can participate in noncontact sports such as swimming, golf, walking, jogging, fishing, and bowling. Football, boxing, hockey, soccer, and rugby are strongly discouraged because the risk of injury outweighs the physical and psychosocial benefits of participating in these sports (National Hemophilia Foundation and American Red Cross, 2005; Scott and Montgomery, 2007).

To prevent oral bleeding, some readjustment in dental hygiene may be needed to minimize trauma to the gums, such as using a water irrigating device, softening the toothbrush in warm water before brushing, or using a sponge-tipped disposable toothbrush. If a regular toothbrush is used, it should be soft bristled and small. Adolescents also need to be advised of the dangers of using safety razors with blades and should use an electric shaver.

Because any trauma can lead to a bleeding episode, all persons caring for these children must be aware of their disorder. These children should wear medical identification, and the nurse should encourage older children to recognize situations in which disclosing their condition is important, such as during dental extractions or injections. Health personnel need to take special precautions to prevent the use of procedures such as intramuscular injection. The subcutaneous route is substituted for intramuscular injection whenever possible. Venipunctures for blood samples are usually preferred by children. There is usually less bleeding after venipuncture than after finger or heel puncture. Neither aspirin nor any aspirin-containing compound should be used. Acetaminophen is a suitable aspirin substitute, especially for use during control of pain at home.

Recognize and Control Bleeding

The earlier a bleeding episode is recognized, the more effectively it can be treated. Factor replacement therapy should be instituted according to established medical protocol, and supportive measures may be implemented, such as RICE, which consists of (1) rest, (2) ice, (3) compression, and (4) elevation. When parents and older children learn such measures beforehand, they can be prepared to initiate immediate treatment before blood loss is excessive. Keep plastic bags of ice or cold packs in the freezer for such emergencies. However, such measures should not take the place of factor replacement.

Prevent Crippling Effects of Bleeding

As a result of repeated episodes of hemarthrosis, incompletely absorbed blood in the joints and limitation of motion, bone and muscle changes occur that may result in flexion contractures and joint fixation. Obviously prevention of bleeding is the ideal goal. However, because spontaneous bleeding is not uncommon in persons with severe hemophilia, definitive measures, including replacement therapy and physical therapy, are necessary to limit joint damage.

During bleeding episodes the joint is elevated and immobilized. Active range-of-motion exercises are usually instituted after the acute phase. This allows the child to control the degree of exercise according to the level of discomfort. Physical therapy is beneficial to promote maximum function of the joint and unaffected body parts. Success of a physical therapy plan involves control of pain by administering analgesics before therapy and adjusting the dose to provide maximum benefit.

If an exercise program is initiated in the home, a physical therapist or public health nurse may need to supervise compliance with the regimen. Rarely, orthopedic intervention, such as casting, application of traction, or aspiration of blood, may be necessary to preserve joint function. Diet is also an important consideration because excessive body weight can increase the strain on affected joints, especially the knees, and predispose the child to hemarthrosis. Consequently, children need calories that meet their energy requirements.

Support the Family and Prepare for Home Care

The development of factor concentrates has greatly changed the outlook for these children. Bleeding can be minimized, and the child can live a much more normal, unrestricted life. Children should learn to take responsibility for their disease at an early age. They learn their limitations, preventive measures, and self-administration of the factor replacement.

The needs of families who have children with hemophilia are best met through a comprehensive team approach involving physicians (pediatrician, hematologist, orthopedist), nurse practitioner, nurse, social worker, and physical therapist.

Parent-group discussions with similarly affected families are beneficial and address certain needs better than health care providers could. For example, with the improved prognosis for these children, adolescents with hemophilia and their parents face vocational and financial problems in addition to concern over future childbearing. Once children reach 21 years of age, many insurance companies will no longer insure them. This can be disastrous because of the cost of treatment, which can exceed $100,000 per year. The National Hemophilia Foundation* and the Canadian Hemophilia Society† provide numerous services and publications for both health care providers and families.

Individuals who have become infected with HIV through transfusions and factor replacement products face the consequences of this dreaded disease. Consequently they need the support of health professionals, especially with regard to instruction in safe sexual practices to avoid disease transmission and public education regarding AIDS and ways to deal with public reactions to those who have AIDS. (See Nursing Care Plan: The Child with Hemophilia, in Wilson and Hockenberry, 2008.)

Identify Persons at Risk

Genetic counseling is essential as soon as possible after diagnosis. Unlike in many other disorders in which both parents carry the trait, the feeling of responsibility for this condition usually rests with the mother. Unless she has an opportunity to discuss her feelings, the couple's relationship may suffer. Prenatal DNA testing can identify affected fetuses and identify carriers in most cases.

VON WILLEBRAND DISEASE

vWD is a hereditary bleeding disorder characterized by a deficiency of or defect in a protein called von Willebrand factor (vWF). The vWF protein contributes to the adherence of platelets to damaged endothelium and serves as a carrier protein for factor VIII (De Meyer, Deckmyn, and Vanhoorelbeke, 2009; Montgomery, Gill, and Di Paola, 2009). This results in prolonged bleeding time because platelets fail to adhere to the walls of the ruptured vessel to form a platelet plug. In many centers, testing using a platelet function analyzer (PFA 100) has replaced measurement of bleeding time as the most sensitive screening

*116 W. 32nd St., 11th floor, New York, NY 10001; 212-328-3700, 800-424-2634; fax: 212-328-3777; e-mail: handi@hemophilia.org; www.hemophilia.org.
†400-1255 University St., Montreal, Quebec, Canada H3B 3B6; 514-848-0503, 800-668-2686; fax: 514-848-9661; e-mail: chs@hemophilia.ca; www.hemophilia.ca.

test for detection of platelet dysfunction and vWD (Cariappa, Wilhite, and Parvin, 2003; Brown, 2005; Scott and Montgomery, 2007) (see Table 35-5). The disease can cause mild, moderate, or severe bleeding. Most cases of vWD are mild and require intervention only for dental and surgical procedures.

The most characteristic clinical feature of vWD is an increased tendency toward bleeding from mucous membranes. The most common symptom is frequent nosebleeds, followed by gingival bleeding, easy bruising, and excessive menstrual bleeding (menorrhagia) in females. Unlike hemophilia, vWD affects both males and females because its inheritance shows an autosomal dominant pattern. However, the treatment and final outcome are similar in both disorders. Treatment of bleeding is with DDAVP and/or a specially concentrated clotting factor known as Humate-P.

Nursing Care Management

The nursing goals are similar to those for hemophilia, with special considerations related to epistaxis. Nosebleeds are often a frightening experience for the child and parents. A calm, reassuring manner can alleviate anxiety and promote the child's cooperation. Because most of the nosebleeding originates in the anterior part of the nasal septum, bleeding can be controlled by applying pressure to the nose with the thumb and forefinger (see Emergency Treatment box). During this time the child breathes through the mouth. If local measures are not successful at stopping the bleeding, a single dose of DDAVP is usually effective. DDAVP increases vWF and factor VIII secretion from storage in the endothelial cells (Brown, 2005; Scott and Montgomery, 2007; Sharathkumar and Pipe, 2008).

✚ EMERGENCY TREATMENT

Epistaxis

- Have child sit up and lean forward (not lie down).
- Apply continuous pressure to nose with thumb and forefinger for at least 10 minutes.
- Insert cotton or wadded tissue into each nostril and apply ice or cold cloth to bridge of nose if bleeding persists.
- Keep child calm and quiet.

For menorrhagia, factor replacement therapy or the administration of DDAVP may be beneficial on the first day of the menstrual cycle to lessen the flow. Teaching the adolescent methods to prevent embarrassing accidents during menstruation, such as wearing plastic-lined underpants and using double sanitary pads, helps her adjust to the inconvenience. Interestingly, these females frequently do not experience excessive bleeding at the time of delivery (Pavlovich-Danis, 2001; Montgomery, Gill, and Di Paola, 2009). This is thought to be because of increased levels of factor VIII during pregnancy. Decisions regarding childbearing are difficult because of the dominant pattern of inheritance.

IDIOPATHIC THROMBOCYTOPENIC PURPURA

Idiopathic thrombocytopenic purpura (ITP) is an acquired hemorrhagic disorder that is characterized by (1) excessive destruction of platelets (thrombocytopenia), (2) purpura (a discoloration caused by petechiae beneath the skin), and (3) normal bone marrow with a usual increase in large, young platelets. Although the cause is unknown, the disorder is believed to represent an autoimmune response to disease-related antigens. The most common thrombocytopenia of childhood accounts for 70% to 80% of cases in children younger than 10 years of age, who recover completely within 6 months (Scott and Montgomery, 2007; Wilson, 2009).

The disease occurs in one of two forms: an acute, self-limiting course or a chronic course (>6 months' duration). The acute form occurs most commonly after upper respiratory tract infections; after the childhood diseases of measles, rubella, mumps, or chickenpox; or after infection with human parvovirus.

Clinical symptoms include petechiae, bruising, bleeding from mucous membranes, and prolonged bleeding from abrasions. Symptomatic bleeding does not usually occur until the platelet count is lower than 20,000/mm³. Fatal hemorrhages have been reported in less than 1% of all patients.

Diagnostic Evaluation

In ITP the platelet count is reduced to less than 20,000/mm³; therefore results of tests that depend on platelet function, such as the tourniquet test, bleeding time, and clot retraction time, are abnormal. There is no definitive test that establishes a diagnosis of ITP; several tests are usually performed to rule out other disorders of which thrombocytopenia is a manifestation, such as systemic lupus erythematosus, lymphoma, and leukemia.

Therapeutic Management

Management of ITP is primarily supportive, since the disease is self-limiting in the majority of cases. Activity is restricted at the onset while the platelet count is low and while active bleeding or progression of lesions is occurring. Treatment for acute presentation is symptomatic and has included prednisone, IV immune globulin (IVIG), and anti-D antibody. These are not curative therapies. Some experts suggest that no therapy is necessary for asymptomatic patients because there is no difference in the recovery time of platelet counts with and without treatment (Neunert, Buchanan, Imbach, et al, 2008; Scott and Montgomery, 2007; Wilson, 2009). Anti-D antibody is a plasma-derived immunoglobulin that causes a transient hemolytic anemia in Rh(D)-positive patients with ITP. With the clearance of antibody-coated RBCs, there is prolonged survival of platelets due to the anti-D antibody blockade of the Fc receptors on the reticuloendothelial cells. The platelet count usually increases approximately 48 hours after an infusion of anti-D antibody; therefore it is not appropriate therapy for patients who are actively bleeding. The benefits of choosing anti-D antibody IV therapy over prednisone or IVIG is that anti-D antibody can be given in one dose over a period of 5 to 10 minutes and is significantly less expensive than IVIG. Historically patients who were treated with prednisone first underwent a bone marrow examination to rule out leukemia, but this is now controversial because leukemia rarely manifests with a low platelet count alone (Scott and Montgomery, 2007; Wilson, 2009). Therefore the use of

anti-D antibody and IVIG alleviates the need for a bone marrow examination. Before receiving the initial dose of anti-D antibody, patients must meet certain criteria. Premedication with acetaminophen 5 to 10 minutes before infusion is recommended.

> ### ⚡ DRUG ALERT
> #### Anti-D Antibody
>
> After administration of anti-D antibody, observe the child for a minimum of 1 hour and maintain a patent IV line. Obtain baseline vital sign measurements before the infusion and again 5, 20, and 60 minutes after beginning the infusion. If fever, chills, or headache occurs during or shortly after the infusion, the nurse should administer acetaminophen, diphenhydramine (Benadryl), and/or hydrocortisone (Solu-Cortef). Observe the patient for an additional hour after the anti-D antibody infusion is complete.

Splenectomy is for patients who have chronic severe ITP that is not responsive to pharmacologic management and have increased risk of severe hemorrhage. It is the only treatment associated with long-term remission for majority of these children and therefore removes the risk of hemorrhage (Scott and Montgomery, 2007; Wilson, 2009). Before splenectomy is considered, it is generally recommended to wait until the child is older than 5 years of age because of the increased risk of bacterial infection. Administration of pneumococcal, meningococcal, and *H. influenzae* vaccines before splenectomy is recommended (if they were not previously administered). The child also receives penicillin prophylaxis after splenectomy. The appropriate length of prophylactic therapy is controversial, but in general, a minimum of 3 years of therapy is recommended.

Prognosis

The majority of children with ITP have a self-limiting course without major complications. Some children develop chronic ITP and require ongoing therapy. A splenectomy may modify the disease process, and the child may be asymptomatic.

Nursing Care Management

Nursing care is largely supportive and should include teaching regarding the possible side effects of therapy and limitation in activities while the child's platelet count is lower than 100,000/mm³. Children with ITP should not participate in any contact sports, bike riding, skateboarding, in-line skating, gymnastics, climbing, or running. Encourage parents to engage their children in quiet activities and to prevent any injuries to the child's head (e.g., by having the child wear protective headgear and lining the crib with protective padding). Instruct the parents to obtain prompt medical evaluation if the child sustains head or abdominal trauma. As with any condition with an uncertain outcome, the family needs emotional support.

> **QUALITY PATIENT OUTCOMES: ITP**
> - Serious bleeding episode prevented
> - Activities that increase risk for serious bleeding avoided
> - Treatment administered without serious side effects

DISSEMINATED INTRAVASCULAR COAGULATION

DIC, also known as consumption coagulopathy, is not a primary disease but a secondary disorder of coagulation that complicates a number of pathologic processes (e.g., hypoxia, acidosis, shock, and endothelial damage [burns]) and many severe systemic disease states (e.g., congenital heart disease, necrotizing enterocolitis, gram-negative bacterial sepsis, rickettsial infections, and some severe viral infections). The hallmarks of this disorder are bleeding and clotting, which occur simultaneously.

Pathophysiology

DIC occurs when the first stage of the coagulation process is abnormally stimulated (Fig. 35-7). Although there is no well-defined sequence of events, two distinct phases can be identified. First, when the clotting mechanism is triggered in the circulation, thrombin is generated in greater amounts than the body neutralize. Consequently, there is rapid conversion of fibrinogen to fibrin with aggregation and destruction of platelets. Local and widespread fibrin deposition occurs in blood vessels. The thrombi impede the blood flow with eventual necrosis of tissues. Concurrently, the fibrinolytic mechanism is activated, which causes extensive destruction of clotting factors. With a deficiency of clotting factors, the child is vulnerable to uncontrollable hemorrhage into vital organs. An additional complication is damage to and hemolysis of RBCs.

Clinical Manifestations

The signs and symptoms of DIC are the same as those of many other diseases, which often confuses the diagnosis. There is evidence of bleeding—petechiae, purpura, bleeding from openings in the skin (e.g., a venipuncture site or surgical incision), hypotension, and dysfunction of organs from infarction and ischemia.

Diagnostic Evaluation

DIC is suspected when there is an increased tendency to bleed (Box 35-7). Hematologic findings include prolonged prothrombin, partial thromboplastin, and thrombin times. There is a profoundly depressed platelet count, fragmented RBCs, and depleted fibrinogen levels.

Therapeutic Management

Direct treatment toward control of the underlying or initiating cause, which in most instances stops the coagulation problem spontaneously. Administration of platelets and fresh frozen plasma may be needed to replace lost plasma components, especially in the child whose underlying disease remains uncontrolled. The extremely ill newborn infant may require exchange transfusion with fresh blood. The administration of IV heparin to inhibit thrombin formation is most often restricted to cases in which there has been no response to treatment of the underlying disease or replacement of coagulation factors and platelets.

Nursing Care Management

The goals of nursing care are to be aware of the possibility of DIC in the severely ill child and to recognize signs that might indicate its presence. The skills needed to monitor IV infusion and blood transfusions and to administer heparin are the same as for any child receiving these therapies. Because the child is usually cared for in an intensive care unit, the special needs of the family must be considered. (See Chapter 26.)

OTHER HEMATOLOGIC DISORDERS

NEUTROPENIA

Neutropenia is a reduction in the number of circulating neutrophils and is usually defined as an ANC of less than $1000/mm^3$ in infants 2 weeks to 1 year of age or less than $1500/mm^3$ in children older than 1 year of age. African-Americans have ANCs that are 200 to $600/mm^3$ lower than those of Caucasians (Dinauer and Newburger, 2009; Segel and Halterman, 2008).

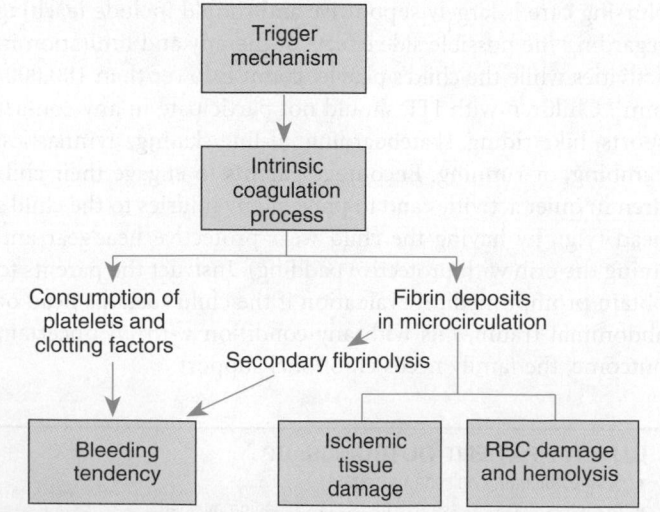

Fig. 35-7 Effects of disseminated intravascular coagulation. *RBC,* Red blood cell.

BOX 35-7   CLINICAL MANIFESTATIONS OF DISSEMINATED INTRAVASCULAR COAGULATION

Petechiae
Purpura
Bleeding from openings in the skin
  • Venipuncture site
  • Surgical incision
Bleeding from umbilicus, trachea (newborn)
Evidence of gastrointestinal bleeding
Hypotension
Organ dysfunction from infarction and ischemia

TABLE 35-8 CLINICAL AND HEMATOLOGIC FEATURES OF SOME CONGENITAL NEUTROPENIAS

FEATURE	SEVERE CONGENITAL NEUTROPENIA (KOSTMANN DISEASE)	FAMILIAL BENIGN NEUTROPENIA	CHRONIC BENIGN NEUTROPENIA; IDIOPATHIC AUTOIMMUNE NEUTROPENIA	RETICULAR DYSGENESIS
Etiology	Autosomal recessive (occasionally autosomal dominant) inheritance pattern	Dominant inheritance pattern	Antineutrophil antibodies detected in almost all cases	Failure of stem cells to produce myeloid and lymphoid cells
Severity	Severe illness Life-threatening pyogenic infections in first months of life	Variable; benign to severe infections	Benign	Severe, fatal thymic dysplasia; lymphoid hypoplasia
Clinical findings	Skin infection Aphthous ulcers Septicemia Meningitis Peritonitis Lung abscess Lymphadenopathy Splenomegaly (20%)	Less troublesome infection to severe infection	Paronychia Gingivitis Impetigo—mild infections, localized	Severe bacterial and viral infection Neonatal death
Hematologic findings	Anemia Neutropenia, <200/mm³ Monocytosis Eosinophilia Risk of leukemia	Neutropenia, usually <300/mm³ Monocytosis	No anemia Absent mature PMN Some band forms Monocytosis	Neutropenia Lymphopenia
Marrow findings	↑ Promyelocytes Absent MM, B, PMN ↑ Monocytes ↑ Eosinophils ↑ Plasma cells	↓ MM, B, PMN "Maturation arrest"	Absent PMN Normal myeloid cells to band stage; lymphocytes increased	Absent myeloid and absent lymphoid cells Normal thrombopoiesis and erythropoiesis
Treatment	Antibiotics Supportive measures G-CSF Bone marrow transplantation	No therapy G-CSF, if indicated	Antibiotics, as indicated G-CSF, if indicated	Bone marrow transplantation

Modified from Lanzkowsky P: *Manual of pediatric hematology and oncology*, San Diego, 2005, Academic Press.
B, Bands; MM, metamyelocytes; PMN, polymorphonuclear leukocytes; G-CSF, granulocyte colony-stimulating factor.

The ANC is calculated by multiplying the total WBC count by the percentage of neutrophils and bands in the differential count (see Table 35-1). When the ANC is less than 500/mm³, the risk of life-threatening infection is high (Boxer, 2007; Segel and Halterman, 2008). Several different types of neutropenia occur in children (Table 35-8). This discussion focuses on the most common type: chronic benign neutropenia.

Diagnostic Evaluation

Chronic benign neutropenia generally represents disorders characterized by mild to moderate neutropenia that are not associated with an increase in infections and often have spontaneous remissions (Boxer, 2007; Segel and Halterman, 2008). Neutropenia is often detected as an incidental finding during the evaluation of a child with fever. The ANC is usually below 500/mm³, and the only physical findings (if any) are those related to infection. Oral ulcerations and skin infections are the most common manifestation of chronic benign neutropenia. However, most children have no infections despite the markedly reduced ANC. Examination of bone marrow aspirates shows normal cellularity with absence of mature neutrophils. Antineutrophil antibodies are usually present, but their absence does not exclude the diagnosis.

To determine a child's neutrophil response during times of infection, a steroid stimulation test may be performed. The child is given a dose of IV steroid, and the neutrophil count is measured at hourly intervals for 4 to 5 hours. If the ANC increases to more than 1000/mm³ after the dose of steroid, the child will have the same response during times of infection. Failure of the ANC to rise is an indication for increased vigilance and medical attention if the child develops fever of 38.3° C (101° F) or higher. These children may require hospitalization and aggressive treatment with broad-spectrum IV antibiotics, depending on the severity of the illness.

Therapeutic Management

Therapy to increase the ANC is rarely required. Children who have recurrent or severe infections, however, may benefit from the administration of G-CSF.

CSFs are a naturally occurring group of glycoproteins. They were first discovered and characterized because of their effect on growth and differentiation of marrow cells. Recombinant DNA technology has enabled the production of large quantities of highly purified CSFs that are nearly identical to the naturally occurring substances and have successfully increased the neutrophil count in a wide variety of neutropenic conditions (Boxer, 2007; Segel and Halterman, 2008).

Children with chronic benign neutropenia have normal cellular immunity; therefore they should receive their routine childhood immunizations.

Nursing Care Management

The care of the child with neutropenia primarily focuses on educating the parents. Instruct parents to keep their child away from large indoor crowds (e.g., grocery store on Saturday morning, movie theaters, daycare centers, church nursery) and individuals who are ill. Parents also need to seek medical attention if their child has a fever of 38.3° C (101° F) or higher, or if skin lesions develop. Because G-CSF is administered parenterally only, parents need to know how to administer subcutaneous injections.

Support the Family

Neutropenia can have many effects on family life. Some parents must quit their jobs to avoid sending their child to daycare. Provide financial counseling as indicated. Parents of children with neutropenia need a listening ear for their frustrations and continued reassurance that these children usually recover by the age of $4\frac{1}{2}$ years.

HENOCH-SCHÖNLEIN PURPURA

Henoch-Schönlein purpura (HSP), also referred to as allergic vasculitis, allergic purpura, and anaphylactoid purpura, is a relatively common acquired disorder in children characterized by a nonthrombocytopenic purpura, arthritis, nephritis, and abdominal pain.

The etiology is unknown, but the disease often follows an upper respiratory tract infection, and allergy or drug sensitivity plays a role in some instances. The disease occurs in children ages 6 months to 16 years but more frequently in children ages 2 to 11 years. It is observed more often in Caucasian children than in those of other races and almost twice as often in boys than in girls.

Pathophysiology

The disease is characterized by inflammation of small blood vessels, and the manifestations observed are influenced by the size and distribution of the affected vessels. A generalized vasculitis of dermal capillaries (and to a lesser extent small arterioles and veins), causing extravasation of RBCs, produces the petechial skin lesions. Inflammation and hemorrhage may also occur in the gastrointestinal tract, synovium, glomeruli, and central nervous system.

Clinical Manifestations

The onset of the disease may be abrupt, with the simultaneous appearance of several manifestations, or gradual, with the sequential appearance of different manifestations. The primary feature, however, is a symmetric purpura that involves the buttocks and lower extremities but may extend to include the extensor surfaces of the upper extremities and, less commonly, the upper trunk and face. The rash may be associated with maculopapular lesions, urticaria, and erythema. There is often

marked edema of the scalp, eyelids, lips, ears, and dorsal surfaces of the hands and feet, especially in infants and younger children. In severe cases the skin may slough, leaving denuded areas that are similar in appearance and treatment to partial-thickness burns.

Arthritic effects are evident in two thirds of affected children and range from asymptomatic swelling around a single joint to painful, tender swelling of several joints, most often the knees and ankles. The involvement is periarticular and resolves in a few days without permanent damage or deformity.

Two thirds of affected children have gastrointestinal involvement manifested by recurrent colicky midabdominal pain, often associated with nausea and vomiting. The stools contain gross or occult blood and mucus.

Renal involvement occurs in up to 50% of affected children and is potentially the most serious long-term complication. Initially the nephritis is manifested as blood, casts, and protein in the urine. Although the majority of children with renal involvement recover completely, some develop chronic renal disease with eventual renal failure.

Diagnostic Evaluation

Diagnosis is usually established on the basis of the history and clinical manifestations. Laboratory tests are used to assess gastrointestinal and renal involvement and to determine adequacy of hemostatic function. Tests for occult blood in the stool are performed. Increased levels of immunoglobulin A are a frequent finding.

Therapeutic Management

Management is primarily supportive, with close observation for signs of renal or gastrointestinal involvement. Edema, rash, malaise, and arthralgia are usually managed with appropriate analgesics such as NSAIDs and mild sedation if necessary. Corticosteroids may be prescribed for relief of more severe edema, arthralgia, and colicky abdominal pain. The nephropathy requires careful monitoring of fluid and electrolyte balance, salt intake, and blood pressure. Antihypertensive agents may be needed.

The majority of children recover without the need for hospitalization, and in most instances a single acute episode clears spontaneously within a month. Others may have periodic recurrences for as long as 2 to 3 years before attaining permanent remission from symptoms. Rarely, death occurs from severe gastrointestinal complications, acute renal failure, or central nervous system involvement. Children with HSP nephritis should receive long-term follow-up because renal involvement is evident in 40% of the patients, many of whom exhibit severe proteinuria (Wilson, 2009).

Nursing Care Management

Nursing care of the child hospitalized with HSP is primarily supportive, with vigilant observation for signs of complications. Measure vital signs and record them at regular intervals, obtain specimens for laboratory examination, and administer medication as prescribed. Carefully observe urine and stools for fresh and occult blood.

If the child suffers from joint pain, then proper positioning, careful movement, and administration of analgesics, including opioids, helps to reduce discomfort. More severe involvement, such as gastrointestinal symptoms and nephritis, is managed as for any such disorder.

Concern about the unsightly appearance of the rash is common. Inform the child and parents that it is only a temporary phenomenon, and that the child can wear clothing that helps hide the rash, such as long-sleeved shirt, long pants, or a robe. Emphasizing good grooming and attractive apparel helps promote a more positive self-image. If the skin surface is denuded, treatment may involve débridement and dressing changes similar to that in the care of burns. (See Chapter 29.)

IMMUNOLOGIC DEFICIENCY DISORDERS

A number of disorders can cause profound, often life-threatening alterations in the body's immune system. The most serious are those conditions that completely depress immunity, such as severe combined immunodeficiency disease (SCID). However, the one disorder that generates the most anxiety in both the family and the community is HIV infection and the subsequent development of AIDS.

Several classifications of immune dysfunction exist. For example, AIDS, SCID, and Wiskott-Aldrich syndrome are disorders in which the body is unable to mount an immune response. The immune response can also be misdirected. In autoimmune disorders, antibodies, macrophages, and lymphocytes attack healthy cells. Some such disorders and their target organs are myasthenia gravis (muscle cells), Graves disease (thyroid cells), and type 1 diabetes (B cells in the pancreas). AIDS, SCIDS, and Wiskott-Aldrich syndrome are discussed here; the other disorders are covered elsewhere in this book.

MECHANISMS INVOLVED IN IMMUNITY

The function of the immune system is to differentiate "self" from "nonself" and to initiate a response to eliminate the "nonself" or foreign substance, known as an antigen. All cells in the body have specific cell surface markers unique to the individual. These cell surface markers are known as the **major histocompatibility complex (MHC)**. Because the markers were first identified on human leukocytes, they are commonly referred to as **human leukocyte antigens (HLAs)**.

The body's protective mechanisms consist of complex, overlapping defense systems. Intact skin serves as the first line of protection for the body. Body secretions such as saliva, sweat, and tears contain chemicals that can kill many organisms. The stomach contains acids that can destroy swallowed pathogens. Organisms trapped in the mucus of the nose and mouth are expelled by sneezing or coughing. If the foreign substance has penetrated these barriers, cellular elements are mobilized.

The immune system is composed of the primary lymphoid organs (thymus, bone marrow, and probably liver) and the secondary lymphoid organs (lymph nodes, spleen, and gut-associated lymphoid tissue). The immune system has two types of function: nonspecific and specific. Nonspecific immune defenses are activated on exposure to any foreign substance but react similarly regardless of the type of antigen; they are unable to identify the antigen, except to know that it is "nonself." The principal activity of this system is phagocytosis, the process of ingesting and digesting foreign substances. Phagocytic cells include neutrophils and monocytes (see p. 1415). Specific defenses are discussed in the following section.

Specific Immune Mechanisms

Specific (adaptive) defenses are those that have the ability to recognize the antigen and respond selectively. The components of adaptive immunity are humoral immunity and cell-mediated immunity. The cells responsible for these two forms of immunity are the lymphocytes, specifically B lymphocytes and T lymphocytes.

Humoral immunity involves antibody production and complement and is concerned with immune processes occurring outside the cells, such as on cell surfaces or in body fluids. The principal cell involved in antibody production is the B lymphocyte, which is probably produced in the bone marrow. When challenged with an antigen, B cells divide and differentiate into plasma cells. The plasma cells produce and secrete large quantities of antibodies specific to the antigen. Five classes of immunoglobulin (Ig) antibodies have been identified: IgG, IgM, IgA, IgD, and IgE, each serving a specific function.

On initial exposure to an antigen, the B-lymphocyte system begins to produce antibody, predominantly IgM, which appears in 2 to 3 days. This process is referred to as the primary antibody response. With subsequent exposure to the antigen, a secondary antibody response occurs. Specific IgG antibodies are formed within 4 to 10 days. An example of the secondary response is the response that occurs with repeat administration of an immunization agent, often called a booster. Memory B cells allow the immune system to recognize the same antigen for months or years.

When antibody reacts with antigen, they bind to form an antigen-antibody complex. This binding serves several functions. Antibody aids in the phagocytosis of antigen by sensitizing it in such a manner that it is more readily destroyed by phagocytes, a process known as opsonization.

Antibody also activates or fixes complement, the second component of humoral immunity. The complement system is a series of proteins (C1 to C9) present in serum that results in a cascade of enzymatic actions and death of a viable antigen. After being activated by antibody, complement produces a chemotactic factor that summons T lymphocytes and macrophages to the antigen site.

Cell-mediated immunity involves a variety of specific functions mediated by the T lymphocyte and occurs within the cell. T lymphocytes do not carry typical immunoglobulins on their surfaces as do the B cells. Microscopically T cells appear identical; however, they are functionally heterogeneous, and there are several subsets, including cytotoxic T cells, helper T cells, and suppressor T cells. T cells may also be classified structurally by the distinctive molecules on their surfaces, known as cluster designations (CDs). Once mature, T cells carry markers known as T2 (CD2), T3 (CD3), T5 (CD5), and T7 (CD7). Helper T cells carry a T4 (CD4) marker and a suppressor, and cytotoxic T cells carry a T8 (CD8) marker.

Specific functions of cell-mediated immunity include (1) protection against most viral, fungal, and protozoan infections and slow-growing bacterial infections, such as tuberculosis; (2) rejection of histoincompatible grafts; (3) mediation of cutaneous delayed hypersensitivity reactions, such as in tuberculin testing; and (4) probably immune surveillance for malignant cells. In addition, T lymphocytes also have regulatory functions within the immune system. For example, helper T lymphocytes help B lymphocytes and other types of T cells to mount an optimum immune response. The cellular immune response is initiated when a T lymphocyte is sensitized by antigen. In response to this contact, the T cell releases numerous humoral factors called lymphokines, which eventually bring about the death of the antigen. Interferons are a group of proteins secreted by leukocytes and infected host cells that nonspecifically inhibit viral replication, promote phagocytosis, and stimulate the killer activity of sensitized lymphocytes.

HUMAN IMMUNODEFICIENCY VIRUS INFECTION AND ACQUIRED IMMUNODEFICIENCY SYNDROME

HIV infection and AIDS have generated intense investigation and constitute one of the major medical, public health, and social issues of our time (Ezekowitz, 2009). In the early 1980s the first cases of AIDS were identified in adult men in urban coastal communities; eventually AIDS affected women and children and broader social and geographic groups. Advances in research and major improvements in the treatment and management of HIV infection have stabilized the incidence of new HIV infections and AIDS globally, with disproportionate distribution of HIV infections and AIDS deaths occurring among people of sub-Saharan Africa (United Nations Programme on HIV/AIDS, 2008).

Worldwide, in 1999 to 2002, it was estimated that 60% of the 42 million HIV-infected individuals were women, and 2.7 million children younger than 15 years of age were living with HIV/AIDS (Centers for Disease Control and Prevention, 2003). The estimated rate of persons living with HIV/AIDS in 2007 declined to 33 million HIV-infected individuals; over 16 million of these were women, and 2 million were children younger than 15 years of age, 90% of whom live in sub-Saharan Africa (Kline, Ferris, Jones, et al, 2009; United Nations Programme on HIV/ AIDS, 2008). In 2001, it was estimated that 800,000 children younger than 15 years of age became newly infected with HIV, compared with an estimated 370,000 children younger than 15 years who became infected with HIV in 2007 (United Nations Programme on HIV/AIDS, 2008). In 2007 an estimated 270,000 HIV-infected children younger than 15 years died because of AIDS; the vast majority of them were from sub-Saharan Africa (Kline, Ferris, Jones, et al, 2009; United Nations Programme on HIV/AIDS, 2008).

The Centers for Disease Control and Prevention estimated that 100 to 200 infants with HIV infection are born in the United States annually (Paintsil and Andiman, 2009). More than ninety percent of these children acquired the disease perinatally from their mothers. The rate of mother-to-child transmission of HIV continues to decrease due to such interventions as increase HIV testing of pregnant women, elective cesarean, use of antiretroviral prophylaxis, and avoidance of breast feeding (Paintsil and Andiman, 2009; Vergidis, Falagas, and Hamer, 2009). In 2006 only about 28 HIV-infected infants

were born in the United States (Noble, 2009). Transmission from mother to child can be reduced from 25% to less than 2% by the use of the preventive interventions, especially antiretroviral therapy during pregnancy, labor, and the neonatal period (Ezekowitz, 2009).

Children of minority populations in the United States are disproportionately affected by the HIV epidemic. Of the children diagnosed with AIDS, the majority were African-American, followed by Hispanic and Caucasian. Since 1996, HIV/AIDS has no longer been listed among the 10 leading causes of death for young children in the United States, regardless of nationality (Palfrey and Richmond, 2005).

Although adolescents ages 13 to 24 years of age with AIDS account for only approximately 5% of the cumulative total of AIDS cases in the United States, they are one of the fastest-growing groups of newly infected persons in the country (Yogev and Chadwick, 2007). The rising AIDS rate among adolescents may be attributed to increased participation in high-risk behaviors such as unprotected sexual contact and IV drug use.

Etiology

HIV is the primary cause of AIDS. There are different strains of HIV. HIV-2 is prevalent in Africa, whereas HIV-1 is the more common form in the United States and elsewhere. Horizontal transmission of HIV occurs through intimate sexual contact or parenteral exposure to blood or body fluids containing visible blood. Vertical (perinatal) transmission occurs when an HIV-infected pregnant woman passes the infection to her infant. There is no evidence that casual contact between infected and uninfected individuals can spread the virus.

The majority of children with HIV infection are younger than 7 years of age. Children with HIV fall into two subpopulations: infants born to HIV-infected women, and adolescents infected as a result of high-risk behaviors.

Perinatal transmission accounts for more than 90% of the AIDS cases to date in children (United Nations Programme on HIV/AIDS, 2008). This is a direct consequence of the increasingly large number of infected women. The transmission of HIV can occur in utero, intrapartum, or after delivery through breast-feeding. Maternal risk factors (e.g., viral load, stage of disease) influence the rate of perinatal transmission, which can range from 15% to 30%. Clinical trials demonstrated a significant decrease in perinatal transmission with zidovudine therapy alone or in combination with lamivudine and nevirapine monotherapy, elective cesarean delivery, and avoidance of breast-feeding for HIV-infected mothers and their newborns (Suksomboom, Poolsup, and Ket-aim, 2007; Vergidis, Falagas, and Hamer, 2009). Nevirapine administered to the mother at labor and to the infant within 48 to 72 hours of life is the most popular regimen in the developing world because of its ease of administration and low cost (Paintsil and Andiman, 2009). The World Health Organization has recommended that pregnant women be treated with an antiretroviral regimen appropriate for their own health if possible (Yogev and Chadwick, 2007). Culturally appropriate opportunities for HIV testing, diagnosis, and access to early treatment and prevention services to reduce further HIV transmission are key to reducing new infections and ultimately decreasing HIV prevalence in the United States and globally (Centers for Disease

Control and Prevention, 2008; United Nations Programme on HIV/AIDS, 2008).

Transfusion of infected blood or blood products has accounted for 3% to 6% of all pediatric AIDS cases to date (Yogev and Chadwick, 2007). Before donor blood started to be routinely tested for HIV in 1985, children with hemophilia were especially at risk because factor concentrates were prepared from pooled plasma. Since the initiation of donor blood screening and development of purification techniques for factor concentrates, transfusion-associated HIV infection has become virtually nonexistent. By 1988, major advances in screening and testing of the blood supply in the United States had reduced the risk of receiving a contaminated single transfusion to 1 in 250,000 (Bove, 1987).

Sexual contact is the leading source of exposure to HIV in the United States. In the young pediatric population this is an infrequent route of transmission; a small number of children have been infected through sexual abuse. In contrast, sexual activity is a major cause of HIV infection in adolescents. Given that the average time from HIV infection to the development of AIDS in adults is 10 years, most people in their twenties with AIDS were likely infected in their teen years. Adolescents commonly take risks and experiment; participation in high-risk behaviors, including IV drug use and unsafe sexual practices, increases their risk of becoming infected with HIV.

Pathophysiology

HIV primarily infects a specific subset of T lymphocytes, the CD4 T cells, but it can also invade cells of the monocyte-macrophage lineage. The virus takes over the machinery of the CD4 lymphocyte, using it to replicate itself and rendering the CD4 cell dysfunctional. Such suppression of cell-mediated immunity places a person at risk for opportunistic infections. HIV also causes dysfunction of B cells and antigen-presenting cells, which results in suppression of humoral immunity.

Although the course of HIV infection varies among individuals, a common progression of events has been recognized. Immediately after primary infection, there is dissemination of virus and seeding of lymphoid organs, along with a transient decrease in the number of CD4 lymphocytes in peripheral blood. An immune response follows, and the resulting level of plasma virus is generally maintained for years. A period of clinical latency ensues that may be longer than 10 years in adults. The CD4 lymphocyte count gradually decreases over time; at some point, physical symptoms appear. The count eventually reaches a critical level below which there is substantial risk of opportunistic illnesses followed by death.

A more rapid progression of disease occurs in perinatally infected children. This is primarily due to the naiveté and immaturity of the developing immune system. Rapid progression of HIV infection in infants and children is also correlated with higher viral burden and faster depletion of infected CD4 lymphocytes than in adults (Yogev and Chadwick, 2007). Perinatally acquired HIV has declined with the use of preventive measures such as HIV counseling, voluntary testing practices, and highly active antiretroviral therapy (HAART). HAART, typically a combination of two nucleoside analog reverse transcriptase inhibitors and a protease inhibitor, is the current gold standard for HIV-infected pregnant women and

---

BOX 35-8 **COMMON CLINICAL MANIFESTATIONS OF HUMAN IMMUNODEFICIENCY VIRUS INFECTION IN CHILDREN**

- Lymphadenopathy
- Hepatosplenomegaly
- Oral candidiasis
- Chronic or recurrent diarrhea
- Failure to thrive
- Developmental delay
- Parotitis

BOX 35-9 **COMMON DEFINING CONDITIONS FOR ACQUIRED IMMUNODEFICIENCY SYNDROME IN CHILDREN**

- *Pneumocystis carinii* pneumonia
- Lymphoid interstitial pneumonitis
- Recurrent bacterial infections
- Wasting syndrome
- Candidal esophagitis
- Human immunodeficiency virus encephalopathy
- Cytomegalovirus disease
- *Mycobacterium avium-intracellulare* complex infection
- Pulmonary candidiasis
- Herpes simplex disease
- Cryptosporidiosis

---

has significantly reduced the transmission of HIV (Cibulka, 2006; Gaum and Yogen, 2002; Garcia-Tejedor, Maiques, Perales, et al, 2009).

Clinical Manifestations

The majority of infants with perinatally acquired HIV infection are clinically normal at birth. Clinical manifestations (Box 35-8) vary and include such signs as lymphadenopathy, hepatosplenomegaly, and unexplained diarrhea. Diarrhea may be a result of pathogens or HIV itself due to malabsorption of carbohydrate, protein, and fat (Anabwani, Woldetsadik, and Kline, 2005; Yogev and Chadwick, 2007). HIV-infected children often do not grow normally; they may be proportionally smaller in both length and weight for age.

The diagnosis of AIDS in children is based on the occurrence of certain illnesses or conditions (Centers for Disease Control and Prevention, 2008). Box 35-9 lists the most common AIDS-defining conditions observed among American children. Recurrent bacterial infections, parotitis, lymphoid interstitial pneumonitis (LIP), and early onset of progressive neurologic deterioration are characteristic of children with HIV infection but are rarely seen in affected adults. Kaposi sarcoma, one of the hallmarks of adult disease, is found in fewer than 1% of affected children. *Pneumocystis carinii* pneumonia (PCP), a frequent cause of death, is common in both age-groups.

Central nervous system abnormalities considered to be the direct effects of HIV infection occur in most children with AIDS. Secondary infections with opportunistic and common pathogens are infrequent in this population. Either global or specific neuropsychologic deficits may occur at random intervals. Many affected children display evidence of developmental disability. Deficits in motor skills, communication, and behavioral functioning are common. Expressive language (use of language) is more frequently impaired than receptive language (understanding of language).

Diagnostic Evaluation

For children 18 months of age and older, the HIV enzyme-linked immunosorbent assay and Western blot immunoassay are performed to detect HIV infection. In infants born to HIV-infected mothers, results of these assays are positive because of the presence of maternal antibodies derived transplacentally. Maternal antibodies may persist in the infant for up to 18 months. Therefore other diagnostic tests are employed: virus culture; polymerase chain reaction for detection of proviral DNA; and p24 antigen detection, which is HIV specific. With these techniques more than 95% of infected infants can be diagnosed by 1 to 3 months of age. Positive results on two separate tests performed on separate blood specimens are required for the diagnosis of HIV infection. Infants born to HIV-infected women are also considered HIV infected if they meet the Centers for Disease Control and Prevention surveillance case definition for AIDS. Before testing, provide counseling to the parent or guardian, including an explanation of HIV infection, the reason for the test, implications of positive test results, confidentiality issues, risk reduction behaviors, and beneficial effects of early intervention.

The Centers for Disease Control and Prevention (1994) has developed a classification system to describe the spectrum of HIV disease in children (Table 35-9). The system indicates the severity of clinical signs and symptoms and the degree of immunosuppression. Mild signs and symptoms include lymphadenopathy, parotitis, hepatosplenomegaly, and recurrent or persistent sinusitis or otitis media. Moderate signs and symptoms include LIP and a variety of organ-specific dysfunctions or infections. Severe signs and symptoms include AIDS-defining illnesses with the exception of LIP. Children with LIP have a better prognosis than those with other AIDS-defining illnesses.

The clinical and immunologic classification categories are mutually exclusive. Once classified, an infant or child may not be reclassified into a less severe category, even if clinical or immunologic status improves in response to antiretroviral therapy or other factors. For children whose HIV infection is not yet confirmed, the letter E (for "vertically exposed") is placed in front of the classification. The immune categories are based on CD4 lymphocyte counts and percentages. Age adjustment of these numbers is necessary because normal counts, which are relatively high in infants, decline steadily until 6 years of age, when they reach adult norms.

Therapeutic Management

The goals of therapy for HIV infection include slowing the growth of HIV, promoting or restoring normal growth and development, preventing complicating infections and cancers, improving quality of life, and prolonging survival. Antiretroviral drugs work at various stages of the HIV life cycle to prevent reproduction of functional new virus particles. Antiretroviral therapy regimens are continually evolving. Classes of antiretroviral agents include nucleoside reverse transcriptase inhibitors (e.g., zidovudine, didanosine, stavudine, lamivudine, abacavir); nonnucleoside reverse transcriptase inhibitors (e.g., nevirapine, delavirdine, efavirenz); and protease inhibitors (e.g., indinavir, saquinavir, ritonavir, nelfinavir, amprenavir, lopinavir, ritonavir). Combinations of antiretroviral drugs are used to stall the emergence of drug resistance, which has been observed historically in some children who received a single drug. In addition, investigational drugs are available through pediatric clinical trials. Although antiretroviral drugs are not a cure, they can delay progression of the disease (Centers for Disease Control and Prevention, 2008; Bhaskaran, Hamouda, Sannes, et al, 2008; Henry, Tebas, and Lane, 2006).

Strict scheduling requirements, side effects, and need for multiple medications, which at times are not very palatable, make it difficult for children and adolescents to take their medications at the right time and in proper coordination with their meals. Yet adhering to the medication schedule is critical to preventing the development of resistant forms of HIV (Anabwani, Woldetsadik, and Kline, 2005; Yogev and Chadwick, 2007). Clinical improvements include weight gain in children with previous growth retardation, decreased hepatosplenomegaly, improvement in symptoms of HIV-associated encephalopathy, and improvement in immune system function.

PCP is the most common opportunistic infection in children infected with HIV. It occurs most frequently between 3 and 6 months of age, when HIV status may be unclear. Therefore all

TABLE 35-9	PEDIATRIC HUMAN IMMUNODEFICIENCY VIRUS INFECTION CLASSIFICATION*			
IMMUNOLOGIC CATEGORY	N: NO SIGNS/ SYMPTOMS	A: MILD SIGNS/ SYMPTOMS	B: MODERATE SIGNS/ SYMPTOMS†	C: SEVERE SIGNS/ SYMPTOMS†
No evidence of suppression	N1	A1	B1	C1
Evidence of moderate suppression	N2	A2	B2	C2
Severe suppression	N3	A3	B3	C3

From Centers for Disease Control and Prevention: 1994 Revised classification system for human immunodeficiency virus infection in children less than 13 years of age, *MMWR Recomm Rep* 43(RR-12):1-10, 1994.

*Children whose human immunodeficiency virus infection status is not confirmed are classified by using the above table with the letter *E* (for perinatally exposed) placed before the appropriate classification code (e.g., EN2).

†Both category C and lymphoid interstitial pneumonitis in category B are reportable to state and local health departments as acquired immunodeficiency syndrome.

infants born to HIV-infected women should receive prophylaxis during the first year of life, according to the guidelines set by the American Academy of Pediatrics (2000). For children older than 1 year of age, the need for prophylaxis depends on the presence of severe immunosuppression or a history of PCP. Trimethoprim-sulfamethoxazole is the agent of choice. If adverse effects are experienced with this medication, dapsone, atovaquone, or pentamidine may be used.

Prophylaxis is often given for other opportunistic infections, such as disseminated *Mycobacterium avium-intracellulare* complex infection, candidiasis, and herpes simplex. However, prophylaxis may be discontinued if the patients have experienced sustained (>6 months' duration) immune reconstitution with HAART, regardless of a history of opportunistic infection (Yogev and Chadwick, 2007). Administration of IVIG has been helpful in preventing recurrent or serious bacterial infections in some HIV-infected children (Spector, Gelber, McGrath, et al, 1994; Yogev and Chadwick, 2007).

Immunization against common childhood illnesses, including the pneumococcal and influenza vaccines, is recommended for all children exposed to and infected with HIV. The varicella and measles-mumps-rubella (MMR) vaccine can be administered if there is no evidence of severe immunocompromise (Yogev and Chadwick, 2007; Centers for Disease Control and Prevention, 1999). Because antibody production to vaccines may be poor or decrease over time, immediate prophylaxis after exposure to several vaccine-preventable diseases (e.g., measles, varicella) is warranted. Children receiving IV gamma globulin prophylaxis may not respond to the MMR vaccine (Centers for Disease Control and Prevention, 2003).

HIV infection often leads to marked failure to thrive and multiple nutritional deficiencies. Nutritional management may be difficult because of recurrent illness, diarrhea, and other physical problems. The nurse should implement intensive nutritional interventions if the child's growth begins to slow or weight begins to decrease.

Prognosis

Early recognition and improved medical care have changed HIV infection from a rapidly fatal disease to a chronic one. Children diagnosed with AIDS in the first year of life, particularly with opportunistic infections such as PCP, are more likely to have a shorter life expectancy. Progressive encephalopathy also carries a poor prognosis. In contrast, LIP, lymphadenopathy, hepatosplenomegaly, and parotitis are associated with a later onset of symptoms and prolonged survival.

The most accurate prognostic indicators of a poor outcome are a CD4 lymphocyte percentage of less than 15% and a high viral load of more than 100,000 copies/ml (Yogev and Chadwick, 2007). The high AIDS mortality rate should be the focus of developed countries in their unrelenting efforts to provide access to HIV testing to all women and preventive antiretroviral treatment for all HIV-infected women and children, thereby changing a fatal disease to chronic disease for children worldwide (Paintsil and Andiman, 2009).

Nursing Care Management

Education concerning the transmission and control of infectious diseases, including HIV infection, is essential for children with HIV infection and anyone involved in their care. The nurse should present basic information about Standard Precautions in an age-appropriate manner, with careful consideration of the educational level of the individual. (See Infection Control, Chapter 27.) It is important to also emphasize safety issues, including appropriate storage of special medications and equipment (e.g., needles and syringes). Unfortunately, relatives, friends, and others in the general public are fearful of contracting HIV infection. Criticism and ostracism of the child and family are common. In an effort to protect the child and deal with the community's fear, the family may limit the child's activities outside the home. Although certain precautions are justified in limiting exposure to sources of infections, these must be tempered with concern for the child's normal developmental needs. Both the family and the community need ongoing education about HIV to dispel many of the myths that have been perpetuated by uninformed persons.

Prevention is a key component of HIV education. Educating adolescents about HIV is essential in preventing HIV infection in this age-group. Education should include information on the routes of transmission, the hazards of IV and other recreational drug use, and the value of sexual abstinence and safe sex practices (American Academy of Pediatrics, 2001; Yogev and Chadwick, 2007). Such education should be a part of anticipatory guidance provided to all adolescent patients. Nurses can also encourage adolescents at risk to undergo HIV counseling and testing. In addition to identifying infected teenagers and getting them into care, such counseling affords adolescents an opportunity to learn about, and possibly change, their risk behaviors.

QUALITY PATIENT OUTCOMES: HIV
- Early recognition of signs and symptoms of HIV
- HIV infection slowed or maintained
- Growth and development promoted
- No infectious complications or cancer development
- Adherence to antiretroviral therapy
- Prolonged survival
- Quality of life supported

The nurse's role in the care of the child with HIV is multifaceted. The nurse serves as educator, direct care provider, case manager, and advocate. As with all children with chronic illnesses, these children have much involvement with the health care system. Clinic visits and hospitalizations may become frequent as the disease progresses. The physiologic care of the child is directed at minimizing exposure to infections; delaying the development of viral resistance; supplying nutritional support; providing comfort measures, including pain management; and assessing and recognizing changes in status that may indicate new complications. The scope of nursing care changes with new symptoms, changes in treatment, and disease progression. Psychologic interventions vary with the unique circumstances of each child and family.

Common psychosocial concerns include disclosing the diagnosis to the child, making custody plans when the parent is infected, and anticipating the loss of a family member. Other stressors may include financial difficulties, HIV-associated stigma, attempts to keep the diagnosis a secret, infection of other family members, and any losses associated with HIV. Most mothers of these children are single mothers who are also HIV infected. As primary caretakers, they often attend to the needs of their child first, neglecting their own health in the process. The nurse can encourage the mother to receive regular health care. Family members are often involved in the care of the child, particularly if the mother has symptomatic illness. The nurse is an integral part of the multidisciplinary team necessary for the successful management of the complex medical and social problems of these families.

The multiple complications associated with HIV disease are potentially painful (Ezekowitz, 2009). Aggressive pain management is essential for these children to have an acceptable quality of life. Their pain may be due to infections (e.g., otitis media, dental abscess), encephalopathy (e.g., spasticity), adverse effects of medications (e.g., peripheral neuropathy), or an unknown source (e.g., deep musculoskeletal pain). Pain is related not only to disease processes, but also to the various treatments these children often undergo, including venipunctures, lumbar punctures, biopsies, and endoscopies. Ongoing assessment of pain is crucial and is most easily accomplished in older children who are able to communicate. Nonverbal and developmentally delayed children are more difficult to assess. The nurse should be alert for other signs of pain: emotional detachment, lack of interactive play, irritability, and depression. Effective pain management depends on the appropriate use of pharmacologic agents, including EMLA or LMX cream, acetaminophen, NSAIDs, muscle relaxants, and opioids. Tolerance to opioids may indicate the need for increased dosing; monitoring of use ensures safety. Nonpharmacologic interventions (guided imagery, hypnosis, relaxation, and distraction techniques) are useful adjuncts.

Children with HIV infection attend daycare centers and school. It is well established that the risk of HIV transmission in school settings is minimal. These institutions are required to follow the guidelines for infection control measures as established by the Centers for Disease Control and Prevention and Occupational Safety and Health Administration. Standard Precautions describing proper management of blood and body fluids are followed. It is recommended that school personnel receive current HIV information and include it in the health education curriculum from kindergarten through twelfth grade (American Academy of Pediatrics, 2000, 1999). School nurses play a vital role in educating the school staff, students, and parents. They also are invaluable in monitoring the needs of known affected children.

Confidentiality is another major issue in daycare and school attendance. Parents and legal guardians have the right to decide whether they inform a school or daycare agency of a child's HIV diagnosis.* Unfortunately, myths about HIV infection continue to exist, and the family often wishes to avoid any potential criticism or ostracism of the child.

---

*Additional information is available from the AIDS hotline, 800-232-4636.

WISKOTT-ALDRICH SYNDROME

Wiskott-Aldrich syndrome (WAS) is a congenital X-linked recessive disorder characterized by a triad of abnormalities: (1) thrombocytopenia with small platelets, (2) eczema, and (3) immunodeficiency involving selective functions of B and T lymphocytes.

Pathophysiology

The abnormal gene, on the proximal arm of the X chromosome, has been identified and designated as the WAS protein (Buckley, 2007; Bonilla and Geha, 2009). The exact defect is unknown. A variety of pathologic findings are evident. The platelets are abnormally small and have a shortened life span, possibly because of a metabolic defect in their synthesis. The primary immunologic defect consists of the inability of phagocytes (macrophages) to process foreign antigens, particularly polysaccharides such as pneumococci. As a result, immunologically competent cells fail to produce normal immunoglobulin patterns. The level of IgM is diminished early in the course of the disease, whereas levels of IgG, IgA, and IgE may be elevated initially and then gradually decline (Bonilla and Geha, 2009). Typically isohemagglutinins (anti-A and anti-B agglutinins in the blood) are decreased or absent. There is a defect in antibody production that progresses to an antibody deficiency with a decrease in T suppressor lymphocytes that explains the increased susceptibility to opportunistic infections (Bonilla and Geha, 2009; Fleisher, 2006).

The thymus and lymph nodes are normal at birth but become progressively dysfunctional with age until a profound cellular immunodeficiency results. Consequently these children are highly susceptible to infection and malignancy, especially lymphoma and leukemia.

Clinical Manifestations

At birth the major effect of the disorder is increased bleeding because of the thrombocytopenia, especially bleeding at the circumcision site or bloody diarrhea, which may be the presenting feature (Bonilla and Geha, 2009). As the child grows older, recurrent infection and eczema become more severe, and the bleeding becomes less frequent.

The eczema is typical of the allergic type and readily becomes superinfected. Chronic infection with herpes simplex is a frequent problem and may lead to chronic keratitis with loss of vision. From infection, chronic pulmonary disease, sinusitis, and otitis media result. In those children who survive the bleeding episodes and overwhelming infections, malignancy presents an additional threat to survival.

Diagnostic Evaluation

The diagnosis can usually be made during the neonatal period because of the thrombocytopenia. Specific tests for immunologic function confirm the diagnosis. Carrier detection is also possible.

Therapeutic Management

Medical treatment primarily involves (1) counteracting the bleeding tendencies with platelet transfusions, (2) giving IVIG to provide passive immunity, (3) administering prophylactic antibiotics to prevent and control infection, and (4) providing aggressive local therapy for the eczema (Bonilla and Geha, 2009; Buckley, 2004). Splenectomy may improve the platelet count, although the risk of asplenic sepsis in these infants is extremely high. These children require the same prophylactic antibiotics and appropriate immunizations as does any child with asplenia. Despite their immunodeficiency, they are able to mount an adequate immunologic response to the inactivated vaccines. When an HLA-matched donor exists, HSCT is the treatment of choice. The lack of suitable therapeutic options for most WAS patients has prompted investigations into gene therapy (Notarangelo and Mori, 2005).

Nursing Care Management

Because of the poor prognosis for these children, the main nursing consideration is supporting the family in the care of a fatally ill child. (See Chapter 23.) Direct physical care at controlling the problems imposed by the disorder. The measures used to control bleeding are similar to those used in hemophilia and vWD. Another major goal is to prevent or control infection. Because eczema is a troublesome problem, nursing measures specific to this condition are especially important.

The genetic implications of this X-linked recessive disorder differ little from those for any other X-linked disease. However, the multiplicity of defects tends to affect emotional adjustment and physical care to a greater degree than in other X-linked disorders. The nurse can be especially supportive by providing short-term goals during periods of hospitalization and by focusing on long-range needs through coordinated efforts with a public health nurse.

SEVERE COMBINED IMMUNODEFICIENCY DISEASE

SCID is a defect characterized by the absence of both humoral and cell-mediated immunity (Bonilla and Geha, 2009; Buckley, 2007). The terms *Swiss-type lymphopenic agammaglobulinemia,* which refers to the autosomal recessive form of the disease, and *X-linked lymphopenic agammaglobulinemia* have been used to describe this disorder, which, as the names imply, can follow either mode of inheritance.

Pathophysiology

The exact cause of SCID is unknown. The theories include (1) a defective stem cell that is incapable of differentiating into B or T cells; (2) defects in the organs responsible for the differentiating process, primarily the thymus and lymphoid complex; or (3) an enzymatic defect that suppresses lymphocytic cell function.

The consequence of the immunodeficiency is an overwhelming susceptibility to infection and to the graft-versus-host reaction, which can occur when any histoincompatible (unmatched) tissue from an immunocompetent donor is infused into the immunodeficient recipient. Because of its immunodeficiency, the body is unable to reject the foreign, incompatible tissue. Therefore the antigenic donor cells attack the host's tissues. The graft-versus-host reaction is a serious complication in the treatment of SCID with HSCT.

Clinical Manifestations

The most common manifestation is susceptibility to infection early in life, most often in the first month. Specifically, the disorder in children is characterized by chronic infection, failure to completely recover from an infection, frequent reinfection, and infection with unusual agents. In addition, the history reveals no logical source of infection. Failure to thrive is a consequence of the persistent illness.

If the child should receive blood products containing viable lymphocytes, signs of graft-versus-host reaction, such as fever, skin rash, alopecia, hepatosplenomegaly, and diarrhea, are expected (Bonilla and Geha, 2009). Because tissue damage does not become evident in the reaction for 7 to 20 days, the symptoms may be mistaken for an infection. However, the presence of a graft-versus-host reaction increases the child's susceptibility to overwhelming infection and therefore is a grave complication.

Diagnostic Evaluation

Diagnosis is usually based on a history of recurrent, severe infections from early infancy; a familial history of the disorder; and specific laboratory findings, which include lymphopenia, lack of lymphocyte response to antigens, and absence of plasma cells in the bone marrow. Documentation of immunoglobulin deficiency is difficult during infancy because of the normally delayed response of infants in producing their own immunoglobulins and maternal transfer of IgG.

Therapeutic Management

The definitive treatment is a histocompatible HSCT. If the condition is diagnosed at birth or within the first 3 months of life, more than 95% of cases can be treated successfully with HLA-identical or T-cell depleted haploidentical (half-matched) related bone marrow stem cells (Bonilla and Geha, 2009; Buckley, 2007). The most suitable donor is a sibling with HLA-matched bone marrow. Because SCID is inherited, an identical twin, who usually is a perfect donor, is not a candidate because he or she would also display the disorder.

Other approaches to the management of SCID include providing passive immunity with IVIG and maintaining the child in a sterile environment. The latter is effective only if the measure is instituted before any infectious process takes hold in the infant, and it represents an extreme effort to prevent life-threatening infections. Other transplant procedures include nonidentical-HLA bone marrow grafting and fetal liver or thymus transplantation. The results of these procedures are still uncertain, although they provide potential hope for future children born with the disorder. Recent success in treating X-linked SCID by gene therapy in Europe offers hope that gene therapy will eventually be the treatment of choice for cases of SCID in which researchers have identified the molecular bases (Bonilla and Geha, 2009; Buckley, 2007).

Nursing Care Management

Nursing care depends on the type of therapy used. If bone marrow transplantation is attempted, the care is consistent with that needed by patients undergoing bone marrow transplantation for any condition. (See Chapter 36.) To prevent infection, implement all interventions aimed at protecting the immunocompromised child. However, even with exacting environmental control, these children are prone to opportunistic infection. Chronic fungal infections of the mouth and nails with *Candida albicans* are frequent problems despite vigorous efforts at prevention or treatment. A hoarse voice may result from repeated esophageal and vocal cord erosions from the fungus. It is important to stress to parents that such conditions are not a result of laxity on their part in preventing them but are a result of the severe immunologic disorder. Encourage parents to immediately notify a physician regarding any evidence of a worsening infection.

Because the prognosis for a child with SCID is very poor if a compatible bone marrow donor is not available, direct nursing care at supporting the family in caring for a child with a fatal illness. (See Chapter 23.) Genetic counseling is essential because of the modes of transmission in either form of the disorder.

KEY POINTS

- Major functions of the hematologic system include production of cells, oxygenation, distribution of nutrients to the cells, immune protection, heat regulation, and waste collection from the cells.
- The major blood-forming organs of the body are red bone marrow, the lymphatic system, and the reticuloendothelial system.
- Anemia is defined as a reduction in the number of RBCs and/or hemoglobin concentration compared with age-matched normal values. The anemias are classified by etiology, physiology, or morphology.
- The nurse's role in treatment of anemia is to assist in establishing a diagnosis, prepare the child for laboratory tests, administer prescribed medications, decrease tissue oxygen needs, implement safety precautions, and observe for complications.
- The main nursing goal in prevention of nutritional anemia is parent education regarding well-balanced meals and correct feeding practices.
- SCA is a hereditary hemoglobinopathy in which normal adult HgbA is partly or completely replaced by sickle hemoglobin (HgbS).
- Nursing care of the child with SCA focuses on teaching the family how to prevent and recognize sickle cell complications and helping the child and parents adjust to a lifelong chronic disease.
- Nursing care of the child with thalassemia includes observing for complications of multiple blood transfusions, assisting the child in coping with the effects of illness, and fostering parent-child adjustment to long-term illness.
- Causes of acquired aplastic anemia include irradiation, drugs, industrial and household chemicals, infections, and infiltration and replacement of myeloid elements; however, the majority of cases are idiopathic.
- Clotting depends on the processes of vascular spasm, platelet aggregation, coagulation, and clot formation.
- Nursing care of the child with hemophilia involves preventing bleeding by decreasing the risk of injury, recognizing bleeding and managing it with factor replacement, preventing the crippling effects of joint degeneration, and preparing the child and family for and supporting them in home care.
- Immunodeficiency disorders render the affected individual unable to fight infectious organisms.
- HIV infection is primarily acquired in infancy from a parent with HIV infection and in adolescence from engaging in high-risk behaviors.

REFERENCES

Akinyanju OO, Otaigbe AI, Ibidapo MOO: Outcome of holistic care in Nigerian patients with sickle cell anaemia, *Clin Lab Haematol* 27:195-199, 2005.

Akman M, Cebecci D, Okur V, et al: The effects of iron deficiency on infant's developmental test performance, *Acta Paediatr* 93:1391-1396, 2004.

Altucher K, Rasmussen KM, Barden EM, et al: Predictors of improvement in hemoglobin concentration among toddlers enrolled in the Massachusetts WIC program, *J Am Diet Assoc* 105(5):709-715, 2005.

American Academy of Pediatrics, Committee on Pediatric AIDS and Committee on Adolescence: Adolescents and human immunodeficiency virus infection: the role of the pediatrician in prevention and intervention, *Pediatrics* 107(1):188-190, 2001.

American Academy of Pediatrics, Committee on Pediatric AIDS: Identification and care of HIV-exposed and HIV-infected infants, children and adolescents in foster care, *Pediatrics* 106(1):149-153, 2000.

American Academy of Pediatrics, Committee on Nutrition: Iron fortification of infant formulas, *Pediatrics* 104(1):119-123, 1999.

Anabwani MG, Woldetsadik EA, Kline MW: Treatment of human immunodeficiency virus (HIV) in children using antiretroviral drugs, *Semin Pediatr Infect Dis* 16:116-124, 2005.

Andrews NC, Ullrich CK, Fleming MD: Disorders of iron metabolism and sideroblastic anemia. In Orkin SH, Nathan DG, Ginsburg D, et al, editors: *Nathan and Oski's hematology of infancy and childhood*, ed 7, Philadelphia, 2009, Saunders.

Armstrong-Wells J, Grimes S, Sidney D, et al: Utilization of TCD screening for primary stroke prevention in children with sickle cell disease, *Neurology* 72:1316-1321, 2009.

Bell MD: Red blood cell transfusions, *Pediatr Rev* 28(8):299-304, 2007.

Beyer JE: Judging the effectiveness of analgesia for children and adolescents during vaso-occlusive events of sickle cell disease, *J Pain Symptom Manage* 19(1):63-72, 2000.

Bhaskaran K, Hamouda O, Sannes M, et al: Changes in the risk of death after HIV seroconversion compared with mortality in the general population, *JAMA* 300(1):51-59, 2008.

Bolarman Z, Kadikoylu G, Yukselen V, et al: Oral versus intramuscular cobalamin treatment in megaloblastic anemia: a single-center, prospective, randomized, open-label study, *Clin Ther* 25:124-134, 2003.

Bonilla FA, Geha RS: Primary immunodeficiency diseases. In Orkin SH, Nathan DG, Ginsburg D, et al, editors: *Nathan and Oski's hematology of infancy and childhood*, ed 7, Philadelphia, 2009, Saunders.

Bove JR: Transfusion-associated hepatitis and AIDS: what is the risk? *N Engl J Med* 317:242-245, 1987.

Boxer LA: Leukopenia. In Kliegman RM, Jenson HB, Behrman RE, et al, editors: *Nelson textbook of pediatrics*, ed 18, Philadelphia, 2007, Saunders.

Brodsky R, Jones R: Aplastic anaemia, *Lancet* 365:1647-1656, 2005.

Brown DL: Congenital bleeding disorders, *Curr Probl Pediatr Adolesc Health Care* 35:38-62, 2005.

Brown K, Subramony C, May W, et al: Hepatic iron overload in children with sickle cell anemia on chronic transfusion therapy, *J Pediatr Hematol Oncol* 31(5):309-312, 2009.

Brugnara C, Oski FA, Nathan DG: Diagnostic approach to the anemic patient. In Orkin SH, Nathan DG, Ginsburg D, et al, editors: *Nathan and Oski's hematology of infancy and childhood*, ed 7, Philadelphia, 2009, Saunders.

Buchanan GR, DeBaun MR, Quinn CT, et al: Sickle cell disease, *Hematology Am Soc Hematol Educ Program* 35-47, 2004.

Buckley RH: Evaluation of the immune system. In Kliegman RM, Jenson HB, Behrman RE, et al, editors: *Nelson textbook of pediatrics*, ed 18, Philadelphia, 2007, Saunders.

Buckley RH: A historical review of bone marrow transplantation for immunodeficiencies, *J Allergy Clin Immunol* 113:793-800, 2004.

Bulas D: Screening children for sickle cell vasculopathy: guidelines for transcranial Doppler evaluation, *Pediatr Radiol* 35:235-241, 2005.

Butler CC, Vidal-Alaball J, Cannings-John R, et al: Oral vitamin B_{12} versus intramuscular vitamin B_{12} for vitamin B_{12} deficiency: a systemic review of randomized control trials, *Fam Pract* 23(3):279-285, 2006.

Butler RB, Schultz JR, Forsberg AD, et al: Promoting safer sex among HIV-positive youth with haemophilia: theory, intervention, and outcome, *Hemophilia* 9(2):214-222, 2003.

Cariappa R, Wilhite TR, Parvin CA: Comparison of PFA-100 and bleeding time testing in pediatric patients with suspected hemorrhagic problems, *J Pediatr Hematol Oncol* 25(6):474-479, 2003.

Centers for Disease Control and Prevention: HIV Prevalence Estimates—United States, *MMWR* 57(39):1073-1076, 2008.

Centers for Disease Control and Prevention: Increases in HIV diagnoses—29 states, 1999-2002, *MMWR* 52(47):1145-1148, 2003.

Centers for Disease Control and Prevention: Prevention of varicella: updated recommendations of the Advisory Committee on Immunization Practices (ACIP), *MMWR Recomm Rep* 48(RR-6):1-5, 1999.

Centers for Disease Control and Prevention: 1994 Revised classification system for human immunodeficiency virus infection in children less than 13 years of age, *MMWR Recomm Rep* 43(RR-12):1-10, 1994.

Chiocca EM: Sickle cell crisis: severe pain and potential tissue necrosis are the major concerns, *AJN* 96(9):49, 1996.

Cibulka NJ: Mother-to-child transmission of HIV in the United States, *AJN* 106(7):56-63, 2006.

Cohen AR, Galanello R, Rennell DJ, et al: Thalassemia, *Hematology Am Soc Hematol Educ Program* 14-34, 2004.

Cohen AR, Glimm E, Porter JB: Effect of transfusional iron intake on response to chelation therapy in β-thalassemia major, *Blood* 111(2):583-587, 2008.

Cunningham MJ: Update on Thalassemia: clinical care and complications, *Pediatr Clin North Am* 55:447-460, 2008.

Cunningham MJ, Sankaran VG, Nathan DG, et al: The Thalassemias. In Orkin SH, Nathan DG, Ginsburg D, et al, editors: *Nathan and Oski's hematology of infancy and childhood*, ed 7, Philadelphia, 2009, Saunders.

Curry H: Bleeding disorder basics, *Pediatr Nurs* 30(5):402-405, 2004.

DeBaun MR, Vichinsky E: Hemoglobinopathies. In Kliegman RM, Jenson HB, Behrman RE, et al, editors: *Nelson textbook of pediatrics*, ed 18, Philadelphia, 2007, Saunders.

De Meyer SF, Deckmyn H, Vanhoorelbeke K: von Willebrand factor to the rescue, *Blood* 113(21):5049-5057, 2009.

Diaz M, Rosado JL, Allen LH, et al: The efficacy of a local ascorbic acid–rich food in improving iron absorption from Mexican diets: a field study using stable isotopes, *Am J Clin Nutr* 78:436-440, 2003.

Dinauer MC, Newburger PE: The phagocyte system and disorders of granulopoiesis and granulocyte function. In Orkin SH, Nathan DG, Ginsburg D, et al, editors: *Nathan and Oski's hematology of infancy and childhood*, ed 7, Philadelphia, 2009, Saunders.

Driscoll MC: Sickle cell disease, *Pediatr Rev* 28:259-268, 2007.

Ezekowitz RAB: Hematologic manifestations of systemic diseases. In Orkin SH, Nathan DG, Ginsburg D, et al, editors: *Nathan and Oski's hematology of infancy and childhood*, ed 7, Philadelphia, 2009, Saunders.

Fleisher, TA: Primary immune deficiencies: windows into the immune system, *Pediatr Rev* 27(10):363-372, 2006.

Garcia-Tejedor A, Maiques V, Perales A, et al: Influence of highly active antiretroviral treatment (HAART) on risk factors for vertical HIV transmission, *Acta Obstet Gynecol* 88(8):882-887, 2009.

Gaum PJ, Yogen R: The role of protease inhibitor therapy in children with HIV, *Pediatr Drugs* 4:581-607, 2002.

Glader B: The anemias. In Kliegman RM, Jenson HB, Behrman RE, et al, editors: *Nelson textbook of pediatrics*, ed 18, Philadelphia, 2007a, Saunders.

Glader B: Anemias of inadequate production. In Kliegman RM, Jenson HB, Behrman RE, et al, editors: *Nelson textbook of pediatrics*, ed 18, Philadelphia, 2007b, Saunders.

Grace RF, Lux SE: Disorders of the red cell membrane. In Orkin SH, Nathan DG, Ginsburg D, et al, editors: *Nathan and Oski's hematology of infancy and childhood*, ed 7, Philadelphia, 2009, Saunders.

Gribbons D, Zahr LK, Opas SR: Nursing management of children with sickle cell disease: an update, *J Pediatr Nurs* 10(4):232-242, 1995.

Gulbis B, Haberman D, DuFour D, et al: Hydroxyurea for sickle cell disease in children and for prevention of cerebrovascular events: the Belgian experience, *Blood* 205(7):2685-2690, 2005.

Haining WN, Duncan C, Lehmann LE: Principles of bone marrow and stem cell transplantation. In Orkin SH, Nathan DG, Ginsburg D, et al, editors: *Nathan and Oski's hematology of infancy and childhood*, ed 7, Philadelphia, 2009, Saunders.

Hankins J, Aygun B: Pharmacotherapy in sickle cell disease—state of the art and future prospects, *Br J Haematol* 145(3):296-308, 2009.

Hankins J, Jeng M, Harris S, et al: Chronic transfusion therapy for children with sickle cell disease and recurrent acute chest syndrome, *J Pediatr Hematol Oncol* 27(3):158-161, 2005.

Heeney M, Dover GJ: Sickle cell disease. In Orkin SH, Nathan DG, Ginsburg D, et al, editors: *Nathan and Oski's hematology of infancy and childhood*, ed 7, Philadelphia, 2009, Saunders.

Heeney M, Ware RE: Hydroxyurea for children with sickle cell disease, *Pediatr Clin North Am* 55:483-501, 2008.

Henry WK, Tebas P, Lane HC: Explaining, predicting, and treating HIV-associated CD4 cell loss, *JAMA* 296(12):1523-1525, 2006.

Hord JD: The acquired pancytopenias. In Kliegman RM, Jenson HB, Behrman RE, et al, editors: *Nelson textbook of pediatrics*, ed 18, Philadelphia, 2007, Saunders.

Howard J, Davies SC: Sickle cell disease in North Europe, *Scand J Clin Lab Invest* 67:27-38, 2007.

Hubbard J: Megaloblastic and nonmegaloblastic macrocytic anemias. In McKenzie SB, editor: *Clinical laboratory hematology*, Upper Saddle River, NJ, 2004, Pearson, Prentice Hall.

Kaferle J, Strzoda CE: Evaluation of macrocytosis, *Am Fam Physician* 79(3):203-208, 2009.

Khoury H, Grimsley E: Oxygen inhalation in nonhypoxic sickle cell patients during vasoocclusive crisis, *Blood* 86(10):3998, 1995.

Kline MW, Ferris MG, Jones DC, et al: The pediatric AIDS corps: responding to the African HIV/AIDS health professional resource crisis, *Pediatrics* 123:134-136, 2009.

Lanzkowsky P: *Manual of pediatric hematology and oncology*, ed 4, San Diego, 2005, Academic Press.

Lucarelli G, Gaziev J: Advances in the allogeneic transplantation for thalassemia, *Blood Rev* 22:53-63, 2008.

Mabry-Hernandez IR: Screening for iron deficiency anemia—including iron supplementation for children and pregnant women, *Am Fam Physician* 79(10):897-898, 2009.

Manco-Johnson MJ, Abshire TC, Shapiro AD, et al: Prophylaxis versus episodic treatment to prevent joint disease in boys with severe hemophilia, *N Engl J Med* 357:535-544, 2007.

Marsh JCW: Management of acquired aplastic anaemia. *Blood Rev* 19:143-151, 2005.

McKenzie SB: Introduction to anemia. In McKenzie SB, editor: *Clinical laboratory hematology*, Upper Saddle River, NJ, 2004, Pearson, Prentice Hall.

Miller ST, Sleeper LA, Pegelow CH, et al: Prediction of adverse outcomes in children with sickle cell disease, *N Engl J Med* 342:83-89, 2000.

Montgomery RR, Gill JC, Di Paola J: Hemophilia and von Willebrand disease. In Orkin SH, Nathan DG, Ginsburg D, et al, editors: *Nathan and Oski's hematology of infancy and childhood*, ed 7, Philadelphia, 2009, Saunders.

Naithani R, Chandra J, Sharma S: Safety of oral iron chelator deferiprone in young thalassaemics, *Eur J Haematol* 74:217-220, 2005.

National Hemophilia Foundation, American Red Cross: *Playing it safe: bleeding disorders, sports and exercise*, New York, 2005, The Foundation.

National Institutes of Health, National Heart, Lung, and Blood Institute, Division of Blood Disease and Resources: *The management of sickle cell disease*, NIH pub no 02-2117, Bethesda, Md, 2002, National Heart, Lung, and Blood Institute, Health Information Network.

Nead KG, Halterman JS, Kaczorowski JM, et al: Overweight children and adolescents: a risk group for iron deficiency, *Pediatrics* 114(1):104-108, 2004.

Nelson M, Poulter J: Impact of tea drinking on iron status in the UK: a review, *J Hum Nutr Dietet* 17:43-54, 2004.

Neufeld EJ: Oral chelators deferasirox and deferiprone for transfusional iron overload in thalassemia major: new data, new questions, *Blood* 107(9):3436-3441, 2008.

Neunert CE, Buchanan GR, Imbach P, et al: Severe hemorrhage in children with newly diagnosed immune thrombocytopenia purpura, *Blood* 112(10):4003-4008, 2008.

Nienhuis AW: Development of gene therapy for blood disorders, *Blood* 111(9):4431-4444, 2008.

Noble R: *United States statistics summary*, 2009, available at www.avert.org/usa-statistics.htm (accessed July 3, 2009).

Notarangelo LD, Mori L: Wiskott-Aldrich syndrome: another piece in the puzzle, *Clin Exp Immunol* 139:173-175, 2005.

Olivieri NF: The β-thalassemias, *N Engl J Med* 341(2):99-109, 1999.

Pack-Mabien A, Haynes J Jr: A primary care provider's guide to prevention and acute care management of adults and children with sickle cell disease, *J Am Acad Nurse Pract* 21:250-257, 2009.

Paintsil E, Andiman WA: Update on successes and challenges regarding mother-to-child transmission of HIV, *Curr Opin Pediatr* 21:94-101, 2009.

Palfrey JS, Richmond JB: Health services past, present and future. In Cosby AG, Greenberg RE, Southward LH, et al, editors: *About children: authoritative resource on the state of childhood today*, Elk Grove Village, Ill, 2005, American Academy of Pediatrics.

Pavlovich-Danis S: Update on von Willebrand's disease, *Clin Advisor*, Nov-Dec, 28-32, 37-39, 2001.

Perkins S: Disorders of hematopoiesis. In Collins RD, Swerdlow SH, editors: *Pediatric hematopathology*, Philadelphia, 2001, Churchill Livingstone.

Pesce MA: Reference ranges for laboratory tests and procedures. In Kliegman RM, Jenson HB, Behrman RE, et al, editors: *Nelson textbook of pediatrics*, ed 18, Philadelphia, 2007, Saunders.

Platt OS: Prevention and management of stroke in sickle cell anemia, *Hematology Am Soc Hematol Educ Program*, pp 54-57, 2006.

Pongtanakul B, Das PK, Charpentier K, et al: Outcome of children with aplastic anemia treated with immunosuppressive therapy, *Pediatr Blood Cancer* 50:52-57, 2008.

Raphael JL, Bernhardt MB, Mahoney DH, et al: Oral iron chelation and the treatment of iron overload in a pediatric hematology center, *Pediatr Blood Cancer* 52:616-620, 2009.

Redding-Lallinger R, Knoll C: Sickle cell disease—pathophysiology and treatment, *Curr Probl Pediatr Adolesc Health Care* 36(10):346-376, 2006.

Renda M, Fischer P: Vegetarian diets in children and adolescents, *Pediatr Rev* 30:e1-e8, 2009.

Richardson M: Microcytic anemia, *Pediatr Rev* 28:5-14, 2007.

Scott JP, Montgomery RR: Hemorrhagic and thrombotic diseases. In Kliegman RM, Jenson HB, Behrman RE, et al, editors: *Nelson textbook of pediatrics*, ed 18, Philadelphia, 2007, Saunders.

Segel GB: Hereditary spherocytosis. In Kliegman RM, Jenson HB, Behrman RE, et al, editors: *Nelson textbook of pediatrics*, ed 18, Philadelphia, 2007, Saunders.

Segel GB, Halterman JS: Neutropenia in pediatric practice, *Pediatr Rev* 29:12-24, 2008.

Shah S, Vega R: Hereditary spherocytosis, *Pediatr Rev* 25(5):166-170, 2004.

Shaiova L, Wallenstein D: Outpatient management of sickle cell pain with chronic opioid pharmacotherapy, *J Natl Med Assoc* 96(7):984-986, 2004.

Sharathkumar AA, Pipe SW: Post-thrombotic syndrome in children: a single center experience, *J Pediatr Hematol Oncol* 30(4):261-266, 2008.

Spector SA, Gelber RD, McGrath N, et al: A controlled trial of intravenous immune globulin for the prevention of serious bacterial infections in children receiving zidovudine for advanced human immunodeficiency virus infection, *N Engl J Med* 331(18):1181-1187, 1994.

Stainsby D, Jones H, Wells AW, et al on behalf of the SHOT Steering Group: Adverse outcomes of blood transfusion in children: analysis of UK reports to the serious hazards of transfusion scheme 1996-2005, *Br J Haematol* 141:73-79, 2008.

Steen RG, Fineberg-Buchner C, Hankins G, et al: Cognitive deficits in children with sickle cell disease, *J Child Neurol* 20(2):102-107, 2005.

Suksomboom N, Poolsup N, Ket-aim S: Systematic review of the efficacy of antiretroviral therapies for reducing the risk of mother-to-child transmission of HIV infection, *J Clin Pharm Therap* 32:293-311, 2007.

Telfer PT, Lahoz C, Ali K, et al: Intranasal diamorphine for acute sickle cell pain, *Arch Dis Child* 94(12):979-980, 2009.

Thankachan P, Walczyk T, Muthayya S, et al: Iron absorption in young Indian women: the interaction of iron status with the influence of tea and ascorbic acid, *Am J Clin Nutr* 87:881-886, 2008.

Trigg M: Hematopoietic stem cells, *Pediatrics* 113(4):1051-1057, 2004.

United Nations Programme on HIV/AIDS: *Status of the global HIV epidemic: 2008 report on the global AIDS epidemic*, 2008, available at http://data.unaids.org/pub/globalReport/2008/jc1510_2008_global_report_pp29_62_en.pdf (accessed May 11, 2009).

US Department of Health and Human Services, Agency for Healthcare Research and Quality: *Guide to clinical preventive services: recommendations of the U.S. Preventive Services Task Force, 2009* (AHRQ Publication No. 09-IP006), Rockville, Md, August 2009, The Agency, available at www.ahrq.gov/clinic/pocketgd09 (accessed April 16, 2010).

Vergidis PI, Falagas ME, Hamer DH: Meta-analytical studies on the epidemiology, prevention, and treatment of human immunodeficiency virus infection, *Infect Dis Clin North Am* 23:295-308, 2009.

Vichinsky EP, Haberkern CM, Neumayr L, et al: A comparison of conservative and aggressive transfusion regimens in the perioperative management of sickle cell disease, *N Engl J Med* 332(4):206-213, 1995.

Vichinsky E, Styles L: Sickle cell disease: pulmonary complications, *Hematol Oncol Clin North Am* 10(6):1275-1286, 1996.

Watkins D, Whitehead VM, Rosenblatt DS: Megaloblastic anemia. In Orkin SH, Nathan DG, Ginsburg D, et al, editors: *Nathan and Oski's hematology of infancy and childhood*, ed 7, Philadelphia, 2009, Saunders.

White KC: Anemia is a poor predictor of iron deficiency among toddlers in the United States: for heme the bell tolls, *Pediatrics* 115(2):315-320, 2005.

Wilson DB: Acquired platelet defects. In Orkin SH, Nathan DG, Ginsburg D, et al, editors: *Nathan and Oski's hematology of infancy and childhood*, ed 7, Philadelphia, 2009, Saunders.

Wilson D, Hockenberry MJ: *Wong's clinical manual of pediatric nursing*, ed 7, St Louis, 2008, Mosby.

Yalsh HM: *Thalassemia*, New York, 2009, Medscape, available at http://emedicine.medscape.com/article/958850-overview (accessed April 16, 2010).

Ye L, Chang JC, Lin C, et al: Induced pluripotent stem cells offer approach to therapy in thalassemia and sickle cell anemia and option in prenatal diagnosis in genetic diseases, 2009, available at www.pnas.org/cg/doi/10.1073/pnas.0904689106 (accessed June 21, 2009).

Yogev R, Chadwick EG: Acquired immunodeficiency syndrome (human immunodeficiency virus). In Kliegman RM, Jenson HB, Behrman RE, et al, editors: *Nelson textbook of pediatrics*, ed 18, Philadelphia, 2007, Saunders.

Young NS, Calado RT, Scheinberg P: Current concepts in the pathophysiology and treatment of aplastic anemia, *Blood* 108(8):2509-2519, 2006.

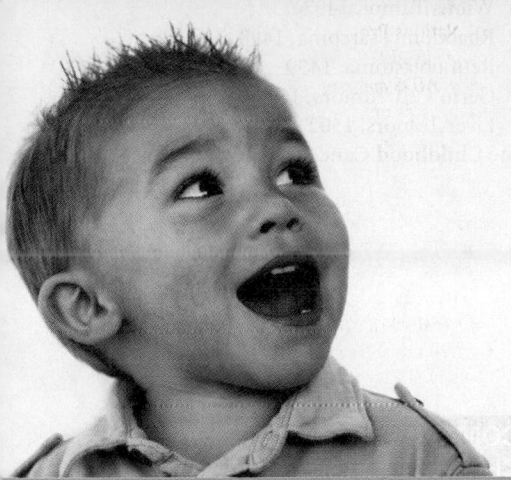

The Child with Cancer

Valerie J. Groben

⊖volve WEBSITE

RELATED TOPICS

Administration of Medication, **Ch. 27**
Anaphylaxis, **Ch. 29**
Anemia, **Ch. 35**
Biologic Development (Adolescence), **Ch. 19**
Bone Marrow Aspiration or Biopsy, **Ch. 27**
The Child with Cerebral Dysfunction, **Ch. 37**
Dental Health, **Ch. 14**
Drug Reactions, **Ch. 18**
Epistaxis (Nosebleeding), **Ch. 35**
Family-Centered Care of the Child with Chronic Illness or
   Disability, **Ch. 22**
Family-Centered Care of the Child During Illness and
   Hospitalization, **Ch. 26**
Family-Centered End-of-Life Care, **Ch. 23**
Immunizations, **Ch. 12**
Infection Control, **Ch. 27**
Lumbar Puncture, **Ch. 27**
Pain Assessment; Pain Management, **Ch. 7**
Physical Examination, **Ch. 6**
Preparation for Diagnostic and Therapeutic Procedures, **Ch. 27**
Stomatitis, **Ch. 16**
Sunburn, **Ch. 18**
Surgical Procedures, **Ch. 27**
Venous Access Devices, **Ch. 28**

CHAPTER OUTLINE

CANCER IN CHILDREN

Few situations in nursing exceed the challenges of caring for a child with cancer. Despite the dramatic improvements in survival rates for these children, the family's needs are tremendous as they cope with a serious physical illness and the fear that the child will not be cured. Nurses should base support of patients and their families on the premise that communication promotes understanding and clarity. With understanding, fear diminishes and hope emerges, and in the presence of hope, anything is possible.

This chapter summarizes the clinical presentation and nursing care issues for the most common types of pediatric cancer. Chapter 22 discusses the general psychologic needs of these children and their families in terms of chronic illness. Chapter 23 discusses situations when the disease is life threatening and death is a possibility.

EPIDEMIOLOGY

Childhood cancer is rare; approximately 12,400 cases of cancer are diagnosed in children younger than 20 years of age in the United States each year. Despite the relatively low incidence, approximately 1600 children under the age of 15 years die from their disease each year, making cancer the leading cause of death from disease in this age-group. The incidence of cancer in children and adolescents is approximately 15 per 100,000 children (Ries, Smith, Gurney, et al, 1999).

The incidence of specific subtypes of childhood cancer can vary according to age, sex and race. For example, males have a higher overall incidence of cancer compared with females, with a ratio of 1.2:1. This is due to the higher incidence of acute lymphoblastic leukemia (ALL), lymphoma, and medulloblastoma—the most common types of childhood cancer—in young boys. Unlike adults, Caucasian children have an overall higher incidence of cancer compared to African-American children. This is accounted for by the higher incidence in ALL and central nervous system (CNS) tumors in Caucasian children. The incidence of childhood cancer is more pronounced during the first year of life with a second peak from ages 2 to 3 years, followed by declining rates until age 9. Although each specific type of cancer has its own age distribution, overall incidence steadily rises from age 9 through adolescence (Scheurer, Bondy, and Gurney, 2011) (see Table 36-1 and Research Focus box).

TABLE 36-1	COMMON FORMS OF CHILDHOOD MALIGNANCY WITH INCIDENCE IN THE UNITED STATES AND PEAK AGE AT DIAGNOSIS	
MALIGNANCY	**PEAK AGE (yr)**	**RATE (per million/yr)**
Leukemia		
Acute lymphoblastic	2-5	24.7
Acute nonlymphoblastic	Constant	5.0
Lymphomas		
Non-Hodgkin	6-16	9.3
Hodgkin	>10	7.5
Central Nervous System Tumors		
Gliomas	Constant	13.4
Medulloblastomas	5-10	4.9
Ependymoma	<5	2.1
Solid Tumors		
Neuroblastomas	<3	8.0
Wilms tumor	<5	6.9
Retinoblastoma	<3	3.0
Rhabdomyosarcoma	2-6 and 14-18	3.7
Ewing sarcoma (primitive neuroectodermal tumor)	10-18	2.1
Osteosarcoma	10-18	3.1
Hepatoblastoma	<2	1.6
Germ cell tumors	<2 and >14	0.4

Adapted from Herrera JM, Krebs A, Harris P, et al: Childhood tumors, *Surg Clin North Am* 80(2):748, 2000.

RESEARCH FOCUS

Childhood Cancer Survival Rates

Childhood cancer survival has dramatically increased over the past 4 decades. In the 1960s, the overall survival rate of childhood cancer was 28% compared to 3-year survival rates now exceeding 80% (Scheurer, Bondy, and Gurney, 2011). The cancers demonstrating the greatest improvement in survival rates are acute leukemia, central nervous system tumors, non-Hodgkin lymphoma, bone tumors, and Wilms tumor. There has been a lack of progress in survival among the adolescent group compared with progress in younger age-groups. The typical definition of "cure" in childhood cancer includes completion of all therapy, clinical and radiologic evidence of no disease, and a period of 5 years since diagnosis.

ETIOLOGY

Often one of the first questions parents of newly diagnosed children with cancer ask is, "How did my child get this and did I do something to cause it?" Parents are also understandably concerned with the question of the likelihood that their other children will get cancer. The cause of cancer is not known. Although there are numerous hypotheses concerning its origin, the most enduring theory is that some genetic alteration results in the unregulated proliferation of cells. Significant advances have been made in our understanding of cell proliferation, programmed cell death (**apoptosis**), genes that activate tumor growth (**oncogenes**), and genes that keep tumor growth in check (**tumor suppressor genes**). Cancer is the result of multiple genetic events but is not necessarily hereditary. Overall, the incidence of cancers caused by direct inheritance is low.

In the early 1970s Alfred Knudson described the "two-hit hypothesis." This explanation of cancer inheritance is best described in retinoblastoma. Like most genes, the retinoblastoma gene *(Rb)* is present in two copies on each cell. It is a tumor suppressor gene, responsible for controlling cell growth. When just one of these copies is lost—the "first hit"—the cell remains normal. However, when the second copy is lost—"second hit"—abnormal cell proliferation occurs and retinoblastoma develops (Knudson, Hethcote, and Brown, 1975). A child can inherit one altered copy of the retinoblastoma gene from a mother or father. Therefore it takes only one more hit for retinoblastoma to develop. Retinoblastoma can be either inherited or sporadic. Familial retinoblastoma manifests earlier and is more commonly bilateral. Population studies of siblings and offspring of children with cancer suggest that there is not, in general, a strong constitutional genetic component for childhood cancers other than retinoblastoma (MacDonald and Lessick, 2000).

Perhaps the most well-known inherited cancer predisposition syndrome is Li-Fraumeni syndrome, which is mainly due to constitutional (in all cells) mutation in the tumor suppressor gene, *p53*. This syndrome is characterized by early incidence of sarcomas, brain tumors, premenopausal breast cancer, and multiple primary tumors. However, other tumors have also been described within the spectrum of this syndrome.

Chromosome abnormalities have been identified in many childhood malignancies and are important in the development of various types of cancer. Chromosome abnormalities can be confined to the tumor or can be present in all cells; the latter are called **germ-line mutations**. Chromosome abnormalities can be due to **translocations** (a rearrangement of information between two chromosomes) or abnormal numbers of chromosomes. For example, many well-established chromosome translocations have been identified in childhood leukemia and solid tumors (see Research Focus box).

Other genetic syndromes that can affect genes or chromosomes and are associated with a predisposition to cancer include Fanconi anemia, Bloom syndrome, Beckwith-Weidemann syndrome, neurofibromatosis type 1, ataxia-telangiectasia, and Klinefelter syndrome.

Children with immunodeficiencies, such as Wiskott-Aldrich syndrome or acquired immunodeficiency syndrome, or children whose immune system has been suppressed, such as

---

RESEARCH FOCUS
Chromosome Abnormalities and Cancer

The Philadelphia chromosome was the first chromosome abnormality to be found in a malignancy. It occurs as a result of a translocation between chromosomes 9 and 22 and is observed in almost all patients with chronic myelogenous leukemia (Altman and Fu, 2011). In addition, children with certain types of congenital chromosome abnormalities, especially those syndromes caused by abnormal numbers of chromosomes, have an increased incidence of cancer. For example, children with Down syndrome (trisomy 21) have a much higher risk of developing leukemia when compared with the general population (Plon and Malkin, 2011; Taub, 2001).

---

following transplant procedures, are at a greater risk for developing various cancers. Of major concern is the increased risk of secondary cancers in some children successfully treated for their primary malignancy.

Risk Factors

Lifestyle-related risks are the main factors that increase the risk of cancer in adults, but have little to no effect on childhood cancer. There is relatively little information to support a strong environmental role in the development of childhood cancer. However, some risk factors are well established. Known risk factors include exposure to ionizing radiation, carcinogenic drugs, immunosuppressive therapy, infections such as Epstein Barr virus, race, and genetic conditions (as previously described).

Although drugs, particularly those containing radioisotopes and immunosuppressive agents, can increase the risk of developing childhood cancer, the one drug most recognized for its carcinogenic effect is diethylstilbestrol. This drug has not been given in the United States since 1971. In the past, large doses of this hormone given to pregnant women to prevent abortion caused adenocarcinoma of the vagina in a significant proportion of the female offspring when they reached adolescence and early adulthood (Hatch, Herbst, Hoover, et al, 2000).

Prevention

Knowledge of the risk factors that increase the likelihood of cancer holds the promise of prevention. Unfortunately, in children the known carcinogens are limited. Therefore at present there is really no known prevention.

Health professionals do have two roles, however. One is aimed at preventing adult type of cancers by educating parents and children about the hazards of known carcinogens, particularly the effects of cigarette smoking and excessive exposure to sunlight. Lung cancer is the leading cause of death from cancer in adults, and malignant melanoma is the leading cause of death from diseases of the skin. Children at higher risk for skin cancer are those with light-colored eyes, complexion, and hair; those who sunburn easily; those who live near the equator; and those with freckles associated with sunburn (Cercato, Nagore, Ramazzotti, et al, 2008). Not only these children but all children should be protected from overexposure to the sun. (See Chapter 18.) In addition, to provide early detection of other types of cancer, males should learn testicular self-examination, and female adolescents should learn breast self-examination and seek periodic health examinations, including a Papanicolaou smear.

BOX 36-1   CARDINAL SYMPTOMS OF CANCER IN CHILDREN

- Unusual mass or swelling
- Unexplained paleness and loss of energy
- Sudden tendency to bruise
- Persistent, localized pain or limping
- Prolonged, unexplained fever or illness
- Frequent headaches, often with vomiting
- Sudden eye or vision changes
- Excessive, rapid weight loss

Data from Hockenberry MJ, Kline NE: Nursing support of the child with cancer. In Pizzo PA, Poplack DP, editors: *Principles and practices of pediatric oncology*, ed 6, Philadelphia, 2011, Lippincott.

Second, health care professionals need to be aware of the cardinal symptoms of childhood cancer (Box 36-1). Unfortunately, fever and pain are manifestations of common childhood disorders and, without a high index of suspicion, may be attributed to minor ailments. The other signs are subtle and easily missed. If parents suspect an abnormality, their concerns must be taken seriously. The greatest weapons against all forms of cancer are early detection and treatment.

DIAGNOSTIC EVALUATION

The evaluation of a child suspected of having cancer may take several days to complete. Specific signs and symptoms depend on the type of cancer and its location. The essential components of a comprehensive evaluation for childhood cancer include complete history and review of symptoms, physical examination, laboratory tests, diagnostic imaging, diagnostic procedures (lumbar puncture [LP], bone marrow aspirate, and biopsy), and surgical pathology.

Complete History

History of present illness—Onset of symptoms, severity and duration, alleviating or potentiating factors

History of previous illnesses—Communicable diseases, infections, medication history, previous hospitalizations or surgeries, exposure to blood products, immunization status

Family history—Family members with prior cases of cancer: type, age at diagnosis, treatment, and outcome

Present health status of family members—History of illness or disease in other family members

Developmental factors—Milestones obtained, recent regression in any milestones

Psychosocial factors—Include family concerns or problems

Review of Symptoms

Skin—History of bruising or bleeding, lesions, lumps, open sores

Head, eyes, ears, nose, and throat (HEENT)—History of trauma, vision disturbances, proptosis, pupil discoloration, unequal pupils, eye muscle weakness, infection, difficulty swallowing

Heart—History of murmur or thrill

Lungs—History of infection, asthma or reactive airway disease, cough, wheezing, shortness of breath, dyspnea

Abdomen—History of abdominal swelling, pain, mass, change in bowel or bladder patterns

Musculoskeletal—History of weakness in extremities, limited range of motion, tenderness or swelling, joint pain

Neurologic—Loss of developmental milestones, altered consciousness, decreased sensations, abnormal reflexes, abnormal cerebellar functions, headaches, seizures

Lymphatic—History of enlarged lymph nodes, frequent infections

Hematologic—History of bruising, nosebleeds or gum bleeding, paleness, fatigue, bloody or tarry-colored stools

Physical Examination

See Physical Examination, Chapter 6.

General—Orientation, general state of health

Skin—Petechiae or ecchymosis, lesions or sores, presence of blood from gum or nose, color of skin

HEENT—Macrocephaly, bulging fontanel, evidence of infection, proptosis, pupil discoloration, anisocoria, extraocular movements not intact, limited peripheral vision, nystagmus, leukocoria

Heart—Murmur or thrill, peripheral pulses

Lungs—Evidence of infection, rales or rhonchi, decreased breath sounds, dyspnea, tachypnea

Abdomen—Hepatosplenomegaly, mass, decreased bowel sounds, striae

Neurologic—Altered consciousness, altered sensation, abnormal reflexes, abnormal cerebellar functions, unstable gait, dysarthria, cranial nerve deficits

Lymphatic—Enlarged lymph nodes

Laboratory Tests

Several laboratory tests must be performed to accurately diagnose and treat children with cancer. The majority of patients have a complete blood count, serum chemistries, liver function tests, coagulation studies, and urinalysis done on initial presentation. For example, patients with leukemia often have a low hemoglobin; low platelet count; and low, normal, or high white blood counts. In addition, these patients may have elevated lactate dehydrogenase, creatinine, and uric acid, which require close monitoring when therapy is initiated. Frequent complete blood counts are necessary to monitor effects of therapy and in some hematologic malignancies, response to therapy.

Blood chemistry yields important information with regards to kidney, liver, bone function, and electrolyte balance. These tests are important to help detect the extent of disease and also to monitor for side effects during therapy. For example, a patient with bone metastasis may have elevated alkaline phosphatase. Elevations in blood urea nitrogen and creatinine may reflect kidney damage from chemotherapy agents. Consequently, regular blood chemistries and urinalysis are standard procedures through the course of the disease.

Diagnostic Procedures

An LP is a routine test employed in leukemia, brain tumors, and other cancers that may metastasize to the CNS. An LP is also used to administer intrathecal drugs in patients with various malignancies such as leukemia.

A bone marrow test is performed by aspirating marrow with a large or fine bore needle. A bone marrow biopsy is performed by obtaining a piece of bone through a special type of needle. These tests are performed to determine the presence or absence of tumor or response to therapy in this specific location. For example, the specific type of leukemia can be identified by examination of the patient's bone marrow and core biopsy. Also, patients with other solid tumors, like neuroblastoma, may have spread of disease to the bone marrow, which can be determined by these procedures.

Diagnostic Imaging

Modern day diagnostic imaging has greatly improved our ability to accurately diagnose childhood cancers. The most commonly employed modes of imaging include chest x rays, computed tomography (CT), magnetic resonance imaging (MRI). More recently, positron emission tomography (PET) is being used increasingly in a variety of pediatric malignancies such as Hodgkin disease and sarcomas. Interventional radiology is playing an increasing role in the diagnosis and management of pediatric malignancies.

Pathologic Evaluation

A biopsy is necessary to establish the diagnosis of a malignancy. Beyond, telling us what type of cancer the patient has, this tissue sample can also be sent for various biologic studies that define the patient's prognosis and allow health care providers to tailor therapy according to the risk group. For example, a bone marrow biopsy determines whether the patient has acute lymphocytic leukemia or acute myelocytic leukemia, but also tells what specific subtype of leukemia the patient has and how aggressively it should be treated. Similarly, patients with neuroblastoma undergo a biopsy of the tumor to establish the diagnosis and to evaluate the tumor for *N-myc* amplification, which determines the type of treatment they receive.

TREATMENT MODALITIES

The use of multimodal therapy consisting of surgery, chemotherapy, and radiotherapy; enrollment of large numbers of children in cooperative group clinical trials or protocols; and improvements in supportive care have greatly increased the survival of children with cancer. Eighty percent of these patients are now expected to be cured of their disease.

Current efforts are aimed at increasing the survival of patients with high-risk tumors, decreasing the acute and long-term side effects of treatment, and studying the biology of the diseases to better identify patients who are at different risk levels for disease recurrence and can therefore benefit from risk-adapted therapies.

Surgery

The main goal of surgery, besides obtaining biopsies, is to remove all traces of tumor and restore normal body functioning. Surgery is most successful when the tumor is encapsulated and localized (confined to the site of origin). It may only be palliative when the cancer is regional (metastasized to an area adjacent to the original site) or advanced (widespread

throughout the body). Obviously the best prognosis is directly related to early detection of the tumor.

Because the majority of pediatric cancers respond well to chemotherapy, more conservative surgical excision is increasingly used in a variety of tumors in an attempt to preserve function and cosmesis. For example, in some types of bone cancer, such as osteosarcoma, patients are successfully treated with resection of the diseased portion of the bone rather than amputation. There is an increasing emphasis on the use of combination drug therapy and radiotherapy after limited surgical intervention.

Chemotherapy

Chemotherapy may be the primary form of treatment, or it may be an adjunct to surgery or radiotherapy. The majority of chemotherapy agents work by interfering with the function or production of nucleic acids, deoxyribonucleic acid (DNA), or ribonucleic acid (RNA). Although several drugs with antineoplastic capabilities have been effective in treating different forms of cancer, the remarkable survival rates have been the result of improved combination drug regimens. Combining drugs allows for optimum cell cycle destruction with minimum toxic effects and decreased resistance by the cancer cells to the agent. For example, VAC (vincristine [Oncovin], doxorubicin [Adriamycin], and cyclophosphamide [Cytoxan]) combines complementary cytotoxic effects with nonsimilar side effects. Doxorubicin and cyclophosphamide are myelosuppressive, whereas vincristine is neurotoxic.

In addition to more effective combinations of drugs, several advances in the administration of chemotherapy have permitted continuous or intermittent IV administration without multiple venipunctures. The use of venous access devices (catheters and implantable infusion ports) has greatly facilitated safe and effective drug administration with minimum discomfort for the child. (See Chapter 28.) Continuous infusions over an extended period using syringe pumps have made possible the administration of certain drugs, such as cytosine arabinoside, in higher doses with less toxicity than when the drug is administered intermittently.

Chemotherapeutic agents can be classified according to their primary mechanism of action. Alkylating agents replace a hydrogen atom of a molecule by an alkyl group. The irreversible combination of alkyl groups with nucleotide chains, particularly DNA, causes unbalanced growth of unaffected cell constituents so that the cell eventually dies. These agents have a steep dose-response curve and, for this reason, can be used in high-dose therapy regimens. Examples of alkylating agents include cyclophosphamide, ifosfamide, cisplatin (Platinol), and dacarbazine. Antimetabolites resemble essential metabolic elements needed for cell growth but are sufficiently altered in molecular structure to inhibit further synthesis of DNA or RNA; their maximum effect occurs in cells that are actively producing DNA. Examples of antimetabolites include methotrexate and mercaptopurine. Plant alkaloids arrest cells in metaphase (a phase of mitosis) by binding to microtubular protein needed for spindle formation. Examples include vincristine and vinblastine. Antitumor antibiotics are natural products that interfere with cell division by reacting with DNA in such a way as to prevent further replication of DNA and transcription of RNA. Examples include doxorubicin and daunomycin.

Both adrenal and gonadal hormones have antineoplastic properties. The precise mechanism of action is still unclear. Adrenocorticosteroids, in theory, bind with DNA and alter the transcription process. Although there are a number of cortisone preparations, prednisone and dexamethasone are most frequently used.

A number of agents are not categorized according to the preceding classifications. For example, L-asparaginase is an enzyme isolated from extracts of bacterial cultures of *Escherichia coli* or *Erwinia carotovora*. It hydrolyzes L-asparagine, an amino acid, to L-aspartic acid, which prevents the cell from synthesizing protein needed for DNA and RNA synthesis. Because L-asparagine is synthesized by normal cells but must be exogenously supplied to certain leukemic and lymphoma cells, administration of the enzyme destroys the essential exogenous supply while sparing normal cells of untoward effects.

An understanding of the actions and side effects of these drugs is essential to nursing care of children with cancer. Unfortunately, almost all drugs are not selectively cytotoxic for malignant cells, and other cells with a high rate of proliferation, such as the bone marrow elements and hair, skin, and epithelial cells of the gastrointestinal tract, are also affected. Frequently the problems related to the destruction of these normal cells require more nursing care than the disease itself.

More recently, a number of targeted agents called tyrosine kinase inhibitors have been developed and are being used in a variety of pediatric and adult malignancies. Examples of some of these agents include imatinib, sunitinib, and sorafenib.

Precautions in Administering and Handling Chemotherapeutic Agents

Many chemotherapeutic agents are **vesicants** (sclerosing agents) that can cause severe cellular damage if even minute amounts of the drug infiltrate surrounding tissue. Only nurses experienced with chemotherapeutic agents should administer vesicants (Fig. 36-1). Guidelines are available* and must be followed meticulously to prevent tissue damage to patients. Interventions for extravasation vary, but each nurse should be aware of the institution's policies before giving any vesicant and implement them at once if indicated.

> ### ! NURSING ALERT
>
> Chemotherapeutic drugs must be given through a free-flowing intravenous (IV) line. The infusion is stopped immediately if any sign of infiltration (pain, stinging, swelling, or redness at needle site) occurs.

In addition to extravasation, a potentially fatal complication is anaphylaxis, especially from L-asparaginase, bleomycin, cisplatin, and etoposide (VP-16). (See Chapter 29.) Hypersensitivity reactions to these chemotherapeutic agents are characterized by

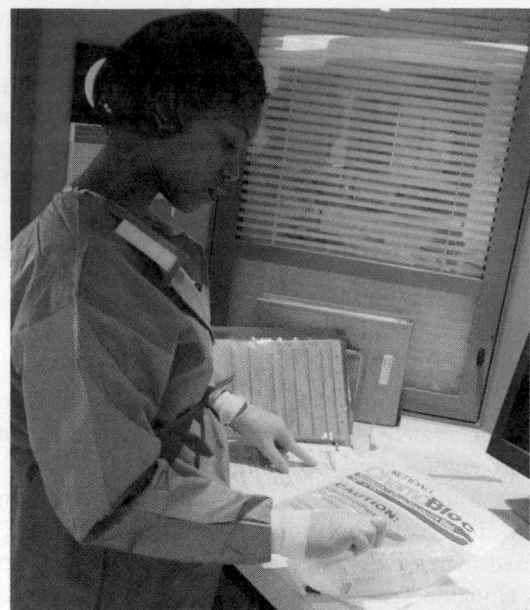

Fig. 36-1 Nurses caring for children with cancer require expertise in the safe administration of chemotherapy.

urticaria, angioedema, flushing, rashes, difficulty breathing, hypotension, and nausea or vomiting. Nursing responsibilities include prevention of, recognition of, and preparation for serious reactions. Prevention begins with a careful history of known allergies and education of the patient and family regarding signs and symptoms to report. (See Chapter 6.)

> ### ! NURSING ALERT
>
> When chemotherapeutic and immunologic agents with known anaphylactic potential are given, it is standard practice to observe the child for 1 hour after the infusion for signs of anaphylaxis (rash, urticaria, hypotension, wheezing, nausea, vomiting). Emergency equipment (especially blood pressure monitor, bag and valve mask, and suction) and emergency drugs (especially oxygen, epinephrine, antihistamine, aminophylline, corticosteroids, and vasopressors) must be readily available.

If a reaction is suspected, the nurse discontinues the drug, flushes the IV line and maintains with saline, and monitors the child's vital signs and subsequent responses.

In addition to the nurse's many responsibilities nurses in regard to the child and family, nurses must also use safeguards to protect themselves. Handling chemotherapeutic agents may present risks to handlers and to their offspring, although the exact degree of risk is not known. The Oncology Nursing Society has published comprehensive guidelines for safe practice issues related to administration of chemotherapy.† They have also established safe management procedures for chemotherapy administered in the home (Oncology Nursing Society, 2004). Basic nursing guidelines are in the Nursing Care Guidelines box.

---

*Giving Cancer Drugs Intravenously: Some Guidelines is available from the American Cancer Society, 1599 Clifton Road, NE, Atlanta, GA 30329; 404-320-3333 (headquarters), 800-ACS-2345 (for general cancer information); www.cancer.org.

†Cancer Chemotherapy Guidelines can be obtained from the Oncology Nursing Society, 125 Enterprise Drive, Pittsburgh, PA 15275; 866-257-4667, 412-859-6100; www.ons.org.

Handling Chemotherapeutic Agents

- Use great care and strict aseptic technique in handling chemotherapeutic agents to prevent any physical contact with the substance.
- Prepare drugs in a properly ventilated room or biologic safety cabinet (which incorporates a protective front panel and vertical laminar airflow to reduce potential for inhalation during preparation).
- Wear disposable gloves and protective clothing and discard in special container after each use.
- Use a sterile gauze pad when priming intravenous (IV) tubing, connecting and disconnecting tubing, inserting syringes into vials, breaking glass ampules, or performing any other procedure in which antineoplastic drugs may be inadvertently discharged.
- Dispose of all contaminated needles, syringes, IV tubing, and other contaminated equipment in a leakproof and puncture-resistant container; do not recap or break needles.

Radiotherapy

Radiotherapy is frequently used in the treatment of childhood cancer, usually in conjunction with chemotherapy or surgery. It can be used for curative purposes and for palliation to relieve symptoms by shrinking the size of the tumor. Recent advances in radiotherapy have optimized its beneficial effects and minimized many of the undesirable side effects, although high-dose irradiation is associated with many serious late effects.

Ionizing radiation is cytotoxic in at least three different ways: (1) damaging the pyrimidine bases cytosine, thymine, and uracil, needed for the synthesis of nucleic acids; (2) causing single-strand breaks in the DNA or RNA molecule; or (3) causing double helical–strand breaks in these molecules. The effect of disturbing cellular metabolic and reproductive functions is either sublethal or lethal damage. Lethal damage refers to the death of the cell. Sublethal damage refers to injured cells that may subsequently be repaired. Many of the acute side effects are the result of lethal damage to radiosensitive tissue, particularly proliferating cells such as those of the bone marrow, gastrointestinal tract, and hair follicles. Late effects are usually the result of cell death.

The acute untoward reactions from radiotherapy depend primarily on the area to be irradiated. Total-body irradiation is associated with the most severe reactions and is employed to prepare the immune system for bone marrow transplantation (BMT). Table 36-2 summarizes the acute effects of radiotherapy and nursing interventions that may be helpful in mitigating

TABLE 36-2	EARLY SIDE EFFECTS OF RADIOTHERAPY	
SITE	**EFFECTS**	**NURSING INTERVENTIONS**
Gastrointestinal tract	Nausea and vomiting	Give antiemetic around the clock. Measure amount of emesis to assess for dehydration.
	Anorexia	Encourage fluids and foods best tolerated, usually light, soft diet and small, frequent meals. Monitor weight loss.
	Mucosal ulceration	Use frequent mouth rinses and oral hygiene to prevent mucositis.
	Diarrhea	Control with antispasmodics and kaolin pectin preparations. Observe for signs of dehydration.
Skin	Alopecia (within 2 wk; hair may regrow by 3-6 mo)	Introduce idea of wig. Stress necessity of scalp hygiene and need for head covering in cold weather.
	Dry or moist desquamation	Do not refer to skin change as a "burn" (implies use of too much radiation). Keep skin clean. Wash daily, using soap (e.g., Tone, Dove) sparingly. Do not remove skin marking for radiation fields. Avoid exposure to sun. For dryness, apply lubricant. For desquamation, consult practitioner for skin hygiene and care.
Head	Nausea and vomiting (from stimulation of vomiting center in brain)	Same as for gastrointestinal tract
	Alopecia	Same as for skin
	Mucositis	Encourage regular dental care, fluoride treatments.
	Potential effects: • Parotitis • Sore throat • Loss of taste	Provide analgesics as needed to relieve discomfort.
	• Xerostomia (dry mouth)	Combat severe dryness of mouth with oral hygiene and liquid diet.
Urinary bladder	Rarely cystitis	Cystitis is more likely to occur with concomitant use of cyclophosphamide. Encourage liberal fluid intake and frequent voiding. Evaluate for hematuria.
Bone marrow	Myelosuppression	Observe for fever (temperature >38.3° C [101° F]). Initiate workup for sepsis as ordered. Administer antibiotics as prescribed. Avoid use of suppositories, rectal temperatures. Institute bleeding precautions. Observe for signs of anemia.

or preventing them. In limited areas of the country, proton beam radiation is available. Protons are positively charged subatomic particles. Protons deposit energy differently than x-ray beams. There is no "exit dose" beyond the tumor involved in proton radiotherapy. Therefore the potential benefit is in long-term effects to organs surrounding the target area. For example, some brain tumor patients receive radiation to the spine. With traditional forms of radiotherapy, long-term effect to nearby vital organs like the heart and lungs are possible. Although research on the potential beneficial effects of proton therapy is still in the early stages, theoretically these organs would not be affected with the use of proton therapy (Lee, Bilton, Famigletti, et al, 2005).

Biologic Response Modifiers

Biologic response modifiers (BRMs) modify the relationship between tumor and host by therapeutically changing the host's biologic response to tumor cells. These agents or interventions may affect the host's immunologic mechanisms (immunotherapy); have direct antitumor activity; or stimulate cell growth, reducing the hematologic toxicity associated with chemotherapy (Smith, 2011). Much of the current work in biotherapy is directed toward the use of monoclonal antibodies in the diagnosis and treatment of cancers. Through a complex process, special cells are fused to form a hybrid clone, or hybridoma, that produces antibodies that recognize a single specific antigen—hence the term *monoclonal antibody* (*mono* meaning one and *clone* meaning exact duplicate). These clones are then frozen, maintained in culture, or grown as tumors in mice to produce large quantities of the antibody in ascites fluid (Trahan, Green, and Murray, 2001). Although monoclonal antibodies have many prospective uses, their current role has been in diagnosing subclasses of leukemia cells to enhance understanding of which types of leukemia respond to different treatments and to determine whether the subclass is related to the prognosis. Researchers have also used monoclonal antibodies to deplete allogeneic bone marrow of T cells to reduce graft-versus-host disease (GVHD) and to selectively eliminate malignant cells from autologous marrow for transplanting back into the patient (Smith, 2011). Results from these studies have been encouraging, but further work is needed to define the role monoclonal antibodies and other BRMs will have in cancer care.

Bone Marrow Transplantation

Another approach to the treatment of childhood cancer is BMT. Candidates for transplantation are children who have malignancies that are unlikely to be cured by other means (see Family-Centered Care box). BMT allows for administration of lethal doses of chemotherapy, often combined with radiotherapy, to rid the body of all cancer cells (Locatelli, Giorgiani, Di-Cesare-Merlone, 2008). Once the body is free of malignant cells and the immune system is suppressed to prevent rejection of the transplanted marrow, the donor marrow or stem cells or the cells previously stored from the patient are given to the patient by IV transfusion. The newly transfused marrow or stem cells begin to produce functioning nonmalignant blood cells. In essence, the recipient accepts a new blood-forming organ.

FAMILY-CENTERED CARE
Decision for a Bone Marrow Transplant

A family's decision for a child to undergo a bone marrow transplant (BMT) may be fraught with challenges. Often the child faces certain death from the malignancy without the BMT. The preparation of the child for the transplant also places the patient at great medical risk.

Once the preparatory regimen begins and the child's immune system is destroyed, there is no turning back. Unlike kidney transplantation, BMT does not have a "rescue" procedure, such as dialysis, for supportive therapy. If the donor is a sibling, the expectation that his or her marrow will "save" the brother or sister can be a concern, especially if the transplant fails. Parents often must leave home to stay at the transplant center and encounter additional stressors such as arranging child care, taking leave from work, and managing finances. The patient faces the greatest stress: fear of BMT failure or life-threatening complications.

The selection process for a suitable donor and the potential complications in transplantation are related to the human leukocyte antigen (HLA) system complex. Some of the major HLA antigens are A, B, C, D, and DR. There is a wide diversity for each of these HLA loci. For example, more than 20 different HLA-A antigens and more than 40 different HLA-B antigens can be inherited. The genes are inherited as a single unit, or haplotype. A child inherits one unit from each parent; thus a child and each parent have one identical and one nonidentical haplotype. Because the possible haplotype combinations among siblings follow the laws of mendelian genetics, there is a 1 in 4 chance that two siblings have two identical haplotypes and are perfectly matched at the HLA loci.

The importance of HLA matching is to prevent the serious complication of GVHD. Because the child's immune system is essentially rendered nonfunctional, the recipient is unlikely to reject the bone marrow. However, the donor's marrow may contain antigens not matched to the recipient's antigens, which begin attacking body cells. The more closely the HLA systems match, the less likely GVHD is to develop. However, it can occur even with a perfect HLA match because of unidentified and thus unmatched histocompatibility antigens (Bollard, Krance, and Heslop, 2011).

Different types of BMT are now performed in children with cancer. Allogeneic BMT involves matching a histocompatible donor with the recipient. However, allogeneic BMT is limited by the presence of a suitable marrow donor. Because of the limited numbers of patients having HLA-identical siblings, other types of allogeneic transplants have been developed. Umbilical cord blood stem cell transplantation is a new source of hematopoietic stem cells for use in children with cancer (Rocha, Wagner, Sobocinski, et al, 2000). Because stem cells can be found with high frequency in the circulation of newborns, cord blood transplantation has become an alternative for some children (Rocha, Wagner, Sobocinski, et al, 2000). The benefit of using umbilical cord blood is the blood's relative immunodeficiency at birth, allowing for partially matched, unrelated cord blood transplants to be successful, with a lower risk of GVHD-related problems (Frey, Guess, Allison, et al, 2009).

Autologous BMTs use the patient's own marrow that was collected from disease-free tissue, frozen, and sometimes treated to remove malignant cells. Children with solid tumors such as neuroblastoma, Hodgkin disease, non-Hodgkin lymphoma

(NHL), rhabdomyosarcoma, Ewing sarcoma, and Wilms tumor have been treated with autologous BMTs.

Peripheral stem cell transplants (PSCTs) are also used in children with cancer. PSCT, a type of autologous transplant, differs in the way stem cells are collected from the patient. Colony-stimulating factor (CSF) is first given to stimulate the production of many stem cells (Lanzkowsky, 2005; Matsubara, Makimoto, Takayama, et al, 2001). Once the white blood cell count is high enough, the stem cells are collected by an apheresis machine. This machine filters out peripheral stem cells from whole blood and returns the remainder of the blood cells and plasma to the child. Stem cells have been collected without problems in very small children weighing 20 kg (44 lb) or less (Sevilla, Gonzalez-Vicent, Madero, et al, 2002). The peripheral stem cells are then frozen until the patient is ready for the PSCT.

COMPLICATIONS OF THERAPY

Although tremendous advances have been achieved through current modes of cancer therapy, the successes are not without consequences. Numerous side effects are expected with chemotherapy and radiotherapy (see Nursing Care Plan, pp. 1470-1472). Other complications that are less common but generally more serious are described here.

Pediatric Oncologic Emergencies
Tumor Lysis Syndrome
Life-threatening conditions may develop in children with cancer as a result of the malignancy and or aggressive treatment modalities. Acute tumor lysis syndrome has hallmark metabolic abnormalities that are the direct result of rapid release of intracellular contents during the lysis of malignant cells. This typically occurs in patients with ALL or Burkitt lymphoma during the initial treatment period but may occur spontaneously before onset of therapy. Tumor lysis syndrome may also occur in other malignancies that have a large tumor burden, are very sensitive to chemotherapy, or have a rapid proliferative rate. The hallmark metabolic abnormalities of tumor lysis syndrome include hyperuricemia, hypocalcemia, hyperphosphatemia, hyperkalemia, and uremia. The crystallization of uric acid in the renal tubules can also lead to acute renal failure and death (Coiffier, Altman, Pui, et al, 2008).

Risk factors for development of tumor lysis syndrome include high white blood cell count at diagnosis, large tumor burden, sensitivity to chemotherapy, and high proliferative rate. In addition to the described metabolic abnormalities, children may develop a spectrum of clinical symptoms, including flank pain, lethargy, nausea and vomiting, oliguria, pruritus, tetany, and altered level of consciousness.

Management of tumor lysis syndrome consists of early identification of patients at risk, prophylactic measures, and early interventions. Patients at risk for tumor lysis syndrome should have serum chemistries and urine pH monitored frequently, strict record of intake and output, and aggressive IV fluids. Medications to reduce uric acid formation and promote excretion of by-products of purine metabolism, such as allopurinol, are often used. If tumor lysis syndrome occurs, IV hydration continues and the specific metabolic abnormalities are treated. Hyperuricemia is now effectively treated with recombinant urate oxidase, or rasburicase. This medication converts uric acid to allantoin, which is more soluble in urine. Exchange transfusions are sometimes necessary to reduce the metabolic consequences of massive tumor lysis, especially in children with a high tumor burden.

Hyperleukocytosis
Hyperleukocytosis, defined as a peripheral white blood cell count greater than $100,000/mm^3$, can lead to capillary obstruction, microinfarction, and organ dysfunction. Children experience respiratory distress and cyanosis. They also experience neurologic changes, including altered level of consciousness, visual disturbances, agitation, confusion, ataxia, and delirium. Management consists of rapid cytoreduction by chemotherapy, hydration, urinary alkalinization, and allopurinol. Leukophoresis or exchange transfusion may be necessary.

Superior Vena Cava Syndrome
Obstruction may create an oncologic emergency for a child with cancer. Space-occupying lesions located in the chest, especially from Hodgkin disease and NHL, may cause superior vena cava syndrome (SVCS) (compression of mediastinal structures), leading to airway compromise and potentially to respiratory failure. SVCS has also occurred with central venous catheters from the formation of a thrombus or a fibrotic reaction (McCloskey, 2002).

Children are initially seen with cyanosis of the face, neck, and upper chest; facial and upper extremity edema; and distended neck veins. They may have dyspnea from airway obstruction. Management consists of airway protection and alleviation of respiratory distress. Rapid treatment is initiated, and symptoms typically improve with as the disease is effectively treated.

Spinal Cord Compression
Different malignancies can invade or impinge on the spinal cord, causing acute symptoms of cord compression. Symptoms can include pain, sensation change, extremity weakness, loss of bowel and bladder function, and respiratory insufficiency. Children with primary CNS tumors can have tumors that originate or spread to the spinal cord. Other solid tumors, like neuroblastoma or rhabdomyosarcoma, can metastasize to the spinal cord and cause compression. Careful physical examination is essential in early detection of symptoms. Treatment may include corticosteroids to reduce associated edema and alleviate symptoms and rapid initiation of treatment such as emergent radiation or laminectomy if indicated.

Disseminated Intravascular Coagulation
Overwhelming infections in the immunocompromised child constitute an emergency situation. Gram-negative sepsis can result in numerous complications, including disseminated intravascular coagulation (DIC), created by bacteria or fungus causing damage to the endothelial system. Life-threatening hemorrhage can occur from DIC in combination with thrombocytopenia (platelet count of $20,000/mm^3$) and leukocytosis (leukocyte count of $100,000/mm^3$). Leukocytosis can cause intracranial bleeding from increased viscosity of the blood. The resulting leukocytosis leads to vascular damage and subsequent hemorrhage.

NURSING CARE MANAGEMENT

This section presents an overview of general nursing concepts that apply to most childhood cancers. Specific nursing care for children with a particular type of cancer is discussed under each disease section later in this chapter. This discussion focuses on the physical aspects of care (see Nursing Care Plan). Chapter 22 (chronic illness) and in Chapter 23 (terminal illness) present the emotional aspects.

QUALITY PATIENT OUTCOMES: The Child with Cancer
- Child and family educated on disease and treatment
- Treatment administered on schedule with appropriate drug doses
- Side-effects of treatment managed
- Treatment complications prevented
- Child and family coping skills supported
- Quality of life during treatment maintained
- Child and family adjusted to chronic illness
- Growth and development maintained during treatment

SIGNS AND SYMPTOMS OF CANCER IN CHILDREN

Early detection is critical to early treatment and eventual cure. Cancers in children are often difficult to recognize. Therefore being alert to the persistence of unusual symptoms is essential (see Box 36-1). This chapter discusses some of the more significant clues to pediatric cancer.

Pain may be an early or late initial sign of cancer and requires a careful history of its onset, characteristics, location, intensity, and alleviating factors. Pain may be generalized or present at a specific location. For example, bone pain occurs in approximately 20% of children with leukemia. Pain, swelling, and tenderness at the tumor site may be the initial sign in bone tumors.

Fever is a frequent occurrence during childhood and is caused by numerous illnesses, including cancer. The major cause of fever in cancer patients is infection, especially related to neutropenia. The malignant process itself can also cause fever. This is often referred to as tumor-associated fever. The exact mechanism as to how the malignancy causes a fever is not known. There are multiple theories, including the release of pyrogens or toxins by the tumor or the hypersensitivity reaction response to tumors that activates other body cells to release pyrogens.

A careful skin assessment will reveal signs and symptoms of a low platelet count. Ecchymosis and petechiae are most commonly found on the child's extremities, and gum or nose bleeding may occur when the platelet count falls below 20,000/mm³.

The child with malignant invasion of the bone marrow often appears pale, with symptoms of lethargy, weight loss, and generalized malaise. These symptoms may be attributed to anemia caused by the replacement of normal cells with malignant cells in the bone marrow. The nurse should assess for signs and symptoms of anemia. (See Chapter 35.)

An abdominal mass is a typical finding in children with Wilms tumor and neuroblastoma. An abdominal mass in a child must be evaluated for a malignancy.

NURSING CARE PLAN

The Child with Cancer

NURSING DIAGNOSIS	NURSING DIAGNOSIS	NURSING INTERVENTIONS	RATIONALE
Risk for Injury related to chemotherapy treatment	Child will exhibit no complications of chemotherapy.	Administer chemotherapeutic agents using established guidelines.	To minimize inappropriate administration techniques
Child's/Family's Defining Characteristics (Subjective and Objective Data)	Child will receive prompt, appropriate treatment of complications.	Assist with procedures for administration of chemotherapeutic agents.	To comply with the cancer treatment protocol
Anaphylaxis: wheezing, hypotension, urticaria, cyanosis	**The Following NOC Concept Applies to These Outcomes**	Administer medications around the clock to prevent nausea and vomiting before chemotherapy.	To minimize side effects of nausea and vomiting
Nausea, vomiting	Risk Control	Administer IV fluid as prescribed.	To maintain hydration
Intravenous (IV) infiltration: pain, redness, swelling at IV infusion site		Encourage frequent intake of fluids in small amounts.	To improve toleration of fluids
		Observe for signs of infiltration of IV site: pain, stinging, swelling, redness.	To prevent infiltration when possible
		Institute policies to treat infiltration if it occurs.	To prevent complications
		Observe child for 20 minutes after infusion of drugs that present a risk for anaphylaxis.	To observe for signs of anaphylaxis
		Stop infusion of drug and flush IV line with normal saline if reaction is suspected.	To prevent further reaction
		Have emergency equipment and emergency drugs readily available.	To avoid delay in treatment
		The Following NIC Concepts Apply to These Interventions Chemotherapy Management Nausea Management	

NURSING CARE PLAN—cont'd

The Child with Cancer

NURSING DIAGNOSIS	NURSING DIAGNOSIS	NURSING INTERVENTIONS	RATIONALE
Risk for Infection related to depressed body defenses **Child's/Family's Defining Characteristics (Subjective and Objective Data)** Fever Altered vital signs Lethargy Change in behavior Septic shock	Child will not exhibit signs of infection. Child will not come in contact with infected persons. **The Following NOC Concepts Apply to These Outcomes** Risk Control Immune Status Infection Status	Use good hand-washing technique. Screen all visitors and staff for signs of infection. Use aseptic technique for all invasive procedures. Monitor temperature. Evaluate needle puncture sites, mucosa for ulceration, and minor abrasions for possible sites of infection. Provide nutritionally complete diet. Avoid giving live attenuated virus vaccines. Give inactivated virus vaccines. Administer antibiotics as prescribed. Administer granulocyte colony-stimulating factor as prescribed. **The Following NIC Concepts Apply to These Interventions** Infection Protection Infection Control Immunization/Vaccination Management	To minimize exposure to infective organisms To decrease chance of infection spread To detect possible infection To detect possible infection To support body's natural defenses To avoid causing overwhelming infection with vaccines To prevent specific infections and avoid placing the child at risk for acquiring the illness To treat a specific infection To promote production of infection-fighting cells
NURSING DIAGNOSIS	NURSING DIAGNOSIS	NURSING INTERVENTIONS	RATIONALE
Imbalanced Nutrition: Less Than Body Requirements related to loss of appetite **Child's/Family's Defining Characteristics (Subjective and Objective Data)** Weight loss Lack of appetite Nausea	Child will have adequate nutritional intake. **The Following NOC Concept Applies to These Outcomes** Nutritional Status: Food and Fluid Intake Nutritional Status: Nutrient Intake	Encourage parents to relax pressure placed on eating. Allow child any food tolerated. Explain expected increase in appetite if child will be taking steroids. Fortify foods with nutritious supplements. Allow child to be involved in food preparation and selection. Make food appealing. Monitor child's weight. **The Following NIC Concepts Apply to These Interventions** Nutrition Management Nutrition Therapy	To promote acceptance of loss of appetite as a consequence of chemotherapy To promote nutrition, knowing that quality of food selections can improve once appetite increases To prepare child and family for changes with taking steroids To maximize quality of intake To encourage eating To monitor child's status
NURSING DIAGNOSIS	NURSING DIAGNOSIS	NURSING INTERVENTIONS	RATIONALE
Pain related to diagnosis, treatment, physiologic effects of cancer **Child's/Family's Defining Characteristics (Subjective and Objective Data)** Crying Withdrawal Fear of procedures Reluctance to move Change in vital signs	Child will experience no pain or reduction of pain to level acceptable to the child. **The Following NOC Concepts Apply to These Outcomes** Pain Level Pain: Disruptive Effects Pain Control	Use pharmacologic and nonpharmacologic interventions before painful procedures. Assess pain with each vital sign measurement. Evaluate effectiveness of pain relief. Administer analgesics as prescribed on preventive schedule (around the clock) when needed. **The Following NIC Concept Applies to These Interventions** Pain Management	To minimize discomfort To determine level of pain To enable adjustments to increase effectiveness of pain relief if necessary To prevent pain from recurring

Continued

◉ **NURSING CARE PLAN—cont'd**

The Child with Cancer

NURSING DIAGNOSIS	NURSING DIAGNOSIS	NURSING INTERVENTIONS	RATIONALE
Fear related to diagnostic tests, procedures, treatment	Child will have reduced fear related to diagnostic procedures and treatment.	Explain procedures carefully at child's level of understanding.	To reduce fear of unknown
Child's/Family's Defining Characteristics (Subjective and Objective Data)	**The Following NOC Concepts Apply to These Outcomes**	Explain what will take place and what child will feel, see, and hear.	To provide a sense of control
Worry and anxiety before procedures	Fear Control	Comply with child's special requests when possible.	To encourage cooperation
Withdrawal	Pain Control	Provide child with some means of involvement with procedures (e.g., holding a piece of equipment, helping put on bandage, counting).	To provide a sense of control, encourage cooperation, and support child's coping skills
Lack of control			
Outbursts			
Anger		Implement distraction techniques and pain reduction interventions.	To reduce pain
Lack of cooperation			
Nausea		**The Following NIC Concept Applies to These Interventions** Pain Management	

NURSING DIAGNOSIS	NURSING DIAGNOSIS	NURSING INTERVENTIONS	RATIONALE
Disturbed Body Image related to changes caused by cancer and treatment	Child will exhibit positive coping skills.	Encourage child to decide how he or she will cope with hair loss (e.g., wig, cap, scarf, no covering).	To promote early adjustment and preparation for hair loss
Child's/Family's Defining Characteristics (Subjective and Objective Data)	**The Following NOC Concepts Apply to These Outcomes** Body Image	Provide adequate covering during exposure to sunlight, wind, or cold.	To provide protection, since natural hair protection is lost with alopecia
Sadness		Explain that hair begins to regrow in 3 to 6 months, and may be a different color and texture.	To prevent anxiety about hair loss
Depression			
Withdrawal		Encourage good hygiene and grooming.	To lower risk for infection
Anger		Encourage rapid return to peer group and friends.	To promote peer support
		Encourage visits from friends before discharge.	To prepare child for reactions of others
		The Following NIC Concepts Apply to These Interventions Counseling Body Image Enhancement	

NURSING DIAGNOSIS	NURSING DIAGNOSIS	NURSING INTERVENTIONS	RATIONALE
Interrupted Family Processes related to having a child with a life-threatening disease	Child and family will demonstrate understanding of the disease and treatment.	Teach parents and child about the disease.	To promote understanding
		Explain all procedures.	
Child's/Family's Defining Characteristics (Subjective and Objective Data)	**The Following NOC Concepts Apply to These Outcomes**	Advise family of expected side effects and toxicities; clarify which demand medical evaluation.	To prevent delay in treatment
	Family Functioning		
Lack of understanding of disease and treatment	Family Coping Family Normalization	Reassure family that reactions are complications of treatment.	To provide support
Inability to identify side effects of treatment	Knowledge: Illness Care	Prepare family for what to do when side effects occur.	To prevent delay in treatment
Inability to understand child's treatment plan		Interpret prognostic statistics carefully, realizing family's level of understanding.	To promote understanding
Lack of family support		Schedule time for family to be together without interruptions.	To encourage communication and expression of feelings
		Help family plan for future.	To promote child's development
		Encourage family to discuss feelings regarding child's disease.	To encourage expression of feelings
		The Following NIC Concepts Apply to These Interventions Counseling Family Support	

Swollen lymph glands are another common finding in children. However, enlarged, firm, lymph nodes in a child with fever for more than 1 week, a recent history of weight loss, or an abnormal chest x-ray film may indicate a serious disease and should be evaluated further.

The presence of a white reflection as opposed to the normal red pupillary reflex in the pupil of a child's eye is the classic sign of retinoblastoma. Squinting, strabismus, or swelling can indicate other solid tumors of the eye.

The child with a brain tumor develops signs and symptoms according to the exact area of the brain involved. The nurse must perform a thorough assessment to identify the specific area of tumor involvement (see Table 36-4).

MANAGING SIDE EFFECTS OF TREATMENT

Cancer care encompasses more than treatments aimed at eliminating the malignant cells. Because of the delicate balance between killing malignant cells and preserving functional cells, supportive therapy is frequently needed during those times that serious damage occurs to normal body tissues.

Infection

A major concern for the child receiving treatment for cancer is the risk for the development of complications secondary to the treatment. Major complications include fever, bleeding, and anemia.

The nurse caring for the child with fever must be aware of the signs and symptoms of septic shock, as discussed in Chapter 29. The child with fever who has an absolute neutrophil count (ANC) lower than 500/mm³ is at risk for (see Nursing Care Guidelines box):

- Overwhelming infection
- General malaise
- Dehydration
- Seizures (young infants and children)
- Invasion of organisms producing secondary infections

 NURSING CARE GUIDELINES

Calculating the Absolute Neutrophil Count (ANC)

1. Determine the total percentage of neutrophils ("polys, or segs," and "bands").
2. Multiply white blood cell (WBC) count by percentage of neutrophils.
   Example: WBC = 1000/mm³, neutrophils = 7%, nonsegmented neutrophils (bands) = 7%
   Step 1: 7% + 7% = 14%
   Step 2: 0.14 × 1000 = 140/mm³ ANC

The child with fever is evaluated for potential sites of infection, such as from a needle puncture, mucosal ulceration, minor abrasion, or skin tears (e.g., a hangnail). Although the body may not be able to produce an adequate inflammatory response to the infection and the usual clinical signs of infection may be partially expressed or absent, fever will occur. Therefore monitor the temperature closely. To identify the source of infection, the health care team takes blood, stool, urine, and nasopharyngeal cultures and chest x-ray films.

Once infection is suspected, broad-spectrum IV antibiotic therapy is begun before the organism is identified and may be continued for 7 to 10 days. If the child does not have a venous access device, a heparin lock should be inserted to prevent the inconvenience of multiple venipunctures in maintaining a patent IV line and to avoid limitations in activity caused by the IV line.

The organisms most lethal to these children are (1) viruses, particularly varicella (chickenpox), herpes zoster, herpes simplex, measles, rubella, mumps, and poliomyelitis; (2) *Pneumocystis carinii* (a protozoan); (3) fungi, especially *Candida albicans*; (4) gram-negative bacteria, such as *Pseudomonas aeruginosa, E. coli,* and *Proteus* and *Klebsiella* organisms; and (5) gram-positive bacteria, especially *Staphylococcus aureus, Staphylococcus epidermidis,* and group A β-hemolytic streptococci (Quadri and Brown, 2000). As prophylaxis against these various organisms, broad-spectrum antibiotics are usually prescribed. Ensuring compliance with this long-term regimen is an important nursing responsibility.

Prophylaxis against *P. carinii* is routinely given to most children during treatment for cancer (American Academy of Pediatrics, 2006). Trimethoprim-sulfamethoxazole (Bactrim, Septra) is usually given three times a week during treatment.

CSFs, a family of glycoprotein hormones that regulate the reproduction, maturation, and function of blood cells, are now routinely used as supportive measures to prevent the side effects caused by low blood counts. CSFs promote stem cell proliferation and stimulate a more rapid maturation of the cells, allowing them to enter the bloodstream earlier. G-CSF (filgrastim [Neupogen], pegfilgrastim [Neulasta]) directs granulocyte development and can decrease the duration of neutropenia following immunosuppressive therapy. This reduces the incidence and duration of infection in children receiving treatment for cancer. G-CSF is also being used to decrease the bone marrow recovery time after BMT (Matsubara, Makimoto, Takayama, et al, 2001). G-CSF is usually administered intravenously or subcutaneously 24 hours after chemotherapy is discontinued and is given for 10 to 14 days. G-CSF is discontinued when the ANC surpasses 10,000/mm³. The pegylated or long-acting form of G-CSF, pegfilgrastim, is given only once after completion of therapy and typically has its peak efficacy (highest white blood cell count) about 8 to 10 days after administration. During G-CSF therapy, children may experience bone pain, fever, rash, malaise, and headaches.

Prevention of infection continues as a priority after discharge from the hospital. Some institutions allow the child to return to school when the ANC is above 500/mm³. Other institutions place no restrictions on the child, regardless of the blood count. If the level falls below this value, cautious isolation from crowded areas, such as shopping centers or subways, is advisable. At all times, encourage family members to practice good hand washing to avoid introducing pathogens into the home (see Critical Thinking Exercise).

Hemorrhage

Before the use of transfused platelets, hemorrhage was a leading cause of death in children with some types of cancer. Now most bleeding episodes can be prevented or controlled with judicious administration of platelet concentrates or platelet-rich plasma.

Fever and Neutropenia

Billy Wright, 9 years old, is undergoing chemotherapy for high-risk acute lymphoblastic leukemia (ALL) but has recently been hospitalized with a fever of 39.5° C (103° F). He last received chemotherapy 10 days ago with vincristine, doxorubicin, and PEG-L-asparaginase and is currently taking oral dexamethasone for 21 days. His current white blood cell count is 0.1/mm³ with an absolute neutrophil count (ANC) of 0. His platelet count is 31,000/mm³, and his hemoglobin is 8.1 g/dl. He has noticeable petechiae on his arms and legs with multiple bruises in various stages of healing.

After your morning report, you visit him, start your assessment, and note the following: alert and oriented 9-year-old Caucasian boy. His tongue and oral mucosa are covered with a white plaque. Vital signs are as follows: temperature, 39.2° C (102.6° F), axial; respiratory rate, 24 breaths/min; heart rate, 140 beats/min; blood pressure, 100/56 mm Hg. Further observation of the patient and his surroundings reveals (1) a sign over his bed that reads "no needle punctures"; (2) he is currently getting 6 L of oxygen via nasal cannula; (3) the portacath is accessed with intravenous fluids infusing, and the dressing is clean and dry; and (4) a tympanic thermometer is in the room.
1. Evidence—Is there sufficient evidence to draw any conclusions about Billy's condition at this time?
2. Assumptions—Describe some underlying assumptions about the following:
    a. Normal blood counts in children and adolescents
    b. Effect of chemotherapy on the hematopoietic system
    c. Effects of chemotherapy on the gastrointestinal system
3. What implications and priorities for nursing care can be drawn at this time?
4. Does the evidence objectively support your conclusion?

Severe spontaneous internal hemorrhage varies, but usually does not occur until the platelet count is 10,000/mm³ or less (Hockenberry and Kline, 2011; Rossetto and McMahon, 2000).

Because infection increases the tendency toward hemorrhage, and because bleeding sites become more easily infected, take special care to avoid performing skin punctures whenever possible. When performing finger sticks, venipunctures, intramuscular injections, and bone marrow tests, employ aseptic technique with continued observation for bleeding. Meticulous mouth care is essential, since gingival bleeding with resultant mucositis is a frequent problem. Because the rectal area is prone to ulceration from various drugs, hygiene is essential. To prevent additional trauma, avoid rectal temperatures and suppositories. Frequent turning and the use of a pressure-reducing mattress under bony prominences prevent development of pressure sores and decubital ulcers.

Platelet transfusions are generally reserved for active bleeding episodes that do not respond to local treatment and that may occur during induction or relapse therapy. Epistaxis and gingival bleeding are the most common. The nurse teaches parents and other children measures to control nosebleeding. Applying pressure at the site without disturbing clot formation is the general rule. Two of the problems with multiple platelet transfusions are the risk of febrile reactions and decreased life span of the platelets. Platelet concentrates normally do not have to be cross-matched for blood group or type. However, because platelets contain specific antigen components similar to blood group factors, children who receive multiple transfusions may become sensitized to a platelet group other than their own. Therefore platelets are cross-matched with the donor's blood components whenever possible.

Transfused platelets generally survive in the body for 1 to 3 days. The peak effect is reached in about 2 hours and decreased by half in 24 hours. Therefore, after a transfusion, the nurse observes and records the approximate time when hemostasis of bleeding sites occurs. Delayed hemostasis is evidence of platelet destruction. For long-term patients, multiple transfusion therapy becomes progressively less effective.

During bleeding episodes the parents and child need much emotional support (see Critical Thinking Exercise). The sight of oozing blood is upsetting. Often parents request a platelet transfusion, unaware of the necessity of trying local measures first. The nurse can help calm their anxiety by explaining the reason for delaying a platelet transfusion until absolutely necessary. Because compatible donors decrease the risk of antigen formation in the recipient, the nurse should encourage parents to locate suitable donors for eventual blood use.

Bleeding

Paul Jones, 14 years old, is undergoing chemotherapy for non-Hodgkin lymphoma but has recently been hospitalized with an infection. He last received chemotherapy 12 days ago. His current platelet count is 28,000/mm³. He has noticeable petechiae on his arms and legs with multiple bruises in various stages of healing. After your morning report, you visit him, start your assessment, and note the following: alert and oriented 14-year-old Caucasian boy. The right sclera has a hemorrhage, and multiple petechiae and bruises are on the arms and legs. Petechiae are noted on the buccal mucosa and palate. Further observation of the patient and his surroundings reveals (1) a sign over his bed reads "no needle punctures"; (2) he is currently getting 6 L of oxygen via nasal cannula; (3) the portacath is accessed with intravenous fluids infusing, and the dressing is clean and dry; and (4) a tympanic thermometer is in the room.
1. Evidence—Is there sufficient evidence to draw any conclusions about Paul's condition at this time?
2. Assumptions—Describe some underlying assumptions about the following:
    a. Normal platelet counts in children and adolescents
    b. Effect of chemotherapy on hematopoietic system
3. What implications and priorities for nursing care can be drawn at this time?
4. Does the evidence objectively support your conclusion?

Children at home who have low platelet counts (usually <100,000/mm³) should avoid activities that might cause injury or bleeding, such as riding bicycles or skateboards, roller skating or in-line skating, climbing trees or playground equipment, and contact sports such as football or soccer. Once the platelet count rises, these restrictions are not necessary. In addition, aspirin and aspirin-containing products are not used; for mild pain or significantly elevated temperature, acetaminophen is substituted.

Anemia

Initially anemia may be profound from complete replacement of the bone marrow by cancer cells. During induction therapy, blood transfusions with packed red blood cells may be necessary to raise the hemoglobin to levels approaching 10 g/dl. The usual precautions in caring for the child are instituted. (See Chapter 35.)

Anemia is also a consequence of drug-induced myelosuppression. Although not as severely affected as the white blood cells, erythrocyte production may be delayed. Because children have an amazing capacity to withstand low hemoglobin levels, the best approach is to allow the child to regulate activity with reasonable adult supervision. It may be necessary for the parents to alert the schoolteacher to the child's physical limitations, particularly in terms of strenuous activity.

Nausea and Vomiting

The nausea and vomiting that occur shortly after administration of several of the drugs and as a result of cranial or abdominal irradiation can be profound. 5-Hydroxytryptamine-3 receptor antagonists are the antiemetics of choice to manage nausea and vomiting caused by chemotherapy and radiotherapy (Culy, Bhana, and Plosker, 2001). The advantage of these agents over conventional drugs is that they produce no extrapyramidal side effects, such as difficulty speaking or swallowing, shuffle walk, slow movements, trembling, stiffness of the arms and legs, or loss of balance. Multiple studies have shown ondansetron (Zofran) to be effective for patients receiving cisplatin, cyclophosphamide, ifosfamide, and anthracyclines (Anastasia, 2000). Ondansetron in combination with dexamethasone has been more effective than ondansetron alone (Culy, Bhana, and Plosker, 2001) and has been superior to metoclopramide (Reglan) for cisplatin-induced emesis (Culy, Bhana, and Plosker, 2001; American Society of Health-System Pharmacists, 1999).

For mild to moderate vomiting, phenothiazine-type drugs remain the mainstay of therapy. Promethazine (Phenergan), chlorpromazine (Thorazine), prochlorperazine (Compazine), or trimethobenzamide (Tigan) may be effective agents. Metoclopramide is a more effective antiemetic for severe vomiting. Unfortunately, the drug causes a number of side effects in children, particularly extrapyramidal reactions, such as muscle tremors or twitching, agitation, grimacing, dysarthria, and oculogyric crisis (fixation of eyes in one position for minutes or hours). Metoclopramide should be administered with dexamethasone or diphenhydramine (Benadryl) (Krane, Casillas, and Zeltzer, 2011).

Synthetic cannabinoids are now being used in children undergoing chemotherapy. A drug that has yielded promising results is tetrahydrocannabinol, or dronabinol. Dronabinol helps control nausea and vomiting and also is an effective appetite stimulant (Lohr, 2008).

The most beneficial regimen for antiemetic control has been the administration of the antiemetic before the chemotherapy begins (30 minutes to 1 hour before) and regular (not as-needed) administration every 2, 4, or 6 hours for at least 24 hours after chemotherapy. The goal is to prevent the child from ever experiencing nausea or vomiting, since this can prevent the development of anticipatory symptoms (the conditioned response of developing nausea and vomiting before receiving the drug). Other nonpharmacologic interventions (similar to those discussed for pain management in Chapter 7) can be useful in controlling posttherapy and anticipatory nausea and vomiting. Giving the antineoplastic drug with a mild sedative at bedtime is also helpful for some children, and there is evidence that nighttime administration of drugs such as

---

BOX 36-2 CRITERIA FOR NUTRITION INTERVENTION IN CHILDREN WITH MALIGNANCIES

- Interval or total weight loss >5% of the preillness body weight
- Relative weight-for-height of ≤90% or weight-for-height ≤10th percentile (according to National Center for Health Statistics growth chart)
- Serum albumin level <3.2 mg/dl
- Arm fat area or subscapular skinfolds <5th percentile for age and sex
- Current percentile for weight or height that is 2 percentile channels less than preillness percentile

Modified from Kumar S, Marwaha RK, Bhalla AK, et al: Protein energy malnutrition and skeletal muscle wasting in childhood acute lymphoblastic leukemia, *Indian Pediatr* 37(7):720-726, 2000.

---

methotrexate and 6-mercaptopurine may be more effective cytotoxically than morning administration.

Altered Nutrition

Altered nutrition is a common side effect of treatment. Continued assessment of the child's nutritional status must occur throughout treatment. Record regular evaluation of the child's intake. The child's height, weight, and head circumference (for children <3 years of age) must be measured routinely during visits to the hospital or clinic. When appropriate, monitor energy reserves, evaluated by skinfold measurements. Biochemical assays may be helpful in some children and include serum prealbumin, transferrin, and albumin (Han-Markey, 2000; Nitenberg and Raynard, 2000). Box 36-2 lists criteria for nutrition intervention in children with cancer.

! NURSING ALERT

Some children develop aversions to certain foods if they are eaten during chemotherapy. It is best to refrain from offering the child's favorite foods while the child is receiving chemotherapy.

Nutritional status is important to maintain because it compromised nutritional status can contribute to reduced tolerance to treatment, altered metabolism of chemotherapy drugs, prolonged episodes of neutropenia, and increased risk for infection.

Supportive nutrition measures include oral supplements with high-protein and high-calorie foods. Ways to increase calories include substituting cream for milk, adding tofu (high in protein) to most meals, and serving full-fat yogurt and ice cream instead on nonfat or low-fat items. Cooking with butter; putting sugar on cereal; and making high-calorie snacks such as trail mix, peanut butter, or dried fruit readily available for the child are other ways to increase calories. Enteral feeding may be necessary when children are unable to maintain the necessary calories to prevent weight loss. The use of parenteral hyperalimentation is used most frequently for children who have digestive problems, after surgery, or with BMT. Chapter 27 discusses these interventions in more detail.

Despite such approaches, some children still do not eat. Theories to explain persistent anorexia include that it is (1) a physical effect related to the cancer that is nonspecific; (2) a conditioned aversion to food from nausea and vomiting during treatment; (3) a response to stress in the environment, related to eating or to the child's condition; (4) a result of depression; (5) a control mechanism when so much else has been imposed on the child; and (6) an opportunity to express anger at parents and punish them for "allowing" the child to become sick. When loss of appetite and weight persists, the nurse should investigate the family situation to determine whether any of these variables are contributing to the problem.

Mucosal Ulceration

One of the most distressing side effects of several drugs is gastrointestinal mucosal cell damage, which results in ulcers anywhere along the alimentary tract. Oral ulcers (stomatitis) are red, eroded, painful areas in the mouth or pharynx. (See Stomatitis, Chapter 16.) Similar lesions may extend along the esophagus and occur in the rectal area. They greatly compound anorexia because eating is extremely uncomfortable.

When oral ulcers develop, the following interventions are helpful: (1) a bland, moist, soft diet; (2) use of a soft sponge toothbrush (Toothette) or cotton-tipped applicator; (3) frequent mouth rinses with normal saline (using a solution of 1 tsp of table salt and 1 pint of water) or sodium bicarbonate and salt mouth rinses (using a solution of 1 tsp of baking soda and ½ tsp of table salt in 1 quart of water); and (4) local anesthetics without alcohol, such as a solution of diphenhydramine and Maalox (aluminum and magnesium hydroxide) or UlcerEase (Velez, Tamara, and Mintz, 2004; Scully, Epstein, and Sonis, 2004). Although local anesthetics are effective in temporarily relieving the pain, many children dislike the taste and numb feeling they produce.

> **! NURSING ALERT**
>
> Viscous lidocaine is not recommended for young children. If applied to the pharynx, it may depress the gag reflex, increasing the risk of aspiration. Seizures have also been associated with the use of oral viscous lidocaine, most likely as a result of the rapid absorption into the bloodstream via the oral lesions (Cho, Cheng, and Cheng, 2000).

Oral preparations used to prevent or treat mucositis include UlcerEase, which is used to soothe mucositis and gum irritations; chlorhexidine gluconate (Peridex) is effective against candidal and bacterial infections (Velez, Tamara, and Mintz, 2004; Scully, Epstein, and Sonis, 2004). Antifungal troches (lozenges) or mouth rinse is typically used prophylactically in patients with myelosuppression, especially for children who have undergone BMT.

> **! NURSING ALERT**
>
> Avoid agents such as lemon glycerin swabs, hydrogen peroxide, and milk of magnesia because of the drying effects on the mucosa. In addition, lemon may irritate eroded tissue and can decay the teeth (Scully, Epstein, and Sonis, 2004).

Administering mouth care is particularly difficult in infants and toddlers. A satisfactory method of cleaning the gums is to wrap a piece of gauze around a finger; soak it in saline or plain water; and swab the gums, palate, and inner cheek surfaces with the finger. Mouth rinses are best accomplished with plain water or saline because the child cannot gargle or spit out excess fluid. Children should perform mouth care routinely before and after any feeding and as often as every 2 to 4 hours to rid mucosal surfaces of debris, which becomes an excellent medium for bacterial and fungal growth.

Dental hygiene can become a serious problem if the child wears an orthodontic appliance. The accumulated debris on braces is difficult to remove without vigorous brushing, and the appliance itself traumatizes the gums. Sometimes braces are removed during chemotherapy.

Difficulty eating is a major problem with stomatitis and may warrant hospitalization if the child refuses fluids. The child usually chooses the foods that are best tolerated. Surprisingly, some children prefer salty foods to bland ones. Drinking can usually be encouraged if a straw is used to bypass the ulcerated oral mucosa. The nurse should encourage parents to relax any eating pressures because the anorexia accompanying stomatitis is well justified. In addition, because it is a temporary condition, once the ulcers heal, the child can resume good food habits. Ordinarily, severe mucosal ulceration indicates a need for decreased chemotherapy until complete healing takes place, usually within a week. Analgesics, including opioids, may be needed when treatment cannot be altered, such as during BMT.

If rectal ulcers develop, meticulous toilet hygiene, warm sitz baths after each bowel movement, and an occlusive ointment applied to the ulcerated area promote healing; the use of stool softeners is necessary to prevent further discomfort. Parents should record bowel movements because the child may voluntarily avoid defecation to prevent discomfort. Rectal temperatures and suppositories are avoided because they may further traumatize the affected area.

Neurologic Problems

Vincristine, and to a lesser extent vinblastine, can cause various neurotoxic effects, one of the more common of which is severe constipation from decreased bowel innervation. Opioids further aggravate constipation. The nurse advises parents to record bowel movements and to notify the practitioner of a change in stool habits. Physical activity and stool softeners are helpful in preventing the problem, but laxatives, such as MiraLax, or enemas are often necessary to stimulate evacuation. Dietary changes such as increased fiber may not be effective, since the increased bulk tends to increase fecal distention and discomfort without producing the necessary mechanical stimulation.

Footdrop and weakness and numbness of the extremities may cause difficulty in walking or in fine hand movement. The nurse should look for these problems and warn parents of these side effects, which are reversible once the drug is stopped. If the child is on bed rest, a footboard is used to preserve proper alignment. If weakness occurs while the child is attending school, a temporary alteration of activity may be necessary. Parents should inform the teacher of the situation to avoid unrealistic expectations of the child's abilities.

Another side effect that can be severe is jaw pain. Analgesics may help relieve the discomfort. Children may avoid movement by not talking or chewing, although continuous chewing, such as with gum, may actually reduce the pain. Because the pain is temporary, usually lasting for a day or two, the child can be given fluids through a straw.

A neurologic syndrome, postirradiation somnolence, may develop 5 to 8 weeks after CNS irradiation and last for 4 to 15 days. It is characterized by somnolence with or without fever, anorexia, and nausea and vomiting. Parents should be warned of the possibility of such symptoms and encouraged to seek medical evaluation, since somnolence may be an early indicator of long-term neurologic sequelae after cranial irradiation.

Hemorrhagic Cystitis

Sterile hemorrhagic cystitis is a side effect of chemical irritation to the bladder from chemotherapy or radiotherapy. It can be prevented by (1) a liberal oral or parenteral fluid intake (at least one and a half times the recommended daily fluid requirement [2 L/m^2/day]); (2) frequent voiding immediately after feeling the urge, including immediately before bed and after arising (may include one nighttime void); (3) administration of the drug early in the day to allow for sufficient fluids and frequent voiding; and (4) administration of mesna, a drug that inhibits the urotoxicity of cyclophosphamide and ifosfamide (Lanzkowsky, 2005).

> **! NURSING ALERT**
>
> If signs of cystitis such as burning on urination occur, prompt medical evaluation is needed. Hemorrhagic cystitis warrants a full workup and prompt intervention.

In most cases IV fluids are given before, during, and after the drug to ensure adequate hydration, thereby eliminating the need for the child's drinking large amounts of fluid. If oral home administration is prescribed, the family needs specific instructions on exactly how much fluid the child must have.

Alopecia

Hair loss is a side effect of several chemotherapeutic drugs and cranial irradiation. Not all children lose their hair during drug therapy. However, retaining hair is the exception rather than the rule. It is better to warn children and parents of this side effect than to allow them to think it is only a remote possibility.

The family should know that the hair falls out in clumps, causing patchy baldness. To lessen the trauma of seeing large amounts of hair on bed linen or clothing, the child can wear a disposable surgical cap to collect the shed hair during the period of greatest hair loss, or the hair can be cut short. Families should also be aware that wigs are tax deductible and that hair regrows in 3 to 6 months. The hair frequently is darker, thicker, and curlier than before.

> **NURSING TIP** Encouraging children to choose a wig similar to their own hairstyle and color before the hair falls out is helpful in fostering later adjustment to hair loss.

If the child chooses not to wear a wig, attention to some type of head covering is important, especially in cold or sunny climates. Scalp hygiene is also important. The scalp should be washed regularly as with any other body part.

Many children demonstrate increased tolerance to hair loss on reinduction therapy. Rather than complete baldness, the child may experience thinning of the hair. If the hair is cut short, kept clean, and blow-dried with an electric hair drier, it usually can look full enough to make a wig unnecessary. This can be a tremendous psychologic boost to the child who is already depressed about learning of a relapse and the need for additional chemotherapy.

Steroid Effects

Short-term steroid therapy produces no acute toxicities and often results in two beneficial reactions: increased appetite and a sense of well-being. However, it does produce physical changes and alterations in body image, which, although not clinically significant, can be extremely distressing to older children. One of these is cushingoid appearance. The child's face becomes rounded and puffy. (See Fig. 38-5.) Unlike hair loss, little can be done to camouflage this obvious change, although careful avoidance of salt and salt-containing foods can help reduce fluid accumulation. It is not unusual for other children to make fun of the child. It is helpful to reassure the child that, after cessation of the drug, the facial contours will return to normal. If the child resumes activity early in the course of treatment, the change may be less noticeable to peers than after a long absence. Also, the use of loose-fitting clothes, such as warm-up outfits, can help camouflage the change in weight.

In contrast, parents may appreciate the full, rounded appearance because it simulates the look of a well-nourished, healthy child. Because of their own needs, they may be less able to understand the child's misery over altered body image. The nurse can foster a better understanding between the parents and child by encouraging both parties to openly discuss their feelings.

Children receiving steroid therapy do look healthy. The moon face, red cheeks, supraclavicular fat pads, protuberant abdomen, and fluid retention indicate weight gain. However, the actual weight gain resulting from increased muscle mass and subcutaneous tissue may be small. Therefore the nurse should evaluate weight gain by observing the extremities and measuring skinfold thickness and arm circumference during steroid therapy to determine whether the weight gain is a result of increased dietary intake.

Shortly after beginning steroid therapy, children may experience a number of mood changes, which range from feelings of well-being and euphoria to depression and irritability. If parents are unaware of these drug-induced changes, they may become unduly concerned. Therefore the nurse should warn them of the reactions and encourage them to discuss the behavioral changes with each other and the child.

NURSING CARE DURING BONE MARROW TRANSPLANTATION

Many of the side effects previously discussed occur in the child undergoing BMT. However, because of the aggressive preconditioning programs used to remove the marrow and the use of growth factors to promote engraftment of transplanted stem cells, these children are usually hospitalized for several weeks after BMT. Because of the risk of infection, the unit may employ such measures as strict hand washing, screening visitors, laminar airflow rooms, and institutional isolation policies.

BMT patients must have numerous procedures performed, such as the insertion of a venous access device, administration of intensive chemotherapy and irradiation, and continued meticulous personal hygiene. During the period after transplantation and before the new marrow begins adequately replacing granulocytes, the child is extremely susceptible to infection. Interstitial or nonbacterial pneumonia is another serious complication with a high mortality rate.

However, the most common complication in allogeneic transplants is GVHD, which can affect the skin, gastrointestinal tract, liver, heart, lungs, lymphoid tissue, and marrow. GVHD is characterized by a hardening of the tissues and drying of the mucous membranes. The severity of the manifestations varies, but once vital organs are affected, death can ensue. Treatment involves the use of steroids or azathioprine (Imuran). However, these immunosuppressive drugs further increase the risk of infection. All blood products should be irradiated to minimize the introduction of additional antigens.

Another unfortunate posttransplant possibility is recurrence of the malignancy after engraftment. Emphasis is now placed on the prevention of GVHD, using various agents such as cyclosporine, methotrexate, and steroids (Bollard, Krance, and Heslop, 2011).

Skin breakdown and delayed wound healing frequently occur in the patient undergoing BMT. Preventive interventions to minimize pressure on dependent areas of the skin include the use of pressure-relieving or pressure-reducing beds or mattresses and frequent turning. Measures to promote healing when breakdown occurs include frequent sitz baths for the perianal area; transparent dressings, such as Tegaderm, over bony prominences; and protective skin barriers, such as hydrocolloid dressings or occlusive ointments. Throughout this long ordeal the family is concerned about successful engraftment and fears fatal complications. Consequently nurses need to provide sensitive care and maintain a supportive attitude during the many crises that may arise. If the procedure is not successful, the care needed by these families is consistent with that required by the family of any child with a life-threatening disorder. (See Chapter 23.)

PREPARATION FOR PROCEDURES

Children in particular need psychologic preparation for the various treatment modalities, which often involve surgery, IV injections, bone marrow aspiration, and LP. The diagnostic procedures initially employed to confirm the diagnosis and those that are repeated to monitor treatment are often a source of discomfort and stress to the child and family. Even noninvasive procedures such as imaging and radiologic tests are frightening to a young child. Many of these tests require the child to lie absolutely motionless for a prolonged time in a confined space with little or no communication with a supportive adult. Consequently infants and young children are usually sedated, and older children need an explanation of what to expect and reminders during the test of how much longer

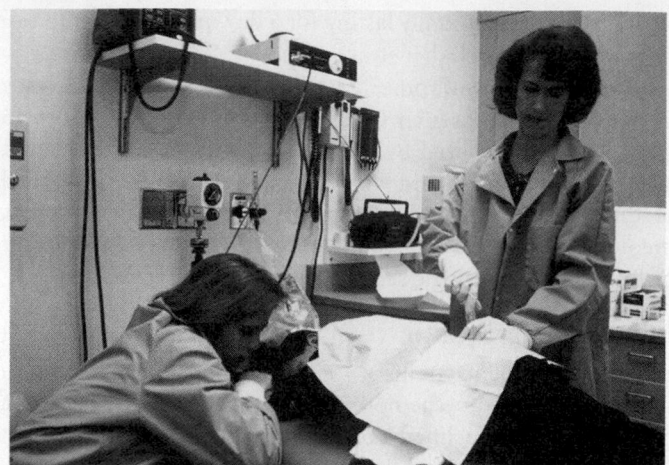

Fig. 36-2 Child with leukemia undergoing bone marrow aspiration.

they must remain still. The same principles for preparing children for procedures that are discussed in Chapter 27 apply here, including the option of having parents stay with the child whenever possible. (See Nursing Care Guidelines box, p. 1001.) Children who undergo repeated tests need additional preparation and emotional support to decrease their stress.

Two procedures, bone marrow studies and LPs, are so commonly performed in many types of childhood cancer that they deserve special consideration in preparing children (Fig. 36-2). Both tests can be frightening to children because they are done behind the child's field of vision. Professionals caring for children with cancer recommend the use of sedation for the initial procedures and subsequent developmentally appropriate support using both pharmacologic and nonpharmacologic approaches. (See Chapter 27).

Lidocaine 4% preparations adequately penetrate intact skin and are used as a local anesthetic before intrusive procedures, including venipunctures, implanted port access, LPs, and subcutaneous or intramuscular injections of growth factors or other drugs (Hockenberry and Kline, 2011). (See Fig. 27-7.) Local intradermal anesthesia is frequently used for LP and bone marrow examination. To reduce the stinging sensation from lidocaine, sodium bicarbonate should be added. (See Pain Management, Chapter 7.) Deeper infiltration of the muscle and periosteum of the bone with buffered lidocaine further reduces the pain from the large-bore aspiration or biopsy needle entering the bone.

For bone marrow studies, LPs, and other procedures, children of preschool age and beyond should be prepared beforehand. If this is not possible, the nurse should explain each step of the procedure as it occurs, stressing what will be done and what it will feel like. If each step is explained beforehand, having the child recall the next step during the procedure can be a distraction mechanism.

Physical care after the procedures is minimum. A small pressure bandage is applied to the bone marrow puncture site, and an adhesive bandage is applied to the LP site. No activity restriction is necessary after the bone marrow test, although the site is usually sore and the child may prefer to remain quiet. Recommendations after LP vary. If medication was instilled, the child may be placed in a slight Trendelenburg position to facilitate circulation of the medicated spinal fluid.

PAIN MANAGEMENT

Nurses must be knowledgeable about the basic pathophysiology of cancer pain and treatment-related side effects. The World Health Organization's three-step analgesic pain ladder should be incorporated into the approach to pain management for every child with cancer (McMain, 2008; Hellsten, 2000). Nurses must acquire extensive knowledge of nonopioid and opioid analgesics used in pediatric pain management. (See Chapter 7.) Interdisciplinary pain management teams are used in many pediatric cancer centers. These teams serve as consultants and provide expertise in the assessment and management of pain. The nurse often serves as the coordinator of care, playing a key role in cancer pain management.

Chapter 7 discusses pharmacologic management of disease-related pain, which involves a variety of methods. It may take more than a trial of one type of medication to find the appropriate agent to manage a patient's pain. The route of administration must be considered as well. Providing "pain relief" by administering painful intramuscular injections, as an alternative to the IV route, is not appropriate therapy because many oral preparations are now available with comparable efficacy. Nonsteroidal antiinflammatory drugs (NSAIDs), acetaminophen with codeine, oxycodone, and morphine are commonly used agents in the management of disease-related pain (Kumar, Rajagopal, and Naseema, 2000). All are available in the oral form, and morphine and the NSAID ketorolac (Toradol) are available as IV preparations. Appropriate dosing is imperative. Doses are titrated to increase the amount of analgesia and minimize side effects.

HEALTH PROMOTION

Children with cancer require the same basic health supervision as any child. Sometimes the overwhelming needs and demands placed on the family, coupled with the singular concern focused on the cancer by both family and practitioners, result in a lack of attention to normal health care needs. Nurses should monitor the type of primary care the child receives, using as a guideline recommendations for health supervision. Areas of particular concern are growth, physical and cognitive development, and neurologic status. Two other areas are also important: (1) dental care because of potential side effects from treatment, and (2) immunizations because of concern with live virus vaccines and immunosuppression.

Dental Care

Irradiation to the head and neck can cause a number of late complications (Armenian, Meadows, and Bhatia, 2011). Some are irreversible, such as facial asymmetry, but those affecting the teeth and gums (caries, periodontal disease) benefit from excellent oral hygiene, including regular use of systemic and topical fluoride. (See Dental Health, Chapter 14.) There is also evidence of delayed or absent development of the permanent teeth (Armenian, Meadows, and Bhatia, 2011; Oeffinger, Eshelman, Tomlinson, et al, 2000). Depending on the child's age, this can be a source of acute psychologic distress, especially during early school-age years, when "losing a tooth" is a status symbol. Children need to be aware of this possibility and need help to explain the delay to peers.

Daily toothbrushing and flossing are encouraged in children with granulocyte counts in excess of 500/mm³ and platelet counts above 40,000/mm³. Fluoride rinses are used as discussed in Chapter 14. Oral hygiene for children whose counts are below these parameters is limited to wiping the teeth with moistened gauze sponges or Toothettes.

Immunizations

Viral replication after the administration of live vaccine for polio, measles, rubella, and mumps can cause serious disease in immunocompromised children. The child receiving chemotherapy for cancer should not receive live, attenuated vaccines. Inactivated vaccines can be given to immunosuppressed children, but the immune response is likely to be suboptimum, so delaying vaccinations is usually recommended (American Academy of Pediatrics, 2006). Children who are immunosuppressed should not receive the varicella vaccine (American Academy of Pediatrics, 2006). Siblings and other family members can receive the live measles, mumps, and rubella vaccine and the varicella vaccine without risk to the child who is immunosuppressed.

An important indication for isolation is an outbreak of childhood disease, especially chickenpox. Ideally the school nurse should work with the treating practitioner to decide the optimum time for school reattendance. If the child has been exposed to the varicella virus, varicella-zoster immune globulin given within 72 hours may favorably alter the course of the disease, or antiviral agents, such as acyclovir, may be given if the child develops varicella. These antiviral agents are effective in preventing serious disease if given during the first 3 days of the appearance of symptoms (American Academy of Pediatrics, 2006). Without treatment, death from disseminated varicella (about 7%) is usually caused by pneumonia; other serious although nonfatal complications include hepatitis, pancreatitis, meningitis, and bacterial skin infections. (See also Immunizations, Chapter 12.)

> **! NURSING ALERT**
>
> Children vaccinated 2 weeks before or during chemotherapy should be considered unimmunized and should be revaccinated or receive live virus vaccines 3 months after chemotherapy has stopped (American Academy of Pediatrics, 2006). Most institutions have individual guidelines regarding vaccinations in a child undergoing immunosuppressive therapy. The nurse should be aware of these guidelines and educate patients and families.

FAMILY EDUCATION

Nurses working with children who have cancer have a significant supportive role in helping the family understand the various therapies, preventing or managing expected side effects or toxicities, and observing for late effects of treatment. Education is a constant feature of the nursing role, especially in terms of new treatments, clinical trials, and home care. Because of the anxiety generated by the diagnosis of cancer, some families may resort to unproven methods of treatment. These unorthodox approaches may produce unnecessary harm by themselves or, if benign, render injury because other proven modes of therapy are avoided. In many instances this causes financial burden and emotional strife among family members.

Nurses are instrumental in helping families avoid the trap of seeking unproven and potentially unsafe "remedies" by encouraging the families to discuss concerns and questions openly with their health care provider. Some families feel pressure from well meaning friends and relatives to "leave no stone unturned" or "try everything." Communicating openly and effectively with families about the diagnosis and forms of therapy and discussing alternative therapies is essential to building a trusting relationship with a patient and his or her family. This will help ensure that the family discusses any possible treatments they are considering, and their physician can guide them regarding the efficacy and safety. Nurses must be fortified with knowledge to substantiate present treatment protocols and to discredit unauthorized methods. The American Cancer Society and local and state medical societies are reliable sources of information concerning research on investigational versus quack methods of cancer therapy. The Association of Pediatric Hematology/Oncology Nurses* has developed numerous educational materials for family and child teaching. The American Childhood Cancer Organization† is an international organization providing support, education, and advocacy programs for children with cancer and their families.

Instruction regarding home care frequently involves teaching about medication schedules, observing for side effects or toxicities that require further evaluation, taking measures to prevent or manage these problems, and caring for special devices such as central venous catheters.‡ Compliance is an important issue, since poor adherence to drug regimens can result in a relapse. Every effort must be made to ensure that the family understands the importance of adhering to the prescribed treatment schedule and measures to improve compliance. (See Chapter 27.)

CESSATION OF THERAPY

Care does not end when the child completes therapy. With the increasing awareness of late effects, nurses play an important role in the assessment of the child for problems such as delayed growth, secondary malignancies, and disturbances in any body system. The family needs to be aware of the importance of continued medical supervision. Other health care professionals caring for the child, such as school nurses, family physicians, and dentists, should be informed of the child's cancer diagnosis. As children reach adulthood, they may benefit from genetic counseling regarding cancers that are likely to be inherited. If the possibility of sterility exists, pretreatment sperm banking may be offered to adolescent boys, which allows additional

*4700 W. Lake Ave., Glenview, IL 60025-1485; 847-375-4724; fax: 847-375-6478; www.aphon.org.

†PO Box 498, Kensington, MD 20895; 800-366-2223 or 301-962-3520; fax: 301-962-3521; www.candlelighters.org.

‡Home care instructions for giving medications to children and caring for a central venous catheter are available in Wilson D, Hockenberry MJ: *Wong's clinical manual of pediatric nursing*, ed 7, St Louis, 2008, Mosby.

options regarding family planning in adulthood (see Nursing Care Plan, pp. 1470-1472). The Children's Oncology Group in collaboration with the American Academy of Pediatrics (2009) has developed guidelines for long term follow-up care for pediatric cancer survivors. Nurses involved with these children should be familiar with these guidelines and use all opportunities to teach patients and families regarding needed continued care.

CANCERS OF THE BLOOD AND LYMPH SYSTEMS

LEUKEMIAS

Acute Leukemias

Leukemia is a broad term given to a group of malignant diseases of the bone marrow and lymphatic system. It is a complex disease of varying heterogeneity. Consequently classification has become increasingly complex, sophisticated, and essential because identification of the subtype of leukemia has therapeutic and prognostic implications. The following is an overview of the major classification systems currently used.

Morphology

In children, two forms are generally recognized: acute lymphoblastic leukemia (ALL) and acute myelogenous leukemia (AML). Synonyms for ALL include lymphatic, lymphocytic, lymphoid, and lymphoblastoid leukemia.

ALL is the most common form of childhood cancer. The annual incidence is 3 or 4 cases per 100,000 Caucasian children (Margolin, Rabin, Steuber, et al, 2011). It occurs more frequently in boys than in girls and in Caucasians than in African-Americans. The peak onset is between 2 and 5 years of age. It is one of the forms of pediatric cancer that has demonstrated dramatic improvements in survival rates. Before the use of antileukemic agents in 1948, a child with ALL lived 2 to 3 months. Current long-term disease-free survival rates for children with ALL approach 80% in major research centers.

AML accounts for about 20% of all cases of childhood leukemia and has an annual incidence of 5 to 7 cases per million. The incidence is similar for males and females, and higher rates are seen during the first 2 years of life. Approximately 40% to 50% of children with AML can be cured of their disease.

Classification

Because of the confusion and inconsistency in classifying the leukemias, ALL and AML are further subdivided according to another system known as the French-American-British (FAB) system. In the FAB system the subtypes are determined after a thorough study of the morphology (structure) and cytochemical reactivity of the leukemic cells. Accordingly, ALL is morphologically classified into three subtypes: L1, L2, and L3. L1 is the most common subtype (Landier, 2001; Margolin, Rabin, Steuber, et al, 2011). AML is classified into eight subtypes.

Cytochemical Markers

Leukemic cells demonstrate different reactions when they are exposed to certain chemicals. For example, terminal deoxynucleotidyl transferase is able to provide excellent differentiation between ALL and AML. Several other chemicals are available to further differentiate various cell types.

Chromosome Studies

Chromosome analysis of leukemic cells has become an important tool in the diagnosis and management of patients with ALL and AML. For example, children with trisomy 21 have 20 times the risk of other children for developing ALL (Plon and Malkin, 2011). Children with more than 50 chromosomes (DNA index >1.16) have a better prognosis. Similarly, patients with ALL and trisomies of chromosomes 4 and 10 have a good prognosis with a low risk of treatment failure (Margolin, Rabin, Steuber, et al, 2011).

In addition, several structural changes (translocations) in the leukemic cells have been identified and are associated with clinical outcome. For example, the presence of a t(12;21) (p13;q22) translocation is associated with a good clinical outcome in ALL. The t(9;22)(q34;p11) translocation, known as the Philadelphia chromosome, is found in approximately 5% of children with ALL and is associated with a poor prognosis. For patients with AML, cytogenetic classification plays an important role in the prognosis and therapy. For example, patients with a t(8;21)(q22;q22) or t(15;17)(q22;q12) have a favorable prognosis.

Cell-Surface Immunologic Markers

Most childhood leukemias are of B-cell lineage. Early pre–B-cell (common) ALL, characterized by the presence of cytoplasmic immunoglobulins, is the most frequent type of cancer found in children. Most (>80%) of these children have the common acute lymphocytic leukemia antigen (CALLA) on their cell surface (Margolin, Rabin, Steuber, et al, 2011). Children with ALL who are CALLA positive have better survival rates.

Other subtypes of ALL include B-cell ALL that secretes immunoglobulin on the cell surface and T-cell ALL (revealed by the presence of T-cell surface antigens and heat-stable rosette formation in the presence of sheep red blood cells). Some groups of patients have a characteristic combination of surface markers that usually correlates with a specific subtype of leukemia.

Pathologic and Related Clinical Manifestations

Leukemia is an unrestricted proliferation of immature white blood cells in the blood-forming tissues of the body. Although not a "tumor" as such, the leukemic cells demonstrate the neoplastic properties of solid cancers. Thus the resultant pathologic and clinical manifestations of the disease are caused by infiltration and replacement of any tissue of the body with nonfunctional leukemic cells. Highly vascular organs, such as the spleen and liver, are most severely affected.

To understand the pathophysiology of the leukemic process, it is important to clarify two common misconceptions. First, although leukemia is an overproduction of white blood cells, most often in the acute form the leukocyte count is low. Instead, the peripheral blood smear and, more definitively, the bone marrow examination reveal greatly elevated counts of immature cells, or blasts. Second, these immature cells do not deliberately attack and destroy the normal blood cells or vascular tissues. Cellular destruction occurs through the process of infiltration and subsequent competition for metabolic elements. The following discussion elaborates on the pathologic process and related clinical manifestations in the most susceptible organs of the body (Fig. 36-3).

Bone Marrow Dysfunction

In all types of leukemia the proliferating cells depress bone marrow production of the formed elements of the blood by competing for and depriving the normal cells of the essential nutrients for metabolism. The three main consequences are (1) anemia from decreased erythrocytes, (2) infection from neutropenia, and (3) bleeding from decreased platelet production.

The invasion of the bone marrow with leukemic cells gradually causes a weakening of the bone and a tendency toward fractures. As leukemic cells invade the periosteum, increasing pressure causes severe pain. The most frequent presenting signs and symptoms of leukemia are a result of infiltration of the bone marrow. These include fever, pallor, fatigue, anorexia, hemorrhage (usually petechiae), and bone and joint pain. In the presence of neutropenia the body's normal bacterial flora can become aggressive pathogens. Any break in the skin is a potential site of infection. Frequently, vague abdominal pain is caused by areas of inflammation from normal flora within the intestinal tract.

Disturbance of Involved Organs

The spleen, liver, and lymph glands demonstrate marked infiltration, enlargement, and eventually fibrosis. Hepatosplenomegaly is typically more common than lymphadenopathy.

The next most important site of involvement is the CNS. Less than 5% of patients with ALL and about 20% of patients with AML have CNS involvement. The use of prophylactic CNS intrathecal therapy has dramatically decreased the incidence of CNS relapse in these patients.

The usual effect of leukemic infiltration of the meninges is increased intracranial pressure (ICP). The pathogenesis is presumably attributable to invasion of the arachnoid by proliferating cells, which then interfere with the flow of cerebrospinal fluid in the subarachnoid space and at the base of the brain. The increased fluid pressure causes dilation of all four ventricles and consequently the signs and symptoms normally associated with this condition, such as severe headache, vomiting, papilledema, irritability, lethargy, and eventually coma. Irritation of the meninges also causes pain and stiffness in the neck and back.

Additional sites of involvement may be the cranial nerves (most often cranial nerve VII, or the facial nerve) and spinal nerves, particularly of the lumbosacral plexus, hypothalamus, and cerebellum. Clinical manifestations for these sites are directly related to the area involved. For example, with lumbosacral invasion, the patient has weakness in the lower extremities, pain radiating down the legs to the feet, and difficulty in voiding. Although such signs may suggest a brain tumor, the absence of localized signs often leads to the discovery of CNS involvement in leukemia.

Other sites that may become invaded with leukemic cells include the kidneys, testes, prostate, ovaries, gastrointestinal tract, and lungs. With long-term survivors becoming

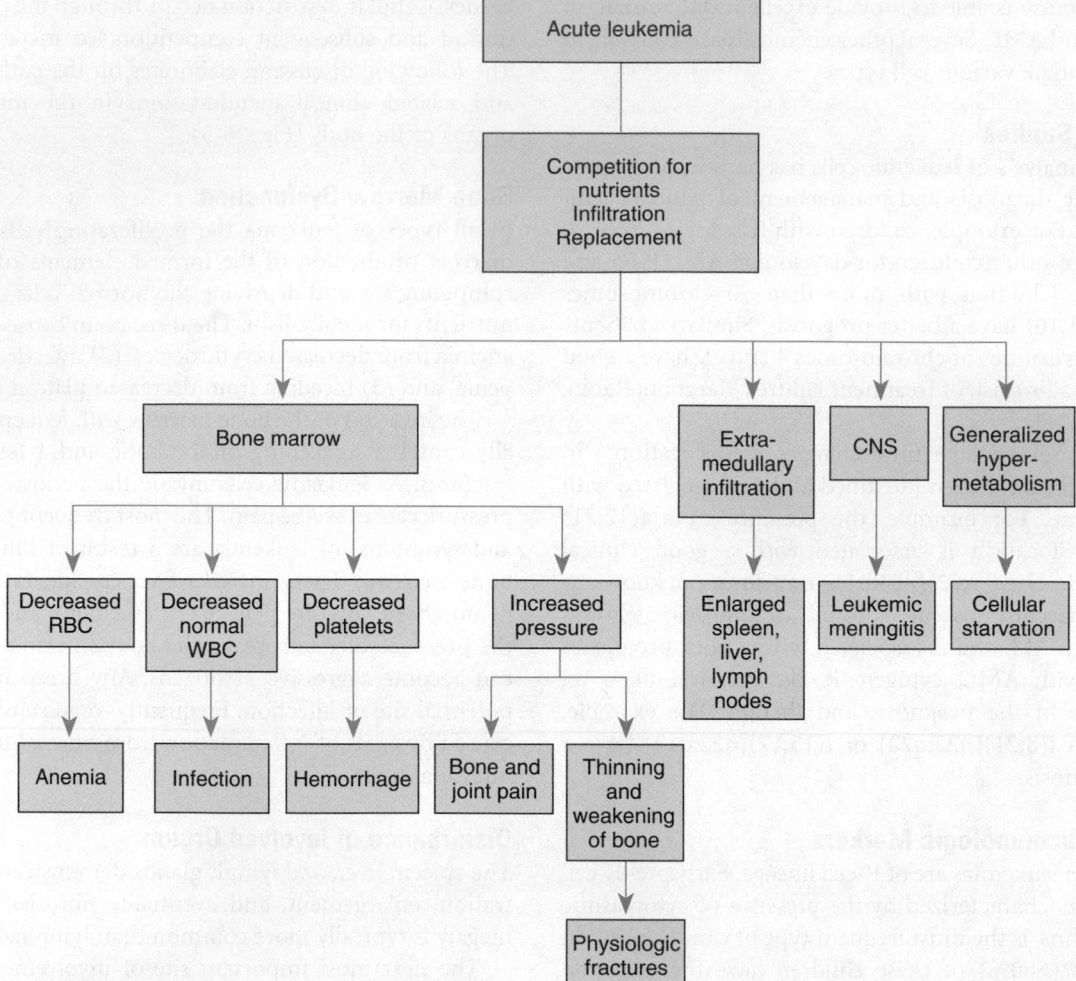

Fig. 36-3 Principal sites of tissue involvement in leukemia. *CNS,* Central nervous system; *RBC,* red blood cells; *WBC,* white blood cells.

increasingly common, such extramedullary sites of leukemic invasion, especially the testes, are becoming more important clinically.

Onset

The onset of leukemia varies from acute to insidious. In most instances the child displays remarkably few symptoms. For example, leukemia may be diagnosed when a minor infection, such as a cold, fails to completely disappear. The child continues to be pale, listless, irritable, febrile, and anorexic. Parents often suspect some underlying problem when they observe the weight loss, petechiae, bruising without cause, and continued complaints of bone and joint pain.

At other times leukemia is diagnosed after an extended history of signs and symptoms mimicking such conditions as rheumatoid arthritis or mononucleosis. In some cases the diagnosis of leukemia accompanies some totally unrelated event, such as a routine physical examination or injury.

The history not only yields valuable medical information regarding the subsequent course of the illness, but also bears heavily on the parents' emotional reaction to the diagnosis. In most instances the diagnosis is an unexpected revelation of catastrophic proportion.

TABLE 36-3	FAVORABLE PROGNOSTIC FACTORS FOR ACUTE LYMPHOBLASTIC LEUKEMIA
FACTOR	**CRITERIA**
Leukocyte count	<50,000/mm³
Age	2-10 yr
Immunologic subtype	CALLA-positive, early pre–B-cell
FAB morphology	L_1
Cytogenetics	Hyperdiploid (>50 chromosomes, DNA index >1.16); trisomies 4 and 10 and translocations t(12/21) (p21/q22)
Sex	Female
Leukemia cell burden	Minimal

CALLA, Common acute lymphocytic leukemia antigen; *DNA,* deoxyribonucleic acid; *FAB,* French-American-British (classification system).

Staging and Prognostic Factors

The most important prognostic factors in determining long-term survival for children with ALL are the initial white blood cell count, the patient's age at diagnosis, cytogenetics, the immunologic subtype, and the child's sex (Table 36-3).

For children with AML, prognostic factors associated with a poorer prognosis include certain chromosome abnormalities (monosomy 7), a high white blood cell count (100,000/mm³), and AML developing after a myelodysplastic syndrome. The absence of Auer rods in the M1 subtype of AML has also been correlated with a low remission rate (Smith, Hasle, Cooper, 2011).

From the time of diagnosis, the nurse has some idea of the expected course the disease will follow. However, in some instances, because of the variety of cell types observed and the marked undifferentiation of immature cells, a definitive classification cannot be made or the diagnosis may be changed. Be aware of the importance of such events in counseling and supporting family members.

Diagnostic Evaluation

Leukemia is usually suspected from the history; physical manifestations; and a peripheral blood smear that contains immature forms of leukocytes, frequently in combination with low blood counts. Definitive diagnosis is based on bone marrow aspiration or biopsy. Typically the bone marrow shows a monotonous infiltrate of blast cells. Once the diagnosis is confirmed, an LP is performed to determine whether there is any CNS involvement, although a small number of children have CNS involvement and most are asymptomatic.

Therapeutic Management

Treatment of leukemia involves the use of IV and intrathecal chemotherapeutic agents. Cranial radiation is sometimes used for resistant CNS disease or testicular relapse. Typically leukemia treatment is divided into phases: (1) induction, which achieves a complete remission or clinical disappearance of leukemic cells; (2) intensification, or consolidation, therapy, which further decreases the total tumor burden; and (3) maintenance, which consists of further chemotherapy to ensure the disease stays in remission. Although the combination of drugs and possibility of irradiation may vary according to the institution, the patient's prognostic or risk characteristics, and the type of leukemia being treated, the following general principles for each phase are consistently employed.

Remission Induction

Almost immediately after confirmation of the diagnosis, induction therapy is begun and lasts for 4 to 6 weeks (Margolin, Rabin, Steuber, et al, 2011). The principal drugs used for induction in ALL are the corticosteroids (prednisone or dexamethasone), vincristine, and L-asparaginase, with or without doxorubicin. Oral steroids are administered daily in divided doses to maintain consistently high blood levels. Vincristine is given by IV infusion once a week for a total of four to six doses, and L-asparaginase or doxorubicin is given at various schedules. A complete remission is determined by the absence of clinical signs or symptoms of the disease and the presence of less than 5% blast cells in the bone marrow. With AML the drug therapies differ from those used for lymphoblastic leukemia. The principal drugs used for induction therapy in AML are doxorubicin or daunomycin and cytosine arabinoside; various other drugs may be added.

Because many of the drugs also cause myelosuppression of normal blood elements, the period immediately after a remission can be critical. The body is defenseless against invading organisms (especially normal bacterial flora) and highly susceptible to spontaneous hemorrhage. Consequently, supportive therapy during this time is essential.

Intensification, or Consolidation, Therapy

Intensification, or consolidation, therapy is used to further decrease the number of leukemic cells in the child's body. Intensification therapy incorporates some of the following agents: L-asparaginase, high-dose methotrexate or intermediate-dose methotrexate with leucovorin rescue, vincristine, doxorubicin, steroids, cytarabine, intramuscular or oral methotrexate, and 6-mercaptopurine. The intensification phase consists of pulses of these agents given periodically during the first 6 months of treatment. The specific agents used for intensification therapy depend on the type of leukemia and the child's risk factors.

Maintenance

The goal of maintenance therapy is to preserve remission and further reduce the number of leukemic cells. Combined drug regimens have been more successful in maintaining remissions and preventing drug resistance. A variety of agents are used during maintenance therapy, including a daily dose of oral 6-mercaptopurine, weekly doses of methotrexate, and intermittent pulses of steroids and vincristine, which are standard in most treatment regimens.

During maintenance therapy, weekly or monthly complete blood counts are taken to evaluate the marrow's response to the drugs. If myelosuppression becomes severe (usually indicated by an ANC <1000/mm³), or if toxic side effects occur, therapy is temporarily stopped or the dose decreased.

Central Nervous System Prophylactic Therapy

Children with leukemia are at risk for invasion of the CNS by the leukemic cells. For this reason, all children receive CNS prophylactic therapy. Before the 1980s children with ALL received cranial-spinal irradiation. Because of the concern regarding late effects of cranial irradiation and secondary malignancies, this mode of therapy is now generally reserved for high-risk patients or those with resistant CNS disease. Depending on protocol, intrathecal methotrexate or triple intrathecal chemotherapy (consisting of methotrexate, cytarabine, and hydrocortisone) is used during induction, intensification, and maintenance therapy to prevent CNS disease.

Duration of therapy has been based on clinical experience comparing survival rates for various time intervals and is concerned with preventing deleterious effects of excessive treatment. Although the optimum time for discontinuing therapy is not known, current practice is to continue treatment for 2½ to 3 years. All children after cessation of therapy require regular medical evaluation for surveillance of relapse and long-term sequelae of treatment. Most relapses (16%) occur during the first year off therapy, about 2% to 3% of the relapses occur during each of the next 3 years, and very few relapses occur after 6 years (Margolin, Rabin, Steuber, et al, 2011).

Reinduction After Relapse

For many children, additional therapy becomes necessary when a relapse occurs, as evidenced by the presence of leukemic cells within the bone marrow. Usually reinduction for ALL includes the use of prednisone and vincristine with a combination of other drugs not previously used. Although remissions may be achieved after more than one relapse, each relapse indicates an increasingly poor prognosis. However, more long-term second and subsequent remissions are occurring, and these may have better outlooks than previously thought.

A site that is resistant to chemotherapy and is responsible for leukemic relapse is the testes. A minority of males experience relapses during maintenance therapy or have occult disease after cessation of therapy. Treatment for testicular disease includes bilateral testicular irradiation, intensive systemic chemotherapy, and CNS prophylactic therapy (Landier, 2001).

Bone Marrow Transplantation

BMT has been used successfully in treating some children with ALL and AML. In general, BMT is not recommended for children with ALL during the first remission because of the excellent results possible with chemotherapy. The group with the best results has been those with ALL who received the graft during the second remission (Bollard, Krance, and Heslop, 2011). Because of the poorer prognosis in children with AML, transplantation may be considered during the first remission when a suitable donor is available (Bollard, Krance, and Heslop, 2011).

Prognosis

The majority of children with newly diagnosed leukemia who receive effective multiagent chemotherapy will survive. More than 80% of the children achieved long-term disease-free survival, and the majority of these children developed no obvious health problems from the leukemia or its treatment (Margolin, Rabin, Steuber, et al, 2011). Prognosis after transplantation varies with the timing of the procedure and the type of leukemia; reported ranges for long-term survival are between 25% and 50% (Bollard, Krance, and Heslop, 2011). However, because many of these children faced almost certain death without transplantation, even these low figures represent a major advance. Still, the use of BMT remains controversial.

Nursing Care Management

Nursing care of the child with leukemia is directly related to the regimen of therapy. Myelosuppression, drug toxicity, and leukemic infiltration cause secondary complications that necessitate supportive physical care. This discussion focuses on supportive interventions for the child with leukemia and the family. General aspects of care appropriate for the child with leukemia are discussed earlier under Nursing Care of the Child with Cancer.

Prepare the Family for Diagnostic and Therapeutic Procedures

From the time before diagnosis to cessation of therapy, children must undergo several tests, the most traumatic of which are bone marrow aspiration or biopsy and LP. Multiple finger sticks and venipunctures for blood analysis and drug infusion are common occurrences for several years after the diagnosis. Therefore the child needs an explanation of why each procedure is done and what can be expected. (See Preparation for Diagnostic and Therapeutic Procedures, Chapter 27.)

Depending on the child's age, one way of beginning diagnostic preparation is to explain the tests, procedures, and treatment plan.* Using a drawing or letting the child look at a drop of blood under a microscope not only teaches, but also fosters trust between the nurse and the child. It also allows the nurse to assess the child's level of understanding. An error many health professionals make is to overestimate children's knowledge about their bodies. For example, a bone marrow aspiration makes sense only when it is clarified that the center of a bone is hollow and contains the cells that later become "working" blood cells or leukemic cells.

Provide Continued Emotional Support

Nursing care of the child with leukemia is based on typical problems the family confronts during the treatment phases. It is not unusual for a child who discontinues therapy after 2 or 3 years and maintains a permanent remission to experience many side effects. Therefore the nurse's role is one of continual support, guidance, clarification, and judgment. Parents need to know how to recognize symptoms that demand medical attention. Although some of the reactions discussed are expected, parents should still report them to their practitioner. Warning parents of their possible occurrence beforehand also allows parents to prepare. At the same time, it reassures them that these reactions are not caused by a return of leukemic cells.

The nurse must also use judgment in recognizing which side effects are normal reactions and which indicate toxicity. Frequently it is the office or clinic nurse who screens such telephone calls and gives advice, when appropriate. Usually nausea and vomiting are not indications for drug cessation. However, severe vomiting may require immediate intervention to prevent dehydration. Signs of infection, mucosal ulceration, hemorrhagic cystitis, peripheral neuropathy, and constipation require medical evaluation.

Another aspect of continued emotional support involves prognosis. Leukemia is not invariably fatal, but present statistics must be correctly interpreted. Although more than 95% of children with ALL achieve an initial remission and almost 80% of them live 5 years or longer, remember that these are average estimates and apply to those children treated with the most successful protocols since diagnosis (Shusterman and Meadows, 2000). For the low-risk child the chances may be better, but for the high-risk child they may be significantly poorer. Of those who do survive after discontinuing therapy, a portion will relapse. At present only the passage of time is positive confirmation that the child is "cured" of the disease.

The nurse must be familiar with these statistics to interpret them correctly to parents. At the same time, the nurse must realize that a realistic understanding of the chances for survival requires an adjustment period. For example, it is not unusual for parents to interpret the "95% remission" as the probability

---

*Especially recommended is Dorfman E: *The C-word: teenagers and their families living with cancer*, ed 2, Portland, 1998, New Sage Press.

for a cure. When a relapse occurs, parents may for the first time be able to "hear" the facts.

Statistics are numbers. Sometimes they bring hope, and at other times they bring despair. Although they are important in terms of research, better treatment, and identification of high- or low-risk populations, they present a general picture of what to expect. The nurse who is working with family members must individualize the numbers to relate to the people. An understanding of each member's emotional needs, as well as competent care of physical ones, is essential to the positive, growth-promoting support of the family. Chapter 23 discusses comprehensive emotional support for the family through all phases of the illness.

LYMPHOMAS

The lymphomas, a group of neoplastic diseases that arise from the lymphoid and hematopoietic systems, are divided into Hodgkin disease and NHL. These diseases are further subdivided according to tissue type and extent of disease (staging). In children NHL is more common than Hodgkin disease. Although Hodgkin disease is extremely rare before 5 years of age, there is a striking increase in children ages 15 to 19 years, when it occurs with almost the same frequency as leukemia.

Hodgkin Disease

Hodgkin disease affects about 5 in 1 million children, mostly adolescents. The malignancy originates in the lymphoid system and primarily involves the lymph nodes. It predictably metastasizes to nonnodal or extralymphatic sites, especially the spleen, liver, bone marrow, lungs, and mediastinum (mass of tissues and organs separating the lungs, including the heart and its vessels, trachea, esophagus, thymus, and lymph nodes), although no tissue is exempt from involvement (Fig. 36-4). It is classified according to four histologic types: (1) lymphocytic predominance, (2) nodular sclerosis, (3) mixed cellularity,

and (4) lymphocytic depletion. With present treatment protocols the histologic stage of the disease has less prognostic significance.

Clinical Staging and Prognosis

Accurate staging of the extent of disease is the basis for treatment protocols and expected prognosis. More than one staging system exists; Box 36-3 shows the Ann Arbor Staging Classification.

Each stage is further subdivided into A or B. A denotes absence of associated general symptoms. B indicates presence of symptoms, such as night sweats, fever (38° C [100.4° F]), or weight loss of 10% or more during the preceding 6 months. In stages II and III, subtype B has a significantly poorer prognosis than subtype A.

The prognosis for patients with Hodgkin disease has improved dramatically, largely as a result of the systematic staging procedure and improved treatment protocols. The prognosis is excellent in children with localized disease. The overall 10-year survival rate is as high as 90%. For relapses, complete remission may occur in 20% to 40% of patients; BMT may represent hope for a cure (Lanzkowsky, 2005). Even in those with disseminated disease, long-term remissions are possible in more than half the patients. Fortunately, now there is a trend toward response-based therapy, and often when radiation is used, it involves field radiotherapy.

Clinical Manifestations

Hodgkin disease is characterized by painless enlargement of lymph nodes. The most common finding is enlarged, firm, nontender, movable nodes in the supraclavicular or cervical area. In children the sentinel node located near the left clavicle may be the first enlarged node. Enlargement of axillary and inguinal lymph nodes is less frequent (see Fig. 36-4).

Other signs and symptoms depend on the extent and location of involvement. Mediastinal lymphadenopathy may cause a persistent, nonproductive cough. Enlarged retroperitoneal nodes may produce unexplained abdominal pain. Systemic symptoms include low-grade or intermittent fever (Pel-Ebstein disease), anorexia, nausea, weight loss, night sweats, and pruritus. Generally, such symptoms indicate advanced lymph node and extralymphatic involvement.

Diagnostic Evaluation

The history and physical examination often yield important clues to the disease, such as fevers; night sweats; weight loss;

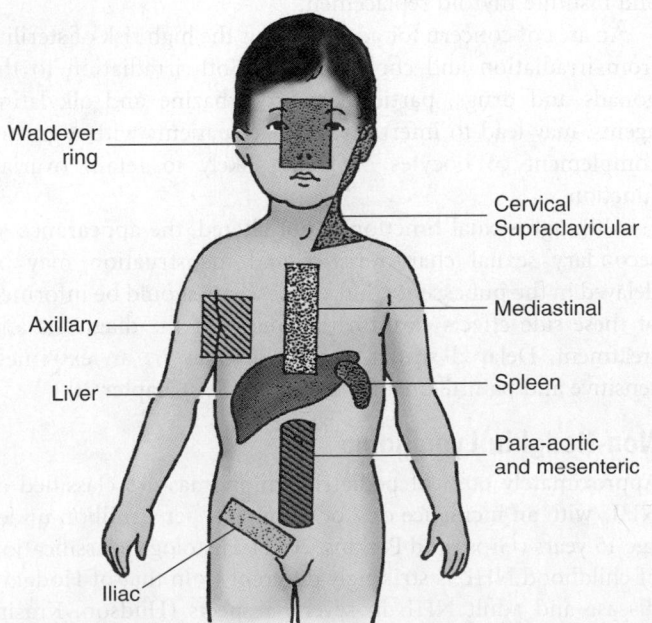

Waldeyer
ring

Cervical
Supraclavicular

Mediastinal

Axillary

Liver

Spleen

Para-aortic
and mesenteric

Iliac

Fig. 36-4 Main areas of lymphadenopathy and organ involvement in Hodgkin disease.

BOX 36-3 STAGING OF HODGKIN DISEASE

Stage I—Lesions are limited to one lymph node area or only one additional extralymphatic site (I-E), such as the liver, lungs, kidney, or intestines.

Stage II—Two or more lymph node regions on the same side of the diaphragm or one additional extralymphatic site or organ (II-E) on the same side of the diaphragm is involved.

Stage III—Lymph node regions on both sides of the diaphragm, or one extralymphatic site (III-E), spleen (III-S), or both (III-SE), are involved.

Stage IV—Cancer has metastasized diffusely throughout the body to one or more extralymphatic sites with or without involvement of associated lymph nodes.

and enlarged lymph nodes, spleen, or liver. Because of the multiple organs that can become involved, diagnosis consists of several tests to confirm the presence of Hodgkin disease and to assess the extent of involvement for accurate staging. Tests include complete blood count, uric acid levels, liver function tests, erythrocyte sedimentation rate or C-reactive protein, alkaline phosphatase, and urinalysis. Radiographic tests include CT scans of the neck, chest, abdomen, and pelvis; a gallium or PET scan (to identify metastatic or recurrent disease); a chest x-ray film; and, if clinically indicated, a bone scan to detect metastasis.

A lymph node biopsy is essential to establish histologic diagnosis and staging. The presence of Sternberg-Reed cell is considered diagnostic of Hodgkin disease because it is absent in the other lymphomas; however, it may occur in infectious mononucleosis. A bone marrow aspiration or biopsy is also usually performed. With the advent of the CT and gallium scans to identify metastatic disease and multiagent chemotherapy and radiotherapy to eradicate metastatic disease, a laparotomy is avoided except in selected cases.

Therapeutic Management

The primary modalities of therapy are chemotherapy and irradiation. Each may be used alone or in combination based on the clinical staging. The goal of treatment is obviously a cure; however, aggressive therapy increases the chances of complications in the disease-free state and can seriously compromise the quality of life. Consequently, numerous research studies are currently investigating treatment options to minimize long-term complications. Because of the diversity of approaches to treatment, the following is an overview of general principles that may not apply to all children. One of the major concerns with combined radiation and antineoplastic drug therapy is the serious late effects in children with an excellent prognosis.

Radiation may entail involved field radiation, extended field radiation (involved areas plus adjacent nodes), or total nodal irradiation (the entire axial lymph node system), depending on the extent of involvement. In stage IV disease, chemotherapy is the primary form of treatment, although limited irradiation may be given to areas of bulky disease. The most effective combination of chemotherapy widely used in the past has been MOPP (mechlorethamine [Mustargen], vincristine [Oncovin], prednisone, and procarbazine), alternating with ABVD (doxorubicin [Adriamycin], bleomycin, vinblastine, and dacarbazine). However, this therapy combination of MOPP and ABVD caused severe late effects, including secondary malignancies. For this reason care providers are now using other drug combinations such as BEACOPP (bleomycin, etoposide, doxorubicin [Adriamycin], cyclophosphamide, vincristine [Oncovin], procarbazine, and prednisone) or ABVD (Hudson, Krasin, Metzger, et al, 2011).

Follow-up care of children no longer receiving therapy is essential to identify relapse and second malignancies. In children with splenectomy because of laparotomy, prophylactic antibiotics are administered for an indefinite period. Also, immunizations against pneumococci and meningococci are recommended before the splenectomy. (See Chapter 12.)

Nursing Care Management

Nursing care involves (1) preparation for diagnostic and operative procedures, (2) explanation of treatment side effects, and (3) child and family support (see Nursing Care Plan, pp. 1470-1472). Once the child is hospitalized for suspected Hodgkin disease, a battery of diagnostic tests is ordered. The family needs an explanation of why each test is performed, since many of them, such as bone marrow aspiration and lymph node biopsy, are invasive procedures. (See Chapter 27.)

Explanations of chemotherapeutic reactions vary with the specific drug regimen. The most common side effects, such as nausea and vomiting, body image changes, neuropathy, and mucosal ulceration, are discussed under Nursing Care of the Child with Cancer. Radiation results in few side effects, sometimes consisting only of a mild skin reaction. With external field radiation to the chest and abdomen, nausea and vomiting, weight loss, and mucosal ulceration (esophagitis, gastric ulcers) are common. The usual measures for providing relief are discussed on p. 1473 and outlined in Table 36-2.

The most common side effect of extensive irradiation is malaise, which may result from damage to the thyroid gland, causing hypothyroidism. Lack of energy is particularly difficult for adolescents because it prevents them from keeping up with their peers. Sometimes adolescents push themselves to the point of physical exhaustion rather than admit fatigue and succumb to the decreased activity tolerance. Parents should observe for such behavior, such as extreme fatigue at the end of the day, falling asleep at the dinner table, inability to concentrate on homework, or an increased susceptibility to infection. Regular bedtimes and periodic rest times are important for these children, especially during chemotherapy, when myelosuppression increases the risk of infection and debilitation. Before discharge, the nurse should discuss a feasible school schedule with the parents and child. If alterations are necessary, such as elimination of strenuous physical education, they are discussed with the teacher, school nurse, and principal. Follow-up care is essential to diagnose hypothyroidism early and institute thyroid replacement.

An area of concern for adolescents is the high risk of sterility from irradiation and chemotherapy. Both irradiation to the gonads and drugs, particularly procarbazine and alkylating agents, may lead to infertility. Younger patients with a greater complement of oocytes are more likely to retain ovarian function.

Although sexual function is not altered, the appearance of secondary sexual characteristics and menstruation may be delayed in the pubescent child. Adolescents should be informed of these side effects early in the course of the diagnosis and treatment. Delayed sexual maturation may be an extremely sensitive and painful area for children. (See Chapter 20.)

Non-Hodgkin Lymphoma

Approximately 60% of pediatric lymphomas are classified as NHL, with an incidence of 7 or 8 children per 1 million under age 15 years (Gross and Perkins, 2011). Histologic classification of childhood NHL is strikingly different from that of Hodgkin disease and adult NHL in several respects (Hudson, Krasin, Metzger, et al, 2011):

- The disease is usually diffuse rather than nodular.
- The cell type is either undifferentiated or poorly differentiated.
- Dissemination occurs earlier, more often, and more rapidly.
- Mediastinal involvement and invasion of meninges typically occur.

Staging and Prognosis

NHL is heterogeneous, exhibiting a variety of morphologic, cytochemical, and immunologic features, not unlike the diversity seen in leukemia. Classification is based on the pattern of histologic presentation: (1) lymphoblastic, (2) Burkitt or non-Burkitt, or (3) large cell. Immunologically these cells are also classified as T cells; B cells (an example of which is Burkitt lymphoma); or non-T, non-B cells, which lack specific immunologic properties.

The clinical staging system used in Hodgkin disease is of little value in NHL, although that system has been modified for NHL and other systems have been developed. A favorable prognosis is defined by (1) lymph node involvement only and limitation to one or two adjacent lymphatic regions (excluding the mediastinum); (2) an extranodal site in the nasopharynx, oropharynx, or other isolated extranodal site, with or without regional lymphadenopathy; or (3) gastrointestinal involvement, with or without regional lymphadenopathy, limited to the mesentery (Gross and Perkins, 2011). Box 36-4 presents the most commonly used staging system.

The use of aggressive combination chemotherapy has had a major impact on the survival rates of children with NHL. The most effective treatment regimens result in cure in almost all children with limited disease involvement; 75% to 90% of children with extensive disease are cured (Gross and Perkins, 2011; Kavan, Kabickova, Gajdos, et al, 1999).

Clinical Manifestations

Clinical manifestations depend on the anatomic site and extent of involvement. Many of the manifestations seen in Hodgkin disease may be present in NHL, although rarely does a single symptom give rise to the diagnosis. Rather, metastasis to the bone marrow or CNS may produce signs and symptoms typical of leukemia. Lymphoid tumors compressing various organs may cause intestinal or airway obstruction, cranial nerve palsies, or spinal paralysis.

The exception to the usual presentation of NHL is Burkitt lymphoma, a type of cancer that is rare in the United States but endemic in parts of Africa. It is a rapidly growing neoplasm that is most commonly seen as a mass in the jaw, abdomen, or orbit. However, no anatomic site appears exempt from involvement. Peripheral lymphadenopathy, hepatosplenomegaly, or signs of conversion to leukemia are rarely seen.

Diagnostic Evaluation

Because most children with NHL have widespread disease at diagnosis, thorough pathologic staging is unnecessary. Current recommendations for staging include a surgical biopsy for histopathologic confirmation of disease with immunophenotyping and cytogenetic evaluation; bone marrow aspiration; radiologic studies, especially CT scans of the lungs and gastrointestinal organs; and LP.

Therapeutic Management

The present treatment protocols for NHL include an aggressive approach using irradiation and chemotherapy. Similar to leukemic therapy, the protocols include induction, consolidation, and maintenance phases, some with intrathecal chemotherapy. At present the differentiation between lymphoblastic lymphoma and all other lymphomas is widely used as a way to categorize patients for specific treatment regimens (Gross and Perkins, 2011). Children with lymphoblastic lymphoma are treated with several drug protocols, most containing several chemotherapeutic agents. One of the most commonly used regimens includes cyclophosphamide or ifosfamide, vincristine, intrathecal chemotherapy, prednisone, daunomycin, 6-thioguanine, cytosine arabinoside, carmustine (BCNU), and L-asparaginase.

Children with nonlymphoblastic lymphoma are treated with cyclic drug combinations, including cyclophosphamide and intermediate- or high-dose methotrexate (Gross and Perkins, 2011). Most protocols also include an anthracycline. These children receive CNS prophylaxis with combination intrathecal chemotherapy. These multiagent regimens are administered for 6 to 24 months.

Nursing Care Management

Nursing care of the child with NHL is similar to the care discussed under Nursing Care of the Child with Cancer. Because of the intensive chemotherapy protocol, nursing care is primarily directed toward managing the side effects of these agents.

NERVOUS SYSTEM TUMORS

BRAIN TUMORS

Tumors of the CNS account for about 20% of all childhood cancers and have an annual incidence of 2.4 per 100,000 children under 15 years of age. About 60% of the tumors are **infratentorial** (below the tentorium cerebelli), which means that they occur in the posterior part of the brain, primarily in the cerebellum or brainstem. This anatomic distribution accounts for the frequency of symptoms resulting from increased ICP. The other tumors are **supratentorial** or lie within the midbrain structures. Fig. 36-5 outlines major brain tumors of childhood.

BOX 36-4	STAGING OF NON-HODGKIN LYMPHOMA

Stage I—Single tumor at a single site

Stage II—Single tumor with regional involvement on same side of diaphragm

Stage III—Tumor on both sides of abdomen; also, all primary thoracic, intraabdominal, and paraspinal or epidural tumors

Stage IV—Any of the involvement in stages I and II, with central nervous system or bone marrow involvement

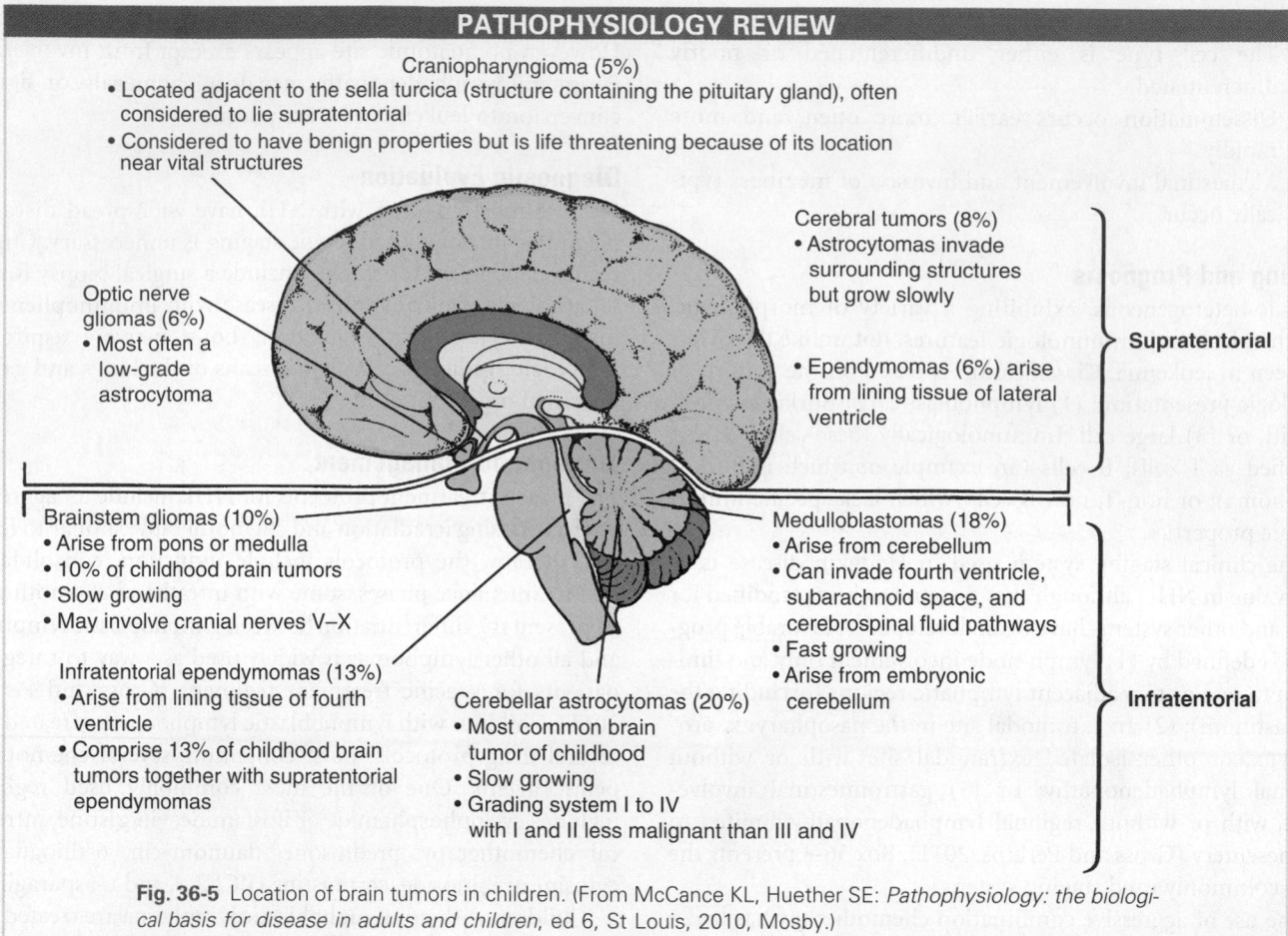

PATHOPHYSIOLOGY REVIEW

Craniopharyngioma (5%)
- Located adjacent to the sella turcica (structure containing the pituitary gland), often considered to lie supratentorial
- Considered to have benign properties but is life threatening because of its location near vital structures

Optic nerve gliomas (6%)
- Most often a low-grade astrocytoma

Cerebral tumors (8%)
- Astrocytomas invade surrounding structures but grow slowly
- Ependymomas (6%) arise from lining tissue of lateral ventricle

Supratentorial

Brainstem gliomas (10%)
- Arise from pons or medulla
- 10% of childhood brain tumors
- Slow growing
- May involve cranial nerves V–X

Infratentorial ependymomas (13%)
- Arise from lining tissue of fourth ventricle
- Comprise 13% of childhood brain tumors together with supratentorial ependymomas

Cerebellar astrocytomas (20%)
- Most common brain tumor of childhood
- Slow growing
- Grading system I to IV with I and II less malignant than III and IV

Medulloblastomas (18%)
- Arise from cerebellum
- Can invade fourth ventricle, subarachnoid space, and cerebrospinal fluid pathways
- Fast growing
- Arise from embryonic cerebellum

Infratentorial

Fig. 36-5 Location of brain tumors in children. (From McCance KL, Huether SE: *Pathophysiological: the biological basis for disease in adults and children*, ed 6, St Louis, 2010, Mosby.)

Because the neoplasms can arise from any cell within the cranium, it is possible to have tumors originating from the glial cells, nerve cells, neuroepithelium, cranial nerves, blood vessels, pineal gland, and hypophysis. Within each of these structures, specific cells may be involved to provide a histologic classification of the major tumors found in children. Astrocytes, cells that form most of the supportive tissue for the neurons, may form astrocytomas, the most common glial tumor (Strickler and Phillips, 2000). Brain tumors may be benign or malignant, although the designation of any tumor in the brain as "benign" should be done cautiously given the vital functions the brain controls.

Clinical Manifestations

The signs and symptoms of brain tumors are directly related to their anatomic location and size and to some extent the child's age. For instance, in infants whose sutures are still open, a bulging fontanel indicates hydrocephalus. Head circumference measurements allow for detection of increased head size. Even in older children, clinical manifestations may be nonspecific. However, the most common symptoms of infratentorial brain tumors are headache, especially on awakening, and vomiting that is not related to feeding. Tumors in this area of the brain often obstruct the flow of cerebrospinal fluid, causing increased ICP and the symptoms mentioned above. In addition, patients may have symptoms related to the specific structure involved. Tumors of the cerebellum often cause nystagmus, ataxia, dysarthria, and dysmetria (Blaney, Haas-Kogan, Young-Pouissant,

et al, 2011; Strickler and Phillips, 2000). Supratentorial symptoms more commonly include seizures, personality or behavioral changes, and contralateral weakness. Tumors involving the structures of the midbrain, including the hypothalamus and pituitary gland, may cause endocrinopathies such as diabetes insipidus, delayed or precocious puberty, and growth failure. Table 36-4 presents the common presenting symptoms of brain tumors.

Diagnostic Evaluation

Diagnosis of a brain tumor is based on presenting clinical signs and diagnostic imaging. Because the signs and symptoms may be vague and easily overlooked, early diagnosis necessitates a high index of suspicion during history taking. A number of tests may be employed in the neurologic evaluation (see Table 37-2), but the gold standard diagnostic procedure is MRI, which permits early diagnosis of brain tumors and assessment of tumor growth during or after treatment. Magnetic resonance (MR) angiography can be performed during the same session as MRI to determine the vascularity of the tumor (Brunelle, 2000). Another test is CT, which permits direct visualization of the brain parenchyma, ventricles, and surrounding subarachnoid space. Through the IV injection of radiographic contrast agents, intracranial blood vasculature can be demonstrated (Blaney, Haas-Kogan, Young-Pouissant, et al, 2011). MR spectroscopy is a new radiographic technique that is able to differentiate between malignant tumors and areas of necrosis (Brunelle, 2000; Lanzkowsky, 2005).

TABLE 36-4 CLINICAL MANIFESTATIONS AND ASSESSMENT OF BRAIN TUMORS

SIGNS AND SYMPTOMS	ASSESSMENT
Headache Recurrent and progressive In frontal or occipital areas Usually dull and throbbing Worse on arising, less during day Intensified by lowering head and straining, such as during bowel movement, coughing, sneezing	Record description of pain, location, severity, and duration. Use pain rating scale to assess severity of pain. (See Chapter 7.) Note changes in relation to time of day and activity. Observe changes in behavior in infants (persistent irritability, crying, head rolling).
Vomiting With of without nausea or feeding Progressively more projectile More severe in morning Relieved by moving about and changing position	Record time, amount, and relationship to feeding, nausea, and activity.
Neuromuscular Changes Incoordination or clumsiness Loss of balance (use of wide-based stance, falling, tripping, banging into objects) Poor fine motor control Weakness Hyporeflexia or hyperreflexia Positive Babinski sign Spasticity Paralysis	Test muscle strength, gait, coordination, and reflexes. (See Chapter 6.)
Behavioral Changes Irritability Decreased appetite Failure to thrive Fatigue (frequent naps) Lethargy Coma Bizarre behavior (staring, automatic movements)	Observe behavior regularly. Compare observations with parental reports of normal behavioral patterns. Monitor growth and food intake. Monitor activity and sleep.
Cranial Nerve Neuropathy Cranial nerve involvement varied according to tumor location Most common signs: • Head tilt • Visual defects (nystagmus, diplopia, strabismus, episodic "graying out" of vision, visual field defect)	Assess cranial nerves, especially VII (facial), IX (glossopharyngeal), X (vagus), V (trigeminal, sensory roots), and VI (abducens). (See Chapter 6.) Assess visual acuity, binocularity, and peripheral vision. (See Chapter 6.)
Vital Sign Disturbances Decreased pulse and respiration Increased blood pressure Decreased pulse pressure Hypothermia or hyperthermia	Measure vital signs frequently. Monitor pulse and respirations for 1 full min. Record pulse pressure (difference between systolic and diastolic blood pressure).
Other Signs Seizures Cranial enlargement* Tense, bulging fontanel at rest* Nuchal rigidity Papilledema (edema of optic nerve)	Record seizure activity. (See Chapter 37.) Measure head circumference daily (infant and young child). Perform funduscopic examination if skilled in procedure.

*Present only in infants and young children.

When a positive CT scan is obtained, angiography may be done to provide information about the tumor's blood supply and degree of vascularity, which may assist the surgeon in planning the operative approach. Other tests may include an MRI of the spine, functional MRI, and electroencephalography. LP is dangerous in the presence of increased ICP because of possible brainstem herniation after sudden release of pressure.

Definitive diagnosis is based on tissue specimens obtained during surgery. Occasionally, special techniques are required for determining the cell type. This period of waiting is one of anxiety for family members, who are aware of the link between cell type and prognosis. Because of the location of some brain tumors, such as brainstem tumors, a biopsy is not possible and the diagnosis is made by imaging findings alone.

Therapeutic Management

Treatment may involve the use of surgery, radiotherapy, and chemotherapy. All three may or may not be used, depending on the type of tumor. The treatment of choice is total removal of the tumor without residual neurologic damage. Patients with the most complete tumor removal have the greatest chance of survival. Several surgical advances have allowed the biopsy and removal of tumors in areas previously considered too dangerous for traditional operative techniques. Stereotactic surgery involves the use of CT and MRI in conjunction with other special computer techniques to reconstruct the tumor in three dimensions. With computer-assisted instruments, removal is sometimes possible. Stereotactic biopsy is performed with CT or MRI computer guidance for inserting the biopsy needle. This procedure has the benefit of a short hospital stay and a lower morbidity and mortality rate in comparison with an open craniotomy (Blaney, Haas-Kogan, Young-Pouissant, et al, 2011). Other procedures include the use of lasers to vaporize tumor tissue and brain mapping to determine the precise location of critical brain areas to avoid during surgery.

Radiotherapy is used to treat most tumors and to shrink the size of the tumor before attempting surgical removal. The use of chemotherapy has emerged in the past decades with an increasingly important role, either in combination with irradiation or alone. The drugs most commonly used are vincristine, cisplatin, carboplatin, cyclophosphamide, and etoposide (Strickler and Phillips, 2000). The problems of treatment are compounded by the serious late effects of all three modes of therapy. Surgery can cause injury to important areas of the brain, especially when the surgeon is attempting to remove invasive tumors. Irradiation has serious long-term consequences, which may include tissue necrosis, secondary malignancies, endocrine dysfunction, and behavioral or intellectual deficits. For these reasons, the use of irradiation is deferred for as long as possible in young children. Although there is limited information regarding a "safe age" for giving radiation, most centers consider it to be over age 3 years, but focal radiation is often given at a younger age (Mainprize, Taylor, and Rutka, 2000).

Nursing Care Management

Nursing care of the child with a brain tumor is similar regardless of the type of intracranial lesion. Because a brain tumor is potentially fatal, the reader is urged to incorporate the psychologic interventions discussed in Chapter 23 with those elaborated on in this section. However, remember that many brain tumors are curable. Medulloblastoma, for instance, has a survival rate of more than 80% in those patients without metastatic disease. Despite the grave nature of some brain tumors, it is important to realize the hope that new standard therapies and emerging therapies have brought to the families of many pediatric brain tumor patients.

Assess for Signs and Symptoms

A child admitted to the hospital with neurologic dysfunction is often suspected of having a brain tumor, even though the actual diagnosis is not yet confirmed. Establishing a baseline of data for comparing preoperative and postoperative changes is an essential step toward planning physical care and preventing complications. It also allows the nurse to assess the degree of physical incapacity and the family's emotional reaction to the diagnosis. For example, children with cerebellar astrocytoma may have displayed vague cerebellar symptoms for several years before a tumor is suspected. For these parents the revelation of a neoplasm may be more of a shock than for those who witnessed a rapid deterioration in their child's abilities. Table 36-4 summarizes common presenting signs and assessment procedures to document significant changes in the child's condition.

Prepare the Family for Diagnostic and Operative Procedures

The suspected diagnosis of a brain tumor is always a crisis. Despite the fact that some tumors are removed with excellent results, the physician can rarely give definitive answers regarding the prognosis until after surgery. Therefore parents and older children require much emotional support to face the diagnostic procedures and a craniotomy.

How the child is prepared for the diagnostic tests depends on the child's age and experience. Because most of the tests involve x-ray equipment, the child may be familiar with the procedure. Chapter 27 discusses preparing children for an MRI or a CT scan. Once surgery is scheduled, the child needs an explanation of what to expect. By the time most children are late preschoolers, they know that the head and brain are important parts of their body. It may be helpful to have children draw their concept of the brain to clarify misconceptions and base the explanation on their level of understanding. Although it may be tempting to justify the surgery by stating that removing the tumor will take away various symptoms, the nurse should refrain from emphasizing this point too strenuously. Postsurgical headaches and cerebellar symptoms, such as ataxia, may be aggravated rather than improved. Surgery may not improve vision. With optic gliomas the child will be blind in one eye if the tumor is fully resected. Finally, surgical removal of the mass may be impossible, and after surgery functioning may temporarily deteriorate or result in permanent damage. Being honest before surgery most often makes honesty after the procedure easier because no false hopes were created.

It is best to deliver information in small amounts to let the child pursue additional answers. For example, some children ask about what happens when part of the tumor is left. An honest reply is that after surgery the physician will try to shrink the tumor with special x rays and medicines. Delay a further explanation of irradiation or chemotherapy until a decision regarding these treatments is made.

The hair is usually shaved in the operating room just before surgery, or sometimes in the child's room, usually the night before surgery. When shaving is done with the child awake, the procedure is approached in a sensitive, positive way. If the child's hair is long, braid it so that the long swatch can be saved. Showing children how they look at different stages of the process helps them prepare for the final appearance.

Once the hair is clipped short or shaved, give the child a cap or scarf to camouflage the baldness. Take every precaution to provide privacy during the procedure and to protect the child from teasing or ridicule by other children before surgery. Also emphasize that the hair will regrow shortly after surgery. Depending on the child's immediate adjustment to the hair loss, the nurse may introduce the idea of wearing a wig until the hair grows in, particularly if additional irradiation or chemotherapy is anticipated.

Also tell children about the size of the dressing. Usually the entire scalp is covered to maintain tight wound closure, even if a small incision is made. Infratentorial head dressings may be attached to the upper back and extend forward to the neck to maintain slight extension and alignment as a precaution against wound rupture. Applying a similar dressing or "special hat" to a doll is often a less traumatic way of demonstrating the physical appearance.

Children also need a brief explanation of how they will feel after surgery and where they will be. Ordinarily they will return to a special intensive care unit, which they may visit beforehand depending on hospital policy. They should be aware that they may be sleepy for some time after surgery and that a headache is likely, although it should last only a few days.

Parents need similar explanations before surgery, especially in terms of special equipment used in the intensive care unit, dressings, and their child's behavior. For example, they should know that it is not unusual for the child to be lethargic for a few days after surgery. The nurse may wish to encourage less frequent visiting during this period so that parents can rest and be able to support their child when the child is awake.

The nurse should participate in preoperative conferences with the physician and parents. The nurse needs to know what information the parents have been given in order to provide further explanations or emotional support when necessary.

> **! NURSING ALERT**
>
> Report sluggish, dilated, or unequal pupils immediately because they may indicate increased ICP and potential brainstem herniation—a medical emergency.

Prevent Postoperative Complications

Usually the surgeon prescribes specific orders for taking vital signs, positioning, regulating fluids, and administering medication. These vary somewhat depending on the location of the craniotomy. The following are general principles of care for infratentorial or supratentorial surgery. Chapter 37 discusses additional aspects of care, such as care of the child with seizures and care of the unconscious child in terms of respiratory status and neurologic assessment.

Assessment

Vital signs are taken as often as every 15 to 30 minutes until the patient is stable. Temperature measurement is particularly important because of hyperthermia resulting from surgical intervention in the hypothalamus or brainstem and from some types of general anesthesia. To prepare for this reaction, a cooling blanket may be placed on the bed before the child returns to the unit, or it may be used when needed. Because the temperature control centers are affected and hypothermia can occur suddenly, the nurse monitors body temperature often when any cooling measures are employed.

> **! NURSING ALERT**
>
> To keep an accurate account of drainage, circle the soiled area with a pen every hour or so to identify continuous bleeding. The presence of colorless drainage is reported immediately because it most likely is cerebrospinal fluid leaking from the incisional area. A foul odor from the dressing may indicate an infection. Such a finding is reported, and a culture is taken.

The most likely types of infection are meningitis and respiratory tract infection. The probable cause of meningitis is wound contamination. The risk of respiratory tract infections is high because of the imposed immobility, danger of aspiration, and possible depression from the brainstem. The usual precautions of deep breathing and turning as allowed are instituted. Regular pulmonary assessments are performed to identify adventitious sounds or any areas of diminished or absent breath sounds. Blood pressure is also taken at frequent intervals. The deflated cuff is left on the arm between readings to allow for the least movement and disturbance of the child. Ocular signs are recorded at least every hour.

Observations for function are not instituted until the child regains consciousness. However, as soon as possible the nurse should begin testing reflexes, hand grip, and functioning of the cranial nerves. Muscle strength is usually less after surgery because of general weakness but should improve daily. Ataxia may be significantly worse with cerebellar intervention, but it slowly improves. Edema near the cranial nerves may depress important functions such as the gag, blink, or swallowing reflex.

Neurologic checks are an essential aspect of care and include pupillary reaction to light, level of consciousness, sleep patterns, and response to stimuli. Although children may be comatose for a few days, once they regain consciousness, there should be a steady increase in alertness. Regression to a lethargic, irritable state indicates increasing pressure, possibly caused by meningitis, hemorrhage, or edema.

Dressings are observed for evidence of drainage. If soiled, the dressing is not removed but reinforced with dry sterile gauze. The approximate amount of drainage is estimated and recorded.

Once the younger child is alert, the arms may need to be restrained to preserve the dressing. Even a child who has been cooperative before surgery must be closely supervised during the initial stages of regaining consciousness, when disorientation and restlessness are common. Elbow restraints are satisfactory to prevent the hands from reaching the head, although additional restraint may be necessary to preserve an infusion line and maintain a specific position.

Positioning

Correct positioning after surgery is critical to prevent pressure against the operative site, reduce ICP, and avoid the danger of aspiration. If a large tumor was removed, the child is not placed on the operative side, since the brain may suddenly shift to that cavity, causing trauma to the blood vessels, linings, and the brain itself. The nurse confers with the surgeon to be certain of the correct position, including the degree of neck flexion. The first 24 to 48 hours after brain surgery are critical. If positioning is restricted, notice of this is posted above the head of the bed. When the child is turned, every precaution is used to prevent jarring or misalignment to prevent undue strain on the sutures. Two nurses, one supporting the head and the other the body, are needed. The use of a turning sheet may facilitate turning a heavy child.

The child with an infratentorial procedure is usually positioned flat and on either side. Pillows should be placed against the child's back, not head, to maintain the desired position. Ordinarily the head and neck are kept in midline with the body and slightly extended. In a supratentorial craniotomy the head is usually elevated above the heart to facilitate cerebrospinal fluid drainage and decrease excessive blood flow to the brain to prevent hemorrhage.

Fluid Regulation

With an infratentorial craniotomy the child is allowed nothing by mouth for at least 24 hours or longer if the gag and swallowing reflexes are depressed or the child is comatose. With a supratentorial procedure, feeding may be resumed soon after the child is alert, sometimes within 24 hours. Clear water is always started first because of the danger of aspiration. If the child vomits, stop oral liquids. Vomiting not only predisposes the child to aspiration, but also increases ICP and the risk for incisional rupture.

IV fluids are continued until fluids are well tolerated. Because of the cerebral edema postoperatively and the danger of increased ICP, fluids are carefully monitored and usually infused at one half the maintenance rate. If drugs, such as prophylactic antibiotics, are given intravenously, the medication amount is calculated as part of the IV fluid. For example, if the child is to receive 20 ml/hr and the diluted drug is 5 ml, the IV solution is reduced to 15 ml for that hour.

A hypertonic solution such as mannitol or dextrose may be necessary to remove excess fluid. These drugs cause rapid diuresis. After surgery the child may have a Foley catheter in place. Urinary output is monitored after administration of these drugs to evaluate their effectiveness.

When able to take fluids, the child should be fed to conserve strength and minimize movement. If there is any sign of facial paralysis, the child is fed slowly to prevent choking or aspiration. Scrupulous mouth care is essential to prevent oral infection. Sometimes gavage feeding is necessary when body functions are too depressed to permit safe oral feedings or the child refuses to eat or drink. In the latter instance the nurse should employ every measure to encourage acceptance of fluids or solids. (See Chapter 27 for nursing interventions.)

Comfort Measures

Headache may be severe and is largely the result of cerebral edema. Measures to relieve some of the discomfort include providing a quiet, dimly lit environment; restricting visitors; preventing any sudden jarring movement, such as banging into the bed; and preventing an increase in ICP. The last is most effectively achieved by proper positioning and prevention of straining, such as during coughing, vomiting, or defecating. Placing an ice bag on the forehead may also provide some headache relief, especially if facial edema is severe. The use of opioids, such as morphine, to relieve pain is controversial because it is thought that they may mask signs of altered consciousness or depress respirations. However, they can be given safely because naloxone can be used to reverse opioid effects, such as sedation or respiratory depression. Acetaminophen and codeine are also effective analgesics. Regardless of the drugs used, adequate dosage and regular administration are essential to provide optimum pain relief. (See Pain Assessment and Pain Management, Chapter 7.)

Monitor bowel movements to prevent constipation. Stool softeners may be given as soon as liquids are tolerated to facilitate easy passage of stool.

Brain edema may severely depress the gag reflex, necessitating suctioning of oral secretions. Facial edema may also be present, necessitating eye care if the lids remain partially open. Ice compresses applied to the eyes for short periods help relieve the edema. A depressed blink reflex also predisposes the corneas to ulceration. Irrigating the eyes with saline drops and covering them with eye dressings are important steps in preventing this complication.

Support the Family

The family's emotional needs are great when the diagnosis is a brain tumor, and the extent of surgery, any neurologic deficits, the prognosis, and additional therapy influence these feelings. Because few definitive answers can be given before surgery, the surgeon's report is a significant finding that can vary from a completely benign, resected neoplasm to a highly malignant, invasive, and only partially removed tumor. Although parents try to prepare themselves for a potentially fatal diagnosis, it is understandably a shock for them.

Ideally, a nurse who will be involved in the continuing care of this child should be with the family when the physician discusses the prognosis and plan of therapy. Although parents may hear only a fraction of what they are told, they can begin to put the future into perspective. Regardless of the future prospects, direct the parents' thinking toward helping the child recover and resume a normal life to his or her fullest potential. Providing the opportunity for the family to share their concerns and questions with other families who have a child with a brain tumor may help the family cope.*

It is also a time to encourage parents to verbalize their feelings about the diagnosis. Often they express guilt for attributing the insidious onset of symptoms, such as ataxia, visual difficulty, or headache, to minor "complaints" by the child. Parents may have punished their child for clumsiness, mistaking it for carelessness, or for their declining performance in school. The nurse listens to such statements, emphasizing the normalcy of the parents' reactions. Sometimes it may be helpful to start a discussion with a statement such as "It is difficult to know when a child's complaints are significant because so often they are caused by minor ailments and you would never have imagined they were a result of a brain tumor." The nurse avoids any comments that insinuate the parents should have sought medical advice sooner, since such remarks only add to the parents' guilt feelings.

---

*Information about support groups is available from the National Brain Tumor Society, 22 Battery St., Suite 612, San Francisco, CA 94111; 800-934-CURE, 415-834-9970; e-mail: info@braintumor.org; www.braintumor.org.

During this period the nurse should also discuss with parents what they plan to tell the child. If the child was prepared honestly, as described previously, the diagnosis can be expressed in a similar manner, such as "The surgeon removed most of the tumor, and the rest will be treated with special drugs and x-ray treatments." During recovery the child needs additional explanation about the treatment and the reason for residual neurologic effects, such as ataxia or blindness. Because the hair was shaved before surgery, hair loss from treatment is less of a concern, although its regrowth will be delayed, depending on the length of therapy. At this point it is advisable to reintroduce the idea of a wig.

Promote Return to Optimum Functioning

The ultimate goal is a cured child who has optimum functioning. As soon as possible, the child should resume usual activities within tolerable limits, especially returning to school.* Until the skull is completely healed, the child may need to wear a helmet when engaging in any active sport. This decision is made by the child's neurosurgeon. The school nurse and teacher should confer with the parents on activity restrictions, such as physical education, and the reactions of schoolmates to the child's appearance.

After discharge the family needs continuing medical and emotional support from health personnel. Even with children who are long-term survivors after treatment for a brain tumor, residual disabilities, such as growth retardation, cranial nerve palsies, sensory defects, motor abnormalities (especially ataxia), intellectual deficits, dysphagia, dysgraphia, and behavioral problems, may occur (Blaney, Haas-Kogan, Young-Pouissant, et al, 2011; Loring and Meador, 2000; Riva and Giorgi, 2000). It is difficult to assess the exact cause of the nonphysical disabilities, since numerous variables influence the child's total rehabilitation. However, the high frequency of late effects attests to the tremendous need for follow-up care despite successful treatment of the tumor.

The vast realm of possible consequences after the diagnosis of a brain tumor is not discussed here. Rather, the reader is referred to other sections of the text that deal with possible outcomes, such as the paralyzed, visually impaired, or unconscious child or the child with a ventricular shunt, seizure disorder, or meningitis. Numerous physical problems can occur with progression of the tumor that may necessitate additional procedures. For example, frequent vomiting, anorexia, and nausea may require nonoral routes of feeding, such as gastrostomy or parenteral alimentation. Trials with chemotherapy may necessitate the use of central venous access devices. Whenever these procedures are instituted, the nurse may be responsible for teaching the family appropriate home care to allow the child the highest quality of life for the longest time. (See discussion of discharge planning and home care in Chapter 25 and Nursing Care Plan: The Child with a Brain Tumor.†)

---

*Excellent publications, including the pamphlet, *When Your Child Is Ready to Return to School*, are available from the American Brain Tumor Association, 2720 River Road, Des Plaines, IL 60018; 847-827-9910; fax: 847- 827-9918; e-mail: info@abta.org; www.abta.org.

†In Wilson D, Hockenberry MJ: *Wong's clinical manual of pediatric nursing*, ed 7, St Louis, 2008, Mosby.

NEUROBLASTOMA

Neuroblastoma is the most common extracranial solid tumor of childhood and the most common cancer diagnosed in infancy. It occurs in about 1 in 7000 live births. The median age at diagnosis is 19 months, and it is slightly more prevalent in males. These tumors originate from embryonic neural crest cells that normally give rise to the adrenal medulla and the sympathetic nervous system. Consequently the majority of the tumors arise from the adrenal gland or from the retroperitoneal sympathetic chain. The primary site is within the abdomen; other sites include the head and neck region, chest, and pelvis.

Clinical Manifestations

The signs and symptoms of neuroblastoma depend on the location and stage of the disease. With abdominal tumors, the most common presenting sign is a firm, nontender, irregular mass in the abdomen that crosses the midline (in contrast to Wilms tumor, which is usually confined to one side). Compression of the kidney, ureter, or bladder may cause urinary frequency or retention.

Distant metastasis frequently causes supraorbital ecchymosis, periorbital edema, and proptosis (exophthalmos) from invasion of retrobulbar soft tissue. Lymphadenopathy, hepatomegaly and skeletal pain are also present in patients with disseminated disease. Vague symptoms of widespread metastasis include pallor, weakness, irritability, anorexia, and weight loss.

Other primary tumor sites may cause significant clinical effects such as neurologic impairment, respiratory obstruction from a thoracic mass, or varying degrees of paralysis from compression of the spinal cord. Infrequently a child may have symptoms of increased catecholamine excretion, such as flushing, hypertension, tachycardia, and diaphoresis (Weinstein, Katenstein, and Cohn, 2003).

Diagnostic Evaluation

Diagnostic evaluation is aimed at locating the primary site and areas of metastasis. A CT of the abdomen, pelvis, or chest is the preferred imaging modality to locate the primary tumor. A bone scan and MIBG (iodine-131 metaiodobenzylguanidine) scan should be performed to evaluate for the presence of skeletal metastases. Examination of the bone marrow with bilateral aspirates and biopsies should be performed in all patients. Neuroblastomas, particularly those arising on the adrenal glands or from a sympathetic chain, excrete the catecholamines epinephrine and norepinephrine. Urinary excretion of catecholamines is detected in approximately 95% of children with adrenal or sympathetic tumors. Analyzing the breakdown products that are normally excreted in the urine, namely, vanillylmandelic acid, homovanillic acid, dopamine, and norepinephrine, permits detection of a suspected tumor both before and after medical-surgical intervention. Amplification of the *N-myc* gene and abnormalities in chromosomes have been associated with a poorer prognosis (Grosfeld, 2000; Lau, Tai, Weitzman, et al, 2004). Increased ferritin and neuron-specific enolase are also seen in neuroblastoma.

BOX 36-5   STAGING OF NEUROBLASTOMA

Stage I—Localized tumor with complete gross excision, with or without microscopic residual disease; representative ipsilateral lymph nodes negative for tumor microscopically (nodes that are attached to and removed with the primary tumor may be positive)

Stage II-A—Localized tumor with incomplete gross resection; representative ipsilateral nonadherent lymph nodes negative for tumor microscopically

Stage II-B—Localized tumor with or without complete gross excision, with ipsilateral nonadherent lymph nodes positive for tumor; enlarged contralateral lymph nodes must be negative microscopically

Stage III—Unresectable unilateral tumor infiltrating across the midline, with or without regional lymph node involvement; or localized unilateral tumor with contralateral regional lymph node involvement; or midline tumor with bilateral extension by infiltration (unresectable) or by lymph node involvement

Stage IV—Dissemination of tumor to distant lymph nodes, bone, bone marrow, liver, skin and/or other organs

Stage IV-S—Localized primary tumor (as defined for stage I, II-A or II-B) with dissemination limited to liver, skin, or bone marrow but not to bone

Staging and Prognosis

Neuroblastoma is a "silent" tumor. In more than 70% of cases, diagnosis is made after metastasis occurs, with the first signs caused by involvement in the nonprimary site, usually the lymph nodes, bone marrow, skeletal system, skin, or liver. Because of the frequency of invasiveness, the prognosis for neuroblastoma is generally poor.

The child's age and the stage of the disease (Box 36-5) at diagnosis are important prognostic factors. Survival is inversely correlated with age. If all stages are grouped together, the survival rates are 75% for children under 1 year of age and less than 50% for children over 1 year of age. This marked difference in survival rates by age is partly accounted for by the larger proportion of very young children with stage I, II, or IV-S disease and the absence of the *N-myc* gene amplification (Brodeur, Hogarty, Mosse, et al, 2011).

Infants who remain free of disease for 1 year after treatment are usually cured, but older children have experienced relapses several years after cessation of treatment. Surgical resection of the tumor in stage I infants diagnosed by ultrasonography done for other reasons appears to be almost 90% curative (Grosfeld, 2000). Neuroblastoma is one of the few tumors that demonstrate spontaneous regression (especially stage IV-S), possibly as a result of maturity of the embryonic cell or development of an active immune system.

Therapeutic Management

Accurate clinical staging is important for establishing initial treatment. Therefore the purpose of surgery is both to remove as much of the tumor as possible and to obtain biopsies. In stages I and II, complete surgical removal of the tumor is the treatment of choice. If the tumors are large, partial resection is attempted, with a course of irradiation postoperatively to shrink the tumor in the hope of complete removal at a later date. Surgery is usually limited to biopsy in stages III and IV because of the extensive metastasis, although additional surgery to assess tumor regression or remove a regressed tumor is not unlikely.

The precise role of radiotherapy is unclear. It does not appear to be of any benefit in children with stage I and II disease. It is commonly used with stage III disease, although it may not improve survival expectancy. It may make a large tumor operable. Radiotherapy provides emergency management of a massive neuroblastoma causing spinal cord compression (Nguyen, Sallah, Ludin, et al, 2000). It also offers palliation for metastatic lesions in bones, lungs, liver, or brain.

Chemotherapy is the mainstay of therapy for extensive local or disseminated disease. The drugs of choice are vincristine, doxorubicin, cyclophosphamide, cisplatin, etoposide, ifosfamide, and carboplatin; they are administered in a variety of combinations according to specific protocols. In addition, the use of consolidative myeloablative therapy using autologous marrow or peripheral stem cells followed by 13-*cis*-retinoic acid has improved the outcome of patients with high-risk disease.

Nursing Care Management

Nursing care management is similar to that discussed under Nursing Care of the Child with Cancer, including psychologic and physical preparation for diagnostic and operative procedures; prevention of postoperative complications for abdominal, thoracic, or cranial surgery; and explanation of chemotherapy and radiotherapy and their side effects (see Tables 36-2 and 36-3).

Because this tumor carries a poor prognosis for many children, evaluate and address the needs of the family in terms of coping with a life-threatening illness. (See Chapter 23.) Because of the high degree of metastasis at the time of diagnosis, many parents suffer guilt for not having recognized signs earlier. Often the guilt is expressed as anger toward professionals for not diagnosing it sooner. Parents need much support in dealing with these feelings and expressing them to the appropriate people.

BONE TUMORS

GENERAL CONSIDERATIONS

Bone tumors account for about 6% of all malignant neoplasms in children. Approximately 90% of all primary malignant bone tumors in children are either osteogenic sarcoma or Ewing sarcoma; osteosarcoma, the most common, occurs in 56% of all cases. The peak age for pediatric bone tumors is 15 years, and they occur more often in males.

Clinical Manifestations

Most malignant bone tumors produce localized pain in the affected site, which may be severe or dull and may be attributed to trauma or the vague complaint of "growing pains." The pain is often relieved by a flexed position, which relaxes the muscles overlying the stretched periosteum. Frequently it draws attention when the child limps, curtails physical activity, or is unable to hold heavy objects. A palpable mass is also a common manifestation of bone tumors, but systemic symptoms such as fever and other clinical symptoms such as spinal cord compression and respiratory distress are more frequent in patients with Ewing sarcoma.

Diagnostic Evaluation

Diagnosis begins with a thorough history and physical examination. A primary objective is to rule out causes such as trauma or infection. Careful questioning regarding pain is essential in attempting to determine the duration and rate of tumor growth. Physical assessment focuses on functional status of the affected area; signs of inflammation; size of the mass; and any systemic indication of generalized malignancy, such as anemia, weight loss, and frequent infection.

Definitive diagnosis is based on radiologic studies, such as plain films and CT or MRI of the primary site, CT of the chest, and radioisotope bone scans to evaluate metastasis and bone marrow examination in patients with Ewing sarcoma. A needle or surgical biopsy is necessary to establish the diagnosis. Ewing sarcoma most commonly involves the pelvis, long bones of the lower extremities, and chest wall and radiographically involves the diaphysis with detachment of the periosteum from the bone (Codman triangle). In osteosarcoma, lesions are most commonly located in the metaphyseal region of the bone, often involving the long bones. Radial ossification in the soft tissue gives the tumor a "sunburst" appearance on plain radiograph.

Prognosis

A better understanding of the biology of neoplastic growth has resulted in more aggressive treatment and an improved prognosis. The natural history of osteogenic sarcoma and Ewing sarcoma suggests that multiple submicroscopic foci of metastatic disease are present at the time of diagnosis despite clinical evidence of localized involvement. Before the use of aggressive multimodal therapy, pulmonary metastasis appeared in the majority of patients who were treated with surgical excision alone (Gorlick, Bielack, Teot, et al, 2011). With current therapies that include surgery and chemotherapy for osteosarcoma and surgery, radiotherapy, and chemotherapy for Ewing sarcoma, more than two thirds of patients with localized disease can be cured.

OSTEOSARCOMA

Osteosarcoma (osteogenic sarcoma) is the most common bone cancer in children and most commonly affects patients in the second decade of life during their growth spurt. It presumably arises from bone-forming mesenchyme, which gives rise to malignant osteoid tissue. Most primary tumor sites are in the diametaphyseal region (wider part of the shaft, adjacent to the epiphyseal growth plate) of long bones, especially in the lower extremities. More than half occur in the femur, particularly the distal portion, with the rest involving the humerus, tibia, pelvis, jaw, and phalanges.

Therapeutic Management

Optimum treatment of osteosarcoma includes surgery and chemotherapy. The surgical approach consists of surgical biopsy followed by either limb salvage or amputation. To ensure local control, all gross and microscopic tumors must be resected. A limb salvage procedure involves en bloc resection of the primary tumor with prosthetic replacement of the involved bone. For example, with osteosarcoma of the distal femur, a total femur and joint replacement is performed. Frequently children undergoing a limb salvage procedure receive preoperative chemotherapy in an attempt to decrease the tumor size and make surgery more manageable (Lanzkowsky, 2005; Gorlick, Bielack, Teot, et al, 2011).

Chemotherapy plays a vital role in treatment of osteosarcoma. Antineoplastic drugs, such as high-dose methotrexate with citrovorum factor rescue, doxorubicin, cisplatin, ifosfamide, and etoposide, may be administered singly or in combination and may be employed both before or after surgical resection of the tumor. The use of postoperative chemotherapy after amputation has comparable results to trials using preoperative chemotherapy followed by limb salvage surgery. Preoperative chemotherapy allows for examination of the surgical specimen at the time of definitive surgery, which predicts clinical outcome. When pulmonary metastases are found, thoracotomy and chemotherapy have resulted in prolonged survival and potential cure. These combined-modality approaches have significantly improved the prognosis in osteosarcoma to approximately 78% for nonmetastatic patients (Lanzkowsky, 2005). Newer trials have recently been completed and have incorporated muramyl tripeptide phosphatidylethanolamine to eradicate micrometastases by stimulating macrophages to kill tumor cells not eliminated by chemotherapy (Lanzkowsky, 2005).

Nursing Care Management

Nursing care depends on the type of surgical approach. Obviously the family may have more difficulty adjusting to an amputation than a limb salvage procedure. In either instance, preparation of the child and family is critical. Straightforward honesty is essential in gaining the child's cooperation and trust. The diagnosis of cancer should not be disguised with falsehoods such as "infection." To accept the need for radical surgery, the child must be aware of the lack of alternatives for treatment. Although the responsibility of telling the child is generally left to the physician, the nurse should be present at the discussion or be aware of exactly what is said. The child should be told a few days before surgery to allow him or her time to think about the diagnosis and consequent treatment and to ask questions. (See Nursing Care Plan: The Child with a Bone Tumor.*)

Sometimes children have many questions about the prosthesis, limitations on physical ability, and prognosis in terms of cure. At other times they react with silence or with a calm manner that belies their concern and fear. Either response must be accepted, since it is part of the grieving process of a loss. For those who desire information, it may be helpful to introduce them to another amputee before surgery or to show them pictures of the prosthesis.† However, the nurse must be careful not to overwhelm children with information. A sound approach is to answer questions without offering additional information. For those who do not pursue additional information, the nurse expresses a willingness to talk.

---

*In Wilson D, Hockenberry MJ: *Wong's clinical manual of pediatric nursing*, ed 7, St Louis, 2008, Mosby.
†Information about prostheses can be obtained from the National Amputation Foundation, 40 Church St., Malverne, NY 11565; 516-887-3600; www.nationalamputation.org.

The child is also informed of the need for chemotherapy and its side effects before surgery. Exercise caution about offering too much information at one time. When discussing hair loss, emphasize positive aspects, such as wearing a wig. Because bone tumors affect adolescents and young adults, it is not unusual for them to become angry over all the radical body alterations.

If an amputation is performed, the child is usually fitted with a temporary prosthesis immediately after surgery, which permits early functioning and fosters psychologic adjustment. If this is not done, the child requires stump care, which is the same as for any amputee. A permanent prosthesis is usually fitted within 6 to 8 weeks. During hospitalization the child begins physical therapy to become proficient in the use and care of the device.

Phantom limb pain may develop after amputation. This symptom is characterized by sensations such as tingling, itching, and, more frequently, pain felt in the amputated limb. The child and family need to know that the sensations are real, not imagined. Amitriptyline (Elavil) has been used successfully in children to decrease the pain (Olsson, 1999). In addition, an epidural is often used preoperatively as a nerve block in an effort to decrease or eliminate the occurrence of phantom limb pain. Much research is needed to further delineate the best care for these patients (Ong, Arneja, and Ong, 2006).

Discharge planning must begin early in the postoperative period. Once the child has begun physical therapy, the nurse should consult with the therapist and practitioner to evaluate the child's physical and emotional readiness to reenter school. It is an opportune time to involve a community nurse in the child's home care. Every effort is made to promote normalcy and gradual resumption of realistic preamputation activities.* Role-playing in anticipation of such experiences is beneficial in preparing the child for the inevitable confrontation by others. Environmental barriers, such as stairs, are assessed in terms of the accessibility in the school and home, especially because the child may need to use crutches or a wheelchair before complete healing and prosthetic competency are achieved.

The nurse encourages the child to select clothing that best camouflages the prosthesis, such as pants or long-sleeved shirts. Well-fitted prostheses are so natural looking that girls can usually wear sheer stockings without revealing the device. Emphasizing feminine or masculine apparel helps the child regain a feeling of self-identity. Even during the postoperative period, encouraging the child to wear blue jeans and a T-shirt may distract attention from the deformity and focus it on familiar aspects of appearance.

The family and child need much support in adjusting not only to a life-threatening diagnosis but also to alteration in body form and function. Because loss of a limb entails a grieving process, those caring for the child need to recognize that the reactions of anger and depression are normal and necessary. Often parents view the anger as a direct affront to them for allowing the amputation to occur, or they see the depression as

rejection. These are not personal attacks but the child's attempts to cope with a loss.

EWING SARCOMA (PRIMITIVE NEUROECTODERMAL TUMOR OF THE BONE)

Ewing sarcomas, or the Ewing sarcoma family of tumors which includes primitive neuroectodermal tumor of the bone, are the second most common malignant bone tumor (after osteosarcoma) in childhood (Lanzkowsky, 2005). Ewing sarcoma arises in the marrow spaces of the bone rather than from osseous tissue. The tumor originates in the shaft of long and trunk bones, most often affecting the pelvis, femur, tibia, fibula, humerus, ulna, vertebra, scapula, ribs, and skull. It occurs almost exclusively in individuals under age 30 and affects Caucasians much more often than other races.

Therapeutic Management

Limb salvage procedures might be feasible in extremity lesions, and amputation may be considered if the results of radiotherapy render the extremity useless or deformed (e.g., from retarded growth in young children). The treatment of choice for the majority of lesions is involved field radiotherapy and chemotherapy. A widely used drug regimen includes vincristine, doxorubicin, cyclophosphamide alternating with ifosfamide, and etoposide. The addition of ifosfamide and etoposide has increased the 3-year survival to 78% for patients with localized disease (Lanzkowsky, 2005).

Nursing Care Management

The psychologic adjustment to Ewing sarcoma is typically less traumatic than it is to osteosarcoma because of the preservation of the affected limb. Many families accept the diagnosis with a sense of relief in knowing that this type of bone cancer does not necessitate amputation, and initially they may not be aware of the damaging effects on the irradiated site. Consequently they need preparation for the various diagnostic tests, including bone marrow aspiration and surgical biopsy, and adequate explanation of the treatment regimen. High-dose radiotherapy often causes a skin reaction of dry or moist desquamation followed by hyperpigmentation. The child should wear loose-fitting clothes over the irradiated area to minimize additional skin irritation. Because of increased sensitivity, protect the area from sunlight and sudden changes in temperature, such as from heating pads or ice packs. Encourage the child to use the extremity as tolerated. Occasionally the physical therapist may plan an active exercise program to preserve maximum function.

The child needs the same considerations for adjusting to the effects of chemotherapy as any other patient with cancer. The drug regimen usually results in hair loss, severe nausea and vomiting, peripheral neuropathy, and possibly cardiotoxicity. Make every effort to outline a treatment plan that allows the child maximum resumption of a normal lifestyle and activities. (See Nursing Care Plan: The Child with a Bone Tumor.†)

---

*Information about special programs for children with amputations is available from the American Childhood Cancer Organization (see footnote, p. 1480).

†In Wilson D, Hockenberry MJ: *Wong's clinical manual of pediatric nursing*, ed 7, St Louis, 2008, Mosby.

OTHER SOLID TUMORS

In addition to the cancers already discussed, several other types of solid tumors may occur in children. Wilms tumor, rhabdomyosarcoma, and retinoblastoma are unique in that they tend to be diagnosed early, typically before 5 years of age. Wilms tumor and retinoblastoma are also unusual in that they are among the few types of cancer that may occur in both hereditary and nonhereditary forms.

WILMS TUMOR

Wilms tumor, or nephroblastoma, is the most common kidney tumor of childhood (Skoldenberg, Christiansson, Sandstedt, et al, 2001). Its frequency is estimated to be 8 cases per 1 million children less than 15 years of age (Lanzkowsky, 2005). Eighty percent of patients with Wilms tumor are diagnosed under 5 years of age, and it has a peak incidence between 3 and 4 years of age (Lanzkowsky, 2005). Wilms tumor may be associated with several congenital malformation syndromes, including WAGR (Wilms tumor, aniridia, genitourinary anomalies, and cognitive impairment [mental retardation]) and Beckwith-Wiedemann syndrome (hemihypertrophy, macroglossia, omphalocele, and visceromegaly) (Lanzkowsky, 2005). About 2% of Wilms tumors are familial.

Clinical Manifestations

The most common presenting sign is painless swelling or mass within the abdomen. The mass is characteristically firm, nontender, confined to one side, and deep within the flank. If it is on the right side, it may be difficult to distinguish from the liver, although, unlike that organ, it does not move with respiration. Parents usually discover the mass during routine bathing or dressing of the child.

Other clinical manifestations are the result of compression from the tumor mass, metabolic alterations secondary to the tumor, or metastasis. Hematuria occurs in less than one fourth of children with Wilms tumor. Anemia, usually secondary to hemorrhage within the tumor, results in pallor, anorexia, and lethargy. Hypertension, probably caused by secretion of excess amounts of renin by the tumor, occurs occasionally. Other effects of malignancy include weight loss and fever. If metastasis has occurred, symptoms of lung involvement, such as dyspnea, cough, shortness of breath, and pain in the chest, may be evident.

Diagnostic Evaluation

In a child suspected of having Wilms tumor, special emphasis is placed on the history and physical examination for the presence of congenital anomalies; a family history of cancer; and signs of malignancy, such as weight loss, enlarged liver and spleen, indications of anemia, and lymphadenopathy. Specific tests include radiographic studies, such as abdominal ultrasound, CT, and MRI of the abdomen; CT of the chest to look for metastases in the lung; and Doppler ultrasound of the inferior vena cava. Laboratory studies should include a complete blood count (polycythemia is sometimes present if the tumor secretes excess erythropoietin), biochemical studies, and urinalysis. Studies to demonstrate the relationship of the tumor to the ipsilateral kidney and the presence of a normally functioning kidney on the contralateral side are essential.

BOX 36-6	STAGING OF WILMS TUMOR

Stage I—Tumor is limited to kidney and completely resected.
Stage II—Tumor extends beyond kidney but is completely resected.
Stage III—Residual nonhematogenous tumor is confined to abdomen.
Stage IV—Hematogenous metastases; deposits are beyond stage III, namely, to lung, liver, bone, and brain.
Stage V—Bilateral renal involvement is present at diagnosis.

Staging and Prognosis

Wilms tumor probably arises from a malignant, undifferentiated metanephrogenic blastoma (a cluster of primordial cells capable of initiating the regeneration of an abnormal structure). Its occurrence slightly favors the left kidney, which is advantageous because surgically this kidney is easier to manipulate and remove. Although the tumor may become large, it remains encapsulated for an extended period. During surgery the tumor is staged to maximize the effectiveness of treatment protocols (Box 36-6).

The histology of the tumor cells is also identified and classified according to two groups: favorable histology (FH) and unfavorable histology (UH). Only about 12% of Wilms tumors demonstrate UH, which is associated with a poorer prognosis and demands a more aggressive treatment protocol, regardless of the clinical stage.

Survival rates for Wilms tumor are one of the highest among all childhood cancers. Children with localized tumor (stages I and II) have a 90% chance of cure with multimodal therapy. For those children who relapse, a better expectancy of disease-free survival is associated with FH of the tumor, more than 12 months elapsing from the first complete remission, and nonabdominal recurrence (Dome, Liu, Krasin, et al, 2002; Plesko, Kramarova, Stiller, et al, 2001).

Therapeutic Management

Combined treatment with surgery and chemotherapy, with or without irradiation, is based on the clinical stage and histologic pattern. In unilateral disease a large transabdominal incision is performed for optimum visualization of the abdominal cavity. The tumor, affected kidney, and adjacent adrenal gland are removed. Great care is taken to keep the encapsulated tumor intact because rupture can seed cancer cells throughout the abdomen, lymph channel, and bloodstream. The contralateral kidney is carefully inspected for evidence of disease or dysfunction. Regional lymph nodes are inspected, and a biopsy is performed when indicated. Any involved structures, such as part of the colon, diaphragm, or vena cava, are removed. Metal clips are placed around the tumor site for exact marking during radiotherapy.

If both kidneys are involved, the child may be treated with radiotherapy or chemotherapy preoperatively to shrink the tumor, allowing more conservative therapy (Graf, Tournade, and deKraker, 2000; Lanzkowsky, 2005). In some cases a partial nephrectomy is performed on the less affected kidney, with a total nephrectomy performed on the opposite side. When a transplant is feasible, such as from a twin, sibling, or parent, bilateral nephrectomy is considered as a last resort.

Postoperative radiotherapy is indicated for children with large tumors, metastasis, residual disease at the primary tumor site, UH, or recurrence. Chemotherapy is indicated for all stages. The most effective agents for treating Wilms tumor are actinomycin D and vincristine; doxorubicin and cyclophosphamide may be used for UH or advanced-stage disease (Fernandez, Geller, Ehrlich, et al, 2011; Lanzkowsky, 2005). The duration of therapy ranges from 6 to 15 months.

Nursing Care Management

The nursing care of the child with Wilms tumor is similar to that of other cancers treated with surgery, irradiation, and chemotherapy. However, some significant differences are discussed for each phase of nursing intervention.

Preoperative Care

As with many of the other cancers, the diagnosis of Wilms tumor is a shock. Frequently the child has no physical indication of the seriousness of the disorder other than a palpable abdominal mass. Because the parents usually discover the mass, the nurse needs to take into account their feelings regarding the diagnosis. Whereas some parents are grateful for their detection of the tumor, others feel guilty for not finding it sooner or anger toward the practitioner for missing it on earlier examinations.

The preoperative period is one of swift diagnosis. Typically, surgery is scheduled within 24 to 48 hours of admission. The nurse is faced with the challenge of preparing the child and parents for all laboratory and operative procedures. Because of the little time available, keep explanations simple and repeat them often with attention to what the child will experience. In addition to usual preoperative observations, monitor blood pressure, since hypertension from excess renin production is a possibility.

There are several special preoperative concerns, the most important of which is to not palpate the tumor unless absolutely necessary because manipulation of the mass may cause dissemination of cancer cells to adjacent and distant sites.

> **! NURSING ALERT**
>
> To reinforce the need for caution, it may be necessary to post a sign on the bed that reads "Do not palpate abdomen." Careful bathing and handling are also important in preventing trauma to the tumor site.

Because radiotherapy and chemotherapy are usually begun immediately after surgery, parents need an explanation of what to expect, such as major benefits and side effects, although the timing of the information should be considered to avoid overwhelming the family. Ideally the nurse should be present during physician-parent conferences to answer questions as they arise.

Postoperative Care

Despite the extensive surgical intervention necessary in many children with Wilms tumor, the recovery period is usually rapid. The major nursing responsibilities are those following any abdominal surgery. (See Nursing Care Plan: The Child Undergoing Surgery, on the Evolve website.) Because these children are at risk for intestinal obstruction from vincristine-induced adynamic ileus, radiation-induced edema, and postsurgical adhesion formation, the nurse monitors gastrointestinal activity, such as bowel movements, bowel sounds, distention, and vomiting. Other considerations are frequent evaluation of blood pressure and observation for signs of infection, especially during chemotherapy. Because of the myelosuppression from the drugs, institute pulmonary hygiene measures in the immediate postoperative period to prevent complications.

Support the Family

The postoperative period is frequently difficult for parents. The shock of seeing their child immediately after surgery may be the first realization of the seriousness of the diagnosis. From surgery, the stage and pathology of the tumor is determined. The physician discusses this information with the parents. The nurse's presence during this conversation is important to provide additional support and assess the parents' understanding of this information.

Older children need an opportunity to deal with their feelings concerning the many procedures to which they have been subjected in rapid succession. Therapeutic play can be beneficial in helping children of any age understand what they have undergone and express their feelings.

RHABDOMYOSARCOMA

Rhabdomyosarcoma (*rhabdo*, striated) is the most common soft tissue sarcoma in children. Striated (skeletal) muscle is found almost anywhere in the body, so these tumors occur in many sites, the most common of which are the head and neck, especially the orbit. The disease occurs in children in all age-groups but is most common in children younger than 5 years of age. Its incidence is approximately 8.5 per 1 million for Caucasian children but only 4.0 per 1 million for African-American children in the age-group from 2 to 19 years (Lanzkowsky, 2005).

Rhabdomyosarcoma arises from embryonic mesenchyme. Three subtypes are recognized (Box 36-7). Soft tissue sarcomas are the fourth most common type of solid tumors in children. These malignant neoplasms originate from undifferentiated mesenchymal cells in muscles, tendons, bursae, and fascia, or in fibrous, connective, lymphatic, or vascular tissue. They derive their name from the specific tissue(s) of origin, such as myosarcoma (*myo*, muscle).

> **BOX 36-7 SUBTYPES OF RHABDOMYOSARCOMA**
>
> **Embryonal**—Most common type; most frequently found in the head, neck, abdomen, and genitourinary tract
> **Alveolar**—Second most common type; most often seen in deep tissues of the extremities and trunk
> **Pleomorphic**—Rare in children (adult form); most often occurs in soft parts of extremities and trunk

TABLE 36-5	CLINICAL MANIFESTATIONS OF RHABDOMYOSARCOMA ACCORDING TO TUMOR SITE
LOCATION	**SIGNS AND SYMPTOMS**
Orbit	Rapidly developing unilateral proptosis
	Ecchymosis of conjunctiva
	Loss of extraocular movements (strabismus)
Nasopharynx	Stuffy nose (earliest sign)
	Nasal obstruction—dysphagia, nasal voice (obstruction of posterior nasal conches), serous otitis media (obstruction of eustachian tube)
	Pain (sore throat and ear)
	Epistaxis
	Palpable neck nodes
	Visible mass in oropharynx (late sign)
Paranasal sinuses	Nasal obstruction
	Local pain
	Discharge
	Sinusitis
	Swelling
Middle ear	Signs of chronic serous otitis media
	Pain
	Sanguinopurulent drainage
	Facial nerve palsy
Retroperitoneal area (usually a "silent" tumor)	Abdominal mass
	Pain
	Signs of intestinal or genitourinary obstruction
Perineum	Visible superficial mass
	Bowel or bladder dysfunction (from tumor compression)

Clinical Manifestations

The initial signs and symptoms are related to the site of the tumor and compression of adjacent organs (Table 36-5). Some tumor locations, such as the orbit, manifest early in the course of the illness. Other tumors, such as those of the retroperitoneal area, only produce symptoms when they are relatively big and compress adjacent organs. Unfortunately, many of the signs and symptoms attributable to rhabdomyosarcoma are vague and frequently suggest a common childhood illness, such as "earache" or "runny nose." Rarely, the site of the primary tumor site is never identified.

Diagnostic Evaluation

Diagnosis begins with a careful history and physical examination. Radiographic studies to delineate the primary tumor site should include CT or MRI. Metastatic evaluation should include a CT of the chest, bone scan, and bilateral bone marrow aspirates and biopsies. For patients with tumors in the parameningeal area, perform an LP to examine the spinal fluid. An excisional biopsy or surgical resection of the tumor, when possible, is done to confirm the diagnosis.

Staging and Prognosis

Careful staging is extremely important for planning treatment and determining the prognosis. The Intergroup Rhabdomyosarcoma Study has developed a surgicopathologic staging system, shown in Box 36-8 (Lanzkowsky, 2005; Helman, 2011).

BOX 36-8	STAGING OF RHABDOMYOSARCOMA

Group I—Localized disease; tumor completely resected and regional nodes not involved
Group II—Localized disease with microscopic residual, or regional disease with no residual or with microscopic residual
Group III—Incomplete resection or biopsy with gross residual disease
Group IV—Metastatic disease present at diagnosis

With the use of contemporary multimodal therapy, more than 80% of patients with nonmetastatic disease are expected to survive (Lanzkowsky, 2005; Helman, 2011). If relapse occurs, the prognosis for long-term survival is poor.

Therapeutic Management

All rhabdomyosarcomas are high-grade tumors with the potential for metastases. Therefore multimodal therapy is recommended for all patients. Complete removal of the primary tumor is advocated whenever possible. However, because the tumor is chemosensitive, radical procedures with high morbidity should be avoided. In the majority of cases, a biopsy is followed by chemotherapy, irradiation, or both. Patients with embryonal tumors and group I disease can be treated with chemotherapy alone, whereas all others require chemotherapy and radiotherapy. Drugs that are used most often for the treatment of rhabdomyosarcoma include vincristine, actinomycin D, cyclophosphamide (VAC), ifosfamide, topotecan, irinotecan, and doxorubicin, which are administered for about 1 year (Lanzkowsky, 2005).

Nursing Care Management

The nursing responsibilities are similar to those for other types of cancer, especially the solid tumors when surgery is employed. Specific objectives include (1) careful assessment for signs of the tumor, especially during well-child examinations; (2) preparation of the child and family for the multiple diagnostic tests (see p. 1478); and (3) supportive care during each stage of multimodal therapy. The reader is urged to review the Nursing Care Management section for cancer and Chapter 23 for emotional support of the family in the event of a poor prognosis.

RETINOBLASTOMA

Retinoblastoma, which arises from the retina, is the most common intraocular malignancy of childhood (Tsinopoulos, Papadopoulou, Papandroudis, et al, 2001). Approximately 3.8 cases per 1 million children occur annually, but it accounts for 11% of all cancers seen in children during the first year of life. The average age of the child at the time of diagnosis is 2 years; it is usually diagnosed earlier in hereditary cases and later in nonhereditary types. Of all cases of retinoblastoma, 60% are unilateral and nonhereditary, 25% are bilateral and hereditary, and 15% are unilateral and hereditary.

Retinoblastoma may be caused by various genetic alterations of the *Rb* gene, including (1) a somatic mutation in nonhereditary cases, (2) a germ-line mutation in hereditary cases, or (3) a chromosomal deletion involving chromosome 13. A "two-hit hypothesis" was developed to explain genetic and sporadic cases. Almost all bilateral retinoblastomas are considered hereditary, and 15% of individuals with unilateral disease have the hereditary form (Hurwitz, Shields, Shields, et al, 2011; Tsinopoulos, Papadopoulou, Papandroudis, et al, 2001). Hereditary retinoblastomas are transmitted as an autosomal dominant trait, with 90% penetrance (Lanzkowsky, 2005). Consequently 10% of gene carriers remain unaffected.

Children who have chromosome aberrations and retinoblastoma also often have an increased incidence of cognitive impairment and congenital malformations, although the vast majority of children with retinoblastomas apparently have normal chromosomes and intelligence.

Clinical Manifestations

Retinoblastoma has few grossly obvious signs. Typically the parents are the ones who first observe a whitish "glow" in the pupil, known as the cat's eye reflex, or leukocoria (Fig. 36-6). The reflex represents visualization of the tumor as the light momentarily falls on the mass. When a tumor arises in the macular region (area directly at the back of the retina when the eye is focused straight ahead), a white reflex may be visible when the tumor is small. It is best observed when a bright light is shining toward the child as the child looks forward. Sometimes parents accidentally discover it when taking a photograph of their child using a flash attachment.

When the tumor arises in the periphery of the retina, it must grow to a considerable size before light can strike it sufficiently to produce the cat's eye reflex. In this situation it is visible only when the child looks in certain directions (sideways) or if the observer stands at an oblique angle to the child's face as the child looks straight ahead. The fleeting nature of the reflex often results in a delayed diagnosis because health care professionals fail to appreciate the ominous significance of the parents' findings.

The next most common sign is strabismus resulting from poor fixation of the visually impaired eye, particularly if the tumor develops in the macula, the area of sharpest visual acuity. Blindness is usually a late sign, but it frequently is not obvious unless the parent consciously observes for behaviors indicating loss of sight, such as bumping into objects, slowed motor development, or turning of the head to see objects lateral to the affected eye. Other signs and symptoms include heterochromia (different color of the iris), glaucoma, and pain.

Diagnostic Evaluation

A detailed family history and recording of eye symptoms is essential. Children suspected of having this disorder are referred to an ophthalmologist; the diagnosis is usually based on indirect ophthalmoscopy, ultrasound, and CT scans.

Metastatic disease at the time of retinoblastoma diagnosis is rare (Singh, Shields, and Shields, 2000); therefore staging procedures such as bone marrow aspiration, bone scan, and LP are not routinely performed.

Staging and Prognosis

Staging of retinoblastomas is done under indirect ophthalmoscopy before surgery to accurately determine the tumor size (measured in disc diameters [DD]) and location (according to an imaginary line called the equator drawn on the midplane of the eye) (Hurwitz, Shields, Shields, et al, 2011; Lanzkowsky, 2005).

Various classification systems have been used to stage retinoblastoma. The Reese-Ellsworth system (Box 36-9) classifies

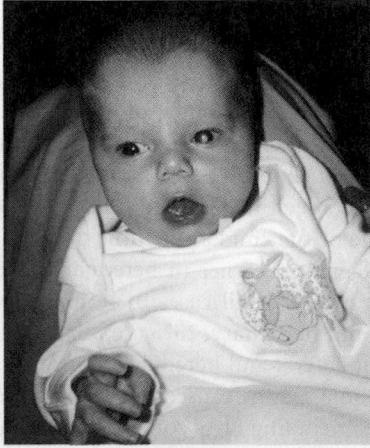

Fig. 36-6 Cat's eye reflex. Whitish appearance of lens is produced as light falls on tumor mass in left eye.

BOX 36-9   INTERNATIONAL CLASSIFICATION FOR INTRAOCULAR RETINOBLASTOMA

Group A—Small intraretinal tumors away from foveola and disc
- All tumors are 3 mm or smaller in greatest dimension, confined to the retina *and*
- All tumors are located farther than 3 mm from the foveola and 1.5 mm from the optic disc

Group B—All remaining discrete tumors confined to the retina
- All other tumors confined to the retina not in group A
- Tumor-associated subretinal fluid less than 3 mm from the tumor with no subretinal seeding

Group C—Discrete local disease with minimal subretinal or vitreous seeding
- Tumor(s) are discrete
- Subretinal fluid, present or past, without seeding involving up to one fourth of retina
- Local fine vitreous seeding may be present close to discrete tumor
- Local subretinal seeding less than 3 mm (2DD) from the tumor

Group D—Diffuse disease with significant vitreous or subretinal seeding
- Tumor(s) may be massive or diffuse
- Subretinal fluid present or past without seeding, involving up to total retinal detachment
- Diffuse or massive vitreous disease may include "greasy" seeds or avascular tumor masses
- Diffuse subretinal seeding may include subretinal plaques or tumor nodules

Group E—Presence of any one or more of these prognostic features:
- Tumor touching the lens
- Tumor anterior to anterior vitreous face, involving ciliary body or anterior segment
- Diffuse infiltrating retinoblastoma
- Neovascular glaucoma
- Opaque media from hemorrhage
- Tumor necrosis with aseptic orbital cellulites
- Phthisis bulbi

Adapted from Shields CL, Shields JA: Basic understanding of current classification and management of retinoblastoma, *Curr Opin Ophthalmol* 17(3):228-234, 2006.

patients according to five groups and predicts survival when patients are treated with radiotherapy. A new classification system is designed based on the extent and location of the intraocular tumor and better predicts globe salvage using contemporary treatments. Cure rates for survival are much better than for retention of useful vision. The overall 10-year survival rate is nearly 90% for unilateral and bilateral tumors (Hurwitz, Shields, Shields, et al, 2011; Singh, Shields, and Shields, 2000). Retinoblastoma is one of the tumors that may spontaneously regress.

Of major concern in long-term survivors is the development of secondary tumors, especially osteosarcoma. Children with bilateral disease (hereditary form) are more likely to develop secondary cancers than are children with unilateral disease. Currently providers think these individuals are predisposed to developing cancer, and radiation increases their risk.

Therapeutic Management

Treatment of retinoblastoma is complex. Enucleation may be used to treat advanced disease with optic nerve invasion in which there is no hope for salvage of vision. Irradiation can be used when there is vitreous seeding. Chemotherapy has been used to decrease the tumor size to allow treatment with local therapies such as plaque brachytherapy (surgical implantation of an iodine-125 applicator on the sclera until the maximum radiation dose has been delivered to the tumor), photocoagulation (use of a laser beam to destroy retinal blood vessels that supply nutrition to the tumor), and cryotherapy (freezing of the tumor, which destroys the microcirculation to the tumor and the cells themselves through microcrystal formation). Vincristine, carboplatin, and etoposide are the agents most commonly used.

The use of chemotherapy in advanced disease, even in group V, is controversial and has not shown improved survival. Drugs that may be used in the treatment of metastatic disease include vincristine, cyclophosphamide, doxorubicin, cisplatin, carboplatin, and etoposide. In the case of CNS disease, intrathecal chemotherapy may be administered (Hurwitz, Shields, Shields, et al, 2011; Lanzkowsky, 2005).

Nursing Care Management
Prepare the Family for Diagnostic and Therapeutic Procedures and Home Care

Because the tumor is usually diagnosed in infants or very young children, most of the preparation for diagnostic tests and treatment involves parents. After indirect ophthalmoscopy the child may not see clearly, or the eyes may be sensitive to light because of pupillary dilation. Make parents aware of these normal reactions before the procedure.

Once the disease is staged, the physician confers with the parents regarding treatment. In most cases, enucleation can be avoided. In the event that an enucleation is performed, tell parents about the procedure and the benefits of a prosthesis. Parents often believe the procedure is bloody and mutilating, envisioning that the eye is "ripped out of its socket." Actually, the surgery is similar to scooping a nut out of its shell. All the adnexal structures of the eye, such as the lids, lashes, and tear glands, are left undisturbed.

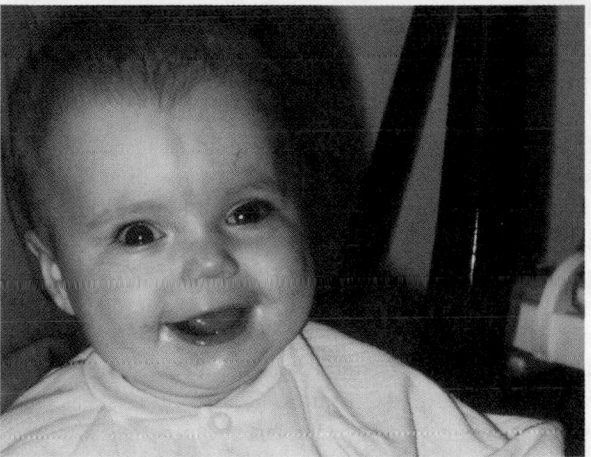

Fig. 36-7 Infant with left prosthetic eye.

Showing parents pictures of another child with an artificial eye may help them adjust to the thought of disfigurement (Fig. 36-7). Although the loss of vision is distressing, most parents seem to realize that there is no alternative. Emphasizing that the unaffected eye retains normal vision and that the affected eye is probably already blind is particularly helpful in promoting acceptance of the imposed impairment.

After surgery the parents need to be prepared for the child's facial appearance. An eye patch is in place, and the child's face may be edematous or ecchymotic. Parents often fear seeing the surgical site because they imagine a cavity in the skull. On the contrary, the lids are usually closed, and the area does not appear sunken because a surgically implanted sphere maintains the shape of the eyeball. The implant is covered with conjunctiva, and when the lids are open, the exposed area resembles the mucosal lining of the mouth. Once the child is fitted for a prosthesis, usually within 3 weeks, the facial appearance returns to normal.

After an uneventful recovery from enucleation, plans can be made for discharge from the hospital, usually within 3 to 4 days postoperatively. Parents need instruction regarding care of the surgical site and preparation for any additional therapy. They should be given the opportunity to see the socket as soon after surgery as possible. A good time to do this without unduly pressuring them is during dressing changes. They should then be encouraged to participate in the dressing changes.

Care of the socket is minimal and easily accomplished. The wound itself is clean and has little or no drainage. If an antibiotic ointment is prescribed, it is applied in a thin line on the surface of the tissues of the socket. To cleanse the site, an irrigating solution may be ordered and is instilled daily or more frequently if necessary, before application of the antibiotic ointment. The dressing consists of an eye pad changed daily. Self-adhesive eye pads can also be used as dressings. Once the socket has healed completely, a dressing is no longer necessary, although there are several reasons for having the child continue to wear an eye patch. Infants and toddlers explore their environment with their hands, and without an eye patch in place, the socket is available to exploring fingers. Although there is little danger of the child injuring the socket, parents may feel more secure with the socket covered. This also helps prevent infection.

The ocularist, who fits and manufactures the prosthesis, gives initial instructions for care of the device. Once in place, the prosthesis need not be removed unless cleaning is necessary, in which case it is taken out by gently pulling down on the lower lid, which frees the lower edge of the prosthesis, and applying pressure to the upper lid. If the child resists by forcing the lids shut, a small rubber instrument resembling a plunger can be used to facilitate removal and reinsertion. The end of the plunger is moistened and placed on top of the prosthetic iris. The lower eyelid is retracted, and the prosthesis is pulled out with a downward motion.

The prosthesis is cleaned by placing it in hot water and soaking it for several minutes. Reinsertion is easier if the prosthesis remains wet. To reinsert the prosthesis, the lids are separated, and with the prosthesis held in the correct position (it should be marked to indicate the nasal side), it is pushed up under the upper lid, allowing the lower lid to cover its lower edge.

Because the prosthesis is easily removed, the child may accidentally dislodge it. Children's reactions vary from fear that they have "lost" their eye to matter-of-fact acceptance. The first time can be disturbing to both parents and child, but it is just one part of the child's adjusted lifestyle. If children are old enough to understand, parents can explain that they have a "special" eye that can accidentally fall out but that can also be quickly put back in place.

Safety is a major concern to prevent damage to the unaffected eye. Safety measures should be practiced at all times, and children should avoid rough contact sports or wear protective eye wear.

Support the Family

The diagnosis of retinoblastoma presents some special concerns in addition to those raised by any type of cancer. Families with a history of the disorder may feel guilt for transmitting the defect to their offspring, especially if they knowingly "played the odds" and parented an affected child. Conversely, when parents are aware of the probability and have an affected child, early treatment results in such favorable outcomes that parental adjustment may be rapid. In families with no history of retinoblastoma, the diagnosis is a shock, frequently complicated by guilt for not having discovered it sooner. Because parents frequently are the first to observe the cat's eye reflex, they may be angry at themselves or others, especially professionals, for delaying a more thorough examination. Consider each of these variables while offering supportive care to the family.

Other concerns also relate to the hereditary aspects of the disease. Of great importance to parents is the risk of retinoblastoma in their subsequent offspring and in the offspring of the surviving affected child. With improving prognoses for these children, genetic counseling to prevent transmission of the disease is assuming greater importance. (See Chapter 5 for a discussion of the nurse's role in genetic counseling.) Determining the risk of transmission is possible through DNA/RNA studies of the tumor cells. If a germinal mutation is found, blood samples from family members can be analyzed to see if they carry the mutation (Hurwitz, Shields, Shields, et al, 2011; Smith, Murray, Fulton, et al, 2000).

Encourage these families to seek regular follow-up care for the affected child to detect secondary tumors, and all subsequent offspring of unaffected parents and survivors should undergo regular ophthalmoscopy to detect retinoblastoma at its earliest stage (Shields and Shields, 2001) (see Nursing Care Plan, pp. 1470-1472).

GERM CELL TUMORS

Germ cell tumors account for about 1% of all childhood tumors and can arise in gonadal and extragonadal sites. Sacrococcygeal teratoma is the most common germ cell tumor and accounts for 40% of all germ cell tumors in childhood. The most common ovarian tumors are teratomas, followed by dysgerminomas and yolk sac tumors. The most common testicular tumors are yolk sac tumors, followed by teratomas. In general, most teratomas and localized gonadal tumors that are surgically resected can be observed without the need for further therapy. For patients with more advanced disease, the use of chemotherapy with cisplatin, etoposide, and bleomycin has produced excellent results.

Nursing Care Management

To supplement routine health assessment, every adolescent male should know how to perform frequent testicular self-examination (TSE) to familiarize himself with his own anatomy and to ensure early detection of any abnormality. Ideally self-examination should be performed once a month beginning when physical development reaches Tanner stage 3, usually about age 13 or 14 years. (See Fig. 19-6.) Each testicle is examined individually, preferably after a warm bath or shower (when scrotal skin is more relaxed), using the thumbs and fingers of both hands and applying a small amount of firm, gentle pressure. The normal testicle is a firm organ with a smooth egg-shaped contour. The epididymis can be palpated as a raised swelling on the superior aspect of the testicle and should not be confused with an abnormality. The efficacy of teaching TSE to adolescent males has been tested, and it has been found to be successful (Han and Peschel, 2000).

LIVER TUMORS

Liver tumors account for 1% of all childhood cancers; the most common histologic subtype is hepatoblastoma. Surgical resection is the treatment of choice for these tumors but can only be accomplished in about 50% of cases. For this reason, chemotherapy with vincristine, 5-fluorouracil, cisplatin, and doxorubicin is commonly used in an attempt to decrease the size of the tumor so that it can be surgically resected. Liver transplantation can be used in unresectable tumors. About 70% of patients with hepatoblastoma can be cured with current therapies (Meyers, 2007).

THE CHILDHOOD CANCER SURVIVOR

Survival for children with cancer has greatly improved over the past 20 years. The 5-year survival rate is now about 80%. As more and more children survive, we are able to better learn about the long-term effects they experience into adulthood.

Care of long-term survivors is an area of growing research, since many resources are needed to reduce the complications of treatment and enhance the survivor's overall quality of life. Long-term effects of treatments, including surgery, chemotherapy, and radiation, can result in a multitude of effects such as neurocognitive impairment, endocrinopathy, risk for second malignancy, and major organ dysfunction (liver failure, kidney failure).

Treatment, as well as the disease, may also affect psychosocial, cognitive, emotional, and physical development. Table 36-6 describes the systemic late effects caused by cancer treatment that require careful nursing assessment.

TABLE 36-6 LATE EFFECTS OF CANCER TREATMENT

SYSTEMIC EFFECTS AND CLINICAL MANIFESTATIONS	ASSOCIATED MODE OF TREATMENT
Central Nervous System (CNS)	
Leukoencephalopathy (syndrome ranging from lethargy, dementia, and seizures to quadriplegia and death)	Methotrexate or CNS irradiation
Mineralizing microangiopathy (headaches, focal seizures, incoordination, gait abnormalities)	Methotrexate or CNS irradiation
Peripheral neuropathy (footdrop, incoordination)	Vincristine
Cognitive deficits (intelligence, nonlanguage skills)	Intrathecal chemotherapy or cranial irradiation (especially before age 3 yr)
Cardiovascular	
Cardiomyopathy (tachycardia, tachypnea, dyspnea, shortness of breath, edema, palpitations)	Anthracyclines (doxorubicin and daunorubicin) or irradiation to heart; High-dose cyclophosphamide
Pericardial damage (pleural effusion, cardiomegaly)	Mediastinal irradiation
Respiratory	
Pneumonitis (dyspnea, nonproductive cough, fever)	Lung irradiation, alkylating agents, possibly bleomycin, vinblastine, cisplatin
Pulmonary fibrosis (dyspnea, restrictive ventilation, decreased exercise tolerance)	
Gastrointestinal	
Chronic enteritis (colic, abdominal pain, vomiting, diarrhea, obstipation, bleeding)	Abdominal irradiation, methotrexate, cytosine arabinoside
Hepatic fibrosis (jaundice, hepatomegaly)	Methotrexate, 6-mercaptopurine
Urinary	
Hemorrhagic cystitis (chronic microscopic hematuria to gross hemorrhage)	Cyclophosphamide; ifosfamide; irradiation, especially with radiomimetic chemotherapeutic agents (e.g., doxorubicin and daunorubicin)
Bladder fibrosis (decreased bladder capacity, ureteral reflux)	Cisplatin
Tubular necrosis (decreased creatinine clearance)	
Endocrine	
Growth retardation (abnormal growth velocity)	Irradiation to thyroid, pituitary gland, testes, ovaries
Thyroid dysfunction (see Chapter 38)	
Gonadal dysfunction (see Reproductive)	
Reproductive	
Possible gonadal damage, both sexes (amenorrhea, decreased sperm counts, increased follicle-stimulating and luteinizing hormones, decreased testosterone or estrogen)	Alkylating agents; Irradiation to pituitary gland, testes, ovaries
Skeletal	
Linear growth retardation (short stature)	Irradiation, long-term steroids
Spinal deformities, scoliosis, kyphosis, asymmetric growth, pathologic fractures	Irradiation
Immune	
Asplenia (overwhelming infection, fever)	Splenectomy (Hodgkin disease)
Sensory Organs	
Cataracts (opacity over pupil)	Cranial irradiation, high-dose steroids
Hearing (decreased hearing associated with high-frequency loss)	Cisplatin
Additional Effects	
Dental Problems	
Increased caries, periodontal disease, hypoplastic teeth, hypodontia (delayed or absent tooth development)	Irradiation to maxilla and mandible
Second Malignancies	
Bone and soft tissue tumors	Irradiation, alkylating agents
Leukemia	
Nonlymphoblastic leukemia	

Vigorous treatment of childhood cancers has resulted in dramatically improved survival rates. However, treatment programs combining surgery, irradiation, and chemotherapy are not without their complications. Some may occur immediately, such as loss of a limb from surgical amputation. However, current concern is with late effects—adverse changes related to treatment modalities, interactions between modes of treatment, individual characteristics of the child, and the disease process that may appear months to years after lifesaving treatment. Because more children are being cured and surviving into adulthood, increasing documentation of late effects is emerging (see Table 36-6). Almost no organ is exempt, and almost every antineoplastic agent (especially irradiation) is responsible for some adverse effect. Many factors influence the development of late effects from irradiation; some of the more important ones include the total cumulative dose given, the child's age (the younger the child, the more radiosensitive the body organs are), and the tumor's location.

Radiotherapy to growing bones or reproductive glands responsible for growth-related hormones can delay or stunt growth. Nurses must document growth by assessing height and weight at each visit. Any decrease in growth velocity should be further evaluated. Further assessment includes documenting parental heights, obtaining a wrist x-ray film to predict further growth potential, and assessing gonadal development and pituitary function.

Radiotherapy and the alkylating agents can cause hormonal dysfunction, decreased fertility, and sterility. The potential for gonadal dysfunction depends on the child's age and sex, the type of treatment, and the duration and total doses of treatment. Nursing assessment must begin with careful documentation of the child's sexual development using the Tanner staging scale. (See Pubertal Sexual Maturation, Chapter 19.)

Irradiation to developing bone and cartilage may cause numerous abnormalities. Assessment includes close observation of the irradiated bone for defects, such as spinal kyphoscoliosis, leg length discrepancy, and skull and facial disfigurement.

Irradiated bones are more fragile than other bones and may fracture easily, have functional limitations, and heal slowly in the presence of infection. Osteoporosis may develop. Children who have received irradiation to the mandibular area are at risk for dental caries, arrested tooth development, and incomplete dental calcification. A careful assessment of the oral cavity in children who have received irradiation to the mandible is performed at each clinic visit.

KEY POINTS

- Cure in childhood cancer can be defined as a disease free state 5 years from time of initial diagnosis.
- Although the cure rate for most types of childhood cancer has improved, the late effects of treatment are of increasing concern.
- The major modes of cancer therapy are surgery, chemotherapy, radiotherapy, immunotherapy, and BMT.
- Chemotherapeutic agents are classified according to their cytotoxic action: alkylating agents, antimetabolites, plant alkaloids, antitumor antibiotics, and hormones.
- Types of BMTs are allogeneic and autologous.
- Nursing goals in the care of the child with cancer are to prepare the family for diagnostic and therapeutic procedures, prevent complications of myelosuppression (e.g., infection, hemorrhage, anemia), manage problems of irradiation and drug toxicity (e.g., nausea and vomiting, anorexia, mucosal ulceration, neuropathy, hemorrhagic cystitis, alopecia, moon face, mood changes), and provide continued emotional support.

- Leukemia is the most common form of childhood cancer. Current 5-year survival rates exceed 80% in major research centers, and the majority of these children will be cured.
- The lymphomas include Hodgkin disease and NHL; Hodgkin disease affects primarily adolescents.
- Nursing care of the child with a brain tumor includes observing for signs and symptoms related to the tumor, preparing the child and family for diagnostic tests and operative procedures, preventing postoperative complications, planning for discharge, and promoting a return to optimum health.
- The treatment of osteosarcoma is limb salvage or amputation followed by chemotherapy.
- Rhabdomyosarcoma may occur almost anywhere in the body, but the most common sites are the head and neck.
- Common presenting signs in retinoblastoma are leukocoria; strabismus; and red, painful eye.
- Male adolescents should be taught to perform monthly TSEs to detect testicular tumors. Female adolescents should be taught to do monthly breast-self examination.

ANSWERS TO CRITICAL THINKING EXERCISES

Fever and Neutropenia

1. **Yes,** there is sufficient evidence to arrive at conclusions.
2. **a.** It is important to note that approximately 10 days after administration of chemotherapeutic agents, patients hit their nadir (time at which their blood counts are at the lowest). At this time in the patient's treatment it is crucial that parents call with any fever (as defined by the treating institution), since this may be the only sign of an infection. Other areas of concern include the appearance of the central line site and

dressing. Is there any drainage on the dressing, foul odors, bleeding at the site, or erythema and pain at the site?

b. Physical assessment reveals that the patient is febrile and has a potential source of infection (mucositis). Chemotherapeutic agents work on all rapidly dividing cells, including the hematopoietic cells, hair, cells that line the gastrointestinal (GI) tract from the mouth to the anus, and the rapidly dividing cancer cells. As the blood counts drop, particularly the neutrophils, patients are at risk for developing infections.

c. Rapidly dividing cells are killed at a rate much quicker than they typically die on their own, which results in a delay in the repair to the mucosa. Mucositis has been defined as an inflammation or an ulceration of the mucous membranes of the GI lining. Because of the presence of bacteria in the mouth and the breaks in the mucosa, the patient is at risk for developing infections.

3. Initially medications and laboratory tests ordered should be reviewed for an acetaminophen order, for antibiotic or antifungal agents, and for parameters on how often blood should be drawn and cultures obtained. Any missing orders should be brought to the attention of the provider (physician or nurse practitioner). If a blood culture is required, it should be drawn before acetaminophen administration. Avoid use of aspirin- or ibuprofen-based medications. It is important with each assessment to pay careful attention to the signs of sepsis, which include fever or hypothermia, unexplained tachycardia, or tachypnea. A late sign of sepsis or septic shock is a drop in the patient's blood pressure. Report any changes in the patients' condition to the provider.

4. **Yes,** the documented vital signs and physical assessment support the need for careful assessment of infection and for continued monitoring for sepsis.

Bleeding

1. **Yes,** there is sufficient evidence to arrive at some possible conclusions.

2. a. Normal platelet counts are typically between 150,000 and 450,000/mm^3 with some minor variations from laboratory to laboratory. Patients are at risk for spontaneous bleeding when the platelet count falls below 20,000/mm^3. In some patients spontaneous bleeding from the nose, gums, or rectal area can occur at any time regardless of the platelet count. Certain medications such as ibuprofen- or aspirin-based products can interfere with platelet function regardless of the actual platelet count.

b. Physical assessment reveals sites of spontaneous bleeding (buccal mucosa, sclera). Chemotherapeutic agents work on all rapidly dividing cells, which include the hematopoietic cells, hair, cells that line the gastrointestinal tract from the mouth to the anus, and the rapidly dividing cancer cells. As the platelet count drops, patients are at risk for bleeding.

3. The immediate intervention would include assessing whether the oxygen is humidified. The nose is vascular and can bleed easily if the mucosa is dried by oxygen. Inspect the length and placement of the nasal prongs and the nasal mucosa for any signs of irritation. Other interventions include transfusing platelets as ordered by a physician or nurse practitioner and having the patient use a soft toothbrush or Toothette (sponge toothbrush) for oral care.

4. **Yes,** the laboratory results, timing of chemotherapy, and expected nadir support these conclusions; since we know that Paul received therapy 10 days ago, we would expect to see his counts drop to their lowest point around this time.

REFERENCES

Altman AJ, Fu C: Chronic leukemias of childhood. In Pizzo PA, Poplack DG, editors: *Principles and practices of pediatric oncology*, ed 6, Philadelphia, 2011, Lippincott.

American Academy of Pediatrics: Long term follow-up care for pediatric cancer survivors, *Pediatrics* 123:906-915, 2009.

American Academy of Pediatrics, Pickering LK, editor: *2006 Red book: report of the Committee on Infectious Diseases*, ed 27, Elk Grove Village, Ill, 2006, The Academy.

American Society of Health-System Pharmacists, Commission of Therapeutics: ASHP therapeutic guidelines on the pharmacologic management of nausea and vomiting in adult and pediatric patients receiving chemotherapy or radiation therapy or undergoing surgery, *Am J Health Syst Pharm* 56:729-764, 1999.

Anastasia PJ: Effectiveness of oral 5-HT3 receptor antagonists for emetogenic chemotherapy, *Oncol Nurs Forum* 27(3):483-493, 2000.

Armenian SH, Meadows AT, Bhatia S: Late effects of childhood cancer and its treatment. In Pizzo PA, Poplack DG, editors: *Principles and practices of pediatric oncology*, ed 6, Philadelphia, 2011, Lippincott.

Blaney SM, Haas-Kogan D, Young-Pouissant T, et al: Tumors of the central nervous system. In Pizzo PA, Poplack DG, editors: *Principles and practices of pediatric oncology*, ed 6, Philadelphia, 2011, Lippincott.

Bollard CM, Krance RA, Heslop HE: Hematopoietic stem cell transplantation in pediatric oncology. In Pizzo PA, Poplack DG,
editors: *Principles and practices of pediatric oncology*, ed 6, Philadelphia, 2011, Lippincott.

Brodeur GM, Hogarty MD, Mosse YP, et al: Neuroblastoma. In Pizzo PA, Poplack DG, editors: *Principles and practices of pediatric oncology*, ed 6, Philadelphia, 2011, Lippincott.

Brunelle F: Noninvasive diagnosis of brain tumours in children, *Childs Nerv Syst* 16(10-11):731-734, 2000.

Cercato MC, Nagore E, Ramazzotti V, et al: Self- and parent-assessed skin cancer risk factors in school-age children, *Prev Med* 47(1):133-135, 2008.

Cho S, Cheng AC, Cheng MCK: Oral care for children with leukaemia, *Hong Kong Med J* 6(2):203-208, 2000.

Coiffier B, Altman A, Pui CH, et al: Guidelines for the management of pediatric and adult tumor lysis syndrome: An evidence-based review, *J Clin Oncol* 26(16):2767-2768, 2008.

Culy CR, Bhana N, Plosker GL: Ondansetron: a review of its use as an antiemetic in children, *Paediatric Drugs* 3(6):441-479, 2001.

Dome JS, Liu T, Krasin M, et al: Improved survival for patients with recurrent Wilms tumor: the experience at St Jude Children's Research Hospital, *J Pediatr Hematol Oncol* 24(3):192-198, 2002.

Fernandez C, Geller JI, Ehrlich PF, et al: Renal tumors. In Pizzo PA, Poplack DG, editors: *Principles and practices of pediatric oncology*, ed 6, Philadelphia, 2011, Lippincott.

Frey MA, Guess C, Allison J, et al: Umbilical cord stem cell transplantation, *Semin Oncol Nurs* 25(2):115-119, 2009.

Gorlick R, Bielack S, Teot L, et al: Osteosarcoma: biology, diagnosis, treatment and remaining challenges. In Pizzo PA, Poplack DG, editors: *Principles and practices of pediatric oncology*, ed 6, Philadelphia, 2011, Lippincott.

Graf N, Tournade MF, deKraker JD: The role of preoperative chemotherapy in the management of Wilms' tumor, *Urol Clin North Am* 27(3):443-454, 2000.

Grosfeld JL: Risk-based management of solid tumors in children, *Am J Surg* 180(5):322-327, 2000.

Gross TG, Perkins SL: Malignant non-Hodgkin lymphomas in children. In Pizzo PA, Poplack DG, editors: *Principles and practices of pediatric oncology*, ed 6, Philadelphia, 2011, Lippincott.

Han S, Peschel RE: Father-son testicular tumors: evidence for genetic anticipation? *Cancer* 88(10):2319-2325, 2000.

Han-Markey T: Nutritional considerations in pediatric oncology, *Semin Oncol Nurs* 16(2):146-151, 2000.

Hatch E, Herbst A, Hoover R, et al: Incidence of squamous neoplasia of the cervix and vaginas in DES-exposed daughters, *Ann Epidemiol* 10(7):467-470, 2000.

Hellsten MB: All the king's horses and all the king's men: pain management from hospital to home, *J Pediatr Oncol Nurs* 17(3):149-159, 2000.

Helman LJ: Rhabdomyosarcoma and the undifferentiated sarcomas of childhood. In Pizzo PA, Poplack DG, editors: *Principles and practices of pediatric oncology*, ed 6, Philadelphia, 2011, Lippincott.

Hockenberry MJ, Kline NE: Nursing support of the child with cancer. In Pizzo PA, Poplack DG, editors: *Principles and practices of pediatric oncology*, ed 6, Philadelphia, 2011, Lippincott.

Hudson MM, Krasin M, Metzger M, et al: Hodgkin lymphoma. In Pizzo PA, Poplack DG, editors: *Principles and practices of pediatric oncology*, ed 6, Philadelphia, 2011, Lippincott.

Hurwitz RL, Shields CL, Shields JA, et al: Retinoblastoma. In Pizzo PA, Poplack DG, editors: *Principles and practices of pediatric oncology*, ed 6, Philadelphia, 2011, Lippincott.

Kavan P, Kabickova E, Gajdos P, et al: Treatment of pediatric B-cell non Hodgkin's lymphomas at the Motol Hospital in Prague, Czech Republic: results based on NHL BFM 90 protocols, *Pediatr Hematol Oncol* 16(3):201-212, 1999.

Knudson AG, Hethcote HW, Brown BW: Mutation and childhood cancer: a probabilistic model for the incidence of retinoblastoma, *Proc Natl Acad Sci* 72(12):5116-5120, 1975.

Krane EJ, Casillas J, Zeltzer LK: Pain and symptom management. In Pizzo PA, Poplack DG, editors: *Principles and practices of pediatric oncology*, ed 6, Philadelphia, 2011, Lippincott.

Kumar KS, Rajagopal MR, Naseema AM: Intravenous morphine for emergency treatment of cancer pain, *Palliat Med* 14:183-188, 2000.

Landier W: Childhood acute lymphoblastic leukemia: current perspectives, *Oncol Nurs Forum* 28(5):823-833, 2001.

Lanzkowsky P: *Manual of pediatric hematology and oncology*, ed 4, San Diego, 2005, Academic Press.

Lau L, Tai D, Weitzman S, et al: Factors influencing survival in children with recurrent neuroblastoma, *J Pediatr Hematol Oncol* 26(4):227-232, 2004.

Lee CT, Bilton SD, Famiglietti RM, et al: Treatment planning with protons for pediatric retinoblastoma, medulloblastoma, and pelvic sarcoma: how do protons compare with conformal techniques? *Intl J Radiat Oncol Biol Phys* 63(2):362-372, 2005.

Locatelli F, Giorgiani G, Di-Cesare-Merlone A: The changing role of stem cell transplantation in childhood, *Bone Marrow Transplant* 41(Suppl 2):S3-S7, 2008.

Lohr L: Chemotherapy-induced nausea and vomiting, *Cancer* 14(2):85-93, 2008.

Loring DW, Meador KJ: Corticosteroids and cognitive function in humans: methodological considerations, *J Pediatr Hematol Oncol* 22(3):193-196, 2000.

MacDonald DJ, Lessick M: Hereditary cancers in children and ethical and psychosocial implications, *J Pediatr Nurs* 15(4):217-225, 2000.

Mainprize TG, Taylor MD, Rutka JT: Pediatric brain tumors: a contemporary prospectus, *Clin Neurosurg* 47:259-302, 2000.

Margolin JF, Rabin KR, Steuber CP, et al: Acute lymphoblastic leukemia. In Pizzo PA, Poplack DG, editors: *Principles and practices of pediatric oncology*, ed 6, Philadelphia, 2011, Lippincott.

Matsubara H, Makimoto A, Takayama J, et al: Possible clinical benefits of the use of peripheral blood stem cells over bone marrow in the allogeneic transplantation setting for the treatment of childhood leukemia, *Jpn J Clin Oncol* 31(1):30-34, 2001.

Meyers RL: Tumors of the liver in children, *Surg Oncol* 16:195-203, 2007.

McCloskey DJ: Catheter related thrombosis in pediatrics, *Pediatr Nurse* 28(2):97-102, 105-106, 2002.

McMain L: Principles of acute pain management, *J Perioper Pract* 18(11):472-478, 2008.

Nguyen NP, Sallah S, Ludin A, et al: Neuroblastoma producing spinal cord compression: rapid relief with low dose of radiation, *Anticancer Res* 20(6c):4687-4690, 2000.

Nitenberg G, Raynard B: Nutritional support of the cancer patient: issues and dilemmas, *Crit Rev Oncol Hematol* 34(3):137-168, 2000.

Oeffinger KC, Eshelman DA, Tomlinson GE, et al: Providing primary care for long-term survivors of childhood acute lymphoblastic leukemia, *J Fam Pract* 49(12):1133-1146, 2000.

Olsson GL: Neuropathic pain in children. In McGrath PJ, Finley GA, editors: *Chronic and recurrent pain in children and adolescents*, Seattle, 1999, IASP Press.

Oncology Nursing Society: New approaches in safe handling of hazardous drugs, *ONS News* 19(Suppl):31-32, 2004.

Ong BY, Arneja A, Ong EW: Effects of anesthesia on pain after lower-limb amputation, *J Clin Anesth* 18(8):600-604, 2006.

Plesko I, Kramarova E, Stiller CA, et al: Survival of children with Wilms tumor in Europe, *Eur J Cancer* 37(6):736-743, 2001.

Plon SE, Malkin D: Childhood cancer and heredity. In Pizzo PA, Poplack DG, editors: *Principles and practices of pediatric oncology*, ed 6, Philadelphia, 2011, Lippincott.

Quadri TL, Brown AE: Infectious complications in the critically ill patient with cancer, *Semin Oncol* 27(3):335-346, 2000.

Ries LAG, Smith MA, Gurney JG, et al, editors: *Cancer incidence and survival among children and adolescents: United States SEER Program 1975-1995*, NIH Pub. No. 99-4649, Bethesda, Md, 1999, National Cancer Institute.

Riva D, Giorgi C: The neurodevelopmental price of survival in children with malignant brain tumors, *Childs Nerv Syst* 16(10-11):751-754, 2000.

Rocha V, Wagner JE, Sobocinski KA, et al: Graft-versus-host disease in children who have received a cord-blood or bone marrow transplant from an HLA-identical sibling, *N Engl J Med* 342(25):1846-1854, 2000.

Rossetto CL, McMahon JE: Current and future trends in transfusion therapy, *J Pediatr Oncol Nurs* 17(3):160-173, 2000.

Scheurer ME, Bondy ML, Gurney JG: Epidemiology of childhood cancer. In Pizzo PA, Poplack DG, editors: *Principles and practices of pediatric oncology*, ed 6, Philadelphia, 2011, Lippincott.

Scully C, Epstein J, Sonis S: Oral mucositis: a challenging complication of radiotherapy, chemotherapy and radiochemotherapy, part 2, Diagnosis and management of mucositis, *Head Neck* 26(1):77-84, 2004.

Sevilla J, Gonzalez-Vicent M, Madero L, et al: Peripheral blood progenitor cell collection in low weight children, *J Hematol Stem Cell Res* 11(4):633-642, 2002.

Shields JA, Shields CL: Pediatric ocular and periocular tumors, *Pediatr Ann* 30(8):491-501, 2001.

Shusterman S, Meadows AT: Long term survivors of childhood leukemia, *Curr Opin Hematol* 7(4):217-222, 2000.

Singh AD, Shields CL, Shields JA: Prognostic factors in retinoblastoma, *J Pediatr Ophthalmol Strabismus* 37(3):134-141, 2000.

Skoldenberg EG, Christiansson J, Sandstedt B, et al: Angiogenesis and angiogenic growth factors in Wilms tumor, *J Urol* 165(6, Pt 2 of 2 Suppl):2274-2279, 2001.

Smith FO, Hasle H, Cooper T: Acute myelogenous leukemia, myeloproliferative and myelodysplastic disorders. In Pizzo PA, Poplack DG, editors: *Principles and practices of pediatric oncology*, ed 6, Philadelphia, 2011, Lippincott.

Smith JH, Murray TG, Fulton L, et al: Siblings of retinoblastoma patients: are we underestimating their risk? *Am J Ophthalmol* 129(3):396-398, 2000.

Smith MA: Molecularly targeted therapies and biotherapeutics. In Pizzo PA, Poplack DG, editors: *Principles and practices of pediatric oncology*, ed 6, Philadelphia, 2011, Lippincott.

Strickler R, Phillips ML: Astrocytomas: the clinical picture, *Clin J Oncol Nurs* 4(4):153-158, 2000.

Taub JW: Relationship of chromosome 21 and acute leukemia in children with Down syndrome, *J Pediatr Hematol Oncol* 23(3):175-178, 2001.

Trahan RP, Green M, Murray JL: Monoclonal antibodies: applications in solid tumors and other diseases. In Rieger PT, editor: *Biotherapy: a comprehensive overview*, ed 2, Boston, 2001, Jones & Bartlett.

Tsinopoulos I, Papadopoulou V, Papandroudis A, et al: Retinoblastoma with an unusual presentation in a child with polydactyly: clinical associations and genetic implications, *Acta Ophthalmol Scand* 79(1):79-80, 2001.

Velez I, Tamara LA, Mintz S: Management of oral mucositis induced by chemotherapy and radiotherapy: an update, *Quintessence Int* 35(2):129-136, 2004.

Weinstein JL, Katenstein HM, Cohn SL: Advances in the diagnosis and treatment of neuroblastoma, *Oncologist* 8(3):278-292, 2003.

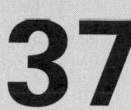

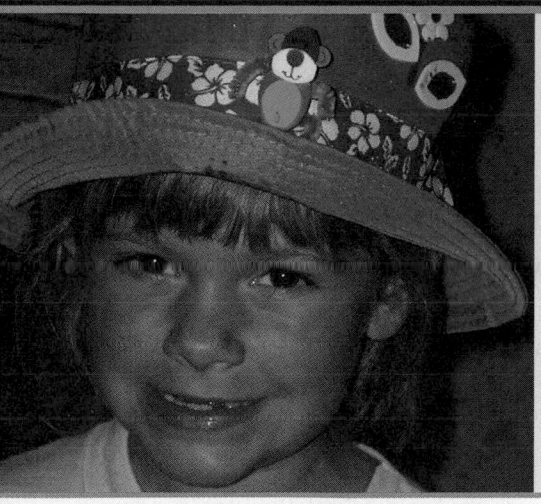

The Child with Cerebral Dysfunction

Rebecca J. Schultz and Marilyn J. Hockenberry

evolve WEBSITE

http://evolve.elsevier.com/wong/ncic

Animations
 Brain Anatomy
 Blood Flow to Brain
 Brain Lobes
 Cerebral Perfusion
 Cervical Nerve Examination
 Meningitis
 Seizure, Generalized
 Subdural Hematoma
Case Study
 Meningitis
Critical Thinking Case Study
 Head Injury
Critical Thinking Exercise
 Seizures
Key Points Audio Summaries
NCLEX Review Questions
Nursing Care Plans
 The Child with Bacterial Meningitis
 The Child with Seizure Disorder
 The Unconscious Child
Skill
 Implementing Seizure Precautions
Spanish/English Translations
WebLinks

RELATED TOPICS

Administration of Medication, **Ch. 27**
Anencephaly, **Ch. 11**
Brain Tumors, **Ch. 36**
Controlling Elevated Temperatures, **Ch. 27**
Cranial Deformities, **Ch. 11**
Family-Centered Home Care, **Ch. 25**
High Risk Related to Neurologic Disturbance, **Ch. 10**
Human Immunodeficiency Virus Infection and Acquired
 Immunodeficiency Syndrome, **Chs. 20 and 35**
Hydrocephalus, **Ch. 11**
Infection Control, **Ch. 27**
Injuries—The Leading Killer, **Ch. 1**
Maintaining Healthy Skin, **Ch. 27**
Neurologic Assessment, **Ch. 6**
Pain Assessment; Pain Management, **Ch. 7**
Preparation for Diagnostic and Therapeutic Procedures, **Ch. 27**

CHAPTER OUTLINE

CEREBRAL STRUCTURE AND FUNCTION

The nervous system is made up of three intimately connected and functioning parts: the central nervous system (CNS), the peripheral nervous system, and the autonomic nervous system. The CNS is composed of two cerebral hemispheres, the brainstem, the cerebellum, and the spinal cord. The peripheral nervous system is composed of the cranial nerves (CNs) that arise from or travel to the brainstem and the spinal nerves that travel to or from the spinal cord and that may be motor (efferent) or sensory (afferent). The autonomic nervous system is composed of the sympathetic and parasympathetic systems, which provide automatic control of vital functions.

This chapter is concerned primarily with disturbances of the brain. Chapter 40 discusses the structure and function of the spinal cord and autonomic nervous system in more detail.

DEVELOPMENT OF THE NEUROLOGIC SYSTEM

In contrast to other body tissues, which grow rapidly after birth, the nervous system grows proportionately more rapidly before birth. Two periods of rapid brain cell growth occur during fetal life. At 15 to 20 weeks of gestation there is a dramatic increase in the number of neurons. Another increase in growth rate begins at 30 weeks of gestation and extends to 1 year of age. This rapid growth during infancy continues during early childhood and slows to a more gradual rate during later childhood and adolescence. Brain volume is readily reflected in head circumference, which increases six times as much during the first year as during the second year of life. One half of the postnatal brain growth is achieved by age 1 year, 75% by age 3, and 90% by age 6. Cerebral blood flow (CBF) and oxygen consumption in childhood (up to age 6 years) is almost twice that of adults, which reflects an increased metabolic requirement consistent with growth and development.

The growth and final form of the brain depend on the development and multiplication of neurons. Creation of new cells occurs, in theory, only during the first 100 days of gestation. During the remainder of gestation, cells divide and multiply at the astonishing rate of 250,000 per minute. It is believed that no new nerve cells appear after the sixth month of fetal life. Postnatal growth consists of increasing the amount of cytoplasm around the nuclei of the 10 billion existing cells, increasing the number and intricacy of communications with other cells, and advancing their peripheral axons to keep pace with expanding body dimensions.

The brain constitutes 12% of the body weight at birth. It doubles its weight in the first year, and by age 5 or 6 years its weight at birth has tripled. Thereafter growth slows until in adulthood the brain is only about 2% of the total body weight. The surface configuration of the brain also changes with development. The early embryonic brain surface is smooth, but the sulci deepen with advancing development. This process continues throughout childhood. At birth the cortex is only about one half of its adult thickness, although all the major surface features are present. There is little cortical control over body movements at birth, with movements guided principally by primitive reflexes. (See Chapter 8.) With advancing development and maturation, the brain, through association pathways, exercises increasing control over much of the reflex activity. This allows the growing child to perform progressively complex tasks that require coordinated movements. Persistence of primitive reflexes may suggest defective cortical development.

Cortical control is closely associated with the acquisition of a myelin coating on the nerves. Although nerve fibers are able to conduct impulses without this myelin sheath, the impulses travel at a slower rate and with more likelihood of diffusion. Myelinization of the various nerve tracts in the CNS, which allows progressive neuromotor function, follows the cephalocaudal (head-to-toe) and proximodistal (near-to-far) sequence. It appears first with the fibers of the spinal cord and cranial nerves, then in the brainstem and corticospinal tracts.

Development of the nervous system proceeds on a continuum and generates the most complex structures within the embryo. The brain and spinal cord are among the first of the major organ systems to be recognized in the embryo and one of the last to finish significant development after birth. The rate of myelogenesis accelerates rapidly after birth. In general, the pathways concerned with sensation are myelinated early, before the motor pathways. The acquisition of motor skills depends on the maturation and myelination of the nervous system, and no amount of special training or practice will hasten the process. Most of an infant's advancing performance is a direct result of brain development indirectly influenced by environmental stimuli.

CENTRAL NERVOUS SYSTEM

The bony skull forms the strongest covering and provides the primary protection to the brain. It is an expansible structure in the infant and young child due to incomplete ossification of the bones of the skull, but becomes rigid in the older child and adolescent. Blood is supplied to the dura mater by the middle meningeal artery, a branch of the external carotid artery. It enters the skull at a point inferior to the temporal bone, then branches over the surface of the dura, usually encased in a groove in the temporal and parietal bones after 2 years of age. Damage to this artery or to its branches is a common cause of an epidural hematoma.

Brain Coverings

Within the skull, three membranes (the meninges) cover and protect the brain: the dura mater, arachnoid membrane, and pia mater (Fig. 37-1). The tough outer membrane, the dura

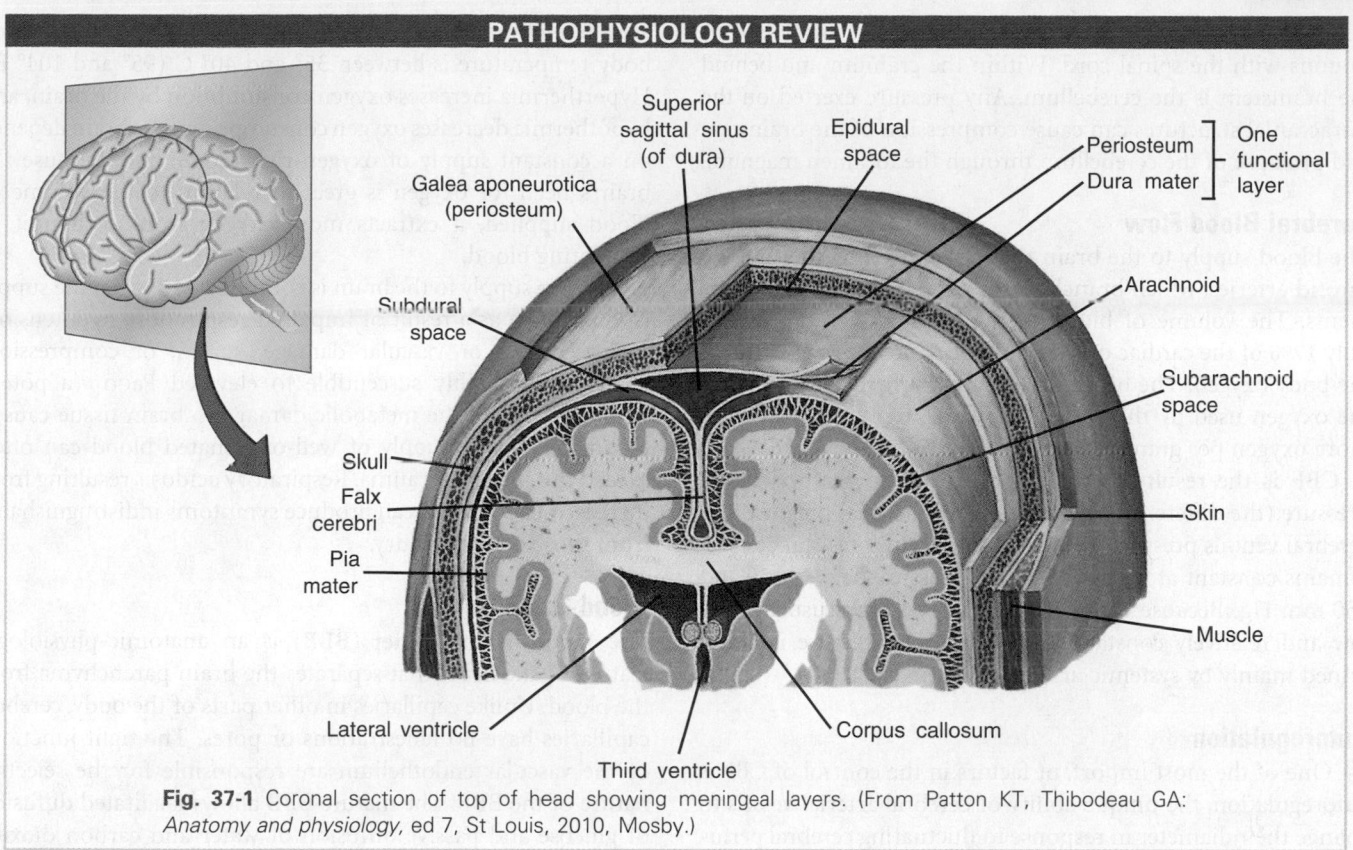

Fig. 37-1 Coronal section of top of head showing meningeal layers. (From Patton KT, Thibodeau GA: *Anatomy and physiology*, ed 7, St Louis, 2010, Mosby.)

mater, is a double layer that serves as the outer meningeal layer and the inner periosteum of the cranial bones. These two layers are separated by the epidural space. The dura is closely attached to the skull in infancy, causing slower spread of blood in epidural hemorrhage. Because of this adherence, epidural hemorrhages are uncommon in the first 2 years of life.

Between these layers of dura inside the skull lie large venous sinuses. Sheets of the dura mater also extend downward and inward to form partitions within the cranium. Projecting downward into the longitudinal fissure is a sheet of dura called the falx cerebri, which separates the cerebral hemispheres, and the falx cerebelli, which separates the cerebellar hemispheres. Another segment is a tentlike structure, the tentorium, which separates the cerebellum from the occipital lobe of the cerebrum. The large gap through which the brainstem passes is the tentorial hiatus, the site of herniation in untreated intracranial pressure (ICP).

The middle meningeal layer, the arachnoid membrane, is a delicate, avascular, weblike structure that loosely surrounds the brain. Between the arachnoid and the dura mater lies the subdural area, a potential space that normally contains only enough fluid to prevent adhesion between the two membranes. During cerebral trauma the fine blood vessels that bridge the subdural space are stretched and ruptured, causing venous blood to escape and spread freely, forming a subdural hemorrhage. The subdural space is small in children; therefore small amounts of blood can increase intracranial hemorrhage significantly.

The innermost covering layer, the pia mater, is a delicate, transparent membrane that, unlike the other coverings, adheres closely to the outer surface of the brain, conforming to the folds (gyri) and furrows (sulci). Within the pial layer lie the arteries and veins of the brain. Between the pia mater and the arachnoid membrane is the subarachnoid space. Cerebrospinal fluid (CSF) fills the entire subarachnoid space surrounding the brain and spinal cord and acts as a protective cushion for the brain tissue. Fibrous filaments known as arachnoid trabeculae provide further protection and help anchor the brain. When the head receives a blow, these attachments allow the arachnoid to slide on the dura, preventing excessive movement.

The Brain

Each section of the brain plays a vital role in regulation and control of body function. Each hemisphere is artificially divided into lobes. Pressure on or damage to these lobes produces observable signs or symptoms directly related to the area of pathology. These signs provide clues to the location of the damage.

The two large cerebral hemispheres that occupy the anterior and medial fossae of the skull are separated in the upper part by the longitudinal fissure. This separation is complete anteriorly and posteriorly, but centrally the hemispheres are joined by the block of fibers known as the corpus callosum, the largest fiber bundle in the brain. These fibers interconnect cortical areas of the right and left hemispheres. Destruction of the corpus callosum causes hemispheric independence, or "split brain."

Situated deeply within each hemisphere and on each side of the midline are the basal ganglia (or cerebral nuclei), which serve as vital sorting areas for messages passing to and from the hemispheres. Connected to the hemispheres by thick bunches of nerve fibers is the brainstem, through which all nerve fibers traverse as they pass from the hemispheres to the cerebellum and spinal cord. The brainstem extends from the base of the hemispheres through the foramen magnum, where it is continuous with the spinal cord. Within the cranium and behind the brainstem is the cerebellum. Any pressure exerted on the intracranial structures can cause compression of the brainstem and prolapse of the cerebellum through the foramen magnum.

Cerebral Blood Flow

The blood supply to the brain tissue is carried by the internal carotid arteries, which branch to supply the various brain segments. The volume of blood to the brain, which constitutes only 17% of the cardiac output, supplies the brain with 20% of the body oxygen. The brain, an "inactive" organ, uses 10 times the oxygen used by the body as a whole. Only the heart uses more oxygen per gram of tissue.

CBF is the result of two opposing forces: cerebral blood pressure (the difference between systemic arterial pressure and cerebral venous pressure) and cerebral vascular resistance. CBF remains constant at a cerebral blood pressure between 50 and 150 mm Hg. Because cerebral venous pressure is usually very low and relatively constant, cerebral blood pressure is determined mainly by systemic arterial pressure.

Autoregulation

One of the most important factors in the control of CBF is autoregulation, the unique ability of cerebral arterial vessels to change their diameter in response to fluctuating cerebral perfusion pressure (CPP). The CPP is the mean arterial pressure (MAP) minus the ICP:

$$CPP = MAP - ICP$$

As a result, cerebral vessels maintain a constant blood flow during alterations in blood pressure and perfusion caused by body posture, increased ICP, decreased cardiac output, or narrowing or occlusion in the major blood vessels of the neck. Autoregulation fails when the limits of cerebrovascular dilation are reached; at this point CBF decreases, causing clinical symptoms of ischemia (nausea, fainting, dizziness, dim vision). Conversely, increased MAP leads to "breakthrough of autoregulation," with increased CBF leading to microhemorrhages and cerebral edema. Autoregulation may be impaired locally or globally as a result of trauma or ischemia.

Changes in arterial oxygen pressure (Pao_2) or arterial carbon dioxide pressure ($Paco_2$) have a profound effect on autoregulation. Hypercapnia ($Paco_2 > 40$ mm Hg) or increased levels of lactic acid have a pronounced dilating effect on cerebral arterioles, which increases CBF and thus cerebral volume. Hypocapnia ($Paco_2$ of 25 to 30 mm Hg) constricts cerebral arterioles and decreases CBF. Pao_2 values between 70 and 100 mm Hg have little effect on the cerebrovascular system. Profound hypoxia ($Pao_2 < 50$ mm Hg) dramatically increases CBF. Consequently maintenance of the airway and effective hyperventilation are of primary importance in the initial management of the neurologically impaired patient. CPP is the most important physiologic determinant because the brain relies on the delivery of oxygen and nutrients to function.

Oxygen

Metabolic requirements for oxygen by the brain are not affected by rest or sleep, but they are reduced by narcosis and coma and are altered by changes in temperature. CBF is not altered when body temperature is between 35° and 40° C (95° and 104° F). Hyperthermia increases oxygen consumption by the brain, and hypothermia decreases oxygen consumption. The brain depends on a constant supply of oxygen-rich blood, and, because the brain's need for oxygen is great in relation to the volume of blood supplied, it extracts more oxygen from each unit of circulating blood.

Oxygen supply to the brain is compromised when the supply is inadequate as a result of impaired respiration, hypotension, increased ICP or vascular damage, spasm, or compression. Neurons are highly susceptible to elevated $Paco_2$ (a potent vasodilator), and the metabolic damage to brain tissue caused by an inadequate supply of well-oxygenated blood can often exceed the effects of trauma. Respiratory acidosis resulting from increased $Paco_2$ levels can produce symptoms indistinguishable from those of head injury.

Blood-Brain Barrier

The blood-brain barrier (BBB) is an anatomic-physiologic feature of the brain that separates the brain parenchyma from the blood. Unlike capillaries in other parts of the body, cerebral capillaries have no fenestrations or pores. The tight junctions of the vascular endothelium are responsible for the selective nature of the BBB. The mature BBB allows facilitated diffusion of glucose and passive diffusion of water and carbon dioxide but is impermeable to protein and does not permit passage of many active substances. However, the BBB of the fetus and newborn is normally indiscriminately permeable, allowing protein and other large and small molecules to pass freely between the cerebral vessels and the brain. Conditions that cause cerebrovascular dilation (hypertension, hypercapnia, hypoxia, acidosis) disrupt the BBB. Hyperosmotic fluids, which cause shrinkage of vascular endothelium and widen the vascular junctions, also disrupt the BBB.

INCREASED INTRACRANIAL PRESSURE

The brain, tightly enclosed in the solid bony cranium, is well protected but highly vulnerable to pressure that may accumulate within the enclosure. Its total volume—brain (80%), CSF (10%), and blood (10%)—must remain approximately the same at all times. A change in the proportional volume of one of these components (e.g., increase or decrease in intracranial blood) must be accompanied by a compensatory change in another (e.g., decrease or increase in CSF). In this way the volume and pressure normally remain constant. Examples of compensatory changes are reduction in blood volume, decrease in production of CSF, increase in CSF absorption, or shrinkage of brain mass by displacement of intracellular and extracellular fluid.

Children with open fontanels compensate for increased volume by skull expansion and widened sutures. However, at any age the capacity for spatial compensation is limited. An increase in ICP may be caused by tumors or other space-occupying lesions, accumulation of fluid within the ventricular system, bleeding, or edema of cerebral tissues. Once compensation is exhausted, any further increase in volume results in a rapid rise in ICP.

BOX 37-1 CLINICAL MANIFESTATIONS OF INCREASED INTRACRANIAL PRESSURE IN INFANTS AND CHILDREN

Infants
Tense, bulging fontanel
Separated cranial sutures
Macewen (cracked-pot) sign
Irritability and restlessness
Drowsiness
Increased sleeping
High-pitched cry
Increased frontooccipital circumference
Distended scalp veins
Poor feeding
Crying when disturbed
Setting-sun sign

Children
Headache
Nausea
Forceful vomiting
Diplopia, blurred vision
Seizures
Indifference, drowsiness
Decline in school performance
Diminished physical activity and motor performance
Increased sleeping
Inability to follow simple commands
Lethargy

Late Signs in Infants and Children
Bradycardia
Decreased motor response to command
Decreased sensory response to painful stimuli
Alterations in pupil size and reactivity
Extension or flexion posturing
Cheyne-Stokes respirations
Papilledema
Decreased consciousness
Coma

The early signs and symptoms of increased ICP are often subtle, such as headache, vomiting, personality changes, irritability, and fatigue (Box 37-1). In older children subjective symptoms are headache, especially when lying flat (e.g., on awakening in the morning) or when coughing, sneezing, or bending over, and nausea and vomiting. The child may complain of double vision or blurred vision with movement of the head. Seizures may occur. In children whose cranial sutures have not closed, there is an increase in head circumference and tense or bulging fontanels. Cranial sutures may become diastatic or may split; head circumference can enlarge until the child is 5 years of age if the condition progresses slowly. As pressure increases, the pupils become progressively sluggish in reaction and eventually become fixed and dilated. The level of consciousness progressively deteriorates from drowsiness to eventual coma. Problems related to increased ICP are discussed later in this chapter in relation to head injury. (See Brain Tumors, Chapter 36, and Hydrocephalus, Chapter 11.)

Physiologic and biochemical changes within the cerebral vasculature serve to complicate the primary causes of increased ICP. Especially in cases of trauma, blood flow often initially increases as a result of venous congestion or vasomotor paralysis. If cerebral hypoxia is associated with the cerebral dysfunction, the compensatory vasodilation caused by oxygen deficiency will tend to increase the cerebral flow. However, blood flow is reduced as ICP progressively increases, with diminished blood supply to the brain tissues. The classic responses observed in adults (widening pulse pressure, increased blood pressure) rarely occur in children or are very late signs. Periodic or irregular breathing is an ominous sign of brainstem (especially medullary) dysfunction that often precedes apnea.

EVALUATION OF NEUROLOGIC STATUS

Earlier chapters discuss methods to evaluate neurologic function in relation to numerous aspects of child care. The neurologic examination is an integral part of the health assessment (see Chapter 6) and newborn assessment (see Chapter 8). Chapter 40 discusses some of the tests used to differentiate neuromuscular disorders. The assessment tools and examinations in this chapter are primarily those used to assess intracranial integrity.

ASSESSMENT: GENERAL ASPECTS

Children younger than 2 years of age require special evaluation because they are unable to respond to directions designed to elicit specific neurologic responses. Early neurologic responses in infants are primarily reflexive; these responses are gradually replaced by meaningful movement in the characteristic cephalocaudal direction of development. This evidence of progressive maturation reflects more extensive myelinization and changes in neurochemical and electrophysiologic properties.

Most information about infants and small children comes from observation of spontaneous and elicited reflex responses. As they develop increasingly complex gross and fine motor skills and communication skills, more sophisticated techniques are used to assess acquisition of developmental milestones. Delay or deviation from expected milestones helps to identify high-risk children. Persistence or reappearance of primitive reflexes indicates a pathologic condition. In evaluating the infant or young child, it is important to obtain the history of the pregnancy, delivery, respiratory status at birth, and neonatal health to determine the possible impact of intrauterine and extrauterine environmental influences known to affect the orderly maturation of the CNS. These influences include maternal infections, chemicals, trauma, medication, illicit drug use, and metabolic insults.

History

A family history can sometimes offer clues regarding possible genetic disorders with neurologic manifestations. A review of family members often identifies conditions that might otherwise be overlooked, especially increased number of miscarriages or siblings or relatives who died at an early age. The nurse asks questions regarding specific neurologic problems, such as intellectual and developmental disabilities, deafness, epilepsy, blindness, unusual movements, weakness, ataxia, stroke, and progressive mental deterioration. History of consanguinity is also important.

A health history provides valuable clues regarding the cause of neurologic dysfunction. Is there a history of injury with loss of consciousness, febrile illness, an encounter with an animal or insect, ingestion of neurotoxic substances, inhalation of chemicals, past illness, or known diabetes mellitus or sickle cell disease? Sudden or progressive alterations in movement or mental abilities may provide clues for investigation. It is also important to ascertain the chronologic course of the illness.

Physical Examination

Physical examination includes observation of the size and shape of the head (particularly in the infant and young child), spontaneous activity and postural reflex activity, and sensory responses. Note whether the patient is lethargic, drowsy, stuporous, alert, active, or irritable. The nurse also observes the overall tone, noting whether there is a normal flexed posture or one of extreme extension, opisthotonos, or hypotonia. Symmetry of movement is also assessed.

Facial features may suggest a specific syndrome. A high-pitched, piercing cry in an infant is often associated with CNS disorders. An abnormal respiratory cycle, such as prolonged apnea, ataxic breathing, paradoxic chest movement, and hyperventilation, may be the result of a neurologic problem.

Older children can be evaluated by the usual methods used in a neurologic examination. In addition, an estimation of the level of development provides essential information about neurologic function. This assessment is discussed throughout the book in relation to evaluation for specific disorders such as intellectual and developmental disabilities, failure to thrive, attention deficit hyperactivity disorder, cerebral palsy, cerebral tumors, and other physical or behavioral problems. Developmental screening tests can assess developmental progress in the young child. (See Appendix A.)

Muscular activity and coordination, including ocular movements and gait, are valuable sources of information. Ocular movements, pupillary response, facial movements, and mouth functions provide clues regarding CNS involvement or impingement. (See Chapter 6 for CNS and reflex testing, p. 176.) Testing reflexes, strength, and coordination and for the presence and location of tremors, twitching, tics, or other unusual movements is also an aspect of the neurologic assessment (Box 37-2). Box 37-3 describes abnormalities of gait that indicate cerebral dysfunction.

ALTERED STATES OF CONSCIOUSNESS

Consciousness implies awareness—the ability to respond to sensory stimuli and have subjective experiences. Consciousness has two aspects: alertness, an arousal-waking state that includes the ability to respond to stimuli; and cognitive power, which includes the ability to process stimuli and produce verbal and motor responses.

An altered state of consciousness usually refers to varying states of unconsciousness that may be momentary or may last for hours, days, or indefinitely. Unconsciousness is depressed cerebral function—the inability to respond to sensory stimuli and have subjective experiences. Coma is defined as a state of

---

BOX 37-2 ABNORMAL INVOLUNTARY MUSCULAR MOVEMENTS

Ataxia—Gross incoordination that may become worse with the eyes closed

Spasm—Involuntary contraction of a muscle

Spasticity—Prolonged and steady contraction of a muscle characterized by clonus (alternating relaxation and contraction of the muscle) and exaggerated reflexes

Rigidity—Inability to flex or extend a joint

Tremors—Constant small involuntary movements

Twitching—Spasmodic movements of short duration

Tic—Involuntary, compulsive, stereotyped movement of an associated group of muscles

Choreiform movements—Quick, jerky, grossly uncoordinated, irregular movements that may disappear on relaxation

Athetosis—Slow, writhing, wormlike, constant, grossly uncoordinated movements that increase on voluntary activity and decrease on relaxation

Dystonia—Slow twisting movements of limbs or trunk

Associated movements—Voluntary movement of one muscle accompanied by involuntary movement of another muscle

Mirroring movements—Same as associated movements except with symmetric muscle groups

---

BOX 37-3 ABNORMALITIES OF GAIT THAT INDICATE CEREBRAL DYSFUNCTION

Ataxia—Impaired ability to coordinate movements; staggering gait and postural imbalance.

Spastic paraplegic gait—Narrow-based gait with a tendency to walk on toes, along with flexion at knees and hips, and shuffling. Hips are adducted, and knees may strike each other with each step; in younger children a "scissoring" position results when lower limbs cross because of increased adductor tone. Patients walk stiffly; take slow, deliberate steps; and have difficulty when attempting to walk on heels or run.

Spastic hemiplegic gait—Involved leg extended, circumducted, plantar flexion. The affected arm is flexed and adducted and does not swing.

Cerebellar gait—Staggering, unsteadiness, wide-based gait; tendency to veer in one lateral direction; often accompanied by swaying of the trunk.

Extrapyramidal gait—Rigidity, few automatic movements, and bradykinesia (slowness of all movements) with associated bending of trunk and head, arms adducted at shoulders and flexed at elbows and wrists, fingers extended; festination (upper body moving forward in advance of lower part), causing rapid steps and risk of falling.

---

unconsciousness from which the patient cannot be aroused, even with powerful stimuli.

⚠ NURSING ALERT

Lack of response to painful stimuli is abnormal and must be reported immediately.

The seat of consciousness, or "alerting area," of the brain is in the reticular formation—the central core of the brainstem. The reticular formation extends from the midbrain to the medulla. The reticular activating system receives collaterals from and is stimulated by every major somatic and special sensory pathway in the brain. Disturbances of consciousness may occur when any part of the reticular, thalamic, hypothalamic, and cortical circuits is sufficiently impaired. However, the effects may vary according to the areas involved. For example, small lesions of the reticular or hypothalamic regions produce a profound effect, whereas extensive impairment of the cortex is required to produce quantitatively similar results.

Etiology

An altered state of consciousness may be the outcome of several processes that affect the CNS. Impaired neurologic function can result from a direct or indirect cause. Some altered states, such as the diffuse changes observed in encephalitis, are directly related to cerebral insult. Others are the result of dysfunction in other organs or processes. For example, biochemical changes can impair neurologic function without morphologic findings, as in hypoglycemia.

Level of Consciousness

Assessment of level of consciousness (LOC) remains the earliest indicator of improvement or deterioration in neurologic status. LOC is determined by observations of the child's responses to the environment. Other diagnostic tests, such as motor activity, reflexes, and vital signs, are more variable and do not necessarily directly parallel the depth of the comatose state. The most consistently used terms are described in Box 37-4.

Coma Assessment

Diminished alertness as a result of pathologic conditions occurs on a continuum and is designated as the comatose state, which extends from somnolence at one end to deep coma at the other. To produce coma, one of the following must occur: (1) extensive, diffuse, bilateral cerebral hemispheric destruction (the brainstem may be intact), (2) a lesion in the diencephalon, or (3) destruction of the brainstem down to the level of the lower pons.

Several scales have been devised in an attempt to standardize the description and interpretation of the degree of depressed consciousness. The most popular of these is the Glasgow Coma Scale (GCS), which consists of a three-part assessment: eye opening, verbal response, and motor response. The GCS was created to meet a clinical need to identify criteria for the consciousness level. For clinical purposes, the primary role of observation of the LOC is to detect a life-threatening complication such as cerebral edema. The GCS requires observational skills and is readily reproducible between observers.

A pediatric version of the GCS recognizes that expected verbal and motor responses must be related to the child's age (Fig. 37-2). The pediatric coma scale does not assess verbal responses as such but records smiling, crying, and interaction. It uses a 6-point motor scale that is inappropriate for children below the age of 6 months. In children under 5 years of age, speech is understood to be any sound at all, even crying. Young children demonstrate orientation by identifying their parents correctly or giving their own names. When assessing LOC in young children, the nurse may find it helpful to have a parent present to help elicit a desired response. An infant or child may not respond in an unfamiliar environment or to unfamiliar voices.

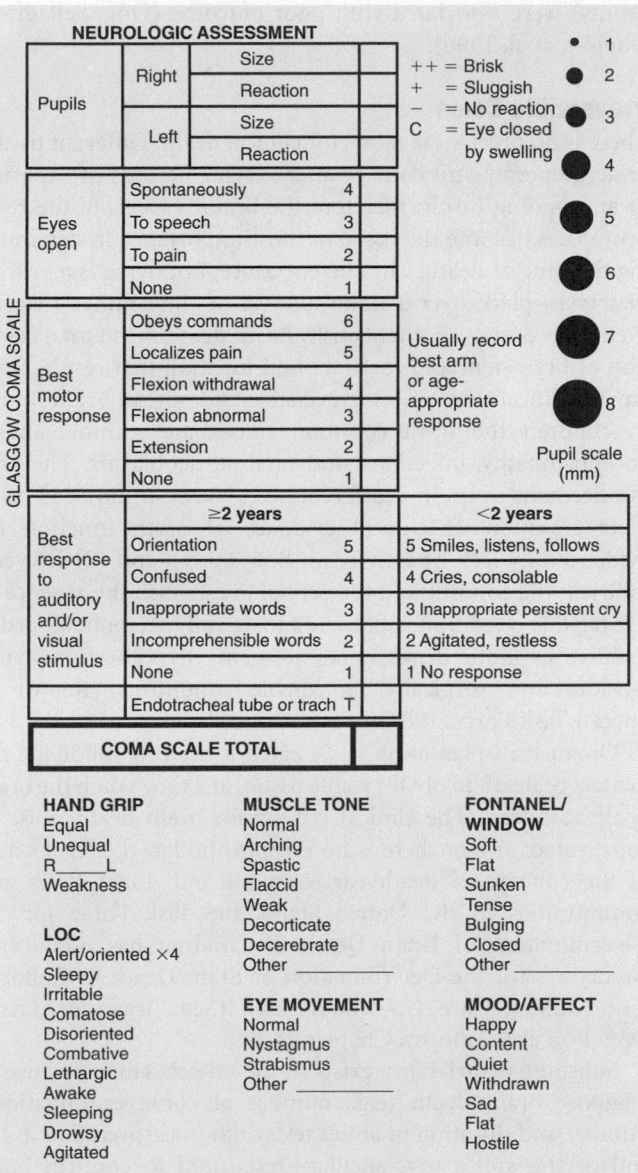

Fig. 37-2 Pediatric coma scale.

BOX 37-4   LEVELS OF CONSCIOUSNESS

Full consciousness—Awake and alert, orientated to time, place, and person; behavior appropriate for age.

Confusion—Impaired decision making.

Disorientation—Confusion regarding time, place; decreased level of consciousness.

Lethargy—Limited spontaneous movement, sluggish speech, drowsy, falling asleep quickly.

Obtundation—Arousable with stimulation.

Stupor—Remaining in a deep sleep, slow response to vigorous and repeated stimulation or moaning responses to stimuli.

Coma—No motor or verbal response or extension posturing to noxious (painful) stimuli.

Persistent vegetative state (PVS)—Permanently lost function of the cerebral cortex. Eyes follow objects only by reflex or when attracted to the direction of loud sounds; all four limbs are spastic but can withdraw from painful stimuli; hands show reflexive grasping and groping; the face can grimace, some food may be swallowed, and the child may groan or cry but utter no words.

Modified from Seidel HM, Ball JW, Dains JE, et al, editors: *Mosby's guide to physical examination*, ed 5, St Louis, 2003, Mosby.

Numeric values are assigned to the levels of response in each category. The sum of these numeric values provides an objective measurement of the patient's LOC. The lower the score, the deeper the coma. A person with an unaltered LOC would score the highest, 15; a score of 8 or below is generally accepted as a definition of coma; the lowest score, 3, indicates deep coma or death.

The GCS in itself is not sufficient to determine the responses of all children. For example, because a child with quadriplegia cannot respond to commands physically, the child can score very low but be cerebrally intact. Nevertheless, the GCS provides a more objective method for evaluating the state of consciousness in most cases. Severely injured children (GCS ≤ 8) may have a consistent grading of motor response, verbal response, and eye opening.

The GCS at admission is predictive of abnormal neurologic findings at discharge only when profoundly depressed (≤6); otherwise the GCS is not useful as a prognostic tool when used alone (White, Farukhi, Bull, et al, 2001). GCS scores of less than 8 in combination with other abnormal findings (e.g., hypoxia on admission and abnormal computed tomography [CT] results) were associated with poor outcome (Ong, Selladurai, Dhillon, et al, 1996).

Irreversible Coma

There is no precise diagnosis for clinical death. Different tissues undergo permanent damage after varying periods of exposure to an ongoing insult; therefore the brain (especially the cerebrum) has become the tissue of most importance in determining the time of death. The current concept of dying is a process that takes place over a finite interval of time rather than an event that occurs spontaneously. Brain death is the total cessation of brainstem and cortical brain function that results from any condition that causes irreversible widespread brain injury. In children the most common causes are trauma, anoxic encephalopathy, infections, and cerebral neoplasms. The pronouncement of brain death requires two conditions: (1) complete cessation of clinical evidence of brain function (as evidenced by lack of activity on flow study), and (2) irreversibility of the condition. It is essential to establish the absence of a reversible condition, especially a toxic and metabolic disorder, sedative-hypnotic drugs, paralytic agents, hypothermia, hypotension, and surgically remediable conditions (Report of Special Task Force, 1987).

Organ transplantation has created a need to subdivide the process of death to obtain viable tissues at a time when the brain is already dead. The clinical criteria for brain death must be constituted so that there is no error. Although the legal status of the concept of death varies among individual states and communities in the United States, the Task Force for the Determination of Brain Death in Children has established Guidelines for the Determination of Brain Death in Children (see Nursing Care Guidelines box). (See Organ or Tissue Donation and Autopsy, Chapter 23.)

Substantial variability exists in the criteria clinicians use to diagnose brain death (e.g., number of coma examinations, number and duration of apnea tests, P_{CO_2} measurements at the end of the apnea test, ancillary tests used to confirm brain

---

NURSING CARE GUIDELINES
Establishing Brain Death in Children

Coma and apnea must coexist. Child must exhibit complete loss of consciousness, vocalization, and volitional activity.

Brainstem function must be absent, as defined by:
- Midposition or fully dilated pupils that do not respond to light. Drugs may influence and invalidate pupillary assessment.
- Absence of spontaneous eye movements and those induced by oculocephalic and caloric (oculovestibular) testing.
- Absence of movement of bulbar musculature, including facial and oropharyngeal muscles. The corneal, gag, cough, sucking, and rooting reflexes are absent.
- Absence of respiratory movements when child is removed from respirator. Apnea testing using standardized methods can be performed but is done after other criteria are met.

Child must not be significantly hypothermic or hypotensive for age.

Flaccid tone and absence of spontaneous or induced movements, including spinal cord events such as reflex withdrawal or spinal myoclonus, should exist.

Examination should remain consistent with brain death throughout the observation and testing period.

Observation periods according to age:
7 days to 2 months—Two separate examinations and two electroencephalograms (EEGs), separated by at least 48 hours
2 months to 1 year—Two separate examinations and two EEGs, separated by at least 24 hours
Over 1 year—Two separate examinations separated by at least 12 hours; if irreversible cause exists, no laboratory testing needed; if difficult to assess extent of reversibility of brain damage, observation indicated for at least 24 hours

Modified from Task Force for the Determination of Brain Death in Children: Guidelines for the determination of brain death in children, *Ann Neurol* 21:616, 1987; Janakiraman N: Brain death, *Indian J Pediatr* 65:525-527, 1998; and Lutz-Dettinger N, de Jaeger A, Kerremans I: Care of the potential pediatric organ donor, *Pediatr Clin North Am* 48:715-749, 2001.

---

death, organ procurement, and reasons for nonprocurement) (DeVita, 2001; Mathur, Petersen, Stadtler, et al, 2008).

NEUROLOGIC EXAMINATION

The purpose of the neurologic examination is to establish an accurate, objective baseline of neurologic function. Therefore it is essential that the neurologic examination be documented in a descriptive and detailed fashion, thereby enhancing the ability to detect subtle changes in neurologic status over time. Descriptions of behaviors should be simple, objective, and easily interpreted—for example, "Drowsy but awake and conversationally rational/oriented"; "Sleepy but arousable with vigorous physical stimuli. Pressure to nail base of right hand results in upper extremity flexion/lower extremity extension."

Vital signs, observation of posture and movement (both spontaneous and elicited), eye examination, CN testing, and reflex testing all provide valuable clues regarding the LOC, the site of involvement, and the probable cause, but they do not necessarily parallel the depth of a comatose state.

Vital Signs

Pulse, respiration, and blood pressure provide information regarding the adequacy of circulation and the possible underlying cause of altered consciousness. Autonomic activity is most intensively disturbed in deep coma and in brainstem lesions. Body temperature is often elevated; sometimes the elevation is extreme. High temperature is most often a sign of an acute infectious process or heatstroke, but may be caused by ingestion of some drugs (especially salicylates, alcohol, and barbiturates) or by intracranial bleeding, especially subarachnoid hemorrhage. Hypothalamic involvement may cause elevated or decreased temperature. Serious infection may produce hypothermia.

The pulse is variable and may be rapid, slow and bounding, or feeble. Blood pressure may be normal, elevated, or very low. The Cushing reflex, or pressor response that causes a slowing of the pulse and an increase in blood pressure, is uncommon in children; when it does occur, it is a very late sign of increased ICP. Medications can also affect vital signs. For assessment purposes, actual changes in pulse and blood pressure are more important than the direction of the change.

Respirations are more often slow, deep, and irregular. Slow and deep breathing often occurs in the heavy sleep caused by sedatives, after seizures, or in cerebral infections. Slow, shallow breathing may result from sedatives or opioids. Hyperventilation (deep and rapid respirations) is usually the result of metabolic acidosis or abnormal stimulation of the respiratory center in the medulla caused by salicylate poisoning, hepatic coma, or Reye syndrome (RS). A pattern of alternating hyperventilation and breath holding during wakefulness is common in Rett syndrome.

Breathing patterns have been described with a number of terms (e.g., *apneustic, cluster, ataxic, Cheyne-Stokes*). However, it is better to describe what is being observed rather than placing a label on it because the terms are often used and interpreted incorrectly. Periodic or irregular breathing is a sign of brainstem (especially medullary) dysfunction. This is an ominous sign that often precedes complete apnea. The odor of the breath may provide additional clues (e.g., the fruity and acetone odor of ketosis, the foul odor of uremia, the fetid odor of hepatic failure, or the odor of alcohol).

Skin

The skin may offer clues to the cause of unconsciousness. The body surface should be examined for injury, needle marks, petechiae, bites, and ticks. Evidence of toxic substances may be found on the hands, face, mouth, and clothing—especially in small children.

Eyes

Assess pupil size and reactivity (Fig. 37-3). Pupils either react or do not react to light. Pinpoint pupils are commonly observed in poisoning (e.g., opiate or barbiturate poisoning) or in brainstem dysfunction. Widely dilated and reactive pupils are often seen after seizures and may involve only one side. Widely dilated and fixed pupils suggest paralysis of CN III (oculomotor nerve) secondary to pressure from herniation of the brain through the tentorium. A unilateral fixed pupil usually suggests a lesion on the same side. Bilateral fixed pupils usually imply brainstem damage if present for more than 5 minutes. Dilated and nonreactive pupils also occur in hypothermia, anoxia, ischemia, poisoning with atropine-like substances, or prior instillation of mydriatic drugs. Some of the therapies used (e.g., barbiturates) can alter pupil size and reaction.

The description of eye movements should indicate whether one or both eyes are involved and how the reaction was elicited. Ask the parents if the child has strabismus, which will cause the eyes to appear normal under compromise.

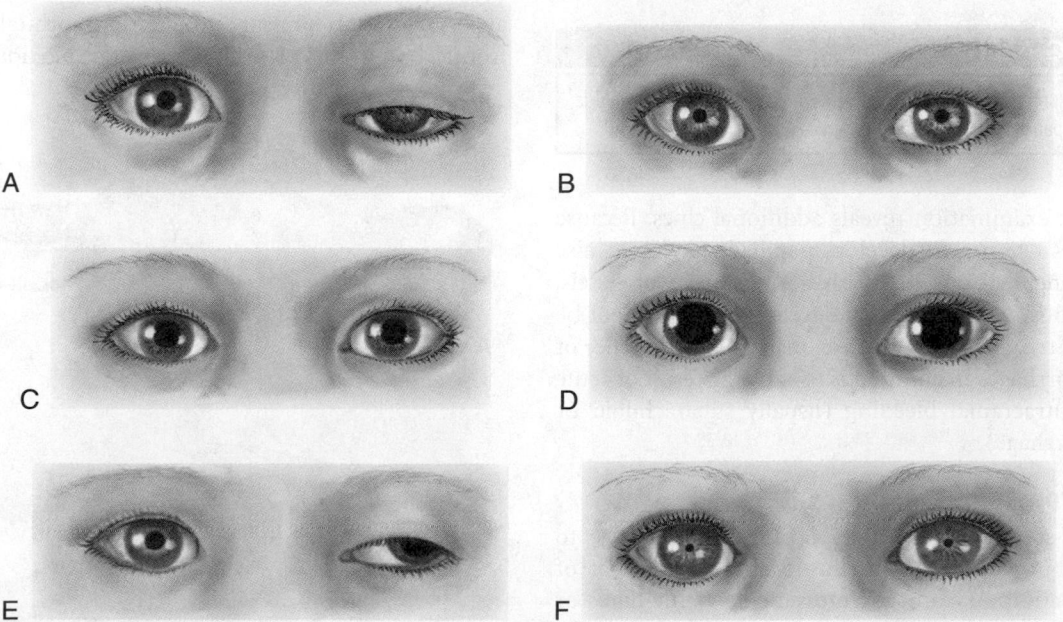

Fig. 37-3 Variations in pupil size with altered states of consciousness. **A,** Ipsilateral pupillary constriction with slight ptosis. **B,** Bilateral small pupils. **C,** Midposition, light fixed to all stimuli. **D,** Bilateral dilated and fixed pupils. **E,** Dilated pupils, left eye abducted with ptosis. **F,** Pinpoint pupils.

Blinking observed at rest or in response to a sudden loud noise or bright light implies that the pontine reticular formation is intact. The corneal reflex, blinking of the eyelids when the cornea is touched with a wisp of cotton or a camel hair pencil, can test the integrity of the ophthalmic division of CN V (trigeminal nerve). Posttraumatic strabismus indicates CN VI (abducens nerve) damage.

Eye movements are assessed by the doll's head maneuver, in which the child's head is rotated quickly to one side and then to the other. When the brainstem centers for eye movement are intact, there is conjugate (paired or working together) movement of the eyes in the direction opposite the head rotation. Absence of this response suggests dysfunction of the brainstem or CN III. Downward or lateral deviation is often observed in association with pupillary dilation in dysfunction of CN III.

The caloric test, or oculovestibular response, is elicited by irrigating the external auditory canal with 10 ml of ice water over a period of approximately 20 seconds (with the head of bed elevated at a 30-degree angle). This test normally causes movement of the eyes toward the side of stimulation. This response is lost when the pontine centers are impaired and thus provides important information in assessment of the comatose patient.

Funduscopic examination reveals additional clues. Because it takes 24 to 48 hours to develop, papilledema (optic disc swelling, indistinct margins, hemorrhages, tortuosity of vessels, absence of venous pulsations), if it develops at all, will not be evident early in the course of unconsciousness. The presence of preretinal hemorrhages in children is usually the result of acute trauma with intracranial bleeding (usually subarachnoid or subdural hemorrhage).

Motor Function

Observation of spontaneous activity, posture, and response to painful stimuli provides clues to the location and extent of cerebral dysfunction. Asymmetric movements of the limbs or the absence of movement suggests paralysis. In hemiplegia the affected limb lies in external rotation and falls uncontrollably when lifted and allowed to drop. Observations should be described rather than labeled.

In the deeper comatose states the child has little or no spontaneous movement, and the musculature tends to be flaccid. There is considerable variability in motor behavior in lesser degrees of coma. For example, the child may be relatively immobile or restless and hyperkinetic; muscle tone may be increased or decreased. Tremors, twitching, and spasms of muscles are common observations. The patient may display purposeless plucking or tossing movements. Combative or negativistic behavior is not uncommon. Hyperactivity is more common in acute febrile and toxic states than in cases of increased ICP. Seizures are common in children and may be present in coma as a result of any cause. Any repetitive or seizure movements are described.

Posturing

Primitive postural reflexes emerge as cortical control over motor function is lost in brain dysfunction. These reflexes are evident in posturing and motor movements directly related to the area of the brain involved. Posturing reflects a balance between the lower exciting and the higher inhibiting influences, and strong muscles overcome weaker ones. Flexion posturing (Fig. 37-4, *A*) occurs with severe dysfunction of the cerebral cortex or with lesions to corticospinal tracts above the brainstem. Typical flexion posturing includes rigid flexion, with arms held tightly to the body; flexed elbows, wrists, and fingers; plantar flexed feet; legs extended and internally rotated; and possibly fine tremors or intense stiffness. Extension posturing (Fig. 37-4, *B*) is a sign of dysfunction at the level of the midbrain or lesions to the brainstem. It is characterized by rigid extension and pronation of the arms and legs, flexed wrists and fingers, clenched jaw, extended neck, and possibly an arched back. Unilateral extension posturing is often caused by tentorial herniation.

Posturing may not be evident when the child is quiet but can usually be elicited by applying painful stimuli, such as a blunt object pressed on the base of the nail. Nurses should avoid applying thumb pressure to the supraorbital region of the frontal bone (risk of orbital damage). Noxious stimuli (e.g.,

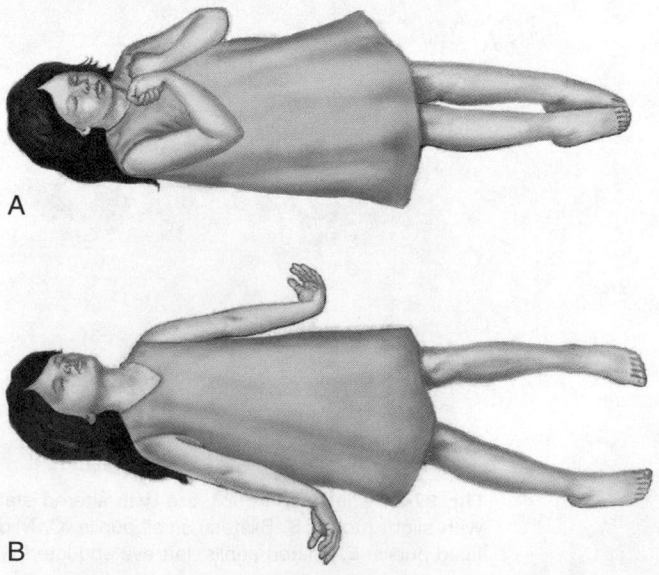

Fig. 37-4 A, Flexion posturing. **B,** Extension posturing.

suctioning) will elicit a response, as may turning or touching. When the nurse is describing posturing, the stimulus needed to provoke the response is as important as the reaction.

Reflexes

Testing of certain reflexes, such as those present in an intact spinal cord, may be of limited value. (See Chapter 6.) In general, the corneal, pupillary, muscle-stretch, superficial, and plantar reflexes tend to be absent in deep coma. The state of reflexes is variable in lighter grades of unconsciousness and depends on the underlying pathologic process and the location of the lesion. The doll's eye reflex maneuver, described previously, reflects paralysis of CN III. The absence of corneal reflexes (CN V) and the presence of a tonic neck reflex are associated with severe brain damage. The Babinski reflex, in which the lateral portion of the foot is stroked, may be of value if it is found to be present consistently in children older than 1 year. A positive Babinski reflex is significant in the assessment of pyramidal tract lesions when it is unilateral and associated with other pyramidal signs. A fluctuating Babinski reflex is often observed after seizures. (See Fig. 8-10, *B*, p. 250.)

NURSING TIP Three key reflexes that demonstrate neurologic health in young infants are the Moro, tonic neck, and withdrawal reflexes.

SPECIAL DIAGNOSTIC PROCEDURES

Numerous diagnostic procedures are used for assessment of cerebral function. Laboratory tests that may help determine the cause of unconsciousness include blood glucose, urea nitrogen, and electrolyte (pH, sodium, potassium, chloride, calcium, and bicarbonate) tests; clotting studies, hematocrit, and a complete blood count; liver function tests; blood cultures if there is fever; and sometimes studies to detect lead or other toxic substances, such as drugs.

An electroencephalogram (EEG) may provide important information. For example, generalized random, slow activity suggests suppressed cortical function, and localized slow activity suggests a space-occupying lesion. A flat tracing is one of the criteria used as evidence of brain death. Examination of spinal fluid is carried out when toxic encephalopathy or infection is suspected. Lumbar puncture is ordinarily delayed if intracranial hemorrhage is suspected, and is contraindicated in the presence of ICP because of the potential for brainstem herniation.

Auditory and visual evoked potentials are sometimes used in neurologic evaluation of very young children. Brainstem auditory evoked potentials are useful for evaluating the continuity of brainstem auditory tracts and are particularly useful for detecting demyelinating disease and neoplasms of the brainstem, and for distinguishing between brainstem and cortical lesions. For example, a normal evoked potential in a comatose patient suggests involvement of the cerebral hemispheres.

Highly sophisticated tests are carried out with specialized equipment. Two imaging techniques, CT and magnetic resonance imaging (MRI) (Fig. 37-5), assist in diagnosis by scanning both soft tissues and solid matter. Most of these tests are listed in Table 37-1. Because such tests can be threatening to

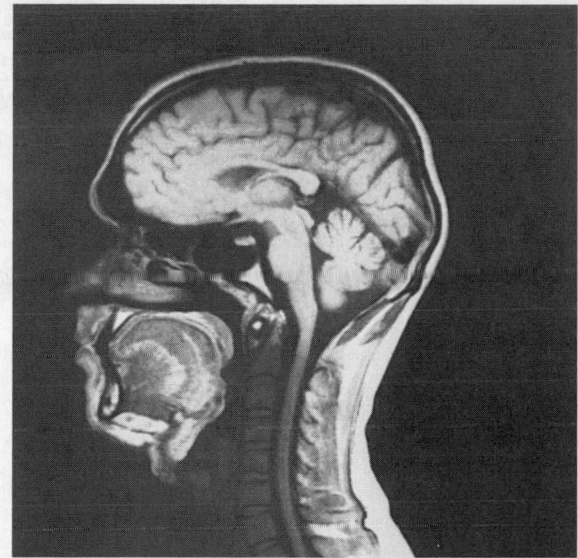

Fig. 37-5 Magnetic resonance imaging. Midsagittal image produces excellent anatomic detail. Note clear delineation of structures such as pituitary gland, brainstem, spinal cord, cerebellum, corpus callosum, and sylvian aqueduct. (Courtesy Philips Medical Systems. From Nolte J: *The human brain: an introduction to its functional anatomy*, ed 3, St Louis, 1993, Mosby.)

children, the nurse needs to prepare patients for the tests and provide support and reassurance during the tests. (See Preparation for Diagnostic and Therapeutic Procedures, Chapter 27.)

Children who are old enough to understand require careful explanation of the procedure, why it is being done, what they will experience, and how they can help. School-age children usually appreciate a more detailed description of why contrast material is injected. The importance of lying still for tests needs to be stressed. Children unfamiliar with the machines can be shown a picture beforehand. Although radiographic examinations are not painful, the machinery often appears so frightening that the child protests because of anxiety.

This is especially true of CT and MRI, both of which require that the child's head be placed within a special immobilizing device. Chin and cheek pads are sometimes used to prevent the slightest head movement, and straps are applied to the body to prevent a slight change in body position. The nurse can explain these events to a frightened child by comparing them to an astronaut's preparation for a space flight. It is important to emphasize to the child that at no time is the procedure painful.

It is helpful for nurses to become acquainted with the equipment and the general environment in which the test will take place so they can better explain the procedure to children at their level of understanding. Written material describing the procedure should be available for parents and may be appropriate to share with children. Equipment is often strange and ominous to children and may be perceived as a frightening monster. They need constant reassurance from a trusted companion. Because children are particularly frightened of needles, they need to be informed of any medication or contrast medium that will be administered intravenously.

The nurse should not expect cooperation from a young child. Sedation may be required. Many different agents are

TABLE 37-1 NEUROLOGIC DIAGNOSTIC PROCEDURES

TEST	DESCRIPTION	PURPOSE	COMMENTS
Lumbar puncture (LP)	Spinal needle is inserted between L3-L4 or L4-L5 vertebral spaces into subarachnoid space; cerebrospinal fluid (CSF) pressure is measured, and sample is collected for examination.	Measures spinal fluid pressure, obtains CSF for laboratory analysis Injection of medication	Contraindicated in patients with increased intracranial pressure (ICP) or infected skin over puncture site.
Subdural tap	Needle is inserted into anterior fontanel or coronal suture (midline to pupil).	Helps rule out subdural effusions Removes CSF to relieve pressure	Place infant in semierect position after subdural tap to minimize leakage from site; prevent child from crying if possible. Check site frequently for evidence of leakage.
Ventricular puncture	Needle is inserted into lateral ventricle via coronal suture (midline to pupil).	Removes CSF to relieve pressure	Risk of intracerebral or ventricular hemorrhage.
Electroencephalography (EEG)	EEG records changes in electrical potential of brain. Electrodes are placed at various points to assess electrical function in a particular area. Impulses are recorded by electromagnetic pen or digitally.	Detects spikes, or bursts of electrical activity that indicate the potential for seizures Used to determine brain death	Patient should remain quiet during procedure; may require sedation. Minimize external stimuli during procedure.
Nuclear brain scan	Radioisotope is injected intravenously, then counted and recorded after fixed time intervals. Radioisotope accumulates in areas where blood-brain barrier is defective.	Identifies focal brain lesions (e.g., tumors, abscesses) Positive uptake of material with encephalitis and subdural hematoma Visualizes CSF pathways	Requires intravenous (IV) access; patient may require sedation. In normal children or noncommunicating hydrocephalus, no retrograde filling of ventricles occurs. Areas of concentrated uptake of material are termed *hot spots*.
Endocephalography	Pulses of ultrasonic waves are beamed through head; echoes from reflecting surfaces are recorded graphically.	Identifies shifts in midline structures from their normal positions as a result of intracranial lesions May show ventricular dilation	Simple, safe, rapid procedure. Fontanel must be patent.
Real-time ultrasonography (RTUS)	RTUS is similar to CT but uses ultrasound instead of ionizing radiation.	Allows high-resolution anatomic visualization in variety of imaging planes	Produces images similar to CT scan. Especially useful in neonatal central nervous system problems. Anterior fontanel must be patent.
Radiography	Skull films are taken from different views—lateral, posterolateral, axial (submentoventricular), half-axial.	Shows fractures, dislocations, spreading suture lines, craniostenosis Shows degenerative changes, bone erosion, calcifications	Simple, noninvasive procedure.
Computed tomography (CT) scan	Pinpoint x-ray beam is directed on horizontal or vertical plane to provide series of images that are fed into computer and assembled in image displayed on video screen. CT uses ionizing radiation.	Visualizes horizontal and vertical cross section of brain in three planes (axial, coronal, sagittal) Distinguishes density of various intracranial tissues and structures—congenital abnormalities, hemorrhage, tumors, demyelinating and inflammatory processes, calcification	Requires IV access if contrast agent is used. Patient may require sedation. Rapid.
Magnetic resonance imaging (MRI)	MRI produces radiofrequency emissions from elements (e.g., hydrogen, phosphorus), which are converted to visual images by computer.	Permits visualization of morphologic feature of target structures Permits tissue discrimination unavailable with many techniques	MRI is noninvasive procedure except when IV contrast agent is used. No exposure to radiation occurs. Patient may require sedation. Parent or attendant can remain in room with child. MRI does not visualize bone detail or calcifications. No metal can be present in scanner.
Positron emission tomography (PET)	PET involves IV injection of positron-emitting radionucleotide; local concentrations are detected and transformed into visual display by computer.	Detects and measures blood volume and flow in brain, metabolic activity, biochemical changes within tissue	Requires lengthy period of immobility. Minimum exposure to radiation occurs. Patient may require sedation.
Digital subtraction angiography (DSA)	Contrast dye is injected intravenously; computer "subtracts" all tissues without contrast medium, leaving clear image of contrast medium in vessels studied.	Visualizes vasculature of target tissue Visualizes finite vascular abnormalities	Safe alternative to angiography. Patient must remain still during procedure; may require sedation.
Single-photon emission computed tomography (SPECT)	SPECT involves IV injection of photon-emitting radionuclide; radionuclides are absorbed by healthy tissue at different rate than diseased or necrotic tissue; data are transferred to computer that converts image to film.	Provides information regarding blood flow to tissues; analyzing blood flow to organ may help determine how well it is functioning	Requires lengthy period of immobility. Minimum exposure to radiation occurs. Patient may require sedation.

currently used for sedation of children undergoing neurologic diagnostic procedures. Chloral hydrate or benzodiazepines have been used for decades as short-term sedative agents and remain safe methods of pediatric outpatient sedation (Wetzell, 2009). Chloral hydrate is used alone for sedating children for procedures such as MRI. In recent years other sedative agents have been used safely, alone and in combination, for children in the outpatient setting. These include intravenous (IV) sodium pentobarbital (Nembutal), IV fentanyl (Sublimaze), IV midazolam (Versed) (Wetzell, 2009), and intranasal midazolam (Ljungman, Kreuger, Andreasson, et al, 2000; Lloyd, Alredy, and Lloyd, 2000). (See Pain Management, Chapter 7.)

Physical preparation for the diagnostic test may involve administration of a sedative. If so, children should be helped through the preparation and administration and assured that someone will remain with them (if this is possible). Children need continual support and reinforcement during procedures in which they remain conscious. Vital signs and physiologic responses to the procedure are monitored throughout. Many diagnostic procedures performed on an outpatient basis require sedation, and children need recovery time and observation. The nurse should review written instructions with parents if the child is discharged after a procedure. Children who have undergone a procedure with a general anesthetic require postanesthesia care, including positioning to prevent aspiration of secretions and frequent assessment of the vital signs and LOC. In addition, other neurologic functions such as pupillary responses, motor strength, and movement are tested at regular intervals. Any surgical wound resulting from the test is checked for bleeding, CSF leakage, and other complications. Children who undergo repeated subdural taps should have their hematocrit monitored to detect excessive blood loss from the procedure.

Consider children's emotional reactions to the procedure. They should be allowed and encouraged to express their feelings about the experience through verbal expression and therapeutic play. Parents also seek an explanation of the results of tests and procedures performed on their children. Nurses are in a unique position to provide support and education to parents regarding procedures.

THE CHILD WITH CEREBRAL COMPROMISE

NURSING CARE OF THE UNCONSCIOUS CHILD

The unconscious child requires nursing attendance with observation, recording, and evaluation of changes in objective signs. These observations provide valuable information regarding the patient's progress and often serve as a guide to diagnosis and treatment. Therefore careful and detailed observations are essential for the child's welfare. In addition, vital functions must be maintained and complications prevented through conscientious and meticulous nursing care. The outcome of unconsciousness is variable and ranges from early and complete recovery, to death within a few hours or days, or persistent and permanent unconsciousness, or recovery with varying degrees of residual mental or physical disability. The outcome and recovery of the unconscious child may depend on the level of nursing care and observational skills.

Direct emergency measures toward ensuring a patent airway, breathing, and circulation (ABCs); stabilizing the spine when indicated; treating shock; and reducing ICP (if present). Delayed treatment often leads to increased damage. Therapies for specific causes of unconsciousness begin as soon as emergency measures have been implemented; in many cases they occur concurrently. Because nursing care is closely related to the medical management, both are considered here.

Continual observation of the LOC, pupillary reaction, and vital signs is essential to management of CNS disorders. Regular assessment of neurologic status and vital signs is an integral part of the nursing care of unconscious children. The frequency depends on the cause of unconsciousness, the LOC, and the progression of cerebral involvement. Intervals between observations may be as short as every 15 minutes or as long as every 2 hours. Significant alterations are reported immediately.

The temperature is measured every 2 to 4 hours, depending on the child's condition. An elevated temperature may occur in children with CNS dysfunction; therefore a light covering may be sufficient. Vigorous efforts, such as tepid sponge baths or application of a hypothermia blanket, are needed to prevent brain damage if the rectal temperature exceeds 40° C (104° F).

The LOC is assessed periodically, including pupillary size, equality, and reaction to light. Signs of meningeal irritation, such as nuchal rigidity, need to be assessed. Assessment of LOC also includes response to vocal commands, spontaneous behavior, resistance to care, and response to painful stimuli. Note any abnormal movements, changes in muscle tone or strength, and body position. If a seizure occurs, describe the seizure, including the body areas involved from the beginning to the end of the seizure, and the duration of seizure (see Box 37-11 and Critical Thinking Exercise, p. 1560).

Pain management for the unconscious child requires astute nursing observation and management. Signs of pain include changes in behavior (e.g., increased agitation and rigidity) and alterations in vital signs and perfusion (usually, an increased heart rate, respiratory rate, and blood pressure; and decreased oxygen saturation). Because these findings are not specific for pain, the nurse should be alert for their appearance during times of induced or suspected pain, and for their disappearance after the inciting procedure or the administration of analgesia. A pain assessment record is used to document indications of pain and the effectiveness of interventions. (See Pain Assessment, Chapter 7.) The use of opioids, such as morphine, to relieve pain is controversial because they can mask signs of altered consciousness or depress respirations. However, unrelieved pain activates the stress response, which can elevate ICP. To block the stress response, some authorities advocate the use of analgesics, sedatives, and, in some cases such as head injury, paralyzing agents via continuous IV infusion. A commonly used combination is fentanyl, midazolam, and vecuronium (Norcuron). If there are concerns about assessing the LOC or respiratory depression, naloxone can be used to reverse the opioid effects. Acetaminophen and codeine may also be effective analgesics for mild to moderate pain. Regardless of the drugs used, adequate dosage and regular administration are essential to provide optimum pain relief.

Other measures to relieve discomfort include providing a quiet, dimly lit environment; limiting visitors; preventing any sudden, jarring movement, such as banging into the bed; and preventing an increase in ICP. The latter is most effectively achieved by proper positioning and prevention of straining, such as during coughing, vomiting, or defecating. (See Pain Management, Chapter 7.)

Antiepileptic drugs, such as fosphenytoin (Cerebyx) or phenobarbital, may be ordered for control of seizure activity.

Respiratory Management

Respiratory effectiveness is the primary concern in the care of the unconscious child, and establishment of an adequate airway is always the first priority. Carbon dioxide has a potent vasodilating effect and will increase CBF and ICP. Cerebral hypoxia at normal body temperature that lasts longer than 4 minutes nearly always causes irreversible brain damage.

Children in lighter stages of coma may be able to cough and swallow, but those in deeper states of coma are unable to manage secretions, which tend to pool in the throat and pharynx. Dysfunction of CN IX and X (glossopharyngeal and vagus nerves) places the child at risk of aspiration and cardiac arrest. Therefore position the child with the head and body to the side to prevent aspiration of secretions, and empty the stomach to reduce the likelihood of vomiting. In infants, the blockage of air passages from secretions can happen in seconds. In addition, upper airway obstruction from laryngospasm is a common complication in comatose children.

An oral airway can be used for the child who is suffering a temporary loss of consciousness, such as after a contusion, seizure, or anesthesia. For children who remain unconscious for a longer time, a nasotracheal or orotracheal tube is inserted to maintain the open airway and facilitate removal of secretions. A tracheostomy is performed in cases in which laryngoscopy for introduction of an endotracheal tube would be difficult or dangerous, or for a child who needs long-term ventilatory support. Suctioning is used only as needed to clear the airway, exerting care to prevent increasing ICP. Respiratory status is observed and evaluated regularly. Signs of respiratory distress may indicate a need for ventilatory assistance.

Mechanical ventilation is usually indicated when the respiratory center is involved. (See Chapter 31.) Blood gas analysis is performed regularly, and oxygen is administered when indicated. Moderately severe hypoxia and respiratory acidosis are often present, but are not always evident from clinical manifestations. Hyperventilation often accompanies unconsciousness and may lead to respiratory alkalosis, or it may represent the

body's attempt to compensate for metabolic acidosis. Therefore blood gas and pH determinations are essential guides for electrolyte therapy. Chest physiotherapy is carried out on a regular basis, and the child's position is changed at least every 2 hours to prevent pulmonary complications.

Intracranial Pressure Monitoring

The selection of the type of ICP monitor should be guided by the clinical presentation and the therapeutic strategy chosen for each child. Indications for inserting an ICP monitor are (1) GCS evaluation of less than 7, (2) GCS evaluation of less than 8 with respiratory assistance, (3) deterioration of condition, and (4) subjective judgment regarding clinical appearance and response.

Four major types of ICP monitors are (1) intraventricular catheter with or without fibroscopic sensors attached to a monitoring system, (2) subarachnoid bolt (Richmond screw), (3) epidural sensor, and (4) anterior fontanel pressure monitor. Transducers for both ventricular and subarachnoid monitoring should be set up without the use of a flush device. Direct ventricular pressure measurement remains the gold standard of ICP monitoring.

The catheter method involves introduction of a catheter into the lateral ventricle on the nondominant side, if known, or placement in the subdural space. The catheter has the advantage of providing a means of extraventricular (or continuous) drainage of CSF to reduce pressure. A drainage bag attached to the system is kept at the level of the ventricles and can be lowered to decrease ICP. This device requires full penetration of the brain, requires skill and experience with placement, and carries the risk of infection.

With the bolt method the end of the bolt is placed into the subarachnoid space. The bolt cannot be adequately secured in a small child's pliant skull, although special modifications have been developed for children under 6 years of age. The placement of the bolt is not adjusted by anyone except the neurosurgeon who placed the device. The neurosurgeon is notified if a satisfactory wave form is not observed.

An epidural sensor can be placed between the dura and the skull through a burr hole and connected to a stopcock assembly and a transducer, which provides a readout of the pressure. Although less invasive, the epidural sensor may have inconsistent correlation of pressure readings. In infants a fontanel transducer can be used to detect impulses from a pressure sensor and convert them to electrical energy. The electrical energy is then converted to visible waves or numeric readings on an oscilloscope. ICP measurement from the anterior fontanel is noninvasive but may prove to be inaccurate if the equipment is poorly placed or inconsistently recalibrated. Use of the intraparenchymal pressure monitoring device (e.g., Camino) uses fiberoptic technology and performs reliably.

ICP can be increased by direct instillation of solutions; therefore antibiotics are administered systemically if a positive CSF culture is obtained. However, ICP monitoring rarely causes infection. CSF is a body fluid; therefore implement Standard Precautions according to hospital policy. (See Infection Control, Chapter 27.)

Nurses caring for patients with intracranial monitoring devices must be acquainted with the system, assist with insertion, interpret the monitor readings, and be able to distinguish between danger signals and mechanical dysfunction. Because systemic blood pressure, ICP, and therefore CPP are normally lower in children, the child's age must be taken into account when deciding what constitutes abnormally high ICP or abnormally low CPP.

Several medical measures are available to treat increased ICP resulting from cerebral edema. These include sedation, CSF drainage, and osmotic diuretics. Osmotic diuretics may provide rapid relief of ICP in emergency situations. Although their effect is transient, lasting only about 6 hours, they can be lifesaving in emergencies. These substances are rapidly excreted by the kidneys and carry with them large quantities of sodium and water. Mannitol (or sometimes urea) administered intravenously is the drug most commonly used for rapid reduction of ICP. The infusion is generally given slowly but may be pushed rapidly if there is herniation or impending herniation. Because of the profound diuretic effect of the drug, an indwelling catheter is inserted to ensure bladder emptying. $Paco_2$ should be maintained at 25 to 30 mm Hg to produce vasoconstriction, which reduces CBF, thereby decreasing ICP. Recording and analyzing the child's volume state, plasma sodium concentration, and serum osmolarity can avert potential fluid and electrolyte problems. Administration of adrenocorticosteroids is not recommended for cerebral edema secondary to head trauma.

Nursing Activities

In cases of high levels of increased ICP, nursing procedures tend to trigger reactive pressure waves in many children. For example, increased intrathoracic or abdominal pressure will be transmitted to the cranium. The goals of monitoring a child who is neurologically compromised include maintaining CPP; controlling ICP, cerebral edema, and factors that increase cerebral metabolism (fever, seizures); and maintaining hemodynamic stability. Take particular care in positioning these patients to avoid neck vein compression that may further increase ICP by interfering with venous return.

> **! NURSING ALERT**
>
> Elevate the head of the bed 15 to 30 degrees, and position the child so that the head is maintained in midline to facilitate venous drainage and avoid jugular compression. Turning side to side is contraindicated because of the risk of jugular compression.

Sandbags or other support devices can help maintain correct head position. The child can be propped to one side or the other, and the use of a pressure-relieving or pressure-decreasing mattress decreases the chance of prolonged pressure to vulnerable skin areas. Frequent clinical assessment of the child cannot be replaced by an ICP monitoring device.

It is important to avoid activities that may increase ICP by causing pain or emotional stress. Individualizing nursing activities and minimizing environmental stimuli by decreasing noxious procedures help to control ICP (El Bashir, Laundy, and Booy, 2003). Range-of-motion exercises can be carried out gently, but should not be performed vigorously. Nontherapeutic touch can cause an increase in ICP. Any disturbing procedures to be performed should be scheduled to take advantage of therapies that reduce ICP, such as osmotherapy and sedation. Make efforts to minimize or eliminate environmental noise. Assessment and intervention to relieve pain are important nursing functions to decrease ICP.

Suctioning and percussion are poorly tolerated; therefore these procedures are contraindicated unless the child has concurrent respiratory problems. Hypoxia and the Valsalva maneuver associated with cough acutely elevate ICP. Vibration, which does not increase ICP, accomplishes excellent results and should be tried first if treatment is needed. If suctioning is necessary, it should be used judiciously and preceded by hyperventilation with 100% oxygen, which can be monitored during suctioning with a pulse oxygen sensor reading to determine oxygen saturation.

Nutrition and Hydration

In the unconscious child, fluids and calories are supplied initially by the IV route. (See Chapter 28.) An IV infusion is started early, and the type of fluid administered depends on the patient's general condition. Fluid therapy requires careful monitoring and adjustment based on neurologic signs and electrolyte determinations. Often, unconscious children cannot tolerate the same amounts of fluid as when they are healthy. Overhydration must be avoided to prevent fatal cerebral edema. When cerebral edema is a threat, fluids may be restricted to reduce the chance of fluid overload. Examine skin and mucous membranes for signs of dehydration. Adjustments to fluid administration are based on urinary output, serum electrolytes and osmolarity, blood pressure, and arterial filling pressure. Observation for signs of altered fluid balance related to abnormal pituitary secretions is a part of nursing care.

Provide long-term nutrition in a balanced formula given by nasogastric or gastrostomy tube. The nasogastric tube is usually taped in place, with care taken to prevent pressure on the nares. Most children have continuous feedings, but if bolus feedings are used, the tube is rinsed with water after each feeding. Tubes are replaced according to institutional policy. Irritation of the nasal mucosa is prevented by alternating nares each time the nasogastric tube is replaced.

Avoid overfeeding to prevent vomiting and the associated risk of aspiration. Stomach contents are aspirated with a syringe and measured before feeding to ascertain the amount remaining in the stomach. The removed contents are refed. If the residual volume is excessive (depending on the child's size), consult the dietitian and physician regarding the composition

TABLE 37-2	EFFECTS OF ALTERED PITUITARY SECRETION	
MEASUREMENT	DIABETES INSIPIDUS	SYNDROME OF INAPPROPRIATE ANTIDIURETIC HORMONE SECRETION
Urinary output	Increased	Decreased
Specific gravity	Decreased	Increased
Serum sodium	Increased (hypernatremia)	Decreased (hyponatremia)

and amount of formula and whether changes are required to provide the needed calories and nutrients in a smaller volume.

Altered Pituitary Secretion

An altered ability to handle fluid loads is attributed in part to the syndrome of inappropriate antidiuretic hormone (SIADH) and diabetes insipidus (DI) resulting from hypothalamic dysfunction. (See Chapter 38.) SIADH often accompanies CNS diseases such as head injury, meningitis, encephalitis, brain abscess, brain tumor, and subarachnoid hemorrhage. In the child with SIADH, scant quantities of urine are excreted, electrolyte analysis reveals hyponatremia and hyposmolality, and manifestations of overhydration are evident. It is important to evaluate all parameters because the reduced urinary output might be erroneously interpreted as a sign of dehydration. The treatment of SIADH consists of fluid restriction until serum electrolytes and osmolality return to normal levels. SIADH often occurs in children who have meningitis.

DI may occur after intracranial trauma. In DI there is increased urinary volume and the accompanying danger of dehydration. See Table 37-2 for comparison of fluid changes in SIADH and DI. Adequate replacement of fluids is essential, and observation of electrolyte balance is necessary to detect signs of hypernatremia and hyperosmolality. Exogenous vasopressin may be administered.

Medications

The cause of unconsciousness determines specific drug therapies. Children with infectious processes are given antibiotics appropriate to the disease and the infecting organism. Corticosteroids are prescribed for inflammatory conditions and edema. Cerebral edema is an indication for osmotic diuretics. Antiepileptic medications are prescribed for seizure activity. Sedation in the combative child provides amnesic and anxiolytic properties in conjunction with a paralytic agent. This combination decreases ICP and allows treatment of cerebral edema. Usual drugs include morphine, midazolam, and pancuronium (Pavulon). Midazolam is attractive because of its short half-life.

Deep coma induced by the administration of barbiturates is controversial in the management of ICP. Barbiturates are currently reserved for the reduction of increased ICP when all else has failed. Barbiturates decrease the cerebral metabolic rate for oxygen and protect the brain during times of reduced CPP. Barbiturate coma requires extensive monitoring, including EEG monitoring to assess for seizure activity, cardiovascular and respiratory support, and ICP monitoring to assess response

to therapy. Paralyzing agents such as pancuronium also may be needed to aid in performing diagnostic tests, improving effectiveness of therapy, and reducing the risks of secondary complications. Elevation of ICP or heart rate in patients who are being given paralyzing agents or are under sedation may indicate the need for another dose of either or both medications.

Thermoregulation

Hyperthermia often accompanies cerebral dysfunction; if it is present, the nurse implements measures to reduce the temperature to prevent brain damage from hyperthermia and to reduce metabolic demands generated by the increased body temperature. Antipyretics are the method of choice for fever reduction; cooling devices are used for hyperthermia. (See Controlling Elevated Temperatures, Chapter 27.) Laboratory tests and other methods help determine the cause, if any, of the hyperthermia. Treatment with hypothermia and barbiturates increases the risk of iatrogenic complications.

Elimination

A urinary catheter is usually inserted in the acute phase, but diapers may be used and weighed to record urinary output. The child who previously had bowel and bladder control is generally incontinent. If the child remains comatose for a long period, the indwelling catheter may be removed and periodic bladder emptying accomplished by intermittent catheterization. Stool softeners are usually sufficient to maintain bowel function, but suppositories or enemas may be needed occasionally for adequate elimination and to prevent fecal impaction. The passage of liquid stool after a period of no bowel activity is usually a sign of impaction. To avoid this preventable problem, daily recording of bowel activity is essential.

Hygienic Care

Routine measures for cleansing and maintaining skin integrity are an integral part of nursing care of the unconscious child. Skinfolds require special attention to prevent excoriation. The child who is unable to move is prone to develop tissue breakdown and necrosis; therefore the child is placed on a resilient appliance (e.g., alternating-pressure or water-filled mattress) to prevent pressure on prominent areas of the body. The goal is prevention by regular change of position and inspection of vulnerable areas (e.g., the ankle, heels, trochanter, sacrum, and shoulder). Unconscious children undergo numerous invasive procedures, and the skin sites used for these procedures require special assessment and intervention to promote healing and prevent infection. Keep bed linen and any clothing dry and free of wrinkles. Rubbing the back and extremities with lotion stimulates circulation and helps prevent drying of the skin. However, to prevent further tissue damage, do not massage reddened and nonblanching skin. (See Maintaining Healthy Skin, Chapter 27.) If the child requires surgery or radiography, the nurse checks all dressings, bony sites, catheters, and IV access lines before and after the procedure.

Mouth care is performed at least twice daily, since the mouth tends to become dry or coated with mucus. The teeth are carefully brushed with a soft toothbrush or cleaned with gauze saturated with saline. Commercially prepared cleansing devices, such as Toothettes, are convenient for cleansing the mouth and teeth. Lips are coated with ointment to protect them from drying, cracking, or blistering.

The unconscious child is also prone to eye irritation. The corneal reflexes are absent; therefore the eyes are easily irritated or damaged by linen, dust, or other substances that may come in contact with them. Excessive dryness results from incomplete closure of the lids and/or decreased secretions, especially if the child is undergoing osmotherapy to reduce or prevent brain edema.

> **! NURSING ALERT**
>
> The eyes are examined regularly and carefully for early signs of irritation or inflammation. Artificial tears (methylcellulose) are placed in the eyes every 1 to 2 hours. Eye patches may be required to protect the eyes from possible damage.

Keep the child's hair combed and secure to prevent tangling. Keep the scalp clean with dry or wet shampoos as needed. The child's head may need to be shaved for tests or surgical procedures. If so, the hair should be saved, if possible, and given to the family.

Positioning and Exercise

The unconscious child is positioned to minimize ICP and to prevent aspiration of saliva, nasogastric secretions, and vomitus. The head of the bed is elevated, and the child is placed in a side-lying or semiprone position. A small, firm pillow is placed under the head, and the uppermost limbs are flexed and supported with pillows. The weight of the body should not rest on the dependent arm. In the semiprone position the child lies with the dependent arm at the side behind the body; the opposite side is supported on pillows, and the uppermost arm and leg are flexed and resting on the pillows. This position prevents undue pressure on the dependent extremities. The dependent position of the face encourages drainage of secretions and prevents the flaccid tongue from obstructing the airway.

Normal range-of-motion exercises help maintain function and prevent contractures of joints. Perform exercises gently to minimize increasing ICP, and with full range of motion. Place a small rolled pad in the palms to help maintain proper positioning of fingers. Footboards or high-top shoes (e.g., running or tennis shoes) can help prevent footdrop, and in some cases splinting is needed to prevent severe contractures of the wrist, knee, or ankle in children.

Stimulation

Sensory stimulation is as important in the care of the unconscious child as it is in the care of the alert child. For the temporarily unconscious or semiconscious child, sensory stimulation helps arouse the child to the conscious state and orient the child in terms of time and place. Auditory and tactile stimulation are especially valuable. Tactile stimulation is not appropriate for a child in whom it may elicit an undesirable response. However, for other children tactile contact often has a relaxing and calming effect. When the child's condition permits, holding or rocking the child is soothing and provides the body contact needed by young children.

The auditory sense is often intact in a state of coma. Hearing is the last sense to be lost and the first one to be regained; therefore speak to the child as any other child. Conversation around the child should not include thoughtless or derogatory remarks. Soft music is often used to provide auditory stimulation. Singing the child's favorite songs or reading a favorite story is a strategy used to maintain the child's contact with a familiar world. Playing songs or favorite stories recorded in the parents' voices can provide a continuous source of familiar stimulation.

Family Support

Helping the parents of an unconscious child cope with the situation is especially difficult. They may demonstrate all the guilt, fear, hostility, and anxiety of any parent of a seriously ill child. (See Chapter 23.) In addition, these parents face the uncertain outcome of the cerebral dysfunction. The fear of death, cognitive impairment, or permanent physical disability is present. Nursing intervention with parents depends on the nature of the pathologic condition, the parents' personality, and the parent-child relationship before injury or illness (see Family-Centered Care box).

> **👪 FAMILY-CENTERED CARE**
>
> ### Understanding the Child's Recovery from a Comatose State
>
> Recovering from coma is a complex process and may be confusing for parents and family members, who are already anxious and overwhelmed. Understanding the stages of recovery may assist parents in coping with the situation. It is important to remember that comatose children may not complete all stages of the recovery process and that they may manifest characteristics of more than one stage at a time.
>
> **Level 1: No response**—Child does not respond to stimuli but may be able to hear what is said in the room.
>
> **Level 2: Generalized response**—Child responds to painful or unpleasant stimuli; responses may not be consistent and may be delayed.
>
> **Level 3: Localized response**—Child responds purposefully to painful or unpleasant stimuli by trying to pull away; turns toward sounds; responds to simple commands.
>
> **Level 4: Confused, agitated**—Child becomes restless, aggressive, frustrated; exhibits abnormal behavior; forgets answers to frequently asked questions.
>
> **Level 5: Confused, inappropriate, nonagitated**—Child behaves more calmly; behavior starts to normalize but child may become frustrated; voice and face lack expression; follows simple commands; performs simple tasks.
>
> **Level 6: Confused, appropriate**—Child is less frustrated and is able to concentrate for longer periods (up to 30 minutes); short-term memory is improving; responses to questions are more appropriate but may not be correct.
>
> **Level 7: Automatic, appropriate**—Child's memory continues to improve, although details may not be clear; continues to have difficulty concentrating; preexisting behavioral or learning problems may be worse than before the comatose state.
>
> **Level 8: Purposeful**—Child's basic thinking skills will have recovered to the maximum extent; incidental changes in social skills, memory, and concentration may continue for months; child will fully understand what happened and may grieve over how things have changed.

Modified from *A booklet for parents: recovering from brain injury*, Toronto, 1996, Hospital for Sick Children. Stages for recovery are based on the Rancho Los Amigos Scale, copyright Rancho Los Amigos, 1989; revised by CJ Wright, MSN, RNC, Children's Hospital Trauma Center.

Awakening from a coma is a gradual process; however, some children regain consciousness within a short time. If there is little or no residual effect, the child is discharged home fairly soon. The parents need the most intensive nursing intervention during the period of crisis and uncertainty. During the recovery phase the nurse gives them information, clarifies it as needed, and encourages them to become involved in the child's care. Often the child's hospitalization is brief; however, some children require extended hospitalization for intensive therapy and rehabilitation. The parents of children who die require support and guidance to cope with the reality of the death and to resolve their grief. (See Chapter 23.)

Probably the most difficult situations are those that involve children who never regain consciousness. Unlike losing a child through death, these children lack finality, which often leaves them in a state of suspended grief. Like parents of dying children, parents of comatose children search for any signs of hope. Well-meaning friends and relatives relate instances of miraculous recoveries. The parents seek confirmation and support for such possibilities and assign erroneous meanings to any sign in the child that might be interpreted as evidence of recovery (e.g., reflexive muscle contractions).

At these times nurses need to respond with compassion and honesty. They can acknowledge that miraculous recoveries do occur but are rare. The important message is to maintain open communication with the family.

Like parents who lose a child through death, the parents of a child who is unconscious attempt to construct a representation of the child. They bring items that belong to the child, such as favorite toys or music. This may be interpreted as an attempt to provide stimulation for the child in the hope of eliciting a response, to let the hospital staff know the child as the unique individual he or she was, and to reconstitute an image of the child "lost" to them and for whom they mourn. The nurses' recognition and understanding of these behaviors and coping mechanisms is important to support the parents in their grief process.

In addition to the process of grieving for the "lost" child, the parents may face difficult decisions. When the child's brain is so severely damaged that vital functions must be maintained by artificial means, the parents must make the final decision whether to remove the life-support systems. Since this decision is so difficult for parents, the practitioner is frequently placed in a position of making the decision indirectly. After providing the parents with information about what removal from life-support means, the practitioner may suggest that the child be removed from life support to "see if the child can make it without help." This approach relieves the parents of the decision and can be effective, but it is based on an evaluation of the parents' intellectual level and emotional state. Sometimes parents may choose to refuse treatment if they believe doing so is best for the child and the family (informed dissent). At other times parents request that "everything possible" be done for the child.

When the child has survived the cerebral insult but is physically and/or mentally limited, either minimally or severely, families must cope with and make decisions about the rehabilitation process and uncertain outcome. The family may need to make decisions whether to place their child in a chronic care facility or to care for their child at home. The drain on financial, emotional, and social resources can be enormous.

For parents who choose to care for their child at home, planning begins early in the recovery process. Family members should become involved with the child's care as soon as they indicate an interest and ability to do so. They need education and support in learning to care for the child, regular follow-up observation and assessment of the home management, and planning for respite care. Parents need to understand that it is important to plan for periodic relief from the continuous care of the child. (See Discharge Planning and Home Care, Chapter 26, and Family-Centered Home Care, Chapter 25.)

HEAD INJURY

Head injury is a pathologic process involving the scalp, skull, meninges, or brain as a result of mechanical force. According to national statistics and Safe Kids Worldwide,* injuries are the number one health risk for children and the leading cause of death in children older than 1 year of age. Each year, one child in four in the United States suffers an injury serious enough to require medical attention.

Etiology

The three major causes of brain damage in childhood, in order of importance, are falls, motor vehicle injuries, and bicycle injuries (Fig. 37-6). Neurologic injury accounts for the highest mortality rate, with boys usually affected twice as often as girls. Falls are the major source of all head injuries in children between the ages 0 to 4 years (Langlois, Rutland-Brown, and Thomas, 2005; Marsh and Whitehead, 2005). In motor vehicle accidents children younger than 2 years of age are almost exclusively injured as passengers, whereas older children may also be injured as pedestrians or cyclists. The majority of deaths from brain trauma caused by bicycle injuries occur between the ages

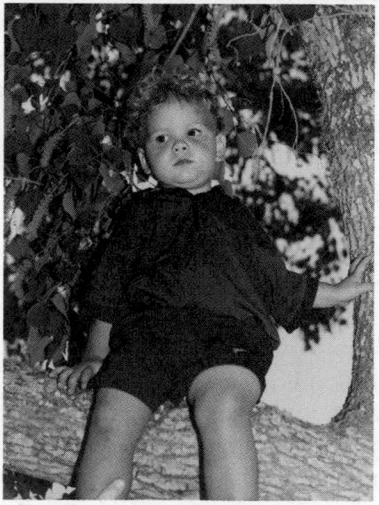

Fig. 37-6 Children possess a sense of adventure and wonder; however, falls remain the leading cause of head injury in children under 5 years of age.

*1301 Pennsylvania Ave., NW, Suite 1000, Washington, DC 20004-1707; 202-662-0600; www.safekids.org.

of 5 and 19 years. Bicycle helmet laws have effectively reduced the risk of head injury by 85% and brain injury by 88% (Rivara and Grossman, 2009).

Many of the physical characteristics of children predispose them to craniocerebral trauma. For example, infants are often left unattended on beds, in high chairs, and in other places from which they can fall. Because the head of an infant or toddler is proportionately large and heavy in relation to other body parts, it is the most likely to be injured. Incomplete motor development contributes to falls at young ages, and the natural curiosity and exuberance of children increase their risk for injury.

Pathophysiology

The pathology of brain injury is directly related to the force of impact. Intracranial contents (brain, blood, CSF) are damaged because the force is too great to be absorbed by the skull and musculoligamentous support of the head. Although nervous tissue is delicate, it usually requires a severe blow to cause significant damage.

A child's response to head injury is different from that of adults. The larger head size in proportion to body size and insufficient musculoskeletal support render the very young child particularly vulnerable to acceleration-deceleration injuries.

Primary head injuries are those that occur at the time of trauma and include skull fractures, contusions, intracranial hematomas, and diffuse injuries. Subsequent complications include hypoxic brain injury, increased ICP, and cerebral edema. The predominant feature of a child's brain injury is the diffuse amount of swelling that occurs. Hypoxia and hypercapnia threaten the energy requirements of the brain and increase CBF. The added volume across the BBB along with the loss of autoregulation exacerbates cerebral edema. Pressure inside the skull that is greater than arterial pressure results in inadequate perfusion. Because the cranium of very young children has the ability to expand and the thin skull is more compliant, they may tolerate increases in ICP better than older children and adults.

Physical forces act on the head through acceleration, deceleration, or deformation. Acceleration or deceleration is more descriptive of the circumstances responsible for most head injuries. When the stationary head receives a blow, the sudden acceleration causes deformation of the skull and mass movement of the brain. Continued movement of the intracranial contents allows the brain to strike parts of the skull (e.g., the sharp edges of the sphenoid or the irregular surface of the anterior fossa) or the edges of the tentorium.

Although the brain volume remains unchanged, significant distortion and cavitation occur as the brain changes shape in response to the force transmitted from the impact to the skull. This deformation can cause bruising at the point of impact (coup) or at a distance as the brain collides with the unyielding surfaces opposite or far removed from the point of impact (contrecoup) (Fig. 37-7). Thus a blow to the occipital region can cause severe injury to the frontal and temporal areas of the brain.

When a moving head strikes a stationary surface, such as during a fall, sudden deceleration occurs and causes the greatest cerebral injury at the point of impact. Deceleration is responsible for most severe brainstem injuries.

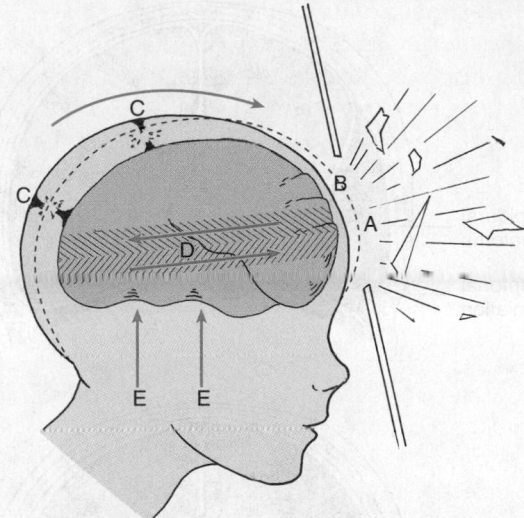

Fig. 37-7 Mechanical distortion of cranium during closed head injury. *A,* Preinjury contour of skull. *B,* Immediate postinjury contour of skull. *C,* Torn subdural vessels. *D,* Shearing forces. *E,* Trauma from contact with floor of cranium. (Redrawn from Grubb RL, Coxe WS: Central nervous system trauma: cranial. In Eliasson SG, Presky AL, Hardin WB, editors: *Neurological pathophysiology,* New York, 1974, Oxford University Press.)

Children with an acceleration-deceleration injury demonstrate diffuse generalized cerebral swelling produced by increased blood volume or by a redistribution of cerebral blood volume (cerebral hyperemia) rather than by the increased water content (edema).

Another effect of brain movement is shearing forces, which are caused by unequal movement or different rates of acceleration at various levels of the brain. A shearing force may tear small arteries that travel from the cerebral surfaces through the meninges to the dural sinuses and cause subdural hemorrhages. Shearing or stretching effects can also be transmitted to nerve fibers. Maximum stress from the shearing force occurs at the interface between structures of different density so that the gray matter (cell body) rapidly accelerates while the white matter (axons) tends to lag behind. Although shearing forces are maximum at the cerebral surface and extend toward the center of rotation within the brain, the most serious effects are often in the area of the brainstem.

Another source of damage occurs when severe compression of the skull causes the brain to be forced through the tentorial opening. This can produce irreparable damage to the brainstem (Fig. 37-8).

Patients with mild head injuries have a GCS evaluation of 13 to 15, and those with moderate head injuries have a GCS of 9 to 12; a GCS value of 8 or less indicates severe injury (Marcin and Pollack, 2002).

Concussion

The most common head injury is **concussion,** an alteration in mental status with or without loss of consciousness, which occurs immediately after a head injury (Lee, 2007). The hallmarks of a concussion are confusion and amnesia. These are often not preceded by loss of consciousness and may occur immediately after the injury or several minutes later. The belief

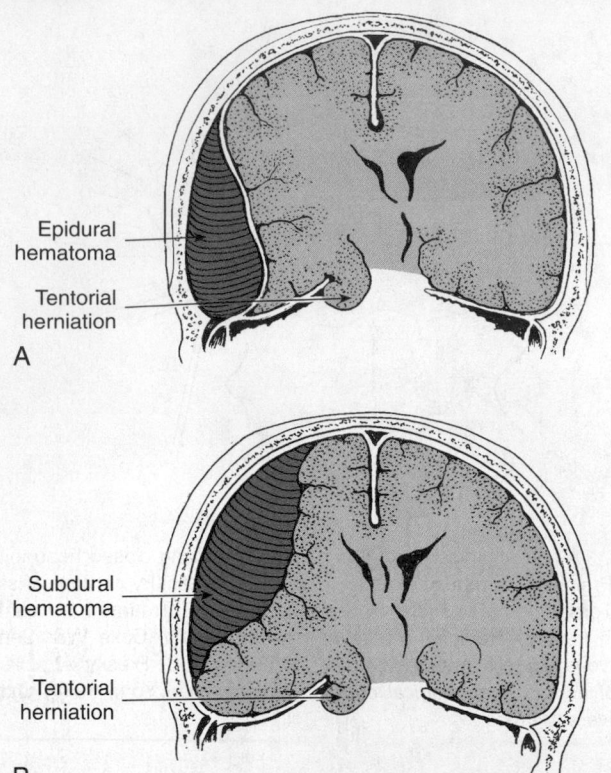

Fig. 37-8 A, Epidural (extradural) hematoma and compression of temporal lobe through tentorial herniation. **B,** Subdural hematoma.

that loss of consciousness is the hallmark of concussion is a common misconception. Blinman, Houseknecht, Snyder, and colleagues (2009) found that fatigue and headache were the most common symptoms after mild traumatic brain injury in a group of 116 children.

The pathogenesis of concussion is still unclear, but it may be a result of shearing forces that cause stretching, compression, and tearing of nerve fibers, particularly in the area of the central brainstem, the seat of the reticular activating system. It has also been suggested that the anatomic alterations of nerve fibers cause the release of large quantities of acetylcholine into the CSF and a reduction in oxygen consumption with increased lactate production.

Contusion and Laceration

The terms *contusion* and *laceration* are used to describe actual bruising and tearing of cerebral tissue. Contusions represent petechial hemorrhages or localized bruising along the superficial aspects of the brain at the site of impact (coup injury) or a lesion remote from the site of direct trauma (contrecoup injury). In serious accidents there may be multiple sites of injury.

The major areas of the brain susceptible to contusion or laceration are the occipital, frontal, and temporal lobes. Also, the irregular surfaces of the anterior and middle fossae at the base of the skull are capable of producing bruises or lacerations on forceful impact. Contusions may cause focal disturbances in strength, sensation, or visual awareness. The degree of brain damage in the contused areas varies according to the extent of vascular injury. Signs vary from mild, transient weakness of a limb to prolonged unconsciousness and paralysis. However, the

signs and symptoms may be clinically indistinguishable from those of concussion.

Infants who are roughly shaken (shaken baby syndrome) can sustain profound neurologic impairment, seizures, retinal hemorrhages (usually bilateral), and intracranial subarachnoid or subdural hemorrhages (McCabe and Donahue, 2000; Bechtel, Stoessel, Leventahal, et al, 2004). In addition to these classic injuries, other skeletal fractures and injuries may occur (Castiglia, 2001; DiCarlo and Frankel, 2009).

Cerebral lacerations are generally associated with penetrating or depressed skull fractures. However, they may occur without fracture in small children. When brain tissue is actually torn, with bleeding into and around the tear, more severe and prolonged unconsciousness and paralysis usually occur, leaving permanent scarring and some degree of disability.

Fractures

Skull fractures result from a direct blow or injury to the skull and are often associated with intracranial injury. Skull fractures after minor head injury are not uncommon, particularly in children younger than 2 years of age. Infants are at increased risk of skull fractures from minor trauma. Falls are the most common cause of head injury. Many of the falls that resulted in a skull fracture in children younger than 2 years of age involved short distances of less than 3 feet, such as falls from infant carrier car seats (Greenberg, Bolte, and Schunk, 2009).

The types of skull fractures that occur are linear, comminuted, depressed, open, basilar, and growing fractures. As a rule, the faster the blow, the greater the likelihood of a depressed fracture; a low-velocity impact tends to produce a linear fracture.

Linear skull fractures are a single fracture line that starts at the point of maximum impact and spread; however, they do not cross suture lines. Linear skull fractures constitute the majority of childhood skull fractures and typically occur in the parietal bone. Most linear skull fractures are associated with an overlying scalp hematoma, particularly in infants younger than 1 year of age and in the parietal or temporal region (Greenes and Schutzman, 2001). Comminuted fractures consist of multiple associated linear fractures. They usually result from intense impact, often from repeated blows against an object. They may suggest child abuse, particularly if they occur in the occipital bone.

Depressed fractures are those in which the bone is locally broken, usually into several irregular fragments that are pushed inward. The greater the depression, the higher the risk of a tear in the dura or cortical laceration. Depressed skull fractures may be associated with direct underlying parenchymal damage and should be suspected when a child's head appears misshapen. Surgery may be needed to elevate the depressed bone fragment if there is an associated intracranial hematoma and if the depression is greater than 1 cm (0.4 inch).

Open fractures result in a communication between the skull and the scalp or the mucosa of the upper respiratory tract. The risk of CNS infection is increased with open fractures. Compound fractures consist of a skin laceration overlying the bone fracture. Open fractures that involve the paranasal sinuses or middle ear may lead to leakage of CSF (rhinorrhea or otorrhea). Prophylactic antibiotics are recommended to prevent osteomyelitis.

Basilar fractures involve the bones at the base of the skull in either the posterior or the anterior region. The bones involved are the ethmoid, sphenoid, temporal, or occipital bones and usually result in a dural tear. Because of the proximity of the fracture line to structures surrounding the brainstem, a basal skull fracture is a serious head injury. Approximately 80% of the cases have distinct clinical features. These include leakage of CSF from the nose (CSF rhinorrhea) or from the ear (CSF otorrhea), blood behind the tympanic membrane (hemotympanum), subcutaneous bleeding over the mastoid process that is located posterior to the ear (Battle sign), and subcutaneous bleeding around the orbit (raccoon eyes). CN palsies may occur and primarily involve CN I (olfactory nerve), VIII (vestibulocochlear nerve), VII (facial nerve), and VI (abducens nerve). The diagnosis of basilar fractures is difficult to make from radiographs because of the complex structure of the base of the skull. Therefore a nonenhanced CT is the recommended diagnostic method. Meningitis, although rare, is always a potential risk with CSF leakage. The use of prophylactic antibiotics is controversial, and the trend has been to treat only documented cases of meningitis.

> **! NURSING ALERT**
>
> Suspect posttraumatic meningitis in children with increasing drowsiness and fever who also have basilar skull fractures.

Growing fractures result from a skull fracture with an underlying tear in the dura that fails to heal properly. The enlargement may be caused by a leptomeningeal cyst, dilated ventricles, or herniated brain. The parietal bone is the most common location. The majority of growing skull fractures occur before 3 years of age (Vignes, Jeelani, Jeelani, et al, 2007). Physical examination can reveal the development of a pulsatile mass or enlarging and sunken skull defect. Clinical neurologic symptoms may be delayed for months to years after the initial skull fracture and include headache, seizures, or asymmetric cranial growth.

Complications

The major complications of trauma to the head are hemorrhage, infection, edema, and herniation through the brainstem. Infection is always a hazard in open injuries, and edema is related to tissue trauma. Vascular rupture may occur even in minor head injuries, causing hemorrhage between the skull and cerebral surfaces. Compression of the underlying brain produces effects that can be rapidly fatal or insidiously progressive.

Epidural Hematoma

Epidural (extradural) hematoma is a hemorrhage into the space between the dura and the skull. As the hematoma enlarges, the dura is stripped from the skull; this accumulation of blood results in a mass effect on the brain, forcing the underlying brain contents downward and inward as it expands (see Fig. 37-8, *A*). Epidural hematomas occur infrequently in infants and children, but may occur after a low-velocity fall (Rocchi,

Caroli, Raco, et al, 2005). Child abuse accounts for a significant number of cases of epidural hematomas in infants and children, whereas motor vehicle accidents account for most epidural hematomas in adolescents.

An epidural hemorrhage is usually arterial in origin, most often as a result of a skull fracture that penetrates the groove in the skull occupied by the middle meningeal artery. The low incidence of epidural hematoma in childhood has been attributed to the fact that the middle meningeal artery is not embedded in the bone surface of the skull until approximately 2 years of age. Therefore a fracture of the temporal bone is less likely to lacerate the artery. However, a child's skull can be indented with sufficient force to tear the middle meningeal artery without causing a fracture. Hemorrhage can also originate from dural veins or the dural sinuses, especially in infants and small children, due to the abundance of dural vasculature in areas of rapid bone growth. In 20% to 40% of children a skull fracture is not detectable.

Because bleeding is generally arterial, brain compression occurs rapidly. Most often the expanding hematoma is located in the parietotemporal region, which forces the medial portion of the temporal lobe under the edge of the tentorium, where it places pressure on nerves and blood vessels. Pressure on the arterial supply and venous return to the reticular formation causes loss of consciousness; pressure on CN III produces dilation and (later) fixation of the ipsilateral pupil. Pressure on the fibers of the pyramidal tract is evidenced by contralateral weakness or paralysis and increased deep tendon reflexes. Extreme pressure may cause brain herniation and death. Expanding epidural hemorrhages may be better tolerated in young children with open sutures that allows for expansion of the skull. In addition, young children have larger subarachnoid and extracellular spaces, which provide space for the expanding hematoma without compression on the brain parenchyma.

The classic clinical picture of an epidural hemorrhage is a lucid interval (momentary unconsciousness) followed by a normal period for several hours, then lethargy or coma due to blood accumulation in the epidural space and compression of the brain (Case, 2008). The child may be seen with varying degrees of impaired consciousness depending on the severity of the traumatic injury. Common symptoms in a child with no neurologic deficit are irritability, headache, and vomiting. In infants less than 1 year of age the most common symptoms are irritability, pallor with anemia, and cephalhematoma. Infants may also have hypotonia, seizures, vomiting, a bulging anterior fontanel, and lethargy.

An epidural hematoma can be detected by an initial CT scan. If the severity of the child's symptoms is not recognized, herniation and death will result. **Cushing triad** (systemic hypertension, bradycardia, and respiratory depression) is a late sign of impending brainstem herniation. See Table 37-3 for a comparison of epidural and subdural hematomas.

> **! NURSING ALERT**
>
> Children with a subdural hematoma and retinal hemorrhages should be evaluated for the possibility of child abuse, especially shaken baby syndrome.

TABLE 37-3	FEATURES OF ACUTE EPIDURAL AND SUBDURAL HEMATOMAS	
FEATURE	**EPIDURAL**	**SUBDURAL**
Supratentorial		
Frequency	Less frequent	More frequent than epidural
Skull fracture	70% of cases	30% of cases
Source of hemorrhage	Arterial or venous	Almost always venous
Age	Usually >2 yr	Usually <1 yr
Location	Usually temporoparietal	Usually frontoparietal
Laterality	Usually unilateral	75% bilateral
Seizures	<25%	75%
Preretinal or retinal hemorrhages	Uncommon	Very frequent
Increased ICP	Present	Present
CT configuration	Usually lenticular	Curvilinear or crescentic
Mortality	Relatively high	Usually lower
Morbidity	Low	High
Infratentorial		
Skull fracture	Almost always	Less common
Source of hemorrhage	Venous	Venous
Impaired consciousness	Frequent	Frequent
Acute hydrocephalus, medullary compression	Variable	Variable
Other posterior fossa signs	Variable	Variable

From Swaiman KF: *Pediatric neurology: principles and practice*, ed 3, St Louis, 1999, Mosby.
CT, Computed tomography; *ICP*, intracranial pressure.

Subdural Hemorrhage

A subdural hemorrhage is bleeding between the dura and the arachnoid membrane, which overlies the brain and the subarachnoid space. The hemorrhage may be from two sources: (1) tearing of the veins that bridge the subdural space, and (2) hemorrhage from the cortex of the brain caused by direct brain trauma (see Fig. 37-8, *B*). Subdural hematomas are much more common than epidural hematomas and occur most often in infancy, with a peak incidence at 6 months (Myhre, Grogaard, Dyb, et al, 2007).

Unlike epidural hemorrhage, which develops inwardly against the less resistant brain tissue, subdural hemorrhage tends to develop more slowly and spreads thinly and widely, crossing cranial sutures, until it is limited by the dural barriers—the falx and the tentorium. Subdural hematoma is fairly common in infants, often as a result of birth trauma, falls, assaults, or violent shaking. The small subdural space and the dura, which is firmly attached to the skull in this area, are highly vulnerable to increased ICP.

Subdural hemorrhage can cause either acute or chronic subdural hematoma. Acute subdural hematoma may be associated with contusions or lacerations and develops within minutes or hours of injury. Chronic subdural hematoma is more common. The clinical course and manifestations vary, depending on the damage sustained by the brain and the child's age.

Presenting signs of acute hematoma include irritability, vomiting, increased head circumference, bulging anterior fon-

tanel (in the infant), lethargy, coma, or seizures. In infants with open fontanels, large amounts of intracranial blood may accumulate causing hemorrhagic shock or fever before there are any changes in the neurologic examination (Case, 2008). Retinal hemorrhages and skull and skeletal fractures are suggestive of physical abuse. An infant who has an altered LOC and in whom the CT scan shows subarachnoid hemorrhage or subdural hematoma may have been physically abused. A child with a GCS of 12 or less requires emergency consultation with the neurosurgeon.

Closely observe older children for signs of neurologic deterioration, including altered mental status, vomiting, papillary changes, and signs of increased ICP. Hemiparesis, hemiplegia, and anisocoria (unequal pupils) are signs of brainstem compression and require emergency treatment targeted at decreasing ICP. The surgical management of subdural hematomas depends on the physical examination, size of the hematoma, and presence of other abnormalities on the CT scan. Not all children require surgery or are candidates for surgery. Subdural taps are sometimes the primary treatment in infants or in children with chronic subdural hematomas (Proctor, 2003).

Other Hemorrhagic Lesions

A subarachnoid hemorrhage is bleeding within the subarachnoid space, which is normally filled with CSF. Nontraumatic intracranial hemorrhages are rare in children. The most common risk factors for intracranial hemorrhages are arteriovenous malformations, congenital heart disease, and brain tumors (Lo, Lee, Rusin, et al, 2008). Sudden onset of a severe headache is the hallmark symptom.

Cerebral Edema

Some degree of brain edema is expected after craniocerebral trauma and often accompanies any of the previously mentioned disorders. Cerebral edema peaks at 24 to 72 hours after injury and may account for changes in a child's neurologic status. Cerebral edema associated with traumatic brain injury may be a result of two different mechanisms: cytotoxic edema or vasogenic edema. Cytotoxic edema is a result of direct cell injury and is caused by intracellular swelling. In many cases the brain cells are irreversibly damaged. Vasogenic edema is due to increased permeability of capillary endothelial cells, resulting in increased intracellular fluid. In vasogenic edema the nerve cells are not primarily injured. Either mechanism can result in increased ICP as a result of increased intracranial volume and changes in CBF as a result of loss of autoregulation and/or hypercapnia or hypoxia. Children at risk for deterioration can be identified by abnormalities seen on admitting noncontrast CT scans (Marcoux, 2005).

Posttraumatic Syndromes

Postconcussion syndrome is a sequela to brain injury with or without loss of consciousness. Controversy exists regarding the definition and pathophysiology of postconcussion syndrome. It typically occurs after a mild head injury but may also occur after moderate to severe head injury. It is a symptom complex that includes headaches, dizziness, fatigue, irritability, anxiety, insomnia, loss of concentration, and memory impairment (Baandrup and Jensen, 2005; Paniak, Reynolds, Phillips, et al,

2002; Yeates, Taylor, Rusin, et al, 2009). Symptoms typically develop within days of the injury and resolve within 3 months. Clinical symptoms of loss of consciousness, posttraumatic amnesia, GCS score of less than 15, disorientation, and other mental status changes are strongly associated with postconcussion syndrome (Yeates, Taylor, Rusin, et al, 2009).

Posttraumatic headaches may occur within 1 week to 3 months after a mild traumatic brain injury. They occur in 25% to 75% of individuals and are typically classified as either tension or migraine headaches (Baandrup and Jensen, 2005).

Posttraumatic seizures occur in a number of children who survive a head injury and are more common in younger children than those over 16 years of age (Baandrup and Jensen, 2005) (see Critical Thinking Exercise). Seizures are more likely to occur in children with severe head injury and usually occur within the first day (Chiaretti, DeBenedictis, Polidori, et al, 2000).

 CRITICAL THINKING EXERCISE

Postconcussion Syndrome

Two weeks ago 4-year-old Thomas attempted to climb the shelves of a storage cabinet in the garage of his home. The shelves and Thomas fell to the concrete floor. Thomas cried immediately. Because of the large occipital hematoma and a vomiting episode, the parents took their son to an emergency department within 1 hour of the incident. He was released after a negative computed tomography (CT) scan, suturing of his occipital scalp laceration, and a Glasgow Coma Scale score of 15.

At his 2-week follow-up visit, his mother reports changes in Thomas's behavior that include enuresis, crying episodes, vomiting in the morning, a poor appetite, and an increased desire to be held.

1. Evidence—Is there sufficient evidence to draw conclusions about Thomas's behavior changes?
2. Assumptions—Describe an underlying assumption about each of the following:
   a. Four-year-old boy who climbed the shelves in a garage
   b. Four-year-old falling from the shelves and striking his head against the concrete floor
   c. Four-year-old boy with behavior changes 2 weeks after a fall
3. What priorities for nursing care should be established for Thomas?
4. Does the evidence support your nursing intervention?

Structural complications may occur as a result of head injuries. Hydrocephalus is seen when there has been subarachnoid hemorrhage or infection. Normal-pressure hydrocephalus is a complication of traumatic brain injury. The clinical signs and symptoms include cognitive deterioration, gait changes, and incontinence. These signs are also seen during posttraumatic amnesia, making early recognition of this syndrome difficult. Focal deficits, including optic atrophy, CN palsies, motor deficits, DI, or aphasia, may be seen. The type of residual effect depends on the location and nature of the trauma.

Diagnostic Evaluation

A detailed health history, both past and present, is essential in evaluating the child with craniocerebral trauma. Certain disorders such as drug allergies, hemophilia, diabetes mellitus, or epilepsy may produce similar symptoms. Even a minor traumatic injury can aggravate a preexisting disease process, thereby producing neurologic signs out of proportion to the injury.

BOX 37-5   CLINICAL MANIFESTATIONS OF ACUTE HEAD INJURY

Minor Injury
May or may not lose consciousness
Transient period of confusion
Somnolence
Listlessness
Irritability
Pallor
Vomiting (one or more episodes)

Signs of Progression
Altered mental status (e.g., difficulty arousing child)
Mounting agitation
Development of focal lateral neurologic signs
Marked changes in vital signs

Severe Injury
Signs of increased intracranial pressure (see Box 37-1)
Bulging fontanel (infant)
Retinal hemorrhages
Extraocular palsies (especially cranial nerve III)
Hemiparesis
Quadriplegia
Elevated temperature
Unsteady gait
Papilledema

Associated Signs
Scalp trauma
Other injuries (e.g., to extremities)

After a minor injury, initial unconsciousness (if present) is brief, and the child ordinarily exhibits a transient period of confusion, somnolence, and listlessness; this period is most often accompanied by irritability, pallor, and one or more episodes of vomiting. A severe head injury requires immediate evaluation and treatment. Because head injuries are often accompanied by injuries in other areas (spine, viscera, extremities), the examination is performed with care to avoid further damage. Box 37-5 lists manifestations of head injury.

 NURSING ALERT

Stabilize the spine after head injury until spinal cord injury is ruled out.

Initial Assessment

Priorities in the initial phase in the care of a child with a head injury include assessment of the ABCs (airway, breathing, circulation); neurologic examination focusing on mental status, papillary responses, and motor responses; and assessment for spinal cord injury. The assessment is carried out quickly in relation to vital signs (see Emergency Treatment box).

 NURSING ALERT

Deep, rapid, periodic, or intermittent and gasping respirations; wide fluctuations or noticeable slowing of the pulse; and widening pulse pressure or extreme fluctuations in blood pressure are signs of brainstem involvement. Marked hypotension may represent internal injuries.

➕ **EMERGENCY TREATMENT**

Head Injury

1. Assess child:
   - A—Airway
   - B—Breathing
   - C—Circulation
   - Neurologic and thermoregulatory status
2. Stabilize neck and spine immediately. Use jaw thrust to open airway, not chin lift.
3. Clean any abrasions with soap and water.
   - Apply clean dressing.
   - If child is bleeding, apply ice to relieve pain and swelling.
4. Keep child NPO (nothing by mouth) until instructed otherwise.
5. Give no analgesics or sedatives.
6. Check pupillary reaction every 4 hours (including twice during night) for 48 hours.
7. Awaken two times during night to check level of consciousness.
8. Seek medical attention for any of the following:
   - Injury sustained at high speed (e.g., auto)
   - Fall from a significant distance (height greater than that of the child)
   - Injury sustained from great force (e.g., baseball bat)
   - Injury sustained under suspicious circumstances
   - Loss of consciousness
   - Discomfort (crying) more than 10 minutes after injury
   - Headache that is severe, worsens, interferes with sleep, or lasts more than 24 hours
   - Vomiting three or more times or that begins or continues 4 to 6 hours after injury
   - Swelling in front of or above earlobe or swelling that increases in size
   - Drainage from ears or nose; blackened eyes
   - Confusion or abnormal behavior
   - Difficulty arousing child from sleep
   - Difficulty speaking
   - Blurring of vision or diplopia
   - Unsteady gait
   - Difficulty using extremities; weakness or incoordination
   - Neck pain or stiffness
   - Pupils dilated, fixed, or unequal
   - Infant with bulging fontanel
   - Seizures

Ocular signs such as fixed, dilated, and unequal pupils; fixed and constricted pupils; and pupils that are poorly reactive or unreactive to light and accommodation indicate increased ICP or brainstem involvement. It is important to remain with the patient who demonstrates fixed and dilated pupils, since these are ominous signs with the probability of respiratory arrest. Dilated, nonpulsating blood vessels indicate increased ICP before the appearance of papilledema. Retinal hemorrhages often occur with acute head injuries, specifically with shaken baby syndrome.

❗ **NURSING ALERT**

Observation of asymmetric pupils or one dilated, unreactive pupil in a comatose child is a neurologic emergency.

Funduscopic examination should be performed routinely to detect retinal hemorrhages in a child with CNS trauma. Cortical blindness, defined as a complete bilateral visual loss associated with normal pupillary responses to light, can be a brief or transient consequence of minor head trauma (Hoyt, 2007). Theories

of possible causes are vasospasm or localized cerebral edema. Transient blindness after mild head trauma may not be obvious in children unless this diagnosis is considered and evaluated.

Less urgent but important assessments include examination of the scalp for lacerations, widely separated sutures, and the size and tension of fontanels, which indicate intracranial hemorrhage or rapidly developing cerebral edema. Scalp lacerations may require surgical intervention. A significant amount of blood loss can occur from scalp lacerations. An underlying skull fracture should be ruled out by CT scan.

❗ **NURSING ALERT**

Bleeding from the nose or ears needs further evaluation, and a watery discharge from the nose (rhinorrhea) that is positive for glucose (as tested with reagent strips [e.g., Dextrostix]) suggests leaking of CSF from a skull fracture.

An accurate assessment of clinical signs provides baseline information. Serial evaluations, preferably by a single observer, help detect changes in the neurologic status. Alterations in mental status, evidenced by increased difficulty in rousing the child, mounting agitation, development of focal neurologic signs, or marked changes in vital signs, usually indicate extension or progression of the basic pathologic process.

Evaluation of reflexes provides information about cerebral and pyramidal involvement, although transient abnormalities of the abdominal reflexes and Babinski sign may be present in children with mild head trauma. Conscious, cooperative children are examined for cerebellar signs such as ataxia. Children may display unsteadiness, clumsiness, or tremor with intentional movement after head injury. Temperature may be moderately elevated for 1 or 2 days following an initial mild hypothermia after injury. A persistent fever may indicate subarachnoid hemorrhage or infection.

Special Tests

After a thorough clinical examination, a variety of diagnostic tests are helpful in providing a more definitive diagnosis of the type and extent of the trauma. A hematocrit and urinalysis are typically done. Serum electrolytes and glucose may also be measured in children with severe head injuries; hyperglycemia and disseminated intravascular coagulation are associated with a poor prognosis. The severity of a head injury may not be apparent on clinical examination of the child but is detectable on a CT scan. Whenever the child has a history consistent with a serious head injury (as with an unrestrained occupant in a severe motor vehicle accident or a fall), it is important to perform a scan even if the child initially appears alert and oriented. All children with head injuries who have any alteration of consciousness, headache, vomiting, skull fracture, seizure, or predisposing medical condition should undergo CT scanning.

MRI may be done to further assess cerebral edema or other structural brain abnormalities. A neurobehavioral assessment after early head injury may be useful in documenting cognitive impairment. Skull radiographs are of little benefit in diagnosing skull fractures. Other radiographic tests may be indicated depending on the severity or cause of the trauma.

Electroencephalography is not helpful for diagnosis of a head injury but is useful for defining seizures. Lumbar puncture is rarely used for craniocerebral trauma and is contraindicated in the presence of increased ICP because of the possibility of herniation.

Therapeutic Management

The majority of children with mild traumatic brain injury who have not lost consciousness can be cared for and observed at home after careful examination reveals no serious intracranial injury. The nurse should give parents both verbal and written instructions of signs and symptoms that warrant concern and the need for reevaluation. These include persistent or worsening headaches, vomiting, change in mental status or behavior, unsteady gait, or seizure. Parents should bring the child in for examination in 1 or 2 days. The manifestations of epidural hematoma in children do not generally appear until 24 hours or more after injury (see Family-Centered Care box and Emergency Treatment box, p. 1530).

FAMILY-CENTERED CARE

Maintaining Contact with Parents After Head Injury

Maintaining contact with parents for continued observation and reevaluation of the child, when indicated, facilitates early diagnosis and treatment of possible complications from head injury, such as hematoma, cerebral edema, and posttraumatic seizures. Children are generally hospitalized for 24 to 48 hours of observation if their family lives far from medical facilities or lacks transportation or a telephone, which would provide access to immediate help. Other circumstances, such as language or other communication barriers or even emotional trauma, may hinder learning and make it difficult for families to feel confident caring for their child at home.

! NURSING ALERT

If a child loses consciousness or vomits more than three times, medical attention should be sought.

Children with severe injuries, those who have lost consciousness for more than a few minutes, and those with prolonged and continued seizures or other focal or diffuse neurologic signs must be hospitalized until their condition is stable and their neurologic signs have diminished. The child is maintained on NPO status (nothing by mouth) or restricted to clear liquids (if able to take fluids by mouth) until it is determined that vomiting will not occur. IV fluids are indicated in the child who is comatose, displays dulled sensorium, or is persistently vomiting.

The volume of IV fluid is carefully monitored to minimize the possibility of overhydration in case of SIADH and cerebral edema. However, damage to the hypothalamus or pituitary gland may produce DI with its accompanying hypertonicity and dehydration. Fluid balance is closely monitored by daily weight, strict intake and output measurement, and serum osmolality (to detect early signs of water retention).

Sedating drugs are usually withheld in the acute phase. Headache is usually controlled with acetaminophen, although opioids may be needed (see p. 1519). Antiepileptics are used for seizure control. Antibiotics are administered if there are lacerations or penetrating injuries. Prophylactic tetanus toxoid is given as appropriate. (See Chapter 12.) Cerebral edema is managed as described for the unconscious child. Hyperthermia is controlled with a hypothermia blanket.

Surgical Therapy

Scalp lacerations are sutured after careful examination of underlying bone. Depressed fractures require surgical reduction and removal of bone fragments. Torn dura is also sutured (see Atraumatic Care box). A skull fracture depressed more than the thickness of the skull or an intracranial hematoma that causes more than 5 mm (0.2 inch) midline shift is an indication for surgery. Direct pressure should not be applied to a depressed skull fracture. Ping-Pong ball skull fractures in very young infants can correct themselves within a few weeks or may require surgical elevation (Hung, Liao, and Huang, 2005).

ATRAUMATIC CARE

Noninvasive Local Anesthesia

The use of topical lidocaine, epinephrine, and tetracaine (LET) or phenylephrine and tetracaine provides noninvasive, equally effective anesthesia for suturing (Zeltzer and Krell, 2009). Both of these preparations provide an acceptable alternative to tetracaine, adrenaline, and cocaine (TAC), which is more expensive, is a restricted narcotic, and carries a higher potential for toxicity.

Prognosis

The outcome of craniocerebral trauma depends on the extent of injury and complications. However, the outlook is generally more favorable for children than for adults. More than 90% of children with concussions or simple linear fractures recover without symptoms after the initial period. Compared with adults, children have a significantly higher percentage of good outcomes, a lower mortality rate, and a lower incidence of surgical mass lesions after severe head trauma. However, their thinner, softer brain may sustain greater long-term damage than previously suggested.

The concern regarding outcome is increasingly focused on cognitive, emotional, or mental problems. Children may experience a higher frequency of psychologic disturbances after head injury, whereas adults are more prone to complaints of a physical nature. Children may be more vulnerable than adults to long-term cognitive and behavioral dysfunction after diffuse brain injury.

True coma (not obeying commands, eyes closed, and not speaking) usually does not last more than 2 weeks. A child's eventual outcome can range from brain death to a persistent vegetative state to complete recovery. However, even the best recovery may be associated with personality changes, including mood lability and loss of confidence, impaired short-term memory, headaches, and subtle cognitive impairments. Many children are left with significant disabilities after head injury that appear months later as learning difficulties, behavioral changes, or emotional disturbances (Anderson, Catroppa, Haritou, et al, 2001, 2005; Ewing-Cobbs, Prasad, Kramer, et al, 2006). In general, 90% of the long-term neurologic outcome has been achieved within 6 months to 1 year after the injury.

Nursing Care Management

The hospitalized child requires careful neurologic assessment and evaluation (see p. 1511) repeated as frequently as every 15 minutes to establish a correct diagnosis, identify signs and symptoms of increased ICP, determine clinical management, and prevent many complications. The goals of nursing management of the child with a head injury are to maintain adequate ventilation, oxygenation, and circulation; to monitor and treat increased ICP; to minimize cerebral oxygen requirements; and to support the child and family during the recovery phases.

QUALITY PATIENT OUTCOMES: Acute Head Injury
- Early recognition of signs and symptoms of increased ICP
- Adequate ventilation, oxygenation, and circulation maintained
- Cerebral oxygen requirements minimized
- Sedation and analgesia provided while allowing for neurologic assessment

---

The child is placed on bed rest, usually with the head of the bed elevated slightly and the head in midline position. Appropriate safety measures, such as side rails kept up and seizure precautions, are implemented. If the child is extremely restless, hard surfaces may be padded and restraints used to prevent further injury. Individualize care according to the child's specific needs.

A key nursing role is to provide sedation and analgesia for the child. The conflict between the need to promote the child's comfort and relieve anxiety versus the need to assess for neurologic changes presents a dilemma. Both goals can be achieved with close observation of the child's LOC and response to analgesics (using a pain assessment record) and effective communication with the practitioner. Decreasing restlessness after administration of an analgesic most likely reflects pain control rather than a decreasing LOC. (See Pain Assessment and Pain Management, Chapter 7.)

Children may be restless and irritable, but more often their reaction is to fall asleep when left undisturbed. A quiet environment helps reduce the restlessness and irritability. Bright lights are irritating. This often makes checking the ocular responses more difficult and more aggravating to the child.

Frequent examinations of vital signs, neurologic signs, and LOC are extremely important nursing observations. When possible, they should be performed by a single observer to better detect subtle changes that may indicate worsening of neurologic status. Pupils are checked for size, equality, reaction to light, and accommodation. After the initial elevations usually seen after injury, the vital signs generally return to normal unless there is brainstem involvement.

The most important nursing observation is assessment of the child's LOC. In the progression of an injury, alterations in consciousness appear earlier than alterations of vital signs or focal neurologic signs (see p. 1512 for evaluation of responsiveness). Frequent examinations of alertness are fatiguing to the child; therefore the child often desires to fall asleep, which may be confused with depressed consciousness. When left alone, the child goes to sleep. It is not uncommon to observe ocular divergence through the partially closed eyelids.

Observations of position and movement provide additional information. Note any abnormal posturing and whether it occurs continuously or intermittently. Questions nurses might ask include:
- Are the child's hand grips strong and equal in strength?
- Are there any signs of extension or flexion posturing?
- What is the child's response to stimulation?
- Is movement purposeful, random, or absent?
- Are movement and sensation equal on both sides or restricted to one side only?

The child may complain of headache or other discomfort. The child who is too young to describe a headache may be fussy and resist being handled. The child who suffers from vertigo often vigorously resists being moved from a position of comfort. Forcible movement causes the child to vomit and display spontaneous nystagmus. Seizures are relatively common in children at the time of head injury and may be of any type. Carefully observe any seizure activity and describe it in detail. Children in postictal states are more lethargic, with sluggish pupils.

Document drainage from any orifice. Bleeding from the ear suggests the possibility of a basal skull fracture. Clear nasal drainage is suggestive of an anterior basal skull fracture. Observe the amount and characteristics of the drainage.

! NURSING ALERT

Suctioning through the nares is contraindicated because there is a risk of the catheter entering the brain through a fracture in the skull.

Head trauma is often accompanied by other undetected injuries; therefore any bruises, lacerations, or evidence of internal injuries or fractures of the extremities are noted and reported. Associated injuries are evaluated and treated appropriately.

The child with a normal LOC is usually allowed clear liquids unless fluid is restricted. If the child has an IV infusion, it is maintained as prescribed. The diet is advanced to that appropriate for the child's age as soon as the condition permits. Intake and output are measured and recorded, and any incontinence of bowel or bladder is noted for the child who has been toilet trained.

Observe the child for any unusual behavior, but interpretation of behavior is made in relation to the child's normal behavior. For example, urinary incontinence during sleep would be of no consequence in a child who routinely wets the bed but would be highly significant for one who is always dry. Parents are invaluable resources in evaluating objective behaviors of their children. Information obtained from parents at, or shortly after, admission is essential in evaluating the child's behavior (e.g., the ease with which the child is roused normally, the usual sleeping position, how much the child sleeps during the day, the child's motor activities [rolling over, sitting up, climbing], hearing and visual acuity, appetite, and manner of eating [spoon, bottle, cup]). There would be less concern about a child who falls asleep several times during the day if this is consistent with the child's usual behavior.

When the child is discharged, advise the parents of probable posttraumatic symptoms that may be expected, such as behavioral changes, sleep disturbances, phobias, and seizures. They should understand observations they need to make and how to contact the practitioner or health facility in case the child develops any unusual signs or symptoms. Emphasize the importance of follow-up evaluation.

Family Support

The emotional and educational support of the family presents a challenge. Witnessing the parents' grief and helplessness on seeing their child in an intensive care unit connected to monitoring equipment and in an altered state evokes empathy. The nurse can encourage the family to be involved in the child's care, to bring in familiar belongings, or to make a tape recording of familiar voices and sounds. Parents may need a demonstration on how to touch or cuddle their child and may want to talk about their grief. The nurse can listen attentively, reinforce what is being done to assist the child, and direct parents toward signs and symptoms of recovery to instill hope without promises. Honesty and kindness, along with consistent and competent care, can help families through this difficult time.

Rehabilitation

Rehabilitation and management of the child with permanent brain injury are essential aspects of care. Rehabilitation begins as soon as possible and usually involves the family and a rehabilitation team. The nurse makes a careful assessment of the child's capabilities, limitations, and probable potential as early as possible, and implements appropriate interventions to maximize the residual capacities. The Brain Injury Association of America* provides information and listings of rehabilitation services and support groups throughout the country.

Pediatric trauma rehabilitation is a national concern. Coordinating care and services for early rehabilitation involves identifying the child's and family's response to the traumatic injury and disability, securing available resources, and recognizing the parents' role in the process.

The child with a disability resulting from head trauma requires assessment on a physical, cognitive, emotional, and social level. The child has experienced separation, pain, sensory deprivation and overload, changes in circadian cycle, and fear of the unknown. Recovery and transition require new coping strategies at the same time that regressive and acting-out behaviors may start. Parents and children need honest communication for decision making. Rehabilitation is recommended when the child is making progress beyond what can be provided in a hospital setting. The Rancho Los Amigos Scale provides a systematic assessment of the progress that a child with a severe head injury may achieve. (See Family-Centered Care box, p. 1523.)

Pediatric rehabilitation focuses on the child's strengths and needs. The rehabilitation team should include physical medicine; rehabilitation nursing; nutritional counseling; physical, occupational, and speech therapy; special education; and psychologic, neuropsychologic, child life, and social services. Families need to know what to look for when visiting a pediatric rehabilitation center. Before the child's transfer, the hospital team should provide a detailed care plan of the child's needs and abilities, especially communication skills, and a description of the child's usual schedule, nursing care interventions, and the family's concerns and needs. To augment the care plan, a videotape introducing the child and family and showing any unique aspects of their care can be sent to the rehabilitation center.

Prevention

Preventive strategies are underused in almost all cases of accidental childhood injury. Head injuries occur in the most serious accidents—especially motor vehicle accidents, sports, and falls.

Tremendous strides have been taken in the prevention of cerebral damage after head injury in children. New developments are directed toward the prevention of cellular injury or the primary insult. The roles of calcium, oxyradicals, and prostaglandins are being investigated. However, the greatest benefit lies in prevention of head injuries. Nurses can exert a valuable influence on behalf of children through education. Accidents occur that are preventable because unnecessary risks go unchecked. Inadequate supervision combined with a child's natural sense of curiosity and exploration can lead to lethal results. Nurses are in the unique position of influencing caregivers in terms of growth and development. Banning the use of infant walkers is an example. This equipment does not help develop motor skills but places infants at risk for head and neck injuries from falls, especially down steps. Public education coupled with legislative support can prevent childhood injuries.

For extensive discussions of childhood injuries, see the information on injury prevention in Chapters 12, 14, 15, 17, and 19.

SUBMERSION INJURY

Submersion injury is a major cause of unintentional injury-related death in children ages 1 to 14 years. The term *near-drowning* is no longer used; instead, the term *submersion injury* should be used up until the time of drowning-related death (American Heart Association, 2005). Multiple definitions to describe submersion injury or near-drowning exist in the literature (Papa, Hoelle, and Idris, 2005). In 2003 guidelines were established for a uniform definition and reporting for submersion injury incidents (Idris, Berg, Bierens, et al, 2003).

Most cases of submersion injury are accidental, usually involving children who are helpless in water, such as inadequately attended children in or near swimming pools or infants in bathtubs; small children who fall into ponds, streams, and flooded excavations, usually near home; occupants of pleasure boats who fail to wear life preservers; children who have diving accidents; and children who are able to swim but overestimate their endurance. Accidental submersion injury occurs predominantly in males; 40% of children are younger than 5 years, and 90% of cases occur in private swimming pools (Kallas, 2009) (Fig. 37-9).

Submersion injury can take place in any body of water, including such unlikely places as a pail of water or a toilet bowl. Top-heavy toddlers fall headfirst into a pail of water, their arms become trapped, and they are unable to free themselves. Hot tubs and whirlpool spas have been implicated in childhood submersion injury. The suction created at the outlet is strong enough to trap even larger children underwater. Submersion

---

*1608 Spring Hill Road, Suite 110, Vienna, VA 22182; 703-761-0750; fax: 703-761-0755; www.biausa.org.

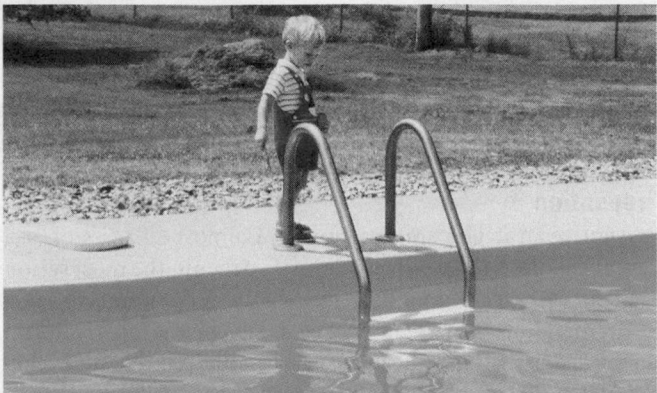

Fig. 37-9 Water is fascinating for children; however, drowning is the second leading cause of accidental death in unsupervised situations.

injury as a form of fatal child abuse also occurs. Homicidal submersion injuries are not witnessed, usually occurring in the home, and the victims are either infants or toddlers.

Pathophysiology

Physiologically most organ systems are affected, especially the pulmonary, cardiovascular, and neurologic systems. The major pulmonary changes that occur in submersion injury are directly related to the length of submersion (regardless of the type and amount of fluid aspirated), the victim's physiologic response, and the development and degree of immersion hypothermia. Cerebral hypoxia is a major component of morbidity and mortality in these individuals. Therefore early and aggressive resuscitation are imperative.

Physiologic factors that influence the extent of damage from immersion include resistance to asphyxia and anoxia, which shows some individual variation. The temperature of the water plays an important role in developing hypoxemia. Cold water decreases metabolic demands, thereby decreasing the effects of hypoxemia. Cold water also activates the diving reflex. This is a primitive neurologic response, often seen in children, of bradycardia and breath-holding. This neurologic response is triggered by immersion of the face in cold water. Blood is shunted away from the periphery to vital organs (i.e., the brain and heart). Submerged children struggle initially to stay above water, and often breath-hold leads to air hunger. Reflex inspiration eventually occurs, which leads to aspiration or reflex laryngospasm due to water contacting the lower respiratory tract (Salomez and Vincent, 2004). Cardiopulmonary arrest is secondary to hypoxemia and hypothermia.

Pathophysiologic features in submersion injuries are hypoxia, aspiration, and hypothermia. Hypoxia is the primary problem because it results in global cell damage, with different cells tolerating variable lengths of anoxia. Neurons, especially cerebral cells, sustain irreversible damage after 4 to 6 minutes of submersion. The heart and lungs can survive up to 30 minutes. Regardless of the amount of water aspirated, the victim suffers arterial hypoxemia (resulting from atelectasis and shunting of blood through the nonventilated alveoli), combined respiratory acidosis (resulting from retained carbon dioxide), and metabolic acidosis (caused by buildup of acid metabolites because of anaerobic metabolism). Although electrolyte imbalances are contributing factors, they are not the

major causes of morbidity and mortality. The pathologic events are directly related to the duration of submersion. The major difficulty is acute ventilatory insufficiency. Approximately 10% of submersion injury victims die without aspirating fluid but succumb from acute asphyxia as a result of prolonged reflex laryngospasm (see Research Focus box).

! NURSING ALERT

All children who have a submersion injury should be admitted to the hospital for observation. Although many patients do not appear to have suffered adverse effects from the event, complications (e.g., respiratory compromise, cerebral edema) may occur 24 hours after the incident.

Aspiration of fluid occurs in the majority of submersion injuries. The aspirated fluid results in pulmonary edema, atelectasis, airway spasm, and pneumonitis, which aggravates hypoxia. It was previously thought that the physiologic response differed between submersion in salt water and fresh water. However, there is no clinically significant difference in human survivors, and the type of water does not alter the therapy or outcome. The duration of submersion and severity of the hypoxia are the main factors that determine outcome (American Heart Association, 2005).

Hypothermia occurs rapidly in infants and children, partly because of their large surface area relative to size and partly as a result of the cold water itself. Profound hypothermia is usually evidence of lengthy submersion.

Clinical Manifestations

Clinical manifestations are directly related to the duration of loss of consciousness and neurologic status after rescue and resuscitation.

Therapeutic Management

With rapid treatment some children can be saved. Resuscitative measures should begin at the scene, and the victim should be transported to the hospital with maximum ventilatory and circulatory support. Many victims need care for some time after aspiration of fluid. In the hospital intensive pulmonary care is implemented and continued according to the patient's needs.

In general, management of the victim with a submersion injury is based on the degree of cerebral insult. The first priority is to restore oxygen delivery to the cells and prevent further hypoxic damage. A spontaneously breathing child does well in an oxygen-enriched atmosphere; the more severely affected child requires endotracheal intubation and mechanical ventilation. Blood gases and pH are monitored at frequent intervals as a guide to oxygen, fluid, and electrolyte therapies. Rewarming the hypothermic patient is initiated. Seizures may occur due to hypoxia and cerebral edema. Seizures result in increased cerebral oxygen consumption. Therefore it is imperative to aggressively control seizure activity. In addition, blood glucose should be monitored; both hypoglycemia and hyperglycemia are harmful to the brain.

All children who have a submersion injury should be hospitalized for 12 to 48 hours for observation. Although some children do not appear to have sustained adverse effects from the event, respiratory compromise or cerebral edema may occur within 24 hours after the incident. Aspiration pneumonia is a common complication that occurs approximately 48 to 72 hours after the episode. Bronchospasm, alveolar-capillary membrane damage, atelectasis, abscess formation, and acute respiratory distress syndrome are other complications that occur after aspiration of fluid.

Prognosis

The best predictors of a good outcome are length of submersion in nonicy water (5° C [41° F]) of less than 5 minutes and the presence of sinus rhythm, reactive pupils, and neurologic responsiveness at the scene. The worst outcomes—death or severe neurologic impairment—are for children submerged for more than 10 minutes and not responding to advanced life support within 25 minutes. All children without spontaneous purposeful movement and normal brainstem function 24 hours after sustaining a submersion injury suffered severe neurologic deficits or death (Kallas, 2009).

Nursing Care Management

Nursing care depends on the child's condition. A child who survives may need intensive respiratory nursing care with attention to vital signs, mechanical ventilation or tracheostomy, blood gas determination, chest physiotherapy, and IV infusion. Often the child has sustained a hypoxic insult and requires the same care as an unconscious child.

A difficult aspect in the care of the child who sustained a submersion injury is helping the parents cope with severe guilt reactions. Given the magnitude of the event, parents need repeated assurance that everything possible is being done to treat their child.

If the child dies, the sudden, unexpected nature of the death and the particular circumstances of the accident, especially in terms of guilt for not preventing it, compound the grief. (See Chapter 23.) The parents of the child who is saved from death face the anxiety of not knowing the final outcome—to what extent will their child recover? This situation generates such intense feelings of loneliness and guilt, it is important for families to know they are not alone. They should be reminded frequently that there are people to assist them through this crisis. Additional sources of support that can be recommended include psychiatric and social work consultants, community services, and religious support. Self-help groups are excellent if available in the community.

Nurses often have difficulty relating to the parents if obvious neglect has precipitated the accident and subsequent problems; therefore it is important for those who care for these children and their families to assess their own feelings about the situation, in addition to assessing the family's coping abilities and

resources. Caring for victims of a submersion injury and their families requires the nurse to be sensitive to the needs of the child and the family and to recognize his or her own reactions and emotions.

Prevention

Most submersion injuries are preventable. The most common cause of submersion injury in infants and small children is inadequate adult supervision. Children with known risk factors such as epilepsy and autism require increased surveillance. In general, children are not developmentally ready for formal swimming lessons until after their fourth birthday. All parents and swimming pool owners should be familiar with basic cardiopulmonary resuscitation (CPR). Rapid, basic CPR is one of the keys to improving the outcome (Salomez and Vincent, 2004). Water safety and survival training should be required for all school-age children. Private pools should be fenced on all four sides. Nurses can be active advocates in their communities. Nurses are also in a position to emphasize the importance of adequate adult supervision when children are in or near the water (Kallas, 2009). (See Injury Prevention, Chapters 12, 14, 15, 17, and 19.)

INTRACRANIAL INFECTIONS

The nervous system is subject to infection by the same organisms that affect other organs of the body. However, the nervous system is limited in the ways in which it responds to injury. Laboratory studies are needed to identify the causative agent. The inflammatory process can affect the meninges (meningitis) or brain (encephalitis).

Meningitis can be caused by a variety of organisms, but the three main types are (1) bacterial, or pyogenic, caused by pus-forming bacteria, especially meningococci, pneumococci, and group B streptococci; (2) viral, or aseptic, caused by a wide variety of viral agents; and (3) tuberculous, caused by the tuberculin bacillus. The majority of children with acute febrile encephalopathy have either bacterial meningitis or viral meningitis as the underlying cause.

BACTERIAL MENINGITIS

Bacterial meningitis is an acute inflammation of the meninges and CSF. The advent of antimicrobial therapy has had a marked effect on the course and prognosis. The introduction of conjugate vaccines against *Haemophilus influenzae* type b (Hib vaccine) in 1990 and *Streptococcus pneumoniae* (pneumococcus) in 2000 has led to dramatic changes in the epidemiology of bacterial meningitis (see Evidence-Based Practice box). Today, *H. influenzae* type b infection has been virtually eradicated among young children in areas in the world where the Hib vaccine is administered routinely (Yogev and Guzman-Cottrill, 2005). Since the introduction of widespread vaccination for *S. pneumoniae,* the incidence of pneumococcal meningitis in children in the United States has decreased by 55% to 60%. Nonetheless, *S. pneumoniae* remains an important and frequent cause of bacterial meningitis in children (Kaplan, Mason, Wald, et al, 2004; Nigrovic, Kuppermann, and Malley, 2008).

S. pneumoniae remains the most common cause of bacterial meningitis in children between 3 months and 10 years of age

---

EVIDENCE-BASED PRACTICE

Children with Bacterial Meningitis and Preventive Vaccines

ASK THE QUESTION

In children and adolescents with bacterial meningitis, has the administration of *Haemophilus influenzae* type b (Hib), pneumococcal, and meningococcal preventive vaccines reduced the incidence and mortality associated with bacterial meningitis?

SEARCH FOR THE EVIDENCE

Search strategies
Search selection criteria included English-language publications within past 15 years, research-based articles (level 3 or lower), children and adult populations.

Databases used
PubMed, Cochrane Collaboration, MDConsult

CRITICALLY ANALYZE THE EVIDENCE

GRADE criteria: Evidence quality strong; recommendation strong (Guyatt, Oxman, Vist, et al, 2008)

- Laval, Pimenta, de Andrade, and colleagues (2003) conducted a systematic review of several studies done in developed and developing countries that compared the effect of the conjugate of the Hib vaccine in the early 1990s to the more recent use of the heptavalent pneumococcal and the serogroup C meningococcal vaccines of today. The researchers concluded that all the vaccines mentioned have contributed directly to the decline in acute bacterial meningitis.
- Data trends on *Streptococcus pneumoniae* infections from the Bacterial Core Surveillance of the Centers for Disease Control and Prevention were evaluated from 1998 to 2001. After being licensed in early 2000, the pneumococcal conjugate vaccine significantly reduced the number of invasive pneumococcal cases, with the largest decline in young children less than 2 years of age (Whitney, Farley, Hadler, et al, 2003).
- Haddy, Perry, Chacko, and colleagues (2005) compared the incidence of *S. pneumoniae* disease before and after the introduction of conjugated pneumococcal vaccine from 1999 to 2002. The trend in the rates of invasive pneumococcal disease cases showed significant declines during the study period for all ages after the introduction of the heptavalent *S. pneumoniae* protein conjugate vaccine.
- Children's Hospital of Pittsburgh reported the occurrence of bacterial meningitis before and after the licensure of the Hib conjugate vaccine. Two hundred and twenty-one children, ages 1 month to 18 years, diagnosed with bacterial meningitis were identified from 1988 to 1998. *H. influenzae* was the organism responsible for approximately 58% of cases of bacterial meningitis. The absolute number of cases of bacterial meningitis caused by *H. influenzae* declined to 2.5 cases per year after introduction of the Hib conjugate vaccine (Neuman and Wald, 2001).
- Data from an outbreak of meningococcal disease in northern Ghana in 1997 was used to assess the potential effect of different vaccination strategies. Vaccination was conducted between February and April, which covered 72% of the high-risk population and prevented approximately 23% of the meningitis cases and 18% of the deaths related to meningitis. Routine childhood and adult immunization would have prevented 61% of cases had this same rate of vaccine coverage been achieved and maintained before the epidemic. This study suggests that the prevention of the meningococcal disease epidemic in West Africa will be difficult unless long-lasting conjugate meningococcal vaccines are incorporated into routine infant immunization schedules (Woods, Armstrong, Sackey, et al, 2000).
- A double-blind randomized trial in Gambia was conducted to assess the efficacy of an Hib conjugate vaccine for the prevention of meningitis, pneumonia, and other invasive diseases caused by *H. influenzae*. From March 1993 to October 1995, 42,848 infants were randomly administered the conjugate vaccine Hib polysaccharide tetanus protein (PRP-T) mixed with diphtheria-tetanus-pertussis vaccine (DTP), or DTP alone at age 2 months, 3 months, and 4 months. Three doses of the vaccine were 95% effective in the prevention of meningitis and pneumonia caused by *H. influenzae* in the group of infants receiving the Hib vaccine (Mulholland, Hilton, Adegbola, et al, 1997).

APPLY THE EVIDENCE: NURSING IMPLICATIONS

The epidemiology studies strongly suggest that all children should be immunized against the most common organisms responsible for bacterial meningitis (i.e., *H. influenzae* type b, *S. pneumoniae*, and *Neisseria meningitidis*) as preventive vaccines to decrease the incidence of bacterial meningitis. The nurse should stress to the parents, children, adolescents, and young adults the importance of adhering to the immunization schedule to protect against serious childhood diseases.

References

Guyatt GH, Oxman AD, Vist GE, et al: GRADE: an emerging consensus on rating quality of evidence and strength of recommendations, *BMJ* 336:924-926, 2008.

Haddy RI, Perry K, Chacko CE, et al: Comparison of incidence in invasive *Streptococcus pneumoniae* disease among children before and after introduction of conjugated pneumococcal vaccine, *Pediatr Infect Dis J* 24(4):320-330, 2005.

Laval CA, Pimenta FC, de Andrade JG, et al: Progress towards meningitis prevention in the conjugate vaccines era, *Braz J Infect Dis* 7(5):315-324, 2003.

Mulholland K, Hilton S, Adegbola R, et al: Randomised trial of *Haemophilus influenzae* type-b tetanus protein conjugate for prevention of pneumonia and meningitis in Gambian infants, *Lancet* 349(9060):1186-1187, 1997.

Neuman HB, Wald ER: Bacterial meningitis in childhood at the Children's Hospital of Pittsburgh: 1988-1998, *Clin Pediatr (Phila)* 40(11):595-600, 2001.

Whitney CG, Farley MM, Hadler J, et al: Decline in invasive pneumococcal disease after the introduction of protein–polysaccharide conjugate vaccine, *N Engl J Med* 348(18):1737-1746, 2003.

Woods CW, Armstrong G, Sackey SO, et al: Emergency vaccination against epidemic meningitis in Ghana: implications for the control of meningococcal disease in West Africa, *Lancet* 355(9197):30-33, 2000.

---

despite appropriate treatment. In children older than 1 month and less than 3 months, group B streptococci and gram-negative bacilli were the most frequent pathogens causing bacterial meningitis (Nigrovic, Kuppermann, and Malley, 2008).

Etiology

A variety of bacterial agents can cause bacterial meningitis. Since the introduction of new vaccinations (Hib and PCV7), the pathogens responsible for meningitis have changed. Currently *S. pneumoniae* and *Neisseria meningitidis* are the leading causes of bacterial meningitis in children between 3 months and 19 years. *S. pneumoniae* is the leading cause in children between 3 months and 10 years, and *N. meningitidis* is the leading cause in children between 10 and 19 years. The distribution of causative pathogens differs in children between 1 and 3 months. The leading causes of neonatal meningitis are group B streptococci (39%) and gram-negative bacilli (32%) (Nigrovic, Kuppermann, and Malley, 2008).

Meningococcal meningitis occurs in epidemic form and is the only type readily transmitted by droplet infection from nasopharyngeal secretions. Although this condition may develop at any age, the risk of meningococcal infection increases with the number of contacts; therefore it occurs predominantly in school-age children and adolescents. There appear to be some seasonal variations. Meningitis caused by pneumococcal and meningococcal infections can occur at any time, but is more common in later winter or early spring.

Maternal factors, such as premature rupture of fetal membranes and maternal infection during the last week of pregnancy, are major causes of neonatal meningitis. Risk factors for children developing meningitis include recent exposure to someone with meningococcal meningitis; recent ear or sinus infection; travel to areas where bacterial meningitis is common such as sub-Saharan Africa; penetrating head trauma; cochlear implant devices; and anatomic defects such as a dermal sinus, urinary tract anomaly, or recent placement of a ventricular shunt (Chavez-Bureno and McCracken, 2005).

Pathophysiology

The most common route of infection is vascular dissemination from a focus of infection elsewhere. For example, organisms from the nasopharynx invade the underlying blood vessels, cross the BBB, and multiply in the CSF. Invasion by direct extension from infections in the paranasal and mastoid sinuses is less common. Organisms also gain entry by direct implantation after penetrating wounds, skull fractures that provide an opening into the skin or sinuses, lumbar puncture or surgical procedures, anatomic abnormalities such as spina bifida, or foreign bodies such as an internal ventricular shunt or an external ventricular device. Once implanted, the organisms spread into the CSF, by which the infection spreads throughout the subarachnoid space.

The infective process is like that seen in any bacterial infection: inflammation, exudation, white blood cell accumulation, and varying degrees of tissue damage. The brain becomes hyperemic and edematous, and the entire surface of the brain is covered by a layer of purulent exudate that varies with the type of organism. For example, meningococcal exudate is most marked over the parietal, occipital, and cerebellar regions; the thick, fibrinous exudate of pneumococcal infection is confined chiefly to the surface of the brain, particularly the anterior lobes; and the exudate of streptococcal infections is similar to that of pneumococcal infections, but thinner.

As infection extends to the ventricles, thick pus, fibrin, or adhesions may occlude the narrow passages and obstruct the flow of CSF.

Clinical Manifestations

The clinical manifestations of acute bacterial meningitis depend to a large extent on the child's age. The type of organism, the effectiveness of therapy for antecedent illness, and whether it occurs as an isolated entity or as a complication of another illness or injury also influence the clinical manifestation (Box 37-6).

Children and Adolescents

The onset of illness may be abrupt and rapid, or develop progressively over one or several days and may be preceded by a

---

BOX 37-6 CLINICAL MANIFESTATIONS OF BACTERIAL MENINGITIS

Children and Adolescents
Usually abrupt onset
Fever
Chills
Headache
Vomiting
Alterations in sensorium
Seizures (often the initial sign)
Irritability
Agitation
May develop:
- Photophobia
- Delirium
- Hallucinations
- Aggressive behavior
- Drowsiness
- Stupor
- Coma

Nuchal rigidity; may progress to opisthotonos
Positive Kernig and Brudzinski signs
Hyperactivity but variable reflex responses
Signs and symptoms peculiar to individual organisms:
- Petechial or purpuric rashes (meningococcal infection), especially when associated with a shocklike state
- Joint involvement (meningococcal and *Haemophilus influenzae* infection)
- Chronically draining ear (pneumococcal meningitis)

Infants and Young Children
Classic picture (above) rarely seen in children between 3 months and 2 years of age
Fever
Poor feeding
Vomiting
Marked irritability
Frequent seizures (often accompanied by a high-pitched cry)
Bulging fontanel
Nuchal rigidity possible
Brudzinski and Kernig signs not helpful in diagnosis
Difficult to elicit and evaluate in this age-group
Subdural empyema (*H. influenzae* infection)

Neonates
Specific Signs
Extremely difficult to diagnose
Manifestations vague and nonspecific
Child well at birth but within a few days begins to look and behave poorly
Refuses feedings
Poor sucking ability
Vomiting or diarrhea
Poor tone
Lack of movement
Weak cry
Full, tense, and bulging fontanel may appear late in course of illness
Neck usually supple

Nonspecific Signs That May Be Present
Hypothermia or fever (depending on the infant's maturity)
Jaundice
Irritability
Drowsiness
Seizures
Respiratory irregularities or apnea
Cyanosis
Weight loss

febrile illness (Feigin and Perlman, 2004). Most children with meningitis are seen with fever, chills, headache, vomiting, irritability, and nuchal rigidity that are associated with or quickly followed by alterations in sensorium. Some children are initially seen after having a seizure or have a seizure within the first 48 hours of admission to the hospital (Feigin and Perlman, 2004). The child is extremely irritable and agitated and may develop photophobia, confusion, hallucinations, aggressive behavior, drowsiness, stupor, or coma.

The child resists flexion of the neck (nuchal rigidity). Kernig and Brudzinski signs are positive. Reflex responses are variable, although they show hyperactivity. (See Reflexes, Chapter 6.) The skin may be cold and cyanotic with poor peripheral perfusion.

Other signs and symptoms may appear that are specific to individual organisms. Petechial or purpuric rashes occur in 50% of cases and indicate a meningococcal infection (meningococcemia), especially when the eruption is associated with a septic shock–like state. Joint involvement is seen in meningococcal and *H. influenzae* infection. A chronically draining ear commonly accompanies pneumococcal meningitis. *Escherichia coli* infection may be associated with a congenital dermal sinus that communicates with the subarachnoid space.

Infants and Young Children

Between 3 months and 2 years of age the illness is characterized by fever or hypothermia, poor feeding, vomiting, marked irritability, restlessness, seizures, and a bulging or tense fontanel, which are often accompanied by a high-pitched cry.

Neonates

Meningitis in newborn and premature infants is extremely difficult to diagnose. The vague and nonspecific manifestations, which are characteristic of all neonatal sepsis, bear little resemblance to the findings in older children. These infants are usually well at birth but within a few days begin to appear ill. They refuse feedings, have poor sucking ability, and may vomit or have diarrhea. They display poor muscle tone and lack of movement and have a poor cry. Other nonspecific signs that may be present include hypothermia or fever (depending on the infant's maturity), jaundice, irritability, drowsiness, seizures, respiratory irregularities or apnea, cyanosis, and weight loss. The full, tense, and bulging fontanel may or may not be present until late in the course of the illness, and the neck is usually supple. Untreated, the child's condition will decline to cardiovascular collapse, seizures, and apnea.

Complications

The incidence of complications from acute bacterial meningitis has been significantly reduced with early diagnosis and vigorous antimicrobial therapy. If infection extends to the ventricles, thick pus, fibrin, or adhesions may occlude the narrow passages, thereby obstructing the flow of CSF and causing obstructive hydrocephalus. Subdural effusions often occur, and thrombosis may occur in meningeal veins or venous sinuses. Destructive changes may take place in the cerebral cortex, and brain abscesses may form by direct extension of the infection or by vascular dissemination. Extension of the infection to the areas of the cranial nerves or compression necrosis from

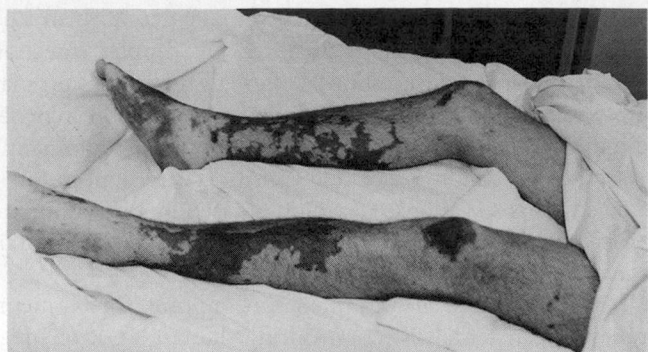

Fig. 37-10 Purpura of the lower extremities of child suffering from meningococcemia.

increased pressure may cause deafness, blindness, or weakness or paralysis of facial or other muscles of the head and neck.

One of the most dramatic and serious complications usually associated with meningococcal infections is meningococcal sepsis, or meningococcemia. When the onset is severe, sudden, and rapid, it is known as the Waterhouse-Friderichsen syndrome. The syndrome is characterized by overwhelming septic shock, disseminated intravascular coagulation, massive bilateral adrenal hemorrhage, and purpura (Fig. 37-10). Meningococcemia requires immediate emergency treatment, hospitalization, and intensive care because of the high mortality rate (Feigin and Perlman, 2004; Woods, 2009).

> **! NURSING ALERT**
>
> Any child who is ill and develops a purpuric or petechial rash may have (overwhelming) meningococcemia and must receive medical attention immediately.

Other acute complications of meningitis include SIADH (see Chapter 38), subdural effusions, seizures, cerebral edema and herniation, and hydrocephalus. Obstruction to the flow of CSF occurs during the acute phase of illness by clumping of purulent material in the drainage channels and during the chronic phase by adhesive arachnoiditis or fibrotic obstruction through any of the ventricular foramina. Postmeningitic complications in neonates include ventriculitis, which results in cystic, walled-off areas of the brain with fluid accumulation and pressure.

Extension of the inflammation to cranial nerves or compression and destruction of the nerves from ICP can produce permanent impairment of vision or hearing and other nerve palsies. CN VIII damage is usually followed by permanent deafness. Other long-term complications include cerebral palsy, cognitive impairments, learning disorder, attention deficit hyperactivity disorder, and seizures.

Hemiparesis and quadriparesis may result from damage caused by arteritis or thrombosis or other mechanisms. Behavioral changes occur in some children. Evidence indicates that psychometric and behavioral defects may be a significant concomitant sign of meningitis in childhood, although it is difficult to determine the degree to which meningitis affects the intelligence of young children. Meningitis in the neonatal period is more likely to cause lifelong impairments, including moderate to severe developmental delay, blindness, deafness, and epilepsy (de Louvois, Halket, and Harvey, 2005).

Diagnostic Evaluation

A lumbar puncture is the definitive diagnostic test. The fluid pressure is measured and samples are obtained for culture, Gram stain, blood cell count, and determination of glucose and protein content. The findings are usually diagnostic. Culture and sensitivity are needed to identify the causative organism. Spinal fluid pressure is usually elevated, but interpretation is often difficult when the child is crying. Sedation with fentanyl and midazolam can alleviate the child's pain and fear associated with this procedure (see Atraumatic Care box). If there is evidence or suspicion of increased ICP (papilledema, focal neurologic deficits, coma, presence of a CSF shunt, history of hydrocephalus), a CT scan of the head may be warranted before the procedure (Tunkel, Hartman, Kaplan, et al, 2004).

ATRAUMATIC CARE

Lumbar Puncture

LMX (4% lidocaine) or EMLA cream (a eutectic mixture of lidocaine and prilocaine), both topical anesthetics, may be applied to the skin overlying L3 to L5 to reduce pain before lumbar puncture. For maximum effect, apply EMLA cream at least 1 hour before the procedure or LMX 30 minutes beforehand.

The patient generally has an elevated white blood cell count, often predominantly polymorphonuclear leukocytes. The glucose level is reduced, generally in proportion to the duration and severity of the infection. The relationship between the CSF glucose and serum glucose levels is important in evaluating the glucose content of CSF; therefore a serum glucose sample is drawn approximately one half hour before the lumbar puncture. Protein concentration is usually increased.

A blood culture is advisable for all children suspected of having meningitis and occasionally will be positive when CSF culture is negative. Nose and throat cultures may provide helpful information in some cases.

Therapeutic Management

Acute bacterial meningitis is a medical emergency that requires early recognition and immediate therapy to prevent death and avoid residual disabilities. The initial therapeutic management includes:

- Isolation precautions
- Initiation of antimicrobial therapy
- Maintenance of hydration
- Maintenance of ventilation
- Reduction of increased ICP
- Management of systemic shock
- Control of seizures
- Control of temperature
- Treatment of complications

The child is isolated from other children, usually in an intensive care unit for close observation. An IV infusion is started to facilitate administration of antimicrobial agents, fluids, antiepileptic drugs, and blood, if needed. The child is placed on a cardiac monitor and in respiratory isolation.

Drugs

Until the causative organism is identified, the choice of antibiotic is based on the known sensitivity of the organism most likely to be the infective agent. After identification of the organism, antimicrobial agents are adjusted accordingly.

⚡ DRUG ALERT

Dexamethasone Use in Meningitis

Dexamethasone may play a role in the initial management of increased ICP and cerebral herniation, but its ability to reduce long-term complications of bacterial meningitis remains controversial. There is evidence that dexamethasone therapy decreases the risk of neurologic sequelae in children with *H. influenzae* type b meningitis and should be considered for use in other bacterial types of meningitis (American Academy of Pediatrics, 2006; Prober, 2009). It should not be used if aseptic or nonbacterial meningitis is suspected (Bonthius and Karacay, 2002).

Signs of gastrointestinal hemorrhage or secondary infection may complicate steroid administration. Antibiotic treatment with cephalosporins demonstrates superiority for promptly sterilizing the CSF and reducing the incidence of severe hearing impairment.

Nonspecific Measures

Maintaining hydration is a prime concern, and the patient's condition determines whether IV fluids are needed and the type and amount of fluid. The optimum hydration involves correction of any fluid deficits followed by fluid restriction as ordered to prevent cerebral edema. Cerebral edema and electrolyte disturbances are associated with poor neurologic outcome after bacterial meningitis (Bonthius and Karacay, 2002). Children with bacterial meningitis must be monitored for signs of increased ICP. If needed, measures to decrease ICP are implemented (see p. 1520).

Complications are treated appropriately, such as aspiration of subdural effusion in infants and treatment for disseminated intravascular coagulation syndrome. Shock is managed by restoration of circulating blood volume and maintenance of electrolyte balance. Seizures can occur during the first few days of treatment. These are controlled with the appropriate antiepileptic drug. Hearing loss is not uncommon. The patient should undergo auditory evaluation 6 months after the illness has resolved.

Lumbar puncture is carried out as needed to determine the effectiveness of therapy. The patient is evaluated neurologically during the convalescent period.

Prognosis

Ten percent to 15% of cases of bacterial meningitis are fatal (Centers for Disease Control and Prevention, 2000). The child's age, duration of illness before antibiotic therapy, rapidity of diagnosis after onset, type of organism, prolonged or complicated seizures, low CSF glucose concentration, and adequacy of therapy are important in the prognosis of bacterial meningitis (see Research Focus box). Bacterial meningitis can result in brain damage, hearing loss, or learning disability (Centers for Disease Control and Prevention, 2000; Prober, 2009).

RESEARCH FOCUS

Meningitis in the Neonate

Neonatal meningitis carries the highest mortality. However, with the development of new antibiotics and the advent of aggressive supportive care measures, the mortality rate for bacterial meningitis in children caused by *Haemophilus influenzae* type b, *Streptococcus pneumoniae*, and *Neisseria meningitidis* is less than 10% in most studies (Prober, 2009).

DRUG ALERT

Antibiotic Use in Meningitis

A major priority of nursing care of a child suspected of having meningitis is to administer antibiotics as soon as they are ordered. The child is placed on respiratory isolation for at least 24 hours after initiation of antimicrobial therapy.

The sequelae of bacterial meningitis occur most often when the disease occurs in the first 2 months of life and least often in children with meningococcal meningitis. The residual deficits in infants are primarily a result of communicating hydrocephalus and the greater effects of cerebritis on the immature brain. In older children the residual effects are related to the inflammatory process itself or result from vasculitis associated with the disease. Bacterial meningitis continues to cause substantial morbidity in infants and children. The mortality rate and incidence of poor neurologic outcome is highest in patients with pneumococcal meningitis (Prober, 2009).

Hearing impairment is the most common sequela of this disease. Evaluation of CN VIII is needed for at least a 6-month follow-up period to assess for possible hearing loss.

Prevention

Vaccines are available for types A, C, Y, and W-135 meningococci and *H. influenzae* type b. Routine meningococcal polysaccharide vaccination of children is licensed for use only in children 2 years and older (Pichichero, 2005). Routine vaccinations for *H. influenzae* type b are recommended for all children beginning at 2 months of age. (See Immunizations, Chapter 12.) Pneumococcal conjugate vaccine is now recommended for all children beginning at 2 months of age (Centers for Disease Control and Prevention, 2009).

Nursing Care Management

Nurses should take the necessary precautions to protect themselves and others from possible infection. Teach parents the proper procedures and supervise them in their application.

Keep the room as quiet as possible, and keep environmental stimuli at a minimum, since most children with meningitis are sensitive to noise, bright lights, and other external stimuli. Most children are more comfortable without a pillow and with the head of the bed slightly elevated. A side-lying position is more often assumed because of nuchal rigidity. The nurse should avoid actions that cause pain or increase discomfort, such as lifting the child's head. Evaluating the child for pain and implementing appropriate relief measures are important during the initial 24 to 72 hours. Acetaminophen with codeine is often used. Measures are used to ensure safety because the child is often restless and subject to seizures.

The nursing care of the child with meningitis is determined by the child's symptoms and treatment (see Box 37-6). Observation of vital signs, neurologic signs, LOC, urinary output, and other pertinent data is carried out at frequent intervals. The child who is unconscious is managed as described previously (see pp. 1519-1524), and all children are observed carefully for signs of the complications just described, especially increased ICP, shock, or respiratory distress. Frequent assessment of the open fontanels is needed in the infant because subdural effusions and obstructive hydrocephalus can develop as a complication of meningitis.

Administration of fluids and nourishment is determined by the child's status. The child with dulled sensorium is usually given nothing by mouth. Other children are allowed clear liquids initially and, if tolerated, progress to a diet suitable for their age. Careful monitoring and recording of intake and output are needed to determine deviations that might indicate impending shock or increasing fluid accumulation, such as cerebral edema or subdural effusion.

One of the most difficult problems in the nursing care of children with meningitis is maintaining IV infusion for the length of time needed to provide adequate antimicrobial therapy (usually 10 days). Because continuous IV fluids are usually not necessary, an intermittent infusion device is used. In some cases children who are recovering uneventfully are sent home with the device, and the parents are taught IV drug administration.

QUALITY PATIENT OUTCOMES: Bacterial Meningitis
- Early recognition of signs and symptoms of meningitis
- Antibiotics administered as soon as diagnosis is established
- Cerebral edema prevented
- Exposure prevented by early isolation
- Side effects managed
- Neurologic sequelae prevented

Family Support

The sudden nature of the illness makes emotional support of the child and parents extremely important (see Family-Centered Care box). Parents are upset and concerned about their child's condition and often feel guilty for not having suspected the seriousness of the illness sooner. They need much reassurance that the natural onset of meningitis is sudden and that they acted responsibly in seeking medical assistance when they did. The nurse encourages the parents to openly discuss their feelings to minimize blame and guilt. The nurse also keeps them informed of the child's progress and of all procedures, results, and treatments. In the event that the child's condition worsens, they need the same psychologic care as other parents facing the possible death of their child. (See Chapter 23.)

TABLE 37-4	VARIATION OF CEREBROSPINAL FLUID ANALYSIS IN BACTERIAL AND VIRAL MENINGITIS	
MANIFESTATIONS	**BACTERIAL***	**VIRAL**
White blood cell count	Elevated; increased polys	Slightly elevated; increased lymphs
Protein content	Elevated	Normal or slightly increased
Glucose content	Decreased	Normal
Gram stain; bacteria culture	Positive	Turbid or cloudy
Color	Clear or slightly cloudy	Negative

*Results may vary in the neonate.

NONBACTERIAL (ASEPTIC) MENINGITIS

Many different viruses cause aseptic meningitis. The onset may be abrupt or gradual. The initial manifestations are headache, fever, malaise, and gastrointestinal symptoms. Signs of meningeal irritation develop 1 or 2 days after the onset of illness. Onset is more insidious in infants and toddlers. Signs and symptoms are vague and are often thought to be associated with a minor illness.

Diagnosis is based on clinical features and CSF findings. Table 37-4 lists variations in CSF values in bacterial and viral meningitis. It is important to differentiate this self-limiting disorder from the more serious forms of meningitis.

Treatment is primarily symptomatic, such as acetaminophen for headache and muscle pain, maintenance of hydration, and positioning for comfort. Until a definitive diagnosis is made, antimicrobial agents may be administered and isolation enforced as a precaution against the possibility that the disease might be of bacterial origin. Nursing care is similar to the care of the child with bacterial meningitis.

TUBERCULOUS MENINGITIS

Tuberculous meningitis must be considered, especially in persons traveling or living in, and in immigrants from, developing countries. The advent of drug-resistant tuberculosis may lead to infections in an increasing number of children. Tuberculous meningitis is more likely to be disseminated (including CNS involvement) in very young or immunosuppressed children.

Ischemic infarction can occur with tuberculous meningitis. The most common clinical findings are meningeal signs, fever, alteration of consciousness, CN involvement, seizures, and focal neurologic deficit.

Early diagnosis of tuberculous meningitis in the child can significantly reduce the disability caused by hydrocephalus, a common complication of this type of meningitis. Nursing care is similar to the care of the child with bacterial meningitis and involves administration of medications, support of the child, control of pain, and neurologic monitoring.

BRAIN ABSCESS

Intracerebral abscesses form when pyogenic organisms gain access to neural tissue by way of the bloodstream from foci of infection or from direct inoculation of organisms from meningitis, penetrating trauma, or surgical procedures. Chronic ear infection, mastoiditis, sinusitis, and cyanotic congenital heart disease are the most common predisposing factors for children with brain abscesses. Meningitis and ventriculitis are dominant causes in infants. The majority (70%) of brain abscesses are caused by a single organism (Haslam, 2009). The most common pyogenic organisms include staphylococci, streptococci, and *Proteus* organisms. However, many children with brain abscesses have no discernible source of infection.

The most common sites of intracerebral abscesses are the temporal and frontal lobes between the gray and white matter. Early signs of the disease are vague; however, the most common symptom is a severe headache. Other symptoms may include vomiting, lethargy, fever, seizures, and progression to coma. Specific neurologic signs are related to the area invaded by the infectious process and, as this area enlarges, resemble those produced by an intracranial tumor. Cerebellar abscesses produce signs and symptoms associated with any posterior fossa mass. (See Brain Tumors, Chapter 36.) Because mortality rates from brain abscesses may exceed 20%, a prompt diagnosis is critical. Successful management consists of surgical drainage and antibiotic therapy. Surgical drainage is necessary if medical therapy does not resolve the abscess. Where possible, the source of the infection is eradicated. Children may experience epilepsy as a long-term complication.

ENCEPHALITIS

Encephalitis is an inflammatory process of the CNS that is caused by a variety of organisms, including bacteria, spirochetes, fungi, protozoa, helminths, and viruses. Most infections are associated with viruses, and this discussion is limited to those agents.

Etiology

Encephalitis can occur as a result of (1) direct invasion of the CNS by a virus or (2) postinfectious involvement of the CNS after a viral disease. Often the specific type of encephalitis may not be identified. The cause of more than half the cases reported in the United States is unknown. The majority of cases of known etiology are associated with the childhood diseases of measles, mumps, varicella, and rubella and, less often, with the enteroviruses, herpesviruses, and West Nile virus.

BOX 37-7 CLINICAL MANIFESTATIONS OF ENCEPHALITIS

Onset
Malaise
Fever
Headache
Dizziness
Apathy
Lethargy
Nuchal rigidity

Severe Cases
High fever
Stupor

Seizures
Disorientation
Nausea and vomiting
Ataxia
Tremors
Hyperactivity
Speech difficulties—mutism
Altered mental status
Spasticity
Coma (may proceed to death)
Ocular palsies
Paralysis

Herpes simplex encephalitis is an uncommon disease, but 30% of cases involve children. The initial clinical findings are nonspecific (fever, altered mental status), but most cases evolve to demonstrate focal neurologic signs and symptoms. Children may experience focal seizures. The CSF is abnormal in most cases. Because of a rise in the number of children with herpes simplex encephalitis, suspected cases require prompt attention, especially because the diagnosis can be difficult. CSF polymerase chain reaction (PCR) testing can confirm the clinical diagnosis rapidly. The early use of IV acyclovir reduces mortality and morbidity. Empiric therapy with acyclovir is given before precise virologic diagnosis has been established.

The multiplicity of causes of viral encephalitis makes diagnosis difficult. Most are those involved with arthropod vectors (togaviruses and bunyaviruses) and those associated with hemorrhagic fevers (arenaviruses, filoviruses, and hantaviruses). In the United States the vector reservoir for most agents pathogenic for humans is the mosquito (St. Louis or West Nile encephalitis); therefore most cases of encephalitis appear during the hot summer months and subside during the autumn.

Clinical Manifestations

The clinical features of encephalitis are similar regardless of the agent involved. Manifestations can range from a mild benign form that resembles aseptic meningitis, lasts a few days, and is followed by rapid and complete recovery, to a rapidly progressing encephalitis with severe CNS involvement. The onset may be sudden or may be gradual with malaise, fever, headache, dizziness, apathy, nuchal rigidity, nausea and vomiting, ataxia, tremors, hyperactivity, and speech difficulties (Box 37-7). In severe cases the patient has high fever, stupor, seizures, disorientation, spasticity, and coma that may proceed to death. Ocular palsies and paralysis also may occur.

Diagnostic Evaluation

The diagnosis is made on the basis of clinical findings and, where possible, identification of the specific virus. Early in the course of encephalitis, CT scan results may be normal. Later, hemorrhagic areas in the frontotemporal region may be seen. Togaviruses (some of which were formerly labeled arboviruses) are rarely detected in the blood or spinal fluid, but viruses of herpes, mumps, measles, and enteroviruses may be found in the CSF. Serologic testing may be required. The first blood sample should be drawn as soon as possible after onset, with the second sample drawn 2 or 3 weeks later.

Therapeutic Management

Patients suspected of having encephalitis are hospitalized promptly for observation. Treatment is primarily supportive and includes conscientious nursing care, control of cerebral manifestations, and adequate nutrition and hydration, with observations and management as for other cerebral disorders. Viral encephalitis can cause devastating neurologic injury. Cerebral hyperemia occurs in severe viral encephalitis, and ICP monitoring to reduce the pressure may be needed (Prober, 2009). Follow-up care with periodic reevaluation and rehabilitation is important for patients who develop residual effects of the disease.

The prognosis for the child with encephalitis depends on the child's age, the type of organism, and residual neurologic damage. Very young children (<2 years of age) may exhibit increased neurologic disability, including learning difficulties and epilepsy.

Nursing Care Management

Nursing care of the child with encephalitis is the same as for any unconscious child and for the child with meningitis. Additional nursing interventions include observation for deterioration in consciousness. Isolation of the child is not necessary; however, follow good hand-washing technique. A main focus of nursing management is the control of rapidly rising ICP. Neurologic monitoring, administration of medications, and support of the child and parents are the major aspects of care.

QUALITY PATIENT OUTCOMES: Encephalitis
- Early recognition of signs and symptoms of meningitis
- Cerebral edema prevented
- Side effects managed
- Neurologic sequelae prevented

RABIES

Rabies is an acute infection of the nervous system caused by a virus that is almost invariably fatal if left untreated. It is transmitted to humans by the saliva of an infected mammal and is introduced through a bite or skin abrasion. After entry into a new host, the virus multiplies in muscle cells and is spread through neural pathways without stimulating a protective host immune response.

Approximately 88% of rabies cases come from wild animals and 12% from domestic animals. Carnivorous wild animals (skunks, raccoons, and bats) are the animals most often infected with rabies and the cause of most indigenous cases of human rabies in the United States (Centers for Disease Control and Prevention, 2006). The likelihood of human exposure to a rabid domestic animal has decreased greatly.

The circumstances of a biting incident are important. An unprovoked attack is more likely than a provoked attack to indicate a rabid animal. Bites inflicted on a child attempting to feed or handle an apparently healthy animal can generally be regarded as provoked. Any child bitten by a wild animal is assumed to be exposed to rabies.

> ⚠ **NURSING ALERT**
>
> Unusual behavior in an animal is cause for suspicion; children should be warned to beware of wild animals that appear to be friendly.

Although rabies is common among wildlife species, human rabies is rarely acquired. Modern-day prophylaxis is nearly 100% successful. The highest incidence occurs in children under age 15 years. The incubation period usually ranges from 1 to 3 months but may be as short as 10 days or as long as 8 months. Only 10% to 15% of persons bitten develop the disease, but once symptoms are present, rabies progresses to a fatal outcome. In the United States, human fatalities associated with rabies occur in people who fail to seek medical attention, usually because they are unaware of their exposure.

The disease is characterized by a period of nonspecific flulike symptoms including general malaise, anorexia, fever, and sore throat, followed by a phase of excitement that features hypersensitivity and increased reaction to external stimuli, seizures, fluctuating consciousness, hypersalivation, and choking (Box 37-8). Attempts at swallowing may cause spasms of respiratory muscles so severe that they produce apnea, cyanosis, and anoxia—the characteristics from which the term *hydrophobia* was derived.

Diagnosis is made on the basis of history and clinical features.

Therapeutic Management

Treatment is of little avail once symptoms appear, but the long incubation period allows time for the induction of active and passive immunity before the onset of illness. Two types of immunizing products are available for use in humans: (1) the inactivated rabies vaccines, which induce an active immune response; and (2) the globulins, which contain preformed antibodies. The two types of products should be used concurrently for rabies postexposure treatment when prophylaxis is indicated.

The current therapy for a rabid animal bite consists of thorough cleansing of the wound and passive immunization with human rabies immunoglobulin as soon as possible after exposure to provide rapid, short-term passive immunity (Centers for Disease Control and Prevention, 2008).

Postexposure active immunity is conferred by administration of the human diploid cell rabies vaccine. The first intramuscular injection of the vaccine is given at the same time as the immunoglobulin (day 0) and is followed by injections at 3, 7, 14, and 28 days after the first dose (Centers for Disease Control and Prevention, 2008). The World Health Organization recommends an additional dose in 90 days. Before antirabies prophylaxis is initiated, consult the local or state health department.

Nursing Care Management

Parents and children are frightened by the urgency and seriousness of the situation. They need anticipatory guidance for the therapy and support and reassurance regarding the efficacy of the preventive measures for this dreaded disease. The vaccine is well tolerated by children, although they need preparation for the series of injections. Mass immunization is unnecessary and unlikely to be implemented. In areas in which rabies is rare, the schedule given is sufficient. However, certain circumstances may warrant preexposure vaccination, such as when a child is being taken to an area of the world where rabies in stray dogs is still a problem.

REYE SYNDROME

RS is a disorder defined as a metabolic encephalopathy associated with other characteristic organ involvement. It is characterized by fever, profoundly impaired consciousness, and disordered hepatic function.

The etiology of RS is not well understood, but most cases follow a common viral illness, typically influenza or varicella. RS is a condition characterized pathologically by cerebral edema and fatty changes of the liver. The onset of RS is notable for profuse vomiting and varying degrees of neurologic impairment, including personality changes and deterioration in consciousness (Pugliese, Beltramo, and Torre, 2008). The cause of RS is a mitochondrial insult induced by different viruses, drugs, exogenous toxins, and genetic factors. Elevated serum ammonia levels tend to correlate with the clinical manifestations and prognosis.

Definitive diagnosis is established by liver biopsy. The staging criteria for RS are based on liver dysfunction and on neurologic signs that range from lethargy to coma. As a result of improved diagnostic techniques, children who in the past would have been diagnosed with RS are now diagnosed with other illnesses such as viral or inborn metabolic errors affecting organic acid, ammonia, and carbohydrate metabolism. Cases of unrecognized, drug-induced encephalopathy by antiemetics given to children during viral illnesses have symptoms similar to those of RS.

BOX 37-8	**CLINICAL MANIFESTATIONS OF RABIES**

Initial Signs
General malaise
Fever
Anorexia
Sore throat

Excitement Phase
Hypersensitivity
Increased reaction to external stimuli
Seizures
Fluctuating consciousness
Choking

Severe Spasm of Respiratory Muscles*
Apnea
Cyanosis
Anoxia

*From attempts at swallowing (characteristics from which the term *hydrophobia* was derived).

The potential association between aspirin therapy for the treatment of fever in children with varicella or influenza and the development of RS precludes its use in these patients. However, by the time the FDA required aspirin product labeling in 1986, most of the decline in RS incidence had already occurred.

Nursing Care Management

The most important aspect of successful management of the child with RS is early diagnosis and aggressive therapy. Cerebral edema with increased ICP represents the most immediate threat to life. Recovery from RS is rapid and usually without sequelae if the diagnosis was made and therapy implemented early. In about one third of patients, RS causes death or long-term neurologic sequelae (Pugliese, Beltramo, and Torre, 2008).

Care and observations are implemented as for any child with an altered state of consciousness (see p. 1512) and increasing ICP. Accurate and frequent monitoring of intake and output is essential for adjusting fluid volumes to prevent both dehydration and cerebral edema. Because of related liver dysfunction, monitor laboratory studies to determine impaired coagulation, such as prolonged bleeding time.

Keep the parents of children with RS informed of the child's progress and explain diagnostic procedures and therapeutic management. They also need concerned and sympathetic support.*

⚡ DRUG ALERT

Salicylates

Families need to be aware that salicylates, the alleged offending ingredient in aspirin, are contained in other products (e.g., Pepto-Bismol). Parents should refrain from administering any product for influenza-like symptoms without first checking the label for "hidden" salicylates.

HUMAN IMMUNODEFICIENCY VIRUS ENCEPHALOPATHY

Documented routine human immunodeficiency virus (HIV) testing and counseling for all pregnant women in the United States is recommended. Consent is obtained before testing. The use of zidovudine (AZT) by HIV-infected pregnant women significantly reduces the chance that the mother will pass the virus on to her infant.

HIV infection is acquired through direct exposure to blood, semen, or vaginal fluid or via breast milk. The majority of pediatric HIV cases worldwide are acquired vertically from an infected mother. HIV deoxyribonuclease polymerase chain reaction can identify HIV infection in more than 90% of infected newborns at 1 month of age. In the United States, antiretroviral therapy is recommended for all HIV-infected infants less than 1 year of age.

*National Reye's Syndrome Foundation, PO Box 829, Bryan, OH 43506; 800-233-7393; e-mail: nrsf@reyessyndrome.org; www.reyessyndrome.org.

Children with HIV infection can develop neurologic manifestations, including progressive multifocal encephalopathy, microcephaly, epilepsy, peripheral neuropathy, and developmental delay or regression. Changes on CT examination, including generalized brain atrophy, and bilateral calcifications of the basal ganglia, may be seen (see Research Focus box).

🔍 RESEARCH FOCUS

Therapies Delay Onset of Neurologic Changes in Children with HIV

A cohort of 722 antiretroviral therapy–naive children with symptomatic human immunodeficiency virus (HIV) infection were assessed at study entry and at later intervals. Assessments included neurodevelopmental testing, neuroradiologic imaging, and neurologic examination of motor function. HIV-infected children with an intelligence quotient (IQ) of less than 70 at baseline have the highest risk for disease progression (56%), compared with those whose functioning is borderline low (IQ 70 to 89, 26%) or average to above average (IQ >90, 18%). Motor dysfunction at study entry is also a predictor of early disease progression (Pearson, McGrath, Nozyce, et al, 2000). The advent of highly active antiretroviral therapy has reversed, stopped, or delayed the onset of neurologic changes in many children with HIV (Kline, 2001; Yogev and Chadwick, 2009).

SEIZURES AND EPILEPSY

Seizures are caused by excessive and disorderly neuronal discharges in the brain. The manifestation of seizures depends on the region of the brain in which they originate and may include unconsciousness or altered consciousness; involuntary movements; and changes in perception, behaviors, sensations, and posture. Seizures are the most common treatable neurologic disorder in children and can occur with a wide variety of conditions involving the CNS. The Nursing Care Guidelines box provides seizure terminology.

📋 NURSING CARE GUIDELINES

Terminology for Seizures

Many words are used synonymously with the terms *seizure, epilepsy,* and *seizure disorder.* Epilepsy used to belong to the medical discipline of psychiatry, and therefore words such as *attacks* and *fits* are sometimes used to describe seizure events. These words, however, still create images of medieval superstitions, evil spirits, and the horrors of mental institutions. Parents are often hesitant to inform caregivers and the school that their child has a seizure disorder for fear of prejudice and misunderstandings.

The words *convulsion, convulsive disorder,* and *anticonvulsive drugs* are often used to cover all seizure types and antiepileptic drugs. However, the word *convulsion* conjures up images of a raving, wild person who is out of control and possibly dangerous. Therefore the wisdom of referring to all seizures as convulsions is questionable, since most seizures are not convulsive in nature. In this chapter the word *event, episode,* or *experience* is used to describe a seizure; likewise, medications are referred to as *antiepileptic drugs.*

In working with families, health professionals should consider the words they use to discuss epilepsy and seizures. Correct terminology can help lessen the stigma and fear often associated with epilepsy and seizures.

EPILEPSY

⊖ Epilepsy is a condition characterized by two or more unprovoked seizures and can be caused by a variety of pathologic processes in the brain. Seizures are a symptom of an underlying disease process. A single seizure event should not be classified as epilepsy and is generally not treated with long-term antiepileptic drugs. Some seizures may result from an acute medical or neurologic illness and cease once the illness is treated. In other cases, children may have a single seizure without the cause ever being known.

Once it is determined that the child has had a seizure, it is important to classify the seizure, according to the International Classification of Epileptic Seizures, and assign it to the appropriate epilepsy syndrome, according to the International Classification of Epilepsies and Epileptic Syndromes. Optimum treatment and prognosis require an accurate diagnosis and a determination of the cause whenever possible.

Etiology

Seizures in children have many different causes. Seizures are classified not only according to type, but also according to etiology. The International League Against Epilepsy guidelines classify seizures as acute symptomatic, remote symptomatic, cryptogenic, or idiopathic (Commission on Epidemiology and Prognosis of International League Against Epilepsy, 1993). Acute symptomatic seizures are associated with an acute insult such as head trauma or meningitis. Remote symptomatic seizures are those without an immediate cause but with an identifiable prior brain injury such as major head trauma, meningitis or encephalitis, hypoxia, stroke, or a static encephalopathy such as cognitive impairment or cerebral palsy. Cryptogenic seizures are those occurring with no clear cause. Idiopathic seizures are genetic in origin. Box 37-9 presents a partial list of causative factors.

Incidence

Epilepsy and seizures affect about 2.3 million Americans. At least 8% of the general population experience one or more seizures in a lifetime. Approximately 1% develop epilepsy, that is, recurring seizures. Epilepsy affects people of all ages, but particularly the very young and the elderly. The onset of epilepsy in children is highest during the first few months of life. The causative factors associated with childhood seizures are often related to the child's age. In very young infants the most common causes are birth injuries (e.g., intracranial trauma, hemorrhage, or anoxia, and congenital defects of the brain). Acute infections are a common cause of seizures in late infancy and early childhood but become an uncommon cause in middle childhood. In children older than 3 years, the most common cause is idiopathic epilepsy.

Pathophysiology

Regardless of the etiologic factor or type of seizure, the basic mechanism is the same. Abnormal electrical discharges (1) may arise from central areas in the brain that affect consciousness; (2) may be restricted to one area of the cerebral cortex, producing manifestations characteristic of that particular anatomic focus; or (3) may begin in a localized area of the cortex and spread to other portions of the brain; if sufficiently extensive, this produces generalized seizure activity.

Seizure activity is caused by spontaneous electrical discharges initiated by a group of hyperexcitable cells referred to

---

BOX 37-9   ETIOLOGY OF SEIZURES IN CHILDREN

Nonrecurrent (Acute)
Febrile episodes
Intracranial infection
Intracranial hemorrhage
Space-occupying lesions (cyst, tumor)
Acute cerebral edema
Anoxia
Toxins
Drugs
Tetanus
Lead encephalopathy
Shigella, Salmonella organisms
Metabolic alterations:
- Hypocalcemia
- Hypoglycemia
- Hyponatremia or hypernatremia
- Hypomagnesemia
- Alkalosis
- Disorders of amino acid metabolism
- Deficiency states
- Hyperbilirubinemia

Recurrent (Chronic)
Idiopathic epilepsy
Epilepsy secondary to:
- Trauma
- Hemorrhage
- Anoxia
- Infections
- Toxins
- Degenerative phenomena
- Congenital defects
- Parasitic brain disease
- Hypoglycemia injury
Epilepsy—sensory stimulus
Epilepsy-stimulating states
- Narcolepsy and catalepsy
- Psychogenic
- Tetany from hypocalcemia, alkalosis
Hypoglycemic states
- Hyperinsulinism
- Hypopituitarism
- Adrenocortical insufficiency
- Hepatic disorders
Uremia
Allergy
Cardiovascular dysfunction or syncopal episodes
Migraine

---

as the **epileptogenic focus**. As evidenced on EEG tracings, these cells display increased electric excitability but may remain quiescent over time while discharging intermittently. Normally these discharges are restrained from spreading beyond the focal area by normal inhibitory mechanisms.

In response to physiologic stimuli, such as cellular dehydration, severe hypoglycemia, electrolyte imbalance, sleep deprivation, emotional stress, and endocrine changes, these hyperexcitable cells activate normal cells in surrounding areas and in distant, synaptically related cells. A generalized seizure develops when the neuronal excitation from the epileptogenic focus spreads to the brainstem, particularly the midbrain and reticular formation. These centers within the brainstem, known as the centrencephalic system, are responsible for the spread of the epileptic potentials. The discharges can originate spontaneously in the centrencephalic system or be triggered by a focal area in the cortex. On the basis of these characteristic neuronal discharges (as recorded by the EEG), seizures are designated as partial, generalized, and unclassified epileptic seizures (Menkes and Sankar, 2000). In a large proportion of children focal seizures spread to other areas, ultimately becoming generalized with loss of consciousness.

Seizure Classification and Clinical Manifestations

There are many different types of seizures, and each has unique clinical manifestations. Seizures are classified into three major categories: (1) partial seizures, which have a local onset and involve a relatively small location in the brain; (2) general-ized seizures, which involve both hemispheres of the brain and are without local onset; and (3) unclassified epileptic seizures (Box 37-10).

Partial Seizures

Partial seizures may arise from any area of the cerebral cortex, but the frontal, temporal, and parietal lobes are most often affected and are characterized by localized motor symptoms; somatosensory, psychic, or autonomic symptoms; or a combination of these. The abnormal EEG discharges remain unilateral and are evident as focal spikes or sharp waves. Partial seizures are subdivided into three types:

Simple partial seizures—Elementary or simple symptoms and no alteration of consciousness (also called an aura; see discussion under Complex Partial Seizures, p. 1548). These are caused by a focal cortical discharge that results

---

BOX 37-10 CLASSIFICATION AND CLINICAL MANIFESTATIONS OF SEIZURES

Partial Seizures

Simple Partial Seizures with Motor Signs

Characterized by:

- Localized motor symptoms
- Somatosensory, psychic, autonomic symptoms
- Combination of these
- Abnormal discharges remaining unilateral

Manifestations

- Aversive seizure (most common motor seizure in children)—Eye or eyes and head turn away from the side of the focus; awareness of movement or loss of consciousness
- Rolandic (Sylvan) seizure—Tonic-clonic movements involving the face, salivation, arrested speech; most common during sleep
- Jacksonian march (rare in children)—Orderly, sequential progression of clonic movements beginning in a foot, hand, or face and moving, or "marching," to adjacent body parts

Simple Partial Seizures with Sensory Signs

Uncommon in children younger than 8 years of age

Characterized by various sensations, including:

- Numbness, tingling, prickling, paresthesia, or pain originating in one area (e.g., face or extremities) and spreading to other parts of the body
- Visual sensations or formed images
- Motor phenomena such as posturing or hypertonia

Complex Partial Seizures (Psychomotor Seizures)

Observed more often in children from 3 years through adolescence

Characterized by:

- Period of altered behavior
- Amnesia for event (no recollection of behavior)
- Inability to respond to environment
- Impaired consciousness during event
- Drowsiness or sleep usually following seizure
- Confusion and amnesia possibly prolonged
- Complex sensory phenomena (aura)—Most frequent sensation is strange feeling in the pit of the stomach that rises toward the throat and is often accompanied by odd or unpleasant odors or tastes, complex auditory or visual hallucinations, ill-defined feelings of elation or strangeness (e.g., déjà vu, a feeling of familiarity in a strange environment), strong feelings of fear and anxiety, distorted sense of time and self, and in small children emission of a cry or attempt to run for help

Patterns of motor behavior:

- Stereotypic
- Similar with each subsequent seizure

- May suddenly cease activity, appear dazed, stare into space, become confused and apathetic, and become limp or stiff or display some form of posturing
- May be confused
- May perform purposeless, complicated activities in a repetitive manner (automatisms), such as walking, running, kicking, laughing, or speaking incoherently, most often followed by postictal confusion or sleep; may exhibit oropharyngeal activities, such as smacking, chewing, drooling, swallowing, and nausea or abdominal pain followed by stiffness, a fall, and postictal sleep; rarely manifests actions such as rage or temper tantrums; aggressive acts uncommon during seizure

Generalized Seizures

Tonic-Clonic Seizures (Formerly Known as Grand Mal)

Most common and most dramatic of all seizure manifestations

Occur without warning

Tonic phase lasts approximately 10 to 20 seconds

Manifestations:

- Eyes roll upward
- Immediate loss of consciousness
- If standing, falls to floor or ground
- Stiffens in generalized, symmetric tonic contraction of entire body musculature
- Arms usually flexed
- Legs, head, and neck extended
- May utter a peculiar piercing cry
- Apneic, may become cyanotic
- Increased salivation and loss of swallowing reflex

Clonic phase: lasts about 30 seconds but can vary from only a few seconds to a half hour or longer

Manifestations:

- Violent jerking movements as the trunk and extremities undergo rhythmic contraction and relaxation
- May foam at the mouth
- May be incontinent of urine and feces

As event ends, movements less intense, occurring at longer intervals, then ceasing entirely

Status epilepticus—Series of seizures at intervals too brief to allow the child to regain consciousness between the time one event ends and the next begins

- Requires emergency intervention
- Can lead to exhaustion, respiratory failure, and death

Postictal state:

- Appears to relax
- May remain semiconscious and difficult to arouse

BOX 37-10   CLASSIFICATION AND CLINICAL MANIFESTATIONS OF SEIZURES—cont'd

- May awaken in a few minutes
- Remains confused for several hours
- Poor coordination
- Mild impairment of fine motor movements
- May have visual and speech difficulties
- May vomit or complain of severe headache
- When left alone, usually sleeps for several hours
- On awakening is fully conscious
- Usually feels tired and complains of sore muscles and headache
- No recollection of entire event

Absence Seizures (Formerly Called Petit Mal or Lapses)
Characterized by:
- Onset usually between 4 and 12 years of age
- More common in girls than in boys
- Usually cease at puberty
- Brief loss of consciousness
- Minimum or no alteration in muscle tone
- May go unrecognized because of little change in child's behavior
- Abrupt onset; suddenly develops 20 or more attacks daily
- Event often mistaken for inattentiveness or daydreaming
- Events possibly precipitated by hyperventilation, hypoglycemia, stresses (emotional and physiologic), fatigue, or sleeplessness

Manifestations:
- Brief loss of consciousness
- Appear without warning or aura
- Usually last about 5 to 10 seconds
- Slight loss of muscle tone may cause child to drop objects
- Ability to maintain postural control; seldom falls
- Minor movements such as lip smacking, twitching of eyelids or face, or slight hand movements
- Not accompanied by incontinence
- Amnesia for episode
- May need to reorient self to previous activity

Atonic and Akinetic Seizures (Also Known as Drop Attacks)
Characterized by:
- Onset usually between 2 and 5 years of age
- Sudden, momentary loss of muscle tone and postural control
- Events recurring frequently during the day, particularly in the morning hours and shortly after awakening

Manifestations:
- Loss of tone causing child to fall to the floor violently
- Unable to break fall by putting out hand
- May incur a serious injury to the face, head, or shoulder
- Loss of consciousness only momentary

Myoclonic Seizures
A variety of seizure episodes
May be isolated as benign essential myoclonus
May occur in association with other seizure forms
Characterized by:
- Sudden, brief contractures of a muscle or group of muscles
- Occur singly or repetitively
- No postictal state
- May or may not be symmetric
- May or may not include loss of consciousness

Infantile Spasms
Also called infantile myoclonus, massive spasms, hypsarrhythmia, salaam episodes, or infantile myoclonic spasms
Most commonly occur during the first 6 to 8 months of life
Twice as common in boys as in girls
Numerous seizures during the day without postictal drowsiness or sleep
Poor outlook for normal intelligence
Manifestations:
- Possible series of sudden, brief, symmetric, muscular contractions
- Head flexed, arms extended, and legs drawn up
- Eyes sometimes rolling upward or inward
- May be preceded or followed by a cry or giggling
- May or may not include loss of consciousness
- Sometimes flushing, pallor, or cyanosis

Infants who are able to sit but not stand:
- Sudden dropping forward of the head and neck with trunk flexed forward and knees drawn up—the *salaam* or *jackknife* seizure

Less often: alternate clinical forms
- Extensor spasms rather than flexion of arms, legs, and trunk, and head nodding
- Lightning events involving a single, momentary, shocklike contraction of the entire body

---

in clinical manifestations related to the area of cerebral involvement, without impairment of consciousness. Simple partial seizures may consist of motor, sensory, autonomic, or psychic symptoms.

Complex partial seizures—Complex symptoms and impairment of consciousness.

Simple or complex seizures secondarily generalized—Simple or complex partial seizures that evolve into generalized seizures, usually a tonic-clonic event.

Partial seizures exhibit manifestations related to where they occur in the brain. A clear description of the seizure (ictal state) by an eyewitness is a valuable aid in localizing the brain area involved. The initial event may provide the best clue for assessing the type of seizure and its localization. Correctly localizing the area of the brain involved during a seizure event is crucial for diagnostic and therapeutic reasons, since many antiepileptic drugs are specific for each type of seizure.

In addition to the initial event, the circumstances that precipitated the episode are important. Identifying and eliminating triggering factors may be the only treatment needed (see p. 1559). The postictal state (the period following a seizure) may be varied. The child may be drowsy, be uncoordinated, have transient aphasia or confusion, and display some sensory or motor impairment. Document neurologic changes. Weakness, hypotonia, or inactivity of a body part may indicate an epileptogenic focus in the corresponding contralateral cortical region.

Simple Partial Seizures. Simple partial seizures with motor signs originate from the primary motor cortex, located in the temporal lobe, which is the area of the brain that controls muscle movement. They are the most frequent type of simple partial seizure. The simplest form of simple partial seizures with motor signs is clonus, the rhythmic alternating contraction and relaxation of muscle groups.

Eye movements provide clues to the focus or origin of the seizure. Discharge in the cortex of one hemisphere tends to cause the eyes to deviate to the opposite side. Bilateral discharges tend to cause the eyes to move upward or straight ahead. When the child's eyes are closed during the seizure episode, a gentle attempt to open them may provide valuable information.

Simple partial seizures with sensory symptoms are usually described as numbness, tingling, or pins and needles. This may be the only symptom of a seizure, or it may spread to involve an adjacent sensory cortex or motor cortex. Auditory seizures may manifest as humming, buzzing, or hissing. Visual seizures typically manifest as flashes of light or colors.

Simple partial seizures with autonomic symptoms may consist of feelings of epigastric rising, flushing or pallor, sweating, or pupil dilation.

Simple partial seizures with psychic symptoms may include speech arrest or vocalizations, the sensation that an experience has occurred before (déjà vu), fear, displeasure, anger, or irritability. The affective symptoms associated with partial seizures last only a few minutes and are unprovoked.

Complex Partial Seizures. The main feature of complex partial seizures is impairment of consciousness. During the period of impaired consciousness the child may look vacant, dazed, or frightened and be unable to respond when spoken to or to follow instructions. Complex partial seizures are the most difficult to diagnose and control. These are the most common type of seizures. Complex partial seizures are observed more often in children from 3 years of age through adolescence. These seizures may begin with an aura—a simple partial seizure that is usually a sensation or sensory phenomenon that reflects the complicated connections and integrative functions of that area of the brain. The most common sensation is a strange feeling at the bottom of the stomach that rises toward the throat. This feeling may be accompanied by odd or unpleasant odors or taste, complex auditory or visual hallucinations, or ill-defined feelings of elevation or strangeness (e.g., déjà vu). Small children may emit a cry as a manifestation of an aura. Strong feelings of fear and anxiety and a disturbed sense of time can be associated with an aura. The aura is part of the seizure event and is associated with EEG changes.

Another feature of a complex partial seizure may be automatisms (repetitive involuntary activities without purpose, carried out in a dreamy state). The predominant observations may be oropharyngeal activities such as lip smacking, chewing, drooling, or swallowing; ambulatory activities such as wandering or running; and verbal manifestations such as repeating words ("please, please," "help, help," or "oh, oh"). These automatisms may be exhibited by antisocial behaviors, such as removing clothes in public or attempting to open the door of

a moving car. The child may begin walking or running and may unknowingly run out into traffic or into obstacles. It is important to realize that the child's consciousness is impaired and that these actions are not deliberate. It is sometimes difficult to determine whether such behavior is related to the seizure activity or to a behavioral deviation. If the behavior results from seizure activity, all attempts to control such behavior with counseling or behavior plans are ineffective. The child may suddenly cease activity, appear dazed, stare into space, become confused or apathetic, become limp or stiff, or display some form of posturing. The term *psychomotor seizure* was formerly used because of the frequent association of psychic symptoms and motor automatisms with complex partial seizures.

If the seizure involves areas of the brain that control motor function, the child exhibits movements such as jerking of the hands and arms. Complex partial seizures generally last only a few minutes. After the seizure the postictal period occurs, with signs of confusion and lack of recollection of the ictal period. Depending on the brain area involved during the episode, the child may sleep for time. (See Table 37-5 for a comparison of simple partial, complex partial, and absence seizures.)

Partial Seizures That Generalize. Simple or complex partial seizures may spread and become generalized, usually into a tonic-clonic seizure. In such cases the partial seizure is considered the primary seizure event, and the generalized seizure is considered the secondary one. Thus it would be stated that the tonic-clonic seizure was not generalized at the onset but was a partial seizure that secondarily generalized.

Generalized Seizures

Generalized seizures without a focal onset appear to arise in the reticular formation, and the clinical observations indicate that the initial involvement is from both hemispheres. Loss of consciousness and impairment of motor function occur from the outset. Unlike partial seizures that become generalized, there is no aura. Seizures occur at any time, day or night, and the interval between events may be minutes, hours, weeks, or even years.

Tonic-Clonic Seizures. The generalized tonic-clonic seizure, formerly known as *grand mal*, is the most dramatic of all seizure manifestations of childhood (Wiederholt, 2000). The seizure usually occurs without warning and consists of two distinct phases: tonic and clonic.

In the tonic phase the person rolls the eyes upward and immediately loses consciousness. If standing, the child falls to the ground. The musculature stiffens in a generalized and

TABLE 37-5	COMPARISON OF SIMPLE PARTIAL, COMPLEX PARTIAL, AND ABSENCE SEIZURES		
CLINICAL MANIFESTATIONS	**SIMPLE PARTIAL**	**COMPLEX PARTIAL**	**ABSENCE**
Age of onset	Any age	Uncommon before age 3 yr	Uncommon before age 3 yr
Frequency (per day)	Variable	Rarely over 1-2 times	Multiple
Duration	Usually <30 sec	Usually >60 sec, rarely <10 sec	Usually <10 sec, rarely >30 sec
Aura	May be sole manifestation of seizure	Frequent	Never
Impaired consciousness	Never	Always	Always, brief loss of consciousness
Automatisms	No	Frequent	Frequent
Clonic movements	Frequent	Occasional	Occasional
Postictal impairment	Rare	Frequent	Never
Mental disorientation	Rare	Common	Unusual

symmetric tonic contraction of the entire body. The arms usually flex, and the legs, head, and neck extend. The mouth snaps shut and the tongue may be bitten. The thoracic and abdominal muscles contract and sometimes produce a "tonic cry" as air is forced over the vocal cords. Parents often misinterpret this as an expression of pain. The average tonic phase lasts 10 to 30 seconds, during which the child is apneic and may become cyanotic. Autonomic phenomena that may be observed include increased blood pressure, increased heart rate, flushing, and increased salivation (Browne and Holmes, 2004).

In the clonic phase the tonic rigidity is replaced by intense jerking movements as the trunk and extremities undergo rhythmic contraction and relaxation. During this time the child cannot control oral secretions and may be incontinent of urine and feces. As the seizure ends, the movements become less intense and occur at less frequent intervals until they cease entirely. The average clonic phase lasts 30 to 50 seconds.

In the postictal phase the child may remain semiconscious and difficult to arouse. The average duration of the postictal phase is from 1 to 15 minutes (Browne and Holmes, 2004). The child may remain confused or sleep for several hours. He or she may have mild impairment of fine motor movements. The child may have visual and speech difficulties and may vomit or complain of headache. On awakening, he or she is fully conscious but usually feels tired and may complain of sore muscles and a headache. The child has no recollection of the event.

Absence Seizures. Absence seizures, formerly called *petit mal* or *lapses*, are generalized seizures. They have a sudden onset and are characterized by a brief loss of consciousness, a blank stare, and automatisms. Absence seizures are divided into typical and atypical. These seizures almost always first appear during childhood. In most instances the onset occurs between 5 and 12 years of age, and they often stop spontaneously in the teenage years (Browne and Holmes, 2004).

The onset of typical absence seizures is abrupt, with the child suddenly experiencing 20 or more events daily. Characteristically the brief loss of consciousness appears without warning and usually lasts approximately 5 to 10 seconds. The child has a motionless blank stare, which may be confused with inattentiveness or daydreaming. Slight loss of muscle tone may cause the child to drop objects, but he or she seldom falls. There may be automatisms such as lip smacking, twitching of the eyelids or face, or fumbling with the clothes. The sudden arrest of activity and consciousness is not accompanied by incontinence, and the child will not remember the episode. There is no postictal sleepiness, but the child may be momentarily confused. Atypical absence seizures have a less abrupt onset than typical absence seizures, and there is a greater loss of tone. Atypical absence seizures, unlike typical absence seizures, may last several minutes.

Hyperventilation is a potent precipitator of absence seizures. Photic stimulation may also precipitate absence seizures but is less likely to do so than hyperventilation (Browne and Holmes, 2004). If the child is involved in a group activity, such as classroom reading or discussion, he or she may need help to catch up with the group after the seizure. Frequent episodes can result in slowed intellectual processes and deterioration in schoolwork and behavior. This is often the first indication of the problem. It is important that the absence seizure be distinguished from daydreaming, attention deficit hyperactivity disorder, and complex partial seizures.

Atonic Seizures. Atonic seizures are manifested as a sudden, momentary loss of muscle tone. The onset is usually between 2 and 5 years of age. During a mild seizure the child may simply experience several sudden brief head drops. During a more severe episode the child suddenly falls to the ground (generally face down), loses consciousness briefly, and after a few seconds gets up as if nothing happened. Because of the sudden loss of tone, the child is unable to break the fall by putting out a hand, and so suffers injuries to the head, face, or shoulder. Therefore, if a child has frequent atonic seizures, he or she should wear a helmet with a face guard to prevent injury to the face and teeth.

Myoclonic Seizures. Myoclonic seizures are characterized by sudden, brief contractions of a muscle or group of muscles. The seizures may involve only the face and trunk or one or more extremities. They may occur singly or repetitively. The seizures may or may not be symmetric. Myoclonic seizures often occur in combination with other seizure types. Myoclonic seizures should not be confused with myoclonic jerks that can occur normally in the course of falling asleep.

The myoclonic seizure can be confused with the exaggerated startle reflex but may be distinguished by placing one's palm against the back of the child's head. If it is possible to push the child's head forward, this indicates an exaggerated startle reflex. In the case of a myoclonic seizure, the child's head resists attempts to bring the head forward.

Tonic Seizures. Tonic seizures are characterized by a sudden onset of increased tone. The child falls if standing. The child may cry out because of contraction of the respiratory and abdominal muscles. Tonic seizures are longer than myoclonic seizures, with an average duration of 10 seconds. Postictal confusion, tiredness, and headache are common. Tonic seizures are uncommon and typically begin between 1 and 7 years of age (Browne and Holmes, 2004).

Clonic Seizures. Clonic seizures are characterized by loss of consciousness and decreased tone followed by jerking movements of the extremities. These movements may be more predominant in one extremity. The duration is typically from 1 to several minutes and may be followed by a rapid recovery or may have a prolonged period of postictal confusion (Browne and Holmes, 2004).

Unclassified Epileptic Seizures

Unclassified epileptic seizures are seizures that lack sufficient information to classify. In addition to the seizures listed in the International Classification of Epileptic Seizures, several types of epileptic syndromes display a group of signs and symptoms that collectively characterize or indicate a particular condition (Commission on Classification and Terminology of International League Against Epilepsy, 1985). Several syndromes associated with epilepsy occur in infants and children. Two of these are West syndrome and Lennox-Gastaut syndrome (LGS).

West Syndrome. Infantile spasms are a rare disorder that has an onset within the first 6 to 8 months of life. The underlying cause of infantile spasms is often not found. The pathophysiology is poorly understood. Nearly all children with infantile spasms have some degree of cognitive impairment (Shields, 2000).

This disorder is also known as *massive spasms, salaam seizures, flexion spasms, jackknife seizures, massive myoclonic jerks,* or *infantile myoclonic spasms.* It is twice as common in boys as in girls. There are three types of seizures in infantile spasms: flexor, extensor, and mixed flexor-extensor. Flexor spasms consist of brief contractions of the neck, trunk, arms, and legs. The arms may either adduct or abduct with the arms flexed at the elbow. Extensor spasms consist predominantly of extensor contractions resulting in abrupt extension of the neck and trunk with extensor adduction or abduction of the arms and legs. Eye deviation or nystagmus often occurs with infantile spasms. Infantile spasms may occur as a single event or in clusters with as many as 150 seizures within a cluster. The infant often cries or is irritable during or after a cluster of spasms.

Adrenocorticotropic hormone (ACTH) is used to treat infantile spasms, but it is associated with significant adverse effects (e.g., immunosuppression, hypertension) (Haberlandt, Weger, Sigl, et al, 2010). Vigabatrin (Sabril) is also for infantile spasms and refractory complex partial seizures but is associated with irreversible visual field deficits (Riikonen, 2010; Willmore, Abelson, Ben-Menachem, et al, 2009). Vigabatrin acts to increase levels of the neurotransmitter γ-aminobutyric acid and thus decreases seizure activity. A Cochrane review of 11 randomized controlled studies found no single treatment proved to be more efficacious than any other in the treatment of infantile spasms, except for vigabatrin in the treatment of infantile spasms in tuberous sclerosis (Hancock and Osborne, 2003).

Lennox-Gastaut Syndrome. Many children who have infantile spasms eventually develop LGS. LGS is diagnosed on the evidence of mixed seizure types (atonic, myoclonic, tonic, and atypical absence), slow mental development, poor response to treatment, and typical EEG changes (diffuse slow spike waves at 1.5 to 2.0 Hz while awake or burst of fast rhythms [10 Hz] while asleep). Onset of LGS is between 1 and 7 years of age, after which it is far less common. Children with LGS typically have multiple seizures daily. Tonic seizures are the most common seizure type in this syndrome. There are many causes of LGS; about one third are idiopathic and two thirds are symptomatic. In addition to cognitive impairments, many of these children develop other problems, including hyperactivity, aggression, or autistic features (van Rijckevorsel, 2008).

Treatment is difficult, and most cases do not respond to therapy. Drugs are chosen according to the types of seizures. Valproic acid (valproate) continues to be the drug of choice for LGS. Other drugs include benzodiazepines, especially clonazepam and nitrazepam. Felbamate has been an effective treatment for LGS, but it is associated with a considerable risk of aplastic anemia and hepatotoxicity (Yoon and Jagoda, 2000). Lamotrigine may also be beneficial. In addition, the ketogenic diet may be efficacious for some of these children. ACTH and steroids may be beneficial, but because of the potential for significant side effects they are infrequently used.

The prognosis is typically poor (van Rijckevorsel, 2008). Additional family support is often required to maintain the child at home.

Diagnostic Evaluation

Establishing a diagnosis is critical for establishing a prognosis and planning the proper treatment. The process of diagnosis in a child suspected of having epilepsy includes (1) determining whether epilepsy or seizures exist and not an alternative diagnosis; and (2) defining the underlying cause, if possible. The assessment and diagnosis rely heavily on a thorough history, skilled observation, and several diagnostic tests.

It is especially important to differentiate epilepsy from other brief alterations in consciousness or behavior. Clinical entities that mimic seizures include migraine headaches, toxic effects of drugs, syncope (fainting), breath-holding spells in infants and young children, movement disorders (tics, tremor, chorea), prolonged Q-T syndrome, sleep disturbances (sleepwalking, night terrors), psychogenic seizures, rage attacks, and transient ischemic attacks (rare in children) (Browne and Holmes, 2004). Cocaine intoxication should be considered in the differential diagnosis of new-onset seizure activity in newborn infants.

It is unusual to observe the child during a seizure; therefore obtain a complete, accurate, and detailed history from a reliable and knowledgeable informant. The history involves prenatal, perinatal, and neonatal periods, including any episodes of infection, apnea, colic, or poor feeding and any previous accidents or serious illnesses.

The history of the seizure should be equally detailed, including the type of seizure or description of the child's behavior during the event, the age at onset, and the time at which the seizure occurs (e.g., early morning, before meals, while awake, or during sleep). Any factors that may have precipitated the seizure are important, including fever, infection, head trauma, anxiety, fatigue, sleep deprivation, menstrual cycle, alcohol, and activity (e.g., hyperventilation or exposure to strong stimuli such as bright flashing light or loud noises). If the child can describe any sensory phenomena, record them. Also record the duration and progression of the seizure (if any) and the post-ictal feelings and behavior (e.g., confusion, inability to speak, amnesia, headache, and sleep). It is important to determine whether more than one seizure type exists. It is often more informative to ask parents to mime the seizure rather than rely on their oral description. Miming often reveals features, such as head turning, that would otherwise go unrecognized. Some seizures are overlooked by parents. For example, some parents may not identify brief head nods or brief single jerks as seizures unless specifically asked whether their child has these symptoms. The family history should include whether other family members have had a seizure, cognitive impairments, cerebral palsy, or other neurologic disorders. A family history can offer clues to paroxysmal disorders such as migraine headaches, breath-holding spells, febrile seizures, or neurologic diseases.

A complete physical and neurologic examination, including developmental assessment of language, learning, behavior, and motor abilities, may provide clues to the etiology of the seizures. A number of laboratory and neuroimaging tests may be ordered depending on the child's age, whether this is a new-onset seizure, the characteristics of the seizure, and the history. Laboratory studies that may prove to be of value include a venous lead level if the history warrants or white blood cell count (for signs of infection). Blood glucose may give evidence of hypoglycemic episodes, and serum electrolytes, blood urea nitrogen, calcium, serum amino acids, lactate, ammonia, and urine organic acids may indicate metabolic disturbances. Blood for chromosomal analysis may also be done if a genetic etiology is suspected. A toxic screen may be done if alcohol or drug abuse or withdrawal is suspected. Lumbar puncture can confirm a suspected diagnosis of meningitis. CT may be done to detect a cerebral hemorrhage, infarctions, and gross malformations. MRI provides greater anatomic detail and is used to detect developmental malformations, tumors, and cortical dysplasias (Kuzniecky, 2001).

The EEG is obtained for all children with seizures and is the most useful tool for evaluating a seizure disorder. The EEG confirms the presence of abnormal electrical discharges and provides information on the seizure type and the focus. The EEG is carried out under varying conditions—with the child asleep, awake, awake with provocative stimulation (flashing lights, noise), and hyperventilating. Stimulation may elicit abnormal electrical activity, which is recorded on the EEG. Various seizure types produce characteristic EEG patterns: high-voltage spike discharges are seen in tonic-clonic seizures, with abnormal patterns in the intervals between seizures; a three-per-second spike and wave pattern is observed in an absence seizure; and absence of electrical activity in an area suggests a large lesion, such as an abscess or subdural collection of fluid.

A normal EEG does not rule out seizures because the EEG is only a surface recording and only represents approximately 1 hour of time and, therefore, may show normal interictal activity. If there is concern about whether a child has seizures or the seizure type cannot be determined, then a long-term video EEG may be done to record the child during wakefulness and sleep. The full body image is recorded on video, with selected EEG channels displayed on the same screen for simultaneous recording and viewing. EEG monitoring is also available in digital EEG and digital video imaging, which allows for greater selection of EEG channels and is available in both routine and long-term EEGs. Polygraph equipment may also be used to monitor physiologic data such as respiratory effort, eye movements, heart rate, and systemic blood pressure. These techniques can be used concurrently and are especially valuable in differentiating epileptic activity from paroxysmal behavior or nonepileptic motor events.

Therapeutic Management

The goal of treatment of seizure disorders is to control the seizures or to reduce their frequency and severity, discover and correct the cause when possible, and help the child live as normal a life as possible. If the seizure activity is a manifestation of an infectious, traumatic, or metabolic process, the seizure therapy is instituted as part of the general therapeutic regimen. Management of epilepsy has four treatment options: drug therapy, the ketogenic diet, vagus nerve stimulation, and epilepsy surgery.

Drug Therapy

It is known that persons predisposed to epilepsy have seizures when their basal level of neuronal excitability exceeds a critical point; no event occurs if the excitability is maintained below this threshold. The administration of antiepileptic drugs serves to raise this threshold and prevent seizures. Consequently, the primary therapy for seizure disorders is the administration of the appropriate antiepileptic drug or combination of drugs in a dosage that provides the desired effect without causing undesirable side effects or toxic reactions. Antiepileptic drugs exert their effect primarily by reducing the responsiveness of normal neurons to the sudden, high-frequency nerve impulses that arise in the epileptogenic focus. Thus the seizure is effectively suppressed; however, the abnormal brain waves may or may not be altered. Complete control can be achieved in 80% of children with epilepsy (Curatolo, Moavero, Lo Castro, et al, 2009). Table 37-6 outlines the drugs used for control of seizures.

Therapy begins with a single drug known to be effective and have the lowest toxicity, that is, the safest side effect profile for the child's particular type of seizure. The dosage is gradually increased until the seizures are controlled or the child develops side effects. If the drug is effective but does not sufficiently control the seizures, a second drug is added in gradually increasing doses. Once seizures are controlled, the first drug may be tapered to reduce the potential adverse effects of polytherapy. However, this decision is individualized for each child (Browne and Holmes, 2004). Monotherapy remains the treatment method of choice for epilepsy, but polypharmacy may be a viable alternative for children who cannot attain seizure control with only one agent (Leppik, 2000).

> ### ⚡ DRUG ALERT
> #### Drug Therapy for Epilepsy
>
> Measurement of blood levels of the drug is important if the seizures continue once the child is on a therapeutic dose of medication, to adjust the dosage, and to assist in determining which medication may be causing the side effects if the child is on multiple antiepileptic medications. Some possible causes of low serum blood concentrations are noncompliance, poor absorption, and drug interactions. The dosage needs to be increased as the child grows. Blood cell counts, urinalysis, and liver function tests are obtained at frequent intervals in children receiving particular antiepileptic medications that can affect organ function.

If complete seizure control is maintained on an anticonvulsant drug for 2 years, it is safe for patients with no risk factors to discontinue the drug. Risk factors include age greater than 12 years at onset, history of neonatal seizures, numerous seizures before control is achieved, and presence of a neurologic dysfunction (i.e., motor handicap or cognitive impairment). Up to 25% of children whose medications are discontinued experience seizure recurrence. Recurrence occurs most frequently within 6 months of discontinuation (Johnston, 2009).

When seizure medications are discontinued, the dose is decreased gradually over several weeks. Sudden withdrawal of a drug is not recommended because it can cause an increase in the number and severity of seizures.

Complications of Drug Therapy. The side effects of continued use of antiepileptic medications are sometimes distressing to the child and the family. Most side effects are transient and dose related, but drug reactions warrant immediate attention. Dose-related side effects such as dizziness, headache, ataxia, and sleepiness often disappear over time or when drug dosages are reduced. Drug reactions require clinical evaluation and may require monitoring of serum drug levels. Combination therapy,

TABLE 37-6 COMMON ANTIEPILEPTIC MEDICATIONS

DRUG	INDICATIONS	HALF-LIFE (hr)	MAINTENANCE DOSE (mg/kg/day)	THERAPEUTIC LEVELS (mcg/ml)	ADVERSE EFFECTS
Carbamazepine	Partial, secondary generalized	14-27 (children) 8-28 (neonates)	10-30	4-12	Allergic rashes, nausea, diplopia, blurry vision, dizziness, drowsiness, hypersensitivity syndrome, aplastic anemia
Phenytoin	Partial, tonic-clonic	5-14 (children) 10-60 (neonates) (nonlinear kinetics)	5-8	10-25 (occasionally lower)	Rashes, sedation, nystagmus, ataxia, hirsutism, gingival hyperplasia, coarse features, folate deficiency
Valproic acid	Primary generalized, absence, myoclonic, akinetic, febrile, infantile spasms, some partial	10-15, 6-8 with carbamazepine, phenobarbital, or primidone	30-80	50-100 (150 if tolerated)	Nausea, tremor, weight gain, hair loss, thrombocytopenia, hepatic failure, pancreatitis
Phenobarbital	Neonatal, febrile, partial, generalized tonic-clonic	36-73	3-5 (<1 yr) 2-4 (≥1 yr)	10-40	Sedation, inattention, hyperactivity, irritability, cognitive impairment, rash, rare hypersensitivity reactions
Ethosuximide	Absence, myoclonic	20-60	15-40	40-100	Nausea, abdominal discomfort, drowsiness, rash, leukopenia
Primidone	Partial, simple and complex; generalized tonic-clonic	5-11	12-25	5-12	Sedation, dysphoria, irritability, psychomotor slowing, rash, rare hematologic and hypersensitivity reactions
Clonazepam	Absence, atypical absence, atonic, myoclonic	20-40	0.1-0.3	0.02-0.08	Sedation, irritability, tolerance, ataxia, diplopia
Felbamate	Partial and generalized (reserved for severe epilepsy such as Lennox-Gastaut syndrome)	20 (in monotherapy)	15-45 (maximum 3600 mg)	Not established	Anorexia, weight loss, nausea, insomnia, headache, fatigue Black box warning: aplastic anemia, hepatic toxicity
Gabapentin	Partial, with or without secondary generalized seizures in patients >12 yr	Not established	30-100	Not established	Somnolence, dizziness, ataxia, fatigue, diplopia, weight gain
Lamotrigine	Partial, absence, atypical absence, atonic, myoclonic	7 with enzyme-inducing antiepileptic drugs; 20 for drugs with no interaction; 45-60 for valproic acid	5 for enzyme inhibitor; 10 for enzyme inhibitor and inducers; 5-15 for enzyme inducers	Not established	Somnolence, dizziness, diplopia, tremor, rash (risk increased if on valproic acid and with rapid titration of dose)
Topiramate	Partial, primary generalized, tonic, atonic	10-15; 6-8 with carbamazepine, phenobarbital, or primidone	5-9	Not established	Somnolence, anorexia, weight loss, fatigue, difficulty with concentration, kidney stones
Tiagabine	Partial	Not established	1-2	Not established	Dizziness, somnolence, headache, tremor, difficulty with concentration, depression
Oxcarbazepine	Partial, secondarily generalized	5-8	30	Not established	Somnolence, headache, dizziness, nausea, ataxia
Levetiracetam	Partial	6-8	10-50	Not established	Drowsiness, dizziness, behavioral problems
Zonisamide	Partial, generalized	50-69	4-8	Not established	Somnolence, dizziness, anorexia, nausea, oligohidrosis, kidney stones

Modified from Browne TR, Holmes GL: *Handbook of epilepsy*, Philadelphia, 2004, Lippincott Williams & Wilkins.

such as with barbiturates and carbamazepine, can potentiate drug levels. Knowledge of drug-to-drug interactions, including other medications such as antibiotics, is critical in caring for the child with epilepsy. Knowledge of potential adverse effects is also imperative. Severe, potentially life-threatening side effects can occur with specific antiepileptic medications. For example, carbamazepine, phenytoin, and lamotrigine may cause a severe, life-threatening rash. Valproic acid may cause liver toxicity, particularly in a child less than 2 years of age. To avoid possible complications of tissue damage and difficulties with administration of IV phenytoin, fosphenytoin should be used. Therefore critical thinking and careful monitoring are necessary in providing optimum care to the child with epilepsy.

⚡ DRUG ALERT

Fosphenytoin

Fosphenytoin is often used to treat seizures instead of IV phenytoin because of possible complications and drug interactions associated with IV phenytoin. If IV phenytoin is used, it should be administered via slow IV push and at a rate that does not exceed 50 mg/min. Because phenytoin precipitates when mixed with glucose, only normal saline is used to flush the tubing or catheter. Fosphenytoin may be given in saline or glucose solutions at a rate of up to 150 mg PE (phenytoin equivalent)/min, and it may be given intramuscularly if necessary.

Chronic treatment with phenytoin may cause gum hypertrophy. Surgical removal of the excess tissue may be needed in severe cases. Enlargement of the tonsillar and adenoidal tissue can cause partial airway obstruction, which produces snoring during sleep. Chronic treatment with antiepileptic medications has been associated with decreased bone mineral density that does not correlate with serum vitamin D levels. However, no guidelines have been established for monitoring bone mineral density in individuals on antiepileptic medications (Farhat, Yamout, Mikati, et al, 2002).

Ketogenic Diet

The ketogenic diet is a high-fat, low-carbohydrate, and adequate-protein diet (Kossoff, Zupec-Kania, and Rho, 2009). Consumption of such a diet forces the body to shift from using glucose as the primary energy source to using fat, and the individual develops a state of ketosis. The diet is rigorous. All foods and liquids the child consumes must be carefully weighed and measured. The diet is deficient in vitamins and minerals; therefore vitamin supplements are necessary. Potential side effects of the diet are constipation, weight loss, lethargy, and kidney stones. There are reports of increased blood lipids in children on the ketogenic diet; the long-term effects of which are unknown (Levy and Cooper, 2003) (see Research Focus box).

🔆 RESEARCH FOCUS

The Ketogenic Diet

The ketogenic diet may be effective in controlling seizures. In the past decade, four major meta-analyses of the efficacy of the ketogenic diet have shown that the diet reduced seizures by more than 90% in a third of the patients and by more than 50% in half of them (Kossoff, Zupec-Kania, and Rho, 2009).

Vagus Nerve Stimulation (Interrupts seizure)

Vagus nerve stimulation uses an implantable device that reduces seizures in individuals who have not had effective control with drug therapy. It is currently indicated as adjunctive therapy in patients 12 years and older with partial onset seizures (with or without secondary generalization). A programmable signal generator is implanted subcutaneously in the chest. Electrodes tunneled underneath the skin deliver electrical impulses to the left vagus nerve (CN X). The device is programmed noninvasively to deliver a precise pattern of stimulation to the left vagus nerve. The patient or caregiver can activate the device using a magnet at the onset of a seizure. Studies show a median reduction in seizures of 35% to 45% after 1 year of therapy (Saillet, Langlois, Feddersen, et al, 2009).

Surgical Therapy

When seizures are caused by a hematoma, tumor, or other cerebral lesion, surgical removal is the treatment. Surgery is reserved for children who suffer from incapacitating, refractory seizures. Refractory seizures are usually defined as the persistence of seizures despite adequate trials of three antiepileptic medications, alone or in combination (Browne and Holmes, 2004).

There are several types of surgical interventions. In resective surgery the focal area of the seizure activity is excised with the expectation that the surgery will not produce serious deficits or increase existing deficits. The use of intraoperative electrocorticography helps localize anatomic areas of focal seizure onset, guide the extent of surgery, map cortical anatomy, and predict epilepsy surgical outcome (Gallentine and Mikati, 2009). Surgical excision of the epileptogenic focus may not eliminate the need for drug therapy. A hemispherectomy to remove all or most of one hemisphere is typically used in patients who have severe epilepsy and who already have hemiparesis or nonfunctional hand use. Patients with Rasmussen syndrome or Sturge-Weber syndrome may benefit from this procedure. Corpus callosotomy involves the separation of the connections between the two hemispheres of the brain and is used in some generalized seizures. In multiple subpial transection, horizontal fibers of the motor cortex are divided to reduce seizures, whereas the vertical fibers are spared to allow for function (Browne and Holmes, 2004).

Status Epilepticus

Status epilepticus is a continuous seizure that lasts more than 30 minutes or a series of seizures from which the child does not regain a premorbid level of consciousness (Shorvon and Walker, 2005; Treiman and Walker, 2006). No consensus has been reached on the duration of seizure required to qualify as status epilepticus (Chen and Wasterlain, 2006). Direct the initial treatment toward support and maintenance of vital functions, that is, the ABCs of life support, administration of oxygen, and gaining of IV access, immediately followed by IV administration of antiepileptic agents.

Rectal diazepam is a simple, effective, and safe treatment for home or prehospital management (Pellock and Shinnar, 2005). It is available in a prefilled rectal gel syringe (Diastat) for easy administration. Rectal diazepam is not associated with respiratory depression when used as recommended (Pellock and

Shinnar, 2005). Midazolam has been given successfully by intranasal route for treatment of acute epileptic seizures (Fisgin, Gurer, Senbil, et al, 2000; Kutlu, Yakinci, Dogrul, et al, 2000; Scheepers, Scheepers, Clarke, et al, 2000). Intranasal midazolam not only is safe and effective for stopping seizures, but also is easier to administer than rectal diazepam (Harbord, Kyrkou, Kyrkou, et al, 2004).

For in-hospital management of status epilepticus, IV diazepam or lorazepam (Ativan) is the first-line drug of choice (Browne and Holmes, 2004). Lorazepam may be replacing IV diazepam as the drug of choice. It has a longer duration of action and causes less respiratory depression in children over 2 years of age. Concurrent IV loading with fosphenytoin is usually necessary for sustained control of seizures. Valproic acid has also been effective in status epilepticus when given rectally or intravenously (Yamamoto and Yim, 2000). The child must be closely monitored during administration to detect early alterations in vital signs that may indicate impending respiratory depression (see Evidence-Based Practice box). When diazepam is ineffective, fosphenytoin or phenobarbital is given intravenously as the next line of treatment. This combination of therapy places the child at high risk for apnea, and therefore respiratory support is generally necessary.

Children who continue to have seizures despite the above drug treatment may be given anesthetizing doses of midazolam, propofol, or pentobarbital (Morrison, Gibbons, and Whitehouse, 2006; van Gestel, Blusse van Oud-Alblas, Malingre, et al, 2005). Sodium valproate has also been studied for control of refractory status epilepticus in children (Mehta, Singhi, and Singhi, 2007). In this situation, continuous EEG monitoring is typically done to detect and treat electrographic seizures.

⚡ DRUG ALERT

Diazepam

Diazepam is incompatible with many drugs. To give intravenously, inject slowly and directly into the vein or through tubing as close as possible to the vein insertion site.

EVIDENCED-BASED PRACTICE   *Quinn Franklin*

Use of Benzodiazepines and the Associated Risk for Respiratory Depression

ASK THE QUESTION
In children with convulsive episodes of status epilepticus (CSE), what are the predictors for respiratory depression when treated with a benzodiazepine?

SEARCH FOR THE EVIDENCE
Search strategies
Search criteria included English-language publications within the past 10 years (1998-2008), research-based articles (level 3 or lower) on children with status epilepticus (SE).

Databases used
PubMed, Cochrane, UpToDate, University of Michigan, Cincinnati Children's Hospital Medical Center, Canadian Medical Association, Scottish Intercollegiate Guidelines Network, New Zealand Guideline Group, National Guideline Clearinghouse (AHRQ), Joanna Briggs Institute

CRITICALLY ANALYZE THE EVIDENCE
GRADE criteria: Evidence quality very low; recommendation strong (Guyatt, Oxman, Vist, et al, 2008)

A review of the literature revealed six studies that examined the most effective, timely and safe benzodiazepine to be used as first-line therapy (Appelton, MacLeod, and Martland, 2008; Prasad, Al-Roomi, Krishnan, et al, 2005; Mahmoudian and Zadeh, 2004; Chin, Neville, Peckham, et al, 2008; Chin, Verhulst, Neville, et al, 2004). Two of the studies specifically identified the predictors of respiratory depression after first-line therapy (Chin, Neville, Peckham, et al, 2008; Chin, Verhulst, Neville, et al, 2004).

- A retrospective, cross-sectional study of children admitted to the intensive care unit (ICU) with a diagnosis of SE or related diagnosis was examined to identify the characteristics of this population (Chin, Verhulst, Neville, et al, 2004). In the 98 episodes (median age: 2.2 years), diazepam or lorazepam was the most commonly used benzodiazepine as first-line therapy. Children who were initially treated in prehospital setting were more likely to receive more than two doses of benzodiazepine and to have respiratory depression. The results indicated the importance of considering prehospital treatment in the management of children with SE.
- Chin, Neville, Peckham, and colleagues (2008) found in a prospective, population-based study of children treated for CSE before being transported to the emergency department that no prehospital treatment was associated with episodes that lasted longer than 60 minutes ($N = 240$ episodes, median age: 3.24 years). In addition, administration of two or more doses of benzodiazepines was associated with respiratory depression. Diazepam and lorazepam continued to be the most commonly used benzodiazepine as first-line therapy; however, intravenous lorazepam was found to be associated with a greater likelihood of seizure termination in comparison to rectal diazepam without an increased risk for respiratory depression.

APPLY THE EVIDENCE: NURSING IMPLICATIONS
- Children receiving more than two doses of benzodiazepine are more likely to have respiratory depression than those receiving fewer or no doses.
- Appropriate prehospital treatment for children with SE is essential to prevent respiratory depression.

References
Appleton R, MacLeod S, Martland T: Drug management for acute tonic-clonic convulsions including convulsive status epilepticus in children, *Cochrane Database Syst Rev* (3):CD001905. DOI:10.1002/14651858.CD001905.pub2, 2008.

Chin RFM, Neville BGR, Peckham C, et al: Treatment of community-onset, childhood convulsive status epilepticus: a prospective, population-based study, *Lancet Neurol* 7(8):696-703, 2008.

Chin RFM, Verhulst L, Neville BGR, et al: Inappropriate emergency management of status epilepticus in children contributes to need for intensive care, *J Neurol Neurosurg Psychiatry* 75(11):1584-1588, 2004.

Guyatt GH, Oxman AD, Vist GE, et al: GRADE: an emerging consensus on rating quality of evidence and strength of recommendations, *BMJ* 336:924-926, 2008.

Mahmoudian T, Zadeh MM: Comparison of intranasal midazolam with intravenous diazepam for treating acute seizures in children, *Epilepsy Behav* 5(2):253-255, 2004.

Prasad K, Al-Roomi K, Krishnan PR, et al: Anticonvulsant therapy for status epilepticus, *Cochrane Database Syst Rev* (4):CD003723. DOI: 10.1002/14651858.CD003723.pub2, 2005.

Nursing care of a child with status epilepticus includes, in addition to the ABCs of life support, monitoring blood pressure and body temperature. During the first 30 to 45 minutes of the seizure the blood pressure may be elevated. Thereafter the blood pressure typically returns to normal but may be decreased, depending on the medications being administered for seizure control. Hyperthermia requiring treatment may occur as a result of increased motor activity.

Status epilepticus is a medical emergency that requires immediate intervention to prevent possible brain injury or death. As imperative as halting the tonic-clonic movement is correct diagnosis of the underlying problem. The outcome is related to the etiology and duration of the status epilepticus.

Prognosis

Most children who experience a second seizure will experience additional seizures. Therefore a history of two seizures is sufficient to diagnose epilepsy (Shinnar, Berg, O'Dell, et al, 2000). Epidemiologic studies using population- or community-based cohorts show that the etiology and specific epilepsy syndromes are the most important factors affecting prognosis. Children who have cognitive impairments or cerebral palsy are at the highest risk for developing epilepsy. Seizures remit in more than two thirds of children with childhood onset of seizure. Mortality is increased in children with epilepsy; those with neurologic abnormalities or seizures that are refractory to treatment are at the highest risk (Browne and Holmes, 2004).

Convulsive status epilepticus is convincingly related to serious morbidity and mortality and is often associated with a severe neurologic abnormality, uncontrolled seizure disorder, or concurrent serious illness or infection. In one study, 79% of children who suffered status epilepticus had neurologic abnormalities. The highest morbidity was in patients with a nonidiopathic, nonfebrile cause (Barnard and Wirrell, 1999).

Nursing Care Management

An important nursing responsibility is to observe the seizure episode and accurately document the events. Record and note any alterations in behavior preceding the seizure and the characteristics of the episode, such as sensory-hallucinatory phenomena (e.g., an aura), motor effects (e.g., eye movements, muscular contractions), alterations in consciousness, and postictal state (Box 37-11). Describe only what is observed, rather than trying to label a seizure type. Note the time that the seizure began and the duration of the seizure.

Generalized seizures and other types with clear manifestations are easy to detect, but absence seizures may present more difficulties. They are easily misinterpreted as inattention. Any unusual behavior, even seemingly inconsequential, such as a momentary interruption of activity, staring, or mental blankness, should be described. The more detailed these descriptions, the more valuable they are for assessment (see Nursing Care Plan).

QUALITY PATIENT OUTCOMES: Seizures
- Etiology of seizure determined
- Seizures controlled or reduced in frequency and severity
- Family and child receive education to manage seizures
- Child adhering to treatment
- Side-effects of treatment minimized

BOX 37-11   GENERAL OBSERVATIONS

The Child During A Seizure

Observations During Seizure

Describe
Order of events (before, during, and after)
Duration of seizure
- Tonic-clonic—from first signs of event until jerking stops
- Absence—from loss of consciousness until consciousness is regained
- Complex partial—from first sign of unresponsiveness, motor activity, automatisms until there are signs of responsiveness to environment

Onset
Time of onset
Significant precipitating events—missed medication dosage, illness, stress, sleep deprivation, menses

Behavior
Change in facial expression
Cry or other sound
Stereotypic or automatous movements
Random activity (wandering)
Position of eyes, head, body, extremities
Unilateral or bilateral posturing of one or more extremities

Movement
Change of position, if any
Site of commencement—hand, thumb, mouth, generalized
Tonic phase—length, parts of body involved
Clonic phase—twitching or jerking movements, parts of body involved, sequence of parts involved, generalized, change in character of movements
Lack of movement or muscle tone of body part or entire body

Face
Color change—pallor, cyanosis, flushing
Perspiration
Mouth—position, deviating to one side, teeth clenched, tongue bitten, frothing at mouth, flecks of blood or bleeding
Lack of expression
Asymmetric expression

Eyes
Position—straight ahead, deviation upward or outward, conjugate or divergent gaze
Pupils—change in size, equality, reaction to light

Respiratory Effort
Presence and length of apnea

Other
Incontinence

Postictal Observations
Duration of postictal period
State of consciousness
Orientation
Arousability
Motor ability
- Any change in motor function
- Ability to move all extremities
- Paresis or weakness
Speech
Sensations
- Complaint of discomfort or pain
- Any sensory impairment
- Recollection of preseizure sensations or aura

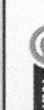

◎ **NURSING CARE PLAN**

The Child with Seizures

NURSING DIAGNOSIS	EXPECTED PATIENT OUTCOMES	NURSING INTERVENTIONS	RATIONALE
Risk for Injury related to CNS dysfunction and inability to control self (motor) secondary to type of seizure	Child will not experience physical injury as a result of seizure activity.	Administer antiepileptic drugs (AEDs).	To prevent seizure activity
		Teach family and child, as appropriate, the purpose of AEDs, expected response and action, potential side effects, timing, dosage, route of administration, and how to monitor effects.	To promote understanding of chronic condition
Child's/Family's Defining Characteristics (Subjective and Objective Data)	**The Following NOC Concepts Apply to These Outcomes** Risk Control		To prevent seizure activity and encourage self-care
Change in LOC	Safety Behavior: Personal	Monitor for side effects of AEDs and therapeutic levels according to child's growth, illness factors that affect metabolism, and effects of drug.	To prevent secondary effects of AEDs and to prevent seizures from occurring because of subtherapeutic drug levels
Disorientation	Safety Behavior: Home Physical Environment		
Clonic movements	Safety Status: Falls Occurrence		
Automatisms		Stress importance of adherence to medication regimen even if child has no evidence of seizure activity.	To prevent seizure activity
Aura			
Postictal impairment (dependent on the type of seizure)		Teach patient and family to identify and avoid situations that are known to precipitate a seizure (e.g., blinking lights, sleep deprivation, excess activity or exercise, physical factors).	To prevent seizure activity
		Initiate seizure precautions in the hospital: • Pad side rails of bed, crib, or wheelchair. • Keep bed relatively free of objects. • Set up suction and oxygen in room.	To prevent physical harm
		Educate family to initiate seizure precautions at home: • Bathroom safety includes taking showers instead of baths to prevent drowning. Use shower seat if falls occur during typical seizure. Leave bathroom door unlocked. • Kitchen safety includes cooking when someone else is nearby, using back burners of the stove to prevent accidental burns, and using shatterproof containers as much as possible. • Sports safety includes wearing protective equipment, having others nearby, not climbing higher than 10 feet without special equipment.	To prevent physical harm
		Teach family seizure first aid: • If child is at risk of falling at beginning of episode, ease child to floor. • Loosen tight or restrictive clothing. • Turn the child into side-lying position. • Prevent child from hitting head on objects. • Time the seizure. • Allow seizure to end spontaneously. • Reassure the child when awakening from seizure. • Do not put anything in child's mouth. • Do not attempt to restrain child or use force. • Call EMS (see Emergency Treatment box, p. 1530) if seizure persists more than 5 minutes, for repeated seizures, or if the child does not wake up after the movements have stopped.	To prepare the family for emergencies
		Counsel females of childbearing age about contraception and birth defects associated with AEDs.	To prevent birth defects
		The Following NIC Concepts Apply to These Interventions Area Restriction Surveillance Safety Environmental Management: Safety Medication Administration Teaching: Medication Administration Emergency Care Oxygen Administration Seizure Precautions	

NURSING CARE PLAN—cont'd

The Child with Seizures

NURSING DIAGNOSIS	EXPECTED PATIENT OUTCOMES	NURSING INTERVENTIONS	RATIONALE
Risk for Aspiration, and Ineffective Breathing Pattern, related to impaired motor activity, LOC, and loss of airway protection (tonic-clonic seizure)	Child's airway will remain patent. Child will have effective ventilation.	In the event of a seizure, place child in a side-lying position on a flat surface such as floor or bed.	To prevent aspiration and choking
		Remain with patient.	To protect the airway
	The Following NOC Concepts Apply to These Outcomes	Remove secretions, food, and liquids from mouth when seizure subsides.	To prevent aspiration
Child's/Family's Defining Characteristics (Subjective and Objective Data)	Aspiration Control Respiratory Status: Airway Patency Respiratory Status: Ventilation	In postictal state monitor oxygenation status.	To determine the need for oxygen
Decreased LOC		Administer oxygen as necessary.	To prevent hypoxia
Depressed cough reflex		Administer rescue breaths if spontaneous respirations do not resume shortly after seizure subsides.	To prevent hypoxia
Apnea			
Decreased inspiratory pressure		Administer medications intended to stop seizure longer than 5 minutes (rectal diazepam, IV dilantin, IV lorazepam)	To prevent continued seizure activity
		The Following NIC Concepts Apply to These Interventions	
		Risk Identification Aspiration Control Oxygen Administration Medication Administration	

NURSING DIAGNOSIS	EXPECTED PATIENT OUTCOMES	NURSING INTERVENTIONS	RATIONALE
Anxiety/Fear, Parent, related to child having life-threatening and incapacitating seizure activity*	Parent will cope with child's condition and receive adequate support.	Allow parent to remain with child during seizure.	To decrease fear of unknown and allow parent to see measures taken to protect child
Child's/Family's Defining Characteristics (Subjective and Objective Data)	**The Following NOC Concepts Apply to These Outcomes**	Instruct parent on proper protection interventions during child's seizure activity: positioning, safety, airway maintenance, reassurance techniques, emergency medication administration.	To promote parent participation and to foster sense of control over situation
Anguish	Anxiety Control Coping Fear Control	Provide information regarding nature (type) of seizure, therapeutic interventions, and lifestyle modifications.	To promote knowledge of condition, parental intervention, and sense of control
Fear			
Feelings of inadequacy and hopelessness		Encourage family involvement in daily care of child with goal of normalization and promotion of optimum growth and development.	To provide hope and promote family functioning and coping
Worry, apprehension			
Report of apprehension		Involve parents in discussion of fears, anxieties, and resources and support options available to family.	To promote family integrity and functioning
Panic			
Excitement		**The Following NIC Concepts Apply to These Interventions**	
		Support Group Coping Enhancement Anxiety Reduction Family Process Maintenance Active Listening Counseling Decision-Making Support Family Involvement Promotion	

CNS, Central nervous system; *EMS*, emergency medical services; *IV*, intravenous; *LOC*, level of consciousness.
*Nursing diagnosis may also apply to child in the postictal phase, depending on type of seizure and child's understanding and cognition level.

The child must be protected from injury during the seizure. Nursing observations made during the event provide valuable information for diagnosis and management of the disorder (see Emergency Treatment box).

It is impossible to halt a seizure once it has begun, and no attempt should be made to do so. The nurse must remain calm, stay with the child, and prevent the child from sustaining any harm during the seizure. If possible, isolate the child from the view of others by closing a door or pulling screens. A seizure can be upsetting to the child, other visitors, and their families. If other persons are present, reassure them that everything is being done for the child. After the seizure, they can be given a simple explanation about the event as needed.

If the nurse is able to reach the child in time, a child who is standing or seated in a chair (including a wheelchair) is eased to the floor immediately. During (and sometimes after) the

✚ EMERGENCY TREATMENT
Seizures

Tonic-Clonic Seizure
During the Seizure
Remain calm.
Time seizure episode.
If child is standing or seated, ease child down to the floor.
Place pillow or folded blanket under child's head.
Loosen restrictive clothing.
Remove eyeglasses.
Clear area of any hazards or hard objects.
Allow seizure to end without interference.
If vomiting occurs, turn child to one side.
Do not:
- Attempt to restrain child or use force.
- Put anything in child's mouth.
- Give any food or liquids.

After the Seizure
Time postictal period.
Check for breathing. Check position of head and tongue.
Reposition if head is hyperextended. If breathing is not present, give rescue breathing and call emergency medical services (EMS).
Keep child on side.
Remain with child.
Do not give food or liquids until child is fully alert and swallowing reflex has returned.
Call EMS when necessary.
Look for medical identification, and determine what factors occurred before onset of seizure that may have been triggering factors.
Check head and body for possible injuries.
Check inside of mouth to see if tongue or lips have been bitten.

Complex Partial Seizure
During the Seizure
Do not restrain.
Remove harmful objects from area.
Redirect to safe area.
Do not agitate; instead, talk in calm, reassuring manner.
Do not expect child to follow instructions.
Watch to see if seizure generalizes.

After the Seizure
Stay with child and reassure until fully conscious.

Call Emergency Medical Service If
Child stops breathing.
There is evidence of injury or child is diabetic or pregnant.
Seizure lasts for more than 5 minutes (unless seizures typically last >5 minutes) and written medical order is present.
Status epilepticus occurs.
Pupils are not equal after seizure.
Child vomits continuously 30 minutes after seizure has ended (sign of possible acute problem).
Child cannot be awakened and is unresponsive to pain after seizure has ended.
Seizure occurs in water.
This is child's first seizure.

Modified from *Seizure recognition and first aid*, Landover, Md, 2001, Epilepsy Foundation, available at www.epilepsyfoundation.org/about/firstaid/seizurespecial.cfm (accessed May 7, 2010).

tonic-clonic seizure, the swallowing reflex is lost, salivation increases, and the tongue is hypotonic. Therefore the child is at risk for aspiration and airway occlusion. Placing the child on the side facilitates drainage and helps maintain a patent airway. Suctioning of the oral cavity and posterior oropharynx may be

necessary. Take vital signs, and allow the child to rest if at school or away from home. When feasible, the child is integrated into the environment as soon as possible. Sending a child with a chronic seizure disorder home from school is not necessary unless requested by the parents.

❗ NURSING ALERT

Do not move or forcefully restrain the child during a tonic-clonic seizure, and do not place a solid object between the teeth.

Seizure precautions are required for children who are known to have seizures or who are under observation for seizures. The extent of these measures depends on the type and frequency of the seizure (Box 37-12).

Long-Term Care
Care of the child with epilepsy involves physical care and instruction regarding the importance of the drug therapy and, probably more significant, the problems related to the emotional aspects of the disorder. Few diseases generate as much anxiety among relatives as epilepsy. Fears and misconceptions about the disease and its treatment are common. For many, it represents the archetype of severe hereditary affliction. Direct nursing care toward educating the child and family about epilepsy and helping them develop strategies to cope with the psychologic and sociologic problems related to epilepsy.

Physical Aspects
Children with epilepsy are prescribed antiepileptic medications, which are administered at regular intervals to maintain adequate levels in the blood. The nurse can help the parents plan the administration of the medication at convenient times to disrupt the family routine as little as possible. The dosage schedule is based on the drug's half-life (the time required to reduce to one-half the amount of unchanged drug that is in the body) and the child's age. Drugs with longer half-lives are given less frequently, and a missed dose will have less of a negative effect than with a drug with a short half-life. The younger child may need a more frequent dosing schedule because of more rapid metabolism. The aim is to simplify the medication routine

BOX 37-12 SEIZURE PRECAUTIONS

The extent of precautions depends on type, severity, and frequency of seizures. They may include:
- Side rails raised when child is sleeping or resting
- Side rails and other hard objects padded
- Waterproof mattress or pad on bed or crib

Appropriate precautions during potentially hazardous activities may include:
- Swimming with a companion
- Showers preferred; bathing only with close supervision
- Use of protective helmet and padding during bicycle riding, skateboarding, in-line skating
- Supervision during use of hazardous machinery or equipment

Have child carry or wear medical identification.
Alert other caregivers to need for any special precautions.
Child may not drive or operate hazardous machinery or equipment unless seizure free for designated period (varies by state).

as much as possible and incorporate it into the parents' and child's daily activities. This also increases the likelihood of compliance. The most convenient times for administration seem to be with meals or at bedtime.

⚡ DRUG ALERT

Vitamin D and Folic Acid Deficiency

> Children taking phenobarbital or phenytoin should receive adequate vitamin D and folic acid, since deficiencies of both have been associated with these drugs. Phenytoin should not be taken with milk.

It is important to impress on the family the necessity of giving the antiepileptic medication regularly and for as long as required. In general, antiepileptic medications are continued until the child has been seizure free for 2 years (Johnston, 2009). The medication is then slowly tapered over a period of weeks to avoid the possibility of precipitating a seizure. It is sometimes easy to skip doses or omit them for a variety of reasons, especially when the child is free of seizures most of the time. This is particularly so when the child is older and assumes responsibility for his or her medication. The seizure threshold may be lowered during any illness, but particularly with fever. Therefore parents should be aware that if their child has an illness, he or she is at increased risk for seizures. Parents should contact their health professional if their child misses medications during an illness because of vomiting.

⚡ DRUG ALERT

Rectal Antiepileptic Medications

> Rectal preparations of some antiepileptic medications are highly effective when a child is unable to take oral medications because of repeated vomiting, gastrointestinal surgery, or status epilepticus. Parents can learn to administer rectal antiepileptic medication for home treatment. Rectal diazepam is a useful adjunctive home treatment for children at risk for prolonged seizures or clusters of seizures. It also minimizes hospitalization and enhances parental confidence.

Educate the child and parents about the possible adverse reactions to the medications used to treat seizures. Parents should understand the common side effects and be encouraged to report their observations to their health care provider. Parents should understand that the child needs periodic physical assessment and laboratory studies. Possible adverse effects on the hematopoietic system, liver, and kidneys may be reflected in symptoms such as fever, sore throat, enlarged lymph nodes, jaundice, and bleeding (e.g., easy bruising, petechiae, ecchymoses, epistaxis). A common factor in status epilepticus is inadequate blood levels of antiepileptic drugs.

Parents need to be aware of possible behavioral changes associated with some antiepileptic medications. Changes in personality, indifference to school activities and family, hyperactivity, or even psychotic behavior may sometimes be observed. If so, the parents should contact their health care provider. The potential effects of antiepileptic drugs on learning and behavior should also be considered. Progressive intellectual deterioration

in a child with epilepsy requires investigation of the present medication plus the role of the underlying cerebral pathologic condition.

Although children with epilepsy are at increased risk for injury, few limitations should be placed on activities. The degree to which activities are restricted is individualized for each child and depends on the type, frequency, and severity of the seizures; the child's response to therapy; and the length of time the seizures have been controlled. Children are encouraged to engage in most normal activities; participation in competitive sports is determined on an individual basis. With encouragement, most older children can accept the restrictions placed on activities. To avoid accentuating differences when possible, only the essential restrictions are placed on children regarding sports and peer activity; these restrictions are approached in a positive way in terms of what the child can do rather than what he or she cannot do. Parents sometimes limit the child's activities more than necessary, which may lead to impaired self-esteem.

To prevent head injuries, children should wear appropriate safety devices, such as helmets, and should avoid activities involving heights. Although bike riding is safe for most children, children with frequent seizures in whom impairment of consciousness occurs should avoid bike riding. Skating, rollerblading, and skateboarding should be restricted only in children with frequent seizures. Helmets must be worn while participating in these activities.

Children with epilepsy are at higher risk for submersion injury than children without epilepsy. Young children should never be left alone in the bathtub, even for a few seconds. Older children and adolescents should be encouraged to use a shower and reminded not to lock the bathroom door when showering. They should never swim unsupervised.

All children should avoid open fires, hot stoves and ovens, and dangerous machinery. Parents must assume that a seizure could occur at any time and should not allow a child to be in a situation where a seizure could be deadly.

Because the child is encouraged to attend school, camp, and other normal activities, the school nurse and teacher should be made aware of the child's condition and therapy. They can help ensure regularity of medication administration and provision of any special care the child might need. Teachers, child care providers, camp counselors, youth organization leaders, coaches, and other adults who assume responsibility for children should be instructed regarding care of the child during a seizure so that they can act in a calm manner for the child's welfare and influence the attitude of the child's peers.*

Triggering Factors

Careful and detailed documentation of seizures over time may indicate a pattern. In such cases the nurse or responsible adult may intervene to identify the triggering factors and alter the

---

*Excellent resources are Santilli N, Dodson WE, Walton AV: *Students with seizures: a manual for school nurses*, Landover, Md, 1991, Epilepsy Foundation; and Schachter SC, Montouris GD, Pellock JM: *The brainstorms family: epilepsy on our terms—stories by children with seizures and their parents*, Philadelphia, 1996, Lippincott Williams and Wilkins.

environment to prevent or decrease seizure frequency. Often the necessary changes are simple but can make an enormous difference in the lives of the child and family (see Critical Thinking Exercise).

❓ CRITICAL THINKING EXERCISE

Seizures

Jane is a 14-year-old girl with cryptogenic localization-related epilepsy with complex partial seizures. Her seizures have been well controlled for the past 6 years on monotherapy with only an occasional breakthrough seizure every 3 or 4 months, often in association with an intercurrent illness. Six months ago she entered high school. She is active on the drill team, which practices for 2 hours after school each day. In addition, she is taking honors English and math classes, both of which have daily homework. Jane typically does homework until midnight and gets up at 6 AM for school. For the past 3 months she has had an increasing number of seizures and is now having at least one seizure per week. She has not had any recent illnesses. Her physical and neurologic examination is normal.

1. Evidence—Is there sufficient evidence to draw any conclusions about Jane's increased seizure frequency?
2. Assumptions—Describe an underlying assumption about the following:
   a. A 14-year-old girl with cryptogenic localization-related epilepsy with complex partial seizures that were previously well controlled on medication
   b. A teenager whose seizures are no longer controlled on the current dose of medication
   c. Triggering factors for seizures
3. What implications and priorities for nursing care can be drawn at this time?
4. Does the evidence objectively support your conclusion?

The most common factors that may trigger seizures in children include emotional stress, sleep deprivation, fatigue, fever, and illness (Frucht, Quigg, Schwaner, et al, 2000; Nakken, Solaas, Kjeldsen, et al, 2005). Other precipitating factors include sleep, flickering lights, menstrual cycle, alcohol, heat, hyperventilation, and fasting (Frucht, Quigg, Schwaner, et al, 2000). Some individuals have pattern-sensitive epilepsy, that is, seizures precipitated by changes in dark-light patterns, such as those that occur with a flash on a camera, automobile headlights, reflections of light on snow or water, or rotating blades on a fan (see Research Focus box).

🔍 RESEARCH FOCUS

Effect of Video Games on Seizure Development

A study by Radhakrishnan, St Louis, Johnson, and colleagues (2005) was conducted to determine the electroclinical features of patients with pattern-sensitive epilepsy. Most of these individuals had absence, myoclonic, or generalized tonic-clonic seizures. Some children have seizures while playing video games. These children are sensitive to intermittent photic stimulation that can trigger an epileptic episode (Shoja, Tubbs, Malekian, et al, 2007). However, the overwhelming majority of children with epilepsy can play video or computer games and watch television without the risk of seizures.

Family Support

Parental attitudes and management of a child with a seizure disorder vary. Whether the seizures result from illness, injury, or unknown cause, the parents may feel guilt, anxiety, and even humiliation. They want to know if the seizures will affect their child's mental capacities. Many persons erroneously associate epilepsy with mental deficiency. Seizures do commonly accompany other manifestations of severe brain damage from disease or injury, but children with seizures, like any population of healthy children, display a wide range of intelligence.

Parents also wonder how the illness will affect their child's future. The answer to this question depends on the cause of the seizures and other comorbid conditions. In many cases parents can be reassured that the illness will not shorten their child's life and that their child can attend school, marry, and elect to have children. The child may need vocational guidance, and the parents need to become familiar with the laws in their state regarding any limitations imposed on people with epilepsy. For children who are severely impaired, the family needs to become familiar with local early childhood programs. The nurse should emphasize that the seizures can be controlled or greatly reduced in the large majority of affected children. Parents need reassurance that less stigma is attached to the condition than in the past.

Encourage a healthy attitude toward the child and the condition, and help the parents feel competent in their ability to meet their responsibilities to their child. The child should be reared in the same manner as any normal child, with natural concern tempered by understanding of the need not to overprotect. Many parents refrain from correcting or punishing their child, especially if the child has had a seizure after being disciplined. The child must not be made to feel different in any way. Encourage parents to be honest and open about the disorder with their child and with others. Some parents try to conceal the nature of their child's illness because of their belief that the disorder is shameful or a disgrace to the family.

Educational materials and support groups may prove beneficial for families. The Epilepsy Foundation* is a national organization that works for the welfare of persons with epilepsy and their families; helps with employment and legal problems; and provides education to patients, families, and communities.

The Child with Epilepsy

The child who is provided the security of a loving family, rewards and punishments no different from those of other children, and support in acquiring self-esteem is more likely to have a positive attitude toward the condition. Children derive their self-concept and self-esteem from observations of others' reactions to them and from their own perceptions of their capabilities. The suddenness and unpredictability of the seizures and the reactions of others further influence their feelings. When others consider children to be different, inferior, or objects of ridicule, the children come to view themselves in the same light.

Children with epilepsy need to learn about their condition and how medication contributes to their prolonged well-being. As soon as they are old enough, children should assume responsibility for taking their own medication and should carry medical identification with pertinent information about their

---

*8301 Professional Place, Landover, MD 20785-7223; 800-332-1000; www.efa.org. In Canada: Epilepsy Canada, 2255B Queen St. E., Suite 336, Toronto, Ontario, Canada M4E 1G3; 877-734-0873; www.epilepsy.ca.

condition. Planning activities with children and emphasizing those in which they can engage, rather than those which are restricted, help them succeed and gain satisfaction in their achievements. They should be offered opportunities and encouraged to exercise judgment in their daily lives.

The adolescent period may prove to be a trying time for the child with epilepsy. Limits imposed on the young person's activities at a time when freedom and independence are desired may bring the disability into sharp focus. For example, all U.S. states have a defined seizure-free period before a driver's license can be obtained.

Epilepsy should not be a severe impairment to most youngsters. The nurse can help provide positive outcomes for the child and family by assuming the role of patient advocate, helping educate the public about the condition, working to make opportunities available to persons with the disorder, and lobbying for legislation that recognizes the needs of individuals with seizure disorders.

FEBRILE SEIZURES

Febrile seizure is "a seizure in association with a febrile illness in the absence of a central nervous system infection or acute electrolyte imbalance in children older than 1 month of age without prior afebrile seizures" (Ostergaard, 2009). Febrile seizures are one of the most common neurologic conditions of childhood, affecting approximately 3% of children. Most febrile seizures occur after 6 months of age and usually before age 3 years, with the average age of onset between 18 and 22 months. They are unusual after 5 years of age. Boys are affected about twice as often as girls, and there appears to be an increased familial susceptibility.

The cause of febrile seizures is still uncertain. Both animal and human studies demonstrate an age-specific susceptibility to seizures induced by fever and that it is the peak temperature that is important, not the rapidity of the temperature elevation (Ostergaard, 2009). The temperature usually exceeds 38.8° C (101.8° F), and the seizure occurs during the temperature rise rather than after a prolonged elevation. Sometimes it constitutes the dramatic beginning of an illness, often an upper respiratory tract or gastrointestinal infection.

> **! NURSING ALERT**
>
> If a febrile seizure lasts more than 5 minutes, parents should seek medical attention right away. Instruct them to call for emergency assistance (911) and not to place the child who is actively having a seizure in the car.

Most febrile seizures have stopped by the time the child is taken to a medical facility. However, if the seizure continues, treatment consists of controlling the seizure with IV or rectal diazepam and reducing the temperature with acetaminophen. Antiepileptic prophylaxis is not indicated. Parental education and emotional support are important interventions. Parents need reassurance regarding the benign nature of febrile seizures. Several large studies show no difference in intelligence, behavior, or academic performance in children with febrile seizures compared with either population or sibling controls

(Verity, Greenword, and Golding, 1998). Parents also need education on how to protect the child from harm and observe exactly what happens to the child during the event. Attempts to lower the temperature will not prevent a seizure. Tepid sponge baths are not recommended for several reasons: they are ineffective in significantly lowering the temperature, the shivering effect further increases metabolic output, and cooling causes discomfort to the child.

Long-term antiepileptic therapy is usually not required for children with simple febrile seizures. Antipyretic therapy during febrile illness offers symptomatic relief for fever-associated symptoms but appears to be ineffective in preventing a seizure (Ostergaard, 2009).

HEADACHE

Headaches are a common complaint of children and are associated with different pathologic conditions, including extracranial disease, intracranial disease, vascular abnormalities, psychogenic disorders, or a combination of the above (Table 37-7). Headaches are classified according to the International Headache Society classification system (Headache Classification Subcommittee of the International Headache Society, 2004).

ASSESSMENT

It is important to determine the pattern of the headache—single acute episode, paroxysmal, acute and recurrent, chronic and progressive, chronic nonprogressive, or mixed. Other assessment information includes the presence of seizures, ataxia, lethargy, weakness, nausea or vomiting, or any personality changes. Factors related to early development and past illnesses and a family history of headaches may also be pertinent. A "headache diary," which includes time of onset and termination of headaches, intensity, associated events, and actions taken and their effects, can be helpful for the patient and practitioner.

Clues to etiology may be found in the family history, including information about the home or social situation (e.g., divorce, separation, alcoholism, school avoidance). Box 37-13 lists specific questions that often elicit needed information. Thorough physical and neurologic examinations are performed, and further diagnostic tests (e.g., CT, MRI, or EEG) are ordered if indicated.

> **! NURSING ALERT**
>
> During the health history and neurologic assessment, the following abnormal signs require immediate follow-up for children:
> - The headache progresses in frequency and severity over a brief period (2 to 3 weeks).
> - It awakens the child from sleep (may also be migraine).
> - It occurs in early morning.
> - It is worse on arising.
> - It is characterized by persistent, occipital, or frontal pain.
> - It is accompanied by unexplained vomiting.
> - It is associated with a change in gait, personality, or behavior.
> - It is exacerbated by Valsalva maneuver (intensified by lowering head and straining, such as during a bowel movement, coughing, or sneezing).

TABLE 37-7 CHARACTERISTICS OF HEADACHES

TYPE OF HEADACHE	CHARACTERISTICS
Acute	
Acute sinusitis (may also be classified as inflammatory)	Usually accompanied by fever and tenderness over involved sinuses: *Ethmoid sinuses*—Referred pain to orbital and temporal areas *Frontal sinuses*—Pain above the eyes
Ocular abnormalities	Headaches usually occurring late in day, precipitated by schoolwork, driving, or television viewing
Dental disorders (may be classified as inflammatory)	Frontal or temporal headaches caused by malocclusion, caries, abscess, temporomandibular joint (TMJ) dysfunction TMJ headaches sometimes exacerbated by chewing or stress
Respiratory infections (pharyngitis, otitis media)	Pain localized to affected structures
Viral infections or febrile illnesses (may also be classified as vascular)	Headache caused by viral infections such as influenza or bacterial infections such as streptococcal pharyngitis
Inflammatory illness (meningitis, encephalitis)	Global headache usually accompanied by nuchal rigidity, fever, mental status changes
Trauma	Localized to area of trauma; related to nerve and tissue injury Postconcussion syndrome
Acute Recurrent	
Migraine (see migraine classification, Box 37-14)	Intermittent attacks of vasoconstriction Paroxysmal Nausea, vomiting, fatigue, pallor Positive family history May be triggered by stress, fatigue, trauma, exercise, menses, medications, diet, sleep deprivation, environmental factors
Chronic Progressive	
Intracranial abnormalities	Symptoms of increased ICP
Tumors	Early morning headaches primarily
Hydrocephalus	Bulging fontanel, suture splitting in infants and young children, symptoms of increased ICP
Subdural hematoma	Usually results from trauma Seizures and focal neurologic deficits more common than headaches
Brain abscess	Rare but may be associated with chronic otitis media or sinusitis, cyanotic heart disease, and immunosuppression
Pseudotumor cerebri	Increased ICP without obstruction of CSF
Chronic Nonprogressive	
Tension type	Common in children Adjustment reaction, anxiety related
Psychiatric	Conversion reaction (anxiety converted to somatic symptoms)

CSF, Cerebrospinal fluid; *ICP,* intracranial pressure.

BOX 37-13 QUESTIONS FOR EVALUATING HEADACHES

1. Do you have more than one type of headache?
2. How did the headache begin? Trauma? Infection?
3. How long has it been present?
4. Are the symptoms getting worse or staying the same?
5. How often do they occur?
6. How long do they last?
7. Do they occur at any special time or when certain things happen?
8. Do you have warning signs?
9. Where does it hurt?
10. How does the pain feel? Pounding? Sharp?
11. Do you feel sick in other ways during the headache? Abdominal pain? Nausea, vomiting?
12. Do you stop what you are doing during the headache?
13. Do you have any other health problems?
14. Are you taking any medicines regularly?
15. Are there some things you do that make the headache worse or better?
16. Does any one medicine make the headache better?
17. Does anyone else in your family have headaches?
18. What do you think is causing your headaches?

Modified from Rothner AD: Management of headaches in children and adolescents, *J Pain Symptom Manage* 8(2):81-86, 1993.

Tension headaches are common in children. They are typically frontal, and the pain is described as a pressing tightness; it is nonthrobbing in character and is not typically accompanied by nausea or vomiting. Simple analgesics, including acetaminophen and ibuprofen, are usually the most effective pharmacologic intervention. Biofeedback and relaxation techniques may be useful nonpharmacologic interventions in children with recurrent tension headaches (Haslam, 2009; Rowley, 2005).

MIGRAINE HEADACHE

Migraine headaches occur in children as well as adults. Migraine headaches can have their onset in very young children, including infants, although this is uncommon. The onset tends to be earlier in boys than girls, with a male prevalence until age 10 to 14 years of age after which time more females are affected (Bigal, Lipton, Winner, et al, 2007).

The exact pathophysiology of migraines continues to be researched. It is postulated that migraine headaches have a genetic and multifactorial etiology. However, no consistent genetic etiology for migraines has been established except for familial hemiplegic migraine, which has autosomal dominant inheritance (Ducros, Tournier-Lasserve, and Bousser, 2002). Previously, it was thought that migraine headaches were caused by dilatation of cerebral blood vessels. However, this is no longer thought to be correct. Although vasodilation appears to play a role in the throbbing pain of migraine, this is likely a secondary symptom. Rather, the primary cause of migraine headaches is now thought to be a neuronal dysfunction that leads to a sequence of changes in blood flow to specific regions of the brain and the release of various polypeptides that cause pain and vasodilation of cranial vessels (Bolay, Reuter, Dunn, et al, 2002).

Revisions in the classification of migraine headaches introduced some new terms and eliminated, renamed, or reclassified

BOX 37-14 MIGRAINE PATTERNS

Migraine with Aura

Aura may be: visual (most common); hemiparethetic (tingling and numbness of lips, lower face (second most common); hemiparetic; hemiplegic; or aphasic

Aura duration less than 1 hour and completely resolves. Followed by throbbing, unilateral or bilateral headache coupled with nausea, vomiting, photophobia, and phonophobia.

Migraine Without Aura

Prodrome that consists of, pallor, alteration in personality, or change in appetite or thirst

Unilateral or bilateral headache coupled with nausea and/or vomiting, photophobia, and phonophobia

Pulsating quality

Moderate or severe pain intensity

Sporadic Hemiplegic Migraine

Migraine with aura

Motor weakness

No first- or second-degree relative who also has migraine with aura and motor weakness

Basilar-Type Migraine

Recurrent attacks

Headache typically occipital

Symptoms may include dysarthria, vertigo, diplopia, vomiting, and altered consciousness

others. Migraine headaches are now classified as migraine without aura and migraine with aura; the latter category includes the following subtypes: auras and prodrome, familial hemiplegic migraine, sporadic hemiplegic migraine, and basilar-type migraine (Box 37-14) (Headache Classification Subcommittee of the International Headache Society, 2004).

The headaches are paroxysmal. The symptoms of migraine headaches vary depending on age. Typical symptoms include nausea, vomiting, and abdominal pain, which are relieved by sleep. Toddlers may be seen with episodic pallor, decreased activity, and vomiting. The onset of a migraine headache in a young child is typically in the afternoon and may be bifrontal, temporal, and bilateral or unilateral. Children may vomit repetitively during a migraine headache. A family history of migraine is elicited in 70% of children with migraine; 5% of all children who have migraines experience a headache before age 15 years. Before the onset of puberty, migraines are more common in boys; this trend reverses after puberty.

Migraine headaches are managed with general measures (education, a headache diary to identify and eliminate precipitating factors, and documented response to treatment), abortive treatment, and prophylactic treatment. At the onset of the headache, the child should rest or sleep in a quiet, dark room when feasible. Migraine therapy, if administered early in the course of the headache, may provide rapid relief. Acetaminophen or ibuprofen is often effective if given early.

⚡ DRUG ALERT

Triptans

Triptans are serotonin agonists and are effective in the abortive treatment of migraines. Although they are widely used, the FDA has not approved many of the triptans for use in children. Sumatriptan nasal spray may be considered for use in adolescents more than 12 years of age (Lewis, Ashwal, Hershey, et al, 2004). For children who experience frequent (more than four times per month) or refractory migraines, prophylactic medications such as cyproheptadine, propranolol, or amitriptyline may be used.

The outlook for a child with migraine is good, but the child and parents should be informed that predisposition to the headaches may be lifelong. Severe headaches can adversely affect the child's routine activities of daily living, including family relations and school.

KEY POINTS

- The CNS is composed of the brain and spinal cord.
- Gait abnormalities that may indicate cerebral dysfunction include ataxia, spastic paraplegic gait, hemiplegic gait, cerebellar gait, and extrapyramidal gait.
- LOC is the most important indicator of neurologic health; altered levels include sleep, confusion, delirium, and comatose states.
- Complete neurologic examination includes LOC; gait, motor, sensory, CN, and reflex testing; and vital signs.
- Nursing care of the unconscious child focuses on respiratory management, neurologic assessment, increased ICP monitoring, adequate nutrition and hydration, drug therapy, promotion of elimination, maintenance of hygiene, positioning and exercise, stimulation, and family support.
- Primary head injury involves events that occur at the time of trauma, including fractured skull, contusions, intracranial hematoma, and diffuse injury. Secondary complications include hypoxic brain damage, increased ICP, infection, cerebral edema, and posttraumatic syndromes.
- The young child's response to head injury is different because of a larger head size in proportion to body; larger blood volume to the brain; small subdural spaces; and thinner, softer brain tissue.
- Fractures resulting from head injuries can be classified as linear, depressed, compound, basilar, and diastatic.
- Problems resulting from submersion injuries are caused by hypoxia and include asphyxiation, aspiration, and hypothermia.
- Nursing care of the child with meningitis includes administration of antibiotics; vital signs monitoring; IV therapy; and promotion of fluid, nutritional status, and family support.
- Routine immunization of infants against *H. influenzae* type b and *S. pneumoniae* infection has reduced the incidence of bacterial meningitis.
- Encephalitis may result from direct invasion of the CNS by a virus or from postinfectious involvement of the CNS after viral illness.

- A seizure is a symptom of underlying pathologic condition and may be manifested by sensory-hallucinatory phenomena, motor effects, sensorimotor effects, or impaired or loss of consciousness.
- Partial seizures are categorized as simple (without associated impairment of consciousness) or complex; both types may become generalized.
- Generalized seizures are categorized as tonic-clonic, absence, atonic, or myoclonic.
- Long-term care of the child with epilepsy involves teaching caregivers appropriate interventions during a seizure, emphasizing the importance of antiepileptic therapy,

giving practical advice regarding drug administration and scheduling, and helping the child and family cope with diagnosis.
- Febrile seizures are the most common type of childhood seizure. The most important nursing intervention is to reassure parents of their benign nature and educate parents regarding protection of their child and meaningful observation during the event.
- A child's complaint of headache requires a thorough history and physical examination with a neurologic assessment. Stress is the most common cause of recurrent headache in children.

ANSWERS TO CRITICAL THINKING EXERCISES

Postconcussion Syndrome

1. **Yes.** Thomas's behavior 2 weeks after a fall, consisting of enuresis, crying episodes, early morning vomiting, decreased appetite, and a desire to be held, are all signs of increased intracranial pressure (ICP).
2. **a.** Preschoolers have increased curiosity and are unaware of safety measures.
   b. A fall predisposes a preschooler to develop posttraumatic insidious brain injury even after an initial negative CT scan.
   c. Behavioral changes 2 weeks after a fall may be signs of ICP because of postconcussion syndrome.
3. The nurse should immediately notify the medical provider because of the worsening postconcussion symptoms and signs of increased ICP, then obtain vital signs and assess Thomas's neurologic status.
4. **Yes.** The preschooler's signs of ICP approximately 2 weeks after head trauma (fall) support the nurse's actions.

Seizures

1. **Yes.** Jane is a teenager with previously well-controlled seizures who is now having frequent seizures. However, until further assessment is performed, the exact reason is not known.

2. **a.** Seizures may change during brain maturation and either become easier or more difficult to control.
   b. Further evaluation is needed in any child whose seizures have been well controlled and then increase in frequency. The child and family should be advised to seek medical reevaluation.
   c. Seizures have many triggering factors. Jane's history is suggestive of several, including sleep deprivation, fatigue, and stress. Further assessment is required to elicit the possibility of others, including poor medication compliance, relation to menses, and alcohol intake.
3. Nursing care should focus on educating Jane and her family on the avoidance of triggering factors for seizures and maintaining healthy lifestyle habits (e.g., getting adequate sleep, taking medications as prescribed, avoiding alcohol).
4. **Yes,** the history and physical assessment support these conclusions. Additionally, knowledge of triggering factors for seizures supports this conclusion. It is not within the scope of nursing practice to change the antiepileptic medication or dosage.

REFERENCES

American Academy of Pediatrics, Committee on Infectious Diseases, Pickering L, editor: *Red book: report of the Committee on Infectious Diseases*, ed 27, Elk Grove Village, Ill, 2006, The Academy.

American Heart Association: Part 10.3 drowning, *Circulation* 112:IV133-IV135, 2005, available at http://circ.ahajournals.org/cgi/content/full/112/24_suppl/IV-133 (accessed May 17, 2009).

Anderson VA, Catroppa C, Haritou F, et al: Identifying factors contributing to child and family outcome 30 months after traumatic brain injury in children, *J Neurol Neurosurg Psychiatry* 76:401-408, 2005.

Anderson VA, Catroppa C, Haritou F, et al: Predictors of acute child and family outcome following traumatic brain injury in children, *Pediatr Neurosurg* 34:138-148, 2001.

Baandrup L, Jensen R: Chronic post-traumatic headache: a clinical analysis in relation to the

International Headache Classification 2nd edition, *Cephalalgia* 25:132, 2005.

Barnard C, Wirrell E: Does status epilepticus cause developmental deterioration and development of epilepsy? *J Child Neurol* 14(12):787-794, 1999.

Bechtel K, Stoessel K, Leventahal JM, et al: Characteristics that distinguish accidental from abusive injury in hospitalized young children with head trauma, *Pediatrics* 114(1):165-168, 2004.

Bigal ME, Lipton RB, Winner P, et al: Migraine in adolescents: association with socioeconomic status and family history, *Neurology* 69(1):16-25, 2007.

Blinman TA, Houseknecht E, Snyder C, et al: Postconcussive symptoms in hospitalized pediatric patients after mild traumatic brain injury, *J Pediatr Surg* 44(6):1223-1228, 2009.

Bolay H, Reuter U, Dunn AK, et al: Intrinsic brain activity triggers trigeminal meningeal

afferents in a migraine model, *Nature Med* 8(2):136-142, 2002.

Bonthius DJ, Karacay B: Meningitis and encephalitis in children: an update, *Neurol Clin* 20(4):1013-1038, 2002.

Browne TR, Holmes GL: *Handbook of epilepsy*, ed 3, Philadelphia, 2004, Lippincott Williams & Wilkins.

Case ME: Accidental traumatic head injury in infants and young children, *Brain Pathol* 18(40):583-589, 2008.

Castiglia PT: Shaken baby syndrome, *J Pediatr Health Care* 15:78-80, 2001.

Centers for Disease Control and Prevention: General Recommendation on Immunization, 2009, available at www.cdc.gov/vaccines/pubs/ACIP-list.htm (accessed June 13, 2009).

Centers for Disease Control and Prevention: Human rabies prevention: United States, 2008, *MMWR Early Release* 57:1-27, 2008.

Centers for Disease Control and Prevention: U.S. Rabies Surveillance Data, 2006, available at www.cdc.gov/rabies/epidemiology.html (accessed June 13, 2009).

Centers for Disease Control and Prevention: Meningococcal disease, 2000, available at www.cdc.gov/ncidod/dbmd/diseaseinfo/meningococcal_t.htm (accessed May 2, 2010).

Chavez-Bureno S, McCracken GH Jr: Bacterial meningitis in children, *Pediatr Clin North Am* 52(3):795-810, 2005.

Chen JWY, Wasterlain CG: Status epilepticus: pathophysiology and management in adults, *Lancet Neurol* 5:246-256, 2006.

Chiaretti A, DeBenedictis R, Polidori G, et al: Early post-traumatic seizures in children with head injury, *Childs Nerv Syst* 16(12):862-866, 2000.

Cohen RH, Matter KC, Sinclair SA, et al: Unintentional pediatric submersion-injury–related hospitalizations in the United States, 2003, *Inj Prev* 14(2):131-135, 2008.

Commission on Classification and Terminology of International League Against Epilepsy: Proposal for classification of epilepsies and epileptic syndromes, *Epilepsia* 26(3):268-278, 1985.

Commission on Epidemiology and Prognosis of International League Against Epilepsy: Guidelines for epidemiologic studies on epilepsy, *Epilepsia* 34(4):592-596, 1993.

Curatolo P, Moavero R, Lo Castro A, et al: Pharmacotherapy of idiopathic generalized epilepsies, *Exp Opin Pharmacother* 10(1):5-17, 2009.

de Louvois J, Halket S, Harvey D: Neonatal meningitis in England and Wales: sequelae at 5 years of age, *Eur J Pediatr* 164(12):730-734, 2005.

DeVita MA: The death watch: certifying death using cardiac criteria, *Prog Transplant* 11(1):58-66, 2001.

DiCarlo JV, Frankel LR: Scoring systems and predictors of mortality. In Behrman RE, Kliegman RM, Jenson HB, editors: *Nelson textbook of pediatrics*, ed 18, Philadelphia, 2009, Elsevier.

Ducros A, Tournier-Lasserve E, Bousser MG: The genetics of migraine, *Lancet Neurol* 1(5):285-293, 2002.

El Bashir H, Laundy M, Booy R: Diagnosis and treatment of bacterial meningitis, *Arch Dis Child* 88(7):814-819, 2003.

Ewing-Cobbs L, Prasad JR, Kramer L, et al: Late intellectual and academic outcomes following traumatic brain injury sustained during early childhood, *J Neurosurg*, 105(4 Suppl Pediatr):287-296, 2006.

Farhat G, Yamout B, Mikati MA, et al: Effect of antiepileptic drugs on bone density in ambulatory patients, *Neurology* 58:1348-1353, 2002.

Feigin RD, Perlman E: Bacterial meningitis beyond the neonatal period. In Feigin RD, Cherry JD, editors: *Textbook of pediatric infectious diseases*, ed 5, Philadelphia, 2004, Saunders.

Fisgin T, Gurer Y, Senbil N, et al: Nasal midazolam effects on childhood acute seizures, *J Child Neurol* 15(12):833-835, 2000.

Frucht MM, Quigg M, Schwaner C, et al: Distribution of seizure precipitants among epilepsy syndromes, *Epilepsia* 41(12):1543-1549, 2000.

Gallentine WB, Mikati MA: Intraoperative electrocorticography and cortical stimulation in children, *J Clin Neurophysiol* 26(2):95-108, 2009.

Greenberg RA, Bolte RG, Schunk JE: Infant carrier-related falls: an unrecognized danger, *Pediatr Emerg Care* 25(2):66-68, 2009.

Greenes DS, Schutzman SA: Clinical significance of scalp abnormalities in asymptomatic head-injured infants, *Pediatr Emerg Care* 17(2):88-92, 2001.

Haberlandt E, Weger C, Sigl SB, et al: Adrenocorticotropic hormone versus pulsatile dexamethasone in the treatment of infantile epilepsy syndromes, *Pediatr Neurol* 42(1):21-27, 2010.

Hancock E, Osborne J: Treatment of infantile spasms, *Cochrane Database Syst Rev* (3):CD001770.DOI: 10.1002/14651858. CD001770, 2003.

Harbord JG, Kyrkou NE, Kyrkou MR, et al: Use of intranasal midazolam to treat acute seizures in paediatric community settings, *J Pediatr Child Health* 40(9-10):556-558, 2004.

Haslam RH: Brain abscess. In Behrman RE, Kliegman RM, Jenson HB, editors: *Nelson textbook of pediatrics*, ed 18, Philadelphia, 2009, Elsevier.

Headache Classification Subcommittee of the International Headache Society: The International Classification of Headache Disorders, ed 2, *Cephalalgia* 24(Suppl 1):9-160, 2004.

Hoyt CS: Brain injury and the eye, *Eye* 21(10):1285-1289, 2007.

Hung KL, Liao HT, Huang JS: Rational management of simple depressed skull fractures in infants, *J Neurosurg* 103(1 Suppl):69-72, 2005.

Idris AH, Berg RA, Bierens J, et al: Recommended guidelines for uniform reporting of data from drowning: the "Ustein style," *Circulation* 108(20):2565-2574, 2003.

Johnston MV: Seizures in childhood. In Behrman RE, Kliegman R, Jenson HB, editors: *Nelson textbook of pediatrics*, ed 18, Philadelphia, 2009, Elsevier.

Kallas HJ: Drowning and submersion injury. In Behrman RE, Kliegman R, Jenson B, editors: *Nelson textbook of pediatrics*, ed 18, Philadelphia, 2009, Elsevier.

Kaplan SL, Mason EO Jr, Wald ER, et al: Decrease of invasive pneumococcal infections in children among eight children's hospitals in the United States after the introduction of 7-valent pneumococcal conjugate vaccine, *Pediatrics* 113(3 Pt 1):443-449, 2004.

Kline N: *Neurologic manifestations of HIV-infection (HIV nursing curriculum)*, Houston, 2001, Baylor College of Medicine.

Kossoff EH, Zupec-Kania BA, Rho HM: Ketogenic diets: an update for child neurologists, *J Child Neurol* 24(8):979-988, 2009.

Kutlu NO, Yakinci C, Dogrul M, et al: Intranasal midazolam for prolonged convulsive seizures, *Brain Dev* 22(6):359-361, 2000.

Kuzniecky RI: Neuroimaging in pediatric epilepsy. In Pellock JM, Dodson WE, Bourgeois BFD, editors: *Pediatric epilepsy: diagnosis and therapy*, New York, 2001, Demos.

Langlois JA, Rutland-Brown W, Thomas KE: The incidence of traumatic brain injury among children in the United States, *J Head Trauma Rehabil* 20(3):229-238, 2005.

Lee LK: Controversies in the sequelae of pediatric mild traumatic brain injury, *Pediatr Emerg Care* 23(8):580-583, 2007.

Leppik IE: Monotherapy and polypharmacy, *Neurology* 55(Suppl 3):525-529, 2000.

Levy R, Cooper P: Ketogenic diet for epilepsy, *Cochrane Database Syst Rev* (3):CD001903. DOI: 10.1002/14651858.CD001903, 2003.

Lewis D, Ashwal S, Hershey A, et al: Practice parameter: Pharmacological treatment of migraine headache in children and adolescents, *Neurology* 63: 2215-2224, 2004.

Ljungman G, Kreuger A, Andreasson S, et al: Midazolam nasal spray reduces procedural anxiety in children, *Pediatrics* 105(1 Pt 1):73-78, 2000.

Lloyd CJ, Alredy T, Lloyd JC: Intranasal midazolam as an alternative to general anaesthesia in the management of children with oral and maxillofacial trauma, *Br J Oral Maxillofac Surg* 38(6):593-595, 2000.

Lo WD, Lee J, Rusin, J, et al: Intracranial hemorrhages in children: an evolving spectrum, *Arch Neurol* 65(12):1629-1633, 2008.

Marcin, JP, Pollack MM: Triage scoring systems, severity of illness measures, and mortality prediction models in pediatric trauma, *Crit Care Med* 30(11 Suppl):S457-S467, 2002.

Marcoux KK: Management of increased intracranial pressure in the critically ill child with an acute neurological injury, *AACN Clin Issues* 16(2):212-231, 2005.

Marsh N, Whitehead G: Skull fracture during infancy: a 5 year follow-up, *J Clin Experiment Neuropsychol* 27:352-366, 2005.

Mathur M, Petersen L, Stadtler M, et al: Variability in pediatric brain death determination and documentation in Southern California, *Pediatrics* 121: 988-993, 2008.

McCabe CF, Donahue SP: Prognostic indicators for vision and mortality in shaken baby syndrome, *Arch Ophthalmol* 118(3):373-377, 2000.

Mehta V, Singhi P, Singhi S: Intravenous sodium valproate versus diazepam infusion for the control of refractory status epilepticus in children: a randomized controlled trial, *J Child Neurol* 22(10):1191-1197, 2007.

Menkes JH, Sankar R: Paroxysmal disorders. In Menkes JH, Sarnat HB, editors: *Child neurology*, Philadelphia, 2000, Lippincott Williams & Wilkins.

Morrison G, Gibbons E, Whitehouse WP: High-dose midazolam therapy for refractory status epilepticus in children, *Intensive Care Med* 32(12):2070-2076, 2006.

Myhre S, Grogaard JB, Dyb GA, et al: Traumatic head injury in infants and toddlers, *Acta Paediatr* 96(8):1159-1163, 2007.

Nakken KO, Solaas MH, Kjeldsen MJ, et al: Which seizure-precipitating factors do patients with epilepsy most frequently report? *Epilepsy Behav* 6(1):85-89, 2005.

Nigrovic LE, Kuppermann N, Malley R: Children with bacterial meningitis presenting to the emergency department during the pneumococcal conjugate vaccine era, *Acad Emerg Med* 15(6):522-528, 2008.

Ong I, Selladurai BM, Dhillon MK, et al: The prognostic value of the Glasgow Coma Scale: hypoxia and computerized tomography in outcome prediction of pediatric head injury, *Pediatr Neurosurg* 24(6):285-291, 1996.

Ostergaard JR: Febrile seizures, *Acta Paediatr* 98(5):771-773, 2009.

Paniak D, Reynolds S, Phillips K, et al: Patient complaints within 1 month of mild traumatic brain injury: a controlled study, *Arch Clin Neuropsychol* 17(4):319-334, 2002.

Papa L, Hoelle R, Idris A: Systematic review of definitions for drowning incidents, *Resuscitation* 65(3):255-264, 2005.

Pearson DA, McGrath NM, Nozyce M, et al: Predicting HIV disease progression in children using measures of neuropsychological and neurological functioning, Pediatric AIDS Clinical Trials 152 Study Team, *Pediatrics* 106(6):E76, 2000.

Pellock JM, Shinnar S: Respiratory adverse events associated with diazepam rectal gel, *Neurology* 64(10):1768-1770, 2005.

Pichichero M: Meningococcal immunization update: a new conjugated vaccine, *Consultant for Pediatricians* 4(6):1-2, 2005.

Prober CG: Central nervous system infections. In Behrman RE, Kliegman RM, Jenson HTS, et al, editors: *Nelson textbook of pediatrics*, ed 18, Philadelphia, 2009, Elsevier.

Proctor MB: Neurosurgical aspects of nonaccidental trauma in children. In Loftus G, editor, *Neurological surgery principles and practice*, Philadelphia, 2003, Lippincott Williams & Wilkins.

Pugliese A, Beltramo T, Torre D: Reye's and Reye's-like syndromes, *Cell Biochem Funct* 26(7):741-746, 2008.

Radhakrishnan K, St Louis EK, Johnson JA, et al: Pattern-sensitive epilepsy: electroclinical characteristics, natural history, and delineation of the epileptic syndrome, *Epilepsia* 46(1):48-58, 2005.

Report of Special Task Force: Guidelines for the determination of brain death in children, *Pediatrics* 80(2):298-300, 1987.

Riikonen RS: Favourable prognostic factors with infantile spasms, *Eur J Paediatr Neurol* 14(1):13-18, 2010.

Rivara FP, Grossman D: Injury control. In Behrman RE, Kliegman RM, Jenson HTS, editors: *Nelson textbook of pediatrics*, ed 18, Philadelphia, 2009, Elsevier.

Rocchi G, Caroli E, Raco A, et al: Traumatic epidural hematoma in children, *J Child Neurol* 20(7):569-572, 2005.

Rowley SM: Headaches in children and adolescents. A blueprint for pharmacologic and nonpharmacologic approaches, *Adv Nurse Pract* 13(2):31-43, 2005.

Saillet S, Langlois M, Feddersen B, et al: Manipulation the epileptic brain using stimulation: a review of experimental and clinical studies, *Epileptic Disord* 11(2): 100-112, 2009.

Salomez F, Vincent JL: Drowning: a review of epidemiology, pathophysiology, treatment and prevention, *Resuscitation* 63(3):261-268, 2004.

Scheepers M, Scheepers B, Clarke M, et al: Is intranasal midazolam an effective rescue medication in adolescents and adults with severe epilepsy? *Seizure* 9(6):417-422, 2000.

Shields WD: Catastrophic epilepsy in childhood, *Epilepsia* 41(Suppl 2):52-56, 2000.

Shinnar S, Berg AT, O'Dell C, et al: Predictors of multiple seizures in a cohort of children prospectively followed from the time of their first unprovoked seizure, *Ann Neurol* 48(2):140-147, 2000.

Shoja MM, Tubbs RS, Malekian A, et al: Video game epilepsy in the twentieth century: a review, *Childs Nerv Syst* 23(3):265-267, 2007.

Shorvon S, Walker M: Status epilepticus in idiopathic generalized epilepsy, *Epilepsia* 46(Suppl 9):73-79, 2005.

Treiman DM, Walker MC: Treatment of seizure emergencies: convulsive and non-convulsive status epilepticus, *Epilepsy Res* 68S:S77-S82, 2006.

Tunkel AR, Hartman BJ, Kaplan SL, et al: Practice guidelines for the management of bacterial meningitis, *Clin Infect Dis* 39(9):1267-1284, 2004.

van Gestel P, Blusse van Oud-Alblas HJ, Malingre M, et al: Propofol and thiopental for refractory status epilepticus in children, *Neurology* 65(4):591-592, 2005.

van Rijckevorsel K: Treatment of Lennox-Gestaut syndrome: overview and recent findings, *Neuropsychiatr Dis Treat* 4(6):1001-1019, 2008.

Verity CM, Greenword R, Golding J: Longterm intellectual and behavioral outcomes of children with febrile convulsions, *N Engl J Med* 338(24):1723-1728, 1998.

Vignes JR, Jeelani NU, Jeelani A, et al: Growing skull fracture after minor closed-head injury, *J Pediatrics* 151(3):316-318, 2007.

Wetzell RC: Anesthesia and perioperative care. In Behrman RE, Kliegman RM, Jenson HB, editors: *Nelson textbook of pediatrics*, ed 18, Philadelphia, 2009, Elsevier.

White JR, Farukhi Z, Bull C, et al: Predictors of outcome in severely head-injured children, *Crit Care Med* 29(7):534-540, 2001.

Wiederholt WC: *Neurology for non-neurologists*, ed 4, Philadelphia, 2000, Saunders.

Willmore LJ, Abelson MB, Ben-Menachem E, et al: Vigabatrin: 2008 update, *Epilepsia* 50(2):163-173, 2009.

Woods C: Neisseria meningitidis. In Behrman RE, Kliegman RM, Jenson HB, editors: *Nelson textbook of pediatrics*, ed 18, Philadelphia, 2009, Elsevier.

Yamamoto LG, Yim GK: The role of intravenous valproic acid in status epilepticus, *Pediatr Emerg Care* 16(4):296-298, 2000.

Yeates KO, Taylor HG, Rusin J, et al: Longitudinal trajectories of postconcussive symptoms in children with mild traumatic brain injuries and their relationship to acute clinical status, *Pediatrics* 123:735-743, 2009.

Yogev R, Chadwick EG: Acquired immunodeficiency syndrome (human immunodeficiency virus). In Behrman RE, Kliegman RM, Jenson HTS, editors: *Nelson textbook of pediatrics*, ed 18, Philadelphia, 2009, Elsevier.

Yogev R, Guzman-Cottrill J: Bacterial meningitis in children: critical review of current concepts, *Drugs* 65(8):1097-1112, 2005.

Yoon U, Jagoda A: New antiepileptic drugs and preparations, *Emerg Med Clin North Am* 18(4):755-765, 2000.

Zeltzer LK, Krell H: Pediatric pain management. In Behrman RE, Kliegman RM, Jenson HTS, editors: *Nelson textbook of pediatrics*, ed 18, Philadelphia, 2009, Elsevier.

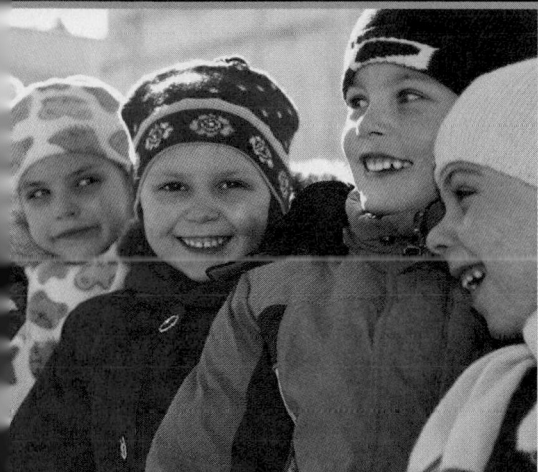

The Child with Endocrine Dysfunction

Elizabeth Record, Linda Ballard, and Amy Barry

evolve WEBSITE

http://evolve.elsevier.com/wong/ncic

Animations
    Adrenal Function
    Insulin Injection
Case Study
    Diabetes Mellitus
Critical Thinking Case Study
    Diabetes Insipidus
Critical Thinking Exercise
    Hypothyroidism
Evidence-Based Practice
    Medication Safety and Insulin Therapy
Key Points Audio Summaries
NCLEX Review Questions
Nursing Care Plans
    The Child with Diabetes Mellitus
    The Child with Diabetic Ketoacidosis
    The Child with Growth Failure
Spanish/English Translations
WebLinks

RELATED TOPICS

Abnormal Sexual Development, **Ch. 11**
Administration of Medication, **Ch. 27**
Family-Centered Home Care, **Ch. 25**
Genetic Evaluation and Counseling, **Ch. 5**
Hypocalcemia, **Ch. 9**
Hypoglycemia, **Ch. 9**
Single-Gene Disorders, **Ch. 5**

CHAPTER OUTLINE

THE ENDOCRINE SYSTEM

The endocrine system consists of three components: (1) the cell, which sends a chemical message by means of a hormone; (2) the target cells, or end organs, which receive the chemical message; and (3) the environment through which the chemical is transported (blood, lymph, extracellular fluids) from the site of synthesis to the sites of cellular action. The endocrine system controls or regulates metabolic processes governing energy production, growth, fluid and electrolyte balance,

Pituitary gland (hypophysis cerebri)—A pea-sized gland that lies within a deep bony depression at the base of the cranium (the sella turcica) and is attached to the hypothalamus on the undersurface of the brain by a slender infundibulum, or pituitary stalk

Thyroid gland—Two large lateral lobes and a connecting portion, the isthmus, situated on the anterior aspect of the neck just below the larynx

Parathyroid glands—Four or five (more or less) small round bodies attached to the posterior surfaces of the lateral lobes of the thyroid gland

Adrenal glands—Pyramid-shaped glands situated atop the kidneys, fitting like caps over these organs

Ovaries—Glands located in the female pelvis on each side of the uterus at the fimbriated end of the fallopian tubes

Testes—Oval-shaped glands situated within the male scrotum

Islets of Langerhans—Small clusters of endocrine cells within the pancreas situated between the acinar or exocrine-secreting portions of the gland

Structures Sometimes Considered Endocrine Glands

Pineal body (epiphysis cerebri)—A gland located in the cranial cavity behind the midbrain and third ventricle, the functions of which are largely speculative

Thymus—A gland situated behind the sternum and below the thyroid gland; plays an important role in immunity but only during fetal life and early childhood

Gastrointestinal glands—Mucosal lining of the gastrointestinal tract containing cells that produce hormones that play important roles in controlling and coordinating secretory and motor activities of digestion

Placenta—A body that secretes ovarian hormones and chorionic gonadotropin during gestation; only a temporary endocrine gland

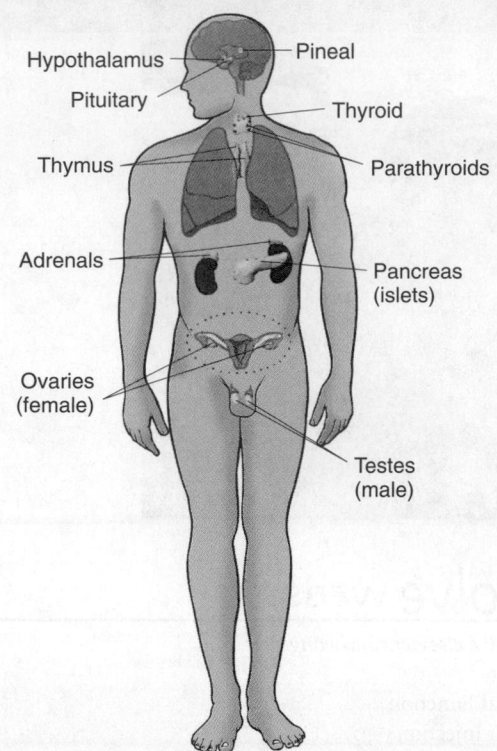

Fig. 38-1 Location of the endocrine glands and structures sometimes considered endocrine glands. (From Thibodeau GA, Patton KT: *Structure and function of the body*, ed 13, St Louis, 2008, Mosby.)

response to stress, and sexual reproduction (Baxter and Ribeiro, 2004).

The endocrine glands, which are distributed throughout the body, are listed in Box 38-1; also listed are several additional structures sometimes considered endocrine glands, although they are not usually included.

HORMONES

A **hormone** is a complex chemical substance produced and secreted into body fluids by a cell or group of cells that exerts a physiologic controlling effect on other cells (Behrman, Kliegman, Jenson, et al, 2009). Some are local hormones, creating their effect near the point of secretion. For example, acetylcholine, released at the parasympathetic and skeletal nerve endings, mediates the synaptic activity of the nervous system; secretin, a digestive hormone secreted by certain cells lining the duodenum, stimulates the pancreas to release a watery secretion; and the prostaglandins, or tissue hormones, secreted by a wide variety of organs (including the seminal vesicles, kidneys, lungs, iris, brain, and thymus), usually diffuse only a short distance to integrate activities of neighboring cells.

General hormones are produced in one organ or part of the body and are carried through the bloodstream to a distant part, or parts, of the body where they initiate or regulate physiologic activity of an organ or group of cells. Some of these hormones (such as thyroid hormone [TH] and growth hormone [GH]) affect most cells of the body, whereas others (such as the tropic hormones) produce their effects on specific tissues, called **target tissues**. For example, the pituitary hormones stimulate the adrenal glands and the thyroid gland to secrete adrenocortico-

tropic hormone (ACTH) and thyroid-stimulating hormone (TSH), respectively.

Control of Hormone Secretion

Hormones are released by endocrine glands into the bloodstream, where they are carried to responsive tissues (Fig. 38-1). These responsive, or target, tissues may be another endocrine gland, an organ, or tissue (Baxter and Ribeiro, 2004). Regulation of hormonal secretion is based on negative feedback. As a rule, endocrine glands have a tendency to oversecrete their particular hormones. However, once the hormone's physiologic effect has been achieved, this information is transmitted to the producing gland, either directly or indirectly, to inhibit further secretion. If the gland undersecretes, the inhibition is relieved, and the gland increases production of the hormone. As a result, the hormone is secreted according to the amount needed. This is the primary function of the tropic hormones.

The endocrine gland primarily responsible for stimulation and inhibition of target glandular secretions is the anterior pituitary, or "master gland." Tropic (which literally means "turning") hormones secreted by the anterior pituitary regulate the secretion of hormones from various target organs (Fig. 38-2). As blood concentrations of the target hormones reach normal levels, a negative message is sent to the anterior pituitary to inhibit release of the tropic hormone. For example, TSH responds to low levels of circulating TH. As blood levels of TH reach normal concentrations, a negative feedback message is sent to the anterior pituitary, resulting in diminished release of TSH.

The pituitary gland is, in turn, controlled by either hormonal or neuronal signals from the hypothalamus. Two types of

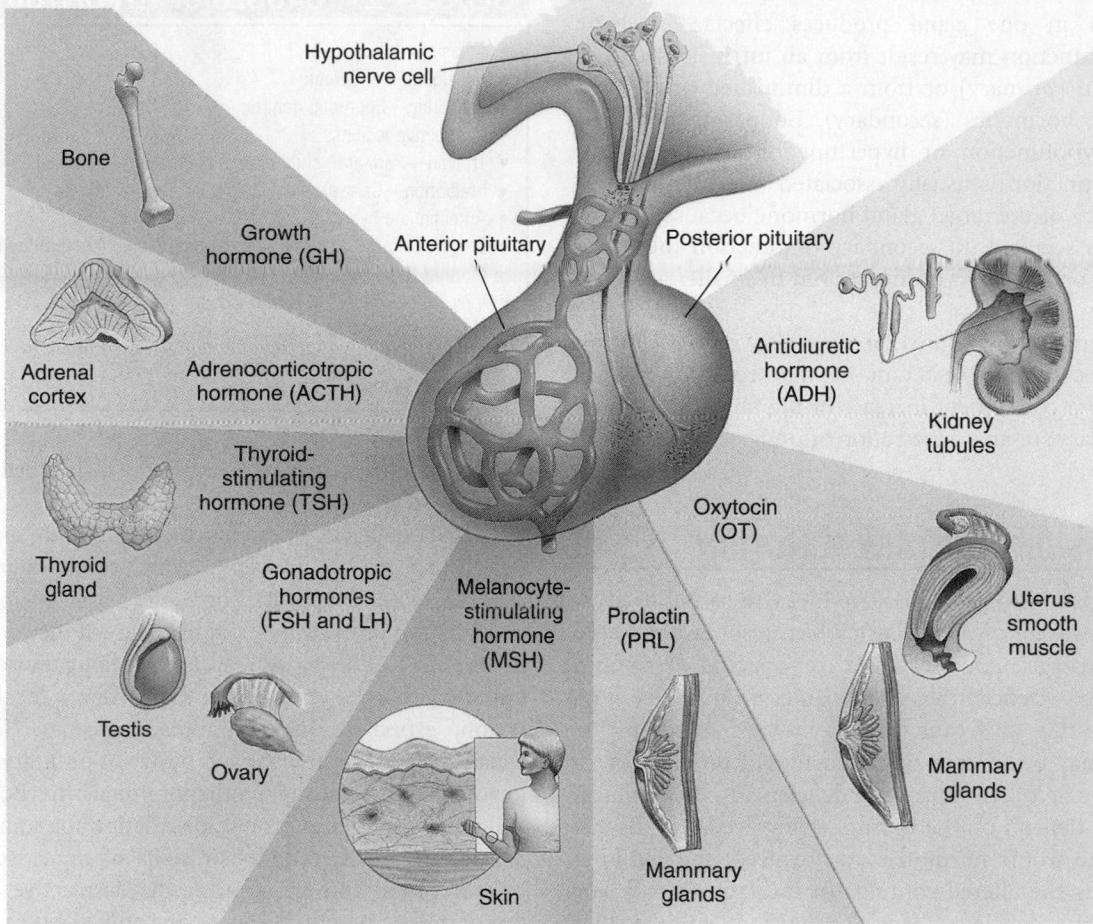

Fig. 38-2 Principal anterior and posterior pituitary hormones and their target organs. (From Thibodeau GA, Patton KT: *Structure and function of the body*, ed 13, St Louis, 2008, Mosby.)

substances are secreted from the hypothalamus: (1) releasing hormones and (2) inhibitory hormones, which are secreted within the hypothalamus and transported by way of the pituitary portal system to the anterior pituitary, where they stimulate the secretion of tropic hormones. An example of this is the secretion of corticotropin-releasing factor (CRF) by the hypothalamus, which stimulates the pituitary to secrete ACTH. In this instance the anterior pituitary is the target of the hypothalamus and secondarily affects a response from another target gland, the adrenals. The adrenals in turn secrete glucocorticoids, which have multiple target sites throughout the body. Pituitary hormones that lack feedback control from the product of a target tissue (GH, prolactin, and melanocyte-stimulating hormone) require hypothalamic inhibitors and stimulators for their control.

Not all hormones depend on other hormones for their release. For example, insulin is secreted in response to blood glucose concentrations. Other glandular hormones that are not under the control of the pituitary gland are glucagon, parathyroid hormone (parathormone, PTH), antidiuretic hormone (ADH), and aldosterone.

NEUROENDOCRINE INTERRELATIONSHIPS

Two regulatory systems maintain hemostasis: the endocrine and the autonomic nervous systems (collectively known as the neuroendocrine system) (Baxter and Ribeiro, 2004). The autonomic nervous system consists of the sympathetic and parasympathetic systems, which control nonvoluntary functions, specifically of smooth muscle, myocardium, and glands. The parasympathetic system is primarily involved in regulating digestive processes, whereas the sympathetic system functions to maintain homeostasis during stress.

The higher autonomic centers, located in the hypothalamus and limbic system, help control the functioning of both autonomic systems. Both sympathetic and parasympathetic nerve fibers secrete neurotransmitting substances: acetylcholine, released by cholinergic fibers, and norepinephrine, released by adrenergic fibers. Release of norepinephrine into the plasma produces the same effects as secretion of this substance by the adrenal medulla. Thus the interrelatedness between the two systems is demonstrated.

The neuroendocrine system acts by synthesizing and releasing various chemical substances that regulate body functions. Information is carried by means of neural impulses in the autonomic system and by the blood in the endocrine system. In general, neural responses are more rapid and localized; endocrine responses are more lasting and widespread. The two systems function synergistically because neural impulses transmitted to the central nervous system (CNS) stimulate the hypothalamus to manufacture and release several releasing or inhibiting factors.

Because of the interdependent relationship of these glands, a malfunction in one gland produces effects elsewhere. Endocrine dysfunction may result from an intrinsic defect in the target gland (primary) or from a diminished or elevated level of tropic hormones (secondary). Endocrine problems occur from hypofunction or hyperfunction of the glands. Primary hypofunction is usually associated with a more profound deficiency of the target gland hormone because little or no hormone is secreted. In secondary dysfunction the target glands secrete some of their hormones but in smaller amounts and less rapidly.

Hyperfunction or hypofunction may also result from an increase or decrease in secretion of the tropic hormones (primary) with a consequent increase in the target gland hormones (secondary) or an oversecretion or undersecretion of the target glands.

DISORDERS OF PITUITARY FUNCTION

The pituitary gland is divided into two lobes; the anterior pituitary and the posterior pituitary. Each lobe is responsible for the production, storage, and secretion of specific hormones (Hanberg, 2005). Deficiencies of the anterior pituitary hormones may be due to organic defects or have an idiopathic etiology and may occur as a single hormonal problem or in combination with other hormonal deficiencies. The clinical manifestations depend on the hormones involved and the age of onset. If the tropic hormones are involved, the resulting disorder reflects the altered stimulus to the target gland. For example, if TSH is deficient, TH is also deficient, and the child displays the manifestations of hypothyroidism.

An overproduction of the anterior pituitary hormones can result in gigantism (caused by excess GH production during childhood), hyperthyroidism, hypercortisolism (Cushing syndrome), and precocious puberty from excessive gonadotropins. Overproduction may be caused by hyperplasia of the pituitary cells—which may eventually progress to a tumor (adenoma)—or a primary hypothalamic defect that results in an excess of the hormone's releasing factor. Although the initial clinical manifestations are a result of pituitary oversecretion, eventually pituitary insufficiency occurs, and the signs of panhypopituitarism become evident. Panhypopituitarism is often defined clinically as the loss of all anterior pituitary hormones, leaving only posterior pituitary function intact (Toogood and Stewart, 2008).

> **! NURSING ALERT**
>
> Children with panhypopituitarism should wear medical identification, such as a bracelet.

HYPOPITUITARISM

Hypopituitarism is diminished or deficient secretion of pituitary hormones. The consequences of the condition depend on the degree of dysfunction. It often leads to:

- Gonadotropin deficiency with absence or regression of secondary sexual characteristics

> **BOX 38-2 CAUSES OF HYPOPITUITARISM**
>
> - Aplasia or hypoplasia
> - Developmental defects
> - Idiopathic—Sporadic; genetic
> - Destructive lesions
> - Trauma—Perinatal; child abuse; basal skull fracture
> - Irradiation—Central nervous system, eye, middle ear
> - Autoimmune hypophysitis
> - Surgery—Removal of pharyngeal pituitary, ablation of craniopharyngioma or other tumor
> - Vascular—Aneurysm, infarct
> - Functional deficiency
> - Psychosocial dwarfism
> - Anorexia nervosa

- GH deficiency, in which children display retarded somatic growth
- TSH deficiency, which produces hypothyroidism
- Corticotropin deficiency, which results in manifestations of adrenal hypofunction

Hypopituitarism can result from any of the conditions listed in Box 38-2. The most common organic cause of pituitary undersecretion is tumors in the pituitary or hypothalamic region, especially the craniopharyngiomas. These tumors usually invade the anterior and posterior pituitary lobes and the hypothalamus, causing panhypopituitarism (Box 38-3). The child may experience growth retardation for some time before developing any symptoms or signs of increased intracranial pressure, local compression, or the destructive effects of the tumor. Other potential causes of panhypopituitarism include encephalitis, radiation to the head or neck, head trauma, and congenital hypoplasia of the hypothalamic area (Hanberg, 2005; Darzy, 2009).

Congenital hypopituitarism, or congenital GH deficiency, can be seen in newborn infants, often as a result of birth trauma. Symptoms of hypoglycemia and seizure activity often manifest within the first 24 hours after birth (Toogood and Stewart, 2008).

Idiopathic hypopituitarism, or idiopathic pituitary growth failure, is usually related to GH deficiency, which inhibits somatic growth in all cells of the body (Miller and Zimmerman, 2004). Growth failure is defined as an absolute height of less than −2 SD for age, or a linear growth velocity consistently less than −1 SD for age. When this occurs without the presence of hypothyroidism, systemic disease, or malnutrition, then an abnormality of the GH–insulin-like growth factor (IGF) axis should be considered (Richmond and Rogol, 2008).

Although most children with hypopituitarism are normal at birth, they show growth patterns that progressively deviate from the normal growth rate, often beginning in infancy. The chief complaint in most instances is short stature. Of those who seek help, boys outnumber girls three to one. The extent of idiopathic GH deficiency may be complete or partial, but the cause is unknown. It is frequently associated with deficiencies of other pituitary hormone, such as TSH and ACTH; thus it is theorized that the disorder is probably secondary to hypothalamic deficiency. It has also been observed that there is a higher than average frequency in some families, which indicates a possible genetic origin in a number of instances.

BOX 38-3   CLINICAL MANIFESTATIONS OF PANHYPOPITUITARISM

Growth Hormone
Short stature but proportional height and weight
Delayed epiphyseal closure
Retarded bone age proportional to height
Premature aging common in later life
Increased insulin sensitivity

Thyroid Stimulating Hormone
Short stature with infantile proportions
Dry, coarse skin; yellow discoloration, pallor
Cold intolerance
Constipation
Somnolence
Bradycardia
Dyspnea on exertion
Delayed dentition, loss of teeth

Gonadotropins
Absence of sexual maturation or loss of secondary sexual characteristics
Atrophy of genitalia, prostate gland, breasts
Amenorrhea without menopausal symptoms
Decreased spermatogenesis

Adrenocorticotropic Hormone
Severe anorexia, weight loss
Hypoglycemia
Hypotension
Hyponatremia, hyperkalemia
Adrenal apoplexy, especially in response to stress
Circulatory collapse

Antidiuretic Hormone
Polyuria
Polydipsia
Dehydration

Melanocyte-Stimulating Hormone
Decreased pigmentation

Not all children with short stature have GH deficiency. In most instances the cause of short stature is either familial short stature or a simple constitutional growth delay. *Familial short stature* refers to otherwise healthy children who have ancestors with adult height in the lower percentiles, and whose height during childhood is appropriate for genetic background. Fig. 38-3 provides an overview of the possible causes of short stature in children.

Constitutional growth delay refers to individuals (usually boys) with delayed linear growth, generally beginning as a toddler, and skeletal and sexual maturation that is behind that of age-mates (Miller and Zimmerman, 2004; Halac and Zimmerman, 2004). Typically these children will reach normal adult height. Often a history of a similar pattern of growth is found in one of the parents or other family members of children with constitutional growth delay. The untreated child proceeds through normal changes as expected on the basis of bone age. These changes, although occurring later than in the average child, appear in normal sequence and manner, and treatment with GH is not usually indicated. However, its use has become controversial, especially in relation to parental and child requests for treatment to accelerate growth.

Clinical Manifestations

Children with hypopituitarism generally grow normally during the first year and then follow a slowed growth curve that is below the 3rd percentile. In children with a partial GH deficiency, the growth retardation is less marked than in children with complete GH deficiency. Height may be retarded more than weight because, with good nutrition, these children can become overweight or even obese. Their well-nourished appearance is an important diagnostic clue to differentiation from other disorders such as failure to thrive.

Skeletal proportions are normal for the age, but these children appear younger than their chronologic age. However, later in life premature aging is common. The appearance of fine wrinkles about the eyes and mouth gives these children a peculiar impression of immaturity combined with presenility. They are no less active than other children if directed to size-appropriate sports, such as swimming, wrestling, gymnastics, soccer, or ballet. Bone age is nearly always retarded but is closely related to height age; the degree of retardation depends on the duration and extent of the hormonal deficiency. Children with diminished function of recent onset may show little retardation in skeletal age, whereas children with a longstanding deficiency may evidence a skeletal age only 40% to 50% of their chronologic age. It is difficult to predict their eventual height. Because the period of growth is prolonged past adolescence into the third or fourth decade, many of them reach a permanent height of 1.2 to 1.5 m (4 to 5 ft).

Usually, primary teeth appear at the expected age, but the eruption of the permanent teeth is delayed. Because of the underdeveloped jaw, the teeth are overcrowded and malpositioned. Sexual development is usually delayed but is otherwise normal. Even without GH replacement, adults with GH deficiency are able to reproduce normal offspring. However, if the gonadotropins are deficient, sexual maturation is absent.

Most of these children have normal intelligence. In fact, during early childhood they often appear precocious in their learning because their ability seems to exceed their small size. However, emotional problems are not uncommon, especially as they near puberty, when their smallness becomes increasingly apparent in comparison with their peers. Height discrepancy has been significantly correlated with emotional adjustment problems and may be a valuable predictor of the extent to which GH-delayed children will experience difficulty with anxiety, social skills, and positive self-esteem (Sandberg, Kranzler, Bukowski, et al, 1999). Academic problems are also common. A history often reveals repeated classes or enrollment in classes for children with learning disabilities. These children are usually not pushed to perform at their chronologic age but at their height age.

Diagnostic Evaluation

Only a small number of children with delayed growth or short stature have hypopituitary dwarfism. In the majority of instances the cause is constitutional delay. Diagnostic evaluation is aimed at isolating organic causes, which, in addition to GH deficiency, may include hypothyroidism, oversecretion of cortisol, gonadal aplasia, chronic illness, nutritional inadequacy, Russell-Silver dwarfism, or hypochondroplasia.

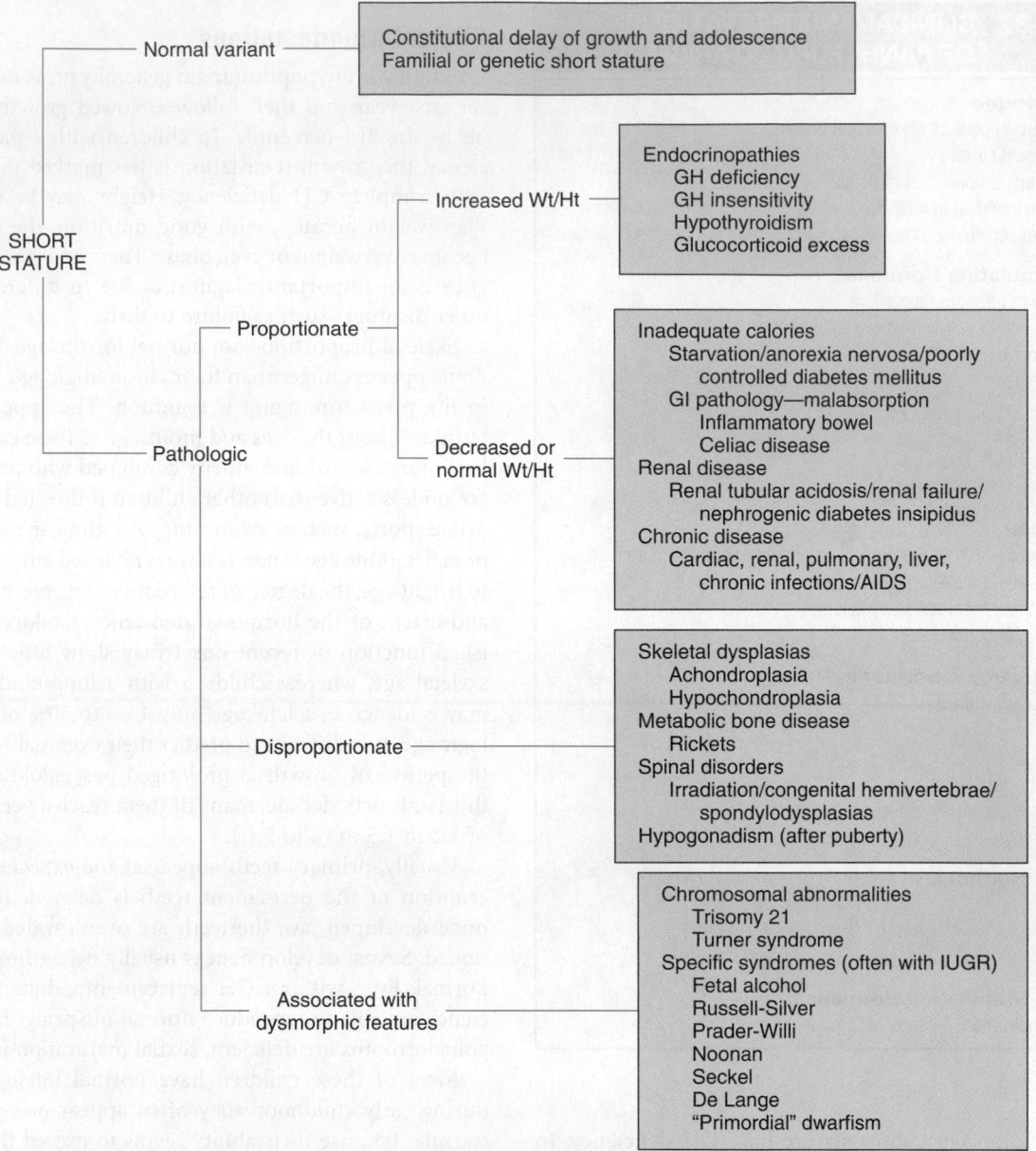

Fig. 38-3 Causes of short stature. *AIDS,* Acquired immunodeficiency syndrome; *GI,* gastrointestinal; *GH,* growth hormone; *IUGR,* intrauterine growth restriction; *Wt/Ht,* weight-to-height ratio. (From Vogiatzi MG, Copeland KC: The short child, *Pediatr Rev* 19(3):92-99, 1998.)

A complete diagnostic evaluation should include a family history, a history of the child's growth patterns and previous health status, physical examination, psychosocial evaluation, radiographic surveys, and endocrine studies.

Family History

A family history is of utmost importance in relating short stature to genetic background. The midparental height is an important prognosticator of the child's ultimate adult height. Normal adult height should fall within 5 cm (2 inches) of midparental height (Miller and Zimmerman, 2004). Children with constitutional delays frequently are the products of parents who experienced similar slow growth patterns and delayed sexual maturation. A small percentage of those with hypopituitarism demonstrate an autosomal recessive inheritance pattern. Height and weight of siblings should be compared with the child's growth patterns at comparable age periods.

Child's History

The child's history should include a thorough prenatal history to rule out maternal disorders that may have influenced growth, such as malnutrition. Compare birth height and weight with gestational age. Children with hypopituitarism are usually of normal size and normal gestational age at birth.

Investigate the child's health history for evidence of chronic illness that may have influenced growth patterns, although a chronic illness, such as congenital heart disease, malabsorptive disorders, severe anemia, or neurologic impairments, usually is identified long before the growth problem becomes a concern. Signs and symptoms suggesting a tumor, such as visual disturbances, headache, and signs of increasing intracranial pressure, are important. Such symptoms often precede retarded growth but may not have been regarded as significant. With lesions involving the hypothalamus, the history may also reveal characteristic manifestations of dysfunction such as somnolence,

Ensure reliability of measurements—Accurately obtain and plot height and weight measurements.

Determine absolute height—The child's absolute height bears some relationship to the likelihood of a pathologic condition. However, the majority of children who have a height below the lowest percentile (either 3rd or 5th percentile on the height curve) do not have a pathologic growth problem.

Assess height velocity—The most important aspect of a growth evaluation is the observation of a child's height over time, or height velocity. Accurate determination of height velocity requires at least 4 and preferably 6 months of observation. A substantial deceleration in height velocity (crossing several percentiles) between 3 and 12 or 13 years of age indicates a pathologic condition until proven otherwise.

Determine weight-to-height relationship—Determination of the weight-to-height ratio has some diagnostic value in ascertaining the cause of growth retardation in a short child.

Project target height—The height of a child can be judged inappropriately short only in the context of his or her genetic potential. Determine the target height of the child with the formula: [Father's height (cm) + Mother's height (cm) + 13]/2 for boys or [Father's height (cm) ?+ Mother's height (cm) − 13]/2 for girls. Most children achieve an adult stature within approximately 10 cm (4 inches) of the target height.

Modified from Vogiatzi MG, Copeland KC: The short child, *Pediatr Rev* 19(3):92-99, 1998.

Bone age refers to a method of assessing skeletal maturity by comparing the appearance of representative epiphyseal centers obtained on x-ray examination with age-appropriate published standards.

Most conditions that cause poor linear growth also cause a delay in skeletal maturation and a retarded bone age. Observation of even a profoundly delayed bone age is never diagnostic or even indicative of a specific diagnosis. A delayed bone age merely indicates that the associated short stature is to some extent "partially reversible," since linear growth will continue until epiphyseal fusion is complete. In comparison, a bone age that is not delayed in a short child is of much greater concern and may, in fact, be of some diagnostic value under certain circumstances.

Modified from Vogiatzi MG, Copeland KC: The short child, *Pediatr Rev* 19(3):92-99, 1998.

thermodysregulation, epilepsy, and polyphagia, resulting in obesity. Because a craniopharyngioma can affect the secretion of any of the pituitary hormones, assessment for hypothyroidism, hypoadrenalism, and hypoaldosteronism should also be included.

Whenever possible, evaluate the child's growth patterns since birth, especially growth velocity, and compare them with standard measurements. The age of onset of short stature provides a significant diagnostic clue. When the clinician evaluates the results of plotting height and weight, upward or downward changes in height velocity in children older than 3 years may indicate a growth abnormality (Halac and Zimmerman, 2004). Progressive retardation in height and weight since early childhood suggests idiopathic hypopituitary dwarfism, whereas a recent change from normal growth is more characteristic of a tumor. In addition, these children are usually well nourished, ruling out other causes of growth failure.

Physical Examination

Accurate measurement of height (using a calibrated stadiometer) and weight and comparison with standard growth charts are essential (Box 38-4). Multiple height measures reflect a more accurate assessment of abnormal growth patterns (Hall, 2000). Other measurements may include crown-to-pubis and pubis-to-heel length to compare body proportions, and sexual development should be assessed and compared with age-appropriate development. Observation of general appearance yields valuable clues, especially signs of premature aging and infantile facial features. Perform a funduscopic examination and testing for visual acuity to detect evidence of ocular damage from a tumor.

Radiographic Surveys

A skeletal survey in children less than 3 years of age and radiographic examination of the hand-wrist for centers of ossification (bone age) (Box 38-5) in older children are important in evaluating growth. Epiphyseal maturation is retarded in hypopituitarism but consistent with retardation in height. This is in contrast to hypothyroidism, in which bone maturation is greatly retarded, or gonadal dysplasia, such as Turner syndrome, in which bone age is near normal. Radiographic studies should also include a skull series, which helps in identifying abnormalities such as an abnormally small sella turcica or evidence of a space-occupying lesion such as craniopharyngioma. Magnetic resonance imaging (MRI), computed tomography (CT), radionuclear scans, or carotid angiograms may be needed to establish diagnosis and localization of lesions (Stanhope, 2004).

Endocrine Studies

Definitive diagnosis of GH deficiency is based on absent or subnormal reserves of pituitary GH. Measuring a single GH level is inaccurate due to the pulsatile secretion of this hormone (Richmond and Rogol, 2008). Exercise is a natural and benign stimulus for GH release, and elevated levels can be detected after 20 minutes of strenuous exercise in normal children. Also, GH levels are elevated 45 to 90 minutes after the onset of sleep.

GH levels are normally so low in children that differentiation from abnormal concentrations is unreliable, GH secretion should be stimulated, followed by measurement of blood levels. Initial assessment of the serum IGF-I and IGF binding protein 3 (IGFBP3) indicates a need for further evaluation of GH dysfunction if levels are lower than −1 SD below the mean for age. It is recommended that GH stimulation tests be reserved for children with low serum IGF-I and IGFBP3 levels and poor growth who do not have other endocrine or nonendocrine causes for short stature (Aimaretti, Bellone, Baldelli, et al, 2004; Richmond and Rogol, 2008). However, although IGF-1 test is useful in detecting severe GH insensitivity, it may not be accurate in detecting less severe cases of idiopathic short stature (Cohen, Rogol, Deal, et al, 2008).

GH stimulation, or provocative testing, involves the use of pharmacologics to provoke the release of GH either directly or indirectly. Provocative testing involves the use of neuromodulators such as levodopa or agents such as clonidine, arginine, insulin, propranolol, or glucagon (Behrman, Kliegman, Jenson, et al, 2009; Richmond and Rogol, 2008). The GH stimulation test of choice is currently country dependent (Cohen, Rogol, Deal, et al, 2008). Studies have shown that traditional GH stimulation test results can be less reliable than previously accepted. Currently, findings in a child of poor linear growth, delayed bone age, and peak levels of GH at less than 10 ng/ml in two stimulation tests are consistent with GH deficiency (Behrman, Kliegman, Jenson, et al, 2009). New reference standards that decrease the lower limit of normal GH levels have been proposed (Cohen, Rogol, Deal, et al, 2008). GH-releasing hormone (GHRH), in combination with an agent that can stimulate GH response to GHRH, has also been used to detect GH deficiency (Aimaretti, Bellone, Baldelli, et al, 2004; Hilczer, Smyczynska, and Lewinski, 2006). The use of GHRH may be more accurate in detecting GH deficiency caused by hypothalamic disorders (Behrman, Kliegman, Jenson, et al, 2009). GH-dependent growth factors may be more sensitive indicators of GH deficiency than GH stimulation tests. Increasingly sensitive radioimmunoassays for GH levels have also been developed.

Therapeutic Management

Treatment of GH deficiency caused by organic lesions is directed toward correction of the underlying disease process (e.g., surgical removal or irradiation of a tumor). The definitive treatment of GH deficiency is replacement of GH, which is successful in 80% of affected children. For more than 20 years cadaver-derived human growth hormone (HGH) was used successfully to enhance linear growth in short children. In 1985 the U.S. Food and Drug Administration stopped use of the hormone in response to reported deaths resulting from Creutzfeldt-Jakob disease (CJD) in three former HGH recipients. Patients have been identified who both received HGH and became infected with CJD, a rare and fatal neurodegenerative condition iatrogenically transmitted through human tissue (Wetterau and Cohen, 2000). Donation of organs or tissues from HGH recipients for transplantation should be prohibited because of the inability to test for infection with CJD. Blood banks do not accept donations from former HGH recipients. Biosynthetic GH prepared by recombinant deoxyribonucleic acid (DNA) technology (and without the risk of CJD) is now available and is the therapy of choice (Miller and Zimmerman, 2004).

In the United States the recommended dosage range of recombinant GH is 0.037 to 0.18 mg/kg/week, divided into six or seven daily subcutaneous doses (Behrman, Kliegman, Jenson, et al, 2009; Cohen, Rogol, Deal, et al, 2008). Growth velocity increases in the first year of treatment and is often above the 95th percentile. With each consecutive year of treatment, growth rates decline (Behrman, Kliegman, Jenson, et al, 2009). A recent meta-analysis of the GH literature concluded that, although GH may improve growth velocity in children, individuals who receive treatment remain shorter than their peers (Bryant, Baxter, Cave, et al, 2007). For children to achieve their genetic growth potential, early diagnosis of and intervention for growth disorders are essential (Leschek, Rose, Yanovski, et al, 2004).

The child, family, and health care team make the decision jointly to stop GH therapy. Growth rates of less than 1 inch/yr and a bone age of more than 14 years in girls and more than 16 years in boys are often used as criteria to stop GH therapy (Behrman, Kliegman, Jenson, et al, 2009). Children with other hormone deficiencies require replacement therapy to correct the specific disorders. This may involve administration of thyroid extract, cortisone, testosterone, or estrogens and progesterone. The sex hormones are usually begun during adolescence to promote normal sexual maturation.

Nursing Care Management

The principal nursing consideration is identifying children with growth problems. Despite the fact that the majority of growth problems are not a result of organic causes, any delay in normal growth and sexual development poses special emotional adjustments for these children.

The nurse may be a key person in helping establish a diagnosis. For example, if serial height and weight records are not available, the nurse can question parents about the child's growth compared with that of siblings, peers, or relatives. Investigating clothing sizes is often helpful in determining growth at different ages. Parents may comment that the child wears out clothes before growing out of them or that, if the clothing fits the body, it often is too long in the sleeves or legs.

QUALITY PATIENT OUTCOMES: Growth Hormone Deficiency
- Early recognition of growth problems
- Accurate diagnosis of GH deficiency
- GH effective in stimulating growth
- Child and family able to cope with diagnosis and treatment

Because the behavioral or physical changes that suggest a tumor are insidious, they are frequently overlooked. It is important to correlate the onset of any positive findings with the initial evidence of growth retardation. For example, visual problems and headache are not uncommon in school-age children and can coincidentally occur after a growth problem is recognized. In fact, headache may represent the emotional trauma caused by short stature rather than be a symptom of a tumor. Pursue this line of questioning cautiously to avoid alarming parents unduly about the possibility of a brain tumor.

Part of a nurse's role in helping establish a diagnosis is assisting with diagnostic tests. Preparation of the child and family is especially important if a number of tests are being performed, and the child requires particular attention during provocative testing. Blood samples are usually taken every 30 minutes for a 3-hour period. Children also have difficulty overcoming hypoglycemia generated by tests with insulin, so carefully observe them for signs of hypoglycemia. Those receiving glucagon are at risk of nausea and vomiting. Patients receiving clonidine require close blood pressure monitoring. Nursing administration of intravenous (IV) fluids may be required if hypotension is detected. The use of arginine is often well tolerated by children, but may cause hypoglycemia in some infants and toddlers. Therefore close monitoring for hypoglycemia is necessary.

Child and Family Support

Once an organic cause of the problem has been confirmed, the parents and child need an opportunity to express their thoughts and feelings. Frequently a growth problem that was present since birth is missed until adolescence, at which time the child's difference in body development becomes dramatically evident in comparisons with peers. Family members may feel anger and resentment toward members of the health staff for not detecting the problem sooner. Parents may experience guilt for not seeking medical attention earlier, especially if the child has been miserable from the ridicule and criticism of peers. Appropriate emotional support from the nurse can include an affirmation of each person's justified feelings, such as anger or guilt, and emphasis on the treatment plan and prospects for improvement in the future.

⚡ DRUG ALERT

Growth Hormone

GH is most effective when it is administered at bedtime. Physiologic release is more normally stimulated as a result of pituitary release of GH during the first 45 to 90 minutes after the onset of sleep.

Even when hormone replacement is successful, these children attain their eventual adult height at a slower rate than their peers; therefore they need assistance in setting realistic expectations regarding improvement. Both sexes need guidance toward appropriate vocational goals. Because these children appear younger than their chronologic age, others frequently relate to them in infantile or childish ways. Children having school problems need special counseling. Parents and teachers benefit from guidance directed toward setting realistic expectations for the child based on age and abilities. For example, in the home such children should have the same age-appropriate responsibilities as their siblings. As they approach adolescence, encourage them to participate in group activities with peers. They should wear styles that accentuate their actual age, not their size. If abilities and strengths are emphasized rather than physical size, such children are more likely to develop a positive self-image.

Professionals and families may find research, education, support, and advocacy from the Human Growth Foundation.* The treatment is expensive—up to $20,0000 to $30,0000 per year, depending on the dosage (Radetti, Buzi, Paganini, et al, 2003; Lee, Davis, Clark, et al, 2006). Usually the cost is partially covered by insurance if the child has a documented deficiency, and some pharmaceutical companies offer copay assistance.

PITUITARY HYPERFUNCTION

Excess GH before closure of the epiphyseal shafts results in proportional overgrowth of the long bones until the individual reaches a height of 2.4 m (8 feet) or more. Vertical growth is accompanied by rapid and increased development of muscles

*997 Glen Cove Ave., Suite 5, Glen Head, NY 11545; 800-451-6434; e-mail: hgf1@hgfound.org; **www.hgfound.org**.

and viscera. Weight is increased but is usually in proportion to height. Proportional enlargement of head circumference also occurs and may result in delayed closure of the fontanels in young children. Children with a pituitary-secreting tumor may also demonstrate signs of increasing intracranial pressure, especially headache.

If oversecretion of GH occurs after epiphyseal closure, growth is in the transverse direction, producing a condition known as acromegaly. Typical facial features include:

- Overgrowth of the head, lips, nose, tongue, jaw, and paranasal and mastoid sinuses
- Separation and malocclusion of the teeth in the enlarged jaw
- Disproportion of the face to the cerebral division of the skull
- Increased facial hair; thickened, deeply creased skin
- Increased tendency toward hyperglycemia and diabetes mellitus (DM)

Excessive secretion of GH by a pituitary adenoma causes most cases of acromegaly. Acromegaly can develop slowly, with patients being diagnosed as much as 10 years after their symptoms first appear. Left untreated, these patients have a higher mortality rate due to potential cardiovascular, metabolic, and pulmonary complications (Katznelson, 2007; Natchtigall, Delgado, Swearingen, et al, 2008).

Diagnostic Evaluation

Diagnosis is based on a history of excessive growth during childhood and evidence of increased levels of GH. Radiographic studies may reveal a tumor in an enlarged sella turcica, normal bone age, enlargement of bones (such as the paranasal sinuses), and evidence of joint changes. Endocrine studies to confirm excess of other hormones, specifically thyroid, cortisol, and sex hormones, should also be included in the differential diagnosis.

Therapeutic Management

If a lesion is present, surgical treatment by cryosurgery or hypophysectomy is performed to remove the tumor when possible. External radiation or radioactive implants may be used to destroy GH-secreting tissue. New pharmacologic agents have evolved and may be used in combination with other therapies to treat this disease (Natchtigall, Delgado, Swearingen, et al, 2008). Depending on the extent of surgical extirpation and degree of pituitary insufficiency, hormone replacement with thyroid extract, cortisone, and sex hormones may be necessary.

Nursing Care Management

The primary nursing consideration is early identification of children with excessive growth rates. Although medical management is unable to reduce growth already attained, further growth can be retarded. The earlier the treatment, the greater the chances of attaining a normal adult height. Nurses in ambulatory settings who are frequently involved in growth screening should refer children who demonstrate excessive linear growth for a medical evaluation. They should also observe for signs of a tumor, especially headache, and evidence of concurrent hormonal excesses, particularly the gonadotropins, which cause sexual precocity.

Children with excessive growth rates require as much emotional support as those with short stature. However, girls may suffer from the effects of excessive height much more than boys, although, like boys, they may find the tallness an asset when pursuing sports such as basketball. Children and their parents need an opportunity to express their thoughts. A compassionate nurse can be supportive to these children, especially before adolescence when they are larger than their peers. The nurse can emphasize to a tall girl that as boys grow older, they become taller and she will not always be looking down at them. Because early adolescence is a time of idol worship, the nurse can point out marriages of celebrities in which the woman is taller than the man to help the girl realize that not all heterosexual relationships follow stereotypic models.

PRECOCIOUS PUBERTY

Manifestations of sexual development before age 9 years in boys or age 8 years in girls have traditionally been considered precocious development, and these children were recommended for further evaluation (Kaplowitz, 2009), but guidelines on this have changed (see Research Focus box).

🔍 RESEARCH FOCUS

Precocious Puberty

Recent examination of the age limit for defining when puberty is precocious reveals that the onset of puberty in girls is occurring earlier than previous studies have documented (Biro, Huang, Crawford, et al, 2006). Mean onset of puberty was 10.2 and 9.6 years in Caucasian and African-American girls, respectively. Based on these findings, precocious puberty evaluation for a pathologic etiology should be performed for Caucasian girls younger than 7 years of age or for African-American girls younger than 6 years of age. No change in the guidelines for evaluation of precocious puberty in boys is recommended. However, recent data suggest that boys may be beginning maturation earlier as well (Herman-Giddens, 2006).

Normally the hypothalamic-releasing factors stimulate secretion of the gonadotropic hormones from the anterior pituitary at the time of puberty. In the male, interstitial cell–stimulating hormone stimulates Leydig cells of the testes to secrete testosterone. In the female follicle-stimulating hormone and luteinizing hormone stimulate the ovarian follicles to secrete estrogens. This sequence of events is known as the **hypothalamic-pituitary-gonadal axis**. If for some reason the cycle undergoes premature activation, the child displays evidence of advanced or precocious puberty. Box 38-6 lists the causes of precocious puberty.

Isosexual precocious puberty is more common among girls than boys. Approximately 50% of children with precocious puberty have central precocious puberty (CPP), in which pubertal development is activated by the hypothalamic gonadotropin-releasing hormone (GnRH). This produces early maturation and development of the gonads with secretion of sex hormones, development of secondary sexual characteristics, and sometimes production of mature sperm and ova (Lee,

---

BOX 38-6 CAUSES OF PRECOCIOUS PUBERTY

Central Precocious Puberty
Idiopathic, with or without hypothalamic hamartoma
Secondary
- Congenital anomalies
- Postinflammatory—Encephalitis, meningitis, abscess, granulomatous disease
- Radiotherapy
- Trauma
- Neoplasms
After effective treatment of longstanding pseudoisosexual precocity

Peripheral Precocious Puberty
Familial male-limited precocious puberty
Albright syndrome
Gonadal or extragonadal tumors
Adrenal
- Congenital adrenal hyperplasia
- Adenoma, carcinoma
- Glucocorticoid resistance
Exogenous sex hormones
Primary hypothyroidism

Incomplete Precocious Puberty
Premature thelarche
Premature menarche
Premature pubarche or adrenarche

Modified from Root AW: Precocious puberty, *Pediatr Rev* 21(1):10-19, 2000.

1999; Root, 2000). CPP occurs more frequently in girls and is usually idiopathic, with 95% demonstrating no causative factor (Nebesio and Eugster, 2007; Greiner and Kerrigan, 2006; Root 2000; Carel and Leger, 2008). A CNS insult or structural abnormality occurs in more than 90% of boys with CPP (Root, 2000).

Peripheral precocious puberty (PPP) includes early puberty resulting from hormone stimulation other than the hypothalamic GnRH–stimulated pituitary gonadotropin release. Isolated manifestations that are usually associated with puberty may be seen as variations in normal sexual development (Greiner and Kerrigan, 2006). They appear without other signs of pubescence and are probably caused by unusual end-organ sensitivity to prepubertal levels of estrogen or androgen. Included are premature thelarche (development of breasts in prepubertal girls), premature pubarche (premature adrenarche, early development of sexual hair), and premature menarche (isolated menses without other evidence of sexual development).

Therapeutic Management

Direct treatment of precocious puberty toward the specific cause when known. In 50% of cases, precocious pubertal development regresses or stops advancing without any treatment (Carel and Leger, 2008). If CPP progresses, it can be managed with monthly injections of a synthetic analog of luteinizing hormone–releasing hormone, which regulates pituitary secretions (Carel and Chaussain, 1999; Lee, 1999). A slow-release formulation of leuprolide acetate (Lupron Depot) is given in a dosage of 0.2 to 0.3 mg/kg intramuscularly q 4 wk. A longer lasting preparation may be given intramuscularly every 3 months and has also been successful in the treatment of CPP in a majority of patients. Although expensive, the GnRH analog (GnRHa) histrelin has been formulated as a subdermal implant and may be beneficial for some patients who would like to avoid injections (Kaplowitz, 2009).

After initiation of treatment, breast development regresses or does not advance, and growth returns to normal rates, enhancing predicted height. Some patients, however, do not attain adult targeted height during therapy. Researchers have taken different approaches to address this issue, proposing the use of GH and, more recently, conducting trials of a nonaromatizable anabolic steroid to improved adult height (Carel and Leger, 2008; Kaplowitz, 2009). Treatment is discontinued at a chronologically appropriate time, allowing pubertal changes to resume. Psychologic management of the patient and family is an important aspect of care. Both parents and the affected child should learn the injection procedure.

Nursing Care Management

Psychologic support and guidance of the child and family are the most important aspects of management. Parents and children need anticipatory guidance, support and information resources, and reassurance of the benign nature of the condition (Greiner and Kerrigan, 2006). Dress and activities for the physically precocious child should be appropriate to the chronologic age. Sexual interest is not usually advanced beyond the child's chronologic age, and parents need to understand that the child's mental age is congruent with the chronologic age and that the child's normal, overt manifestations of affection are age appropriate and do not represent sexual advances.

Despite the early sexual development, maturation of the gonads and the appearance of secondary sexual characteristics proceed in the usual order. The most difficult time for the child is usually the school years before adolescence. After puberty, physical differences from peers are no longer present.

Although the child's sexual behavior may be appropriate for the chronologic age, the nurse should emphasize to parents that the child may be fertile. Usually no form of contraception is necessary unless the child is sexually active. In this situation proper counseling is important because hormonal forms of birth control, such as estrogen pills, prematurely initiate epiphyseal closure, resulting in stunted linear growth.

DIABETES INSIPIDUS

The principal disorder of posterior pituitary hypofunction is diabetes insipidus (DI), also known as neurogenic DI, resulting from undersecretion of ADH, or vasopressin, and producing a state of uncontrolled diuresis (Makaryus and McFarlane, 2006). This disorder is not to be confused with nephrogenic DI, a rare hereditary disorder affecting primarily males and caused by unresponsiveness of the renal tubules to the hormone. (See Chapter 30.)

Neurogenic DI may result from a number of different causes. Primary causes are familial or idiopathic; of the total cases, approximately 45% to 50% are idiopathic. Secondary causes include trauma (accidental or surgical), tumors, granulomatous disease, infections (meningitis or encephalitis), and

vascular anomalies (aneurysm). Certain drugs, such as alcohol or phenytoin (diphenylhydantoin), can cause a transient polyuria. DI may be an early sign of an evolving cerebral process (De Buyst, Massa, Christophe, et al, 2007).

Clinical Manifestations

The cardinal signs of DI are polyuria and polydipsia. In the older child, signs such as excessive urination accompanied by a compensatory insatiable thirst may be so intense that the child does little more than go to the toilet and drink fluids (Cheetham and Baylis, 2002). Frequently the first sign is enuresis. In the infant the initial symptom is irritability that is relieved with feedings of water but not milk. The infant is also prone to dehydration, electrolyte imbalance, hyperthermia, azotemia, and potential circulatory collapse.

Dehydration is usually not a serious problem in older children, who are able to drink larger quantities of water. However, any period of unconsciousness, such as after trauma or anesthesia, may be life threatening because the voluntary demand for fluid is absent. During such instances careful monitoring of urine volumes, blood concentration, and IV fluid replacement is essential to prevent dehydration.

> **! NURSING ALERT**
>
> The child with DI complicated by congenital absence of the thirst center must be encouraged to drink sufficient quantities of liquid to prevent electrolyte imbalance.

Diagnostic Evaluation

The simplest test used to diagnose this condition is the water deprivation test, which restricts oral fluids and observes changes in urine volume and concentration. Normally, reducing fluids results in concentrated urine and diminished volume. In DI, fluid restriction has little or no effect on urine formation but causes weight loss from dehydration. Accurate results from this procedure require strict monitoring of fluid intake and urinary output, measurement of urine concentration (specific gravity or osmolality), and frequent weight checks. A weight loss between 3% and 5% indicates significant dehydration and requires termination of the fluid restriction.

> **! NURSING ALERT**
>
> Small children require close observation during fluid deprivation to prevent them from drinking, even from toilet bowls, flower vases, or other unlikely sources of fluid.

If this test is positive, the child should be given a test dose of injected aqueous vasopressin (Pitressin), which should alleviate the polyuria and polydipsia. Unresponsiveness to exogenous vasopressin usually indicates nephrogenic DI. A rise by more than 50% in urine osmolality after vasopressin administration indicates central DI (Carr and Gill, 2007).

An important diagnostic consideration is differentiating DI from other causes of polyuria and polydipsia, especially DM.

Other tests used in the diagnostic evaluation include CT of the brain or MRI to detect a tumor, kidney function tests, urine osmolality tests and blood electrolyte levels to assess renal failure, and specific endocrine studies to isolate associated problems (Carr and Gill, 2007). In rare instances a psychologic consultation may be warranted to confirm the possibility of compulsive water drinking related to psychogenic causes.

Therapeutic Management

The usual treatment is hormone replacement, either with an intramuscular or subcutaneous injection of vasopressin tannate in peanut oil or with a nasal spray of aqueous lysine vasopressin (Verbalis, 2003; Makaryus and McFarlane, 2006). The injectable form has the advantage of lasting for 48 to 72 hours, which affords the child a full night's sleep. However, it has the disadvantage of requiring frequent injections and proper preparation of the drug.

⚡ DRUG ALERT

Vasopressin

To be effective, vasopressin must be thoroughly mixed in the oil by being held under warm running water for 10 to 15 minutes and shaken vigorously before being drawn into the syringe. If this is not done, the oil may be injected minus the ADH. Small brown particles, which indicate drug dispersion, must be seen in the suspension.

The nasal spray has the benefit of being a simple, painless route of administration. However, applications must be repeated every 8 to 12 hours to prevent recurrence of symptoms. To provide longer relief during the night, a cotton pledget moistened with the spray can be inserted into the nostril. However, mucous membrane irritation caused by a cold or allergy renders this route unreliable. Although the vaginal and buccal mucosae are substitute routes for the spray, this can be inconvenient. Desmopressin acetate (DDAVP), a long-acting analog of arginine vasopressin, which has fewer side effects, is administered intranasally by way of a flexible tube to achieve adequate control. The child's response pattern is variable, with duration ranging from 6 to 24 hours (Verbalis, 2003; Makaryus and McFarlane, 2006). It is usually administered twice daily—at bedtime to allow the child to sleep through the night and in the morning to allow fewer interruptions in the school day. Some "breakthrough" urination is allowed during the evening hours as a precaution against overmedication. The signs of overmedication are similar to manifestations associated with syndrome of inappropriate ADH (SIADH). (See next section.)

Nursing Care Management

The initial objective is identification of the disorder. Because an early sign may be sudden enuresis in a child who is toilet trained, excessive thirst with bed-wetting is an indication for further investigation. Another clue is persistent irritability and crying in an infant that is relieved only by bottle-feedings of water. After head trauma or certain neurosurgical procedures, the development of DI can be anticipated; therefore closely monitor these patients.

QUALITY PATIENT OUTCOMES: Diabetes Insipidus
- Early recognition of signs and symptoms of DI
- Differentiation of DI from other causes of polyuria and polydipsia (e.g., DM)
- Effective hormone replacement

Assessment includes measurement of body weight, serum electrolytes, blood urea nitrogen, hematocrit, and urine specific gravity taken before surgery and every other day after the procedure. Carefully measure and record fluid intake and output. Alert patients are able to adjust intake to urine losses, but unconscious or very young patients require closer fluid observation. In children who are not toilet trained, collection of urine specimens may require application of a urine-collecting device.

After confirmation of the diagnosis, parents need a thorough explanation regarding the condition with specific clarification that DI is a different condition from DM. They must realize that treatment is lifelong. If children are to receive the injectable vasopressin, ideally two caregivers should learn the correct procedure for preparation and administration of the drug. Once children are old enough, encourage them to assume full responsibility for their care.

For emergency purposes, these children should wear medical alert identification. Older children should carry the nasal spray with them for temporary relief of symptoms. School personnel need to be aware of the problem so they can grant children unrestricted use of the lavatory. Failure to permit this may result in embarrassing accidents that often result in a child's unwillingness to attend school.

SYNDROME OF INAPPROPRIATE ANTIDIURETIC HORMONE

The disorder that results from oversecretion of the posterior pituitary hormone, or ADH, is known as SIADH. It occurs with increased frequency in a variety of conditions, especially those involving infections, tumors, or other CNS disease or trauma, and is the most common cause of hyponatremia in the pediatric population (Lin, Liu, and Lim, 2005; Rivkees, 2008).

The manifestations are directly related to fluid retention and hypotonicity. Excess ADH causes most of the filtered water to be reabsorbed from the kidneys back into central circulation. Serum osmolality is low, and urine osmolality is inappropriately elevated. When cells in the brain are exposed to too much water as opposed to sodium, swelling occurs (Rivkees, 2008). When serum sodium levels are diminished to 120 mEq/L, affected children display anorexia, nausea (and sometimes vomiting), stomach cramps, irritability, and personality changes. With progressive reduction in sodium, other neurologic signs, stupor, and convulsions may be evident. The symptoms usually disappear when the underlying disorder is corrected.

The immediate management consists of restricting fluids. Subsequent management depends on the cause and severity. Fluids continue to be restricted to one-fourth to one-half maintenance. When there are no fluid abnormalities but SIADH can be anticipated, fluids are often restricted expectantly at two-thirds to three-fourths maintenance.

Nursing Care Management

The first goal of nursing management is recognizing the presence of SIADH from symptoms described in patients at risk, especially those in the pediatric intensive care unit.

QUALITY PATIENT OUTCOMES: Syndrome of Inappropriate Antidiuretic Hormone
- Early recognition of signs and symptoms of SIADH
- Fluid overload prevented
- Seizures prevented

! NURSING ALERT

Nausea, vomiting, and malaise may precede the onset of more severe stages such as disorientation, confusion, coma, and seizures (Majzoub and Muglia, 2003).

Accurately measuring intake and output, noting daily weight, and observing for signs of fluid overload are primary nursing functions, especially in the child receiving IV fluids. Seizure precautions are implemented, and the child and family need education regarding the rationale for fluid restrictions. The rare child with chronic SIADH is placed on long-term ADH-antagonizing medication, and the child and family require instructions for its administration.

DISORDERS OF THYROID FUNCTION

The thyroid gland secretes two types of hormones: TH, which consists of the hormones thyroxine (T_4) and triiodothyronine (T_3), and calcitonin. The secretion of thyroid hormones is controlled by TSH from the anterior pituitary, which in turn is regulated by thyrotropin-releasing factor (TRF) from the hypothalamus as a negative feedback response. Consequently, hypothyroidism or hyperthyroidism may result from a defect in the target gland or from a disturbance in the secretion of TSH or TRF. Because the functions of T_3 and T_4 are qualitatively the same, the term *thyroid hormone* (TH) is used throughout the discussion (Box 38-7).

The synthesis of TH depends on available sources of dietary iodine and tyrosine. The thyroid is the only endocrine gland capable of storing excess amounts of hormones for release as needed. During circulation in the bloodstream, T_4 and T_3 are bound to carrier proteins (thyroxine-binding globulin). They must be unbound before they are able to exert their metabolic effect.

The main physiologic action of TH is to regulate the basal metabolic rate and thereby control the processes of growth and tissue differentiation, as outlined in Box 38-7. Unlike GH, TH is involved in many more diverse activities that influence the growth and development of body tissues. Therefore a deficiency of TH exerts a more profound effect on growth than that seen in hypopituitarism.

Calcitonin helps maintain blood calcium levels by decreasing the calcium concentration. Its effect is the opposite of that of

---

BOX 38-7 PHYSIOLOGIC EFFECTS OF THYROID HORMONE

- Regulates metabolic rate of all cells; protein, fat, and carbohydrate catabolism; and nitrogen excretion
- Regulates body heat production and heat-dissipating mechanisms
- Regulates protein synthesis and catabolism, amino acid incorporation into protein, and transcription of messenger ribonucleic acid
- Increases gluconeogenesis and peripheral utilization of glucose
- Maintains appetite and secretion of gastrointestinal substances
- Maintains calcium mobilization
- Stimulates cholesterol synthesis and hepatic mechanisms that remove cholesterol from the circulation; stimulates lipid turnover and free fatty acid release
- Regulates hepatic conversion of carotene to vitamin A
- Maintains growth hormone secretion, skeletal maturation, and tissue differentiation
- Is necessary for muscle tone and vigor and normal skin constituents
- Maintains cardiac rate, force, and output
- Affects respiratory rate, depth of oxygen utilization, and carbon dioxide formation
- Affects central nervous system development and cerebration during first 2 to 3 years
- Affects milk production during lactation and menstrual cycle fertility
- Maintains sensitivity to insulin and insulin degradation
- Affects red cell production
- Affects cortisol secretion, probably by directly affecting the adrenal glands and by increasing adrenocorticotropic hormone secretion

---

PTH in that it inhibits skeletal demineralization and promotes calcium deposition in the bone.

JUVENILE HYPOTHYROIDISM

Hypothyroidism is one of the most common endocrine problems of childhood. It may be either congenital (see Chapter 9) or acquired and represents a deficiency in secretion of TH (Foley, 2001). Hypothyroidism from dietary insufficiency of iodine is now rare in the United States, since iodized salt is a readily available source of the nutrient.

Beyond infancy, a number of defects may cause primary hypothyroidism. For example, a congenital hypoplastic thyroid gland may provide sufficient amounts of TH during the first year or two but be inadequate when rapid body growth increases demands on the gland. A partial or complete thyroidectomy for cancer or thyrotoxicosis can leave insufficient thyroid tissue to furnish hormones for body requirements. Radiotherapy for Hodgkin disease or other malignancies may lead to hypothyroidism (Hudson, Krasin, Metzger, et al, 2011). Infectious processes may cause hypothyroidism. It can also occur when dietary iodine is deficient.

Clinical manifestations depend on the extent of dysfunction and the child's age at onset. Primary congenital hypothyroidism is characterized by low levels of circulating thyroid hormones and raised levels of TSH at birth. If left untreated, congenital hypothyroidism causes decreased mental capacity. Improvements in newborn screening have led to earlier detection and prevention of cognitive dysfunction in many children (American Academy of Pediatrics, Rose, Section on Endocrinology and Committee on Genetics of the American

Thyroid Association, et al, 2006). The presenting symptoms are decelerated growth from chronic deprivation of TH or thyromegaly. Growth and development are less impaired when hypothyroidism is acquired at a later age, and, because brain growth is nearly complete by 2 to 3 years of age, intellectual disability and neurologic sequelae are not associated with juvenile hypothyroidism. Some clinical manifestations of hypothyroidism in a child are myxedematous skin changes (dry skin, puffiness around the eyes, sparse hair), dry skin, constipation, sleepiness, lethargy, and mental decline. Growth failure, delayed puberty, and excessive weight gain can also be seen.

Therapy is TH replacement, the same as for hypothyroidism in the infant, although the prompt treatment needed in the infant is not required in the child. In children with severe symptoms, the restoration of euthyroidism is achieved more gradually with administration of increasing amounts of L-thyroxine over a period of 4 to 8 weeks to avoid symptoms of hyperthyroidism, which can occur with treatment of chronic hypothyroidism. Researchers have found that children treated early continue to have mild delays in reading, comprehension, and arithmetic but catch up by grade 6 (Rovet and Ehrlich, 2000). However, adolescents may demonstrate problems with memory, attention, and visuospatial processing.

Nursing Care Management

The importance of early recognition in the infant is discussed in Chapter 9. Growth cessation or retardation in a child whose growth has previously been normal should alert the observer to the possibility of hypothyroidism. After diagnosis and implementation of thyroxine therapy, the importance of compliance and periodic monitoring of response to therapy should be stressed to parents. Children should learn to take responsibility for their own health as soon as they are old enough, at about 9 or 10 years of age.

GOITER

A goiter is an enlargement or hypertrophy of the thyroid gland. It may occur with deficient (hypothyroid), excessive (hyperthyroid), or normal (euthyroid) TH secretion. It can be congenital or acquired. Congenital disease usually occurs as a result of maternal administration of antithyroid drugs or iodides during pregnancy. Acquired disease can result from increased secretion of pituitary TSH in response to decreased circulating levels of TH or from infiltrative neoplastic or inflammatory processes. In areas where dietary iodine (essential for TH production) is deficient, goiter can be endemic.

Enlargement of the thyroid gland may be mild and noticeable only when there is an increased demand for TH (e.g., during periods of rapid growth). Where iodine deficiency is severe, a large percentage of the population display goiters. Enlargement of the thyroid at birth can be sufficient to cause severe respiratory distress. Sporadic goiter is usually caused by lymphocytic thyroiditis, and intrinsic biochemical defects in synthesis of the hormones are associated with goiters. TH replacement is necessary to treat the hypothyroidism and reverse the TSH effect on the gland.

Nursing Care Management

Large goiters are identified by their obvious appearance. Smaller nodules may be evident only on palpation. Nurses in ambulatory settings need to be aware of the possibility of goiters and report such findings. Benign enlargement of the thyroid gland may occur during adolescence and should not be confused with pathologic states. Nodules rarely are caused by a cancerous tumor but always require evaluation. Include questions regarding exposure to radiation in the assessment.

> **! NURSING ALERT**
>
> If an infant is born with a goiter, immediately begin precautions for emergency ventilation, such as having supplemental oxygen and a tracheostomy set nearby. Hyperextension of the neck often facilitates breathing.

Immediate surgery to remove part of the gland may be lifesaving in infants born with a goiter. When thyroid replacement is necessary, parents have the same needs regarding its administration as discussed for the parents of children who have hypothyroidism. (See Chapter 9.)

LYMPHOCYTIC THYROIDITIS

Lymphocytic thyroiditis (Hashimoto disease, juvenile autoimmune thyroiditis) is the most common cause of thyroid disease in children and adolescents and accounts for the largest percentage of juvenile hypothyroidism (Szymborska and Staroszczyk, 2000). It accounts for many of the enlarged thyroid glands formerly designated as thyroid hyperplasia of adolescence or adolescent goiter. Although it can occur during the first 3 years of life, it occurs more frequently after age 6. It reaches a peak incidence during adolescence, and there is evidence that the disease is self-limiting. The presence of a goiter and elevated thyroglobulin antibody with progressive increase in both thyroid peroxidase antibody and TSH may be predictive factors for future development of hypothyroidism (Radetti, Gottardi, Bona, et al, 2006).

Pathophysiology

There is a strong genetic predisposition to the development of lymphocytic thyroiditis, although no mode of inheritance has been delineated and the basic stimulus or autoimmune defect is unknown. In families this disease is closely related to other thyroid disorders (Graves disease, idiopathic hypothyroidism, idiopathic myxedema) and autoimmune disorders (pernicious anemia, Addison disease, type 1 DM, and hypoparathyroidism).

The disease is characterized by lymphocytic infiltration of the gland, germinal center inflammation, and, in many patients, replacement with fibrous tissue. In the early stages there may be only hyperplasia. A defect in autoregulation allows the persistence of a T-cell clone, which induces a cell-mediated immune response. Several antithyroid antibodies have been recognized in patients with thyroiditis.

Clinical Manifestations

The practitioner usually detects the enlarged thyroid gland during a routine examination, although parents may notice it when the youngster swallows. In most children the entire gland is enlarged symmetrically (but may be asymmetric) and is firm, freely movable, and nontender. There may be manifestations of moderate tracheal compression (sense of fullness, hoarseness, and dysphagia), but it is extremely rare for a nontoxic diffuse goiter to enlarge to the extent that it causes mechanical obstruction. Most children are euthyroid, but some display symptoms of hypothyroidism. Others have signs suggestive of hyperthyroidism, such as nervousness, irritability, tachycardia, increased sweating, or hyperactivity.

Diagnostic Evaluation

Thyroid function tests are usually normal, although TSH levels may be slightly or moderately elevated. With progressive disease the T_4 decreases, followed by a decrease in T_3 levels and an increase in TSH. A variety of abnormalities in radioactive iodine uptake may be noted. The majority of children have serum antibody titers to thyroid antigens, but fewer children have a positive red blood cell hemagglutination test result. When both tests are used, almost all children with thyroid autoimmunity are detected. However, levels in children are lower than in adults; therefore repeated measurements may be needed in doubtful cases, since titers may increase later in the disease.

Therapeutic Management

In many cases the goiter is transient and asymptomatic and regresses spontaneously within a year or two. Therapy of a nontoxic diffuse goiter is usually simple, uncomplicated, and effective. Oral administration of TH decreases the size of the gland significantly and provides the feedback needed to suppress TSH stimulation, and the hyperplastic thyroid gland gradually regresses in size. Surgery is contraindicated in this disorder. Evaluate untreated patients periodically.

Nursing Care Management

Nursing care consists of identifying the youngster with thyroid enlargement, reassuring the child that the condition is probably only temporary, and reinforcing instructions for thyroid therapy.

HYPERTHYROIDISM

The largest percentage of hyperthyroidism in childhood is caused by Graves disease, which is usually associated with an enlarged thyroid gland and exophthalmos (Streetman and Khanderia, 2004; Thompson, 2002). Most cases of Graves disease in children occur between the ages 6 and 15 years, with a peak incidence at 12 to 14 years of age, but the disease may be present at birth in children of thyrotoxic mothers. The incidence is five times higher in girls than in boys.

The hyperthyroidism of Graves disease is apparently caused by an autoimmune response to TSH receptors, but no specific etiology has been identified. There is definitive evidence for familial association, with a high concordance incidence in twins. Patients with Graves disease possess the histocompatibility antigens A1, B8, and DR3 (Dallas and Foley, 2003; Simmonds, Howson, Heward, et al, 2005). Currently, there is no cure for Graves disease, but blocking the production of autoantibodies responsible for overstimulating the thyroid gland is being investigated (Siarkowski, 2005).

Clinical Manifestations

The development of manifestations is highly variable. Signs and symptoms develop gradually, with an interval between onset and diagnosis of approximately 6 to 12 months. The principal clinical features are excessive motion—irritability, hyperactivity, short attention span, tremors, insomnia, and emotional lability. Gradual weight loss despite a voracious appetite occurs in half the cases. Linear growth and bone age are usually accelerated. Muscle weakness often occurs. Hyperactivity of the gastrointestinal tract may cause vomiting and frequent stooling. Cardiac manifestations include a rapid, pounding pulse even during sleep; widened pulse pressure; systolic murmurs; and cardiomegaly. Dyspnea occurs during slight exertion, such as climbing stairs. The skin is warm, flushed, and moist. Heat intolerance may be severe and is accompanied by diaphoresis. The hair is unusually fine and unable to hold a wave.

Exophthalmos (protruding eyeballs), observed in many children, is accompanied by a wide-eyed staring expression, increased blinking, lid lag, lack of convergence, and absence of wrinkling of the forehead when looking upward. As protrusion of the eyeball increases, the child may not be able to completely cover the cornea with the lid. Visual disturbances may include blurred vision and loss of visual acuity. Ophthalmopathy can develop long before or after the onset of hyperthyroidism. A consistent pathogenic link between them has not been identified. It is now thought that Graves ophthalmopathy is a disorder of autoimmune origin caused by a complex interplay of endogenous and environmental factors (Bartalena, Tanda, Piantanida, et al, 2003).

Diagnostic Evaluation

The presence of a thyroid mass in a child requires a thorough history, including inquiry into prior irradiation to the head and neck and exposure to a goitrogen. The diagnosis is established on the basis of increased levels of T_4 and T_3. TSH is suppressed to unmeasurable levels. Other tests are rarely indicated.

Therapeutic Management

Therapy for hyperthyroidism is controversial, but all methods are directed toward retarding the rate of hormone secretion. The three acceptable modes available are the antithyroid drugs, which interfere with the biosynthesis of TH, including propylthiouracil (PTU) and methimazole (MTZ, Tapazole); subtotal thyroidectomy; and ablation with radioiodine (^{131}I iodide) (Streetman and Khanderia, 2004; Rivkees and Cornelius, 2003). Each is effective, but each has advantages and disadvantages.

When affected children exhibit signs and symptoms of hyperthyroidism (e.g., increased weight loss, pulse, pulse pressure, and blood pressure), their activity should be limited to classwork only. Vigorous exercise is restricted until thyroid levels are decreased to normal or near-normal values.

The American Thyroid Association* has an extensive website with information relation to prevention, treatment, and cure of thyroid disease.

Drug Therapy

Most centers favor drugs as an initial therapy. An effective response to these drugs occurs after a latent period because they inhibit production of additional TH but do not retard secretion of stored supplies. Generally, some improvement is noted within the first 2 weeks, with evidence of decreased nervousness, less fatigue, increased strength, a lowered pulse, and weight gain. In many children an initial treatment course of 1 to 2 years is followed by a complete remission of the disorder. Those who relapse may benefit from a second course of therapy but may also be candidates for surgical intervention or radioiodine therapy (Siarkowski, 2005).

Disadvantages include toxic drug reactions requiring alternate therapy, chronic dependency on the drug, and failure to produce remission in a large number of patients. The most serious side effect of these antithyroid drugs is agranulocytosis (severe leukopenia), which generally occurs within the initial weeks or months of therapy. It is usually accompanied by a sore throat and fever. Treatment involves immediate discontinuation of the drug, social isolation of the child, and administration of antibiotics and glucocorticoids until symptoms resolve.

Thyroidectomy

Surgical treatment involves surgical ablation of the thyroid (thyroidectomy). Although this approach has the advantage of being a long-lasting form of therapy without the need for multiple-dose drug therapy, it has a number of serious disadvantages, including an increased incidence of hypothyroidism and the need for thyroxine therapy, infrequent recurrent laryngeal nerve palsy and permanent hypoparathyroidism, keloid formation of the anterior cervical scar, and (rarely) surgical mortality. Therefore surgery in most centers is reserved for children who do not respond to or comply with the use of antithyroid drugs or who are prone to recurrences.

Radioiodine Therapy

Radioiodine may be a therapy of choice in young patients with Graves disease who relapse after medical treatment (Cheetham, Hughes, Barnes, et al, 1998). Radioiodine therapy has become an even more acceptable option since it has become apparent that lifelong thyroxine replacement is required after either surgery or radioiodine therapy.

Thyrotoxicosis

Thyrotoxicosis (thyroid "crisis" or thyroid "storm") may occur from sudden release of the hormone. Although thyrotoxicosis is unusual in children, a crisis can be life threatening. These "storms" are evidenced by the acute onset of severe irritability

and restlessness, vomiting, diarrhea, hyperthermia, hypertension, severe tachycardia, and prostration. There may be rapid progression to delirium, coma, and even death. A crisis may be precipitated by acute infection, surgical emergencies, or discontinuation of antithyroid therapy. Treatment in addition to antithyroid drugs is administration of β-adrenergic blocking agents (propranolol), which provide relief from the adrenergic hyperresponsiveness that produces the disturbing side effects of the reaction. Therapy is usually required for 2 to 3 weeks.

Nursing Care Management

The initial nursing objective is identification of children with hyperthyroidism. Because the clinical manifestations often appear gradually, the goiter and ophthalmic changes may not be noticed, and the excessive activity may be attributed to behavioral problems. Nurses in ambulatory settings, particularly schools, need to be alert to signs that suggest this disorder, especially weight loss despite an excellent appetite, academic difficulties resulting from a short attention span and inability to sit still, unexplained fatigue and sleeplessness, and difficulty with fine motor skills such as writing. Exophthalmos may develop long before the signs and symptoms of hyperthyroidism and may be the only presenting sign (Thompson, 2002). Exophthalmos is less common in adults than children (Jospe, 2001).

Much of these children's care is related to treating physical symptoms before a response to drug therapy is achieved. These children need a quiet, unstimulating environment that is conducive to rest. Sometimes hospitalization is necessary during the immediate treatment phase to remove a child from a troubled home. A regular routine is beneficial in providing frequent rest periods, minimizing the stress of coping with unexpected demands, and meeting the children's needs promptly. Physical activity is restricted. For example, school physical education classes are discontinued.

QUALITY PATIENT OUTCOMES: Hyperthyroidism
- Early recognition of signs and symptoms of hyperthyroidism
- Physical symptoms managed
- Regular routine established for child during recovery period
- Adherence to antithyroid drugs as prescribed

Because the manifestations often interfere with schoolwork, a consultation with the child's teachers is important to advise them of the medical reason for the problem and suggest ways of helping the child adjust. For example, the child may benefit from a shortened school day or at least study periods in a quiet area. Limiting demands on the child, such as reciting in class or participating in extracurricular activities, may help conserve strength for academic studies. Despite the excessive activity of these children, they tire easily, experience muscle weakness, and are unable to relax to recover their strength.

Emotional lability is often manifested by sudden episodes of crying or elation. Such behavior, coupled with irritability, disrupts interpersonal relationships, creating difficulties within and outside the home. Parents need help in understanding the uncontrollable nature of these outbursts and ways of minimiz-

---

*6066 Leesburg Pike, Suite 550, Falls Church, VA 22041; 800-THYROID, 703-998-8890; e-mail: thyroid@thyroid.org; **www.thyroid.org**.

ing them through decreased environmental stimulation, stress, and frustration. Encourage the child to express feelings about behavior and its effect on others. The nurse can encourage the child to concentrate on friendship with one special peer rather than a group until the condition is stabilized.

Heat intolerance may produce considerable family conflict. Preferring a cooler environment than others, the child is likely to open windows, complain about the heat, wear minimum clothing, and remove blankets while sleeping. Although the child should dress in accordance with climatic conditions, the use of light cotton clothing in the home, good ventilation, air conditioning or fans, frequent baths, and adequate hydration is helpful in providing comfort. Stress hygiene because of excessive sweating.

Adjust dietary requirements to meet the child's increased metabolic rate. Although the need for calories is increased, these should be provided in wholesome foods rather than "junk" foods. The child may require vitamin supplements to meet daily requirement. Rather than three large meals, the child's appetite may be better satisfied by five or six moderate meals throughout the day. Family members should refrain from making remarks about the child's appetite because the child may voluntarily restrict his or her eating to avoid such attention.

Once therapy begins, the nurse explains the drug regimen, emphasizing the importance of observing for side effects of antithyroid drugs. Harmful effects of PTU and related compounds include urticarial rash, fever, arthritis, or arthralgia. There may be enlargement of the salivary and cervical lymph glands, a diminished sense of taste, hepatitis, and edema of the lower extremities. Parents should also be aware of the signs of hypothyroidism, which can occur from overdose of the drugs. The most common indications are lethargy and somnolence.

⚡ DRUG ALERT

Propylthiouracil and Methimazole

Children being treated with PTU or MTZ must be carefully monitored for side effects of the drug. Because sore throat and fever accompany the grave complication of leukopenia, these children should be seen by a practitioner if such symptoms occur. Parents and children should learn to recognize and report symptoms immediately.

Surgical Care

If surgery is anticipated, iodine is usually administered for a few weeks before the procedure. Because oral iodine preparations are unpalatable, they should be mixed with a strong-tasting fruit juice, such as grape or punch flavors, and be given through a straw. Compliance with iodine therapy is essential to avoid the danger of thyroid crisis after sudden discontinuation.

Psychologic preparation of children for thyroidectomy is similar to that for any other surgical procedure. (See Chapter 27.) However, of special consideration is the site of the incision. The fear of having the throat cut is very real and in older children is associated with death. The nurse should explain that the throat is not cut, only the skin, to remove the gland. Showing children a picture of the anatomic location of the thyroid around the trachea is often helpful. Children should be pre-

pared for the dressing around the neck and the possibility of an endotracheal or "breathing" tube after surgery.

Postoperative care involves positioning with the neck slightly flexed to avoid strain on the sutures and observation for bleeding and complications. The children learn to support the neck in this position when they sit up. Damage to the laryngeal nerve is evidenced by severe stridor or hoarseness, although some hoarseness is expected. **Laryngospasm**, a spasmodic contraction of the larynx, can be a life-threatening complication of thyroidectomy. Signs of laryngospasm are stridor, hoarseness, and a feeling of tightness in the throat. Place a tracheostomy set near the bed for emergency use. The nurse should observe for signs of hypoparathyroidism, which causes hypocalcemia, in the immediate postoperative period.

⚠ NURSING ALERT

The earliest indication of hypoparathyroidism may be anxiety and mental depression, followed by paresthesia and evidence of heightened neuromuscular excitability, such as:

Chvostek sign—Facial muscle spasm elicited by tapping the facial nerve in the region of the parotid gland

Trousseau sign—Carpal spasm elicited by pressure applied to nerves of the upper arm

Tetany—Carpopedal spasm (sharp flexion of wrist and ankle joints), muscle twitching, cramps, seizures and stridor

---

DISORDERS OF PARATHYROID FUNCTION

The parathyroid glands secrete PTH, the main function of which, along with vitamin D and calcitonin, is homeostasis of serum calcium concentration (Perheentupa, 2003). The effect of PTH on calcium is opposite that of calcitonin. Box 38-8 lists the principal effects of PTH on its target sites.

The net result of the integrated action of PTH and vitamin D is maintenance of serum calcium levels within a narrow normal range and the mineralization of bone. Secretion of PTH is controlled by a negative feedback system involving the serum calcium ion concentration. Low ionized calcium levels stimulate PTH secretion, causing absorption of calcium by the target tissues; high ionized calcium concentrations suppress PTH.

HYPOPARATHYROIDISM

Hypoparathyroidism is a spectrum of disorders that result in deficient PTH. Congenital hypoparathyroidism may be caused by a specific defect in the synthesis or cellular processing of PTH or by aplasia or hypoplasia of the gland (Perheentupa, 2003).

Hypoparathyroidism can occur secondary to other causes. Postoperative hypoparathyroidism may follow thyroidectomy

---

BOX 38-8 PHYSIOLOGIC EFFECTS OF PARATHYROID HORMONE

Bones—Increases osteoclastic activity, causing phosphate-producing bone demineralization

Kidneys—Increases absorption of calcium and excretion of phosphate

Gastrointestinal tract—Promotes calcium absorption

with acute or gradual onset and be transient or permanent. Two forms of transient hypoparathyroidism may be present in the newborn, both of which are the result of a relative PTH deficiency. One type is caused by maternal hyperparathyroidism or maternal DM. A more common, later form appears almost exclusively in infants fed a milk formula with a high phosphate-to-calcium ratio.

Clinical Manifestations

Symptoms vary from none to significant morbidity if treatment is not initiated. Mild deficiency may be identified through laboratory studies. Muscle cramps are an early symptom, progressing to numbness, stiffness, and tingling in the hands and feet. A positive Chvostek or Trousseau sign or laryngeal spasms may be present. Convulsions with loss of consciousness may occur. These episodes may be preceded by abdominal discomfort, tonic rigidity, head retraction, and cyanosis. Headaches and vomiting with increased intracranial pressure and papilledema may occur and may suggest a brain tumor (Behrman, Kliegman, Jenson, et al, 2009).

Children with longstanding deficiency may have dry, scaly, coarse skin with eruptions often caused by *Candida* organisms (Behrman, Kliegman, Jenson, et al, 2009). Dental and enamel hypoplasia often occurs. Cataracts develop in patients with untreated disease. Because hypoparathyroidism results in decreased bone resorption and inactive osteoclastic activity, skeletal growth is retarded.

Diagnostic Evaluation

The diagnosis of hypoparathyroidism is made on the basis of clinical manifestations associated with decreased serum calcium and increased serum phosphorus. Levels of plasma PTH are low in idiopathic hypoparathyroidism but high in pseudohypoparathyroidism. End-organ responsiveness is tested by the administration of PTH with measurement of urinary cyclic adenosine monophosphate. Kidney function tests are included in the differential diagnosis to rule out renal insufficiency. Although bone radiographs are usually normal, they may demonstrate increased bone density and suppressed growth.

Therapeutic Management

The objective of treatment is to maintain normal serum calcium and phosphate levels with minimum complications. Acute or severe tetany is corrected immediately by IV and oral administration of calcium gluconate and follow-up daily doses to achieve normal levels. Twice-daily serum calcium measurements are taken to monitor the efficacy of therapy and prevent hypercalcemia. When diagnosis is confirmed, vitamin D therapy is begun. Vitamin D therapy is somewhat difficult to regulate because the drug has a prolonged onset and a long half-life. Some authorities advocate beginning with a lower dose with stepwise increases and careful monitoring of serum calcium until stable levels are achieved. Others prefer rapid induction with higher doses and rapid reduction to lower maintenance levels.

Long-term management consists of administration of massive doses of vitamin D, and oral calcium supplementation may be useful in maintaining adequate serum calcium levels, although it is not essential. Blood calcium and phosphorus are monitored frequently until the levels have stabilized; they are then monitored monthly and less often until the child is seen at 6-month intervals. Renal function, blood pressure, and serum vitamin D levels are measured every 6 months. Serum magnesium levels are measured every 3 to 6 months to permit detection of hypomagnesemia, which may raise the requirement for vitamin D.

Nursing Care Management

The initial objective is recognition of hypocalcemia. Unexplained convulsions, irritability (especially to external stimuli), gastrointestinal symptoms (diarrhea, vomiting, cramping), and positive signs of tetany should lead the nurse to suspect this disorder. Much of the initial nursing care is related to the physical manifestations and includes institution of seizure and safety precautions; reduction of environmental stimuli (e.g., avoiding sudden or loud noise, bright lights, stimulating activities); and observation for signs of laryngospasm such as stridor, hoarseness, and a feeling of tightness in the throat. A tracheostomy set and injectable calcium gluconate should be located near the bedside for emergency use. The administration of calcium gluconate requires precautions against extravasation of the drug and tissue destruction.

After initiation of treatment, the nurse discusses with the parents the need for continuous daily administration of calcium salts and vitamin D. Because vitamin D toxicity can be a serious consequence of therapy, parents should watch for signs that include weakness, fatigue, lassitude, headache, nausea, vomiting, and diarrhea. Polyuria, polydipsia, and nocturia are signs of early renal impairment.

HYPERPARATHYROIDISM

Hyperparathyroidism is rare in childhood but can be primary or secondary. The most common cause of primary hyperparathyroidism is adenoma of the gland (Behrman, Kliegman, Jenson, et al, 2009). The most common causes of secondary hyperparathyroidism are chronic renal disease, renal osteodystrophy, and congenital anomalies of the urinary tract. The common factor is hypercalcemia. Box 38-9 lists the manifestations of hyperparathyroidism.

Diagnostic Evaluation

Blood studies to identify elevated calcium and decreased phosphorus levels are routinely performed. Measurement of PTH,

---

BOX 38-9   CLINICAL MANIFESTATIONS OF HYPERPARATHYROIDISM

Gastrointestinal—Nausea, vomiting, abdominal discomfort, and constipation

Central nervous system—Delusions, confusion, hallucinations, impaired memory, lack of interest and initiative, depression, and varying levels of consciousness

Neuromuscular—Weakness, easy fatigability, muscle atrophy (especially proximal muscles of the lower limbs), twitching of the tongue, and paresthesias in extremities

Skeletal—Vague bone pain, subperiosteal resorption of phalanges, spontaneous fractures, and absence of lamina dura around the teeth

Renal—Polyuria and polydipsia, renal colic, and hypertension

as well as several tests to isolate the cause of the hypercalcemia, such as renal function studies, should be included. Other procedures used to substantiate the physiologic consequences of the disorder include electrocardiography and radiographic bone surveys.

Therapeutic Management

Treatment depends on the cause of hyperparathyroidism. The treatment of primary hyperparathyroidism is surgical removal of the tumor or hyperplastic tissue. Parathyroidectomy may cause recurrent laryngeal nerve damage, voice impairment, hypoparathyroidism, hypocalcemia, and tetany (Wang, Roman, and Sosa, 2008). Treatment of secondary hyperparathyroidism is directed at the underlying contributing cause, which subsequently restores the serum calcium balance. However, in some instances such as in chronic renal failure the underlying disorder is irreversible. In this case treatment is aimed at raising serum calcium levels to inhibit the stimulatory effect of low levels on the parathyroids. This includes oral administration of calcium salts, high doses of vitamin D to enhance calcium absorption, a low-phosphorus diet, and administration of a phosphorus-mobilizing aluminum hydroxide to reduce phosphate absorption.

Nursing Care Management

The initial nursing objective is recognition of the disorder. Because secondary hyperparathyroidism is a consequence of chronic renal failure, the nurse is always alert to signs that suggest this complication, especially bone pain and fractures. Because urinary symptoms are the earliest indication, assessment of other body systems for evidence of high calcium levels is indicated when polyuria and polydipsia coexist. Clues to the possibility of hyperparathyroidism include change in behavior, especially inactivity; unexplained gastrointestinal symptoms; and cardiac irregularities.

Much of the initial nursing care is related to the physical symptoms and prevention of complications. To minimize renal calculi formation, hydration is essential. Encourage the child to drink fruit juices that maintain a low urinary pH, such as cranberry or apple juice, since acidity of body fluids promotes calcium absorption. All urine should be strained for evidence of renal casts.

Safety precautions, such as keeping side rails in place at all times and assisting with ambulation, are instituted because of the tendency toward fractures and muscular weakness. Children with renal rickets (osteodystrophy) may wear braces to minimize skeletal deformities. These should be worn as prescribed. If the child is confined to bed, the nurse should consult with the physical therapist regarding proper use of orthopedic appliances.

Vital signs should be taken frequently, and the pulse should be counted for 1 full minute to detect irregularities. Report a decrease in pulse rate, since it may signal severe bradycardia and cardiac arrest. The diet needs supervision to ensure compliance with low-phosphate foods, particularly dairy products. The nurse should instruct parents regarding foods to avoid and the necessity of administering calcium and vitamin D.

If surgery is anticipated, care is similar to that discussed for the child with hyperthyroidism. Because hypocalcemia is a potential complication, observing for signs of tetany, instituting seizure precautions, and having calcium gluconate available for emergency use are part of the nursing care.

DISORDERS OF ADRENAL FUNCTION

ADRENAL HORMONES

The adrenal glands consist of two distinct portions: the cortex, or outer section, and the medulla, or inner core. The adrenal cortex secretes hormones, collectively called steroids, which are essential to life. The adrenal medulla produces the catecholamines, epinephrine and norepinephrine. Because these chemicals are also produced by the sympathetic nervous system, absence of the adrenal supply is compatible with life.

Adrenal Cortex

The cortex secretes three groups of hormones that are classified according to their biologic activity: (1) glucocorticoids (cortisol, corticosterone), (2) mineralocorticoids (aldosterone), and (3) sex steroids (androgens, estrogens, and progestins). The glucocorticoids and mineralocorticoids influence metabolic regulation and stress adaptation. The sex steroids influence sexual development but are not essential because the gonads secrete the major supply of these hormones.

Glucocorticoids

The most important glucocorticoids in humans are cortisol and corticosterone, the principal effects of which are listed in Box 38-10. Normally the hypothalamus secretes CRF, which causes the pituitary gland to produce ACTH, which stimulates the adrenal glands to synthesize glucocorticoids (primarily cortisol). The switch that controls this feedback is cortisol. When blood levels of cortisol are low, the system turns on. When blood levels of cortisol rise, the system turns off.

In times of stress the anterior pituitary is stimulated by CRF from the hypothalamus, which causes the release of increased amounts of ACTH. Stressful stimuli capable of provoking this response include trauma; anesthesia; surgical intervention; sepsis; acute anoxia; hypothermia; hypoglycemia; and emotional states, especially panic, anxiety, or anger.

BOX 38-10 PHYSIOLOGIC EFFECTS OF GLUCOCORTICOIDS

- Stimulation of gluconeogenesis by the liver (a hyperglycemic effect)
- Increased protein catabolism with resulting reduction in protein stores (except in the liver)
- Increased mobilization and utilization of fatty acids for energy
- Increased storage of adipose tissue in certain sites
- Decreased inflammatory and allergic reactions
- Regulation of fluid and electrolytes by promoting sodium retention and potassium excretion by the kidneys and by water diuresis through direct antagonistic action against antidiuretic hormone
- Increased gastric acid and pepsin production
- Suppression of lymphocytes, eosinophils, and basophils, but elevation of neutrophils, erythrocytes, and thrombocytes

Body rhythms also regulate secretion of the glucocorticoids. Blood levels of cortisol demonstrate a typical diurnal or circadian pattern. In individuals who follow a regular routine of nighttime sleeping, cortisol levels are highest in the early morning hours after arising and lowest in the evening hours before bedtime.

Mineralocorticoids

The most important mineralocorticoid is aldosterone. Like cortisol, it promotes sodium retention and potassium excretion in the renal tubules. The effect of aldosterone is many times more potent than that of the glucocorticoids in maintaining extracellular fluid volume, acid-base balance, and normal potassium levels.

Aldosterone synthesis is regulated primarily by the renin-angiotensin system of the kidney. A block in aldosterone synthesis causes high plasma renin activity levels (Huether, 2000). The juxtaglomerular cells of the kidney respond to decreased arterial pressure or blood volume and to decreased sodium concentrations by secreting the enzyme renin into the blood. Renin in turn converts angiotensinogen to angiotensin I and then to angiotensin II. Increased levels of angiotensin stimulate the adrenal cortex to secrete aldosterone, which preserves sodium, thereby retaining water. The renin-angiotensin mechanism also results in increased blood pressure.

Sex Steroids

Except for the first few days of life, the sex hormones are normally secreted in only minimum amounts until adolescence, at which time they play a role in pubertal changes. Their actions are the same as those of the gonadal hormones on internal and external sexual structures and skeletal growth.

Adrenal Medulla

The adrenal medulla secretes the catecholamines epinephrine and norepinephrine. Both hormones have essentially the same effects on different organs as those caused by direct sympathetic stimulation, except that the hormonal effects last several times longer. Their major actions are listed in Box 38-11.

Although the catecholamines evoke similar responses from target sites, there are some important differences. Epinephrine has a greater effect on cardiac activity than norepinephrine, but it causes only weak constriction of the blood vessels of muscles in comparison with the effect of norepinephrine. As a result, norepinephrine elevates blood pressure, whereas epinephrine increases cardiac output. Another important difference is their

---

BOX 38-11   PHYSIOLOGIC EFFECTS OF CATECHOLAMINE SECRETION

- Increased cardiac activity
- Vasoconstriction of blood vessels (elevation of blood pressure)
- Increased rate and depth of respirations
- Bronchial dilation
- Inhibition of gastrointestinal activity
- Increased muscular contraction
- Pupillary dilation
- Increased metabolic rate
- Heightened sensory awareness
- Diaphoresis

---

effect on metabolism. Epinephrine increases the metabolic rate to a much greater extent than norepinephrine. These differences in action have been attributed to the catecholamines' effects on α- or β-adrenergic receptors. Supposedly norepinephrine can only affect those effector cells that contain α-receptors, which are mostly excitatory (constriction and contraction). Epinephrine, however, can affect both α- and β-receptors, and β-receptors are mostly inhibitory (dilation and relaxation). Control of secretion of catecholamines, primarily in response to physiologic or emotional stress, is through the hypothalamus. Also, stimulation of the sympathetic nervous system results in the release of epinephrine and norepinephrine from the sympathetic nerves and adrenal medulla. Both systems support each other, and one can be substituted for the other. For this reason no condition is attributable to hypofunction of the adrenal medulla. Even in bilateral adrenalectomy, catecholamine replacement is not necessary because the sympathetic release of these chemicals is sufficient to meet all the physiologic functions required to cope with stressful events.

Catecholamine-secreting tumors are the primary cause of adrenal medullary hyperfunction. In children the most common neoplasms of this type are pheochromocytoma (see p. 1593), neuroblastoma, and ganglioneuroma. Ganglioneuromas are neuroblastomas that have undergone maturation into a benign tumor composed of ganglion cells. These tumors are associated with less abnormal catecholamine secretion than the other two types, but persons with ganglioneuromas may have a clinical picture of chronic diarrhea, failure to thrive, skin rash, hypokalemia, persistent cough, and abdominal distention. The exact reason for these symptoms is unknown, although they are attributable to the tumor because they disappear after surgical removal of the mass.

ACUTE ADRENOCORTICAL INSUFFICIENCY

The acute form of adrenocortical insufficiency (adrenal crisis) may have a number of causes during childhood. Although a rare disorder, some of the more common etiologic factors include hemorrhage into the gland from trauma, which may be caused by a prolonged, difficult labor and rapidly progressing infections, such as meningococcemia, which result in hemorrhage and necrosis (Waterhouse-Friderichsen syndrome). Abrupt withdrawal of exogenous sources of cortisone or failure to increase endogenous supplies during stressor congenital adrenogenital hyperplasia of the salt-losing type can also cause adrenal crisis.

Clinical Manifestations

Early symptoms of adrenocortical insufficiency include increased irritability, headache, diffuse abdominal pain, weakness, nausea and vomiting, and diarrhea. Generalized hemorrhagic manifestations are present in Waterhouse-Friderichsen syndrome. Abnormal serum electrolyte levels include hyponatremia and hyperkalemia. Fever increases as the condition worsens and is accompanied by signs of CNS involvement, such as nuchal rigidity, convulsions, stupor, and coma. The child is in a shocklike state with a weak, rapid pulse; decreased blood pressure; shallow respirations; cold, clammy skin; and cyanosis. Circulatory collapse is the terminal event.

In the newborn, adrenal crisis is accompanied by extreme hyperpyrexia (high temperature), tachypnea, cyanosis, and seizures. Usually there is no evidence of infection or purpura. However, hemorrhage into the adrenal gland may be evident as a palpable retroperitoneal mass.

Diagnostic Evaluation

There is no rapid, definitive test for confirmation of acute adrenocortical insufficiency. Samples for measurement of plasma cortisol and ACTH levels should be sent for analysis, but this is too time-consuming to be practical for initial diagnosis. Therefore diagnosis is usually made based on clinical presentation, especially when a fulminating sepsis is accompanied by hemorrhagic manifestations and signs of circulatory collapse despite adequate antibiotic therapy. Serum electrolytes can be helpful in narrowing the diagnosis as well. Because there is no real danger in administering a cortisol preparation for a short period, institute treatment immediately. Improvement with cortisol therapy confirms the diagnosis.

Therapeutic Management

Treatment involves replacement of cortisol, replacement of body fluids to combat dehydration and hypovolemia, administration of glucose solutions to correct hypoglycemia, and specific antibiotic therapy in the presence of infection. Initially IV hydrocortisone (Solu-Cortef) is administered as a bolus, followed by a continuous infusion for 24 hours. Normal saline containing 5% glucose is given parenterally to replace lost fluid, electrolytes, and glucose. Persistent hyperkalemia that is associated with electrocardiographic changes may require the use of insulin and glucose or Kayexalate to reduce the potassium levels. If hemorrhage has been severe, whole blood may be replaced. In the event that these measures do not reverse the circulatory collapse, vasopressors are used for immediate vasoconstriction and elevation of blood pressure.

Once the child's condition is stabilized, oral doses of cortisone, fluids, and salt are given, similar to the regimen used for chronic adrenal insufficiency. To maintain sodium retention, synthetic salt-retaining steroids replace aldosterone.

Nursing Care Management

Because of the abrupt onset and potentially fatal outcome of this condition, prompt recognition is essential. Vital signs and blood pressure are taken every 15 minutes to monitor the hyperpyrexia and shocklike state. Seizure precautions are instituted, since convulsions from the elevated temperature are not uncommon. As soon as therapy is instituted, the nurse should monitor the child's response to fluid and cortisol replacement. Too rapid administration of fluids can precipitate cardiac failure, whereas overdosage with cortisol produces hypotension and a sudden fall in temperature.

QUALITY PATIENT OUTCOMES: Acute Adrenocortical Insufficiency

- Early recognition of signs and symptoms of acute adrenal crisis
- Hypokalemia or hyperkalemia prevented
- Fluid balance maintained
- Sufficient cortisol replacement

The nurse should regulate IV infusions carefully to guard against too rapid administration of drugs. The nurse should also record intake and urinary output and monitor electrolytes frequently.

Once the acute phase is over and the hypovolemia is corrected, give the child oral fluids, such as small quantities of ginger ale, fruit juice, or ice pops. Too rapid ingestion of oral fluids may induce vomiting, which increases dehydration. Therefore the nurse should plan a gradual schedule for reintroducing liquids. For children who refuse to drink, the prospect of having the IV infusion removed once oral fluids are increased is often a motivating factor.

! NURSING ALERT

Monitor serum electrolyte levels and observe for signs of hypokalemia or hyperkalemia (e.g., weakness, poor muscle control, paralysis, cardiac dysrhythmias, and apnea). The condition is rapidly corrected with IV or oral potassium replacement.

⚡ DRUG ALERT

Oral Potassium

When an oral potassium preparation is given, mix it with a small amount of strongly flavored fruit juice to disguise its bitter taste.

The sudden, severe nature of this disorder necessitates a great deal of emotional support for the child and family. The child may be placed in an intensive care unit where the surroundings are strange and frightening. Despite the need for emergency intervention, the nurse must be sensitive to the family's psychologic needs and prepare them for each procedure, even if this is as brief as a statement such as "The IV infusion is necessary to replace fluid that the child is losing." Because recovery within 24 hours is often dramatic, the nurse should keep the parents apprised of the child's condition, emphasizing signs of improvement, such as a lowered temperature and normal blood pressure.

If treatment needs to be continued past the acute stage, parents require the same preparation as in the case of children with chronic adrenal insufficiency. Preparation for discharge should begin as soon as possible after the child's condition has stabilized.

CHRONIC ADRENOCORTICAL INSUFFICIENCY (ADDISON DISEASE)

Chronic adrenocortical insufficiency is rare in children. Causes include infections (fungal, human immunodeficiency virus, tuberculosis), destructive lesions of the adrenal gland or neoplasms, and autoimmune processes, or the cause is idiopathic. At one time, generalized tuberculosis was the leading cause of adrenal gland destruction.

Evidence of this disorder is usually gradual in onset, since 90% of adrenal tissue must be nonfunctional before signs of insufficiency are manifested. However, during periods of stress, when demands for additional cortisol are increased, symptoms of acute insufficiency may appear in a previously well child (Table 38-1).

TABLE 38-1	CLINICAL MANIFESTATIONS OF ADRENOCORTICAL INSUFFICIENCY	
SIGNS AND SYMPTOMS	**CLINICAL MANIFESTATIONS**	
Glucocorticoid		
Fasting hypoglycemia	Headache, diaphoresis, weakness, trembling, hunger, seizures (rare)	
Decreased gastric acidity	Anorexia, nausea, vomiting	
Fatigue	Increased sleeping, listlessness	
Psychologic symptoms	Irritability, apathy, negativism	
Mineralocorticoid		
Muscle weakness	Generalized weakness that is aggravated by slight additional exertion or minor illness	
Weight loss	Dehydration and anorexia	
Fatigue	Increased sleeping, listlessness	
Gastrointestinal symptoms	Nausea, vomiting, anorexia	
Nutritional symptoms	Salt craving	
Circulatory symptoms	Hypotension, small heart size, syncope (fainting), dizziness	
Electrolyte imbalances	Hyperkalemia, hyponatremia, acidosis	
Psychologic symptoms	Irritability, apathy, negativism	
Androgen Deficiency (Older Children and Adults)		
Integumentary changes	Decreased pubic and axillary hair	
Psychologic symptoms	Decreased libido	
Increased ACTH and β-Lipotropin		
Dermatologic changes	Hyperpigmentation (elbow, knees, waist), pigmentary changes of previous scars, palmar creases	

ACTH, Adrenocorticotropic hormone.

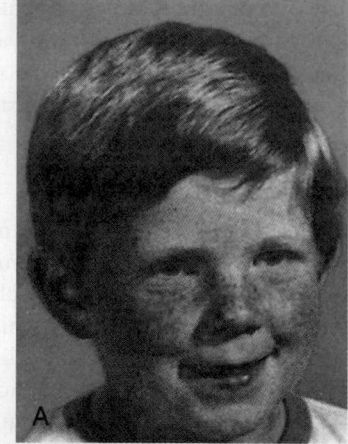
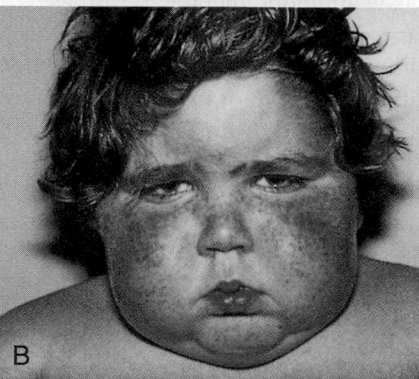

Fig. 38-4 A, Boy before development of Cushing syndrome. **B,** Same boy 4 months after onset of Cushing syndrome. (From Zitelli BJ, Davis HW: *Atlas of pediatric physical diagnosis*, ed 5, St Louis, 2007, Mosby.)

The initial step in the laboratory diagnosis of adrenal insufficiency is measurement of a fasting serum cortisol and ACTH in the early morning. An ACTH stimulation test can confirm the diagnosis. The cortisol and urinary 17-hydroxycorticosteroid levels are low and fail to rise, whereas plasma ACTH levels are elevated with corticotropin (ACTH) stimulation, the definitive test for the disease.

Therapeutic Management

Treatment involves replacement of glucocorticoids (cortisol) and mineralocorticoids (aldosterone). Some children are able to be maintained solely on oral supplements of cortisol (cortisone or hydrocortisone preparations) with a liberal intake of salt. During stressful situations, such as fever, infection, emotional upset, or surgery, the dosage must be tripled to accommodate the body's increased need for glucocorticoids. Failure to meet this requirement will precipitate an acute crisis. Overdosage produces appearance of cushingoid signs (Fig. 38-4).

Children with more severe states of chronic adrenal insufficiency require mineralocorticoid replacement to maintain fluid and electrolyte balance. Other forms of therapy include monthly injections of desoxycorticosterone acetate or implantation of desoxycorticosterone acetate pellets subcutaneously every 9 to 12 months.

Nursing Care Management

Once the disorder is diagnosed, parents need guidance concerning drug therapy. They must be aware of the continuous

need for cortisol replacement. Sudden termination of the drug because of inadequate supplies or inability to ingest the oral form because of vomiting places the child in danger of an acute adrenal crisis. Therefore parents should always have a spare supply of the medication in the home. Ideally they will have a prefilled syringe of hydrocortisone and be instructed in proper technique for intramuscular administration of the drug in case of crisis. Unnecessary administration of cortisone will not harm the child, but if it is needed, it may be lifesaving. Report any evidence of acute insufficiency to the practitioner immediately.

Parents also need to be aware of side effects of the drugs. Undesirable side effects of cortisone include gastric irritation, which is minimized by ingestion with food or the use of an antacid; increased excitability and sleeplessness; weight gain that may require dietary management to prevent obesity; and, rarely, behavioral changes, including depression or euphoria. Parents should be aware of signs of overdose and report these to the practitioner. In addition, the drug has a bitter taste, which creates a challenge for nurses and parents in its administration.

NURSING TIP Taste a drop of the different preparations of cortisone; some are less bitter than others. Although using the concentrated form means a smaller volume of liquid to ingest, this form is also the most bitter.

⚡ DRUG ALERT
Mineralocorticoids

The side effects of mineralocorticoids are primarily caused by overdosage and include generalized edema, which is first noticed around the eyes; hypertension, which may cause headaches; cardiac arrhythmias; and signs of hypokalemia. Evaluate the child periodically for evidence of excessive medication. Emphasizing the importance of routine follow-up care is a significant nursing responsibility.

BOX 38-12   ETIOLOGY OF CUSHING SYNDROME

Pituitary—Cushing syndrome with adrenal hyperplasia, usually attributed to an excess of adrenocorticotropic hormone (ACTH)

Adrenal—Cushing syndrome with oversecretion of glucocorticoids, generally the result of adrenocortical neoplasms

Ectopic—Cushing syndrome with autonomous secretion of ACTH, most often caused by extrapituitary neoplasms

Iatrogenic—Frequently the result of administration of large amounts of exogenous corticosteroids

Food dependent—Inappropriate sensitivity of adrenal glands to normal postprandial increases in secretion of gastric inhibitory polypeptide

Because the body cannot supply endogenous sources of cortical hormones during times of stress, the home environment should be stable and relatively unstressful. Parents need to be aware that during periods of emotional or physical crisis the child requires additional hormone replacement. The child should wear medical identification, such as a bracelet, to permit medical personnel to adjust requirements during emergency care.

CUSHING SYNDROME

Cushing syndrome is a characteristic group of manifestations caused by excessive circulating free cortisol. It can result from a variety of causes, which generally fall into one of five categories (Box 38-12 and Table 38-2). Cushing syndrome in young children may be due to an adrenal tumor (Moshang, 2003).

Cushing syndrome is uncommon in children. When seen, it is often caused by excessive or prolonged steroid therapy that produces a cushingoid appearance (see Fig. 38-4). This condition is reversible once the steroids are gradually discontinued. Abrupt withdrawal precipitates acute adrenal insufficiency. Gradual withdrawal of exogenous supplies is necessary to allow the anterior pituitary an opportunity to secrete increasing amounts of ACTH to stimulate the adrenals to produce cortisol.

Clinical Manifestations

Because the actions of cortisol are widespread, clinical manifestations are equally profound and diverse (see Table 38-2). Those symptoms that produce changes in physical appearance occur early in the disorder and are of considerable concern to school-age and older children (Fig. 38-5). The physiologic disturbances, such as hyperglycemia, susceptibility to infection, hypertension, and hypokalemia, may have life-threatening consequences unless recognized early and treated successfully.

TABLE 38-2   CLINICAL MANIFESTATIONS OF CUSHING SYNDROME

SIGNS AND SYMPTOMS	PHYSIOLOGIC CAUSE

Centripetal fat distribution
  Truncal obesity
  Supraclavicular fat pads
  Fat pads on neck and back (buffalo hump)
Rounded or "moon" face
	Increased appetite and deposition of fat

Muscular wasting
  Thin extremities
  Pendulous abdomen
  Muscle weakness
Thin skin and subcutaneous tissue
Poor wound healing
	Increased protein catabolism resulting in negative nitrogen balance

Increased frequency of infection Decreased inflammatory response	Decreased production and circulating levels of antibodies by lysis of fixed plasma cells and lymphocytes
Excessive bruising Petechial hemorrhages Facial plethora ("red cheeks") Reddish purple abdominal striae	Capillary weakness resulting from loss of protein Thin skin that allows capillary blood to be visible; increased color from polycythemia
Hypertension—arteriosclerosis	Increased salt and water retention (hypervolemia)
Hypokalemia Alkalosis	Increased excretion of potassium and hydrogen ions

Osteoporosis
  Compression fractures of vertebrae
  Kyphosis
  Backache
  Retarded linear growth (short stature)
  Delayed bone age
	Increased glomerular filtration rate and excretion of calcium and decreased absorption of calcium from intestinal tract
	Increased levels of cortisol interfering with action of growth hormone

Hypercalciuria—renal calculi	Excessive amount of calcium in urine

Psychoses
  Irritability
  Insomnia
  Euphoria
  Depression
  Frank psychoses
	Cause unknown

Peptic ulcer	Increased production of hydrochloric acid and pepsin and decreased gastric mucus production
Hyperglycemia Glycosuria	Increased gluconeogenesis by liver and decreased rate of glucose utilization by cells
Latent or overt diabetes	Overstimulation of islets of Langerhans

Virilization
  Hirsutism (excessive body hair)
  Acne
  Deepening of voice
  Clitoral enlargement
  Tendency toward male physique in female
  Amenorrhea
  Impotence
	Excess production of androgens

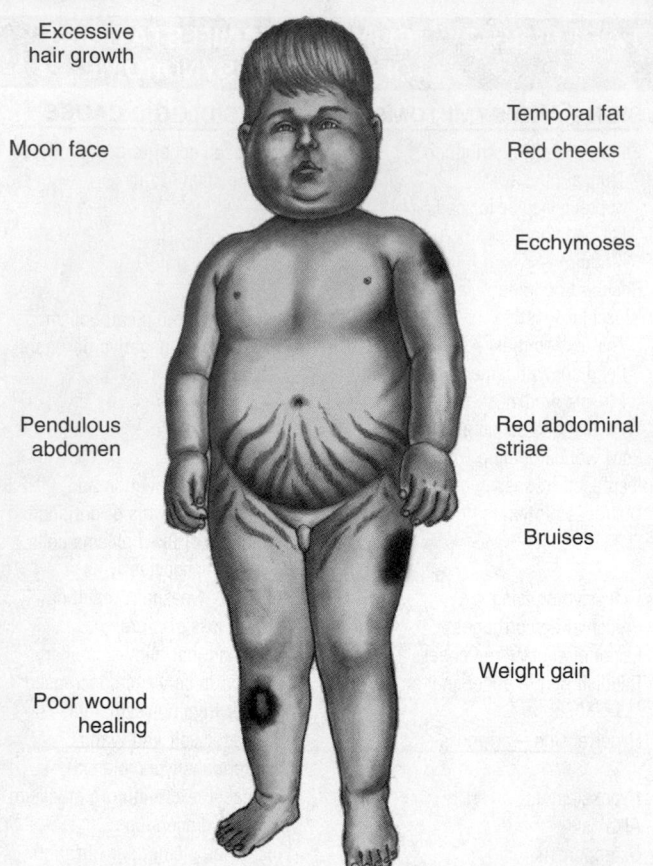

Excessive hair growth

Moon face

Temporal fat

Red cheeks

Ecchymoses

Pendulous abdomen

Red abdominal striae

Bruises

Weight gain

Poor wound healing

Fig. 38-5 Characteristics of Cushing syndrome.

Children with short stature may be responding to increased cortisol levels, resulting in Cushing syndrome. Cortisol inhibits the action of GH.

Diagnostic Evaluation

Several tests are helpful in confirming Cushing syndrome. Serum cortisol levels should be measured at midnight and in the morning, along with corticotropin hormone, urinary free cortisol, fasting blood glucose levels for hyperglycemia, serum electrolyte levels for hypokalemia and alkalosis, and 24-hour urinary levels of elevated 17-hydroxycorticoids and 17-ketosteroids. Imaging of the pituitary and adrenal glands to assess for tumors, bone density studies for evidence of osteoporosis, and skull x-rays examination to determine enlargement of the sella turcica may also aid in the diagnosis. Another procedure used to establish a more definitive diagnosis is the dexamethasone (cortisone) suppression test (Batista, Riar, Keil, et al, 2007). Administration of an exogenous supply of cortisone normally suppresses ACTH production. However, in individuals with Cushing syndrome, cortisol levels remain elevated. This test is helpful in differentiating between children who are obese and those who appear to have cushingoid features.

Therapeutic Management

Treatment depends on the cause. In most cases surgical intervention involves bilateral adrenalectomy and postoperative replacement of the cortical hormones (the therapy for this is the same as that outlined for chronic adrenal insufficiency). If a pituitary tumor is found, surgical extirpation or irradiation

may be chosen. In either of these instances, treatment of panhypopituitarism with replacement of GH, thyroid extract, ADH, gonadotropins, and steroids may be necessary for an indefinite period.

Nursing Care Management

Nursing care also depends on the cause. When cushingoid features are caused by steroid therapy, the effects may be lessened with administration of the drug early in the morning and on an alternate-day basis. Giving the drug early in the day maintains the normal diurnal pattern of cortisol secretion. If given during the evening, it is more likely to produce symptoms because endogenous cortisol levels are normally low and the additional supply exerts more pronounced effects. An alternate-day schedule allows the anterior pituitary an opportunity to maintain more normal hypothalamic-pituitary-adrenal control mechanisms.

If an organic cause is found, nursing care is related to the treatment regimen. Although a bilateral adrenalectomy permanently solves one condition, it reciprocally produces another syndrome. Before surgery, parents need to be adequately informed of the operative benefits and disadvantages. Postoperative teaching regarding drug replacement is the same as discussed in the previous section.

> **! NURSING ALERT**
>
> Postoperative complications of adrenalectomy are related to the sudden withdrawal of cortisol. Observe for shocklike symptoms (e.g., hypotension, hyperpyrexia).

Anorexia and nausea and vomiting are common and may be improved with the use of nasogastric decompression. Muscle and joint pain may be severe, requiring use of analgesics. The psychologic depression can be profound and may not improve for months. Parents should be aware of the physiologic reasons behind these symptoms in order to be supportive of the child.

CONGENITAL ADRENAL HYPERPLASIA

Congenital adrenal hyperplasia (CAH) is a family of disorders caused by decreased enzyme activity required for cortisol production in the adrenal cortex. The most common defect (accounting for >90% of cases) is 21-hydroxylase deficiency (American Academy of Pediatrics, 2000 [reaffirmed 2005]). This deficiency is an autosomal recessive disorder that results in improper steroid hormone synthesis. It occurs in approximately 1 per 12,000 to 15,000 births. In its most severe form, it can be life threatening (Glatt, Garzon, and Popovic, 2005).

Pathophysiology

Interference in the biosynthesis of cortisol during fetal life results in an increased production of ACTH, which stimulates hyperplasia of the adrenal gland. Depending on the enzymatic defect, increased quantities of cortisol precursors and androgens are secreted. There are six major types of biochemical defects. The most common is partial or complete 21-hydroxylase deficiency. With partial deficiency, enough aldosterone is produced to preserve sodium, and adequate cortisol is produced to prevent signs of adrenocortical insufficiency.

In the complete, or salt-losing, form, insufficient amounts of aldosterone and cortisol are produced. If salt-losing CAH is not diagnosed and treated at birth, infants will exhibit symptoms of failure to thrive, weakness, vomiting, and dehydration, and a salt-losing crisis will ensue (Behrman, Kliegman, Jenson, et al, 2009). In 11-hydroxylase deficiency there is an increase in the mineralocorticoid 11-desoxycorticosterone, which leads to hypertension. In each of these types excess production of androgens causes ambiguous genitalia in females and precocious genital development in males. Other forms of CAH do not result in excess production of androgens but cause various degrees of hypoaldosteronism or hyperaldosteronism.

Clinical Manifestations

Excessive androgens cause masculinization of the urogenital system at approximately the tenth week of fetal development. The most pronounced abnormalities occur in the female, who is born with varying degrees of ambiguous genitalia. Masculinization of external genitalia causes the clitoris to enlarge so that it appears as a small phallus. Fusion of the labia produces a saclike structure resembling the scrotum without testes. However, no abnormal changes occur in the internal sexual organs, although the vaginal orifice is usually closed by the fused labia. (See also Ambiguous Genitalia, Chapter 11.) The label **ambiguous genitalia** should be applied to any infant with hypospadias or micropenis and no palpable gonads, and a diagnostic evaluation for CAH should be contemplated. Males do not display genital abnormalities at birth (New and Ghizzoni, 2003), so it may go undetected.

Increased pigmentation of skin creases and genitalia caused by increased ACTH may be a subtle sign of adrenal insufficiency. A salt-wasting crisis frequently occurs, usually within the first few weeks of life (Behrman, Kliegman, Jenson, et al, 2009). Infants fail to gain weight, and hyponatremia and hyperkalemia may be significant. Cardiac arrest can occur.

Untreated CAH results in early sexual maturation, with enlargement of the external sexual organs; development of axillary, pubic, and facial hair; deepening of the voice; acne; and marked increase in musculature with changes toward an adult male physique. However, in contrast to precocious puberty, breasts do not develop in the female, and she remains amenorrheic and infertile. In the male the testes remain small, and spermatogenesis does not occur. In both sexes linear growth is accelerated, and epiphyseal closure is premature, resulting in short stature by the end of puberty.

Diagnostic Evaluation

Clinical diagnosis is initially based on congenital abnormalities that lead to difficulty in assigning sex to the newborn and on signs and symptoms of adrenal insufficiency. Newborn screening is currently done in all 50 U.S. states by measurement of the cortisol precursor 17-hydroxyprogesterone. Definitive diagnosis is confirmed by evidence of increased 17-ketosteroid levels in most types of CAH (American Academy of Pediatrics, 2000 [reaffirmed 2005]). In complete 21-hydroxylase deficiency, blood electrolytes demonstrate loss of sodium and chloride and elevation of potassium. In older children bone age is advanced,

and linear growth is increased. DNA analysis for positive sex determination and to rule out any other genetic abnormality (e.g., Turner syndrome) is done in any case of ambiguous genitalia.

Another test that can be used to visualize the presence of pelvic structures is ultrasonography, a noninvasive imaging technique that does not require anesthesia or sedation. It is especially useful in CAH because it readily identifies the presence of female reproductive organs or male testes in a newborn or child with ambiguous genitalia. Because ultrasonography yields immediate results, it has the advantage of determining the child's gender before the more complex laboratory results for chromosome analysis or steroid levels are available.

Therapeutic Management

After diagnosis is confirmed, medical management includes administration of glucocorticoids to suppress the abnormally high secretions of ACTH and adrenal androgens (Glatt, Garzon, and Popovic, 2005). If cortisone begins early enough, it is very effective. Cortisone depresses the secretion of ACTH by the adenohypophysis, which in turn inhibits the secretion of adrenocorticosteroids, which stems the progressive virilization. The signs and symptoms of masculinization in the female gradually disappear, and excessive early linear growth is slowed. Puberty occurs normally at the appropriate age.

The recommended oral dosage is divided to simulate the normal diurnal pattern of ACTH secretion. Because these children are unable to produce cortisol in response to stress, it is necessary to increase the dosage during episodes of infection, fever, or other stresses. Acute emergencies require immediate IV or intramuscular administration. Emergency situations include bacterial and viral infections, vomiting, surgery, fractures, major injuries, and sometimes insect stings.

Children with the salt-losing type of CAH require aldosterone replacement, as outlined under chronic adrenal insufficiency, and supplementary dietary salt. Frequent laboratory tests are conducted to assess the effects on electrolytes, hormonal profiles, and renin levels. The frequency of testing is individualized to the child.

Gender assignment and surgical intervention in the newborn with ambiguous genitalia is complex and controversial. It is a significant stress for families, who need support and education from a multidisciplinary team of experienced specialists. Factors that influence gender assignment include genetic diagnosis, genital appearance, surgical options, fertility, and family and cultural preferences. Generally, genetically female (46XX) infants should be raised as girls. Early reconstructive surgery should be considered only in the case of severe virilization (Lee, Houk, Ahmed, et al, 2006). Emphasis is on functional rather than cosmetic outcomes, and surgery can often be delayed. Reports concerning sexual satisfaction after partial clitoridectomy indicate that the capacity for orgasm and sexual gratification is not necessarily impaired. Male infants may require phallic reconstruction by an experienced surgeon.

Unfortunately, not all children with CAH are diagnosed at birth and raised in accordance with their genetic sex. Particularly in the case of affected females, masculinization of the external genitalia may have led to sex assignment as a male. In children with milder forms of CAH, especially males, diagnosis may be delayed until early childhood, when signs of virilism appear. In these situations it is usually advisable to continue rearing the child as a male in accordance with assigned sex and phenotype. Hormone replacement may be required to permit linear growth and to initiate male pubertal changes. Surgery is usually indicated to remove the female organs and reconstruct the phallus for satisfactory sexual relations. These individuals are not fertile.

Nursing Care Management

Of major importance is early recognition of ambiguous genitalia and diagnostic confirmation in newborns. As with any congenital defect, the parents require an adequate explanation of the condition and time to grieve for the loss of perfection. In this instance they may also need to grieve for the loss of the desired-sex child. For example, the birth of a phenotypically male infant may fulfill their wish for a son. Knowledge of the child's actual sex may leave them disappointed. Such situations may also lead them to discuss the possibility of raising the child as a boy despite the actual sex. This is a difficult question that requires thoughtful discussion among the parents and members of the health team.

In general, rearing the genetically female child as a girl is preferred because of the success of surgical intervention and the satisfactory results with hormones in reversing virilism and providing a prospect of normal puberty and the ability to conceive. This is in contrast to the choice of rearing the child as a boy, in which case the child is sterile and may never be able to function satisfactorily in heterosexual relationships. If the parents persist in their decision to assign a male sex to a genetically female child, request a psychologic consultation to explore their motivations and ensure their understanding of the future consequences for the child.

Parents need an explanation regarding this disorder that helps them explain it to others. When referring to the external genitalia, it is preferable to refer to them as sex organs and to emphasize the similarity between the penis-clitoris and scrotum-labia during fetal development. Explain that the sex organs were overdeveloped because of too much male hormone secretion. Using a correct vocabulary allows parents to explain the abnormalities to others in a straightforward manner, just as if the defect involved the heart or an extremity.

Parents often fear that the infant will retain "male behavioral characteristics" because of prenatal masculinization and will not be able to develop female characteristics. It is important to stress that gender identity and psychosexual development depend on multiple influences. Because the prognosis for normal sexual development is excellent after early treatment, the nurse should foster identification with the child as one sex only. Ambiguous genitalia have no relationship to sexual preference for partners later in life.

As soon as the sex is determined, inform parents of the findings and encourage them to choose an appropriate name and identify the child as a male or female, with no reference to ambiguous sex. If the appearance of the enlarged genitalia in a girl concerns the parents, encourage them to discuss their feelings. Suggesting ways to avoid questioning remarks from visitors, such as diapering the child in a separate room, is also helpful. If surgery is anticipated, showing parents before-and-after photographs of reconstruction helps to reinforce the expected cosmetic benefits.

Nursing care management regarding cortisol and aldosterone replacement are the same as those discussed for chronic adrenocortical insufficiency. A follow-up visit by a home health nurse may be desirable to ensure that parents understand and comply with the treatment regimen. Nurses in well-child facilities should assume responsibility for guidance and supervision regarding this aspect of care during each visit. Monitor vital signs closely for early signs of hypertension due to cortisol therapy.

Because infants are especially prone to dehydration and salt-losing crises, parents need to be aware of signs of dehydration and the urgency of immediate medical intervention to stabilize the child's condition. Parents should have injectable hydrocortisone available and know how to prepare and administer the intramuscular injection. (See Chapter 27.) Parents, and later the child, need to understand that the medical regimen must be a lifelong commitment; therefore provide them with the education and counseling that is most likely to ensure informed and willing compliance. They also need to know that growth retardation that may have occurred before therapy cannot be overcome and that normal stature is not a realistic expectation, even though growth velocity may improve with medication. Assess males for development of testicular tumors.

In the unfortunate situation in which the sex is erroneously assigned and the correct sex determined later, parents need a great deal of help in understanding the reason for the incorrect sex identification and the options for sex reassignment or medical-surgical intervention.

> ⚠ **NURSING ALERT**
>
> Advise the parents that there is no physical harm in treating for suspected adrenal insufficiency that is not present, whereas the consequence of not treating acute adrenal insufficiency can be fatal.

Because the hereditary form of adrenal hyperplasia is an autosomal recessive disorder, refer parents for genetic counseling before they conceive another child. The nurse's role is to ensure that parents understand the probability of transmitting the trait or disorder with each pregnancy. Prenatal diagnosis and treatment for CAH are available. Affected offspring also require genetic counseling, since both sexes are generally able to reproduce. (See Chapter 5 for recurrence risks and genetic counseling.)

HYPERALDOSTERONISM

Excessive secretion of aldosterone may be caused by an adrenal tumor or, in some types of adrenogenital syndromes, result from enzymatic deficiency. The signs and symptoms are caused by increased sodium levels, water retention, and potassium loss. Hypervolemia causes hypertension and resultant headaches. Paradoxically, funduscopic changes resulting from increased blood pressure and edema from water retention are minimal. Hypokalemia results in muscular weakness, paresthesia, episodes of paralysis, and tetany and may be responsible for polyuria and consequent polydipsia.

The clinical diagnosis is suspected when there are findings of hypertension, hypokalemia, and polyuria that fail to respond to ADH administration. Renin and angiotensin titers are abnormally low. Urinary levels of 17-hydroxycorticosteroids and 17-ketosteroids are normal in primary hyperaldosteronism caused by an aldosterone-secreting tumor but are usually abnormal in adrenogenital syndrome.

Therapeutic Management

Temporary treatment of the disorder involves replacement of potassium and administration of spironolactone (Aldactone), a diuretic that blocks the effects of aldosterone, thereby promoting excretion of sodium and water while preserving potassium. Definitive treatment is similar to that for chronic adrenocortical insufficiency.

Nursing Care Management

An important nursing consideration is recognition of the syndrome, particularly in children with high blood pressure. Other clues include bed-wetting, excessive thirst, and unexplained weakness. After the diagnosis, nursing care is related to the treatment regimen. If diuretics are used, they should be administered in the morning to avoid accidents during the night. Children need unrestricted restroom privileges at school. Potassium supplements should be mixed with fruit juice such as grape juice to increase their acceptability, and potassium-rich foods should be encouraged. Parents need to be aware of the signs of hypokalemia and hyperkalemia. After an adrenalectomy, nursing care is similar to that for chronic adrenocortical insufficiency.

PHEOCHROMOCYTOMA

Pheochromocytoma is a rare tumor characterized by secretion of catecholamines. The tumor most commonly arises from the chromaffin cells of the adrenal medulla but may occur wherever these cells are found, such as along the paraganglia of the aorta or thoracolumbar sympathetic chain. Approximately 10% of these tumors are located in extraadrenal sites. In children they are frequently bilateral or multiple and are generally benign. Often there is a familial transmission of the condition as an autosomal dominant trait (Behrman, Kliegman, Jenson, et al, 2009).

Clinical Manifestations

The clinical manifestations of pheochromocytoma are caused by an increased production of catecholamines, producing hypertension, tachycardia, headache, decreased gastrointestinal activity with resultant constipation, increased metabolism with anorexia, weight loss, hyperglycemia, polyuria, polydipsia, hyperventilation, nervousness, heat intolerance, and diaphoresis. In severe cases, signs of congestive heart failure are evident.

Diagnostic Evaluation

The clinical manifestations mimic those of other disorders, such as hyperthyroidism or DM. Tests specific to these conditions may be performed as part of the differential diagnosis. In a small number of instances a palpable tumor suggests the diagnosis. Usually the tumor is identified by a CT scan or MRI.

Definitive tests include 24-hour measurement of urinary levels of the catecholamine metabolites; histamine stimulation, which provokes a hypertensive attack from sudden release of large amounts of catecholamines; and α-adrenergic blocking agents, which produce a hypotensive episode by inhibiting the action of circulating catecholamines.

Therapeutic Management

Definitive treatment consists of surgical removal of the tumor. In children the tumors may be bilateral, requiring a bilateral adrenalectomy and lifelong glucocorticoid and mineralocorticoid therapy. The major complications that can occur during surgery are severe hypertension, tachyarrhythmias, and hypotension. The first two are caused by excessive release of catecholamines during manipulation of the tumor, and the latter results from catecholamine withdrawal and hypovolemic shock.

Preoperative medication to inhibit the effects of catecholamines is begun 1 to 3 weeks before surgery to prevent these complications. The major group of drugs used is the α-adrenergic blocking agents with or without β-adrenergic blocking agents. The most commonly used α-adrenergic blocker is phenoxybenzamine (Dibenzyline), a longer-acting medication given orally every 12 hours. The shorter-acting phentolamine (Regitine) is equally effective but less satisfactory for long-term use, although it is useful for acute hypertension. To control catecholamine release when α-adrenergic blocking agents are inadequate, the child is given β-adrenergic blocking agents.

Success of therapy is judged by lowering of blood pressure to normal, absence of hypertensive attacks (flushing or blanching, fainting, headache, palpitations, tachycardia, nausea and vomiting, profuse sweating), heat tolerance, decrease in perspiration, and disappearance of hyperglycemia. A disadvantage of these drugs is their inability to block the effects of catecholamines on β-receptors.

Nursing Care Management

An initial nursing objective is identification of children with this disorder. Outstanding clues are hypertension and hypertensive attacks. Because of behavioral changes (nervousness, excitability, overactivity, even psychosis), increased cardiac and respiratory activity may appear to be related to an acute anxiety attack. Therefore a careful history of the onset of symptoms and association with stressful events is helpful in distinguishing between an organic and a psychologic cause for the symptoms.

Preoperative nursing care involves frequent monitoring of vital signs and observation for evidence of hypertensive attacks and congestive heart failure. Therapeutic effects are evidenced by normal vital signs and absence of glycosuria. Note daily blood glucose levels and urine acetone; report any signs of hyperglycemia immediately.

The environment is made conducive to rest and free of emotional stress. This requires adequate preparation during hospital admission and before surgery. Encourage parents to room-in with their child and to participate in care. Play activities need to be tailored to the child's energy level without being overly strenuous or challenging because these can increase metabolic rate and promote frustration and anxiety.

> ⚠ **NURSING ALERT**
>
> Do not palpate the mass. Preoperative palpation of the mass releases catecholamines, which can stimulate severe hypertension and tachyarrhythmias.

After surgery observe the child for signs of shock from removal of excess catecholamines. If a bilateral adrenalectomy was performed, the nursing interventions are those discussed for chronic adrenocortical insufficiency.

DISORDERS OF PANCREATIC HORMONE SECRETION

DIABETES MELLITUS

DM is a chronic disorder of metabolism characterized by a partial or complete deficiency of the hormone insulin. It is the most common metabolic disease, resulting in metabolic adjustment or physiologic change in almost all areas of the body. Approximately one in three children born in the United States will develop diabetes. The odds are higher for African-American and Hispanic children: nearly 50% of them will develop diabetes (Urrutia-Rojas and Menchaca, 2006). The age of presentation of childhood-onset type 1 DM has a bimodal distribution, with one peak at 4 to 6 years of age and another at early puberty (10 to 14 years of age) (Felner, Klitz, Ham, et al, 2005). The incidence in boys is slightly higher than girls (1:1 to 1.2:1).

Type 1 DM is more prominent in Caucasians, with an incidence of 24 per 100,0000 (Dabelea, Bell, and D'Agostino, 2007). The incidence in African-Americans is 11 per 100,0000; the incidence in Hispanics is 15.2 per 100,0000; and the incidence in Cubans is 2.6 per 100,0000. Native Americans tend to develop type 2 DM rather than type 1 DM, even when diagnosed in childhood. The Pima Tribe reports a greater than 55% incidence of type 2 DM.

Classification

Traditionally DM had been classified according to the type of treatment needed. The old categories were insulin-dependent diabetes mellitus (IDDM), or type I; and non–insulin-dependent diabetes mellitus (NIDDM), or type II. In 1997 these terms were eliminated because treatment can vary (some people with NIDDM require insulin) and because the terms do not indicate the underlying problem. The new terms are type 1 and type 2, using Arabic symbols to avoid confusion (e.g., type II could be read as type eleven) (American Diabetes Association, 2001). The characteristics of type 1 DM and type 2 DM are compared in Table 38-3.

Type 1 diabetes is characterized by destruction of the pancreatic beta cells, which produce insulin; this usually leads to absolute insulin deficiency (Fig. 38-6). Type 1 diabetes has two forms. Immune-mediated DM results from an autoimmune destruction of the beta cells; it typically starts in children or young adults who are slim, but it can arise in adults of any age. Idiopathic type 1 refers to rare forms of the disease that have no known cause.

TABLE 38-3	CHARACTERISTICS OF TYPES 1 AND 2 DIABETES MELLITUS	
CHARACTERISTIC	**TYPE 1**	**TYPE 2**
Age at onset	<20 yr	Increasingly occurring in younger children
Type of onset	Abrupt	Gradual
Sex ratio	Males slightly more than females	Females outnumber males
Percentage of diabetic population	5%-8%	85%-90%
Heredity:		
Family history	Sometimes	Frequently
Human leukocyte antigen	Associations	No association
Twin concordance	25%-50%	90%-100%
Ethnic distribution	Primarily Caucasians	Increased incidence in Native Americans, Hispanics, African-Americans
Presenting symptoms	3 Ps common: polyuria, polydipsia, polyphagia	May be related to long-term complications
Nutritional status	Underweight	Overweight
Insulin (natural):		
Pancreatic content	Usually none	>50% normal
Serum insulin	Low to absent	High or low
Primary resistance	Minimum	Marked
Islet cell antibodies	80%-85%	<5%
Therapy:		
Insulin	Always	20%-30% of patients
Oral agents	Ineffective	Often effective
Diet only	Ineffective	Often effective
Chronic complications	>80%	Variable
Ketoacidosis	Common	Infrequent

Type 2 diabetes usually arises because of insulin resistance, in which the body fails to use insulin properly, combined with relative (rather than absolute) insulin deficiency. People with type 2 can range from predominantly insulin resistant with relative insulin deficiency to predominantly deficient in insulin secretion with some insulin resistance. It typically occurs in those who are over 45, are overweight and sedentary, and have a family history of diabetes.

Several other specific types of DM have been defined, such as those resulting from genetic defects of beta cell function, pancreatic diseases (e.g., cystic fibrosis), and defects in insulin action. **Maturity-onset diabetes of the young (MODY)** is associated with monogenetic defects in beta cell function that are characterized by impaired insulin secretion with minimum or no defects in insulin action. The disease is inherited as an autosomal dominant pattern, and the onset of hyperglycemia occurs at an early age (generally before age 25 years).

Etiology

The clinical syndrome of DM results from a large variety of etiologic and pathogenic mechanisms. Type 1 DM is an autoimmune disease that arises when a person with a genetic predisposition is exposed to a precipitating event, such as a viral infection. Type 2 DM is more likely to be influenced by stronger, but as yet unknown, genetic factors. Thus its origin is considered to be polygenic.

PATHOPHYSIOLOGY REVIEW

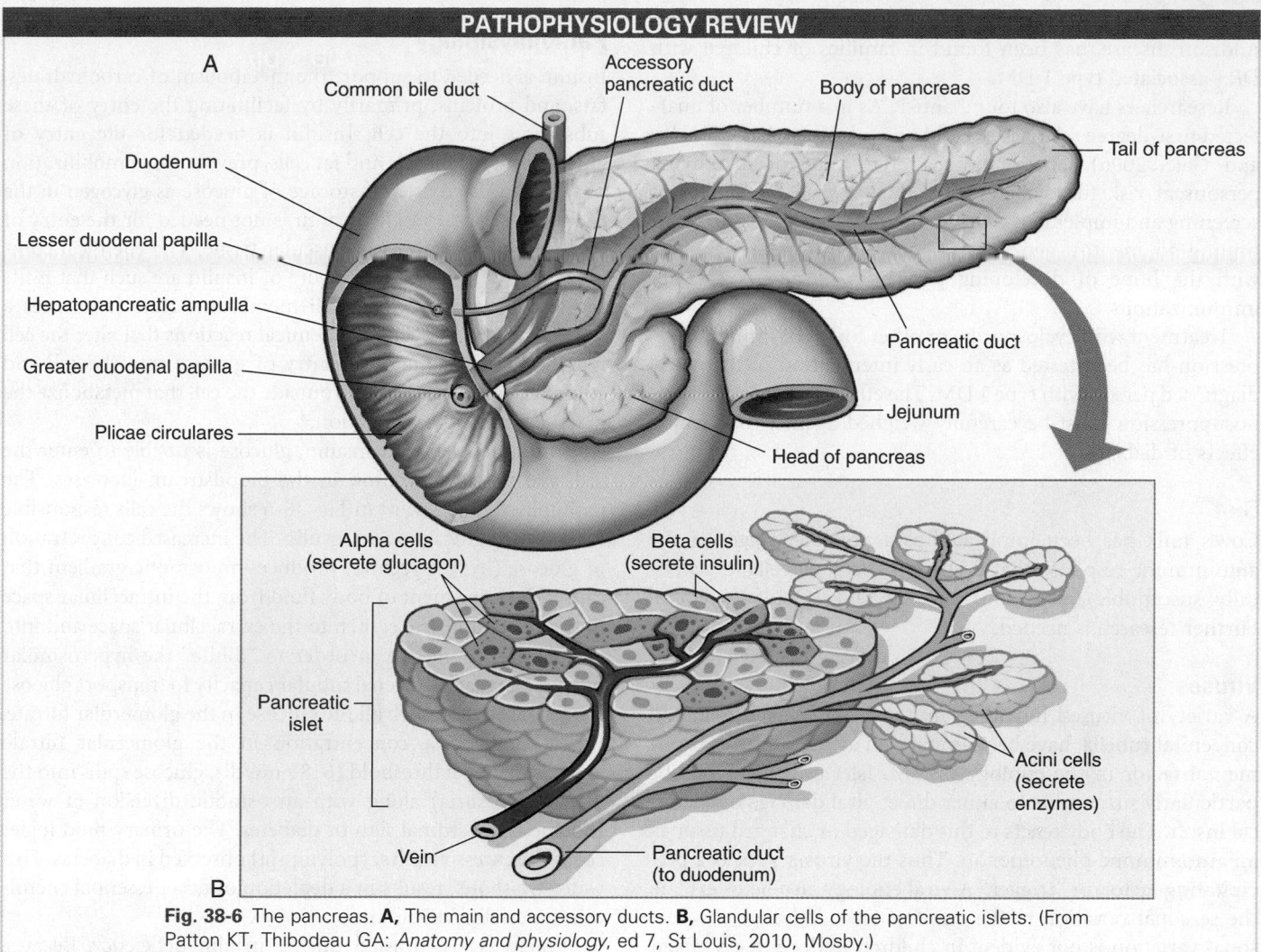

Fig. 38-6 The pancreas. **A,** The main and accessory ducts. **B,** Glandular cells of the pancreatic islets. (From Patton KT, Thibodeau GA: *Anatomy and physiology*, ed 7, St Louis, 2010, Mosby.)

Genetic Factors

Type 1 DM is not inherited, but heredity is a prominent factor in the etiology. In more than 40 rare genetic syndromes, diabetes is a major feature (Harris, 2003). No simple mendelian pattern is found for DM. Children born to fathers with type 1 DM are about three times more likely to develop type 1 DM (approximately 7% frequency) than children born to mothers with type 1 DM (approximately 2% frequency) (see Research Focus box).

RESEARCH FOCUS

Genetic Factors and Diabetes

Studies of type 2 diabetes mellitus (DM) in identical twins demonstrate a 100% concordance throughout the life span, whereas studies of type 1 DM in identical twins demonstrate a 30% to 50% concordance rate, suggesting that both environmental and genetic factors are important in the development of type 1 DM (Stephenson, 2003). Children diagnosed with type 1 diabetes before 5 years of age may have different autoimmune and genetic characteristics related to their diabetes than older children (Hathout, Hartwick, Fagoaga, et al, 2003).

At least 60% of the genetic susceptibility to type 1 diabetes is conferred by human leukocyte antigen (HLA) on chromosome 6. Several alleles have been implicated, including *DR3*, *DR4*, and *DQ8*. The highest-risk alleles *(DR3* and *DR4)* are found in 95% of patients with diabetes. Only 50% of nondiabetic persons have these alleles. Certain alleles, such as *DR2*, may actually protect the individual from diabetes (Barker and Eisenbarth, 2003).

Autoimmune Mechanisms

Pancreatic islet cell antibodies (ICAs) are found in about 70% to 85% of patients newly diagnosed with type 1 DM. The antibodies disappear by 1 year after diagnosis in most persons, but in some they may persist for years. The current theory is that the presence of the HLA genes causes a defect in the immune system that renders the possessor susceptible to a trigger event, which can be a dietary source, a virus, bacteria, or a chemical irritant. The predisposing factor initiates an autoimmune process that gradually destroys beta cells. Without beta cells, the body cannot produce insulin. It is unclear whether the ICAs are a result of the inflammatory process or a significant aspect of the beta cell destruction. Controversy exists regarding whether the autoimmune response is primarily mediated by the lymphocyte response or the humoral (antibody) response or is a result of the two.

There is a strong association between type 1 DM and other autoimmune endocrine disorders. An increased incidence of other autoimmune endocrine disorders, such as thyroiditis and Addison disease, has been found in families of children with *DR3*-associated type 1 DM.

Researchers have also found anti-ICAs in a number of unaffected first-degree relatives of children with type 1 DM (Bingley and Gale, 2006). These findings offer hope of identifying persons at risk for diabetes with the eventual possibility of screening and implementation of therapy. Research is also continuing to identify genetic risk and environmental triggers with the hope of developing prevention strategies such as immunizations.

Treatment with cyclosporine or other forms of immunosuppression has been tested as an early intervention in the newly diagnosed person with type 1 DM. The effects of lifelong immunosuppression must be carefully weighed against the lifelong effects of diabetes.

Diet

Cow's milk has been implicated as a possible trigger of the autoimmune response that destroys pancreatic cells in genetically susceptible hosts, thus causing DM (Goldfarb, 2008). Further research is needed.

Viruses

A variety of viruses, including mumps, coxsackievirus B, and congenital rubella, have been implicated as the prime environmental factor in the etiology of DM. Islet cells appear to be particularly susceptible to either direct viral damage or chemical insult. The body reacts to this damaged or changed tissue in an autoimmune phenomenon. Thus the virus serves as a precipitating factor, or "trigger." A viral etiology also helps explain the seasonal variation in the onset of DM. Although this seasonal variation is not evident in children under 5 years of age, the marked increase in older children during the winter months strongly suggests an infectious disease relationship in either cause or expression of diabetes in children.

Type 2 Diabetes

Type 1 DM is the predominant form of diabetes in the pediatric age-group. However, changes in food consumption and exercise patterns have increased the rate of type 2 DM in children and adolescents in the Unites States (Ramchandani, 2004; Kiess, Bottner, Raile, et al, 2003; Steinberger and Daniels, 2003; Stephenson, 2003). The disturbed carbohydrate metabolism of type 2 DM may be a result of a sluggish or insensitive secretory response in the pancreas or a defect in body tissues that requires unusual amounts of insulin, or it may be that the insulin secreted is rapidly destroyed, inhibited, or inactivated in affected persons. Children with type 2 diabetes often have other features of insulin resistance syndrome: polycystic ovary syndrome and acanthosis nigricans (AN). AN is found in as many as 90% of children with type 2 diabetes and is characterized by velvety hyperpigmented areas in skinfolds. Risk factors include non-European ancestry, family history of type 2 DM, obesity, insulin resistance, and older age (American Diabetes Association, 2007). While performing routine scoliosis screenings, school nurses often identify AN on the child's neck. Refer such children to their primary care provider for further metabolic evaluation.

Pathophysiology

Insulin is needed to support the metabolism of carbohydrates, fats, and proteins, primarily by facilitating the entry of these substances into the cell. Insulin is needed for the entry of glucose into the muscle and fat cells, prevention of mobilization of fats from fat cells, and storage of glucose as glycogen in the cells of liver and muscle. Insulin is not needed for the entry of glucose into nerve cells or vascular tissue. The chemical composition and molecular structure of insulin are such that it fits into receptor sites on the cell membrane. Here it initiates a sequence of poorly defined chemical reactions that alter the cell membrane to facilitate the entry of glucose into the cell and stimulate enzymatic systems outside the cell that metabolize the glucose for energy production.

With a deficiency of insulin, glucose is unable to enter the cell, and its concentration in the bloodstream increases. The pathophysiology review in Fig. 38-6 shows the cells responsible for secreting glucagon and insulin. The increased concentration of glucose (hyperglycemia) produces an osmotic gradient that causes the movement of body fluid from the intracellular space to the interstitial space, then to the extracellular space and into the glomerular filtrate in order to "dilute" the hyperosmolar filtrate. Normally the renal tubular capacity to transport glucose is adequate to reabsorb all the glucose in the glomerular filtrate. When the glucose concentration in the glomerular filtrate exceeds the renal threshold (6180 mg/dl), glucose spills into the urine (glycosuria) along with an osmotic diversion of water (polyuria), a cardinal sign of diabetes. The urinary fluid losses cause the excessive thirst (polydipsia) observed in diabetes. This water "washout" results in a depletion of other essential chemicals, especially potassium.

Protein is also wasted during insulin deficiency. Because glucose is unable to enter the cells, protein is broken down and converted to glucose by the liver (glucogenesis); this glucose then contributes to the hyperglycemia. These mechanisms are similar to those seen in starvation when substrate (glucose) is absent. The body is actually in a state of starvation during insulin deficiency. Without the use of carbohydrates for energy, fat and protein stores are depleted as the body attempts to meet its energy needs. The hunger mechanism is triggered, but increased food intake (polyphagia) enhances the problem by further elevating blood glucose (Fig. 38-7).

Ketoacidosis

When insulin is absent or there is altered insulin sensitivity, glucose is unavailable for cellular metabolism, and the body chooses alternate sources of energy, principally fat. Consequently fats break down into fatty acids, and glycerol in the fat cells is converted by the liver to ketone bodies (β-hydroxybutyric acid, acetoacetic acid, acetone). Any excess is eliminated in the urine (ketonuria) or the lungs (acetone breath). The ketone bodies in the blood (ketonemia) are strong acids that lower serum pH, producing ketoacidosis.

Ketones are organic acids that readily produce excessive quantities of free hydrogen ions, causing a fall in plasma pH. Then chemical buffers in the plasma, principally bicarbonate, combine with the hydrogen ions to form carbonic acid, which readily dissociates into water and carbon dioxide. The

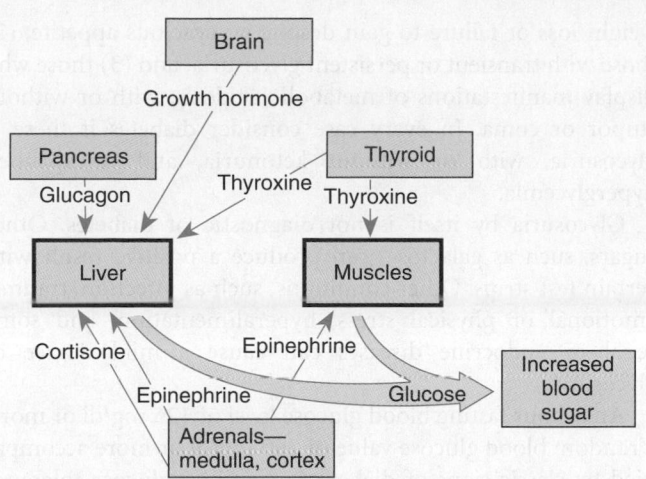

Fig. 38-7 Body systems respond to hypoglycemia in various ways to increase blood glucose level.

respiratory system attempts to eliminate the excess carbon dioxide by increased depth and rate—**Kussmaul respirations**, or the hyperventilation characteristic of metabolic acidosis. Sodium and potassium in the plasma buffer the ketones. The kidney attempts to compensate for the increased pH by increasing tubular secretion of hydrogen and ammonium ions in exchange for fixed base, thus depleting the base buffer concentration.

With cellular death, potassium is released from the cell (intracellular fluid) into the bloodstream (extracellular fluid) and excreted by the kidney, where the loss is accelerated by osmotic diuresis. The total body potassium is then decreased, even though the serum potassium level may be elevated as a result of the decreased fluid volume in which it circulates. Alteration in serum and tissue potassium can lead to cardiac arrest.

If insulin therapy in combination with correction of the fluid deficiency and electrolyte imbalance does not reverse these conditions, progressive deterioration occurs with dehydration, electrolyte imbalance, acidosis, coma, and death. **Diabetic ketoacidosis (DKA)** should be diagnosed promptly in a seriously ill patient and therapy instituted in an intensive care unit.

Long-Term Complications

Long-term complications of diabetes involve both the microvasculature and the macrovasculature. The principal microvascular complications are nephropathy, retinopathy, and neuropathy. Microvascular disease develops during the first 30 years of diabetes, beginning in the first 10 to 15 years after puberty, with renal involvement evidenced by proteinuria and clinically apparent retinopathy.

With poor diabetic control, vascular changes can appear as early as $2\frac{1}{2}$ to 3 years after diagnosis; however, with good to excellent control, changes can be postponed for 20 or more years. Intensive insulin therapy appears to delay the onset and slow the progression of clinically important retinopathy, including vision-threatening lesions, nephropathy, and neuropathy, by 35% to more than 70%, according to studies on treatment and complications of type 1 DM (American Diabetes Association, 2002).

The postpubertal duration, not the total duration, of type 1 DM is implicated as a risk factor for the development of microvascular disease. The process appears to be one of glycosylation, wherein proteins from the blood become deposited in the walls of small vessels (e.g., glomeruli), where they become trapped by "sticky" glucose compounds (glycosyl radicals). The buildup of these substances over time causes narrowing of the vessels, with subsequent interference with microcirculation to the affected areas (Rosenson and Herman, 2008). Macrovascular disease develops after 25 years of diabetes and creates the predominant problems in patients with type 2 DM.

Other complications have been observed in children with type 1 DM. Hypertension and atherosclerotic cardiovascular disease also contributes to the mortality and morbidity of type 1 DM (Karik, Fields, and Shannon, 2007). Hyperglycemia appears to influence thyroid function, and altered function is frequently observed at the time of diagnosis, as well as in poorly controlled diabetes. Limited mobility of small joints of the hand occurs in 30% of 7- to 18-year-old children with type 1 DM and appears to be related to changes in the skin and soft tissues surrounding the joint as a result of glycosylation.

Mild Diabetes

Although most cases of childhood diabetes are recognized during the rapid initial deterioration in carbohydrate metabolism, other cases with more benign disease are being identified with increasing frequency. A few are detected accidentally by urinalysis before overt symptoms occur. MODY, for instance, is a rare genetic type of diabetes resulting from mutations at one of five genes and transmission by an autosomal dominant inheritance (Fajans and Bell, 2003). Children with this type of diabetes phenotypically resemble type 2 DM but are usually not obese. MODY is characterized by beta cell dysfunction and is often treated similarly to type 2 DM.

Clinical Manifestations

The symptomatology of diabetes is more readily recognizable in children than in adults, so it is surprising that the diagnosis may sometimes be missed or delayed. Diabetes is a great imitator; influenza, gastroenteritis, and appendicitis are the conditions most often diagnosed when it turns out that the disease is really diabetes. Diabetes should be suspected in children with a strong family history of diabetes, especially if another child in the family has the disease.

The sequence of chemical events described previously results in hyperglycemia and acidosis, which produce weight loss and the three "polys" of diabetes—polyphagia, polydipsia, and polyuria—the cardinal symptoms of the disease. In type 2 DM the insulin values are elevated. Eighty percent to 90% of this population are overweight, and fatigue and frequent infections (such as candidal infections in females) are often present.

> **! NURSING ALERT**
>
> Recurrent vaginal and urinary tract infections, especially with *Candida albicans*, are often an early sign of type 2 DM, especially in adolescents.

The variability of clinical manifestations in type 1 DM at diagnosis is best understood if the autoimmune destruction of

---

BOX 38-13 CLINICAL MANIFESTATIONS OF TYPE 1 DIABETES MELLITUS

Polyphagia
Polyuria
Polydipsia
Weight loss
Enuresis or nocturia
Irritability; "not himself" or "herself"
Shortened attention span
Lowered frustration tolerance
Fatigue
Dry skin
Blurred vision
Poor wound healing
Flushed skin
Headache
Frequent infections
Hyperglycemia
- Elevated blood glucose levels
- Glucosuria
Diabetic ketosis
- Ketones and glucose in urine
- Dehydration in some cases
Diabetic ketoacidosis
- Dehydration
- Electrolyte imbalance
- Acidosis
- Deep, rapid breathing (Kussmaul)

---

islet cells is considered an ongoing process (Box 38-13). Symptoms of hyperglycemia may be apparent only during stress (such as an illness) in early stages of disease because of near-normal levels of insulin production. Progressive islet cell destruction of later stages produces more obvious signs and symptoms. By the time there are overt diabetic symptoms, 80% to 90% of islet cell function has been destroyed. Frequently identified symptoms of overt diabetes include enuresis, irritability, and unusual fatigue.

Abdominal discomfort is common. Weight loss, though observable on the charts, may be a less frequent presenting complaint because the family might not have noticed the change over time. Another outstanding feature of diabetes is thirst. One couple reported that their child, during a trip from California to Kansas, drank the contents of a gallon jug of water between each gas station stop. As abdominal discomfort and nausea increase, the child may actually refuse fluid and food, increasing the state of dehydration and malnutrition. Other symptoms include dry skin, blurred vision, and sores that are slow to heal. More commonly in children, fatigue and bed-wetting are the chief complaints that prompt parents to take their child for evaluation.

At diagnosis, the child may be hyperglycemic, with elevated blood glucose levels and glucose in the urine; ketotic, with ketones measurable in the blood and urine, with or without dehydration; or suffering from DKA, with dehydration, electrolyte imbalance, and acidosis.

Diagnostic Evaluation

Three groups of children who are candidates for diabetes are (1) children who have glycosuria, polyuria, and a history of weight loss or failure to gain despite a voracious appetite; (2) those with transient or persistent glycosuria; and (3) those who display manifestations of metabolic acidosis, with or without stupor or coma. In every case consider diabetes if there is glycosuria, with or without ketonuria, and unexplained hyperglycemia.

Glycosuria by itself is not diagnostic of diabetes. Other sugars, such as galactose, can produce a positive result with certain test strips. Other conditions, such as infection, trauma, emotional or physical stress, hyperalimentation, and some renal or endocrine diseases can cause a mild degree of glycosuria.

An 8-hour fasting blood glucose level of 126 mg/dl or more, a random blood glucose value of 200 mg/dl or more accompanied by classic signs of diabetes, or an oral glucose tolerance test (OGTT) finding of 200 mg/dl or more in the 2-hour sample is almost certain to indicate diabetes (American Diabetes Association, 2005). Postprandial blood glucose determinations and the traditional OGTTs have yielded low detection rates in children and are not usually necessary for establishing a diagnosis. Serum insulin levels may be normal or moderately elevated at the onset of diabetes; delayed insulin response to glucose indicates the presence of impaired glucose tolerance.

Ketoacidosis must be differentiated from other causes of acidosis or coma, including hypoglycemia, uremia, gastroenteritis with metabolic acidosis, salicylate intoxication encephalitis, and other intracranial lesions. DKA is a state of relative insulin insufficiency and may include the presence of hyperglycemia (blood glucose level 330 mg/dl), ketonemia (strongly positive), acidosis (pH 7.30 and bicarbonate 15 mmol/L), glycosuria, and ketonuria (Dunning, 2009). Tests used to determine glycosuria and ketonuria are the glucose oxidase tapes (Keto-Diastix).

Therapeutic Management

The management of the child with type 1 DM consists of a multidisciplinary approach involving the family; the child (when appropriate); and professionals, including a pediatric endocrinologist, diabetes nurse educator, nutritionist, and exercise physiologist. Often psychologic support from a mental health professional is also needed. Communication among the team members is essential and extends to other individuals in the child's life, such as teachers, school nurse, school guidance counselor, and coach (see Community Focus box).

The definitive treatment is replacement of insulin that the child is unable to produce. However, insulin needs are also affected by emotions, nutritional intake, activity, and other life events such as illnesses and puberty. The complexity of the disease and its management requires that the child and family incorporate diabetes needs into their lifestyle. Medical and nutritional guidance are primary, but management also includes continuing diabetes education, family guidance, and emotional support.

Insulin Therapy

Insulin replacement is the cornerstone of management of type 1 DM. Insulin dosage is tailored to each child based on home blood glucose monitoring. The goal of insulin therapy is maintaining near-normal blood glucose values while avoiding

🏠 COMMUNITY FOCUS

The Adolescent with Type 1 Diabetes Mellitus

As a nurse caring for adolescents with type 1 diabetes mellitus (DM), I am constantly aware of the wide range of adolescent behaviors that affect the course of this disease. Education of the child and the parents can often make the difference between a disease in control of the teen and a teen in control of the disease.

I have cared for many adolescent girls who have episodes of hyperglycemia at the time of menstruation that can result in diabetic ketoacidosis. I have found that education regarding sick-day protocol with sliding-scale regular insulin instituted at the first sign of hyperglycemia, which may occur 1 to 2 days before onset of menses, can keep the adolescent girl out of the intensive care unit and in control of her diabetes.

Eating disorders, such as bulimia or anorexia nervosa, in the teenager with type 1 DM pose a serious health hazard (Mannucci, Rotella, Recca, et al, 2005). Also, insulin manipulation or omission has been identified as a weight loss method used by some adolescent girls (Hoffman, 2001). Nurses working with these adolescents, especially females, must be aware of the hazards and openly discuss the risks with the young person. A referral for specialized intervention may be needed.

Another group of adolescents with diabetes who are at risk are those who drink alcohol. I have found that confusion about the effects of alcohol on blood glucose is common. Teens may believe that alcohol will increase blood glucose levels, when in fact the opposite occurs. Ingestion of alcohol inhibits the release of glycogen from the liver, thereby resulting in hypoglycemia. Teens with diabetes who drink alcohol may become hypoglycemic but be treated as though they were inebriated. Behaviors may be similar, such as shakiness, combativeness, slurred speech, and loss of consciousness.

Education regarding the effects of alcohol is important and must be included in a teaching plan. If teens insist on drinking alcohol, they can be cautioned to use sweetened mixers or eat snacks when consuming alcoholic beverages.

Episodes of hyperglycemia or hypoglycemia may become a serious issue for adolescents who are leaving home for the first time. One teenager confided that her mother always recognized her combative, antisocial behavior as impending hypoglycemia and treated her with the appropriate intervention. The teen feared that a college roommate might be offended by the behavior and leave her alone with impending hypoglycemia.

One young man realized he could not live alone when he took a nap because he "felt tired" and woke up 4 days later in the hospital. Fortunately, his family realized he was in a coma and summoned emergency medical service. The fatigue signaled the beginning of a viral infection, which led to a blood glucose level of 410 mg/dl. Nurses need to address these fears openly and facilitate ways in which the teen can enlist the aid of significant peers who may be available during hyperglycemic or hypoglycemic episodes.

Susan Zekauskas, RN, MSN, PNP

BOX 38-14 TYPES OF INSULIN

There are four types of insulin, based on the following criteria:
- How soon the insulin starts working (onset)
- When the insulin works the hardest (peak time)
- How long the insulin lasts in the body (duration).

However, each person responds to insulin in his or her own way. That is why onset, peak time, and duration are given as ranges.
- Rapid-acting insulin (lispro) reaches the blood within 15 minutes after injection. The insulin peaks 30 to 90 minutes later and may last as long as 5 hours.
- Short-acting (regular) insulin usually reaches the blood within 30 minutes after injection. The insulin peaks 2 to 4 hours later and stays in the blood for about 4 to 8 hours.
- Intermediate-acting (NPH and Lente) insulins reach the blood 2 to 6 hours after injection. The insulins peak 4 to 14 hours later and stay in the blood for about 14 to 20 hours.
- Long-acting (Ultralente) insulin takes 6 to 14 hours to start working. It has no peak or a very small peak 10 to 16 hours after injection. The insulin stays in the blood between 20 and 24 hours.

Some insulins come mixed together. For example, you can buy regular insulin and NPH insulins already mixed in one bottle, which makes it easier to inject two kinds of insulin at the same time. However, you cannot adjust the amount of one insulin without also changing how much you get of the other insulin.

Insulin Preparations. Insulin is available in highly purified pork preparations and in human insulin biosynthesized by and extracted from bacterial or yeast cultures. Most clinicians suggest human insulin as the treatment of choice. Insulin is available in rapid-, intermediate-, and long-acting preparations, and all are packaged in the strength of 100 units/ml. Some insulins are available as premixed insulins, such as 70/30 and 50/50 ratios, the first number indicating the percentage of intermediate-acting and the second number the percentage of rapid-acting insulin. Box 38-14 lists the different types of insulin.

Lispro-H (Humalog) and insulin aspart (NovoLog) are human insulin analogs. One unit of the analog has the same glucose-lowering effect as 1 unit of human rapid-acting insulin, but the effect is even more rapid and of shorter duration. One benefit is a decreased risk of hypoglycemia, since the peak effect is reached in 1 to 1½ hours. Because of its rapid onset, each of the analogs must be injected within 15 minutes before eating.

⚡ DRUG ALERT

Insulin Preparations

The human insulins from various manufacturers may be interchangeable, but human insulin and pork insulin or pure pork insulin should never be substituted for one another.

Dosage. Conventional management is a twice-daily insulin regimen combining rapid-acting (regular) and intermediate-acting (NPH or Lente) insulin drawn up into the same syringe and injected before breakfast and before the evening meal. The amount of morning regular insulin is determined by patterns in the late morning and lunchtime blood glucose values. The morning intermediate-acting dosage is determined by patterns

---

too frequent episodes of hypoglycemia. Insulin is administered as two or more injections per day or as continuous subcutaneous infusion using a portable insulin pump.

Healthy pancreatic cells secrete insulin at a low but steady basal rate with superimposed bursts of increased secretion that coincide with intake of nutrients. Consequently insulin levels in the blood increase and decrease coincidentally with rise and fall in blood glucose levels. In addition, insulin is secreted directly into the portal circulation; therefore the liver, which is the major site of glucose disposal, receives the largest concentration of insulin. No matter which method of insulin replacement is used, this normal pattern cannot be duplicated. Subcutaneous injection results in absorption of the drug into the general circulation, thus reducing the concentrations of insulin to which the liver is exposed.

in the late afternoon and supper blood glucose values. Fasting blood glucose patterns at breakfast help determine the evening dose of intermediate insulin, and the blood glucose patterns at bedtime help determine the evening dose of rapid-acting (regular) insulin. For some children, better morning glucose control is achieved by a later (bedtime) injection of intermediate-acting insulin.

Regular insulin is best administered at least 30 minutes before meals. This allows sufficient time for absorption and results in a significantly greater reduction in the postprandial rise in blood glucose than if the meal were eaten immediately after the insulin injection. Intensive therapy consists of multiple injections throughout the day with a once- or twice-daily dose of long-acting (Ultralente) insulin to simulate the basal insulin secretion and injections of rapid-acting insulin before each meal. A multiple daily injection program reduces microvascular complications of diabetes in young, healthy patients who have type 1 DM. The precise dose of insulin needed cannot be predicted. Therefore the total dosage and percentage of regular- to intermediate-acting insulin should be determined empirically for each child. Usually 60% to 75% of the total daily dose is given before breakfast, and the remainder before the evening meal. Furthermore insulin requirements do not remain constant but change continuously during growth and development; the need varies according to the child's activity level and pubertal status. For example, less insulin is required during spring and summer months, when the child is more active. Illness also alters insulin requirements. Some children require more frequent insulin administration. This includes children with difficult-to-control diabetes and children undergoing the adolescent growth spurt.

Methods of Administration. Daily insulin is administered subcutaneously by twice-daily injections, by multiple-dose injections, or by means of an insulin infusion pump. The insulin pump is an electromechanical device designed to deliver fixed amounts of regular or lispro insulin continuously (basal rate), thereby more closely imitating the release of the hormone by the islet cells (Olohan and Zappitelli, 2003). Although the pump delivers a programmed amount of basal insulin, the child or parent must program a dose for the pump to deliver before each meal.

The system consists of a syringe to hold the insulin, a plunger, and a computerized mechanism to drive the plunger. The insulin flows from the syringe through a catheter to a needle inserted into subcutaneous tissue (the abdomen or thigh), and the lightweight device is worn on a belt or a shoulder holster. The child or parent changes the needle and catheter every 48 to 72 hours, using aseptic technique, and tapes it in place.

Although the pump provides more consistent insulin delivery, it has certain disadvantages. Pump therapy is expensive and requires commitment from the parent and child. A certain level of math skills is required to calculate infusion rates. It should not be removed for more than 1 hour at a time, which may limit some activities. Skin infections are common; and, as with any other mechanical device, it is subject to malfunction. However, the pumps are equipped with alarms that signal problems that may arise, such as a depleted battery, an occluded needle or tubing, or a microprocessor malfunction.

Future Therapies

Islet cell or whole pancreas transplantation may offer hope to patients in the future. Viable insulin-producing cells have been injected into the portal vein, where they are transported via the circulation to the liver and eventually produce up to two thirds of the required insulin. The major use of transplants has been in persons who have serious complications, particularly those whose deteriorating kidneys have required renal transplantation and who are receiving immunosuppressive therapy. However, islet cell and pancreatic transplants tend not to be sustainable over time despite continuation of therapy. The use of nonhuman islet cells encapsulated in immunoprotective, semipermeable membranes may have a future in the treatment of type 1 DM (Campbell, 2004).

Other routes for insulin administration are being studied. Inhaled insulin, for instance, has been an effective and safe means to control postprandial glucose levels (Garg, Rosenstock, Silverman, et al, 2006).

Monitoring

Daily monitoring of blood glucose levels is an essential aspect of appropriate DM management.

Blood Glucose. Self-monitoring of blood glucose (SMBG) has improved diabetes management and is used successfully by children from the onset of their diabetes. By testing their own blood, children are able to change their insulin regimen to maintain their glucose level in the euglycemic (normal) range of 80 to 120 mg/dl. Diabetes management depends to a great extent on SMBG. In general, children tolerate the testing well. Table 38-4 lists plasma blood glucose and hemoglobin A_{1c} goal ranges.

Glycosylated Hemoglobin. The measurement of glycosylated hemoglobin (hemoglobin A_{1c}) levels is a satisfactory method for assessing the control of the diabetic patient. As red blood cells circulate in the bloodstream, glucose molecules gradually attach to the hemoglobin A molecules and remain there for the lifetime of the red blood cell, approximately 120 days. The attachment is not reversible; therefore this glycosylated hemoglobin reflects the average blood glucose levels over the previous 2 to 3 months. The test is a satisfactory method for assessing control, detecting incorrect testing, monitoring effectiveness of changes in treatment, defining patients' goals, and detecting nonadherence. Nondiabetic hemoglobin A_{1c} values are generally between 4% and 6% but can vary by laboratory. Diabetes control for children depends on age, with hemoglobin A_{1c} levels of 6.5% to 8% indicating a slightly elevated but acceptable result (American Diabetes Association, 2005). Table 38-5 gives comparisons of hemoglobin A_{1c} to blood glucose levels.

Urine. Urine testing for glucose is no longer used for diabetes management. There is poor correlation between simultaneous glycosuria and blood glucose concentrations. However, urine testing can be carried out to detect evidence of ketonuria.

❗ NURSING ALERT

It is recommended that urine be tested for ketones every 3 hours during an illness or whenever the blood glucose level is over 240 mg/dl when illness is not present.

TABLE 38-4	PLASMA BLOOD GLUCOSE AND HEMOGLOBIN A₁c GOALS FOR TYPE 1 DIABETES MELLITUS BY AGE-GROUP			
AGE	VALUE* BEFORE MEALS (mg/dl)	VALUE* AT BEDTIME/ OVERNIGHT (mg/dl)	HEMOGLOBIN A₁c (%)	RATIONALE FOR RESULTS
Toddlers and preschoolers (<6 yr)	100-180	110-200	≤8.5% (but ≥7.5%)	High risk and vulnerability to hypoglycemia
School age (6-12 yr)	90-180	100-180	<8%	Risks of hypoglycemia and relatively low risk of complications before puberty
Adolescents (>12 yr) and young adults	90-130	90-150	<7.5%	Risk of hypoglycemia Developmental and psychologic issues

Modified from American Diabetes Association: Standards of medical care in diabetes, *Diabetes Care* 28(Suppl):S4-S36, 2005.
*Plasma blood glucose goal range.

TABLE 38-5	COMPARISON OF HEMOGLOBIN BLOOD GLUCOSE LEVELS TO HEMOGLOBIN A₁c		
HEMOGLOBIN A₁c LEVELS	HEMOGLOBIN A₁c (%)	MEAN BLOOD GLUCOSE (mg/dl)	MEAN BLOOD GLUCOSE (mmol/L)
Severely elevated	14	360	20
	13.5		
	13	330	18.3
	12.5		
	12	300	16.7
	11.5		
	11	270	15
	10.5		
Elevated	10	240	13.3
	9.5		
	9	210	11.7
	8.5		
Slightly elevated	8	180	10
	7.5		
	7	150	8.3
	6.5		
Normal	6	120	6.7
	5.5		
	5	90	5
	4.5		
	4	60	3.3

Modified from American Diabetes Association: Standards of medical care in diabetes: clinical practice recommendations, *Diabetes Care* 28(Suppl):S4-S36, 2005.

Nutrition

Essentially the nutritional needs of children with diabetes are no different from those of healthy children. Children with diabetes need no special foods or supplements. They need sufficient calories to balance daily expenditure for energy and to satisfy the requirement for growth and development. Unlike the child without diabetes, whose insulin is secreted in response to food intake, insulin injected subcutaneously has a relatively predictable time of onset, peak effect, duration of action, and absorption rate depending on the type of insulin used. Consequently the timing of food consumption must be regulated to correspond to the time and action of the insulin prescribed.

Meals and snacks must be eaten according to peak insulin action, and the total number of calories and proportions of basic nutrients must be consistent from day to day. The constant release of insulin into the circulation makes the child prone to hypoglycemia between the three daily meals unless a snack is provided between meals and at bedtime. Calculate the distribution of calories to fit the activity pattern of each child. For example, a child who is more active in the afternoon needs a larger snack at that time. This larger snack might also be split to allow some food at school and some food after school. Food intake should be altered to balance food, insulin, and exercise. Extra food is needed for increased activity.

The food intake may be planned in a variety of ways but is based on a balanced diet that incorporates six basic food groups: milk, meat, vegetables, fat, fruit, and starch. There are several meal-planning approaches, including the exchange system and carbohydrate counting. The exchange system from the American Diabetes Association groups foods by nutrient content. Within each group, portion sizes of foods are calculated to give an equivalent amount of the nutrient. In the fruit list, for instance, one small apple has the equivalent amount of carbohydrate as a half banana. In the exchange system, food groups are important: fruits exchange with fruits, starches exchange with starches.

Carbohydrate counting has been popular since the Diabetes Control and Complications Trial. Portion sizes are still important, but all carbohydrates are considered equivalent. In this system, food groups are not as important as carbohydrate content. For example, one small apple and one slice of bread have the same carbohydrate amount (15 g) and may be used interchangeably.

Concentrated sweets are discouraged, and because of the increased risk for atherosclerosis in persons with DM, fat is reduced to 30% or less of the total caloric requirement. Dietary fiber has become increasingly important in dietary planning because of its influence on digestion, absorption, and metabolism of many nutrients. It has been found to diminish the rise in blood glucose after meals.

Correctly used, the diet allows for flexibility and the incorporation of preferred foods in most instances. For the growing child, never use food restriction for diabetic control, although caloric restrictions may be imposed for weight control if the child is overweight. In general, the child's appetite should be the guide for the amount of calories needed, with the total

BOX 38-15 NUTRITIONAL MANAGEMENT IN TYPE 1 DIABETES MELLITUS

Goal
Attain metabolic control of glucose and lipid levels

Objectives
Appropriate meal and snack planning:
- Achieve a dietary balance of carbohydrates, fats, and proteins.
- Provide extra food during periods of exercise.
- Time meals consistently to prevent hypoglycemia.
- Avoid high-sugar, high-carbohydrate foods to prevent hyperglycemia.

Develop an appropriate insulin regimen and physical activity program:
- Administer insulin as directed before eating.
- Increase insulin dose or activity level when extra food is eaten.
- Decrease insulin dose during periods of strenuous activity.

caloric intake adjusted to appetite and activity. Box 38-15 outlines basic principles of diet management.

Exercise

Exercise is encouraged and never restricted unless indicated by other health conditions. Exercise lowers blood glucose levels, depending on the intensity and duration of the activity. Consequently exercise should be included as part of diabetes management, and the type and amount of exercise should be planned around the child's interests and capabilities. However, in most instances children's activities are unplanned, and the resulting decrease in blood glucose can be compensated for by providing extra snacks before (and, if the exercise is prolonged, during) the activity. In addition to a feeling of well-being, regular exercise aids in utilization of food and often results in a reduction of insulin requirements.

Physical training tends to increase tissue sensitivity to insulin, even in the resting state. Consequently it is especially important to understand the relationship between the activity and the diabetic regimen. Vigorous muscular contraction increases regional blood flow and accelerates the absorption and circulation of insulin that is injected into the area, which can contribute to development of hypoglycemia. If exercise involving leg muscles is planned, it is recommended that non-exercised sites (arm or abdomen) be used for insulin injection. This practice may replace the need for further increased carbohydrate intake or a reduced insulin dose (or both) to avoid exercise-induced hypoglycemia.

Children with poorly controlled diabetes are particularly at risk for hyperglycemia with exercise, or exercise may actually stimulate ketoacid production. Therefore discourage the child who has marked hyperglycemia (blood glucose level >240 mg/dl) and ketonuria from strenuous physical activity until the diabetes is controlled by appropriate adjustments of insulin and diet.

Athletes and youngsters who regularly participate in organized sports should adjust their insulin dosage in anticipation of sustained physical activity during the part of the day devoted to strenuous exercise. Team sports may encourage overexertion and subsequent hypoglycemia. Insulin dosages are decreased for participation in organized sports or prolonged activities, such as swimming for several hours. It is important that the patient consult with the practitioner for advice on insulin dose adjustment.

Hypoglycemia

Occasional episodes of hypoglycemia are an integral part of insulin therapy, and an objective of diabetes management is to achieve the best possible glycemic control while minimizing the frequency and severity of hypoglycemia. Even with good control, a child may frequently experience mild symptoms of hypoglycemia. If the signs and symptoms are recognized early and promptly relieved by appropriate therapy, the child's activity should be interrupted for no more than a few minutes

! NURSING ALERT

Hypoglycemic episodes most commonly occur before meals, or when the insulin effect is peaking.

The most common causes of hypoglycemia are bursts of physical activity without additional food, or delayed, omitted, or incompletely consumed meals. Reglycosylation of muscles may occur over the ensuing 24 hours. Particular vigilance related to hypoglycemia may be necessary during the night after vigorous exertion. Occasionally, hypoglycemic reactions occur unexpectedly and without apparent cause. They may be the result of an inadvertent or deliberate error in insulin administration.

Gastroenteritis, in which there is gastric stasis, may impede the absorption of food, even though the child is eating reasonably well. It can also occur when the blood glucose level is so low that it causes stasis. Then the child may eat a meal or snack and still have an insulin reaction. Continued feeding does not seem to alter the blood glucose level because the simple glucose or sugar remains in the stomach.

The signs and symptoms of hypoglycemia are caused by both increased adrenergic activity and impaired brain function. The increased adrenergic nervous system activity plus increased secretion of catecholamines produces nervousness, pallor, tremulousness, palpitations, sweating, and hunger. Weakness, dizziness, headache, drowsiness, irritability, loss of coordination, seizures, and coma are more severe responses and reflect CNS glucose deprivation and the body's attempts to elevate the serum glucose levels.

It is often difficult to distinguish between hyperglycemia and a hypoglycemic reaction (Table 38-6). Because the symptoms are similar and usually begin with changes in behavior, the simplest way to differentiate the two is to test the blood glucose level. The blood glucose level is low in hypoglycemia, whereas in hyperglycemia the glucose level is significantly elevated. Urinary ketones may be present after hypoglycemia as a result of starvation ketone production. In doubtful situations it is safer to give the child some simple carbohydrate. This will help alleviate the symptoms in the case of hypoglycemia but will do little harm if the child is hyperglycemic.

Children are usually able to detect the onset of hypoglycemia, but some are too young to implement treatment. Parents should become adept at recognizing the onset of symptoms—for example, a change in a child's behavior, such as tearfulness

TABLE 38-6	COMPARISON OF MANIFESTATIONS OF HYPOGLYCEMIA AND HYPERGLYCEMIA	
VARIABLE	HYPOGLYCEMIA	HYPERGLYCEMIA
Onset	Rapid (min)	Gradual (days)
Mood	Labile, irritable, nervous, weepy	Lethargic
Mental status	Difficulty concentrating, speaking, focusing, coordinating Nightmares	Dulled sensorium Confusion
Inward feeling	Shaky feeling, hunger Headache Dizziness	Thirst Weakness Nausea and vomiting Abdominal pain
Skin	Pallor Sweating	Flushed Signs of dehydration
Mucous membranes	Normal	Dry, crusty
Respirations	Shallow, normal	Deep, rapid (Kussmaul)
Pulse	Tachycardia, palpitations	Less rapid, weak
Breath odor	Normal	Fruity, acetone
Neurologic	Tremors	Diminished reflexes Paresthesia
Ominous signs	Late: hyperreflexia, dilated pupils, seizure Shock, coma	Acidosis, coma
Blood:		
Glucose	Low: <60 mg/dl	High: ≥250 mg/dl
Ketones	Negative	High, large
Osmolarity	Normal	High
pH	Normal	Low (≤7.25)
Hematocrit	Normal	High
Bicarbonate	Normal	<20 mEq/L
Urine:		
Output	Normal	Polyuria (early) to oliguria (late)
Glucose	Negative	Enuresis, nocturia
Ketones	Negative or trace	High
Visual	Diplopia	Blurred vision

When in doubt, it is best to assume hypoglycemia and treat, but overtreatment could result in hyperglycemia. The treatment may be repeated in 10 to 15 minutes if the initial response is not satisfactory. Rest and the addition of food should be part of the plan.

An insulin reaction is often the most feared aspect of diabetes because severe brain symptoms may develop. In a severe reaction the various areas of the brain respond in sequence: the forebrain with increased drowsiness and perspiration, the hypothalamus and thalamus with tachycardia and loss of consciousness, the midbrain with seizure activity that may be started from stimulation initially from the hypothalamus, and finally the hindbrain with responses of deeper coma and decreasing reflexes. The treatment of choice for severe hypoglycemia is 50% glucose administered intravenously.

Glucagon is sometimes prescribed for home treatment of hypoglycemia. It is available as an emergency kit that must be mixed at the time of use and is administered intramuscularly or subcutaneously. Glucagon functions by releasing stored glycogen from the liver and requires about 15 to 20 minutes to elevate the blood glucose level.

❗ NURSING ALERT

Vomiting may occur after administration of glucagon; therefore take precautions against aspiration (e.g., placing the child on the side), since the child will be unconscious.

Once the child is responsive, the lost glycogen stores are replaced by small amounts of sugar-containing fluid administered frequently until the child feels comfortable about trying solid foods.

Morning Hyperglycemia. The management of elevated morning blood glucose levels depends on whether the increase is a true dawn phenomenon, insulin waning, or a rebound hyperglycemia (the Somogyi effect). Insulin waning is a progressive rise in blood glucose levels from bedtime to morning. It is treated by increasing the nocturnal insulin dose. The true dawn phenomenon shows a relatively normal blood glucose level until about 3 AM, when the level begins to rise. The Somogyi effect may occur at any time but often entails an elevated blood glucose level at bedtime and a drop at 2 AM with a rebound rise following. The treatment for this phenomenon is decreasing the nocturnal insulin dose to prevent the 2 AM hypoglycemia. The rebound rise in the blood glucose level is a result of counterregulatory hormones (epinephrine, GH, and corticosteroids), which are stimulated by hypoglycemia. More frequent blood monitoring (especially at times of anticipated peak insulin action) usually identifies these conditions. Trace amounts of urinary ketones aid in identifying undetected hypoglycemia.

Illness Management

Illness alters diabetes management, and maintaining control is usually related to the seriousness of the illness. In the well-controlled child an illness runs its course as it does in the unaffected child.

The goals during an illness are to restore euglycemia, treat urinary ketones, and maintain hydration. Monitor blood

or euphoria. In the majority of cases, 10 to 15 g of simple carbohydrate, such as 1 tbsp of table sugar, will elevate the blood glucose level and alleviate the symptoms. The simpler the carbohydrate, the more rapidly it will be absorbed (8 oz of milk equals 15 g of carbohydrate). The rapid-releasing sugar is followed by a complex carbohydrate such as a slice of bread or a cracker and by a protein such as peanut butter or milk.

For a mild reaction, milk or fruit juice is good to use in children. Milk supplies them with lactose or milk sugar, as well as a more prolonged action from the protein and fat (helps decrease absorption). Other glucose sources include Insta-Glucose (cherry-flavored glucose), carbonated drinks (not sugarless), sherbet, gelatin, or cake icing. All children with diabetes should carry with them glucose tabs, Insta-Glucose, sugar cubes, or sugar-containing candy such as LifeSavers or Charms. A difficulty with candies or icing is that the child may learn to fake a reaction to get the sweets; therefore commercial treatment products such as Insta-Glucose or glucose tabs may be preferred.

glucose levels and urinary ketones every 3 hours. Some hyperglycemia and ketonuria are expected in most illnesses, even with diminished food intake, and are an indication for increased insulin. Insulin should never be omitted during an illness, although dosage requirements may increase, decrease, or remain unchanged, depending on the severity of the illness and the child's appetite. Often the child needs supplemental insulin between usual dose times. If the child vomits more than once, if blood glucose levels remain above 240 mg/dl, or if urinary ketones remain high, notify the health care practitioner. Simple carbohydrates may be substituted for carbohydrate-containing exchanges in the meal plan. Although insulin and diet are important tools in sick-day care, fluids are the most important intervention. Fluids must be encouraged to prevent dehydration and to flush out ketones.

Surgery

The physiologic and emotional stresses related to surgery require careful adjustment of insulin. Because the child receives IV glucose during surgery and the stress of the surgery itself also raises the blood glucose level, the risk of an insulin reaction is slight. Short-acting insulins should be continued until the child is able to tolerate oral feedings and return to the routine pattern of insulin administration.

Prevention

Major advances have been made in the ability to detect susceptibility to type 1 DM, and animal studies indicate that the disease can be prevented by various immunologic interventions (Skyler and Marks, 2003). Early immunosuppression may preserve long-term endogenous insulin secretion in individuals with type 1 DM.

Cyclosporine, mycophenolic acid, and nicotinamide have shown promise in delaying beta cell destruction or lowering the incidence of type 1 DM in relatives of children with the disease. Much progress has been made in the identification of islet cell antigens targeted by the immune response. Many potential treatments to prevent type 1 DM have appeared, and human trials have begun.

Therapeutic Management: Diabetic Ketoacidosis

DKA, the most complete state of insulin deficiency, is a life-threatening situation. Management consists of rapid assessment, adequate insulin to reduce the elevated blood glucose level, fluids to overcome dehydration, and electrolyte replacement (especially potassium).

DKA constitutes an emergency situation; therefore the child should be admitted to an intensive care facility for management. The priority is to obtain venous access for administration of fluids, electrolytes, and insulin. The child should be weighed, measured, and placed on a cardiac monitor. Blood glucose and ketone levels are determined at the bedside, and samples are obtained for laboratory measurement of glucose, electrolytes, blood urea nitrogen, arterial pH, Po_2, Pco_2, hemoglobin, hematocrit, white blood cell count and differential, calcium, and phosphorus.

Oxygen may be administered to patients who are cyanotic and in whom arterial oxygen is less than 80%. Gastric suction is applied to unconscious children to avoid the possibility of pulmonary aspiration. Antibiotics may be administered to febrile children after appropriate specimens are obtained for culture. A Foley catheter may or may not be inserted for urine samples and measurement. Unless the child is unconscious, a collection bag is usually sufficient for accurate assessments.

Fluid and Electrolyte Therapy

All patients with DKA suffer from dehydration (10% of total body weight in severe ketoacidosis) because of the osmotic diuresis, accompanied by depletion of electrolytes, sodium, potassium, chloride, phosphate, and magnesium. Serum pH and bicarbonate reflect the degree of acidosis. Prompt and adequate fluid therapy restores tissue perfusion and suppresses the elevated levels of stress hormones.

The initial hydrating solution is 0.9% saline solution. Traditionally deficits have been replaced at a rate of 50% over the first 8 to 12 hours and the remaining 50% over the next 16 to 24 hours. Current trends suggest more cautious fluid management to reduce the risk of cerebral edema. Consequently, the recommendations now are to replace the deficit evenly over 36 to 48 hours (Cooke and Plotnick, 2004).

> ### ⚡ DRUG ALERT
> **Potassium and Serum Potassium levels**
>
> Potassium must never be given until the serum potassium level is known to be normal or low and urinary voiding is observed. All maintenance IV fluids should include 30 to 40 mEq/L of potassium unless the potassium concentration is elevated or urinary output is absent (Cooke and Plotnick, 2004). Never give potassium as a rapid IV bolus, or cardiac arrest may result.

Serum potassium levels may be normal on admission, but after fluid and insulin administration the rapid return of potassium to the cells can seriously deplete serum levels, with the attendant risk of cardiac arrhythmias. As soon as the child has established renal function (is voiding at least 25 ml/hr) and insulin has been given, vigorous potassium replacement is implemented. The cardiac monitor is used as a guide to therapy, and the nurse should observe the configuration of T waves every 30 to 60 minutes to determine changes that might indicate alterations in potassium concentration (widening of the Q-T interval and the appearance of a U wave following a flattened T wave indicate hypokalemia; an elevated and spreading T wave and shortening of the Q-T interval indicate hyperkalemia).

Insulin should not be given until after obtaining urine ketones and a blood glucose level. Continuous IV regular insulin is given at a dosage of 0.1 units/kg/hr. Insulin therapy should be started after the initial rehydration bolus, since serum glucose levels fall rapidly after volume expansion. Blood glucose levels should decrease by 50 to 100 mg/dl/hr. When blood glucose levels fall to 250 to 300 mg/dl, dextrose is added to the IV solution. The goal is to maintain blood glucose levels between 120 and 240 mg/dl by adding 5% to 10% dextrose. Sodium bicarbonate is used conservatively; it is used for pH less than 7.0, severe hyperkalemia, or cardiac instability. Because sodium bicarbonate has been associated with increased risk for cerebral edema, children receiving this substance must be carefully monitored for changes in level of consciousness (Brown, 2004).

If bicarbonate treatment is necessary, 1 to 2 mEq/kg should be added to the IV fluids to run over 1 to 2 hours (Cooke and Plotnick, 2004).

When the critical period is over, the task of regulating insulin dosage in relation to diet and activity is started. Children should be actively involved in their own care and are given responsibility according to their ability and the guidance of the nurse.

> ⚡ **DRUG ALERT**
>
> **Insulin and Tubing**
>
> Because insulin can chemically bind to plastic tubing and in-line filters, thereby reducing the amount of medication reaching the systemic circulation, an insulin mixture is run through the tubing to saturate the insulin-binding sites before the infusion is started.

Nursing Care of the Child with Diabetes Mellitus: Acute Care

Children with DM may be admitted to the hospital at the time of their initial diagnosis; during illness or surgery; or for episodes of ketoacidosis, which may be precipitated by any of a variety of factors. Many children are able to keep the disease under control with periodic assessment and adjustment of insulin, diet, and activity as needed under the supervision of a practitioner. Under most circumstances these children can be managed well at home and require hospitalization only for a serious illness or upset (see Research Focus box).

> 🔍 **RESEARCH FOCUS**
>
> **Outpatient Treatment of Type 1 Diabetes**
>
> A Cochrane systematic review of seven studies evaluating whether children newly diagnosed with type 1 diabetes should be admitted to a hospital or treated in the outpatient setting found no disadvantages to allowing the child to remain as an outpatient. Studies evaluated metabolic control, acute diabetic complications and hospitalizations, psychosocial variables and behavior, and total care costs (Clar, Waugh, and Thomas, 2007).

However, a small number of children with diabetes exhibit a degree of metabolic lability and have repeated episodes of DKA that require hospitalization, which interferes with education and social development. These children appear to display a characteristic personality structure. They tend to be unusually passive and nonassertive and to come from families that are inclined to smooth over conflicts without resolution. Children in this type of setting experience emotional arousal with little, if any, opportunity or ability to resolve it. Other children from psychosocially dysfunctional families display behavioral and personality problems. This emotional stress causes an increased production of endogenous catecholamines, which stimulate fat breakdown, leading to ketonemia and ketonuria.

Loving discipline is a supportive measure for any child; however, children with poorer diabetic control come from predominantly disruptive family units with little or no discipline. Lack of control is psychologically harmful. Because many of the psychosocial problems are not immediately apparent, psychosocial assessment by professionals is required, together with ongoing emotional support and counseling to reverse the patterns of ketoacidosis (Wolsdorf, Glaser, and Sperling, 2006).

Hospital Management

The child with DKA requires intensive nursing care. Observe vital signs and record them frequently. Hypotension caused by the contracted blood volume of the dehydrated state may cause decreased peripheral blood flow, which can be particularly hazardous to the heart, lungs, and kidneys. An elevated temperature may indicate infection and should be reported so that treatment can be implemented immediately.

Maintain careful and accurate records, including vital signs (pulse, respiration, temperature, and blood pressure), weight, IV fluids, electrolytes, insulin, blood glucose level, and intake and output. Use a urine collection device or retention catheter to obtain the urine measurements, which include volume, specific gravity, and glucose and ketone values. The volume relative to the glucose content is important because 5% glucose in a 300-ml sample is a significantly greater amount than a similar reading from a 75-ml sample. A diabetic flow sheet maintained at the bedside provides an ongoing record of the vital signs, urine and blood tests, amount of insulin given, and intake and output. Assess the level of consciousness and record it at frequent intervals. The comatose child generally regains consciousness fairly soon after initiation of therapy but is managed like any unconscious child during that time.

When the critical period is over, the task of regulating insulin dosage to diet and activity begins. The same meticulous records of intake and output, urine glucose and acetone levels, and insulin administration are maintained. Capable children should be actively involved in their own care and are given responsibility for keeping the intake and output record, testing the blood and urine, and, when appropriate, administering their own insulin—all under the nurse's supervision and guidance (see Nursing Care Plan).

Nursing Care of the Child with Diabetes Mellitus: General Care

Diabetes management involves a constant state of assessment. Daily monitoring of blood glucose levels; periodic urinalysis for ketones; and observation for signs of hypoglycemia, hyperglycemia, or other complications are part of the daily life of children with diabetes and their families. Suspect diabetes in any child who exhibits the manifestations of hypoglycemia or hyperglycemia, and refer the child for further assessment and appropriate testing.

> **QUALITY PATIENT OUTCOMES: Diabetes Mellitus**
> - Blood glucose levels maintained within normal range
> - HbA$_{1c}$ range from 6.5% to 8%
> - DKA prevented

The nurse should be alert to evidence of complications, although these are usually not manifested until adulthood. Assessment of skin for evidence of breakdown is important so that appropriate care can be implemented to facilitate healing and prevent infection. Because illnesses, such as respiratory

◎ **NURSING CARE PLAN**

The Child with Diabetes Mellitus

NURSING DIAGNOSIS	EXPECTED PATIENT OUTCOMES	NURSING INTERVENTIONS	RATIONALE
Risk for Injury related to insulin deficiency **Child's/Family's Defining Characteristics** (Subjective and Objective Data) See Box 38-13.	Child will demonstrate normal blood glucose levels. **The Following NOC Concept Applies to These Outcomes** Blood Glucose Control	Obtain blood glucose level. Administer insulin as prescribed. Understand the action of insulin: differences in composition, time of onset, and duration of action for the various preparations. Employ aseptic techniques when preparing and administering insulin. Rotate sites. **The Following NIC Concepts Apply to These Interventions** Health Education Hyperglycemia Management Hypoglycemia Management	To determine most appropriate dose of insulin To maintain normal blood glucose level To ensure accurate insulin administration To prevent infection To enhance absorption of insulin

NURSING DIAGNOSIS	EXPECTED PATIENT OUTCOMES	NURSING INTERVENTIONS	RATIONALE
Risk for Injury related to hypoglycemia **Child's/Family's Defining Characteristics** (Subjective and Objective Data) Shaky feeling Hunger Headache Dizziness Difficulty concentrating, speaking, and focusing Tremors Tachycardia Shallow respirations Can lead to convulsion, shock, and coma	Child will exhibit no evidence of hypoglycemia. **The Following NOC Concept Applies to These Outcomes** Blood Glucose Control	Recognize signs of hypoglycemia early. Be alert at times when blood glucose levels are lowest (before meals and snacks; 2 to 4 AM; after bursts of physical activity without additional food; or with delayed, omitted, or incompletely consumed meal or snack). Test blood glucose. Offer 10 to 15 g of readily absorbed carbohydrates, such as orange juice, hard candy, or milk. Follow with complex carbohydrate and protein, such as bread or cracker spread with peanut butter or cheese. Administer glucagons to unconscious or combative child. **The Following NIC Concepts Apply to These Interventions** Health Education Hypoglycemia Management	To prevent hypoglycemia To evaluate glucose level To elevate blood glucose level and alleviate symptoms of hypoglycemia To maintain blood glucose level To elevate blood glucose level

NURSING DIAGNOSIS	EXPECTED PATIENT OUTCOMES	NURSING INTERVENTIONS	RATIONALE
Deficient Knowledge (diabetes management) related to care of a child with newly diagnosed diabetes mellitus **Child's/Family's Defining Characteristics** (Subjective and Objective Data) Lack of understanding Inability to prepare and administer insulin Inability to follow meal planning guidelines Difficulty describing treatment plan	Child and family will have attitude conducive to learning. Child and family will demonstrate understanding and proficiency related to meal planning, administering insulin, testing blood glucose level, managing hyperglycemia and hypoglycemia, and practicing proper hygiene. **The Following NOC Concepts Apply to These Outcomes** Blood Glucose Control Knowledge: Medication Knowledge: Treatment Regimen	Select methods, vocabulary, and content appropriate to learners' level. Allow time for family and child to begin to adjust to initial impact of the diagnosis. Select an environment conducive to learning. Involve all senses and employ a variety of teaching strategies, especially participation. Provide pamphlets or other supplementary materials. Emphasize relationship between normal nutritional needs and the disease. Become familiar with family's culture and food preferences. Teach or reinforce learners' understanding of the basic food groups and the prescribed meal plan.	To maximize learning To allow child and family to set pace To promote learning To use most effective methods for learning To promote learning To encourage sense of normalcy To include culture preference in meal planning To reinforce existing knowledge base

NURSING CARE PLAN—cont'd

The Child with Diabetes Mellitus

NURSING DIAGNOSIS	EXPECTED PATIENT OUTCOMES	NURSING INTERVENTIONS	RATIONALE
		Help child and family estimate portion sizes by volume.	To teach a method of meal planning that is more practical than weighing food
		Suggest low-carbohydrate snack items.	To foster appropriate food choices
		Guide family in assessing labels of food products for carbohydrate content.	To foster consistency in carbohydrate portions
		Teach child and family the characteristics of the insulins prescribed.	To increase understanding that there are several insulin preparations
		Teach proper mixing of insulins.	To prevent child and family from contaminating the vials
		Teach injection procedure.	To promote appropriate administration
		Teach basic techniques using an orange or similar item.	To build confidence
		Use demonstration and return demonstration techniques on another before injecting child.	To reduce stress for the child
		Help families and child work out a set rotational pattern.	To ensure maximum absorption of insulin and prevent hypertrophy at injection site
		Teach proper care of insulin and equipment.	To prevent contamination and minimize complications
		Teach family and child, if old enough, blood glucose monitoring or use of equipment, interpretation of results, and care and maintenance of equipment.	To ensure that child and family learn how to adjust insulin based on blood glucose level
		Instruct learners in how to recognize signs of hyperglycemia and hypoglycemia.	To prevent delay of treatment
		Explain relationship of insulin needs to illness, activity, and intense emotion.	To ensure appropriate treatment
		Teach how to adjust food, activity, and insulin at times of illness and during other situations that alter blood glucose levels.	To ensure appropriate treatment
		Suggest carrying source of carbohydrate, such as sugar cubes or hard candy in pocket.	To prevent delay of treatment
		Instruct parents and child in how to treat hypoglycemia with food, simple sugars, or glucagons.	To prevent delay of treatment
		Emphasize importance of personal hygiene.	To establish health practices that last a lifetime
		Encourage regular dental care and yearly ophthalmologic examinations.	To detect vision problems caused by diabetes
		Teach proper care of cuts and scratches.	To minimize risk of infection
		Teach proper foot care.	To prevent infection related to poor circulation

**The Following NIC Concepts Apply
to These Interventions**
Health Education
Hyperglycemia Management
Hypoglycemia Management

tract infections or gastrointestinal upsets, complicate the diabetes management, they should be detected early.

Education is the cornerstone of diabetes management and the major responsibility in diabetes nursing care. This includes education and reinforcement of information for the family and for children who are old enough to participate in self-management of the disease. With younger children, parents must supervise and manage their therapeutic program, but children should assume some responsibility for self-management as soon as they are capable. Children can assist with blood glucose testing at a relatively young age, and most should be able to administer their own insulin at about 9 years of age. In situations in which the parents are inconsistent or unreliable, the child can learn self-care at an earlier age. However, education programs cannot be conducted as one-time activities with the expectation that they will achieve permanent behavior changes. Education is an ongoing nursing activity as family and patient needs change and new findings are applied.

Concepts of Child and Family Education

Children and their families vary in educational background and the capacity to learn and understand the various aspects of the therapeutic program. Some families respond best to simple explanations and directions, whereas others expect thorough, in-depth information about the physiologic processes and responses associated with the disease and its therapy. All the principles of teaching and learning are applied in the educational process; therefore, before beginning, the nurse must determine the optimum time, place, method, and content to be taught. Self-management, the ultimate goal for children with diabetes, is more likely to occur when children understand the disease and the care it requires. Properly educated and motivated, most families should be able to follow a program of regulated control satisfactorily.

When to teach a family and child is best judged by their psychologic state and emotional readiness. When a child is newly diagnosed, the psychologic adjustment to the disease can block the learning process completely. For example, in a follow-up visit family members may state that they are hearing a certain bit of information for the first time even though the material had been covered several times in the course of teaching.

Certainly the first 3 or 4 days after diagnosis are not an optimum time for complex learning. In fact, the later the more complex material is presented, the better. For example, one successful program teaches only essential, or survival, information first and intense information a month later. Another program advocates teaching 1 week after diagnosis followed by a review of survival techniques 2 weeks after discharge. Probably the worst time for teaching is the day or so after diagnosis, when the education must be compressed into a few hours or days so that the child can be discharged early.

Regardless of the teaching plan, the nurse must accurately assess individual ability to learn. This includes assessment of the individuals' educational background and emotional stability and the use of appropriate measurement tools, such as a pretest or an objective assessment of the learners' educational level. The stepped approach to patient education employs the method of simple to complex. The stepped approach involves (1) using good interpersonal skills, (2) teaching about the illness and regimen, and (3) overcoming obstacles to behavior change.

The setting for the educational process can facilitate learning. If the child must be hospitalized, bedside education may be necessary in some cases, but the coming and going of a number of people is distracting. At times in the educational process individual instruction is needed, but contact with other children or parents can assist in adjustment to the reality of the disease and the implications of having a chronic condition.

A child learns best when sessions are short, no more than 15 to 20 minutes. The parents do best with periods of 45 to 60 minutes, or longer if they are inquisitive. Education should involve all the senses. Although visual aids are valuable tools, participation is the most effective method for learning. For example, to teach blood glucose testing, the nurse explains the technique, demonstrates the procedure, and allows the learner to perform the procedure; this is followed by a review of the material using visual aids, with learning validated by some testing method that includes feedback. A variety of teaching methods and teaching aids can be used. Some visual aids may be beautifully illustrated but miss a major point; therefore materials should be previewed for accuracy and appropriateness. Varying the presentation with a variety of audiovisual materials, including films, slide-tape programs, and books, stimulates the senses and helps the individual learn.

Several organizations are prepared to assist with education and dissemination of knowledge about diabetes. The American Diabetes Association,* Canadian Diabetes Association,† Juvenile Diabetes Research Foundation International,‡ and American Association of Diabetes Educators§ are valuable resources for a wide variety of educational materials. The National Institute of Diabetes and Digestive and Kidney Diseases¶ publishes a number of comprehensive annotated bibliographies, including "Educational Materials for and About Young People with Diabetes," a compilation of resource materials for children, siblings, parents, teachers, and health professionals; and "Sports and Exercise for People with Diabetes."

The content of the educational course must include all aspects of the disease as they relate to the individual child. Many aspects of the disease may not be covered in an initial educational course but can be postponed until subsequent office or clinic visits or can be done through referral sources such as the American Diabetes Association. The minimum information needed should help the family manage from one day to the next; expanded information helps the individual with long-term adjustment to the disease. The more the family understands about the disease in relation to body needs, the better they are able to maintain a high degree of control. Important content needed for minimum management is discussed briefly in the following sections.

Identification

One of the first things the nurse should call to the parents' attention is the need for the child to wear some means of medical identification. Usually recommended is the Medic-Alert identification, a stainless steel, silver, or gold-plated identification bracelet that is visible and immediately recognizable.

---

*1701 N. Beauregard St., Alexandria, VA 22311; 800-342-2383; www. diabetes.org.
†1400-522 University Ave., Toronto, Ontario, Canada M5G 2R5; 800-226-8464; www.diabetes.ca.
‡26 Broadway, 14th Floor, New York, NY 10004; 800-533-2873; www. jdf.org.
§200 W. Madison St., Suite 800, Chicago, IL 60606; 800-338-3633; www.aadenet.org.
¶Office of Communications and Public Liaison, NIDDK, NIH, Building 31, Room 9A06, 31 Center Dr., MSC 2560, Bethesda, MD 20892-2560; 301-496-3583; www.niddk.nih.gov.

It contains a collect telephone number that medical personnel can call around the clock for medical records and personal information.

Nature of Diabetes

The better the parents understand the pathophysiology of diabetes and the function and action of insulin and glucagon in relation to caloric intake and exercise, the better they will understand the disease and its effects on the child. Parents need answers to a number of questions (voiced or unvoiced) to increase their confidence in coping with the disease. For example, they may want to know about the various procedures performed on their child and treatment rationale, such as what is being put in the IV bottle and the expected effect.

Meal Planning

Normal nutrition is a major aspect of the family education program. The nutritionist usually conducts diet instruction, with reinforcement and guidance from the nurse. The emphasis is on adequate intake for age, consistent menus, complex carbohydrates, and consistent eating times. The family learns how the meal plan relates to the requirements of growth and development, the disease process, and the insulin regimen. Meals and snacks are modified based on the child's preferences and current menu, preserving cultural patterns and preferences as much as possible. Extensive exchange lists are available that include foods compatible with most lifestyles.

Learning about foods within specific food groups helps in making choices. Weights and measures of foods are used as eye-training devices for defining serving sizes and should be practiced for about 3 months, with gradual progression to estimation of food portions. Even when the child and family become competent in estimating portion sizes, reassessment should take place weekly or monthly and when there is any change of brands.

Family members should also be guided in reading labels for the nutritional value of foods and food content. They need to become familiar with the carbohydrate content of food groups. Substitution with foods of equal carbohydrate content is the skill needed for successful carbohydrate counting. Substitution might be necessary if a food is not available in sufficient quantity or for the teenager who wishes to eat fast food with peers. The use of a multiple daily injection program lends flexibility to the timing of meals.

Educating children or teenagers to make healthy food choices is an ongoing task. Teach younger children to choose from a special treat box stocked with sugar-free items when others bring high-sugar treats to the classroom. Discussions with school-age children might include situations encountered at school or parties, such as choosing food in the cafeteria or bringing substitute treats to parties. Role-playing and discussion help teenagers deal with food choices when on dates, with friends, or on a food break after school.

Lists of popular fast-food items and items served at the major fast-food chains can be obtained from the restaurants to help guide food selections. It is important that the child know the nutritional value of these items (the major chains are remarkably uniform), but the child should be cautioned to avoid high-fat, high-sugar, and high-carbohydrate items. For example, the child could choose a plain hamburger instead of a double cheeseburger.

Children should use sugar substitutes with moderation in items such as soft drinks. Artificial sweeteners have been shown to be safe, but if there is any question about amounts, the physician, dietitian, or nurse specialist can provide guidelines based on body weight. Sugar-free chewing gum and candies made with sorbitol may be used in moderation by children with DM. Although sorbitol is less cariogenic than other varieties of sugar substitutes, it is an alcohol sugar that is metabolized to fructose and then to glucose. Furthermore, large amounts can cause osmotic diarrhea. Most dietetic foods contain sorbitol. They are more expensive than regular foods. Also, although a product may be sugar free, it is not necessarily carbohydrate free.

Traveling

Traveling requires advance planning, especially when a trip involves crossing time zones. A number of tips are included in pamphlets available free of charge. Suggestions for traveling encompass what will be needed from the practitioner before leaving, what and how much to take along, needs in transit, what to consider at the destination, and planning for when the child returns home. Planning is needed no matter what type of travel is considered—automobile, plane, bus, or train.

Insulin

Families need to understand the treatment method and the insulin prescribed, including the effective duration, onset, and peak action. They also need to know the characteristics of the various types of insulins, the proper mixing and dilution of insulins, and how to substitute another type when their usual brand is not available (insulin is a nonprescription drug). Insulin need not be refrigerated but should be maintained at a temperature between 15° and 29.5° C (59° and 85° F). Freezing renders insulin inactive.

Insulin bottles that have been "opened" (i.e., the stopper has been punctured) should be stored at room temperature or refrigerated for up to 28 to 30 days. After 1 month these vials should be discarded. Unopened vials should be refrigerated and are good until the expiration date on the label. Diabetic supplies should not be left in a hot environment.

Injection Procedure

Learning to give insulin injections is a source of anxiety for both parents and children. It is helpful for the learner to know that this important aspect of care will become as routine as brushing the teeth. First, the basic injection technique is taught, using an orange or similar item and sterile normal saline for practice. To gain children's confidence, the nurse can demonstrate the technique by giving a skillful injection to the parent and then having the parent return the demonstration by giving the nurse an injection. With practice and confidence, the parents soon are able to give the insulin injection to their children, and their children trust them. Another effective strategy is to instruct the children and then have them teach the technique to the parents while the nurse observes. Both parents should participate, and as little time as possible should elapse between instruction and the actual injection, especially with parents and teenage learners.

Animation—Insulin Injection

TABLE 38-7	ONSET AND DURATION OF ACTION RELATED TO INJECTION SITE			
	SITE OF INJECTION			
	ABDOMEN	**ARM**	**LEG**	**BUTTOCK**
Rate	Very fast	Fast	Slow	Very slow
Duration	Very short	Short	Long	Very long

From Albisser AM, Sperlich M: Adjusting insulins, *Diabetes Educ* 18(3):211-218, 1992.

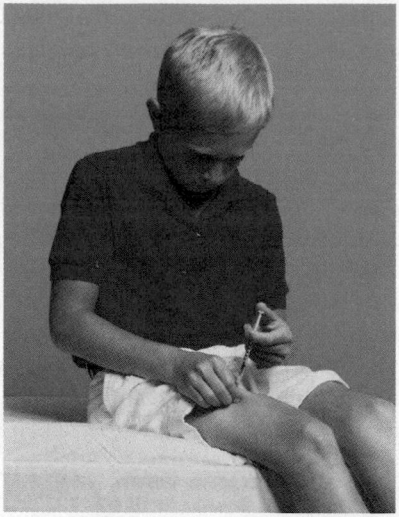

Fig. 38-8 School-age children are able to administer their own insulin.

Insulin can be injected into any area in which there is adipose (fat) tissue over muscle; the drug is injected at a 90-degree angle. Newly diagnosed children may have lost adipose tissue, and care should be exerted not to inject intramuscularly. The pinch technique is the most effective method for tenting the skin to allow easy entrance of the needle to subcutaneous tissues in children. The site selected sometimes depends on whether children or parents administer the insulin. The arms, thighs, hips, and abdomen are usual injection sites for insulin. The children can reach the thighs, abdomen, and part of the hip and arm easily but may require help to inject other sites. For example, a parent can pinch a loose fold of skin of the arm while the child injects the insulin.

The parents and child are helped to work out a rotation pattern to various areas of the body to enhance absorption, since insulin absorption is slowed by fat pads that develop in overused injection areas. The most efficient rotation plan involves giving about four to six injections in one area (each injection about 2.5 cm [1 inch] apart, or the diameter of the insulin vial from the previous injection) and then moving to another area.

Remember that the absorption rate varies in different parts of the body (Table 38-7). Methodically using one anatomic area and then moving to another (as described in the previous paragraph) minimizes variations in absorption rates. However, vigorous exercise, which enhances absorption from exercised muscles, also alters absorption. Therefore it is recommended that a site be chosen other than the exercising extremity (e.g., avoiding legs and arms when playing in a tennis tournament).

Injection sites for an entire month can be determined in advance on a simple chart. For example, the "paper doll" (body outline) described on p. 138 can be constructed and insulin sites marked by the child. After injection, the child places the date on the appropriate site. To keep in practice, it is a good idea for the parent to give two or three injections a week in areas that are difficult for the child to reach.

The same basic methodology is used when teaching children to give their own insulin injections (Fig. 38-8). They should practice first on an orange or a doll, building courage gradually. The first attempt is usually awkward because children tend to slowly push the needle through the skin rather than using a quick approach. It is best not to pressure them into assuming this responsibility until they are ready. When children participate in a group learning situation or have an opportunity to observe their peers giving their own injections, they may become more motivated. Warn parents that at some time children will give themselves an uncomfortable injection at home

and that they will need parental support and encouragement. Otherwise children may not wish to give themselves injections for some time.

Other devices are available for insulin injection and may offer advantages to some children. Children who do not wish to give themselves injections can learn to use a syringe-loaded injector (Inject-Ease). With the device, puncture is always automatic. Adolescents respond well to a self-contained and compact device resembling a fountain pen (NovoPen), which eliminates conventional vials and syringes. Preloaded pens may also improve adherence to intensive insulin regimens, improve lifestyle flexibility, and decrease pain (Rex, Jensen, and Lawton, 2006).

Teaching includes the proper way to equalize pressure in the bottle by injecting an amount of air equal to the amount of solution withdrawn and how to remove air bubbles from the syringe. When insulin doses are small, an air bubble in the syringe can displace a significant amount of medication. Since the introduction of the 0.5-ml and 0.3-ml syringes, the risk of incorrect dosage has diminished. Advise patients who have small doses of mixed insulins to use one of these syringes. Insulin syringes should be compared for accuracy, comfort, and strength. The family and child should be able to choose both "their" insulin and "their" syringe from a variety of samples. The needle length and gauge are also factors to consider from the point of view of comfort (e.g., use the shortest and smallest-gauge needle available). Some brands of syringes may be more comfortable than others. When currently available syringes are used, insulin injections of less than 2 units of U100 may have an unacceptably large error. Diluted insulin is sometimes used if the prescribed dose is less than 2 units. Special diluent is available from the insulin manufacturers (Eli Lilly, 2007).

When the child's dosage requires the injection of both short- and intermediate-acting insulin at the same time, most families prefer to mix the two and use a single injection. Insulin can be premixed and stored in the refrigerator for later use. Commercially prepared insulin mixtures are also available (e.g., 70/30 and 50/50). To obtain maximum benefit from mixing insulins, the recommended practice is to (1) inject the measured amount of air (equivalent to the dosage) into the long-acting insulin; (2) inject the measured amount of air into the rapid-acting (clear) insulin and, without removing the needle; (3) withdraw the clear insulin; and (4) insert the needle (already containing the clear insulin) into the long-acting (cloudy) insulin and then withdraw the desired amount.

⚡ **DRUG ALERT**

Mixing Insulin

When mixing types of insulin, always withdraw the clear, rapid-acting insulin into the syringe first, then the long-acting insulin. This avoids contaminating the short-acting insulin with the longer-acting insulin.

Inject the mixture either less than 5 minutes after mixing (before the zinc content of the long-acting insulin affects the action time of the short-acting insulin) or 15 or more minutes after mixing (to allow the insulins to resume long-acting and short-acting properties).

Nurses should also teach proper disposal of equipment after use in the home. Although not standard practice in the hospital, the use of a needle clipper is recommended to safely remove and house the used needle. The syringe plunger can be broken before disposal. An excellent means for syringe disposal is in an opaque, puncture-resistant container, such as an empty coffee can, bleach bottle, or milk carton. The container is labeled "biohazardous waste" and is discarded with similar material only, not with household refuse and consistent with local regulations.

Continuous Subcutaneous Insulin Infusion. Some children are candidates for use of a portable insulin pump, and even some young children with unsatisfactory metabolic control can benefit from its use. The child and the parents learn to operate the device, including the mechanics of the pump, battery changes, and alarm systems. A number of devices are available on the market that vary in the basal rates they are able to deliver and in the cost of the equipment. Families can investigate the various devices and select the model that best suits their needs. Product information is available from pump manufacturers and distributors.

Parents and children learn (1) the technical aspects of the pump and self-monitoring of blood glucose; (2) prevention and treatment for hyperglycemia, sick-day management, and meal planning; (3) the effects of exercise, stress, and diet on blood glucose levels; and (4) decision-making strategies to evaluate blood glucose patterns and how to make adjustments in all aspects of the regimen.

Numerous blood glucose measurements (at least four times per day) are an essential part of infusion pump use. Intensive education and supervision are critical to obtaining maximum efficiency and control. This is particularly important if the family has been accustomed to a conventional insulin regimen. They must realize that simply wearing the pump will not normalize blood glucose. The pump is merely an insulin delivery device, and frequent, routine blood glucose determinations are necessary to adjust the insulin delivery rate.

The major problem with use of the insulin pump is inflammation from irritation or infection at the insertion site. The site should be cleaned thoroughly before the needle is inserted and then covered with a transparent dressing. The site is changed and rotated every 48 to 72 hours (this may vary) or at the first sign of inflammation. Nurses working where pumps are part of the therapeutic regimen should become familiar with the operation of the specific device being used and the protocol of disease management. Others should be aware of this management technique and be prepared to assist patients using the pump.

Monitoring

Nurses should also be prepared to teach and supervise blood glucose monitoring. SMBG is associated with few complications, and although it does not necessarily lead to improved metabolic control, it provides a more accurate assessment of blood glucose levels than can be obtained with the historical urine testing. Blood glucose monitoring has the added advantage that it can be performed anywhere (see Atraumatic Care box).

ATRAUMATIC CARE

Minimizing Pain of Blood Glucose Monitoring

- To enhance blood flow to the finger, hold it under warm water for a few seconds before the puncture.
- When obtaining blood samples, use the ring finger or thumb (blood flows more easily to these areas), and puncture the finger just to the side of the finger pad (more blood vessels and fewer nerve endings).
- To prevent a deep puncture, press the platform of the lancet device lightly against the skin and avoid steadying the finger against a hard surface.
- Use lancet devices with adjustable-depth tips. Begin with the shallowest setting.
- Use glucose monitors that require small blood samples (e.g., Ascensia Elite) to avoid repeated punctures.

Blood for testing can be obtained by two different methods: manually or with a mechanical bloodletting device. A mechanical device is recommended for children, although the child and family should learn to use both methods in the event of mechanical failure. Several lancet devices are available from which to choose, and each provides a means for obtaining a large drop of blood for testing (Fig. 38-9).

❗ **NURSING ALERT**

Caution children not to allow anyone else to use their lancet because of the risk of contracting hepatitis B virus or human immunodeficiency virus infection.

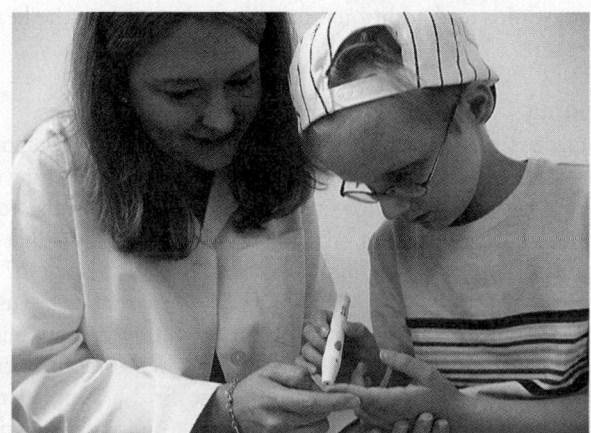

Fig. 38-9 Child using finger-stick device to obtain blood sample.

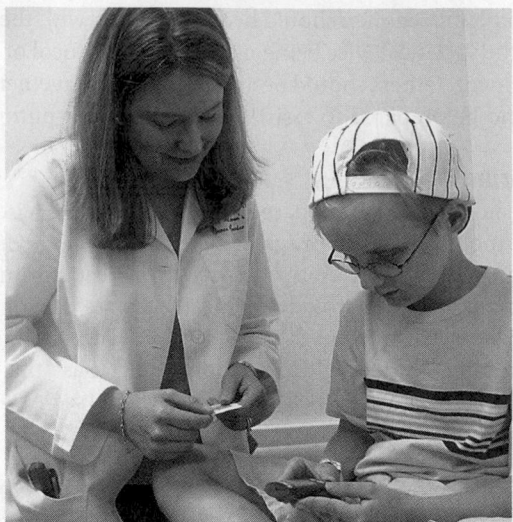

Fig. 38-10 Child using blood glucose monitor and reagent strips to test blood for glucose.

The blood sample may be obtained from fingertips or alternate sites such as the forearm. Alternate site testing requires a meter that can test a small volume of blood. Not all meters are capable of this.

The practitioner should examine signs of redness and soreness at the site of finger puncture. It may be evidence of poor technique, poor hygiene, or poor skin healing relative to poor control. Many types of blood-testing meters are available for home use. Newer technology has brought about improvements in meter size and ease of use. The family should be shown features of several meters, including advantages and disadvantages, and allowed to choose equipment that best meets their needs.

The least expensive testing method uses a reagent strip to which blood is applied (Fig. 38-10). After blotting, the color change is compared to a color scale for an estimation of the blood glucose level. The strips can be cut in half (although not all professionals recommend this) to obtain two readings per strip. This method is not accepted practice but may be necessary for some families or situations.

Urine Testing. Testing for urinary ketones is recommended during times of illness or when blood glucose values are elevated. Information on a specific ketone-testing product should include correct procedure, storage, and product expiration. Families need a clear understanding of home management of ketones: fluids and additional insulin as directed by the health care team.

Shopping

Diabetic maintenance is an expensive necessity. Families should investigate all sources of obtaining supplies for managing the disease. Prices are often lower when supplies are purchased in volume; however, it is not advisable to buy bulk items that are unfamiliar, since the new items may not be satisfactory for the individual child or may become outdated before they are used. Costs vary considerably among pharmacies and other suppliers, including the numerous discount mail-order establishments. When buying by mail, it is important to find a supplier that responds to the family's satisfaction and to allow ample time for delivery to avoid running out of supplies. Parents are also

cautioned not to substitute insulins or the type of insulin syringe (e.g., a 1-ml syringe for the low-dose type) simply to save money. Parent groups and the local American Diabetes Association can offer some suggestions for investigation. Most states have legislation mandating that insurance companies cover the cost of diabetes supplies and education.

Hyperglycemia

Severe hyperglycemia is most often caused by illness, growth, emotional upset, or missed insulin doses. Emotional stress from school finals or examinations or physical response to immunizations are examples of causes of hyperglycemia. With careful glucose monitoring, any elevation can be managed by adjustment of insulin or food intake. Parents should understand how to adjust food, activity, and insulin at the time of illness or when the child is treated for an illness with a medication known to raise the blood glucose level (e.g., steroids). The hyperglycemia is managed by increasing insulin soon after the increased glucose level is noted.

Hypoglycemia

Hypoglycemia is caused by imbalances of food intake, insulin, and activity. Ideally hypoglycemia should be prevented, and parents need to be prepared to prevent, recognize, and treat the problem. They should be familiar with the signs of hypoglycemia and instructed in treatment, including care of the child with seizures. (See Chapter 37.) Early signs are adrenergic, including sweating and trembling, which help raise the blood glucose level, much like the reaction when an individual is startled or anxious. The second set of symptoms that follow an untreated adrenergic reaction are neuroglycopenic (also called brain hypoglycemia). These symptoms typically include difficulty with balance, memory, attention, or concentration; dizziness or lightheadedness; and slurred speech. Severe and prolonged hypoglycemia leads to seizures, coma, and possible death (Cryer, 2003). In particular, infants are at an increased risk because of the developing brains' vulnerability to the potential neurotoxic insult of hypoglycemia (Cooke and Plotnick, 2004). Hypoglycemia can be managed effectively (see Emergency Treatment box).

✚ EMERGENCY TREATMENT

Hypoglycemia

Mild Reaction: Adrenergic Symptoms
Give child 10 to 15 g of a simple, high-carbohydrate substance (preferably liquid, e.g., 3 to 6 oz of orange juice).
Follow with starch-protein snack.

Moderate Reaction: Neuroglycopenic Symptoms
Give child 10 to 15 g of a simple carbohydrate as above.
Repeat in 10 to 15 minutes if symptoms persist.
Follow with larger snack.
Watch child closely.

Severe Reaction: Unresponsive, Unconscious, or Seizures
Administer glucagon as prescribed.
Follow with planned meal or snack when child is able to eat, or add a snack of 10% of daily calories.

Nocturnal Reaction
Give child 10 to 15 g of a simple carbohydrate.
Follow with snack of 10% of daily calories.

It is advisable for parents to plan for anticipated excitement or exercise. In addition, gastroenteritis may decrease insulin needs slightly as a result of poor appetite, vomiting, or diarrhea. If the blood glucose level is low but urinary ketones are present, the family should be aware of the increased need for simple carbohydrates and liquids.

Hygiene

All aspects of personal hygiene should be emphasized for the child with diabetes. Caution the child against wearing shoes without socks, wearing sandals, or walking barefoot. Correct nail and extremity care tailored to the individual child (with the guidance of a podiatrist) can begin health practices that last a lifetime. Eyes should be checked once a year unless the child wears glasses, and then as directed by the ophthalmologist. Regular dental care is emphasized, and cuts and scratches should be treated with plain soap and water unless otherwise indicated. Diaper rash in infants and candidal infections in teens may indicate poor diabetes control.

Exercise

Exercise is an important component of the treatment plan. If the child is more active at one time of the day than at another time, food or insulin can be altered to meet that activity pattern. Food should be increased in the summer, when children tend to be more active. Decreased activity on return to school may require a decrease in food intake or increase in insulin dosage. The child who is active in team sports needs a snack about a half hour before the anticipated activity. Races or other competition may call for a slightly higher food intake than practice times.

Food intake usually needs to be repeated for prolonged activity periods, often as frequently as every 45 minutes to 1 hour. Families should be informed that if increased food is not tolerated, decreased insulin is the next course of action. If the timing of the exercise is changed so that the supper meal is delayed, the insulin in the second or third dose of the day may be moved back to precede the mealtime. Sugar may sometimes be needed during exercise periods for quick response. Elevated blood glucose levels after extreme activity may represent the body's adrenergic response to exercise. If the blood glucose level is elevated (>240 mg/dl) before planned exercise, urine ketones should be checked and the activity may need to be postponed until the blood glucose is controlled.

Without adequate insulin levels the cells are unable to receive glucose, the preferred fuel, despite the high level of blood glucose. The low insulin level allows glucagon to act, uninhibited, to increase hepatic glucose production, further raising the blood glucose level with no means to use sugar at the muscle site. Breakdown of fat (lipolysis) is the alternative, and the end product of lipolysis is ketone body production (Cooke and Plotnick, 2008).

! **NURSING ALERT**

Ketonuria in the presence of hyperglycemia is an early sign of ketoacidosis and a contraindication to exercise.

Record Keeping

Home records are an invaluable aid to diabetes self-management. The nurse and family devise a method to chart insulin administered, blood glucose values, urine ketone results, and other factors and events that affect diabetes control. The child and family should observe for patterns of blood glucose responses to events such as exercise. If lapses in management occur (such as eating a candy bar), the child should be encouraged to note this and not be criticized for the transgression.

Complications

The nurse should present the implications of the disease in a tactful, clear, and nonthreatening manner. Knowledge of the complications of diabetes and their relationship to control provides a basis for knowledgeable decision making. Eye and kidney diseases are the greatest threats, with neurologic complications close behind. Clear explanations of these problems clarify false information often given by well-meaning friends. The information should include discussion of research so that the family is left with the positive impression that others are concerned about finding answers and preventing complications. It also gives them hope that somehow, some way, a prevention or cure will be possible.

Self-Management

Self-management is the key to close control. Being able to make changes when they are needed rather than waiting until the next contact with health care professionals is important for self-management and gives the individual and family the feeling they have control over the disease. Psychologically this helps family members feel they are useful and participating members of the team. Allowing the child to learn to look at records objectively promotes independence in self-management support. As children grow and assume more responsibility for self-management, they develop confidence in their ability to manage their disease and confidence in themselves as persons. They learn to respond to the disease and to make more accurate interpretations and changes in treatment when they become adults.

Self-management techniques to be mastered are the testing and adjustment of insulin and diet with alterations in day-to-day activities and anticipation of unusual occurrences. However, the nurse should provide guidelines regarding when to consult with the health care professionals. For instance, the degree of metabolic control before an illness is a determining factor in seeking medical help during the illness. In an individual with poor control, it takes only a few hours before the trouble is severe, whereas if control is good before the illness, several days may elapse before help is needed. Also caution patients and families to seek assistance if glucose levels are elevated and urine is not clear of ketones after 24 hours of self-management.

Child and Family Support

Just as the physiologic responses affect the child, the parents and other family members of the child with newly diagnosed DM experience various emotional responses to the crisis. Care in the acute setting is short but may create fears and frustrations. The prospect of a chronic illness in their child engenders all the feelings and concerns that are faced by parents of children with other chronic illnesses. (See Chapter 22.) The threat of complications and death is always present, as well as the continuing drain on emotional and financial resources.

Certain fears may develop as a result of past experiences with the disease. A severe insulin reaction with seizures can contribute to fear of repetition. Once parents observe a seizure or the adolescent has one in a public place, the desire to maintain better control is reinforced. They must understand how to prevent problems and how to handle problems calmly and coolly if they occur, and they must understand the complexities of the body, the disease, and its complications. Young children usually adjust well to problems related to the disease. With toddlers and preschoolers, insulin injections and glucose testing may be difficult at first. However, they usually accept the procedures when the parents use a matter-of-fact approach without calling attention to a "hurt" and treat the procedure like any other routine part of the child's life. After the injection, time with some special and positive attention, such as reading, talking, or another pleasant activity, is one way to convert children who initially refuse injections to those who accept them.

In the years before adolescence children probably accept their condition most easily. They are able to understand the basic concepts related to their disease and its treatment. They are able to test blood glucose and urine; recognize food groups; give injections; keep records; and distinguish between fear, excitement, and hypoglycemia. They understand how to recognize, prevent, and treat hypoglycemia. However, they still need considerable parental involvement.

> **NURSING TIP** Ongoing motivation to adhere to a regimen is difficult. An older child and parent (or another caregiver) may enjoy negotiating a day off when the responsibility for testing and recording blood glucose is delegated from the child to the caregiver (or vice versa).

Adolescents appear to have the most difficulty adjusting. Adolescence is a time of stress in trying to be perfect and like one's peers, and no matter what others say, having diabetes is being different. Some adolescents are more upset about not being able to have a candy bar than about injections, diet, and other aspects of management. If children can accept the difference as a part of life—in other words, that each person is different in some way—then with adequate parental support they should be able to adjust well.

Problems of adjustment to diabetes are especially difficult for the young person whose disease is diagnosed in adolescence. Denial is sometimes expressed by omitting insulin, not performing tests, and eating incorrectly, although denial of the disease usually diminishes during this period as the adolescent with DM begins to feel competent and worthy. Diabetes makes the teenager different when conformity and sameness are desired; having the disease emphasizes vulnerability and imperfection when the search for identity is the foremost developmental task of adolescence. It is often difficult for the adolescent to know what to tell friends.

Camping and other special groups are useful. At diabetes camp, children learn that they are not alone. As a result, they become more independent and resourceful in other settings.

Useful information about such camps and organizations can be obtained from the American Diabetes Association. A list of accredited camps specifically for children and teenagers with diabetes is also available from the American Camp Association.*

Puberty is associated with decreased sensitivity to insulin that normally would be compensated for by an increased insulin secretion. Health care professionals should anticipate that pubertal patients will have more difficulty maintaining glycemic control. Insulin doses commonly need to be increased, often dramatically (Tfayli and Arslanian, 2007). Patients should learn to give themselves additional doses of rapid-acting insulin (5% to 10% of their daily dose) when their blood glucose levels are increased. The use of supplemental rapid-acting insulin is preferred to withholding food in the adolescent.

Eating disorders, such as bulimia or anorexia nervosa, in the teenager with type 1 DM (see Chapter 21) pose a serious health hazard (Ackard, Vik, Neumark-Sztainer, et al, 2008). The nurse should be alert to a history of preoccupation with weight, food faddism, excessive caloric restriction, or unexplained hypoglycemia. Moreover, insulin manipulation or omission has been identified as a weight loss tool used by some female adolescents (Tierney, Deaton, Webb, et al, 2008).

Inaccurate doses of insulin may occur inadvertently or, if they occur frequently, may be an attention-seeking device; in a number of cases they may demonstrate adolescent depression and, more seriously, a subconscious but socially accepted method of suicide. Excessive intake of food leads to obesity and may also be symptomatic of depression. Psychiatric counseling may be needed if suicidal tendencies are amplified by the diabetes.

Rehospitalizations are most often related to poor control of the disease, although they may be indirectly related to poor coping and are a method of avoiding the pressures caused by family and peers. The hospital may represent an environment that is peaceful and free of stress. The goal for this problem is to determine the cause of the hospitalization. It may be related to poor control, poor self-management, or the need for better supportive management at home. Evaluation should be based on the physiologic and psychologic adjustment of the child and family.

Parents. Parents develop guilt feelings when they have a child with any chronic disease, especially one with a hereditary component. They cope with these feelings in a number of ways. For example, they may be overprotective or neglectful. Guilt-ridden parents may blame themselves for the disease, consciously or subconsciously. Nevertheless, they must come to realize through education and counseling that they could not have done anything to prevent the disease and it was not their fault, since both environmental and hereditary factors may be involved in the development of diabetes.

Parents who are overprotective of the child suffer from feelings of guilt and fear of the unknown. Overprotection is a mechanism that alters the guilt responses to justify the parents' own needs—for example, "If the child is in my sight, nothing

---

*5000 State Road 67 N., Martinsville, IN 46151; 765-342-8456; www.ACAcamps.org.

worse will happen than getting diabetes." The overprotective parent becomes the smothering parent, one who hampers the child's growth, development, and maturation.

The neglectful parent, on the other hand, has a different problem. This response is a mechanism developed to block feelings that give pain and provide relief from feelings of guilt—"This is your disease, and I have no responsibilities related to your disease; therefore, if anything bad happens to you as a result of this disease, it is not my fault." The neglectful parent assigns responsibilities to the child before the child is mature enough to accept them.

Threatened parents look at the disease as a way to keep the child tied to them. If the child learns to be independent, as is expected during a camping experience, the parent may feel threatened and place obstacles in the child's path to independent development. Problems in the parental response provide a challenge for the nurse to assist by counseling or, if severe enough, by referring the parents to resources designed to help them alter their behavior (see Critical Thinking Exercise).

Children who are sufficiently mature may be seen alone by the health care professional, although the parents should not be made to feel left out. Time should be set aside during the child's health visit or afterward to meet the parents' needs. Parents should also be included in special sessions to keep them abreast of the child's management, to help them continue to participate in the child's care, and to provide an opportunity to express their feelings concerning their own or their child's adjustment to the disease. The amount of information that they offer at this time can give clues to their level of support of the child and assist in decisions concerning therapeutic management. This helps guide the child through the most disruptive time of life—the teenage years.

Health care professionals must be aware of parents who voice support and appear to be supporting the child to the optimum level but who, with more in-depth interviewing, are found not to be supportive. These parents seldom see the need for following through from verbalizing to meeting the child's real needs, and they unknowingly place obstacles in the child's path. They may be helping the child grow up too fast and therefore insecurely. These parents urgently need counseling so they can realize how their behavior affects the child. The classroom experience, group therapy, or parenting programs can guide the parents' relationships with their children. All parents should be helped to recognize that, as children grow and develop, they are children first and children with diabetes second. The ultimate goal for these parents is to be supportive of their children, to communicate more effectively with them, and to help their children develop in an acceptable manner (Wysocki, Harris, Buchloh, et al, 2006).

CRITICAL THINKING EXERCISE

Type 1 Diabetes Mellitus

Rebecca, a 15-year-old with a 3-year history of type 1 diabetes mellitus (DM), has been admitted to the pediatric intensive care unit for treatment of diabetic ketoacidosis (DKA). This is her fifth hospital admission for DKA in the past year. Rebecca's parents are divorced, and she has four younger siblings, none of whom has diabetes. Rebecca's mother has maintained two jobs for the past 5 years and frequently leaves Rebecca in charge of the household. In anticipation of her discharge you are planning a patient education program for Rebecca and her mother. What important issues regarding Rebecca's unstable diabetes management must you consider to plan the education program?

1. Evidence—Is there sufficient evidence to draw conclusions about Rebecca's recurrent episodes of DKA?
2. Assumptions—Describe an underlying assumption about each of the following:
   a. Type 1 DM in adolescence
   b. Type 1 DM and menses
   c. Emotional stress and elevated blood glucose levels
   d. Blood glucose monitoring for insulin management
3. What priorities for nursing care should be established for Rebecca?
4. Does the evidence support your nursing intervention?

KEY POINTS

- The endocrine system has three components: the cell, which sends a chemical message via a hormone; target cells, which receive the message; and the environment through which the chemical is transported from the site of synthesis to the sites of cellular action.
- Pituitary dysfunction is manifested primarily by growth disturbance.
- The main physiologic action of TH is to regulate the basal metabolic rate and control the processes of growth and tissue differentiation.
- Disorders of thyroid function include hypothyroidism, autoimmune thyroiditis, goiter, and hyperthyroidism.
- Therapy for hyperthyroidism is directed at retarding the rate of hormone secretion and may include drug therapy, thyroidectomy, or radioiodine therapy.
- Classic forms of hypoparathyroidism in childhood are idiopathic (deficient production of PTH) and pseudohypoparathyroidism (increased PTH production with end-organ unresponsiveness to PTH).

- The adrenal cortex secretes three important groups of hormones: glucocorticoids, mineralocorticoids, and sex steroids.
- Disorders of adrenal function include acute adrenocortical insufficiency, chronic adrenocortical insufficiency, Cushing syndrome, CAH, and hyperaldosteronism.
- Five categories of Cushing syndrome are pituitary, adrenal, ectopic, iatrogenic, and food dependent.
- Management of CAH includes assignment of a sex according to genotype, administration of cortisone, and, possibly, reconstructive surgery.
- The focus of type 1 DM is insulin replacement, diet, and exercise.
- Education of families includes explanation of diabetes, meal planning, administering insulin injections, monitoring general hygiene practices, promoting exercise, record keeping, and observing for complications.

ANSWERS TO CRITICAL THINKING EXERCISE

Type 1 Diabetes Mellitus

1. **Yes.** Rebecca has had five hospital admissions for DKA in the past year. Numerous factors must be involved with her unstable disease.

2. **a.** The normal tasks of adolescence can play a significant role in blood glucose instability.

   b. Adolescent girls with diabetes have frequent fluctuations of blood glucose levels immediately before, during, or after their menses.

   c. Rebecca's personal loss from the divorce, her mother's absence because of a heavy work schedule, and the added responsibilities of the household may cause significant stress, resulting in elevated blood glucose levels.

   d. Careful, frequent, consistent monitoring of blood glucose levels is essential for effective insulin management during adolescence.

3. The first priority would be to focus directly on the issues of hyperglycemia. Determination of Rebecca's practice of monitoring and management of her diabetes at home is essential. Areas of diabetes management that should be emphasized include careful dietary management, an appropriate exercise program, conscientious self-testing of blood glucose, appropriate administration of daily insulin, and adherence to sliding-scaling insulin therapy. Discussion of the emotional stressors she identifies at this time is appropriate.

4. **Yes,** Rebecca's history of DKA over the past year supports her inability to monitor and manage her diabetes.

REFERENCES

Ackard D, Vik N, Neumark-Sztainer D, et al: Disordered eating and body dissatisfaction in adolescent with type 1 diabetes: a population based comparison sample: comparative prevalence and clinical implications, *Pediatr Diab* 9(4 Part 1):312-319, 2008.

Aimaretti G, Bellone S, Baldelli R, et al: Growth hormone stimulation tests in pediatrics, *Endocrinologist* 14(4):216-221, 2004.

American Academy of Pediatrics, Section on Endocrinology and Committee on Genetics: Technical report: congenital adrenal hyperplasia, *Pediatrics* 106(6):1511-1518, 2000. Reaffirmation statement published 2005.

American Academy of Pediatrics, Rose SR, Section on Endocrinology and Committee on Genetics of the American Thyroid Association, et al: Update of newborn screening and therapy for congenital hypothyroidism, *Pediatrics* 117(6):2290-2303, 2006.

American Diabetes Association: Standards of Medical Care in Diabetes—2007, *Diabetes Care* 30(Suppl):S4-S41, 2007.

American Diabetes Association: Care of children and adolescents with type 1 diabetes, *Diabetes Care* 28:186-212, 2005.

American Diabetes Association: Implications of the diabetes and control and complications trial, *Diabetes Care* 25:S25-S27, 2002.

American Diabetes Association: Report of the Expert Committee on the Diagnosis and Classification of Diabetes Mellitus, *Diabetes Care* 24(Suppl 1):S5-S20, 2001.

Barker J, Eisenbarth G: The natural history of autoimmunity in type 1A diabetes mellitus. In Le Roith D, Taylor S, Olefsky J, editors: *Diabetes mellitus: a fundamental and clinical text*, ed 3, Philadelphia, 2003, Lippincott Williams & Wilkins.

Bartalena L, Tanda ML, Piantanida E, et al: Oxidative stress and Graves' ophthalmopathy: in vitro studies and therapeutic implications, *Biofactors* 19(3-4):155-163, 2003.

Batista DL, Riar J, Keil M, et al: Diagnostic tests for children who are referred for the investigation of Cushing syndrome, *Pediatrics* 120(3):2007:e575-e586.

Baxter JD, Ribeiro RCJ: Introduction to endocrinology. In Greenspan FS, Gardner DG, editors: *Basic and clinical endocrinology*, ed 7, New York, 2004, Lange Medical Books/McGraw-Hill.

Behrman RE, Kliegman RM, Jenson HB, et al: *Nelson textbook of pediatrics*, ed 18e, Philadelphia, 2009, Elsevier.

Bingley PJ, Gale EAM: Progression to type I diabetes in islet cell antibody–positive relatives in the ENDIT: the role of additional immune, genetic and metabolic markers of risk, *Diabetologia* 49:881-890, 2006.

Biro FM, Huang B, Crawford PB, et al: Pubertal correlates in black and white girls, *J Pediatr* 148(2):234-240, 2006.

Brown TB: Cerebral edema in childhood diabetic ketoacidosis: Is treatment a factor? *Emerg Med J* 21:141-144. 2004.

Bryant J, Baxter L, Cave CB, et al: Recombinant growth hormone for idiopathic short stature in children and adolescents, *Cochrane Database Syst Rev* 18(3):CD004440, 2007.

Campbell S: Request for applications: islet cell replacement in type 1 diabetes, *Cell Biochem Biophys* 40(3 Suppl):23-24, 2004.

Carel JC, Chaussain JL: Gonadotropin releasing hormone against treatment for central precocious puberty, *Horm Res* 51(Suppl 3):64-69, 1999.

Carel JC, Leger J: Precocious puberty, *N Engl J Med* 358:2366-2377, 2008.

Carr M, Gill D: Polyuria, polydipsia, polypopsia: "Mummy I want a drink," *Arch Dis Child Educ Pract* 92:139-143, 2007.

Cheetham T, Baylis PH: Diabetes insipidus in children: pathophysiology, diagnoses and management, *Paediatr Drugs* 4(12):785-796, 2002.

Cheetham TD, Hughes IA, Barnes ND, et al: Treatment of hyperthyroidism in young

people, *Arch Dis Child* 78(3):207-209, 1998.

Clar C, Waugh N, Thomas S: Routine hospital admission vs outpatient or home care in children at diagnosis of type 1 diabetes mellitus, *Cochrane Database Syst Rev* 18(2):CD004099, 2007.

Cohen P, Rogol AD, Deal CL, et al: Consensus statement on the diagnosis and treatment of children with idiopathic short stature: a summary of the Growth Hormone Research Society, the Lawson Wilkins Pediatric Endocrine Society, and the European Society for Paediatric Endocrinology works, *J Clin Endocrinol Metab* 93(11):4210-4217, 2008.

Cooke D, Plotnick L: Management of diabetic ketoacidosis in children and adolescents, *Pediatr Rev* 29:431-436, 2008.

Cooke D, Plotnick L: Management of type 1 diabetes mellitus. In Pescovitz OH, Eugster EA, editors: *Pediatric endocrinology: mechanisms, manifestations and management*, Philadelphia, 2004, Lippincott Williams & Wilkins.

Cryer P: Glucose counterregulatory hormones: physiology, pathophysiology, and relevance to clinical hypoglycemia. In Le Roith D, Taylor S, Olefsky J, editors: *Diabetes mellitus: a fundamental and clinical text*, ed 3, Philadelphia, 2003, Lippincott Williams & Wilkins.

Dabelea D, Bell RA, D'Agostino RB: SEARCH for diabetes in youth study group: incidence of diabetes in the United States, *JAMA* 297:2716-2724, 2007.

Dallas JS, Foley TP: Hyperthyroidism. In Lifshitz F, editor: *Pediatric endocrinology*, ed 4, New York, 2003, Marcel Dekker.

Darzy KH: Radiation-induced hypopituitarism after cancer therapy: who, how and when to test, *Natl Clin Pract Endocrinol Metab* 5(2):88-99, 2009.

De Buyst J, Massa G, Christophe C, et al: Clinical, hormonal and imaging findings in 27 children with central diabetes insipidus, *Eur J Pediatr* 166(1):43-49, 2007.

Dunning, T: *Care of people with diabetes: A manual of nursing practice*, ed 3, Oxford, 2009, Blackwell.

Eli Lilly: *Humalog package insert*, Indianapolis, May 1, 2007, Eli Lilly.

Fajans S, Bell G: Maturity-onset diabetes of the young: a model for genetic studies of diabetes mellitus. In Le Roith D, Taylor S, Olefsky J, editors: *Diabetes mellitus: a fundamental and clinical text*, ed 3, Philadelphia, 2003, Lippincott Williams & Wilkins.

Felner EI, Klitz W, Ham M, et al: Genetic interaction among three genomic regions creates distinct contributions to early and late onset type 1 diabetes mellitus, *Pediatr Diab* 6(4):213-220, 2005.

Foley TP: Hypothyroidism. In Hoekelman RA, Adam HM, Nelson NM, et al, editors: *Primary pediatric care*, ed 4, St Louis, 2001, Mosby.

Garg S, Rosenstock J, Silverman BL, et al: Efficacy and safety of preprandial human insulin inhalation powder versus injectable insulin in patients with type 1 diabetes, *Diabetologia* 49(5):891-899, 2006.

Glatt K, Garzon DL, Popovic J: Congenital adrenal hyperplasia due to 21-hydroxylase deficiency, *J Soc Pediatr Nurs* 10(3):104-114, 2005.

Goldfarb MF: Relation of time of introduction of cow milk protein to an infant and risk of type I diabetes mellitus, *J Proteome Res* 7(5):2165-2167, 2008.

Greiner MV, Kerrigan JR: Puberty: timing is everything, *Pediatr Ann* 35(12):916-922, 2006.

Halac I, Zimmerman D: Evaluating short stature in children, *Pediatr Ann* 33(3):171-176, 2004.

Hall DMB: Growth monitoring, *Arch Dis Child* 82(1):10-15, 2000.

Hanberg A: Common disorders of the pituitary gland: hyposecretion versus hypersecretion, *J Infus Nurs* 28(1):36-44, 2005.

Harris M: Definition and classification of diabetes mellitus and the new criteria for diagnosis. In Le Roith D, Taylor S, Olefsky J, editors: *Diabetes mellitus: a fundamental and clinical text*, ed 3, Philadelphia, 2003, Lippincott Williams & Wilkins.

Hathout EH, Hartwick N, Fagoaga OR, et al: Clinical, autoimmune, and HLA characteristics of children diagnosed with type 1 diabetes before 5 years of age, *Pediatrics* 111(4):860-863, 2003.

Herman-Giddens ME: Recent data on pubertal milestones in United States children: the secular trend toward earlier development, *Int J Androl* 29(1):241-246, 2006.

Hilczer M, Smyczynska J, Lewinski A: Limitations of clinical utility of growth hormone stimulating tests in diagnosing children with short stature, *Endocrinol Regul* 40(3):69-75, 2006.

Hoffman RP: Eating disorders in adolescents with type 1 diabetes: a closer look at a complicated condition, *Postgrad Med* 109(4):67-69, 73-74, 2001.

Hudson MM, Krasin M, Metzger M, et al: Hodgkin lymphoma. In Pizzo PA, Poplack DG, editors: *Principles and theories of pediatric oncology*, Philadelphia, 2011, Lippincott Williams & Wilkins.

Huether SE: Fluids and electrolytes, acids and bases. In Huether SE, McCance KL, editors: *Understanding pathophysiology*, ed 2, St Louis, 2000, Mosby.

Jospe N: Hyperthyroidism. In Hoekelman RA, Adam HM, Nelson NM, et al, editors: *Primary pediatric care*, ed 4, St Louis, 2001, Mosby.

Kaplowitz PB: Treatment of central precocious puberty, *Curr Opin Endocrinol Diabetes Obes* 16:31-36, 2009.

Karik AA, Fields AV, Shannon RP: Diabetic cardiomyopathy, *Curr Hypertens Rep* 9(6):467-473, 2007.

Katznelson L: Current thinking on the management of the acromegalic patient, *Curr Opin Endocrinol Diabetes Obes* 14:311-316, 2007.

Kiess W, Bottner A, Raile K, et al: Type 2 diabetes in children and adolescents: a review from a European perspective, *Horm Res* 59(Suppl 1):77-84, 2003.

Lee JM, Davis MM, Clark SJ, et al: Estimated cost-effectiveness of growth hormone therapy for idiopathic short stature, *Arch Pediatr Adolesc Med* 160:263-269, 2006.

Lee PA: Central precocious puberty: an overview of diagnosis, treatment, and outcome, *Endocrinol Metab Clin North Am* 28(4):901-918, 1999.

Lee PA, Houk CP, Ahmed SF, et al: Consensus Statement on Management of Intersex Disorders, *Pediatrics* 118:e488, 2006.

Leschek EW, Rose SR, Yanovski JA, et al: Effect of growth hormone treatment on adult height in peripubertal children with idiopathic short stature: a randomized, double blind, placebo-controlled trial, *J Clin Endocrinol Metab* 89(7):3140-3148, 2004.

Lin M, Liu SJ, Lim IT: Disorders of water imbalance, *Emerg Med Clin North Am* 23(3):749-770, 2005.

Majzoub JA, Muglia LJ: Disorders of water homeostasis. In Lifshitz F, editor: *Pediatric endocrinology*, ed 4, New York, 2003, Marcel Dekker.

Makaryus AN, McFarlane SI: Diabetes insipidus: Diagnosis and treatment of a complex disease, *Cleveland Clin J Med* 73(1):65-71, 2006.

Mannucci E, Rotella F, Recca V, et al: Eating disorders in patients with type I diabetes: a meta analysis, *J Endocrinol Invest* 28(5):417-419, 2005.

Miller BS, Zimmerman D: Idiopathic short stature in children, *Pediatr Ann* 33(3):177-181, 2004.

Moshang T: Cushing's disease, 70 years later ... and the beat goes on (editorial), *J Clin Endocrinol Metab* 88(1):31-33, 2003.

Natchtigall L, Delgado A, Swearingen B, et al: Extensive clinical experience: changing patterns in diagnosis and therapy of acromegaly over two decades, *J Clin Endocrinol Metab* 93(6):2035-2041, 2008.

Nebesio TD, Eugster EA: Current concepts in normal and abnormal puberty, *Curr Prob Pediatr Adolesc Health Care* 37(2):50-72, 2007.

New MI, Ghizzoni L: Update on congenital adrenal hyperplasia. In Lifshitz F, editor: *Pediatric endocrinology*, ed 4, New York, 2003, Marcel Dekker.

Olohan K, Zappitelli D: The insulin pump, *Am J Nurs* 103(4):48-56, 2003.

Perheentupa J: Hypoparathyroidism and mineral homeostasis. In Lifshitz F, editor: *Pediatric endocrinology*, ed 4, New York, 2003, Marcel Dekker.

Radetti G, Buzi F, Paganini C, et al: Treatment of GH-deficient children with two different GH doses: effect on final height and cost-benefit implications, *Eur J Endocrinol* 148(5):515-518, 2003.

Radetti G, Gottardi E, Bona G, et al: Study Group for Thyroid Diseases of the Italian Society for Pediatric Endocrinology and Diabetes (SIEDP/ISPED): the natural history of euthyroid Hashimoto's thyroiditis in children, *J Pediatr* 149(6):827-832, 2006.

Ramchandani N: Type 2 diabetes in children, *Am J Nurs* 104(3):65-68, 2004.

Rex J, Jensen KH, Lawton SA: A review of 20 years experience with the NovoPen family of insulin injection devices, *Clin Drug Invest* 26(7):367-401, 2006.

Richmond EJ, Rogol AD: Growth hormone deficiency in children, *Pituitary* 11:115-120, 2008.

Rivkees SA: Differentiating appropriate antidiuretic hormone secretion, inappropriate antidiuretic hormone secretion and cerebral salt wasting: the common, uncommon and misnamed, *Curr Opin Pediatr* 20:448-452, 2008.

Rivkees SA, Cornelius EA: Influence of iodine-131 dose on the outcome of hyperthyroidism in children, *Pediatrics* 111(4):745-748, 2003.

Root AW: Precocious puberty, *Pediatr Rev* 21(1):10-19, 2000.

Rosenson RS, Herman WH: Glycated proteins and cardiovascular disease in glucose intolerance and type II diabetes, *Curr Cardiovasc Risk Rep* 2(1):43-46, 2008.

Rovet JF, Ehrlich R: Psychoeducational outcome in children with early-treated congenital hypothyroidism, *Pediatrics* 105(3):515-522, 2000.

Sandberg DE, Kranzler J, Bukowski WM, et al: Psychosocial aspects of short stature and growth hormone therapy, *J Pediatr* 135(1):133-134, 1999.

Siarkowski K: Advances in assessment, diagnosis, and treatment of hyperthyroidism in children, *J Pediatr Nurs* 20(4):119-126, 2005.

Simmonds MJ, Howson JM, Heward JM, et al: Regression mapping of association between the human leukocyte antigen region and Graves disease, *Am J Human Genet* 76(1):157-163, 2005.

Skyler J, Marks J: Immune intervention. In Le Roith D, Taylor S, Olefsky J, editors: *Diabetes mellitus: a fundamental and clinical text*, ed 3, Philadelphia, 2003, Lippincott Williams & Wilkins.

Stanhope R: Transition from paediatric to adult endocrinology: hypopituitarism, *Growth Horm IGF Res* 14:s85-s88, 2004.

Steinberger J, Daniels SR: Obesity, insulin resistance, diabetes and cardiovascular risk in children: an American Heart Association scientific statement from the Atherosclerosis, Hypertension, and Obesity in the Young Committee (Council on Cardiovascular Disease in the Young) and the Diabetes Committee (Council on Nutrition, Physical Activity, and Metabolism), *Circulation* 107:1448-1453, 2003.

Stephenson M: Type 2 diabetes: a growing epidemic in children, *Infect Dis Child* 16(4):34-37, 2003.

Streetman DD, Khanderia U: Diagnosis and treatment of Graves disease, *Am J Nurse Pract* 8(1):27-36, 2004.

Szymborska M, Staroszczyk B: Thyroiditis in children, *Med Wieku Rozwoj* IV(4):383-391, 2000.

Tfayli H, Arslanian S: The challenge of adolescence: hormonal changes and sensitivity to insulin, *Diabetic Voice* 52:28-30, 2007.

Thompson GB: Surgical management in Graves' disease, *Panminerva Med* 44(4):287-293, 2002.

Tierney S, Deaton C, Webb K, et al: Isolation, motivation and balance: living with type 1 or cystic fibrosis-related diabetes, *J Clin Nurs* 17(7B):235-243, 2008.

Toogood AA, Stewart PM: Hypopituitarism: clinical features, diagnosis, and management, *Endocrinol Metab Clin North Am* 37:235-261, 2008.

Urrutia-Rojas X, Menchaca J: Prevalence of risk for type 2 diabetes in school children, *J Sch Health* 76(5):189-194, 2006.

Verbalis JG: Diabetes insipidus, *Rev Endocr Metab Disord* 4(2):177-185, 2003.

Wang TS, Roman SA, Sosa JA: Predictors of outcomes following pediatric thyroid and parathyroid surgery, *Curr Opin Oncol* 21:23-28, 2008.

Wetterau L, Cohen P: New paradigms for growth hormone therapy in children, *Horm Res* 53(Suppl 3):31-36, 2000.

Wolsdorf J, Glaser N, Sperling MD: Diabetic ketoacidosis in infants, children and adolescents, *Diabetes Care* 29:150-159, 2006.

Wysocki T, Harris MD, Buchloh LM, et al: Effects of behavioral family systems therapy for diabetes on adolescent family relationship, treatment adherence and metabolic control, *J Pediatr Psychol* 31(9):928-938, 2006.

The Child with Musculoskeletal or Articular Dysfunction

David Wilson and Martha Curry

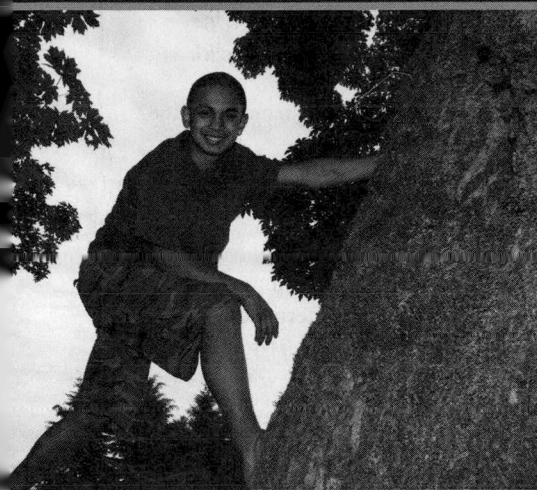

evolve WEBSITE

http://evolve.elsevier.com/wong/ncic

Animations
  Bone Fractures
  Osteomyelitis
  Spine Structure
Case Studies
  Fractures
  Osteomyelitis
Critical Thinking Case Studies
  Legg-Calvé-Perthes Disease
  Scoliosis
Key Points Audio Summaries
NCLEX Review Questions
Pediatric Assessment Video Clip
Skill
  Monitoring Neurovascular Status
Spanish/English Translations
WebLinks

RELATED TOPICS

CHAPTER OUTLINE

THE CHILD AND TRAUMA

TRAUMA MANAGEMENT

Epidemiology of Trauma

Trauma is a leading cause of death in children older than age 1 year (see Chapter 1) and an important cause of disability during childhood and adolescence. In many ways, childhood trauma differs little from trauma in adults. However, the child's developmental stage affects many aspects of injury, including the type of injury incurred and the physiologic response to injury. The Centers for Disease Control and Prevention estimated that 9.2 million children ages 0 to 19 years visited an emergency department annually between 2000 and 2006 for treatment of an unintentional injury (Borse, Gilchrist, Dellinger, et al, 2008).

Unintentional Injury

Among the leading causes of morbidity in children are medical problems resulting from traumatic injury that occurs at home or at school, in an automobile, or in association with recreational activities. Children's everyday activities include vigorous play that may involve such things as climbing, falling, running into immovable objects, and receiving blows to any part of the body. All of these activities make them prone to injury. School-age children and adolescents are vulnerable to multiple and severe trauma because they are mobile on bikes and motorcycles and in automobiles; they are also active in sports. Speed and congested surroundings often increase the chance of injury.

Young children and adolescents usually do not calculate risks as they learn to manipulate their environment and achieve developmental goals. Therefore accidents are a part of many childhood experiences. Fortunately, when children fall or are hit, their body's resilience protects them from serious damage to soft tissue, the musculoskeletal system, or other body organs. Their bones are more flexible than those of adults and therefore do not offer the rigid resistance to external forces that are likely to cause fractures (as occurs in more mature bones).

Child Abuse Injury

Unfortunately, careless handling of an infant or child (in some instances intentional physical abuse) is not uncommon. A multitude of different types of bone and soft tissue injury are inflicted on children by adults, and smaller children who are unable to protect themselves are most vulnerable. It is estimated that 25% to 50% of fractures in children younger than 3 years of age are the result of child abuse.

A traumatic incident that produces physical injury to an infant or child may be the outcome of an accident that was no one's fault, or it may be associated with child abuse. A well-documented history and a careful examination are essential to determine the cause of the injury. Emergency department and pediatric office personnel should be alert to situations in which the child's injuries are not congruent with the parent's description of the incident; in which the child's behaviors, such as fearful mannerisms or lack of crying, are not the expected ones; or in which radiographs show multiple healed fractures. Accounts of injury inconsistent with developmental abilities can alert the provider to possible abuse. For example, a 6-month-old infant cannot "climb out of the crib and break her leg." Reporting these incidents will aid in securing help for the child and family. (See Community Focus box; also see Physical Abuse, Chapter 16.)

🏠 COMMUNITY FOCUS

Distinguishing Unintentional from Intentional Fractures

Distinguishing abusive from unintentional fractures can be challenging. The history, location of the injury, x-ray data, and associated injuries must be carefully considered. Details of the history to consider include delay in seeking medical care and an inappropriate clinical history or the report of a change in the child but no report of injury.

The child's age was determined to be a factor in one study. The demographics in children most likely to suffer abuse requiring orthopedic treatment were less than 1 year of age, 1 to 2 years of age, and Medicaid as primary payer; winter and weekday presentation was also a strong predictor of child abuse presentation in this study (Bullock, Koval, Moen, et al, 2009). Loder and Feinberg (2007) found that the most common fractures in nonaccidental trauma involved the femur and humerus, and most of these fractures occurred in infants less than 2 years of age.

Although not diagnostic of an intentional injury, the location of a fracture can raise suspicions about the actual cause. In an infant, midshaft or metaphyseal humerus fractures and radius-ulna, tibia-fibula, and femur fractures are not common and raise suspicion about the likelihood of abuse. Rib fractures, scapular fractures, bilateral fractures, complex skull fractures, and vertebral fractures or subluxations are also suspicious. In contrast, in children older than 1 year of age, supracondylar humerus fractures and fractures of the clavicle, distal extremity, and femur are most frequently related to an unintentional or accidental injury.

In children of all ages, radiographic evidence of previous fractures at different stages of healing may indicate repeated trauma and raise concern about intentional injuries. The presence of bruises, burns, and additional soft tissue injuries in children may also prompt further evaluation to determine whether the child has been subjected to intentional harm. One mnemonic used to prompt consideration of the possibility of intentional physical abuse is B-5: bumps, bruises, breaks, burns, and anything that happens in the bathroom.

Childhood Characteristics

Certain developmental characteristics of children at various ages render them more susceptible to injury. For example, the large head of infants and toddlers predisposes them to head injury, especially in falls or motor vehicle injuries. Also, the relatively large spleen and liver and the broad costal arch make these structures prone to direct trauma. Because of their light weight and small size, infants and small children are easily thrown around in a moving vehicle. Their natural curiosity and their propensity for using large muscles lure them to attempt potentially hazardous activities.

Later, in school-age children and adolescents, whose bone growth outstrips muscle growth, difficulty controlling movement can contribute to physical injury. This is also a time when many children attempt to engage in activities beyond their physical capabilities to keep up with more agile companions and to meet the expectations of adults and older siblings. They are also vulnerable to a "dare." Risk taking compounded by a feeling of invulnerability is also characteristic of adolescence. Children of school-age and early adolescence may also be encouraged to continue engaging in sports activities after suffering a contusion or sprain and are therefore subject to repetitive sprain injuries.

Prevention of Injury

Increasingly, health care providers are recognizing the importance of injury prevention efforts in preserving the health and well-being of children. Nurses have an important role to play in these efforts.

Leading causes of injury to children include falls, being struck by or against an object, motor vehicle accidents, fires, pedestrian-vehicle accidents, drowning, and firearms. Falls were the leading cause of nonfatal injury among children ages 0 to 15 years. Motor vehicle collisions were the leading cause of nonfatal injury in adolescents ages 15 to 19 years of age (Borse, Gilchrist, Dellinger, et al, 2008). Poisonings also occur in young children, especially those between 1 and 4 years of age, and sports injuries occur in school-age children and adolescents.

Unintentional, preventable injury is the primary cause of pediatric mortality and a significant contributor to morbidity, including permanent disability. Both morbidity and mortality could be reduced dramatically by improved efforts at injury prevention. Studies have indicated a general lack of public awareness regarding risks, causes, and prevention of injury to children. Studies also show that injury prevention counseling is effective both in reducing hazards in the home and in increasing car seat use. Nurses can be active in legislative efforts, public awareness campaigns, group classes on injury prevention, and individual prevention counseling with children and families.

Many injury prevention strategies have been suggested for nurses. Nursing history or hospital admission forms can include screening questions about safety issues. Discharge planning or primary care visits might be a time to provide a family with information on safety practices. Well-child visits to the practitioner for physicals and immunizations are an excellent time to visit with children and parents about injury prevention in the home and the community. Home health care nurses can easily assist a family in conducting a home safety assessment. School nurses can develop safety education programs for different age-groups and discuss injury prevention with children that is applicable to their specific age-group. Additional resources for discussing injury prevention with adolescents include automobile insurance companies and the police and first-rescue

personnel.* Nurses in emergency department and outpatient clinic settings can provide instructions related to injury prevention on an individual basis as developmentally appropriate.

Accident prevention among adolescents presents a unique challenge to all health care workers. For accident prevention to be effective, adolescents must perceive the specific interventions as having an impact on their lives. Adolescents are concerned with body image and often feel indestructible unless their own life or the life of a close friend is touched by a catastrophic debilitating injury or death. With increased emphasis in society on having fun and enjoying life to its fullest (today) regardless of the consequences (tomorrow), it is difficult for adolescents to understand the need to follow the rules laid down by authority figures.

Concern is also increasing about injuries to older school-age children and adolescents from the use of all-terrain motor vehicles (for which many states have no laws on minimum age for riders), snowmobiles, personal water craft such as wave runners, in-line skates, trampolines, scooters, and motor vehicles. Activities involving such vehicles and equipment, although safe in and of themselves when conducted according to safety guidelines (of the manufacturer), may be dangerous for children and adolescents who are unable to appreciate the risks involved, not only to self but to others as well.

ASSESSMENT OF TRAUMA

The site of the injury usually influences the order of priority of interventions when emergency care is being instituted. Consider the safety of both the victim and the "Good Samaritan" rescuers to prevent further injury.

> **! NURSING ALERT**
>
> Always consider personal safety a top priority, since the victim cannot be helped if the rescuer is injured.

For example, removing a child from a burning building or the bottom of a swimming pool is an obvious, logical action, but anxious rescuers may not consider their own safety to be of prime importance. The major reason for thinking through the steps to be taken in an emergency before an incident actually occurs is to have preplanned actions available at a stimulus-response level.

Emergency Management

The Emergency Treatment box outlines guidelines for care of the child at the scene of an injury. After level of consciousness is assessed, the concerns are for airway, breathing, and circulation (ABC), after which other injuries are managed as indicated by the assessment. When spinal trauma is a possibility, open the airway using the modified jaw thrust maneuver, which is accomplished by grasping the angles of the victim's lower jaw and lifting with both hands, one on each side, and displacing the mandible upward and outward (without head

---

*SafeKids USA is an excellent resource for those interested in child safety; www.usa.safekids.org.

tilt or chin lift). Otherwise a head tilt–chin lift maneuver is effective in opening the victim's airway. (See Cardiopulmonary Resuscitation, Chapter 31.)

✚ EMERGENCY TREATMENT

Trauma

Before entering trauma area, observe for potential threats or dangers to rescuers and bystanders. Be aware of potential for further injuries to child.

Observe scene for signs and mechanism of injury (e.g., head-on motor vehicle injury), which helps to determine proper course of action for treating child's injuries.

Do not move child before arrival of emergency medical services (EMS) personnel unless child is in danger of further injury. If it is necessary to move child, follow appropriate steps to prevent further injury (e.g., stabilize cervical spine to avoid exacerbation of spinal injury during movement).

Primary Assessment and Intervention

Assess level of consciousness. Use the AVPU method:

A—Child is alert.

V—Child responds to verbal stimulus.

P—Child responds to painful stimulus.

U—Child is unresponsive to any stimulus.

Open airway, using appropriate method.

- In child with head, trunk, or multisystem trauma, modified jaw thrust is preferred method (see p. 1213).
- At this point, cervical spine should be manually immobilized and held in alignment with rest of spinal column and should not be released until EMS personnel have immobilized child with appropriate equipment.

Activate the EMS system if child appears to be 8 years old or older. If child is less than 8, perform 2 minutes of cardiopulmonary resuscitation (CPR) (as per assessment); then activate EMS. (See Cardiopulmonary Resuscitation, Chapter 31.)

Assess for breathing. If necessary, begin rescue breathing.

Assess for circulation. If necessary, begin chest compressions.

- Palpate carotid artery in children 1 year or older.
- Palpate brachial artery in infants younger than 1 year.

Observe for hemorrhage. Control bleeding with a gloved or protected hand:

1. Apply direct pressure to wound site.
2. Elevate wound site.
3. Apply pressure to appropriate arterial pressure point.
4. Apply tourniquet only as a last resort. Once a tourniquet is applied, it should not be loosened.

Assess for further injury.

Do not remove objects protruding from child's body.

Check for evidence of decreased motor or sensory function in extremities:

- Infant and young child—Observe spontaneous movement in extremities.
- Older child—Ask if able to wiggle extremities.

Evaluate pain—Present, absent; severe, mild.

- Attempt to alleviate with nonpharmacologic techniques.
- Encourage use of analgesics when EMS personnel arrive.

Assess pulses in extremity distal to injury.

- Check color and temperature of extremities.

Manage any injuries appropriately (e.g., splint fractures) (see Emergency Treatment box, p. 1639).

Maintain body heat.

Identify child.

Obtain information regarding the injury from witnesses, if any.

Spinal cord injury cannot be assessed adequately in the prehospital setting. Radiography, computed tomography (CT), or magnetic resonance imaging (MRI) is required for diagnosis. Spinal cord injury is always suspected in a patient with head, trunk, or multisystem trauma. Only in a fully equipped trauma center with radiography and other diagnostic testing can spinal cord injury be ruled out. Therefore the patient is treated as if injury were present. Immobilize the cervical spine by maintaining the head in a neutral position and not allowing movement of the head or body in any direction.

❗ NURSING ALERT

In any situation in which spinal cord injury is suspected or is a possibility, the child should be calmed, reassured, and told not to move. *No one should be allowed to move the child unless the entire spine is stabilized.* A rigid cervical collar is used to immobilize the cervical spine, and the child is placed supine on a rigid immobilization board. Infants and small children are removed in their car seats; no attempt should be made to take them out of their seats.

Breathing is assessed after the airway is opened. If the child is not breathing, rescue breaths are given at a rate of 20 breaths/min. Oxygen should be provided when possible. Circulation is assessed only after the airway has been maintained and breathing is established. In children younger than 1 year of age, a brachial pulse is assessed. In those older than 1 year of age, a carotid pulse is palpated. Chest compressions should be initiated if necessary. (See Cardiopulmonary Resuscitation, Chapter 31.)

Control of bleeding is first attempted by application of direct pressure with a gloved hand. If this does not work, a pressure dressing is applied. The next step is to elevate the body part and then attempt to control hemorrhage by pressing on arterial pressure points. A tourniquet is used only when the bleeding cannot be controlled with a pressure dressing (Laskowski-Jones, 2002). If used, the tourniquet should be applied only to control bleeding. Once applied, it should not be removed or loosened. Below the tourniquet site, skin and tissue necrosis begins. If the tourniquet is loosened or removed, the toxins can be released into the circulation in high concentrations and may induce a systemic, deadly, tourniquet shock. With the tourniquet in place, the patient has a better chance of survival, even though it may mean the loss of a limb. Tourniquet use in prehospital settings has been shown to be safe (Doyle and Taillac, 2008; Lee, Porter, and Hodgetts, 2007).

Assessment of the child involves observation from head to toe, since infants and young children are unable to communicate except by crying and other behaviors. Therefore pinpointing areas of pain is difficult. To check for any motor or sensory dysfunction in the extremities, the nurse should note any spontaneous movement, which provides the best clue in infants and young children. Older children are able to follow directions to wiggle toes or fingers, demonstrate a grasp, "push down on the gas pedal," or lift legs off the bed. The child is identified as soon as feasible by anyone who knows the child. It is important to determine whether the child has any existing health problems that might have implications for the circumstances of the injury and for therapeutic management. Ask any witnesses for details about the incident to aid in assessment of the child's emotional responses.

In the prehospital setting the nurse's role consists of contacting emergency medical services (EMS) and providing basic life support until EMS personnel arrive on the scene. The nurse's role is limited to basic life support because the nurse has no standing orders or protocols under which to work in the pre-hospital setting (see Emergency Treatment box). Call EMS as soon as possible so that the patient can receive advanced life support before and during transport. A pediatric trauma triage system with personnel designated to care for an injured child is essential to provide excellent trauma patient care.

A paramedic-level ambulance provides at least one para-medic with skills in advanced cardiac life support, pediatric advanced life support, and neonatal resuscitation. A paramed-ic's skills include electrocardiogram interpretation and defibril-lation, advanced airway management (including endotracheal intubation, as well as intravenous [IV] and pharmacologic therapy), placement of a pneumatic antishock garment (PASG), pleural decompression (with a chest tube), and placement of a nasogastric tube and Foley catheter. Other advanced life support skills include expertise in spinal immobilization, extrication, management of fractures and bleeding, and emergency scene management. The paramedic remains in constant contact with the emergency department physician by means of a radio or cellular telephone for situations requiring medical control. Attempting to transport a child by automobile wastes valuable time in obtaining help. Transportation by EMS is recom-mended. Services in most large communities can institute advanced life support immediately or en route to a medical facility.

> **! NURSING ALERT**
>
> It is imperative that EMS be called to respond as soon as possible. Family, friends, or strangers should *not* transport the trauma victim.

Systematic Assessment

Several factors can affect a child's response to trauma. An unde-tected congenital anomaly can contribute to a complicated injury. Acute gastric distention occurs frequently in children because of the crying and screaming that accompany an injury. The temperature of young children is unstable because of their large surface area in relation to body mass, and temperature maintenance is critical in trauma management. Children also experience rapid metabolic changes. When they are ill, children are really ill; but as they recover, they change very rapidly. In addition, children have a small volume of blood in absolute terms. Whereas blood volume is 60% of total body weight in the adult, it is 70% to 85% in the child.

The first priority on admission to an emergency facility is rapid assessment of ABC status. Because the overwhelming majority of childhood injuries are the result of blunt-impact trauma, multiple organ involvement is a common finding. Therefore it is essential to perform a systematic assessment of the trauma victim.

The secondary survey is a systematic head-to-toe search for any additional injuries not originally addressed in the primary survey. However, children are often an exception to the head-to-toe approach. It may be preferable to complete the second-ary survey on the injured child in a toe-to-head direction. This approach may allow the rescuer to gain the child's trust as the survey progresses and the rescuer moves gradually into the

child's personal space. The Nursing Care Guidelines box gives an example of a complete secondary survey. Throughout the assessment, the nurse observes for areas of deformity, edema, ecchymosis, bleeding, hematoma, paralysis, or pain.

> **NURSING CARE GUIDELINES**
>
> ### Assessing Trauma
>
> **Primary Assessment**
> **Respirations**—Assess rate and quality; auscultate lung sounds.
> **Pulse**—Assess rate and quality.
> **Blood pressure**—If available, obtain baseline on all children regardless of age.
> **Skin**—Assess color, temperature, and condition. Treat for shock if mecha-nism of injury and vital signs indicate possible need. Administer high-flow oxygen if available. Elevate lower extremities (if no possibility of spinal injury). Maintain body temperature.
>
> **Systematic Head-to-Toe (or Toe-to-Head) Assessment**
> **Neck and cervical spine**—Palpate for point tenderness; observe for stoma, distended neck veins, tracheal shift, medical alert tags.
> - Immobilize neck with rigid cervical collar and towel rolls and/or foam head blocks (to prevent lateral neck movement) if available. (Manual cervical spine immobilization should still be in effect from emergency assessment and intervention.)
>
> **Scalp and skull**—Palpate for indentations, deformity, etc. Observe for cere-brospinal fluid in ears, Battle sign (bruising behind ears, which indicates possible skull fracture).
> **Face**—Observe for deformity, cerebrospinal fluid in nose.
> **Eyes**—Observe for pupillary response, equality.
> **Mouth**—Observe for possible obstructions, breath odor, loose teeth.
> **Chest and ribs**—Palpate for possible fractures, deformity; observe and feel for equal expansion, asymmetry.
> **Abdomen**—Auscultate, then palpate all quadrants for deformity, rigidity (indicating possible intraabdominal bleed).
> **Lumbar spine**—Palpate for deformity, tenderness. Reassess airway patency and level of consciousness.
> **Pelvis and hips**—Perform three-way compression test for possible fracture without rocking the hip (contraindicated if known pelvic fracture).
> **Groin**—Observe for bleeding, priapism (indicating possible severe spinal injury).
> **Extremities**—Palpate and observe all extremities for deformity; crepitus; bleeding; sensory, motor, and circulatory function; medical alert tags.
> Reevaluate treatment for shock, and reassess airway patency, breathing, circulation, level of consciousness, bleeding control, and vital signs.

THE IMMOBILIZED CHILD

IMMOBILIZATION

One of the most difficult aspects of illness is the immobility it often imposes on a child. Children's natural tendency to be mobile influences all elements of growth and development—physical, social, psychologic, and emotional. Impaired physical mobility related to disability or imposed activity restrictions presents a definite challenge to the child, staff, and parents providing care.

Causes of Immobilization

The usual reason for immobilizing or restricting the activity of a child without disabilities is illness or injury. Bed rest or mechanical restraining devices are frequently prescribed to aid in the healing and restorative processes. When children are ill, they are content to remain quiet, and most of them instinctively reduce their activity. It is children who are forced to remain inactive because of physical limitations or therapy who display the multiple effects of restricted movement.

The most frequent reasons for immobility are congenital defects (e.g., spina bifida); neuromuscular conditions (e.g., muscular dystrophy, spinal muscular atrophy); the need for prolonged mechanical ventilation and sedation; and infections or injuries that impair the integumentary system (severe burns), the musculoskeletal system (complex fractures or osteomyelitis), or the neurologic system (spinal cord injury, Guillain-Barré syndrome, or traumatic brain injury and coma). Sometimes therapies such as traction and spinal fusion are responsible for prolonged immobilization, although the trend is toward early mobilization, early discharge, and outpatient care.

Physiologic Effects of Immobilization

Many clinical studies, including space program research, have documented predictable consequences that occur after immobilization and the absence of gravitational force. Functional and metabolic responses to restricted movement occur in most of the body systems. Each has a direct influence on the child's growth and development, since homeostatic mechanisms thrive on normal use and need feedback to maintain dynamic equilibrium. Inactivity leads to a decrease in the functional capabilities of the whole body as dramatically as the lack of physical exercise leads to muscle weakness.

Although children usually become mobile once they feel well, the effects of immobility may be offset by a process termed **prehabilitation**, in which the individual's functional capacity is enhanced before prolonged immobility to help withstand the stress on the body's vital function. Prehabilitation has been implemented for adult patients in the intensive care unit and for those undergoing coronary artery bypass graft, knee arthroplasty, or orthopedic surgery who require prolonged immobilization; it could also be used for children anticipating

immobility. Athletes use prehabilitation to decrease the incidence of injuries and increase vital functioning of the cardiorespiratory system, muscles, and metabolism.

Most of the pathologic changes that take place during immobilization arise from decreased muscle strength and mass, decreased metabolism, and bone demineralization. The three are closely interrelated, with one change leading to or affecting another. Some results of immobilization are primary and produce a direct effect; other pathophysiologic consequences occur frequently but seem to be more indirect and are therefore secondary effects. Many pathophysiologic changes affect more than one body system, with the primary or secondary effect being demonstrated in multiple systems.

Children who are confined to bed during an illness or traumatic injury are usually restricted in movement for a relatively short time or are sufficiently active to avoid the physical consequences of immobility.

The major effects of immobilization (Fig. 39-1) are related directly or indirectly to decreased muscle activity, which produces numerous primary changes in both muscular and bone structures along with secondary alterations in the cardiovascular, respiratory, metabolic, and renal systems. The major consequences are:

- Significant loss of muscle strength, endurance, and muscle mass (atrophy)
- Bone demineralization leading to osteoporosis
- Loss of joint mobility and contracture

The larger the portion of the body immobilized and the longer the immobilization, the greater the hazards of immobility.

Muscular System

Inactive muscle loses strength at the rate of 3% per day, and several weeks or months are sometimes required for function to be regained when there is no primary neuromuscular deficit. Stretching can occur as muscle loses its tone or as excessive strain is put on weakened muscle (e.g., stretching by tight bed

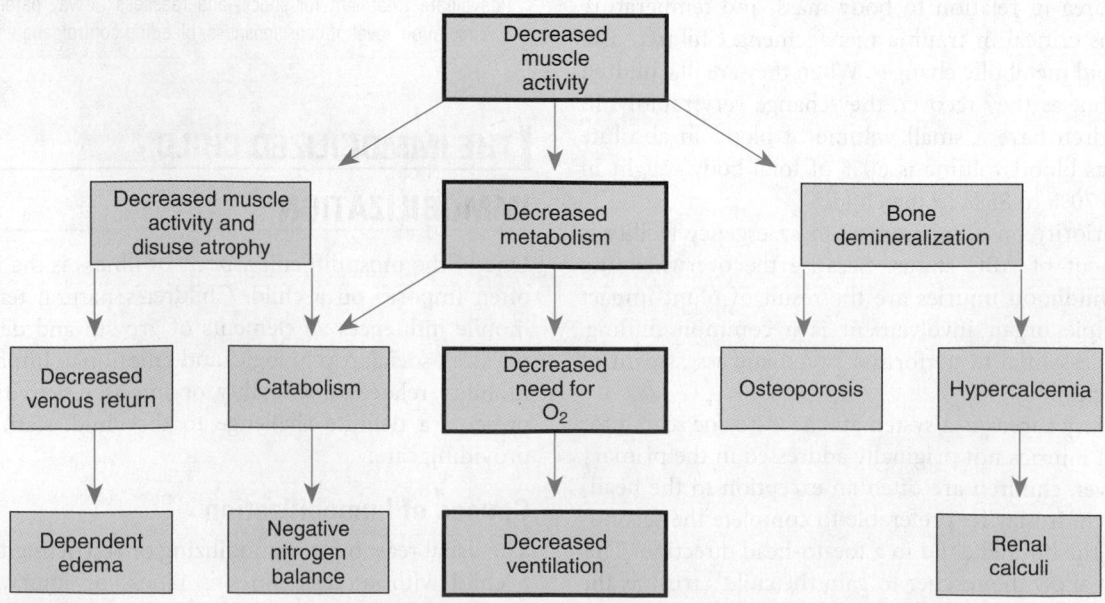

Fig. 39-1 Physiologic effects of immobilization.

covers or poor body position that produces footdrop as experienced by some children with disability). The disuse leads to tissue breakdown and loss of muscle mass (**atrophy**). The chief intracellular muscle enzyme, creatine, is released into the serum as the muscle atrophies; therefore serum levels provide an indication of the amount of muscle mass undergoing degeneration. Muscle inactivity also affects the cardiovascular system by decreasing venous return and cardiac output. In general, muscle atrophy causes decreased strength and endurance. Passive or active range-of-motion exercise and proper positioning can prevent joint stiffness and joint and intraarticular dysfunction.

Skeletal System

The daily stresses on bone created by motion and weight bearing maintain the balance between bone formation (**osteoblastic** activity) and bone resorption (**osteoclastic** activity). When these stresses are diminished, bone formation ceases, but bone destruction continues, so that the state of equilibrium is disrupted. Bone calcium becomes severely depleted, and secretion of phosphorus and nitrogen is increased. This demineralization of the bone (**osteopenia**) makes the skeletal structures prone to pathologic fractures and increases calcium ion concentration in the blood (hypercalcemia).

In children who have limited mobility, such as children who are unconscious or partially or fully paralyzed, joint mobility becomes restricted. In the absence of normal structural stretching, collagen fibers generated within the joint become fibrotic and further limit movement. This tissue fibrosis creates shortening of the muscles and contracture of the joint. Any decrease in circulation to the joint caused by edema, inflammation, or restrictive positioning contributes to further fibrotic changes. The problem rapidly becomes cyclic as the contracture leads to muscle fatigue and pain, which causes the child to protect the site, thus leading to more fibrosis. This process is further exaggerated because body flexor muscles are stronger than extensor muscles, and unless range of motion is reestablished within 3 to 7 days, contractures will develop. Frequent disabling contractures are hip flexion, knee flexion, shoulder stiffness, and plantar flexion of the feet.

Cardiovascular System

Immobility has three major cardiovascular consequences: **orthostatic intolerance**, increased workload of the heart, and thrombus formation. During movement, muscle contraction causes pressure on peripheral veins, which in turn causes the venous valves to close and thus assists in return of the blood to the heart when the individual is in an upright position. In the absence of this assistance, blood tends to pool in the dependent areas, reducing the blood supply to the trunk and brain. In addition, direct reflex stimulation to the splanchnic and peripheral vessels causes them to constrict when a person is upright. Impairment of this neurovascular orthostatic reflex activity from lack of motion causes further interference with venous return. The individual displays signs of excessive autonomic activity (e.g., pallor, sweating, and restlessness, which are frequently followed by fainting). The child with a spinal cord injury has unique problems with orthostatic intolerance, which is discussed in Chapter 40.

> **! NURSING ALERT**
>
> Carefully evaluate sudden chest pain and dyspnea; sudden onset of shortness of breath; air hunger; or pain and swelling in the lower extremities, which sometimes indicates deep vein thrombosis.

Changes in vascular resistance caused by the horizontal position and immobility alter the distribution of blood within the body. The reduction in gravity pressure to the extremities causes much of the total blood volume to be redistributed from lower extremities to other parts of the body. Consequently there is an increase in the venous return and the volume of blood to be handled by the heart, which is reflected in elevated blood pressure. As a result, cardiac output and stroke volume are increased, and a progressive increase in heart rate occurs. When immobilization extends over time, there is a compensatory decrease in blood volume and a decrease in heart rate and blood pressure.

Without muscle contraction, venous stasis and increased intravascular pressure in the extremities often lead to dependent edema. If undue pressure is exerted on the major veins by positioning or mechanical devices, the likelihood of interstitial edema is increased. Edematous tissue, especially tissue located over an area that receives much of the body's weight, is prone to skin breakdown.

Circulatory stasis combined with hypercoagulability of the blood, which results from factors such as damage to the endothelium of blood vessels (Virchow triad), can lead to thrombus and embolus formation. **Deep vein thrombosis (DVT)** involves the formation of a thrombus in a deep vein such as the iliac and femoral veins and can cause significant morbidity if it remains undetected and untreated. DVT may develop with prolonged venous stasis in conditions such as obesity, chronic heart failure, prolonged surgical procedure, long trips without exercise, or prolonged immobilization (Wipke-Tevis and Rich, 2007).

The state of deconditioned cardiac function, caused by skeletal muscle inactivity, can produce a variety of secondary problems in other systems. However, the major clinical manifestation is increased pulse and heart rate in response to an active exercise program. After prolonged immobility the child should build up activity tolerance slowly to allow the heart to regain optimum capabilities.

Respiratory System

Initially the effects of immobilization are compensatory or adaptive. The basal metabolic rate is decreased because with reduced expenditure of energy the cells require less oxygen and produce less carbon dioxide. Lessened demand for oxygen–carbon dioxide exchange causes the respirations to become slower and more shallow. Chest expansion may be limited by the supine posture; by abdominal distention caused by accumulation of feces, gas, or fluid; and by mechanical restriction such as from a body cast, brace, or tight binders. Reduced muscle power and coordination secondary to altered innervation can also hinder respiratory movement. More effort is required to expand the lungs in the supine position.

Prolonged immobility also reduces the normal movement of secretions from the tracheobronchial tree, particularly in the presence of impaired muscle function and without positional changes that normally facilitate removal of secretions. A weak and ineffectual cough reflex contributes to stasis of secretions and the possibility of airway obstruction in the smaller airways of children. Shallow respirations and obstruction of the airway with thick mucus are factors in the development of secondary complications such as atelectasis and pneumonia.

Gastrointestinal System

Prolonged immobility produces a state of negative nitrogen balance resulting from the increased catabolic activity related to muscle atrophy. This and the reduced energy requirements contribute to a diminished appetite and a resulting decrease in ingestion of nutrients (anorexia). Eating and feeding become more difficult with immobility, and the risk of aspiration is increased. Associated psychologic factors further influence intake.

The process of elimination depends on the integration of smooth and skeletal muscle activity and on visceral reflex patterns. Immobility may interfere with these mechanisms, as well as with the gravitational effect on stool passing through the intestines. Slowing of stool in the colon causes the feces to become hard, and the bowel wall is not stimulated to further its peristaltic movement down the tract to the rectum. Weakened muscles used in defecation (diaphragmatic and abdominal muscles) are unable to produce the intraabdominal pressure needed for elimination. Sometimes embarrassment in using a bedpan or bedside commode may be the cause of not responding to the urge to defecate.

Renal System

The urinary system is designed to function in an upright posture. When the gravitational force is altered by the reclining position, the peristaltic contractions of the ureters are insufficient to overcome gravitational resistance. Consequently there may be stasis of urine in the kidney pelves, and any particulate matter that settles in the calyces may serve as nuclei for calculi formation or as foci for infection.

In the horizontal position the individual has difficulty relaxing the perineal musculature and external sphincter sufficiently to initiate the integrated reflex micturition mechanism, which involves the external sphincter, the internal sphincter, and the detrusor muscle of the bladder wall. If adequate intraabdominal pressure is exerted, voiding can occur, but if the individual does not respond to the sensation to void, bladder distention leads to stasis, and its complications add to embarrassing overflow incontinence. In time, reflux and back pressure may impair renal function, and urinary tract infection is always a hazard with urine retention.

Normally the kidney is able to handle the increased metabolites from protein breakdown and bone demineralization. However, the increased level of calcium excreted may predispose the person to calculus formation. Formation of calculi (kidney stones) is further favored by urinary stasis, infection, and an alkaline urine caused by the decreased production of the acid by-products of metabolism. Hematuria may be the only clue to the diagnosis.

Metabolism

Immobility or severe restriction of activity is often accompanied by decreased or inappropriate nutritional intake, which frequently leads to a decreased basal metabolic rate, a negative nitrogen balance associated with catabolism, and a high serum calcium level.

All body systems are influenced by a decrease in metabolism. The altered energy level leads to further fatigue and lack of motivation for moving. Immobilized persons often feel sluggish and have a poor appetite, particularly for protein foods. The protein breakdown in the body related to a loss of muscle and other tissues is more apt to be severe after injury or surgery. Protein breakdown produces nitrogenous wastes, and on the fifth or sixth day of catabolic protein metabolism, an increase in urinary nitrogen level develops that contributes to anemia and delayed healing.

Another metabolic problem is hypercalcemia associated with bone catabolism. Completely immobilized children or adolescents are especially prone to hypercalcemia. Symptoms, which include nausea and vomiting, polydipsia, polyuria, and lethargy, usually appear 4 to 8 weeks after immobilization. In tetraplegia, symptoms may occur within 10 days and last for as long as 6 months. The accelerated rate of bone metabolism in children makes the bone demineralization a greater hazard. Larger amounts of calcium are released into the blood than the kidney can excrete, and calcium continues to accumulate in serum. High levels of serum calcium decrease neuronal permeability, which can lead to a depression of the central and peripheral nervous systems. Symptoms, including smooth and skeletal muscle fatigue, diminished reflexes, and atony of the gastrointestinal tract, are a result of the depressed nervous system.

A child with bone demineralization may not develop hypercalcemia, but the excess amount of calcium that the kidneys are required to excrete may produce a negative calcium balance, with more calcium than citric acid lost in the urine. This imbalance causes the urine to become alkaline, with the potential danger of renal calculi, especially if there is an accompanying retention of urine.

Integumentary System

Circulation to the skin is reduced during inactivity and may be further impeded by dependent edema. Circulation is especially compromised in places where the bone surface is near the skin, such as areas over the sacrum, occiput, trochanter, and ankle, and continued impairment causes rapid necrosis with ulcer formation. Friction and mechanical irritation from appliances, such as straps, rods, and ropes, and the friction of bedclothes during turning or other movement can produce skin breakdown. Healing capacity is also impaired by poor circulation, negative nitrogen balance, and anemia. Immobilization often makes it difficult to carry out adequate cleansing and hygienic measures, which may also contribute to tissue breakdown in areas that are difficult to reach. Guard children with neurologic deficit against extremes of heat and cold in direct contact with the skin.

Cellular breakdown caused by prolonged pressure has several characteristics. Normally when pressure is applied to the skin, the skin appears pale but becomes very red, or hyperemic, after

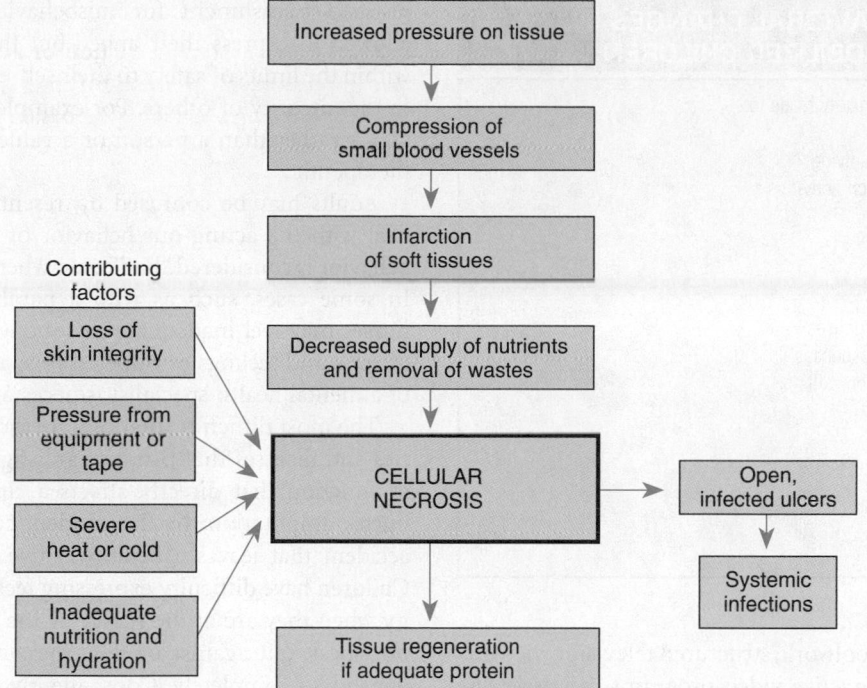

Contributing factors

Fig. 39-2 Sequence of events in tissue breakdown.

the pressure is removed. This reactive **hyperemia** should disappear within 5 to 15 minutes. Prolonged redness (>30 minutes) indicates that a pressure area is developing and treatment should begin. Other manifestations of tissue ischemia include an increase in temperature in the area, blistering, swelling, and dark purple or black areas. The pressure area may be limited to the skin and subcutaneous layers or may be deeper and more extensive. The skin changes observed may represent the top of a cone-shaped area with widespread tissue destruction, beneath which tissue rapidly ulcerates and creates a large pressure ulcer that sometimes extends to the bone. Fig. 39-2 illustrates the sequence of events in tissue breakdown. (See also Maintaining Healthy Skin, Chapter 27.)

Neurosensory System

Studies indicate that immobilization does not produce neurosensory consequences directly; however, two occurrences—loss of innervation and sensory and perceptual deprivation—are common.

Peripheral nerves, in contrast to skeletal muscles, do not degenerate with disuse, but loss of innervation takes place if nerves are damaged by pressure or if their blood supply is disrupted. Improper body positioning, poorly applied casts or restraints, or fluid buildup within a compartment (**compartment syndrome**) can place excessive pressure on nerves and blood vessels that can lead to ischemia and nerve degeneration. Frequent sites of nerve compression phenomenon are the peroneal nerve, where pressure results in footdrop, and the radial nerve, where pressure leads to wristdrop. These complications significantly interfere with attempts to regain functional use of the extremities, but they can be prevented by conscientious nursing assessment and intervention. Preventing pressure on vulnerable areas and avoiding extreme positions of flexion and extension that apply inappropriate pressure on nerves and blood vessels reduce the likelihood of compression injury. Periodic plantar flexion and dorsiflexion of the feet and hands by passive or active range of motion will stimulate circulation and keep nerves from becoming pinched. Numbness, tingling, change in sensation, and loss of motion are symptoms of neurologic impairment and should be evaluated immediately.

Psychologic Effects of Immobilization

For children, one of the most difficult aspects of illness is immobilization. Throughout childhood, physical activity is an integral part of daily life and is essential for physical growth and development. It also serves children as an instrument for communication and expression and as a means for learning about and understanding their world. Activity helps them deal with a variety of feelings and impulses and provides a mechanism by which they can exert control over inner tensions. Children respond to anxiety with increased activity. Removal of this power deprives them of necessary input and a natural outlet for their feelings and fantasies. Through movement children also gain sensory input, which provides an essential element for developing and maintaining a body image.

Active children have many opportunities for input from a wide variety of settings. When they are immobilized by disease or as a part of a treatment regimen, they experience diminished environmental stimuli with a loss of tactile, vestibular, and proprioceptive input and an altered perception of themselves and their environment. Sudden or gradual immobilization narrows the amount and variety of environmental stimuli they receive by means of all their senses: touch, sight, hearing, taste, smell, and proprioception. This sensory deprivation frequently leads to feelings of isolation, boredom, and being forgotten, especially by peers. Nursing interventions involving the use of

---

BOX 39-1   BEHAVIORAL CHANGES IN IMMOBILIZED CHILDREN

Higher than normal level of anxiety leads to:
- Restlessness
- Difficulty with problem solving
- Inability to concentrate on activities
- Depression
- Regression
- Egocentrism

Monotony leads to:
- Sluggish intellectual responses
- Sluggish psychomotor responses
- Decreased communication skills
- Increased fantasizing
- Hallucinations
- Disorientation
- Dependence
- Acting-out behavior
- Depression

---

diversional activities, schoolwork, structured television viewing, computer games, or interactive video programs can assist the child in maintaining usual activities. (See Chapter 26.)

The struggle for independence is thwarted by imposed immobility. For toddlers, exploration and imitative behaviors are essential to developing a sense of autonomy; preschoolers' expression of initiative is evidenced by their penchant for vigorous physical activity; school-age children's development is strongly influenced by physical achievement and competition; and adolescents rely on mobility to achieve independence. The quest for mastery at every stage of development is related to mobility. To children, the inability to move is threatening to self-preservation and reactivates the struggle between activity and passivity, and between dependence and independence.

Behavioral changes occur when children experience prolonged sensory deprivation. Some of these behaviors are indications of a higher-than-normal level of anxiety (Box 39-1). Children are likely to become depressed over their loss of ability to function or the marked changes in body image. Significant others often notice regressive behavior and a greater reliance on them for tasks the children are able to perform. Children seek their attention by reverting to earlier developmental behaviors, such as wanting to be fed, bed-wetting, and baby talk. In many ways immobilized children are realistically dependent on others; therefore intelligent and sensitive care is required to prevent major developmental regressions during the period of immobility.

Limbs that are immobilized by casts, traction, or paralysis transmit less sensory data than normally. Sensory impairment may be a concomitant problem of the involved part. Numbness or loss of feeling markedly alters proprioception. Children who have limited ability to feel others touching them not only experience less tactile stimulation in a physical sense but are also deprived of warm, loving feelings that arise from being touched. The loss of feeling from touch can further add to their sense of being isolated and unwanted.

Children often react to immobility with active protest, anger, and aggressive behavior, or they may become quiet, passive, and submissive. Often children believe that the immobilization is a justified punishment for misbehavior. Children should be allowed to express their anger, but this expression should be within the limits of safety to their self-esteem and not damaging to the integrity of others. For example, providing an object to attack rather than a person or a valued possession is safe and therapeutic.

Adults may be confused by, resent, and find it difficult to deal with the acting-out behavior of children. Too often this behavior is considered "bad" even when it is a release of tension. In some cases, such as with a paralyzed child, parents and nurses may feel inadequate to cope with the child's profound distress and feelings of hopelessness, and the professional help of a mental health specialist is necessary.

The most difficult situations are those involving major injuries and diseases that produce a disfigurement or a severe loss of function that directly affects a child's self-image, such as burns; amputation; or the sudden, catastrophic effects of an accident that leaves a healthy, active child paralyzed for life. Children have difficulty expressing feelings of anger and hostility when they are at the mercy of the environment. They dare not speak out against or defy the authorities on whom they depend so completely. Consequently their aggression may be masked by cheerfulness or rigidity. When they are unable to express their anger, the aggression is often displayed inappropriately through regressive behavior and outbursts of crying or temper tantrums over insignificant irritations. Adolescents and older school-age children should vary their daily routine to fit their needs for independence; allowing this age-group to stay up late at night and sleep in during the daytime (within reasonable limits to accommodate treatment needs) may help decrease struggles over other inconsequential matters and at the same time allow a daily pattern of life. Encourage parents to continue setting limits and not abandon disciplinary measures with children who are confined to bed due to trauma or illness.

Effects of Immobilization on Families

Brief periods of child immobilization have few effects on the family; however, a child's catastrophic illness or disability may severely tax their resources. The need for instruction concerning medical and nursing care, community resources to contact, and emotional support are paramount. Many families have unmet needs, operate from crisis to crisis, and are unable to use outside help appropriately. For these families the new situation can be disruptive; therefore the rehabilitation team must help the family members identify unmet needs and solve problems. The following are commonly occurring problems:

- Financial strains may decrease or totally eliminate the family's resources.
- Attention is focused, at least temporarily, on the affected member; therefore other members of the family, especially siblings, may feel that they are being neglected or that their needs may not be met.
- The family may have difficulty accepting the child's altered body condition.
- Individual family members may be unable to express their feelings and may have difficulty coping with the crisis.
- Parents often experience guilt over their child's condition and need for immobilization. Their perception of failing

to protect the child forms the basis for their difficulty coping.

The family's needs often must be met through the services of a multidisciplinary team, and nurses play a key role in anticipating the services the family will need and in coordinating appropriate care. In preparation for the child's discharge from the hospital, home visits are recommended, and home management is frequently planned weeks in advance of the actual discharge, including special provisions for meeting cultural, economic, physical, and psychologic needs. A child with a severe disability is dependent, and caregivers need rest periods to revitalize themselves. Individual and group counseling is beneficial for problem-solving situations and provides an emotional support system. Parent groups are also helpful and often allow nonthreatening social contact. The families of children with permanent disabilities need long-term resources, since some of the most difficult problems arise as they try to sustain high-quality care for many years. (See Chapters 25 and 22.)

Nursing Care Management

Assessment

Physical assessment of the child who is immobilized as a result of an injury or a degenerative disease includes a focus not only on the injured part (e.g., fracture or damaged joint), but also on the functioning of other systems that may be affected secondarily—the circulatory, renal, respiratory, muscular, and gastrointestinal systems.

Encourage children to be as active as their condition and restrictive devices allow. This usually poses few problems for children, whose innate ingenuity and natural inclination toward mobility provide them with the impetus for physical activity. They need the opportunity, the materials or objects to stimulate activity, and the encouragement and participation of others. Those who are unable to move will need passive exercise and movement, often in consultation with a physical therapist. An occupational therapist and child life specialist may also assist in planning activities to decrease boredom and to help regain lost skills such as self-feeding. A child psychologist may be consulted to discuss with the child and family issues such as depression, anger management, and the effects of the illness on family function.

Children who require prolonged total immobility and are unable to move themselves in bed should be placed on a pressure reduction mattress to prevent skin breakdown. Frequent position changes also help prevent dependent edema and stimulate circulation, respiratory function, gastrointestinal motility, and neurologic sensation. Children at higher risk for skin breakdown include those with prolonged immobilization; those who use orthotic and prosthetic devices, including wheelchairs; those who have plaster casts; and children requiring intensive care. Additional risk factors include poor nutrition, friction (from bed linen with traction), and moist skin (from urine or perspiration) (Fig. 39-3). Nursing care of children at risk includes proactive strategies for preventing skin breakdown when such conditions are present. The Modified Braden Q Scale is a reliable, objective tool the nurse can use in assessing for pressure ulcer development in children who are acutely ill or who are at risk for skin breakdown from neurologic conditions and immobilization (Curley, Razmus, Roberts, et al, 2003).

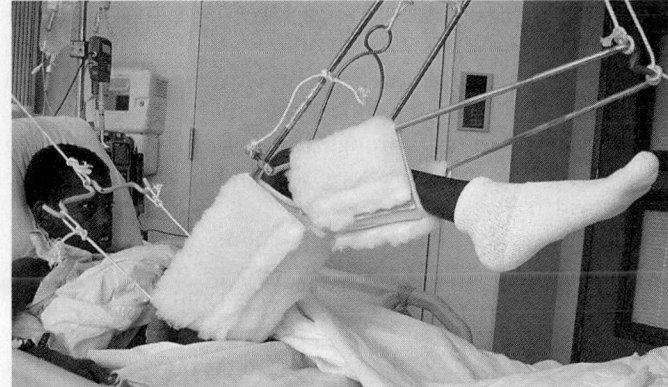

Fig. 39-3 Immobilized child. (Courtesy Eufemia Jacob, Texas Children's Hospital, Houston.)

Circulatory stasis and DVT development are prevented by instructing patients to change positions frequently, dorsiflex their feet and rotate the ankles, sit in a bedside chair periodically, or ambulate several times daily. The use of antiembolism stockings or intermittent compression devices prevents circulatory stasis and dependent edema in the lower extremities and the development of DVT. Anticoagulant therapy may also be implemented with low-molecular-weight heparin, vitamin K antagonists, or unfractionated heparin. Children who are unable to move should have passive range-of-motion exercises of the upper and lower extremities to increase circulation and minimize stasis.

Transporting the child by stretcher, wheelchair, stroller, or wagon outside the confines of the room whenever possible increases environmental stimuli and provide social contact with others. While hospitalized, the child benefits from frequent visitors, accessibility of clocks and calendars, and a program of diversional therapy to help the child function more normally. A child life specialist should be consulted for recreational planning. An activity center or slanting tray can be helpful for the child with limited mobility to use for drawing, coloring, writing, and playing with small toys such as trucks and cars. A child is able to express frustration, displeasure, and anger through play, which is helpful in the child's recovery. As soon as possible, the child should wear street clothes and resume school and preinjury hobbies. Play is the most useful tool of nursing (see Chapter 26), and activities should be selected on the basis of interest, ability, and limitations. They should include some form of physical activity that encourages the use of uninvolved muscles and joints. Any activity that is tolerated (e.g., turning in bed or changing the position of the bed in the room) helps to alter the monotony of immobilization and dissipates tension and frustration. Allow a parent or siblings to room in with the hospitalized child to prevent the effects of family disruption from hospitalization. Make every effort to minimize family disturbance resulting from the hospitalization. Although most of the suggestions discussed relate to hospital care, the same consultations (physical therapist, occupational therapist, child life specialist, speech/language pathologist) and environment may be considered in the home as well to help the child to gain independence and the family to achieve normalization.

Using dolls or a stuffed animal such as a bear to illustrate and explain the restraining method is a valuable tool for small children. Placing a cast, tubing, or other restraining device on the doll or stuffed animal offers the child a nonthreatening opportunity to express, through the doll, feelings concerning the restrictions and feelings toward the nurse and other health care providers.

Children typically dislike hospital food, which is usually not tailored to their age. In some institutions food services are geared toward children's preferences with child-friendly menus and smaller food portions served. Allow parents and friends to bring in favorite foods from home or other sources such as fast food places, provided they meet necessary requirements for the illness. This enables children to have more control of their environment and will decrease resistance to treatments and schedules, which is common behavior evidenced when adults and children are not given any choices in an acute care setting.

One of the most useful interventions to help children cope with immobility is participation in their own care. Self-care to the maximum extent possible is usually well received by children. They can help plan their daily routine; select their diet (when possible); and choose the clothes they are to wear, including innovative adornment, such as a baseball cap, brightly colored stockings, or other items that express their autonomy and individuality. Encourage them to do as much for themselves as they are able to keep muscles active and their interest alive. If feasible, they should be placed where they can benefit from the company of other children, which assures them that they are not being singled out for this medical treatment.

It is important for children to understand behavioral limitations or rules. Their questions should be answered. For example, children need to know the reasons for medical, nursing, occupational, and physical therapy and to know that some schedules are necessary. In some areas they have a choice; in others they do not. They may or may not be permitted to sleep late, but they can choose their own clothing. Most of children's activities of daily living are play; therefore therapies that incorporate play are more apt to gain their cooperation.

Visits from significant persons, such as family members and friends from school or the neighborhood, offer occasions for emotional support and also provide opportunities for learning how to care for the child. If a traumatic incident caused the child's disability, guilt feelings may be displayed overtly or masked behind regressive or aggressive behavior. The feeling that "I must have been bad to receive this fate" is common, and honest feedback, such as "It just happened—it was an accident," needs repeating many times. Additional aspects of grieving are involved if there was a loss of another person or if permanent disability occurred as a result of the accident. All these feelings need to be brought out and dealt with. In addition, professionals working with these children must not "baby" or overprotect them but must help them to cope with their altered body image and reestablish their self-esteem.

For a child with greatly restricted movement (e.g., a child with tetraplegia or a child with a large bilateral hip spica cast), creativity in nursing care is often required to keep the child stimulated and prevent the effects of immobilization. These situations may require long-term care in the hospital, a rehabilitation center, or, increasingly, at home. Wherever the care occurs, consistent planning and coordination of activities with professionals and significant others is vital.

Nursing assessment includes gathering psychosocial data, in addition to assessing physical manifestations, since long-term immobilization has a profound effect on the child and the family. Nursing approaches are evaluated frequently and continued, discontinued, or modified to meet the changing problems and goals. Table 39-1 summarizes the physical effects of immobilization and appropriate nursing care management. With the increased trend toward early mobilization, early discharge, and home health care, many children are discharged home after a few days of hospitalization. Follow-up treatment may take place in the home or in an outpatient ambulatory facility.

MOBILIZATION DEVICES

Orthotics and Prosthetics

Developments in the fields of **orthotics** (fabrication and fitting of braces) and **prosthetics** (fabrication and fitting of artificial limbs) have resulted in lighter and better-fitting devices and thus greater patient compliance in using them. Orthoses are often used to prevent deformity, increase the energy efficiency of the gait, and control alignment. Braces that facilitate walking can sometimes stabilize paralyzed or markedly weakened extremities. Special joint hinges permit the hip, knee, and ankle to flex while sitting, whereas the leg is held rigid during ambulation. Well-fitted orthoses promote ambulation, whereas ill-fitting braces throw off the child's balance and frequently cause muscle stress and tissue breakdown. In the growing child braces need frequent adjustment and replacement by the orthotist if long-term use is necessary.

A standing frame or a parapodium (a standing frame on a circular base) helps small children to assume an upright position and begin mobilization. Children learn to use their arms and shift their weight to swivel the base of the parapodium to mobilize. Four common types of orthoses are used in older children and are described based on the joints controlled by the orthosis. The ankle-foot orthosis (AFO) is used to prevent footdrop due to bed rest, trauma to the foot, or paralysis of muscles that flex the foot; to prevent heel cord tightening after heel cord–lengthening surgery; or to support the foot in proper position for standing and walking (Fig. 39-4). AFOs are now available in patterns and colors.

The knee-ankle-foot orthosis (KAFO) is used to prevent buckling of the knee, to support the extremity when there is paralysis or marked weakness of the knee extension or quadriceps muscle, or to protect the limb when the bone structure is weak (Fig. 39-5). The hip-knee-ankle-foot orthosis (HKAFO) is used to provide various types of control for the knee and ankle joints (as described earlier), as well as the hip (e.g., flail lower limb and paralysis). The reciprocal gait orthosis (RGO) is a type of HKAFO that has a mechanism allowing children with significant paraplegia to walk in a reciprocal fashion on a flat surface. RGOs are used in children with spinal cord injury, sacral agenesis, and spina bifida.

The thoracolumbosacral orthosis (TLSO) is custom molded and fits snugly around the trunk of the body to exert pressure on the ribs and back to support the spine in a straight position

TABLE 39-1	SUMMARY OF PHYSICAL EFFECTS OF IMMOBILIZATION WITH NURSING INTERVENTIONS*	
PRIMARY EFFECTS	**SECONDARY EFFECTS**	**NURSING CONSIDERATIONS**
Muscular System		
Decreased muscle strength, tone, and endurance	Decreased venous return and decreased cardiac output	Use antiembolism stockings or intermittent compression devices to promote venous return (monitor circulatory and neurovascular status of extremities when such devices are used).
	Decreased metabolism and need for oxygen	Plan play activities to use uninvolved extremities.
	Decreased exercise tolerance	Place in upright posture when possible.
	Bone demineralization	
Disuse atrophy and loss of muscle mass	Catabolism	Have patient perform range-of-motion, active, passive, and stretching exercises.
	Loss of strength	
Loss of joint mobility	Contractures, ankylosis of joints	Maintain correct body alignment.
		Use joint splints as indicated to prevent further deformity.
		Maintain range of motion.
Weak back muscles	Secondary spinal deformities	Maintain body alignment.
Weak abdominal muscles	Impaired respiration	See nursing care for respiratory system.
Skeletal System		
Bone demineralization—osteoporosis, hypercalcemia	Negative bone calcium uptake	With paralysis, use upright posture on tilt table.
	Pathologic fractures	Handle extremities carefully when turning and positioning.
	Calcium deposits	Administer calcium-mobilizing drugs (diphosphonates) and normal saline infusions if ordered.
	Extraosseous bone formation, especially at hip, knee, elbow, and shoulder	Ensure adequate intake of fluid; monitor output.
	Renal calculi	Acidify urine.
		Promptly treat urinary tract infections.
Negative bone calcium uptake	Life-threatening electrolyte imbalance	Monitor serum levels of calcium.
		Provide electrolyte replacement as indicated.
Metabolism		
Decreased metabolic rate	Slowing of all systems	Mobilize as soon as possible.
	Decreased food intake	Have patient perform active and passive resistance exercises and deep-breathing exercises.
		Ensure adequate food intake.
		Provide a high-protein diet.
Negative nitrogen balance	Decline in nutritional state	Encourage small, frequent feedings with protein and preferred foods.
	Impaired healing	Prevent pressure areas.
Hypercalcemia	Electrolyte imbalance	See nursing care for skeletal system.
Decreased production of stress hormones	Decreased physical and emotional coping capacity	Identify causes of stress.
		Implement appropriate interventions to lower physical and psychosocial stresses.
Cardiovascular System		
Decreased efficiency of orthostatic neurovascular reflexes	Inability to adapt readily to upright position (orthostatic intolerance)	Monitor peripheral pulses and skin temperature changes.
	Pooling of blood in extremities in upright posture	Use antiembolism stockings or intermittent compression devices to decrease pooling when upright.
Diminished vasopressor mechanism	Orthostatic intolerance with syncope, hypertension, decreased cerebral blood flow, tachycardia	Provide abdominal support.
		In severe cases, use antigravitational pants.
		Position horizontally.
Altered distribution of blood volume	Increased cardiac workload	Monitor hydration, blood pressure, and urinary output.
	Decreased exercise tolerance	
Venous stasis	Pulmonary emboli or thrombi	Encourage and assist with frequent position changes.
		Elevate extremities without knee flexion.
		Ensure adequate fluid intake.
		Have patient perform active or passive exercises or movement as needed.
		Prescribe routine wearing of antiembolism stockings or intermittent compression devices.
		Monitor for signs of pulmonary embolism—sudden dyspnea, chest pain, respiratory arrest.
		Promptly intervene to maintain adequate oxygenation if signs and symptoms of pulmonary emboli are noted.
		Measure circumference of extremities periodically.
		Give anticoagulant drugs as prescribed.

*Individualize care according to child's needs; interventions may vary in different institutions.

Continued

TABLE 39-1 SUMMARY OF PHYSICAL EFFECTS OF IMMOBILIZATION WITH NURSING INTERVENTIONS*—cont'd

PRIMARY EFFECTS	SECONDARY EFFECTS	NURSING CONSIDERATIONS
Cardiovascular System—cont'd		
Dependent edema	Tissue breakdown and susceptibility to infection	Administer skin care.
		Turn every 2-4 hr.
		Monitor skin color, temperature, and integrity.
		Use pressure-reduction surface as necessary to prevent skin breakdown. (See Chapter 27.)
Respiratory System		
Decreased need for oxygen	Altered oxygen–carbon dioxide exchange and metabolism	Promote exercise as tolerated.
Decreased chest expansion and diminished vital capacity	Diminished oxygen intake	Position for optimum chest expansion.
	Dyspnea and inadequate arterial oxygen saturation; acidosis	Use prone positioning without pressure on abdomen to allow gravity to aid in diaphragmatic excursion.
		Ensure that patient maintains proper alignment when sitting to prevent pressure on respiratory mechanism.
Poor abdominal tone and distention	Interference with diaphragmatic excursion	Avoid restriction of chest and abdominal musculature.
		Supply torso support to promote chest expansion.
Mechanical or biochemical secretion retention	Hypostatic pneumonia	Change position frequently.
	Bacterial and viral pneumonia	Carry out percussion, vibration, and drainage (or suctioning) as necessary.
	Atelectasis	Monitor breath sounds.
Loss of respiratory muscle strength	Poor cough	Encourage coughing and deep breathing.
		Support chest wall by splinting with pillow when patient coughs.
		Use incentive spirometer.
		Observe for signs of respiratory distress with pulse oximetry or blood gas measurement as necessary.
	Upper respiratory tract infection	Prevent contact with infected persons.
		Provide adequate hydration.
		Administer immunizations as necessary (pneumococcal, meningococcal).
Gastrointestinal System		
Distention caused by poor abdominal muscle tone	Interference with respiratory movements	Monitor bowel sounds.
		Encourage small, frequent feedings.
	Difficulty in feeding in prone position	Have patient sit in upright position if possible.
No specific primary effect	Possible constipation caused by gravitational effect on feces through ascending colon or weakened smooth muscle tone	Carry out bowel training program with hydration, stool softeners, increased fiber intake, and mild laxatives if necessary.
	Anorexia	Stimulate appetite with favored foods.
Urinary System		
Alteration of gravitational force	Difficulty in voiding in prone position	Position as upright as possible to void.
Impaired ureteral peristalsis	Urinary retention in calyces and bladder	Hydrate to ensure adequate urinary output for age.
	Infection	Collect specimens as needed.
	Renal calculi	Stimulate bladder emptying with warm running water, as necessary.
		Catheterize only for severe urinary retention.
		Administer antibiotics as indicated.
Integumentary System		
Altered tissue integrity	Decreased circulation and pressure leading to tissue injury	Turn and position at least every 2-4 hr.
		Frequently inspect total skin surface.
		Eliminate mechanical factors causing pressure, friction, or irritation.
	Difficulty with personal hygiene	Assess ability to perform hygienic care and assist with bathing, grooming, and toileting as needed.
		Encourage self-care to potential ability.
		Ensure adequate intake of protein, vitamins, and minerals.

*Individualize care according to child's needs; interventions may vary in different institutions.

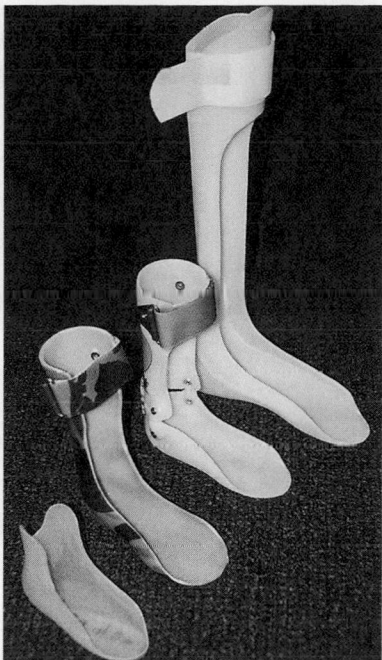

Fig. 39-4 *Left to right:* Supramalleolar ankle-foot orthosis (AFO), solid ankle AFO, articulating ankle AFO, floor reaction AFO.

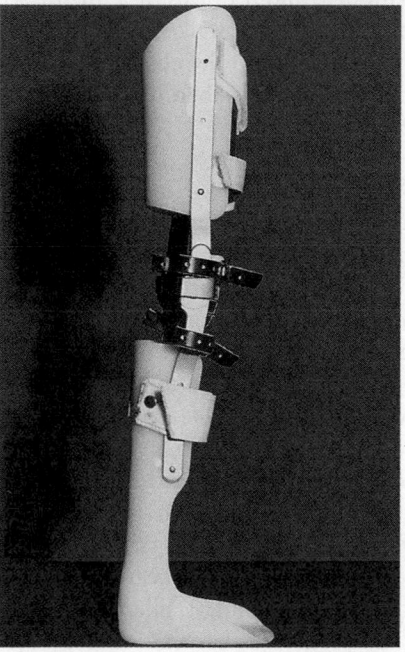

Fig. 39-5 Knee-ankle-foot orthosis (KAFO).

(Fig. 39-6). The Boston brace is an underarm orthosis customized from prefabricated plastic shells, with corrective forces for each patient supplied by lateral pads. These braces may prevent the progression of curves in the spine, such as scoliosis, or provide needed torso support in a child with paraplegia. The Jewett-Taylor brace is sometimes used to support the spine and trunk during ambulation to prevent compression after fracture of the spinal column.

An orthosis must fit each body curvature to avoid undue pressure on tissues and imbalance between muscle groups. Bony prominences where a brace has contact, such as along the spine, chin, and iliac crests, are observed closely for pressure or irritation and are padded as necessary.

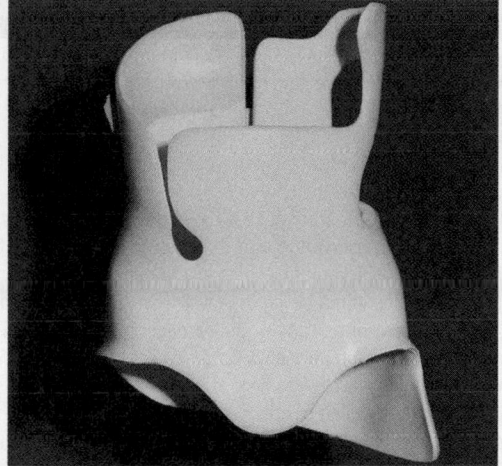

Fig. 39-6 Thoracolumbosacral orthosis (TLSO).

BOX 39-2	TYPES OF AMPUTATION

Syme—Ankle disarticulation
BK—Below knee
KD—Knee disarticulation
AK—Above knee
HD—Hip disarticulation
WD—Wrist disarticulation
BE—Below elbow
ED—Elbow disarticulation
AE—Above elbow
SD—Shoulder disarticulation

When prostheses are prescribed, the provider considers many factors: level of amputation, age, weight, activity, agility, and skin condition. Each prosthesis is custom made or fabricated of various plastic and foam materials. The style of the prosthesis depends on the most distal joint involved in the amputation or prosthetic fitting. Common abbreviations used to describe types of amputations are listed in Box 39-2.

Advances are constantly occurring in both the fabrication and fitting of prosthetics. Development of myoelectric devices, use of new cosmetic materials in terminal gloves and feet, and socket construction using computer-aided design and computer-aided manufacturing are but a few of the recent changes with positive effects for patients who require prostheses.

Nursing Care Management

Meticulous skin care under a brace is necessary. At times, protective clothing should be worn under braces to protect the skin from friction and pressure. Assessment of all areas that make contact with the brace every 2 to 4 hours for the first few days after application is recommended. If any area is reddened, the brace should be removed for ½ to 1 hour. If the redness does not disappear, the nurse should notify the practitioner or orthotist (see Family-Centered Care box).

Before a prosthesis is applied, the condition of the skin must be assessed, with special note taken of areas of redness or breaks in the integrity of the skin. Prevention of skin breakdown is best accomplished through good hygiene of the residual limb, proper fitting of the artificial limb, and prosthetic training (see Family-Centered Care box).

FAMILY-CENTERED CARE

Orthoses

Care of Skin

AFO, KAFO

If the child has decreased sensation in the legs, check the skin condition more frequently than every 4 hours.

If the child complains of a burning sensation under the brace, remove the brace promptly and observe the skin for any reddened areas. If the child complains of burning several times, contact the physician or orthotist.

If a small blister or open area develops, cover it with a sterile bandage and check the skin more often. Do not put alcohol on open areas. The child should avoid wearing the device until the skin heals.

Sometimes open areas are slow to heal. If no sign of healing occurs after 3 days, contact the physician or orthotist.

Lotions and creams will soften the skin and should be used only if the skin is dry.

TLSO

Because the device works by pressing against the body and is kept very snug by straps and buckles, some skin pinkness is to be expected. The skin at the brace edges and under the pads should be inspected carefully and frequently, especially in the initial period when the child or adolescent is getting accustomed to the device. Any red mark that does not fade within 20 minutes, or any area that appears raw and sore, should be reported to the orthotist.

Have the child wear a cotton undershirt under the brace to protect the skin; keeping it clean, dry, and free of wrinkles will help prevent skin problems.

Care of Orthoses

TLSO

Clean the brace with soap and water, followed by a good rinsing with water, on a weekly basis. Thoroughly dry the brace before it is put on. It is also important to avoid leaving it in hot places, such as in direct, strong sunlight or by a warm heater.

AFO, KAFO, HKAFO

Clean the plastic sections of the brace with soap and water and dry them thoroughly.

Keep the joints of the brace well oiled; 3-in-One oil is a good lubricant.

Check all screws periodically to make certain that they are tight.

If the brace is broken, out of alignment, or causing skin problems, notify the orthotist.

AFO, Ankle-foot orthoses; *HKAFO*, hip-knee-ankle-foot orthoses; *KAFO*, knee-ankle-foot orthoses; *TLSO*, thoracolumbosacral orthoses.

 FAMILY-CENTERED CARE

Prostheses

Care of Residual Limb

Wash with mild, nonperfumed soap, rinse, and dry thoroughly daily.

A small amount of powder may be used on the skin, but no alcohol.

Check skin for redness, sensitive areas, or signs of infection.

Care of Prosthesis

Routinely wash the socket with water and mild soap, rinse, and dry thoroughly.

Check straps and rubber bands with each application.

Check joints to ensure that they operate smoothly.

Replace worn or broken parts (heels, soles, straps) as needed.

Use 100% cotton stump socks to absorb perspiration, prevent skin friction, and provide comfort.

Change socks daily and wash and dry following instructions provided by prosthetist.

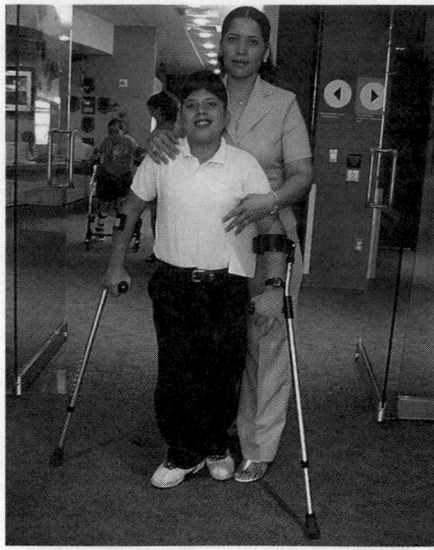

Fig. 39-7 Adolescent using forearm crutches for ambulation. (Courtesy Texas Children's Hospital, Houston.)

Safety is another important consideration. Parallel bars provide secure hand rails on both sides as the child learns to walk again with or without braces or a prosthesis. As the child becomes more proficient, a walker with or without wheels is substituted for the bars, and the child is no longer confined to a limited territory. The child then progresses to crutches if age and condition permit it.

Crutches and Canes

Crutches are used when children are not allowed to bear weight; need support for balance while walking in braces; or can place only part of their body weight on an extremity, such as with most lower leg injuries. There are many types of crutches, and the selection depends on the child's individual needs. Axillary swing-through crutches are used most frequently as temporary assistance. Forearm crutches (Fig. 39-7) are the usual selection for children who anticipate permanent use, such as paraplegic children who are able to use braces. In children with limited hand and arm strength or function, the use of trough crutches allows the weight to be assumed by the elbow. For habilitating small children who have not yet learned to walk or who are unsteady, front- or rear-rolling walkers are typically used until the children can progress to crutches (Fig. 39-8).

Children must be properly fitted with a crutch or cane to prevent both poor posture and crutch pressure on the axilla during ambulation. A physical therapist usually measures the child for crutches and teaches crutch and cane use; however, nurses in some areas such as the emergency department do teach children crutch walking. Nurses also supervise the use of crutches and canes in pediatric units and in the home. The type of crutch gait taught to a child depends on how stable the child is on crutches, whether or not the knees can be flexed, how much weight bearing is allowed, and what specific goal is established for the child.

Performing upper body strengthening exercises to condition and strengthen arms and shoulders before crutch use is important if immobilization has been prolonged. The child gains confidence in ambulating by wearing a safety belt held by the

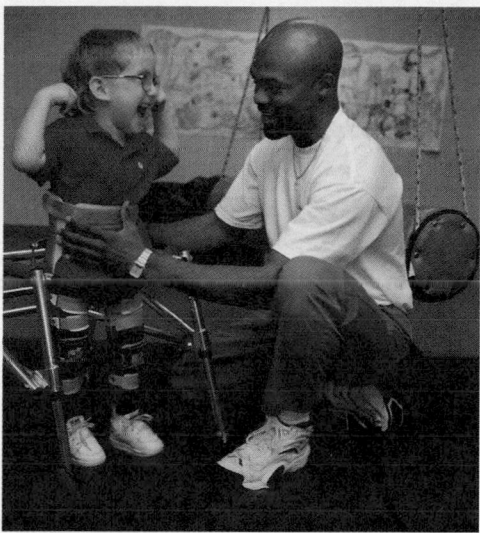

Fig. 39-8 Young child with rear-rolling walker. (Courtesy Paul Vincent Kuntz, Texas Children's Hospital, Houston.)

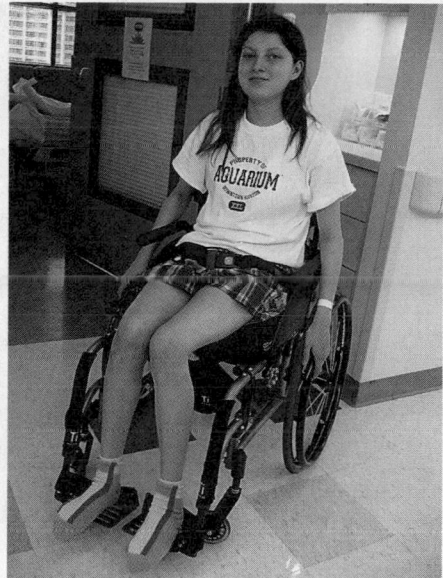

Fig. 39-10 Wheelchair allows adolescent mobility and independence. (Courtesy Texas Children's Hospital, Houston.)

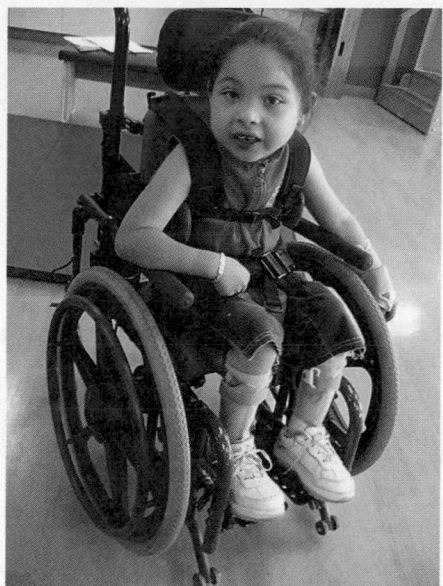

Fig. 39-9 Child in wheelchair, which should be scaled appropriately to child's size. Note ankle-foot orthoses and left wrist splint to prevent contractures. (Courtesy Texas Children's Hospital, Houston.)

therapist. The types of gaits used and instructions given to children are similar to those for adults. Instructions are conveyed in language children understand and with a demonstration. Most children adapt to the techniques readily.

Wheelchairs

Wheelchairs are used temporarily or permanently as a means of transportation. A wheelchair for temporary use should fit the child and contain any adaptations needed, such as an elevating leg rest or reclining back. The child learns how to transfer in and out of the chair and how to move it safely. Prescribing a wheelchair for permanent use is the joint responsibility of the physician and therapist after an assessment of home and surroundings. A wheelchair should be neither too small nor too large and preferably should be adaptable as the child grows (Fig. 39-9).

Detachable or rotating armrests, which permit easy transfer in and out, are needed for children with spinal cord injuries. Other desirable features are detachable and swing-away footrests and detachable desk arms. Elevating leg rests are required for children who are prone to contractures, and a reclining back rest is needed for those who may have poor trunk balance. A pressure-relief cushion should be provided for a child who has decreased sensation. Hand-rim and brake-lever projections are helpful for children with upper extremity weakness. For children who have the use of only one arm, a special "one-arm drive" wheelchair is available. Children with paraplegia require upper arm strengthening exercises and instruction on transfer techniques before wheelchair mobilization (Fig. 39-10). Often a tilt table is used to overcome the problem of orthostatic intolerance before the child is able to tolerate wheelchair sitting.

Various motorized chairs are available for children with marked upper extremity weakness, and mouth- or cheek-operated models are obtainable for children who do not have the use of upper extremities so that they can operate the wheelchairs independently. Very small children who have permanent paralysis of the lower extremities are provided with specially designed units that allow independent mobility. A detachable handle on these units permits their conversion to strollers.

Bicycles and tricycles (Figs. 39-11 and 39-12) can be modified for children with limited ambulatory mobility; these also promote muscle strengthening and prevent disuse contractures. Gait training may be accomplished with a number of special devices (Fig. 39-13).

THE CHILD WITH A FRACTURE

The process of ossification, the gradual conversion of precursor substances (i.e., cartilage) to bony structures, begins in the embryo and continues until the child is 18 to 21 years of age. In long bones this process progresses outward from the diaphysis, the hard, shaftlike portion that constitutes the major part

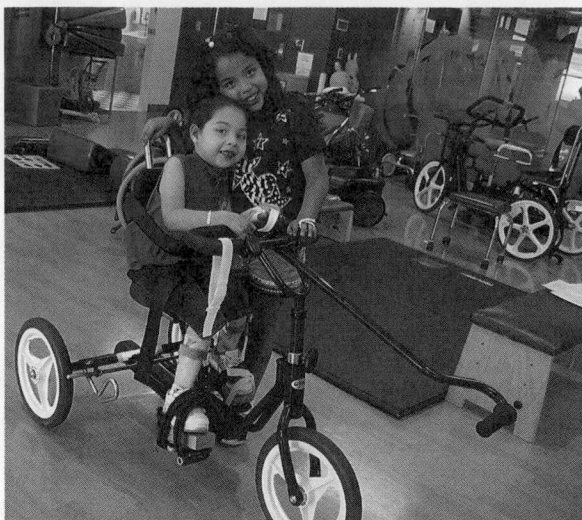

Fig. 39-11 Tricycle used to provide mobility and to strengthen leg muscles. (Courtesy Texas Children's Hospital, Houston.)

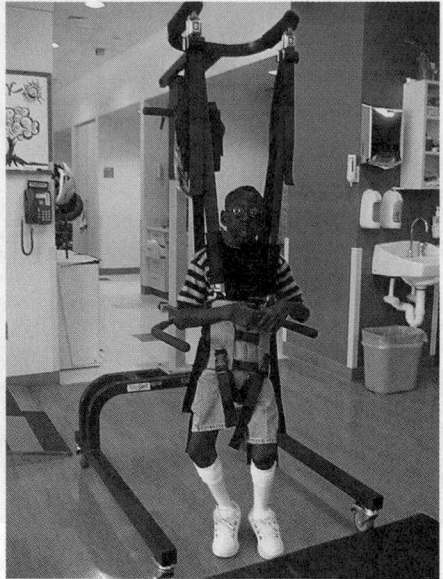

Fig. 39-13 Gait walker with suspension belts for balance and gait training. (Courtesy Texas Children's Hospital, Houston.)

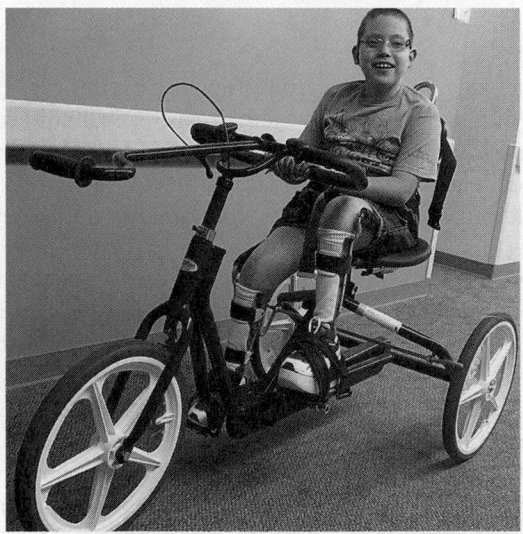

Fig. 39-12 Bike walker used to provide mobility and to enhance leg muscle strength. (Courtesy Texas Children's Hospital, Houston.)

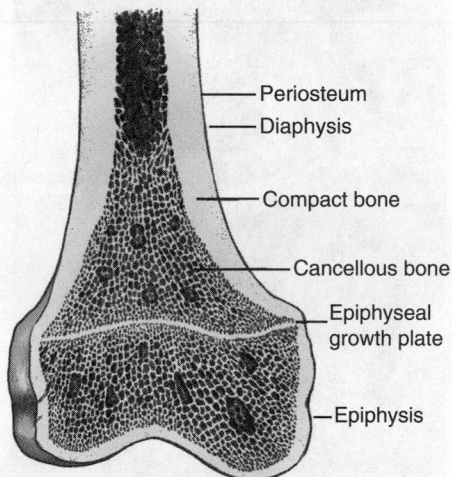

Fig. 39-14 Diagram of bone showing relationships of compact and cancellous bone, epiphysis, epiphyseal plate, and diaphysis. (From Thompson JM, McFarland GK, Hirsch JE, et al: *Mosby's clinical nursing*, ed 4, St Louis, 1997, Mosby.)

of the bone. Within this hard, compact shaft is the hollow medullary canal composed of the bone marrow.

The **epiphyses**, located at the ends of long bones, consist of layers of cartilage, subchondral bone, and spongelike cancellous bone. Situated between the diaphysis and the epiphysis is the epiphyseal plate, which plays a major role in the longitudinal growth of the developing child (Fig. 39-14). The **periosteum**, the thin, tough membrane covering all bones, contains blood vessels that nourish the living bone. Damage to this thin membrane can be a major problem in bone growth and healing.

FRACTURES

Bones fracture when the resistance of the bone against the stress being exerted yields to the stress force. Fractures are a common injury at any age but are more likely to occur in children and the elderly. Their natural tendency toward active mobility and their limited gross motor coordination make children susceptible to physical injury.

Etiology

The causes of fracture injuries in children are those described for general traumatic injuries in childhood. Fractures in infancy are more often the result of birth trauma, injury, or child abuse. Aside from motor vehicle injuries, true accidents causing fracture are uncommon in infancy; therefore injuries in children in this age-group warrant further investigation. Most often, early bone trauma in infants consists of periosteal bleeding in the long bones of the arms and legs, usually caused by rough handling, twisting, and pulling, which is not evident on radiographic examination until 3 to 6 weeks after the injury. Any investigation of fractures in infants, particularly multiple fractures, should include the suspicion of osteogenesis imperfecta (OI) (see p. 1675). In any small child, radiographic evidence of fractures at various stages of healing, with few exceptions, indicates physical abuse (see Community Focus box, on p. 1620).

Periosteum
Diaphysis
Compact bone
Cancellous bone
Epiphyseal growth plate
Epiphysis

Case Study—Fractures

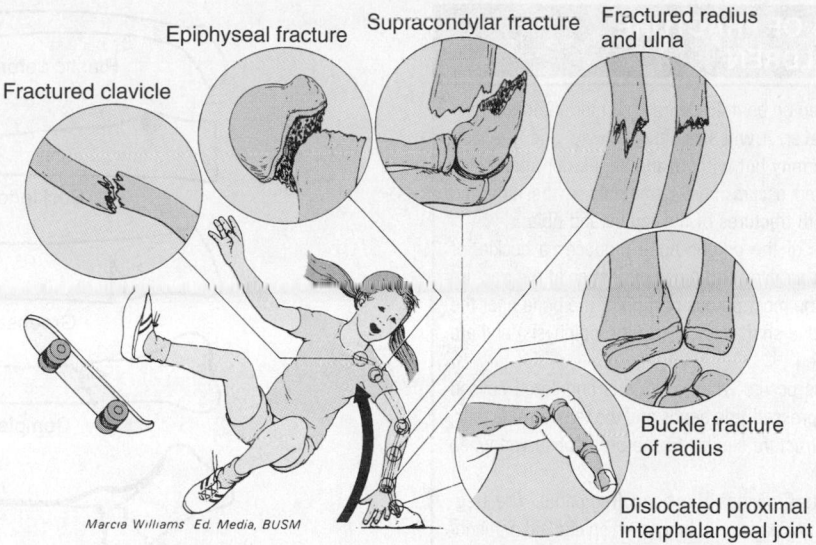

Fractured clavicle · Epiphyseal fracture · Supracondylar fracture · Fractured radius and ulna · Buckle fracture of radius · Dislocated proximal interphalangeal joint

Marcia Williams Ed. Media, BUSM

Fig. 39-15 Trauma resulting from progression of force in fall on outstretched hand. (From Segal D: Pediatric orthopedic emergencies, *Pediatr Clin North Am* 26(4):793-802, 1979.)

Fractures of the forearm are common bone injuries in childhood and are usually caused when the child extends the palm of the hand to break a fall. The force resulting from a fall on the outstretched hand progresses up the length of the extremity with the possibility of injury to the finger, wrist, elbow, shoulder, or clavicle (Fig. 39-15). DiFazio and Atkinson (2005) report that upper extremity fractures are more common in children than in adults. The radius is the most commonly fractured bone of the upper extremity, followed by the bones in the hand. The clavicle is another frequently broken bone in children; approximately half of clavicle fractures occur in children younger than 10 years of age. Many such fractures occur at birth. Hip fractures are uncommon in children and require a great deal of force to produce. A femoral neck fracture may be sustained in children 6 or 7 years of age as a result of pedestrian-automobile accidents because in these children the hip is at the same level as an automobile bumper. In older children the femur is the most likely target; in adolescents knee injuries are common.

Children fall from heights (e.g., trees, roofs, playground equipment) as their insatiable curiosity and immature judgment lure them to places of danger. Fractures in school-age children are often the result of bicycle-automobile collisions or skateboard injuries. Sports are a frequent cause of injury in the school-age child and adolescent.

At all ages motor vehicle mishaps are a frequent cause of bone injury. Most children who are hit by an automobile are between 4 and 7 years of age and sustain a triad of injuries, which must be kept in mind when making an assessment: (1) the child's femur, which is at the level of the bumper, is fractured; (2) the hood of the automobile produces injuries to the child's trunk; and (3) a contralateral head injury is usually sustained when the child is thrown to the ground by the impact. Therefore a child with any one of these injuries who was struck by an automobile should be examined for evidence of the other two.

Pathophysiology

The anatomic, biomechanical, and physiologic nature of children's skeletons causes differences from adults in the

BOX 39-3   FEATURES OF FRACTURES IN CHILDREN

- The growth plate, a thick, elastic portion of bone where growth takes place, serves to absorb shock and protect joint surfaces from injury and is the means by which the limb is able to grow and to straighten itself. Growth is stimulated by a fracture in the diaphysis, whereas damage to the growth plate can cause shortening and often a progressive angular deformity.
- The periosteum of a child's bone is thicker and stronger and has more active osteogenic potential than that of an adult's bone.
- The pliable bones of the growing child are more porous than those of the adult, which allows them to bend, buckle, and break in a "greenstick" manner. The greater porosity increases the flexibility of the bone and dissipates and absorbs a significant amount of the force on impact.
- Healing is more rapid in children, and the rapidity is inversely related to the child's age. The younger the child, the more rapid the healing process. Nonunion of bone fragments is uncommon except in severe injuries in children.
- Stiffness is unusual and, unlike in adults, an uninjured joint in a child can be immobilized for a long period without producing stiffness that lasts longer than a few minutes. Injured joints do become stiff, however, and the current trend is toward early mobilization and active range-of-motion exercises as preventive measures.
- Children only complain when something is wrong. Unreasonable crying, restlessness, and calling for the parents are usually indications that something is amiss and requires investigation.

patterns of fracture, the problems of diagnosis, and the methods of treatment. The bones of the adult are strong and require a violent traumatic force to fracture, which is accompanied by massive injury to surrounding soft tissues. In children the bones are more easily injured, and fractures may result from minor falls or twists and are less likely to be accompanied by soft tissue damage. Features of children's fractures not observed in adults are listed in Box 39-3.

Types of Fracture

A fractured bone consists of fragments: the fragment closest to the midline, or the proximal fragment, and the fragment farthest from the midline, or the distal fragment. When fracture fragments are separated, the fracture is **complete**; when

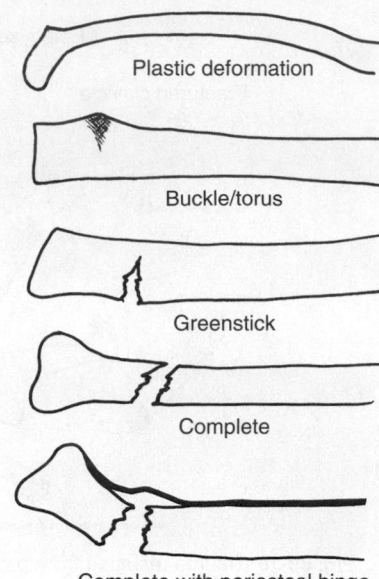

Fig. 39-16 Common types of fracture in children. Note that there are subclassifications of complete fractures based on characteristics of the fracture line.

> **BOX 39-4** **TYPES OF FRACTURE IN CHILDREN**
>
> **Bend**—A child's flexible bone can be bent 45 degrees or more before breaking. If the bone is bent, however, it will straighten slowly, and not completely, to produce some deformity but without the angulation that exists when the bone breaks. A bend occurs more commonly in the ulna and fibula, often in association with fractures of the radius and tibia.
>
> **Buckle fracture**—Compression of the porous bone produces a buckle, or torus, fracture. This appears as a raised or bulging projection at the fracture site. Torus fractures occur in the most porous portion of the bone near the metaphysis (the part of the bone shaft adjacent to the epiphysis) and are more common in young children.
>
> **Greenstick fracture**—This type occurs when a bone is angulated beyond the limits of bending. The compressed side bends and the tension side fails, which causes an incomplete fracture similar to the break observed when a green stick is broken.
>
> **Complete fracture**—This fracture divides the bone fragments. The fragments often remain attached by a periosteal hinge, which can aid or hinder reduction. Complete fractures are subclassified according to the form of the fracture line as transverse, spiral, oblique, comminuted (multiple fractures at the site), or butterfly (a large, central fragment at the site).

fragments remain attached, the fracture is said to be **incomplete**. The fracture line can be any of the following:

Transverse—Crosswise, at right angles to the long axis of the bone

Oblique—Slanting but straight, between a horizontal and a perpendicular direction

Spiral—Slanting and circular, twisting around the bone shaft

All fractures affect the entire cross section of the bone. The twisting of an extremity while the bone is breaking results in a spiral fracture. If the fracture injury does not produce a break in the skin, it is a **simple**, or closed, fracture. Open, or **compound**, fractures are those with an open wound through which the bone protrudes. If the bone fragments cause damage to other organs or tissues (e.g., the lung or bladder), the injury is said to be **complicated**. When small fragments of bone are broken from the fractured shaft and lie in the surrounding tissue, the fracture is called **comminuted**. This type of fracture is rare in children. The types of fracture that occur most often in children are shown in Box 39-4.

Epiphyseal (or Physeal) Injuries

The weakest point of long bones is the cartilage growth plate, or epiphyseal plate. Consequently, this is a frequent site of damage during trauma. Under most conditions, fractures in this area proceed along the zone of degenerating cartilage cells, before the cartilage begins to ossify, without injury to the growth plate and thus cause little damage. Healing is usually prompt. When fracture lines deviate from a transverse direction through the degenerating cells, more serious damage to the epiphysis and the plate may occur. Fig. 39-16 illustrates the types of epiphyseal injury in order of increasing risk of permanent epiphyseal damage and possible growth disturbance. The Salter-Harris classification is typically used to describe epiphyseal injuries, as indicated in Fig. 39-17.

Detection of epiphyseal injuries is sometimes difficult, and they may be mistaken for dislocations or ligamentous injuries.

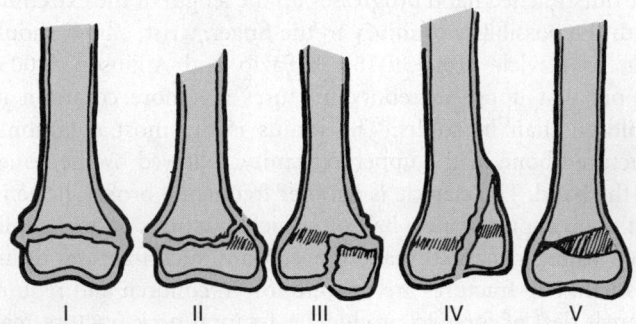

Fig. 39-17 Types of epiphyseal injury in order of increasing risk. The injuries are classified as follows: type I, separation or slip of growth plate without fracture of the bone; type II, separation of growth plate and breaking off of section of metaphysis; type III, fracture of epiphysis extending through joint surface; type IV, fracture of growth plate, epiphysis, and metaphysis; type V, crushing injury of epiphysis (can be diagnosed only in retrospect). This classification of epiphyseal injuries was developed by orthopedists RB Salter and WR Harris. (First published in Salter RB, Harris WR: Injuries involving the physeal plate, *J Bone Joint Surg Am* 45[3]:587-622, 1963.)

Fractures involving the epiphysis or epiphyseal plate present special problems in determining whether bone growth will be affected. Early and correct assessment is essential to prevent longitudinal growth problems and angular deformities. The medical and surgical management of these injuries is different from that for other fractures because open reduction and internal fixation are often employed to prevent complications. If the affected limb is shorter, epiphyseal surgery is performed either to stimulate the involved epiphysis or to restrict growth in the unaffected leg.

Associated Problems

Immediately after a fracture occurs, the muscles contract and physiologically splint the injured area. This phenomenon accounts for the muscle tightness observed over a fracture site and the deformity that is produced as the muscles pull the bone ends out of alignment. This muscle response must be overcome by traction or complete muscle relaxation (i.e., anesthesia) in order for the distal bone fragment to be realigned to the proximal bone fragment.

Contusions of the soft tissues often accompany a fracture, especially of the femur or pelvis, and severe hemorrhage into the tissues is not uncommon. Both the bleeding and the pain are major contributors to shock associated with this injury; therefore suspected musculoskeletal injury should be treated as a fracture until radiographic confirmation can be obtained. The surrounding tissue will be swollen, and a hematoma is usually present. The soft tissue injury must be treated as any other contusion. Because the injury may cause damage to essential structures, the circulatory and neurologic status of tissues distal to the fracture is carefully assessed, especially for fractures of the femur and supracondylar fractures of the elbow.

> ! **NURSING ALERT**
>
> A fracture should be strongly suspected in a small child who refuses to walk or crawl. However, the fact that a child walks on a suspected fractured extremity does not rule out a fracture.

Clinical Manifestations

Children demonstrate the usual signs of injury: generalized swelling, pain or tenderness, and diminished functional use of the affected part. There may be bruising, severe muscular rigidity, and sometimes crepitus (a grating sensation at the fracture site), which are also frequent signs in adults. More often the fracture is remarkably stable because of the usually intact periosteum. The child may even be able to use an affected arm or walk on a fractured leg.

Although neurologic and vascular damage is much less frequent in children than in adult patients, the integrity of these structures must be thoroughly assessed. This is often difficult in infants and young children, who are unable to cooperate. Vascular injury is most likely to occur with supracondylar fractures of the humerus and femur. Femoral and popliteal vessels and the sciatic nerve are prone to trauma in femoral fractures. Humeral fractures may cause damage to the medial, ulnar, or radial nerves and to the brachial artery.

During the assessment, include examination for the five Ps of ischemia from a vascular injury: pain, pallor, pulselessness, paresthesia, and paralysis.

Nursing Assessment

Nurses often conduct the initial assessment of a child with a suspected fracture (see Emergency Treatment box). The child and the parents are frightened and upset; the child is in pain; and, because some fractures are obvious, the parents and frequently the child are already convinced of the diagnosis. As a first step, the injured limb should be supported in some manner. Then, if the child is alert and there is no evidence of hemorrhage, direct the initial nursing interventions toward calming and reassuring the child and parents so that a thorough assessment is easier to accomplish.

> ✚ **EMERGENCY TREATMENT**
> *Fracture*
>
> Assess the extent of injury—5 *P*s:
> - Pain and point of tenderness
> - Pulselessness—distal to the fracture site (late and ominous sign)
> - Pallor
> - Paresthesia—sensation distal to the fracture site
> - Paralysis—movement distal to the fracture site
>
> Determine the mechanism of injury.
> Move the injured part as little as possible.
> Cover open wounds with sterile or clean dressing.
> Immobilize the limb, including the joints above and below the fracture site; do not attempt to reduce the fracture or push protruding bone under the skin.
> - Soft splint (with pillow or folded towel)
> - Rigid splint (rolled newspaper or magazine)
> - Uninjured leg can serve as splint for leg fracture if no splint is available
>
> Reassess neurovascular status.
> Apply traction if circulatory compromise is present.
> Elevate the injured limb if possible.
> Apply cold to the injured area (no longer than 20 minutes with each application).
> Call emergency medical services or transport to medical facility.

Maintaining a calm manner, the nurse can ask the parents to describe what happened and what they think about it. As long as the limb is supported in some manner, this minute or two does not delay or endanger the treatment. It is best not to touch children initially but to ask them to point to the painful area and wiggle their fingers or toes distal to the injury. Previous experiences with injury and health care personnel will influence a child's anxiety. However, children need to be told what will happen and what they can do to help. The affected limb need not be palpated and should not be moved unless properly splinted. A temporary splint should be applied carefully if the child must be transported to a hospital or clinic or to the radiology department.

Diagnostic Evaluation

A history of the injury or events leading up to the injury may be lacking for childhood injuries. Infants and toddlers are unable to clearly communicate the details of what occurred. Older children may not be reliable informants or volunteer information (even under direct questioning) if the injury occurred during questionable activities. In cases of child abuse, parents or caregivers may deliberately give false information to protect themselves. Whenever possible, it is helpful to get information from someone who witnessed the injury.

Radiography

Radiographic examination is the most useful diagnostic tool for assessing skeletal trauma. The calcium deposits in mature bone make the entire structure radiopaque. However, during normal growth and development, much of the skeleton of infants and young children is composed of radiolucent growth cartilage that does not appear on radiographs. In addition, the epiphyseal cartilage and undisplaced separations of the epiphysis (which are common) are not easily detected on x-ray films.

Radiographs are sometimes less reliable than gross deformity and point tenderness in predicting extremity fractures.

Practitioners often obtain a film of the uninjured limb for a direct comparison to help identify minor alterations in alignment and configuration of the epiphysis and associated injuries that might be missed. Radiographic films are also taken after fracture reduction and in some situations may be taken during the healing process to confirm satisfactory progress.

Therapeutic Management

The goals of fracture management are:

- To reestablish alignment and length of the bony fragments (**reduction**)
- To retain alignment and length (immobilization)
- To restore function to the injured parts
- To prevent further injury

Some conditions may require immediate medical attention. These include open fractures, compartment syndrome with and without fracture, fractures associated with vascular or nerve injuries, and joint dislocations that cannot be reduced (DiFazio and Atkinson, 2005). Some fractures may be splinted to immobilize and protect the fractured (or suspected fractured) extremity (see Research Focus box), and pain management is initiated with nonsteroidal antiinflammatory drugs (NSAIDs) such as ibuprofen, oxycodone, or acetaminophen with codeine (Friday, Kanegaye, McCaslin, et al, 2009; Koller, Myers, Lorenz, et al, 2007). In one study ibuprofen was as effective as acetaminophen with codeine for the treatment of musculoskeletal trauma in children (Clark, Plint, Correll, et al, 2007), whereas another study reported no difference among these agents in reducing pain in a group of children with fractures (Drendel, Lyon, Bergholte, et al, 2006).

RESEARCH FOCUS

Removable Splints

Plint, Perry, Correll, and colleagues (2006) treated radius and/or ulna buckle fractures in children with a removable splint for 3 to 4 weeks, instead of using a short arm cast. The children treated with removable splints had better wrist function, had adequate bone healing, and experienced less inconvenience for bathing compared with the group of children placed in a short arm cast.

In children the bone fragments are usually realigned and immobilized by traction or by closed manipulation and casting until adequate callus is formed. Internal and external fixation is also used. Weight bearing and active movement for the purpose of regaining function can begin after the fracture site is stable. The child's natural tendency to be active is usually sufficient to restore normal mobility, and physical therapy is usually required only with more complex traumatic injuries. Open reduction is seldom required and is limited to fractures that cannot be maintained by conservative methods and cases in which there is interposed tissue or injury to arteries or nerves, such as in a motor vehicle accident or other major trauma. In the majority of cases children's fractures can be managed by closed reduction and immobilization with plaster or fiberglass; this is often done on an outpatient basis with reevaluation in 7 to 10 days.

For many fractures closed reduction may be carried out in the emergency department with administration of procedural sedation drugs such as midazolam (Versed), fentanyl (Sublimaze), and morphine (Cimpello, Khine, and Avner, 2004); a local or regional nerve block; fentanyl and midazolam; ketamine (Ketalar) and midazolam; or a combination of nitrous oxide and local or regional anesthesia (Kennedy, Luhmann, and Luhmann, 2004). Etomidate is a rapid-acting sedative that induces unconsciousness and is cleared rapidly from the system. This hypnotic drug may be used for procedural sedation; however, it does not have analgesic properties (Meredith, O'Keefe, and Galwankar, 2008). With any fracture appropriate pain management should be implemented in all children. Studies have shown that historically children have been inadequately treated for pain during procedures in the emergency department and pain scores have been underused (Brown, Klein, Lewis, et al, 2003).

Children are most frequently hospitalized for fractures of the femur and the supracondylar area of the distal humerus. If simple reduction cannot be achieved or a neurovascular problem is detected after injury, observation in a hospital unit is indicated. Severe contusions with profound swelling cannot be treated with a cast, which would act as a tourniquet on the extremity, and badly malaligned fractures may require traction for a time before a cast is applied. The trend, however, is to avoid hospitalization. Some malaligned fractures respond to treatment with external pinning and traction or, more commonly, the use of an Ilizarov external fixator (see p. 1650). Several factors determine the method of fracture reduction (Box 39-5).

Medical interventions to manage a fracture injury involve the physician, the nurse, and the family (Box 39-6). Specific interventions and nursing responsibilities associated with the care of a child with a fracture are discussed later in the chapter.

BOX 39-5 FACTORS IN DETERMINING THE REDUCTION METHOD FOR FRACTURES

- Age of child
- Degree of displacement
- Amount of overriding
- Degree of edema
- Condition of skin and soft tissue
- Sensation and circulation distal to fracture

BOX 39-6 MEDICAL INTERVENTIONS FOR FRACTURE INJURY

- Control of pain, hemorrhage, and edema
- Relief of muscle spasms
- Realignment of fracture fragments
- Promotion of bone healing
- Immobilization of fracture until adequate healing has begun
- Prevention of secondary complications
- Limitation of disuse syndrome
- Restoration of function

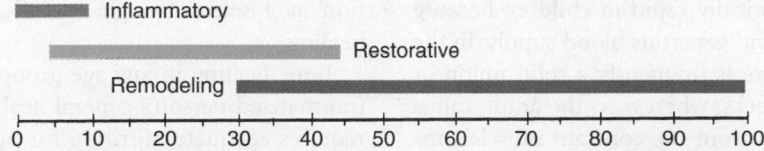

Fig. 39-18 Approximate time spent in inflammatory, restorative, and remodeling phases of bone healing. Scale indicates percentage of healing time.

TABLE 39-2	STAGES OF BONE HEALING
TIME*	**PHYSIOLOGIC EVENTS**

Stage 1: Hematoma Formation

Impact	Fracture occurs.
	Injury to soft tissue envelops site.
	Periosteal tissue tears.
	Vessels rupture.
3-5 min	Bleeding occurs from bone and tissues into area between and around bone fragments.
First 24 hr	Hematoma forms and clots; fibrin assists in clotting periosteal membrane to aid in repair.
	Clot provides fibrin network for cellular invasion.
	Granulation tissue forms by fibroblasts and new capillaries.
	Osteoblastic activity stimulated.

Stage 2: Cellular Proliferation

After 24 hr	Blood supply increases, bringing available calcium, phosphate, and fibroblasts.
	Cells proliferate at ends of bone fragments and differentiate into cartilage and connective tissue.
Next few days	Hematoma becomes granulation tissue, which develops into a framework for bone-forming substances.
	Fibroblasts convert to osteoblasts (bone marrow–forming cells).
2-3 days	*Halisteresis* (softening of bone ends) occurs for ⅛ to ¼ inch; bone cells are resorbed.

Stage 3: Callus Formation

6-10 days	Fibroblasts form in granulation tissue; form bone in areas adjacent to surface of bone shaft; form cartilage at surfaces more distal to blood supply.
	Provisional callus develops, bridging fracture ends; holds bone together but will not support body weight.
14-21 days	*True callus* develops, seen on radiographs; more than needed is formed, but with remodeling, excess callus is resorbed.
	Cartilage differentiates to bone tissue.

Stage 4: Ossification

3-10 wk	Callus forms into bone, which grows beneath periosteum of fragments; fuses (knits together) fracture defect.
	Also called *union stage*.

Stage 5: Consolidation and Remodeling

After 9 mo	Bone marrow cavity is restored.
	Compact bone forms according to stress patterns.
	Remodeling occurs according to Wolff's law.
	Fracture line is always visible on radiographs.

*Healing time more rapid in infants and in cancellous (spongy) bone; may be delayed if complications occur.

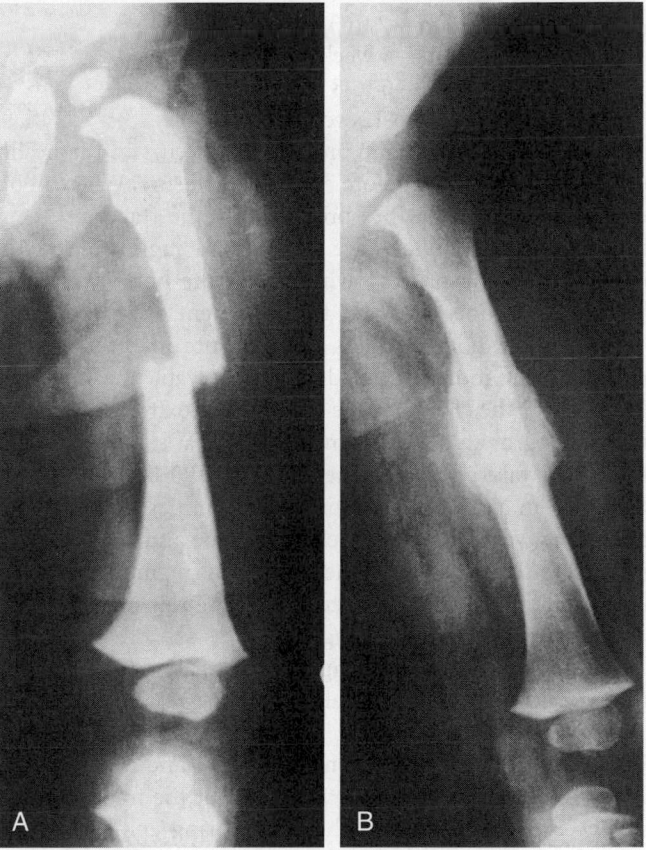

Fig. 39-19 Fractured femur. Most fractured femurs in childhood are of the spiral type shown here. Note comparison of **A,** original x-ray film, with **B,** 6-month postfracture film showing callus formation. (Courtesy Henrietta Egleston Hospital for Children, Atlanta. From Hilt NE, Schmitt EW: *Pediatric orthopedic nursing,* St Louis, 1975, Mosby.)

Bone Healing and Remodeling

Bone healing follows a patterned sequence. Fig. 39-18 shows three broad overlapping phases: inflammatory, restorative, and remodeling. Bone healing can be described more definitively in terms of five stages (Table 39-2). When the bone breaks, the envelope of subcutaneous tissue, muscle, and periosteal tissue surrounding the site is torn, blood vessels rupture, and a hematoma forms. The ends of the fractured bone segments, deprived of circulation, die as far back as the nearest collateral circulation. Necrotic tissue accumulates, and an inflammatory response takes place at the site, with its characteristic vasodilation, plasma exudation, and edema. The organization and reabsorption of the hematoma proceeds, and the restorative phase begins with the reestablishment of local circulation. Repair requires an adequate blood supply and immobilization of the fracture fragments.

When there is a break in the continuity of bone, the periosteal and intraosseous osteoblasts are in some way stimulated to maximum activity. New osteoblasts are formed in immense numbers almost immediately after the injury and begin building a bridge, as evidenced by a bulging growth of osteoblastic tissue and new bone matrix between the fractured bone fragments. This is followed by deposition of calcium salts to form callus, which provides stability (Fig. 39-19, *B*).

Bone healing is characteristically rapid in children because of the thickened periosteum and generous blood supply. In the young child, for example, there is frequently a solid union of the femoral shaft in 3 to 4 weeks, whereas in the adult, callus sufficient to avoid deformities from the constant muscle contraction associated with movement may not form in fewer than 10 to 16 weeks. The approximate healing times for a femoral shaft fracture are as follows:

- Neonatal period—2 to 3 weeks
- Early childhood—4 weeks
- Later childhood—6 to 8 weeks
- Adolescence—8 to 12 weeks

Remodeling is a unique process that occurs in the healing of long bone fractures before epiphyseal closure. When a bone remodels, the irregularities produced by the fracture become indistinct because hollows are filled in and angles are rounded off in the healing process, which gives the bone a straighter appearance. It does not alter the alignment of the bone. The buildup of new bone or callus restores a portion of the normal bone structure in most cases despite observable malalignment. The younger the child and the closer the proximity of the fracture to the growth plate, the more likely that spontaneous correction will take place. In some instances a 90-degree angle will straighten in a year, but rotational deformities do not correct themselves. Various factors such as the type and location of the fracture, the child's age, and the amount of fragment angulation or rotation influence the degree of correction in alignment that can be obtained by remodeling.

The position of the bone fragments in relation to one another influences the rapidity of healing and the residual deformity. For example, a gap between fragments delays (or prevents) healing (Fig. 39-20, A). Healing is prompt and complete with end-to-end apposition (Fig. 39-20, B), but the fracture stimulates accelerated growth of the neighboring epiphysis, which causes bony overgrowth and increased length of the extremity. Angulation deformity caused by an incomplete fracture (Fig. 39-20, C) may remodel in the young child, but the degree of residual deformity depends on the relationship of the angulation of the bone fragments to the angle of the joint. This requires careful evaluation and reduction to prevent permanent deformity.

Wolff's law is applied in treating children with orthopedic problems. Paraphrased, it states that bone will grow in the direction in which stress is placed on it. Examples of the use of this law are the hip spica cast with an abduction bar for treating developmental hip dysplasias and application of casts or trac-

tion at a selected angle to influence the direction of bone healing.

Bone healing in any age-group is greatly influenced by the traumatized person's general health. The child with a fracture requires adequate nutrition for optimum bone healing. When nutritional intake is insufficient, vitamin and mineral supplementation may be necessary. No special dietary changes need to be made except to correct any existing nutritional deficiencies. Monitoring for fluid and electrolyte balance, renal function, and possible anemia is equally important to promote the child's wellness.

THE CHILD IN A CAST

The completeness of the fracture, the type of bone involved, and the amount of weight that can be placed on the limb influence how much of an extremity must be included in a cast to immobilize the fracture site completely. In most situations the joints above and below the fracture are immobilized to eliminate the possibility of movement that might cause displacement at the fracture site. Three major types of cast are used for immobilization of fractures: upper extremity to immobilize the wrist or elbow, lower extremity to immobilize the ankle or knee, and spica to immobilize the hip and knee (Fig. 39-21). Fig. 39-22 shows a full spica cast with a hip abductor, and Fig. 39-23 shows a single spica cast.

The Cast
Casting Materials

Casts are constructed from gauze strips and bandages impregnated with plaster of Paris or synthetic lighter-weight, water-resistant materials (e.g., fiberglass and polyurethane resin). The lightweight casts are being used more often for casting in children. They are available in colors and prints. Plaster casts are usually reserved for situations that require close conformity, such as "total contact" casting for wounds or small, irregularly shaped areas such as the hand. Table 39-3 compares the relative merits of plaster and synthetic casts.

Cast Application

A nurse may assist in cast application by holding the extremity in alignment. Special cast tables that hold the child's body are used for applying large hip spica casts.

Consider the child's developmental age before the cast is applied. For preschoolers who fear bodily harm and fantasize the loss of an extremity, use a plastic doll or stuffed animal to explain the procedure beforehand. Toddlers and preschoolers do not have easily defined body boundaries. If an extremity is wrapped in a bandage, cast, or splint, to the young child the extremity ceases to exist. Explain to the child that some synthetic cast material will become warm but will not burn. During the application of the cast, use various distraction methods, including discussing favorite pets or activities at school and blowing bubbles. In this age-group explanations such as "This will help your arm get better" are futile because the child has no concept of causality.

Before the cast is applied, check the extremities for any abrasions, cuts, or other alterations in the skin surface and for the

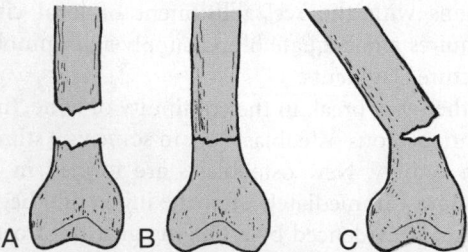

Fig. 39-20 Relationships of fracture fragments. **A,** Gap between fragments. **B,** End-to-end apposition. **C,** Angulation of incomplete fracture.

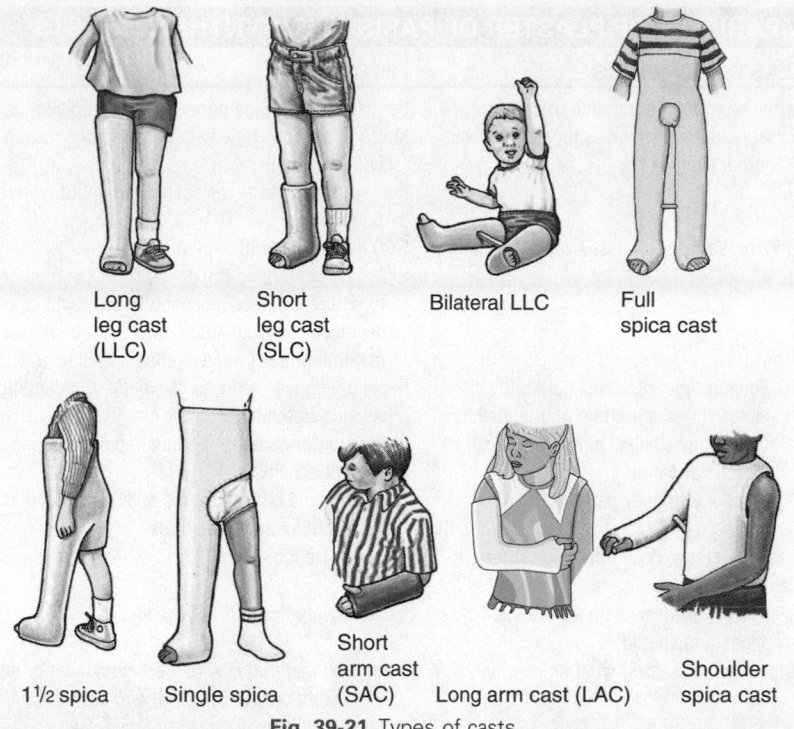

Long
leg cast
(LLC)

Short
leg cast
(SLC)

Bilateral LLC

Full
spica cast

1½ spica

Single spica

Short
arm cast
(SAC)

Long arm cast (LAC)

Shoulder
spica cast

Fig. 39-21 Types of casts.

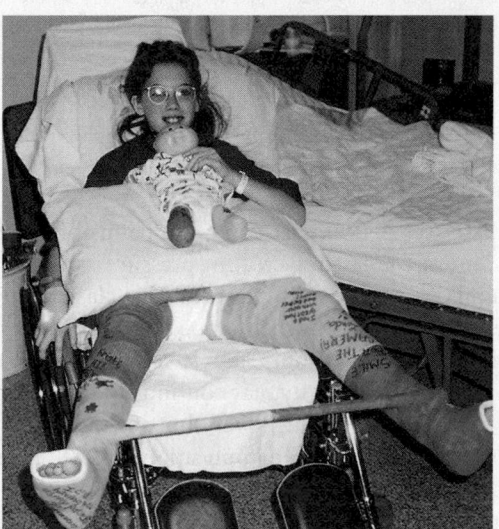

Fig. 39-22 Spica cast with hip abductor. Note casts on doll as well.

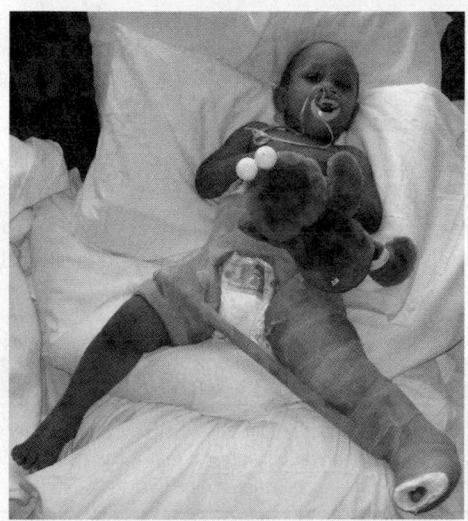

Fig. 39-23 Single spica cast. Note diaper to maintain dryness. (Courtesy Texas Children's Hospital, Houston.)

presence of rings or other items that might cause constriction with swelling; such objects are removed.

To apply a plaster cast, a tube of stockinette is stretched over the area to be casted, and bony prominences are padded with soft cotton sheeting. Some practitioners use a special plastic material or Gore-Tex under a spica cast to prevent skin break-down. Dry rolls of gauze impregnated with plaster of Paris are immersed in a pail of tepid water with the open end of the roll angled downward to allow soaking of the bandage. The wet plaster rolls are applied in bandage fashion and molded to the extremity. A heat-producing chemical reaction occurs between the plaster and water as the plaster becomes a crystalline gypsum. During application of the cast, the underlying

stockinette is pulled over the raw edges of the cast and secured with a layer of wet plaster 1 to 2.5 cm (0.5 to 1 inch) below the rim to form a smooth, padded edge to protect the skin.

If the operator does not form such a protective edge with the stockinette, the raw edges of the cast can be protected by creating a "petaled" edge. Small pieces approximately 5 to 7.5 cm (2 to 3 inches) long are cut from moleskin or adhesive tape 2.5 to 4 cm (1 to 1.5 inches) wide. The edges are rounded with scissors, and the individual "petals" are placed over the edge of the cast, with each petal slightly overlapping the previous one to form a smooth, neat edge. It is easier to apply the petal to the underside of the cast first and then bring the unadhered edge to the front, pressing firmly so the edges remain

TABLE 39-3 **COMPARISON OF PLASTER OF PARIS AND SYNTHETIC CASTS**

	PLASTER OF PARIS	SYNTHETIC
Composition and preparation	Cotton tape permeated with calcium sulfate crystals that interlock as tape dries (tepid water activated)	Polyester-cotton tape permeated with polyurethane resin (cool water activated) Knitted fiberglass tape with polyurethane resin (tepid water activated or photoactivated) Knitted thermoplastic polyester fabric (hot water activated)
Setting time	3-8 min	3-15 min
Drying time	10-72 hr (varies with cast size)	5-20 min (varies with type of cast) NOTE: The more rapid the drying time, the greater the likelihood of burning; therefore it is recommended to use tepid or cool water to slow drying time and decrease chemical heat produced; the warmer the water, the faster the material dries or hardens (Boyd, Benjamin, and Asplund, 2009).
Indentations	Slow drying time increases possibility of indentations or alteration of intended fit	Rapid drying time reduces likelihood of indentations; allows rapid use (see previous statement)
Weight	Relatively heavy; bulky; makes it difficult to wear regular clothing	Lightweight; less bulky; permits regular clothing to be worn; allows for greater range of activity
Conformity	Molds readily to body part	Does not mold easily to some body parts such as fingers and toes; may be unsuitable for some fractures
Surface	Smooth exterior; does not snag clothing or scratch furniture	Smooth exterior
Cost	Relatively inexpensive; an advantage if cast changes anticipated	Inexpensive unless Gore Tex added
Stability	Relatively stable; cast must be kept dry	Some cast material may tolerate being wet or immersed in water with permission from practitioner *(only those with use of nonabsorbent synthetic lining)*; can be cleaned with small amount of mild soap and water, dried with towel followed by blow dryer on cool or warm setting; takes considerable time to dry if immersed
Miscellaneous	Child may feel uncomfortable warming or burning sensation under cast while it dries (chemical reaction) Skin under cast may become irritated Cast must be protected when around water (bathing)	Child may feel uncomfortable warming or burning sensation under cast while it dries (chemical reaction) but this lasts only a few minutes (see Drying Time) Skin under cast may become macerated from inadequate drying after water immersion

securely attached. Adhesive strip bandages can be used instead of tape petals for quicker preparation and a slightly padded cast edge.

 NURSING ALERT

Heated fans or dryers are not used because they cause the plaster cast to dry on the outside and remain wet beneath, so that it can become moldy. They also cause burns from heat conduction by the cast to the underlying tissue.

Nursing Care Management

The complete evaporation of the water from a hip spica cast can take 24 to 48 hours when plaster materials are used. Drying occurs within minutes with fiberglass materials. The cast must remain uncovered to allow it to dry from the inside out. Turning the child in a plaster cast at least every 2 hours will help to dry a body cast evenly and prevent complications related to immobility. Use of a regular fan or a hair dryer on the cool setting to circulate air may be helpful when the humidity is high.

 NURSING ALERT

Immediately report any observations that include the five *P*s of ischemia: pain, especially with passive range of motion; pallor; pulselessness (an ominous and late sign); paresthesia; and paralysis.

Handle a wet plaster cast using the palms of the hands to avoid indenting the cast and creating pressure areas, and support it with a pillow covered with plastic. A dry plaster of Paris cast produces a hollow sound when tapped with the finger.

During the first few hours after a cast is applied, the chief concern is that the extremity may continue to swell to the extent that the cast becomes a tourniquet, shutting off circulation and producing neurovascular complications. One measure to reduce the likelihood of this problem is to elevate the body part and thereby increase venous return. If edema is excessive, casts are bivalved (i.e., cut to make anterior and posterior halves that are held together with an elastic bandage). The cast and the involved extremity are observed frequently to assess neurovascular integrity and detect any signs of compromise. Within 6 to 8 hours permanent muscle and tissue damage can occur, for which nurses can be held liable. Once the cast has dried, "hot spots" felt on the cast surface or foul-smelling areas of the cast may indicate infection underneath and should be further evaluated. Often the cast is windowed over the area of suspicion to directly observe and treat the area if necessary.

When a cast is applied to an extremity that has sustained an open fracture, a window is often left over the wound area to allow for observation and dressing of the wound.

Usually the child is discharged to home care after a cast is applied in the emergency department or clinic. Parents need instructions on drying and caring for the cast and checking for signs and symptoms that indicate the cast is too tight (see

Family-Centered Care box). They should also know to take the child to the health care professional for attention if the cast becomes too loose, since a loose cast no longer serves its purpose. A cast may represent a badge of honor for the child and serves as visible evidence of an otherwise invisible injury.

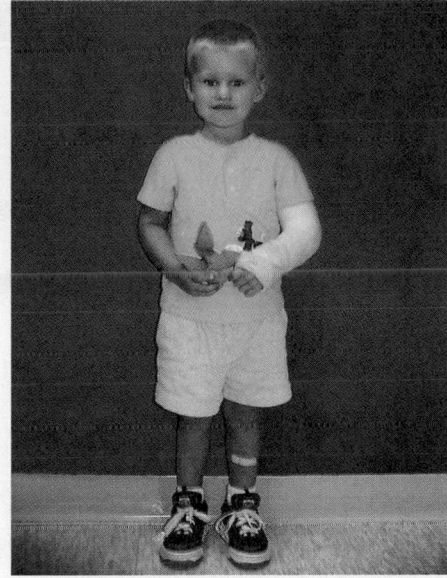

Fig. 39-24 Young children come to regard a cast as part of their body. They usually adapt well but may fear its removal.

FAMILY-CENTERED CARE

Cast Care

- Expose the plaster cast to air until dry.
- Keep the casted part of the body elevated on pillows or similar support for the first day or as directed by the health care professional.
- The wet plaster cast should be lifted and supported with the palms of the hands only, to avoid indenting with the fingers.
- Observe the fingers or toes for any evidence of swelling or discoloration (darker or lighter than a comparable extremity), and contact the health care professional immediately if either is noted.
- Check the movement and sensation of the visible fingers or toes frequently, and contact the health care professional regarding any changes noted.
- Encourage frequent rest for a few days, and elevate the injured arm or leg while resting.
- Do not allow the affected limb to hang in a dependent position for more than 30 minutes (to prevent swelling and circulatory stasis).
- Keep an injured arm or hand elevated (e.g., in a sling) most of the time; supporting it on pillows at chest level is helpful.
- Elevate an injured leg when the child is sitting, and have the child avoid standing for more than 30 minutes.
- Do not allow the child to put anything inside the cast.
- Keep small items that might be placed inside the cast away from young children.
- Examine the skin at the cast edges to detect irritation or breakdown, and pad the cast accordingly.
- Relieve itching by an ice pack and administration of medication as recommended by the practitioner.
- Instruct the child and parents to avoid placing the cast in water (e.g., tub, shower, swimming pool).
- If the patient is incontinent, protect the cast with waterproof tape and plastic. Use diapers, pull-ups, or other guards.

Cast Removal

Cutting the cast to remove it or to relieve tightness is frequently a frightening experience for children. They fear the sound of the cast cutter and are terrified that their flesh, as well as the cast, will be cut. Because it works by vibration, a cast cutter cuts only the hard surface of the cast. This can be demonstrated by the person removing the cast. The oscillating blade vibrates back and forth very rapidly and will not cut when placed lightly on the skin. Children have described it as producing a "tickly" sensation. The vibration also generates heat that the child may feel. Explain both of these sensations to the child.

Preparation for the procedure helps reduce anxiety, especially if the nurse has established a trusting relationship with the child. Many young children come to regard the cast as part of themselves, which intensifies their fear of removal (Fig. 39-24). They need continual reassurance that all is going well and that their behavior is accepted.

Home care of children in casts can create problems, especially with large casts (e.g., a hip spica cast). Common situations (e.g., returning the child home safely and comfortably) become problematic. Standard seat belts and car seats are not readily adapted for use by children in casts. (See Developmental

Dysplasia of the Hip, Chapter 11.) Sitting can be impossible in a spica cast, and leg casts require extra space in a small room, under a table, and in a bathroom. Children in spica casts may experience difficulty with feeding, and the bed or wheelchair may need to be elevated for feeding; alternatively, they may manage a semisitting position in bed or in a wheelchair (see Figs. 39-22 and 39-23). Use of a conventional toilet is almost impossible for a child in a spica cast. Small bedpans or other containers offer alternatives for elimination. The use of a Gore-Tex pantaloon, a protective skin barrier, and absorbent pads is a way of reducing urine burns and heat rash and improving hygiene with a hip spica cast.

Nurses can help families adapt the child's environment to accommodate the temporary encumbrance of a cast (e.g., devise plastic wraps for waterproofing casts for a shower). Baths are possible only if the plaster cast is kept out of the water and covered to prevent it from becoming wet from splashes. Some synthetic casts are waterproof, but skin can become irritated if water collects beneath the cast.

After the cast is removed, the skin surface is caked with desquamated skin and sebaceous secretions. Simple soaking in a bathtub is usually sufficient for their removal, but it may take several days to completely eliminate accumulation. The parents and child should not pull or forcibly remove this material with vigorous scrubbing, since this may cause excoriation and bleeding.

THE CHILD IN TRACTION

When bone fragments cannot be reduced with simple traction and stabilization with a cast, the extended pulling force obtained with continuous traction may be required. Traction is also used for other purposes (Box 39-7).

With the increased emphasis on outpatient treatment of acute and chronic illnesses to cut health care costs, developmental and social considerations, immobilization problems, and newer surgical techniques, traction is used with decreasing

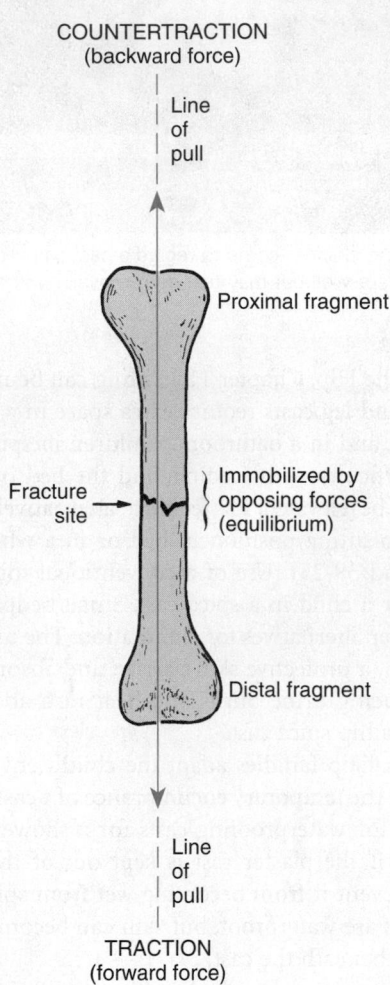

Fig. 39-25 Application of traction for maintaining equilibrium.

frequency. Skeletal fixation (internal or external) and early ambulation of the child have replaced the use of traction in many instances.

Purposes of Traction

When two forces of given direction and magnitude act on an object at the same point simultaneously from opposite directions, the object either changes its state of rest or motion or remains in equilibrium. The use of traction in the management of fractures is the direct application of such forces to produce equilibrium at the fracture site. A forward force (**traction**) is produced by attaching weight to the distal bone fragment. This force is balanced by the backward force of the muscle pull (**countertraction**) and the frictional force between the patient and the bed (Fig. 39-25).

To reduce or realign a fracture site, traction is provided by weights applied to the distal bone fragment; body weight provides countertraction. By adjusting the line of pull upward or downward or by adducting or abducting the extremity, the operator uses these forces to align the distal and proximal bone fragments. To attain equilibrium, the amount of forward force is adjusted by adding weight to or subtracting weight from the traction, or countertraction is increased by elevating the foot of the bed to create a greater gravitational pull in the backward force.

The three primary purposes of traction for reduction of fractures are:

1. To fatigue the involved muscle and reduce muscle spasm so that bones can be realigned
2. To position the distal and proximal bone ends in the desired realignment to promote satisfactory bone healing
3. To immobilize the fracture site until realignment has been achieved and sufficient healing has taken place to permit casting or splinting

In some cases traction may be used to treat a pathologic joint condition such as developmental hip dysplasia. The muscle is fatigued by applying constant stress to the muscle so that the buildup of lactic acid will produce muscle relaxation. The all-or-none law, which characterizes muscle contractility, applies to muscle relaxation as well. When the muscle is stretched, muscle spasm ceases, which permits the realignment of the bone ends. The continuous maintenance of traction is important during this phase, since releasing the traction allows the muscle to contract normally and again cause malpositioning of the bone ends.

The realignment of the bone fragments is a gradual process that is achieved more rapidly in infants, who have limited muscle tone, than in muscular teenagers. The line of pull and callus formation are checked periodically by radiographic examination. The traction pull to some degree immobilizes the fracture site; however, adjunct immobilizing devices such as splints or casts are sometimes used with skeletal traction. In injuries in which there is severe soft tissue swelling or vascular and nerve damage, it is customary to use traction until these complications have been resolved and it is safe to apply a cast. Immobilization with traction is maintained until the bone ends are in satisfactory realignment, after which a less-confining type of immobilization, usually a cast, is applied.

Types of Traction (General)

The two main types of traction are skin traction and skeletal traction. The pull needed for traction can be applied to the distal bone fragment in several ways (Box 39-8). The type of traction applied is determined primarily by the child's age, the condition of the soft tissues, and the type and degree of displacement of the fracture. Fractures most commonly treated by application of traction are those involving the humerus, femur, and vertebrae.

Upper extremity traction is rarely used because of the urgency in management. Fractures of the humerus, which are usually the result of a fall with the arm in extension, frequently involve the supracondylar portion. Three major complications are associated with this injury: Volkmann contractures (p. 1651); traumatic injury to the median, ulnar, or radial nerve;

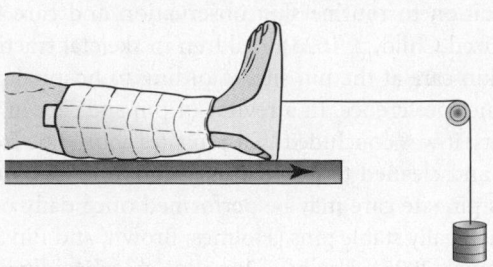

Fig. 39-20 Buck traction. (From Lewis SL, Heitkemper MM, Dirksen S, et al, editors: *Medical-surgical nursing: assessment and management of clinical problems,* ed 7, St Louis, 2007, Mosby.)

BOX 39-8 TYPES OF TRACTION

Manual traction—Traction applied to the body part by the hand placed distal to the fracture site. Nurses frequently provide manual traction during cast application to realign bone fragments. It is used in uncomplicated arm or leg fractures in which there is little overriding of the bones and minimum muscle pull to overcome.

Skin traction—Pull applied directly to the skin surface and indirectly to the skeletal structures. The pulling mechanism is attached to the skin with adhesive material, an elastic bandage, or a soft boot. In these cases the mechanism is applied over soft foam-backed traction straps to distribute the traction pull. Skin traction is applied when there is minimum displacement and little muscle spasticity, but it is contraindicated when there is associated skin damage. There are specific limits to the weight that can be applied using skin traction without causing tissue breakdown.

Skeletal traction—Pull applied directly to the skeletal structure by means of a pin or wire inserted into or through the diameter of the bone distal to the fracture. It is used when significant traction pull must be applied to achieve realignment and immobilization. When a pin or wire is inserted into the bone, the stress is placed on the bone, not on the surrounding tissue. With cervical traction (using tongs inserted into the skull), the traction is maintained on the cervical vertebrae, not the skull. In this case the skull serves as a stabilization anchor for the traction rods.

---

and angulation deformities. The fracture must be carefully reduced with the child sedated or under anesthesia. Because of the danger of complications, children with closed reduction of supracondylar fractures are often hospitalized for observation.

In cases of upper extremity fracture the child is sedated, and treatment by closed reduction is attempted in the emergency department. Closed reduction with percutaneous pinning or open reduction with internal fixation is performed in the operating room as indicated.

The common site for a femoral fracture is the middle one third of the shaft (see Fig. 39-19, *A*). With such a fracture there is significant overriding but minimal displacement. In a fracture in the lower one third of the shaft, the pull of the gastrocnemius muscle causes the distal fragment to become downwardly displaced. The severity of the fracturing force and the ability of the muscles to hold the fracture out of alignment determine the fracture type and the amount of overriding of the fragments. The periosteum may remain intact, which helps maintain alignment.

Buck extension traction is a type of skin traction applied with the legs in an extended position (Fig. 39-26). Buck extension traction is used primarily for short-term immobilization, such as preoperative management of a child with a dislocated

hip, or for correction of contractures or bone deformities, such as in Legg-Calvé-Perthes disease. A side-lying position may be permissible if the leg is stable.

Russell traction uses skin traction on the lower leg and a padded sling under the knee. Two lines of pull, one along the longitudinal axis of the lower leg and one perpendicular to the leg, are produced. This combination of pulls allows realignment of the lower extremity and immobilizes the hip and knee in a flexed position. The hip flexion must remain at the prescribed angle to prevent fracture malalignment, since there is no direct support under the fracture and the skin traction may slip. Because the traction is set up to have two ropes pulling in the same direction at the foot plate, the traction pull is twice the amount of weight at the end of the bed.

A common skeletal traction is 90-degree–90-degree traction (90-90 traction). The lower leg is put in a boot cast or supported in a sling, and a skeletal Steinmann pin or Kirschner wire is placed in the distal fragment of the femur. From a nursing standpoint, this type of traction facilitates position changes, toileting, and prevention of traction complications. This traction also:

- Achieves the desired line of pull for reducing the fracture by means of the skeletal traction
- Allows a 90-degree flexion of both the hip and the knee
- Supports the lower extremity in a desired position with good venous return
- Provides adequate immobilization of the fracture site

Balanced suspension traction may be used with or without skin or skeletal traction. Unless it is combined with another type of traction, balanced suspension traction merely holds the leg in a desired flexed position to relax the hip and hamstring muscles and does not exert any traction directly on a body part. A Thomas splint extends from the thigh to midair above the foot, and a Pearson attachment supports the lower leg. Towels or pieces of felt covered with stockinette are clipped or pinned to the splints for leg support. Ropes are attached to create a balanced traction. When the child is lifted from the bed, the traction lifts as well, with no loss of alignment (see Fig. 39-3).

The Pearson attachment stays wherever it is positioned. Many times the practitioner puts a rope between the end of the Pearson attachment and the end of the Thomas splint to prevent any alteration in knee flexion when the child is moved. This type of traction requires very careful checking of splints and ropes to make certain that no slippage or fraying has occurred. This mode of traction is of great value when lifting the older and heavier child for care.

The cervical area is a vulnerable site for flexion or extension injuries to muscles, vertebrae, or the spinal cord. Cervical muscle trauma without other complications is treated with a cervical soft or hard collar to relieve the weight of the head on the fracture site. Intermittent cervical skin traction using a head halter and weight might be employed to decrease muscle spasms. Injuries limited to cervical muscles can be uncomfortable but, with prompt medical care, usually resolve with conservative treatment.

When a child's cervical vertebra is displaced or fractured, the site must be reduced and immobilized with cervical skeletal traction. The spinal cord runs through the intravertebral canal, and dislocation or fracture of the vertebrae can also cause spinal

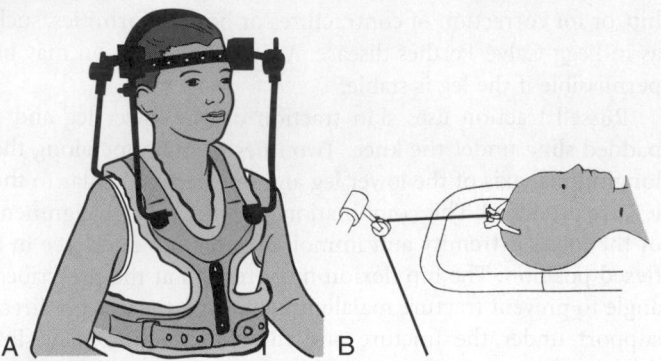

Fig. 39-27 A, Halo vest. **B,** Gardner-Wells traction. (**B,** Redrawn from Hilt NE, Schmitt EW: *Pediatric orthopedic nursing,* St Louis, 1975, Mosby.)

cord trauma. Physical examination, especially a neurologic assessment, and radiographic studies are essential diagnostic aids to determine:

- The presence of a vertebral fracture
- The degree of vertebral dislocation
- Displacement of an intervertebral disk
- Compression of the spinal cord and other neurologic structures
- Sensory, motor, and autonomic nerve deficits

Cervical traction may be accomplished with halo ring traction, a halo vest (Fig. 39-27, *A*), or Gardner-Wells tongs (Fig. 39-27, *B*) (Fisher, Williams, and Levine, 2008). Gardner-Wells tongs are spring loaded, so making burr holes and shaving hair are not required; a local anesthetic may be used during application. The head is placed in a hyperextended position, and, as the neck muscles fatigue with constant traction pull, the vertebral bodies gradually are pulled apart and the cord is no longer pinched between the vertebrae. Immobilization until fracture healing can occur is an essential goal of cervical traction. If the injury has been limited to a vertebral fracture without neurologic deficit, a halo vest permits earlier ambulation (see Fig. 39-27, *A*). Halo vest devices are also used preoperatively and postoperatively to stabilize the cervical spine.

! NURSING ALERT

Skeletal traction is never released by the nurse (except under direct supervision by the practitioner). This precaution includes not lifting the weights that are applying traction (e.g., for moving the child in bed, for repositioning).

Nursing Care Management

To assess the child in traction, it is essential to know the purpose for which the traction is being applied. Regular assessment of both the child and the traction apparatus is required (see Nursing Care Guidelines box). The nurse also assesses the child for evidence of adverse effects of immobilization (see pp. 1624-1629).

Evaluating the therapeutic effects and possible negative consequences of traction is essential to good patient care. Many of the nursing problems associated with traction in a child are related to immobility. However, a number of physical needs related to traction require attention and vigilance.

In addition to routine skin observation and care (see The Immobilized Child, p. 1623), children in skeletal traction need special skin care at the pin site according to hospital policy or practitioner preference. In a review of pin site care in children and adults, it was concluded that pin sites should be frequently assessed and cleaned to prevent infection; after the first 48 to 72 hours pin site care may be performed once daily or weekly for mechanically stable pins (Holmes, Brown, and Pin Site Care Expert Panel, 2005). Use of a 2 mg/ml chlorhexidine solution has been proposed as best-practice care for skeletal pin sites by the National Association of Orthopaedic Nurses (Holmes, Brown, and Pin Site Care Expert Panel, 2005). Before the child's discharge, teach parents and family pin site care, including how to observe for infection or pin instability, using a return demonstration method (Holmes, Brown, and Pin Site Care Expert Panel, 2005). A pressure reduction device, such as a foam overlay or an alternating-pressure mattress placed beneath the hips and back, reduces the chance of skin breakdown in these vulnerable areas.

When the child is first placed in traction, discomfort commonly increases because the traction pull fatigues the muscle. Muscle relaxants may be administered for muscle spasms. Orthopedic conditions are associated with a higher-than-average number of painful events and a higher percentage of bodily symptoms than other common conditions. Analgesics, including opioids, and muscle relaxants help during this phase of care and should be administered liberally.

Helping children cope with the confinement and new experience requires more than medications. Give an explanation about what is happening and why the child must remain in the device according to each child's level of development. Reassure children that someone will always be available to aid them in adjusting to the traction and coping with the problems of immobilization.

Some devices assist children in performing activities independently. An overhead trapeze, which children can use to help lift themselves, facilitates hygiene and repositioning and provides exercise for uninvolved muscles. Encourage the child to move in bed as much as possible while maintaining the primary function of the device. Encourage active range of motion on unaffected joints and extremities and frequent repositioning.

Later, when traction is released, muscle spasms can be quite severe. Pain assessment and pain management should be a part of care at this phase. (See Chapter 7.)

DISTRACTION

Unlike traction, which helps bones realign and fuse properly, distraction is the process of separating opposing bone to encourage generation of new bone in the created space. Distraction can be used when limbs are of unequal lengths and new bone is needed to elongate the shorter limb.

EXTERNAL FIXATION

The Ilizarov external fixator (Fig. 39-28) is the most common external fixation device. It uses a system of wires, rings, and telescoping rods that permits limb lengthening to occur by manual distraction. In addition to lengthening bones, the

NURSING CARE GUIDELINES

Traction Care

Understand Therapy
Understand purpose of traction.
Understand function of traction in each specific situation.

Maintain Traction
Check desired line of pull and relationship of distal fragment to proximal fragment.
Check whether fragment is being directed upward, adducted, or abducted.
Check function of each component:
- Position of bandages, frames, splints, specialized boot
- Ropes—In center track of pulley, taut, no fraying, knots tied securely
- Pulleys—In original position on attachment bar; have not slid from original site; wheels freely movable
- Weights—Correct amount of weight, hanging freely, in safe location

Check bed position—Head or foot elevated as directed for desired amount of pull and countertraction.
Do not remove skeletal traction or adhesive traction straps on skin traction.
Assess for pain or discomfort from traction.

Maintain Alignment
Observe for correct body alignment with emphasis on alignment of shoulder, hip, and leg.
Check after child has moved.
Maintain correct angles at joints.
Maintain hip alignment (prevent external rotation) with rolled blanket, pillow, or sandbag against greater trochanter region of femur.

Provide Care for Skin Traction
Replace nonadhesive straps or elastic bandage on skin traction when permitted or absolutely necessary, but make certain that traction on limb is maintained by someone during procedure.
Assess straps or bandages to ascertain whether they are correctly applied (diagonal or spiral) and not too loose or too tight, which could cause slippage and malalignment of traction.
Assess traction boot to ensure it has not slipped and is not causing compression of the foot, thus impairing the circulation.

Provide Care for Skeletal Traction
Check pin sites frequently for signs of bleeding, inflammation, and infection.
Cleanse and dress pin sites as per protocol or as ordered.
Apply topical antiseptic or antibiotic to pin sites daily per protocol or orders.
Cover ends of pins with protective padding to prevent child's being scratched by pin.
Note pull of traction on pin; pull should be even.

Check pin screws to be certain that screws are tight in metal clamp that attaches traction apparatus to pin.

Prevent Skin Breakdown
Provide alternating-pressure mattress underneath hips and back.
Make total body skin checks for redness or breakdown, especially over areas that receive greatest pressure.
Wash and dry skin at least daily.
Use a skin breakdown assessment such as Modified Braden Q.
Inspect pressure points daily or more often if risk for breakdown is observed.
Stimulate circulation with gentle massage only over healthy skin.
Avoid skin friction with bed linens or traction device.
Keep skin dry and free from moisture such as sweat or urine.
Change position at least every 2 hours to relieve pressure. (See Maintaining Healthy Skin, Chapter 27.)
Encourage increase in intake of oral fluids (state intake goal).
Provide and encourage eating a balanced diet, including vegetables and fruit as age appropriate.

Prevent Complications
Check pulse in affected area and compare with pulses in contralateral side.
Assess circular dressings for excessive tightness.
Assess restrictive bandages or devices used to maintain traction on affected limb:
- Make certain that they are not too loose or too tight.
- Remove periodically and check for skin breakdown or pressure areas.

Encourage deep breathing, coughing, use of incentive spirometry.
Note any neurovascular changes, such as alterations in:
- Color in skin and nail beds
- Capillary refill
- Sensation, increased pain
- Motor ability
- Skin temperature
- Presence or absence of pulses

Take immediate action to correct problem or report to practitioner if neurovascular changes are found.
Record findings of neurovascular changes.
Carry out passive, active, or active-with-resistance exercises of uninvolved joints.
Note if any tightness, weakness, or contractures are developing in uninvolved joints and muscles.
Take measures to correct or prevent further development of weakness, such as applying foot board or athletic shoe or foam boot to prevent footdrop.
Check beneath child for small objects (e.g., food, toys, candy).

---

device can be used to correct angular or rotational defects or to immobilize fractures. It allows earlier mobilization and earlier hospital discharge, and it obviates the need for traction. The device is attached surgically by securing a series of external full or half rings to the bone with wires. External telescoping rods connect the rings to each other. Manual distraction is accomplished by manipulating the rods to increase the distance between the rings. A percutaneous osteotomy is performed when the device is applied to create a false growth plate. In a special osteotomy or corticotomy, only the cortex of the bone is cut, and its blood supply, bone marrow, endosteum, and periosteum are preserved. Capillary blood flow to the transected area is essential for proper bone growth. Cut bone ends typically grow at a rate of 1 cm (0.4 inch) per month. Use of

the external fixator can result in a gain in length of up to 15 cm (5.9 inches).

Other types of external fixation are used in the management of certain types of fractures—for example, fracture of a distal radius or a tibia in an adolescent. Mandibular distraction may be used within external fixation for Pierre Robin sequence. (See Chapter 11.)

Nursing Care Management

Successful use of external fixation depends on the child's and family's cooperation; therefore, before surgery, they must be fully informed about the appearance of the device, the way it accomplishes bone growth, required alterations in activities, and home and follow-up care. Children are involved in learning

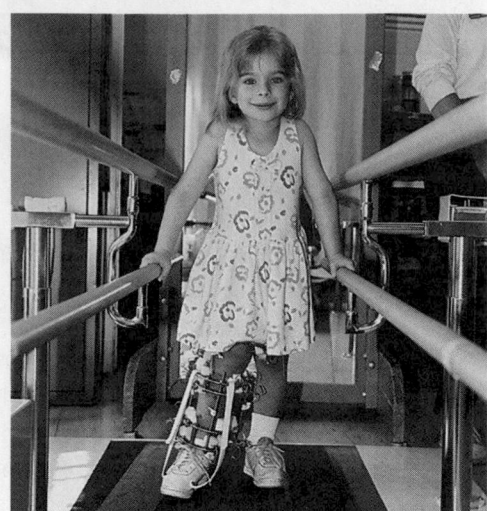

Fig. 39-28 Child with Ilizarov external fixator (on right leg) during physical therapy on parallel bars.

Skill—Monitoring Neurovascular Status

to adjust the device to accomplish distraction. Children who participate actively in their own care report less discomfort. With lower extremity fixation such as an Ilizarov fixator, partial weight bearing is allowed, and the child needs to learn to walk with crutches. Alterations in activity include modifications at school and in physical education. Full weight bearing is not allowed until the distraction is completed and bone consolidation has occurred. Instruct parents in pin care, including observation for infection and loosening of pins. Follow-up care is essential to maintain appropriate distraction until the desired leg length is achieved. The child may need to use crutches or have a cast for 4 to 6 weeks after removal of the device.

INTERNAL FIXATION

Internal fixation methods require surgery and include screw and plate fixation and intramedullary fixation. When surgical intervention is necessary to realign a fracture, the child needs physical and psychologic preparation. The preoperative teaching is the same as for any other surgical procedure, except that orthopedic surgery uses a variety of rods, screws, staples, and plates, and the child and family need to know that these objects will allow proper bone growth and repair to occur. The fixating devices are made of substances that do not act as proteins foreign to the body and therefore are not rejected.

Usually rods are driven down the shaft of the long bones, whereas screws and plates are attached to the sides of the bone shaft. Postoperatively the bone healing takes place with callus formation, as it does in a new fracture. Generally, after placement of an internal fixation device, the child sits in a chair and walks with a walker or crutches within a few hours or days. The most common postoperative complication is infection. The nurse's responsibility includes close monitoring of neurovascular changes in the involved extremity and the prevention of postanesthesia problems. Alert the family to signs of infection and instruct them regarding appropriate weight-bearing and activity plans. Occasionally, supplemental casting or bracing is needed.

> **! NURSING ALERT**
>
> When circulatory impairment is evident (absence of pulse, discoloration, swelling, pain), the nurse takes quick action to relieve the problem by reporting the situation immediately. If the practitioner is unable to come and release the pressure, the nurse or orthopedic technician must be able to cut the cast in half to form a bivalve cast or make a large window in it to decrease the pressure.

FRACTURE COMPLICATIONS

Circulatory Impairment

If the trauma or immobilizing device restricts blood flow in veins or arteries of the affected extremity, bone healing will be seriously impaired. Careful assessment of the pulses, capillary refill, skin color, and temperature is an important nursing responsibility. After injury, swelling of tissues occurs more rapidly in the child than in the adult. In the upper extremity, brachial, radial, ulnar, and digital pulses are felt. In the leg, femoral, popliteal, posterior tibial, and dorsalis pedis pulses are checked.

Closely associated with an inadequate blood supply is a low hematocrit value, which can result from the initial blood loss or surgically induced anemia. Although the blood flow may be adequate, a lowered amount of hemoglobin will not provide a sufficient supply of oxygen for tissue repair.

Nerve Compression Syndromes

Nerve damage can occur at the time of injury, develop in the process of realignment, or arise as a complication of use of an immobilizing apparatus. The syndromes are classified according to the anatomic area affected and can involve the median nerve (carpal tunnel syndrome), ulnar nerve (at wrist or elbow), radial nerve, posterior tibial nerve (tarsal tunnel syndrome), common peroneal nerve, or sciatic nerve. Peroneal nerve damage can result in footdrop, and radial nerve impairment produces wristdrop. Both these disabilities can significantly interfere with activities of daily living.

Sensory testing with touch and pinprick and evaluation of motor strength by asking the child to move the unaffected joint distal to the injury are common means of determining neurologic involvement. Subjective symptoms are pain or discomfort, muscular weakness, a burning sensation, limitation of motion, and altered sensation. Because the fear of pain limits the child's cooperation, play can be the nurse's most valuable tool.

Treatment is alleviation of pressure on the nerve. The practitioner determines whether correcting the alignment will alleviate pressure on the nerve or whether surgical intervention is necessary. At times sensory or motor changes indicate ischemia, and the treatment is correction of the vascular disturbance.

Compartment Syndromes

A compartment is a group of muscles surrounded by tough, inelastic fascial tissue. Compartment syndrome occurs when pressure within this closed space increases and compromises circulation to the muscles and nerves within the space. Muscles and nerves of both upper and lower extremities are enclosed within such compartments. The most frequent causes of compartment syndrome are tight dressings or casts, skin traction, hemorrhage, trauma, burns, and surgery. Other causes include an increase in compartment contents (hemorrhage, venous obstruction, infiltrated IV infusion, exudate) and externally applied pressure, such as lying on the affected limb. Intraarterial medication administration through an arterial line and prolonged operation time may also contribute to compartment syndrome (Green and Swiontkowski, 2008).

> **! NURSING ALERT**
>
> Assessing for compartment syndrome includes monitoring for the five *P*s of ischemia (pain, pallor, pulselessness, paresthesia, and paralysis), plus the sixth *P* of pressure.

Signs and symptoms of compartment syndrome reflect a deficit in or deterioration of neuromuscular status in the anatomic area surrounding the involved structures. These include motor weakness and pain that is out of proportion to the injury and requires opioids for control (Lucas and Davis, 2005). Clinical manifestations may be difficult to recognize in small children or in those who have a head injury. A palpable peripheral pulse and brisk capillary refill may be present despite increasing compartmental pressure. Sensory deficit in the affected limb is reported to be the most reliable physical finding in compartment syndrome (Green and Swiontkowski, 2008). Clinical manifestations of compartment syndrome may occur as early as 30 minutes after the ischemia develops. Tenseness may be noted on palpation of the area. Because early detection is important in preventing permanent damage to tissues, in certain high-risk situations specialists may recommend continuous monitoring of compartment pressures by way of a small, slit-tip catheter; Wick catheter; or needle inserted into the compartment. Treatment of compartment syndrome is immediate relief of pressure, which sometimes requires fasciotomy.

Volkmann contracture (ischemic muscular atrophy) is a serious, persistent flexion contraction of the forearm and hand caused by massive infarction of muscle. Pressure caused by a cast or tight bandage or by swelling from the injury in the area of the elbow begins with arterial occlusion and then progresses to muscle anoxia and reflex vasospasms. Finally, the lack of blood supply leads to muscle necrosis and replacement with fibrous tissue, which produces paralysis and a clawlike hand contracture. Any fracture that requires excessive traction can be complicated by Volkmann contracture; however, it occurs most often in the elbow.

The neuromuscular symptoms are severe pain (although pain is not always a manifestation), pallor or cyanosis, edema, absence of pulses in the extremity, and loss of sensitivity. Unrelieved, the occlusive hypoxic process can cause some contracture if ischemia lasts as little as 6 hours. A great deal of muscle damage occurs after 12 to 24 hours; 48 hours of ischemia produces severe deformity, with muscle fibrosis and contractures in 5 to 10 days. If not treated, the contracture leads to severe deformity and paralysis.

The immediate treatment is to remove any mechanically obstructive materials, such as tight bandages, and extend the joint to free blood vessels. If the symptoms do not improve within a few hours, arteriography is done in anticipation of a possible need for surgical intervention (fasciotomy) to decrease arterial spasms and to improve the blood supply by separation of the fascial sheaths of the involved muscles. Elevation of the affected extremity is not recommended and may further decrease blood flow to the area (Green and Swiontkowski, 2008).

Epiphyseal Damage

Growth of bone originates from the epiphyseal plate, and damage to this structure can result in unequal lengths of the extremities. Surgical intervention involving the epiphysis on the affected extremity or the epiphyseal line on the opposite extremity is the usual treatment.

Nonunion

Bone healing and callus formation can span and repair only a limited space between bone fragments. When bone fragments cannot be maintained in correct alignment for repair due to inadequate reduction, poor immobilization, or a damaged or softened cast, bone healing is impaired. The factors most likely to interfere with bone healing and cause delayed union or nonunion, based on the physiologic needs for bone healing, are listed in Box 39-9.

The hematoma, which becomes the matrix for bone deposition in the break, must be free of infection or bits of adipose or connective tissue. The constant supply of nutrients and bone-forming cells brought to the area by way of the bloodstream provides the vital ingredients for repair.

Sometimes artificial means are employed to facilitate bone healing. Bone grafting becomes necessary when bone nonunion occurs. The donor site is usually the tibia or the iliac crest. Bleeding of bone ends may need to be artificially stimulated, and at times holes are drilled near the bone ends in an attempt to increase circulation. Postsurgical immobilization of the recipient area is crucial to the success of the graft. The Ilizarov external fixator and protocol for care are frequently used to assist bone healing in patients with nonunion (see p. 1650).

Malunion

Malunion is fracture union with increased angulation or deformity at the fracture site. It can be detected at any stage in the

> **BOX 39-9   FACTORS THAT INTERFERE WITH BONE HEALING**
>
> - Separation of bone fragments at fracture site
> - Interposition of tissue between bone fragments
> - Loss of bone tissue, especially from necrosis
> - Infection
> - Poor nutrition
> - Interruption of blood supply
> - Diseases that influence calcium metabolism (e.g., thyroid disorder)
> - Bone cancer
> - Administration of steroids

healing process or after complete healing. Unsatisfactory reduction is the usual reason for malunion. A cast or splint that allows fracture movement will also likely result in malunion. Periodic radiographic examinations help detect this complication and prevent it from becoming a major problem over a long period.

Excessive deformity can be corrected during the healing process through realignment and reimmobilization. However, attempts at correction may cause delayed union or nonunion; therefore the degree of deformity is carefully evaluated in light of these complications. The probability that sufficient spontaneous alignment will occur with growth and continuation of the healing process also is considered. Correction of the malunion when healing is near completion requires surgical intervention.

Infection

Osteomyelitis, infection of the bone, is often secondary to a bloodstream infection but is a potential problem when the fracture is an open one, when pressure ulcers develop, or when bone surgery has been performed. Any bacterial organism can cause this infectious process; however, Staphylococcus aureus is the pathogen most frequently identified (see p. 1673 for a discussion of osteomyelitis).

Kidney Stones

Although uncommon in children, development of renal calculi is a potential risk whenever the child has a limb that is non–weight bearing for a long time, especially if the circumstances also produce urinary stasis. Measures to prevent the formation of renal calculi include maintaining optimal hydration, mobilizing the child as much as possible, and checking closely the amount and characteristics of urinary output. Any urinary tract infection should be treated promptly with appropriate antimicrobials and urine acidification, since the nucleus of a calculus is often composed of bacterial debris or calcium and the buildup of stone is precipitated by alkaline urine. An associated problem, hypercalcemia, was reviewed in the section on problems of the immobilized child.

Pulmonary Emboli

Blood, air, or fat emboli can be a hazard to the child with a fracture. As postinjury bleeding and clotting occur, a small piece of the clot can travel to vital organs, such as the lung, heart, or brain, and produce a life-threatening vascular obstruction and ischemia. Generally the pulmonary system is the most frequent site of emboli deposition, but it may not occur until 6 to 8 weeks after the injury.

> **! NURSING ALERT**
>
> Pulmonary embolism should be suspected in a child with a history of recent surgery, major trauma, or prolonged immobilization who suddenly develops chest pain and dyspnea. The severe dyspnea must be treated immediately by elevating the head when possible and administering oxygen by means of a mask or nasal cannula. This is a medical emergency.

Fat emboli are the greatest threat in an individual with multiple fractures, particularly fractures of the long bones such as the femur. Fat droplets from the marrow are transferred to the general circulation by the venous-arterial route, where they can be transported to the lung or brain. This type of embolism occurs within the first 24 hours, generally in the second 12 hours after the injury occurs. Adolescents are those usually affected in the pediatric age-groups.

Intermittent compression devices are used to prevent venous pooling in the lower extremities when prolonged immobilization is required. These devices are inflatable sleeves that allow cyclic emptying and filling of leg veins; the devices are used in children with spinal cord injury once mobilization is initiated to decrease the effects of orthostatic intolerance. Anticoagulant drug therapy, passive and active range of motion, and early mobilization are also used to decrease venous stasis and prevent thrombus development.

AMPUTATION

A child may be born with the congenital absence of a body part, experience a traumatic loss of an extremity, or require a surgical amputation for a pathologic condition such as osteogenic sarcoma. With today's surgical technology and the quick thinking of bystanders who save a traumatically amputated body part, some children have had fingers and arms sewn back on with variable degrees of functional use regained. A severed part should be rinsed in saline; wrapped gently but completely in sterile gauze; and placed in a watertight bag labeled with the child's name, the date, and the time. The bag should then be placed in ice water to keep the limb chilled but not frozen. The part should not be packed in ice, since damage to the tissue may make reimplantation impossible.

Surgical amputation or the surgical repair of a permanently severed limb focuses on constructing an adequately nourished stump. For lower extremities the presence of a smooth, healthy, padded stump, free of nerve endings, is important for prosthesis fitting and subsequent ambulation. In some situations in which there is no vascular or neurologic deficit, a cast is applied to the stump immediately after the procedure, and a pylon, metal extension, and artificial foot are attached so that the patient can walk on the temporary prosthesis within a few hours.

> **! NURSING ALERT**
>
> For a traumatically amputated limb or body part, do the following:
> 1. Rinse limb in saline.
> 2. Loosely wrap limb in sterile gauze.
> 3. Place in a watertight bag.
> 4. Chill bag, without freezing, in ice water.
> 5. Transport patient and limb by EMS to trauma center.

Nursing Care Management

Lower extremity stump shaping is done postoperatively with special elastic bandaging using a figure-8 compression bandage, which applies pressure in a conical fashion. This technique decreases stump edema, controls hemorrhage, and aids in developing desired contours so that the child will bear weight on the posterior aspect of the skin flap rather than on the end of the stump. When appropriate, a stump shrinker, in addition to an elastic wrap, may be used. Some surgeons apply a prosthetic device in surgery after the amputation to reduce edema and promote early ambulation.

The stump may be elevated for the first 24 hours, but after this time the extremity should not be left in this position because contractures in the proximal joint will develop and seriously hamper ambulation. Monitoring proper body alignment further decreases the risk of flexion contractures. Postoperatively, children who undergo amputation of a lower extremity should be turned not only from side to side but also from front to back. Postoperative complications for which the nurse should be vigilant include hemorrhage and infection of the operative site. As the child progresses, encourage him or her to lie prone at least three times a day, increasing the time prone to tolerance of an hour at a time.

For older children and adolescents, arm exercises, bed pushups, and exercises with parallel bars (which are used in prosthesis training programs) help to build up the arm muscles necessary for walking with crutches. An overhead trapeze bar enhances mobilization and upper body strength building in the early postoperative period when a lower limb has been amputated. Full range-of-motion exercises of joints above the amputation must be performed several times daily, using active and isotonic exercises. Young children are spontaneously active and require little encouragement.

Depending on the child's age, the child or parents need to learn stump care, including careful washing with soap and water every day and checking for skin irritation, breakdown, or infection. A tube of stockinette or talcum powder is used to make the prosthesis slide on more easily. A careful skin check must be performed every time the prosthesis is removed, and prosthesis tolerance time must be adjusted to prevent skin breakdown.

Evaluate limb pain, especially pain that increases with ambulation, to check for a possible neuroma at the free nerve endings in the stump or a poorly fitting prosthesis. Chronic pain may also be related to weakness or joint instability, injury to the nerve, or fibrosis of soft tissues. Pain in the contralateral extremity may result from asymmetric weight bearing.

For children who have had an amputation, phantom limb pain is an expected experience because the nerve-brain connections are still present. Phantom pain is real pain and should be treated appropriately with analgesics and other pain-relieving measures. Gradually these sensations fade, although in many amputees they persist for years. Preoperative discussion of this phenomenon helps a child understand these feelings and not hide the experience from others.

INJURIES AND HEALTH PROBLEMS RELATED TO SPORTS PARTICIPATION

Adolescents probably spend more time and energy practicing and participating in sports activities than members of any other age-group. The practice of sports and games contributes significantly to growth and development, to the education process, and to good health. It provides exercise for growing muscles, interactions with peers, and a socially acceptable means of enjoying stimulation and conflict. In addition, competitive activities help the older child and adolescent engage in self-appraisal and develop self-respect and concern for others.

Every sport has some potential for injury to the participant—whether the young person participates in serious competition or purely for enjoyment. Serious injury is not limited to the athlete who competes in rough contact sports; a large number of severe or fatal injuries occur to persons who engage in milder physical activity but are not physically prepared for it. For example, a person's body build may not be suited to the sport, muscles and support systems (respiratory and cardiovascular) may not have been sufficiently conditioned to withstand the rigors of the physical stress, or the child or adolescent may not possess the insight and judgment to recognize when an activity is beyond his or her capabilities. Rapidly growing bones, muscles, joints, and tendons are especially vulnerable to unusual strain.

The awkward and inexperienced child or adolescent may suffer more injury than the more skilled and experienced one. Strong muscles are less easily damaged than weak ones and provide better protection to the joints they cross. Fatigue significantly impairs muscle function and judgment. More injuries occur during recreational sports participation than in organized athletic competition. Likewise, most injuries occur in practices rather than in games. Although team sports give rise to frequent injuries, serious injuries resulting from recreational and individual sports are generally more common. The increase in strength and vigor in adolescence may tempt children to overextend themselves. This is especially true of boys who are egged on by teammates or coaches or are stimulated by the admiration of female observers.

Not only does the activity itself pose a hazard of greater or lesser degree, but the environment and the sports or recreational equipment present additional risks. Adolescents participate in physical activities in a variety of environments, both indoors and outdoors, on floors, on the ground, on snow, on or beneath water surfaces, and sometimes in free air space. These activities frequently involve equipment that intensifies the risk.

PREPARATION FOR SPORTS

Among adolescents of the same age, the degree of physical maturation varies greatly, and many of the physical characteristics important in sports are related to hormone production. Consequently, physical strength, coordination, endurance, and size vary considerably among children and adolescents who wish to compete against each other. Sports competition between young people who differ markedly in strength and agility is unfair and hazardous. Matching of candidates for sports should be based on physical maturity, height, weight, and physical fitness and skills, particularly in sports involving rigorous body contact. Age is a less important consideration.

The American Academy of Pediatrics (Rice and Council on Sports Medicine and Fitness, 2008) has developed a classification that categorizes sports according to probability of collision and strenuousness (Box 39-10). Collision sports such as tackle football, basketball, hockey, and soccer have the highest injury rates, followed by other contact sports (Figs. 39-29 and 39-30). In addition, the American Academy of Pediatrics (Rice and

BOX 39-10 CLASSIFICATION OF SPORTS

Contact Sports
Contact or Collision
Basketball
Boxing*
Cheerleading
Diving
Extreme sports
Field hockey
Football (tackle)
Gymnastics
Ice hockey†
Lacrosse
Martial arts
Rodeo
Rugby
Ski jumping
Skiing, downhill
Snowboarding
Soccer
Team handball
Ultimate Frisbee
Water polo
Wrestling

Limited Contact or Collision
Adventure racing
Baseball
Bicycling
Canoeing or kayaking (white water)
Fencing
Field (high jump, pole vault)
Football (flag or touch)
Handball
Horseback riding
Skateboarding

Skating (ice, roller, in-line)
Skiing (cross country, water)
Snowboarding
Softball
Squash
Volleyball
Weight lifting
Windsurfing or surfing

Noncontact Sports
Aerobic dancing
Archery
Badminton
Body building
Bowling
Canoeing and kayaking (flat water)
Curling
Dancing (ballet, modern, jazz)
Field (discus, javelin, shot put)
Golf
Hunting
Orienteering
Race walking
Riflery
Rope jumping
Rowing
Running
Sailing
Scuba diving
Swimming
Table tennis
Tennis
Track
Walking
Weight lifting

Modified from Rice SG, American Academy of Pediatrics, Committee on Sports Medicine and Fitness: Medical conditions affecting sports participation, *Pediatrics* 121(4):841-848, 2008.
NOTE: This categorization does not reflect the relative risk of injury.
*Participation not recommended by American Academy of Pediatrics.
†American Academy of Pediatrics recommends limiting amount of body checking allowed in players younger than 15 years.

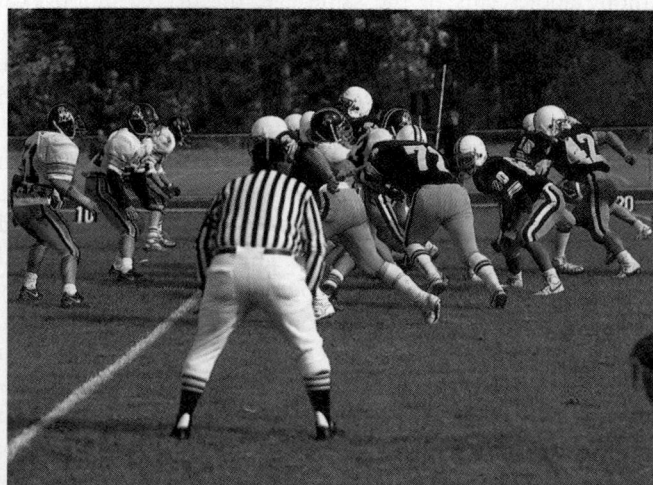

Fig. 39-29 Football is an example of a strenuous collision sport with a high risk of serious injury.

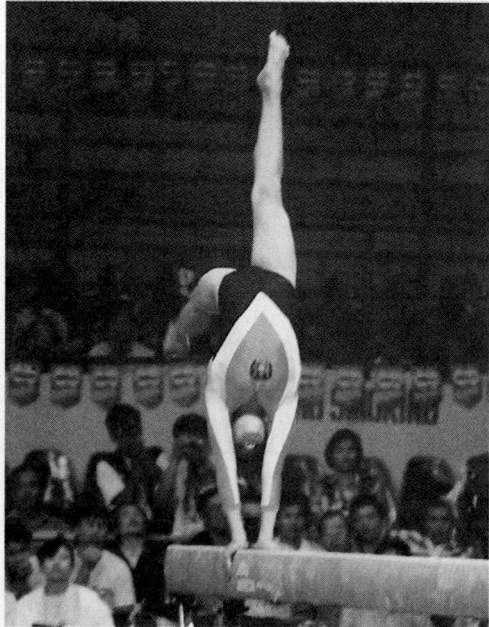

Fig. 39-30 Gymnastics is an example of a strenuous limited contact, limited collision sport with a high risk of serious injury.

Council on Sports Medicine and Fitness, 2008) has developed and published guidelines that provide criteria for determining inclusion or exclusion of the young athlete based on common medical and surgical conditions and relative risks in various sports categories. This serves as a useful guideline for the health professional in counseling youth regarding sports activities.

The American Academy of Pediatrics (2000a; Brenner and Council on Sports Medicine and Fitness, 2007) encourages sports participation by young persons and encourages adults close to sports activities to be aware of the early warning signs of fatigue, dehydration, and injury. Athletes should seek assistance when an injury is suspected and not "work through" injuries caused by overuse (shin splints, stress fractures, tendinitis, and apophysitis).

The role of health care professionals, specifically nurses, in relation to sports injuries focuses on prevention, treatment, and rehabilitation. Of these areas, prevention is perhaps the most important. It is difficult to "sell" prevention, however, especially to children. Anticipatory guidance is an important aspect of preventive counseling for sports injuries, since many injuries occur when children are tired and are not concentrating on their activities; injuries are also more common when participants are distracted by events off the field of play, such as not really wanting to play or thinking about personal problems.

Everyone wants to play the game, but not necessarily to practice. Often, if an 8- to 15-minute warm-up is suggested, adolescents and children warm up for 30 seconds and say they are ready to go. Youth who are actively involved in athletic programs need to undergo medical evaluation as a prerequisite to participation and to receive education in sports skills using correct training and conditioning methods. Tactics that are dangerous beyond the ordinary risk associated with the specific sport should be omitted. In addition, children should use appropriate protective equipment, properly maintained and suited to the individual. The sports environment should make maximum provision for safety and availability of first-aid and medical services.

The same protective principles apply to enthusiasts in non-competitive sports. They need the same education in basic safety precautions, encouragement to acquire proper instruction in the skills required for performing the activity (such as water safety, skiing techniques), and proper maintenance of equipment.

TYPES OF INJURY

The injuries sustained in sports or recreational activities can involve any part of the body and range from relatively minor cuts, bruises, and abrasions to severe closed head injuries such as concussion or totally incapacitating central nervous system injuries or death. Some of these injuries are discussed in chapters devoted to the major topic (e.g., spinal cord injuries [Chapter 40] and head injuries [Chapter 37]). Fractures are discussed earlier in this chapter.

Some sports are particularly dangerous for children and adolescents. Snowmobiling, snowboarding, use of all-terrain motor vehicles, in-line skating, skateboarding, motorcycle riding, full contact hockey, bicycle riding, wave running, and trampoline use are examples of sports and recreational activities

that can lead to significant injuries in connection with inappropriate use, failure to wear protective equipment, or participation by children who are under age. According to the American Academy of Orthopaedic Surgeons (2007), sports injuries account for approximately 20% of visits to the emergency department for injury. Basketball and pedal cycling account for the majority of injuries, followed by football, baseball or softball, and skate boarding or in-line skating. One study reported a high incidence of injuries in high school football athletic competition; boys' soccer had a high rate of head, neck, and face injuries; and high rates of concussion injuries occurred in boys' soccer (Rechel, Yard, and Comstock, 2008). Ankle injuries are the most common competitive sports-related injuries, with significant numbers occurring in boys' and girls' basketball (Nelson, Collins, Yard, et al, 2007).

A variety of injuries can result when an external force is applied that causes severe stress on tissue, muscle, and skeletal structures (Fig. 39-31). The body structures attempt to absorb the force, but when they are unable to do so, injuries occur. Two general types of injury are recognized. The first is **acute trauma**, which is defined as a sudden, acute injury from a major force. Among such injuries are fractures of long bones and the axial skeleton; sprains of joint ligaments; strains of muscle tendon units; and contusions, including those of muscle tendon units and overlying soft tissue. The second type is repetitive **overuse injuries**, or microtrauma, which result from repetitive injury to tissue over a long period. Overuse injuries include stress fractures, bursitis, tendonitis, apophysitis of tendon insertions, and at times injuries of the joint surface.

More than 95% of sports injuries involve the soft tissues, not the bony skeleton. About two thirds of these consist of strains

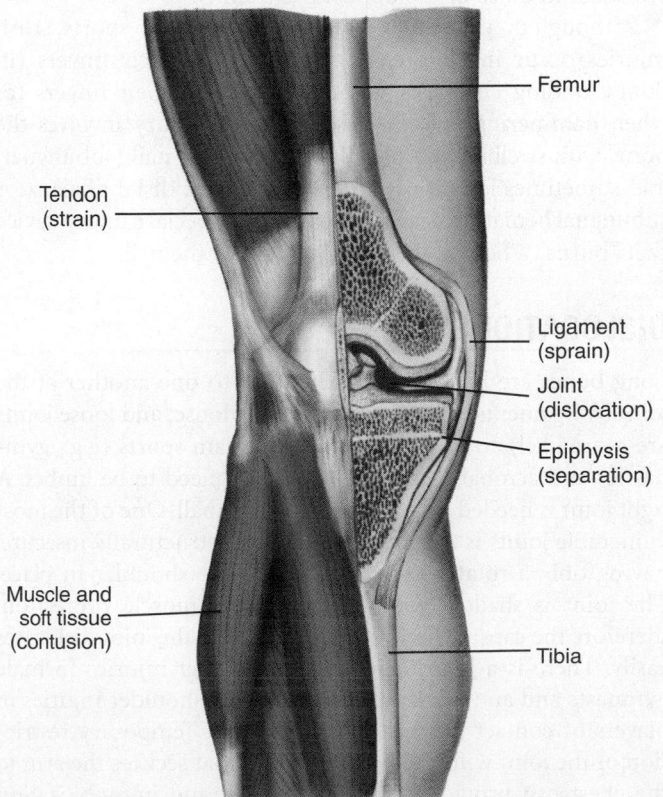

Fig. 39-31 Sites of injury to bones, joints, and soft tissues.

and sprains, and most injuries involve the extremities. Acute overload injuries are those that occur suddenly during an activity and produce immediate symptoms. They can be caused by a blow or overstretching, twisting, or any other forces that cause a sudden stress to tissues.

CONTUSIONS

Contusions are probably the most common sports injuries and are often considered to be "part of the game." A contusion is damage to the soft tissue, subcutaneous structures, and muscle. The tearing of these tissues and small blood vessels and the ensuing inflammatory response lead to hemorrhage, edema, and associated pain when the child or adolescent attempts to move the injured part. The escape of blood into the tissues is observed as ecchymosis, a black-and-blue discoloration.

The most serious contusions are those involving the quadriceps; they are common in strenuous, collision-type sports and usually result from being kicked or kneed in the thigh. Large contusions cause gross swelling, pain, and disability and usually receive immediate attention from health care personnel. The less spectacular smaller injuries may go unnoticed, so that continued participation is allowed. They can become disabling after rest, however, because of pain and muscle spasm. The young athlete is frequently instructed to "work it out" or disregard the pain. *Myositis ossificans* may occur from deep contusions to the biceps or quadriceps muscles; this condition may result in a restriction of flexibility of the affected limb.

Immediate treatment of a contusion consists of application of cold for no more than 20 to 30 minutes, as in the treatment of sprains described below. Return to participation is allowed when the strength and range of motion of the affected extremity are equal to those of the opposite extremity.

Although they are not always directly related to sports, crush injuries occur in children when they slam their fingers (in doors, folding chairs, or equipment) or hit their fingers (as when hammering a nail). A severe crush injury involves the bone, with swelling and bleeding beneath the nail (subungual) and sometimes laceration of the pulp of the distal phalanx. A subungual hematoma can be released by a special cautery device that "burns" a hole at the proximal end of the nail.

DISLOCATIONS

Long bones are held in approximation to one another at the joint by ligaments. Joints can be tight or loose, and loose joints are more likely to be dislocated. For certain sports (e.g., gymnastics and acrobatic dancing) the joints need to be limber. A tight joint is needed for sports such as football. One of the most vulnerable joints is the shoulder, which is structurally insecure, having only a rotator cuff to maintain the shoulder in place. The joint is shallow with relatively little muscle protection; therefore the capsule becomes stretched and the joint dislocates easily. There is a high incidence of shoulder injuries in male gymnasts and an even greater incidence of shoulder injuries in players of contact sports, such as football. Temporary restriction of the joint with a sling or bandage that secures the arm to the chest can provide sufficient comfort and immobilization until the individual receives medical attention.

Dislocations are less common in children than in older persons, but some types are specific to the younger age-groups. Before final closure of the epiphyses, injuries to the joints are more likely to cause epiphyseal separation than dislocation. For example, shoulder dislocation occurs most often in older adolescents, and dislocation unaccompanied by fracture is rare. Dislocations of the phalanges are the most common type seen in children, followed by elbow dislocations. Injury to the hip causes dislocation more frequently than femoral neck fracture (often experienced by persons in the older age-groups).

In children younger than 5 years of age, the hip can be dislocated by a fall. The greatest risk after this injury is the potential loss of blood supply to the head of the femur. Children with naturally lax joints, such as those with Down syndrome, are more prone to recurrent dislocation of the hip.

A dislocation occurs when the force of stress on the ligament is great enough to disrupt the normal position of the opposing bone ends or the bone end and its socket. The predominant symptom is pain that increases with attempted passive or active movement of the extremity. In dislocations there may be an obvious deformity and inability to move the joint. Temporary restriction of the joint with a sling or bandage that secures the arm to the chest in a shoulder dislocation provides sufficient comfort and immobilization until the child or adolescent can receive medical help.

In hip dislocation the best chance for prevention of damage to the head of the femur is to relocate the hip within 60 minutes after the injury occurs. As the length of time between injury and hip relocation increases, the risk of irreparable damage increases. Simple dislocations should be reduced as soon as possible with the child under mild sedation and often local anesthesia. Sedative agents such as midazolam or propofol (Diprivan), and analgesics such as ketamine or fentanyl, can be used to produce partial or complete analgesia during the reduction. Increased swelling, which makes reduction difficult and increases the risk of neurovascular problems, can complicate an unreduced dislocation. Treatment depends on the severity of the injury.

Dislocation of the patella occurs spontaneously in some children; in others it is a result of injury. It is common among adolescent girls. The patella is always dislocated laterally. Most dislocations are reduced either spontaneously or by a companion before the child is seen by a practitioner. Therapy is immobilization for 3 to 4 weeks. Surgery may be needed to treat recurrent dislocations.

The most common dislocation injury is subluxation or partial dislocation of the radial head in the elbow, also called *pulled elbow* or *nursemaid's elbow*. In the vast majority of cases the injury occurs in a child between ages 1 and 3 years who receives a sudden longitudinal pull or traction at the wrist while the arm is fully extended and the forearm pronated. It usually occurs when an adult is holding the child by the hand or wrist and gives a sudden jerk to prevent a fall or attempts to lift the child by pulling the wrist, or the child suddenly pulls away by dropping to the floor (or ground). The child has an anxious expression, whines, complains of pain in the elbow and wrist, refuses to move the arm, and holds it with the opposite hand and in a slightly flexed and pronated position against his or her body.

BOX 39-11 CLASSIFICATION OF SPRAINS

Grade I—Mild injury; involves overstretching or microscopic tearing but without hemorrhage or increased instability of the involved joint. Swelling may develop later.

Grade II—Moderate injury; involves partial, overt tearing of the ligament with at least some ligamentous continuity remaining; usually immediate pain and swelling with decreased function.

Grade III—Severe injury; total loss of ligamentous continuity (i.e., disruption of one or more ligaments or the musculotendinous unit). Pain is immediate but subsides because none of the pain fibers is being stretched. Swelling may be minimal because hemorrhage extravasates outside of the area into soft tissues.

The practitioner manipulates the arm by applying firm finger pressure to the head of the radius and then supinates and flexes the forearm to return the bone structures to normal alignment. A click or clunk may be heard or felt, and functional use of the arm returns within minutes. Immobilization of the arm is not necessary (Cornwall, 2007). The longer the subluxation is present, however, the longer it takes for the child to recover mobility after treatment. A radiograph may be needed if attempts to reduce the dislocation are not successful.

SPRAINS AND STRAINS

A sprain occurs when trauma to a joint is so severe that a ligament is either stretched or partially or completely torn by the force created as a joint is twisted or wrenched. This is often accompanied by damage to associated blood vessels, muscles, tendons, and nerves. As a guideline for management and prognosis, sprains are classified according to the degree of injury (Box 39-11). Because of the number of ligaments required to maintain knee stability, the knee is one of the joints most commonly injured in sports. It is also the largest joint and consequently is more prone to injury. Ankle sprains in children account for approximately 75% of all ankle injuries; these injuries are common in individuals who participate in sports, especially in the pediatric age-group (Chorley, 2005).

The presence of joint laxity is the most valid indicator of the severity of a sprain. With a severe injury the athlete complains that the joint "feels loose" or as if "something is coming apart" and may describe hearing a "snap," "pop," or "tearing." Pain is seldom the principal subjective symptom. There is a rapid onset with swelling, often diffuse, accompanied by immediate disability and appreciable reluctance to use the injured joint.

A strain is a microscopic tear to the musculotendinous unit and has features in common with sprains. The area is painful to the touch and is swollen. The severity is evaluated as grade I, II, or III, as for sprains, except that the degree of laxity does not apply. Even with severe grade III injuries, complaints of laxity are rare. Most strains happen over time rather than suddenly, and the rapidity of the appearance provides clues regarding severity. In general the more rapidly the strain occurs, the more severe the injury. When the strain involves the muscular portion, there is more bleeding, often palpable soon after injury and before edema obscures the hematoma.

Therapeutic Management

The first 6 to 12 hours is the most critical period for virtually all soft tissue injuries. Basic principles for managing sprains and other soft tissue injuries are summarized in the acronyms RICE and ICES:

R—Rest	**I**—Ice
I—Ice	**C**—Compression
C—Compression	**E**—Elevation
E—Elevation	**S**—Support

The trend with ankle sprains is to encourage early mobilization and rehabilitation rather than prolonged immobilization and rest. The acronym PRICEMMS is used to describe measures to implement early mobilization and prevent chronic ankle instability and pain (Chorley, 2005):

P—Proprioception or balance exercises
R—Rest, alteration of activity, use of crutches, progressive weight bearing
I—Icing
C—Compression wrap or brace
E—Elevation
M—Medication for analgesia
M—(Range of) Motion exercises (active or passive)
S—Strengthening exercises, isometric or with movable resistance

Soft tissue injuries should be iced immediately. This is best accomplished using crushed ice wrapped in a towel or encased in a screw-top ice bag or plastic bag (e.g., a resealable storage bag). A wet elastic wrap is applied to provide compression and to keep the ice pack in place. A single layer of the wrap or cloth is placed over the injured area to protect the skin under the ice pack, and the remainder of the bandage secures the pack in place. The wet wrap transfers the cold better than a dry wrap. Athletic trainers often keep wet elastic wraps refrigerated for ready use.

There is still controversy over whether heat or ice should be used during the rehabilitative phase of management. Regardless of the method used, it is accompanied by appropriate exercise, depending on the severity of the injury, and carried out under the direction of a competent professional experienced in the care of sports injuries.

Ice has a rapid cooling effect on tissues that reduces pain and the magnitude of the stretch reflex by decreasing muscle spindle response, afferent nerve discharge, and the afferent loop response (monosynaptic reflex). Secondary effects are achieved by vasoconstriction, decrease in muscle nerve velocity, and increase in muscle viscosity. Also, the decreased temperature slows metabolism, which reduces tissue oxygen requirements. Edema formation is reduced when fewer histamine-like substances are released. Nine to 15 minutes of ice exposure produces deep-tissue vasodilation without increased metabolism. However, the effects last up to 7 hours. Ice therapy should be intermittent, and ice should never be applied for more than 30 minutes at a time to prevent tissue damage.

Elevating the extremity uses gravity to facilitate venous return and reduce edema formation in the damaged area (see Research Focus box). The point of injury must be kept several inches above the level of the heart for therapy to be effective (Fig. 39-32). Several pillows can be used effectively for

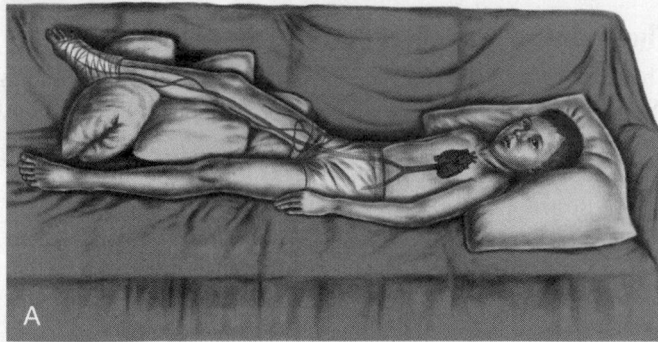

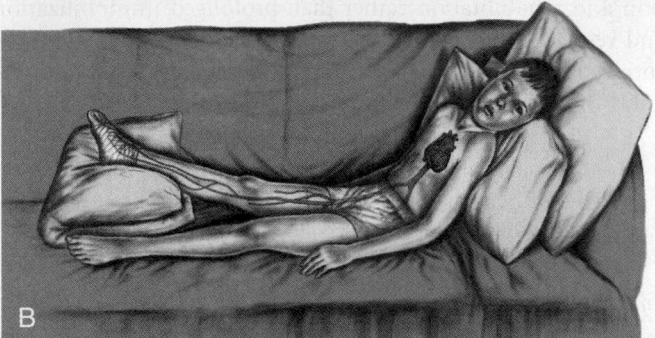

Fig. 39-32 Correct and incorrect methods for elevating a lower extremity. **A,** Correct method: lower leg elevated on pillows; ankle above heart level. **B,** Incorrect positioning: ankle below level of heart.

elevation. Allowing the extremity to be dependent causes excessive fluid accumulation in the area of injury, which delays healing and causes painful swelling. Ivins (2006) recommends a 72-hour rest period for a sprained ankle to allow ligament healing.

🔒 RESEARCH FOCUS

Ankle Support After a Sprain

A semirigid lace-up ankle support was more effective than tape or elastic bandage in providing ankle stability after a sprain in adults; the lace-up support also decreased edema and skin irritation compared with tape or elastic bandage (Ivins, 2006; Kerkhoffs, Struijs, Assendelft, et al, 2002).

Major sprains or tears to the ligamentous tissue rarely occur in growing children. Ligaments are stronger than bone, and the epiphysis and growth plate are the weakest areas of the bone; therefore the more usual site of injury is at the growth plate (see Fractures, p. 1636). Torn ligaments, especially those in the knee, are usually treated by immobilization with a knee immobilizer or range-of-motion brace until the child is able to walk without a limp. Crutches are used for mobility to rest the affected extremity. Passive leg exercises, gradually increased to active ones, begin as soon as sufficient healing has taken place. Caution parents and children against using any form of liniment or other heat-producing preparation before examination. If the injury requires casting or splinting, the heat generated in the enclosed space can produce extreme discomfort and may even cause tissue damage. In some cases torn knee ligaments are managed with arthroscopy and ligament repair or reconstruction as necessary, depending on the extent of the tear, the

ligaments involved, and the child's age. Surgical reconstruction of the anterior cruciate ligament may be performed in young athletes who wish to continue in active sports.

Postoperative mobilization of the affected joint is implemented immediately using a continuous passive motion device. This device provides passive range-of-motion exercise to the injured extremity and decreases postoperative complications related to restricted mobility. The patient often is ambulatory within hours on crutches and is discharged late on the day of surgery or the following day.

OVERUSE INJURY

To excel in sports, the young athlete is forced to train longer, harder, and earlier in life than previously. The rewards are an increased level of fitness, better performance, faster times, and the satisfaction of attaining a personal goal. With the increase in the number of children participating in a wide variety of sports year-round, more overuse injuries are being seen in the pediatric age-group (Brenner and Council on Sports Medicine and Fitness, 2007).

The risk of overuse injury is always present and can be related to several factors: training errors, muscle-tendon imbalance, anatomic malalignment (e.g., femoral anteversion, excessive lumbar lordosis, tibial torsion), incorrect footwear or playing surface, an associated disease state, and growth (growth cartilage is less resistant to microtrauma). Athletes who run extensively frequently experience shin splints. The ligaments tear away from the tibial shaft, and this creates the pain. Ice, rest, and NSAIDs, such as ibuprofen or naproxen, are the usual treatment. Shin splints are rarely serious.

Chronic pain in athletes is often associated with overuse injury, which can occur at any level of athletic participation. The common feature in overuse injuries is the repetitive microtrauma that occurs to a particular anatomic structure (Brenner and Council on Sports Medicine and Fitness, 2007). Performing the same movements time and time again can cause several types of injury: (1) frictional, or rubbing of one structure against another; (2) tractional, or repeated pull on a ligament or tendon; and (3) cyclic, or repetitive loading of impact forces (stress fractures). The end result is inflammation of the involved structure with complaints of pain, tenderness, swelling, and disability.

Bursae, tendons, muscles, ligaments, joints, and bones are all subject to overuse. Table 39-4 outlines some of the common overuse syndromes. Plantar fasciitis is common in athletes, and Osgood-Schlatter disease often occurs in children who do a lot of jumping. The occurrence of overuse-type injuries, such as sore shoulders and strained elbows, may indicate that too much is being asked of the child in too short a period.

Stress Fractures

Given the intensity and duration of sports training, many young athletes suffer stress fractures, especially after a recent increase in training regimens. These fractures occur as a result of repeated muscle contraction and occur most often in sports involving repetitive weight bearing such as running, gymnastics, and basketball. They occur less often in swimming (in the upper extremities). Tibial fractures are most common.

TABLE 39-4	SELECTED OVERUSE INJURIES	
DISORDER	**CAUSE**	**MANIFESTATIONS**
Plantar fasciitis	Repetitive stretching of the plantar fascia (calcaneus to metatarsal heads)	Pain in arch or heel
Achilles tendinitis	Repeated forcible traction on short tendon	Pain on palpation; pain with plantar flexion against resistance
Sever disease	Epiphysitis of the calcaneus	Pain over insertion of Achilles tendon into tip of calcaneus
Anterior leg pain (shin splints)	Irritation of posterior tibial muscle in unconditioned athlete or one not conditioned to a new sport	Pain in leg along anterior or medial edge of midshaft or distal third of tibia
Osgood-Schlatter disease	Traction apophysitis of tibial tubercle	Pain and tenderness; overprominence of involved tubercle
Sinding-Larsen-Johansson syndrome (jumper's knee)	A variant of Osgood-Schlatter disease; traction apophysitis on inferior pole of patella	Same as above; pain slightly lower than in Osgood-Schlatter disease
Patellofemoral syndromes	Malalignment of extensors, increased patellar compression, and increased training intensity	Chronic knee pain, especially following forced leg extension from flexion or after running
Tennis elbow	Lateral epicondylitis from repetitive strain on elbow	Pain in elbow, aggravated by use
Little League elbow	Osteochondritis of the capitellum; tendinitis of flexor-origin medial epicondyle from repetitive valgus strain to elbow from throwing	Pain in elbow that increases with activity
Little League shoulder	Microfracture of proximal humeral growth plate from repetitive throwing	Pain and characteristic contracture; loss of internal rotation and increased external rotation
Swimmer's shoulder	Supraspinatus tendinitis from repetitive shoulder movement	Pain in shoulder that increases with activity

The most common symptom of stress fracture is a sharp, persistent, progressive pain or a deep, persistent dull ache located over the bone. Sometimes there is pain on impact (heel strike), but the most important clinical sign is pain over the involved bony surface. Diagnosis is based on clinical observation. Plain radiographs are rarely diagnostic of stress fractures during the initial few weeks, since callus formation is not yet evident. Occasionally a bone scan will indicate a "hot spot."

Therapeutic Management

Inflammation is common to all overuse syndromes; therefore management involves rest or alteration of activities, physical therapies, and medication. Rest is the primary therapy, usually interpreted as reduced activity and the use of alternative exercise—not bed rest or immobilization with casting. The main purpose is to alleviate the repetitive stress that initiated the symptoms. It is important to keep the child or adolescent mobile, and training can be continued. Alternative exercise is selected that maintains conditioning without aggravating the injury. For example, pool running (treading water in the deep end of a pool) can use the same movements as running but without the weight bearing; bicycling, swimming, and rowing are viable alternatives.

Other modalities include cryotherapy and cold whirlpool baths, and sometimes taping, bracing, splinting, and other orthoses are employed, depending on the injury. Medications such as NSAIDs (see Table 7-4) are sometimes prescribed to reduce inflammation and pain. Topical medications are of questionable value.

EXERCISE-INDUCED HEAT STRESS

Infants, children, and adolescents are at greater risk for heat-related illness than adults (American Academy of Pediatrics, 2000a). Several characteristics of infants and children render them more vulnerable to heat stress. The greater ratio of surface area to body mass in infants and young children leads to increased transfer of heat between the body and the environment. Children produce more metabolic heat for body mass during exercise and have a reduced capacity to convey heat from the body core to the skin. Also, children do not have the sweating capacity of adults and take longer to become acclimated to hot conditions. Young children may not feel the need to drink a sufficient amount of fluid during extended exercise.

Heat cramps are caused by sodium depletion, which in turn potentiates the effects of calcium on skeletal muscle. They most often occur as a result of strenuous exercise in a hot environment. Cramps most frequently involve the leg muscles. Vital signs are usually normal, but the core temperature may be elevated. The child sweats profusely, but mentation is normal. Treatment is rest and replacement of fluid and electrolytes. Ingestion of dilute sports drinks or electrolyte replacement liquids is helpful. Electrolyte replacement solutions are now available as popsicles and gelatin (like Jell-O), which are well tolerated with less vomiting. Replacement electrolyte strips that easily dissolve in the mouth are also available; small sips of a clear fluid such as water can be taken as tolerated.

Heat exhaustion, or heat stress, is a common condition that usually occurs during vigorous exercise in a hot environment. It results from excessive loss of fluids, especially in poorly acclimated and dehydrated children. The onset may be gradual, with initial complaints that include thirst, headache, fatigue, dizziness, anxiety, or nausea and vomiting. The child usually has a clear sensorium but may be somewhat disoriented. The temperature can be normal or mildly elevated; sweating is profuse. Tachycardia, hypotension (usually postural), and syncope may be observed secondary to intravascular volume depletion. Treatment is to move the child to a cool environment, provide rest, and replace fluid volume. The child with a clear sensorium can receive oral replacement fluids, but often IV fluids are required due to vomiting. External cooling methods are not necessary.

Heatstroke represents a failure of normal thermoregulatory mechanisms. Heatstroke usually occurs during or immediately after physical activity, especially in the unacclimated adolescent who is exercising vigorously. The onset is rapid with initial symptoms of headache, weakness, and disorientation. Central nervous system manifestations may be agitation, confusion, and lethargy. Loss of consciousness may occur without warning and may be accompanied by nuchal rigidity, posturing, and convulsions. Sweating may not be present. The temperature is typically higher than 40° C (104° F), and there is severe volume depletion. Immediate care is relocation to a cool environment, removal of clothing, application of cool water (wet towels or immersion), and use of fans. The child is transported to the hospital by EMS for intensive care.

Acute care includes rapid cooling until core temperature reaches 38.9° C (102° F) to prevent overcooling. Antipyretics are not used because they are metabolized by the liver, which is already not functioning properly. Renal and liver failure are common sequelae to heatstroke. Treatment includes careful monitoring of temperature and other vital signs, supportive care such as supplemental oxygen administration, and cautious fluid and electrolyte replacement. Prevention remains the best treatment for hyperthermia. If the temperature is elevated, time in the sun should be decreased. Activity should be stopped if the humidity is elevated as well. The athlete should drink plenty of fluids, preferably with low sugar content.

Nonexertional, or classic, heatstroke has a slow onset with insidious development of anorexia, nausea, vomiting, headache, mental manifestations, and loss of intravascular volume. Classic heatstroke occurs primarily in children with abnormal thermoregulation (e.g., children with cystic fibrosis) and infants subjected to prolonged neglect in a hot environment.

HEALTH CONCERNS ASSOCIATED WITH SPORTS

Nutrition

Some athletes are motivated to enhance their performance by any and all means available. They are eager to learn about nutrition, and many are influenced by misconceptions, fads, and superstitions regarding certain foods. Physical performance is affected by energy and body composition. The young athlete must maintain a diet that provides sufficient nutrients and energy to meet metabolic needs for optimum functioning. Physical training increases the need for energy and for more nutrients that convert food energy into chemical energy for physical performance.

There is no evidence to indicate that food supplements, extra vitamins, sports bars, or high-protein diets are needed to meet the demands of heavy physical exercise or improve physical performance. In addition, there are no scientific data, other than anecdotal reports, supporting the benefits of such supplements in increasing physical performance. Athletes should be given accurate information regarding the lack of proven safety for such supplements (Rodriguez, DiMarco, Langley, et al, 2009). Young athletes need considerably more calories than the recommended dietary allowance (RDA). When the basic requirements for growth and activity are met by a balanced diet

of protein, grains and cereals, fruits and vegetables, and dairy products,* the additional calories needed for the extra exertion can be selected as desired. The athlete can obtain these extra calories by eating additional helpings from any of the basic four food groups, but many of the additional calories are provided by complex carbohydrates found in foods such as vegetables, pastas, and bread.

The recommended dietary energy intake for adolescents involved in sports is at least 50% of caloric intake from carbohydrates (6 to 10 g/kg/day), protein intake of 1.2 to 1.4 g/kg/day, and 25% to 30% from fat (American Academy of Pediatrics, 2009). It should be noted, however, that energy requirements vary depending on the sport and the child's age and body build. Adolescent athletes need additional iron and calcium intake from appropriate food sources to meet growth and developmental needs and to replace amounts lost in competition. Box 39-12 presents nutrition pointers for young athletes.

Water and Electrolytes

Considerable water is lost from the body through perspiration, urination, and evaporation from the respiratory tract. Water losses, especially from the skin, increase as the duration and intensity of exercise increase and as environmental temperature rises. Although thirst is experienced early in dehydration, it is unreliable as an indicator of fluid deficit. Athletes should hydrate with water regardless of thirst during strenuous exercise or activity. Water is recommended as *the best drink* for most athletes, and current recommendations are to take 5 to 8 oz of water every 15 to 20 minutes (150 ml for 40 kg [88 lb] athletes and 250 ml for athletes >40 kg); fluids should never be restricted during activity. A flavored, colored sports beverage containing 6% to 8% carbohydrate, however, may be preferred by children for the taste (American Academy of Pediatrics, 2009). Drinking carbonated beverages is discouraged. Athletes participating in multiple daily exercise sessions in warm environments are at risk for dehydration and should receive all the water they desire.

Very little water is exchanged in the stomach, and it must reach the intestines for absorption. The best fluids for rapid gastric emptying are cold, have low osmolality, and have a large volume. Gatorade and other sports drinks contain excess carbohydrate (6% to 8%); they should be diluted with one or two parts water to one part drink for children, but older adolescents may tolerate the carbohydrate load. New sports drinks are commercially available that reportedly boost physical performance. These new carbohydrate-electrolyte drinks, as well as other commercially available carbohydrate-electrolyte drinks, may cause dental enamel erosion, although the research results vary (Venables, Shaw, Jeukendrup, et al, 2005). Studies outlining the effects of these newer sports drinks on actual physical performance and their untoward effects in adolescent athletes have

---

*Basic guidelines for dietary intake can be accessed at www.choosemy plate.gov. This interactive site allows the individual to enter her or his age, sex, and average exercise pattern to see the types of food and total estimated number of calories that should be consumed. Athletes may use this site as a basis for formulating a balanced diet and add the recommended number of calories for athletic activity.

BOX 39-12 FIFTEEN STEPS TO GOOD SPORTS NUTRITION

1. A well-balanced diet consists of elements from the MyPlate food guide. The recommended percentages of major nutrients are 55% to 75% carbohydrates, 25% to 30% fat, and 15% to 20% protein.*

2. Athletes should take water at regular intervals (every 15 to 20 minutes) during exercise.

3. For each pound of fluid lost through exercise, the athlete should consume 16 oz of water.

4. Any athlete who loses more than 3% of body weight in an exercise session should not return to activity until the fluid is restored. Monitoring body weight can prevent chronic dehydration.

5. Beverages with small amounts of simple sugars or glucose polymers with little or no electrolytes are acceptable alternatives to water.

6. Use of salt tablets should be avoided and may actually do harm by increasing dehydration.

7. Glycogen loading is of value only for endurance exercises that take longer than 1 hour, such as marathons and cross-country ski races. It is not recommended for children.

8. Protein and amino acid supplements are potentially harmful and should be discouraged.

9. Vitamin supplements are usually unnecessary and a waste of money; excessive doses may be harmful. One daily multivitamin is not harmful for children who do not consume well-balanced meals.

10. Mineral supplements are usually not needed, except by young athletes, especially menstruating females, who develop a specific deficiency such as iron deficiency.

11. Any weight loss program should be designed to produce primarily loss of body fat and not of lean body tissue or water. The goal should be to achieve a certain percentage of body weight as fat.

12. Athletes should not lose more than 1 to 2 lb per week. They should not reduce daily caloric intake to fewer than 1200 calories for girls and 1500 calories for boys.

13. Athletes who wish to gain weight can do so by combining increased caloric intake with muscle work (i.e., weight training). Nutritional supplements are not usually needed.

14. Athletes should gain weight no more rapidly than 1 to 2 lb per week. They should be monitored for percentage of body fat.

15. The pregame meal should be eaten at least 2.5 hours before competition. It should consist primarily of carbohydrates and not foods that are slowly digested (fats) or that have excessive concentrated sugars (desserts).

Modified from Primos WA, Landry GL: Fighting the fads in sports nutrition, *Contemp Pediatr* 6(9):14-50, 1989; and American Academy of Pediatrics, Section on Sports Medicine and Fitness: *Guidelines for pediatricians: nutrition and sports,* August 2001, issue 6, pp. 1-2, The Academy, available online at **www.aap.org/sections/sportsmedicine/PDFs/SportsShorts_06.pdf** (accessed August 15, 2009).
*Note that percentages may vary according to different authorities and should take into consideration the athlete's energy expended, body build, and age.

yet to receive adequate attention in the medical and scientific community.

Small amounts of electrolytes, especially sodium and chloride, are lost during exercise. Because sweat is quite dilute relative to plasma, excessive perspiration can result in excessive loss of water and an increase in plasma concentrations of sodium chloride. Therefore it is more important to replace water than sodium and chloride. Children should be well hydrated before beginning strenuous exercise or sports, especially in warm climates or environments. Periodic drinking breaks are encouraged, and adults or other team members should be alert to the child who has complaints such as headache, cramping, nausea, or vertigo. The use of salt tablets or table salt is unnecessary and may actually be harmful. Athletes usually derive sufficient salt replacement from the diet.

Minerals

The basic diet does not satisfy the iron requirement of 10% to 15% of female athletes, most of whom are teenage girls who tend to become iron depleted after menarche. Young boys who are experiencing rapid adolescent growth and who have irregular and inadequate diets also are at risk of iron depletion. These children need iron supplements.

Adequate calcium intake during puberty is essential to promote mineralization of the growing skeleton. The recommended dietary reference intake (DRI) for calcium in adolescents ages 13 to 18 years is 1300 mg/day, yet few adolescents meet this goal. Calcium plays a vital role in nerve transmission, muscle contraction, and blood coagulation. Female athletes who engage in intensive training may develop amenorrhea, with subsequent decreased bone mineral density, osteopenia, and osteoporosis. Although the last two conditions may not

occur immediately, stress fractures and impaired muscle contractions may be seen with low calcium intake. The best sources of additional calcium for athletes are nonfat dairy products. In addition, foods such as regular or low-fat yogurt and cheese, calcium-fortified orange juice, low-fat chocolate milk, and pudding may help meet daily calcium requirements. Consider the amount of calcium in the following: 1 glass of calcium-fortified orange juice contains 200 to 250 mg of calcium; 1 cup of skim milk has 300 mg of calcium; and 8 oz of yogurt contains approximately 410 mg of calcium. A well-balanced diet can provide the necessary calcium intake if adolescent athletes are made aware of the requirements and of the long-term consequences of poor nutrition.

Glycogen

Energy comes primarily from glycogen previously stored in muscles and the liver. Energy for prolonged exercise is derived from high-carbohydrate foods (e.g., bread, cereals, pancakes, potatoes, rice, spaghetti) consumed 24 to 48 hours before the activity, not from a meal eaten just before the activity. The meal before a physical contest should be eaten at least 2 to 4 hours before the exertion and should consist mainly of carbohydrates. Carbohydrate (glycogen) loading is a technique reserved for competition in prolonged aerobic endurance events and requires dietary changes a week before the competitive event. For more information regarding carbohydrate loading and other techniques for improving athletic performance, the reader is directed to texts on sports medicine and sports training.

Weight

Control of body weight by restricting water or food intake or increasing sweat loss is dangerous. Weight loss should not exceed 1.5% of total body weight per week (or 1 to 2 lb/wk) (American Academy of Pediatrics, 2009). Young athletes need appropriate information about nutrition to dispel the allure of fads and fallacies about diet and performance. A sports nutritionist should be consulted for determining an optimal diet based on amount of energy expenditure and energy requirements. The optimum diet for an athlete is one that contains the essential food groups and that is adjusted to the energy requirements of the sport in which the child or adolescent is engaged. Such a dietary plan should provide adequate nutrition for top physical efficiency and performance, maintenance of physical fitness and desirable body weight, and optimum function of all organ systems.

Considerations for the Female Athlete

The syndrome known as female athlete triad consists of amenorrhea, osteoporosis, and disordered eating (American Academy of Pediatrics, 2009). The triad was originally described in athletes in sports for which thinness was desired (gymnasts, ballet dancers, figure skaters, and long distance runners) but is now recognized in virtually all sports. The phenomenon has been attributed to a complex interplay of physical, genetic, hormonal, nutritional, psychologic, and environmental factors that include the stress of competition, decreased protein consumption, and altered lean-to-fat body ratio.

Amenorrhea has been reported among girls who engage in strenuous exercise. Except in swimmers, menarche is attained later in athletes than in nonathletes. Gymnasts, figure skaters, and ballet dancers have the latest mean ages of menarche; track athletes have less of a delay in maturity than do gymnasts and ballet dancers, who also tend to be smaller, lighter, and leaner than other female athletes. Swimmers, who tend to be larger, have a mean age of menarche that approximates that for nonathletes. Also, there appears to be an association between delayed menarche and more advanced competitive levels; that is, athletes at more advanced levels have a greater delay than those at lower competitive levels.

One topic for counseling of the female athlete with delayed menarche is pregnancy. Sexually active teenagers, regardless of menstrual status, need to consider contraceptive precautions. Most teenage girls erroneously believe that if they do not menstruate, they cannot become pregnant.

Osteoporosis from decreased levels of estrogen in these athletes, complicated by poor nutritional intake, leads to loss of bone density and stress fractures. The peak of bone density is reached in late adolescence and is related to circulating estrogen levels. Girls with diminished estrogen secretion in delayed menarche will reach late adolescence with low bone density and will be subject to stress fractures and osteoporosis. Hypoestrogenic bone loss greatly increases the risk of injury. It is recommended that bone density (DEXA scan) be evaluated in the athlete who has been amenorrheic for more than 6 months (Joy, Van Hala, and Cooper, 2009).

Disordered eating is less severe and more subtle than eating disorders such as anorexia and bulimia. Disordered eating includes food restrictions, rigid food patterns, fasting, vomiting, and the use of diet pills and laxatives. The goal is to achieve a specific body image that is seen as desirable for the sport and is influenced by others such as a coach, teammates, or peers.

Disordered eating results in poor protein intake, low fat intake, and inadequate caloric intake. Adolescent females should increase calcium intake to four to six servings per day of low-fat dairy products (1500 mg of calcium and 400 to 800 international units of vitamin D are the RDAs for amenorrheic athletes [American Academy of Pediatrics, 2000b]) (see Nutrition, p. 1660). In addition, they should consume adequate protein and calories to meet the energy and metabolic needs of exercise. Trainers and coaches also need to be aware of the potentially long-term results of intensive, prolonged exercise in pubertal girls.

Treatment may be long term and often involves development of an appropriate nutritional plan with a registered dietitian, decrease in exercise, behavioral change therapy, and nutritional supplementation aimed at preventing osteoporosis (Waldrop, 2005). However, education alone may not provide adequate incentive to change behavior, and further psychologic health interventions may be required.

An excellent source of further information for parents, coaches, and athletes regarding nutrition for female athletes is "Female Athlete Triad."*

Substance Misuse by Athletes

Young athletes have used various performance-enhancing substances in an attempt to augment their athletic performance. These substances, also known as *ergogenic aids,* are believed by athletes to increase strength and endurance, delay the onset of fatigue, increase the ability to concentrate, and decrease sensitivity to pain. Although use of these substances is prohibited in international Olympic competition, there are no means at present to enforce a prohibition on their use in other sports settings.

Examples of substances used by athletes include psychomotor stimulants (e.g., amphetamines), anabolic-androgenic steroids (AAS), ephedra, androstenedione (andro), dehydroepiandrosterone (DHEA), creatine, guarana, ginseng, amino acid and protein supplements, and excess amounts of vitamins (niacin, vitamin A, vitamin B_6). Because many of these substances are considered natural, many people willingly use them without further investigating potential hazards. The belief is that anything "natural," even if consumed in excess of the DRI (see Chapter 6), must be perfectly fine for the body because it will be rapidly metabolized and excreted without causing harm. This is not necessarily true for all substances, however, and parents, coaches, trainers, athletes, and health care workers should be knowledgeable about the effects of such substances. Rather than prohibiting their use, a better approach, especially for adolescents, is to provide open, informed discussion on the availability of appropriate substitutes that exist in foods that are indeed healthy to consume yet provide beneficial effects for athletic performance. Schools may include such discussions in existing curricula for their athletes and encourage participation in these educational programs.

Amphetamines and related drugs, such as methylphenidate (Ritalin), as well as caffeine and ephedra or other stimulants,

---

*American Academy of Pediatrics: Female athlete triad, *Sports Shorts,* Issue 8, July 2002, available at www.aap.org/sections/sportsmedicine/SportsShorts.cfm.

may be taken to provide a sense of increased alertness and relief of fatigue; however, obscuring fatigue may permit participants to exceed their limits and precipitate a sudden collapse. Some stimulants such as ephedra are used to burn fat when used in combination with caffeine. These substances can also make the users more aggressive, which can contribute to injuries to themselves and others.

Other misused drugs include stimulants intended for bronchodilation, decongestants, agents for weight gain or loss, physiologic agents used to enhance oxygen-carrying capacity, and nutritional supplements taken in doses greater than required (American Academy of Pediatrics, 2005). Anabolic steroids are a source of concern to health professionals. The majority of these drugs are no longer manufactured in the United States by legitimate companies. Black market supplies of anabolic steroids are of poor quality and potency. In an attempt to enhance muscle strength, these drugs may be administered to athletes by coaches, managers, athletic trainers, and even physicians. The user develops larger-appearing muscles and increased body weight and body water, but reports on the side effects of these drugs outweigh any benefits for performance during athletic competition (Gregory and Fitch, 2007). Although the psychologic effect may be beneficial, many valid studies have failed to demonstrate any improvement in performance (Calfee and Fadale, 2006).

The precise incidence of anabolic steroid use by adolescent athletes remains debatable but may range from 5% to 11% of high school athletes. Middle-school children are reporting an increased use of anabolic steroids to enhance athletic performance. Coaches and health professionals who work with youth report a trend toward increased use of these agents. Adolescents and young adults rely on poor sources of information about the potential hazards of steroid use (friends, television, muscle magazines) and are generally poorly informed about their potential negative side effects. Health care professionals need to be aware of the clinical manifestations of steroid use. Clinical signs such as severe acne, a sudden increase in strength and muscle mass, a sudden decrease in body fat, a male pattern of baldness, and water retention are common. In females a male pattern of hair growth and a deepening voice are significant observations.

The dangers of continued use are well known and include virilization in females; oligospermia, prostatic hypertrophy, myocardial infarction, stroke, testicular atrophy, infertility, and gynecomastia in males; and premature closure of the epiphyses, acne, increased blood cholesterol levels, hypertension, and hepatocellular carcinoma in both genders. Mood changes have been observed, including aggressiveness, changes in libido, depression, anxiety, and psychosis (Gregory and Fitch, 2007). Health hazards outweigh any potential gain that the drug might provide.

Other drugs that are often misused include nutritional aids, local anesthetic agents, narcotic analgesics such as nalbuphine (Nubain), growth hormone, erythropoietin, creatine, beta blockers (to reduce levels of circulating catecholamines and thus reduce anxiety related to the somatic type of stress), antiinflammatory drugs such as dimethyl sulfoxide (DMSO) (which is not approved for use and is available only as a veterinary or an industrial preparation), and corticosteroids. The possibility of their use by the adolescent athlete should be considered when performing a health assessment.

The American Academy of Pediatrics (2005) recommends that parents and coaches be involved in educating athletes about the adverse effects of performance-enhancing substances and that schools and other sports organizations discourage the use of such substances among athletes. In addition, it is recommended that interventions for encouraging substance-free competition that are positive, rather than punitive, are promoted and encourage sound nutrition and training practices. The pressure to win at all costs is high, and athletes face pressures not only from peers and immediate authority figures but also from others who promise financial gain and potential fame. The problem is often compounded by the existence of poor role models in professional sports activities who earn thousands or even millions of dollars yearly and are known by their colleagues to take performance-enhancing substances yet deny the practice.

Sudden Death

A death associated with sports produces renewed anxiety in both parents and health care professionals. The term *sudden* or *instantaneous death* is applied to death that occurs within minutes of the onset of the cause of death or within 24 hours of the episode. *Sudden cardiac arrest* is also a term used to describe the athlete who experiences a sudden death. The incidence of sudden death among high school athletes has been estimated to be 1 per 200,000 per year (Maron, Gohman, and Aeppli, 1998; Maron, 2003). Maron, Doerer, Haas, and colleagues (2009) reported that between 1980 and 2006 most causes of sudden death in athletes occurred as a result of cardiovascular disease (56%), followed by blunt trauma (22%), commotio cordis (3%), and heat stroke (2%). One study of sudden cardiac deaths in young athletes reported an average of 69 cases per year during the years 2000 to 2006 (Drezner, Chun, Harmon, et al, 2008). Overall survival rates for young athletes experiencing sudden cardiac arrest during an athletic event between 2000 and 2006 were 11%, with a trend toward improved survival in the latter years of the study. More males (83%) than females (17%) experienced sudden cardiac arrest, and females were more likely to survive the arrest than were males (Drezner, Chun, Harmon, et al, 2008).

Causes of sudden death are related to three main risk factors: (1) sports with a high inherent risk for sports-related sudden death, (2) recognized or unknown underlying medical problems in child participants, and (3) the sports environment (e.g., the rules, equipment, practice fields or areas of sport participation, and ambient temperature of the geographic area). (Chapter 23 discusses the impact of sudden death on the family and relevant nursing interventions.)

Sports

Sports associated with the greatest risk of sudden death are those involving collision and frequent body contact. Examples of collision sports are football, ice hockey, rugby, and boxing. There is a high potential for serious injury or fatality in sports such as mountain or rock climbing and hang gliding. Sports that involve high-velocity objects, such as baseball and ice hockey, may result in death from serious head or chest injuries.

Riding vehicles such as snowmobiles, mopeds, water jet skis, all-terrain vehicles, snowboards, minibikes, and motorcycles can also be considered high-risk sports.

Medical Conditions

The most frequent medical causes of sudden death during sports activity are cardiac abnormalities, especially idiopathic hypertrophic subaortic stenosis (hypertrophic cardiomyopathy). Manifestations suggestive of hypertrophic cardiomyopathy include a typical triad of severe chest pain, dizziness, and dyspnea. Unfortunately some affected individuals never display signs of disease until they collapse during a sports event. A history of sudden death of a relative or relatives in the second or third decade of life often offers a clue to recognition.

Well-trained athletes often display evidence of hypertrophic cardiomyopathy, the so-called athlete's heart, but the condition is not pathologic. Congenital coronary artery malformation is the second most common cause of sudden death in athletes. Additional causes include valvular heart disease, atherosclerotic coronary artery disease, dilated cardiomyopathy, Marfan syndrome, and myocarditis. Children with systemic hypertension, some types of cardiac arrhythmias such as prolonged QT syndrome, and some forms of heart block will face restrictions in the type and amount of exercise they can tolerate safely. **Commotio cordis** is a common cause of sudden death in athletes without previous history of heart disease. This occurs following a blunt, nonpenetrating blow to the chest, which produces ventricular fibrillation. Commotio cordis is more common in children and adolescents, with a mean age at occurrence of 13 years, and the blow may not be perceived as being that unusual or significant enough to produce such drastic results.

Appropriate use of an automatic external defibrillator (AED) by civilian bystanders or health care workers may save the life of an athlete who experiences a life-threatening cardiac emergency. A school-based AED program provides a high survival rate for student athletes and nonathletes who experience sudden cardiac arrest on school grounds (Drezner, Rao, Heistand, et al, 2009). (See also Cardiopulmonary Resuscitation, Chapter 31.)

Environmental Causes

Environmental factors that are potential causes of death include playing conditions, clothing, equipment, rules used by officials governing a sport, and outdoor temperature. Heatstroke and hypothermia (see Chapter 18) are the most serious environment-related causes of death in athletes.

The American Academy of Pediatrics has introduced an emergency response plan for schools that includes training teachers and school workers in cardiopulmonary resuscitation and first aid, collecting data to evaluate the risk for injuries in the school environment, and acting to reduce such risk (Hazinski, Markenson, Neish, et al, 2004). Encourage nurses in school programs and in the community to become involved in the establishment of such programs and to assist in training and in planning and implementation of effective risk prevention strategies designed to minimize child deaths in schools and local communities.

The American Academy of Pediatrics also recommends implementing a lay rescuer AED program in schools and that communication regarding the location of such equipment be properly managed (Hazinski, Markenson, Neish, et al, 2004). A consensus statement was developed the National Athletic Trainers' Association in conjunction with 15 national health care organizations for emergency preparedness and response in the event of sudden cardiac arrest in young athletes. This statement includes recommendations for those involved in high school and collegiate athletics for the prompt recognition and treatment of sudden cardiac arrest, including the use of an AED (Drezner, Courson, Roberts, et al, 2007).

NURSE'S ROLE IN CHILDREN'S SPORTS

Nurses may become involved in children's sports activities in preparation and evaluation of children for activities, provision of anticipatory guidance and counseling about athletic competition and nutrition, prevention of injuries, treatment of injuries, and rehabilitation after injuries. Selecting an appropriate sport for both recreation and competition is a joint effort of the child or adolescent, parents, and health professionals. Children are introduced to sports as part of family activities, neighborhood games, and school physical education programs, and both parents and children are influenced by media exposure to a variety of sports. Children are highly influenced by the popularity of and exposure afforded athletics in the school setting, especially in high school.

The best approach to counseling children and parents regarding sports participation is to encourage activities that are most likely to provide pleasure and physical benefits throughout childhood and into adulthood. Exposure to a variety of sports activities is probably better for young children than limitation to only one sport. Caution parents against overprogramming children to allow ample time for other activities and associations. Burnout among children and adolescents who continuously participate in sports is increasing in the United States. Children and adolescent are encouraged to take periodic breaks from such activities to allow physical healing, refresh the mind, and work on strength and conditioning (Brenner and Council on Sports Medicine and Fitness, 2007).

Nurses are sometimes members of a sports medicine team. Although certified sports trainers and other specialists in sports medicine usually manage training and rehabilitation, the nurse should have input regarding injury prevention. Nurses should be able to provide emergency treatment for most types of injuries and know when to refer the injured child for evaluation and care. Sports injuries can occur in free play as well as in organized athletic programs, and a school nurse is often the first person who attends an injured child.

When children sustain athletic injuries, nurses are often responsible for instructing the children and their parents regarding care and rehabilitation. Instructions regarding, for example, the need and schedule for follow-up appointments, application of ice, and any restrictions in activity should be delivered clearly and preferably accompanied by written directions. Emphasize the importance of taking medications as prescribed, since they may be needed for an extended period and compliance may be difficult. For children continuing with activities, nonnarcotic pain medication administration an hour before practice or competition is advantageous.

Prevention of sports injuries is probably the most important aspect of any athletic program. Nurses collaborate with coaches and athletic trainers to ensure that safety measures are carried out. Stretching exercises, warming-up and cooling-down activities, and an appropriate training program are only some of the requisites for safe participation. Protective measures, such as padding, taping, wrapping, or use of other devices, are employed for areas at risk. Nurses are also on the alert for environmental safety risks.

Participation of youth in sports programs has grown significantly in the past several decades. This trend toward greater participation by both genders has been encouraged because of its demonstrated effect in reducing obesity, lowering blood pressure, and lowering cholesterol and lipid levels.

For some athletes, their whole life revolves around sports participation. When a serious injury occurs, the athlete's self-esteem and self-image may suffer a devastating blow. Nursing assessment may reveal an athlete who appears to have difficulty dealing with this event and actually rejects any positive reinforcement. The nurse may help the child and family in establishing a support system. The athlete may need to learn new coping skills and explore other avenues to foster feelings of increased self-worth and a sense of accomplishment.

Lack of participation, exercise aversion, and declining interest in sports are sometimes the aftermath of participation during the school years and adolescence. Motivation can be altered or permanently destroyed by failure to appreciate the child's or adolescent's needs related to sports activities. Ridicule or derogation during acquisition of motor skills can shatter a child's or adolescent's self-esteem, producing anxiety and self-doubt that may result in a lifelong aversion to sports. Every child should have the opportunity to develop a strong sense of personal worth through the process of motor learning and acquisition of skills. All participants should have the opportunity to participate and be rewarded with positive encouragement for their contribution, no matter how small; all participants should be rewarded for what they do right.

MUSCULOSKELETAL DYSFUNCTION

TORTICOLLIS

Torticollis (wry neck), which can be either congenital or acquired, is a condition of limited neck motion in which the neck is flexed and the head is drawn or tilted laterally to the affected side while the chin is pointed toward the opposite side. It is a manifestation rather than a disease entity and may be associated with a number of conditions, including congenital abnormality of the cervical spine or a traumatic lesion of the sternocleidomastoid muscle. Congenital muscular torticollis may occur as a result of abnormal positioning in utero, which causes contracture of the sternocleidomastoid muscle (Spiegel, Hosalkar, Dormans, et al, 2007). Infants with positional plagiocephaly may have muscular torticollis as well, which can be successfully treated with neck stretching exercises (Graham, Gomez, Halberg, et al, 2005; Persing, James, Swanson, et al, 2003).

In early infancy a firm, nontender mass may be felt in the midportion of the muscle. The mass regresses and is replaced by fibrous tissue. If the condition remains untreated, permanent limitation of neck movement results, and the head and face become asymmetric, probably because of impaired blood supply to the depressed side of the head. Plagiocephaly and facial asymmetry often occur as a result of the contractured sternocleidomastoid muscle. Patients may have other associated musculoskeletal conditions, including calcaneovalgus foot deformity and metatarsus adductus (Spiegel, Hosalkar, Dormans, et al, 2007).

Treatment of simple torticollis consists of gentle stretching exercises. The face is turned toward the affected muscle while the head is tilted in the opposite direction with the neck extended. A physical therapist typically establishes the treatment regimen to be followed by the nurse and family. The exercises are best performed by two persons—one to control the torso and one to manipulate the head. If stretching exercises are unsuccessful, surgical release of the sternocleidomastoid muscle may be needed. Increasingly, surgical correction by age 12 to 18 months is recommended to prevent muscle contractures and further progression of plagiocephaly. Other forms of torticollis occur in infancy or may develop at a later age but are not discussed in this text.

Nursing Care Management

Nurses should be alert to the possibility of torticollis in infants with limited head movement. After diagnosis it is frequently the nurse's responsibility to teach the exercises and supervise the family in performing them. The exercises require very explicit instructions to the family, and compliance is mandatory. The nurse should also suggest that the child be placed in the crib or playpen in a way that encourages turning the head away from the deformity to observe activities and interesting items. Parents can encourage the child to turn the head in the direction desired for correction through feeding and playing with the child.

LEGG-CALVÉ-PERTHES DISEASE

Legg-Calvé-Perthes disease, sometimes called coxa plana or osteochondritis deformans juvenilis, is a self-limiting disorder in which there is aseptic necrosis of the femoral head. The disease affects children ages 2 to 12 years, but most cases occur as an isolated event in boys between 4 and 8 years of age. In approximately 10% of cases the involvement is bilateral; most of the affected children have a skeletal age significantly below their chronologic age (Hosalkar, Horn, Friedman, et al, 2007). The male/female ratio is 4:1 or 5:1. Caucasian children are affected 10 times more frequently than African-American children.

Pathophysiology

The cause of the disease is unknown. A disturbance of circulation to the femoral capital epiphysis produces an ischemic aseptic necrosis of the femoral head. During middle childhood, circulation to the femoral epiphysis is more tenuous than at other ages, being supplied almost entirely by lateral retinacular vessels. This circulatory impairment appears to extend to the epiphysis and acetabulum as well. The pathologic events seem to take place in four stages (Box 39-13), although there is controversy regarding prognostic classification. The entire disease

---

BOX 39-13 STAGES OF LEGG-CALVÉ-PERTHES DISEASE

Stage I—Aseptic necrosis or infarction of the femoral capital epiphysis with degenerative changes producing flattening of the upper surface of the femoral head (the avascular stage)

Stage II—Capital bone resorption and revascularization with fragmentation (vascular resorption of the epiphysis) that gives a mottled appearance on radiographs (the fragmentation, or revascularization stage)

Stage III—New bone formation, which is represented on radiographs as calcification and ossification or increased density in the areas of radiolucency; this filling-in process appears to take place from the periphery of the head centrally (the reparative stage)

Stage IV—Gradual reformation of the head of the femur without radiolucency and, it is hoped, to a spherical form (the regenerative stage)

---

process may encompass as few as 18 months or continue for several years. The reformed femoral head may be severely altered or appear entirely normal.

Clinical Manifestations

The onset of Legg-Calvé-Perthes disease is usually insidious, and the history may reveal only intermittent appearance of a limp on the affected side or a symptom complex, including hip soreness, ache, or stiffness that can be constant or intermittent. The parents may report seeing the child limping, and the limp becomes more pronounced with increased activity. The pain may be experienced in the hip, along the entire thigh, or in the vicinity of the knee joint. The pain and limp are usually most evident on arising and at the end of a long day of activities. The pain is usually accompanied by joint dysfunction and limited range of motion. There may be a vague history of trauma. The diagnosis is established by radiographic examination, with the definitive diagnosis being made by MRI, which demonstrates osteonecrosis.

Therapeutic Management

Because deformity occurs early in the disease process, the aims of treatment are to eliminate hip irritability; restore and maintain adequate range of hip motion; prevent capital femoral epiphyseal collapse, extrusion, or subluxation; and ensure a well-rounded femoral head at the time of healing. Treatment varies according to the child's age at the time of diagnosis and the appearance of the femoral head vasculature and position within the acetabulum. Nonsurgical containment of the femoral head may be accomplished with abduction casts, whereas a pelvic or femoral osteotomy may be used to contain the femoral head. Activity causes microfractures of the soft ischemic epiphysis, which tend to induce synovitis, stiffness, and adductor contracture. The initial therapy is rest and non–weight bearing, which help reduce inflammation and restore motion. Later, active motion is encouraged. In some cases traction is applied to stretch tight adductor muscles.

Containment can be accomplished in several ways. One is the use of non–weight-bearing devices, such as an abduction brace (e.g., Atlanta Scottish Rite orthosis), leg casts, or a leather harness sling, which prevent weight bearing on the affected limb. Another includes the use of various weight-bearing appliances, such as abduction-ambulation braces or casts after a period of bed rest and traction. A third option consists

of surgical reconstruction and containment procedures. Conservative therapy must be continued for 2 to 4 years, although braces constructed from lightweight materials allow the child to maintain a nearly normal activity level. Surgical correction, although subjecting the child to additional risks (e.g., from anesthesia, infection, blood transfusion), returns the child to normal activities in 3 to 4 months. The use of home traction has also been explored.

The disease is self-limiting, but the ultimate outcome of therapy depends on early and efficient treatment and the child's age at the onset of the disorder. Children 5 years and younger, whose epiphyses are more cartilaginous, have the best prognosis for complete recovery. Children over 9 years old have a significant risk for degenerative arthritis, especially if they have femoral head deformity at the time of diagnosis (Hosalkar, Horn, Friedman, et al, 2007). The later the diagnosis is made, the more femoral damage will have occurred before treatment is implemented. In many cases, with good patient compliance, the prognosis is excellent.

Nursing Care Management

Nurses are often the first health care professionals to identify affected children and to refer them for medical evaluation. Because these children are largely cared for on an outpatient basis, the major emphasis of nursing care is on teaching the family the required care. The family needs to learn the purpose, function, application, and care of the corrective device and the importance of compliance with the prescribed regimen to achieve the desired outcome.

One of the most difficult aspects of the disorder is the need to cope with normally active children who feel well but must remain relatively inactive. It is important to emphasize that children should continue to attend school and engage in former activities that can be adapted to the therapeutic appliance. Adaptation of school activities may need to be arranged with school personnel.

Suitable activities must be devised to meet the needs of the child in the process of developing a sense of initiative or industry. Activities that fulfill the creative urges are well received. This is also an opportune time to encourage the child to begin a hobby such as assembling collections, building models, or engaging in crafts.

SLIPPED CAPITAL FEMORAL EPIPHYSIS

Slipped capital femoral epiphysis (SCFE), or coxa vara, refers to the spontaneous displacement of the proximal femoral epiphysis in a posterior and inferior direction. It develops most frequently shortly before or during accelerated growth and the onset of puberty (children between the ages of 10 and 16 years; median age, 13 for boys, 12 for girls) and is most frequently observed in boys and obese children. Bilateral involvement occurs in up to 60% of cases. Osteonecrosis is a common complication of SCFE and is reported to occur in 17% to 47% of all patients (Hosalkar, Horn, Friedman, et al, 2007).

Pathophysiology

Most cases of SCFE are idiopathic, although it can be associated with endocrine disorders, renal osteodystrophy, and radiotherapy. The cause of idiopathic SCFE is multifactorial and includes obesity, physeal architecture and orientation, and pubertal hormone changes that affect physeal strength. Approximately 65% of patients with SCFE are above the 90th percentile in weight-for-age profiles; therefore obesity is believed to play a significant role in the development of the condition (Hosalkar, Horn, Friedman, et al, 2007). Although obesity stresses the physeal plate, SCFE can also occur in children who are not obese. Radiographs show medial displacement of the epiphysis and uncovered upper portion of the femoral neck adjacent to the physis. There is a widened growth plate and irregular metaphysis. The capital femoral epiphysis remains in the acetabulum, but the femoral neck slips, deforming the femoral head and stretching blood vessels to the epiphysis.

Clinical Manifestations

The following different types of clinical manifestation have been observed: (1) an episode of minor trauma in which the epiphysis is acutely displaced in a previously functional joint; (2) gradual displacement without definite injury, with progressively increased hip disability; (3) intermittent bouts of displacement alternating with periods of well-being, with the gradual appearance of symptoms associated with ambulation (e.g., external rotation); and (4) a combined gradual and traumatic displacement in which there is gradual slippage, with further displacement caused by injury.

SCFE is suspected when an adolescent or preadolescent, especially one who is obese or tall and lanky, begins to limp and complains of pain in the hip continuously or intermittently. The pain is frequently referred to the groin, anteromedial aspect of the thigh, or knee. Physical examination reveals early restriction of internal rotation on adduction and external rotation deformity with loss of abduction and internal rotation as the severity increases. The child or adolescent often lies still with the lower extremity flexed, abducted, and externally rotated because of the intense pain; any attempts to move the limb are met with significant resistance (Loder, 2006). The diagnosis is confirmed by radiographic examination.

Therapeutic and Nursing Care Management

The treatment goals of SCFE are to (1) prevent further slipping until physeal closure, (2) avoid further complication such as avascular necrosis, and (3) maintain adequate hip function (Loder, 2006). Once the diagnosis is established, the child should be made completely non–weight bearing to prevent further slippage. Surgical treatment varies with the degree of displacement. Traditional methods included presurgery bed rest and traction followed by surgical pinning. Some surgeons prefer to take the child to surgery within 24 hours of the onset of acute symptoms and avoid further risk for avascular necrosis (Loder, 2006). Surgical pinning involves the placement of a single pin or alternatively two cannulated screws through the femoral neck into the proximal femoral epiphysis to prevent further slippage (Hart, Grottkau, and Albright, 2007; Loder, 2006). Several other surgical treatment options are also available and are described in the Loder (2006) reference. Postsurgical care includes non–weight bearing with crutch ambulation until acceptable, painless range of motion is achieved.

SCFE is an emergency and requires early diagnosis and treatment to increase the likelihood of a satisfactory cure. The two most severe complications of SCFE are avascular necrosis of the proximal femoral physis and chondrolysis, which involves the loss of articular cartilage, decreased range of motion, and pain (Hart, Grottkau, and Albright, 2007). Avascular necrosis is a complication of an unstable hip, which may result in degenerative hip disease in later life (Loder, 2006).

Nursing care involves preparing the child and family for the surgical procedure and recovery. The child may be placed on a patient-controlled analgesia (PCA) pump for postoperative pain management and should receive appropriate instructions preoperatively for activating the dosing by the pump. If traction is used preoperatively, nursing care is the same as that for a child in traction, as discussed earlier in this chapter. Postoperative care involves hemodynamic stabilization and assessment for complications. The adolescent is taught the proper use of crutches and the importance of avoiding any weight bearing on the affected hip (if unilateral). The adolescent may be involved in building upper body strength during the convalescent period to increase mobility from bed to wheelchair, as appropriate. Self-care and performance of activities of daily living to capability are encouraged to promote confidence and decrease a sense of helplessness.

Pain management is essential, and observation for major complications associated with major surgery and immobilization (thrombus, pneumonia, constipation) is an important part of nursing care.

KYPHOSIS AND LORDOSIS

The spine, which consists of numerous segments, can acquire deformation curves of three types: kyphosis, lordosis, and scoliosis (Fig. 39-33).

Kyphosis is an abnormally increased convex angulation in the curvature of the thoracic spine (see Fig. 39-33, *B*). It can occur secondary to disease processes such as tuberculosis, chronic arthritis, osteodystrophy, or compression fractures of the thoracic spine. The most common form of kyphosis is postural. Children, especially during the time when skeletal growth outpaces growth of muscle, are prone to exaggeration of a tendency toward kyphosis. This is particularly common in self-conscious adolescent girls who assume a round-shouldered slouching posture in an attempt to hide their developing breasts and increasing height. Scheuermann kyphosis is a thoracic curve of greater than 45 degrees with wedging of more than 5 degrees of at least three adjacent vertebral bodies and vertebral irregularity.

Postural kyphosis is almost always accompanied by a compensatory postural lordosis, an abnormally exaggerated concave lumbar curvature. Treatment of kyphosis consists of exercises to strengthen shoulder and abdominal muscles and bracing for more marked deformity. With adolescents who are significantly self-conscious about their appearance, the best approach is to emphasize the cosmetic value of corrective therapy and to place the responsibility on the adolescent for carrying out an exercise program at home, with regular visits to and assessments by a physical therapist. Treatment with a brace may be indicated until skeletal maturity; surgical spinal fusion may be considered

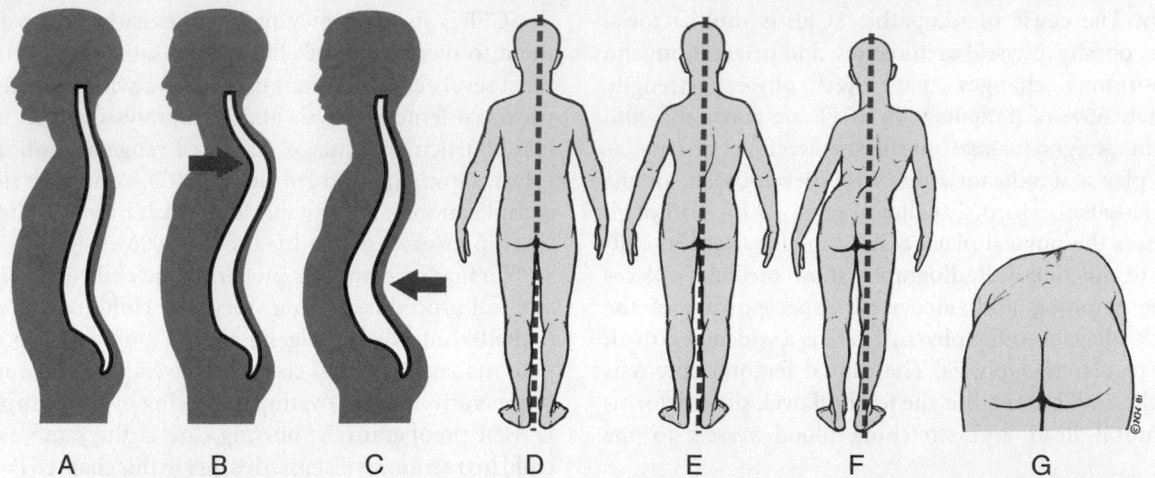

Fig. 39-33 Defects of spinal column. **A,** Normal spine. **B,** Kyphosis. **C,** Lordosis. **D,** Normal spine in balance. **E,** Mild scoliosis in balance. **F,** Severe scoliosis not in balance. **G,** Rib hump and flank asymmetry seen in flexion caused by rotary component. (Redrawn from Hilt NE, Schmitt EW: *Pediatric orthopedic nursing,* St Louis, 1975, Mosby.)

for severe, painful, or progressive deforming thoracic curves such as Scheuermann kyphosis.

Lordosis is an accentuation of the lumbar curvature beyond physiologic limits (see Fig. 39-33, *C*). It may be a secondary complication of a disease process, the result of trauma, or idiopathic. Lordosis is a normal observation in toddlers, and in older children it is often seen in association with flexion contractures of the hip, obesity, congenital dislocated hip, and SCFE. During the pubertal growth spurt, lordosis of varying degrees is observed in teenagers, especially girls. In obese children the weight of the abdominal fat alters the center of gravity, which causes a compensatory lordosis. Unlike kyphosis, severe lordosis is usually accompanied by pain.

Treatment involves management of the predisposing cause when possible, such as weight loss and correction of any existing orthopedic or neuromuscular conditions. Postural exercises or support garments are helpful in relieving symptoms in some cases; however, these do not usually effect a permanent cure.

Spondylolisthesis is the forward slipping of one vertebral body on another ("slipped disk"). It usually involves L5 and S1. Retrospondylolisthesis, or retrolisthesis, is the posterior slipping or displacement of one vertebral body on another. Either condition can have multiple causes, including congenital deficiency or fracture of part of the vertebra. The condition may be asymptomatic, or it may cause lower back pain or neurologic compromise. Spondylolisthesis can usually be treated nonsurgically, although spinal fusion may be indicated in cases of severe, progressive slip.

IDIOPATHIC SCOLIOSIS

Scoliosis is a complex spinal deformity in three planes, usually involving lateral curvature, spinal rotation causing rib asymmetry, and thoracic hypokyphosis (see Fig. 39-33, *E-G,* and Fig. 39-34). It is the most common spinal deformity and can be further classified according to age of onset: *congenital,* occurs in fetal development; *infantile,* at birth or up to 3 years

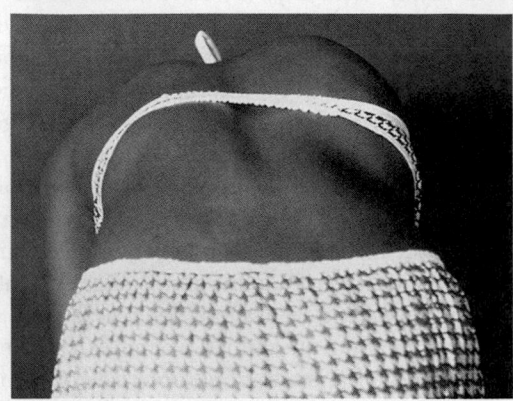

Fig. 39-34 Moderate thoracic idiopathic adolescent scoliosis. Forward flexion reveals a mild rib hump deformity. (From Zitelli BJ, Davis HW: *Atlas of pediatric physical diagnosis,* ed 4, St Louis, 2002, Mosby.)

of age; childhood (*juvenile*), occurs in children ages 4 to 10 years of age; or *adolescent,* during the growth spurt of early adolescence (the most common type). Scoliosis can be caused by a number of conditions and may occur alone or in association with other diseases, particularly neuromuscular conditions (neuromuscular scoliosis). In most cases, however, there is no apparent cause, hence the name *idiopathic scoliosis.* The following discussion involves the adolescent type, which is often called adolescent idiopathic scoliosis. There appears to be a genetic component to the etiology of idiopathic scoliosis; however, the exact relationship has yet to be established.

Clinical Manifestations

Idiopathic scoliosis is most noticeable during the preadolescent growth spurt. Parents frequently bring a child for follow up on an abnormal school scoliosis screening or because of ill-fitting clothes, such as poorly fitting jeans. School screening is somewhat controversial, since there are no controlled studies to demonstrate improved outcomes and a reported number of false positives lead to referrals (Bunnell, 2005). The American

Academy of Orthopaedic Surgeons and the American Academy of Pediatrics have recently published a joint statement favoring scoliosis screening for preadolescents and adolescents either in the school, physician's office, or nurses' clinic (Richards and Vitale, 2008). According to the American Academy of Orthopaedic Surgeons (Richards and Vitale, 2008), girls should be screened at ages 10 and 12 years, whereas boys should be screened once either at age 13 or 14 years. The benefits of early detection, referral, and medical treatment are considered to be significant, but the persons performing the screenings must be educated in the detection of spinal deformity.

Diagnostic Evaluation

The standing child, wearing only underpants and viewed from behind, may exhibit asymmetry of shoulder height, scapular or flank shape, or hip height, or may demonstrate pelvic obliquity. Cutaneous changes may also be observed. When the child bends forward at the waist so that the trunk is parallel with the floor and the arms hang free (the Adams position), asymmetry of ribs and flanks may also be appreciated (see Figs. 39-33, *G*, and 39-34). A scoliometer is also used in the initial screening to measure truncal rotation (as does the Adams test). Often a primary curve and a compensatory curve will place the head in alignment with the gluteal cleft. With an uncompensated curve, however, the head and hips are not aligned. By stabilizing the pelvis and asking the child to twist to both sides, the practitioner can evaluate the flexibility of the curve.

Definitive diagnosis is made by radiographs of the child in the standing position and use of the Cobb technique (standard measurement of angle curvature), which establishes the degree of curvature. The Risser scale is used to evaluate skeletal maturity on the radiographs. This scale assists in making a determination of the likely progression of the spinal angulature as the child's bones mature. The Tanner maturity rating is also used to evaluate the risk of curve progression in adolescents. Not all spinal curvatures are scoliosis. A curve of less than 10 degrees is considered a postural variation. Curves of less than 20 degrees are mild and, if nonprogressive, do not require treatment.

Intraspinal conditions or other disease processes that can cause scoliosis must be ruled out. The presence of pain, sacral dimpling or hairy patches, cutaneous vascular changes, absent or abnormal reflexes, bowel or bladder incontinence, or left thoracic curve may indicate an intraspinal abnormality such as syringomyelia, diastematomyelia, or tethered cord syndrome. An MRI scan is usually obtained for evaluation.

Therapeutic Management

Current management options include observation with regular clinical and radiographic evaluation, orthotic intervention (bracing), and surgical spinal fusion (Fig. 39-35). Treatment decisions are based on the magnitude, location, and type of curve; the age and skeletal maturity of the child or adolescent; and any underlying or contributing disease process.

Bracing and Exercise

For many curves in the growing child and adolescent, bracing may be the treatment of choice. It is important to realize that *bracing is not curative*, but that it may slow the progression of the curvature to allow skeletal growth and maturity. The two

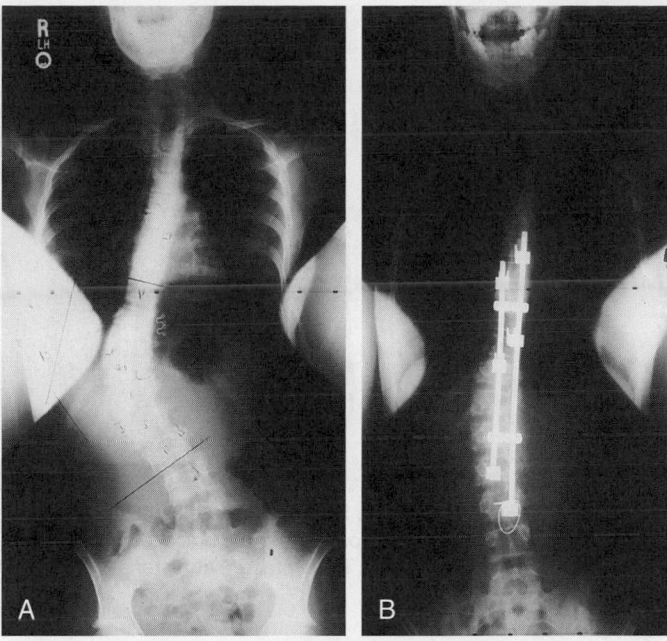

Fig. 39-35 Radiographs showing severe scoliosis before surgical correction **(A)** and after surgical correction of scoliosis, including internal fixation **(B)**.

most common types of bracing are (1) the Boston and Wilmington braces, which are underarm orthoses customized from prefabricated plastic shells, with corrective forces for each patient using lateral pads and decreasing lumbar lordosis; and (2) a TLSO, which is an underarm orthosis made of plastic that is custom molded to the body and then shaped to correct or hold the deformity (Fig. 39-36). The Milwaukee brace, which is an individually adapted brace that includes a neck ring, is rarely used in scoliosis but is sometimes used in the treatment of kyphosis. The Charleston nighttime bending brace is worn only when the child is in bed because it prevents walking because of the severity of the trunk bend.

Bracing, although used as the gold standard treatment for mild to moderate curvatures, has not proved to be entirely effective in the treatment of scoliosis. Compliance in wearing the brace is difficult because of the adolescent's age and preoccupation with body image and appearance. In addition, bracing was historically intended to be a 23-hour treatment. In some cases treatment may involve bracing at nighttime only, since this may enhance compliance in adolescents with scoliosis (Jarvis, Garbedian, and Swamy, 2008). Experts recognize that brace treatment in some children with significant scoliosis may help avoid surgical intervention by slowing curve progression; however, further studies are needed to clarify the effectiveness of bracing (Richards and Vitale, 2008).

Exercises alone and chiropractic treatment are rarely of value in managing scoliosis; transcutaneous electrical nerve stimulation has also proved to be an ineffective treatment for this condition. Exercises are of benefit when used in conjunction with bracing to maintain and increase the strength of spinal and abdominal muscles during treatment.

Operative Management

Surgical intervention may be required for correction of severe curves (see Fig. 39-35, *A*) (usually 45 degrees or more in

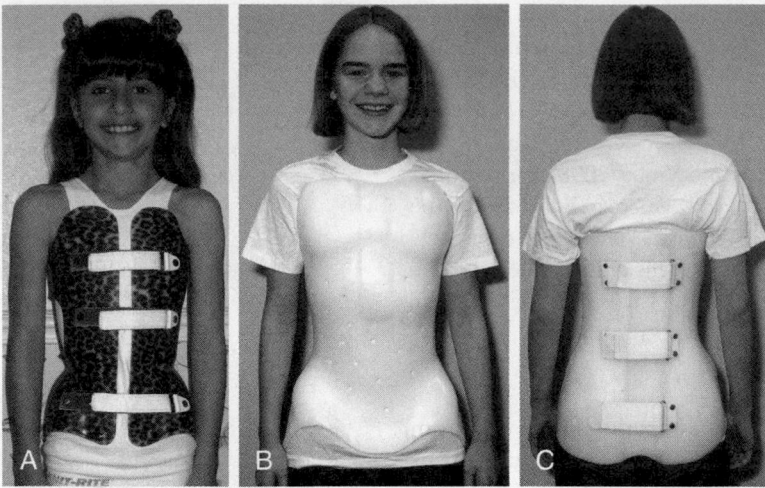

Fig. 39-36 A, Standard thoracolumbosacral orthosis (TLSO) brace for idiopathic scoliosis. Note the color and design incorporated into the brace to make it more acceptable to children and adolescents. **B** and **C,** Variation of a standard TLSO brace that fastens in the back to provide needed support for the spinal curvature.

skeletally immature patients and 50 to 55 degrees or more in the skeletally mature [Spiegel, Hosalkar, and Dormans, 2007]). The degree of curvature and the cause determine the decision regarding surgery. Bracing and exercise have been universally disappointing in treating curves greater than 40 degrees, and paralytic and congenital curves, which eventually progress, are best treated with early surgical stabilization if the child's health status will allow major surgery. The child's age and location of the curvature influence the decision for surgery, and any progressive or severe curve that does not respond to more conservative orthotic measures requires surgical correction. Difficulties with balance or seating, respiratory excursion, or pain are also considered.

A number of surgical techniques are now available. One surgical technique consists of realignment and straightening with internal fixation and instrumentation combined with bony fusion (**arthrodesis**) of the realigned spine. The goals of surgical intervention are to correct the curvatures on the sagittal and coronal planes and to provide a solid, pain-free fusion in a well-balanced torso, with maximum mobility of the remaining spinal segments.

Many instrumentation systems, including Harrington, Dwyer, Zielke, Luque, Cotrel-Dubousset, Isola, TSRH (Texas Scottish Rite Hospital), and Moss Miami, are available. Selection of the system is individualized according to the patient's needs and surgeon's preference. Posterior or anterior surgical approaches can be used.

The Harrington system, the first internal spinal instrumentation device, consists of distraction and compression rods, hooks, and nuts. The posterior elements are decorticated, and bone from the iliac crest or donor bone is placed across the vertebrae to provide fusion. Postoperatively the child is logrolled to prevent spinal motion, and a molded plastic jacket is used to stabilize the spine until the fusion is solid.

The Luque-rod segmental spinal instrumentation provides segmental stability by the use of wires and L-shaped rods. By way of a posterior approach, the wires are threaded beneath the lamina of each vertebra and tightened around the rods resting along the transverse processes to stabilize the spine. Bone from

the iliac crest or donor bone is used to fuse the spine. The advantage of this method is that the patient can be mobile within a few days and requires no postoperative immobilization. The disadvantage is the risk of nerve damage.

The Cotrel-Dubousset instrumentation combines the Harrington and L-rod approaches by using bilateral rods and hooks at many sites. Anterior approaches using the Dwyer or Zielke instrumentation involve screws into the vertebral bodies connected by a cable or rod. These systems require postoperative immobilization with a custom-fitted plastic jacket.

Advances in surgical technology currently being evaluated include thoracoscopic spinal fusion and placement of implants; metallic staples may also be placed into the vertebral bodies to achieve spinal fusion and to correct the deformity (Spiegel, Hosalkar, and Dormans, 2007). The use of minimally invasive surgery techniques such as video assisted thoracoscopic surgery has gained widespread acceptance for its decreased recovery time, decreased pain, fewer intraoperative and postoperative complications, small incision, less impact on pulmonary function, and less chest wall disruption (Lonner, 2007).

Nursing Care Management

Treatment for scoliosis extends over a significant portion of the affected child's period of growth. In adolescents this period is the one in which their identity, physical and psychologic, is formed. The identification of scoliosis as a "deformity," in combination with unattractive appliances and a significant surgical procedure, can have a negative effect on the already fragile adolescent body image. The adolescent and family require excellent nursing care to meet not only physical needs, but also psychologic needs associated with the diagnosis, surgery, postoperative recovery, and eventual rehabilitation (Slote, 2002).

Although these adolescents are encouraged to participate in most peer activities, necessary therapeutic modifications are likely to make them feel different and apart. Nursing care of the adolescent who is facing scoliosis surgery, potential social isolation, pain, and uncertainty, not to mention misunderstood emotions and body image issues, must be evaluated from the adolescent's perspective to be successful in meeting the individual's needs (Napierkowski, 2007).

When a child or adolescent first faces the prospect of a prolonged period in a brace, jacket, or other device, the therapy program and the nature of the device must be explained thoroughly to both the child and the parents so that they will understand the anticipated results, how the appliance corrects the defect, the freedoms and constraints imposed by the device, and what they can do to help achieve the desired goal. The management involves the skills and services of a team of specialists, including the orthopedist, physical therapist, orthotist (a specialist in fitting orthopedic braces), nurse, social worker, and sometimes a thoracic or pulmonary specialist.

It is difficult for a child to be restricted at any phase of development, but the adolescent needs continual positive reinforcement, encouragement, and as much independence as can be safely assumed during this time. Guidance and assistance regarding anticipated problems, such as selection of clothing and participation in social activities, are appreciated by adolescents. Socialization with peers is strongly encouraged, and every effort is expended to help the adolescent feel attractive and worthwhile.

Preoperative Care

The preoperative workup usually involves a radiographic series, including bending and traction films, pulmonary function studies, and a number of routine laboratory studies (including prothrombin, partial thromboplastin, and bleeding times; blood count; electrolyte levels; urinalysis and urine culture; and blood levels of any medications). Because spinal surgery usually involves considerable blood loss, several options are considered preoperatively to maintain or replace blood volume. These options include autologous blood donations obtained from the patient before the surgery; intraoperative blood salvage; intraoperative hemodilution; erythropoietin administration; and controlled induced hypotension, which must be carefully monitored at all times to prevent physiologic instability (Newton and Wenger, 2001).

Surgery for spinal fusion is complex, and often adolescents who require the procedure because of idiopathic scoliosis are not familiar with medical terms or procedures. Preoperative teaching is critical for the adolescent to be able to cooperate and participate in his or her treatment and recovery. Because the surgery is extensive, the patient is taught how to manage his or her own PCA pump; how to log-roll; and the use and function of other equipment, such as a chest tube (for anterior repair) and Foley catheter. It is recommended that the child or adolescent bring a favorite toy (age dependent) or personal items such as a favorite stuffed animal, laptop computer, cellular phone (for web surfing, texting, and e-mailing), movie player, MP3 player, or portable compact disc player for postoperative use. Meeting with a peer who has undergone a similar surgery is also valuable (Slote, 2002).

Postoperative Care

After surgery, patients are monitored in an acute care setting and log-rolled when changing position to prevent damage to the fusion and instrumentation. In some cases an immobilization brace or cast is used postoperatively depending on the type of surgical intervention. Skin care is important, and pressure-relieving mattresses or beds may be needed to prevent pressure wounds. (See Maintaining Healthy Skin, Chapter 27.)

In addition to the usual postoperative assessments of wound, circulation, and vital signs, the neurologic status of the patient's extremities requires special attention. Prompt recognition of any neurologic impairment is imperative because delayed paralysis may develop that requires surgical intervention. Common postoperative problems after spinal fusion include neurologic injury or spinal cord injury, hypotension from acute blood loss, wound infection, syndrome of inappropriate antidiuretic hormone, atelectasis, pneumothorax, ileus, delayed neurologic injury, and implanted hardware complications (Freeman, 2007; Newton and Wenger, 2001). Superior mesenteric artery syndrome may occur several days after spinal surgery; this involves duodenal compression by the aorta and superior mesenteric artery and may result in acute partial or complete duodenal obstruction. Clinical manifestations include epigastric pain, nausea, copious vomiting, and eructation; symptoms are aggravated in the supine position and often relieved with the patient in a left lateral decubitus or prone position.

The adolescent usually has considerable pain for the first few days after surgery and requires frequent administration of pain medication, preferably opioids administered intravenously on a regular schedule. For children able to understand the concept, PCA is recommended. (See Pain Assessment; Pain Management, Chapter 7.) In most cases the patient begins walking as soon as possible. Depending on the instrumentation used and the surgical approach, most patients are walking by the second or third postoperative day and are discharged by 1 week. In addition to pain management, the patient is evaluated for skin integrity, adequate urinary output, fluid and electrolyte balance, and ileus (Slote, 2002). Discharge planning should include a timetable for follow-up with the practitioner and resumption of regular activities.

All patients are started on physical therapy as soon as they are able, beginning with range-of-motion exercises on the first postoperative day and many of the activities of daily living in the following days. Self-care, such as washing and eating, is always encouraged. Throughout the hospitalization, age-appropriate activities and contact with family and friends are important parts of nursing care and planning (see Immobilization, p. 1623).

Encourage the family to become involved in the patient's care to facilitate the transition from hospital to home management (see Nursing Care Plan). An organization that provides education and services to both families and professionals is the National Scoliosis Foundation.* The American Academy of Orthopaedic Surgeons† and Scoliosis Research Society,‡ an organization of physicians and scientists, have published an excellent book, *Scoliosis,* and the Scoliosis Research Society has educational information on its website.

---

*Five Cabot Place, Stoughton, MA 02072; 800-673-6922; www. scoliosis.org.
†6300 N. River Road, Rosemont, IL 60018-4262; 847-823-7186; www.aaos.org.
‡555 E. Wells St., Suite 1100, Milwaukee, WI 53202; 414-289-9107; www.srs.org.

NURSING CARE PLAN

The Adolescent with Scoliosis

NURSING DIAGNOSIS	EXPECTED PATIENT OUTCOME	NURSING INTERVENTIONS	RATIONALE
Disturbed Body Image related to diagnosis of scoliosis and subsequent therapy and perceived defect in body structure	Adolescent will cope effectively with therapy.	Allow adolescent to verbalize feelings about wearing brace and how it affects her lifestyle.	To promote expression of negative feelings
Child's/Family's Defining Characteristics (Subjective and Objective Data)	**The Following NOC Concepts Apply to These Outcomes**	Discuss a plan of action for participation in activities with peers.	To encourage participation and prevent self-isolation
Verbalization of change in lifestyle	Psychosocial Adjustment: Life Change	Discuss implications of not wearing brace and impact on appearance.	To provide information related to noncompliance
Expression of negative feelings about body	Self-Esteem	Emphasize positive aspects of participation in activities of daily living with brace.	To promote positive reinforcement of treatment plan
Verbalization of perceptions that reflect an altered view of one's body in appearance, structure, or function		Encourage self-care regarding activities of daily living; address with adjustments related to restrictions with brace, adjusting and removing brace.	To promote self-care
		Encourage meeting periodically with other female adolescents who must wear brace.	To gain perspective and support of others like her who are affected by wearing brace
		Encourage meeting with peers as before and performing activities as tolerated with peers.	To promote acceptance by peers and self
		Assist parents and siblings with discussion of feelings about daughter's diagnosis, wearing of brace, and family's and siblings' feelings regarding therapy.	To provide emotional support
		Discuss with family and siblings how they can support adolescent through therapy.	To promote family functioning
		The Following NIC Concepts Apply to These Interventions Body Image Enhancement Socialization Enhancement Family Involvement Promotion Mutual Goal Setting Anticipatory Guidance	

NURSING DIAGNOSIS	EXPECTED PATIENT OUTCOME	NURSING INTERVENTIONS	RATIONALE
Risk for Injury (postoperatively) related to neurologic surgical intervention on spinal column	Adolescent will be injury free and regain capability for ambulation.	Log roll with assistance.	To prevent injury
		Implement aspiration precautions.	To prevent aspiration while supine
Child's/Family's Defining Characteristics (Subjective and Objective Data)	**The Following NOC Concepts Apply to These Outcomes**	Administer pain medications and/or assist with patient-controlled analgesia pump infusion of pain medications.	To promote comfort
Spinal immobilization	Risk Control	Encourage isometric exercises of lower extremities as allowed.	To promote muscle movement and tone
Tissue and bone trauma	Personal Safety Behavior	Assess neurologic signs as warranted or per protocol.	To assess signs indicating further intervention required to prevent neurologic injury
	Neurological Status: Spinal Sensory/Motor Function	Assist patient to a sitting position on side of bed and in ambulation as allowed as soon as possible (depending on type of instrumentation and surgery performed); medicate for pain 30 to 45 minutes before ambulation.	To prevent side effects of immobilization
		Encourage patient to ambulate and assist with ambulation.	To prevent immobilization complications
		Assess pressure points if patient is immobile for long period, and provide appropriate interventions (massage, special mattress, turning).	To prevent skin breakdown
		The Following NIC Concepts Apply to These Interventions Risk Identification Environmental Management: Safety Exercise Promotion Positioning Surveillance Vital Signs Monitoring Postanesthesia Care Skin Surveillance	

ORTHOPEDIC INFECTIONS

OSTEOMYELITIS

Osteomyelitis, an infectious process in the bone, can occur at any age but most frequently is seen in children 10 years of age or younger. *S. aureus* is the most common causative organism (Box 39-14). Neonates are also likely to have osteomyelitis caused by group B streptococci. Since the advent of *Haemophilus influenzae* type b immunization in the late 1980s, *H. influenzae* has become a less common causative pathogen. Children with sickle cell anemia may develop osteomyelitis from *Salmonella* organisms as well as *S. aureus*. *Neisseria gonorrhoeae* is a potential causative organism in the sexually active adolescent.

Acute hematogenous osteomyelitis results when a blood-borne bacterium causes an infection in the bone. Common foci include infected lesions, upper respiratory tract infections, otitis media, tonsillitis, abscessed teeth, pyelonephritis, and infected burns. Exogenous osteomyelitis is acquired from direct inoculation of the bone from a puncture wound, open fracture, surgical contamination, or adjacent tissue infection. Subacute osteomyelitis has a longer course and may be caused by less virulent microbes with a walled-off abscess or Brodie abscess, typically in the proximal or distal tibia. Chronic osteomyelitis is a progression of acute osteomyelitis and is characterized by the presence of dead bone, bone loss, and drainage and sinus tracts. Generally healthy bone is not likely to become infected. Factors that contribute to infection include inoculation with a large number of organisms, presence of a foreign body, bone injury, high virulence of an organism, immunosuppression, and malnutrition. Certain types and locations of bone are also more vulnerable to infection.

Pathophysiology

In acute osteomyelitis bacteria adhere to bone, causing a suppurative infection with inflammatory cells, edema, vascular congestion, and small-vessel thrombosis; the result is bone destruction, abscess formation, and dead bone (sequestra). Infection within the bone can rupture through the cortex into the subperiosteal space, stripping loose periosteum and forming an abscess. As dead bone is resorbed, new bone is formed along the live bone and infection borders. This surrounding sheath of live bone is called an **involucrum**. Sinus tracts from perforations in the involucrum may drain pus through soft tissue to the skin.

The pathology of osteomyelitis is different in infants, children older than 1 year of age, and adults. In infants blood vessels cross the growth plate into the epiphysis and joint space, which allows infection to spread into the joint. In children the infection is contained by the growth plate, and joint infection is less likely (unless the infection is intracapsular) (Fig. 39-37). Adults have no growth plate to contain infection, and again the joint is compromised. Adult periosteum is attached to bone; consequently, rupture through the periosteum and sinus drainage is more common in adults.

Clinical Manifestations

In children severe pain, fever, irritability, and tenderness with or without local signs of inflammation suggest osteomyelitis. The extremity is tender, and the child may hold it in semiflexion and resist movement. In infants these symptoms may be

BOX 39-14 CAUSATIVE MICROORGANISMS OF OSTEOMYELITIS ACCORDING TO AGE

Newborns
Staphylococcus aureus
Group B streptococcus
Gram-negative enteric rods

Infants
S. aureus (methicillin-sensitive *S. aureus* 70, methicillin-resistant *S. aureus* 30)
Haemophilus influenzae

Older Children
S. aureus
Pseudomonas organisms
Salmonella organisms
Neisseria gonorrhoeae

Adolescents and Adults
Pseudomonas organisms
Mycobacterium tuberculosis

From McCance KL, Huether SE: *Pathophysiology: the biological basis for disease in adults and children,* ed 6, St Louis, 2010, Mosby.

PATHOPHYSIOLOGY REVIEW

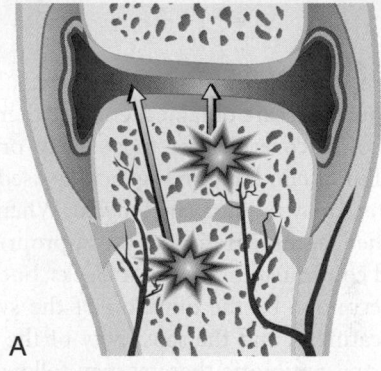

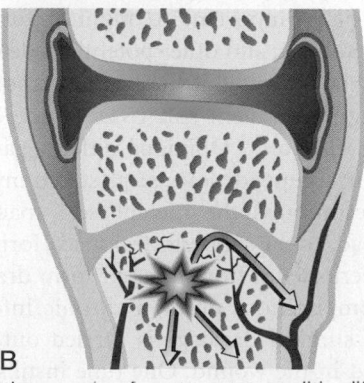

Fig. 39-37 Pathogenesis of acute osteomyelitis differs with age. **A,** In infants younger than 1 year the epiphysis is nourished by penetrating arteries through the physis, allowing development of the condition within the epiphysis. **B,** In children up to 15 years of age the infection is restricted to below the physis because of interruption of the vessels. (From McCance KL, Huether SE: *Pathophysiology: the biological basis for disease in adults and children,* ed 6, St Louis, 2010, Mosby.)

Case Study—Osteomyelitis

Animation—Osteomyelitis

minimal or absent, and pain may be difficult to localize. The infant may demonstrate pain with movement of the extremity or hold it immobile. Fever is uncommon in infants, and they often do not appear to be ill (Lampe, 2007). Infants may have an adjacent joint effusion. Typically the metaphysis of long bones, the tibia and femur, is involved. In a small portion of children more than one bone may be affected.

Diagnostic Evaluation

Organism identification and antibiotic susceptibility testing are essential for effective therapy. Obtain cultures of aspirated sub-periosteal pus along with cultures of blood, joint fluid, and infected skin samples. Bone biopsy is indicated if blood culture results and radiographic findings are not consistent with osteomyelitis. Supporting evidence for osteomyelitis includes leukocytosis and elevated erythrocyte sedimentation rate. Radiographic signs, except for soft tissue swelling, are evident only after 2 to 3 weeks. A three-phase technetium bone scan can show areas of increased blood flow, such as occurs in early stages in infected bone, and is useful in locating multiple sites; however, it is not a diagnostic test. CT can detect bone destruction, and MRI provides anatomic details useful in delineating the area of involvement, especially if surgical intervention is planned. The differential diagnosis includes trauma, malignant lesions, leukemia, juvenile rheumatoid arthritis, and acute rheumatic fever. Sometimes the osteomyelitis may be unrecognized if it occurs as a complication of a severe toxic and debilitating disease.

Therapeutic Management

After culture specimens are obtained, empiric therapy is started with IV antibiotics covering the most likely organisms. For *S. aureus* nafcillin or clindamycin is generally used; methicillin-resistant *S. aureus* may require vancomycin. When the infective agent is identified, administration of the appropriate antibiotic is initiated and continued for at least 4 weeks, but the length of therapy is determined by the duration of the symptoms, the response to treatment, and the sensitivity of the organism. In selected cases oral antibiotic therapy may follow a shorter IV course. Because of the prolonged duration of high-dose antibiotic therapy, it is important to monitor for hematologic, renal, hepatic, ototoxic, and other potential side effects.

Surgery may be indicated if there is no response to specific antibiotic therapy, persistent soft tissue abscess, or infection that spreads to the joint. Opinions differ regarding surgical intervention, but many advocate sequestrectomy and surgical drainage to decompress the metaphyseal space before pus erupts and spreads to the subperiosteal space, forming abscesses that strip the periosteum from bone or form draining sinuses. When these complications occur, a chronic infection usually persists. When surgical drainage is carried out, polyethylene tubes are placed in the wound. One tube instills an antibiotic solution directly into the infected area by gravity, and the other, connected to a suction apparatus, provides drainage. (See Chapter 18 for a discussion of wound care.)

Nursing Care Management

During the acute phase of illness, any movement of the affected limb causes discomfort to the child; therefore the child is posi-

tioned comfortably with the affected limb supported. Moving and turning are carried out carefully and gently to minimize discomfort. The child may require pain medication (see Chapter 7) or sedation. Take vital signs and record them frequently, and implement measures to reduce a significant temperature elevation.

Antibiotic therapy requires careful observation and monitoring of the IV equipment and site. Because more than one antibiotic is usually administered, the compatibility of the drugs must be determined and care taken to avoid mixing incompatible drugs. The stability of the drugs and their toxic nature are also considered when determining the rate of administration. The infusion device must be well situated in the vein to ensure that the drug does not infiltrate into surrounding tissues, where it may produce tissue damage. For long-term antibiotic therapy, a venous access device, such as a peripherally inserted central catheter, is the preferred method of IV administration. (See Chapter 28.)

Standard Precautions are put in effect for children with open wounds, depending on the institution's policies. The wound is managed according to the practitioner's directions. Administration of antibiotic solution directly into the wound is most efficiently accomplished using a regular infusion setup that is prepared and regulated in the same manner as for any IV infusion. Intake and output are measured and recorded, and the character of both the wound and drainage is noted. The amount and character of drainage on the wound dressing are also noted.

As the infection subsides, physical therapy is instituted to ensure restoration of optimum function. The child is usually discharged on a regimen of oral antibiotics, and progress is followed closely for some time.

SEPTIC ARTHRITIS

Septic (suppurative) arthritis is a bacterial infection in the joint. It usually results from hematogenous spread or from direct extension of an adjacent cellulitis or osteomyelitis. Direct inoculation from trauma accounts for 15% to 20% of septic arthritis cases. The most common causative organism is *S. aureus* (Lampe, 2007). Community-acquired methicillin-resistant *S. aureus* is commonly a cause of septic arthritis (Gutierrez, 2005). In addition to *S. aureus*, pathogens seen in neonates include group B streptococci, *Escherichia coli,* and *Candida albicans.* In children 2 months to 5 years of age, *S. aureus, Streptococcus pyogenes, Streptococcus pneumoniae,* and *Kingella kingae* are the primary organisms causing infection, whereas children older than 5 years are more likely to be infected by *S. aureus* and *S. pyogenes;* sexually active adolescents may be infected by *N. gonorrhoeae* (Gutierrez, 2005).

Knees, hips, ankles, and elbows are the most commonly affected joints. Clinical manifestations include severe joint pain, swelling, warmth of overlying tissue, and occasionally erythema. The child is resistant to any joint movement. Features of systemic illness such as fever, malaise, headache, nausea, vomiting, and irritability may also be present.

Therapeutic and Nursing Care Management

The affected joint is aspirated and the specimen evaluated by Gram stain, culturing (including separate cultures for

H. influenzae and *N. gonorrhoeae*), and determination of leukocyte count. In addition, perform blood culture and obtain complete blood count with differential and erythrocyte sedimentation rate or C-reactive protein level. Early radiographic findings are limited to soft tissue swelling but may reveal a foreign body, and such films always provide a baseline for comparison. Technetium scans reveal areas of increased blood flow but will not differentiate between sites. MRI and CT scans provide more detailed images of cartilage loss, joint narrowing, erosions, and ankylosis of progressive disease. An infection involving the hip, however, is considered a surgical emergency to prevent compromised blood supply to the head of the femur (Lampe, 2007).

Treatment is IV antibiotic therapy based on Gram stain results and the clinical presentation. The benefits of serial aspirations to demonstrate sterility of synovium fluid and reduce pressure or pain are controversial. Pain management is an important aspect of nursing care, particularly with involvement of a large joint such as the hip. Surgical intervention may also be required if there was a penetrating wound or a foreign object was possibly involved. Physical therapy may be initiated for the child who is immobilized in a cast or traction to prevent flexion contractures. Additional nursing care is the same as for osteomyelitis.

SKELETAL TUBERCULOSIS

In children tubercular infection of the bones and joints is acquired by lymphohematogenous spread at the time of primary infection. Occasionally it is from chronic pulmonary tuberculosis. Skeletal tubercular infection is not common in the United States but should be considered in communities with high tuberculosis case rates. The infection is most likely to involve the vertebrae, causing a tubercular spondylitis. If the infection is progressive, it causes Pott disease with destruction of the vertebral bodies and results in kyphosis. Symptoms are insidious. The child may report persistent or intermittent pain. Other findings include joint swelling and stiffness; fever and weight loss are not common. Tubercular arthritis can also affect single joints such as a knee or hip and tends to cause severe destruction of adjacent bone. Infection in the fingers causes spina ventosa, a tuberculous dactylitis.

As with pulmonary tuberculosis, the index case should be located. A family and environmental history needs to be obtained and skin tests performed. (See also Tuberculosis, Chapter 32.) Results of tuberculin skin tests are positive for the majority of children with tuberculous arthritis; however, the results are not diagnostic, and the clinical and laboratory features do not differentiate tubercular arthritis from a nontubercular septic arthritis. Diagnosis requires isolation of *Mycobacterium tuberculosis* from the site. Patients with the susceptible organism start treatment with combined antituberculosis chemotherapy (isoniazid, rifampin, and pyrazinamide); directly observed therapy is preferred.

Nursing care depends on the site and extent of infection. Tuberculous spondylitis and hip infection may require immobilization, casting, and fusion. Nursing care is the same as for osteomyelitis with the addition of isolation requirements.

SKELETAL AND ARTICULAR DYSFUNCTION

OSTEOGENESIS IMPERFECTA

OI is the most common osteoporosis syndrome in children, characterized by excessive fractures and bone deformity. There are at least five types of OI, accounting for significant disease variability. Clinical features include varying degrees of bone fragility, deformity, and fracture; blue sclerae; hearing loss; and dentinogenesis imperfecta (hypoplastic discolored teeth). The inheritance pattern is autosomal dominant in the majority of cases, although the most severe form demonstrates autosomal recessive inheritance.

Most types of OI have defects in the *COL1A1* or *COL1A2* genes, which code for polypeptide chains in type 1 procollagen, a precursor of type 1 collagen, a major structural component of bone. The error results in faulty bone mineralization, abnormal bone architecture, and increased susceptibility to fracture.

Classifications for OI are based on clinical features and patterns of inheritance (Box 39-15). Clinically, type I is the most common, with wide variability of bone fragility; some affected family members have significant deformity and disability, whereas others lead agile, active lives. Type II variants are the most severe and are considered lethal in infancy. Type III OI is characterized by multiple fractures, bone deformity, and severe disability; affected individuals rarely live to 30 years of age. Type IV is similar to type I with blue or white sclerae. Another variant, or type V, has been described in which those affected have a hyperplastic callus, a radiodense metaphyseal band, and calcification of the interosseous membrane of the forearm; no collagen mutations are noted in this group (Marini, 2007). A type VI has been described with a characteristic mineralization defect, which does not respond to pamidronate therapy as do

---

BOX 39-15 CLASSIFICATION OF OSTEOGENESIS IMPERFECTA

Type I*
  A—Mild bone fragility; blue sclerae; normal teeth; hearing loss (occurs between ages 20 and 30 years); autosomal dominant inheritance
  B—Same as A except dentinogenesis imperfecta instead of normal teeth
  C—Same as B but no bone fragility
Type II—Lethal; stillborn or die in early infancy; severe bone fragility, multiple fractures at birth; 10% of cases of osteogenesis imperfecta (OI); autosomal recessive inheritance
Type III—Severe bone fragility leading to severe progressive deformities; normal sclerae; marked growth failure; most autosomal recessive inheritance, with a few autosomal dominant inheritance
Type IV
  A—Mild to moderate bone fragility; normal sclerae; normal teeth; short stature; variable deformity; autosomal dominant inheritance
  B—Same as A except dentinogenesis imperfecta instead of normal teeth; approximately 6% of cases of OI
Type V—Clinically similar to type IV; hyperplastic callus; collagen mutation is negative
Type VI—Sclerae and dentition normal; moderate to severe bone fragility; diagnosis by bone biopsy because of similarities to other types; only identified in eight persons to date (Land, Rauch, Travers, et al, 2007)

*Two thirds of cases are type I.

types I to V (Land, Rauch, Travers, et al, 2007). Children affected with this type have no dental involvement and normal sclerae; a bone biopsy is the only way to establish a diagnosis because of the similarities to other types.

Therapeutic Management

The treatment for OI is primarily supportive, although patients and families are optimistic about new research advances. Bone marrow transplant for severe OI was first reported in 1999 with positive results; however, this is still considered an experimental treatment. Bisphosphonate therapy with pamidronate, olpadronate, neridronate, or alendronate to promote increased bone density and prevent fractures has become standard therapy for many children with OI. Bisphosphonate therapy reportedly is more beneficial for increasing vertebral bone density but is considered less effective for long bones (Marini, 2007). Others report effectiveness of pamidronate in children with moderate to severe OI (Alharbi, Pinto, Finidori, et al, 2009). Bachrach and Ward (2009) suggest data are inadequate to recommend the use of bisphosphonate therapy in children with OI for sole treatment of bone mineral density reduction. Oral risedronate has been reported to be mildly effective in treating children with type I OI, but is not superior to pamidronate therapy (Rauch, Munns, Land, et al, 2009).

The rehabilitative approach to management is directed to preventing (1) positional contractures and deformities, (2) muscle weakness and osteoporosis, and (3) malalignment of lower extremity joints prohibiting weight bearing. Lightweight braces and splints help support limbs, prevent fractures, and aid in ambulation. Physical therapy helps prevent disuse osteoporosis and strengthens muscles, which in turn improves bone density. Surgery is sometimes used to help treat the manifestations of the disease. Surgical techniques are used to correct deformities that interfere with bracing, standing, or walking. For the child with recurrent fractures, inserting an intramedullary rod provides stability to bones.

Because there is a 50% risk of an affected individual passing the gene to an offspring, genetic counseling is recommended.

Nursing Care Management

Infants and children with this disorder require careful handling to prevent fractures. They must be supported when they are being turned, positioned, moved, and held. Even changing a diaper may cause a fracture in severely affected infants. These children should never be held by the ankles when being diapered but should be gently lifted by the buttocks or supported with pillows.

Children with current fractures or healing fractures should be screened for OI; the assumption that abuse or neglect is the cause of fractures in children must be carefully evaluated by a multidisciplinary team. A detailed history, no evidence of associated soft-tissue injury, and the presence of other symptoms related to OI help determine the diagnosis.

Both parents and the affected child need education regarding the child's limitations and guidelines in planning suitable activities that promote optimum development and protect the child from harm. Realistic occupational planning and genetic counseling are part of the long-term goals of care. The parents can obtain educational materials and information from the Osteogenesis Imperfecta Foundation, Inc.* which also has a network that can put a family in contact with other families with a similar problem.

JUVENILE IDIOPATHIC ARTHRITIS (JUVENILE RHEUMATOID ARTHRITIS)

Juvenile idiopathic arthritis (JIA), also commonly called *juvenile rheumatoid arthritis (JRA),* refers to chronic childhood arthritis. JIA is gradually replacing JRA in the research literature and is increasingly used in clinical practice; consequently, both JIA and JRA classifications are discussed here. The revision of JRA nomenclature to JIA was due in part to the minimally applicable reference to "rheumatoid" in childhood arthritis, which is relevant to only a small proportion of affected children yet burdens the family with images of disfiguring adult rheumatoid arthritis. Furthermore, the old subtyping of JRA into systemic, pauciarticular, and polyarticular disease reflects disease onset and not disease progression, which is of greater importance (Warren, Perez, Curry, et al, 2001).

JIA is a group of idiopathic chronic inflammatory diseases affecting the joints and other tissues in approximately 1 in 1000 children. Some theories speculate that the disorder arises when an infectious agent activates an autoimmune inflammatory process in a genetically predisposed child. Although a genetic susceptibility to JIA is known, such as human leukocyte antigen (HLA) polymorphisms and the *PTPN22* gene, this accounts for less than half of the genetic susceptibility; additional genetic factors are being researched (Prahalad and Glass, 2008). There is a female predominance of 2:1 and two peak ages of onset: between 1 and 3 years and 8 and 10 years of age.

Pathophysiology

The disease process is characterized by a chronic inflammation of the synovium with joint effusion and eventual erosion, destruction, and fibrosis of the articular cartilage. Adhesions between joint surfaces and ankylosis of joints occur if the process persists.

Clinical Manifestations

Whether a single joint or multiple joints are involved, stiffness, swelling, and loss of motion develop in the affected joints. They are swollen and warm to the touch but seldom red. The swelling results from edema, joint effusion, and synovial thickening. The affected joints may be tender and painful to the touch or relatively painless. The limited motion early in the disease is a result of muscle spasm and joint inflammation; later it is caused by ankylosis or soft tissue contracture. Morning stiffness, or "gelling," of the joint(s) is characteristic and present on arising in the morning or after inactivity. Infections, injuries, and surgical procedures often precipitate a flare-up of the arthritis; therefore prompt recognition and treatment of infections are necessary.

In severe, long-standing cases growth is significantly restricted. Corticosteroid therapy is also a contributing factor. There may be growth disturbances, either overgrowth or

---

*804 W. Diamond Ave., Suite 210, Gaithersburg, MD 20878; 800-981-2663; www.oif.org.

undergrowth, adjacent to the inflamed joints (e.g., altered leg length after knee involvement) and micrognathia (receding chin) from temporomandibular arthritis.

Classification

The older JRA classification has been replaced in pediatric rheumatology centers and in research by JIA, but in many pediatrician offices, the term *JRA* remains in use; consequently the JRA classification is still pertinent for review. JRA is a variable disease with three major disease courses: systemic onset, pauciarticular (involving few joints, usually less than five), and polyarticular (involving four or more joints simultaneously). The International League of Associations for Rheumatology classification of JIA, developed in 1997, revised and published in 1998, and revised again in 2001, lists seven disease categories, each with its own set of criteria and exclusions: systemic arthritis, oligoarthritis, rheumatoid factor (RF)–negative polyarthritis, RF-positive arthritis, psoriatic arthritis, enthesitis-related arthritis, and undifferentiated arthritis (Petty, Southwood, Baum, et al, 1998; Petty, Southwood, Manners, et al, 2004) (Box 39-16).

Course and Prognosis

The outcome of JIA is variable and unpredictable. Even in severe forms, the disease is rarely life threatening and is significantly different from adult rheumatoid arthritis. Features that distinguish JIA from adult disease include onset before 16 years of age; a negative test result for RF (in 90% of cases); classic symptoms of systemic arthritis such as quotidian fever, rash, and pericarditis; development of uveitis (inflammation of the iris and ciliary body) as a complication (in 8% to 20% of cases); and a tendency for the arthritis to become inactive.

The arthritis tends to wax and wane and eventually becomes inactive in approximately 60% of the cases. These children may have severe or minimal joint damage remaining when active arthritis abates. Forty percent of the children have progressive arthritis into adulthood. Their arthritis can cause significant joint deformity and functional disability requiring medication, physical therapy, and perhaps future joint replacement. Chronic and acute uveitis is an extraarticular complication of JIA that may cause permanent vision loss if undiagnosed and not aggressively treated. Although many children have minimal arthritis, it can produce severe physical, functional, and emotional impairment.

Diagnostic Evaluation

JIA and JRA are diagnoses of exclusion; there are no definitive tests. Both diagnoses are based on the clinical criteria of age of onset before 16 years, arthritis in one or more joints for 6 weeks or longer, and exclusion of other causes (Petty, Southwood, Manners, et al, 2004). Laboratory test results may provide supporting evidence of disease. An elevated sedimentation rate or C-reactive protein may or may not be present. Leukocytosis is frequently present during flares of systemic disease. Tests for RF give positive results in only 10% of the children with JIA. The presence of antinuclear antibodies is common in JIA, but they are not specific for arthritis; however, their presence helps to identify children with pauciarticular disease, who are at greater risk for uveitis.

BOX 39-16 **INTERNATIONAL LEAGUE OF ASSOCIATIONS FOR RHEUMATOLOGY CLASSIFICATION OF JUVENILE IDIOPATHIC ARTHRITIS**

Systemic Arthritis
Definition—Arthritis in one or more joints with or preceded by fever for at least 2 weeks' duration that is documented to be daily for at least 3 days, and accompanied by one or more of the following: evanescent (nonfixed) erythematous rash, generalized lymph node enlargement, hepatomegaly and/or splenomegaly, serositis.
Exclusions—a, b, c, d*

Oligoarthritis
Definition—Arthritis affecting one to four joints during the first 6 months of disease. Two subcategories are recognized: (1) persistent oligoarthritis, which never extends over four affected joints during disease course; and (2) extended oligoarthritis, which affects more than four joints after 6 months of disease.
Exclusions—a, b, c, d, e*

Polyarthritis (Rheumatoid Factor Negative)
Definition—Arthritis affecting five or more joints during the first 6 months of the disease and a negative rheumatoid factor.
Exclusions—a, b, c, e*

Polyarthritis (Rheumatoid Factor Positive)
Definition—Arthritis affecting five or more joints during the first 6 months of disease and two or more positive rheumatoid factor tests at least 3 months apart during the first 6 months of disease.
Exclusions—a, b, c, e*

Psoriatic Arthritis
Definition—Arthritis and psoriasis, or arthritis and at least two of the following: (1) dactylitis, (2) nail pitting or onycholysis, and (3) psoriasis in a first-degree relative.
Exclusions—b, c, d, e*

Enthesitis-Related Arthritis
Definition—Arthritis and enthesitis (inflammation at a tendon insertion site), or arthritis or enthesitis with at least two of the following: (1) presence or history of sacroiliac joint tenderness and/or inflammatory lumbosacral pain; (2) presence of HLA-B27 antigen; (3) onset of arthritis in a male over 6 years of age; (4) symptomatic anterior uveitis; and (5) a history of ankylosing spondylitis, enthesitis-related arthritis, sacroiliitis with inflammatory bowel disease, Reiter syndrome, or acute anterior uveitis in a first-degree relative.
Exclusions—a, d, e*

Undifferentiated Arthritis
Definition—Arthritis that fulfills criteria in no category or in two or more of the above categories.
HLA, Human leukocyte antigen.

From Petty RE, Southwood TR, Manners P, et al: International League of Associations for Rheumatology classification of juvenile idiopathic arthritis: second revision, Edmonton, 2001, *J Rheumatol* 31(2):390-392, 2004.
*Exclusions: (a) Psoriasis or a history of psoriasis in the patient or first-degree relative; (b) arthritis in an HLA-B27–positive male beginning after the sixth birthday; (c) ankylosing spondylitis, enthesitis-related arthritis, sacroiliitis with inflammatory bowel disease, Reiter syndrome, or symptomatic anterior uveitis, or a history of one of these disorders in a first-degree relative; (d) the presence of immunoglobulin M rheumatoid factor on at least two occasions at least 3 months apart; (e) the presence of systemic juvenile idiopathic arthritis in the patient (Petty, Southwood, Manners, et al, 2004).

Therapeutic Management

There is no cure for JIA. The major goals of therapy are to control pain, preserve joint range of motion and function, minimize the effects of inflammation such as joint deformity, and promote normal growth and development. Achievement of these goals requires a family-centered approach with collaboration among the child, the family, and the health care team. The team includes the primary care physician; pediatric rheumatologist; rheumatology nurse educator; social worker; physical and occupational therapists; subspecialists (e.g., pediatric ophthalmologist); and a community of friends, relatives, and teachers. The treatment plan is individualized and varies, but it can be complicated and intrusive, including medications, physical and occupational therapy, slit-lamp eye examinations, splints, comfort measures, dietary management, modification of school activities, and psychosocial support.

Outpatient care is the mainstay of therapy; lengthy hospital admissions for rehabilitation used to be common but are now limited in the era of managed care. Chronic uveitis can cause permanent vision loss, glaucoma, and cataracts. Slit-lamp ophthalmologic examinations at regular intervals are required to diagnose chronic anterior uveitis (iridocyclitis), inflammation of the anterior segments of the eye, iris, and ciliary body. The majority of affected children have a relatively good visual prognosis if the inflammation is detected and treated early; however, most cases are asymptomatic. Consequently, routine slit-lamp examinations are critical. The children at greatest risk for development of uveitis have pauciarticular disease and a positive antinuclear antibody (Cassidy, Kivlin, Lindsley, et al, 2006; American Academy of Pediatrics, 1993).

Medications

A variety of antirheumatic drugs are available, and most are effective in suppressing the inflammatory process and relieving pain. The drugs may be given alone or in combination. NSAIDs are the first drugs used. Common NSAIDs include ibuprofen, naproxen, tolmetin, diclofenac, indomethacin, and meloxicam. (See Table 7-4.) Aspirin, once the initial drug of choice, is seldom used in children. NSAIDs offer an immediate analgesic effect, but the antiinflammatory effect requires larger doses and more time to achieve. The child must take an NSAID for at least 3 weeks before effectiveness can be evaluated. Patient and family education regarding potential gastrointestinal, renal, and hepatic side effects and reduced clotting is essential. Parents should monitor the child for abdominal pain and blood in the stool. Naproxen has the potential side effect of skin fragility in individuals with fair skin so families need to take precautions regarding sun exposure and report unusual skin lesions.

Additional medication is required in approximately 65% of children with arthritis. The agents used are **slower-acting antirheumatic drugs (SAARDs)** and include methotrexate, sulfasalazine, and hydroxychloroquine. Weekly low-dose methotrexate therapy is usually the first SAARD regimen used. Families may be overwhelmed by the potential adverse effects, including liver disease, bone marrow suppression, gastrointestinal disturbance, teratogenic effects, and the alarming but unconfirmed risk of carcinogenesis. Methotrexate is effective, however, and the potential benefits outweigh the potential risks. Methotrexate therapy has also improved uveitis in children with uveitis resistant to steroid treatment (Foeldvari and Wierk, 2005). Laboratory monitoring of liver enzyme levels and blood counts is crucial. A daily folic acid supplement can help reduce the occurrence of oral ulcers. Taking methotrexate at bedtime may help reduce nausea.

Frank discussion about sexual activity and birth defects is critical. Sexually active teenagers need effective birth control and documented periods, as well as pregnancy tests if periods are not regular. As a precaution, pregnant caregivers and those trying to conceive need to avoid contact with methotrexate.

Alcohol consumption is another sensitive topic that needs to be discussed honestly because it increases the risk of hepatotoxicity. Most children require both an NSAID and methotrexate, and parents may be notified by pharmacists about combination toxicity. This is a known interaction of which the rheumatologist is aware; however, instruct patients to avoid additional over-the-counter NSAIDs and to take acetaminophen for episodes of fever. They should also avoid sulfa antibiotics and other bone-marrow–suppressing drugs. Parents should always discuss methotrexate drug interactions with providers prescribing medications for interval illness. During some illnesses, especially varicella, methotrexate should be discontinued because it can suppress the immune response. Sulfasazaline may be selected as the first SAARD in children with axial arthritis, a positive test result for HLA-B27, or symptoms of inflammatory bowel disease, given this drug's success in these select groups of patients.

Corticosteroids are the most potent antiinflammatory agents; however, they will not cure arthritis, and the significant adverse effects of long-term steroid use are undesirable. Steroids are administered when other medications have failed to control a disease flare and the child has substantial physical disability. Prednisone is given orally in a burst or at the lowest effective dosage. Use of an alternate-day schedule may help reduce side effects. High-dose IV steroids may provide sustained improvement for children with severe arthritis and pericarditis associated with systemic disease. Intraarticular injections of long-acting steroids have proven effective in treating limited arthritis with minimal adverse effects. Children may require conscious sedation or general anesthesia, which affects risk-benefit considerations, but it is critical to have a cooperative patient for good procedure outcome.

Biologic Agents. Etanercept and adalimumab are approved for use in children with JIA. Biologic agents are typically used in children with moderate to severe arthritis after unsuccessful treatment with NSAIDs and methotrexate. Etanercept blocks the binding of tumor necrosis factor (TNF) with cell surface receptors, thereby reducing proinflammatory activity. Adalimumab is a monoclonal antibody TNF blocking agent, which also reduces the proinflammatory response that promotes arthritis. Studies have shown etanercept and adalimumab to be effective and well tolerated (Lovell, Giannini, Reiff, et al, 2003; Lovell, Ruperto, Goodman, et al, 2008).

Although etanercept and adalimumab have been found safe and effective, parents need to inform providers of any unusual symptoms in the child given the relatively limited experience with these drugs and the potential for long-term side effects

(Lovell, Reiff, Ilowite, et al, 2008; Burmester, Mease, Dijkmans, et al, 2009). The potential for malignancy, particularly lymphoma, is continuing to be monitored in children on TNF blockers. Increased infection risk is the most common adverse effect. Parents should withhold etanercept and adalimumab during a concurrent infection and promptly report symptoms of infection to their provider for assessment and treatment. A negative tuberculin skin test should to be obtained before starting etanercept and adalimumab; yearly follow-up skin testing has been suggested. Other biologic agents that interrupt cytokine activity are approved by the U.S. Food and Drug Administration for the adult rheumatoid arthritis population and are available off label and may be useful in treating children with JIA (Ilowite, 2008).

The cytotoxic agents cyclophosphamide, azathioprine, cyclosporine, and chlorambucil have been used to treat severe refractory arthritis that has not responded to other medications. Experience is limited with these drugs, and the toxicity risks and potential benefits are not well defined.

Physical Management

Programs of physical management are individualized for each child and are designed to reach the ultimate goal of preserving function and preventing deformity. Physical therapy is directed toward specific joints and focuses on strengthening muscles, mobilizing restricted joints, and preventing or correcting deformities. Occupational therapists assume responsibility for increasing general mobility and improving performance of activities of daily living.

General treatment and maintenance programs vary. Physical therapists may be involved several times weekly to monthly in management of a home program, or their visits may be limited to infrequent review of the home program for compliance, effectiveness, and need. Muscle strength is frequently lost around the involved joints, and inactivity leads to generalized weakness. However, performance of the normal activities of daily living and the child's natural tendency to be active are usually sufficient to maintain muscle strength and joint mobility. Unless there is a specific risk of injury related to arthritis, the child should not be restricted from regular play, dance, exercise programs, and even individual and team sports. Activity modifications may be needed to accommodate joint limitations, but exercise should be encouraged; a sedentary lifestyle contributes to a deconditioned state, which further limits physical activity and ultimately influences the child's quality of life (Klepper, 2008).

Exercising in a pool is excellent because it allows freedom of movement with support. When joints are inflamed, heavy resistance aggravates the pain. At such times, simple isometric or tensing exercises that do not involve joint movement are generally tolerated and should be encouraged. Range-of-motion exercises are an important aspect of therapy and are continued after evidence of disease has disappeared in order to detect any signs of recurrence.

Practitioners may recommend splinting and positioning during rest to help minimize pain and prevent or reduce flexion deformity. Joints most frequently splinted are knees, wrists, and hands. Positioning during rest is also important. The child should rest on a firm mattress with no pillow or a very low one.

Loss of extension in the knee, hip, and wrist causes special problems. Vigilance is required to detect the earliest signs of involvement, and vigorous attention must be given to specialized passive stretching, positioning, and resting splints to prevent deformity.

Surgery

The benefits of synovectomy, an established preventive and therapeutic procedure in adults, are questionable in children with arthritis. Synovectomy is used primarily in pauciarticular disease. In cases of synovitis, intraarticular steroid injection is an alternative to synovectomy and may be tried once or twice before surgery is performed. Joint replacement is proving to be successful in older children who are fully grown.

Nursing Care Management

Nursing care of children with JIA involves assessment of their general health, the status of involved joints, and their emotional responses to all of the ramifications of the disease—pain; physical restrictions; therapies; and self-concept, especially in preadolescents and adolescents.

The effects of the disease are manifested in every aspect of the child's life, including physical activities, social experiences, and personality development. Children's adjustment to the stresses and demands of the disease and the level of functioning they achieve are related largely to the reaction and support they receive from their family and the health care professionals involved in their care and management (see Nursing Care Plan).

Relieve Pain

Multiple factors influence the pain of arthritis: disease severity, functional status, individual pain threshold, family variables, and psychologic adjustment. Although complete pain relief is desirable, it is probably unrealistic. The aim is to provide as much relief as possible with antiinflammatory medication and other therapies to help children tolerate the pain and complete the activities of daily living. At present, opioid administration is not a routine therapy for the chronic pain of arthritis. Nonpharmacologic modalities such as relaxation may be helpful. (See Pain Management, Chapter 7.)

Promote General Health

Diet and Exercise. The general health of children with arthritis and their siblings must be considered but may be overlooked as parents and health personnel concentrate on the disease. Maintenance of a well-balanced diet and assessment of nutritional status are integral parts of health supervision. A daily children's complete multivitamin with iron is a reasonable dietary supplement, but there is no "arthritis diet" or foods to avoid that are specifically associated with arthritis. Unfortunately children with arthritis have not been spared the nationwide obesity epidemic. After assessing the child growth chart, make a referral to a dietitian for children who are underweight or overweight due to malnutrition. Excessive weight causes additional strain on inflamed joints. Joint pain during or after exercise impedes active play, which perpetuates the vicious cycle of inactivity and weight gain. Encourage daily physical exercise, starting with a gradual program of

NURSING CARE PLAN

The Child with Arthritis

NURSING DIAGNOSIS	EXPECTED PATIENT OUTCOME	NURSING INTERVENTIONS	RATIONALE
Chronic Pain related to joint inflammation	Child will be able to move (joints) and complete activities of daily living with no or minimal discomfort.	Use pain rating scale to evaluate pain (discomfort) level.	To provide objective assessment of pain level
Child's/Family's Defining Characteristics (Subjective and Objective Data)	**The Following NOC Concepts Apply to These Outcomes**	Administer nonsteroidal antiinflammatory drugs (NSAIDs) promptly on report of pain and around the clock when discomfort is acute.	To manage pain and prevent breakthrough pain
Verbal report of pain	Comfort Level	Administer other rheumatic drugs such as slow-acting antirheumatic drugs.	To provided relief from inflammation
Guarding behavior	Pain Control		
Change in sleep pattern	Anxiety Self-Control	Schedule routine rest periods throughout the day.	
	Coping	Encourage child to eat a well-balanced diet and exercise daily.	To prevent obesity and promote wellness
		Help child set up a routine of daily exercise.	To prevent further joint stiffness
		Encourage nonpharmacologic pain relief remedies such as use of heat pad, moist heat, and pool therapy.	To promote mobility of joints and relieve painful stiff joints
		Encourage child to discuss effect of pain on lifestyle and activities.	To provide outlet for emotions such as anger, frustration, and depression at having a chronic illness
		The Following NIC Concepts Apply to These Interventions	
		Analgesic Administration	
		Sleep Enhancement	
		Exercise Promotion	
		Medication Management	
		Environmental Management: Comfort	

NURSING DIAGNOSIS	EXPECTED PATIENT OUTCOME	NURSING INTERVENTIONS	RATIONALE
Impaired Physical Mobility related to pain and swelling in joints	Child will engage in activities of daily living to capability level.	Encourage ambulation and performance of activities of daily living to maximum potential every day.	To keep joints limber and prevent disuse contractures
Child's/Family's Defining Characteristics (Subjective and Objective Data)	**The Following NOC Concepts Apply to These Outcomes**	Assist with range-of-motion exercises for child who is severely limited.	To promote muscle movement and keep joints limber
Limited ability to perform fine and gross motor skills	Ambulation	Encourage child to be as active as tolerated.	To promote independence
	Body Mechanics Performance		
	Rest		
Limited range of motion	Joint Movement: Ankle	Assist with planning and encourage rest periods during the day.	To prevent fatigue
Verbal report of pain	Joint Movement: Spine		
Measurable pain on pain scale	Joint Movement: Wrist	Encourage child to take pain medication such as NSAIDs before ambulation and activity.	To promote activity with minimal pain
	Joint Movement: Knee		
	Joint Movement: Hip	Use nonpharmacologic pain adjuncts such as heat pad, hydrotherapy.	To decrease pain and encourage mobility of joints
	Joint Movement: Elbow		
	Joint Movement: Fingers	Encourage child to be active in self-care activities to maximum potential.	To enhance self-worth and independence
		The Following NIC Concepts Apply to These Interventions	
		Energy Management	
		Exercise Promotion: Stretching	
		Exercise Therapy: Joint Mobility	
		Self-Care Assistance	
		Teaching: Prescribed Activity/Exercise	

walking and slowly advancing to more active play as tolerated. During the school year this can be accomplished with participation in physical education classes as tolerated. When school is out, parents and children should devise a family plan for exercise that includes a variety of options such as games, sports, dance, yoga, swimming, bike riding, and walking. This builds good habits for an active lifestyle for the entire family.

Sleep and Rest. Children with JIA report frequent disrupted nighttime sleep, daytime sleepiness, fatigue, and sleep anxiety (Bloom, Owens, McGuinn, et al, 2002). Restorative sleep is essential. Children should get 8 to 10 hours of nighttime sleep.

Daytime naps are discouraged, especially because inactivity provokes stiffness and prolonged naps can interfere with sleepiness at bedtime. Fatigue should be handled with rest rather than sleep. Thirty to 60 minutes of relaxation—viewing television, reading, playing video games, using the computer, or listening to music—is refueling and less likely to disrupt nighttime sleep than a nap. Use of a firm mattress to maintain alignment of spine, hips, and knees is recommended. A thin pillow or no pillow better aligns the spine. Lying prone during rest is encouraged to straighten the hips and knees. Children with joint contractures may wear nighttime splints, which may take some time to get used to but should not be painful and should not hamper falling asleep.

Encourage School Attendance

School-aged children should attend school, even on days when there is joint pain. Staying home and lying around will not improve arthritis. If joint pain and stiffness prevent school attendance, the rheumatologist should be notified and the child assessed. The rheumatology team can make recommendations to the school to maximize attendance and participation. Enlisting the school nurse to administer scheduled medications and as-needed analgesics such as acetaminophen for pain rescue will help keep the child at school. Requesting one set of books for use at home and one for the classroom eliminates the need for heavy backpacks and the subsequent strain on arthritic joints. The child's participation in the physical education program as tolerated is another way to maximize attendance and performance. If more extensive modifications to the school routine are indicated, the development of an individualized education plan for the school setting (see Chapter 24) may ensure that the child's needs are met. Examples of provisions included in such plans are half-day programs, special transportation, and in-school physical therapy. Although home teaching is rarely indicated, in some circumstances it is necessary; it is initiated with the goal of returning the child to the classroom as soon as possible.

Facilitate Compliance

For any medical or physical plan of therapy to be effective, the family must agree to it and understand the benefits of treatment and the problems associated with noncompliance. Review a simple written list of exercise benefits and complications of joint immobility. At the outset, elicit barriers to a plan from the child and parents. If a child cannot swallow pills or refuses injections, the given modality is not acceptable. If parents know they cannot monitor or enforce a complicated medication and physical therapy schedule, the plan needs to be simplified to honestly reflect the actual care that is being provided. If joint range-of-motion exercises are too painful and emotionally difficult for parents to implement despite use of pretherapy analgesics and comfort measures, then physical therapy home visits or outpatient physical therapy sessions need to be considered.

In addition to developing a plan that is attainable, recognizing a child's compliance by providing inexpensive weekly or monthly rewards fosters goal setting and ultimately boosts self-esteem. It is not just the child who needs therapy rewards; the nonprimary child care provider needs to step in and offer relief to the primary caregiver to prevent burnout, as well as to verbally acknowledge the extra parenting responsibilities being performed.

Everyone needs reminders; a simple written schedule of medications and physical therapy exercises should be provided and reviewed with the family at each visit.

Encourage Comfort Measures and Activities of Daily Living

Application of heat has been beneficial to children with arthritis. Moist heat is best for relieving pain and stiffness, and the most efficient and practical method is via the bathtub. The temperature and duration of the bath are specified by the therapist but usually do not exceed 10 minutes at 37.8° C (100° F). Sometimes a daily whirlpool bath, paraffin bath, or hot packs may be used as needed for temporary relief of acute swelling and pain. Hot packs are easily applied at home using a towel that is wrung out after being immersed in hot water or heated in a microwave oven, applied to the area, and covered with plastic for 20 minutes. Painful hands or feet can be immersed in a pan of water for 10 minutes two or three times daily as an adjunct to tub baths.

Pool therapy is the easiest method for exercising a large number of joints. Swimming activities strengthen muscles and maintain mobility in larger joints. Very small children who are frightened of the water can perform their exercises in the bathtub. Small children love to splash, kick, and throw things in the water.

Activities of daily living provide satisfactory exercise for older children to maintain maximum mobility with minimum pain. These children should be encouraged in their efforts and patiently allowed to dress and groom themselves, to assume daily tasks, and to care for their belongings. It is often difficult for stiff fingers to manipulate buttons, comb or brush hair, and turn faucets, but parents and other caregivers should not readily offer assistance. In addition, children should be helped to understand why others do not assist them. Many helpful devices, such as self-adhering fasteners, tongs for manipulating difficult items, and grab bars installed in bathrooms for safety, can be used to facilitate tasks. An elevated toilet seat often makes the difference between dependent and independent toileting, since weak quadriceps muscles and sore knees inhibit the ability to raise the body from a low sitting position.

A child's natural affinity for play offers many opportunities for incorporating therapeutic exercises. Throwing or kicking a ball, hanging from monkey bars, and riding a tricycle (with the seat raised to achieve maximum leg extension) are excellent moving and stretching exercises for a young child whose daily living activities are physically limited.

An effective approach to beginning the day's activities is to awaken children early to give them their medication and then allow them to sleep for an hour. On arising, children take a hot bath (or shower) and perform a simple ritual of limbering-up exercises, after which they commence the activities of the day, such as going to school. Exercise, heat, and rest are spaced throughout the remainder of the day according to individual needs and schedules. Instruct parents in exercises that fit the needs of the child.

The Arthritis Foundation and the American Juvenile Arthritis Organization* (an organization within the Arthritis Foundation) provide information and services for both parents and professionals, and nurses can refer families to these agencies as an added resource.

The Child. Arthritis affects every aspect of the child's daily life. The physical pain and limitations interfere with performance of normal tasks and provision of self-care. Even simple tasks, such as dressing, combing the hair, using the bathroom, cutting food, climbing stairs, manipulating doors and faucets, and using public transportation, are difficult or impossible. The child may have school difficulties related to transportation to and from school, stair climbing, and loss of time as a result of exacerbations and hospitalization. Physical limitations interfere with participation in many activities, both curricular and extracurricular, which limits peer contacts and interaction and increases social isolation. These problems are especially critical for adolescents, for whom peer acceptance and relationships are vital to personality development (see Family-Centered Care box). Many children with arthritis increasingly turn to solitary activities and to the family at a time when they are expected to move into greater independence and relationships with peers.

👥 FAMILY-CENTERED CARE

Juvenile Rheumatoid Arthritis/Juvenile Idiopathic Arthritis

As a nurse, and mother of a child with juvenile rheumatoid arthritis (juvenile idiopathic arthritis [JRA/JIA]), I believe it is important for nurses always to keep in mind the feelings and emotions of children with JRA/JIA.

Emotionally, I think preadolescent and adolescent children with JRA/JIA have the most questions and concerns about their disease. Children, including my daughter, often ask, "Why me?" Adolescence-preadolescence is an age of socialization and change. These children want to be part of the social scene, to be included. Often these children are limited in their activities. Nurses need to emphasize to their patients, as well as the patients' families, the positive accomplishments these children have made. They need to know that we, as nurses, parents, and doctors, don't know why they have the arthritis, but that we will help and encourage them as much as possible in all aspects of their lives.

Disfigurement of joints, weight gain, weight loss, bloating, and physical impairments are all important in the eyes of a preteen or teenager. They must understand and accept themselves for who they are and not what they look like or appear to look like.

Communication with my daughter was and still is very essential. Nurses have an opportunity to reinforce positive attitudes and encourage open communication with their patients. I believe it is important for nurses to always keep in mind that nursing skills are essential, but that communication with patients and families is equally important. It is the key to nursing assessment.

Sandra L. Guyette, RN
Shriners Hospital
Springfield, Massachusetts

---

*PO Box 7669, Atlanta, GA 30357; 800-283-7800; www.arthritis.org. In Canada: The Arthritis Society, 393 University Ave., Suite 1700, Toronto, Ontario, Canada M5G 1E6; 416-979-7228; fax: 416-979-8366; www.arthritis.ca.

Changes in personality may accompany JIA, as with any chronic illness. These changes may be temporary, such as demanding, irritable behavior, or may be persistent, such as passive hostility, uncommunicativeness, and manipulativeness. Families need confirmation that adjusting to a chronic illness is difficult. Consider and encourage support referrals to social workers, counselors, and psychologists. (See Chapter 22.)

The Family. The beginning of the disease is often sudden and frightening for the family, and its variable course with cycles of remission and exacerbation is discouraging. Many parents become susceptible to experimenting with unorthodox cures advanced by advertisers and well-meaning friends. Access to the Internet and more than 200 sites dedicated to arthritis provides families a welcome relief to the isolation of living with arthritis, but the Internet is also a bottomless source of unsubstantiated information that necessitates frank discussion and review with the family to help them sort out what is opinion versus fact, and safe versus dangerous. Sometimes health care providers do not know the benefits or risks of a nutritional, herbal, or other complementary therapy. It is hoped that the new surge of legitimate scientific investigations of these remedies will provide future answers. Carefully evaluate these therapies. Obviously harmless measures such as wearing a copper bracelet need not be discouraged, but dissuade parents from engaging in questionable or obviously harmful practices. Parents' understanding of the disease and their attitude toward the child can determine the success or failure of a treatment program, and major focuses of nursing intervention are parental education and support.

Nurses should be alert to cues that signal undue anxiety and guilt, which may lead to unhealthy overprotection, such as preoccupation with causative factors, constant analysis of the effects of various therapies, experimentation with diets, and continual searching for a magical cure. Parental overprotection and overindulgence can be especially harmful to the child's progress. Sometimes parents avoid prescribed medications, keep the child home from school unnecessarily, restrict interaction with age-mates, do not discipline the child, and assume self-care activities that are best performed by the child.

Parents and patients need to hear that nurses promote independence. The child's participation in extracurricular activities, including play with friends, scouting, youth groups, dancing, and sports, is recommended. Nurses also support assigning children family chores and allowing older children to hold a part-time job, which foster self-reliance.

Most of the reactions, problems, and concerns of families of a child with JIA are those of any parents of a child with a chronic illness or disability. The impact of the diagnosis is felt most acutely by the parents, who demonstrate anxiety, guilt, and all the manifestations of the grief process. The concerns and needs of these families are discussed extensively in Chapter 22, and the reader is directed to this chapter for additional guidance in planning care.

SYSTEMIC LUPUS ERYTHEMATOSUS

Systemic lupus erythematosus (SLE) is a chronic multisystem autoimmune disease of the blood vessels and connective issue. The Lupus Foundation of America (2009) estimates 1.5

million individuals have lupus, and 10% to 15% of these adults were diagnosed with SLE as children or adolescents. It typically manifests between the ages of 10 and 19 years, and onset before age 5 years is unusual. There is a 5:1 female/male predominance.

Its course and symptoms are variable and unpredictable, with mild to life-threatening complications. SLE in children tends to be more severe at onset and has a more aggressive clinical course than adult-onset disease. Other types of lupus erythematosus include chronic cutaneous lupus erythematosus (discoid lupus erythematosus), drug-induced lupus erythematosus, subacute cutaneous lupus erythematosus, and neonatal lupus erythematosus. Neonatal lupus erythematosus occurs when maternal autoantibodies cross the placenta and cause transient lupuslike symptoms in the newborn, with the potential lethal complication of heart block. The remaining discussion focuses on SLE.

Etiology

The cause of SLE is not known. It appears to result from a complex interaction of genetics with an unidentified trigger that causes the disease to activate. Suspected triggers include exposure to ultraviolet light, estrogen, pregnancy, infections, and drugs. Although a specific gene or genes have not yet been identified as the cause of SLE, an expanding volume of genetic research has identified specific loci associated with SLE.

There is a documented genetic predisposition to SLE as evidenced by an increased concordance rate in twins (tenfold), increased incidence within family members (10% to 16%), an increased frequency of certain gene alleles in population-based studies, and increased risk of autoimmune disease in first-degree relatives of individuals with SLE (Priori, Medda, Conti, et al, 2003; Tsao and Wu, 2007). The incidence of pediatric SLE is also increased in Hispanic, Asian, and African-American pediatric populations.

Pathophysiology

SLE is the result of an abnormal immune response causing production of abnormal antibodies and formation of immune complexes. These immune complexes are deposited in tissues, causing inflammation and inciting other proinflammatory mediators that result in tissue injury and damage. Immune complex deposition in the glomerulus of the kidney causes lupus nephritis, a life-threatening complication of SLE. Almost any tissue in the body can be damaged by this abnormal inflammatory response, including the brain, heart, lungs, liver, gastrointestinal tract, spleen, joint tissues, muscles, and skin.

Clinical Manifestations

The onset of SLE can be insidious, with intermittent constitutional symptoms such as fever, fatigue, weight loss, and arthralgia. However, rapid involvement of vital organs, primarily the kidneys, can herald an accelerated course with potentially fatal outcome. Recent reports suggest that survival rates in children with SLE have significantly improved; 5-year survival rates are said to be almost 100%, and 10-year survival rates are close to 90% (Ravelli, Ruperto, and Martini, 2005).

Box 39-17 lists the manifestations related to the various tissues involved.

BOX 39-17   MANIFESTATIONS OF SYSTEMIC LUPUS ERYTHEMATOSUS

Constitutional—Fever, fatigue, weight loss, anorexia

Cutaneous—Erythematosus butterfly rash over bridge of nose and across cheeks, discoid rash, photosensitivity, mucocutaneous ulceration, alopecia, periungual telangiectasias

Musculoskeletal—Arthritis, arthralgia, myositis, myalgia, tenosynovitis

Neurologic—Headache, seizure, forgetfulness, behavior change, change in school performance, psychosis, chorea, stroke, cranial and peripheral neuropathy, pseudotumor cerebri

Pulmonary and cardiac—Pleuritis, basilar pneumonitis, atelectasis, pericarditis, myocarditis, and endocarditis

Renal—Glomerulonephritis, nephrotic syndrome, hypertension

Gastrointestinal—Abdominal pain, nausea, vomiting, blood in stool, abdominal crisis, esophageal dysfunction, colitis

Hepatic, splenic, and nodal—Hepatomegaly, splenomegaly, lymphadenopathy

Hematologic—Anemia, cytopenia

Ophthalmologic—Cotton wool spots, papilledema, retinopathy

Vascular—Raynaud phenomenon, thrombophlebitis, livedo reticularis

---

Rash is a common feature in SLE. The erythematous malar "butterfly" rash that spares the nasolabial fold is a suggestive feature but not pathognomonic. Maculopapular rashes are frequent and can occur anywhere but typically are found on sun-exposed skin. Nails and hair can be involved, with red, cracked cuticles; periungual telangiectasia; and patchy or diffuse alopecia. Raynaud phenomenon, or spasm of the blood vessels, causes cool hands and feet with pain and a characteristic tricolor (purple or blue–white-red) change. Raynaud phenomenon usually appears as a response to cold exposure and can cause significant tissue damage. In addition to color changes in the extremities, vascular necrosis and digital ulceration can occur. Arthritis and tenosynovitis are common in SLE. The arthritis is usually painful and typically of short duration; joint deformity is unusual.

Renal involvement is a serious complication caused primarily by deposition of circulating immune complexes in the glomerular basement membrane with cellular infiltrates. Lupus nephritis is usually asymptomatic; consequently, monitoring of urine and renal function is required to detect disease. Kidney biopsy is required for lupus nephritis classification. There are six classes depending on the type and extent of the renal lesion. Specific treatment is based on the class of nephritis. Although outcomes have improved for children with renal disease, the course is difficult to predict. Some children get better, whereas some remain the same or progress to renal failure requiring dialysis and transplantation.

Neuropsychiatric lupus is another serious complication found in approximately 25% of pediatric SLE patients. The majority of these children manifest central nervous system involvement within the first year of diagnosis (Benseler and Silverman, 2007). Symptoms can vary from manifestations as subtle as inability to concentrate to frank psychosis and seizure. Assess school performance and emotional stability at each visit as possible indicators of central nervous system involvement.

Cardiovascular disease results in significant mortality and morbidity in lupus. Young women with SLE ages 35 to 45

BOX 39-18 CLASSIFICATION CRITERIA FOR SYSTEMIC LUPUS ERYTHEMATOSUS*

Malar rash—Fixed malar erythema
Discoid rash—Patchy erythematous lesions
Photosensitivity—Rash with sunlight exposure
Oronasal ulcers—Painless ulcers in mouth and nose
Arthritis—Swelling, tenderness, or effusion in two or more peripheral joints (nonerosive)
Serositis—Pleuritis, pericarditis
Renal disorder—Proteinuria, casts in urine
Neurologic disorder—Psychosis, seizures
Hematologic disorder—Hemolytic anemia, thrombocytopenia, leukopenia, lymphopenia
Immunologic disorder—Anti–double-stranded deoxyribonucleic acid, anti-Sm, antiphospholipid antibodies; lupus anticoagulant; false-positive result on syphilis test (rapid plasma reagin)
Antinuclear antibodies

*The presence of four criteria is required for classification as systemic lupus erythematosus.

years are 50 times more like to have a myocardial infarction compared with population controls (Manzi, Meilahn, Rairie, et al, 1997). The immune dysregulation of SLE directly contributes to premature atherosclerosis. Children with SLE have an increased rate of dyslipidemia (Hayata, Borba, Bonfa, et al, 2005). Treatment includes exercise and dietary changes to promote a healthy weight, cardiovascular fitness, and management of hypertension. Studies are currently underway to assess the usefulness of statins in pediatric lupus for future evidence-based treatment of premature atherosclerosis in SLE (Sandborg, Ardoin, and Schanberg, 2008).

Diagnostic Evaluation

SLE is a clinical diagnosis supported by specific abnormal results on laboratory tests. The American College of Rheumatology criteria for the classification of SLE in adults has a sensitivity of 96% and a specificity of 96% if 4 of the 11 criteria are present (Box 39-18). The SLE workup includes an extensive history taking and physical examination with inquiry about school performance and behavior change. Initial laboratory tests include complete blood count with differential; comprehensive metabolic chemistry panel; microscopic urinalysis; rapid plasma reagin test; quantitative determination of immunoglobulin levels; and tests for antinuclear antibodies, anti–deoxyribonucleic acid antibodies, complement 3 (C3), complement 4 (C4), lupus anticoagulant, and antiphospholipid antibodies.

A diagnosis of lupus should not be made without consideration of all medications being taken and their side effects. Some commonly used drugs such as minocycline, procainamide, hydralazine, and chlorpromazine can cause lupuslike symptoms. Minocycline, a common acne treatment, may not be considered important by the teenager and omitted from the history, so an accurate recent past and present medication history is essential for treatment. Drug-induced lupus resolves with time after the triggering medication has been discontinued (Tucker, 2007).

Therapeutic Management

There is no cure for SLE; the management goal is to reverse or minimize disease activity with appropriate medications while helping the child and family cope with the complications of the disease and treatment.

Medications

Since the 1950s, corticosteroids have been the mainstay of SLE therapy. They are effective antiinflammatory and immunosuppressive agents. Unfortunately, the use of steroids is hampered by side effects, which include growth delay, decreased resistance to infection, osteoporosis, weight gain, hypertension, development of cushingoid features and cataracts, and diabetes risks. Generally, a dosage sufficient to control symptoms is prescribed, and then the dosage is tapered to the lowest level possible to achieve an acceptable balance between disease activity and steroid side effects. For severe disease IV pulse (high-dose) steroids are given on an intermittent schedule, which may allow reduction in the daily steroid dose with better compliance and fewer cushingoid features (Klein-Gitelman and Pachman, 1998). Topical steroids are used for cutaneous lesions, but prolonged therapy thins the skin; consequently, facial application needs to be brief or with medication of lower concentration. Because of increased immunosuppression with steroid use, a tuberculin skin test should be performed before starting steroid therapy, especially in high-risk communities. A medical identification tag should be worn by children undergoing chronic steroid therapy so that administration of stress steroids can be considered in emergency situations.

Other medications used include NSAIDs such as naproxen and ibuprofen for pain associated with arthritis, arthralgia, and myalgia. Nurses need to instruct patients to take NSAIDs with food to help prevent gastrointestinal side effects. Hydroxychloroquine, an antimalarial drug, is an effective therapy for skin and joint manifestations. Possible untoward effects include skin, gastrointestinal, and retinal toxicity. A complete ophthalmologic examination is indicated before treatment begins and every 6 months thereafter. Methotrexate may be used in patients with stubborn arthritis that has not responded to NSAIDs and hydroxychloroquine and allows a lower dose of glucocorticoids to be used. Azathioprine, another steroid sparer, has been useful in treatment of SLE thrombocytopenia. Both methotrexate and azathioprine have significant potential adverse effects, including potential for increased infection, malignancy risks, liver and lung toxicity, and birth defects. Well-documented discussions of these risks with patients and parents are required.

Cyclophosphamide, a potent immunosuppressive chemotherapy agent, used in combination with corticosteroids, is effective in treating proliferative lupus nephritis and neuropsychiatric lupus. A detailed cyclophosphamide education session should be held for patient and family to clearly describe potential benefits and risks, including infertility and future malignancy.

Mycophenolate mofetil, a purine inhibitor, has been used with success in adult lupus nephritis and is currently being used as a steroid-sparing agent in active pediatric lupus and as maintenance therapy after standard cyclophosphamide treatment for lupus nephritis. It is also being evaluated as an alternative to standard treatment of lupus nephritis with cyclophosphamide (Paredes, 2007). Mycophenolate mofetil is an attractive alternative, if successful, because it is less toxic and better tolerated than cyclophosphamide; however, it is not without potential side effects, including increased infection risk, liver toxicity, and birth defects.

New biologic treatments are being developed that focus on the immune dysregulation in SLE, cancer, and other autoimmune diseases. Rituximab is a monoclonal antibody that eliminates CD20-positive B cells without affecting early B cells or plasma cells. This results in decreased antibody formation and has been used off label in pediatric lupus patients who have not responded to standard therapy (Nwobi, Abitbol, Chandar, et al, 2008).

General Measures

In addition to medication, treatment includes general measures such as patient and family education, rest and exercise, proper diet, sun avoidance, and social support.

SLE is complex and requires ongoing patient education. Families and patients need up-to-date, understandable information so they can become informed decision makers and participate in disease management. Nurses are duty bound to discuss information families bring to appointments from the Internet, friends, and family. As health care providers critically evaluate disease information with families, families learn the skills needed to become self-advocates. Families also want to hear about the impact of SLE on growth and development, childbearing, schooling, and career choice. The message should be optimistic and clear, with few exceptions: "Prepare for the future; you will attend school, graduate, have children, and work."

Diet, exercise, and rest are the daily elements under direct patient control. The family needs to maximize the power of these normal functions to their benefit. There is no specific SLE diet, but a balanced diet that does not exceed calorie expenditure is essential for maintaining appropriate weight on corticosteroid therapy. A low-salt diet may be required if the patient becomes nephrotic or hypertensive. A low-fat diet is indicated in children with dyslipidemia. Maximizing peak bone mass in adolescent SLE is essential, especially since both SLE and its treatment with glucocorticoids increase the risk of osteoporosis. A diet rich in calcium and vitamin D is essential to prevent osteoporosis. If dietary calcium is not sufficient, calcium and vitamin D supplements need to be recommended. Consultation with a registered dietitian will help the family develop an individualized diet that meshes with their lifestyle.

The benefits of a regular exercise program include weight maintenance, cardiovascular fitness, and osteoporosis prevention, all of which help minimize SLE complications and corticosteroid side effects. Unfortunately many children stop participation in sports after diagnosis. Children with SLE report more fatigue and have lower aerobic fitness (Houghton, Tucker, Potts, et al, 2008). Encourage continuation of sports and recreational activities, if possible; if not, try to modify the activity or find alternatives to encourage the child and parents to view

daily exercise as an essential part of the treatment plan and a continuation of the child's normal lifestyle. Additional rest is necessary during disease exacerbations but not to the extent that it interferes with regular sleep patterns.

Given the frequency of photosensitive rash, the dangers of excessive ultraviolet A and B light exposure (including exposure to uncovered fluorescent lights) need to be stressed. This can be a sensitive topic for sun-loving teenagers and outdoor athletes. Discuss the use of sunscreen (with an SPF [sun protection factor] ≥30), hats, and protective clothing. Cosmetics and moisturizers that contain sunscreen are attractive options for adolescent girls. One useful rule to share with the adolescent who may be surrounded by peers who regularly seek out sun exposure is the "slip, slop, slap" rule: slip on a shirt, slop on sunscreen, and slap on a hat before going out in the sun. (See Chapter 18.) Scheduling outdoor activities in the morning and evening can reduce exposure without limiting participation in recreational activities. Make every effort to encourage children to participate in peer activities and to make sun-shielding modifications as inconspicuous as possible.

Social support from family, friends, teachers, counselors, and professional social workers and therapists can help the child and family through difficult times and promote adaptation to an illness that is not going to go away. Destructive coping mechanisms need to be identified and replaced with behaviors that enhance adaptation and healthy outcomes. Organizations that can help children and families learn about and adjust to the disease are the Lupus Foundation of America* and the Arthritis Foundation† (see p. 1682).

Nursing Care Management

Fostering adaptation and self-advocacy is the primary nursing goal. Patient and family acceptance and understanding of this life-threatening and therapeutically intrusive disease are big challenges for any nurse. Patient education is started at diagnosis and continued at every opportunity; repetition is good. Encourage family members to call with questions and concerns. Advise patients to write down their questions so they are prepared during the appointment. Consider adolescent development, with heightened concerns about body image and looking different. The nurse should be open about this. Skin care, cosmetics, and unobtrusive moisturizers with sunscreen and sun block should be discussed.

Weight gain is an emotional issue, and it must be approached honestly with a workable plan for family dietary changes and a realistic exercise program. The nurse should work with a dietitian and a trainer or physical therapist to individualize a nutrition and fitness program for the child. A parent or sibling should be involved in the program, so the child does not feel that restrictions are punitive.

With older children, sexual activity and birth control must be discussed, especially because pregnancy is a potential trigger

---

*2000 L St. NW, Suite 710, Washington, DC 20036; 202-349-1155; fax: 202-349-1156; www.lupus.org.
†A recommended booklet available from the Arthritis Foundation is *Meeting the Challenge: A Young Person's Guide to Living with Lupus.*

for disease flare. Honest discussion about healthy, responsible reproductive choices with both the teenager and parents is important for establishing communication. The parents and teenager should know that the teenager can come to the nurse with reproductive concerns. Because estrogen can trigger disease flare, low-dose estrogen or progestin-only oral contraceptives are preferred. Some teenagers choose the compliance-friendly Depo-Provera (medroxyprogesterone) 3-month injections. Again, frank discussion about risks and benefits is essential.

Prevention of infection includes hand washing (especially at school) and preprocedure antibiotic coverage for routine events such as dental cleaning. Immunization vaccinations should be maintained in SLE, except live and attenuated vaccines should be withheld in patients on immunosuppressive therapy.

To compensate for the side effects of some drugs such as the corticosteroids, teenagers often go on fad or starvation diets. It is critical that nutritional counseling be available to ensure that the adolescent understands the role that a healthy diet plays in the management of SLE. School attendance may decrease because of loss of self-esteem, depression, feelings of inadequacy, or poor academic performance. Assessment of common adolescent risk taking behaviors, including tobacco and recreational drug use, needs to be performed as it would for any teenage patient. Treatment compliance is a significant issue in adolescence, especially given the medication side effects and restrictions on sun exposure. Adolescents need to understand what the function of each drug is, how each drug helps to manage the disease, and what effect missing doses may have on their health. The nurse needs to keep track of prescription refills to evaluate compliance and medication efficacy. Barriers to medication compliance should be investigated, and patients should be helped to devise a workable plan. If friends are going to the beach, the patient should consider going late in the day with a beach umbrella, sun block, and a wide-brim hat. Give instructions to reapply sun block after swimming and to limit time in direct sun. (See Chapter 18.)

Teaching patients how to find ways to adapt positively to SLE with normal growth and development as the goal will give them self-advocacy skills. Nurses should apply the principles of adjusting to a chronic illness that are discussed in Chapter 22.

KEY POINTS

- Trauma is the leading cause of death in children and is caused by accidental injury, child abuse injury, and birth injury.
- Immobility has a profound effect on all elements of growth and development.
- The major consequences of immobilization are loss of muscle strength, endurance, and muscle mass; bone demineralization leading to osteoporosis; circulatory stasis and thrombus formation; loss of joint mobility; and contractures.
- In the care of the immobilized child, nurses are concerned with position changes, adequate dietary intake, adequate hydration, promotion of activity, and involvement of the child in self-care.
- Features of children's bones not observed in those of adults include presence of a growth plate, a thicker and stronger periosteum, greater bone porosity, more rapid healing, and less joint stiffness.
- Types of fractures seen in children include bend, buckle, greenstick, and complete fractures.
- Goals of fracture management in children are to reestablish alignment and length of the bony fragments, retain alignment and length, and restore function to injured parts.
- The method of fracture reduction is determined by the child's age, the degree of displacement, the amount of overriding bone, the amount of edema, the condition of the skin and soft tissues, and the integrity of sensation and circulation distal to the fracture.
- The primary purposes of traction are to fatigue involved muscle and reduce muscle spasm, to realign bone ends, and to immobilize the fracture site until realignment has been achieved to permit casting or splinting.
- Complications of fractures are circulatory impairment, nerve compression syndromes, compartment syndromes, epiphyseal damage, nonunion, malunion, infection, kidney stones, and pulmonary emboli.
- Participation in sports predisposes adolescents to acute injuries, such as contusions, dislocations, sprains, and strains, and to overuse syndromes, such as stress fractures.
- Health concerns associated with sports include menstrual dysfunction, substance misuse, and sudden death from sudden cardiac arrest.
- Musculoskeletal disorders in children include torticollis, Legg-Calvé-Perthes disease, SCFE, kyphosis, lordosis, and scoliosis.
- Observation for idiopathic scoliosis is an important part of a routine physical assessment.
- Management of idiopathic scoliosis includes bracing or surgery.
- Postoperative nursing care of the child with idiopathic scoliosis demands careful attention to peripheral neurovascular function, respiratory function, pain control, and skin care.
- Nursing care of the child with osteomyelitis is directed at positioning for comfort, administering antibiotics, monitoring IV equipment and site, and ensuring adequate nutrition.
- Osteomyelitis is acquired by direct or secondary invasion or hematogenous spread of infectious organisms.
- Goals of therapy for arthritis in children are to control pain, preserve joint range of motion and function, minimize the effects of inflammation such as joint deformity, and promote normal growth and development.
- Nursing care of the child with arthritis consists of relieving pain, promoting general health, preventing deformity, preserving optimum function, and encouraging self-care and maximum involvement in school and other activities.
- SLE is a chronic multisystem autoimmune disorder that affects the blood vessels and connective tissues of the body.

REFERENCES

Alharbi M, Pinto G, Finidori G, et al: Pamidronate treatment of children with moderate-to severe osteogenesis imperfect: a note of caution, *Horm Res* 71(1):38-44, 2009.

American Academy of Orthopaedic Surgeons: Keep injured high school athletes out of the game, *Your Orthopaedic Connection*, 2007, available at http://orthoinfo.aaos.org/topic. cfm?topic=A00048 (accessed August 1, 2009).

American Academy of Pediatrics, Committee on Nutrition: *Pediatric nutrition handbook*, ed 6, Elk Grove Village, Ill, 2009, The Academy.

American Academy of Pediatrics: Use of performance-enhancing substances, *Pediatrics* 115(4):1103-1106, 2005.

American Academy of Pediatrics, Committee on Sports Medicine and Fitness: Climatic heat stress and the exercising child and adolescent, *Pediatrics* 106(1):158-159, 2000a.

American Academy of Pediatrics, Committee on Sports Medicine and Fitness: Medical concerns in the female athlete, *Pediatrics* 106(3):610-613, 2000b.

American Academy of Pediatrics, Section on Rheumatology and Section on Ophthalmology: Guidelines for ophthalmologic examinations in children with juvenile rheumatoid arthritis, *Pediatrics* 92(2):295-296, 1993.

Bachrach LK, Ward LM: Clinical review 1: bisphosphonate use in childhood osteoporosis, *J Clin Endocrinol Metab* 94(2):400-409, 2009.

Benseler SM, Silverman ED: Neuropsychiatric involvement in pediatric systemic lupus erythematosus, *Lupus* 16(3):564-571, 2007.

Bloom BJ, Owens JA, McGuinn M, et al: Sleep and its relationship to pain, dysfunction and disease activity in juvenile rheumatoid arthritis, *J Rheumatol* 29(1):169-173, 2002.

Borse NN, Gilchrist J, Dellinger AM, et al: *CDC childhood injury report: patterns of unintentional injuries among 0-19 year olds in the United States, 2000-2006*, Atlanta, 2008, Centers for Disease Control and Prevention.

Boyd AS, Benjamin HJ, Asplund C: Principles of casting and splinting, *Am Fam Physician* 79(1):16-22, 23-24, 2009.

Brenner JS, Council on Sports Medicine and Fitness: Overuse injuries, overtraining, and burnout in child and adolescent athletes, *Pediatrics* 119(6):1242-1245, 2007.

Brown JC, Klein EJ, Lewis CW, et al: Emergency department analgesia for fracture pain, *Ann Emerg Med* 42(2):197-205, 2003.

Bullock DP, Koval KJ, Moen KY, et al: Hospitalized cases of child abuse in America: who, what, when, and where, *J Pediatr Orthop* 29(3):231-237, 2009.

Bunnell WP: Selective screening for scoliosis, *Clin Orthop Relat Res* 434:40-45, 2005.

Burmester GR, Mease PJ, Dijkmans BA, et al: Adalimumab safety and mortality rates from global clinical trials of six immune-mediated inflammatory diseases, *Ann Rheum Dis* 68(12):1863-1869, 2009.

Calfee R, Fadale P: Popular erogenic drugs and supplements in young athletes, *Pediatrics* 117(3):e577-e589, 2006.

Cassidy J, Kivlin J, Lindsley C, et al: Ophthalmologic Examinations in Children with juvenile rheumatoid arthritis, *Pediatrics* 117(5):1843-1845, 2006.

Chorley JN: Ankle sprain discharge instructions from the emergency department, *Pediatr Emerg Care* 21(8):498-501, 2005.

Cimpello LB, Khine H, Avner JR: Practice patterns of pediatric versus general emergency physicians for pain management of fractures in pediatric patients, *Pediatr Emerg Care* 20(4):228-232, 2004.

Clark E, Plint AC, Correll R, et al: A randomized, controlled trial of acetaminophen, ibuprofen, and codeine for acute pain relief in children with musculoskeletal trauma, *Pediatrics* 119(3):460-467, 2007.

Cornwall R: Upper limb. In Kliegman RM, Behrman RE, Jenson HB, et al, editors: *Nelson textbook of pediatrics*, ed 18, Philadelphia, 2007, Saunders.

Curley MA, Razmus IS, Roberts KE, et al: Predicting pressure ulcer risk in pediatric patients: the Braden Q Scale, *Nurs Res* 52(1):22-33, 2003.

DiFazio R, Atkinson CC: Extremity fractures in children: when is it an emergency? *J Pediatr Nurs* 20(4):298-304, 2005.

Doyle GS, Taillac PP: Tourniquets: a review of current use with proposals for expanded prehospital use, *Prehosp Emerg Care* 12(2):241-256, 2008.

Drendel AL, Lyon R, Bergholte J, et al: Outpatient pediatric pain management practices for fractures, *Pediatr Emerg Care* 22(2):94-99, 2006.

Drezner JA, Chun JS, Harmon KG, et al: Survival trends in the United States following exercise-related cardiac arrest in the youth, 2000-2006, *Heart Rhythm* 5(6):794-799, 2008.

Drezner JA, Courson RW, Roberts WO, et al: Inter Association Task Force recommendations on emergency preparedness and management of sudden cardiac arrest in high school and college athletic programs: a consensus statement, *Prehosp Emerg Care* 11(3):253-271, 2007.

Drezner JA, Rao AL, Heistand J, et al: Effectiveness of emergency response planning for sudden cardiac arrest in United States high schools with automated external defibrillators, *Circulation* 120(6):518-525, 2009.

Fisher TJ, Williams SL, Levine AM: Spinal orthosis. In Browner BD, Jupiter JB, Levine AM, et al, editors: *Skeletal trauma: basic science, management, and reconstruction*, ed 4, Philadelphia, 2008, Saunders.

Foeldvari I, Wierk A: Methotrexate is an effective treatment for chronic uveitis associated with juvenile idiopathic arthritis, *J Rheumatol* 33(2):362-365, 2005.

Freeman BL III: Scoliosis and kyphosis. In Canale ST, Beaty JH, editors: *Campbell's operative orthopaedics*, ed 11, Philadelphia, 2007, Mosby.

Friday JH, Kanegaye JT, McCaslin I, et al: Ibuprofen provides analgesia equivalent to acetaminophen-codeine in the treatment of acute pain in children with extremity injuries: A randomized clinical trial, *Acad Emerg Med* 16(8):711-716, 2009.

Graham JM, Gomez M, Halberg A, et al: Management of deformational plagiocephaly: repositioning versus orthotic therapy, *J Pediatr* 146(2):258-262, 2005.

Green NE, Swiontkowski MF: *Skeletal trauma in children*, ed 4, Philadelphia, 2008, Mosby/ Elsevier.

Gregory AJM, Fitch RW: Sports medicine: performance-enhancing drugs, *Pediatr Clin North Am* 54(4):797-806, 2007.

Guticrrcz K: Bone and joint infections in children, *Pediatr Clin North Am* 52(3):779-794, 2005.

Hart ES, Grottkau BE, Albright MB: Slipped capital femoral epiphysis: don't miss this pediatric hip disorder, *Nurs Pract* 32(3):14, 16-18, 21, 2007.

Hayata AL, Borba EF, Bonfa E, et al: The frequency of high/moderate lipoprotein risk factor for coronary artery disease is significant in juvenile-onset systemic lupus erythematosus, *Lupus* 14(8):613-617, 2005.

Hazinski MF, Markenson D, Neish S, et al: Response to cardiac arrest and selected life-threatening medical emergencies: the medical emergency response plan for schools: a statement for healthcare providers, policymakers, school administrators, and community leaders, *Pediatrics* 113(1):155-168, 2004.

Holmes SB, Brown SJ, Pin Site Care Expert Panel: Skeletal pin site care: National Association of Orthopaedic Nurses guidelines for orthopaedic nursing, *Orthop Nurs* 24(2):99-107, 2005.

Hosalkar HS, Horn D, Friedman J, et al: The hip. In Kliegman RM, Behrman RE, Jenson HB, et al, editors: *Nelson textbook of pediatrics*, ed 18, Philadelphia, 2007, Saunders.

Houghton KM, Tucker LB, Potts JE, et al: Fitness, fatigue, disease activity, and quality of life in pediatric lupus, *Arthritis Rheum* 59(4):537-545, 2008.

Ilowite, NT: Update on biologics in juvenile idiopathic arthritis, *Curr Opin Rheumatol* 20(5):613-618, 2008.

Ivins D: Acute ankle sprain: an update, *Am Fam Physician* 74(10):1714-1720, 1723-1724, 1725-1726, 2006.

Jarvis J, Garbedian S, Swamy G: Juvenile idiopathic scoliosis: the effectiveness of part-time bracing, *Spine (Phila 1976)* 33(10):1074-1078, 2008.

Joy EA, Van Hala S, Cooper L: Health-related concerns of the female athlete: a lifespan approach, *Am Fam Physician* 79(6):489-495, 2009.

Kennedy RM, Luhmann JD, Luhmann SJ: Emergency department management of pain and anxiety related to orthopedic fracture care: a guide to analgesic techniques and procedural sedation in children, *Pediatr Drugs* 6(1):11-31, 2004.

Kerkhoffs GM, Struijs PA, Assendelft WJ, et al: Different functional treatment strategies for acute lateral ankle ligament injuries in adults, *Cochrane Database Syst Rev* (3):CD002938, 2002.

Klein-Gitelman MS, Pachman LM: Intravenous corticosteroids: adverse reactions are more variable than expected in children, *J Rheumatol* 25(10):1995-2002, 1998.

Klepper SE: Exercise in pediatric rheumatic diseases, *Curr Opin Rheumatol* 20(5):619-624, 2008.

Koller DM, Myers AB, Lorenz D, et al: Effectiveness of oxycodone, ibuprofen, or the combination in the initial management of orthopedic injury-related pain in children, *Pediatr Emerg Care* 23(9):627-633, 2007.

Lampe RM: Osteomyelitis and suppurative arthritis. In Kliegman RM, Behrman RE, Jenson HB, et al, editors: *Nelson textbook of pediatrics*, ed 18, Philadelphia, 2007, Saunders.

Land C, Rauch F, Travers R, et al: Osteogenesis imperfecta type VI in childhood and adolescence: effects of cyclical intravenous pamidronate treatment, *Bone* 40(3):638-644, 2007.

Laskowski-Jones L: Responding to an out-of-hospital emergency, *Nursing 2002* 32(9):36-42, 2002.

Lee C, Porter KM, Hodgetts TJ: Tourniquet use in the civilian prehospital setting, *Emerg Med J* 24(8):584-587, 2007.

Loder RT: Controversies in slipped capital femoral epiphysis, *Orthop Clin North Am* 37(2):211-221, 2006.

Loder RT, Feinberg JR: Orthopaedic injuries in children with nonaccidental trauma: demographics and incidence from the 2000 kids' inpatient database, *J Pediatr Orthop* 27(4):421-426, 2007.

Lonner BS: Emerging minimally invasive technologies for the management of scoliosis, *Orthop Clin North Am* 38(3):431-440, 2007.

Lovell DJ, Giannini EH, Reiff A, et al: Long-term efficacy and safety of etanercept in children with polyarticular juvenile rheumatoid arthritis: interim results from an ongoing multicenter, open-label, extended-treatment trial, *Arthritis Rheum* 48(1):218-226, 2003.

Lovell DJ, Reiff A, Ilowite NT, et al: Safety and efficacy of up to 8 years of continuous etanercept therapy in patients with juvenile rheumatoid arthritis, *Arthritis Rheum* 58(5):1496-1503, 2008.

Lovell DJ, Ruperto N, Goodman S, et al: Adalimumab with or without methotrexate in juvenile rheumatoid arthritis, *N Engl J Med* 359(8):810-820, 2008.

Lucas B, Davis PS: Why restricting movement is important. In Kneale JD, Davis PS, editors: *Orthopaedic and trauma nursing*, ed 2, London, 2005, Elsevier.

Lupus Foundation of America: *About lupus: what is lupus?* Washington, DC, 2009, The Foundation, accessed April 25, 2010, at www.lupus.org/webmodules/webarticlesnet/templates/new_learnunderstanding.aspx?articleid=2232&zoneid=523.

Manzi S, Meilahn EN, Rairie JE, et al: Age-specific incidence rates of myocardial infarction and angina in women with systemic lupus erythematosus: comparison with the Framingham study, *Am J Epidemiol* 145(5):408-414, 1997.

Marini JC: Osteogenesis imperfect. In Kliegman RM, Behrman RE, Jenson HB, et al, editors: *Nelson textbook of pediatrics*, ed 18, Philadelphia, 2007, Saunders.

Maron BJ: Medical progress: sudden death in young athletes, *N Engl J Med* 349(11):1064-1075, 2003.

Maron BJ, Doerer JJ, Haas TS, et al: Sudden deaths in young competitive athletes: analysis of 1866 deaths in the United States, 1980-2006, *Circulation* 119(8):1085-1092, 2009.

Maron BJ, Gohman TE, Aeppli D: Prevalence of sudden cardiac death during competitive sports activities in Minnesota high school athletes, *J Am Coll Cardiol* 32(7):1881-1884, 1998.

Meredith JR, O'Keefe KP, Galwankar S: Pediatric procedural sedation and analgesia, *J Emerg Trauma Shock* 1(2):88-96, 2008.

Napierkowski DB: Scoliosis: a case study in an adolescent boy, *Orthop Nurs* 26(3):147-153, 2007.

Nelson AJ, Collins CL, Yard EE, et al: Ankle injuries among United States high school sports athletes, 2005-2006, *J Athl Train* 42(3):381-387, 2007.

Newton PO, Wenger DR: Idiopathic and congenital scoliosis. In Morrissy RT, Weinstein SL, editors: *Lovell and Winter's pediatric orthopaedics*, Philadelphia, 2001, Williams & Wilkins.

Nwobi O, Abitbol CL, Chandar J et al: Rituximab therapy for juvenile-onset systemic lupus erythematosus, *Pediatr Nephrol* 23(3):413-419, 2008.

Paredes A: Can mycophenolate mofetil substitute cyclophosphamide treatment of pediatric lupus? *Pediatr Nephrol* 22(8):1077-1082, 2007.

Persing J, James H, Swanson J, et al: Prevention and management of positional skull deformities in infants, *Pediatrics* 112(1):199-202, 2003.

Petty RE, Southwood TR, Baum J, et al: Revision of the proposed classification criteria for juvenile idiopathic arthritis: Durban, 1997, *J Rheumatol* 25(10):1991-1994, 1998.

Petty RE, Southwood TR, Manners P, et al: International League of Associations for Rheumatology classification of juvenile idiopathic arthritis: second revision, Edmonton, 2001, *J Rheumatol* 31(2):390-392, 2004.

Plint AC, Perry JJ, Correll R, et al: A randomized, controlled trial of removable splinting versus casting for wrist buckle fractures in children, *Pediatrics* 117(3):691-697, 2006.

Prahalad S, Glass DN: A comprehensive review of the genetics of juvenile idiopathic arthritis, *Pediatr Rheumatol* 11(6), 2008, available at www.ped-rheum.com/content/6/1/11 (accessed April 24, 2009).

Priori R, Medda E, Conti F, et al: Familial autoimmunity as a risk factor for systemic lupus erythematosus and vice versa: a case-control study, *Lupus* 12(10):735-740, 2003.

Rauch F, Munns CF, Land C, et al: Risedronate in the treatment of mild pediatric osteogenesis imperfecta: a randomized placebo-controlled study, *J Bone Miner Res* 24(7):1282-1289, 2009.

Ravelli A, Ruperto N, Martini A: Outcome in juvenile onset lupus erythematosus, *Curr Opin Rheumatol* 17(5):568-573, 2005.

Rechel JA, Yard EE, Comstock RD: An epidemiologic comparison of high school sports injuries sustained in practice and competition, *J Athl Train* 43(2):197-204, 2008.

Rice SG, Council on Sports Medicine and Fitness: Medical conditions affecting sports participation, *Pediatrics* 121(4):841-848, 2008.

Richards BS, Vitale MG: Screening for idiopathic scoliosis in adolescents: an information statement, *J Bone Joint Surg* 90(1):195-198, 2008.

Rodriguez NR, DiMarco NM, Langley S, et al: Position of the American Dietetic Association, Dietitians of Canada, and the American College of Sports Medicine: nutrition and athletic performance, *J Am Diet Assoc* 109(3):509-527, 2009.

Sandborg C, Ardoin SP, Schanberg L: Therapy insight: cardiovascular disease in pediatric systemic lupus erythematosus, *Nat Clin Pract Rheumatol* 4(5):258-265, 2008.

Slote RJ: Psychological effects of caring for the adolescent undergoing spinal fusion for scoliosis, *Orthop Nurs* 21(6):19-28, 2002.

Spiegel DA, Hosalkar HS, Dormans JP, et al: The neck. In Kliegman RM, Behrman RE, Jenson HB, et al, editors: *Nelson textbook of pediatrics*, ed 18, Philadelphia, 2007, Saunders.

Spiegel DA, Hosalkar HS, Dormans JP: Bone and joint disorders: the spine. In Kliegman RM, Behrman RE, Jenson HB, et al, editors: *Nelson textbook of pediatrics*, ed 18, Philadelphia, 2007, Saunders.

Tsao BP, Wu H: Genetics of human lupus. In Wallace DJ, Hahn BH, editors: *Dubois' Lupus Erythematosus*, ed 7, Philadelphia, 2007, Lippincott Williams & Wilkins.

Tucker LB: Making the diagnosis of systemic lupus erythematosus in children and adolescents, *Lupus* 12(8):546-549, 2007.

Venables MC, Shaw L, Jeukendrup AE, et al: Erosive effect of a new sports drink on dental enamel during exercise, *Med Sci Sports Exerc* 37(1):39-44, 2005.

Waldrop J: Early identification and interventions for female athlete triad, *J Pediatr Health Care* 19(4):213-220, 2005.

Warren RW, Perez MD, Curry MR, et al: Juvenile idiopathic arthritis (juvenile rheumatoid arthritis). In Koopman WJ, editor: *Arthritis and allied conditions*, Philadelphia, 2001, Lippincott Williams & Wilkins.

Wipke-Tevis DD, Rich K: Vascular disorders. In Lewis SL, Heitkemper MM, Dirksen S, et al, editors: *Medical-surgical nursing: assessment and management of clinical problems*, ed 7, St Louis, 2007, Mosby.

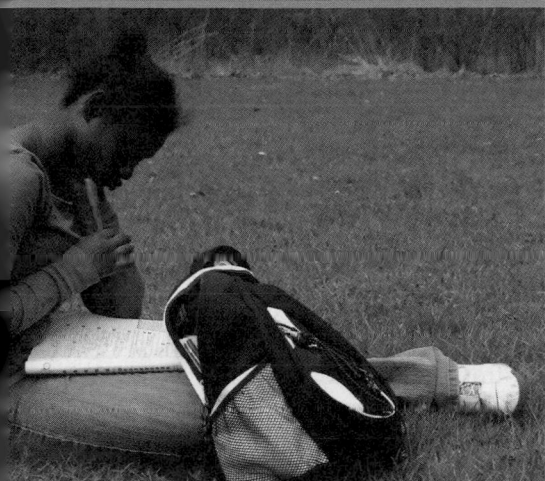

The Child with Neuromuscular or Muscular Dysfunction

David Wilson

ⓔvolve WEBSITE

http://evolve.elsevier.com/wong/ncic

Animation
   Guillain-Barré Syndrome
Critical Thinking Case Study
   Cerebral Palsy
Critical Thinking Exercise
   Guillain-Barré Syndrome
Key Points Audio Summaries
NCLEX Review Questions
Nursing Care Plan
   The Child with Cerebral Palsy
Spanish/English Translations
WebLinks

RELATED TOPICS

CHAPTER OUTLINE

NEUROMUSCULAR DYSFUNCTION

Weakness or abnormal performance of skeletal muscle may represent a defect in the muscle itself or reflect a pathologic disorder at some point along the neural pathway from the cortex of the brain to the neuromuscular junction. The identification of the source of muscular dysfunction includes not only the testing of muscle function but also the systematic elimination of possible disorders of neural structures on which muscle function depends for its stimulus. In a few disorders muscle disease may be accompanied by a neural disorder.

Some clinical features are shared by muscle disease (myopathy), which differs in many ways from muscular dysfunction resulting from disorders of neuronal structures—brain, cranial nerve nuclei, long nerve tracts, anterior horn cells of the spinal cord, and peripheral nerves. Motor function is accomplished by means of the simple reflex arcs or by way of impulses transmitted from the cerebral cortex and other centers in the brain through the various nerve pathways of the central nervous system (CNS). The upper motor neurons consist of cells that lie in the cerebral cortex and fibers that traverse the brainstem and spinal cord to terminate at their synapses with the anterior horn cells. The lower motor neurons consist of the anterior horn cells, axons, and peripheral nerve branches. The motor unit consists of the lower motor neuron, the neuromuscular (or myoneural) junction, and the muscle fibers it supplies

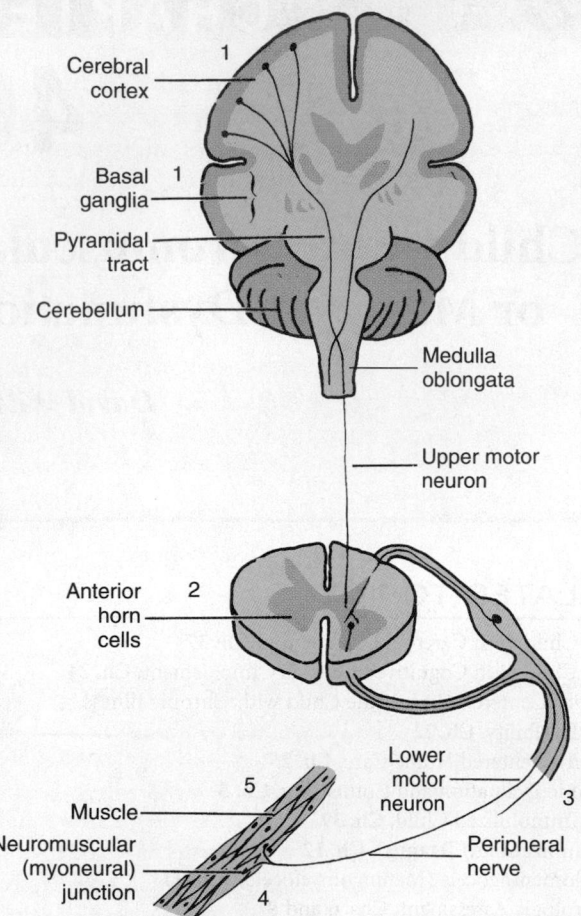

Fig. 40-1 Site of origin for neuromuscular disorders. *1,* Cerebral palsy; *2,* poliomyelitis, spinal muscular atrophy; *3,* mononeuropathies, polyneuropathies; *4,* myasthenia gravis, neurotoxic disorders; *5,* muscular dystrophies.

(Fig. 40-1). The upper motor neuronal pathways from the cerebrum to the lower motor neuron are described as (1) pyramidal—those whose fibers extend from the cortex, come together in the medulla, cross from one side to the other, then extend down the cord to synapse with anterior horn motor neurons; and (2) extrapyramidal—a complex network of motor neurons that comprise relays between motor areas of the cortex, basal ganglia, thalamus, cerebellum, and brainstem.

CLASSIFICATION AND DIAGNOSIS

The site of pathologic disturbance determines the type of muscular dysfunction. In general, upper motor neuron lesions produce weakness associated with spasticity, increased deep tendon reflexes, and abnormal superficial reflexes. The primary disorder of upper motor neuron dysfunction is cerebral palsy (CP). Lower motor neuron lesions interrupt the reflex arc, causing weakness and atrophy of the skeletal muscles involved with associated hypotonia or flaccidity, which eventually progress to atrophy with varying degrees of contracture deformity. A disorder of the extrapyramidal pathway and the cerebellum rarely produces muscle weakness.

Lower motor neuron involvement is usually symmetric (except that of poliomyelitis and single peripheral nerve disease), whereas disorders of the pyramidal tract are more often asymmetric. Muscle wasting is characteristic of lower motor neuron lesions and more marked than in diseases of muscles. Deep tendon reflexes are briskly active in upper motor neuron disease, are diminished or absent in lower motor neuron disease, and depend on the progress of muscle degeneration in the myopathies.

These disorders can also be categorized according to onset: those in which there is acute onset of flaccid paralysis and those with more gradual onset and progressive degeneration. In most instances the sudden appearance of flaccid paralysis in a previously healthy child is due to an infectious process. Neurotoxins (e.g., botulism, tick paralysis, or heavy metal poisoning), pressure on the spinal cord from tumors or abscesses, and spinal cord injury (SCI) are less likely causes. Hereditary factors and metabolic disease are more often responsible for muscular weakness and atrophy of gradual onset.

Classification

The most useful classification of neuromuscular disorders is one that defines the site of origin of the pathologic lesion: the anterior horn cells of the spinal cord, the peripheral nerves, the neuromuscular junction, and the muscles.

Diseases of Anterior Horn Cells

Diseases and disorders that affect the anterior horn cells are the result of destruction or atrophy of the anterior horn of the spinal column along with the inability to transfer impulses from sensory neurons to motor neurons. Enteroviruses, which have a worldwide distribution, are prominent etiologic agents that selectively affect anterior horn cells. These include the polioviruses, of which there are three types: coxsackieviruses, groups A and B, and the enterocytopathogenic human orphan (ECHO) viruses. Inherited disorders, primarily the spinal muscular atrophies, cause degeneration of the anterior horn cells.

Neuropathies

Disorders affecting peripheral nerves may be mononeuropathies, which involve a single nerve and the muscles it innervates, or polyneuropathies, which involve multiple nerves and the muscles they supply. Neuropathies are caused by a number of hereditary diseases, traumatic injuries, infections, poisons, and (secondarily) some metabolic diseases. Polyneuropathy can be restricted to specific areas (as in diabetes mellitus). Some hereditary diseases involve skeletal muscles extensively. The distal limbs (feet and hands) are usually affected first, with gait disturbance and footdrop being early manifestations. The involvement gradually progresses proximally as the disorder becomes more severe.

In some polyneuropathies there is segmented or patchy loss of the myelin sheath of nerve fibers; in others the primary process appears to be progressive degeneration of nerve fibers. Examples of acute and chronic polyneuropathies are infectious polyneuritis and peroneal atrophy, respectively.

Neuromuscular Junction Disease

Disorders involving a neurohormonal deficiency interfere with transmission of nerve impulses to muscles at the neuromuscular junction. Normally nerve impulses are transmitted to skeletal muscles across the neuromuscular junction by acetylcholine.

This is accomplished in three steps: (1) acetylcholine is released from vesicles in the terminal nerve endings; (2) it then diffuses across the junction and contacts receptor sites in the muscle membrane, stimulating the muscle to contract; and (3) it is removed by the action of cholinesterase. Interference at any of these three steps will block transmission of nerve impulses and prevent muscular contraction.

Several toxic substances act at the neuromuscular junction to inhibit nerve impulses to the skeletal muscles. Examples of toxins that prevent the release of acetylcholine are those that produce the paralysis of botulism and tick paralysis. Action at receptor sites is also blocked by the drug curare. Paralysis resulting from inhibition of cholinesterase release is caused by poisoning with organic phosphate insecticides.

Diseases of Muscles

Diseases of skeletal muscles can be inflammatory (such as polymyositis), the result of endocrine dysfunction (such as hypothyroidism and hyperthyroidism), or the result of congenital defects (e.g., absence of muscle, periodic paralysis, and the various muscular dystrophies [MDs] and myotonias). Inflammation occurs in a number of infectious illnesses such as trichinosis, toxoplasmosis, and those caused by the coxsackieviruses.

Diagnostic Tools

Several general diagnostic tools aid in differentiating diseases with similar manifestations. In addition, a number of more definitive tests are used to establish a specific diagnosis. The neurologic examination is a basic test that helps assess the extent of motor and sensory function.

The electromyogram (EMG) measures the electric potentials generated in individual muscles. A small metal disk is placed on the skin overlying the muscle to be tested, or a sterile needle electrode is inserted directly into the muscle. The electric activity generated in the skeletal muscles is measured at rest, with slight voluntary contraction, and with maximum contraction. The electric activity is amplified and displayed on a cathode ray oscilloscope. Needle electrodes are sensitive enough to pick up the activity of a single muscle fiber; thus this is usually the method of choice. However, the procedure is traumatic for children. It is often not useful because it requires cooperation. A topical anesthetic such as EMLA (eutectic mixture of local anesthetics) or LMX4 (4% lidocaine) applied to the EMG sites can decrease the amount of pain.

Nerve conduction velocity, or the velocity of electric impulse conduction along motor or sensory nerves, is often measured in conjunction with the EMG. Certain diseases affect the peripheral nerves, prolonging the conduction time from the point of stimulation of the nerve to the muscle and increasing the duration of the evoked potential of the muscle.

Muscle biopsy is the most useful laboratory examination to confirm and classify muscle disorders. The vastus lateralis is the most commonly sampled muscle. Procedural sedation may be accomplished with a number of medications used singly or in combination: midazolam and morphine; ketamine and midazolam; pentobarbital; etomidate; inhaled nitrous oxide; or midazolam and fentanyl. (See Surgical Procedures, Chapter 27.) Serum enzyme measurements are helpful in diagnosing and monitoring the course of muscular disease, but these are used as adjuncts in the diagnosis of most neuromuscular diseases. The intracellular enzyme creatine (phosphokinase) kinase (CK) is present in muscle tissues, including cardiac muscle, and the brain. It is released in large amounts in some muscular diseases, such as MD. CK is not elevated in neurogenic disease.

CEREBRAL PALSY

A new definition describes CP as a "group of permanent disorders of the development of movement and posture, causing activity limitation, that are attributed to nonprogressive disturbances that occurred in the developing fetal or infant brain" (Rosenbaum, Paneth, Leviton, et al, 2007). In addition to motor disorders, the condition often involves disturbances of sensation, perception, communication, cognition, and behavior; secondary musculoskeletal problems; and epilepsy (Rosenbaum, Paneth, Leviton, et al, 2007). The cause, clinical features, and course are variable and are characterized by abnormal muscle tone and coordination as the primary disturbances. It is the most common permanent physical disability of childhood, and the incidence is reported to range from 2.4 to 3.6 in 1000 live births in various studies in the United States (Hirtz, Thurman, Gwinn-Hardy, et al, 2007; Yeargin-Allsopp, Van Naarden Braun, Doernberg, et al, 2008). In the 1960s the prevalence of CP rose approximately 20%, which most likely reflected the improved survival of extremely low–birth-weight (ELBW) and very low–birth-weight (VLBW) infants. However, in the past two decades there has been a decrease in the incidence of CP among ELBW and VLBW infants (Hack and Costello, 2008).

Etiology

A variety of prenatal, perinatal, and postnatal factors contribute to the development of CP, singly or multifactorially (Box 40-1). The human brain undergoes development during the prenatal period and up to 2 years of age. A brain insult or injury occurring during this period may result in CP.

Although the prevalent traditional hypothesis has been that CP results from perinatal problems, especially birth asphyxia, it is now believed that CP results more often from existing *prenatal* brain abnormalities. However, the exact cause of these abnormalities remains unknown. It has been estimated that as many as 70% to 80% of the cases of CP are caused by unknown prenatal factors (Krigger, 2006). Intrauterine exposure to maternal chorioamnionitis is associated with an increased risk of CP in infants of normal birth weight and preterm infants (Hermansen and Hermansen, 2006); however, not all term infants exposed to chorioamnionitis develop CP (Grether, Nelson, Walsh, et al, 2003; Wu, Escobar, Grether, et al, 2003).

In general, infants exposed to maternal and perinatal infections are at increased risk for the development of CP as a result of the effects on the developing brain. Although CP occurs in term births, preterm birth of ELBW and VLBW infants continues to be the single most important risk factor for CP. Still, in some cases no identifiable cause is determined. Periventricular leukomalacia and intracerebral hemorrhage in low-birth-weight infants are significant risk factors in the development of CP. Perinatal ischemic stroke is also associated with a later diagnosis of CP (Golomb, Saha, Garg, et al, 2007). White matter abnormalities such as focal lesions are present in a large number of preterm infants subsequently diagnosed with CP (Johnston, 2007). Damage occurring as a result of shaken baby syndrome may also result in CP in survivors. Additional factors that may contribute to the development of CP postnatally include bacterial meningitis, viral encephalitis, motor vehicle accidents, and child abuse (Krigger, 2006). In summary, as many as 80% of the total cases of CP may be linked to a perinatal or neonatal brain lesion or brain maldevelopment, regardless of the cause (Krageloh-Mann and Cans, 2009).

A number of biochemical disorders may cause motor abnormalities often seen in CP and may be initially misdiagnosed as CP (Nehring, 2010).

Pathophysiology

It is difficult to establish a precise location of neurologic lesions on the basis of etiology or clinical signs because there is no characteristic pathologic picture. In some cases there are gross malformations of the brain. In others there may be evidence of vascular occlusion, atrophy, loss of neurons, and laminar degeneration that produce narrower gyri, wider sulci, and low brain weight. Anoxia appears to play the most significant role in the pathologic state of brain damage, which is often secondary to other causative mechanisms.

There are a few exceptions. In some cases the manifestations or etiology are related to anatomic areas. For example, CP associated with preterm birth is usually spastic diplegia caused by hypoxic infarction or hemorrhage with periventricular leukomalacia in the area adjacent to the lateral ventricles. The athetoid (extrapyramidal) type of CP is most likely to be associated with birth asphyxia but can also be caused by kernicterus and metabolic genetic disorders such as mitochondrial disorders and glutaricaciduria (Johnston, 2007). Hemiplegic (hemiparetic) CP is often associated with a focal cerebral infarction (stroke) secondary to an intrauterine or perinatal thromboembolism, usually a result of maternal thrombosis or hereditary clotting disorder (Johnston, 2007). Cerebral hypoplasia and, sometimes, severe neonatal hypoglycemia are related to ataxic CP. Generalized cortical and cerebral atrophy often cause severe quadriparesis with cognitive impairment and microcephaly.

Clinical Classification

A revision of the Winter classification was proposed in 2005 to reflect the child's actual clinical problems and their severity, an assessment of the child's physical and quality-of-life status across time, and long-term support needs (Bax, Goldstein, Rosenbaum, et al, 2005; Nehring, 2010). The proposed new definition has four major dimensions of classification (Bax, Goldstein, Rosenbaum, et al, 2005):

Motor abnormalities—Nature and typology of the motor disorder; functional motor abilities

Associated impairments—Seizures; hearing or vision impairment; attentional, behavioral, communicative, and/or cognitive deficits; oral motor and speech function

Anatomic and radiologic findings—Anatomic distribution or parts of the body affected by motor impairments or limitations; radiologic findings sometimes including white matter lesions or brain anomaly noted on com-

BOX 40-2	CLINICAL CLASSIFICATION OF CEREBRAL PALSY

Spastic (Pyramidal)

Characterized by persistent primitive reflexes, positive Babinski reflex, ankle clonus, exaggerated stretch reflexes, eventual development of contractures

Seventy percent to 80% of all cases of cerebral palsy (CP)

Diplegia—All extremities affected; lower more than upper (30% to 40% of spastic CP)

Tetraplegia—All four extremities involved: legs and trunk, mouth, pharynx, and tongue (10% to 15% of spastic CP)

Triplegia—Three limbs involved

Monoplegia—Only one limb involved

Hemiplegia—Motor dysfunction on one side of the body; upper extremity more affected than lower (20% to 30% of spastic CP)

Hypertonicity with poor control of posture, balance, and coordinated motion

Impairment of fine and gross motor skills

Dyskinetic (Nonspastic, Extrapyramidal)

Athetoid—Chorea (involuntary, irregular, jerking movements); characterized by slow, wormlike, writhing movements that usually involve the extremities, trunk, neck, facial muscles, and tongue

Dystonic—Slow, twisting movements of the trunk or extremities; abnormal posture

Involvement of the pharyngeal, laryngeal, and oral muscles causing drooling and dysarthria (imperfect speech articulation)

Ataxic (Nonspastic, Extrapyramidal)

Wide-based gait

Rapid, repetitive movements performed poorly

Disintegration of movements of the upper extremities when the child reaches for objects

Mixed Type

Combination of spastic CP and dyskinetic CP

May be labeled *mixed* when no specific motor pattern is dominant; however, this term losing favor to more precise descriptions of motor function and affected area of brain involved (Rosenbaum, Paneth, Leviton, et al, 2007)

Data from Nehring W: Cerebral palsy. In Allen PJ, Vessey JA, Schapiro NA (editors): *Primary care of the child with a chronic condition*, ed 5, St Louis, 2010, Mosby; Jones MW, Morgan E, Shelton JE, et al: Cerebral palsy: introduction and diagnosis, part 1, *J Pediatr Health Care* 21(3):146-152, 2007; and National Institute of Neurologic Disorders and Stroke: *Cerebral palsy: hope through research*, 2006, available at www.ninds.nih.gov/disorders/cerebral_palsy/detail_cerebral_palsy.htm (accessed July 9, 2007).

BOX 40-3	TYPES OF SPASTIC CEREBRAL PALSY

Hemiparesis—One side of body affected
- Most common form of spastic cerebral palsy
- Motor deficit usually greater in upper extremity; most children able to walk; underdevelopment of affected limbs
- Pattern of spasticity
  Leg—Increased tone of calf, hamstring, and hip adductor muscles
  Gait—Walk with foot inverted and plantar flexed, knee flexed, and leg adducted
  Arm—Increased tone in shoulder adductor and internal rotator muscles, elbow flexor and pronator muscles, and wrist and finger flexor muscles
- Parietal lobe syndrome—Impairment of cortical sensory function (absence or inability to recognize size, shape, or texture of objects held in affected hand); impaired two-point discrimination and position sense

Quadriparesis (or tetraparesis)—All four extremities involved; lower affected more than upper limbs
- Highest incidence of severe disability
- One fourth only mildly affected with minimum functional limitations on ambulation, self-care, and other activities; one half moderately impaired and handicapped in self-care and independent living capability; and one fourth severely damaged and require almost total care
- Delay in attaining developmental milestones proportionate to degree of motor deficit
- Speech dysarthric; swallowing possibly impaired; tongue protrusion incomplete
- In some children emotions more labile, with inappropriate laughing or crying

Diplegia—Similar parts on both sides of the body involved, such as both arms
- Spasticity in legs greater than in arms
- Late attainment of gross motor milestones, sitting, standing, and walking; development of hand skills generally appropriate for age

Monoplegia*—Involving only one extremity

Triplegia*—Involving three extremities

Paraplegia*—Pure cerebral paraplegia of lower extremities

*Rare occurrences.

puted tomography (CT) or magnetic resonance imaging (MRI)

Causation and timing—Identification of a clearly identified cause such as a postnatal event (e.g., meningitis, traumatic brain injury)

CP has four primary types of movement disorders: spastic, dyskinetic, ataxic, and mixed (Box 40-2) (Nehring, 2010). The most common clinical type, spastic CP, represents an upper motor neuron muscular weakness. See Box 40-3 for types of spastic CP. The reflex arc is intact, and the characteristic physical signs are increased stretch reflexes, increased muscle tone, and (often) weakness. Early neurologic manifestations are usually generalized hypotonia or decreased tone that lasts for a few weeks or may extend for months or even as long as a year.

Clinical Manifestations

The alert observer may suspect CP when a child demonstrates some of the following groups of manifestations (Box 40-3).

Delayed Gross Motor Development

Delayed gross motor development is a universal manifestation of CP. The child shows a delay in all motor accomplishments, and the discrepancy between motor ability and expected achievement tends to increase with successive developmental milestones as growth advances. It is especially significant if other developmental behaviors, such as language and personal-social achievement, are normal. Delayed development of the ability to balance may also slow the progression of milestones.

Abnormal Motor Performance

Neuromotor dysfunction is particularly evident in motor performance. An early sign is preferential unilateral hand use that may be apparent at approximately 6 months of age. Hand dominance does not normally develop until the preschool years. Abnormal crawling with propulsion by hand movements only and with lower extremities and hips hiked along, much like a "bunny hop," occurs in diplegia. Children with hemiplegia have an asymmetric crawl, using the unaffected arm and leg to propel themselves on either the buttocks or the abdomen. Spasticity may cause the child to stand or walk on the toes. Uncoordinated or involuntary movements are characteristic of dyskinetic CP, and facial grimacing and writhing movements of the tongue, fingers, and toes are signs of athetosis. Other significant signs of motor dysfunction are poor sucking and feeding difficulties, with persistent tongue thrust. Head staggering, tremor on reaching, and truncal ataxia are also common. Hand preference in the first 2 years of life is reported to be a sign of hemiplegic CP (Berker and Yalçin, 2008).

Alterations of Muscle Tone

Increased or decreased resistance to passive movements is a sign of abnormal muscle tone. The child may exhibit opisthotonic postures (exaggerated arching of the back) and may feel stiff on handling or dressing. Also, there is difficulty in diapering because of spasticity of the hip adductor muscles and lower extremities. When pulled to a sitting position, the child may extend the entire body and be rigid and unbending at the hip and knee joints. This is an early sign of spasticity.

Abnormal Posture

Children with spastic CP assume abnormal postures at rest or when their position is changed. From an early age, a child lying in a prone position will maintain the hips higher than the trunk with the legs and arms flexed or drawn under the body. In the supine position spasticity is evident by scissoring (legs in crossed position; knees, hips, and ankles stiff) and extension of the legs, with the feet plantar flexed. This posture is exaggerated when the child is suspended vertically or when others try to make the child bear weight. Depending on the degree of impairment, spasticity may be mild or severe. A persistent infantile resting and sleeping posture (i.e., arms abducted at shoulders, elbows flexed, and hands fisted) is a sign of spasticity when it remains constant after 4 to 5 months of age. The hemiparetic child may rest with the affected arm adducted and held against the torso, with the elbow pronated and slightly flexed and the hand closed.

Reflex Abnormalities

Persistence of primitive reflexes is one of the earliest clues to CP (e.g., obligatory tonic neck reflex at any age or nonobligatory persistence beyond 6 months of age, and the persistence or even hyperactivity of the Moro, plantar, and palmar grasp reflexes). Hyperreflexia, ankle clonus, and stretch reflexes can be elicited from many muscle groups on fast passive movements (e.g., resistance to passive abduction when the hips are suddenly separated [adductor catch]).

Associated Disabilities and Problems

Some of the disabilities associated with CP are visual impairment, hearing impairment, behavioral problems, communication and speech difficulties, seizures, and intellectual impairment. Additional sensory deficits such as hypersensitivity, hyposensitivity, and balance difficulties may occur in children with CP (Nehring, 2010).

Intellectual impairment is a concern, although children with CP have a wide range of intelligence and 50% to 60% are within normal limits. Speech difficulties are often interpreted as a sign of cognitive impairment. Assessing the intelligence of a child with CP is often difficult because of the motor and sensory deficits. Tests carried out periodically over time should determine the degree of intelligence. Many persons with CP who have severely limiting physical involvement actually have the least intellectual impairment. As a group, children with athetosis and ataxia are intellectually superior to those with other types of CP. The incidence of severe or profound impairment is highest in rigid, atonic, and quadriparetic CP.

The manifestations of attention deficit hyperactivity disorder may occur in children with CP. The primary presenting symptoms are poor attention span, marked distractibility, hyperactive behavior, and defects of integration. (See Chapter 18.) Seizures are more likely to accompany postnatally acquired hemiplegia. They are an unusual finding in ataxia and diplegia. The most common types of seizures are generalized tonic-clonic seizures and minor motor types (Nehring, 2010).

Poor control of oral musculature may contribute to a number of problems. Abnormal posture and motor performance and alterations in muscle tone affect chewing, swallowing, and talking. Occupational and speech-language therapy interventions may be necessary to assist some children with feeding and speech. Coughing and choking, especially while eating, may predispose the child with CP to aspiration, which may not be readily apparent. Respiratory problems may result from and coexist with feeding difficulties in children with CP; respiratory symptoms observed during feedings include apnea, dyspnea, tachypnea, coughing and choking, and hypoxemia (Nehring, 2010). Many children with CP may also have gastroesophageal reflux.

Motor impairment associated with CP contributes to other problems. Children with CP who are nonambulatory have an increased risk of developing orthopedic complications such as unilateral or bilateral hip dislocations, scoliosis, and joint contractures resulting from unbalanced muscle tone. A variety of factors, including decreased mobility, decreased fluid intake, a fear of toileting, poor positioning on the toilet, and lack of fiber intake may be responsible for constipation (Nehring, 2010). Stool softeners, laxatives, and a bowel management program may be required to prevent chronic constipation.

Increased incidence of dental caries results from (1) improper dental hygiene, (2) congenital enamel defects (hypoplasia of primary teeth), (3) high carbohydrate intake and retention, (4) dietary imbalance with poor nutritional intake, (5) inadequate fluoride, and (6) difficulty in mouth closure and drooling. Spastic or clonic movements can cause gagging or biting down on the toothbrush, thus interfering with cleaning techniques. Oral hypersensitivity is also common, which causes the child to resist dental hygiene. Malocclusion can occur in as many as 90% of these children. Gingivitis is secondary to inadequate dental hygiene and may be further complicated by the use of antiepileptic drugs (AEDs) such as phenytoin (Nehring, 2010).

Skin breakdown may occur with prolonged positioning, especially with underweight children with bony prominences and those who are unable to reposition themselves or who may have insensate areas of skin.

Nystagmus and amblyopia are common and may require surgery, corrective lenses, or both. Hearing impairment is also common in children with CP. Some loss is caused by sensorineural involvement. Affected infants may spend increased amounts of time lying flat. This predisposes them to otitis media, which may result in conductive hearing loss. (See Chapter 24.)

Diagnostic Evaluation

Infants at risk according to known etiologic factors associated with CP warrant careful assessment during early infancy to identify the signs of muscular dysfunction as early as possible. The neurologic examination and history are the primary modalities for diagnosis. Neuroimaging of the child with suspected brain abnormality and CP is now recommended for diagnostic assessment, with MRI being the preferred method to identify the lesions or abnormalities associated with CP (Ashwal, Russman, Blasco, et al, 2004). Metabolic and genetic testing is recommended if no structural abnormality is identified by neuroimaging; laboratory tests are no longer recommended in the diagnostic process for CP (Ashwal, Russman, Blasco, et al, 2004).

Early recognition is made more difficult by the lack of reliable neonatal neurologic signs. However, the nurse should monitor infants with known etiologic risk factors and evaluate them closely in the first 2 years of life. Box 40-4 lists some warning signs, but these are not diagnostic. Because cortical control of movement does not occur until later in infancy, motor impairment associated with voluntary control is usually not apparent until after 2 to 4 months of age at the earliest. More often the diagnosis cannot be confirmed until the age of 2 years because motor tone abnormalities may be indicative of another neuromuscular illness. In addition, some children who show signs consistent with CP before 2 years do not demonstrate such signs after 2 years (Nehring, 2010). However, there is no consensus regarding an age cut-off for the onset of symptoms (Ashwal, Russman, Blasco, et al, 2004).

Establishing a diagnosis may be easier with the persistence of primitive reflexes: (1) either the asymmetric tonic neck reflex or persistent Moro reflex (beyond 4 months of age), and (2) the crossed extensor reflex. The tonic neck reflex normally disappears between 4 and 6 months of age. An obligatory response is considered abnormal. This is elicited by turning the infant's head to one side and holding it there for 20 seconds. When a crying infant is unable to move from the asymmetric posturing of the tonic neck reflex, it is considered obligatory and an abnormal response. The crossed extensor reflex, which normally disappears by 4 months, is elicited by applying a noxious stimulus to the sole of one foot with the knee extended. Normally the contralateral foot responds with extensor, abduction, and then adduction movements. The possibility of CP is suggested if these reflexes occur after 4 months.

A number of assessment instruments are now available to evaluate muscle spasticity (Modified Ashworth Scale); functional independence in self-care, mobility, and cognition (Functional Independence Measure and WeeFIM [specific to children]); self-initiated movements over time (Gross Motor Function Measure); and capability and performance of functional activities in self-care, mobility, and social function (Pediatric Evaluation of Disability Inventory) (Krigger, 2006).

A thorough knowledge of normal variations of motor development is required for detecting abnormal progress, and a careful history is necessary to detect possible etiologic factors. Observe the child's spontaneous movements and behavior, including posture; attitude; and muscle size, function, and tone. Because children with CP often have sensory deficits, it is appropriate to evaluate the child for hearing and vision deficits.

Therapeutic Management: General Concepts

The goals of therapy for children with CP are early recognition and promotion of an optimum developmental course to enable affected children to attain their potential within the limits of their dysfunction. The disorder is permanent, and therapy is chiefly symptomatic and preventive.

The beneficial influences of a habilitation program on both child and family are based on recognizing the disability as early as possible and implementing treatment. Parents are essential to a treatment program. Consider their goals and desires, their cooperation, and their confidence in all aspects of management. With early diagnosis parents can begin to provide the sensorimotor experiences essential to cognitive development, since CNS structures depend on stimulation and use to attain and maintain their functional integrity.

The broad aims of therapy are to (1) establish locomotion, communication, and self-help; (2) gain optimum appearance and integration of motor functions; (3) correct associated defects as early and effectively as possible; (4) provide educational opportunities adapted to the individual child's needs and capabilities; and (5) promote socialization experiences with other affected and unaffected children. Each child is evaluated and managed on an individual basis. The plan of therapy may involve a variety of settings, facilities, and specially trained persons. The scope of the child's needs requires multidisciplinary planning and care coordination among professionals and the child's family (Box 40-5). The outcome for the child and family with CP is normalization and promotion of self-care activities that empower the child and family to achieve maximum potential.

Mobilizing Devices

Many children with CP wear ankle-foot orthoses (AFOs) (braces) and a variety of orthotics. Orthotics are molded to fit

---

BOX 40-4 POSSIBLE SIGNS OF CEREBRAL PALSY

Physical Signs
Poor head control after 3 months of age
Stiff or rigid arms or legs
Pushing away or arching back
Floppy or limp body posture
Cannot sit up without support by 8 months
Uses only one side of the body, or only the arms to crawl
Clenched hands after 3 months
Persistence of primitive reflexes such as Moro and atonic neck past 6 months
Hand preference demonstrated before 18 months
Leg scissoring
Seizures
Sensory impairment (hearing, vision)
After 6 months of age, persistent tongue thrusting

Behavioral Signs
Extreme irritability or crying
Feeding difficulties
Little interest in surroundings
Excessive sleeping

BOX 40-5 THERAPEUTIC INTERVENTIONS FOR CEREBRAL PALSY

Interdisciplinary developmental and physical assessment with recommendations may include the following:

Physical Therapy
Orthotic Devices
Braces
Splints
Casting
Molded orthoses

Adaptive Equipment
Scooters, bicycles, and tricycles
Wheelchairs
Boards
Standing devices

Occupational Therapy
Adaptive Equipment
Utensils for functional use (e.g., eating, writing)
Switches
Computers

Speech-Language Therapy
Oral-motor skills
Adaptive communication techniques

Special Education
Early intervention programs
Specialized learning programs and support services in school
Socialization to promote self-concept development

Surgical Intervention
Orthopedic (e.g., tendon transfers, muscle lengthening, spinal deformities)
Neurologic (e.g., neurectomies)
Selective dorsal rhizotomy
Feeding (e.g., gastrostomy)
Dental

Medication Therapy
Medications to treat:
• Spasticity
• Pain
• Secondary conditions (e.g., seizure disorder, chronic constipation, urinary tract infections, gastroesophageal reflux)
Primary care for health supervision and acute childhood illnesses

Behavioral Therapy
Functional (neuromuscular) electrical stimulation

Care Coordination
Care coordination of specialized services and community resources in collaboration with the child's family

Modified from Nehring WM: Cerebral palsy. In Jackson PL, Vessey JA, Schapiro NA, editors: *Primary care of the child with a chronic illness,* ed 5, St Louis, 2010, Mosby.

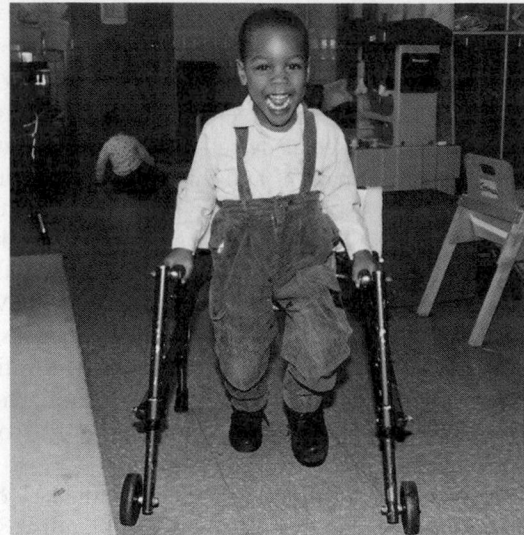

Fig. 40-2 Child ambulating with use of assistive device.

the feet and are worn inside the shoes. Devices are often used to help prevent or reduce deformity, increase the energy efficiency of gait, and control alignment. Some of the more commonly used mobility devices include wheeled scooter boards that allow children to propel themselves while the abdomen or total body is supported and the legs are positioned with wedges to prevent scissoring. Wheeled go-carts provide good sitting balance and serve as an early "wheelchair" experience for young children. Strollers can be equipped with custom seats for dependent mobilization. Special devices for independent mobilization that may or may not allow the upper extremities to remain free are particularly valuable for children with lower extremity involvement (Fig. 40-2). A number of wheelchairs can be customized to meet the needs and preferences of older children. (See Mobilization Devices, Chapter 39.)

Surgery

Surgical intervention is usually reserved for the child who does not respond to the more conservative measures such as orthotics, but it is also indicated for the child whose spasticity causes progressive deformities. Orthopedic surgery may be required to correct contracture or spastic deformities, to provide stability for an uncontrollable joint, to address bone malalignment (e.g., lever arm dysfunction), and to provide balanced muscle power. This includes tendon-lengthening procedures (especially heel-cord lengthening), release of spastic wrist flexor muscles, and correction of hip and adductor muscle spasticity or contracture to improve locomotion. Orthopedic surgery is generally not performed until after the child is 6 years of age (Nehring, 2010). Surgery is used primarily to improve function rather than for cosmetic purposes and is followed by physical therapy. Surgery may also be performed to improve feedings, correct gastroesophageal reflux disease, and correct associated dental problems (Nehring, 2010).

Neurosurgical procedures are used only in selected cases. Selective dorsal rhizotomy has provided marked improvement in some children with CP (Nordmark, Josenby, Lagergren, et al, 2008). However, achieving the benefits from the surgery requires intensive physical therapy and family commitment. Because the procedure results in flaccid muscles, the child must relearn to sit, stand, and walk.

Medication

Intense pain may occur with muscle spasms in patients with CP. Children with CP may also experience pain as a result of painful procedures such as injection with botulinum toxin type A (Botox), surgical procedures intended to reduce contracture deformities, abdominal pain related to position and gastroesophageal reflux, and pain associated with physical therapy (McKearnan, Kieckhefer, Engel, et al, 2004). Therefore pain management is an important aspect of the care of the child with CP.

Inhaled nitrous oxide or oral midazolam may be used for sedation during botulinum toxin A injections. In one study children who received inhaled nitrous oxide had fewer side effects than those receiving midazolam (Zier, Rivard, Krach, et al, 2008).

Pharmacologic agents given orally (dantrolene sodium [Dantrium], baclofen [Lioresal], and diazepam [Valium]) have had little effectiveness in improving muscle coordination in children with CP. However, they are effective in decreasing overall spasticity. The most common side effects of these agents include hepatotoxicity (dantrolene), drowsiness, fatigue, and muscle weakness. Less commonly, diaphoresis and constipation may occur with oral baclofen; other possible complications include hallucinations, mood changes, seizures, nausea, and urinary incontinence. Diazepam is used frequently but should be restricted to older children and adolescents.

Botulinum toxin A is also used to reduce spasticity in targeted muscles of the upper and lower extremities (Lukban, Rosales, and Dressler, 2009). Botulinum toxin A is injected into a selected muscle (commonly the quadriceps, gastrocnemius, or medial hamstrings), where it acts to inhibit the release of acetylcholine into a specific muscle group, thereby preventing muscle movement. When it is administered early in the course of the illness, this may prevent affected muscle contractures, particularly in lower extremities, thus avoiding surgical procedures with possible adverse effects. The goal is to allow stretching of the muscle as it relaxes and permits ambulation with an AFO. The major reported adverse effects of botulinum toxin A injection include pain at the injection site and a temporary weakness (Lukban, Rosales, and Dressler, 2009; Roscigno, 2002). Prime candidates for botulinum toxin A injections are children with spasticity confined to the lower extremities. The onset of action occurs within 24 to 72 hours, with a peak effect observed at 2 weeks and a duration of action of 3 to 6 months (Green, Greenberg, and Hurwitz, 2003).

The neurosurgical and pharmacologic approach to managing the spasticity associated with CP involves the implantation of a pump to infuse baclofen directly into the intrathecal space surrounding the spinal cord to provide relief of spasticity. High doses of oral baclofen are associated with significant side effects, including drowsiness and confusion, yet are often unable to provide adequate relief of spasticity. Direct infusion of baclofen into the intrathecal space provides relief without as many side effects (Krach, 2001).

Patients may be screened before pump placement by the infusion of a "test dose" of intrathecal baclofen delivered via a lumbar puncture. Close monitoring for side effects (hypotonia, somnolence, seizures, nausea, vomiting, headache, and catheter- or pump-related problems) (Albright, Gilmartin, Swift, et al, 2003) and relief of spasticity occurs for several hours after the infusion. If a positive effect occurs, the patient is considered a candidate for pump placement.

The pump is placed in the subcutaneous space of the midabdomen. An intrathecal catheter is tunneled from the lumbar area to the abdomen and connected to the pump. The pump is filled with baclofen and programmed to provide a set dose using a telemetry wand and a computer. The patient remains hospitalized for 3 to 7 days to adjust the dosage and ensure proper healing. Outpatient visits to refill the pump and make dosage adjustments occur about every 4 to 6 weeks, depending on the patient's response to the treatment. Benefits of intrathecal baclofen include fewer systemic side effects, dosage titration for maximizing effects, and reversibility of therapy with removal of the pump if so desired. Abrupt withdrawal of intrathecal baclofen, especially at high doses, may result in adverse effects such as rebound spasticity, pruritus, hyperthermia, rhabdomyolysis, disseminated intravascular coagulation, multiorgan failure, and death; in some cases intrathecal baclofen withdrawal may mimic sepsis (Zuckerbraun, Ferson, Albright, et al, 2004). Treatment of withdrawal centers on reestablishing the medication dosage, with improvements observed within 1 to 2 hours. Hospitalization and surgery may be required for withdrawal as a result of pump or catheter failure.

AEDs such as carbamazepine (Tegretol), divalproex (valproate sodium and valproic acid; Depakote), oxcarbazepine (Trileptal), and lamotrigine (Lamictal) are prescribed routinely for children who have seizures. Gabapentin (Neurontin) has been used in adults with SCI to decrease spasticity with success. No studies are available on the effectiveness of the drug in children (Krach, 2001). The α_2-adrenergic agonists clonidine (Catapres) and tizanidine (Zanaflex) have been used to decrease spasticity in adults with SCI and multiple sclerosis; however, their use in children does not appear to have gained widespread acceptance in the United States. Oral tizanidine given in conjunction with botulinum type A has been reported to be more effective than oral baclofen and botulinum type A in one study of children with CP (Dai, Wasay, and Awan, 2008). Monitor all medications for maintenance of therapeutic levels and avoidance of subtherapeutic or toxic levels.

QUALITY PATIENT OUTCOMES: Seizures
- No physical injury as a result of seizure activity
- Prevention of seizure activity

Children with CP have been treated with a number of complementary and alternative medicine strategies, including Chinese herbs, acupuncture, growth hormone therapy, aquatic exercise, equine-assisted therapy, and hyperbaric oxygen (Nehring, 2010). Gasalberti (2006) reported some alternative therapies being used in children with disabilities that the practitioner may overlook during a health history but that may be beneficial to such children. These include pet therapy, massage, hippotherapy (horse riding), music, and color-light therapy. Other alternative therapies that may be used by families with children with disabilities include vitamins, prayer, meditation, hypnosis, and guided imagery.

Technical Aids

A wide variety of technical aids are available to improve the functioning of children with CP. These include electromechanical toys that employ the concept of biofeedback and operate from a head unit. The toy is manipulated only when the head and trunk are in correct alignment. Computerized toys and games can also enhance eye-hand coordination.

Microcomputers combined with voice synthesizers help children with speech difficulties to "speak." These and other devices print messages onto screen monitors and paper. These devices have made it apparent that some children have been erroneously considered to be cognitively impaired. Microcomputers have also increased the possibilities for increased mobility via wheelchairs and specially designed mobilization devices.

Many other electronic devices allow independent functioning. Sensors can be activated and deactivated using a head-stick, a voluntary muscle such as the tongue, or any other voluntary muscle movement over which the child has control. (See Figs. 24-4 and 24-5.) The application of this technology makes it possible for older persons with CP to eventually function in their own apartments and can be extended into the workplace.

Associated Problems

Children with CP often have sensory deficits, which require the attention of appropriate specialists. Speech-language therapy involves the services of a speech-language pathologist (SLP) who may also assist with feeding problems. (See Chapter 24.) Dental care is especially important for children with CP and often is overlooked. Regular visits to the dentist and dental prophylaxis, including brushing, fluoride, and flossing (after several teeth are present), should begin as soon as the teeth erupt. This is especially important for children given phenytoin, who often develop gum hyperplasia. Additional problems common among children with CP include constipation caused by neurologic deficits and lack of exercise; poor bladder control and urinary retention; chronic respiratory tract infections and aspiration pneumonia, which occur as a result of gastroesophageal reflux, abnormal muscle tone, immobility, and altered positioning; and skin problems as a result of altered positioning, poor nutrition, and immobility. Hip dislocation occurs often in children with CP. Latex allergy has also been reported in children with CP (Nehring, 2010).

Therapeutic Management: Therapies, Education, Recreation

Physical Therapy

Physical therapy is one of the most commonly used treatment modalities in children with CP. In general, physical therapy is directed toward good skeletal alignment for the child with spasticity; training in purposeful acts, even in the face of involuntary motion, for the child with athetosis; and gait training and maximum development of proprioceptive sense for the child with ataxia.

An active therapy program involves the family, the physical therapist (PT), the occupational therapist (OT), and other members of the health care team. Developing a treatment program that can be carried out at home is of utmost importance. The major approach uses traditional types of therapeutic exercises that consist of stretching, passive, active, and resistive movements applied to specific muscle groups or joints to maintain or increase range of motion, strength, or endurance.

No therapeutic approach is able to achieve spectacular changes in the ultimate outcome of motor disability. Early efforts focus on alleviating abnormal postures by positioning and range-of-motion exercises. Passive range-of-motion exercises, stretching, and elongation exercises are valuable at any age, even when the child is too young to cooperate. Some active extension can be performed when the child is old enough to cooperate, with passive motion applied to complete joint extension. Prevention of contracture deformity is a prime function of physical therapy. Seating and mobility are other key goals.

Functional and Adaptive Training (Occupational Therapy)

Training in manual skills and activities of daily living (ADLs) proceeds along developmental lines and according to the child's functional level. Sitting, balancing, crawling, and walking are encouraged at appropriate ages and are accompanied by stimulation of protective extension and equilibrium reactions. Hand activities are begun early to improve motor function and provide the child with sensory experiences and information about the environment. As the child progresses from simple feeding and self-care activities, training is extended to include other tasks (e.g., cooking or use of keyboard or computer mouse) that are within the child's developmental and functional capabilities.

Incorporating play into the therapeutic program often requires great ingenuity and inventiveness from those involved in the child's care. Objects and toys are chosen to provide needed sensory input using a variety of shapes, forms, and textures. Nurses can help parents integrate therapy into play activities in natural ways.

Children with CP may need considerable help (and patience) in learning to feed and dress themselves and care for personal hygiene needs. A feeding program may be developed by an OT in conjunction with an SLP. Children should be fed in the normal eating position. When they have difficulty sucking and swallowing, it is tempting to hold them in a semireclining posture to make use of gravity flow. However, this method does not promote active swallowing, and the neck hyperextension may even interfere with swallowing. A more flexed sitting position, with the arms brought forward to decrease the tendency toward back and neck extension, is more natural during bottle- or spoon-feeding and encourages active swallowing.

Because jaw control is compromised, more normal control can be achieved if the feeder stabilizes the oral mechanism from the side or front of the face. When directed from the front, the middle finger of the nonfeeding hand is placed posterior to the bony portion of the chin, the thumb is placed below the bottom lip, and the index finger is placed parallel to the child's mandible (Fig. 40-3). Manual jaw control from the side assists with head control, correction of neck and trunk hyperextension, and jaw stabilization. The middle finger of the nonfeeding hand is placed posterior to the bony portion of the chin, the index finger is placed on the chin below the lower lip, and the thumb is placed obliquely across the cheek to provide lateral jaw stability (Fig. 40-4).

In all ADLs it is important to capitalize on the child's assets and compensate for liabilities. The level of expected independence is related to both gross and fine motor manipulation. Even when complete independence in a specific activity is not realistic, the child should learn any part of the task that he or

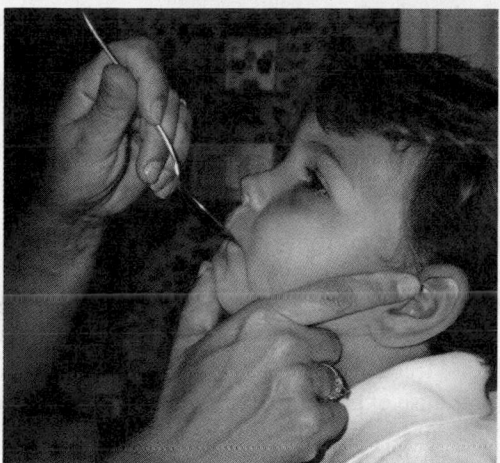

Fig. 40-3 Manual jaw control provided anteriorly.

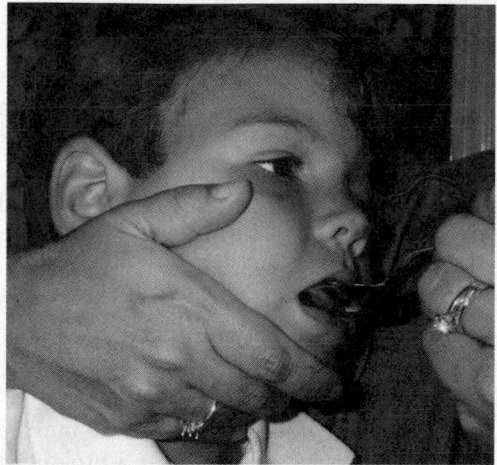

Fig. 40-4 Manual jaw control provided from the side.

she can master. However, motor function is not the sole purpose of learning to be as independent as possible. Any accomplishment promotes self-reliance and self-esteem for healthier personality development.

Speech Therapy

Speech training under the supervision of an SLP begins early, before the child learns poor habits of communication. Parents and others can help by following the directions of the speech therapist and by talking to the child slowly while using pictures or handling objects about which the adult is speaking. Feeding techniques such as forcing the child to use the lips and tongue in eating facilitate speech. An example of this technique is placing food at the side of the tongue, first one side, then the other; making the child use the lips to take food from a spoon rather than placing it directly on the tongue. If severe dysarthria prevents articulate speech and the child has reasonable intelligence, the child learns nonverbal communication (e.g., sign language). (See Chapter 24.)

Education

As in all aspects of care, educational requirements are determined by the child's needs and potential. This includes the severity of the child's disease and the presence and degree of associated conditions that affect learning and participation,

such as learning impairment, abnormal actions or behavior, impaired vision or hearing, and seizures. Children with mild to moderate involvement are generally able to participate, for varying amounts of time, in regular classes. Resource rooms are available in most schools to provide more individualized attention to a child's particular needs. Integration of these children into regular classrooms should be the initial goal. Teachers' assistants often work one-on-one with children in both settings. A training program may be appropriate for those children who are unable to benefit from formal education. Prevocational and vocational counseling and guidance are arranged at adolescence. Education is geared toward the child's assets at any phase or in any setting. Nurses should be aware of early intervention programs and provisions for special education and related services for children (see Box 24-3) and should support parents in their efforts to obtain appropriate educational services for the child.

Recreation

Recreational activities are also a necessary part of growing up. Recreational outlets and after-school activities should be an option for the child who is unable to participate in regular athletic and other peer activities. Some can compete in athletic and artistic endeavors, and many games and pastimes are suited to their capabilities. Sports, physical fitness, and recreation programs are encouraged for children with CP, and young children should be exposed to all physical activities available to children without disabilities. Individual sports such as the martial arts (e.g., TaeKwonDo) in which groups are small and the emphasis is on discipline and balance are also enjoyable to many children with CP. Many states mandate adaptive physical education classes.

Numerous developmental centers have facilities for indoor and outdoor activities designed to appeal to children of all ages. If these are not available, they should be developed. However, such programs require adequate supervision to avoid any harmful effects. Recreational activities serve to stimulate children's interest and curiosity, help them adjust to their disability, improve their functional abilities, and build self-esteem. Competitive sports are also becoming increasingly available to children with disabilities and offer an added dimension to physical activities. For more information access the United Cerebral Palsy website (**www.ucp.org**) and go to the Sports and Leisure link.

Prognosis

The prognosis for the child with CP depends largely on the type and severity of the condition. Children with mild to moderate involvement (85%) have the capability of achieving ambulation between the ages of 2 and 7 years (Berker and Yalçin, 2008). If the child does not achieve independent ambulation by this time, chances are poor for ambulation and independence. Approximately 30% to 50% of individuals with CP have significant cognitive impairments, and an even higher percentage have mild cognitive and learning deficits (Green, Greenberg, and Hurwitz, 2003; Liptak and Accardo, 2004). However, many children with severe spastic tetraplegic CP have normal intelligence. Individuals with CP and severe cognitive impairment had lower survival rates in an Australian study (Blair, Watson,

Badawi, et al, 2001). Growth is affected in children with spastic tetraplegia, and many children remain below the 5th percentile for age and sex.

As children with CP become adults, about 30% remain in the home and are cared for by a parent or caregiver; 50% of individuals with spastic tetraplegia live in independent settings and function at appropriate social levels considering their disability (Green, Greenberg, and Hurwitz, 2003). Vocational rehabilitation and higher education are possible for adults with CP. One study found that 53% of all persons with CP were able to work outside the home in regular jobs; one third of the severely disabled adults with CP worked outside the home (Murphy, Molnar, and Lankasky, 2000). Children with severe CP mobility impairment and feeding problems often succumb to respiratory tract infection in childhood. The few survival rate studies on children or adults with CP show that survival is influenced by existing comorbidities (Nehring, 2010).

> **QUALITY PATIENT OUTCOMES: Pain**
> - Acceptable pain threshold experienced as defined by patient or caregiver, or a pain score of 4 or less

Nursing Care Management

Assessment

Nursing assessment includes risk identification of infants with etiologic factors that are associated with CP. Ongoing assessment of infants for abnormal muscle tone, inability to achieve developmental milestones, and persistence of neonatal reflexes alert the nurse to investigate further.

Reinforce Therapeutic Plan and Assist in Normalization

Because children are being treated at an earlier age, parents are participating at an earlier stage in treatment programs for their disabled child. They learn the proper handling and home care of young children with CP and need carefully programmed steps so that their expanded parental role can be melded into the established relationship. Close work with other multidisciplinary team members is essential. Nurses reinforce the therapeutic plan and assist the family in devising and modifying equipment and activities to continue the therapy program in the home. (See also Chapter 24.)

Some children have difficulty keeping their heads upright. Because of this, they can neither explore much of their environment nor process the information. Parents need to be complimented on their efforts to provide a stimulating environment for these children. These infants are at risk for delayed development in holding up their heads, righting their shoulders and trunks for stable posture, sitting, pulling, standing, and crawling. Most parents of children with impaired movements benefit from support and practical suggestions for feeding, moving, holding, and encouraging the infant to explore hands and feet and to play. Helping parents incorporate therapeutic suggestions into typical daily activities is an important normalizing strategy. (See Chapter 22 for a discussion of normalization.)

Although practical advice is important, the nurse, OT, or PT should offer suggestions at a pace that can be absorbed by the parents. Encourage the parents to define their concerns,

acknowledge the concerns as genuine, and ask the parents what approach(es) they have tried and for how long. In this way the nurse is able to find out what works, what does not work, and what the parents would like to try next. Give the parents positive feedback for their observations of the infant, the progress they note, and how they differentiate the child's needs.

Address Health Maintenance Needs

Because children with CP expend so much energy in their efforts to accomplish ADLs, more frequent rest periods should be arranged to avoid the fatigue that may aggravate their limited capabilities. Meeting the child's nutritional needs may be a challenge because of gastroesophageal reflux, feeding and swallowing difficulties, chronic constipation and subsequent anorexia, and absence or diminished ability to independently feed himself or herself (Jones, Morgan, and Shelton, 2007). As a result of being ELBW or VLBW in combination with these feeding problems, children with CP are at risk for growth failure (failure to thrive), and the nurse must ensure an adequate caloric intake. Children with spasticity expend more energy and often require more energy intake than same age counterparts to maintain adequate growth. Nutritional supplements such as high-calorie milk products (e.g., Pediasure, Ensure, Boost) may be necessary to provide adequate caloric intake. Additional nutritional concerns include providing adequate intake of fruits and fiber to enhance gastrointestinal motility, routinely monitoring child's growth on a standardized growth chart, and avoiding overfeeding and obesity (Jones, Morgan, and Shelton, 2007).

Routine assessment of skin status is imperative in children with CP who are limited in movement or who must remain in assistive devices such as a wheelchair for a prolonged period. The overall nutritional status may also be a risk factor for skin breakdown. Care must be taken to ensure that adequate objective skin assessments are routinely performed. If skin breakdown does occur, consult a skin and wound specialist for treatment and further prevention.

Gastrostomy feedings may be necessary to supplement regular feedings and ensure adequate weight gain, particularly in children at risk for growth failure and chronic malnutrition, those with severe CP and subsequent oral feeding difficulties, and children whose well-being is affected by illness and decreased fluid or medication intake (Rogers, 2004). Oral feedings may be continued to maintain oral motor skills. Weight gain is perceived as an important measure of adequate oral feeding efficiency (Rogers, 2004).

Parents may need assistance and advice with medication administration through a gastrostomy tube to prevent clotting. Pills may be crushed and mixed with small amounts of water but not other liquids, such as formula or elixir medications, since these may act together to form a sludge that can interfere with gastrostomy tube function. When crushed pills or tablets are administered, flush the feeding tube with more water after instilling the dissolved pill in water. The pharmacist can provide information regarding crushed pills and tablets and elixirs, which should not be mixed together when administered via gastrostomy or nasogastric tube. A skin-level gastrostomy is particularly suited for the child with CP. (See also Gastrostomy Feeding, Chapter 27.)

Safety precautions are implemented, such as having children wear protective helmets if they are subject to falls or capable of injuring their heads on hard objects. Because the child with CP is at risk for altered proprioception and subsequent falls, parents should adapt the home and play environment to the child's particular needs to prevent bodily harm. Transportation of the child with motor problems and restricted mobility may be especially challenging for the family and child. Attention must be given to the child's safety when riding in a motor vehicle; a federally approved safety restraint should be used at all times. Lovette (2008) recommends that children with CP ride in a rear-facing position as long as possible because of their poor head, neck, and trunk control. This author also provides a list of options for special car restraint systems for children with CP, including several restraints that are suitable for children with a hip spica cast.

Appropriate immunizations should be administered to prevent childhood illnesses and protect against respiratory tract infections such as influenza. Depending on the level of involvement, dental problems may be more common in children with CP, which creates a need for meticulous attention to all aspects of dental care.

Support the Family

The nursing interventions that are probably most valuable to the family are support and help in coping with the emotional aspects of the chronic disorder, many of which are discussed in Chapter 22. Initially the parents need information and support in understanding the implications of the diagnosis and all the feelings it engenders. Later they need clarification regarding what they can expect from the child and from health care professionals. Educating families in the principles of family-centered care and parent-professional collaboration is essential. The family also may require help modifying the home environment for care of the child. (See Chapter 25.) Transportation to the practitioner's office and other health care agencies often requires special considerations.

Care management for the child and family with CP is an important nursing role. In many cases the family assumes complete care of the child and becomes quite adept at caring for her or his individual needs. The home health nurse or case manager has an important role in the support and encouragement of families who assume the primary care of a child with CP. Having a child with CP implies numerous problems of daily management and changes in family life, and the nurse can stress principles of normalization. (See Normalization, Chapter 22.)

The nurse can support the parents by acknowledging and addressing their concerns and frustrations and by noting and appreciating their problem-solving skills and their approaches to helping the child. Siblings of a child with a disability are also affected and may respond with overt or less evident behavioral problems. The family needs a relationship with nurses who can provide continued contact, support, and encouragement through the long process of habilitation.

Parents can also find help and support from parent groups, where they can share experiences, accomplishments, problems, and concerns while deriving comfort and practical information. For example, parents can understand from others what it is like to have a child with CP. United Cerebral Palsy* has branches in most communities and provides a variety of services for children and families.

Care of the Hospitalized Child

CP is not a disorder that requires hospitalization; therefore when children with CP are hospitalized, they are usually admitted for an associated illness or for corrective surgery.

To facilitate the care and management of hospitalized children with CP, the therapy program should be continued (insofar as their condition allows) while they are hospitalized. This should be incorporated into the multidisciplinary care plan, with every effort expended to make certain the ground that has been so laboriously gained is not lost. Encouraging the parent to room-in and actively participate in the child's care facilitates a continuation of the home therapy program and helps the child adjust to an unfamiliar environment. However, it is equally important to remember that a hospitalization may be the first time a parent can defer care to a nurse and not be the primary caregiver. This respite may be crucial to the parent's well-being. Respect the parent's preference in this regard (see Nursing Care Plan).

HYPOTONIA

Decreased muscle tone may be observed in the neonatal period and is one of the most common presenting symptoms in neuromuscular disorders. Hypotonia in neonates born before 37 weeks may be due to neuromuscular immaturity or perinatal maternal medications. (See also Chapter 10.) Monitor such infants over time for neuromuscular tone and make further evaluation if physiologic immaturity is not determined to be a contributing factor. Hypotonia may also indicate a variety of systemic conditions. Common causes are cerebral trauma or perinatal hypoxia, but most neuromuscular disorders with hypotonia as the presenting symptom, especially Down syndrome and infantile spinal muscular atrophy (SMA), are genetically determined.

Clinical Manifestations

Hypotonia is marked by diminished muscle tone and weakness in both spontaneous and passive motion and reflex testing. The affected infant, when placed in a supine position, assumes a characteristic "frog-leg posture" or lies in some other unusual position at rest. Normally the neonate or infant who is held in horizontal suspension (i.e., with the examiner's hand supporting the infant under the chest) responds by slightly raising the head with the back relatively straight, the arms flexed and slightly abducted, and the knees partly flexed. The hypotonic infant droops over the supporting hand with head and extremities hanging loosely, resembling an inverted U. The muscles feel atrophied when palpated, and there is marked head lag when the infant is pulled to a sitting position. Poor sucking may be noted. *Floppy infant syndrome* was the term traditionally used to describe infants with hypotonia.

*1660 L St., NW, Suite 700, Washington, DC 20036; 800-872-5827; fax: 202-776-0414; e-mail: info@ucp.org; **www.ucp.org**. The website also has links to each state's United Cerebral Palsy organization.

Diagnostic Evaluation

The infant with hypotonia presents a diagnostic challenge. The child's and family's history and the physical examination offer important clues to the general category of causes, such as central or motor neuron disorders. Laboratory diagnosis may include a CK level specific for skeletal muscle. Molecular deoxyribonucleic acid (DNA) analysis may eliminate the need for additional invasive tests when a definitive diagnosis is made for a hereditary myopathy or neuropathy (Sarnat, 2007). Nerve conduction velocity, EMG, and muscle biopsy may be used in diagnostic testing. Accurate diagnosis is essential for appropriate treatment, genetic implications, and family counseling.

Therapeutic and Nursing Care Management

The management of an infant with hypotonia is determined by the cause of the hypotonia. It is a nursing responsibility to record and report findings that suggest hypotonia in an infant so that further evaluation can be carried out and therapeutic measures implemented if indicated.

◎ NURSING CARE PLAN
The Child with Cerebral Palsy

NURSING DIAGNOSIS	PATIENT OUTCOMES	NURSING INTERVENTIONS	RATIONALE
Impaired Physical Mobility related to neuromuscular impairment	The infant or toddler will demonstrate active muscle movement.	Carry out and teach family to perform stretching exercises on affected muscles.	To prevent muscle contractures
Child's/Family's Defining Characteristics (Subjective and Objective Data)	The child will have adequate mobility to perform activities of daily living to maximum potential.	Use assistive devices such as wheelchair, ankle-foot orthoses (AFOs), and wrist splints.	To increase mobility and prevent contractures
Postural instability during performance of routine activities of daily living	**The Following NOC Concepts Apply to These Outcomes**	Administer medications (specify) intended to decrease muscle spasticity.	To minimize pain and decrease spasticity
Limited ability to perform gross motor skills	Body Mechanics Performance		
Limited range of motion	Ambulation: Wheelchair	Encourage and teach parent(s) to use jaw control during feedings.	To facilitate eating
Limited ability to perform fine motor skills	Joint Movement: Elbow, Wrist, Neck, Knee, Hip, Ankle	Position child semiupright during feedings.	To decrease chance of aspiration and facilitate mobilization of food and fluids through esophagus
Gait changes	Mobility		
Movement-induced tremor		Encourage play exercises that involve joint movement and promote fine and gross motor skill acquisition and repetition.	To promote joint movement
Persistence of primitive reflexes			To promote achievement of developmental milestones
		The Following NIC Concepts Apply to These Interventions	
		Exercise Therapy: Joint Mobility	
		Exercise Promotion: Stretching	
		Self-Care Assistance	

NURSING DIAGNOSIS	PATIENT OUTCOMES	NURSING INTERVENTIONS	RATIONALE
Risk for Injury related to mobility limitation, neuromuscular impairment, and perception and cognition impairment	Child will remain injury free. Home physical environment will be safe.	Educate family regarding child's physical limitations that place him or her at greater risk for injury.	To prevent accidental injury during mobilization
Child's/Family's Defining Characteristics (Subjective and Objective Data)	**The Following NOC Concepts Apply to These Outcomes**	Instruct family in steps to avoid injury: padded furniture, lowered bed or side rails as appropriate, gates on stairs, avoidance of throw rugs, thick carpeting.	To promote family involvement in injury prevention
Physical factors: altered mobility	Personal Safety Behavior		
Neuromuscular factors:	Falls Occurrence		
• Limited perception of danger		Position child in semiupright position after feedings.	To prevent aspiration
• Uncontrollable muscular movements		Use jaw support as needed during feedings.	To prevent choking
		Use appropriate mobilization devices and ensure they are safe for child's age.	To prevent muscle contractures
		Encourage mobilization and play activities that stretch muscles.	To promote personal safety
		Teach child which activities of daily living are safe and appropriate to perform without assistance of another person.	To promote self-care
		The Following NIC Concepts Apply to These Interventions	
		Risk Identification	
		Environmental Management: Safety	
		Surveillance: Safety	
		Physical Restraint	
		Parent Education: Childrearing, Family	

⊚ **NURSING CARE PLAN—cont'd**

The Child with Cerebral Palsy

NURSING DIAGNOSIS	PATIENT OUTCOMES	NURSING INTERVENTIONS	RATIONALE
Pain (chronic) related to involuntary muscle movements (spasticity) and treatments for muscle spasticity	Child's optimum comfort level will be maintained.	Administer medications to control spasticity (specify).	To prevent muscle spasm pain
Child's/Family's Defining Characteristics (Subjective and Objective Data)	**The Following NOC Concepts Apply to These Outcomes**	Perform stretching exercises after pain medication has been administered (60 minutes for oral medications).	To control pain impulses during exercises
Observed evidence of guarded behavior, grimace, crying, restlessness	Comfort Level	Administer pain medications (specify) such as nonsteroidal antiinflammatory drugs.	To minimize pain
Atrophy of involved muscle group	Pain: Disruptive Effects	For treatments such as botulinum toxin A (Botox) injections, assist with administration of appropriate pain medications and monitoring child for pain sensation (specify).	To decrease pain of injection at site
Altered ability to continue previous activities	Depression Level	For postoperative pain, administer pain medications on an around-the-clock schedule for 48 to 72 hours; use patient-controlled analgesia pump as child's cognitive and motor skills allow.	To promote personal physical comfort
		Use objective pain scale to assess pain level.	To provide objective measure of pain for intervention
		Encourage child to verbalize effects of pain on activities of daily living.	To provide outlet for frustration related to chronic pain experience
		Use assistive devices such as AFOs and knee-ankle-foot orthoses.	To decrease muscle spasticity and contractures.
		Teach parent(s) and child appropriate positions to assume while sitting and recumbent to minimize effects of muscle spasticity.	To promote self-care
		The Following NIC Concepts Apply to These Interventions Medication Administration Analgesic Administration Emotional Support Splinting Environmental Management: Comfort Exercise Promotion	

INFANTILE SPINAL MUSCULAR ATROPHY (WERDNIG-HOFFMANN DISEASE)

Progressive infantile SMA (Werdnig-Hoffmann disease), or SMA type 1, is a disorder characterized by progressive weakness and wasting of skeletal muscles caused by degeneration of anterior horn cells. It is inherited as an autosomal recessive trait and is the most common paralytic form of the floppy infant syndrome. The sites of the pathologic condition are the anterior horn cells of the spinal cord and the motor nuclei of the brainstem, but the primary effect is atrophy of skeletal muscles.

Clinical Manifestations

The age of onset is variable, but the earlier the onset, the more disseminated and severe the motor weakness. The disorder may be manifested early—often at birth or in utero—and almost always before 6 months of age; death may occur as a result of respiratory failure by age 2 years (Iannaccone and Burghes, 2002; Lunn and Wang, 2008). The manifestations (Box 40-6) and prognosis are categorized according to the age of onset, severity of weakness, and clinical course; some children may fluctuate between exhibiting symptoms of types 1 and 2 or

between types 2 and 3 in terms of clinical function (Sarnat, 2007). Some experts also categorize SMA according to the highest level of motor function (Lunn and Wang, 2008); type 1 would be "nonsitters," type 2 "sitters," and type 3 "walkers" (Iannaccone, 2007). A severe rare fetal form of SMA, classified as type 0, is reported to be lethal in the perinatal period (Sarnat, 2007).

Diagnostic Evaluation

The diagnosis is the molecular genetic marker for the survival motor neuron gene, which is located on chromosome 5q13. Prenatal diagnosis may be made by genetic analysis of circulating fetal cells in maternal blood (Beroud, Karliova, Bonnefont, et al, 2003) or circulating fetal cells in amniotic fluid. Maternal report of decreased fetal movements may also be suggestive of SMA (Markowitz, Tinkle, and Fischbeck, 2004). The risk of subsequent affected offspring in carriers of the mutant gene or in families with known cases of SMA may also be evaluated genetically. Further diagnostic studies include muscle EMG, which demonstrates a denervation pattern, and muscle biopsy; however, the genetic analysis has become the gold standard for diagnosis of the condition. Newborn screening is possible yet is

BOX 40-6 CLINICAL MANIFESTATIONS OF SPINAL MUSCULAR ATROPHY

Type 1 (Werdnig-Hoffmann Disease)
Clinical manifestations within first few weeks or months of life
Onset within 6 months of life
Inactivity the most prominent feature
Infant lying in a frog-leg position with legs externally rotated, abducted, and flexed at knees
Generalized weakness
Absent deep tendon reflexes
Limited movements of shoulder and arm muscles
Active movement usually limited to fingers and toes
Diaphragmatic breathing with sternal retractions (diaphragmatic paralysis may occur)
Abnormal tongue movements (at rest)
Weak cry and cough
Poor suck reflex
Tires quickly during feedings (if breast-fed, may lose weight before noticeable)
Failure to thrive (nutritional)
Alert facies
Normal sensation and intellect
Affected infants not able to sit alone, roll over, or walk
Early death possible from respiratory failure or infection

Type 2 (Intermediate Spinal Muscular Atrophy)
Onset before age 18 months
   Early—Weakness confined to arms and legs
   Later—Becomes generalized
Legs usually involved to greater extent than arms
Prominent pectus excavatum
Movements absent during complete relaxation or sleep
Some infants able to sit if placed in position, but few can ambulate
For most, life span varies from 7 months to 7 years, although many have normal life expectancy

Type 3 (Kugelberg-Welander Syndrome; Mild Spinal Muscular Atrophy)
Onset of symptoms after 18 months of age
Normal head control and ability to sit unassisted by 6 to 8 months of age
Thigh and hip muscles weak
Scoliosis common
Failure to walk a common presentation
In those who manage to walk:
- Waddling gait
- Genu recurvatum
- Protuberant abdomen
- Ambulation becoming increasingly difficult
- Confined to a wheelchair by second decade
Deep tendon reflexes may be present early but disappear

Type IV (Adult Spinal Muscular Atrophy)
Rare, adult-onset SMA usually in second or third decade of life; muscle weakness is first symptom.

NOTE: These classifications are general, but some research suggests there may be variations in life span and other characteristics (Iannaccone and Burghes, 2002; Russman, Iannaccone, Buncher, et al, 1992; Lunn and Wang, 2008; Russman, 1996).

not available on a widespread basis, possibly because there is no treatment (Lunn and Wang, 2008).

Therapeutic Management

There is no cure for the disease, and treatment is symptomatic and preventive, primarily preventing joint contractures and treating orthopedic problems, the most serious of which is scoliosis; hip subluxation and dislocation may also occur. Many children benefit from powered chairs, lifts, special pressure-adjustable mattresses, and accessible environmental controls. Muscle and joint contractures require careful attention and care to prevent further complications. Nutritional failure to thrive may occur in infants and toddlers as a result of poor feeding; supplemental gastrostomy feedings may be required to maintain adequate nutritional status and maintain weight gain (Iannaccone and Burghes, 2002). The use of lower extremity orthoses may assist with ambulation, but eventually the child may be confined to a wheelchair as muscle atrophy progresses.

Restrictive lung disease is the most serious complication of SMA (Iannaccone, 2007). Upper respiratory tract infections often occur and are treated with antibiotic therapy; they are the cause of death in many children. Sleep-disordered breathing is common in children with SMA and often requires noninvasive mechanical ventilation (Iannaccone and Burghes, 2002; Iannaccone, 2007). A polysomnogram may be performed to determine optimal therapeutic intervention with supplemental oxygen or noninvasive ventilation modes. Noninvasive ventilation methods such as bilevel positive airway pressure (BiPAP) have decreased the morbidity and increased the survival rate of children with SMA types 1 and 2. A significant number of infants with SMA require a tracheotomy, and associated medical conditions in survivors include gastroesophageal reflux, scoliosis, early-onset puberty, hip dysplasia, and recurrent oral candidiasis (Bach, 2007).

A number of clinical trials are currently in progress with existing drugs (e.g., valproic acid, phenylbutyrate, creatine) aimed at increasing the SMN mRNA and thus decreasing muscle wasting (Lunn and Wang, 2008).

Nursing Care Management

The infant or small child with progressive muscle weakness requires nursing care similar to that of the immobilized patient. However, the underlying goal of treatment is to assist the child and family in dealing with the illness while progressing toward a life of normalization within the child's capabilities.

Infants who are able to feed may require special nutritional considerations during breast- and bottle-feeding. Such infants tire easily and may be difficult to feed as a result of a weak suck and an unprotected airway, which cause choking and aspiration. Skin care needs must be addressed because the infant or child is not able to turn over and requires turning to prevent skin breakdown. A compromised nutritional status may further threaten skin integrity.

Preventing muscle and joint contractures, promoting independence in performance of ADLs, and incorporating the child into the mainstream of school when possible should be the focal points of care. In addition, parents need support and resources to be able to provide for the child and remain an intact family. Because children with neuromuscular disease have abnormal breathing patterns that often contribute to early death, it is important to ensure adequate ventilation and oxygenation, especially during sleep when breathing is shallow and hypoxemia may develop. Home pulse oximetry may be used to assess the child during sleep and provide supplemental oxygenation treatment as necessary (Young, Lowe, and Fitzgerald, 2007;

Bush, Fraser, and Jardine, 2005) (see section on Duchenne muscular dystrophy [DMD], later in this chapter, for respiratory management). Supportive care also includes management of orthoses and other orthopedic equipment as required.

Because children with SMA are intellectually normal, verbal, tactile, and auditory stimulation are important aspects of developmental care. Supporting them so that they can see the activities around them and transporting them in appropriate devices (e.g., wagon, power wheelchair) for a change of environment provide stimulation and a broader scope of contacts.

Children who are able to sit require proper support and attention to alignment to prevent deformities and other complications. Children who survive beyond infancy need attention to educational needs and opportunities for social interaction with other children. The parents of a child who is chronically ill require much support and encouragement.* (See Chapters 22 and 23.) Parents who have not sought genetic counseling should be encouraged to do so to evaluate further risk potential. (See Chapter 5.)

JUVENILE SPINAL MUSCULAR ATROPHY (KUGELBERG-WELANDER DISEASE)

Juvenile SMA (Kugelberg-Welander disease, or SMA type 3, juvenile proximal hereditary muscular atrophy) is also the result of anterior horn cell and motor nerve degeneration. The disease is characterized by a pattern of muscular weakness similar to that of infantile SMA. Several modes of inheritance have been reported for the disease: autosomal recessive, autosomal dominant, and a rare X-linked recessive form.

The onset occurs from younger than 1 year of age into adulthood, with symptoms resembling those of type 3 infantile SMA. Individuals with type 3 SMA may demonstrate a wide range of clinical symptoms (Lunn and Wang, 2008). Proximal muscle weakness (especially of the lower limbs) and muscular atrophy are the predominant features. The disease runs a slowly progressive course. Some children lose the ability to walk 8 to 9 years after the onset of symptoms, but many can still walk after 30 years or more. Many affected persons have a normal life expectancy (Iannaccone, 1998; Lunn and Wang, 2008).

Therapeutic and Nursing Care Management

Management is primarily symptomatic and supportive and related to maintaining mobility as long as possible, preventing complications, and providing child and family support. The discussion of family support in the section for DMD is also applicable to families of children with SMA.

GUILLAIN-BARRÉ SYNDROME

Guillain-Barré syndrome (GBS), also known as infectious polyneuritis, is an uncommon acute demyelinating polyneuropathy with a progressive, usually ascending flaccid paralysis. The hallmark of GBS is acute peripheral motor weakness. The paralysis usually occurs approximately 10 days after a nonspecific viral infection (Sarnat, 2007). Several subtypes of GBS include acute inflammatory demyelinating neuropathy, acute motor axonal neuropathy, acute motor sensory axonal neuropathy, and Miller Fisher syndrome. Children are less often affected than adults; among children, those between ages 4 and 10 years have higher susceptibility. The male/female ratio is reported to be 1.5:1. Two peak periods with an increased incidence of GBS have been identified: late adolescence and young adulthood.

Congenital GBS is rare yet may occur in the neonatal period and consists of hypotonia, weakness, and decreased or absent reflexes. Maternal neuromuscular disease may or may not be present. Diagnosis is established by the same criteria as in older children, but the symptoms gradually subside over the first few months of life and disappear by 12 months (Sarnat, 2007).

Concerns over the incidence of GBS in those vaccinated for swine influenza in the 1970s prompted a study of the incidence of influenza vaccine–associated GBS in adults. From 1990 through 2003 the incidence of vaccine-associated GBS in adults decreased significantly (fourfold) from 0.17 cases per 100,000 vaccines in 1993 to 1994 to 0.04 per 100,000 vaccines in 2002 to 2003 (Haber, DeStefano, Angulo, et al, 2004). Twenty-two cases of GBS were reported in adolescents ages 11 to 19 years who had received the meningococcal vaccine MCV4 between June 2005 and October 2007. The American Academy of Pediatrics (2009) indicates that there is no conclusive evidence of MCV4 causing GBS, yet suggests that children receive MPSV4 if they have had GBS. The Centers for Disease Control and Prevention notes that since the 1976 swine influenza–associated cases of GBS, there have been no significant increases noted in cases of GBS related to influenza vaccine administration (Fiore, Shay, Broder, et al, 2009). The Centers for Disease Control recommends influenza vaccination for all children ages 6 months to 18 years but cautions against vaccinating persons with GBS or those who have had GBS in the previous 6 weeks.

Pathophysiology

GBS is an immune-mediated disease often associated with a number of viral or bacterial infections or the administration of vaccines. It has been associated with infectious mononucleosis, measles, mumps, *Campylobacter jejuni* (gastroenteritis), cytomegalovirus, *Borrelia burgdorferi* (Lyme disease), Epstein-Barr virus, *Helicobacter pylori,* and *Mycoplasma* and *Pneumocystis* infections. Previous infection with *C. jejuni* is associated with a severe form of GBS.

Pathologic changes in spinal and cranial nerves consist of inflammation and edema with rapid, segmented demyelination and compression of nerve roots within the dural sheath. Nerve conduction is impaired, producing ascending partial or complete paralysis of muscles innervated by the involved nerves. GBS has three phases (Newswanger and Warren, 2004):

1. **Acute or progressive**—This phase begins with onset of symptoms and continues until new symptoms stop appearing or deterioration ceases; may last as long as 4 weeks.

---

*Family resources include Families of SMA, 925 Busse Road, Elk Grove Village, IL 60007; 800-886-1762; www.fsma.org. In Canada: Families of Spinal Muscular Atrophy Canada, PO Box 97, Rivers, Manitoba, Canada R0K 1X0; 800-866-0016; www.curesma.ca. Muscular Dystrophy Association–USA, 3300 E. Sunrise Drive, Tucson, AZ 85718; 800-572-1717; www.mda.org.

Critical Thinking Exercise—Guillain-Barré Syndrome

Animation—Guillain-Barré Syndrome

2. **Plateau**—Symptoms remain constant without further deterioration; may last from days to weeks.
3. **Recovery**—Patient begins to improve and progress to complete recovery; usually lasts a few weeks to a few months.

Clinical Manifestations

A mild influenza-like illness or sore throat usually precedes the paralytic manifestations of GBS. The onset can be rapid, reaching peak activity within 24 hours, or there may be a gradual progression of symptoms over days or weeks. Neurologic symptoms initially involve muscle tenderness that sometimes is accompanied by paresthesia and cramps. Proximal muscle weakness progressing to paralysis usually occurs before distal weakness, and there is a tendency toward symmetric involvement. In most patients paralysis ascends from the lower extremities, often involving the muscles of the trunk and upper extremities and those supplied by cranial nerves. The seventh cranial (facial) nerve is often affected.

Tendon reflexes are depressed or absent, and paralysis is flaccid. Paralysis may involve facial, extraocular, labial, lingual, pharyngeal, and laryngeal muscles. Evidence of intercostal and phrenic nerve involvement includes breathlessness in vocalizations and shallow, irregular respirations. There may be variable degrees of sensory impairment. Most patients complain of muscle tenderness or sensitivity to slight pressure. Lower limb pain and back pain are common in children with GBS. Urinary incontinence or retention and constipation are often present. Abdominal pain and fatigue have also been reported in children with GBS (Lyons, 2008).

Autonomic nervous system disturbances may occur in children and adolescents with severe muscle involvement and respiratory muscle paralysis. These include orthostatic hypotension; hypertension; and vagal responses such as bradycardia, asystole, and heart block (Laskowski-Jones, 2007).

Diagnostic Evaluation

Diagnosis is based on the paralytic manifestations and on EMG. Motor nerve conduction velocities are greatly reduced. Sensory nerve conduction time is often slowed. Cerebrospinal fluid analysis reveals an elevated protein concentration, and normal glucose level, but other laboratory studies are noncontributory. The symmetric nature of the paralysis helps differentiate this disorder from spinal paralytic poliomyelitis, which usually affects sporadic muscles.

Therapeutic Management

Treatment of GBS is primarily supportive. In the acute phase, patients are hospitalized because respiratory and pharyngeal involvement may require assisted ventilation, sometimes with a temporary tracheotomy. Treatment modalities include aggressive ventilatory support, intravenous (IV) administration of immunoglobulin (IVIG), and steroids; plasmapheresis and immunosuppressive drugs may also be used. Plasmapheresis has been shown to decrease the length of recovery in patients with severe GBS yet is expensive, and side effects include hypotension, fever, bleeding disorders, chills, urticaria, and bradycardia. Further evidence reports equal benefits to treatment of GBS with IVIG administration or plasmapheresis; both sped up

recovery time in studies reviewed (Hughes and Cornblath, 2005). There is evidence of significant improvement in children with IVIG therapy (versus supportive treatment alone), and IVIG therapy is more cost-effective than plasmapheresis (Harel and Schoenfeld, 2005; Hughes, Raphael, Swan, et al, 2006; Tsai, Wang, Liu, et al, 2007). IVIG is now recommended as the primary treatment of GBS when administered within 2 weeks of diseases onset (Hughes, 2008). Corticosteroids alone do not decrease the symptoms or shorten the duration of the disease.

Medications that may be administered during the acute phase include a low-molecular-weight heparin to prevent deep vein thrombosis (DVT), a mild laxative or stool softener to prevent constipation, pain medication such as acetaminophen, and a histamine-antagonist to prevent stress ulcer formation. Chronic neuropathic pain following GBS may be treated with gabapentin, which is reported to be more effective than carbamazepine (Sarnat, 2007).

Rehabilitation after the acute phase may involve physical therapy, occupational therapy, and speech therapy. Additional consideration should be given to problems of general weakness and retraining for toileting and feeding (Lyons, 2008).

Prognosis

Recovery usually begins within 2 to 3 weeks, and most patients regain full muscle strength. The recovery of muscle strength progresses in the reverse order of onset of paralysis, with lower extremity strength being the last to recover. There are few long-term outcome studies in children, but in one study 23% of the children had a residual weakness in at least one muscle group (Vajsar, Fehlings, and Stephens, 2003). Poor prognosis with subsequent residual effects in children is reportedly associated with cranial nerve involvement, extensive disability at time of presentation, and intubation (Sarnat, 2007).

The rate of recovery is usually related to the degree of involvement, which may extend from a few weeks to months. The greater the degree of paralysis, the longer the recovery phase.

Nursing Care Management

Nursing care is essentially supportive and is the same as that required for the child with immobilization and respiratory compromise. The emphasis of care is on close observation to assess the extent of paralysis and on prevention of complications, including aspiration, atelectasis, DVT, pressure ulcer, fear and anxiety, autonomic dysfunction, and pain.

During the acute phase of the disease the nurse should carefully observe the child's condition for possible difficulty in swallowing and respiratory involvement. Closely monitor the child's respiratory function, and keep the oxygen source, appropriate-sized insufflation bag and mask, endotracheal intubation and suctioning equipment, tracheotomy tray, and vasoconstrictor drugs available. Monitor vital signs frequently, including neurologic signs and level of consciousness. For the child who develops respiratory impairment, the care is the same as that for any child with respiratory distress requiring mechanical ventilation.

Respiratory care, should intubation be required, requires close monitoring of oxygenation status (usually by pulse oximetry and sometimes arterial blood gases), maintenance of an open airway with suctioning, and postural changes to prevent pneumonia. Children with oral and pharyngeal involvement may be fed via a nasogastric or gastrostomy tube to ensure adequate feeding. Immobilization, which occurs with GBS, decreases gastrointestinal function; therefore attention to problems such as decreased gastric emptying, constipation, and feeding residuals require nursing assessment and appropriate collaborative interventions. Temporary urinary catheterization may be required; urinary retention is not uncommon, and appropriate assessment of urinary output is vital. Sensory impairment and paralysis in the lower extremities make the child susceptible to skin breakdown; therefore attention should be given to meticulous skin care. Passive range-of-motion exercises and application of orthoses to prevent muscle contractures are important when paralysis is present. Prevention of DVT is accomplished with pneumatic compression (antiembolism) devices, administration of a low-molecular-weight heparin, and early mobilization and ambulation. Autonomic dysfunction may be life threatening; thus close monitoring of vital signs in the acute phase is essential.

A key to recovery in the child with GBS is the prevention of muscle and joint contractures, so passive range-of-motion exercises must be carried out routinely to maintain vital function. Although the child may have a generalized paralysis, cognitive function remains intact; therefore it is important for nursing care to involve communication with the child regarding procedures and treatments that may be frightening, especially if mechanical ventilation is required. Encourage parents to talk to the child and make eye and physical contact as much as possible to reassure the child during the illness.

Pain management is crucial in the care of children with GBS. Although neuromuscular impairment may make pain perception more difficult to accurately evaluate, use objective pain scales. Carbamazepine and gabapentin may be used to manage neuropathic pain in patients with GBS.

Physical therapy may be limited to passive range-of-motion exercises during the evolving phase of the disease. Later, as the disease stabilizes and recovery begins, an active physical therapy program is implemented to prevent contracture deformities and facilitate muscle recovery. This may include active exercise, gait training, and bracing.

Throughout the course of the illness, child and parent support is paramount. The usual rapidity of the paralysis and the long recovery period greatly tax the emotional reserves of all family members. The parents and child benefit from repeated reassurance that recovery is occurring and from realistic information regarding the possibility of permanent disability. In the event of a residual disability, the family needs assistance in accepting and adjusting to the loss of function. (See Chapter 22.) The GBS/CIDP Foundation International* is a nonprofit organization devoted to support, education, and research. It provides families with support from recovered persons, publishes informational literature and a newsletter, and maintains a list of practitioners experienced with the disease.

*The Holly Building, 104½ Forrest Ave., Narberth, PA 19072; 610-667-0131, 866-224-3301; http://gbs-cidp.org.

TETANUS

Tetanus, or lockjaw, is an acute, preventable, but sometimes fatal disease caused by an exotoxin produced by the anaerobic, spore-forming, gram-positive bacillus *Clostridium tetani*. It is characterized by painful muscular rigidity primarily involving the masseter and neck muscles. The development of tetanus has four requirements: (1) presence of tetanus spores or vegetative forms of the bacillus, (2) injury to the tissues, (3) wound conditions that encourage multiplication of the organism, and (4) a susceptible host.

Tetanus spores are found in soil, dust, and the intestinal tracts of humans and animals, especially herbivorous animals. The organisms are more prevalent in rural areas but are readily carried to urban areas by wind. They enter the body by way of wounds, particularly a puncture wound, burn, or crushed area. In the newborn, infection may occur through the umbilical cord, usually in situations in which infants are delivered in contaminated surroundings and the mother has not been properly immunized against tetanus. The disease has the greatest incidence during months in which persons are more involved in outdoor activities.

Prevention

Primary prevention is key and occurs through immunization and boosters (American Academy of Pediatrics, 2009). Once an injury has occurred, further preventive measures are based on the child's immune status and the nature of the injury. Specific prophylactic therapy after trauma is administration of either tetanus toxoid or tetanus antitoxin. A dose of tetanus toxoid is not necessary for clean, minor wounds in children who have completed the immunization series (see Chapter 12) or who have received a booster within the previous 10 years. Protective levels of antibody are maintained for at least 10 years. Therefore antitoxin is not indicated for the fully immunized child. Children with more serious wounds (e.g., contaminated, puncture, crush, or burn wounds) are given a tetanus toxoid booster prophylactically as soon as possible after injury.

The unprotected or inadequately immunized child who sustains a "tetanus-prone" wound (including wounds contaminated with dirt, feces, soil, and saliva; puncture wounds; avulsions; and wounds resulting from missiles, crushing, burns, and frostbite) should receive tetanus immunoglobulin (TIG). Concurrent administration of both TIG and tetanus toxoid at separate sites is recommended both to provide protection and to initiate the active immune process (American Academy of Pediatrics, 2009). Completion of active immunization is carried out according to the usual pattern. Proper surgical cleansing and débridement of contaminated wounds reduce the chance of infection.

Pathophysiology

When prevention efforts are not effective and conditions are favorable, the organisms multiply and form two exotoxins: (1) tetanospasmin, a potent toxin that affects the CNS to produce the clinical manifestations of the disease; and (2) tetanolysin, which appears to have no significance. The ideal conditions for growth of the organisms are devitalized tissues without access to air (e.g., puncture wounds); wounds that have not been washed or kept clean; and those that have crusted over, trapping pus beneath. The exotoxin appears to reach the CNS by way of either the neuron axons or the vascular system. The toxin becomes fixed on nerve cells of the brainstem and the anterior horn of the spinal cord. The toxin acts at the neuromuscular junction to produce muscular stiffness and to lower the threshold for reflex excitability.

The incubation period is 3 days to 3 weeks and averages 8 days. Most cases occur within 14 days; in neonates it is usually 5 to 14 days. Shorter incubation periods have been associated with more heavily contaminated wounds, more severe disease, and a worse prognosis (American Academy of Pediatrics, 2009).

Clinical Manifestations

There are several forms of the disease. Local tetanus is a less common but severe form characterized by persistent rigidity of muscles near the inoculation site, which may persist for weeks or months. Some cases resolve without sequelae. Neonatal tetanus results from contamination of the umbilical cord, which is rare in the United States but is common and often fatal in developing countries. The first symptom is difficulty in sucking, progressing to total inability to suck, excessive crying, irritability, and nuchal rigidity.

Generalized tetanus is the most common and dangerous form of the disease. The manner of onset varies, but the initial symptoms are usually a progressive stiffness and tenderness of the muscles in the neck and jaw. The characteristic difficulty in opening the mouth (**trismus**), which is caused by sustained contraction of the jaw-closing muscles, is evident early and gives the disease its common name, lockjaw. Spasm of facial muscles produces the so-called sardonic smile (**risus sardonicus**). Progressive involvement of the trunk muscles causes opisthotonos and a boardlike rigidity of abdominal and limb muscles. The patient has difficulty swallowing and is highly sensitive to external stimuli. The slightest noise, a gentle touch, or bright light triggers convulsive muscular contractions that last seconds to minutes. The paroxysmal contractions recur with increased frequency until they become almost continuous.

Mentation is unaffected; the patient remains alert, and pain and distress are reflected in a rapid pulse, sweating, and an anxious expression. Laryngospasm and tetany of respiratory muscles and accumulated secretions predispose the child to respiratory arrest, atelectasis, and pneumonia. Fever is usually absent or mild and generally indicates a poor prognosis. As the child recovers from the disease, the paroxysms become less frequent and gradually subside. Survival beyond 4 days usually indicates recovery, but complete recovery may take weeks.

Therapeutic Management

The unprotected or inadequately immunized child who sustains a "tetanus-prone" wound (as described above) should receive TIG. Concurrent administration of both TIG and tetanus toxoid at separate sites is recommended both to provide protection and to initiate the active immune process. Completion of active immunization is carried out according to the usual pattern (American Academy of Pediatrics, 2009). Antibiotic treatment with penicillin G (or erythromycin or tetracycline in older children with allergy to penicillin) is impor-

tant in the management of tetanus as an adjunct against clostridia (Arnon, 2007).

Aggressive supportive care is necessary to treat tetanus in the acute phase. The acutely ill child is best treated in an intensive care facility, where close and constant observation and equipment for monitoring and respiratory support are readily available.

General supportive care is indicated, including maintaining adequate airway and fluid and electrolyte balance, providing pain management, and ensuring adequate caloric intake. Indwelling oral or nasogastric feedings may be required to maintain adequate fluid and caloric intake; continued laryngospasm may necessitate total parenteral nutrition or gastrostomy feeding. Severe or recurrent laryngospasm or excessive secretions may require advanced airway management such as endotracheal intubation; in some cases a tracheotomy may be performed to provide an adequate airway.

TIG therapy to neutralize toxins is the most specific therapy for tetanus. In countries where TIG is not available, equine tetanus antitoxin (not available in the United States) should be administered. Antibiotics are administered to control the proliferation of the vegetative forms of the organism at the site of infection. When the child recovers, active immunization should take place, since contraction of the disease does not confer a permanent immunity. Standard Precautions for the child with tetanus are recommended; isolation is not recommended.

Local care of the wound by surgical débridement and cleansing with an antiseptic solution helps reduce the number of proliferating organisms at the site of injury. The cleansing should be repeated several times during the first 48 hours. Deep, infected lacerations are usually exposed and débrided.

Diazepam is the drug of choice for seizure control and muscle relaxation (Arnon, 2007), but lorazepam (Ativan) may be used in some cases. Other AEDs may be administered as well. Intrathecal baclofen, magnesium sulfate, dantrolene sodium, and midazolam may also be used in the management of tetanus; intrathecal baclofen may cause apnea and should only be used in the intensive care setting (Arnon, 2007). Patients with severe tetanus and those who do not respond to other muscle relaxants may require the administration of a neuromuscular blocking agent, such as rocuronium or vecuronium. Because of their paralytic effect on respiratory muscles, use of these drugs requires mechanical ventilation with endotracheal intubation or tracheotomy and constant cardiopulmonary monitoring. Endotracheal tube insertion or tracheotomy is often indicated and should be performed before severe respiratory distress develops. Despite the absence of pain manifestation with these drugs, it is important to administer adequate analgesia.

The administration of corticosteroids has met with success in some cases.

Nursing Care Management

The care of the child with tetanus requires supportive management with particular attention to airway and breathing. Carefully evaluate respiratory status for any signs of distress, and keep appropriate emergency equipment available at all times. The location and extent of muscle spasms and the assessment of their severity are important nursing observations. Muscle relaxants, opioids, and sedatives that may be prescribed can also cause respiratory depression; therefore assess the child for excessive CNS depression, apnea, and respiratory failure. At times it may be necessary to completely paralyze the child with a muscle relaxant because of the intensity of the muscle spasms. Attention to hydration and nutrition involves monitoring an IV infusion, monitoring nasogastric or gastrostomy feedings, providing oral hygiene, and suctioning oropharyngeal secretions when indicated.

In caring for the child with tetanus, make every effort to control or eliminate stimulation from sound, light, and touch. A quiet environment is desirable to reduce the amount of stimuli on the CNS. Although a darkened room is ideal, sufficient light is essential so the child can be carefully observed. Light appears to be less irritating than vibratory or auditory stimuli.

If a potent muscle relaxant such as rocuronium or vecuronium is used, total paralysis (including respirations) makes oral communication impossible. The drug is not a sedative, however, and anxiolysis should be considered in children who are intubated. Fentanyl and midazolam may be used to manage pain and anxiety in such children. The nurse must anticipate all of the child's needs and carefully explain the procedures beforehand to the child and family.

Additional care is focused on preventing the complications associated with prolonged immobility: decreased bowel and bladder tone and subsequent constipation, anorexia, DVT, pneumonia, and skin breakdown.

Because their mental status is often clear, intubated children are aware of what is happening to them and are often extremely anxious. Parents should stay with the child to offer security and support. They also need support, information, and reassurance from the nurse.

BOTULISM

Botulism is serious food poisoning that results from ingestion of the preformed toxin produced by the anaerobic bacillus *Clostridium botulinum*. Botulism toxin exerts its effect by inhibiting the release of acetylcholine at the neuromuscular junction, thereby impairing motor activity of the muscles innervated by the affected nerves. The disease has a wide variation in severity, from constipation to progressive sequential loss of neurologic function and respiratory failure. Human botulism is caused by neurotoxins A, B, E, and rarely F (American Academy of Pediatrics, 2009). Types A and B are the most common causes of infant botulism.

Types of Botulism

Several forms of botulism are recognized: food borne, infant, wound, man made (for bioterrorism), and botulism from undetermined causes. This chapter only covers the first three forms.

Food-Borne Botulism

This classic form of the disease usually occurs in adults but may occur in children and adolescents. The most common source of the toxin is improperly sterilized home-canned foods (see Community Focus box). CNS symptoms appear abruptly approximately 12 to 36 hours after ingestion of contaminated food and may or may not be preceded by acute digestive disturbance. Early symptoms include blurred vision, diplopia, weakness, dizziness, difficulty talking and speaking, vomiting, and dysphagia. These are followed by descending paralysis and dyspnea. Progressive respiratory paralysis is life threatening.

🏠 COMMUNITY FOCUS

Preventing Botulism

Home assessment and education regarding possible modes of infection (such as the use of honey as formula sweetener) are nursing responsibilities. Because the prime sources of food-borne botulism toxin are inadequately cooked or improperly canned food, families are advised about the danger of home-canned foods, especially vegetables, fruits, fish, and condiments. Boiling is not always adequate, particularly at high altitudes, where water boils at a lower temperature, which does not destroy the organisms. Encourage parents to avoid giving honey to infants less than 12 months old.

Infant Botulism

Infant botulism, unlike the disease in older persons, is caused by ingestion of spores or vegetative cells of *C. botulinum* and the subsequent release of the toxin from organisms colonizing the gastrointestinal tract. *C. botulinum* types A and B are the most common causative strains of infant botulism. This form of botulism has become more prevalent than any other form. Many cases of infant botulism occur in breast-fed infants who are being introduced to nonhuman milk substances (American Academy of Pediatrics, 2009). There appears to be no common food or drug source of the organisms; however, the *C. botulinum* organisms have been found in honey. Botulism may occur in infants from 1 week to 12 months of age, with peak incidence between 2 and 4 months of age.

The severity of the disease varies widely, from mild constipation to progressive sequential loss of neurologic function and respiratory failure. The affected infant is usually well before the onset of symptoms. Constipation is a common presenting symptom, and almost all infants exhibit generalized weakness and a decrease in spontaneous movements. Deep tendon reflexes are usually diminished or absent. Cranial nerve deficits are common, as evidenced by loss of head control, difficulty in feeding, weak cry, and reduced gag reflex. SMA type 1 and metabolic disorders are often mistaken for infant botulism in the initial diagnostic phase because of the similarities in clinical manifestations of hypotonia, lethargy, and poor feeding (Francisco and Arnon, 2007). Presenting clinical signs also often mimic those of sepsis in young infants. Botulism toxin exerts its effect by inhibiting the release of acetylcholine at the myoneural junction, thereby impairing motor activity of muscles innervated by affected nerves.

Wound Botulism

Wounds contaminated with *C. botulinum* and subsequent elaboration of the toxin produce classic symptoms approximately 4 to 14 days after tissue trauma. The disease has been described in a small number of adolescents and adults, and most wounds are sustained in open fields or on farms.

Diagnosis and Therapeutic Management

Diagnosis is made on the basis of the clinical history, physical examination, and laboratory detection of the organism in the patient's stool and, less commonly, blood. However, isolation of the organism may take several days; therefore suspicion of botulism by clinical presentation should require emergent treatment (Arnon, 2007). EMG may be helpful in establishing the diagnosis; however, results may be normal early in the course of the illness.

Treatment consists of immediate administration of botulism immune globulin intravenously (BIG-IV [BabyBIG]) (Francisco and Arnon, 2007), without waiting for laboratory diagnosis. Early administration of BIG-IV neutralizes the toxin and stops the progression of the disease. The human-derived botulism antitoxin (BIG-IV) has been evaluated and is now available nationwide for use only in infant botulism. In one study infants treated with BIG-IV experienced a mean length of hospitalization decrease from 5.7 to 2.6 weeks and also had decreased time spent in intensive care, decreased mean duration of mechanical ventilation, and decreased mean duration of tube or IV feeding. In addition, the infants did not experience any adverse events related to BIG-IV. Most infants received BIG-IV treatment within 3 to 18 days of hospitalization for botulism (Arnon, Schechter, Maslanka, et al, 2006). Studies indicate that treatment with BIG-IV decreased length of hospital stay in affected infants an average of 17 days; infants with botulism requiring mechanical ventilation also had shorter hospitalizations when treated with BIG-IV (Thompson, Filloux, Van Orman, et al, 2005). Potential complications of BIG-IV include hypotension and anaphylaxis (Cirillo, 2008).

Approximately 50% of affected infants require intubation and mechanical ventilation; therefore respiratory support is crucial, as is nutritional support, since the infant is unable to feed. Trivalent equine botulinum antitoxin and bivalent antitoxin, used in adults and older children, is not administered to infants. Antibiotic therapy is not part of the management because the botulinum toxin is an intracellular molecule and antibiotics would not be effective; aminoglycosides in particular should not be administered because they may potentiate the blocking effects of the neurotoxin (Arnon, 2007).

The prognosis is generally good if the patient is adequately treated, although recovery may be slow, requiring a few weeks after severe illness. The average length of stay for infant botulism is 44 days, and the fatality rate is reported to be less than 2%. Untreated patients may require a longer hospitalization.

Nursing Care Management

Nursing responsibilities include observing, recognizing, and reporting signs of poor feeding, constipation, and muscle impairment in the infant with botulism and providing intensive nursing care when an infant is hospitalized. (See Nursing Care Management for the infant with SMA, p. 1704, and Nursing Care of High-Risk Newborns, Chapter 10.) Parental support and reassurance are important. Most infants recover when the disorder is recognized and BIG-IV therapy is implemented. Nursing care of the infant on mechanical ventilation requires observation of oxygenation status and vigilance for any complications. Parents should be aware that, during recovery, infants fatigue easily when muscular action is sustained. This has important implications for timing the resumption of feedings because of the risk of aspiration. They should also be advised that normal bowel activity may not return for several weeks. Therefore a stool softener can be beneficial.

MYASTHENIA GRAVIS

Myasthenia gravis (MG) is relatively uncommon in childhood. The incidence in children under 18 years is 1 per 1 million in North America (Cirillo, 2008). Juvenile MG appears to be identical to that seen in adults and usually has its onset after age 10 years, but it may appear as early as age 2 years. Girls are affected three times more than boys. Juvenile and adult forms of the disease are autoimmune disorders associated with the attack of circulating antibodies on the acetylcholine receptors on the muscle end plate, which blocks their function.

Clinical Manifestations

The most common symptoms are general paralysis of the optic muscles with ptosis and diplopia. Difficulty swallowing, chewing, and speaking are also prominent and are accompanied by weakness and paralysis of all skeletal muscles. The signs and symptoms are more pronounced in the late afternoon and evening. Rest can help relieve the symptoms, but exercise and stress worsen them.

Diagnostic Evaluation

The diagnosis is made on the basis of the characteristic distribution of muscle weakness and the progressive weakness on repeated or sustained muscular contraction. The definitive diagnosis is established on the basis of an EMG, which demonstrates a decrease in muscle potentials with repetitive nerve stimulation (Sarnat, 2007). A clinical diagnosis may be established by observation of the response to the anticholinesterase drugs. IV administration of a small test dose of edrophonium (Tensilon) produces a beneficial effect in 1 minute, but the effect lasts less than 5 minutes. Electrophysiologic studies are helpful in diagnosis and help document transmission failure at the neuromuscular junction. Antibodies to human muscle acetylcholine are detected in the serum of almost one third of affected individuals.

Therapeutic Management

Treatment consists of the administration of cholinesterase-inhibiting drugs, such as neostigmine (Prostigmin), given intramuscularly or as oral neostigmine bromide. Pyridostigmine (Mestinon) may be administered because it is considered less toxic, but a higher dose is required to achieve the same results as neostigmine. The starting dosage of neostigmine is usually 0.04 mg/kg, administered intramuscularly every 4 to 6 hours; oral doses may be well tolerated (Sarnat, 2007). The dosage is gradually increased until a satisfactory result is obtained. The child must be observed for signs of parasympathetic stimulation from overmedication. These signs include lacrimation, salivation, abdominal cramps, sweating, diarrhea, vomiting, bradycardia, and weakness of respiratory muscles.

Other therapies directed at the immunologic mechanism include thymectomy (removal of the thymus), IVIG, long-term corticosteroid treatment, and plasmapheresis. Thymectomy may be curative for some individuals, but is not effective for familial and congenital forms of MG.

⚡ **DRUG ALERT**

Atropine Sulfate

Atropine sulfate (0.01 mg/kg) is the antidote for neostigmine and pyridostigmine.

⚡ **DRUG ALERT**

Neuromuscular-Blocking Agents

Avoid neuromuscular-blocking agents such as pancuronium or succinylcholine in patients with MG because they may induce paralysis that can last for weeks. Avoid aminoglycoside antibiotics such as gentamicin because they potentiate MG symptoms (Sarnat, 2007).

The prognosis for juvenile MG is relatively good. However, the course of the disease is marked by fluctuating remissions and exacerbations.

Nursing Care Management

Children with MG need ongoing medical and nursing supervision. Teach the parents the importance of accurate administration of medications, with special emphasis on recognizing side effects, including the dangers of choking, aspiration, and respiratory distress.

Counsel parents to promote a lifestyle that minimizes stress and maximizes relaxation. Discourage strenuous activity. Also warn them of the possibility of a sudden exacerbation of symptoms during times of physical or emotional stress (myasthenia crisis), which requires immediate medical attention. They should receive instruction in providing respiratory assistance until help arrives or the child can be transported to medical aid.

Neonatal Myasthenia Gravis

A transient form of MG occurs in approximately 10% to 20% of infants born to mothers with MG, who may not know they have the disease. The muscular weakness results from transplacentally acquired maternal acetylcholine receptor antibodies. These infants display generalized muscular weakness and hypotonia at birth with a depressed Moro reflex, ptosis, ineffective sucking and swallowing reflexes, and weak cry. Some infants may require short-term mechanical ventilation (Sarnat, 2007). Symptoms may be evident within a few hours of birth, following a period of normal appearance after delivery. There is no evidence of neurologic damage. Cholinesterase inhibitors may be given on a short-term basis to improve feeding ability. Symptoms usually disappear within 2 to 3 weeks. Infants with transient neonatal MG regain strength once maternal antibodies clear the system, and they are not at increased risk of MG later in life (Cirillo, 2008; Sarnat, 2007).

Congenital Myasthenia Gravis

Congenital MG is a rare familial abnormality of neuromuscular transmission that is not immunologically mediated. It appears indistinguishable from the transient form, but the mother usually does not have the disease. The disease persists throughout life, and more than one sibling may be affected, which suggests a genetic etiology. Gender distribution is equal. The disorder is relatively resistant to drug therapy, and the eyelid and extraocular muscles seem to be the muscles most severely affected.

The prognosis in congenital MG is usually good. Despite gradual worsening of symptoms with age, the life span is not affected significantly.

SPINAL CORD INJURIES

SCIs with major neurologic involvement are not a common cause of physical disability in children. However, many children with these injuries are admitted to major medical centers, and because of the increased survival rate as a result of improved management, nurses have an important role in the care of children with SCI.

The principles of management and nursing care of the child with a spinal cord lesion apply regardless of cause. In addition to care related to the immobilized child, as discussed in Chapter 39, children with damage to the spinal cord present additional problems—specifically, complications related to the neuropathology of the central and autonomic nervous systems. The extent of paralysis is determined by both neurologic and clinical assessment. Although the majority of children with SCI are paraplegic, some are tetraplegic (quadriplegic). Some children with tetraplegia are able to move only their face and neck muscles, whereas others are able to lift and bend their arms but are unable to perform fine hand movements. Almost every physiologic system is disrupted in a child with high-level tetraplegia. Not only are the central and peripheral nerves impaired, but there is also autonomic nervous system dysfunction. Vital structures such as blood vessels, lungs, bladder, and bowel are affected. Therefore an understanding of neuromuscular physiology is essential to effectively care for the child with damage or injury to the spinal cord.

More males than females experience SCI as children. Cirak, Ziegfeld, Knight, and colleagues (2004) found that the mean age of children with SCI was 9.48 years. Motor vehicle crashes (MVCs) accounted for the majority of infants injured, whereas toddlers and school-aged children up to 9 years were more likely to suffer SCI as a result of a fall. Almost one half (46%) of the pediatric injuries in this study were high cervical injuries. In the United States football injuries accounted for a high percentage of sport-related injuries in adolescents, whereas in Canada such injuries were associated with ice hockey (Mathison, Kadom, and Krug, 2008).

Essential Neuromuscular Physiology

The spinal cord extends from the medulla oblongata to the lower border of the first lumbar vertebra and contains millions of nerve fibers. However, because of its protected location, a considerable amount of direct trauma is required to cause injury. Posteriorly the cord is protected by the spinous processes, which are stabilized by related ligaments and muscles. It is further protected by the spinal fluid, which surrounds it and absorbs some of the shock.

Spinal Nerves

The 31 nerves of the spinal cord are divided into five segments (Fig. 40-5). The cervical cord segments lie within the first seven

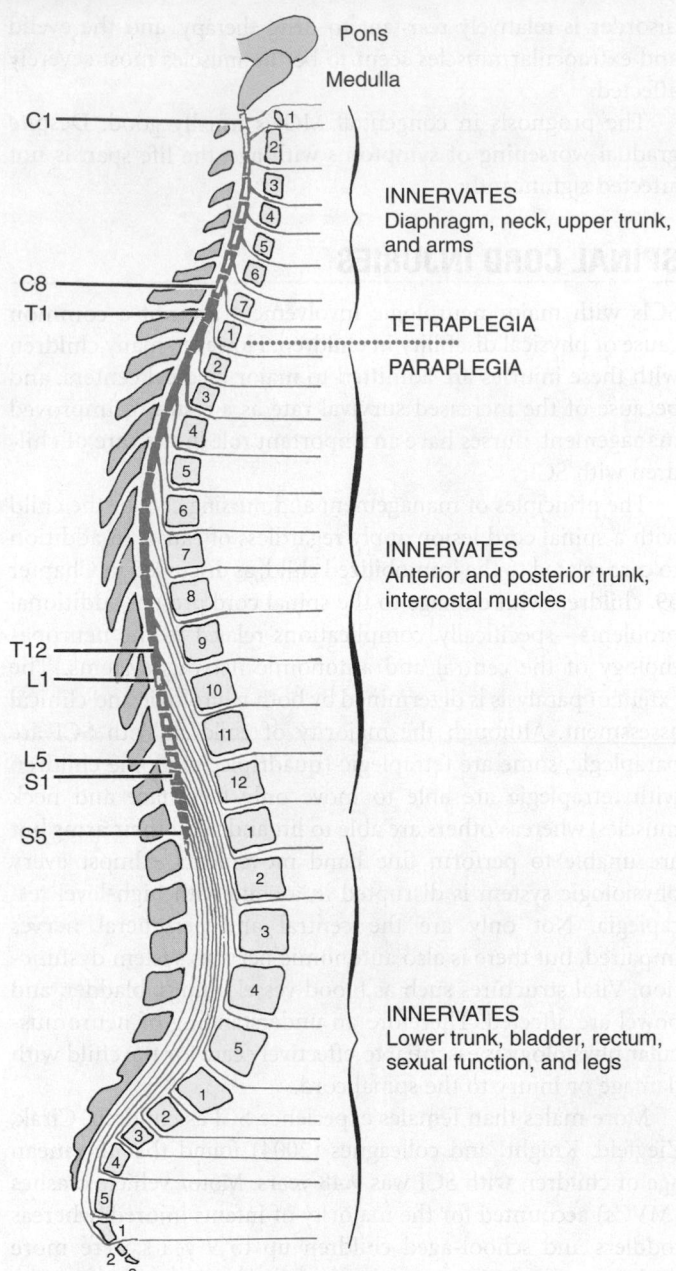

Fig. 40-5 Relationships of spinal cord segments and spinal nerves to vertebral bodies. Cervical nerves exit through intervertebral foramina above their respective vertebral bodies (seven cervical vertebrae and eight cervical nerves). Spinal cord ends at L1-L2 vertebral level.

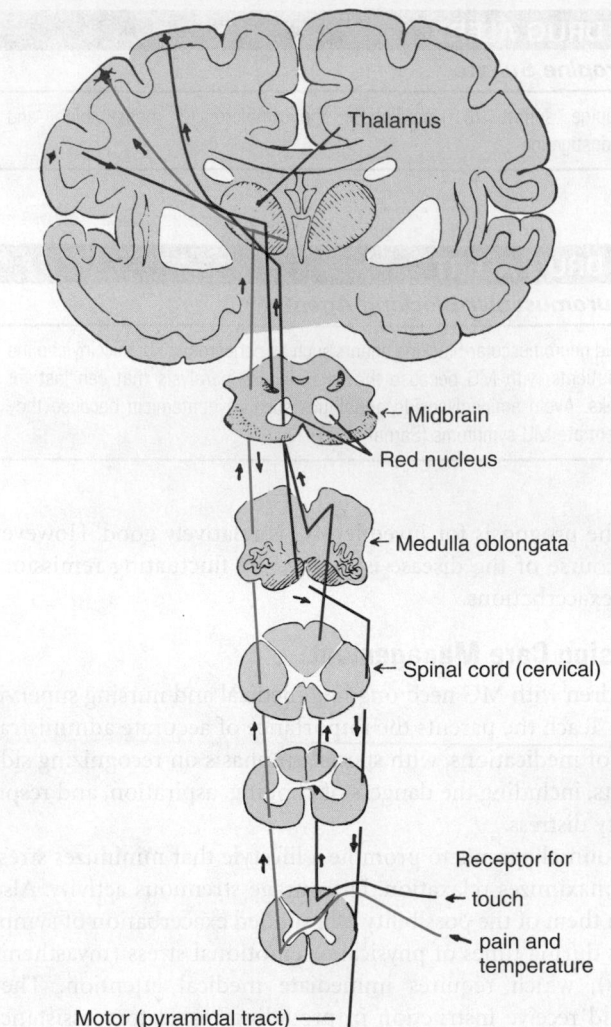

Fig. 40-6 Main motor and sensory pathways. Perception of touch, passive motion, position, and vibration is transmitted through posterior tract in spinal cord through medial lemniscus in brainstem to thalamus and through internal capsule to cortex (pathway is represented by *solid red line*). Pain and temperature sensations are transmitted through anterolateral tract and lateral lemniscus to thalamus, then through internal capsule to cortex *(blue line)*. Motor impulses are transmitted by pyramidal tract, descending from cerebral cortex, crossing in medulla to opposite side, and continuing to anterior horns of spinal cord *(black line)*. (From Conway BL: *Carini and Owens' neurological and neurosurgical nursing*, ed 7, St Louis, 1978, Mosby.)

vertebrae. The remaining cord segments—thoracic (12), lumbar (5), sacral (5), and coccygeal (1)—extend from the first thoracic vertebra to the lower level of the first lumbar vertebra. Therefore the cord constituents do not anatomically match by number the 33 associated vertebrae. However, nerves that arise from the spinal cord exit from the spinal column at the numerically corresponding vertebrae. In describing injuries to the spinal cord, the highest point at which there is normal function is referred to in relation to the vertebra; for example, an intact cord at the sixth cervical vertebra is designated a C6 injury.

Certain areas of the curved vertebral column are less stable and more prone to damage from severe flexion and twisting. These sites are the cervical area and the junction of the thoracic and lumbar regions. The cervical vertebrae are fractured most

often, and this high level of injury causes extensive paralysis and many associated neurologic problems (Table 40-1). Also, traumatic tearing or embolic occlusion of the arteries supplying these areas can markedly jeopardize the cord tissue. Impaired blood supply often produces severe neurologic deficit, which can extend to complete loss of cord function at the level of injury.

Cell bodies of interneurons and motor neurons within the spinal cord are identified as H-shaped gray matter surrounded by columns of white myelinated nerve fibers. Each column serves as a route for a specific type of impulse, such as touch, vibration, pain, and temperature (Fig. 40-6). Nerve pathways in the spinal cord transmit sensory and motor impulses between peripheral receptors and the brain, conduct impulses

TABLE 40-1	FUNCTIONAL SIGNIFICANCE OF SPINAL CORD LESIONS		
HIGHEST INTACT CORD SEGMENT	**MUSCLE INNERVATION**	**FUNCTIONAL CAPACITY**	**FUNCTIONAL GOALS**
Tetraplegia			
C1-C3	None below chin, including phrenic nerve to diaphragm	No voluntary control below chin Respiratory paralysis complete May cause bradycardia or tachycardia, vomiting	Mechanical ventilation; can be taught glossopharyngeal breathing to be used for short periods Electric wheelchair Adaptive equipment for special tasks in bed or wheelchair using mouth stick
C4	Intact sternocleidomastoid, trapezius, upper cervical paraspinal muscle	No voluntary function of upper extremities, trunk, or lower extremities All neck movements Mechanical ventilation dependent	Electric wheelchair Externally powered devices and adaptive equipment for special tasks in bed or wheelchair with mouth stick, such as turning pages, using computer Totally dependent for activities of daily living
C5	Partial deltoid, biceps, major muscles of rotator cuffs at shoulders Diaphragm	Abduction, flexion, and extension of arm Flexion and extension of forearm Unable to roll over or attain sitting position Abdominal respiration Poor respiratory reserve	Electric wheelchair Requires attendant to assist in moving and transfer to wheelchair Adaptive devices for self-feeding, grooming, using computer Vocational potential with adaptive devices
C6	Pectoralis major, serratus anterior, latissimus dorsi muscles Complete deltoid and brachioradialis muscles Partial triceps muscle	Significant increase in function over that with lesion at C5 level Adduction and medial rotation of arm Wrist extension Good elbow flexion	Cuff strapped to hand to permit use of implements for self-care and other activities Able to assist in dressing and transfer Hand rim extension to permit independence in wheelchair
C7	Triceps and finger flexion and extensor muscle Shoulder depressor muscles Still nerve disruption to intercostal muscles	With elbow stabilized in extension and intact shoulder depressor muscles, able to lift body weight Grasp and release still weak; dexterity lacking	Almost complete independence within limitations of wheelchair Requires some assistance in transfer and lower extremity dressing Hand splints helpful Can roll over in bed, sit up in bed, and eat independently Homebound employment possible; outside work usually not feasible
Paraplegia			
T1-T10	Full innervation of upper extremity muscles	Full use of upper extremities, including intrinsic muscles of hand Trunk balance poor—may have difficulty lifting trunk sufficiently to put on lower extremity clothing Considerable energy expenditure to put on long leg braces with extensive attachments	Completely wheelchair dependent Trunk balance benefits from training Able to drive automobile with hand controls May be braced for standing May hold job away from home Can manage adapted public transportation
T10-L2	Full abdominal and upper back muscle control	Good trunk balance Good respiratory reserve Can accomplish moderate hip hiking using external oblique and latissimus dorsi muscles	Ambulation with bilateral long braces using four-point or swing-through crutch gait Usually able to negotiate curbs Some able to use regular public transportation Few vocational limitations as long as does not require much walking or standing
L3-L4	Quadriceps muscle Partial gluteus and hamstring muscles	May have lumbar lordosis Floppy ankles	Ambulates well, often with short leg braces with or without cane Difficulty in getting out of wheelchair May never require wheelchair

through the reflex arc, and convey sympathetic and parasympathetic nerve impulses from the brain to peripheral structures.

Sensory transmission begins when peripheral receptors pick up a wide variety of stimuli and transfer the impulses, by means of peripheral nerves, to the spinal nerves, where they make ganglionic connections and enter the cord posteriorly. At this point the impulses travel in two directions: (1) across the interneuron connection and then to the motor neurons (reflex arc), or (2) up the spinal cord to predetermined areas of the brain. Motor impulses are transmitted from the cerebral cortex to the medulla (where nerve tracts cross) and proceed down descending motor pathways to the desired level within the spinal cord. Here they connect with the anterior horn cells

---

BOX 40-7   THE THREE MAJOR PLEXUSES

Cervical plexus (C1-C4)—Innervates the neck and diaphragm
Brachial plexus (C4-T1)—Supplies the shoulders, chest, and arms
Lumbosacral plexus (L1-S4)—Transmits impulses to the lower trunk and legs

---

BOX 40-8   DIFFERENCES IN CLINICAL MANIFESTATIONS BETWEEN UPPER AND LOWER MOTOR NEURON SYNDROMES

Upper Motor Neuron Syndrome
Spastic paralysis in muscle groups below lesion (intact reflex arcs below lesion)
Hyperreflexia with tendon reflexes exaggerated, Babinski reflex present
No wasting of muscle mass because of increased muscle tone
Flexion contractures and spasms of muscle groups below lesion level common
No skin or tissue changes

Lower Motor Neuron Syndrome
Flaccid paralysis caused by muscle atonia (reflex arcs permanently damaged)
Reflex with associated muscle response absent
Marked atrophy of atonic muscle
Fasciculations (local twitching of muscle groups) common
No flexor spasms
Loss of hair
Skin and tissue changes
Cornified nails

BOX 40-9   SIGNIFICANT EFFECTS OF AUTONOMIC DISRUPTION

- Decreased muscle tone and impairment of vasoconstrictive effects of sympathetic innervation cause venous pooling; diminished venous return to the heart; decreased cardiac output; and hypotension, especially orthostatic hypotension (orthostatic intolerance).
- Thermoregulatory disruption in the hypothalamus and skin receptors causes blood vessels to remain dilated during the initial stage, an inability to sweat in response to increased environmental temperature, and a possible rapid elevation in body temperature.
- Voluntary bowel and bladder function is lost because of damage to nerve fibers that innervate these organs.
- Altered sexual function (lack of erection, ejaculation, and orgasm) results from interference with numerous autonomic nerve fibers and plexuses.

---

and are transmitted to the muscle fibers by means of the lower motor neurons to complete a meaningful movement.

A network of nerves that serves the major muscle groups constitutes a plexus. Total involvement of any one of these plexuses seriously impairs function to the areas it innervates. Box 40-7 describes the three major plexuses.

Upper Versus Lower Motor Neurons

Upper motor neurons extend from cerebral centers to cells in the spinal column; lower motor neurons consist of anterior horn cells and spinal and peripheral nerves. Motor fibers of the reflex arc are lower motor neurons. This is an important point because relative dominance of the CNS over reflex arcs suppresses some reflex responses. When the higher centers no longer exert an influence in SCI, spastic responses are observed in muscles innervated by the intact lower motor neurons. Most SCIs involve upper motor neurons; children born with spinal cord defects have primarily lower motor neuron deficits (see Fig. 40-1). Box 40-8 outlines manifestations of upper and lower motor neuron syndromes.

Effect on Sensory and Motor Tracts

Voluntary muscle control is lost after complete transection of the cord. In partial transection, function is altered to varying degrees depending on the areas innervated by involved nerves. The crossing of motor tracts at various levels makes it possible for an injured person to have motor paralysis in one leg but retain pain and temperature sensation in that leg, while the opposite leg retains its motor function but loses pain and temperature sensation.

Although a transected cord injury leads to sensory loss, it is not uncommon for the injured person to experience pain. For example, smooth or skeletal muscle spasms, destruction of the myelin sheath (impulses cross to adjacent nerves), and scar formation or irritation of nerve endings may cause pain. Pain suffered by a person with tetraplegia or paraplegia is often intensified because of loss of sensation in other parts. Severe and prolonged pain should be medically evaluated for a treatable pathologic condition.

Effect on Autonomic System

Sympathetic and parasympathetic systems receive both excitatory and inhibitory stimuli from autonomic centers in the cerebral cortex, limbic system, and hypothalamus. The stimuli are transmitted by means of a feedback mechanism within the ascending fibers of the cord that normally controls descending input. Axons of the many CNS neurons synapse with autonomic preganglionic fibers and thus are able to alter their patterned responses. Box 40-9 describes the most significant effects of autonomic disruption.

Etiology

The most common cause of serious spinal cord damage in children is trauma involving MVCs (including automobile-bicycle, all-terrain vehicles, and snowmobiles), sports injuries (especially from diving, trampoline activities, gymnastics, and football), birth trauma, and child abuse. The increased use of recreational activities involving motorized vehicles such as jet water skis and motorcycles has increased the incidence of SCIs in children.

Congenital defects of the spine such as myelomeningocele (see Chapter 11) also may, in some cases, produce the effects of SCI. Transverse myelitis (inflammation of the spinal cord) has been reported to develop from inadvertent intraarterial administration of long-acting penicillin injected into the buttocks. Damage can be extensive enough to result in paraplegia or even lower limb amputation.

In MVCs most SCIs in children are a result of indirect trauma caused by sudden hyperflexion or hyperextension of the neck, often combined with a rotational force. Trauma to the spinal cord without evidence of vertebral fracture or dislocation (SCI without radiographic abnormality, or SCIWORA) is particularly likely to occur in an MVC when proper safety restraints are not used. An unrestrained child becomes a projectile during sudden deceleration and is subject to injury from contact with a variety of objects inside and outside the vehicle. Individuals who use only a lap seat belt restraint are at greater risk of SCI than those who use a combination lap and shoulder restraint. High cervical spine injuries have been reported in children less than 2 years of age who are restrained in forward-facing car seats. Infants who are improperly restrained in an infant car seat may experience cervical trauma in a car crash. Small children may also be severely injured by front seat air bags. (See Chapter 12.)

Falling from heights occurs less often in children than in adults, but vertebral compression of the spine from blows to the head or buttocks occurs in water sports (diving and surfing) or falls from horses or other athletic injuries. Birth injuries may occur in breech delivery from excessive traction force and rotation on the cord during delivery of the head and shoulders. When shaken, infants commonly sustain cervical cord damage, as well as subdural hematoma and retinal hemorrhage; cognitive impairment and death may occur subsequent to the traumatic event. Infants have weak neck muscles, and during vigorous shaking their large and heavy heads rapidly wobble back and forth. An increasing number of adolescents receive SCIs secondary to gunshot wounds, stabbings, or other violent inflicted injury.

Because of the marked mobility of the neck, fracture or subluxation (partial dislocation) is the most common immediate cause of SCI, particularly in the lower cervical region. Although unusual in adults, SCI without fracture is not uncommon in the child, whose spine is suppler, weaker, and more mobile than that of the adult. Therefore the force is more easily dissipated over a larger number of segments. Upper cervical injuries account for as many as 80% of the SCIs in children under the age of 2 years (Haslam, 2007). In children the vertebral column is composed of cartilaginous rings and is capable of considerable elongation, whereas the cord itself, its meninges, and its vascular supply are unable to withstand the same degree of traction.

The injury sustained can affect any of the spinal nerves; the higher the injury, the more extensive the damage. The child can be left with complete or partial paralysis of the lower extremities (paraplegia) or with damage at a higher level and without functional use of any of the four extremities (tetraplegia). A high cervical cord injury that affects the phrenic nerve paralyzes the diaphragm and leaves the child dependent on mechanical ventilation.

A mild but equally frightening form of cord trauma is spinal cord compression, a temporary neural dysfunction without visible damage to the cord. Complete tetraplegia can result but initially may not be differentiated from serious cord injury.

Pathophysiology

The severity of the force, the mechanisms of the injury, and the degree of the individual's muscular relaxation at the time of the injury greatly influence the extent of the trauma. SCIs are classified as either complete or incomplete. In a complete injury there is no motor or sensory function more than three segments below the neurologic level of the injury (Mathison, Kadom, and Krug, 2008). Incomplete lesions have several typical characteristics (Mathison, Kadom, and Krug, 2008):

BOX 40-10 ASIA IMPAIRMENT SCALE

A—Complete: No motor or sensory function is preserved in the sacral segments S4-S5.

B—Incomplete: Sensory but not motor function is preserved below the neurologic level and includes the sacral segments S4-S5.

C—Incomplete: Motor function is preserved below the neurologic level, and more than half of key muscles below the neurologic level have a muscle grade less than 3.

D—Incomplete: Motor function is preserved below the neurologic level, and at least half of key muscles below the neurologic level have a muscle grade of 3 or more.

E—Normal: Motor and sensory function are normal.

Clinical Syndromes (Optional)
Central cord
Brown-Séquard
Anterior cord
Conus medullaris
Cauda equina

Used with permission, American Spinal Injury Association, 2006.

Central cord syndrome—Central gray matter destruction and preservation of peripheral tracts; tetraplegia with sacral sparing common; some motor recovery gained

Anterior cord syndrome—Complete motor and sensory loss with trunk and lower extremity proprioception and sensation of pressure

Posterior cord syndrome—Loss of sensation, pain, and proprioception with normal cord function, including motor function; able to move extremities but have difficulty controlling such movements

Brown-Séquard syndrome—Unilateral cord lesion with a motor deficit on the opposite side of the body from the primary insult; absence of pain and temperature sensation on the opposite side from the injury

Spinal cord concussion—Transient loss of neural function below the level of the acute spinal cord lesion, resulting in flaccid paralysis and loss of tendon, autonomic, and cutaneous reflex activity; may last hours to weeks

The American Spinal Injury Association (2009) Standards for neurologic classification of SCI worksheet is available online at **www.asia-spinalinjury.org/publications/2006_Classif_worksheet.pdf**. The ASIA Impairment Scale (Box 40-10) combines motor and sensory function and is used to determine the severity of impairment from the injury (complete or incomplete). It may also be used to measure neurologic changes and functional goals for rehabilitation (Mathison, Kadom, and Krug, 2008).

Clinical Manifestations

It is often difficult to determine the extent and severity of damage at first. Immediate loss of function is caused by both anatomic and impaired physiologic function, and improved function may not be evident for weeks or even months. Manifestation of the initial response to acute SCI is flaccid paralysis below the level of the damage. This stage is often referred to as spinal shock syndrome and is caused by the sudden disruption of central and autonomic pathways. Local effects of cord edema and ischemia produce a physiologic transection with or without an anatomic severance. Most children with an SCI experience some spinal shock. Manifestations include the absence of reflexes at or below the cord lesion, with flaccidity or limpness of the involved muscles, loss of sensation and motor function, and autonomic dysfunction (symptoms of hypotension, low or high body temperature, loss of bladder and bowel control, and autonomic dysreflexia).

Autonomic paralysis also affects thermoregulatory functions. Afferent impulses from temperature receptors in the skin are not integrated; therefore the patient is subject to temperature increases or decreases in response to alterations in environmental temperature. Hyperthermia can result from excessive ambient temperature, such as too many covers.

Except in the situations previously mentioned, flaccid paralysis is replaced by spinal reflex activity and increasing spasticity or, in incomplete lesions, greater or lesser degree of neurologic recovery.

The paralytic nature of autonomic function is replaced by autonomic dysreflexia, especially when the lesions are above the midthoracic level. This autonomic phenomenon is caused by visceral distention or irritation, particularly of the bowel or bladder. Sensory impulses are triggered and travel to the cord lesion, where they are blocked, which causes activation of sympathetic reflex action with disturbed central inhibitory control. Excessive sympathetic activity is manifested by a flushing face, sweating forehead, pupillary constriction, marked hypertension, headache, and bradycardia. The precipitating stimulus may be merely a full bladder or rectum or other internal or external sensory input. It can be a catastrophic event unless the irritation is relieved.

Additional clinical findings of SCI may include numbness, tingling, or burning; priapism; weakness; and loss of bowel and bladder control (Hayes and Arriola, 2005).

Neurogenic shock occurs as a result of a disruption in the descending sympathetic pathways with loss of vasomotor tone and sympathetic innervations to the cardiovascular system (Hayes and Arriola, 2005). Hypotension, bradycardia, and peripheral vasodilation occur as a result of neurogenic shock.

Children with suspected SCI may have suffered multiple injuries (e.g., MVC); therefore multiple clinical manifestations may occur that may mask those of an SCI.

In the final stage neurologic signs are stabilized in terms of loss and recovery of function. The major emphasis is on rehabilitation. A problem unique to injury in childhood is progressive spinal deformity usually not seen in adults or in adolescents near the end of the growth period. Scoliosis develops in the majority of children with high thoracic and cervical lesions and is almost certain to occur in children with tetraplegia whose injury occurred in infancy or early childhood.

Diagnostic Evaluation

A history of the injury provides valuable clues regarding the possible type of damage incurred and directions for further assessment without the risk of additional damage. A complete neurologic examination determines whether damage was incurred and, if so, the level and extent of any nerve impairment. A neurologic unit of the CNS is considered normal if reflex arcs are functioning, sensory tracts are intact when each dermatome is examined separately, and voluntary motor response demonstrates an ability to move a body part against gravity on command.

Testing a reflex arc is accomplished by stimulating the peripheral receptors at a specific site, such as eliciting the patellar reflex. Symmetric testing is performed to determine unilateral or bilateral neurologic deficit. A sufficient number of reflexes are examined to test motor function thoroughly. The blunt end of a safety pin is used to assess pressure sensitivity, and the sharp point is used to elicit pain. Hot and cold water, a tuning fork, and cotton may also be used to determine specific sensory loss (e.g., temperature, vibration, and light touch).

The ASIA dermatome classification worksheet is used to determine the extent of neurologic damage (Fig. 40-7). Body surface zones, or dermatomes, accurately correspond to the spinal cord segment receiving the sensory input from the peripheral nerves in that zone. Systematically pinpricking the body surface in each zone determines intactness of sensory pathways. Figure 40-7 illustrates the zones and the spinal cord segments they represent. The examiner tests for each specific sensory fiber in the dermatome areas in which neurologic deficit is suspected.

Matching cord level to vertebra is more difficult in infants and young children than it is in older children and adults because the sacral and several lower lumbar cord segments lie at a lower position, especially during the first 2 years of life. The spinal anatomy approaches adult configuration by the time the child reaches age 7 or 8 years; by late adolescence the conus medullaris has usually reached the level of L1.

Motor system evaluation includes observing gait if the child is able to walk; noting balance maintenance with the child's eyes open and closed; and noting the ability to lift, flex, and extend the arms and legs. Testing muscle strength with and without resistance and against gravity provides clues to the specific nature and degree of motor dysfunction. The number of muscles in any muscle group that remain completely intact in the upper extremities makes a marked difference in the individual's ability to provide self-care, especially at high injury levels. Hip movement is necessary for ambulation with braces and crutches.

The degree to which supportive aids are needed for ambulation is determined by the strength, stability, and movement of the pelvis, trunk, hip flexor muscles, and quadriceps muscles. A general guideline for determining the capacity for self-help is that a person with paraplegia who has function down to and including the quadriceps muscle or muscle function below the L3 level will have little difficulty in learning to walk with or without braces and crutches. It is especially vital that children with lumbar levels of injury be taught to walk functionally so that they are weight bearing at least part of the time; this minimizes the risk of osteoporosis and hypercalcemia. The functional significance of the spinal cord lesion level is given in Table 40-1.

If a CNS pathologic disorder is detected, a body system assessment is performed to determine the degree of autonomic impairment. Because the cord and CNS directly influence the function of the autonomic nerves, the specific sympathetically related organ systems are examined for skeletal muscle and vascular tone and body temperature regulation. For example,

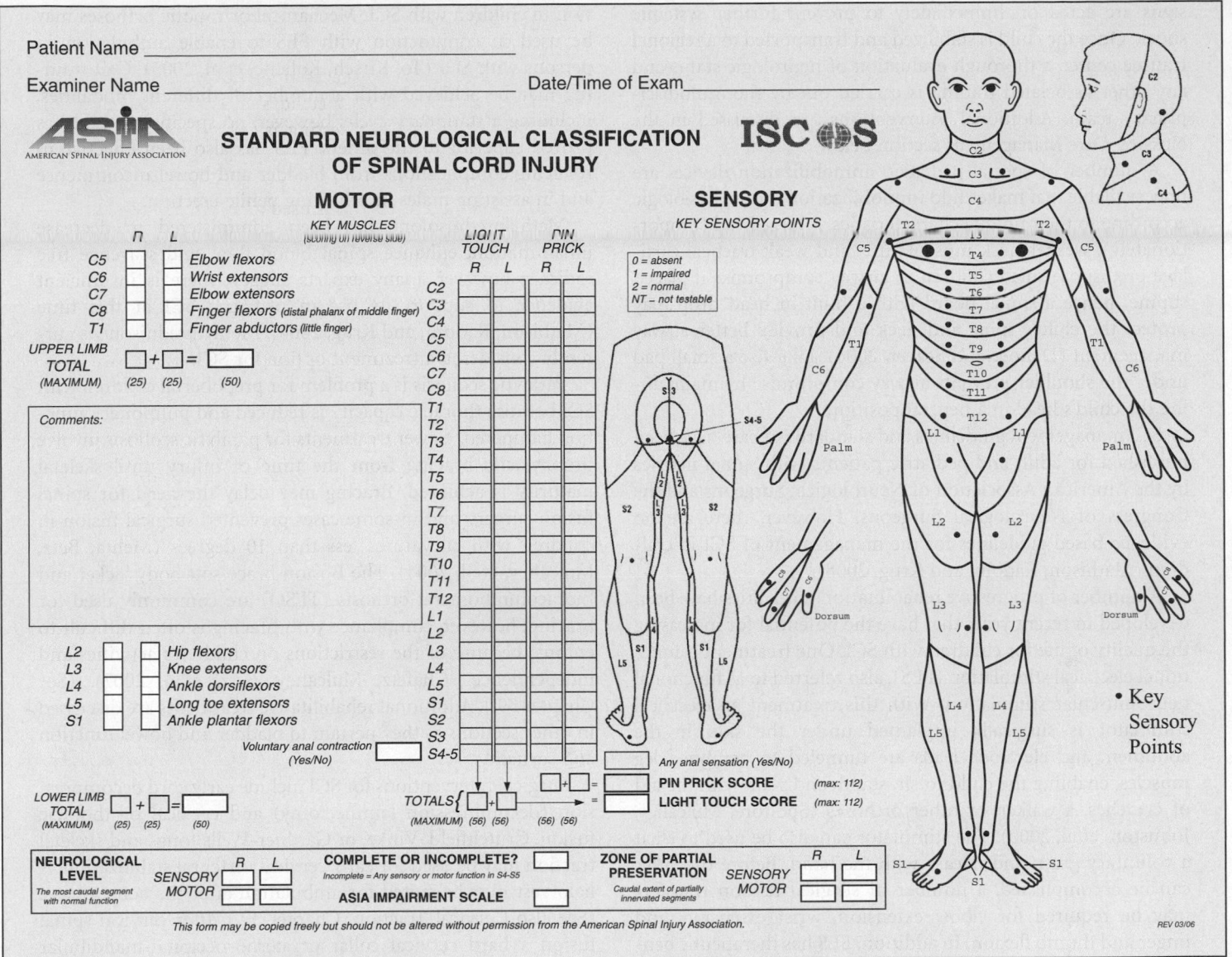

Fig. 40-7 ASIA classification of spinal cord injury. (Used with permission, American Spinal Injury Association, 2006.)

bladder and gastrointestinal function has sympathetic and parasympathetic innervation and local reflexes.

CT and MRI scans are important for localizing the lesion, but the nature of the spine in childhood often creates difficulty in interpretation. Small children often have no radiographic evidence of vertebral or spinal injury despite significant injuries ranging from complete transection with major hemorrhage to minor hemorrhage, edema, or normal neural findings (Pang, 2004). This condition, SCIWORA, is reported to occur in 19% to 34% of all pediatric SCIs (Mathison, Kadom, and Krug, 2008; Launay, Leet, and Sponseller, 2005). Pang (2004) reports a mean incidence of 34.8% for SCIWORA in children from birth to 17 years. SCIWORA is a common finding in very young children who are victims of abuse (primarily shaken baby syndrome) because of the elasticity and incomplete ossification of the vertebrae. SCIWORA is more common in children under the age of 8 years and injury to the cervical spine is common. Diagnostic scans must be taken carefully and with sufficient help to prevent further damage to the spine.

Therapeutic Management

Initial care begins at the scene of the accident with proper immobilization of the cervical, thoracic, and lumbar spine. Because of the complexity of these injuries, it is usually recommended that these persons be transported to a spinal injury center for care by specially trained health care personnel as soon as possible after the injury for appropriate diagnostic evaluation and intervention. (See The Child and Trauma, Chapter 39.)

The initial management of the child with a suspected SCI should begin with an assessment of the ABCs: airway, breathing, and circulation. Guidelines for the child who is found unconscious with an unknown cause are discussed in Chapter 31 (Cardiopulmonary Resuscitation). The airway should be opened using the jaw-thrust technique to minimize damage to the cervical spine. The child is monitored for cardiovascular instability, and measures are taken to support systemic blood pressure and maintain optimal cardiac output. Because MVC and other trauma in children may involve internal organ damage and potential bleeding, abdominal distention or other signs are acted on immediately to prevent further systemic shock. Once the child is stabilized and transported to a regional trauma center, a thorough evaluation of neurologic status and any other associated trauma is carried out by the multidisciplinary team. Additional interventions are discussed in the Nursing Care Management section below.

A number of special pediatric immobilization devices are now available that make child immobilization more physiologic according to their unique characteristics. A large head (proportionately), weaker neck musculature, and weak tracheal cartilage predispose small children to airway compromise if placed supine; hence a spinal board with a built-in head drop may protect the child's spine and neck and provide better airway management (DeBoer and Seaver, 2004). Likewise a small pad under the shoulder prevents airway compromise by maintaining the child's head in a neutral position.

SCI management guidelines and standards of care have been published for adult and pediatric patients with spinal injuries by the American Association of Neurological Surgeons and the Congress of Neurological Surgeons. However, there are no evidence-based guidelines for the management of SCI in children (Mathison, Kadom, and Krug, 2008).

A number of progressive rehabilitation modalities have been developed in recent years that have the potential for increasing the quality of life for children with SCI. One treatment is functional electrical stimulation (FES), also referred to as functional neuromuscular stimulation. With this treatment an electrical stimulator is surgically implanted under the skin in the abdomen, and electrode leads are tunneled to paralyzed leg muscles, enabling the child to sit, stand, and walk with the aid of crutches, a walker, or other orthoses (Spoltore, Mulcahey, Johnston, et al, 2000). The stimulator can also be used to elicit a voluntary grasp and release with the hand. Before the latter can be accomplished, a number of surgical tendon transfers may be required for elbow extension, wrist extension, and finger and thumb flexion. In addition, FES has therapeutic benefits, which include increased muscle strength, improved gait function, and increased cardiovascular fitness (Thrasher and Popovic, 2008). Tendon transfers have been shown to be successful in enhancing hand function, increasing pinch force, and facilitating independence in ADLs (Spoltore, Mulcahey, Johnston, et al, 2000). Restoration of hand and arm function enables children with SCI to perform self-catheterization and achieve greater independence in personal hygiene.

FES is reported to have many benefits for children with SCI, including cardiovascular conditioning, decreasing pressure ulcers, and increasing blood flow (Merenda, Spoltore, and Betz, 2000). Implanted FES has also been reported to enhance bowel function in adolescents with SCI. Subjects were also able to stand independently from a wheelchair and walk 6 m (20 feet) when using the FES (Johnston, Betz, Smith, et al, 2005).

Administration of pharmacologic agents such as clonidine hydrochloride may improve ambulation in patients with partial SCIs, and exercise therapy through interactive locomotor training has helped some individuals with SCI regain ambulatory function (Kalb, 2003).

A number of orthoses or ambulation aids such as crutches may still be necessary to achieve upright mobility, yet, as robotic technology advances, so do the chances for improved mobiliza-

tion in children with SCI. Mechanical or robotic orthoses may be used in conjunction with FES to enable ambulation in persons with SCI (To, Kirsch, Kobetic, et al, 2005). Gait training may be achieved with a number of different modalities, including a stationary cycle; however, no specific method has proved superior to the others. FES has also been effective in reducing complications from bladder and bowel incontinence and in assisting males in achieving penile erection.

Methylprednisolone has been administered to decrease inflammation, enhance spinal blood flow, and scavenge free radicals; however, many experts suggest there is insufficient evidence to support its use in pediatric SCI at this time (Mathison, Kadom, and Krug, 2008). Methylprednisone is currently considered a treatment option for SCI.

Paralytic scoliosis is a problem for prepubertal children with SCI because thoracic capacity is reduced and pulmonary function hampered. Newer treatments for paralytic scoliosis involve prophylactic bracing from the time of injury until skeletal maturity is achieved. Bracing may delay the need for spinal fusion surgery and in some cases prevented surgical fusion in children with curvatures less than 10 degrees (Mehta, Betz, Mulcahey, et al, 2004). The Boston brace soft body jacket and thoracolumbosacral orthosis (TLSO) are commonly used for bracing; however, compliance with bracing is often difficult to enforce because of the restrictions on children's activities and independence (Chafetz, Mulcahey, Betz, et al, 2007). (See Chapter 39.). Additional rehabilitative treatments are discussed in other sections as they pertain to bladder and bowel function and sexuality.

Surgical interventions for SCI include early cord decompression (decompression laminectomy) and cervical or thoracic fusion. Crutchfield, Vinke, or Gardner-Wells tongs and skeletal traction may be used for early cervical vertebral stabilization. A halo vest may be suited for ambulation after the acute phase. (See also Cervical Traction, Chapter 39.) After cervical spinal fusion a hard cervical collar or sterno-occipital-mandibular immobilizer brace may be worn until the fusion is solidified.

Prognosis

The ultimate outlook for spinal cord function after injury depends on the completeness of the cord transection, site of injury, complicating damage to the neuronal tissue, and success of treatment regimens aimed at recovery of lost muscle movement and ability. Healing of the injury and the return of neurologic function are related to two factors:

1. Although individual nerve fibers do regenerate, they do not necessarily reconnect or make synaptic connections with the distal portion of the severed fibers; the chance of numerous fibers reconnecting is highly unlikely.
2. The damage resulting from cord ischemia produces necrosis in the gray and white matter of the cord tissue, which does not regenerate if the axon cylinder is not intact.

In children the prognosis for recovery is considered better than in adults because children have rapid healing of bone and ligaments and increased potential for nervous system regeneration. Paraplegia is more common in children under 12 years, whereas older children and adolescents tend to have incomplete injuries (Mathison, Kadom, and Krug, 2008). In one study the mortality rate was 4% and associated injuries contributed to the majority of deaths; cerebral injury was a common factor in the cause of death in this study (Cirak, Ziegfeld, Knight, et al, 2004). Another study reported a mortality rate of 28%, with 66% having long-term neurologic deficits (Platzer, Jaindl, Thalhammer, et al, 2007). Shavelle, DeVivo, Paculdo, and colleagues (2007) reported an increased likelihood of mortality among children less than 16 years of age who suffered an SCI in comparison to adults with similar injuries. Children with incomplete injuries (and who are not ventilator dependent) had a projected 83% chance of normal life expectancy, whereas those with high-level cervical injuries who are not ventilator dependent had a 50% chance of having a normal life expectancy.

In general, recovery of motor function in children with thoracic lesions is variable. Cervical injuries are also variable in the extent of damage. Incomplete lesions produce hemiplegia, whereas complete transection implies some involvement of all extremities—from partial use of the upper extremities to complete paralysis, including the need for some type of assisted ventilation. Lumbar injury may involve partial or complete loss of function in the lower extremities and bladder. With rapidly advancing surgical technology, use of microcomputers in medicine, and newer treatment modalities such as FES, there is increasing hope and evidence that functional mobility and independence can be restored in children with SCI.

QUALITY PATIENT OUTCOMES: Neurologic Impairment
- Neurologic status maintained or improved
- No further injuries

Nursing Care Management

The nursing care of the child affected by SCI is complex and challenging. A multidisciplinary SCI team is equipped to manage the acute phase of the injury, and some members, including the nurse, may follow the patient to eventual recovery. Nursing management is concerned with ensuring adequate initial stabilization of the entire spinal column with a rigid cervical collar with supportive blocks on a rigid backboard (Barker and Saulino, 2002). The traumatic event causing the injury may or may not be recalled if the child lost consciousness; such events are extremely frightening to the child. The young child may also be frightened by the immobilization process and the inability to move extremities; therefore it is important to reassure and comfort the child during this process.

During the acute phase of the injury it is imperative that airway patency be ensured, complications prevented, and function maintained. Evaluate the extent of the neurologic damage early to establish a baseline for neurologic function. Continual assessment of sensory and motor function should occur to prevent further deterioration of neurologic status as a result of spinal cord edema. The ASIA Impairment Scale can be used to assess neurologic function on a routine basis during the patient's recovery. Once the patient is admitted, further evaluation of his or her ability to perform ADLs and need for assistance during recovery can be made with the Functional Independence Measure scale (Barker and Saulino, 2002).

Nursing care during the acute phase should also focus on frequent monitoring of neurologic signs to determine any changes in neurologic function that require further intervention (e.g., level of consciousness using the Glasgow Coma Scale). In addition to airway maintenance, the nurse monitors for changes in hemodynamic status that may require immediate medical attention. Neurogenic shock consists of hypotension, bradycardia, and vasodilation. Inotropic medications may be required to maintain adequate perfusion. Renal function is closely monitored by measuring urinary output and fluids administered. The child with a head injury may experience elevated intracranial pressure; therefore changes in neurologic status are reported to the practitioner. Fluid restriction may be required if intracranial pressure is elevated, so fluid intake should be closely monitored.

Although care of the child with an SCI is, in most aspects, the same as that of any immobilized child, some important differences are discussed here. (See The Immobilized Child, Chapter 39.) Additional aspects of care that should be addressed on an individual basis include hypercalcemia in adolescent males, DVT, latex sensitization, and sleep disordered breathing (Vogel, Hickey, Klaas, et al, 2004).

Respiratory Care

The child with a high-level cervical injury (C3 and above) requires continuous ventilatory assistance. In most instances a tracheostomy is the method of choice for greater ease in clearing secretions and for less trauma to tissues during long-term ventilatory dependence. Patient-triggered synchronous intermittent mandatory ventilation (SIMV–assist/control mode) may be required to maintain adequate oxygenation. In an acute care center, respiratory therapy personnel are often responsible for establishing and maintaining the equipment, but the nurse must understand how it works and recognize mechanical malfunction and deviations from the prescribed rate and volume. In case of malfunction the nurse must be prepared to maintain respirations manually with a self-inflating bag-valve-mask device. In many home care situations the family is responsible for the care of ventilatory assistance devices; therefore adequate family training and availability of the nurse (or durable medical equipment representative) for questions related to the equipment and evaluation of the child's breathing are essential. For some children, breathing pacemaker devices (phrenic nerve stimulators) are implanted to stimulate the phrenic nerve and produce diaphragmatic contractions and lung expansion without assisted ventilation.

Children with lesions below the C4 level are seldom ventilator dependent, but pulmonary vital capacity is significantly reduced. Position them for optimum chest expansion, and use a variety of breathing exercises and assistive devices to stimulate deep breathing. Chest physiotherapy is performed as needed to mobilize secretions, and flow-by oxygen may be needed occasionally. Regular monitoring of breath sounds to assess for adequate ventilation in all lung fields is part of routine care.

The cough reflex may be markedly diminished, which, combined with weak intercostal muscles, may mean the child has difficulty with secretions. Increasing the elastic qualities of the lung by breathing exercises, mechanical cough assist techniques, and incentive spirometry helps the child achieve a productive cough. (See discussion of airway management and airway clearance devices under Muscular Dystrophies: Therapeutic Management.)

Cardiovascular Care

Children with SCI may experience cardiovascular instability as a result of loss of vagal tone, vagal stimulation during procedures such as oral suctioning or insertion of a nasogastric tube, turning, and endotracheal suctioning. Close monitoring of heart rate and blood pressure is essential to detect any signs of decreased cardiac output. Pneumothorax may occur, resulting in a mediastinal shift and decreased cardiac output. Autonomic dysreflexia may occur and result in decreased cardiac output (see discussion below).

The child with loss of muscle tone and prolonged immobility may be at high risk for the development of DVT. In addition, major reparative surgery for associated injuries and spinal decompression place the child at risk for thrombus formation. DVT is prevented with the use of pneumatic compression devices and low-molecular-weight heparin during the acute phase of care. Fluid and electrolyte balance may be impaired as a result of trauma and associated injuries or decreased fluid intake during the recovery period. Fluid intake should be closely monitored, especially with regard to the development of pulmonary edema and intracranial pressure. The child may require nasogastric tube feedings due to anorexia and immobility.

Temperature Regulation

Temperature regulation usually creates few problems, although environmental conditions can influence body temperature. During the spinal shock stage the dilated capillaries conducting body heat to the subcutaneous tissues cause heat loss. Without the capacity to sweat, the body retains heat in hot weather. An elevated temperature that cannot be corrected by environmental measures should be evaluated to rule out urinary or upper respiratory tract infection. However, excessive perspiration observed in sentient areas usually indicates an elevated ambient temperature. Because the skin is a less reliable indicator in these children, the oral or aural (ear) route is usually the preferred method of temperature measurement.

Skin Care

Children with SCI have unique needs in relation to skin care. Because of decreased sensation and impaired mobility, they depend on others to assess and assist in the management of intact skin. Skin care practices are the same as those for any child who is immobilized. A skin score scale such as the Braden Q Scale can objectively evaluate risks for skin breakdown and skin conditions (Curley, Razmus, Roberts, et al, 2003). Keep an alternating-pressure mattress or other pressure relief/reduction device underneath the child, and inspect the skin thoroughly at least twice a day for signs of pressure, especially over bony prominences. Prevention of skin breakdown is much easier than treatment. A number of factors contribute to the risk of skin breakdown in these children: decreased sensation, inadequate nutrition, muscle spasticity, impaired peripheral circulation, diaphoresis, mechanical shearing from assistive devices, and improper positioning. (See Maintaining Healthy Skin, Chapter 27.)

The areas most likely to be affected are the sacrum, scapulae, heels, and occiput when the child is supine; the trochanters and the lateral aspect of the ankles, heels, and knees when the child is in a side-lying position; and the ischial tuberosities when the child is sitting. The pressure wound may begin in deeper tissues and be visible on the surface only at a later stage. Therefore areas that feel firm, irregular, or warm or that appear to be only slightly reddened require careful evaluation. (See Wounds, Chapter 18.) Keeping the skin clean and dry is particularly important in these children, especially those who are incontinent of urine or stool. When there is any evidence of skin breakdown, treatment to prevent further breakdown is implemented promptly. When orthotic devices such as AFOs and braces are used, skin care and vigilance for pressure areas are also important in the prevention of pressure ulcers. Prolonged use of wheelchairs without special sacral protection may also lead to skin ulceration.

The child who is heavily sedated or who is being given muscle paralytics should receive appropriate eye care to prevent corneal damage (artificial tears, ointment, and impermeable eye shield). Additional nursing care may involve the administration of histamine blockers and proton pump inhibitors to prevent stress ulcer by reducing the secretion of hydrochloric acid.

Physical Therapy

Maintaining proper body alignment, preventing pressure from bed linens, providing proper support, applying splints, and using padded devices such as foam boots to hold the feet in correct position are important in daily care. Range-of-motion, passive, and active exercises are carried out under the guidance of a PT. In children with upper motor neuron involvement, the spasticity that develops may require administration of an antispasmodic medication such as diazepam. Baclofen is considered the drug of choice for reducing muscle spasticity. Gabapentin may be used to treat neuropathic pain (Hayes and Arriola, 2005; Vogel, Hickey, Klaas, et al, 2004). Botulinum toxin type A and α_2-adrenergic agonists may be used in older children with SCI to decrease muscle spasticity (see p. 1697).

Unless there are contraindications, exercises during the period of immobilization are aimed at maintaining and increasing the strength of the child's intact musculature. Upper extremity strengthening is especially important to the paraplegic child, who must rely on these muscle groups for turning, transferring, dressing, parallel bar walking, gait training, and other activities. Children are usually eager to use their muscles and respond to interesting and innovative activities.

Neurogenic Bladder

When the bladder is denervated, as in the acute stage of spinal shock syndrome or after lower motor neuron damage, the bladder wall is flaccid. Lack of muscle tone inhibits the bladder's ability to respond to changes in passive pressure, causing overdistention. Therefore it is important to prevent distention by periodic emptying, even though there may be dribbling between emptying.

In contrast, an upper motor neuron lesion causes increased bladder tone and contractions that often include the urinary sphincter. Thus, although the bladder empties periodically by reflex action, complete emptying is prevented, resulting in urinary retention and ureteral reflux. Administration of an anti-cholinergic drug such as dicyclomine (Bentyl) relaxes bladder musculature and promotes increased bladder capacity and more adequate emptying. Intervals of urination depend on many factors, including patterns of fluid intake and perspiration.

In school-age children and adolescents, achieving bladder and bowel continence is a significant developmental issue related to self-esteem and perception of self in relation to peers. Therefore it is imperative to consider options that best meet the child's physiologic and emotional needs.

Surgical options for children with neurogenic bladder include the creation of a urinary stoma, made possible by removing the appendix and creating a urinary diversion from the bladder to the exterior, usually the umbilicus, thus making self-catheterization more private, especially with the recovery of hand and elbow movement (with tendon transfers). Other options include surgical bladder augmentation to increase capacity and FES to restore micturition on command without a urinary catheter (Merenda and Hickey, 2005; Spoltore, Mulcahey, Johnston, et al, 2000).

Emptying the bladder by clean intermittent catheterization (CIC) is also an option for children with SCI; older children who are functionally capable can learn to perform self-catheterization. Encourage the child to adhere to a schedule for CIC and to maintain a regular pattern of fluid intake throughout the day; they should avoid large intakes of fluid without considering the need for more frequent CIC. Caffeinated beverages and other caffeinated foods are used sparingly to avoid bladder overdistention with increased urine formation (Francis, 2007). Latex catheters should be avoided to prevent the development of latex allergy (if it is not already present). Bladder-training programs usually begin with intermittent bladder emptying at regular intervals that are gradually increased. (See Management of Genitourinary Function under Myelomeningocele [Meningomyelocele], Chapter 11.) The Credé method (applying suprapubic pressure) for emptying the bladder may be used by some individuals with SCI, but this may result in high intravesical pressures, causing further bladder complications (Francis, 2007).

Urinary tract infections are common due to urinary stasis. A regular schedule of CIC may help prevent such infections. Encourage the child to increase fluid intake by approximately 240 ml/day and use CIC every 3 to 4 hours.

Maintenance of bladder dynamics and control of urinary tract infections are of utmost importance. Pyelonephritis and renal failure are the most significant causes of death in long-standing paraplegia.

Bowel Training

The loss of bowel function is considered to be one of the most stressful events when quality-of-life issues are considered in persons with SCI; however, successful bowel training is easier to institute than bladder management. The aim is to control defecation until an appropriate time and place are found. Merenda and Hickey (2005) propose four components in a successful bowel management program: desired stool consistency (i.e., a soft stool), a regular evacuation pattern, upright positioning for planned evacuation, and motivation and commitment from the child and family.

A diet with sufficient fiber (approximately 15 g/day) for adequate stool bulk and insertion of a glycerin or bisacodyl (Dulcolax) suppository at a convenient time, either morning or evening, are often all that are necessary to induce a bowel movement within a short time. The probability of an accident between times diminishes once the bowel is completely evacuated. The key to adequate bowel training is to maintain consistency in the time of day for evacuation. Stool softeners, such as docusate sodium (Colace) and senna (Senokot), may be prescribed, and manual anal stimulation may help initiate evacuation, especially in spastic paraplegia. Sometimes an oral laxative such as bisacodyl may be necessary. Once an appropriate regimen is established, little modification is required.

One surgical option is the antegrade continence enema, which involves the creation of a stoma whereby colonic washouts may be performed with the child sitting on the toilet (Francis, 2007). FES has also been used successfully in some children with SCI to achieve bowel training (Johnston, Betz, Smith, et al, 2005).

Autonomic Dysreflexia

Children with high-level lesions are susceptible to the development of autonomic dysreflexia, which requires prompt action to prevent encephalopathy and shock. Clinical manifestations of autonomic dysreflexia include an increase in systemic blood pressure, headache, bradycardia, profuse diaphoresis, cardiac arrhythmias, flushing, piloerection, blurred vision, nasal congestion, anxiety, spots on the visual field, or absent or minimum symptoms (Vogel, Hickey, Klaas, et al, 2004). A quick assessment may rule out other causes, such as orthostatic intolerance. After that, vital signs, including blood pressure, are taken while the bladder is checked for distention (the usual precipitating cause). The bladder is drained slowly; if this does not relieve symptoms, any tight clothing is loosened, and the bowel is checked for the pressure of impacted feces.

Other potential causes of autonomic dysreflexia in SCI children include bowel impaction and abdominal distention, pressure ulcers, tight clothing, burns, DVT, menses, trauma, fractures, pregnancy, labor, surgery or invasive procedures, any painful stimulus, and hyperthermia (Vogel, Hickey, Klaas, et al, 2004). If removal of the causative agent is unsuccessful in controlling the syndrome, IV administration of an antihypertensive drug is indicated, followed by oral maintenance doses. Antispasmodics may also be administered.

Remobilization

As soon as the condition warrants doing so, the child is moved from a reclining to an upright position. Cardiovascular deconditioning and impaired autonomic responses below the level of injury will cause pooling of blood in the extremities (because of peripheral vasodilation); a drop in blood pressure; and a feeling of lightheadedness, dizziness, or fainting on sudden assumption of an upright posture, often referred to as **orthostatic intolerance**. Therefore an upright position must be accomplished gradually by first placing the child (who is secured by passive restraint) on a head-up tilt table. The table is slowly elevated from a horizontal to a 30-degree semireclining position. This is performed twice daily for 20 to 30 minutes, with the angle gradually increased until the vertical angle is reached.

During the procedure the vital signs are monitored, and the child's behavior is observed for subjective symptoms of syncope. The pooling of blood is reduced by using elastic antiembolism stockings and sequential pneumatic compression devices, which consist of inflatable sleeves that fit on the legs and compress the leg muscles for cyclic emptying and filling of leg veins. The process of achieving an upright posture may require several weeks. After tolerance is achieved, the child will be ready to begin using a wheelchair. Getting the child up should be accomplished slowly by gradually elevating the bed over 20 to 30 minutes before placing the child in the wheelchair and then gradually lowering the legs after the child has been in the chair a short time.

All adaptive devices help children increase their mobility, function, and endurance. The child with some lower extremity function progresses to parallel bars and then to a walker. The child with tetraplegia learns to use a wheelchair—among the most valuable aids available to the child with an SCI. The wheelchair should be selected carefully in relation to where it will be used, the architectural barriers, and the child's functional capacity. For lower extremity paralysis, the wheelchair described on p. 1635 is applicable. For children with severe upper extremity paralysis, a variety of motorized wheelchairs are used; however, the more complex they are, the greater their cost, weight, and tendency to break down. Wheelchair tolerance is gained over time and is accompanied by measures to prevent orthostatic hypotension and pressure sores.

A variety of orthoses and other appliances can be adapted for use by many children. The primary purpose of lower extremity bracing in the child with an SCI is for ambulation, although correction of deformities may be attempted. However, the efficacy is limited because of the tendency to develop pressure lesions over insensate areas. The higher the lesion, the more support required, with the accompanying difficulties of getting into the orthosis and the greater energy expended in using the appliance. The energy required in walking with crutches and braces is two to four times greater than that required for normal walking.

Children, with their natural and overwhelming desire for mobility, usually attain or even surpass the maximum expectation in ambulation. However, as they approach adulthood, the increasing weight and energy cost usually cause them to resort to predominant use of the wheelchair for mobility and the pursuit of more intellectual and vocational interests. Wheelchair mobility has the advantages of requiring no more energy than normal walking and allowing the person with paraplegia to maintain the speed of other pedestrians on level ground.

Physical Rehabilitation

The process of physical rehabilitation usually begins once the child is medically stable and associated problems have been managed. The major aims of physical rehabilitation are to prepare the child and family to achieve normalization and resume life at home and in the community. Additional goals of rehabilitation in children with SCI are to promote independence in mobility and self-care skills, academic achievement, independent living, and employment (Box 40-11).

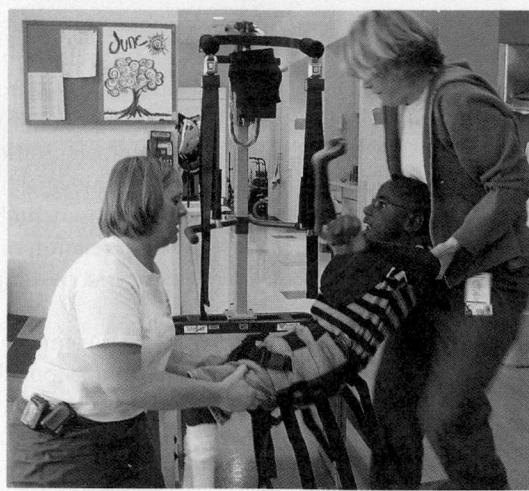

Fig. 40-8 Training in a rehabilitation facility can promote achievement and encourage the child to strive to reach his maximum physical abilities. (Courtesy E. Jacob, Texas Children's Hospital, Houston.)

BOX 40-11 **GOALS OF REHABILITATION FOR THE CHILD WITH A SPINAL CORD INJURY**

- Maximizing motor function and minimizing the disabling effects of the pathologic condition
- Assisting the child and family in setting realistic goals for the child, learning to be good problem solvers, and using the child's assets
- Helping the child to cope with the stigma of being different and to build a positive self-image

---

Members of the multidisciplinary rehabilitation team cooperate with each other and the family to identify the child's needs and to plan realistic interventions. Integration of activities is coordinated by one team member, most often a specialist in physical medicine and rehabilitation. Members of the team attempt to achieve their collaborative goals through mutual trust, good communication, professional respect, and sincere interest in the child and family. Training in the rehabilitation center promotes maximum achievement commensurate with each child's physical capacities (Fig. 40-8). Instruction for home routine is stressed and includes all the precautions and management implemented in the acute care center (e.g., skin care, nutrition, bladder and bowel training, gait training) and an exercise program.

Inpatient physical rehabilitation of children with tetraplegia takes approximately 2 to 4 months; children with paraplegia can achieve these goals in 1 to 3 months but require constant vigilance to avoid complications. Emotional adjustments take longer, especially in older children and adolescents. In most children the outlook is favorable unless the life-threatening consequences of urinary pathologic condition are severe or the emotional adjustment is poor.

Psychosocial Rehabilitation

Early-acquired or congenital disability is usually more readily accepted by children than paralysis that appears later in childhood. Rehabilitation efforts should include not only the child's emotional responses but also those of the persons closest to the child. Intensive education is important so that family members understand the nature of the disability, the therapeutic regimen, and complications and are able to provide the physical and emotional support the child needs.

As with any disability, treat children as normally as possible and encourage them in developmental tasks at the age at which they would typically be expected to acquire abilities and perform activities. However, the goals must be realistic, and children should not be forced beyond their capabilities. Vogel, Hickey, Klaas, and colleagues (2004) emphasize the need for children and adolescents with SCI to assume responsibility for their own care. When this is not physically possible, they should direct others in their care. Encouraging self-care is important in the emotional and physical rehabilitation of the child or adolescent with SCI.

Severe depression can be emotionally and intellectually immobilizing, but it indicates that the child is no longer hiding behind denial. In rehabilitation it is desirable for the child to begin to express negative feelings toward the situation because these feelings, redirected by efforts of the rehabilitation team, are the ones that will motivate the child toward learning a new way of life. Anxiety and depression in young children and adolescents with SCI are associated with a poorer quality of life (Anderson, Kelly, Klaas, et al, 2009).

The responses to loss are discussed in Chapter 23; the multiple problems related to altered self-image, especially in older children and adolescents, are discussed in relation to children with disabilities in Chapter 22. Children with severe disabilities need to alter certain concepts about self and social roles. If they perceive adults as persons with complete control over their bodies and the ability to do what they want when they want, they will need to develop a more realistic definition of interdependent adult living.

The needs of young children and adolescents who are permanently disabled must be reevaluated periodically by the total rehabilitation team, including the children and their families. Vocational rehabilitation is important for helping these adolescents find meaningful work activities and enroll in formal educational programs as desired.

The outlook for children and adolescents with SCI is increasingly favorable for integration into society. Increased awareness of the needs of persons with disabilities has removed many structural and occupational barriers. The success of a rehabilitation program is judged not by how well children and adolescents manage within the rehabilitation setting but by how well they function on the outside. In addition to agencies that offer assistance to children with disabilities in general, some agencies provide specific assistance to paralyzed persons, including children.*

---

*Information about organizations and resources can be found through Spinal Cord Injury and Disease Resources, www.makoa.org/sci.htm; and New Mobility, www.newmobility.com. Other helpful resources for families are Spinal Cord Injury Information Network, www.spinalcord.uab.edu; and the Christopher and Dana Reeve Foundation, www.christopherreeve.org.

Sexuality

Issues related to loss of sexual function also apply to adolescents with debilitating neuromuscular diseases such as DMD and SMA. The problems of self-image are particularly significant when children with SCI reach puberty, especially if the disability was acquired during early adolescence. Sexual development and awareness and changing perceptions of body image are prominent aspects of adolescence; a loss that affects these areas is often devastating. Development of secondary sexual characteristics does not seem to be altered by SCIs, and it is now believed that with comprehensive rehabilitation, motivated young people can look forward to successful participation in marital and family activities.

In females, if the injury occurs after the onset of menstruation, there is usually a temporary cessation and irregularity in menstrual flow, but menstruation resumes in the majority of cases. Ovulation and conception are possible, but only about 50% of females experience vaginal or clitoral orgasms, although they can learn to use other erogenous zones for a sexual experience. This is important to emphasize in sex education, since many females have the misconception that they are unable to conceive because they lack sensation. FES may help some women with SCI achieve orgasm. Education is important because the pregnant paraplegic or tetraplegic patient may be unaware that she is in labor, and those with a high-level injury are subject to autonomic dysreflexia during labor.

More attention has been focused on rehabilitating male sexual function (erection and ejaculation) than female sexual function until the last two decades. A number of pharmacologic (prostaglandin E_1) and mechanical devices (penile implants, vacuum devices) now make it possible for males to participate in sexual intercourse and produce offspring, provided that fertility has not been affected by associated complications. Penile injections with vasoactive substances (prostaglandin E_1) are reported to be effective in 90% of men (DeForge, Blackmer, Garritty, et al, 2006). However, sildenafil (Viagra) is now considered the treatment of choice for the sexually active male. Adolescents with SCI should be counseled regarding condom use and the symptoms of latex allergy.

As soon as adolescent males become aware of their functional loss, they will be concerned about sexual capacities, regardless of the type of sexual activities experienced before the SCI. The health care professional should take the initiative in discussing sexuality with adolescents and their families. Parents of younger children may want to know about their children's sexual and reproductive potential. As their interest and understanding increase, adolescents need to know the specifics of physiology, the prognosis, and sexual techniques related to their particular problems. The practitioner should provide them with information about what can be expected regarding erection, ejaculation, and other sexual experiences.

A knowledgeable rehabilitation team is valuable to adolescents as they experience concerns regarding loss as a sexual being. This is especially true in paraplegia or tetraplegia. Most sexual counseling for adolescents with SCI focuses on developing the idea that sex means different things to different people. Most rehabilitation teams have an active counseling program to help adolescents learn intimacy and how to function sexually within their limitations. Through individual and group counseling they gain new attitudes concerning sexuality and experiences exclusive or inclusive of intercourse.

Transition to Adulthood

With the ultimate goal of making an effective transition to adulthood, adolescents with SCI often face challenges similar to others with chronic and debilitating conditions. Issues such as housing, education, personal assistance care, transportation, medical care, and specialized medical care must be addressed in a coordinated transition program (Vogel, Hickey, Klaas, et al, 2004). The concepts of care coordination for children and adolescents requiring home care also apply to adolescents making the transition to adulthood, since different health care services may be needed or requirements may change for benefits for those no longer dependent on parents. (See Chapter 25.)

MUSCULAR DYSFUNCTION

JUVENILE DERMATOMYOSITIS

Juvenile dermatomyositis (JDM) is a relatively rare systemic autoimmune vasculopathy that often occurs after a triggering event such as infection with group A β-hemolytic streptococci, enterovirus (coxsackievirus B), or parvovirus. An environmental trigger such as excessive sun exposure has also been proposed in some children. In children one of the human leukocyte antigens (DQA1*0501, B8, DRB*0301, or DQA1*0301) is present on chromosome 6 and may be associated with increased susceptibility to the disease (Feldman, Rider, Reed, et al, 2008; Pachman, 2007). Caucasian girls are twice as likely to be affected as boys. The average age at onset is 6.9 years. Children with onset before age 7 may experience milder symptoms.

The diagnosis is often established through clinical presentations of bilateral symmetric proximal weakness, a characteristic malar rash (described below), elevated serum enzymes (aldolase, creatine kinase, transaminase, and lactate dehydrogenase), altered EMG, and abnormal muscle biopsy. An alternative to muscle biopsy is an MRI. Nailfold capillaroscopy shows decreased capillary density and presence of disease activity and may be used to diagnose the condition (Feldman, Rider, Reed, et al, 2008).

For approximately half of affected children, the disease is acute and progresses rapidly. Children under 6 years of age often are seen initially with fever and signs of an upper respiratory tract illness. There is proximal limb and trunk muscle weakness and loss of reflexes. Consequently, the child may not be able to rise from the floor to a standing position without walking the hands up the legs (Gower sign). The disease often affects the neck muscles, and the child may have difficulty lifting the head or supporting it in an upright position. Muscles tend to be stiff and sore. A generalized vasculitis of small arteries and capillaries is one prominent feature of the disease. Masseter involvement with atrophy may occur, which makes it difficult to chew food during the active stage of the disease. Soft palate dysfunction may make speech difficult and interfere with breathing. Distal muscle strength and reflex responses remain unaffected. JDM is characterized by a red erythematous rash over the malar areas and nose and a violet discoloration of the eyelids. The skin over extensor muscle surfaces may be erythematous, scaly, and atopic. Calcium deposits develop in muscle tissues as the disease progresses. Dystrophic calcifications may develop over areas exposed to pressure, including the elbows, knees, digits, and buttocks. These lesions may result in skin ulceration with subsequent infection, pain, and functional disability from joint contractures. The vasculitis may cause gastrointestinal, renal, cardiac, and ophthalmologic symptoms as the disease progresses. A common problem in JDM is aspiration pneumonia, and measures should be taken to ensure the child has an adequate airway at all times. If the child has difficulty feeding, a gastrostomy may be used to supplement caloric intake until the drug regimen controls the symptoms.

JDM responds to high-dose oral corticosteroid therapy and methotrexate; in some children high-dose intermittent intravenous methylprednisone may be required. All children with JDM should use a sunscreen to protect against ultraviolet A and B rays. Vitamin D and adequate dietary intake of calcium are also recommended to increase and maintain bone density and minimize osteopenia (Feldman, Rider, Reed, et al, 2008; Pachman, 2007). Some children may respond to cyclophosphamide if methotrexate and IV corticosteroid therapy are not effective (Pachman, 2007). IVIG has been effective in some children who were intolerant of high-dose corticosteroids. Other treatments that have been effective in adult myositis and in isolated cases of JDM include hydroxychloroquine, systemic tacrolimus, etanercept or infliximab, rituximab, and cyclosporin (Feldman, Rider, Reed, et al, 2008).

Physical therapy is essential to prevent contracture deformity and to rebuild muscle strength. Meticulous skin care is an important nursing consideration in the care of these patients.

Although the prognosis for survival has steadily improved, JDM remains a serious chronic illness. Death can occur in the acute phase as a result of myocarditis, progressive unresponsive myositis, perforation of the bowel, or, occasionally, lung involvement. The current mortality rate is approximately 1% (Pachman, 2007).

MUSCULAR DYSTROPHIES

The MDs constitute the largest and most important single group of muscle diseases of childhood (Table 40-2). They have a genetic origin in which there is gradual, progressive degeneration of muscle fibers, and they are characterized by progressive weakness and wasting of symmetric groups of skeletal muscles, with increasing disability and deformity. In all forms of MD there is insidious loss of strength, but each differs in regard to the muscle groups affected, age of onset, rate of progression, and inheritance patterns.

The basic defect in MD is unknown but appears to be caused by a metabolic disturbance unrelated to the nervous system. Initial sites of muscle involvement are illustrated in Fig. 40-9.

Treatment of the MDs consists mainly of providing supportive measures (including physical therapy; orthopedic procedures to minimize deformity; and ventilatory support, including airway clearance techniques) and assisting the affected child in meeting the demands of daily living. Duchenne muscular dystrophy is discussed in the following sections. Other forms of MD include myotonic dystrophy, scapulohumeral

TABLE 40-2   CHARACTERISTICS OF MAJOR MUSCULAR DYSTROPHIES

PRIMARY MYOPATHY AND INHERITANCE PATTERN	AGE OF ONSET	INITIAL MANIFESTATIONS	PROGRESSION	THERAPY
Duchenne X-linked recessive, sporadic	Early childhood; ages 3-5 yr	Lordosis Waddling gait Frequent falls Toe walking Difficulty in rising from floor and climbing stairs Fat deposits replace wasted gastrocnemius muscles	Rapid Ultimately involves all voluntary muscles Death usually occurs at ages 15-30 yr	Supportive Physical therapy to prevent disuse atrophy of unaffected muscles
Becker X-linked recessive, sporadic	>7 yr of age	Same as Duchenne	Much slower progression than Duchenne	Same as Duchenne
Myotonic MD Autosomal dominant Second most common MD in United States and Europe	Early infancy, except for severe congenital form	Facial wasting and hypotonia	Progressive muscle wasting into adolescence and adulthood; affects multiple organs	Treatment of cardiac, ocular, endocrine, and GI complications
Limb-girdle Autosomal recessive (usually, but 16 genetic forms are recognized and some are autosomal dominant)	Late childhood or adolescence; >8 yr of age	Weakness of proximal muscles of both pelvic and shoulder girdles	Variable but usually slow Most become incapacitated within 20 yr of onset; in some, disability may remain slight	Supportive Physical therapy to prevent disuse atrophy of unaffected muscles
Facioscapulohumeral (Landouzy-Dejerine) Autosomal dominant	Early adolescence; >8 yr of age	Lack of facial mobility Difficulty raising arms over head Forward slope of shoulders	Very slow May be intervals with no progression Considerable disability in time, but life span unaffected	Supportive

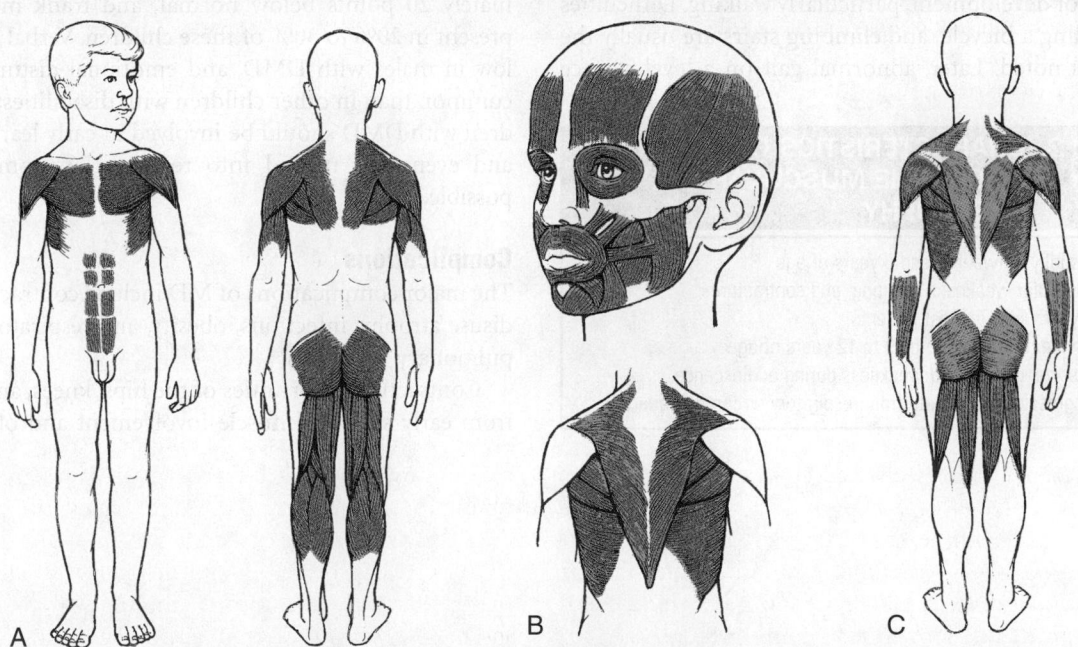

Fig. 40-9 Initial muscle groups involved in muscular dystrophies. **A,** Pseudohypertrophic (Duchenne). **B,** Facioscapulohumeral. **C,** Limb-girdle.

MD, limb-girdle MD, fascioscapulohumeral MD, and congenital MD (Sarnat, 2007).

DUCHENNE MUSCULAR DYSTROPHY

DMD is the most severe and most common MD of childhood. It is inherited as an X-linked recessive trait, and the single-gene defect is located on the short arm of the X chromosome. DMD has a high mutation rate, with a negative family history in approximately 65% to 75% of all cases; therefore genetic counseling is an important aspect of the care of the family. Approximately 30% of DMD patients are *new* mutations and the mother is *not* the carrier (Sarnat, 2007).

As in all X-linked disorders, males are affected almost exclusively. The female carrier may have an elevated serum CK, but muscle weakness is usually not a problem; however, about 10%

of female carriers develop cardiomyopathy (Manzur, Kinali, and Muntoni, 2008). In rare instances a female may be identified with DMD disease yet with muscular weakness that is milder than in boys (Sarnat, 2007). The incidence is approximately 1 in 3600 male births for the Duchenne form and approximately 1 in 30,000 live births for the Becker type, a milder variant (Sarnat, 2007). Box 40-12 describes the characteristics of DMD.

At the genetic level, both DMD and Becker MD result from mutations of the gene that encodes dystrophin, a protein product in skeletal muscle. Dystrophin is absent from the muscle of children with DMD and is reduced or abnormal in children with Becker MD. The absence of dystrophin leads to a number of problems in muscle, including muscle fiber degeneration. A deficiency of dystrophin isoforms in brain tissue causes cognitive and intellectual impairment (Manzur, Kinali, and Muntoni, 2008). Children with Becker MD have a later onset of symptoms, which are usually not as severe as those seen in DMD. There is a strong correlation between the clinical severity of these disorders and the type of genetic mutation and dystrophin protein alterations.

Clinical Manifestations

Most children with DMD reach the appropriate developmental milestones early in life, although they may have mild, subtle delays. Evidence of muscle weakness usually appears during the third to seventh year, although there may have been a history of delay in motor development, particularly walking. Difficulties in running, riding a bicycle, and climbing stairs are usually the first symptoms noted. Later, abnormal gait on a level surface

---

BOX 40-12 CHARACTERISTICS OF DUCHENNE MUSCULAR DYSTROPHY

- Early onset, usually between 3 and 5 years of age
- Progressive muscular weakness, wasting, and contractures
- Calf muscle hypertrophy in most patients
- Loss of independent ambulation by 9 to 12 years of age
- Slowly progressive, generalized weakness during adolescence
- Relentless progression until death from respiratory or cardiac failure

---

becomes apparent. In the early years, rapid developmental gains may mask the progression of the disease. Questioning the parents may reveal that the child has difficulty in rising from a sitting or supine position. Occasionally the parents notice enlarged calves.

Typically, affected boys have a waddling gait and lordosis, fall frequently, and develop a characteristic manner of rising from a squatting or sitting position on the floor (Gower sign) (Fig. 40-10). Lordosis occurs as a result of weakened pelvic muscles, and the waddling gait is a result of weakness in the gluteus medius and maximus muscles (Battista, 2010). Muscles, especially in the calves, thighs, and upper arms, become enlarged from fatty infiltration and feel unusually firm or woody on palpation. The term *pseudohypertrophy* is derived from this muscular enlargement. Profound muscular atrophy occurs in the later stages; contractures and deformities involving large and small joints are common complications as the disease progresses. Ambulation usually becomes impossible by 12 years of age. The loss of mobilization further increases the spectrum of complications, which may include osteoporosis, fractures, constipation, skin breakdown, and psychosocial and behavioral problems. Atrophy of facial, oropharyngeal, and respiratory muscles does not occur until the advanced stage of the disease. Ultimately the disease process involves the diaphragm and auxiliary muscles of respiration, and cardiomegaly is common.

Mild to moderate mental impairment is commonly associated with MD. The mean intelligence quotient (IQ) is approximately 20 points below normal, and frank mental deficit is present in 20% to 30% of these children. Verbal IQ is markedly low in males with DMD, and emotional disturbance is more common than in other children with disabilities; however, children with DMD should be involved in early learning programs and eventually moved into regular classrooms as much as possible.

Complications

The major complications of MD include contractures, scoliosis, disuse atrophy, infections, obesity, and respiratory and cardiopulmonary problems.

Contracture deformities of the hips, knees, and ankles occur from early selective muscle involvement and often exaggerate

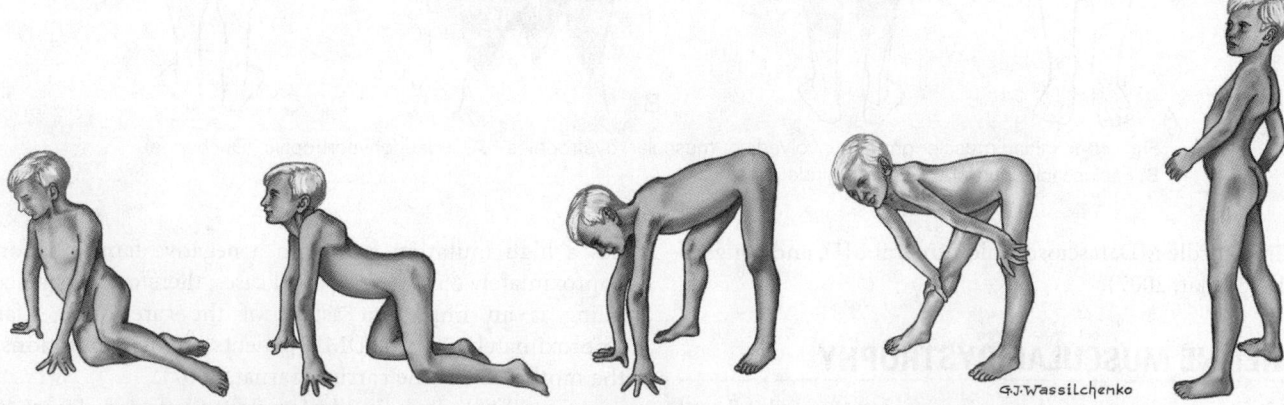

Fig. 40-10 Child with Duchenne muscular dystrophy attains standing posture by kneeling, then gradually pushing his torso upright (with knees straight) by "walking" his hands up his legs (Gower sign). Note marked lordosis in upright position.

the weakness. Passive range-of-motion exercises, stretching, and active exercises under the supervision of a PT are effective in treating reducible contractures. Nonreducible contractures require wedge casting or surgical reduction. Scoliosis caused by muscle imbalance is common in children who lose ambulatory capability and tends to progress even when the child becomes dependent on a wheelchair. Bracing with an orthosis may be required, but in many cases spinal fusion surgery is performed to prevent complications associated with cardiac and pulmonary restriction.

Atrophy of disuse from prolonged inactivity occurs readily when children are immobilized or confined to bed with illness, injury, or surgery. To minimize this complication, physical therapy should begin if bed rest extends beyond a few days. To maintain muscle strength, a daily goal for well children with moderate disability should be at least 3 hours of ambulation.

Pulmonary infections become increasingly frequent as the dystrophic process produces a progressive decrease in pulmonary vital capacity as a result of weakness of the primary, secondary, and associated muscles of respiration. Consequently even minor upper respiratory tract infections may become serious in these children. The eventual cause of death is usually respiratory tract infection or cardiac failure; however, much progress has been made in providing ventilatory methods to prolong and maintain quality of life. Prompt and vigorous antibiotic therapy, supplemented by postural drainage and aggressive airway clearance methods, is effective. Because of the respiratory musculature weakness, these children are unable to cough effectively and secretions collect easily.

Obesity is a common complication that contributes to premature loss of ambulation. Children who have restricted opportunities for physical activity and who suffer from boredom easily consume calories in excess of their needs. This may be compounded by overfeeding by well-meaning family and friends. Proper dietary intake and a diversified recreational program help reduce the likelihood of obesity and enable children to maintain ambulation and functional independence for a longer time.

Cardiac manifestations are usually late events but may occur in ambulatory children. The most significant of these, cardiac failure, is difficult to correct in advanced cases, but treatment with digoxin and diuretics is often beneficial in the early stages of the disease.

Diagnostic Evaluation

MD is suspected on the basis of clinical manifestations (see Box 40-12) and confirmed by molecular genetic detection of deficient dystrophin by DNA analysis from peripheral blood or in muscle tissue obtained by biopsy. The diagnosis of DMD is primarily established by blood polymerase chain reaction (PCR) for the dystrophin gene mutation (Sarnat, 2007). Diagnostic techniques such as multiplex PCR have made it possible to diagnose 98% of the DMD mutations. Prenatal diagnosis is also possible as early as 12 weeks of gestation. However, ethical questions exist regarding diagnosing a condition in the fetus when no treatment exists.

Serum enzyme measurement, muscle biopsy, and EMG may also be used in establishing the diagnosis. Serum CK levels are extremely high in the first 2 years of life, before the onset of clinical weakness. If the child demonstrates the usual characteristics, has a positive family history for DMD, and the PCR is positive, the muscle biopsy may be deferred.

Muscle biopsy reveals degeneration of muscle fibers, with fibrosis and fatty tissue replacement. EMG readings show a decrease in amplitude and duration of motor unit potentials.

Therapeutic Management

Currently no effective treatment exists for childhood MD. Increased muscle bulk and muscle power have been reported after a course of corticosteroids. Several clinical trials demonstrated increased muscle strength and improved performance and pulmonary function, with significant decrease in the progression of weakness, when prednisone was administered for 6 months to 2 years (Manzur, Kuntzer, Pike, et al, 2008). Corticosteroid administration also prolonged ambulation, preserved respiratory function, and decreased the incidence of scoliosis and cardiomyopathy (Manzur, Kinali, and Muntoni, 2008). Major side effects in these studies included weight gain and a cushingoid facial appearance. The American Academy of Neurology has published a practice parameter for the administration of corticosteroids in the treatment of DMD (Moxley, Ashwal, Pandya, et al, 2005).

Maintaining optimum function in all muscles for as long as possible is the primary goal; secondary is the prevention of contractures. In general, children who remain as active as possible are able to avoid wheelchair confinement for a longer time. Maintenance of function often includes stretching exercises, strength and muscle training, breathing exercises and use of incentive spirometry to increase and maintain vital lung capacity, airway clearance, range-of-motion exercises, surgery to release contracture deformities, bracing, and performance of ADLs. Knee-ankle-foot orthoses have been shown to prolong ambulation for 18 to 24 months beyond the termination of independent ambulation. Serial casting of ankles has proved more effective than surgical release of Achilles tendons in many children with DMD to prevent contractures (Manzur, Kinali, and Muntoni, 2008).

Parents should always be involved in making decisions about the child's care, and teaching regarding home safety and prevention of falls is important as well (Metules, 2002). Also encourage parents to have the child keep follow-up appointments for medical care and physical and occupational therapy. Because respiratory tract infections are most troublesome in these children, encourage regular influenza and pneumococcal vaccines and avoidance of contact with persons with respiratory tract infections as much as possible. Baseline pulmonary function testing, electrocardiograms, and echocardiograms are also recommended (Metules, 2002).

Eventually, respiratory and cardiac problems become the central focus of the debilitating illness. The child and parents should be involved in a discussion of long-term ventilation options. Cardiac and respiratory assessment during wake-sleep cycles is imperative. Children with neuromuscular disease eventually develop abnormal breathing patterns, particularly during rapid-eye-movement sleep, and hypoxia occurs as a result of inadequate oxygenation. The sleep-disordered breathing of DMD results in symptoms such as frequent night awakenings, morning headache, and daytime sleepiness.

Polysomnography should be performed once daytime symptoms of sleep-disordered breathing occur. Noninvasive positive pressure ventilation should be considered in such children to prevent further hypoventilation and cardiorespiratory deterioration (Culebras, 2008). Respiratory care for children with neuromuscular conditions such as SMA and DMD may involve the use of noninvasive ventilation with BiPAP on a temporary or full-time basis, mechanically assisted coughing (MAC), or tracheotomy and relief of airway obstruction with coughing and suctioning devices; the tracheotomy, however, is associated with more complications (Simonds, 2006; Young, Lowe, and Fitzgerald, 2007). Home pulse oximetry may be used to monitor oxygenation during sleep or to aid in decision making regarding the use of MAC to clear the airways. A polysomnogram may be used to evaluate the effectiveness of supplemental oxygen and noninvasive ventilation devices.

Several devices are available for children with neuromuscular disease to assist in clearing the airway when the cough reflex is ineffective or diminished. The mechanical cough in-exsufflator (MIE) (also referred to as cough assist) has been found to be safe and effective in the daily management of respiratory function (Kravitz, 2009; Miske, Hickey, Kolb, et al, 2004). The MIE delivers positive inspiratory pressures at a set rate, followed by negative pressure exsufflation coordinated with the patient's own breathing rhythm. The exsufflation is designed to mimic a cough reflex so mucus can be effectively cleared. Airway suctioning after exsufflation is accomplished as necessary to clear the airways. In children the MIE device may be connected directly to a tracheostomy or used with a mouthpiece or face mask. The Boitano (2009) reference contains a variety of equipment options, including various masks that can be used to deliver noninvasive positive pressure.

Manual cough-assisting techniques include glossopharyngeal breathing or air stacking (frog breathing); the abdominal thrust, which is similar to the Heimlich maneuver (Kravitz, 2009); and manual hyperinflation with a self-inflating resuscitation bag (without oxygen) and a mouthpiece. Hyperinflation may be used in conjunction with abdominal thrusts to improve peak cough flows (Boitano, 2009).

The use of routine chest physiotherapy for DMD has not been adequately evaluated for its effectiveness in clearing the airway of mucus except when there is focal atelectasis and mucus plugging the airways (Kravitz, 2009).

Survival in individuals with DMD may be prolonged several years with the use of noninvasive ventilation and airway clearance devices such as cough assist as alternatives to tracheotomy and airway suctioning (Simonds, 2006). The American Thoracic Society (2004) has published extensive guidelines for respiratory monitoring and care of children and adults with DMD. See the Finder (2009) reference for an elaboration on the 2004 American Thoracic Society statement.

The American Academy of Pediatrics (2005) recommends an extensive cardiac evaluation of the child diagnosed with either DMD or Becker MD. Patients with neuromuscular conditions may not have the typical signs and symptoms of cardiac dysfunction. Therefore symptoms such as weight loss, nausea and vomiting, cough, increased fatigue on performance of ADLs, and orthopnea should be carefully evaluated to detect early signs of cardiomyopathy.

Research evaluating a number of treatments for DMD is in progress. These include clinical trials with glutamine and creatine monohydrate to preserve muscle strength; utrophin, a protein that is similar to dystrophin and in large quantities may counteract the effects of the dystrophin deficiency (Chakkalakal, Thompson, Parks, et al, 2005; Miura and Jardin, 2006); and the enzyme CT GalNAc transferase, which blocks muscle wasting in mice (Metules, 2002). Oral albuterol administered daily for 12 weeks increased lean body mass and decreased fat mass in a group of 14 ambulatory boys with Becker and DMD; however, overall muscle strength improvement was not observed (Skura, Fowler, Wetzel, et al, 2008).

Genetic counseling is recommended for parents, sisters, and maternal aunts and their daughters. (See Chapter 5.) Long-term care, end-of-life care, and palliative care options are issues that the health care team must discuss with the child and family affected by MD (Finder, 2009). Professional counseling is necessary in some cases to allow frank discussion of these issues, and referrals should be made as appropriate (Finder, Birnkrant, Carl, et al, 2004). (See Chapter 23.)

Nursing Care Management

The care and management of a child with MD involve the combined efforts of a multidisciplinary health care team. Nurses can help clarify the roles of these health care professionals to family and others. The major emphasis of nursing care is to assist the child and family in coping with the progressive, incapacitating, and fatal nature of the disease; to help design a program that will afford a greater degree of independence and reduce the predictable and preventable disabilities associated with the disorder; and to help the child and family deal constructively with the limitations the disease imposes on their daily lives. Because of advances in technology, children with MD may live into early adulthood; therefore the goals of care should also involve decisions regarding quality of life, achievement of independence, and transition to adulthood.

Working closely with other team members, nurses assist the family in developing the child's self-help skills to give the child the satisfaction of being as independent as possible for as long as possible. It is tempting for parents to overprotect their affected children. Children derive pleasure and build self-esteem from performing actions that visibly please their parents. Therefore parents must be helped to develop a balance between limiting the child's activity because of muscular weakness and allowing the child to accomplish things alone. This requires continual evaluation of the child's capabilities, which are often difficult to assess. Most children with MD instinctively recognize the need to be as independent as possible and strive to do so.

Practical difficulties faced by families are the physical limitations of housing, transportation, and mobility. Housing accommodations must be made so the wheelchair-bound child can be mobile in the home setting. Transportation in a car restraint seat adapted for the child with weakened neck and back musculature will be necessary, and eventually a wheelchair-accessible vehicle will be required. Discuss diet, nutritional needs, and nutrition modification according to the needs of the individual child and family. Nutritional needs decrease once the child becomes wheelchair bound, and dietary modifications should be made in conjunction with a pediatric dietitian to ensure the child is receiving an adequate amount of the necessary nutrients to maintain bone health and prevent constipation.

Parents' social activities may be restricted, and the family's activities must be continually modified to meet the needs of the affected child. (See Chapter 22.) When the child becomes increasingly incapacitated, the family may consider home care to provide the care needed. The nurse as case manager can assist the family in making this difficult transition. Unless the child is severely incapacitated, he or she should also be involved in the decisions regarding such care. Nurses can assist with decision making by exploring all available options and resources and supporting the child and family in the decision.

Each child's therapy program is tailored to individual needs and capabilities, and family members should be active participants. Parents often need assistance with the physical therapy program and education regarding a home regimen of exercises and activity. Many parents erroneously believe that by exerting sufficient effort, the child can overcome the weakness and prevent progression of the disease process. They should also be advised to notify the nurse or other designated person when the child becomes even temporarily bedridden so that the exercise program can be modified and continued during this time.

Children with MD tend to become socially isolated as their physical condition deteriorates to the point that they can no longer keep up with friends and classmates. Their physical capabilities diminish, and their dependency increases at the age at which most children are expanding their range of interests and relationships. To gain peer associations, they often learn and employ behaviors that bring them the rewards of other children's company. These friends are often children who have been rejected by more able-bodied classmates.

Older boys with MD may also need psychiatric or psychologic counseling to deal with issues such as depression, anger, and quality of life (Bothwell, Dooley, Gordon, et al, 2002). Parents need encouragement to become involved in support groups, since there is evidence that adequate social support from family, community, and other parents is crucial to appropriate coping in families with children with chronic illness (Bothwell, Dooley, Gordon, et al, 2002).

Regardless of the success of the program and how well the family adapts to the disorder, superimposed on the physical and emotional problems associated with the child's long-term disability is the constant specter of the disease's ultimate outcome. These families encounter all the manifestations of the child with a chronic and fatal illness. (See Chapter 23.)

Nurses are especially valuable health care professionals as they come to know the family and the family's challenges. Nurses can be alert to the problems and needs of the families and make necessary referrals when supplementary services are indicated. The Muscular Dystrophy Association–USA* has branches in most communities to provide assistance to families that have a member with MD.

---

*3300 E. Sunrise Drive, Tucson, AZ 85718; 800-572-1717 e-mail: mda@mdausa.org; www.mda.org. In Canada: Muscular Dystrophy Canada, 2345 Yonge St., Suite 900, Toronto, Ontario, Canada M4P 2E5; 866-MUSCLE-8; fax: 416-488-7523; www.muscle.ca.

KEY POINTS

- Upper motor neuron lesions produce weakness associated with spasticity, increased deep tendon reflexes, and abnormal superficial reflexes; lower motor neuron lesions interrupt the reflex arc, causing weakness and atrophy of the skeletal muscles.
- The most useful classification of neuromuscular disorders defines the source of the lesion: cerebral cortex, anterior horn cells of the spinal cord, peripheral nerves, neuromuscular junction, and muscles.
- Clinical manifestations of CP include delayed gross motor development; abnormal motor performance; alterations of muscle tone; abnormal posture; reflex abnormalities; and associated disabilities such as developmental and cognitive impairment, seizures, behavioral disorder, speech problems, feeding and growth problems, chronic constipation, and sensory impairment.
- Therapy for CP takes into account the nature of the physical disability, defects associated with the disorder, and interpersonal and social influences encountered by the affected child.
- Werdnig-Hoffmann disease is characterized by progressive weakness and wasting of skeletal muscles caused by degeneration of anterior horn cells.
- Nursing care of the child with GBS consists of monitoring vital signs, monitoring respiratory status, ensuring alignment and positioning, providing physical therapy, managing pain, and providing support to the family.

- Tetanus occurs when tetanus spores or vegetative bacilli enter a wound and multiply in a susceptible host.
- Infant botulism results from toxins produced by *C. botulinum*; constipation is often a presenting symptom in infants, followed by generalized weakness and poor feeding.
- Management of MG includes administering oral anticholinesterase drugs, ensuring adequate rest periods, and preventing MG crises.
- SCIs represent a major debilitating health problem that is largely preventable in children and adolescents by instituting and following safety measures such as proper car safety restraints and avoiding alcohol ingestion before driving a motor vehicle.
- SCIs usually involve four interrelated pathologic changes: cellular damage to cord tissue; hemorrhage and vascular damage; structural changes of white and gray matter related to vascular disruption, inflammation, and edema; and local biochemical response to trauma.
- Therapeutic management of SCI is directed toward preventing further neuronal damage, managing associated complications, and maintaining vital functions.
- The goals of rehabilitation in SCI are to maximize functional mobility; to help the child cope with the dysfunction and build a positive self-image; to promote independence in performing ADLs (including self-care and hygiene); and to

- promote education, employment, social relationships, and independent living.
- MDs are the largest and most important group of debilitating muscular dysfunctions in childhood.

- The major complications of MD include contractures, disuse atrophy, respiratory infections, scoliosis, obesity, respiratory compromise, and cardiac failure.

REFERENCES

Albright AL, Gilmartin R, Swift D, et al: Long-term intrathecal baclofen therapy for severe spasticity of cerebral origin, *J Neurosurg* 98(2):291-295, 2003.

American Academy of Pediatrics, Committee on Infectious Diseases, Pickering L, editor: 2009 *Red book: report of the Committee on Infectious Diseases*, ed 28, Elk Grove Village, Ill, 2009, The Academy.

American Academy of Pediatrics: Cardiovascular health supervision for individuals affected by Duchenne or Becker muscular dystrophy, *Pediatrics* 116(6):1569-1573, 2005.

American Spinal Injury Association: *Standard neurological classification of spinal cord injury*, 2009, The Association, available at www.asia-spinalinjury.org/publications/2006_Classif_worksheet.pdf (accessed April 29, 2010).

American Thoracic Society: Respiratory care of the patient with Duchenne muscular dystrophy: ATS consensus statement, *Am J Respir Crit Care Med* 170(4):456-465, 2004.

Anderson CJ, Kelly EM, Klaas SJ, et al: Anxiety and depression in children and adolescents with spinal cord injuries, *Dev Med Child Neurol* 51(10):826-832, 2009.

Arnon SS: Tetanus (*Clostridium tetani*). In Kliegman RM, Behrman RE, Jenson HB, et al, editors: *Nelson textbook of pediatrics*, ed 18, Philadelphia, 2007, Saunders.

Arnon SS, Schechter R, Maslanka SE, et al: Human botulism immune globulin for the treatment of infant botulism, *N Engl J Med* 354(5):462-471, 2006.

Ashwal S, Russman BS, Blasco PA, et al: Practice parameter: diagnostic assessment of the child with cerebral palsy: report of the Quality Standards Subcommittee of the American Academy of Neurology and the Practice Committee of the Child Neurology Society, *Neurology* 62(6):851-863, 2004.

Bach JR: Medical considerations of long-term survival of Werdnig-Hoffmann disease, *Am J Phys Med Rehabil* 86(5):349-355, 2007.

Barker E, Saulino MF: Special report: first-ever guidelines for spinal cord injuries, *RN* 65(10):32-37, 2002.

Battista V: Muscular dystrophy, Duchenne. In Jackson PL, Vessey JA, Schapiro NA, editors: *Primary care of the child with a chronic illness*, ed 5, St Louis, 2010, Mosby.

Bax M, Goldstein M, Rosenbaum P, et al: Proposed definition and classification of cerebral palsy, *Dev Med Child Neurol* 47(8):571-576, 2005.

Berker AN, Yalçin MS: Cerebral palsy: orthopedic aspects and rehabilitation, *Pediatr Clin North Am* 55(5):1209-1225, 2008.

Beroud C, Karliova M, Bonnefont JP, et al: Prenatal diagnosis of spinal muscular atrophy by genetic analysis of circulating fetal cells, *Lancet* 361(9362):1013-1014, 2003.

Blair E, Watson L, Badawi N, et al: Life expectancy among people with cerebral palsy in Western Australia, *Dev Med Child Neurol* 43(8):508-515, 2001.

Boitano LJ: Equipment options for cough augmentation, ventilation, and noninvasive interfaces in neuromuscular respiratory management, *Pediatrics* 123(Suppl 4):S226-S230, 2009.

Bothwell JE, Dooley JM, Gordon KE, et al: Duchenne muscular dystrophy: parental perceptions, *Clin Pediatr* 41(2):105-109, 2002.

Bush A, Fraser J, Jardine E: Respiratory management of the infant with type 1 spinal muscular atrophy, *Arch Dis Child* 90(7):709-711, 2005.

Chafetz RS, Mulcahey MJ, Betz RR, et al: Impact of prophylactic thoracolumbosacral bracing on functional activities and activities of daily living in the pediatric spinal cord injury population, *J Spinal Cord Med* 30(Suppl 1):S178-S183, 2007.

Chakkalakal JV, Thompson J, Parks RJ, et al: Molecular, cellular, and pharmacological therapies for Duchenne/Becker muscular dystrophies, *FASEB J* 19(8):880-891, 2005.

Cirak B, Ziegfeld S, Knight VM, et al: Spinal injuries in children, *J Pediatr Surg* 39(4):607-612, 2004.

Cirillo ML: Neuromuscular emergencies, *Clin Pediatr Emerg Med* 9(2):88-95, 2008.

Culebras A: Sleep-disordered breathing in neuromuscular disease, *Sleep Med Clin* 3(3):377-386, 2008.

Curley MAQ, Razmus IS, Roberts KE, et al: Predicting pressure ulcer risk in pediatric patients: the Braden Q Scale, *Nurs Res* 52(1):22-33, 2003.

Dai AI, Wasay M, Awan S: Botulinum toxin type A with oral baclofen versus oral tizanidine: a randomized pilot comparison in patients with cerebral palsy and equines foot deformity, *J Child Neurol* 23(12):1464-1466, 2008.

DeBoer SL, Seaver M: Pediatric spinal immobilization: C-spines, car seats, and color-coded collars, *J Emerg Nurs* 30(5):481-484, 2004.

DeForge D, Blackmer J, Garritty C, et al: Male erectile dysfunction following spinal cord injury: a systematic review, *Spinal Cord* 44(8):465-473, 2006.

Feldman BM, Rider LG, Reed AM, et al: Juvenile dermatomyositis and other idiopathic inflammatory myopathies of childhood, *Lancet* 371(9631):2201-2212, 2008.

Finder JD: A 2009 perspective on the 2004 American Thoracic Society statement, "Respiratory care of the patient with Duchenne muscular dystrophy," *Pediatrics* 123(Suppl 4): S239-S241, 2009.

Finder JD, Birnkrant D, Carl J, et al: Respiratory care of the patient with Duchenne muscular dystrophy: ATS consensus statement, *Am J Respir Crit Care Med* 170(4):456-465, 2004.

Fiore AE, Shay DK, Broder K, et al: Prevention and control of seasonal influenza with vaccines, *MMWR Early Release* 58(Early release):1-52, 2009.

Francis R: Physiology and management of bladder and bowel continence following spinal cord injury, *Ostomy Wound Manage* 53(12):18-27, 2007.

Francisco AM, Arnon SS: Clinical mimics of infant botulism, *Pediatrics* 119(4):826-828, 2007.

Gasalberti D: Alternative therapies for children and youth with special health care needs, *J Pediatr Health Care* 20(2):133-136, 2006.

Golomb MR, Saha C, Garg BP, et al: Association of cerebral palsy with other disabilities in children with perinatal arterial ischemic stroke, *Pediatr Neurol* 37(4):245-249, 2007.

Green L, Greenberg GM, Hurwitz E: Primary care of children with cerebral palsy, *Clin Fam Pract* 5(2):1-21, 2003.

Grether JK, Nelson KB, Walsh E, et al: Intrauterine exposure to infection and risk of cerebral palsy in very preterm infants, *Arch Pediatr Adolesc Med* 157(1):26-32, 2003.

Haber P, DeStefano F, Angulo FJ, et al: Guillain-Barré syndrome following influenza vaccination, *JAMA* 292(20):2478-2481, 2004.

Hack M, Costello DW: Trends in the rates of cerebral palsy associated with neonatal intensive care of preterm children, *Clin Obstet Gynecol* 51(4):763-774, 2008.

Harel M, Schoenfeld Y: Intravenous immunoglobulin and Guillain-Barré syndrome, *Clin Rev Allergy Immunol* 29(3):281-287, 2005.

Haslam RHA: Spinal cord injuries. In Kliegman RM, Behrman RE, Jenson HB, et al, editors: *Nelson textbook of pediatrics*, ed 18, Philadelphia, 2007, Saunders.

Hayes JS, Arriola T: Pediatric spinal injuries, *Pediatr Nurs* 31(6):464-467, 2005.

Hermansen MC, Hermansen MG: Perinatal infections and cerebral palsy, *Clin Perinatol* 33(2):315-333, 2006.

Hirtz D, Thurman DJ, Gwinn-Hardy K, et al: How common are the "common" neurologic disorders? *Neurology* 68(5):326-337, 2007.

Hughes R: The role of IVIG in autoimmune neuropathies: the latest evidence, *J Neurol* 255(Suppl 3):7-11, 2008.

Hughes RA, Cornblath DR: Guillain-Barré syndrome, *Lancet* 366(9497):1653-1666, 2005.

Hughes RA, Raphael JC, Swan AV, et al: Intravenous immunoglobulin for Guillain-Barré syndrome, *Cochrane Library* (1):CD002063, 2006.

Iannaccone ST: Modern management of spinal muscular atrophy, *J Child Neurol* 22(8):974-978, 2007.

Iannaccone ST: Spinal muscular atrophy, *Semin Neurol* 18(1):19-26, 1998.

Iannaccone ST, Burghes A: Spinal muscular atrophies, *Adv Neurol* 88:83-98, 2002.

Johnston MV: Cerebral palsy. In Kliegman RM, Behrman RE, Jenson HB, et al, editors: *Nelson textbook of pediatrics*, ed 18, Philadelphia, 2007, Saunders.

Johnston TE, Betz RR, Smith BT, et al: Implantable FES system for upright mobility and bladder and bowel function for individuals with spinal cord injury, *Spinal Cord* 43(12):713-723, 2005.

Jones MW, Morgan E, Shelton JE: Primary care of the child with cerebral palsy: a review of systems (part II), *J Pediatr Health Care* 21(4):226-237, 2007.

Kalb RG: Getting the spinal cord to think for itself, *Arch Neurol* 60(6):805-808, 2003.

Krach LE: Pharmacotherapy of spasticity: oral medications and intrathecal baclofen, *J Child Neurol* 16(1):31-36, 2001.

Krageloh-Mann I, Cans C: Cerebral palsy update, *Brain Dev* 31(7):537-544, 2009.

Kravitz RM: Airway clearance in Duchenne muscular dystrophy, *Pediatrics* 123(Suppl 4):S231-S235, 2009.

Krigger KW: Cerebral palsy: an overview, *Am Fam Physician* 73(1):91-100, 101-102, 2006.

Laskowski-Jones L: Peripheral nerve and spinal cord problems. In Lewis SL, Heitkemper MM, Dirksen SR, et al, editors, *Medical-surgical nursing: assessment and management of clinical problems*, ed 7, St Louis, 2007, Mosby/Elsevier.

Launay F, Leet AI, Sponseller PD: Pediatric spinal cord injury without radiographic abnormality: a meta-analysis, *Clin Orthop Related Res* 433:166-170, 2005.

Liptak GS, Accardo PJ: Health and social outcomes of children with cerebral palsy, *J Pediatr* 145(Suppl):S36-S41, 2004.

Lovette B: Safe transportation for children with special needs, *J Pediatr Health Care* 22(5):323-328, 2008.

Lukban MB, Rosales RL, Dressler D: Effectiveness of botulinum toxin A for upper and lower limb spasticity in children with cerebral palsy: a summary of evidence, *J Neural Transm* 116(3):319-331, 2009.

Lunn MR, Wang CH: Spinal muscular atrophy, *Lancet* 371(9630):2120-2133, 2008.

Lyons R: Elusive belly pain and Guillain-Barré syndrome, *J Pediatr Health Care* 22(5):310-314, 2008.

Manzur AY, Kinali M, Muntoni F: Update on the management of Duchenne muscular dystrophy, *Arch Dis Child* 93(11):986-990, 2008.

Manzur AY, Kuntzer T, Pike M, et al: Glucocorticoid corticosteroids for Duchenne muscular dystrophy, *Cochrane Database Syst Rev* 23(1): CD003725, 2008.

Markowitz JA, Tinkle MB, Fischbeck KH: Spinal muscular atrophy in the neonate, *JOGNN* 33(1):12-20, 2004.

Mathison DJ, Kadom N, Krug SE: Spinal cord injury in the pediatric patient, *Clin Pediatr Emerg Med* 9(2):106-123, 2008.

McKearnan KA, Kieckhefer GM, Engel JM, et al: Pain in children with cerebral palsy: a review, *J Neurosci Nurs* 36(5):252-259, 2004.

Mehta S, Betz RR, Mulcahey MJ, et al: Effect of bracing on paralytic scoliosis secondary to spinal cord injury, *J Spinal Cord Med* 27(Suppl 1):S88-S92, 2004.

Merenda LA, Hickey K: Key elements of a bladder and bowel management for children with spinal cord injuries, *Sci Nurs* 22(1):8-14, 2005.

Merenda LA, Spoltore TA, Betz RR: Progressive treatment options for children with spinal cord injury, *Sci Nurs* 17(3):102-109, 2000.

Mctules T: Duchenne muscular dystrophy, *RN* 65(10):39-47, 2002.

Miske LJ, Hickey EM, Kolb SM, et al: Use of the mechanical in-exsufflator in pediatric patients with neuromuscular disease and impaired cough, *Chest* 125(4):1406-1412, 2004.

Miura P, Jardin BJ: Utrophin upregulation for treating Duchenne or Becker muscular dystrophy: how close are we? *Trends Mol Med* 12(3):122-129, 2006.

Moxley RT, Ashwal S, Pandya S, et al: Practice parameter: corticosteroid treatment on Duchenne dystrophy, *Neurology* 64(1):13-20, 2005.

Murphy KP, Molnar GE, Lankasky K: Employment and social issues in adults with cerebral palsy, *Arch Phys Med Rehabil* 81:807-811, 2000.

Nehring WM: Cerebral palsy. In Jackson PL, Vessey JA, Schapiro NA, editors: *Primary care of the child with a chronic illness*, ed 5, St Louis, 2010, Mosby.

Newswanger DI, Warren CR: Guillain-Barré syndrome, *Am Fam Physician* 69(10):2405-2410, 2004.

Nordmark E, Josenby AL, Lagergren J, et al: Long-term outcomes 5 years after selective dorsal rhizotomy, *BMC Pediatr* 8:54, 2008.

Pachman LM: Juvenile dermatomyositis. In Kliegman RM, Behrman RE, Jenson HB, et al, editors: *Nelson textbook of pediatrics*, ed 18, Philadelphia, 2007, Saunders.

Pang D: Spinal cord injury without radiographic abnormality in children: two decades later, *Neurosurg Online* 55(6):1325-1343, 2004.

Platzer P, Jaindi M, Thalhammer G, et al: Cervical spine injuries in pediatric patients, *J Trauma* 62(2):389-396, 2007.

Rogers B: Feeding method and health outcomes of children with cerebral palsy, *J Pediatr* 145(2 Suppl):S28-S32, 2004.

Roscigno CI: Addressing spasticity-related pain in children with spastic cerebral palsy, *J Neurosci Nurs* 34(3):123-131, 2002.

Rosenbaum P, Paneth N, Leviton A, et al: A report: the definition and classification of cerebral palsy April 2006, *Dev Med Child Neurol* 49(S109):1-44, 2007.

Russman BS: Function changes in spinal muscular atrophy II and III: the DCN/SMA Group, *Neurology* 47(4):973-976, 1996.

Russman BS, Iannaccone ST, Buncher CR, et al: Spinal muscular atrophy: new thoughts on the pathogenesis and classification schema, *J Child Neurol* 7(4):347-353, 1992.

Sarnat HB: Neuromuscular disorders. In Kliegman RM, Behrman RE, Jenson HB, et al, editors: *Nelson textbook of pediatrics*, ed 18, Philadelphia, 2007, Saunders.

Shavelle RM, DeVivo MJ, Paculdo DR, et al: Long-term survival after childhood spinal cord injury, *J Spinal Cord Med* 30(Suppl 1):S48-S54, 2007.

Simonds AK: Recent advances in respiratory care for neuromuscular disease, *Chest* 130(6):1879-1886, 2006.

Skura CL, Fowler EG, Wetzel GT, et al: Albuterol increases lean body mass in ambulatory boys with Duchenne or Becker muscular dystrophy, *Neurology* 70(2):137-143, 2008.

Spoltore T, Mulcahey MJ, Johnston T, et al: Innovative programs for children and adolescents with spinal cord injury, *Orthop Nurs* 19(3):55-61, 2000.

Thompson JA, Filloux FM, Van Orman CB, et al: Infant botulism in the age of botulism immune globulin, *Neurology* 64(12):2029-2032, 2005.

Thrasher TA, Popovic MR: Functional electrical stimulation of walking: function, exercise and rehabilitation, *Ann Readapt Med Phys* 51(6):452-460, 2008.

To CS, Kirsch RF, Kobetic R, et al: Simulation of a functional neuromuscular stimulation powered mechanical gait orthosis with coordinated joint locking, *IEEE Trans Neural Syst Rehabil Eng* 13(2):227-235, 2005.

Tsai CP, Wang KC, Liu CY, et al: Pharmacoeconomics of therapy for Guillain-Barré syndrome: plasma exchange and intravenous immunoglobulin, *J Clin Neurosci* 14(7):625-629, 2007.

Vajsar J, Fehlings D, Stephens D: Long-term outcome in children with Guillain-Barré syndrome, *J Pediatr* 142(3):305-309, 2003.

Vogel LC, Hickey KJ, Klaas SJ, et al: Unique issues in pediatric spinal cord injury, *Orthop Nurs* 23(5):300-308, 2004.

Wu YW, Escobar GJ, Grether JK, et al: Chorioamnionitis and cerebral palsy in term and near-term infants, *JAMA* 290(20):2677-2684, 2003.

Yeargin-Allsopp M, Van Naarden Braun K, Doernberg NS, et al: Prevalence of cerebral palsy in 8-year-old children in three areas of the United States in 2002: a multisite collaboration, *Pediatrics* 121(3):547-554, 2008.

Young HK, Lowe A, Fitzgerald DA: Outcome of noninvasive ventilation in children with neuromuscular disease, *Neurology* 68(3):198-201, 2007.

Zier JL, Rivard PF, Krach LE, et al: Effectiveness of sedation using nitrous oxide compared with enteral midazolam for botulinum toxin A injections in children, *Dev Med Child Neurol* 50(11):854-858, 2008.

Zuckerbraun NS, Ferson SS, Albright AL, et al: Intrathecal baclofen withdrawal: emergent recognition and management, *Pediatr Emerg Care* 20(11):759-764, 2004.

Developmental/Sensory Assessment

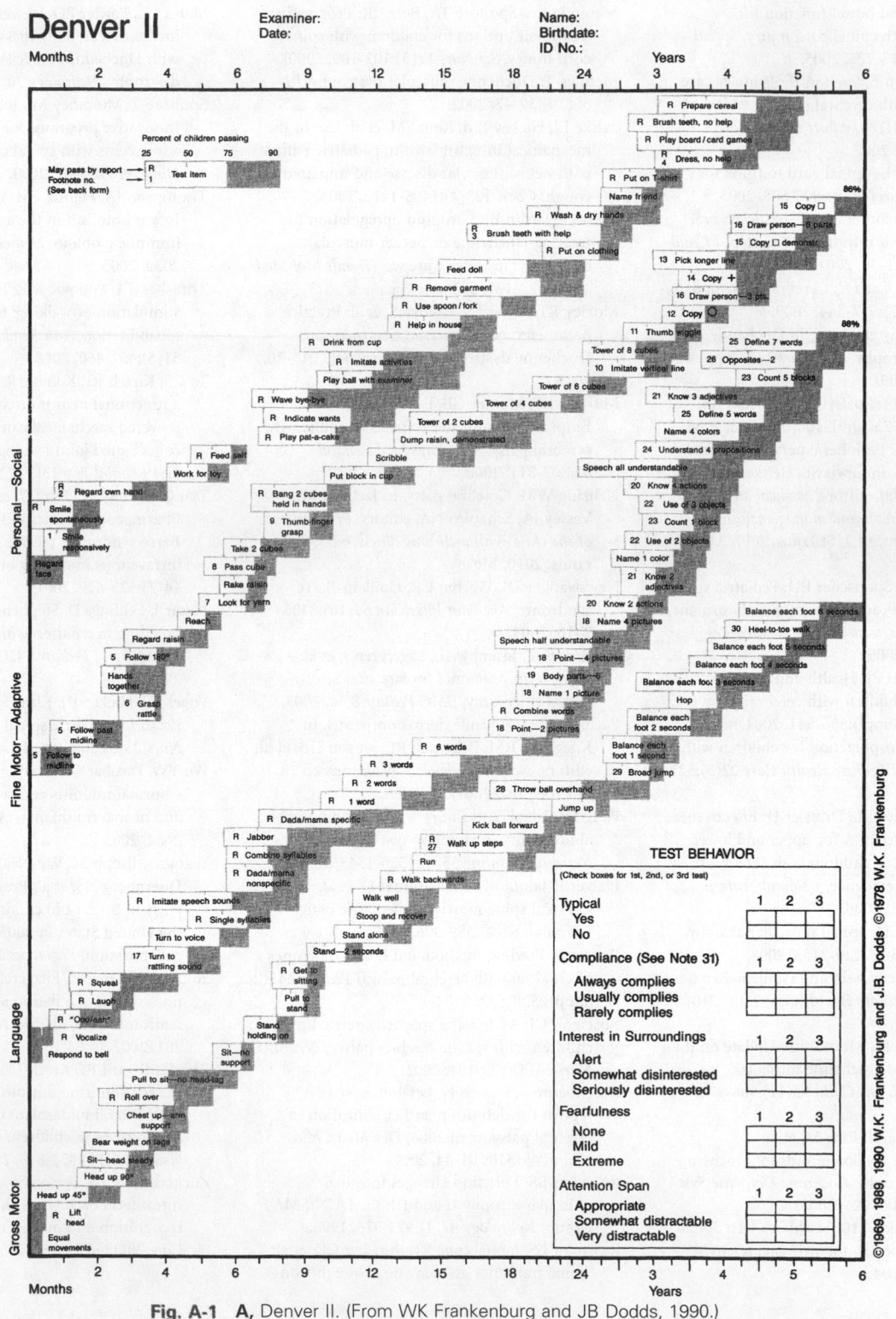

Fig. A-1 **A,** Denver II. (From WK Frankenburg and JB Dodds, 1990.)

DIRECTIONS FOR ADMINISTRATION

1. Try to get child to smile by smiling, talking or waving. Do not touch him/her.
2. Child must stare at hand several seconds.
3. Parent may help guide toothbrush and put toothpaste on brush.
4. Child does not have to be able to tie shoes or button/zip in the back.
5. Move yarn slowly in an arc from one side to the other, about 8" above child's face.
6. Pass if child grasps rattle when it is touched to the backs or tips of fingers.
7. Pass if child tries to see where yarn went. Yarn should be dropped quickly from sight from tester's hand without arm movement.
8. Child must transfer cube from hand to hand without help of body, mouth, or table.
9. Pass if child picks up raisin with any part of thumb and finger.
10. Line can vary only 30 degrees or less from tester's line.
11. Make a fist with thumb pointing upward and wiggle only the thumb. Pass if child imitates and does not move any fingers other than the thumb.

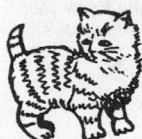
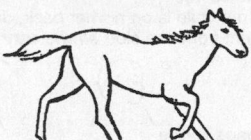
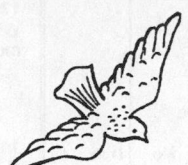
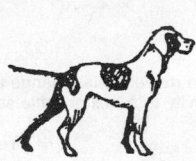

12. Pass any enclosed form. Fail continuous round motions.
13. Which line is longer? (Not bigger.) Turn paper upside down and repeat. (pass 3 of 3 or 5 of 6)
14. Pass any lines crossing near midpoint.
15. Have child copy first. If failed, demonstrate.

When giving items 12, 14, and 15, do not name the forms. Do not demonstrate 12 and 14.

16. When scoring, each pair (2 arms, 2 legs, etc.) counts as one part.
17. Place one cube in cup and shake gently near child's ear, but out of sight. Repeat for other ear.
18. Point to picture and have child name it. (No credit is given for sounds only.)
    If less than 4 pictures are named correctly, have child point to picture as each is named by tester.

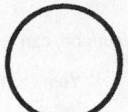
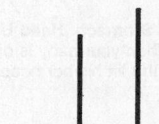
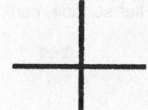
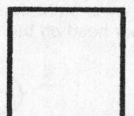
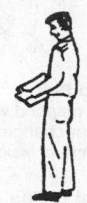

19. Using doll, tell child: Show me the nose, eyes, ears, mouth, hands, feet, tummy, hair. Pass 6 of 8.
20. Using pictures, ask child: Which one flies?... says meow?... talks?... barks?... gallops? Pass 2 of 5, 4 of 5.
21. Ask child: What do you do when you are cold?... tired?... hungry? Pass 2 of 3, 3 of 3.
22. Ask child: What do you do with a cup? What is a chair used for? What is a pencil used for?
    Action words must be included in answers.
23. Pass if child correctly places <u>and</u> says how many blocks are on paper. (1, 5).
24. Tell child: Put block **on** table; **under** table; **in front of** me, **behind** me. Pass 4 of 4.
    (Do not help child by pointing, moving head or eyes.)
25. Ask child: What is a ball?... lake?... desk?... house?... banana?... curtain?... fence?... ceiling? Pass if defined in terms of use, shape, what it is made of, or general category (such as banana is fruit, not just yellow). Pass 5 of 8, 7 of 8.
26. Ask child: If a horse is big, a mouse is __? If fire is hot, ice is __? If the sun shines during the day, the moon shines during the __? Pass 2 of 3.
27. Child may use wall or rail only, not person. May not crawl.
28. Child must throw ball overhand 3 feet to within arm's reach of tester.
29. Child must perform standing broad jump over width of test sheet (8 1/2 inches).
30. Tell child to walk forward, ⚬⚬⚬⚬⚬➔ heel within 1 inch of toe. Tester may demonstrate.
    Child must walk 4 consecutive steps.
31. In the second year, half of normal children are non-compliant.

B **OBSERVATIONS:**

Fig. A-1, cont'd B, Directions for administration of numbered items on Denver II.

0-9 MONTHS (R-PDQ)

REVISED DENVER PRESCREENING DEVELOPMENTAL QUESTIONNAIRE

Child's Name _____

Person Completing R-PDQ: _____

Relation to Child: _____

For Office Use

Today's Date: _____ yr _____ mo _____ day

Child's Birthdate: _____ yr _____ mo _____ day

Subtract to get Child's Exact Age: _____ yr _____ mo _____ day

R-PDQ Age: (_____ yr _____ mo _____ completed wks)

CONTINUE ANSWERING UNTIL 3 "NOs" ARE CIRCLED | For Office Use

1. Equal Movements
When your baby is lying on his/her back, can (s)he move each of his/her arms as easily as the other and each of the legs as easily as the other? Answer No if your child makes jerky or uncoordinated movements with one or both of his/her arms or legs.
Yes No (0) FMA

2. Stomach Lifts Head
When your baby is on his/her stomach on a flat surface, can (s)he lift his/her head off the surface?
Yes No (0-3) GM

3. Regards Face
When your baby is lying on his/her back, can (s)he look at you and watch your face?
Yes No (1) PS

4. Follows To Midline
When your child is on his/her back, can (s)he follow your movement by turning his/her head from one side to facing directly forward?
Yes No (1-1) FMA

5. Responds To Bell
Does your child respond with eye movements, change in breathing or other change in activity to a bell or rattle sounded outside his/her line of vision?
Yes No (1-2) L

6. Vocalizes Not Crying
Does your child make sounds other than crying, such as gurgling, cooing, or babbling?
Yes No (1-3) L

7. Smiles Responsively
When you smile and talk to your baby, does (s)he smile back at you?
Yes No (1-3) PS

8. Follows Past Midline
When your child is on his/her back, does (s)he follow your movement by turning his/her head from one side *almost all the way to the other side*?
Yes No (2-2) FMA

9. Stomach, Head Up 45°
When your baby is on his/her stomach on a flat surface, can (s)he lift his/her head 45°?
Yes No (2-2) GM

10. Stomach, Head Up 90°
When your baby is on his/her stomach on a flat surface, can (s)he lift his/her head 90°?
Yes No (3) GM

11. Laughs
Does your baby laugh out loud without being tickled or touched?
Yes No (3-1) L

12. Hands Together
Does your baby play with his/her hands by touching them together?
Yes No (3-3) FMA

13. Follows 180°
When your child is on his/her back, does (s)he follow your movement from one side *all the way* to the other side?
Yes No (4) FMA

14. Grasps Rattle
It is important that you follow instructions carefully. Do *not* place the pencil in the palm of your child's hand. When you touch the pencil to the back or tips of your baby's fingers, does your baby grasp the pencil for a few seconds?
Yes No (4) FMA

TRY THIS   NOT THIS

(Please turn page)   ©Wm. K. Frankenburg, M.D., 1975, 1986

Fig. A-2 Revised Denver Prescreening Developmental Questionnaire (sample of first page only). (Reprinted with permission of William K. Frankenburg. Copyright 1975, 1986, WK Frankenburg.)

Snellen Screening*

Preparation

1. Hang the Snellen chart on a light-colored wall so that the 20- to 30-foot lines are at eye level when children 6 to 12 years old are tested in the standing position (Fig. A-3).

2. Secure the chart to the wall with double-stick tape on the back side of all four corners. If the chart must be reversed for use of letter or E chart, secure it at the top and bottom with tacks. Make certain that the chart does not swing when in place.

3. The illumination intensity on the chart should be 10 to 30 footcandles, without any glare from windows or light fixtures. The illumination should be checked with a light meter.

4. Mark an exact 20-foot distance from the chart. Mark the floor with a piece of tape or "footprints" positioned so that the heels touch the 20-foot line.

*Modified from recommendations of the National Society to Prevent Blindness: *Guide to testing distance visual acuity*, Schaumburg, Ill, 1988, The Society.

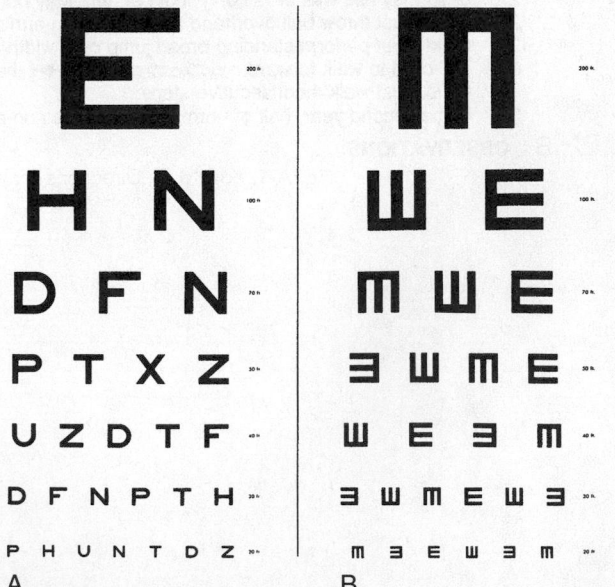

Fig. A-3 Snellen chart. **A,** Letter (alphabet) chart. **B,** Symbol E chart. (From National Society to Prevent Blindness, Inc., Schaumburg, Illinois.)

Procedure

1. Place the child at the 20-foot mark, with the heel edging the line if the child is standing or with the back of the chair placed at the marker if the child is seated.
2. If the E chart is used, accustom the child to identifying which direction the "legs of the E" are pointing. Use a demonstration E card for this purpose.
3. Teach the child to use the occluder to cover one eye. Instruct the child to keep both eyes open during the test. Provide a clean cover card for each child and then discard after use.
4. If the child wears glasses, test only with glasses on.
5. Test both eyes together, then the right eye, then the left eye.
6. Begin with the 40- or 30-foot line and proceed with the test to include the 20-foot line.
7. With a child suspected of low vision, begin with the 200-foot line, and proceed until child can no longer correctly read three out of four or four out of six symbols on a line.
8. Use covers on the Snellen chart to expose only one symbol or one line at a time. When screening kindergarten or older children, expose one line but use a pointer to point to one symbol at a time.

Recording and Referral

1. Record the last line the child read correctly (three out of four or four out of six symbols).
2. Record visual acuity as a fraction. The numerator represents the distance from the chart, and the denominator represents the last line read correctly. For example, 20/30 means that the child read the 30-foot line at a 20-foot distance.
3. Observe the child's eyes during testing and record any evidence of squinting, head tilting, thrusting the head forward, excessive blinking, tearing, or redness.
4. Only make referrals after a second screening has been made on children who are potential candidates for referral.
5. The following children should be referred for a complete eye examination:
   a. Three-year-old children with vision in either eye of 20/50 or less (inability to correctly identify one more than half the symbols on the 40-foot line) *or* a two-line difference in visual acuity between the eyes in the passing range (e.g., 20/20 in one eye and 20/40 in the other)
   b. All other ages and grades with vision in either eye of 20/40 or less (inability to correctly identify one more than half the symbols on the 30-foot line)
   c. All children who consistently show any of the signs of possible visual disturbances, regardless of visual acuity

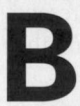
Growth Measurements

Body Mass Index Formula

English Formula

$$BMI = [Weight\ in\ pounds \div Height\ in\ inches \div Height\ in\ inches] \times 703$$

Fractions and ounces must be entered as decimal values.

FRACTION	OUNCES	DECIMAL
1/8	2	0.125
1/4	4	0.25
3/8	6	0.375
1/2	8	0.5
5/8	10	0.625
3/4	12	0.75
7/8	14	0.875

Example: A 33-lb, 4-oz child is 37⅞ inches tall.

$$[(33.25\ lb \div 37.625\ in) \div 37.625\ in] \times 703 = 16.5$$

Metric Formula

$$BMI = Weight\ in\ kilograms \div [Height\ in\ meters]^2$$

or

$$BMI = [(Weight\ in\ kilograms \div Height\ in\ cm) \div Height\ in\ cm] \times 10,000$$

Example: A 16.9-kg child is 105.2 cm tall.

$$[(16.9\ kg \div 105.2\ cm) \div 105.2\ cm] \times 10,000 = 15.3$$

From Kuczmarski RJ, et al: *CDC growth charts: United States: advance data from vital and health statistics,* no 314, Hyattsville, Md, June 8, 2000, National Center for Health Statistics; retrieved from www.cdc.gov/nchs/about/major/nhanes/growthcharts/fullreport.htm.

HEIGHT AND WEIGHT MEASUREMENTS FOR BOYS

| | HEIGHT BY PERCENTILES | | | | | | WEIGHT BY PERCENTILES | | | | | |
| | 5 | | 50 | | 95 | | 5 | | 50 | | 95 | |
AGE*	cm	inches	cm	inches	cm	inches	kg	lb	kg	lb	kg	lb
Birth	46.4	18¼	50.5	20	54.4	21½	2.54	5½	3.27	7¼	4.15	9¼
3 mo	56.7	22¼	61.1	24	65.4	25¾	4.43	9¾	5.98	13¼	7.37	16¼
6 mo	63.4	25	67.8	26¾	72.3	28½	6.20	13¾	7.85	17¼	9.46	20¾
9 mo	68.0	26¾	72.3	28½	77.1	30¼	7.52	16½	9.18	20¼	10.93	24
1	71.7	28¼	76.1	30	81.2	32	8.43	18½	10.15	22½	11.99	26½
1½	77.5	30½	82.4	32½	88.1	34¾	9.59	21¼	11.47	25¼	13.44	29½
2†	82.5	32½	86.8	34¼	94.4	37¼	10.49	23¼	12.34	27¼	15.50	34¼
2½†	85.4	33½	90.4	35½	97.8	38½	11.27	24¾	13.52	29¾	16.61	36½
3	89.0	35	94.9	37¼	102.0	40¼	12.05	26½	14.62	32¼	17.77	39¼
3½	92.5	36½	99.1	39	106.1	41¾	12.84	28¼	15.68	34½	18.98	41¾
4	95.8	37¾	102.9	40½	109.9	43¼	13.64	30	16.69	36¾	20.27	44¾
4½	98.9	39	106.6	42	113.5	44¾	14.45	31¾	17.69	39	21.63	47¾
5	102.0	40¼	109.9	43¼	117.0	46	15.27	33¾	18.67	41¼	23.09	51
6	107.7	42½	116.1	45¾	123.5	48½	16.93	37¼	20.69	45½	26.34	58
7	113.0	44½	121.7	48	129.7	51	18.64	41	22.85	50¼	30.12	66½
8	118.1	46½	127.0	50	135.7	53½	20.40	45	25.30	55¾	34.51	76
9	122.9	48½	132.2	52	141.8	55¾	22.25	49	28.13	62	39.58	87¼
10	127.7	50¼	137.5	54¼	148.1	58¼	24.33	53¾	31.44	69¼	45.27	99¾
11	132.6	52¼	143.3	56½	154.9	61	26.80	59	35.30	77¾	51.47	113½
12	137.6	54¼	149.7	59	162.3	64	29.85	65¾	39.78	87¾	58.09	128
13	142.9	56¼	156.5	61½	169.8	66¾	33.64	74¼	44.95	99	65.02	143¼
14	148.8	58½	163.1	64¼	176.7	69½	38.22	84¼	50.77	112	72.13	159
15	155.2	61	169.0	66½	181.9	71½	43.11	95	56.71	125	79.12	174½
16	161.1	63½	173.5	68¼	185.4	73	47.74	105¼	62.10	137	85.62	188¾
17	164.9	65	176.2	69¼	187.3	73¾	51.50	113½	66.31	146¼	91.31	201¼
18	165.7	65¼	176.8	69½	187.6	73¾	53.97	119	68.88	151¾	95.76	211

Modified from National Center for Health Statistics, Health Resources Administration, Department of Health, Education and Welfare, Hyattsville, Md.

Conversion of metric data to approximate inches and pounds by Ross Laboratories.

*Years unless otherwise indicated.

†Height data include some recumbent length measurements, which make values slightly higher than if all measurements had been of stature (standing height).

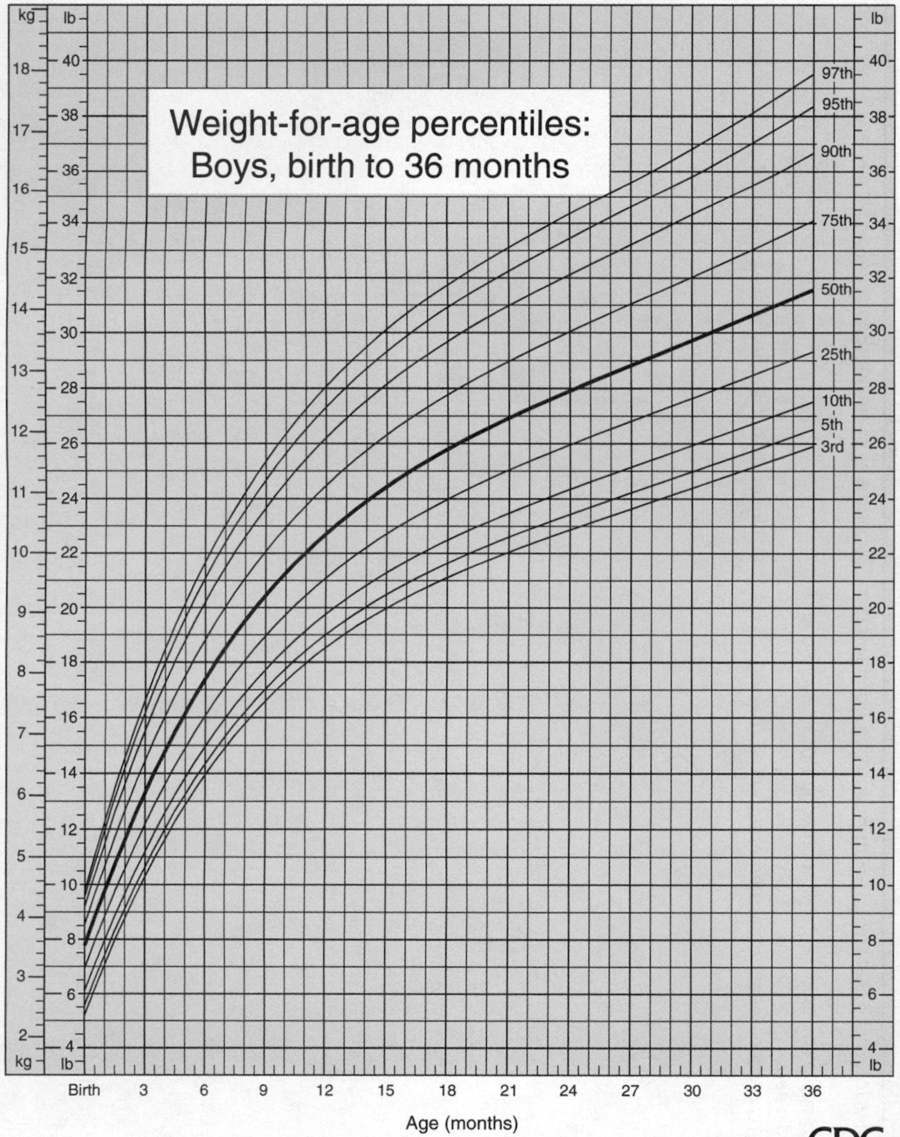

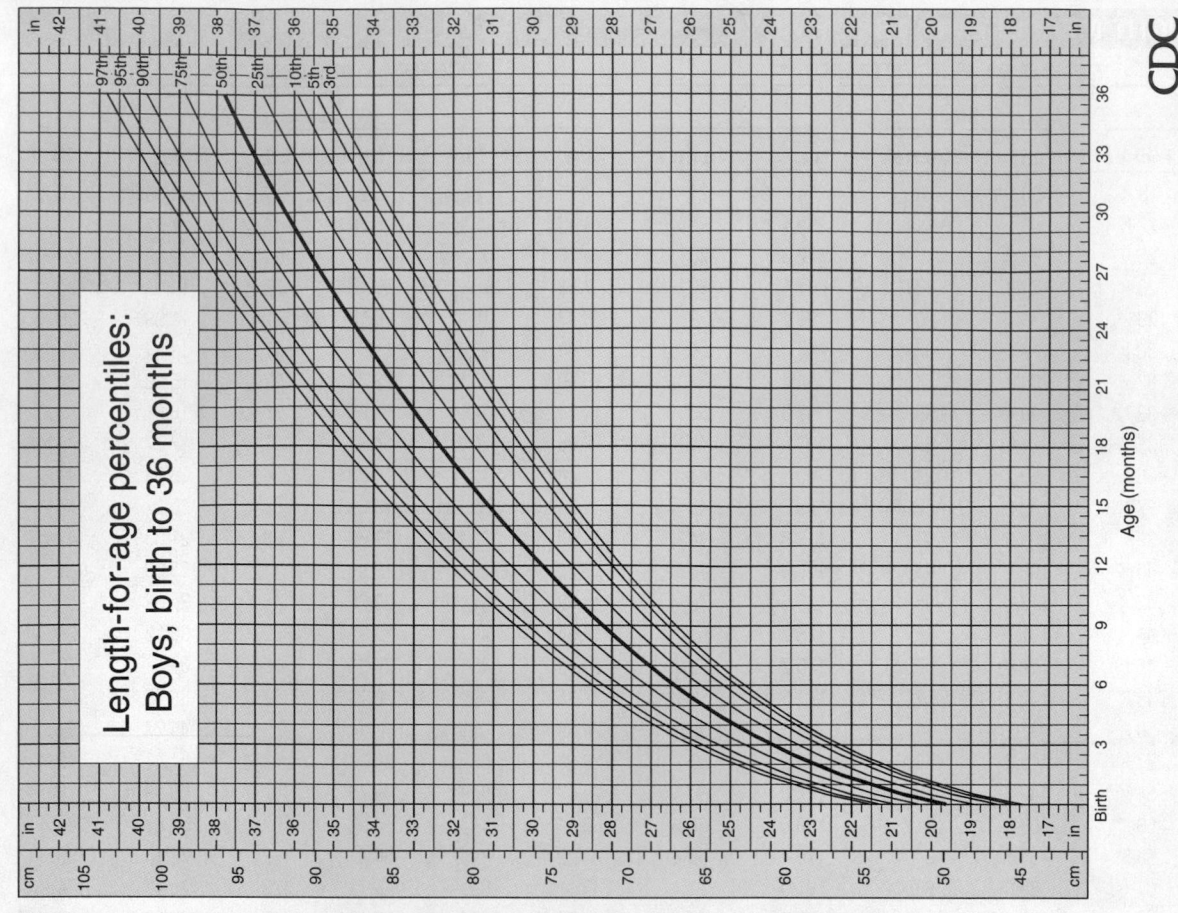

Fig. B-1 Weight-for-age percentiles, boys, birth to 36 months, CDC growth charts: United States. (Developed by the National Center for Health Statistics in collaboration with the National Center for Chronic Disease Prevention and Health Promotion, 2000.)

Fig. B-2 Length-for-age percentiles, boys, birth to 36 months, CDC growth charts: United States. (Developed by the National Center for Health Statistics in collaboration with the National Center for Chronic Disease Prevention and Health Promotion, 2000.)

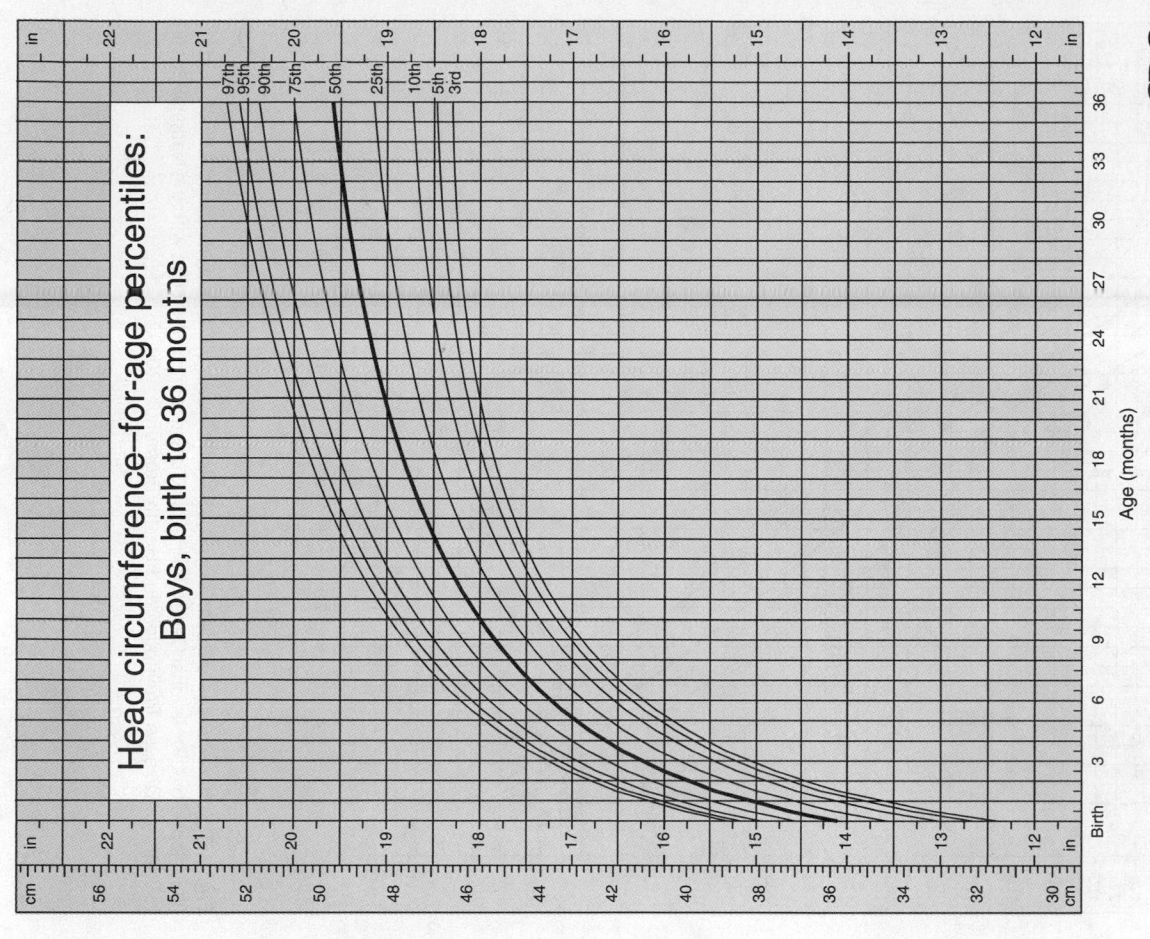

Fig. B-4 Head circumference-for-age percentiles, boys, birth to 36 months, CDC growth charts: United States. (Developed by the National Center for Health Statistics in collaboration with the National Center for Chronic Disease Prevention and Health Promotion, 2000.)

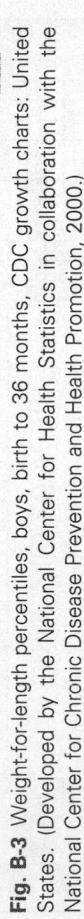

Fig. B-3 Weight-for-length percentiles, boys, birth to 36 months, CDC growth charts: United States. (Developed by the National Center for Health Statistics in collaboration with the National Center for Chronic Disease Prevention and Health Promotion, 2000.)

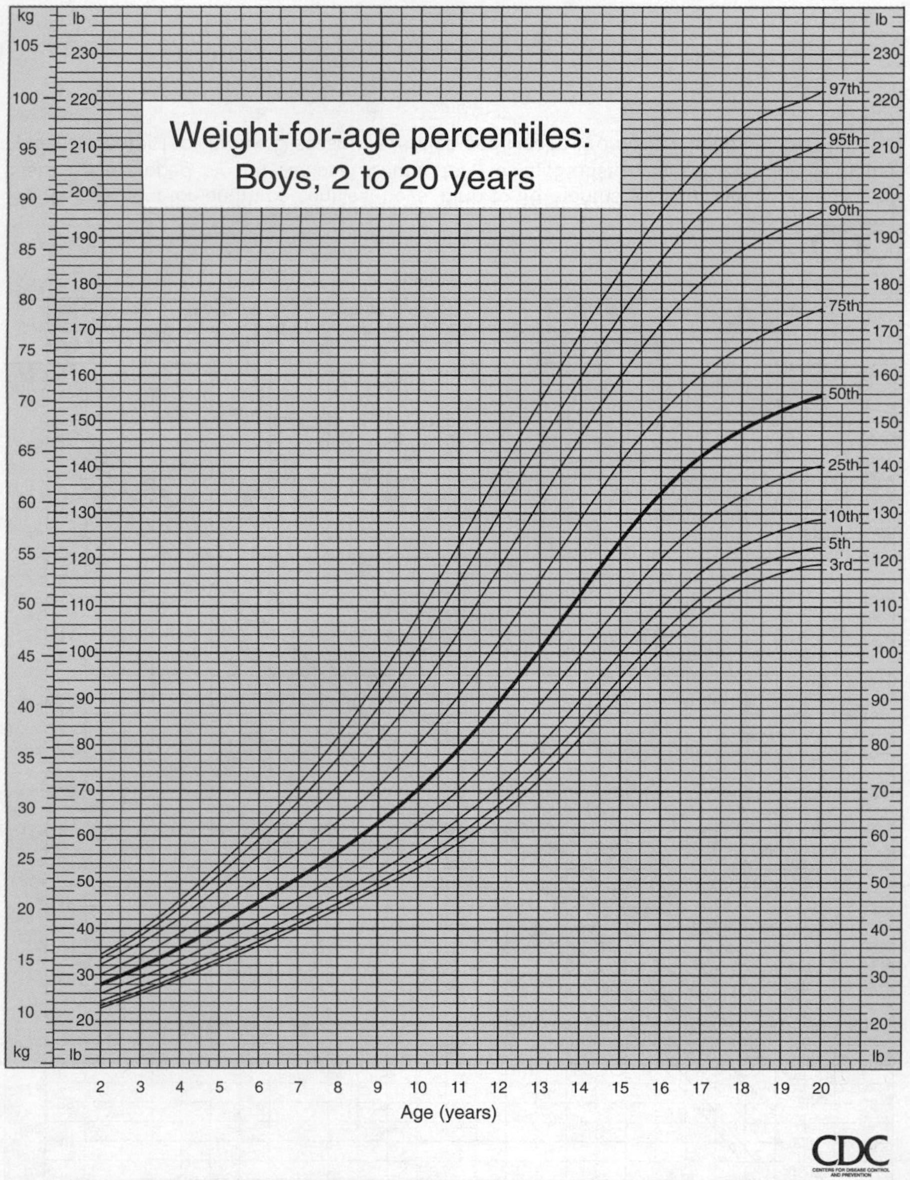

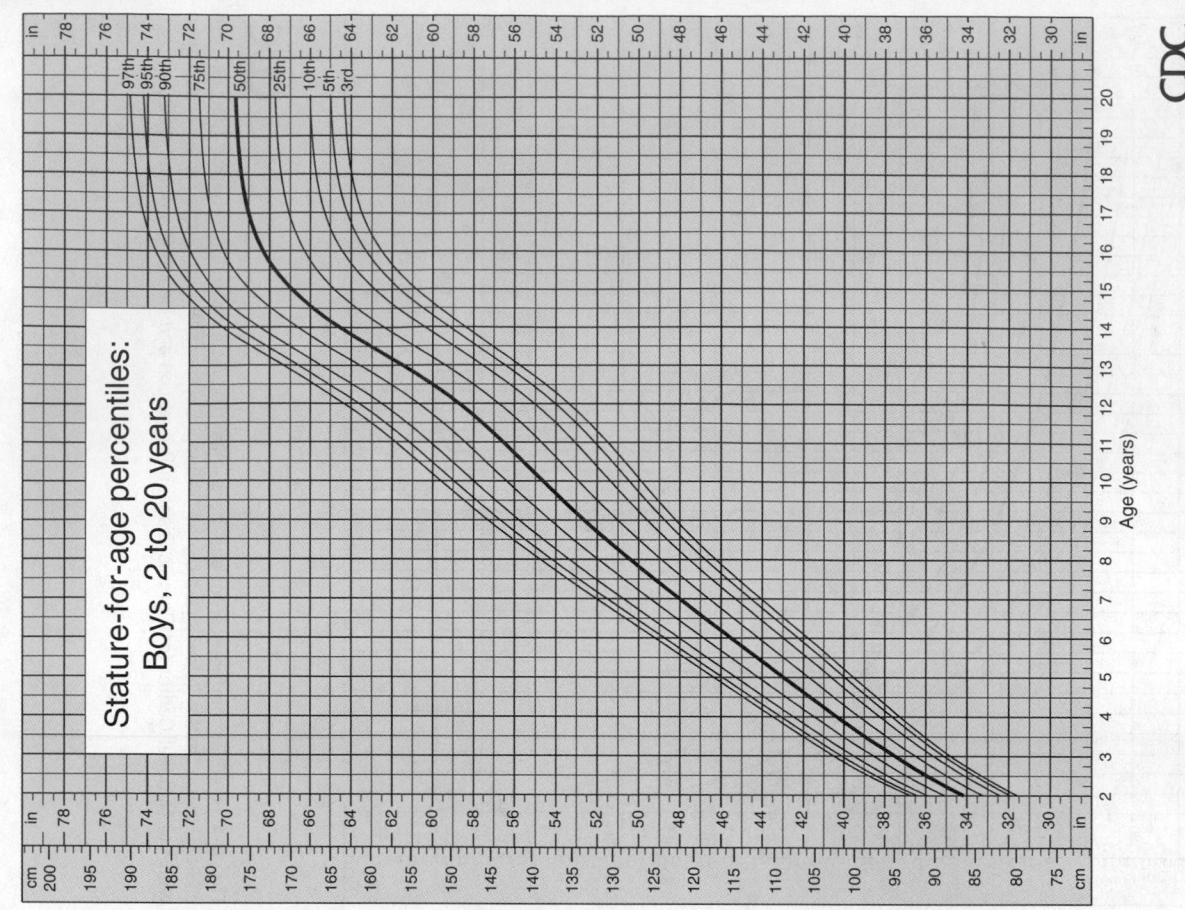

Fig. B-5 Weight-for-age percentiles, boys, 2 to 20 years, CDC growth charts: United States. (Developed by the National Center for Health Statistics in collaboration with the National Center for Chronic Disease Prevention and Health Promotion, 2000.)

Fig. B-6 Stature-for-age percentiles, boys, 2 to 20 years, CDC growth charts: United States. (Developed by the National Center for Health Statistics in collaboration with the National Center for Chronic Disease Prevention and Health Promotion, 2000.)

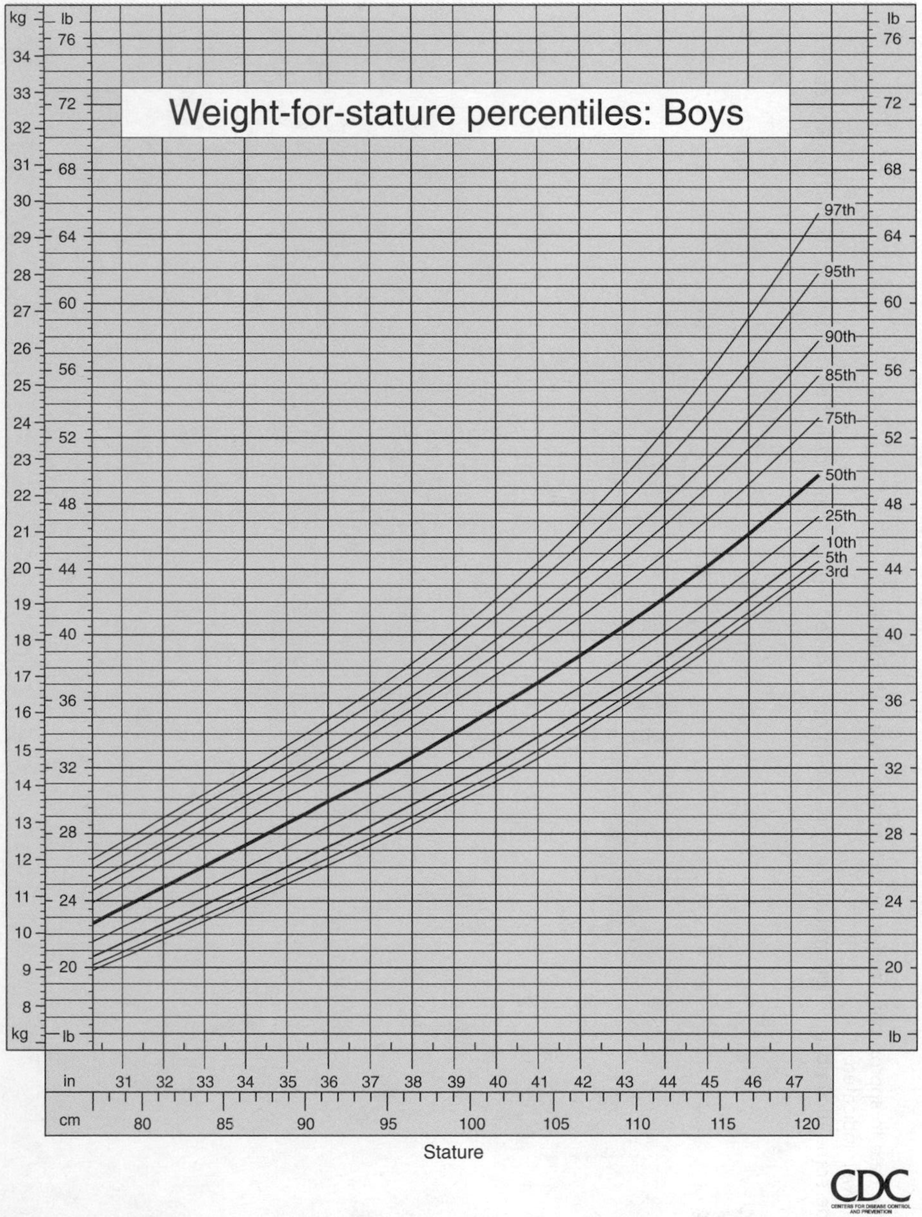

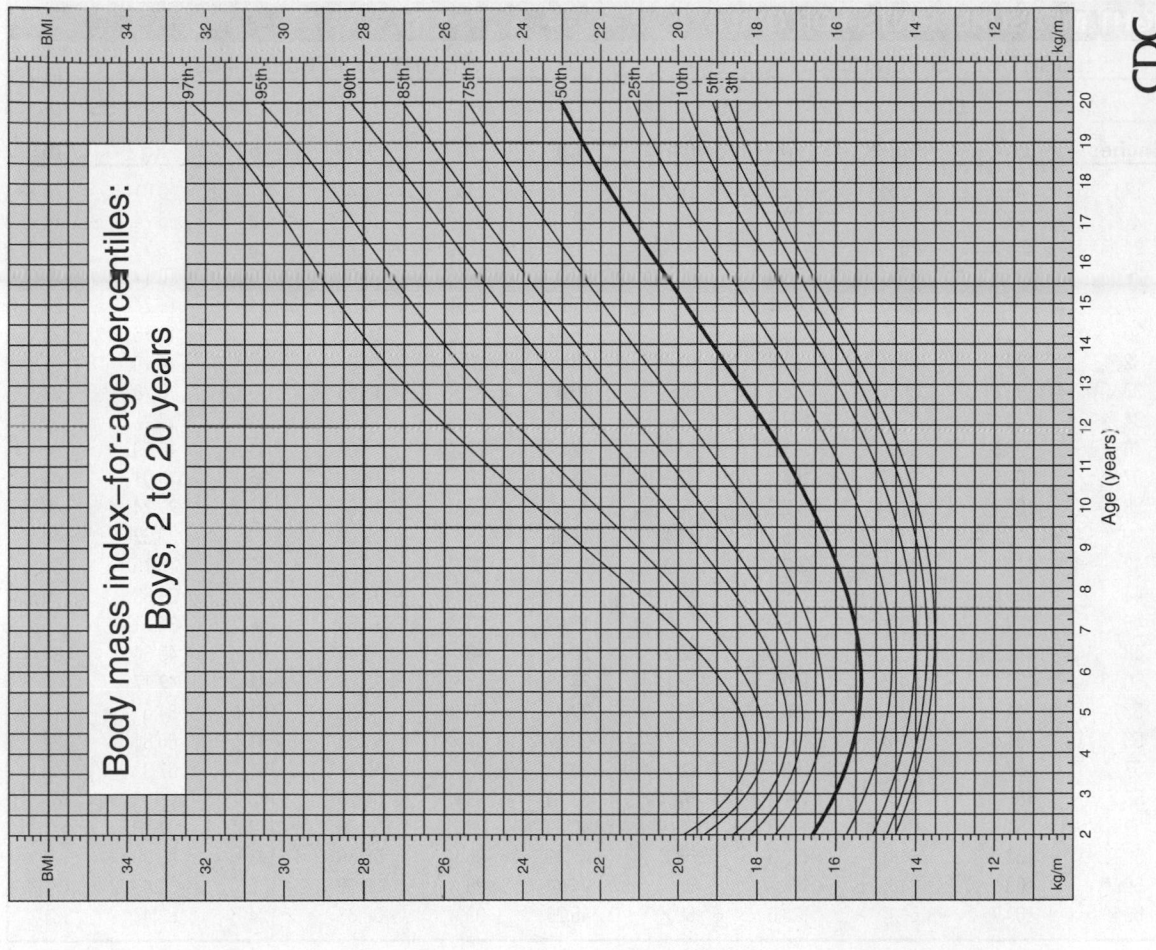

Fig. B-8 Body mass index–for-age percentiles, boys, 2 to 20 years, CDC growth charts: United States. (Developed by the National Center for Health Statistics in collaboration with the National Center for Chronic Disease Prevention and Health Promotion, 2000.)

Fig. B-7 Weight-for-stature percentiles, boys, CDC growth charts: United States. (Developed by the National Center for Health Statistics in collaboration with the National Center for Chronic Disease Prevention and Health Promotion, 2000.)

HEIGHT AND WEIGHT MEASUREMENTS FOR GIRLS

	HEIGHT BY PERCENTILES						WEIGHT BY PERCENTILES					
	5		50		95		5		50		95	
AGE*	cm	inches	cm	inches	cm	inches	kg	lb	kg	lb	kg	lb
Birth	45.4	17¾	49.9	19¾	52.9	20¾	2.36	5¼	3.23	7	3.81	8½
3 mo	55.4	21¾	59.5	23½	63.4	25	4.18	9¼	5.4	12	6.74	14¾
6 mo	61.8	24¼	65.9	26	70.2	27¾	5.79	12¾	7.21	16	8.73	19¼
9 mo	66.1	26	70.4	27¾	75.0	29½	7.0	15½	8.56	18¾	10.17	22½
1	69.8	27½	74.3	29¼	79.1	31¼	7.84	17¼	9.53	21	11.24	24¾
1½	76.0	30	80.9	31¾	86.1	34	8.92	19¾	10.82	23¾	12.76	28¼
2†	81.6	32¼	86.8	34¼	93.6	36¾	9.95	22	11.8	26	14.15	31¼
2½†	84.6	33¼	90.0	35½	96.6	38	10.8	23¾	13.03	28¾	15.76	34¾
3	88.3	34¾	94.1	37	100.6	39½	11.61	25½	14.1	31	17.22	38
3½	91.7	36	97.9	38½	104.5	41¼	12.37	27¼	15.07	33¼	18.59	41
4	95.0	37½	101.6	40	108.3	42¾	13.11	29	15.96	35¼	19.91	44
4½	98.1	38½	105.0	41¼	112.0	44	13.83	30½	16.81	37	21.24	46¾
5	101.1	39¾	108.4	42¾	115.6	45½	14.55	32	17.66	39	22.62	49¾
6	106.6	42	114.6	45	122.7	48¼	16.05	35½	19.52	43	25.75	56¾
7	111.8	44	120.6	47½	129.5	51	17.71	39	21.84	48¼	29.68	65½
8	116.9	46	126.4	49¾	136.2	53½	19.62	43¼	24.84	54¾	34.71	76½
9	122.1	48	132.2	52	142.9	56¼	21.82	48	28.46	62¾	40.64	89½
10	127.5	50¼	138.3	54½	149.5	58¾	24.36	53¾	32.55	71¾	47.17	104
11	133.5	52½	144.8	57	156.2	61½	27.24	60	36.95	81½	54.0	119
12	139.8	55	151.5	59¾	162.7	64	30.52	67¼	41.53	91½	60.81	134
13	145.2	57¼	157.1	61¾	168.1	66¼	34.14	75¼	46.1	101¾	67.3	148¼
14	148.7	58½	160.4	63¼	171.3	67½	37.76	83¼	50.28	110¾	73.08	161
15	150.5	59¼	161.8	63¾	172.8	68	40.99	90¼	53.68	118¼	77.78	171½
16	151.6	59¾	162.4	64	173.3	68¼	43.41	95¾	55.89	123¼	80.99	178½
17	152.7	60	163.1	64¼	173.5	68¼	44.74	98¾	56.69	125	82.46	181¾
18	153.6	60½	163.7	64½	173.6	68¼	45.26	99¾	56.62	124¾	82.47	181¾

Modified from National Center for Health Statistics, Health Resources Administration, Department of Health, Education and Welfare, Hyattsville, Md.

Conversion of metric data to approximate inches and pounds by Ross Laboratories.

*Years unless otherwise indicated.

†Height data include some recumbent length measurements, which make values slightly higher than if all measurements had been of stature.

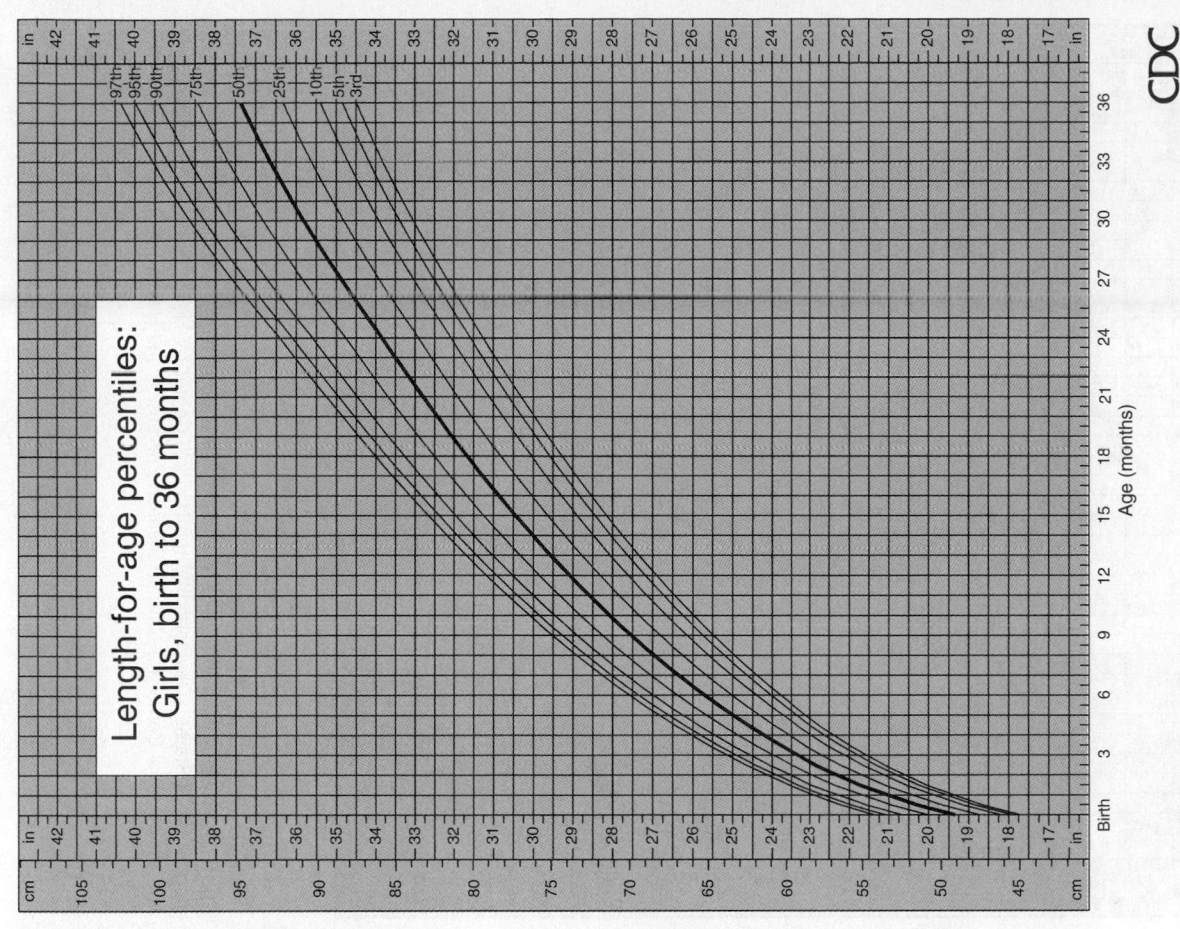
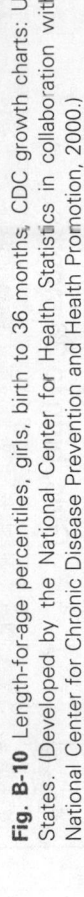

Fig. B-10 Length-for-age percentiles, girls, birth to 36 months, CDC growth charts: United States. (Developed by the National Center for Health Statistics in collaboration with the National Center for Chronic Disease Prevention and Health Promotion, 2000.)

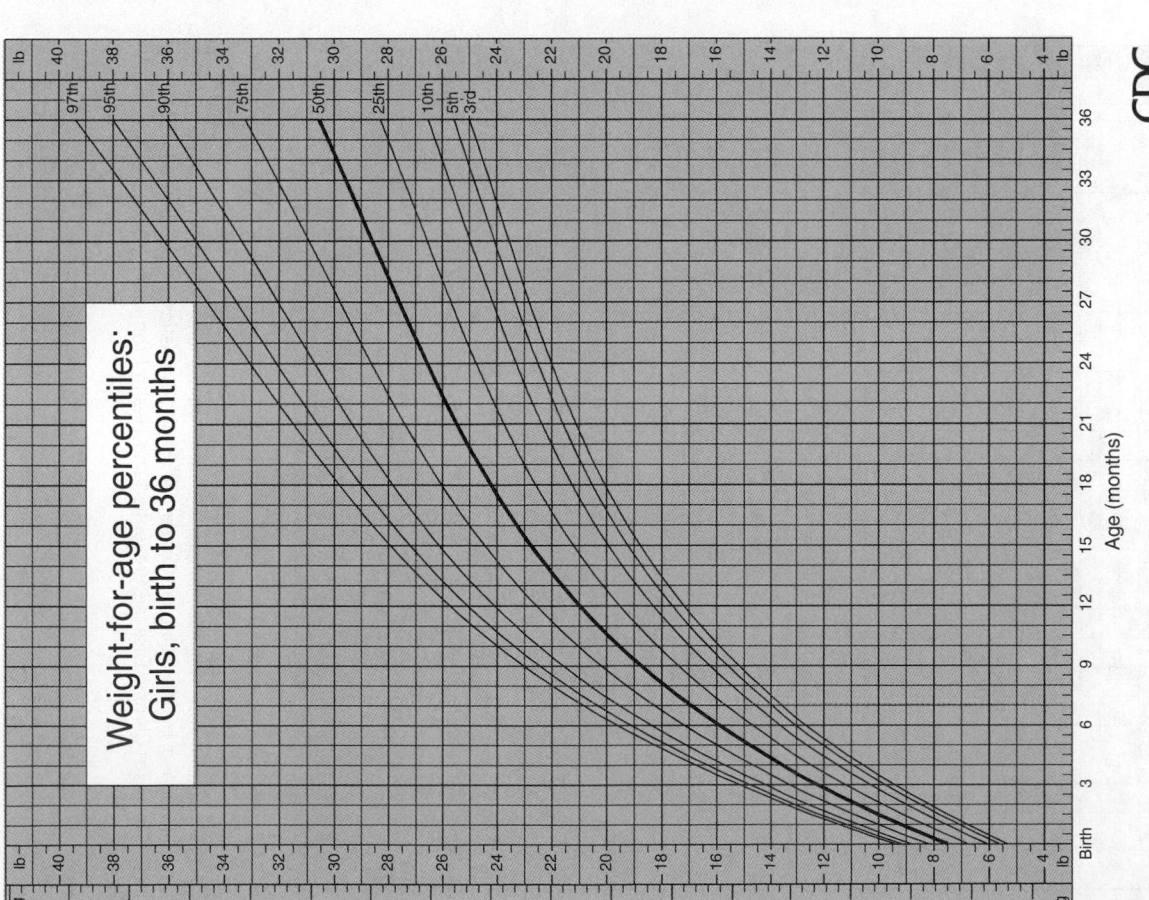

Fig. B-9 Weight-for-age percentiles, girls, birth to 36 months, CDC growth charts: United States. (Developed by the National Center for Health Statistics in collaboration with the National Center for Chronic Disease Prevention and Health Promotion, 2000.)

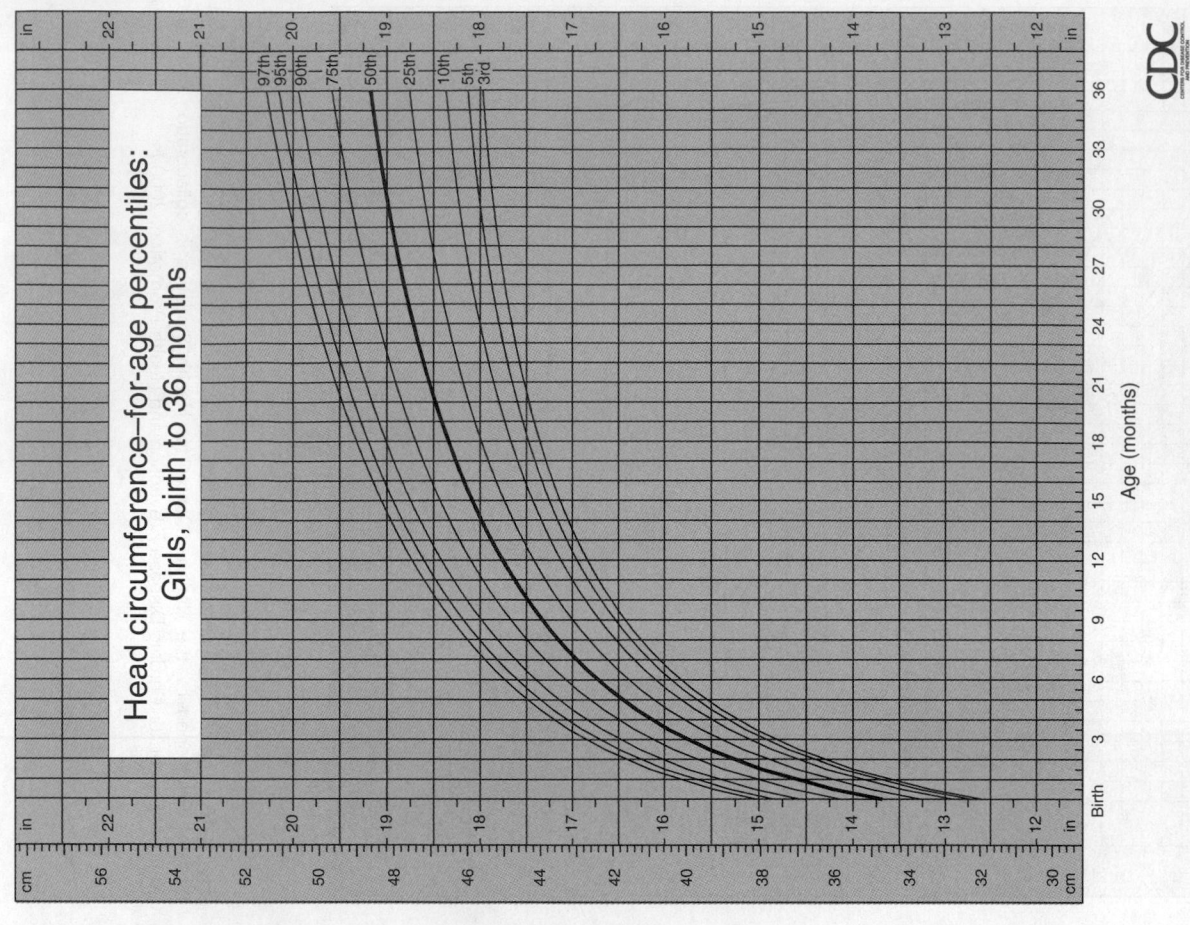

Fig. B-11 Weight-for-length percentiles, girls, birth to 36 months, CDC growth charts: United States. (Developed by the National Center for Health Statistics in collaboration with the National Center for Chronic Disease Prevention and Health Promotion, 2000.)

Fig. B-12 Head circumference-for-age percentiles, girls, birth to 36 months, CDC growth charts: United States. (Developed by the National Center for Health Statistics in collaboration with the National Center for Chronic Disease Prevention and Health Promotion, 2000.)

Head circumference–for–age percentiles:
Girls, birth to 36 months

Weight-for-length percentiles:
Girls, birth to 36 months

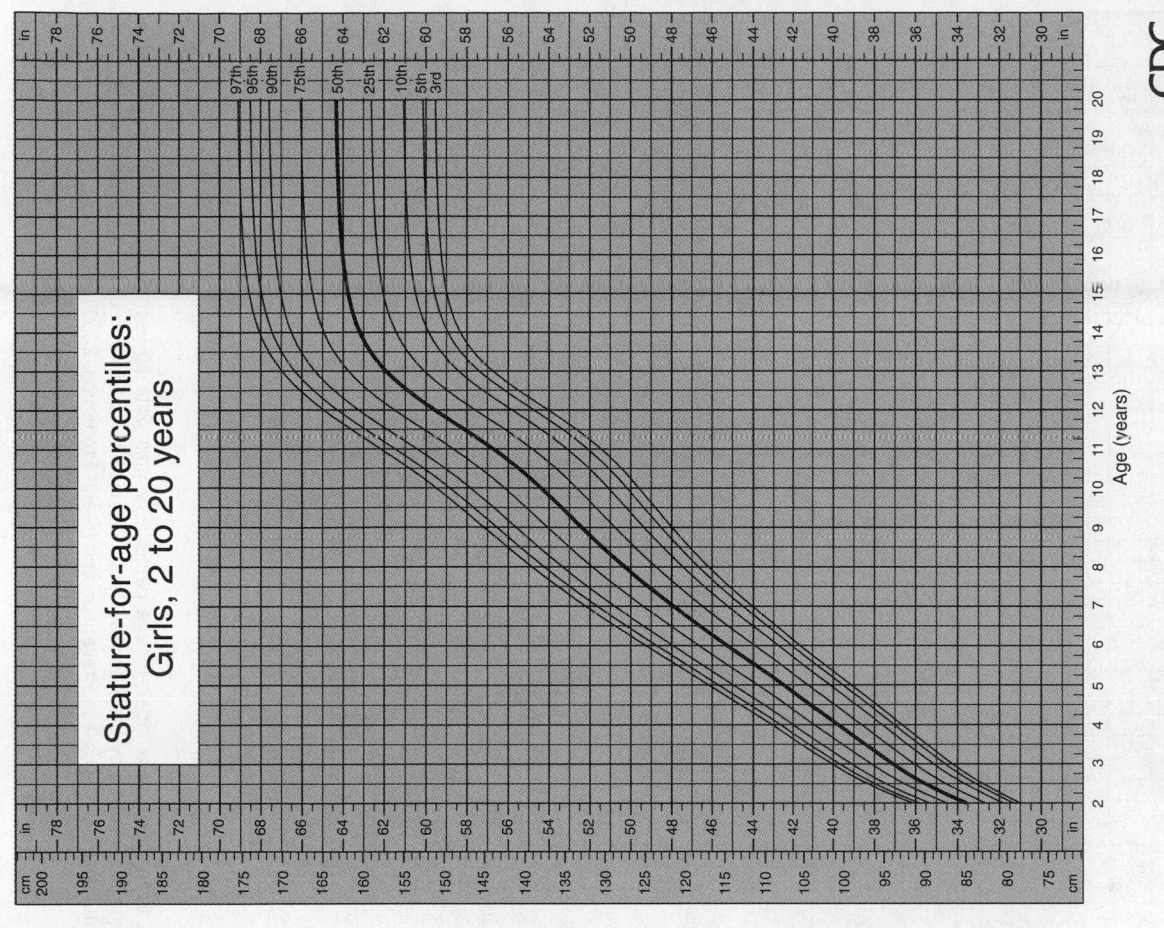

Fig. B-14 Stature-for-age percentiles, girls, 2 to 20 years, CDC growth charts: United States. (Developed by the National Center for Health Statistics in collaboration with the National Center for Chronic Disease Prevention and Health Promotion, 2000.)

Fig. B-13 Weight-for-age percentiles, girls, 2 to 20 years, CDC growth charts: United States. (Developed by the National Center for Health Statistics in collaboration with the National Center for Chronic Disease Prevention and Health Promotion, 2000.)

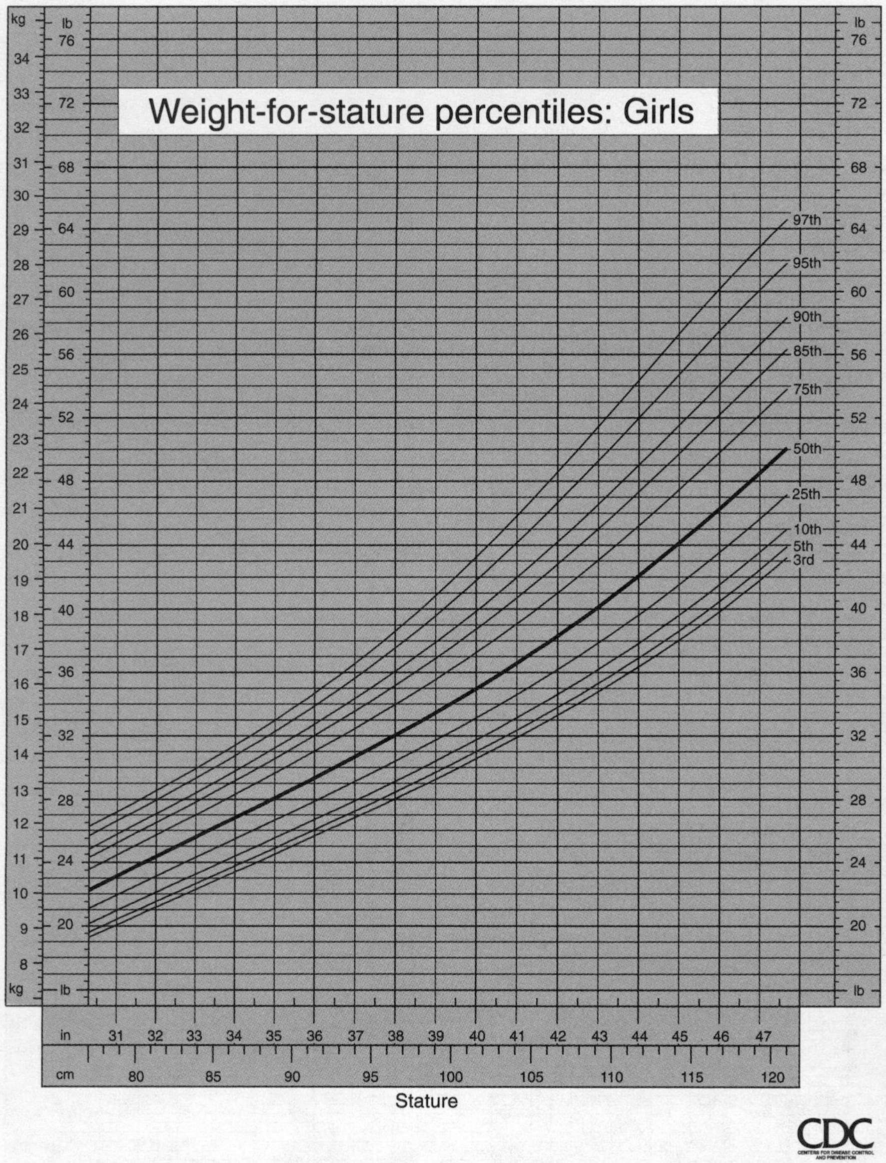

Body mass index–for–age percentiles: Girls, 2 to 20 years

Age (years)

BMI

kg/m²

97th
95th
90th
85th
75th
50th
25th
10th
5th
3rd

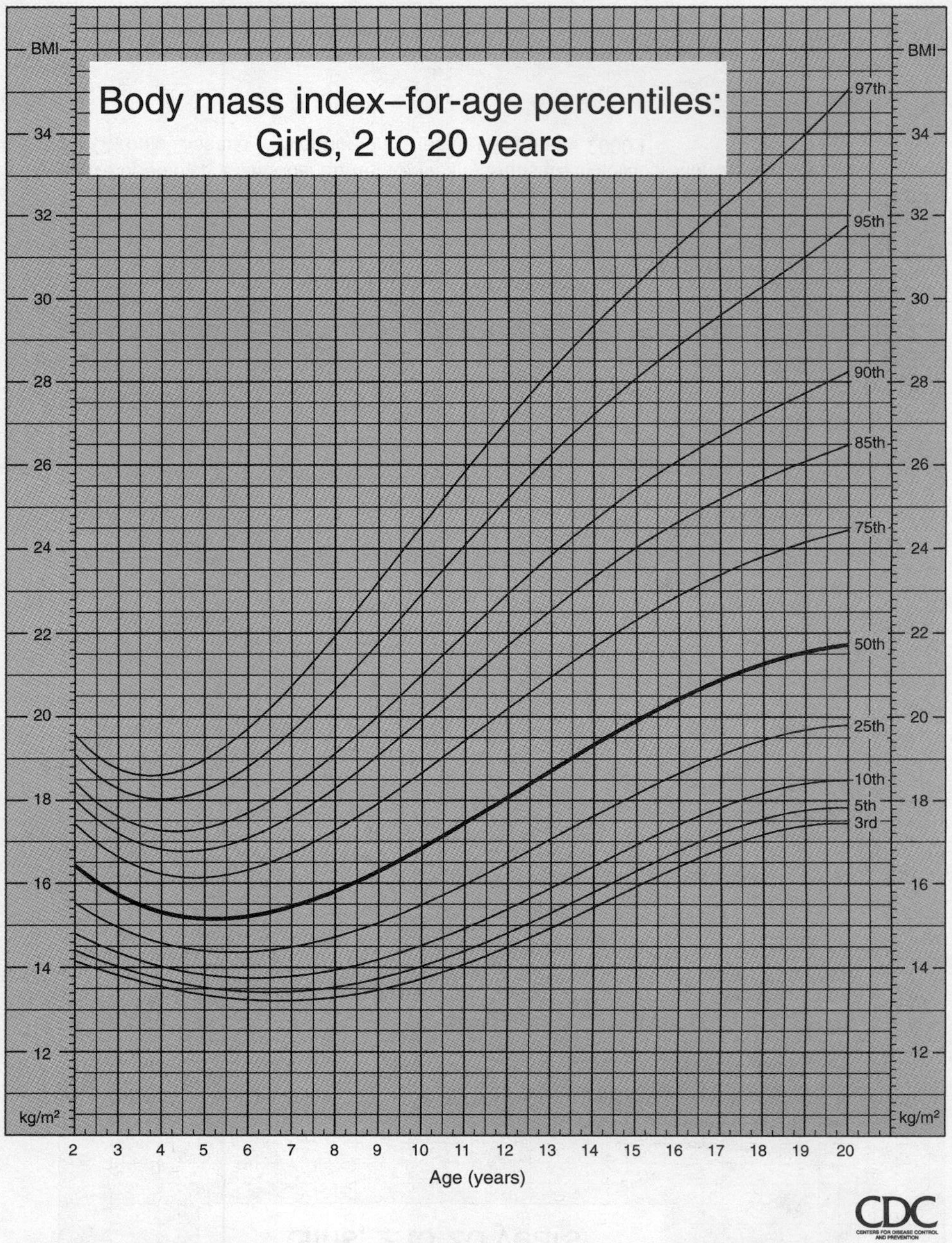

Fig. B-16 Body mass index-for-age percentiles, girls, 2 to 20 years, CDC growth charts: United States. (Developed by the National Center for Health Statistics in collaboration with the National Center for Chronic Disease Prevention and Health Promotion, 2000.)

Weight-for-stature percentiles: Girls

Stature

97th
95th
90th
85th
75th
50th
25th
10th
5th
3rd

Fig. B-15 Weight-for-stature percentiles, girls, CDC growth charts: United States. (Developed by the National Center for Health Statistics in collaboration with the National Center for Chronic Disease Prevention and Health Promotion, 2000.)

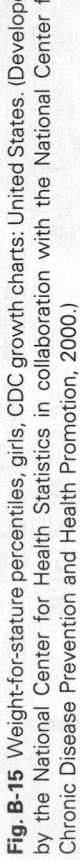

Common Laboratory Tests

COMMON LABORATORY TESTS AND TESTS RESULTS*

TEST/SPECIMEN	AGE/GENDER/REFERENCE	NORMAL RANGES			
		CONVENTIONAL UNITS		INTERNATIONAL UNITS (SI)	
Acetaminophen					
Serum or plasma	Therap. conc.	10-30 mcg/ml		66-200 µmol/L	
	Toxic conc.	>200 mcg/ml		>1300 µmol/L	
Ammonia nitrogen					
Plasma or serum	Newborn	90-150 mcg/dl		64-107 µmol/L	
	0-2 wk	79-129 mcg/dl		56-92 µmol/L	
	>1 mo	29-70 mcg/dl		21-50 µmol/L	
	Thereafter	0-50 mcg/dl		0-35.7 µmol/L	
Antistreptolysin O titer (ASO)					
Serum	2-4 yr	<160 Todd units			
	School-age children	170-330 Todd units			
Base excess					
Whole blood	Newborn	(−10)-(−2) mEq/L		(−10)-(−2) mmol/L	
	Infant	(−7)-(−1) mEq/L		(−7)-(−1) mmol/L	
	Child	(−4)-(+2) mEq/L		(−4)-(+2) mmol/L	
	Thereafter	(−3)-(+3) mEq/L		(−3)-(+3) mmol/L	
Bicarbonate (HCO_3)					
Serum	Arterial	21-28 mEq/L		21-28 mmol/L	
	Venous	22-29 mEq/L		22-29 mmol/L	
Bilirubin, total		**Premature** (mg/dl)	**Full term** (mg/dl)	**Premature** (µmol/L)	**Full term** (µmol/L)
Serum	Cord	<2.0	<2.0	<34	<34
	0-1 d	<8.0	<6.0	<137	<103
	1-2 d	<12.0	<8.0	<205	<137
	2-5 d	<16.0	<12.0	<274	<205
	Thereafter	<20.0	<10.0	<340	<171
Bilirubin, direct (conjugated)					
Serum		0.0-0.2 mg/dl		0-3.4 µmol/L	
Bleeding time					
Blood from skin puncture					
Ivy	Normal	2-7 min		2-7 min	
	Borderline	7-11 min		7-11 min	
Simplate (G-D)		2.75-8 min		2.75-8 min	
Blood volume					
Whole blood	Male	52-83 ml/kg		0.052-0.083 L/kg	
	Female	50-75 ml/kg		0.050-0.075 L/kg	
C-reactive protein (CRP)					
Serum	Cord	52-1330 ng/ml		52-1330 mcg/L	
	2-12 yr	67-1800 ng/ml		67-1800 mcg/L	
Calcium, ionized					
Serum, plasma, or whole	Cord	5.0-6.0 mg/dl		1.25-1.50 mmol/L	
blood	Newborn, 3-24 hr	4.3-5.1 mg/dl		1.07-1.27 mmol/L	
	24-48 hr	4.0-4.7 mg/dl		1.00-1.17 mmol/L	
	Thereafter	4.8-4.92 mg/dl or 2.24-2.46 mEq/L		1.12-1.23 mmol/L	

Continued

COMMON LABORATORY TESTS AND TESTS RESULTS—cont'd

TEST/SPECIMEN	AGE/GENDER/REFERENCE	NORMAL RANGES	
		CONVENTIONAL UNITS	**INTERNATIONAL UNITS (SI)**
Calcium, total			
Serum	Cord	9.0-11.5 mg/dl	2.25-2.88 mmol/L
	Newborn, 3-24 hr	9.0-10.6 mg/dl	2.3-2.65 mmol/L
	24-48 hr	7.0-12.0 mg/dl	1.75-3.0 mmol/L
	4-7 d	9.0-10.9 mg/dl	2.25-2.73 mmol/L
	Child	8.8-10.8 mg/dl	2.2-2.70 mmol/L
	Thereafter	8.4-10.2 mg/dl	2.1-2.55 mmol/L
Carbon dioxide, partial pressure (P_{CO_2})			
Whole blood, arterial	Newborn	27-40 mm Hg	3.6-5.3 kPa
	Infant	27-41 mm Hg	3.6-5.5 kPa
	Thereafter: Male	35-48 mm Hg	4.7-6.4 kPa
	Female	32-45 mm Hg	4.3-6.0 kPa
Carbon dioxide, total (tCO_2)			
Serum or plasma	Cord	14-22 mEq/L	14-22 mmol/L
	Premature (1 wk)	14-27 mEq/L	14-27 mmol/L
	Newborn	13-22 mEq/L	13-22 mmol/L
	Infant, child	20-28 mEq/L	20-28 mmol/L
	Thereafter	23-30 mEq/L	23-30 mmol/L
Cerebrospinal fluid (CSF)			
Pressure		70-180 mm H_2O	70-180 mm H_2O
Volume	Child	60-100 ml	0.06-0.10 L
	Adult	100-160 ml	0.10-0.16 L
Chloride			
Serum or plasma	Cord	96-104 mEq/L	96-104 mmol/L
	Newborn	97-110 mEq/L	97-110 mmol/L
	Thereafter	98-106 mEq/L	98-106 mmol/L
Sweat	Normal (homozygote)	<40 mEq/L	<40 mmol/L
	Marginal (e.g., asthma, Addison disease, malnutrition)	45-60 mEq/L	45-60 mmol/L
	Cystic fibrosis	>60 mEq/L	>60 mmol/L
Cholesterol, total			
Serum or plasma†	Acceptable	<170 mg/dl	<4.4 mmol/L
	Borderline	170-199 mg/dl	4.4-5.1 mmol/L
	High	≥200 mg/dl	≥5.2 mmol/L
Clotting time (Lee-White)			
Whole blood		5-8 min (glass tubes)	5-8 min
		5-15 min (room temp)	5-15 min
		30 min (silicone tube)	30 min
Creatine kinase (CK, CPK)			
Serum	Cord	70-380 U/L	70-380 U/L
	5-8 hr	214-1175 U/L	214-1175 U/L
	24-33 hr	130-1200 U/L	130-1200 U/L
	72-100 hr	87-725 U/L	87-725 U/L
	Adult	5-130 U/L	5-130 U/L
Creatinine			
Serum	Cord	0.6-1.2 mg/dl	53-106 µmol/L
	Newborn	0.3-1.0 mg/dl	27-88 µmol/L
	Infant	0.2-0.4 mg/d	18-35 µmol/L
	Child	0.3-0.7 mg/dl	27-62 µmol/L
	Adolescent	0.5-1.0 mg/dl	44-88 µmol/L
	Adult: Male	0.6-1.2 mg/dl	53-106 µmol/L
	Female	0.5-1.1 mg/dl	44-97 µmol/L
Urine, 24 hr	Premature	8.1-15.0 mg/kg/24 hr	72-133 µmol/kg/24 hr
	Full term	10.4-19.7 mg/kg/24 hr	92-174 µmol/kg/24 hr
	1.5-7 yr	10-15 mg/kg/24 hr	88-133 µmol/kg/24 hr
	7-15 yr	5.2-41 mg/kg/24 hr	46-362 µmol/kg/24 hr
Creatinine clearance (endogenous)			
Serum or plasma and urine	Newborn	40-65 ml/min/1.73 m²	
	<40 yr: Male	97-137 ml/min/1.73 m²	
	Female	88-128 ml/min/1.73 m²	

COMMON LABORATORY TESTS AND TESTS RESULTS—cont'd

TEST/SPECIMEN	AGE/GENDER/REFERENCE	NORMAL RANGES	
		CONVENTIONAL UNITS	INTERNATIONAL UNITS (SI)
Digoxin			
Serum, plasma; collect at least 12 hr after dose	Therap. conc.		
	CHF	0.8-1.5 ng/ml	1.0-1.9 nmol/L
	Arrhythmias	1.5-2.0 ng/ml	1.9-2.6 nmol/L
	Toxic conc.		
	Child	>2.5 ng/ml	>3.2 nmol/L
	Adult	>3.0 ng/ml	>3.8 nmol/L
Eosinophil count			
Whole blood, capillary blood		50-250 cells/mm^3 (μl)	50-250 $\times$ 10^6 cells/L
Erythrocyte (RBC) count			
Whole blood	Cord	3.9-5.5 million/mm^3	3.9-5.5 $\times$ 10^{12} cells/L
	1-3 d	4.0-6.6 million/mm^3	4.0-6.6 $\times$ 10^{12} cells/L
	1 wk	3.9-6.3 million/mm^3	3.9-6.3 $\times$ 10^{12} cells/L
	2 wk	3.6-6.2 million/mm^3	3.6-6.2 $\times$ 10^{12} cells/L
	1 mo	3.0-5.4 million/mm^3	3.0-5.4 $\times$ 10^{12} cells/L
	2 mo	2.7-4.9 million/mm^3	2.7-4.9 $\times$ 10^{12} cells/L
	3-6 mo	3.1-4.5 million/mm^3	3.1-4.5 $\times$ 10^{12} cells/L
	0.5-2 yr	3.7-5.3 million/mm^3	3.7-5.3 $\times$ 10^{12} cells/L
	2-6 yr	3.9-5.3 million/mm^3	3.9-5.3 $\times$ 10^{12} cells/L
	6-12 yr	4.0-5.2 million/mm^3	4.0-5.2 $\times$ 10^{12} cells/L
	12-18 yr: Male	4.5-5.3 million/mm^3	4.5-5.3 $\times$ 10^{12} cells/L
	Female	4.1-5.1 million/mm^3	4.1-5.1 $\times$ 10^{12} cells/L
Erythrocyte sedimentation rate (ESR)			
Whole blood			
Westergren (modified)	Child	0-10 mm/hr	0-10 mm/hr
	<50 yr: Male	0-15 mm/hr	0-15 mm/hr
	Female	0-20 mm/hr	0-20 mm/hr
Wintrobe	Child	0-13 mm/hr	0-13 mm/hr
	Adult: Male	0-9 mm/hr	0-9 mm/hr
	Female	0-20 mm/hr	0-20 mm/hr
Fibrinogen			
Plasma	Newborn	125-300 mg/d	1.25-3.00 g/L
	Thereafter	200-400 mg/dl	2.00-4.00 g/L
Galactose			
Serum	Newborn	0-20 mg/dl	0-1.11 mmol/L
	Thereafter	<5 mg/dl	<0.28 mmol/L
Urine	Newborn	≤60 mg/dl	≤3.33 mmol/L
	Thereafter	<14 mg/24 hr	<0.08 mmol/d
Glucose			
Serum	Cord	45-96 mg/dl	2.5-5.3 mmol/L
	Newborn, 1 d	40-60 mg/dl	2.2-3.3 mmol/L
	Newborn, >1 d	50-90 mg/dl	2.8-5.0 mmol/L
	Child	60-100 mg/dl	3.3-5.5 mmol/L
	Thereafter	70-105 mg/dl	3.9-5.8 mmol/L
Whole blood	Adult	65-95 mg/dl	3.6-5.3 mmol/L
CSF	Adult	40-70 mg/dl	2.2-3.9 mmol/L
Urine (quantitative)		<0.5 g/d	<2.8 mmol/d
Urine (qualitative)		Negative	Negative

Glucose tolerance test (GTT), oral
Serum

Dosages		**Normal**	**Diabetic**	**Normal**	**Diabetic**
Adult: 75 g	Fasting	70-105 mg/dl	≥126 mg/dl	3.9-5.8 mmol/L	≥7.0 mmol/L
Child: 1.75 g/kg of ideal	60 min	120-170 mg/dl	≥200 mg/dl	6.7-9.4 mmol/L	≥11 mmol/L
weight up to maximum	90 min	100-140 mg/dl	≥200 mg/dl	5.6-7.8 mmol/L	≥11 mmol/L
of 75 g	120 min	70-120 mg/dl	≥200 mg/dl	3.9-6.7 mmol/L	≥11 mmol/L

Growth hormone (GH, somatotropin)

Plasma	1 d	5-53 ng/ml	5-53 mcg/L
	1 wk	5-27 ng/ml	5-27 mcg/L
	1-12 mo	2-10 ng/ml	2-10 mcg/L
	Fasting child/adult	<0.7-6.0 ng/ml	<0.7-6.0 mcg/L

Continued

COMMON LABORATORY TESTS AND TESTS RESULTS—cont'd

TEST/SPECIMEN	AGE/GENDER/REFERENCE	NORMAL RANGES	
		CONVENTIONAL UNITS	INTERNATIONAL UNITS (SI)
Hematocrit (HCT, Hct)			
Whole blood	1 d (cap)	48%-69%	0.48-0.69 vol fraction
	2 d	48%-75%	0.48-0.75 vol fraction
	3 d	44%-72%	0.44-0.72 vol fraction
	2 mo	28%-42%	0.28-0.42 vol fraction
	6-12 yr	35%-45%	0.35-0.45 vol fraction
	12-18 yr: Male	37%-49%	0.37-0.49 vol fraction
	Female	36%-46%	0.36-0.46 vol fraction
Hemoglobin (Hb)			
Whole blood	1-3 d (cap)	14.5-22.5 g/dl	2.25-3.49 mmol/L
	2 mo	9.0-14.0 g/dl	1.40-2.17 mmol/L
	6-12 yr	11.5-15.5 g/dl	1.78-2.40 mmol/L
	12-18 yr: Male	13.0-16.0 g/dl	2.02-2.48 mmol/L
	Female	12.0-16.0 g/dl	1.86-2.48 mmol/L
Hemoglobin A			
Whole blood		>95% of total	>0.95 fraction of Hb
Hemoglobin F			
Whole blood	1 d	63%-92% HbF	0.63-0.92 mass fraction HbF
	5 d	65%-88% HbF	0.65-0.88 mass fraction HbF
	3 wk	55%-85% HbF	0.55-0.85 mass fraction HbF
	6-9 wk	31%-75% HbF	0.31-0.75 mass fraction HbF
	3-4 mo	<2%-59% HbF	<0.02-0.59 mass fraction HbF
	6 mo	<2%-9% HbF	<0.02-0.09 mass fraction HbF
	Adult	<2.0% HbF	<0.02 mass fraction HbF
Immunoglobulin A (IgA)			
Serum	Cord	1.4-3.6 mg/dl	14-36 mg/L
	1-3 mo	1.3-53 mg/dl	13-530 mg/L
	4-6 mo	4.4-84 mg/dl	44-840 mg/L
	7-12 mo	11-106 mg/dl	110-1060 mg/L
	2-5 yr	14-159 mg/dl	140-1590 mg/L
	6-10 yr	33-236 mg/dl	330-2360 mg/L
	Adult	70-312 mg/dl	700-3120 mg/L
Immunoglobulin D (IgD)			
Serum	Newborn	None detected	None detected
	Thereafter	0-8 mg/dl	0-80 mg/L
Immunoglobulin E (IgE)			
Serum	Male	0-230 IU/ml	0-230 kIU/L
	Female	0-170 IU/ml	0-170 kIU/L
Immunoglobulin G (IgG)			
Serum	Cord	636-1606 mg/dl	6.36-16.06 g/L
	1 mo	251-906 mg/dl	2.51-9.06 g/L
	2-4 mo	176-601 mg/dl	1.76-6.01 g/L
	5-12 mo	172-1069 mg/dl	1.72-10.69 g/L
	1-5 yr	345-1236 mg/dl	3.45-12.36 g/L
	6-10 yr	608-1572 mg/dl	6.08-15.72 g/L
	Adult	639-1349 mg/dl	6.39-13.49 g/L
Immunoglobulin M (IgM)			
Serum	Cord	6.3-25 mg/dl	63-250 mg/L
	1-4 mo	17-105 mg/dl	170-1050 mg/L
	5-9 mo	33-126 mg/dl	330-1260 mg/L
	10-12 mo	41-173 mg/dl	410-1730 mg/L
	2-8 yr	43-207 mg/dl	430-2070 mg/L
	9-10 yr	52-242 mg/dl	520-2420 mg/L
	Adult	56-352 mg/dl	560-3520 mg/L
Iron			
Serum	Newborn	100-250 mcg/dl	18-45 μmol/L
	Infant	40-100 mcg/dl	7-18 μmol/L
	Child	50-120 mcg/dl	9-22 μmol/L
	Thereafter: Male	65-170 mcg/dl	12-30 μmol/L
	Female	50-170 mcg/dl	9-30 μmol/L
	Intoxicated child	280-2550 mcg/dl	50.12-456.5 μmol/L
	Fatally poisoned child	>1800 mcg/dl	>322.2 μmol/L

COMMON LABORATORY TESTS AND TESTS RESULTS—cont'd

TEST/SPECIMEN	AGE/GENDER/REFERENCE	NORMAL RANGES		
		CONVENTIONAL UNITS		INTERNATIONAL UNITS (SI)
Iron-binding capacity, total (TIBC)				
Serum	Infant	100-400 mcg/dl		17.90-71.60 μmol/L
	Thereafter	250-400 mcg/dl		44.75-71.60 μmol/L
Lead				
Whole blood	Child	<10 mcg/dl		<0.48 μmol/L
Urine, 24 hr		<80 mcg/L		<0.39 μmol/L
Leukocyte count (WBC count)		×1000 cells/mm³ (μl)		×10⁹ cells/L
Whole blood	Birth	9.0-30.0		9.0-30.0
	24 hr	9.4-34.0		9.4-34.0
	1 mo	5.0-19.5		5.0-19.5
	1-3 yr	6.0-17.5		6.0-17.5
	4-7 yr	5.5-15.5		5.5-15.5
	8-13 yr	4.5-13.5		4.5-13.5
	Adult	4.5-11.0		4.5-11.0
		×1000 cells/mm³ (μl)		×10⁶ cells/L
CSF (cell count)	Premature	0-25 mononuclear		0-25
		0-10 polymorphonuclear		0-10
		0-1000 RBC		0-1000
	Newborn	0-20 mononuclear		0-20
		0-10 polymorphonuclear		0-10
		0-800 RBC		0-800
	Neonate	0-5 mononuclear		0-5
		0-10 polymorphonuclear		0-10
		0-50 RBC		0-50
	Thereafter	0-5 mononuclear		0-5
Leukocyte differential count				
Whole blood	Myelocytes	0%	0 cells/mm³ (μl)	Number fraction 0
	Neutrophils—"bands"	3%-5%	150-400 cells/mm³ (μl)	Number fraction 0.03-0.05
	Neutrophils—"segs"	54%-62%	3000-5800 cells/mm³ (μl)	Number fraction 0.54-0.62
	Lymphocytes	25%-33%	1500-3000 cells/mm³ (μl)	Number fraction 0.25-0.33
	Monocytes	3%-7%	285-500 cells/mm³ (μl)	Number fraction 0.03-0.07
	Eosinophils	1%-3%	50-250 cells/mm³ (μl)	Number fraction 0.01-0.03
	Basophils	0%-0.75%	15-50 cells/mm³ (μl)	Number fraction 0-0.0075
Mean corpuscular hemoglobin (MCH)				
Whole blood	Birth	31-37 pg/cell		0.48-0.57 fmol/cell
	1-3 d (cap)	31-37 pg/cell		0.48-0.57 fmol/cell
	1 wk–1 mo	28-40 pg/cell		0.43-0.62 fmol/cell
	2 mo	26-34 pg/cell		0.40-0.53 fmol/cell
	3-6 mo	25-35 pg/cell		0.39-0.54 fmol/cell
	0.5-2 yr	23-31 pg/cell		0.36-0.48 fmol/cell
	2-6 yr	24-30 pg/cell		0.37-0.47 fmol/cell
	6-12 yr	25-33 pg/cell		0.39-0.51 fmol/cell
	12-18 yr	25-35 pg/cell		0.39-0.54 fmol/cell
	18-49 yr	26-34 pg/cell		0.40-0.53 fmol/cell
Mean corpuscular hemoglobin concentration (MCHC)				
Whole blood	Birth	30%-36% Hb/cell or g Hb/dl RBC		4.65-5.58 mmol Hb/L RBC
	1-3 d (cap)	29%-37% Hb/cell or g Hb/dl RBC		4.50-5.74 mmol Hb/L RBC
	1-2 wk	28%-38% Hb/cell or g Hb/dl RBC		4.34-5.89 mmol Hb/L RBC
	1-2 mo	29%-37% Hb/cell or g Hb/dl RBC		4.50-5.74 mmol Hb/L RBC
	3 mo–2 yr	30%-36% Hb/cell or g Hb/dl RBC		4.65-5.58 mmol Hb/L RBC
	2-18 yr	31%-37% Hb/cell or g Hb/dl RBC		4.81-5.74 mmol Hb/L RBC
	>18 yr	31%-37% Hb/cell or g Hb/dl RBC		4.81-5.74 mmol Hb/L RBC
Mean corpuscular volume (MCV)				
Whole blood	1-3 d (cap)	95-121 μm³		95-121 fl
	0.5-2 yr	70-86 μm³		70-86 fl
	6-12 yr	77-95 μm³		77-95 fl
	12-18 yr: Male	78-98 μm³		78-98 fl
	Female	78-102 μm³		78-102 fl

Continued

COMMON LABORATORY TESTS AND TESTS RESULTS—cont'd

		NORMAL RANGES	
TEST/SPECIMEN	**AGE/GENDER/REFERENCE**	**CONVENTIONAL UNITS**	**INTERNATIONAL UNITS (SI)**
Osmolality			
Serum	Child, adult	275-295 mOsm/kg H_2O	
Urine, random		50-1400 mOsm/kg H_2O, depending on fluid intake; after 12-hr fluid restriction: >850 mOsm/kg H_2O	
Urine, 24 hr		≅300-900 mOsm/kg H_2O	
Oxygen, partial pressure (PO_2)			
Whole blood, arterial	Birth	8-24 mm Hg	1.1-3.2 kPa
	5-10 min	33-75 mm Hg	4.4-10.0 kPa
	30 min	31-85 mm Hg	4.1-11.3 kPa
	>1 hr	55-80 mm Hg	7.3-10.6 kPa
	1 d	54-95 mm Hg	7.2-12.6 kPa
	Thereafter (decreased with age)	83-108 mm Hg	11-14.4 kPa
Oxygen saturation (SaO_2)			
Whole blood, arterial	Newborn	85%-90%	Fraction saturated 0.85-0.90
	Thereafter	95%-99%	Fraction saturated 0.95-0.99
Partial thromboplastin time (PTT)			
Whole blood (Na citrate)			
Nonactivated		60-85 s (Platelin)	60-85 s
Activated		25-35 s (differs with method)	25-35 s
pH			H^+ concentration
Whole blood, arterial (must be corrected for body temperature)	Premature (48 hr)	7.35-7.50	31-44 nmol/L
	Birth, full term	7.11-7.36	43-77 nmol/L
	5-10 min	7.09-7.30	50-81 nmol/L
	30 min	7.21-7.38	41-61 nmol/L
	>1 hr	7.26-7.49	32-54 nmol/L
	1 d	7.29-7.45	35-51 nmol/L
	Thereafter	7.35-7.45	35-44 nmol/L
Urine, random	Newborn/neonate	5-7	0.1-10 μmol/L
	Thereafter	4.5-8 (average ≅6)	0.01-32 μmol/L (average ≅1.0 μmol/L)
Stool		7.0-7.5	31-100 nmol/L
Phenylalanine			
Serum	Premature	2.0-7.5 mg/dl	120-450 μmol/L
	Newborn	1.2-3.4 mg/dl	70-210 μmol/L
	Thereafter	0.8-1.8 mg/dl	50-110 μmol/L
Urine, 24 hr	10 d—2 wk	1-2 mg/d	6-12 μmol/d
	3-12 yr	4-18 mg/d	24-110 μmol/d
	Thereafter	Trace—17 mg/d	Trace—103 μmol/d
Plasma volume			
Plasma	Male	25-43 ml/kg	0.025-0.043 L/kg
	Female	28-45 ml/kg	0.028-0.045 L/kg
Platelet count (thrombocyte count)			
Whole blood (EDTA)	Newborn (after 1 wk, same as adult)	$84\text{-}478 \times 10^3/mm^3$ (μl)	$84\text{-}478 \times 10^9$/L
	Adult	$150\text{-}400 \times 10^3/mm^3$ (μl)	$150\text{-}400 \times 10^9$/L
Potassium			
Serum	Newborn	3.0-6.0 mEq/L	3.0-6.0 mmol/L
	Thereafter	3.5-5.0 mEq/L	3.5-5.0 mmol/L
Plasma (heparin)		3.4-4.5 mEq/L	3.4-4.5 mmol/L
Urine, 24 hr		2.5-125 mEq/d (varies with diet)	2.5-125 mmol/L
Protein			
Serum, total	Premature	4.3-7.6 g/dl	43-76 g/L
	Newborn	4.6-7.4 g/dl	46-74 g/L
	1-7 yr	6.1-7.9 g/dl	61-79 g/L
	8-12 yr	6.4-8.1 g/dl	64-81 g/L
	13-19 yr	6.6-8.2 g/dl	66-82 g/L
Total			
Urine, 24 hr		1-14 mg/dl	10-140 mg/L
		50-80 mg/d (at rest)	50-80 mg/d
		<250 mg/d (after intense exercise)	<250 mg/d (after intense exercise)
CSF		Lumbar: 8-32 mg/dl	80-320 mg/L

COMMON LABORATORY TESTS AND TESTS RESULTS—cont'd

TEST/SPECIMEN	AGE/GENDER/REFERENCE	NORMAL RANGES	
		CONVENTIONAL UNITS	INTERNATIONAL UNITS (SI)
Prothrombin time (PT)			
One-stage (Quick)			
Whole blood (Na citrate)	In general	11-15 s (varies with type of thromboplastin)	11-15 s
	Newborn	Prolonged by 2-3 s	Prolonged by 2-3 s
Two-stage modified (Ware and Seegers)			
Whole blood (sodium citrate)		18-22 s	18-22 s
RBC count: see Erythrocyte (RBC) count			
Red blood cell volume			
Whole blood	Male	20-36 ml/kg	0.020-0.036 L/kg
	Female	19-31 ml/kg	0.019-0.031 L/kg
Reticulocyte count			
Whole blood	Adults	0.5%-1.5% of erythrocytes or 25,000-75,000/mm³ (µl)	0.005-0.015 (number fraction) or 25,000-75,000 × 10⁶/L
Capillary	1 d	0.4%-6.0%	0.004-0.060 (number fraction)
	7 d	<0.1%-1.3%	<0.001-0.013 (number fraction)
	1-4 wk	<0.1%-1.2%	<0.001-0.012 (number fraction)
	5-6 wk	<0.1%-2.4%	<0.001-0.024 (number fraction)
	7-8 wk	0.1%-2.9%	0.001-0.029 (number fraction)
	9-10 wk	<0.1%-2.6%	<0.001-0.026 (number fraction)
	11-12 wk	0.1%-1.3%	0.001-0.013 (number fraction)
Salicylates			
Serum, plasma	Therap. conc.	15-30 mg/dl	1.1-2.2 mmol/L
	Toxic conc.	>30 mg/dl	>18.5 mmol/L
Sedimentation rate: see Erythrocyte sedimentation rate (ESR)			
Sodium			
Serum or plasma	Newborn	134-146 mEq/L	134-146 mmol/L
	Infant	139-146 mEq/L	139-146 mmol/L
	Child	138-145 mEq/L	138-145 mmol/L
	Thereafter	136-146 mEq/L	136-146 mmol/L
Urine, 24 hr		40-220 mEq/L (diet dependent)	40-220 mmol/L
Sweat	Normal	<40 mEq/L	<40 mmol/L
	Indeterminate	45-60 mEq/L	45-60 mmol/L
	Cystic fibrosis	>60 mEq/L	>60 mmol/L
Specific gravity			
Urine, random	Adult	1.002-1.030	1.002-1.030
	After 12-hr fluid restriction	>1.025	>1.025
Urine, 24 hr		1.015-1.025	
Theophylline			
Serum, plasma	Therap. conc.		
	Bronchodilator	10-20 mcg/ml	56-110 µmol/L
	Premature apnea	5-10 mcg/ml	28-56 µmol/L
	Toxic conc.	>20 mcg/ml	>110 µmol/L
Thrombin time			
Whole blood (Na citrate)		Control time ±2 s when control is 9-13 s	Control time ±2 s when control is 9-13 s
Thyroxine, total (T₄)			
Serum	Cord	8-13 mcg/dl	103-168 nmol/L
	Newborn	11.5-24 mcg/dl (lower in low-birth-weight infants)	148-310 nmol/L
	Neonate	9-18 mcg/dl	116-232 nmol/L
	Infant	7-15 mcg/dl	90-194 nmol/L
	1-5 yr	7.3-15 mcg/dl	94-194 nmol/L
	5-10 yr	6.4-13.3 mcg/dl	83-172 nmol/L
	Thereafter	5-12 mcg/dl	65-155 nmol/L
	Newborn screen (filter paper)	6.2-22 mcg/dl	80-284 nmol/L

Triglycerides (TG)		**Male** (mg/dl)	**Female** (mg/dl)	**Male** (g/L)	**Female** (g/L)
Serum, after ≥2-hr fast	Cord	10-98	10-98	0.10-0.98	0.10-0.98
	0-5 yr	30-86	32-99	0.30-0.86	0.32-0.99
	6-11 yr	31-108	35-114	0.31-1.08	0.35-1.14
	12-15 yr	36-138	41-138	0.36-1.38	0.41-1.38
	16-19 yr	40-163	40-128	0.40-1.63	0.40-1.28

Continued

COMMON LABORATORY TESTS AND TESTS RESULTS—cont'd

TEST/SPECIMEN	AGE/GENDER/REFERENCE	NORMAL RANGES	
		CONVENTIONAL UNITS	INTERNATIONAL UNITS (SI)
Triiodothyronine (T₃), free			
Serum	Cord	20-240 pg/dl	0.3-3.7 pmol/L
	1-3 d	200-610 pg/dl	3.1-9.4 pmol/L
	6 wk	240-560 pg/dl	3.7-8.6 pmol/L
	Adults (20-50 yr)	230-660 pg/dl	3.5-10.0 pmol/L
Triiodothyronine, total (T₃-RIA)			
Serum	Cord	30-70 ng/dl	0.46-1.08 nmol/L
	Newborn	72-260 ng/dl	1.16-4 nmol/L
	1-5 yr	100-260 ng/dl	1.54-4 nmol/L
	5-10 yr	90-240 ng/dl	1.39-3.70 nmol/L
	10-15 yr	80-210 ng/dl	1.23-3.23 nmol/L
	Thereafter	115-190 ng/dl	1.77-2.93 nmol/L
Urea nitrogen			
Serum or plasma	Cord	21-40 mg/dl	7.5-14.3 mmol/L
	Premature (1 wk)	3-25 mg/dl	1.1-9 mmol/L
	Newborn	3-12 mg/dl	1.1-4.3 mmol/L
	Infant/child	5-18 mg/dl	1.8-6.4 mmol/L
	Thereafter	7-18 mg/dl	2.5-6.4 mmol/L
Urine volume			
Urine, 24 hr	Newborn	50-300 ml/d	0.05-0.3 L/d
	Infant	350-550 ml/d	0.35-0.5 L/d
	Child	500-1000 ml/d	0.5-1 L/d
	Adolescent	700-1400 ml/d	0.7-1.4 L/d
	Thereafter: Male	800-1800 ml/d	0.8-1.8 L/d
	Female	600-1600 ml/d (varies with intake and other factors)	0.6-1.6 L/d

WBC: see Leukocyte count (WBC count)

Modified from Kliegman RM, Behrman RE, Jenson HB, et al, editors: *Nelson textbook of pediatrics*, ed 18, Philadelphia, 2007, Saunders; McMillan JA, Deangelis CD, Feigin RD, and others, editors: *Oski's pediatrics: principles and practice*, ed 3, Philadelphia, 1999, Lippincott Williams & Wilkins; and Fischbach F: *A manual of laboratory and diagnostic tests,* ed 6, Philadelphia, 2000, Lippincott Williams & Wilkins.
*For a description of abbreviations, see p. 1755.
†From National Cholesterol Education Program: Report of the expert panel on blood cholesterol levels in children and adolescents, *Pediatrics* 89(3 pt 2):527, 1992.

ABBREVIATIONS USED IN LABORATORY TESTS

ABBREVIATION	TERM
cap	capillary
CHF	congestive heart failure
conc.	concentration
CSF	cerebrospinal fluid
d	day; diem
EDTA	ethylenediaminetetraacetate
g	gram
H^+	hydrogen ion
Hb	hemoglobin
hr	hour
IU	International unit
L	liter
m	meter
mEq	milliequivalent
min	minute
mm	millimeter
mm Hg	millimeters of mercury
mm H_2O	millimeters of water
mm^3	cubic millimeter
mo	month
mol	mole
mOsm	milliosmole
Na	sodium
Pa	pascal
RBC	red blood cells
s	second
temp	temperature
therap.	therapeutic
U	international unit of enzyme activity
vol	volume
WBC	white blood cells
wk	week
yr	year
>	greater than
≥	greater than or equal to
<	less than
≤	less than or equal to
±	plus/minus
≅	approximately equal to

PREFIXES DENOTING DECIMAL FACTORS

PREFIX	SYMBOL	AMOUNT
deci	d	one tenth (10^{-1})
centi	c	one hundredth (10^{-2})
milli	m	one thousandth (10^{-3})
micro	mc, μ	one millionth (10^{-6})
nano	n	one billionth (10^{-9})
pico	p	one trillionth (10^{-12})
femto	f	one quadrillionth (10^{-15})

Translations of Wong-Baker FACES Pain Rating Scale*

	0	1	2	3	4	5
0-5 coding	0	1	2	3	4	5
0-10 coding	0	2	4	6	8	10
English	No Hurt	Hurts Little Bit	Hurts Little More	Hurts Even More	Hurts Whole Lot	Hurts Worst
Spanish	No duele	Duele un poco	Duele un poco más	Duele mucho	Duele mucho más	Duele el máximo
French	Pas mal	Un petit peu mal	Un peri plus mal	Encore plus mal	Très mal	Très mal
Italian	Non fa male	Fa male un poco	Fa male un po di piu	Fa male ancora di piu	Fa molto male	Fa maggiormente male
Portuguese	Não doi	Doi um pouco	Doi um pouco mais	Doi muito	Doi muito mais	Doi o máximo
Bosnian	Ne boli	Boli samo malo	Boli malo više	Boli još više	Boli puno	Boli najviše
Vietnamese	Không dau	Hòi dau	Dau hòn chút	Dau nhiêu hòn	Dau thât nhiêu	Dau qúa dô
Chinese†	無痛	微痛	較痛	更痛	很痛	劇痛
Greek	Δεν Ποναΐ	Πονιΐ Λιγο	Πονιΐ Λιγο Πιο Πολν	Πονιΐ Πολν	Πονιΐ Πιο Πολν	Πονιΐ Παρα Πολν
Romanian	No doare	Doare puțin	Doare un pic mai mult	Doare şi mai mult	Doare foarte tare	Doare cel mai mult

Brief Word Instructions (Above)

Point to each face using the words to describe the pain intensity. Ask person to choose face that best describes own pain and record the appropriate number. Rating scale can be used with people 3 years and older.

NOTE: In a study of 148 children ages 4 to 5 years, there were no differences in pain scores when children used the original or brief word instructions. (In Wong D, Baker C: *Reference manual for the Wong-Baker FACES Pain Rating Scale*, Duarte, Calif, 1998, City of Hope Mayday Pain Resource Center; retrieved from http://evolve.elsevier.com/Wong/essentials.)

---

*Wong-Baker FACES Pain Rating Scale:** Available at no charge from The Purdue Frederick Company, 100 Connecticut Ave., Norwalk, CT 06850-3590; www.partnersagainstpain.com. Spanish and Portuguese translations by Ellen Johnsen; French translation from Wong DL: *Soins infirmiers pediatrie*, Quebec, 2002, Editions Etudes Vivantes, Groupe Educalivres, Inc.; Italian translation by Madeline Mitchko; Bosnian translation by Barbara Bogomolov; Vietnamese translation by Yen B. Isle; Chinese translation by Hung-Shen Lin; Greek translation by Nicholas Mamalis; Romanian translation by Bogdan R. Dinu.

Original Instructions

English. Explain to the person that each face is for a person who feels happy because he has no pain (hurt) or sad because he has some or a lot of pain. **Face 0** is very happy because he doesn't hurt at all. **Face 1** hurts just a little bit. **Face 2** hurts a little more. **Face 3** hurts even more. **Face 4** hurts a whole lot. **Face 5** hurts as much as you can imagine, although you don't have to be crying to feel this bad. Ask the person to choose the face that best describes how he or she is feeling.

Rating scale is recommended for persons ages 3 years and older.

Spanish. Expliquele a la persona que cada cara representa una persona que se siente feliz porque no tiene dolor o triste porque siente un poco o mucho dolor. **Cara 0** se siente muy feliz porque no tiene dolor. **Cara 1** tiene un poco de dolor. **Cara 2** tiene un poquito más de dolor. **Cara 3** tiene más dolor. **Cara 4** tiene mucho dolor. **Cara 5** tiene el dolor más fuerte que usted pueda imaginar, aunque usted no tiene que estar llorando para sentirse asi de mal. Pidale a la persona que escoja la cara que mejor describe su proprio dolor.

Esta escala se puede usar con personas de tres años de edad o más.

French. Expliquez à la personne que chaque visage représent une personne qui est heureux parce qu'elle n'a pas point du mal ou triste parce qu'elle a un peu ou beaucoup du mal. **Visage 0** est trés heureux parce qu'elle n'a pas point du mal. **Visage 1** a un petit peu de mal. **Visage 2** a plus du mal. **Visage 3** a encore plus du mal. **Visage 4** a beaucoup du mal. **Visage 5** a autant mal que vous pouvez imaginer, bien que ces mauvais sentiments ne finissent pas nécessairement a vous faire pleurer. Demandez à la personne de choisir le visage qui convient le mieux avec ses sentiments.

Ces evaluations sont recommendés pour des personnes de trois ans et davantage.

Italian. Spiegare a la persona che ogni facien è per una persona che si sente felice perchè non tiene dolore oppure triste perchè ha poco o molto dolore. **Faccia O** è molto felice perchè non tiene dolore. **Faccia 1** tiene poco dolore. **Faccia 2** tiene un po più di dolore. **Faccia 3** tiene più dolore. **Faccia 4** tiene molto dolore. **Faccia 5** tiene molto dolore che non puoi immaginare però non devi piangere per tenere dolore. Domandi ala persona di scegliere quale faccia meglio descrive come si sente.

Grado scale è raccomandata a la persona di tre anni in sù.

Portuguese. Explique a pessoa que cada face representa uma pessoa que está feliz porque não têm dor, ou triste por ter um pouco ou muita dor. **Face 0** está muito feliz porque não têm nenhuma dor. **Face 1** têm apenas um pouco de dor. **Face 2** têm um pouco mais de dor. **Face 3** têm ainda mais dor. **Face 4** têm muita dor. **Face 5** têm uma dor máxima, apesar de que nem sempre provoca o choro. Peça a pessoa que escolhe a face que melhor descreve como ele se sente.

Esta escala é aplicável a pessoas de tres anos de idade ou mais.

Romanian. Explicati copilului că fiecare desen (figură) corespunde unei persoane care este veselă, pentru ca nu are nici o durere, sau unei persoane care este tristă, pentru că are dureri. **Figura 0** este foarte fericită pentru că nu are nici o durere. **Figura 1** arată că doare doar un pic. **Figura 2** arată că doare ceva mai mult. **Figura 3** arată că doare şi mai mult. **Figura 4** arată că doare foarte tare. **Figura 5** arată că doare atât de tare cât se poate

imagina, chiar dacă nu este însotita neapărat de lacrimi. Cereti copilului (persoanei) să indice figura care exprimă cel mai bine cum se simte el.

Scala de evaluare a durerii este recomandată pentru copiii în vârstuă de trei ani şi peste.

Bosnian. Objasnite osobi da je svako lice namjenjeno za osobu koja se osjeća sretnom jer ne osjeća bol ili tužnom jer osjeća malo ili puno boli. **Lice 0** je sretno jer ne osjeća nikakvu bol. **Lice 1** osjeća samo malu bol. **Lice 2** osjeća malo više boli. **Lice 3** osjeća još veću bol. **Lice 4** osjeća puno boli. **Lice 5** osjeća onoliku bol koju je moguće zamisliti, što ne znaći da osoba koja osjeća tu bol mora plakati. Upitajte osobu da izabere lice koje najbolje opisuju kako se osjeća. Skala procijene bola se preporučuje za osobe starosti 3 godine ili više.

Upirati prstom na svako lice objašnjavajući rijećima intensitet boli. Pitajte dijete da izabere lice koje najbolje opisuje njihovu bol i zabiljezue odgovarajući broj.

German. Erläutern Sie dem Kind, daß jedes Gesicht zu einer Person gehört, die froh darüber ist, keine Schmerzen zu haben, oder die sehr traurig ist, weil sie mäßige bis starke Schmerzen hat. **Gesicht 0** ist sehr froh, weil es keine Schmerzen hat. **Gesicht 1** sagt, es tut ein bißchen weh. **Gesicht 2** hat ein bißchen mehr Schmerzen. **Gesicht 3** sagt, es tut noch mehr weh, und **Gesicht 4,** es tut ziemlich weh. **Gesicht 5** leidet unter so starken Schmerzen, wie Du Dir nur vorstellen kannst, auch wenn dabei nicht unbedingt Tränen fließen müssen. Bitten Sie das Kind, das Gesicht auszuwählen, das seinem Empfinden am besten entspricht.

Empfohlen für Kinder ab drei Jahren.

Vietnamese

Xin cắt nghĩa cho mỗi người, từng khuôn mặt của một người cảm thấy vui vẻ tại vì không có sự đau đớn hoặc, buồn vì có chút ít hay rất nhiều sự đau đớn.

Cái **mặt** với số 0 thì rất là vui tại vì mặt ấy không có sự đau đớn. **Mặt số** 1 chỉ đau một chút thôi. **Mặt số** 2 hơi đau hơn một chút nữa. **Mặt số** 3 đau hơn chút nữa. **Mặt số** 4 đau thật nhiều. **Mặt số** 5 đau không thể tưởng tượng, mặc dù người ta không cần phải khóc mới cảm thấy được sự buồn khổ như thế.

Bạn hỏi từng người tự chọn khuôn mặt nào diễn tả được sự đau đớn của chính mình.

Japanese

3歳以上の患者に望ましい。それぞれの顔は、患者の痛み(pain, hurt)がないのでご機嫌な感じ、または、ある程度の痛み・沢山の痛みがあるので悲しい感じを表現していることを説明して下さい。0＝痛みがまったくないから、とても幸せな顔をしている、1＝ほんの少し痛い、2＝もう少し痛い、3＝もっと痛い、4＝とっても痛い、5＝痛くて涙を流す必要はないけれども、これ以上の痛みは考えられないほど痛い。今、どのように感じているか最もよく表わしている顔を選ぶよう、患者に求めて下さい。

Chinese

解釋給人聽用每張臉譜來代表著一個人的感覺是因為沒有疼痛〔傷痛〕而感快樂或是因為些許疼痛或者是許多疼痛而感傷心。第零張臉是很快樂的因為他一點也不覺得疼痛。第一張臉只痛一丁點兒。第二張臉又痛多了一些。第三張臉痛得更多了。第四張臉是非常痛了。第五張臉是為人們所能想到的劇痛即使感到這樣難過，卻不一定哭出來。請這人選擇出最能代表他現在感覺的一張臉譜。此量表適用於三歲以上的人。

INDEX

Page numbers followed by *f* indicate figures; *t*, tables; *b*, boxes.

1758

Please see next page for blood pressure levels for girls.

Blood Pressure (BP) Levels for Boys by Age and Height Percentile

AGE (yr)	BP PERCENTILE	SYSTOLIC BP (mm Hg) PERCENTILE OF HEIGHT							DIASTOLIC BP (mm Hg) PERCENTILE OF HEIGHT						
		5th	10th	25th	50th	75th	90th	95th	5th	10th	25th	50th	75th	90th	95th
1	50th	80	81	83	85	87	88	89	34	35	36	37	38	39	39
	90th	94	95	97	99	100	102	103	49	50	51	52	53	53	54
	95th	98	99	101	103	104	106	106	54	54	55	56	57	58	58
	99th	105	106	108	110	112	113	114	61	62	63	64	65	66	66
2	50th	84	85	87	88	90	92	92	39	40	41	42	43	44	44
	90th	97	99	100	102	104	105	106	54	55	56	57	58	58	59
	95th	101	102	104	106	108	109	110	59	59	60	61	62	63	63
	99th	109	110	111	113	115	117	117	66	67	68	69	70	71	71
3	50th	86	87	89	91	93	94	95	44	44	45	46	47	48	48
	90th	100	101	103	105	107	108	109	59	59	60	61	62	63	63
	95th	104	105	107	109	110	112	113	63	63	64	65	66	67	67
	99th	111	112	114	116	118	119	120	71	71	72	73	74	75	75
4	50th	88	89	91	93	95	96	97	47	48	49	50	51	51	52
	90th	102	103	105	107	109	110	111	62	63	64	65	66	66	67
	95th	106	107	109	111	112	114	115	66	67	68	69	70	71	71
	99th	113	114	116	118	120	121	122	74	75	76	77	78	78	79
5	50th	90	91	93	95	96	98	98	50	51	52	53	54	55	55
	90th	104	105	106	108	110	111	112	65	66	67	68	69	69	70
	95th	108	109	110	112	114	115	116	69	70	71	72	73	74	74
	99th	115	116	118	120	121	123	123	77	78	79	80	81	81	82
6	50th	91	92	94	96	98	99	100	53	53	54	55	56	57	57
	90th	105	106	108	110	111	113	113	68	68	69	70	71	72	72
	95th	109	110	112	114	115	117	117	72	72	73	74	75	76	76
	99th	116	117	119	121	123	124	125	80	80	81	82	83	84	84
7	50th	92	94	95	97	99	100	101	55	55	56	57	58	59	59
	90th	106	107	109	111	113	114	115	70	70	71	72	73	74	74
	95th	110	111	113	115	117	118	119	74	74	75	76	77	78	78
	99th	117	118	120	122	124	125	126	82	82	83	84	85	86	86
8	50th	94	95	97	99	100	102	102	56	57	58	59	60	60	61
	90th	107	109	110	112	114	115	116	71	72	72	73	74	75	76
	95th	111	112	114	116	118	119	120	75	76	77	78	79	79	80
	99th	119	120	122	123	125	127	127	83	84	85	86	87	87	88
9	50th	95	96	98	100	102	103	104	57	58	59	60	61	61	62
	90th	109	110	112	114	115	117	118	72	73	74	75	76	76	77
	95th	113	114	116	118	119	121	121	76	77	78	79	80	81	81
	99th	120	121	123	125	127	128	129	84	85	86	87	88	88	89
10	50th	97	98	100	102	103	105	106	58	59	60	61	61	62	63
	90th	111	112	114	115	117	119	119	73	73	74	75	76	77	78
	95th	115	116	117	119	121	122	123	77	78	79	80	81	81	82
	99th	122	123	125	127	128	130	130	85	86	86	88	88	89	90
11	50th	99	100	102	104	105	107	107	59	59	60	61	62	63	63
	90th	113	114	115	117	119	120	121	74	74	75	76	77	78	78
	95th	117	118	119	121	123	124	125	78	78	79	80	81	82	82
	99th	124	125	127	129	130	132	132	86	86	87	88	89	90	90
12	50th	101	102	104	106	108	109	110	59	60	61	62	63	63	64
	90th	115	116	118	120	121	123	123	74	75	75	76	77	78	79
	95th	119	120	122	123	125	127	127	78	79	80	81	82	82	83
	99th	126	127	129	131	133	134	135	86	87	88	89	90	90	91
13	50th	104	105	106	108	110	111	112	60	60	61	62	63	64	64
	90th	117	118	120	122	124	125	126	75	75	76	77	78	79	79
	95th	121	122	124	126	128	129	130	79	79	80	81	82	83	83
	99th	128	130	131	133	135	136	137	87	87	88	89	90	91	91
14	50th	106	107	109	111	113	114	115	60	61	62	63	64	65	65
	90th	120	121	123	125	126	128	128	75	76	77	78	79	79	80
	95th	124	125	127	128	130	132	132	80	80	81	82	83	84	84
	99th	131	132	134	136	138	139	140	87	88	89	90	91	92	92
15	50th	109	110	112	113	115	117	117	61	62	63	64	65	66	66
	90th	122	124	125	127	129	130	131	76	77	78	79	80	80	81
	95th	126	127	129	131	133	134	135	81	81	82	83	84	85	85
	99th	134	135	136	138	140	142	142	88	89	90	91	92	93	93
16	50th	111	112	114	116	118	119	120	63	63	64	65	66	67	67
	90th	125	126	128	130	131	133	134	78	78	79	80	81	82	82
	95th	129	130	132	134	135	137	137	82	83	83	84	85	86	87
	99th	136	137	139	141	143	144	145	90	90	91	92	93	94	94
17	50th	114	115	116	118	120	121	122	65	66	66	67	68	69	70
	90th	127	128	130	132	134	135	136	80	80	81	82	83	84	84
	95th	131	132	134	136	138	139	140	84	85	86	87	87	88	89
	99th	139	140	141	143	145	146	147	92	93	93	94	95	96	97

The 90th percentile is 1.28 SD, the 95th percentile is 1.645 SD, and the 99th percentile is 2.326 SD over the mean.

Please see previous page for blood pressure levels for boys.

Blood Pressure (BP) Levels for Girls by Age and Height Percentile

AGE (yr)	BP PERCENTILE	SYSTOLIC BP (mm Hg) PERCENTILE OF HEIGHT							DIASTOLIC BP (mm Hg) PERCENTILE OF HEIGHT						
		5th	10th	25th	50th	75th	90th	95th	5th	10th	25th	50th	75th	90th	95th
1	50th	83	84	85	86	88	89	90	38	39	39	40	41	41	42
	90th	97	97	98	100	101	102	103	52	53	53	54	55	55	56
	95th	100	101	102	104	105	106	107	56	57	57	58	59	59	60
	99th	108	108	109	111	112	113	114	64	64	65	65	66	67	67
2	50th	85	85	87	88	89	91	91	43	44	44	45	46	46	47
	90th	98	99	100	101	103	104	105	57	58	58	59	60	61	61
	95th	102	103	104	105	107	108	109	61	62	62	63	64	65	65
	99th	109	110	111	112	114	115	116	69	69	70	70	71	72	72
3	50th	86	87	88	89	91	92	93	47	48	48	49	50	50	51
	90th	100	100	102	103	104	106	106	61	62	62	63	64	64	65
	95th	104	104	105	107	108	109	110	65	66	66	67	68	68	69
	99th	111	111	113	114	115	116	117	73	73	74	74	75	76	76
4	50th	88	88	90	91	92	94	94	50	50	51	52	52	53	54
	90th	101	102	103	104	106	107	108	64	64	65	66	67	67	68
	95th	105	106	107	108	110	111	112	68	68	69	70	71	71	72
	99th	112	113	114	115	117	118	119	76	76	76	77	78	79	79
5	50th	89	90	91	93	94	95	96	52	53	53	54	55	55	56
	90th	103	103	105	106	107	109	109	66	67	67	68	69	69	70
	95th	107	107	108	110	111	112	113	70	71	71	72	73	73	74
	99th	114	114	116	117	118	120	120	78	78	79	79	80	81	81
6	50th	91	92	93	94	96	97	98	54	54	55	56	56	57	58
	90th	104	105	106	108	109	110	111	68	68	69	70	70	71	72
	95th	108	109	110	111	113	114	115	72	72	73	74	74	75	76
	99th	115	116	117	119	120	121	122	80	80	80	81	82	83	83
7	50th	93	93	95	96	97	99	99	55	56	56	57	58	58	59
	90th	106	107	108	109	111	112	113	69	70	70	71	72	72	73
	95th	110	111	112	113	115	116	116	73	74	74	75	76	76	77
	99th	117	118	119	120	122	123	124	81	81	82	82	83	84	84
8	50th	95	95	96	98	99	100	101	57	57	57	58	59	60	60
	90th	108	109	110	111	113	114	114	71	71	71	72	73	74	74
	95th	112	112	114	115	116	118	118	75	75	75	76	77	78	78
	99th	119	120	121	122	123	125	125	82	82	83	83	84	85	86
9	50th	96	97	98	100	101	102	103	58	58	58	59	60	61	61
	90th	110	110	112	113	114	116	116	72	72	72	73	74	75	75
	95th	114	114	115	117	118	119	120	76	76	76	77	78	79	79
	99th	121	121	123	124	125	127	127	83	83	84	84	85	86	87
10	50th	98	99	100	102	103	104	105	59	59	59	60	61	62	62
	90th	112	112	114	115	116	118	118	73	73	73	74	75	76	76
	95th	116	116	117	119	120	121	122	77	77	77	78	79	80	80
	99th	123	123	125	126	127	129	129	84	84	85	86	86	87	88
11	50th	100	101	102	103	105	106	107	60	60	60	61	62	63	63
	90th	114	114	116	117	118	119	120	74	74	74	75	76	77	77
	95th	118	118	119	121	122	123	124	78	78	78	79	80	81	81
	99th	125	125	126	128	129	130	131	85	85	86	87	87	88	89
12	50th	102	103	104	105	107	108	109	61	61	61	62	63	64	64
	90th	116	116	117	119	120	121	122	75	75	75	76	77	78	78
	95th	119	120	121	123	124	125	126	79	79	79	80	81	82	82
	99th	127	127	128	130	131	132	133	86	86	87	88	88	89	90
13	50th	104	105	106	107	109	110	110	62	62	62	63	64	65	65
	90th	117	118	119	121	122	123	124	76	76	76	77	78	79	79
	95th	121	122	123	124	126	127	128	80	80	80	81	82	83	83
	99th	128	129	130	132	133	134	135	87	87	88	89	89	90	91
14	50th	106	106	107	109	110	111	112	63	63	63	64	65	66	66
	90th	119	120	121	122	124	125	125	77	77	77	78	79	80	80
	95th	123	123	125	126	127	129	129	81	81	81	82	83	84	84
	99th	130	131	132	133	135	136	136	88	88	89	90	90	91	92
15	50th	107	108	109	110	111	113	113	64	64	64	65	66	67	67
	90th	120	121	122	123	125	126	127	78	78	78	79	80	81	81
	95th	124	125	126	127	129	130	131	82	82	82	83	84	85	85
	99th	131	132	133	134	136	137	138	89	89	90	91	91	92	93
16	50th	108	108	110	111	112	114	114	64	64	65	66	66	67	68
	90th	121	122	123	124	126	127	128	78	78	79	80	81	81	82
	95th	125	126	127	128	130	131	132	82	82	83	84	85	85	86
	99th	132	133	134	135	137	138	139	90	90	90	91	92	93	93
17	50th	108	109	110	111	113	114	115	64	65	65	66	67	67	68
	90th	122	122	123	125	126	127	128	78	79	79	80	81	81	82
	95th	125	126	127	129	130	131	132	82	83	83	84	85	85	86
	99th	133	133	134	136	137	138	139	90	90	91	91	92	93	93

The 90th percentile is 1.28 SD, the 95th percentile is 1.645 SD, and the 99th percentile is 2.326 SD over the mean.